Immunologic Disorders in Infants & Children

Immunologic Disorders in Infants & Children

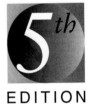

5th EDITION

E. Richard Stiehm, MD
Professor of Pediatrics
David Geffen School of Medicine at UCLA
Attending Physician
Mattel Children's Hospital at UCLA
UCLA Center for Health Sciences
Los Angeles, California

Hans D. Ochs, MD
Professor of Pediatrics
University of Washington School of Medicine
Seattle, Washington

Jerry A. Winkelstein, MD
Eudowood Professor of Pediatrics
Professor of Medicine and Pathology
Johns Hopkins University School of Medicine
Baltimore, Maryland

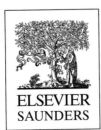

ELSEVIER
SAUNDERS

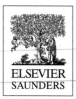

ELSEVIER
SAUNDERS

The Curtis Center
170 S Independence Mall W 300E
Philadelphia, Pennsylvania 19106

NOTICE

Pediatric immunology is an ever-changing field. Standard safety precautions must be followed, but
as new research and clinical experience broaden our knowledge, changes in treatment and drug
therapy may become necessary or appropriate. Readers are advised to check the most current
product information provided by the manufacturer of each drug to be administered to verify the
recommended dose, the method and duration of administration, and contraindications. It is the
responsibility of the licensed prescriber, relying on experience and knowledge of the patient, to
determine dosages and the best treatment for each individual patient. Neither the publisher nor the
author assumes any liability for any injury and/or damage to persons or property arising from this
publication.

Previous editions copyrighted 1996, 1989, 1980, 1973

Library of Congress Cataloging-in-Publication Data
Immunologic disorders in infants & children / [edited by] E. Richard Stiehm, Hans D.
Ochs, Jerry A. Winkelstein.–5th ed.
    p. ; cm.
  ISBN 0-7216-8964-7
    1. Immunologic diseases in children. 2. Developmental immunology. I. Title:
Immunologic disorders in infants and children. II. Stiehm, E. Richard, III. Ochs, Hans D.,
IV. Winkelstein, Jerry A.
    [DNLM: 1. Immunologic Diseases–Child. 2. Immunologic Diseases–Infant. WD 300 1324 2004]
  RJ385.146 2004
  618.92'97–dc21

                                                                    2003045649

Executive Editor: Judith Fletcher
Editorial Assistant: Dana Lamparello
Publishing Services Mananger: Joan Sinclair
Project Manager: Mary Stermel

Printed in the United States of America

Last digit is the print number: 9 8 7 6 5 4 3 2

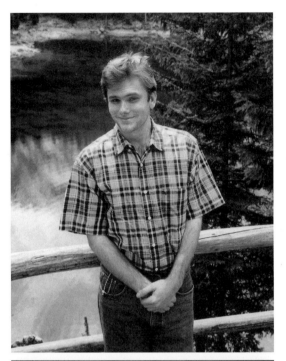

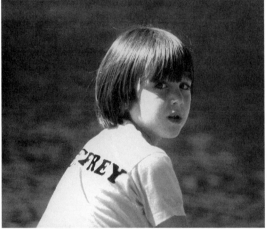

Dedication

To

John G. Boyle and Jeffrey Modell—
the children of Marcia and John Boyle
and Vicki and Fred Modell,
whose children's illness inspired them to establish
The Immune Deficiency Foundation
and the Jeffrey Modell Foundation,
both dedicated to improving
the lives of patients with immunodeficiency.

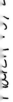

Preface to the First Edition

Twenty-five years ago, the thymus was a mystery organ that was irradiated for respiratory stridor, organ transplantation was science fiction, a gamma globulin determination was a sophisticated research effort, the function of the lymphocyte was not known, and the immunodeficiencies were not yet discovered. Since then a bountiful harvest of immunologic information has been gathered by the combined efforts of physicians, biochemists, microbiologists, pathologists, and other scientists. A significant portion has relevance to human health and disease and has been collected under the heading of clinical immunology. This book is concerned with the clinical immunology of infancy and childhood.

Like other specialty fields, clinical pediatric immunology is primarily concerned with a specific group of related illnesses necessitating special investigative procedures—the primary immunodeficiency diseases. Unlike most other specialties, pediatric immunology widens its horizons to include such related areas as collagen diseases, infectious diseases, allergies, transplantation, and immunization procedures. Further, the field encompasses many aspects of endocrine, hematologic, renal, neurologic, gastrointestinal, and malignant diseases, and thus it is especially attractive to the physician who enjoys the entire scope of pediatric medicine. In sum, pediatric immunology has some relevance and contribution to the whole of pediatrics.

This book has been written by men and women from 18 universities in North America and Europe whose own careers have been devoted to some aspect of clinical immunology. Writing with both the specialist and the generalist in mind, the contributors have combined the basic knowledge of the immunologic system with clinical descriptions of immunologic disorders.

The book begins with the development and biology of the immune response and the components of the immunologic system (Part One), continues with a detailed exposition of the immunodeficiencies (Part Two), and concludes with a group of chapters detailing the immunologic aspects of various pediatric disorders (Part Three). Included in Part One is a review by Dr. Robert Good of the major experiments in nature which have served as the impetus for the advances in clinical immunology.

The terminology employed for the immunoglobulin classes, complement components, and immunodeficiencies is that recommended by the World Health Organization. The terminology for the primary immunodeficiencies has only recently been codified, and since many eponyms are well established in the literature (e.g., Wiskott-Aldrich syndrome), we have added these to avoid ambiguity. Except in the section on immunodeficiences (Part Two), no attempt has been made to present complete bibliographies. In the other sections, key references to summary and review articles are often used.

A suitable subtitle for a primarily American work on pediatric immunology might be "A Tale of Two Cities." The cities are not London and Paris in the 1780's but Minneapolis and Boston in the 1960's. The pediatric departments of the University of Minnesota and Harvard, under the leadership of Good, Janeway, and Gillin, have provided much of the information in this volume and served as the training grounds for many of the contributors. Others, including the editors, have indirectly benefited from the stimulation from these centers. In 1859 Dickens stated about the 1780's that "It was the best of times, it was the worst of times." In 1973, it is the best of times for physicians concerned with the exciting and challenging aspects of immunologic disorders; for most patients, it is still the worst of times, because, with rare exceptions, therapy is unrewarding. The outlook should be bright; one large cloud is the diminution of support for the further exposition of this subject.

The skilled secretarial assistance of Mrs. Paulette Stroehnisch and Mrs. Donna Keller is acknowledged. The editorial guidance of Mr. Albert Meier and Mr. Michael Jackson of the W. B. Saunders Company is greatly appreciated.

E. Richard Stiehm
Vincent A. Fulginiti

Preface to the Fifth Edition

The history of this text begins and ends with Robert A. Good. Dr. Good authored the first chapter of the first edition published in 1973. Titled "Crucial experiments of nature that have guided analysis of the immunologic apparatus," it summarizes a theme that reverberates throughout his long and amazing career. He died on Friday, June 13, 2003, at the age of 81, the exact day that the final chapter of this fifth edition was sent to the publisher. Although the efforts of many have contributed to pediatric immunology, Dr. Good's contributions are unmatched in their timeliness, inclusiveness, and mentorship.

Since the last edition was published in 1996, advances in both basic and clinical immunology have accelerated. Isaac Newton said "to explain all nature is too difficult a task for any one man or even for any one age." Thus this text, although outlining many new diagnostic techniques, previously unrecognized illnesses, and therapeutic successes (e.g., therapeutic monoclonal antibodies, gene therapy), will be seriously outdated by the year 2010, when the next edition is scheduled to be published. We must be content to summarize the current information deemed most significant to the science of immunology relevant to pediatric patients. Thus this book is for pediatric specialists, general pediatricians, fellows, residents, and medical students

The increasing complexity of the field has led to increased collaboration among doctors, basic scientists, laboratories, institutions, and countries. A single-authored report such as Dr. Ogdon Bruton's 1952 article on Agammaglobulinemia is now as rare as a multi-authored novel. Several organizations throughout the world facilitate this interaction; examples include the International Union of Immunologic Scientists (IUIS), the Clinical Immunology Society, the European Society for Immunodeficiencies, and the Pan-American Society for Immunodeficencies—all of which facilitate this interaction by sponsorship of meetings, workshops, summer schools, registries, and position papers.

Equally important has been the work of two foundations, the Immune Deficiency Foundation, founded in 1980, and the Jeffrey Modell Foundation, founded in 1987, to promote awareness, scholarship, patient information and education, collaborative studies, centers of excellence, guest lectureships, and lobbying efforts. The dedication of this volume to the children of Marcia and John Boyle and Vickie and Fred Modell honors their continuing contributions.

This fifth edition has undergone extensive revision. Part I, Development and Function of the Immune System, includes new chapters on the natural defense system and the immunology of pregnancy. As in the rest of the book, there are several new authors, and the others have made extensive revisions of their previous chapter.

Part II, Primary Immunodeficiencies, now includes four chapters (15 through 18) on combined and isolated cellular (T-cell) immunodeficiencies—previously covered in one chapter. These chapters reflect much of the new information on these complex immunodeficiencies. A new chapter on apoptosis syndromes has been added as well. All told, a discussion of more than 100 primary immunodeficiencies is included.

Part III, Secondary Immunodeficiencies, includes a new chapter on genetic syndromes with immunodeficiency (e.g., syndromic immunodeficiencies). The immunodeficiencies of malnutrition, splenic deficiency, surgical and anesthetic stress, and burns have been expanded. The immunodeficiencies of immaturity and HIV infection, two fast-moving areas, have been expanded and updated.

Part IV, Immunologic Aspects of Pediatric Illness, presents a new chapter on periodic fever and an updated review of bone marrow and solid organ transplantation.

Two co-editors and 70 new authors, many from Europe and other areas of the world, have been added. Particular thanks are extended to authors Alexander Lawton, Jane Schaller, and Rebecca Buckley, who have contributed to all five editions, and to Arthur Ammann who agreed at a late date to rewrite the chapter on HIV infection.

The editors would like to acknowledge the patience and support of our families, the assistance of our divisional assistants, and the guidance of our Medical Editor Judith Fletcher.

E. Richard Stiehm
Hans D. Ochs
Jerry A. Winkelstein

Contributors

Arthur J. Ammann, MD
Clinical Professor of Pediatrics
University of California
San Francisco Medical Center
San Francisco, California
Pediatric Human Immunodeficiency Virus Infection

Jintanat Ananworanich, MD
Clinical Trials Physician
The HIV Netherlands Australia Thailand Research
  Collaboration (HIV-NAT)
The Thai Red Cross AIDS Research Center
Bangkok, Thailand
Immune Responses in Malnutrition; Immune Deficiency
  in Metabolic Diseases

Bernard M. Babior, MD, PhD
Professor
The Scripps Research Institute
San Diego, California
The Polynuclear Leukocyte System

Mark Ballow, MD
Professor, Department of Pediatrics
SUNY School of Medicine and Biomedical Sciences
Director, Allergy/Clinical Immunology Fellowship
  Training Program
Chief, Allergy/Clinical Immunology and Pediatric
  Rheumatology Division
Women & Children's Hospital of Buffalo
Buffalo, New York
Stress-Related Immunodeficiencies: Trauma, Surgery,
  Anesthesia, Burns, Exercise, and Splenic Deficiencies

Laurie O. Beitz, BA, MD
Assistant Professor of Pediatrics
University of Washington School of Medicine
Attending Physician, Department of Rheumatology
Children's Hospital and Regional Medical Center
Seattle, Washington
Rheumatic Disorders

Melvin Berger, MD, PhD
Professor of Pediatrics and Pathology
Case Western Reserve University
Allergy-Immunology Division
Department of Pediatrics
Rainbow, Babies and Children's Hospital
University Hospitals Health System
Cleveland, Ohio
The Serum Complement System

Jack J.H. Bleesing, MD, PhD
Assistant Professor of Pediatrics
University of Arkansas for Medical Sciences
Attending Physician, Division of Allergy and
  Immunology
Arkansas Children's Hospital
Little Rock, Arkansas
Autoimmune Lymphoproliferative Syndrome (ALPS)

John F. Bohnsack, MD
Professor of Pediatrics
Adjunct Professor of Pathology
University of Utah School of Medicine
Salt Lake City, Utah
The Natural (Innate) Defense System

Athos Bousvaros, MD, MPH
Assistant Professor of Pediatrics
Harvard Medical School
Associate Director, Inflammatory Bowel Disease
  Center
Children's Hospital
Boston, Massachusetts
Gastroenterologic and Liver Disorders

Rebecca H. Buckley, MD
J. Buren Sidbury Professor of Pediatrics
Professor of Immunology
Duke University School of Medicine
Durham, North Carolina
Other Well-Defined Immunodeficiency Syndromes;
  Transplantation

Fabio Candotti, MD
Head, Disorders of Immunity Section
Senior Investigator, Genetics and Molecular Biology
    Branch
National Human Genome Research Institute
National Institutes of Health
Bethesda, Maryland
    Combined Immunodeficiencies

James D. Cherry, MD, MSc
Professor of Pediatrics
David Geffen School of Medicine at UCLA
Member, Division of Infectious Diseases
Mattel Children's Hospital at UCLA
Los Angeles, California
    Infection in the Compromised Host

Javier Chinen, MD, PhD
Staff Clinician
National Human Genome Research Institute
National Institutes of Health
Bethesda, Maryland
    Immunosuppression Induced by Therapeutic Agents
        and Environmental Conditions

James E. Crowe, Jr., MD
Associate Professor of Pediatrics, Infectious Diseases,
    and Microbiology and Immunology
Vanderbilt University Medical Center
Nashville, Tennessee
    Ontogeny of Immunity

Charlotte Cunningham-Rundles, MD, PhD
Professor, Medicine, Pediatrics, Immunobiology
Mount Sinai Medical School
Attending Physician
Mount Sinai Medical Center
New York, New York
    Antibody Deficiencies; Disorders of the IgA System

Susanna Cunningham-Rundles, PhD
Vice Chair for Academic Affairs
Professor of Immunology
Department of Pediatrics
Cornell University Weill Medical College
New York, New York
    Immune Responses in Malnutrition

Maite de la Morena, MD
Assistant Professor of Pediatrics
Washington University School of Medicine
St. Louis Children's Hospital
St. Louis, Missouri
    The Immunology of Pregnancy

Genevieve de Saint-Basile, MD, PhD
Director of Research
Inserm Unit 429
University Hospital, Necker
Paris, France
    Other Well-Defined Immunodeficiency Syndromes

Jean-Pierre de Villartay, PhD
Director of Research
University Hospital, Necker
Paris, France
    Combined Immunodeficiencies

Jaime G. Deville, MD
Assistant Clinical Professor of Pediatrics
David Geffen School of Medicine at UCLA
UCLA School of Medicine
Attending Physician, Division of Pediatric Infectious
    Diseases
Mattel Children's Hospital at UCLA
Attending Physician, UCLA Maternal-Child
    Immunology Clinic
Los Angeles, California
    Infection in the Compromised Host

Steven D. Douglas, MD
Professor of Pediatrics and Microbiology
Associate Chair, Academic Affairs, Department of
    Pediatrics
University of Pennsylvania School of Medicine
Chief, Section of Immunology, Division of Allergy and
    Immunology
Director, Clinical Immunology Laboratories
The Children's Hospital of Philadelphia
Philadelphia, Pennsylvania
    The Mononuclear Phagocytic, Dendritic Cell, and Natural Killer
        Cell Systems

Anne Durandy, MD, PhD
Director of Research
Inserm Unit 429
Hopital Necker Enfants Malades
Paris, France
    Antibody Deficiencies

Kurt H. Edelmann, PhD
The Viral-Immunobiology Laboratory
The Scripps Research Institute
La Jolla, California
    The T-Lymphocyte System

Kathryn M. Edwards, MD
Professor of Pediatrics
Vanderbilt University School of Medicine
Vice Chair for Clinical Research
Vanderbilt Children's Hospital
Nashville, Tennessee
    Periodic Fever Syndromes

Alain Fischer, MD, PhD
Professor
Necker Medical Faculty
Université Paris
Director, Inserm Unit 429
Necker University Hospital
Paris, France
Combined Immunodeficiencies

Thomas A. Fleisher, MD
Chief, Department of Laboratory Medicine
Clinical Center
National Institutes of Health, Department of Health
and Human Services
Bethesda, Maryland
Autoimmune Lymphoproliferative Syndrome (ALPS)

John O. Fleming, MD
Professor, Vice Chair, Neurology
Professor, Medical Microbiology and Immunology
University of Wisconsin School of Medicine
Attending Neurologist
University of Wisconsin Hospital and Clinics
Madison, Wisconsin
Immunologic Disorders of the Nervous System

Michael M. Frank, MD
Professor of Pediatrics, Immunology and Medicine
Duke University Medical Center
Durham, North Carolina
The Serum Complement System

Eleonora Gambineri, MD
Researcher
University of Florence, Department of Pediatrics
"A. Meyer" Children's Hospital
Florence, Italy
Other Well-Defined Immunodeficiency Syndromes

Roberto P. Garofalo, MD
Professor, Department of Pediatrics and Sealy Center
for Vaccine Development
Professor, Department of Microbiology and
Immunology
The University of Texas Medical Branch
Galveston, Texas
The Mucosal Defense System

Jonathan David Gitlin, MD
Helene B. Roberson Professor of Pediatrics
Professor of Pathology and Immunology
Washington University School of Medicine
St. Louis, Missouri
The Immunology of Pregnancy

Randall M. Goldblum, MD
Professor, Department of Pediatrics and Human
Biological Chemistry and Genetics
University of Texas Medical Branch
Galveston, Texas
The Mucosal Defense System

John M. Graham, Jr., MD, ScD
Professor of Pediatrics
David Geffen School of Medicine at UCLA
UCLA School of Medicine
Director of Clinical Genetics and Dysmorphology
Cedars Sinai Medical Center
Los Angeles, California
Genetic Disorders, Including Syndromic Immunodeficiencies

Barbara Grospierre, PhD
Director of Research
Inserm Unite 429
University Hospital Necker
Paris, France
Combined Immunodeficiencies

Anna Virginia Gulino, MD
Visiting Fellow
National Institutes of Health
National Cancer Institute, Metabolism Branch
Bethesda, Maryland
Other Well-Defined Immunodeficiency Syndromes

Jon M. Hanifin, MD
Professor of Dermatology
Oregon Health & Science University
Portland, Oregon
Dermatologic Disorders

Michael Hershfield, MD
Professor of Medicine and Biochemistry
Duke University Medical Center
Durham, North Carolina
Combined Immune Deficiencies Due to Purine Enzyme Defects

Harry R. Hill, MD
Professor of Pathology, Pediatrics, and Medicine
University of Utah School of Medicine
Salt Lake City, Utah
The Natural (Innate) Defense System

Wenzhe Ho, MD
Associate Professor of Pediatrics
University of Pennsylvania School of Medicine
Director, Retrovirology Laboratory, Division of Allergy
    and Immunology
The Children's Hospital of Philadelphia
Philadelphia, Pennsylvania
    The Mononuclear Phagocytic, Dendritic Cell, and Natural Killer
    Cell Systems

Steven M. Holland, MD
Chief, Immunopathogenesis Section
Laboratory of Host Defenses
National Institute of Allergy and Infectious Diseases
National Institutes of Health
Bethesda, Maryland
    Other Well-Defined Immunodeficiency Syndromes; Phagocyte
    Disorders

Alex Y.C. Huang, MD, PhD
Post-Doctoral Fellow
Lymphocyte Biology Section, Laboratory of
    Immunology
National Institute of Allergy and Infectious Diseases
National Institutes of Health
Bethesda, Maryland
    The Immune Response: Generation, Regulation, and
    Maintenance

Richard A. Insel, MD
Executive Vice President of Research
Juvenile Diabetes Research Foundation International
    (JDRF)
New York, New York
    The B-Lymphocyte System: Fundamental Immunology

Richard B. Johnston, Jr., MD
Professor of Pediatrics
University of Colorado School of Medicine and
    National Jewish Medical and Research Center
Associate Dean for Research Development
University of Colorado School of Medicine
Denver, Colorado
    The Polymorphonuclear Leukocyte System

Stanley C. Jordan, MD
Professor of Pediatrics
David Geffen School of Medicine at UCLA
Medical Director, Kidney Transplant Program
Director, Division of Nephrology and Transplant
    Immunology
Cedars-Sinai Medical Center
Los Angeles, California
    Immune-Mediated Renal Diseases

Reuben Kapur, PhD
Professor of Pediatrics
Indiana University School of Medicine
Cancer Research Institute
Indianapolis, Indiana
    The Mononuclear Phagocytic, Dendritic Cell, and Natural Killer
    Cell Systems

Charles H. Kirkpatrick, MD
Professor of Medicine
Director, Adult Immune Deficiency Program
University of Colorado Health Sciences Center
Denver, Colorado
Attending Physician
University of Colorado Hospital
Aurora, Colorado
    Other Well-Defined Immunodeficiency Syndromes

Mark W. Kline, MD
Professor of Pediatrics
Head, Section of Retrovirology
Baylor College of Medicine
Attending Physician
Texas Children's Hospital
Houston, Texas
    Active and Passive Immunization in the Prevention of Infectious
    Diseases

Thomas J. Kunicki, PhD
Associate Professor, Department of Molecular and
    Experimental Medicine
The Scripps Research Institute
La Jolla, California
    Immune-Mediated Hematologic and Oncologic Disorders

Timothy R. La Pine, MD
Adjunct Assistant Professor of Pediatrics and
    Pathology
University of Utah School of Medicine
Salt Lake City, Utah
    The Natural (Innate) Defense System

Martin F. Lavin, BSc (Hons), PhD
Professor of Molecular Oncology
University of Queensland
Senior Principal Research Fellow
Queensland Institute of Medical Research
Brisbane, Australia
    Chromosomal Breakage Syndromes Associated with
    Immunodeficiency

Alexander R. Lawton, MD
Edward C. Stahlman Professor of Pediatric Physiology
    and Cell Metabolism
Professor of Microbiology and Immunology
Vanderbilt University School of Medicine
Nashville, Tennessee
    Ontogeny of Immunity; Periodic Fever Syndromes

Howard M. Lederman, MD, PhD
Professor of Pediatrics and Medicine
Johns Hopkins University School of Medicine
Director of Immunodeficiency Clinic
Director of Pediatric Immunology Laboratory
Johns Hopkins Hospital
Baltimore, Maryland
    Antibody Deficiencies; Chromosomal Breakage Syndromes
    Associated with Immunodeficiency

David B. Lewis, MD
Associate Professor, Department of Pediatrics and
    Immunology
Stanford University School of Medicine
Stanford, California
Attending Physician
Lucile Salter Packard Children's Hospital
Palo Alto, California
    The Physiologic Immunodeficiency of Immaturity

Maria Ines Garcia Lloret, MD
Clinical Instructor of Pediatrics
Mattel Children's Hospital at UCLA
Los Angeles, California
    Other Well-Defined Immunodeficiency Syndromes

R. John Looney, MD
Professor, Department of Medicine, Allergy,
    Immunology, Rheumatology Unit
University of Rochester
Rochester, New York
    The B-Lymphocyte System: Fundamental Immunology

Katherine Luzuriaga, MD, MS
Professor of Pediatrics
University of Massachusetts Medical School
Worcester, Massachusetts
    Immune Mechanisms in Infectious Disease

Kenneth J. Mack, MD, PhD
Associate Professor
Mayo Medical School
Consultant
Mayo Clinic
Rochester, Minnesota
    Immunologic Disorders of the Nervous System

Kenneth L. McClain, MD, PhD
Professor of Pediatrics
Baylor College of Medicine
Texas Children's Cancer Center/Hematology Service
Houston, Texas
    Proliferative and Histiocytic Disorders

David F. McNeeley, MD, MPHTM
Associate Director, Global Clinical Research
J & J Pharmaceutical Research
Raritan, New Jersey
    Immune Responses in Malnutrition

Jeffrey D. Merrill, MD
Assistant Professor of Pediatrics
University of Pennsylvania School of Medicine
Medical Director, Intensive Care Nursery
Hospital of the University of Pennsylvania
Philadelphia, Pennsylvania
    The Mononuclear Phagocytic, Dendritic Cell, and Natural Killer
    Cell Systems

Laurie C. Miller, MD
Tufts University School of Medicine
Associate Professor of Pediatrics
Division of Pediatric Rheumatology
New England Medical Center
Boston, Massachusetts
    Rheumatic Disorders

Jeffrey E. Ming, MD, PhD
Assistant Professor of Pediatrics
Division of Human Genetics
The Children's Hospital of Philadelphia and The
    University of Pennsylvania School of Medicine
Philadelphia, Pennsylvania
    Genetic Disorders, Including Syndromic Immunodeficiencies

Lynne H. Morrison, MD
Assistant Professor of Dermatology
Oregon Health & Science University
Staff Physician
Portland VA Medical Center
Portland, Oregon
    Dermatologic Disorders

Asha Moudgil, MD
Assistant Professor of Pediatrics
George Washington University
Director, Kidney Transplant
Children's National Medical Center
Washington, DC
    Immune-Mediated Renal Diseases

David L. Nelson, MD
Chief, Immunophysiology Section
Metabolism Branch, Center for Cancer
Research National Cancer Institute
National Institutes of Health
Bethesda, Maryland
    Other Well-Defined Immunodeficiency Syndromes

Karin Nielsen, MD, MPH
Assistant Clinical Professor of Pediatrics
David Geffen School of Medicine at UCLA
Attending Physician, Division of Pediatric Infectious
    Diseases
Mattel Children's Hospital at UCLA
Attending Physician, Maternal Child Immunology
    Clinic/Care 4 Kids
Los Angeles, California
    Other Well-Defined Immunodeficiency Syndromes

Luigi D. Notarangelo, MD
Professor of Pediatrics
School of Medicine
University of Brescia
Head, Department of Pediatrics
Children's Hospital, Spedali Civili
Brescia, Italy
Antibody Deficiencies; Combined Immunodeficiencies; Other
Well-Defined Immunodeficiency Syndromes

Diane J. Nugent, MD
Director of Hematology
Director of Molecular Medicine Core and Pediatric
Hemostasis Research
Children's Hospital of Orange County
Orange, California
Immune-Mediated Hematologic and Oncologic Disorders

Hans D. Ochs, MD
Professor of Pediatrics
University of Washington School of Medicine
Seattle, Washington
Immunodeficiency Disorders: General Considerations; Antibody
Deficiencies; Other Well-Defined Immunodeficiency
Syndromes

Fabienne Dayer Pastore, MB, BS
Assistant Professor of Pediatrics
Section of Allergy and Immunology
Department of Pediatrics
Baylor College of Medicine
Houston, Texas
Proliferative and Histiocytic Disorders

Yves Pastore, MD
Assistant Professor
Section of Allergy and Immunology
Department of Pediatrics
Baylor College of Medicine
Houston, Texas
Proliferative and Histiocytic Disorders

John K. Pfaff, MD
Medical Director, Respiratory Services
Department of Pulmonary Medicine
Cook Children's Medical Center
Fort Worth, Texas
Pulmonary Disorders

Susan F. Plaeger, PhD
Chief, Pathogenesis & Basic Research Branch
Division of AIDS
National Institute of Allergy & Infectious Diseases
National Institutes of Health, Department of Health &
Human Services
Bethesda, Maryland
Cluster Designation Nomenclature for Human Leukocyte
Differentiation Antigens; Principal Human Cytokines and
Chemokines

Alessandro Plebani, MD
Professor in Pediatrics
University of Brescia
Medical Doctor, Chief Section of Pediatric
Immunology and Rheumatology
Spedali Civili
Brescia, Italy
Combined Immunodeficiencies

Jennifer M. Puck, MD
Chief, Genetics and Molecular Biology Branch
Division of Intramural Research
National Human Genome Research Institute
National Institutes of Health
Senior Staff Physician
Warren Magnusen Clinical Center
National Institutes of Health
Bethesda, Maryland
Autoimmune Lymphoproliferative Syndrome (ALPS)

David J. Rawlings, MD, BS
Head, Section of Immunology/Rheumatology,
Department of Pediatrics
Associate Professor of Pediatrics and Immunology
University of Washington, School of Medicine
Seattle, Washington
Antibody Deficiencies

Mark R. Rigby, MD, PhD
Assistant Professor, Department of Pediatrics
McKelvey Scholar, Emory Transplant Center
Emory University School of Medicine
Attending Physician, Critical Care Medicine
Children's Healthcare of Atlanta at Egleston
Atlanta, Georgia
The Immune Response: Generation, Regulation, and
Maintenance

Gail S. Rodich, MD
Assistant Professor of Pediatrics
David Geffen School of Medicine at UCLA
Attending Pediatric Nephrologist
Cedars-Sinai Medical Center
Los Angeles, California
Immune-Mediated Renal Diseases

Chaim M. Roifman, MD
Professor of Pediatrics and Immunology
Donald and Audrey Campbell Chair of Immunology
University of Toronto
Head, Division of Immunology/Allergy
Head, Infection Immunity, Injury and Repair Program
The Hospital for Sick Children
Toronto, Canada
Antibody Deficiencies

Sergio D. Rosenzweig, MD
Immunopathogenesis Section, Laboratory of Host
  Defenses
National Institute of Allergy and Infectious Diseases
National Institutes of Health
Bethesda, Maryland
Servicio de Inmunologia
Hospital de Pediatria J. P. Garrahan
Beunos Aires, Argentina
  Other Well-Defined Immunodeficiency Syndromes; Phagocyte
    Disorders

Gary J. Russell, MD
Assistant Professor of Pediatrics
Harvard Medical School
Associate Pediatrician
Pediatric Gastroenterology and Nutrition
Massachusetts General Hospital
Boston, Massachusetts
  Gastroenterologic and Liver Disorders

Hugh A. Sampson, MD
Professor of Pediatrics & Immunology
Chief, Pediatric Allergy & Immunology
Director, Jaffe Food Allergy Institute
Director of General Clinical Research Center
Mount Sinai School of Medicine
New York, New York
  Allergic Diseases

Jane G. Schaller, MD
Karp Professor of Pediatrics Emerita
Tufts University School of Medicine
Chief, Division of Pediatric Rheumatology
Floating Hospital for Children
Boston, Massachusetts
  Rheumatic Disorders

Heidi Schwarzwald, MD, MPH
Assistant Professor of Pediatrics
Baylor College of Medicine
Attending Physician
Texas Children's Hospital
Houston, Texas
  Active and Passive Immunization in the Prevention of Infectious
    Diseases

William T. Shearer, MD, PhD
Professor of Pediatrics and Immunology
Baylor College of Medicine
Chief of Allergy and Immunology Service
Texas Children's Hospital
Houston, Texas
  Immune Deficiency in Metabolic Diseases; Proliferative and
    Histiocytic Disorders; Immunosuppression Induced by
    Therapeutic Agents and Environmental Conditions

Scott H. Sicherer, MD
Associate Professor of Pediatrics
Jaffe Food Allergy Institute
Mount Sinai School of Medicine
New York, New York
  Allergic Diseases

Maria Rita Signorino, MD
Physician
Pediatric Department
University of Catania
Catania, Italy
  Autoimmune Endocrinopathies

E. Richard Stiehm, MD
Professor of Pediatrics
David Geffen School of Medicine at UCLA
Attending Physician
Mattel Children's Hospital at UCLA
UCLA Center for Health Sciences
Los Angeles, California
  The B-Lymphocyte System: Clinical Immunology;
    Immunodeficiency Disorders: General Considerations;
    Antibody Deficiencies; Other Well-Defined Immunodeficiency
    Syndromes

John L. Sullivan, MD
Professor of Pediatrics and Molecular Medicine
Director, Office of Research
University of Massachusetts Medical School
Worcester, Massachusetts
  Other Well-Defined Immunodeficiency Syndromes; Immune
    Mechanisms in Infectious Disease

Kathleen E. Sullivan, MD, PhD
Associate Professor
University of Pennsylvania School of Medicine
Associate Physician
Children's Hospital of Philadelphia
Philadelphia, Pennsylvania
  Other Well-Defined Immunodeficiency Syndromes; Deficiencies
    of the Complement System

Troy R. Torgerson, MD, PhD
Senior Fellow, Pediatric Rheumatology/Immunology
University of Washington
Children's Hospital Regional Medical Center
Seattle, Washington
  Other Well-Defined Immunodeficiency Syndromes

Wenwei Tu, MD, PhD
Research Associate
Stanford University School of Medicine
Stanford, California
  The Physiologic Immunodeficiency of Immaturity

Gülbû Uzel, MD
Assistant Professor of Pediatrics
Division of Immunology and Rheumatology
Children's Memorial Hospital
Feinberg School of Medicine, Northwestern University
Chicago, Illinois
    Phagocyte Disorders

W. Allan Walker, MD
Conrad Taff Professor of Nutrition and Pediatrics
Director, Division of Nutrition
Harvard Medical School
Director, Mucosal Immunology and Development
    Gastroenterology Laboratories
Massachusetts General Hospital
Boston, Massachusetts
    Gastroenterologic and Liver Disorders

Christopher B. Wilson, MD
Professor and Chair, Department of Immunology
Professor of Pediatrics
University of Washington School of Medicine
Seattle, Washington
    The T-Lymphocyte System

Jerry A. Winkelstein, MD
Eudowood Professor of Pediatrics
Professor of Medicine and Pathology
Johns Hopkins University School of Medicine
Baltimore, Maryland
    Immunodeficiency Disorders: General Considerations; Antibody
    Deficiencies; Deficiencies of the Complement System

William E. Winter, MD
University of Florida
Medical Director for Clinical Chemistry
Shands Hospital
Gainesville, Florida
    Autoimmune Endocrinopathies

Mervin C. Yoder, Jr., MD
Professor of Pediatrics, Biochemistry and Molecular
    Biology
Indiana University School of Medicine
Cancer Research Institute
Indianapolis, Indiana
    The Mononuclear Phagocytic, Dendritic Cell, and Natural Killer
    Cell Systems

Contents

part

Development and Function of the Immune System

Ontogeny of Immunity

Alexander R. Lawton and James E. Crowe, Jr.

INTRODUCTION

The cells of the immune system are derived from a relatively small pool of pluripotential hematopoietic stem cells (HSCs) present in the fetal liver, the omentum, and ultimately the bone marrow. In response to inductive signals from specialized microenvironments, HSCs enter one of two major differentiation pathways. One pathway generates several lineages of specialized effector cells, which constitute the innate immune system. These cells include the professional phagocytes (polymorphonuclear leuko-cytes, monocytes, and macrophages), specialized antigen-presenting cells (dendritic cells of germinal centers, Langerhans cells of skin), natural killer (NK) cells, and purveyors of the mediators of inflammation (mast cells, basophils, and eosinophils). The second pathway generates the two major classes of lymphocytes, T cells and B cells, which form the adaptive immune system.

Collectively the lymphocytes of the adaptive immune system have the capacity to recognize specifically an almost limitless number of antigens; individually each cell expresses one receptor (in the case of T cells, perhaps two receptors [Padovan et al., 1993]). In addition to having unique receptors, mature lymphoid cells have distinct effector functions ranging from the secretion of antibodies to the direct killing of other cells. Lymphocytes express a variety of membrane molecules that determine their migration patterns and communicate signals to and from other lymphocytes. They also secrete soluble cytokines that regulate the functions of the cells of the innate immune system and of other lymphocytes. The result is a network of interacting cells that resembles the central nervous system in its organizational complexity and capacity for learning.

Each step in the developmental process that generates the lymphoid system is genetically controlled. The number of structural and regulatory genes involved is quite large; therefore, the potential for genetic defects resulting in abnormal function of the immune system is great. Just as the elucidation of enzymatic defects responsible for inborn errors of metabolism depends on the identification of each step in a metabolic pathway, understanding lymphoid differentiation defects requires appreciation of the sequence and regulation of normal lymphoid development. The study of the ontogeny of lymphocytes offers the great advantage of isolating some of the early events of their differentiation from the complex regulatory interactions occurring in mature animals.

In this chapter we describe the major steps in the development of T and B lymphocytes. We briefly discuss the maturation of the integrated functions of these cells and the characteristics that distinguish the immune responses of the fetus and newborn from those of older children or adults.

T- AND B-CELL SYSTEMS

Lymphoid development occurs along two distinct pathways, leading to populations of cells that have different functions and phenotypic markers. The thymus is the induction site for T cells, which are responsible for those effector functions termed *cell-mediated immunity*. B cells, which are collectively responsible for the synthesis and secretion of humoral antibodies, constitute the second major limb of the lymphoid system. The name is derived from their primary developmental sites, the bursa of Fabricius in birds or the bone marrow in mammals.

Surface Markers

Hematopoietic cells, including T and B cells, are identified and characterized in blood and tissues by labeled monoclonal antibodies that recognize some unique component of the cell membrane. An international committee assigns *cluster of differentiation* (CD) numbers to markers recognized by several different monoclonal antibodies that have uniform physical characteristics and cellular distribution. The number of CD molecules is increasing rapidly, as is knowledge of their structure and function. A list of CD designations and descriptions of the proteins they represent is included in the Appendix at the end of this book.

B lymphocytes are classically distinguished by the presence of surface immunoglobulin (Ig), predominantly of the IgM and IgD isotypes, and the B-cell–specific glycoproteins CD19 and CD20. A number of membrane proteins recognized by widely available monoclonal antibodies are used to identify T cells. The predominant T-cell receptor (TCR) consists of a heterodimeric antigen recognition unit of α and β chains linked to a multichain signaling complex recognized by CD3 monoclonal antibodies.

Included in this complex are co-receptor molecules CD4 and CD8 and the tyrosine phosphatase CD45. The last marker is found on all hematopoietic cells, but it is of particular importance because the expression of different isoforms distinguishes naïve T cells from memory T cells (Janeway, 1992). A much smaller T-cell population has an antigen recognition unit consisting of δ and γ chains and generally lacks CD4 and CD8.

A third class of lymphoid cells can be defined by the use of monoclonal antibodies. These are variously called null cells, NK cells, or large granular lymphocytes. These cells are nonphagocytic and lack the antigen-specific receptors of T or B cells, but they share markers and some functions with macrophages and T cells. The ability to efficiently lyse antibody-coated target cells (antibody-dependent cellular cytotoxicity) and the capacity to kill certain target cells without prior sensitization (NK activity) are the important functions of these cells. NK cells have lectin receptors that recognize a variety of cell surface carbohydrate molecules and trigger cytolytic function. Other receptors recognizing self major histocompatibility complex (MHC) class I molecules inhibit killing of normal cells (Lanier, 1998). Tumor cells or virus-infected cells may become NK targets if expression of class I MHC is altered.

B and T cells are developmentally independent, have distinctive cell membrane characteristics, occupy different areas in lymphoid tissues, have different patterns of recirculation, and can be grouped into effectors of humoral and cellular immunity, respectively. This distinctiveness should not obscure the fact that these two systems use related gene families and common mechanisms for the generation of diverse receptors and are remarkably interrelated in terms of their functions. A discussion of the extent and mechanisms of these interactions is beyond the scope of this chapter. Nevertheless, we briefly outline some of the phenomena that are relevant to an understanding of the ontogeny of immunity.

T-Cell Subsets

T cells with $\alpha\beta$ receptors are divided into two nonoverlapping classes distinguished by expression of either CD4 or CD8 on the cell membrane. CD4 binds to conserved sites on MHC class II proteins; CD8 binds to class I MHC molecules.

The receptors of CD4$^+$ T cells recognize foreign peptides derived from extracellular antigens that have been ingested and processed by professional antigen-presenting cells and are presented bound to MHC class II molecules. CD8$^+$ T cells recognize peptides bound to MHC class I molecules; these peptides are usually derived from proteins synthesized by the presenting cell. CD4$^+$ T cells perform as helpers for the differentiation of B cells and of cytotoxic T cells and as activators of various cells of the innate immune system, such as macrophages and eosinophils. CD8$^+$ cells function as cytotoxic effectors. Because MHC class I molecules are expressed by all nucleated cells and are associated on the cell surface with endogenously synthesized peptides, CD8$^+$ cells are particularly suited to recognize and destroy virus-infected cells and perhaps tumor cells.

CD4$^+$ cells are divisible into functional subsets based on the patterns of cytokines they produce. Cells designated T-helper 1 (Th1) produce interleukin (IL-2) and interferon-γ (IFN-γ) as predominant cytokines and mediate delayed-type hypersensitivity reactions. T-helper 2 (Th2) cells produce mostly IL-4 and IL-5 and serve as helpers for B-cell differentiation. The development of Th1 and Th2 cells from precursor Th0 cells is a postthymic, antigen-driven differentiation process. The type of T cell emerging from an encounter appears to be determined by properties of the antigen, the antigen-presenting cells, the cytokine environment, and the genetic background of the host (Mosmann and Coffman, 1989; Prescott et al., 1999; Sher and Coffman, 1992).

B- and T-Cell Cooperation

With few exceptions, the production of specific antibodies requires an interactive collaboration among antigen-presenting cells, T cells, and B cells. Professional antigen-presenting cells (phagocytic macrophages, follicular dendritic cells in the germinal centers of lymph nodes, and Langerhans cells in the skin) ingest protein antigens and digest them into peptides. Relevant peptides are bound intracellularly to nascent class II MHC proteins and exported to the cell membrane. B lymphocytes are able to process soluble protein antigens and are extremely efficient in presenting the antigens recognized by their receptors (Lanzavecchia, 1990).

T cells become activated when their receptors bind to peptides residing in the groove of MHC molecules. Full activation of CD4[+] T cells requires a co-stimulatory signal delivered when the T-cell molecule CD28 binds to the related B7.1 (CD80) or B7.2 (CD86) molecules expressed by professional antigen-presenting cells and activated B cells (Freeman et al., 1993; Linsley and Ledbetter, 1993).

Activated CD4[+] T cells transiently express a surface glycoprotein antigen CD154 (also called CD40 ligand or CD40L), which binds to CD40 on B cells. The ligation of CD40 transmits a signal to B cells that makes them competent to proliferate, undergo isotype switching, and differentiate to antibody-secreting plasma cells (Noelle et al., 1992; Purkerson and Isakson 1992). These last steps are driven by various cytokines, and it is these cytokines that determine which isotypes will be produced. For example, IL-4 directs switching to IgG1 and IgE, and IL-10 is needed for IgA synthesis (Defrance et al., 1992; Purkerson and Isakson, 1992).

T-cell regulation of the antibody response is also exerted in a negative sense. Mechanisms for T-cell suppression have eluded molecular definition, although the phenomenon is reproducible. One mechanism may be the secretion of cytokines that inhibit T-cell activation, such as IL-10 and TGF-β (Kamradt and Mitchison, 2001).

B cells and their products, the antibody molecules, also serve both immunoregulatory and effector functions. A landmark in immunologic thought occurred with the publication in 1974 of Jerne's network theory of immune regulation (Jerne, 1974). The network consists of idiotypes (unique antigenic determinants associated with the combining site of antibody molecules) and successive generations of auto–anti-idiotypic antibodies that they may provoke. The idea that immunization results in the production not only of antibodies but also of autologous anti-idiotypic antibodies and T cells has been verified in several species (Paul and Bona, 1982), including humans (Colley et al., 1999; Geha, 1983).

Idiotypic regulation may be responsible for the amplification or the suppression of immune responses and is clearly one of the mechanisms by which T-cell immunity and B-cell immunity are linked. The expression of anti-idiotypic antibodies occurs in certain autoimmune diseases. For example, antibodies to the acetylcholine receptor found in patients with myasthenia gravis seem regularly to stimulate an anti-idiotypic response (Dwyer et al., 1983).

The importance of understanding these humoral and cellular interactions is potentially immense. There is much evidence that immunoregulatory abnormalities occur in immunodeficiency diseases, and autoimmunity is such a disorder by definition. Unraveling the mechanisms by which T-cell and B-cell interactions are responsible for the induction and maintenance of tolerance should eventually lead to ways of inducing specific tolerance to cellular antigens in humans; such an accomplishment would be an unparalleled advance in the field of organ transplantation. How some of these relationships play a role in the maturation of the immunologic capacity of the human fetus and newborn is discussed at the end of this chapter.

Stem Cell Compartment

All cells of the immune system are derived from pluripotential hematopoietic stem cells, which are first found within the blood islands of the yolk sac. During embryogenesis, they migrate to other sites of hematopoiesis: the liver, spleen, and bone marrow. The bone marrow is the major repository of HSCs during adult life. Human HSCs express the CD34 glycoprotein. They are present in small numbers in peripheral blood of adults and in relatively higher numbers in neonates. Techniques for mobilization of CD34[+] cells from bone marrow in sufficient numbers for autologous transplantation have been developed.

HSCs from the same highly enriched population can generate both T-cell and B-cell lineages following migration to the thymus or bone marrow, respectively. It remains to be established whether there is a committed lymphoid stem cell incapable of myeloid differentiation and whether independent precursors for T- and B-cell development exist (Ikuta et al., 1992).

T-CELL DEVELOPMENT

T-Cell Receptor Diversity

The role of central lymphoid organs is the generation and education of large numbers of T and B cells having an immensely diverse repertoire of receptors for antigens. This process occurs throughout life but is the defining element of the ontogeny of immunity. The mechanisms for the generation of receptor diversity are described briefly here and in greater detail in Chapters 2 and 3.

T-cell and B-cell receptors for antigen are the products of related but distinct clusters of genes belonging to the large Ig gene superfamily. Receptor diversity is generated from relatively small sets of germline genes by DNA rearrangement mediated by recombinase. The same recombinase enzyme creates functional TCR and Ig receptor genes by a *looping out mechanism*, whereby the DNA separating two segments to be joined is deleted as a circle (Schatz et al., 1992). Seven extended loci of similarly organized genes arranged in tandem are involved in this recombinational process.

TCRs are of two types, αβ and γδ. The αβ types are expressed on the great majority of T cells. T cells with γδ receptors are the first to appear in the thymus and may serve specialized functions. With regard to organization of their constituent genes, the α and γ chains are similar to Ig light chains and the β and δ chains resemble heavy chains. The genes for the 90-kd TCR polypeptides are formed by recombination of gene segments called variable (V), diversity (D), joining (J), and constant (C). The β gene family consists of approximately 20 Vβ genes, a set of Dβ genes, and two sets of several Jβ genes, each associated with a Cβ gene. The last are called Cβ1 and Cβ2. The α and γ gene families lack D genes but are otherwise similarly organized. The γ and δ families contain many fewer V genes than do the α and β families.

Functional genes are generated by sequential rearrangements. To form a β gene, for example, a Dβ gene is translocated and joined to one of the Jβ genes. A second recombination links a Vβ gene to that DJ segment and generates a functional transcriptional unit. Depending on the J gene used, the chain will be of either the β1 or β2 type. A single VJ joining event creates functional γ and δ genes.

Receptor diversity is created at several levels of this process, which is common to the TCR and Ig gene families. The V, D, and J genes inherited in the germline all contribute to the structure of the antigen-binding site, so that each possible combination of these units may produce a different specificity. The splice sites of DJ and VDJ joints are imprecise and are also subject to the addition of random nucleotides by the enzyme terminal deoxynucleotidyltransferase (TdT). This mechanism, called N diversity, makes a particularly large contribution to the generation of diverse TCRs of the αβ type. Finally, different combinations of α with β or of γ with δ chains produce distinct receptor specificities. The γδ TCRs have a restricted repertoire because there are relatively few germline V genes in these families and because they do not use the N diversity mechanism (discussed in the next section).

These mechanisms create an immensely diverse repertoire of receptor specificities from relatively few inherited genes. Imprecise splicing of gene segments and the random addition of untemplated nucleotides produce diversity at the cost of generating a high proportion of defective genes resulting from changes in reading frames or from the introduction of stop codons. This cost is easily met by the production of an excess number of lymphocytes in the thymus and bone marrow. More than 95% of thymocyte production is eliminated by apoptosis prior to circulation.

Another certain consequence of these random processes is the production of receptors with specificity for antigenic determinants of self. The clones of lymphocytes bearing such receptors are subject to deletion at their sites of origin but are also regulated in peripheral lymphoid tissues if they escape the central negative selection process. The occasional development of serious autoimmune disease may be counted as an unavoidable cost of having an immune system sufficiently diverse to recognize virtually any foreign antigen. Finally, these mechanisms suggest that selective pressures during evolution have acted primarily to increase diversity rather than preserve particular useful receptor specificities. This idea is supported by the many different strategies that are successfully used to create antibody and TCR diversity in different species (McCormack et al., 1991).

Thymic Development

The thymus is derived from elements of three primitive germ layers: the endoderm of the third pharyngeal pouch; the ectoderm of the third brachial cleft; and mesenchymal elements (at least a portion of which are of neural crest origin) (Anderson et al., 1996; Bockman and Kirby, 1984). These tissue elements migrate caudally to their eventual location in the anterior mediastinum. Beginning in about the seventh week of gestation in humans, blood-borne stem cells enter the thymus and are induced to begin lymphoid differentiation.

In birds (Jotereau and Le Douarin, 1982) and mice (Ikuta et al., 1992), the thymus initially becomes receptive to the immigration of circulating HSCs in cyclic periods that last a few days and are separated by somewhat longer periods during which it is refractory. This pattern appears to be due to chemotactic activity generated by the thymus epithelium. In birds a soluble form of β2-microglobulin has been identified as a stem cell chemotactic factor (Dunon et al., 1990).

The earliest waves of HSCs to populate the mouse thymus express distinct developmental programs. T cells generated at 14 to 17 days' gestation have a homogeneous TCR consisting of Vγ5 and Vδ1 polypeptides. These cells are precursors of dendritic epidermal T cells of the skin (Havran and Allison, 1990; Ikuta et al., 1992). The next wave of T cells expresses Vγ6 and Vδ1 and migrates to mucosa of the reproductive tract. Precursors rearranging Vγ1, 2, 4, and 7 gene segments develop later, continuously rather than in waves. An additional developmentally determined characteristic of the TCR is the junctional diversity at the VJ and VDJ joints. The fetal Vγ5 and Vγ6 lack inserted nucleotides at these joints, whereas abundant N nucleotides are an important source of diversity in adult γδ TCRs.

The same HSCs give rise to the late-developing γδ TCR and αβ TCR cells. Mature αβ T cells usually have defective rearrangements of γ and δ genes while some γδ T cells have productively rearranged β genes. Determination of TCR type may depend on whether in-frame rearrangements of both γ and δ genes occur before successful rearrangement of a β chain gene and its expression with pre-Tα. Expression of the pre–T-cell receptor (β:pTα) causes β chain rearrangements to cease and triggers a period of rapid proliferation. At the end of this burst of cell division, rearrangements of α chain genes begin. Because there are many Vα and Jα segments, sequential rearrangements can eliminate out-of-frame VJ joints. Thus each β chain is likely to be paired with a number of different α chains. These events are associated with transition of developing thymocytes from CD3⁻, CD4⁻, CD8⁻ "double-negative" precursors to CD3⁺, CD4⁺, CD8⁺ "double-positive" cells subject to positive and negative selection. A more detailed description of this process is given in Chapter 2.

Early development of the human thymus was described by Haynes and colleagues (Haynes et al., 1988, 1989; Lobach et al., 1985) and by Campana and coworkers (1989). Figure 1-1 summarizes the main steps in this pathway. CD7, a marker present on mature T cells, is expressed by hematopoietic cells before the beginning of thymic lymphopoiesis. CD7⁺ cells, which also contain cytoplasmic CD3, accumulate in prethymic mesenchyme from 7 to 8 weeks' gestation. These investigators postulated that because the epithelial thymus is poorly vascularized at this time, the CD7⁺ cells migrate directly into the epithelial rudiment. CD7⁺ cells from thorax or liver cultured with IL-2 and other cytokines generated progeny with markers of mature thymocytes: CD2, CD3, CD4, CD8, and αβ TCRs. The same population cultured under different conditions could give rise to myeloid colonies, indicating their pluripotential nature. In a subsequent study, a population of CD7⁺CD3⁻CD4⁻CD8⁻ cells isolated from postnatal thymus generated γδ TCR and CD8⁺ cells on culture (Denning et al., 1989).

Campana and colleagues (1989) have delineated several stages of T-cell differentiation in human fetal thymus. The least mature proliferating cell population is marked by membrane CD7 and cytoplasmic CD3. Before 18 weeks' gestation, these cells are TdT negative; after this time, they are TdT positive. These cells subsequently express cytoplasmic TCR β chain, CD4, CD8, and CD1. The next stage is marked by membrane

expression of CD3 and αβ TCR and by loss of TdT. Finally, the mature medullary cells lose CD4 or CD8 and are no longer in cycle. Cells expressing the γδ TCR are infrequent in humans at all stages of development.

Shaping the T-Cell Repertoire

The sequential processes of positive and negative selection that shape the T-cell repertoire have been discovered through very elegant experiments, a few of which are briefly described here. The central fact that T cells are educated in the thymus to distinguish self from nonself major histocompatibility determinants was established using bone marrow chimeras. If a mouse of strain A is lethally irradiated and given bone marrow cells from an AxB F1 mouse, the T cells derived from the marrow donor will recognize antigen presented by antigen-presenting cells from strain A but not strain B. The converse is true if the chimera is made by injecting AxB F1 marrow cells into a strain B host. Thymic stromal epithelial cells are responsible for positive selection, as shown by experiments in which athymic AxB mice engrafted with A or B thymus epithelium are recipients of AxB marrow cells. Mature T cells from such animals recognize antigen only when the antigen-presenting cell expresses MHC molecules of the type present on the thymus epithelial graft.

Studies using TCR transgenic mice have provided a remarkably detailed view of the major functional events of intrathymic T-cell development. The genes encoding TCR α and β chains from a T cell of known specificity and MHC restriction, including the regulatory elements

THYMOCYTE DIFFERENTIATION

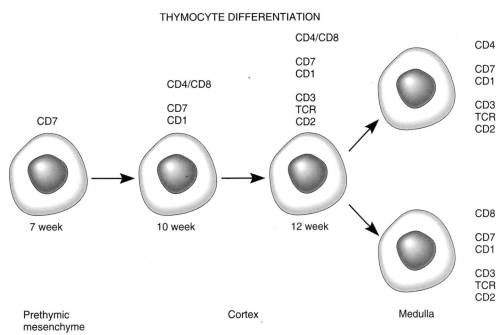

Figure 1-1 · T-cell development within the thymus. The locations and cluster of differentiation (CD) markers for the major steps in thymocyte differentiation are indicated. Both positive and negative selection occur at the double-positive CD4⁺CD8⁺ stage (see text).

that ensure the expression of this TCR by most or all developing thymocytes, are introduced into the germline to create these animals. Selective breeding is then used to manipulate the environment in which these cells develop. These studies have been performed by several groups, but the most important results are particularly well illustrated by the elegant experiments of Von Boehmer and colleagues (Von Boehmer, 1990). The TCR used in these studies recognized the HY antigen, expressed by male but not female mice of the same strain, in association with the class I H-2D^b MHC antigen. Transgenic mice were backcrossed to alter the MHC background, or alternatively backcrossed to mice with severe combined immunodeficiency (SCID) to silence the expression of any endogenous TCR. The SCID mouse has a defective recombinase enzyme that cannot make the gene rearrangements needed to create either T-cell or Ig receptors. Generation of both T and B cells is severely compromised.

The αβ transgenic mice had accelerated fetal development of thymocytes bearing CD3, CD4, and CD8, indicating that expression and proliferation of cells with these co-receptors is dependent on TCR expression. When introduced into SCID mice, the αβ transgene restored normal production of thymocytes. Transfer of only the β transgene raised thymocyte numbers moderately while permitting expression of CD4 and CD8. Rearrangement and expression of the complete αβ TCR is thus necessary for the generation of an expanded population of CD4$^+$CD8$^+$ thymocytes.

The H-2D^b restricted transgenes were derived from a CD8$^+$ T-cell clone. Female transgenic mice of this MHC haplotype had increased numbers of CD4$^-$CD8$^+$ thymocytes and reduced numbers of mature CD4$^+$CD8$^-$ cells. The latter population expressed endogenous α chains in combination with the transgenic β chain, whereas the former expressed the transgenic αβ TCR. In transgenic females of the D^d haplotype, there was no such selection for CD8$^+$ T cells; both CD8$^+$ and CD4$^+$ mature cells expressed endogenous α genes with the β transgene. Thus T cells having a receptor specific for a self-MHC molecule (in this case, T cells with the complete αβ transgene) are positively selected in the thymus. The MHC molecule determines whether the CD4$^+$CD8$^+$ T-cell will retain CD8 (for class I MHC) or CD4 (for class II MHC).

The fate of T cells bearing the transgenic TCR in male mice of D^b haplotype was quite different. Their thymuses contained 10-fold fewer cells than those of females, and virtually all T-cells expressed the transgenic TCR but neither CD4 nor CD8. In control D^d mice, the thymuses of male and female mice were indistinguishable. These results indicate that T cells having receptors that bind avidly to self-antigens are eliminated in the thymus. Deletion by apoptosis occurs at the immature CD4$^+$CD8$^+$ cell stage and therefore affects both CD4$^+$ and CD8$^+$ mature subsets.

Experiments with radiation chimeras have demonstrated that positive selection is dependent on thymus epithelium, whereas expression of the restricting MHC molecule on bone marrow–derived cells is sufficient for negative selection to occur. It has recently been shown that some tissue-restricted self-antigens, including pancreatic β cell proteins, are synthesized in the thymus from fetal through adult life. These self-peptides are expressed by specialized macrophages and dendritic cells in the thymus medulla, around which are found clusters of apoptotic thymocytes apparently undergoing negative selection. Antigen-presenting cells with diabetes-associated autoantigens were also found in peripheral lymphoid tissue (Pugliese et al., 2001).

Determinants of Thymic Development

The identification of the defective gene in X-linked SCID uncovered a role for specific cytokines in thymus development. The defective gene encoded a protein then known only as the γ chain of the IL-2 receptor (Noguchi et al., 1993). The investigators who made the discovery immediately suspected additional functions for this protein because inability to produce IL-2 caused a form of SCID in which T cells were present in normal numbers (Weinberg and Parkman, 1990). Additional experiments have demonstrated that this polypeptide, renamed common γ chain, is a component of the receptors for IL-4, IL-7, and IL-15 (Noguchi et al., 1993; Russell et al., 1993). The factors that drive thymocyte proliferation and differentiation may include several cytokines acting in concert.

Ontogeny of Peripheral T Cells

CD7$^+$ cells with cytoplasmic expression of CD3 appear in fetal liver and perithymic mesenchyme at 7 to 10 weeks' gestation. T cells with membrane αβ TCR and CD3 begin to accumulate in fetal liver at about 10 weeks' gestation and are subsequently found in other lymphoid tissues. Cells with γδ TCR have not been found in human fetal liver and are rare in the thymus (Campana et al., 1989). Specific responses to histocompatibility antigens are demonstrable in the thymus by 12 weeks and in the spleen by 15 weeks (Toivanen et al., 1978).

The ability of infants born at 24 weeks' gestation to survive in the hostile environment of the intensive care nursery suggests that a heterogeneous population of functional T cells is present by this time. T-cell receptor heterogeneity was analyzed by comparing the diversity of expressed Vβ CDR3 regions from 24- to 41-week fetuses with that of adults (Schelonka et al., 1998). At 24 weeks, all Vβ families were represented and had size heterogeneity equivalent to that found in adult TCRs. Fetal CDR3 segments increased in length as a function of age. Oligoclonal expansions of particular Vβ TCR were more common among fetal T cells at 29 to 33 weeks' gestation than adult T-cell populations and were found in both CD4 and CD8 cells. It seems likely that these clones are generated by limited antigen exposure.

The functional capabilities of neonatal T cells, which are discussed in a following section and in Chapter 22,

GENERATION OF ISOTYPE DIVERSITY

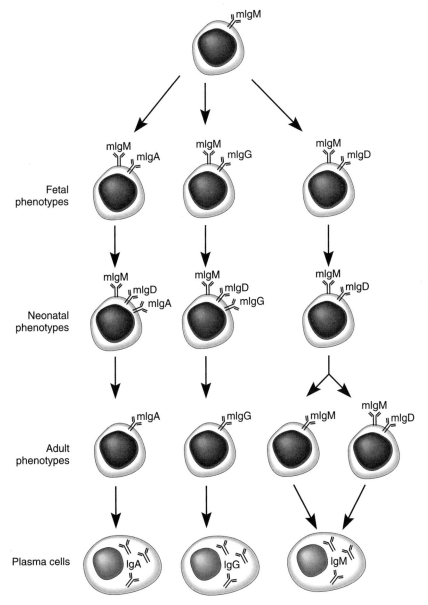

Figure 1-3 · Development of intraclonal isotype diversity. The expression of multiple cell surface isotypes (other than IgM and IgD) is characteristic of immature B cells.

capacity to produce antibodies of the IgG or IgA classes to protein antigens or antibodies of any class to carbohydrate antigens. One of the goals of the study of ontogeny has been to understand, and perhaps learn to circumvent, these impediments to effective immunization against serious infectious diseases of infancy. Neonatal immunity is discussed in depth in Chapter 22.

Neonatal B Cells

The first problem became particularly interesting with the discovery of the long gap between the development of B lymphocytes bearing IgG or IgA isotypes on their membranes late in the first trimester and the expression

of adult concentrations of these isotypes in serum in middle to late childhood (Buckley et al., 1968; Stiehm and Fudenberg, 1966).

The mechanism underlying the observation that newborn B lymphocytes were able to synthesize and express these isotypes on their membranes but not differentiate into secretory plasma cells became a focus of ontogenetic investigation. The later observation that fetal B cells share an immature phenotype with B cells from patients with common variable immunodeficiency and isolated IgA deficiency (Conley and Cooper, 1982; Fiorilli et al., 1986) made this problem even more interesting. Functional studies comparing in vitro responses of neonatal B and T cells with those of adult cells implicated both T and B cells in the impaired capacity to produce IgG and IgA.

In addition to providing poor helper function, neonatal T cells were active suppressors (Hayward and Lawton, 1977). The inability of neonatal B cells to efficiently produce IgG or IgA isotypes was confirmed through the use of polyclonal stimulants that were completely (pokeweed mitogen), partially (*Nocardia* water-soluble mitogen), or not (Epstein-Barr virus) T-cell dependent (Andersson et al., 1981; Miyawaki et al., 1981; Tosato et al., 1980).

All these studies are technically flawed because the stimulants used address only a small fraction of the total B-cell population—that is, preactivated cells that have recently been stimulated by antigen, which are unlikely to be present in neonatal blood (Anderson et al., 1988). Investigations that have used an efficient culture system in which B-cell differentiation is initiated by direct contact with anti-CD3–activated T cells (capable of inducing plasma cell differentiation in 50% to 90% of peripheral blood B cells) have nevertheless confirmed the earlier results (Splawski et al., 1991). Neonatal lymphocytes of both T and B lineages were induced to proliferate, and the T cells produced as much IL-2 as adult cells; however, little or no Ig was produced. In co-culture experiments neonatal T cells could initiate proliferation of adult B cells, but little Ig was produced. Adult T cells provided help for IgM production, but not IgG or IgA production, by neonatal B cells.

Neonatal Cytokine Production

The functional deficits of neonatal cells can be overcome by the addition of exogenous IL-2 and either IL-4 or IL-6. The effect of IL-2 is critical, because antibodies to the IL-2 receptor eliminate Ig production in the presence of any of these lymphokines. No cytokine-specific patterns of isotype secretion were observed in these experiments (Splawski and Lipsky, 1991). These results indicate that neonatal B cells require both a competence signal provided by direct contact with activated T cells and higher concentrations of IL-2 and IL-4 or IL-6 than do adult B cells to undergo differentiation into plasma cells. Neonatal T cells produce sufficient IL-2 to drive T-cell proliferation, but they do not provide the additional cytokines required to support optimal B-cell differentiation.

Differential expression of isoforms of the tyrosine phosphatase CD45 distinguish adult CD4+ T cells with helper activity (CD45RO) from those with suppressor/inducer function (CD45RA). CD45RO cells, which constitute 50% of adult but only 5% of neonatal CD4+ cells, appear to represent a memory population derived from virgin CD45RA cells. These CD45RA cells account for 90% of neonatal CD4+ cells (Clement et al., 1988, 1990; Janeway, 1992). The small number of CD45RO+CD4+ cells present in neonatal blood has helper activity equivalent to the same population of adult cells, whether stimulated by pokeweed mitogen or anti-CD3.

The reciprocal CD45RA+ neonatal T-cell population actively suppresses the helper function of CD45RO cells. This radiation-sensitive suppressor activity is absent from adult CD45RA+ cells. Neonatal CD45RA+ cells stimulated by mitogen and cultured for long periods with IL-2 lose suppressor activity, become CD45RA−, and acquire helper function (Clement et al., 1988; Clement et al., 1990).

Early studies suggested that neonatal T cells produce quantities of IL-2 and tumor necrosis factor α and β similar to those made by adult cells but made little or no IFN-γ, IL-3, IL-4, IL-5, IL-6, or granulocyte-macrophage colony-stimulating factor (Ehlers and Smith, 1991; Lewis et al., 1991; Wilson et al., 1991). Neonatal T cells, however, can produce reasonably similar quantities and profiles of cytokines to T cells of adults under certain conditions (Delespesse et al., 1998). The quantitative differences in cytokine secretion that have been observed are due to reduced numbers of activated cells making a given cytokine. For example, IFN-γ was produced by 40% of adult T cells but only 3% of neonatal T cells analyzed by in situ hybridization (Lewis et al., 1991).

The synthesis of diverse cytokines by T cells is linked to their activation. For example, the frequency of adult CD4+ cells containing mRNA for IFN-γ or for IL-4 was highest in the CD45RO fraction, intermediate in unfractionated cells, and extremely low in CD45RA cells (Wilson et al., 1991). Neonatal cell populations are low in cells with memory markers and have an altered threshold of responsiveness to cytokines. Neonatal cells stimulated by anti-CD3 and cultured with IL-2 for 7 to 10 days produced an adult pattern of cytokine expression (Ehlers and Smith, 1991).

This requirement for post-thymic differentiation, almost certainly an antigen-driven process in vivo, must contribute to the deficiencies in neonatal helper function. Another factor contributing to the poor production of IFN-γ by neonatal cells is the meager production of IL-12 by cord blood mononuclear cells (Joyner et al., 2000).

Th1 and Th2 Cells

Studies on the pathogenesis of atopic disease are making an important contribution toward understanding the maturation of the immune system. T cells from infants with a family history of atopic disease make less of the Th1 cytokine IFN-γ than cells from control infants (Holt et al., 1992; Rinas et al., 1993). Prescott and colleagues studied responses of cord blood mononuclear cells to purified allergens (Prescott et al., 1998). They observed that 83% of 60 samples mounted proliferative responses to one or more allergens (e.g., ovalbumin, dust mite extract or *Der* p 1 major determinant, *Fel* d 1 cat antigen, or β-lactoglobulin) as compared with a 3% response rate to tetanus toxoid. Allergen-specific T-cell clones were shown to be of fetal origin by microsatellite typing of DNA. Allergen-stimulated cultures had increased synthesis of the Th2 cytokines IL-4, IL-5, IL-9, and particularly IL-10 and IL-13. The latter two cytokines could easily be detected as proteins in bulk culture. These studies were carried out after 24 hours of stimulation to exclude the in vitro maturation phenomenon (Ehlers and Smith, 1991).

Serial studies from birth to 2 years of babies with high and low genetic risk for development of allergic disease have been reported (Prescott et al., 1999). Infants destined to be atopic had lower levels of both Th1 and Th2 cytokine responses at birth and did not switch to a Th1 pattern, as did the nonatopic babies. Purified CD4 cells from cord blood of nonatopic babies produced more IFN-γ than those from babies destined to become atopic when stimulated with anti-CD3, which does not require antigen-presenting cells. At least with respect to environmental allergens, T-cell priming in utero is common and seems invariably to result in a Th2-skewed response pattern.

Isotype Switching

Discovery of the gene defect in X-linked immunodeficiency with hyper-IgM type 1 (HIGM1) has provided a model for the functional immaturity of neonatal B cells (see Chapter 13). Data from two early studies indicated that B cells from hyper-IgM1 patients could not produce IgG or IgA when co-cultivated with normal T cells stimulated by pokeweed mitogen, whereas patients' T cells provided help for secretion of these isotypes by normal B cells (Geha et al., 1979; Levitt et al., 1983). A subsequent study had concordant results for co-cultures of normal T with patients' B cells but described a leukemic T cell that could induce hyper-IgM B cells to produce IgG and IgA (Mayer et al., 1986).

An explanation for the conflicting results came with the discovery of CD154 (e.g., CD40 ligand) and the gene responsible for this disease. CD154 is not expressed on activated T cells from most affected males. B cells from these patients activated by cross-linking of CD40 with antibody or with cells constitutively expressing CD154 are able to switch to synthesis of diverse isotypes (Allen et al., 1993; Aruffo et al., 1993; Kroczek et al., 1994). B cells from hyper-IgM1 patients cannot be stimulated to undergo isotype switching by normal T cells because the CD154 is expressed transiently; the same B cells will undergo class switch when exposed to cells that express CD154 constitutively.

Neonatal T cells, like adult T cells, transiently express CD154 (Splawski et al., 1996). Together these data suggest that either prolonged or repeated signaling through CD40 is required to bring B cells to a state of full differentiation and competence. The lack of such stimulation is a logical explanation for the functional immaturity of neonatal B cells.

Response to Polysaccharide Antigens

The inability of newborn animals and humans to respond to carbohydrate antigens remains an enigma (Davie, 1985). Might the characteristic restrictions in expression of V_H genes constrain diversity to the extent that important epitopes of carbohydrate antigens are not recognized?

The developmental period during which the murine B-cell repertoire exhibits restricted diversity occupies approximately one prenatal and two postnatal weeks; even very young mice exhibit considerable clonal diversity (Cancro et al., 1979). Based on the histologic appearance of lymphoid tissues and the relative numbers of peripheral T and B cells, the immune system of the newborn mouse is at a developmental stage equivalent to that of the human newborn at 12 to 16 weeks. Given the mechanisms for the generation of diversity and the long gestational period in humans, it is not clear that diversity is a principal limiting factor. This theoretical view is supported by the excellent responses of young infants to protein-carbohydrate conjugate vaccines (Adderson et al., 1992).

DEVELOPMENT OF THE ANTIGEN-SPECIFIC ANTIBODY REPERTOIRE

Antibody Genes

Many studies have examined the role of variable gene repertoire bias in restriction of functional fetal and neonatal immune responses. Murine neonatal studies must be compared carefully with neonatal human immune studies because the developmental stage of the two is not equivalent at a specified postnatal age. It has been estimated that B cells are capable of producing approximately 10^{15} different variable regions, but it is not clear what proportion of these potential combining sites are ever generated or maintained in vivo.

Although diversity of the antibody repertoire results from a series of apparently random gene rearrangement and mutational events, the mature B-cell population uses a restricted set of genetic elements to express antigen-specific antibodies. The protein structure of the antibody-combining site is determined by the complexity and length of the CDRs). The amino acids comprising the heavy-chain CDRs are encoded by the V_H, D_H, and J_H segments and the light-chain CDRs from the $V_κ$ or $V_λ$ and J gene segments.

Antibody gene expression in naïve circulating B cells of fetuses or adult humans is highly biased toward the expression of a limited set of V_H genes, a restriction also noted in the usage of D and J_H segments (Brezinschek et al., 1995; Schroeder et al., 1987). Once surface Ig is expressed, positive and negative selection for antigens plays an important role in molding the mature B-cell repertoire (Rajewsky, 1996).

Microbial Antibodies

The genetic origins of microbial-specific antibodies exhibit a further level of restriction. Narrow Ag-specific repertoires with preferred V_H regions have been identified in human responses to the polysaccharide antigens of

Hemophilus influenzae type B, *Streptococcus pneumoniae*, and the yeast *Cryptococcus neoformans*. Antibody responses to these antigens are T-cell independent. These studies suggest that, for simple antigens with a limited diversity of structure, the number of structurally ideal antibody combining sites in the germline is limited. Additional V-gene biases are observed in special populations of humans. V_H region biases change with age, and these biases may contribute to impaired functional antibody responses to infection and immunization in fetuses and the elderly. V_H gene usage is also altered in human immunodeficiency virus (HIV) infection, with negative biases against V_H3 family usage in peripheral blood lymphocytes from acquired immunodeficiency syndrome (AIDS) patients. A concomitant preferential usage of V_H gene families 1 and 4 in HIV-infected individuals has been noted in many studies (Scamurra et al., 2000; Wisnewski et al., 1996).

The precise role of the bias toward particular gene segments in response to infections is not well understood. It is likely that structural and biochemical aspects of germline antibodies expressed by certain V, D, and J genes allows a "best-fit" starting structure for binding to conformations of a particular microbial epitope. Studies with polysaccharide antibodies suggest that the strongest biases are likely to be observed in V_H usage; however, other segments can dominate binding to antigen in certain cases. For example, Messmer and colleagues isolated two IgM mAbs from B cells of two umbilical cord blood samples that both recognize a conformational epitope of lactoferrin. The antibodies use different families of V_H, J_H, and V_K gene cassettes but an identical J_K segment (Messmer et al., 1999). These findings underscore the potential for any of the segments to determine antigen binding.

Other Factors Influencing the Antibody Repertoire

Antigen-specific selection at the mature B-cell stage is based on physical forces associated with the amino acids in the combining site that regulate antigen binding, such as hydrogen bonds, electrostatic attractions, hydrophobic forces, and Van der Waals contacts. Unlike the genes for TCRs, the genes specifying BCRs undergo a process of somatic hypermutation during proliferation in the germinal centers of secondary lymphoid tissues. Somatically mutated virus-specific antibodies for a single epitope may share multiple amino acid positions in the rearranged heavy and light chains, even when the genetic origins of the V, D, and J regions are disparate (Bagley et al., 1994).

Germline antibodies in the peripheral repertoire that are expressed before exposure to antigen may provide a starting point for binding, but most of these so-called natural antibodies are polyreactive IgM antibodies that display low-affinity interactions with antigens and often little functional activity against pathogens (Llorente et al., 1999). The dominant model of specific antibody acquisition is that clones with an adequate binding for antigen specified by certain V genes improve with

prolonged or recurrent exposure to antigen due to somatic hypermutation within those V genes. V-region gene replacement (receptor editing) with somatic hypermutation is sufficient to enable B-cell repertoire diversification and antibody responses.

Experimental evidence exists for the contribution of V-gene replacement to the generation of antibody responses in quasi-monoclonal mice with a nitrophenyl specificity that were infected with vesicular stomatitis virus, lymphocytic choriomeningitis virus, or poliovirus (Lopez-Macias et al., 1999).

SUMMARY

The generation of clonal diversity of T and B cells begins early in gestation and proceeds at a rapid rate by parallel mechanisms. The lack of precision of the VDJ recombinase enzyme in making coding joints for Ig and TCR genes and the creation of nontemplated nucleotides at joints through the action of TdT stand in striking contrast to the fidelity of other enzymes involved in DNA replication and repair, emphasizing the evolutionary advantage of diversity in the immune system. Efficient mechanisms for the elimination of inevitable autoreactive clones of both T and B cells have been developed.

The long-recognized immaturities of neonatal T and B cells are beginning to achieve molecular definition. The new findings emphasize the importance of maturation events occurring in the peripheral rather than central lymphoid organs, and further study may lead to new strategies for immunization of the very young infant.

REFERENCES

Adderson EE, Johnston JM, Shackelford PG, Carroll WL. Development of the human antibody repertoire. Pediatr Res 32:257–263, 1992.

Allen RC, Armitage RJ, Conley ME, Rosenblatt H, Jenkins A, Copeland NG, Bedell MA, Edelhoff S, Disteche CM, Simoneaux DK, Fanslow WC, Belmont J, Spriggs MK. CD40 ligand gene defects responsible for X-linked hyper-IgM syndrome. Science 259:990–993, 1993.

Alt FW, Oltz EM, Young F, Groman J, Taccioli G, Chen J. VDJ recombination. Immunol Today 13:306–314, 1992.

Andersson U, Bird AG, Britton S, Palacios R. Humoral and cellular immunity in humans studied at the cell level from birth to two years of age. Immunol Rev 57:5–38, 1981.

Anderson SJ, Hummell DS, Lawton AR. Differentiation of human B lymphocyte subpopulations induced by an alloreactive helper T cell clone. J Clin Immunol 8:275–284, 1988.

Anderson G, Moore NC, Owen JJ Jenkinson EJ. Cellular interactions in thymocyte development. Annu Rev Immunol 14:73–99, 1996.

Aruffo A, Farrington M, Hollenbaugh D, Li X, Milatovich A, Nonoyama S, Bajorath J, Grosmaire LS, Stenkamp R, Neubauer M, Roberts RL, Noelle RJ, Ledbetter JA, Francke U, Ochs HD. The CD40 ligand gp39 is defective in activated T cells from patients with X-linked hyper-IgM syndrome. Cell 72:291–300, 1993.

Banchereau J, Bazan F, Blanchard D, Brière F, Galizzi JP, Van Kooten C, Liu YJ, Rousset F, Saeland S. The CD40 antigen and its ligand. Annu Rev Immunol 12:881–922, 1994.

Bockman DE Kirby ML. Dependence of thymus development on derivatives of the neural crest. Science 223:498–500, 1984.

Bofill M, Janossy G, Janossa M, Burford GD, Seymour GJ, Wernet P, Kelemen E. Human B cell development. II. Subpopulations in the human fetus. J Immunol 134:1531–1538, 1985.

Brière F, Servet-Delprat C, Bridon JM, Saint-Remy JM, Bancereau J. Human interleukin 10 induces naive sIgD+ B cells to secrete IgG1 and IgG3. J Exp Med 179:757–762, 1994.

Buckley RH, Dees SC O'Fallon WM. Serum immunoglobulins. I. Levels in normal children and in uncomplicated childhood allergy. Pediatrics 41:600–611, 1968.

Callard RE, Armitage RJ, Fanslow WC, Spriggs MK. CD40 ligand and its role in X-linked hyper IgM syndrome. Immunol Today 14:559–564, 1993.

Campana D, Janossy G, Coustan-Smith E, Amlot PL, Tian WT, Ip S, Wong L. The expression of T cell receptor-associated proteins during T cell ontogeny in man. J Immunol 142:57–66, 1989.

Cancro MP, Wylie DE, Gerhard W, Klinman NR. Patterned acquisition of the antibody repertoire: diversity of the hemagglutinin-specific B-cell repertoire in neonatal BALB/c mice. Proc Natl Acad Sci USA 76:6577–6581, 1979.

Casali P, Notkins AL. Probing the human B cell repertoire with EBV: polyreactive antibodies and CD5+ B lymphocytes. Annu Rev Immunol 7:513–535, 1989.

Casellas R, Shih TA, Kleinewietfeld M, Rakonjac J, Nemazee D, Rajewsky K, Nussenzweig MC. Contribution of receptor editing to the antibody repertoire. Science 291:1541–1544, 2001.

Caton AJ. A single pre-B cell can give rise to antigen-specific B cells that utilize distinct immunoglobulin gene rearrangements. J Exp Med 172:815–825, 1990.

Chen C, Prak EL, Weigert M. Editing disease-associated autoantibodies. Immunity 6:97–105, 1997.

Clement LT, Vink PE, Bradley GE. Novel immunoregulatory functions of phenotypically distinct subpopulations of CD4+ cells in the human neonate. J Immunol 145:102–108, 1990.

Clement LT, Yamashita N, Martin AM. The functionally distinct subpopulations of human CD4+ helper/inducer T lymphocytes defined by anti-CD45R antibodies derive sequentially from a differentiation pathway that is regulated by activation-dependent post-thymic differentiation. J Immunol 141:1464–1470, 1988.

Colley DG, Montesano MA, Freeman GL, Secor WE. Infection-stimulated or perinatally initiated idiotypic interactions can direct differential morbidity and mortality in schistosomiasis. Microbes Infect 1:517–524, 1999.

Conley ME, Cooper MD. Immature IgA B cells in IgA-deficient patients. N Engl J Med 305:495–497, 1981.

Cook GP, Tomlinson IM. The human immunoglobulin VH repertoire. Immunol Today 16:237–242, 1995.

Cooper MD, Burrows PD. B cell differentiation. In Honjo T, Alt FW, Rabbits TH, eds. Immunoglobulin Genes. San Diego, Academic Press, 1990, pp 1–21.

Cooper MD, Kincade PW, Lawton AR. Thymus and bursal function in immunologic development. A new theoretical model of plasma cell differentiation. In Kagan BM, Stiehm ER, eds. Immunologic Incompetence. Chicago Year Book, 1971, pp 81–104.

Cooper MD, Peterson RDA, South MA, Good RA. The functions of the thymus system and bursa system in the chicken. J Exp Med 123:75–102, 1966.

Cuisinier AM, Gauthier L, Boubli L, Fougereau M, Tonnelle C. Mechanisms that generate human immunoglobulin diversity operate from the 8th week of gestation in fetal liver. Eur J Immunol 23:110–118, 1993.

Davie JM. Antipolysaccharide immunity in man and animals. In Sell SH, Wright PF, eds. Hemophilus Influenzae: Epidemiology, Immunology, and Prevention of Disease. New York, Elsevier Biomedical, 1985, pp 129–134.

Defrance T, Vanbervliet B, Briere F, Durand I, Rousset F, Banchereau J. Interleukin 10 and transforming growth factor beta cooperate to induce anti-CD40-activated naive human B cells to secrete immunoglobulin A. J Exp Med 175:671–682, 1992.

Delespesse G, Yang LP, Ohshima Y, Demeure C, Shu U, Byun DG, Sarfati M. Maturation of human neonatal CD4+ and CD8+ T lymphocytes into Th1/Th2 effectors. Vaccine 161:415–1419, 1998.

Denning SM, Kurtzberg J, Leslie DS Haynes BF. Human postnatal CD4-CD8-CD3-thymic T cell precursors differentiate in vitro into T cell receptor delta-bearing cells. J Immunol 142:2988–2997, 1989.

Dunon D, Kaufman J, Salomonsen J, Skjoedt K, Vainio O, Thiery JP, Imhof BA. T cell precursor migration towards beta 2-microglobulin is involved in thymus colonization of chicken embryos. EMBO J 9:3315–3322, 1990.

Dwyer DS, Bradley RJ, Urquhart CK, Kearney JF. Naturally occurring anti-idiotypic antibodies in myasthenia gravis patients. Nature 301:611–614, 1983.

Ehlers S, Smith KA. Differentiation of T cell lymphokine gene expression: the in vitro acquisition of T cell memory. J Exp Med 173:25–36, 1991.

Ehlich A, Schaal S, Gu H, Kitamura D, Müller W, Rajewsky K. Immunoglobulin heavy and light chain genes rearrange independently at early stages of B cell development. Cell 72:695–704, 1993.

Fayette J, Dubois B, Vandenabeele S, Bridon JM, Vanbervliet B, Durand I, Banchereau J, Caux C, Briere F. Human dendritic cells skew isotype switching of CD40-activated naive B cells towards IgA1 and IgA2. J Exp Med 185:1909–1918, 1997.

Fiorilli M, Crescenzi M, Carbonari M, Tedesco L, Russo G, Gaetano C, Aiuti F. Phenotypically immature IgG-bearing B cells in patients with hypogammaglobulinemia. J Clin Immunol 6:21–25, 1986.

Freeman GJ, Gribben JG, Boussiotis VA, Ng JW, Restivo VA Jr., Lombard LA, Gray GS, Nadler LM. Cloning of B7-2: a CTLA-4 counter-receptor that costimulates human T cell proliferation. Science 262:909–911, 1993.

Gandini M, Kubagawa H, Gathings WE, Lawton AR. Expression of three immunoglobulin isotypes by individual B cells during development: implications for heavy chain switching. Am J Reprod Immunol 1:161–163, 1981.

Gascan H, Gauchat JF, Roncarolo MG, Yssel H, Spits H, de Vries JE. Human B cell clones can be induced to proliferate and to switch to IgE and IgG4 synthesis by interleukin 4 and a signal provided by activated CD4+ T cell clones. J Exp Med 173:747–750, 1991.

Gathings WE, Lawton AR, Cooper MD. Immunofluorescent studies of the development of pre-B cells, V-genes and immunoglobulin isotype diversity in humans. Eur J Immunol 7:804–810, 1977.

Geha RS. Presence of circulating anti-idiotype-bearing cells after booster immunization with tetanus toxoid (TT) and inhibition of anti-TT antibody synthesis by auto-anti-idiotypic antibody. J Immunol 130:1634–1639, 1983.

Geha RS, Hyslop N, Alami S, Farah F, Schneeberger EE, Rosen FS. Hyper immunoglobulin M immunodeficiency. (Dysgammaglobulinemia). Presence of immunoglobulin M-secreting plasmacytoid cells in peripheral blood and failure of immunoglobulin M-immunoglobulin G switch in B-cell differentiation. J Clin Invest 64:385–391, 1979.

Goodnow CC. Transgenic mice and analysis of B-cell tolerance. Annu Rev Immunol 10:489–518, 1992.

Gupta S, Pahwa R, O'Reilly RO, Good RA, Siegal FP. Ontogeny of lymphocyte subpopulations in human fetal liver. Proc Natl Acad Sci USA 73:919–922, 1976.

Griffioen AW, Toebes EA, Zegers BJ, Rijkers GT. Role of CR2 in the human adult and neonatal in vitro antibody response to type 4 pneumococcal polysaccharide. Cell Immunol 143:11–22, 1992.

Havran WL, Allison JP. Origin of Thy-1+ dendritic epidermal cells of adult mice from fetal thymic precursors. Nature 344:68–70, 1990.

Hayakawa K, Hardy RR. Development and function of B-1 cells. Curr Opin Immunol 12:346–353, 2000.

Haynes BF, Denning SM, Singer KH, Kurtzberg J. Ontogeny of T-cell precursors: a model for the initial stages of human T-cell development. Immunol Today 10:87–91, 1989.

Haynes BF, Martin ME, Kay HH, Kurtzberg J. Early events in human T cell ontogeny. Phenotypic characterization and immunohistologic localization of T cell precursors in early human fetal tissues [published erratum appears in J Exp Med 169:603]. J Exp Med 168:1061–1080, 1988.

Hayward AR, Ezer G. Development of lymphocyte populations in human thymus and spleen. Clin Exp Immunol 17:169–178, 1974.

Hayward AR, Lawton AR. Induction of plasma cell differentiation of human fetal lymphocytes: evidence for functional immaturity of T and B cells. J Immunol 119:1213–1217, 1977.

Hillson JL, Oppliger IR, Sasso EH, Milner EC, Wener MH. Emerging human B cell repertoire. Influence of developmental stage and interindividual variation. J Immunol 149:3741–3752, 1992.

Holt PG, Clough JB, Holt BJ, Baron-Hay MJ, Rose AH, Robinson BW, Thomas WR. Genetic 'risk' for atopy is associated with delayed postnatal maturation of T-cell competence. Clin Exp Allergy 22:1093–1099, 1992.

Honjo T. Immunoglobulin genes. Annu Rev Immunol 1:499–528, 1983.

Ikuta K, Uchida N, Friedman J, Weissman IL. Lymphocyte development from stem cells. Annu Rev Immunol 10:759–783, 1992.

Jabara HH, Fu SM, Geha RS, Vercelli D. CD40 and IgE: synergism between anti-CD40 monoclonal antibody and interleukin 4 in the induction of IgE synthesis by highly purified human B cells. J Exp Med 172:1861–1864, 1990.

Janeway CA Jr. The T cell receptor as a multicomponent signalling machine: CD4/CD8 coreceptors and CD45 in T cell activation. Annu Rev Immunol 10:645–674, 1992.

Jerne NK. Towards a network theory of the immune system. Ann Immunol (Inst Pasteur) 125C:373–389, 1974.

Jotereau FV, Le Douarin NM. Demonstration of a cyclic renewal of the lymphocyte precursor cells in the quail thymus during embryonic and perinatal life. J Immunol 129:1869–1877, 1982.

Joyner JL, Augustine NH, Taylor KA, La Pine TR, Hill HR. Effects of group B streptococci on cord and adult mononuclear cell interleukin-12 and interferon-gamma mRNA accumulation and protein secretion. J Inf Dis 182:974–977, 2000.

Kamradt T, Mitchison NA. Tolerance and Autoimmunuty. N Engl J Med 344:655–664, 2001.

Kamps WA, Cooper MD. Microenvironmental studies of pre B and B cell development in human and mouse fetuses. J Immunol 129:526–531, 1982.

Kipps TJ, Robbins BA, Carson DA. Uniform high frequency expression of autoantibody-associated crossreactive idiotypes in the primary B cell follicles of human fetal spleen. J Exp Med 171:189–196, 1990.

Kitamura D, Kudo A, Schaal S, Müeller W, Melchers R, Rajewsky K. A critical role of λ5 protein in B cell development. Cell 69:823–831, 1992.

Kraj P, Rao SP, Glas AM, Hardy RR, Milner EC, Silberstein LE. The human heavy chain Ig V region gene repertoire is biased at all stages of B cell ontogeny, including early pre-B cells. J Immunol 158:5824–5832, 1997.

Kroczek RA, Graf D, Brugnoni D, Giliani S, Korthuer U, Ugazio A, Senger G, Mages HW, Villa A, Notarangelo LD. Defective expression of CD40 ligand on T cells causes "X-linked immunodeficiency with hyper-IgM (HIGM1)." Immunol Rev 138:39–59, 1994.

Kubagawa H, Cooper MD, Carroll AJ, Burrows PD. Light-chain gene expression before heavy-chain rearrangement in pre-B cells transformed by Epstein-Barr virus. Proc Natl Acad Sci USA 86:2356–2360, 1989.

Lanier LL. NK cell receptors. Annu Rev Immunol 16:359–393, 1998.

Lassoued K, Nuñez CA, Billips L, Kubagawa H, Monteiro RC, LeBien T, Cooper MD. Expression of surrogate light chain receptors is restricted to a late stage in pre-B cell differentiation. Cell 73:73–86, 1993.

Lanzavecchia A. Receptor-mediated antigen uptake and its effect on antigen presentation to class II-restricted T lymphocytes. Annu Rev Immunol 8:773–793, 1990.

Lawton AR. Ontogeny of B cells: relations to immunodeficiency diseases. Clin Immunol Immunopathol 40:5–12, 1986.

Lawton AR, Cooper MD. Modification of B lymphocyte differentiation by anti-immunoglobulins. In Cooper MD, Warner NL, eds. Contemporary Topics in Immunobiology, vol 3. New York, Plenum Publishing, 1974, pp 193–225.

Le Douarin NM, Houssaint E, Jotereau FV, Belo M. Origin of haemopoietic stem cells in the embryonic bursa of Fabricius and bone marrow studied through interspecies chimaeras. Proc Natl Acad Sci USA 72:2701–2705, 1975.

Levitt D, Haber P, Rich K, Cooper MD. Hyper IgM immunodeficiency. A primary dysfunction of V-gene isotype switching. J Clin Invest 72:1650–1657, 1983.

Lewis DB, Yu CC, Meyer J, English BK, Kahn SJ, Wilson CB. Cellular and molecular mechanisms for reduced interleukin 4 and interferon-gamma production by neonatal T cells. J Clin Invest 87:194–202, 1991.

Linsley PS, Ledbetter JA. The role of the CD28 receptor during T cell responses to antigen. Annu Rev Immunol 11:191–212, 1993.

Lobach DF, Hensley LL, Ho W, Haynes BF. Human T cell antigen expression during the early stages of fetal thymic maturation. J Immunol 135:1752–1759, 1985.

Malisan F, Brière F, Bridon JM, Harindranath N, Mills FC, Max EE, Banchereau J, Martinez-Valdez H. IL-10 induces IgG isotype switch recombination in human CD40-activated naive V-genes. J Exp Med 183:937–947, 1996.

Matsuda DF, Ishii K, Bourvagnet P, Kuma Ki, Hayashida H, Miyata T, Honjo T. The complete nucleotide sequence of the human immunoglobulin heavy chain variable region locus. J Exp Med 188:2151–2162, 1998.

Mayer L, Kwan SP, Thompson C, Ko HS, Chiorazzi N, Waldmann T, Rosen F. Evidence for a defect in "switch" T cells in patients with immunodeficiency and hyperimmunoglobulinemia M. N Engl J Med 314:409–413, 1986.

McCormack WT, Tjoelker LW, Thompson CB. Avian B-cell development: generation of an immunoglobulin repertoire by gene conversion. Annu Rev Immunol 9:219–241, 1991.

Milili M, Schiff C, Fougereau M, Tonnelle C. The VDJ repertoire expressed in human preB cells reflects the selection of bona fide heavy chains. Eur J Immunol 26:63–69, 1996.

Miyawaki T, Moriya N, Nagaoki T, Taniguchi N. Maturation of B-cell differentiation ability and T-cell regulatory function in infancy and childhood. Immunol Rev 57:61–87, 1981.

Mond JJ, Lees A, Snapper CM. T cell-independent antigens type 2. Annu Rev Immunol 13:655–692, 1995.

Mortari F, Wang JY, Schroeder HW Jr. Human cord blood antibody repertoire: mixed population of V_H gene segments and CDR 3 distribution in the expressed Cα and Cγ repertoires. J Immunol 150:1348–1357, 1993.

Mosmann TR, Coffman RL. TH1 and TH2 cells: different patterns of lymphokine secretion lead to different functional properties. Annu Rev Immunol 7:145–173, 1989.

Noelle RJ, Roy M, Shepherd DM, Stamenkovic I, Ledbetter JA, Aruffo A. A 39-kDa protein on activated helper T cells binds CD40 and transduces the signal for cognate activation of B cells. Proc Natl Acad Sci USA 89:6550–6554, 1992.

Noguchi M, Yi H, Rosenblatt HM, Filipovich AH, Adelstein S, Modi WS, McBride OW, Leonard WJ. Interleukin-2 receptor gamma chain mutation results in X-linked severe combined immunodeficiency in humans. Cell 73:147–157, 1993.

Nossal GJV, Szenberg A, Ada GL, Austin CM. Single cell studies on 19S antibody production. J Exp Med 119:485–502, 1964.

Osmond DG. Proliferation kinetics and the lifespan of B cells in central and peripheral lymphoid organs. Curr Opin Immunol 3:179–185, 1991.

Padovan E, Casorati G, Dellabona P, Meyer S, Brockhaus M, Lanzavecchia A. Expression of two T cell receptor alpha chains: dual receptor T cells. Science 262:422–424, 1993.

Lawton AR, Asofsky R, Hylton MD, Cooper MD. Suppression of immunoglobulin class synthesis in mice: I. Effects of treatment with antibody to f chain. J Exp Med 135:277–297, 1972.

Pascual V, Verkruyse L, Casey ML, Capra JD. Analysis of Ig H chain gene segment utilization in human fetal liver. J Immunol 151:4164–4172, 1993.

Paul WE, Bona, C. Regulatory idiotypes and immune networks: an hypothesis. Immunol Today 3:230–234, 1982.

Pelanda R, Schwers S, Sonoda E, Torres RM, Nemazee D, Rajewsky K. Receptor editing in a transgenic mouse model: site, efficiency, and role in B cell tolerance and antibody diversification. Immunity 7:765–775, 1997.

Perlmutter RM, Kearney JF, Chang SP, Hood LE. Developmentally controlled expression of immunoglobulin V_H genes. Science 227:1597–1601, 1985.

Prescott SL, Macaubas C, Holt BJ, Smallacombe TB, Loh R, Sly PD, Holt PG. Transplacental priming of the human immune system to environmental allergens: universal skewing of initial T cell responses toward the Th2 cytokine profile. J Immunol 160: 4730–4737, 1998.

Prescott SL, Macaubas C, Smallacombe T, Holt BJ, Sly PD Holt PG. Development of allergen-specific T-cell memory in atopic and normal children. Lancet 353:196–200, 1999.

Pugliese A. Self-antigen-presenting cells expressing diabetes-associated autoantigens exist in both thymus and peripheral lymphoid organs. J Clin Invest 107:555-564, 2001.

Purkerson J, Isakson P. A two-signal model for regulation of immunoglobulin isotype switching. FASEB J 6:3245–3252, 1992.

Raaphorts FM, Timmers E, Keuter MJH. Restricted utilization of germ line V_H3 genes and short diverse third complementarity-determining regions (CDR3) in human fetal B lymphocyte immunoglobulin heavy chain gene rearrangements. Eur J Immunol 22:247–251, 1992.

Rao SP, Riggs JM, Friedman DF, Scully MS, LeBien TW, Silberstein LE. Biased VH gene usage in early lineage human B cells: evidence for preferential Ig gene rearrangement in the absence of selection. J Immunol 163:2732–2740, 1999.

Rinas U, Horneff G, Wahn V. Interferon-gamma production by cord-blood mononuclear cells is reduced in newborns with a family history of atopic disease and is independent from cord blood IgE-levels. Pediatr Allergy Immunol 4:60–64, 1993.

Rousset F, Garcia E, Banchereau J. Cytokine-induced proliferation and immunoglobulin production of human V-genes triggered through their CD40 antigen. J Exp Med 173:705–710, 1991.

Russell SM. Interleukin-2 receptor gamma chain: a functional component of the interleukin-4 receptor. Science 262:1880–1883, 1993.

Sandel PC, Monroe JG. Negative selection of immature B cells by receptor editing or deletion is determined by site of antigen encounter. Immunity 10:289–99, 1999.

Schatz DG, Oettinger MA, Schlissel MS. V(D)J recombination: molecular biology and regulation. Annu Rev Immunol 10: 359–383, 1992.

Schelonka RL, Raaphorst FM, Infante D, Kraig E, Teale JM, Infante AJ. T cell receptor repertoire diversity and clonal expansion in human neonates. Pediatr Res 43:396–402, 1998.

Schroeder HW Jr, Hillson JL, Perlmutter RM. Early restriction of the human antibody repertoire. Science 238:791–793, 1987.

Schroeder HW Jr, Wang JY. Preferential utilization of conserved immunoglobulin heavy chain variable gene segments during human fetal life. Proc Natl Acad Sci USA 87:6146–6150, 1990.

Schroeder HW Jr, Mortari F, Shiokawa S, Kirkham PM, Elgavish RA, Bertrand FE III. Developmental regulation of the human antibody repertoire. Ann NY Acad Sci 764:242–260, 1995.

Sher A, Coffman RL. Regulation of immunity to parasites by T cells and T cell-derived cytokines. Annu Rev Immunol 10:385–409, 1992.

Sigal NH, Pickard AR, Metcalf ES, Gearhart PJ, Klinman NR. Expression of phosphorylcholine specific B cells during murine development. J Exp Med 146:933–948, 1977.

Solvason N, Kearney JF. The human fetal omentum: a site of B cell generation. J Exp Med 175:397–404, 1992.

Splawski JB, Jelinek DF, Lipsky PE. Delineation of the functional capacity of human neonatal lymphocytes. J Clin Invest 87: 545–553, 1991.

Splawski JB, Lipsky PE. Cytokine regulation of immunoglobulin secretion by neonatal lymphocytes. J Clin Invest 88:967–977, 1991.

Splawski JB, Nishioka J, Nishioka Y, Lipsky PE. CD40 ligand is expressed and functional on activated neonatal T cells. J Immunol 156:119–127, 1996.

Stiehm ER, Fudenberg HH. Serum levels of immune globulins in health and disease: a survey. Pediatrics 37:715–727, 1966.

Timens W, Boes A, Rozeboom-Uiterwijk T, Poppema S. Immaturity of the human splenic marginal zone in infancy. Possible contribution to the deficient infant immune response. J Immunol 143:3200–3206, 1989.

Toivanen P, Asantila T, Granberg C, Leino A, Hirvonen T. Development T cell repertoire in the human and the sheep fetus. Immunol Rev 42:185–201, 1978.

Tosato G, Magrath IT, Koski IR, Dooley NJ, Blaese RM. B cell differentiation and immunoregulatory T cell function in human cord blood lymphocytes. J Clin Invest 66:383–388, 1980.

Tsubata T, Reth M. The products of the pre-B cell specific genes ($\lambda 5$ and VpreB) and the immunoglobulin μ chain form a complex that is transported to the cell surface. J Exp Med 172:973–976, 1990.

Tucker PW. Transcriptional regulation of IgM and IgD. Immunol Today 6:181–182, 1985.

Vakil M, Kearney J. Functional characterization of monoclonal auto-anti-idiotype antibodies isolated from the early B cell repertoire of BALB/c mice. Eur J Immunol 16:1151–1158, 1986.

Vakil M, Sauter H, Paige C, Kearney, J. In vivo suppression of perinatal multispecific B cells results in a distortion of the adult B cell repertoire. Eur J Immunol 16:1159–1165, 1986.

Van Parijs L, Abbas AK. Homeostasis and self-tolerance in the immune system: turning lymphocytes off. Science 280:243–248, 1998.

Von Boehmer H. Developmental biology of T cells in T cell-receptor transgenic mice. Annu Rev Immunol 8:531–556, 1990.

Weinberg K, Parkman R. Severe combined immunodeficiency due to a specific defect in the production of interleukin-2. N Engl J Med 322:1718–1723, 1990.

Willems van Dijk K, Milner LA, Sasso EH, Milner ECB. Chromosomal organization of the heavy chain variable region gene segments comprising the human fetal antibody repertoire. Proc Natl Acad Sci USA 89:10403–10434, 1992.

Wilson CB, Lewis DB, English BK. T cell development in the fetus and neonate. Adv Exp Med Biol 310:17–27, 1991.

The T-Lymphocyte System

Christopher B. Wilson and Kurt H. Edelmann

INTRODUCTION

T lymphocytes, which are commonly referred to as T cells, are so named because the vast majority originate in the thymus, and along with B lymphocytes they comprise the adaptive or antigen-specific immune system. T lymphocytes play a central role in immunity because they both mediate antigen-specific cellular immunity and play a critical role in facilitating antigen-specific, B-cell–dependent humoral immunity.

The role of the thymus in the generation of T lymphocytes was first demonstrated through experimental thymectomy in neonatal mice, and was later confirmed through studies in irradiated, thymectomized adult mice that received bone marrow transplants and through the identification of the immune defects in athymic, or nude, mice. Subsequently, the development of monoclonal antibodies to proteins and glycoproteins unique to T lymphocytes has played an essential role in the elucidation of their development and functional differentiation. Using these tools, studies of humans and experimental animals with naturally occurring genetic immunodeficiency disorders helped to define key T-lymphocyte developmental checkpoints and functions and later the molecular basis for these processes.

The development of procedures for the propagation, cloning, and biochemical and genetic manipulation of T lymphocytes in vitro, and of systems to study T-cell development in fetal thymic organ culture, provided tools through which important processes and principles could be readily tested in more simple and tractable systems. All this provided a foundation for the explosion in information provided through the genetic manipulation of mice and most recently by the complete sequencing of the human (Fahrer et al., 2001; Lander et al., 2001; Sachidanadam et al., 2001; Venter et al., 2001) and mouse genomes.

This chapter seeks to summarize the information derived from these sources and thereby to provide a framework for understanding the molecular and cellular basis for normal and abnormal T-lymphocyte biology.

T-CELL RECOGNITION

T-Cell Receptor Complex and MHC Restriction

Antigen-specific T-cell receptors (TCRs) are heterodimeric molecules composed either of α and β chains ($\alpha\beta$-TCR) or γ and δ chains ($\gamma\delta$-TCR). The amino-terminal portion of each of these chains is variable and involved in antigen recognition. As discussed later, the highly variable nature of this portion of the TCR is generated, in large part, as a result of TCR gene segment recombination. In contrast, the carboxy-terminal region of each of the four TCR chains is monomorphic, or constant. The TCR on the cell surface is invariably associated with the nonpolymorphic complex of CD3 proteins (Fig. 2-1) (Clevers et al., 1988; Kane et al., 2000). The cytoplasmic domains of proteins of the CD3 complex include immunoreceptor tyrosine-based activation motifs (ITAMs), which serve as docking sites for intracellular tyrosine kinases that transduce activation signals to the interior of the cell after the TCR has been engaged by antigen (see later discussion).

$\alpha\beta$- and $\gamma\delta$-T Cells

Nearly all T cells that bear an $\alpha\beta$-TCR, hereafter referred to as $\alpha\beta$-T cells, also express on their surface CD4 or CD8 co-receptors, which are expressed in a mutually exclusive manner. The cytoplasmic domain of these co-receptors associates with the Lck tyrosine kinase, which plays an essential role in the development and function of $\alpha\beta$-T cells (see following discussion).

Nearly all $\alpha\beta$-T cells recognize protein antigen in the form of peptide fragments bound to classical major histocompatibility complex (MHC) molecules (i.e., MHC class I or MHC class II molecules). As a consequence of a rigorous selection process that occurs in the thymus, the recognition of antigenic peptide–MHC complexes by mature $\alpha\beta$-T cells is MHC restricted; that is, there is preferential recognition by the $\alpha\beta$-TCR of peptides bound to self MHC class I or class II as opposed to non-self MHC alleles.

By contrast to $\alpha\beta$-T cells, the majority of T cells that express $\gamma\delta$-TCR (hereafter referred to as $\gamma\delta$-T cells) appear to recognize either stress-induced, nonclassical MHC molecules directly or nonpeptide antigens, such as host or pathogen-derived lipids, bound to these nonclassical MHC molecules.

Antigen Presentation by MHC Class I Molecules

Classical MHC class I molecules consist of a polymorphic α or heavy chain, which is associated with a monomorphic light chain, β_2-microglobulin (Fig. 2-2) (York and Rock, 1996). There are three major types of MHC class I heavy chains in humans, HLA-A, HLA-B, and HLA-C, which are encoded by three genes clustered on chromosome 6, in a region known as the MHC locus. MHC molecules have a special cleft for presenting antigenic peptides. In MHC class I molecules, this cleft is formed by the $\alpha1$ and $\alpha2$ domains of the heavy chain (York and Rock, 1996). Peptides bound to MHC class I are preferentially recognized by the CD8 subset rather than the CD4 subset of $\alpha\beta$-T cells. This is due, at least in part, to an affinity of the CD8 molecule for the $\alpha3$ domain of the heavy chain, which is distinct from that involved in binding peptide (Salter et al., 1990).

Most peptides bound to MHC class I molecules are derived from proteins synthesized de novo within host cells (see Fig. 2-2) (Pamer and Cresswell, 1998; York and Rock, 1996). In uninfected cells these are derived from normal host proteins; that is, they are self-peptides. After intracellular infection, such as with a virus, peptides derived from viral proteins endogenously synthesized within the cell bind to and are presented by MHC class I. Antigenic peptides are predominantly derived by enzymatic cleavage of proteins in the cytoplasm by a specialized organelle called the proteasome.

A specific peptide transporter or pump, the transporter associated with antigen processing (TAP), then shuttles peptides formed in the cytoplasm to the endoplasmic reticulum, where peptides are able to bind to recently synthesized MHC class I molecules. Peptide binding stabilizes the association of the heavy chain with β_2-microglobulin in this compartment and allows the complex to transit to the cell surface.

Peptides bound to MHC class I molecules in vivo are typically 8 to 10 amino acids in length (Pamer and Cresswell, 1998; Wilson and Bjorkman, 1998; York and Rock, 1996). The peptide binding groove is closed at both ends so that larger peptides cannot be accommodated. For a given MHC allele, certain positions (anchor residues) within the peptide can be encoded only by specific amino acids for effective binding to the cleft. Amino acid residues at other more variable positions point out of the cleft and are recognized by the TCR (epitope residues). The antigen recognition process clearly imposes significant restrictions on the ability of peptides from a particular protein to be immunogenic, because the peptide must both bind to the MHC molecule *and* be recognized by the TCR.

HLA-A, HLA-B, and HLA-C

These constraints on peptide immunogenicity are offset by the availability of the three different types of MHC class I molecules (HLA-A, HLA-B, and HLA-C), each of which is highly polymorphic. The human HLA-A,

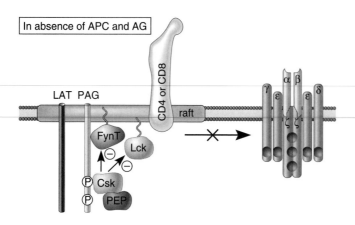

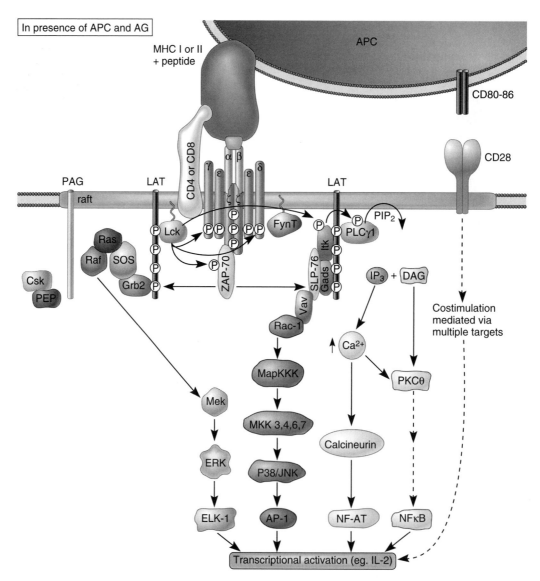

Figure 2-1 · TCR/CD3 complex, co-receptors, and downstream signaling pathways. Activation results in the recruitment of the TCR/CD3 complex into lipid rafts within the plasma membrane, which facilitates downstream signaling events. On the top, the αβ-TCR heterodimer is shown complexed with the CD3γδε₂ζ₂ complex, with cytosolic immunoreceptor tyrosine-based activation motifs (ITAMs) shown as shaded boxes. Engagement of the TCR by antigenic peptide-MHC complexes on APCs induces the translocation of the TCR/CD3 complex to plasma membrane rafts (also known as glycolipid-enriched microdomains [GEMs]) and initiates signaling cascades leading to T-cell activation. DAG = diacylglycerol; PAG = phosphoprotein associated with GEMs; SOS = son of sevenless. See text for discussion and references.

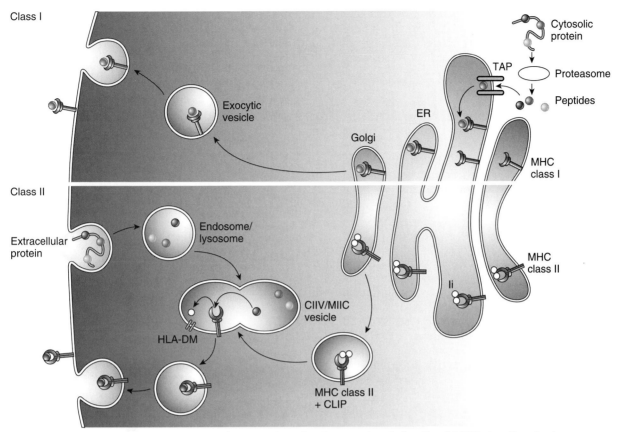

Figure 2-2 · Processing and presentation of antigens on MHC class I and MHC class II molecules proceeds through distinct pathways. See text for discussion.

HLA-B, and HLA-C heavy-chain genes have at least 86, 185, and 45 different molecularly defined alleles, respectively, with the greatest degree of polymorphism found in the region encoding the antigenic cleft (Mason and Parham, 1998). MHC polymorphism ensures that at the individual and population level, MHC molecules are able to bind and present a variety of peptides to T cells. It has been proposed that populations in which the MHC alleles are less polymorphic (e.g., Native Americans) may be at greater risk for certain infections due to limitations in the diversity of antigenic peptides that can be presented (Black, 1992).

MHC class I molecules and the cell components required for peptide generation, transport, and MHC class I binding are virtually ubiquitous in the cells of vertebrates (Daar et al., 1984; Vogel et al., 1999). The advantage to the host is that this allows cytotoxic CD8 T cells to recognize and lyse cells infected with intracellular pathogens in most tissues. Neuronal cells are one of the few cell types that constitutively lack MHC class I (Griffin et al., 1992). Because neurons are predominantly postmitotic cells, lack of MHC class I molecules may help to limit immune-mediated destruction of a cell type with a limited capacity to be replaced. MHC class I molecules are expressed by some populations of fetal neuronal cells, suggesting that these molecules may play a role in processes distinct from

antigen presentation during early development (Corriveau et al., 1998).

MHC class I HLA-A, HLA-B, and HLA-C molecules are also absent from the trophoblast of the human placenta, which may serve to limit the recognition of fetal-derived trophoblast cells as foreign by maternal T cells, as discussed later. The trophoblast does express two alternative HLA molecules, HLA-E and HLA-G (Hunt et al., 2000; King et al., 2000; Rouas-Freiss et al., 2000), which may protect the placenta from attack by natural killer (NK) cells (see Chapter 11). The abundance of MHC class I molecules is increased by exposure to interferons, which can also induce the expression of modest amounts of MHC class I molecules on cell types that normally lack expression, including neuronal cells.

Antigen-Presenting Cells

Certain types of cells express MHC class I molecules in high abundance and also constitutively express MHC class II molecules, which endows them with enhanced capacity to present antigenic peptides to T cells. Such cells are commonly referred to as antigen-presenting cells (APCs) and include dendritic cells (DCs), macrophages, and B lymphocytes. DCs, which not only express high amounts of MHC class I and class II molecules but also other molecules that allow them to effectively present antigen to naïve CD8 (and CD4) αβ-T cells, play a critical role in the initiation of primary antigen-specific T-cell responses (Banchereau et al., 2000) (see later discussion).

Antigen Cross-Presentation

DCs also appear to be unique in their ability to present antigenic peptides on MHC class I molecules by an additional pathway, known as cross-presentation, in which extracellular proteins that are taken up as large particles (phagocytosis), small particles (macropinocytosis), or in soluble form (micropinocytosis) are then transferred from endocytic vesicles to the cytoplasm and then are loaded onto MHC class I molecules via TAP (Larsson et al., 2001). Phagocytosis of apoptotic cells or blebs from apoptotic cells appears to be a particularly efficient source of antigens for cross-presentation (Larsson et al., 2001). Cross-presentation is essential for the induction of primary CD8 T-cell responses directed toward antigens not synthesized in APCs or antigens from viruses that disrupt MHC class I presentation in the cells that they infect, as do a number of viruses, including those of the herpes family and human immunodeficiency virus (HIV) (Lorenzo et al., 2001; Ploegh, 1998).

Antigen Presentation by MHC Class II Molecules

In MHC class II molecules, an α and β chain each contribute to the formation of the groove in which antigenic peptides bind (see Fig. 2-2) (Busch and Mellins, 1996; Busch et al., 2000). MHC class II peptide complexes are recognized primarily by αβ-T cells of the CD4 but not the CD8 subset. This is due, at least in part, to an affinity of the CD4 molecule for a domain of the MHC class II β chain distinct from the region that forms part of the peptide-binding groove (Konig et al., 1992). In contrast to MHC class I, peptides that bind to MHC class II proteins are mostly derived from phagocytosis or endocytosis of soluble or membrane-bound proteins (see Fig. 2-2) (Busch and Mellins, 1996). In the absence of foreign proteins, the majority of peptides bound to MHC class II molecules are self-peptides derived from proteins found either on the cell surface or secreted by the cell itself (Chicz et al., 1992; Rudensky et al., 1991).

Newly synthesized MHC class II molecules associate in the endoplasmic reticulum with a protein called the invariant chain, which impedes their binding of endogenous peptides in this compartment. The loading of exogenously derived peptides and the removal of invariant chain from MHC class II are facilitated by HLA-DM (see Fig. 2-2), a relatively nonpolymorphic heterodimeric protein that is encoded in the MHC locus (Busch and Mellins, 1996; Busch et al., 2000). This appears to occur in a specialized endocytic compartment, known as class II vesicles or MHC class II compartment (CIIV or MIIC), effectively separating

peptides binding to MHC class I and to class II into two separate pools (Busch and Mellins, 1996).

Unlike the MHC class I cleft, the MHC class II cleft is open at both ends, allowing the binding of larger peptides than in the case of MHC class I. Most MHC class II peptides are from 14 to 18 amino acids in length, although they can be substantially longer. As for MHC class I molecules, the genes that encode the α and β chains of the three major human MHC class II molecules, HLA-DR, HLA-DP, and HLA-DQ, are located on chromosome 6 and are highly polymorphic, particularly in the region encoding the peptide-binding cleft (Marsh, 1998).

The distribution of MHC class II in uninflamed tissues is much more restricted than MHC class I (Daar et al., 1984), with constitutive MHC class II mainly limited to APCs, such as DCs, mononuclear phagocytes, and B cells. Limiting MHC class II expression in most situations to these cell types makes teleologic sense, because the major function of these professional APCs is to process foreign antigen for recognition by CD4 T cells.

Other cell types can be induced to express MHC class II and, in some cases, present antigen to CD4 T cells, as a consequence of tissue inflammation or exposure to cytokines, particularly IFN-gamma (IFN-γ), but also tumor necrosis factor (TNF) or granulocyte-macrophage colony-stimulating factor (GM-CSF) (Table 2-1).

Nonclassical MHC Molecules Recognized by T Cells

Also found at the MHC locus on chromosome 6 are the nonclassical MHC molecules, HLA-E and HLA-G, which appear to function as surrogate MHC class I molecules to prevent lysis of cells by NK cells (Hunt et al., 2000; King et al., 2000; Rouas-Freiss et al., 2000); this may be particularly important on tissues that normally express little or no classical MHC class I molecules. Other nonclassical MHC molecules are recognized by unique subsets of T cells.

MHC Class I–Related Chains

MHC class I–related chains A and B (MICA and MICB), the genes for which are also found at the MHC locus, have limited but clear homology with conventional MHC class I molecules (Bahram and Spies, 1996; Groh et al., 2001; Li et al., 1999; Steinle et al., 1998). However, in contrast to conventional MHC class I, they lack a binding site for CD8, are not associated with β2-microglobulin, and do not appear to be involved with the presentation of peptide antigens. Instead, these molecules are expressed on stressed intestinal epithelial cells, such as those experiencing heat shock, and are recognized by γδ-T cells that bear Vδ1-containing γδ-TCR.

MICA and MICB are also induced on other cell types in response to infection with cytomegalovirus and probably with other types of viruses. MICA and MICB

TABLE 2-1 · CYTOKINES PRODUCED BY OR INFLUENCING T LYMPHOCYTES

Cytokine	Receptor/Receptor Complex	Principal Sources of Cytokine	Major Actions
Regulation of T-Cell Growth and Survival			
IL-2	IL-2Rαβγ$_c$	Naïve/Th1 T cells	T-cell replication, acquisition of effector function, sensitization to apoptosis
IL-7	IL-7Rαγ$_c$	Stromal cells	Essential for T- (and B-) cell development, naïve T-cell survival
IL-15	IL-15Rα/IL-2Rβγ$_c$	Stromal cells, activated monocytes and DCs	NK T-cell development, memory CD8 T-cell survival
Th1 Effector Responses			
IFN-γ	IFN-γRI/R2	Th1 and Tc1 T cells, NK T cells, NK cells	Induces macrophage activation/cellular immunity, enhances MHC class I and II expression and antigen presentation, enhances Th1, and inhibits Th2 responses; B-cell class switch to complement fixing IgG classes
IL-12 p70 (p40/p35 heterodimer)	IL-12Rβ1β2	Activated/mature DCs, macrophages	Enhances IFN-γ production, Th1, Tc1 differentiation, NK responses
IL-18	IL-18Rαβ	Activated/mature DCs, macrophages, others	Works in concert with IL-12 to induce IFN-γ production, Th1, and Tc1 responses; can induce Th2 responses in absence of IL-12
IL-23 (IL-12p40/p19 heterodimer)	IL-12Rβ1 (not IL-12Rβ2 chain)	Activated/mature DCs, macrophages	Similar to IL-12
Th2 Effectors			
IL-4	IL-4Rαγ$_c$	Th2 T cells, NK T cells, mast cells	Master regulator of Th2 T-cell differentiation; inhibits Th1 responses; enhances B-cell growth and MHC class II expression, class switching to IgE; enhances mast cell growth
IL-5	IL-5α/β; β chain is shared with GM-CSFR/IL-3R	Th2 cells, mast cells	Eosinophil differentiation, growth and survival
IL-9	IL-9Rαγ$_c$	Th2 cells, mast cells	Growth factor for subset of Th2 cells and for mast cells
IL-13	IL-4Rα/IL-13Rα	Th2 cells, mast cells	Similar to IL-4, but T cells lack IL-13Rα and do not respond
T Regulatory/Suppressor Cytokines			
IL-10	IL-10R1R2	Treg, macrophages, B cells, others	Blocks macrophage activation and DC maturation and cytokine production, inhibits T-cell responses, particularly Th1
TGF-β	TGF-βR1/RII	Treg/Th3 T cells, macrophages, others	Inhibit cytokine synthesis, cell replication
TNF Family*			
Tumor necrosis factor	TNFRI/II	T cells, macrophages, NK cells	Fever, inflammatory responses, acute phase responses, maturation of DCs
Lymphotoxin (LT) α and β	LT-α3 uses TNFRI/II; LT-α1β2 and LT-α2β1 use LT-βR	LT-α by Th1 cells, B cells and NK cells; LT-β by naïve T cells and blood progenitor cells	LT-α3 similar to TNF LT-α1β2 and LT-α2β1; formation of lymph nodes, Peyer's patches, and germinal centers
Fas ligand	Fas (CD95)	T and NK cells	Induction of apoptosis in cells expressing Fas
CD40 ligand (CD154)	CD40	CD4 T cells, higher on effector/ memory than naïve	Mediates B-cell help, replication, Ig class switching, and affinity maturation; DC maturation and IL-12 production
4-1BB ligand (CD137)	4-1BB	Activated B cells, macrophages, mature DCs	Co-stimulates responses of activated T cells, particularly CD8 T-cell responses
OX40 ligand	OX40 (CD134)	Activated B cells and mature DCs, some T cells, others	Co-stimulates CD4 T-cell responses, particularly T-cell help for B cells
Hematopoietic Growth Factors			
IL-3	IL-3α/β; β chain is shared with GM-CSFR/IL-5R	T cells	Growth factor for early hematopoietic progenitors, lymphoid DCs
GM-CSF	GM-CSFα/β; β chain is shared with IL-3R/IL-5R	T cells	Growth factor for granulocytes, monocytes, and myeloid DCs; enhances macrophage and neutrophil function and viability

*TNF proteins function as trimers. TNF homotrimers are expressed on the plasma membrane and secreted; LT forms include secreted LT-α3, and plasma membrane–associated LT-α1β2 and LT-α2β1; LT-α3 binds to TNF-RI; LT-α1β2 and LT-α2β1 bind to LT-βR; Fas ligand, CD40 ligand, OX40 ligand, and 4-1BB ligand are homotrimers primarily expressed on the plasma membrane.

are also ligands for the activating CD94/NKG2D receptor found on most NK cells and on some CD8 T cells and γδ-T cells, which can either activate or act in concert with TCR-mediated signals to activate these cells (McMahon and Raulet, 2001; Raulet et al., 2001).

CD1 Locus Genes

The human CD1 locus includes four nonpolymorphic genes, CD1a through CD1d (Jayawardena-Wolf and Bendelac, 2001; Porcelli et al., 1998). CD1 molecules associate with β_2-microglobulin but have limited structural homology with either MHC class I or class II proteins. In humans they are mainly expressed on APCs, including DCs (Banchereau et al., 2000). CD1b efficiently binds and presents highly hydrophobic lipoglycan molecules of mycobacteria, such as lipoarabinomannans, mycolic acid, and glucose monomycolate and some self-lipids, such as GM1 ganglioside (Jayawardena-Wolf and Bendelac, 2001; Porcelli et al., 1998).

Mycobacterial lipoglycans undergo processing and loading onto CD1b in an endosomal compartment that is similar or identical to the compartment where peptides are loaded onto MHC class II molecules. CD1c may be involved in the presentation of lipidated bacterial polysaccharides, such as the polyribosylribitol phosphate component of the capsule of *Haemophilus influenzae* type b (Fairhurst et al., 1998). Subsets of CD8 T cells and of the rare CD4−CD8− αβ-T cells respond to microbial lipids on CD1b and CD1c molecules, and a subset of γδ-T cells recognizes as yet uncharacterized antigens on CD1c molecules (Jayawardena-Wolf and Bendelac, 2001).

CD1d, the only member of the human CD1 cluster that is also expressed in the mouse, appears to be specialized for the presentation of hydrophobic nonpeptide molecules, such as the glycosylphosphatidylinositol (GPI) moiety of GPI-linked proteins (Jayawardena-Wolf and Bendelac, 2001). Such GPI-linked proteins are found at particularly high levels on the surface of certain protozoa pathogens, such as *Plasmodium* and *Trypanosoma*. However, it is as yet uncertain that GPI from these pathogens is actually presented, and the current data favors the notion that endogenous lipids or glycolipids may be presented on CD1d.

As in the case of CD1b, loading of antigens onto CD1d is apparently accomplished in a late endosomal compartment similar or identical to the compartment where peptides are loaded onto MHC class II molecules. A unique subset of αβ-T cells, which are autoreactive to CD1d in vitro, are commonly referred to as NK T cells (see later discussion); NK T cells are CD4−CD8− and express a canonical TCR alpha chain (Vα24JαQ).

Studies in mice indicate that other molecules with some homology to MHC class I are specialized for the presentation of peptides containing N-formyl-methionine derived from the amino terminus of bacterial proteins (Lindahl et al., 1997). However, there is no evidence to date for a homologous or orthologous protein in humans.

INTRATHYMIC DEVELOPMENT OF T LYMPHOCYTES

Thymic Ontogeny

With the exception of a subset of the T lymphocytes found in the gut and perhaps the liver (Dejbakhsh-Jones et al., 1995; Ohteki et al., 1992; Ohteki et al., 1996), T lymphocytes develop from hematopoietic stem cells within the unique microenvironment of the thymus. The thymus arises from the ventral portions of the third and fourth pharyngeal pouches. Both ectoderm and mesoderm contribute to the formation of this tissue.

Defects in the development of the thymus accompany DiGeorge syndrome/velocardiofacial syndrome, which is associated with haploinsufficiency of a variable portion of chromosome 22 q11.2 (see Chapter 17). In mice, haploinsufficiency of the transcription factor TBX1, which is contained within the syntenic region, reproduces the cardiac but not the thymic phenotype of DiGeorge syndrome, whereas homozygous deficiency also results in thymic aplasia and perinatal lethality (Jerome and Papaioannou, 2001; Merscher et al., 2001). This suggests that TBX1 deficiency is at least in part responsible for the thymic defect in DiGeorge syndrome. Formation of the thymus is disrupted by the *nude* defect in mice, which results from a mutation of the whn transcription factor (Nehls et al., 1994). Other induced gene defects have also been associated with abnormal thymus development in mice (reviewed in Berg and Kang, 2001).

By approximately 7 weeks' gestation in humans, the thymic rudiment is seeded by CD34+ hematopoietic stem cells derived from the liver. Mature T cells bearing the TCR, CD3, and CD4 or CD8 are first detected 1 week later (Haynes and Heinly, 1995). By 12 weeks' gestation, a clear distinction between the cortex and medulla of the thymus is evident, and Hassall's corpuscles are detected in the medulla soon thereafter (Gilhus et al., 1985; Horst et al., 1990). By 14 weeks' gestation, all T-cell developmental intermediates, also called thymocyte subsets, are present and reside within the appropriate compartments (see following discussion). By mid-gestation, the bone marrow replaces the liver as a source of hematopoietic progenitors seeding the thymus.

Thymic cellularity increases dramatically during the last trimester of gestation and continues to do so postnatally. Relative to body mass, the thymus is largest at birth, but the absolute thymic mass is greatest at about 10 years of age. When complete thymectomy is performed during the first year of life, subsequent numbers of CD4 and CD8 T cells are decreased in the circulation, indicating the importance of postnatal production of thymocytes for the peripheral T-cell compartment (Ramos et al., 1996).

The thymus gradually involutes after puberty, and the cortex and medulla are progressively replaced with fat. Although reduced in magnitude, thymic output continues throughout life, as indicated by recent studies in which TCR excision circles and in vivo labeling studies have been used to assess thymic output (Douek and Koup, 2000; McCune et al., 2000).

Throughout life, the thymus retains the capacity to increase the output of T cells in response to severe T-cell lymphopenia (e.g., following intense cytoablative chemotherapy and in patients with HIV following treatment with highly active antiretroviral therapy [HAART]); however, the magnitude of this response appears to diminish with age (Douek and Koup, 2000; Douek et al., 2000; Mackall et al., 1995; McCune et al., 2000).

Intrathymic Development of T Lymphocytes Is an Ordered Process

T lymphocytes mature from hematopoietic progenitors through an ordered process in which sequential cell fate decisions are made and the majority of cells are discarded. Monoclonal antibodies to cell surface antigens and other key reagents have been used to define in detail these sequential stages, and there is an extensive literature on the role of specific genes in this process (Berg and Kang, 2001; Candotti et al., 2002). The delineation of these stages and the genes and proteins involved have come both from human and murine studies. Although certain cell surface markers that define specific stages differ between humans and mice, the major cell surface markers and checkpoints that determine whether a cell adopts one or another fate have been validated in both systems. We use the human cell markers in this discussion, as outlined in the recent review by Res and Spits (1999); the paralogous murine markers can be found in other reviews (Berg and Kang, 2001; Pénit et al., 1995; Shortman and Wu, 1996).

The major stages of T-cell development can be delineated by the expression of CD4, CD8, and the TCR/CD3 complex on the plasma membrane of thymic lymphocytes, also called thymocytes. In Figure 2-3, maturation of thymocytes is shown from left to right. The most immature subsets are TCR/CD3$^-$CD4$^-$CD8$^-$ and are often referred to collectively as **double-negative (DN,** because they lack both the CD4 and CD8 coreceptors) or triple-negative (TN, because they lack TCR/CD3, CD4, and CD8) thymocytes; herein they are referred to as DN thymocytes. DN thymocytes mature sequentially into cells that are CD4$^+$CD8$^+$ **double-positive (DP),** then CD4$^+$ or CD8$^+$ **single-positive (SP).** In general, the immature DN thymocytes are found in the subcapsular region, the DP thymocytes in the cortex, and the SP thymocytes in the medulla (see Fig. 2-3).

DN thymocytes can be further divided based on cell surface markers and their developmental potential. The most immature DN cell expresses the hematopoietic stem cell marker CD34 but little or no CD5, CD1a, CD38, or IL-7 receptor α chain. These cells remain multipotent, because they can give rise to T, B, NK, and dendritic cells. Sequential changes in cell surface marker expression lead to the gradual loss of CD34 and the acquisition of CD5, then Cd1a and CD4. In parallel, these populations become progressively committed to the T-cell lineage, such that CD34$^{-/low}$CD5$^+$CD1a$^+$ cells are restricted to the T-cell fate.

Thereafter these cells make sequential cell fate choices: αβ-TCR vs. γδ-TCR, then, among the αβ-T cell lineage, between CD4 or CD8. These cell fate decisions are associated with the initiation and completion of TCR rearrangement and require that cells successfully complete the processes of positive and negative selection.

Generation of the TCR and TCR Diversity

As noted previously, T (and B) lymphocytes undergo a unique developmental event, the generation of antigen receptors through DNA recombination, a process referred to as V(D)J recombination. This is a highly ordered process and is controlled at multiple levels (Agrawal et al., 1998; Gellert, 1996; Hiom et al., 1998).

Recombination-Activating Genes

The restriction of this process to cells of the T and B lineage is controlled by the unique expression in their precursors of two **recombination-activating genes,** *RAG-1* and *RAG-2*. RAG proteins mediate V(D)J recombination in concert with a series of proteins that, unlike RAG proteins, are expressed ubiquitously and are involved in the process of double-stranded DNA break repair by the **nonhomologous end-joining (NHEJ)** pathway (Hoeijmakers, 2001). The RAG proteins are critically involved in the initiation of the recombination process—they recognize and cleave conserved sequences flanking each V, D, and J segment (see Fig. 2-3). The subsequent alignment of the segments generated by RAG-mediated cleavage is mediated by the catalytic subunit of the double-stranded DNA-dependent protein kinase (DNA-PK$_{cs}$) and its associated Ku70 and Ku80 proteins, and the aligned ends are then joined by DNA ligase IV and its associated XRCC4 protein (Frank et al., 1998; Gao et al., 1998; Gu et al., 1997; Sekiguchi and Frank, 1999).

RAG Defects

Because T-cell and B-cell development depends on the surface expression of rearranged TCR and immunoglobulin genes, respectively, humans (and mice) with genetic deficiency of either RAG-1 or RAG-2 have a form of severe combined immunodeficiency (SCID) in which T and B cells are absent or markedly reduced but NK cells are normal (T$^-$B$^-$NK$^+$ SCID) (Fischer, 2000; Fischer and Malissen, 1998) (see Chapter 15). Similarly, SCID in mice results from a naturally occurring mutation in the DNA-PKcs (Blunt et al., 1995) or induced mutations in Ku70 or Ku80 (Frank et al., 1998; Gu et al., 1997). Because these latter defects also impair processes of general importance to DNA repair, these defects, but not RAG deficiency, also result in increased sensitivity to radiation-induced DNA damage and cancer.

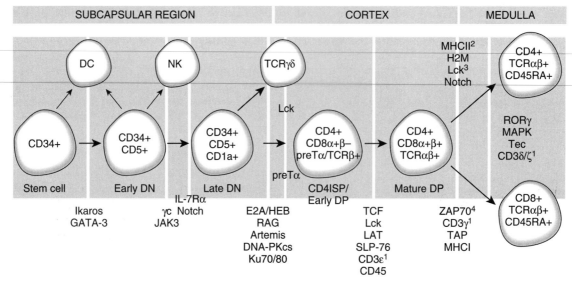

Figure 2-3 · Intrathymic T-lymphocyte development. The pathway of development is shown schematically from left to right, with the most immature hematopoietic stem cell from which lymphoid progenitors are derived shown on the left and the most mature CD4+ or CD8+ single-positive (SP) thymocyte shown on the right. We have used the markers for human early developmental stages described in Rees and Spits (1999), and matched them based on other features with murine stages reviewed in Berg and Kang (2001). For purposes of simplicity, some of the early developmental intermediates before the CD4+CD8+ double-positive (DP) stage have been omitted, including the common lymphoid progenitor cell that is an intermediate between the CD34+ stem cell and the early double-negative (DN) stage. Naturally occurring and induced mutations that result in a marked (>75%) reduction in subsequent developmental stages are indicated next to a line where the block occurs; factors shown in bold have been demonstrated in humans with primary immunodeficiency; factors shown in plain type have been identified only in mice. In some cases, different phenotypes are observed between mice and humans with defects in the same gene, and in these cases, only the human phenotype is indicated: (1) Mice with deficiencies in CD3γ or ε have a block in development of DP thymocytes, whereas mice with deficiencies of CD3δ or ζ have a block at the DP to SP transition (Wang et al, 1999). Humans with single gene defects in CD3ε or CD3γ have incomplete blocks in T-cell development predominantly at the DP stage and in the generation of CD8 SP cells, respectively, and their mature T cells have reduced surface expression of TCR/CD3 and defects in activation (Arnaiz-Villena et al., 1995; Kappes et al., 1995). (2) The genes shown adjacent to CD4 or CD8 SP cells result in a selective block in generation of the respective subset; genes shown between these two subsets impair the generation of both. (3) Reduced but not absent expression of Lck due to an exon 7 splice defect selectively impaired the generation of CD4 SP cells (Goldman et al., 1998), whereas complete loss of Lck in mice blocks the generation of αβ-T–cell lineage cells at the DP stage and γδ-T cells. The finding in the human patient is compatible with reports in mice expressing varying amounts of Lck, which suggest that low expression favors the generation of CD8 vs. CD4 SP cells (reviewed in Berg and Kang, 2001). (4) ZAP-70 deficiency in mice results in a block in the generation of DP thymocytes and in humans in a block in generation of CD8 SP thymocytes, paralleling the difference in the effects of CD3γ deficiency in humans vs. mice.

Artemis Defect

Recently a defect in the gene encoding a newly discovered protein, Artemis, was shown to account for a subset of human T−B−NK+ SCID patients (Moshous et al., 2001) (see Chapter 15). Cells from these patients, like murine SCID cells, show both increased radiosensitivity and a specific defect in repair of the coding junctions (but not the excised signal junctions). Artemis forms a complex with DNA-PKcs, which leads to the phosphorylation of Artemis; this complex is then able both to cleave the hairpin DNA structure formed at the coding ends of the DNA by RAG-mediated cleavage and to participate in the joining of the coding ends through nonhomologous DNA end repair (Ma et al., 2002).

Nonhomologous End-Joining Defects

Finally, other forms of incomplete human combined immune deficiency, which exhibit increased radiosensitivity and defects outside the immune system, are associated with defects in sensor genes that help to activate the NHEJ pathway—ataxia telangiectasia, Nijmegen breakage syndrome, MRE11 deficiency, and ligase IV deficiency (Hoeijmakers, 2001; O'Driscoll et al., 2001) (see Chapter 18).

Restriction of Rearrangement

The interrupted V, D, and J segments of the TCR and immunoglobulin variable domains (Fig. 2-4) appear to

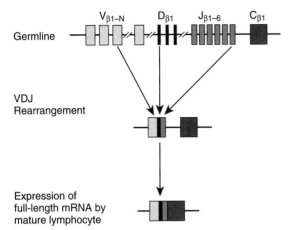

Figure 2-4· TCR-β V(D)J recombination. Shown is a schematic of the TCR-β locus, recombination of V(D)J segments with deletion of the intervening introns giving rise to a single VDJ exon juxtaposed to the TCR-β constant region (C) exon. Following transcription, the intron between the VDJ and C exons is spliced out, yielding an in-frame mRNA encoding TCR-β. A similar process occurs at the TCR-α, TCR-δ and TCR-γ loci.

have been created in a vertebrate ancestor by RAG-mediated transposition, which interrupted a putative single primordial receptor variable region exon, followed by diversification through gene duplication (Agrawal et al., 1998; Hiom et al., 1998; Melek et al., 1998). Although V(D)J recombination is restricted to T- (and B-) cell progenitors, because only they express the *RAG* genes, this is not sufficient to explain the restriction of TCR rearrangement and expression to T cells, immunoglobulin rearrangement and expression to B cells, the ordered rearrangement and expression of receptor heavy chains before light chains, and allelic exclusion (see following discussion). Rather, both the expression of the *RAG* genes and the structure of chromatin at the TCR and immunoglobulin loci are regulated, such that V(D)J recombination is restricted to specific TCR and immunoglobulin loci in a manner specific to the cell lineage and developmental stage (Krangel, 2001; Sleckman et al., 1996).

Sequence of Rearrangement of TCR-β

The unrearranged human TCR-β chain gene, which spans 685 kilobases of DNA on human chromosome 7, consists of 46 potentially functional variable (V) gene segments located upstream of two constant (C) regions, each associated with one diversity (D) and six joining (J) segments (see Fig. 2-4) (Rowen et al., 1996). The D segment first rearranges to a downstream J segment, with the deletion of intervening DNA. This is followed by rearrangement of a V segment to the DJ segment, resulting in a contiguous VDJ β-chain exon. If this VDJ exon lacks premature translation stop codons, its transcript will be spliced in frame to the constant (C) region-encoding exon, and the TCR-β chain protein can then be expressed on the thymocyte surface in association with a pre-TCR-α chain protein (pre-Tα) and the CD3 complex (Malissen et al., 1999; von Boehmer et al., 1999).

RAG gene expression, and therefore the potential to rearrange TCR genes, commences in the CD5[+], CD1a[+], DN thymocyte subset and is active in these cells and in the subsequent CD5[+], CD1a[+], CD4[+] stage (CD4 ISP thymocytes) (Res and Spits, 1999; Trigueros et al., 1998). Expression of RAG proteins in these thymocyte subsets is associated with the rearrangement of TCR-β (or TCR-γ and TCR-δ) genes—TCR-α genes remain in the germline configuration. Cells not generating a productive TCR-β gene either die, or those that productively rearrange TCR-γ and TCR-δ chains mature along the alternative γδ-T–cell pathway. The factors that dictate commitment of immature thymocytes to the γδ-T–cell vs. the αβ-T–cell lineage are incompletely defined (see following).

Cessation of Rearrangement

Expression of TCR-β along with pre-Tα generates a signal that triggers multiple rounds of proliferation, the induction of CD8 expression and upregulation of CD4 expression, and maturation to the DP stage. Concomitantly, the TCR-β signal extinguishes further V(D)J rearrangement at the TCR-β locus, thereby assuring that a productive TCR-β chain is retained. This also excludes productive V(D)J rearrangement and expression of a second TCR-β in that cell. In this way allelic exclusion of TCR-β is achieved, such that a given T cell rearranges a complete in-frame TCR-β V(D)J variable region (with rare exceptions) (Padovan et al., 1995) on only one of the two possible alleles. This is also associated with the reinduction of RAG expression, a change in chromatin structure at the TCR-α locus, and rearrangement of TCR-α.

Rearrangement of TCR-α

Rearrangement of the TCR-α gene involves the joining of V segments directly to J segments, without intervening D segments. The human TCR-α chain gene locus contains approximately 100 V segments and 50 to 100 J segments (Clark et al., 1995). Allelic exclusion is relatively ineffective for the TCR-α chain gene, and it is estimated that as many as one third of human peripheral αβ-T cells may express two types of TCR-α chains (Padovan et al., 1993). RAG protein expression normally ceases in cortical thymocytes, limiting gene rearrangement to early thymocyte development.

Recent experiments using mice bearing an αβ-TCR encoded by a transgene suggest that peripheral T cells may also have the capacity to re-express the RAG proteins and undergo secondary TCR-β chain gene rearrangement (McMahan and Fink, 1998). Whether this process, known as TCR editing, occurs in human T cells or in genetically unmanipulated mice, and whether it is biologically significant, is not known.

TCR Diversity Generation

TCR diversity is generated by the largely random use of V, D, and J segments in assembling the TCR-α and TCR-β chain genes (Davis et al., 1997). The third complementarity determining region (CDR3), where the distal portion of the V segment joins the (D)J segment, appears to be a particularly important source of diversity in peptide-MHC recognition for the αβ-TCR. In addition to this combinatorial diversity, several other mechanisms increase potential diversity at the junctions between V, D, and J. First, the recombinase is imprecise in cleaving the ends of the V, D, and J segments, so that variable numbers of nucleotides are lost (Gellert, 1996; Gellert, 1997).

Second, **terminal deoxynucleotidyl transferase (TdT)**, an enzyme expressed at high levels in TCR gene-rearranging thymocytes, randomly adds nucleotides (called N-nucleotides) to the ends of segments undergoing rearrangement (Komori et al., 1993; Siu et al., 1984). TdT addition is a particularly important mechanism for diversity generation because every three additional nucleotides encodes an additional codon, potentially increasing repertoire diversity by a factor of 20. Finally, one or two nucleotides that are palindromic to the end of the gene segment (termed P nucleotides) can be added (Lewis, 1994).

Together these mechanisms for generating diversity can theoretically result in as many as 10^{15} types of αβ-TCR. However, actual αβ-TCR diversity is likely to be less than this theoretical maximal value, because particular V, D, and J segments may be used less often than would be predicted on a random basis (Jores and Meo, 1993). The reasons for this deviation from random segment usage remain unclear, but it may be due to differences among segments in their accessibility to the protein complex involved in the recombination process.

Positive and Negative Selection and Thymocyte Maturation

DP thymocytes that have successfully rearranged and expressed αβ-TCR on the cell surface are subject to a stringent selection process. Those cells with an αβ-TCR that interacts weakly (but with sufficient strength to allow them to recognize foreign antigenic peptides in association with self MHC molecules) are positively selected and survive. Positive selection appears to require that cortical epithelial cells present to DP thymocytes a diverse group of self-peptides bound to MHC molecules (Barton and Rudensky, 1999). The αβ-TCR interacts not only with the MHC-associated peptide but also regions of the MHC molecule that form the peptide-binding groove (Garcia and Teyton, 1998), for which it has an intrinsic affinity (Zerrahn et al., 1997).

Positive selection is also influenced by interactions between MHC molecules and the CD4 and CD8 molecules. As mentioned previously, MHC class I and MHC class II molecules have constant domains located outside their peptide-binding grooves that have affinity for CD8 and CD4, respectively. As a result of these interactions, nearly all CD4 SP thymocytes (and CD4 T cells) recognize peptides bound to MHC class II molecules, and CD8 SP thymocytes (and CD8 T cells) recognize peptides bound to MHC class I molecules. Positive selection also extinguishes *RAG* gene expression, terminating further α-TCR rearrangement.

Conversely, cells expressing a αβ-TCR that does not interact, or that interacts with an unacceptably high affinity, with self MHC molecules undergo apoptosis in processes commonly referred to as death by neglect and negative selection, respectively. Thymic epithelial cells found in the medulla may express a diverse array of self-antigens, such as insulin and myelin basic protein, which help in this elimination (Farr and Rudensky, 1998), but negative selection appears to be most efficiently mediated by medullary DCs (Laufer et al., 1996). Negative selection helps eliminate αβ-T cells with TCRs that are potentially autoreactive, and has an important influence on the final TCR repertoire (van Meerwijk et al., 1997).

Cells that both are positively selected and avoid negative selection upregulate surface expression of αβ-TCR and downregulate either CD4 or CD8 (Jameson and Bevan, 1998; Kearse et al., 1995; Kisielow and Von Boehmer, 1995), becoming SP thymoyctes. As a result of the stringency of positive and negative selection, only 2% to 3% of the initial hematopoietic lymphoid precursors that enter the thymus emerge as SP thymocytes (Jameson and Bevan, 1998).

As thymocytes mature from the DP to SP stage, they change their pattern of chemokine receptor expression (see below), downregulating the expression of CCR9 and upregulating the expression of CCR7. This probably accounts for their migration from the thymic medulla into the blood, where, as naïve T cells, they preferentially migrate to the secondary lymphoid organs (Campbell and Butcher, 2000).

Checkpoints and Fate Choices during Intrathymic T-Lymphocyte Development

The cell fate choices described previously, and the subsequent maturation, survival, and proliferation following each developmental fate choice, are governed in concert by transcription factors, cytokines, and key signal transduction molecules, such that defects in their expression lead to aberrant T-cell development (see Fig. 2-3) (Berg and Kang, 2001; Fischer, 2000; Fischer and Malissen, 1998; Res and Spits, 1999).

Most of the findings have been deduced from studies in mice with genetically engineered defects, and in some cases in humans with similar defects. In some cases there are differences in the phenotype observed between mice and humans, and these are noted. In the absence of this, the stage at which a specific gene defect exerts a block or aberration in T-cell development in the mice has been imposed on the pathway of developmental cell surface markers as defined in the human thymus (Res and Spits, 1999). However, the reader should recognize that the effects in humans of such a defect might not be exactly those observed in mice.

Generation of a Common Lymphoid Progenitor

The first cell fate checkpoint is the generation of common lymphoid progenitor (CLP) cells from pluripotent hematopoietic stem cells. In mice the generation of all lymphoid lineages is dependent on the transcription factor Ikaros (Cortes et al., 1999). An early block in T-cell development is also seen in the absence of GATA-3 and Notch-1 (Berg and Kang, 2001; Radtke et al., 2000; Van Esch et al., 2000), but global defects produce embryonic lethality in mice deficient in these genes. Thereafter, further development of T cells (and NK cells) is dependent on signaling through the **common cytokine receptor γ chain (γc)** (Di Santo and Rodewald, 1998; Fischer, 2000; Fischer and Malissen, 1998), which is a component of the IL-2, IL-4, IL-7, IL-9, and IL-15 cytokine receptor complexes (see Table 2-1) (Di Santo and Rodewald, 1998).

Human Defects of T-Cell Development

Individuals with X-linked SCID, due to a defect in expression of γc, lack T and NK cells (Fischer, 2000; Fischer and Malissen, 1998). A similar phenotype is observed in autosomal recessive SCID due to a defect in Jak3, which transduces signals downstream of γc (Notarangelo et al., 2000). Experimental evidence in mice indicates that the defect in NK cells is likely to be due to the loss of IL-15 signaling, whereas the lack of T cells recapitulates the T-cell phenotype of IL-7 receptor α deficiency in humans, which produces a form of T-NK$^+$B$^+$ SCID (Puel and Leonard, 2000; Roifman et al., 2000); notably, IL-7 receptor α-deficient mice also have a profound block in B-cell development not seen in humans. These disorders are discussed in Chapter 15.

αβ- and γδ-T Cell Development

After cells become committed to T-cell development, the next major cell fate decision is between the αβ- vs. γδ-T cell lineages. The basis for this decision is unclear (Robey and Fowlkes, 1998; Zorbas and Scollay, 1993), but E2A and the related transcription factor HEB may contribute. Deficiency of HEB impairs αβ-T cell development at the DN stage but, unlike E2A deficiency, does not affect the development of γδ-T cells. E2A-deficient mice also invariably develop T-cell lymphomas. Both E2A and HEB may act in part by facilitating TCR V(D)J recombination, and a specific role of IL-7 in facilitating recombination at the TCR-γ locus has been shown in mice (Durum et al., 1998; Schlissel et al., 2000).

Notch also appears to contribute to this decision, in that murine precursors with reduced Notch expression preferentially develop into γδ-T cells (Robey and Fowlkes, 1998; Washburn et al., 1997), but how this is mediated is uncertain. In any case, productive rearrangement of either TCR-γ and TCR-δ or of TCR-β is required at this stage, which leads to the expression of the γδ-TCR or pre-Tα/TCR-β, respectively, along with the CD3 complex, on the cell surface.

Thus individuals or mice lacking components of the recombinase machinery (see previous discussion) are unable to achieve this, resulting in a block of T-cell development at the late DN stage (see Fig. 2-3); in humans, defects in RAG1, RAG2, and Artemis have been reported to cause SCID, in which T-cell development is blocked at the late DN thymocyte stage (Fischer, 2000; Fischer and Malissen, 1998; Moshous et al., 2001).

CD3/TCR Complex Defects

Expression of the TCR/CD3 complex allows late DN thymocytes to pass this critical developmental check point, at which time they both proliferate (particularly those expressing pre-Tα/TCR-β) and mature. In mice, deficiency of TCF1, a transcription factor in the Wnt signaling pathway, markedly impairs the proliferation that normally occurs following the expression of pre-Tα/TCR-β and thereby impairs the generation of adult but not neonatal DP thymocytes (Clevers et al., 1988; Verbeek et al., 1995).

As discussed in greater detail later, the CD3 complex in concert with CD4 and CD8 co-receptors on αβ-T cells is linked to a complex signal transduction pathway that is necessary for the proliferation of late DN thymocytes and their maturation into DP thymocytes. The proximal elements of this pathway include the CD3 complex itself and the downstream tyrosine kinases and adaptor proteins that form links to other signaling molecules. CD3γδε, Lck and ZAP70 tyrosine kinases, and two adaptor proteins, SLP-76 and LAT, are essential for transmitting the signal from the pre-Tα/TCR-β receptor, and deficiencies of these proteins lead to severe impairment in the maturation of late DN to DP thymocytes in mice (reviewed in Berg and Kang, 2001).

Unlike mice, complete deficiency of ZAP-70 in humans blocks CD8 but not CD4 T cell development (Berg and Kang, 2001; Elder et al., 1994; Roifman, 1995, 2000); the difference between humans and mice may reflect a compensatory role for the related Syk kinase that allows the development of CD4 T cells in humans, which nonetheless are dysfunctional (Elder et al., 1994; Roifman, 1995).

Similarly, humans with isolated CD3ε or CD3γ deficiency or partial deficiency of Lck have partial blocks in T-cell development (see Fig. 2-3) and impaired T-cell function (Arnaiz-Villena et al., 1995; Kappes et al., 1995).

CD4 and CD8 Lineage Selection

To survive and mature further, DP thymocytes must undergo positive selection, escape negative selection, and adopt either the CD4 or CD8 T-cell fate. Positive selection is dependent on signals transduced through the Ras-Raf-MAP kinase pathway (reviewed in Berg and Kang, 2001). As a consequence, mice with a complete deficiency of p44 MAPK have approximately a 50% reduction in the number of SP thymocytes and T cells, and the T cells also have a defect in activation-induced proliferation (Pages et al., 1999); surprisingly, there is no obvious nonlymphoid defect in these mice.

Selection into the CD4 lineage requires the expression of MHC class II molecules, HLA-DM (H2M in the mouse) and CD4, whereas selection into the CD8 lineage requires expression of MHC class I molecules, TAP and CD8. Furthermore, differences in the strength of signals transduced through Lck and MAPK may influence the choice between the CD4 and CD8 lineage, with more robust signals favoring development of CD4 SP cells. Deficiency of the orphan nuclear hormone receptor RORγ leads to a selective approximately 50% loss of DP and SP thymocytes due to a failure in expression of the antiapoptotic Bcl-x$_L$ protein in DP thymocytes (Sun et al., 2000); those cells maturing to the SP stage emigrate to the blood and spleen and function normally, but these mice also lack lymph nodes or Peyer's patches due to a defect in fetal lymphoid progenitors.

MIGRATION OF T CELLS TO THE PERIPHERY

Thymocyte Emigration

SP thymocytes emigrate from the thymus via the blood to the secondary lymphoid tissues, which consist of the lymph nodes, spleen, and mucosal-associated lymphoid tissues. Development of lymph nodes and Peyer's patches in mice is dependent on signaling by members of the TNF cytokine gene family through the lymphotoxin-β (LT-β) receptor (see Table 2-1) (Fu and Chaplin, 1999; Futterer et al., 1998; Rennert et al., 1998).

The failure of the anlage of these tissues to be seeded in fetal life by CD3$^-$CD4$^+$CD45$^+$IL-7 receptor α$^+$CLP cells correlates with the lack of these organs in LT-β–deficient mice, and the failure of these fetal CLP cells to develop in mice lacking Id2 and RORγ is associated with the absence of lymph nodes and Peyer's patches (Sun et al., 2000; Yokota et al., 1999). In mice, LT-β receptors are also required for the proper formation of lymphoid compartments within the spleen, including germinal centers (see following) but not for the formation of the spleen itself. Formation of the spleen requires Hox 11, a homeobox gene (Fu and Chaplin, 1999).

The migration of leukocytes, including T cells, is mediated by a combinatorial and multistep process determined by the pattern of expression on the cell surface of adhesion molecules and chemokine receptors and by the local patterns and gradients of adhesion molecule and chemokine receptor ligands in tissues (Table 2-2).

Role of Chemokines

Chemokines constitute a cytokine superfamily with more than 50 members known at the present time, most of which are secreted and of relatively low molecular weight (reviewed in Mackay, 2001; Rossi and Zlotnik,

TABLE 2-2 · CHEMOKINES AND ADHESION MOLECULES GOVERNING T-CELL MIGRATION INTO SPECIFIC TISSUES/ORGANS

Site	Cell Type	Initial Binding	Chemokine-Chemokine Receptor	Firm Adhesion	Tissue Zones
Peripheral lymph node	Naïve T cell	L-selectin-PNAd*	CCR7 – SLC (CCL21)‡	LFA-1-ICAM-1	CCR7– ELC(CCL19) in T-cell zones
Peripheral lymph node	Central memory T cell	L-selectin-PNAd	CCR7 – SLC (CCL21)	LFA-1-ICAM-1	CCR7–ELC(CCL19) in T-cell zones
Peripheral lymph node	Follicular B helper T cells				CXCR5–BLC (CXCL13) in B-cell zones
Small intestinal lamina propria	Gut effector/ effector memory T cells	α4β7 integrin-MAdCAM1	CCR9-TECK (CCL25)	LFA-1-ICAM1 α4β7 integrin-MAdCAM1	
Inflamed skin tissues	Skin effector/effector memory T cells	CLA†-E-selectin α4β1-VCAM-1	CCR4-TARC(CCL17) CCR10-CTACK (CCL27)	LFA-1-ICAM-1 α4β1-VCAM-1	
Various	Th1/Tc1 effector T cells	Varies with tissue	CCR5-MIP-1α/ MIP-1β/RANTES (CCL3/CCL4/CCL5) CXCR3-IP10/MIG/ I-TAC (CXCL10, CXCL9, CXCL11)	Variable	
Various	Th2/Tc2 effector T cells	Varies with tissue	CCR2, CCR3, CCR8-MCP-4, Eotaxin-1,2,3, I309 (CCL13, CCL11,24,26, CCL1)	Variable	

*Peripheral lymph node addressin
†Cutaneous lymphocyte antigen.
‡In parentheses are the numbers of the chemokine ligand (CCL or CXCC) corresponding to the common name of the chemokine(s); for example, SLC = CCL1.

2000). Chemokines are produced by a large number of cell types and selectively attract various leukocyte populations, which bear the appropriate G-protein–linked chemokine receptors.

Chemokines can be divided into four families based on their pattern of N-terminal cysteine residues: CC, CXC, C, and CX_3C (X represents a noncysteine amino acid between the cysteines). A nomenclature for the chemokines and their receptors has been recently adopted, in which the family is first given (e.g., CC), followed by *L* for *ligand* (the chemokines itself) and a number or followed by *R* (for *receptor*) and a number. Functionally, chemokines can also be defined by their principal function—in homeostatic or inflammatory cell migration—and by the subsets of cells on which they act (Moser and Loetscher, 2001).

Departure of naïve T cells from the thymus and entry into the secondary lymphoid tissues coincide with and are mediated in part by a change in the expression of chemokine receptors on their surface (Cyster, 1999; Mackay, 2001; Moser and Loetscher, 2001). As they enter the medulla, SP thymocytes begin to lose expression of CCR9 and to gain expression of CCR7. As explained later, this allows them to leave the thymic medulla, where chemokines binding to CCR9 (TECK, CCL25) are found, and enter the secondary lymphoid tissues, where chemokines that bind to CCR7 are found.

Role of Adhesion Molecules

There are two major families of adhesion molecules that govern leukocyte migration: the selectins and the integrins. There are three selectins, L-selectin (CD62L), which is constitutively expressed on many types of leukocytes, including naïve and certain subsets of memory T cells, and E-(CD62E) and P-selectin (CD62P), both of which are expressed on activated vascular endothelium; the latter is also expressed on activated platelets (Butcher and Picker, 1996; Springer, 1995).

Selectins bind to multivalent carbohydrate ligands, which are displayed on specific protein or lipid backbones on the cell surface. The other major adhesion molecules are the integrins, which are heterodimers composed of different combinations of α and β chains. All T cells express $\alpha_1\beta_2$ integrin, also known as LFA-1, and subsets of T cells express other integrins, including $\alpha_4\beta_1$ (VLA-4) and $\alpha_4\beta_7$. Integrins bind to members of the immunoglobulin superfamily: LFA-1 binds to ICAM-1, ICAM-2, ICAM-3, and VLA-4 binds to vascular cell adhesion molecule 1 (VCAM-1), which is induced on activated endothelial cells. MAdCAM-1, expressed on endothelial cells in the gut, is a ligand for both L-selectin and the $\alpha_4\beta_7$ integrin. Many integrins also bind to components of the extracellular matrix, which is thought to contribute to leukocyte migration in the tissues after cells migrate across the vascular endothelium.

Leukocyte Movement in Vessels and Lymph Nodes

The initial interaction of leukocytes with the vascular endothelium is mediated by selectins and their ligands (Butcher and Picker, 1996; Springer, 1995). This low-affinity, high valency interaction is facilitated by the display of selectins on the tips of microvilli, where they are positioned to sample the endothelial surface. If ligand is displayed, leukocytes are induced to roll along the endothelium, which allows them to survey for the presence of chemokines. In the case of naïve T cells, surface expression of L-selectin (CD62L) allows them to bind to the peripheral lymph node addressin, which is expressed on the surface of the specialized high endothelium of the postcapillary venules (HEV) in the peripheral lymph nodes, Peyer's patches, and tonsils (Campbell and Butcher, 2000).

Tethered to the surface of the HEV is the chemokine, SLC (CCL21), which binds to CCR7 on the surface of naïve T cells. SLC, and another CCR7 ligand, ELC (CCL19), are produced by stromal cells and perhaps some APCs in the lymph node. The engagement of CCR7 on naïve T cells by SLC triggers signals leading to an increase in the affinity of LFA-1, allowing the naïve T cells to bind avidly to the LFA-1 ligand, ICAM-1 and ICAM-2 on the vascular endothelium. This arrests T-cell rolling, thereby allowing T cells to diapedese across the endothelium and enter the T-cell zones of the lymph node. There ELC is produced by DCs, resulting in the juxtaposition of naïve T cells and DCs.

If naïve T cells encounter DCs presenting cognate peptide-MHC complexes, they stop migrating and remain in the lymph node. If not, they migrate through the lymph node to the efferent lymph and through this return to the bloodstream. Thus naïve T cells continually circulate between the blood and secondary lymphoid tissues, allowing them the opportunity to continuously sample APCs for their cognate antigen. Because they regulate this homeostatic recirculation of naïve T cells, SLC and ELC are referred to as homeostatic chemokines.

Survival of Naïve T Cells

Studies in mice indicate that the survival of naïve T cells in the periphery is dependent on two major exogenous factors (Fig. 2-5). The first is continuous interaction with self-peptide–MHC complexes; current evidence suggests that the self-peptides involved include those that mediated positive selection in the thymus. In the absence of these self-peptide–MHC complexes, the normal approximately 6-month life span of naïve T cells in mice is markedly reduced (Surh and Sprent, 2000).

The second major factor appears to be signals provided through the common cytokine receptor γ chain (γc). In the absence of γc, naïve T cells appear to survive for fewer than 5 days (Lantz et al., 2000). It appears that the role of γc is primarily if not solely to transduce signals in response to IL-7 through the IL-7R α/γc receptor

PATHWAYS TO INDUCE DC MATURATION

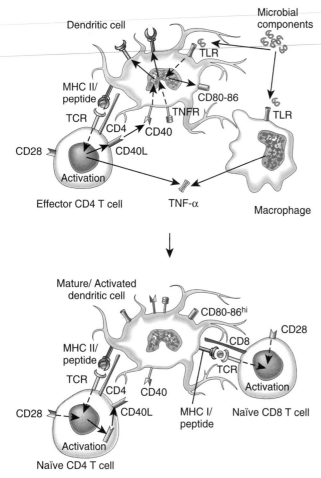

Figure 2-5 · Dendritic cell maturation and function. Immature DCs mature in response to stimulation via toll-like receptors (TLRs) that recognize pathogen-associated molecular patterns (PAMPs); inflammatory cytokines produced by other cells (e.g., TNF), like macrophages; or CD40 ligand expressed on effector CD4 T cells. Maturation is associated with the increased expression of MHC and co-stimulatory molecules, including CD80-86 (B7-1, B7-2). This allows them to present antigen effectively to naïve T cells. See text for additional discussion.

complex (Schluns et al., 2000). By contrast, once naïve T cells are activated in response to cognate peptide-MHC complexes, homeostasis is maintained by different mechanisms, which are discussed later.

Finally, resting T cells express a transcription factor, LKLF, that is necessary for the maintenance of their quiescent phenotype and survival (Kuo and Leiden, 1999; Kuo et al., 1997). T cells lacking LKLF develop normally in the thymus but thereafter develop an activated phenotype in the periphery and undergo apoptosis, leading to a marked reduction in T-cell numbers in these mice.

DENDRITIC CELLS: MIGRATION, MATURATION, AND FUNCTION

DCs are often referred to as the sentinels of the immune system; they provide a critical bridge between the innate and adaptive immune response (Banchereau et al., 2000). DCs are the most efficient APCs for activating naïve T cells during their initial encounter with antigen and for inducing B-cell responses to T-cell–dependent antigens, such as intact proteins. The unique efficiency of DCs as APCs reflects the expression of MHC class I and MHC class II molecules and antigen-processing machinery in high abundance and the expression of accessory factors that facilitate T-cell activation and influence the quality and magnitude of the T-cell response (Fig. 2-6).

Recent studies have identified in humans and in mice two distinct lineages of DCs: myeloid and plasmacytoid/lymphoid DCs (Liu, 2001; Patterson, 2000). In their resting state, myeloid DCs are found in epithelia, as well as the interstitium of solid organs, such as the heart and kidney. By contrast, resting plasmacytoid DCs appear to reside principally in the circulation.

Although the precise relationship between DCs and less mature precursor cells in vivo is incompletely understood, cells with the appearance, function, and surface expression of proteins characteristic of myeloid DCs can be derived from pluripotent stem cells of the bone marrow, monocytes, or their immediate precursors by incubation with various combinations of cytokines (e.g., GM-CSF and IL-4).

Myeloid Dendritic Cells

Myeloid DCs are commonly defined by their morphology, high expression of MHC molecules, and the expression of the myeloid CD11b and CD11c antigens, which are the $\alpha_2\beta_2$ and $\alpha_3\beta_2$ integrins. By contrast, plasmacytoid DC lack myeloid; B-, T-, or NK-cell lineage markers, with the exception of CD4; and express receptors for the cytokine IL-3 (CD123), which can be used to support them in culture. Flt3-ligand, a cytokine produced by stromal cells within the bone marrow microenvironment, is a particularly potent inducer of both types of DC after administration in vivo (Patterson, 2000).

Resting (also called immature) myeloid DC progenitors express the chemokines receptors CCR1, CCR2, CCR5, CCR6, and CXCR2, which allows them to migrate from the blood preferentially into epithelial and the interstitial space of solid organs, where they are found at a low frequency and are poised to encounter invading microbes. DC that initially encounter potential antigens in epithelial and the solid organs appear to be specialized for the initiation of the process of antigen presentation in that they are highly phagocytic but lack high levels of MHC molecules on the cell surface. Some DCs in the spleen may also serve this function.

Phagocytosis by DCs, in contrast to phagocytosis by monocytes and macrophages, is not markedly enhanced by the binding of antibody or complement to the target particle (opsonophagocytosis) and may occur independently of such binding (Austyn, 1996). DCs also express high levels of carbohydrate-specific receptors that may enhance glycoprotein uptake and entry into intracellular antigen-presentation compartments. They are also

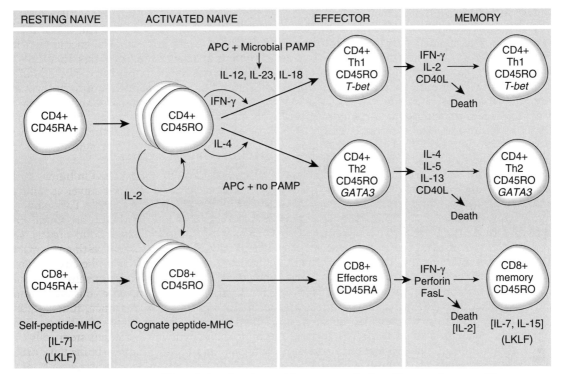

Figure 2-6 · **Activation, differentiation, function, and homeostasis of naïve, effector, and memory T lymphocytes.** In response to primary stimulation with antigenic peptide-MHC complexes on effective APCs, like DCs, naïve T cells secrete IL-2, express IL-2 receptors, divide, and differentiate. In the presence of IL-12, IL-18 and IL-23 produced by DCs activated by microbial pathogen associated molecular patterns (PAMPs) (or by inflammatory cytokines or CD40 ligand [not shown]), CD4 T cells differentiate into Th1 effector T cells. Conversely, in the absence of these cytokines and in the presence of IL-4, they differentiate into Th2 effector T cells. Most effector T cells die by apoptosis, either due to deprivation of survival-enhancing cytokines or due to activation-induced cell death through a Fas-mediated mechanism; IL-2 sensitizes activated effectors to Fas-mediated killing. A small fraction of effectors persist as memory T cells. The factors that sustain survival of naïve T cells and memory CD8 T cells are shown along the bottom of the figure. Shown inside the cells are the isoforms of CD45 expressed at each stage, and for Th1 and Th2 T cells the deterministic transcription factors, T-bet and GATA-3. The default (Tc1) pathway of CD8 T-cell differentiation is shown.

highly efficient at taking up extracellular fluid by macropinocytosis and micropinocytosis. Finally, DCs efficiently phagocytose apoptotic cells or blebs from apoptotic cells (Larsson et al., 2001). Proteins derived from these sources can enter into the MHC class II pathway and can be cross-presented by MHC class I by a TAP-dependent mechanism (den Haan et al., 2000).

DCs that encounter infectious pathogens or injured host cells interpret these encounters as signals of threat or danger (Matzinger, 1994) and are stimulated to mature and to migrate from the tissues to the regional lymph nodes (Banchereau et al., 2000). DC maturation and migration can be triggered by proinflammatory stimuli, such as bacterial peptides, cell walls, or DNA; host proinflammatory cytokines, such as IL-1 and TNF; or CD40 ligand expressed on activated CD4 T cells (see Fig. 2-5).

The initial step of maturation results in the loss of phagocytic activity and the secretion of proinflammatory chemokines and cytokines, such as MIP-1α and TNF. This facilitates the recruitment of monocytes, DCs, and memory T cells to the sites of infection or injury. The maturing DCs then downregulate the expression of receptors (e.g., CCR5) for inflammatory chemokines present in the tissues and modulate the expression of adhesion molecules, thereby facilitating their exit from the tissues. Concomitantly, maturing DCs begin to express the CCR7 chemokine receptor, which binds SLC (CCL21) and ELC (CCL19), produced by cells in the secondary lymphoid tissues (Lanzavecchia and Sallusto, 2001b); this directs DC to the T-cell zones of the draining lymph nodes. DC undergoing this migration have a unique cytologic appearance and are known as veiled cells.

Concomitant with migration to the regional lymph nodes, maturing DC increase surface expression of MHC class II molecules and accessory or co-stimulatory factors (Lanzavecchia and Sallusto, 2001b). This markedly enhances their ability to trigger the activation of those naïve T cells that express TCR-recognizing peptide-MHC complexes on these mature DC (Lanzavecchia and Sallusto, 2001a, 2001b; Pulendran et al., 2001). These accessory factors include adhesins, co-stimulatory molecules (e.g., CD80 and CD86, also known as

B7-1 and B7-2), CD40, chemokines that attract naïve T cells expressing CCR7, and chemokine receptors that facilitate DC–T-cell interactions and T-cell activation (Table 2-3).

The production of the cytokine IL-12 in response to engagement of the CD40 molecule on the DC by CD40 ligand on the T cell (see Fig. 2-5) may be particularly important for the T cells to acquire the capacity to produce IFN-γ and mature into Th1 effector T cells (see later discussion). This sequence of events has been best documented for Langerhans DC of the skin, but it is likely that a similar process occurs for DC found in the other epithelia or in solid organs.

Plasmacytoid Dendritic Cells

Plasmacytoid DC were originally defined by their appearance in pathologic analysis of inflamed lymph nodes. Initial studies with these cells suggested that they preferentially supported the generation of Th2 effector T cells (see following), whereas myeloid DC preferentially supported the generation of Th1 effector T cells. However, recent data indicate that the state of maturation and presence or absence of relevant microbial or endogenous factors affecting cytokine production by myeloid and lymphoid DC, not the type of DC, determines whether a Th1 or Th2 effector T cell response is induced.

Plasmacytoid DC are potent producers of type I IFNs (IFN α/β) and TNF in response to viral infection (Cella et al., 2000; Liu, 2001). These cytokines promote the survival and maturation of plasmacytoid DC. Maturation is associated with the upregulation of MHC and co-

stimulatory molecules and downregulation of CD62L and CXCR3 expression. The latter receptors likely contribute to the migration of plasmacytoid DC from blood to lymph nodes draining sites of inflammation; once in inflamed lymph nodes, loss of CD62L and CXCR3 may facilitate juxtaposition of mature plasmacytoid DC to naïve T cells.

MECHANISMS OF T-CELL ACTIVATION

Activation Signals via the TCR/CD3 Complex

The TCR/CD3 complex is linked to an intricate and highly interconnected complex of kinases, phosphatases, and adapter molecules that transduces signals in response to engagement of the TCR and, in αβ-T cells, the appropriate CD4 or CD8 co-receptor by cognate peptide-MHC complexes (see Fig. 2-1). A proximal event in this pathway is the activation of the src-family tyrosine kinase, Lck (Judd and Koretzky, 2000; Latour and Veillette, 2001; Leo and Schraven, 2001); the Fyn kinase is also activated but plays a less critical role in T-cell activation. Lck is associated with the cytoplasmic domains of CD4 and CD8 and upon activation via the TCR phosphorylates tyrosine residues in the immunoreceptor tyrosine-based activation motifs (ITAMs) in the cytoplasmic domains of the CD3 proteins (Malissen et al., 1999), in particular those in CD3ε and CD3ζ.

This allows the recruitment of a cytosolic tyrosine kinase, ZAP-70, which in turn phosphorylates tyro-

TABLE 2-3 · PAIRS OF SURFACE MOLECULES INVOLVED IN THE INTERACTIONS BETWEEN T CELLS AND APCs

T-Cell Surface Molecule	T-Cell Distribution	Corresponding Ligand(s) on APC	APC Distribution
CD2	Most T cells, higher on memory/effector T cells	LFA-3 (CD58), CD59	Leukocytes
CD4	Subset of αβ-T cells with predominantly helper activity	Class II MHC β chain	DCs, macrophages, B cells, others (see text)
CD5	All T cells	CD72	B cells, macrophages
CD8	Subset of αβ-T cells with predominantly helper activity	MHC class I heavy chain	Ubiquitous
LFA-1 (CD11a/CD18)	All T cells; higher on memory/effector T cells	ICAM-1 (CD54)	Leukocytes (ICAM-3 > ICAM-1, ICAM-2) and endothelium (ICAM-1 and ICAM-2); ICAM-1 is increased by TNF, IL-1
		ICAM-2 (CD102) ICAM-3 (CD50)	
CD28	Most CD4 T cells; naïve and memory (not effector) CD8 T cells	B7-1 (CD80) B7-2 (CD86)	Mature DCs, macrophages, activated B cells Mature DCs, macrophages, activated B cells
CTLA-4 (CD152)	Activated T cells, Treg	B7-1 (CD80) B7-2 (CD86)	
ICOS	Activated and memory CD4 T cells	B7RP-1 (B7h)	B cells; variable on DCs and monocytes
PD-1	Activated T cells	PD-L1 (B7-H1), PD-L2	DCs, monocytes, tissue cells
CD40 ligand (CD154)	Activated CD4 T cells; higher on activated memory/effector	CD40	DCs, macrophages, B cells, thymic epithelial cells
VLA-4 (CD49d/CD29)	Memory/effector T cells	VCAM-1 (CD106)	Activated or inflamed endothelium (increased by TNF, IL-1, and IL-4)
ICAM-1 (CD54)	All T cells; higher on memory/effector T cells	LFA-1 (CD11a/CD18)	Leukocytes

sine residues in a transmembrane adapter protein LAT. LAT then nucleates the formation of a trimolecular complex, consisting of LAT and two cytosolic adapter proteins, SLP-76 and GADS. LAT is constitutively localized in regions of the plasma membrane known as lipid rafts or GEMs, so the formation of this complex leads to the localization of the TCR/CD3/co-receptor complex to these regions, which form important signaling domains that are juxtaposed to the immunologic synapse between the T cell and APC (see following).

The CD45 tyrosine phosphatase also plays an essential role in the tyrosine kinase pathway just described, which may reflect its role in the dephosphorylation of the negative regulatory tyrosine on Lck.

It is thought that lipid rafts play a critical role in facilitating the assembly of signaling complexes at specific regions of the plasma membrane; these complexes in turn recruit other adapters and signal transducing proteins (Latour and Veillette, 2001; Xavier et al., 1998). Recruited proteins include phospholipase Cγ1, which acts on membrane lipids to generate inositol triphosphate (IP3) and diacylglycerol (DAG), leading to the release of intracellular calcium stores, entry of extracellular calcium via capacitance calcium channels, and activation of protein kinase C.

In parallel, the Ras-Raf-Erk/MAPK pathway is activated via its recruitment to tyrosine-phosphorylated LAT. Sustained elevation of intracellular calcium leads to the activation of calcineurin and the translocation of NFAT transcription factors from the cytosol to the nucleus, and activation of the ERK/MAPK pathway enhances activation of other transcription factors. The phosphoinositide 3 kinase (PI3K) pathway is activated in part through its association with TRIM, a transmembrane adapter that associates with the CD3 complex. This leads to the activation of protein kinase B/Akt, which facilitates the induction of genes involved in cell survival (Ward and Cantrell, 2001).

In turn, this leads to the generation of phosphoinositide 3 phosphate (PIP3), which provides a membrane anchor for Itk and Tec, members of the Tec family of cytosolic tyrosine kinases. Activation of Itk/Tec enhances calcium entry and helps to sustain elevated intracellular calcium concentrations. Members of the c-Jun N-terminal kinase (JNK)/p38 kinase MAPK family are also activated; this leads to the activation of AP-1/ATF transcription factors.

Collectively, these transcription factors induce the transcription of genes encoding key proteins for activation, such as cytokines, cell cycle regulators, and, in cytotoxic T cells, proteins involved in killing other cells, such as perforins. The expression of more than 100 genes is altered as a result of the activation process (Alizadeh et al., 2000; Feske et al., 2001).

T-Cell Activation vs. Anergy

For full T-cell activation that leads to both cytokine production and commitment of the cell to proliferate, signaling through the trimolecular TCR-peptide-MHC complex and through accessory or co-stimulatory signaling pathways must exceed a specific threshold. The nature and magnitude of the signal transmitted via the TCR/CD3 complex is a function of the affinity of the TCR for the peptide-MHC complex and the duration of their interaction (Jelley-Gibbs et al., 2000; Lanzavecchia and Sallusto, 2001a). Alterations in the amino acids comprising the epitope of the antigenic peptide that alter the affinity of the interaction with the TCR can result in partial activation (e.g., cytokine production but not cell proliferation) or in anergy (Jameson et al., 1994).

Anergic T cells fail to proliferate when subsequently exposed to the wild-type peptide-MHC complexes under conditions that normally would lead to full activation. This reflects the inability of anergic T cells to produce IL-2 , and in many cases anergic T cells can be "rescued" by the addition of exogenous IL-2 (Kundig et al., 1996; Schwartz, 1997). Anergy is thought to contribute to the maintenance of tolerance by mature T cells to certain self-antigens, in particular those that are not expressed in the thymus in sufficient abundance to induce negative selection.

From in vitro experiments, it has been estimated that naïve CD4 T cells require sustained TCR signaling for 20 to 24 hours to become activated. Surprisingly, recent studies suggest that a much shorter period of TCR-peptide-MHC interaction is required to activate naïve CD8 T cells—as little as 2 hours is sufficient for cells to commit to proliferation (Kaech and Ahmed, 2001; Van Stipdonk et al., 2001). However, like naïve CD4 T cells, cell division does not commence for approximately 24 hours after the initiation of signaling. The basis for this difference between naïve CD4 and CD8 T cells is not known.

In any case, optimal signals provided through TCR-peptide-MHC interactions are generally not sufficient to fully activate either naïve CD4 or CD8 T cells—additional co-stimulatory signals play an important role in allowing naïve T cells to commit to cytokine production and proliferation. By contrast, memory T cells have a lower activation threshold, are less dependent on these co-stimulatory signals, and can commit to proliferate following engagement of their TCR for as little as 1 hour (Coyle and Gutierrez-Ramos, 2001; Lanzavecchia and Sallusto, 2001a, 2001b).

Co-stimulatory Interactions Facilitate T-Cell Activation

Although signals transmitted via the CD3 complex in response to engagement of the TCR by peptide-MHC complexes on APCs are necessary for T-cell activation, many argue that these signals, commonly referred to collectively as signal 1, are rarely sufficient for full activation of naïve T cells under most physiologic conditions. Rather, it appears that the immune system has evolved a strategy by which to tune down the response of naïve T cells compared with memory T cells, thereby rendering naïve T cells dependent on secondary co-stimulatory signals (signal 2) provided by other molecular interactions between APCs and T cells. Signal 2 alone does not lead to T-cell activation, but acts in concert with signal 1 provided through TCR/CD3 to facilitate full T-cell activation rather than anergy. Co-stimulatory signals (signal 2) appear to be particularly important if the abundance and duration of antigenic peptide-MHC complexes are limiting.

CD28 Interaction with CD80 and CD86

The best characterized co-stimulatory signal is provided by the engagement of CD28 on the T cell with CD80 (B7-1) or CD86 (B7-2) on the APC (see Table 2-3) (Coyle and Gutierrez-Ramos, 2001; Lenschow et al., 1996). CD80 and CD86 are related proteins belonging to the immunoglobulin superfamily, which are expressed at low levels on immature DC, macrophages, and B cells. The expression of both CD80 and CD86 can be induced on APCs by a variety of factors, such as lipopolysaccharide (LPS), B-cell receptor crosslinking, and CD40 signaling (see Fig. 2-5). Thus APCs primed by these factors, and in particular mature DC, express high amounts of CD80 and CD86. The kinetics of expression of these two proteins differs; CD86 is expressed early after induction and CD80 later, with maximal expression occurring after 48 hours.

CD80 and CD86 both bind to CD28, which is constitutively expressed on T cells. Signaling through CD28 lowers the strength or duration of TCR signaling needed to fully activate T cells, which is particularly important for naïve T cells in which the threshold for full activation is high compared with memory and effector T cells (Lanzavecchia and Sallusto, 2001a, 2001b; Margulies, 2001). This effect of CD28 is due in part to its ability to enhance the transcription and stability of IL-2 mRNA (Lenschow et al., 1996). CD28 signals lead to the activation of the PI3 kinase–protein kinase B/Akt pathway and thereby induce the pro-survival factor Bcl-x_L (Burr et al., 2001). In addition, co-stimulatory interactions may induce increased expression of surface molecules on the APC that further augment co-stimulation or adhesion. For example, the engagement of the CD40 molecule on the APC increases expression of CD80 and CD86 (Edelmann and Wilson, 2001; Yang, 1996).

Other Co-stimulatory Interactions

The genome project has contributed to the identification of a family of related co-stimulatory molecules that collectively constitute the B7 superfamily (Coyle and Gutierrez-Ramos, 2001). These co-stimulatory molecules may play a role in selective enhancement of certain types of T-cell responses. For example, B7-H3 appears to favor the production of IFN-γ, whereas B7RP-1 and its receptor on T cells (the inducible co-stimulator [ICOS]) favor the production of IL-4 and B-cell help (Coyle and Gutierrez-Ramos, 2001). Other members of the family may act to dampen the T-cell response by inducing T-cell apoptosis.

In addition to these co-stimulatory interactions, a number of molecules on the T-cell and APC surfaces can bind to ligands on the other cell type (see Table 2-3) and enhance T-cell activation as a result of stabilizing the interaction between the T cell and APC. Such adhesive interactions may be physiologically important because the affinity of the TCR for peptide-MHC complexes appears relatively low (Davis et al., 1997).

Immunologic Synapse Orchestrates Signals from the TCR and Co-stimulatory Receptors

Based on studies in vitro (which have not yet been confirmed in vivo), T-cell signaling molecules appear not to be randomly distributed at the point of interaction between the T cell and APC, but form an *immunologic synapse*, which is the term used to describe the highly ordered junction that forms between the APC and the T cell during antigenic stimulation. This structure resembles a doughnut, in which the TCR-peptide-MHC, CD4 or CD8 co-receptors, and CD28 molecules are aggregated in the central zone of the synapse, whereas CD2 and LFA-1 localize to the outer perimeter of the synapse (Bromley et al., 2001).

The large extracellular domain of CD45 leads to its exclusion from the synapse, which may be important in allowing the tyrosine kinase signaling cascade to be initiated (Bromley et al., 2001; Johnson et al., 2000). However, recent evidence suggests that the lower molecular weight forms of CD45 (e.g., CD45R0) found on memory T cells may gain access to the synapse over time and help to terminate signaling (Bromley et al., 2001; Johnson et al., 2000; Majeti et al., 2000).

The organized structure of the synapse promotes sustained signaling by concentrating TCRs and some co-stimulatory molecules together in one area of high adhesion. CD28 appears to play an important role in mediating the reorganization of the membrane microdomains (Bromley et al., 2001), which facilitate the creation of this synapse, thereby decreasing the time required to achieve efficient T-cell activation.

Gene Defects in T-Cell Signaling

In mice, defects in most of the known aspects of the proximal signal transduction mechanisms have been created by gene targeting (Judd and Koretzky, 2000; Latour and Veillette, 2001; Leo and Schraven, 2001; Noraz et al., 2000; Sun et al., 2000; Yoder et al., 2001). These result in variable defects in T-cell development and in the function of T cells that do develop. Defects in T-cell activation resulting from deficiency of CD3ε or CD3γ and in T-cell activation due to a defect in extracellular calcium flux have been described in humans. Individuals with CD3ε or CD3γ defects also have incomplete blocks in T-cell development predominantly at the DP stage and in the generation of CD8 SP cells (see Fig. 2-2), respectively (Arnaiz-Villena et al., 1995;

Kappes et al., 1995). One of two patients with CD3γ deficiency and the patient with a defect in extracellular calcium flux have clinically significant T-cell dysfunction (Feske et al., 2001).

Individuals with a total lack of CD45 (Kung et al., 2000) or partial loss of Lck expression due to a splicing defect (Goldman et al., 1998) also have been described, which have signaling defects and incomplete T$^+$B$^+$NK$^+$ SCID; in the patient with the partial Lck defect the numbers of CD4 T cells are selectively reduced. Conversely, human ZAP-70 deficiency is associated with a selective absence of CD8 T cells, but the CD4 T cells have profound defects in T-cell activation, resulting in SCID (Elder et al., 1994; Roifman, 1995).

CONSEQUENCES OF T-CELL ACTIVATION

Proliferation and Functional Differentiation of Naïve CD4 T Cells

When naïve CD4 T cells first encounter foreign peptide-MHC complexes during a primary immune response, they extinguish expression of LKLF, a transcription factor that maintains naïve T cells in a resting state (Buckley et al., 2001; Kuo and Leiden, 1999; Kuo et al., 1997), and produce a limited number of cytokines, including IL-2 in robust amounts and CD40-ligand in modest amounts (see Fig. 2-6). They also are induced to express high-affinity IL-2 receptor complexes composed of the IL-2Rα and β chains and the common cytokine receptor γ chain (γc).

IL-2 Receptor Engagement

Engagement of the IL-2 receptor complex by IL-2, acting both as an autocrine and paracrine growth factor, triggers T cells to undergo multiple rounds of proliferation, thereby expanding the numbers of antigen-specific T cells, and to differentiate into effector T cells (see Fig. 2-6) (Dubey et al., 1996; Jelley-Gibbs et al., 2000; Reiner and Seder, 1999). They also express on their surface CD69 and Fas molecules (Miyawaki et al., 1992) and downregulate expression of Bcl-2, an intracellular protein that protects against apoptosis (Akbar et al., 1993). Downregulation of Bcl-2 sensitizes these cells to apoptosis, which is countered by signals via the IL-2 receptor complex; this makes effector T cells dependent for their survival on IL-2 (or other cytokines that signal through γc) to induce the expression of Bcl-x$_L$, which, like Bcl-2, inhibits apoptosis (Nelson and Willerford, 1998). Thus when concentrations of IL-2 become limiting, effector T-cell attrition occurs, dampening the immune response. Conversely, IL-2 signals may sensitize T cells to Fas-mediated activation-induced cell death. Thus the relative importance of the different functions of IL-2 in the expansion, survival, or death of effector T cells will represent a balance of these effects.

In this regard, it is notable that recent studies suggest that antigen-induced proliferation of murine CD4 T cells in vivo, in striking contrast to findings in vitro, does not require signals via the IL-2 receptor or other receptor complexes that contain γc (Lantz et al., 2000); whether this is also true for CD8 T cells and in humans is not known. Although these results do not exclude a role for IL-2 in antigen-induced proliferation of CD4 T cells, they reinforce the observation that the dominant effect observed in humans with IL-2 receptor α chain deficiency and in mice that lack IL-2 or IL-2 receptor α or β is lymphocytic infiltration and autoimmunity (Nelson and Willerford, 1998; Roifman, 2000). The basis for this is not certain but may reflect defects in activation-induced cell death via Fas-Fas ligand and defects in regulatory T cells (Suzuki et al., 1999).

CD40 Engagement

CD40 ligand, a member of the TNF ligand family (see Tables 2-1 and 2-3), engages the CD40 molecule on B cells, DCs, and mononuclear phagocytes (Foy et al., 1996; Grewal and Flavell, 1998; Lanzavecchia, 1998). CD40 engagement on the B-cell surface transduces intracellular signals that promote the expression of antibody isotypes and differentiation of B cells into memory cells. CD40 ligand is also an important activator of the microbicidal activity of mononuclear phagocytes in some infections, such as *Pneumocystis carinii*, and is also important in the initial priming, expansion, and differentiation of naïve CD4 T cells into effector T cells.

In vivo, CD40 appears to play an important role in expansion of CD4 T cells during a primary immune response and a less critical role in the expansion of CD8 T cells (Edelmann and Wilson, 2001; Whitmire and Ahmed, 2000). As mentioned previously, CD40 engagement may also induce DCs to produce IL-12 and other cytokines (see Fig. 2-5) and to express increased levels of CD80 and CD86, which modulate the development and function of effector T cells, as described in the following section.

Th1 and Th2 Effector CD4 T Cells

T-Cell–Derived Cytokines

The functions of effector T cells, particularly those of the CD4 subset, are mediated in large part by the multiple additional cytokines not produced by naïve T cells. Most of these cytokines are secreted, although some may be predominantly expressed on the T-cell surface. These cytokines include IL-3, IL-4, IL-5, IL-9, IL-10, IL-13, IFN-γ, GM-CSF, CD40 ligand, TNF, and Fas ligand (Liles and Van Voorhis, 1995; Spellberg and Edwards, 2001). Table 2-1 summarizes the major immunomodulatory effects of T-cell–derived cytokines and of cytokines produced by other cell types that act on T cells. Some key effects of cytokines in T-cell proliferation, differentiation, and effector function, and in B-cell, NK-cell, and mononuclear phagocyte function, are discussed next.

Two major types of CD4 effector T cells, Th1 and Th2, were initially described in mice, and similar profiles of polarized cytokine expression have subsequently been confirmed in other species, including humans (Asnagli and Murphy, 2001; Fearon and Locksley, 1996; Glimcher and Murphy, 2000; Romagnani et al., 1997). IFN-γ is the signature cytokine produced by Th1 effector cells, which also produce substantial amounts of IL-2, lymphotoxin-α, and TNF but little or no IL-4, IL-5, and IL-13. By contrast, IL-4 is the signature cytokine of Th2 cells, which also produce IL-5, IL-9, and IL-13 but little or no IFN-γ or IL-2.

Th0 Cells

In humans, there may be more overlap or variability in patterns of cytokine production than in mice. Cells producing effector cytokines of both types are commonly referred to as Th0 cells, which are often seen following vaccination with protein antigens or following viral infections, such as influenza or cytomegalovirus (CMV) (Rowe et al., 2001; Toellner et al., 1998). Generation of Th0 cells in vitro seems to be favored by the presence of large amounts of IL-2 in the absence of cytokines that polarize differentiation toward either Th1 or Th2 effector cells (Fearon and Locksley, 1996; Grogan et al., 2001; O'Garra, 1998). An alternative possibility is that Th0 cells have undergone less proliferation and differentiation and for this reason have not yet become committed Th1 or Th2 cells (Lanzavecchia and Sallusto, 2001a, 2001b).

In addition to their differing cytokine profiles, Th1 and Th2 cells also differ in chemokine receptor and cell adhesion molecule expression (see Table 2-2) (Campbell and Butcher, 2000; Campbell et al., 2001; Kim et al., 2001; Mackay, 2001; Moser and Loetscher, 2001). This may allow Th1 and Th2 cells to differentially localize to particular tissues; for instance, Th2 cells are often found in the mucosa.

Factors Regulating Th1 and Th2 Cell Generation

Factors contributing to the generation of Th1 vs. Th2 cells include the strength of the activating signals, the nature and abundance of co-stimulatory molecules on APCs, and the cytokine milieu, with the latter playing the dominant role (Fearon and Locksley, 1996; Glimcher and Murphy, 2000; O'Garra, 1998). Th1 effector development is favored by the exposure of CD4 T cells during their initial activation to high levels of IL-12, IL-18, and IL-23 produced by APCs and to IFN-γ produced by NK cells and other T cells (see Fig. 2-6). In humans but not in mice, IFN-α also is a potent inducer of Th1 cells (Asnagli and Murphy, 2001; Glimcher and Murphy, 2000). Chemokines may affect Th1 vs. Th2 differentiation (Luther and Cyster, 2001).

The importance of these cytokines in the development of robust Th1 responses and of IFN-γ in human host defense is demonstrated by the increased susceptibility of patients with genetic defects in IL-12, IL-12 receptors, and IFN-γ receptors to infection with intracellular pathogens, particularly mycobacteria and *Salmonella* (Jouanguy et al., 1999).

Th2 development is favored when CD4 T cells are initially activated in the presence of IL-4 and/or in the absence of IL-12, IL-18, IL-23, IFN-α, or IFN-γ (see Fig. 2-6). The source of IL-4 in a primary CD4 T-cell response leading to the generation of Th2 cells is uncertain. It is possible that in the absence of cytokines favoring Th1 development, the low levels of IL-4 produced by naïve T cells are sufficient (Grogan et al., 2001), but NK T cells, mast cells, or basophils also produce IL-4 and may contribute in some situations. High amounts of co-stimulation through CD86 (Schweitzer and Sharpe, 1998) and the engagement of OX40 on the T cell by OX40 ligand, a member of the TNF ligand superfamily expressed by B cells, also may favor Th2 rather than Th1 CD4 T-cell development (Flynn et al., 1998).

Regulation of Mouse Th1 and Th2 Cells by Transcription Factors: Implication for Humans

Recent evidence in the mouse suggests that the development and propagation of Th1 and Th2 T cells is not only influenced by these exogenous factors but is determined by the expression within CD4 T cells of opposing transcription factors that dictate the Th1 vs. Th2 development (see Fig. 2-6) (Asnagli and Murphy, 2001; Glimcher and Murphy, 2000). GATA-3 appears to be a master regulator of Th2 T-cell development. The expression of GATA-3 is sufficient to override the other influences described previously and to reinforce its own expression through a positive feedback loop. Conversely, T-bet induces the development of Th1 cells. GATA-3 inhibits the expression of T-bet (Mullen et al., 2001), and it has been proposed but not yet shown that the reciprocal is also true.

Exactly how these master regulatory factors are induced is not yet certain. It appears that activation of naïve T cells may lead to their induction and that signals via cytokines that influence Th1 vs. Th2 development may then alter the relative balance of T-bet vs. GATA-3 expression (Asnagli and Murphy, 2001; Glimcher and Murphy, 2000; Mullen et al., 2001). For example, binding of IL-12 to its receptor leads to the activation of the STAT4 transcription factor, which inhibits GATA-3 expression, whereas, binding of IL-4 to its receptor induces STAT6, which inhibits T-bet expression. GATA-3 and T-bet may act by affecting the accessibility of Th1 and Th2 cytokine loci to engagement by transcription factors induced in response to T-cell activation and cytokine receptor ligation, rather than or in addition to directly regulating the active transcription of IFN-γ and IL-4, respectively.

The studies in the mice from which these findings have been derived have yet to be replicated in humans, but they raise the possibility that immunologic disorders in humans may result from alterations in T-cell autonomous mechanisms governing patterns of Th1 vs. Th2 cytokine production.

T cells and their secondary effector progeny (Hu et al., 2001; Lanzavecchia and Sallusto, 2001a; Sprent and Tough, 2001).

Regulatory T Cells

Historical Background: Suppressor T Cells

The phenomenon of T-cell–mediated immune suppression—dominant inhibition of the response of one subset of T cells by another—was observed many years ago, and the cells mediating the inhibition were referred to as suppressor T cells (Hodes, 1989). Initial studies in the mouse suggested that suppression was mediated predominantly by the CD8 subset, giving rise to the description of this subset as cytotoxic/suppressor T cells. However, considerable difficulty arose in trying to clone such cells and to define the molecular mechanisms by which they mediated suppression, casting doubt on the validity of these observations. Nonetheless, a large body of data attested to the validity of the phenomenon of antigen-induced suppression of the immune response as a mechanism, along with clonal deletion and anergy, for maintaining self-tolerance.

Phenotype of Regulatory T Cells

In the mid-1990s, studies by Sakaguchi and colleagues in mice and Roncarolo and her colleagues in humans provided evidence that a subset of CD4 T cells were involved in the active suppression of autoimmunity. (Roncarolo and Levings, 2000; Sakaguchi, 2000; Shevach, 2000; Shevach et al., 2001). The characterization of these cells was aided by the observation that cells mediating suppression were present within the small fraction of CD4 T cells that are $CD25^+CD45RO^+$. Although not all cells of this phenotype mediate suppression, many do. These cells are now referred to as **regulatory T cells (Treg)**. Treg are generated in the thymus during the normal process of positive and negative selection and can also be induced by activation of naïve peripheral CD4 T cells in the presence of certain cytokines, including (in humans) IL-10 and type I IFNs (Levings et al., 2001). Suppression requires activation through the TCR (e.g., antigenic peptide-MHC), but thereafter their actions are not antigen specific.

Mechanisms of Suppression

Different mechanisms of inhibition have been described, including the production of IL-10 or TGF-β; some investigators categorize cells that mediate suppression through different mechanisms as Treg subsets, such as IL-10-dependent Treg or Tr1 cells. However, contact-dependent inhibition of the activation of other T cells through an APC-independent process appears to be the major mechanism by which they mediate suppression, although the molecular basis for this is not known. Through characterization of these cells, we have also gained some insight into the basis for the failure of earlier studies to generate T suppressor clones: Treg are anergic and cannot be expanded readily by culturing them in vitro in the presence of IL-2 and APCs.

NATURAL KILLER T CELLS

A small population of circulating αβ-T cells express NKR-P1A, the human homologue of the mouse NK1.1 protein, and lack expression of CD4 or CD8. These T cells express other cell surface antigens commonly found on NK cells (NKR-P1A, CD56, and CD57), and, like NK cells, their development and survival are dependent on IL-15 (Ohteki et al., 1997). For this reason they are often referred to as NK T cells or natural T cells.

Like murine T cells expressing NK1.1, human NK T cells have a highly restricted repertoire of αβ-TCR and mainly recognize antigens presented by the non-classical MHC molecule, CD1d, rather than by MHC class I or class II. These antigens include certain lipids or highly hydrophobic peptides. NK T cells also have the ability to produce high levels of IL-4, IFN-γ, and Fas ligand upon primary stimulation, a capacity that is not observed with most αβ-T cells.

The function of NK T cells remains controversial. In mice, NK T cells appear to provide help to B cells, presumably in the form of cytokines, for the production of antibodies against glycosyl-phosphatidylinositol (GPI)–linked proteins (Godfrey et al., 2000; Schofield et al., 1999). These proteins are found in particularly high amounts on the surface of malarial parasites and trypanosomes, but it remains unclear if NK T cells play an important role in host defense against these pathogens.

In addition to their role in host defense, NK T cells may act as negative regulators of certain T-cell–mediated immune responses, such as those involved in the pathogenesis of insulin-dependent diabetes mellitus (Hammond et al., 2001; Wilson et al., 1998).

CLINICAL EVALUATION OF T LYMPHOCYTES AND THEIR FUNCTION

Screening Tests

The total lymphocyte count derived from the white blood cell count and differential count may offer a clue to the presence of a cellular immune defect. Lymphopenia should be further explored utilizing lymphocyte subsets (see Chapter 12).

Although delayed-type hypersensitivity skin tests provide a measure of antigen-specific T-cell function and of APC–T-cell collaboration, the value of this approach is limited by problems with technical proficiency, variations in the quality of antigens, and poor responsiveness of normal infants and children younger than age 2.

Thus flow cytometry and measures of T-cell function in vitro are more useful measures in current clinical practice.

Enumeration of Lymphocyte Subsets

Delineation of the numbers of lymphocytes as part of a complete blood cell count, coupled with the determination of the fraction of specific lymphocyte subsets by flow cytometry, is the most useful initial method to screen for defects involving T lymphocytes. Because T lymphocytes represent approximately two thirds of the lymphocytes in normal individuals, a deficiency of T-cell numbers is often suggested by the finding of a persistent, absolute lymphopenia. It is important to note that the absolute numbers of lymphocytes and of T cells is greatest early in infancy and declines slowly thereafter, so it is important to be aware of age-related normal values (see Chapter 12 on General Aspects of Immunodeficiency and Chapter 22 on the Immunodeficiency of Immaturity), because cases of combined immunodeficiency may be missed by failing to recognize that values that are normal for adults (≥1500 lymphocytes) may represent lymphopenia in infants.

High-quality monoclonal antibodies allow the precise definition of T-lymphocyte numbers, the enumeration of specific T-lymphocyte subsets, and the detection of concomitant defects in B or NK cells. In general, the initial evaluation should include antibodies to detect all T cells (anti-CD3), CD4 and CD8 T-cell subsets, B lymphocytes (CD19 or CD20), and NK cells (anti-CD16 or CD56; note that young infants have CD16+ NK cells that are CD56−).

The inclusion of antibodies to detect B and NK cells is valuable because they may provide a clue to the cause of T lymphopenia: The absence of T and B cells but normal numbers of NK cells suggests a defect in one of the RAG genes or one of the proteins involved in DNA repair (e.g., Artemis or ligase IV), whereas the absence of T and NK cells but not B cells suggests a defect in γc or Jak3, and selective reduction of T cells but not of B or NK cells suggests a defect in IL-7Rα.

In general, CD45 is used as a reference antibody to ensure that the cells analyzed are of hematopoietic origin; deficiency of CD45, which results in a functional T-cell (and combined) immunodeficiency, will be detected through this as a matter of routine. Screening evaluations should also include antibodies to detect MHC class II, expression of which is defective in the bare lymphocyte syndrome, and MHC class I, which is reduced in TAP deficiency.

Lymphocyte Proliferation

T lymphocytes may be activated in vitro and responses evaluated through several different measures, most commonly through assessment of proliferation. Cells may be activated by mitogens, including plant lectins or monoclonal antibodies to the TCR/CD3 complex, alloantigens, or exogenous antigens.

Mitogenic lectins bind to multiple cell surface molecules, including components of the TCR/CD3 complex, and to molecules on APCs, crosslinking and triggering signals in T cells that mimic those initiated in response to antigens. The majority of T cells, including naïve and memory/effector T cells, respond to these nonspecific activators. Like the response to antigen, APCs are required, but prior contact with specific antigens is not, so responses to mitogens are present throughout life and do not measure directly the capacity to mount antigen-specific responses.

For human T cells, phytohemagglutinin (PHA) is generally the most potent mitogenic lectin, followed by concanavalin A (Con A) and pokeweed mitogen (PWM). PWM also activates T-cell–dependent B-cell responses. Mitogenic monoclonal antibodies to CD3 also can be used to activate T cells. Because only the TCR/CD3 complex is engaged, the response to such stimulation is more stringent—naïve T cells or T cells with partial signaling defects may be less effectively activated than in response to PHA. Defects in proximal cell signaling can be bypassed by stimulating cells with a calcium ionophore (e.g., ionomycin) and phorbol myristate acetate (PMA), which together are mitogenic for T and B cells.

Mitogens provide a good initial screen for T-cell responses and complement flow cytometric enumeration of T-cell subsets. Stimulation with allogeneic cells in the one-way mixed leukocyte reaction (MLR) activates T cells that express TCR that are reactive to the allogeneic MHC molecules expressed on blood lymphocytes from other individuals; on average approximately 5% of T cells are alloreactive against a given MHC type. MLR are often used as one measure to evaluate risk for graft-versus-host disease, when hematopoietic stem cell transplantation is being considered.

The response to recall antigens—that is, antigens to which the individual has been exposed or immunized—provides the most stringent screening test of general T-cell responses. To detect a response to antigen in vivo, memory/effector T cells must be present in the blood of the individual in sufficient numbers that a measurable response to the antigen can be detected. In practice, tetanus toxoid and *Candida* extracts make useful antigens, because both contain highly antigenic proteins to which normal individuals mount robust responses following two or more immunizations with tetanus toxoid and normal exposure to *Candida* during the first year or two of life, respectively. Other antigens, such as purified protein derivative (PPD) and diphtheria, may be useful in immunized individuals.

The most common readout of a functional lymphocyte response is assessment of lymphocyte proliferation. This requires that the cell transduce signals leading to the expression of IL-2 and the IL-2 receptor complex and transduce signals through the IL-2 receptor that drive proliferation. The test is done by culturing cells in the presence of one or more of the stimuli described earlier, including a set of cells that are not stimulated as a control, then measuring the uptake of ^{3}H-thymidine after an interval of 3 to 7 days; peak responses with mitogens are generally obtained by 3 days, whereas the peak response to antigens is later. It is important to include cells from normal controls that have been processed and stimulated in parallel on each day. Each laboratory should also develop a range of normal values for the assay done under their conditions, to which patient and daily control results are compared.

Expression of Cytokines and Other Activation-Induced Proteins

Alternative and complementary assessments of lymphocyte responses can be obtained by assessment of cytokine production. Activated T cells normally produce IL-2, a substantial fraction of which is consumed to drive T-cell proliferation, and other cytokines, including IFN-γ, IL-4, IL-5, TNF, and GM-CSF. In the first 24 to 48 hours of activation, naïve T cells produce IL-2 and little else, so in neonates and young infants in which most of the T cells are naïve, production of these other cytokines is commonly less than that by older individuals.

Cytokine production can be assessed either by measuring their abundance in culture supernatants, most commonly using readily available enzyme-linked immunosorbent assay (ELISA) kits, or by flow cytometry after trapping the cytokines within the cell using reagents that block Golgi transport and staining with fluorochrome-labeled, anticytokine antibodies.

Expression on the activated T-cell surface of CD40 ligand, Fas, and Fas ligand can also be determined by flow cytometry. Similarly, perforin can be detected by intracellular staining of activated effector T cells. It is worth noting that individuals with mutations that do not affect expression but do affect the function of the protein may not be detected if only monoclonal antibodies are used to detect the protein; for some proteins, such as CD40 ligand, one can specifically assess functional protein by using a fluorochrome-labeled ligand for that protein (Seyama et al., 1998).

Cytotoxic T-Cell Function

When directly isolated from the blood, most CD8 T cells are in a resting state and not able to mediate cytolysis. The exception is individuals with active systemic viral infections, and in particular individuals with HIV infection. The rapid clearance of HIV during resolution of the acute infection is associated with the presence of circulating CTLs that are able to lyse HIV-infected or HIV peptide-pulsed APCs in an MHC class I–restricted manner (Posnett et al., 1999). In other individuals, cytotoxic T-cell function is most readily assessed after initial stimulation with allogeneic cells in an MLR. During the MLR, both CD4 and CD8 T cells become activated and proliferate and CD8 T cells differentiate into CTL capable of lysing the allogeneic targets (or cells of the same MHC class I type) used to stimulate them.

Mutation Analysis

In current practice, clinical and screening laboratory testing is used to detect the presence of a numeric or functional T-cell defect and to provide clues regarding the possible molecular nature of the defect. Thereafter, the most direct and definitive approaches are methods that identify mutations in the gene encoding the suspect protein, either by sequencing of the cDNA or of the gene itself, with or without the use of screening methods that help to detect mutations in the gene. A more complete description of these approaches is contained in Chapter 12.

ACKNOWLEDGMENT

We thank David B. Lewis who contributed to earlier versions of some of this material.

REFERENCES

Agrawal A, Eastman QM, Schatz DG. Transposition mediated by RAG1 and RAG2 and its implications for the evolution of the immune system. Nature 394:744–751, 1998.

Ahmed R, Gray D. Immunological memory and protective immunity: understanding their relation. Science 272:54–60, 1996.

Akbar AN, Salmon M, Savill J, Janossy G. A possible role for bcl-2 in regulating T-cell memory—a 'balancing act' between cell death and survival. Immunol Today 14:526–532, 1993.

Algeciras-Schimnich A, Griffith TS, Lynch DH, Paya CV. Cell cycle-dependent regulation of FLIP levels and susceptibility to Fas-mediated apoptosis. J Immunol 162:5205–5211, 1999.

Alizadeh AA, Eisen MB, Davis RE, Ma C, Lossos IS, Rosenwald A, Boldrick JC, Sabet H, Tran T, Yu X, Powell JI, Yang L, Marti GE, Moore T, Hudson J Jr, Lu L, Lewis DB, Tibshirani R, Sherlock G, Chan WC, Greiner TC, Weisenburger DD, Armitage JO, Warnke R, Staudt LM, et al. Distinct types of diffuse large B-cell lymphoma identified by gene expression profiling. Nature 403, 503–511, 2000.

Ameratunga R, Lederman HM, Sullivan KE, Ochs HD, Seyama K, French JK, Prestidge R, Marbrook J, Fanslow WC, Winkelstein JA. Defective antigen-induced lymphocyte proliferation in the X-linked hyper-IgM syndrome. J Pediatr 131:147–150, 1997.

Arnaiz-Villena A, Rodriguez-Gallego C, Timon M, Corell A, Pacheco A, Alvarez-Zapata D, Madrono A, Iglesias P, Regueiro JR. Diseases involving the T-cell receptor/CD3 complex. Crit Rev Oncol Hematol 19:131–147, 1995.

Asnagli H, Murphy K. Stability and commitment in T helper cell development. Curr Opin Immunol 13:242–247, 2001.

Austyn JM. New insights into the mobilization and phagocytic activity of dendritic cells. J Exp Med 183:1287–1292, 1996.

Badovinac VP, Tvinnereim AR, Harty JT. Regulation of antigen-specific CD8+ T cell homeostasis by perforin and interferon-gamma. Science 290:1354–1358, 2000.

Bahram S, Spies T. The MIC gene family. Res Immunol 147: 328–333, 1996.

Bancereau J, Briere F, Caux C, Davoust J, Lebecque S, Liu Y-J, Pulendran B, Palucka K. Immunobiology of dendritic cells. Annu Rev Immunol 18:767–812, 2000.

Barton GM, Rudensky AY. Requirement for diverse, low-abundance peptides in positive selection of T cells. Science 283:67–70, 1999.

Berg LJ, Kang J. Molecular determinants of TCR expression and selection. Curr Opin Immunol 13:232–241, 2001.

Black FL. Why did they die? Science 258:1739–1740, 1992.

Blunt T, Finnie NJ, Taccioli GE, Smith GC, Demengeot J, Gottlieb TM, Mizuta R, Varghese AJ, Alt FW, Jeggo PA, et al. Defective DNA-dependent protein kinase activity is linked to V(D)J recombination and DNA repair defects associated with the murine scid mutation. Cell 80:813–823, 1995.

Bromley SK, Burack WR, Johnson KG, Somersalo K, Sims TN, Sumen C, Davis MM, Shaw AS, Allen PM, Dustin ML. The immunological synapse. Annu Rev Immunol 19:375–936, 2001.

Buckley AF, Kuo CT, Leiden JM. Transcription factor LKLF is sufficient to program T cell quiescence via a c-Myc–dependent pathway. Nat Immunol 2:698–704, 2001.

Burr JS, Savage ND, Messah GE, Kimzey SL, Shaw AS, Arch RH, Green JM. Cutting edge: distinct motifs within CD28 regulate T cell proliferation and induction of Bcl-XL. J Immunol 166:5331–5335, 2001.

Busch R, Doebele RC, Patil NS, Pashine A, Mellins ED. Accessory molecules for MHC class II peptide loading. Curr Opin Immunol 12:99–106, 2000.

Busch R, Mellins ED. Developing and shedding inhibitions: how MHC class II molecules reach maturity. Curr Opin Immunol 8: 51–58, 1996.

Butcher EC, Picker LJ. Lymphocyte homing and homeostasis. Science 272:60–66, 1996.

Callan MF, Tan L, Annels N, Ogg GS, Wilson JD, O'Callaghan CA, Steven N, McMichael AJ, Rickinson AB. Direct visualization of antigen-specific CD8+ T cells during the primary immune response to Epstein-Barr virus in vivo. J Exp Med 187:1395–1402, 1998.

Campbell JJ, Butcher EC. Chemokines in tissue-specific and microenvironment-specific lymphocyte homing. Curr Opin Immunol 12, 336–341, 2000.

Campbell JJ, Murphy KE, Kunkel EJ, Brightling CE, Soler D, Shen Z, Boisvert J, Greenberg HB, Vierra MA, Goodman SB, Genovese MC, Wardlaw AJ, Butcher EC, Wu L. CCR7 expression and memory T cell diversity in humans. J Immunol 166:877–884, 2001.

Candotti F, Notarangelo L, Visconti R, O'Shea J. Molecular aspects of primary immunodeficiencies: lessons from cytokine and other signaling pathways. J Clin Invest 109:1261–1269, 2002.

Cella M, Facchetti F, Lanzavecchia A, Colonna M. Plasmacytoid dendritic cells activated by influenza virus and CD40L drive a potent TH1 polarization. Nat Immunol 1:305–310, 2000.

Chambers CA, Allison JP. CTLA-4—the costimulatory molecule that doesn't: regulation of T-cell responses by inhibition. Cold Spring Harb Symp Quant Biol 64:303–312, 1999.

Champagne P, Ogg GS, King AS, Knabenhans C, Ellefsen K, Nobile M, Appay V, Rizzardi GP, Fleury S, Lipp M, Forster R, Rowland-Jones S, Sekaly RP, McMichael AJ, Pantaleo G. Skewed maturation of memory HIV-specific CD8 T lymphocytes. Nature 410:106–111, 2001.

Chan KF, Siegel MR, Lenardo JM. Signaling by the TNF receptor superfamily and T cell homeostasis. Immunity 13:419–422, 2000.

Chicz RM, Urban RG, Lane WS, Gorga JC, Stern LJ, Vignali DA, Strominger JL. Predominant naturally processed peptides bound to HLA-DR1 are derived from MHC-related molecules and are heterogeneous in size. Nature 358:764–768, 1992.

Clark SP, Arden B, Kabelitz D, Mak TW. Comparison of human and mouse T-cell receptor variable gene segment subfamilies. Immunogenetics 42:531–540, 1995.

Clement LT. Isoforms of the CD45 common leukocyte antigen family: markers for human T-cell differentiation. J Clin Immunol 12:1–10, 1992.

Clevers H, Alarcon B, Wileman T, Terhorst C. The T cell receptor/CD3 complex: a dynamic protein ensemble. Annu Rev Immunol 6:629–662, 1988.

Corriveau RA, Huh GS, Shatz CJ. Regulation of class I MHC gene expression in the developing and mature CNS by neural activity. Neuron 21:505–520, 1998.

Cortes M, Wong E, Koipally J, Georgopolous K. Control of lymphocyte development by the Ikaros gene family. Curr Opin Immunol 11, 1999.

Coyle AJ, Gutierrez-Ramos, J. C. The expanding B7 superfamily: increasing complexity in costimulatory signals regulating T cell function. Nat Immunol 2:203–209, 2001.

Cyster JG. Chemokines and cell migration in secondary lymphoid organs. Science 286:2098–2102, 1999.

Daar AS, Fuggle SV, Fabre JW, Ting A, Morris PJ. The detailed distribution of HLA-A, B, C antigens in normal human organs. Transplantation 38:287–292, 1984.

Daar AS, Fuggle SV, Fabre JW, Ting A, Morris PJ. The detailed distribution of MHC Class II antigens in normal human organs. Transplantation 38:293–298, 1984.

Davis MM, Lyons DS, Altman JD, McHeyzer-Williams M, Hampl J, Boniface JJ, Chien YT. Cell receptor biochemistry, repertoire selection and general features of TCR and Ig structure. Ciba Found Symp 204:94–100, 1997.

Dejbakhsh-Jones S, Jerabek L, Weissman IL, Strober S. Extrathymic maturation of alpha beta T cells from hemopoietic stem cells. J Immunol 155:3338–3344, 1995.

Den Haan JM, Lehar SM, Bevan MJ. CD8(+) but not CD8(−) dendritic cells cross-prime cytotoxic T cells in vivo. J Exp Med 192:1685–1696, 2000.

Di Santo JP, Rodewald HR. In vivo roles of receptor tyrosine kinases and cytokine receptors in early thymocyte development. Curr Opin Immunol 10:196–207, 1998.

Douek DC, Koup RA. Evidence for thymic function in the elderly. Vaccine 18:1638–1641, 2000.

Douek DC, Vescio RA, Betts MR, Brenchley JM, Hill BJ, Zhang L, Berenson JR, Collins RH, Koup RA. Assessment of thymic output in adults after haematopoietic stem-cell transplantation and prediction of T-cell reconstitution. Lancet 355:1875–1881, 2000.

Dubey C, Croft M, Swain SL. Naïve and effector CD4 T cells differ in their requirements for T cell receptor versus costimulatory signals. J Immunol 157:3280–3289, 1996.

Durum SK, Candeias S, Nakajima H, Leonard WJ, Baird AM, Berg LJ, Muegge K. Interleukin 7 receptor control of T cell receptor γ gene rearrangement: role of receptor-associated chains and locus accessibility. J Exp Med 188:2233–2241, 1998.

Edelmann KH, Wilson CB. Role of CD28/CD80-86 and CD40/CD154 costimulatory interactions in host defense to primary herpes simplex virus infection. J Virol 75:612–621, 2001.

Elder ME, Lin D, Clever J, Chan AC, Hope TJ, Weiss A, Parslow TG. Human severe combined immunodeficiency due to a defect in ZAP-70, a T cell tyrosine kinase. Science 264:1596–1599, 1994.

Fairhurst RM, Wang CX, Sieling PA, Modlin RL, Braun J. CD1 presents antigens from a gram-negative bacterium, Haemophilus influenzae type B. Infect Immun 66:3523–3526, 1998.

Farr AG, Rudensky A. Medullary thymic epithelium: a mosaic of epithelial "self"? J Exp Med 188:1–4, 1998.

Fearon DT, Locksley RM. The instructive role of innate immunity in the acquired immune response. Science 272:50–53, 1996.

Feske S, Giltnane J, Dolmetsch R, Staudt LM, Rao A. Gene regulation mediated by calcium signals in T lymphocytes. Nat Immunol 2:316–24, 2001.

Fischer A. Severe combined immunodeficiencies (SCID). Clin Exp Immunol 122:143–149, 2000.

Fischer A, Malissen B. Natural and engineered disorders of lymphocyte development. Science 280:237–243, 1998.

Flynn S, Toellner KM, Raykundalia C, Goodall M, Lane P. CD4 T cell cytokine differentiation: the B cell activation molecule, OX40 ligand, instructs CD4 T cells to express interleukin 4 and upregulates expression of the chemokine receptor, Blr-1. J Exp Med 188:297–304, 1998.

Foy TM, Aruffo A, Bajorath J, Buhlmann JE, Noelle RJ. Immune regulation by CD40 and its ligand GP39. Annu Rev Immunol 14:591–617, 1996.

Frank KM, Sekiguchi JM, Seidl KJ, Swat W, Rathbun GA, Cheng HL, Davidson L, Kangaloo L, Alt, FW. Late embryonic lethality and impaired V(D)J recombination in mice lacking DNA ligase IV. Nature 396:173–177, 1998.

Fu YX, Chaplin DD. Development and maturation of secondary lymphoid tissues. Annu Rev Immunol 17:399–433, 1999.

Futterer A, Mink K, Luz A, Kosco-Vilbois MH, Pfeffer K. The lymphotoxin beta receptor controls organogenesis and affinity maturation in peripheral lymphoid tissues. Immunity 9:59–70, 1998.

Gao Y, Sun Y, Frank KM, Dikkes P, Fujiwara Y, Seidl KJ, Sekiguchi JM, Rathbun GA, Swat W, Wang J, Bronson RT, Malynn BA, Bryans M, Zhu C, Chaudhuri J, Davidson L, Ferrini R, Stamato T, Orkin SH, Greenberg ME, Alt FW. A critical role for DNA end-joining proteins in both lymphogenesis and neurogenesis. Cell 95:891–902, 1998.

Garcia KC, Teyton L. T-cell receptor peptide-MHC interactions: biological lessons from structural studies. Curr Opin Biotechnol 9:338–343, 1998.

Gellert M. A new view of V(D)J recombination. Genes Cells 1: 269–275, 1996.

Gellert M. Recent advances in understanding V(D)J recombination. Adv Immunol 64:39–64, 1997.

Gilhus NE, Matre R, Tonder O. Hassall's corpuscles in the thymus of fetuses, infants and children: immunological and histochemical aspects. Thymus 7:123–135, 1985.

Glimcher LH, Murphy KM. Lineage commitment in the immune system: the T helper lymphocyte grows up. Genes Dev 14: 1693–1711, 2000.

Godfrey DI, Hammond KJ, Poulton LD, Smyth MJ, Baxter AG. NKT cells: facts, functions and fallacies. Immunol Today 21: 573–583, 2000.

Goldman FD, Ballas ZK, Schutte BC, Kemp J, Hollenback C, Noraz N, Taylor N. Defective expression of p56lck in an infant with severe combined immunodeficiency. J Clin Invest 102:421–429, 1998.

Greenwald RJ, Boussiotis VA, Lorsbach RB, Abbas AK, Sharpe AH. CTLA-4 regulates induction of anergy in vivo. Immunity 14: 145–155, 2001.

Grewal IS, Flavell RA. CD40 and CD154 in cell-mediated immunity. Annu Rev Immunol 16:111–135, 1998.

Griffin DE, Levine B, Tyor WR, Irani DN. The immune response in viral encephalitis. Semin Immunol 4:111–119, 1992.

Grogan JL, Mohrs M, Harmon B, Lacy DA, Sedat JW, Locksley RM. Early transcription and silencing of cytokine genes underlie polarization of T helper cell subsets. Immunity 14:205–15, 2001.

Groh V, Rhinehart R, Randolph-Habecker J, Topp MS, Riddell SR, Spies T. Costimulation of CD8alphabeta T cells by NKG2D via engagement by MIC induced on virus-infected cells. Nat Immunol 2:255–260, 2001.

Gu Y, Seidl KJ, Rathbun GA, Zhu C, Manis JP, Van der Stoep N, Davidson L, Cheng HL, Sekiguchi JM, Frank K, Stanhope-Baker P, Schlissel MS, Roth DB, Alt FW. Growth retardation and leaky SCID phenotype of Ku70-deficient mice. Immunity 7:653–665, 1997.

Hamann D, Baars, PA, Rep MH, Hooibrink B, Kerkhof-Garde SR, Klein MR, Van Lier RA. Phenotypic and functional separation of memory and effector human CD8+ T cells. J Exp Med 186: 1407–1418, 1997.

Hamann D, Kostense S, Wolthers KC, Otto SA, Baars PA, Miedema F, Van Lier RA. Evidence that human CD8+CD45RA+CD27-cells are induced by antigen and evolve through extensive rounds of division. Int Immunol 11:1027–1033, 1999.

Hammond KJ, Pellicci DG, Poulton LD, Naidenko OV, Scalzo AA, Baxter AG, Godfrey DI. CD1d-restricted NKT cells: an interstrain comparison. J Immunol 167:1164–1173, 2001.

Haynes BF, Heinly CS. Early human T cell development: analysis of the human thymus at the time of initial entry of hematopoietic stem cells into the fetal thymic microenvironment. J Exp Med 181:1445–1458, 1995.

Hiom K, Melek M, Gellert M. DNA transposition by the RAG1 and RAG2 proteins: a possible source of oncogenic translocation. Cell 94:463–470, 1998.

Hodes RJ. T-cell-mediated regulation: help and suppression. In Paul WE, ed. Fundamental Immunology. New York, Raven Press, 1989.

Hoeijmakers JHJ. Genome maintenance mechanisms for preventing cancer. Nature 411:366, 2001.

Horst E, Meijer CJ, Duijvestijn, AM, Hartwig N, Van der Harten HJ, Pals ST. The ontogeny of human lymphocyte recirculation: high endothelial cell antigen (HECA-452) and CD44 homing receptor expression in the development of the immune system. Eur J Immunol 20:1483–1489, 1990.

Hu H, Huston G, Duso D, Lepak N, Roman E, Swain SL. CD4(+) T cell effectors can become memory cells with high efficiency and without further division. Nat Immunol 2:705–710, 2001.

Hunt JS, Petroff MG, Morales P, Sedlmayr P, Geraghty DE, Ober C. HLA-G in reproduction: studies on the maternal-fetal interface. Hum Immunol 61:1113–1117, 2000.

Jackson CE, Puck JM. Autoimmune lymphoproliferative syndrome, a disorder of apoptosis. Curr Opin Pediatr 11:521-527, 1999.

Jameson SC, Bevan MJ. T-cell selection. Curr Opin Immunol 10:214–219, 1998.

Jameson SC, Hogquist KA, Bevan MJ. Specificity and flexibility in thymic selection. Nature 369:750–752, 1994.

Jayawardena-Wolf J, Bendelac A. CD1 and lipid antigens: intracellular pathways for antigen presentation. Curr Opin Immunol 13:109–113, 2001.

Jelley-Gibbs DM, Lepak NM, Yen M, Swain SL. Two distinct stages in the transition from naïve CD4 T cells to effectors, early antigen-dependent and late cytokine-driven expansion and differentiation. J Immunol 165:5017–5026, 2000.

Jenkins MK, Khoruts A, Ingulli E, Mueller DL, McSorley SJ, Reinhardt RL, Itano A, Pape KA. In vivo activation of antigen-specific CD4 T cells. Annu Rev Immunol 19:23–45, 2001.

Jerome LA, Papaioannou VE. DiGeorge syndrome phenotype in mice mutant for the T-box gene, Tbx1. Nat Genet 27:286–291, 2001.

Johnson KG, Bromley SK, Dustin ML, Thomas ML. A supramolecular basis for CD45 tyrosine phosphatase regulation in sustained T cell activation. Proc Natl Acad Sci USA 97: 10138–10143, 2000.

Jores R, Meo T. Few V gene segments dominate the T cell receptor beta-chain repertoire of the human thymus. J Immunol 151: 6110–6122, 1993.

Jouanguy E, Doffinger R, Dupuis S, Pallier A, Altare F, Casanova JL. IL-12 and IFN-gamma in host defense against mycobacteria and salmonella in mice and men. Curr Opin Immunol 11: 346–351, 1999.

Judd BA, Koretzky GA. Antigen specific T lymphocyte activation. Rev Immunogenet 2:164–174, 2000.

Kaech SM, Ahmed R. Memory CD8+ T cell differentiation: initial antigen encounter triggers a developmental program in naïve cells. Nat Immunol 2:415–422, 2001.

Kaech SM, Wherry EJ, Ahmed R. Effector and memory T-cell differentiation: implications for vaccine development. Nature Rev Immunol 2:251–262, 2002.

Kane LP, Lin J, Weiss A. Signal transduction by the TCR for antigen. Curr Opin Immunol 12:242–249, 2000.

Kappes DJ, Alarcon B, Regueiro JR. T lymphocyte receptor deficiencies. Curr Opin Immunol 7:441–447, 1995.

Kearse KP, Takahama Y, Punt JA, Sharrow SO, Singer, A. Early molecular events induced by T cell receptor (TCR) signaling in immature CD4+CD8+ thymoyctes: increased synthesis of TCR-α protein is an early response to TCR signaling that compensates for TCR-α instability, improves TCR assembly, parallels other indicators of positive selection. J Exp Med 181:193–202, 1995.

Kim CH, Kunkel EJ, Boisvert J, Johnston B, Campbell JJ, Genovese MC, Greenberg HB, Butcher EC. Bonzo/CXCR6 expression defines type 1-polarized T-cell subsets with extralymphoid tissue homing potential. J Clin Invest 107:595–601, 2001.

King A, Allan DS, Bowen M, Powis SJ, Joseph S, Verma S, Hiby SE, McMichael AJ, Loke YW, Braud VM. HLA-E is expressed on trophoblast and interacts with CD94/NKG2 receptors on decidual NK cells. Eur J Immunol 30:1623–1631, 2000.

Kisielow P, Von Boehmer, H. Development and selection of T cells: facts and puzzles. Adv Immunol 58:87–209, 1995.

Komori T, Okada A, Stewart V, Alt FW. Lack of N regions in antigen receptor variable region genes of TdT-deficient lymphocytes. Science 261:1171–1175, 1993.

Konig R, Huang LY, Germain RN. MHC class II interaction with CD4 mediated by a region analogous to the MHC class I binding site for CD8. Nature 356:796–798, 1992.

Krangel MS. V(D)J recombination becomes accessible. J Exp Med 193:F27–F30, 2001.

Ku CC, Murakami M, Sakamoto A, Kappler J, Marrack P. Control of homeostasis of CD8+ memory T cells by opposing cytokines. Science 288:675–678, 2000.

Kundig TM, Shahinian A, Kawai K, Mittrucker HW, Sebzda E, Bachmann MF, Mak TW, Ohashi PS. Duration of TCR stimulation determines costimulatory requirement of T cells. Immunity 5:41–52, 1996.

Kung C, Pingel JT, Heikinheimo M, Klemola T, Varkila K, Yoo LI, Vuopala K, Poyhonen M, Uhari M, Rogers M, Speck SH, Chatila T, Thomas ML. Mutations in the tyrosine phosphatase CD45 gene in a child with severe combined immunodeficiency disease. Nat Med 6:343–345, 2000.

Kuo CT, Leiden JM. Transcriptional regulation of T lymphocyte development and function. Annu Rev Immunol 17:149–187, 1999.

Kuo CT, Veselits ML, Leiden JM. LKLF: A transcriptional regulator of single-positive T cell quiescence and survival. Science 277: 1986–1990, 1997.

Lantz O, Grandjean I, Matzinger P, Di Santo JP. Gamma chain required for naïve CD4+ T cell survival but not for antigen proliferation. Nat Immunol 1:54–58, 2000.

Lanzavecchia A. Licence to kill. Nature 393:413–414, 1998.

Lanzavecchia A, Sallusto F. Antigen decoding by T lymphocytes: from synapses to fate determination. Nat Immunol 2:487–492, 2001a.

Lanzavecchia A, Sallusto F. Regulation of T cell immunity by dendritic cells. Cell 106:263–266, 2001b.

Larsson M, Fonteneau JF, Bhardwaj N. Dendritic cells resurrect antigens from dead cells. Trends Immunol 22:141–148, 2001.

Latour S, Veillette A. Proximal protein tyrosine kinases in immunoreceptor signaling. Curr Opin Immunol 13, 299–306, 2001.

Laufer TM, DeKoning J, Markowitz JS, Lo D, Glimcher LH. Unopposed positive selection and autoreactivity in mice expressing class II MHC only on thymic cortex. Nature 383:81–85, 1996.

Lenschow DJ, Walunas TL, Bluestone JA. CD28/B7 system of T cell costimulation. Annu Rev Immunol 14, 233–258, 1996.

Leo A, Schraven B. Adapters in lymphocyte signalling. Curr Opin Immunol 13, 307–16, 2001.

Levings MK, Sangregorio R, Galbiati F, Squadrone S, De Waal Malefyt R, Roncarolo MG. IFN-alpha and IL-10 induce the differentiation of human type 1 T regulatory cells. J Immunol 166:5530–5539, 2001.

Lewis SM. P nucleotides, hairpin DNA and V(D)J joining: making the connection. Semin Immunol 6:131–141, 1994.

Li P, Willie ST, Bauer S, Morris DL, Spies T, Strong RK. Crystal structure of the MHC class I homolog MIC-A, a gammadelta T cell ligand. Immunity 10:577–584, 1999.

Liles WC, Van Voorhis WC. Review: nomenclature and biologic significance of cytokines involved in inflammation and the host immune response. J Infect Dis 172:1573–1580, 1995.

Lindahl KF, Byers DE, Dabhi VM, Hovik R, Jones EP, Smith GP, Wang CR, Xiao H, Yoshino M. H2-M3, a full-service class Ib histocompatibility antigen. Annu Rev Immunol 15, 851–879, 1997.

Liu Y, Wenger RH, Zhao M, Nielsen PJ. Distinct costimulatory molecules are required for the induction of effector and memory cytotoxic T lymphocytes. J Exp Med 185:251–262, 1997.

Liu YJ. Dendritic cell subsets and lineages, their functions in innate and adaptive immunity. Cell 106:259–262, 2001.

Locksley RM, Killeen N, Lenardo MJ. The TNF and TNF receptor superfamilies: integrating mammalian biology. Cell 104:487–501, 2001.

Lorenzo ME, Ploegh HL, Tirabassi RS. Viral immune evasion strategies and the underlying cell biology. Semin Immunol 13:1–9, 2001.

Luther SA, Cyster, J. G. Chemokines as regulators of T cell differentiation. Nat Immunol 2:102–107, 2001.

Ma Y, Pannicke U, Schwarz K, Lieber MR. Hairpin opening and overhang processing by an Artemis/DNA-dependent protein kinase complex in nonhomologous end joining and V(D)J recombination. Cell 108:781–794, 2002.

Mackall CL, Fleisher TA, Brown MR, Andrich MP, Chen CC, Feuerstein IM, Horowitz ME, Magrath IT, Shad AT, Steinberg SM, et al. Age, thymopoiesis, and CD4+ T-lymphocyte regeneration after intensive chemotherapy. N Engl J Med 332, 143–149, 1995.

Mackay CR. Chemokines: immunology's high impact factors. Nat Immunol 2:95–101, 2001.

Majeti R, Xu Z, Parslow TG, Olson JL, Daikh DI, Killeen N, Weiss A. An inactivating point mutation in the inhibitory wedge of CD45 causes lymphoproliferation and autoimmunity. Cell 103:1059–1070, 2000.

Malissen B, Ardouin L, Lin SY, Gillet A, Malissen M. Function of the CD3 subunits of the pre-TCR and TCR complexes during T cell development. Adv Immunol 72:103–148, 1999.

Margulies DH. TCR avidity: it's not how strong you make it, it's how you make it strong. Nat Immunol 2:669–670, 2001.

Marsh SG. HLA class II region sequences, 1998. Tissue Antigens 51:467–507, 1998.

Mason PM, Parham P. HLA class I region sequences, 1998. Tissue Antigens 51:417–466, 1998.

Masopust D, Vezys V, Marzo AL, Lefrancois L. Preferential localization of effector memory cells in nonlymphoid tissue. Science 291:2413–2417, 2001.

Matzinger P. Tolerance, danger, the extended family. Annu Rev Immunol 12:991–1045, 1994.

McCune JM, Hanley MB, Cesar D, Halvorsen R, Hoh R, Schmidt D, Wieder E, Deeks S, Siler S, Neese R, Hellerstein M. Factors influencing T-cell turnover in HIV-1-seropositive patients. J Clin Invest 105, R1–8, 2000.

McMahan CJ, Fink PJ. RAG reexpression and DNA recombination at T cell receptor loci in peripheral CD4+ T cells. Immunity 9:637–647, 1998.

McMahon CW, Raulet DH. Expression and function of NK cell receptors in CD8(+) T cells. Curr Opin Immunol 13:465–470, 2001.

McMichael AJ, Callan M, Appay V, Hanke T, Ogg G, Rowland-Jones S. The dynamics of the cellular immune response to HIV infection: implications for vaccination. Philos Trans R Soc Lond B Biol Sci 355:1007–10011, 2000.

Melek M, Gellert M, Van Gent DC. Rejoining of DNA by the RAG1 and RAG2 proteins. Science 280:301–303, 1998.

Merscher S, Funke B, Epstein JA, Heyer J, Puech A, Lu MM, Xavier RJ, Demay MB, Russell RG, Factor S, Tokooya K, Jore BS, Lopez M, Pandita RK, Lia M, Carrion D, Xu H, Schorle H, Kobler JB, Scambler P, Wynshaw-Boris A, Skoultchi AI, Morrow BE, Kucherlapati R. TBX1 is responsible for cardiovascular defects in velo-cardio-facial/DiGeorge syndrome. Cell 104:619–629, 2001.

Miyawaki T, Uehara T, Nibu R, Tsuji T, Yachie A, Yonehara S, Taniguchi N. Differential expression of apoptosis-related Fas antigen on lymphocyte subpopulations in human peripheral blood. J Immunol 149:3753–3758, 1992.

Mongkolsapaya J, Jaye A, Callan MF, Magnusen AF, McMichael AJ, Whittle HC. Antigen-specific expansion of cytotoxic T lymphocytes in acute measles virus infection. J Virol 73:67–71, 1999.

Moser B, Loetscher P. Lymphocyte traffic control by chemokines. Nat Immunol 2:123–128, 2001.

Moshous D, Callebaut I, De Chasseval R, Corneo B, Cavazzana-Calvo M, Le Deist F, Tezcan I, Sanal O, Bertrand Y, Philippe N, Fischer A, De Villartay JP. Artemis, a novel DNA double-strand break repair/V(D)J recombination protein, is mutated in human severe combined immune deficiency. Cell 105:177–186, 2001.

Mullen AC, High FA, Hutchins AS, Lee HW, Villarino AV, Livingston DM, Kung AL, Cereb N, Yao TP, Yang SY, Reiner SL. Role of T-bet in commitment of TH1 cells before IL-12-dependent selection. Science 292:1907–1910, 2001.

Nehls M, Pfeifer D, Schorpp M, Hedrich H, Boehm T. New member of the winged-helix protein family disrupted in mouse and rat nude mutations. Nature 372:103–107, 1994

Nelson BH, Willerford DM. Biology of the interleukin-2 receptor. Adv Immunol 70:1–81, 1998.

Noraz N, Schwarz K, Steinberg M, Dardalhon V, Rebouissou C, Hipskind R, Friedrich W, Yssel H, Bacon K, Taylor N. Alternative antigen receptor (TCR) signaling in T cells derived from ZAP-70-deficient patients expressing high levels of Syk. J Biol Chem 275:15832–15838, 2000.

Notarangelo LD, Giliani S, Mazza C, Mella P, Savoldi G, Rodriguez-Perez C, Mazzolari E, Fiorini M, Duse M, Plebani A, Ugazio AG, Vihinen M, Candotti F, Schumacher RF. Of genes and phenotypes: the immunological and molecular spectrum of combined immune deficiency. Defects of the gamma(c)-JAK3 signaling pathway as a model. Immunol Rev 178:39–48, 2000.

O'Driscoll M, Cerosaletti KM, Girard PM, Dai Y, Stumm M, Kysela B, Hirsch B, Gennery A, Palmer SE, Seidel J, Gatti RA, Varon R, Oettinger MA, Neitzel H, Jeggo PA, Concannon P. DNA ligase IV mutations identified in patients exhibiting developmental delay and immunodeficiency. Mol Cell 8:1175–1185, 2001.

O'Garra A. Cytokines induce the development of functionally heterogeneous T helper cell subsets. Immunity 8:275–283, 1998.

Ohteki T, Ho S, Suzuki H, Mak TW, Ohashi PS. Role for IL-15/IL-15 receptor beta-chain in natural killer 1.1+ T cell receptor-alpha beta+ cell development. J Immunol 159:5931–5935, 1997.

Ohteki T, Okuyama R, Seki S, Abo T, Sugiura K, Kusumi A, Ohmori T, Watanabe H, Kumagai K. Age-dependent increase of extrathymic T cells in the liver and their appearance in the periphery of older mice. J Immunol 149:1562–1570, 1992.

Ohteki T, Wilson A, Verbeek S, MacDonald HR, Clevers H. Selectively impaired development of intestinal T cell receptor gamma delta+ cells and liver CD4+ NK1+ T cell receptor alpha beta+ cells in T cell factor-1-deficient mice. Eur J Immunol 26:351–355, 1996.

O'Shea JJ, Notarangelo LD, Johnston JA, Candotti F. Advances in the understanding of cytokine signal transduction: the role of Jaks and STATs in immunoregulation and the pathogenesis of immunodeficiency. J Clin Immunol 17:431–447, 1997.

Ostrowski MA, Justement SJ, Ehler L, Mizell SB, Lui S, Mican J, Walker BD, Thomas EK, Seder R, Fauci AS. The role of CD4+ T cell help and CD40 ligand in the in vitro expansion of HIV-1-specific memory cytotoxic CD8+ T cell responses. J Immunol 165:6133–6141, 2000.

Padovan E, Casorati G, Dellabona P, Meyer S, Brockhaus M, Lanzavecchia A. Expression of two T cell receptor alpha chains: dual receptor T cells. Science 262:422–424, 1993.

Padovan E, Giachino C, Cella M, Valitutti S, Acuto O, Lanzavecchia A. Normal T lymphocytes can express two different T cell receptor β chain: implications for the mechanism of allelic exclusion. J Exp Med 181:1587–1591, 1995.

Pages G, Guerin S, Grall D, Bonino F, Smith A, Anjuere F, Auberger P, Pouyssegur J. Defective thymocyte maturation in p44 MAP kinase (Erk 1) knockout mice. Science 286:1374–1377, 1999.

Pamer E, Cresswell P. Mechanisms of MHC class I–restricted antigen processing. Annu Rev Immunol 16:323–358, 1998.

Patterson S. Flexibility and cooperation among dendritic cells. Nat Immunol 1:273–274, 2000.

Pénit C, Lucas B, Vasseur F. Cell expansion and growth arrest phases during the transition from precursor (CD4–8–) to immature (CD4+8+) thymocytes in normal and genetically modified mice. J. Immunol 154:5103–5113, 1995.

Perez-Melgosa M, Ochs HD, Linsley PS, Laman JD, Meurs M, Flavell RA, Ernst RK, Miller SI, Wilson CB. Carrier-mediated enhancement of cognate T cell help: the basis for enhanced immunogenicity of meningococcal outer membrane protein polysaccharide conjugate vaccine. Eur J Immunol 31:2373–2381, 2001.

Ploegh HL. Viral strategies of immune evasion. Science 280:248–253, 1998.

Porcelli SA, Segelke BW, Sugita M, Wilson IA, Brenner MB. The CD1 family of lipid antigen-presenting molecules. Immunol Today 19:362–368, 1998.

Posnett DN, Edinger JW, Manavalan JS, Irwin C, Marodon G. Differentiation of human CD8 T cells: implications for in vivo persistence of CD8+ CD28– cytotoxic effector clones. Int Immunol 11:229–241, 1999.

Puel A, Leonard WJ. Mutations in the gene for the IL-7 receptor result in T(-)B(+)NK(+) severe combined immunodeficiency disease. Curr Opin Immunol 12:468–473, 2000.

Pulendran B, Palucka K, Banchereau J. Sensing pathogens and tuning immune responses. Science 293:253–256, 2001.

Radtke F, Ferrero I, Wilson A, Lees R, Aguet M, MacDonald HR. Notch1 deficiency dissociates the intrathymic development of dendritic cells and T cells. J Exp Med 191:1085–1094, 2000.

Ramesh N, Geha RS, Notarangelo LD. CD40 ligand and the hyper-IgM syndrome. In Ochs HD, Smith CIE, Puck JM, eds. Primary Immunodeficiency Diseases: a Molecular and Genetic Approach. New York, Oxford University Press, 1999, pp. 233–249.

Ramos SB, Garcia AB, Viana SR, Voltarelli JC, Falcao RP. Phenotypic and functional evaluation of natural killer cells in thymectomized children. Clin Immunol Immunopathol 81:277–281, 1996.

Raulet DH, Vance RE, McMahon CW. Regulation of the natural killer cell receptor repertoire. Annu Rev Immunol 19:291–330, 2001.

Reiner SL, Seder RA. Dealing from the evolutionary pawnshop: how lymphocytes make decisions. Immunity 11:1–10, 1999.

Rennert PD, James D, Mackay F, Browning JL, Hochman PS. Lymph node genesis is induced by signaling through the lymphotoxin beta receptor. Immunity 9:71–79, 1998.

Res P, Spits H. Developmental stages in the human thymus. Semin Immunol 11:39–46, 1999.

Robey E, Fowlkes BJ. The alpha beta versus gamma delta T-cell lineage choice. Curr Opin Immunol 10:181–187, 1998.

Roifman CM. Human IL-2 receptor alpha chain deficiency. Pediatr Res 48:6–11, 2000.

Roifman CM. A mutation in zap-70 protein tyrosine kinase results in a selective immunodeficiency. J Clin Immunol 15, 52S–62S, 1995.

Roifman CM, Zhang J, Chitayat D, Sharfe N. A partial deficiency of interleukin-7R alpha is sufficient to abrogate T-cell development and cause severe combined immunodeficiency. Blood 96:2803–2807, 2000.

Romagnani S, Parronchi P, D'Elios MM, Romagnani P, Annunziato F, Piccinni MP, Manetti R, Sampognaro S, Mavilia C, De Carli M, Maggi E, Del Prete GF. An update on human Th1 and Th2 cells. Int Arch Allergy Immunol 113:153–156, 1997.

Roncarolo MG, Levings MK. The role of different subsets of T regulatory cells in controlling autoimmunity. Curr Opin Immunol 12:676–683, 2000.

Rossi D, Zlotnik A. The biology of chemokines and their receptors. Annu Rev Immunol 18:217–242, 2000.

Rouas-Freiss N, Paul P, Dausset J, Carosella ED. HLA-G promotes immune tolerance. J Biol Regul Homeost Agents 14:93–98, 2000.

Rowe J, Macaubas C, Monger T, Holt BJ, Harvey J, Poolman JT, Loh R, Sly PD, Holt PG. Heterogeneity in diphtheria-tetanus-acellular pertussis vaccine-specific cellular immunity during infancy: relationship to variations in the kinetics of postnatal maturation of systemic th1 function. J Infect Dis 184:80–88, 2001.

Rowen L, Koop BF, Hood L. The complete 685-kilobase DNA sequence of the human beta T cell receptor locus. Science 272:1755–1762, 1996.

Rudensky A, Preston-Hurlburt P, Hong SC, Barlow A, Janeway CA Jr. Sequence analysis of peptides bound to MHC class II molecules. Nature 353:622–627, 1991.

Sakaguchi S. Regulatory T cells: key controllers of immunologic self-tolerance. Cell 101:455–458, 2000.

Salter RD, Benjamin RJ, Wesley PK, Buxton SE, Garrett TP, Clayberger C, Krensky AM, Norment AM, Littman DR, Parham P. A binding site for the T-cell co-receptor CD8 on the alpha 3 domain of HLA-A2. Nature 345:41–46, 1990.

Sanders ME, Makgoba MW, Sharrow SO, Stephany D, Springer TA, Young HA, Shaw S. Human memory T lymphocytes express increased levels of three cell adhesion molecules (LFA-3, CD2, and LFA-1) and three other molecules (UCHL1, CDw29, and Pgp-1) and have enhanced IFN-gamma production. J Immunol 140:1401–1407, 1988.

Schlissel MS, Durum SD, Muegge K. The interleukin 7 receptor is required for T cell receptor gamma locus accessibility to the V(D)J recombinase. J Exp Med 191:1045–1050, 2000.

Schluns KS, Kieper WC, Jameson SC, Lefrancois, L. Interleukin-7 mediates the homeostasis of naïve and memory CD8 T cells in vivo. Nat Immunol 1:426–432, 2000.

Schofield L, McConville MJ, Hansen D, Campbell AS, Fraser-Reid B, Grusby MJ, Tachado SD. CD1d-restricted immunoglobulin G formation to GPI-anchored antigens mediated by NKT cells. Science 283:225–229, 1999.

Schwartz RH. T cell clonal anergy. Curr Opin Immunol 9:351–357, 1997.

Schweitzer AN, Sharpe AH. Studies using antigen-presenting cells lacking expression of both B7-1 (CD80) and B7-2 (CD86) show distinct requirements for B7 molecules during priming versus restimulation of Th2 but not Th1 cytokine production. J Immunol 161:2762–2771, 1998.

Sekiguchi J, Frank K. V(D)J recombination. Curr Biol 9:R835, 1999.

Seyama K, Nonoyama S, Gangsaas I, Hollenbaugh D, Pabst HF, Aruffo A, Ochs HD. Mutations of the CD40 ligand gene and its effect on CD40 ligand expression in patients with X-linked hyper IgM syndrome. Blood 92:2421–2434, 1998.

Shevach EM. Regulatory T cells in autoimmunity. Annu Rev Immunol 18:423–449, 2000.

Shevach EM, McHugh RS, Thornton AM, Piccirillo C, Natarajan K, Margulies DH. Control of autoimmunity by regulatory T cells. Adv Exp Med Biol 490:21–32, 2001.

Shortman K, Wu L. Early T lymphocyte progenitors. Annu Rev Immunol 14:29–47, 1996.

Siu G, Kronenberg M, Strauss E, Haars R, Mak TW, Hood L. The structure, rearrangement and expression of D beta gene segments of the murine T-cell antigen receptor. Nature 311:344–350, 1984.

Sleckman BP, Gorman JR, Alt FW. Accessibility control of antigen-receptor variable-region gene assembly: Role of cis-acting elements. Annu Rev Immunol 14:459–481, 1996.

Spellberg B, Edwards JE Jr. Type 1/Type 2 immunity in infectious diseases. Clin Infect Dis 32:76–102, 2001.

Sprent J, Tough DF. T cell death and memory. Science 293:245–248, 2001.

Springer TA. Traffic signals on endothelium for lymphocyte recirculation and leukocyte emigration. Annu Rev Physiol 57: 827–872, 1995.

Steinle A, Groh V, Spies T. Diversification, expression, and gamma delta T cell recognition of evolutionarily distant members of the MIC family of major histocompatibility complex class I-related molecules. Proc Natl Acad Sci USA 95:12510–12515, 1998.

Sun Z, Arendt CW, Ellmeier W, Schaeffer EM, Sunshine MJ, Gandhi L, Annes J, Petrzilka D, Kupfer A, Schwartzberg PL, Littman DR. PKC-theta is required for TCR-induced NF-kappaB activation in mature but not immature T lymphocytes. Nature 404:402–407, 2000.

Sun Z, Unutmaz D, Zou YR, Sunshine MJ, Pierani A, Brenner-Morton S, Mebius RE, Littman DR. Requirement for RORgamma in thymocyte survival and lymphoid organ development. Science 288:2369–2373, 2000.

Surh CD, Sprent J. Homeostatic T cell proliferation: how far can T cells be activated to self-ligands? J Exp Med 192:F9–F14, 2000.

Suzuki H, Zhou YW, Kato M, Mak TW, Nakashima I. Normal regulatory alpha/beta T cells effectively eliminate abnormally activated T cells lacking the interleukin 2 receptor beta in vivo. J Exp Med 190:1561–1572, 1999.

Takeda K, Tanaka T, Shi W, Matsumoto M, Minami M, Kashiwamura S, Nakanishi K, Yoshida N, Kishimoto T, Akira S. Essential role of Stat6 in IL-4 signalling. Nature 380:627–630, 1996.

Tan LC, Gudgeon N, Annels NE, Hansasuta P, O'Callaghan CA, Rowland-Jones S, McMichael AJ, Rickinson, AB, Callan MF. A re-evaluation of the frequency of CD8+ T cells specific for EBV in healthy virus carriers. J Immunol 162:1827–1835, 1999.

Toellner KM, Luther SA, Sze DM, Choy RK, Taylor DR, MacLennan IC, Acha-Orbea HT helper 1 (Th1) and Th2 characteristics start to develop during T cell priming and are associated with an immediate ability to induce immunoglobulin class switching. J Exp Med 187:1193–1204, 1998.

Trigueros C, Ramiro AR, Carrasco YR, De Yebenes VG, Albar JP, Toribio ML. Identification of a late stage of small noncycling pTalpha pre-T cells as immediate precursors of T cell receptor alpha/beta+ thymocytes. J Exp Med 188:1401–1412, 1998.

Van Esch H, Groenen P, Nesbit MA, Schuffenhauer S, Lichtner P, Vanderlinden G, Harding B, Beetz R, Bilous RW, Holdaway I, Shaw NJ, Fryns JP, Van de Ven W, Thakker RV, Devriendt, K. GATA3 haplo-insufficiency causes human HDR syndrome. Nature 406:419–422, 2000.

Van Meerwijk JP, Marguerat S, Lees RK, Germain RN, Fowlkes BJ, MacDonald HR. Quantitative impact of thymic clonal deletion on the T cell repertoire. J Exp Med 185:377–383, 1997.

Van Parijs L, Abbas AK. Homeostasis and self-tolerance in the immune system: turning lymphocytes off. Science 280, 243–248, 1998.

Van Stipdonk MJ, Lemmens EE, Schoenberger SP. Naïve CTLs require a single brief period of antigenic stimulation for clonal expansion and differentiation. Nat Immunol 2:423–429, 2001.

Verbeek S, Izon D, Hofhuis F, Robanus-Maandag E, Te Riele H, Van de Wetering M, Oosterwegel M, Wilson A, MacDonald HR, Clevers H. An HMG-box-containing T-cell factor required for thymocyte differentiation. Nature 374:70–74, 1995.

Vogel TU, Evans DT, Urvater JA, O'Connor DH, Hughes AL, Watkins DI. Major histocompatibility complex class I genes in primates: co-evolution with pathogens. Immunol Rev 167: 327–337, 1999.

Von Boehmer H, Aifantis I, Feinberg J, Lechner O, Saint-Ruf C, Walter U, Buer J, Azogui O. Pleitropic changes controlled by the pre-T-cell receptor. Curr Opin Immunol 11:135–142, 1999.

Wang B, Wang N, Whitehurst CE, She J, Chen J, Terhorst C. T lymphocyte development in the absence of CD3 epsilon or CD3 gamma delta epsilon zeta. J Immunol 162:88–94, 1999.

Ward SG, Cantrell DA. Phosphoinositide 3-kinases in T lymphocyte activation. Curr Opin Immunol 13, 332–338, 2001.

Washburn T, Schweighoffer E, Gridley T, Chang D, Fowlkes BJ, Cado D, Robey E. Notch activity influences the alphabeta versus gammadelta T cell lineage decision. Cell 88:833–843, 1997.

Watts TH, DeBenedette MA. T cell co-stimulatory molecules other than CD28. Curr Opin Immunol 11:286–293, 1999.

Weng NP, Levine BL, June CH, Hodes RJ. Human naïve and memory T lymphocytes differ in telomeric length and replicative potential. Proc Natl Acad Sci USA 92:11091–11094, 1995.

Whitmire JK, Ahmed R. Costimulation in antiviral immunity: differential requirements for CD4(+) and CD8(+) T cell responses. Curr Opin Immunol 12:448–455, 2000.

Wilson IA, Bjorkman PJ. Unusual MHC-like molecules: CD1, Fc receptor, the hemochromatosis gene product, and viral homologs. Curr Opin Immunol 10:67–73, 1998.

Wilson SB, Kent SC, Patton KT, Orban T, Jackson RA, Exley M, Porcelli S, Schatz DA, Atkinson MA, Balk SP, Strominger JL, Hafler DA. Extreme Th1 bias of invariant Valpha24JalphaQ T cells in type 1 diabetes. Nature 391:177–181, 1998.

Xavier R, Brennan T, Li Q, McCormack C, Seed B. Membrane compartmentation is required for efficient T cell activation. Immunity 8:723–732, 1998.

Yang YW, JM. CD40 ligand-dependent T cell activation: requirement of B7-CD28 signaling through CD40. Science 273:1862–1864, 1996.

Yoder J, Pham C, Iizuka YM, Kanagawa O, Liu SK, McGlade J, Cheng AM. Requirement for the SLP-76 adaptor GADS in T cell development. Science 291:1987–1991, 2001.

Yokota Y, Mansouri A, Mori S, Sugawara S, Adachi S, Nishikawa S, Gruss P. Development of peripheral lymphoid organs and natural killer cells depends on the helix-loop-helix inhibitor Id2. Nature 397:702–706, 1999.

York IA, Rock KL. Antigen processing and presentation by the class I major histocompatibility complex. Annu Rev Immunol 14: 369–396, 1996.

Young JL, Ramage JM, Gaston JS, Beverley PC. In vitro responses of human CD45R0brightRA- and CD45R0-RAbright T cell subsets and their relationship to memory and naïve T cells. Eur J Immunol 27:2383–2390, 1997.

Zerrahn J, Held W, Raulet DH. The MHC reactivity of the T cell repertoire prior to positive and negative selection. Cell 88: 627–636, 1997.

Zorbas M, Scollay R. Development of gamma delta T cells in the adult murine thymus. Eur J Immunol 23:1655–1660, 1993.

CHAPTER

3

The B-Lymphocyte System: Fundamental Immunology

Richard A. Insel and R. John Looney

INTRODUCTION

B lymphocytes are the subset of lymphocytes that synthesize, express on their surface, and differentiate to secrete immunoglobulins, which encompass the extensive repertoire of antigen-specific antibodies. The B designation arises from their origin in the bone marrow of humans and other mammals and in the bursa of Fabricius in birds.

This chapter reviews the structure and function of immunoglobulin, generation of immunoglobulin diversity, antigen-independent or early B-cell development, antigen-dependent or late B-cell development, and regulation of B-cell activation. Clinical aspects of the topic are interspersed in this and the next chapter and further detailed in other chapters of this book.

IMMUNOGLOBULIN STRUCTURE AND FUNCTION

Antibodies are the antigen-specific proteins produced by B lymphocytes and synthesized and secreted by plasma cells, which arise from terminally differentiated B cells (Padlan, 1994). Antibodies are Y-shaped molecules. The two arms of the Y (F(ab) portion) bind antigen and the stem of the Y (Fc portion) binds effector molecules or cells. The antigen-binding or variable (V) regions vary extensively among antibodies of different specificity. The remainder of the antibody molecule is its constant (C) region and has much more limited diversity. The family of plasma proteins containing antibodies is known as immunoglobulins.

Antibodies are a critical component of host defenses. By themselves, antibodies are often able to neutralize toxins and viruses or prevent colonization by pathogenic organisms. In addition, bacteria and fungi opsonized with antibodies can bind to phagocytic cells expressing immunoglobulin receptors to activate their ingestion and subsequent destruction. Antibodies are also able to activate the complement cascade, which enhances opsonization and may directly lyse gram-negative bacteria.

Basic Structure of Immunoglobulins

Chains

Two pairs of identical heavy and light chains form immunoglobulins (Fig. 3-1). There are five classes of immunoglobulins, IgM, IgD, IgG, IgA, and IgE, based on differences in the constant regions of the μ, δ, γ, α, and ε heavy chains, respectively. There are also two types of light chains—κ and λ chains. Each type of light chain can pair with each class of heavy chain. The immunoglobulin on the B-cell surface exists as a monomer composed of two pairs of heavy and light chains (Fig. 3-2).

In the plasma, however, some types of immunoglobulin exist in other forms. IgM in the plasma occurs primarily as a pentamer where five monomer units of two paired heavy and light chains are joined together by disulfide bonds and by an additional polypeptide, the joining (J) chain. In the absence of J chain, IgM forms a hexamer with six units of IgM. Plasma IgA can occur as a polymer with two monomer subunits in combination with a J chain (Fig. 3-3). Secretory IgA is found in gastrointestinal, respiratory, and vaginal secretions as a complex of two IgA monomers, a J chain, and **secretory component (SC)**, which is a fragment of the polymeric immunoglobulin receptor that transports polymeric IgA through the epithelial cells of exocrine glands.

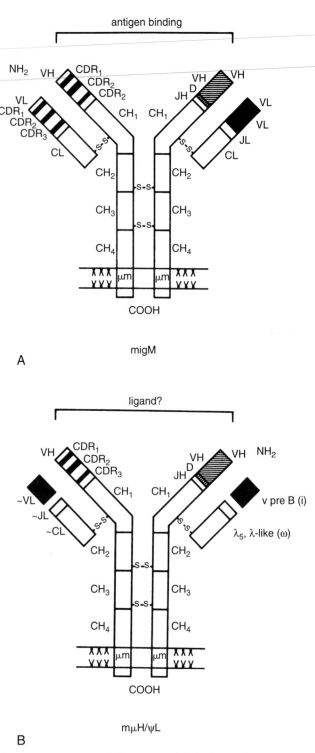

Figure 3-2 · Diagram of the immunoglobulin heavy-chain receptors found on mature or pre-B cells. **A.** Disulfide-linked heavy (H) and light (L) chains form a membrane IgM molecule with two identical antigen-binding sites. Within the μ-H chain, intracellular, transmembrane (μm), four constant (C_H1-C_H4), and three complementary-determining regions (CDR1–CDR3) are indicated relative to the V, D, and J segments. **B.** In pre-B cells, the μ-H chain chains are associated with the surrogate light chain, which is composed of covalently linked λ5 (14.1) and noncovalently linked V pre-B. Both receptors are associated with the signal transducing molecules Igα (CD79a) and Igβ (CD79b). (From Van Noesel CJM, Van Lier RAW. Architecture of the human B-cell antigen receptors. Blood 82:363–373, 1993.)

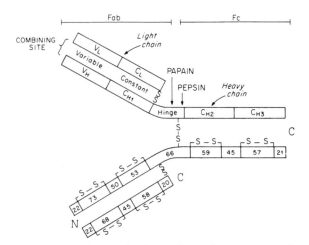

Figure 3-1 · **Typical IgG molecule.** N indicates the amino terminal end and C the carboxyl terminal end. The intrachain and interchain disulfide bonds are indicated by —S—S—. Papain splits the molecule at the hinge region, so that two Fab fragments and one Fc fragment result. Pepsin splits the molecule at the hinge region, so that an F(ab′)₂ fragment results (Braun and Stiehm, 1996).

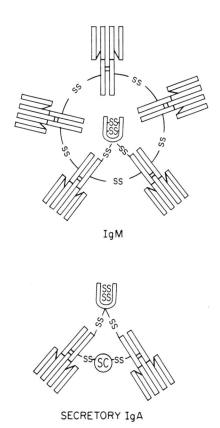

IgM

SECRETORY IgA

Figure 3-3· Structural models of polymeric serum IgM and secretory IgA. The U-shaped chain is the J chain, common to all polymeric immunoglobulins. SC is the secretory component of the secretory IgA molecule that is generated from the polymeric immunoglobulin receptor. The disulfide bonds (—S—S—) of the monomeric units are indicated by lines between the chains (Braun and Stiehm, 1996).

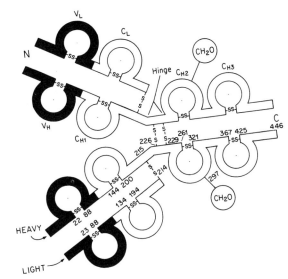

Figure 3-4· Details of the structural composition of human IgG immunoglobulin. The shaded areas of the chains are the V regions, and the unshaded areas are the C regions. Within each region are 60 amino acid loops stabilized by disulfide bonds (—S—S—), termed domains. The numbers refer to the amino acid positions of the cysteine residues that form disulfide bonds or are the attachment sites of carbohydrate (Braun and Stiehm, 1996).

Domains

Each heavy and light chain consists of globular segments, or domains, and linear sequences linking the globular domains (Fig. 3-4). Light chains have two domains, and heavy chains have either four or five. Each immunoglobulin domain is a globular structure with several strands of the polypeptide chain forming two antiparallel beta sheets held together by a disulfide bond. This immunoglobulin fold is a type of beta barrel or sandwich.

All the globular domains of the heavy and light chains share amino acid sequences needed for formation of this immunoglobulin fold. Antigen binding is conferred by the amino terminal variable or V region domains of both the heavy chain and light chain (V_H and V_L, respectively). The remaining globular domains are the constant or C regions (C_L and C_{H1} to C_{H4}). The two domains of a light chain are complexed to the two amino terminal domains of a heavy chain. Pairing of two light chain/heavy chain heterodimers forms the characteristic Y shape of immunoglobulins.

Hinge Region

The region between C_{H1} and C_{H2} consists of the hinge region. It is longer than the other linear sequences link-ing the globular domains and contains disulfide bonds that covalently link the two heavy chains.

Fragments

Digestion of IgG with the protease papain cleaves the heavy chains just before the disulfide bonds in the hinge region, creating two **Fab fragments** (Fragment *a*ntigen *b*inding) composed of V_L + C_L complexed with V_H + C_{H1}, and one **Fc fragment** (C_{H2} + C_{H3} from both heavy chains complexed with each other) (see Fig. 3-1).

The Fab fragments retain antigen-binding activity, and the Fc (Fragment *c*rystallizable) fragments are easily crystallized.

The Fc portion of immunoglobulins is responsible for effector functions, such as fixing complement and opsonizing particles, interacting with the transport mechanisms of the placenta and epithelial cells of exocrine glands, and regulating immunoglobulin half-life in plasma.

Digestion of IgG with the protease pepsin cleaves the hinge region just after the disulfide bonds, creating an **F(ab')₂ fragment**—that is, two Fab fragments connected by a portion of the hinge region. An F(ab')₂ fragment retains antigen-binding activity and is dimeric, permitting agglutination or precipitation of antigen, but lacks effector function.

Recombinant DNA technology can be used to generate a small single **Fv fragment** (Fragment *v*ariable), which is composed of the V_H joined to the V_L by a synthetic peptide linker. Because of their small size and short half-life, Fvs coupled to toxins or radionucleotides are being used experimentally to target cells for the diagnosis and therapy of human diseases, such as cancer.

Antigen Binding of Immunoglobulins

In each immunoglobulin domain, there are amino acid loops connecting the polypeptide strands that form the β sheets. These loops are relatively unconstrained by structural requirements. In the variable region domains, three of the flexible loops can directly interact with antigen and are largely responsible for determining antigen-binding specificity. The amino acid sequence of the three variable domain loops that interact with antigen varies extensively, and thus these loops are also known as the hypervariable regions. The rest of the variable region sequences are constrained by the necessity of forming the immunoglobulin fold; therefore they are relatively less variable and are known as the framework regions.

The heavy- or light-chain variable region consists of three hypervariable regions (**HV1–3**) and four framework regions (**FR1–4**). Both the heavy-chain and light-chain variable regions can contribute to antigen binding. The three hypervariable regions of the heavy chain can pair with the three hypervariable regions of the light chain, forming three pairs of hypervariable regions, termed complementary-determining regions (**CDR1–3**), that act in concert to bind antigen (see Fig. 3-2). The genetic machinery that creates variability in the variable region of immunoglobulins is discussed elsewhere in this chapter.

The juxtaposition of the CDRs of the heavy and light chains creates an antibody surface that interacts with a specific antigen through this antigen-binding or antibody-combining site (Alzari et al., 1988; Getzoff et al., 1988). For small-molecular-weight antigens, the antibody variable region may form a pocket or groove. For large-molecular-weight antigens, the variable region may form a flat, concave, undulating, or convex surface that complements the surface of the antigen. The antibody molecule has flexibility to allow it to accommodate to the topography of the antigen.

Antigens, Epitopes, Immunogens

Antibodies bind a variety of different substances termed **antigens** (Berzofsky and Berkower, 1999; Davies and Cohen, 1996). Antigens are most commonly proteins or polysaccharides but can be peptides, nucleic acids, lipids, and small-molecular-weight chemicals.

The regions of a molecule specifically recognized by antibodies are antigenic determinants or **epitopes.** Linear epitopes are determined by the primary sequence of the molecule. Conformational epitopes are formed by segments of a molecule that are discontinuous in the primary sequence but are brought together because of the conformation of the three-dimensional structure of the molecule. Antibodies to native proteins often recognize conformational epitopes that may be destroyed by denaturation or proteolytic digestion. Conversely, antibodies generated to linear epitopes using peptide fragments or synthetic peptides may fail to bind the native protein.

Antigens that are able to induce an immune response are termed **immunogens.** All immunogens are antigens but not all antigens are immunogens. In particular,

small-molecular-weight molecules called **haptens** may be recognized by antibodies but are unable to induce an immune response by themselves. Haptens must be covalently linked to carrier proteins to become complete antigens—that is, immunogens.

Antigen Binding

Antibodies bind to antigen noncovalently, and therefore binding is reversible. The forces involved in antigen binding include ionic bonds, hydrogen bonding, Van der Waals forces, and hydrophobic interactions. The overall contribution of each force to binding depends on the specific antibody and antigen pair. Antibody-antigen interactions can be disrupted using extremes of pH, high salt concentration, detergents, or chaotropic agents such as urea. The strength of interaction between antigen and antibody can sometimes be gauged by the concentration of denaturing agent needed to dissociate antibody from antigen but can more accurately be measured using Scatchard plots.

All antibodies have at least 2 antigen-binding regions, and polymeric IgM can have as many as 10. Therefore an antibody may be able to bind antigen at several sites simultaneously. The strength of interaction between a single antigen-binding region and antigen is termed affinity, and the overall strength of interaction due to binding antigen at one or more sites is termed avidity. Thus polymeric IgM in a primary immune response may make up for relatively low affinity by binding antigen at multiple sites and thus still have a reasonably high avidity.

Immunoglobulin Diversity

Isotypes

A total of 18 different isotypes or classes and subclasses of immunoglobulins are present in plasma or expressed on the surface of B lymphocytes. They are composed of five classes of heavy-chain isotypes (μ, δ, γ, α, and ε chains), which include four subclasses of γ chain (γ1, γ2, γ3, and γ4) and two classes of α chain (α1 and α2), that pair with two types (κ and λ) of light chains.

Allotypes

Allotypes are genetic differences (**alleles**) in constant region sequences that were originally identified serologically and can be identified today by molecular approaches. There are 18 γ-chain alleles (**Gm**), 2 α-chain alleles (**Am**), 1 ε-chain allele (**Em**), and 3 κ-chain alleles (**Km**). These are discussed further in Chapter 4.

Idiotypes

Idiotypes are individual unique epitopes in the V region that distinguish one antibody from another and that can be identified with antibodies (anti-idiotypes) or by molecular approaches.

Membrane and Secreted Immunoglobulins

Each isotype of immunoglobulin is generated in two major forms in the B cell—a membrane protein expressed on the surface of B lymphocytes and a smaller protein, identical in its variable region sequence and most of its constant region, that is secreted by the B cell after activation and differentiation. The membrane form of an immunoglobulin has both a hydrophobic transmembrane domain and a cytoplasmic region at its carboxy terminus that are not present in the secreted form. Conversely, the secreted form has a peptide tail not present in the membrane form (Fig. 3-5). The size of the carboxy cytoplasmic tail is 3 amino acids for IgM and IgD, 14 amino acids for IgA, and 28 amino acids for IgG and IgE, respectively.

The transmembrane and secreted immunoglobulins are derived by alternative RNA processing from the same heavy-chain primary RNA transcript that then dictates where the transcript is polyadenylated (see Fig. 3-5). With B-cell differentiation to a plasma cell, not only is immunoglobulin transcription dramatically increased, but the ratio of secreted versus membrane exon usage is increased by about 100-fold above that of resting B cells through the regulation of alternative RNA splicing.

Membrane immunoglobulin is a monomer of immunoglobulin that is a component of the multiprotein **B-cell receptor (BCR)**. Signal transduction through the BCR does not occur through the short cytoplasmic tail of transmembrane immunoglobulin but through two transmembrane protein components of the BCR, Igα and Igβ, encoded by the mb-1 and B29 genes, that are noncovalently bound to surface immunoglobulin (see p. 75,

B-Lymphocyte Signaling and Activation). The BCR is initially composed of IgM, but the same V region can be expressed with other isotypes through a process of isotype or class switch recombination (as detailed on p. 65, Class Switch Recombination [Isotype Switching] of Immunoglobulin Heavy Chains).

Alternative processing of the primary RNA transcript for the heavy chain allows naïve B lymphocytes to also express both IgD and IgM, as detailed later, and during heavy-chain switching, more than one heavy chain may be produced and expressed for a brief time on the B-cell surface. With these two exceptions, each mature B lymphocyte otherwise expresses a single immunoglobulin isotype.

DISTRIBUTION AND METABOLISM OF IMMUNOGLOBULINS

Immunoglobulins are synthesized and secreted by plasma cells that are located in secondary lymphoid tissue, mucosal sites, and bone marrow. Plasma cells producing IgA and IgE are enriched at mucosal sites. The light chains of human serum immunoglobulin consist of 60% κ and 40% λ light-chain types. The serum concentration of each isotype and IgG subclass is age related throughout childhood.

IgG

IgG is distributed equally between the intravascular and extravascular compartments (Tables 3-1 and 3-2). The mean half-life for IgG is the longest of any plasma

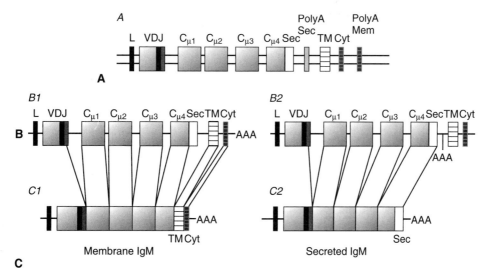

Figure 3-5· Alternative RNA processing generates membrane or secreted immunoglobulin. **A.** Genomic DNA of an IgM heavy-chain immunoglobulin rearrangement (VDJ) encoding the variable region and the constant region (Cμ1–4). Potential sites for polyadenylation (polyA) of the transcript to generate membrane (Mem) or secreted (Sec) IgM exist in the genomic DNA. **B** and **C.** A primary immunoglobulin transcript is alternatively spliced at the C terminal or 3′ end. Differential splicing and polyA site selection dictate which form is generated. Membrane immunoglobulin is composed of a transmembrane (TM) region and a cytoplasmic (Cyt) exon that are spliced together. Secreted immunoglobulin is composed of an extra coding region that is contiguous with the last heavy-chain constant region (C). B-cell differentiation to plasma cells is associated with increased expression of the secreted form of immunoglobulin.

TABLE 3-1 · PROPERTIES OF IMMUNOGLOBULINS

Characteristic	Immunoglobulin Class				
	IgG	IgM	IgA	IgD	IgE
Chains					
Heavy	γ	μ	α	δ	ε
Light	κ, λ	κ, λ	κ, λ	κ, λ	κ, λ
Monomer units	1	5	1–3	1	1
Molecular weight	150,000	900,000	160–500,000	180,000	200,000
Percent carbohydrate	3	12	7.5–11	12–18	12
Serum concentration					
Adult mean (mg/dl)	1,200	120	200	3	0.01
Percent of total	70–80	5–10	10–15	<1	<0.01
Heat lability	±	++	+	++++	+++
Number of subclasses	4	1	2	1	1
Biologic half-life (days)	23	5	7	2.8	2.3
Distribution (% intravascular)	45	80	45	75	50
Placental transfer	+	–	–	–	–

protein, approximately 23 days. Moreover, the half-life or fractional catabolic rate of IgG is not fixed but varies inversely with the concentration of IgG. Thus the half-life of IgG in patients with agammaglobulinemia may be greater than 35 days, but it may be as short as 10 days in patients with hypergammaglobulinemia. IgG1, IgG2, and IgG4 all have a 23-day half-life, but the half-life of IgG3 is only 9 days (see Chapter 4).

Regulation of IgG Half-Life: Role of FcRn

The long half-life of IgG and its unique relationship to serum levels are due to the **FcRn,** or Fc receptor of the neonate (Ghetie and Ward; 2000, Simister and Story, 1997), which was originally described on neonatal intestinal epithelium in animals, where it mediates uptake of colostral IgG from the gut. The heterodimeric receptor is composed of one polypeptide chain related to major histocompatibility complex (MHC) class I proteins and one chain composed of β2-microglobulin.

There is continuous and ongoing pinocytosis of IgG from the plasma into cells (Fig. 3-6). FcRn, which is present on the membrane of a variety of cells and enriched on vascular endothelial cells, is simultaneously taken into the cell with pinocytosis. The FcRn and IgG enter endocytic vesicles, where they bind to each other in this acidified environment. This binding of IgG to FcRn prevents the degradation of IgG in lysosomes in the cell. IgG bound to FcRn is then transported back to the cytoplasmic surface of the plasma membrane of the cell, where neutralization of the pH releases IgG from the FcRn. The IgG then egresses by reverse pinocytosis from the intracellular environment to the plasma.

When levels of IgG are high, the capacity of FcRn to rescue IgG from degradation is overwhelmed and the rate of IgG catabolism increases. Conversely, with lower levels of IgG, there is less competition for FcRn binding and IgG catabolism decreases. Administration of high doses of IgG accelerates the destruction of normal and pathogenic (e.g., autoantibodies) IgG antibodies by this mechanism, accounting for some of the beneficial effect of intravenous immunoglobulin therapy in antibody-mediated autoimmune disease.

IgA and Secretory IgA

IgA is synthesized primarily by plasma cells located in the lamina propria just below the basement membrane of the epithelium at surfaces of exocrine glands and mucous membranes. Some of the IgA, mostly in a monomeric form, enters the blood and circulates as serum IgA, with a half-life of about 9 days.

In other plasma cells, two monomeric IgA molecules bind through their carboxy end to the 15 kD **J chain** (see Fig. 3-3). Dimeric IgA, associated with the J chain, is secreted by the plasma cell and binds to the **polymeric immunoglobulin receptor** (poly-Ig receptor) receptor on the basolateral surface of mucosal epithelial cells. Binding of the IgA results in its internalization and

TABLE 3-2 · PROPERTIES OF IgG SUBCLASSES

Property	IgG1	IgG2	IgG3	IgG4
Molecular weight	146,000	146,000	165,000	146,000
Mean adult serum level (mg/dl)	840	240	80	40
Percentage of total IgG	70	20	7	3
Biologic half-life (days)	23	23	9	23
Placental transport	++	+	++	++
Complement activation via classical pathway	++	+	++	–

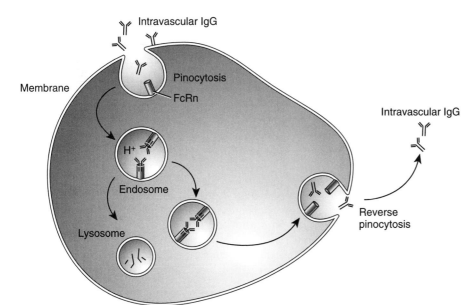

Figure 3-6·Regulation of serum IgG half-life by FcRn. Serum IgG is pinocytosed spontaneously by cells, such as endothelial cells, that express the Fc receptor FcRn. In the acidified environment of an endosome, IgG binds to FcRn, which rescues IgG from entering a lysosome and undergoing degradation. The endosome migrates back to the membrane and the IgG dissociates from FcRn at neutral pH and is then delivered to the extracellular space by reverse pinocytosis. With elevated IgG levels, the IgG half-life is shortened because FcRn is saturated. In contrast, with decreased IgG levels, the half-life of IgG is increased because IgG will be more completely bound by FcRn and rescued from destruction.

transport in a transcytotic vesicle to the apical (luminal) surface of the epithelial cell. At the apical surface, the extracellular, ligand-binding portion of the poly-Ig receptor is enzymatically cleaved and becomes the secretory component (SC) that remains covalently attached to secretory IgA. Secretory IgA is then released from the cell into the mucosal site. The 80 kD SC renders secretory IgA resistant to proteolytic cleavage at this location

IgM

IgM antibodies are the first antibodies produced during an immune response. For most immune responses, the IgM response wanes as IgG or other isotypes are produced. However, persistent IgM responses may be seen for polysaccharides (isohemagglutinins) or lipopolysaccharides (antiendotoxins) and with certain autoantibodies (cold agglutinins and the rheumatoid factors in cryoglobulinemia). IgM may exist as a pentamer with disulfide bonding of IgM monomers to each other and to J chain (see Fig. 3-3) or as a hexamer in the absence of J chain. IgM is an excellent agglutinin and activator of complement, and its 10 antigen binding sites may provide high avidity even when the affinity of each site is low. The majority of IgM (80%) is intravascular, and its half-life is 5 days.

IgE

IgE mediates type 1 hypersensitivity allergic reactions. Plasma levels of IgE are normally very low (1/100,000 of that for IgG) but can be markedly increased in certain allergic conditions, such as bronchopulmonary aspergillosis, or with parasitic diseases, such as schistosomiasis. IgE plasma cells are present in mucosal areas, especially in the respiratory tract, where it mediates allergic reactions, and the gastrointestinal tract, where it may mediate expulsion

of parasitic worm infestations. The half-life of IgE in plasma is only 2 to 3 days but is prolonged to 2 to 3 weeks after IgE binds to the Fc receptor FcεRI on the surface of mast cells, basophils, or dendritic cells.

COMPLEMENT BINDING OF IMMUNOGLOBULIN

Complement was originally described as a heat-labile component of serum that allowed antibodies to opsonize bacteria or to lyse gram-negative bacteria. Thus the heat-labile component was able to "complement" the activity of bacteria-specific antibodies.

Complement is made up of a large number of plasma proteins that act in a cascading series of reactions to opsonize particles, lyse microorganisms, attract phagocytes, and activate leukocytes or mast cells (see Chapter 7). After binding of antigen, antibodies activate the complement system through the classical pathway of complement activation. Complement activation is initiated when C1q, the first protein in the classical complement pathway, binds the Fc portion of IgM or IgG antibodies bound to multiple sites on the surface of a target antigen.

IgG1, IgG3, and to a lesser degree IgG2 are effective at activating complement through the classical pathway. IgG4 does not activate complement. IgA does not activate complement via the classical pathway, but IgA complexes may activate complement through the alternative pathway.

Fc RECEPTORS AND BINDING TO IMMUNOGLOBULINS

Although antibody by itself or through the action of complement activation may neutralize certain toxins, viruses, or bacteria, many infections require the recruitment of additional protective mechanisms provided by accessory effector cells bearing receptors for the Fc portion of immunoglobulins (FcRs) (Daeron, 1997; Heyman, 2000) (Fig. 3-7).

Effector mechanisms activated via FcRs include phagocytosis by macrophages and neutrophils and secretion of stored mediators by **natural killer cells (NK cells)**, eosinophils, mast cells, and basophils. Further, negative signaling to cells by signaling through FcRs can downregulate antibody production, anaphylaxis, or phagocytosis. Although FcRs for all five heavy-chain classes have been reported, this chapter focuses on the FcRs for IgG, IgE, and IgA. FcRs are members of the immunoglobulin superfamily. Signaling is mediated by **immunoreceptor transmembrane activation motifs (ITAMS)** on the cytoplasmic domain of the receptor itself or of an associated accessory chain, such as the γ chain of FcγRI.

FcγRs

There are three types of FcγRs: FcγRI (CD64), FcγRII (CD32), and FcγRIII (CD16) (Ravetch and Bolland, 2001). FcγRI has a relatively high affinity for IgG (compared with FcγRII and FcγRIII); it binds well to IgG1 and IgG3, poorly to IgG4, and not at all to IgG2. FcγRI occurs constitutively on macrophages and monocytes and is upregulated on these cells, neutrophils, and eosinophils by interferon-γ. Engaging FcγRI triggers phagocytosis, respiratory burst, secretion, and **antibody-dependent cellular cytotoxicity (ADCC)**. FcγRI has a very short cytoplasmic domain and forms a complex with the signaling γ chain. When FcγRI is engaged, the ITAMs in the γ chain recruit and activate Src-family tyrosine kinases.

There are three forms of FcγRII—FcγRIIa, FcγRIIb1, and FcγRIIb2. FcγRIIa occurs constitutively on macrophages, neutrophils, eosinophils, platelets, and dendritic cells. Engaging FcγRIIa stimulates phagocytosis, respiratory burst, secretion, ADCC, and platelet activation. FcγRIIa binds IgG3 > IgG1 = IgG2 > IgG4. However, there is an allele of FcγRIIa that binds IgG2 very poorly. The cytoplasmic domain of FcγRIIa contains ITAM motifs that engage Src-family tyrosine kinases. FcγRIIb2 occurs on macrophages, eosinophils, and macrophages, and FcγRIIb1 occurs on B lymphocytes and mast cells. FcγRIIb1 differs from FcγRIIb2 by an insertion in the cytoplasmic domain, which arises from alternative RNA processing, that prevents receptor-mediated endocytosis. FcγRIIb1 and FcγRIIb2 bind IgG3 > IgG1 > IgG4 >> IgG2.

The cytoplasmic domains of FcγRIIb1 and FcγRIIb2 contain **immunoreceptor transmembrane inhibitory motifs (ITIMs)** that inhibit cellular activation by recruiting the tyrosine phosphatase **SHP-1** and the 5′ inositol phosphatase **SHIP**. Binding of antigen-IgG complexes to FcγRIIb1 on B cells downregulates BCR-induced B-cell activation and terminates the B-cell antibody response to provide a feedback to the B cell to regulate its activation.

Experimental evidence in the mouse suggests that the therapeutic effect of intravenous immunoglobulins in models of autoimmune disease is mediated by FcγRII activation of ITIMs that inhibit cellular activation and release of inflammatory cytokines from macrophages, as well as B lymphocytes (Samuelsson et al., 2001). These experimental models also suggest that FcγRII may inhibit the release of inflammatory mediators from mast cells to attenuate anaphylactic reactions.

FcγRIII occurs as a transmembrane protein (FcγRIIIa) on NK cells, macrophages, and some monocytes, and as a **glycosylphosphatidyl-inositol (GPI)–linked receptor** (FcγRIIIb) on neutrophils. FcγRIIIa is complexed to the γ chain (or the closely related ζ chain) and activates phagocytosis, respiratory burst, secretion, and ADCC. FcγRIIIb, the nontransmembrane receptor, does not induce ADCC. FcγRIII binds IgG1 = IgG3 >>> IgG2 or IgG4.

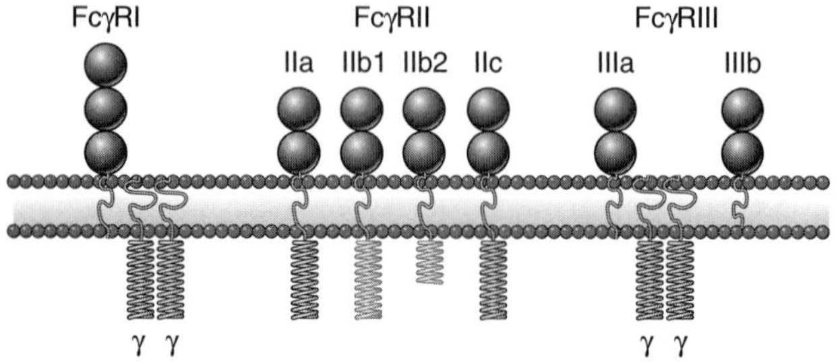

FcεRs

There are two types of FcεRs, the **high-affinity FcεRI** on mast cells, basophils, and dendritic cells, and the **low-affinity FcεRII**, which is expressed on a wide range of cells, including B cells, eosinophils, activated macrophages, and platelets.

FcεRI has a very high affinity for IgE monomer, such that most IgE is surface bound rather than circulating in the plasma. FcεRI consists of three chains: the α chain, which binds IgE; the β chain, which regulates levels of receptor expression and signal transduction; and the γ chain, which possesses ITAMs to allow recruitment of Src-family tyrosine kinases. Crosslinking FcεRI on mast cells and basophils releases histamine, leukotrienes, and cytokines involved in type I hypersensitivity reactions (immediate hypersensitivity) such as urticaria, asthma, and anaphylaxis (see Chapter 4). FcεRI on accessory cells such as dendritic cells does not express the β chain

Figure 3-7 · Human FcγRs. The external domains consist of two or three immunoglobulin-like domains that bind IgG. FcγRI and FcγRIIIa are multichain receptors that associate with γ-chain dimers. (FcγRIIIa on natural killer cells can also associate with ζ-chain dimers or γζ heterodimers.) The γ and ζ chains and the cytoplasmic domains of FcζRIIa and FcζRIIc contain immunoreceptor tyrosine-based activation motifs (ITAMs). In contrast, FcγRIIb1 and FcγRIIb2 contain immunoreceptor tyrosine-based inhibitory motifs (ITIMs). FcγRIIIb is glycosylphosphatidyl inositol (GPI) linked.

and is involved in receptor-mediated endocytosis of allergens for presentation to T cells.

FcεRII (**CD23**), a type II protein of the C-type lectin family, has a lower affinity for IgE than FcεRI and binds additional ligands such as CD21 (Conrad, 1990). FcεRII can occur in a soluble form and act as a B-cell cytokine. FcεRII also allows eosinophils to kill IgE-coated parasites such as *Schistosoma mansoni*.

FcαR

FcαR (**CD89**) occurs on neutrophils, macrophages, eosinophils, and some B and T lymphocytes. Like FcγRI, FcγRIII, and FcεRI, FcαR is complexed with a γ chain that is responsible for signal transduction. FcαR binds IgA1 = IgA2, and crosslinking FcαRs induces phagocytosis, respiratory burst, secretion, and ADCC. IgA that is bound to SC fails to bind FcαR.

ONTOGENY OF IMMUNOGLOBULINS

Transplacental Transport

Only the IgG isotype of immunoglobulin is transported across the placenta. IgG antibody of all subclasses can cross the placenta via binding to the FcRn receptor, as detailed previously (Ghetie and Ward, 2000). IgG1 subclass antibodies cross the placenta more efficiently than IgG2 subclass antibodies. At birth, levels of IgG1 in the full-term newborn are greater than maternal levels and levels of IgG2 are approximately comparable to or slightly lower than the mother's. Placental transfer of IgG begins in the second trimester, but transfer does not reach maximal levels until the third trimester (Fig. 3-8). Therefore premature infants have significantly lower levels of protective IgG antibodies than full-term infants.

After birth, levels of maternal IgG begin to decrease and the infant's active synthesis of IgG fails to maintain the total IgG level bestowed at birth. A nadir of total IgG level is observed at approximately 4 months of age, a condition sometimes termed **physiologic hypogammaglobulinemia of infancy.** Although the total IgG may have reached its nadir, the level of many protective antibodies continues to fall during the first year of life unless the infant is immunized or becomes infected. IgG does not reach adult levels until around 6 years of age. IgG1 and IgG3 subclasses reach adult levels at an earlier age than do IgG2 and IgG4 subclasses.

The fetus synthesizes small amounts of IgM, which at birth reach approximately 10% of adult levels. After birth, IgM synthesis increases and reaches about 50% of adult levels by 6 months, 75% by 12 months of age, and adult levels by approximately 2 years of age. IgA synthesis is even more delayed, reaching only 20% to 25% of adult levels by 1 year of age and not attaining adult levels until adolescence.

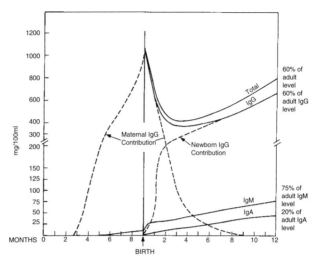

Figure 3-8 · Immunoglobulin (IgG, IgM, and IgA) levels in the fetus and infant in the first year of life. The IgG of the fetus and newborn infant is solely of maternal origin. The maternal IgG disappears by the age of approximately 9 months, by which time endogenous synthesis of IgG by the infant is well established. The IgM and IgA of the neonate are entirely endogenously synthesized because maternal IgM and IgA do not cross the placenta (Braun and Stiehm, 1996).

GENERATION OF ANTIBODY DIVERSITY

The variable regions (**V regions**) of the immunoglobulin light (L) and heavy (H) chains are generated by somatic genetic recombination or rearrangement of single **variable** (**V**) and **joining** (**J**) gene segments for the V_L and of V_H, J_H, and **diversity** (**D**) gene segments for V_H (Honjo, 1983; Honjo and Alt, 1996) (Fig. 3-9). The genetic loci for the immunoglobulin heavy chain, the kappa light chain, and lambda light chain are located on human chromosome 14, 2, and 22, respectively. The immunoglobulin heavy chain (IgH) locus is composed of approximately 50 functional variable or V_H region gene segments, each about 300 base pairs in length, separated from other V genes by intron sequences and classified into seven V_H families (Cook and Tomlinson, 1995; Matsuda and Honjo, 1996; Pascual and Capra, 1991).

There are approximately 30 diversity or D_H region elements and six joining or J_H gene segments. The V, D, and J gene segments are located upstream or 5' of nine constant IgH region C_H genes in the heavy-chain locus. The kappa IgL locus is composed of approximately 40 functional Vκ genes, representing seven families, five functional Jκ genes, and one Cκ gene. The lambda IgL locus is composed of approximately 30 functional Vλ genes, representing eight families, and three functional Jλ genes, each expressed with its corresponding unique Cλ gene.

In addition to the generation of antibody diversity in early B-lymphocyte development by rearrangement of heavy- and light-chain variable region gene segments, there is alteration of variable region expression in antigen-dependent, late B-cell development by somatic hypermutation. Immunoglobulin heavy-chain constant

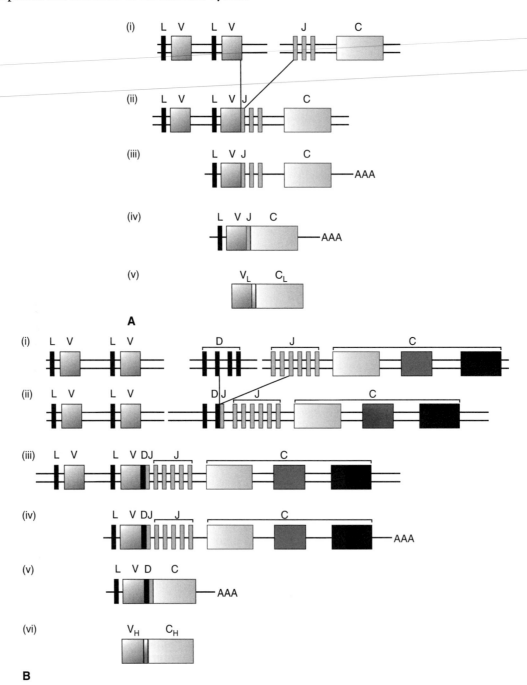

Figure 3-9 · Immunoglobulin gene rearrangement and RNA processing and expression to generate a light-chain (A) or heavy-chain (B) immunoglobulin molecule. At the genomic DNA level (A, B, i), the light-chain loci on chromosome 2 (κ) and 22 (λ) are comprised of multiple V-region and J-region genes and the heavy-chain locus on chromosome 14 is composed of V-, J-, and D-region genes. A light-chain V-region exon is formed by rearrangement of a single V and J gene segment (A, ii), and a heavy-chain V region is formed by initial rearrangement of a D and J gene segment (B, ii) followed by rearrangement of a V gene segment to the DJ rearrangement (B, iii). Recombination signal sequences (RSS) composed of a heptamer, nonamer, and a spacer of either 12 or 23 base pairs (bp) flank the immunoglobulin gene segments, with joining of segments flanked by 12-bp RSS to segments flanked by 23-bp RSS. The V_L and J_L segments are flanked by RSS with 12 and 23 bp spacers, and the V_H and J_H gene segments are flanked by 23-bp RSS and the D segment with 12-bp RSS. The primary RNA transcript (A, iii; B, iv) includes a leader (L) exon, a VJ or VDJ exon, and constant (C) region exons. This primary transcript is processed (A, iv; B, v) with splicing of the introns and then translated to generate a light- and heavy-chain (A, v; B, vi) protein that initially joins noncovalently and then disulfide bonds to form an intact immunoglobulin molecule.

region or isotype expression is altered by isotype or class switch recombination.

Immunoglobulin Gene Rearrangement

Overview

Generation of an antibody molecule involves the combinatorial productive rearrangement of single gene segments to generate a continuous V(D)J exon in the genome that is in the correct reading frame (Honjo and Alt, 1996) (see Fig. 3-9). The diversity of the immunoglobulin repertoire arises from this combinatorial process of selection of individual gene segments, imprecision of the joining of these gene segments, and subsequent pairing of the immunoglobulin heavy- and light-chain gene rearrangements to form an intact antibody.

Rearrangement is an ordered process. In the majority of B-cell precursors, Ig heavy-chain precedes light-chain rearrangement, DJ_H precedes $V_H DJ_H$ rearrangement, and VJ rearrangement at the κ-L chain locus precedes VJ rearrangement at the λ-L chain locus. If the first κ allele fails to generate a productive rearrangement, the cell undergoes rearrangement at the second κ gene locus, and if this rearrangement is nonproductive, then a rearrangement occurs at the λ locus. A functional VDJ or VJ productive rearrangement at one chromosomal allele inhibits rearrangement on the other allele, a process termed allelic exclusion, to guarantee that a B cell produces immunoglobulin from only one IgH allele. As detailed later, antigen-independent B-cell development requires generation of a functional pre-B–cell receptor, composed of a μ-IgH chain, the signal-transducing Igα/β heterodimer, and λ 5 and Vpre-B of the **surrogate light chain (SLC)**.

Mechanism of Immunoglobulin Gene Rearrangement

With immunoglobulin gene rearrangement, variable-region DNA segments or exons on the genome that are separated become recombined with deletion of the intervening sequences. Recombination requires regulatory elements called **recombination signal sequences (RSSs)**, which are composed of a conserved, palindromic heptamer and an AT-rich nonamer sequence that flank nonconserved 12 or 23 base pair (bp) spacers. The 12/23 bp rule dictates that a gene segment with a 12-nucleotide spacer RSS must join to a gene segment with a complementary 23-nucleotide spacer RSS.

Thus the D_H gene segment that is flanked by RSS with 12 bp spacers can join to a V_H gene segment at one end and to a J_H gene segment at its other end because both V_H and J_H genes are flanked by RSS with 23 bp spacers. With V(D)J recombination, the 12 bp–spaced and 23 bp–spaced RSS are juxtaposed. The intervening DNA is then looped out followed by ligation of the signal and the coding joints. The signal joints are generated by a precise blunt-end ligation of the heptamers without nucleotide loss or addition. In contrast, joining

of the coding segments is imprecise with nucleotide addition or deletion, which generates the high degree of antibody diversity observed in the CDR3 of the variable region.

Immunoglobulin gene rearrangement and transcription require that the locus be accessible to lymphoid-specific **recombination-activating enzymes RAG-1 and RAG-2** and the transcriptional machinery, consisting of RNA polymerase and ubiquitous and cell-specific transcription factors (Hempel et al., 1998). The locus becomes accessible by transcription-factor–induced alteration in histone acetylation, which leads to chromatin remodeling. Binding of transcription factors and regulation of RAG expression is controlled by the immunoglobulin gene enhancer located in the μ intron between the VDJ and Cμ and the 3′ immunoglobulin enhancer located 3′ downstream of the C_H region genes.

V(D)J recombination consists of three major stages (Fugmann et al., 2000; Gellert, 1997; Hesslein and Schatz, 2001) (Fig. 3-10). The first stage is the formation of a cleavage complex that generates DNA **double-strand breaks (DSBs)** located precisely at the border of the RSS heptamer and the adjacent coding region of each immunoglobulin gene segment. This is followed by a second stage of processing of the ends of the DSBs. In the third stage, the DSBs are joined to generate a coding and signal end joint. DNA excision and recombination is mediated by the enzymes RAG-1 and RAG-2, which bind as a complex to the RSS. Binding and cleavage by the RAG enzymes is facilitated by the DNA binding and bending **high mobility group proteins-1 and-2 (HMG-1, HMG-2)**.

Initially the RAG complex binds to the two RSSs and brings them into juxtaposition or synapsis. Then the RAGs generate two single-strand DNA breaks or nicks between the coding segment sequence and 5′ of the heptamer at each RSS. The nick-generated, free 3′-hydroxyl group at the end of each coding segment hydrolyzes the phosphodiester bond on the complementary strand in a transesterification reaction to create a DSB with a covalently sealed hairpin coding end and a 5′-phosphorylated blunt signal end. The two coding ends and the two signal ends are held together by the RAG complex. The signal ends are joined by a precise blunt head-to-head ligation of the heptamers, but the hairpin coding region must first be processed.

The hairpin is nicked randomly by RAGs with a contribution from activity of a **DNA-dependent protein kinase (DNA-PK)** holoenzyme complex, which is composed of the DNA-PK catalytic subunit (PKcs), Ku70 (XRCC6), and Ku80 (XRCC5), to generate a single-stranded break with 5′ or 3′ overhangs. The Ku proteins increase the affinity of binding of DNA-PKcs to the DSBs where DNA-PKcs phosphorylates several proteins required for DSB repair. The hairpin end is then modified by polymerases, nucleases, and the lymphocyte-specific enzyme **terminal deoxynucleotidyl transferase (TdT)**. The 3′ overhangs are excised by exonuclease activity, and the 5′ overhangs are filled in by polymerases. The DNA DSBs are repaired and ligated by **nonhomologous end-joining (NHEJ)** DSB repair that is

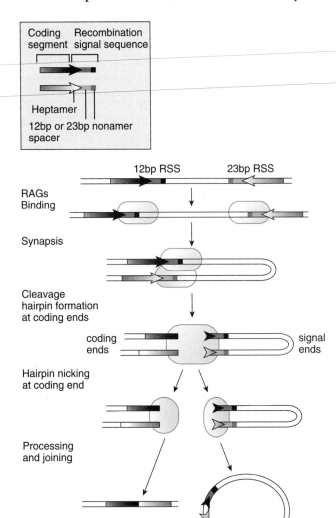

Figure 3-10 · Stages of immunoglobulin gene rearrangement. The RAG-1 and RAG-2 enzymes *(ovals)* bind as a complex to RSS with a 12- and 23-bp spacer *(arrows)* and bring them into juxtaposition or synapsis. The RAGs then generate a DNA double-strand break precisely between the RSS and the flanking immunoglobulin gene coding elements that results in generation of a covalently sealed hairpin at the coding end and 5'-phosphorylated signal ends. The double-strand breaks are then processed. The hairpin at the coding end is opened by generation of a nick or single-strand break that is imprecise and leads to nucleotide base deletion or addition, which occurs by formation of P nucleotides or by terminal deoxytidylnucleotide-mediated N-region addition. This imprecision of coding end formation leads to diversification of the antibody repertoire. The signal joint is a precise blunt-end ligation of the heptamers of the RSS. The double-strand breaks are joined by nonhomologous end-joining (NHEJ) repair to form the coding and signal joints.

mediated by the DNA-PK complex and a heterodimer of **XRCC4** and **DNA ligase IV** (Weaver, 1995).

This filling in of the coding sequence creates P-nucleotide palindromes or P-region sequences. Nontemplated GC-rich **nucleotide regions (N-regions)** are added to the coding ends by activity of TdT. This variable processing of the coding ends at the V-J or V-D-J junctions generates the extensive diversity conferred by the CDR3 of antibodies.

Outcome of Immunoglobulin Gene Rearrangement

Approximately two thirds of the time, a nonproductive rearrangement is generated because the reading frame of the coding sequence is disrupted because of imprecision of joining of gene segments. Based on the transcriptional orientation of the gene segment on the chromosome, rearrangement leads to either deletion of the intervening gene segments, joined at the signal sequences by excision of an excisional circle from the chromosome, or to an inversion with retention of the intervening sequences in the chromosome upstream of the new coding joint.

The rearrangement process generates the high degree of diversity of the antibody repertoire that can exceed 10^{11} unique molecules. Immunoglobulin diversity arises from **combinatorial diversity,** generated by VDJ rearrangement of single immunoglobulin gene segments, and **junctional diversity,** which arises from imprecision of the DNA joins of the coding ends that leads to nucleotide deletion and addition. Also contributing to the high degree of diversity of CDR3 is the ability of D genes to rearrange by inversion or deletion, rearrange in one of three reading frames, and undergo D-D gene fusion. The pairing of individual H and L chains in the B cell to generate an intact antibody then adds further diversity. As described later, further diversification of the V(D)J rearrangement occurs after naïve B cells are activated by antigen through a process of somatic hypermutation of the V regions.

Somatic Hypermutation of Immunoglobulin Variable Regions

Overview

The preimmune or naïve antibody repertoire generated in bone marrow early B cells is further diversified in lymphoid germinal centers after immunization with antigen by hypermutation of the germline-encoded V(D)J rearrangement (Kocks and Rajewsky, 1989). Mutations are introduced into the V region by a unique process termed **somatic hypermutation.** An antigen selection process occurs in the germinal center to preserve B cells expressing mutated surface immunoglobulin with increased affinity for the immunogen to lead to affinity maturation of the antibody response.

Mutations that give rise to an amino acid replacement that confers increased antigen binding are selected and come to predominate in the CDRs through this affinity selection. In contrast, replacement mutations in the **framework region (FR)** that alter the basic structure of the immunoglobulin molecule are negatively selected. Thus the replacement to silent mutation ratio (R/S) is high in the CDRs and low in the FRs.

The mutations are primarily single-point substitutions that are targeted to the rearranged heavy- and light-chain variable region with a sharp upstream boundary in the middle of the leader intron and an approximately 1.5 kb imprecise downstream boundary in the J-C intron (Wagner and Neuberger, 1996). The majority of mutations are located within 500 bp of the V gene promoter in the V(D)J exon.

The rate of mutation has been estimated to be 10^3 to 10^4 mutations per base pair per generation, which is the highest rate of mutation observed in the eukaryotic genome and about 5 to 6 logs higher than the background mutation rate that occurs with normal DNA replication. Mutations involving **transitions** (purine to purine or pyrimidine to pyrimidine) are favored over **transversions** (purine to pyrimidine or vice versa) and may preferentially occur at so-called hot spots, such as RGYW (A/G, G, C/T, A/T). Mutations can target either DNA strand. Although the majority of mutations are single-point mutations, about 5% of the mutations are deletions and 1% are duplications.

Mechanism of Somatic Hypermutation

The mechanism of somatic hypermutation of immunoglobulin genes at a cellular or molecular level is not well understood (Jacobs and Bross, 2001). Error-prone DNA polymerases or error-prone repair processes have been invoked (Poltoratsky et al., 2000). A role for mismatch repair proteins in the accumulation of mutations has been suggested but not fully established. The mutation process is linked to transcription of the immunoglobulin gene and appears to require the immunoglobulin intronic enhancers but does not require the V gene sequence or the specific V region promoter per se.

Somatic hypermutation involves the generation of DNA DSBs, especially occurring at the RGYW motif, that may be undergoing repair in an error-prone homologous end-joining DSB repair process. The enzyme **activation-induced cytidine deaminase (AID)**, which is defective in a form of autosomal recessive **hyper-IgM syndrome** (HIGM2) and required for isotype switching, as described later, is required for somatic hypermutation (Honjo et al., 2002). However, its role in the mutation process is not well understood.

AID may be the catalytic subunit of an RNA-editing complex that edits a transcript whose expression is involved in a unique DNA repair process or a transcript that encodes an endonuclease or hypermutator. Alternatively, and more likely, AID may initiate cytidine deamination at the DNA level at the Ig locus with repair associated with an error-prone, low-fidelity, nonprocessive DNA polymerase.

Class Switch Recombination (Isotype Switching) of Immunoglobulin Heavy Chains

Overview

A human IgH transcript is expressed with one of five classes of heavy chain constant regions, four subclasses of IgG, or two subclasses of IgA. These C_H genes are ordered as H-chain constant region exons in a linear array downstream or 3' from the heavy-chain V_H region elements in the IgH locus on chromosome 14. The V_HDJ_H rearrangement is separated by a large intron from the exons that encode the constant region genes, and C_H exons are separated from each other by introns (Fig. 3-11). The locus consists of a 5' or V_H-proximal region composed of μ, $\gamma3$, $\gamma1$, $\alpha1$, $\psi\epsilon$, and a more 3' distal region composed of $\gamma2$, $\gamma4$, $\alpha2$, and ϵC_H genes.

The primary IgH transcript is a long transcript composed of VDJ and C_H genes that is spliced to excise the intron between the V_HDJ_H rearrangement and the most proximal C_H gene(s) to bring together into continuous linear array the exons coding for the complete H chain. A V_HDJ_H rearrangement may recombine with any of the downstream heavy-chain coding elements, resulting in acquisition of new immunoglobulin constant region effector function with preservation of the VDJ-encoded variable region and thus of antigenic specificity.

In the developing B cell, the first isotype generated is IgM. As a mature B cell is generated, both IgM and IgD are produced. The B cell generates a long RNA transcript that includes both the $C\mu$ and $C\delta$ exons with an upstream VDJ. This transcript is then alternatively spliced to give rise to an IgM μ-H or IgD δ-H chain transcript (Fig. 3-12). The relative levels of production of IgM and IgD are controlled by regulation of splicing, whose molecular mechanism is not completely understood.

Mechanism of Class Switch Recombination

Isotype switching from IgM to a downstream C_H gene occurs with B-cell activation during an immune response (Coffman et al., 1993). Switching requires a unique looping-out deletion recombination event, termed **class switch recombination (CSR)**, that juxtaposes the VDJ region to a different C-region exon (see Fig. 3-11). When IgM switches to IgG isotypes, both the $C\mu$ and $C\delta$ genes are deleted. Switching can continue to occur sequentially to 3' or downstream C_H genes with looping out of the intervening DNA. CSR occurs on both the productive and nonproductive immunoglobulin alleles.

The mechanism of CSR is distinct from V(D)J recombination. With CSR, there is recombination between the **switch (S) regions** flanking each C_H gene at their 5' end and another located in the intron between the J_H and $C\mu$. The S regions are composed of tandem repeats with palindromes that can generate a loop secondary structure. There is initial selection of the target S region to be recombined with the $S\mu$ region. Targeting to a particular S region is regulated by germline transcripts that initiate from an **intronic (I) promoter** lying 5' of each S loop, runs through the S region, and is polyadenylated downstream of the C_H exon. The transcript is then processed with deletion of the S-region sequence and fusing of the I and C_H exons.

Cytokines dictate the S region targeted for CSR and therefore the subsequent immunoglobulin isotype or class that will be expressed by activating specific intronic promoters. Both cognate and noncognate T-cell

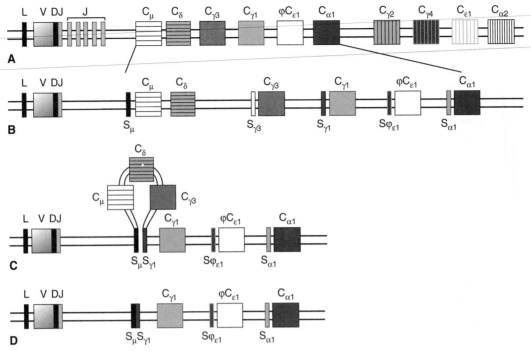

Figure 3-11 · Immunoglobulin heavy-chain class switch recombination. A. The human heavy-chain locus on chromosome 14 is organized into a 5′ or V-proximal region of the Cμ, Cδ, Cγ3, Cγ1, Cα1, and Cψε constant regions and a 3′ or V-distal region composed of $C_{\gamma 2}$, $C_{\gamma 4}$, $C_{\alpha 2}$, and C_{ε} constant regions. **B.** Switch (S) regions lie upstream or 5′ of each constant region gene. **C.** The S regions recombine. **D.** The intervening DNA is then looped out by the action of a putative class switch recombinase. The initial switch involves Sμ joining to another S region. Sequential switching can occur between the recombined Sμ-S fusion and a 3′ or downstream S region.

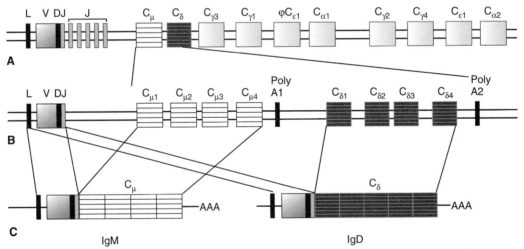

Figure 3-12 · Expression of IgM and IgD in the B cell. A and B. Genomic DNA at the human heavy-chain locus on chromosome 14 comprises a polyadenylation site (polyA) 3′ of both the IgM (Cμ) and IgD (Cδ) constant region genes. **C.** A primary transcript is generated that includes both Cμ and Cδ exons. This primary transcript is then alternatively processed by cleaving, polyadenylation, and splicing to generate either a Cμ or Cδ transcript. Processing is developmentally regulated.

help is required for class switch recombination with signaling via CD40, the B-cell receptor, and cytokine receptors, as detailed later. Cytokines regulating switching to specific isotypes include interleukin-4 (IL-4) directing switching to IgE, and transforming growth factor-β (TGF-β) directing switching to IgA.

After selection of the specific S region, cleavage is activated. It is believed that germline S-region transcription renders the site susceptible to cleavage by formation of transient heteroduplexes or R loops with single-stranded DNA regions that serve as a recognition site for the cleaving enzyme. DNA recombination occurs between the S regions with looping-out deletion of the intervening DNA with its C_H genes to lead to juxtaposition of the VDJ to a new downstream C_H region.

The DSBs generated from the cleavage step are then repaired and ligated by NHEJ repair that is mediated by the DNA-PKcs complex, composed of Ku70, Ku80, and DNA-PKcs, and an XRCC4-DNA ligase IV complex. NHEJ also requires a complex composed of Rad50, Mre11, and the **Nijmegen breakage syndrome protein** (**Nbs1**). Thus DSBs are generated with V(D)J recombination, somatic hypermutation, and CSR.

Activation-Induced Cytidine Deaminase and Hyper-IgM Syndrome Type 2

A putative class switch recombinase distinct from RAG-1 and RAG-2 that has not yet been identified mediates CSR. Although this **CSR recombinase** has not been identified, the **activation-induced cytidine deaminase** (**AID**) gene, which is defective in one form of **autosomal recessive hyper-IgM syndrome**, is required for CSR. It is not understood how AID regulates CSR, but it is postulated that AID may be the catalytic subunit of an RNA-editing complex that edits the transcript encoding a nicking endonuclease specific to stem-loop structures (Honjo et al., 2002; Okazaki et al., 2002) or alternatively, and more likely, by cytidine deamination that generates uracils in the switch region at the DNA level. Although AID is required for both somatic hypermutation and CSR, they can occur as independent events. IgM antibodies may exhibit extensive somatic hypermutation with abundant mutations, and conversely, isotype switching occurs in the absence of somatic hypermutation in naïve B cells in the extrafollicular region of lymph nodes. AID deficiency is discussed in Chapter 13.

OVERVIEW OF HUMAN B-LYMPHOCYTE DEVELOPMENT

B-cell development can be divided into an **antigen-independent stage,** which occurs in the bone marrow in humans after birth, and an **antigen-dependent stage,** which occurs in germinal centers of secondary lymphoid organs, such as the spleen and lymph nodes. During the antigen-independent stage, a stem cell undergoes B-cell lineage specification that is then followed by a defined commitment to the B-cell lineage. The committed B cell undergoes successive stages of development characterized by ordered expression of genes, cell surface markers, and immunoglobulin gene rearrangement events.

Immunoglobulin gene rearrangement events occur at the heavy and light chain immunoglobulin gene loci to produce an intact immunoglobulin molecule that is expressed on the surface of the naïve B cell. This antigen-independent stage of B-cell development generates the primary or preimmune antibody repertoire of naïve B cells.

This primary repertoire is then diversified in an antigen-dependent phase of B-cell development in germinal centers in peripheral secondary lymphoid organs activated by antigen binding to the surface immunoglobulin (sIg) of the B-cell receptor (BCR) and by signaling from activated T lymphocytes or antigen-presenting cells. The immunoglobulin genes of the activated B cell undergo a process of somatic hypermutation to give rise to mutated immunoglobulin molecules on the surface of the B cell that are selected for higher affinity binding to antigen. During this antigen-dependent or late stage of B-cell development, the B cell differentiates to become either a **memory B cell** or a terminally differentiated antibody-secreting **plasma cell**.

ANTIGEN-INDEPENDENT B-LYMPHOCYTE DEVELOPMENT

Stages of Antigen-Independent B-Lymphocyte Development

B-cell development is divided into distinct stages characterized by an ordered rearrangement of immunoglobulin H- and L-chain genes and expression of cell surface marker and genes (Ghia et al., 1998). Outside of fetal life, early B-cell development occurs normally only in the bone marrow. As depicted in Figure 3-13, B-lineage development proceeds through successive stages, including a **progenitor (pro) B cell**, an IgM H-chain (μ)–expressing **precursor (pre) B cell**, a surface IgM (sIgM)–expressing **immature B cell** that has undergone both H- and L-chain loci rearrangements, and an sIgM, sIgD–expressing **mature B cell** (LeBien, 1998). With B-cell development, initially there is lineage specification with progressive narrowing of the potential to generate non–B-cell lineages. This is then followed by a stage of commitment to the B-cell lineage. Both lineage specification and commitment are mediated by transcription factors.

Common Lymphoid Progenitor and Pro-B Cells

The earliest identifiable cell committed to the B-cell lineage is a pro-B cell that expresses on its surface CD19, as well as CD34, CD45RA, CD38, CD24, and CD10, and intracellularly terminal deoxynucleotidyl transferase (TdT) and RAG-1 and RAG-2. The IgH- and IgL-chain loci are in germline configuration at this stage of development. The pro-B cell is thought to derive from a CD19−,CD34+, interleukin-7 receptor (IL-7R)α+, TdT+ common lymphoid progenitor (CLP), which has the potential to give rise to B cells, T cells, dendritic cells, and NK cells (Kondo et al., 1997).

The progenitor for the CLP is a pluripotent hematopoietic stem cell. Another postulated progenitor of the B-cell lineage is a common lymphoid- and myeloid-restricted progenitor that can give rise to either lymphoid or macrophage-myeloid cells (Katsura, 2002).

B-cell lineage specification and then subsequent B-cell commitment are regulated by several transcription factors that limit differentiation capability to the B-cell

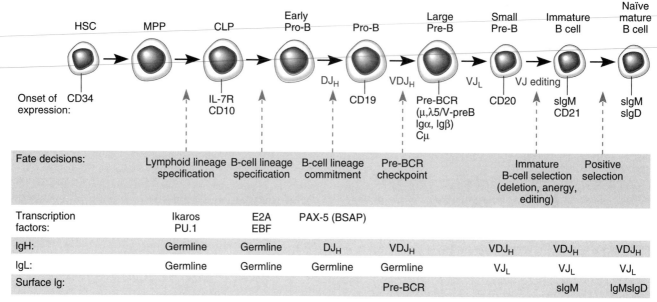

Figure 3-13 · Antigen-independent B-cell development.

lineage and prevent differentiation to other lymphoid and nonlymphoid cell lineages, as detailed later (Henderson and Calame, 1998; Kee and Murre, 2001; O'Riordan and Grosschedl, 2000). Lineage specification with expression of lymphocyte-associated genes occurs initially at the CLP and early pro-B–cell stage. B-cell lineage commitment subsequently occurs at the pro-B–cell stage.

Pre-B Cells

With differentiation, the pro-B cell undergoes initially DJ_H and then VDJ_H rearrangements. The L-chain loci remain in germline form. The pro-B cell differentiates to become a $CD34^-$,$CD19^+$ cytoplasmic IgM heavy chain ($c\mu^+$) large pre-B cell that expresses a productive VDJ_H rearrangement. Large pre-B cells may express on their surface a **pre-B–cell receptor (pre-BCR)** consisting of μ heavy chain linked to an SLC, which is composed of the λ5 human homologue 14.1 and Vpre-B.

The signal transducing molecules Igα (**CD79a**) and Igβ (**CD79b**), which will serve ultimately as the signaling components of the B-cell receptor (BCR) of the mature B cell, are also a component of the pre-BCR (Karasuyama et al., 1996). At this pre-B–cell stage, the cell is actively cycling and RAG-1 and RAG-2 are not expressed.

Only pre-B cells that have made a functional μ heavy-chain gene rearrangement that can bind to the SLC and generate a pre-BCR enter the cell cycle and undergo further development. It is unclear whether there exists a natural ligand for the pre-BCR, or alternatively and more likely, that formation of the receptor serves as a checkpoint for generation of a productive H-chain VDJ rearrangement that is capable of pairing successfully with an L chain at later stages of B-cell development.

It is believed that the productive pairing of IgH and the SLC, even in the absence of ligand, signals through the protein **tyrosine kinases Syk and Btk** to downregulate the expression of RAG and TdT, which leads to loss of accessibility and allelic exclusion at the IgH locus (Melchers et al., 1999b). Signaling also leads to the proliferation of large pre-B cells. The proliferation at this stage ultimately leads to mature B cells that share the same immunoglobulin heavy chain but express different light chains.

Btk is the tyrosine kinase defective in **X-linked agammaglobulinemia**, which in humans is associated with arrest of B-cell development. It is unclear which Btk-dependent molecules or signaling pathways are critical for early B-cell development (see Chapter 13).

Arrest of B-cell development is also observed at the pro-B– to pre-B–cell stage in C_H, λ5, or Igβ knockout mice and in human immunodeficiency disorders involving the same molecules. A paucity of large cycling pre-B cells is observed in these immunodeficiency disorders, suggesting that expression of a functional pre-BCR is required to activate pre-B–cell proliferation and progression of B-cell development.

Immature and Mature B Cells

The large cycling pre-B cell transitions to the next stage of a small, noncycling pre-B cell that begins L-chain rearrangement and ceases proliferation. At this stage, there is upregulation of RAG-1 and RAG-2 and downregulation of Vpre-B and loss of SLC expression. After L-chain gene rearrangement, an immature $CD20^+CD21^+$B cell is generated that expresses sIgM but fails to express sIgD. The immature B cell fails to proliferate or differentiate after antigenic stimulation but is susceptible to negative selection or induction of tolerance if exposed to a self-antigen, as described later.

At the final stage, the immature B cell then differentiates either in the bone marrow or in peripheral lymphoid tissues to become an sIgD$^+$sIgM$^+$ mature B cell. With B-cell development in the bone marrow, B-cell precursors move from the subendosteum at the inner bone surface toward the center of the marrow cavity, where they egress from sinuses in the marrow to secondary lymphoid tissues in the periphery.

After egress from the bone marrow to the periphery, B cells undergo a maturation process that is associated with expression of higher levels of surface IgD and lower levels of surface IgM. The majority of these newly **emergent B cells** die in the periphery within a few days unless they are selected into the pool of long-lived **mature B cells,** as detailed next.

B-Lymphocyte Survival and Selection into the Repertoire

Selection into the Long-Lived B-Cell Pool

Most B cells leaving the bone marrow die after a few days in the periphery (MacLennan and Chan, 1993). In the periphery, the immature **naïve B cells** enter the spleen through the central arterioles, enter the marginal zone, migrate along the outer zone of the **periarteriolar lymphoid sheath (PALS)**, and attempt to enter primary follicles. The immature B cell must compete for access to lymphoid follicles with the 10 to 20 times more abundant long-lived peripheral B cells. Cells that migrate successfully into the follicles receive a survival/maturation signal that maintains their lifespan for approximately 4 months.

Only 3% to 10% of the naïve immature B cells become part of the peripheral long-lived, mature naïve B-cell pool. The nature of this survival/maturation signal is not completely understood, but the BCR, the **tumor necrosis factor receptor (TNF-R)** family member **B-cell activation factor receptor (BAFF-R or BR3)**, the tyrosine phosphatase **CD45,** and the **tyrosine kinase Syk** are required. Thus some form of signaling to the B cell is involved in positive selection into the long-lived pool. It is unclear whether natural self-ligands engaging the BCR of immature, naïve B cells help mediate this selection.

Checkpoints to Censor Self-reactive B Cells

Not only is there cell loss as B cells egress from the bone marrow, but at each stage of B-cell development there is also extensive cell death (Goodnow et al., 1995; Melchers et al., 1995). B cells that fail to generate a functional pre-B cell and a B-cell receptor die from apoptosis. Only one third of pre-B cells express a productive IgH rearrangement, and then only some of these cells proceed to generate a functional L-chain rearrangement. B cells with successful productive IgH and IgL rearrangements are then censored to prevent the emergence of B cells that express a BCR that binds at high affinity to self-antigens.

Generation of a self-reactive BCR in the bone marrow leads to **clonal deletion** by apoptosis, induction of anergy, or activation of receptor editing of the BCR. The type and amount of antigen and the affinity of the BCR for self-antigens dictate which event occurs (Nemazee, 2000b). Cell surface and multivalent self-antigens activate apoptosis and thus clonal B-cell deletion. In contrast, soluble antigens tend to render the self-reactive B cell anergic and unresponsive to signals through the BCR. Anergic cells egress from the bone marrow but are short-lived in the periphery and fail to enter the long-lived circulating B-cell pool because of absence of basal signaling through the BCR and failure to migrate through lymphoid follicles, where they receive T-cell help.

Receptor Editing in Self-Reactive B Cells

A process termed **receptor editing** is also activated in self-reactive immature B cells (Nemazee, 2000a). With receptor editing, the original BCR is replaced by a new BCR through activation of a secondary light chain rearrangement. Receptor editing occurs because RAGs are still expressed in the pre-B cell after light-chain rearrangement and there exist nonrearranged V and J gene segments flanking the original self-reactive VJ light-chain gene rearrangement. With binding of a soluble self-antigen, the immature B cell maintains RAG expression and undergoes successive rearrangements at either the κ or λ immunoglobulin light-chain locus in an attempt to generate a non–self-reactive BCR. Receptor editing diversifies the repertoire.

Sites and Ontogeny of Antigen-Independent B-Lymphocyte Development

Hematopoietic development begins in the human fetus in the first month of life in the blood islands of the extra-embryonic yolk sac (Bofill et al., 1985; Kamps and Cooper, 1982; Lawton, 1986). By the second month of fetal life, hematopoiesis and lymphopoiesis are detected in the liver and by the end of the first trimester begin in the bone marrow.

Development of the B-lymphocyte lineage is not detected until approximately 7 to 8 weeks' gestation, when both pro-B and pre-B cells are first detected in the fetal liver. Immature sIgM$^+$sIgD$^-$ B lymphocytes are detected approximately 2 weeks later, and sIgD$^+$ mature B cells are detected at approximately 12 weeks' gestation. Mature B cells expressing surface IgG or IgA are detected shortly thereafter and simultaneously express sIgM and sIgD, in contrast to the sIgG- or sIgA-expressing B cells of older children or adults. By 12 weeks' gestation, the ratio of pro-/pre-B cells to immature and mature B cells in the fetal liver is 2:1.

The fetal liver remains a site of B-cell lymphopoiesis until about 30 weeks' gestation. At about 12 weeks' gestation, the fetal bone marrow becomes a site of B-cell development, and by midgestation the bone marrow becomes and remains throughout life the major site of B-cell development. B cells are not detected in the peripheral blood or other organs until about 12 weeks' gestation, but by 15 weeks' gestation they attain levels comparable to postnatal life. Population of primary lymphoid follicles by B lymphocytes becomes detectable in the tonsils and lymph nodes, intestinal lamina propria, and spleen by approximately 24 weeks' gestation, but germinal centers in these sites are not detected until after birth.

Although it is believed that fetal liver stem cells give rise to bone marrow stem cells, the origin of the pluripotent hematopoietic stem cell that migrates to the fetal liver to give rise to definitive B lymphopoiesis has been controversial. It has not been resolved whether the precursor to fetal liver B-cell development arises from the embryo proper, which in the mouse occurs in the **para-aortic splanchnopleura (P-Sp)** and its derived **aorta-gonad-mesonephros (AGM)** region or in humans in an equivalent region in the ventral endothelium of the aorta, or alternatively arises from the blood islands of the extra-embryonic fetal yolk sac.

B-cell lymphopoiesis continues in the bone marrow throughout life, with a relatively constant ratio of pre-B to immature B cells. After birth, B cells represent approximately 10% to 20% of peripheral blood and thoracic duct lymphocytes; 20% to 30% of the lymphocytes of the spleen, lymph nodes, and the mucosal lamina propria; and the majority of the lymphocytes of the bone marrow, palatine tonsil, and intestinal Peyer's patches and appendix. Microanatomic sites in these organs where B cells are concentrated include the follicles, germinal centers, and medullary cords of lymph nodes; the follicles, germinal centers, marginal zone, and red pulp of spleen; and the central follicles of Peyer's patches. B cells in the marginal zone, which are described in greater detail later, are not fully populated until after 2 years of age.

Approximately 5% to 20% of lymphocytes in the peripheral blood are CD19+ B cells. In the adult, about 60% to 70% of circulating B cells are IgD+CD27- naïve B cells and the remainder are IgD-CD27+ memory B cells that express either IgM, IgG, or IgA. The percentage of memory B cells increases during childhood to reach these adult levels.

Transcriptional Regulation of Antigen-Independent B-Lymphocyte Development

Several transcription factors are critical for initial lymphoid lineage specification (Schebesta et al. 2002). The **zinc-finger DNA-binding Ikaros** family members function to repress myeloid cell gene expression and to activate genes required for B-cell lineage development (Georgopoulos et al., 1997; Georgopoulos, 2002). The *ets* **family transcription factor PU.1,** acts on a common lymphoid-myeloid progenitor to determine whether lymphoid or myeloid/macrophage development occur (DeKoter and Singh, 2000; Simon, 1998). A low concentration of PU.1 induces a B-cell fate by activating transcription of the gene encoding the IL-7R α chain and downregulating the expression of the **c-fms gene,** which encodes a receptor for macrophage colony-stimulating factor (**M-CSF**). Conversely, a high concentration of PU.1 promotes myeloid differentiation and blocks B-cell development.

B-cell lineage specification is also critically regulated by the **basic helix-loop-helix (bHLH)** transcription factors **E12** and **E47,** generated by alternative splicing of transcripts of the *E2A* gene. These form B-cell lineage–specific homodimeric complexes that regulate expression of the immunoglobulin heavy- and light-chain loci and expression of RAGs (Rothenberg, 2000). A target of E12/E47 is the transcriptional activator **early B-cell factor (EBF),** which with cooperation from E12/E47 regulates the **mb-1** and **B29** genes encoding the Igα (CD79a) and Igβ (CD79b) signaling components of the pre-B cell and B-cell receptor (Gisler et al., 2000), immunoglobulin locus accessibility to RAG-1 and RAG-2, and expression of λ5 and VpreB of the SLC. Both E12/E47 and EBF also regulate the transcription factor Pax-5, which as described below then regulates B-cell lineage commitment. Another signal that determines fate decisions is Notch-1, which promotes T-cell development at the expense of B-cell development by inhibiting transcription induced by E12/E47.

Commitment specifically to the B-cell lineage is regulated by the paired-domain transcription factor **BSAP,** which is encoded by the **Pax-5 gene** (Busslinger et al., 2000; Morrison et al., 1998). BSAP/Pax-5 is expressed in all B-lineage cells except plasma cells, and its expression is regulated by E12/E47 and EBF. BSAP activates B-cell specific genes and represses transcription of lineage-inappropriate genes to suppress the development of myeloid, NK, or T-cell lineages (Busslinger et al., 2000; Kee and Murre, 2001).

The B-cell specific genes regulated by BSAP include CD19, the prototypic B-cell marker that is associated with B-lineage commitment, Vpre-B and λ5, both components of the pre B-cell receptor, Igα(CD79a), and BLNK (SLP-65), an adapter molecule required for signaling at the pro-B–cell stage (Neurath et al., 1995). BSAP simultaneously downregulates non-B–lineage genes, such as the M-CSF receptor and myeloperoxidase, both of which are associated with myeloid development. Pax-5$^{-/-}$ knockout mice lack lymphocytes that have undergone VDJ rearrangement, express CD19, or can be activated by soluble IL-7.

Regulation of B-Cell Development by Chemokines, Cytokines, and Accessory Cells

B-cell development is regulated by the interaction of B cells with stromal cells, membrane-bound and secreted lymphokines, adhesion molecules, and extracellular matrix components (Rossi and Zlotnik, 2000; Yoshie et al., 2001). The **chemokine stromal cell-derived factor-1**

The B-Lymphocyte System: Fundamental Immunology / 71

(SDF-1, CXCL-12, pre-B–cell growth-stimulating factor [PBSF]) is produced by bone marrow stromal cells and binds to the **chemokine receptor CXCR4** on B-cell precursors (Nagasawa et al., 1999). CXCL-12/CXCR4 interactions are required for the earliest stages of pro-B–cell development. In early fetal life these interactions retain developing B cells in the fetal liver and then in the bone marrow in late fetal and adult life. At the stages of the immature and mature B cell, there is loss of responsiveness to CXCL-12, which allows egress of the B cell from the bone marrow.

Other important stromal-derived signals regulating B cell precursor development include **stem cell factor,** which interacts with the cell-surface receptor **tyrosine kinase Kit;** vascular cell adhesion molecule-1 (VCAM-1), which interacts with the VLA-4 integrin of pre-B cells; flt3 ligand; and IL-7. In vitro, the earliest B-cell precursors respond to stromal cells, whereas more mature B-cell precursors respond to both stromal cells and IL-7; with Pax-5 expression, the pro-B cell responds to IL-7 alone. IL-7/IL-7 receptor interactions are required for pro-B– and pre-B–cell development. After egress of immature or transitional B cells from the marrow, B-cell signaling through its TNF receptor superfamily member BAFF-R (BR3) creates a requisite survival signal for the cell.

B-cell homing to follicles is also regulated by chemokine/chemokine receptor interactions. The G-protein–coupled **chemokine receptor, lymphoma CXCR5 (Burkitt's receptor 1 [BLR1]),** is newly expressed on mature recirculating B cells, required for B-cell homing to follicles in the spleen and Peyer's patches, and is

attracted to the **B-lymphocyte chemoattractant (BLC, BCA-1, CXCLL-13)** generated by stromal and follicular dendritic cells in these sites.

ANTIGEN-DEPENDENT B-LYMPHOCYTE DEVELOPMENT

Sites and Mechanisms of Antigen-Dependent B-Lymphocyte Development

Late or antigen-dependent human B-cell development occurs in secondary lymphoid organs after encounter with antigen to generate either a terminally differentiated antibody-secreting plasma cell or a memory B cell, which responds quickly after reimmunization with the production of high-affinity antibodies (MacLennan, 1994; Rajewsky, 1996) (Figs. 3-14 and 3-15).

Lymphocyte Activation in Extrafollicular Sites in Secondary Lymphoid Organs

In secondary lymphoid organs, B cells are activated by both antigen and T-cell help in the extrafollicular PALS to differentiate to become either a short-lived plasma cell, which secretes germline-encoded immunoglobulin, or a germinal center "founder" B cell, which migrates to primary lymphoid follicles.

Antigen-specific B cells first encounter antigen in lymph nodes near the **high endothelial venules (HEV)**

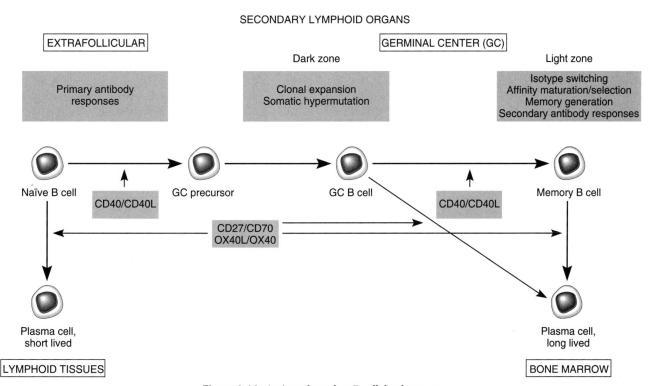

Figure 3-14 · Antigen-dependent B-cell development.

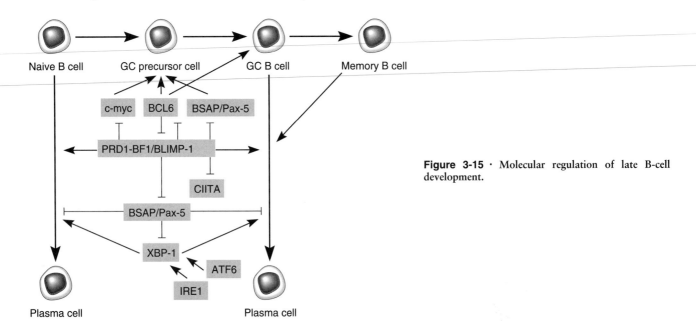

Figure 3-15 · Molecular regulation of late B-cell development.

and redirect their migration to the boundary of the B-cell and T-cell zones. Antigen binding activates arrest of B-cell migration by the engagement and activation of adhesion molecules or chemokine receptors on the B cell, including the chemokine receptor CCR7, which binds the **Epstein-Barr virus–induced molecule and ligand chemokine (ELC), macrophage inflammatory protein-3α (MIP-3α),** and **secondary lymphoid tissue chemokine** (Cyster, 1999; Melchers et al., 1999a). SDF-1/CXCR4 chemokine interactions may also be important in arresting B-cell migration.

The activated B cell also produces chemokines to attract CD4+ helper T (Th) cells that have been activated by antigen presented by interdigitating dendritic cells in the PALS. Both cognate T-cell interactions that signal through CD40 and CD80 and CD86 (B7.1 and B7.2) on the B cell and the release from T cells of soluble cytokines activate the B cell, as follows.

A primary, localized focus of activated antigen-specific B cells and T cells forms in the PALS that is associated with both B-cell proliferation and differentiation to antibody-secreting plasma cells. It is believed that the plasma cells generated at this site are usually short lived. The activated B cells also develop into germinal center precursor cells that are attracted to primary follicles. The **B-lymphocyte chemoattractant or chemokine (BLC, also known as BCA-1 or CXCLL-13),** generated by follicular dendritic cells in the follicle, attracts the cells by binding to the B-cell CXCR5 chemokine receptor. There is cross-stimulation between the B cell and follicular dendritic cell. The activated B cells produce lymphotoxin-α, lymphotoxin-β, and TNF-α to mature the follicular dendritic cell and increase their expression of BLC.

The decision for activated B cells to progress toward the antibody-secreting versus germinal center cell pathway is dictated by the state of maturation of the naïve B cell versus the memory B cell and the degree and type of T-cell help (Liu and Banchereau, 1997). Memory

B cells, in contrast to naïve B cells, differentiate preferentially to plasma cells after activation. T-cell/B-cell signaling between TNF superfamily members OX40 (CD134)/OX40 ligand(CD134L) promotes plasma cell development, whereas signaling between CD40L (CD154)/CD40 activates germinal center precursor formation (see Fig. 3-14).

B-Lymphocyte Development in Germinal Centers

The germinal center founder cells migrate to primary follicles, where they form germinal centers, characterized by an accumulation of proliferating cells at one pole of the germinal center termed the **dark zone** (Kelsoe, 1996). These proliferating cells, termed centroblasts, have a cell cycle time as short as 6 to 8 hours. Up to 10 B-cell clones may populate a germinal center, but there is an outgrowth of only 3 to 5 of these clones. The centroblasts have downregulated expression of their surface immunoglobulin and are also undergoing somatic hypermutation of their immunoglobulin V regions to diversify the primary antibody repertoire, a process detailed earlier (Kocks and Rajewsky, 1989).

Centroblasts then develop into nonproliferating centrocytes that accumulate in the **light zone** of the germinal center, where they are interspersed within a network of **follicular dendritic cells (FDCs)** and CD4 T cells. In the light zone, the centrocytes undergo positive selection of those B cells that express surface immunoglobulin with mutations that confer higher-affinity binding for antigen that is presented on the surface of the FDC. The centrocytes that receive a positive rescue signal from the FDC then continue to migrate through the light zone, where they interact with germinal center CD4 Th cells that recognize the FDC-derived antigen on the surface of the centrocyte. Those centrocytes that are positively selected then differentiate to become either memory

B cells, which populate secondary lymphoid tissues and circulate, or long-lived plasma cells, which egress from the lymph nodes or spleen as a plasmablast and populate the bone marrow.

Most of the B cells in the light zone do not differentiate into plasma cells or memory B cells but die from apoptosis. Positive selection and rescue from apoptosis is mediated by multiple receptor-ligand interactions between the centrocytes and FDC and antigen-specific Th cells. Antigen is presented to the centrocyte as antigen-antibody immune complexes that are deposited on the surface of the FDC through binding to either Fc or complement receptors. The native antigen can then be transferred from the surface of the FDC to the B cell, where it is internalized, processed, and presented, bound to MHC class II molecules, to CD4 Th cells, which then direct signals specifically to the antigen-presenting B cell.

Prominent among the diverse T-cell/B-cell interactions are CD40L/CD40 interactions, which stimulate memory B-cell formation and inhibit B-cell terminal differentiation to plasma cells. Conversely, OX40/OX40L and CD70/CD27 interactions activate differentiation to plasma cells. In addition to signaling the centrocyte through antigen, the FDC co-stimulates upregulation of surface MHC class II and B7.2 (CD86) expression on the B cell, which helps activate CD4$^+$ Th cells. FDC-B–cell interactions occur through multiple adhesion molecules, including **leukocyte function-associated molecule (LFA-1)** and **very late antigen-4 (VLA-4)** on the B-cell surface. The germinal center Th cells secrete cytokines that stimulate the B cell, including IL-2, IL-4, IL-10, IFN-γ, and TNF-α.

Expression of Cell Surface Markers

Late B-cell differentiation is characterized by changes in surface expression of B-cell receptors. Subpopulations of B cells can be identified in human secondary organs based on the surface markers—sIgD, CD38, CD23, and CD77, including IgD$^+$CD38$^-$CD23$^-$ naïve B cells, IgD$^+$CD38$^-$CD23$^+$ activated B-cells, sIgM$^+$sIgD$^+$CD38$^+$ germinal center founder B cells, sIgD$^-$CD38$^+$CD77$^+$ centroblasts, sIgD$^-$CD38$^+$CD77$^-$ centrocytes, and sIgD$^-$CD38$^-$CD27$^+$ memory B cells (Liu et al., 1996). Surface immunoglobulin expression changes with differentiation. The centroblasts in the dark zone downregulate surface immunoglobulin expression, which is later re-expressed with development of centrocytes in the light zone.

During terminal differentiation to plasma cells, the B cell shifts from expression of membrane to secreted immunoglobulin. The isotype of surface immunoglobulin changes during late B-cell differentiation. The IgD expression of the naïve B cell is lost with B-cell activation and isotype switching. Class switch recombination occurs both outside germinal centers in the PALS, where it occurs in the absence of somatic hypermutation, and within the light zone of germinal centers, where it occurs after somatic hypermutation has ensued.

Elimination of Self-Reactive B Lymphocytes

B cells that have become self-reactive through mutation of their sIg are either rendered anergic or die from apoptosis. Negative selection of B cells in the light zone of germinal centers occurs through **Fas-ligand-Fas (CD95L)/Fas(CD95)** T-cell/B-cell interactions that activate B-cell apoptosis, a pathway detailed later. Fas-mediated cell death is prevented by B-cell activation from antigen crosslinking of the B-cell receptor, CD40L activation, and B-cell signaling from the FDC. Self-reactive B cells that bind antigen in the absence of T-cell help undergo apoptosis. Therefore there are multiple checkpoints in secondary lymphoid organs to prevent the development of self-reactive B cells and to positively select B cells that express surface immunoglobulin receptors with high-affinity antigen binding.

Memory B Cells

Memory B cells are sIgD$^-$CD38$^-$CD27$^+$ B cells that express on their surface mutated immunoglobulin and increased levels of co-stimulatory molecules such as B7.1 (CD80) and B7.2 (CD86) and persist long term in the host. They are located in the circulation, marginal zone of the spleen, or mucosal epithelium, such as under the dome of Peyer's patches or in crypts of the palantine tonsil. Differentiation toward the memory cell pathway is promoted by CD40-CD40L interactions. The requirements to activate memory B cells are less stringent than for naïve B cells. In part, this reflects the upregulation of co-stimulatory molecules (CD80, CD86) on the memory B cell (see later discussion). When activated, memory B cells, in comparison to naïve B cells, are more prone to generate a plasma cell rather than a germinal center reaction, but some memory cells are maintained for future antigen responses. The differentiation of memory B cells to plasma cells is activated by CD70-CD27 interactions between CD4$^+$ Th cells and memory B cells.

Whether antigen must persist in the host to maintain the long-term viability of memory B cells has been debated (Gray, 1993, 2002). Protein antigens can in fact persist for prolonged periods after immunization as antigen-antibody complexes bound to the surface of follicular dendritic cells in lymphoid tissues. Although B-cell memory can be maintained for a prolonged period in mice in the absence of antigen (Maruyama et al., 2000), antigen can potentiate the persistence of long-term memory.

As described earlier, memory B cells arise after multiple cycles of B-cell proliferation in germinal centers. Proliferation in germinal centers is associated with the induction of expression of the ribonucleoprotein telomerase (Hu et al., 1997), which is expressed normally only by stem cells or germ cells and maintains the telomere length that is shortened with each cell division by approximately 50 to 100 bp. Telomere length acts as a mitotic clock with a critical short size of the telomere signaling cellular senescence. The upregulation of telomerase in germinal centers can preserve telomere length, longevity of the memory B cell, and immunologic memory.

Terminal B-Lymphocyte Differentiation to Plasma Cells

Activated naïve or memory B lymphocytes can terminally differentiate to an antibody-secreting plasma cell. The plasma cell is characterized by an eccentric nucleus with clumped chromatin around its periphery, abundant rough endoplasmic reticulum, a prominent perinuclear Golgi apparatus, and secretory vacuoles. The plasma cell has shifted from expression of membrane to secreted immunoglobulin messenger RNA (mRNA) and may devote as much as 20% of its protein synthesis to antibody production.

Plasma cells are detected in the mucosal lamina propria, perivascular sinuses of bone marrow, splenic red pulp, and lymph node medulla. Plasma cells that develop in the mesenteric lymph node or Peyer's patches primarily populate the lamina propria of the gastrointestinal tract rather than the bone marrow. The majority of serum immunoglobulin arises from plasma cells in the bone marrow. The isotype secreted by plasma cells in human tonsil is mainly IgG with smaller amounts of IgA and IgM. IgA secretion predominates in the plasma cells in the lamina propria of the gastrointestinal tract, Peyer's patches, and mesenteric lymph nodes.

With B-cell terminal differentiation to plasma cells, there is marked increased in immunoglobulin synthesis and secretion with loss of surface immunoglobulin, CD19, MHC class II, and CXCR5 chemokine receptor expression and upregulation of surface expression of **syndecan-1 (CD138)**, which binds to the extracellular matrix, and of the **CXCR4 chemokine receptor,** which is attracted to bone marrow stromal chemokine **CXCL-12** (Hargreaves et al., 2001). This represents a recapitulation of the lymphoid cell–stromal cell chemokine-chemokine receptor interactions observed with early B-cell development.

Plasma cell development is stimulated by OX40/OX40L and CD70/CD27 T-cell/B-cell interactions (Lens et al., 1998) and the cytokines IL-2, IL-6, and IL-10 (see Fig. 3-14). Plasma cells may be either short- or long-lived antibody-secreting cells (McHeyzer-Williams and Ahmed, 1999). The molecular basis for this difference is not well understood, but short-lived plasma cells are both activated and tend to reside in the extrafollicular foci of secondary lymphoid organs, whereas long-lived plasma cells are generated in the germinal center and reside in the bone marrow and other lymphoid tissues. Plasma cells do not respond to secondary immunization directly but must be regenerated from memory B cells.

Transcriptional Regulation of Antigen-Dependent B-Lymphocyte Differentiation

Late B-cell differentiation is regulated by multiple transcription factors that initially control B-cell proliferation in the germinal center and inhibit terminal differentiation (see Fig. 3-15) (Calame, 2001; Schebesta et al. 2002). Other transcription factors arrest the cell cycle and initiate terminal differentiation. The **zinc-finger Kruppel transcriptional repressor BCL-6** plays a prominent and critical role in germinal center B-cell development and function (Shaffer et al., 2000). In the absence of BCL-6, the activated, extrafollicular B cell differentiates to a plasma cell. BCL-6 is a repressor of the gene encoding the zinc-finger–containing transcription factor **B-lymphocyte–induced maturation protein-1 (BLIMP-1, human homologue PRDI-BF1)**, a master gene regulator of terminal B-cell differentiation. BLIMP-1 activates genes whose expression is associated with plasma cells and represses genes whose expression is associated with germinal center B cells (Angelin-Duclos et al., 2000; Turner et al., 1994).

Terminal differentiation to immunoglobulin-secreting plasma cells is associated with activation of both BLIMP-1 and the basic region **leucine zipper transcription factor X-box–binding protein-1 (XBP-1)** (Morrison et al., 1998). BLIMP-1 represses transcription of *c-Myc* and other genes regulating cellular proliferation to signal the B cell to exit the cell cycle. Other genes transcriptionally repressed by BLIMP-1 are genes regulating B-cell function and identity, including the promoter that regulates the **MHC class II transactivator (CIITA)** to decrease MHC class II expression on the plasma cell and BSAP/Pax-5, which leads to induction of J-chain and IgH transcription in the plasma cell and decrease of CD19 expression on the plasma cell. BLIMP-1 is also a transcriptional repressor of BCL-6 (Calame, 2001), which feeds back to completely downregulate BCL-6 expression.

Terminal differentiation to an immunoglobulin-secreting plasma cell with its typical morphology requires increased expression of the **XBP-1 transcription factor,** whose expression is activated by IL-6. XBP-1 is a major component of the so-called **unfolded protein response (UPR)** pathway that is activated with endoplasmic reticulum stress as arises in plasma cells from high levels of antibody synthesis. The UPR pathway activates expression of both the **transcriptional regulator ATF6,** which activates XBP-1 expression, and the **endoribonuclease IRE1,** which generates an XBP-1 spliced transcript that is more efficiently translated and produces a more stable XBP-1 protein.

The UPR pathway signals the production of various **protein chaperones** that preserve high-output immunoglobulin folding, assembly, and secretion. Thus there exists a feedback loop whereby early plasmablasts that synthesize and secrete high amounts of antibody induce ATF6 and IRE1, which then activates higher levels and activity of XBP-1 for preservation and progression of terminal B-cell differentiation with high-output antibody secretion.

The paired-domain transcription factor BSAP/Pax-5 controls B-cell proliferation and class switch recombination by activating germline immunoglobulin gene transcription. BSAP/Pax-5 also is a negative regulator of the immunoglobulin 3′ enhancer and represses J-chain gene expression. Therefore a network of transcription factor interactions occurs (see Fig. 3-15), with down-regulation of BCL-6 gene leading to BLIMP-1 expression; this then downregulates Pax-5 expression, which leads to increased expression of XBP-1. BLIMP-1 also represses BCL-6 expression to re-enforce the pathway, leading to full loss of BSAP/Pax-5 expression and higher levels of XBP-1 expression to allow terminal B-cell differentiation with high levels of immunoglobulin production and secretion.

B-LYMPHOCYTE SIGNALING AND ACTIVATION

The B cell is activated by antigen binding to the BCR and by co-stimulation from both cognate or cell contact signals from antigen-presenting cells (APCs) and T cells and noncognate or soluble signals, such as cytokines (Banchereau and Rousset, 1992; Craxton et al., 1999).

B-cell activation involves several discrete steps, including (1) binding of ligands to surface receptors, (2) crosslinking and clustering of receptors, (3) signal transduction from the extracellular environment to the cytoplasm, (4) activation of multiple intracellular signaling pathways, and finally (5) alteration in gene expression to lead to cellular proliferation, differentiation, or maturation.

The extent and duration of engagement of antigen by the BCR determines which signaling pathways are acti-vated and to what extent. Decisions for B-cell activation, anergy, or apoptosis are dictated by the strength of the signal, the presence or absence of co-stimulation, and the state of maturation of the B cell. The BCR signals differently at various times in its development. In the absence of some basal level of signaling through the BCR, the B cell undergoes apoptosis. Multiple B-cell co-receptors influence signaling, including the BCR, CD19/CD21, CD40, CD80, and CD86, as well as receptors for multiple cytokines (e.g., IL-2, IL-4, IL-6, and IL-10), as detailed later.

B-Cell Receptor Activation

The major receptor for signaling throughout all stages of B-cell development is the BCR or pre-BCR (Fig. 3-16). The BCR is composed of discrete components that are noncovalently linked in the plasma membrane for both recognition and binding of antigens (IgH and IgL) and for transducing engagement of the BCR to activation of intracellular **protein tyrosine kinases (PTKs)**. The activation of multiple intracellular pathways leads to alteration in gene expression that signals expression of various transcription factors.

The signaling components of the BCR are composed of Igα (CD79a) and Igβ (CD79b), which are encoded by the mb-1 and B29 genes. On the surface of the B cell, there is expressed a ratio of one Igα/Igβ heterodimer per

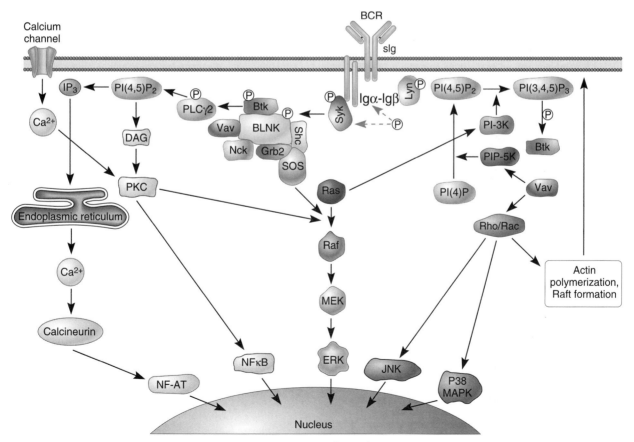

Figure 3-16 · B-cell signaling.

single immunoglobulin molecule (Matsuuchi and Gold, 2001; Reth and Wienands, 1997).

Both Igα and Igβ have a cytoplasmic domain with ITAMs, which have two YXXL (Y = tyrosine, L = leucine) motifs separated by six to eight amino acids. ITAMs are sites of tyrosine phosphorylation by specific receptor-associated Src-family tyrosine kinases and interact with intracellular signaling molecules. In the pre-B cell, Igα and Igβ are associated with the μ heavy-chain protein and the SLC, which consists of Vpre-B and λ5.

In addition to binding antigen and activating several intracellular pathways, the BCR also plays an active role in capturing protein antigens for processing and presentation by the B cell to T cells. B cells capture antigen from dendritic cells or other APCs through their BCR. Synapse formation occurs between the B cell and the APC with concentration of the BCR at the synapse (Batista et al., 2001). This process enhances presentation and transfer of antigen to the B cell, especially when antigen is present at low concentration. The antigen is then internalized by endocytosis to enter the cytoplasm. Crosslinking the BCR leads to receptor clustering and accelerates endocytosis of antigen in the form of BCR aggregates.

After endocytosis, antigen is processed in endocytic vesicles and presented as MHC class II–restricted peptides to antigen-specific T cells. The interval between capture and presentation of antigen may be as short as 20 minutes. The internalized antigen undergoes sorting through early endosomes, which requires the presence of the Igα and Igβ components of the BCR and the recruited PTK Syk. Properly sorted vesicles are then transported into specialized **lysosome-associated protein-1⁺(Lamp-1⁺)** late endosomes referred to as the MHC class II–enriched compartment.

Processing of antigen then takes place in the acidified environment of the late endosome to generate peptides that are loaded onto MHC class II molecules by displacement of the invariant chain (Ii) from the peptide-binding cleft. The nonclassical MHC molecule HLA-DM facilitates peptide loading, and another nonclassical MHC molecule, HLA-DO, which is expressed specifically in B cells at this location, negatively regulates loading and inhibits MHC class II–restricted antigen processing and presentation. The peptide–MHC class II complex is then expressed on the B-cell surface and recruits and activates CD4 T cells, which deliver cognate and noncognate signals to activate B-cell proliferation and differentiation.

The linked recognition of T-cell and B-cell responses to T-cell dependent (TD) antigens is exploited clinically with immunization of infants with the *Haemophilus influenzae* b (Hib) conjugate vaccines, composed of the Hib capsular polysaccharide covalently linked to a carrier protein. The vaccine can bind to Hib capsular polysaccharide-specific B cells and activate endocytosis of the conjugate. After processing, carrier-derived peptides are presented by the B cell to activate peptide-specific CD4 Th cells. The activated Th cells then stimulate B-cell proliferation, antipolysaccharide antibody pro-duction, and maturation of the naïve B cell to respond to the unconjugated Hib polysaccharide (Insel and Anderson, 1986).

B-Cell Receptor Signaling

B-Cell Engagement

Engagement and crosslinking of the BCR by antigen activates a cascade of intracellular PTKs that result in activation of B-cell proliferation, differentiation, cytoskeletal reorganization, and cell surface changes (see Fig. 3-16) (Cambier et al., 1994; Campbell, 1999; Hsueh and Scheuermann, 2000; Kurosaki, 1999). The cascade of signaling involves activation of Src-family kinases that in turn leads to ITAM tyrosine phosphorylation. Syk family tyrosine kinases are recruited to the phosphorylated ITAMs and are then subsequently activated. Adaptors are then recruited to the membrane and are tyrosine phosphorylated to lead to activation of downstream signaling molecules and ultimately the activation of transcription factors that alter gene expression in the nucleus.

With BCR engagement, four types of nonreceptor PTKs—Src, Syk, Tec, and Csk family members—are activated and redistributed in the cell. PTK activation is physically organized in the membrane of the B cell. With BCR crosslinking, there is a rapid topographic reorganization or translocation of B-cell membrane proteins that concentrates the ligated BCR into association with Src-family PTKs to promote phosphorylation and initiate signaling (Cherukuri et al., 2001b; Langlet et al., 2000; Satterthwaite and Witte, 1996).

Raft Formation

After BCR crosslinking, **glycolipid-enriched microdomains (GEMs)** of the membrane, termed **lipid rafts,** are generated, which include the BCR and multiple signaling proteins (Lyn, Syk, Btk, Vav, PLC-γ2, PI3-kinase, and BLNK) described later and exclude simultaneously most membrane proteins, including the phosphatases CD22 and CD45, which inhibit signaling from PTKs (Pierce 2002). In addition to facilitating the initiation of signaling and the optimal phosphorylation of ITAMS, raft formation also promotes endocytosis of antigen bound to the BCR.

Lipid raft formation is affected by the stage of B-cell differentiation and activation (Cheng et al., 2001). The BCR of immature B cells, in contrast to mature B cells, is excluded from rafts with signaling leading to apoptosis rather than B-cell activation. In anergic or unresponsive B cells, the BCR is also excluded from rafts, which leads to failure of transmission of an effective signal. In contrast to the BCR, the pre-BCR of the immature B cell is constitutively raft associated. This may explain why at this stage of development pre-B–cell proliferation is activated spontaneously after the generation of a μ heavy-chain protein that is capable of binding to the surrogate light chain.

Signaling Cascade

With BCR crosslinking and clustering, Src family PTK Lyn, as well as Blk and Fyn, in the lipid rafts phosphorylate each other and phosphorylate the tyrosine-containing ITAMs located on the cytoplasmic tail of Igα and Igβ of the BCR (see Fig. 3-16). The PTK Syk is then recruited through its tandem **Src homology 2 (SH$_2$)** domains to the tyrosine-phosphorylated ITAMs, where it becomes activated by phosphorylation mediated by Src kinases. Phosphorylated Syk amplifies and propagates signaling by phosphorylating the **cytoplasmic adapter protein BLNK (SLP-65, BASH)** (Leo and Schraven, 2001; Minegishi et al., 1999) and PLCγ2. BLNK integrates PTK activation with multiple downstream signaling pathways. These interactions are occurring in the concentrated microenvironment of the lipid rafts.

With activation of the BCR, the lipid kinase phosphatidylinositol 3-OH kinase (PI3-kinase) is activated and generates 3'-phosphorylated phosphoinositides, such as phosphatidylinositol-3,4,5-triphosphate (PI[3,4,5]P$_3$) from phosphatidylinositol-4,5-biphosphate PI[4,5]P$_2$, which facilitates recruitment to the membrane and activation of the Tec PTK, Btk, which is mutated in X-linked agammaglobulinemia. Btk is also phosphorylated by Src-family PTKs. Activated Btk binds to Syk-phosphorylated BLNK through its SH$_2$ domains, and BLNK and Btk recruit the phosphorylated lipid phospholipase C-γ$_2$ (PLCγ$_2$) from the cytoplasm to the membrane.

Activated and membrane-directed PLC-γ$_2$ enzymatic cleaves phosphatidylinositol-4,5-biphosphate (PI[4,5]P$_2$), located on the inner surface of the plasma membrane, to produce inositoltriphosphate (IP$_3$) and diacylglycerol (DAG). The IP$_3$ diffuses away from the membrane and activates the release of calcium (Ca^{2+}) into the cytosol from the endoplasmic reticulum via IP$_3$-gated channels. With depletion of Ca^{2+} in the endoplasmic reticulum, calcium channels in the plasma membrane open and sustain the increased intracellular Ca^{2+} concentration in a process termed capacitive calcium entry.

The quantity of IP3 generated by PLC-γ$_2$ dictates whether endoplasmic reticulum Ca^{2+} stores are emptied to generate a sustained flux of Ca^{2+} entry into the cell. The increased intracellular calcium activates Ca^{2+}-dependent enzymes, such as calcineurin, a serine/threonine protein phosphatase that dephosphorylates and activates the **transcription factor NF-AT (nuclear factor of activated T cells)**. DAG remains membrane associated where it attracts and activates, in the presence of increased Ca^{2+}, the serine/threonine **protein kinase C (PKC)**. This then activates the transcription factor NF-κB and other pathways.

BLNK also couples BCR activation to the **extracellular signal-related kinase (ERK)**, **c-Jun N-terminal kinase (JNK)**, and p38 mitogen-activated protein kinase (MAPK) pathways. BLNK binds to multiple other SH2-containing elements, including **Vav** and Grb2. Vav is a **guanine-nucleotide exchange factor (GEF)** that activates Rho-family GTPases (Rac-1, Rho-A, Cdc 42) by displacing bound GDP with GTP to activate downstream effectors such as PIP-5 kinase, and JNK and MAPK

pathways (Fig. 3-17; see Fig. 3-16). PIP-5 kinase replenishes PI(4,5)P$_2$ from PI(4)P. The PI(4,5)P$_2$ serves as a substrate for PI3-kinase, which generates PI(3,4,5)P$_3$, and for PLC-γ$_2$, which generates IP$_3$ and DAG, described earlier.

Activation of Rho-family GTPases also regulates polymerization of the actin cytoskeleton, which alters membrane structure and may enhance raft formation. BCR crosslinking also activates formation of Grb2-SOS complexes, which activates the Ras pathway. Ras then activates PI3-kinase, which generates PI(3,4,5)P$_3$ from PI(4,5)P$_2$, and activates ERK.

Signaling leads to the activation of various transcription factors, including AP-1, a heterodimer of Jun and Fos, NF-κB, NF-AT, and the **octamer-binding protein Oct-2** and its **co-activator OCA-B (Bob-1, OBF-1)**, all of which regulate gene expression critical for the antigen-dependent phase of B-cell development.

Modulation of BCR Signaling by Co-Receptors

Several co-receptors either enhance or inhibit signaling from the BCR (see Fig. 3-17). CD19 acts synergistically to enhance signaling through the BCR by reducing the threshold for B-cell activation (Fearon and Carroll, 2000). On the B-cell surface, CD19 is expressed as a noncovalent complex with CD21 (complement receptor 2, CR2), CD81 (TAPA-1), and Leu 13. Co-ligation of the CD19-CD21 complex with the BCR, as occurs when the B cell binds antigen or antigen-antibody complexes coated with the C3d fragment of complement, enhances B-cell signaling by recruiting the CD19-CD21 complex along with the BCR into the lipid rafts (Carroll, 1998; Cherukuri et al., 2001a; Fearon and Carroll, 2000). The CD19-CD21 complex prolongs signaling through lipid rafts by physically tethering the BCR in the rafts and preventing its internalization and degradation. This leads to sustained tyrosine phosphorylation of CD19 and other proteins within the rafts and thus prolongs signaling.

Phosphorylated CD19 recruits Src-family kinases and the **lipid kinase phosphatidylinositol 3-OH kinase (PI3-kinase)**, which generates PI(3,4,5)P$_3$ from PI(4,5)P$_2$, and recruits the adapter GEF Vav to the membrane complex. Vav activates small GTP-binding proteins such as Rac that stimulate the JNK pathway and result in activation of Jun, which binds to Fos to form the AP-1 transcription factor. Vav also acts to replenish PI(4,5)P$_2$ from PI(4)P by activating PIP-5 kinase. The PI(4,5)P$_2$ is a substrate for phosphorylated CD19-activated PI3-kinase to generate PI(3,4,5)P$_3$ and also for PLC-γ$_2$ to generate IP$_3$ and DAG, as described earlier. Coupling of C3d to an antigen enhances immunogenicity approximately 1000-fold to 10,000-fold by providing this dual recognition through both the BCR and the CD19-CD21 complex.

B-cell binding of soluble antigen-antibody complexes that do not contain C3d leads to co-inhibitory signaling by co-aggregation of the BCR, bound to antigen, and

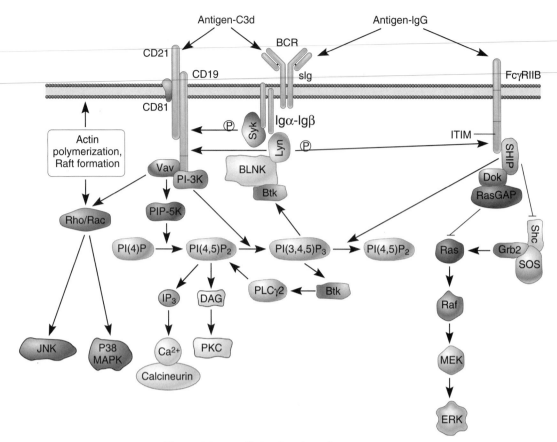

Figure 3-17· B-cell signaling through co-receptors.

FcγRIIb receptors, bound to the Fc of the antibody (Coggeshall, 1998) (see Fig. 3-17). With co-aggregation of the BCR and FcγRIIb, the phosphorylated ITIM of FcγRIIb recruits SH2 domain-containing inositol 5′-phosphatase (SHIP) and SHP-1. These dephosphorylate phosphatidylinositol triphosphate PI(3,4,5)P$_3$ to PI(3,4)P$_2$ and downregulate BCR signaling by altering the pool of phosphoinositides available for activating PLCγ$_2$ and Btk (Tamir et al., 2000). In addition, co-aggregation of the BCR and FcγRIIb results in tyrosine phosphorylation of the inhibitory RasGAP-binding adapter Dok. Phosphorylated Dok inhibits Ras activation both through SHIP and by recruiting Shc away from the Grb2-SOS complex.

FcγRIIb-activated signaling provides a mechanism for feedback inhibition by secreted antibody to the B cell and helps explain the induction of tolerance by passively administered intravenous immunoglobulin or specific antibodies, such as the prevention of hemolytic disease of the newborn with Rh immunoglobulin.

Other ITIM-containing inhibitory co-receptors on the B cell include **CD22** (Tedder et al., 1997) and the **paired immunoglobulin-like receptors (PIR-B)**. With BCR activation, the Lyn-phosphorylated ITIM of CD22 provides a docking site for SHP-1, which can dephosphorylate Lyn and Syk and inhibit signaling.

B-Cell Activation by T-Cell–Dependent Antigens

Full activation of the B cell requires simultaneous signaling through both the BCR and co-stimulatory receptors that engage either cell surface ligands or soluble cytokines (Table 3-3). For T-dependent antigens, co-stimulation is provided by contact-mediated or cognate signals and cytokine or noncognate signals from activated T lymphocytes (Bishop and Hostager, 2001). Upon binding to the B cell, the activated T cell forms a tight junction with the B cell and reorients its cytoskeleton and Golgi apparatus to localize its secretion of cytokines toward the B cell.

Contact-mediated signaling prevents promiscuous activation of self-reactive B cells, which are not eliminated as effectively as self-reactive T cells, and the physical contact between the T cell and B cell increases the efficiency of B-cell signaling by soluble T-cell cytokines. Engagement of the BCR primes the B cell to respond to T-cell activation signals by enhancing the expression of B-cell surface receptors for these T-cell signals.

Multiple TNF-R family members mediate B-cell co-stimulation and either promote cell death (e.g., CD95) or activate cell survival and oppose cell death (e.g., CD40L, BAFF-R, TACI, APRIL). Typical TNF receptor

TABLE 3-3 · B-CELL RECEPTOR AND LIGAND INTERACTIONS

B-Cell Receptor	T-Cell Ligand	B-Cell Effector Function
CD40	CD154 (CD40L)	Proliferation, differentiation, isotype switching, cytokine production, protection from apoptosis, germinal center and memory response development
CD80 (B7.1)/CD86(B7.2)	CD28/CD152 (CTLA4)	Co-stimulation
B7h (B7RP-1)	ICOS	Co-stimulation
Class II MHC	TCR; CD4	Proliferation, differentiation, enhanced antigen presentation
CD27	CD70	Differentiation into plasma cells
CD134L/OX40L	CD134/OX40	Stimulation, differentiation, and enhancement of IgG response
CD95/Fas	CD95L/FasL	Programmed cell death
CD30/CD153	CD153/CD30	Inhibition of B-cell responses, such as isotype switching and plasma cell differentiation
CD72	CD100	Production of high-affinity IgG, enhanced antigen presentation
CD137L/4-1BBL	CD137/4-1BB	Stimulation of T cells
CD11a-CD18/CD54	CD54/CD11a-CD18	Cell adhesion, enhanced antigen presentation, enhanced activation
LFA-3	CD2	Cell adhesion
ICAM-1, ICAM-2, ICAM-3	LFA-1	Cell adhesion
B-cell receptor	Non–T-cell ligand	B-cell effector function
TACI	BAFF > APRIL	Prevention of apoptosis, T-cell independent (TI) responses, B-cell proliferation and differentiation
BCMA	APRIL > BAFF	Prevention of apoptosis
BAFF-R	BAFF	Prevention of apoptosis of transitional, immature cells

family members contain several modules with six cysteines that form three disulfide bonds in their extracellular region. CD40 is a constitutively expressed TNF-R on the B cell that binds membrane-bound CD40 ligand (CD154, CD40L) on activated T cells (Banchereau et al., 1994).

CD40L engagement of B cell CD40 activates B-cell proliferation, antibody secretion, cytokine production, upregulation of surface molecules, isotype switching, development of germinal centers, and memory B-cell responses. Abnormal expression or function of CD40L occurs in **X-linked hyper-IgM syndrome (HIGM-1)** (Callard et al., 1993) and of CD40 or its signaling pathway in various forms of **autosomal recessive hyper-IgM syndrome**. These immunodeficiency diseases are characterized by poor IgG memory antibody responses.

Signaling by CD40 occurs through binding of its cytoplasmic carboxy terminus to cytoplasmic adapter **TNF-R–associated factors (TRAFs)**, which can associate with various kinases through its TRAF and zinc-binding domains (Grammar and Lipsky, 2000). Multiple kinases and signaling pathways are activated through TRAFs, including the JNK and p38 MAPK pathway, phosphatidylinositol 3-OH kinase (PI3-kinase), and the NF-κB–inducing kinase (NIK). Activation of these kinases leads to **IκB kinase (IKK)** activation, which phosphorylates IκB that is bound to cytoplasmic NF-κB (Fig. 3-18). This leads to ubiquitination and proteolytic degradation of IκB and subsequent release of NF-κB to permit its translocation to the nucleus where its induces gene transcription.

The B and T cells mutually signal each other in a stepwise manner with successive upregulation of various surface signaling ligands or receptors. CD40L activation of B-cell CD40 upregulates both B-cell CD86 (B7-2), which is constitutively expressed and is further upregulated quickly with B-cell activation, and B-cell CD80 (B7-1), which becomes newly and more slowly expressed after B-cell activation. CD28, which is constitutively expressed on T cells, then binds to CD80 and CD86 (Hathcock and Hodes, 1996; Lenschow et al., 1996) and signals increased production of T-cell cytokines and Th cell commitment to either Th1 or Th2 cell subsets.

Multiple cytokines (IL-2, IL-4, IL-5, IL-6, IL-10, IL-13) are generated by the activated T cell and promote B-cell proliferation, differentiation, or isotype switching. T-cell **cytotoxic T-lymphocyte–associated protein-4 (CTLA4)**, expressed by the activated T cell, later binds to B-cell CD80/CD86 and downregulates the activated T cell. With initial B-cell or APC activation of the T cell, the **inducible co-stimulatory molecule (ICOS)**, a CD28 homologue, becomes expressed on T cells that have been activated through both CD28 and the T-cell antigen receptor. ICOS can bind to B7h (B7RP-1), which has homology to CD80/CD86, on the B cell and also signal B-cell activation, isotype switching, and germinal center formation. The interaction between ICOS and B7RP-1 appears to be particularly important for activating IgE production for allergic responses.

B-Cell Activation by T-Cell–Independent Antigens

T-cell–independent antigens are polymeric, repetitive antigens that induce the proliferation and differentiation of B cells in the absence of T-cell help (Mond et al., 1995). Multiple bacterial polysaccharides, which have a polymeric structure, appear to require less or alternative forms of T-cell help (Vos et al., 2000). It is conceivable that raft formation is readily facilitated by the repetitive epitopes of polymeric antigen that efficiently crosslink the BCR. The status of T-independent antigens in humans, however, is not as clear as in mice.

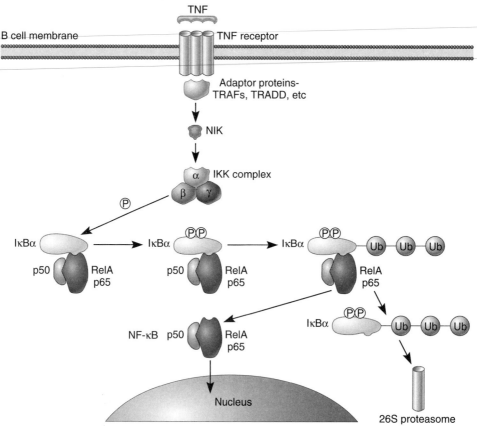

Figure 3-18 · Activation of the NF-κB pathway. Signaling through TNF receptors activates the NF-κB–inducing kinase (NIK) that activates the trimeric I Kappa B (IκB) Kinase (IKK) enzyme complex. IKK then phosphorylates I κBα, which leads to its modification with ubiquitin (Ub) groups and subsequent degradation by the 26S proteasome. Release of IκBα frees NF-κB, composed of its RelA and p50 subunits, to move to the nucleus where it activates target genes.

B cells in the marginal zone of the spleen, a microanatomic site located around the mantle zone in the periphery of the splenic white pulp, respond efficiently to polysaccharides and other antigens (Martin et al., 2001; Spencer et al., 1998). The B cells in the marginal zone include a distinct population of noncirculating naïve B cells that differ from follicular B cells in higher levels of surface complement receptors (CD21), sIgM, and basal and induced levels of B7-1 and B7-2, lower levels of surface IgD and CD23, and their ability to rapidly differentiate into plasma cells after activation. Marginal zone B cells develop slowly in life and do not reach the number observed in the adult until approximately 3 to 5 years of age.

The marginal zone is perfused with blood from the central arterioles and thus encounters antigen early with antigen entry into the bloodstream. Antigen with bound complement components C3 and C4 are targeted to marginal zone macrophages that express receptors for these components of complement (CR3, CR4). Antigen with bound C3d, the activation product of the third component of complement, binds simultaneously to the BCR and to the CD19-CD21 complex on marginal zone B cells to enhance B-cell signaling. In mice, CD5+ B1 B cells are a major source of natural antibodies, but the role of CD5+ B cells in humans is unclear.

Rapidly after encounter with antigen, marginal zone B cells generate germline-encoded antibodies that display low-affinity, multireactive specificity. These so-called **natural antibodies** play a role in the initial handling of infectious agents that enter the bloodstream by neutralizing a pathogen or forming antigen-antibody complexes, which promote antigen clearance by complement-mediated lysis or uptake by cells, including follicular dendritic cells in germinal centers of secondary lymphoid organs. B cells that can generate a specific, high-affinity antibody response, such as follicular B cells, are activated by the complement-bound antigen through co-activation of the BCR and the CD19-CD21 complex on the B-cell surface.

Activation of marginal zone B cells and other B cells by T-cell–independent antigens requires co-stimulatory signals generated by APCs, such as dendritic cells and macrophages. Prominent among these co-stimulatory signals are TNF superfamily members **B-cell activation factor BAFF** (also known as **BLyS, TALL-1, THANK,** or **zTNF4**) and the proliferation-inducing ligand **APRIL**, which are expressed on and secreted by APCs such as macrophages, monocytes, and dendritic cells (Khare and Hsu, 2001). BAFF and APRIL bind to the TNF-R family members **transmembrane activator and calcium modulator and cyclophilin ligand interactor**

(TACI) and **B-cell maturation antigen (BCMA) receptors,** which are constitutively expressed on B cells. BAFF binds better to the TACI receptor and APRIL to the BCMA receptor. BAFF but not APRIL also binds to a third TNF-R, the BAFF-R (BR3), which prevents apoptosis of transitional, immature B cells. TNF-R engagement by BAFF and APRIL activates intracellular TNF-R associated factors, so-called TRAF proteins that then activate NFκB and antiapoptotic pathways (see Fig. 3-18).

Signaling through the TACI receptor is essential for responses to some T-cell–independent antigens and through the BAFF-R for responses to T-dependent antigens and for survival of immature or transitional B cells to become long-lived, mature follicular and marginal zone B cells. Antigen signaling through the BCR in the absence of BAFF or APRIL signaling leads to apoptosis or programmed cell death. The combination of BCR and BAFF/APRIL signaling therefore is required to activate the B cell and prevent apoptosis. Self-reactive B cells that fail to receive BAFF or APRIL co-stimulation die from apoptosis. T-cell–independent antigens probably require co-stimulation from both BCR crosslinking and simultaneous BAFF signaling through the TACI receptor.

Death Signals for B Cells

Apoptosis occurs in B cells that fail to generate a functional BCR, generate a self-reactive BCR, fail to be recruited into the long-lived circulating pool, fail to be rescued by antigen and T-cell help in germinal centers, or become self-reactive after somatic hypermutation of their immunoglobulin genes. B cells require continuous signaling through the BCR to avoid cell death from neglect.

Fas-Mediated Apoptosis

TNF-R family members promote either cell survival or cell death. The TNF-R family member Fas (CD95, APO-1) on B cells is a cell death receptor that signals apoptosis of self-reactive B cells after binding to the Fas ligand (CD95L), expressed on the surface of activated T cells (Arch and Thompson, 1999; Matiba et al., 1997) (Fig. 3-19). Fas signaling activates *c*ysteine proteases with *asp*artic acid specificity, so-called **caspases,** that signal sequentially to mediate apoptosis. Target proteins of the caspases include cell structural proteins, kinases, signaling proteins, cell cycle control proteins, and DNA repair proteins.

After Fas ligand binds to and trimerizes Fas on the B-cell surface, a **death-inducing signaling complex (DISC)** is recruited to the trimerized Fas composed of the adapter protein **Fas-associated death domain (FADD/MORT-1)** and **procaspase-8 (Fas-associated death-domain–like interleukin-1-beta converting enzyme [ICE] or FLICE),** a member of the ICE family of proteases (see Fig. 3-19) (Rathmell and Thompson, 1999). FADD binds through its death domain to the death domain of Fas and through its death effector domain to one of the death effector domains of procaspase-8.

With binding and clustering by FADD, procaspase-8 is transactivated and converted from its proenzyme form to its hetero-tetrameric active form. Activated caspase-8 then initiates a cascade of ICE family protease activation that culminates in activation of the effector caspase-3, which cleaves multiple proteins required for cell survival, death-inducing substrates, and I-CAD, an inhibitor of the **caspase-activated DNAse/DNA fragmentation factor (CAD)** that digests nuclear DNA.

Autoimmune Lymphoproliferative Syndrome

Signaling through the BCR or CD40 inhibits the Fas signaling pathway by upregulating the **cellular FLICE-inhibitory protein (c-FLIP),** which is composed of death effector domains that can bind to FADD or pro-caspase-8 to prevent the formation of a functional DISC and thus inhibit activation of caspase-8. Deficiency of Fas signaling, which may occur secondary to dysfunction at several steps in the signaling pathway, occurs in the **autoimmune lymphoproliferative syndrome (ALPS),** characterized by B-cell proliferation, lymphoid hyperplasia, hypergammaglobulinemia, lymphomas, and autoimmune disease (Straus et al., 1999) (see Chapter 19).

Mitochondrial Apoptosis

A second pathway of apoptosis may also be initiated at the mitochondrial level by the release of cytochrome c from the mitochondrial intermembranous space (see Fig. 3-19). The cytosolic cytochrome c binds to the *apoptotic protease-activating factor* Apaf-1 to generate an Apaf-1/cytochrome-c complex that recruits pro-caspase-9. Caspase-9 is generated from autoproteolysis of pro-caspase-9. Caspase-3 is then activated by caspase-9. The two pathways of apoptosis are interconnected. Caspase-8 activation through the Fas pathway leads to cleavage and activation of the Bcl-2 family member Bid to form an activated, truncated Bid (tBid), which promotes release of cytochrome c by inhibiting Bcl-2 in the outer membrane of the mitochondria, as described later.

Regulation of Apoptosis

Activation of apoptosis is regulated by the Bcl-2 gene family, which includes the apoptosis-inhibiting genes Bcl-2 and Bcl-X_L and the apoptosis-promoting genes Bax and Bad (Newton and Strasser, 2000; Rathmell and Thompson, 1999). Bcl-2 and Bcl-X_L prevent apoptosis by binding to the outer membrane of mitochondria, where they generate cation-specific channels and prevent the release of cytochrome c. Bcl-2 plays a prominent role in preventing apoptosis in antigen-independent or early B-cell development, and Bcl-X_L takes on a greater role in antigen-dependent or late B-cell development that occurs in the germinal center. Regulation of the pathways is also mediated by inhibitors of caspase activity, such as **inhibition of apoptosis proteins (IAP).**

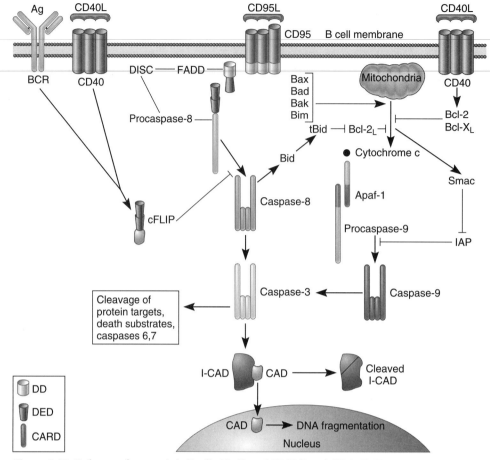

Figure 3-19·Pathways of apoptosis in B cells. Binding of CD95 ligand (CD95L) (FasL) trimerizes CD95 (Fas) and attracts through it death domain (DD), the FADD protein that in turn through its death effector domain (DED) attracts procaspase-8 (also known as Fas-associated death-domain–like interleukin-1-beta–converting enzyme [FLICE]). This complex of CD95, FADD, and procaspase-8 forms the death-inducing signaling complex (DISC) that oligomerizes and activates procaspase-8 to the heterotetrameric caspase-8. Caspase-8 in turn activates downstream effector caspases, including caspase-3, that cleave multiple proteins required for cell viability, including the inhibitor of the caspase-activatable DNAse/DNA fragmentation factor (I-CAD). A second intrinsic pathway of apoptosis occurs at a mitochondrial level from release of cytochrome c, which complexes with apoptotic-protease–activating factor-1 (Apaf-1) and binds to procaspase-9 through its caspase recruiting domain (CARD). Procaspase-9 is converted to caspase-9, which in turn activates caspase-3. The two pathways are linked through caspase-8 activation of Bid. Regulation of the pathways can occur at the level of cellular-FLICE–inhibitory proteins (c-FLIP), which inhibit activation of caspase-8 and are activated by CD40 or BCR signaling. The antiapoptotic members of the Bcl-2 family (Bcl-2 and Bcl-X_L) inhibit release of cytochrome c from the mitochondria.

R E F E R E N C E S

Alzari PM, Lascombe, MB, Poljak RJ. Three-dimensional structure of antibodies. Annu Rev Immunol 6:555–580, 1988.

Angelin-Duclos C, Cattoretti G, Lin KI, Calame K. Commitment of B lymphocytes to a plasma cell fate is associated with Blimp-1 expression in vivo. J Immunol 165:5462–5471, 2000.

Arch RH, Thompson CB. Lymphocyte survival—the struggle against death. Annu Rev Cell Develop Biol 15:113–140, 1999.

Bancereau J, Bazan F, Blanchard D, Briere F, Galizzi JP, Van K, Liu YJ, Rousset F, Saeland S. The CD40 antigen and its ligand. Annu Rev Immunol 12:881–922, 1994.

Bancereau J, Rousset F. Human B lymphocytes: phenotype, proliferation, and differentiation. Adv Immunol 52:125–262, 1992.

Batista FD, Iber D, Neuberger MS. B cells acquire antigen from target cells after synapse formation. Nature 411:489–494, 2001.

Berzofsky JA, Berkower IJ. Immunogenicity and antigen structure. In Paul WE, ed. Fundamental Immunology, ed 4. Philadelphia, Lippincott-Raven Publishers, 1999, pp 651–699.

Bishop GA, Hostager BS. B lymphocyte activation by contact-mediated interactions with T lymphocytes. Curr Opin Immunol 13:278–285, 2001.

Bofill M, Janossy G, Janossa M, Burford GD, Seymour GJ, Wernet P, Kelemen E. Human B cell development. II. Subpopulations in the human fetus. J Immunol 134:1531–1538, 1985.

Braun J, Stiehm ER. The B-lymphocyte system. In Stiehm ER, ed. Immunologic Disorders in Infants and Children, ed 4. Philadelphia, WB Saunders, 1996, pp 35–74.

Busslinger M, Nutt SL, Rolink AG. Lineage commitment in lymphopoiesis. Curr Opin Immunol 12:151–158, 2000.

Calame KL. Plasma cells: finding new light at the end of B cell development. Nat Rev Immunol 2:1103–1108, 2001.

Callard RE, Armitage RJ, Fanslow WC, Spriggs MK. CD40 ligand and its role in X-linked hyper-IgM syndrome. Immunol Today 14:559–564, 1993.

Cambier JC, Pleiman CM, Clark MR. Signal transduction by the B cell antigen receptor and its coreceptors. Annu Rev Immunol 12:457–486, 1994.

Campbell KS. Signal transduction from the B-cell antigen receptor. Curr Opin Immunol 11:256–264, 1999.

Carroll, MC. The role of complement and complement receptors in induction and regulation of immunity. Annu Rev Immunol 16:545–568, 1998.

Cheng PC, Cherukuri A, Dykstra M, Malapati S, Sproul T, Chen MR, Pierce SK. Floating the raft hypothesis: the roles of lipid rafts in B cell antigen receptor function. Semin Immunol 13:107–114, 2001.

Cherukuri A, Cheng PC, Sohn HW, Pierce SK. The CD19/CD21 complex functions to prolong B cell antigen receptor signaling from lipid rafts. Immunity 14:169–179, 2001a.

Cherukuri A, Dykstra M, Pierce SK. Floating the raft hypothesis: lipid rafts play a role in immune cell activation. Immunity 14:657–660, 2001b.

Coffman RL, Lebman DA, Rothman P. Mechanism and regulation of immunoglobulin isotype switching. Adv Immunol 54:229–270, 1993.

Coggeshall KM. Inhibitory signaling by B cell Fc gamma RIIb. Curr Opin Immunol 10:306–312, 1998.

Conrad DH. Fc epsilon RII/CD23: the low affinity receptor for IgE. Annu Rev Immunol 8:623–645, 1990.

Cook GP, Tomlinson IM. The human immunoglobulin V-H repertoire. Immunol Today 16:237–242, 1995.

Craxton A, Otipoby KL, Jiang A, Clark EA. Signal transduction pathways that regulate the fate of B lymphocytes. Adv Immunol 73:79–152, 1999.

Cyster JG. Chemokines and cell migration in secondary lymphoid organs. Science 286:2098–2102, 1999.

Daeron M. Fc receptor biology. Annu Rev Immunol 15:203–234, 1997.

Davies DR, Cohen GH. Interactions of protein antigens with antibodies. Proc Natl Acad Sci USA 93:7–12, 1996.

DeKoter RP, Singh H. Regulation of B lymphocyte and macrophage development by graded expression of PU.1. Science 288:1439–1441, 2000.

Fearon DT, Carroll MC. Regulation of B lymphocyte responses to foreign and self-antigens by the CD19/CD21 complex. Annu Rev Immunol 18:393–422, 2000.

Fugmann SD, Lee AI, Shockett PE, Villey IJ, Schatz DG. The RAG proteins and V(D)J recombination: complexes, ends, and transposition. Annu Rev Immunol 18:495–527, 2000.

Gellert M. Recent advances in understanding V(D)J recombination. Adv Immunol 64:39–64, 1997.

Georgopoulos K. Haematopoietic cell-fate decisions, chromatin regulation and ikaros. Nat Rev Immunol 2:162–174, 2002.

Georgopoulos K, Winandy S, Avitahl N. The role of the Ikaros gene in lymphocyte development and homeostasis. Annu Rev Immunol 15:155–176, 1997.

Getzoff ED, Tainer JE, R. Lerner RA, Geysen HM. The chemistry and mechanism of antibody binding to protein antigens. Adv Immunol 43:1–98, 1988.

Ghetie V, Ward ES. Multiple roles for the major histocompatibility complex class I-related receptor FcRn. Annu Rev Immunol 18:739–766, 2000.

Ghia P, Ten Boekel E, Rolink AG, Melchers F. B-cell development: a comparison between mouse and man. Immunol Today 19:480–485, 1998.

Gisler R, Jacobsen SE, Sigvardsson M. Cloning of human early B-cell factor and identification of target genes suggest a conserved role in B-cell development in man and mouse. Blood 96:1457–1464, 2000.

Goodnow CC, Cyster JG, Hartley SB, Bell SE, Cooke MP, Healy JI, Akkaraju S, Rathmell JC, Pogue SL, Shokat KP. Self-tolerance checkpoints in B lymphocyte development. Adv Immunol 59:279–368, 1995.

Grammer AC, Lipsky PE. CD40-mediated regulation of immune responses by TRAF-dependent and TRAF-independent signaling mechanisms. Adv Immunol 76:61–178, 2000.

Gray D. Immunological memory. Annu Rev Immunol 11:49–77, 1993.

Gray D. A role for antigen in the maintenance of immunological memory. Nat Rev Immunol 2:60–65, 2002.

Hargreaves DC, Hyman PL, Lu, TT, Ngo, N, Bidgol A, Suzuki G, Zou YR, Littman DR, Cyster, JG. A coordinated change in chemokine responsiveness guides plasma cell movements. J Exper Med 194:45–56, 2001.

Hathcock KS. and Hodes RJ. Role of the CD28–B7 costimulatory pathways in T cell–dependent B cell responses. Adv Immunol 62:131–166, 1996.

Hempel WM, Leduc I, Mathieu N, Tripathi RK, Ferrier P. Accessibility control of V(D)J recombination: lessons from gene targeting. Adv Immunol 69:309–352, 1998.

Henderson A, Calame K. Transcriptional regulation during B cell development. Annu Rev Immunol 16:163–200, 1998.

Hesslein DG, Schatz DG. Factors and forces controlling V(D)J recombination. Adv Immunol 78:169–232, 2001.

Heyman B. Regulation of antibody responses via antibodies, complement, and Fc receptors. Annu Rev Immunol 18:709–737, 2000.

Hondo M, Weissman IL, Akashi K. Identification of clonogenic common lymphoid progenitors in mouse bone marrow. Cell 91:661–672, 1997.

Honjo T. Immunoglobulin genes. Annu Rev Immunol 1:499–528, 1983.

Honjo T, Alt FW, eds. Immunoglobulin Genes, ed 2. London, Academic Press, 1996.

Honjo T, Kinoshita K, Muramatsu M. Molecular mechanisms of class switch recombination: Linkage with somatic hypermutation. Annu Rev Immunol 20:165–196, 2002.

Hsueh RC. and Scheuermann RH. Tyrosine kinase activation in the decision between growth, differentiation, and death responses initiated from the B cell antigen receptor. Adv Immunol 75:283–316, 2000.

Hu BT, Lee SC, Marin E, Ryan DH, Insel RA. Telomerase is up-regulated in human germinal center B cells in vivo and can be re-expressed in memory B cells activated in vitro. J Immunol 159:1068–1071, 1997.

Insel RA, Anderson PW. Oligosaccharide-protein conjugate vaccines induce and prime for oligoclonal IgG antibody responses to the Haemophilus influenzae b capsular polysaccharide in human infants. J Exp Med 163:262–269, 1986.

Jacobs H, Bross L. Towards an understanding of somatic hypermutation. Curr Opin Immunol 13:208–218, 2001.

Kamps WA, Cooper MD. Microenvironmental studies of pre-B and B cell development in human and mouse fetuses. J Immunol 129:526–531, 1982.

Karasuyama H, Rolink A, Melchers F. Surrogate light chain in B cell development. Adv Immunol 63:1–41, 1996.

Katsura Y. Redefinition of lymphoid progenitors. Nat Rev Immunol 2:1–6, 2002.

Kee BL, Murre C. Transcription factor regulation of B lineage commitment. Curr Opin Immunol 13:180–185, 2001.

Kelsoe G. The germinal center: a crucible for lymphocyte selection. Semin Immunol 8:179–184, 1996.

Khare SD, Hsu H. The role of TALL-1 and APRIL in immune regulation. Trends Immunol 22:61–63, 2001.

Kocks C, Rajewsky K. Stable expression and somatic hypermutation of antibody V regions in B-cell developmental pathways. Annu Rev Immunol 7:537–559, 1989.

Kurosaki T. Genetic analysis of B cell antigen receptor signaling. Annu Rev Immunol 17:555–592, 1999.

Langlet C, Bernard AM, Drevot P, He HT. Membrane rafts and signaling by the multichain immune recognition receptors. Curr Opin Immunol 12:250–255, 2000.

Lawton AR. Ontogeny of B cells and pathogenesis of humoral immunodeficiencies. Clin Immunol Immunopathol 40:5–12, 1986.

LeBien TW. B-cell lymphopoiesis in mouse and man. Curr Opin Immunol 10:188–195, 1998.

Lens SM, Tesselaar K, Van Oers, MH, Van Lier RA. Control of lymphocyte function through CD27–CD70 interactions. Semin Immunol 10:491–499, 1998.

Lenschow DJ, Walunas TL, Bluestone JA. CD28/B7 system of T cell costimulation. Annu Rev Immunol 14:233–258, 1996.

Leo A, Schraven B. Adapters in lymphocyte signalling. Curr Opin Immunol 13:307–316, 2001.

Liu YJ, Arpin C, De Bouteiller O, Guret C, Banchereau J, Martinez VH, Lebecque S. Sequential triggering of apoptosis, somatic mutation and isotype switch during germinal center development. Semin Immunol 8:169–177, 1996.

Liu YJ, Banchereau J. Regulation of B-cell commitment to plasma cells or to memory B cells. Semin Immunol 9:235–240, 1997.

MacLennan I, Chan E. The dynamic relationship between B-cell populations in adults. Immunol Today 14:29–34, 1993.

MacLennan IC. Germinal centers. Annu Rev Immunol 12:117–139, 1994.

Martin F, Oliver AM, Kearney JF. Marginal zone and B1 B cells unite in the early response against T-independent blood-borne particulate antigens. Immunity 14:617–629, 2001.

Maruyama M, Lam KP, Rajewsky K. Memory B-cell persistence is independent of persisting immunizing antigen. Nature 407:636–642, 2000.

Matiba B, Mariani SM, Krammer PH. The CD95 system and the death of a lymphocyte. Semin Immunol 9:59–68, 1997.

Matsuda F, Honjo T. Organization of the human immunoglobulin heavy-chain locus. Adv Immunol 62:1–29, 1996.

Matsuuchi L, Gold MR. New views of BCR structure and organization. Curr Opin Immunol 13:270–277, 2001.

McHeyzer-Williams MG, Ahmed R. B cell memory and the long-lived plasma cell. Curr Opin Immunol 11:172–179, 1999.

Melchers F, Rolink A, Grawunder U, Winkler TH, Karasuyama H, Ghia P, Andersson, J. Positive and negative selection events during B lymphopoiesis. Curr Opin Immunol 7:214–227, 1995.

Melchers F, Rolink AG, Schaniel C. The role of chemokines in regulating cell migration during humoral immune responses. Cell 99:351–354, 1999a.

Melchers F, Ten Boekel E, Yamagami T, Andersson J, Rolink A. The roles of preB and B cell receptors in the stepwise allelic exclusion of mouse IgH and L chain gene loci. Semin Immunol 11:307–317, 1999b.

Minegishi Y, Rohrer J, Coustan-Smith E, Lederman HM, Pappu R, Campana D, Chan AC, Conley ME. An essential role for BLNK in human B cell development. Science 286:1954–1957, 1999.

Mond JJ, Lees A, Snapper CM. T cell-independent antigens type 2. Annu Rev Immunol 13:655–692, 1995.

Morrison AM, Nutt SL, Thevenin C, Rolink A, Busslinger M. Loss- and gain-of-function mutations reveal an important role of BSAP (Pax-5) at the start and end of B cell differentiation. Semin Immunol 10:133–142, 1998.

Nagasawa T, Tachibana K, Kawabata K. A CXC chemokine SDF-1/PBSF: a ligand for a HIV coreceptor, CXCR4. Adv Immunol 71:211–228, 1999.

Nemazee D. Receptor editing in B cells. Adv Immunol 74:89–126, 2000a.

Nemazee D. Receptor selection in B and T lymphocytes. Annu Rev Immunol 18:19–51, 2000b.

Neurath MF, Stuber ER, Strober W. BSAP: a key regulator of B-cell development and differentiation. Immunol Today 16:564–569, 1995.

Newton K, Strasser A. Cell death control in lymphocytes. Adv Immunol 76:179–226, 2000.

Okazaki IM, Kinoshita K, Muramatsu M, Yoshikawa K, Honjo T. The AID enzyme induces class switch recombination in fibroblasts. Nature 416:340–345, 2002.

O'Riordan M, Grosschedl R. Transcriptional regulation of early B-lymphocyte differentiation. Immunol Rev 175:94–103, 2000.

Padlan EA. Anatomy of the antibody molecule. Mol Immunol 31:169–217, 1994.

Pascual V, Capra JD. Human immunoglobulin heavy-chain variable region genes: organization, polymorphism, and expression. Adv Immunol 49:1–74, 1991.

Pierce SK. Lipid rafts and B-cell activation. Nat Rev Immunol 2:96–105, 2002.

Poltoratsky V, Goodman MF, Scharff MD. Error-prone candidates vie for somatic mutation. J Exper Med 192:F27–F30, 2000.

Rajewsky K. Clonal selection and learning in the antibody system. Nature 381:751–758, 1996.

Rathmell JC, Thompson CB. The central effectors of cell death in the immune system. Annu Rev Immunol 17:781–828, 1999.

Ravetch JV, Bolland S. IgG Fc receptors. Annu Rev Immunol 19:275–290, 2001.

Reth M, Wienands J. Initiation and processing of signals from the B cell antigen receptor. Annu Rev Immunol 15:453–479, 1997.

Rossi D, Zlotnik A. The biology of chemokines and their receptors. Annu Rev Immunol 18:217–242, 2000.

Rothenberg EV. Stepwise specification of lymphocyte developmental lineages. Curr Opin Genet Dev 10:370–379, 2000.

Samuelsson A, Towers TL, Ravetch JV. Anti-inflammatory activity of IVIG mediated through the inhibitory Fc receptor. Science 291:484–486, 2001.

Satterthwaite A, Witte O. Genetic analysis of tyrosine kinase function in B cell development. Annu Rev Immunol 14:131–154, 1996.

Schebesta M, Heavey B, Busslinger M. Transcriptional control of B-cell development. Curr Opin Immunol 14:216–223, 2002.

Shaffer AL, Yu X, He Y, Boldrick J, Chan EP, Staudt LM. BCL-6 represses genes that function in lymphocyte differentiation, inflammation, and cell cycle control. Immunity 13:199–212, 2000.

Simister NE, Story CM. Human placental Fc receptors and the transmission of antibodies from mother to fetus. J Reprod Immunol 37:1–23, 1997.

Simon MC. PU.1 and hematopoiesis: lessons learned from gene targeting experiments. Semin Immunol 10:111–118, 1998.

Spencer J, Perry ME, Dunn-Walters DK. Human marginal-zone B cells. Immunol Today 19:421–426, 1998.

Straus SE, Sneller M, Lenardo J, Puck JM, Strober W. An inherited disorder of lymphocyte apoptosis: the autoimmune lymphoproliferative syndrome. Ann Intern Med 130:591–601, 1999.

Tamir I, Dal Porto JM, Cambier JC. Cytoplasmic protein tyrosine phosphatases SHP-1 and SHP-2: regulators of B cell signal transduction. Curr Opin Immunol 12:307–315, 2000.

Tedder TF, Tuscano J, Sato S, Kehrl JH. CD22, a B lymphocyte-specific adhesion molecule that regulates antigen receptor signaling. Annu Rev Immunol 15:481–504, 1997.

Turner CAJ, Mack DH, Davis MM. Blimp-1, a novel zinc finger-containing protein that can drive the maturation of B lymphocytes into immunoglobulin-secreting cells. Cell 77:297–306, 1994.

Vos Q, Lees A, Wu ZQ, Snapper CM, Mond JJ. B-cell activation by T-cell-independent type 2 antigens as an integral part of the humoral immune response to pathogenic microorganisms. Immunol Rev 176:154–170, 2000.

Wagner SD, Neuberger MS. Somatic hypermutation of immunoglobulin genes. Annu Rev Immunol 14:441–457, 1996.

Weaver DT, V(D)J recombination and double-strand break repair. Adv Immunol 58:29–85, 1995.

Yoshie O, Imai T, Nomiyama H. Chemokines in immunity. Adv Immunol 78:57–110, 2001.

C H A P T E R

4

The B-Lymphocyte System:
Clinical Immunology

E. Richard Stiehm

THE IMMUNOGLOBULIN SYSTEM

Components

The B-lymphocyte (B-cell) system is composed of the cells capable of immunoglobulin (Ig) synthesis (B cells and plasma cells), the precursors of these cells (stem cells, pro-B cells, and pre-B cells), and the products of these cells, the immunoglobulins. The entire system is directed toward one result, the production of a vast array of Ig molecules with different specificities (antibodies) that comprise the humoral immune system.

Although different types (classes and subclasses) of Ig exist, they make up a single effector system that arises from a spectrum of B cells. This is in contrast to the T-cell system (see Chapter 2), which develops into several divergent and distinct effector systems.

The preceding chapter delineates the development of the B cells, the mechanisms by which they are able to synthesize antibodies with thousands of specificities, and the structure and biology of the immunoglobulins. This chapter focuses on the function of immunoglobulins in health and disease, the methods used to assess them, and their value in diagnosis and therapy.

Definition

The immunoglobulins, also termed immune globulins or gamma globulins, are proteins endowed with known antibody activity and certain proteins related to them by chemical and antigenic structure. These related proteins are clearly immunoglobulins, but antibody activity has simply not been demonstrated for them—for example, myeloma proteins, Bence Jones proteins, and naturally occurring subunits of the immunoglobulins such as gamma-chain fragments in gamma-chain disease (World Health Organization [WHO], 1964).

The immunoglobulins, as the mediators of humoral or antibody-mediated immunity, are present as free molecules in the bloodstream, tissues, and exocrine secretions. Immunoglobulins also exist as integral membrane proteins on B-cell surfaces and therein serve the additional function of antigen recognition for the B cell–immunoglobulin system.

The functions of free Ig are (1) to combine with antigen (e.g., show specific antibody activity) and (2) to participate in adjunctive biologic functions such as opsonization, neutralization, complement fixation, transport into secretions, and immune complex formation. Different portions of the antibody molecule are involved in each; antigen binding is a property of the Fab, or *variable*, region of the molecule, and adjunctive biologic functions are properties of the Fc, or *constant*, region.

Immunoglobulin Heterogeneity

In the 1930s, the plasma proteins were separated by salt fractionation into albumin and globulins. In 1937 Tiselius introduced electrophoresis, which separates proteins on the basis of electrical charge. This technique permitted resolution of the globulins into four fractions: gamma, beta, alpha-2, and alpha-1. At a pH of 8.6, the gamma fraction migrates the slowest and the alpha-1 migrates the fastest, adjacent to albumin. Immunoglobulins from serum are primarily located in the gamma fraction, but some are also present in the beta and the alpha-2 fractions. The distribution of different immunoglobulin classes in serum is illustrated in Figure 4-1.

Subsequently, extensive chemical, serologic, and molecular studies have indicated that antibodies (immunoglobulins) possess considerable heterogeneity and make up a group of related proteins. Immunoelectrophoresis has been especially valuable in delineating this heterogeneity (Fig. 4-2). Immunoelectrophoresis combines the migration of a protein solution (such as serum) in an electrical field (electrophoresis), followed by immune precipitation in agar by an antiserum to the protein(s). The antiserum is placed in a trough parallel with the path of the electrophoretic migration to which the serum was subjected. The antiserum then diffuses toward the electrophoretically separated serum components. Where a protein that reacts with the antiserum is encountered, a distinct arc of precipitation is formed.

Immunoelectrophoresis of normal human serum discloses 25 or more separate proteins; three of these—IgG, IgM, and IgA—have antibody activity and are missing in the serum of patients with agammaglobulinemia (see Fig. 4-2). In addition to these three antigenically distinct immunoglobulin classes, two other immunoglobulins, IgD and IgE, are present in normal serum but are below the level of detection of immunoelectrophoresis.

Other techniques are used to further define immunoglobulin heterogeneity and structure. Starch-gel or acrylamide-gel electrophoresis, which separates similarly charged proteins on the basis of size by their different rates of migration through the gels, has been used to separate immunoglobulins and their subunits into multiple fractions. The molecular weight (MW) of immunoglobulins can be estimated using ultracentrifugation or filtra-

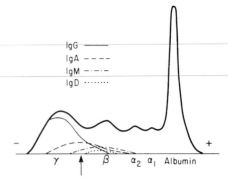

Figure 4-1 · **Electrophoretic distribution of the immunoglobulins.** There is an approximate correlation between the gamma globulin on electrophoresis and the total of the immunoglobulins measured immunochemically. Immunoglobulin E (IgE) is present in such small concentrations that it contributes insignificantly to the gamma globulin on electrophoresis.

tion through dextran gels such as Sephadex, which separates large-molecular-weight immunoglobulins (e.g., IgM) from other immunoglobulins.

Immunoglobulin structure can be visualized by use of the electron microscope. X-ray diffraction studies have been used to define the three-dimensional structure of immunoglobulin molecules (Nisonoff et al., 1975a). For this technique, however, pure crystallizable proteins or subunits, which are only occasionally available, are required.

Techniques to determine the exact amino acid sequence of proteins and peptides have been utilized to arrive at the primary structure of several myeloma proteins (Nisonoff et al, 1975b). Most recently the ability to clone the DNA sequences for the various constant region heavy- and light-chain genes has allowed the exact determination of the C-region composition (both the DNA sequence and thereby the amino acid sequence) for all the immunoglobulins.

Nomenclature

The nomenclature of the immunoglobulin classes and their structural units, codified by the World Health Organization (WHO, 1964, 1970) is presented in Table 4-1. All immunoglobulins are designated Ig, and the

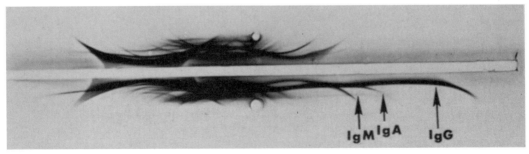

Figure 4-2 · **Immunoelectrophoretic analysis of an agammaglobulinemic serum** *(top)* **and a normal serum** *(bottom)*. The trough contains a rabbit antiserum to normal human serum. Each of the precipitin arcs that is formed represents a unique protein. The normal serum demonstrates the three immunoglobulins (IgG, IgM, and IgA) that are missing from the serum of the agammaglobulinemic individual.

TABLE 4-1 · CHAIN STRUCTURES OF THE HUMAN IMMUNOGLOBULIN CLASSES

Immunoglobulin Class	Heavy Chain	Light Chain	Other Chain(s)	Chain Formula
IgG	γ	κ		$\gamma_2\kappa_2$
		λ		$\gamma_2\lambda_2$
IgM	μ	κ	J	$(\mu_2\kappa_2)_5$-J
		λ	J	$(\mu_2\lambda_2)_5$-J
IgD	δ	κ		$\delta_2\kappa_2$
		λ		$\delta_2\lambda_2$
IgE	ε	κ		$\varepsilon_2\kappa_2$
		λ		$\varepsilon_2\lambda_2$
IgA	α	κ		$\alpha_2\kappa_2$
		λ		$\alpha_2\lambda_2$
Secretory IgA	α	κ	J, SC	$(\alpha_2\kappa_2)_2$-SC-J
		λ	J, SC	$(\alpha_2\lambda_2)_2$-SC-J

J = joining; SC = secretory component.

five classes are designated IgG, IgM, IgA, IgD, and IgE, all of which are present in normal adult serum (WHO, 1964, 1970). The class of immunoglobulin is determined by the heavy chain (mu, delta, gamma, epsilon, or alpha) for IgM, IgD, IgG, IgE, and IgA, respectively.

Each immunoglobulin molecule is composed of two pairs of polypeptide chains: one pair of identical heavy chains and one pair of identical light chains (see Table 4-1 and Fig. 3-1). There are two types of light chains, termed kappa (κ) and lambda (λ). Immunoglobulin molecules have two κ chains or two λ chains, never one of each. These two light-chain types are common to all immunoglobulin classes; the heavy-chain pair is different in each immunoglobulin class.

IgM primarily exists as a pentamer of five monomeric units of paired light and heavy chains, with an additional single-polypeptide molecule, the joining (J) chain (see Fig. 3-3). The J chain is common to all polymeric immunoglobulins (IgM and some IgA molecules). Secretory IgA present in exocrine gland secretions also is a polymeric molecule containing two and occasionally three IgA molecules, a J chain, and a secretory component (SC) (Tomasi, 1972) (see Fig. 3-3). Based on the chain structure of the immunoglobulin, the molecular composition of each of the immunoglobulin classes can be formulated (see Table 4-1).

Isotypes, Allotypes, and Idiotypes

Immunoglobulin molecules can be divided into three subcategories based on antigen differences within their structural subunits.

The *isotypes* are all present in normal individuals and include (1) the five major immunoglobulin classes, based on major antigenic and physicochemical differences in their heavy (H) chain (see Table 4-1); (2) the four IgG and two IgA subclasses, based on subtle antigenic variability within the H chains of IgG and IgA, respectively (Fig. 4-3); (3) the two light (L) chain types (κ and λ); and (4) several λ-chain subtypes. The latter are dependent on the presence or absence of certain nonexclusive antigenic determinants termed Oz, Mz,

Kern, and Mcg, initially identified on λ-chain Bence Jones proteins (Solomon, 1976). Other λ subtypes may also exist (Schanfield and Van Loghem, 1988).

The *allotypes* are genetic markers present on certain H- and L-chain isotypes that are inherited in typical mendelian fashion. Thus only certain individuals carry these antigenic determinants. The allotypes associated with the γ heavy chain are designated Gm (gamma marker). The allotypes associated with the α and ε heavy chains are designated Am and Em, respectively; those associated with the κ light chain are designated Km. No allotypes of IgM or λ light chain have been identified.

The *idiotypes* are unique antigenic determinants present on a single homogeneous antibody or an antibody

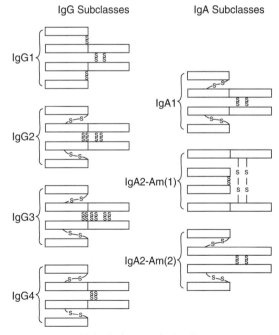

Figure 4-3 · Disulfide linkages of the human IgG and IgA immunoglobulin subclasses. The heavy-chain cysteine residue of IgG 1 forming the heavy-light disulfide bond is considerably closer to the C-terminal end than in the other IgG subclasses. The IgA2Am(1) molecule lacks the heavy-light disulfide bonds, which are linked by covalent bonds.

clone (M component). These are generally on the variable regions of the immunoglobulin molecule and, when involving the antibody combining site, the hypervariable region. Different classes or subclasses of antibodies with similar specificity may be directed against the same unique determinant (the isotype) and thus be of an identical idiotype.

Mouse and human monoclonal Abs are laboratory-derived idiotypic antibodies directed against a single antigenic determinant. A pathologic M component will generally have a unique antigenic specificity not shared by other immunoglobulins, directed against a usually unidentified antigen.

Idiotypes can themselves be immunogenetic. Following a normal immune response, anti-idiotypic antibodies are produced that may regulate and limit the immune response. Jerne's network theory (Jerne, 1974) states that a large number of idiotype–anti-idiotype interactions form a dynamic idiotypic network, which is essential for the development and control of the normal antibody response. Human immunoglobulin for therapeutic purposes contains multiple anti-idiotypes; their presence may be one reason why large doses of intravenous immunoglobulin neutralize or suppress auto-antibodies.

IgG and IgA Subclasses

The four IgG subclasses were initially defined by antigenic differences among the heavy chains of IgG myeloma proteins (Grey and Kunkel, 1964; Terry and Fahey, 1964). These antigenic differences among subclasses are less profound than among classes, so that rabbit antisera to IgG cannot distinguish between them. Mouse monoclonal antibodies from animals immunized with isolated myeloma proteins produce the best antisera for distinguishing between the IgG subclasses. In addition to their antigenic differences, IgG subclasses differ in their structural, chemical, and biologic properties (see Table 3-2 and Fig. 4-3).

Two subclasses of IgA—IgA1 and IgA2—have been recognized. Normal serum IgA has 93% IgA1 and 7% IgA2 (Vaerman et al., 1968). Only IgA2 has the A2m(1) and A2m(2) genetic markers. There is a considerably increased amount of IgA2 in the secretions (60% IgA2, 40% IgA1) as contrasted to the 9:1 ratio of IgA1 to IgA2 in the serum; this may confer resistance to secretory IgA-splitting enzymes known to be produced by bacteria in the gastrointestinal tract (Plaut et al., 1974).

Immunoglobulin Allotypes

Further variation in the immunoglobulins is based on the presence or absence of genetic inherited differences in immunoglobulin amino acid sequences. These were first described by Grubb in 1956. These inherited markers, termed Gm, Am, and Km, are allotypes (genetic alternatives within the same species controlled by allelic

genes) and are present in only certain individuals as determined by mendelian genetics.

The nomenclature and a list of genetic immunoglobulin factors are presented in Table 4-2. The recommended nomenclature (WHO, 1965, 1976) labels the allotypes first by class and subclass (e.g., G1m) and then by allele (in parenthesis). These factors are inherited in accordance with typical mendelian genetics (Natvig and Kunkel, 1973). There are at least 23 genetic factors recognized to date (Schanfield and Van Loghem, 1986).

Three groups of genetic factors are recognized:

· Gm factors, present on the γ heavy chain of IgG and thus limited to IgG classes
· Am factors, present on the α2 heavy chain of IgA
· Km factors, present on the κ light chain and thus represented in all classes of immunoglobulins

In addition, allotypy has been described for IgE (Em) by Van Loghem and others (1984) using a monoclonal antibody.

Methods of Detection

The original method of detection of Ig allotypy is cumbersome, as shown in Figure 4-4. Human O Rh-positive (D) erythrocytes are exposed to an incomplete Rh antibody (an IgG immunoglobulin), which will coat but not agglutinate them. This antibody is generally obtained from an Rh-negative multiparous woman sensitized by an Rh-positive fetus. The coated red cells will be agglutinated by human sera with rheumatoid factor (an IgM antibody

TABLE 4-2 · GENETIC FACTORS OF HUMAN IMMUNOGLOBULINS

Genetic Factor	Subclass or Chain Location
Factors at the Gm Locus	
G1m(1)	IgG1
G1m(2)	IgG1
G1m(3)	IgG1
G1m(17)	IgG1
G2m(23)	IgG2
G3m(5)	IgG3
G3m(6)	IgG3
G3m(10)	IgG3
G3m(11)	IgG3
G3m(13)	IgG3
G3m(14)	IgG3
G3m(15)	IgG3
G3m(16)	IgG3
G3m(21)	IgG3
G3m(24)	IgG3
G3m(26)	IgG3
G3m(27)	IgG3
G3m(28)	IgG3
Factors at the Am Locus	
A2m(1)	IgA2
A2m(2)	IgA2
Factors at the Km Locus	
Km(1)	κ
Km(2)	κ
Km(3)	κ

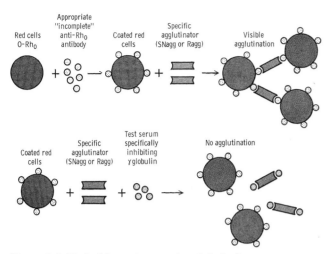

Figure 4-4 · Method for typing genetic γ globulin factors. (From Engle RL Jr, Wallis LA. Immunoglobulinopathies. Springfield, Ill., Charles C Thomas, 1969.)

that reacts with an IgG immunoglobulin) when the rheumatoid factor is directed toward the immunoglobulin allotype of the coat. This agglutination reaction between the rheumatoid factor (agglutinator) and the IgG-coated erythrocyte can be inhibited by a serum whose IgG has the same genetic determinant to which the rheumatoid factor is directed. If the added serum does not have the genetic determinant, no inhibition occurs and the rheumatoid factor will agglutinate the coated erythrocyte. Thus serum from an individual of G1m(1) type will inhibit the agglutination of an anti-G1m(1) rheumatoid factor with a G1m(1)-coated erythrocyte.

The sera of frequently transfused individuals may also contain antibodies to immunoglobulin allotypes (because of exposure of allotypes of immunoglobulin that the individual lacks) and can be used as agglutinators instead of rheumatoid factors. These sera are generally preferable because they have a higher degree of specificity (e.g., a narrower spectrum). The latter type of agglutinator is often called a serum normal agglutinin (SNagg) and is usually an IgG globulin; a rheumatoid factor is often called a rheumatoid agglutinin (Ragg) and is usually an IgM globulin (Fudenberg, 1963).

The inhibition of the agglutination system so described necessitates a pair of human serum reagents: a coat consisting of an incomplete Rh antibody, or myeloma protein, and a specific antibody (the SNagg and Ragg agglutinator) reactive to it for each factor to be tested. Newer techniques such as polymerase chain reaction (PCR) and monoclonal antibodies are increasingly being used (Grubb et al, 1995).

Gm Factors

The Gm groups are the most widely studied (see Table 4-2) (Nisonoff et al., 1975c). They are localized to the constant region of the δ heavy chain, and each is located on one of the four subclasses. Many of the Gm factors are inherited together; for example, G1m(1) and G1m(3) are either both present or both absent in any

individual. Others seem to be identical, including G1m(3) and G1m(4) and G3m(5) and G3m(12) (Steinberg, 1969). In many instances, the exact amino acid substitution is known; for example, G3m(21) and nG3m(21) differ as a result of a single amino acid substitution at position 296 of the C_{H3} region; G3m(21) has tyrosine and nG3m(21) has phenylalanine at this position.

Although Gm factors are present on the heavy chain, G1m(3) and G1m(17) require the presence of light chains for their expression, probably because of conformational change when the light chain is separated from the heavy chain.

Isoallotypes are Gm determinants that are allotypic variants in one subclass of IgG but are present in all molecules of at least one other subclass. These isoallotypes, or nonmarkers, are designated by the letter *n* or a minus sign before the allelic factor notation. The notation indicates the allotype present when other subclasses are absent. The nG1m(1) is an allele on IgG1 molecules but is also present on all IgG2 and IgG3 molecules.

Biologic Significance of Gm Allotypes

Levels of specific IgG subclasses, IgD, and possibly the antibody response to certain antigens may be related to the Gm or Km type (Kunkel and Kindt, 1975). For example, normal subjects of IgG allotype G3m(5) have twice the IgG3 level as those of G3m(21). The antibody response to the polysaccharide capsule of *Haemophilus influenzae* of children with the Km(1) allotype is fivefold to tenfold greater than these children who lack this determinant (Granoff et al., 1984).

Gene deletions governing the Gm alleles may occur and may result in low levels of an IgG subclass; for example, when G3m(21) and G3m(5) are deleted, low levels of IgG1 occur. In one symptomatic patient with hypogammaglobulinemia, a heterozygous gene deletion of IgG1 from one parent and a heterozygous gene deletion of IgG3 from the other were present, resulting in very low levels of both IgG1 and IgG3 (Yount et al., 1970). (See Chapter 13.)

Certain populations have a high incidence of specific Gm factors that are absent or low in other populations, thus making Gm typing useful in anthropologic studies (Steinberg, 1969). For example, G1m(3) is present in 90% of whites but is very rare in blacks; G3m(6) is present in 25% to 50% of blacks but rare (less than 1%) in whites. These observations can be used to determine the degree of racial admixture (e.g., there is approximately 30% white admixture among U.S. blacks), as well as tribal migration patterns. Antibodies of certain genetic types may offer superior protection to microorganisms indigenous to various regions, thus explaining the marked variability of the Gm types from population to population.

Am Factors

A2m(1), one of the two allotypes of the IgA2 subclass, is unique among the immunoglobulins, inasmuch as the heavy and light chains are not joined by disulfide bonds; indeed, the two light chains are linked by disulfide bonds (Fig. 4-3). The other allele of the IgA2 subclass, A2m(2), has the usual disulfide bond arrangement. The A2m(1) factor is present in 98% of whites and 51% of blacks. No relation between the Am type and the Gm or Km types exists (Vyas and Fudenberg, 1969).

Km Factors

Three allelic markers on the κ light chain—Km(1), Km(2), and Km(3)—have been described. Individuals who express Km(2) activity always express Km(1) activity. The amino acid substitutions responsible for this allotypy have been described (Solomon, 1976).

Antiallotypic Antibodies

Anti-Gm antibodies may appear after multiple blood or gamma globulin administration (Allen and Kunkel, 1966) and, under normal circumstances, in some newborns transiently exposed to maternal IgG different from their own (Steinberg and Wilson, 1963). Also, in one instance an anti-Gm factor developed in a pregnant mother as a result of exposure to her infant's paternally derived Gm factor (Fudenberg and Fudenberg, 1964); this is analogous to sensitization of an Rh-negative mother by an Rh-positive infant. Anti-Gm antibodies are not a source of transfusion reactions. Maternal anti-Gm antibodies do not inhibit the synthesis of IgG by the fetus even when they are IgG antibodies and cross the placenta (Nathenson et al., 1971).

Summary of Immunoglobulin Variation

Immunoglobulin heterogeneity is summarized in Table 4-3. There are 9 variants of heavy chain (1 for each of 4 IgG subclasses, 2 IgA subclasses, and 1 for IgM, IgD, and IgE classes), 1 light-chain type (κ chain), and

TABLE 4-3 · SUMMARY OF IMMUNOGLOBULIN CHAIN STRUCTURES AND VARIANTS

Classes: IgG, IgM, IgA, IgD, IgE

Chains: Heavy, light

Heavy chain:
    Classes and subclasses: γ1, γ2, γ3, γ4, α1, α2, μ, δ, ε
    Variable region families: V_H1, V_H2, V_H3, V_H4, V_H5, V_H6, V_H7
    Allotypes of γ chains: Gm (18 types)
    Allotypes of α chains: Am (2 types)
    Allotypes of ε chains: Em (2 types)

Light chain:
    Types: κ, λ
    Constant regions: C_κ, $C_\lambda1$, $C_\lambda2$, $C_\lambda3$, $C_\lambda7$
    Variable regions: $V_\kappa I$–$V_\kappa IV$; $V_\lambda I$–$V_\lambda IX$
    Allotypes of κ chains: Km (3 types)

Surrogate light chain (ψL):
    Constant regions: 14.1, 16.1, 16.2, $C_\lambda1$
    Variable region: Vpre-B

at least 10 subtypes of λ chains, thus resulting in multiple varieties of immunoglobulin molecules. Further variation results from allotypic and idiotypic differences.

Fc RECEPTORS

Definition

Fc receptors (FcRs) are molecules on the surface of multiple cells and tissues that bind to the Fc portion of immunoglobulin, leaving the antibody site able to attach to antigen and thus enabling antibodies to undertake biologic functions independent of the antigenic-binding site; the immunoglobulin serves as a ligand between the antigen and the Fc-bearing cell. FcRs have been identified (Table 4-4) for all the immunoglobulin classes except for IgD (Van de Winkel and Capel, 1993).

Most FcRs belong to the immunoglobulin supergene family (an exception is FcεRII) and thus show structural homology with each other and their Ig ligands (see Figure 4-10). FcRs serve crucial function in triggering cytotoxicity, secreting mediators, permitting phagocytes, initiating oxidative burst, and regulating antibody production (Table 4-5).

Several types and subtypes of Fc receptors can be defined depending on their immunoglobulin ligand and their physicochemical, immunologic, and antigenic properties (see Table 4-4). Most are characterized by an extracellular region, a transmembrane region, and a cytoplasmic tail, as discussed in Chapter 3 and shown in Figure 3-7. Soluble forms of the Fc receptors also exist; they lack the transmembrane and cytoplasmic tail. These may be shed from activated leukocytes or synthesized de novo. These soluble receptors may have important immunoregulatory rates such as control of Ig synthesis. The extracellular regions consist of two or three disulphide-bonded domains similar to those present in immunoglobulin. Multiple genes control their synthesis; they are located on the long arm of chromosome 21. Separate genes control each of the Fc receptors (Ravetch and Kinet, 1991).

Molecules similar or identical to FcRs may be present on certain parasites, bacteria (notably staphylococcal protein A), and viral-infected cells, so that immunoglobulin binds to them nonspecially.

Fc receptors for IgG (FcγRs)

Three types of FcγR exist. FcγRI (CD64) is distinguished primarily by its high affinity for monomeric IgG and is expressed constitutively only on monocytes and macrophages. It is also expressed on interferon-γ–activated neutrophils and eosinophils. This receptor binds strongly with IgG1 and IgG3, slightly with IgG4, and not at all with IgG2.

Four isoforms of FcγR1 exist: FcγRIa, sFcγRIb1, FcγRIb2, and FcγRIc. The sFcγRIb2 is the soluble receptor.

TABLE 4-4 · CHARACTERISTICS OF HUMAN Fc RECEPTORS

Receptor	FcR Type	Ligand	CD	Molecular Weight (kD)	Cell Distribution
FcγRI	IgG high affinity	Monomeric IgG	CD64	72	Monocytes and macrophages Activated neutrophils and eosinophils
FcγRII	IgG low affinity	Complexed IgG	CD32	40	Monocytes and macrophages Neutrophils, basophils, eosinophils B cells, T-cell subset Langerhans cells Placental and endothelial cells
FcγRIII	IgG low affinity	Complexed IgG	CD16	50–70	K/NK cells Neutrophils Activated monocytes and macrophages T-cell subset Placental trophoblast Mesangial cells
FcεRI	IgE high affinity	IgE	—	50/32/7	Mast cells and basophils
FcεRII	IgE low affinity	IgE	CD23	45	Monocytes and macrophages Eosinophils B-cell subset Platelets
FcαR	IgA	IgA	—	50–70	Monocytes and macrophages Neutrophils T-cell subset B-cell subset NK cells Erythrocytes
FcμR	IgM	IgM	—	90	B cells Glandular epithelium Hepatocytes

CD = cluster of differentiation; K = killer cell; kD = kilodalton; NK = natural killer.

FcγRII (CD32) is a family of molecules encoded by three genes with six isoforms (FcγRIIa1, sFcγRIIa2, FcγRIIb1, FcγRIIb2, FcγRIIb3, and FcRIIc) and binds primarily to complexed or aggregated IgG. It is expressed on multiple cells and is a low-affinity receptor.

Genetic polymorphism exists for FcγRIIa. One allotype, FcRIIa1 is present on monocytes and reacts with a mouse IgG1 monoclonal antibody (41H16). Individuals with a proliferative response to this antibody are designated high responders (HRs), and individuals who do not react are designated low responders (LRs) (Gosselin et al., 1990). Other nonallelic polymorphisms exist for the FcRII isoforms.

FcγRIII is a low-affinity FcR, binding to complexed IgG and identified as the CD16 antigen. Two forms of FcγRIII exist; one is present on monocytes/macrophages, natural killer cells, and some T cells (FcγRIIIa), and a second form is present on neutrophils (FcγRIIIb). The latter is distinct, inasmuch as instead of a transmembrane anchoring domain, there is a phosphatidylinositol linkage to the neutrophil. FcγRIIIb does not mediate antibody-dependent cellular cytotoxicity (ADCC), probably because signal transduction does not occur. FcγRIIIa is the main FcR involved in ADCC of antibody-coated platelets in immune thrombocytopenic purpura.

Genes on chromosome 1 control FcγRIII synthesis; several polymorphic variants have been identified for both FcγRIIIa and FcγRIIIb. The latter include the allelic neutrophil antigens NA1 and NA2, sometimes involved in immune neutropenias.

Clinical Aspects of FcγRs

One mode of action of interferon-γ used in the therapy of chronic granulomatous disease may be to induce FcγRs on neutrophils and eosinophils and enhance their expression on monocytes, thus increasing their antimicrobial activity.

The LR form of FcγRII may work synergistically with IgG2 antibodies to certain organisms, and individuals lacking this FcγRII (i.e., those with the HR phenotype) may be more susceptible to certain encapsulated bacteria, such *Haemophilus influenzae* and pneumococci (Van de Winkel and Capel, 1993).

Neutrophils from patients with paroxysmal nocturnal hemoglobinuria lack FcγIIIb on their neutrophils

TABLE 4-5 · BIOLOGIC FUNCTIONS TRIGGERED BY FcγR ENGAGEMENT

Phagocytosis
Superoxide generation
Antibody-dependent cellular cytotoxicity (ADCC)
Cytokine release
Enhanced antigen presentation
Regulation of immunoglobulin production
Placental transport of IgG
Clearance of immune complexes

but have this receptor on their natural killer cells (Selvaraj et al., 1988).

FcRγ function may require interaction with other receptors. For example, leukocyte adhesion defect-1 (LAD-1) patients lacking CD11b/CD18 may fail to trigger FcR-mediated phagocytosis and the oxidative burst. Individuals totally lacking FcRγI have been reported, and they are apparently healthy (Ceuppens et al., 1988).

Fc Receptors for IgM, IgA, and IgE

The FcαR (CD89) is present on the surface of a variety of leukocytes, as well as on erythrocytes. The FcαR can induce reactive oxygen intermediates (Shen and Collins, 1989) and bacterial phagocytosis of neutrophils (Weisbart et al., 1988). It differs from the poly-IgA receptor that transports IgA into the glandular lumen.

The FcμR is present on activated B cells but not on other cells (Ohno et al., 1991). Little is known about its function.

The high-affinity FcεR1 is expressed on mast cells and circulating basophils (Metzger, 1986). When bound IgE molecules are crosslinked by antigen, allergic mediators are released from the mast cells and basophils to initiate the allergic response.

The low-affinity FcεRII (CD23) is expressed on a broad range of cells and serves to regulate IgE responses. It is a 45-kD type II protein of the C-type lectin family and is thus distinct in its structure from the other major Fc receptor proteins (Kikutani et al., 1986). A distinct second ligand for this receptor is CD21. RcεRII is often released as a soluble receptor and acts as a cytokine for B cells through its avidity for its alternative ligand, B-cell CD21 (Aubry et al., 1992). CD23 on B cells is a differentiation antigen.

Further discussion of FcR structure is presented in Chapter 3.

IMMUNOGLOBULIN SYNTHESIS AND METABOLISM

Sites of Synthesis

Plasma cells and, to a much smaller extent, the less differentiated cells of the B-lymphocyte lineage, synthesize immunoglobulins. These immunoglobulin-synthesizing cells are scattered throughout the body but are concentrated in the spleen, lymph nodes, liver, bone marrow, and lymphatic tissue of the gastrointestinal and respiratory tract and exocrine glands. Each cell synthesizes only one class or subclass of heavy chain and one type of light chain. The number of cells producing each class or subclass of immunoglobulin is proportional to the percentage of each immunoglobulin class within the body. Essentially all the circulating Ig is derived from plasma cells.

IgM-producing plasma cells are morphologically distinct from immunoglobulin-producing cells of other classes. These cells have scant cytoplasm and a poorly developed endoplasmic reticulum; because they resemble a large lymphocyte, they often are termed *lymphocytoid plasma cells*. This morphologic difference permits a distinction between Waldenström's macroglobulinemia and multiple myeloma. There are no morphologic differences between plasma cells producing the other classes of immunoglobulins; multiple myelomas of the IgA, IgG, IgD, and IgE varieties are not distinguishable morphologically.

IgA production mainly occurs in mucosal sites as a result of homing properties of the B- and T-cell subsets committed to the immunoregulatory process required for IgA expression (Berlin et al., 1994; Platts-Mills, 1979). Local mucosal plasma cells are the source of IgA used by mucosal epithelium for complexing with secretory component and for luminal transport. These cells are also the predominant source of serum IgA. Similarly, IgE-producing plasma cells are located mainly in the lymphoid tissue associated with the respiratory mucosa and the gastrointestinal tract.

Immunoglobulin is synthesized on the ribosomes within the plasma cell by the endoplasmic reticulum (Askonas and Williamson, 1966). Newly synthesized immunoglobulin is localized between the membranes of the endoplasmic reticulum (Fig. 4-5A) and may accumulate in inclusions called *Russell bodies* (Fig. 4-5B).

Heavy and light chains are synthesized separately and combined before release, carbohydrate being added last. Polymeric IgM and IgA also follow this pattern; shortly before secretion, the J chain is added. The entire process takes only 30 minutes.

There is not an exact balance between heavy-chain and light-chain synthesis. Normally, a slight excess of light chains is synthesized, resulting in the presence of small numbers of free light chains.

It is estimated that each immunoglobulin-producing cell can synthesize 2000 molecules of immunoglobulin per second and 1.7×10^8 molecules per day. Based on an IgG synthetic rate of 35 mg/kg/day, there are 9.4×10^{18} immunoglobulin molecules produced per day by 5.5×10^{10} cells. The volume of this number of cells is only 10 ml (Engle and Wallis, 1969).

Distribution and Destruction

Although immunoglobulin theoretically could be stored in the plasma cells after synthesis, kinetic studies have shown that it is rapidly secreted from the cell. Because plasma cells release their immunoglobulins into the circulatory system, it is unnecessary for them to be concentrated in any particular region of the body. However, the production of IgA along the gastrointestinal tract and the synthesis of IgE adjacent to the respiratory mucosa are two examples of regional immunoglobulin synthesis that can thereby effect an increased local concentration. Indeed, there is selective secretion of IgA into the gut and respiratory fluids, whereas IgE is concentrated in the nasal washings.

Immunoglobulin destruction occurs within granulocytes (after phagocytosis of immunoglobulin-coated bac-

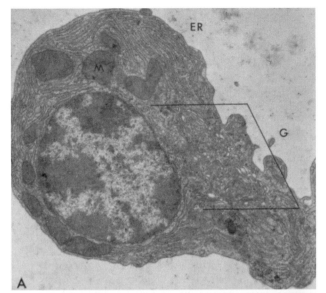

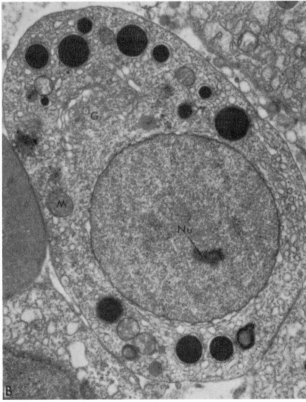

Figure 4-5 · Ultrastructure of the plasma cell. **A.** An electron micrograph shows the extensive development of the rough-surfaced endoplasmic reticulum (ER) and the large area occupied by the Golgi zone *(bracket).* A material of homogeneous density is seen in the tubules of the ER, presumably representing γ globulin (× 13,000). **B.** An electron micrograph shows Russell bodies of varying sizes. M = mitochondria; G = Golgi zone; Nu = nucleolar mass with irregular outline (× 15,600). (A and B from Zucker-Franklin D. Multiple myeloma. Semin Hematol 1:165–198, 1964.)

teria and particles), in the cells of the reticuloendothelial system (particularly in the liver), and in the gastrointestinal tract. As much as 40% of the immunoglobulin may be broken down within the intestinal lumen. Small quantities of immunoglobulin are also lost via the kidney.

Immunoglobulin Metabolism

Studies of immunoglobulin metabolism were facilitated by techniques to isolate and purify the immunoglobulin classes and trace-label them, usually with radioactive iodine (^{131}I or ^{125}I) (Waldmann and Strober, 1969). Because of the difficulty in isolating normal IgM, IgA, IgD, and IgE in an undenatured state, most metabolic studies have been done with the purified M-components. Even under optimal isolation conditions, some denaturation may occur, resulting in a spuriously rapid turnover.

By measuring the dilution of a known quantity of trace-labeled immunoglobulin, its rate of disappearance from the serum, and its rate of excretion in the urine and stools, one can calculate the half-life in the circulation, as well as the intravascular and extravascular distribution, the total body pool, the synthetic rate, and the amount of the total body pool synthesized per day (fractional catabolic rate) (Waldmann and Strober, 1969). These data are presented in Table 4-6.

Immunoglobulin metabolism has also been studied by the turnover of in vivo–labeled immunoglobulin (obtained by administering radioactive precursor compounds such as ^{14}C-labeled amino acids) or by the disappearance rate of passively administered immunoglobulin or antibody. These studies have confirmed the findings obtained by the in vitro isotopic studies.

IgG

The synthetic rate of IgG is 35 mg/kg/day under normal conditions, equivalent to 2 g of IgG synthesized per day by a 70-kg adult. The mean half-life of IgG as a class is about 23 days and is the longest of any plasma protein. There is no difference in catabolic rate between autologous and homologous IgG. The half-life of IgG3 subclass is considerably shorter (i.e., 9 days) than the other

TABLE 4-6 · METABOLIC PROPERTIES OF THE IMMUNOGLOBULIN CLASSES

	IgG	IgM	IgA	IgD	IgE
Mean adult serum concentration (mg/dl)	1200	120	200	3	0.01
Percentage of total immunoglobulin	70–80	5–10	10–15	<1	<0.01
Biologic half-life (days)	23	5	7	2.8	2.3
Distribution (percentage intravascular)	45	80	45	75	50
Total body pool (mg/kg)	1150	49	230	1.5	0.04
Synthetic rate (mg/kg/day)	35	7	25	0.4	0.02
Placental transfer	+	–	–	–	–
Fractional catabolic rate (percent of body content catabolized/day)	3	14	12	35	89

IgG subclasses (see Table 4-6). The metabolic studies of normal IgG reflect a mean of all four subclasses.

IgG metabolism is regulated by the serum level of IgG, so that there is an increase in the fractional catabolic rate at higher IgG levels and a decrease at low levels. The long half-life and its regulation of IgG is in part due to FcRn function, as described in Chapter 3. Thus the IgG half-life in patients with agammaglobulinemia is prolonged to 35 to 40 days; by contrast, the IgG half-life is shortened in multiple myeloma and other hypergammaglobulinemic states. High levels of other immunoglobulins or albumin do not influence IgG turnover. The shortest IgG half-lives are in protein-losing states (see Chapter 25).

IgA

The IgA half-life of 7 days is significantly shorter than that of IgG, despite similar size and distribution (see Table 4-6). The lower serum level (mean, 200 mg/dl in adults) compared with IgG and its rapid catabolism results in a synthetic rate of 25 mg/kg/day, nearly equivalent to that of IgG. Additional IgA, synthesized as secretory IgA in tears, saliva, gastrointestinal fluid, and so forth, makes IgA the immunoglobulin with the largest total synthesis. The catabolic rate of IgA (and of IgE and IgM) is independent of the level of IgA, IgE, or IgM.

IgM, IgD, and IgE

IgM is found primarily (75%) in the intravascular compartment. This feature, combined with its early appearance after antigenic stimulation and its opsonic and complement-fixing properties, suggests that IgM is a first line of defense against organisms entering the bloodstream. The synthetic rate of IgM (7 mg/kg/day) is considerably less than that of IgG or IgA, whereas its half-life (5 days) is similar to that of IgA.

Both IgD and IgE have short serum half-lives (2.8 and 2.3 days, respectively) and correspondingly large fractional catabolic rates. As pointed out earlier, there is evidence for local synthesis of IgE at the mucosal surfaces, particularly of the upper respiratory tract. Although IgE has a measurable serum half-life, there are two pools of IgE—IgE in the circulation and IgE attached to mast cells/basophils. Such cytophilic IgE has a half-life of 2 to 3 weeks.

Placental Transfer

Placental transfer from mother to infant occurs only for IgG. The role of the FcRn in this process has been defined (see Chapter 3). The rate of maternal-fetal transfer is a function of maternal and fetal IgG levels, as well as of age of the placenta (Gitlin, 1971). At low levels of maternal IgG, there is little IgG transfer; at higher levels of maternal IgG, transfer occurs in proportion to the maternal IgG level. Because of an immature placenta, premature infants at birth have low serum levels

of IgG in inverse proportion to the gestational age (Hyvarinen et al., 1973).

The other immunoglobulins (IgM, IgA, IgD, and IgE) are not transferred across the placenta, with the result that certain antibodies present in the maternal circulation are absent in the infant. This is disadvantageous in some instances, because most antibodies to gram-negative organisms are IgM globulins; on the other hand, maternal IgM isoagglutinins, which could cause ABO hemolytic disease of the newborn, and maternal IgE antibodies, which could cause allergic reactions, do not have access to the infant's circulation.

Clinical Implications

Commercial gamma globulin preparations (e.g., intravenous immune globulins [IVIGs]), while containing some Igs of all classes, are essentially all IgG from the point of view of therapeutic benefit. The biologic half-life of both the intravenous and intramuscular forms of IgG is somewhat less than 23 days in normal patients because of some denaturation during processing. However, because of the feedback on IgG catabolism by the serum level of IgG, the actual half-life in patients with hypogammaglobulinemia is generally prolonged beyond 23 days. The difficulty in isolating IgM and IgA, as well as their short half-lives, makes IgM and IgA preparations impractical for therapeutic use, despite theoretical advantages for individuals who lack IgM or IgA. Plasma can be used to supply IgM and IgA; however, the IgM and IgA content is relatively low and therapeutic levels are not sustained for a significant period.

Several disorders of immunoglobulin metabolism are known. These include Wiskott-Aldrich syndrome (see Chapter 17), in which there is hypercatabolism of IgG, and myotonic dystrophy (see Chapters 24 and 40). In addition, increased loss can occur through the gastrointestinal tract (e.g., in protein-losing enteropathy) and through the genitourinary tract (e.g., in nephrotic syndrome) (see Chapter 25).

BIOLOGIC PROPERTIES OF IMMUNOGLOBULINS

IgG and IgG Subclasses

The biologic properties of the immunoglobulin classes are summarized in Table 4-7. IgG, normally representing about 80% of the serum immunoglobulin, is the chief component of the body's serologic defenses and contains most of the antibacterial, antiviral, antiprotozoal, and antitoxic activity of the serum. Although IgG probably does little if any direct killing, IgG can activate the complement system, promote opsonization, and participate in antibody-dependent cytolytic reactions. The distribution of IgG within the tissues, because of its small size, makes IgG the primary Ig participating in extravascular immune reactions. IgG can be thought of as guarding the tissues (including the alveoli) from bac-

TABLE 4-7 · BIOLOGIC PROPERTIES OF THE IMMUNOGLOBULIN CLASSES AND IgG SUBCLASSES

Property	IgG1	IgG2	IgG3	IgG4	IgM	IgA	IgD	IgE	Secretory IgA
First detectable antibody	–	–	–	–	+	–	–	–	–
Major part of secondary response	+	+	+	+	–	–	–	–	–
Placental transport	+ +	+	+ +	+ +	–	–	–	–	–
Complement activation via									
Classical pathway	+ +	+	+ +	–	–	–	–	–	–
Alternate pathway	–	–	–	–*	–	+ +	±	+	+
Reacts with *Staphylococcus aureus*									
Protein A	+ +	+ +	–	+ +	–	–	–	–	–
Agglutination	+	+	+	+	+ +	–	–	–	–
Opsonization	+	+	+	+	+ +	–	–	–	–
Virus neutralization	+	+	+	+	+	–	–	–	+
Hemolysis	+	+	+	+	+ +	–	–	–	–
Anaphylactic activity	–	–	–	–	–	–	–	+ +	–
Present in exocrine secretions	+	+	+	+	+	+	–	+	+ +
Cytophilic for									
Macrophages	+ +	±	+ +	±	–	–	–	+	–
Lymphocytes	+	±	+	±	–	–	–	–	–
Neutrophils	+	+	+	+	+	+	±	±	–
Platelets	+	+	+	+	–	–	–	–	–
Mast cells	–	–	–	–	–	–	–	+	–
Binding to Fc Receptors									
FcγRI	+ +	±	+ +	+	–	–	–	–	–
FcγRII	+ +	+	+ +	±	–	–	–	–	–
FcγRIII	+ +	±	+ +	±	–	–	–	–	–
FcαR	–	–	–	–	–	+	–	–	+
FcμR	–	–	–	–	+	–	–	–	–
FcεRI and FcεRII	–	–	–	–	–	–	–	+	–

++ = Very strong; + = strong ± = equivocal; – = absent.
*Aggregated IgG4 may activate alternate pathway.

terial infection. Passage across the placenta provides the full-term newborn with passive immunity for about 6 months.

An IgG antibody response after initial antigenic challenge is associated with the development of immunologic memory; upon subsequent challenge, the anamnestic response is predominantly an IgG response. Most of the antibody following repetitive antigenic challenge is IgG. The long half-life of IgG and its association with the anamnestic response make it the ideal immunoglobulin for durable host immunity.

IgG antibodies are potent inhibitors and competitors of other immune responses. The inhibition of Rh sensitization by passive administration of IgG anti-Rh antibodies is used clinically in the prevention of Rh hemolytic disease of the newborn. Successful allergy desensitization in part results when highly avid blocking antibodies are developed that can prevent an allergen from reacting with an IgE-coated mast cell. This is particularly true of the blocking antibodies protective against systemic reactions such as that seen with stinging insects. Blocking antibodies are predominantly but not exclusively IgG antibodies.

All subclasses of IgG can fix complement except for IgG4. It alone is unable to bind to C1q and initiate the complement cascade. IgG1, IgG2, and IgG3 can promote phagocytosis, initiate chemotaxis, release anaphylatoxin, and lyse target cells.

IgG immunoglobulins have strong cytophilic properties and can interact with macrophages, neutrophils, lymphocytes, and platelets via Fc receptors on these cells (see Table 4-7). This interaction occurs via specific receptors for the Fc portion of the IgG subclasses found on these various cellular elements. The presence of specific IgG on target cells (tumor cells, heterologous erythrocytes, allogeneic lymphocytes) may permit antibody-dependent cytotoxicity by lymphocytes, neutrophils, and macrophages with Fc receptors.

IgG antibodies participate in various immunopathologic reactions. IgG rarely may be involved in *anaphylactoid reactions* (resembling type I [anaphylactic] reactions), in which large amounts of IgG antibody may bind antigen in the circulation and activate anaphylatoxins from the complement cascade, as in transfusion reactions to IgA. More commonly, IgG is involved in *cytotoxic reactions* (type II), such as hemolytic anemia, or *immune complex reactions* (type III), such as serum sickness. Some investigators have attempted to ascribe reaginic properties (IgE-like) to IgG4, but the weight of evidence is that IgG4 subclass antibodies contain protective antibodies against immediate hypersensitivity reactions rather than being their instrument (Urbanek, 1988).

Antibody activity differs among the IgG subclasses. Most treponemal antibodies are IgG1. Rh antibodies are usually of the IgG1 and IgG3 subclasses, occasionally of IgG4, but never of the IgG2 subclass (Frame et al., 1970). Coagulation factor VIII (antihemophiliac globulin) antibodies are limited to the IgG4 subclass (Anderson and Terry, 1968). Antibodies to polysaccharide antigens, such as antidextran and antilevan, generally belong to the IgG2 subclass. The ability of IgG to combine with staphylococcal protein A, a property of the Fc portion of the molecule, is present in IgG1, IgG2, and IgG4 subclasses but is lacking in IgG3 (Kronvall and Williams, 1969).

Patients with low levels of one or more IgG subclasses may demonstrate increased susceptibility to infection. Some patients with selective IgA deficiency have associated selective IgG2 deficiency (Oxelius et al, 1981). Patients with IgG2 deficiency may have defective antibody responses to polysaccharide antigens. Beck and Heiner (1981) have suggested that some patients with selective IgG4 have recurrent pulmonary infection, but most such patients are asymptomatic. Most patients with clinically significant subclass deficiencies show slightly decreased total IgG levels and poor antibody responses. The subclass deficiencies are discussed in Chapter 13.

Therapeutic Use of IgG

Antibody, both human and animal, has been used for over a century for the prevention and treatment of certain infectious diseases. Human immunoglobulin has been used for half a century in the treatment of antibody immunodeficiencies, both primary and secondary. High-dose human immunoglobulin (e.g., IVIG) has been used for a quarter of a century as an immunomodulatory agent for a variety of autoimmune and inflammatory diseases.

Several types of antibody preparations are used for therapeutic purposes. These include (1) standard human immune serum globulin (HISG) for general use, available in two forms—intramuscular immune globulin (IG) and intravenous immune globulin (IVIG); (2) special IGs with a known antibody content for specific illnesses; (3) animal sera and antitoxins from immunized animals; and (4) monoclonal antibodies. These are listed in Table 4-8.

A discussion of the use of various Ig preparations for treatment of antibody deficiencies is presented in Chapter 12. The side effects are also presented. The use of antibody in the prevention and treatment of infectious diseases is presented in Chapter 42 and in a review by Keller and Stiehm (2000).

Use of IVIG as an Immunomodulator

The value of IVIG as an immunomodulator was first observed by Imbach and colleagues (1981), who noted that the platelet count of patients with immune thrombocytopenic purpura could be rapidly increased with large infusions of IVIG. Since that time, numerous illnesses, as listed in Table 4-9, have been treated with IVIG, some with clear therapeutic benefit, others with suggestive benefit, and still others with little or no benefit. As a result of these multiple indications, their occurrence in adults (with their larger weight) and the need for large (and often repeated) doses, more than half the IVIG used is for these illnesses. IVIG costs $25 to $50 per gram, so that a 2 g/kg dose

for a 70-kg adult costs $3,500 to $7,000, plus infusion costs.

High-dose IVIG may work by one or more of the following mechanisms (Ballow, 1997; Dwyer, 1992; Silvestris et al., 1994; Takéi et al., 1993).

1. IVIG inhibits antibody synthesis by direct effect on proliferating B cells, probably through ligation of the FcRII receptor (Samuelsson et al., 2001). This may be the mechanism in illnesses associated with a pathologic antibody such as myasthenia gravis and coagulopathy with a factor VIII inhibitor.
2. IVIG contains anti-idiotypic antibodies, which can combine with autoimmune antibodies and remove them rapidly from the circulation. This may be the mechanism by which IVIG reduces anti-HLA antibodies in transplant patients.
3. IVIG combines with Fc receptors, causing an Fc-receptor blockade, thus reducing the destruction of antibody-coated cells in the spleen or the liver. This is the mechanism for the rapid response to IVIG noted in patients with immune thrombocytopenic purpura.
4. IVIG combines with other cell surface receptors to inhibit cellular activation; for example, in toxic epidermal necrolysis, IVIG prevents Fas-mediated cell death of keratinocytes by blocking the Fas receptor (Viard et al., 1998).
5. IVIG downregulates immune activation by decreasing inflammatory cytokine release or action. In Kawasaki disease, there is immediate dampening of the cytokine "storm" that occurs with this illness.
6. IVIG antibodies neutralize bacterial superantigens and prevent them from activating T cells. This is the likely mechanism for the beneficial effect of toxic shock syndrome (Takei et al., 1993).
7. IVIG combines with complement components to prevent complement-mediated tissue injury. An example is inhibition of complement-mediated myocyte damage in dermatomyositis.
8. IVIG neutralizes viral or bacterial antigens that may trigger or cause the disease. An example may be neutralization of *Escherichia coli* antigens in hemolytic-uremic syndrome.

The illnesses for which IVIG may be of benefit are often of unknown cause, refractory to standard treatment, somewhat responsive to steroids, and associated with local or generalized immune activation with fever, inflammatory cells, and cytokine release. Large doses of IVIG are necessary (e.g., usually 1 to 2 g/kg/day, which may need to be repeated at weekly intervals). All immune globulin preparations are seemingly equivalent in their action. If a favorable response does not occur immediately or within a few weeks, it probably will not occur later. Proof of efficacy requires a double-blind study (e.g., as done for Kawasaki disease) or dramatic reversal of progressive severe disease (e.g., as noted in toxic shock syndrome).

TABLE 4-8 · ANTIBODY PREPARATIONS AVAILABLE FOR PASSIVE IMMUNITY IN THE UNITED STATES

Product	Abbreviations or Brand Names	Principal Use
Standard Human Immune Serum Globulins	HISG, gamma globulin	
Immune globulin, intravenous	IVIG, IGIV	Treatment of antibody deficiency, immune thrombocytopenic purpura, Kawasaki disease, other immunoregulatory and inflammatory diseases
Immune globulin, intramuscular	IG, ISG	Treatment of antibody deficiency; prevention of measles, hepatitis A
Special Human Immune Serum Globulins for Intramuscular or Subcutaneous Use		
Hepatitis B immune globulin	HBIG	Prevention of hepatitis B
Varicella-zoster immune globulin	VZIG	Prevention or modification of chickenpox
Rabies immune globulin	RIG	Prevention of rabies
Tetanus immune globulin	TIG	Prevention or treatment of tetanus
Vaccinia immune globulin*	VIG	Prevention or treatment of vaccinia, prevention of smallpox
Rho(D) immune globulin	RhoGAM	Prevention of Rh hemolytic disease
Botulinum immune globulin	BIG	Treatment of newborn botulism
Special Human Intravenous Immunoglobulins		
Cytomegalovirus (CMV) immune globulin	CMV-IVIG, CMVIG CytoGam	Prevention or treatment of cytomegalovirus infection
Respiratory syncytial virus (RSV) immune globulin	RSV-IVIG, RSVIG RespiGam	Prevention of RSV infection
Rho(D) immune globulin-IV	WinRho SD	Treatment of immune thrombocytopenic purpura
Animal Serums and Globulins		
Tetanus antitoxin (equine)	TAT	Prevention or treatment of tetanus (when TIG unavailable)
Diphtheria antitoxin (equine)*	DAT	Treatment of diphtheria
Botulinum antitoxin (equine)*		Treatment of botulism
Lactrodectus mactans antivenin (equine)		Treatment of black widow spider bites
Crotalidae polyvalent antivenin (equine)		Treatment of most snake bites
Crotalidae polyvalent Immune Fab (ovine)		Treatment of most snake bites
Micrurus fulvius antivenin (equine)		Treatment of coral snake bites
Digoxin immune Fab fragments (ovine)	Digibind, DigiFab	Treatment of digoxin or digitoxin overdose
Lymphocyte/thymocyte immune globulin (equine)	Equine ATG, Atgam	Immunosuppression
Lymphocyte/thymocyte immune globulin (rabbit)	Rabbit ATG, Thymoglobulin	Immunosuppression
Monoclonal Antibodies†		
Muromonab (Anti-CD3)	OKT3	Immunosuppression
Daclizamab (Anti-IL-2Rγ)	Zenapak	Immunosuppression
Basiliximab (Anti-IL-2Rα)	Simulect	Immunosuppression
Infliximab (Anti-TNF-α)	Remicade	Treatment of inflammatory bowel disease, rheumatoid arthritis
Adalimumab (anti-TNFα)	Humira	Treatment of rheumatoid arthritis
Trastuzumab (Anti-p185)	Herceptin	Treatment of breast cancer
Rituximab (Anti-CD20)	Rituxin	Treatment of B-cell lymphoma
Ibritumab Tiuxetan (radioactive anti-CD20)‡	Zevalin	Treatment of refractory B-cell lymphoma
Gemtuzamab (anti-CD33)	Mylotarg	Treatment of acute myelocytic leukemia
Alemtuzumab (Anti-CD52)	Campath	Treatment of chronic lymphocytic leukemia
Abciximab (Anti-GPIIb/IIIa)	ReoPro, Cento Rx	Prevention of thrombosis
Palivizumab (Anti-RSV-F)	Synagis	Prevention of RSV infection
Omalizumab (Anti-IgE)	Xolair	Prevention and treatment of allergic disorders

*Available from the U.S. Centers for Disease Control and Prevention (404/635-3670).
†All are humanized mouse monoclonal antibodies except for muromonab, which is a mouse monoclonal antibody.
‡Conjugated with either indium-111 or yttrium-90.

Special Immune Globulins and Monoclonal Antibodies

Special preparations of IG for intramuscular use are available for the prevention and treatment of certain infectious diseases (Keller and Stiehm, 2000). These include varicella-zoster immunoglobulin (VZIG), rabies immunoglobulin (RIG), tetanus immunoglobulin (TIG), hepatitis B immunoglobulin (HBIG), botulism immune globulin (BIG) for neonatal botulism, and Rh immune globulin for prevention of Rh disease (see Table 4-8). Three special IVIG preparations are also available, cytomegalovirus immune globulin (CMV-IVIG, CytoGam), respiratory syncytial virus immune globulin (RSV-IVIG, RespiGam), and Rho immune globulin (WinRho) for immune thrombocytopenic purpura. These have been prepared from immunized or convalescing donors, and their antibody content has been

TABLE 4-9 · AUTOIMMUNE AND INFLAMMATORY DISEASES TREATED WITH IVIG

Proven Benefit*
1. Kawasaki disease
2. Immune thrombocytopenic purpura (e.g., idiopathic)
3. Dermatomyositis
4. Neurologic diseases
   a. Guillain-Barré syndrome
   b. Chronic inflammatory demyelinating polyneuropathy
   c. Multifocal motor neuropathy
   d. Lambert-Eaton myasthenia syndrome

Probable Benefit†
1. Postinfectious thrombocytopenic purpura
2. Neonatal isoimmune or autoimmune thrombocytopenic purpura
3. Pregnancy associated with antiplatelet antibodies
4. Autoimmune or isoimmune neutropenia
5. Autoimmune hemolytic anemia
6. Toxic epidermal necrolysis
7. Neurologic diseases
   a. Myasthenia gravis
   b. Polymyositis

Possible Benefit‡
1. Toxic shock syndrome
2. Anticardiolipin antibody syndrome
3. Coagulopathy with factor VIII inhibitor
4. Bullous pemphigoid
5. Churg-Strauss vasculitis
6. Vasculitis with antineutrophil cytoplasmic antibodies
7. Other vasculitides
8. Graves' ophthalmopathy
9. Uveitis
10. Stevens Johnson syndrome
11. Solid-organ transplantation
    a. Highly HLA-sensitized patients awaiting transplantation
    b. Prevention of antibody-mediated rejection
    c. Prevention of allograft rejection in high-risk patients
    d. Treatment of delayed rejection

12. Neurologic diseases
    a. Multiple sclerosis
    b. Rasmussen's syndrome
    c. Intractable pediatric epilepsy
    d. Demyelinating neuropathy with IgM monoclonal gammopathy or anti-GAM antibodies
    e. Acute disseminated encephalomyelitis
    f. Cerebral infarction with antiphospholipid antibodies
    g. HTLV-1 associated myelopathy
    h. Lumbosacral or brachial plexitis
    i. Stiff-man syndrome
    j. PANDAS syndrome

Unproven or no benefit§
1. Steroid-dependent asthma
2. Atopic dermatitis
3. Epidermolysis bullosa acquisita
4. Recurrent abortion
5. Hemolytic-uremic syndrome
6. Thrombotic thrombocytopenic pupura
7. Pure red cell or white cell aplasia
8. Acquired Von Willebrand's disease
9. Chronic fatigue syndrome
10. Infantile autism
11. Acute myocarditis
12. Type I diabetes mellitus
13. Rheumatoid arthritis
14. Lupus erythematosus
15. Inflammatory bowel disease
16. Neurologic diseases
    a. Inclusion body myositis
    b. Amyotrophic lateral sclerosis
    c. POEMS syndrome
    d. Paraneopastic cerebellar degeneration, sensory neuropathy, encephalitis

*Controlled studies demonstrate efficacy.
†Several case reports or uncontrolled series are convincing.
‡Preliminary studies are encouraging but incomplete.
§Preliminary studies are limited, equivocal, or negative.
HTLV = human T lymphocytotrophic virus.

standardized. Pharmacologically, these preparations are identical to standard IG or IVIG preparations (see Chapter 41 for indications and dosage).

Monoclonal antibodies specific for a single antigenic epitope have been available for laboratory use for several decades and are being rapidly developed as therapeutic agents (see Table 4-8). The first monoclonal antibody, introduced in 1984, was a murine antilymphocyte antibody (anti-CD3[OKT3]) used for immunosuppression in transplant patients. Since then other monoclonals for treatment have been licensed and many others are under study in the United States and abroad.

Most licensed monoclonal antibodies are humanized murine monoclonal antibodies, containing the antibody-combining site of a mouse antibody, hybridized to a human IgG1 molecule (95% of the molecule), thus making it less antigenic and with the long half-life of a human IgG molecule. One of these antibodies, palivizumab (Synagis) is used in the prevention of RSV in high-risk infants (see Chapter 41). Monoclonal antibodies against microbial antigens and inflammatory

mediators will play an important role in tomorrow's battle with infectious pathogens.

IgM

IgM antibodies are the earliest antibodies identified in phylogeny and in the developing fetus; they also are the first antibody class formed after antigenic stimulation. IgM antibodies appear within 4 days but do not persist; durable immunity is associated with IgG antibody. Indeed, if only an IgM response occurs, immunologic memory is not acquired. Presence of IgM antibodies to an infectious agent can often be used as an indicator of recent infection. The presence of IgM antibodies in a newborn infant indicates congenital or perinatal infection; such antibodies cannot be acquired from the mother because of lack of transplacental passage.

IgM antibodies are excellent agglutinating antibodies, are unusually avid because of their multimeric nature, and are complement fixing. The majority of IgM (80%) is localized within the intravascular system. IgM thus primarily assists the reticuloendothelial system in clearing the bloodstream of bacteria and particles by opsonization and agglutination. The aggregating action is enhanced by the 10 combining sites on each polymeric IgM molecule. IgM is a strong activator of the classic pathway of complement by means of its interaction with C1; the 19S IgM molecule has 15 times the complement-activating activity of monomeric IgM or IgG1. The predominant intravascular localization, the ability to fix complement and act as an efficient opsonin, and the early appearance after antigenic challenge enable IgM to serve as the first serologic line of defense to bacterial infection. Individuals who lack IgM are susceptible to rapid, overwhelming sepsis.

Certain antigens stimulate a persistent IgM antibody response, resulting in serum antibody that is of the IgM class. These include (1) antibodies to polysaccharide antigens, such as anti-A and anti-B isoagglutinins; (2) the Wassermann and heterophile antibodies; (3) typhoid O antibodies; and (4) antibodies to endotoxins of gram-negative organisms. Rheumatoid factors, cold agglutinins, and certain other autoantibodies also are predominantly IgM. These IgM antibodies do not depend (or depend little) on T-cell effects for their expression and therefore are often called T-independent responses.

IgM antibodies participate in cytotoxic hypersensitivity (type II) reactions, such as autoimmune hemolytic anemia. However, the clinical manifestations may be different from those seen with IgG antibodies and are often accentuated by the enhanced ability of IgM to activate complement. Likewise, IgM antibodies participate in immune complex (type III) formation and disease states.

IgM Monomers

Naturally occurring 7S IgM monomers may be present in normal serum and in cord serum (Bush et al., 1969). High concentration of monomeric IgM occurs in hypergammaglobulinemic states such as lupus erythematosus, rheumatoid arthritis, and Waldenström's macroglobulinemia. Monomeric IgM has also been noted in certain immunodeficiencies, notably ataxia-telangiectasia, and in dysgammaglobulinemia (Metzger, 1970). The IgM monomers may have antibody activity against blood group substances and cell nuclei. The IgM monomers are synthesized de novo and are not a result of the breakdown of polymeric IgM (Solomon and McLaughlin, 1970).

IgM monomers are the predominant form of IgM that is present on the surface of or within B cells. The attachment of the J chain and resulting polymerization may be defective in states in which monomeric IgM is present in excessive amounts.

IgA

Serum IgA globulin contains several varieties of antibodies, including isoagglutinins, antibrucella, antidiphtheria, antiinsulin, and antipoliomyelitis antibodies. Serum IgA antibodies provide no known unique defense mechanism; indeed, most individuals who lack IgA are not unusually susceptible to systemic infections. Isolated IgA deficiency is a common abnormality occurring in one of 700 normal subjects (see Chapter 14). Although IgA antibodies are found both in the circulation and in the tissues, their primary defense role is at mucosal surfaces after transport into local secretions.

Engagement of the Fc receptor for IgA (FcαR) on neutrophils and monocytes and other cells by IgA-coated bacteria may initiate phagocytosis (Weisbart et al., 1988) or superoxide generation (Shen and Collins, 1989).

IgA antibodies do not activate the classic pathway of complement but can activate the alternate pathway. This may aid in phagocytosis and killing of certain organisms. IgA has some bactericidal activity, particularly when combined with lysozyme and complement. IgA molecules may serve to combine with tissue antigens (from damaged organs) or exogenous protein antigens (coming in primarily from the gastrointestinal tract) and prevent them from stimulating an immune response. By so doing, IgA antibodies prevent such antigens from provoking an antibody or cell-mediated response that may be harmful. In individuals who lack IgA, there is a high incidence of autoantibodies to antigens such as thyroglobulin, adrenal tissue, DNA, and bovine milk proteins, as well as an increased risk of autoimmune disorders.

The serum monomeric IgA (molecular weight [MW] 160,000) is structurally different from the dimeric secretory IgA (MW 500,000) found in exocrine secretions, and the latter contains a secretory piece and a J chain. The majority of serum IgA (90%) is IgA1; the majority of secretory IgA (60%) is IgA2, but this varies from secretion to secretion. IgA2, but not IgA1, is resistant to bacterial IgA protease. This resistance to proteolytic digestion makes IgA1 particularly suited for defense of mucosal surfaces.

Serum IgA is not specifically transported from the serum to the exocrine glands (Tomasi, 1972). However, a large portion of the serum IgA is produced in the plasma cells of the exocrine glands, where instead of being excreted as secretory IgA, it diffuses into the circulation. Thus the serum IgA will have the antibody specificities of the secretory IgA molecules, which is the chief antibody providing antiviral and antibacterial activity on mucous surfaces. Individuals who lack secretory IgA generally lack serum IgA. Such persons may experience increased infections involving primarily the upper respiratory system and sinuses. The structure and role of secretory IgA are further detailed in Chapter 9.

IgD

IgD was discovered by the finding of a new myeloma protein unrelated to IgG, IgA, or IgM (Rowe and Fahey, 1965). It had the clinical and structural characteristics of an immunoglobulin, and with the use of monospecific antisera to this protein, it was possible to demonstrate small quantities of IgD in all normal adult serum (mean, 3 mg/dl). Although IgD has been shown to have some antibody activity (to benzylpenicilloyl acid, diphtheria toxoid, bovine gamma globulin, and cell nuclei) (Heiner and Rose, 1970), its primary biologic function is not, as for the other Ig classes, as a soluble effector molecule. This is highlighted by its low concentration in serum or secretions and by its inability to fix complement, cross the placenta, or interact with neutrophils or mast cells.

An important clue to the biologic role of IgD was the observation that IgD made up a disproportionately high percentage (up to 10%) of immunoglobulin bound to the membrane of B cells from newborns (Rowe et al., 1973). This is in marked contrast to the low levels of IgD in serum, particularly in cord serum. Subsequent studies have identified IgD as being present on the majority of normal B lymphocytes, usually with surface IgM. This led to the proposal that IgD and IgM serve as antigen receptors on the lymphocyte surface, particularly during immune development. Further evidence for this has come from experiments showing that interaction with antibody to the IgD on B cells can dramatically alter the ability of those cells to develop a normal antibody response. Thus IgD appears to primarily function as an antigen receptor (along with membrane Ig on B cells) involved in regulation of B-cell development.

A few individuals have been identified with polyclonal hyperimmunoglobulin-D with periodic fevers (Drenth et al., 1994; Van der Meer, 1984) (see Chapter 36).

IgE

IgE, the anaphylactic or reaginic antibody, was the last immunoglobulin discovered (Ishizaka et al., 1966) and the one present in the smallest concentration. Its elucidation was greatly facilitated by finding two patients with IgE myeloma, which permitted its isolation, structural analysis, and measurement by immunoassay. Like IgM and unlike IgG, IgD, or IgA, it has one extra heavy-chain segment and lacks a hinge region. It has a molecular weight of 190,000 daltons.

Reaginic Activity

IgE functions primarily as a trigger for immediate hypersensitivity (type I) reactions. This occurs because IgE binds to basophils and mast cells located in the lungs, skin, peripheral blood, tonsils, and gastrointestinal tract. IgE binds to the high-affinity Fc receptor (FcεRI) for such cells. Allergens (antigens) combine with IgE to initiate cell activation, leading to release of chemical mediators such as histamine and leukotrienes. For this to occur, crosslinking of the IgE bound to the cell surface must occur. Such a reaction requires a bivalent antibody (isolated Fab fragments of IgE will not work) and a multivalent antigen (Ishizaka, 1974). Anti-IgE antisera can also be used to initiate the reaction, because it will bridge two bound IgE molecules.

IgE has a strong affinity for basophils and mast cells scattered throughout the body and persists for weeks on such cells. Triggering of the bound antigen-specific IgE results in varied hypersensitivity reactions such as anaphylactic shock, bronchoconstriction, nasal mucosal rhinorrhea, urticaria, and gastrointestinal disturbances, depending on the site and degree of the reaction. Complement is not involved in these reactions, although aggregated IgE in vitro can activate the alternate complement system.

IgE is synthesized in the central lymphoid tissue (e.g., lymph nodes, spleen, bone marrow), the tonsils, and the exocrine glands. The majority of IgE-containing plasma cells are found in lymphoid tissue associated with the respiratory or gastrointestinal tract. IgE antibodies are not specifically secreted in exocrine fluids, as they do not contain secretory component. Although IgE is found in higher than expected levels in fluids such as nasal washings, this primarily results from increased local production and diffusion (Platts-Mills, 1979).

IgE Regulation

Considerable study has examined the stimulus for IgE production by B cells (Leung, 1993). The first signal is T-cell–secreted IL-4, which switches Ig gene synthesis to the ε locus. The second signal, delivered by IL-4 along with contact with antigen-activated T cells, activates mRNA and IgE synthesis. T-cell contact in vivo can be replaced in vitro by Epstein-Barr virus, hydrocortisone, or a monoclonal antibody to CD40, a differentiation receptor on T cells. Certain cytokines (e.g., IL-4, IL-5, IL-6) amplify IgE synthesis, whereas others (e.g., IFN-α, IFN-γ, TGF-β) suppress IL-4–stimulated IgE synthesis. It is of note that one type of T helper cells (Th1 cells) secretes IL-2 and IFN-γ, which inhibit IgE synthesis, whereas another type (Th2 cells) secretes IL-4, IL-5, and IL-6, which promote IgE synthesis. Th1 cells facilitate delayed hypersensitivity reactions, and Th2 cells facilitate antibody responses. IL-4 also promotes the expression of low-affinity FcεRII (CD23) on B cells and monocytes of patients with hyper-IgE states, such as eczema and hyper-IgE syndrome (Vercelli and Geha, 1992).

IgE antibody responses are regulated by T lymphocytes to a degree greater than are the other Ig classes (Hamaoka et al., 1973). Patients with profound antibody and cellular immunodeficiencies lack serum IgE, but several partial cellular immunodeficiencies syndromes are characterized by elevated levels of IgE, including DiGeorge syndrome, Wiskott-Aldrich syndrome, and Hodgkin's disease. In experimental animals, IgE levels increase following thymectomy, whole-body irradiation, or the administration of antithymocyte serum or other immunosuppressive drugs. Similarly, following bone marrow transplantation, IgE levels may rise precipitously, particularly in the presence of graft-versus-host disease.

Beneficial Effects of IgE

A protective biologic role for IgE antibodies has been sought, because it is unlikely that a totally harmful immunoglobulin would persist in evolution. The high incidence of allergy in the general population suggests some survival advantage. A possible clue to a beneficial biologic role of IgE is the repeated observation of marked elevation of serum IgE levels in the presence of intestinal parasitism.

Experimental work in rats infected with the intestinal parasite *Nippostrongylus brasiliensis* suggests one beneficial role (Bloch, 1972). When worms enter the gastrointestinal tract, IgE antiworm antibodies are formed. These may damage the worm and result in the release of more worm antigen and stimulation of more IgE antibody. Worm antigen reacts with IgE antibodies on the mast cell or eosinophil to release pharmacologic mediators; these in turn cause enlargement of the villi, edema of the intestinal wall, leakage of serum proteins into the gastrointestinal tract (including other immunoglobulins and complement), and worm expulsion. Treatment with antihistamines inhibits worm expulsion.

Thus IgE may serve as a mechanism for defending against parasitism, inhibiting the attachment and entry of the invading organism by binding to the parasite; by IgE-mediated mast cell release, causing a flushing effect on the mucosal surface; and by increased local delivery of other defense effectors, such as IgG, complement, macrophages, lymphocytes, and particularly eosinophils.

Another beneficial effect of IgE has been shown with experimental schistosomiasis in rats. The schistosomes that penetrate the skin and migrate through the blood vessels are attacked by macrophages, which interact with the parasite in the presence of IgE antibodies. The macrophage FcεRII then binds to the parasite and brings about its destruction (Capron et al., 1975).

A third beneficial effect of IgE antibody may be the potentiation of an IgG antitoxic reaction. At the site of an allergic skin reaction induced by IgE antibody and antigen, considerably more diphtheria toxin is neutralized by serum antitoxin than at a nonsensitized site (Steinberg et al., 1974). The mechanism appears to be increased cutaneous permeability, permitting more serum antitoxin to diffuse into the reaginic area and to neutralize more toxin.

It has been noted that in developing countries the incidence of allergy in children seemingly is low, despite high levels of IgE. Although it was thought that the high levels of IgE due to parasitism might compete for all the IgE sites on mast cells and in so doing inhibit other allergic reactions, this is not the case. Indeed, when such individuals are exposed to a more urban environment, the incidence of allergy approaches that of the more developed countries.

The absence of detectable IgE (<1 IU/ml) does not appear to be associated with an enhanced susceptibility to infection, at least in more industrialized countries.

ASSESSMENT OF B CELLS AND IMMUNOGLOBULINS

Enumeration and Analysis of B Cells

Estimation of peripheral blood B-, T-, and other lymphocyte subpopulations is of value in many clinical sit-uations, particularly immunodeficiency. Generally this is done by flow cytometry using monoclonal antibody-stained cells. Manual immunofluorescence techniques can also be used to enumerate the stained cells, but this is laborious and imprecise. As noted in Figure 3-13, B cells have several distinct antigens that can be used.

In general, CD19 or CD20 are used to measure total B cells. These are B-cell markers that react with all B cells (pan-B markers) and react with no other types of cells. Other B-cell markers (see Table 11-2) react with some T cells (e.g., CD10) or with B cells at a limited developmental stage (CD21) and thus are less valuable for B-cell enumeration. Normal values for peripheral blood B cells at various ages are given in Table 11-9.

B cells can also be identified by detecting immunoglobulin on the lymphocyte membrane by immunofluorescent techniques (WHO/IARC, 1974). With antisera directed against light chains or against heavy-chain determinants, 10% to 20% of the peripheral blood lymphocytes show an immunofluorescent pattern indicating the presence of surface membrane immunoglobulin (sIg). When monovalent antisera specific for one or another Ig classes or subclass are used, the relative percentages of B-cell subtypes can be estimated.

B cells have receptors for the Fc portion (FcR) of immunoglobulin and the third component of complement, C3, and can thus form rosettes with sheep erythrocytes coated with IgG antibody (EA rosettes) or with antibody and complement (EAC rosettes). Because monocytes and certain lymphocytes lacking sIg (non-B cells) have Fc and C3 receptors, this method for B-cell enumeration is not generally employed.

Enumeration of B cells is indicated in evaluation of immunodeficiency and lymphoproliferative disorders. However, B-cell quantitation in immunodeficiency is rarely indicated if immunoglobulin levels are normal. In autoimmune disorders and other immunologic disorders in which B-cell dysfunction is suspected, B-cell quantitation occasionally may be of value. B cells likewise can be quantitated in tissue sections of lymph nodes, spleen, and other tissues.

Pre-B cells are evaluated by staining bone marrow cells for cytoplasmic μ chains in the absence of light-chain staining. This is generally done only in the evaluation of certain humoral immunodeficiencies and lymphoid malignancy. Although plasma cells may be quantitated by immunohistologic techniques, they are generally measured by routine histologic staining.

It is also possible to use DNA analysis (Southern blotting technique) to determine the nature of the DNA rearrangements in proliferating cells. This will determine whether the cells are of B-cell origin, and, if so, whether they represent a monoclonal (malignant) or polyclonal (reactive) proliferation. For a monoclonal (lymphoproliferative) disorder, this type of analysis will also reveal the stage of maturation of the B cells. This has been particularly revealing in acute lymphoblastic and chronic myelogenous leukemias in blast crisis, both of which represent B-cell neoplasms (Korsmeyer et al., 1983).

Low levels of B cells are decreased in some but not all antibody deficiency disorders. Particularly, in hypogammaglobulinemia with thymoma, the number of both pre-B cells and B cells is diminished; in X-linked agammaglobulinemia, B cells are very low but pre-B cells are present in normal numbers; and in common variable immunodeficiency, both B cells and pre-B cells are normal in number. High percentages and absolute levels of B cells are found in B-cell neoplasms (lymphoid malignancies). Monoclonality is suggested by the presence of a single light-chain or heavy-chain type. Molecular techniques are also used to supplement or supplant this approach.

The numbers of T, B, and natural killer (NK) cells, monocytes, or Ig-secreting plasma cells in body fluids (e.g., cerebrospinal or synovial fluid) or tissues (e.g., synovium or kidney) may help to define the immunologic mechanisms occurring in specific diseases. This has been applied particularly to the mononuclear cells derived from the lungs by bronchoalveolar lavage, a technique that provides insights into the immunopathophysiology of hypersensitivity pneumonitis and sarcoidosis.

Measurement of Ig synthesis by isolated B cells and assay of the effect on their Ig synthetic rate by other cells (suppressor and helper T cells), serum factors, or growth factors are of value in certain immunodeficiency disorders and assessing the value of new therapeutic agents used to stimulate Ig synthesis (see Chapter 12).

Immunoglobulin Assessment

Immunoglobulin levels and antibody function are assessed in many illnesses. Synthetic deficiencies of the immunoglobulins must initially be differentiated from loss of serum proteins. When the latter occurs, the total serum protein and other serum proteins (such as albumin and transferrin) are usually simultaneously reduced and lymphopenia may be present. However, as a result of its low fractional catabolic rate, IgG may be decreased out of proportion to other serum proteins under conditions of extracorporal loss.

Electrophoresis

Serum electrophoresis, either on paper, gel, or cellulose acetate, is sometimes used for detecting abnormalities of the serum proteins. There is some correlation between the electrophoretic gamma globulin level and the sum of the individually measured immunoglobulins. This correlation is not absolute, because most IgM and IgA molecules, and some IgG molecules, migrate in the beta and alpha-2 regions of the electrophoretic field. Nevertheless, it is unusual to find hypogammaglobulinemia if the gamma globulin level is normal by serum electrophoresis and if results of screening tests for antibody function are normal. However, isolated deficiency of IgA and IgM will not be detected by electrophoresis.

Serum electrophoresis is also of value in hypergammaglobulinemic states. A broad increase in the gamma globulin fraction is the usual finding, which indicates an increase in several immunoglobulin classes and subclasses. This polyclonal hypergammaglobulinemia is a nonspecific finding seen in chronic infection, inflammatory disorders, and liver diseases. In contrast to this pattern, a sharp (monoclonal) spike in the gamma globulin region (or occasionally in the alpha and beta globulins) denotes an increase of a single clone of immunoglobulin, an M-component. Monoclonal hypergammaglobulinemia is characteristically present in multiple myeloma or Waldenström's macroglobulinemia (Fig. 4-6).

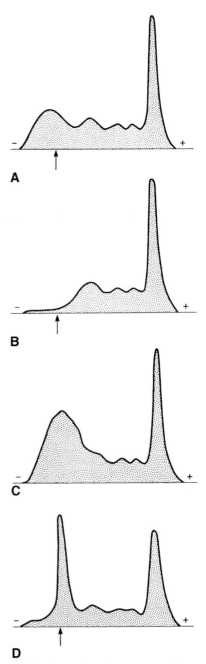

Figure 4-6 · A. Electrophoretic pattern of normal serum. B. Agammaglobulinemic serum. C. Diffuse hypergammaglobulinemic serum. D. M-component hypergammaglobulinemic serum. The arrow indicates the point of application of the serum.

Immunoelectrophoresis

Immunoelectrophoresis is a qualitative test for individual serum proteins that can be used to demonstrate the presence or absence of IgG, IgM, or IgA immunoglobulins (see Fig. 4-2). It also is useful for identifying the presence and class of M-components. Immunoelectrophoresis is not a very sensitive technique, so that proteins present in low concentrations (less than 10 to 20 mg/dl) may not be detected. In pediatric diagnosis, immunoelectrophoresis is generally an unnecessary intermediate procedure because it must be followed by quantitative immunoglobulin determinations.

Immunoglobulin Quantitation

Quantitative immunoglobulin determinations to measure levels of IgG, IgM, IgA, IgE, and IgD (the latter is not usually performed routinely) are available for evaluation of patients with frequent infections, allergy, and related disorders. Quantitative immunoglobulin determinations are often done by the radial diffusion technique, but this has now been replaced in large centers by laser nephelometry, radioimmunoassay (RIA), or enzyme-linked immunosorbent assay (ELISA). Because levels of immunoglobulins change with age, especially in the first year, the results must be compared with those of normal age-matched controls. Levels of immunoglobulins are generally reported in milligrams per deciliter (mg/100 ml), although milligrams per milliliter is also used. The use of International Units (except for IgD and IgE) is not yet widely accepted. One International Unit of IgD = .14 mg and 1 IU of IgE = 2.4 ng. Normal levels of immunoglobulins are given in Chapter 12.

Immunoglobulin Subclasses and Allotypes

Although antisera for determination of some IgG subclasses are commercially available, reliable determinations must be done in research or reference laboratories performing these on a regular basis. Normal levels of IgG subclasses are given in Chapter 12.

Assay for Ig allotypes is a research procedure with little current clinical relevance.

Immunoglobulins in Secretions and Fluids

The immunoglobulin content of the spinal fluid, joint fluid, urine, and exocrine gland secretions is often of clinical interest. Because these fluids are more dilute than serum, they often must be concentrated before analysis with radial diffusion techniques. However, the immunoassay in current use for immunoglobulin levels is capable of measuring these levels directly in most of the specimens. We have used tears to measure the immunoglobulins of external secretions; others have used saliva, nasal fluid, or gastric juice. Levels of IgG in cerebrospinal fluid are of considerable diagnostic value in multiple sclerosis.

Other Procedures

Other laboratory procedures available to evaluate immunoglobulins include the following:

· Erythrocyte sedimentation rate (ESR)
· Bence Jones urinary protein test
· Sia water test
· Cryoglobulin test

The ESR is elevated in active inflammation or tissue necrosis and is associated primarily with an increase in fibrinogen and secondarily with elevated gamma globulin levels. The ESR may be low in the presence of agammaglobulinemia despite the presence of infection.

Monoclonal free light chains are excreted in the urine of some patients with multiple myeloma or Waldenström's macroglobulinemia. Urinary light chains from some patients precipitate when the urine is heated to 56°C, redissolve at higher temperatures, and reprecipitate with cooling. Light chains having these characteristics are called *Bence Jones proteins*. Because not all urinary monoclonal light chains protein have these characteristics, a more reliable method for their detection in a concentrated (100×) sample of urine is the demonstration of a monoclonal spike on electrophoresis or a light-chain paraprotein arc on immunoelectrophoresis. The urinary protein will react with antiserum to either κ or λ light chains but not to both.

The *Sia water test* is a bedside test for high concentrations of euglobulin (a globulin insoluble at low ionic strength) and is characteristically positive in Waldenström's macroglobulinemia. A drop of serum is added to a cylinder of distilled water, and a flocculent precipitate or dense coagulum is noted immediately. Although characteristic of M-components, test results are occasionally positive in polyclonal hypergammaglobulinemias associated with chronic infection. This test is primarily of historical interest.

Cryoglobulins are serum immunoglobulins that precipitate in the cold and redissolve at room temperature. Three general forms of cryoglobulins occur: (1) monoclonal proteins (M-components), generally of the IgG or IgM classes; (2) mixed cryoglobulins composed of an array of normal immunoglobulins; and (3) cryoglobulins composed of a single clone of cold-reactive immunoglobulin but without a monoclonal gammopathy. Generally, the latter two forms of cryoglobulins are associated with high levels of anti-immunoglobulin (rheumatoid factor) activity. When cryoglobulins are present in high concentrations, Raynaud's disease, cold urticaria, microthromboses, and peripheral gangrene may result.

Immunoglobulin Alterations in Health and Disease

Immunoglobulin Alterations with Age

Marked alterations in the levels of immunoglobulins occur during intrauterine life and the neonatal period (see Fig. 3-8). The full-term newborn synthesizes little immunoglobulin at the time of birth but receives an adult level of IgG as a result of active transplacental transport from the mother (Stiehm and Fudenberg, 1966). Placental IgG transport begins at about 3 months' gestation. By term (40 weeks) the IgG level in the infant is slightly greater (110%) than the IgG level in the mother (Kohler and Farr, 1966). The cord blood level of IgG can be used to estimate the gestational age of the fetus (Yeung and Hobbs, 1968).

After birth, the IgG level in the infant decreases as a result of the normal catabolism of maternal IgG and the delay in the infant's own IgG synthesis. During this physiologic hypogammaglobulinemia, the IgG level generally falls to 300 to 500 mg/dl by 4 months. After 4 months, IgG synthesis increases slowly, and 60% of the adult IgG level of 1200 mg/dl is attained by 1 year. Adult levels are reached by age 10 years.

The physiologic dip in IgG levels to hypogamma-globulinemic levels (by adult standards) from age 2 to 6 months is a period that coincides with the peak incidence of many serious infections, such as *Haemophilus influenzae* meningitis, and of sudden, unexplained death in infancy. Because of their lower cord IgG levels, premature infants have a more prolonged and severe physiologic hypogammaglobulinemia and are more susceptible to neonatal infections.

Levels of IgG are slightly higher in postmature infants than in term infants. Further, IgA is occasionally elevated in postmature infants (above 5 mg/dl in 25% of the cases described by Ackerman and colleagues [1969]). In infants with Down syndrome, IgG levels are decreased at birth, averaging 80% of the maternal concentrations (Miller et al., 1969).

IgM does not cross the placenta, but because of some in utero synthesis it is present in infants with a mean level of 10 mg/dl (adult mean, 125 mg/dl). Within a week of birth, IgM synthesis accelerates, with the result that IgM is the chief immunoglobulin synthesized by the newborn infant. The stimulus for the accelerated IgM synthesis is probably the bacterial flora of the recently colonized gastrointestinal tract; thus immature infants, regardless of gestational age, demonstrate a similarly accelerated IgM synthesis immediately after birth. IgM levels reach 50% of adult values by age 6 months and 80% by 1 year.

Because most antibodies to gram-negative bacteria are IgM globulins, infants are not passively protected by transplacental antibodies to these organisms (Gitlin et al., 1963). Conversely, maternal IgG antibodies pass the placenta readily; thus the infant acquires passive protection to many bacterial and viral diseases for the first 6 months of life. In some circumstances, active immunization (e.g., to measles) will be inhibited by this passive maternal IgG antibody, so that certain immunizations should be delayed until after the child is 15 months of age.

IgA, IgD, and IgE neither cross the placenta nor are synthesized in significant quantities by the newborn. Cord levels of these immunoglobulins are very low and rise slowly in the first year (Fig. 4-7; see Fig. 3-8), achieving levels of 10% to 25% of adult levels by

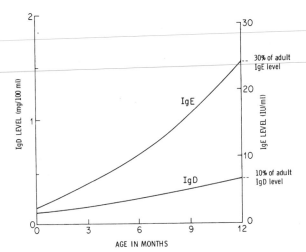

Figure 4-7· Immunoglobulin IgD and IgE levels in the first 12 months of life. Neither IgD nor IgE crosses the placenta, so these immunoglobulins are synthesized solely by the newborn. Note the different scales for IgD (mg/dl) and IgE (IU/ml) (1 IU = 2.4 ng).

12 months. Adult levels are achieved by about age 15. The levels for each age are given in Chapter 12.

Immunoglobulins in Congenital Infection

In congenital infection, cord blood IgM levels are increased, usually to levels exceeding 20 mg/dl (Stiehm et al., 1966). In about 1% to 3% of all infants, cord IgM is elevated. Although it is not always possible to identify an infection in these infants, they should be regarded as a high-risk group and watched carefully for infection. In infants with congenital rubella, toxoplasmosis, cytomegalic inclusion disease, and syphilis, IgM levels are usually, but not invariably, elevated; in infants with cytomegalovirus, IgA levels may also be elevated.

Elevated levels of IgM in cord blood may also occur as a result of leakage of blood from mother to fetus, resulting in a false-positive IgM test for congenital infection. Maternal-fetal leakage is responsible for about 5% to 10% of instances of elevated IgM and can be suspected if the cord IgA exceeds the cord IgM (because maternal IgA is higher than maternal IgM). It can be confirmed by repeat assay of infant IgM and IgA levels; maternally derived IgM and IgA will decrease after 3 or 4 days because of their rapid half-lives. By contrast, levels of IgM and IgA synthesized by the infant will increase or will be maintained.

Immunoglobulins in Antibody Immunodeficiencies

Several chapters of this text are devoted to the antibody deficiency disorders; most of these are associated with deficiency of one or more of the immunoglobulins. There are unusual instances in which immunoglobulin levels are normal but the immunoglobulins function poorly as antibodies. Thus tests for antibody function should be included in the evaluation of a patient with suspected immunodeficiency (see Chapter 12).

In most patients with antibody immunodeficiency, synthesis of immunoglobulins is defective. However, in certain disorders, hypogammaglobulinemia (total immunoglobulin levels less than 400 mg/dl or an IgG globulin less than 200 mg/dl) is due to excessive loss as a result of extracorporal loss, such with nephrotic syndrome, protein-losing enteropathy, or hypercatabolism. In these disorders, levels of many serum proteins are decreased, not just those of the immunoglobulins. The IgG globulin survival is markedly shortened, in contrast to the normal or prolonged IgG survival in most antibody immunodeficiencies. Replacement of IgG is generally not indicated, because it will be rapidly lost. Furthermore, patients with these conditions usually do not experience the same degree of serious infection seen in conditions with defective immunoglobulin synthesis.

M-Components and Paraproteins

Considerable information about immunoglobulin structure has been derived from the study of individuals with excess amounts of a single serum or urinary immunoglobulin, termed an M-component or paraprotein. These proteins are characteristically found in patients with multiple myeloma or Waldenström's macroglobulinemia. An M-component is a homogeneous immunoglobulin present in large quantities produced by a single clone of neoplastic cells. This monoclonal protein results in a single, sharp spike on electrophoresis (see Fig. 4-6). This single peak, in contrast to the relatively broad peak of normal immunoglobulins, occurs as a result of the electrophoretic homogeneity of the component. Monoclonal antibodies produced by hybridema techniques are laboratory-derived M-components limited to a single antigenic specificity.

The presence of large quantities of single M-components permits their isolation and characterization and led to many important observations about the immunoglobulins. For example, recognition of the IgD and IgE immunoglobulin classes resulted from the study of individuals with previously undefined M-components. The entire amino acid sequence of a number of myeloma proteins has been established (Nisonoff et al., 1975a, 1975b).

M-component disorders are mostly of theoretic interest to the pediatrician, because multiple myeloma and macroglobulinemia have not been described in children. The incidence of M-components increases with age; in older individuals, low levels of M-component may occur without associated illness and their serum concentration remains relatively stable for years. This disorder has been termed benign monoclonal gammopathy. M-components have been noted in some pediatric patients with combined immunodeficiency (DeFazio et al., 1975; Geha et al., 1974) and transiently in some patients following immunologic reconstitution by bone marrow transplantation (Rádl et al., 1971).

Myeloma or Macroglobulinemia M-Components

An M-component can belong to any immunoglobulin class. Multiple myeloma is associated with IgG, IgA, IgD, or IgE M-components, whereas Waldenström's macroglobulinemia is associated with an IgM M-component. A myeloma M-component contains either κ or λ light chains, not both. If it is an IgG or IgA myeloma, it contains a heavy chain belonging to only one of the respective subclasses. Some myeloma cells produce κ or λ light chains only and therefore have light-chain M-components. M-components have limited allotypic determinants and idiotypic antigenic characteristics, indicating molecular homogeneity.

Bence Jones protein is an M-component found in the urine (rarely in the serum) of patients with multiple myeloma or macroglobulinemia. Often there is an associated serum M-component. The Bence Jones proteins are dimers of either two κ or two λ light chains with a molecular weight of 40,000 daltons. The light-chain type is the same as the light-chain type of the corresponding serum M-component, because the Bence Jones protein results simply from excess synthesis of light chains not incorporated into intact immunoglobulin molecules.

The frequency of M-components among the classes of immunoglobulins reflects their relative serum concentration. IgG myeloma proteins are the most common, followed by IgA myeloma and IgM macroglobulinemia. IgD myelomas are extremely rare, and IgE myelomas have been found in only eight patients.

Heavy-Chain M-Components

The M-components of heavy-chain disease are homogeneous proteins completely lacking light chains (Franklin, 1976; Franklin and Frangione, 1975). Three types of heavy-chain disease have been identified involving the γ, μ, or α heavy chain, called γ, μ, and α heavy-chain disease. Clinically, the disorder resembles a lymphoreticular neoplasm. Gamma heavy-chain disease affects elderly individuals who manifest lymphadenopathy (particularly that of Waldemeyer's ring) and hepatosplenomegaly. Alpha heavy-chain disease occurs in younger individuals in areas around the Mediterranean Sea. It is generally associated with Mediterranean lymphoma, a malignant infiltration of the gastrointestinal tract, giving rise to diarrhea, malabsorption, and steatorrhea. Mu heavy-chain disease generally occurs with chronic lymphocytic leukemia; prominent features include vacuolated plasma cells and marked visceral involvement.

In all these patients, there is an M-protein in the serum, and occasionally in the urine, that reacts with heavy-chain antisera. There is no associated light chain seen in γ or α heavy-chain disease. Structural studies on these proteins indicate that all the molecules have, in addition to absence of light chains, internal deletions of variable size, including deletions of the variable region, the constant region, and the hinge region. The heavy-chain fragments are the product of synthesis of protein from aberrant DNA rearrangements in the abnormal B cells rather than the product of degradation of normal heavy chains.

Amyloid

Amyloidosis, an extravascular deposition of homogeneous eosinophilic protein throughout the body, is a common complication of multiple myeloma, or it may exist as a primary disorder. Analysis of the amyloid protein in myeloma patients indicates that it is made up of homogeneous light chains, related to Bence Jones protein. These light chains have the ability to fold into the characteristic β pleated sheets of *amyloid L* (AL). In other patients, the amyloid protein is not a portion of the immunoglobulin molecule but is due to the deposition of a reactive serum protein, *amyloid A* (AA).

Hypergammaglobulinemic Disorders

An immunoglobulin level greater than two standard deviations above the mean for age-matched controls is considered abnormally elevated. Some causes of selective immunoglobulin elevations are noted in Table 4-10. In certain immunodeficiencies, elevated levels of one or more immunoglobulins are noted, especially in the immunodeficiencies with hyper-IgM (see Chapter 13) and in Wiskott-Aldrich syndrome (high IgA and IgE) (see Chapter 17). Patients with acquired immunodeficiency syndrome (AIDS), even before multiple opportunistic infections, often have elevated IgG and IgA levels with normal IgM. All pediatric patients with a total Ig level greater than 2000 mg/dl should be screened for HIV antibodies.

Other chronic infections are associated with high levels of IgG, as well as other immunoglobulins. By contrast, infectious mononucleosis, kala-azar, and trypanosomiasis are often associated with selected elevation of IgM levels. Hamano and colleagues (2001) described markedly elevated IgG4 subclass levels in 20 patients with sclerosing pancreatitis.

In many collagen diseases, diffuse hypergammaglobulinemia is present. The degree of hypergammaglobulinemia reflects the duration and severity of the illness and is correlated with the degree of elevation of the ESR. Certain families may have hypergammaglobulinemia and a high incidence of collagen disease. In liver diseases, high immunoglobulin levels are also observed; in chronic active hepatitis, the total Ig may exceed 4000 mg/dl. Patients with Down syndrome, especially institutionalized patients, have high levels of immunoglobulins, particularly of the IgG and IgA classes (Stiehm and Fudenberg, 1966).

Chronic exposure to exogenous antigenic stimulation, as in hypersensitivity pneumonitis (such as pigeon breeder's lung), may also give rise to hypergammaglobulinemia. The finding of elevated levels of immunoglobulins, of itself, is not associated with unusual ability to fight infection.

TABLE 4-10 · SOME NONMALIGNANT CAUSES OF IMMUNOGLOBULIN ELEVATIONS IN CHILDREN

High Levels of One or Two Immunoglobulins

Immunodeficiency diseases
Hyper-IgM immunodeficiency (↑ IgM)
Wiskott-Aldrich syndrome (↑ IgA, ↑ IgE)
Job's syndrome (↑ IgE)
Buckley's syndrome (↑ IgE)

Infections
Congenital infection (↑ IgM)
Infectious mononucleosis (↑ IgM)
Trypanosomiasis (↑ IgM)
Malaria (↑ IgM)
Kala-azar (↑ IgM)

Miscellaneous
Anaphylactoid purpura (↑ IgA)
Extrinsic allergy (↑ IgE)
Eczema (↑ IgE)
Kawasaki syndrome (↑ IgE)
Periarteritis nodosa (↑ IgE)
Cold agglutinin disease (↑ IgM)

High Levels of All Immunoglobulins

Immunodeficiencies
Chronic granulomatous disease
Acquired immunodeficiency syndrome

Infections
Intestinal parasitism (↑ ↑ IgE)
Visceral larva migrans
Chronic bacterial infections (osteomyelitis, endocarditis, abscesses, tuberculosis)

Collagen-vascular diseases
Rheumatic fever
Rheumatoid arthritis
Lupus erythematosus
Ulcerative colitis
Regional enteritis

Liver diseases
Acute hepatitis
Chronic active hepatitis
Cirrhosis

Miscellaneous
Down syndrome
Hyperglobulinemic purpura
Pulmonary hypersensitivity diseases
Illicit intravenous drug use
Cystic fibrosis
Sarcoidosis

REFERENCES

Ackerman BD, Taylor WF, O'Loughlin BJ. Serum immunoglobulin levels in postmature infants. Pediatrics 43:956–962, 1969.

Allen JC., and Kunkel HG. Antibodies against gamma-globulin after repeated blood transfusions in man. J Clin Invest 45:29–39, 1966.

Anderson BR, Terry WD. Gamma G4-globulin antibody causing inhibition of clotting factor VIII. Nature (London) 217:174–175, 1968.

Askonas BA, Williamson AR. Biosynthesis of immunoglobulins on polyribosomes and assembly of the IgG molecule. Proc Roy Soc London (Biol) 166:232–243, 1966.

Aubry J-P, Pochon S, Grabar P, Jansen KU, Bonnefoy J-Y. CD21 is a ligand for CD23 and regulates IgE production. Nature 358:505–507,1992.

Ballow M. Mechanisms of action of intravenous immune serum globulin in autoimmune and inflammatory diseases. J Allergy Clin Immunol, 100:151–157, 1997.

et al., 2000; Orkin, 2000). In humans, bone marrow and blood stem cells can generate hepatocytes (Alison et al., 2000). The therapeutic potential of stem cell transplantation is obvious (Weissman, 2000).

More than 40 different growth factors, cytokines, and chemokines interact with stem and progenitor cells through specific receptors to regulate proliferation, differentiation, and cell fate (Watowich et al., 1996). Among these, granulocyte colony-stimulating factor (G-CSF) has emerged as the most clinically useful. G-CSF specifically promotes neutrophil proliferation and maturation, and it enhances neutrophil microbicidal activity when administered in vivo (Liles et al., 1997; Root and Dale, 1999). It is available for clinical application in mobilizing stem cells from the marrow for transplantation purposes, for treatment of some types of neutropenia, and as adjunctive therapy for treatment of serious bacterial and fungal infections in nonneutropenic patients (American Society of Clinical Oncology, 1996; Root and Dale, 1999). It is relatively nontoxic and can protect against the septic consequences of infection such as acute respiratory distress syndrome (ARDS) and other organ failures, perhaps at least in part because it stimulates production of anti-inflammatory factors such as interleukin-1 (IL-1) receptor antagonist and soluble tumor necrosis factor (TNF) receptor (Nelson et al., 1998; Root and Dale, 1999).

Cell-cell and cell-extracellular matrix interactions through perhaps as many 20 different adhesion receptors also play a major role in hematopoiesis (Prosper and Verfaille, 2001). These receptors modulate the retention in the marrow of stem cells and hematopoietic progenitor cells, their homing to the marrow when transplanted, and their survival, proliferation, and differentiation.

Associated with their short life span, neutrophils have poorly developed protein synthetic machinery. However, neutrophils maintain active genes that program their unique activities. A profile of genes actively expressed in human granulocytes, when compared with such profiles from other cells or tissues, revealed several genes that appeared to be unique to granulocytes (Itoh et al., 1998), although the function of many of these genes is not known.

Granule Content and Function

Initial descriptions of the histology of the polymorphonuclear leukocyte in the late nineteenth century emphasized the obviously prominent granules, and these were assumed to play a role in killing microorganisms (Fig. 5-2). This concept was substantiated in the mid twentieth century by the work of DeDuve defining lysosomal granules as packets of enzymes and that of Hirsch and Cohn demonstrating that neutrophil granules fuse with the plasma membrane surrounding internalized bacteria (the phagocytic vacuole) and rupture into the vacuole (Cohn and Hirsch, 1960; Zucker-Franklin and Hirsch, 1964). We now know that this degranulation is necessary but may not be sufficient to

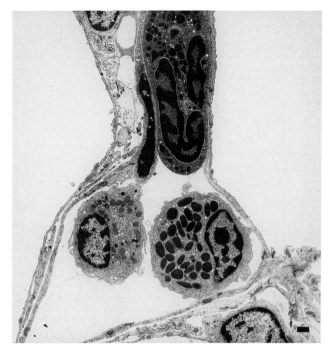

Figure 5-2 · Transmission electron micrograph (EM) of small blood vessel in alveolar parenchyma. A neutrophil is shown at top in full cross-section, a monocyte at the lower left, and an eosinophil with distinctive large granules in the lower right. Magnification ×4000. Bar represents 1 μm. (Courtesy Jan E. Henson.)

kill most bacteria, at least in large numbers, and that neutrophils must also convert oxygen to toxic oxidative metabolites to achieve full bactericidal activity (see following discussion).

It is now clear that four distinct subpopulations of granules can be identified in human neutrophils (azurophil, specific, gelatinase, and secretory granules or vesicles). These subpopulations can be distinguished by size, morphology, density, ease of mobilization, and, perhaps most meaningfully, the proteins they contain. Yet they may be viewed as a continuum that reflects the differences in the time of biosynthesis of the various granule proteins (Borregaard and Cowland, 1997; Borregaard et al., 2001; Cowland and Borregaard, 1999). These organelles play a varied and fundamental role in the biology of neutrophils. In fact, the sequential steps by which neutrophils participate in host defense and inflammation—adherence to endothelium, diapedesis, chemotaxis, phagocytosis, and killing—all depend at least partially on the contents and mobilization of granules. The composition of neutrophil granules and their membranes is summarized in Table 5-1.

Azurophil Granules

Azurophil granules are identified by their myeloperoxidase content but contain many hydrolytic enzymes and bactericidal proteins that are important to neutrophil function. These include elastase and cathepsin G, implicated in bacterial killing and tissue degradation, and the antimicrobial proteins defensins, cathelicidins,

TABLE 5-1 · COMPOSITION OF HUMAN NEUTROPHIL GRANULES AND SECRETORY VESICLES

Azurophil Granules	Specific Granules	Gelatinase Granules	Secretory Vesicles
Membrane	**Membrane**	**Membrane**	**Membrane**
CD63	CD11b	CD11b	Alkaline phosphatase
CD68	CD15 antigens	Cytochrome b_{558}	CR1
V-type H$^+$-ATPase	CD66	Diacylglycerol-deacylating enzyme	Cytochrome b_{558}
	CD67	FMLP-R	CD11b
	Cytochrome b_{558}	SCAMP	CD14
	FMLP-R	Urokinase-type plasminogen	CD16
	Fibronectin-R	activator-R	FMLP-R
	G-protein subunit	VAMP-2	SCAMP
	Interleukin-10-R	V-type H$^+$-ATPase	Urokinase-type
	Laminin-R		plasminogen activator-R
	NB-1 antigen		V-type H$^+$-ATPase
	19-kd protein		VAMP-2
	155-kd protein		CD10, CD13, CD45
	Rap1, Rap2		C1q-R
	SCAMP		DAF
	Thrombospondin-R		
	TNF-R		
	Urokinase-type		
	plasminogen activator-R		
	VAMP-2		
	Vitronectin-R		
Matrix	**Matrix**	**Matrix**	**Matrix**
Acid	β_2-Microglobulin	Acetyltransferase	Plasma proteins (including
mucopolysaccharide	Collagenase	β-Microglobulin	albumin and tetranectin)
α_1-Antitrypsin	Gelatinase	Gelatinase	
α-Mannosidase	hCAP-18	Lysozyme	
Azurocidin/CAP37/	Histaminase		
heparin-binding protein	Heparanase		
Bactericidal permeability	Lysozyme		
increasing protein	Lactoferrin		
β-Glycerophosphatase	NGAL		
β-Glucuronidase	Properdin		
Cathepsins	Sialidase		
Defensins	SGP28		
Elastase	Urokinase-type plasminogen		
Lysozyme	activator		
Myeloperoxidase	Vitamin B$_{12}$-binding protein		
N-acetyl-β-glucosaminidase			
Proteinase-3			
Sialidase			
Ubiquitin-protein			

ATP = adenosine triphosphate; CAP = cationic antimicrobial protein; CD = cluster of differentiation (antigen); CR = complement receptor; DAF = decay accelerating factor; FMLP = formyl-met-leu-phe; hCAP = human CAP (cathelicidin); NB-1 = neutrophil antigen B-1; NGAL = neutrophil gelatinase-associated lipocalin; R = receptor; SCAMP = secretory carrier membrane protein; SGP = specific granule protein; TNF = tumor necrosis factor; VAMP = vesicle-associated membrane protein.
Modified from Borregaard N, Cowland JB. Granules of the human neutrophilic polymorphonuclear leukocyte. Blood 89:3503–3521, 1997.

bactericidal/permeability-increasing protein (BPI), and lysozyme (Belaaouaj et al., 2000; Borregaard and Cowland, 1997; Lehrer et al., 1991; Risso, 2000; Spitznagel, 1990; Weiss and Olsson, 1987; Yang et al., 2001). Defensins are cationic peptides that exhibit antimicrobial activity in vitro against bacteria, fungi, and enveloped viruses. They comprise 5% of total neutrophil protein and 30% to 50% of azurophil granule protein (Lehrer et al., 1993).

Defensins and other antimicrobial peptides are also synthesized and released by epithelial cells in human skin, airway, small intestine, kidney, and reproductive tract (Ganz, 1999; Huttner and Bevins, 1999; Scott and Hancock, 2000). Neutrophil and epithelial antimicrobial peptides offer broad-spectrum and highly effective protection against microbial invasion and represent a central component of the *innate immune system* (see Chapter 9). These cationic peptides are noninflammatory because they preferentially disrupt microbial membranes, which are rich in negatively charged (anionic) phospholipids compared with mammalian cell membranes (Ganz, 1999). Neutrophil defensins and cathelicidins are chemotactic for CD4 and CD8 T cells, immature dendritic cells, monocytes, and in some cases, other neutrophils. Thus they represent a mechanism by which innate and adaptive antimicrobial immunity may be linked (Yang et al., 2001). Upregulation of mammalian defensin genes occurs during infection and inflammation through stimulation of signal transduction pathways common to other innate immune responses, including nuclear factor-κB (NF-κB) and NF IL-6 (Kaiser and Diamond, 2000).

BPI has structural homology to serum lipopolysaccharide (LPS)–binding protein; it binds bacterial LPS and is cytotoxic to gram-negative bacteria (Elsbach et al., 1999; Weiss et al., 1992). Mouse neutrophils lack BPI and defensins (Elsbach et al., 1999) and differ in other significant ways (Nauseef, 2001), emphasizing that findings with normal or gene-manipulated mouse neutrophils must be extrapolated cautiously to their human counterpart. Neutrophil antimicrobial peptides, including BPI, are beginning to be studied in patients as treatment for infection (Hancock, 1999).

Proteinase 3, a cationic proteinase contained primarily in azurophil granules, is also expressed in active form on the neutrophil cell surface, especially after exposure of the cell to cytokines and chemoattractants (Campbell et al., 2000). Proteinase 3 is the most common antigenic target for the antineutrophil antibodies that characterize Wegener's granulomatosis (Jenette et al., 1990). MPO and BPI are other target antigens of antineutrophil autoantibodies that are present in certain conditions of vasculitis or chronic inflammation (Schultz et al., 2001).

Specific Granules

Specific granules are characterized by lactoferrin content; but they are rich in enzymes, and their limiting membranes serve as a reservoir of many proteins whose upregulation to the plasma membrane is essential for normal host defense. These include receptors, other proteins involved in adherence and signal transduction, and both pieces of cytochrome b_{558} (gp91phox and p22phox), which is the central component of the respiratory burst oxidase (see Table 5-1). In response to contact with an opsonized microbe (coated with antibody and complement component 3 (C3) or mannose-binding lectin-C3), granules move to and fuse with the plasma membrane, allowing incorporation of the cytochrome and subsequent binding of the cytoplasmic constituents of the oxidase. The neutrophil alloantigen NB-1, present on the membrane of specific granules and the plasma membrane, can induce maternal sensitization and neonatal neutropenia (Goldschmeding et al., 1992; Lalezari et al., 1971).

Gelatinase Granules

Gelatinase granules, defined by their high gelatinase B content, are mobilized more readily than specific granules, which in turn are mobilized more readily than azurophil granules (Borregaard and Cowland, 1997). This hierarchy is maintained when neutrophils isolated from blood are stimulated and when exudate neutrophils from skin window chambers are analyzed and stimulated further (Sengelov et al., 1995). Gelatinase granules also contain 20% to 25% of the neutrophil's cytochrome b_{558} (Kjeldsen et al., 1994). Gelatinase B is a matrix metalloproteinase (MMP-9) that can degrade extracellular matrix and truncate, and thereby activate 10-fold, the neutrophil chemotactic factor IL-8 (Opdenakker et al., 2001; Van den Steen et al., 2000).

Thus gelatinase granules may play an important part in the movement of neutrophils into sites of infection and inflammation.

Secretory Vesicles

The most rapidly mobilizable intracellular organelles in neutrophils are the secretory vesicles, which appear to represent unique endocytic vesicles that can be triggered to exocytose by inflammatory stimuli (Borregaard et al., 1992; Robinson et al., 1999). Their membrane is rich in alkaline phosphatase and various receptors (see Table 5-1). Their discovery followed the observation that β_2-integrin (CD11b/CD18, Mac-1) becomes incorporated into the plasma membrane without corresponding exocytosis of granule contents. Their only known content is plasma, indicating that they are formed by endocytosis (Bainton, 1999; Borregaard and Cowland, 1997).

Exposure of neutrophils to LPS or inflammatory cytokines moves a receptor for IL-10 from specific granules to the cell surface (Elbim et al., 2001). Subsequent interaction with IL-10 can then downregulate many of the neutrophil's inflammatory activities, including the respiratory burst (Cassatella, 1999; Elbim et al., 2001).

Secretion of Inflammatory Proteins

Until recently, mature neutrophils were considered to be terminally differentiated cells that could not synthesize RNA or protein. It is now clear that exposure of neutrophils to bacteria increases expression of several hundred RNA species (Subrahmanyam et al., 2001) and that neutrophils can release a variety of pro- and antiinflammatory polypeptides that contribute to host defense and disease expression (reviewed in Cassatella, 1999). These include the proinflammatory cytokines TNF-α, IL-1, and IL-12; the antiinflammatory cytokines IL-1 receptor antagonist and transforming growth factor-β (TGF-β); chemokines, including IL-8; and the growth factor G-CSF. The capacity of neutrophils to respond to and secrete cytokines lends support to the argument that they play an important role in immunosurveillance against some tumors (DiCarlo et al., 2001) and in linking innate immunity to the adaptive response to infection (Yamashiro et al., 2001).

Adhesion and Emigration

During the inflammatory response, neutrophils are stimulated to leave the marrow by IL-8, fragments cleaved from C3, and other blood-borne microbial and host factors. Certain local factors influence this egress, including movement of more mature neutrophils closer to the marrow sinus endothelial cells and induction of gaps between these endothelial cells (Opdenakker et al., 1998). Once out of the marrow, neutrophils get a brief ride in the circulation, then undergo a coordinated series of adhesive events that begin to guide the cells toward their target, the source of inflammation.

Adhesion, then *diapedesis* (emigration from the bloodstream across the endothelial barrier) and *chemotaxis* (movement toward the center of a chemical gradient), are all orchestrated by release of a variety of chemical factors from microorganisms or from activated or damaged host tissue (Fig. 5-3).

Under conditions that are not influenced by inflammation, about half the neutrophils within the circulation are riding with the flow and half are sequestered so that they are not accessible by phlebotomy, such as in the spleen and along vessel walls. Cells can be mobilized from this *marginating pool* by infection/inflammation, labor and childbirth, emotional or physical stress, or injection of epinephrine. When a focus of infection or tissue damage emerges, neutrophils entering a postcapillary venule in an adjacent area begin to adhere loosely and reversibly to the endothelial surface in a process termed *rolling*. The *selectins*, a family of leukocyte and endothelial cell lectins (carbohydrate-binding proteins), appear primarily responsible for this initial interaction

(Anderson and Smith, 2001; Muller, 1999). L-selectin (CD62L) is expressed constitutively on neutrophils and other leukocytes; E-selectin and P-selectin are not constitutively expressed by endothelial cells but are upregulated by stimulation with cytokines (IL-1, TNF) or with histamine, respectively.

The selectins bind particular types of carbohydrate ligands, including an oligosaccharide that characterizes the sialylated Lewis X blood group, generally referred to as sialyl Lewis X (sLeX) (Varki, 1994). sLeX-bearing ligands are expressed constitutively at high levels on neutrophils, and these bind to E- and P-selectin on endothelial cells (Varki, 1997). Conversely, L-selectin on neutrophils can bind sLeX-like molecules on endothelial cells (Anderson and Smith, 2001).

The importance of the adhesive interactions between neutrophil sLeX-bearing ligands and endothelial selectins is emphasized by the disorder leukocyte adhesion deficiency (LAD) type II (Etzioni et al., 1992). Patients with LAD II have recurrent bacterial infections,

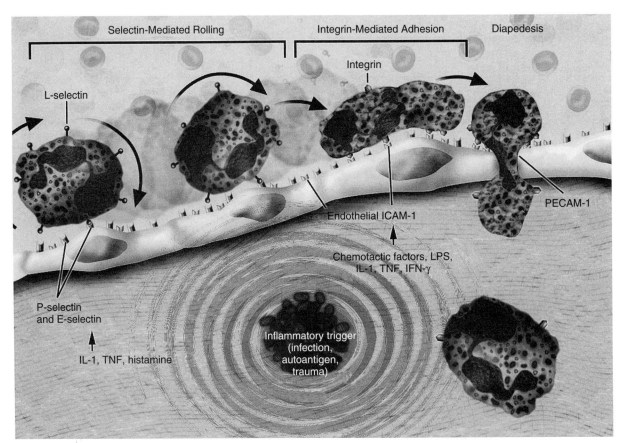

Figure 5-3· **The neutrophil response to inflammation—rolling, adhesion, diapedesis, and chemotaxis.** As neutrophils move along the blood vessel wall, they can be activated by exposure to cytokines, chemokines, chemotactic factors, and microbial products released at a site of inflammation. In the initial phase (rolling), the neutrophils adhere loosely and reversibly through binding of L-selectin on the neutrophil to E- and P-selectins on the endothelial cell. As contact increases, L-selectin is rapidly shed and integrins (Mac-1 and LFA-1) are upregulated on the neutrophil plasma membrane. The binding of integrins to ICAM-1 on the endothelial cell induces the neutrophil to flatten, adhere tightly, and then migrate across the endothelial barrier, using integrin/ICAM-1 and platelet-endothelial cell adhesion molecule-1 (PECAM-1) binding for traction. Once into the tissue, neutrophils move along a gradient of chemotactic factors toward the source of the inflammatory response, which they can then remove by phagocytosis. (Illustration by Boyd Jacobson.)

striking neutrophilia in the presence or absence of infection, and decreased neutrophil rolling, adhesion, and emigration (Etzioni, 1996). Their leukocytes fail to express sLeX and do not bind to E-selectin in vitro (Etzioni, 1996; Karsan et al., 1998) (see Chapter 20).

In human granulocytic ehrlichiosis, a tickborne febrile illness characterized by reduced neutrophil and platelet counts, the causative agent uses sLeX to bind to and penetrate granulocytes (Goodman et al., 1999). The organism, *Ehrlichia phagocytophila*, is the only microbe known to replicate within human granulocytes. Cryptococcal polysaccharides can cause shedding of neutrophil L-selectin, and in disseminated cryptococcosis this may prevent neutrophils from effectively attaching to endothelial cells and penetrating to sites of cryptococcal infection (Dong and Murphy, 1996).

The next step in the movement of neutrophils toward the focus of inflammation depends on the neutrophil *integrins* Mac-1 (complement receptor-3 [CR-3], CD11b/CD18) and lymphocyte-function-associated antigen-1 (LFA-1, CD11a/CD18) (Anderson and Smith, 2001; Springer, 1995). As the rolling neutrophil slows, it comes into contact with chemotactic factors that are expressed on the surface of endothelial cells. Neutrophil L-selectin is subsequently downregulated and Mac-1 is upregulated (Kishimoto et al., 1989). Intercellular adhesion molecule-1 (ICAM-1, CD54) is the principal ligand on endothelial cells for these integrins (see Fig. 5-3). ICAM-1 is constitutively expressed on venular endothelial cells and is markedly upregulated by exposure of these cells to inflammatory cytokines (IL-1, TNF, interferon-γ [IFN-γ]).

As a result of the integrin–ICAM-1 interaction, the neutrophils stop rolling, flatten, and then migrate across the endothelial barrier (Fig. 5-4) using integrins for traction, as well as homophilic binding between platelet–endothelial cell adhesion molecule-1 (PECAM-1) expressed both on neutrophils and on the intercellular junctions of endothelial cells (see Fig. 5-3) (Bogen et al., 1994; Delves and Roitt, 2000; Muller, 1999; Vaporciyan et al., 1993). Neutrophil gelatinase B is thought to play a role in digesting the basement membrane, allowing entrance into the tissue (Opdenakker et al., 2001) (see Fig. 5-4). Neutrophils from humans, cattle, or dogs that have markedly reduced or absent expression of CD18 integrins (LAD type I) exhibit profound deficiency in emigration to sites of infection and inflammation (see Chapter 20).

Chemotaxis

The direction of emigration and of movement once in the tissues depends on cues from chemotactic factors. Neutrophils can sense a chemoattractant concentration difference of 1% across their diameter and move steadily toward the greater concentration (Springer, 1995). Neutrophils are the fastest cells in the human body, moving at speeds of up to 30μm per minute when optimally attracted (Stossel, 1994a, 1994b).

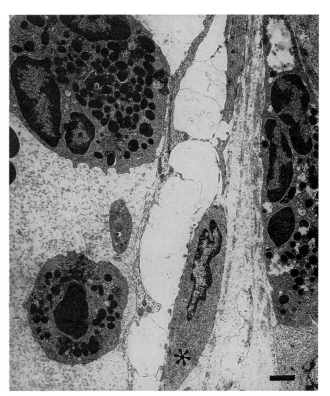

Figure 5-4 · Transmission EM of two rabbit neutrophils closely apposed to vascular endothelium in an area of lung inflammation. The asterisk indicates the endothelial cell, which shows cytoplasmic blebbing characteristic of a damaged cell. A platelet sits between the two neutrophils. A third neutrophil (right) has penetrated beneath the basal lamina of the vessel toward the area of inflammation. Magnification ×7000. Bar represents 1 μm. (Courtesy Jan E. Henson.)

Classical chemoattractants for granulocytes act broadly on neutrophils, eosinophils, and basophils (Table 5-2). A relatively recently described, and still growing, family of chemoattractant cytokines termed *chemokines,* now numbering more than 40 proteins, have some specificity for granulocyte subsets (Luster, 1998; Zlotnick and Yoshie, 2000). Chemokines have been divided into two major subfamilies on the basis of arrangement of the N-terminal cysteine residues, CXC and CC, depending on whether the first two cysteine residues have an amino acid between them (CXC) or are adjacent (CC). The specificity for different leukocyte subtypes is directed by the chemokine receptors they display. At least 18 receptors for chemokines are expressed variably across leukocyte types (Loetscher and Clark-Lewis, 2001; Luster, 1998). In the relatively new standardized nomenclature, the two major groups of the chemokines, as ligands, are designated CXCL and CCL and the receptors are termed CXCR and CCR (Loetscher and Clark-Lewis, 2001; Zlotnick and Yoshie, 2000). For example, IL-8 becomes CXCL8, which binds to CXCR1 and CXCR2 on neutrophils. Certain CXC chemokines share similar biochemical characteristics with defensins, including being cationic, and can induce direct antibacterial activity (Cole et al., 2001) (see Appendix).

TABLE 5-2 · MAJOR CHEMOTACTIC FACTORS FOR GRANULOCYTES

Chemoattractant	Origin	Responding Granulocytes		
		Neutrophils	Eosinophils	Basophils
C5a	Complement activation	+	+	+
Leukotriene B4	Arachidonate metabolism	+		
Platelet-activating factor	Phosphatidylcholine metabolism	+	+	
N-formyl peptides	Bacteria	+	+	+
CXC chemokines (e.g., IL-8 [CXCL8])	T cells, monocytes, endothelial/epithelial cells, fibroblasts, neutrophils, others	+		+
CC chemokines (e.g., eotaxins [CCL11, CCL24])	T cells, monocytes, endothelial cells, dendritic cells, fibroblasts, platelets		+	+

Role of Actin and Myosin

The mechanism of neutrophil movement toward a focus of inflammation depends on the highly regulated assembly and disassembly of actin filaments within the cell (Condeelis, 1993; Stossel, 1994a, 1994b, 1999). In an unstimulated cell, actin, which constitutes 10% of the neutrophil's total cell protein, concentrates in the cell cortex bound to regulatory proteins that prevent assembly of actin subunits into filaments. Ligation of chemotactic factor receptors at the protruding edge of the cell (lamella or pseudopodium) elicits a series of steps in signal transduction that lead to the freeing of the regulatory proteins from the actin subunits, which then polymerize into filaments.

Interaction with actin-binding protein permits filaments to form a gel, a more rigid three-dimensional lattice, to which myosin is attached. The Ca^{2+} fluxes associated with cell activation, as well as guanosine triphosphatase (GTPase) activity, promote myosin interaction with actin (Stossel, 1999). Actin-myosin interaction contracts the microfilament gel, new cortical cytoplasm is pushed forward, and the cell crawls closer to its target. The trailing edge of the actin network must be disassembled or the cell will be stuck fast. Gelsolin converts the trailing edge of the actin gel to a sol by blocking the addition of actin subunits to the filaments and by breaking the bonds between the actin subunits already in the filament (Stossel, 1999).

Neutrophil microtubules, made up of polymers of the protein tubulin, can be seen as strands radiating from organizing centers (centrioles) situated between the nucleus and leading edge of the cell (Anderson et al., 1982; Malech et al., 1977). This system organizes delivery of cytoplasmic granules to the leading edge of the cell during chemotaxis and phagocytosis and may otherwise organize and stabilize the cell.

Familial Mediterranean Fever

Familial Mediterranean fever (FMF) is characterized by massive infiltration of neutrophils into inflammatory sites, apparently as an abnormally vigorous response to a suboptimal signal. Pyrin, the protein product of the gene that is abnormal in FMF, has been located in association with actin filaments in lamellae and with microtubules, suggesting that FMF may result from an abnormality in the cytoskeletal regulation of chemotaxis (Mansfield et al., 2001).

Phagocytosis

The term *endocytosis* refers to the interiorization of extracellular material, either fluid or solid. With either type material, a portion of the plasma membrane pinches off from the cell surface to form an endosome, a membrane-bound cytoplasmic compartment. In *pinocytosis*, soluble material is taken into a pinocytic vesicle. Receptors may be involved, such as for hormones, cholesterol in lipoprotein particles, or nutrients such as vitamin B_{12} bound to transcobalamin II. The receptor-ligand complexes are concentrated into small invaginations in the plasma membrane termed coated pits because of their appearance on electron microscopy. The protein clathrin is prominent in the pit walls. These clathrin-coated pits pinch off and become coated vesicles (Fig. 5-5).

Phagocytosis refers to internalization of large particles, particularly microorganisms, cell debris, or foreign material. Mycoplasma, with a diameter of about 0.5 μm, is the smallest microbe known to stimulate phagocytosis (Marshall et al., 1995). Chlamydia, the next smallest, and viruses enter cells by nonphagocytic mechanisms (Greenberg, 1999; Gregory et al., 1979). In contrast to pinocytosis, phagocytosis cannot occur at temperatures less than 13°C to 18°C (Greenberg, 1999).

At physiologic temperatures, pseudopodia extend from the phagocytic cell over the surface of the particle until it is surrounded within a plasma membrane–bound *phagosome* (phagocytic vesicle). Cytoplasmic granules fuse with the phagosome and release their contents in on the captured material, creating a *phagolysosome* in which killing and digestion can occur. Pseudopodia formation and phagocytosis depend on the same processes of actin polymerization-depolymerization and interaction with myosin that underlie the chemotactic response (Greenberg, 1999). Cytosolic free Ca^{2+}, which is critical for regulating many cellular systems, including actin-myosin interaction, becomes concentrated in the filamentous actin-rich pseudopodia surrounding the ingested particle (Stendahl et al., 1994).

The triggers for chemotaxis and phagocytosis differ. In contrast to the soluble factors that serve as chemoat-

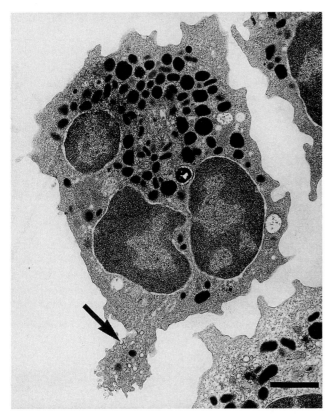

Figure 5-5 · **Transmission EM of neutrophil.** Coated pits can be seen as invaginations of the plasma membrane in the cytoplasmic projection at the lower left (arrow). Coated vesicles are visible in adjacent cytoplasm. Magnification ×13,400. Bar represents 1 μm. (Courtesy Jan E. Henson.)

TABLE 5-3 · PRINCIPAL RECEPTORS FOR PHAGOCYTOSIS EXPRESSED ON NEUTROPHILS AND EOSINOPHILS

Receptor	Ligand	Cell Type	
		Neutrophils	Eosinophils
FcγRI	Fc portion of IgG	+	+
FcγRIIA	Fc portion of IgG	+	+
FcγRIIIA	Fc portion of IgG	+	+
FcαRI	Fc portion of IgA	+	+
FcεRI and II	Fc portion of IgE		+
CR1	C3b > C4b > iC3b	+	+
CR3	iC3b	+	+
CR4	iC3b	+	+
C1qR	Clq	+	

From Greenberg, 1999; Indik et al., 1995; Monteiro and van de Winkel, 2003; Ravetch, 1994; Rosenberg, 1999; Underhill and Ozinsky, 2002.

tractants (see Table 5-2), phagocytosis by neutrophils is triggered when serum opsonins (from the Greek meaning "to prepare food for" or "cater") bound to the foreign material or microorganism encounter their specific receptors on the phagocyte. IgG antibodies and activated (cleaved) forms of C3 (C3b and iC3b) are the principal serum opsonins, and the receptors for these opsonins (Fc receptors and complement receptor 3 [CR3]) are central to the phagocytic process in granulocytes (Table 5-3) (Greenberg, 1999; Indik et al., 1995; Monteiro and van de Winkel, 2003; Ravetch, 1994; Rosenberg, 1999; Underhill and Ozinsky, 2002). The receptor for C1q might also promote bacterial uptake under some conditions (Eggleton et al., 1994). The function of the various forms of the Fc receptor for IgG appears to be at least partially redundant, in that a single class of Fcγ receptors (I, II, or III) can mediate phagocytosis in the absence of other Fc receptors (Indik et al., 1995).

Two general classes of Fcγ receptors are now recognized on most effector cells involved in host defense: activation receptors, FcγRI, RIIA, and RIIIA; and an inhibitory receptor, FcγRIIB (reviewed in Ravetch and Bolland, 2001). These bind IgG with reasonably comparable affinity and specificity and are usually coexpressed on the same cell surface. The cytoplasmic domain that is associated with each receptor type deter-

mines signaling for an activating or an inhibitory effect. The inhibitory FcγRIIB does not induce phagocytosis in neutrophils. It mediates an apoptotic response in B cells (Pearse et al., 1999), but its modulatory function in neutrophils has not been fully defined (Ravetch and Bolland, 2001).

In addition to binding opsonic C3 fragments, CR3 can serve as a *pattern recognition receptor* in that it can bind extracellular matrix proteins such as fibronectin and it can act as a lectin and bind a variety of carbohydrates (Sengelov, 1995). Neutrophils can use CR3 as a nonopsonic phagocytic receptor for pathogenic mycobacteria when CR3 sits in cholesterol-rich microdomains (rafts) in the plasma membrane (LeCabec et al., 2000; Peyron et al, 2000). Neutrophils that ingest mycobacteria of the *Mycobacterium avium* complex can kill them (Hartmann et al., 2001). However, this neutrophil mycobactericidal capacity is not sufficient to protect the host fully, judged by the fact that nontuberculous mycobacterial disease occurs characteristically in individuals with abnormal macrophage or T-cell function (e.g., acquired immunodeficiency syndrome [AIDS]) but presumably normal neutrophil function.

Oxygen-Dependent Killing of Microorganisms

The Respiratory Burst and Other Sources of Microbicidal Oxidants

Neutrophils use oxygen for the destruction of a wide range of pathogens. The association between phagocytosis and oxygen metabolism was first made by Baldridge and Gerard (1933), who found that phagocytosis was accompanied by a large increase in oxygen uptake, a "respiratory burst." This was originally attributed to an increase in oxygen uptake required to provide energy for phagocytosis through oxidative phosphorylation; but Sbarra and Karnovsky (1959) in a classic study showed that the respiratory burst was unaffected by cyanide, ruling out mitochondrial respiration as the cause of the burst of oxygen uptake. The crucial role of the respiratory burst in microbial killing was finally appreciated in 1967, when it was shown that patients with chronic granulomatous disease (CGD) failed to express a respiratory burst (Holmes et al., 1967; Quie et al., 1967).

The respiratory burst is manufactured by neutrophils, monocytes, macrophages, and eosinophils and results in the production of superoxide (O_2^-), which is oxygen reduced by a single electron, according to the following reaction (Babior et al., 1976):

$$2 O_2 + NADPH \xrightarrow{NADPH\ oxidase} 2 O_2^- + NADP^+ + H^+$$

The electron comes from NADPH, which in turn is produced in the hexosemonophosphate (HMP) shunt in a reaction catalyzed by glucose-6-phosphate dehydrogenase (G6PD) (Karnovsky and Badwey, 1983):

$$glucose\text{-}6\text{-}phosphate + NADP^+ \xrightarrow{G6PD} 6\text{-}phosphogluconate + NADPH + H^+$$

$$6\text{-}phosphogluconate + NADP^+ \rightarrow ribulose\text{-}5\text{-}phosphate + CO_2 + NADPH + H^+$$

X-linked deficiency of G6PD is expressed in erythrocytes and less severely in leukocytes. When leukocyte G6PD activity is less than about 5% of normal, the respiratory burst is reduced to the point that CGD develops, probably because there is insufficient NADPH to supply electrons for oxygen reduction to superoxide (Baehner et al., 1972; Gray et al., 1973).

Superoxide anion generated in the respiratory burst interacts with itself in a dismutation reaction to form H_2O_2:

$$2 O_2^- + 2 H^+ \rightarrow H_2O_2 + O_2$$

The reaction is greatly accelerated by the enzyme superoxide dismutase, which exists in the cytosol and mitochondria of phagocytes (and all mammalian cells).

STRUCTURE OF NADPH OXIDASE

NADPH oxidase is the enzyme responsible for production of O_2^-. It is a complex enzyme that assembles in the membrane under the stimulation of phagocytosis. In the resting cell its components are distributed between two cellular compartments, cytosol and membranes (Babior, 1999). The membranes contain two components: gp91phox, a 91 kDa protein that contains flavin adenine dinucleotide (FAD) and an iron-containing, oxygen-binding heme, and p22phox, a 22 kDa protein. Together these two proteins are called cytochrome b_{558}. gp91phox is thought to be the electron carrier of the oxidase (Cross et al., 1982), and its deficiency leads to the most common, X-linked form of CGD (Johnston, 2001).

The cytosol contains three components. One, p47phox, becomes heavily phosphorylated when the phagocyte is activated and is involved in the assembly of the complete oxidase (Lopes et al., 1999). Evidence suggests that its phosphorylation is necessary for oxidase activation. A second component, p67phox, is a protein whose function is unknown but that is essential for oxidase function. The function of the third cytosolic component, p40phox, is unclear, but it does not appear to be necessary for oxidase activity. When the cell is activated by the binding to its surface of a microorganism opsonized with antibody, complement, or both, the components assemble on the membrane to form the complete oxidase (Babior, 1999). Absence or a defect in any of the cytosolic components (except p40phox) gives rise to autosomal recessive CGD (Johnston, 2001) (see Chapter 17).

In addition to the components just described, activation of the oxidase requires the action of certain low-molecular-weight guanosine triphosphate–cleaving enzymes (GTPases, G proteins). These include Rac1 and Rac2, which are cytosolic G proteins, and rap1A, a membrane-associated G protein that co-purifies with p22phox (Ambruso et al., 2000; Bokoch, 1994; M'Rabet et al., 1998). In human neutrophils, Rac2 accounts for more than 96% of Rac protein.

A boy with a dominant negative Rac2 mutation, which inhibited all Rac function in his neutrophils, had abnormal neutrophil actin assembly, migration, degranulation, and oxidant production and a clinical phenotype of severe bacterial infections (Ambruso et al., 2000).

OTHER SOURCES OF REACTIVE OXYGEN SPECIES

Production of reactive oxygen species, including O_2^- and H_2O_2, has been detected in a variety of nonphagocytic cells, but it has not been clear whether their only source is mitochondrial respiration (Finkel and Holbrook, 2000; Lambeth et al., 2000). It is now recognized that homologs of gp91phox exist in many cell types, and these have been grouped as the NADPH oxidase (Nox) family of enzymes (Cheng et al., 2001; Finkel, 1998; Lambeth et al., 2000). Their principal function appears to be the control of cell growth through production of H_2O_2, which activates intracellular signaling pathways (Bae et al., 1997; Cheng et al., 2001; Finkel, 1998; Lambeth et al., 2000; Suh et al., 1999; Sundaresan et al., 1995).

Myeloperoxidase (MPO) and inducible nitric oxide synthase (iNOS) are other enzymes involved in oxygen-dependent microbial killing. MPO is a green protein that catalyzes the oxidation of halides (Andrews and Krinsky, 1981):

$$Cl^- + H_2O_2 \xrightarrow{MPO} HOCl + OH^-$$

MPO can also oxidize Br^- and I^-, though Cl^- is the preferred substrate, the microbicidal product being hypochlorous acid (HOCl) (Furtmuller et al., 1998).

iNOS is a 130 kDa enzyme with a complex assortment of cofactors that manufactures nitric oxide (NO·), a free radical–like superoxide, in the reaction (Griffith and Stuehr, 1995):

$$arginine + NADPH + O_2 \rightarrow NO\cdot + citrulline + NADPH + H_2O$$

Neutrophils make very little NO· compared with monocytes and macrophages, but iNOS in neutrophils can be upregulated by bacterial infection (Wheeler et al., 1997).

TABLE 5-4 · MAJOR PRODUCTS OF BASOPHILS AND MAST CELLS

Product	Basophils	Mast Cells
Mediators stored in granules	Histamine, chondroitin sulfates, elastase, cathepsin G, β-glucuronidase, MBP, lysophospholipase (Charcot-Leyden crystal protein)	Histamine, heparin and/or chondroitin sulfates, tryptase with/without chymase, acid hydrolases, cathepsin G, carboxypeptidase
Lipid mediators	LTC_4	LTB_4, LTC_4, PGD_2, PAF
Cytokines	IL-4, IL-13	IL-4, IL-5, IL-6, IL-8, IL-13, TNF-α, bFGF
Chemokines	MIP-1α (CCL3)	MIP-1α (CCL3)

bFGF = basic fibroblast growth factor; LT = leukotriene; MBP = major basic protein; PAF = platelet-activating factor; PG = prostaglandin.
Data from Costa JJ, Weller PF, Galli SJ. The cells of the allergic response: mast cells, basophils, and eosinophils. JAMA 278:1815–1822, 1997; Falcone FH, Haas H, Gibbs BF. The human basophil: a new appreciation of its role in immune responses. Blood 96:4028–4038, 2000; Nilsson G, Costa JJ, Metcalfe DD. Mast cells and basophils. In Gallin JI, Synderman R, eds. Inflammation: Basic Principles and Clinical Correlates, ed 3. Philadelphia, Lippincott Williams and Wilkins, 1999, pp 97–117; Schroeder JT, MacGlashan DW Jr, Lichtenstein LM. Human basophils: mediator release and cytokine production. Adv Immunol 77:93–122, 2001.

and elevated blood counts (Costa et al., 1997; Denburg et al., 1992).

Tissue Basophils

Basophils infiltrate tissues as a part of the allergic response, often in association with eosinophils and Th2 lymphocytes (Guo et al., 1994). Basophils exposed to IgE-specific allergen upregulate surface integrin adhesion molecules (LFA-1 and Mac-1) and adhere more firmly to vascular endothelium (Bochner et al., 1989). Basophil chemoattractants include IL-3; GM-CSF; several chemokines, including RANTES (CCL5) and MCP-3 (CCL7); C3a and C5a; LTB_4; and platelet-activating factor (PAF) (reviewed in Nilsson et al., 1999).

Once in the tissues, basophils have the potential to secrete an array of multifunctional cytokines and mediators. A comparison of major secreted products of basophils and mast cells is shown in Table 5-4. When these cells are activated, they release mediators that function in both the early phase of immediate hypersensitivity (vascular reaction and exudation) and the late phase response (leukocyte accumulation and extension of inflammation). Either cell can be activated by binding of antigen-IgE complexes to the high-affinity IgE receptor (FcεRI) or by exposure to complement-derived "anaphylatoxins" (C3a, C4a, C5a), the neuropeptide substance P, radiocontrast medium, or a variety of other agents (Costa et al., 1997; Nilsson et al., 1999).

Just as with eosinophils, it is reasonable to question what evolutionary advantage basophils offer. It is certainly clear that basophil products contribute to the clinical manifestations of allergy and asthma. These are unpleasant at best and fatal in the extreme, but they are assumed to be a byproduct of defense against parasitic infection. Some role in protection against helminth infection and ectoparasites such as ticks does seem likely (Damonneville et al., 1986; Klion et al., 1999; Ridel et al., 1988). Moreover, it is now understood that basophils produce large amounts of the cytokines IL-4 and IL-13, which regulate IgE synthesis, and that they constitutively express cell surface CD40 ligand, which allows B-cell signaling (reviewed in Falcone et al., 2000, Nilsson et al., 1999; Schroeder et al., 2001; and

Yanagihara et al., 1998). The breadth of functions expressed by basophils suggests that these cells could play a central role in both innate and acquired immunity, but this needs to be defined more clearly.

Thus it is the case with all three types of granulocytes that fundamental questions of cell physiology remain to be answered. And with each cell type, the more we have learned, the more intriguing and uncomfortable our ignorance has become.

REFERENCES

Alison MR, Poulsom R, Jeffery R, Dhillon AP, Quaglia A, Jacob J, Novelli M, Prentice G, Williamson J, Wright NA. Hepatocytes from non-hepatic adult stem cells. Nature 406:257, 2000.

Ambruso DR, Knall C, Abell AN, Panepinto J, Kurkchubasche A, Thurman G, Gonzalez-Aller C, Heister A, De Boer M, Harbeck RJ, Oyer R, Johnson GL, Roos D. Human neutrophil immunodeficiency syndrome is associated with an inhibitory Rac2 mutation. Proc Natl Acad Sci USA 97:4654–4659, 2000.

American Society of Clinical Oncology. Update of recommendations for the use of hematopoietic colony-stimulating factors: evidence-based clinical practice guidelines. J Clin Oncol 14:1957–1960, 1996.

Anderson DC, Smith CW. Leukocyte adhesion deficiencies. In Scriver CR, Beaudet AL, Sly WS, Valle D, eds. The Metabolic and Molecular Basis of Inherited Disease, ed 8. New York, McGraw-Hill, 2001, pp 4829–4856.

Anderson DC, Wible LJ, Hughes BJ, Smith CW, Brinkley BR. Cytoplasmic microtubules in polymorphonuclear leukocytes: effects of chemotactic stimulation and colchicine. Cell 31:719–729, 1982.

Andrews PC, Krinsky NI. The reductive cleavage of myeloperoxidase in half, producing enzymically active hemi-myeloperoxidase. J Biol Chem 256:4211–4218, 1981.

Arlandson M, Decker T, Roongta VA, Bonilla L, Mayo KH, MacPherson JC, Hazen SL, Slungaard A. Eosinophil peroxidase oxidation of thiocyanate: characterization of major reaction products and a potential sulfhydryl-targeted cytotoxicity system. J Biol Chem 276:215–224, 2001.

Babior BM. NADPH oxidase: an update. Blood 93:1464–1476, 1999.

Babior BM, Curnutte JT, McMurrich BJ. The particulate superoxide-forming system from human neutrophils: properties of the system and further evidence supporting its participation in the respiratory burst. J Clin Invest 58:989–996, 1976.

Bae YS, Kang SW, Seo MS, Baines IC, Tekle E, Chock PB, Rhee SG. Epidermal growth factor (EGF)-induced generation of hydrogen peroxide: role in EGF receptor-mediated tyrosine phosphorylation. J Biol Chem 272:217–221, 1997.

Baehner RL, Boxer LA, Allen JM, Davis J. Autooxidation as a basis for altered function by polymorphonuclear leukocytes. Blood 50:327–335, 1977.

Baehner RL, Johnston RB Jr, Nathan DG. Comparative study of the metabolic and bactericidal characteristics of severely glucose-6-phosphate dehydrogenase-deficient polymorphonuclear leukocytes and leukocytes from children with chronic granulomatous disease. J Reticuloendothel Soc 12:150–159, 1972.

Baehner RL, Johnston RB, Jr. Metabolic and bactericidal activities of human eosinophils. Br J Haematol 20:277–285, 1971.

Bainton DF. Developmental biology of neutrophils and eosinophils. In Gallin JI, Snyderman R, eds. Inflammation: Basic Principles and Clinical Correlates, ed 3. Philadelphia, Lippincott Williams and Wilkins, 1999, pp 13–34.

Baldridge CW, Gerard RW. The extra respiration of phagocytosis. Am J Physiol 103:235–236, 1933.

Bandeira-Melo C, Sugiyama K, Woods LJ, Weller PF. Eotaxin elicits rapid vesicular transport-mediated release of preformed IL-4 from human eosinophils. J Immunol 166:4813–4817, 2001.

Beckman JS, Koppenol WH. Nitric oxide, superoxide, and peroxynitrite: the good, the bad, and the ugly. Am J Physiol Cell Physiol 271:C1424–C1437, 1996.

Belaaouaj AA, Kim KS, Shapiro SD. Degradation of outer membrane protein A in Escherichia coli killing by neutrophil elastase. Science 289:1185–1187, 2000.

Bjornson CR, Rietze RL, Reynolds BA, Magli MC, Vescovi AL. Turning brain into blood: a hematopoietic fate adopted by adult neural stem cells in vivo. Science 283:534–537, 1999.

Bochner BS, MacGlashan DW Jr, Marcotte GV, Schleimer RP. IgE-dependent regulation of human basophil adherence to vascular endothelium. J Immunol 142:3180–3186, 1989.

Bogen S, Pak J, Garifallou M, Deng X, Muller WA. Monoclonal antibody to murine PECAM-1 (CD31) blocks acute inflammation in vivo. J Exp Med 179:1059–1064, 1994.

Bokoch GM. Regulation of the human neutrophil NADPH oxidase by the Rac GTP-binding proteins. Curr Opin Cell Biol 6:212–218, 1994.

Borregaard N, Kjeldsen L, Rygaard K, Bastholm L, Nielsen MH, Sengelov H, Bjerrum OW, Johnsen AH. Stimulus-dependent secretion of plasma proteins from human neutrophils. J Clin Invest 90:86–96, 1992.

Borregaard N, Cowland JB. Granules of the human neutrophilic polymorphonuclear leukocyte. Blood 89:3503–3521, 1997.

Borregaard N, Theilgaard-Monch K, Sorensen OE, Cowland JB. Regulation of human neutrophil granule protein expression. Curr Opin Hematol 8:23–27, 2001.

Boxer LA, Oliver JM, Spielberg SP, Allen JM, Schulman JD. Protection of granulocytes by vitamin E in glutathione synthetase deficiency. N Engl J Med 301:901–905, 1979.

Boyce JA, Friend D, Matsumoto R, Austen KF, Owen WF. Differentiation in vitro of hybrid eosinophil/basophil granulocytes: autocrine function of an eosinophil developmental intermediate. J Exp Med 182:49–57, 1995.

Breton-Gorius J, Coquin Y, Guichard J. Cytochemical distinction between azurophils and catalase-containing granules in leukocytes. Lab Invest 38:21–34, 1978.

Buhring H-J, Simmons PJ, Pudney M, Muller R, Jarrossay D, van Agthoven A, Willheim M, Brugger W, Valent P, Kanz L. The monoclonal antibody 97A6 defines a novel surface antigen expressed on human basophils and their multipotent and unipotent progenitors. Blood 94:2343–2356, 1999.

Bujak JS, Root RK. The role of peroxidase in the bactericidal activity of human blood eosinophils from normal human blood. Infect Immun 53:192–198, 1986.

Campbell EJ, Campbell MA, Owen CA. Bioactive proteinase 3 on the cell surface of human neutrophils: quantification, catalytic activity, and susceptibility to inhibition. J Immunol 165:3366–3374, 2000.

Campbell MS, Lovell MA, Gorbsky GJ. Stability of nuclear segments in human neutrophils and evidence against a role for microfilaments or microtubules in their genesis during differentiation of HL60 myelocytes. J Leukoc Biol 58:659–666, 1996.

Cassatella MA. Neutrophil-derived proteins: selling cytokines by the pound. Adv Immunol 73:369–509, 1999.

Chai YC, Ashraf SS, Rokutan K, Johnston RB Jr, Thomas JA. S-thiolation of individual human neutrophil proteins including actin by stimulation of the respiratory burst: evidence against a role for glutathione disulfide. Arch Biochem Biophys 310:273–281, 1994.

Cheng G, Cao Z, Xu X, van Meir EG, Lambeth JD. Homologs of gp91phox: cloning and tissue expression of Nox3, Nox4, and Nox5. Gene 269:131–140, 2001.

Cohen AJ, Steigbigel RT. Eosinophilia in patients infected with human immunodeficiency virus. J Infect Dis 174:615–618, 1996.

Cohn ZA, Hirsch JG. The isolation and properties of the specific cytoplasmic granules of rabbit polymorphonuclear leukocytes. J Exp Med 112:983–1004, 1960.

Cole AM, Ganz T, Liese AM, Burdick MD, Liu L, Strieter RM. IFN-inducible ELR⁻ CXC chemokines display defensin-like antimicrobial activity. J Immunol 167:623–627, 2001.

Collins PD, Marleau S, Griffiths-Johnson DA, Jose PJ, Williams TJ. Cooperation between interleukin-5 and the chemokine eotaxin to induce eosinophil accumulation in vivo. J Exp Med 182:1169–1174, 1995.

Condeelis J. Life at the leading edge: the formation of cell protrusions. Annu Rev Cell Biol 9:411–444, 1993.

Costa JJ, Weller PF, Galli SJ. The cells of the allergic response: mast cells, basophils, and eosinophils. JAMA 278:1815–1822, 1997.

Cotter TG, Fernandes RS, Verhaegen S, McCarthy JV. Cell death in the myeloid lineage. Immunol Rev 142:93–112, 1994.

Cowland JB, Borregaard N. The individual regulation of granule protein mRNA levels during neutrophil maturation explains the heterogeneity of neutrophil granules. J Leukoc Biol 66:989–995, 1999.

Cronkite EP, Vincent PC. Granulocytopoiesis. Ser Haematol 2:3–43, 1969.

Cross AR, Jones OTG, Garcia R, Segal AW. The association of FAD with the cytochrome b-245 of human neutrophils. Biochem J 208:759–763, 1982.

Culley FJ, Brown A, Conroy DM, Sabroe I, Pritchard DI, Williams TJ. Eotaxin is specifically cleaved by hookworm metalloproteases preventing its action in vitro and in vivo. J Immunol 165:6447–6453, 2000.

Damonneville M, Auriault C, Verwaerde C, Delanoye A, Pierce R, Capron A. Protection against experimental Schistosoma mansoni schistosomiasis achieved by immunization with schistosomula relased products antigens (SRP-A):role of IgE antibodies. Clin Exp Immunol 65:244–252, 1986.

David JR, Butterworth AE, Vadas MA. Mechanism of interaction mediating killing of Schistosoma mansoni by human eosinophils. Am J Trop Med Hyg 29:842–848, 1980.

DeChatelet LR, Shirley PS, McPhail LC, Huntley CC, Muss HB, Bass DA. Oxidative metabolism of the human eosinophil. Blood 50:525–535, 1977.

Delves PJ, Roitt IM. The immune system. N Engl J Med 343:37–49, 2000.

Denburg JA. Basophil and mast cell lineages in vitro and in vivo. Blood 79:846–860, 1992.

Desreumaux P, Capron M. Eosinophils in allergic reactions. Curr Opin Immunol 8:790–795, 1996.

Di Carlo E, Forni G, Lollini PL, Colombo MP, Modesti A, Musiani P. The intriguing role of polymorphonuclear neutrophils in antitumor reactions. Blood 97:339–345, 2001.

Domachowske JB, Dyer KD, Bonville CA, Rosenberg HF. Recombinant human eosinophil-derived neurotoxin/RNase 2 functions as an effective antiviral agent against respiratory syncytial virus. J Infect Dis 177:1458–1464, 1998.

Dong ZM, Murphy JW. Cryptococcal polysaccharides induce L-selectin shedding and tumor necrosis factor receptor loss from the surface of human neutrophils. J Clin Invest 97:689–698, 1996.

Dvorak AM, Ackerman SJ, Weller PF. Subcellular morphology and biochemistry of eosinophils. In Harris JR, ed. Blood Cell Biochemistry, vol 2. New York, Plenum Press, 1990, pp 237–244.

Dvorak AM, Letourneau L, Login GR, Weller PF, Ackerman SJ. Ultrastructural localization of the Charcot-Leyden crystal protein (lysophospholipase) to a distinct crystalloid-free granule population in mature human eosinophils. Blood 72:150–158, 1988.

Egesten A, Calafat J, Knol EF, Janssen H, Walz TM. Subcellular localization of transforming growth factor-α in human eosinophil granulocytes. Blood 87:3910–3918, 1996.

Eggleton P, Ghebrehiwet B, Coburn JP, Sastry KN, Zaner KS, Tauber AI. Characterization of the human neutrophil C1q receptor and functional effects of free ligand on activated neutrophils. Blood 84:1640–1649, 1994.

Elbim C, Reglier H, Fay M, Delarche C, Andrieu V, El Benna J, Gougerot-Pocidalo M-A. Intracellular pool of IL-10 receptors in specific granules of human neutrophils: differential mobilization by proinflammatory mediators. J Immunol 166:5201–5207, 2001.

Elsbach P, Weiss J, Levy O. Oxygen-independent Antimicrobial Systems of Phagocytes. Baltimore, Lippincott Williams and Wilkins, 1999, pp 801–817.

Etzioni A. Adhesion molecules—their role in health and disease. Pediatr Res 39:191–198, 1996.

Etzioni A, Frydman M, Pollack S, Avidor I, Phillips ML, Paulson JC, Gershoni-Barugh R. Recurrent severe infections caused by a novel leukocyte adhesion deficiency. N Engl J Med 327:1789–1792, 1992.

Fadok VA, Bratton DL, Konowal A, Freed PW, Westcott JY, Henson PM. Macrophages that have ingested apoptotic cells in vitro inhibit proinflammatory cytokine production through autocrine/paracrine mechanisms involving TGF-β, PGE2, and PAF. J Clin Invest 101:890–898, 1998.

Fadok VA, Bratton DL, Rose DM, Pearson A, Ezekewitz RAB, Henson PM. A receptor for phosphatidylserine-specific clearance of apoptotic cells. Nature 405:85–90, 2000.

Fadok VA, Bratton DL, Guthrie L, Henson PM. Differential effects of apoptotic versus lysed cells on macrophage production of cytokines: role of proteases. J Immunol 166:6847–6854, 2001a.

Fadok VA, de Cathelineau A, Daleke DL, Henson PM, Bratton DL. Loss of phospholipid asymmetry and surface exposure of phosphatidylserine is required for phagocytosis of apoptotic cells by macrophages and fibroblasts. J Biol Chem 276:1071–1077, 2001b.

Falcone FH, Haas H, Gibbs BF. The human basophil: a new appreciation of its role in immune responses. Blood 96:4028–4038, 2000.

Feng D, Nagy JA, Pyne K, Dvorak HF, Dvorak AM. Neutrophils emigrate from venules by a transendothelial cell pathway in response to FMLP. J Exp Med 187:903–915, 1998.

Fenna R, Zeng J, Davey C. Structure of the green heme in myeloperoxidase. Arch Biochem Biophys 316:653–656, 1995.

Finkel T, Holbrook NJ. Oxidants, oxidative stress and the biology of ageing. Nature 408:239–247, 2000.

Finkel T. Oxygen radicals and signaling. Curr Opin Cell Biol 10:248–253, 1998.

Fridovich I. Superoxide radical: an endogenous toxicant. Annu Rev Pharmacol Toxicol 23:239–257, 1983.

Furtmuller PG, Burner U, Obinger C. Reaction of myeloperoxidase compound I with chloride, bromide, iodide, and thiocyanate. Biochemistry 37:17923–17930, 1998.

Ganz T. Defensins and host defense. Science 286:420–421, 1999.

Goldschmeding R, vanDalen CM, Faber N, Calafat J, Huizinga TWJ, van der Schoot CE, Clement LT, von dem Borne AEGK. Further characterization of the NB 1 antigen as a variably expressed 56-62kD GPI-linked glycoprotein of plasma membranes and specific granules of neutrophils. Br J Haematol 81:336–345, 1992.

Goodman JL, Nelson CM, Klein MB, Hayes SF, Weston BW. Leukocyte infection by the granulocytic ehrlichiosis agent is linked to expression of a selectin ligand. J Clin Invest 103:407–412, 1999.

Gray GR, Stamatoyannopoulos G, Naiman SC, Kilman MR, Klebanoff SJ, Austin T, Yoshida A, Robinson GCF. Neutrophil dysfunction, chronic granulomatous disease, and nonspherocytic hemolytic anemia caused by complete deficiency in glucose-6-phosphate dehydrogenase. Lancet 2:530–534, 1973.

Greenberg S. Biology of phagocytosis. In Gallin JI, Snyderman R, eds. Inflammation: Basic Principles and Clinical Correlates. Philadelphia, Lippincott Williams and Wilkins, 1999, pp. 681–701.

Gregory WW, Byrne GI, Gardner M, Moulder JW. Cytochalasin B does not inhibit ingestion of Chlamydia psittaci by mouse fibroblasts (L cells) and mouse peritoneal macrophages. Infect Immun 25:463–466, 1979.

Griffith OW, Stuehr DJ. Nitric oxide synthases: properties and catalytic mechanism. Annu Rev Physiol 57:707–736, 1995.

Guo C-B, Liu MC, Galli SJ, Bochner BS, Kagey-Sobotka A, Lichtenstein LM. Identification of IgE-bearing cells in the late-phase response to antigen in the lung as basophils. Am J Respir Cell Mol Biol 10:384–390, 1994.

Haisch K, Gibbs BF, Körber M, Ernst M, Grage-Griebenow E, Schlaak M, Haas H. Purification of morphologically and functionally intact human basophils to near homogeneity. J Immunol Methods 226:129–137, 1999.

Hamann KJ, Gleich GJ, Checkel JL, Loegering DA, McCall JW, Barker RL. In vitro killing of microfilariae of Brugia pahangi and Brugia malayi by eosinophil granule proteins. J Immunol 144:3166–3173, 1990.

Hancock RE. Host defense (cationic) peptides. Drugs 57:469–473, 1999.

Harrison AM, Bonville CA, Rosenberg HF, Domachowske JB. Respiratory syncytial virus-induced chemokine expression in the lower airways: eosinophil recruitment and degranulation. Am J Respir Crit Care Med 159:1918–1924, 1999.

Hartmann P, Becker R, Franzen C, Schell-Frederick E, Römer J, Jacobs M, Fätkenheuer G, Plum G. Phagocytosis and killing of Mycobacterium avium complex by human neutrophils. J Leukoc Biol 69:397–404, 2001.

Heinecke JW. Eosinophil-dependent bromination in the pathogenesis of asthma. J Clin Invest 105:1331–1332, 2000.

Hengartner MO. The biochemistry of apoptosis. Nature 407:770–776, 2000.

Henson PM, Johnston RB Jr. Tissue injury in inflammation: oxidants, proteinases, and cationic proteins. J Clin Invest 79:669–674, 1987.

Hochstenbach PFR, Scheres JMJC, Hustinx TWJ, Wieringa B. Demonstration of X chromatin in drumstick-like nuclear appendages of leukocytes by in situ hybridization on blood smears. Histochemistry 84:383–386, 1986.

Holmes B, Page AR, Good RA. Studies of the metabolic activity of leukocytes from patients with a genetic abnormality of phagocytic function. J Clin Invest 46:1422–1432, 1967.

Huttner KM, Bevins CL. Antimicrobial peptides as mediators of epithelial host defense. Pediatr Res 45:785–794, 1999.

Indik ZK, Park J-G, Hunter S, Schreiber AD. The molecular dissection of Fcγ receptor mediated phagocytosis. Blood 86:4389–4399, 1995.

Itoh K, Okubo K, Utiyama H, Hirano T, Yoshii J, Matsubara K. Expression profile of active genes in granulocytes. Blood 92:1432–1441, 1998.

Jennette JC, Hoidal JR, Falk RJ. Specificity of anti-neutrophil cytoplasmic autoantibodies for proteinase 3. Blood 75:2263–2264, 1990.

Johnston RB Jr. Biochemical defects of polymorphonuclear and mononuclear phagocytes associated with disease. In Sbarra AJ, Strauss R, eds. The Reticuloendothelial System, vol 2. New York, Plenum Press, 1980, pp 397–421.

Johnston RB Jr. Clinical aspects of chronic granulomatous disease. Curr Opin Hematol 8:17–22, 2001.

Johnston RB Jr. Pathogenesis of pneumococcal pneumonia. Rev Infect Dis 13:S509–517, 1991.

Johnston RB Jr, Lehmeyer JE. Elaboration of toxic oxygen by-products by neutrophils in a model of immune complex disease. J Clin Invest 57:836–841, 1976.

Johnston RB Jr, Keele BB Jr, Misra HP, Lehmeyer JE, Webb LS, Baehner RL, Rajagopalan KV. The role of superoxide anion generation in phagocytic bactericidal activity: studies with normal and chronic granulomatous disease leukocytes. J Clin Invest 55:1357–1372, 1975.

Juhlin L. Basophil leukocyte differential in blood and bone marrow. Acta Haematol 29:89–95, 1963.

Kaiser V, Diamond G. Expression of mammalian defensin genes. J Leukoc Biol 68:779–784, 2000.

Karnovsky ML, Badwey JA. Determinants of the production of active oxygen species by granulocytes and macrophages. J Clin Chem Clin Biochem 21:545–553, 1983.

Karsan A, Cornejo CJ, Winn RK, Schwartz BR, Way W, Lannir N, Gershoni-Baruch R, Etzioni A, Ochs HD, Harlan JM. Leukocyte adhesion deficiency type II is a generalized defect of de novo GDP-fucose biosynthesis: endothelial cell fucosylation is not required for neutrophil rolling on human nonlymphoid endothelium. J Clin Invest 101:2438–2445, 1998.

Kazura JW, Grove DI. Stage-specific antibody-dependent eosinophil-mediated destruction of *Trichinella spiralis*. Nature 274:588–589, 1978.

Kempuraj D, Saito H, Kaneko A, Fukagawa K, Nakayama M, Toru H, Tomikawa M, Tachimoto H, Ebisawa M, Akasawa A, Miyagi T. Kimura H, Nakajima T, Tsuji K, Nakahata T. Characterization of mast cell-committed progenitors present in human umbilical cord blood. Blood 93:3338–3346, 1999.

Kerr JFR, Wyllie AH, Currie AR. Apoptosis: a basic biological phenomenon with wide-ranging implications in tissue kinetics. Br J Cancer 26:239–257, 1972.

Kilgore KS, Todd RF III, Lucchesi BR. Reperfusion injury. In Gallin JI, Snyderman R, eds. Inflammation: Basic Principles and Clinical Correlates, ed 3. Philadelphia, Lippincott Williams and Wilkins, 1999, pp 1047–1060.

Kirshenbaum AS, Goff JP, Semere T, Foster B, Scott LM, Metcalfe DD. Demonstration that human mast cells arise from a progenitor cell population that is CD34+, c-kit+, and expresses aminopeptidase N (CD13). Blood 94:2333–2342, 1999.

Kishimoto TK, Jutila MA, Berg EL, Butcher EC. Neutrophil Mac-1 and MEL-14 adhesion proteins inversely regulated by chemotactic factors. Science 245:1238–1241, 1989.

Kita H, Gleich GJ. Chemokines active on eosinophils: potential roles in allergic inflammation. J Exp Med 183:2421–2426, 1996.

Kjeldsen L, Sengelov H, Lollike K, Nielsen MH, Borregaard N. Isolation and characterization of gelatinase granules from human neutrophils. Blood 83:1640–1649, 1994.

Klion AD, Armant MA, Nutman TB. Role of immunoglobulin E and eosinophils in mediating protection and pathology in parasitic helminth infections. In Gallin JI, Snyderman R, eds. Inflammation: Basic Principles and Clinical Correlates, ed 3. Philadelphia, Lippincott Williams and Wilkins, 1999, pp 929–936.

Krammer PH. CD95's deadly mission in the immune system. Nature 407:789–795, 2000.

Lagasse E, Connors H, Al-Dhalimy M, Reitsma M, Dohse M, Osborne L, Wang X, Finegold M, Weissman IL, Grompe M. Purified hematopoietic stem cells can differentiate into hepatocytes in vivo. Nature Med 6:1229–1234, 2000.

Lalezari P, Murphy GB, Allen FH Jr. NB1, a new neutrophil-specific antigen involved in the pathogenesis of neonatal neutropenia. J Clin Invest 50:1108–1115, 1971.

Lambeth JD, Cheng G, Arnold RS, Edens WA. Novel homologs of gp91phox. Trends Biochem Sci 25:459–461, 2000.

Le Cabec V, Cols, C, Maridonneau-Parini I. Nonopsonic phagocytosis of zymosan and *Mycobacterium kansasii* by CR3 (CD11b/CD18) involves distinct molecular determinants and is or is not coupled with NADPH oxidase activation. Infect Immun 68:4736–4745, 2000.

Lehrer RI, Ganz T, Selsted ME. Defensins: endogenous antibiotic peptides of animal cells. Cell 64:229–230, 1991.

Lehrer RI, Lichtenstein AK, Ganz T. Defensins: antimicrobial and cytotoxic peptides of mammalian cells. Annu Rev Immunol 11:105–128, 1993.

Li L, Li Y, Reddel SW, Cherrian M, Friend DS, Stevens RL, Krilis SA. Identification of basophilic cells that express mast cell granule proteases in the peripheral blood of asthma, allergy, and drug-reactive patients. J Immunol 161:5079–5086, 1998.

Liles WC, Huang JE, van Burik JAH, Bowden RA, Dale DC. Granulocyte colony-stimulating factor administered in vivo augments neutrophil-mediated activity against opportunistic fungal pathogens. J Infect Dis 175:1012–1015, 1997.

Limaye AP, Abrams JS, Silver JE, Ottesen EA, Nutman TB. Regulation of parasite-induced eosinophilia: selectively increased interleukin-5 production in helminth-infected patients. J Exp Med 172:399–402, 1990.

Loetscher P, Clark-Lewis I. Agonistic and antagonistic activities of chemokines. J Leukoc Biol 69:881–884, 2001.

Lopes LR, Hoyal CR, Knaus UG, Babior BM. Activation of the leukocyte NADPH oxidase by protein kinase C in a partially recombinant cell-free system. J Biol Chem 274:15533–15537, 1999.

Luster AD. Chemokines—chemotactic cytokines that mediate inflammation. N Engl J Med 338:436–445, 1998.

MacPherson JC, Comhair SAA, Erzurum SC, Klein DF, Lipscomb MF, Kavuru MS, Samoszuk MK, Hazen SL. Eosinophils are a major source of nitric oxide-derived oxidants in severe asthma: characterization of pathways available to eosinophils for generating reactive nitrogen species. J Immunol 166:5763–5772, 2001.

Malech HL, Root RK, Gallin JI. Structural analysis of human neutrophil migration: centriole, microtubule and microfilament orientation and function during chemotaxis. J Cell Biol 75:666–693, 1977.

Mansfield E, Chae JJ, Komarow HD, Brotz TM, Frucht DM, Aksentijevich I, Kastner DL. The familial Mediterranean fever protein, pyrin, associates with microtubules and colocalizes with actin filaments. Blood 98:851–859, 2001.

Marmont AM, Damasio E, Zucker-Franklin D. Neutrophils. In Zucker-Franklin D, Greaves MF, Grossi CE, Marmont AM, eds. Atlas of Blood Cells: Function and Pathology, ed 2. Philadelphia, Lea and Febiger, 1988, pp 157–246.

Marodi L, Forehand JR, Johnston RB Jr. Mechanisms of host defense against *Candida* species II. Biochemical basis for the killing of *Candida* by mononuclear phagocytes. J Immunol 146:2790–2794, 1991.

Marshall AJ, Miles RJ, Richards L. The phagocytosis of mycoplasmas. J Med Microbiol 43:239–250, 1995.

Martensson J, Jain A, Stole E, Frayer W, Auld PAM, Meister A. Inhibition of gluthathione synthesis in the newborn rat: a model for endogenously produced oxidative stress. Proc Natl Acad Sci USA 88:9360–9364, 1991.

Martin SJ. Apoptosis. In Delves PJ, Roitt IM, eds. Encyclopedia of Immunology, ed 2. San Diego, Academic Press, 1998, pp 220–227.

McCormick ML, Metwali A, Railsback MA, Weinstock JV, Britigan BE. Eosinophils from schistosome-induced hepatic granulomas produce superoxide and hydroxyl radical. J Immunol 157:5009–5015, 1996.

Meister A. Glutathione-ascorbic acid antioxidant system in animals. J Biol Chem 269:9397–9400, 1994.

Monteiro RC, van de Winkel JGH. Ig A Fc receptors, Annu Rev Immunol 21: 177–204, 2003.

M'Rabet L, Coffer P, Zwartkruis F, Franke B, Segal AW, Koenderman L, Bos JL. Activation of the small GTPase rap 1 in human neutrophils. Blood 92:2133–2140, 1998.

Muller WA. Leukocyte-endothelial cell adhesion molecules in transendothelial migration. In Gallin JI, Snyderman R, eds. Inflammation: Basic Principles and Clinical Correlates, ed 3. Philadelphia, Lippincott Williams and Wilkins, 1999, pp 585–592.

Nauseef WM. The proper study of mankind. J Clin Invest 107:401–403, 2001.

Nelson S, Belknap SM, Carlson RW, Dale D, DeBoisblanc B, Farkas S, Fotheringham N, Ho H, Marrie T, Movahhed H, Root R, Wilson J. A randomized controlled trial of filgrastim as an adjunct to antibiotics for treatment of hospitalized patients with community-acquired pneumonia. J Infect Dis 178:1075–1080, 1998.

Newman SL, Henson JE, Henson PM. Phagocytosis of senescent neutrophils by human monocyte-derived macrophages and rabbit inflammatory macrophages. J Exp Med 156:430–442, 1982.

Nilsson G, Costa JJ, Metcalfe DD. Mast cells and basophils. In Gallin JI, Synderman R, eds. Inflammation: Basic Principles and Clinical Correlates, ed 3. Philadelphia, Lippincott Williams and Wilkins, 1999, pp 97–117.

Opdenakker G, Fibbe WE, Van Damme J. The molecular basis of leukocytosis. Immunol Today 19:182–189, 1998.

Opdenakker G, Van den Steen PE, Dubois B, Nelissen I, Van Coillie E, Masure S, Proost P, Van Damme J. Gelatinase B functions as regulator and effector in leukocyte biology. J Leukoc Biol 69:851–859, 2001.

Orkin SH. Stem cell alchemy. Nature Med 6:1212–1213, 2000.

Parry MF, Root RK, Metcalf JA, Delaney KK, Kaplow LS, Richar WJ. Myeloperoxidase deficiency: prevalence and clinical significance. Ann Intern Med 95:293–301, 1981.

Pearse RN, Kawabe T, Bolland S, Guinamard R, Kurosaki T, Ravetch JV. SHIP recruitment attenuates FcγRIIB-induced B cell apoptosis. Immunity 10:753–760, 1999.

Peters MS, Rodriguez M, Gleich GJ. Localization of human eosinophil granule major basic protein, eosinophil cationic protein, and eosinophil-derived neurotoxin by immunoelectron microscopy. Lab Invest 54:656–662, 1986.

Peyron P, Bordier C, N'Diaye E-N, Maridonneau-Parini I. Nonopsonic phagocytosis of *Mycobacterium kansasii* by human neutrophils depends on cholesterol and is mediated by CR3 associated with glycosylphosphatidylinositol-anchored proteins. J Immunol 165:5186–5191, 2000.

Prosper F, Verfaillie CM. Regulation of hematopoiesis through adhesion receptors. J Leukoc Biol 69:307–316, 2001.

Quie PG, White JG, Holmes B, Good RA. In vitro bactericidal capacity of human polymorphonuclear leukocytes: diminished activity in chronic granulomatous disease of childhood. J Clin Invest 46:668–679, 1967.

Ravetch JV. Fc receptors: rubor redux. Cell 78:553–560, 1994.

Ravetch JV, Bolland S. IgG Fc receptors. Annu Rev Immunol 19:275–290, 2001.

Ravichandran V, Seres T, Moriguchi T, Thomas JA, Johnston RB Jr. S-thiolation of glyceraldehyde-3-phosphate dehydrogenase induced by the phagocytosis-associated respiratory burst in blood monocytes. J Biol Chem 269:25010–25015, 1994.

Resnick MB, Weller PF. Mechanisms of eosinophil recruitment. Am J Respir Cell Mol Biol 8:349–355, 1993.

Rich T, Allen RL, Wyllie AH. Defying death after DNA damage. Nature 407:777–783, 2000.

Ridel P-R, Auriault C, Darcy F, Pierce RJ, Leite P, Santoro F, Neyrinck J-L, Kusnierz J-P, Capron A. Protective role of IgE in immunocompromised rat toxoplasmosis. J Immunol 141:978–983, 1988.

Risso A. Leukocyte antimicrobial peptides: multifunctional effector molecules of innate immunity. J Leukoc Biol 68:785–792, 2000.

Robinson JM, Kobayashi T, Seguchi H, Takizawa T. Evaluation of neutrophil structure and function by electron microscopy: cytochemical studies. J Immunol Methods 232:169–178, 1999.

Roos D, Weening RS, Voetman AA, Van Schaik MLJ, Bot AM, Meerhof LJ, Loos JA. Protection of phagocytic leukocytes by endogenous glutathione: studies in a family with glutathione reductase deficiency. Blood 53:851–866, 1979.

Roos D, Weening RS, Wyss SR, Aebi E. Protection of human neutrophils by endogenous catalase: studies with cells from catalase-deficient individuals. J Clin Invest 65:1515–1522, 1980.

Root RK, Dale DC. Granulocyte colony-stimulating factor and granulocyte-macrophage colony-stimulating factor: comparisons and potential for use in the treatment of infections in nonneutropenic patients. J Infect Dis 179(Suppl 2):S342–352, 1999.

Rosenberg HF. Eosinophils. In Gallin JI, Snyderman R, eds. Inflammation: Basic Principles and Clinical Correlates, ed 3. Philadelphia, Lippincott Williams and Wilkins, 1999, pp 61–76.

Rothenberg ME. Eosinophilia. N Engl J Med 338:1592–1600, 1998.

Sanderson CJ. Interleukin-5, eosinophils, and disease. Blood 79:3101–3109, 1992.

Savill J, Fadok V. Corpse clearance defines the meaning of cell death. Nature 407:784–788, 2000.

Savill JS, Wyllie AH, Henson JE, Walport MJ, Henson PM, Haslett C. Macrophage phagocytosis of aging neutrophils in inflammation: programmed cell death in the neutrophil leads to its recognition by macrophages. J Clin Invest 83:865–875, 1989.

Sbarra AJ, Karnovsky ML. The biochemical basis of phagocytosis. I. Metabolic changes during the ingestion of particles by polymorphonuclear leukocytes. J Biol Chem 234:1355–1362, 1959.

Schroeder JT, MacGlashan DW Jr, Lichtenstein LM. Human basophils: mediator release and cytokine production. Adv Immunol 77:93–122, 2001.

Schultz H, Weiss J, Carroll SF, Gross WL. The endotoxin-binding bactericidal/permeability-increasing protein (BPI): a target antigen of autoantibodies. J Leukoc Biol 69:505–512, 2001.

Scott MG, Hancock REW. Cationic antimicrobial peptides and their multifunctional role in the immune system. Crit Rev Immunol 20:407–431, 2000.

Sengelov H, Follin P, Kjeldsen L, Lollike K, Dahlgren C, Borregaard N. Mobilization of granules and secretory vesicles during in vivo exudation of human neutrophils. J Immunol 154:4157–4165, 1995.

Sengelov H. Complement receptors in neutrophils. Crit Rev Immunol 15:107–131, 1995.

Seres T, Ravichandran V, Moriguchi T, Rokutan K, Thomas JA, Johnston RB Jr. Protein S-thiolation and dethiolation during the respiratory burst in human monocytes: a reversible post-translational modification with potential for buffering the effects of oxidant stress. J Immunol 156:1973–1980, 1996.

Seres T, Knickelbein RG, Warshaw JB, Johnston RB Jr. The phagocytosis-associated respiratory burst in human monocytes is associated with increased uptake of gluthathione. J Immunol 165:3333–3340, 2000.

Simon HU, Yousefi S, Schranz C, Schapowal A, Bachert C, Blaser K. Direct demonstration of delayed eosinophil apoptosis as a mechanism causing tissue eosinophilia. J Immunol 158:3902–3908, 1997.

Simpson AJ, Maxwell AI, Govan JRW, Haslett C, Sallenave J-M. Elafin (elastase-specific inhibitor) has anti-microbial activity against Gram-positive and Gram-negative respiratory pathogens. FEBS Lett 452:309–313, 1999.

Simpson AJ, Wallace WAH, Marsden ME, Govan JRW, Porteous DJ, Haslett C, Sallenave J-M. Adenoviral augmentation of elafin protects the lung against acute injury mediated by activated neutrophils and bacterial infection. J Immunol 167:1778–1786, 2001.

Skiest DJ, Keiser P. Clinical significance of eosinophilia in HIV-infected individuals. Am J Med 102:449–453, 1997.

Spielberg SP, Boxer LA, Oliver JM, Allen JM, Schulman JD. Oxidative damage to neutrophils in glutathione synthetase deficiency. Br J Haematol 42:215–223, 1979.

Spitznagel JK. Antibiotic proteins of human neutrophils. J Clin Invest 86:1381–1386, 1990.

Springer TA. Traffic signals on endothelium for lymphocyte recirculation and leukocyte emigration. Annu Rev Physiol 57:827–872, 1995.

Stendahl O, Krause K-H, Krischer J, Jerstrom P, Theler J-M, Clark RA, Carpentier J-L, Lew DP. Redistribution of intracellular Ca2+ stores during phagocytosis in human neutrophils. Science 265:1439–1441, 1994.

Stossel TP. The machinery of blood cell movements. Blood 84:367–379, 1994a.

Stossel TP. The machinery of cell crawling. Scientific American, pp 54–63, 1994b.

Stossel TP. Mechanical responses of white blood cells. In Gallin JI, Snyderman R, eds. Inflammation: Basic Principles and Clinical Correlates, ed 3. Philadelphia, Lippincott Williams and Wilkins, 1999, pp 661–679.

Subrahmanyam YVBK, Yamaga S, Prashar Y, Lee HH, Hoe NP, Kluger Y, Gerstein M, Goguen JD, Newburger PE, Weissman SM. RNA expression patterns change dramatically in human neutrophils exposed to bacteria. Blood 97:2457–2468, 2001.

Suh YA, Arnold RS, Lassegue B, Shi J, Xu X, Sorescu D, Chung AB, Griendling KK, Lambeth JD. Cell transformation by the superoxide-generating oxidase Mox1. Nature 401:79–82, 1999.

Sundaresan M, Yu Z-X, Ferrans VJ, Irani K, Finkel T. Requirement for generation of H_2O_2 for platelet-derived growth factor signal transduction. Science 270:296–299, 1995.

Swerdloff JN, Filler SG, Edwards JE Jr. Severe candidal infections in neutropenic patients. Clin Infect Dis 17:S457–467, 1993.

Taliaferro WH, Sarles MP. The cellular reactions in the skin, lungs, and intestine of normal and immune rats after infection with *Nippostrongylus brasiliensis*. J Infect Dis 64:157–192, 1939.

Tischendorf FW, Brattig NW, Buttner DW, Pieper A, Lintzel M. Serum levels of eosinophil cationic protein, eosinophil-derived neurotoxin and myeloperoxidase in infections with filariae and schistosomes. Acta Trop 62:171–182, 1996.

To LB, Haylock DN, Simmons PJ, Juttner CA. The biology and clinical uses of blood stem cells. Blood 89:2233–2258, 1997.

Underhill DM, Ozinsky A. Phagocytosis of microbes: complexity in action. Annu Rev Immunol 20: 825-852, 2002.

Valent P, Schmidt G, Besemer J, Mayer P, Zenke G, Liehl E, Hinterberger W, Lechner K, Maurer D, Bettelheim P. Interleukin-3 is a differentiation factor for human basophils. Blood 73:1763–1769, 1989.

Van den Steen PE, Proost P, Wuyts A, VanDamme J, Opdenakker G. Neutrophil gelatinase B potentiates interleukin-8 tenfold by aminoterminal processing, whereas it degrades CTAP-III, PF-4, and GRO-α and leaves RANTES and MCP-2 intact. Blood 96:2673–2681, 2000.

Vaporciyan AA, Delisser HM, Yan H-C, Mendiguren II, Thom SR, Jones ML, Ward PA, Albelda SM. Involvement of platelet-endothelial cell adhesion molecule-1 in neutrophil recruitment in vivo. Science 262:1580–1582, 1993.

Varki A. Selectin ligands. Proc Natl Acad Sci USA 91:7390–7397, 1994.

Varki A. Selectin ligands: will the real ones please stand up? J Clin Invest 99:158–162, 1997.

Walker RI, Willemze R. Neutrophil kinetics and the regulation of granulopoiesis. Rev Infect Dis 2:282–292, 1980.

Wallace PJ, Packman CH, Lichtman MA. Maturation-associated changes in the peripheral cytoplasm of human neutrophils: a review. Exp Hematol 15:34–45, 1987.

Walsh GM. Eosinophil granule proteins and their role in disease. Curr Opin Hematol 8:28–33, 2001.

Watowich SS, Wu H, Socolovsky M, Klingmuller U, Constantinescu SN, Lodish HF. Cytokine receptor signal transduction and the control of hematopoietic cell development. Annu Rev Cell Dev Biol 12:91–128, 1996.

Weber C, Katayama J, Springer TA. Differential regulation of β1 and β2 integrin avidity by chemoattractants in eosinophils. Proc Natl Acad Sci USA 93:10939–10944, 1996.

Wein M, Sterbinsky SA, Bickel CA, Schleimer RP, Bochner BS. Comparison of human eosinophil and neutrophil ligands for P-selectin: ligands for P-selectin differ from those for E-selectin. Am J Respir Cell Mol Biol 12:315–319, 1995.

Weiss J, Elsbach P, Shu C, Castillo J, Grinna L, Horwitz A, Theofan G. Human bactericidal/permeability-increasing protein and a recombinant NH2-terminal fragment cause killing of serum-resistant gram-negative bacteria in whole blood and inhibit tumor necrosis factor release induced by the bacteria. J Clin Invest 90:1122–1130, 1992.

Weiss J, Olsson I. Cellular and subcellular localization of the bactericidal/permeability-increasing protein of neutrophils. Blood 69:652–659, 1987.

Weissman IL. Translating stem and progenitor cell biology to the clinic: barriers and opportunities. Science 287:1442–1446, 2000.

Weller PF, Bubley GJ. The idiopathic hypereosinophilic syndrome. Blood 83:2759–2779, 1994.

Weller PF, Marshall WL, Lucey DR, Rand TH, Dvorak AM, Finberg RW. Infection, apoptosis, and killing of mature human eosinophils by human immunodeficiency virus-1. Am J Respir Cell Mol Biol 13:610–620, 1995.

Werns SW, Lucchesi BR. Myocardial ischemia and reperfusion: the role of oxygen radicals in tissue injury. Cardiovasc Drugs Ther 2:761–769, 1989.

Wheeler MA, Smith SD, Garcia-Cardena G, Nathan CF, Weiss RM, Sessa WC. Bacterial infection induces nitric oxide synthase in human neutrophils. J Clin Invest 99:110–116, 1997.

Wu W, Samoszuk MK, Comhair SAA, Thomassen MJ, Farver CF, Dweik RA, Kavuru MS, Erzurum SC, Hazen SL. Eosinophils generate brominating oxidants in allergen-induced asthma. J Clin Invest 105:1455–1463, 2000.

Yamashiro S, Kamohara H, Wang J-M, Yang D, Gong W-H, Yoshimura T. Phenotypic and functional change of cytokine-activated neutrophils: inflammatory neutrophils are heterogeneous and enhance adaptive immune responses. J Leukoc Biol 69:698–704, 2001.

Yanagihara Y, Kajiwara K, Basaki Y, Ikizawa K, Ebisawa M, Ra C, Tachimoto H, Saito H. Cultured basophils but not cultured mast cells induce human IgE synthesis in B cells after immunologic stimulation. Clin Exp Immunol 111:136–143, 1998.

Yang D, Chertov O, Oppenheim JJ. Participation of mammalian defensins and cathelicidins in anti-microbial immunity: receptors and activities of human defensins and cathelicidin (LL-37). J Leukoc Biol 69:691–697, 2001.

Yazdanbakhsh M, Tai PC, Spry CJ, Gleich GJ, Roos D. Synergism between eosinophil cationic protein and oxygen intermediates in killing of schistosomula of Schistosoma mansoni. J Immunol 138:3443–3447, 1987.

Yazdanbakhsh M, Eckmann CM, Bot AAM, Roos D. Bactericidal action of eosinophils from normal human blood. Infect Immun 53:192–198, 1986.

Young JD-E, Peterson CGB, Venge P, Cohn ZA. Mechanism of membrane damage mediated by human eosinophil cationic protein. Nature 321:613–616, 1986.

Zlotnick A, Yoshie O. Chemokines: a new classification system and their role in immunity. Immunity 12:121–127, 2000.

Zucker-Franklin D, Hirsch JG. Electron microscopic studies on the degranulation of rabbit peritoneal leukocytes during phagocytosis. J Exp Med 120:569–576, 1964.

C H A P T E R

6

The Mononuclear Phagocytic, Dendritic Cell, and Natural Killer Cell Systems

Steven D. Douglas, Reuben Kapur, Jeffrey D. Merrill, Mervin C. Yoder, Jr., and Wenzhe Ho

THE MONONUCLEAR PHAGOCYTIC CELL SYSTEM

Overview

Since the modern study of mammalian phagocytes began with Metchnikoff in the nineteenth century, classification of these cells with respect to structure-function relationships has been controversial. Studies of phagocytic cells in animals have led to the concept of the mononuclear phagocyte system (MPS), which identifies a specific lineage of hematopoietic cells that share certain morphological, cytochemical, and functional characteristics (Van Furth et al., 1975). The MPS, as presently defined, consists of bone marrow *promonocytes*, circulating blood *monocytes*, and both mobile and fixed tissue *macrophages* (Table 6-1). MNP share common functional characteristics, including the following:

1. Phagocytosis and digestion of microorganisms and tissue debris
2. Secretion of inflammatory mediators and regulators
3. Antigen processing and interaction with lymphocytes in the generation of the immune response
4. Extracellular killing, as of some tumor cells
5. Performance of specialized functions specific for macrophages of particular organs or tissues

Fibroblasts, vascular endothelial cells, and lymphoid reticular cells are not included, although terms used in the past, such as the *reticuloendothelial system*, denoted these cells as mononuclear phagocytes (MNPs) collectively. These cells do not display the above characteristics and cannot be demonstrated to share a common hematopoietic precursor with members of the MPS. Although dendritic cells differ in several morphological, cytochemical, and functional characteristics, evidence indicates that dendritic cells are derived from the same bone marrow hematopoietic progenitor cells as circulating monocytes and macrophages and deserve inclusion within the MPS.

Although many investigations of MNP function in experimental animals have used tissue macrophages, in the belief that these are the most important functional elements in the MPS, human tissue macrophages are not routinely accessible and are difficult to obtain. The circulating blood monocyte, however, is easily isolated. After in vitro culture for 5 to 7 days, the monocyte develops macrophage-like properties (Zuckerman et al., 1979). The in vitro study of human MNP biology has been a useful model for examining macrophage physiology and function (Ackerman et al., 1981).

TABLE 6-1 · CELLS BELONGING TO THE MONONUCLEAR PHAGOCYTE SYSTEM

Bone Marrow	Tissues	Body Cavities
Monoblasts	Macrophages occurring in	Pleural macrophages
Promonocytes	Connective tissue (histiocytes)	Peritoneal macrophages
Monocytes	Skin (histiocytes; Langerhans cells?)	
	Liver (Kupffer cells)	**Inflammation**
Blood	Spleen (red pulp macrophages)	Exudate macrophages
Monocytes	Lymph nodes (free and fixed macrophages;	Epithelioid cells
	interdigitating cells?)	Multinucleated giant cells
	Thymus	
	Bone marrow (resident macrophages)	
	Bone (osteoclasts)	
	Synovia (Type A cell)	
	Lung (alveolar and tissue macrophages)	
	Mucosa-associated lymphoid tissues	
	Gastrointestinal tract	
	Genitourinary tract	
	Endocrine organs	
	Central nervous system (macrophages,	
	[reactive] microglia, CSF macrophages)	

CSF = cerebrospinal fluid.
From Van Furth R. Development and distribution of mononuclear phagocytes in the normal steady state and inflammation. In Gallin JI, Goldstein IM, Synderman R, eds. Inflammation: Basic Principles and Clinical Correlates. New York, Raven Press, 1988, p 291.

Origin and Development

During the third week of embryogenesis, primitive macrophages are the first hematopoietic cells to appear in the yolk sac. By the fifth week of gestation, hematopoiesis appears in the fetal liver, which becomes the predominant hematopoietic organ by the second month of gestation (Kelemen, 1979). Initially 70% of the blood cells in the liver are macrophages but decrease to 1% to 2% of the total differentiated cell population, with erythroblasts predominating (Kelemen and Janossa, 1980). Hematopoiesis appears in the bone marrow by the eighth week of gestation (Kelemen and Calvo, 1982), and after birth, throughout childhood and adult life, hematopoiesis occurs in the bone marrow.

All lymphohematopoietic cells arise from lineage-committed hematopoietic progenitor cells and ultimately from a pool of self-renewing pluripotent stem cells. One committed progenitor cell, the granulocyte-macrophage colony-forming unit (GM-CFU), is supported in its differentiation along granulocytic or mononuclear phagocyte pathways by colony-stimulating factors (CSFs). Human CSFs influencing MNP production include interleukin-3 (IL-3), granulocyte-macrophage CSF (GM-CSF), and macrophage CSF (M-CSF) (Bartocci et al., 1987; Broxmeyer, 1986; Clark and Kamen, 1987; Metcalf, 1986; Sieff, 1987). In addition, numerous lineage-restricted transcription factors regulate patterns of gene expression in hematopoietic cells, affecting hematopoietic progenitor cell proliferation and differentiation (Shivdasani and Orkin, 1996; Valledor et al., 1998).

High concentrations of CFU-GM are present in the fetal liver and circulation by mid-gestation (Moore and Williams, 1973; Porcellini, 1980). Circulating levels of CFU-GM decline near term gestation and decrease rapidly after birth (Christensen et al., 1986, 1987; Porcellini et al., 1983).

After commitment to the MNP lineage (Fig. 6-1) occurs in the bone marrow, the *monoblast*, the MNP bone marrow precursor cell, differentiates to the promonocyte and subsequently to the mature circulating monocyte (Douglas and Musson, 1986). The monoblast is a small, round cell that actively incorporates thymidine, is esterase and peroxidase negative, contains lysozyme, and has receptors for complement and immunoglobulin G (IgG). The promonocyte contains specific monocyte enzymes, has complement and IgG receptors, and is capable of phagocytosing particles. The promonocyte is also an actively dividing cell that undergoes several intramarrow mitoses before differentiating into the monocyte, at which time it moves into the intravascular compartment. Blood monocytes circulate for 1 to 4 days, then migrate into tissues. Some of the circulating blood monocytes bind to blood vessel walls, and this marginating pool represents approximately 75% of the total intravascular monocyte pool (Van Furth, 1980).

The resident tissue macrophages are replaced from the blood monocyte pool with defined turnover and exist as both fixed and free macrophages. Free macrophages are found in pleural, synovial, peritoneal, and alveolar spaces and in inflammatory sites. The generally less motile fixed tissue macrophages are present in splenic sinusoids, in the liver as Kupffer cells, in reticulum cells of the bone marrow, in the lamina propria of the gastrointestinal tract, in specific sites in lymph nodes, in bone as osteoclasts, and as microglia in the central nervous system (Van Furth, 1980). In pathologic sites, tissue macrophages may undergo cell fusion and form multinucleated giant cells, which are the source of epitheliod cells in chronic granulomata (Adams, 1976).

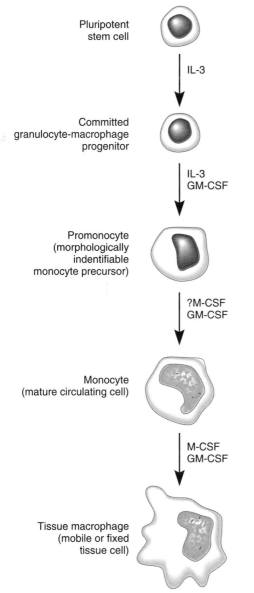

Pluripotent
stem cell

IL-3

Committed
granulocyte-macrophage
progenitor

IL-3
GM-CSF

Promonocyte
(morphologically
indentifiable
monocyte precursor)

?M-CSF
GM-CSF

Monocyte
(mature circulating cell)

M-CSF
GM-CSF

Tissue macrophage
(mobile or fixed
tissue cell)

Figure 6-1 · **Mononuclear phagocyte cell lineage.** (From Yoder M, Douglas SD. Mononuclear Phagocyte Systems. In Polin RA, Fox WW, eds. Fetal and Neonatal Physiology, vol 2, ed 2. Philadelphia, WB Saunders, 1998, pp 1931–1954.)

Cell Kinetics

The cell kinetics of human monocytes have been actively studied by in vivo pulse labeling and by auto-transfusion of radiolabeled monocytes (Meuret and Hoffman, 1973; Meuret et al., 1971, 1974a, 1975; Whitlaw, 1972). The total blood monocyte pool is made up of both a circulating monocyte pool and a marginal monocyte pool, with a circulating monocyte pool–to–marginal monocyte pool ratio of approximately 1:3.5 in normal individuals. The circulating monocyte pool is made up predominantly of cells in a G_1 state, which are released into the circulation following a maturation time in the bone marrow of between

50 and 60 hours. Under normal conditions, the bone marrow promonocyte pool produces approximately 7×10^6 monocytes/kg/hr. The half-disappearance time of labeled monocytes from the blood is considerably longer than for granulocytes (monocytes, approximately 70 hours; granulocytes, approximately 7 hours) (Athens et al., 1961; Meuret et al., 1974a, 1974b; Whitlaw, 1972). The mean absolute monocyte count in peripheral blood ranges from 1100/mm³ during the first 2 weeks of life (when there is a relative monocytosis) to between 350/mm³ and 700/mm³ during the remainder of childhood (Yoder et al., 1992). The blood monocyte counts in normal subjects oscillate in a cycle that varies between 3 and 6 days. This is shorter than the cycle for polymorphonuclear leukocytes, platelets, and reticulocytes.

Monocytes may undergo spontaneous apoptosis, or programmed cell death, after leaving the circulation. Apoptosis may be inhibited by adherence to endothelial cells and induced by microbial products; growth factors such as GM-CSF; and proinflammatory cytokines, including IL-1, tumor necrosis factor-α (TNF-α), and interferon-γ (IFN-γ) (Kiener et al., 1997; Managan et al., 1991). In addition, interaction between the CD40 receptor on monocytes and the CD40 ligand on activated T cells may rescue monocytes from spontaneous apoptosis (Grewel and Flavell; 1997).

In addition to the normal cyclical variation, perturbations in the monocyte count can occur following the injection of a number of different materials, as well as in response to inflammation and disease (see Chapter 16). Usually, monocytopenia develops during endotoxin or steroid administration.

The tissue macrophage does not usually undergo division. It has a life span that has been estimated to range from 60 days to many years; however, an extremely small proportion (less than 5%) of tissue macrophages were found to synthesize DNA and divide locally in the tissues (Van Furth et al., 1985). The macrophage does not return to the peripheral circulation; however, its ultimate fate is not precisely known.

Morphology

Monoblasts and promonocytes are the precursors of monocytes. Monoblasts bear finely dispersed nuclear chromatin and nucleoli when observed in stained films of the blood or bone marrow but lack distinctive features and are indistinguishable by light microscopy from the neutrophilic precursor, the myeloblast. Promonocytes are 12 to 18 μm in diameter and have characteristic deeply indented, irregularly shaped nuclei with condensed chromatin and numerous cytoplasmic microfilaments (Nichols and Bainton, 1973; Nichols et al., 1971).

Monocytes are found both in the blood and in tissues and body cavities, in which they exhibit morphologic variation. In the stained blood film, the diameter is 12 to 15 μm. The nucleus occupies about half the area of the cell in a film and is usually eccentrically placed. The nucleus is most often reniform but may be round or irregular. It contains a characteristic chromatin net with fine strands bridging small chromatin clumps. Chromatin aggregates are arranged along the internal aspect of the nuclear membrane. The nuclear chromatin pattern has been called "raked" because of its fine-stranded appearance. The cytoplasm is spread out, stains grayish-blue with Wright's stain, and contains a variable number of fine, pink-purple granules that at times are sufficiently numerous to give the entire cytoplasm a pink hue. Clear cytoplasmic vacuoles and a variable number of larger azurophilic granulations are often encountered in these cells.

The monocyte generally assumes a triangular shape as it moves, with one point trailing behind and the other two points advancing before the cell. It adheres to and spreads on glass surfaces (Bessis, 1955; Fedorko and Hirsch, 1970; North, 1970). The spread form of the monocyte is characteristic, with the nucleus and granulations located centrally and the abundant hyaloplasm around the periphery of the cell, terminating in a fringed border that displays characteristic undulating movement. The small monocyte may be difficult to distinguish from the large lymphocyte when examined by phase-contrast microscopy, although the two cells can be differentiated by the ability of small monocytes to adhere to glass surfaces (Fig. 6-2).

Under examination by scanning electron microscopy, there is extensive ruffling of the monocyte plasma membrane (Bumol and Douglas, 1977) (Fig. 6-3). The monocyte is both motile and phagocytic, and for these functions to be accomplished, there must be physical contact with fibers or cell surfaces, which occurs through plasma membrane ruffling. Reduction in the radius of curvature of the cell surface by formation of ruffles or microvilli may decrease repulsive forces when

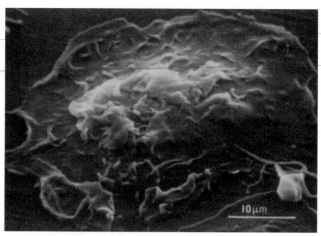

Figure 6-3 · Blood monocyte cultured 1 hour in vitro. The cell is flattened against the substratum and possesses prominent surface ruffles. (Scanning electron micrograph, ×2750.) (From Ackerman SK, Douglas SD. Morphology of Monocytes and Macrophages. In Carr I, Daems WT, eds. Reticuloendothelial System: Morphology. New York, Plenum Press, 1980, pp 297–327.)

surface negative-charge groups on the cell approach and contact a negatively charged substratum or cell (Van Oss et al., 1975). Also, redundancy of the cell membrane may provide reserve membrane required for locomotion and for phagocytosis.

The ultrastructural morphology of the monocyte consists of a relatively small quantity of endoplasmic reticulum and a variable quantity of ribosomes and polysomes. The mitochondria are usually numerous, small, and elongated. The Golgi complex is well developed. Centrioles and filamentous centriolar satellites can often be visualized. Microtubules and microfibrils are numerous (DePetris et al., 1962).

Many dense, homogeneous cytoplasmic granules are present, measuring approximately 0.05 to 0.2 μm. These granules contain acid phosphatase and arylsulfatase and are therefore primary lysosomes (Axline, 1970). After endocytosis, lysosomes fuse with the phagosome, forming secondary lysosomes (North, 1970). Monocyte granules may give a positive reaction for peroxidase, although in a large proportion of monocytes this reaction is negative (Breton-Gorius and Cuichard, 1969; Nichols et al., 1971; Nichols and Bainton, 1973).

A morphologic transformation of peripheral blood monocytes into mature macrophages may be seen within in vitro culture and is characterized by an increase in cell size, an increase in lysosomal granules, an enlargement of the Golgi complex, an increase in the size and number of mitochondria, and the appearance of large vacuoles called phagosomes (Ackerman and Douglas, 1983).

Macrophages are heterogeneous in size and shape, ranging from 25 to 70 μm in diameter and appearing as oval, stellate, or spindle-shaped cells. The nucleus is eccentrically placed and contains finely dispersed chromatin and prominent nucleoli. Numerous granules and vacuoles are present near the cell periphery (Zuckerman et al., 1979), characteristic of pinocytic cells (Fig. 6-4).

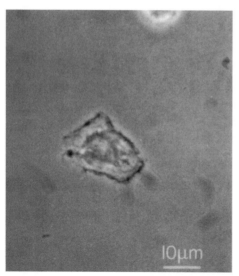

Figure 6-2 · Human blood monocyte after in vitro culture for 1 hour. Note phase-dense thickening at the peripheral region of the cell, signifying ruffling of the membrane. (Phase-contrast micrograph, original magnification ×400.) (From Ackerman SK, Douglas SD. Morphology of Monocytes and Macrophages. In Carr I, Daems WT, eds. Reticuloendothelial System: Morphology. New York, Plenum Press, 1980, pp 297–327.)

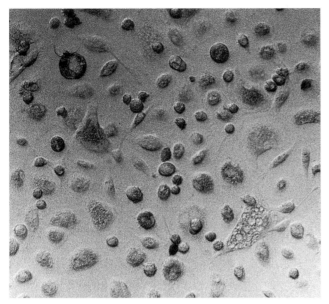

Figure 6-4 · Human peripheral blood monocyte-derived macrophages maintained in vitro for 7 days. (Light microscopy, ×250.)

Ultrastructural features of macrophages include numerous electron-dense lysosomes along the cell surface, a well-developed Golgi zone, an extensive endoplasmic reticulum, and lipid vacuoles (Fig. 6-5). Collections of microfilaments are present underneath the plasma membrane near sites of cell attachment either to a substratum or to ingestable particles (Reaven and Axline, 1973). The cell surface is characterized by numerous microvilli and vesicles of micropinocytosis.

Histochemistry

Macrophages contain a variety of hydrolytic enzymes that are synthesized in the rough endoplasmic reticulum and are packaged in units of membrane-bound vesicles known as lysosomes. Lysozyme, β-glucuronidase, acid

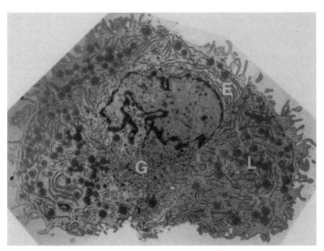

Figure 6-5 · Monocyte-derived macrophage cultured 17 days in vitro. Note the presence of a Golgi zone (G) with scattered endoplasmic reticulum (E) and lipid vacuoles (L). (Transmission electron micrograph, ×6000.)

phosphatase, cathepsins, hydrolases, and esteroproteases have all been described in macrophages (Axline and Cohn, 1970; Solotorovsky and Soderberg, 1972). These enzymes play an important role in intracellular digestion of phagocytized material and in the development and maintenance of inflammatory reactions. They also may be involved in microbial killing.

Nonspecific esterase is an enzyme on the external side of the plasma membrane (ectoenzyme) on alveolar macrophages (Jaubert et al., 1978) and blood monocytes (Bozdech and Bainton, 1981). Nonspecific esterases are present in many cell types (Braunsteiner and Schmalzl, 1968, 1970; Li et al., 1973; Wachstein and Wolfe, 1958). Monocyte esterases are inhibited by sodium fluoride, whereas the esterases of the granulocytic series are not. The nonspecific esterase reaction is positive in promyelocytes and myelocytes, and therefore analysis of fluoride inhibition is necessary to distinguish marrow monocytes from early myelocytes (Braunsteiner and Schmalzl, 1968). As monocytes mature into differentiated macrophage, additional nonspecific esterase isoenzymes resistant to sodium fluoride are expressed.

Monocytes, neutrophils, and lymphocytes differ in hydrolytic enzyme content (Braunsteiner and Schmalzl, 1968, 1970; Li et al., 1973; Wachstein and Wolfe, 1958). Human marrow promonocytes and blood monocytes contain granules that make up two functionally distinct populations (Nichols and Bainton, 1973; Nichols et al., 1971). One population contains the enzymes acid phosphatase, arylsulfatase, and in humans but not in rabbits, peroxidase; these granules are therefore modified primary lysosomes and are analogous to the azurophil granules of the neutrophil. The monocyte azurophil granule population is heterogeneous with respect to cytochemical reactivity for peroxidase, acid phosphatase, and arylsulfatase (Nichols and Bainton, 1975; Bodel et al., 1977). Moreover, primary granules that are morphologically identical with other vesicles may be identified cytochemically as lysosomes. The content of the other population of monocyte granules is unknown; however, they lack alkaline phosphatase (Nichols and Bainton, 1975) and hence are not strictly analogous to the specific granules of neutrophils. The function of the lysosomal granule is presumably digestive; the purpose of the second population is not known.

About 10% of granules in normal human blood monocytes stain with reagents that identify complex acid carbohydrates, or *acid mucosubstances* (Parmley et al., 1978). These substances are found in leukemic monocyte granules and in granules of normal neutrophils (Horn and Spicer, 1964), and their function is unknown. Monocytes also have a weak but positive periodic acid-Schiff (PAS) reaction (for polysaccharides) and Sudan black B reaction (for lipids).

Cell Surface Antigens

The MNP cell surface is rich in antigenic markers that have been studied with a variety of monoclonal antibodies. Studies of the expression of these antigens on human MNPs have led to better understanding of the origin, differentiation, and functions of MNPs (Todd and Schlossman, 1982; Dimitriu-Bona et al., 1983; Andreesen et al., 1986; Auger and Ross, 1992; Ho et al., 1992). Table 6-2 lists many of the antigenic determinants of MNP cells that are recognized as *clusters of differentiation* (CD) by the International Workshop on Human Leukocyte Differentiation Antigens (adapted from Barclay et al., 1993). These cell surface antigens function as cell recognition or adhesion molecules, enzymes, or receptors for immunoglobulins, complement components, cytokines, chemokines, growth factors, hormones, opioids, lipids, extracellular matrix molecules, and lectins (Gordon et al., 1988, Snyderman 1989); some antigens are not sufficiently characterized to be assigned a specific cellular function.

Most of these antigens are not expressed exclusively by MNP; however, unique patterns of antigen expression have been useful in defining developmentally regulated or tissue-specific MNP phenotypes (Andreesen et al., 1988, 1990; Buckley, 1991; Ho et al., 1992; Terstappen et al., 1990; Todd and Schlossman, 1984). CD14 antigen expression, for example, appears after 15 weeks gestation on human fetal blood monocytes, and the intensity of expression on human neonatal cord blood monocytes at birth is equal to that in adults (Rainaut, 1987). CD11a, CD11b, and CD11c antigens, however, are expressed at a lower density on human neonatal cord blood monocytes as compared with adults (Marwitz 1988). In addition, most primary blood monocytes express high levels of CD14 yet variably express the CD16 antigen. Monocyte-derived macrophages in vitro, however, have decreased expression of CD14 and CD11b and increased expression of CD16 (Ziegler-Heitbrock and Ulevitch, 1993).

Metabolism

The metabolic activities of MNPs vary, depending on their degree of development, site of origin, and state of activation or stimulation (Cline, 1965; Cohn, 1968; Karnovsky et al., 1973; Nelson, 1969). The monocyte uses active aerobic glycolysis as a source of energy, whereas mature macrophages derive their energy from both glycolytic and aerobic pathways (Cline and Lehrer, 1968; Cohn, 1968). There is a developmental effect on energy metabolism. Studies have demonstrated that term and preterm cord blood MNP have decreased glycolysis and little metabolic response to lectin stimulation, decreased pyruvate kinase activity, and decreased adenosine triphosphate (ATP) concentrations as compared with adult peripheral blood MNP, which may relate to observed neonatal immune dysfunction (Das, 1979) (see Chapter 22).

The degree to which macrophages depend on either aerobic or anaerobic processes appears to differ with their tissue site. Pulmonary macrophages manifest a high degree of oxygen consumption, gaining energy through oxidative phosphorylation (Hocking and Golde, 1979; Rossman and Douglas, 1988). Peritoneal macrophages, in contrast, utilize anaerobic glycolysis

as their main energy source (Oren, 1963). These different characteristics appear to represent distinct functional advantages for the macrophages at each particular anatomic site. For example, the capacity of nonalveolar macrophages to be metabolically active under anaerobic conditions is crucial to their ability to function optimally at sites of inflammation, where oxygen tension may be low. The dependence of the alveolar macrophage on aerobic sources of energy may represent a logical anatomic adaptation. However, this may be a disadvantage in situations of compromised pulmonary function, because these cells have shown reduced phagocyte capacity under conditions of low oxygen tension (Cline, 1970).

Biochemistry

Respiratory Burst

Stimulation of MNP with soluble chemoattractants or through cell surface receptor-ligand interactions is associated with a dramatic increase in MNP oxygen consumption. This respiratory burst is not required for energy production but is necessary for superoxide anion, hydrogen peroxide, and hydroxyl radical production. A plasma membrane–bound enzyme complex (NADPH oxidase), along with several cytosolic proteins, converts molecular oxygen to superoxide anion. The reactive oxygen intermediates produced are further metabolized to free radicals and hypohalous acid and are used to kill ingested bacterial and fungal pathogens (Nathan, 1982, 1983). Respiratory burst activity diminishes as monocytes differentiate into macrophages, and tissue macrophages may rely more on oxygen-independent means to kill pathogens. MNP derived from neonatal cord blood have a respiratory burst, when quantified in vitro, equivalent to adult peripheral blood MNP (Speer, 1986). Likewise, monocyte-derived macrophages from cord blood and adult MNP have equal superoxide anion generation when stimulated with soluble agents, but peak generation with lypopolysaccharide priming is less in neonatal MNP as compared with adults (Speer, 1985).

Lysosomes

Lysosomes are intracellular granular compartments composed of numerous enzymes and proteases. The primary function of these granules appears to be degradation of ingested materials. Acid hydrolases, lipases, ribonucleases, phosphatases, sulfatases, and neutral proteases are some of the constituents of lysosomes. Many of these proteins are not restricted to lysosomes and are secreted by MNPs on cytokine or complement stimulation, engagement of IgG-opsonized material through Fc receptors, or exposure to bacteria (Lasser, 1983; Pantalone and Page, 1975).

Synthesis and Secretion of Growth Factors and Cytokines

Among the mechanisms used by MNPs to influence local and systemic immune responses are the biosynthesis and

TABLE 6-2 · CD ANTIGENS ON MONONUCLEAR PHAGOCYTE CELLS

CD Group	Molecule	Distribution on Hematopoietic Cells
4	T$_4$	Thymocytes, T cells, monocytes, macrophages
11a	LFA-1	All leukocytes
11b	CR3, OKM-1, Mac-1	Neutrophils, monocytes, platelets
11c	p150, 95	Monocytes, neutrophils, cells
w12	p 150–160	Monocytes, neutrophils, platelets
13	gp 150	Monocytes, neutrophils, some macrophages
14	LPS receptor	Monocytes, macrophages, dendritic cells, some neutrophils
15	Lewis X (Le^x)	Neutrophils, eosinophils, monocytes, myeloid leukemia cells
16	FcγRIII	NK cells, macrophages, some monocytes
w17	Lactosylceramide	Neutrophils, monocytes, platelets
18	Integrin β2	Most leukocytes
23	FcεRII	B cells, activated macrophages, monocytes, platelets
25	IL-2 receptor	T and B cells, monocytes
26	DPP IV	Macrophages, lymphocytes
29	VLA-1	All leukocytes
31	PECAM-1	Monocytes, platelets, neutrophils
32	FcγRII	Monocytes, neutrophils, B cells
33	p67	Monocytes, progenitor cells, myeloid leukemia cells
34	p105–120	Progenitor cells, myeloid and lymphoid leukemia cells
35	CR1	Erythrocytes, monocytes, macrophages, neutrophils
36	Platelet glycoprotein IV	Monocytes
40	TNFR family	Monocytes, macrophages, lymphocytes
43	Leukosialin	T cells, monocytes, macrophages, platelets
44	Phagocytic glycoprotein-1	T and B cells, monocytes, thymocytes, erythrocytes
45	B220, T200, Ly-5	All leukocytes
46	Membrane co-factor protein	T and B cells, NK cells, monocytes, platelets
48	gp41	Most leukocytes
49	Integrin α$^{1-6}$ chains	Most leukocytes
w50	p148/108, ICAM-3	T and B cells, monocytes
w52	CAMPATH-1	Monocytes, lymphocytes, neutrophils
53	gp21–28	Thymocytes, T and B cells, monocytes, osteoclasts
54	ICAM-1	Activated B and T cells, monocytes
55	DAF	Hematopoietic cells
58	LFA-3	Macrophages, B cells, thymocytes
59	MIRh	Hematopoietic cells
61	Integrin β$_3$	Macrophages, osteoclasts, platelets
62L	L-selectin	Monocytes, lymphocytes, neutrophils
63	gp53	Platelets, monocytes, macrophages, B and T cells
64	FcγRI	Monocytes, macrophages, activated neutrophils
w65	Ceramide dodecasaccharide 4c	Monocytes, activated neutrophils
68	p110	Macrophages, monocytes, neutrophils
71	Transferrin receptor	Activated monocytes, neutrophils, B and T cells
74	MHC II-associated invariant chain	B cells, monocytes
80	B7.1	Monocytes, macrophages
w84	MAX.3	Macrophages, lymphocytes
85	VMP55, GH1/75, ILT2	Monocytes, lymphocytes, NK cells
86	B7.2	Monocytes, macrophages
87	uPAR	Monocytes, lymphocytes, neutrophils
88	C5aR	Macrophage, neutrophils
89	FcαR	Monocytes, lymphocytes, neutrophils
91	LRP, α2 macroglobulin R	Monocytes
95	Fas, APO-1	Monocytes, lymphocytes
102	ICAM-2	Monocytes
w116	GM-CSFR	Monocytes, neutrophils, progenitor cells
117	CSFR	Monocytes, macrophages, progenitor cells
119	IFN-γR	Monocytes, macrophages
120a	TNF-αR	Hematopoietic cells
120b	TNF-αR	Hematopoietic cells
121b	IL-1R, type 2	Monocytes, macrophages
123	IL-3R	Monocytes
124	IL-4R	Hematopoietic cells
126	IL-6R	Most leukocytes
w130	gp130 subunit	Most leukocytes

CD = cluster of differentiation; CR = complement receptor; ICAM = intercellular adhesion molecule; gp = glycoprotein; LFA = leukocyte function antigen; LPS = lipopolysaccharide; Mac = macrophage; MHC = major histocompatibility complex; NK = natural killer; p = protein; PECAM = platelet endothelial cell adhesion molecule; T$_4$ = thyroxine.

TABLE 6-3 · CYTOKINES SECRETED BY MONONUCLEAR PHAGOCYTES

Cytokine	Stimuli for Production	Biological Action
IFN-α	Viruses, bacteria	Antiviral; antimitotic; MHC class II ($\uparrow$), NK activity ($\uparrow$); decreased c-*myc* expression
M-CSF	LPS, IL-1, IFN-γ, TNF-α, TNF-β, IL-3, IL-4, GM-CSF	Macrophage colonies; antimicrobial, induces PGE$_2$, plasminogen activator, IL-1, IFN-γ, TNF-α, G-CSF, osteoclast progenitors
GM-CSF	LPS, IL-1, TNF, retroviral infection	Granulocyte, eosinophil, macrophage colonies, radioprotection, protection from bacterial and parasitic infections; enhances neutrophil and eosinophil functions, PGE$_2$, IL-1, TNF, and O$_2$ induction
G-CSF	LPS, IL-1	Granulocyte colonies; terminal differentiation of myeloid cells; enhancement of neutrophil function
TNF-α	LPS and other microbial products, IL-2, GM-CSF, IL-1	Necrosis of tumors; endotoxic shock–like syndrome; cachexia; fever; IL-1; acute-phase protein response; antiparasitic; in vitro induction of ICAM-1, IL-1, GM-CSF, IL-6; upregulation of MHC I and II expression
IL-1	Microbial products, TNF, GM-CSF, IL-2, antigen presentation	Immunoregulation (induction of IL-2, IL-4, IL-6, TNF); fever; acute-phase protein response; hypotension; slow wave sleep; induction of collagenase and PGE$_2$, bone and cartilage resorption in culture
IL-6	IL-1, TNF, PDGF	Proliferation of myeloma cell lines, hemopoietic cells (GM-CSF and IL-3–like action); induces IL-2R in T cells; induces Ig production in B cells; induces acute-phase protein production by hepatocytes; fever
IL-8	LPS, IL-1, TNF-α	Neutrophil chemoattractant; increases neutrophil activation, adhesion, and transendothelial migration
IL-10	LPS, viruses, bacteria	Macrophage deactivation; decreases APC MHC class II expression; suppresses T-cell activation and antigen-specific proliferation; inhibits of proinflammatory cytokine release
IL-12	Bacteria, intracellular pathogens, APC–T-cell interaction via CD40	Th1 cell maturation; augments Th1-mediated proinflammatory response, increases proliferation, cytotoxicity, and IFN-γ release of T and NK cells
IL-15	LPS, microbial infection	Augments proliferation and differentiation of monocytes, macrophages, lymphocytes, and NK cells; augments NK-cell activation, cytotoxicity, and IFN-γ release; increases phagocytosis and delays apoptosis;
IL-18	LPS, microbial products	Augments Th1-mediated proinflammatory response, synergizes with IL-12 to augment Th1 maturation; induces IFN-γ, IL-1β, IL-8, TNF-α, GM-CSF release; increases adhesion molecule expression
TGF-β		Inhibition of IL-2 effects; role in fibrosis and wound healing in vivo; antiproliferative effects on hepatocytes, epithelial cells, T and B cells; influences integrin expression and differentiation; inhibits proliferative actions of EGF, PDGF, IL-2, and FGF
Basic FGF		Endothelial cell chemotaxis and growth; IFN-γ, IFN-β, PGE$_2$, LDL-receptor, c-myc, c-fos, amino acid transport; neutrophil activation; intracellular actin reorganization; augments synthesis of collagen; chemotaxis and proliferation of mesenchymal cells
EGF		Proliferation and differentiation of basal layer in epithelia; angiogenic; wound healing

APC = antigen presenting cell; EGF = epidermal growth factor; FGF = fibroblast growth factor; G-CSF = granulocyte colony-stimulating factor; ICAM = intracellular adhesion molecule; LDL = low-density lipoprotein; LPS = lipopolysaccharide; MHC = Major histocompatibility complex; NK = natural killer; PDGF = platelet-derived growth factor; PGE =; TGF = transforming growth factor; Th1 = T-helper type I.
Adapted from Auger MJ, Ross JA. The biology of the macrophage. In Lewis CE, McGee JO, eds. The Macrophage. Oxford, England, IRL Press, 1992, pp 1–74.

secretion of numerous cytokines and growth factors (Table 6-3; Fig. 6-6). MNP production and release of proinflammatory cytokines, such as IL-1, IL-6, IL-8, and IL-12, are modulated by infectious and noninfectious stimuli and depend on the state of MNP activation (Dinarello, 1996; Trinchieri and Gerosa, 1996; Vignola, 1998). These regulatory molecules have pleiotropic effects that affect nearly all cell types, allowing for cell-to-cell communication among immune and nonimmune cells. IL-12, produced by MNP and other antigen-presenting cells in a T-cell–independent (stimulation by bacteria or intracellular parasites) or T-cell–dependent fashion, increases IFN-γ production by T and natural killer (NK) cells, enhances NK cytotoxicity, and induces T-helper 1 (Th1) cell phenotype of proinflammatory cytokine production. The increased production of IFN-γ by T and NK cells in turn increases macrophage activation and antimicrobial and tumoricidal activity (Takenaka et al., 1997; Trinchieri and Gerosa, 1996).

Techniques have been developed to assay for the biosynthesis and secretion of growth factors and cytokines by human MNPs. Usually, growth factor and cytokine assays have been performed on isolated peripheral blood monocytes or monocyte-derived macrophages cultured and stimulated in vitro. Comparisons between reports of cytokine secretion from MNPs must consider the following:

1. Method and site of MNP isolation
2. Purity of the isolated population
3. State of differentiation of the isolated cells
4. Whether the cells were studied in suspension or adherent to tissue culture plates
5. Sensitivity and specificity of the assays
6. Whether messenger RNA (mRNA) or protein is measured
7. Quantification of secreted or cell-associated protein
8. Whether recombinant or native cytokines were used for stimulation of MNP secretion of additional cytokines
9. Medium and serum concentration used in the assay

Cytokines produced by MNP (IL-10) and by other immune cells (IL-4, IL-13) have anti-inflammatory, sup-

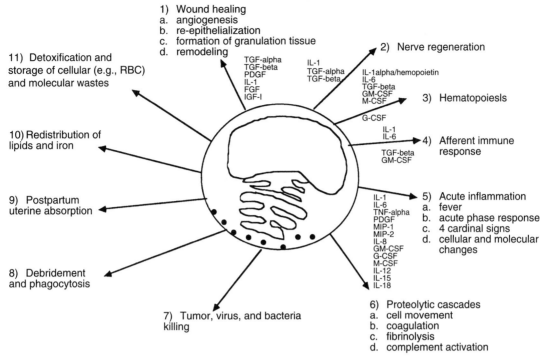

Figure 6-6 · Growth factors produced by mononuclear phagocytes correlated with specific macrophage functions. FGF = fibroblast growth factor; IGF = insulin-like growth factor; MIP = macrophage inflammatory protein; PDGF = platelet-derived growth factor; RBC = red blood cells; TGF = transforming growth factor. (Modified from Rappolee DA, Werb Z. Macrophage-derived growth factors. Curr Top Microbiol Immunol 181:87–140, 1992.)

pressive effects and modulate MNP phenotype and function. For example, IL-10 inhibits the expression of major histocompatibility complex (MHC) type II co-stimulatory surface molecules on antigen-presenting cells and inhibits IL-6–, IL-12–, and IFN-γ–induced intercellular cell adhesion molecule-1 (ICAM-1) gene transcription (De Waal-Malefyt et al., 1992; Donnelly et al., 1999; Vignola, 1998). IL-10 and IL-13 inhibit chemoattractant (macrophage inflammatory protein-1α [MIP-1α]) production and release by MNP. In addition, IL-13 decreases glucocorticoid receptor binding affinity and may contribute to impaired glucocorticoid responsiveness during inflammatory disease states (De Vries and Zurawaski, 1995). Neonatal MNP production of various cytokines, including IL-6, IL-8, and IL-10, are decreased compared with adult MNP cells and may contribute to the diminished immune response seen in newborns (Johnston, 1998; Kotiranta-Ainamo et al., 1999).

Systemic and local events may be influenced by MNP cytokine secretion. Thus normal homeostatic mechanisms such as core body temperature maintenance may be overridden in times of acute inflammation by the secretion of macrophage pyrogen IL-1, TNF-α, and IL-6 (see Table 6-3). These same cytokines alter liver metabolism and protein biosynthesis, resulting in liver secretion of acute-phase reactant proteins (Heinrich, 1990). B and T lymphocytes are activated to proliferate and differentiate in response to MNP secretion of IL-1 and IL-6 and the hematopoietic colony-stimulating

factors M-CSF-1, GM-CSF, and granulocyte colony-stimulating factor (G-CSF). The T-lymphocyte–derived cytokines IL-6, G-CSF, and GM-CSF have positive feedback loops and further stimulate MNP secretion of growth factors and regulatory molecules and increase bone marrow production of immature MNPs and granulocytes (Metcalf, 1987).

Other MNP-derived growth factors, such as basic fibroblast growth factor, platelet-derived growth factor, and epidermal growth factor, promote mesenchymal and epithelial cell growth and differentiation, whereas MNP secretion of transforming growth factor-β (TGF-β) has immunosuppressive and antiproliferative effects on a variety of immune and nonimmune cells (Carpenter, 1987; Lobb et al., 1986; Massague, 1987; Rappolee and Werb, 1992; Ross, 1987). Several anticytokine molecules have been identified in human MNPs. IL-1 receptor antagonist (IL-1Ra) and TNF-soluble receptor-binding protein are secreted by MNP and serve to inhibit the effects of IL-1 and TNF, respectively, during acute and chronic inflammatory states (Arend et al., 1989; Seckinger et al., 1987, 1988).

Other Secretory Products

More than 100 MNP secretory products have been studied (Nathan, 1987). Certain products are released on a constitutive basis and are little influenced by the tissue of origin or state of activation of the MNP (Davies, 1981). Other products are dependent on the activity of the cell in vitro or the site of origin in vivo (Rappolee and Werb, 1989). Table 6-4 lists some of the classes of MNP secretory products. Although some of these products are unique to the MNP, many are produced by other secretory cells (Nathan, 1987).

Motility

An effective macrophage response to infection is predicated on the ability to migrate and accumulate at an infection site. Macrophages, like neutrophils, are capable of both *random* and *directed* movement. Random migration is nondirected movement that occurs in the absence of attracting substances. Directed movement, or *chemotaxis*, refers to macrophage migration that occurs in response to identifiable chemotactic factors or stimuli and that is mediated by different types of receptors on phagocyte cell surfaces (Snyderman and Pike, 1989).

Chemotaxis

Chemotaxis plays a major role in macrophage accumulation at the site of an infection. This process of cellular attraction is mediated by a number of chemotactic substances that either are produced as a result of activation of the complement system and the fibrinolytic and kinin-generating systems or are secreted by leukocytes (Gallin and Wolff, 1976). The complement pathway and the fibrinolytic and kinin-generating systems can be activated by a variety of substances, including antigen-antibody complexes, endotoxin, and even enzymes from macrophages and neutrophils released during the phagocytic process. C5a is the complement component that manifests chemotactic activity.

Plasminogen activator and kallikrein are chemotactic factors produced by the fibrinolytic and kinin-generating systems, respectively (Gallin and Kaplan, 1974). During the acute inflammatory response, leukotriene B4, platelet-activating factor, and neutrophil-derived chemotactic factor, produced by activated neutrophils, and platelet factor 4, platelet-derived growth factor, and TGF-β, produced by activated platelets, are potent chemotactic factors for human monocytes (Verghese and Snyderman, 1989).

Lymphocytes exposed to antigenic stimulation also produce substances that are capable of attracting MNPs (Ward et al., 1970). These lymphokines include lymphocyte-derived chemotactic factor (Altman et al., 1973), TNF-α and -β, and GM-CSF (Verghese and Snyderman, 1989). Certain compounds produced as a result of bacterial growth in vitro (Ward, 1968) also possess chemotactic activity for mononuclear phagocytes. In addition, classes of proinflammatory chemoattractants, named chemokines, have been isolated that direct MNP migration, and play a role in cellular activation and leukocyte effector function. Members of the Monocyte Chemotactic Protein family (MCP-1, MCP-2, MCP-3) are produced by many cell types and are a major chemoattractant of CD4+ cells, CD8+ cells and monocytes. MIP-1, which is secreted by MNP, serves as a chemoattractant of MNP and lymphocytes. RANTES, produced by macrophage, fibroblasts, and T lymphocytes, also regulates MNP chemotaxis. Dexamethasone and prostaglandin E suppress MNP migration by blocking induction and release of various chemokines (reviewed in Vignola, 1998).

In addition to substances that stimulate macrophage motility, a number of biologically active inhibitors of mononuclear cell movement and inactivators of chemotactic factors have been described (Gallin and Wolff, 1976). Inhibition of MNP motility appears to play a significant role in accumulation of MNPs at sites of infection and inflammation. An important mediator of this phenomenon may be migration inhibition factor, a lymphokine released by antigen-stimulated lymphocytes that inhibits macrophage migration in vitro (David, 1973).

MNP migration has been evaluated in the newborn. Most reports suggest that cord blood MNP random migration is equivalent to adult peripheral blood MNP (Klein, 1977; Marodi, 1980; Weston, 1977). Chemotactic mobility, however, is decreased in neonatal cord blood and peripheral blood MNP as compared with adults. Monocyte chemotactic mobility increases gradually over childhood and is equivalent to adult MNP by 5 to 6 years of age (Raghunathan, 1982; Yegin, 1983).

Adherence

Migration of MNPs into areas of inflammation in tissues requires multiple receptor-ligand interactions between the MNP and capillary endothelial cells. In the systemic circulation, monocyte extravasation from postcapillary venules occurs in three stages (Butcher, 1991). Initially, monocytes rolling along the vascular endothelium make transient focal contact with the endothelial cells through a family of adhesion molecules called *selectins* (Fig. 6-7) (Lasky, 1992). *L-selectin* is constitutively expressed on the cell surface of monocytes and recognizes several types of carbohydrate molecules present on endothelial cell surface glycoproteins. *E-selectin* and *P-selectin* are adhesion molecules that are expressed only by activated

---

TABLE 6-4 · SECRETORY PRODUCTS OF MONONUCLEAR PHAGOCYTES

Polypeptide hormones
Complement (C) components
Coagulation factors
Enzymes
Chemokines
Neuropeptides
Inhibitors of enzymes and cytokines
Protease inhibitors
Proteins of extracellular matrix or cell adhesion
Other binding proteins
Bioactive oligopeptides
Bioactive lipids
Sterol hormones
Purine and pyrimidine products
Reactive oxygen intermediates
Reactive nitrogen intermediates

Modified from Nathan CF. Secretory products of macrophages. J Clin Investigation 319–326, 1987.

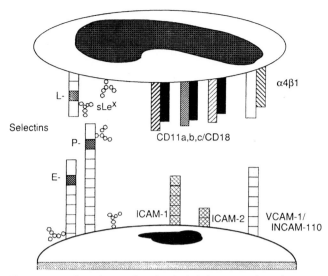

Figure 6-7· Selected examples of endothelial-mononuclear phagocyte adhesion molecules. Mononuclear phagocytes express cell surface carbohydrate and integrin (CD11a,b,c/CD18 and α4β1) molecules that can interact with ligand counter-receptors on endothelial cells. Thus adhesion of mononuclear phagocytes to endothelial cells is mediated by carbohydrate-selectin, integrin-ICAM, and integrin–vascular cell adhesion molecule-1 (VCAM-1)/intercellular cell adhesion molecule-110 (INCAM-110) interactions. (From Bevilacqua MP. Endothelial-leukocyte adhesion molecules. Annu Rev Immunol 11:767–804.)

endothelial cells (Carlos et al., 1991; Hakkert et al., 1991, Sanders et al., 1992). These selectins recognize several types of carbohydrate molecules expressed on monocyte cell surface glycoproteins.

Inhibition of Rolling

The second phase of monocyte extravasation results in inhibition of monocyte rolling, with firm attachment of the monocyte to the activated endothelial cell (Carlos and Harlan, 1990). Adherence to endothelium is associated with overall activation of the monocyte and requires interaction of adhesion molecules of the integrin family on the monocyte with members of the immunoglobulin family on the endothelial cell (see Fig. 6-7). Specifically, heterodimeric monocyte cell surface CD11a/CD18, CD11b/CD18, and CD11c/CD18 molecules bind to endothelial cell surface ICAM-1 or ICAM-2 (Arnaout, 1990; Makgoba et al., 1988; Springer, 1990; Staunton et al., 1989). Monocytes also express another heterodimeric integrin family member composed of α4 and β1 chains that interacts with endothelial cell surface vascular cell adhesion molecule-1 (VCAM-1) and is associated with monocyte-endothelial adhesion on endothelial cell activation (Rice et al., 1990, 1991; Wellicome et al., 1990). Monocyte adherence to endothelial cells is modulated by endothelin-1 and vascular endothelium growth factor (VEGF) (Vignola, 1998).

Emigration into Tissues

The final step in monocyte extravasation involves transendothelial monocyte migration and emigration into the tissue toward the nidus of inflammation. Passage across the endothelial lining into the site of inflammation involves platelet endothelial cell adhesion molecule-1 (PECAM-1), expressed both on monocytes and endothelial cells. In addition, C-C class chemokines selectively regulate expression and affinity of various integrins and may facilitate transendothelial mobility (Muller and Randolph, 1999; Van Furth, 1998).

Several studies on the mechanisms that control pseudopod formation during macrophage movement have been performed. Actin is an abundant cytoplasmic protein that organizes into a three-dimensional network in the macrophage cortical cytoplasm (Hartwig and Stossel, 1985). Actin filaments attach to specific cell surface receptors (e.g., fibronectin receptors) that induce a change in cytoplasmic actin assemblies on binding to fibronectin. Myosin filaments that are present in macrophage cytoplasm control the contractility of the cells. Other proteins have been described, including gelsolin (Yin et al., 1981) and acumentin (Southwick and Hartwig, 1982), that serve to regulate actin filament assembly and macrophage mobility (Stossel, 1989). The observation that there is defective mononuclear phagocytic chemotaxis in a number of disease states emphasizes the importance of an intact mononuclear phagocytic migratory response in host defense against infection and perhaps malignancy.

Endocytosis: Pinocytosis and Phagocytosis

The ability of macrophages to ingest a variety of materials is crucial to their immunologic function. Endocytosis is important in antigen processing, antimicrobial resistance, antineoplastic activity, removal of senescent cells and other "debris," and a number of other monocyte and macrophage functions. Two forms of endocytosis occur: pinocytosis and phagocytosis. The distinction between these two processes is related to the difference in the size and type of particles being ingested; the basic mechanisms are believed to be similar. *Pinocytosis* refers to the ingestion of microscopic fluid droplets. *Phagocytosis* describes the ingestion of larger particulate matter. Both processes involve interiorizing the respective materials in the cytoplasm.

The ingested material becomes progressively surrounded by the plasma membrane through either invagination or engulfment by membrane extensions or microvilli. In this way the particle comes to lie within a vesicle that is formed by the exterior plasma membrane of the cell. This vesicle becomes detached from the cell membrane and moves, apparently propelled by the undulating motion of the plasma membrane and cytoplasm, in a centripetal fashion toward the peri-Golgi region of the cell. En route these vesicles often fuse to form phagocytic vacuoles, or *phagosomes*. Phagosomes in turn fuse with the hydrolytic enzyme containing primary lysosomes and form *phagolysosomes*, in which the ultimate digestion process takes place (Cohn, 1968; Gordon and Cohn, 1973).

Particulate material is not ingested without first becoming attached to the MNP cell surface membrane. Microorganisms that have been opsonized by complement, Ig, or both are more readily sequestered by the MNP cell surface membrane and ingested through cell surface receptors for complement component C3 products (C3b and C3bi) and the Fc portion of immunoglobulin (Horwitz, 1982; Ross et al., 1989). MNP receptors for the Fc domain of IgG (FcγR) belong to the immunoglobulin superfamily and are grouped in three primary classes; at least 12 isoforms of these molecules may be synthesized in humans (Van de Winkel and Capel, 1993) (see Chapter 3 and 4).

Role of Fc Receptors

The receptor expressed by monocytes and macrophages that recognizes monomeric IgG is FcγRI (CD64). This high-affinity receptor allows the MNP to bind and ingest bacteria with low concentrations of IgG that may not be recognized by neutrophils. A second receptor, FcRII (CD32), is expressed by many leukocytes, including MNPs, and this receptor binds aggregated or complexed IgG. Neutrophils utilize FcγRII as the primary receptor in ingesting IgG-opsonized microorganisms. A third receptor, FcγRIII (CD16), appears in two forms, derived from two distinct genes. FcγRIIIa is an intermediate-high–affinity receptor present on monocytes/macrophages and NK cells. FcγRIIIb is a low-affinity receptor present on neutrophils.

There are cell type–specific differences in glycosylation that affect receptor binding affinty (Edberg and Kimberly, 1997). FcγRIIIa/CD16 receptor is expressed on less than 10% of circulating monocytes (Ziegler-Heitbrock et al., 1993), and functionally these cells resemble tissue macrophages (Weber et al., 2000). The FcγRIIIa receptor on monocytes/macrophages has an important function in immune complex capture, mediating clearance of IgG-coated platelets and erythrocytes, as well as antibody-dependent cellular cytotoxicity (ADCC) (Edberg and Kimberly, 1997; Unkeless, 1989). Circulating subsets of monocytes expressing FcγRIIIa/CD16 are expanded in several clinical conditions (e.g., sepsis, autoimmune disease, and acquired immunodeficiency syndrome [AIDS]) (Ancuta et al., 2000, Weber et al., 2000).

Role of Complement Receptors

Receptors expressed by MNPs bind fragments of complement (Law, 1988). Complement receptor 1 (CR1 [CD35]), expressed by monocytes and macrophages, binds C3b, C4b, and iC3b. CR3 (CD11b/CD18) binds iC3b and is the primary MNP receptor used in binding serum-opsonized particles (Wright and Detmers, 1988). Neither CR1 or CR3 receptors on MNP can mediate phagocytosis of opsonized particles unless the MNP has been previously stimulated with phorbol esters or fibronectin (Brown, 1986; Wright and Griffin, 1985). The role of CR4 (CD11c/CD18) in mediating complement-opsonized material by MNPs remains unclear (see Chapter 7).

Role of Mannose/Fucose Receptors

Monocytes and macrophages also express cell surface receptors that bind specific carbohydrate moieties on the surface of microorganisms. Human macrophages express a receptor that binds proteins conjugated with *mannose* (Ezekowitz et al., 1990). This receptor is not expressed by monocytes but appears during monocyte-macrophage differentiation (Lennartz et al., 1989; Mokoena and Gordon, 1985). Because L-*fucose*–terminated proteins are bound by the mannose receptor, this receptor is often called the *mannose/fucose receptor* (Shepherd et al., 1982). Macrophages utilize the mannose receptor to directly recognize, bind, and ingest a variety of microorganisms, including *Candida albicans* and *Pneumocystis carinii* (Ezekowitz, 1992; Ezekowitz et al., 1990). Macrophage mannose receptor expression and function is downregulated by IFN-γ exposure but is increased in dexamethasone- or vitamin D–pretreated cells (Mokoena and Gordon, 1985; Stahl, 1990).

Role of Other Receptors

MNPs also express a β-glucan receptor (Czop and Austen, 1985), as well as receptors that recognize the end products of nonenzymatic glycosylation of proteins (Vlassara et al., 1988, 1989), termed *advanced glycation end products* (AGE). AGE binding to MNP results in cellular activation, induction of MNP migration, and release of cytokines, including GM-CSF, IL-6, TNF-α, and platelet-derived growth factor (Moroshi et al., 1995; Sasaki et al., 1999; Schmidt et al., 1993). AGE binding activates cell adhesion molecules (ICAM-1 and β2 integrins) on endothelial and MNP and may be responsible for enhanced MNP adhesion to and migration through vessel walls. AGE are identified as mediators of late diabetic vascular complications (Kyurkchiev et al., 1997).

Microbicidal Activity

Several different antimicrobial mechanisms have been identified in MNPs. These are generally divided into oxygen-independent and oxygen-dependent mechanisms. To this must be added reactive nitrogen reactions.

Oxygen-Independent Mechanisms

Several antimicrobial proteins and enzymes are present within the lysosomes of MNPs. Cathepsin G, azurocidin, proteinase 3, elastase, collagenase, arginase, ribonuclease deoxyribonuclease, defensins, and lysozyme are constituents of lysosomes that may account for the bacteriolytic activity of these intracellular organelles (Selsted et al., 1985; Thorne et al., 1976). Most of these proteins are active at neutral pH. The initial rise in pH to 7.0 to 8.0 in phagocytic vacuoles may create an optimal working environment for these antimicrobial proteins, and as the pH in the phagosome becomes acidic, these proteins become generally ineffective and acid hydrolases predominate (Thorne et al., 1976).

Oxygen-Dependent Mechanisms

Oxygen-dependent mechanisms also are important in tissue damage to a variety of cells and are linked to secretory responses and to other intracellular events. Reactive *oxygen* and *nitrogen intermediates* have a direct role in the killing of certain microorganisms. Microbicidal activity for certain organisms is decreased under conditions of anaerobiosis (Cline, 1970; Miller, 1971), emphasizing the role of oxygen-dependent killing.

Stimulated peripheral blood monocytes exhibit a brisk respiratory burst and elaboration of reactive oxygen intermediates, initiated through a transmembrane electron transport system involving a reduced pyridine nucleotide, extracellular or phagosomal oxygen, and additional plasma membrane enzymes and co-factors (Babior 1978). Superoxide anion is the initial product and may be directly toxic to proteins and membrane components; however, it is often converted to hydrogen peroxide (H_2O_2), catalyzed by superoxide dismutase. H_2O_2 is highly toxic to a number of pathogenic organisms and tumor cells (Baehner and Johnston, 1972; Klebanoff and Hamon, 1973). Toxicity can be enhanced using H_2O_2 as a substrate to generate various oxidants, including diffusible radical species, reactive halogens, and aldehydes, catalyzed by myeloperoxidase (Chisolm et al., 1999; Nathan, 1986).

Monocytes from patients with chronic granulomatous disease have defective generation of H_2O_2 and manifest decreased microbicidal activity for catalase-forming bacteria (Davis et al., 1968; Dinauer and Orkin, 1992; Klebanoff, 1988; Nathan et al., 1969).

The in vitro differentiation of monocytes into macrophages is associated with a decrease in oxygen-dependent microbiocidal mechanisms. The magnitude of the respiratory burst decreases, and the peroxidase-containing granules are lacking in mature macrophage (Nakagawara, 1981; Van Furth and Cohn, 1968). H_2O_2 remains an important microbiocidal agent; however, given the lack of lysosomal peroxidase, the mature macrophage appears unable to amplify the toxicity of this molecule endogenously. Ingestion of peroxidase released from other degranulating phagocytes may help amplify the H_2O_2 toxicity (Heifets et al., 1986).

Reactive Nitrogen Intermediates

Another oxygen-dependent antimicrobial system functioning in MNPs is derived from the oxidation of L-arginine to nitrate with the formation of reactive nitrogen intermediates (Nathan and Gabay, 1992). Nitric oxide, nitrogen dioxide, and nitrosamines are the bioactive antimicrobial molecules produced by this pathway when MNPs are appropriately stimulated (Nathan, 1991). Reactive nitrogen intermediate synthesis, as with synthesis of reactive oxygen intermediates, is highly regulated, being induced and inhibited by numerous cytokines (Ding et al., 1988; Lioy et al., 1993). Normal macrophages require both a priming signal, such as IFN-γ or IFN-β, and an activating signal, such as lipopolysaccharide, muramyl dipeptide, or TNF-α, to fully induce production of reactive nitrogen intermediate from the L-arginine pathway (Hibbs et al., 1992).

Cytotoxicity

Macrophages are involved in the host defense against malignancy (Alexander, 1976; Evans and Hibbs, 1976; Levy and Wheelock, 1974). Macrophages can be activated to function as effector cells that are capable of inhibiting tumor growth. Chronic infection with a variety of organisms or injection of a number of inducing substances, such as endotoxin, lipid A, double-stranded RNA, complete Freund's adjuvant, and pyran co-polymer, will produce tumoricidal macrophages (Alexander, 1976). These nonspecifically cytotoxic macrophages exhibit selectivity in that they express cytotoxicity against transformed but not normal cells (Hibbs, 1973; Hibbs et al., 1972).

Types of Cytotoxicity

In vitro studies show that destruction of tumor cells by macrophages is accomplished by two different mechanisms (Adams and Hamilton, 1984). Antibody-independent cellular cytotoxicity is a highly selective killing of malignant cells, usually nonphagocytic, and most often requires cell-to-cell contact (Adams and Hamilton, 1992). Evidence exists indicating a role for TNF-α, IFN-γ, reactive oxygen, or nitric oxide intermediates and cytotoxic proteases (Adams and Hamilton, 1987; Adams et al., 1980; Beutler and Cerami, 1986; Higuchi et al., 1990; Keller et al., 1990; Nathan, 1982; Steuhr and Nathan, 1989; Urban et al., 1986).

MNP-mediated ADCC, in contrast, is rapid and specific. The immunoglobulin-bound target interacts with the Fc surface receptor on MNPs (Adams and Nathan, 1983). The initial binding of the antibody-coated target is necessary but not sufficient for destruction of the targets (Adams and Hamilton, 1992). Reactive oxygen intermediates, in particular H_2O_2, are the major secretory products of MNP that lyse target cells (Nathan, 1983).

Role of Lymphokines

Lymphocytes may play a cooperative role in the induction of tumoricidal macrophages. Lymphokines produced by nonspecific stimulation of lymphocytes in vitro can induce macrophages to become cytotoxic for syngeneic tumor cells (Piessens et al., 1975). In addition, the prolonged maintenance of nonspecific cytotoxic potential in an in vitro culture system requires a factor produced by an interaction between inducing antigen and sensitized lymphocytes (Hibbs, 1974). Under different experimental conditions, lymphocytes produce a *specific macrophage arming factor*, which renders macrophages specifically cytotoxic to the tumor to which the lymphocytes were originally sensitized (Evans and Alexander, 1971).

Antigen Processing and Presentation

A complex interaction exists between lymphocytes and macrophages during a primary immune response (Fig. 6-8). Immunoregulatory molecules, including IFN-γ and IL-1, modulate the interactions between lymphocytes and macrophages (Unanue and Allen, 1987a). Cells serving in antigen presentation have been shown to process antigen, express human leukocyte antigen (HLA) class II glycoprotein (Ia) on their surfaces, and secrete IL-1 (Rosenthal, 1978).

Initially, proteins enter the antigen-presenting cell (APC) following their interaction with plasma membrane. After uptake by macrophages, degradation of protein occurs in acid vesicles, enabling the generation of an immunogenic fragment complexed with the major histocompatibility determinant. Following protein degradation, some fragments proceed to the lysosome vesicles, whereas others complex directly with HLA class II molecules and appear on the cell surface (Geuze et al., 1983). The density of expression of HLA class II on different populations of macrophages correlates with their ability to present antigen to T cells (Beller, 1984).

Several lymphokines regulate HLA class II expression on the macrophage surface. IFN-γ increases HLA class II expression (Basham and Merigan, 1983); prostaglandins of the E class (Snyder et al., 1982), α-fetoprotein (Lu et al., 1984), and glucocorticoids (Snyder and Unanue, 1982) inhibit HLA class II expression. Similarly, IL-1 plays an important role in macrophage antigen presentation (Chu et al., 1984). IL-1 is secreted by macrophages after the T cell interacts with macrophage cell surface HLA class II antigens. The binding of IL-1 to its receptor on T-cell surfaces induces

T-cell proliferation, most likely through stimulation of IL-2 synthesis and release. Studies have identified a membrane-bound form of IL-1 required for antigen presentation by macrophages (Kurt-Jones et al., 1985). This membrane IL-1 is an integral membrane protein, distinct from the soluble IL-1 nonspecifically bound or fixed to the macrophage membrane.

Tissue Remodeling and Wound Healing

Macrophages are necessary for injured tissues and organs to heal properly (Leibovich and Ross, 1975; Riches, 1988). During the earliest phases of wound repair, monocytes are recruited to the injury site and, along with the resident tissue macrophages, participate in the debridement of the damaged tissue. Although macrophages secrete enzymes competent to degrade connective tissue matrices in vitro (Banda et al., 1985; Werb et al., 1980), endocytosis of matrix fragments leading to activation of the macrophages and IL-1 secretion may have a more widespread effect on damaged matrix dismantling by increasing collagenase synthesis and secretion by fibroblasts (Huybrechts-Godin et al., 1985; Postlethwaite et al., 1983).

Macrophages further contribute in three general ways to heal the debrided wound and remodel the site to a preinjured state. Macrophages secrete numerous potent growth factors (see Fig. 6-6) for fibroblasts and mesenchymal cells. These factors promote the production of the loose connective tissue and new blood capillaries that constitute granulation tissue, the provisional matrix utilized by fibroblasts to deposit structural matrix molecules (Greenburg and Hunt, 1978; Polverini et al., 1977).

A direct role in provisional extracellular matrix synthesis has been demonstrated in macrophages by Brown and colleagues (1993); wound macrophages synthesized embryonic isoforms of fibronectin before fibroblast synthesis of these important elements of granulation tissue. Later in the wound-healing process, macrophages secrete factors that modulate fibroblast collagen production and, in cutaneous wounds, re-epithelialization (Rappolee and Werb, 1992; Schultz et al., 1987). Macrophages may also participate in the exaggerated deposition of fibroblast-derived matrix materials, leading to tissue fibrosis (Wong and Wahl, 1989).

Activation

Macrophages obtained from animals that have become immune following sublethal infection manifest an impressive morphologic, metabolic, and functional metamorphosis and are said to be activated. These cells are larger, have an increased tendency to spread (North, 1978); adhere more avidly to glass; and have more lysosomes, a more elaborate Golgi apparatus, and more ribosomes. Such activated macrophages also have increased metabolic and mitotic rates and are capable of increased pinocytosis and phagocytic activity (Cohn,

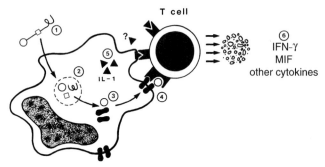

Figure 6-8 · Events involved in macrophage processing and presentation of antigen to T lymphocytes. Most protein antigens (1) require internalization and phagolysosomal processing (2) and physical association with newly synthesized MHC class II molecules (3) before presentation to T cells at the cell surface of the mononuclear phagocyte. IL-1 (5) production in conjunction with antigen presentation (4) activates the T cell to release numerous cytokines, including IFN-γ, macrophage migration inhibitory factor (MIF), and other cytokines (6), that further activate macrophages, B cells, and T cells. (Modified from Yoder MC, Hassan NF, Douglas SD. Mononuclear phagocyte system. In Polin RA, Fox WW, eds. Fetal and Neonatal Physiology, vol 2. Philadelphia, WB Saunders, 1992, pp 1438–1461.)

1978; Karnovsky and Lazdins, 1978). One of the more important functional correlates of these metabolic changes is the observation that activated macrophages are capable of enhanced microbicidal activity. Mackaness (1962) observed that following sublethal *Listeria,* challenge mice were temporarily resistant to subsequent rechallenge with a much larger number of *Listeria* organisms.

This increased resistance was in large part due to the fact that the macrophages from such animals had become "activated" and consequently were much more efficient in the killing of *Listeria.* However, macrophage activation is a nonspecific phenomenon, in that macrophages activated by infection with one intracellular organism express increased microbicidal activity toward antigenically different organisms. For example, animals infected with *Brucella abortus* become resistant to infection with *Listeria* (Blaese, 1975).

In addition to enhanced microbicidal activity, a number of other macrophage functions are stimulated by the activation process. For example, activated macrophages are known to have increased tumoricidal capacity (Alexander, 1973), accelerated movement (Poplack et al., 1976), the ability to produce a number of important biologically active substances (Wahl et al., 1975), and an enhanced ability to collaborate with immunocompetent cells in the production of specific antibody (Blaese, 1975). Thus the activation process itself, although invoked in the macrophage response to infection, is important in a variety of macrophage functions.

IFN-γ, produced by activated T cells and NK cells, is one of the primary macrophage activators (Murray, 1988). IFN-γ production by cord blood T lymphocytes is diminished a compared with adults. Concomitantly, neonatal cord blood MNPs have decreased activation and less enhanced killing (Marodi et al., 1994; Wilson and Westall, 1985).

Activation of the macrophage may not always lead to increases in tumoricidal or antimicrobial activity. The term *activation* is used to describe the effects of any stimulus on MNP morphology, physiology, or function. Thus activation may refer to a change in the level of expression of one specific cell surface membrane receptor or to a change in the size of the cell without invoking any change in a complex function, such as tumor cell killing or phagocytosis and killing of microbes. Adams and Hamilton (1992) have proposed that the term *macrophage activation* refer to macrophage acquisition of competence to complete some complex cell function.

THE DENDRITIC CELL SYSTEM

Definition

Dendritic cells are a distinct lineage of migratory leukocytes that primarily serve as accessory cells in initiation of primary immune responses. Members of this family share certain morphologic, kinetic, and functional characteristics and can be identified in discrete locations in lymphoid and nonlymphoid organs (Inaba et al., 1983; Steinman and Cohn, 1973; Tew et al., 1982).

Although dendritic cells express certain cell surface antigenic features that resemble those of MNPs, they demonstrate poor phagocytic activity and weak or no adhesion to tissue culture surfaces and generally lack nonspecific esterase activity—three universal characteristics of mononuclear phagocytes (Tew et al., 1982). Nevertheless, there is compelling evidence for a common hematopoietic progenitor for cells of the dendritic cell system and the MNP system. The origin, kinetics, characterization, and tissue distribution of dendritic cells, along with several well-recognized functions of these potent APCs, are reviewed.

Cell Origin and Kinetics

Dendritic cells (DCs) are derived from bone marrow hematopoietic progenitor cells (Katz et al., 1979; Reid et al., 1990; Volk-Platzer et al., 1984). During embryologic development, dendritic cells and macrophages have been identified as early as week 6 in the yolk sac (Janossy et al., 1986). By 12 weeks' gestation, dendritic cells are present in thymus, lymph nodes, spleen, and many nonlymphoid organs. In these tissues, dendritic cells occupy distinct sites that differ from the location of macrophages (Hofman et al., 1984; Janossy et al., 1986). The question of whether dendritic cells originate from a separate lineage or belong to the monocyte/macrophage family remains unresolved.

A common precursor for MNPs and dendritic cells was suggested by the presence of CFU-like clusters containing both macrophages and dendritic cells and a single peak of thymidine incorporation in the macrophage-dendritic cultures (Santiago-Schwarz et al., 1992). Dendritic cells can be generated in vitro from hematopoietic progenitor cells in the bone marrow (Inaba et al., 1992; Szaboks et al., 1998), placental blood (Santiago-Schwartz et al., 1992; Rosenzwaijg et al., 1996), and CD14+ blood monocytes (Hashimoto et al., 1999; Peters et al., 1993; Zhou et al., 1995) if the cells are incubated with GM-CSF, IL-4, and TNF-α (Peters et al., 1993; Zhou et al., 1996).

Whether dendritic cells generated from these sources differ from circulating dendritic cells and dendritic cells in tissues with respect to morphology, phenotype, and function remain to be investigated. The observation that the transition from monocytes to dendritic cells can be induced under physiologic conditions in vitro indicates that similar regulatory events may take place in vitro, giving rise to the many variations among macrophages observed at different sites, as a consequence of different functional demands, and at different stages of maturation. Dendritic cells have been considered as the terminal stage of monocyte differentiation (Palucka et al., 1998) (Fig. 6-9).

A probable common bone marrow and peripheral blood hematopoietic precursor of MNPs and dendritic cells has been identified in adult human subjects (Reid et al., 1990; Thomas et al., 1993). In methylcellulose colony assays, pure colonies of dendritic-appearing cells and mixed colonies containing dendritic cells and

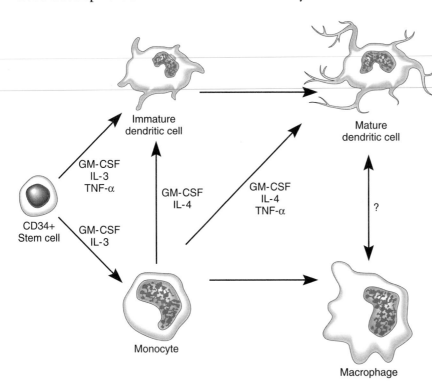

Figure 6-9 · Dendritic cell development pathway. CD and monocytes are not only from a similar progenitor cell but also have a pathway that allows a transition from monocytes to dendritic cells. The possible interconversions between DCs and macrophages are areas of current investigation.

macrophages were cultured from human adult bone marrow and peripheral blood mononuclear cells. The dendritic cells strongly expressed MHC class II antigens, lacked nonspecific esterase, expressed some cell surface markers of skin Langerhans cells, and stimulated allogeneic mixed leukocyte reactions—all characteristic features of freshly isolated dendritic cells (Reid et al., 1990; Thomas et al., 1993). Although these findings strongly suggest a common myeloid origin for MNPs and dendritic cells, conclusive evidence using genetic markers is lacking.

The kinetics of dendritic cell production are not well delineated in humans, but mice and rat dendritic cells have a short life span. Murine splenic dendritic cells live an estimated 8 to 11 days, with similar turnover times for lymph node dendritic cells in rats. Some rat dendritic cells in nonlymphoid tissues live 2 to 4 weeks, and in one experiment human skin dendritic cells lived more than 9 weeks after transplantation to immunodeficient mice (Fossum, 1989). Some investigators propose heterogeneity in dendritic cell turnover, with rapidly and slowly dividing populations of cells in spleen and skin (Chen et al., 1986; Steinman, 1991). The ultimate fate of dendritic cells in lymphoid and nonlymphoid tissues is not known; most dendritic cells do not leave the organs they enter and are presumed to die in situ (Fossum, 1989; Steinman, 1991).

Morphology

Dendritic cells from human peripheral blood have an irregular cell surface outline with an eccentrically placed, elongated, and often lobulated nucleus. These peripheral blood cells are of a size similar to circulating monocytes and have a nuclear-cytoplasmic ratio between 1:2 and

1:4 (Kamperdijk et al., 1989). Circulating dendritic cells have few cytoplasmic vacuoles, but those vacuoles present are located near the cell surface.

Tissue dendritic cells vary greatly in morphology, reflecting site-specific morphologic features (Fossum, 1989). Circulating dendritic cells display a "veiled," extensively folded plasma membrane that becomes partitioned into numerous blunt pseudopodia that extend for varying lengths from the body of the cell (Fig.

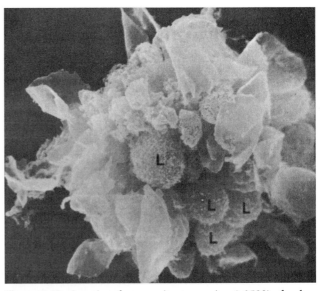

Figure 6-10 · Scanning electron microscope view (×2500) of a dendritic cell clustering with several lymphocytes (L). The numerous dendritic cell surface membrane and cytoplasmic projections in the shape of sheets, pseudopods, and dendrites are characteristic of these cells. (From Steinman RM et al. Dendritic cells. In Zucker-Franklin D, Greaves MF, Grossi CE, Marmont AM, eds. Atlas of Blood Cells: Function and Pathology, ed 2. Philadephia, Lea & Febiger, 1988, p 360.)

6-10); these dendritic processes give rise to the name for this family of leukocytes (Tew et al., 1982). Ultrastructurally, the nuclear material is euchromatic; the cytoplasm contains mitochondria and strands of rough and smooth endoplasmic reticulum. Few granules are evident, and phagolysosomes are not present (Kamperdijk et al., 1989). Epidermal Langerhans cells contain unique organelles, called *Birbeck granules*, that are lost with in vitro culture (Austyn, 1987).

Histochemistry

Dendritic cells lack many of the enzymes that express in monocytes/macrophages. Nonspecific esterase activity is weak or nonexistent in dendritic cells. Dendritic cells, such as Langerhans cells, express acid phosphatase, adenosine triphosphatase (ATPase), 5'-nucleotidase, and aminopeptidase N (Stachura, 1989). These cells also express S100 protein, a product that is found in Schwann cells and melanocytes (Romani et al., 1991). Dipeptidyl aminopeptidase I and cathepsin B activity are low in human peripheral blood dendritic cells (Thomas et al., 1993).

Cell Surface Antigens

No unique cell surface antigenic determinants have been identified that can be utilized to isolate and characterize human dendritic cells (Steinman, 1991). All human dendritic cells express 30- to 100-fold more HLA class II antigens (DP, DQ, DR) than the level expressed by resting MNPs (Steinman, 1991). Human dendritic cell precursors strongly express MHC class I and II molecules; moderately express CD11a,b,c/CD18, CD40, CD44, CD54, CD64, CD32, CD33, and CD34; and weakly express CD14 (Thomas et al., 1993). These purported precursors lack CD16, CD19, CD3, or CD1 (Thomas et al., 1993). Mature dendritic cells express both MHC class I and class II molecules, as well as CD1, CD4, CD8, CD11a,b,c/CD18, CD25, CD40, CD54, and CD58, and weakly express CD23 and 32 (Steinman, 1991). Two new markers have been identified for distinguishing mature from less mature dendritic cells. These are CD83, a member of the Ig superfamily, and P55 or fascin, a presumptive actin bundling protein (Steinman et al., 1997). Dendritic cells also express CD48, CD148 (a molecule with phosphatase activity), and several other non–lineage-restricted markers (Hart et al., 1997; Zhou et al., 1998). CD13 is expressed in blood dendritic cell precursors but not in more differentiated dendritic cells (Thomas et al., 1994; Wood et al., 1992). In contrast, tissue macrophages are CD13 positive (Hogg et al., 1987).

Types of Dendritic Cells

Dendritic cells are found in almost all types of tissue and comprise 0.5% to 4% of cells in various tissue. Steinman (1991) has suggested that the dendritic cell system can be categorized in three groups by location: nonlymphoid organ cells (Langerhans and interstitial dendritic cells), circulating cells (afferent lymph veiled and blood dendritic cells), and lymphoid organ cells (dendritic and interdigitating cells).

Langerhans Cells

Langerhans cells are the best-studied nonlymphoid dendritic cells. These cells, which are probably derived from blood dendritic precursors, are capable of leaving the dermis and migrating through afferent lymph fluid to local lymph nodes (Hoefsmit et al., 1982; Silberberg-Sinakin et al., 1976). Langerhans cells have the ability to acquire foreign proteins by phagocytosis or pinocytosis and reduce them to an array of antigens ready for presentation on the cell surface (Austyn et al., 1996). Dendritic cells are present in the interstitium of nearly all organs except the brain (Hart and McKenzie, 1990). In the lung, dendritic cells are present in the alveolar septa and just beneath the tracheobronchial epithelial cells, where the capture of aerosolized particulates is facilitated (Toews, 1991).

Circulating Dendritic Cells

Afferent but not efferent lymph contains dendritic cells that can capture antigens throughout the body and carry the material to lymphoid tissues (Bujdoso et al., 1989). Dendritic cells in blood are a minor population (less than 0.1%) that may be difficult to identify morphologically from peripheral blood monocytes by light microscopy. If viewed by video microscopy, blood dendritic cells are unique in repeatedly protruding and retracting lamellipodia, or "veils" (Steinman, 1991). The role of the blood dendritic cells is unclear. These cells may be en route from bone marrow to nonlymphoid organs or may have left nonlymphoid organs to migrate to the spleen (Thomas et al., 1993).

Lymphoid Dendritic Cells

In lymphoid tissues, dendritic cells are positioned to have maximal interaction with the T lymphocytes. Interdigitating dendritic cells are found clustered with T cells in lymph nodes. In the spleen, dendritic cells reside as interdigitating cells in the periarterial sheaths and are present in the periphery of T-cell areas, interrupting the marginal zone of macrophages (Fossum, 1989). Because T cells and antigenic material must traverse the marginal zone on leaving the arterial system, dendritic cells present a cellular barrier through which the T cells and antigens pass; thus cell-to-cell communication between dendritic cells, T cells, and antigen is anatomically intimate (Steinman, 1991).

Antigen Processing and Presentation

Whereas macrophages, B cells, and dendritic cells can serve as APCs, dendritic cells are the primary presenters of antigen to antigen-specific T cells after antigen administration (Bujdoso et al., 1989; Crowley et al., 1990). The ability of dendritic cells to take up antigen and process it is highly dependent on the stage of dendritic cell differentiation. In vivo, this is related to dendritic cell location. In vitro, it relates to the time in culture, degree of activation, and antigen/T-lymphocyte exposure (Hart et al., 1997). APCs need not express large amounts of the antigen to stimulate effective T-cell responses, although the number of MHC-antigen complex required to stimulate T cells is likely to vary with the APC source (Demotz et al., 1990). Dendritic cells are highly efficient in ingesting material by endocytosis, move the material into acidic lysosomal compartments, combine newly synthesized MHC class II invariant chain with the liberated antigenic peptides, and present the MHC class II peptide material on the cell surface to the appropriate antigen-specific T cell (Steinman, 1991).

Macrophage antigen processing and presentation are characterized by degradation of large quantities of material into antigenic peptides, rapid loss of antigen-presenting activity after pulsing with antigen, and a requirement for additional adjuvants to prime T cells in situ after antigen priming (Steinman, 1991). Dendritic cells are nearly 100 times more potent at antigen presentation and T-cell activation than macrophages (Romani et al., 1989). The prolonged (1 to 2 days) capacity to present antigen after pulsing and the ability to directly activate T cells in situ after antigen pulsing are unique features of dendritic cells (Inaba et al., 1990).

Transport of Captured Antigen

Dendritic cells are professional antigen-presenting cells that efficiently capture antigens in the peripheral tissues and process these antigens to form MHC-peptide complex. Dendritic cells are also uniquely capable of transporting immunogenic material to lymphoid tissues. As dendritic cells travel, they mature and alter their profile of cell surface molecules to attract resting T cells and present their antigen load (Adema et al., 1997; Banchereau et al., 1998). Some examples of in situ antigen capture and transport include T-cell stimulation by dendritic cells isolated from afferent lymph after intradermal administration of antigen (Bujdoso et al., 1989), T-cell activation by lymph node dendritic cells after application of a contact allergen (Macatonia et al., 1987), and in situ activation of CD4+ T cells in the draining lymph nodes of mice injected in the foot pads with splenic dendritic cells exposed to antigenic material in vitro (Inaba et al., 1990). Contact between dendritic cells and resting T cells is necessary to initiate a primary immune response. However, how this initial contact between dendritic cells and resting T cells is established and regulated is still largely unknown.

Role of DC-SIGN

Recently a novel dendritic cell–specific ICAM-3 receptor (DC-SIGN) has been identified to play a critical role in supporting primary immune response (Geijtenbeek et al., 2000a, 2000b). DC-SIGN, originally described in 1992 as a C-type lectin, binds to human immunodeficiency virus (HIV) surface protein, gp120 (Curtis et al., 1992). DC-SIGN is a dendritic cell–specific adhesion receptor that mediates dendritic T-cell clustering and dendritic cell–induced proliferation of resting T-cell response (Geijtenbeek et al., 2000a, 2000b). The DC-SIGN molecule is used by HIV to attach to dendritic cells in the genitourinary tract and rectum (Geijtenbeek et al., 2000a, 2000b). Without allowing HIV entry, DC-SIGN retains the attached virus in an infectious state for days and then transmits them to replication-permission T cells (Geijtenbeek et al., 2000a, 2000b). In addition, expression of DC-SIGN on cells that also express the HIV receptors enhance infection (Lee et al., 2001). It is possible that other pathogens are also transmitted via dendritic cells, and in particular via DC-SIGN, because the glycan ligands for DC-SIGN could be present on other viral envelopes, the cell walls of other microbes, or even tumor cells (Steinman, 2000). Hepatitis C virus glycoproteins interact with DC-SIGN (Pöhlmann et al., 2003).

Activation of T-Lymphocyte Growth and Effector Function

Dendritic cells in lymph and blood preferentially home to T-cell areas of lymphoid organs. The mechanisms of homing are poorly understood, but dendritic cells express several cell surface molecules that have been implicated in leukocyte homing (Steinman, 1991; Thomas et al., 1993). Dendritic cells are also capable of tightly clustering with resting T cells in initiation of primary immune responses; macrophages and B cells are unable to do so (Inaba and Steinman, 1985, 1986). The cluster formation requires an intact dendritic cell cytoskeleton and protein kinase C activation (Scheeran et al., 1991).

In some cases, dendritic cells bind T cells in an antigen-independent fashion that may facilitate subsequent antigen-specific interactions between APCs and clustered T cells (Inaba and Steinman, 1986). The dendritic cells and T-lymphocyte interaction are stabilized by adhesion molecules (Prickett et al., 1992; Starling et al., 1995). ICAM-3, which is constitutively expressed on dendritic cells in high concentrations, provides the predominant initial adhesion interaction with leukocyte function antigen-1 (LFA-1) on T lymphocytes (Starling et al., 1995). LFA-3 on dendritic cells may also increase cluster stability by binding the CD2 ligand on T lymphocytes (Prickett et al., 1992).

Role of Cytokines and Chemokines

Because the lack of purity of some dendritic cell preparations may have allowed significant cytokine release from contaminating other cell populations, conflicting data have been reported. In addition, different states of differentiation and activation influence dendritic cell cytokine production. Neither IL-1α nor IL-1β is produced in significant amounts by human tonsil or blood dendritic cells (Hart et al., 1997; Vakkila et al., 1990). Although human blood dendritic cells express low levels of TNF-α mRNA, no biologically detectable TNF-α was produced by the cells (Zhou et al., 1995). Although IL-6 protein is not produced by blood dendritic cells, viral exposure induces IL-6 secretion (Ghanekar et al., 1996). Unstimulated dendritic cells do not produce IFN-α or IFN-γ (Zhou et al., 1995, 1994). However, HIV infection induces high levels of dendritic cell IFN-α production (Ferbas et al., 1994).

Dendritic cells also produce chemokines that facilitate the migration of leukocytes. Expression of β-chemokine (MIP-1α, MIP-1β, and RANTES) mRNA has been described (Zhou et al., 1995; Sallusto et al., 1999). Langerhans cells also produce MIP-1α, MIP-1β, RANTES, and MIP-3φ148

(Dieu et al., 1998). In addition, immature dendritic cells express chemokine receptors, principally CCR5 and CCR6. Human Langerhans cells dendritically express functional CD4, CCR5, and CXCR4 (Lee et al., 1999; Rubbert et al., 1998; Zaitseva et al., 1997), the primary receptors for HIV entry into macrophages and CD4+ T lymphocytes.

THE NATURAL KILLER CELL SYSTEM

Definition

NK cells are lymphocytes that do not undergo genetic recombination events to increase their affinity for particular ligands, and are thus considered part of innate immunity against viruses, intracellular bacteria, and parasites. In addition, NK cells have spontaneous cytotoxicity against most cultured cell lines, immature hematopoietic cells, and tumor cells. NK cells secrete cytokines such as IFN-α and IFN-γ during infection and inflammation. NK cells play an important role in modulating host adaptive immune defense, comparable to the mononuclear phagocyte and dendritic cell systems. They may bridge innate and adaptive immune responses (Fig. 6-11). Although NK cells display some features of peripheral blood lymphocytes, these cells comprise a distinct lineage as evidenced by normal NK cell development in mice that are genetically deficient in B and T cells (Dorschkind et al., 1985, Mombaerts et al., 1992).

Origin

As with all hematopoietic cells, the bone marrow is considered to be the site of postnatal NK cell production. NK cell progenitors are enriched in those cord blood, adult peripheral blood, and bone marrow CD34+ hematopoietic progenitors that express CD7 or CD38 but do not express other mature lineage specific antigens (Miller et al., 1994). The close relationship between T-cell and NK cell development is noted in those human fetal liver NK progenitor cells that express

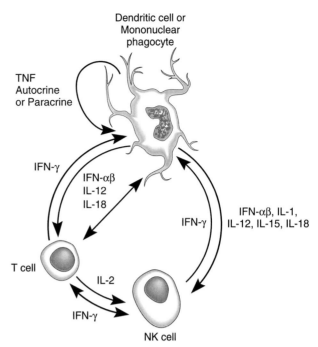

Figure 6-11 · NK-cell interactions with effectors of the innate immune system (mononuclear phagocytes and dendritic cells) and acquired immune system (T cells) via secreted cytokines. NK cells activate mononuclear phagocytes and dendritic cells via IFN-γ secretion. These activated phagocytes demonstrate increased microbicidal activity against intracellular phathogens. The phagocytes secrete numerous cytokines, which in turn activate NK cells, inducing additional IFN-γ secretion. IFN-γ from NK cells and IFN-αβ, IL-12, and IL-18 from mononuclear phagocytes promote T-cell differentiation along the TH1 pathway.

the CD3ε and CD3δ chains found on T cells. Currently the developmental sequence of cell surface antigen expression that most closely mirrors the maturational sequence of marrow-derived NK cells is CD161, CD56, CD16, and CD2, respectively (Blom et al., 1998). Although several cytokines stimulate NK cell differentiation and activation, IL-15 and the IL-15 receptor appear essential for NK cell development (Lodolce et al., 1998; Ogasawara et al., 1998).

NK cells comprise 5% to 15% of circulating lymphocytes. NK cells in the unactivated state do not circulate in lymph and are rare in unstimulated lymph nodes. NK cells constitute 5% to 10% of splenic lymphocytes and have been identified in low concentration in the lungs, gastrointestinal tract, and liver. Hepatic NK cells are unique in expressing CD1 (Lanier et al., 1994, Lantz and Bendelac, 1994). These cells have been termed NK T cells.

Morphology

Human peripheral blood NK cells display features of large granular lymphocytes including a high cytoplasmic/nucleus ratio, indented nucleus, and azurophilic granules (Timonen et al., 1979). By transmission electron microscopic analysis of NK cells, the cells appear as medium-sized lymphocytes with condensed chromatin and unusually prominent nucleoli. NK cells have abundant cytoplasm with a well-developed Golgi apparatus, prominent centrioles and associated microtubules, abundant mitochondria, and a number of lysosomal organelles (Babcock and Phillips, 1983). NK cells also contain numerous pinocytic vesicles and endocytic vacuoles (Huhn et al., 1982).

The granules of NK cells contain those enzymes typically identified in primary lysosomes, including numerous glycoproteins, acid phosphatase, trimetaphosphatase, arylsulfatase, and β-glucuronidase (Kang et al., 1987). Some NK cell granules also exhibit naphthol AS-D chloroacetate esterase activity, which is generally a characteristic of neutrophilic granulocytes (Babcock and Phillips, 1983). Likewise, the α-naphthyl acetate and α-naphthyl butyrate esterases generally expressed by mononuclear phagocytes are also present in some NK cell granules and as an ectoenzyme on the cell surface (Grossi et al., 1982). This fluoride-inhabitable esterase activity is only routinely detected at the electron microscopic level in NK cells.

Cell Surface Antigens

NK cells were originally identified based on their ability to mediate spontaneous cytotoxicity against a variety of target cells, but this function is shared by mononuclear phagocytes and some T cells. Attempts at purifying NK cells have been significantly advanced in the past 20 years by moving from morphologic and buoyant density isolation techniques to monoclonal antibodies and flow cytometry (Trinchieri, 1989). NK cells express a variety of cell surface molecules that in combination permit high enrichment from peripheral blood, tissues, and organs.

T-Cell Antigens

Although NK cells have the appearance of cytotoxic T cells, NK cells do not express the CD3/T-cell receptor or CD5 (Seaman, 2000). NK cells do not express CD4 but 30% to 50% express the α/α form of CD8. Additional molecules expressed in common by T and NK cells include CD2, CD16, CD56, CD57, CD161, and 2B4 (Lanier, 1998; Seaman, 2000). CD16 is a component of the FcγIIIB receptor. CD16 is activated by binding IgG-coated target cells and permits NK cells to lyse the target cells (Ojo and Wigzell, 1978). This form of target cell killing is called antibody-dependent cell-mediated cytotoxicity and differs from the natural killing mechanisms utilized primarily by NK cells (see below). CD56 is a form of neural cell adhesion molecule, which does not appear to play a direct role in NK cytotoxicity. Furthermore, a decreased level of CD16 and higher level of CD56 cell surface expression correlate with lower levels of cytotoxicity (Nagler et al., 1989). NK cells utilize the 2B4 molecule to bind to hematopoietic cells expressing CD48. This cell-to-cell

interaction may be important in NK-mediated natural killing of transplanted hematopoietic cells.

NK-Specific Antigens

Three recently identified receptors, NKp46, NKp44, NKp30, may play important roles in NK biology. NKp46 and NKp30 are uniquely expressed by NK cells, and experimental blockade of these receptors impairs target cell lysis (Seaman, 2000). The ligands for these NK cell surface receptors are unknown.

Mechanisms of NK Cytotoxicity

T and B lymphocytes recognize foreign antigenic material via clonally restricted cell surface receptors generated by gene rearrangement during cellular differentiation from lineage-specific progenitor cells in the thymus (T cell) and liver or bone marrow (B cell). NK cells recognize foreign antigenic material through receptors that are not clonally generated or even restricted to NK cells (Lanier, 2000a). A further unique aspect of NK cell recognition of foreign material is that NK responses to foreign antigens are modulated by the presence of inhibitory NK receptors recognizing MHC class I antigens.

Human MHC I antigens include the classic molecules HLA-A, HLA-B, and HLA-C and the nonclassic molecules HLA-E and HLA-G. Class I MHC inhibits NK cytotoxicity by binding to cell surface molecules that generate inhibitory signals blocking NK cytotoxicity (Karre et al., 1986). Although NK cells express HLA self and nonself molecules, all NK cells express at least one inhibitory receptor for self HLA antigen, thus preventing the NK cell from lysing host cells in an autoimmune fashion. Such restriction of target cell lysis by class I MHC expression has been called the "missing-self" hypothesis of Karre and colleagues (1986). If NK cells are spontaneously ready to kill cells but are prevented by target cell expression of self MHC class I antigen, the loss of self-antigen, as occurs in many malignancies or postviral infections, now permits NK killing of the host cells. Thus T- and B-lymphocyte activation requires exposure to foreign material for initiation. In contrast, NK cells must be continually held in restraint from attacking not only foreign material but host cells by expression of self HLA molecules.

In addition to killing cells by antibody-dependent cell cytotoxicity (see earlier discussion), NK cells use several "natural" cytotoxic mechanisms. Upon NK cell activation, granules containing perforin, a target cell pore-forming protein, are released in a calcium-dependent fashion (Podack, 1995). Additional cell damage is inflicted by release of granules containing the proteinases granzyme A and B, which enter the target cell and induce DNA fragmentation. NK cells also contain Fas ligand (FasL) in secretory granules that are released upon NK activation and induce apoptosis in Fas-expressing target cells (Bossi and Griffiths, 1999). NK cells constitutively express TNF-related apoptosis-inducing ligand (TRAIL) and induce apoptosis in target cells expressing the TRAIL receptor (Zamai, et al., 1998). Of all the mechanisms discussed here, perforin-mediated cell injury is thought to be the predominant mechanism of NK cell cytotoxicity.

During the early response to viral infections, NK cells are a potent source of IFN-γ and TNF (Biron et al., 1999). These cytokines promote differentiation of CD4 T cells into Th1 effector cells. Production of IL-1, IL-2, IL-12, IL-15, and IL–18 by mononuclear phagocytes, dendritic cells, and activated T cells further stimulates NK cells to produce MIP-1α and -1β, along with other chemokines. These molecules augment recruitment of additional mononuclear phagocytes to the site of NK cytotoxicity (Biron et al., 1999). NK T cells are distinct from NK cells in possessing the capacity to produce IL-4, a cytokine that promotes a Th2 response that may encourage enhanced defenses against parasitic infection (Yoshimoto and Paul, 1994). Like classical NK cells, NK T cells can be induced to produce substantial amounts of IFN-γ upon stimulation. Additionally, NK T cells are unique in their activation after recognition of lipid structures, such as bacterial cell wall components, via cell surface CD1-expressed receptors.

NK-Cell Function

NK cells have an important role in the control of certain infectious agents, malignancy, graft-versus-host disease (GVHD), and hematopoietic graft rejection (Biron et al., 1999; Lanier, 2000b; Seaman 2000; Trinchieri, 1989).

Role in Infection

The significance of a particular lineage of cells in sustaining an effective immune defense is often best illustrated when that particular lineage is genetically or functionally decimated. Several human subjects with NK cell deficiency have been noted to suffer life-threatening infections with certain viruses, particularly γ herpesviruses (Biron et al., 1999; Joncas et al., 1989) (see Chapter 17). Mice deficient in NK cells also reveal diminished killing of herpesviruses and the intracellular pathogens *Listeria monocytogenes*, *Toxoplasma gondii*, and *Leishmania* (Lanier, 2000a).

Role in Malignancy

NK cells were originally identified by the capacity to kill tumor cells in vitro and in vivo. Experimental depletion of NK cells in tumor-bearing mice facilitates tumor growth (Seaman et al., 1987). Administration of IL-2 augments NK-mediated tumor cell killing in vitro and in vivo. However, the role of NK cells in host protection against development of malignancy remains unproven. Although some support for the clinical use of activated NK cells in the treatment of malignancy has been gathered, the toxicity of the therapy has limited its widespread use (Lotze et al., 1990).

Role in Graft-Versus-Host Disease

A clear role for NK cell modulation of GVHD in human subjects has not been determined. Murine models of GVHD have revealed a role for NK and NK T cells. IL-2–activated donor NK cells suppress GVHD under certain conditions, purportedly via TGF-β production (Asai et al., 1998). Recently, donor NK T cells have been shown to suppress GVHD in mice, whereas T cells from the same donor produce the disease. NK T cells may alter GVHD through the release of IL-4 (Zeng et al., 1999).

Role in Hematopoietic Graft Rejection

In rodent models of marrow transplantation, NK cells may present a barrier against histoincompatible donor cell engraftment (Kumar et al., 1997). Offspring of two different inbred strains of mice will reject bone marrow grafts from either parent. Although the offspring express the parental MHC on their endogenous marrow cells, inhibitory NK receptors recognize these MHC as self-antigens. Transplantation of marrow from one parent, however, will activate NK cells in the offspring that are only inhibited by MHC molecules from the other parent, and the activated NK cells will kill the transplanted hematopoietic cells. The role of NK cells in marrow graft rejection in human patients is not as well delineated (Valiante and Parham, 1997).

REFERENCES

Ackerman SK, Douglas SD. Morphology of monocytes and macrophages. In Williams WJ, Beutler E, Erslev A, Rundles W, eds. Haematology, ed 3. New York, McGraw-Hill, 1983, pp 837–847.

Ackerman SK, Zuckerman SH, Douglas SD. Isolation and culture of human blood monocytes. In Douglas SD, Quie PG, eds. Practical Methods in Clinical Immunology: Investigation of Phagocytes in Disease. London, Churchill Livingstone, 1981, pp 66–75.

Adams DO. The granulomatous inflammatory response. Am J Pathol 84:164–191, 1976.

Adams DO, Hamilton TA. Molecular basis of macrophage activation: diversity and its origins. In Lewis CE, McGee JO, eds. The Macrophage. Oxford, UK, Oxford University Press, 1992, pp 75–114.

Adams DO, Hamilton TA. Molecular transductional mechanisms by which IFN-γ and other signals regulate macrophage development. Immunol Rev 97:5–27, 1987.

Adams DO, Hamilton TA. Phagocytic cells: cytotoxic activities of macrophages. In Gallin JI, Goldstein IM, Snyderman R, eds. Inflammation: Basic Principles and Clinical Correlates. New York, Raven Press, 1988, pp 471–492.

Adams DO, Hamilton TA. The cell biology of macrophage activation. Annu Rev Immunol 2:283–318, 1984.

Adams DO, Kao KJ, Farb R, Pizzo SV. Effector mechanisms of cytolytically activated macrophages. J Immunol 124:292–300, 1980.

Adams DO, Nathan CF. Molecular mechanisms in tumor-cell killing by activated macrophages. Immunol Today 4:166–170, 1983.

Adema GJ, Hartgers F, Verstraten R, de Vries E, Marland G, Menon S, Foster J, Xu Y, Nooyen P, McClanahan T, Bacon KB, and Figdor CG. A dendritic-cell-derived C-C chemokine that preferentially attracts naïve T cells. Nature 387:713–717, 1997.

Alexander P. Activated macrophages and the anti-tumor action of BCG. Natl Cancer Inst Monograph 39:127–133, 1973.

Alexander P. The functions of the macrophage in malignant disease. Annu Rev Med 27:207–224, 1976.

Altman LC, Snyderman R, Oppenheim JJ, Mergenhagen SE. A human mononuclear leukocyte chemotactic factor: characterization, specificity, and kinetics of production by homologous leukocytes. J Immunol 110:801–810, 1973.

Ancuta P, Weiss L, Haeffner-Cavaillon N. CD14+CD16+ cells derived in vitro from peripheral blood monocytes exhibit phenotypic and functional dendritic cell-like characteristics. Eur J Immunol 30:1872–1883, 2000.

Andreesen R, Bross KJ, Osterholz J, Emmrich F. Human macrophage maturation and heterogeneity: analysis with a newly generated set of monoclonal antibodies to differentiation antigens. Blood 67:1257–1264, 1986.

Andreesen R, Brugger W, Scheibenbogen C, Kreutz M, Leser H, Rebin A, Lohr GW. Surface phenotype analysis of human monocyte to macrophage differentiation. J Leuk Biol 47:490–497, 1990.

Andreesen R, Gadd S, Costabel U, Leser HG, Speth V, Cesnik B, Atkins RC. Human macrophage maturation and heterogeneity: restricted expression of late differentiation antigens in situ. Cell Tissue Res 253:271–279, 1988.

Arend WP, Joslin FG, Thompson RC, Hannum CH. An interleukin-1 inhibitor from human monocytes: production and characterization of biological properties. J Immunol 143:1851–1858, 1989.

Arnaout MA. Structure and function of the leukocyte adhesion molecules CD11/CD18. Blood 75:1037–1050, 1990.

Asai O, Longo DL, Tian Z-G, Hornung RL, Taub DD, Ruscetti F, Murphy WJ: Suppression of graft-versus-host disease and amplification of graft-versus-tumor effects by activated natural killer cells after allogeneic bone marrow transplantation. J Clin Invest 101:1835–1842, 1998.

Athens JW, Haab OP, Raab SO, Mauer AM, Aslenbrucker H, Cartwright GE, Wintrobe MM. Leukokinetic studies. III. The total blood, circulating and marginal granulocyte pools, and the granulocyte turnover rate in normal subjects. J Clin Invest 40:989–995, 1961.

Auger MJ, Ross JA. The biology of the macrophage. In Lewis CE, McGee JO, eds. The Macrophage. Oxford, UK, Oxford University Press, 1992, pp 1–74.

Austyn JM. Lymphoid dendritic cells. Immunol 62:161–170, 1987.

Austyn JM. New insights into the mobilization and phagocytic activity of dendritic cells. J Exp Med 183:1287–1292, 1996.

Axline SG. Functional biochemistry of the macrophage. Semin Hematol 7:142–160, 1970.

Axline SG, Cohn ZA. In vitro induction of lysosomal enzymes by phagocytosis. J Exp Med 131:1239–1260, 1970.

Babcock G, Phillips J: Human NK cells: light and electron microscopic characteristics. Surv Immunol Res 2:88–101, 1983.

Babior BM. Oxygen-dependent microbial killing by phagocytes. N Engl J Med 298:659–668, 1978.

Baehner RL, Johnston RB. Monocyte function in children with neutropenia and chronic infection. Blood 40:31–41, 1972.

Banchereau J, Steinman RM. Dendritic cells and the control of immunity. Nature 392:245–252, 1998.

Banda MJ, Clark EJ, Werb Z. Macrophage elastase: regulatory consequences of the proteolysis of non-elastin substrates. In Van Furth R, ed. Mononuclear Phagocytes. Dordrecht, Netherlands, Martinus Nijhoff, 1985, pp 295–300.

Barclay NA, Birkeland ML, Brown MH, Beyers AD, Davis SJ, Somoza C, Williams AF. The Leukocyte Antigen Facts Book. Orlando, Fla, Harcourt Brace Jovanovich, 1993, pp 1–269.

Bartocci A, Mastrogiannis DS, Migliorati G, Stockert RJ, Wolkoff AW, Stanley ER. Macrophages specifically regulate the concentration of their own growth factor in the circulation. Proc Natl Acad Sci USA 84:6179–6183, 1987.

Basham TY, Merigan TC. Recombinant interferon-gamma increases HLA-DR synthesis and expression. J Immunol 130:1492–1494, 1983.

Beller DI. Functional significance of the regulation of macrophage Ia expression. Eur J Immunol 14:138–143, 1984.

Bessis M. Cytologic aspects of immunohematology: a study with phase contrast cinematography. Ann NY Acad Sci 59:986–995, 1955.

Beutler B, Cerami A. Cachectin and tumor necrosis factor as two sides of the same biological coin. Nature 320:584–588, 1986.

Biron C, Byron K, Sullivan J: Severe herpes virus infections in an adolescent without natural killer cells. N Engl J Med 320:1731–1735, 1989.

Biron C, Nguyen K, Pien G, Cousens L, Salazar-Mather T: Natural killer cells in antiviral defense: function and regulation by innate cytokines. Annu Rev Immunol 17:189–220, 1999.

Blaese RM. Macrophages and the development of immunocompetence. In Bellanti JA, Dayton DA, eds. The Phagocytic Cell in Host Resistance. New York, Raven Press, 1975, pp 309–320.

Blom B, Res P, Spits H: T cell precursors in man and mice. Crit Rev Immunol 18:371–388, 1998.

Bodel PT, Nichols BA, Bainton DF. Appearance of peroxidase reactivity within the rough ER of blood monocytes after surface adherence. J Exp Med 145:264–274, 1977.

Bossi G, Griffiths G: Degranulation plays an essential part in regulating cell surface expression of Fas ligand in T cells and natural killer cells. Nat Med 5:90–96, 1999.

Bozdech MJ, Bainton DF. Identification of α-naphthyl butyrate esterase as a plasma membrane ectoenzyme of monocytes and as a discrete intracellular membrane-bounded organelle in lymphocytes. J Exp Med 153:182–185, 1981.

Braunsteiner H, Schmalzl F. Cytochemistry of monocytes and macrophages. In Van Furth R, ed. Mononuclear Phagocytes. Oxford, Blackwell Scientific Publications, 1970, pp 62–81.

Braunsteiner H, Schmalzl F. Étude cytochemique des monocytes: mise en evidence d'une esterase caracteristique. Nouv Rev Fr Hematol 9:678–687, 1968.

Breton-Gorius J, Guichard J. ?tude au microscope ?lectronique de la localisation des peroxidases dans les cellules de la moelle asseuse humaine. Nouv Rev Fr Hematol 9:678–687, 1969.

Brown EJ. The role of extracellular matrix protein in the control of phagocytosis. J Leuk Biol 39:579–591, 1986.

Brown LF, Dubin D, Lavikgne L, Logan B, Dvorak HF, Van de Water L. Macrophages and fibroblasts express embryonic fibronectins during cutaneous wound healing. Am J Pathol 142:793–801, 1993.

Broxmeyer HE. Biomolecule-cell interactions and the regulation of myelopoiesis. Int J Cell Cloning 4:378–405, 1986.

Buckley PJ. Phenotypic subpopulations of macrophages and dendritic cells in human spleen. Scan Electron Microsc 5:147–158, 1991.

Bujdoso R, Hopkins J, Dutra BM, Young P, McConnell I. Characterization of sheep afferent lymph dendritic cells and their role in antigen carriage. J Exp Med 170:1285–1302, 1989.

Bumol TF, Douglas SD. Human monocyte cytoplasmic spreading in vitro: early kinetics and scanning electron microscopy. Cell Immunol 34:70–78, 1977.

Butcher EC. Leukocyte-endothelial cell recognition: three (or more) steps to specificity and diversity. Cell 67:1033–1037, 1991.

Carlos TM, Harlan JM. Membrane proteins involved in phagocytic adherence to endothelium. Immunol Rev 114:5–28, 1990.

Carlos T, Kovach N, Schwartz B, Rosa M, Newman B, Wayner E, Benjamin C, Osborn L, Labb R, Harlan J. Human monocytes bind to two cytokine-induced adhesive ligands on cultured human endothelial cells: endothelial-leukocyte adhesion molecule-1 and vascular cell adhesion molecule-1. Blood 77:2261–2271, 1991.

Carpenter G. Receptors for epidermal growth factor and other polypeptide mitogens. Annu Rev Biochem 56:881–914, 1987.

Caux C, Dezutter-Dambuyant C, Schmitt D, Banchereau J. GM-CSF and TNF-α cooperate in the generation of dendritic Langerhans cells. Nature 360:258–261, 1992.

Chen H-D, Ma C, Yuan J-T, Wang Y-K, Silvers WK. Occurrence of donor Langerhans cells in mouse and rat chimeras and their replacement in skin grafts. J Invest Dermatol 86:630–633, 1986.

Chisolm GM, Hazen SL, Fox PL, Cathcart MK. The oxidation of lipoproteins by monocytes-macrophages: Biochemical and biological mechanisms. J Biol Chem 274:25959–25962, 1999.

Christensen RD, Harper TE, Rothstein G. Granulocyte-macrophage progenitor cells in term and preterm neonates. J Pediatr 109:1047–1051, 1986.

Christensen RD. Circulating pluripotent hematopoietic progenitor cells in neonates. J Pediatr 110:623–625, 1987.

Chu E, Rosenwasser LJ, Dinarello CA, Lareau M, Geha RS. Role of interleukin-1 in antigen-specific T cell proliferation. J Immunol 132:1311–1316, 1984.

Clark SC, Kamen R. The human hematopoietic colony-stimulating factors. Science 236:1229–1237, 1987.

Cline MJ. Bactericidal activity of human macrophages: analysis of factors influencing the killing of listeria monocytogenes. Infect Immun 2:156–161, 1970.

Cline MJ. Metabolism of the circulating leukocyte. Physiol Rev 45:674–720, 1965.

Cline MJ, Lehrer RI. Phagocytosis by human monocytes. Blood 32:423–435, 1968.

Cohn ZA. The activation of mononuclear phagocytes: fact, fancy, and future. J Immunol 121:813–816, 1978.

Cohn ZA. The structure and function of monocytes and macrophages. Adv Immunol 9:163–214, 1968.

Cohn ZA, Benson B. The differentiation of mononuclear phagocytes: morphology, cytochemistry, and biochemistry. J Exp Med 121:153–170, 1965.

Crowley M, Inaba K, Steinman RM. Dendritic cells are the principal cells in mouse spleen bearing immunogenic fragments of foreign proteins. J Exp Med 172:383–386, 1990.

Curtis BM, Scharmowske S, Watson AJ. Sequencing and expression of a membrane-associated C-type lectin that exhibits CD4-independent binding of human immunodeficiency virus envelope glycoprotein gp120. Proc Natl Acad Sci USA 89:8356, 1992.

Czop JK, Austen KF. A glucan-inhibitable receptor on human monocytes: its identity with the phagocytic receptor for particulate activators of the alternative complement pathway. J Immunol 134:2588–2593, 1985.

Das M, Henderson T, Feig SA. Neonatal mononuclear cell metabolism: further evidence for diminished monocyte function in the neonate. Pediatr Res 13:632–634, 1979.

David JR. Lymphocyte mediators and cellular hypersensitivity. N Engl J Med 288:143–149, 1973.

Davies P. Secretory functions of mononuclear phagocytes: overview and methods for preparing conditioned supernatants. In Adams DO, Edelson PJ, Koren H, eds. Methods for Studying Mononuclear Phagocytes. New York, Academic Press, 1981, pp 549–560.

Davis WC, Huber H, Douglas SD, Fudenberg HH. A defect in circulating mononuclear phagocytes in chronic granulomatous disease of childhood. J Immunol 101:1093–1095, 1968.

Demotz S, Grey HM, Sette A. The minimal number of class II MHC-antigen complexes needed for T cell activation. Science 249:1029–1030, 1990.

DePetris S, Karlsbad G, Pernis B. Filamentous structures in the cytoplasm of normal mononuclear phagocytes. J Ultrastruct Res 7:39–55, 1962.

De Vries JE, Zurawski G. Immunoregulatory properties of IL-13: Its potential role in atopic disease. Int Arch Allergy Immunol 106:175–179, 1995.

De Waal-Malefyt R, Yssel H, Roncarolo MG, Spits H, de Vries JE. Interleukin-10. Curr Opin Immunol 4:314–320, 1992.

Dieu MC, Vanbervliet B, Vicari A, Bridon JM, Oldham E, Ait-Yahia S, Biere F, Zlotnik A, Lebecque S, Caux C. Selective recruitment of immature and mature dendritic cells by distinct chemokines expressed in different anatomic sites. J Exp Med 188:373–386, 1998.

Dimitriu-Bona A, Burmester GR, Waters SJ, Winchester RJ. Human mononuclear phagocyte differentiation antigens. I. Patterns of antigenic expression on the surface of human monocytes and macrophages defined by monoclonal antibodies. J Immunol 130:145–152, 1983.

Dinarello CA. Biologic basis for interleukin-1 in disease. Blood 87:2095–2147, 1996.

Dinauer MC, Orkin SH. Chronic granulomatous disease. Annu Rev Med 43:117–124, 1992.

Ding A, Nathan CF, Stuehr DJ. Release of reactive nitrogen intermediates and reactive oxygen intermediates from mouse peritoneal macrophages: comparison of activating cytokines and evidence for independent production. J Immunol 141:2407–2412, 1988.

Donnelly RP, Dickensheets H, Finbloom DS. The interleukin-10 signal transduction pathway and regulation of gene expression in mononuclear phagocytes. J Interferon Cytokine Res 19:563–573, 1999.

Dorschkind K, Pollack S, Bosma M, Phillips R: Natural killer (NK) cells are present in mice with severe combined immunodeficiency (scid). J Immunol 134:3798–3801, 1985.

Douglas SD. Alterations in intramembrane particle distribution during interaction of erythrocyte-bound ligands with immunoprotein receptors. J Immunol 120:131–157, 1978.

Douglas SD. Human monocyte spreading in vitro: inducers and effects on Fc and C3 receptors. Cell Immunol 21:344–349, 1976.

Douglas SD, Musson RA. Phagocytic defects: monocytes/macrophages. Clin Immunol Immunopathol 40:62–68, 1986.

Edberg JC, Kimberly RP. Cell type-specific glycoforms of FcγRIIIa (CD16): Differential ligand binding. J Immunol 159:3849–3857, 1997.

Evans R, Alexander P. Mechanisms of extracellular killing of nucleated mammalian cells by macrophages. In Nelson DS, ed. Immunobiology of the Macrophage. New York, Academic Press, 1976, pp 536–576.

Evans R, Alexander P. Rendering macrophages specifically cytotoxic by a factor released from immune lymphoid cells. Transplantation 12:227–229, 1971.

Ezekowitz RAB. The mannose receptor and phagocytosis. In Van Furth R, ed. Mononuclear Phagocytes. Dordrecht, Netherlands, Kluwer Academic Publishers, 1992, pp 208–213.

Ezekowitz RAB, Sostry K, Bailly P, Warner A. Molecular characterization of the human macrophage receptor: demonstration of multiple carbohydrate recognition-like domains and phagocytosis of yeasts in Cos-1 cells. J Exp Med 172:1785–1794, 1990.

Fedorko M, Hirsch JG. Structure of monocytes and macrophages. Semin Hematol 7:109–124, 1970.

Ferbas JJ, Toso JF, Logar AJ, Navratil JS, Rinaldo CR: CD4+ blood dendritic cells are potent producers of IFN-α in response to in vitro HIV infection. J Immunol 152:4649, 1994.

Fossum S. The life history of dendritic leukocytes (DL). Curr Topics Pathol 79:101–124, 1989.

Gallin JI, Kaplan AP. Mononuclear cell chemotactic activity of kallikrein and plasminogen activator and its inhibition by C1 inhibitor and ?2 macroglobulin. J Immunol 113:1928–1934, 1974.

Gallin JI, Wolff SM. Leucocyte chemotaxis: physiological considerations and abnormalities. Clin Haematol 4:567–607, 1976.

Geijtenbeek TBH, Kwon DS, Torensma R, van Vliet SJ, van Duijnhoven GCF, Middel J, Cornelissen ILMHA, Nottet HSLM, KewalRamani VN, Littman DR, et al. DC-SIGN: a dendritic cell-specific HIV-1 binding protein that enhances trans-infection of T cells. Cell 100:587, 2000a.

Geijtenbeek TBH, Torensma R, van Vliet S, van Duijnhoven GCF, Adema GL, van Kooyk Y, Figdor CG. Identification of DC-SIGN, a novel dendritic cell-specific ICAM-3 receptor that supports primary immune responses. Cell 100:575–585, 2000b.

Geuze HJ, Slot JW, Strous GJAM, Lodish HF, Schwartz AL. Intracellular site of asialoglycoprotein receptor-ligand uncoupling: double-label immunoelectron microscopy during receptor-mediated endocytosis. Cell 323:277–287, 1983.

Ghanekar S, Zheng L, Logar A, Navratil J, Browski L, Gupta P, Rinaldo C. Cytokine expression by human peripheral blood dendritic cells stimulated in vitro with HIV-1 and herpes simplex virus. J Immunol 157:4028, 1996.

Gordon S, Cohn SA. The macrophage. Int Rev Cytol 36:171–214, 1973.

Gordon S, Perry VH, Rabinowitz S, Chung L, Rosen H. Plasma membrane receptors of the mononuclear phagocyte system. J Cell Sci (Suppl 9):1–26, 1988.

Greenburg GB, Hunt TK. The proliferation response in vitro of vascular endothelial and smooth muscle cells exposed to wound fluid and macrophages. J Cell Physiol 97:353–360, 1978.

Grewal IS, Flavell RA. The CD40 ligand: at the center of the universe? Immunol Res 16:59–70, 1997.

Grossi C, Cadorti A, Zicca A, Leprini A, Ferrarini M: Large granular lymphocytes in human peripheral blood: Ultrastructural and cytochen-dcal characterization of the granules. Blood 59:277–283, 1982.

Hakkert BC, Kuijpers TW, Leewenberg JFM, Van Mourik JA, Ross D. Neutrophil and monocyte adherence to and migration across monolayers of cytokine-activated endothelial cells: the contribution of CD18, ELAM-1, VLA-4. Blood 78:2721–2726, 1991.

Hamilton JA. Colony-stimulating factors, cytokines, and monocyte-macrophages: some controversies. Immunol Today 14:18–24, 1993.

Hart DNJ, McKenzie JL. Interstitial dendritic cells. Int Rev Immunol 6:128–149, 1990.

Hart J. Dendritic cells: unique leukocyte populations which control the primary immune response. Blood 90:3245–3287, 1997.

Hartwig JH, Stossel TP. Macrophage movement. In Van Furth R, ed. Mononuclear Phagocytes: Characteristics, Physiology and Function. Dordrecht, Netherlands, Martinus Nijhoff Publishers, 1985, pp 329–335.

Hashimoto SI, Suzuki T, Dong HY, Nagai S, Yamazaki N, Matsushima K. Serial analysis of gene expression in human monocyte-derived dendritic cells. Blood 94:845–852, 1999.

Heifets, L, Imai K, Goren MB. Expression of peroxidase-dependent iodination by macrophages ingesting neutrophil debris. J Reticuloendothel Soc 28:391–404, 1980.

Heinrich PC. Interleukin-6 and the acute phase protein response. Biochem J 265:621–636, 1990.

Hibbs JB. Heterocytolysis by macrophages activated by bacillus Calmette-Guerin: lysosome exocytosis into tumor cells. Science 184:471, 1974.

Hibbs JB. Macrophage nonimmunologic recognition of target cell factors related to contact inhibition. Science 180:868–870, 1973.

Hibbs JB. Role of activated macrophages in nonspecific resistance to neoplasia. J Reticuloendothel Soc 20:223–231, 1976.

Hibbs JB, Granger DL, Krahenbuhl JL, Adams LB. Synthesis of nitric oxide from L arginine: a cytokine-inducible pathway with antimicrobial activity. In Van Furth R, ed. Mononuclear Phagocytes. Dordrecht, Netherlands, Kluwer Academic Publishers, 1992, pp 279–292.

Hibbs JB, Lambert LH, Remington JS. In vitro nonimmunologic destruction of cells with abnormal growth characteristics by adjuvant-activated macrophages. Proc Soc Exp Biol Med 139:1049–1052, 1972.

Higuchi M, Higachi N, Taki H, Osawa T. Cytolytic mechanisms of activated macrophages. Tumor necrosis factor and L-arginine-dependent mechanisms act synergistically as the major cytolytic mechanisms of activated macrophages. J Immunol 144:1425–1431, 1990.

Ho W-Z, Lioy J, Song L, Cutilli JR, Polin RA, Douglas SD. Infection of cord blood monocyte-derived macrophages with human immunodeficiency virus type 1. J Virol 66:573–579, 1992.

Hocking WG, Golde DW. The pulmonary-alveolar macrophage. N Engl J Med 301:580–587, 1979.

Hoefsmit ECM, Duijverstyn AM, Kamperdijk WA. Relation between Langerhans cells, veiled cells, and interdigitating cells. Immunobiology 161:255–265, 1982.

Hofman FM, Danilous JA, Taylor CR. HLA-DR (Ia)-positive dendritic-like cells in human fetal nonlymphoid tissues. Transplantation 37:590–594, 1984.

Hogg N. Human mononuclear phagocyte molecules and the use of monoclonal antibodies in their detection. Clin Exp Immunol 69:687, 1987.

Horn RG, Spicer SS. Sulfated mucopolysaccharide and basic protein in certain granules of rabbit leukocytes. Lab Invest 13:1–15, 1964.

Horwitz MA. Phagocytosis of microorganisms. Rev Infect Dis 4:104–123, 1982.

Huhn D, Huber C, Gastl G: Large granular lymphocytes: morphological studies. Eur J Inununol 12:985–988, 1982.

Huybrechts-Godin G, Peeters-Joris C, Voes G. Partial characterization of the macrophage factor that stimulates fibroblasts to produce collagenase and to degrade collagen. Biochim Biophys Acta 846:51–54, 1985.

Inaba K, Inaba M, Romani N, Aya H, Deguchi M, Ikehara S, Muratsu S, Steinman RM. Generation of large numbers of dendritic cells from mouse bone marrow cultures supplemented with granulocyte/macrophage colony-stimulating factor. J Exp Med 176:1693–1702, 1992.

Inaba K, Metlay JP, Crowley MT, Steinman RM. Dendritic cells pulsed with protein antigens in vitro can prime antigen-specific MHC-restricted T cells in situ. J Exp Med 172:631–640, 1990.

Inaba K, Steinman RM. Accessory cell-T lymphocyte interactions: antigen-dependent and independent clustering. J Exp Med 163:247–261, 1986.

Inaba K, Steinman RM. Protein-specific helper T lymphocyte formation initiated by dendritic cells. Science 229:475–479, 1985.

Inaba K, Steinman RA, Van Voorhis WC, Muramatsu S. Dendritic cells are critical accessory cells for thymus-dependent antibody responses in mouse and man. Proc Natl Acad Sci USA 80:6041–6049, 1983.

Janossy G, Bofiel M, Pouler LW, Rawlings E, Burford GD, Navarette C, Ziegler A, Keleman E. Separate ontogeny of two macrophage-like accessory cell populations in the human fetus. J Immunol 136:4354–4360, 1986.

Jaubert F, Monnel JP, Danel C, Cretien J, Nezelof C. The location of nonspecific esterase in human lung macrophages. Histochemistry 59:141–147, 1978.

Johnston RB. Function and cell biology of neutrophils and mononuclear phagocytes in the newborn infant. Vaccine 16:1363–1368, 1998.

Joncas J, Monczak Y, Ghibu F, Alfieri C, Bonin A, Ahronheim G, Rivard G: Brief report: killer cell defect and persistent immunological abnormalities in two patients with chronic active Epstein-Barr virus infection. J Med Virol 28:110–117, 1989.

Kamperdijk EWA, Bos HJ, Bellen RHJ, Hoefsmit ECM. Morphology and ultrastructure of dendritic cells. In Zembala M, Asherson GL, eds. Human Monocytes. London, Academic Press, 1989, pp 17–25.

Kang Y, Carl M, Grimley P, Serrate S, Yaffe L: Immunoultrastructural studies of human NK cells. 1. Ultracytochemistry and comparison with T cell subsets. Anat Rec 217:274289, 1987.

Karnovsky ML, Lazdins JK. Biochemical criteria for activated macrophages. J Immunol 121:809–813, 1978.

Karnovsky ML, Lazdins JK, Simmons SR. Metabolism of activated mononuclear phagocytes at rest and during phagocytosis. In Van Furth R, ed. Mononuclear Phagocytes in Immunity, Infection and Pathology. Oxford, UK, Blackwell Scientific Publications, 1973, pp 423–439.

Karre K, Ljunggren H, Piontek G, Kiessling R: Selective rejection of H-2-deficient lymphoma variants suggest alternative immune defense strategy. Nature 319:675–678, 1986.

Katz SI, Tamaki K, Salles D. Epidermal Langerhans cells are derived from cells originating in bone marrow. Nature 282:324–327, 1979.

Kelemen E, Calvo W. Prenatal hematopoiesis in human bone marrow and its developmental antecedents, In Trubowitz S, Davis S, eds. The Human Bone Marrow: Anatomy, Physiology, and Pathophysiology. Boca Raton, Fla, CRC Press 1982, pp 3–42.

Kelemen E, Calvo W, Fleidner TM. Atlas of Human Hematopoietic Development. New York, Springer-Verlag, 1979, pp 1–261.

Kelemen E, Janossa M. Macrophages are the first differentiated blood cells formed in human embryonic liver. Exp Hematol 8:996–1000, 1980.

Keller R. Susceptibility of normal and transformed cell lines to cytostatic and cytocidal effects exerted by activated macrophages. J Natl Cancer Inst 56:369–374, 1976.

Keller R, Geiges M, Keist R. L-Arginine-dependent reactive nitrogen intermediates as mediators of tumor cell killing by activated macrophages. Cancer Res 50:1421–1425, 1990.

Kiener PA, Davis PM, Starling GC, Mehlin C, Klebanoff SJ, Ledbetter JA, Liles WC. Differential induction of apoptosis by fas-fas ligand interactions in human monocytes and macrophages. J Exp Med 185:1511–1516, 1997.

Klebanoff SJ. Phagocytic cells: products of oxygen metabolism. In Gallin JI, Goldstein IM, Snyderman R, eds. Inflammation: Basic Principles and Clinical Correlates. New York, Raven Press, 1988, pp 391–444.

Klebanoff SJ, Hamon CB. Antimicrobial systems of mononuclear phagocytes. In Van Furth R, ed. Mononuclear Phagocytes in

Immunity, Infection and Pathology. Oxford, Blackwell Scientific Publications, 1973, pp 507–531.

Klein RB, Fischer TJ, Gard SE, Biberstein M, Rich KC, Stiehm ER. Decreased mononuclear and polymorphonuclear chemotaxis in human newborns, infants and young children. Pediatrics 60:467–472, 1977.

Kotiranta-Ainamo A, Rautonen J, Rautonen N. Interleukin-10 production by cord blood mononuclear cells. Pediatr Res 41:110–113, 1999.

Kumar V, George T, Yu Y, Liu J, Bennett M. Role of murine NK cells and their receptors in hybrid resistance. Curr Opin Immunol 9:52–56, 1997.

Kurt-Jones EA, Beller DI, Mizel SB, Unanue ER. Identification of a membrane-associated interleukin 1 in macrophages. Proc Natl Acad Sci USA 82:1204–1208, 1985.

Kyurkchiev S, Ivanov G, Manolova V. Advanced glycosylated end products activate the functions of cell adhesion molecules on lymphoid cells. Cell Mol Life Sci 53:911–916, 1997.

Lanier L. NK cell receptors. Annu Rev Immunol 16:359–393, 1998.

Lanier L. The origin and functions of natural killer cells. Cell Immunol 95:S14–S18, 2000a.

Lanier L. Turning on natural killer cells. J Exp Med 191:1259–1262, 2000b.

Lanier L, Chang C, Phillips J. Human NKR-PLA: a disulfide-linked homodimer of the C-type lectin superfamily expressed by a subset of NK and T lymphocytes. J Immunol 153:2417–2428, 1994.

Lantz O, Bendelac A. An invariant T cell receptor a chain is used by a unique subset of major histocompatibility complex class I-specific CD4+ and CD4-8-T cells in mice and humans. J Exp Med 180:1097–1106, 1994.

Lasky LA. Selectins: interpreters of cell-specific carbohydrate information during inflammation. Science 258:964–969, 1992.

Lasser A. The mononuclear phagocyte system: a review. Hum Pathol 14:108–126, 1983.

Law SKA. C3 receptors on macrophages. J Cell Sci (Suppl 9):67–97, 1988.

Lee B, Leslie G, Soilleux E, O'Doherty U, Baik S, Levroney E, Flummerfelt K, Swiggard W, Coleman N, Malim M, Doms RW. Cis expression of DC-SIGN allows for more efficient entry of human and simian immunodeficiency viruses via CD4 and a coreceptor. J Virol 75:12028-12038, 2001.

Lee B, Sharron M, Montaner LJ, Weissman D, Doms RW. Quantification of CD4, CCR5, and CXCR4 levels on lymphocyte subsets, dendritic cells, and differentially conditioned monocyte-derived macrophages. Proc Natl Acad Sci USA 96:5215–5220, 1999.

Leibovich SJ, Ross R. The role of the macrophage in wound repair. A study with hydrocortisone and antimacrophage serum. Am J Pathol 78:71–100, 1975.

Lennartz MR, Cole FS, Stahl P. Biosynthesis and processing of the mannose receptor in human macrophages. J Biol Chem 264:2385–2390, 1989.

Levy MH, Wheelock EF. The role of macrophages in defense against neoplastic disease. Adv Cancer Res 20:131–163, 1974.

Li CY, Lam KW, Yam LT. Esterases in human leukocytes. J Histochem Cytochem 21:1–12, 1973.

Lioy J, Ho W-Z, Cutilli JR, Polin RA, Douglas SD. Thiol suppression of human immunodeficiency virus type 1 replication in primary cord blood monocyte-derived macrophages in vitro. J Clin Invest 91:495–498, 1993.

Lobb RR, Harper JW, Fett JW. Purification of heparin-binding growth factors. Ann Biochem 154:1–14, 1986.

Lodolce J, Boone D, Chai S, Swain RE, Dassopoulos T, Trettin S, Ma A: IL-15 receptor maintains lymphoid homeostasis by supporting lymphocyte homing and proliferation. Immunity 9:669–676, 1998.

Lotze M, Ciuster M, Bolton E, Wiebke E, Kawakami Y, Rosenberg S: Mechanisms of immunologic antitumor therapy: Lessons from the laboratory and clinical applications. Human Inununol 28:198–207, 1990.

Lu CY, Changelian PS, Unanue ER. Alpha-Fetoprotein inhibits macrophage expression of Ia antigen. J Immunol 132:1722–1727, 1984.

Macatonia SE, Knight SC, Edwards AJ, Griffiths S, Fryer P. Localization of antigen on lymph node dendritic cells after exposure to the contact sensitizer fluorescein isothiocyanate. J Exp Med 166:1654–1667, 1987.

Mackaness GB. Cellular resistance to infection. J Epidemiol Med 116:381–406, 1962.

Makgoba MW, Sanders ME, Luce G, Dustin ML, Springer TA, Clark EA, Mannoni P, Shaw S. ICAM-1a ligand for LFA-1-dependent adhesion of B, T, and myeloid cells. Nature 331:86–88, 1988.

Managan DF, Welch GR, Wahl SM. Lipopolysaccharide, tumor necrosis factor-α, and IL-1β prevent programmed cell death (apoptosis) in human peripheral blood monocytes. J Immunol 146:1541–1546, 1991.

Marodi L, Csorba S, Nagy B. Chemotatic and random movement of human newborn monocytes. Eur J Pediatr 135:73–75, 1980.

Marodi L, Kaposzta R, Campbell DE, Polin RA, Csongor J, Johnston RB. Candidacidal mechanisms in the human neonate. Impaired IFN-gamma activation of macrophages in newborn infants. J Immunol 153:5643–5649, 1994.

Marwitz PA, Van Arkel-Vigna E, Rijkers GT, Zegers BJ. Expression and modulation of cell surface determinants on human adult and neonatal monocytes. Clin Exp Immunol 72:260–266, 1988.

Massague J. The TGF-beta family of growth and differentiation factors. Cell 49:437–438, 1987.

Metcalf D. The molecular biology and functions of the granulocyte-macrophage colony-stimulating factors. Blood 67:257–267, 1986.

Metcalf D. The molecular control of normal and leukemic granulocytes and macrophages. Proc R Soc Lond (Biol) 230:389–423, 1987.

Meuret G, Bammert J, Hoffman G. Kinetics of human monocytopoiesis. Blood 44:801–816, 1974a.

Meuret G, Bremer C, Bammert J, Ewen J. Oscillation of blood monocyte counts in healthy individuals. Cell Tissue Kinet 7:223–230, 1974b.

Meuret G, Detel V, Kilz HP, Senn HJ, Van Lessen H. Human monocytopoiesis in acute and chronic inflammation. Acta Haemat 54:328–335, 1975.

Meuret G, Djawari D, Berlet R, Hoffmann G. Kinetics, cytochemistry, and DNA synthesis of blood monocytes in man. In DiLuzio NR, Flemming K, eds. The Reticulo-endothelial System and Immune Phenomena. New York, Plenum Press, 1971, pp 33–46

Meuret G, Hoffman G. Monocyte kinetic studies in normal and disease states. Br J Haematol 24:275–285, 1973.

Miller J, Alley K, McGlave P: Differentiation of natural killer (NK) cells from human primitive marrow progenitors in a stroma-based long-term culture system: identification of a CD34+7+ NK progenitor. Blood 83:2594–2601, 1994.

Miller TE. Metabolic events involved in the bactericidal activity of normal mouse macrophages. Infect Immun 3:390–397, 1971.

Mokoena T, Gordon S. Human macrophage activation modulation of mannosyl, fucosyl receptor in vitro by lymphokines, gamma and alpha interferons, and dexamethasone. J Clin Invest 75:624–635, 1985.

Mombaerts P, Iacomini J, Johnson R, Herrup K, Tonegawa S, Papaioannou V: RAG-1-deficient mice have no mature B and T lymphocytes. Cell 68:869–877, 1992.

Moore MA, Williams N. Analysis of proliferation and differentiation of foetal granulocyte– macrophage progenitor cells in haemopoietic tissue. Cell Tissue Kinet 6:461–476, 1973.

Morohoshi M, Fujisawa K, Uchimura I, Numano F. The effect of glucose and advanced glycosylation end products on Il-6 production by human monocytes. Ann N Y Acad Sci 748:562–570, 1995.

Muller WA, Randolph GJ. Migration of leukocytes across endothelium and beyond: molecules involved in the transmigration and fate of monocytes. J Leukoc Boil 66:698–704, 1999.

Murray HW. Interferon-gamma, the activated macrophage, and host defense against microbial challenge. Ann Intern Med 108:595–608, 1988.

Nagler A, Lanier L, Cwirla S, Phillips J: Comparative studies of human FcRIII-positive and negative natural killer cells. J Immunol 143:3183–3191, 1989.

Nakagawara A, Nathan CF, Cohn ZA. Hydrogen peroxide metabolism in human monocytes during differentiation in vitro. J Clin Immunol 68:1243–1252, 1981.

Nathan CF. Mechanisms and modulation of macrophage activation. Behring Inst Mitt 888:200–207, 1991.

Nathan CF. Mechanisms of macrophage antimicrobial activity. Trans R Soc Trop Med Hyg 77:620–630, 1983.

Nathan CF. Secretion of oxygen intermediates: role in effector functions of activated macrophages. Fed Proc 41:2206–2211, 1982.

Nathan CF. Secretory products of macrophages. J Clin Invest 79:319–326, 1987.

Nathan CF, Gabay J. Antimicrobial mechanisms of macrophages. In Van Furth R, ed. Mononuclear Phagocytes. Dordrecht, Netherlands, Kluwer Academic Publishers, 1992, pp 259–267.

Nathan CF, Tsunawaki S. Secretion of toxic oxygen products by macrophages: regulatory cytokines and their effects on the oxidase. Ciba Found Symp 118:211–230, 1986.

Nathan DG, Baehner RL, Weaver DK. Failure of nitroblue tetrazolium reduction in the phagocytic vacuoles of leukocytes in chronic granulomatous disease. J Clin Invest 48:1895–1904, 1969.

Nelson DS. Macrophages and Immunity. Amsterdam, North-Holland Publishing, 1969.

Nichols BA, Bainton DF. Differentiation of human monocytes in bone marrow and blood: sequential formation of two granule populations. Lab Invest 29:27–40, 1973.

Nichols BA, Bainton DF. Ultrastructure and cytochemistry of mononuclear phagocytes. In Van Furth R, ed. Mononuclear Phagocytes in Immunity, Infection and Pathology. Oxford, UK, Blackwell Scientific Publications, 1973, pp 17–55.

Nichols BA, Bainton DF, Farquhar MG. Differentiation of monocytes: origin, nature and fate of their azurophil granules. J Cell Biol 50:498–515, 1971.

North RJ. Endocytosis. Semin Hematol 7:161–171, 1970.

North RJ. The concept of the activated macrophage. J Immunol 121:806–808, 1978.

Ogasawara K, Hilda S, Azimi N, Tagaya Y, Sato T, Yokochi-Fukuda T, Waldmann T, Taniquchi T, Taki S: Requirement for IRF-1 in the microenvironment supporting development of natural killer cells. Nature 391:700–703, 1998.

Ojo E, Wigzell H: Natural killer cells may be the only cells in normal mouse lymphoid cell populations endowed with cytolytic ability for antibody-coated tumour target cells. Scand J Immunol 7:297–306, 1978.

Oren R, Farnham AE, Saito K, Milofsky E, Karnovsky ML. Metabolic patterns in three types of phagocytizing cells. J Cell Biol 17:487–501, 1963.

Palucka KA, Taquet N, Sanchez-Chapuis F, Gluckman JC. Dendritic cells as the terminal stage of monocyte differentiation. J Immunol 160:4587–4595, 1998.

Pantalone RM, Page RC. Lymphokine-induced production and release of lysosomal enzymes by macrophages. Proc Natl Acad Sci USA 72:2091–2094, 1975.

Parmley RT, Spicer SS, O'Dell RF. Ultrastructural identification of acid complex carbohydrate in cytoplasmic granules of normal and leukaemic human monocytes. Br J Haematol 39:33–39, 1978.

Piessens WF, Churchill WH, David JR. Macrophages activated in vitro with lymphocyte mediators kill neoplastic but not normal cells. J Immunol 114:293–299, 1975.

Ploem JS. Reflection contrast microscopy as a tool in investigation of the attachment of living cells to glass surface. In Van Furth R, ed. Mononuclear Phagocytes in Immunity, Infection and Pathology. London, Blackwell Scientific Publications, 1973, pp 405–422.

Podack E: Perforin, killer cells, and gene transfer immunotherapy for cancer. Curr Top Microbiol Immunol 198:121–130, 1995.

Pöhlmann S, Zhang J, Baribaud F, Chen Z, Leslie GJ, Lin G, Granelli-Piperno A, Doms RW, Rice CM, McKeating JA. Hepatitis C virus glycoproteins interact with DC-SIGN and DC-SIGNR. J Virol 77:4070–4080, 2003.

Polverini PJ, Cotran RS, Gimbrone MA, Unanue ER. Activated macrophages induce vascular proliferation. Nature 269:804–806, 1977.

Poplack DG, Sher NA, Chaparas SD, Blaese RM. The effect of mycobacterium bovis (bacillus Calmette-Guerin) on macrophage random migration, chemotaxis, and pinocytosis. Cancer Res 36:1233–1237, 1976.

Porcellini A. In vitro culture of granulocytic colonies from liver, spleen and bone marrow of human fetuses. In Lucarelli G, Fliedner TM, Gale RP eds. Fetal Liver Transplantation. Amsterdam, Exerpta Medica, 1980, pp 29–38.

Porcellini A, Manna A, Manna M, Talevi N, Delfini C, Moretti L, Rizzoli V. Ontogeny of granulocyte-macrophage progenitor cells in the human fetus. Int J Cell Cloning 1:92–104, 1983.

Postlethwaite AE, Lachman LB, Mainardi CL, Kang AH. Interleukin 2 stimulation of collagenase production by cultured fibroblasts. J Exp Med 157:801–806, 1983, pp 49–86.

Prickett TCR, McKenzie JL, Hart DNJ. Adhesion molecules on human tonsil dendritic cells. Transplantation 53:483, 1992.

Raghunathan R, Miller ME, Everett S, Leake RD. Phagocyte chemotaxis in the perinatal period. J. Clin Immunol 2:242–245, 1982.

Rappolee DA, Werb Z. Macrophage-derived growth factors. Curr Top Microbiol Immunol 181:87–140, 1992.

Rappolee DA, Werb Z. Macrophage secretions: a functional perspective. Bull Inst Pasteur 87:361–394, 1989.

Rainaut M, Pagniez M, Hercend T, Daffos F, Forestier F. Characterization of mononuclear cell subpopulations in normal fetal peripheral blood. Hum Immunol 18:331–337, 1987.

Reaven EP, Axline SG. Subplasmalemmal microfilaments and microtubules in resting and phagocytizing cultivated macrophages. J Cell Biol 59:12–27, 1973.

Reid CDL, Fryer PR, Clifford C, Kirk A, Tikerpae J, Knight SC. Identification of hematopoietic progenitors of macrophages and dendritic Langerhans cells (DL-CFU) in human bone marrow and peripheral blood. Blood 76:1139–1149, 1990.

Rice GE, Munro JM, Bevilacqua MP. Inducible cell adhesion molecule 110 (INCAM-110) is an endothelial receptor for lymphocytes. A CD11/CD18-independent adhesion mechanism. J Exp Med 171:1369–1374, 1990.

Rice GE, Munro JM, Corless C, Bevilacqua MP. Vascular and nonvascular expression of INCAM-110. A target for mononuclear leukocyte adhesion in normal and inflamed human tissues. Am J Pathol 138:385–393, 1991.

Riches DWH. The multiple roles of macrophages in wound healing. In Clark RAF, Henson PM, eds. The Molecular and Cellular Biology of Wound Repair. New York, Plenum Press, 1988, pp 213–239.

Romani N, Korde S, Crowley M, Witmer-Pack M, Livingstone AM, Fathman CG, Inaba K, Steinman RM. Presentation of exogenous protein antigens by dendritic cells to T cell clones: intact protein is presented best by immature epidermal Langerhans cells. J Exp Med 169:1169–1178, 1989.

Romani N, Fritsch P, Schuler G. Identification and phenotype of Langerhans cells. In Schuler G, ed. Epidermal Langerhans Cells. Boca Raton, Fla., CRC Press, 1991.

Romani N, Gruner S, Brang D, Kampgen E, Lenz A, Trockenbacher B, Konwalinka G, Fritsch PO, Steinman RM, Schuler G. Proliferating dendritic cell progenitors in human blood. J Exp Med 180:83–93, 1994.

Rosenthal AS. Determinant selection and macrophage function in genetic control of the immune response. Immunol Rev 40:136–152, 1978.

Ross GD, Walport MJ, Hogg N. Receptors for IgG Fc and fixed C3. In Zembala M, Asherson GL, eds. Human Monocytes. London, Academic Press, 1989, pp 123–140.

Ross R. Platelet-derived growth factor. Annu Rev Med 38:71–79, 1987.

Rossman MD, Douglas SD. The alveolar macrophage-receptors and effector cells function. In Daniele RP, ed. Pulmonary Immunology and Immunologic Diseases of the Lung. London, Blackwell Scientific Publications, 1988, pp 168–183.

Rosenzwaig M, Canque B, Gluckman JC. Human dendritic cell differentiation pathway from CD34[+] hematopoietic precursor cells. Blood 87:535–544, 1996.

Rubbert A, Combadiere C, Ostrowski M, Arthos J, Dybul M, Machado E, Cohn MA, Hoxie JA, Murphy PM, Fauci AS, Weissman D. Dendritic cells express multiple chemokine receptors used as coreceptors for HIV entry. J Immunol 160:3533–41, 1998.

Sallusto F, Palermo B, Lenig D, Miettinen M, Matikainen S, Julkunen I, Forster R, Burgstahler R, Lipp M, Lanzavecchia A. Distinct patterns and kinetics of chemokine production regulate dendritic cell function. Eur J Immunol 29:1617–1625, 1999.

Sanders WE, Wilson RW, Ballantyne CM, Beaudet AL. Molecular cloning and analysis of in vivo expression of murine P-selectin. Blood 80:795–800, 1992.

Santiago-Schwarz F, Belilos E, Diamond B, Carson SE. TNF in combination with GM-CSF enhances the differentiation of neonatal cord blood stem cells into dendritic cells and macrophages. J Leukoc Biol 52:274–281, 1992.

Sasaki T, Horiuchi S, Yamazaki M, Yui S. Induction of GM-CSF production of macrophages by advanced glycation end products of the Maillard reaction. Bio Biotech Biochem 63:2011–2013, 1999.

Schmidt AM, Yan SD, Brett J, Mora R, Nowygrod R, Stern D. Regulation of human mononuclear phagocyte migration by cell surface-binding proteins for advanced glycation end products. J Clin Invest 91:2155–2168, 1993.

Schultz GS, White M, Mitchell R, Brown G, Lynch J, Twardzik DR, Todaro GJ. Epithelial wound healing enhanced by transforming growth factor-β and vaccinia growth factor. Science 235:350–3542, 1987.

Seaman W. Natural killer cells and natural killer T cells. Arth Rheu 43:1204–1217, 2000.

Seaman W, Sleisenger M, Eriksson E, Koo G. Depletion of natural killer cells in mice by monoclonal antibody NK1.1: reduction in host defense against malignancy without loss of cellular or humoral immunity. J Immunol 138:4539–4544, 1987.

Seckinger P, Isaaz S, Dayer JM. A human inhibitor of tumor necrosis factor-α. J Exp Med 167:1511–1516, 1988.

Seckinger P, Williamson K, Balavione J-F, Mach B, Mazzi G, Shaw A, Dayer JM. A urine inhibitor of interleukin-1 activity affects both interleukin-1α and 1β but not tumor necrosis factor-α. J Immunol 139:1541–1545, 1987.

Selsted ME, Szklarek D, Ganz T, Lehrer RI. Activity of rabbit leukocyte peptides against Candida albicans. Infect Immun 49:202–207, 1985.

Scheeren RA, Koopman G, Van der Baan S, Meijer CJLM, Pals ST. Adhesion receptors involved in clustering of blood dendritic cells and T lymphocytes. Eur J Immunol 21:1101, 1991.

Shepherd V, Campbell E, Senior R, Stahl P. Characterization of the mannose/fucose receptor on human mononuclear phagocytes. J Reticuloendothel Soc 32:423–431, 1982.

Shivdasani RA, Orkin SH. The transcriptional control of hematopoiesis. Blood 87:4025–4039, 1996.

Sieff CA. Hematopoietic growth factors. J Clin Invest 79:1549–1557, 1987.

Silberberg-Sinakin I, Thorbecke G, Baer RL, Rosenthal SA, Berezowsky V. Antigen-bearing Langerhans cells in skin, dermal lymphatics and in lymph nodes. Cell Immunol 25:137–151, 1976.

Snyder DD, Unaue ER. Corticosteroids inhibit murine macrophage Ia expression and interleukin-1 production. J Immunol 129:1803–1805, 1982.

Snyder DS, Beller DI, Unanue ER. Prostaglandins modulate macrophage Ia expression. Nature 229:163–165, 1982.

Snyderman R, Pike MC. Structure and function of monocytes and macrophages. In McCarty DJ, ed. Arthritis and Allied Conditions. Philadelphia, Lea & Febiger, 1989, pp 306–335.

Solotorovsky M, Soderberg L. Host-parasite interactions with macrophages in culture. In Laskin AI, Lechavalier H, eds. Macrophages and Cellular Immunity. Cleveland, CRC Press, 1972, pp 77–123.

Southwick FS, Hartwig JH. Acumentin, a protein in macrophages which caps the pointed ends of actin filaments. Nature 297:303, 1982.

Speer CP, Ambruso DR, Grimsley J, Johnston RB. Oxidative metabolism in cord blood monocytes and monocyte-derived macrophages. Infect Immun 50:919–921, 1985.

Speer CP, Wieland M, Ulbrich R, Gahr M. Phagocytic activities in neonatal monocytes. Eur J Pediatr 145:418–421, 1986.

Springer TA. Adhesion receptors of the immune system. Nature 346:425–434, 1990.

Stachura J. Cytochemistry of monocytes and macrophages. In Zembala M, Asherson GL, eds. Human Monocytes. London, Academic Press, 1989, pp 27–36.

Stahl P. The macrophage mannose receptor: current status. Am J Respir Cell Mol Biol 2:317–318, 1990.

Starling GC, Egner W, McLellan AD, Fawcett J, Simmons DL, Hart DNJ. Intercellular adhesion molecule-3 is a costimulatory ligand for LFA-1 expressed on human blood dendritic cells. Eur J Immunol 25:2528, 1995.

Staunton DE, Dustin ML, Springer TA. Functional cloning of ICAM-2, a cell adhesion ligand for LFA-1 homologous to ICAM-1. Nature 339:61–64, 1989.

Steinman RM. DC-SIGN: a guide to some mysteries of dendritic cells. Cell 100:491–494, 2000.

Steinman RM. The dendritic cell system and its role in immunogenicity. Annu Rev Immunol 9:271–296, 1991.

Steinman RM, Cohn ZA. Identification of a novel cell type in peripheral lymphoid organs of mice. J Exp Med 137:1142–1147, 1973.

Steinman RM, Pack M, Inaba K. Dendritic cell development and maturation. In Ricciardi-Castagnoli, ed. Dendritic Cells in Fundamental and Clinical Immunology. New York, Plenum Press, 1997, p 1.

Stossel TP. From signal to pseudopod: how cells control cytoplasmic actin assembly. J Biol Chem 264:18261–18264, 1989.

Stuehr DJ, Nathan CF. Nitric oxide: a macrophage product responsible for cytostasis and respiratory inhibition in tumor target cells. J Exp Med 169:1543–1545, 1989.

Szabolcs P, Avigan D, Gezelter S, Ciocon DH, Moore MAS, Steinman RM, Young JW. Dendritic cells and macrophages can mature independently from a human bone marrow-derived, post-colony-forming unit intermediate. Blood 87:4520–4530, 1996.

Takenaka H, Maruo S, Yamamoto N, Wysocka M, Ono S, Kobayashi M, Yagita H, Okumura K, Hamaoka T, Trinchieri G, Fujiwara H. Regulation of T cell–dependent and –independent IL-12 production by the three TH2-type cytokines IL-10, IL-6, and IL-4. J Leukoc Biol 61:80–87, 1997.

Terstappen LWMM, Hollander Z, Meiners H, Loken MR. Quantitative comparison of myeloid antigens on five lineages of mature peripheral blood cells. J Leuk Biol 48:138–148, 1990.

Tew JG, Thorbecke J, Steinman RM. Dendritic cells in the immune response. Characteristics and recommended nomenclature. J Reticuloendothel Soc 31:371–380, 1982.

Thomas R, Davis LS, Lipshy PE. Isolation and characterization of human peripheral blood dendritic cells. J Immunol 150:821–834, 1993.

Thomas R, Lipsky PE. Human peripheral blood dendritic cell subsets: Isolation and characterization of precursor and mature antigen producing cells. J Immunol 153:4016, 1994.

Thorne KJI, Oliver RC, Barnet AJ. Lysis and killing of bacteria by lysosomal proteinases. Infect Immun 14:555–563, 1976.

Timonen T, Saksela E, Ranki A, Hayry P: Fractionation, morphological, and functional characterization of effector cells responsible for human natural killer activity against cell line targets. Cell Immunol 48:133–148, 1979.

Todd RF III, Schlossman SF. Analysis of antigenic determinants on human monocytes and macrophages. Blood 59:775–786, 1982.

Todd RF III, Schlossman SF. Utilization of monoclonal antibodies in the characterization of monocyte-macrophage differentiation antigens. In Bellanti JA, Herscowitz HB, eds. The Reticuloendothelial System. New York, Plenum Publishing, 1984, pp 87–112.

Toews GB. Pulmonary dendritic cells: sentinels of lung-associated lymphoid tissues. Am J Resp Cell Mol Biol 4:204–205, 1991.

Trinchieri G. Biology of natural killer cells. Adv Immunol 47:187–376, 1989.

Trinchieri G, Gerosa F. Immunoregulation by interleukin-12. J Leukoc Biol 59:505–511, 1996.

Unanue ER, Allen PM. The basis for the immunoregulatory role of macrophages and other accessory cells. Science 236:551–557, 1987a.

Unanue ER, Allen PM. The immunoregulatory role of the macrophage. Hosp Pract 22:63–80, 1987b.

Unkeless JC. Function and heterogeneity of human Fc receptors for immunoglobulin G. J Clin Invest 83:355–361, 1989.

Urban JL, Shepard HM, Rothstein JL, Sugarman BJ, Schreiber H. Tumor necrosis factor: a potent effector molecule for tumor cell killing by activated macrophages. Proc Natl Acad Sci USA 83:5233–5237, 1986.

Vakkila J, Sihvola M, Hurme M. Human peripheral blood-derived dendritic cells do not produce IL-1α, IL-1β or IL-6. Scand J Immunol 31:345, 1990.

Valiante N, Parham P. Natural killer cells, HLA class I molecules, and marrow transplantation. Biol Blood & Marrow Transplant 3:229–235, 1997.

Valledor AF, Borras FE, Cullell-Young M, Celada A. Transcription factors that regulate monocyte/macrophage differentiation. J Leuk Biol 63:405–417, 1998.

Van de Winkel JGJ, Capel PJA. Human IgG Fc receptor heterogeneity: molecular aspects and clinical implications. Immunol Today 14:215–221, 1993.

Van Furth R. Cells of the mononuclear phagocyte system: nomenclature in terms of sites and conditions. In Van Furth R, ed. Mononuclear Phagocytes. Functional Aspects. Dordrecht, Netherlands, Martinus Nijhoff Publishers, 1980, pp 1–40.

Van Furth R. Human monocytes and cytokines. Res Immunol 149:719–720, 1998.

Van Furth R, Cohn ZA. The origin and kinetics of mononuclear phagocytes. J Exp Med 128:415–435, 1968.

Van Furth R, Diesselhoff den Dulk MMC, Sluiter W, Van Dissel JT. New perspective on the kinetics of mononuclear phagocytes. In Van Furth R, ed. Mononuclear Phagocytes: Characteristics, Physiology and Function. Dordrecht, Netherlands, Martinus Nijhoff Publishers, 1985, pp 201–209.

Van Furth R, Langevoort HL, Schaberg A. Mononuclear phagocytes in human pathology. Proposal for an approach to improved classification. In Van Furth R, ed. Mononuclear Phagocytes in Immunity, Infection and Pathology. London, Blackwell Scientific Publications, 1975, pp 1–16.

Van Oss CJ, Gillman CF, Neuman AW. Phagocytic Engulfment and Adhesiveness as Cellular Surface Phenomena. New York, Marcel Dekker, 1975, pp 1–153.

Verghese MW, Snyderman R. Chemotaxis and chemotactic factors. In Zembala M, Asherson GL, eds. Human Monocytes. Oxford, UK, Oxford University Press, 1989, pp 167–176.

Vignola AM, Gjomarkaj M, Arnoux B, Bousquet J. Update on cells and cytokines: monocytes. J Allergy Clin Immunol 101:149–52, 1998.

Vlassara H, Brownlee IM, Manogue KR, Dinarillo CA, Pasagian A. Cachectin/TNF and IL-1 induced by glucose-modified proteins: role in normal tissue remodeling. Science 240:1546–1548, 1988.

Vlassara H, Moldawer L, Chan B. Macrophage/monocyte receptor for nonenzymatically glycosylated proteins is upregulated by cachectin/tumor necrosis factor. J Clin Invest 84:1813–1820, 1989.

Volk-Platzer B, Stingl G, Wolff K, Hinterberg W, Schnedl W. Cytogenetic identification of allogeneic epidermal Langerhans cells in a bone marrow-graft recipient. N Engl J Med 310:1123–1127, 1984.

Wachstein M, Wolfe G. The histochemical demonstration of esterase activity in human blood and bone marrow smears. J Histochem Cytochem 6:457, 1958.

Wahl LM, Wahl SM, Mergenhagen SE, Martin GR. Collagenase production by lymphokine-activated macrophages. Science 187:261–263, 1975.

Ward PA. Chemotaxis of mononuclear cells. J Exp Med 128:1201–1221, 1968.

Ward PA, Remold HG, David JR. The production by antigen-stimulated lymphocytes of a leukotactic factor distinct from migratory inhibitory factor. Cell Immunol 1:162–174, 1970.

Weber C, Belge KU, Von Hundelshausen P, Draude G, Steppich B, Mack M, Frankenberger M, Weber KS, Ziegler-Heitbrock HWL. Differential chemokine receptor expression and function in human monocyte subpopulations. J Leukoc Biol 67:699–704, 2000.

Weinstein RS, Khoudadad JK, Steck TL. Ultrastructural characterization of proteins at the natural surfaces of the red cell membrane. In Brewer GJ, ed. The Red Cell. New York, Alan R Liss, 1978, pp 413–427.

Wellicome SM, Thornhill MH, Pitzalis C, Thomas DS, Lanchburg JSS, Panayi GS, Haskard DO. A monoclonal antibody that detects a novel antigen on endothelial cells that is induced by tumor necrosis factor, IL-1, or lipopolysaccharide. J Immunol 144:2558–2565, 1990.

Werb Z, Banda MJ, Jones PA. Degradation of connective tissue matrices by macrophages. I. Proteolysis of elastin, glycoproteins, and collagen by proteinases isolated from macrophages. J Exp Med 152:1340–1357, 1980.

Weston WL, Carson BS, Barkin RM, Slater GD, Dustin RD, Hecht SK. Monocyte-macrophage function in the newborn. Am J Dis Child 131:1241–1242, 1977.

Whitlaw DW. Observations on human monocyte kinetics after pulse labeling. Cell Tissue Kinet 5:3111–3117, 1972.

Wilson CB, Westall J. Activation of neonatal and adult human macrophages by alpha, beta and gamma interferons. Infect Immun 49:351–356, 1985.

Wong HL, Walh SM. Tissue repair and fibrosis. In Zembala M, Asherson GL, eds. Human Monocytes. London, Academic Press, 1989, pp 383–394.

Wood GS, Freudenthal RS. CD5 monoclonal antibody reacts with human peripheral blood dendritic cells. Am J Pathol 141:789, 1992.

Wright SD, Detmer PA. Adhesion-promoting receptors on phagocytes. J Cell Sci 9(Suppl):99–120, 1988.

Wright SD, Griffin FM. Activation of phagocytic cells' C3 receptors for phagocytosis. J Leuk Biol 38:327–339, 1985.

Yegin O. Chemotaxis in childhood. Pediatr Res 17:183–187, 1983.

Yin HL, Hartwig JH, Maruyama K, Stossel TP. Ca^{2+} control of actin filament length. Effect of macrophage gelsolin on actin polymerization. J Biol Chem 256:9693–9697, 1981.

Yoder MC, Hassan SF, Douglas SD. Mononuclear phagocyte system. In Polin RA, Fox WW, eds. Fetal and Neonatal Physiology. Philadelphia, WB Saunders, 1992, pp 1438–1461.

Yoshimoto T, Paul W. CD4+, NK1.1+ T cells promptly produce interleukin 4 in response to in vivo challenge with anti-CD3. J Exp Med 179:1285–1295, 1994.

Zaitseva M, Blauvelt A, Lee S, Lapham CK, Klaus-Kovtun V, Mostowski H, Manischewitz J, Golding H. Expression and function of CCR5 and CXCR4 on human Langerhans cells and macrophages: implications for HIV primary infection. Nature Med 3:1369, 1997.

Zamai L, Ahamad M. Bennett 1, Azzoni L, Alnemri E, Perussia B. Natural killer (NK) cell-mediated cytotoxicity: differential use of TRAIL and Fas ligand by immature and mature primary human NK cells. J Exp Med 188:2375–2380, 1998.

Zeng D, Lewis D, Dejbakhsh-Jones S, Lan F, Garcia-Ojeda M, Sibley R, Strober S. Bone marrow NK1.1 (–) and NK1.1 (+) T cells reciprocally regulate acute graft versus host disease. J Exp Med 189:1073–1081, 1999.

Zheng Z, Takahashi M, Narita M, Toba K, Liu A, Furukawa T, Koike T, Aizawa Y. Generation of dendritic cells from adherent cells of cord blood by culture with granulocyte-macrophage colony-stimulating factor, Interleukin-4 and tumor necrosis factor-α. J Hematother Stem Cell Res 9:453–464, 2000.

Zhou L, Tedder TF. A distinct pattern of cytokine gene expression by human CD83+ blood dendritic cells. Blood 86:3295, 1995.

Zhou L, Tedder TF. CD14+ blood monocytes can differentiate into functionally mature CD83 dendritic cells. Proc Natl Acad Sci USA 93:2588, 1996.

Zhou L, Tedder TF. Human blood dendritic cells selectively express CD83, a member of the immunoglobulin superfamily. J Immunol 154:3821, 1995.

Ziegler-Heitbrock HWL, Fingerle GN, Ströbel M, Schraut W, Stelter F, Schüt C, Passlick B, Pforte A. The novel subset of CD14+/CD16+ blood monocytes exhibits features of tissue macrophages. Eur J Immunol 23:2053–2058, 1993.

Ziegler-Heitbrock HWL, Ulevitch RJ. CD14: Cell surface receptor and differentiation marker. Immunol Today 14:121–125, 1993.

Zuckerman SH, Ackerman SK, Douglas SD. Long-term peripheral blood monocyte cultures: establishment and morphology of primary human monocyte-macrophage cell culture. Immunology 38:401–411, 1979.

7

The Serum Complement System

Melvin Berger and Michael M. Frank

INTRODUCTION AND HISTORY

The complement system was originally described at the end of the nineteenth century, when it was discovered that there were heat-labile proteins in plasma that were able to lyse antibody-sensitized gram-negative bacteria, as well as cholera vibrios. Later it was found that these proteins could lyse erythrocytes sensitized with the heat-stable, specific component now recognized as antibody. Early in the twentieth century, it became apparent that the bactericidal activity of plasma or serum required the sequential activation of multiple factors or components. With sensitized erythrocytes used as a model target for complement attack, the lytic process was studied in detail and characterized mathematically (Borsos and Rapp, 1970; Mayer, 1961). With modern biochemical technology, the individual proteins of this classical, antibody-dependent pathway of activation were isolated and characterized and the basis of complement activity came to be understood on a molecular level.

In the 1950s a second pathway of complement activation was described by Pillemer and colleagues (1954). Initially termed the *properdin system,* it is now referred to as the *alternative* or *alternate pathway* because it is activated by an alternative series of proteins that bypass the early components of the classical pathway. The alternative pathway does not require specific antibody but is activated by interaction of the plasma complement protein, C3, with certain types of surfaces, including the surface of many microbes, as well as a yeast cell wall particle, called *zymosan,* which is often used as a model target. The proteins that constitute this pathway have also been isolated and characterized, and their relationships to the classical pathway components have been defined (Müller-Eberhard and Schreiber, 1980). More recently a third pathway, activated by recognition of polysaccharides by mannose-binding lectin, has also been described (Turner and Hamvas, 2000).

The components of these activation pathways, together with their important regulatory factors, thus comprise more than 25 unique serum and membrane proteins. The properties of many of these proteins are summarized in Table 7-1. The originally described activity of the complement system, lysis of bacteria or erythrocytes, is still its most commonly recognized function. However, many other functions have subsequently been attributed to this complex system of proteins. These include the generation of peptide fragments that serve as potent mediators of inflammation and attractants for phagocytic cells. They also include the formation of opsonins, proteins that coat pathogens and facilitate phagocytosis, which have essential functions in the host defense against infection. Complement also plays critical roles in solubilization and clearance of immune complexes by the reticuloendothelial system and in immunologic homeostasis, such as initiating antibody responses, modulating lymphocyte activation, and establishing immunologic memory. Thus understanding the mechanisms of complement activation, its biologic effects, and its regulation has become a major endeavor of modern immunologic research.

More detailed discussions of the complement system are available in a comprehensive series of reviews edited by Müller-Eberhard (1983/1984), a textbook by Volanakis and Frank (1998), and a recent review of current concepts of complement physiology (Walport, 2001).

TABLE 7-1 · PHYSICOCHEMICAL PROPERTIES OF COMPLEMENT COMPONENTS AND INHIBITOR PROTEINS

Component	Molecular Weight	Serum Concentration, µg/ml	Chain Structure
Classical Pathway			
C1q	390,000	190	6 each α, β, γ
C1r	95,000	100	1 chain
C1s	85,000	80	1 chain
C4 (β_{1E})	209,000	430	α, β, γ
C2	117,000	30	1 chain
C3 (β_{1C})	190,000	1400	α, β
C5	206,000	75	α, β
C6	95,000	60	1 chain
C7	120,000	55	1 chain
C8	163,000	80	α, β, γ
C9	79,000	160	1 chain
Alternative Pathway			
P (properdin)	223,000	25	4 identical chains
D (C3 proactivator convertase)	25,000	1–5	1 chain
B (C3 proactivator, glycine-rich β-glycoprotein)	100,000	200	1 chain
Mannan Binding Lectin Pathway			
Mannan Binding Lectin	32,000	0.5 ng-5 µg/ml	3 identical chains per unit circulates as assembly of 2-8 units
MASP 1	90,000	1.6–7.5 µg/ml	1 chain
MASP 2	74,000	?	1 chain
Control Proteins			
C1 esterase inhibitor (C1EI, C1 INH)	105,000	180	1 chain
C4 binding protein	570,000	?	8 identical chains
I (C3b/C4b inactivator, C3 INA)	100,000	50	α, β
H (β_{1H} globulin)	150,000	520	1 chain
S protein (vitronectin)	80,000	600	1 chain
Membrane Bound Control Proteins*		**CD Designation**	
Decay accelerating factor (DAF)	70–80,000	CD55	1 chain
Membrane cofactor protein (MCP)	48–68,000	CD46	1 chain
Complement receptor type 1 (CR1)	190–220,000	CD35	1 chain
Protectin, membrane inhibitor of reactive lysis (MIRL)	18–25,000	CD59	1 chain
Homologous restriction factor (HRF), C8 binding protein	65,000	Not assigned	1 chain

*Absent in serum; present on multiple cells identified by monoclonal antibodies to specific surface antigens.
CD = cluster of differentiation; MASP = Mannose-binding lectin-associated serine proteins.

COMPLEMENT AS AN INNATE RECOGNITION SYSTEM

Although early studies centered on the ability of the complement proteins to lyse bacteria and foreign cells once they had been specifically recognized by the immune system and antibody had been formed, phylogenetic studies have made it clear that proteins of the complement system evolved before the appearance of specific adaptive immunity. The ability to make antibody appears phylogenetically at the level of the lower fish, but by that point almost all the elements of the complement system are established. It has become clear that complement plays a primitive host defense function very early in phylogeny, even in invertebrates. Invasion by infectious agents is a major problem for all living organisms, and the complement proteins appear to have evolved as a primitive form of protection even in the absence of antibody and specific immune recognition per se.

Three major pathways of complement activation have now been identified and are described in more detail later. Two of these pathways are able to function in the absence of antibody: the lectin pathway and the alternative complement pathway. The evolution of antibody appears to provide more accurate specificity and the ability to amplify activation of complement's defense functions at far lower complement protein concentrations. The lectin pathway utilizes a specific protein, mannan-binding lectin (MBL), that binds to specific polysaccharides present on the surface of some microorganisms and then activates a series of proteases that engage the complement proteins. MBL and the proteases of the lectin pathway may be viewed as serving an adapter role to activate complement in the presence of these polysaccharides, which is analogous to that of C1q and the proteases of the early classical pathway in activating complement in the presence of the appropriate bound antibody.

Alternative pathway function is dependent on the unusual chemical structure of one of the complement proteins, C3. This protein has an internal thioester bond buried in its structure and protected from contact with the milieu. The thioester bond slowly hydrolyses, momentarily exposing a site that can form a covalent bond with many structures in the vicinity, such as the surface of a microorganism. A conformational change in the C3 structure occurs on hydrolysis that allows for the binding of other complement proteins. Once an organism has been tagged by C3, additional complement proteins may assemble on its surface and the organism can thereby be opsonized or destroyed. Obviously, such a primitive mechanism of activation can lead to tagging of one's own cells, and many mechanisms have evolved to regulate the activity of C3. This includes the presence of a series of regulatory proteins that inactivate C3 when it becomes bound to one's own cells or tissues. These various mechanisms are described in detail later.

Thus the lectin pathway recognizes and helps destroy organisms with foreign-looking sugars on their surface.

The alternative pathway helps deal with a range of organisms that lack the sugars needed for lectin pathway activity but do not have the same surface characteristics as one's own cells.

The classical pathway, the last to evolve, is composed of building blocks that are analogous to those of the two other pathways and has evolved to provide a far more specific and powerful mechanism to destroy these foreign invaders. It uses specific antibody to identify invaders; then adapter proteins (C1q) amplify and focus complement activation on their surface.

NOMENCLATURE

A uniform set of symbols for the components and intermediates involved in complement activation has been adopted by the World Health Organization and is now in general use (Alper et al., 1981; Austen et al., 1968). The classical pathway proteins (components) are assigned numbers in the order of their discovery and are thus designated C1 through C9. They also act in numeric sequence except for C4, which is the second protein in the cascade. The alternative pathway components or factors are referred to by the letters B, D, and P, which correspond to the previously used names listed in Table 7-1. The two soluble control proteins that regulate activation of this pathway have also been assigned letters: H and I. The proteins that control the earliest steps of the classical activation pathway retain their original names: C1 inhibitor and C4 binding protein. C1 is composed of three distinct and separate subunits denoted by C1q, C1r, and C1s. None of the other components have distinct subunits, but for those that contain more than one peptide chain, the first three letters of the Greek alphabet are used to designate the separate chains: α denoting the largest, β the next, and γ the smallest.

Most laboratory studies of the function of complement components employ hemolytic assays using sheep erythrocytes as the particle to be lysed. The target erythrocyte is denoted by E and the specific antibody by A. As complement components bind to the surface, their number (or letter in the case of alternative pathway components) is added (i.e., EAC1 or EAC142). Many of the activation steps involve limited proteolytic cleavages, and the cleavage products are usually denoted by lowercase letters (e.g., C3a and C3b). The actual polypeptide chains cleaved are designated with a prime mark, so that upon cleavage, the α chain of native C3 becomes the α' chain of C3b. Enzymatically active intermediates or complexes are denoted by a bar over the fragments involved, as in $\overline{C3bBb}$, the alternative pathway C3 convertase. Proteins that have lost their ability to act as convertases are given the lowercase letter i, as in iC3b. This designation is important because even though iC3b is not active in convertases, it still plays an important role in opsonization by binding to its specific receptor, CR3 (discussed later).

COMPLEMENT ACTIVATION

Classical Pathway

C142 Activation

The classical pathway is initiated when C1 binds to an antigen-antibody complex and becomes activated. C1 normally circulates in the blood as a macromolecular complex held together in the presence of calcium. C1q itself has a molecular weight of 410,000 and is composed of 18 polypeptide chains of three types (six each of α, β, and γ). These are bound together to form six triple-helical collagen-like strands with a globular structure at the end of each one, giving the appearance under an electron microscope of a bunch of tulips (Porter and Reid, 1978). The strandlike domains of C1q are rich in glycine, hydroxylysine, and hydroxyproline and can be digested by collagenase. Because of these structural features, C1q is considered a member of a family of collagen-like lectins or collectins (Thiel and Reid, 1989) that also includes MBL (discussed later). The globular domains contain the sites that bind to the Fc domains of antibody molecules. Although monomeric immunoglobulin (IgG) can interact weakly with C1q, activation requires binding of more than one of the globular domains of a single C1q molecule to individual Fc portions of immunoglobulin.

IgM is an efficient activator of C1, presumably because the five Fc portions of this molecule are all linked together and provide a good binding site for the multiple globular domains of C1q. A single IgM molecule is thus sufficient to activate the classical pathway, although studies suggest that more than one of the antigen-binding sites of the IgM molecule must be engaged for activation to occur.

Activation by IgG requires two or more molecules to be brought into close proximity, as in an antigen-antibody complex or on a cell surface. In hemolytic systems or with particulate activators in general, this requirement for a doublet of IgG means that many thousands of IgG molecules must be deposited on an erythrocyte or bacterium for two of them to be close enough to bind with and activate a single C1 molecule. Human IgG subclasses 1, 2, and 3 can activate C1, but IgG4, IgA, IgD, and IgE cannot. The C1q interacts noncovalently with the CH_2 domain of the immunoglobulin molecule, but it is not clear whether a conformational change is induced in this domain when the immunoglobulin binds antigen, which then promotes C1q binding, or whether antigen binding is required just to bring multiple Fc fragments into appropriate proximity to form a C1 fixing site.

Macromolecular C1 contains two molecules each of C1r and C1s in addition to the C1q. Each C1r is a single polypeptide chain with a molecular weight of 85,000 daltons, and each C1s is a single chain of similar molecular weight (Cooper, 1983; Reid and Porter, 1981; Ziccardi, 1981). These subunits are globular and associate with the stalk region of the C1q molecule. C1r and C1s are activated when the globular ends of the C1q bind to antibody molecules, probably by conformational changes in C1q that are transmitted down the stalks when multiple globular heads interact with the immunoglobulins. During activation, each of the C1r chains is cleaved into fragments of approximately 57,000 and 27,000 daltons. The smaller fragment contains an active site serine and has protease activity. These active proteases then carry out similar cleavages on C1s to form the active $\overline{C1s}$ molecules (Sim, 1981). The $\overline{C1s}$ then acts as the protease that cleaves and activates C4 and C2, the next plasma proteins to act in the complement sequence; but it can also cleave synthetic esters. Hence it is sometimes referred to as C1 esterase because this activity is easily studied in the laboratory.

After binding and activation of C1, the $\overline{C1s}$ subunit can cleave and activate the next protein in the sequence, C4 (see Fig. 7-1). This component is made up of three chains: α, with a molecular weight of 93,000; β, with a molecular weight of 75,000; and γ, with a molecular weight of 33,000. Activation is accomplished by cleavage at a single site on the α chain, giving rise to C4a, a small fragment (molecular weight 9000) that diffuses away; and C4b, the remainder of the molecule, which can continue the activation cascade. C4 activation is biochemically similar to C3 activation (discussed later), and the major fragment, C4b, is transiently able to bind covalently to the cell surface or immune complex. A single active $\overline{C1}$ complex can cleave multiple C4 molecules so that many C4b molecules may cluster around a single original C1 fixing site, providing the first amplification step of the complement cascade.

The bound C4b molecules have no enzymatic activity per se but provide binding sites for C2, the next protein in the sequence (see Fig. 7-1). C2 bound to C4b is a substrate for $\overline{C1s}$, which again cleaves at a single site, uncovering the enzymatic activity that is carried on the larger fragment, $\overline{C2a}$. The interaction of $\overline{C2a}$ with C4b is stabilized by C2b (Nagasawa and Stroud, 1977). This complex then functions as the C3 convertase, with C4b providing the binding site for native C3 and $\overline{C2a}$, the proteolytic active site, which is serine dependent. The $\overline{C4b2a}$ complex is held together by weak, noncovalent interactions and decays spontaneously with loss of the C2a (see Fig. 7-1). Each C4b can promote cleavage of multiple C2 molecules by $\overline{C1s}$. Activation is thus more efficient on a surface where the C1 complex and C4b remain bound in close proximity. In the fluid phase, diffusion makes it difficult to sustain the multiple protein-protein interactions necessary for $\overline{C1s}$ to cleave C2.

C3 Activation

Activation of C3 by the classical pathway C3 convertase $\overline{C4b2a}$ also involves a single specific proteolytic cleavage (see Fig. 7-1). C3 has the highest concentration in serum of any of the complement components, 1.0 to 1.5 mg/ml, and it plays central roles in the classical, alternative, and lectin pathways of activation. It also

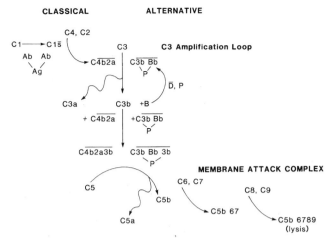

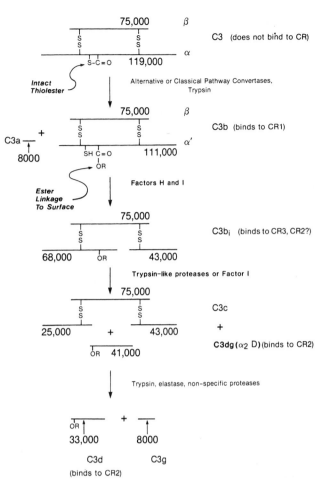

Figure 7-1 · Complement activation pathways. Note the analogous function of C4b2a, the classical pathway C3 convertase, and C3bBb, the alternative pathway C3 convertase. Addition of another molecule of C3b to each of these leads to formation of the respective C5 convertases. The alternative pathway convertases are shown here in their properdin (P) stabilized forms. The MBL pathway is not shown in this figure. After the interaction of MBL with appropriate polysaccharides, MBL-associated serine protease-1 and -2 (MASP-1 and MASP-2) are activated and can cleave C4 and C3 like C1s and C2a. Note that only the active fragments, C3a and C5a, are indicated; inactive cleavage fragments are not shown. (Modified from Berger M, Frank MM. Complement. In Wedgwood RJ, Davis SD, Ray CG, Kelley VC, eds. Infections in Children. Philadelphia, JB Lippincott, 1982, pp 86–108.)

has important biologic activities in opsonization and immune complex clearance and is thus the focal point of much complement research.

Native C3 is a glycoprotein (molecular weight, 195,000) composed of an α chain (molecular weight, 120,000) linked by disulfide bonds to a β chain (molecular weight, 75,000) (Fig. 7-2). Activation of C3 by C4b2a, by the alternative pathway C3 convertase, or by other serine proteases activated by the lectin pathway appears to be identical, with release of C3a, a 77 amino acid fragment from the NH$_2$ terminal of the α chain. This small fragment has anaphylatoxin activity (discussed later). The remaining large fragment, C3b, undergoes a complex conformational change exposing an internal thioester in the C3d region of the α′ chain, remote from the initial cleavage site (see Fig. 7-2). Studies by Tack and colleagues led to the discovery of this unusually reactive chemical structure, which is shared by C4 and α$_2$-macroglobulin, and accounts for the ability of these proteins to bind covalently to their targets (Harrison et al., 1981; Tack et al., 1980; Thomas et al., 1982).

The peptide chain that contains this bond has the following sequence

$$\text{S}\underline{\hspace{3cm}}\text{C}=0$$
—Gly—Cys*—Gly—Glu—Glu*—Asn—Met—

The asterisks indicate the cysteine residue that provides the thiol and the glutamate residue that provides the acyl moiety of the thioester. This group is usually protected in a hydrophobic pocket in the native mole-

Figure 7-2 · Schematic polypeptide chain structure of C3 and its cleavage fragments. Note that the site of cleavage by the convertases is toward the NH$_2$-terminal of the α chain, remote from the thioester site. This activation step may be accompanied by a transesterification reaction, resulting in surface-bound C3b (shown), or the thioester may react with H$_2$O, in which case the carboxyl moiety would be COOH, resulting in fluid-phase C3b. A conformational change accompanies this process and allows C3b to bind to CR1. Further cleavage by factor I in the presence of factor H or CR1 leads to production of iC3b, which binds to CR3, then to release of C3c, which is actually a three chain molecule with a molecular weight of 145,000. Cleavage by factor I stops at this point, leaving α$_2$D in serum or C3dg bound. Additional cleavage by nonspecific proteases releases a small fragment (C3g), leaving C3d bound. (Modified from Harrison RA, Lachmann PJ. The physiological breakdown of the third component of complement. Mol Immunol 17:9–20, 1980; and Ross GD, et al. Generation of three different fragments of bound C3 with purified factor I or serum. II. Location of binding sites in the C3 fragments for factors B and H, complement receptors, and bovine conglutinin. J Exp Med 158:334–352, 1983.)

cule. Upon exposure, however, it is subject to nucleophilic attack and thus becomes highly reactive. This unique structure can then participate in transesterification reactions in which the acyl moiety is transferred from the thiol to another electron-rich acceptor, forming a new covalent bond (Hostetter et al., 1982; Sim et al., 1981).

Acceptors can include the oxygen atoms of hydroxyl groups on cell surface carbohydrates, glycoprotein side chains, or amino acid side chains, leading to the formation of an ester linkage (Law et al., 1979). The thioester may also react with amino groups, forming amide linkages. If the thioester does not react with a suitable acceptor within a very brief half-life, the oxygen atom of water will provide the necessary pair of electrons, resulting in hydrolysis and the formation of fluid-phase C3b. Because the thioester remains available for a matter of only milliseconds before reacting with water, the newly cleaved C3b is referred to as *nascent* and the thioester as the *labile* binding site (because its ability to bind to biologic targets is only transient).

Once the thioester has reacted with water, the fluid-phase C3b is no longer capable of covalent interactions with targets. Biologic acceptors for C4b and C3b binding include cell surface carbohydrates of red cells and bacteria, as well as antibody molecules (Brown et al., 1983; Campbell et al., 1980; Goers and Porter, 1978). Chemicals that can disrupt the hydrophobic pocket of native C3 and C4 or low-molecular-weight nucleophiles that can diffuse in and react directly with the thioester will inactivate these components, thus explaining the sensitivity of the complement system to inactivation by thiocyanate, ammonia, and hydrazine.

During complement activation, many C3 molecules are cleaved. Some are hydrolyzed and remain in free solution, but many are deposited on the cell surface. Some of these are too far from their activation site to participate in furthering the activation sequence. These molecules may nevertheless have important biologic activity in opsonization, one of the major functions of the complement system, as well as activating the alternative pathway (discussed later).

C5 to C9 Activation

Those C3b molecules that do bind in close proximity to $C\overline{4b2a}$ serve as binding sites for C5 and thus transform the C3 convertase function of $C\overline{4b2a}$ into the C5 convertase, $C\overline{4b2a3b}$, with $C\overline{2a}$ again providing the proteolytic active site (Rawal and Pangburn, 2001). The cleavage of C5 is analogous to that of C4 and C3 in that an NH_2-terminal fragment of the α chain is released. Designated C5a, it has a molecular weight of 11,000 and potent anaphylatoxin activity. In addition, it is a chemoattractant and activator of neutrophils (see below). In contrast to C4 and C3, with which it shares several common molecular characteristics, C5 does not contain an internal thioester and does not bind covalently to cells.

C5b is unstable and rapidly loses activity unless it binds to C6. On interaction with C6 and C7, the hydrophobic properties of C5b increase, and the complex is capable of inserting into cell membranes and lipid bilayers in much the same way that detergents interact with lipids. Similar to C6 and C7, the remaining components, C8 and C9, are activated in numeric sequence without requiring proteolytic cleavage. These reactions increase their lipophilicity and C5 to C9 together form the *membrane attack complex* that can insert into and lyse biologic membranes (see Membrane Attack Complex and Cytolysis).

Mannan-Binding Lectin Pathway

The more recently recognized but important mannan-binding lectin pathway of complement activation is also being defined at a molecular level (Chen and Wallis, 2001; Rossi et al 2001; Turner and Hamvas, 2000). This pathway is initiated by a plasma protein, MBL, which has many structural similarities to C1q and is also considered a member of the *collectin* family (Thiel and Reid, 1989) (see Chapter 9). Its basic unit structure is that of a collagen-like helix of three protein chains, like C1q, that ends in a globular domain. In the case of C1, the globular domain binds to the Fc fragment of IgG or IgM. In the case of MBL, the globular domain has lectin activity and can bind to certain polysaccharide structures best exemplified by mannan. Like C1q, MBL is a polymer, but unlike C1q, which is composed of 6 basic trimeric units, the MBL polymer can consist of a variable number of basic units, from 2 to 8.

The MBL can bind directly to certain sugars on the surface of many microorganisms. This binding leads to the activation of serine proteases, which are associated with MBL analogous to the way that C1r and C1s are associated with C1q. In the case of MBL, the proteases are termed MBL-associated serine proteases (MASPs).

Three MASPS have been identified and may be isolated from plasma as a large complex with MBL, together with an additional 19,000 molecular weight protein that lacks enzymatic activity, and is designated MAp 19. The different MASPs and MAp19 appear to be alternatively spliced products of two related genes (Schwaeble et al., 2001). MASP-1 is believed to cleave and activate MASP-2 in a manner analogous to the activation of C1s by C1r. In vitro studies have shown that isolated MASP 1 and 3 can cleave C3 directly (Rossi et al., 2001; Vorup-Jensen et al 1998). However, it is now believed that physiologically MASP 2 functions like C1s, and that it cleaves and activates C4 and C2, forming a C3 convertase which is identical to that formed by the classical pathway (Chen and Wallis, 2001; Rossi et al., 2001; Schwaeble et al., 2002).

The MBL pathway is thus able to bypass C1 and activate the classical pathway before specific antibody has been formed. Like the early classical pathway proteases C1r and C1s, the activities of MASP-1 and MASP-2 are limited by C1 inhibitor (discussed later) (Matsushita et al, 2000; Petersen et al., 2000; Rossi et al., 2001). The importance of the Mannan-Binding Lectin pathway in the host defenses is illustrated by the occurrence of increased bacterial infections in patients who are deficient in MBL or MASP2 (see Chapter 21).

Alternative Pathway

The alternative pathway of complement activation also involves the formation of convertases analogous to those described for the classical pathway (Müller-Eberhard and Schreiber, 1980). The major difference is that specific antibody is not required to initiate the process. As discussed, this pathway appears to be phylogenetically older than the classical pathway and can provide natural resistance in the early stages of infection, before the immune system has had time to respond by synthesizing specific antibody. Bacterial and other polysaccharides, endotoxins, yeast cell wall particles, and aggregated immunoglobulins, including IgA, are all capable of activating the alternative pathway. The chemical nature of the surface that initiates activation partly determines this capability (discussed in Role of the Surface/Substrate later in this chapter).

Alternative pathway activation is initiated by C3b, which may be produced by classical or MBL pathway activation, or by nonspecific proteolytic attack. Thus the alternative pathway may serve as a potent amplifier of initial signals generated by those pathways. The alternative pathway can also be activated by a form of C3 (C3-H_2O) that has not been activated by proteolytic cleavage but resembles C3b because its thioester has been hydrolyzed by water (see earlier discussion) (Pangburn and Müller-Eberhard, 1980). Hydrolysis of C3 by water probably goes on continuously at a slow rate in plasma and accounts for the previously observed fluid-phase C3 "tickover," providing a basal level of activity that can be rapidly amplified in the presence of a suitable surface without the need for additional recognition or initiating factors. Thioester hydrolyzed C3 (C3-H_2O) or C3b play a role analogous to that of the C4b in the classical pathway and serve as binding sites for factor B, which is biochemically and functionally homologous to C2.

When factor B is bound to C3b, it becomes susceptible to activation by a single specific proteolytic cleavage carried out by factor D. Factor D is a low-molecular-weight (25,000) serine protease that apparently circulates in its active form in plasma at all times but at very low concentration, 1 to 5 µg/ml. D can cleave B only when it is bound to C3b or C3-H_2O. After cleavage, a small fragment (Ba) diffuses away and the large fragment ($\overline{Bb}$) remains associated with C3b to form the alternative pathway C3 convertase (C3$\overline{bBb}$). In this enzyme the C3b continues to function like C4b by providing a binding site for additional C3 molecules, and $\overline{Bb}$ functions like C$\overline{2a}$ in providing the proteolytically active site. The alternative pathway convertase, C3b$\overline{Bb}$, binds and cleaves additional molecules of C3 to form C3a and C3b.

An additional molecule, called *properdin* or P, which does not have an analog in the classical pathway, is important in activity of the alternative pathway, which was in the past sometimes called the properdin pathway in recognition of its role. P binds to and stabilizes the alternative pathway C3 and C5 convertases, which could otherwise lose activity by dissociation of Bb, which would then diffuse away. Inappropriate stabilization of alternate pathway convertases, and therefore excessive activation of complement, may occur pathologically in the presence of C3 nephritic factor (C3NeF), an autoantibody that stabilizes C3$\overline{bBb}$ by binding to certain sites on C3b exposed only in that convertase (Davis et al., 1977).

Once again, the nascent C3b has a number of different fates. A few C3b molecules bind very closely to the

C3$\overline{bBb}$ convertase and complex with it, providing a binding site for C5. This transforms the C3 convertase to a C5 convertase just as in the classical pathway, and $\overline{Bb}$ is thus able to cleave the C5 (Rawal and Pangburn, 2001). After activation of C5 by this enzyme, the later components continue to act in sequence exactly as in classical pathway activation, resulting in the formation of the membrane attack complex and leading to cell lysis.

Membrane Attack Complex and Cytolysis

In contrast to host defense activities such as opsonization, which require the interaction of complement components with phagocytic cells, the complement system can generate direct cytolytic activity by the formation of the membrane attack complex.

The first step in formation of this complex is the activation of C5 by the classical or alternative pathway C5 convertases. After release of the smaller glycopeptide C5a, the large fragment, C5b, undergoes conformational changes that increase its lipophilicity and allow it to complex with the next component in the sequence, C6. The C5b is stabilized by binding to C6, and the C5b6 complex can insert into lipid membranes at a distance from the C5 convertase.

In some cases the C5b6 can diffuse far enough to deposit on another cell (Hammer et al., 1976). C5b6 then acts as an acceptor for C7, which can bind either on the cell surface or in the fluid phase, forming a C5b67 trimolecular complex. This complex is highly hydrophobic and readily inserts into lipid membranes. It can also react with plasma lipoproteins or protein S, also known as *vitronectin*, presumably through hydrophobic interactions, in which case it no longer interacts with cell membranes.

The C5b67 complex is the binding site for C8. If this interaction occurs in the fluid phase, the attachment of C8 reduces the ability of the complex to bind to lipid membranes and thus inhibits its activity (Nemerow et al., 1979). Binding of C8 to membrane-bound C5b67, however, forms an active complex that can cause erythrocyte lysis even in the absence of C9. This complex can bind phospholipids and apparently disrupts the integrity of the phospholipid bilayer to increase the permeability of the cell. At this step in the lytic sequence, there is no morphologically recognizable membrane lesion or pore (Podack and Tschopp, 1984; Podack et al., 1979).

The assembled membrane attack complex as extracted from membranes is composed of one molecule each of C5b, C6, C7, and C8 and up to 12 C9 molecules. Thus the C5b-8 complex serves as a nidus for polymerization of C9 (Mayer et al., 1981; Müller-Eberhard, 1984; Podack and Tschopp, 1984; Podack et al., 1982).

Isolated C9 can also polymerize when incubated at elevated temperatures or for a prolonged time. These polymers appear under electron microscopy as hollow rings or donuts that resemble the membrane attack complex; both structures appear to contain disulfide-linked

C9 dimers (Podack and Tschopp, 1984; Ware and Kolb, 1981). Binding to C5b-8 causes the C9 molecules to elongate and unfold, exposing previously hidden hydrophobic domains and allowing disulfide exchange to occur. Evidence in favor of conformational changes in C9 is provided by the development of a monoclonal antibody that reacts with a "neoantigen" exposed on polymerized C9 and the membrane attack complex, which is not recognizable on native C9 or other native complement components (Falk et al., 1983).

Because the steps recognized in formation of the membrane attack complex beyond the cleavage of C5 do not involve enzymatic cleavage by earlier components, any cell on which C5b6 deposits, even if the C5 was cleaved by a convertase on a different cell, can in theory be lysed by the activity of the later components C7 through C9. This phenomenon of *bystander* or *reactive lysis* may be an important mechanism of tissue injury in infectious and immunologic diseases, particularly those in which soluble antigen-antibody complexes are thought to be pathogenic.

The membrane attack complex, as extracted from a membrane in which it has formed, appears as an annulus, 15 to 20 nm in diameter, that sits above the membrane; it is connected to a somewhat smaller diameter cylindrical stalk, 15 to 16 nm long, that spans the hydrophobic bilayer of the membrane (Bhakdi and Tranum-Jensen, 1979). When this complex is formed in a cell membrane, it functions as an open channel allowing an influx of water into the cell and leading to osmotic lysis with release of the cellular contents into the medium. In some nucleated cells, the initial membrane damage can be repaired, but with erythrocytes a single complement hole is sufficient for lysis. Hence the process may be described as a "one-hit" phenomenon.

C9 deficiency is associated with a mild increase in meningitis and other infections with *Neisseria*; patients deficient in C5, C6, C7, or C8 have recurrent *Neisserial* infection suggesting that the membrane attack complex may be necessary for defense against some gram-negative bacteria even in the presence of normal opsonization and phagocytosis (Densen, 1998).

Control of Membrane Attack Complex Formation

Studies with monoclonal antibodies to neoantigens on the membrane attack complex suggest that it is formed in vivo during complement activation in a variety of inflammatory processes; however, there are also plasma- and membrane-associated proteins that protect autologous cells against damage by this lytic activity. These proteins are discussed in Regulation of Complement Activation.

Nonimmunologic Complement Activation

Nonimmunologic activation of complement can occur when plasma comes into contact with a number of materials or when certain substances, including some radiographic contrast materials, are injected into the bloodstream. C1 can be activated directly by complexes of heparin with protamine, certain bacterial lipopolysaccharides, and other repeating-charge polymers. In addition, many serine proteases have overlapping specificity, so that plasmin or trypsin is capable of directly activating C1s and C3. Activation by plasmin may be important when the fibrinolytic system is activated in vivo, and activation by trypsin has been an important tool for in vitro studies.

An excellent example of nonimmunologic activation of the alternative pathway occurs when blood is passed through cellulose membranes during hemodialysis or in certain pump oxygenators. This commonly results in transient leukopenia and pulmonary dysfunction, which have been shown to be caused by activation of the alternative pathway by the cellulose. This leads to release of C5a, which can interact with and activate circulating neutrophils (Chenowith et al., 1981; Craddock et al., 1977; Jacob et al., 1980). These leukocytes then aggregate and plug pulmonary capillaries, and additional vasoactive substances may be released. Although the symptoms are usually mild, severe hypoxia and cardiovascular decompensation may occur in patients with preexisting cardiovascular or pulmonary impairment. Similar mechanisms probably contribute to the severe pulmonary dysfunction that occurs in the acute respiratory distress syndrome (ARDS) (Hammerschmidt et al., 1980).

Another condition in which nonimmunologic activation of the alternative pathway may have pathologic consequences is in the rare disease porphyria cutanea tarda, in which ultraviolet irradiation apparently causes photoactivation of abnormal circulating porphyrins. These porphyrins then react with skin proteins, transforming them into activators of the alternative pathway. This leads to local complement activation, which generates anaphylatoxins and causes inflammatory damage to the involved skin (Lim et al., 1984).

Burns, and ischemia followed by reperfusion, also may lead to structural changes in tissue proteins and exposure of intracellular structures or release of cellular proteases. Activation of the classical or alternative pathway, or both, often occurs in those situations, leading to formation of membrane attack complexes, vascular leakage, attraction of neutrophils, and enhanced tissue damage.

REGULATION OF COMPLEMENT ACTIVATION

Complement Regulatory Molecules

Activation of the complement system can lead not only to lytic and other cell-damaging activities but also to the production of potent mediators of inflammation. It is now recognized that complement activity is also necessary for proper trafficking and disposal of antigen-antibody complexes and that this system is important in the afferent arm of the immune response (reviewed by Davies and Walport, 1998; and Walport, 2001). Regulators of complement activity are thus necessary to prevent excessive or inappropriate complement activation and to ensure that the required components are present when needed.

The degree of complement activation at any site and time first depends on the amounts of native precursor proteins present. This in turn is determined not only by their concentrations in plasma and local vascular permeability but also by local synthesis, particularly in inflamed tissues (see Sites of Synthesis). Thus in addition to the liver serving as the major site of synthesis of the circulating components, local synthesis in lung, synovium, and other inflammatory sites has been clearly documented (Ruddy and Colten, 1974).

An inherent limit on activation is imposed by the requirements for the various proteins to act in sequence and the limited stability of activated proteins and protein complexes before they spontaneously lose activity. In some situations, as in the case of the thioester in nascent C3b and C4b, the activated molecules combine with water if they do not bind covalently to the target. In other cases, such as the multimolecular enzymatically active complexes (i.e., $C\overline{4b2a}$ or $Bb\overline{3b}$), there is dissociation or decay. Because complement is a self-amplifying system, there is a critical dependence on the density of the enzymatically active intermediates at a given site and time. The need to hold together multimolecular assemblies long enough to turn over several molecules of substrate (the next component in the activation sequence) probably explains why activation is much more efficient on the surface of a cell or large immune complex than in free solution.

The inefficiency of sustained sequential activation in free solution is illustrated by the lack of marked consumption of C3 in patients with hereditary angioedema (C1 inhibitor deficiency). This is even true during attacks, when the C4 and C2 may become quite low, indicating marked activation by $C\overline{1}$. The chemical nature and physical characteristics of the antigen-antibody complex initiating the sequence and the surface on which complement activation occurs are important

determinants of the amounts of various complement components activated and assembled.

Additional regulation of complement activation and function is provided by specific inhibitor proteins (Table 7-2). These may be found in solution, as well as on cell surfaces, and inhibit complement activity at multiple critical points.

C1 inhibitor (C1 INH), formerly called C1 esterase inhibitor, a single-chain molecule with an apparent molecular weight on gels of 105,000, is one of the group of proteins termed *serpins*, serine protease inhibitors. This single-chain molecule resembles a substrate for several different proteases, including $C\overline{1r}$ and $C\overline{1s}$, because it has a highly reactive arginine at position 444. The protease cleaves the inhibitor, just like its usual substrates, between this arginine and the next residue (threonine).

Following cleavage, the inhibitor springs apart, revealing a highly interactive chemical group buried in its native conformation, which interacts covalently with the enzymatic site on the protease (Patston et al., 1991). It is believed that C1 inhibitor is composed of a flat beta sheet made up of five segments, with a sixth segment protruding out of the sheet surface and containing the protease-sensitive site (Davis, 1998). On cleavage, this sixth segment can align with the other five segments to form a completed beta sheet and thus a thermodynamically favored configuration. The protein springs apart upon cleavage because the native inhibitor is held in an unstable form until it is cleaved and then forms the more stable configuration.

C1 INH was first described as an inhibitor of $C\overline{1r}$ and $C\overline{1s}$, two serine proteases of the classical pathway, but it is known that it inhibits activated Hageman factor and its fragments, as well as factor XIa, plasmin, and kallikrein of the coagulation, fibrinolytic, and kinin generating pathways. Recently it has been shown that C1 INH also is a regulator of the alternative pathway. A reduced level of C1 INH is found in the condition known as hereditary angioedema and in related conditions in which the deficiency may be acquired (see Davis, 1998; and Chapter 21).

TABLE 7-2 · PROTEIN REGULATORS OF COMPLEMENT ACTIVATION

Protein	Abbreviation	Molecular Weight	Number of Short Consensus Repeats (SCRs)	Dissociation of C3 and C5 Convertases		Factor I Co-factor Activity for	
				Alternative	Classical	C3b	C4b
Factor H, β_{1H} (p)*	H	150,000	20	+	−	+	−
C4 binding protein (p)	C4bp	570,000 (Octomer)	8	−	+	−	+
Decay accelerating factor (CD55)	DAF	70,000–80,000	4	+	+	−	−
Membrane co-factor protein (CD46)	MCP	45,000–70,000	4	−	−	+	+
Complement receptor type 1 C3b/C4b receptor (CD35)	CR1	205,000–250,000	30	+	+	+	+
Complement receptor type 2 C3d receptor (CD21)	CR2	145,000	15/16	−	−	−	−

*p indicates plasma proteins; membrane proteins are indicated by CD number.
Adapted from Ahearn JM, Fearon DT. Structure and function of the complement receptors, CR1 (CD35) and CR2 (CD21). Adv Immunol 46:183–219, 1989; Weisman HF, Bartow T, Leppo MK, et al. Soluble human complement receptor type 1: in vivo inhibitor of complement suppressing post-ischemic myocardial inflammation and necrosis. Science 249:146–151, 1990.

The activity of C4b and the formation of the classical pathway C3 convertase are regulated by a specific protein called C4 binding protein (C4bp). Binding of this protein to C4b promotes dissociation of C$\overline{2a}$ from the enzyme and facilitates further cleavage of C4b by a distinct control protein, which is itself a proteolytic enzyme called the C4b/C3b inactivator or, more commonly, factor I. Action of factor I on the α' chain of C4b results in the loss of the ability of C4b to serve its role in the C3 convertase and, after additional cleavages at specific sites, the release of most of the C4b molecule, leaving only the C4d fragment bound to the surface or immune complex, in a manner similar to that shown for C3d in Figure 7-2 (Fujita et al., 1978).

C3 Control Proteins, Regulation of the Alternative Pathway, and the C3 Amplification Loop

Besides its own important activities in host defense and immune complex clearance, C3 sits at a critical juncture in several complement activation sequences: the convergence of the alternative, classical, and lectin-binding activation pathways. It is an essential part of the convertases required for the cleavage of C5, which leads to the formation of the membrane attack complex. Control of cleavage of C3 and the activities of its major product, C3b, is thus a major target of the regulatory functions of the complement system. The first step in regulating C3 is regulating its convertases. Just as activity of the classical pathway C3 convertase is intrinsically controlled by dissociation of its two components, C4b and C$\overline{2a}$, the C3 convertase of the alternative pathway may also lose activity (or decay) by dissociation of its homologous components, C3b and $\overline{Bb}$.

A system of additional proteins has been identified whose major role is regulation of the activity of this critical component. Their names and properties are summarized in Table 7-2. In controlling the alternative pathway, the protein factor H acts analogously to C4 binding protein and promotes dissociation of Bb by binding to C3b. If the C3bBb complex decays spontaneously, the C3b may continue to serve as a binding site for additional molecules of B, allowing further alternative pathway activation and amplifying the initial number of C3b molecules formed.

When factor H binds to C3b, however, it promotes cleavage of the C3b by the same enzyme that cleaves C4b, factor I. The "inactive" iC3b that remains after initial cleavage by factor I still has opsonic activity and will bind to a receptor on phagocytes termed CR3 (see Complement Receptors). However, iC3b no longer promotes binding and activation of B or C5. This combined action of factors H and I is important in limiting the rate of spontaneous activation or "tickover" of C3.

Patients who are deficient in H or I have continuous activation of the alternative pathway, resulting in depletion of native C3 and conversion to circulating and erythrocyte bound C3b. This hypercatabolism of C3 leaves them with an increased susceptibility to bacterial infection, which resembles that seen in patients with primary C3 deficiency.

Membrane Regulators of C3

In addition to the soluble proteins that regulate complement activation at the convertase level, a family of structurally related membrane proteins has similar regulatory activities (see Table 7-2). These proteins play an important role in protecting body cells against activation and binding of autologous complement on their membranes. This may occur in autoimmune diseases or when extrinsic antigens are passively adsorbed onto their surfaces. Like the soluble proteins, these membrane proteins inhibit complement activation either by binding to one component of a convertase (e.g., C4b or C3b) and displacing a noncovalently bound component (e.g., C$\overline{2a}$ or $\overline{Bb}$), thus inactivating the convertase; or by acting as a co-factor for cleavage of the cell-bound component (e.g., C4b or C3b). Because the convertase activity decays spontaneously when the noncovalently bound components dissociate naturally, the former function of the regulatory molecules is referred to as *accelerating decay* of the convertase.

Besides accelerating decay, the regulatory molecules (H or C4bp) also serve as co-factors that enable factor I to cleave and inactivate the C3b or C4b to which they have bound. This prevents the C3b or C4b from participating in the formation of any new convertase complexes and also generates new fragments of C3 that bind to a different array of receptors (see Complement Receptors). As reviewed in Table 7-2, different members of the regulatory protein family are capable of either or both of these regulatory functions.

Complement receptor type 1 (CR1, CD35) has both decay acceleration and co-factor activities. The 70,000-dalton protein known as *decay-accelerating factor* (DAF, CD55) promotes dissociation of the classical and alternative pathway convertases but does not serve as a co-factor for factor I–mediated cleavage reactions. This protein is not a true transmembrane protein but is anchored in the cell membrane by phosphatidyl-inositol glycolipid (PIG) (Rosse, 1997). It has been speculated that this linkage increases the lateral mobility of DAF in the plane of the membrane, allowing it to move quickly to any site of C3b deposition and thereby protect the cell from amplification of complement attack sites initiated by errant C3b molecules. The importance of DAF is suggested by the observations that tumor cells that express high levels of DAF are resistant to immunologic attack and complement-mediated lysis (Cheung et al., 1988) and that overexpression of DAF transgenes protects organs from rejection when they are subsequently used for transplantation (see Transplantation).

In contrast to DAF, the 48,000- to 68,000-dalton protein termed *membrane co-factor protein* (MCP, CD46) facilitates cleavage of C4b and C3b by factor I but by itself does not interfere with binding of the enzymatically active subunits of the convertases, C$\overline{2a}$ or $\overline{Bb}$. Nor does it promote their dissociation from active convertases. Presumably, differences in the specific sites on C3b to which the different control proteins bind, and differences in the overall configuration of the complex of the control protein with C3b or C4b, determine which activities—co-factor for I versus acceleration of decay—will be manifested by any given control protein.

Structural Homology of C3b and C4b Regulatory Proteins: The Regulators of Complement Activation Gene Family

All the proteins discussed earlier that regulate complement activation by binding to C3b or C4b (including DAF, MCP, factor H, and C4 binding protein) share a high degree of structural homology. This is not surprising, because the C3b or C4b to which they bind are themselves homologous proteins. CR1 (CD35) and CR2 (CD21), which bind to C3b and C3d, respectively, also share structural homology with these regulatory proteins. CR1 possesses both decay-accelerating and cofactor activity (see Membrane Regulators of C3), whereas CR2 apparently has neither activity but promotes further cleavage of iC3b into products further down the degradation sequence (see Table 7-2). The genes for all these proteins are clustered together in band q32 on human chromosome 1 in what has been termed the *regulators of complement activation* (RCA) gene cluster (Bora et al., 1989; Carroll et al., 1988).

The basic structural unit of these proteins is a highly conserved short consensus repeat (SCR) of 60 to 65 amino acids, which contains two disulfide bonds that give it a double-looped structure. The individual proteins contain different numbers of these SCRs (see Table 7-2) grouped into long homologous repeats that form the C4b or C3b binding sites. Slight variations in the sequences determine the relative affinity for binding of C3b versus C4b. It seems likely that they have all evolved from a common primordial gene corresponding to a single SCR. For this reason, the proteins themselves are regarded as constituting a distinct family, although other membrane receptors, not related to the complement system (e.g., the interleukin-2 [IL-2] receptor), also contain domains that are highly homologous with the complement regulatory protein SCRs.

Role of the Surface/Substrate in Regulating C3 Function

As noted earlier, complement plays a major role in innate immunity by providing an important recognition system that can distinguish self from nonself upon initial exposure of the body to a foreign substance, such as a microorganism, without the assistance of specific antibodies. Part of the ability of complement to recognize nonself surfaces is a result of the surface influencing the competition between factors H and B for binding to C3b molecules, which are always being generated in the fluid phase and that randomly deposit on all types of cells and surfaces. The binding of H versus B (Fig. 7-3) in turn determines whether the C3b will be inactivated by factor I–mediated cleavage (after H binding), stopping alternative pathway activation, or

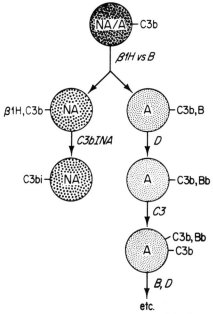

Figure 7-3· Control of alternative pathway activation by competition between B and H (β1H) for binding to membrane-associated C3b. C3b binds to both nonactivating (NA) and activating (A) cell surfaces, and discrimination between these surfaces by the alternative pathway occurs after this step. On a nonactivating cell, certain membrane constituents, such as sialic acid, promote the binding of β$_{1H}$ (factor H), which facilitates conversion of C3b to C3bi by factor I, the C3b inactivator (C3bINA). On an activating cell, binding of B leads to formation of C3bBb, which catalyzes deposition of more C3b, allowing activation of the C3 amplification loop. (From Fearon DT, Austen KF. The alternative pathway of complement: a system for host resistance to microbial infection. N Engl J Med 303:259–263, 1980.)

whether it will become part of a convertase that can cleave additional molecules of C3 (after B binding) (Kazatchkine et al., 1979).

Surfaces or chemical substrates that favor the latter therefore serve as activators of the alternative pathway. Because the additional molecules of C3b that are formed can also deposit on these surfaces, which further allows alternative pathway activation, a positive feedback loop is established and marked amplification can occur. Antibody molecules often provide protected sites where C3b cannot be bound by H or attacked by I (Fries et al., 1984). Thus a small amount of initial classical pathway activation induced by antibody may be amplified by the alternative pathway employing these mechanisms. On surfaces or acceptors for C3b that favor the binding of factor H, cleavage and inactivation of C3b by factor I will be promoted and alternative pathway activation will not occur.

Role of Sialic Acid

An important determinant of whether a surface will be an activator of the alternative pathway is its sialic acid content, because exposed sialic acid residues promote the binding of factor H to C3b (see Fig. 7-3) (Fearon, 1978). Although most human cells bear a considerable amount of sialic acid as a terminal sugar on their membrane glycoproteins and glycolipids, many bacterial polysaccharides, endotoxins, and cell walls are devoid of this sugar. The deposition of a small amount of C3b on most bacteria therefore leads to the rapid and continued activation of this C3 amplification loop in the presence of the alternative pathway components B and D and additional C3 (Fearon and Austen, 1980). This results in extensive opsonization with C3b or activation of the later components and lysis of the microorganism by the membrane attack complex, limiting the pathogenicity of organisms that activate the alternative pathway.

Rabbit erythrocytes do not normally bear sialic acid and are often used to assay the intrinsic activity of the alternative pathway in human serum. Because factor H recognizes surfaces that have characteristics in common with normal human cells and inhibits activation of the alternative pathway on them, bacteria and other organisms that have evolved capsules or endotoxin side chains bearing sialic acid mimic human cells. These often become dangerous pathogens because they do not support alternative pathway activation or amplification of complement's protective functions, such as opsonization or lysis. Those strains of *Escherichia coli* and group B streptococcus that are dangerous pathogens for neonates have evolved this method of mimicry to evade human innate defenses and are poor activators of the alternative pathway (Edwards et al., 1982; Stevens et al., 1978).

Role of Antibody

In addition to the ability of IgG and IgM to activate the classical pathway by the interaction of their Fc domains with C1q, F(ab')₂ fragments and other classes of antibody such as IgA can also activate the alternative pathway, even on surfaces that would otherwise be nonactivating (Moore et al., 1981; Winkelstein and Shin, 1974). Antibody molecules provide good acceptor sites for covalent binding of nascent C3b, and it thus is not surprising that C3b bound to antibody might be protected from the action of H and I (Fries et al., 1984). Another likely effect of antibody is to cover up sialic acid residues that would favor factor H binding, such as on the surface of a bacterium. This has been suggested as a function of antibodies against the capsules of group B streptococcus and against pathogenic serotypes of pneumococcus, which have sialic acid moities on their polysaccharides (Edwards et al., 1980).

Control of Membrane Attack Complex Formation

Just as there are soluble and cell surface molecules that protect host cells against deposition of C3 and prevent untimely initiation of the complement activation pathways, there are both circulating and cell surface inhibitors of the lytic activity of the membrane attack complex (Lachmann, 1991; Morgan and Meri, 1994). Several plasma proteins, including lipoproteins; S-protein or vitronectin (Bhakdi et al., 1988), which also regulates the coagulation system (Jenne and Stanley, 1985); and a soluble protein called SP-40,40 or clusterin (O'Bryan et al., 1990), can bind to C5b-6 and C5b-7 in the fluid phase and prevent their attachment to adjacent plasma membranes (Podack and Müller-Eberhard, 1978). This ability to prevent eventual membrane insertion of complexes initiated by formation of C5b in the fluid phase inhibits complement-mediated hemolysis of erythrocytes in vitro and probably plays an important protective function in vivo as well.

Additional membrane proteins can inhibit formation of the complete membrane attack complex as well (Davies and Lachmann, 1993; Miwa and Song, 2001). CD59, also known as *protectin*, is an 18,000-dalton molecule that binds to membrane attack complexes as they are assembling on cells, inhibiting the binding of C9 and preventing C9 that has bound from forming the C9 polymers essential for efficient lysis. The presence of a 65,000-dalton membrane protein called *homologous restriction factor (HRF)* or *C8 binding protein* has also been reported. HRF is thought to act after C8 has become bound to the C5b67 complex, and it prevents formation of full lytic complexes. Both CD59 and HRF are reported to be linked to the cell membrane by PIG anchors, as is DAF (CD55).

In the condition paroxysmal nocturnal hemoglobinuria (PNH), PIG-linked proteins are deficient on affected erythrocytes, which undergo spontaneous intravascular lysis (Rosse, 1997). It is now known that PNH is a disorder in which clones of cells cannot synthesize the glycolipid anchor that holds these proteins in the membrane because of a failure to synthesize the enzyme PIG transferase A (PIG A) (Nishimura et al., 1999; Rosse, 1997).

Conversely, overexpression of these molecules in transgenic animals is one strategy being developed to facilitate xenotransplantation by decreasing complement's participation in rejection of the transplanted organs (see Transplantation and Transgenic Animals with Human Complement Control Proteins).

COMPLEMENT RECEPTORS

Several of the most important physiologic functions of the complement system are mediated by the interaction of complement fragments bound to a target such as an antigen-antibody complex or microorganism with specific receptors on cells of the immune system such as phagocytes or lymphocytes. C3 is the complement component present in the highest concentration in serum, and there are four distinct receptors for different cell-bound fragments of C3 (see Fig. 7-2) (Berger et al., 1982; Ross and Medof, 1985). These are designated CR1 (CD35), CR2 (CD21), CR3 (CD11b/CD18), and CR4 (CD11c/CD18). CR1 and CR3 (and probably CR4 as well) are important in phagocytosis of microorganisms and immune complexes that have been opsonized with C3 fragments, whereas CR2 is important in regulating B-cell activities such as antigen presentation and antibody production.

Upon activation, C3, usually in the form of its major fragment C3b, becomes covalently bound to its target. The degradation fragments formed at different stages of processing of the bound C3b (Harrison and Lachmann, 1980) have differing affinities for receptors expressed on various cell types (see Fig. 7-2). The ability of these various fragments of C3 to direct the target antigen to various cell types depending on the affinity of the various receptors accounts for the major role that complement plays in directing the trafficking of antigens and in the afferent limb of the immune response. Other ligands, such as the Fc fragments of antibody, also influence the traffic patterns and type of cell to which the antigen is delivered, hence determining the fate of the antigen and the body's response to it. Thus antigens bearing C3b and or iC3b, especially if IgG is also present, may be cleared from the circulation or tissues by neutrophils, which are not very effective antigen-presenting cells. On the other hand, antigens bearing C3dg or C3d may be selectively bound to dendritic cells, which may then present the antigen to T cells, or by B cells, whose stimulation by the antigen will be greatly enhanced by the concomitant interaction of the C3d or C3dg with CR2.

Breakdowns in the bloodstream clearance functions of the complement system, as in congenital C3 deficiency, may result in sepsis and other problems with infection due to the lack of opsonins. However, they may also result in diseases caused by deposition of immune complexes in other organs such as the kidney or skin (Berger et al., 1983; Fearon, 1988; Davies and Walport, 1988; Walport, 2001). (This is discussed in detail in the section on CR1.)

In addition to the receptors for the various fragments of C3, there is a receptor for C1q, which may have a role in phagocytic defenses, and there are specific receptors for C3a and C5a, which are important as anaphylatoxins and chemoattractants. The latter two receptors are also discussed in the section on chemoattractants, leukocyte activation and leukocyte migration, and anaphylatoxins.

CR1 (CD35)

Native C3 does not effectively interact with any of the complement receptors, but upon cleavage and formation of C3b, conformational changes take place that result in a more than 1000-fold increase in the affinity with which the C3b binds to CR1 (Berger et al., 1981). C4b can also bind to CR1, a single-chain glycoprotein, which has both structural and quantitative polymorphisms (Dykman et al., 1984; Wong et al., 1983). The most common form of CR1 has a molecular weight of approximately 220,000 daltons. In addition to its presence on phagocytes, and on erythrocytes (only in humans and other primates), on which it plays an important role in transporting and facilitating removal of immune complexes bearing C3b from the circulation (see following discussion), CR1 is also found on glomerular epithelial podocytes, where it participates in retention of certain immune complexes (Gelfand et al., 1975).

CR1 is often clustered in cell membranes rather than being distributed evenly (Paccaud et al., 1990). It is a traditional transmembrane molecule with a short cytoplasmic tail and a single long extracellular domain. The extracellular domain consists of 28 (or more in different allotypes) SCRs of a highly homologous or consensus sequence of 60 to 65 amino acids characteristic of the RCA gene family. The entire receptor resembles an extended chain or string of beads, which may extend more than 1100 Å beyond the outer leaflet of the plasma membrane (Klickstein et al., 1987, 1988). This extended chainlike structure may be important in allowing phagocytes to reach out and catch opsonized microorganisms or immune complexes in the circulation. The SCRs are further organized in groups of seven into long homologous repeats (LHRs) that actually form the C3b and C4b binding sites (Fearon, 1988; Klickstein et al, 1988; Wilson et al., 1987).

A major advance in the recognition of complement receptors and their role in host defense was the description by Nelson in 1953 of the phenomenon called *immune adherence*, referring to the observation that bacteria coated with antibody and complement adhered to erythrocytes, which facilitated their phagocytosis by neutrophils (Nelson, 1953). Studies in monkeys have shown that preformed immune complexes rapidly fix C3b upon injection into the bloodstream and then bind to and are transported by the *immune adherence receptors*, which we now recognize to be CR1, on the erythrocytes. This facilitates their rapid removal from the bloodstream by macrophages in the sinusoidal circulation of the liver (Cornacoff et al., 1983) (see Immune Complex Solubilization and Clearance).

The cytoplasmic tail of CR1 is very short and does not contain any tyrosine residues (Klickstein, 1987), which probably explains why it, by itself, does not seem to play a major role in intracellular signaling or in activating phagocytosis per se. In general, binding of opsonized particles is felt to be the major role of CR1, with phagocytosis depending on a "second signal," often provided by IgG binding to an activating Fc receptor, or by polysaccharides interacting with CR3 (see Opsonization and Phagocytosis).

As noted previously, CR1 can participate in control of complement activation by accelerating decay of C3b- and C4b-containing convertases (Fearon, 1979; Iida and Nussenzweig, 1981), and it can also serve as a co-factor to help promote cleavage of C3b into iC3b and then C3dg by factor I (Medof et al., 1982). Taken together with the requirement for a second signal for phagocytosis of C3b opsonized particles, this suggests that immune complexes bearing only IgM antibody (which cannot provide the second signal because phagocytes do not have receptors for the Fc of IgM) and complement might remain on the surface of the CR1-bearing cell rather than being internalized. Although the complex sits on the surface of the CR1-bearing cell, factor I has a chance to cleave the bound C3b to the C3dg stage because of the co-factor activity provided by the CR1.

Evidence that this activity occurs in vivo is provided by studies of the trafficking of C3-coated erythrocytes that have been sensitized with IgM antibody and C3b but not IgG. These cells are transiently sequestered in the liver but then reappear in the circulation bearing C3d (Frank et al., 1977). Because dendritic cells and B cells express CR2, which binds C3d, this type of processing could play an important role in inducing subsequent IgG responses after initial complement fixation directed by IgM natural antibody.

CR2 (CD21)

Although also a member of the RCA family, and composed of short consensus repeats that resemble those of CR1, CR2 (CD21) is a distinct receptor that binds C3d, C3dg, and to a lesser extent iC3b. CR2 is most prominently expressed on B lymphocytes and plays an important role in stimulating and modulating the activity of these cells (Fearon and Carroll, 2000). CR2 in the cell membrane generally associates with CD19 and a molecule termed TAPA-1. Co-engagement of the B-cell antigen receptor (i.e., surface immunoglobulin) and the CR2-CD19 complex occurs when a C3d-bearing antigen engages the antigen receptor. This can enhance and prolong antigen signaling (Cherukuri et al., 2001a, 2001b). When antigens bearing C3dg fragments are offered to B cells in vitro, less antigen is required to induce any given degree of antibody production compared with antigen that does not bear complement fragments (Dempsey et al., 1996) (see Role in Afferent Arm of Immune Responses).

CR3 (CD11b/CD18)

The initial cleavage of bound C3b by factor I in the presence of H forms iC3b (see Fig. 7-2). This iC3b is inactive in both classical and alternative pathway convertases and has a greatly reduced affinity for CR1. However, this form of the molecule still has important opsonic activity (Stossel et al., 1975) and binds to a distinct receptor called CR3 that is found mainly on phagocytes. CR3 is not a member of the RCA family but is a heterodimer with an α chain of 155,000 daltons (CD11b) and a β chain of 95,000 daltons (CD18).

CR3 belongs to a family of cell surface molecules called *integrins* (because they share this particular β chain, they are referred to as β2-integrins), which are extremely widely distributed throughout nature and which generally are important in cellular adhesion and cell-cell interactions in a variety of cells and circumstances. Within this leukocyte β-integrin family, three different α chains (CD11a, CD11b, CD11c) determine the individual binding activity of each member, whereas the common β chain is responsible for holding the α chains in the membrane (Sanchez-Madrid et al., 1983). Several different monoclonal antibodies, including Mac1, OKM1, Leu15 and Mo1,

have been made against CD11b/CD18. Most of these antibodies block the binding of iC3b-coated erythrocytes to human neutrophils and monocytes and inhibit other functions of these cells as well, emphasizing the multifunctional activity of this class of proteins (Arnaout et al., 1983; Beller et al., 1982; Wright et al., 1983).

Thus, in addition to the site to which iC3b binds, CR3 has additional binding sites that allow it to function as the neutrophils' major adherence protein, playing a critical role in these cells' ability to attach to and migrate along extracellular matrices. This molecule also carries the ability to interact with intracellular endothelial cell adhesion molecule-1 (ICAM-1). This interaction is necessary (in most vascular beds) for the neutrophils to emigrate from the circulation to reach sites of inflammation.

Deficiency of CD18 severely inhibits a number of neutrophil functions besides phagocytosis of iC3b-bearing particles and results in the clinical syndrome leukocyte adhesion deficiency-1 (LAD), discussed later. CR3 and other β-integrins also have lectinlike binding sites and can interact directly with β-glucans, mannans, and other polysaccharides on the surface of bacteria and tumor cells (Thornton et al., 1996) (see Chapter 20).

Integrins are capable of both "outside-in" and "inside-out" signaling. Outside-in signals allow the migrating phagocyte to behave differently on different extracellular matrices, and, when ligated by certain extracellular matrix proteins or bacterial polysaccharides, these integrins can activate phagocytosis in the absence of IgG (Zhou and Brown, 1993). The inside-out signaling that occurs with CR3 is manifested by a marked change in the affinity of the integrin for certain ligands, which occurs transiently when neutrophils are activated (Diamond and Springer, 1994). When the cell is activated, the receptor's affinity is greatly increased and there is also a quick upregulation of the number of CD11b/CD18 molecules expressed on the cell surface, which are rapidly translocated from an intracellular pool.

These two phenomena together account for the increased adhesiveness of activated neutrophils to endothelial cells and surfaces. The transient nature of the increase in affinity of the adhesion site is responsible for the rapid aggregation and disaggregation that occurs when neutrophils in suspension are treated with chemoattractants. Rapid cycles of increased then decreased affinity of the integrins, as well as cycling of internalization and externalization, likely are important in cell movement.

A fully activated neutrophil may express on its plasma membrane 2×10^5 or more CR3 molecules per cell (Berger et al., 1984). The activated neutrophil may also express more than 5×10^4 CR1 molecules. Thus neutrophils can rapidly and firmly bind a large number of targets coated with C3b or iC3b, forming impressive rosettes in in vitro studies. If an appropriate second signal or state of preactivation is also present, the neutrophils will rapidly ingest and in most cases lyse or kill their targets.

CR4 (CD11c/CD18)

There are two other members of the leukocyte β2-integrin family: LFA-1 (CD11a/CD18), which is an important co-stimulatory factor in lymphocyte activation but is not prominently expressed on phagocytes; and a protein, originally called P150/95, which was renamed CR4 and identified as CD11c/CD18 because of its homology with the other members of its family. CR4 has relatively weak affinity for iC3b, C3dg, and C3d, and it is the most prominently expressed member of this family on tissue macrophages (Berger et al., 1994; Myones et al., 1988). Although some researchers have proposed that it helps to promote phagocytosis, neither its exact binding specificity nor its physiologic role is clear. The observation that transiently sequestered sensitized erythrocytes are released from the liver bearing C3d and have normal survival in the circulation (Frank et al., 1977) suggests that CR4-mediated phagocytosis of C3d-coated targets is not of major importance in vivo.

However, studies that show that crosslinking of CD11c on human monocytes by monoclonal antibodies induces cytokine and chemokine synthesis (Rezzonico et al., 2001) suggest that CR4 might play a role in inflammatory responses initiated at sites of complement activation. Dendritic cells may be characterized as belonging to subsets that differ in their degree of CR4 (CD11c) expression, but it is not clear whether the level of CR4 expression correlates with preferential presentation of C3d-bearing antigens or other complement-related functional differences.

C1q Receptors

Several laboratories have reported activation of phagocytes and other cells of the immune system by antigen-antibody complexes bearing C1q or by C1q-coated surfaces, implying the existence of receptors that mediated the observed responses. Enhancement of phagocytosis in the presence of C1q has also been reported. Characterization of the receptors has been made difficult in part because C1q resembles other members of the collectin family, which share homologous features, including multivalency, extended collagen-like domains, and lectinlike activity that generally requires Ca^{++} or other cations for activity and that all bind similar ligands.

Other members of this family include lung surfactant proteins A and D, mannan-binding lectin, and conglutinin (Tenner, 1999; Thiel and Reid, 1989). Many of these proteins play an important role in innate immunity. In addition, C1q seems to react with several different proteins that normally reside intracellularly but that may be released from the cells at sites of inflammatory damage, such as calreticulin, making their role as receptors difficult to define.

A consensus seems to be forming that a heavily glycosylated cell surface molecule exists, which has been termed *C1qRP* (C1q receptor for phagocytosis) and which also appears to bind mannose-binding lectin and surfactant protein A and promotes phagocytosis of targets bearing these collectins (Tenner, 1999). A cDNA clone coding for a protein with 631 amino acids but with a molecular weight of 126,000 daltons because of its glycosylation has been isolated that corresponds with this protein, and monoclonal antibodies against it have been prepared. Crosslinking of the protein on the surface of human monocytes and macrophages with these antibodies or the collectins enhances the phagocytic activity of the cells (Nepomuceno et al., 1999).

Besides this C1qRP, proteins that bind the globular heads of C1q have also been described (Ghebrehiwet and Peerschke, 1998) and are referred to as gC1q-R, but their role in phagocytosis and other physiologic activities of the immune system is less clear. It may be that this binding activity represents synergistic effects of multiple low-affinity interactions of certain proteins with the IgG binding sites or other surface features of the multiple globular domains of C1q.

C3a, C4a, and C5a Receptors

Distinct receptors for C3a and C5a have been identified and cloned (Wetsel, 1995). Both receptors belong to the superfamily of receptors that have seven membrane-spanning segments whose signaling is mediated by their coupling with G proteins. The C5a receptor has been designated CD88, but the C3a receptor has not yet been assigned a CD designation. It is not clear if there is a distinct receptor for C4a or whether its weak activity is due to an ability to bind to the C3a receptor because of its homology with C3a.

These receptors are clearly expressed on cells of myeloid origin, including neutrophils, monocytes, and mast cells, but controversy exists regarding whether they are expressed on nonmyeloid epithelial or parenchymal cells. Most recent studies have shown that although there is messenger RNA (mRNA) and receptor protein expression on uninflamed lung epithelial cells, liver parenchymal cells, and keratinocytes, the expression of both proteins is clearly increased by inflammatory stimuli (Drouin et al., 2001b; Haviland et al., 1995; Rothermel et al., 2000). The presence of C3a and C5a receptors on lung epithelial and smooth muscle cells may provide one explanation for non–histamine-mediated local allergic responses (e.g., bronchoconstriction and increased mucous secretion to antigen exposure) (Drouin et al., 2001a), in addition to the responses induced by mast cell mediators recruited by their anaphylatoxin receptors.

Binding of C3a and C5a to their receptors in some cell types, including keratinocytes, peripheral blood mononuclear cells, and astrocytes, has been reported to either induce or enhance the production of IL-6 by these cells (Fayyazi et al., 1999; Fischer et al., 1999; Sayah et al., 1999; Takabayashi et al., 1998). In this way a locally produced complement fragment could help induce and amplify a systemic response to infection.

COMPLEMENT IN ANTIMICROBIAL DEFENSE

Opsonization and Phagocytosis

The high concentration of C3 in plasma and the presence of multiple different receptors for C3 fragments reflect the importance of this component in facilitating phagocytosis of invading microorganisms, a process termed *opsonization*. Although another important contribution of the complement system to phagocytic host defenses in vivo is generation of C5a, which attracts and activates neutrophils and mononuclear phagocytes (see Anaphylatoxins), it may be argued that the binding of C3 to an organism and the interactions of opsonic fragments of C3 with their receptors on the phagocytes is the most important host defense activity of the complement system.

CR1 and CR3 are the receptors most important in phagocytosis, and C3b and iC3b are, correspondingly, the most important complement opsonins. In most experimental systems, the interactions of these ligands and receptors facilitates adherence, which may be quite tight and stable but is insufficient to induce phagocytosis per se.

Activation of the cellular processes involved in internalizing the adherent target generally requires a second signal, which is most often provided by IgG. Early studies of the quantitative requirements for adherence versus internalization showed that if C3b was present on a test particle such as a sheep erythrocyte, the addition of only a small amount of IgG, which by itself could not even promote adherence, induced rapid and extensive phagocytosis (Ehlenberger and Nusenzweig, 1977). This is due to signaling through activating receptors for the Fc of IgG. However, because there are not similar receptors for the Fc of IgM, that antibody does not provide the necessary activating signal. Similar observations have been made for the clearance of specifically sensitized erythrocytes from the human circulation and in experimental bacteremia in animals (Frank et al., 1977; Joiner et al., 1984).

Particles composed of yeast cell walls (zymosan), as well as some bacteria, are ingested when coated with C3b and or iC3b alone. In those situations the second signal is likely provided by the interaction of β-glucans, mannans, or other repeating polysaccharide units with lectinlike sites on CR3 or other lectinlike receptors on the phagocyte surface. Phagocytes that are adherent to extracellular matrices may be in an already activated state in which the second signal either is not required (Pommier et al., 1983) or is being provided continuously by CR3 in its role as the integrin-adherence protein, in what would be considered an example of outside-in signaling (Zhou and Brown, 1993). The enhanced phagocytosis of C3b-coated particles by mononuclear cells adhering to plates covered with C1q may be an analogous phenomenon.

Similarly, cytokines such as interferon-γ, certain chemoattractants, and chemicals such as phorbol esters may induce a state of partial activation or priming of the phagocytes such that there is no need for a second signal (Bianco et al., 1975; Griffin and Griffin, 1979; Wright and Silverstein, 1982). Several cellular alterations, including increased receptor expression, clustering or other changes in the distribution of the CR1 and CR3 on the surface of the cell, alterations in the linkage of the receptors to cytoskeletal elements, and preassembly of machinery required for internalization, may all occur as part of these priming phenomena.

Chemoattractants, Leukocyte Activation, and Leukocyte Migration

C3a, C5a, and to a lesser extent C4a have anaphylatoxin activity that is mainly manifested by their binding to specific receptors on mast cells. This causes mast cell activation and release of mediators (discussed later). Besides anaphylatoxin activity, C5a and its des-Arg derivative account for most of the chemoattractant and leukocyte stimulating activities of the complement system. Both C5a and C5a des-Arg exert powerful chemoattractant activity for neutrophils, monocytes, and macrophages, which is mediated by a specific receptor, CD88, that links with G proteins to initiate a signaling sequence, culminating in activation of phosphatidyl inositol 3′ kinase and a marked influx of free Ca++ into the cytosol. These in turn mediate translocation to the plasma membrane of intracellular vesicles containing several important receptors, including additional CR1 and CR3 molecules and additional chemoattractant receptors, increasing the response to a subsequent activating stimulus.

Chemotaxis and priming or full activation of the microbicidal oxidase system are also induced by binding of C5a and C5a des-Arg to their receptor. Because the most prominent difference between C5a and its homologs C3a and C4a is the presence of a large polysaccharide moiety (which accounts for 3000 daltons of its 11,000 dalton molecular weight) in C5a only, it seems likely that participation of this polysaccharide is important in the activity of C5a/C5a des-Arg. Although the affinities with which C5a and C5a des-Arg bind to neutrophils are quite high, in the nM range, their binding can be significantly enhanced by the presence of an additional serum protein called Gc-globulin or vitamin D–binding protein. This protein can thus be considered a co-chemotaxin or helper factor for C5a and C5a des-Arg, (Binder et al., 1999; DiMartino et al., 2001). Early reports suggesting that the C5b67 complex was the major complement-derived chemoattractant probably reflect the effects of C5a that had incompletely dissociated from the complex.

Interestingly, several different pathogens have developed adaptations that diminish the ability of neutrophils to respond to C5a/C5a des-Arg, either by cleaving or downregulating expression of the receptor (Jagels et al., 1996; Veldkamp et al., 2000) or by degrading C5a itself (Cheng et al., 2001). C5a/C5a des-Arg–mediated responses have been reported to be decreased in patients with human immunodeficiency virus infection (HIV), which correlates with decreased expression of CD88 (Meddows-Taylor et al., 2001). Although the means by which the HIV infection affects this molecule and other neutrophil functions has not yet been elucidated, it has been suggested that the resulting neutrophil dysfunction may contribute to the increased incidence of bacterial infection that is particularly seen in HIV-infected children.

As alluded to earlier, circulating neutrophils express very few CR1 or CR3 molecules on their surface, but the expression of these molecules increases more than 10-fold within minutes when the cells are activated by chemoattractants or other stimuli (Berger et al., 1984). Preformed receptors are stored intracellularly in "secretory vesicles," which rapidly translocate to the plasma membrane in response to chemoattractants or other activation signals (Sengeløv et al., 1994). In addition, there is transient activation of binding sites on CR3 (CD11b/CD18). The latter is believed to be the major phenomenon responsible for the transient aggregation and then spontaneous disaggregation observed when neutrophils in suspension are exposed to chemoattractants in vitro (Jacob et al., 1980).

Similar aggregation, occurring in response to intravascular complement activation and formation of C5a/C5a des-Arg, may be responsible for neutrophil sequestration in and plugging of pulmonary capillaries, which can contribute to ARDS in a number of situations (Craddock et al., 1977; Jacob et al., 1980). This phenomenon is also responsible for trapping aggregated neutrophils in the pulmonary capillaries during hemodialysis and cardiopulmonary bypass, as discussed in Nonimmunologic Complement Activation.

The neutrophils of newborn babies are partially deficient in CR3 and do not increase expression of this molecule normally when they are activated, although they do increase CR1 expression as well as adults' neutrophils (Abughali et al., 1994; Anderson et al., 1990; Bruce et al., 1987). The deficient CR3 expression likely contributes to decreased adherence, chemotaxis, and phagocytic activity of newborns' cells, markedly increasing their susceptibility to infection.

In addition to the integrin CR3, another class of adhesion molecules, called *selectins*, is also involved in neutrophil-endothelial cell interactions (Cronstein and Weissmann, 1993; Kishimoto and Rothlein, 1994; Tedder et al., 1995). Under normal conditions, circulating neutrophils have only weak interactions with the endothelium, which cause them to roll along the vessel wall, pushed forward by the flow but not adhering firmly. This weak or rolling adherence is caused by the interactions of L-selectin (CD62L) and other neutrophil surface proteins that bear polysaccharides corresponding to the blood group antigen sialyl-Lewis X with the ligands P- and E-selectin (CD62P and CD62E) on the endothelium (Hogg, 1992).

When endothelial cells are activated (i.e., by lipopolysaccharide [LPS], IL-1, tumor necrosis factor [TNF], or other mediators likely to be present in the vicinity of sites of infection or inflammation), they increase expression of P- and E-selectins. This increases their overall adhesiveness for the neutrophils and slows them down, increasing their chances of being activated by C5a, IL-8, or other chemoattractants or cytokines.

Those activation signals in turn cause shedding of the weak adhesion molecule L-selectin (CD62L) from the neutrophil at the same time as they cause increases in the number and affinity of CD11b/CD18 (CR3) molecules on the neutrophil surface (Springer, 1994). The major endothelial ligand for CD11b/CD18 is ICAM-1 (CD54), whose expression is also induced by TNF and IL-1. The interaction between ICAM-1 and β-integrins is quite strong and holds the neutrophil in place despite the shear forces of capillary flow. The rolling movement thus stops, and the neutrophil begins migrating out of the circulation.

ICAM-1 is also a ligand for CD11a/CD18 (LFA-1), and similar interactions are involved in adherence and then extravasation of lymphocytes, monocytes, and eosinophils. These types of cells have an additional type of integrin known as very late after activation antigen (VLA-4), which binds to an endothelial cell ligand called vascular cell adhesion molecule (VCAM). Because VLA-4 is not prominently expressed on neutrophils, the relative expression of ICAM versus VCAM can influence the cellular characteristics of the local inflammatory response. ICAM and VCAM are members of the immunoglobulin superfamily.

The selectins, on the other hand, all contain the types of structural motifs found in CR1 and the other RCA family proteins. Blocking of any of the three types of adhesion molecules—selectins, integrins, or ICAMs/VCAM—by monoclonal antibodies can be used to inhibit or modify immune and inflammatory responses in animal models, and they are being evaluated as new forms of therapy for a variety of immunologic and inflammatory diseases.

Agents that block platelet integrins are already in use to prevent platelet aggregation and clotting after coronary artery angioplasty.

Leukocyte Adhesion Defects

The three different α chains of the leukocyte integrin family of which CR3 (CD11b/CD18) and CR4 (CD11c/CD18) are members are all dependent on the common β chain for proper insertion into the cell membrane. Deficiency of CD18 thus causes an inability to express any of these proteins on the plasma membrane and results in the clinical syndrome LAD-1 (Etzioni and Harlan, 1999). Clinical features include delayed separation of the umbilical cord; persistent leukocytosis, because the cells cannot migrate out of the circulation; and recurrent infections (Arnaout et al., 1982; Bowen et al., 1982; Crowley et al., 1980). Other immunologic abnormalities are also present (see Chapter 20).

Severe and moderate forms of LAD-1 exist, differing in the degree of protein deficiency, which are caused by different mutations. Neutrophils from these patients have diminished ability to bind and ingest iC3b-coated particles and may also be deficient in phagocytosing other particles as well, reflecting the multiple functions and roles in signaling and adherence served by these β-integrins. They also demonstrate decreased adherence to surfaces and chemotaxis in vivo.

Patients with LAD-2 have defects in producing the sialyl-Lewis X polysaccharide component of L-selectin production and an increased susceptibility to infection. Their neutrophils adhere poorly to endothelial surfaces, and their migration to sites of infection is impaired by the absence of this ligand for P- and E-selectin. This confirms the importance of that first step in the overall process of recruitment of neutrophils from the circulation (Etzioni and Harlan, 1999).

Neutrophils from neonates are also partially deficient in L-selectin. This may be due to high levels of granulocyte-macrophage colony-stimulating factor (GM-CSF), which, like other cytokines that activate mature neutrophils, causes shedding of L-selectin (Koenig et al., 1996) (see Chapter 22).

Interactions of Complement with Bacteria

Complement is critically important in defense against both gram-positive and gram-negative organisms (Joiner et al., 1984), and increased susceptibility to bacterial infection is a major problem in patients with complement deficiencies (see Chapter 21). In the case of gram-negative organisms, binding of complement to the organism surface may cause direct lysis of the bacterium. In many cases this is due to activation of complement in the absence of antibody, via the alternative or MBL pathway. In the case of gram-positive organisms, a thick peptidoglycan layer within the cell wall prevents late-acting complement proteins from penetrating to the cell membrane. Thus gram-positive organisms are not susceptible to the lytic action of complement. However, complement-mediated defense plays an essential role in protection against gram-positive organisms by providing opsonins on the organism's surface.

Bacteria have evolved many mechanisms for eluding complement attack, and we see in the development of the adaptive immune system the generation of mechanisms to overcome these microbial changes (Moffitt and Frank, 1994). Thus gram-negative organisms have evolved proteins that bind activated complement proteins and prevent formation of a lytic membrane attack complex or the insertion of the activated membrane attack complex proteins into the cell membrane. In some cases, microbes such as E. coli and T. pallidum have evolved mechanisms to coat their surface with sialic acid, which promotes degradation of opsonically active complement fragments by the complement regulatory factors H and I. Polysaccharide capsules and long side chains on LPS, which project out at some distance from the surfaces of many gram-positive and gram-negative bacteria, may provide docking sites for complement that are far from the bacterial surface. These adaptations thus protect the organism from complement-mediated attack or phagocytosis.

As discussed earlier, the complement system appears phylogenetically at a point before the evolution of specific antibody. We can thus postulate that one function of specific antibody is its ability to recognize the capsule or the surface components of the bacterium and activate complement at that surface, so that the complement fragments will be available to interact with receptors on phagocytes. Interestingly, with many gram-negative organisms, the antibody appears to direct deposition of complement via the classical pathway onto critical points on the bacterial surface, where they can cause lysis. In the absence of antibody, the complement proteins bind to different sites on the bacterium where they do no harm.

In a primitive way, complement provides a chemical system that allows the host to distinguish self from nonself and to selectively attack nonself (see Role of the Surface/Substrate). On the surface of some microorganisms, C3b is often deposited in what is termed a *protected site*, meaning protected from interaction with factors H and I and therefore protected from degradation. The C3b remains hemolytically active and able to activate the alternative pathway, thus promoting further complement attack on the organism. These organisms would be considered good activators of the alternative pathway and are thus not likely to be important pathogens in patients with a normal complement system.

On cells of the body, there are many regulatory molecules and cell membrane structures (see Regulation of Complement Activation) that facilitate the rapid degradation of C3b, so that it can do no harm to normal host cells. The role of membrane sialic acid in facilitating C3b degradation by factors H and I has been detailed earlier. Thus when deposited on self, the complement proteins are degraded, but when deposited on nonself they remain active and cause opsonization or destruction. The distinction between self and nonself by the complement system is primitive, and the adaptive immune response (specific antibody) leads to amplified and directed destruction of microbes in a far more effective way.

Viral Neutralization

In general, viruses must attach to specific docking sites to invade host cells. The binding of complement to viral adhesion proteins may preclude such binding and thereby protect against invasion. It is known that deposition of C1 and C4 on herpes simplex viruses will partially protect against viral attachment and invasion. With enveloped viruses, complement can assemble the membrane attack complex and form a lytic lesion in the surface of the viral envelope, much like the lesion formed in the surface of the cell. This can lead to loss of integrity of the virus and ultimately its destruction.

As in the case with bacteria, antibody can often direct complement attack to sensitive sites on the pathogen (Parren and Burton, 2001). Thus certain viruses will bind complement via activation of the alternative pathway in the absence of antibody, but the complement does little damage. In the presence of specific antibody, the complement attack is directed to critical sites and damage to the virus occurs (Vasantha et al., 1988).

It is of interest that retroviruses may activate complement directly in the absence of antibody via the classical pathway, by direct binding of C1. In general, this nondirected complement activation does not lead to viral neutralization.

Molecular Mimicry of Complement Proteins by Infectious Agents and Other Mechanisms of Evasion of Complement Attack

Microorganisms have evolved virtually every mechanism imaginable for evasion of complement attack and often use mimicry of complement proteins to increase their pathogenicity. Space precludes a detailed discussion, but several reviews are available (Cooper, 1991, 1998). It is fascinating that some viruses have chosen to use complement regulatory proteins as docking sites for invasion of cells or to protect themselves (Fishelson, 1994). Thus measles virus invades cells by binding to membrane co-factor protein (CD46), thereby facilitating entry. Coxsackie and other viruses bind to other complement proteins. Protein M on streptococci binds factor H, thereby helping to protect the organism by facilitating degradation of C3b.

Perhaps even more astonishing is the fact that Epstein-Barr virus (EBV) codes for a 9–amino acid sequence at the amino terminus of a 350-residue surface glycoprotein that is similar to a sequence in human C3. This sequence allows EBV to bind to cells bearing CR2 (CD21, the C3d receptor) (Ahearn and Fearon, 1989; Nemerow et al., 1989). Such cells include B lymphocytes, thereby explaining the propensity for EBV to invade B lymphocytes.

Mycobacteria may become coated with complement and are ingested following interaction with macrophage complement receptors. They are not killed by the macrophages but undergo a complex intracellular process that ultimately leads to the mycobacterium invading and prospering in an intracellular location, to which it gained entry by the cell's own complement receptors.

Protozoa have also evolved mechanisms that allow them to either utilize or prevent complement attack in maintaining their life cycle in the host. Some even bind complement control proteins, such as factor H, when invading the bloodstream, thereby facilitating the degradation of C3 and protecting themselves from opsonization or attack. In general, pathogenic parasites that have a blood stage have evolved mechanisms to resist complement attack. The form of the parasite that invades cells may become susceptible to complement because it no longer needs to resist complement attack and no longer expresses the protein that protected its blood stage.

COMPLEMENT IN INFLAMMATION AND IMMUNE RESPONSES

Anaphylatoxins

As discussed previously, activation of C4, C3, and C5 is accompanied by release of C4a, C3a, and C5a, 74– to 77–amino acid residue peptides from the NH$_2$ end of the α chain of each molecule. These small peptides do not participate in further reactions of the activation sequence but remain in the fluid phase. C4a has a molecular weight of 8650, is nonglycosylated, and has only weak biologic activity (Gorski et al., 1979). C3a is a 9000-dalton peptide released when C3 is cleaved by the convertase of either the classical or alternative pathway. C5a is a similar but glycosylated peptide with a molecular weight of 11,000; it is released by corresponding cleavage of C5. These fragments have similar amino acid sequences and contain a helical portion, as well as several disulfide bonds that form a rigid, complex loop in the peptide chain (Hugli, 1984). The higher molecular weight of C5a is due to the presence of a large carbohydrate moiety that accounts for 25% to 30% of this fragment's weight. These molecules are termed anaphylatoxins because they cause mast cells to release histamine and other mediators and when injected systemically cause a response that resembles anaphylaxis. Their activity is induced by binding to specific receptors for C3a and C5a on the mast cells (see C3a, C4a, and C5a Receptors).

The anaphylatoxin activity of C3a is about 100 times greater than that of C4a when measured by the wheal-and-flare response of normal skin. The degranulation of mast cells responsible for this is independent of IgE and is noncytotoxic for the mast cells. Although many of the responses to the anaphylatoxins are secondary effects of the mast cell–derived mediators, it is believed that some smooth muscle contraction is induced as a direct effect of C3a binding (Hugli and Müller-Eberhard, 1978). In addition, Marom and colleagues (1985) have shown that C3a induces mucus secretion by human lung explants that is not histamine dependent.

The anaphylatoxin activity of C5a is approximately 100- to 200-fold that of C3a in human skin. Besides its anaphylatoxin activity, C5a is an important chemoattractant for neutrophils and monocytes (discussed earlier) (Taylor et al., 2001). C3a is apparently devoid of this activity, and C5a is now believed to be the major chemotactic factor formed during activation of the complement system (see Chemoattractants, Leukocyte Activation, and Leukocyte Migration).

All these anaphylatoxins are rapidly inactivated by serum carboxypeptidase-N, which cleaves an essential carboxyl terminal arginine from each of these peptides. Although these des-Arg forms lose most of their anaphylatoxin activity, C5a des-Arg retains considerable chemoattractant and neutrophil-activating activity for which the carbohydrate moiety is important (Gerard and Hugli, 1981).

Radioimmunoassays for these anaphylatoxins are used as sensitive monitors of complement activation.

The presence of circulating C3a des-Arg most reliably reflects in vivo anaphylatoxin generation because the affinity of C5a for cell surface receptors is so high that this peptide remains in the circulation only transiently (Chenowith and Hugli, 1980). Because release of these highly active factors allows complement activation to mimic classical IgE-mediated anaphylaxis, use of these assays should lead to a marked improvement in understanding a variety of apparently non–IgE-mediated anaphylactoid reactions.

Control of Inflammation

A major contribution of complement to inflammatory responses is provided by the anaphylatoxin and chemoattractant activities of C3a and C5a/C5a des-Arg (see previous section). Classical pathway activation at sites where antibody complexes with antigen on foreign materials or microbes, or where autoantibodies are reacting with self-antigens, leads to the generation of these peptides. As discussed, the peptides bind to specific receptors on tissue mast cells, causing the release of mediators, including histamine and arachidonic acid metabolites, which will increase local vascular permeability and can cause contraction of visceral smooth muscle and glandular secretion. Obviously, in this way the reaction of preformed IgG or IgM antibodies with an inhaled antigen in the airways could mimic an IgE-mediated response to the same antigen.

The syndrome of urticarial vasculitis and other situations in which urticaria is associated with serum sickness or other manifestations of circulating antigen-antibody complexes are also almost certainly due in part to mast cell mediators whose release has been triggered by the complement-derived anaphylatoxins.

Targeted disruption of the gene for the C5a receptor in knockout mice thus results in a marked amelioration of immune complex–mediated lung injury and inhibition of the reverse passive arthus reaction (a model in which antigen and antibody are combined in tissue) in skin and the peritoneal cavity (Hopken et al., 1997). Interestingly, this also results in decreased production of TNF and IL-6. It is likely that production of those cytokines represents contributions from local tissue cells bearing C5a receptors, as well as from the secondary wave of cells migrating into the tissue in response to mast cell–derived chemoattractants and C5a/C5a des-Arg.

Activities such as these, which lead to tissue injury and end organ damage in immune complex models, are really double-edged swords. The same activities—increasing vascular permeability and activating and attracting phagocytes—may be important in protecting the host when the stimulus is infectious. Thus the same C5a receptor knockout mice that are protected from lung injury in immune complex challenges become extremely sensitive to overwhelming lethal infection following intratracheal challenge with inocula of viable *Pseudomonas aeruginosa* that are readily cleared and killed by normal mice (Hopken et al., 1996).

In some knockout mouse models, C3-deficient mice have been shown to have decreased IL-4 production, decreased antigen-specific IgE, decreased airway hyperresponsiveness, and decreased eosinophilic inflammation of the lung in sensitization/challenge protocols used to mimic allergic inflammation or asthma (Drouin et al., 2001a, 2001b). In a different model, in which the C3a receptor gene was knocked out, there was increased lethality after endotoxin challenge, which correlated with increased production of IL-1 (Kildsgaard et al., 2000).

These models provide provocative results implying broader roles of complement in regulation of immune and inflammatory responses than have been previously appreciated. However, it is not clear whether knockout models necessarily indicate direct roles for the complement components or their fragments or indirect roles of already recognized functions of complement (e.g., facilitating clearance of antigens, activating the alternative pathway, and controlling trafficking of immune cells exerting local immunomodulatory effects).

Complement can be activated at sites of tissue and cellular injury, either by exposure of sites to which natural or autoantibodies can bind or exposure of cellular components that support activation of either the classical or alternative pathway. Demonstration of increased circulating levels of C3a des-Arg or increased expression of CR1 and CR3 on circulating neutrophils in burn patients (Moore et al., 1986) and after ischemia/reperfusion injury suggest that this occurs in vivo, as does demonstration of neoantigens associated with formation of the membrane attack complex on vascular endothelial cells in postischemic tissue (Weisman et al., 1990). The increased adhesiveness of neutrophils exposed to circulating C5a/C5a des-Arg and their attraction to sites of tissue damage may be viewed as being beneficial or deleterious, depending on the exact circumstances and the etiology of the inciting stimulus and whether the subsequent response is viewed as being part of healing or injury.

In many ways the normal physiologic function of the complement system results in removal or eradication of stimuli that would be dangerous or injurious if not dealt with properly and efficiently. Thus killing of microorganisms by complement lysis or complement-facilitated phagocytosis will often terminate responses to infectious stimuli. Complement is important in solubilizing antigen-antibody complexes and in directing the trafficking of soluble immune complexes to macrophages of the reticuloendothelial system, which are best equipped to phagocytose and dispose of them without inducing tissue damage. Effective mobilization, removal, and disposal of antigen fragments of killed infectious agents (and perhaps tissue fragments and intracellular proteins that could be autoantigens) are likely important mechanisms by which the complement system may limit or prevent inappropriate inflammation (Davies and Walport, 1998; Walport, 2001).

A well-documented example of the importance of these mechanisms in normal body physiology and immunologic homeostasis is provided by the observation of high levels of circulating antigen-antibody complexes and the renal deposition of antibodies after treatment of sinusitis in a C3-deficient patient, who went on to develop severe glomerulonephritis (Berger et al., 1983). Similar observations have been made in other patients with early classical pathway component or C3 deficiencies, confirming this physiologic role for complement (Walport, 2001).

Immune Complex Solubilization and Clearance

Complexes of antibodies with antigens are often found in the circulation. Antigens enter the body via the gastrointestinal (GI) tract, via infections such as in viral illness, or via invasion following breaks in the skin, for example, and the adaptive immune response produces antibody to deal with these foreign antigens. Immune complexes may be formed in the tissues, at sites of infection, or in the circulation. In the appropriate circumstances, depending on the class of antibody and the stochiometry of the antigen and antibodies combining, they may activate complement. It has been known for many years that such immune complexes may be solubilized by their interaction with complement, disrupting the antigen-antibody lattice and making the complexes smaller and perhaps more easily phagocytosed (Davies and Walport, 1998; Schifferli et al., 1986).

When complement binds to immune complexes, C3b is deposited on the complex. The complex can interact with cells in the blood that bear C3b receptors (CR1, CD35). The most prevalent source of cells in the blood with CR1 is erythrocytes, which have 400 to 1200 CR1 per cell (Cornacoff et al., 1983). Immune complexes coated with C3b bind rapidly to the circulating erythrocytes because of these complement receptors and are effectively removed from the circulation by phagocytes in the reticuloendothelial system (RES), limiting their deposition in tissues. As the red cells circulate to the liver and spleen, they come in contact with RES macrophages that are capable of removing the immune complexes from the surface of the red cells. During this process, the macrophages may remove some of the CR1, as well as the complexes.

Thus patients with lupus erythematosus have a decreased number of complement receptors on their red blood cells. Indeed, normal red cells infused into patients with active lupus will lose their complement receptors. However, following partial loss of their complement receptors, the red cells return to the circulation and have perfectly normal survival (Walport, 2001).

Role in Afferent Arm of Immune Responses

It appears that complement plays a role in multiple aspects of the afferent immune response. Antigens that activate complement, either spontaneously via the alternative pathway or because of the presence of natural antibody that binds to the antigen and then activates the classical pathway, may become coated with C3b, which may then be degraded, leaving the C3d fragment. B lymphocytes and follicular dendritic cells have on their surface receptors (CD21, CR2) for this fragment. As noted earlier, antigens with bound C3d can bind to B lymphocytes or antigen-presenting cells through CR2, as well as antigen-specific receptors, thereby amplifying the antigenic signal by as much as 10,000-fold. Co-engagement of CR2 along with antigen receptor also results in more rapid and efficient production of antigen peptide/class II major histocompatibility complex (MHC) molecule complexes on the B-cell surface than engagement of the antigen receptor alone (Cherukuri et al., 2001a).

Studies demonstrating tyrosine phosphorylation of several different intracellular signaling molecules and activation of phosphatidyl inositol triphosphate kinase upon ligation or crosslinking of CR2 suggest that in addition to focusing or facilitating binding of antigens bearing C3d, direct signaling is an important part of these effects (Barel et al., 2001) and that co-engagement of antigen receptor and CR2 prolongs these signals (Cherukuri et al., 2001b). Antigens and antigen-antibody complexes with bound C3 can localize to follicular dendritic cells of the germinal center and persist there, bound to the surface of these cells, thus providing continuous stimulation of B lymphocytes and contributing to long-term immunologic memory.

Complement-deficient animals have impaired immune memory (Pepys, 1976). C4 deficiency in humans and guinea pigs diminishes the secondary response to reimmunization with phage antigen ϕX-174 and interferes with the normal switch from IgM to IgG production (Jackson et al., 1979). This defect can be corrected by administration of C4 (to the guinea pigs), indicating that it is not a separate linked defect (Ochs et al., 1983). Complement depletion by administration of cobra venom factor to experimental animals also decreases antibody responses, particularly to T-dependent antigens (Pepys, 1976). In this situation, as in C4 deficiency, the anamnestic response and the switch to IgG production are affected more than the primary response.

Finally, complement appears to contribute to the process of negative selection whereby lymphocytes with high affinity for self-antigen are eliminated from the immune repertoire. Many complement-deficient individuals and C1q- and C4-deficient mice have a high degree of autoimmunity and failure of normal tolerance mechanisms (reviewed in Walport, 2001).

MOLECULAR BIOLOGY AND SYNTHESIS

Organization of Genes

The genes for each of the complement proteins, receptors, and control proteins have been identified and sequenced (Crawford and Alper, 2000). Several of the complement components have multiple alleles; these allotypes can be distinguished by variations in their electrophoretic mobility (Alper and Rosen, 1976). Although there are differences in the functions of allotypes of the two C4 loci (discussed later), the allotypes of C3 are similar in functional activity.

The genes for C2, C4, and factor B are on chromosome 6 as part of the MHC (Alper, 1981; Colten et al., 1981). Determination of an individual's *complotype* (the allotype of each polymorphic protein) correlates with the incidence of certain diseases, such as juvenile diabetes mellitus. The reasons for this association are not yet known; however, the increasing information on complement in the afferent immune response makes it likely that this is not a chance association.

There are two separate C4 loci in the genome of humans and animals; alleles at both positions have been described, and in some individuals there are duplications of these alleleles. Interestingly, the protein coded for by one of these genes (C4B) has more hemolytic activity than the other (C4A). Furthermore, C4A tends to form amide bonds with substrates, whereas C4B tends to form ester bonds. These two gene products are related to the Chido and Rogers blood group antigens, which represent fragments of the two different C4 gene products.

The human C3 gene is on chromosome 19, and this protein also has multiple alleles. C3, C4, and C5 are apparently encoded by single genes and synthesized as single-chain polypeptide precursors, which are subsequently cleaved before secretion (Colten et al., 1981; Hall and Colten, 1977). As much as 5% of serum C4 may be in the single-chain pro-C4 form; other incompletely cleaved intermediates have also been described.

Unlike the other multichain components synthesized as single-chain precursors, the three chains of C8 are products of two different, apparently unlinked genes.

The C3b receptor, CR1, also has a number of allotypic structural variants. The quantitative expression of this receptor on erythrocytes is also under genetic control; high- and low-expression genotypes give rise to three patterns of receptor expression: high and low homozygotes and intermediate heterozygotes (Wilson et al., 1982). Although low levels of erythrocyte CR1 expression occur in patients with systemic lupus erythematosus and their families, additional nongenetic factors likely govern quantitative CR1 expression in this situation (see Immune Complex Solubilization and Clearance) (Iida et al., 1982; Wilson et al., 1982).

As noted earlier, many of the proteins that interact with C3b and C4b and regulate their function share structural homology, and their genes are all grouped within a region of chromosome 1 that has become known as the RCA cluster. It is not known whether common control elements coordinate the expression of multiple members of this family (see Regulation of Complement Activation).

Sites of Synthesis

In vitro organ culture and in vivo tissue localization methods indicate that many types of cells synthesize complement components (Colten, 1976). The intestinal epithelial cells are an important source of C1 in the body, and parenchymal cells of the liver are the major synthetic site of C3 and most other components. This was nicely demonstrated by observing shifts in the allotypes of these proteins after liver transplantation (Alper et al., 1969). Most of the complement and the regulatory proteins are synthesized by monocytes and macrophages (Whaley, 1980). Increased production of these components by activated phagocytic cells during inflammatory reactions may partly explain why they are acute-phase reactants. Teleologically it may be advantageous to synthesize complement components locally, so they are available at sites of inflammation. An example is the C3 synthesis by synovial tissue in patients with active rheumatoid arthritis (Ruddy and Colten, 1974).

COMPLEMENT IN THE FETUS AND NEWBORN

Complement synthesis by fetal tissues has been observed as early as $5\frac{1}{2}$ weeks' gestation (Gitlin and Biasucci, 1969; Gitlin and Gitlin, 1975). Studies in complement-deficient mothers and in situations in which the fetus synthesizes an allotype of a given component different from that of its mother indicate that complement proteins do not cross the placenta. C3, C4, and most other components are detectable in fetal serum by 10 weeks; levels increase progressively with gestational age, reaching about 50% to 75% of the maternal levels for most of the proteins at term. Because complement levels in the maternal circulation generally rise during pregnancy, this corresponds to 60% to 80% of normal adult levels. This is true for the CH_{50}, most of the early classical components, and factor B; but the levels of C8 and C9 are lower and may reach only 10% of the maternal concentration at term (Ballow et al., 1978). By contrast, C1 inhibitor is present in full adult concentrations as early as the twenty-eighth week of gestation.

Preterm and low-birth-weight infants have lower complement levels than do full-term babies, but by 3 months of age, most infants' complement levels are within the normal adult range (Fireman et al., 1969; Sawyer et al., 1971). The relatively low levels of C3, factor B, and other components in neonates, particularly low-birth-weight babies, may in part be responsible for the decreased opsonic activity of their serum and may contribute to their increased susceptibility to infection. Lack of the usual febrile response and leukocytosis accompanying infection in some babies may also be related in part to the low complement component levels (see Chapter 22).

Besides the low complement levels, phagocytic host defenses in newborns may be further compromised by the neonatal neutrophils' partial deficiency of CR3, which results in decreased adherence and complement-dependent phagocytosis when the cells are activated (Abughali et al., 1994, Bruce et al., 1987).

COMPLEMENT IN CLINICAL MEDICINE

General Principles

The role of complement in host defense was discussed earlier; there are also several diseases usually thought of as autoimmune in nature in which complement activation plays a major pathogenic role (see Chapter 35). In these illnesses the complement cascade functions appropriately, but activation is induced by antibody directed against a normal body constituent or as part of an immune complex deposited in otherwise normal tissue, such as DNA/anti-DNA complexes in the kidney in lupus. Complement plays multiple important roles in serum sickness and immune complex illnesses that resemble serum sickness, even if the antigens are endogenous (Lawley et al., 1984).

Illnesses in which the complement system itself is defective are rare. Individuals with a genetically controlled deficiency of complement proteins exist but are also quite rare. In general, the deficiency diseases are inherited as autosomal recessive with the exception of properdin deficiency, which is X linked. Besides infection, autoimmunity may also be associated with these deficiencies due to a failure to adequately clear immune complexes or damaged or apoptotic cells, as well as defects in normal tolerance induction (reviewed in Walport, 2001).

Complement deficiencies are discussed in detail in Chapter 21. Examples of deficiency states also include patients with deficiencies of regulatory proteins: C1 inhibitor in hereditary angioedema; factor I deficiency, which results in secondary C3 deficiency due to hypercatabolism; and those associated with the C3 nephritic factor, which causes the alternative pathway to escape from control.

In most acute infections, complement component levels are normal or elevated, reflecting their role as acute-phase reactants. In several autoimmune conditions, in contrast, the rate of synthesis is lower than the rate of consumption, resulting in decreased complement levels. Serum complement determinations may then be used as a laboratory measure of disease activity.

Ischemia, Reperfusion Injury, and Burns

As mentioned in the section on nonimmunologic activation, there are times when newly exposed or partially denatured tissue constituents can activate complement, causing injury to be more extensive than it would be ordinarily (see Gelfand et al., 1982). An example is myocardial infarction, in which ischemic injury is exacerbated during reperfusion. Animal studies have shown that complement is activated and that membrane attack complex neoantigens are deposited in myocardial capillaries after coronary artery ligation. Conversely, administration of recombinant complement inhibitors can limit the deposition of membrane attack complexes in the capillaries and the size of the infarct in these models

(Weisman et al., 1990). Currently, clinical trials of agents that may suppress complement-mediated tissue damage in several diseases are ongoing.

Transplantation

Although kidney transplant rejection is primarily mediated by cellular mechanisms, humoral mechanisms also play a role, particularly in hyperacute rejection (Carpenter, 1974) (see Chapter 43). When a kidney is transplanted into a recipient with preformed antibodies against the donor tissues or when animal tissues are xenografted into humans, all of whom have natural antibody that recognizes the graft endothelium, hyperacute rejection occurs. This is accompanied by severe endothelial damage with local activation of complement and other mediators of inflammation.

In chronic or repeated episodes of rejection, antibody and complement may also play a role. Diminished serum levels of both classical and alternative pathway components are noted and turnover studies confirm increased complement catabolism. Immunofluorescent studies suggest that activation of both the classical and alternative pathways can contribute to allograft rejection (Carpenter, 1974; Fearon et al., 1977). In xenografts, hyperacute rejection can be prevented by inhibition of complement activity (Platt, 2001).

THERAPEUTIC INHIBITION OF COMPLEMENT ACTIVATION AND TISSUE DAMAGE

Inhibition of Complement-Mediated Tissue Damage by IVIG

As noted earlier, IgG can serve as an acceptor for covalent binding of C3b during complement activation. Indeed, a large percentage of the C3b bound to opsonized pneumococci is attached to the IgG rather than to the organism itself (Brown et al., 1983). In vitro studies show that IgG-C3b complexes are resistant to attack by factors H and I and that they are recognized simultaneously by both Fc receptors and CR1, leading to extremely efficient phagocytosis.

In vitro studies show that when complement is activated by antibody-sensitized erythrocytes in the presence of excess nonspecific IgG (intravenous immunoglobulin [IVIG]), less C3b is deposited onto the erythrocytes and lysis is inhibited (Berger et al., 1985). This occurs at concentrations of IgG readily achievable during high-dose IVIG therapy and results from the binding of nascent C3b molecules to fluid-phase IgG molecules rather than to erythrocyte-bound IgG or to the erythrocyte membrane. Decreasing the binding of C3b to blood cells, with subsequent inhibition of reticuloendothelial clearance (Basta et al., 1989b), may be a major mechanism for the therapeutic effects of high-dose IVIG in autoimmune cytopenias.

Animal models of complement-mediated tissue damage also show that IVIG can decrease the deposition of complement within tissues and can ameliorate antibody-induced complement-mediated reactions, including Forssman shock (Basta et al., 1989a). Thus the ability to divert C3b may be an important anti-inflammatory mechanism of IVIG.

C1 Inhibitor as an Anti-Inflammatory Molecule

As described in the section on regulators, C1 INH inhibits a range of proteases and thus has wide-ranging anti-inflammatory function, allowing it to play a regulatory role in a number of inflammatory diseases. It has even been suggested that C1 inhibitor will delay or prevent hyperacute graft-versus-host disease under appropriate circumstances. Its clinical usefulness is still unclear because it has a relatively short half-life in the circulation. The value of C1 inhibitor as an anti-inflammatory agent will be tested (Caliezi et al., 2000) as it is becomes available for human use.

Soluble CR1 Inhibition of Tissue Injury

As noted earlier, nonimmunologic activation of complement can take place in tissues affected by burns (Gelfand et al., 1982) or ischemia (Pemberton et al., 1993; Weisman et al., 1990), presumably because these injuries alter tissue proteins or expose structures that are normally intracellular, thus creating surfaces that activate the classical or alternative pathway.

In searching among the RCA proteins (see Table 7-2) for an inhibitor that might be used therapeutically to ameliorate the effects of complement activation, CR1 seems in many ways ideal. CR1 inhibits the alternative and classical pathway C3 and C5 convertases and has co-factor activity for cleavage of C3b and C4b. A soluble form of CR1 (sCR1), which lacks the transmembrane and cytoplasmic domains of the native protein, has been produced by molecular engineering (Weisman et al., 1990). This recombinant protein decreases both local tissue damage and the systemic complications of complement activation in animal models (Mulligan et al., 1992; Pemberton et al., 1993; Weisman et al., 1990). However, this molecule is rod shaped and disappears rapidly from the circulation. Although it has been available for a decade, it still has not found a place in therapy of human diseases.

Transgenic Animals with Human Control Proteins

Over the years there has been major interest in transplantation of animal tissues into human beings. It is often impossible to find a suitable donor, and, for example, many more heart and lung transplants would be performed if suitable donor tissue were available.

Nonhuman primates are extremely limited in number, and therefore there is relatively little research in this area. It has been apparent for decades that pigs have many anatomic characteristics that would allow their organs to be used in humans, and therefore considerable research has been done with this species.

One of the problems with a porcine xenograft is hyperacute rejection that occurs within minutes after a xenograft is transplanted into humans (Platt, 2001). "Natural" IgM antibodies to xenograft antigens, such as galactosyl α-1-3-galactose, bind to this polysaccharide antigen on the endothelium of the donor organ, activate complement, and trigger release of tissue factor from endothelial cells in the blood vessels of the donor organ, which causes rapid thrombosis and failure of the graft.

It is now possible to genetically engineer human complement control protein genes into pigs, and transgenic pigs have been developed with human DAF and MCP on all their cells. Organs from these animals, when transplanted into nonhuman primates, have far better survival rates, particularly in the early minutes after engraftment. It is likely that over time this technology will become more sophisticated, and such grafts with human genes may play a role in clinical care in the future.

At present there is considerable concern about retroviruses that might be present in pig tissue, which then might activate in humans. Thus work with xenotransplantation proceeds slowly, but if this concern can be put to rest it is likely to proceed rapidly.

MEASUREMENT OF COMPLEMENT COMPONENTS AND ACTIVATION PRODUCTS

The primary clinical use of complement assays is in the diagnosis and assessment of complement activation in disease (e.g., systemic lupus erythematosus). Complement levels are also measured in some patients with increased susceptibility to infection (see Chapters 12 and 21). The serum level of a complement component reflects the balance between its synthetic and catabolic rates. Most complement proteins have rapid catabolic rates, with half-lives of about 1 to 2 days in most individuals (Ruddy et al., 1975). Although a relatively small increase in catabolic rate of a given component might be expected to lead to a rapid decrease in its serum concentration, this is often not the case because the synthetic rate often increases concomitantly.

Several complement components are *acute-phase reactants,* and their blood levels rise during inflammation (Alper, 1974); hence the presence of normal levels does not exclude involvement of complement in a given disorder. The best method to assess complement metabolism is by using turnover studies with purified radioactively labeled components, but such methods are available at only a few research centers. Serum assays for complement fragments that are released during activation, such as C3a des-Arg; for degradation products, such as C3d; and for new antigens formed during activation, such as poly-C9 or complexes such as C1 with C1 INH may be used to assess complement activation independent of the actual concentration of the native components.

Functional Hemolytic Assays

Complement components can be measured by functional methods, usually in hemolytic assays, or by immunochemical methods (Wagner et al., 2001). Hemolytic assays are more sensitive but require special reagents and expertise. In addition, serum specimens for functional assays must be handled carefully because the components lose activity rapidly at room temperature, and if immune complexes or other activators are present, continued consumption of the components may occur after the sample is obtained. Accordingly, chelators such as ethylenediamine tetra-acetic acid (EDTA) are used when the total content of a component is to be assessed immunochemically, but chelators may interfere with functional assays.

The total hemolytic complement activity is measured as the serum dilution that will lyse 50% of a standard preparation of sheep erythrocytes sensitized with specific rabbit antibody. The result is termed the CH_{50} and is usually expressed as the reciprocal of the serum dilution that gives 50% hemolysis. This test is normally used to determine the functional integrity of the classical pathway; however, it is relatively insensitive, and severe depletion of individual components may occur without altering the CH_{50} (see Chapter 20).

A similar assay for the alternative pathway can be performed using unsensitized rabbit erythrocytes, which directly activate the alternative pathway. This is termed the *alternative pathway hemolytic titer–50%* (AP_{50}) and gives comparable information on those components. However, falsely elevated readings are obtained in the presence of antirabbit erythrocyte antibodies, which often occur naturally. A rapid semiquantitative assay of classical or alternative complement activity uses glass slides coated with a thin layer of agarose gel in which sensitized sheep erythrocytes or rabbit erythrocytes have been incorporated. A circular zone of hemolysis occurs around a well in which a serum has been added; the size of the circle is proportional to the hemolytic activity of the serum.

Assays using antigen-antibody complexes bound to multiwell plastic plates, then specific antibodies to detect neoantigens on C9 in the membrane attack complex, are now being used in some laboratories to assess the whole classical pathway with automated enzyme-linked immunosorbent assay (ELISA) technology.

Functional titration of individual components is performed by a variation of the basic hemolytic assay. All components other than the one being assayed are added in excess; dilutions of the serum to be tested are used for the component in question. Often, preformed intermediates, such as EAC14 or EAC142, are used to increase the efficiency and sensitivity of these assays. Sera from humans or animals with isolated single-component deficiencies or reagents prepared by mixing appropriate amounts of isolated purified components can also be used to ensure that only a single component is being measured. The results are expressed as the serum dilution that gives a standard degree of hemolysis under defined conditions.

Immunochemical Assays

Immunochemical methods (e.g., radial immunodiffusion or automated nephelometry) are used by most laboratories to determine serum levels of individual components. Specific antisera are used to measure the total level of the component protein present, and the results are usually expressed as micrograms per unit volume of serum. These immunoassays may be misleading, however, because many of the antisera react with degradation products (e.g., soluble C3c) in addition to intact native components, so the results obtained do not correlate with functional determinations. In the case of C3, crossed immunoelectrophoresis allows direct estimation of the amount of native C3 relative to the amounts of C3c and C3d that might have been formed during activation.

Activation Assays

Commercially available radioimmunoassays have been developed to quantitate anaphylatoxins in serum. The inhibition of binding of ^{125}I-C3a, C4a, or C5a to a fixed amount of antibody by unlabeled anaphylatoxin in the test serum is measured (Chenowith and Hugli, 1980). These assays avoid the problems of crossreactivity of native components and degradation fragments and assess the degree of activation occurring, independent of the total concentration of the component.

Enzyme- or fluorescent-conjugated antibodies to individual components (e.g., C1q, C3, C4, properdin, or factor B) are used to identify sites of complement activation or deposition in tissue sections, and assessment of the pathway by which the activation occurred can sometimes be made. In addition, antibodies to neoantigens exposed during formation of the membrane attack complex have been used to localize deposition of these proteins in a number of diseases (Falk et al., 1983).

Clinical Applications

CH_{50} activity is the best test to indicate whether an individual component of the classical pathway component is lacking and is thus particularly valuable in screening for suspected complement deficiency. In inflammatory or autoimmune diseases, the usual assessment of a patient's complement status, or profile, involves measurement of both CH_{50} and C3 levels. In addition, measurement of factor B or properdin and C4 may allow the determination of which activation pathway is primarily involved. Depression of C4 with a normal factor B indicates that the classical pathway is activated, whereas a normal C4 with depressed factor B or properdin levels indicates alternative pathway activation. In either case the C3 level and probably the CH_{50} level are usually depressed.

Complement Fixation Assays

Complement fixation tests are widely used to detect and quantitate specific antigens and antibodies in biologic fluids. To determine the presence of antibody, for example, a known amount of antigen is incubated with a sample of fresh serum. If antibody is present, immune complexes form and the complement in the serum is activated or "fixed." After suitable incubation, antibody-sensitized sheep erythrocytes are added. Because the complement activated by the antigen-antibody complexes is no longer available to react with the erythrocytes, a diminished amount of lysis is observed. Complement fixation tests are widely used in the diagnosis of infectious diseases because a common set of reagents can be used to measure many antigen-antibody combinations and the amplification provided by the complement system makes the assays quite sensitive.

Immune Complex Assays

Several assays for measuring circulating antigen-antibody or immune complexes assess the binding of complement fragments to the complexes (Lawley and Frank, 1980; Theofilopoulos and Dixon, 1979). The C1q binding assay takes advantage of the ability of the multiple Fc binding sites on the C1q molecule to interact with antigen-antibody complexes. After binding C1q, the complexes are precipitated, leaving free antibodies and nonbound C1q in solution. The use of ^{125}I-C1q permits measurement of the amount of C1q precipitated, which is proportional to the amount of complexed antibody in serum. Only IgG and IgM complexes are detected by this method. In some diseases, such as urticarial vasculitis, antibodies to C1q are formed and will be detected as immune complexes.

Other assays take advantage of the fact that the C3 fragments become bound to the antigen-antibody complexes during complement activation. Thus antibodies to C3 and its fragments are coupled to solid-phase surfaces. Immune complexes containing C3 are allowed to bind. Then, conjugated antihuman immunoglobulin reagents are used to detect the antibodies in the complex with radioactive or enzyme-linked assay systems.

Similar assays can also be performed using conglutinin, a bovine protein that binds to iC3b, or Raji cells, a human lymphoblastoid cell culture line that bears CR2 receptors, to trap the C3-containing complexes. These methods allow the detection of complexes that activate either the classical or alternative pathway.

Another method to measure alternative pathway activation uses ELISA techniques and antiproperdin antibodies to detect complexes containing properdin and C3b (Cooper et al., 1983).

REFERENCES

Abughali N, Berger M, Tosi MF. Deficient total cell content of CR3 (CD11b) in neonatal neutrophils. Blood 83:1086–1092, 1994.

Ahearn JM, Fearon DT. Structure and function of the complement receptors, CR1 (CD35) and CR2 (CD21). Adv Immunol 46:183–219, 1989.

Alper CA. Complement and the MHC. In Dorff ME, ed. The Role of the Major Histocompatibility Locus in Immunobiology. New York, Garland Press, 1981, pp 173–220.

Alper CA. Plasma protein measurements as a diagnostic aid. N Engl J Med 291:287–290, 1974.

Alper CA, Austen KF, Cooper NR, Fearon DT, Gigli I, Hadding U, Lachmann PJ, Lambert PH, Lepow IH, Mayer MM, Müller-Eberhard JH, Nishioka K, Pondman K, Rosen FS, Stroud RM. Nomenclature of the alternative activating pathway of complement. Bull WHO 59:189–191, 1981.

Alper CA, Johnson AM, Birtch AG, Moore FD. Human C3: Evidence for the liver as the primary site of synthesis. Science 162:286–288, 1969.

Alper CA, Rosen FS. Genetics of the complement system. In Harris H, Hirschhorn K, eds. Advances in Human Genetics, vol 7. London, Plenum Press, 1976, pp. 141–188.

Anderson DC, Rothlein R, Marlin SD, Krater SS, Smith CW. Impaired trasendothelial migration by neonatal neutrophils: Abnormalities of Mac-1 (CD11b/CD18)-dependent adherence reactions. Blood 76:2613–2621, 1990.

Arnaout MA, Pitt J, Cohen JH, Melamed J, Rosen FS, Colten HR. Deficiency of a granulocyte membrane glycoprotein (gp 150) in a boy with recurrent bacterial infections. N Engl J Med 306:693–699, 1982.

Arnaout MA, Todd RF, Dana N, Melamed J, Schlossman S, Colten HR. Inhibition of phagocytosis of C3 or IgG coated particles and of C3bi binding with monoclonal antibodies to a monocyte/granulocyte membrane glycoprotein (Mo1). J Clin Invest 72:171–179, 1983.

Austen KF, Becker EL, Biro CE, Borsos T, Dalmasso AP, Dias DA, Silva W, Isliker H, Klein P, Lachmann PJ, Leon MA, Lepow IH, Mayer MM, Müller-Eberhard HJ, Nelson RA, Nilsson U, Nishioka I, Rapp HP, Brosen FS, Trnka Z, Ward PA, Wardlaw AC. Nomenclature of Complement. Bull WHO 39:935–938, 1968.

Ballow M, Fang F, Good RA, Day NK. Developmental aspects of complement components in the newborn. Clin Exp Immunol 18:257–266, 1978.

Barel M, Le Romancer M, Frade R. Activation of the EBV/C3d receptor (CR2, CD21) on human B lymphocyte surface triggers tyrosine phosphorylation of the 95-kDa nucleolin and its interaction with phosphatidylinositol 3 kinase. J Immunol 166:3167–3173, 2001.

Basta M, Kirshbom P, Frank MM, Fries LF. Mechanism of therapeutic effect of high-dose intravenous immunoglobulin. Attenuation of acute, complement-dependent immune damage in a guinea pig model. J Clin Invest 84:1974–1981, 1989a.

Basta M, Langlois PF, Marques M, Frank MM, Fries LF. High-dose intravenous immunoglobulin modifies complement-mediated in vivo clearance. Blood 74:326–333, 1989b.

Beller DI, Springer TA, Schrieber RD. Anti-Mac 1 selectively inhibits the mouse and human type three complement receptor. J Exp Med 156:1000–1009, 1982.

Berger M, Balow JE, Wilson CB, Frank MM. Circulating immune complexes and glomerulonephritis in a patient with congenital absence of the third component of complement. N Engl J Med 308:1009–1012, 1983.

Berger M, Gaither TA, Frank MM. Complement receptors. Clin Immunol Rev 1:471–545, 1982.

Berger M, Gaither TA, Hammer CH, Frank MM. Lack of binding of human C3 in its native state to C3b receptors. J Immunol 127:1329–1334, 1981.

Berger M, Norvell TM, Tosi MF, Emancipator SN, Konstan MW, Schreiber JR. Tissue specific Fc γ and complement receptor expression by alveolar macrophages determines relative importance of IgG and complement in promoting phagocytosis of *Pseudomonas aeruginosa*. Pediatr Res 35:68–77, 1994.

Berger M, O'Shea J, Cross AS, Folks TM, Chused TM, Brown EJ, Frank MM. Human neutrophils increase expression of C3bi as well as C3b receptors upon activation. J Clin Invest 74:1566–1571, 1984.

Berger M, Rosenkranz P, Brown CY. Intravenous and standard immune serum globulin preparations interfere with update of ^{125}I-C3 onto sensitized erythrocytes and inhibit hemolytic complement activity. Clin Immunol Immunopathol 34:227–236, 1985.

Bhakdi S, Käflein R, Halstensen TS, Hugo F, Preissner KT, Mollnes TE. Complement S-protein (vitronectin) is associated with cytolytic membrane-bound C5b-9 complexes. Clin Exp Immunol 74:459–464, 1988.

Bhakdi S, Tranum-Jensen J. Molecular nature of the complement lesion. Proc Natl Acad Sci USA 74:5655–5659, 1979.

Bianco C, Griffin FM Jr, Silverstein SC. Studies of the macrophage complement receptor. Alteration of receptor function upon macrophage activation. J Exp Med 141:1278–1290, 1975.

Binder R, Kress A, Kan G, Herrmann K, Kirschfink M. Neutrophil priming by cytokines and vitamin D binding protein (Gc-globulin): impact on C5a mediated chemotaxis, degranulation and respiratory burst. Mol Immunol 36:885–892, 1999.

Bora NS, Lublin DM, Kumar BV, Hockett RD, Holers VM, Atkinson JP. Structural gene for human membrane cofactor protein (MCP) of complement maps to within 100 kb of the 3' end of the C3b/C4b receptor gene. J Exp Med 169:597–602, 1989.

Borsos T, Rapp HJ. Molecular Basis of Complement Action. New York, Appleton-Century-Crofts, 1970, pp 1–164.

Bowen TJ, Ochs HD, Altman LC, Price TH, van Epps DE, Brautigan DL, Rosin RE, Perkins WD, Babior BM, Klebanoff SJ, Wedgwood RJ. Severe recurrent bacterial infections associated with defective adherence and chemotaxis in two patients with neutrophils deficient in a cell associated glycoprotein. J Pediatr 101:932–940, 1982.

Brown E, Berger M, Joiner K, Frank MM. Classical complement pathway activation by antipneumococcal antibodies leads to covalent binding of C3b to antibody molecules. Infect Immunol 42:594–598, 1983.

Bruce MC, Baley JE, Medvik KA, Berger M. Impaired surface membrane expression of C3bi but not C3b receptors on neonatal neutrophils. Pediatr Res 21:306–311, 1987.

Caliezi C, Wuillemin WA, Zeerleder S, Redondo M, Eisele B, Hack CE. C1-esterase inhibitor: an anti-inflammatory agent and its potential use in the treatment of diseases other than hereditary angiodema. Pharmacol Rev 52:91–112, 2000.

Campbell RD, Dodds AW, Porter RR. The binding of human complement component C4 to antibody-antigen aggregates. Biochem J 189:67–80, 1980.

Carpenter CB. Abnormalities of the complement system in clinical transplantation situations. Transplant Proc 6:83–89, 1974.

Carroll MC, Alicot EM, Katzman PJ, Klickstein LB, Smith JA, Fearon DT. Organization of the genes encoding complement receptors type 1 and 2, decay-accelerating factor, and C4-binding protein in the RCA locus on human chromosome 1. J Exp Med 167:1271–1280, 1988.

Chen CB and Wallis R. Stoichiometry of complexes between mannose-binding protein and its associated serine proteases: defining functional units for complement activation. J Biol Chem 276: 25894-902, 2001.

Cheng Q, Carlson B, Pillai S, Eby R, Edwards L, Olmsted SB, Cleary P. Antibody against surface-bound C5a peptidase is opsonic and initiates macrophage killing of group B streptococci. Infect Immun 69:2302–2308, 2001.

Chenowith DE, Cooper SW, Hugli TE, Stewart RW, Blackstone EM, Kirklin JW. Complement activation during cardiopulmonary bypass. N Engl J Med 304:497–503, 1981.

Chenowith DE, Hugli TC. Techniques and significance of C3a and C5 measurement. In Nakamura RM, ed. Future Perspectives in Clinical Laboratory Immunoassays. New York, Alan R. Liss, 1980, pp. 443–460.

Cherukuri A, Cheng PC, Pierce SK. The role of the CD19/CD21 complex in B cell processing and presentation of complement-tagged antigens. J Immunol 167:163–172, 2001a.

Cherukuri A, Cheng PC, Sohn HW, Pierce SK. The CD19/CD21 complex functions to prolong B cell antigen receptor signaling from lipid rafts. Immunity 14:169–179, 2001b.

Cheung NK, Walter EI, Smith-Mensah WH, Medoff ME. Decay-accelerating factor protects human tumor cells from complement-mediated cytotoxicity in vitro. J Clin Invest 81:1122–1128, 1988.

Colten HR. Biosynthesis of complement. Adv Immunol 22:67–118, 1976.

Colten HR, Alper CA, Rosen FS. Genetics and biosynthesis of complement proteins. N Engl J Med 304:653–656, 1981.

Cooper NR. Activation and regulation of the first complement component. Fed Proc 42:134–138, 1983.

Cooper NR. Complement and viruses. In Volanakis JR and Frank MM, eds. The Human Complement System in Health and Disease. New York, Marcel Dekker, 1998, pp 393–407.

Cooper NR. Complement evasion strategies of microorganisms. Immunol Today 12:327–331, 1991.

Cooper NR, Nemerow GR, Meyes JT. Methods to detect and quantitate complement activation. Springer Semin Immunopathol 6:195–212, 1983.

Cornacoff JB, Hebert LA, Smead WL, VanAman ME, Birmingham DJ, Waxman FJ. Primate erythrocyte-immune complex-clearing mechanism. J Clin Invest 71:236–247, 1983.

Craddock PR, Fehr J, Brigham KL, Kronenberg RS, Jacob HS. Complement and leukocyte-mediated pulmonary dysfunction in hemodialysis. N Engl J Med 296:769–774, 1977.

Crawford K, Alper CA. Genetics of the complement system. Rev Immunogenet 2:323–338, 2000.

Cronstein BN, Weissmann G. The adhesion molecules of inflammation. Arthritis Rheum 36:147–157, 1993.

Crowley CA, Curnutte JT, Rosen RE, Schwartz JA, Gallin JI, Klempner M, Synderman R, Southwick FS, Stossel TP, Babior BM. An inherited abnormality of neutrophil adhesion-genetic transmission and association with a missing protein. N Engl J Med 302:1163–1168, 1980.

Davies A, Lachmann PJ. Membrane defece against complement lysis: The structure and biological properties of CD59. Immunol Res 12:258–275, 1993.

Davies KA, Walport MJ. Processing and clearance of immune complexes by complement and the role of complement in immune complex diseases. Volanakis JE and Frank MM, eds. In The Human Complement System in Health and Disease. New York, Marcel Dekker, 1998, pp 423–454.

Davis AE III. C1 inhibitor gene and hereditary angioedema. Volanakis JE and Frank MM, eds. In The Human Complement System in Health and Disease. New York, Marcel Dekker, 1998, pp 455–480.

Davis AE, Ziegler JB, Gelfand EW, Rosen FS, Alper CA. Heterogeneity of nephritic factor and its identification as an immunoglobulin. Proc Natl Acad Sci USA 74:3980–3983, 1977.

Dempsey PW, Fearon DT. Complement: Instructing the acquired immune system through the CD21/CD19 complex. Res Immunol 147:71–75, 1996.

Densen P. Complement deficiencies and infection. Volanakis JR and Frank MM, eds. In The Human Complement System in Health and Disease. New York, Marcel Dekker, 1998, pp 409–421.

Diamond MS, Springer TA. The dynamic regulation of integrin adhesiveness. Curr Biol 4:506–517, 1994.

DiMartino SJ, Shah AB, Trujillo G, Kew RR. Elastase controls the binding of the vitamin D-binding protein (Gc-globulin) to neutrophils: A potential role in the regulation of C5a co-chemotactic activity. J Immunol 166:2688–2694, 2001.

Drouin SM, Corry DB, Kildsgaard J, Wetsel RA. The absence of C3 demonstrates a role for complement in Th2 effector functions in a murine model of pulmonary allergy. J Immunol 167:4141–4145, 2001a.

Drouin SM, Kildsgaard J, Haviland , Zabner J, Jia HP, McCray PB Jr, Tack BF, Wetsel RA. Expression of the complement anaphylatoxin C3a and C5qa receptors on bronchial epithelial and smooth muscle cells in models of sepsis and asthma. J Immunol 166:2025–2032, 2001b.

Dykman TA, Hatch JA, Atkinson JP. Polymorphism of the human C3b/C4b receptor. J Exp Med 159:691–703, 1984.

Edwards MS, Kasper DL, Jennings HJ, Baker CJ, Nicholson-Weller A. Capsular sialic acid prevents activation of the alternative complement pathway by type III, group B streptococci. J Immunol 128:1278–1283, 1982.

Edwards MS, Nicholson-Weller A, Baker CJ, Kasper DL. The role of specific antibody in alternative complement pathway mediated opsonophagocytosis of type III, group B streptococcus. J Exp Med 151:1275–1287, 1980.

Ehlenberger AG, Nussenzweig V. The role of membrane receptors for C3b and C3d in phagocytosis. J Exp Med 145:357–371, 1977.

Etzioni A, Harlan JM. Cell adhesion and leukocyte adhesion defects. In Ochs MD, Smith CIE and Puck JM, eds. Primary Immunodeficiency Disease. New York, Oxford University Press, 1999, pp 375–388.

Falk RJ, Dalmasso AP, Kim Y, Tsai CH, Scheinman JI, Gewurz H, Michael AF. Neoantigen of the polymerized ninth component of complement: Characterization of a monoclonal antibody and histochemical localization in renal disease. J Clin Invest 72:560–573, 1983.

Fayyazi A, Sandau R, Duong LQ, Gotze O, Radzun JH, Schweyer S, Soruri A, Zwirner J. C5a receptor and interleukin-6 are expressed in tissue macrophages and stimulated keratinocytes but not in pulmonary and intestinal epithelial cells. Am J Path 154:495–501, 1999.

Fearon DT. Complement, C receptors, and immune complex disease. Hosp Pract 15:63–72, 1988.

Fearon DT. Regulation by membrane sialic acid of B1H-dependent decay dissociation of amplification C3 convertase of the alternative complement pathway. Proc Natl Acad Sci USA 75:1971–1975, 1978.

Fearon DT. Regulation of the amplification C3 convertase of human complement by an inhibitory protein isolated from human erythrocyte membrane. Proc Natl Acad Sci USA 76:5867–5871, 1979.

Fearon DT, Austen KF. The alternative pathway of complement: a system for host resistance to microbial infection. N Engl J Med 303:259–263, 1980.

Fearon DT, Carroll MC. Regulation of B lymphocyte responses to foreign and self-antigens by the CD19/CD21 complex. Annu Rev Immunol 18:393–422, 2000.

Fearon DT, Daha MR, Strom TB, Weiler JM, Carpenter CB, Austen RF. Pathways of complement activation in membranoproliferative glomerulonephritis and allograft rejection. Transplant Proc 9:729–739, 1977.

Fireman P, Zuckowski DA, Taylor PM. Development of human complement system. J Immunol 103:25–31, 1969.

Fischer WH, Jagels MA, Hugli TE. Regulation of IL-6 synthesis in human peripheral blood mononuclear cells by C3a and C3a (desArg). J Immunol 162:453–459, 1999.

Fishelson Z. Complement-related proteins in pathogenic organisms. Springer Semin Immunopathol 15:345–368, 1994.

Frank MM, Schrieber AD, Atkinson JP, Jaffe CJ. Pathophysiology of immune hemolytic anemia. Ann Intern Med 87:210–222, 1977.

Fries LF, Gaither TA, Hammer CH, Frank MM. C3b covalently bound to IgG demonstrates a reduced rate of inactivation by factors H and I. J Exp Med 160:1640–1655, 1984.

Fujita T, Gigli I, Nussenzweig V. Human C4 binding protein: II. Role in proteolysis of C4b by C3b inactivator. J Exp Med 148:1044–1051, 1978.

Gelfand JA, Donelan M, Hawiger A, and Burke JF. Alternative complement pathway activation increases mortality in a model of burn injury in mice. J Clin Invest 70:1170–1176, 1982.

Gelfand MC, Frank MM, Green I. A receptor for the third component of complement in the human renal glomerulus. J Exp Med 142:1029–1034, 1975.

Gerard C, Hugli TE. Identification of classical anaphylatoxin as the des-Arg form of the C5a molecule: evidence of a modulator role for the oligosaccharide unit in human des-Arg[71]-C5a. Proc Natl Acad Sci USA 78:1833–1837, 1981.

Ghebrehiwet B, Peerschke EI. Structure and function of gC1q-R: a multiligand binding cellular protein. Immunobiology 199:225–238, 1998.

Gitlin D, Biasucci A. Development of γG, γA, γM, β_{-1C}/β_{-1A}, C′1 esterase inhibitor, ceruloplasmin, transferrin, hemopexin, haptoglobin, fibrinogen, plasminogen, antitrypsin, orosomucoid, β-lipoprotein, α2 macroglobulin and prealbumin in the human conceptus. J Clin Invest 48:1433–1446, 1969.

Gitlin D, Gitlin JD. Fetal and neonatal development of human plasma proteins. In Putnam FE, ed. The Plasma Proteins, ed 2. New York: Academic Press, 1975, pp 263–319.

Goers JWF, Porter RR. The assembly of early components of complement on antibody-antigen aggregates and on antibody-coated erythrocytes. Biochem J 175:675–684, 1978.

Gorski JP, Hugh TE, Müller-Eberhard, HJ. C4a: The third anaphylatoxin of the human complement system. Proc Natl Acad Sci USA 76:5299–5302, 1979.

Griffin JA, Griffin FM Jr. Augmentation of macrophage complement receptor function in vitro. I. Characterization of the cellular interactions required for the generation of a T-lymphocyte product that enhances macrophage complement receptor function. J Exp Med 150:653–675, 1979.

Hall RE, Colten HR. Cell-free synthesis of the fourth component of guinea pig complement (C4): identification of a precursor of serum (Pro-C4). Proc Natl Acad Sci USA 74:1707–1710, 1977.

Hammer CH, Abramovitz AS, Mayer MM. A new activity of complement component C3: cell-bound C3b potentiates lysis of erythrocytes by C5b6 and terminal components. J Immunol 117:830–834, 1976.

Hammerschmidt DE, Weaver LJ, Hudson LD, Craddock PR, Jacob H. Complement activation and elevated plasma C5a with adult respiratory distress syndrome: pathophysiological relevance and possible prognostic value. Lancet 1:947–949, 1980.

Harrison RA, Lachmann PJ. The physiological breakdown of the third component of complement. Mol Immunol 17:9–20, 1980.

Harrison RA, Thomas ML, Tack BF. Sequence determination of the thiolester site of the fourth component of human complement. Proc Natl Acad Sci USA 78:7388–7392, 1981.

Haviland DL, McCoy RL, Whitehead WT, Akama H, Molmenti EP, Brown A, Haviland JC, Parks WC, Perlmutter DH, Wetsel RA. Cellular expression of the C5a anaphylatoxin receptor (C5aR): demonstration of C5aR on nonmyeloid cells of the liver and lung. J Immunol 154:1861–1869, 1995.

Hogg N. Roll, roll, roll your leucocyte gently down the vein . . . . Immunol Today 13:113–115, 1992.

Hopken UE, Lu B, Gerard NP, Gerard C. Impaired inflammatory responses in the reverse arthus reaction through genetic deletion of the C5a receptor. J Exp Med 186:749–756, 1997.

Hopken UE, Lu B, Gerard NP, Gerard C. The C5a chemoattractant receptor mediates mucosal defence to infection. Nature 383:86–89, 1996.

Hostetter MK, Thomas ML, Rosen FS, Tack BF. Binding of C3b proceeds by a transesterification reaction at the thiolester site. Nature 298:72–75, 1982.

Hugli TE. Structure and function of the anaphylatoxins. Springer Semin Immunopathol 7:193–220, 1984.

Hugli TE, Müller-Eberhard HJ. Anaphylatoxins: C3a and C5a. Adv Immunol 26:1–53, 1978.

Iida K, Mornaghi R, Nussenzweig V. Complement receptor (CR1) deficiency in erythrocytes from patients with systemic lupus erythematosus. J Exp Med 153:1427–1438, 1982.

Iida K, Nussenzweig V. Complement receptor is an inhibitor of the complement cascade. J Exp Med 153:1138–1150, 1981.

Jackson CG, Ochs MD, Wedgwood RJ. Immune response of a patient with deficiency of the fourth component of complement and systemic lupus erythematosus. N Engl J Med 300:1124–1129, 1979.

Jacob HS, Craddock PR, Hammerschmidt DE, Moldow CF. Complement induced granulocyte aggregation. N Engl J Med 302:789–794, 1980.

Jagels MA, Travis J, Potempa J, Pike R, Hugli TE. Proteolytic inactivation of the leukocyte C5a receptor by proteinases derived from *Porphyromonas gingivalis*. Infect Immun 64:1984–1991, 1996.

Jenne D, Stanley KK. Molecular cloning of S-protein, a link between complement, coagulation and cell-substrate adhesion. The EMBO J 4:3151–3157, 1985.

Joiner KA, Brown EJ, Frank MM. Complement and bacteria: chemistry and biology in host defense. Ann Rev Immunol 2:461–491, 1984.

Kazatchkine MD, Fearon DT, Austen KF. Human alternative complement pathway: membrane-associated sialic acid regulates the competition between B and B1H for cell bound C3b. J Immunol 122:75–81, 1979.

Kildsgaard J, Hollmann TJ, Matthews KW, Bian K, Murad F, Wetsel RA. Targeted disruption of the C3a receptor gene demonstrates a novel protective anti-inflammatory role for C3a in endotoxin-shock. J Immunol 165:5406–5409, 2000.

Kishimoto TK, Rothlein R. Integrins, ICAMS, and selectins: Role and regulation of adhesion molecules in neutrophil recruitment to inflammatory sites. Adv Pharmacol 25:117–169, 1994.

Klaus CGB, Humphrey JH, Kunkl A, Dongworth DW. The follicular dendritic cell-its role in antigen presentation in the generation of immunological memory. Immunol Rev 59:3–28, 1980.

Klickstein LB, Bartow, TJ, Miuletic V, Rabson LD, Smith JA, Fearon DT. Identification of distinct C3b and C4b recognition sites in the human C3b/C4b receptor (CR1, CD35) by deletion mutagenesis. J Exp Med 168:1699–1717, 1988.

Klickstein LB, Wong WW, Smith JA, Weis JH, Wilson JG, Fearon DR. Human C3b/C4b receptor (CR1). Demonstration of long homologous repeating domains that are composed of the short consensus repeats characteristics of C3/C4 binding proteins. J Exp Med 165:1095–1112, 1987.

Koenig JM, Siomon J, Anderson DC, Smith E, Smith CW. Diminished soluble and total cellular L-selectin in cord blood is associated with its impaired shedding from activated neutrophils. Pediatr Res 39:616–621, 1996.

Lachmann PJ. The control of homologous lysis. Immunol Today 12:312–315, 1991.

Law SK, Lichtenberg NA, Levine RP. Evidence for an ester linkage between the labile binding site of C3b and receptive surfaces. J Immunol 123:1388–1394, 1979.

Lawley TJ, Bielory L, Gascon P, Yancey KB, Young NS, Frank MM. A prospective clinical and immunologic analysis of patients with serum sickness. N Engl J Med 311:1407–1413, 1984.

Lawley TJ, Frank M. Immune complexes and immune complex diseases. In Parker CT, ed. Clinical Immunology. Philadelphia, WB Saunders, 1980, pp 143–172.

Lim HW, Poh-Fitzpatrick MB, Gigli I. Activation of the complement system in patients with porphyrias after irradiation in vivo. J Clin Invest 74:1961–1965, 1984.

Marom Z, Shelhamer J, Berger M, Frank M, Kaliner M. The anaphylatoxin C3a enhances mucous glycoprotein release from human airways in vitro. J Exp Med 161:657–668, 1985.

Matsushita M, Thiel S, Jensenius JC, Terai I, Fujita T. Proteolytic activities of two types of mannose-binding lectin-associated serine protease. J Immunol 165:2637–2642, 2000.

Mayer MM. Complement and complement fixation. In Kabat E, Mayer MF, eds. Experimental Immunochemistry. Springfield, Ill., Charles C. Thomas, 1961, pp 133–240.

Mayer MM, Michaels DW, Ramm LE, Whitlow MB, Willoughby JB, Shin ML. Membrane damage by complement. CRC Crit Rev Immunol 2:133–166, 1981.

Meddows-Taylor S, Pendle S, Tiemessen CT. Altered expression of CD88 and associated impairment of complement 5a-induced neutrophil responses in human immunodeficiency virus type 1-infected patients with and without pulmonary tuberculosis. J Infect Dis 183:662–665, 2001.

Medof ME, Iida K, Mold C, Nussenzweig V. Unique role of the complement receptor CR1 in the degradation of C3b associated with immune complexes. J Exp Med 156:1739–1754, 1982.

Miwa T, Song WC. Membrane complement regulatory proteins: insight from animal studies and relevance to human diseases. Int Immunopharmacol 1:445–459, 2001.

Moffitt MC, Frank MM. Complement resistance in microbes. Springer Seminars Immunopath 15:327–344, 1994.

Moore FD Jr, Davis C, Rodrick M, Mannick JA, Fearon DT. Neutrophil activation in thermal injury as assessed by increased expression of complement receptors. N Engl J Med 314:948–953, 1986.

Moore FD, Fearon DT, Austen KF. IgG on mouse erythrocytes augments activation of the human alternative complement pathway by enhancing deposition of C3b. J Immunol 125:1805–1809, 1981.

Morgan BP, Meri S. Membrane proteins that protect against complement lysis. Springer Semin Immunopathol 15:369–396, 1994.

Müller-Eberhard HJ, ed. Complement: I, II, III. Springer Semin Immunopathol 6:117–258, 259-390; 7:93–270, 1983/1984.

Müller-Eberhard HJ. The membrane attack complex. Springer Semin Immunopathol 7:93–142, 1984.

Müller-Eberhard HJ, Schreiber RD. Molecular biology and chemistry of the alternative pathway of complement. Adv Immunol 29:1–53, 1980.

Mulligan MS, Yeh CG, Rudolph AR, Ward PA. Protective effects of soluble CR1 in complement- and neutrophil-mediated tissue injury. J Immunol 148:1479–1485, 1992.

Myones BL, Dalzell JG, Hogg N, Ross GD. Neutrophil and monocyte cell surface p150,95 has iC3b-receptor (CR4) activity resembling CR3. J Clin Invest 82:640–651, 1988.

Nagasawa S, Stroud RM. Cleavage of C2 and C1s into antigenically distinct fragments C2a and C2b: Demonstration of binding of C2b to C4b. Proc Natl Acad Sci USA 74:2998–3001, 1977.

Nelson RA. The immune adherence phenomenon: An immunologically specific reaction between micro-organisms and erythrocytes leading to enhanced phagocytosis. Science 118:733–737, 1953.

Nemerow GR, Houghten RA, Moore MD, Cooper NR. Identification of an epitope in the major envelope protein of Epstein-Barr virus that mediates viral binding to the B lymphocyte EBV receptor (CR2). Cell 56:369–377, 1989.

Nemerow GR, Yamamoto K, Lint TF. Restriction of complement-mediated membrane damage by the eighth component of complement. A dual role for C8 in the complement attack sequence. J Immunol 123:1245–1252, 1979.

Nepomuceno RR, Ruiz S, Park M, Tenner AJ. C1qRP is a heavily O-glycosylated cell surface protein involved in the regulation of phagocytic activity. J Immunol 162:3583–3589, 1999.

Nishimura J, Murakami Y, Kinoshita T. Paroxysmal nocturnal hemoglobinuria: an acquired genetic disease. Am J Hematol 62:175–182, 1999.

O'Bryan MK, Baker HWG, Saunders JR, Kirszbaum L, Walker ID, Hudson P, Liu DY, Glew MD, d'Apice AJF, Murphy BF. Human Seminal Clusterin (SP-40,40): isolation and Characterization. J Clin Invest 85:1477–1486, 1990.

Ochs MD, Wedgwood RJ, Frank MM, Heller SP, Hosea SW. The role of complement in induction of antibody responses. Clin Exp Immunol 53:208–216, 1983.

Paccaud JP, Carpentier JL, Schifferli JA. Difference in the clustering of complement receptor type 1 (CR1) on polymorphonuclear leukocytes and erthyrocytes: effect on immune adherence. Eur J Immunol 20:283–289, 1990.

Pangburn MK, Müller-Eberhard HJ. Relation of a putative thioester bond in C3 to activation of the alternative pathway and the binding of C3b to biological targets of complement. J Exp Med 152:1102–1114, 1980.

Parren PW, Burton DR. The antiviral activity of antibodies in vitro and in vivo. Adv Immunol 77:195–262, 2001.

Patston PA, Gettins P, Beechem J, Schapira M. Mechanisms of serpin action: evidence that C1 inhibitor function as a suicide substrate. Biochemistry 30:8876–8882, 1991.

Pemberton M, Anderson G, Vetvicka V, Justus DE, Ross GD. Microvascular effects of complement blockade with soluble recombinant CR1 on ischemia/reperfusion injury of skeletal muscle. J Immunol 150:5104–5113, 1993.

Pepys MB. Role of complement in the induction of immunological responses. Transplant Rev 32:93–120, 1976.

Petersen SV, Thiel S, Jensen L, Vorup-Jensen T, Koch C, Jensenius JC. Control of the classical and the MBL pathway of complement activation. Mol Immunol 37:803–811, 2000.

Pillemer L, Blum L, Lepow IH, Ross OA, Todd EW, Wardlaw AC. The properdin system and immunity I. Demonstration and isolation of a new serum protein, properdin, and its role in immune phenomena. Science 120:279–285, 1954.

Platt JL, ed. Xenotransplantation. Washington, DC, ASM Press, 2001.

Podack ER, Biesecker G, Müller-Eberhard HJ. Membrane attack complex of complement: generation of high affinity phospholipid binding sites by fusion of five hydrophilic plasma proteins. Proc Natl Acad Sci USA 76:897–901, 1979.

Podack ER, Müller-Eberhard HJ. Binding of desoxycholate, phosphatidylchol vesicles, lipoprotein and of the S-protein to complexes of terminal complement component. J Immunol 121:1025–1030, 1978.

Podack ER, Tschopp J. Membrane attack by complement. Molec Immunol 21:589–603, 1984.

Podack ER, Tschopp J, Müller-Eberhard HJ. Molecular organization of C9 within the membrane attack complex of complement: induction of circular C9 polymerization by the C5b-8 assembly. J Exp Med 156:268–282, 1982.

Pommier CG, Inada S, Fries LF, Takahashi T, Frank MM, Brown EJ. Plasma fibronectin enhances phagocytosis of opsonized particles by human peripheral blood monocytes. J Exp Med 157:1844–1854, 1983.

Porter RR, Reid KBM. The biochemistry of complement. Nature 275:699–704, 1978.

Rawal N, Pangburn MK. Structure/function of C5 convertases of complement. Int Immunopharm 1:415–422, 2001.

Reid KBM, Porter RR. The proteolytic activation systems of complement. Ann Rev Biochem 50:433–464, 1981.

Rezzonico R, Chicheportiche R, Imbert V, Dayer JM. Engagement of CD11b and CD11c β2 integrin by antibodies or soluble CD23 induces IL-1β production on primary human monocytes through mitogen-activated protein kinase-dependent pathways. Blood 95:3868–3877, 2000.

Ross GD, Medof ME. Membrane complement receptors specific for bound fragments of C3. Adv Immunol 37:217–267, 1985.

Rosse WF. Paroxysmal nocturnal hemoglobinuria as a molecular disease. Medicine 76:63–93, 1997.

Rossi V, Cseh S, Bally I, Thielens NM, Jensenius JC and Arlaud GJ. Substrate specificities of Recombinant Mannan-binding Lectin Associated Serine Proteases-1 and 2. J Biol Chem 276:40880–40887, 2001.

Rothermel E, Gotze C, Zahn S, Schlaf G. Analysis of the tissue distribution of the rat C5a receptor and inhibition of C5a-mediated effects through the use of two MoAbs. Scand J Immunol 52:401–410, 2000.

Ruddy S, Carpenter CB, Chin KW, Knostman JN, Soter NA, Gotze O, Müller-Eberhard HJ, Austen KF. Human complement metabolism: an analysis of 144 studies. Medicine 54:165–178, 1975.

Ruddy S, Colten HR. Rheumatoid arthritis: biosynthesis of complement proteins by synovial tissues. N Engl J Med 290:1284–1288, 1974.

Sanchez-Madrid F, Nagy JA, Robbins E, Simon P, Springer TA. A human leukocyte differentiation antigen family with distinct alpha subunits and a common beta subunit: The lymphocyte function-associated antigen (LFA-1), the C3bi complement receptor (OKM1/Mac-1), and the P150, 95 molecule. J Exp Med 158:1785–1803, 1983.

Sawyer MK, Forman ML, Kuplic LS, Stiehm ER. Development aspects of the human complement system. Biol Neonate 19:148–162, 1971.

Sayah S, Ischenko AM, Zhakhov A, Bonnard AS, Fontaine M. Expression of cytokines by human astrocytomas following stimulation by C3a and C5a anaphylatoxins: specific increase in interleukin-6 mRNA expression. J Neurochem 72:2426–2436, 1999.

Schifferli JA, Ng YC, Peters DK. The role of complement and its receptor in the elimination of immune complexes. N Engl J Med 315:488–495, 1986.

Schwaeble W, Dahl MR, Thiel S, Stover C and Jensenius JC. The mannan-binding lectin associated serine proteases (MASPS) and MAP19: Four components of the lectin pathway activation complex encoded by two genes. Immunobiol 205:455–466, 2002.

Sengeløv H, Kjeldsen L, Kroeze W, Berger M, Borregaard N. Secretory vesicles are the intracellular reservoir of Complement Receptor 1 in human neutrophils. J Immunol 153:804–810, 1994.

Sim RB, Twose TM, Paterson DS, Sim E. The covalent-binding reaction of complement component C3. Biochem J 193:115–127, 1981.

Sim RB. The human complement system serine proteases C1r and C1s and their proenzymes. Methods Enzymol 80:26–42, 1981.

Springer TA. Traffic signals for lymphocyte recirculation and leukocyte emigration: multistep paradigm. Cell 76:301–314, 1994.

Stevens P, Huang SNY, Welch WD, Young LS. Restricted complement activation by E. coli with the K-1 capsular serotype: possible role in pathogenicity. J Immunol 121:2174–2180, 1978.

Stossel TP, Field RJ, Gitlin JD, Alper CA, Rosen FS. The opsonic fragment of the third component of human complement. J Exp Med 141:1329–1347, 1975.

Tack BF, Harrison RA, Janatova J, Thomas ML, Prahl JW. Evidence for presence of an internal thiolester bond in third component of human complement. Proc Natl Acad Sci USA 77:5764–5768, 1980.

Takabayashi T, Vannier E, Burke JF, Thompkins RG, Gelfand JA, Clark BD. Both C3a and C3a (desArg) regulate interleukin-6 synthesis in human peripheral blood mononuclear cells. J Infect Dis 177:1622–1628, 1998.

Taylor SM, Sherman SA, Kirnarsky L, Sanderson SD. Development of response-selective agonists of human C5a anaphylatoxin: conformational, biological and therapeutic considerations. Current Medicinal Chemistry 8:675–684, 2001.

Tedder TF, Steeber DA, Chen A, Engel P. The selectins: Vascular adhesion molecules. FASEB J 9:866–873, 1995.

Tenner AJ. Membrane receptors for soluble defense collagens. Curr Opin Immunol 11:34–41, 1999.

Theil S and Reid KBM. Structures and functions associated with the group of mammalian lectins containing collagen like sequences. FEBS Lett 250:78, 1989.

Theofilopoulos AN, Dixon FJ. The biology and detection of immune complexes. Adv Immunol 28:89–220, 1979.

Thomas ML, Janatova J, Gray WR, Tack BF. Third component of human complement: localization of the internal thiolester bond. Proc Natl Acad Sci USA 79:1054–1058, 1982.

Thornton BP, Vetvicka V, Pitman M, Goldman RC, Ross GD. Analysis of the sugar specificity and molecular location of the beta-glucan-binding lectin site of complement receptor type 3 (CD11b/CD18). J Immunol 156:1235–1246, 1996.

Turner MW, Hamvas RM. Mannose-binding lectin: Structure, function, genetics and disease associations. Reviews in Immunogenetics 2:305–322, 2000.

Vasantha S, et al. Interactions of a nonneutralizing IgM antibody and complement in parainfluenza virus neutralization. Virology 167:433–441, 1988.

Veldkamp KE, Heezius HC, Verhoef J, van Strijp JA, van Kessel KP. Modulation of neutrophil chemokine receptors by Staphylococcus aureus supernate. Infect Immun 68:5908–5913, 2000.

Volanakis JE, Frank MM, eds. The Human Complement System in Health and Disease. New York, Marcel Dekker, 1998.

Vorup-Jensen T, Jensenius JC, Thiel S. MASP-2, the C3 convertase generating protease of the MBLectin complement activating pathway. Immunobiology 199:348–357, 1998.

Wagner E, Jiang H, Frank MM. Complement and kinins: Mediators of inflammation. In Henry JB, ed. Clinical Diagnosis and Management by Laboratory Methods, ed 20. Philadelphia, WB Saunders, 2001, pp 892–913.

Walport MJ. Complement. N Engl J Med 344:1058–1066, 1140–1144, 2001.

Ware CF, Kolb WP. Assembly of the functional membrane attack complex of human complement: formation of disulfide linked C9 dimers. Proc Natl Acad Sci USA 78:6426–6430, 1981.

Weisman HF, Bartow T, Leppo MK, Marsh HC Jr, Carson GR, Concino MF, Boyle MP, Roux KH, Weisfeldt ML, Fearon DT. Soluble human complement receptor type 1: in vivo inhibitor of complement suppressing post-ischemic myocardial inflammation and necrosis. Science 249:146–151, 1990.

Wetsel RA. Structure, function and cellular expression of complement anaphylatoxin receptors. Curr Opin Immunol 7:48–53, 1995.

Whaley K. Biosynthesis of the complement components and the regulatory proteins of the alternative complement pathway by human peripheral blood monocytes. J Exp Med 151:501–516, 1980.

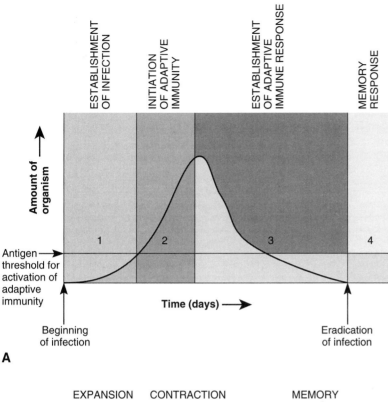

ESTABLISHMENT OF INFECTION

INITIATION OF ADAPTIVE IMMUNITY

ESTABLISHMENT OF ADAPTIVE IMMUNE RESPONSE

MEMORY RESPONSE

Amount of organism

Antigen threshold for activation of adaptive immunity

1   2   3   4

Time (days) →

Beginning of infection

Eradication of infection

A

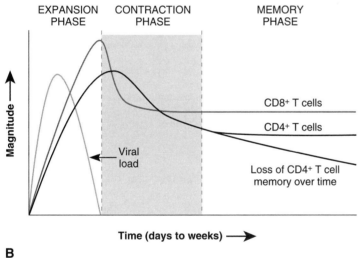

EXPANSION PHASE   CONTRACTION PHASE   MEMORY PHASE

Magnitude →

Viral load

CD8+ T cells

CD4+ T cells

Loss of CD4+ T cell memory over time

Time (days to weeks) →

B

Figure 8-1 · Time course of a typical acute infection.
A. 1, During an acute bacterial or viral infection, the level of infectious agent increases as the pathogen replicates. 2, An immune response is initiated when numbers of the pathogen exceed the threshold dose of antigen required for an adaptive response. At the same time, the pathogen continues to grow, retarded only by the innate and nonadaptive responses. Immunologic memory is also believed to be initiated at this stage. 3, After 4 to 5 days, effector arms of the immune response begin to clear the infection. 4, Upon clearance of the infectious agent and after the dose of antigen falls below the response threshold, the response ceases. However, the presence of antibody, residual effector cells, and immunologic memory provide lasting protection against reinfection in most cases. **B.** During a viral infection, antigen-specific T cells clonally expand during the first phase in the presence of antigen. Soon after the virus is cleared, the contraction phase ensues and the number of antigen-specific T cells decreases due to apoptosis. After the contraction phase, the number of virus-specific T cells stabilizes and can be maintained for great lengths of time (the memory phase). Of note, the magnitude of the CD4+ T-cell response is lower than that of the CD8+ T-cell response, and the contraction phase can be less pronounced than that of CD8+ T cells. The number of memory CD4+ T cells might decline slowly over time. (Adapted from Kaech SM, Wherry EJ, Ahmed R. Effector and memory T-cell differentiation: implications for vaccine development. Nat Rev Immunol 2:251–262, 2002.)

T cells, and APCs in space and time, although such temporal and spatial co-localization may still occur as part of the immune activation process.

Once activated, the effector T cells must be able to leave the secondary lymphoid organ and enter any tissue where pathogens may be present. Activated effector T cells need to interact with other leukocytes such as eosinophils, mast cells, and basophils (in the case of allergic reactions) or macrophages and neutrophils (in the case of delayed-type hypersensitivity reactions) at the local site. In addition, activated Th2 CD4+ T cells need to gain access to the germinal centers, where they can exert their effect on antibody-producing B cells. Finally, memory T cells need to be generated that not only can provide immediate surveillance and protection in tissues against a secondary challenge but also can reach secondary lymphoid organs for further clonal expansion (Fig. 8-4).

Recent evidence indicates that the selectivity and flexibility necessary to regulate cell traffic under homeostatic and inflammatory conditions are provided by a differential tissue distribution of a class of chemicals called chemokines and a regulated expression of chemokine receptors on different leukocyte subsets (Sallusto et al., 2000). The roles these effector T cells play in cell-mediated and humoral immune responses to different pathogens are listed in Table 8-1. As in many cases, both cell-mediated and humoral immunity are

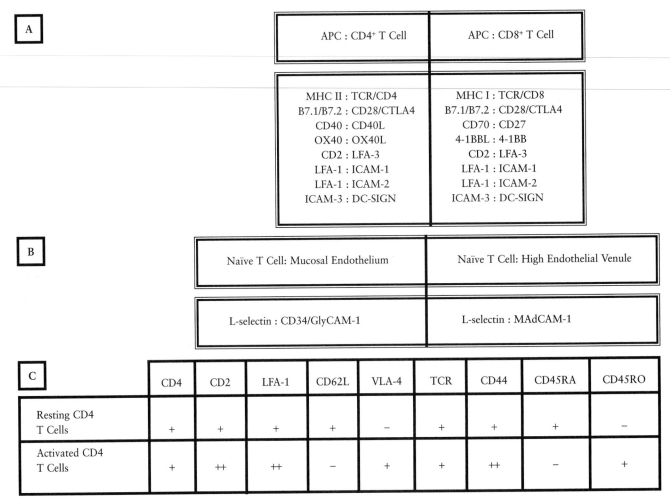

Figure 8-2 · Surface receptor interactions among members of the immune system. A. Cell-surface receptor interactions between APC and T cells. In each receptor pair, those ligands that are expressed on the APC are presented in the left column, and those that are expressed on T cells are presented on the right column. For example, APCs express CD40, whereas T cells express CD40L. Dendritic cell–specific ICAM-grabbing nonintegrin (DC-SIGN) is a C-type lectin. LFA-3 is also known as CD58, intracellular adhesion molecule-1 (ICAM-1), -2, and -3 are CD54, CD102, and CD50, respectively. B7.1 and B7.2 are known as CD80 and CD86, respectively. CD70 is also known as CD27L, 4-1BB as CD137, and OX40 as CD134 **B.** Naïve T cells interaction with endothelial cells. Naïve T cells express L-selectin, which binds sulfated sialyl-Lewis X moieties on the vascular addressins CD34 and GlyCAM-1 on high endothelial venules (HEV) to enter lymph nodes. The addressin MAdCAM-1 is expressed on mucosal endothelium and guides cell entry into mucosal lymphoid tissue. **C.** Expression of surface adhesion molecules on resting and activated CD4+ lymphocytes. Resting naïve T cells express L-selectin (CD62L), which helps them home to lymph nodes. They express relatively low levels of other adhesion molecules, such as CD44, CD2, and LFA-1. Naïve T cells also express the RA isoform of CD45 on the surface. Upon activation, T cells lose expression of CD62L; increase the level of the integrin very late antigen-4 (VLA-4), a homing receptor for vascular endothelium of inflamed tissues; expresses high levels of CD44, LFA-1, and CD2; and express the RO isoform of CD45. The expression of CD45RO sensitizes T cells to stimulation by lower concentrations of MHC/peptide complexes.

involved in the eradication of many infections, such as responses to *Pneumocystis carinii*, which requires antibody for ingestion by phagocytes and macrophage activation for effective destruction of the ingested pathogen.

B-Cell Activation

Detailed biology of B-cell development and activation has been discussed in previous chapters. In general, naïve antigen-specific lymphocytes in adaptive immunity are difficult to activate by antigen alone. This is the case for naïve B cells encountering the antigen for the first time. These cells require accessory signals that can come from either an armed T cell or directly from microbial sources. B cells can receive help from T-helper cells when antigen bound by surface immunoglobulin is internalized and returned to the cell surface as peptides bound to MHC class II molecules (Hasler and Zouali 2001). This peptide/MHC class II complex is then recognized by T-helper cell via surface TCRs, resulting in

THREE-CELL INTERACTION MODEL

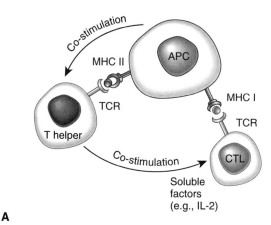

A

SEQUENTIAL TWO-CELL INTERACTION MODEL

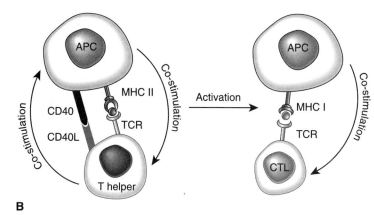

B

Figure 8-3 · Three-cell versus sequential two-cell interaction models of T-cell activation. **A.** During priming phase of a T-cell–mediated immune response, the classical model of activation requires geographic proximity of CD8+ T cell, CD4+ T cells, and APCs. **B.** An alternative model suggests that successful generation of an immune response can occur via subsequent encounter of a CD8+ T lymphocyte with an APC that has been preconditioned by an activated CD4+ T cell through CD40-CD40L interaction. In this model the continuous presence of T-helper cell (CD40L signal) is not necessary for APCs to activate CD8+ T-killer cells, although such temporal and spatial co-localization may occur as part of the immune activation process.

the stimulation of such T cells to produce proteins (e.g., CD40L, IL-4, transforming growth factor-β [TGF-β], IL-4, and IFN-γ) that cause B cells to proliferate and undergo processes of isotype switching, somatic hypermutation, affinity maturation, and differentiation into antibody-producing plasma cells. The presence of the B-cell co-receptor complex, CD19/CD21/CD81, can greatly enhance B-cell responsiveness to an antigen.

Antigens with antibodies already bound to them can activate the complement system, thereby coating the antigen with the complement fragment C3d, the ligand for CD21 (also known as complement receptor 2 [CR2]) (Fearon and Carroll, 2000). B cells can also be activated independently of T-helper cells via microbial constituents, such as bacterial polysaccharides, which induce antibody responses by direct recognition of the bacterial constituents via the B-cell receptor or by a non–thymus-derived accessory cell in conjunction with massive crosslinking of B-cell receptors. This can occur when a B cell binds repeating epitopes on the bacterial cell wall. Yet this form of activation usually is not as complete as when T cells supply help (i.e., there is no isotype switching without T-cell help).

As discussed later, the T-cell–dependent B-cell activation occurs at the interface between T-cell and B-cell zones of the secondary lymphoid organs, leading to for-

mation of primary follicles and germinal centers, as well as providing an environment suitable for the processes of immunoglobulin class switching, somatic hypermutation, and affinity maturation.

GENERATION OF IMMUNOLOGIC MEMORY

As discussed earlier, a critical distinction of adaptive immunity from innate immunity is that adaptive immunity is associated with the host's ability to generate a more rapid and robust response upon re-exposure to the same foreign antigen. In antibody production, immunologic memory involves the rapid production of high-affinity immunoglobulin G (IgG) antibody upon re-exposure to a previously encountered antigen by the host. In T-cell responses, immunologic memory produces more robust cytokine production, faster cell cycling, and greater efficiency of cytotoxicity generation.

The exact mechanisms by which the immune system decides what proportion of cells encountering antigen will end in the generation of memory cells and what proportion of cells result in acquisition of effector function remain an area of active investigation. An important factor in this process is the amount of stimulation

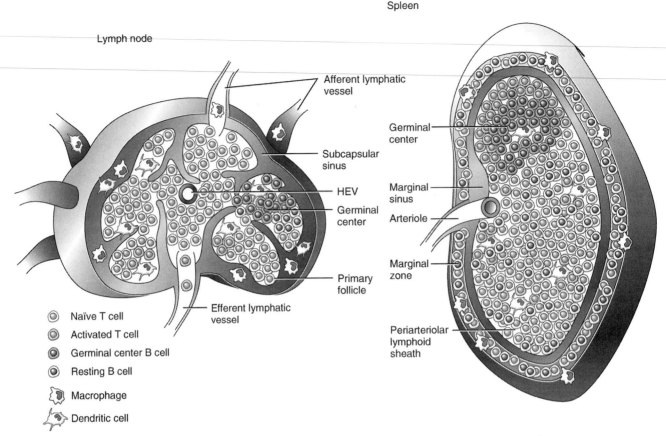

Figure 8-4 · Localization of T and B cells within secondary lymphoid organs. Schematic views of cross-sections through a lymph node and one representative splenic white pulp cord.

as related to antigen dose intensity and amount of co-stimulation encountered by a cohort of responding lymphocytes. For cells that are exposed to high-dose intensity of antigen, the lymphocytes are pushed farther along the differentiation pathway with more robust cell signaling, thus resulting in a terminally differentiated, fully functional effector cell population.

In addition to the fully activated, terminally differentiated, peripherally located effector cells, some subsets of lymphocytes may not differentiate fully into terminal effectors. Rather, they proliferate only modestly and do not acquire full effector function. Instead, they remain

capable of further proliferating and differentiating into effector cells upon future encounter with the same antigen presented by another APC. In effect, these are a subset of memory cells, the so-called *central memory* cells. Another pool of memory T cells is composed of *peripheral memory* cells, which lie between the two previously described populations along the differentiation and self-renewal spectrum (Kaech et al., 2002; Zinkernagel, 2002). Models of memory/effector T-cell generation are shown in Figure 8-5.

Model A proposes a linear-differentiation pathway, whereby memory T cells are direct descendants of effector

TABLE 8-1 · CELL–MEDIATED AND HUMORAL IMMUNITY TO VARIOUS PATHOGENS

	Cell-Mediated Immunity		Humoral Immunity
Effector T Cell	CD8$^+$ cytotoxic T cell	CD4$^+$ Th1 cell	CD4$^+$ Th2/Th1 cell
Source of Antigen	Cytosol	Macrophage vesicles	Extracellular fluid
Antigen Recognition	Peptide: MHC I on infected cell	Peptide: MHC II on macrophages	Peptide: MHC II on antigen-specific B cells
Mechanism of Effector	Killing of infected cell	Activation of infected macrophages	Activation of B cell for antibody production
Examples of Pathogens	Vaccinia virus, Influenza virus, Rabies virus *Listeria*	*Mycobacterium tuberculosis, Mycobacterium leprae, Leishmania donovani, Pneumocystis carinii*	*Clostridium tetani, Staphylococcus aureus, Streptococcus pneumoniae, P. carinii,* Poliovirus

Cell-mediated immune responses involve the destruction of infected cells by CD8$^+$ killer cells or the destruction of intracellular pathogens by macrophages activated by Th1 cells. Th1 cells can also contribute to humoral immunity by inducing antibody production. Th2 cells initiate the humoral response by activating naïve B cells to secrete immunoglobulin M (IgM) and other classes of antibody. All types of antibody contribute to humoral immunity, which is directed principally at extracellular pathogens.

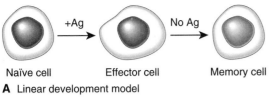

Naïve cell → +Ag → Effector cell → No Ag → Memory cell

A Linear development model

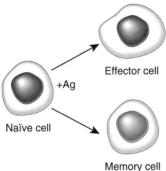

Effector cell

Naïve cell +Ag

Memory cell

B Divergent pathway model

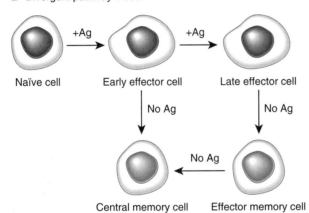

Naïve cell → +Ag → Early effector cell → +Ag → Late effector cell

No Ag

No Ag

Central memory cell ← No Ag ← Effector memory cell

C Memory subset formation model

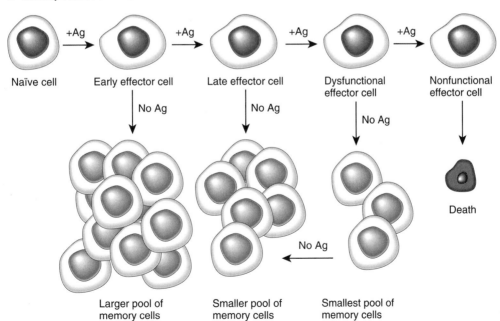

Naïve cell → +Ag → Early effector cell → +Ag → Late effector cell → +Ag → Dysfunctional effector cell → +Ag → Nonfunctional effector cell

No Ag

No Ag

No Ag

Death

Larger pool of memory cells   Smaller pool of memory cells   No Ag   Smallest pool of memory cells

D Decreasing-potential model

Figure 8-5 · Models of effector/memory T-cell generation. A. Model A: linear development model. **B.** Model B: divergent pathway model. **C.** Model C: memory subset formation model. **D.** Model D: decreasing-potential model. (Adapted from Kaech SM, Wherry EJ, Ahmed R. Effector and memory T-cell differentiation: implications for vaccine development. Nat Rev Immunol 2:251–262, 2002.)

cells. This model indicates that memory T-cell development does not occur until antigen is removed or greatly decreased in concentration.

Model B describes a divergent pathway of memory generation, whereby a naïve T cell can give rise to daughter cells that develop into either effector or memory T cells. Such decisions could be either a passive or instructive process. In this particular model, naïve T cells can bypass an effector-cell stage and develop directly into memory T cells.

Model C represents a variation of model A, in which a short duration of antigenic stimulation favors the development of central memory T cells, whereas a longer duration of stimulation favors the differentiation of effector memory T cells. Model D proposes a decreasing-potential hypothesis, which suggests that effector T-cell functions steadily decrease as a consequence of persisting antigen (as is the case in chronic infection). Furthermore, accumulative encounters with antigen lead to increased susceptibility of effector cells to apoptosis and the formation of reduced memory T cell numbers. This model also suggests that T cells might regain function over time following the removal of antigen. The area of effector-memory decision making is under intense investigation, and more information will certainly be forthcoming in the near future. Elucidation of the process of effector and memory cell generation may have important implications for the design of effective vaccine and immunotherapeutic strategies.

CELLULAR TRAFFICKING

Immune responses require timely interaction of multiple cell types within specific microenvironments. As such, leukocyte trafficking represents a key element in the proper regulation of the immune response. As mentioned earlier, the rare T and B lymphocytes specific for the same antigen need to maximize the possibility of encounter with antigen and with each other during primary adaptive immune responses.

Recent evidence suggests that naïve lymphocytes continuously circulate through blood and secondary lymphoid organs, such as lymph nodes and spleen, and do not usually gain access to extravascular space. However, naïve lymphocytes are capable of leaving the circulation via high endothelial venules (HEV) into the spleen and lymph nodes (Jenkins et al., 2001; Kaech et al., 2002) (see Fig. 8-4). It is in these secondary lymphoid organs where a lymphocyte of a particular specificity can come in contact with an antigen-presenting cell that bears such antigen.

T-Cell Traffic

Once circulating T cells encounter APCs bearing the antigen, cellular programs of recognition, proliferation, and differentiation can occur. Depending on the state of activation, the responding T cells have several possible fates (Fig. 8-6A). If a particular antigen is present at an amount that reaches a certain threshold of activation, the corresponding T cells may differentiate into terminal effector cells bearing the machinery capable of carrying out a full range of effector functions, such as cytokine (e.g., IL-4, IFN-γ, IL-2) production or cytotoxic capabilities (e.g., granzyme production) (Table 8-2). These cells also downregulate the expression of chemokine receptors such as CCR7 or CD62L that allow them to leave the secondary lymphoid organ and migrate into tissues where they are needed to fight infections.

In other scenarios, activated T lymphocytes may express surface chemokine receptors (CXCR5) that allow them to migrate to B-cell–rich areas within secondary lymphoid organs, where they can provide "help" for B-cell maturation and antibody production. Figure 8-6B shows a scenario in which inflammation is not accompanied by antigen presentation and the resultant tolerance or ignorance of T cells to such antigen. The exact maturation state of antigen-bearing APCs needed and the microenvironment in which these cell populations were created are subjects of ongoing investigation.

B-Cell Traffic

Recent experiments have shown that antigen-binding B cells are trapped in the T-cell zone of secondary lymphoid tissues when they migrate through HEV. In contrast, most of the non–antigen-binding B cells move quickly through the T-cell zone into the B-cell zone (the primary follicle). This trapping of antigen-binding B cells maximizes the chance of encountering a helper T cell that can activate them, thereby establishing a primary focus of clonal expansion at the border between T-cell and B-cell zones.

After several days of proliferation, some B cells differentiate into antibody-producing plasma cells and migrate to the medullary cords of the lymph node (see Fig. 8-4A) or the red pulp of the spleen (see Fig. 8-4). Some activated T and B cells migrate into a primary lymphoid follicle, where they continue to proliferate and ultimately form a germinal center. Proliferating B cells within the germinal center are surrounded by resting B cells located in the mantle zone. Some of the proliferating B cells in the germinal centers eventually form plasma cells, whereas others go on to become memory B cells.

DOWNMODULATION OF THE IMMUNE RESPONSE

Once the immune system has a chance to respond to the offending agent by proper presentation of foreign antigen by APC to appropriate effector cells, leading to eradication of such agents, the system itself must have a built-in brake to stop the developing immunity from spreading to other self-antigens or undergoing uncontrolled proliferation. There are multiple mechanisms by

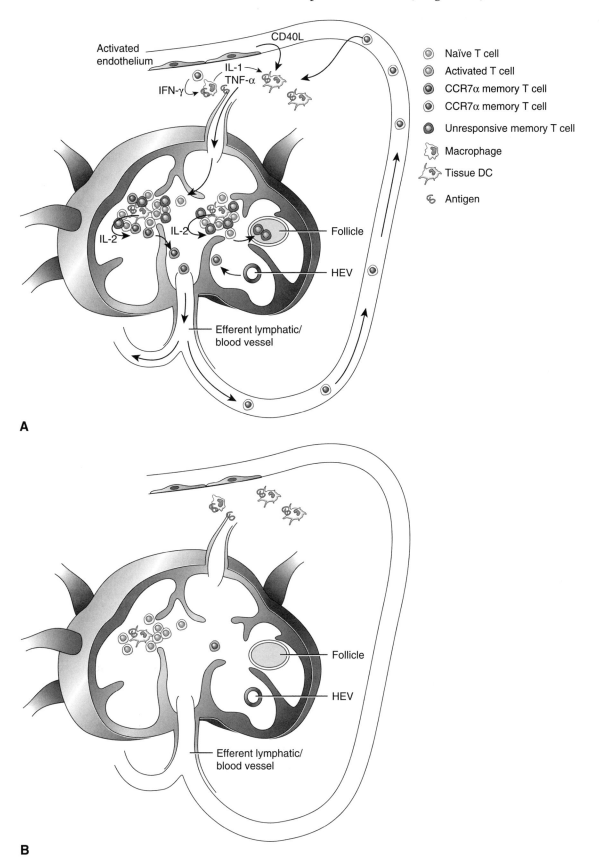

Figure 8-6 · Immune cell trafficking and migration under conditions of immune priming (A) and tolerance (B).

TABLE 8-2 · VARIOUS EFFECTS OF T-CELL–SECRETED CYTOKINES ON CELLS OF THE IMMUNE SYSTEM

| Cytokines | Source | Biologic Effect On | | | | |
		B Cells	T Cells	Macrophages	Hematopoietic Cells	Somatic Cells
IL-2	Th0, Th1, CTL	Growth and J chain synthesis	Growth	—	Stimulates NK growth	—
IFN-γ	Th1, CTL	IgG synthesis	Inhibits Th2	Activation	NK activation	Antiviral
TNF-β	Th1, CTL	Inhibition	Killing	Activation, NO production	Neutrophil activation	Fibroblast and tumor killing
IL-4	Th2	Activation, IgG1 and IgA synthesis	Survival, Growth	Inhibition	Mast cell growth	—
IL-5	Th2	Differentiation, IgA	—	—	Eosinophil growth and differentiation	—
IL-10	Th2	Increase MHC class II	Inhibits Th1	Inhibits cytokine release	Mast cell co-stimulation	—
TNF-α	Th1, Th2, CTL	—	—	Activation	—	Endothelial activation
GM-CSF	Th1, Th2, CTL	Differentiation	Inhibits growth	Activation of DC	Increases myelopoiesis	—
TGF-β	CD4+ T cells	Inhibition of IgA switching	—	Inhibits activation	Neutrophil activation	Mixed effect on growth

In general, each cytokine has multiple biologic effects on different components of the immune system. Combinations of cyokines secreted by a given cell or a host of cells act as a network to exert their effect on the overall immunologic outcome.
CTL = cytotoxic T lymphocytes; NK = natural killer; NO = nitric oxide.

which the immune system downregulates itself after the specific antigenic source has been eliminated. Some of these immunologic mechanisms are discussed briefly in this section. These include antigen-induced cell death, hypoxia-induced anergy, and bystander suppression.

Antigen-Induced Cell Death

It has been described that T cells, following exposure to a viral infection, will experience significant expansion for 3 to 7 days (see Fig. 8-1*B*). These cells subsequently undergo a dramatic contraction of their number with rapid disappearance from secondary lymphoid organs, such as lymph nodes and spleen. Recent analysis using transgenic mice and adoptive transfer techniques have demonstrated that some of the expanded cells undergo antigen-induced apoptosis via actions of surface molecules, Fas-Fas ligand (FasL) interaction. FasL is upregulated on the surface of activated T cells, whereas Fas is upregulated on the surfaces of activated B cells and APCs.

Hypoxia-Induced Cell Death and Anergy

Another proposed immunologic brake comes from recent studies involving tissue damage, hypoxia, and adenosine receptors. T cells, upon receptor engagement, trigger an intracellular signaling cascade, the result of which is transcription, translation, and release of chemokines and cytokines. These secreted molecules cause local inflammation to vascular endothelial and other damaged tissues.

The result of such damage is to cause local accumulation of intracellular and secreted adenosine. This accumulation of adenosine is exacerbated by hypoxia, a condition often found in damaged or inflamed tissues. Hypoxia also causes a decrease in the enzymatic activity of adenosine deaminase, resulting in the decreased conversion of toxic adenosine to nontoxic inosine. Although short lived, extracellular adenosine can bind to subsets of adenosine receptor (A2aR) predominantly found on lymphocytes. It has been postulated that the engagement of A2aR on T cells by adenosine causes an intracellular elevation of cyclic adenosine monophosphate (cAMP), which can downmodulate the effect of receptor engagement on cytokine or chemokine production. The net effect is to downmodulate the previously activated lymphocyte (Aposov et al., 1995).

This model of immune downregulation indicates that agents that block binding of adenosine to A2aR should enhance ongoing immunity and exacerbate conditions that promote autoimmunity. In contrast, agonistic agents binding to A2aR are predicted to cause a downmodulation of the resulting immunity. Indeed, in vivo and in vitro experiments using mice deficient in A2aR by recombinant techniques provides evidence for this mechanism of termination of immune response (Ohta and Sitkovsky, 2001). However, questions remain regarding the timing and duration of such a mechanism and the overall contribution of these and other, yet undescribed pathways to achieving a precise off switch to immunity.

Suppressor T Cells

The idea of suppressor T cells was first postulated in the 1970s as a means by which immune responses can be terminated. These cells were thought to be a subpopulation of lymphocytes that appeared to block or down-

diseases occur at a substantially higher frequency in females than males. This is recapitulated in some animal models of autoimmunity. For example, usually more than 80% of nonobese diabetic (NOD) female mice develop autoimmune diabetes, whereas less than 40% of male mice develop disease (Atkinson and Leiter, 1999). These observations led to the hypothesis that the balance of certain sex hormones may be involved in the predisposition or the initiation of autoimmunity. Castration or female hormone administration in male animals can increase the frequency of autoimmunity (Hawkins et al., 1993). Some epidemiologic evidence suggests that diet, specifically ingestion of cow's milk products, may increase the incidence of TIDM. These observations have not been experimentally substantiated but are reminders that many internal and external factors may affect not only autoimmunity but also proper immune function in general (Greiner et al., 2001).

Genetic Effects

There is evidence that the genetic background of individuals is involved with the expression of and protection from autoimmunity. Some MHC molecules (e.g., human leukocyte antigen [HLA]) occur more commonly in persons with autoimmune diseases than in the general public (Ridgway and Fathman, 1998). The expression of certain HLA molecules (e.g., HLA DR3 or HLA DR4) is associated with a relative risk of certain autoimmune conditions that is approximately 5 to 90 times higher than in those not expressing these molecules.

On the other hand, expression of other MHC molecules, such as HLA-DQ$_b$, may confer protection to other autoimmune states, such as TIDM. It is likely that different HLA molecules hold on to self-antigens in slightly different conformation with different avidities. This may modulate how self-antigen is presented to developing T cells and may alter tolerance induction. Simplistically, if the self-antigen is held in a conformation that enhances TCR–Ag/MHC interaction, tolerance is more likely to occur. On the other hand, poor TCR–Ag/MHC interaction may not promote positive selection of a potentially self-reactive lymphocyte.

Role of T Cells in Autoimmunity

In human and animal models of autoimmunity, autoaggressive T cells and autoantibodies can be isolated, indicating that T and B cells are actively involved in the process (Shlomchik et al., 2001; Zouali, 2002). The effector arm of certain autoimmune diseases seems to favor humoral responses (e.g., Graves' disease and SLE), yet T-cell involvement should not be forgotten. T-cell help is required for full B-cell activation and efficient antibody production and class switching. In most situations, autoimmunity cannot be initiated solely with the transfer of antibodies, yet T cells usually can efficiently transfer disease (Atkinson and Leiter, 1999). On

the other hand, some autoimmune diseases (e.g., multiple sclerosis) seem to result mostly from T-cell effector mechanisms, yet antibody-mediated mechanisms are likely involved also. From this standpoint, autoimmunity is no different from immunity toward a foreign microbe.

The rapidity of the development of clinical autoimmunity depends on the target and the aggressiveness of an immune attack. Destruction of pancreatic islets or thyroid cells occurs over weeks, whereas renal insufficiency and failure in SLE may develop in weeks to years. Progressive and partially remitting exacerbations of neurologic manifestations may take place over years in multiple sclerosis.

SUMMARY

The immune system operates in a highly coordinated, precise, and robust fashion to defend against myriad invading foreign organisms. This defense system comprises mainly two arms: innate immunity, which offers rapid mobilization of the primitive, non–antigen-specific defense system; and adaptive immunity, which can generate potent, antigen-specific immunity with the potential for building a memory response against such organism. Furthermore, the immune system has built-in checks and balances to ensure proper eradication of invading organisms while keeping the responding immunity from being overly aggressive.

In the vast majority of cases, both the innate and adaptive immune responses act in concert to protect the host from microbial takeover. However, there are times when these highly orchestrated interactions break down. Ultimately, we will be able to apply our understanding of these interactions in order to enhance immune responsiveness to fight malignancies, develop tolerance-induction strategies for organ transplantation, design immune reconstitution therapies for congenital and acquired immune deficiencies, and enable immune re-education in autoimmune disorders.

R E F E R E N C E S

Albert ML, Jegathesan M, Darnell RB. Dendritic cell maturation is required for the cross-tolerization of CD8+ T cells. Nat Immunol 2:1010–1017, 2001.

Atkinson MA, Leiter EH. The NOD mouse model of type 1 diabetes: as good as it gets? Nat Med 5:601–604, 1999.

Apasov S, Koshiba M, Redegeld F, Sitkovsky M. Role of extracellular ATP and P1 and P2 classes of purinergic receptors in T-cell development and cytotoxic T lymphocyte effector functions. Immunol Rev 146:5–19, 1995.

Banchereau J, Steinman RM. Dendritic cells and the control of immunity. Nature 392:245–252, 1998.

Bennett SR, Carbone FR, Flavell RA, Heath WR, Karamalis F, Miller JF. Help for cytotoxic-T-cell responses is mediated by CD40 signaling. Nature 393:478–480, 1998.

Boyton RJ, Altmann DM. Transgenic models of autoimmune disease. Clin Exp Immunol 127:4–11, 2002.

Cortesini R, LeMaoult J, Ciubotariu R, Cortesini NS. CD8+CD28− T-suppressor cells and the induction of antigen-specific, antigen-presenting cell-mediated suppression of Th reactivity. Immunol Rev 182:201–206, 2001.

Diehl L, Den Buer AT, Van der Voort EI, Melief C. The role of CD40 in peripheral T cell tolerance and immunity. J Mol Med 78:363–371, 2000.

Fearon DT, Carroll MC. Regulation of B lymphocyte responses to foreign and self-antigens by the CD19/CD21 complex. Annu Rev Immunol 18:393–422, 2000.

Friedl P, Gunzer M. Interaction of T cells with APCs: the serial encounter model. Trends Immunol 22:187–191, 2001.

Gallucci S, Matzinger P. Danger signals: SOS to the immune system. Curr Opin Immunol 13:114–119, 2001.

Gallucci S, Lolkema M, Matzinger P. Natural adjuvants: endogenous activators of dendritic cells. Nat Med 5:1249–1255, 1999.

Germain RN. Antigen Processing and Presentation. Fundamental Immunology, ed 4. Philadelphia, Lippincott Williams and Wilkins, 1999, pp 287–340.

Gorelik L. Flavell RA. Transforming growth factor-beta in T-cell biology. Nat Rev Immunol 2:46–53, 2002.

Greiner DL, Rossini AA, Mordes JP. Translating data from animal models into methods for preventing human autoimmune diabetes mellitus: caveat emptor and primum non nocere. Clin Immunol 100:134–143, 2001.

Hasler P, Zouali M. B cell receptor signaling and autoimmunity. FASEB J 15:2085–2098, 2001.

Hawiger D, Inaba K, Dorsett Y, Guo M, Mahne K, Rivera M, Ravetch JV, Steinman RM, Nussenzweig MC. Dendritic cells induce peripheral T cell unresponsiveness under steady state conditions in vivo. J Exp Med 194:769–779, 2001.

Hawkins T, Gala RR, Dunbar JC. The effect of neonatal sex hormone manipulation on the incidence of diabetes in nonobese diabetic mice. Proc Soc Exp Biol Med 202:201–205, 1993.

Huang FP, MacPherson GG. Continuing education of the immune system—dendritic cells, immune regulation and tolerance. Curr Mol Med 1:457–468, 2001.

Inaba K, Deguchi M, Hagi K, Yasumizu R, Ikehara S, Muramatsu S, Steiman RM. Granulocytes, macrophages, and dendritic cells arise from a common major histocompatibility complex class II–negative progenitor in mouse bone marrow. Proc Natl Acad Sci USA 90:3038–3042, 1993.

Janeway CA Jr. Approaching the asymptote? Evolution and revolution in immunology. Cold Spring Harb Symp Quant Biol 54:1–13, 1989.

Jenkins MK, Khoruts A, Ingulli E, Mueller DL, McSorley SJ, Reinhardt RL, Itaho A, Pape KA. In vivo activation of antigen-specific CD4 T cells. Annu Rev Immunol 19:23–45, 2001.

Kaech SM, Wherry EJ, Ahmed R. Effector and memory T-cell differentiation: implications for vaccine development. Nat Rev Immunol 2:251–262, 2002.

Li XC, Strom TB, Turka LA, Wells AD. T cell death and transplantation tolerance. Immunity 14:407–416, 2001.

Maldonado-Lopez R, Moser M. Dendritic cell subsets and the regulation of Th1/Th2 responses. Sem Immunol 13:275–282, 2001.

Matzinger P. The danger model: a renewed sense of self. Science 296:301–305, 2002.

Medzhitov R, Janeway CJ. Innate immune recognition: mechanisms and pathways. Immunol Rev 173:89–97, 2000.

Mondina A, Khoruts A, Jenkins MK. The anatomy of T-cell activation and tolerance. Proc Natl Acad Sci USA 93:2245–2252, 1996.

Mordes JP, Bortell R, Doukas J, Rigby M, Whalen B, Zipris D, Greiner DL, Rossini AA. The BB/Wor rat and the balance hypothesis of autoimmunity. Diabetes Metab Rev 12:103–109, 1996.

Ohta A, Sitkovsky M. Role of G-protein-coupled adenosine receptors in downregulations of inflammation and protection from tissue damage. Nature 414:916–920, 2001.

Papiernik M. Natural CD4$^+$CD25$^+$ regulatory T cells: their role in the control of superantigen responses. Immunol Rev 182:180–189, 2001.

Ridge JP, Di Rosa F, Matzinger P. A conditioned dendritic cell can be a temporal bridge between a CD4$^+$ T-helper and a T-killer cell. Nature 393:474–478, 1998.

Ridgway WM, Fathman CG. The association of MHC with autoimmune diseases: understanding the pathogenesis of autoimmune diabetes. Clin Immunol Immunopathol 86:3–10, 1998.

Rose NR, Mackay IR. Molecular mimicry: a critical look at exemplary instances in human diseases. Cell Mol Life Sci 57:542–51, 2000.

Rossini AA, Greiner DL, Mordes JP. Induction of immunologic tolerance for transplantation. Physiol Rev 79:99–141, 1999.

Sallusto F, Mackay CR, Lanzavecchia A. The role of chemokine receptors in primary, effector, and memory immune responses. Annu Rev Immunol 18:593–620, 2000.

Salomon B, Bluestone JA. Complexities of CD28/B7: CTLA-4 costimulatory pathways in autoimmunity and transplantation. Annu Rev Immunol 19:225–252, 2001.

Sayegh MH, Turka LA. The role of T-cell costimulatory activation pathways in transplant rejection. N Engl J Med 338:1813–1821, 1998.

Schoenberger SP, Toes RE, Van der Voort EI. Et al. T-cell help for cytotoxic T lymphocyte is mediated by CD40-CD40L interactions. Nature 393:480–483, 1998.

Shevach EM. Regulatory T cells in autoimmunity. Annu Rev Immunol 18:423–449, 2000.

Shlomchik MJ, Craft JE, Mamula MJ. From T to B and back again: positive feedback in systemic autoimmune disease. Nat Rev Immunol 1:147–153, 2001.

Shortman K, Liu YJ. Mouse and human dendritic cell subtypes. Nat Rev Immunol 2:151–161, 2002.

Sprent J, Kishimoto H. The thymus and central tolerance. Transplantation 72:S25–S28, 2001.

Thery C, Smigorena S. The cell biology of antigen presentation in dendritic cells. Curr Opin Immunol 13:45–51, 2001.

Vendetti S, Chai JG, Dyson J, Simpson E, Lombardi G, Lechler R. Anergic T cells inhibit the antigen-presenting function of dendritic cells. J Immunol 165:1175–1181, 2000.

Walker LSK, Abbas AK. The enemy within: keeping self-reactive T cells at bay in the periphery. Nat Rev Immunol 2:11–19, 2002.

Zelenika D, Adams E, Humm S, Lin CY, Waldmann H, Cobbold SP. The role of CD4+ T-cell subsets in determining transplantation rejection or tolerance. Immunol Rev 182:164–179, 2001.

Zinkernagel RM. On differences between immunity and immunological memory. Curr Opin Immunol 14:523–536, 2002.

Zouali M. B cell diversity and longevity in systemic autoimmunity. Mol Immunol 38:895–901, 2002.

C H A P T E R

9

The Mucosal Defense System

Randall M. Goldblum and Roberto P. Garofalo

HISTORICAL BACKGROUND

The mucous membranes that line the body's internal surfaces are constantly exposed to numerous microorganisms and potentially injurious macromolecules. These sites are the major interface between the antigen-laden external environment and the host defense system. Therefore it is not surprising that the mucosal surfaces are also the site of most infections, especially in children. Teleologically, the mucosal epithelium and its secretions should play a major role in local defense. This assumption is supported by numerous studies of experimental bacterial infections, especially of the gastrointestinal tract.

In 1892 Ehrlich showed that newborn mice that were suckled by immunized mothers were protected against the toxic effects of ricin and abrin in the gastrointestinal tract. In 1919 Besredka demonstrated that rabbits were protected against dysentery following oral immunization with Shiga's bacilli. In 1922 Davies showed that patients with dysentery had antibodies in the feces (coproantibodies) several days before antibodies appeared in serum. Later, Burrows and Havens (1948) found that fecal antibodies to *Vibrio cholerae* were not correlated with titers in the serum. Similar studies indicated that antibacterial antibodies are produced locally in the respiratory tract (Bull and McKee, 1929). Subsequent investigations by Fazekas de St. Groth and colleagues (1950, 1951) extended the concept of local immune defense to include viral infections of the respiratory tract; these studies are reviewed by Pierce (1986).

Following the identification of different classes of antibodies, it was shown that the major forms of antibodies of exocrine secretion differed from serum antibodies and that these antibodies were produced locally. Particularly notable was the predominance of immunoglobulin A (IgA) in several external body fluids (Chodirker and Tomasi, 1963) and that this secretory IgA (SIgA) was immunochemically and physicochemically distinct from serum IgA (Hanson, 1961; Hanson and Johansson, 1962; Tomasi et al., 1965).

It was soon recognized that SIgA of the external secretions is made of multiple Ig subunits containing a small joining (J) chain (Halpern and Koshland, 1970;

Mestecky et al., 1971) and a larger glycopeptide, unique to SIgA, called *secretory component* (SC) (Hanson, 1961). These observations accelerated the interest in local immune responses, especially as they related to the control of SIgA formation. Subsequent studies have elucidated the pathways and mechanisms by which antigen stimulation at a mucosal surface results in the production of specific IgA antibodies at several mucosal sites, often with a limited or undetectable serum antibody response.

Other studies indicate that effective defense of the mucosal surfaces also requires T lymphocytes, phagocytes, and innate (nonspecific) immune factors. In addition, the epithelial cells that line the mucosal lumens are now known to be important initiators of local immune responses. Because the humoral immune responses at mucosal surfaces are understood best, they are emphasized here. However, an overview of the role of other mechanisms in host defense, as well as immunologic injury of mucosal tissue, is also included.

The extensive advances in understanding the host defenses of the mucosal surfaces have led to the publication of a complete multiauthor text dedicated to mucosal immunity (Ogra et al., 1999). The goal of this chapter is to provide an overview of the clinically relevant issues in mucosal defenses, particularly as they relate to the health and diseases of infants and children.

MUCOSAL HUMORAL IMMUNE RESPONSES

Components

The machinery for eliciting antigen-specific immune responses at mucosal surfaces consists of the lymphoid and accessory cells distributed throughout the mucosal tissues. In aggregate, the organized lymphoid nodules at mucosal sites, termed *mucosa-associated lymphoid tissue* (MALT) (Biensenstock et al., 1979) contains many more lymphoid cells than the internal, or systemic, immune system. The majority of the MALT is found in the gastrointestinal tract and is called *gut-associated lymphoid tissue* (GALT). Other concentrations of cells are seen in the nasal region and bronchi of the respiratory tract and are termed the *nasal-associated lymphoid tissue* (NALT) and *bronchus-associated lymphoid tissue* (BALT).

In addition to the lymphocytes of the MALT, other immune cells in mucosae are distributed as solitary nodules, diffusely in the lamina propria, and interspersed between epithelial cells. These latter cells are termed *interepithelial lymphocytes* (IELs). Some authors consider lymph nodes draining the mucosal sites (e.g., mesenteric and bronchial lymph nodes) part of the MALT. The MALT seems to employ interconnecting migratory pathways that integrate the mucosal immune responses, both locally and distal to the site of antigenic stimulation. Hence, the whole system for mucosal immune responses has been considered a "common" mucosal immune system.

Although many of the processes in mucosal immunity are similar to those of systemic immunity, one characteristic sets it apart. Because of the extensive antigenic exposure at mucosal sites, there is a need to respond to microorganisms and potentially deleterious macromolecules in a way that minimizes inflammatory injury to the host tissue. This is accomplished largely by displacing the site of interaction between foreign antigens and specific immune reactants into the lumen of the mucosal organ or, at least, to the epithelial surface, where deleterious inflammatory responses are less likely to injure the underlying and internal tissue.

In addition, the host defense mechanisms of the mucosal sites also function largely without inflammatory mechanisms, particularly complement and phagocytes, which are required to eliminate and destroy pathogens that successfully invade the deeper tissues. Thus inflammatory injury to mucosal tissue is usually avoided.

Several major immune mechanisms seem to underlie the differences between the mucosal and systemic immune system. These include unique mechanisms for sampling antigenic material from the lumen of mucosal organs, propensity for IgA-dominance of the humoral immune responses, selective migration of lymphoid cells to mucosal sites, and transport of secretory Igs (SIgs) into secretions. These unique mechanisms are emphasized in this chapter.

Induction of Secretory Immune Responses

Specific mucosal immune responses are usually initiated by antigenic stimulation of specialized lymphoid follicles within certain mucosal tissues (Fig. 9-1). The Peyer's patches of the distal small intestine are the prototype for these organized immunogenic sites. However, anatomically similar lymphoepithelial tissues are present in the appendix (Bockman et al., 1983), tonsils (Owen and Nemanic, 1978), and sometimes in the inflamed bronchi (McDermott et al., 1982). The histology of MALT differs from lymph nodes in that it has no capsule, no medulla, and no afferent lymphatic ducts (Kato and Owen, 1994). This lack of afferent lymphatics suggests that antigens taken up by the epithelium immediately overlying the nodules provide the antigenic stimulation of the follicles.

The epithelium overlying the domelike structure of the Peyer's patches contains cells that differ from the surrounding enterocytes. These cells, which lack microvilli, are therefore termed *membranous* (M) cells. The basolateral aspects of these cells are also unusual because they have invaginations containing lymphocytes and macrophages that have transversed the fenestrated basal lamina below. This unique anatomic configuration may provide for the efficient transfer of antigenic material from the intestine to the juxtaposed immune cells.

Most of the mucosal follicles consist of distinct anatomic regions, including a superficial dome, a

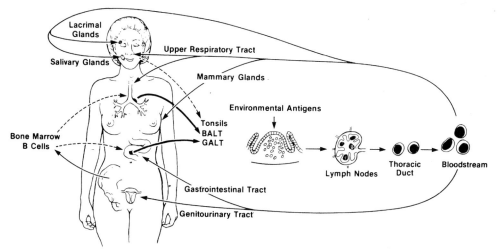

Figure 9-1 · Hypothetical diagram of the common mucosal immune system in humans. Lymphoid cells, presumably from the bone marrow, enter the Peyer's patches (gut-associated lymphoid tissue [GALT]) through high endothelial venules. Under the local influence of T cells and accessory cells, they express surface immunoglobulin A (IgA). Environmental antigens enter Peyer's patches through pinocytotic and phagocytic M cells and interact with resident accessory, T, and B cells. IgA-committed and antigen-sensitized B cells and lymphoblasts leave Peyer's patches and enter the regional lymph nodes, then the lymph and circulation. Finally, such cells populate various exocrine glands and mucosa-associated tissues, where terminal differentiation into IgA-secreting plasma cells occurs. Bronchus-associated lymphoid tissue (BALT) apparently plays a role analogous to that of GALT. It is thought that tonsils may also contribute to the pool of precursor cells that populate the upper aerodigestive tract. (From Mestecky J. The common mucosal immune system and current strategies for induction of immune responses in external secretions. J Clin Immunol 7:265–276, 1987.)

corona, and a central germinal center. The germinal centers of Peyer's patches differ from those in peripheral lymph nodes because 75% to 80% of their B cells have surface IgA (sIgA$^+$). The surrounding cells are mainly CD4$^+$ T cells. These characteristics are in keeping with the role of MALT in the genesis of specific IgA immune responses.

Sampling of Luminal Antigens and Presentation to T Cells

Neutra and Kraehenbuhl (1999) have reviewed the function of the lymphoepithelial structures in sampling and processing luminal antigens for mucosal immune response. The M cells demonstrate some specificity of uptake, probably mediated by a number of receptor-ligand pairs. Viable organisms and particulate material are taken up best (Kato and Owen, 1994). The presence of receptors for Igs on the apical surface of the M cell may enhance the uptake of antigens combined with luminal antibodies (Weltzin et al., 1989).

The site at which the absorbed luminal antigen is processed for presentation has not been definitively identified. However, the M cells, unlike the subepithelial macrophages and interdigitating dendritic cells, express little or no major histocompatibility complex (MHC) class II molecules (Brandtzaeg and Bjerke, 1990). Even though they do have acidic endosomal compartments (Allan et al., 1993; Nagura et al., 1991), which are necessary for antigen processing, this activity may be limited by the small number of M cells and their paucity of MHC class II molecules. As indicated later, there is now

much interest in the role of the mucosal dendritic cells in presenting antigen to the Peyer's patch T cells and helping to induce a population of T cells that support the development of sIgA$^+$ B cells.

Development of IgA Precursor Cells

Antigen-presenting dendritic cells and activated CD4$^+$ T cells are needed to initiate an IgA-predominant mucosal antibody response. However, the details of the pathways by which the microenvironment in lymphoepithelial structures, like the Peyer's patches, promotes IgA preferential humoral immune responses have not been elucidated completely.

McIntyre and Strober (1999) have reviewed the current knowledge concerning the pathways for IgA B-cell development in the GALT. The previous controversy between those who argued that the commitment of Peyer's patch B cells to IgA was due to direct and repeated antigenic stimulation, leading to stepwise B-cell isotype switches, and those who said that soluble factors from local T cells directed the isotype switch to IgA has been largely resolved, in favor of the latter view. Differentiation of B cells into IgA precursor cells requires direct interactions of the antigen-presenting dendritic cells and CD4$^+$ T cells with the B cells.

Antigenic exposure and presentation is required at several steps in this process and may be critical in isotype selection. However, current evidence is strongest for activated T cells and locally secreted cytokines as the mediators of the isotype specificity. Early evidence for this concept was provided by Elson and co-workers'

(1979) demonstration that antigen-activated T cells from Peyer's patches enhance lipopolysaccharide (LPS)-driven IgA synthesis but suppress IgM and IgG synthesis (Elson et al., 1979).

Cell lines containing "switch" T cells (Mayer et al., 1985) and clones derived from them (Benson and Strober, 1988) can induce in vitro production of specific Ig isotypes by activated B cells. Although some commitment of Peyer's patch B cells to IgA may depend on antigen-stimulated, interdigitating dendritic cells, these cells are ineffective in the absence of T cells (Strober and Ehrhardt, 1994).

The soluble T-cell mediators that direct B-cell commitment to IgA have been studied intensively. The sequence and site of the differentiation events are important in this process because some factors enhancing early steps of differentiation may inhibit later steps. All of the steps of differentiation from a virgin (sIgM[+], sIgD[+]) B cell to an IgA-committed cell are thought to take place in the Peyer's patch follicles. Although Peyer's patch is the most important site for the development of B cells that will eventually produce IgA antibodies, there is very little IgA production within the patches. Thus maturation and terminal differentiation to plasma cells must occur in transit to or in the effector site (e.g., gut lamina propria).

The earliest step of B-cell switch to a "downstream" (e.g., IgA) isotype is increased accessibility of the transcriptional enzymes to the deoxyribonucleic acid (DNA) regions which are 5' to the C_H genes (McIntyre and Strober, 1999; Strober and Ehrhardt, 1994). This step seems to depend on both soluble factors and activation of the B cells. The mechanisms involved in this process are still being elucidated. The next step in the differentiation of an IgA B cell is the production of germline transcripts, encoded by $C\alpha$ genes, which have not yet rearranged to a VDJ segment (Stavnezer et al., 1988; Wakatsuki and Strober, 1993).

This transcriptional process suggests that this segment of DNA is also available to the switch recombinase. Stavnezer and colleagues (1988) showed that transforming growth factor-β (TGF-β) induces $C\alpha$ germline transcripts in a B-cell lymphoma. This activity of TGF-β is probably mediated by effects on the promoter upstream from the α heavy chain genes (Nilsson and Paschalis, 1993). The source of the TGF-β that supports this process is thought to be mucosally derived T cells, termed *T-helper 3 (Th3) cells,* which are unusual in their capacity to produce a large amount of TGF-β. However, TGF-β alone is not sufficient to achieve this step. In humans, interleukin 10 (IL-10) and activation via CD40 enhance B-cell switching to IgA (Fayette et al., 1997).

Another requirement for isotype switching is activation of the B cells for a proliferative response, an event required for the switch recombination of DNA that results in productive rearrangements. One effective way to deliver an activation signal for IgA production is through the CD40 membrane structure (Rousset et al., 1991). The natural ligand for CD40 (CD40L) is found on activated T cells.

Further evidence for the requirement of CD40 ligand for IgA (and IgG) production is the deficiencies of these isotypes in patients with X-linked hyper-IgM syndrome (see Chapter 13), a congenital deficiency of CD40L on T cells (Cutler et al., 1993). However, for a complete effect, membranes of activated T cells or anti-CD40 on intact B cells are required (Rousset et al., 1991). This finding suggests that other accessory membrane signals are also needed.

A unifying but unproven concept for commitment of B cells of MALT to IgA production is that the process is regulated by the way in which antigen is presented to the T cells by mucosal dendritic cells that have migrated to the nodules. This mode of antigen presentation, and/or accessory signals from the antigen-presenting cells, may activate T cells to perform as switch cells that drive the local B cells to undergo commitment to IgA isotypes (Weinstein and Cebra, 1991). This process may also initiate B-cell migration to distant mucosal sites. Here the primed B cells, under the influence of memory T cells, differentiate into plasma cells, which produce predominantly polymeric IgA.

Migration, Proliferation, and Differentiation of IgA Cells

The functions of human IgA B cells have been reviewed by Brandtzaeg and Farstad (1999). When antigen-activated IgA-precursor cells leave MALT, they migrate through afferent lymphatics to their regional lymph nodes (see Fig. 9-1). These sites are critical for preparing the B cells for homing to their ultimate effector sites, because the B lymphoblasts from mesenteric lymph nodes migrate preferentially to the gut lamina propria (Phillips-Quagliata et al., 1983).

Activation and proliferation are essential activities that occur in the regional lymph nodes. The activated B cells leave the regional nodes via efferent lymphatics and enter the thoracic duct and eventually the venous blood. Some of the B cells extravasate through the vessels near the intestinal crypt or similar sites near other secretory epithelium. To localize at these sites, the IgA-committed B cells must express on their surface structures that recognize a mucosal vascular addressin cell adhesion molecule 1 (MadCAM-1) on the venules in the lamina propria (Butcher, 1999; Streeter et al., 1988).

The counter receptor, for this ligand expressed on the B cell (and mucosal T cells), appears to be the integrin $\alpha4\beta7$ (Picker, 1994). However, the interaction of other counter receptors, including L-selectin and leukocyte function-associated antigen 1 with their vascular receptors, are also involved in the mucosal homing process. In addition, MadCAM-1 is also expressed on follicular dendritic cells in mucosal lymphoid organs, where it serves to promote the interaction with $\alpha4\beta7$-expressing B cells (Szabo et al., 1997).

The central role for MadCAM-1 in mucosal immune development is further indicated by its selective expression by high endothelial venules of Peyer's patches, where it is involved in migration of immature B cells. In the gut, the IgA-producing cells then localize in the lamina propria, mainly at the level of the crypt openings. Once migration is complete, further antigenic stimulation is necessary for the B cells to proliferate locally (Husband and Dunkley, 1985).

Within the integrated mucosal immune system, there is regional preference for the sites of final migration of IgA-committed B cells. Mesenteric lymph node cells localize preferentially to the small intestine, whereas bronchial lymph node cells preferentially migrate to the lung (McDermott and Bienenstock, 1979). Even within the gut, there is migratory preference between the small intestine and colon (Pierce and Cray, 1982). Activated B cells from human tonsils (part of NALT) may preferentially seed exocrine sites of the upper respiratory tract (Brandtzaeg and Halstensen, 1992). Such preferences may be determined by differences in homing molecules and/or the types of foreign antigens encountered at the various mucosal sites (Brandtzaeg and Farstad, 1999).

The differentiation and migratory pathway through mucosal nodules and regional nodes may not be the only pathway for mucosal IgA precursors. A less well understood lineage of mucosal B cell, arising from the peritoneal cavity, has been described in mice by Herzenberg and associates (1986). These cells, coelomic or B-1 cells, apparently do not migrate through the Peyer's patches (Kroese et al., 1989), and their presence in the lamina propria may be only transient. Reconstitution studies of Kroese and colleagues (1989) suggest that B-1 cells may constitute 30% to 40% of the IgA-producing cells in the murine lamina propria. A similar B-cell population has not been identified in humans.

Terminal Differentiation of B Cells Producing Polymeric IgA

After migration to mucosal effector sites, IgA precursor cells come under the influence of another set of regulatory T cells that, along with direct antigenic exposure, induce B cells to terminally differentiate into IgA-secreting plasma cells. The population of CD4+ T-helper cells responsible for this maturation must differ from those of the Peyer's patches because mucosal IgA synthesis there is much less prominent than that in the lamina propria.

In vitro stimulation of murine B cells with recombinant cytokines, reviewed by Lebman and Coffman (1994), suggests that certain cytokines, namely IL-2, IL-4, IL-5, and IL-6, are responsible for IgA B-cell differentiation. Similar studies in humans are limited and mainly performed on tonsillar B cells. In one system, human B cells were stimulated with a CD40 antibody attached through an Fcγ receptor to human fibroblasts (Rousset et al., 1991), thus providing the membrane signals of activated T cells without the associated T-cell cytokines. By the addition of single or mixtures of recombinant cytokines, it was shown in mice that IL-4, in combination with IL-2, interferon-γ (IFN-γ), or IL-5, increases IgA production; however, only the IL-2/IL-5 combination selectively enhanced IgA production.

The mechanism by which IL-5 induces IgA in this system is not known, but it may selectively stimulate the IgA-committed B cells. IL-10 also strongly enhances IgA production in similar systems (Defrance et al., 1992). The finding that the majority of cytokines involved in this process are produced selectively by Th2 cells suggests that polarization to this helper type should promote mucosal IgA formation (Neurath et al., 2002).

It is difficult to obtain persistent memory in the secretory immune system. Secretory antibodies from the primary response may exclude the antigens of the booster dose, providing a partial explanation. Both animal (Montgomery et al., 1984) and human (Carlsson et al., 1985) studies show that persistent topical stimulation eventually results in a decreased local IgA response, perhaps because of induction of tolerance. With the exception of cholera toxin (Lycke and Holmgrem, 1987), topical induction of a long-lasting secretory immune response requires large and repeated doses of dead antigen (Pierce and Sack, 1977) or the continuous exposure to a replicating antigen (Ogra and Karzon, 1970).

Ogra (1979) found that even 34 months after live oral poliovirus vaccination, there was no decline in nasopharyngeal IgA antibody levels. Similarly, SIgA antibodies against rubella virus persist for several years following live rubella vaccine (Banatvala et al., 1979). On the other hand, SIgA antibodies against poliovirus persist in the saliva without any known re-exposure to antigen other than repeated parenteral injections of inactivated poliovirus vaccine (Carlsson et al., 1985). Functional IgA memory cells have been identified in the Peyer's patches of mice (Lebman et al., 1987).

Studies in dogs and rats demonstrate that parenteral priming and topical boosting is more efficient than topical priming and boosting for the induction of mucosal immune responses (Cebra et al., 1982; Pierce and Gowans, 1975; Pierce and Sack, 1977). Conversely, using Escherichia coli antigens in rats and mice, the best SIgA response was obtained by parenteral boosting after mucosal priming (Hanson et al., 1983b). In agreement with this, parenteral vaccination with poliovirus is more efficient in humans in boosting milk SIgA antibodies than peroral vaccination (Sveennerholm et al., 1981; Carlsson et al., 1985). Such parenteral boosting by cholera vaccine occurred only in individuals who had been previously naturally exposed (Svennerholm et al., 1980).

Together, these findings indicate considerable interaction between MALT and other lymphoid tissues. In addition to practical problems in eliciting local immunity (Waldman and Ganguly, 1975), this is an important aspect to consider when immunoprophylaxis is planned, because parenteral immunization will induce IgG antibodies that may decrease antigen penetrability and thus limit vaccine effectiveness (Brandtzaeg and Tolo, 1977).

Characterization of Immunocytes at Secretory Sites

This topic has also been reviewed in depth by Brandtzaeg and Farstad (1999). All secretory tissues of

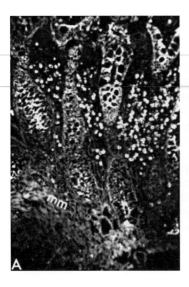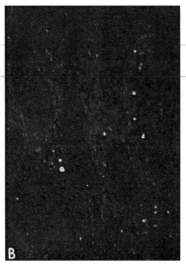

Figure 9-2 · Paired immunohistochemical staining of immunoglobulin A (IgA) (A) and IgG (B) in a section of normal human colon mucosa. The two pictures are from the same field after selective filtration of green and red fluorescence, respectively. Most of the extracellular immunoglobulins had been removed from the tissue by washing, but some IgA was retained in the muscularis mucosae and submucosa. Intracellularly, IgA is present in numerous immunocytes in the lamina propria, in columnar crypt cells, and to a lesser extent in the surface epithelium (at the top). Very few IgG-producing cells are present, and this immunoglobulin is not transported through the columnar epithelial cells. Note that the muscularis mucosae and submucosa are virtually devoid of Ig-producing cells. (×140.)

adults contain a striking preponderance of IgA-producing immunocytes, including plasma cells and their immediate precursors (Fig. 9-2 and Table 9-1). However, the density of such cells varies greatly, being highest in intestinal mucosa and lacrimal glands (Brandtzaeg, 1983b). Almost 10^{10} IgA-producing cells occur per meter of bowel (Brandtzaeg and Baklien, 1976), and thus most of the immunocytes of the secretory immune system are located in the gut. The total size of this Ig-producing cell population is considerably greater than 2.5×10^{10} cells, the estimated total number of immunocytes present in bone marrow, spleen, and lymph nodes combined (Turesson, 1976).

The density of IgA-producing cells correlates with the rate of IgA secretion at various sites. Even though the IgA cell density is not much greater in the lactating human mammary gland than in the parotid, the large size of the former and the local accumulation of IgA between emptying periods explains the large IgA output during milk feedings (Brandtzaeg, 1983b). Although IgM-producing cells contribute significantly to jejunal immunocytes, nasal and bronchial mucosae contain a substantial proportion of IgG-producing cells (see Table 9-1). The reasons for these regional differences

are unknown, but differences in antigenic and mitogenic stimulation by the microbial flora in the intestinal and respiratory tracts may influence the development of the local immunocyte populations (Brandtzaeg, 1994).

Ig-producing cells are not normally present in human intestinal mucosa before 10 days of postnatal age (Perkkio and Savilathi, 1980). However, T and B lymphocytes appear together with dendritic cells in the fetal gut by gestational age of 16 to 19 weeks. IgM and IgD are already expressed at that time (Spencer et al., 1986a, 1986b), suggesting an early capacity for antigenic responses. After birth, a rapid increase in IgM immunocytes occurs; these predominate in the lamina propria for up to 1 month (Brandtzaeg et al., 1991). Blanco and coworkers (1976) found no increase of IgA-producing cells in children after 1 year, although the number of IgM immunocytes decreased. A decrease in intestinal IgM immunocytes with age is associated with an increase of IgA cells even beyond 2 years of age (Maffei et al., 1979; Savilathi, 1972).

Tada and Ishizaka (1970) claim that large numbers of IgE-producing cells are present in mucous membranes and tonsils, but there are many technical problems involved in their identification (Brandtzaeg, 1976b).

TABLE 9-1 · DISTRIBUTION OF Ig-PRODUCING IMMUNOCYTES IN NORMAL ADULT HUMAN GLANDULAR TISSUE

Tissue Site	IgA (%)	IgM (%)	IgG (%)	IgD (%)	Reference
Lacrimal gland	77	7.2	5.8	9.7	Gjeruldsen and Brandtzaeg, 1978
Parotid gland	91	3.0	3.7	2.5	Korsrud and Brandtzaeg, 1978
Nasal concha	67	7.8	15.8	9.2	Brandtzaeg et al., 1979 Brandtzaeg and Berdal, 1973
Bronchial mucosa	74	N.D.	29.0	N.D.	Boye and Brandtzaeg, 1986
Gastric body mucosa	73	13	14	<1.0	Valnes et al., 1986
Gastric antral mucosa	80	8	12	<1.0	Valnes et al., 1986
Jejunum	81	17	2.6	<1.0	Brandtzaeg and Baklien, 1976a
Ileum	83	11	5.0	<1.0	Baklien and Brandtzaeg, 1976
Large bowel	90	6	4.2	<1.0	Baklien and Brandtzaeg, 1975
Lactating mammary gland	68	13	16.0	2.4	Brandtzaeg, 1983a

N.D. = not determined.

Other studies indicate that their numbers in these tissues are extremely low (Ragnum and Brandtzaeg, 1989).

IgD-producing cells are virtually absent from human intestinal mucosa (Brandtzaeg and Baklien, 1976; Brandtzaeg, 1983b). In the tonsils, however, there are about one third as many IgD-producing cells as those containing cytoplasmic IgM (Brandtzaeg et al., 1978), and in the parotid, lacrimal, and nasal glands (see Table 9-1) there are about the same number as the IgM-producing cells (Brandtzaeg et al., 1979; Brandtzaeg, 1983b). This discrepancy is accentuated in IgA deficiency, in which IgA-producing cells are often replaced by IgD immunocytes in the upper aeroalimentary tract, rather than by IgM immunocytes, which predominate in the gut (Brandtzaeg et al., 1979, 1987a).

Secretory IgA Production

Extracellular Immunoglobulins in Mucosal Tissues

Immunohistochemical studies of secretory tissues has shown that despite extensive local production of IgA, IgG predominates in the extravascular space (Brandtzaeg, 1974b, 1976a). This finding is compatible with rapid external transport of the locally produced polymeric IgA. Thus the IgA of the stroma may represent monomeric IgA of local or serum origin. Because local synthesis of IgG is sparse, the intense stromal staining most likely represents serum-derived IgG.

Although 50% to 60% of circulating IgA and IgG is extravascular, only 20% of IgM is extravascular (Waldmann and Strober, 1969). Accordingly, the secretory tissue shows little IgM except in basement membrane zones and vessel walls. With antigenic stimulation, the amount of extracellular IgA and IgM may be substantially increased, as in the mucosa of patients with celiac disease (Brandtzaeg and Baklien, 1977b). IgD and IgE cannot usually be demonstrated extracellularly.

Nature of Locally Formed IgA

As reviewed by Brandtzaeg and Farstad (1999), it was initially believed that IgA immunocytes at secretory sites produced monomers, which were then polymerized by complexing with an epithelial glycoprotein called *secretory piece* or *SC* to form dimeric SIgA. However, the later finding of J chain in most IgA immunocytes in exocrine tissue strongly suggested that the IgA dimers were produced within the plasma cells (Brandtzaeg, 1974b, 1983a). SC-affinity tests on tissue sections substantiated that the J-chain containing IgA, as well as IgM, is assembled within the plasma cells; this finding, however, does not exclude a concomitant production of some IgA monomers by lamina propria immunocytes (Brandtzaeg, 1994).

Analyses of cultured mononuclear cells from human gut mucosa have not demonstrated conclusively the proportion of IgA monomers and dimers produced

(Brandtzaeg, 1985a). However, IgA immunocytes of secretory sites preferentially produce IgA polymers compared with other lymphoid tissues, such as tonsils or cells from inflammatory foci, where little production of J chain takes place (Brandtzaeg and Korsrud, 1984).

A large fraction of IgA immunocytes (35% to 60%) at secretory sites contain the IgA2 subclass, compared with cells of the tonsils and peripheral lymph nodes (Crago and Mestecky, 1984; Jonard et al., 1984). Production of IgA2 is particularly striking in the ileum and large bowel, where mucosal IgA2 immunocytes often predominate (Kett et al., 1986).

Teleologically, this may be advantageous because IgA2 is more resistant to microbial proteases. There is also a relatively high proportion of IgA2 cells in salivary glands (approximately 37%), whereas nasal mucosa contains about 95% IgA1 producers (Kett et al., 1986). Thus IgA2 predominates at sites where the intensity of bacterial exposure is greatest (Brandtzaeg, 1994).

Active Transfer of Immunoglobulin into External Secretions

Despite the high stromal concentration of IgG, secretory epithelial cells are virtually devoid of this isotype. IgD and IgE cannot be detected in epithelia, except for IgE that is carried by mast cells (Brandtzaeg and Korsud, 1984; Brandtzaeg, 1985b). In contrast, IgA is present at the basal and lateral surfaces of the mucosal epithelial cells and intracellularly in serous-type cells, especially in the apical part of colonic and rectal crypt cells (Brandtzaeg, 1974a; Brandtzaeg and Baklien, 1977b).

The epithelial distribution of IgM mimics that of IgA, although it is much less prominent and is readily demonstrable only in the large bowel (Brandtzaeg, 1975). The predominance of polymeric Igs (PIgs) (dimeric IgA and pentameric IgM) within epithelial cells suggested that they are selectively transported into or through these cells.

Polymeric Immunoglobulin Receptor

The selective transport of polymeric Ig into the external secretions is unique to the secretory immune system. This process has been reviewed in depth by Mostov and Keetzel (1999). The specificity and efficiency of secretory Ig formation lie in a receptor-ligand interaction. Unlike most receptor-mediated processes, however, the polymeric Ig receptor (PIgR) remains attached to its ligand (dimeric IgA or pentameric IgM) throughout the transport and secretory process.

A fragment of the PIgR, first recognized by Hanson in 1961 as a unique structural component of SIgA, was initially termed *bound secretory piece* but is now called simply *bound SC*. The PIgR corresponds to the transmembrane form of SC, and a major fragment of this receptor is released to the lumen, either bound to PIgA or alone as free SC, structurally identical to bound SC.

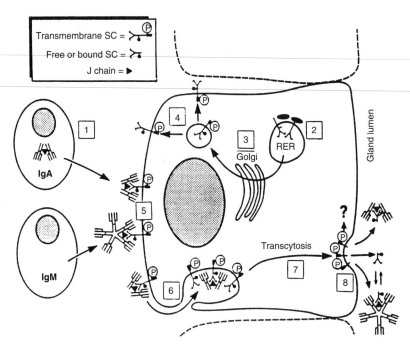

Figure 9-3 · Model for local generation of human secretory immunoglobulin A (SIgA) and SIgM: (1) Production of J chain-containing poly-IgA and pentameric IgM by gland-associated plasma cells. (2) Synthesis and core glycosylation of transmembrane secretory component (SC) in rough endoplasmic reticulum of epithelial cell. (3) Terminal glycosylation in Golgi complex. (4) Phosphorylation at some later step. (5) Complexing of SC with J chain-containing poly-Ig on basolateral cell membrane. (6) Endocytosis of complexed and unoccupied SC. (7) Transcytosis of vesicles. (8) Cleavage and release of SIgA, SIgM, and excess free SC. The cleavage mechanism and the fate of the cytoplasmic tail of transmembrane SC are mostly unknown. During the external translocation, covalent stabilization of the IgA-SC complexes regularly occurs (two disulfide bridges indicated in SIgA), whereas an excess of free SC in the secretion serves to stabilize the noncovalent SIgM complexes (dynamic equilibrium indicated). (From Brandtzaeg P, Halstensen TS, Huitfeldt HS, et al. Epithelial expression of HLA, secretory component [poly-Ig receptor], and adhesion molecules in the human alimentary tract. Ann NY Acad Sci 664:61, 1992.)

STRUCTURE OF PIgR

With few exceptions, PIgR expression is limited to the serous-type secretory epithelial cells (Figs. 9-3 and 9-4). The PIgR is a member of the Ig supergene family, which consists of seven domains, or functional segments (Brandtzaeg, 1994; Mostov et al., 1984). The five N-terminal domains, which bear strong homology with the Ig variable domains, form the extracellular segment of the receptor. After synthesis in the rough endoplasmic reticulum and extensive glycosylation (approximately 20% carbohydrate by weight) in Golgi's complex, the PIgR is selectively targeted to the basal and lateral membranes of the epithelial cells.

The molecular information necessary for this targeting resides in a 17-amino acid segment of the cytoplasmic tail (Casanova et al., 1990). Once inserted in the epithelial cell membrane, the extracellular receptor segment becomes available for binding PIg. Bakos and colleagues (1991) have identified a small segment of the first (N-terminal) domain that is critical for noncovalent

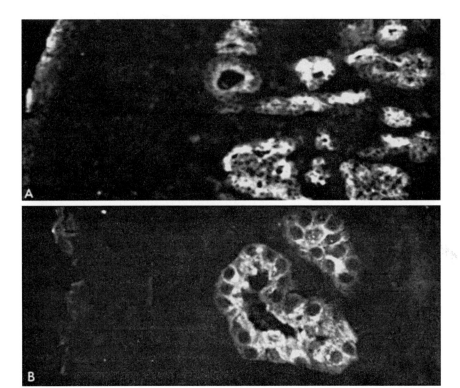

Figure 9-4 · Immunohistochemical localization of secretory component (SC) in normal human nasal mucosa from the concha inferior. **A.** Note fluorescence of serous glandular acini, whereas the surface epithelium (to the left) does not contain SC except in occasional cells where IgA (not shown) is also present. The mucous coat on the surface has not been retained. **B.** In addition to cytoplasmic localization, SC is also present in relation to lateral and basal borders of acinar cells, apparently incorporated into the plasma membrane. Note the absence of SC in the connective tissue, where numerous Ig-producing cells (not shown) are present. (A, ×60; B, ×160.)

binding of Igs (Bakos et al., 1991). However, studies using synthetic peptides representing this region and proteolytic fragments of native PIgR indicate that a more extensive structure is required to achieve specific binding of polymeric IgA and IgM (Baklien and Brandtzaeg, 1974). This finding was confirmed by domain-switching experiments, which indicated that PIgR domains 2 and 3 contribute to IgA, but not IgM binding (Norderhaug et al., 1999).

ROLE OF J CHAIN

The regions of the Ig polymer necessary for binding to the PIgR have been elucidated recently by Hexam and associates (1999). Their finding that an exposed loop on the Cα3 of IgA was responsible for IgA binding to PIgR was confirmed recently (Braathen et al., 2002). That J chain is required for PIgR binding was suggested by the finding that monoclonal polymeric IgA and IgM, which are deficient in J chains, do not bind free SC (Brandtzaeg, 1976a) or the PIgR (Brandtzaeg and Prydz, 1984). Further, antibody to J chain blocks the SC-binding site of IgA dimers (Brandtzaeg, 1976b).

The requirement for J chain in PIgR-mediated transport in vivo was demonstrated in mice in which the J chain had been knocked out (Hendrickson et al., 1996). These mice were able to produce PIgA (devoid of J chain), but PIgR accumulated in the serum and interstitial space, rather than being transported into the secretions. However, J chain is involved only indirectly in receptor binding, because free J chain has little affinity for SC (Brandtzaeg, 1985b). Thus the J chain is probably necessary for establishing or maintaining a conformation of the α chain that is required for IgA to bind avidly and noncovalently to the PIgR.

TRANSCYTOSIS OF PIgR

After Ig binding, the PIgR-PIg complexes are internalized via clathrin-coated pits into intracellular vesicles (see Fig. 9-3). The transport of PIgR through the epithelial cell is called *transcytosis*. The migration of these vesicles across the epithelial cells is regulated by signaling information present in the cytoplasmic tail of the PIgR (Mostov et al., 1984).

At least three steps in the transcytosis are regulated by interrelated, intracellular signaling events, some of which are initiated by the binding of PIg to PIgR. For instance the movement of PIgR from the apical membrane into the transcytotic pathway seems to require masking of the signals that result in the basolateral sorting of newly formed PIgR molecules. In some tissues, the PIgR-ligand complexes accumulate in vesicles near the apical surface of the cell. These complexes may serve as a reservoir of SIg that can be rapidly secreted when needed or may be used within the cell to neutralize viruses.

There appears to be a protein kinase C and intracellular Ca^{++}-dependent pathway that releases PIgR from an apical recycling compartment for exocytosis into the lumen (Song et al., 1994). The final steps of SIg formation entail fusion of the vesicles with the epithelial apical membrane and enzyme cleavage of the extracellular segment of the PIgR within the apical membrane (Musil and Baenziger, 1988). This process releases SIg (polymeric Ig and its bound SC) into the lumen.

PHYSIOLOGIC ROLE OF PIgR

The physiologic role of PIgR and PIgR-mediated Ig secretion has been demonstrated in mice with targeted deletions of J chain (Hendrickson et al., 1996) and mice with PIgR deletion (Johansen et al., 1999). The surprising finding from both models is that the quantity of total IgA in saliva was not decreased. However, in the PIgR-knockout animals the IgA content of the small intestine and fecal pellets were reduced somewhat and strikingly, respectively.

Based on measurements of IgG and albumin in the secretions of PIgR-knockout mice, it is clear that in the absence of PIgR, Igs accumulate in the serum and interstitial space and are "leaked" into the lumen at an increased rate. Despite the normal survival of the PIgR-knockout mice, these finding suggest that PIgR or SIgs are important in the integrity of the mucosal epithelial barrier.

Secretory IgA Formation

Several elements of SIg formation deserve further comment. During transcytosis, a disulfide bond is formed between the PIgA and the PIgR. Only one of the subunits of IgA is involved in this reaction (Garcia-Pardo et al., 1979; Underdown et al., 1977). The intracellular site of this covalent bond formation probably occurs during the later phases of transcytosis (Chintalacharuvu et al., 1994; Lindh and Bjork, 1976). Although intracellular enzymes may be involved in this process, the same bonds can be formed in vitro in the absence of any enzymes (Brandtzaeg, 1977). Interchain disulfide bonds do not form between IgM and SC because of the lack of a free sulfhydryl group on IgM. The importance of the disulfide bond on IgA-SC integrity and function has not been studied in detail, but covalently binding of SC may enhance the resistance of S-IgA against proteolytic degradation.

The process of transcytosis of the PIgR does not require the binding of Ig polymers. In the absence of this ligand, the proteolytic product of PIgR is free SC. This fragment can also be found in the secretions in which SIgA is normally found. This suggests that epithelial transport is constitutive and that PIgR may not be the rate-limiting factor for SIgA formation.

Free SC can be found in secretions of young infants and other patients who are IgA-deficient (South et al., 1966) in amounts similar to the total (free and bound) SC in healthy subjects (Brandtzaeg, 1974b). This suggests that polymers are not necessary for PIgR expression by secretory epithelia. The presence of free SC in body fluids (e.g., amniotic fluid) has been used as a marker for the presence of secretory epithelium capable of SIgA formation (Cleveland et al., 1991).

Secretory Ig formation by epithelial cells is highly regulated at several levels (Mostov and Kaetzel, 1999). The expression of PIgR seems to be regulated, at least in some tissues. Evidence for the enhanced PIgR expression after stimulation by proinflammatory cytokines (TNF-α, IFN-γ, IL-4, IL-1β, and IL-1α) is derived from in vitro studies using multiple epithelial cell lines (Phillips et al., 1990; Mostov and Kaetzel, 1999). A small effect of TGF-β on SC production has also been demonstrated in a rat epithelial cell line (McGee et al., 1991).

The physiologic relevance of PIgR regulation is suggested by the finding of increased epithelial expression of PIgR in several diseases in which these cytokines can be expected to be produced (Brandtzaeg and Halstensen, 1992). Some studies suggest that the modulation occurs at the messenger ribonucleic acid (mRNA) level (Krajci et al., 1993; Piskurich et al., 1993).

In vivo regulation of the PIgR expression may increase SIgA production at sites of mucosal inflammatory responses, thereby focusing the output of the secretory immune system to sites of infection or other injury. Thus increased amounts of SIgA, free SC, or both may indicate enhanced local immunity. Examples include high levels of SIgA in the urine of patients with pyelonephritis (Brandtzaeg, 1993; Fliedner et al., 1986; Greenwell et al., 1995) and in duodenal secretions in untreated celiac disease (Brandtzaeg, 1993). Dysregulation of PIgR expression has been also used as a prognostic indicator in colon carcinomas (Krajci et al., 1996).

Passive Transfer of Immunoglobulin into External Secretions

In addition to selective external transport of PIgA and IgM, passive, intercellular epithelial diffusion contributes to the Ig content of exocrine fluids, as indicated by the immunohistochemical demonstration of IgG in the interstitium of mucosal tissues and secretions. Intercellular epithelial diffusion is more pronounced in respiratory and intestinal surface epithelia than in glandular epithelia. Thus the composition of an exocrine fluid also depends on extraglandular extravasation, which may be influenced by inflammation and local Ig production (Brandtzaeg et al., 1970; Haneberg and Aarskog, 1975).

STRUCTURE AND FUNCTION OF IMMUNOGLOBULINS IN EXOCRINE SECRETIONS

Secretory IgA Structure

Most serum IgA molecules are monomers composed of two identical heavy and two light chains, arranged as in IgG. Only approximately 15% to 20% of normal serum IgA molecules are dimers and larger polymers of IgA (Delacroix and Vaerman, 1983; Neukirk et al., 1983). The proportion of polymeric IgA is considerably higher in infancy (Delacroix et al., 1983; Splawski et al., 1984). Conversely, polymeric forms predominate in the secretions and monomeric IgA makes up only 5% to 20% (Brandtzaeg et al., 1970; Jonard et al., 1984). Variation of the monomer/polymer ratio in different secretions may be due to different degrees to which the IgA is transported by the PIgR or leaks through the epithelium. Both processes are influenced by inflammation and local Ig production (Brandtzaeg et al., 1970; Haneberg and Aarskog, 1975).

SIgA polymers are somewhat heterogeneous in size, but most are dimers. The proportion of larger polymers varies; some authors have found 5% to 20% (Delacroix and Vaerman, 1982; Hurlimann et al., 1969; Tomasi et al., 1965), others found considerably higher percentages (Brandtzaeg et al., 1970). Variable degrees of aggregation following SIgA purification may explain these discrepancies

IgA and IgM polymers also contain a polypeptide J chain of about 15 kD (Halpern and Koshland, 1970; Mestecky et al., 1971). This J chain is disulfide-linked to the penultimate cysteine of the C-terminal octapeptide of the heavy chains (Mestecky, 1976). There is typically one J chain that acts as a clasp connecting only two Ig subunits, whereas the remaining subunits of polymers larger than dimers are mutually connected by inter–heavy-chain disulfide bridges (Bastian et al., 1992; Inman and Mestecky, 1974; Koshland, 1975). However, J chains are prone to degradation, and exact quantification is difficult.

SIgA also differs from serum polymeric IgA by its content of bound SC. The majority of SIgA consists of a dimer of IgA, one or two J chains, and one SC. The resulting molecule has a molecular weight of 375 kD estimated by gel filtration and 390 kD by ultracentrifugation (Hurlimann et al., 1969; Newcomb et al., 1968; Tomasi and Czerwinski, 1968).

SC endows SIgA with unique antigenic properties. Thus antibodies to SC distinguish between the serum IgA and SIgA. These antibodies are used extensively in studies of clinical samples and molecular structure. Degradation of SIgA, followed by antigenic analyses of the split products, provides information about the tertiary and quaternary structure of the intact molecule. Disruption of only the noncovalent bonds results in only minor release of IgA monomers and SC (Brandtzaeg, 1971c; Tomasi and Bienenstock, 1968).

In human SIgA, 70% to 80% of SC is bound by disulfide bridges, secondarily stabilized by noncovalent bonds. Thus when complexed with IgA, part of the SC is inaccessible to antibodies or enzymes. Moreover, formation of SIgA results in extensive configurational changes on SC because most epitopes of free SC are not detectable on SIgA (Bakos et al., 1993; Brandtzaeg, 1971c; Brandtzaeg et al., 1970; Iscaki et al., 1978; Woodard et al., 1984). The enhanced stability and resistance to enzymatic degradation of SIgA may result from masking the labile segments of serum IgA and free SC (Bakos et al., 1993).

Secretory IgA Stability

The external secretions are potentially more destructive to proteins than are the plasma and interstitial tissue spaces. Thus enhanced resistance of SIg to degradation favors protection of the host. Most in vitro studies showing increased resistance of SIgA to proteolytic digestion do not identify whether the effect is due to the presence of a dimeric structure or presence of SC (Ghetie and Mota, 1973; Lindh, 1975; Underdown and Dorrington, 1974).

In either case, these results suggest that SIgA has functional advantage over serum-type IgA found in the protease-containing external secretions. In vivo evidence for this is derived from studies showing that human milk SIgA traverses the infant gut with its antibody activity intact (Gindrat et al., 1972; Haneberg, 1974b; Kenny et al., 1967; Schanler et al., 1986). Most of these studies did not assess the amount of antibody the infants were receiving or other properties of human milk (e.g., its high buffering capacity), but it is believed that SIgA preferentially persists and functions well, even in the harsh environment of the gastrointestinal tract.

Some bacteria can counter the attack of SIgA antibodies. As in the mammalian liver (Hanson et al., 1973), some *Escherichia coli* have nucleotide-dependent reductases that can split colostral IgA (Moore et al., 1964), thus degrading SIgA antibodies attached to *E. coli* bacteria in the intestine. Other pathogenic oral, enteric, and upper respiratory tract bacteria have proteases with high specificity and activity for IgA1, cleaving it to fragment crystallizable (Fc) and fragment antigen binding (Fab) fragments (Kilian and Reinholdt, 1986; Kilian and Russell, 1994; Plaut, 1983).

IgA1 normally constitutes approximately 80% of serum IgA, whereas SIgA consists of 60% to 70% IgA1, depending on the site of production (Brandtzaeg, 1994; Delacroix and Verman, 1982). This IgA2 enrichment in secretions may provide enhanced protection, especially in the colon and mouth, where the IgA2 isotype is highest and bacteria are plentiful. However, *Clostridium ramosum* protease has specificity for both IgA1 and IgA2 (Fujiyama et al., 1985). Furthermore, yeasts of the species *Torulopsis* and *Candida* as well as *Pseudomonas aeruginosa* make proteases that can degrade IgA1, IgA2, and SIgA (Kilian and Russell, 1994; Reinholdt et al., 1987).

Thus the resistance of SIgA to in vivo proteolytic degradation is not absolute. Humans often make SIgA antibody to certain microbial enzymes, thereby inhibiting their activity (Gilbert, 1983). Serum IgA and SIgA are often resistant to IgA proteases as a result of antibodies that neutralize the enzymes (Kobayashi et al., 1987). However, neither fluid contains neutralizing antibodies to the *Clostridium* enzyme that degrades IgA1 and IgA2 (Fujiyama et al., 1985).

The fact that some 20% to 80% of milk SIgA can be recovered undegraded in the stool of breastfed babies (Davidson and Lonnerdal, 1987; Schanler et al., 1986) suggests that the overall balance of this microbe-host defense battle favors the host. The most effective SIgA antibodies are those that bind to the pathogenic microorganisms; however, these may be particularly susceptible to microbial proteases (Kilian and Russell, 1994).

Function of Secretory IgA

The first issue regarding the function of SIgA is whether these antibodies in secretions are indeed protective. Despite evidence that SIgA antibodies appear in the secretions after oral immunization, that their presence is correlated with protection against toxic substances and pathogenic microorganisms, and that most of the Ig produced is released into the secretions, direct evidence that SIgA mediates immune protection is limited. Indeed, most patients with severe isolated IgA deficiency have no obvious increase in mucosal infections. The best explanation for this observation is that SIgA is so important that compensatory mechanisms, including SIgM and certain IgG subclasses, compensate for deficiencies in the SIgA system (see Chapter 14).

Several studies provide evidence for a protective role of SIgA. The most convincing have examined the effects of passively transferred IgA, thus excluding a contribution by other components of the immune system. Glass and coworkers (1983) demonstrated that infants ingesting maternal milk containing cholera antibodies have fewer symptoms after exposure to cholera than infants ingesting maternal milk lacking such antibodies. Other studies have confirmed these findings for other enteric organisms (Carlsson and Hanson, 1994). In most of these studies, IgA antibodies reduced the frequency and severity of symptoms rather than preventing infection.

The efficacy of SIgA antibodies in experimental models also demonstrates that passive transfer of specific polymeric IgA prevents infection following challenge with the live homologous organism. Winner and coauthors (1991) demonstrated serotype-specific protection against oral challenge of mice with *Vibrio cholerae* by subcutaneous implantation of a hybridoma producing polymeric IgA, directed against the LPS of that organism. Renegar and Small (1991) showed that intravenous polymeric IgA but not monomeric IgA antibodies against influenza virus protected against challenge of the respiratory tract with influenza virus.

Similarly, mice bearing hybridoma tumors that produce PIgA specific for a rotavirus are protected against infection (Burns et al., 1996). Interestingly, the protective antibodies were directed against the inner capsid rotavirus protein, suggesting that in this model, the neutralization took place before the assembly of the virus in the intestinal epithelial cell. The role of SIgA in the resolution of ongoing mucosal infections is less clear. In sum, human and animal studies indicate that mucosal antibody responses are effective at preventing mucosal infections.

The next issue is whether SIgA protection is mediated solely by the specificity of the antibodies or whether it requires the unique biochemical properties of SIgA. Kilian and Russell (1999) divide the functions of

SIgA into those mediated solely by (Fab) antigen binding portion and those dependent on Fc and/or secretory specific portions of the SIgA (Kilian et al., 1988). This distinction may be particularly important for SIgA1 in secretions frequently exposed to pathogenic bacteria that produce IgA1 proteases. Despite cleavage into Fc and Fab fragments, some IgA1 antibody functions may be preserved.

The Fab portion of SIgA by itself can neutralize some toxins and virulence enzymes of microorganisms at the mucosal surfaces. Antibodies against cholera toxin (Lycke et al., 1987) and to glucosyltransferase of streptococci that synthesize adherent glucans (Smith et al., 1985) are examples of virulence factors neutralized by the Fab portion of IgA. Single Fab units of IgA may also prevent viral attachment to their cellular receptors.

Most functions of SIgA require the intact molecule. This includes most viral neutralization, inhibition of bacterial adherence, and immune exclusion (Brandtzaeg and Korsrud, 1984; Newby, 1984). SIgA antibodies neutralize viruses efficiently (Hanson and Johansson, 1970; Newcomb and Sutoris, 1974; Taylor and Dimmock, 1985), with a broader antibody specificity than serum antibodies (Shvartzman, 1977; Waldman et al, 1970). This broad neutralizing activity may be advantageous in coping with the antigenic drift of microorganisms growing on mucosal surfaces.

SIgA antibodies may also inhibit internalization or even intracellular replication of certain viruses (Armstrong and Dimmock, 1992). Polymeric IgA may even be able to inhibit replication of viruses that have previously entered cells (Mazanec et al., 1992b). This activity is mediated by polymeric IgA antibodies that enter infected epithelial cells via the PIgR. Thus a virus entering an epithelial cell at its apical (luminal) face might be neutralized by antibodies within the transcytotic pathway, thus extending the range of IgA-mediated protection. Finally, a virus that breaches the epithelial cell may combine with IgA antibodies to form immune complexes that are transported to the lumen by other PIgR-expressing cells (Kaetzel et al., 1991).

Prevention of bacterial adherence and colonization by SIgA is one of its most crucial functions (Svanborg, 1994; Svanborg and Svennerholm, 1978; Tramont, 1977; Williams and Gibbons, 1972). The mechanisms by which SIgA prevents bacterial adherence are multiple. Binding of the surface adherence factors on the bacteria by the Fab region of SIgA may have some neutralizing effects. The hydrophilic nature of the intact IgA provided by the extensive glycosylation of both α chains of IgA2 and SC may also reduce the ability of bacteria to interact with epithelial cell membranes. The multiple combining sites of SIgA polymers promote agglutination of microorganisms and enhance their removal by peristalsis. SIgA may also interact directly with mucin (Clamp, 1977) or, by their hydrophilicity, may make the bacteria more "mucophilic" and susceptible to mucociliary clearance (Magnusson and Stjernstrom, 1982).

In vivo coating of bacteria by SIgA can be demonstrated by immunofluorescence (Fig. 9-5), but this may be mediated, in part, by nonspecific binding of type 1 pili of gram-negative bacteria to mannose residues of SIgA. This binding, which is reversed by mannose, may agglutinate bacteria, thus augmenting mucosal defense (Wold et al., 1988). Moreover, several types of bacteria express Fcα receptors that may bind SIgA.

Immune exclusion refers to the ability of SIgA antibodies to hamper microbial colonization and the penetration of macromolecules through the mucous membranes (Andre et al., 1974; Lim and Rowley, 1982; Stokes et al., 1975; Walker et al., 1972, 1974; Walker et al., 1975). This concept is supported by the observation that IgA-deficient individuals have increased levels of antibodies to dietary antigens and circulating immune complexes containing such antigens (Cunningham et al., 1979) (see Chapter 14). The

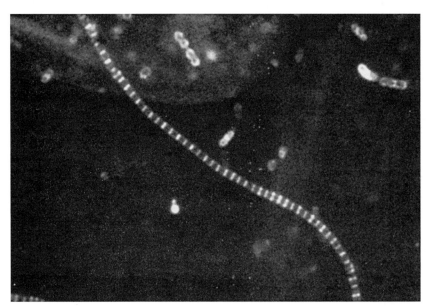

Figure 9-5 · Adsorption of immunoglobulin A (IgA) onto oral bacteria in vivo, as revealed by direct immunofluorescence staining. Salivary sediments were washed, and smears were reacted with a fluorescein-labeled anti–β-chain reagent. Immunofluorescence demonstrated that numerous cocci (mainly diplococci) were coated with IgA and that the immunoglobulin was also bound to the older cell wall segments of streptococci forming long chains. The majority of the bacteria were found in relation to epithelial cells, which were revealed by their autofluorescence (upper and right parts of the field). For further details see Brandtzaeg P, Fjellanger I, Gjeruldsen ST. Adsorption of immunoglobulin A onto oral bacteria in vivo. J Bacteriol 96:242-249, 1968. (×600.)

mechanisms involved in immune exclusion are probably similar to those that inhibit viral and bacterial invasion. The finding that PIgR-knockout mice leak serum proteins into the bowel, discussed previously, suggest an important role for SIgs in intestinal integrity.

In summary, SIgA antibodies act as a "first line of defense" because of their physical attributes and largely their ability to inhibit microbes and antigens from interacting with the mucosa (see Fig. 9-5). Because host-pathogen interactions largely occur in the confines of the luminal space, they can protect the host without risking the injurious effects of tissue inflammation. Certain cells and soluble components of the secretory system may also interact with SIgA, enhancing its protective activity.

Structure and Function of Secretory IgM

Only small amounts of IgM are found in the external secretions of normal adults, but their levels are increased in young infants and in individuals with selective IgA deficiency (Brandtzaeg, 1971a; Brandtzaeg et al., 1968b; Girard and de Kalbermatten, 1970; Mellander et al., 1984, 1985, 1986b; Savilathi, 1973).

It was originally thought that IgM in serum and secretions was identical; later it was shown that 60% to 70% of SIgM contains bound SC (Brandtzaeg, 1975). Pentameric IgM shows better in vitro affinity for SC than does dimeric IgA (Brandtzaeg, 1977, 1985a). This may reflect the fact that IgM probably served the function of protecting mucosal surfaces before the evolution of dimeric IgA (Portis and Coe, 1975). Alternatively, because the SC-IgM complex is not stabilized by disulfide bonds, a higher avidity may be required for survival during transcytosis or in the secretions.

However, both rabbit SIgA of the subclass g, which lacks SC-IgA disulfide bonds (Knight et al., 1975), and human SIgM are sensitive to proteolytic digestion (Haneberg, 1974b). Thus the disulfide bond in human SIgA may have a stabilizing effect that cannot be fully overcome by strong noncovalent binding forces. This property of the disulfide bonds in SIgA may contribute to its evolution as the major secretory antibody in mammals.

Secretory IgM also has antibody activity (Haneberg and Aarskog, 1975; Mellander et al., 1984, 1986b; Ogra et al., 1974) and is extremely efficient at promoting phagocytosis, complement-mediated bacteriolysis, and protection against intestinal infection (Heddle and Rowley, 1975). Some of these effects are markedly enhanced by complement (Girard and de Kalbermatten, 1970). Further, local IgM production in the upper respiratory tract of IgA-deficient patients may confer resistance to infection (Brandtzaeg et al., 1987b). However, SIgM may not be stable enough to provide sufficient antigen exclusion in every IgA-deficient individual. Thus although SIgM may contribute to a first

line of defense for infants and IgA-deficient individuals, it cannot completely replace SIgA (Hanson et al., 1983b).

Other Immunoglobulin Classes in External Secretions

Traces of IgG, IgD, and IgE are found in most normal human secretions. The low concentrations relative to SIgA and even SIgM in mammary and parotid gland secretions and lack of association with SC indicate that the external transfer of these Ig classes is probably passive (Brandtzaeg, 1971a). Fluids collected from surfaces of mucous membranes contain relatively more IgG, indicating their origin from extraglandular, external diffusion. More than 90% of IgG in nasal fluid is of serum origin (Mygind et al., 1975). Such leakage of IgG is enhanced by inflammatory processes (Brandtzaeg et al., 1970). However, there may be preferential local synthesis of certain IgG subclasses (Keller et al., 1983). Even serum-derived IgG may exert some external protective functions, particularly in respiratory secretions. In fact, IgG seems to be the major antibody class of the lower respiratory tract (Newhouse et al., 1976).

Early studies suggested that IgE was actively transported into the external secretions, but this conclusion was based on IgE measurement that overestimated its secretory concentration (Johansson and Deuschl, 1976; Magnusson and Masson, 1985; Turner et al., 1977; Underdown et al., 1976). Moreover, SC shows no affinity for IgE in vitro (Brandtzaeg, 1977) and is not associated with exocrine IgE (Bennich and Johansson, 1971; Newcomb and Ishizaka, 1970). Thus when there is an enrichment of IgE in some exocrine fluids, this is probably due to passive diffusion through the epithelium (Nakajima et al., 1975) combined with local contribution of IgE to some extent synthesized by local plasma cells, but mainly from mast cells armed with IgE in regional lymph nodes (Brandtzaeg, 1985b; Mayrhofer et al., 1976).

The biologic significance of IgE in external secretions is unknown; it is rapidly degraded in intestinal fluid (Brown et al., 1975). In mucosal membranes, IgE is of major importance for defense against parasites, by arming macrophages, platelets, and eosinophils (Capron et al., 1982).

Like IgG and IgE, IgD has no affinity for SC (Brandtzaeg, 1977). Nevertheless, one study indicated preferential appearance of IgD in human colostrum compared with IgG (Keller et al., 1985). The fact that IgD appears in colostrum and saliva but not in intestinal fluid (Sewell et al., 1979) indicates that exocrine IgD is of local origin. Indeed, IgD-producing cells are absent in the gastrointestinal tract, in contrast to other secretory sites (Brandtzaeg, 1983b). Exocrine IgD can exhibit antibody activities (Keller et al., 1985), but its biologic significance is unknown. In some patients with IgA deficiency, a striking increase of IgD-producing immunocytes has been noted in nasal mucosa. This IgD was not transported into the lumen, and these patients, unlike patients with an increase of IgM producing cells, still had frequent infections (Brandtzaeg et al., 1987b).

Quantification of Secretory Immunoglobulins

The biologic activity of an Ig depends on its total quantity, antigenic specificity, and binding affinity. Measurement of Ig production is more difficult in secretions than in serum, because the rates of formation, under basal and stimulated states, must also be considered. An additional problem is the loss during sample storage, particularly pronounced in unstimulated and dilute exocrine fluids (e.g., parotid fluid and urine) (Brandtzaeg, 1971a; Sohl-Akerlund et al., 1977).

Quantification of Total Immunoglobulins in Secretions

Depending on the exocrine site and collection method, the IgA in secretions may vary from essentially all SIgA to a mixture of SIgA and transudated serum IgA. However, because serum IgA and SIgA are antigenically different and dissimilar in size, some immunoassays can specifically quantify SIgA. This approach is preferable for assessment of secretory immunity. Such assays use antibodies against α chain and SC and a purified SIgA standard in successive steps of a solid-phase immunosorbent assay, for example, the enzyme-linked immunosorbent assay (ELISA) (Goldblum and Van Bavel, 1978; Goldblum et al., 1980; Sohl-Akerlund et al., 1977).

Particular care must be taken when testing secretions containing free SC, monomeric IgA, and polymeric IgA with and without bound SC and SIgM. Another assay approach uses monoclonal antibodies, which recognize combinatorial epitopes formed from SC-PIg complexes (Vincent and Revillard, 1988; Woodard et al., 1984). By using such antibodies as the capture phase of the immunoassay, one can avoid competition with nonsecretory Igs and free SC (Vincent and Revillard, 1988). Theoretically, SIgA and SIgM can also be quantified independently by using different isotype-specific detecting reagents. However, it is not possible to obtain a reliable estimate of SIgM because of its lack of covalent association with SC (Feltelius et al., 1994).

Few methodologic studies have evaluated the different assay methods and standards in the quantification of IgM, IgG, IgE, and IgD in secretions. Theoretically, it should be acceptable to use a serum-derived Ig as a reference. However, degradation of these Igs in secretions is common and Ig fragments can interfere in most immunoassays. In addition, quantification in secretions of low Ig levels (such as IgE and IgD) with highly sensitive methods is often subject to nonspecific interference that may lead to overestimation (Johansson and Deuschl, 1976; Magnusson and Masson, 1985; Turner et al., 1977; Underdown et al., 1976).

Quantification of Specific Secretory IgA Antibodies

Many of the same considerations as described for measurement of total SIgA apply to SIgA antibodies. Isotype-specific antibody assays are often based on a solid-phase immunoassay (e.g., ELISA) in which the specific antigen is attached to the solid phase prior to adding dilutions of the secretion. After unbound material is removed by washing, specific antibodies to SC are added. This approach avoids interference from free SC, but does not allow a distinction between SIgA and SIgM (Mellander et al., 1984). These assays are also susceptible to competition for antigen-binding sites by high concentrations of antibodies of other isotypes.

The other major limitation in assessing specific SIgA antibodies is the lack of a good standard. Ideally, affinity-purified human antibodies can be obtained and their quantity determined in an immunoassay for total SIgA. However, this is rarely feasible because of the limited availability of specific antibodies. Often a pool of high-titered biologic fluid is used as the standard, and the antibody concentration in the unknown is expressed as a proportion of the antibody content in that pool. Although it does not provide an absolute measurement, this approach allows comparison of the antibody concentration before and after infection or immunization.

The total SIgA or SIgA antibody concentration may vary, depending on how the sample was obtained. Washings of mucosal membranes are particularly susceptible to differences in the amount of solution applied and the proportion that is recovered. Even with naturally flowing secretions, such as saliva or urine, the concentration of antibody often depends on the flow rate (Brandtzaeg, 1971b). The best way to express the concentration of SIgA antibodies is as a ratio to the total SIgA in the same sample. This provides a measure of the specific activity of the SIgA as an indicator of the intensity of the local immune response.

Variables That Influence Immunoglobulin Concentrations in Secretions

In view of these technical limitations, normal levels of SIgA or SIgA antibodies in various secretions are limited and usually not confirmed by multiple laboratories. Some values for secretions from healthy individuals are presented in Table 9-2. The IgG/IgA ratio in most secretions is much lower than in serum and probably depends on the amount of contamination from transudated serum proteins. The IgG/IgM ratio in colostrum and saliva is also reduced compared with serum. This is more evident in IgA-deficient individuals whose secretions often have increased amounts of IgM, although they may also have elevated levels of IgG (Hanson, 1968; Brandtzaeg, 1971a; Hanson et al., 1983a).

The wide anatomic and functional differences between glandular structures account for part of the variations in the concentrations and proportions of the secreted Ig; additional variations occur as a result

TABLE 9-2 · IMMUNOGLOBULINS IN SERUM AND SECRETIONS FROM HEALTHY ADULTS

Tested Material	Reference	No. of Samples	Immunoglobulin Levels (g/L)			Ratio	
			IgA	IgM	IgG	IgG:IgA	IgG:IgM
Serum	a	pool	3.28	1.32	12.30	3.750	9.32
Colostrum, 1–2 days	a	pool	12.34	0.61	0.10	0.008	0.16
Milk, 2–5 days	c	pool	0.99	0.34	0.08	0.081	0.24
Milk, 5–44 days	c	13	0.468	0.14	0.04	0.085	0.29
Milk, 55–147 days	c	3	0.88	0.14	0.05	0.057	0.36
Stimulated parotid saliva	b	10	0.0149	—	—	—	—
Stimulated parotid saliva	a	9	0.0395	0.00043	0.00036	0.009	0.84
Nasal secretion	d	17	0.846	—	0.304	0.359	—
Urine, adults	b	13	0.00062	—	—	—	—
Duodenal fluid	e	40	0.313	0.207	0.104	0.33	0.50
Jejunal fluid	f	5	0.276	—	0.340	1.230	—
Colonic fluid	f	3	0.827	—	0.860	1.040	—

a. Brandtzaeg et al., 1970 (radial immunodiffusion with correction factor for IgA).
b. Sohl-Åkerlund et al., 1977 (enzyme-linked immunosorbent assay specific for secretory IgA).
c. Wadsworth et al., 1977a (spot immunoprecipitate assay, SIA).
d. Mygind et al., 1975 (radial immunodiffusion).
e. Girard and de Kalbermatten, 1970 (radial immunodiffusion).
f. Bull et al., 1971 (radial immunodiffusion).

of fluctuations in the flow rate. Thus the concentration of IgA in parotid saliva decreases threefold to fourfold after stimulation, although the actual IgA excretion rate increases twofold to threefold (Brandtzaeg, 1971a). The marked diurnal variation in nasal IgA points to the importance of collecting secretions at a fixed time of day (Mygind et al., 1975).

The SIgA concentration in human milk also depends on the flow rate and the volume produced. The high concentration of IgA and specific antibodies in the small volume of colostrum produced during the first few days of lactation rapidly diminishes in parallel with an increase in volume during the transition to mature milk. Consequently, the total daily output of SIgA antibodies stays high and relatively constant throughout lactation (Goldman et al., 1986). During nursing, when the flow rate is high, the concentration is relatively constant (Prentice, 1987; Prentice et al., 1984; Sohl-Akerlund et al., 1977), and the titers of *Escherichia coli* antibodies remain fairly stable. However, Haneberg (1974a) found 30% to 40% higher IgA levels at the end of a feeding than before the infant started to nurse. Per weight of secretory tissue, the IgA output from the lactating breast is similar to that of the parotid gland (Brandtzaeg, 1983b).

INFLUENCE OF AGE

Ontogeny has a striking impact on the Ig levels in secretions. Age-matched controls must therefore be used when studies are performed in young patients (Burgio et al., 1980). The timing of SIgA appearance in the infant has been reviewed by Hanson and associates (1980) and Brandtzaeg and colleagues (1991). In one study, SIgA and SIgM antibodies to *E. coli* and poliovirus were found in the saliva during the first days of life. Although these antibodies may represent maternal IgA and IgM, there was evidence that they may also be of fetal origin.

SIgA antibodies were found in the saliva and meconium of a newborn of a hypogammaglobulinemic mother whose IgA and IgM levels were undetectable (Mellander et al., 1986a).

In developing countries, infants exposed to poliovirus develop salivary SIgA antibodies against poliovirus antigens by 1 month of age, and the antibody concentration reaches adult levels by the age of 6 months (Carlsson et al., 1985). Infants heavily exposed to *E. coli* from the time of birth had significantly increased salivary SIgA antibody levels by 2 to 3 weeks of age, rapidly reaching adult levels (Mellander et al., 1985). In less exposed infants, such levels were not attained until approximately 12 months of age for both SIgA and SIgA antibodies to *E. coli* O antigens. A slower increase in the levels of such antibodies was found by Gleeson and colleagues (1987).

Other studies show that SIgM antibodies predominate in the secretions of infants (Girard and de Kalbermatten, 1970). SIgM antibodies to *E. coli* were consistently found in the saliva of young infants (Mellander et al., 1984, 1985, 1986a, 1986b). As the synthesis and transport of SIgA antibodies into the saliva increased during the first 1 to 3 months of age, levels of the SIgM antibodies decreased in parallel, suggesting competition for the same SC-dependent transfer mechanism or replacement of the local IgM-producing cells by IgA producers.

The perinatal ontogeny of SIg formation in the parotid, as studied immunohistologically by Thrane and coworkers (Brandtzaeg et al., 1991), confirmed that the IgM-producing cells that predominated were replaced by IgA-producing cells during the first 6 months of life. Prenatally, most IgA-producing cells were of the IgA1 isotype and contained J chains. However, IgA2-producing cells reached adult proportions (approximately 40% of IgA producers) soon after birth. The early ability to transport the polymeric Igs into the lumen of the parotid gland was indicated by the prenatal expression of SC. However, anti-SC staining increased rapidly after birth, concomitant with a rapid increase in IgA-producing cells, which suggested that these events are driven by the presence of microbial flora or other antigens.

INFLUENCE OF NUTRITION

The enhanced susceptibility to infections of undernourished children may be explained by impairment in the mucosal immune system (see Chapter 23). SIgA concentrations are more sensitive to malnutrition than are serum IgA, IgG, or IgM. A reduction in IgA concentrations has been reported in duodenal, nasal, and salivary secretions of children with severe protein-calorie malnutrition (Chandra, 1975; McMurray et al., 1977; Reddy et al., 1976; Sirisinha et al., 1975).

Conversely, Beatty and colleagues (1983) have shown that the intestinal immune system of undernourished children responds to bacterial overgrowth with enhanced IgA synthesis and secretion. Furthermore, total salivary SIgA and salivary antibody responses of chronically undernourished children are equal to those of better nourished children (Glass et al., 1986). Renourishment after acute malnutrition rapidly restored the secretory Ig concentration (Reddy et al., 1976).

Severe protein undernutrition in mice resulted in decreased total IgA concentration in intestinal washes, whereas serum IgA levels were increased (McGee and McMurray, 1988). The IgA plaque-forming cell response to an orally administered antigen was unchanged, although this response was decreased in the spleens from the most severely underfed. Refeeding resulted in normalized IgA levels and antibody responses.

In severely undernourished mothers, the titer of SIgA antibodies to *E. coli* in milk were comparable to those of healthy mothers, but because their milk volumes were smaller, their total output of milk SIgA was diminished (Carlsson et al., 1976). The effects of two different levels of protein supplementation on SIgA concentration and daily excretion in milk of undernourished mothers were examined by Herias and coworkers (1993). The higher protein supplementation prevented the fall in SIgA production seen in mothers who received less protein, suggesting that nutritional protein is a rate-limiting factor for SIgA production. Interestingly, there were no differences in the concentrations or avidities of three different specific antibodies between early and late gestation or with the different supplementations (Herias et al., 1993).

There is considerable interest in the effects of vitamin A on the mucosal immune responses. Rats made vitamin A deficient have lower serum and biliary IgA concentrations and markedly reduced IgA responses to oral immunization with cholera toxin (Wiedermann et al., 1993). Most of these effects were reversed by supplementation with vitamin A, which suggested that the immune defects were a direct effect of the vitamin deficiencies rather than a secondary effect of poor food intake. The deficient IgA response was due to a suppression of Th2 cells, associated with an increase in IFN-γ and IL-2 production in vitro, suggesting enhanced Th1 activity (Wiedermann et al., 1993).

Secretory Immunoglobulins in Serum

Trace quantities of SIgA can be detected in human serum (Brandtzaeg, 1971b; Thompson et al., 1969). Studies using solid-phase radioimmunoassay (Delacroix and Vaerman, 1981), an immunofluorescence assay (Goldblum et al., 1980), or ELISA (Iscaki et al., 1979; Kvale and Brandtzaeg, 1986) have produced somewhat discrepant results; however, most indicate that approximately 1% of the serum IgA is normally SIgA. SIgM has also been detected in normal serum (Delacroix and Vaerman, 1982; Kvale and Brandtzaeg, 1986). Elevated serum levels of SIgA and SIgM in patients with various mucosal or liver diseases may have some diagnostic value (Delacroix et al., 1982; Goldblum et al., 1980; Kvale and Brandtzaeg, 1986), but the difficulty of the assays has limited their widespread use.

MUCOSAL T LYMPHOCYTES

T-lymphocyte responses at mucosal surfaces, particularly the gut, have been reviewed by Kelsall and Strober (1999). They suggest dividing the system into inductive sites and effector sites for mucosal immunity. The inductive sites reside predominantly in organized MALT (e.g., Peyer's patches in the small intestine). The effector sites include the lamina propria and epithelium (e.g., intraepithelial T cells, IELs). Recent investigations of the mucosal T-cell responses suggest that intestinal T cells follow a migration pathway similar to that of the IgA-committed B cells. Thus activation and differentiation of CD4+ T cells may be initiated within the T-cell and dendritic cell-rich subepithelial dome or interfollicular region of Peyer's patches (Kelsall and Strober, 1999).

The mucosal T cells are phenotypically and functionally different from those in the blood or systemic lymphoid tissues. These differences are understandable, because mucosal T cells are constantly exposed to foreign antigens and must have their responses muted to prevent chronic, inflammatory tissue injury. This is compatible with the concept that the mucosal immune system must maintain its barrier function without developing deleterious inflammatory reactions. The major populations of mucosal T-lymphocytes are described in the following sections.

Peyer's Patch T Lymphocytes

Peyer's patches are thought to be the major inductive sites for mucosal T lymphocytes. Here CD4+ cells predominate over CD8+ lymphocytes. Because Peyer's patches do not have any afferent lymphatics, all lymphocyte entry is from the blood stream via high endothelial venules in the interfollicular region. The T lymphocytes entering the Peyer's patches are thought to be of thymic origin.

These T cells first encounter antigens that are transported into the subepithelial dome by M cells and presented by either dendritic cells or B cells. From here, some T cells migrate into the B-cell–rich germinal centers, where they produce cytokines required for B-cell differentiation. Other activated T cells migrate out of the Peyer's patch and home to the lamina propria of mucosal tissues, although some also home to peripheral tissues (Kelsall and Strober, 1999).

The ultimate function of the T cells that migrate from the Peyer's patches is thought to depend on the type of stimulus they encounter there. Thus T cells stimulated by soluble antigens or nonpathogenic microorganisms exhibit a Th2-predominant response (Xu-Amano et al., 1993), which supports IgA production. T cells encountering antigens from a pathogenic organism, such as *Salmonella typhimurium*, may make a Th1-predominant response (Karem et al., 1996), which may ultimately protect the intestine against reinfection.

Lamina Propria T Lymphocytes

Lamina propria T lymphocytes consist of predominantly CD4$^+$ cells that are phenotypically different from circulating T cells in that they are mostly memory cells (95% CD45RO$^+$) (Halstensen et al., 1990). Approximately half of the adult blood T cells express this isoform. In addition, approximately 40% of lamina propria T cells express the integrin $\alpha4\beta7$; this marker is present on freshly isolated lymphocytes from other tissue sites (Cerf-Bensussan et al., 1987). However, $\alpha4\beta7$ can be induced on other lymphocyte populations by in vitro activation, which again suggests that the lamina propria T cells are stimulated, perhaps in a tissue-specific fashion (Schieferdecker et al., 1990).

L-selectin, another surface antigen involved in cell migration, is present on approximately half of the blood T cells, but is absent on lamina propria lymphocytes (James and Zeitz, 1994). This finding is consistent with the fact that L-selectin is lost with activation or migration to the lamina propria.

Other markers of T-cell activation, such as IL-2R (CD25) and MHC class II antigens, are also increased on lamina propria T cells (Taguchi et al., 1990). Consistent with inherent priming, lamina propria T cells express more mRNAs for the cytokines IFN-γ, IL-2, IL-4, and IL-5 after nonspecific stimulation than do circulating T lymphocytes.

An intriguing characteristic of lamina propria lymphocytes is their limited capacity to proliferate (Brandtzaeg and Halstensen, 1992) or become cytotoxic killer cells. Lamina propria T cells show weak proliferative responses to specific antigen, mitogens, or even anti-CD3 antibodies. However, after antigenic or pokeweed mitogen stimulation, these T cells can act as helpers for B-cell antibody production (James et al., 1987). This suggests that lamina propria T cells predominantly enhance local Ig production rather than proliferate or injure surrounding structures.

Intraepithelial Lymphocytes

The origin of IELs is independent of Peyer's patches; some IELs are thymic-independent as well. The IELs are strategically located to respond to antigenic stimulation by luminal antigens while minimizing tissue injury. Because epithelial cells are rapidly replenished, immunologic identification and destruction of infected or otherwise abnormal villus cells may protect the internal environment without detrimental effects to normal tissues. Although this is an attractive hypothesis, the exact function of the IEL remains obscure (Lefrancois, 1994).

The origin and function of the IELs are suggested by their surface phenotype, which differs extensively from those of circulating T cells. Similarly, the IEL do not seem to arise from the lamina propria T cells. Unlike the murine (mouse) situation, in which the $\gamma\delta$ form of the T cell receptor (TCR) predominates, most human small intestinal IELs express the $\alpha\beta$ form of TCR, typical of T cells in the blood and lymphoid tissues (Brandtzaeg et al., 1989). However, most IELs express the CD8 marker (Brandtzaeg et al., 1989; Parrott et al., 1983) associated with suppressor and cytotoxic activities. The few IELs that express CD4 co-express CD8. These double-positive cells are extremely rare in other tissues except the thymus. This finding suggests that some of the murine IELs are derived not from the thymus but from a prethymic population that migrates to the gut and differentiates there.

Another characteristic of IELs is the limited repertoire of their TCR (Balk et al., 1991; Van Kerckhove et al., 1992). This is in marked distinction to peripheral T cells, in which essentially each cell has a unique TCR structure. The IEL must recognize a limited number of antigens, perhaps autologous antigens that become expressed when the enterocyte becomes infected or otherwise stressed. The functional activities of IELs, once activated, may be to release cytokines (e.g. IL-2, IL-5, IFN-γ, TGF-β and TNF-α and β), some of which may destroy damaged enterocytes (Lefrancois, 1994).

INNATE IMMUNITY OF MUCOSAL SURFACES

In addition to antigen-specific mucosal immune responses, several other primitive soluble and cellular defense mechanisms protect the mucosal surfaces. These factors may function alone to prevent or control microbial colonization or infections or to initiate or augment T-cell and B-cell immunity at these sites.

Soluble Factors

Lactoferrin, an iron-binding protein present in secretions, inhibits the growth of many pathologic bacteria and fungi. This activity, which is potentiated by antibodies (Bullen et al., 1972), including human milk IgA antibodies (Rogers and Synge, 1978), is probably due to neutralization of iron-binding compounds from the bacteria (Bullen et al., 1974; Griffiths and Humphreys, 1977), thereby further depriving the microorganisms of growth-promoting iron. However, a bactericidal peptide of lactoferrin (lactoferricin) may also be important in mucosal defense by lactoferrin (Bellamy et al., 1992).

External secretions also contain the enzyme *lysozyme* (muramidase), which can cleave the cell wall of gram-positive bacteria. The concentration of lysozyme is particularly high (0.5 to 2 g/L) in human milk, where it persists throughout lactation, (Chandan et al., 1964; Hanson and Johansson, 1970; Goldman et al., 1982a, 1982b, 1983b). SIgA antibodies may become bacteriolytic by activating complement in combination with lysozyme (Adinolfi et al., 1966; Hill and Porter, 1974), but this has not been confirmed (Eddie et al., 1971; Heddle et al., 1975). Indeed, all forms of human IgA, including both subclasses, lack classical complement-activating properties (Johnson et al., 1984; Nikolova et al., 1994; Pfaffenbach et al., 1982; Russel-Jones et al., 1984). In the rat, IgA immune complexes can activate complement via the alternative pathway (Rits et al., 1988).

The *lactoperoxidase* of various secretions may also provide defense against infections (Goldman and Smith, 1973; Gothefors, 1975; Gothefors and Marklund, 1975; Mata and Wyatt, 1971). Lactoperoxidase may not be present in human milk (Moldoveanu et al., 1982). SIgA may enhance the effect of the lactoperoxidase system independently of antibody specificity (Tenovuo et al., 1982).

IFN-α may be another important nonspecific defense factor. Its synthesis is stimulated by infection or viral vaccines. Interferons appear in nasal secretions within 24 hours of viral infections (Danielescu et al., 1975) and therefore may play a decisive role in the initial phase of infection.

Immune reactions at epithelial surfaces may stimulate release of *mucus* from goblet cells, thereby enhancing this mechanical barrier of macromolecules and microorganisms (Walker et al., 1982). Furthermore, the development of goblet cells may depend on functional T lymphocytes in humans (Karlsson et al., 1985) and animals (Ahlstedt et al., 1988; Mayrhofer, 1979). Antigens of immune complexes trapped in the mucous layer are more rapidly degraded by proteolytic enzymes (Walker et al., 1975).

Mucin, a highly glycosylated protein that is present in human milk, protects against experimental rotavirus infections in mice (Yolken et al., 1992). This activity may be crucial, because rotavirus is the most common cause of infectious enteritis in infants and children. Mucins associated with the milk fat globules of human milk may interfere with the binding of S-fimbriated *E. coli* to the infant's mucous membranes (Schroten et al., 1992).

Bacterial Receptor Analogues

Most mucosal infections begin with attachment of the microorganism to epithelial cells, often mediated by specific receptors on the epithelium. For instance, in the urinary tract, Svanborg and coworkers (1983) have shown that the *E. coli* that cause acute pyelonephritis often have fimbrial receptors for the P antigen on urinary epithelium. Receptor analogs, present in exocrine secretions such as milk, may prevent bacterial attachment (Holmgren et al., 1981, 1983; Svanborg et al., 1983; Otnaess et al., 1983; Andersson et al., 1985; Andersson et al., 1986). This topic has been reviewed by Svanborg (1994).

A number of secretions, including human milk, contains glycocompounds that function as analogs to mucosal receptors for bacteria. Bacterial hemagglutination by *V. cholerae* and *E. coli*, as well as enterotoxin-binding, are inhibited by non-Ig fractions of milk, which contain glycoprotein and/or oligosaccharide (Holmgren et al., 1981, 1983). The inhibitory activity of milk on *E. coli* and *V. cholerae* enterotoxin is related to a glycolipid fraction (Otnaess and Orstavik, 1981; Otnaess and Svennerholm, 1982) that resembles the GM_1 ganglioside, the receptor for those toxins (Otnaess et al., 1983). Cleary and colleagues (1983) detected a human milk component, presumably an oligosaccharide, that prevents fluid loss in mice induced by *E. coli* heat-stable enterotoxin. An antisecretory factor found in rat milk that inhibits enterotoxin may be related to this factor (Lange and Lonnroth, 1986).

Prevention of the attachment of pneumococci to pharyngeal cells by human milk is mediated, at least in part, by low-molecular-weight substances that contain the disaccharide N-acetylglucosamine (1→3)-β-galactose, the minimal component of the *Pneumococcus* receptor (Andersson et al., 1986; Hanson et al., 1983a; Svanborg et al., 1983). Mucosal attachment of *Haemophilus influenzae* is inhibited by a high-molecular-weight non-Ig component (Andersson et al., 1985, 1986). A carbohydrate-containing constituent of milk, thought to be a glucosaminoglycan, has been found to inhibit binding of human immunodeficiency virus (HIV) to its lymphocyte CD4 receptor (Newburg et al., 1992). A protective role for receptor analogs is suggested by animal studies (Cleary et al., 1983), but their role in human milk is not established.

Phagocytes

Under normal conditions, few polymorphonuclear leukocytes (PMNs) are present in mucosal tissues; however, certain secretions, notably milk, do contain PMNs. PMNs are critical in the control of microbial colonization at highly contaminated mucosal sites, such as the gingiva. Because PMN function depends on opsonins for optimal phagocytosis, their interaction with IgA is of interest.

The role of SIgA in opsonizing bacteria for phagocytosis is controversial. Fcα receptors are present on human neutrophils (Lawrence et al., 1975) and show much better binding activity for dimeric than for monomeric IgA (Fanger et al., 1980). In vitro phagocytosis-promoting effect of purified SIgA antibodies depends on the presence of lysozyme (Girard and de

Kalbermatten, 1970). In vivo experiments, however, have produced discrepant results (Eddie et al., 1971; Heddle and Rowley, 1975), possibly because of differences in the bacteria or the type of phagocyte involved. In human saliva, IgA coats certain bacteria (see Fig. 9-5), but it is unknown whether the coating is directly bacteriostatic. Growing chains of streptococci occur in the mouth, and some of the IgA-coated bacteria are engulfed by neutrophils mainly derived from the gingival crevices (Brandtzaeg et al., 1968a; Sharry and Drasse, 1960).

A prompt immune-mediated emigration of neutrophils takes place in the gut lumen after epithelial exposure to antigen to which there is serum antibody (Bellamy and Nielsen, 1974). These cells may then limit further antigen penetration. However, the reaction of serum antibodies with luminal antigen may enhance penetration of other macromolecules. This is probably caused by adverse effects on the mucosa exerted by lysosomal enzymes released from the phagocytes (Brandtzaeg and Tolo, 1977; Lim and Rowley, 1982). Formation of immune complexes outside the epithelium does not induce chemotaxis of neutrophils (Bellamy and Nielsen, 1974). Cultured epithelial cells of the respiratory and gastrointestinal tracts infected with viruses or bacteria can induce the production and release of IL-8, a potent chemoattractant for PMNs (Garofalo et al., 1995).

Certain lymphocytes, eosinophils, and monocytes also express Fcα receptors and, in conjunction with IgA, mediate antibody-dependent cellular cytotoxicity (ADCC) against bacteria and parasites to assist in mucosal defense (Lowell et al., 1980). Intraepithelial lymphocytes from the murine gut exert antibacterial ADCC with SIgA antibodies from rabbit intestinal juice (Tagliabue et al., 1984). Bacterial killing by SIgA antibodies and T lymphocytes occurs in the human gut after vaccination against *Salmonella typhi* (Tagliabue et al., 1986).

Physical Factors That Potentiate Mucosal Immunity

The acidity of the gastric juices, the flow of urine in the urinary tract, the flow of saliva in the oral cavity, intestinal peristalsis, the cough reflex, and mucociliary transport in the respiratory tract also contribute to local defense by inactivating or removing microorganisms.

CLINICAL SIGNIFICANCE OF THE MUCOSAL DEFENSE SYSTEM

Immunologic Homeostasis of Mucosa

Immunologic homeostasis is normally maintained in the mucosa through a critical balance between the levels of local antibodies of the various isotypes (Fig. 9-6). Dimeric IgA (and pentameric IgM) may act as the first line of defense by excluding antigen at the mucosal sur-

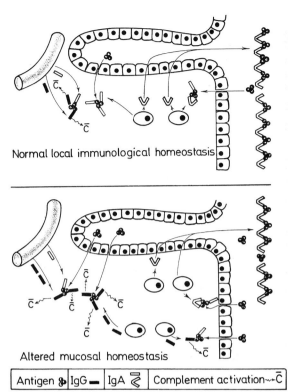

Figure 9-6 · It is postulated (top) that a normal immunologic homeostasis is maintained in the mucosa through a critical balance between humoral available antibodies. Dimeric immunoglobulin A (IgA) acts in a "first line of defense" by antigen exclusion at the mucosal surface (to the right). Antigens that bypass this trapping mechanism may meet corresponding serum-derived IgG antibodies in the lamina propria. The immune complexes formed will activate complement, and inflammatory mediators are thus generated in the mucosa. Such a development is moderated by "blocking" antibody activities in the lamina propria exerted by serum-derived or locally produced monomeric or dimeric IgA. This homeostasis is altered (bottom) when there is undue antigen stimulation because of increased mucosal penetrability or excessive antigen exposure. A "second line of defense" is then set up in the mucosa by local production of IgG as part of the "pathotopic potentiation" of mucosal immunity (see Fig. 9-7) to limit dissemination of foreign substances. However, because of the phlogistic properties of IgG antibodies, a vicious circle may develop with further increase of mucosal antigen penetrability, intensified complement activation and cytotoxic reactions, massive attraction of phagocytic cells, and release of their lysosomal enzymes. This results in aggravation and perpetuation of inflammation and thus leads to disease.

face. Antigens that bypass this trapping mechanism, however, may meet non-IgA antibodies in the lamina propria. Because IgG and IgM antibodies can activate complement and because complement permeates the lamina propria (Baklien and Brandtzaeg, 1974), an inflammatory cascade may be initiated. However, this may be moderated by "blocking" activities of dimeric and monomeric IgA of local or systemic origin (Griffis, 1983; Hall et al., 1971; Nikolova et al., 1994; Russel-Jones et al., 1984).

In vitro studies suggest that immune complexes containing IgA formed in the vicinity of secretory epithelia can be transported externally by the PIg receptor mechanism and released into the lumen (Kaetzel et al., 1991). This transport system may also include mixed immune complexes with IgG and dimeric IgA, acting as a backup for the immune exclusion process (Mazanec et al., 1993).

Conversely, excessive IgG and possibly IgM antibodies may attract phagocytes to mucosal sites (Bellamy and Nielsen, 1974). Release of their lysosomal enzymes may enhance mucosal permeability (Brandtzaeg and Tolo, 1977; Lim and Rowley, 1982). However, leukocyte migration is suppressed by dimeric IgA, which inhibits leukocyte chemotaxis (Kemp et al., 1980; Reed et al., 1979; Van Epps and Williams, 1976). IgA may also inhibit the release of proinflammatory cytokines from mucosal phagocytes and inhibit production of toxic oxygen radicals (Wolf et al., 1994a, 1994b).

In addition to antibodies and complement, beneficial (or detrimental) effects may be mediated by activated T cells, macrophages, mast cells, goblet cells, and natural killer (NK) cells at local tissue sites. The effectiveness of these backup systems for mucosal immunity is evidenced in patients with X-linked agammaglobulinemia and common variable immunodeficiency, most of whom have no clinical, functional, or structural abnormalities in the gut (Eidelman, 1976).

Primary and Secondary Mucosal Defense Lines

Deviations from the normal polymeric Ig-dominant pattern of mucosal defenses may occur transiently or permanently. In most cases, the SIgA response (first line of defense) neutralizes noxious influences and maintains local immunologic homeostasis. Transient shifts to a backup mode may result in proinflammatory mechanisms with deleterious, although reversible, changes of the mucosa, as seen, for example, in celiac disease (Brandtzaeg, 1985b).

However, when the secretory immune system fails to cope with persistent mucosal antigen, a pronounced local IgG response may occur, possibly combined with an IgE response in atopic individuals. The phlogistic properties of these antibodies may contribute to the "pathotopic potentiation" of local immunity (Fig. 9-7). This may be considered the "second line of defense" of the mucosa. However, the local consequence may be severe alteration of mucosal immunologic homeostasis (see Fig. 9-6), with aggravation and perpetuation of an inflammatory reaction. This is probably the underlying mechanism leading to chronic inflammatory disease of mucous membranes.

Antimicrobial Activities of the Mucosal Immune System

Viral Infections

Immune responses to viral infections of the mucosal surfaces have been reviewed by Murphy (1999). Once a viral infection begins, resolution is mediated by cellular

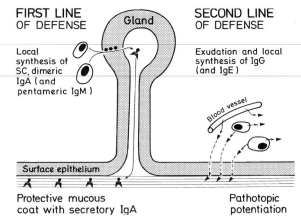

Figure 9-7 · Schematic representation of human nasal mucosa. Two basic principles of antibody protection are visualized. The "first line of defense" primarily consists of secretory immunoglobulin A (IgA), which is produced as J chain–containing dimers by immunocytes adjacent to glandular structures; the dimers are then conjugated with epithelial secretory component during selective transmission through the glandular epithelium and are subsequently included in a protective mucous coat on the surface epithelium. The "second line of defense" is associated with a local inflammatory reaction, giving rise to passive external diffusion of serum-derived and locally produced IgG and perhaps influx of IgE bound to mast cell; the latter events represent "pathotopic potentiation" of local immunity.

mechanisms, including NK cells (Biron et al., 1989), MHC class I restricted CD8+ cytotoxic T cells, and CD4+ helper cells (Murphy, 1994). These cells must recognize the viral or viral-induced structures on the host cell and combat the viral infection by destroying the host cells. For rapidly dividing viruses, specific cellular immunity may not have much effect until after the peak of virus production (Greenberg et al., 1978). Thus other host responses must limit the early phase of viral replication. These include production of IFN by multiple cell types and possibly the intracellular neutralization in secretory epithelial cells by internalized polymeric antibodies, as described earlier (Mazanec et al., 1992a).

Antibodies are more important in prevention of mucosal reinfection. At some sites, notably the lungs and upper respiratory tract, IgG antibodies, which diffuse passively from the systemic circulation provide some protection (Murphy, 1994). In contrast, protection in the gastrointestinal tract is mostly mediated by SIgA. The effectiveness of antibodies in preventing viral reinfection has been demonstrated experimentally by passive administration of antibodies directly on the mucosal surface (Mazanec et al., 1992b) or intravenously as polymeric IgA antibodies (Renegar and Small, 1991).

These experiments indicate that antibodies directed against a virus can prevent or markedly reduce mucosal viral replication. Human breast milk antibodies largely diminish symptoms of natural viral infections (Carlsson and Hanson, 1994; Murphy, 1994). This outcome is similar to the first reinfection with a respiratory virus, when residual levels of endogenous SIgA antibodies are low. Only after multiple infections are titers of mucosal antibodies high enough to prevent subsequent infection (Murphy, 1994).

Bacterial Infections

Mucosal immunity to bacterial infections has been recently reviewed (Holmgren and Rudin, 1999). Secretory antibodies may protect against bacterial infections (Artenstein, 1975; Gay, 1924). The specificity of the secretory antibodies that have been detected reflects the local nature of the antigenic stimulus. Thus gonococcal antibodies are found in genital secretions (Kearns et al., 1973); *Streptococcus pneumoniae* and *Haemophilus influenzae* (Gump et al., 1973), *Mycoplasma pneumoniae* (Biberfeld and Sterner, 1971), and *Neisseria meningitidis* (Wenzel et al., 1973) antibodies are found in respiratory secretions; *Streptococcus mutans* and other oral bacterial antibodies are found in saliva (Arnold et al., 1976). *E. coli* (Girard and de Kalbermatten, 1970) and *Shigella* (Reed and Williams, 1971) antibodies are found in intestinal contents.

The presence of antibodies in the nasal secretions against diphtheria toxoid in individuals with high serum antibody titers indicates some transfer of serum antibodies that may increase during infection (Remington et al., 1964) (see Fig. 9-3). To demonstrate this, it is necessary to use specific methods that distinguish between SIgA and serum IgG responses.

Parasitic Infections

Certain parasites (e.g., *Trichinella spiralis*) can be trapped in mucus by either the complement-conglutinin system or by secretory or serum antibodies (Lee and Ogilvie, 1982). Although IgA antibodies against several parasites are present in secretions, their protective role is unclear. Milk of immunized mothers protects infant mice against *Giardia muris* infection (Andrews and Hewlett, 1981).

ADCC may be of major importance for host defense against parasites (Capron et al., 1982). Eosinophils, neutrophils, and macrophages (but not NK cells) participate in antiparasitic reactions through their IgG and especially IgE Fc receptors. IgE antibodies may also protect against parasites by binding to and activating platelets. Such IgE platelet-mediated hypersensitivity may contribute to the pathogenesis of mucosal atopic reactions (Capron et al., 1987).

Many parasitic infections are immunosuppressive. *T. spiralis* infection, for example, depresses serum antibody responses and Ig-producing cells in the lamina propria following oral immunization with cholera toxin (Ljungstrom et al., 1980). A similar immunosuppression was observed for cellular immune responses during *Nippostrongylus brasiliensis* infection, especially in MALTs (McElroy et al., 1983).

Intestinal infections with some parasites cause local inflammation. Infection with *N. brasiliensis* or *T. spiralis* causes mice to mount a strong Th2 response in the spleens and mesenteric lymph nodes, resulting in increased levels of IL-4 and IL-5 and decreased levels of IFN-γ and IL-2 (Pond et al., 1989). This results in increased levels of circulating eosinophils and IgE, which may contribute to the expulsion of the parasites.

Clearance of some parasites is blocked by the injection of anti-IL-4 antibodies (Urban et al., 1991).

Gastrointestinal Mucosal Immunity

Oral Mucosal Immunity

Oral mucosal immunity has been reviewed by Challacombe and Shirlaw (1999). Both local and systemic immune factors help stabilize the bacterial flora, thus preventing acute infections and chronic oral inflammation of the mouth. The salivary glands are the source of oral SIgA, including the parotid (40%); submandibular (40%); sublingual (10%); and minor salivary glands (10%) (Challacombe and Shirlaw, 1994). Serum-derived components of saliva enter through the junctions between the teeth and the mucosa.

The presence of secretory oral antibodies can be demonstrated by the finding of bacteria coated with IgA (see Fig. 9-5). These antibodies, demonstrated by Brandtzaeg and coworkers (1968b), may prevent bacterial adherence to oral epithelial cells (Williams and Gibbons, 1972) and teeth, thereby promoting the disposal of oral microorganisms. Oral colonization with *Streptococcus mutans*, the major causative organism of dental caries, may be inhibited by salivary SIgA antibodies. These antibodies can be induced in humans by oral immunization (Gregory and Filler, 1987; Mestecky et al., 1978).

The SIgA response in experimental animals may be enhanced by administering antigens or bacteria in liposomes or by adding adjuvants such as muramyl dipeptide (Michalek et al., 1985). In rats, control of caries can be achieved by vaccination. In humans, resistance to dental caries is related to natural salivary IgA antibodies against *S. mutans* (Lehtonen et al., 1984). An efficient and safe caries vaccine is not yet available.

The salivary SIgA may function in the oral cavity through its interactions with local innate immune factors, including mucin, lactoferrin, lysozyme, and lactoperoxidase. In addition, because the phagocytes that enter the saliva have enhanced expression of Fcα receptors, these cells may effectively phagocytize IgA-coated (opsonized) bacteria (Fanger et al., 1980).

INTESTINAL IMMUNITY AND GASTROENTERITIS

The SIgA responses against bacterial and viral infections of the gastrointestinal tract have been examined extensively. In experimental cholera, SIgA antibodies are protective by diminishing the adherence of *V. cholerae* to the intestinal wall (Lange and Holmgren, 1978; Svennerholm et al., 1978). Effective immunity following immunization correlated with a number of lamina propria plasma cells producing antibodies to cholera toxin (Lange et al., 1980). Antibodies against cholera enterotoxin and LPS have a synergistic protective effect (Svennerholm and Holmgren, 1976). Antibacterial antibodies presumably keep bacteria from adhering to the gut epithelium, and antitoxin antibodies neutralize or prevent the toxin from binding to its specific epithelial receptor.

In humans, immunity to cholera can be long-lasting despite a short-lived local SIgA response. This finding may reflect the presence of long-lasting SIgA immunologic memory in the response to cholera toxin (Lange et al., 1980; Lycke and Holmgrem, 1987; Pierce and Cray, 1982). The cholera toxin is a remarkably potent immunogen because of its special binding capability and physiologic activities. Oral toxin induces SIgA as well as serum IgG and IgA responses (Elson and Ealding, 1984). The serum IgA and IgG responses have their origin in Peyer's patches (Dahlgren et al., 1986, 1987; Elson and Ealding, 1984).

The nontoxic receptor-binding beta-subunit of cholera toxin is a good immunogen that efficiently induces toxin-neutralizing antibodies. An oral beta-subunit/whole cell cholera vaccine stimulates a good mucosal antibody response and has been successful in large-scale field trials (Clemens et al., 1986; Svennerholm et al., 1984). This vaccine also protects against E. coli enterotoxin-induced diarrhea (Clemens et al., 1988b). Vaccination results in a decreased diarrheal morbidity and mortality (Clemens et al., 1988a). Oral administration of GM_1 ganglioside, the epithelial cell receptor for cholera toxin, also prevents toxin-induced diarrhea in experimental animals, but this has not been studied in humans (Glass et al., 1984).

Passive transfer of SIgA in animals confirms the efficacy of local SIgA against enteric infection. Winner and associates (1991) implanted mice with hybridoma that produced polymeric IgA antibodies to the LPS of V. cholerae. These mice demonstrated a high level of strain-specific resistance to oral challenge with the cholera organisms. Interestingly, there was no protection with antibodies to the cholera toxin itself (Apter et al., 1991). This difference is presumably due to the ability of the LPS antibodies to prevent colonization or the inability of antitoxin to neutralize locally produced toxin (Neutra and Kraehenbuhl, 1999).

Specific antibody is not the only mechanism against intestinal toxins. Desensitization of intestinal adenylate cyclase occurs after immunization with cholera toxin, presumably because of the production of an "antisecretory factor" found in bile, milk, and intestinal mucosa (Lonnroth and Lange, 1981, 1986). This factor, a 60-kd protein, is induced by hyperosmotic solutions of monosaccharides and amino acids (Lonnroth and Lange, 1987). The protective effects of antisecretory factor may explain the lack of correlation between the protection against toxin and the titers of antitoxin (Lange et al., 1984).

For some enteric bacteria, immune cells may also be involved in the protection. Tagliabue and colleagues (1984) demonstrated SIgA-mediated ADCC against Salmonella strains and Shigella X16 (a hybrid between Shigella flexneri and E. coli). Whereas IgG antibodies were best at arming splenic lymphocytes for ADCC, SIgA functioned better in ADCC with lymphocytes from Peyer's patches, mesenteric lymph nodes, gut epithelium, and lamina propria. Such SIgA antibodies have also been described in humans (Tagliabue et al., 1986).

For intracellular intestinal infections, such as those caused by Salmonella, T-cell mediated mechanisms similar to those that mediate the clearing of other viral infections may be involved. MHC class I-restricted cytotoxic lymphocytes may be crucial in these responses (Kaufmann, 1988).

Liver and Gall Bladder Immunity

Unlike the liver of some animals, the human liver does not efficiently transport polymeric IgA from the circulation into the bile (Brown et al., 1982). This difference is due to the lack of expression of the PIgR by human hepatocytes (Brandtzaeg, 1982, 1985a; Vaerman et al., 1982), although some discrepant information has been reported. Some SC-independent binding of IgA to hepatocytes may take place, and this along with transport through SC-expressing duct epithelium may explain why 50% of the small amounts of polymeric IgA of human bile is derived from the circulation (Brandtzaeg, 1985a; Delacroix and Vaerman, 1983). However, only approximately 2% of injected polymeric IgA appears in the bile after 24 hours (Delacroix and Vaerman, 1983). Thus polymeric IgA (without bound SC) can accumulate in extremely high concentrations (up to 6000 mg/dl) in the blood of patients with excessive intestinal IgA production, even when liver function is normal (Brandtzaeg and Baklien, 1977a).

Although serum IgA is often increased in various liver disorders, it is not known whether this reflects increased IgA production in the intestinal mucosa, decreased hepatic uptake or catabolism of circulating IgA or IgA-containing immune complexes, or reflux of biliary IgA into the blood. In alcoholic liver disease, IgA1 accumulation in the liver may be due to a dysfunction of the asialoglycoprotein receptor on the sinusoidal surface of the hepatocyte (Ashwell and Harford, 1982).

Respiratory Tract Mucosal Immunity

Mucosal immunity is more important in the upper respiratory tract and perhaps in the bronchi than in the lower respiratory tract, notably the lungs, where systemic immunity predominates.

Upper Respiratory Tract Immunity

Mucosal immune responses to respiratory viruses, particularly respiratory syncytial virus (RSV) and influenza, has been studied in detail (Garofalo et al., 1999; Graham et al., 2000; Hussell et al., 1999). SIgA antibodies specific for RSV have been demonstrated after primary infection, but their role in clearing the infection is uncertain (McIntosh et al., 1979). Although systemic administration of IgG antibodies to RSV does not decrease viral shedding in infected infants (Hemming et al., 1987), the presence of neutralizing serum antibodies correlates with resistance to infection

(Hall et al., 1991). Repeated infections also result in accelerated production of local RSV-specific antibodies (Kaul et al., 1980). Thus the relative contributions of local and systemic antibodies to resolution and prevention of reinfection with RSV remains unclear. However, because some individuals with high levels of serum antibodies can become infected (Hall et al., 1991), rapid production of local antibodies after reexposure may be a major determinant in resistance to reinfection.

Renegar and Small (1991) demonstrated that intravenous administration of a monoclonal IgA antibody to influenza virus in mice resulted in resistance to infection after intranasal challenge. Much larger amounts of IgG antibodies were required to achieve the same degree of protection; this suggested that specific polymeric IgA antibodies selectively transported into the respiratory tract are more effective than transduded serum IgG.

Resolving ongoing RSV infections probably depends on the development of specific cytotoxic T cells. Such cells have been demonstrated in the blood of infants at about the time when viral shedding begins to wane (Chiba et al., 1989; Issacs et al., 1987). Indeed, infants lacking T-cell immunity may have persistent infection despite large doses of passive RSV antibody. T cells may be involved in the lung disease that develops in some infants with RSV (Welliver et al., 1979).

Middle Ear Immunity and Otitis Media

The mucosal immunity of the middle ear and eustachian tube have been reviewed recently (Kurono et al., 1999a). The surfaces of the eustachian tube and middle ear are lined largely with ciliated respiratory epithelium, but secretory glands are also found in the proximal eustachian tube and to a lesser extent in the tympanic cavity and antrum (Lim, 1974). Only a few immunocompetent cells are normally associated with the middle ear mucosa (Lim, 1974) and mast cells predominate. In experimental models of middle ear infection, cells of the monocyte/macrophage lineage and T and B lymphocytes accumulate in the middle ear mucosa over a period of weeks (Ichimiya et al., 1990; Takahashi et al., 1992).

The noninfected human middle ear contains minimal fluid. The fluid that accumulates in chronic serous or acute purulent otitis media may contain antibodies to pneumococci and H. influenzae (Howie et al., 1973; Sloyer et al., 1975). Although IgG and IgM antibodies are present, SIgA antibodies dominate. The role of locally produced IgA antibodies in protection against reinfection is unknown, but bacteria were isolated less often from those ear effusions with high levels of SIgA than from those with low titers (Howie et al., 1973).

It has been proposed that the tonsils and adenoids are a major source of the antibody-producing cells of the middle ear (Brandtzaeg and Korsrud, 1984). In guinea pigs, however, systemic priming, followed by intraduodenal or intratracheal challenge, also results in IgA-specific antibodies in the inflamed middle ear (Watanabe et al., 1988).

Serum IgG antibodies may also help to protect against middle ear infection. It has been found that patients with recurrent otitis media had much higher serum IgG titers of strain-specific antibodies than those of the IgM or IgA class. Over time, persistent titers of these type-specific antibodies in the serum correlated with decreased infection. However, these studies did not exclude the possibility that a rapid local response to reexposure in the middle ear mediated the protection. In experimental animal models, serum antibodies and complement can themselves produce otitis media after antigen is introduced into the middle ear (Kurono et al., 1999b).

The bacteria that cause otitis media enter through the eustachian tube after colonization and/or infection of the nasopharynx. Strains of H. influenzae and pneumococci, which are common causes of otitis media, adhere efficiently to retropharyngeal epithelium (Andersson et al., 1981; Porras et al., 1985). Antibodies present in exocrine secretions (such as milk or saliva) may inhibit attachment of the bacteria, decrease colonization, and prevent ear infection (Andersson et al., 1985, 1986). Indeed, breastfeeding seems to reduce nasopharyngeal carriage of these bacteria (Shimamura et al., 1990).

Lower Respiratory Tract Immunity

Locally formed antibodies against several respiratory bacterial pathogens have been demonstrated in humans (Brandtzaeg and Korsrud, 1984). It has been claimed that the presence of local IgA antibodies to M. pneumoniae may confer resistance (Brunner and Chanock, 1973). Antibodies against the P1 protein, which functions as an adhesin for M. pneumoniae to ciliated epithelium, may be protective by blocking its adhesion (Ho et al., 1983). Immunization of the respiratory tract with a streptococcal M protein vaccine may confer local protection against challenge with streptococci (Waldman et al., 1975). Ingestion of H. influenzae can induce IgA and IgG antibodies in exocrine secretions, such as saliva and tears (Clancy et al., 1983).

Acute bacterial infections of the lower respiratory tract frequently follow viral infections. Several different mechanisms have been invoked to explain this relationship, but none are proven (Welliver, 1994). The resolution of bacterial lung infections does not seem to depend on the mucosal immune response. Specific serum antibodies and the complement system seem to be the major factors in resolution of pneumonia and prevention of reinfection. The fact that administration of large doses of IgG can prevent upper and lower respiratory tract infections, including pneumonia, in patients with severe antibody deficiencies suggests that serum IgG can compensate for a lack of both serum and local antibody responses in the lung.

Urogenital Tract Mucosal Immunity

Urinary Tract Infection

Recurrent and chronic infections are common in the urinary tract and in the female and male reproductive tracts. The host mechanisms involved in resolution and prevention of reinfections at these sites are poorly understood. However, the recognition of HIV as a sexually and vertically transmitted infection has expanded the interest in prevention of genital tract infections.

Urinary IgG and especially SIgA antibodies against *E. coli* O and K antigens appear in patients with acute urinary tract infections (Jodal et al., 1974). In noninfected children, SIgA dominates, but during infection, total IgG and monomeric IgA as well as SIgA levels increase (Fliedner et al., 1986; Greenwell et al., 1985; Svanborg et al., 1985; Uehling and Stiehm, 1971). Such urinary SIgA antibodies may prevent *E. coli* adherence to uroepithelial cells (Svanborg et al., 1976). This activity may be of biologic significance, because bacteria with the capacity to adhere are isolated commonly from the urine of patients with acute pyelonephritis, whereas bacteria from patients with "asymptomatic" bacteriuria adhere poorly or not at all (Svanborg et al., 1983).

Urinary antibodies may therefore protect against symptomatic infection. It is possible that antibodies induce changes in the urinary bacteria in patients with long-standing bacteriuria, resulting in less virulent asymptomatic infections (Hanson et al., 1977). However, one study has also shown that girls with normal urinary tracts but recurrent symptomatic bacteriuria have abnormally low levels of urinary SIgA between infections (Fliedner et al., 1986), perhaps leading to recurrent infections.

Local immunity to urinary tract infections can be induced in rats (Hanson et al., 1977; Kaijser et al., 1978). In mice, resistance to ascending urinary tract infection was linked to the LPS response gene, whereas genetic defects in T and B lymphocytes and C5 had little effect on the clearance of bacteria from the kidneys (Hagberg et al., 1984b; Svanborg et al., 1984). These data suggest that the inflammatory mechanisms induced by LPS are important in the host defense against pyelonephritis.

Children with the blood group P_1 were found to be more susceptible to recurrent pyelonephritis in the absence of reflux. This enhanced susceptibility is most likely because the P globoside structure, expressed on the epithelium of the urinary tract, can serve as a receptor for pyelonephritogenic *E. coli* (Lomberg et al., 1983). In the presence of reflux, P-dependent adherence may not be required to induce renal infection. The secretory status of the host may also influence bacterial attachment to the epithelium, because the released A and B glycoconjugates can block binding of bacteria to these receptors (Lomberg et al., 1986a). However, the overrepresentation of nonsecretors among patients with urinary tract infection who have renal scarring (May et al., 1989) and the low frequency of adhering strains in this group of patients, regardless of the presence of reflux (Lomberg et al., 1986b), suggest an altered balance between host and organism unrelated to adherence. Instead, a more generalized host defense defect may be present (Grundbacher, 1972; Waissbluth and Langman, 1971). A wide range of infections have been found to be over represented among nonsecretors (Blackwell et al., 1986; Kilian et al., 1983).

Oligosaccharide analogs for the *E. coli*-specific receptor have been shown to prevent ascending urinary infections in mice (Hagberg et al., 1984a). It is not yet known whether such approaches can be applied in humans.

Genital Tract Infections

Infections of the reproductive tract are uncommon in young children but are an increasing problem of adolescence. The topic of mucosal immunity of the reproductive tracts has been reviewed by Parr and Parr (1999). One of the major dilemmas in understanding the immune mechanisms that induce mucosal immune responses in the female genital tract is that local immunity to sperm and seminal fluid can result in infertility (Bronson et al., 1984). Thus if immune responses are to be stimulated at the vaginal cervical site, they must be limited to organisms that, unlike sperm, penetrate the epithelial barrier. Given the lack of organized lymphoid tissue at these sites, it is likely that vaginal immune responses can be induced more efficiently by antigen stimulation of GALT in the rectum (Forrest et al., 1990) or at more distant mucosal surfaces.

BREAST MILK AND BREASTFEEDING

Breast milk can be considered a specialized mucosal secretion. Its main function is to transfer nutrients from the mother to the infant during a period when the infant is adapting to other sources of nutrition. Mucosal immune factors of the milk are important in protecting the mammary gland and infant against infection. Both roles may enhance the adaptation of the nursing infant to the extrauterine environment. The immunologic role of human milk in protecting the infant has been reviewed by Goldblum and Goldman (1994) and Carlsson and Hanson (1994).

Many of the immunologic factors in human milk are the same as those in other secretions, although the concentration is usually higher in milk. However, these concentrations decline as lactation proceeds, in a temporal relationship with increases in the infant's own production of the same factors. This finding suggests a dynamic regulation tuned to the infant's needs. The immunologic factors in milk are well adapted to protect the mucosal surfaces, where they function without inciting tissue-injuring inflammatory reactions. Human milk also contains growth factors and cytokines that may modulate the development of the infant's immune system.

Breast Milk Immunoglobulins

Secretory IgA in Human Milk

SIgA is the predominant Ig in human milk throughout lactation. Indeed, the observation that mother's milk contained predominantly IgA that differed structurally from serum IgA led to the first descriptions of SIgA (Hanson, 1961; Hodes et al., 1964; Tomasi et al., 1965). Subsequent studies showed that milk SIgA antibodies develop after maternal intestinal antigenic exposure (Allardyce et al., 1974; Bohl and Saif, 1975; Goldblum et al., 1975; Montgomery et al., 1979) and that natural milk SIgA antibodies are directed against intestinal microorganisms and food antigens. Experimental animal studies later demonstrated that lymphoid cells from the Peyer's patches migrate specifically to the lactating mammary gland (Dahlgren et al., 1986, 1987; Roux et al., 1977).

Together this information led to the concept of the enteromammary pathway of secretory immune response (see Fig. 9-1). Additional studies showed that exposure of the mother's respiratory tract to live organisms also resulted in specific SIgA antibodies in the milk (Cumella and Ogra, 1986; Theodore et al., 1982), providing evidence for a similar bronchomammary pathway.

Most milk antibodies are synthesized within the mammary gland. Brandtzaeg (1983a, 1983b) showed that the lactating human mammary gland has sufficient numbers of IgA-producing cells to account for the daily output of milk SIgA. The concentration of Ig in human milk varies throughout breastfeeding (Goldman et al., 1982a; Hanson et al., 1971; McClelland et al., 1978; Ogra and Ogra, 1978; Reddy et al., 1977). The concentration of SIgA is highest in the colostrum but decreases to a relatively stable level, around 1.0 mg/ml, after the first few weeks. Because the milk volumes increase, the fully breast-fed infant obtains at least 500 mg of SIgA per day, corresponding to about 75 to 125 mg/kg/day for the first 4 months of life (Butte et al., 1984). By comparison, this is many times the IgG given intravenously to patients with hypogammaglobulinemia (~100 mg/kg/week).

The high concentrations of SIgA in milk persist, even during a second year of lactation (Butte et al., 1984; Goldman et al., 1983a). During weaning, there is a slight increase in SIgA concentration and S-IgA titers against E. coli O antigens (Goldman et al., 1983b). Lower SIgA levels with increasing parity were observed in Gambian (Prentice et al., 1983) but not British mothers (Lewis-Jones et al., 1985).

Milk from mothers of premature infants has significantly higher concentrations of SIgA than milk from term mothers and shows a further increase toward the twelfth week of lactation, as do specific E. coli SIgA antibodies (Goldman et al., 1982b; Suzuki et al., 1983). Malnutrition may also decrease breast milk SIgA antibodies (see Influence of Nutrition, earlier).

Breast Milk Antibodies and Response to Immunization

Because of the enteromammary pathway, human milk is rich in SIgA antibodies against microorganisms present in the mother's intestine. As a result, infants ingest antibodies against the microorganisms that they are most likely to encounter. Thus the Pakistani infant receives SIgA antibodies against V. cholerae and E. coli enterotoxin from the mother's milk, but the Swedish infant does not (Holmgren et al., 1976).

Typically human milk contains antibodies to the common colonizing bacteria of the species E. coli, Klebsiella, Clostridium, Bacteroides, streptococci, and Lactobacillus and against a number of bacterial pathogens, viruses, fungi, and dietary proteins (Hanson et al., 1983a; Ogra et al., 1983; Pickering and Ruiz-Palacios, 1986). The presence in human milk of SIgA antibodies to bacterial adhesins, such as somatic pili of E. coli (Svanborg et al., 1979) and CFA/I of toxin-producing E. coli (Castrignano et al., 1988), Klebsiella (Davis et al., 1982), and Bordetella (Oda et al., 1985), may be of particular value to the infant, because they may prevent colonization and infection with potentially pathogenic, piliated enterobacteria.

One approach to disease prevention in newborns would be to immunize their lactating mothers, who could provide passive protective antibodies. The nature of the enteromammary immune response limits this approach, particularly following oral immunization. Although parenteral vaccination with cholera vaccine boosts the milk SIgA response (Svennerholm et al., 1977), this occurred only in previously exposed Pakistani mothers, not in unexposed Swedish mothers (Svennerholm et al., 1980). This finding agrees with rodent experiments showing that optimal SIgA responses follow parenteral boosting after mucosal priming (Hanson et al., 1983a). Indeed, oral immunization with polio vaccine during lactation caused an unexplained decrease in the level of SIgA antibody to poliovirus in the milk (Hanson et al., 1979; Sveennerholm et al., 1981). Subcutaneous or intranasal immunization with attenuated rubella virus gave small but consistent milk IgA responses (Losonsky et al., 1982).

Fate of Secretory IgA in Ingested Milk

Because human milk antibodies ingested by the infant are not absorbed into the circulation, the advantages of ingesting SIgA on local immunity were not appreciated until recently. Some milk SIgA passes through the gastrointestinal tract of the infant undigested (see Secretory IgA Stability, earlier). Antibodies have been found in the stool of breast-fed babies (Gindrat et al., 1972; Kenny et al., 1967; Schanler et al., 1986) and as much as 20% to 80% of the milk SIgA can be detected in the stool (Davidson and Lonnerdal, 1987; Ogra et al., 1977; Prentice, 1987; Schanler et al., 1986). Some additional SIgA, not measured in the stool, may be bound to fecal bacteria.

Much of the SIgA that escapes proteolysis in the small intestines is degraded by bacterial IgA proteases and reductases in the colon (Kilian and Reinholdt, 1986; Kilian et al., 1983; Plaut, 1983). Some of the Fab fragments of SIgA produced by these enzymes may still be active, for example against poliovirus (Hanson and Johansson, 1970).

IgG and IgM in Milk

Human milk also contains small amounts of IgG and IgM antibodies. The IgG concentration is less than 3% of the serum IgG value and the IgM is about 10% of the serum IgM level (McClelland et al., 1978). Thus the daily intake of the breastfed infant is never more than 100 mg of IgG and 70 mg of IgM, and these immunoglobulins become undetectable in milk after the 50th day of lactation. Some milk IgG and IgM is locally produced (Brandtzaeg, 1983b; Cox et al., 1985; Dahlgren et al., 1986). Transfer experiments in rats indicate that none of the IgA or IgM antibodies injected into the serum appears in the milk (Dahlgren et al., 1987; Nilsson et al., 1988).

Soluble Immunoregulatory Factors

Clinical and epidemiologic observations suggest that the ability of human milk to modulate the development of the infant's own mucosal and systemic immune systems may be associated with immunoregulatory agents present in colostrum and in mature milk. Several different types of immunomodulatory agents can be identified in human milk, including lactoferrin, lysozyme, cytokines, growth factors, nucleotides, and substances with antioxidant and antiinflammatory properties.

Many of these milk components have other biologic functions, as in the case of hormones or growth factors, and their immunoregulatory properties overlaps with their antimicrobial or antiinflammatory properties. Substances in human milk with proven or potential ability to protect against infections and/or modulate the infant immune response have been reviewed by Garofalo and Goldman (1999) and briefly discussed in the following text.

Lactoferrin

Lactoferrin is a major protein of human milk (1 to 6 mg/ml). Intact lactoferrin found in the urine of breastfed premature infants has its origin in maternal milk (Hutchens et al., 1991), thus indicating that intact lactoferrin is absorbed by the infant gut. In vitro antimicrobial activities of lactoferrin include bacteriostatic, bactericidal, and fungicidal activities alone or in synergy with other antibacterial milk components such as human lysozyme and Ig (Nuijens et al., 1996).

The bacteriostatic activity of lactoferrin depends on its capacity to bind iron, thereby eliminating this as a growth factor for most aerobic bacteria (except lactobacilli). The described synergy between SIgA antibodies and unsaturated lactoferrin in inhibiting the growth of *E. coli* (Adinolfi et al., 1966) may be related to the presence of specific antibodies against the bacterial iron-binding proteins or to the targeting of bacteria by lactoferrin-IgA complexes (Jorieux et al., 1984; Watanabe et al., 1984).

The in vitro anti-inflammatory activities of lactoferrin include inhibition of the formation of hydroxyl radicals by scavenging free iron (see following text), inhibition of cytokine production (Crouch et al., 1992) and binding to the inflammatory mediator LPS (Appelmelk et al., 1994). Lactoferrin has also been shown to promote the growth of intestinal cells in vitro (Nichols et al., 1987), but the in vivo value of this activity is not precisely known.

Lysozyme

The enzyme lysozyme, with activity against the cell wall of gram-positive bacteria, is present in milk throughout lactation (~ 0.1 mg/ml). Unlike other factors, lysozyme concentration increases late in lactation (Goldman et al., 1982a, 1983a, 1983b). The effect of lysozyme in the gastrointestinal tract is not known.

Lipolytic Products

Human milk contains both triglycerides and lipolytic enzymes that combine to produce lipolytic products with antimicrobial activity. The infant's own lingual lipase may be important in initiating lipolysis (Hamosh, 1990). Fatty acids and monoglycerides produced from milk fats by bile salt-stimulated lipases or lipoprotein lipase may prevent intestinal coronavirus infections (Resta et al., 1985). Enveloped viruses may also be disrupted by these products (Issacs et al., 1986; Stock and Francis, 1940; Thromar et al., 1987; Welsh et al., 1979). Killing of *Giardia lamblia* is also dependent on bile salt-stimulated lipase (Gillin et al., 1985), which causes the release of fatty acids (Hernell et al., 1986).

Cytokines and Cytokine Receptors

The effector phases of both natural and specific immunity are largely mediated by cytokines. Several cytokines, chemokines, and colony-stimulating factors have been discovered in human milk over the past years and the list is growing rapidly (Garofalo and Goldman, 1998). Although it is tempting to speculate that cytokines present in milk may interact with mucosal tissues in the upper parts of the respiratory and alimentary tracts, receptor-dependent or independent uptake of cytokines by mucosal barriers during the neonatal period has not been demonstrated.

IL-10, the major immunomodulatory and anti-inflammatory cytokine, is present at very high concentrations in samples of human milk collected during the first 80 hours of lactation (Garofalo et al., 1995). Its bioactive properties were confirmed by the finding that human milk samples inhibited blood lymphocyte proliferation and that this was greatly reduced by the treatment with anti-IL-10 antibody. IL-10 mRNA was found in cultured human mammary epithelial cells, suggesting that the mammary gland may be a source of this molecule.

Among the chemokines that are present in human milk, IL-8, growth-related peptide-α, and RANTES (regulated on activation, normal T expressed and secreted) have been found to be the most potent chemotactic factors for intestinal IEL (Ebert, 1995). Soluble receptors and cytokine receptor antagonists are also potent anti-inflammatory agents. In this regard, human colostrum and mature milk contain the IL-1 receptor antagonist (IL-1Ra) and significant levels of soluble TNF-α receptors I and II (sTNF-α RI and RII) (Buescher and Malinowska, 1996).

Nucleotides

A host of nucleotides in the form of nucleic acids, nucleotides, and nucleosides are present in human milk. Their concentration is higher and qualitatively different than in bovine milk or protein-based infant formula (Gil and Uauy, 1995). Several studies in animal models have shown that nucleotides enhance mucosal development by stimulating growth and maturation of the gastrointestinal tract and intestinal repair after diarrhea (Uauy et al., 1990).

The immunomodulatory activity of nucleotides results in the enhancement of T-cell maturation and function, improvement of delayed cutaneous hypersensitivity and alloantigen-induced lymphoproliferation, and partial resistance to infection with bacteria or other pathogens (Kulkarni et al., 1986). When compared with a nonsupplemented milk formula, infants fed with a formula fortified with nucleotides had enhanced humoral responses to immunization with *Haemophilus influenzae* b and diphtheria vaccines (Pickering et al., 1998). Because these nucleotides can be absorbed and used for pyrimidine and purine synthesis, they may be active systemically as well as locally on the mucosa of the respiratory and alimentary tracts.

Antioxidants

Antioxidants are a significant part of the anti-inflammatory system in human milk (Buescher and Mcilharn, 1992; Garofalo and Goldman, 1999). Peaks of antioxidant activity in colostrum have been shown to be associated with an ascorbate compound and uric acid. In addition, α-tocopherol and β-carotene present in human milk are readily absorbed into the systemic circulation by the gastrointestinal mucosa. These vitamins are potent scavengers of oxygen radicals that may be produced at the mucosal sites in the breastfed infant.

Catalase and glutathione peroxidase, which degrade hydrogen peroxide and prevent lipid peroxidation, respectively, are also present in human milk. Mature human milk shows antioxidant effects qualitatively similar to but quantitatively less than those of colostrum. The lipid fraction of human milk has been reported to inhibit the generation of superoxide anions by human blood neutrophils, but these lipid phase inhibitors have not been identified (Pickering et al., 1980). In this regard, although lactoferrin avidly binds Fe^{3+}, the molecule is largely unsaturated in human milk and therefore it may function as an important antioxidant factor in milk.

The Cells of Breast Milk

Milk differs from most other secretions, in that it contains numerous viable cells, especially during the first few weeks of lactation (Smith and Goldman, 1968). Enumeration of the cells in milk is complicated by the presence of numerous cell-like particles, mainly milk fat globules. The neutrophils and macrophages are difficult to recognize because they contain cytoplasmic vacuoles consisting of phagocytosed milk fat globules and casein micelles (Ho and Lawton, 1978; Paape and Wergin, 1977). These inclusions also make the milk phagocytes difficult to separate (Paape and Keller, 1985).

Colostrum and early milk contain 1 to 3×10^6 leukocytes/ml, falling to about 1×10^5 cells/ml 2 to 3 months later (Goldman et al., 1982a; Ogra, 1979). Of these cells, 18% to 23% are neutrophils, 59% to 63% are monocytes/macrophages, and 7% to 13% are lymphocytes, as determined by conventional and monoclonal antibody staining techniques (Soderstrom et al., 1988).

The mechanism by which leukocytes enter the mammary secretions is poorly understood. The finding that both milk neutrophils and macrophages have markers of cellular activation suggests that their migration may be similar to those present at sites of inflammation. Thus, relative to blood neutrophils, milk neutrophils demonstrate decreased adherence, decreased response to chemotactic factors, decreased motility (Thorpe et al., 1986), and decreased uptake and killing of *Staphylococcus aureus* (Pickering et al., 1980b).

These functional differences may be associated with prior PMN activation (Keeney et al., 1993). By contrast, milk macrophages, which also demonstrate markers of activation (Keeney et al., 1993), are more motile than blood monocytes. In addition, human milk leukocytes contain considerable amounts of SIgA (Pittard et al., 1977), which suggests that they transport some of the SIgA antibodies to the milk. However, the amount of IgA in leukocytes varies considerably (Moro et al., 1983; Clemente et al., 1986) and release of intact IgA remains controversial.

Milk contains small numbers of lymphocytes, 80% of which are T cells (Wirt et al., 1992). Some studies using flow cytometry on unfractionated cells suggest a slight predominance of CD8+ cells (Wirt et al., 1992) in agreement with a finding of a CD4/CD8 ratio of less than 1.0 in 17 of 22 milk samples (Soderstrom et al., 1988). Earlier studies suggested differential antigen reactivity of milk T cells and circulating T cells (Parmely et al., 1976; Richie et al., 1980), but other reports show similarities in antigen responsiveness (Keller et al., 1980) and production of monocyte chemotactic factor and IFN (Emodi and Just, 1974; Keller et al., 1981; Keller et al., 1984). Cytotoxic lymphocytes have been identified in milk, as have cells mediating weak ADCC (Kohl et al., 1980; Steinmetz et al., 1981) and NK cell activity (Moro et al., 1985). As with milk phagocytes, the T cells display surface activation markers (CD45RO, IL-2 receptor and MHC class II antigens) (Wirt et al., 1992).

The lymphocyte fraction may also contain IgA-producing B cells (Murillo and Goldman, 1970; Smith and Goldman, 1968). IgA synthesis was also shown by Goldblum and van Bavel (1978) in some but not all milk cell cultures. However, later papers pointed out that the presence of particles and cell fragments that carry IgA make the agar plaque technique unreliable in assessing IgA production. Other workers could not demonstrate in vitro antibody synthesis by milk lymphocytes (Crago and Mestecky, 1984; Crago et al., 1979; Laven et al., 1981; Moro et al., 1983). However, colostral lymphocytes transformed by Epstein-Barr virus produce IgM, IgA, and IgG (Hanson et al., 1985; Soderstrom et al., 1988). The IgM- and IgA-producing cells contained J chain in high frequency and were of the IgA1 isotype (Soderstrom et al., 1988).

Shinmoto and co-workers (1986) identified an 80-kd factor from human colostrum that provided selective help for IgA production by peripheral lymphocytes. This factor may be responsible for the IgA-enhancing activity of colostrum reported by Pittard and Bill (1979).

In summary, human milk contains IgA-producing cells, has cells containing ingested IgA, and has a factor that stimulates IgA production.

The biologic role of milk phagocytes is not known. They may protect the mammary gland or aid in the infant's host defense. Milk T and B lymphocytes may enhance antigen-specific reactivity of the infant. Several groups have reported that human milk feeding can transfer tuberculin sensitivity from the mother to the infant (Mohr, 1973; Schlesinger and Covelli, 1977), at least temporarily (Ogra et al., 1977). However, because intrauterine transfer of tuberculin sensitivity may also occur (Masters, 1982), transfers of specific cellular sensitivity by humoral factors in the milk (e.g., antiidiotypic antibodies) cannot be excluded.

Immunologic Protection by Breastfeeding

Several epidemiologic studies have demonstrated that breastfeeding prevents infantile infections, particularly those affecting the gastrointestinal and respiratory tract in infection-prone environments such as is present in developing countries (Cunningham et al., 1991). In addition, human milk feeding decreases the incidence and/or severity of diarrhea, lower respiratory infections, otitis media, bacteremia, bacterial meningitis, and urinary tract infections even in middle-class populations of developed countries (American Academy of Pediatrics, 1997).

Soluble factors of milk such as Igs as well as leukocytes provide the essential "passive" component associated with breastfeeding. Specific SIgA antibodies in milk can prevent or attenuate bacterial and viral gastrointestinal infections (Carlsson and Hanson, 1994). Other evidence for protection is derived from epidemiologic studies that compare the frequency of infections in breast and bottle-fed infants. Most of these studies indicate some protective effect of breastfeeding but do not address which component is responsible for its effect.

Avoidance of contaminated foods and reduced exposure to other infants may reduce the incidence of infections in breastfed infants. On the other hand, infants from developing countries often receive foods and fluids that are contaminated with microbes prior to initiation of and during breastfeeding (Ashraf et al., 1993). The inclusion of these infants in the breastfeeding group may reduce the apparent protective effect of breastfeeding. The methodologic problems in the epidemiologic studies of breastfeeding have been reviewed by Kramer (1987).

The major effect of breastfeeding on acute infections is the reduction in frequency and severity of gastroenteritis. These studies indicate that breastfeeding is protective, especially in developing countries and in disadvantaged subpopulations of developed countries (Chandra, 1979; Clemens et al., 1986; Cunningham, 1979; Cunningham et al., 1991; Fergusson et al., 1978, 1981; Forman et al., 1984; Larsen & Homer, 1978; Mata and Urrutia, 1971; Mittal et al, 1983; Rowland et al., 1980). However, protection may be difficult to demonstrate, even in the fully breastfed infants, because of extremely heavy microbial inocula (Hanson et al., 1986; Jalil et al., 1995). Further, breastfeeding in rotavirus gastroenteritis may not result in complete prevention; instead only its severity is reduced (Duffy et al., 1986; Jason et al., 1984).

Human milk may also directly modulate the infant's immunologic development. Breast-fed infants have a reduced incidence of allergic diseases (Saarinen and Kajosaari, 1995) and other disorders of dysregulated immunity, such as Crohn's disease (Koletzko et al., 1989) ulcerative colitis (Koletzko et al., 1991), insulin-dependent diabetes mellitus (Mayer et al., 1988) and some lymphomas (Davis et al., 1988), long after the termination of breastfeeding.

Humoral and cellular immune responses to specific antigens (e.g., vaccines) given during the first year of life appear to develop more vigorously in breastfed than in formula-fed infants. Thus the immature immune system of the newborn infant is enhanced by maternal immunity transferred both transplacentally and via the breast milk without inducing unwanted inflammatory responses (Goldman et al., 1986, 1998).

ACKNOWLEDGMENT

The authors wish to thank Drs. Lars Hanson and Per Brandtzaeg who originally authored and then co-authored this chapter for previous editions of this book. Much of their historical perspective, insights, and extensive references have been retained in this revision.

REFERENCES

American Academy of Pediatrics. Breastfeeding and the use of human milk. Work group on breastfeeding. Pediatrics 103:1150–1157, 1997.

Adinolfi M, Glynn AA, Lindsay M, Milne CM. Serological properties of gamma-A antibodies to *Escherichia coli* present in human colostrum. Immunology 10:517–526, 1966.

Ahlstedt S, Enander I, Johansen K. Immunological regulation of the appearance of goblet cells in the mucosa. Monogr Allergy 24:71–77, 1998.

Allan C H, Mendrick DL, Trier JS. Rat intestinal M cells contain acidic endosomal-lysosomal compartments and express class II major histocompatibility complex determinants. Gastroenterology 104:698–708, 1993.

Allardyce RA, Shearman DJ, McClelland DB, Marwick K, Simpson AJ, Laidlaw RB. Appearance of specific colostrum antibodies after clinical infection with *Salmonella typhimurium*. Br Med J 3:307–309, 1974.

Andersson B, Eriksson B, Falsen E, Fogh A, Hanson LA, Nylen O, Peterson H, Svanborg EC. Adhesion of *Streptococcus pneumoniae* to human pharyngeal epithelial cells in vitro: differences in adhesive capacity among strains isolated from subjects with otitis media, septicemia, or meningitis or from healthy carriers. Infect Immun 32:311–317, 1981.

Andersson B, Porras O, Hanson LA, Lagergard T, Svanborg EC. Inhibition of attachment of *Streptococcus pneumoniae* and *Haemophilus influenzae* by human milk and receptor oligosaccharides. J Infect Dis 153:232–237, 1986.

Andersson B, Porras O, Hanson LA, Svanborg EC, Leffler H. Non-antibody-containing fractions of breast milk inhibit epithelial attachment of *Streptococcus pneumoniae* and *Haemophilus influenzae* [letter]. Lancet 1:643, 1985.

Andre C, Lambert R, Bazin H, Heremans JF. Interference of oral immunization with the intestinal absorption of heterologous albumin. Eur J Immunol 4:701, 1974.

Andrews JS Jr, Hewlett EL. Protection against infection with *Giardia muris* by milk containing antibody to Giardia. J Infect Dis 143:242–246, 1981.

Appelmelk BJ, An YQ, Geerts M, Thijs BG, de Boer HA, MacLaren DM, de Graaff J, Nuijens JH. Lactoferrin is a lipid A-binding protein. Infect Immun 62:2628–2632, 1994.

Apter FM, Lencer WI, Mekalanos JJ, Neutra MR. (abstract) Analysis of epithelial protection by monoclonal IgA antibodies directed against cholera toxin B subunit in vivo and in vitro. J Cell Biol 115:399a, 1991.

Armstrong SJ, Dimmock NJ. Neutralization of influenza virus by low concentrations of hemagglutinin-specific polymeric immunoglobulin A inhibits viral fusion activity, but activation of the ribonucleoprotein is also inhibited. J Virol 66:3823–3832, 1992.

Arnold RR, Mestecky J, McGhee JR. Naturally occurring secretory immunoglobulin A antibodies to *Streptococcus mutans* in human colostrum and saliva. Infect Immun 14:355–362, 1976.

Ashraf RN, Jalil F, Khan SR, Zaman S, Karlberg J, Lindblad BS, Hanson LA. Early child health in Lahore, Pakistan: V. Feeding patterns. Acta Paediatr 390(Suppl 82):47–61, 1993.

Ashwell G, Harford J. Carbohydrate-specific receptors of the liver. Annu Rev Biochem 51:531–554, 1982.

Baklien K, Brandtzaeg P. Letter: Immunohistochemical localization of complement in intestinal mucosa. Lancet 2:1087–1088, 1974.

Bakos MA, Kurosky A, Czerwinski EW, Goldblum RM. A conserved binding site on the receptor for polymeric Ig is homologous to CDR1 of Ig V kappa domains. J Immunol 151:1346–1352, 1993.

Bakos MA, Kurosky A, Goldblum RM. Characterization of a critical binding site for human polymeric Ig on secretory component. J Immunol 147:3419–3426, 1991.

Balk SP, Ebert EC, Blumenthal RL, McDermott FV, Wucherpfennig KW, Landau SB, Blumberg RS. Oligoclonal expansion and CD1 recognition by human intestinal intraepithelial lymphocytes. Science 253:1411–1415, 1991.

Banatvala JE, Best JM, O'Shea S, Harcourt GC. Rubella-immunity gap: is intranasal vaccination the answer? Lancet 1:970, 1979.

Bastian A, Kratzin H, Eckart K, Hilschmann N. Intra- and interchain disulfide bridges of the human J chain in secretory immunoglobulin. A Biol Chem Hoppe Seyler 373:1255–1263, 1992.

Beatty DW, Napier B, Sinclair-Smith CC, McCabe K, Hughes EJ. Secretory IgA synthesis in kwashiorkor. J Clin Lab Immunol 12:31–36, 1983.

Bellamy JE, Nielsen NO. Immune-mediated emigration of neutrophils into the lumen of the small intestine. Infect Immun 9:615–619, 1974.

Bellamy W, Takase M, Yamauchi K, Wakabayashi H, Kawase K, Tomita M. Identification of the bactericidal domain of lactoferrin. Biochem Biophys Acta 1121:130–136, 1992.

Bennich H, Johansson SG. Structure and function of human immunoglobulin E. Adv Immunol 13:1–55, 1971.

Benson EB, Strober W. Regulation of IgA secretion by T cell clones derived from the human gastrointestinal tract. J Immunol 140:1874–1882, 1988.

Besredka A. Du mechanisme de l'infection dysenterique de la vaccination contre la dysenterie par la voie buccale et de la nature de l'immunite antidysenterique. Ann Inst Pasteur 33:301–317, 1919.

Biberfeld G, Sterner G. Antibodies in bronchial secretions following natural infection with Mycoplasma pneumoniae. Acta Pathol Microbiol Scand [B] Microbiol Immunol 79:599–605, 1971.

Biensenstock J, McDermott M, Befus D. A common mucosal immune system. In Ogra PL, Dayton D, eds. Immunology of Breast Milk. New York, Raven Press, 1979, pp 91–107.

Biron CA, Byron KS, Sullivan JL. Severe herpesvirus infections in an adolescent without natural killer cells. N Engl J Med 320:1731–1735, 1989.

Blackwell CC, Jonsdottir K, Hanson MF, Weir DM. Non-secretion of ABO blood group antigens predisposing to infection by *Haemophilus influenzae*. Lancet 2:687, 1996.

Blanco A, Linares P, Andion R, Alonso M, Sanchez VE. Development of humoral immunity of the small bowel. Allergol Immunopathol (Madr.) 4:235–240, 1976.

Bockman DE, Boydston WR, Beezhold DH. The role of epithelial cells in gut-associated immune reactivity. Ann NY Acad Sci 409:129–144, 1983.

Bohl EH, Saif LJ. Passive immunity in transmissible gastroenteritis of swine: immunoglobulin characteristics of antibodies in milk after inoculating virus by different routes. Infect Immun 11:23–32, 1975.

Braathen R, Sorensen V, Brandtzaeg P, Sandlie I, Johansen FE. The carboxyl-terminal domains of IgA and IgM direct isotype-specific polymerization and interaction with the polymeric immunoglobulin receptor. J Biol Chem 277:42755–42762, 2002.

Brandtzaeg P. Human secretory immunoglobulins. 3. Immunochemical and physicochemical studies of secretory IgA and free secretory piece. Acta Pathol Microbiol Scand [B] Microbiol Immunol 79:165–188, 1971a.

Brandtzaeg P. Human secretory immunoglobulins. II. Salivary secretions from individuals with selectively excessive or defective synthesis of serum immunoglobulins. Clin Exp Immunol 8:69–85, 1971b.

Brandtzaeg P. Human secretory immunoglobulins. VII. Concentrations of parotid IgA and other secretory proteins in relation to the rate of flow and duration of secretory stimulus. Arch Oral Biol 16:1295–1310, 1971c.

Brandtzaeg P. Mucosal and glandular distribution of immunoglobulin components. Immunohistochemistry with a cold ethanol-fixation technique. Immunology 26:1101–1114, 1974a.

Brandtzaeg P. Presence of J chain in human immunocytes containing various immunoglobulin classes. Nature 252:418–420, 1974b.

Brandtzaeg P. Human secretory immunoglobulin M. An immunochemical and immunohistochemical study. Immunology 29:559–570, 1975.

Brandtzaeg P. Complex formation between secretory component and human immunoglobulins related to their content of J chain. Scand J Immunol 5:411–419, 1976a.

Brandtzaeg P. Studies on J chain and binding site for secretory component in circulating human B cells. II. The cytoplasm. Clin Exp Immunol 25:59–66, 1976b.

Brandtzaeg P. Human secretory component-VI. Immunoglobulin-binding properties. Immunochemistry. 14:179–188, 1977.

Brandtzaeg P. Review and discussion of IgA transport across mucosal membranes. In Stober W, Hanson L, Sell KW, eds. Recent Advances in Mucosal Immunity. New York, Raven Press, 1982, pp 267–285.

Brandtzaeg P. The oral secretory immune system with special emphasis on its relation to dental caries. Proc Finn Dent Soc 79:71–84, 1983a.

Brandtzaeg P. The secretory immune system of lactating human mammary glands compared with other exocrine organs. Ann NY Acad Sci 409:353–382, 1983b.

Brandtzaeg P. Research in gastrointestinal immunology. State of the art. Scand J Gastroenterol Suppl 114:137–156, 1985a.

Brandtzaeg P. Role of J chain and secretory component in receptor-mediated glandular and hepatic transport of immunoglobulins in man. Scand J Immunol 22:111–146, 1985b.

Brandtzaeg P. Meningitis and septic shock as acute, fatal conditions. Tidsskr Nor Laegeforen 113:1994–1997, 1993.

Brandtzaeg P. Distribution and characteristics of mucosal immunoglobulin-producing cells. In Ogra PL, Mestecky J, Lamm ME, Strober W, McGhee J, Bienenstock J. Handbook of Mucosal Immunology. San Diego, Academic Press, 1994, pp 251-262.

Brandtzaeg P, Baklien K. Immunohistochemical studies of the formation and epithelial transport of immunoglobulins in normal and diseased human intestinal mucosa. Scand J Gastroenterol Suppl 36:1–45, 1976.

Brandtzaeg P, Baklien K. Characterization of the IgA immunocyte population and its product in a patient with excessive intestinal formation of IgA. Clin Exp Immunol 30:77–88, 1977a.

Brandtzaeg P, Baklien K. Intestinal secretion of IgA and IgM: a hypothetical model. Ciba Found Symp 46:77–113, 1977b.

Brandtzaeg P, Bjerke K. Immunomorphological characteristics of human Peyer's patches. Digestion 46(Suppl 2):262–273, 1990.

Brandtzaeg P, Farstad IN. The human mucosal B-cell system. In Ogra PL, Mestecky J, Lamm ME, Strober W, Bienenstock J, McGhee JR, eds. Mucosal Immunology San Diego, Academic Press, San Diego, 1999, pp 439-468.

Brandtzaeg P, Halstensen TS. Immunology and immunopathology of tonsils. Adv Otorhinolaryngol 47:64–75, 1992.

Brandtzaeg P, Korsrud FR. Significance of different J chain profiles in human tissues: generation of IgA and IgM with binding site for secretory component is related to the J chain expressing capacity of the total local immunocyte population, including IgG and IgD producing cells, and depends on the clinical state of the tissue. Clin Exp Immunol 58:709–718, 1984.

Brandtzaeg P, Prydz H. Direct evidence for an integrated function of J chain and secretory component in epithelial transport of immunoglobulins. Nature 311:71–73, 1984.

Brandtzaeg P, Tolo K. Mucosal penetrability enhanced by serum-derived antibodies. Nature 266:262–263, 1977.

Brandtzaeg P, Fjellanger I, Gjeruldsen ST. Adsorption of immunoglobulin A onto oral bacteria in vivo. J Bacteriol 96:242–249, 1968a.

Brandtzaeg P, Fjellanger I, Gjeruldsen ST. Immunoglobulin M: local synthesis and selective secretion in patients with immunoglobulin A deficiency. Science 160:789–791, 1968b.

Brandtzaeg P, Fjellanger I, Gjeruldsen ST. Human secretory immunoglobulins. I. Salivary secretions from individuals with normal or low levels of serum immunoglobulins. Scand J Haematol Suppl 12:3–83, 1970.

Brandtzaeg P, Surjan L, Berdal P. Immunoglobulin systems of human tonsils. I. Control subjects of various ages: quantification of Ig-producing cells, tonsillar morphometry and serum Ig concentrations. Clin Exp Immunol 31:367–381, 1978.

Brandtzaeg P, Gjeruldsen ST, Korsrud F, Baklien K, Berdal P, Ek J. The human secretory immune system shows striking heterogeneity with regard to involvement of J chain-positive IgD immunocytes. J Immunol 122:503–510, 1979.

Brandtzaeg P, Baklien K, Bjerke K, Rognum TO, Scott H, Valnes K. Nature and properties of the human gastrointestinal immune system. In Miller K, Nicklin S, eds. Immunology of the Gastriointesinal Tract. Boca Raton, FL, CRC Press, 1987a, pp 1–85.

Brandtzaeg P, Karlsson G, Hansson G, Petruson B, Bjorkander J, Hanson LA. The clinical condition of IgA-deficient patients is related to the proportion of IgD- and IgM-producing cells in their nasal mucosa. Clin Exp Immunol 67:626–636, 1987b.

Brandtzaeg P, Halstensen TS, Kett K, Krajci P, Kvale D, Rognum TO, Scott H, Sollid LM. Immunobiology and immunopathology of human gut mucosa: humoral immunity and intraepithelial lymphocytes. Gastroenterology 97:1562–1584, 1989.

Brandtzaeg P, Nilssen DE, Rognum TO, Thrane PS. Ontogeny of the mucosal immune system and IgA deficiency. Gastroenterol Clin North Am 20:397–439, 1991.

Bronson RA, Cooper GW, Rosenfeld DL. Sperm antibodies: their role in infertility. Fertil Steril 42:171–183, 1984.

Brown WR, Borthistle BK, Chen ST. Immunoglobulin E (IgE) and IgE-containing cells in human gastrointestinal fluids and tissues. Clin Exp Immunol 20:227–237, 1975.

Brown WR, Smith PD, Lee E, McCalmon RT, Nagura H. A search for an enriched source of polymeric IgA in human thoracic duct lymph, portal vein blood and aortic blood. Clin Exp Immunol 48:85–90, 1982.

Brunner H, Chanock RM. A radioimmunoprecipitation test for detection of Mycoplasma pneumoniae antibody. Proc Soc Exp Biol Med 143:97–105, 1973.

Buescher ES, Malinowska I. Soluble receptors and cytokine antagonists in human milk. Pediatr Res 40:839–844, 1996.

Buescher SE, Mcilharn SM. Colostral antioxidants: separation and characterization of two activities in human colostrum. J Pediatr Gastroenterol Nutr 14:47–56, 1992.

Bull CG, McKee CM. Respiratory immunity in rabbits: resistance to intranasal infection in absence of demonstrable antibodies. Am J Hyg 9:490–499, 1929.

Bullen JJ, Rogers HJ, Griffiths E. Bacterial iron metabolism in infection and immunity. In Neilands JB, ed. Microbial Iron Metabolism. New York, Academic Press, 1974, pp 517-551.

Bullen JJ, Rogers HJ, Leigh L. Iron-binding proteins in milk and resistance to Escherichia coli infection in infants. Br Med J 1:69–75, 1972.

Burgio GR, Lanzavecchia A, Plebani A, Jayakar S, Ugazio AG. Ontogeny of secretory immunity: levels of secretory IgA and natural antibodies in saliva. Pediatr Res 14:1111–1114, 1980.

Burns JW, Siadat-Pajouh M, Krishnaney AA, Greenberg HB. Protective effect of rotavirus VP6-specific IgA monoclonal antibodies that lack neutralizing activity. Science 272:104–107, 1996.

Burrows W, Havens I. Studies on immunity to Asiatic cholera: V. J Infect Dis 82:231–250, 1948.

Butcher EC. Lymphocyte homing and intestinal immunity. In Ogra PL, Mestecky J, Lamm ME, Strober W, Bienenstock J, McGhee JR, eds. Mucosal Immunology. San Diego, Academic Press, San Diego, 1999, pp 507–522.

Butte NF, Goldblum RM, Fehl LM, Loftin K, Smith EO, Garza C, Goldman AS. Daily ingestion of immunologic components in human milk during the first four months of life. Acta Paediatr Scand 73:296–301, 1984.

Capron A, Dessaint JP, Haque A, Capron M. Antibody-dependent cell-mediated cytotoxicity against parasites. Prog Allergy 31:234–267, 1982.

Capron A, Joseph M, Ameisen JC, Capron M, Pancre V, Auriault C. Platelets as effectors in immune and hypersensitivity reactions. Int Arch Allergy Appl Immunol 82:307–312, 1987.

Carlsson B, Hanson L. Immunologic effects of breast-feeding on the infant. In Ogra PL, Lamm ME, McGhee JR, Mestecky J, Strober W, Bienenstock J, eds. Handbook of Mucosal Immunology. San Diego, Academic Press, 1994, pp 653-660.

Carlsson B, Ahlstedt S, Hanson LA, Lidin-Janson G, Lindblad BS, Sultana R. Escherichia coli O antibody content in milk from healthy Swedish mothers and mothers from a very low socio-economic group of a developing country. Acta Paediatr Scand 65:417–423, 1976.

Carlsson B, Zaman S, Mellander L, Jalil F, Hanson LA. Secretory and serum immunoglobulin class-specific antibodies to poliovirus after vaccination. J Infect Dis 152:1238–1244, 1985.

Casanova JE, Breitfeld PP, Ross SA, Mostov KE. Phosphorylation of the polymeric immunoglobulin receptor required for its efficient transcytosis. Science 248:742–745, 1990.

Castrignano SB, Carlsson B, Jalil F, Hanson L. The ontogeny of serum and secretory antibodies to Escherichia coli CCFA/I and other types of pili in Pakistani infants. Personal communications, 1988.

Cebra JJ, Fuhrman JA, Horsfall DJ, Shatin RD. Natural and deliberate priming of IgA responses to bacterial antigens by the mucosal route. In Robbins JB, Hill JC, Sadoff JC, eds. Seminars in Infectious Diseases. Bacterial Vaccines, vol 4. New York, Thieme-Stratton, 1982, pp 6-12.

Cerf-Bensussan N, Jarry A, Brousse N, Lisowska-Grospierre B, Guy-Grand D, Griscelli C. A monoclonal antibody (HML-1) defining a novel membrane molecule present on human intestinal lymphocytes. Eur J Immunol 17:1279–1285, 1987.

Challacombe SJ, Shirlaw PJ. Immunology of diseases of the oral cavity. In Ogra PL, Lamm ME, McGree JR, Mestecky J, Strober W, Bienenstock J, eds. Handbook of Mucosal Immunology. Academic Press, San Diego, 1994, pp 607–624.

Challacombe SJ, Shirlaw PJ. Immunology of diseases of the oral cavity. In Ogra PL, Mestecky J, Lamm ME, Strober W, Bienenstock J, McGhee JR, eds. Mucosal Immunology San Diego, Academic Press, 1999, pp 1313-1337.

Chandan RC, Shahani KM, Holly RG. Lysozyme content of himan milk. Nature 204:76–77, 1964.

Chandra RK. Reduced secretory antibody response to live attenuated measles and poliovirus vaccines in malnourished children. Br Med J 2:583–585, 1975.

Chandra RK. Nutritional deficiency and susceptibility to infection. Bull World Health Organ 57:167–177, 1979.

Chiba Y, Higashidate Y, Suga K, Honjo K, Tsutsumi H, Ogra PL. Development of cell-mediated cytotoxic immunity to respiratory syncytial virus in human infants following naturally acquired infection. J Med Virol 28:133–139, 1989.

Chintalacharuvu KR, Tavill AS, Louis LN, Vaerman JP, Lamm ME, Kaetzel CS. Disulfide bond formation between dimeric immunoglobulin A and the polymeric immunoglobulin receptor during hepatic transcytosis. Hepatology 19:162–173, 1994.

Chodirker WB, Tomasi TB, Jr. Gamma-globulins: quantitative relationships in human serum and nonvascular fluids. Science 142:1080–1081, 1963.

Clamp JR. The relationship between secretory immunoglobulin A and mucus [proceedings]. Biochem Soc Trans 5:1579–1581, 1977.

Clancy RL, Cripps AW, Husband AJ, Buckley D. Specific immune response in the respiratory tract after administration of an oral polyvalent bacterial vaccine. Infect Immun 39:491–496, 1983.

Cleary TG, Chambers JP, Pickering LK. Protection of suckling mice from the heat-stable enterotoxin of Escherichia coli by human milk. J Infect Dis 148:1114–1119, 1983.

Clemens JD, Sack DA, Harris JR, Chakraborty J, Khan MR, Stanton BF, Kay BA, Khan MU, Yunus M, Atkinson W, Svennerholm A-M, Holmgren J. Field trial of oral cholera vaccines in Bangladesh. Lancet 2:124–127, 1986.

Clemens JD, Sack DA, Harris JR, Chakraborty J, Neogy PK, Stanton B, Huda N, Khan MU, Kay BA, Khan MR, Yunus M, Rao MR, Svennerholm AM, Holmgren J. Cross-protection by B subunit-whole cell cholera vaccine against diarrhea associated with heat-labile toxin-producing enterotoxigenic Escherichia coli: results of a large-scale field trial. J Infect Dis 158:372–377, 1988a.

Clemens JD, Sack DA, Harris JR, Chakraborty J, Khan MR, Stanton BF, Ali M, Ahmed F, Yunus M, Kay BA, Khan MR, Yunus M, Rao MR, Svennerholm A-M, Holmgren J. Impact of B subunit killed whole-cell and killed whole-cell-only oral vaccines against cholera upon treated diarrhoeal illness and mortality in an area endemic for cholera. Lancet 1:1375–1379, 1988b.

Clemente J, Leyva-Cobian F, Hernandez M, Garcia-Alonso A. Intracellular immunoglobulins in human milk macrophages. Ultrastructural localization and factors affecting the kinetics of immunoglobulin release. Int Arch Allergy Appl Immunol 80:291–299, 1986.

Cleveland MG, Bakos MA, Pyron DL, Rajaraman S, Goldblum RM. Characterization of secretory component in amniotic fluid. Identification of new forms of secretory IgA. J Immunol 147:181–188, 1991.

Cox DS, Furman S, Muench D. Affinity of antibody at a secretory site in the rat. Immunol Invest 14:151–159, 1985.

Crago SS, Mestecky J. Human colostral cells. II. Response to mitogens. Cell Immunol 86:222–229, 1984.

Crago SS, Prince SJ, Pretlow TG, McGhee JR, Mestecky J. Human colostral cells. I. Separation and characterization. Clin Exp Immunol 38:585–597, 1979.

Crouch SP, Slater KJ, Fletcher J. Regulation of cytokine release from mononuclear cells by the iron-binding protein lactoferrin. Blood 80:235–240, 1992.

Cumella JC, Ogra PL. Pregnancy associated hormonal milieu and bronchomammary cell traffic. In Hamosh M, Goldman AS, eds. Human Lactation. 2. Maternal and Environmental Factors. New York, Plenum Press, pp 507–524.

Cunningham AS. Morbidity in breast-fed and artificially fed infants. II. J Pediatr 95:685–689, 1979.

Cunningham RC, Brandeis WE, Good R, Day NK. Bovine antigens and the formation of circulating immune complexes in selective immunoglobulin A deficiency. J Clin Invest 64:272–279, 1979.

Cunningham AS, Jelliffe DB, Jelliffe EF. Breast-feeding and health in the 1980s: a global epidemiologic review. J Pediatr 118:659–666, 1991.

Cutler A, Armitage R, Conley ME, Rosenblatt H, Jenkins N, Copeland NG, Bedell MA, Edelhoff S, Disteche CM, Simoneaux DK, Fanslow WC, Belmont J, Spriggs MK. CD40 ligand gene defects responsible for X-linked hyper-IgM syndrome. Science 259:990–993, 1993.

Dahlgren UI, Ahlstedt S, Hanson LA. Origin and kinetics of IgA, IgG and IgM milk antibodies in primary and secondary responses of rats. Scand J Immunol 23:273–278, 1986.

Dahlgren UI, Ahlstedt S, Hanson LA. The localization of the antibody response in milk or bile depends on the nature of the antigen. J Immunol 138:1397–1402, 1987.

Danielescu G, Barbu C, Sorodoc Y, Cajal N, Sarateanu D. The presence of interferon and type A immunoglobulins in the nasopharyngeal secretions of volunteers immunized with an inactivated influenza vaccine. Acta Virol 19:245–249, 1975.

Davidson LA, Lonnerdal B. Persistence of human milk proteins in the breast-fed infant. Acta Paediatr Scand 76:733–740, 1987.

Davies A. An investigation on the serological properties of dysentery stools. Lancet 2:1009–1012, 1922.

Davis CP, Houston CW, Fader RC, Goldblum RM, Weaver EA, Goldman AS. Immunoglobulin A and secretory immunoglobulin A antibodies to purified type 1 Klebsiella pneumoniae pili in human colostrum. Infect Immun 38:496–501, 1982.

Davis MK, Savitz DA, Graubard BI. Infant feeding and childhood cancer. Lancet 2:365–368, 1988.

Defrance T, Vanbervliet B, Briere F, Durand I, Rousset F, Banchereau J. Interleukin 10 and transforming growth factor beta cooperate to induce anti-CD40-activated naive human B cells to secrete immunoglobulin A. J Exp Med 175:671–682, 1992.

Delacroix DL, Vaerman JP. A solid phase, direct competition, radioimmunoassay for quantitation of secretory IgA in human serum. J Immunol Methods 40:345–358, 1981.

Delacroix DL, Vaerman JP. Secretory component (SC): preferential binding to heavy (greater than 11S) IgA polymers and IgM in serum, in contrast to predominance of 11S and free SC forms in secretions. Clin Exp Immunol 49:717–724, 1982.

Delacroix DL, Vaerman JP. Function of the human liver in IgA homeostasis in plasma. Ann NY Acad Sci 409:383–401, 1983.

Delacroix DL, Jonard P, Dive C, Vaerman JP. Serum IgM-bound secretory component (SIgM) in liver diseases: comparative molecular state of the secretory component in serum and bile. J Immunol 129:133–138, 1982.

Delacroix DL, Liroux E, Vaerman JP. High proportion of polymeric IgA in young infants' sera and independence between IgA-size and IgA-subclass distributions. J Clin Immunol 3:51–56, 1983.

Duffy LC, Riepenhoff-Talty M, Byers TE, La Scolea LJ, Zielezny MA, Dryja DM, Ogra PL. Modulation of rotavirus enteritis during breast-feeding. Implications on alterations in the intestinal bacterial flora. Am J Dis Child 140:1164–1168, 1986.

Ebert EC. Human intestinal intraepithelial lymphocytes have potent chemotactic activity. Gastroenterology 109:1154–1159, 1995.

Eddie DS, Schulkind ML, Robbins JB. The isolation and biologic activities of purified secretory IgA and IgG anti-Salmonella typhimurium "O" antibodies from rabbit intestinal fluid and colostrum. J Immunol 106:181–190, 1971.

Ehrlich P. Uber Immunitat durch Vereburng and Saugung. S Hyg Infektionskrankheiten 12:183–203, 1892.

Eidelman S. Intestinal lesions in immune deficiency. Hum Pathol 7:427–434, 1976.

Elson CO, Ealding W. Generalized systemic and mucosal immunity in mice after mucosal stimulation with cholera toxin. J Immunol 132:2736–2741, 1984.

Elson CO, Heck JA, Strober W. T-cell regulation of murine IgA synthesis. J Exp Med 149:632–643, 1979.

Emodi G, Just M. Interferon production by lymphocytes in human milk. Scand J Immunol 3:157–160, 1974.

Fanger MW, Shen L, Pugh J, Bernier GM. Subpopulations of human peripheral granulocytes and monocytes express receptors for IgA. Proc Natl Acad Sci USA 77:3640–3644, 1980.

Fayette J, Dubois B, Vandenabeele S, Bridon JM, Vanbervliet B, Durand I, Banchereau J, Caux C, Briere F. Human dendritic cells skew isotype switching of CD40-activated naive B cells towards IgA1 and IgA2. J Exp Med 185:1909–1918, 1997.

Fazekas de St. Groth S, Donnelley M. Studies in experimental immunology of influenza: IV. The protective value of active immunization. Aust J Exp Biol Med Sci 28:61–75, 1950.

Fazekas de St. Groth S, Donnelley M, Graham DM. Studies in experimental immunology of influenza: VIII. Pathotopic adjuvants. Aust J Exp Biol Med Sci 29:323–337, 1951.

Feltelius N, Hvatum M, Brandtzaeg P, Knutson L, Hallgren R. Increased jejunal secretory IgA and IgM in ankylosing spondylitis: normalization after treatment with sulfasalazine. J Rheumatol 21:2076–2081, 1994.

Fergusson DM, Horwood LJ, Shannon FT, Taylor B. Infant health and breast-feeding during the first 16 weeks of life. Aust Paediatr J 14:254–258, 1978.

Fergusson DM, Horwood LJ, Shannon FT, Taylor B. Breast-feeding, gastrointestinal and lower respiratory illness in the first two years. Aust Paediatr J 17:191–195, 1981.

Fliedner M, Mehls O, Rauterberg EW, Ritz E. Urinary sIgA in children with urinary tract infection. J Pediatr 109:416–421, 1986.

Forman MR, Graubard BI, Hoffman HJ, Beren R, Harley EE, Bennett P. The Pima infant feeding study: breast feeding and gastroenteritis in the first year of life. Am J Epidemiol 119:335–349, 1984.

Forrest BD, Shearman DJ, LaBrooy JT. Specific immune response in humans following rectal delivery of live typhoid vaccine. Vaccine 8:209–212, 1990.

Fujiyama Y, Kobayashi K, Senda S, Benno Y, Bamba T, Hosoda S. A novel IgA protease from Clostridium sp. capable of cleaving IgA1 and IgA2 A2m(1) but not IgA2 A2m(2) allotype paraproteins. J Immunol 134:573–576, 1985.

Garcia-Pardo A, Lamm ME, Plaut AG, Franzione B. Secretory component is covalently bound to a single subunit in human secretory IgA. Mol Immunol 16:477–482, 1979.

Garcia-Pardo A, Lamm ME, Plaut AG, Frangione B. J chain is covalently bound to both monomer subunits in human secretory IgA. J Biol Chem 256:11734–11738, 1981.

Garofalo RP, Goldman AS. Cytokines, chemokines, and colony-stimulating factors in human milk: the 1997 update. Biol Neonate 74:134–142, 1998.

Garofalo RP, Goldman AS. Expression of functional immunomodulatory and anti-inflammatory factors in human milk. Clin Perinatol 26:361–377, 1999.

Garofalo R, Chheda S, Mei F, Palkowetz KH, Rudloff HE, Schmalstieg FC, Rassin DK, Goldman AS. Interleukin-10 in human milk. Pediatr Res 37:444–449, 1995.

Garofalo RP, Welliver RC, Ogra PL. Clinical aspects of bronchial reactivity and cell-virus interaction. In Ogra PL, Lamm ME, Bienenstock J, Mestecky J, Strober W, McGhee JR, eds. Mucosal Immunology. San Diego, Academic Press, 1999, pp 1223–1237.

Gay FP. Local resistance and local immunity to bacteria. Physio Rev 4:191–214, 1924.

Ghetie V, Mota G. The decrease of human colostral immunoglobulin A resistance to papain action after gradual release of the secretory component. Immunochemistry 10:839–840, 1973.

Gil A, Uauy R. Nucleotides and related compounds in human and bovine milks. In Jensen RG, ed. Handbook of Milk Compositions. San Diego, Academic Press, 1995, pp 436–464.

Gilbert JV. Inhibition of microbial IgA proteases by human secretory IgA and serum. Mol Immunol 20:1039–1049, 1983.

Gillin FD, Reiner DS, Gault MJ. Cholate-dependent killing of Giardia lamblia by human milk. Infect Immun 47:619–622, 1985.

Gindrat JJ, Gothefors L, Hanson LA, Winberg J. Antibodies in human milk against E. coli of the serogroups most commonly found in neonatal infections. Acta Paediatr Scand 61:587–590, 1972.

Girard JP, de Kalbermatten A. Antibody activity in human duodenal fluid. Eur J Clin Invest 1:188–195, 1970.

Glass RI, Svennerholm AM, Stoll BJ, Khan MR, Hossain KM, Huq MI, Holmgren J. Protection against cholera in breast-fed children by antibodies in breast milk. N Engl J Med 308:1389–1392, 1983.

Glass RI, Holmgren J, Khan MR, Hossain KM, Huq MI, Greenough WB. A randomized, controlled trial of the toxin-blocking effects of B subunit in family members of patients with cholera. J Infect Dis 149:495–500, 1984.

Glass RI, Stoll BJ, Wyatt RG, Hoshino Y, Banu H, Kapikian AZ. Observations questioning a protective role for breast-feeding in severe rotavirus diarrhea. Acta Paediatr Scand 75:713–718, 1986.

Gleeson M, Cripps AW, Clancy RL, Wlodarczyk JH, Dobson AJ, Hensley MJ. The development of IgA-specific antibodies to Escherichia coli O antigen in children. Scand J Immunol 26:639–643, 1987.

Goldblum RM, Goldman AS. Immunological components of milk: formation and function. In Ogra PL, Lamm ME, McGhee JR, Mestecky J, Strober W, Bienenstock J, eds. Handbook of Mucosal Immunology. San Diego, Academic Press, 1994, pp 643–652.

Goldblum RM, Van Bavel J. Immunoglobulin A production by human colostral cells: quantitative aspects. Adv Exp Med Biol 107:87–94, 1978.

Goldblum RM, Ahlstedt S, Carlsson B, Hanson LA, Jodal U, Lidin-Janson G, Sohl-Akerlund A. Antibody-forming cells in human colostrum after oral immunization. Nature 257:797–798, 1975.

Goldblum RM, Powell GK, Van Sickle G. Secretory IgA in the serum of infants with obstructive jaundice. J Pediatr 97:33–36, 1980.

Goldman AS, Garza C, Nichols BL, Johnson CA, Smith EO, Goldblum RM. Effects of prematurity on the immunologic system in human milk. J Pediatr 101:901–905, 1982a.

Goldman AS, Garza C, Nichols BL, Goldblum RM. Immunologic factors in human milk during the first year of lactation. J Pediatr 100:563–567, 1982b.

Goldman AS, Goldblum RM, Garza C. Immunologic components in human milk during the second year of lactation. Acta Paediatr Scand 72:461–462, 1983a.

Goldman AS, Goldblum RM, Garza C, Nichols BL, Obrian SE. Immunologic components in human milk during weaning. Acta Paediatr Scand 72:133–134, 1983b.

Goldman AS, Smith CW. Host resistance factors in human milk. J Pediatr 82:1082–1090, 1973.

Goldman AS, Thorpe LW, Goldblum RM, Hanson LA. Anti-inflammatory properties of human milk. Acta Paediatr Scand 75:689–695, 1986.

Goldman AS, Chheda S, Garofalo R. Evolution of immunologic functions of the mammary gland and the postnatal development of immunity. Pediatr Res 43:155–162, 1998.

Gothefors L. Studies of antimicrobial factors in human milk and bacterial colonization of the newborn. Doctoral dissertation, Umea University, 1975.

Gothefors L, Marklund S. Lactoperoxidase activity in human milk and in saliva of newborn infants. Infect Immun 11:1210–1215, 1975.

Graham BS, Johnson TR, Peebles RS. Immune-mediated disease pathogenesis in respiratory syncytial virus infection. Immunopharmacology 48:237–247, 2000.

Greenberg SB, Criswell BS, Six HR, Couch RB. Lymphocyte cytotoxicity to influenza virus-infected cells: response to vaccination and virus infection. Infect Immun 20:640–645, 1978.

Greenwell H, Bakr A, Bissada N, Debanne S, Rowland D. The effect of Keyes' method of oral hygiene on the subgingival microflora compared to the effect of scaling and/or surgery. J Clin Periodontol 12:327–341, 1985.

Greenwell D, Petersen J, Kulvicki A, Harder J, Goldblum R, Neal DE Jr. Urinary secretory immunoglobulin A and free secretory component in pyelonephritis. Am J Kidney Dis 26:590–594, 1995.

Gregory RL, Filler SJ. Protective secretory immunoglobulin A antibodies in humans following oral immunization with Streptococcus mutans. Infect Immun 55:2409–2415, 1987.

Griffis JM. IgA blocks IgM- and IgG-initiated immune lysis by separate molecular mechanisms. J Immunol 130:2882–2885, 1983.

Griffiths E, Humphreys J. Bacteriostatic effect of human milk and bovine colostrum on Escherichia coli: importance of bicarbonate. Infect Immun 15:396–401, 1977.

Grundbacher FJ. Immunoglobulins, secretor status, and the incidence of rheumatic fever and rheumatic heart disease. Hum Hered 22:399–404, 1972.

Gump DW, Christmas WA, Forsyth BR, Phillips CA, Stouch WH. Serum and secretory antibodies in patients with chronic bronchitis. Arch Intern Med 132:847–851, 1973.

Hagberg L, Hull R, Hull S, McGhee JR, Michalek SM, Svanborg EC. Difference in susceptibility to gram-negative urinary tract infection between C3H/HeJ and C3H/HeN mice. Infect Immun 46:839–844, 1984a.

Hagberg L, Leffler H, Svanborg EC. Non-antibiotic prevention of urinary tract infection. Infection 12:132–137, 1984b.

Hall CB, Walsh EE, Long CE, Schnabel KC. Immunity to and frequency of reinfection with respiratory syncytial virus. J Infect Dis 163:693–698, 1991.

Hall WH, Manion RE, Zinneman HH. Blocking serum lysis of Brucella abortus by hyperimmune rabbit immunoglobulin A. J Immunol 107:41–46, 1971.

Halpern MS, Koshland ME. Noval subunit in secretory IgA. Nature 228:1276–1278, 1970.

Halstensen TS, Scott H, Brandtzaeg P. Human CD8+ intraepithelial T lymphocytes are mainly CD45RA−RO+ and show increased co-expression of CD45R0 in celiac disease. Eur J Immunol 20:1825–1830, 1990.

Hamosh M. Lingual and gastric lipases. Nutrition 6:421–428, 1990.

Haneberg B. Human milk immunoglobulins and agglutinins to rabbit erythrocytes. Int Arch Allergy Appl Immunol 47:716–729, 1974a.

Haneberg B. Immunoglobulins in feces from infants fed human or bovine milk. Scand J Immunol 3:191–197, 1974b.

Haneberg B, Aarskog D. Human faecal immunoglobulins in healthy infants and children, and in some with diseases affecting the intestinal tract or the immune system. Clin Exp Immunol 22:210–222, 1975.

Hanson L. Comparative immunological studies of the immune globulins of human milk and of blood serum. Int Arch Allergy Appl Immunologic 18:241–267, 1961.

Hanson LA. Aspects of the absence of IgA system. In Bergsma D, Good R, eds. Immunologic Deficiency Diseases in Man. Baltimore, Williams & Wilkins, 1968, pp 292–297.

Hanson L, Johansson BG. Immunological characterization of chromatographically separated protein fractions from human colostrum. Int Arch Allergy Appl Immunol 20:65–79, 1962.

Hanson L, Johansson B. Immunological studies of milk. In McKenzie H, ed. Milk Proteins, Chemistry and Molecular Biology. New York, Academic Press, 1970, pp 45–123.

Hanson L, Borssen R, Holmgre J, Jodal U, Johansson BG, Kaijser B. Secretory IgA. In Kagan B, Stiehm ER, eds. Immunologic Incompetence. Chicago, Year Book Medical Publishers, 1971, pp 39–59.

Hanson L, Motas C, Barrett J, Wadsworth C, Jodal U. Studies of the main immunoglobulin of human milk: secretory IgA. In Immunology of Reproduction. Sofia, Bulgarian Academy Science Press, 1973, pp. 687–692.

Hanson LA, Carlsson B, Ahlstedt T, Svanborg C, Kaijser B. Immune defense factors in human milk. In Milk and Lactation. Karger, Basel, 1975, pp 63–72.

Hanson LA, Ahlstedt S, Fasth A, Jodal U, Kaijser B, Larsson P, Lindberg U, Olling S, Sohl-Akerlund A, Svanborg EC. Antigens of Escherichia coli, human immune response, and the pathogenesis of urinary tract infections. J Infect Dis 136(Suppl):S144–S149, 1977.

Hanson L, Carlsson B, Cruz JR, Garcia B, Holmgre J, Khan SR, Lindblad BS, Svennerholm A-M, Svennerholm B, Urrutia JJ. Immune response in the mammary gland. In Ogra PL, Dayton D, eds. Immunology of Breast Milk. New York, Raven Press, 1979, pp 145–157.

Hanson LA, Carlsson B, Dahlgren U, Mellander L, Svanborg ED. The secretory IgA system in the neonatal period. In Excerpta Medica. Amsterdam, Ciba Foundation Symposium, 1980, pp 187–204.

Hanson LA, Ahlstedt S, Andersson B, Carlsson B, Cole MF, Cruz JR, Dahlgren U, Ericsson TH, Jalil F, Khan SR, Mellander L, Schneerson R, Eden CS, Soderstrom T, Wadsworth C. Mucosal immunity. Ann NY Acad Sci 409:1–21, 1983a.

Hanson LA, Bjorkander J, Oxelius V. Selective IgA deficiency. In Chandra R, ed. Primary and Secondary Immunodeficiency Disorders. New York, Churchill Livingstone, 1983b, pp 62–84.

Hanson LA, Ahlstedt S, Andersson B, Carlsson B, Fallstrom SP, Mellander L, Porras O, Soderstrom T, Eden CS. Protective factors in milk and the development of the immune system. Pediatrics 75:172–176, 1985.

Hanson LA, Jalil F, Hasan R, Khan SR, Karlberg J, Carlsson B, Lindblad BS, Adlerbert I, Mellander L, Soderstrom T. Breast-feeding in reality. In Hamosh M, Goldman AS, ed. Human Lactation 2: Maternal Environmental Factors in Human Lactation. New York, Plenum Press, 1986, pp 1–12.

Heddle RJ, Knop J, Steele EJ, Rowley D. The effect of lysozyme on the complement-dependent bactericidal action of different antibody classes. Immunology 28:1061–1066, 1975.

Heddle RJ, Rowley D. Dog immunoglobulins. II. The antibacterial properties of dog IgA, IgM and IgG antibodies to Vibrio cholerae. Immunology 29:197-208, 1975.

Hemming VG, Rodriguez W, Kim HW, Brandt CD, Parrott RH, Burch B, Prince GA, Baron PA, Fink RJ, Reaman G. Intravenous immunoglobulin treatment of respiratory syncytial virus infections in infants and young children. Antimicrob Agents Chemother 31:1882–1886, 1987.

Hendrickson BA, Rindisbacher L, Corthesy B, Kendall D, Waltz DA, Neutra MR, Seidman JG. Lack of association of secretory component with IgA in J chain-deficient mice. J Immunol 157:750–754, 1996.

Herias MV, Cruz JR, Gonzalez-Cossio T, Nave F, Carlsson B, Hanson LA. The effect of caloric supplementation on selected milk protective factors in undernourished Guatemalan mothers. Pediatr Res 34:217–221, 1993.

Hernell O, Ward H, Blackberg L, Pereira ME. Killing of Giardia lamblia by human milk lipases: an effect mediated by lipolysis of milk lipids. J Infect Dis 153:715–720, 1986.

Herzenberg LA, Stall AM, Lalor PA, Sidman C, Moore WA, Parks DR, Herzenberg LA. The Ly-1 B cell lineage. Immunol Rev 93:81–102, 1986.

Hexham JM, White KD, Carayannopoulos LN, Mandecki W, Brisette R, Yang YS, Capra JD. A human immunoglobulin (Ig)A calpha3 domain motif directs polymeric Ig receptor-mediated secretion. J Exp Med 189:747–752, 1999.

Hill IR, Porter P. Studies of bactericidal activity to Escherichia coli of porcine serum and colostral immunoglobulins and the role of lysozyme with secretory IgA. Immunology 26:1239–1250, 1974.

Ho PC, Lawton JW. Human colostral cells: phagocytosis and killing of E. coli and C. albicans. J Pediatr 93:910–915, 1978.

Ho PC, Powell DA, Albright F, Gardner DE, Collier AM, Clyde WA. A solid-phase radioimmunoassay for detection of antibodies against mycoplasma pneumoniae. J Clin Immunol 11:209–213, 1983.

Hodes HL, Berger R, Ainbender E, Hevizy MM, Zepp HD, Kochwa S. Proof that colostrum polio antibody is different from serum antibody. J Pediatr 65:1017–1018, 1964.

Holmgren J, Rudin A. Mucosal immunity and bacteria. In Ogra PL, Mestecky J, Lamm ME, Strober W, Bienenstock J, McGhee, eds. Mucosal Immunology. San Diego, Academic Press, 1999, pp. 685–693.

Holmgren J, Hanson LA, Carlson B, Lindblad BS, Rahimtoola J. Neutralizing antibodies against Escherichia coli and Vibrio cholerae enterotoxins in human milk from a developing country. Scand J Immunol 5:867–871, 1976.

Holmgren J, Svennerholm AM, Ahren C. Nonimmunoglobulin fraction of human milk inhibits bacterial adhesion (hemagglutination) and enterotoxin binding of Escherichia coli and Vibrio cholerae. Infect Immun 33:136–141, 1981.

Holmgren J, Svennerholm AM, Lindblad M. Receptor-like glycocompounds in human milk that inhibit classical and El Tor Vibrio cholerae cell adherence (hemagglutination). Infect Immun 39:147–154, 1983.

Howie VM, Ploussard JH, Sloyer JL, Johnston RB. Immunoglobulins of the middle ear fluid in acute otitis media: relationship to serum immunoglobulin concentrations and bacterial cultures. Infect Immun 7:589–593, 1973.

Hurlimann J, Waldesbuhl M, Zuber C. Human salivary immunoglobulin A. Some immunological and physicochemical characteristics. Biochim Biophys Acta 181:393–403, 1969.

Husband AJ, Dunkley ML. Lack of site of origin effects on distribution of IgA antibody-containing cells. Immunology 54:215–221, 1985.

Hussell T, Pietro P, Sparer TE, Openshaw PJM. Beneficial and harmful immune responses in the respiratory tract. In Ogra PL, Mestecky J, Lamm ME, Strober W, Bienenstock J, McGhee JR, eds. Mucosal Immunology. San Diego, Academic Press, 1999, pp 1215–1221.

Hutchens TW, Henry JF, Yip TT, Hachey DL, Schanler RJ, Motil KJ, Garza C. Origin of intact lactoferrin and its DNA-binding fragments found in the urine of human milk-fed preterm infants. Evaluation by stable isotopic enrichment. Pediatr Res 29:243–250, 1991.

Ichimiya I, Kawauchi H, Mogi G. Analysis of immunocompetent cells in the middle ear mucosa. Arch Otolaryngol Head Neck Surg 116:324–330, 1990.

Inman FP, Mestecky J. The J chain of polymeric immunoglobulins. Contemp Top Mol Immunol 3:111–141, 1974.

Iscaki S, Geneste C, Pillot J. Human secretory component-I. Evidence for a new antigenic specificity. Immunochemistry 15:401–408, 1978.

Iscaki S, Geneste C, d'Azambuja S, Pillot J. Human secretory component. II. Easy detection of abnormal amounts of combined secretory component in human sera. J Immunol Methods 28:331–339, 1979.

Issacs CE, Thromar H, Pessolano T. Membrane-disruptive effect of human milk: inactivation of enveloped viruses. J Infect Dis 154:966–971, 1986.

Issacs D, Bangham C, McMichael AJ. Cell-mediated cytotoxic response to respiratory syncytial virus in infants with bronchiolitis. Lancet 2:769–771, 1987.

James SP, Zeitz M. Human gastrointestinal mucosal T cells. In Ogra PL, Lamm ME, McGhee JR, Mestecky J, Strober W, Bienenstock J, eds. Handbook of Mucosal Immunology. San Diego, Academic Press, 1994, pp 275–286.

James SP, Graeff AS, Zeitz M. Predominance of helper-inducer T cells in mesenteric lymph nodes and intestinal lamina propria of normal nonhuman primates. Cell Immunol 107:372–383, 1987.

Jason JM, Nieburg P, Marks JS. Mortality and infectious disease associated with infant-feeding practices in developing countries. Pediatrics 74:702–727, 1984.

Jodal U, Ahlstedt S, Carlsson B, Hanson LA, Lindberg U, Sohl A. Local antibodies in childhood urinary tract infection: a preliminary study. Int Arch Allergy Appl Immunol 47:537–546, 1974.

Johansen FE, Pekna M, Norderhaug IN, Haneberg B, Hietala MA, Krajci P, Betsholtz C, Brandtzaeg P. Absence of epithelial immunoglobulin A transport, with increased mucosal leakiness, in polymeric immunoglobulin receptor/secretory component-deficient mice. J Exp Med 190:915–922, 1999.

Johansson SG, Deuschl H. Immunoglobulins in nasal secretion with special reference to IgE. I. Methodological studies. Int Arch Allergy Appl Immunol 52:364–375, 1976.

Johnson KJ, Wilson BS, Till GO, Ward PA. Acute lung injury in rat caused by immunoglobulin A immune complexes. J Clin Invest 74:358–369, 1984.

Jonard PP, Rambaud JC, Dive C, Vaerman JP, Galian A, Delacroix DL. Secretion of immunoglobulins and plasma proteins from the jejunal mucosa. Transport rate and origin of polymeric immunoglobulin A. J Clin Invest 74:525–535, 1984.

Jorieux S, Mazurier J, Montreuil J, Spik G. Characterization of lactotransferrin complexes in human milk. In Peeters H, ed. Protides of the Biological Fluids. Oxford, Pergamon Press, Oxford, 1984, pp 115–118.

Kaetzel CS, Robinson JK, Chintalacharuvu KR, Vaerman JP, Lamm ME. The polymeric immunoglobulin receptor (secretory component) mediates transport of immune complexes across epithelial cells: a local defense function for IgA. Proc Natl Acad Sci USA 88:8796–8800, 1991.

Kaijser B, Larsson P, Olling S. Protection against ascending Escherichia coli pyelonephritis in rats and significance of local immunity. Infect Immun 20:78–81, 1978.

Karem KL, Kanangat S, Rouse BT. Cytokine expression in the gut associated lymphoid tissue after oral administration of attenuated Salmonella vaccine strains. Vaccine 14:1495–1502, 1996.

Karlsson G, Hansson HA, Petruson B, Bjorkander J, Hanson LA. Goblet cell number in the nasal mucosa relates to cell-mediated immunity in patients with antibody deficiency syndromes. Int Arch Allergy Appl Immunol 78:86–91, 1985.

Kato T, Owen RL. Structure and function of intestinal mucosal epithelium. In Ogra PL, Lamm ME, McGhee JR, Mestecky J, Strober W, Bienenstock J, eds. Handbook of Mucosal Immunology. San Diego, Academic Press, 1994, pp 11–26.

Kaufmann SH. CD8+ T lymphocytes in intracellular microbial infections. Immunol Today 9:168–174, 1988.

Kaul MN, Misra RC, Agarwal SK, Saha K. Decreased gut-associated IgA levels in patients with typhoid fever. Scand J Immunol 11:623–628, 1980.

Kearns DH, O'Reilly RJ, Lee L, Welch BG. Secretory IgA antibodies in the urethral exudate of men with uncomplicated urethritis due to Neisseria gonorrhoeae. J Infect Dis 127:99–101, 1973.

Keeney SE, Schmalstieg FC, Palkowetz KH, Rudloff HE, Le BM, Goldman AS. Activated neutrophils and neutrophil activators in human milk: increased expression of CD11b and decreased expression of L-selectin. J Leuk Biol 54:97–104, 1993.

Keller MA, Turner JL, Stratton JA, Miller ME. Breast milk lymphocyte response to K1 antigen of Escherichia coli. Infect Immun 27:903–909, 1980.

Keller MA, Kidd RM, Bryson YJ, Turner JL, Carter J. Lymphokine production by human milk lymphocytes. Infect Immun 32:632–636, 1981.

Keller MA, Heiner DC, Kidd RM, Myers AS. Local production of IgG4 in human colostrum. J Immunol 130:1654–1657, 1983.

Keller MA, Kidd R, Reisinger D, Stewart D. PPD-induced monocyte chemotactic factor production by human milk cells. Acta Paediatr Scand 73:465–470, 1984.

Keller MA, Heiner DC, Myers AS, Reisinger DM. IgD in human colostrum. Pediatr Res 19:122–126, 1985.

Kelsall B, Strober W. Gut-associated lymphoid tissue antigen handling and t-lymphocyte responses. In Ogra PL, Lamm ME, McGhee JR, Mestecky J, Strober W, Bienenstock J, eds. Handbook of Mucosal Immunology. San Diego, Academic Press, 1994, pp 293–317.

Kemp AS, Cripps AW, Brown S. Suppression of leucocyte chemokinesis and chemotaxis by human IgA. Clin Exp Immunol 40:388–395, 1980.

Kenny JF, Boesman MI, Michaels RH. Bacterial and viral coproantibodies in breast-fed infants. Pediatrics 39:202–213, 1967.

Kett K, Brandtzaeg P, Radl J, Haaijman JJ. Different subclass distribution of IgA-producing cells in human lymphoid organs and various secretory tissues. J Immunol 136:3631–3635, 1986.

Kilian M, Reinholdt J. Interference with IgA defense mechanisms by extracellular bacterial enzymes. In Easmon G, Jeljaszewics J, eds. Medical Microbiology. London, Academic Press, 1986, pp 173–208.

Kilian M, Russell MW. Function of mucosa immunoglobulins. In Ogra PL, Lamm ME, McGhee JR, Mestecky J, Strober W, Bienenstock J, eds. Handbook of Mucosal Immunology. San Diego, Academic Press, 1994, pp 127–137.

Kilian M, Russell MW. Microbial evasion of IgA functions. In Ogra PL, Mestecky J, Lamm ME, Strober W, Bienenstock J, McGhee JR, eds. Mucosal Immunology. San Diego, Academic Press, 1999, pp 241–251.

Kilian M, Thomsen B, Petersen TE, Bleeg HS. Occurrence and nature of bacterial IgA proteases. Ann NY Acad Sci 409:612–624, 1983.

Kilian M, Mestecky J, Russell MW. Defense mechanisms involving Fc-dependent functions of immunoglobulin A and their subversion by bacterial immunoglobulin A proteases. Microbiol Rev 52:296–303, 1988.

Knight KL, Vetter ML, Malek TR. Distribution of covalently bound and non-covalently bound secretory component on subclasses of rabbit secretory IgA. J Immunol 115:595–598, 1975.

Kobayashi K, Fujiyama Y, Hagiwara K, Kondoh H. Resistance of normal serum IgA and secretory IgA to bacterial IgA proteases: evidence for the presence of enzyme-neutralizing antibodies in both serum and secretory IgA, and also in serum IgG. Microbiol Immunol 31:1097–1106, 1987.

Kohl S, Pickering LK, Cleary TG, Steinmetz KD, Loo LS. Human colostral cytotoxicity. II. Relative defects in colostral leukocyte cytotoxicity and inhibition of peripheral blood leukocyte cytotoxicity by colostrum. J Infect Dis 142:884–891, 1980.

Koletzko S, Sherman P, Corey M, Griffiths A, Smith C. Role of infant feeding practices in development of Crohn's disease in childhood. Br Med J 298:1617–1618, 1989.

Koletzko S, Griffiths A, Corey M, Smith C, Sherman P. Infant feeding practices and ulcerative colitis in childhood. Br Med J 302:1580–1581, 1991.

Koshland ME. Structure and function of the J chain. Adv Immunol 20:41–69, 1975.

Krajci P, Meling GI, Andersen SN, Hofstad B, Vatn MH, Rognum TO, Brandtzaeg P. Secretory component mRNA and protein expression in colorectal adenomas and carcinomas. Br J Cancer 73:1503–1510, 1996.

Krajci P, Tasken K, Kvale D, Brandtzaeg P. Interferon-gamma stimulation of messenger RNA for human secretory component (poly-Ig receptor) depends on continuous intermediate protein synthesis. Scand J Immunol 37:251–256, 1993.

Kramer MD. Breast feeding and child health methodologic issues in epidemiologic research. In Goldman AS, Atkinson SA, Hanson L, eds. Human Lactatin. New York, Plenum Press, 1987, pp 339–360.

Kroese H, Butcher EC, Stall AM, Lalor PA, Adams S, Herzenberg LA. Many of the IgA producing plasma cells in murine gut are from self-replenishing precursors in the peritoneal cavity. Int Immunol 1:75–84, 1989.

Kulkarni AD, Fanslow WC, Rudolph FB, Van Buren CT. Effect of dietary nucleotides on response to bacterial infections. J Parenter Enteral Nutr 10:169–171, 1986.

Kurono Y, Lim DJ, Mogi G. Middle ear and eustachian tube. In Ogra PL, Mestecky J, Lamm ME, Strober W, Bienenstock J, McGhee JR, eds. Mucosal Immunology. San Diego, Academic Press, 1999a, pp 1305–1311.

Kurono Y, Yamamoto M, Fujihashi K, Kodama S, Suzuki M, Mogi G, McGhee JR, Kiyono H. Nasal immunization induces Haemophilus influenzae-specific Th1 and Th2 responses with mucosal IgA and systemic IgG antibodies for protective immunity. J Infect Dis 180:122–132, 1999b.

Kvale D, Brandtzaeg P. An enzyme-linked immunosorbent assay for differential quantitation of secretory immunoglobulins of the A and M isotypes in human serum. J Immunol Methods 86:107–114, 1986.

Lange S, Holmgren J. Protective antitoxic cholera immunity in mice: influence of route and number of immunizations and mode of action of protective antibodies. Acta Pathol Microbiol Scand[C.] 86C:145–152, 1978.

Lange S, Lonnroth I. Bile and milk from cholera toxin treated rats contain a hormone-like factor which inhibits diarrhea induced by the toxin. Int Arch Allergy Appl Immunol 79:270–275, 1986.

Lange S, Nygren H, Svennerholm AM, Holmgren J. Antitoxic cholera immunity in mice: influence of antigen deposition on antitoxin-containing cells and protective immunity in different parts of the intestine. Infect Immun 28:17–23, 1980.

Lange S, Lonnroth I, Nygren H. Intestinal resistance to cholera toxin in mouse. Antitoxic antibodies and desensitization of adenylate cyclase. Int Arch Allergy Appl Immunol 74:221–225, 1984.

Larsen SA, Homer DR. Relation of breast versus bottle feeding to hospitalization for gastroenteritis in a middle-class U.S. population. J Pediatr 92:417–418, 1978.

Laven GT, Crago SS, Kutteh WH, Mestecky J. Hemolytic plaque formation by cellular and noncellular elements of human colostrum. J Immunol 127:1967–1972, 1981.

Lawrence DA, Weigle WO, Spiegelberg HL. Immunoglobulins cytophilic for human lymphocytes, monocytes, and neutrophils. J Clin Invest 55:368–387, 1975.

Lebman DA, Coffman RL. Cytokines in the mucosal immune system. In Ogra PL, Lamm ME, McGhee JR, Mestecky J, Strober W, Bienenstock J, eds. Handbook of Mucosal Immunology. San Diego, Academic Press, 1994, pp 243–250.

Lebman DA, Griffin PM, Cebra JJ. Relationship between expression of IgA by Peyer's patch cells and functional IgA memory cells. J Exp Med 166:1405–1418, 1987.

Lee GB, Ogilvie BM. The intestinal mucus layer in Trichinella spiralis-infected rats. In Strober W, Hanson LA, Sell KW, eds. Recent Advances in Mucosal Immunity. New York, Raven Press, 1982, pp 319–329.

Lefrancois L. Basic aspects of intraepithelial lymphocyte immunobiology. In Ogra PL, Lamm ME, McGhee JR, Mestecky J, Strober W, Bienenstock J, eds. Handbook of Mucosal Immunology. San Diego, Academic Press, 1994, pp 287–297.

Lehtonen P, Grangstromhn EM, Stangstromlberg TH, Laitinen LA. Amount and avidity of salivary and serum antibodies against Streptococcus mutans in two groups of human subjects with different dental caries susceptibility. Infect Immun 43:308–313, 1984.

Lewis-Jones DI, Lewis-Jones MS, Connolly RC, Lloyd DC, West CR. The influence of parity, age and maturity of pregnancy on antimicrobial proteins in human milk. Acta Paediatr Scand 74:655–659, 1985.

Lim DJ. Functional morphology of the lining membrane of the middle ear and Eustachian tube: an overview. Ann Otol Rhinol Laryngol 83(Suppl):26, 1974.

Lim PL, Rowley D. The effect of antibody on the intestinal absorption of macromolecules and on intestinal permeability in adult mice. Int Arch Allergy Appl Immunol 68:41–46, 1982.

Lindh E. Increased resistance of immunoglobulin A dimers to proteolytic degradation after binding of secretory component. J Immunol 114:284–286, 1975.

Lindh E, Bjork I. Binding of secretory component to dimers of immunoglobulin A in vitro. Mechanism of the covalent bond formation. Eur J Biochem 62:263–270, 1976.

Ljungstrom I, Holmgren J, Huldt G, Lange S, Svennerholm AM. Changes in intestinal fluid transport and immune responses to enterotoxins due to concomitant parasitic infection. Infect Immun 30:734–740, 1980.

Lomberg H, Hanson LA, Jacobsson B, Jodal U, Leffler H, Eden CS. Correlation of P blood group, vesicoureteral reflux, and bacterial attachment in patients with recurrent pyelonephritis. N Engl J Med 308:1189–1192, 1983.

Lomberg H, Cedergren B, Leffler H, Nilsson B, Carlstrom AS, Svanborg-Eden C. Influence of blood group on the availability of receptors for attachment of uropathogenic Escherichia coli. Infect Immun 51:919–926, 1986a.

Lomberg H, Hellstrom M, Jodal U, Svanborg EC. Renal scarring and non-attaching Escherichia coli. Lancet 2:1341, 1986b.

Lonnroth I, Lange S. A new principle for resistance to cholera: desensitization to cyclic AMP-mediated diarrhea induced by cholera toxin in the mouse intestine. J Cyclic Nucleotide Res 7:247–257, 1981.

Lonnroth I, Lange S. Intake of monosaccharides or amino acids induces pituitary gland synthesis of proteins regulating intestinal fluid transport. Biochim Biophys Acta 925:117–123, 1987.

Losonsky GA, Fishaut JM, Strussenberg J, Ogra PL. Effect of immunization against rubella on lactation products. I. Development and characterization of specific immunologic reactivity in breast milk. J Infect Dis 145:654–660, 1982.

Lowell GH, Smith LF, Griffiss JM, Brandt BL. IgA-dependent, monocyte-mediated, antibacterial activity. J Exp Med 152:452–457, 1980.

Lycke N, Holmgrem J. Strong adjuvant properties of cholera toxin of gut mucosal immune responses to orally presented antigens. Immunology 59:301–308, 1987.

Lycke N, Eriksen L, Holmgren J. Protection against cholera toxin after oral immunization is thymus-dependent and associated with intestinal production of neutralizing IgA antitoxin. Scand J Immunol 25:413–419, 1987.

Maffei HV, Kingston D, Hill ID, Shiner M. Histopathologic changes and the immune response within the jejunal mucosa in infants and children. Pediatr Res 13:733–736, 1979.

Magnusson CG, Masson PL. A reappraisal of IgE levels in various human secretions by particle counting immunoassay combined with pepsin digestion. Int Arch Allergy Appl Immunol 77:292–299, 1985.

Magnusson KE, Stjernstrom I. Mucosal barrier mechanisms. Interplay between secretory IgA (SIgA), IgG and mucins on the surface properties and association of salmonellae with intestine and granulocytes. Immunology 45:239–248, 1982.

Masters PL. Maternal transmission of skin sensitivity to tuberculin. Lancet 2:276–277, 1982.

Mata LJ, Wyatt RG. The uniqueness of human milk. Host resistance to infection. Am J Clin Nutr 24:976–986, 1971.

Mata LK, Urrutia JJ. Intestinal colonization of breast-fed children in a rural area of low socioeconomic level. Ann NY Acad Sci 176:93–109, 1971.

May SJ, Blackwell CC, Brettle RP, MacCallum CJ, Weir DM. Non-secretion of ABO blood group antigens: a host factor predisposing to recurrent urinary tract infections and renal scarring. FEMS Microbiol Immunol 1:383–387, 1989.

Mayer EJ, Hamman RF, Gay EC, Lezotte DC, Savitz DA, Klingensmith GJ. Reduced risk of IDDM among breast-fed children. The Colorado IDDM Registry. Diabetes 37:1625–1632, 1988.

Mayer L, Posnett DN, Kunkel HG. Human malignant T cells capable of inducing an immunoglobulin class switch. J Exp Med 161:134–144, 1985.

Mayrhofer G. The nature of the thymus dependency of mucosal mast cells. II. The effect of thymectomy and of depleting recirculating lymphocytes on the response to Nippostrongylus brasiliensis. Cell Immunol 47:312–322, 1979.

Mayrhofer G, Bazin H, Gowans JL. Nature of cells binding anti-IgE in rats immunized with Nippostrongylus brasiliensis: IgE synthesis in regional nodes and concentration in mucosal mast cells. Eur J Immunol 6:537–545, 1976.

Mazanec MB, Kaetzel CS, Lamm ME, Fletcher D, Nedrud JG. Intracellular neutralization of virus by immunoglobulin A antibodies. Proc Natl Acad Sci USA 89:6901–6905, 1992a.

Mazanec MB, Lamm ME, Lyn D, Portner A, Nedrud JG. Comparison of IgA versus IgG monoclonal antibodies for passive immunization of the murine respiratory tract. Virus Res 23:1–12, 1992b.

Mazanec MB, Nedrud JG, Kaetzel CS, Lamm ME. A three-tiered view of the role of IgA in mucosal defense. Immunol Today 14:430–435, 1993.

McClelland DB, McGrath J, Samson RR. Antimicrobial factors in human milk. Studies of concentration and transfer to the infant during the early stages of lactation. Acta Paediatr Scand Suppl 1:20, 1978.

McDermott MR, Bienenstock J. Evidence for a common mucosal immunologic system. I. Migration of B immunoblasts into intestinal, respiratory, and genital tissues. J Immunol 122:1892–1898, 1979.

McDermott MR, Befus AD, Bienenstock J. The structural basis for immunity in the respiratory tract. Int Rev Exp Pathol 23:47–112, 1982.

McElroy PJ, Szewczuk MR, Befus AD. Regulation of heterologous IgM, IgG, and IgA antibody responses in mucosal-associated lymphoid tissues of Nippostrongylus brasiliensis-infected mice. J Immunol 130:435–441, 1983.

McGee DW, McMurray DN. The effect of protein malnutrition on the IgA immune response in mice. Immunology 63:25–29, 1988.

McGee DW, Aicher WK, Eldridge JH, Peppard JV, Mestecky J, McGhee JR. Transforming growth factor-beta enhances secretory component and major histocompatibility complex class I antigen expression on rat IEC-6 intestinal epithelial cells. Cytokine 3:543–550, 1991.

McIntosh K, McQuillin J, Gardner PS. Cell-free and cell-bound antibody in nasal secretions from infants with respiratory syncytial virus infection. Infect Immun 23:276–281, 1979.

McIntyre TM, Strober W. Gut-associated lymphoid tissue regulation IgA b-cell development. In Ogra PL, Mestecky J, Lamm ME, Strober W, Bienenstock J, McGhee JR, eds. Mucosal Immunology. San Diego, Academic Press, 1999, pp 319–356.

McMurray DN, Rey H, Casazza LJ, Watson RR. Effect of moderate malnutrition on concentrations of immunoglobulins and enzymes in tears and saliva of young Colombian children. Am J Clin Nutr 30:1944–1948, 1977.

Mellander L, Bjorkander J, Carlsson B, Hanson LA. Secretory antibodies in IgA-deficient and immunosuppressed individuals. J Clin Immunol 6:284–291, 1986a.

Mellander L, Carlsson B, Hanson LA. Appearance of secretory IgM and IgA antibodies to Escherichia coli in saliva during early infancy and childhood. J Pediatr 104:564–568, 1984.

Mellander L, Carlsson B, Hanson LA. Secretory IgA and IgM antibodies to E. coli O and poliovirus type I antigens occur in amniotic fluid, meconium and saliva from newborns. A neonatal immune response without antigenic exposure: a result of anti-idiotypic induction? Clin Exp Immunol 63:555–561, 1986b.

Mellander L, Carlsson B, Jalil F, Soderstrom T, Hanson LA. Secretory IgA antibody response against Escherichia coli antigens in infants in relation to exposure. J Pediatr 107:430–433, 1985.

Mestecky J. Structural aspects of human polymeric IgA. LaRicerca Clin Lab 6:87–95, 1976.

Mestecky J, Zikan J, Butler WT. Immunoglobulin M and secretory immunoglobulin A: presence of a common polypeptide chain different from light chains. Science 171:1163–1165, 1971.

Mestecky J, McGhee JR, Arnold RR, Michalek SM, Prince SJ, Babb JL. Selective induction of an immune response in human external secretions by ingestion of bacterial antigen. J Clin Invest 61:731–737, 1978.

Michalek SM, Morisaki I, Gregory RL, Kimuva S, Harmon CC, Hamada S, Kotani SS, McGhee JR. Oral adjuvants enhance salivary IgA responses to purified Streptococcus mutans antigens. In Peeters H, ed. Protides of the Biological Fluids. Oxford, Pergamon Press, Oxford, 1985, pp 53–56.

Mittal SK, Kanwar A, Varghese A, Ramachandran VG. Gut flora in breast and bottle fed infants with and without diarrhea. Indian Pediatr 20:21–26, 1983.

Mohr JA. The possible induction and-or acquisition of cellular hypersensitivity associated with ingestion of colostrum. J Pediatr 82:1062–1064, 1973.

Moldoveanu Z, Tenovuo J, Mestecky J, Pruitt KM. Human milk peroxidase is derived from milk leukocytes. Biochim Biophys Acta 718:103–108, 1982.

Montgomery PC, Cohen C, Skandera C. Evidence for an IgA anamnestic response in rabbit mammary secretions. In Ogra PL, Dayton D, eds. Immunology of Breast Milk. New York, Raven Press, 1979, pp 115–127.

Montgomery PC, Majumdar AS, Skandera CA, Rockey JH. The effect of immunization route and sequence of stimulation on the induction of IgA antibodies in tears. Curr Eye Res 3:861–865, 1984.

Moore EC, Reichard P, Thelander L. Enzymatic synthesis of deoxyribonucleotides: V. Purification and properties of thioredoxin reductase from Escherichia coli. Br J Biol Chem 239:3445–3452, 1964.

Moro I, Crago SS, Mestecky J. Localization of IgA and IgM in human colostral elements using immunoelectron microscopy. J Clin Immunol 3:382–391, 1983.

Moro I, Abo T, Crago SS, Komiyama K, Mestecky J. Natural killer cells in human colostrum. Cell Immunol 93:467–474, 1985.

Mostov KE, Friedlander M, Blobel G. The receptor for transepithelial transport of IgA and IgM contains multiple immunoglobulin-like domains. Nature 308:37–43, 1984.

Mostov KE, Kaetzel CS. Immunoglobulin transport and the polymeric immunoglobulin receptor. In Ogra PL, Mestecky J, Lamm ME, Strober W, Bienenstock J, McGhee JR, eds. Mucosal Immunology. San Diego, Academic Press, 1999, pp 181–211.

Murillo GJ, Goldman AS. The cells of human colostrum. II. Synthesis of IgA and Beta1c. Pediatr Res 4:71–75, 1970.

Murphy BR. Mucosal immunity to viruses. In Ogra PL, Mestecky J, Lamm ME, Strober W, Bienenstock J, McGhee JR, eds. Handbook of Mucosal Immunology. San Diego, Academic Press, 1994, pp 333–343.

Musil LS, Baenziger JU. Proteolytic processing of rat liver membrane secretory component. Cleavage activity is localized to bile canalicular membranes. J Biol Chem 263:15799–15808, 1988.

Mygind N, Weeke B, Ullman S. Quantitative determination of immunoglobulins in nasal secretion. Int Arch Allergy Appl Immunol 49:99–107, 1975.

Nagura H, Ohtani H, Masuda T, Kimura M, Nakamura S. HLA-DR expression on M cells overlying Peyer's patches is a common feature of human small intestine. Acta Pathol Jpn 41:818–823, 1991.

Nakajima S, Gillespie DN, Gleich GJ. Differences between IgA and IgE as secretory proteins. Clin Exp Immunol 21:306–317, 1975.

Neukirk MM, Klein MH, Katz A, Fishcer MM, Underdown BM. Estimation of polymeric IgA in human serum: an assay based o binding of radiolabelled human secretory component with applications in the study of IgA nephropathy, IgA monoclonal gammopathy, and liver disease. J Pediatr 71:441–445, 1983.

Neurath MF, Finotto S, Glimcher LH. The role of Th1/Th2 polarization in mucosal immunity. Nat Med 8:567–573, 2002.

Neutra MR, Kraehenbuhl JP. Cellular and molecular basis for antigen transport across epithelial barriers. In Ogra PL, Mestecky J, Lamm ME, Strober W, Bienenstock J, McGhee JR, eds. Mucosal Immunology. San Diego, Academic Press, 1999, pp 101–114.

Newburg DS, Viscidi RP, Ruff A, Yolken RH. A human milk factor inhibits binding of human immunodeficiency virus to the CD4 receptor. Pediatr Res 31:22–28, 1992.

Newby TJ. Protective immune responses in the intestinal tract. In Newby TJ, Stokes CR, eds. Immune Responses of the Gut. Boca Raton, FL, CRC Press, 1984, pp 143–198.

Newcomb RW, Ishizaka K. Physicochemical and antigenic studies on human gamma E in respiratory fluid. J Immunol 105:85–89, 1970.

Newcomb RW, Normansell D, Stanworth DR. A structural study of human exocrine IgA globulin. J Immunol 101:905–914, 1968.

Newcomb RW, Sutoris CA. Comparative studies on human and rabbit exocrine IgA antibodies to an albumin. Immunochemistry 11:623–632, 1974.

Newhouse M, Sanchis J, Bienenstock J. Lung defense mechanisms. N Engl J Med 295:1045–1052, 1976.

Nichols BL, McKee KS, Henry JF, Putman M. Human lactoferrin stimulates thymidine incorporation into DNA of rat crypt cells. Pediatr Res 21:563–567, 1987.

Nikolova EB, Tomana M, Russell MW. All forms of human IgA antibodies bound to antigen interfere with complement (C3) fixation induced by IgG or by antigen alone. Scand J Immunol 39:275–280, 1994.

Nilsson L, Paschalis S. The human Ia1 and Ia2 germline promotor elements: proximal positive and distal negative elements may regulate the tissue specific expressions of Ca1 and Ca2 germline transcripts. Int Immunol 5:271–282, 1993.

Norderhaug IN, Johansen FE, Krajci P, Brandtzaeg P. Domain deletions in the human polymeric Ig receptor disclose differences between its dimeric IgA and pentameric IgM interaction. Eur J Immunol 29:3401–3409, 1999.

Nuijens JH, van Berkel PH, Schanbacher FL. Structure and biological actions of lactoferrin. J Mammary Gland Biol Neoplasia 1:285–295, 1996.

Oda M, Cowell JL, Burstyn DG, Thaib S, Manclark CR. Antibodies to Bordetella pertussis in human colostrum and their protective activity against aerosol infection of mice. Infect Immun 47:441–445, 1985.

Ogra PL. Ontogeny of the local immune system. Pediatrics 64:765–774, 1979.

Ogra PL, Karzon DT. The role of immunoglobulins in the mechanism of mucosal immunity to virus infection. Pediatr Clin North Am 17:385–400, 1970.

Ogra PL, Coppola PR, MacGillivray MH, Dzierba JL. Mechanism of mucosal immunity to viral infections in gamma A immunoglobulin-deficiency syndromes. Proc Soc Exp Biol Med 145:811–816, 1974.

Ogra PL, Losonsky GA, Fishaut M. Colostrum-derived immunity and maternal-neonatal interaction. Ann NY Acad Sci 409:82–95, 1983.

Ogra PL, Mestecky J, Lamm ME, Strober W, Bienenstock J, McGhee JR, eds. Mucosal Immunology. San Diego, Academic Press, 1999.

Ogra SS, Ogra PL. Immunologic aspects of human colostrum and milk. I. Distribution characteristics and concentrations of immunoglobulins at different times after the onset of lactation. J Pediatr 92:546–549, 1978.

Ogra SS, Weintraub D, Ogra PL. Immunologic aspects of human colostrum and milk. III. Fate and absorption of cellular and soluble components in the gastrointestinal tract of the newborn. J Immunol 119:245–248, 1977.

Otnaess AB, Laegreid A, Ertresvag K. Inhibition of enterotoxin from Escherichia coli and Vibrio cholerae by gangliosides from human milk. Infect Immun 40:563–569, 1983.

Otnaess AB, Orstavik I. Effect of fractions of Ethiopian and Norwegian colostrum on rotavirus and Escherichia coli heat-labile enterotoxin. Infect Immun 33:459–466, 1981.

Otnaess AB, Svennerholm AM. Non-immunoglobulin fraction of human milk protects rabbits against enterotoxin-induced intestinal fluid secretion. Infect Immun 35:738–740, 1982.

Owen RL, Nemanic P. Antigen processing structures of the mammalian intestinal tract: an SEM study of lymphoepithelial organs. In Becker RP, Johari O, eds. Scanning Electron Microscopy. O'Hare, IL, Inc., 1978, pp 367–378.

Paape MJ, Keller M. Determination of numbers and function of cells in milk. In Jensen RG, Neville MC, eds. Human Lactation. Milk Components and Methodologies. New York, Plenum Press, 1985, pp 53–60.

Paape MJ, Wergin WS. Scanning and transmission electron microscopy of polymorphonuclear leucocytes (PMN) isolated from milk. Fed Proc 36:1201, 1977.

Parmely MJ, Beer AE, Billingham RE. In vitro studies on the T-lymphocyte population of human milk. J Exp Med 144:358–370, 1976.

Parr MB, Parr EL. Female genital tract immunity in animal models. In Ogra PL, Mestecky J, Lamm ME, Strober W, Bienenstock J, McGhee JR, eds. Mucosal Immunology. San Diego, Academic Press, 1999, pp 1395–1409.

Parrott DM, Tait C, MacKenzie S, Mowat AM, Davies MD, Micklem HS. Analysis of the effector functions of different populations of mucosal lymphocytes. Ann NY Acad Sci 409:307–320, 1983.

Perkkio M, Savilathi E. Time of appearance of immunoglobulin-containing cells in the mucosa of the neonatal intestine. Pediatr Res 14:953–955, 1980.

Pfaffenbach G, Lamm ME, Gigli I. Activation of the guinea pig alternative complement pathway by mouse IgA immune complexes. J Exp Med 155:231–247, 1982.

Phillips JO, Everson MP, Moldoveanu Z, Lue C, Mestecky J. Synergistic effect of IL-4 and IFN-gamma on the expression of polymeric Ig receptor (secretory component) and IgA binding by human epithelial cells. J Immunol 145:1740–1744, 1990.

Phillips-Quagliata JM, Roux ME, Arny M, Kelly-Hatfield P, McWilliams M, Lamm ME. Migration and regulation of B-cells in the mucosal immune system. Ann NY Acad Sci 409:194–203, 1983.

Picker LJ. Control of lymphocyte homing. Curr Opin Immunol 6:394–406, 1994.

Pickering LK, Cleary TG, Kohl S, Getz S. Polymorphonuclear leukocytes of human colostrum. I. Oxidative metabolism and kinetics of killing of radiolabeled Staphylococcus aureus. J Infect Dis 142:685–693, 1980b.

Pickering LK, Granoff DM, Erickson JR, Masor ML, Cordle CT, Schaller JP, Winship TR, Paule CL, Hilty MD. Modulation of the immune system by human milk and infant formula containing nucleotides. Pediatrics 101:242–249, 1998.

Pickering LK, Ruiz-Palacios G. Antibodies in milk directed against specific enteropathogens. In Hamosh M, Goldman AS. Human Lactation 2. Maternal Environmental Factors. New York, Plenum Press 1986, pp 499–506.

Pierce AE. Specific antibodies at mucous surfaces. Vet Rev Annot 5:17–36, 1986.

Pierce NF, Cray WC. Determinants of the localization, magnitude, and duration of a specific mucosal IgA plasma cell response in enterically immunized rats. J Immunol 128:1311–1315, 1982.

Pierce NF, Gowans JL. Cellular kinetics of the intestinal immune response to cholera toxoid in rats. J Exp Med 142:1550–1563, 1975.

Pierce NF, Sack RB. Immune response of the intestinal mucosa to cholera toxoid. J Infect Dis 136(Suppl):S113–S117, 1977.

Piskurich JF, France JA, Tamer CM, Willmer CA, Kaetzel CS, Kaetzel DM. Interferon-gamma induces polymeric immunoglobulin receptor mRNA in human intestinal epithelial cells by a protein synthesis dependent mechanism. Mol Immunol 30:413–421, 1993.

Pittard WB III, Bill K. Differentiation of cord blood lymphocytes into IgA-producing cells in response to breast milk stimulatory factor. Clin Immunol Immunopathol 13:430–434, 1979.

Pittard WB, Polmar SH, Fanaroff AA. The breastmilk macrophage: a potential vehicle for immunoglobulin transport. J Reticuloendothel Soc 22:597–603, 1977.

Plaut AG. The IgA1 proteases of pathogenic bacteria. Annu Rev Microbiol 37:603–622, 1983.

Pond L, Wassom DL, Hayes CE. Evidence for differential induction of helper T cell subsets during *Trichinella spiralis* infection. J Immunol 143:4232–4237, 1989.

Porras O, Svanborg EC, Lagergard T, Hanson LA. Method for testing adherence of *Haemophilus influenzae* to human buccal epithelial cells. Eur J Clin Microbiol 4:310–315, 1985.

Portis JL, Coe JE. IgM the secretory immunoglobulin of reptiles and amphibians. Nature 258:547–548, 1975.

Prentice A. Breast feeding increases concentrations of IgA in infants' urine. Arch Dis Child 62:792–795, 1987.

Prentice A, Prentice AM, Cole TJ, Paul AA, Whitehead RG. Breast-milk antimicrobial factors of rural Gambian mothers. I. Influence of stage of lactation and maternal plane of nutrition. Acta Paediatr Scand 73:796–802, 1984.

Prentice A, Prentice AM, Cole TJ, Whitehead RG. Determinants of variations in breast milk protective factor concentrations of rural Gambian mothers. Arch Dis Child 58:518–522, 1983.

Ragnum TO, Brandtzaeg P. IgE-positive cells in human intestinal mucosa are mainly mast cells. Int Arch Allergy Appl Immunol 89:256–260, 1989.

Reddy V, Raghuramulu N, Bhaskaram C. Secretory IgA in protein-calorie malnutrition. Arch Dis Child 51:871–874, 1976.

Reddy V, Bhaskaram C, Raghuramulu N, Jagadeesan V. Antimicrobial factors in human milk. Acta Paediatr Scand 66:229–232, 1977.

Reed WP, Williams RC. Intestinal immunoglobulins in shigellosis. Gastroenterology 61:35–45, 1971.

Reed KJ, Van Epps DE, Williams RC. Inhibition of human eosinophil chemotaxis by IgA paraproteins. Inflammation 3:405–416, 1979.

Reinholdt J, Krogh P, Holmstrup P. Degradation of IgA1, IgA2, and S-IgA by Candida and Torulopsis species. Acta Pathol Microbiol Immunol Scand [C.] 95:265–274, 1987.

Remington JS, Vosti KL, Lietze A, Zimmerman AL. Serum proteins and antibody activity in human nasal secretions. J Clin Invest 43:1613–1624, 1964.

Renegar KB, Small PA. Passive transfer of local immunity to influenza virus infection by IgA antibody. J Immunol 146:1972–1978, 1991.

Resta S, Luby JP, Rosenfeld CR, Siegel JD. Isolation and propagation of a human enteric coronavirus. Science 229:978–981, 1985.

Richie ER, Steinmetz KD, Meistrich ML, Ramirez I, Hilliard JK. T lymphocytes in colostrum and peripheral blood differ in their capacity to form thermostable E-rosettes. J Immunol 125:2344–2346, 1980.

Rits M, Hiemstra PS, Bazin H, Van Es LA, Daha M, Vaerman JP. Activation of rat complement by soluble and insoluble immune complexes of rat IgA. Monogr Allergy 24:129–133, 1988.

Rogers HJ, Synge C. Bacteriostatic effect of human milk on *Escherichia coli*: the role of IgA. Immunology 34:19–28, 1978.

Rousset F, Garcia E, Banchereau J. Cytokine-induced proliferation and immunoglobulin production of human B lymphocytes triggered through their CD40 antigen. J Exp Med 173:705–710, 1991.

Roux ME, McWilliams M, Phillips-Quagliata JM, Weisz-Carrington P, Lamm ME. Origin of IgA-secreting plasma cells in the mammary gland. J Exp Med 146:1311–1322, 1977.

Rowland MG, Cole TJ, Tully M, Dolby JM, Honour P. Bacteriostasis of *Escherichia coli* by milk. VI. The in-vitro bacteriostatic property of Gambian mothers' breast milk in relation to the in-vivo protection of their infants against diarrhoeal disease. J Hyg Lond 85:405–413, 1980.

Russel-Jones GJ, Ey PL, Reynolds BL. The ability of IgA to inhibit complement consumption by complement-fixing antigens and antigen-antibody complexes. Aust J Exp Biol Med Sci 62:567–571, 1984.

Saarinen UM, Kajosaari M. Breastfeeding as prophylaxis against atopic disease: prospective follow-up study until 17 years old. Lancet 346:1065–1069, 1995.

Savilathi E. Immunoglobulin-containing cells in the intestinal mucosa and immunoglobulins in the intestinal juice in children. Clin Exp Immunol 11:415–425, 1972.

Savilathi E. IgA deficiency in children: immunoglobulin-containing cells in the intestinal mucosa, immunoglobulins in secretions, and serum IgA levels. Clin Exp Immunol 13:406, 1973.

Schanler RJ, Goldblum RM, Garza C, Goldman AS. Enhanced fecal excretion of selected immune factors in very low birth weight infants fed fortified human milk. Pediatr Res 20:711–715, 1986.

Schieferdecker HL, Ullrich R, Weiss-Breckwoldt AN, Schwarting R, Stein H, Riecken EO, Zeitz M. The HML-1 antigen of intestinal lymphocytes is an activation antigen. J Immunol 144:2541–2549, 1990.

Schlesinger JJ, Covelli HD. Evidence for transmission of lymphocyte responses to tuberculin by breast-feeding. Lancet 2:529–532, 1977.

Schroten J, Hanisch FF, Plogmann R, Hacker J, Uhlernbruch G, Nobis-Bosch R, Wahn V. Inhibition of adhesion of S-fimbriated *Escherichia coli* to buccal epithelial cells by human milk fat globule membrane components: a novel aspect of the protective function of mucins in the nonimmunoglobulin fraction. Pediatr Res 32:58–63, 1992.

Sewell HF, Matthews JB, Flack V, Jefferis R. Human immunoglobulin D in colostrum, saliva and amniotic fluid. Clin Exp Immunol 36:183–188, 1979.

Sharry JJ, Drasse B. Observations on the origins of salivary leukocytes. Acta Odontol Scand 18:347–358, 1960.

Shimamura K, Shigemi H, Kurono Y, Mogi G. The role of bacterial adherence in otitis media with effusion. Arch Otolaryngol Head Neck Surg 116:1143–1146, 1990.

Shvartzman YS. Formation of secretory and circulating antibodies after immunization with live inactivated influenza virus vaccines. J Infect Dis 135:697–705, 1977.

Sirisinha S, Suskind R, Edelman R, Asvapaka C, Olson RE. Secretory and serum IgA in children with protein-calorie malnutrition. Pediatrics 55:166–170, 1975.

Sloyer JL, Cate CC, Howie VM, Ploussard JH, Johnston RB. The immune response to acute otitis media in children. II. Serum and middle ear fluid antibody in otitis media due to *Haemophilus influenzae*. J Infect Dis 132:685–688, 1975.

Smith DJ, Taubman MA, Ebersole JL. Salivary IgA antibody to glucosyltransferase in man. Clin Exp Immunol 61:416–424, 1985.

Smith HW, Goldman AS. The cells of human colostrum: I. *In vitro* studies of morphology and functions. Pediatr Res 2:103–109, 1968.

Soderstrom T, Lundberg A, Soderstrom R, Hanson LA. Characterization of fresh and Epstein-Barr virus transformed human colostral cells. Unpublished observations, 1988.

Sohl-Akerlund A, Hanson LA, Ahlstedt S, Carlsson B. A sensitive method of specific quantitation of secretory IgA. Scand J Immuno 6:1275–1282, 1977.

Song W, Apodaca G, Mostov K. Transcytosis of the polymeric immunoglobulin receptor is regulated in multiple intracellular compartments. J Biol Chem 269:29474–29480, 1994.

South MA, Cooper MD, Wollheim FA, Hong R, Good RA. The IgA system. I. Studies of the transport and immunochemistry of IgA in the saliva. J Exp Med 123:615–627, 1966.

Spencer J, Dillon SB, Isaacson PG, MacDonald TT. T cell subclasses in fetal human ileum. Clin Exp Immunol 65:553–558, 1986a.

Spencer J, MacDonald TT, Finn T, Isaacson PG. The development of gut associated lymphoid tissue in the terminal ileum of fetal human intestine. Clin Exp Immunol 64:536–543, 1986b.

Splawski JB, Woodard CS, Denney RM, Goldblum RM. Rapid development of polymeric IgA in the serum of infants. Abstract. Clin Res 31:902A, 1984.

Stavnezer J, Radcliffe G, Lin YC, Nietupski J, Berggren L, Sitia R, Severinson E. Immunoglobulin heavy-chain switching may be directed by prior induction of transcripts from constant-region genes. Proc Natl Acad Sci USA 85:7704–7708, 1988.

Stavnezer J, Radcliffe G, Severinson E. Specificity of immunoglobulin heavy chain switching by cultured I.29 B lymphoma cells. Monogr Allergy 24:197–207, 1998.

Steinmetz KD, Kohl S, Richie ER. Separation of cytotoxic leukocyte populations of human peripheral blood and colostrum of PVP-silica (Percoll) density gradients. J Immunol Methods 42:157–170, 1981.

Stock CC, Francis T Jr. The inactivation of the virus of epidemic influenza by soaps. J Exp Med 71:661–681, 1940.

Stokes CR, Soothill JF, Turner MW. Immune exclusion is a function of IgA. Nature 255:745–746, 1975.

Streeter PR, Berg EL, Rouse BT, Bargatze RF, Butcher EC. A tissue-specific endothelial cell molecule involved in lymphocyte homing. Nature 331:41–46, 1988.

Strober W, Ehrhardt RO. Regulation of IgA B cell development. In Ogra PL, Lamm ME, McGhee JR, Mestecky J, Strober W, Bienenstock J, eds. Handbook of Mucosal Immunology. San Diego, Academic Press, 1994, pp 159–176.

Suzuki S, Lucas A, Lucas PJ, Coombs RR. Immunoglobulin concentrations and bacterial antibody titers in breast milk from mothers of 'preterm' and 'term' infants. Acta Paediatr Scand 72:671–677, 1983.

Svanborg EC, Carlsson B, Hanson LA, Jann B, Jann K, Korhonen T, Wadstrom T. Anti-pili antibodies in breast milk. Lancet 2:1235–1979, 1979.

Svanborg EC. Bacterial adherence and mucosal immunity. In Ogra PL, Lamm ME, McGhee J, Mestecky J, Strober W, Bienenstock J, eds. Handbook of Mucosal Immunology. San Diego, Academic Press, 1994, pp 71–75.

Svanborg N, Hedqvist P, Green K. Aspects of prostaglandin action in asthma. Adv Prostaglandin Thromboxane Res 1:439–447, 1976

Svanborg EC, Andersson B, Hagberg L, Hanson LA, Leffler H, Magnusson G, Noori G, Dahmen J, Soderstrom T. Receptor analogues and anti-pili antibodies as inhibitors of bacterial attachment in vivo and in vitro. Ann NY Acad Sci 409:580–592, 1983.

Svanborg EC, Briles D, Hagberg L, McGhee J, Michalec S. Genetic factors in host resistance to urinary tract infection. Infection 12:118–123, 1984.

Svanborg EC, Kulhavy R, Marild S, Prince SJ, Mestecky J. Urinary immunoglobulins in healthy individuals and children with acute pyelonephritis. Scand J Immunol 21:305–313, 1985.

Svanborg EC, Svennerholm AM. Secretory immunoglobulin A and G antibodies prevent adhesion of Escherichia coli to human urinary tract epithelial cells. Infect Immun 22:790–797, 1978.

Svennerholm AM, Holmgren J. Synergistic protective effect in rabbits of immunization with Vibrio cholerae lipopolysaccharide and toxin/toxoid. Infect Immun 13:735–740, 1976.

Svennerholm AM, Holmgren J, Hanson LA, Lindblad BS, Quereshi F, Rahimtoola RJ. Boosting of secretory IgA antibody responses in man by parenteral cholera vaccination. Scand J Immunol 6:1345–1349, 1977.

Svennerholm AM, Lange S, Holmgren J. Correlation between syntheses of specific immunoglobulin A and protection against experimental cholera in mice. Infect Immun 21:1–6, 1978.

Svennerholm AM, Hanson LA, Holmgren J, Lindblad BS, Nilsson B, Quereshi F. Different secretory immunoglobulin A antibody responses to cholera vaccination in Swedish and Pakistani women. Infect Immun 30:427–430, 1980.

Sveennerholm AM, Hanson LA, Holmgren L, Lindblad BS, Khan SR, Nilsson A, Svennerholm B. Milk antibodies to live and killed polio vaccines in Pakistani and Swedish mothers. J Infect Dis 143:707–711, 1981.

Svennerholm AM, Jertborn M, Gothefors L, Karim AM, Sack DA, Holmgren J. Mucosal antitoxic and antibacterial immunity after cholera disease and after immunization with a combined B subunit-whole cell vaccine. J Infect Dis 149:884–893, 1984.

Szabo MC, Butcher EC, McEvoy LM. Specialization of mucosal follicular dendritic cells revealed by mucosal addressin-cell adhesion molecule-1 display. J Immunol 158:5584–5588, 1997.

Tada T, Ishizaka K. Distribution of gamma E-forming cells in lymphoid tissues of the human and monkey. J Immunol 104:377–387, 1970.

Tagliabue A, Boraschi D, Villa L, Keren DF, Lowell GH, Rappuoli R, Nencioni L. IgA-dependent cell-mediated activity against enteropathogenic bacteria: distribution, specificity, and characterization of the effector cells. J Immunol 133:988–992, 1984.

Tagliabue A, Villa L, De Magistris MT, Romano M, Silvestri S, Boraschi D, Nencioni L. IgA-driven T cell-mediated anti-bacterial immunity in man after live oral Ty 21a vaccine. J Immunol 137:1504–1510, 1986.

Taguchi T, McGhee JR, Coffman RL, Beagley KW, Eldridge JH, Takatsu K, Kiyono H. Analysis of Th1 and Th2 cells in murine gut-associated tissues. Frequencies of CD4+ and CD8+ T cells that secrete IFN-gamma and IL-5. J Immunol 145:68–77, 1990.

Takahashi M, Kanai N, Watanabe A, Oshima O, Ryan AF. Lymphocyte subsets in immune-mediated otitis media with effusion. Eur Arch Otorhinolaryngol 249:24–27, 1992.

Taylor HP, Dimmock NJ. Mechanism of neutralization of influenza virus by secretory IgA is different from that of monomeric IgA or IgG. J Exp Med 161:198–209, 1985.

Tenovuo J, Moldoveanu Z, Mestecky J, Pruitt KM, Rahemtulla BM. Interaction of specific and innate factors of immunity: IgA enhances the antimicrobial effect of the lactoperoxidase system against Streptococcus mutans. J Immunol 128:726–731, 1982.

Theodore CM, Losonsky G, Peri B, Fishaut M, Rothberg RM, Ogra PL. Immunologic aspects of colostrum and milk: development of antibody response to respiratory syncytial virus and bovine serum albumin in the human and rabbit mammary gland. In Strober W, Hanson LA, Sell K, eds. Recent Advances in Mucosal Immunity. New York, Raven Press, 1982, pp 393–403.

Thompson RA, Asquith P, Cooke WT. Secretory IgA in the serum. Lancet 2:517–519, 1969.

Thorpe LW, Rudloff HE, Powell LC, Goldman AS. Decreased response of human milk leukocytes to chemoattractant peptides. Pediatr Res 20:373–377, 1986.

Thromar H, Issacs CE, Brown HR, Barshatzky MR, Pessolano T. Inactivation of enveloped viruses and killing of cells by fatty acids and monoglycerides. J Am Soc Microbiol 32:27–31, 1987.

Tomasi TB, Bienenstock J. Secretory immunoglobulins. Adv Immunol 9:1–96, 1968.

Tomasi TB Jr, Czerwinski DS. The secretory IgA system. In Bergsma D, Good RA, eds. Immunologic Deficiency Diseases in Man. Baltimore, William & Wilkins, 1968, pp 270–275.

Tomasi TB Jr, Tan EM, Solomon A, Prendergast RA. Characteristics of an immune system common to certain external secretions. J Exp Med 121:101–124, 1965.

Tramont EC. Inhibition of adherence of Neisseria gonorrhoeae by human genital secretions. J Clin Invest 59:117–124, 1977.

Turesson I. Distribution of immunoglobulin-containing cells in human bone marrow and lymphoid tissues. Acta Med Scand 199:293–304, 1976.

Turner MW, McClelland DB, Medlen AR, Stokes CR. IGE in human urine and milk. Scand J Immunol 6:343–348, 1977.

Uauy R, Stringel G, Thomas R, Quan R. Effect of dietary nucleosides on growth and maturation of the developing gut in the rat. J Pediatr Gastroenterol Nutr 10:497–503, 1990.

Uehling DT, Stiehm ER. Elevated urinary secretory IgA in children with urinary tract infection. Pediatrics 47:40–46, 1971.

Underdown BJ, Dorrington KJ. Studies on the structural and conformational basis for the relative resistance of serum and secretory immunoglobulin A to proteolysis. J Immunol 112:949–959, 1974.

Underdown BJ, Knight A, Papsin F. The relative paucity of IgE in human milk. J Immunol 116:1435–1438, 1976.

Underdown BJ, De Rose J, Plaut A. Disulfide bonding of secretory component to a single monomer subunit in human secretory IgA. J Immunol 118:1816–1821, 1977.

Urban JF, Katona IM, Paul WE, Finkelman FD. Interleukin 4 is important in protective immunity to a gastrointestinal nematode infection in mice. Proc Natl Acad Sci USA 88:5513–5517, 1991.

Vaerman JP, Lemaitre-Coelho I, Limet J, Delacroix DL. Hepatic transfer of polymeric IgA from plasma to bile in rats and other mammals: a survey. In Strober W, Hanson LA, Sell KW, eds. Recent Advances in Mucosal Immunity. New York, Raven Press, 1982, pp 233–250.

Van Epps DE, Williams RC. Suppression of leukocyte chemotaxis by human IgA myeloma components. J Exp Med 144:1227–1242, 1976.

Van Kerckhove C, Russell GJ, Deusch K, Reich K, Bhan AK, DerSimonian H, Brenner MB. Oligoclonality of human intestinal intraepithelial T cells. J Exp Med 175:57–63, 1992.

Vincent C, Revillard JP. Sandwich-type ELISA for free and bound secretory component in human biological fluids. J Immunol Methods 106:153–160, 1988.

Waissbluth JG, Langman JS. ABO blood group, secretor status, salivary protein, and serum and salivary immunoglobulin concentrations. Gut 12:646–649, 1971.

Wakatsuki Y, Strober W. Effect of downregulation of germline transcripts on immunoglobulin A isotype differentiation. J Exp Med 178:129–138, 1993.

Waldman RH, Ganguly R. Techniques for eliciting mucosal immune response. Acta Endocrinol Suppl (Copenh) 194:262–280, 1975.

Waldman RH, Lee JD, Polly SM, Dorfman A, Fox EN. Group A streptococcal M protein vaccine: protection following immunization via the respiratory tract. Dev Biol Stand 28:429–434, 1975.

Waldman RH, Wigley FM, Small PA. Specificity of respiratory secretion antibody against influenza virus. J Immunol 105:1477–1483, 1970.

Waldmann TA, Strober W. Metabolism of immunoglobulins. Prog Allergy 13:1–110, 1969.

Walker WA, Isselbacher KJ, Bloch KJ. Intestinal uptake of macromolecules: effect of oral immunization. Science 177:608–610, 1972.

Walker WA, Isselbacher KJ, Bloch KJ. Immunologic control of soluble protein absorption from the small intestine: a gut-surface phenomenon. Am J Clin Nutr 27:1434–1440, 1974.

Walker WA, Wu M, Isselbacher KJ, Bloch KJ. Intestinal uptake of macromolecules. III. Studies on the mechanism by which immunization interferes with antigen uptake. J Immunol 115:854–861, 1975.

Walker WA, Lake AM, Bloch KJ. Immunologic mechanisms for goblet cell mucous release: possible role in mucosal host defense. In Strober W, Hanson LA, Sell KW, eds. Recent Advances in Mucosal Host Defense. New York, Raven Press, 1982, pp 331–351.

Watanabe T, Nagura H, Watanabe K, Brown WR. The binding of human milk lactoferrin to immunoglobulin A. FEBS Lett. 168:203–207, 1984.

Watanabe N, Yoshimura H, Mogi G. Induction of antigen-specific IgA-forming cells in the middle ear mucosa. Arch Otolaryngol Head Neck Surg 114:758–762, 1988.

Weinstein PD, Cebra JJ. The preference for switching to IgA expression by Peyer's patch germinal center B cells is likely due to the intrinsic influence of their microenvironment. J Immunol 147:4126–4135, 1991.

Welliver RC. Respiratory infections. In Olgra PL, Lamm ME, McGhee JR, Mestecky J, Strober W, Bienenstock J, eds. Handbook of Mucosal Immunology. San Diego, Academic Press, pp 551–559, 1994.

Welliver RC, Kaul A, Ogra PL. Cell-mediated immune response to respiratory syncytial virus infection: relationship to the development of reactive airway disease. J Pediatr 94:370–375, 1979.

Welsh JK, Arsenakis M, Coelen RJ, May JT. Effect of antiviral lipids, heat, and freezing on the activity of viruses in human milk. J Infect Dis 140:322–328, 1979.

Weltzin R, Lucia-Jandris P, Michetti P, Fields BN, Kraehenbuhl JP, Neutra MR. Binding and transepithelial transport of immunoglobulins by intestinal M cells: demonstration using monoclonal IgA antibodies against enteric viral proteins. J Cell Biol 108:1673–1685, 1989.

Wenzel RP, Mitzel JR, Davies JA, Edwards EA, Berling C, McCormick DP, Beam WE. Antigenicity of a polysaccharide vaccine from *Neisseria meningitidis* administered intranasally. J Infect Dis 128:31–40, 1973.

Wiedermann U, Hanson LA, Holmgren J, Kahu H, Dahlgren UI. Impaired mucosal antibody response to cholera toxin in vitamin A-deficient rats immunized with oral cholera vaccine. Infect Immun 61:3952–3957, 1993.

Williams RC, Gibbons RJ. Inhibition of bacterial adherence by secretory immunoglobulin A: a mechanism of antigen disposal. Science 177:697–699, 1972.

Winner L, Mack J, Weltzin R, Mekalanos JJ, Kraehenbuhl JP, Neutra MR. New model for analysis of mucosal immunity: intestinal secretion of specific monoclonal immunoglobulin A from hybridoma tumors protects against Vibrio cholerae infection. Infect Immun 59:977–982, 1991.

Wirt DP, Adkins LT, Palkowetz KH, Schmalstieg FC, Goldman AS. Activated and memory T lymphocytes in human milk. Cytometry 13:282–290, 1992.

Wold AE, Mestecky J, Svanborg EC. Agglutination of *E. coli* by secretory IgA-a result of interaction between bacterial mannose-specific adhesins and immunoglobulin carbohydrate? Monogr Allergy 24:307–309, 1988.

Wolf HM, Fischer MB, Puhringer H, Samstag A, Vogel E, Eibl MM. Human serum IgA downregulates the release of inflammatory cytokines (tumor necrosis factor-alpha, interleukin-6) in human monocytes. Blood 83:1278–1288, 1994a.

Wolf HM, Vogel E, Fischer MB, Rengs H, Schwarz HP, Eibl MM. Inhibition of receptor-dependent and receptor-independent generation of the respiratory burst in human neutrophils and monocytes by human serum IgA. Pediatr Res 36:235–243, 1994b.

Woodard CS, Splawski JB, Goldblum RM, Denney RM. Characterization of epitopes of human secretory component on free secretory component, secretory IgA, and membrane-associated secretory component. J Immunol 133:2116–2125, 1984.

Xu-Amano J, Kiyono H, Jackson RJ, Staats HF, Fujihashi K, Burrows PD, Elson CO, Pillai S, McGhee JR. Helper T cell subsets for immunoglobulin A responses: oral immunization with tetanus toxoid and cholera toxin as adjuvant selectively induces Th2 cells in mucosa associated tissues. J Exp Med 178:1309–1320, 1993.

Yolken RH, Peterson JA, Vonderfecht SL, Fouts ET, Midthun K, Newburg DS. Human milk mucin inhibits rotavirus replication and prevents experimental gastroenteritis. J Clin Invest 90:1984–1991, 1992.

10

The Natural (Innate) Defense System

Harry R. Hill, John F. Bohnsack, and Timothy R. La Pine

INTRODUCTION

The natural, or innate, immune system includes those mechanisms that protect the host against microbial invasion without the need for prior exposure to that microbe (Table 10-1). Unlike the adaptive immune system, the natural immune system does not change or amplify upon re-exposure to that microbe. The natural immune system developed first phylogenetically, appearing in all multicellular organisms, including plants, insects, and animals (Hoffmann et al., 1999; Qureshi et al., 1999).

Natural immunity is the first line of defense against pathogens, active long before the adaptive immune response (antibodies and T cells) can protect the host. Humans can survive for prolonged periods without immunoglobulins or T lymphocytes, but without the normal barriers of the skin (e.g., following a severe burn) or in the absence of neutrophils (e.g., following marrow invasion by leukemia or severe congenital neutropenia), infection ensues rapidly.

The activities of natural immunity must be both rapid (to halt early microbial invasion) and nonspecific (to protect against multiple diverse pathogens). The cells of the innate immune system also play a major role in antigen processing and presentation and augmenting the cells of the adaptive immune system. Thus the adaptive immune system utilizes the effector functions of the natural immune system to eliminate microbes. Antibodies of the adaptive immune system serve as opsonins, but bactericidal activity is derived from nonspecific phagocytic cells. Likewise, cytokines of innate immunity serve as early warning signals of microbial invasion, priming the adaptive immune system. For example, macrophage-derived interleukin-1β (IL-1β) and tumor necrosis factor-alpha (TNF-α) alert and prime multiple cells of microbial invasion.

The natural immune system is composed first of physical barriers that impede entry of organisms. These include the epithelial cells of the skin, mucous

TABLE 10-1 · COMPONENTS OF THE NATURAL IMMUNE SYSTEM

Epithelial and Mucosal Barriers	Cells in Natural Immunity	Natural Antimicrobial Agents	Natural Opsonins	Reactive Oxygen and Nitrogen Species	Carbohydrate Recognition Receptors	Cytokines
Mechanical barriers	Macrophages/	Defensins	Natural	Superoxide	Collectins	IL-1, TNF-α,
Hairs and cilia	dendritic cells	Lactoferrin	antibodies	Hydrogen	Conglutinin	IL-6, IL-8,
Mucin	Neutrophils	Transferrin	Complement	peroxide	MBP	MIP, MCP,
Normal flora	Natural killer	Lysozyme	Fibronectin	Hydroxyl radical	SP-A	IFN-γ, IL-12,
	cells	Myeloperoxidase		Hypochlorite ion	SP-B	IL-15, IL-18,
	Mast cells	Seprocidins		Nitric oxide	Selectins	GM-CSF,
	γδ-T cells				LBP	G-CSF, M-CSF
	B1 lymphocytes				CD14	
					Toll-like receptors	
					BPI factor	

BPI = bacterial permeability increasing; G-CSF = granulocyte colony-stimulating factor; GM-CSF = granulocyte-macrophage colony-stimulating factor; IFN = interferon; IL = interleukin; LBP = lipopolysaccharide-binding protein; MBP = mannose-binding protein; M-CSF = macrophage colony-stimulating factor; MCP = macrophage chemotactic peptide; MIP = macrophage inflammatory proteins; SP = surfactant protein; TNF = tumor necrosis factor.

membranes, respiratory, and gastrointestinal tracts, as well as the secretions and mucins that coat these surfaces. The convoluted airways protected by hairs and cilia physically impede the invasion of microbes.

Second, a variety of different cells function in a non–antigen-specific manner to ingest and kill microbes or produce mediators and cytokines, as well as natural antimicrobial agents or reactive oxygen species that function in innate host resistance.

Third, a number of proteins provide nonspecific opsonic activity derived from naturally occurring immunoglobulin M (IgM), IgG, and IgA antibodies, complement fragments, C reactive protein, and fibronectin that function in innate immunity to promote ingestion, processing, and destruction of bacteria, fungi, and viruses in the naïve host (Ochsenbein et al., 1999).

Fourth, a variety of carbohydrate recognition receptors, such as the collectins (conglutinin, mannose-binding protein, and the surfactant-binding proteins, A and D), lipopolysaccharide-binding protein, CD14, and signal-transducing recognition receptors (such as the Toll-like receptors) recognize and bind pathogen-associated molecular patterns (PAMPs) common to bacteria, yeast, fungi, and some viruses (Medzhitov and Janeway, 2000a, 2000b; Feizi, 2000).

This chapter outlines the important factors in natural immunity and illustrates their critical role in host defense. This includes a description of the human deficiencies in natural immunity that result in recurrent infections or malignancies.

EPITHELIAL AND MUCOSAL BARRIERS

Mechanical Barriers

The three main interfaces of the body with the external environment, and therefore with potential pathogens, are the skin and the epithelial surfaces of the gastrointestinal and respiratory tracts. The presence of a contin-

uous epithelial layer at each of these interfaces serves to physically impede the ingress of microbes. In contrast, loss of integrity in these epithelial layers often results in cutaneous, respiratory, and gastrointestinal infection. Burns, eczema, or traumatic injury to the skin often result in localized infection, cellulitis, or abscess formation. Severe eczema likely contributes to staphylococcal invasion of the skin in allergic individuals. This is particularly true in patients with hyperimmunoglobulinemia-E (Job's) syndrome of recurrent infections, where the eczema, along with poor neutrophil chemotaxis, results in frequent and often deep-seated abscesses (Davis et al., 1966; Hill et al., 1974) (see Chapter 17).

Damage to the respiratory epithelium by smoke inhalation, oxygen toxicity, or other irritants can predispose one to pneumonia. Likewise, enterotoxins, graft-versus-host disease (GVHD), or certain microbial pathogens such as *Salmonella* or *Shigella* can alter the gastrointestinal epithelial lining, leading to invasive microbial diarrhea with tissue or even bloodstream invasion.

A variety of cells of the natural immune system are involved in protection of the epithelial barriers of the body if the integrity of the epithelial cell layer is breached. These include macrophages and their counterparts in different tissues, neutrophils, mast cells, γδ-T cells, and even B1 lymphocytes. These cells may ingest and kill invading pathogens or process antigens for presentation to cells of the adaptive immune system. Alternatively, these cells may produce critical cytokines or reactive oxygen species that can eliminate pathogens at or just below the epithelial barriers. In addition, the cells of the innate immune system may produce natural antibodies and other nonspecific opsonins that promote ingestion and elimination of pathogens.

Hairs and Cilia

The components of natural immunity in the respiratory tract include the hairs of the nasal mucosa; the tortuous passageways of the upper airways, bronchi, and bronchioles; and the cilia present on respiratory epithelium, which either impede respiratory invasion of microbial pathogens or serve to remove or expel them (Zhang et al., 2000). Abnormalities lead to recurrent infections, such as in Kartagener syndrome. These patients suffer chronic bronchitis and bronchiectasis because of a defect in ciliary rods, resulting in immotile cilia. Patients with tracheotomies also suffer from recurrent pulmonary infections because of loss of these immune barriers in the nasopharynx, glottis, and upper trachea.

Mucins and Airway Surface Fluid Components

A major component of the airway surface fluid (ASF) are large mucin glycoproteins that provide viscosity and physically impair the invasion of microbes and inhaled particles deeper into the airways and pulmonary tissues (Diamond et al., 2000; Rose, 1992). The genes for these mucin glycoproteins, MUC2 and MUC5A, are upregulated by lipopolysaccharide (LPS) and by both gram-positive and gram-negative bacteria (Dohrman et al., 1998). These glycoproteins do not possess antimicrobial activity themselves, but the airway surface fluid contains a variety of antimicrobial proteins, such as lysozyme, lactoferrin, and defensins, as well as reactive oxygen and nitrogen species (Diamond et al., 2000; Harbitz et al., 1984; Travis et al., 1999).

The salt or fluid content of the airway surface fluid may also have a role in protection against microbial invasion. High salt content or decreased airway fluid, such as that which is present in cystic fibrosis (resulting from abnormal respiratory epithelial cell chloride channels), may overwhelm the antibacterial activity of other aspects of airway defense (McCray et al., 1999; Travis et al., 1999) and contribute to persistent bacterial colonization and chronic infections seen in these patients.

A variety of inflammatory cells, including macrophages, neutrophils, natural killer cells, and mast cells, as well as cytokines produced by these cells and the respiratory epithelium, also contribute to the antimicrobial activity of airway surface fluid.

NORMAL MICROBIAL FLORA

The normal microbial flora contribute to natural defense at the epithelial and mucosal surfaces (Boman, 2000). Certain animals, such as the hippopotamus and the frog, are literally bathed in water and mud rich in microbes, yet infection is rare, due mostly to innate immunity. Similarly, humans are colonized with a variety of microorganisms, termed normal flora, which hold more pathogenic microbes in check. When the normal flora are suppressed by antimicrobial therapy, such as occurs in intensive care units, invasive pathogens emerge and cause serious illness. The normal flora produce bacteriocins and other antimicrobial agents that suppress the growth of invasive pathogens. In the absence of normal flora, virulent encapsulated bacteria,

yeast, and fungi may emerge on the skin, as well as the gastrointestinal and respiratory epithelium, leading to serious and overwhelming infection.

The moisture content or type of epithelial cell may predispose the host to colonization with invasive pathogens. For example, circumcision decreases the incidence of urinary tract infections (Schoen et al., 2000; Wiswell, 2000). Uncircumcised males are more likely to harbor uropathogenic *Escherichia coli* and *Proteus mirablis* in the urethral meatus and peri-uretheral area than circumcised males (Glennon et al., 1988; Wiswell et al., 1988). Fimbriated *E. coli* adhere better to the inner surface of the foreskin than to the outer keratinized surface (Fussell et al., 1988).

CELLS IN NATURAL IMMUNITY

The cells involved in the natural immune response include monocytes, macrophages, and neutrophils, which ingest or endocytose microbial invaders and kill them. Macrophages and other antigen-presenting cells (e.g., skin Langerhans cells, dendritic cells of lymphoid and nonlymphoid organs, microglial cells of the central nervous system) process ingested antigens for presentation to cells of the adaptive immune system, thus serving as a link between innate and adaptive immunity. Natural killer cells, lymphocytes lacking specific T-cell receptors, are capable of recognizing and killing viral- or tumor-transformed cells, and mast cells, which produce a number of inflammatory mediators, also contribute to natural immunity. These cells produce a variety of cytokines, including IL-1, TNF-α, IL-6, IL-8, IFN-γ, IL-12, IL-15, IL-18, and colony-stimulating factors (CSFs), which have critical roles in both innate and adaptive immunity.

Intraepithelial T Cells

Intraepithelial T cells, which are present in the skin or mucosal epithelium, express antigen receptors of very limited diversity, which are encoded in the germline. These cells, which are often γδ-T cells, are components of the adaptive immune system but function more like cells of the natural immune system. They only recognize a small number of antigens, such as microbial glycolipids, without employing great variation in the complementary-determining regions of their receptors. Upon antigen activation, intraepithelial T cells secrete cytokines and activate other cells of the natural immune system to kill microbes.

B1 lymphocytes, somewhat like γδ-T cells, containing IgM receptors, only recognize polysaccharide and lipid antigens such as lipopolysaccharide and phosphoryl-choline on diverse microbes. These cells produce IgM, and to a lesser extent IgG and IgA, natural antibodies that protect the epithelial barriers of the body's defenses.

The role of these cell types in natural immunity are described later in this chapter, as well as in Chapters 5, 6, and 21.

Macrophages and Dendritic Cells

Macrophages and their precursor monocytes have a central role in natural immunity. These cells appeared first phylogenetically. Even the fruit fly, *Drosophila*, has macrophage-like cells, termed hemocytes, which surround and phagocytize microbes and wall off infection by initiating coagulation (Abbas et al., 2000). Blood monocytes develop in the marrow and are released into the bloodstream, where they may circulate for extended periods (they have a half-life of approximately 70 hours).

The monocytes then enter into tissues and differentiate into macrophages, where they reside in the subepithelial connective tissue and the interstitium of internal organs. Macrophages also line the vascular sinusoids of the spleen, liver, and lymph nodes. Thus they are strategically placed to detect invaders just below the epithelial barriers of the skin, respiratory, and gastrointestinal tracts; at the major filtering sites of the bloodstream (lymph node, spleen, and liver); and in the parenchymal organs.

Macrophage-like cells in the skin are known as Langerhans cells; those of the liver are Kupffer cells; those of the central nervous system, microglial cells; and those of the lung, alveolar macrophages.

Macrophages are avidly phagocytic and can readily kill most pathogens, such as *Streptococcus pneumoniae*, *Hemophilus influenzae*, and *Staphylococcus aureus* (Zhang et al., 2000). Some pathogens, such as *Mycobacteria*, *Nocardia*, and *Legionella*, can survive within macrophages and require cytokines, such as IFN-γ, IL-12, IL-18, and CSFs, to kill these pathogens. Individuals lacking these cytokines or cytokine receptors suffer from serious intracellular infection with these pathogens.

Macrophages employ a variety of pattern recognition receptors (PRRs) to recognize PAMPs (Medzhitov and Janeway, 2000b). These include plasma components such as mannose-binding protein (MBP) and the surfactant proteins, but also cell-bound macrophage mannose receptors and C1q receptors, as well as signaling receptors such as the Toll-like receptors (TLRs). These assist the macrophage in recognizing, phagocytizing, or endocytosing microbes and their products and producing mediators to alert the other cells of the natural and adaptive immune system to microbial invasion.

In addition to phagocytosis and direct killing of microbes by oxygen (O_2^-, H_2O_2, $\cdot OH$) and nitrogen-dependent (NO) reactive molecules, macrophages generate several ligands and proteins that contribute to microbial killing. Ligands include arachidonic acid pathway components such as leukotriene B4. Proteins include lysozyme, lactoferrin, transferrin, and defensins (Zhang et al., 2000). In addition, a number of macrophage-derived mediators initiate the inflammatory response and recruit neutrophils to the local area, including cytokines such as TNF-α, IL-1, granulocyte-macrophage CSF (GM-CSF), granulocyte CSF (G-CSF), IL-12, IFN-γ, and the chemokines and chemotactic peptides IL-8, macrophage inflammatory proteins (MIPs), macrophage chemotactic peptide (MCP), and other related chemokines (Sibille and Reynolds, 1990; Standiford et al., 1996; Zhang et al., 2000).

Thus macrophages located at critical sites throughout the body detect invading microbes, ingest and kill them, and recruit other professional phagocytes and neutrophils. The macrophage alerts the cells of both natural and adaptive immunity to microbial invasion and orchestrates the protective response through the release of cytokines and other critical mediators.

Dendritic Cells

Dendritic cells are macrophage-like cells that are less phagocytic and less adherent than macrophages and lack nonspecific esterase of macrophages (see Chapter 6). These cells may leave the skin and migrate to afferent lymphatics and regional lymph nodes. Interstitial dendritic cells are present throughout the lungs and most organs except the brain. These macrophage-like cells are very efficient at taking up material and microbial antigens by endocytosis and processing these in lysosomal compartments for presentation in the context of class II human leukocyte antigen (HLA) molecules. Thus these cells serve an important role in adaptive immunity.

Neutrophils

Neutrophils are critical components of early natural defenses (Yang et al., 1999) (see Chapter 5). These cells are the first to migrate into a local area of microbial invasion in response to the macrophage-derived mediators and cytokines mentioned earlier, as well as to microbial products such as formylated peptides. These cells possess individual receptors for complement fragments such as C5a, formylated peptides, LTB$_4$, and chemokines such as IL-8. The receptors initiate intracellular responses through α-, β-, and γ-guanosine triphosphate–binding proteins, which, when stimulated, lead to activation of phosphotidylinositol-specific phospholipase C. This enzyme, in turn, converts phosphytidylinositol biphosphate into diacylglycerol and inositol triphosphate, which activates protein kinase C and releases intracellular calcium, respectively.

Through these signaling pathways, binding of inflammatory mediators to their receptors on neutrophils induces changes in their surface charge, membrane potential, ion flux, membrane fluidity, degranulation, and upregulate surface expression of adhesive glycoproteins such as the leukocyte selectin, sialyl-Lewis X, and the integrins, CD11/CD18 (Hill, 1987; Yang et al., 1999). Sialyl-Lewis X promotes the intermittent binding of neutrophils to endothelial cell selectin (E-selectin), causing margination and rolling along the endothelium, whereas the integrins Mac-1 (CD11b/18) and gp-150/95 bind to endothelial cell intracellular adhesion molecule-1 (ICAM-1), resulting in firm binding in the area nearest to the site of microbial invasion.

Movement of neutrophils is initiated when the trimeric G proteins activate additional small G proteins of the Rho family, which, along with calcium binding to calmodulin, activates the contraction of cytoskeleton actin and myosin. This leads to diapedesis and chemotaxis of the cells toward the inflammatory focus along a gradient of inflammatory mediators. Movement is partially dependent on interactions between Mac-1 (CD11b/CD18), as well as the other integrins (Bohnsack, 1992; Bohnsack and Zhou, 1992), and the extracelluar matrix. When the neutrophil arrives at the site of microbial invasion, the cell is surrounded by chemotactic mediators, so that no gradient of these factors exists.

At this point the cells spread out and upregulate several phagocytic receptors, including receptors for the Fc fragment of immunoglobulin and for C3b (complement receptor 1 [CR1]), iC3b (CR3, CD11b/CD18), fibronectin, and other nonspecific receptors of the natural immune system.

Neutrophils ingest microbial invaders opsonized with natural antibodies, complement fragments, or nonspecific opsonins such as fibronectin using the phagocytic receptors mentioned above (Gresham et al., 1986). The pathogens are then killed employing oxygen-dependent or independent processes, as well as oxygen-independent antimicrobial factors (see also Chapters 5 and 22). Phagolysosome fusion permits entry of granule contents into the phagocytic vacuole. Myeloperoxidase from primary or azurophilic granules catalyzes the production of hypochlorite ion from chloride and hydrogen peroxide, which can react with amines to produce toxic chloramines (Zhang et al., 2000). Other components of the azurophilic granules possess strong antibacterial activities, including defensins, lysozyme, bacterial permeability increasing (BPI) protein, and other factors describe later in this chapter (Borregaard and Cowhand, 1997). Lastly, the neutrophil also can produce a number of proinflammatory cytokines, including TNF-α, IL-1β, IL-6, and MIP-2 (Xing, et al., 1994).

In summary, the neutrophil plays a critical early role in natural defense, responding rapidly to microbial invasion in response to inflammatory mediators released at the site of infection. The neutrophil is the cell primarily responsible for the uptake and intracellular killing of most bacterial pathogens and some yeast and fungi and is therefore a critical cell in natural immunity and a major effector cell of adaptive immunity. Patients with congenital and acquired defects in neutrophil (and macrophage) function, as well as neutropenic individuals suffer severe skin, tissue, pulmonary, and even gastrointestinal infections (see Chapter 20).

Natural Killer Cells

Natural killer (NK) cells are non-B, non-T cells (lacking surface immunoglobulins and T-cell antigen receptors) that are essential components of the adaptive immune system (Whiteside and Herberman, 1994) (see Chapter 6). These cells often are larger and more granular than other lymphocytes (sometimes termed large granular lymphocytes), and compose 5% to 20% of the blood mononuclear cells and up to 45% of tissue-infiltrating lymphocytes (Whiteside and Herberman, 1989).

Natural killer cells can recognize and kill cells transformed by viruses or tumors and allogeneic blast cells. Recognition of target cells can be facilitated by antibody coating of the target cell, leading to binding to CD16 (FcγRIIIa), the low-affinity receptor for the Fc fragment of IgG1 and IgG3. This is a function of the adaptive immune system if somatically rearranged antibody is involved and is termed antibody-dependent cellular cytotoxicity (ADCC). Another means by which NK cells recognize target cells is by a reduced expression of class I HLA molecules on the target cell surface, which can result from virus infection or malignancy.

At least two types of receptors exist on NK cells, which inhibit binding in the presence of normal class I HLA expression on target cells: killer inhibitory receptors (KIR) and heterodimers of an invariant protein, CD94. These receptors prevent NK cells from attacking normal cells with normal class I HLA expression. Other molecules involved in attachment of NK cells to target cells include the CD2 antigen and integrin molecules (Abbas et al., 2000).

The exact mechanisms by which NK cells induce cytotoxicity remain controversial. After contact with target cells, there is calcium-dependent organization of intracellular organelles and subsequent granule release. The granule contains perforin and granzyme A, which can induce holes on the target cell surface and subsequent cytolysis (Henkart and Yue, 1988; Kupfer et al., 1985). Granule release, as well as release of cytokines such as TNF-α and TNF-β, promote apoptosis and induce NK cytotoxicity (Richards et al., 1989; Valiante and Trinchieri,1993). Perforin appears to be particularly significant in inducing membrane pores of approximately 50 Å, allowing other granule contents to enter the target cell, and promoting apoptosis with DNA fragmentation (Podack, 1992; Shi et al., 1992; Trapani and Smyth, 1993).

Natural killer cells also release a variety of cytokines, including TNF-α, TNF-β, IFN-γ, GM-CSF, and CSF-l (Seaman,1996). In turn, several cytokines enhance NK activity, notably IL-2, IL-12, IL-15, IFN-α, IFN-β, and IFN-γ.

NK-Cell Deficiencies

Although there is little direct evidence that NK cells reduce the occurrence of malignancies (Seaman, 1996), patients with Chediak-Higashi syndrome have deficient NK activity and an increased incidence of lymphoreticular malignancies (Whiteside and Herberman, 1994) (see Chapter 17). NK cells may participate in natural immunity to viruses. Biron and colleagues (1989) described a patient who lacked NK-cell activity who suffered severe herpesvirus infections, including varicella, cytomegalovirus, and herpes simplex infection. NK activity is decreased in patients with acquired immunodeficiency disease (AIDS) but not in asymptomatic human immunodeficiency virus (HIV) infection (Scott-Algara et al., 1992; Welsh and Vargas-Cortez, 1992).

Other conditions associated with persistently low numbers or activity of NK cells include deficiency of CD11/CD18 adhesive glycoproteins (leukocyte adhesion defect-1 [LAD-1]), X-linked lymphoproliferative syndrome, leukemia, breast cancer at the time of diagnosis, various viral infections, chronic fatigue syndrome, depression, chronic stress, and certain autoimmune disease (Whiteside and Herberman, 1989, 1994) (see Chapter 17). Persistently high NK-cell activity may be seen in chronic or acute large granular lymphocyte proliferation and some hepatic diseases (Hata et al., 1991).

NK Cells in Disease

Natural killer cells also appear to be important in protection against intracellular infections, such as those due to *Listeria monocytogenes* and *Toxoplasma gondii* (Bancroft et al., 1991; Gazzinelli et al., 1993; Tripp et al., 1993). These pathogens induce macrophages to secrete the NK-cell–activating cytokines IL-12 and IL-15, which in turn induce NK cells to produce IFN-γ. This NK-cell–derived IFN-γ then stimulates macrophages to kill these intracellular pathogens. Newborn infants have depressed NK-cell activity, which might contribute to their susceptibility to these two pathogens, as well as to herpesvirus and cytomegalovirus (Ching and Lopez, 1979; Kohl et al., 1981) (see Chapter 22).

NK cells are found in increased numbers in the epithelium of humans with GVHD, where they are in close association with necrotic cells, a hallmark of the disease. This may result from the local production of IL-2 and IFN-γ by CD4+ T cells. NK cells stimulated with IL-2 demonstrate enhanced cytotoxicity for a variety of cells. These lymphokine-activated killer (LAK) cells have been used in treating certain human malignancies (Abbas et al., 2000). They have demonstrated only limited clinical success in treating patients with advanced malignancies.

Mast Cells

Mast cells are the chief effector cells of the allergic response, contributing to the early vascular reaction and exudation phase and to the late phase of leukocyte accumulation (Fearon and Locksley, 1996; Mekori and Metcalfe, 2000). Mast cells also interact with certain microorganisms, leading to mast cell activation, mediator release, and bacterial clearance in certain model systems (Mekori and Metcalfe, 2000). IL-3, c-kit ligand, and stem cell factor (SCF) are the major cytokines involved in mast cell differentiation, maturation, and proliferation. Mast cells are located strategically in tissues that interface with the external environment, where they can react to a variety of stimuli. Recent evidence suggests that mast cells play a central role in both natural and adaptive immunity (Galli et al., 1999).

Mast cells can be activated by IgE-mediated interaction with allergens or in vitro by the addition of anti-IgE antibodies, which crosslinks the IgE and causes aggregation of FcεRI. This in turn initiates the release of mediators, including histamine, arachidonic acid pathway metabolites (leukotriene C4, prostaglandin D2, and platelet-activating factor), proteases, proteoglycans, and cytokines (TNF-α, IL-3, IL-4, IL-5, IL-6, IL-10, IL-13, IL-14, Il-16, GM-CSF, SCF, and certain chemokines) (Mekori and Metcalf, 2000).

Mast cells can also be activated by microbial pathogens, their products, and nonspecific components of the natural immune system. Other small peptide mediators, including substance P, endothelin, and MIP-1, as well as plasma-derived fragments of fibrinogen and fibronectin and the complement-derived anaphylotoxins, C3a and C5a, can also stimulate mast cell activation (Alam et al., 1994; Ansel et al., 1993; Columbo et al., 1996; El-Lati et al., 1994; Wojtecka-Lukasik and Maslinski, 1992; Yamamura et al., 1994).

Mast cell activation by microbes such as *Salmonella typhimurium* and *Schistosoma mansoni* may be opsonin dependent and are mediated by complement fragments, including C3b and iC3b (Sher, 1976; Sher et al., 1979). Bacteria such as *Escherichia coli* and *Klebsiella pneumoniae*, as well as *Leshmania* parasites, may associate with mast cells in an opsonin-independent manner through mast cell pattern receptors and their corresponding ligands on microbes (Arock et al., 1998; Bidri et al., 1997; Malaviya et al., 1994). The pattern recognition receptor on mast cells for the mannose-binding lectin of type 1 fimbriae (FimH) on *E. coli* and other enterobacteria appears to be a mannose-containing receptor molecule, CD48 (Malaviya et al., 1999). In addition, gram-positive bacteria such as *Staphylococcus aureus* and streptococci appear to be able to induce mast cell mediator and cytokine release (Arock et al., 1998).

Mast cell activation mediates leukocyte recruitment and enhances defenses against microbial invasion (Echtenbacher et al., 1996; Malaviya et al., 1996). The effects on leukocyte recruitment are mediated, in part, by TNF-α stimulation of vascular and bronchial ICAM-1, leading to increased adherence of leukocytes in the area of mast cell degranulation. Histamine can upregulate selectins and promote leukocyte rolling along the endothelium. Platelet-activating factor (PAF) may also enhance CD18-dependent leukocyte adhesion (Gaboury et al., 1995). Mast cells may release IL-8 and stimulate migration of neutrophils to sites of microbial invasion.

Mast cells can phagocytize and kill both gram-positive and gram-negative bacteria, employing oxidative and nonoxidative microbicidal mechanisms such as the production of superoxide and hydrogen peroxide and the secretion of granule-associated enzymes (Abraham and Arock, 1998, Arock et al., 1998; Malaviya, 1994). Mast cells can present antigen, in the context of class I or II HLA molecules, to cells of the adaptive immune system (Mecheri and David, 1997). Mast cells or their products play an important role in the defense against parasitic infections (Metcalfe et al., 1997). Mast cell activation and hyperplasia are prominent in intestinal helminthic infections. The cells or their mediators may damage parasites directly or stimulate intestinal contraction and mucus secretion to expel the organisms (Mekori and Metcalfe, 2000).

In spite of animal data indicating a role for mast cells in natural and adaptive immunity, there is no known human disease resulting from a functional defect or absence of mast cells, which leads to recurrent infections (Mekori and Metcalfe, 2000). Mast cells and their products, therefore, may play a secondary role in natural defense that is not essential if other systems are fully operative.

γδ-T Lymphocytes

The late response to viral, bacterial, and parasitic infections includes infiltration with γδ-T lymphocytes (Born et al., 1999). γδ-T cells have a limited diversity of T-cell receptors encoded in the germ line rather than by somatic mutation, unlike αβ-T cells. The γδ-T cell receptors recognize glycolipid antigens present on many microbes and thus function more in the natural immune system than in the adaptive one (Abbas et al., 2000). When located in the epithelial linings of the skin and gastrointestinal and respiratory tracts, they are also termed intraepithelial T lymphocytes. These cells accumulate in the lesions of several autoimmune disorders, including rheumatoid arthritis and multiple sclerosis, where they may downregulate the inflammatory response (Carding and Egan, 2000).

They also accumulate at the site of infections and play a key role in host defense. γδ-T cells are particularly prominent in mycobacterial infection, in which they proliferate and release cytokines (Munk et al., 1991; Kabelitz et al., 1990). A decrease in γδ-T cells reactive to mycobacteria are observed in patients with adrenal disease and positive sputum cultures, both possibly the result of Fas-Fas ligand–mediated apoptosis induced by exposure to mycobacterial products. Carding and Egan (2000) suggest that poor outcome in some patients may result from failure of γδ-T cells to downregulate the inflammatory granulomatous response directly and through the action of cytokines.

B1 Lymphocytes

The peritoneal cavity contains B lymphocytes termed B1 cells, which express the CD5 antigen (Hardy and Hayakawa, 1994). The antigen receptors of these cells are encoded both by the germ line and by somatic mutation but have very limited diversity, much like intraepithelial γδ-T cells (Abbas et al., 2000; Gommerman and Carroll, 2000). B1 cell receptors bind immunoglobulins, mainly IgM, which are reactive with common microbial antigens such as lipopolysaccharide and phosphorylcholine. These cells alone function more in natural than adaptive immunity. B1 lymphocytes produce natural antibodies, which function as preformed opsonins reactive against a variety of microbes likely to penetrate the epithelial barriers. These natural antibodies may also be self-reactive, directed to antigens such as DNA or phosphatidylcholine.

NATURAL OPSONINS

Nonspecific opsonins play a major role in the natural immune system, binding invading microbes to cells of the natural immune system. Without these natural opsonins, pathogens could overwhelm the host before specific opsonic antibody could be generated. These natural opsonins include natural antibodies, complement fragments C3b and iC3b, fibronectin, and C reactive protein.

Natural Antibodies

Natural antibodies are antibodies present in normal sera without specific antigen stimulation (Boyden, 1966). They may be self-reactive or autoreactive or reactive against a variety of viral, fungal, and bacterial pathogens (Avrameas and Ternynck, 1993; Coutinho et al., 1995; Ochsenbein et al., 1999). Natural antibodies are the products of B1 lymphocytes, which develop predominantly during fetal and neonatal development (Hardy and Hayakawa, 1994). They are most often of the IgM isotype but also may be IgG and IgA. The repertoire of these natural antibodies is much more limited because of preferential usage of J_H proximal V_H gene segments and because of the lack of terminal deoxynucleotidyl transferase activity, resulting in less chance of somatic mutation occurring in B-cell ontogeny (Yancopoulos, et al., 1984; Feeney, 1990). A large proportion of these antibodies are reactive to phylogenetically conserved components such as nucleic acids, carbohydrates, phospholipids, and heat shock proteins.

Function of Natural Antibodies

Natural antibodies serve as a second line of defense after an organism has breached the epithelial or mucosal barrier. Because many of these natural antibodies are IgM with 10 antigen-combining sites per molecule, they are excellent activators of the complement system. They also bind well to repeating moieties of polysaccharides. Because many microorganisms share structural polysaccharides and phospholipids, natural antibodies protect against a variety of pathogens. Mice lacking natural antibody have enhanced susceptibility to bacterial peritonitis, reduced cytokine expression (especially TNF-α), and higher mortality rates from infection (Boes et al., 1998). Ochsenbein and colleagues (1999) found that natural antibody–deficient mice have increased replication of vesicular stomatitis virus, lymphocytic choriomeningitis virus, and L. monocytogenes during experimental infection.

Natural antibody prevents viral dissemination to parenchymal organs and directs viruses and bacteria to the lymphoid organs, where subsequent adaptive immune responses come into play. Natural antibodies are present with polyreactive specificities in the serum of normal children at stable concentrations over years (Mirilas et al., 1999). Trauma may activate B1 cells and increase levels of natural antibodies.

Role of Self-Reactive Antibodies and Xenotransplantation

Natural antibodies may play a pathogenic role in autoimmune disease, or they may act, in concert with complement and other factors, to remove autoreactive clones and thus prevent autoimmune disease (Gommerman and Carroll, 2000). Xenoreactive natural antibodies (antibodies against another species) are a major hurdle in xenotransplantation (e.g., pigs to humans); development of methods to inhibit these antibodies is underway (Bracy et al., 1998).

Complement

Complement is an important component of the natural immune system. Chapter 7 describes this complex series of interacting proteins in detail; thus only the role of the complement system in innate immunity is detailed here. The classic complement pathway is triggered primarily by antigen-antibody complexes or aggregated IgG or IgM. Natural IgM and IgG antibodies can trigger the complement system, with classical pathway activation and formation of the inflammatory components C3a, C4a, and C5a, and opsonic fragments C3b and iC3b (Johnston, 1993). Mannose-binding protein, described later, combines with mannose-containing microbial components to activate the complement pathway (Schweinle et al., 1989). C reactive protein can bind directly with C1q to activate the classic pathway.

Complement fragments can also be generated by the alternative pathway, which is triggered by complex polysaccharides, lipopolysaccharides, snake venoms, yeast, bacterial cell wall components, and aggregated IgA and IgE. The alternative pathway is a major source of opsonins for the natural immune system. Phagocytic cells of the natural immune system have receptors for C3b (CR1), iC3b (CR3), and CR4 that allow them to ingest, process, and kill pathogens (Abbas et al., 2000). C1q-coated particles can be ingested by macrophages. The terminal complement components, C5 to C9, can lyse some bacteria, notably *Neisseria* species and some *E. coli*.

Complement also may have a protective role early in viral infections when antibody concentrations are absent or low. When animal RNA viruses interact directly with C1q, activation of the classic pathway result in viral lysis (Johnston, 1993). Thus complement plays an important role in natural and adaptive immunity to bacteria, yeast, and viral pathogens.

Complement Defects

Defects in the complement system (described in Chapter 21) can affect its function in natural immunity. In general, deficiencies of complement components lead either to autoimmune disorders with deposition of immune complexes in the skin, joints, and kidneys (C1, C4, C2) or bacteremia due to inadequate opsonization (C4, C2, C3) or bacteriolysis (C5–C8). The most common bacte-

ria are *Streptococcus pneumoniae, Neisseria meningitidis* or *Neisseria gonorrhea* (Figueroa and Densen, 1991). Newborns have low serum levels of most complement components but especially C9 (Lassiter et al., 1992) and factor B of the alternative pathway (Hill et al., 1977). Patients with nephrotic syndrome lose factor B in their urine and thus are susceptible to polysaccharide-coated bacteria.

Splenectomized individuals, who may have inadequate alternative pathway opsonic activity, as well as absence of an early IgM response, have markedly increased susceptibility to sepsis (see Chapter 30).

Fibronectin

Fibronectin (Fn), fibrinogen, C reactive protein (CRP), and MBP in plasma and tissue fluid bind, in a nonspecific fashion, to certain microbes and enhances their ingestion and killing (Abbas et al., 2000). Fibronectin is a high-molecular-weight glycoprotein (440 kD) that participates in a number of complex processes, including hemostasis, wound healing, cell migration and differentiation, and phagocytosis (Yang et al., 1993).

Fibronectin binds to organisms such as *S. aureus, Staphylococcus epidermidis,* and *Streptococcus pyogenes* to promote their interactions with phagocytic cells, including macrophages and neutrophils (Proctor et al., 1982; Simpson et al., 1982; Yang et al., 1988). Proctor (1987) noted that Fn promotes the binding of *S. aureus* to neutrophils but not ingestion, unless the cell is first activated by a mediator such as fMLP.

Hill and colleagues (1984) reported that Fn increases the uptake of antibody-coated group B streptococci (GBS) by human neutrophils and enhances the survival of mice after GBS infection. Jacobs and co-workers (1985) made similar observations utilizing macrophages. Yang and colleagues (1988) also found that Fn increases the respiratory burst, as well as phagocytosis and intracellular killing of *S. aureus* and *S. epidermidis* by human neutrophils in the absence of antibody, probably through functional binding of organisms to Fn receptors on phagocytic cells. In contrast, GBS and *E. coli* uptake and killing are also enhanced by Fn only in the presence of opsonic antibody.

Fibronectin activates phagocytic cells through integrin receptor binding to an Arg-Gly-Asp (RGD)–containing sequence (Hill et al., 1993). Binding of Fn to this receptor on neutrophils, monocytes, or macrophages enhances the respiratory burst of the cells and alters actin polymerization (Yang et al., 1994) and the release of TNF-α (Peat et al., 1995). Thus Fn serves a role in both natural and adaptive immunity by promoting attachment, uptake, and killing of antibody-coated bacteria.

Fibronectin Deficiency

Subjects with reduced levels of plasma fibronectin include normal newborn infants; neonates with respiratory distress and perinatal asphyxia and sepsis; and patients with severe trauma, septic shock, or severe burns (Akiyama and Yamada, 1983; Barnard and Arthur, 1983; Ganrot, 1972; Gerdes et al., 1983; Hill et al., 1983, 1984; Lanser et al., 1980; Saba et al., 1978, 1986; Yang et al., 1993; Yoder et al., 1983).

Saba and colleagues (1978, 1986) showed that administration of cryoprecipitate containing Fn or purified Fn improves the opsonic deficiency in these patients. Grossman (1987), reviewing six prospective control trials of Fn administration in adults with sepsis, concluded that such therapy increases Fn levels in survivors compared with nonsurvivors but has no significant effect on survival or major organ function. Thus Fn may contribute to the host's susceptibility to infection, but replacing Fn does not improve clinical outcome.

CARBOHYDRATE PATTERN RECOGNITION RECEPTORS

An important feature of the natural immune system is that it recognizes and limits infectious challenge prior to the development of an adaptive immune response. Much work defining this system has come from studies on *Drosophila*, which is uniquely resistant to microbial infections (Hoffmann et al., 1999). This resistance is derived primarily from proteolytic cascades leading to (1) blood clotting and the generation of opsonic fragments; (2) phagocytosis of pathogens; and (3) the synthesis of antimicrobial peptides. Mammals have evolved similar systems, which are phylogenetically related to those of *Drosophilia* (Hoffmann et al., 1999; Imler and Hoffman, 2000).

One important distinction between adaptive and natural immunity is the process of immune recognition. The B-cell immunoglobulin and T-cell receptors in adaptive immunity are generated somatically, resulting in approximately 10^{14} and 10^{18} different specificities, respectively (Medzhitov and Janeway, 2000a). This diversity requires time to develop and expand the multiple specific clones of cells in order to deal with the full spectrum of microbial invasion. In contrast, the natural immune system has many fewer microbial receptors (numbered in the hundreds), which instead of recognizing every possible antigen recognize limited number of highly conserved molecular structures common to many pathogens. These structures, termed PAMPs, are produced only by microbes and not by host cells (Janeway, 1989; Medzhitov and Janeway, 2000a). They serve to distinguish self from nonself for both the innate and adaptive immune system.

PAMPs are often critical to the survival or pathogenicity of many organisms. Gram-positive bacteria would not survive without peptidoglycan to provide structural integrity for its cell wall. Gram-negative bacteria would be much less pathogenic without LPS and its endotoxin properties. Gram-negative and gram-positive bacteria, mycobacteria, and fungi employ LPS, lipoteichoic acid (LTA), lipoarabinomannan, and mannans, respectively, as molecular patterns (Medzhitov

and Janeway, 2000b). Although this model may not work for some viruses, double-stranded RNA is recognized by double-stranded RNA protein kinase employing a pattern recognition mechanism. Viral- or tumor-transformed cells may be recognized by changes in lipid composition or glycosylation patterns on the cell surface.

In response to PAMPs, animals have evolved a series of pattern recognition receptors (PRRs) early during phylogeny, because there are many homologies between *Drosophila* and humans (Medzhitov and Janeway, 2000a; Hoffman et al., 1999). These receptors are expressed on most effector cells of the natural immune system, including macrophages, dendritic cells, and B1 cells, but are also secreted into the plasma or tissue fluid or contained intracellularly as cytoplasmic proteins. PRRs employ a number of different protein domains, including the C-type lectin domains, leucine-rich repeats, and cysteine-rich domains. Secreted PRRs can opsonize pathogens or trigger the complement system, whereas cell-bound or intracellular PRRs may promote uptake of microbes or transmit signals that initiate secretion of cytokines and antimicrobial peptides.

Collectins

The collectins are a family of PPRs, including conglutinin, MBP, and surfactant proteins A and D, which contain collagen and lectin domains and share biologic activities (Hoffmann et al., 1999). They possess an N-terminal cysteine-rich region, a collagen-like region, an α helical coiled neck region, and a carbohydrate recognition domain. The basic structure of the collectin is a trimer of the polypeptide chain held together by the collagen-like component with an α helical coiled neck region (Lawson and Reid, 2000). The collectins include conglutinin (a tetramer), MBP (a tetramer or hexamer), and the surfactant proteins A (a hexamer) and D (a tetramer), which are homotrimeric proteins of the C-type lectin family that bind carbohydrates on bacteria, yeast, and viruses (Feizi, 2000).

Conglutinin

Conglutinin, present in bovine serum, binds preferentially to high-mannose–containing oligosaccharides (Man_8 and Man_9) but also to fucose-containing oligosaccharides and to N-acetylglucosamine–terminating glycans (Solis et al., 1994; Mizuochi et al., 1989). Conglutinin binds to and agglutinates iC3b-coated particles through an interaction with mannose oligosaccharides on the α chain of the molecule (Feizi, 2000).

Mannose-Binding Protein

MBP, or mannose-binding lectin (MBL), is probably the best characterized of the PRR collectins (Turner, 1996). It contains a collagenous domain attached to a calcium-dependent lectin domain that binds to high-mannose N-glycans with five to nine mannose residues

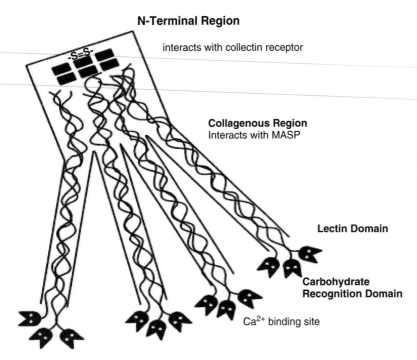

N-Terminal Region

interacts with collectin receptor

Collagenous Region
Interacts with MASP

Lectin Domain

Carbohydrate Recognition Domain

Ca²⁺ binding site

Figure 10-1 · Mannose-binding protein tetramer. MASP = MBP-associated serine protease. (Adapted from Turner MW. Mannose-binding lectin: the pluripotent molecule of the innate immune system. Immunol Today 7:532–540, 1996.)

(Man$_5$ to Man$_9$ N-glycans) (Solis et al., 1994) and to N-acetylglucosamine (Fig. 10-1). It can appear in serum as a dimer, trimer, tetramer, pentamer, and hexamer; human MBPs are mostly trimers, tetramers, and pentamers.

MBPs bind to carbohydrate structures on grampositive and gram-negative bacteria, yeast, parasites, and some viruses (Epstein et al., 1996). The selectivity of human MBP is N-acetylglucosamine > mannose > N-acetylmannosamine and fucose > maltose > glucose and N-acetylgalactosamine. MBP can bind to highmannose N-glycans on the envelope glycoprotein (gp120) of HIV, as well as to influenza virus (Ezekowitz et al., 1989; Hartley et al., 1992), where it may have a role in protection. Antitumor activity has been ascribed to MBP because of its binding to a colorectal carcinoma cell line in vitro. MBP can prolong life in tumor-bearing mice (Ma et al., 1999).

MBP is associated with two serine proteases (MBP-associated serine proteases-1 and -2 [MASP-1 and MASP-2]), which are closely related to the C1r and C1s serine proteases of the classic complement pathway. (Indeed, MBP is structurally related to C1q.) MASP-1 and MASP-2 are activated when MBP binds to microbial ligands, leading to the generation of C3 convertase activity and breakdown of C3 to inflammatory mediators (C3a and C5a), opsonins (C3b and iC3b), and activation of the terminal complement pathway lytic activity (Fig. 10-2) (Epstein et al., 1996; Medzhitov and Janeway, 2000a). Microbial pathogens bound by MBP in the blood or tissue fluid are then opsonized and phagocytocized or lysed by the complement system without the presence of antibody.

MASPs have been identified in lamprey and tunicates (a sea vertebrate), and C3 is present in sea urchins and tunicates, suggesting these may have been the early ancestors of the complement system (Hoffmann et al., 1999).

MBP DEFICIENCY

MBP is encoded on the long arm of chromosome 10, close to the genes for surfactant protein D (SP-D), SP-A1, and SP-A2 (Turner, 1996). Deficiency of MBP is a relatively common disorder associated with increased susceptibility to bacterial, fungal, and viral infections, usually beginning early in life prior to the development of adaptive immunity (Sumiya et al., 1991; Super et al., 1989; Turner, 1996). Individuals with homozygous or heterozygous deficiency of MBP who are infected with HIV have shorter survival times than wild-type genotypes with normal MBP levels (Garred et al., 1997). The disorder is characterized by low serum concentrations of MBP (Madsen et al., 1994; Super et al., 1989; Wallis and Cheng, 1999). Furthermore, the proteins present are not the large oligomeric structures present in normal serum but are low-molecular forms (Lipscombe et al., 1992).

These patients usually suffer from recurrent upper respiratory infections, otitis media, chronic diarrhea of infancy, and failure to thrive in the first year of life (Sumiya et al., 1991; Super et al., 1989). The disorder was first recognized as a defect of yeast opsonization before the molecular basis of the disease was determined (Candy et al., 1980; Miller et al., 1968; Richardson et al., 1983; Soothill and Harvey, 1976). It may be present in as high as 5% to 7% of the general population (Soothill and Harvey, 1976). Deficiency of MBP may also contribute to the severity and progression of infection later in life.

Three different point mutations in the MBP gene have been documented, which result in amino acid substitutions in the N-terminal collagen-like domain of the pro-

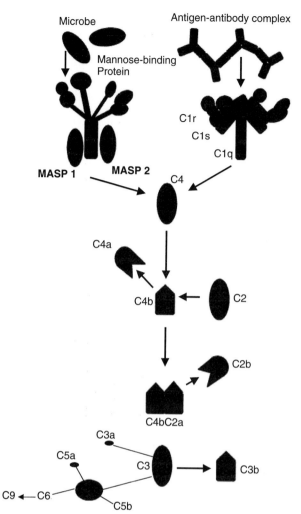

Figure 10-2 · **Activation of the classic complement pathway by MBP and microbes.** (Adapted from Medzhitov R, Janeway C Jr. Innate immunity. N Engl J Med 343:338–344, 2000.)

glycine, resulting in profoundly reduced MBP concentrations with a distorted collagen helix.

A third mutation occurs in codon 52, resulting in a cysteine replacement for arginine, which has less effect on MBP concentrations (reviewed in Turner, 1996).

Deficiency of MBP may represent one of the more common defects of the natural or innate immune system leading to an immune deficiency disorder. Like IgA deficiency, there may be minimal manifestations or marked symptomatic clinical manifestations. MBP levels and MBP polymorphisms should be sought.

The median MBP concentration for 10 children with a functional opsonic defect was 4.9 µg/L (range 2.5–35.0 µg/L), compared with 143 µg/L (range 2.5–880 µg/L) in normal pediatric patients, as determined by a mannose-binding enzyme-linked immunoassay (Super et al., 1989).

Surfactant Proteins

Pulmonary surfactant is a complex mixture of proteins and lipids that promotes normal respiratory function and enhances lung host defense (Crouch, 1999; Lawson and Reid, 2000). Two surfactant proteins, SP-A and SP-D, belong to the PRRs termed collectins. These are products of alveolar type II cells and bronchiolar epithelial cells following stimulation with LPS or lung injury during the third trimester of pregnancy.

Initial reports indicated that surfactant improves macrophage killing of *S. aureus* (LaForce et al., 1973). SP-A and SP-D bind to certain bacteria, viruses, yeast, and fungi to promote their attachment to phagocytic cells via Fc and complement receptors (CR1), thus enhancing their elimination (Geertsma et al., 1994; Lawson and Reid 2000). SP-A and SP-B bind to gram-positive and gram-negative bacteria; *Pneumocystis carinii;* fungi such as *Aspergillus;* yeast, including *Cryptococcus neoformans*, bacteria such as *Hemophilus influenzae*, as well as *Herpes simplex* virus, *Mycobacterium tuberculosis;* and *Mycoplasma pulmonis* (Gaynor et al., 1995; Hickman-Davis et al., 1998; Kabha et al., 1997; Madan et al., 1997a; McNeely and Coonrod, 1994; O'Riordan et al., 1995; Schelenz et al., 1995; Stamme and Wright, 1999; Tino and Wright, 1996; Van Iwaarden et al., 1992; Zimmerman et al., 1992). SP-A and especially SP-D form large aggregates with viruses such as influenza, which may promote its mucociliary clearance (Crouch et al., 2000).

The surfactant collectins stimulate neutrophil and macrophage chemotaxis, actin polymerization, respiratory burst activity, and nitric oxide production. SP-A knockout mice cannot kill mycoplasma via NO-dependent mechanisms. They also have abnormalities in neutrophil recruitment and production of toxic oxygen and nitrogen intermediates and defective phagocytosis and killing of certain organisms (Lawson and Reid, 2000). These knockout mice develop disseminated GBS infection following intratracheal inoculation and have diminished clearance of *S. aureus* and *Pseudomonas aeruginosa*, reversed by administration of SP-A to SP-A (LeVine et al., 1997, 1998, 1999).

tein (Lipscombe et al., 1992, 1995; Madsen et al., 1994; Sumiya et al., 1991). Wallis and Cheng (1999) have created these mutations in rat MBP, which result in alterations in the size of the molecules, disruption of the normal oligomeric state, and decreased ability to interact with complement. The functional defect is dependent on the specific mutation involved. In fact, all the mutations result in abnormal interaction of MBP with the complement system.

In humans, a mutation in codon 54 of the first exon of the MBP gene results in an abnormal protein (aspartic acid for a glycine), which impairs the structural stability of the collagenous region and results in low levels of MBP. This mutation is inherited in an autosomal co-dominant fashion (reviewed in Turner, 1996). Homozygous deficiency is associated with markedly depressed MBP levels, whereas the heterozygotes have levels approximately one eighth of normal (Turner, 1996); both may be susceptible to infections.

Mutations in codon 57 of exon 1 have been identified in symptomatic patients from sub-Saharan Africa. This mutation results in a glutamic-acid substitution for

Lectins on the macrophage bind to N-linked carbohydrates and the collagenous stalks of the SP (Lawson and Reid, 2000). SP-A binds, in order of preference, to N-acetylmannoseamine > L-fucose > maltose > glucose > mannose and dimannose repeating units of gram-negative polysaccharide capsules (Crouch et al., 2000). SP-D binds to maltose > glucose, mannose, fucose >galactose, lactose, glucosamine > N-acetylglucosamine and the glucose-containing core oligosaccharides of gram-negative bacterial LPS. SP-A and SP-D bind rough but not smooth LPS from organisms such as *E. coli, K. pneumoniae,* and *P. aeruginosa.* SP-A and LPS subsequently bind to macrophages via CD14-dependent and -independent mechanisms, increasing TNF-α release (Sano et al., 1999; Stamme and Wright, 1999).

Thus SP-A and SP-D function as molecular flypaper by clumping pathogens and promoting adherence to inflammatory cells (Lawson and Reid, 2000; Acton et al., 1993). Furthermore, they may downregulate T cells and their cytokine responses and suppress the response to inhaled allergens (Madan et al., 1997b; Wang et al., 1998). The human genes for SP-A, SP-A1, SP-A2, and SP-D are located in a tight cluster on chromosome 10 (10q22.2–q23.1).

PULMONARY SURFACTANT DEFICIENCY

Deficiencies of surfactant are observed in premature infants and patients with cystic fibrosis, respiratory syncytial virus infection, and acute respiratory distress syndrome (likely due to destruction of the proteins by neutrophil elastase). Reduced SP-D opsonization has been observed in diabetic mice because of simple competition by free glucose for SP-D binding sites (Lawson and Reid, 2000).

Selectins

Selectins are adhesion molecules that facilitate neutrophil rolling along the vascular endothelium. Selectins include leukocyte selectin (L-selectin or sialyl-Lewis X) and the endothelial selectins, E-selectin and P-selectin, which have lectinlike domains (Bevilacqua and Nelson, 1993). L-selectin binds lipid-linked galactose with sulfate residues. P-selectin binds sulfotyrosine, and E-selectin binds fuco-oligosaccharides present on leukocytes, epithelial cells, and some tumor cells (Feizi, 2000). Deficiency of L-selectin (sialyl-Lewis X) results in LAD-2 (see Chapter 20), which is associated with decreased leukocyte infiltration, resulting in a poor inflammatory response and neurologic and developmental abnormalities.

LPS Binding Protein, CD14, and Toll-Like Signaling Receptors

Bacterial LPS is a major virulence factor of gram-negative bacteria, capable of inducing massive activation and cytokine release from macrophages and other cells. The polysaccharide groups of LPS vary considerably from microbial species to species, and even between strains of the same species, permitting bacteria such as *E. coli* to be serotyped. In contrast, the lipid of LPS is generally highly conserved, allowing binding to phylogenetically developed (Hoffmann et al., 1999), germline–derived PRRs of the natural immune system (Abbas et al., 2000).

The primary cellular receptor for LPS is CD14, a glycosylphosphatidyl inositol–linked protein (Diamond et al., 2000). CD14 was first identified on phagocytic cells but also occurs on many other cells. Binding of LPS to CD14 is markedly potentiated by lipopolysaccharide-binding protein (LBP), a normal component of the serum (Fig. 10-3). Binding of LPS to LBP greatly enhances the sensitivity of effector cells to LPS, allowing activation and cytokine release to occur in subpicomolar LPS concentrations (Hoffmann et al., 1999). LBP also contributes to clearance of LPS-containing bacteria; mice lacking LBP or CD14 are much more susceptible to infection. CD14 has no cytoplasmic domain but is closely associated with signal-transducing receptors known as Toll-like receptors.

The ancestors of these receptors were first described in *Drosophila* (fruit flies) (Rock et al., 1998). *Drosophila* require Toll proteins in order to resist fungal pathogens; flies lacking Toll receptors cannot produce an antifungal peptide, drosomycin (Lemaitre et al., 1996). Flies lacking another Toll-like receptor (18-Wheeler) have increased susceptibility to gram-negative bacteria and failure of synthesis of the anti–gram-negative peptide, attacin (Williams et al., 1997). *Drosophila,* lacking an adaptive immune system, have at least eight Toll-like proteins, which have the ability to respond to different microbial pathogens (Lemaitre et al., 1997; Medzhitov and Janeway, 2000a).

Studies with knockout mice indicate that TLR4 is associated with responses to gram-negative bacteria through recognition of LPS, whereas TLR2 recognizes lipoteichoic acid and peptidoglycan of gram-positive bacteria (Flo et al., 2000; Schwandner et al., 1999; Yoshimura et al., 1999). Other members of the Toll family of receptors probably recognize other PAMPs.

TLRs show structural homology with the type I IL-1 receptor (Gay and Keith, 1991). Engagement of Toll in *Drosophila* activates a transcription factor, Dorsal, which is an analog of nuclear factor κB (NF-κB) in mammals that is activated by LPS (Abbas et al., 2000).

The signal transduction pathway after TLR receptor activation in humans is complex (see Fig. 10-3). First an adaptor protein, MyD88, is recruited to the Toll/IL-1 receptor domain (TIR) of the TLR, where it associates with a protein kinase, IL-1R–associated kinase (IRAK) (Medizhitov et al., 1998; Muzio et al., 1998; Wesche et al., 1997). IRAK is then autophosphorylated, which causes it to disassociate from MyD88 and then associate with tumor necrosis–associated factor (TRAF). TRA, in turn activates an NF-κB–inducing kinase (NIK) and IκB kinase (IKK), which leads to disassociation of NF-κB from IκB. This is followed by nuclear translocation of NF-κB and transcription of many proinflammatory cytokines (reviewed in Diamond et al., 2000;

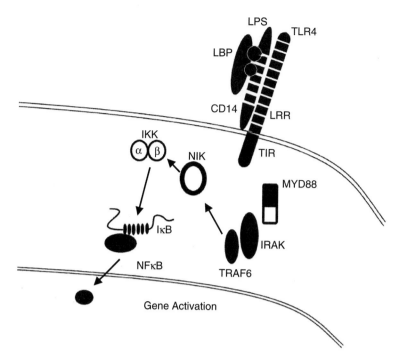

Figure 10-3 · Lipopolysaccharide binding and signaling pathway in macrophages. IKK = IκB kinase; IRAK = IL-1 receptor–associated kinase; LRR = leucine-rich domain; MAP3K = mitogen-activated protein 3 kinase; TIR = Toll/IL-1 receptor domain; TRAF-6 = tumor necrosis factor receptor (TNFR) associated factor 6; MyD88 = adaptor protein. (Adapted from Hoffman et al. Phylogenetic perspectives in innate immunity. Science 234:1313–1318, 1999.)

Medzhitov and Janeway, 2000a). Thus LBP, CD14, TLRs, and the NF-κB pathway are all critical to natural defense against pathogenic microbes.

Bacterial Permeability-Increasing (BPI) Factor

BPI is a 55-kD PRR present in neutrophil granules, which contain two domains, one of which binds with LPS to increase membrane permeability and lysis of gram-negative bacteria, whereas the other promotes opsonization (Hoffmann et al., 1999). Neutrophil BPI functions best in inflamed tissues, where it acts in concert with defensins and the membrane attack complex of complement to cause lysis.

Neonates have reduced release and activity of BPI, perhaps contributing to their enhanced susceptibility to gram-negative bacterial infections (Levy et al., 1999). Recombinant BPI (rBPI) has been used as an adjunct to antimicrobial therapy in children with severe meningococcal sepsis (Levin et al., 2000); 14 of 193 patients with severe meningococcal disease who received rBPI (2 mg/kg over 30 minutes) died, compared with 20 of 203 control infants, an insignificant difference. Among the treated patients, fewer needed severe amputations and more had good functional outcome, suggesting a beneficial effect in decreasing complications. More studies are needed.

NATURAL ANTIMICROBIAL AGENTS

Antimicrobial peptides, first described in insects in 1981 (Steiner et al., 1981), have now been found in all multi-cellular organisms, including, plants, insects, and humans (Hoffmann, 1999). *Drosophila* produces at least seven different peptides with antibacterial and fungal activity, including cecropins, drosocin, diptericin, attacin, drosomycin, and metchnikowin. Humans also express cecropins, but by far the most important antimicrobial peptides are the α and β defensins. These are contained in phagocytic cell primary (or azurophilic) granules, first at the promyelocytic stage, and in secondary or specific granules (Table 10-2).

Defensins

The defensins are strongly cationic, single-chain peptides with molecular weights between 3 and 4.5 kD that share a consensus motif of six cysteines with three intramolecular disulfide bridges. Defensins make up 50% of the protein content of the neutrophil primary granules (Ganz and Weiss, 1997; Zhang et al., 2000). These are divided into α- and β-defensins. These peptides possess broad antimicrobial activity against gram-positive and gram-negative bacteria, fungi, mycobacteria, and some envelop viruses. The defensins create voltage-sensitive pores in microbial membranes, resulting in lysis. Humans have six human α defensins (HD-1 to HD-6) and two human β defensins (HBD-1 and HBD-2).

The α-defensins, HD-1 to HD-6, are made primarily by neutrophils and comprise 30% to 50% of the primary granule content (Harwig et al., 1994). Defensins appear at the site of inflammation. They are present after neutrophil degranulation induced by LPS, IL-8, C5a, and other stimuli. They are also found on the epithelial surfaces of the bronchi and in the bronchial

TABLE 10-2 · CONTENTS OF PRIMARY (AZUROPHILIC) AND SECONDARY (SPECIFIC) GRANULES OF NEUTROPHILS

Primary Granules	Secondary Granules
Myeloperoxidase	Lysozyme
Hydrolases	Lactoferrin and transferrin
Lysozyme	Collagenase
Bacterial permeability–increasing protein	Plasminogen activator
Cathepsin G	Vitamin B_{12}–binding protein
Elastase	Histaminase
Proteinase 3	Adhesion receptors
Azuricidin	Flavocytochrome of NADPH oxidase
Defensins	

lavage fluid of patients with various types of inflammatory lung disease. The antimicrobial activity of defensins are inhibited by high salt content, which may be important in decreasing microbial activity of ASF in cystic fibrosis (Goldman et al., 1997).

The β-defensins are produced by epithelial cells of the respiratory and gastrointestinal tracts (Boman, 2000; Selsted and Ouellette, 1995). HBD-1 is expressed constitutively by epithelial cells in the bronchi and intestine, whereas HBD-2 synthesis is upregulated by inflammatory stimuli, including LPS, TNF-α, bacterial infection, and injury. Thus HBD-1 acts to kill organisms in the absence of inflammation, and HBD-2 acts primarily as part of the inflammatory process.

In inflammatory lung disease, such as chronic bronchitis and chronic obstructive lung disease, both αHD-1 to HD-6 defensins and β HBD-2 may be increased significantly, perhaps contributing to airway inflammation and cell death (Zhang et al., 2000). There are no clinical disorders of defensin production, except that low concentrations are observed in specific granule deficiency. Defensins as potential pharmacologic agents are under study.

Lactoferrin and Transferrin

Lactoferrin and transferrin are iron-binding proteins with antibacterial activity to certain iron-requiring bacteria (Baggiolini et al., 1970). Lactoferrin in lysosomal granules may provide intracellular iron necessary for the generation of hydroxyl radicals by the Haber-Weiss reaction of the respiratory burst. Hydroxyl radical contributes significantly to oxygen-dependent microbicidal activity (see Chapters 5 and 20).

In addition to its role in microbicidal activity, lactoferrin also contributes to leukocyte adherence and chemotaxis (Oseas et al., 1981). Patients with absence of specific granules who lack lactoferrin have impaired neutrophil adherence and chemotaxis, corrected by adding lactoferrin (Boxer et al., 1982; Gallin et al., 1982; Yang et al., 1999). This disorder is apparently transmitted by autosomal recessive inheritance. Lactoferrin may also be directly toxic to some bacteria (Kalmar and Arnold, 1988).

Lysozyme

Lysozyme, present in primary and secondary granules of neutrophils, is an antimicrobial component present in inflammatory exudates, nasal secretions, and alveolar surface fluid. (Diamond et al., 2000). Lysozyme is a small cationic enzyme that hydrolyzes glycosidic bonds and thus disrupts the peptidoglycan structural components of some gram-positive bacterial cell walls. This, along with its strong cationic properties, contributes to the destruction of certain gram-positive bacteria. Lysozyme can be present in concentrations up to 1 mg/ml in sputum and 10 ug/ml in ASF, where it may be an important component of the natural defense system (Harbitz et al., 1984; Travis et al., 1999).

There are no known deficiencies of lysozyme. High concentrations are present in some patients with rapid neutrophil destruction, such as in acute and chronic myelocytic and myelomonocytic leukemia, acute and chronic infections, and autoimmune gastrointestinal disorders.

Myeloperoxidase

Myeloperoxidase is the most abundant enzyme in the primary or azurophilic granules of phagocytes. It catalyzes the reaction between chloride and hydrogen peroxide to form hypochlorite ion, a potent microbicidal agent of the respiratory burst (Yang et al., 1999). Bacterial killing takes almost twice as long if this enzyme is missing.

Myeloperoxidase Deficiency

Both congenital and acquired forms of myeloperoxidase deficiency exist (see Chapter 20). The congenital form may sometimes be associated with disseminated candidiasis (Lehrer and Cline, 1969; Salmon et al., 1970). The gene for myeloperoxidase is located on chromosome 17 (Weil et al., 1987). Myeloperoxidase deficiency may also be observed in monomyelocytic leukemia, which is sometimes associated with recurrent abscesses (Davis et al., 1971). Deficiency of myeloperoxidase in approximately 1 in 2000 individuals may also be asymptomatic.

Chediak-Higashi syndrome (oculocutaneous albinism, recurrent pyogenic infections, and giant lysosomal granules) is associated with a defect in lysosomal membrane fusion (Barbosa et al., 1996; Nagle et al., 1996). The giant granules are primary, azurophilic granules with a high content of myeloperoxidase, which cannot discharge their granule contents. Thus there is a functional deficiency of myeloperoxidase and delayed microbial killing. In addition, these giant granules impede neutrophil migration and chemotaxis (see Chapter 20).

Serprocidins

The serprocidins are a family of cationic proteins present in primary granules with structural homology to serine proteases. These include cathepsin G, a chymotrypsin-like protease, which interferes with the microbial membrane and metabolism of gram-positive and gram-negative bacteria (Odeberg et al., 1975).

Azurocidin is another cationic protein with activity against gram-negative bacteria, potentiated by cathepsin G and elastase (Miyasaki and Bodeau, 1992; Spitznagel, 1990). Elastase and proteinase 3 are other members of the serocidins with antimicrobial activity, alone or in combination with other granule peptides.

LL-37/CAP-18 is a cathelicidin found in alveolar macrophages, ASF, and bronchial epithelial cells (Bals et al., 1998) with broad-spectrum antimicrobial activity.

REACTIVE OXYGEN AND NITROGEN SPECIES

Reactive Oxygen Species

The phagocytic cells of the natural defense system, upon stimulation by microbes or their products (Yang et al., 1999), undergo a respiratory burst through activation of NADPH oxidase; this results in the generation of superoxide (O_2^-). NADPH oxidase consists of a flavocytochrome b_{558} composed of a $gp91^{phox}$ heavy chain and a $p22^{phox}$ light chain, along with two cytosolic proteins, $p47^{phox}$ and $p67^{phox}$, and a small G protein, p21 Rac (Wientjes et al., 1996). The NADPH oxidase transfers a single electron to molecular oxygen, thus forming the highly reactive superoxide anion. Superoxide dismutase converts superoxide to hydrogen peroxide (H_2O_2), which in the presence of iron and myeloperoxidase forms hydroxyl radical (Yang et al., 1999).

Each of these reactive oxygen species possess potent intracellular microbicidal activity but also can escape from the cells to kill organisms in the tissue or damage host tissues. The latter occurs in some infections, reperfusion injury, autoimmunity, and acute respiratory distress syndrome (Lefkowitz et al., 1995; McCord et al., 1994).

Because the respiratory burst requires molecular oxygen, Grief and associates (2000) studied the effect of supplemental oxygen on wound infection. They provided 250 patients undergoing colorectal surgery with 80% O_2 during surgery and for 2 days afterward. A control group was given 30% O_2. There were 13 infections in the 80% O_2 group and 28 infections in the 30% O_2 group, a significant reduction (p = 0.01). Additional studies are needed to confirm these observations, as well as to exclude adverse effects of oxygen toxicity to the retina, central nervous system, and lungs (see Chapter 5).

Defects in the respiratory burst, including chronic granulomatous disease and myeloperoxidase deficiency, are described in detail in Chapter 20 and will not be discussed here except to note that the major oxygen-dependent microbicidal activity of the effector cells of both the innate and adaptive immune system are profoundly affected in these disorders. This can lead to frequent and often overwhelming bacterial and fungal infections at the epithelial surfaces of the skin, respiratory tract, and gastrointestinal tract.

Nitric Oxide

Nitric oxide, an endogenously produced lipophilic free radical, results from the conversion of arginine and oxygen into citrulline through the enzymatic action of nitric oxide synthetase (Hibbs et al., 1987; Michel and Feron, 1997). Nitric oxide synthetase (NOS) has three isoforms: (1) constitutively expressed NOS-1 (nNOS) is present in neuronal tissue; (2) NOS-3 (eNOS) is present in endothelial cells (Bred and Snyder, 1989; Michel and Feron, 1997; Palmer et al., 1988); and (3) NOS-2 inducible (iNOS) is present in many tissues. NOS-1 and NOS-3 are normally present in low amounts to generate NO for neurotransmission and vasodilation (Moncada et al., 1991).

In contrast, the third isoform, NOS-2 (iNOS), can be induced by microbial products (including LPS and gram-positive bacterial superantigens) (Forstermann et al., 1995; Nathan, 1997; Sriskandan et al., 1996) and inflammatory cytokines (including TNF-α, IL-1β, and IFN-γ) and serves as a major bactericidal and tumoricidal agent (Fang, 1997; Hibbs et al., 1987; Liew and Cox, 1991) that can modulate the immune response (Allione et al., 1999; Bingisser et al., 1998). Nitric oxide can also cause tissue damage through release of free radicals and activation of apoptosis (Brune et al., 1995; Cross et al., 1994; Singer et al., 1996).

Nitric oxide has a critical role in adaptive immunity to such intracellular pathogens as M. tuberculosis and L. monocytogenes. Macrophages are unable to kill mycobacteria unless they are stimulated by IFN-γ, derived mostly from CD4 memory T cells. However, natural killer cells, γδ-T cells, and macrophages can produce IFN-γ and induce NO synthesis through iNOS activation. The role of NO in the early phase (1 to 2 days) of the immune response has been studied. Mice infected with K. pneumoniae produce large amounts of NO within 48 hours of infection, which helps to limit bacterial growth. Treatment with a NOS inhibitor, L-arginine methyl ester (L-NAME), increases bacteria in the blood and lungs and decreases survival (Tsai et al., 1997).

NO also enhances the activity of NK cells and changes their responsiveness to an IFN-γ–inducing cytokine, IL-12 (Bogdan et al., 2000). Low concentrations of NO improve the function of the signaling pathway of IL-12 in NK cells by increasing phosphorylation of signal transducer and activator of transcription 4 (STAT4) in response to IL-12. This serves to increase IFN-γ production by NK cells and enhance microbial defenses (Bogdan et al., 2000). Knockout mice lacking iNOS have 15- to 25-fold less IFN-γ messenger RNA (mRNA) production following Leishmania major infection than normal mice (iNOS$^{+/+}$). This defect is present in NK cells but not in T cells. The response to L. major infection in the iNOS$^{-/-}$ mice is also associated with increased production of the immunosuppressive cytokine, TGF-β. In humans, production of IFN-γ in response to staphylococcal and streptococcal super-antigens is also decreased by the iNOS inhibitor N-monomethyl-L-arginine (Sriskandan et al., 1996).

Nitric oxide may also limit cell damage and death in certain autoimmune disorders, such as experimental autoimmune encephalopathy and infection-induced liver damage (Brunet, et al., 1999; O'Brien et al., 1999), probably through its ability to control cytokine production, influence T-cell apoptosis, influence Fas and Fas-ligand interactions, increase corticosteroid production, and improve vascular perfusion.

CYTOKINES

In response to microbial invasion, most cells of the natural and adaptive immune system produce cytokines, which function in an autocrine (affecting the cell producing the cytokine), paracrine (affecting cells nearby), and endocrine (affecting cells at distant sites in the body) fashion. Macrophages, NK cells, neutrophils, mast cells, and γδ-T cells produce cytokines critical in the early response to microbial invasion. Antigen-activated T and B lymphocytes also produce cytokines (lymphokines) that can activate or recruit effector cells of the innate immune system to kill microbes. Lymphocytes, macrophages, and stromal cells of the bone marrow produce CSFs, which promote the growth and differentiation of immature leukocytes (Abbas

et al., 2000; La Pine and Hill, 1994). In this section we consider cytokines that mediate natural immunity (Table 10-3), notably TNF, IFNs, ILs, and CSFs. The appendix lists other cytokines and their function.

Tumor Necrosis Factor

TNF-α and lymphotoxin (TNF-β) are structurally related; they bind to the same receptors with equal affinity and elicit similar biologic effects. TNF-α is synthesized as a 25-kD precursor transmembrane protein that is cleaved and secreted as a 17-kD fragment, which often circulates as a 51-kD homotrimer (Abbas et al., 2000). TNF-α is primarily the product of macrophages and other antigen-presenting cells, NK cells, and activated mast cells of the natural immune system but can be produced by antigen-activated T cells. TNF-β is synthesized by T lymphocytes. Tumor necrosis factor was so named because it was initially reported to cause hemorrhagic necrosis of some tumors (Carswell et al., 1975; Haranaka et al., 1985; Old, 1985). It has also been termed cachexin because it caused cachexia in malignancy, probably through activation of lipoprotein lipase (Beutler et al., 1985; Kawakami and Cerami, 1981).

TNF-α and IL-1 are the major mediators in gram-negative endotoxin shock (Beutler and Cerami, 1986; Movat, 1987; Movat et al., 1987; Tracey et al., 1988). This occurs when TNF-α activates neutrophils, stimulating their adhesion to vascular endothelial cells and

TABLE 10-3 · CYTOKINES OF THE NATURAL IMMUNE SYSTEM

Cytokine	Size	Source	Target Cell and Effect
IL-1	17 kD	MACs, monocytes, endothelial and epithelial cells	Hypothalamus: fever Liver: acute-phase reactants (APR) Endothelial cells: adhesion
TNF-α	17 kD	MACs, monocytes, NK cells, mast cells	Neutrophil and endothelial cell activation Hypothalamus: fever Liver: APR Muscle, fat catabolism Apoptosis
IL-6	26 kD	MACs, monocytes, fibroblasts, endothelial cells	Liver: APR B-cell proliferation Enhances GM-CSF and G-CSF
IL-8	8–10 kD	MACs, monocytes, endothelial cells, fibroblasts	Neutrophil activation and chemotaxis
MCP-1	8–10 kD	MACs, monocytes, endothelial and other cells	Macrophage activation and chemotaxis
MIP-1α	8–10 kD	MACs, monocytes, decidual cells	Macrophage activation and chemotaxis
IFN-α	15–21 kD	MACs, monocytes	Antiviral state in all cells
IFN-β		Fibroblasts	Upregulates class I HLA antigens
IFN-γ	20–25 kD 20–25 kD	NK cells, CD4+ and CD8+ T cells	Activates NK cells Antiviral state, upregulates class I and II HLA antigens, activates MACs, NK cells, neutrophils
IL-12	70 kD	MACs, monocytes, B cells	Enhances IFN-γ production by T cells and NK cells, MAC activation
IL-15		MACs, monocytess	NK cell activation and proliferation, T-cell activation and proliferation
IL-18	17 kD	MACs, monocytes, osteoclasts, keratinocytes	NK cell activation and IFN-γ production by NK and CD4+ T cells
GM-CSF	14–35 kD	T cells, MACs, endothelial cells, fibroblasts	Precursors of monos, MACs, neutrophils, platelets, RBC growth and differentiation
G-CSF	18–22 kD	MACs, endothelial cells, fibroblasts	Neutrophil progenitor, growth and differentiation Activation and function of neutrophils

MACs = macrophages; RBC = red blood cell.

inducing production of toxic oxygen products (Berkow et al., 1987; Koivuranta-Vaara et al., 1987; Salyer et al., 1990; Tsujimoto, et al., 1986; Zhang et al., 2000). If TNF-α production is excessive, toxic oxygen products damage endothelial cells and cause fluid leak and hypovolemia. TNF-α also depresses cardiac contractility, leading to shock. Multiple stimuli induce TNF-α production. These include gram-positive bacteria and their products (including peptidoglycans, lipoteichoic acids, and pyogenic exotoxins) (Fast et al., 1989; Mancuso et al., 1994; Vallejo et al., 1996; Williams et al., 1993); nonspecific mediators, such as fibronectin, C5a, and surfactant proteins (Kremlev and Phelps, 1994; Okusawa et al., 1988; Peat et al., 1995; Schindler et al., 1990); and lactic acid (which is elevated in septic shock) (Steele et al., 1998).

TNF-α knockout mice, or normal mice pretreated with anti–TNF-α monoclonal antibody, have increased susceptibility to experimental bacterial infection. In vitro, human mononuclear cells stimulated by GBS first generate TNF-α, followed by IL-1, IL-6, IL-8, and IFN-γ (Kwak et al., 2000). In experimental models of GBS, anti–TNF-α monoclonal antibody therapy, administered early following infection (but not before), improves survival, probably by limiting the potentially fulminant cytokine cascade (Teti et al., 1993). Use of the TNF-α receptor fusion protein (etanercept) or TNF-α monoclonal antibody (rituximab) in patients with rheumatoid arthritis and inflammatory bowel disease may predispose to sepsis and activation of tuberculosis (Zhang et al., 2000). TNF-α has other properties similar to IL-1 as defined in the next section.

IL-1

IL-1 is produced predominantly by macrophages and macrophage-like cells but also by endothelial and epithelial cells. It was originally described as a co-stimulator of T-cell proliferation, probably because of its ability to upregulate IL-2 receptors on T cells rather than having a direct effect on mitogenesis. Like TNF, IL-1 is synthesized as a 33-kD precursor that is cleaved to generate the biologically active 17-kD protein. There are two forms of IL-1, IL-1α and IL-1β, encoded by two separate genes, which are 30% homologous, but, like the two forms of TNF, bind to the same IL-1 receptors. There are two IL-1 receptors that bind to the two forms of IL-1 with different affinities; these are present on different cells at different concentrations throughout the body.

Unlike TNF-α, IL-1 does not directly activate neutrophils but rather upregulates endothelial expression of adhesive glycoproteins, such as ICAM-1, thus promoting neutrophil attachment and the inflammatory response (Bevilacqua et al., 1985). IL-1 also promotes IL-6, IL-8, and other chemokine production by macrophages. IL-1, along with TNF-α, induces prostaglandin E_2 production in the hypothalamus, raising the body thermostat and increasing the body temperature through peripheral vascular contraction and

induction of shivering. Fever serves a nonspecific protective role against a number of microbes that grow less well at increased temperature.

IL-1, TNF-α, and especially IL-6 (which is produced by macrophages in response to IL-1 and TNF-α) cause production and release of acute-phase reactants by the liver, including α1-antitrypsin, haptoglobin, C reactive protein, serum amyloid P protein, complement components, and fibrinogen. All play roles in natural immunity against infection. As noted, excess production of IL-1 and TNF-α contribute to the production of the septic shock syndrome (Cannon et al., 1990).

IL-1 is the only cytokine with a natural inhibitor, IL-1 receptor antagonist (IL-1Ra), produced by the same cells that produce IL-1, which functions as a competitive antagonist to IL-1. IL-1Ra downregulates the proinflammatory effects of IL-1 and thus may be a potential anti-inflammatory agent. It has been shown to reduce mortality from endotoxin shock in experimental animals (Ohlsson et al., 1990).

IL-6

IL-6 is a 26-kD cytokine produced mainly by macrophages and mononuclear cells but also by fibroblasts and endothelial cells. IL-6 is produced in response to TNF-α, IL-1, and microbes and their products (Abbas et al., 2000; La Pine and Hill, 1994). After cellular activation, IL-1 and TNF-α production occurs, followed by IL-6 synthesis; IL-6 levels may remain elevated longer than these other two cytokines. IL-6 does not activate neutrophils or induce cytotoxicity but does increase the production of acute-phase reactants. IL-6 promotes the growth of B cells, stimulates antibody production, and enhances T-cell proliferation. IL-6 also enhances the activity of hematopoietic growth factors, such as G-CSF and macrophage colony-stimulating factor (M-CSF), thus playing a role in both natural and adaptive immunity.

IL-8

IL-8 is a member of the chemokine family of small cytokines (8 to 10 kD) that induce cell mobility. The chemokines are divided into two groups, depending on if the two amino terminal cysteine residues are adjacent (Cys-Cys) or are separated by an amino acid (Cys-X-Cys) (Baggiolini et al., 1994). This latter group, termed α-chemokines, is produced predominantly by mononuclear phagocytes but also by endothelial cells and fibroblasts. They act predominantly on neutrophils, promoting their activation and movement into inflammatory sites.

IL-8, one of the best-described Cys-X-Cys chemokines, is strongly chemotactic for neutrophils and thus plays an important role in the response of natural immunity to microbial invasion. Richman-Eisenstat and colleagues (1993) noted increased chemotactic activity in the sputum of patients with cystic fibrosis, bronchiectasis, and bronchitis, along with high levels of IL-8. The IL-8–induced chemotactic activity was inhibited by anti–IL-8 monoclonal antibody. Aerosolized inhibitors of IL-8 have been used in cystic fibrosis patients to decrease lung inflammation (Strober and James, 1988; McElvaney et al., 1992). IL-8 is a major factor in recruitment of neutrophils to the lung in bacterial pneumonia, thus serving as a crucial early defense mechanism (Greenberger et al., 1996; Standiford et al., 1996).

Chemokines: MIPs, MAPs, and RANTES

Chemokines of the Cys-Cys structure (β-chemokines) are usually produced by activated T cells and act on T cells and monocytes (Abbas et al., 2000; Baggiolini et al., 1994). One of these is RANTES (an acronym derived from its gene and gene-product properties: *Regulated upon Activation, Normal T Expressed and Secreted*), which is produced by activated T cells and which acts on CD4$^+$ T cells and monocytes (Schall, et al., 1988). These Cys-Cys chemokines are components of the adaptive immune system.

MCP-1 is a chemokine produced by activated macrophages (and endothelial and other tissue cells) and has a chemotactic effect on monocytes. Another β-chemokine, αMIP-1α, attracts and activates monocytes and macrophages (Baggiolini et al., 1994; Dudley et al., 1997). MIP-1α is released when mononuclear or decidual cells are exposed to organisms such as group B streptococci and to bacterial components such as lipoteichoic acid (Danforth et al., 1995; Dudley et al., 1997). Cook and associates (1995), using knockout mice, showed that MIP-1α plays an important role in the inflammatory response to influenza and coxsackie infection.

Interferons

The interferons are cytokines between 18 and 20 kD produced by a variety of cells; they function in both natural and acquired immunity. Interferons are divided into type I interferons, which include IFN-α and IFN-β, and type II or immune IFN (IFN-γ). The type I interferons, IFN-α and -β, share a common receptor, induce similar responses, and are encoded on chromosome 9p21 by a cluster of intronless genes. IFN-α and IFN-β have 30% amino acid homology. In contrast, IFN-γ (type II IFN) has a distinct receptor separate from that of IFN-α and IFN-β. IFN-γ is also structurally distinct from the type I interferons and is encoded on chromosome 12p24.

Type I Interferons (IFN-α, IFN-β)

IFN-α actually consists of a family of 20 structurally related polypeptides encoded by separate genes, whereas IFN-β is a 20-kD polypeptide encoded by a single gene (Abbas et al., 2000). IFN-α is the product of mononuclear phagocytes and has been known as leukocyte IFN, whereas IFN-β is produced by fibroblasts and is known as fibroblast IFN. The major stimuli for type I IFN production are viral infections or experimental exposure to synthetic double-stranded RNA. In addition, the synthesis of both type I IFNs are stimulated by the adaptive immune response to antigens in response to T-cell–derived factors.

IFN-α and IFN-β have identical cellular receptors and identical biologic actions. They inhibit viral replication, probably through stimulation of the production of 2′,5′-oligoadenylate synthetase, which in turn interferes with RNA or DNA replication. Patients who produce IFNs in inadequate amounts suffer severe progressive or fulminant viral disease (Levin and Hahn, 1985). IFNs also inhibit cell proliferation, enhance the lytic potential of NK cells, and increase cellular expression of class I HLA antigens while decreasing expression of class II HLA antigens (Abbas et al., 2000).

IFN-α is used clinically as an antiproliferative and antiviral agent to treat Kaposi's sarcoma (Groopman et al., 1984; Krown et al., 1983; Lane et al., 1988), hairy cell leukemia (Itri, 1992; Quesada et al., 1984), and hepatitis B and C (Davis et al., 1989; Di Bisceglie et al., 1989; Perrillo, 1989).

Type II Interferons (IFN-γ)

IFN-γ (immune IFN) is a 20- to 25-kD glycoprotein (depending on the degree of glycosylation) encoded by a single gene on chromosome 12p24 (Hill, 1993; Hill et al., 1991). It is produced by CD4$^+$ and CD8$^+$ T cells and by NK cells and thus is a component of both the adaptive and the natural immune systems. T-cell IFN-γ production occurs following antigen stimulation in the presence of IL-2, IL-12, and IL-18. IFN-γ also has antiviral and antiproliferative activity and upregulates both class I and class II HLA molecule expression. It enhances cellular cytotoxicity through upregulation of class I molecules and assists in antigen presentation by enhancing class II HLA expression.

Although IFN-γ is produced by T-helper 1 (Th1) CD4$^+$ T cells in response to antigen stimulation, it is also produced by NK cells of the natural immune system. Moreover, activated macrophages can generate cytokines (IL-12, IL-15, and IL-18), which induce NK cell activation and IFN-γ production and enhance macrophage antibacterial activity. This positive feedback of the natural immune system is a key defense mechanism before adaptive immunity commences.

IFN-γ Deficiencies

IFN-γ activates mononuclear phagocytes and neutrophils, resulting in enhanced killing of phagocytized microbes and intracellular pathogens such as *Mycobacteria* and *Listeria*. Patients with defects in IFN-γ receptors suffer severe infections with *Mycobacteria* and related pathogens (Dorman and Holland, 2000; Holland, 2000) (see Chapter 17).

IFN-γ is the key inducer of iNOS in macrophages, resulting in the generation of NO from arginine, an important bactericidal and tumoricidal component. IFN-γ also enhances the chemotactic activity of newborn neutrophils (Hill, 1993; Hill et al., 1991). Newborns have a deficiency in the transcription and production of IFN-γ and IL-12 (Bryson et al., 1980; Wilson et al., 1986; Joyner et al., 2000b).

IFN-γ is also decreased in the hyperimmunoglobulinemia-E (hyper-IgE) syndrome (Davis et al., 1966; Del Prete et al., 1989). Recently, Borges and colleagues (2000) showed that mononuclear cells have decreased IFN-γ responses to staphylococci. Moreover, in vitro incubation of their neutrophils with recombinant human IFN-γ significantly improves their chemotactic responsiveness (Hill, 1993; Jeppson et al., 1991).

In preliminary studies, IFN-γ administration to patients with hyper-IgE syndrome increased neutrophil responsiveness, improved eczema, and decreased respiratory symptoms (Petrak et al., 1994). Severe progressive *Aspergillus* pneumonia has been reversed in a hyper-IgE patient with IFN-γ, surgery, and antifungal therapy.

IFN-γ lowers the incidence of serious infections in patients with chronic granulomatous disease by 70% (ICGDCSG, 1991) without demonstrating an effect on their neutrophil respiratory burst. Its beneficial protective effect may involve enhanced generation of NO by phagocytic cells or increases in other nonoxidative defense mechanisms (see Chapter 20).

IL-12

Mononuclear cell production of IL-12 is an important component of the early response to microbial infection (Trinchieri, 1995). Although monocytes and macrophages are the main source of IL-12, other cells, including B cells, can also produce IL-12. IL-12 is heterodimeric with two covalently linked proteins of 40 kD (p40) and 35 kD (p35) (D'Andrea et al., 1992; Kobayashi et al., 1989). The p35 gene is constitutively expressed by most cells at low levels, whereas expression of the p40 gene and assembly of the active 70-kD heterodimer are confined to activated cells. IL-12 induces IFN-γ production by T cells and NK cells and promotes cellular cytotoxicity and lymphocyte proliferation. It is downregulated by IL-10 (Aste-Amezaga et al., 1998). IL-12 can be induced by exposure of mononuclear cells to microbes or their products, including *S. aureus*, GBS, LPS, and *Candida* (Aste-Amezaga et al., 1998; Cenci et al., 1998; Joyner et al., 2000a, 2000b; Romani et al., 1996; Snijders et al., 1996). The IL-12 receptor, composed of β1 and β2 subunits, binds IL-12 with high affinity (Presky et al., 1996).

Patients with defects in the IL-12R have been identified who develop *Mycobacteria* and *Salmonella* infections (Dorman and Holland 2000; Holland, 2000). Hyper-IgE patients have defective synthesis of IFN-γ in response to exposure to staphylococci and candida, even with added IL-12, suggesting an abnormality in the IL-12/IFN-γ pathway in these patients (Borges et al., 2000).

Decreased transcription and secretion of IL-12 and decreased IFN-γ production by newborn mononuclear cells suggest an abnormality within the IL-12/IFN-γ pathway (see Chapter 22). IL-12 can partially correct the IFN-γ deficiency (Joyner et al., 2000a). IL-12 administration to neonatal mice with group B streptococcal infection significantly improves their survival (Mancuso et al., 1997). The IL-12/IFN-γ pathway is also suppressed in older patients with critical infections (Ertel et al., 1997). In the future, IL-12 may be useful in enhancing natural and adaptive immunity.

IL-15

Interleukin-15 is a 13-kD cytokine produced by monocytes and macrophages; it resembles IL-2 in many of its activities (Abbas et al., 2000; Yoshikai and Nishimura, 2000), including stimulation of T-cell and B-cell proliferation, induction of cytokines, and production of antibodies of the adaptive immune system. It enhances NK cell activity, stimulates neutrophils, and stimulates the growth of mast cells (Yoshkai and Nishimura, 2000).

IL-18

Interleukin-18, produced by monocytes, macrophages, osteoclasts, and keratinocytes, stimulates the production of IFN-γ (Dinarello, 1999). Its structure is similar to that of IL-1β, and it is cleaved from its precursor to its active form by IL-1β–converting enzyme (caspase 1). The IL-18 receptor is also closely related to the IL-1 receptor. Receptor binding of IL-18 to its receptor recruits IRAK and IκB kinase (KIK), resulting in nuclear translocation of NF-κB, in a manner similar to the effect of TNF and IL-1 (Dinarello, 1999). IL-18 stimulates IFN-γ production using a different transcription promoter than that used by IL-12, but IL-12 and IL-18 act in a synergistic manner to enhance IFN-γ production in response to microbes and their products. IL-18 knockout mice have a near but not absolute deficiency of IFN-γ (Takeda et al., 1998), as do mice lacking caspase 1 (Ghayur et al., 1997; Gu et al., 1997).

Stimulation of NK cells with IL-18 markedly enhances their cytotoxic activity (Okamura et al., 1995; Ushio et al., 1996). IL-18 knockout mice have decreased but not absent NK activity (Takeda et al., 1998). IL-18 also stimulates CD4+ T cells and B cells to produce cytokines and antibodies. It also stimulates IL-8 production by mononuclear cells and IFN-γ production by NK cells (Puren et al., 1998). Patients with various types of leukemia have been reported to have increased concentrations of IL-18 (Taniguchi et al., 1997).

Decreased IL-18 production in cord blood mononuclear cells exposed to group B streptococci, along with their deficiency of IL-12 production, contributes to inadequate IFN-γ production and increased susceptibility to infection of human neonates (Hill et al., 2001).

Colony-Stimulating Factors

The production and function of neutrophils and macrophages is regulated in part by glycoprotein colony-timulating factors (Clark and Kamen, 1987; Groopman et al., 1989). GM-CSF is a 14-to 35-kD glycoprotein (the range of molecular weights resulting from different degrees of glycosylation) encoded on chromosome 5q23-31 that stimulates production of neutrophils, macrophages, and eosinophils (Lau et al., 1996; La Pine and Hill, 1994).

G-CSF is an 18- to 22-kD glycoprotein encoded on chromosome 17q11-21 that stimulates neutrophil production. M-CSF is a 21- to 40-kD glycoprotein encoded on chromosome 5q23-31 that stimulates monocyte production.

GM-CSF is produced by activated T cells and mononuclear phagocytes, vascular endothelial cells, and fibroblasts. It promotes the growth and differentiation of monocytes, macrophages, and neutrophils but also, to a lesser extent, platelets and progenitor red blood cells. GM-CSF activates macrophages in much the same fashion as IFN-γ. GM-CSF is produced by macrophages, fibroblasts, and endothelial cells in inflammatory sites but is not present in the circulation.

G-CSF is also produced by macrophages, fibroblasts, and endothelial cells and is present in low concentrations in the bloodstream. Microbes and their products and cytokines such as TNF-α and IL-1β stimulate the production of G-CSF (Zhang et al., 2000). G-CSF acts on neutrophil progenitors, a more mature population than neutrophil precursors stimulated by GM-CSF, to produce neutrophil maturation and release from the marrow. G-CSF also activates and enhances the function of neutrophils and macrophages (Campbell and Edwards, 2000; Hill et al., 1991; La Pine and Hill, 1994; Vadhan Raj et al., 1988; Wolach et al., 2000). G-CSF regulates neutrophil adhesion molecule expression and neutrophil adhesion, chemotaxis, respiratory burst activity, phagocytosis, and intracellular microbial killing (Roilides et al., 1991; Sullivan et al., 1993; Zhang et al., 1998). Pulmonary or systemic infection stimulates the production of G-CSF in the blood, with resultant neutrophilia and enhanced inflammatory response (Kawakami et al., 1990; Pauksen et al., 1994).

Clinical Uses of CSFs

GM-CSF is used therapeutically to stimulate the production of monocytes and neutrophils in patients with advanced malignancies (Antman et al., 1988; Fernandez et al., 2000; Lieschke et al., 1989) and aplastic anemia (Vadhan-Raj et al., 1988). English and co-workers (1992) noted decreased production of GM-CSF by stimulated neonatal mononuclear cells, T cells, and neutrophils, a possible contributing factor to the profound neutropenia that may develop with neonatal bacterial sepsis.

The use of GM-CSF in infected neonates has resulted in increased neutrophil, eosinophil, monocyte, lymphocyte, and platelet counts and some suggestion of a decrease in mortality (Bilgin et al., 2001; Venkateswaran et al., 2000). GM-CSF has also been used to treat patients with AIDS to increase neutrophil counts (Groopman et al., 1987), but there is a concern that macrophage activation could enhance HIV infection.

De Ugarte and colleagues (2002) have used GM-CSF locally to induce wound healing in patients with leukocyte dysfunction.

Congenital agranulocytosis (Kostmann syndrome), a familial disorder of severe neutropenia resulting from a maturation arrest of neutrophil precursors (Wriedt et al., 1970), has been successfully treated with G-CSF (Bonilla et al., 1989; Zeidler et al., 2000). Cyclic neutropenia also responds dramatically to G-CSF (Bonilla et al., 1994; Fink-Puches et al., 1996; Hammond et al., 1989; Heussner et al., 1995).

G-CSF production by neonatal mononuclear cells is decreased (Calhoun and Christensen, 2000; Nesin and Cunningham-Rundles, 2000), leading to the use of G-CSF in the treatment or prevention of infection in newborns. A controlled trial in neonates showed that G-CSF increased neutrophil counts but did not decrease mortality, however (Miura et al., 2001). A decrease in nosocomial infections in the second week after therapy was noted. Additional studies of G-CSF therapy in newborns are underway (see Chapter 22).

REFERENCES

Abbas AK, Lichtman AH, Pober JS: Innate immunity. In Abbas AK, Lichtman AH, Pober JS, eds. Cellular and Molecular Immunology. ed 4. Philadelphia, WB Saunders, 2000, pp 270–290.

Acton S, Resnick D, Freeman M, Ekkel Y, Ashkenas J, Krieger M. The collagenous domains of macrophage scavenger receptors and complement component C1q mediate their similar, but not identical, binding specificities for polyanionic ligands. J Biol Chem 268:3530–3537, 1993.

Abraham SN, Arock M. Mast cell and basophils in innate immunity. Semin Immunol 10:373–381, 1998.

Akiyama SK, Yamada KM. Fibronectin in disease. In Wagner B, Kaufman N, eds. Connective Tissue Diseases. Baltimore, Williams and Wilkins, 1983, pp 55–96.

Alam R, Kumar D, Anderson-Walters D, Forsythe PA. Macrophage inflammatory protein-1a and monocyte chemoattractant peptide-1 elicit immediate and late cutaneous reactions and activate murine mast cells in vivo. J Immunol 152:1298–1303, 1994.

Allione A, Bernabei P, Bosticardo M, Ariotti S, Forni G, and Novelli F. Nitric oxide suppresses human T lymphocyte proliferation through IFN-γ-dependent and IFN-γ-independent induction of apoptosis. J Immunol 163: 4182–4191, 1999.

Ansel JC, Brown JR, Payan DG, Brown MA. Substance P selectively activates TNF-α gene expression in murine mast cells. J Immunol 150: 4478–4485, 1993.

Antman KS, Griffin JD, Elias A, Socinski MA, Ryan L, Cannistra SA, Whitley M, Frei E 3d, Schnipper LE. Effect of recombinant human granulocyte-macrophage colony-stimulating factor on chemotherapy induced myelosuppression. N Engl J Med 319:593–598, 1988.

Arock M, Ross E, Lai-Kuen R: Phagocytic and tumor necrosis factor α response of human mast cells following exposure to gram-negative and gram-positive bacteria. Infect Immun 66:6030–6034, 1998.

Aste-Amezaga M, Ma X, Sartori A, Trinchieri G. Molecular mechanisms of the induction of IL-12 and its inhibition by IL-10[1]. J Immunol 160:5936–5944, 1998.

Avrameas S, Ternynck T: The natural autoantibodies system: between hypotheses and facts. Mol Immunol 30:1133–1142, 1993.

Baggiolini M, De Duve C, Masson PL, Heremans JF. Association of lactoferrin with specific granules in rabbit neutrophil leukocytes. J Exp Med 131:559–570, 1970.

Baggiolini M, Dewald B, Moser B. Interleukin-8 and related chemotactic cytokines—CXC and CC chemokines. Adv Immunol 55:97–179, 1994.

Bals R, Wang X, Zasloff M, Wilson JM. The peptide antibiotic LL-37/hCAP-18 is expressed in epithelia of the human lung where it has broad antimicrobial activity at the airway surface. Proc Natl Acad Sci USA 95:9541–9546, 1998.

Bancroft GJ, Schreiber RD, Unanue ER. Natural immunity: a T-cell-independent pathway of macrophage activation, defined in the scid mouse. Immunol Rev 124:5–24, 1991.

Barbosa MDFS, Nguyen QA, Tchernev VT, Ashley JA, Detter JC, Blaydes SM, Brandt SJ, Chotai D, Hodgman C, Solari RCE, Lovett M, Kingsmore SF. Identification of the homologous beige and Chediak-Higashi syndrome genes. Nature 382:262–265, 1996.

Barnard DR, Arthur MM. Fibronectin (cold insoluble globulin) in the neonate. J Pediatr 102:453–455, 1983.

Berkow RL, Wang D, Larrick JW, Dodson RW, Howard TH. Enhancement of neutrophil superoxide production by preincubation with recombinant human tumor necrosis factor. J Immunol 139:3783–3791, 1987.

Beutler B, Cerami A. Cachectin and tumour necrosis factor as two sides of the same biological coin. Nature 320:584–588, 1986.

Beutler B, Mahoney J, Le Trang NL, Pekala P, Cerami A. Purification of cachectin, a lipoprotein lipase-suppressing hormone secreted by endotoxin induced raw 264.7 cells. J Exp Med 161:984–995, 1985.

Bevilacqua MP, Nelson RM. Selectins. J Clin Invest 91:379–387, 1993.

Bevilacqua MP, Pober MS, Wheeler ME, Cotran RS, Gimbrone MA Jr. Interleukin-1 acts on cultured human vascular endothelium to increase the adhesion of polymorphonuclear leukocytes, monocytes, and related cell lines. J Clin Invest 76:2003–2011, 1985.

Bidri M, Vouldoukis I, Mossalayi MD, Debre P, Guillosson JJ, Mazier M, Arock M. Evidence for direct interaction between mast cells and Leishmani parasites. Parasite Immunol 19:475–483, 1997.

Bilgin KB, Yaramis A, Haspolat K, Tas MA, Gunbey S, Derman O. A randomized trial of granulocyte-macrophage colony-stimulating factor in neonates with sepsis and neutropenia. Pediatrics 107:36–41, 2001.

Bingisser RM, Tilbrook PA, Holt PA, Kees RU. Macrophage-derived nitric oxide regulates T cell activation via reversible disruption of the Jak3/STAT5 signaling pathway. J Immunol 160:5729–5734, 1998.

Biron CA, Byron KS, Sullivan JL. Severe herpesvirus infections in an adolescent without natural killer cells. N Engl J Med 320:1731–1735, 1989.

Boes M, Prodeus AP, Schmidt T, Carroll MC, Chen J. A critical role of natural immunoglobulin M in immediate defense against systemic bacterial infection. J Exp Med 188:2381–2386, 1998.

Bogdan C, Röllinghoff M, Diefenbach A. The role of nitric oxide in innate immunity. Immunol Rev 173:17–26, 2000.

Bohnsack JF. CD11/CD18-independent neutrophil adherence to laminin is mediated by integin VLA-6. Blood 79:1545–1552, 1992.

Bohnsack JF, Zhou X. Divalent cation substitution reveals CD18- and very late antigen-dependent pathways that mediate human neutrophil adherence to fibronectin. J Immunol 149:1340–1347, 1992.

Boman HG. Innate immunity and the normal microflora. Immunol Rev 173:5–16, 2000.

Bonilla MA, Gillio AP, Ruggeiro M, Kernan NA, Brochstein JA, Abboud M, Fumagalli L, Vincent M, Gabrilove JL, Welte K, Souza LM, O'Reilly RJ. Effect of recombinant human granulocyte colony-stimulating factor on neutropenia in patients with congenital agranulocytosis. N Engl J Med 320:1574–1580, 1989.

Bonilla MA, Dale D, Zeidler C, Last L, Reiter A, Ruggeiro M, Davis M, Koci B, Hammond W, Gillio A, Welte K. Long-term safety of treatment with recombinant human granulocyte colony-

stimulating factor (r-metHuG-CSF) in patients with severe congenital neutropenias. Br J Haematol 88:723–730, 1994.

Borges WG, Augustine NH, Hill HR. Defective interleukin-12/inteferon-γ pathway in patients with hyperimmunoglobulinemia E syndrome. J Pediatr 136:176–180, 2000.

Born W, Cady C, Jones-Carson J, Mukasa A, Lahn M, O'Brien R. Immunoregulatory functions of γδ T cells. Adv Immunol 71:77–144, 1999.

Borregaard N, Cowland JB. Granules of the human neutrophilic polymorphonuclear leukocyte. Blood 89:3503–3521, 1997.

Boxer LA, Coates TD, Haak RA, Wolach JB, Hoffstein S, Baehner RL. Lactoferrin deficiency associated with altered granulocyte function. N Engl J Med 307:404–410, 1982.

Boyden SV: Natural antibodies and the immune response. Adv Immunol 5:1–28, 1966.

Bracy JL, Sachs DH, Iacomini J. Inhibition of xenoreactive natural antibody production by retroviral gene therapy. Science 281:1845–1847, 1998.

Bredt DS, Snyder SH. Nitric oxide mediates glutamate-linked enhancement of cGMP levels in the cerebellum. Proc Natl Acad Sci USA 86:9030–9033, 1989.

Brune B, Messmer UK, Sandau K. The role of nitric oxide in cell injury. Toxicol Let 82/83:233–237, 1995.

Brunet LR, Beall M, Dunne DW, Pearce EJ. Nitric oxide and the Th2 response combine to prevent severe hepatic damage during Schistosoma mansoni infection. J Immunol 163:4976–4984, 1999.

Bryson YJ, Winter HS, Gard SE, Fischer TJ, Stiehm ER. Deficiency of immune interferon production by leukocytes of normal newborns. Cell Immunol 55:191–200, 1980.

Calhoun DA, Christensen RD. Human developmental biology of granulocyte colony-stimulating factor. Clin Perinatol 27:559–576, 2000.

Campbell JR, Edwards MS. Cytokines enhance opsonophagocytosis of type III group B streptococcus. J Perinatol 20:225–230, 2000.

Candy DCA, Larcher VF, Tripp JH, Harries JT, Harvey BAM, Soothill JF. Yeast opsonization in children with chronic diarrheal states. Arch Dis Child 55:189–193, 1980.

Cannon JG, Tompkins RG, Gelfand JA, Michie HR, Stanford GG, Van der Meer JW, Endres S, Lonnemann G, Corsetti J, Chernow B, Wilmore DW, Wolff SM, Burke JF, Dinarrello CA. Circulating interleukin-1 and tumor necrosis factor in septic shock and experimental endotoxin fever. J Infect Dis 161:79–84, 1990.

Carding SR, Egan PJ. The importance of γδ T cells in the resolution of pathogen-induced inflammatory immune responses. Immunol Rev 173:98–108, 2000.

Carswell EA, Old LJ, Kassel RL, Green S, Fiore N, Williamson B. An endotoxin-induced serum factor that causes necrosis of tumors. Proc Natl Acad Sci USA 72:3666–3670, 1975.

Cenci E, Mencacci A, Del Sero G, D'Ostiani CF, Mosci P, Bacci A, Montagnoli C, Kopf M, and Romani L. IFN-γ is required for IL-12 responsiveness in mice with Candida albicans infection. J Immunol 161:3543–3550, 1998.

Ching C, Lopez C. Natural killing of herpes simplex virus type 1-infected target cells: normal human responses and influence of antiviral antibody. Infect Immun 26:49–56, 1979.

Clark SC, Kamen R. The human hematopoietic colony-stimulating factors. Science 236:1229–1237, 1987.

Columbo M, Horowitz EM, Kagey-Sobotka A, Lichtenstein LM. Substance P activates the release of histamine from human skin mast cells through a pertussis toxin-sensitive and protein kinase C-dependent mechanism. Clin Immunol Immunopathol 81:68–73, 1996.

Cook DN, Beck MA, Coffman TM, Kirby SL, Sheridan JF, Pragnell IB, Smithies O. Requirement for MIP-1 alpha for an inflammatory response to viral infection. Science 269:1583–1585, 1995.

Coutinho A, Kazatchkine MD, Avrameas S. Natural autoantibodies. Curr Opin Immunol 7:812–818, 1995.

Cross AH, Misko TP, Lin RF, Hickey WF, Trotter JL, Tilton RG. Aminoguanidine, an inhibitor of inducible nitric oxide synthase, ameliorates experimental autoimmune encephalitis. J Clin Invest 93:2684–2690, 1994.

Crouch EC. Modulation of host-bacterial interactions by collectins. Am J Respir Cell Mol Biol 21:558–561, 1999.

Crouch E, Hartshorn K, Ofek I. Collectins and pulmonary innate immunity. Immunol Rev 173:52–65, 2000.

D'Andrea A, Rengaraju M, Valiante NM, Chehimi J, Kubin M, Aste-Amezaga M, Chan SH, Kobayashi M, Young D, Nickbarg E, Chizzonite R, Wolfe, SF, Trinchieri G. Production of natural killer cell stimulatory factor (NKSF/IL-12) by peripheral blood mononuclear cells. J Exp Med 176:1387–1398, 1992.

Danforth JM, Streiter RM, Kunkel SI, Arenberg DA, VanOtteren GM, Standiford TJ. Macrophage inflammatory protein-1α expression in vivo and in vitro: the role of lipoteichoic acid. Clin Immunol Immunopathol 74:77–83, 1995.

Davis AT, Brunning RD, Quie PG. Polymorphonuclear leukocyte myeloperoxidase deficiency in a patient with myelomonocytic leukemia. N Eng J Med 285:789–790, 1971.

Davis GL, Balart LA, Schiff ER, Lindsay K, Bodenheimer HC Jr, Perrillo RP, Carey W, Jacobson IM, Payne J, Dienstag JL, Van Thiel DH, Tamburro C, Lefkowitch J, Albrecht J, Meschievitz C, Ortego TJ, Gibas A. Treatment of chronic hepatitis C with recombinant interferon alpha: A multicenter randomized controlled trial. N Engl J Med 321:1501–1506, 1989.

Davis SD, Schaller J, Wedgwood RJ. Job's syndrome: recurrent "cold" staphylococcal abscesses. Lancet 1: 1013–1015, 1966.

De Ugarte DA, Roberts RL, Lerdluedeeporn P, Stiehm ER, Atkinson JB. Treatment of chronic wounds by local delivery of granulocyte-macrophage colony-stimulating factor in patients with neutrophil dysfunction. Pediatr Surg Int 18:517–520, 2002.

Del Prete G, Tiri A, Maggi E, De Carli M, Macchia D, Parronchi P, Rossi ME, Pietrogrande MC, Ricci M, Romagnani S. Defective in vitro production of γ-interferon and tumor necrosis factor-α by circulating T cells from patients with the hyper-immunoglobulin E syndrome. J Clin Invest 84:1830–1835, 1989.

Diamond G, Legarda D, Ryan LK. The innate immune responses of the respiratory epithelium. Immunol Rev 173: 27–38, 2000.

Di Bisceglie AM, Martin P, Kassianides C, Lisker-Melman M, Murray L, Waggoner J, Goodman Z, Banks SM, Hoofnagle JH. Recombinant interferon alpha therapy for chronic hepatitis C: a randomized, double-blind, placebo-controlled trial. N Engl J Med 321:1506–1510, 1989.

Dinarello CA. IL-18: A Th1-inducing, proinflammatory cytokine and new member of the IL-1 family. J Allergy Clin Immunol 103:11–24, 1999.

Dohrman A, Miyata S, Gallup M, Li JD, Chapelin C, Coste A, Escudier E, Nadel J, Basbaum C. Mucin gene (MUC 2 and MUC 5AC) upregulation by gram-positive and gram-negative bacteria. Biochim Biophys Acta 1406:251–259, 1998.

Dorman SE, Holland SM. Inteferon-gamma and interleukin-12 pathway defects and human disease. Cytokine Growth Factor Rev 11:321–333, 2000.

Dudley DJ, Edwin SS, Van Wagoner J, Augustine NH, Hill HR, Mitchell MD. Regulation of decidual cell chemokine production by group B streptococci and purified bacterial cell wall components. Am J Obstet Gynecol 177:666–672, 1997.

Echtenacher B, Mannel DN, Hultner L. Critical protective role of mast cells in a model of acute septic periotonitis. Nature 381:75–77, 1996.

El-Lati SG, Dahinden CA, Church MK. Complement peptides C3a- and C5a-induced mediator release from dissociated human skin mast cells. J Invest Dermatol 102:803–806, 1994.

English BK, Hammond WP, Lewis DB, Brown CB, Wilson CB. Decreased granulocyte-macrophage colony-stimulating factor production by human neonatal blood mononuclear cells and T cells. Pediatr Res 31:211–216, 1992.

Epstein J, Eichbaum Q, Sheriff S, Ezekowitz RA. The collectins in innate immunity. Curr Opin Immunol 8:29–35, 1996.

Ertel W, Keel M, Neidhardt R, Steckholzer U, Kremer JP, Ungethuem U, Trentz O. Inhibition of the defense system stimulating interleukin-12 interferon-γ pathway during critical illness. Blood 89:1612–1620, 1997.

Ezekowitz RAB, Kuhlman M, Groopman JE, Byrn RA. A human serum mannose-binding protein inhibits in vitro infection by the human immunodeficiency virus. J Exp Med 169:185–196, 1989.

Fang FC. Perspective series: host/pathogen interactions. Mechanisms of nitric oxide-related antimicrobial activity. J Clin Invest 99:2818–2825. 1997.

Fast DJ, Schlievert DJ, Nelson RD. Toxic shock syndrome-associated staphylococcal and streptococcal pyogenic exotoxins are potent inducers of tumor necrosis factor production. Infect Immun 57:291–294, 1989.

Fearon DT, Locksley RM. The instructive role of innate immunity in the acquired immune response. Science 272:50–53, 1996.

Feeney AJ. Lack of N regions in fetal and neonatal mouse immunoglobulin V-D-J junctional sequences. J Exp Med 172:1377–1390, 1990.

Feizi T. Carbohydrate-mediated recognition systems in innate immunity. Immunol Rev 173:79–88, 2000.

Fernandez MC, Krailo MD, Gerbing RR, Matthay KK. A phase I dose escalation of combination chemotherapy with granulocyte-macrophage-colony stimulating factor in patients with neuroblastoma. Cancer 88:2838–2844, 2000.

Figueroa JE, Densen P. Infectious diseases associated with complement deficiencies. Clin Microbiol Rev 4:359–395, 1991.

Fink-Puches R, Kainz JT, Kahr A, Urban C, Smolle J, Kerl H. Granulocyte colony-stimulating factor treatment of cyclic neutropenia with recurrent oral aphthae. Arch Dermatol 132:1399–1400, 1996.

Flo TH, Halaas Ø, Lien E, Ryan L, Teti G, Golenbock DT, Sundan A, Espevik T. Human Toll-like receptor 2 mediates monocyte activation by Listeria monocytogenes, but not by group B streptococci or lipopolysaccharide. J Immunol 164:2064–2069, 2000.

Forstermann U, Kleinert H, Gath I, Schwartz P, Closs E, Dun E. Expression and expressional control of nitric oxide syntheses in various cell types. Adv Pharmacol 37:171–186, 1995.

Fussell EN, Kaack MB, Cherry R, Roberts JA. Adherence of bacteria to human foreskins. J Urol 140:997–1001, 1988.

Gaboury JP, Johnston B, Niu XF, Kubes P. Mechanisms underlying acute mast cell-induced leukocyte rolling and adhesion in vivo. J Immunol 154:804–813, 1995.

Galli SJ, Maurer M, Lantz CS. Mast cells as sentinels of innate immunity. Curr Opin Immunol 11:53–59, 1999.

Gallin JI, Fletcher MP, Seligmann BE, Hoffstein S, Cehrs K, Mounessa N. Human neutrophil-specific granule deficiency: a model to assess the role of neutrophil-specific granules in the evolution of the inflammatory response. Blood 59:1317–1329, 1982.

Ganrot PO. Variation of the concentration of some plasma proteins in normal adults, in pregnant women and in newborns. Scand J Clin Lab Invest 124:83–88, 1972.

Ganz T, Weiss J. Antimicrobial peptides of phagocytes and epithelia. Semin Hematol 34:343–354, 1997.

Garred P, Madsen HO, Balslev U, Hofmann B, Pedersen C., Gerstoft J, Svejgaard A. Susceptibility to HIV infection and progression of AIDS in relation to variant alleles of mannose-binding lectin. Lancet 349:236–240, 1997.

Gay NJ, Keith FJ. Drosophila Toll and IL-1 receptor. Nature 351:355–356, 1991.

Gaynor CD, McCormack FX, Voelker DR, McGowan SE, Schlesinger LS. Pulmonary surfactant protein A mediates enhanced phagocytosis of Mycobacterium tuberculosis by a direct interaction with human macrophages. J Immunol 155:5343–5351, 1995.

Gazzinelli RT, Hieny S, Wynn TA, Wolf S, Sher A. Interleukin 12 is required for the T-lymphocyte-independent induction of interferon gamma by an intracellular parasite and induces resistance in T cell–deficient hosts. Proc Natl Acad Sci USA 90:6115–6119, 1993.

Geertsma MF, Nibbering PH, Haagsman HP, Daha MR, Van Furth R. Binding of surfactant protein A to C1q receptors mediates phagocytosis of Staphylococcus aureus by monocytes. Am J Physiol 267:L578–L584, 1994.

Gerdes JS, Yoder MC, Douglas SD, Polin RA. Decreased plasma fibronectin in neonatal sepsis. Pediatrics 72:877–881, 1983.

Ghayur T, Banerjee S, Hugunin M, Butler D, Herzog L, Carter A, Quintal L, Sekut L, Talanian R, Paskind M, Wong W, Kamen R, Tracey D, Allen H. Caspase-1 processes IFNγ-inducing factor and regulates LPS-induced IFN-γ production. Nature 386:619–623, 1997.

Glennon J, Ryan PJ, Keane CT, Rees JP. Circumcision and periurethral carriage of Proteus mirabilis in boys. Arch Dis Child 63:556–557, 1988.

Goldman MJ, Anderson GM, Stolzenberg ED, Kari UP, Zasloff M, Wilson JM. Human β-defensin-1 is a salt-sensitive antibiotic in lung that is inactivated in cystic fibrosis. Cell 88:553–560, 1997.

Gommerman JL, Carroll MC. Negative selection of B lymphocytes: a novel role for innate immunity. Immunol Rev 173:120–130, 2000.

Greenberger MJ, Strieter RM, Kunkel SL, Danforth JM, Laichalk LL, McGillicuddy DC, Standiford TJ. Neutralization of macrophage inflammatory protein-2 attenuates, neutrophil recruitment and bacterial clearance in murine Klebsiella pneumonia. J Infect Dis 173:159–165, 1996.

Gresham HD, Peters MG, Brown EJ. Pertussis toxin and cholera toxin modulation of human neutrophil Fc-receptor mediated phagocytosis. J Cell Biol 103:215A, 1986.

Grief R, Akça O, Horn EP, Kurz A, Sessler DI. Supplemental perioperative oxygen to reduce the incidence of surgical-wound infection. N Eng J Med 342:161–167, 2000.

Groopman JE, Gottlieb MS, Goodman J, Mitsuyasu RT, Conant MA, Fahey JL, Derezin M, Weinstein WM, Casavante C, Rothman J, Rudnick SA, Volberdling PA. Recombinant alpha-2 interferon therapy for Kaposi's sarcoma associated with acquired immunodeficiency syndrome. Ann Intern Med 100:671–676, 1984.

Groopman JE, Mitsuyasu RT, DeLeo MJ, Oette DH, Golde DW. Effect of recombinant human granulocyte-macrophage colony-stimulating factor on myelopoiesis in the acquired immunodeficiency syndrome. N Engl J Med 317:593–598, 1987.

Groopman JE, Molina JM, Scadden DT. Hematopoietic growth factors. Biology and clinical applications. N Engl J Med 321:1449–1459, 1989.

Grossman JE. Plasma fibronectin and fibronectin therapy in sepsis and critical illness. Rev Infect Dis 9:S420–430, 1987.

Gu Y, Kuida K, Tsutsui H, Ku G, Hsiao K, Fleming MA, Hayashi N, Higashino K, Okamura H, Nakanishi K, Kurimoto M, Tanimoto T, Flavell RA, Sato V, Harding MW, Livingston DJ, Su MS. Activation of interferon-γ inducing factor mediated by interleukin-1β converting enzyme. Science 275:206–209, 1997.

Hammond WP 4th, Price TH, Souza LM, Dale DC: Treatment of cyclic neutropenia with granulocyte colony-stimulating factor. N Engl J Med 320:1306–1311, 1989.

Haranaka K, Satomi N, Sakurai A. Antitumor activity of murine tumor necrosis factor (TNF) against transplanted murine tumors and heterotransplanted human tumors in nude mice. Int J Cancer 34:263–267, 1984.

Harbitz O, Jenssen AO, Smidsrod O. Lysozyme and lactoferrin in sputum from patients with chronic obstructive lung disease. Eur J Respir Dis 65:512–520, 1984.

Hardy RR, Hayakawa K. CD5 B cells, a fetal B cell lineage. Adv Immunol 55:297–339, 1994.

Hartley CA, Jackson DC, Anders EM. Two distinct serum mannose-binding lectins function as β inhibitors of influenza virus: identification of bovine serum β inhibitor as conglutinin. J Virol 66:4358–4363, 1992.

Harwig SSL, Ganz T, Lehrer RI. Neutrophil defensins: purification, characterization and antimicrobial testing. Methods Enzymol 236:160–172, 1994.

Hata K, Van Thiel DH, Herberman RB, Whiteside TL. Natural killer activity of human liver-derived lymphocytes in various liver diseases. Hepatology 14:495–503, 1991.

Henkart P, Yue CC. The role of cytoplasmic granules in lymphocyte cytotoxicity. Prog Allergy 40:82–110, 1988.

Heussner P, Haase D, Kanz L, Fonatsch C, Welte K, Freund M. G-CSF in the long-term treatment of cyclic neutropenia and chronic idiopathic neutropenia in adult patients. Int J Heamtol 62:225–234, 1995.

Hibbs JB Jr, Taintor RR, Vavrin Z. Macrophage cytotoxicity: role for L-arginine deaminase activity and imino nitrogen oxidation to nitrate. Science 235:473–476, 1987.

Hickman-Davis JM, Lindsey JR, Zhu S, Matalon S. Surfactant protein A mediates mycoplasmacidal activity of alveolar macrophages. Am J Physiol 274:L270–L277, 1998.

Hill HR. Biochemical, structural, and functional abnormalities of polymorphonuclear leukocytes in the neonate. Pediatr Research 22:375–382, 1987.

Hill HR. Modulation of host defenses with interferon-γ in pediatrics. J Infect Dis 167:S23–S28, 1993.

Hill HR, Augustine NH, Jaffe HW. Human recombinant interferon γ enhances neonatal polymorphonuclear leukocyte activation and movement, and increases free intracellular calcium. J Exp Med 173:767–770, 1991.

Hill HR, Augustine NH, Williams PA, Brown EJ, Bohnsack JF. Mechanism of fibronectin enhancement of group B streptococcal phagocytosis by human neutrophils and culture-derived macrophages. Infect Immun 61:2334–2339, 1993.

Hill HR, Boline J, Augustine N, Rote NS, Schwartz RS. Fibronectin deficiency: a correctable defect in the neonate's host defense mechanism. Pediatr Res 17:25A, 1983.

Hill HR, Hogan NA, Bale JF, Hemming VG. Evaluation of nonspecific (alternative pathway) opsonic activity by neutrophil chemiluminescence. Internat Arch Allergy Appl Immunol 53:490–497, 1977.

Hill HR, Joyner JL, La Pine TR, Kwak SD, Augustine NH. Defective production of IL-18 by cord blood cells in response to group B streptococci. J Invest Med 49:72A, 2001.

Hill HR, Ochs HD, Quie PG, Clark RA, Pabst HF, Klebanoff SJ, Wedgwood RJ. Defect in neutrophil granulocyte chemotaxis in Job's syndrome of recurrent "cold" staphylococcal abscesses. Lancet 2:617–619, 1974.

Hill HR, Shigeoka AO, Augustine NH, Pritchard D, Lundblad JL, Schwartz RS. Fibronectin enhances the opsonic and protective activity of monoclonal and polyclonal antibody against group B streptococci. J Exp Med 159:1618–1628, 1984.

Hoffmann JA, Kafatos FC, Janeway Jr CA, Ezekowitz RA. Phylogenetic perspectives in innate immunity. Science 284:1313–1318, 1999.

Holland SM. Treatment of infections in the patient with Mendelian susceptibility to mycobacterial infection. Microbes Infect 2:1579–1590, 2000.

Imler JL, Hoffmann JA. Signaling mechanisms in the antimicrobial host defense of Drosophila. Curr Opin Microbiol 3:16–22, 2000.

International Chronic Granulomatous Disease Cooperative Study Group (ICGDCSG). A controlled rail of interferon gamma to prevent infection in chronic granulomatous disease. N Engl J Med 324:509–516, 1991.

Itri LM. The interferons. Cancer 70:940–945, 1992.

Jacobs RF, Kiel DP, Sanders ML, Steele RW. Phagocytosis of type III group B streptococci by neonatal monocytes: enhancement by fibronectin and gammaglobulin. J Infect Dis 152:695–700, 1985.

Janeway CA Jr. Approaching the asymptote? Evolution and revolution in immunology. Cold Spring Harb Symp Quant Biol 54:1–13, 1989.

Jeppson JD, Jaffe HS, Hill HR. Use of recombinant human interferon gamma to enhance neutrophil chemotactic responses in Job syndrome of hyper-immunoglobulin E and recurrent infections. J Pediatr 118:383–387, 1991.

Johnston RB Jr. The complement system in host defense and inflammation: the cutting edges of a double edged sword. Pediatr Infect Dis J 12:933-941, 1993.

Joyner JL, Augustine NH, La Pine TR, Hill HR. Interleukin-12 increases IFNγ production by cord and adult blood mononuclear cells in response to group B streptococci. Pediat Res 47:333A, 2000a.

Joyner JL, Augustine NH, Taylor KA, La Pine TR, Hill HR. Effects of group B streptococci on cord and adult mononuclear cell interleukin-12 and interferon-γ mRNA accumulation and protein secretion. J Infect Dis 182:974–977, 2000b.

Kabelitz D, Bender A, Schondelmaier S, Schoel B, Kaufmann SH. A large fraction of human peripheral blood γδ+ T cells is activated by Mycobacterium tuberculosis but not by its 65-kDa heat shock protein. J Exp Med 171:667–679, 1990.

Kabha K, Schmegner J, Keisari Y, Parolis H, Schlepper-Schaeffer J, Ofek I. SP-A enhances phagocytosis of Klebsiella by interaction with capsular polysaccharides and alveolar macrophages. Am J Physiol 272:L344–L352, 1997.

Kalmar JR, Arnold RR. Killing of Actinobacillus actinomycetemcomitans by human lactoferrin. Infect Immun 56:2552–2557, 1988.

Kawakami M, Cerami A. Studies of endotoxin-induced decrease in lipoprotein lipase activity. J Exp Med 154:631–639, 1981.

Kawakami M, Tsutsumi H, Kumakawa T, Abe H, Hirai M, Kurosawa S, Mori M, Fukushima M. Levels of serum granulocyte colony-stimulating factor in patients with infections. Blood 76:1962–1964, 1990.

Kobayashi M, Fitz L, Ryan M, Hewick RM, Clark SC, Chan S, Loudon R, Sherman F, Perussia B, Trinchieri G. Identification and purification of natural killer cell stimulatory factor (NKSF), a cytokine with multiple biologic effects of human lymphocytes. J Exp Med 170:827–845, 1989.

Kohl S, Frazier JJ, Greenberg SB, Picerking KL, Loo LS. Inteferon induction of natural killer cytotoxicity in human neonates. J Pediatr 98:379–384, 1981.

Koivuranta-Vaara P, Banda D, Goldstein IM. Bacterial-lipopolysaccharide-induced release of lactoferrin from human polymorphonuclear leukocytes: role of monocyte-derived tumor necrosis factor α. Infect Immun 55:2956–2961, 1987.

Kremlev SG, Phelps DS. Surfactant protein A stimulation of inflammatory cytokine and immunoglobulin production. Am J Physiol 267:L712–L719, 1994.

Krown SE, Real FX, Cunningham-Rundles S, Myskowski PL, Koziner B, Fein S, Mittelman A, Oettgen HF, Safai B. Preliminary observations on the effect of recombinant leukocyte A interferon in homosexual men with Kaposi's sarcoma. N Engl J Med 308:1071–1076, 1983.

Kupfer A, Dennert G, Singer SJ. The reorientation of the Golgi apparatus and the microtubule-organizing center in the cytotoxic effector cell is a prerequisite in the lysis of bound target cells. J Mol Cell Immunol 2:37-49, 1985

Kwak DJ, Augustine NH, Borges WG, Joyner JL, Green WF, Hill HR. Intracellular and extracellular cytokine production by human mixed mononuclear cells in response to group B streptococci. Infect Immunity 68:320–327, 2000.

LaForce FM, Kelly WJ, Huber GL. Inactivation of staphylococci by alveolar macrophages with preliminary observations on the importance of alveolar lining material. Am Rev Respir Dis 108:784–790, 1973.

Lane HC, Kovacs JA, Feinberg J, Herpin B, Davey V, Walker R, Deyton L, Metcalf JA, Baseler M, Salzman N, Manischewitz J, Quinnan G, Masur H, Fauci AS. Antiretroviral effects of interferon alpha in AIDS associated Kaposi's sarcoma. Lancet 2:1218–1222, 1988.

Lanser ME, Saba TM, Scovil DW. Opsonic glycoprotein (plasma fibronectin) levels after burn injury. Relationship to extent of burn and development of sepsis. Ann Surg 192:776–782, 1980.

La Pine TR, Hill HR. Immunomodifiers applicable to the prevention and management of infectious diseases in children. In Arnoff SC, ed. Advances in Pediatric Infectious Diseases, vol 9. St Louis, Mosby-Year Book, 1994, pp 37–58.

Lassiter HA, Watson SW, Seifring ML, Tanner JE. Complement factor 9 deficiency in serum of human neonates. J Infect Dis 166:53–57, 1992.

Lau AS, Lehman D, Geertsma FR, Yeung MC. Biology and therapeutic uses of myeloid hematopoietic growth factors and interferons. Pediatr Infect Dis J 15:563–575, 1996.

Lawson PR, Reid KBM. The roles of surfactant proteins A and D innate immunity. Immunol Rev 173:66–78, 2000.

Lefkowitz DL, Mills K, Lefkowitz SS, Bollen A, Moguilevsky N. Neutrophil-macrophage interaction: a paradigm for chronic inflammation. Med Hypotheses 44:58–62, 1995.

Lehrer RI, Cline MJ. Leukocyte myeloperoxidase deficiency and disseminated candidiasis: the role of myeloperoxidase in resistance to Candida infection. J Clin Invest 48:1478–1488, 1969.

Lemaire B, Nicolas E, Michaut L, Reichhart JM, Hoffmann JA. The dorsoventral regulatory gene cassette spatzle/Toll/cactus controls the potent antifungal response in Drosophilia adults. Cell 86:973–983, 1996.

Lemaitre B, Reichhart JM, Hoffmann JA. Drosophilia host defense: differential induction of antimicrobial peptide genes after infection by various classes of microorganisms. Proc Natl Acad Sci USA 94:14614–14619, 1997.

Levin M, Quint PA, Goldstein B, Barton P, Bradley JS, Shemie SD, Yeh T, Kim SS, Cafaro DP, Scannon PJ, Giroir BP, the rBp21 Meningococcal Sepsis Study Group. Recombinant bactericidal/permeability-increasing protein (rBPI21) as adjunctive treatment for children with severe meningococcal sepsis: a randomised trial. Lancet 356:961–967, 2000.

Levin S, Hahn T. Interferon deficiency syndrome. Clin Exp Immunol 60:267–273, 1985.

LeVine AM, Bruno MD, Huelsman KM, Ross GF, Whitsett JA, Korfhagen TR. Surfactant protein A-deficient mice are susceptible to group B streptococcal infection. J Immunol 158:4336–4340, 1997.

LeVine AM, Gwozdz J, Stark J, Bruno M, Whitsett J, Korfhagen T. Surfactant protein-A binds group B streptococcus enhancing phagocytosis and clearance from lungs of surfactant protein-A-deficient mice. Am J Respir Cell Mol Biol 20:279–286, 1999.

LeVine AM, Kurak KE, Wright JR, Watford WT, Bruno MD, Ross GF, Whitsett JA, Korfhagen TR. Surfactant protein-A-deficient mice are susceptible to Pseudomonas aeruginosa infection. Am J Respir Cell Mol Biol 19:700–708, 1998.

Levy O, Martin S, Eichenwald E, Ganz T, Valore E, Carrroll SF, Lee K, Goldmann D, Thorne GM. Impaired innate immunity in the newborn: newborn neutrophils are deficient in bactericidal/permeability-increasing protein. Pediatrics 104:1327–1333, 1999.

Lieschke GJ, Maher D, Cebon J, O'Connor M, Green M, Sheridan W, Boyd A., Rallings M, Bonnem E, Metcalf D, Burges AW, McGrath K, Fox RM, Monstyn G. Effects of bacterially synthesized recombinant human granulocyte-macrophage colony stimulating factor in patients with advanced malignancy. Ann Intern Med 110: 357–364, 1989.

Liew FY, Cox FE. Nonspecific defense mechanism: the role of nitric oxide. Immunol Today 12:A17–A21, 1991.

Lipscombe RJ, Sumiya M, Hill AVS, Lau YL, Levinsky RJ, Summerfield JA, Turner, MW. High frequencies in African and non-African populations of independent mutations in the mannose binding protein gene. Hum Mol Genet 1:709–715, 1992.

Lipscombe RJ, Sumiya M, Summerfield JA, Turner MW. Distinct physiochemical characteristics of human mannose binding protein expressed by individuals of differing genotype. Immunology 85:660–667, 1995.

Ma Y, Uemura K, Oka S, Kozutsumi Y, Kawasaki N, Kawasaki T. Antitumor activity of mannan-binding protein in vivo as revealed by a virus expression system: mannan-biding protein-dependent cell-mediated cytotoxicity. Proc Natl Acad Sci USA 96:371–375, 1999.

Madan T, Eggleton P, Kishore U, Strong P Aggrawal SS, Sarma PU, Reid KB. Binding of pulmonary surfactant proteins A and D to Aspergillus fumigatus conidia enhances phagocytosis and killing by human neutrophils and alveolar macrophages. Infect Immun 65:3171–3179, 1997a.

Madan T, Kishore U, Shah A, Eggleton P, Strong P, Wang JY, Aggrawal SS, Sarma PU, Reid KB. Lung surfactant proteins A and D can inhibit specific IgE binding to the allergens of Aspergillus fumigatus and block allergen-induced histamine release from human basophils. Clin Exp Immunol 110:241–249, 1997b.

Madsen HO, Garred P, Kurtzhals JA, Lamm LU, Ryder LP, Thiel S, Svejgaard A. A new frequent allele is the missing link in the structural polymorphism of the human mannan-binding protein. Immunogenetics 40:37–44, 1994.

Malaviya R, Gao Z, Thankavel K, Van der Merwe PA, Abraham SN. The mast cell tumor necrosis factor α response to FimH-expressing E. coli is mediated by the glycosylphosphatidylinositol-anchored molecule CD48. Proc Natl Acad Sci USA 96:8110–8115, 1999.

Malaviya R, Ikeda T, Ross EA, Abraham SN. Mast cell modulation of neutrophil influx and bacterial clearance at sites of infection through TNF-alpha. Nature 381:77–80, 1996.

Malaviya R, Ross EA, MacGregor JI, Ikeda T, Little JR, Jakschik BA, Abraham SN. Mast cell phagocytosis of FimH-expressing enterobacteria. J Immunol 152:1907–1914, 1994.

Mancuso G, Cusumano V, Genovese F, Gambuzza M, Beninati C, Teti G. Role of interleukin 12 in experimental neonatal sepsis caused by group B streptococci. Infect Immun 65:3731–3735, 1997.

Mancuso G, Tomasello F, Von Hunolstein C, Orefici G, Teti G. Induction of tumor necrosis factor alpha by the group and type-specific polysaccharides form type III group B streptococci. Infect Immun 62:2748–2753, 1994.

McCord JM, Gao B, Leff J, Flores SC. Neutrophil-generated free radicals: possible mechanisms of injury in adult respiratory distress syndrome. Environ Health Perspect 10:57–60, 1994.

McCray PB Jr, Zabner J, Jia HP, Welsh MJ, Thorne PS. Efficient killing of inhaled bacterial in DeltaF508 mice: role of airway surface liquid composition. Am J Physiol 277:L183–L190, 1999.

McElvaney NG, Nakamura H, Birrer P, Hebert CA, Wong WL, Alphonso M, Baker JB, Catalano MA, Crystal RG. Modulation of airway inflammation in cystic fibrosis: In vivo suppression of interleukin-8 levels on the respiratory epithelial surface by aerosolization of recombinant secretory leukoprotease inhibitor. J Clin Invest 90; 1296–1301, 1992.

McNeely TB, Coonrod JD. Aggregation and opsonization of type A but not type B *Hemophilus influenzae* by surfactant protein A. Am J Respir Cell Mol Biol 11:114–122, 1994.

Mecheri S, David B. Unravelling the mast cell dilemma: culprit or victim of its generosity? Immunol Today 18:212–215, 1997.

Medzhitov R, Janeway C Jr. Innate immunity. N Engl J Med 343:338–344, 2000a.

Medzhitov R, Janeway C Jr. Innate immune recognition: mechanisms and pathways. Immunol Rev 173:89–97, 2000b.

Medzhitov R, Preston-Hurlburt P, Kopp E, Stadlen A, Chen C, Ghosh S, Janeway CA Jr. MyD88 is an adaptor protein in the hToll/IL-1 receptor family signaling pathways. Mol Cell 2:253–258, 1998.

Mekori YA, Metcalfe DD. Mast cells in innate immunity. Immunol Rev 173:131–140, 2000.

Metcalfe DD, Baram D, Mekori YA. Mast cells. Physiol Rev 77:1033–1079, 1997.

Michel T, Feron O. Nitric oxide synthases: which, where, how and why? J Clin Invest 100:2146–2152, 1997.

Miller ME, Seals J, Kaye R, Levinsky LC. A familial, plasma associated defect of phagocytosis: a new cause of recurrent bacterial infections. Lancet 2:60–63, 1968.

Mirilas P, Fesel C, Guilbert B, Beratis NG, Avrameas S. Natural antibodies in childhood: development, individual stability, and injury effect indicate a contribution to immune memory. J Clin Immunol 19:109–115, 1999.

Miura E, Procianoy RS, Bittar C, Miura CS, Miura MS, Mello C, Christensen RD. A randomized, double-masked, placebo-controlled trial of recombinant granulocyte colony-stimulating factor administration to preterm infants with the clinical diagnosis of early-onset sepsis. Pediatrics 107:30–35, 2001.

Miyasaki KT, Bodeau AL: Human neutropil azurocidin synergizes with leukocyte elastase and cathespin G in the killing of Capnocytophaga sputigena. Infect Immun 60:4973–4975, 1992.

Mizuochi T, Loveless RW, Lawson AM, Chai W, Lachmann PJ, Childs RA, Thiel S, Feizi T. A library of oligosaccharide probes (neoglycolipids) form N-glycosylated proteins reveals that conglutinin binds to certain complex type as well as high-mannose type oligosaccharide chains. J Biol Chem 264:13834–13839, 1989.

Moncada S, Palmer R, and Higgs E. Nitric oxide: physiology, pathophysiology and pharmacology. Pharmacol Rev 43:109–142, 1991.

Movat HZ. Tumor necrosis factor and interleukin-1: role in acute inflammation and microvascular injury. J Lab Clin Med 110:668–681, 1987.

Movat HZ, Cybulsky MI, Colditz IG, Chan MK, Dinarello CA. Acute inflammation in gram-negative infection: endotoxin, interleukin 1, tumor necrosis factor, and neutrophils. Fed Proc 46:97–104, 1987.

Munk ME, Gatrill AJ, Kaufmann SHE. In vitro activation of human γδ T cells by bacteria: evidence for specific interleukin secretion and target cell lysis. Curr Top Microbiol Immunol 173:159–165, 1991.

Muzio M, Natoli G, Saccani S, Levrero M, Mantovani A. The human Toll signaling pathway: divergence of nuclear factor κβ and JNK/SAPK activation upstream of tumor necrosis factor receptor-associated factor 6 (TRAF6). J Exp Med 187:2097–2101, 1998.

Nagle DL, Karim MA, Woolf EA, Holmgren L, Bork P, Misumi DJ, McGrail SH, Dussault BJ Jr, Perou CM, Boissy RE, Duyk GM, Spritz RA, Moore KJ. Identification and mutation analysis of the complete gene for Chediak-Higashi syndrome. Nat Genet 14:307–311, 1996.

Nathan C. Inducible nitric oxide synthases what difference does it make? J Clin Invest 100:2417–2423, 1997.

Nesin M, Cunningham-Rundles S. Cytokines and neonates. Am J Perinatol 17:393–404, 2000.

O'Brien NC, Charlton B, Cowden WB, Willenborg DO. Nitric oxide plays a critical role in the recovery of Lewis rats from experimental autoimmune encephalomyelitis and the maintenance of resistance to reinduction. J Immunol 163:6841–6847, 1999.

Ochsenbein AF, Fehr T, Lutz C, Suter M Brombacher F, Hengartner H, Zinkernagel RM. Control of early viral and bacterial distribution an disease by natural antibodies. Science 286:2156–2159, 1999.

Odeberg H, Olsson I, Venge P. Antibacterial cationic proteins of human granulocytes. J Clin Invest 56:1118–1124, 1975.

Ohlsson K, Bjork P, Bergenfeldt M, Hageman R, Thompson RC. Interleukin-1 receptor antagonist reduces mortality from endotoxin shock. Nature 348:550–552, 1990.

Okamura H, Tsutsi H, Komatsu T, Yutsudo M, Hakura A, Tanimoto T, Torigoe K, Okura T, Nukada Y, Hattori K, Akita K, Namba M, Tanabe F, Konishi K, Fukuda S, Kurimoto M. Cloning of a new cytokine that induces interferon-γ. Nature 378:88–91, 1995.

Okusawa S, Yancey KB, Van der Meer JWM, Endres S, Lonnemann G, Hefter K, Frank MM, Burke J, Dinarello CA, Gelfand JA. C5a stimulates secretion of tumor necrosis factor from human mononuclear cells in vitro. J Exp Med 168:443–448, 1988.

Old LJ. Tumor necrosis factor (TNF). Science 230:630–632, 1985.

O'Riordan DM, Standing JE, Kwon KY, Chang D, Crouch EC, Limper AH. Surfactant protein D interacts with *Pneumocystis carinii* and mediates organism adherence to alveolar macrophages. J Clin Invest 95:2699–2710, 1995.

Oseas R, Yang HH, Baehner RL, Boxer LA. Lactoferrin: a promoter of polymorphonuclear leukocyte adhesiveness. Blood 57:939–945, 1981.

Palmer R, Ashton D, and Moncada S. Vascular endothelial cells synthesize nitric oxide from L-arginine. Nature 333:664–666, 1988.

Pauksen K, Elfman L, Ulfgren AK, Venge P. Serum levels of granulocyte-colony stimulating factor (G-CSF) in bacterial and viral infections, and in atypical pneumonia. Br J Haematol 88:256–260, 1994.

Peat EB, Augustine NH, Drummond WK, Bohnsack JF, and Hill HR. Effects of fibronectin and group B streptococci on tumour necrosis factor-α production by human culture-derived macrophages. Immunology 84:440–445, 1995.

Perrillo RP. Treatment of chronic hepatitis B with interferon: experience in western countries. Semin Liver Dis 9:240–248, 1989.

Petrak BA, Augustine NH, and Hill HR. Recombinant human interferon gamma treatment of patients with Jobs syndrome of Hyperimmunoglobulin E and recurrent infections. Clin Res 42:1A, 1994.

Podack ER. Perforin: structure, function, and regulation. Curr Top Microbiol Immunol 178:175–184, 1992.

Presky DH, Yang H, Minetti LJ, Chua AO, Nabavi N, Wu CY, Gately MK, Gubler U. A functional interleukin-12 receptor complex is composed of two beta-type cytokine receptor subunits. Proc Natl Acad Sci USA 93:14002–14007, 1996.

Proctor RA. Fibronectin: an enhancer of phagocyte function. Rev Infect Dis 9:S412–S419, 1987.

Proctor RA, Prendergast E, Mosher DF. Fibronectin mediates attachment of *Staphylococcus aureus* to human neutrophils. Blood 59:681–687, 1982.

Puren AJ, Fantuzzi G, Gu Y, Su MS-S, Dinarello CA. Interleukin-18 (IFNγ-inducing factor) induces IL-1β and IL-8 via TNF-α production from non-CD14+ human blood mononuclear cells. J Clin Invest 101:711–724, 1998.

Quesada JR, Reuben J, Manning JT, Hersh EM, Gutterman JU. Alpha interferon for induction of remission in hairy-cell leukemia. N Engl J Med 310:15–18, 1984.

Qureshi ST, Skamene E, Malo D. Comparative genomics and host resistance against infectious diseases. Emerg Infect Dis 5:36–47, 1999.

Richards AL, Dennert G, Pluznick DH, Takagaki Y, Djeu JY. Natural cytotoxic activity in a cloned natural killer cell line is mediated by tumor necrosis factor. Nat Immun Cell Growth Regul 8:76–88, 1989.

Richardson VF, Larcher VF, Price JF. A common congenital immunodeficiency predisposing to infection and atopy in infancy. Arch Dis Child 58:799–802, 1983.

Richman-Eisenstat J, Jorens PG, Herbert CA, Ueki I, Nadel JA. Interleukin-8: an important chemoattractant in the sputum of patients with chronic inflammatory airway diseases. Am J Physiol 264:L413–L418, 1993.

Rock FL, Hardiman G, Timans JC, Kastelein RA, Bazan JF. A family of human receptors structurally related to Drosphila Toll. Proc Natl Acad Sci USA 95:588–593, 1998.

Roilides E, Walsh TJ, Pizzo PA, Rubin M. Granulocyte colony-stimulating factor enhances the phagocytic and bactericidal activity of normal and defective human neutrophils. J Infect Dis 163:579–583, 1991.

Romani L, Bistoni F, Mencacci A, Cenci E, Spaccapelo R, Puccetti P. IL-12 in *Candida albicans* infections. Res Immunol 146:532–538, 1996.

Rose MC. Mucins: structure, function, and role in pulmonary diseases. Am J Physiol 263:L413–L429, 1992.

Saba TM, Blumenstock FA, Scovill WA, Bernard H. Cryoprecipitate reversal of opsonic alpha2 surface binding glycoprotein deficiency in septic surgical and trauma patients. Science 201:622–624, 1978.

Saba TM, Blumenstock FA, Shah DM, Landaburu RH, Hrinda ME, Deno DC, Holman JM Jr, Cho E, Dayton C, Cardarelli PM. Reversal of opsonic deficiency in surgical, trauma, and burn patients by infusion of purified human plasma fibronectin. Am J Med 80:229–240, 1986.

Salmon SE, Cline MJ, Schultz J, Lehrer RI. Myeloperoxidase deficiency. Immunologic study of a genetic leukocyte defect. N Engl J Med 282:250–253, 1970.

Salyer JL, Bohnsack JF, Knape WA, Shigeoka AO, Ashwood ER, Hill HR. Mechanisms of tumor necrosis factor-alpha alteration of PMN adhesion and migration. Am J Pathol 136:831–841, 1990.

Sano H, Sohma H, Muta T, Nomura S, Voelker DR, Kuroki Y. Pulmonary surfactant protein A modulates the cellular response to smooth and rough lipopolysaccharides by interaction with CD14. J Immunol 163:387–395, 1999.

Schall TJ, Jongstra J, Dyer BJ, Jorgensen J, Clayberger C, Davis MM, Kresnky AM. A human T cell-specific molecule is a member of a new gene family. J Immunol 141:1018–1025, 1988.

Schelenz S, Malhotra R, Sim RB, Holmskov U, Bancroft GJ. Binding of host collectins to the pathogenic yeast *Cryptococcus neoformans*: human surfactant protein D acts as an agglutinin for acapsular yeast cells. Infect Immun 63:3360–3366, 1995.

Schindler R, Gelfand JA, Dinarello CA. Recombinant C5a stimulates transcription rather than translation of interleukin-1 (IL-1) and tumor necrosis factor: translational signal provided by lipopolysaccharide or IL-1 itself. Blood 76:1631–1638, 1990.

Schoen EJ, Colby CJ, Ray GT. Newborn circumcision decreases incidence and costs of urinary tract infections during the first year of life. Pediatrics 105:789–793, 2000.

Schwandner R, Dziarski R, Wesche H, Rothe M, Kirschning CJ. Peptidoglycan- and lipoteichoic acid-induced cell activation is mediated by Toll-like receptor 2. J Biol Chem 274:17406–17409, 1999.

Schweinle JE, Ezekowitz RAB, Tenner AJ, Kuhlman M, Joiner KA. Human mannose-binding protein activates the alternative complement pathway and enhances serum bactericidal activity on a mannose-rich isolate of *Salmonella*. J Clin Invest 84:1821–1829, 1989.

Scott-Algara D, Vuillier F, Cayota A, Dighiero G. Natural killer (NK) cell activity during HIV infection: a decrease in NK activity is observed at the clonal level and is not restored after in vitro long-term culture of NK cells. Clin Exp Immunol 90:181–187, 1992.

Seaman WE. Natural killer cells. In Rich RR, Fleisher TA, Schwartz BD, Shearer WT, Strober W, eds. Clinical Immunology: Principles and Practice. St. Louis, Mosby, 1996, pp 282–289.

Selsted ME, Ouellette AJ. Defensins in granules and non-phagocytic cells. Trends Cell Biol 5:114–119, 1995.

Sher A. Complement-dependent adherence of mast cells to schistosomula. Nature 263:334–336, 1976.

Sher A, Hein A, Moser G, Caulfield JP. Complement receptors promote the phagocytosis of bacteria by rat peritoneal mast cells. Lab Invest 41:490–499, 1979.

Shi L, Kraut RP, Aebersold R, Greenberg AH. A natural killer cell granule protein that induces DNA fragmentation and apoptosis. J Exp Med 175:553–566, 1992.

Sibille Y, Reynolds HY. Macrophages and polymorphonuclear neutrophils in lung defense and injury. Am Rev Respir Dis 141:471–501, 1990.

Simpson WA, Hasty DL, Mason JM, Beachey EH. Fibronectin-mediated binding of group A streptococci to human polymorphonuclear leukocytes. Infect Immun 37:805–810, 1982.

Singer II, Kawka DW, Scott S, Weidmer JR, Mumford RA, Riehl TE, Stenson WF. Expression of inducible nitric oxide synthase and nitrotyrosine in clonic epithelium in inflammatory bowel disease. Gastroenterolgy 111:871–885, 1996.

Snijders A, Hilkens CMU, Van der Pouw Kraan CTM, Engel M, Aarden LA, Kapsenberg ML. Regulation of bioactive IL-12 production in lipopolysaccharide-stimulated human monocytes is determined by the expression of the p35 subunit. J Immunol 156:1207–1212, 1996.

Solis D, Feizi T, Yuen CT, Lawson AM, Harrison RA, Loveless RW. Differential recognition by conglutinin and mannan-binding protein of N-glycans presented on neoglycolipids and glycoproteins with special reference to complement glycoprotein C3 and ribonuclease B. J Biol Chem 269:11555–11562, 1994.

Soothill JF, Harvey BAM. Defective opsonization. A common immunity deficiency. Arch Dis Child 51:91–99, 1976.

Spitznagel JK. Antibiotic proteins of human neutrophils. J Clin Invest 86:1381–1386, 1990.

Sriskandan S, Evans TJ, Cohen J. Bacterial superantigen-induced human lymphocyte responses are nitric oxide dependent and mediated by IL-12 and IFN-γ. J Immunol 156:2430–2435, 1996.

Stamme C, Wright JR. Surfactant protein A enhances the binding and deacylation of *E. coli* LPS by alveolar macrophages. Am J Physiol 276:L540–L547, 1999.

Standiford TJ, Kunkel SL, Greenberger MJ, Laichalk LL, Strieter RM. Expression and regulation of chemokines in bacterial pneumonia. J Leukoc Biol 59:24–28, 1996.

Steele PM, Augustine NH, Hill HR. The effect of lactic acid on mononuclear cell secretion of proinflammatory cytokines in response to group B streptococci. J Infect Dis 177:1418–1421, 1998.

Steiner H, Hultmark D, Engström A, Bennich H, Boman HG. Sequence and specificity of two antibacterial proteins involved in insect immunity. Nature 292:246–248, 1981.

Strober W, James SP. The interleukins. Pediatr Res 24:549–557, 1988.

Sullivan GW, Carper HT, Mandell GL. The effect of three human recombinant hepatopoietic growth factors (granulocyte-macrophage colony-stimulating factor, granulocyte colony-stimulating factor, and interleukin-3) on phagocyte oxidative activity. Blood 81:1863–1870, 1993.

Sumiya M, Super M, Tabona P, Levinsky RJ, Arai T, Turner MW, Summerfield JA. Molecular basis of opsonic defect in immunodeficient children. Lancet 337:1569–1570, 1991.

Super M, Thiel S, Lu J, Levinsky RJ, Turner MW. Association of low levels of mannan-binding protein with a common defect of opsonization. Lancet 2:1236–1239, 1989.

Takeda K, Tsutsui H, Yoshimoto T, Adachi O, Yoshida N, Kishimoto K, Okamura H, Nakanishi K, Akira S. Defective NK cell activity and Th1 response in IL-18-deficient mice. Immunity 8:383–390, 1998.

Taniguchi M, Nagaoka K, Kunikata T, Kayano T, Tamauchi H, Nakamura S, Ikeda M, Orita K, Kurimoto M. Characterization of anti-human interleukin-18 (IL-18)/interferon inducing (IGIF) monoclonal antibodies and their application in the measurement of human IL-18 ELISA. J Immunol Methods 206:107–113, 1997.

Teti G, Mancuso G, Tomasello F. Cytokine appearance and effects of anti-tumor necrosis factor alpha antibodies in a neonatal rat model of group B streptococcal infection. Infect Immun 61:227–235, 1993.

Tino MJ, Wright JR. Surfactant protein A stimulates phagocytosis of specific pulmonary pathogens by alveolar macrophages. Am J Physiol 270:L677–L688, 1996.

Tracey KJ, Lowry SF, Cerami A: Cachectin: a hormone that triggers acute shock and chronic cachexia. J Infect Dis 157:413–420, 1988.

Trapani JA, Smyth MJ. Killing by cytotoxic T cells and natural killer cells: multiple granule serine proteases as initiators of DNA fragmentation. Immunol Cell Biol 71:201–208, 1993.

Travis SM, Conway BA, Zabner J, Smith JJ, Anderson NN, Singh PK, Greenberg EP, Welsh MJ. Activity of abundant antimicrobials of the human airway. Am J Respir Cell Mol Biol 20:872–879, 1999.

Trinchieri G. Interleukin-12: a proinflammatory cytokine with immunoregulatory functions that bridge innate resistance and antigen-specific adaptive immunity. Annu Rev Immunol 13:251–276, 1995.

Tripp CS, Wolf SF, Unanue ER. Interleukin 12 and tumor necrosis factor alpha are costimulators of interferon gamma production by natural killer cells in severe combined immunodeficiency mice with liseriosis, and interleukin 10 is a physiologic antagonist. Proc Natl Acad Sci USA 990:3725–3729, 1993.

Tsai WC, Strieter RM, Zisman DA, Wilkowski JM, Bucknell KA, Chen GH, Standiford TJ. Nitric oxide is required for effective innate immunity against Klebsiella pneumoniae. Infect Immun 65:1870–1875, 1997.

Tsujimoto M, Yokota S, Vilcek J, Weissmann G. Tumor necrosis factor provokes superoxide anion generation from neutrophils. Biochem Biophys Res Commun 137:1094–1100, 1986.

Turner MW. Mannose-binding lectin: the pluripotent molecule of the innate immune system. Immunol Today 17:532–540, 1996.

Ushio S, Namba M, Okura T, Hattori K, Nukada Y, Akita K, Tanabe F, Konishi K, Micallef M, Fujii M, Torigoe K, Tanimoto T, Fukuda S, Ikeda M, Okamura H, Kurimoto M. Cloning of the cDNA for human IFNγ-inducing factor, expression in Escherichia coli, and studies on the biologic activities of the protein. J Immunol 156:4274–4279, 1996.

Vadhan-Raj S, Buescher S, Broxmeyer HE, LeMaistre A, Lepe-Zunig JL, Ventura G, Jeha S, Horwitz LJ, Trujillo JM, Gillis S, Hittelman WN, Gutterman JU. Stimulation of myelopoiesis in patients with aplastic anemia by recombinant human granulocyte-macrophage colony-stimulating factor. N Engl J Med 319:1628–1634, 1988.

Valiante NM, Trinchieri G. Identification of a novel signal transduction surface molecule on human cytotoxic lymphocytes. J Exp Med 178:1397–1406, 1993.

Vallejo JG, Baker CJ, Edwards MS. Roles of the bacterial cell wall and capsule in induction of tumor necrosis factor alpha by type III group B streptococci. Infect Immun 64:5042–5046, 1996.

Van Iwaarden JF, Van Strijp JA, Visser H, Haagsman HP, Verhoef J, Van Golde LM. Binding of surfactant protein A (SP-A) to herpes simplex virus type 1-infected cells is mediated by the carbohydrate moiety of SP-A. J Biol Chem 267:25039–25043, 1992.

Venkateswaran L, Wilimas JA, Dancy R, Wang WC, Korones S, Hayden J, Hayes FA. Granulocyte-macrophage colony-stimulating factor in the treatment of neonates with neutropenia and sepsis. Pediatr Hematol Oncol 17: 469–473, 2000.

Wallis R, Cheng JYT. Molecular defects in variant forms of mannose-binding protein associated with immunodeficiency. J Immunol 163:4953–4959, 1999.

Wang JY, Shieh CC, You PF, Lei HY, Reid KB. Inhibitory effect of pulmonary surfactant proteins A and D on allergen-induced lymphocyte proliferation and histamine release in children with asthma. Am J Respir Crit Care Med 158:510–518, 1998.

Weil SC, Rosner GL, Reid MS, Chisholm RL, Farber NM, Spitznagel JK, Swanson MS, cDNA cloning of human myeloperoxidase: decrease in myeloperoxidase mRNA upon induction of HL-60 cells. Proc Natl Acad Sci USA 84: 2057–2061, 1987.

Welsh RM, Vargas-Cortes C. Natural killer cells in viral infection. In Lewis CE, McGee JO'D, eds. The Natural Killer Cell. Oxford, UK, Oxford University Press, 1992.

Wesche H, Henzel WJ, Shillinglaw W, Li S, Cao Z. MyD88: an adapter that recruits IRAK to the IL-1 receptor complex. Immunity 7:837–847, 1997.

Whiteside TL, Herberman RB. Role of human natural killer cells in health and disease. Clin Diagn Lab Immunol 1:125–133, 1994.

Whiteside TL, Herberman RB. The role of natural killer cells in human disease. Clin Immunol Immunopathol 53:1–23, 1989.

Wientjes FB, Panayotou G, Reeves E, Segal AW. Interactions between cytosolic components of the NADPH oxidase: p40phox interacts with both p67 phox and p47 phox. Biochem J 317:919–924, 1996.

Williams MJ, Rodriguez A, Kimbrell DA, Eldon ED. The 18-wheeler mutation reveals complex antibacterial gene regulation in Drosophilia host defense. EMBO J 16:6120–6130, 1997.

Williams PA, Bohnsack JF, Augustine NH, Drummond WK, Rubes CE, Hill HR. Production of tumor necrosis factor by human cells in vitro and in vivo, induced by group B streptococci. J Pediatr 123:292–300, 1993.

Wilson CB, Westall J, Johnston L, Lewis DB, Dower Sk, Alpert AR. Decreased production of interferon-gamma by human neonatal cells: intrinsic and regulatory deficiencies. J Clin Invest 77:860–867, 1986.

Wiswell TE. The prepuce, urinary tract infections, and the consequences. Commentaries Ped 105:860–862, 2000.

Wiswell TE, Miller GM, Gelston HM Jr, Jones SK, Clemmings AF. Effect of circumcision status on periurethral bacterial flora during the first year of life. J Pediatr 113:442–446, 1988.

Wojtecka-Lukasik E, Maslinski S. Fibronectin and fibrinogen degradation products stimulate PMN-leukocyte and mast cell degranulation. J Physiol Pharmacol 43:173–181, 1992.

Wolach B, Gavrieli R, Pomeranz A. Effect of granulocyte and granulocyte macrophage colony stimulating factors (G-CSF and GM-CSF) on neonatal neutrophil functions. Pediatr Res 48:369–373, 2000.

Wriedt K, Kauder E, Mauer AM. Defective myelopoiesis in congenital neutropenia. N Engl J Med 283:1072–1077, 1970.

Xing X, Jordana M, Kirpalani H, Driscoll KE, Schall TJ, Gauldie J. Cytokine expression by neutrophils and macrophages in vivo: endotoxin induces tumor necrosis factor-α, macrophage inflammatory protein-2, interleukin-1β, and interleukin-6 but not RANTES or transforming growth factor-β1 mRNA expression in acute lung inflammation. Am J Respir Cell Mol Biol 10:148–153, 1994.

Yamamura H, Nabe T, Kohno S, Ohata K. Endothelin 1, one of the most potent histamine releasers in mouse peritoneal mast cells. Eur J Pharmacol 265:9–15, 1994.

Yancopoulos GD, Desiderio SV, Paskind M, Kearney JF, Baltimore D, Alt FW. Preferential utilization of the most J_H-proximal V_H gene segments in pre-B-cell lines. Nature 311:727–733, 1984.

Yang KD, Augustine NH, Gonzalez LA, Bohnsack JF, Hill HR. Effects of fibronectin on the interaction of polymorphonuclear leukocytes with unopsonized and antibody-opsonized bacteria. J Infect Dis 158:823–830, 1988.

Yang KD, Augustine NH, Men-Fang S, Bohnsack JF, Hill HR. Effects of fibronectin on actin organization and respiratory burst activity in neutrophils, monocytes, and macrophages. J Cell Physiol 158:347–353, 1994.

Yang KD, Bohnsack JF, Hill HR. Fibronectin in host defense: implications in the diagnosis, prophylaxis and therapy of infectious diseases. Pediatr Infect Dis J 12:234–239, 1993.

Yang KD, Quie PG, Hill HR: Phagocytic system. In Ochs HD, Smith EI, Puck J, eds: Primary Immunodeficiency Diseases. A Molecular and Genetic Approach. New York, Oxford University Press, 1999, pp 82–96.

Yoder MC, Douglas SD, Gerdes J, Kline J, Polin RA. Plasma fibronectin in healthy newborn infants, respiratory distress syndrome and perinatal asphyxia. J Pediatr 102:777–780, 1983.

Yoshikai Y, Nishimura H. The role of interleukin-15 in mounting an immune response against microbial infections. Microbes Infect 2:381–389, 2000.

Yoshimura A, Lien E, Ingalls RR, Tuomanen E, Dziarski R, Golenbock D. Cutting edge: recognition of gram-positive bacterial cell wall components by the innate immune system occurs via Toll-like receptor 2. J Immunol 163:1–5, 1999.

Zeidler C, Boxer L, Dale DC, Freedman MH, Kinsey S, Welte K. Management of Kostmann syndrome in the G-CSF era. Br J Haematol 109:490–495, 2000.

Zhang P, Bagby GJ, Stolz DA, Summer WR, Nelson S. Enhancement of peritoneal leukocyte function by granulocyte colony-stimulating factor in rats with abdominal sepsis. Crit Care Med 26:315–321, 1998.

Zhang P, Summer WR, Bagby GJ, Nelson S. Innate immunity and pulmonary host defense. Immunol Rev 173:39–51, 2000.

Zimmerman PE, Voelker DR, McCormack FX, Paulsrud JR, Martin WJD 2nd. 120-kD surface glycoprotein of *Pneumocystis carinii* is a ligand for surfactant protein A. J Clin Invest 89:143–149, 1992.

11 The Immunology of Pregnancy

Maite de la Morena and Jonathan David Gitlin

INTRODUCTION

Understanding the immunobiology of pregnancy is an important goal of all immunologists interested in defining the mechanisms of immunologic tolerance. Medawar provided three possible explanations for the phenomena of fetal acceptance by the pregnant mother: (1) anatomic separation of the fetus from the mother, (2) antigenic immaturity of the fetus, and (3) immunologic inertness of the mother (Medawar, 1953). Although no clear picture has yet emerged to allow for a complete molecular definition of the complex immunologic processes that underlie human development, our current understanding suggests that elements of all of Medawar's explanations are critical to the healthy outcome of pregnancy.

In this chapter we review the fundamental immunologic principles that determine the immunobiology of pregnancy by focusing on the cellular and molecular interactions known to be involved with immune function during normal gestation. Increased knowledge of the immunobiology of pregnancy allows for elucidation of the immunologic mechanisms leading to infertility and pathologic outcome of pregnancy, as well as gestational complications of autoimmune diseases, and may permit the development of novel therapeutic approaches to manipulate immunologic tolerance during solid organ transplantation.

CONCEPTION AND FERTILIZATION

Fertilization in mammals results from a carefully synchronized sequence of events that includes sperm-oocyte recognition, adhesion, plasma membrane binding and fusion, and egg activation (Table 11-1) (Vacquier, 1998). Chemoattractant molecules released by the egg guide the sperm through the female reproductive tract during the process of sperm cell maturation, termed *capacitation* (Schaefer et al., 1998). Sperm-oocyte recognition occurs via a mechanism involving species-specific proteins (Vacquier, 1998). Adhesion permits the *acrosomal reaction* to occur (defined as an exocytic event with release of hydrolytic enzymes and reorganization of the sperm plasma membrane), enabling subsequent plasma membrane binding and fusion between the sperm and the egg. This cell–cell interaction can be considered analogous to what is observed with receptor-ligand pairs, which guide leukocyte–endothelial cell interactions (Evans, 1999; Geng et al., 1997; Sueoka et al., 1997). In many species the point of entry of the sperm is spatially restricted (Pederson, 2001).

Sperm-specific proteins, which mediate these processes of adhesion and entry, include members of the ADAM (*A Disintegrin and A Metalloprotease*) family. An ADAM protein contains multiple domains, which include recognizable metalloprotease, disintegrin, and epidermal growth factor (EGF)–like transmembrane motifs. Cell adherence is conferred by these proteins through its disintegrin domain and protease activity through the metalloprotease domain (Primakoff and Myles, 2000). These disintegrins are localized to the plasma membrane of mouse and human sperm where they interact with cell surface adhesion molecules, termed *integrins,* on the egg (Almeida, et al., 1995; Bronson and Fusi, 1996). Fertilin, originally known as PH-30, is one of the most extensively studied ADAM proteins known to be involved in fertilization (Primakoff et al., 1987). This protein, composed of two subunits called fertilin-α and fertilin-β, is found in mouse, rat, guinea pig, bovine, macaque, and human sperm. Consistent with a role for this protein in sperm adherence, administration of monoclonal antibodies recognizing fertilin-β inhibits fertilization.

TABLE 11-1 · PROTEINS AND SIGNALING MOLECULES IDENTIFIED DURING MAMMALIAN FERTILIZATION

Stages of Mammalian Fertilization			
I. Sperm-oocyte recognition	Chemoattractant molecules from follicular fluid		
	Species specific proteins	Abalon* sperm lysin	
		Zonadhesin†	
	MHC molecules		
II. Adhesion, plasma membrane binding and fusion	ADAM family: fertilin		
	Integrin molecules: alpha6-beta1 (mouse)		
	Cadherins		
	MHC II–CD4/p56Lck interactions		
III. Egg activation	Nitric oxide		

*A marine mollusk.
†Identified in pigs and mice.
ADAM = A disintegrin and A metalloprotease; MHC = major histocompatibility complex.

The **cadherins** are another well-defined group of ligand-receptor pairs localized to human gametes (Rufas et al., 2000). These molecules belong to a family of glycoproteins that bind with high affinity to a cadherin on an adjacent cell. Cadherins participate in signal transduction, but their role in egg activation has yet to be elucidated.

The fusion step of fertilization is mediated by major histocompatibility complex (MHC) class II molecules, located posteriorly on the sperm head, and CD4/p56Lck complex present on the plasma membrane of the egg (Mori et al., 1992). Gamete binding can be blocked with monoclonal antibodies to the CD4 receptor, as well as antibodies to the monomorphic region of class II molecules (Mori et al., 1991). MHC gene products are fundamental elements in immune recognition that develop within immunocompetent hosts. The MHC gene complex located on human chromosome 6 consists of more than 100 highly polymorphic genes, which are divided into two mayor groups based on the structures of the encoded immunologic molecules.

Class I genes encode both class Ia molecules ubiquitously expressed on all nucleated cells encoded by human leukocyte antigen-A (HLA-A), HLA-B, and HLA-C genes, as well as the class Ib nonclassical MHC proteins encoded by the HLA-E, HLA-F, and HLA-G genes. Class II molecules, encoded by HLA-DP, HLA-DQ and HLA-DR genes, are restricted in their tissue distribution to professional antigen-presenting cells, activated T cells, thymic epithelial cells, and endothelial cells. MHC products have been identified on gametes and trophoblast cells during mammalian fertilization and implantation (Fernandez et al., 1999; Omu et al., 1999; Tsuji et al., 2000).

The first encounter with foreign proteins during the reproductive process is at sexual intercourse, when MHC-expressing spermatozoa and seminal fluid are deposited in the female tract. Sensitization occurs rarely among infertile couples (Coulam and Stern, 1992). MHC class I molecules expressed on mature gametes may be regulated during development, in that HLA-Ia molecules are identified before sperm maturation and are significantly reduced in mature sperm. These data suggest that significant levels of HLA class Ia molecules on either mature spermatozoa or secondary oocytes are not required for successful fertilization. Alternatively, altered expression of MHC class I molecules on murine sperm or oocytes results in both impaired fertility and abnormal development beyond mid-gestation, suggesting a critical role for the expression of these molecules in embryonic survival (Fernandez et al., 1999). MHC class Ib molecules are present in secondary oocytes and embryos at all stages of preimplantation and placental development.

In contrast to the data just noted, antibodies against sperm antigens are associated with infertility (Sargent et al., 1987). Interestingly, distinct immunogenetic backgrounds may contribute to the production of specific antisperm antibodies. For example, homozygosity for HLA-B6, HLA-DR4, and HLA-DR6 appears to be a risk factor for the production of antisperm antibodies (Omu et al., 1999). A higher frequency of HLA-DRB1*0901 and HLA-DQB1*0303 was found in 38 Japanese women with antisperm immobilizing antibodies (Tsuji et al., 2000). In support of another immunologic mechanism for impaired fertility and development, increased fetal loss has been reported when spouses, among a Caucasian religious isolate known as the Hutterites, matched for entire 16-locus haplotypes (Ober, 1999; Ober et al., 1998).

IMPLANTATION

As a consequence of egg activation, a rapid succession of mitotic divisions occurs as the fertilized egg travels along the tubal isthmus. In some species this process of egg activation is dependent on nitric oxide, raising the possibility of specific immunologic mechanisms that may regulate the production and release of this signaling molecule (Kuo et al., 2000). Following these mitotic divisions, a mass of cells termed the *morula* is transformed into the blastocyst as the outer cells produce a fluid-filled cavity. The fertilized ovum reaches the endometrial cavity approximately 3 days following ovulation (Fig. 11-1).

Once the blastocyte reaches the uterine cavity, two different cellular components can be distinguished: the trophoblast, which surrounds the blastocyte, and the inner cell mass, from which the embryo will develop. Implantation is the process by which the embryo adheres to the endometrial epithelium and penetrates until it reaches the stromal tissues, to which it anchors

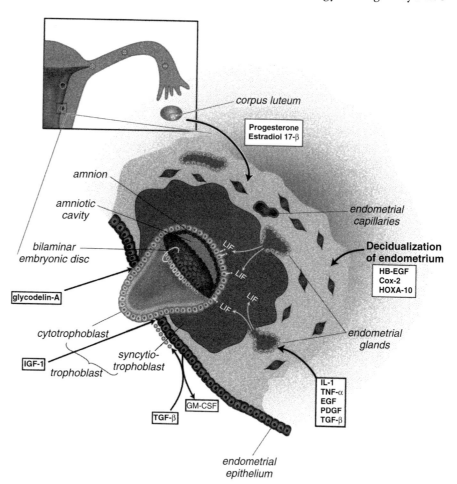

Figure 11-1 · Mechanisms regulating blastocyst implantation. GM-CSF = granulocyte-macrophage colony-stimulating factor; HB-EGF = heparin-binding EGF-like growth factor; IGF = insulin growth factor; IL = interleukin; PDGF = platelet-derived growth factor; TGF = transforming growth factor; TNF = tumor necrosis factor.

and continues its differentiation. The mechanisms that coordinate these events in humans are still poorly understood. In rodents this process of implantation requires both the activation of the blastocyst and conversion of the uterus to a receptive state.

These changes are coordinated by ovarian hormones, including progesterone and estrogen, as well as a network of cytokines that utilize gp130 for signal transduction (Sanchez-Cuenca et al., 1999). Although it is clear that the state of activity of the blastocyst determines the timing for the window of implantation, the precise factors involved in the transformation of a dormant human blastocyst are unknown. A comprehensive review of the biochemical factors associated with implantation and maintenance of early pregnancy reveals the complex interrelationship of hormonal and immunologic factors (Norwitz, 2001).

In murine gestation, the uterus evolves into a receptive state under the direction of ovarian progesterone, estradiol 17β, and endometrial-derived *leukemia inhibitory factor (LIF)* (Delage et al., 1995; Paria et al., 2000). LIF binds to its receptor on trophoblastic cells, which have a 130-glycoprotein transduction chain (King et al., 1995). LIF is constitutively expressed on human endometrial glands and can be induced by interleukin-1 (IL-1), tumor necrosis factor-α (TNF-α), EGF, platelet-derived growth factor (PDGF), and transform-

ing growth factor-β (TGF-β). Mifepristone (RU-486), an antiprogestin contraceptive agent, inhibits the secretory development of the endometrium and downregulates the expression of LIF, as well as several surface integrins (Danielsson et al., 1997). LIF is also a key regulatory element in controlling the invasiveness of trophoblasts by inhibition of metalloprotease secretion and the differentiation of cytotrophoblast into syncytium (Bischof et al., 1995; Harvey et al., 1995). Interestingly, recent data suggest that LIF may also contribute to natural killer (NK) cell recruitment by increasing fibronectin deposition into the extracellular matrix (Sanchez-Cuenca et al., 1999).

In addition to this critical role for LIF in blastocyst implantation, molecular genetic studies have also identified an essential role for EGFs, such as heparin-binding EGF-like growth factor (HB-EGF), cyclo-oxygenase-2 (COX-2), and the *homeobox gene HOXA-10*, in implantation in the mouse (Paria et al., 2000, 2001). Blastocyst attachment occurs as a result of the coordinated interaction of these gene products, which then results in decidualization of the endometrium. In this process, uterine fibroblasts proliferate and form large polyclonal decidual cells with essential endocrine functions for maintenance of pregnancy.

A second cytokine identified as essential in the preparation of the uterus to a receptive state is TGF-β

(Mummery, 2001). The TGF-β superfamily of growth factors is involved in the regulation of cellular growth and differentiation, as well as the expression of adhesion molecules, which mediates both immunoregulatory and anti-inflammatory activity. TGF-β is present in seminal fluid in concentrations of 100 to 200 ng/ml and has been shown to be secreted by the genital tract (Loras et al., 1999; Nocera and Chu, 1995). TFG-β production within the genital tract is enhanced by prostaglandin E_2 (PGE$_2$), which is known to promote T-helper type 2 (Th2) cytokine pattern from dendritic cells via the downregulation of IL-12 (Kapsenberg et al., 1999). Multiple pathways have been described for the activation of TGF-β (Koli et al., 2001), and apparently the acidic environment of the vaginal fluids is permissive for the activation of seminal TGF-β (Loras et al., 1999; Nocera and Chu, 1995).

In addition to the known biologic effects of TFG-β on growth and differentiation cited earlier, this cytokine has been shown to stimulate the release of granulocyte-macrophage colony-stimulating factor (GM-CSF) by rodent uterine epithelial cells following mating (Tremellen et al., 1998). The TGF-β–mediated presence of these cells appears critical for the early immunologic and inflammatory events mediating implantation.

Placental protein 14 (PP14), or *glycodelin A*, is an important immunomodulatory protein essential for the progression of pregnancy. This protein belongs to a family of hydrophobic transporter proteins known as lipocalins. PP14 inhibits sperm-zona interaction and is also important for endometrial preparation prior to blastocyte implantation. Interestingly, this protein can suppress T-cell proliferation and induce apoptosis. These cellular events may contribute to clearance of T lymphocytes potentially reactive with fetal paternal antigens (Mukhopadhyay et al., 2001).

Corticotropin-releasing hormone (CRH) has a role in promoting blastocyst implantation and early maternal tolerance. CRH is produced by trophoblast and maternal decidua and experimental studies indicate that antalarmin, a CRH receptor antagonist, promotes T-cell apoptosis by downregulating FasL expression on these cells. Rats treated with antalarmin demonstrate a marked decrease in implantation and embryo survival, and genetic manipulation reveals that these effects are T-cell dependent. The results of this study suggest that production of CRH in the local environment may promote implantation and tolerance of early pregnancy via directed killing of T lymphocytes (Makrigiannakis et al., 2001).

Gene-targeting technologies have also helped define the functions of genes critical for the implantation process. IL-11–deficient mice experience complete infertility due to defective decidual responses (Robb et al., 1998). Insulin growth factor-1 (IGF-1)–deficient animals demonstrate reduced fertility (Baker et al., 1996). This growth factor is abundantly expressed at the sites of implantation, and administration of purified growth factors leads to local changes in the murine uterus consistent with a role for IGF-1 in uterine preparation for implantation. Further analysis of the signaling pathways involved in these growth factors and cytokines during implantation may increase our understanding of the mechanisms involved with infertility secondary to abnormalities of implantation (Paria et al., 2001).

THE MATERNAL–FETAL INTERFACE

A fundamental immunologic question following the implantation of the blastocyst is whether the maternal immune system is aware of the presence of a fetus and whether this recognition triggers an immunologic response. Although the data are not complete on either question, current data suggest that the maternal immune system does recognize and respond to the fetus (Kotlan et al., 2001; Mellor, 1998; Mellor and Munn, 2000; Tafuri et al., 1995; Van Kampen et al., 2001; Zhou and Mellor, 1998).

Hemolytic disease of the newborn is a classic example of maternal humoral allorecognition. Rh incompatibility triggers a maternal antibody response when fetal Rh-positive blood enters, at delivery, a maternal Rh-negative circulation. Maternal immunoglobulin G (IgG) alloantibodies will cross the placenta, during a subsequent pregnancy, in increasing amounts during the second and third trimester. If the fetus is Rh positive, these antibodies are responsible for hemolysis of fetal red cells, which can result in severe anemia and ultimately hydrops fetalis. Alternatively, blood group O mothers have both IgM and IgG to blood groups A and B in circulation, and the IgG antibodies may cross the placenta with similar but generally less severe consequences. The understanding of this biologic process and its modification by Rh antibody is one of the major advances in clinical medicine of the past century.

Despite experiments comparing the successful pregnancy with an allogeneic solid organ transplant, such comparison represents a naïve interpretation of the complex physiology of the maternal–fetal interface. Classic studies by Beer and Billingham demonstrated that fetal allografts survive within the uterus but are rejected when transplanted in other locations (Beer and Billingham, 1971). Therefore immunologic tolerance alone cannot explain the maternal acceptance of the fetus. Immunologic and biochemical studies indicate that the maternal acceptance of the fetus results in isolation of the embryo in a semipermeable environment that shields the growing fetus from the maternal capacity of the immune system for rejection. This anatomic organization is therefore devoid of classic non–self recognition and is presumed to be dependent instead on maternal recognition, which results in beneficial consequences for the fetus. If this is the case, then these concepts imply that the maternal immune response must be modulated to allow for such recognition, as well as the maintenance of a well-regulated immunologic interaction that results in a viable pregnancy.

In this regard we view the recruitment of inflammatory cells to the maternal–fetal border in the context of maternal innate immune responsiveness. The maternal-fetal interface is also characterized by unique roles of complement regulatory proteins, uterine NK cells, macrophages, and various T-cell phenotypes. Finally, the local environmental cytokine milieu also makes a unique contribution to successful pregnancy outcome.

The Trophoblast

The trophoblast is the mesoectodermal cell layer covering the blastocyst that erodes into the uterine mucosa and contributes to the formation of the placenta. Anchoring processes are served by a core of vascular mesoderm that becomes the chorionic villi. The immunologic characteristics of trophoblast cells include unique HLA expression, as well as apoptotic mechanisms and cytokines that regulate its proliferative and invasive nature of the trophoblast (Table 11-2).

HLA Expression

Following implantation, the trophoblast differentiates into an outer layer, the syncytiotrophoblast, composed of a multinucleated mass (syncytium), and the inner layer, the cytotrophoblast, consisting of cells with intact membranes located next to the mesoderm (see Fig. 11-1). Interestingly, multiple studies now demonstrate that trophoblast cells lack constitutive expression of classical histocompatibility antigens A, B, DR, DQ, and DP. However, these cells do express several non-classical HLA class 1 molecules, including HLA-G and HLA-E, as well as the classical class 1 molecule HLA-C (Hutter et al., 1998). The absence of expression of classical MHC molecules on the trophoblast surface provides a potential explanation for the lack of maternal–fetal rejection.

The molecular mechanisms that regulate HLA gene expression in the cellular trophoblast are under both transcriptional and post-translational control (Torry et al., 1997). Transcription of classical class I gene products is regulated by both cis- and trans-acting mechanisms. Methylation of CpG islands near transcriptional start sites is a known cis-acting mechanism and results in decreased transcription of a gene (Razin and Cedar, 1991). The choriocarcinoma cell line JAR has been shown to undergo in vitro hypermethylation of CpG islands near transcriptional start sites of human class I

genes. Consistent with the data noted earlier, these cells do not express HLA-A, HLA-B, HLA-C, HLA-E, or HLA-G antigens. As studies in human placental tissue reveal demethylation of HLA-G CpG islands, the regulation of HLA expression within the trophoblast likely involves multiple competing molecular mechanisms.

Another regulatory pathway of HLA expression operates through negative regulatory elements upstream of the transcription start site. Nucleotide sequence analysis of HLA-G genes reveals an absence of this consensus-negative regulatory element, suggesting that this difference may directly contribute to the presence of HLA-G molecules on the surface of trophoblast cells (Chiang and Main, 1994; Lefebvre et al., 1999). In vitro studies demonstrate resistance to cytokine-induced upregulation of classical MHC molecules in trophoblast cells, suggesting that expression is either independent of cytokine upregulation or due to an intrinsic characteristic of this cell population (Hunt and Orr, 1992; Hunt et al., 1987).

HLA-G is an MHC class Ib molecule with limited polymorphisms. Six different isoforms exist as a result of alternative splicing, and both membrane and soluble forms have been identified (Carosella et al., 1999). HLA-G is expressed on trophoblast cells during both normal and abnormal embryonic development (Carosella et al., 2000). This molecule lacks the characteristic cytoplasmic tail due to a stop codon in exon 6, which results in truncation of the sequence encoding this specific region (Hunt et al., 2000b).

The precise biologic role of HLA-G molecules remains unknown. Perhaps the most interesting studies in this regard have revealed that the presence of HLA-G on trophoblast cells confers protection from NK-mediated cell lysis and that large granular lymphocyte cell lines transfected with HLA-G are partially protected from lysis by decidual NK cells (Chumbley et al., 1994; Pazmany et al., 1996). The protective effect was determined to be secondary to binding of trophoblast cells to inhibitory receptors on NK cells called *killer inhibitory receptors (KIRs)*. These receptors deliver inhibitory signals that prevent activation of NK cells. A second binding target for membrane-bound HLA-G molecules appears to be the *macrophage inhibitory receptors ILT2 and ILT4* (Long, 1999). Evidence for HLA-G binding to peripheral blood myelomonocytic cells has also been

---

TABLE 11-2 · IMMUNOLOGIC CHARACTERISTICS OF TROPHOBLAST CELLS

		Proposed Mechanism
· Cell-surface HLA expression	Absence of HLA-A, HLA-B, HLA-DR, HLA-DP, HLA-DQ	→ Lack of classic non–self recognition
	Presence of HLA-G, HLA-C, HLA-E	→ Bind to natural killer (NK) cell inhibitory receptors (KIR) preventing NK-mediated lysis
· Control of growth and differentiation	Fas-Fas ligand, p53, Bcl-2, Mcl-1, TNF-α, and IFN-γ	→ Regulate apoptosis
	TNF-α, TGF-β, CSF-1, GM-CSF, IGF-1, p53, and metalloproteases	→ Control trophoblast invasiveness
· Complement regulatory proteins	Expression of DAF, MCP, Crry*	→ Unclear

*Identified in murine pregnancy.
DAF = decay accelerating factor; IFN = interferon; MCP = membrane co-factor protein.

demonstrated; however, the role, if any, for interaction of these molecules with placental/decidual macrophages has not been determined (Allan et al., 1999).

In addition to the membrane-bound form of HLA-G, soluble forms of the molecule have been identified in maternal serum, suggesting a potential immunomodulatory role (Hunt et al., 2000b).

Cell Growth, Differentiation, and Apoptosis

The mechanisms determining trophoblast invasiveness must be tightly regulated to ensure that the endometrial layer of the uterus remains intact and is not breached by the growing placenta. Current studies suggest that the regulation of growth control of the invading trophoblast is mediated at least in part by the selective apoptotic deletion of cells, a process that does not alter the normal architecture of the tissue. Apoptosis is inducible in cultured trophoblast cells and may be developmentally regulated in human placenta, because a higher incidence of this form of cell death is consistently observed in third trimester villi (Smith, 2000; Smith et al., 1997a).

Apoptotic signal transduction occurs via a number of receptor-ligand binding pathways, including Fas–Fas ligand, which in turn lead to activation of a group of enzymes termed *caspases*. These caspases propagate downstream signals leading to DNA fragmentation and cell death. Fas is a surface membrane receptor and a member of the TNF family of receptors. Interactions of Fas with its ligand, FasL (also called *Apo-1L*), have been shown in immunologically privileged sites such as the eye to protect such tissue from immunologic attack (Gao et al., 1998). Fas–FasL interactions also occur in the human placenta throughout fetal development, and Fas ligand–expressing decidual and trophoblast cells are ideally positioned to delete Fas-expressing lymphocytes (Hunt et al., 1997).

In addition to these interactions, cytokines including TNF-α and interferon-γ (IFN-γ) also regulate apoptosis, and each of these is expressed in human placenta (Bulmer et al., 1990; Eades et al., 1988). Uterine epithelium and endometrial lymphocytes produce TNF-α, TGF-β, colony stimulating factor-1 (CSF-1), and GM-CSF, which may be involved in regulating trophoblast invasiveness (Huppertz et al., 2001).

The signaling events leading to apoptosis are also controlled by both proapoptotic (p53) and antiapoptotic (Bcl-2 and Mcl-1) proteins, which are expressed in trophoblast cells (Ho et al., 1999; Quenby et al., 1998). Enhanced expression of p53 in undifferentiated trophoblast could therefore be an additional mechanism for controlling normal trophoblast invasion and proliferation (Levy and Nelson, 2000). Human cytotrophoblast cells are constitutively invasive and produce *matrix metalloproteases (MMPs)*. In vitro studies suggest that IGF-1, the major secretory product of the decidua, stimulates MMP expression. Conversely, TGF-β inhibits the proteolytic activity of cytotrophoblast cells (Bischof et al., 2000). Of potential therapeutic importance, abnormal expression of several of these apoptotic signaling proteins has been detected in placental tissue from patients with preeclampsia and in women whose pregnancies are complicated by fetal growth restrictions (DiFederico et al., 1999; Genbacev et al., 1999; Smith et al., 1997b).

Cellular Components and Complement

Detailed studies of normal leukocyte populations in the human uterus reveal abundant aggregates of T and B cells, as well as cytotoxic T lymphocytes, macrophages, mast cells, and eosinophils. Not unexpectedly, these studies indicate that the constituents of the cell population change with different stages of the menstrual cycle, as well as during the phases of the pregnancy (Hunt et al., 2000a). Following implantation, aggregates of T and B cells disappear, eosinophils and mast cells are rarely seen, and uterine NK cells and macrophages become the predominant cell population.

Natural Killer Cells

NK cells are the most abundant lymphocytes in human and murine implantation sites (Table 11-3) (Croy and Kiso, 1993; King et al., 1996). Indeed, these cells constitute approximately 60% to 70% of maternal lymphocytes isolated from human decidua cell suspensions (Ashkar and Croy, 2001). NK cells are localized mainly within endometrial glandular epithelium and surrounding small arteries. In mice they are found in a poorly defined structure termed the *mesometrial lymphoid aggregate of pregnancy (MLA[p])*. NK cells in the uterus are defined by the presence of surface CD3$^-$/CD16$^-$/CD56$^+$ and KIR and the ability to lyse target K562 cells in the presence of IL-2 (King et al., 1991). Precursors are found in secondary lymphoid tissues, including the spleen and lymph nodes in mice, and both thymus and bone marrow contain progenitor cells with the potential to differentiate into uterine NK cells (Ashkar and Croy, 2001). These maternally derived NK cells increase in number, precede implantation during the luteal phase, differentiate during pregnancy, and decrease substantially in number to near absence by the end of pregnancy (King et al., 1989).

Little is known about the signals that attract these cells to specific sites. Progesterone, through upregulation of fibronectin receptors, may contribute to such recruitment. The characteristic feature of such NK cells is

TABLE 11-3 · CHARACTERISTICS OF UTERINE NATURAL KILLER CELLS

- 60%–70% of maternal lymphocytes within the pregnant uterus
- Localization { Endometrial glandular epithelium / Surrounding small arteries
- Express KIR
- Express perforin and *i*NOS
- Proposed role in vascular remodeling and decidua integrity mediated by IFN-γ
- Secrete GM-CSF, LIF, TGF-β, TNF-α

the expression of high levels of KIRs. These receptors belong to both the immunoglobulin superfamily of receptors (IgG-SF), p58.1/p58.2 and NKB1/p70, and the C-type lectin superfamily, which include CD94/NKG2A. Upon engagement to MHC class I molecules, inhibitory signals are delivered that block activation of the NK cell. CD158A (p58.1), CD158B (p58.2), LIR1, and CD94/NKGA2 recognize HLA-C. HLA-E binds to CD94 and NKG2A, and HLA-G is recognized by LIR-1, CD94/NKG2A, and p49 (Biassoni et al., 1999, 2000; Lee et al., 1998).

Uterine NK cells express membrane lytic molecules such as perforin, as well as inducible nitric oxide synthetase (iNOS). Perforin is a cytolytic, pore-forming molecule responsible for cell-mediated cytotoxicity reactions. Immunohistochemical staining identified abundant perforin-containing cells in the decidua of human pregnancies. Perforin is thought to contribute to the decidual homeostasis by eliminating antigen-presenting cells that are biased toward Th1 cytokine production. This process was readily observed in the infertile murine model resulting from perforin/FasL double deficiency (Rukavina and Podack, 2000). Progesterone produced by human lymphocytes may also contribute to this environmental milieu by resulting in expression of *progesterone-induced blocking factor (PIBF)*, which inhibits NK cytotoxicity via inhibition of the normal upregulation of perforin expression (Faust et al., 1999; Laskarin et al., 1999; Szereday et al., 1997).

A slightly different role for these uterine NK cells has been proposed based on four strains of NK- and T-cell–deficient mice, including tgε26, p56$^{lck-/-}$/IL-2Rβ$^{-/-}$, IL-2Rγ$^{-/-}$, and recombination-activating gene-2 (RAG-2)$^{-/-}$/γ$_c$$^{-/-}$ (Ashkar and Croy, 2001; Colucci et al., 1999; Croy et al., 1997; DiSanto et al., 1996; Guimond et al., 1997). These mice, each of which lack uterine NK cells, have multiple abnormalities, including implantation site anomalies, failure to develop MLAp, and impaired angiogenesis and decidua formation. Importantly, these changes are all reversible by bone marrow transplantation in which only uterine NK cells are restored (using NK$^+$T$^-$B$^-$ severe combined immunodeficiency [SCID] mice as donors). Interestingly, when bone marrow grafts from IFN-γ$^{-/-}$ were utilized as donors into RAG-2$^{-/-}$/γ$_c$$^{-/-}$ recipients, normal numbers of uterine NK were restored in the absence of vascular remodeling or normal decidual integrity.

Taken together, these data suggest that a critical component of uterine NK-cell activity is mediated by IFN-γ (Ashkar and Croy, 2001; Ashkar et al., 2000). In keeping with the accumulated cytokine and growth factor noted earlier, recent work reveals that activated NK cells also secrete GM-CSF, LIF, TGF-β, and TNF-α at specific and different times during normal placental development (Carretero et al., 1997; King et al., 1997).

Macrophages

The number of macrophages remains stable throughout pregnancy, representing 10% to 15% of total cells within the endometrium. Monocytes are activated during pregnancy, and many soluble placental products released into the maternal circulation activate monocytes and suppress lymphocyte proliferation in vitro (Sacks et al., 1999). Monocyte inflammatory protein-1α (MIP-1α) has been isolated from cytotrophoblast-conditioned medium and shown to be an important chemoattractant of both uterine NK and monocytes, directing them toward the maternal–fetal interface (Drake et al., 2001). Many other cytokines and growth factors also participate in cellular recruitment and activation of the monocyte lineage, including LIF, CSF-1, GM-CSF, IFN-γ, TNF-α, IL-4, IL-6, IL-10, and TGF-β. As noted earlier, the sources for these cytokines and growth factors consist of cells in the local environment, including uterine epithelial cells, trophoblast cells, uterine NK cells, and the cells of the decidua and seminal plasma (Haynes et al., 1993; Hunt and Robertson, 1996; Pollard et al., 1991).

Monocytes and macrophages within the uterine endometrium may enhance nonspecific immune responses of the mother by increasing the expression of FcγRI (CD64) and FcγRII (CD32), as well as through the promotion of phagocytosis (Davis et al., 1998). Some fascinating studies suggest that substance P–mediated macrophage and mast cells activation may be responsible for psychic stress–induced abortions in mice (Arck et al., 1995). Importantly, vascular endothelial growth factor (VEGF), a predominant macrophage product, has recently been found to play a critical role in placental angiogenesis via activation of the VEGF tyrosine receptor-2 (Carmeliet et al., 2001; Charnock-Jones et al., 1999; Clark et al., 1996).

Complement

The complement system is a critical component of the innate immune response. This system is evolutionarily conserved and plays a critical role as an early effector system of host defense. One important component of the complement system is a series of circulating effector proteins that target microbes and other antigens within the plasma and extravascular spaces. These proteins are normally inactive, and their expression is tightly regulated. Upon specific proteolytic activation, complement proteins may bind to the surface of foreign organisms and destroy them by damaging the cell membranes.

Another important component of the complement system is a network of regulatory proteins that are necessary to prevent damage to normal cells and tissues and to avoid the release of degradation products that act on adjacent cells, causing tissue damage. Three membrane-bound proteins regulate the activation of the third and fourth components of complement (C3 and C4). These include decay accelerating factor (DAF), membrane co-factor protein (MCP), and, in mice, a protein called *Crry*. The latter regulates the deposition of activated C3 and C4 on cells in vitro.

Crry-deficient animals die in the uterus at about 10 days after conception, thus suggesting that Crry is important for survival of the embryo (Xu et al., 2000). Crry is the only complement regulatory component found on murine trophoblast cells. In Crry-deficient animals, extensive deposition of C3 occurs, and it is hypothesized that the subsequent influx of polymorphonuclear granulocytes leads to the eventual destruction of the embryo. Although DAF and MCP are abundantly expressed in human placenta, an analogous protein to Crry has yet to be found in humans (see Table 11-2). Nevertheless, this mouse model provides a physiologic role for complement regulatory proteins on trophoblast cells, revealing that the absence or dysregulation of such receptors could conceivably result in recurring abortions in a subset of patients.

In this regard, the maternal innate immune response may actively modulate human pregnancy through the activity of uterine NK cells, macrophages, and complement regulatory proteins. The study of cellular immunologic functions in pathologic pregnancy states will clarify such role (Sacks et al., 1999). Recent data supportive of a specific role for T-cell–driven complement activation and inflammation in pregnancy failure have focused on the role of indolamine 2,3-dioxygenase (IDO), known to protect developing fetuses from maternal immune responses (Munn et al., 1998). In these studies an IDO inhibitor was used to demonstrate that protection by IDO results from suppression of T-cell–driven inflammatory responses to fetal alloantigens (Mellor et al., 2001).

T Lymphocytes

T lymphocytes found in the uterus have at least two known functions. First, these cells provide effector/cytotoxic activities in host defense by eliminating noxious antigens of bacteria and viruses. Second, the regulation of these T cells defines the fundamental properties of immunologic tolerance. Thus, within the uterus, T cells may contribute to the local immunosuppressive environment that maintains the survival of the fetus. T lymphocytes are most abundant at the cervix in the nonpregnant uterus. At the beginning of pregnancy the number of T-cell aggregated within the endometrium decreases but rises within the decidua as pregnancy advances. During mid-gestation, T cells represent 20% of lymphocytes within the uterus.

Although the origin of uterine T cells is not known, their recruitment from the maternal circulating T-cell pool is suggested by cell-tracking experiments. The uterus itself may be a site of extrathymic T-lymphocyte maturation (Robertson, 2000). RAG-1 and RAG-2 are present at implantation sites, and the local presence of specific Vα11 T cells in placentas of abortion-primed mice supports the hypothesis that T-lymphocyte maturation may occur in the uterus (Kimura et al., 1995; Yamasaki et al., 2001). Patterns of adhesion molecule expression suggest a direct role for these proteins in T-lymphocyte recruitment to the pregnant uterus. For example, previous studies have demonstrated abundant expression of the adhesin mucosal vascular addressin (MAdCAM-1) in vessels at the leading edge of trophoblast invasion (Burrows et al., 1994; Kruse et al., 1999).

Both αβ-T and γδ-T cells have been identified within the pregnant uterus during human gestation. The role of conventional αβ-T cells in the decidua is unclear. Indolamine 2,3-dioxygenase, an enzyme that catabolizes tryptophan, is expressed by both trophoblast cells and macrophages and appears to play a role in suppression of αβ-T–cell activation in the decidua, as evidenced by rapid T-cell–induced rejection of the conceptus upon pharmacologic inhibition of this enzyme (Munn et al., 1998; Munn et al., 1999). Murine and human γδ-T cells exhibit antigen specificity to trophoblast cells in a nonrestricted manner (Mincheva-Nilsson et al., 1997). These γδ-T cells constitutively synthesize perforin, which is localized to intracellular cytolytic granules. In addition, FasL is detected within the cytoplasm and, on degranulation, translocates to the cell surface. Taken together, these observations suggest that T-cell cytotoxic potential and immunoregulatory functions at the maternal–fetal interface are under complex control.

T lymphocytes within the uterus are also found to be composed of different phenotypes based on cytokine expression. Th1 cells produce IL-2 and IFN-γ, enhancing cell-mediated immunity. IL-4 and IL-10 production characterize the Th2 phenotype or antibody-driven immune response. Th3 cells are the main producers of TGF-β. Th1 cells produce IL-10 and TGF-β and can be further induced by IL-10 (Robertson, 2000). It is also known that Th2 cytokines, and in particular IL-10, can downregulate Th1 responses. Th2 cytokines (IL-4, IL-10) are detectable in freshly isolated decidual and placental cells. IFN-γ (Th1) predominance during the first trimester of pregnancy is barely detectable in the second and is undetectable in the third trimester. Importantly, persistent Th1 phenotypes have been identified in mice strains that experience spontaneous abortions, such as the CBA/J females mated with DBA/2J males (CBA/J X DBA/2J).

Consistent with these observations, administration of TNF-α, IFN-γ, and IL-2 causes spontaneous abortions (Parant, 1990). Likewise, a strong Th1 response such as that needed to clear Leishmania major infection will also result in fetal resorption (Krishnan et al., 1996). These observations have led to the hypothesis that successful pregnancy requires a Th2-dominant situation (Lin et al., 1993; Michie, 1998; Raghupathy, 1997; Wegmann et al., 1993). In support of this hypothesis, administration of IL-10 prevents fetal wastage in abortion-prone mice (Chaouat et al., 1996).

These findings also may help explain the clinical observation that cell-mediated autoimmune diseases such as rheumatoid arthritis, psoriatic arthritis, and ankylosing spondilitis all may improve during pregnancy, whereas patients with antibody-driven processes such as systemic lupus erythematosus (SLE) may experience exacerbation of disease activity while pregnant.

Interestingly, a predominant Th1 environment has been observed in a subset of patients with recurrent abortions. Supernatants from trophoblast-activated peripheral blood mononuclear cells from 244 women with unexplained recurrent abortions were studied for toxic effects on mouse embryos. In 51% of women,

IFN-γ was detected in these supernatants, and this was significantly associated with embryotoxicity. Alternatively, supernatants from reproductively normal women and men were not found to contain Th1-type cytokines (Hill et al., 1995). Women with term pregnancies infected with *Plasmodium falciparum* malaria demonstrated both Th1 and Th2 cytokine patterns from chorionic villi, placental blood, and serum. Although the Th1 pathway was favored, a strong IL-10 response was noted. This observation led the authors to speculate that such response permitted placental protection and therefore allowed these pregnancies to reach term (Fievet et al., 2001).

Although this Th1/Th2 dichotomy may help in explaining the cytokine environments that underlie a successful pregnancy, this hypothesis does not explain the fact that IFN-γ, a known Th1 cytokine, is essential for implantation and early placental development. Furthermore, other investigators have shown that overexpression of Th2 activation can also be associated with pathologic pregnancies (Hayakawa et al., 2000). Curiously, in mice deficient in both IL-4 and IL-10, the absence of these cytokines at either the maternal or fetal-placental side of the interface did not prevent normal breeding (Svensson et al., 2001). These findings suggest that neither of these cytokines is crucial for the completion of allogeneic pregnancy in mice. Obviously, much work remains to be done to elucidate the multiple and complex factors associated with successful pregnancy.

MATERNAL TOLERANCE

Microchimerism is defined by the presence within an individual of a low level of cells derived from a different individual. An important source of chimerism is pregnancy. Male cells can be found in pregnant females as early as 6 weeks' gestation. Maternal cells may also reach the fetal circulation, as initially demonstrated in children with SCID. More recently, such cells have been detected in adult life, suggesting a long-lasting persistence under certain circumstances (Aractingi et al., 2000). The relevance of microchimerism in disease states such as scleroderma is the subject of intense investigation (Nelson, 1999). Because microchimerism is often found in normal individuals, the significance of any observations in this area remains unclear. Nevertheless, understanding how foreign cells may breach a tolerant state may well permit an increased understanding of the mechanisms of autoimmunity.

Maternal T cells recognize fetal alloantigens, as demonstrated by the identification of distinct T-cell clones detectable in maternal blood during pregnancy. By utilizing mice that express a transgenic T-cell receptor (TCR) of known antigenic specificity, the fate of maternal T cells to fetal antigens can be followed throughout gestation. Interestingly, clonal deletion, immunologic unresponsiveness (anergy), and co-receptor downregulation have all been identified as specific mechanisms of peripheral immunologic tolerance during murine pregnancy (Hoger et al., 1996; Jiang and Vacchio, 1998; Rogers et al., 1998; Tafuri et al., 1995; Vacchio and Jiang, 1999).

Although these experiments demonstrate different mechanisms of peripheral tolerance, factors such as the maternal–fetal source of antigen presentation, as well as the precise fetal antigen load, may also contribute to the establishment of one mechanism of peripheral immune tolerance versus another (Vacchio and Jiang, 1999).

IMMUNOMODULATORY STRATEGIES FOR TREATMENT OF RECURRENT PREGNANCY LOSS

Despite advances in reproductive medicine and the understanding of its immunobiology, pregnancy losses continue to be an important complication of human gestation, affecting 15% of women. Although anatomic, hormonal, and chromosomal abnormalities and endometriosis are known etiologic factors, in 40% of cases no cause can be determined. The precise role of immunologic factors contributing to the biologic process of recurrent pregnancy loss remains the subject of much debate. Identification of maternal cytotoxic and blocking antibodies, changes in NK populations, and HLA sharing have been described in women with recurrent abortions of unknown etiology (Jablonowska et al., 2001; Kwat et al., 2000; Rigal et al., 1994). However, the only proven alloimmune mechanism has been demonstrated in those patients in whom antiphospholipid antibodies are associated with recurrent pregnancy loss (Porter et al., 2000). Unfortunately, surrogate markers and specific and sensitive laboratory tests necessary in the clinical setting to diagnose a specific alloimmune process are currently lacking. Despite this, when faced with the desperate clinical entity of recurrent pregnancy losses, therapies known for their immunomodulatory effects in other clinical settings have been tried. Two such therapies worth reviewing include intravenous immunoglobulin (IVIG) infusions and allogeneic leukocyte transfusions.

In the past two decades, IVIG has been used and has benefited a variety of patients with inflammatory and autoimmune conditions. Some proposed mechanisms include an increase in the IgG catabolic rate, the presence of anti-idiotypic antibodies, and influences on cytokine production (Ballow, 1997; Zhiya and Lemon, 1999). Despite theoretical benefits, studies demonstrating IVIG efficacy in recurrent pregnancy loss have been somewhat disappointing. The heterogeneity among studied patients and differences in trial design appear to have contributed to the observed inconclusive therapeutic benefit of IVIG (Clark et al., 2000).

Five pilot studies and one double-blind controlled multicenter study of 236 patients with recurrent pregnancy loss summarized a European experience, where no specific benefit of IVIG was demonstrated despite variable success rates in study patients (Mueller-Eckhardt, 1994). Finally, a systematic review of 10 therapeutic trials involving 627 patients for treatment of antiphospholipid syndrome found a 54% reduction in pregnancy loss with combination therapy of heparin and aspirin; IVIG provided no further added benefit (Empson et al., 2002). Thus consistent therapeutic trials are still necessary to demonstrate the potential efficacy in a yet to be defined subset of patients in whom such therapy may be valuable.

Paternal allogeneic leukocyte transfusion, for treatment of women with recurrent pregnancy loss of unknown etiology, is premised on induction of immunologic tolerance. Blood transfusions, containing allogeneic leukocytes, given prior to solid organ transplantation can result in fewer episodes of acute rejection. Due to the myriad single-center studies, the American Society for Reproductive Immunology sponsored a worldwide collaborative observational study on the use of leukocyte immunotherapy for recurrent spontaneous abortions (RMITG, 1994). A small treatment effect benefited 8% to 10% of affected couples, and subsequent reviews of meta-analysis have confirmed such benefit for a subset of women in whom there was no evidence of autoimmunity, in whom recurrent abortions had occurred after 6 weeks' gestation, and who demonstrated normal karyotype (Clark et al., 2001).

SUMMARY

To further our understanding of immunologic tolerance, immunologists turned to the fundamental biologic process of pregnancy. The knowledge of how the maternal immune system is modulated to allow for the survival of the fetus is provided through insights into both innate and adaptive immune maternal recognition occurring during pregnancy.

In this chapter we reviewed the cellular and molecular immunologic interactions known to contribute to a successful pregnancy. Sperm-specific protein interactions, developmental regulation of MHC molecules on human gametes, and unique immunogenetic backgrounds associated with immunologic mechanisms of infertility provide evidence for the participation of the immune system during the early phases of conception and fertilization. During implantation, cytokines of known immunologic significance, such as LIF, TGF-β, PP14, IL-11, IGF, along with sex hormones, provide optimal conditions for blastocyst apposition, transformation, and penetration into a receptive endometrium.

As gestation evolves, the developing embryo becomes isolated within a semipermeable environment. The anatomic organization of this maternal–fetal interface appears to be critical to the healthy outcome of pregnancy. Absence of classical MHC molecules on trophoblast surface and recognition of nonclassical HLA-G molecules by KIR receptors on uterine NK cells provide examples of cellular recognition at the maternal–fetal interface that results in beneficial consequences to the fetus (Table 11-4).

The unique roles of complement regulatory proteins, uterine NK cells, macrophages, T-cell phenotypes, indolamine 2,3-dioxygenase, and cytokine milieu, along with the demonstration of specific mechanisms of

TABLE 11-4 · PROPOSED MECHANISMS LEADING TO MATERNAL IMMUNE TOLERANCE OF THE FETUS

· Expression of HLA-G, HLA-E, and HLA-C molecules on trophoblast cells
· Control of NK cytolytic activity via inhibitory receptors
· Expression of complement regulatory proteins
· Regulated leukocyte recruitment and cell proliferation at the maternal–fetal interface
· IDO suppression of αβ-T–lymphocyte activation within the decidua
· Evidence of peripheral immune tolerance by clonal deletion, anergy, and co-receptor downregulation during murine pregnancy

peripheral immunologic tolerance, provide a basis for potential therapeutic approaches to pathologic pregnancies, autoimmune diseases, and immunologic manipulations during tissue transplantation.

REFERENCES

Allan DS, Colonna M, Lanier LL, Churakova TD, Abrams JS, Ellis SA, McMichael AJ, Braud VM. Tetrameric complexes of human histocompatibility leukocyte antigen (HLA)-G bind to peripheral blood myelomonocytic cells. J Exp Med 189:1149–1156, 1999.

Almeida EA, Huovila AP, Sutherland AE, Stephens LE, Calarco PG, Shaw LM, Mercurio AM, Sonnenberg A, Primakoff P, Myles DJ, et al. Mouse egg integrin alpha 6 beta 1 functions as a sperm receptor. Cell 81:1095–1094, 1995.

Aractingi, S, Uzan, S, Dausset J, Carosella ED. Microchimerism in human diseases. Immunol Today 21:116–118, 2000.

Arck PC, Merali FS, Stanisz AM, Stead RH, Chaouat G, Manuel J, Clark DA. Stress-induced murine abortion associated with substance P-dependent alteration in cytokines in maternal uterine decidua. Biol Reprod 53:814–819, 1995.

Ashkar AA, Croy BA. Functions of uterine natural killer cells are mediated by interferon gamma production during murine pregnancy. Semin Immunol 13: 235–241, 2001.

Ashkar AA, Di Santo JP, Croy BA. Interferon gamma contributes to initiation of uterine vascular modification, decidual integrity, and uterine natural killer cell maturation during normal murine pregnancy. J Exp Med 192:259–270, 2000.

Baker J, Hardy MP, Zhou J, Bondy C, Lupu F, Bellve AR, Efstratiadis A. Effects of an Igf1 gene null mutation on mouse reproduction. Mol Endocrinol 10:903–918, 1996.

Ballow M. Mechanisms of action of intravenous immune serum globulin in autoimmune and inflammatory diseases. J Allergy Clin Immunol 100:151–157, 1997.

Beer AE, Billingham RE. Immunobiology of mammalian reproduction. Adv Immunol 14:1–84, 1971.

Biassoni R, Bottino C, Millo R, Moretta L, Moretta A. Natural killer cell–mediated recognition of human trophoblast. Semin Cancer Biol 9:13–18, 1999.

Biassoni R, Cantoni C, Falco M, Pende D, Millo R, Moretta L, Bottino C, Moretta A. Human natural killer cell activating receptors. Mol Immunol 37:1015–1024, 2000.

Bischof P, Haenggeli L, Campana A. Effect of leukemia inhibitory factor on human cytotrophoblast differentiation along the invasive pathway. Am J Reprod Immunol 34:225–230, 1995.

Bischof P, Meisser A, Campana A. Mechanisms of endometrial control of trophoblast invasion. J Reprod Fertil Suppl 55: 65–71, 2000.

Bronson RA, Fusi FM. Integrins and human reproduction. Mol Hum Reprod 2:153–168, 1996.

Bulmer JN, Morrison L, Johnson PM, Meager A. Immunohistochemical localization of interferons in human placental tissues in normal, ectopic, and molar pregnancy. Am J Reprod Immunol 22:109–116, 1990.

Burrows TD, King A, Loke YW. Expression of adhesion molecules by endovascular trophoblast and decidual endothelial cells:

implications for vascular invasion during implantation. Placenta 15:21–33, 1994.

Carmeliet P, Moons L, Luttun A, Vincenti V, Compernolle V, De Mol M, Wu Y, Bono F, Devy L, Beck H, Scholz D, Acker T, DiPalma T, Dewerchin M, Noel A, Stalmans I, Barra A, Blacher S, Vandendriessche T, Ponten A, Eriksson U, Plate KH, Foidart JM, Schaper W, Charnock-Jones DS, Hicklin DJ, Herbert JM, Collen D, Persico MG. Synergism between vascular endothelial growth factor and placental growth factor contributes to angiogenesis and plasma extravasation in pathological conditions. Nat Med 7:575–583, 2001.

Carosella ED, Paul P, Moreau P, Rouas-Freiss N. HLA-G and HLA-E: fundamental and pathophysiological aspects. Immunol Today 21:532–534, 2000.

Carosella ED, Rouas-Freiss N, Paul P, Dausset J. HLA-G: a tolerance molecule from the major histocompatibility complex. Immunol Today 20:60–62, 1999.

Carretero M, Cantoni C, Bellon, T, Bottino, C, Biassoni R, Rodriguez A, Perez-Villar JJ, Moretta L, Moretta A, Lopez-Botet M. The CD94 and NKG2-A C-type lectins covalently assemble to form a natural killer cell inhibitory receptor for HLA class I molecules. Eur J Immunol 27:563–567, 1997.

Chaouat G, Menu E, De Smedt D, Khrihnan L, Hui L, Assal Meliani A, Martal J, Raghupathy R, Wegmann TG. The emerging role of IL-10 in pregnancy. Am J Reprod Immunol 35:325–329, 1996.

Charnock-Jones DS, Sharkey AM, Boocock CA, Ahmed A, Plevin R, Ferrara N, Smith SK. Vascular endothelial growth factor receptor localization and activation in human trophoblast and choriocarcinoma cells. Biol Reprod 51:524–530, 1994.

Chiang MH, Main EK. Nuclear regulation of HLA class I genes in human trophoblasts. Am J Reprod Immunol 32:167–172, 1994.

Chumbley G, King A, Robertson K, Holmes N, Loke YW. Resistance of HLA-G and HLA-A2 transfectants to lysis by decidual NK cells. Cell Immunol 155:312–322, 1994.

Clark DA, Coulam CB, Daya S, Chaouat G. Unexplained sporadic and recurrent miscarriages in the new millennium: a critical analysis of immune mechanism and treatments. Human Reprod Updates 7:501–511, 2001.

Clark DE, Smith SK, Sharkey AM, Charnock-Jones S. Localization of VEGF and expression of its receptors flt and KDR in human placenta throughout pregnancy. Hum Reprod 11:1090–1098, 1996.

Colucci F, Soudais C, Rosmaraki E, Vanes L, Tybulewicz VL, Di Santo JP. Dissecting NK cell development using a novel alymphoid mouse model: investigating the role of the c-abl proto-oncogene in murine NK cell differentiation. J Immunol 162:2761–2765, 1999.

Coulam CB, Stern JJ. Evaluation of immunological infertility. Am J Reprod Immunol 27:130–135, 1992.

Croy BA, Ashkar AA, Foster RA, DiSanto JP, Magram J, Carson D, Gendler SJ, Grusby MJ, Wagner N, Muller W, Guimond MJ. Histological studies of gene-ablated mice support important functional roles for natural killer cells in the uterus during pregnancy. J Reprod Immunol 35:111–133, 1997.

Croy BA, Kiso Y. Granulated metrial gland cells: a natural killer cell subset of the pregnant murine uterus. Microsc Res Tech 25:189–200, 1993.

Danielsson KG, Swahn ML, Bygdeman M. The effect of various doses of mifepristone on endometrial leukaemia inhibitory factor expression in the midluteal phase—an immunohistochemical study. Hum Reprod 12:1293–1297, 1997.

Davis D, Kaufmann R, Moticka EJ. Nonspecific immunity in pregnancy: monocyte surface Fc gamma receptor expression and function. J Reprod Immunol 40:119–128, 1998.

Delage G, Moreau FJ, Taupin JL, Freitas S, Hambartsoumian, E, Olivennes F, Fanchin R, Letur-Konirsch H, Frydman R, Chaouat G. In-vitro endometrial secretion of human interleukin for DA cells/leukaemia inhibitory factor by explant cultures from fertile and infertile women. Hum Reprod 10:2483–2488, 1995.

DiFederico E, Genbacev O, Fisher SJ. Preeclampsia is associated with widespread apoptosis of placental cytotrophoblasts within the uterine wall. Am J Pathol 155:293–301, 1999.

DiSanto JP, Guy-Grand D, Fisher A, Tarakhovsky A. Critical role for the common cytokine receptor gamma chain in intrathymic and peripheral T cell selection. J Exp Med 183:1111–1118, 1996.

Drake PM, Gunn MD, Charo IF, Tsou CL, Zhou Y, Huang L, Fisher SJ. Human placental cytotrophoblasts attract monocytes and CD56(bright) natural killer cells via the actions of monocyte inflammatory protein 1alpha. J Exp Med 193:1199–1212, 2001.

Eades DK, Cornelius P, Pekala PH. Characterization of the tumour necrosis factor receptor in human placenta. Placenta 9:247–251, 1988.

Empson M, Lassere M, Craig JC, Scott JR. Recurrent pregnancy loss with antiphospholipid antibody: a systematic review of therapeutic trials. Obstet Gynecol 99:135–144, 2002.

Evans JP. Sperm disintegrins, egg integrins, other cell adhesion molecules of mammalian gamete plasma membrane interactions. Front Biosci 4:D114–131, 1999.

Faust Z, Laskarin G, Rukavina D, Szekeres-Bartho J. Progesterone-induced blocking factor inhibits degranulation of natural killer cells. Am J Reprod Immunol 42:71–75, 1999.

Fernandez N, Cooper J, Sprinks M, AbdElrahman M, Fiszer D, Kurpisz M, Dealtry G. A critical review of the role of the major histocompatibility complex in fertilization, preimplantation development and feto-maternal interactions. Hum Reprod Update 5:234–248, 1999.

Fievet N, Moussa M, Tami G, Maubert B, Cot M, Deloron P, Chaouat G. Plasmodium falciparum induces a Th1/Th2 disequilibrium, favoring the Th1-type pathway, in the human placenta. J Infect Dis 183:1530–1534, 2001.

Gao Y, Herndon JM, Zhang H, Griffith TS, Ferguson TA. Antiinflammatory effects of CD95 ligand (FasL)–induced apoptosis. J Exp Med 188:887–896, 1998.

Genbacev O, DiFederico E, McMaster M, Fisher SJ. Invasive cytotrophoblast apoptosis in pre-eclampsia. Hum Reprod 14:59–66, 1999.

Geng JG, Raub TJ, Baker CA, Sawada GA, Ma L, Elhammer AP. Expression of a P-selectin ligand in zona pellucida of porcine oocytes and P-selectin on acrosomal membrane of porcine sperm cells. Potential implications for their involvement in sperm-egg interactions. J Cell Biol 137:743–754, 1997.

Guimond MJ, Luross JA, Wang B, Terhorst C, Danial S, Croy BA. Absence of natural killer cells during murine pregnancy is associated with reproductive compromise in TgE26 mice. Biol Reprod 56:169–179, 1997.

Harvey MB, Leco KJ, Arcellana-Panlilio MY, Zhang X, Edwards DR, Schultz GA. Proteinase expression in early mouse embryos is regulated by leukaemia inhibitory factor and epidermal growth factor. Development 121:1005–1014, 1995.

Hayakawa S, Fujikawa T, Fukuoka H, Chisima F, Karasaki-Suzuki M, Ohkoshi E, Ohi H, Kiyoshi Fujii T, Tochig M, Satoh K, Shimizu T, Nishinarita S, Nemoto N, Sakurai I. Murine fetal resorption and experimental pre-eclampsia are induced by both excessive Th1 and Th2 activation. J Reprod Immunol 47:121–138, 2000.

Haynes MK, Jackson LG, Tuan RS, Shepley KJ, Smith JB. Cytokine production in first trimester chorionic villi: detection of mRNAs and protein products in situ. Cell Immunol 151:300–308, 1993.

Hill JA, Polgar K, Anderson DJ. T-helper 1-type immunity to trophoblast in women with recurrent spontaneous abortion. JAMA 273:1933–1936, 1995.

Ho S, Winkler-Lowen B, Morrish DW, Dakour J, Li H, Guilbert LJ. The role of Bcl-2 expression in EGF inhibition of TNF-alpha/IFN-gamma–induced villous trophoblast apoptosis. Placenta 20:423–430, 1999.

Hoger TA, Tokuyama M, Yonamine K, Hayashi K, Masuko-Hongo K, Kato T, Kobata T, Mizushima Y, Nishioka K, Yamamoto K. Time course analysis of alpha+ beta+ T cell clones during normal pregnancy. Eur J Immunol 26:834–838, 1996.

Hunt JS, Andrews GK, Wood G. Normal trophoblasts resist induction of class I HLA. J Immunol 138:2481–2487, 1987.

Hunt JS, Orr HT. HLA and maternal-fetal recognition. FASEB J 6:2344–2348, 1992.

Hunt JS, Petroff MG, Burnett TG. Uterine leukocytes: key players in pregnancy. Semin Cell Dev Biol 11:127–137, 2000a.

Hunt JS, Petroff MG, Morales P, Sedlmayr P, Geraghty DE, Ober C. HLA-G in reproduction: studies on the maternal-fetal interface. Hum Immunol 61:1113–1117, 2000b.

Hunt JS, Robertson SA. Uterine macrophages and environmental programming for pregnancy success. J Reprod Immunol 32:1–25, 1996.

Hunt JS, Vassmer D, Ferguson TA, Miller L. Fas ligand is positioned in mouse uterus and placenta to prevent trafficking of activated leukocytes between the mother and the conceptus. J Immunol 158: 4122–4128, 1997.

Huppertz B, Rote NS, Nelson DM, Reister F, Black S, Hunt JS. Apoptosis: molecular control of placental function—a workshop report. Placenta 22: S101–103, 2001.

Hutter H, Hammer A, Dohr G, Hunt JS. HLA expression at the maternal-fetal interface. Dev Immunol 6:197–204, 1998.

Jablonowska B, Palfi M, Ernerudh J, Kjellberg S, Selbing S. Blocking antibodies in blood from patients with recurrent spontaneous abortion in relation to pregnancy outcome and intravenous immunoglobulin treatment. Am J Reprod Immunol 45:226–231, 2001.

Jiang SP, Vacchio MS. Multiple mechanisms of peripheral T cell tolerance to the fetal allograft. J Immunol 160:3086–3090, 1998.

Kapsenberg ML, Hilkens CM, Wierenga EA, Kalinski P. The paradigm of type 1 and type 2 antigen-presenting cells. Implications for atopic allergy. Clin Exp Allergy 29:33–36, 1999.

Kimura M, Hanawa H, Watanabe H, Ogawa M, Abo T. Synchronous expansion of intermediate TCR cells in the liver and uterus during pregnancy. Cell Immunol 162:16–25, 1995.

King A, Balendran N, Wooding P, Carter NP, Loke YW. CD3-leukocytes present in the human uterus during early placentation: phenotypic and morphologic characterization of the CD56++ population. Dev Immunol 1:169–190, 1991.

King A, Burrows T, Loke YW. Human uterine natural killer cells. Nat Immun 15:41–52, 1996.

King A, Jokhi PP, Smith SK, Sharkey AM, Loke YW. Screening for cytokine mRNA in human villous and extravillous trophoblasts using the reverse-transcriptase polymerase chain reaction (RT-PCR). Cytokine 7:364–71, 1995.

King A, Loke W, Chaouat G. NK cells and reproduction. Immunol Today 18:64–66, 1997.

King A, Wellings V, Gardner L, Loke YW. Immunocytochemical characterization of the unusual large granular lymphocytes in human endometrium throughout the menstrual cycle. Hum Immunol 24:195–205, 1989.

Koli K, Saharinen J, Hyytiainen M, Penttinen C, Keski-Oja J. Latency, activation, and binding proteins of TGF-beta. Microsc Res Tech 52:354–362, 2001.

Kotlan B, Fulop V, Padanyi A, Szigetvari I, Reti M, Gyodi E, Feher E, Petranyi G. High anti-paternal cytotoxic T-lymphocyte precursor frequencies in women with unexplained recurrent spontaneous abortions. Hum Reprod 16:1278–1285, 2001.

Krishnan L, Guilbert LJ, Wegmann TG, Belosevic M, Mosmann TR. T helper 1 response against Leishmania major in pregnant C57BL/6 mice increases implantation failure and fetal resorptions. Correlation with increased IFN-gamma and TNF and reduced IL-10 production by placental cells. J Immunol 156:653–662, 1996.

Kruse A, Merchant MJ, Hallmann R, Butcher EC. Evidence of specialized leukocyte-vascular homing interactions at the maternal/fetal interface. Eur J Immunol 29:1116–1126, 1999.

Kuo RC, Baxter GT, Thompson SH, Stricker SA, Patton C, Bonaventura J, Epel D. NO is necessary and sufficient for egg activation at fertilization. Nature 406:633–636, 2000.

Kwat JYH, Kwat FM, Gilman-Sachs A, Beaman KD, Cho DD, Beer AE. Immunoglobulin G infusion treatment for women with recurrent spontaneous abortions and elevated CD56+ natural killer cells. Early Preg 4:154–164, 2000.

Laskarin G, Strbo N, Sotosek V, Rukavina D, Faust Z, Szekeres-Bartho J, Podack ER. Progesterone directly and indirectly affects perforin expression in cytolytic cells. Am J Reprod Immunol 42:312–320, 1999.

Lee N, Llano M, Carretero M, Ishitani A, Navarro F, Lopez-Botet M, Geraghty DE. HLA-E is a major ligand for the natural killer inhibitory receptor CD94/NKG2A. Proc Natl Acad Sci USA 95:5199–5204, 1998.

Lefebvre S, Moreau P, Guiard V, Ibrahim EC, Adrian-Cabestre F, Menier C, Dausset J, Carosella ED, Paul P. Molecular mechanisms controlling constitutive and IFN-gamma-inducible HLA-G expression in various cell types. J Reprod Immunol 43:213–224, 1999.

Levy R, Nelson DM. To be, or not to be, that is the question. Apoptosis in human trophoblast. Placenta 21:1–13, 2000.

Lin H, Mosmann TR, Guilbert L, Tuntipopipat S, Wegmann TG. Synthesis of T helper 2-type cytokines at the maternal-fetal interface. J Immunol 151:4562–4573, 1993.

Long EO. Regulation of immune responses through inhibitory receptors. Annu Rev Immunol 17:875–904, 1999.

Loras B, Vetele F, El Malki A, Rollet J, Soufir JC, Benahmed M. Seminal transforming growth factor-beta in normal and infertile men. Hum Reprod 14:1534–1539, 1999.

Makrigiannakis A, Zoumakis E, Kalantaridou S, Coutifaris C, Margioris AN, Coukos G, Rice KC, Gravanis A, Chrousos GP. Corticotropin-releasing hormone promotes blastocyst implantation and early maternal tolerance. Nat Immunol 2:1018–1024, 2001.

Medawar PB. Some immunological problems raised by the evolution of viviparity in vertebrates. Symp Soc Exp Biol 7:320–338, 1953.

Mellor AL, Munn DH. Immunology at the maternal-fetal interface: lessons for T cell tolerance and suppression. Annu Rev Immunol 18:367–391, 2000.

Mellor AL, Sivakumar J, Chandler P, Smith K, Molina H, Mao D, Munn DH. Prevention of T cell–driven complement activation and inflammation by tryptophan catabolism during pregnancy. Nat Immunol 2:64–68, 2001.

Michie C. Th1 and Th2 cytokines in pregnancy, from a fetal viewpoint. Immunol Today 19:333–334, 1998.

Mincheva-Nilsson L, Kling M, Hamarstrom A, Nagaeva O, Sundqvist KG, Hammarstrom ML, Baranov V. Gamma delta T cells of human early pregnancy decidua: evidence for local proliferation, phenotypic heterogeneity, and extrathymic differentiation. J Immunol 159:3266–3277, 1997.

Mori T, Gou MW, Yoshida H, Saito S, Mori E. Expression of the signal transducing regions of CD4-like and lck genes in murine egg. Biochem Biophys Res Commun 182:527–533, 1992.

Mori T, Wu GM, Mori E. Expression of CD4-like structure on murine egg vitelline membrane and its signal transductive roles through p56lck in fertilization. Am J Reprod Immunol 26:97–103, 1991.

Mueller-Erkhardt, G. Alternative treatment of lymphocyte immunization for treatment of recurrent spontaneous abortion. Immunotherapy with intravenous immunoglobulin for prevention of recurrent pregnancy loss: European experience. Am J Reprod Immunol 32:281–285, 1994.

Mukhopadhyay D, Sundereshan S, Rao C, Karande AA. Placental protein 14 induces apoptosis in T cells but not in monocytes. J Biol Chem 276:28268–28273, 2001.

Mummery CL. Transforming growth factor beta and mouse development. Microsc Res Tech 52:374–386, 2001.

Munn DH, Shafizadeh E, Attwood JT, Bondarev I, Pashine A, Mellor AL. Inhibition of T cell proliferation by macrophage tryptophan catabolism. J Exp Med 189:1363–1372, 1999.

Munn DH, Zhou M, Attwood JT, Bondarev I, Conway SJ, Marshall B, Brown C, Mellor AL. Prevention of allogeneic fetal rejection by tryptophan catabolism. Science 281:1191–1193, 1998.

Nelson JL. Microchimerism and scleroderma. Curr Rheumatol Rep 1(1):15–21, 1999.

Nocera M, Chu TM. Characterization of latent transforming growth factor-beta from human seminal plasma. Am J Reprod Immunol 33:282–291, 1995.

Norwitz ER, Schust DJ, Fisher SJ. Mechanisms of disease: implantation and the survival of early pregnancy. N Engl J Med 345:1400–1408, 2001.

Ober C. Studies of HLA, fertility and mate choice in a human isolate. Hum Reprod Update 5:103–107, 1999.

Ober C, Hyslop T, Elias S, Weitkamp LR, Hauck WW. Human leukocyte antigen matching and fetal loss: results of a 10 year prospective study. Hum Reprod 13:33–38, 1998.

Omu AE, al-Qattan F, Ismail AA, al-Taher S, al-Busiri N. Relationship between unexplained infertility and human leukocyte antigens and expression of circulating autogeneic and allogeneic antisperm antibodies. Clin Exp Obstet Gynecol 26:199–202, 1999.

Parant M. Possible mediators in endotoxin-induced abortion. Res Immunol 141(2):164–168, 1990.

Paria BC, Lim H, Das SK, Reese J, Dey SK. Molecular signaling in uterine receptivity for implantation. Semin Cell Dev Biol 11: 67–76, 2000.

Paria BC, Ma W, Tan TJ, Raja S, Das SK, Dey SK, Hogan BL. Cellular and molecular responses of the uterus to embryo implantation can be elicited by locally applied growth factors. Proc Natl Acad Sci USA 98:1047–1052, 2001.

Pazmany L, Mandelboim O, Vales-Gomez M, Davis DM, Reyburn HT, Strominger JL. Protection from natural killer cell-mediated lysis by HLA-G expression on target cells. Science 274:792–795, 1996.

Pedersen, R. A. Sperm and mammalian polarity. Nature 409:473–474., 2001.

Pollard JW, Hunt JH, Wiktor-Jedrzejczak W, Stanley ER. A pregnancy defect in the osteopetrotic (op/op) mouse demonstrates the requirement for CSF-1 in female fertility. Dev Biol 148:273–283, 1991.

Porter TF, Scott JR. Alloimmune causes of recurrent pregnancy loss. Sem Reprod Med 18:393–400, 2000.

Primakoff P, Hyatt H, Tredick-Kline J. Identification and purification of a sperm surface protein with a potential role in sperm-egg membrane fusion. J Cell Biol 104:141–149, 1987.

Primakoff P, Myles DG. The ADAM gene family: surface proteins with adhesion and protease activity. Trends Genet 16:83–87, 2000.

Quenby S, Brazeau C, Drakeley A, Lewis-Jones DI, Vince G. Oncogene and tumour suppressor gene products during trophoblast differentiation in the first trimester. Mol Hum Reprod 4:477–481, 1998,

Raghupathy R. Th1-type immunity is incompatible with successful pregnancy. Immunol Today 18:478–482, 1997.

Razin A, Cedar H. DNA methylation and gene expression. Microbiol Rev 55: 451–8.1991

Recurrent Miscarriages Immunotherapy Trialists Group (RMITG). Worldwide collaborative observational study and meta-analysis on allogeneic leukocyte immunotherapy for recurrent spontaneous abortions. Am J Reprod Immunol 32:55–72, 1994.

Rigal D, Vermot-Desroches C, Hertz S, Bernaud J, Alfonsi F, Monier JC. Effects of intravenous immunoglobulin (IVIG) on peripheral blood B, NK, T cell populations in women with recurrent spontaneous abortion: Specific effects on LFA-1 and CD56 molecule. Clin Immunol Immunopathol 71:309–314, 1994.

Robb L, Li R, Hartley L, Nandurkar HH, Koentgen F, Begley CG. Infertility in female mice lacking the receptor for interleukin 11 is due to a defective uterine response to implantation. Nat Med 4:303–308, 1998.

Robertson SA. Control of the immunological environment of the uterus. Rev Reprod 5(3):164–174, 2000.

Rogers AM, Boime I, Connolly J, Cook JR, Russell JH. Maternal-fetal tolerance is maintained despite transgene-driven trophoblast expression of MHC class I, and defects in Fas and its ligand. Eur J Immunol 28:3479–3487, 1998.

Rufas O, Fisch B, Ziv S, Shalgi R. Expression of cadherin adhesion molecules on human gametes. Mol Human Reproduc 6:163–169, 2000.

Rukavina D, Podack ER. Abundant perforin expression at the maternal-fetal interface: guarding the semiallogeneic transplant? Immunol Today 21:160–163, 2000.

Sacks G, Sargent I, Redman C. An innate view of human pregnancy. Immunol Today 20:114–118, 1999.

Sanchez-Cuenca J, Martin JC, Pellicer A, Simon C. Cytokine pleiotropy and redundancy—gp130 cytokines in human implantation. Immunol Today 20:57–59, 1999.

Sargent IL, Arenas J, Redman CW. Maternal cell–mediated sensitisation to paternal HLA may occur, but is not a regular event in normal human pregnancy. J Reprod Immunol 10:111–120, 1987.

Schaefer M, Hofmann T, Schultz G, Gudermann T. A new prostaglandin E receptor mediates calcium influx and acrosome reaction in human spermatozoa. Proc Natl Acad Sci USA 95:3008–3013, 1998.

Smith SC. Re: Apoptotic and proliferative activities in first trimester placentae (Placenta [1999], 20, 223–227, C. C. W. Chan, T. T. Lao and A. N. Y. Cheung). Placenta 21:286–288, 2000.

Smith SC, Baker PN, Symonds EM. Placental apoptosis in normal human pregnancy. Am J Obstet Gynecol 177:57–65, 1997a.

Smith SC, Baker PN, Symonds EM. Increased placental apoptosis in intrauterine growth restriction. Am J Obstet Gynecol 177:1395–1401, 1997b.

Sueoka K, Shiokawa S, Miyazaki T, Kuji N, Tanaka M, Yoshimura Y. Integrins and reproductive physiology: expression and modulation in fertilization, embryogenesis, and implantation. Fertil Steril 67:799–811, 1997.

Svensson L, Arvola M, Sallstrom MA, Holmdahl R, Mattsson R. The Th2 cytokines IL-4 and IL-10 are not crucial for the completion of allogeneic pregnancy in mice. J Reprod Immunol 51:3–7, 2001.

Szereday L, Varga P, Szekeres-Bartho J. Cytokine production by lymphocytes in pregnancy. Am J Reprod Immunol 38:418–422, 1997.

Tafuri A, Alferink J, Moller P, Hammerling GJ, Arnold B. T cell awareness of paternal alloantigens during pregnancy. Science 270:630–633, 1995.

Torry DS, McIntyre JA, Faulk WP. Immunobiology of the trophoblast: mechanisms by which placental tissues evade maternal recognition and rejection. Curr Top Microbiol Immunol 222:127–140, 1997.

Tremellen KP, Seamark RF, Robertson SA. Seminal transforming growth factor beta1 stimulates granulocyte-macrophage colony-stimulating factor production and inflammatory cell recruitment in the murine uterus. Biol Reprod 58:1217–1225, 1998.

Tsuji Y, Mitsuo M, Yasunami R, Sakata K, Shibahara H, Koyama K. HLA-DR and HLA-DQ gene typing of infertile women possessing sperm-immobilizing antibody. J Reprod Immunol 46:31–38, 2000.

Vacchio MS, Jiang SP. The fetus and the maternal immune system: pregnancy as a model to study peripheral T-cell tolerance. Crit Rev Immunol 19:461–480, 1999

Vacquier VD. Evolution of gamete recognition proteins. Science 281:1995–1998, 1998.

Van Kampen CA, Versteeg-Van der Voort Maarschalk MF, Langerak-Langerak J, Van Beelen E, Roelen DL, Claas FH. Pregnancy can induce long-persisting primed CTLs specific for inherited paternal HLA antigens. Hum Immunol 62:201–207, 2001.

Wegmann TG, Lin H, Guilbert L, Mosmann TR. Bidirectional cytokine interactions in the maternal-fetal relationship: is successful pregnancy a TH2 phenomenon? Immunol Today 14:353–356, 1993.

Xu C, Mao D, Holers VM, Palanca B, Cheng AM, Molina H. A critical role for murine complement regulator crry in fetomaternal tolerance. Science 287:498–501, 2000.

Yamasaki M, Sasho T, Moriya H, Kanno M, Harada M, Kamada N, Shimizu E, Nakayama T, Taniguchi M. Extrathymic development of V alpha 11 T cells in placenta during pregnancy and their possible physiological role. J Immunol 166:7244–7249, 2001.

Zhiya Y, Lennon VA. Mechanism of intravenous immunoglobulin therapy in antibody-mediated autoimmune diseases. N Engl J Med. 340:227–228, 1999.

Zhou M, Mellor AL. Expanded cohorts of maternal CD8+ T-cells specific for paternal MHC class I accumulate during pregnancy. J Reprod Immunol 40:47–62, 1998.

p a r t

P A R T

II

Primary Immunodeficiencies

CHAPTER

Immunodeficiency Disorders: General Considerations

E. Richard Stiehm, Hans D. Ochs, and Jerry A. Winkelstein

HISTORICAL ASPECTS

Primary immunodeficiency disorders, the naturally occurring defects of the immune system, were not identified until after the introduction of antibiotics, because morbidity and mortality from infection even in normal subjects was so high. Only after the "expectation of cure" of pneumonia, meningitis, cellulitis, and other severe infections with antibiotics could these illnesses be identified.

Nevertheless, several syndromes of immunodeficiency with characteristic clinical features were described before 1940, including mucocutaneous candidiasis by Thorpe and Handley in 1929, ataxia-telangiectasia by Syllaba and Henner in 1926, and Wiskott-Aldrich syndrome (WAS) by Wiskott in 1937.

A patient with defective cellular immunity was initially described by Glanzmann and Riniker in 1950. In 1958 the combination of antibody deficiency with defective cellular immunity was identified in a Swiss infant, Swiss-type agammaglobulinemia (Hitzig et al., 1958).

Two years after Bruton's description of congenital agammaglobulinemia in 1952, acquired agammaglobulinemia (common variable immunodeficiency [CVID]) in an adult was described in 1954 by Sanford and co-workers.

289

A phagocytic immunodeficiency was first described in 1957 as fatal (now chronic) granulomatous disease by Berendes and associates. A complement deficiency (C2 deficiency) was initially described in 1965 by Klemperer and associates.

Treatment milestones include the first use of immune globulin for immune deficiency (Bruton, 1952), the first U.S. trial of intravenous immune globulin (IVIG) (Ammann et al., 1982a), the first successful bone marrow transplant (for severe combined immunodeficiency [SCID]) (Gatti et al., 1968), the first use of a haploidentical transplant (also for SCID) (Reinherz et al., 1982), the first use of a cytokine for treatment (interferon [IFN]-γ) for chronic granulomatous disease [CGD]) (International Chronic Granulomatous Disease Cooperative Study Group, 1991), and the first success of gene therapy (for X-linked severe combined immunodeficiency [XL-SCID]) (Cavazzana-Calvo et al., 2000).

GENERAL CONSIDERATIONS

Definition

The immunodeficiency disorders are a diverse group of illnesses that, as a result of one or more abnormalities of the immune system, increase susceptibility to infection. The primary immunodeficiencies are not associated with other illnesses that impair the immune system, and many are genetic disorders with a characteristic inheritance pattern.

Although the possibility of an immunodeficiency should be considered in any individual with "too many" infections, these are relatively uncommon disorders and it is thus important to consider other conditions that lead to infection (Table 12-1).

A consideration of nonimmunologic causes of recurrent infection is beyond the scope of this volume; most of these conditions can be readily suspected after a careful history and physical examination and can be confirmed by appropriate laboratory tests.

When there is no apparent explanation for the recurrent infections, a primary defect in host defense must be considered. Because the primary immunodeficiencies generally are congenital and hereditary, most newly diagnosed patients are infants or children. However, many more adults are surviving so that the registries of

patients are approximately half adults. The following represents a typical case.

Case Report

A boy, 8 years old, was well until the age of 4 years, when pneumonia with rubeola developed. The birth, developmental history, and family history were normal; a male sibling was well. At age 4½ years, the patient experienced chills, fever, and pain in the left knee. Physical examination was unremarkable except for a few petechiae on the arms and tenderness of the knee. The white blood cell (WBC) count was 16,400/mm³ with 88% neutrophils; blood culture findings were normal. The pain and fever disappeared with administration of penicillin.

Two weeks later, fever recurred; pneumonia was diagnosed, and sulfadiazine was given. Four days later, mumps and gastroenteritis developed, and the boy was admitted to the hospital. He experienced a prolonged febrile course, complicated by recurrent otitis. The throat, blood, and ear cultures were positive for type XIV pneumococcal infection.

After being treated with penicillin for 10 days, the boy improved. Otitis media developed 2 months later. Two days after antibiotics were discontinued for an ear infection, fever and left shoulder pain developed. The WBC count was 25,000/mm³ with 91% neutrophils. Antibiotics were again administered. Six months later, fever recurred, and type XXXIII pneumococci were recovered from the blood stream.

After recovery, a tonsillectomy and adenoidectomy were performed in the hope of decreasing the number of infections. During the next 4 years, however, the patient experienced 15 episodes of high fever resulting from sepsis; on seven occasions, pneumococci specimens from the blood were obtained for culture. He also had two episodes of pneumonia, three episodes of otitis, and two episodes of mumps. Prophylactic sulfadiazine and pneumococcal vaccine were ineffective in controlling the infections.

This is the first recorded case of X-linked agammaglobulinemia (XLA) (Bruton, 1952); it demonstrates many of the major characteristics of this disorder, including male sex, early onset, recurrent major pyogenic infection, and ineffectiveness of most forms of

TABLE 12-1 · DISORDERS WITH INCREASED SUSCEPTIBILITY TO INFECTION AND EXAMPLES

Type of Disorder	Examples
Circulatory disorders	Sickle cell disease, diabetes, congenital cardiac defects
Obstructive disorders	Ureteral or urethral stenosis, bronchial asthma, allergic rhinitis, blocked eustachian tube, cystic fibrosis
Integumental defects	Eczema, burns, skull fracture, midline sinus tracts, ciliary abnormalities
Metabolic disorders	Nephrosis, galactosemia, uremia
Unusual microbiologic factors	Antibiotic overgrowth, chronic infections with resistant organism, continuous reinfection (contaminated water supply, infectious contact, contaminated inhalation therapy equipment)
Foreign bodies	Ventricular shunt, central venous catheter, artificial heart valve, urinary catheter, aspirated peanut
Secondary immunodeficiencies	Malnutrition, prematurity, lymphoma, splenectomy, uremia, immunosuppressive therapy, protein-losing enteropathy
Primary immunodeficiencies	X-linked agammaglobulinemia, DiGeorge anomaly, chronic granulomatous disease, C3 deficiency

therapy and the favorable response to injected immunoglobulin (Ig). The study of antibody immunodeficiencies in pediatric patients and hypergammaglobulinemic states in adults (e.g., multiple myeloma) first served to stimulate the specialty of clinical immunology.

Nomenclature

Since Bruton's description of XLA, well over 100 primary immunodeficiencies have been delineated (Chapel et al., 2003). This chapter lists and classifies these disorders, details common clinical features, discusses some causal mechanisms, outlines laboratory diagnosis, and discusses general approaches to treatment. The latter includes a detailed discussion of the therapeutic use of immune globulin. The rest of this part is devoted to a detailed exposition of each primary immunodeficiency.

Part III covers the many secondary immunodeficiencies. Part IV covers immunologic aspects of other pediatric disorders, including a chapter on transplantation.

The names of the immunodeficiencies were initially based on place of discovery, name of discoverer, Ig patterns, or possible pathogenic mechanisms. In addition, several names were applied to the same disorder, leading to considerable confusion and ambiguity. The terminology for the primary immunodeficiencies, which is continuously being recodified by an International Union of Immunological Societies (IUIS) committee, (formerly the World Health Organization Expert Committee) (Chapel et al., 2003), is used in this book.

It minimizes eponyms, designation of country, numbers based on Ig pattern, and hypothetical pathogenic mechanisms; it stresses the mode of genetic transmission and distinctive features. Thus Bruton's agammaglobulinemia is renamed *X-linked agammaglobulinemia (XLA)*. Because certain eponyms are well established (such as Swiss-type agammaglobulinemia for SCID), they also are provided. The most recent compilation of the IUIS is shown in Table 12-2.

TABLE 12-2 · 2003 MODIFIED IUIS CLASSIFICATION OF PRIMARY AND SECONDARY IMMUNODEFICIENCIES

Groups and Diseases	Inheritance	Groups and Diseases	Inheritance
A. Predominantly Antibody Deficiencies		23. Primary CD7 deficiency	
1. XL agammaglobulinemia	XL	24. IL-2 deficiency	
2. AR agammaglobulinemia	AR	25. Multiple cytokine deficiency	
3. Hyper-IgM syndromes		26. Signal transduction deficiency	
a. XL	XL	**D. Defects of Phagocytic Function**	
b. AID defect		27. Chronic granulomatous disease	
c. CD40 defect	AR	a. XL	XL
d. Other AR defects	AR	b. AR	AR
4. Ig heavy-chain gene deletions	AR	1. p22 phox deficiency	
5. κ chain deficiency mutations	AR	2. P47 phox deficiency	
6. Selective IgG class deficiencies	?	3. P57 phox deficiency	
7. Selective IgA deficiency	Variable	28. Leukocyte adhesion defect 1	AR
8. Antibody deficiency with normal or elevated Igs	?	29. Leukocyte adhesion defect 2	AR
		30. Neutrophil G6PD deficiency	XL
9. Common variable immunodeficiency	Variable	31. Myeloperoxidase deficiency	AR
10. Transient hypogammaglobulinemia of infancy	?	32. Secondary granule deficiency	AR
		33. Schwachman syndrome	AR
B. Combined Immunodeficiencies		34. Severe congenital neutropenia (Kostmann)	*AR*
11. T⁻B⁺ SCID		35. Cyclic neutropenia (elastase defect)	*AR*
a. X-linked (γc deficiency)	XL	36. Leukocyte mycobacterial defects	*AR*
b. Autosomal recessive (Jak3 deficiency)	AR	IFN-γR1 or R2 deficiency	AR
12. T⁻B⁻SCID		IFN-γR1 deficiency	AD
a. RAG-1/2 deficiency	AR	IL-12Rβ1 deficiency	AR
b. ADA deficiency	AR	IL-12p40 deficiency	AR
c. Reticular dysgenesis	AR	STAT1 deficiency	AD
d. Artemis defect	AR	**E. Immunodeficiencies Associated with Lymphoproliferative Disorders**	
13. T⁺B⁻SCID		37. Fas Deficiency	AD
a. Omenn syndrome	AR	38. Fas ligand deficiency	
b. IL-2Rα deficiency	AR	39. FLICE or caspase 8 deficiency	
14. Purine nucleoside phosphorylase deficiency	AR	40. Unknown (caspace 3 deficiency)	
15. MHC class II deficiency	AR	**F. Complement Deficiencies**	
16. MHC class I deficiency caused by TAP-2 defect	AR	41. C1q deficiency	AR
		42. C1r deficiency	AR
17. CD3γ or CD3ε deficiency	AR	43. C4 deficiency	AR
18. CD8 deficiency (ZAP-70 defect)	AR	44. C2 deficiency	AR
C. Other Cellular Immunodeficiencies		45. C3 deficiency	AR
19. Wiskott-Aldrich syndrome	XL	46. C5 deficiency	AR
20. Ataxia-telangiectasia	AR	47. C6 deficiency	AR
21. DiGeorge anomaly	?		
22. Primary CD4 deficiency			

Continued

TABLE 12-2 · 2003 MODIFIED IUIS CLASSIFICATION OF PRIMARY AND SECONDARY IMMUNODEFICIENCIES—cont'd

Groups and Diseases	Inheritance	Groups and Diseases	Inheritance
F. Complement Deficiencies—cont'd		71. Growth retardation, facial anomalies, and immunodeficiency	
48. C7 deficiency	AR	72. Progeria (Hutchinson-Gilford syndrome)	
49. C8α deficiency	AR	IMMUNODEFICIENCY WITH DERMATOLOGIC DEFECTS	
50. C8β deficiency	AR	73. Partial albinism	
51. C9 deficiency	XL	74. Dyskeratosis congenita	
52. C1 inhibitor	AD	75. Netherton syndrome	
53. Factor I deficiency	AR	76. Acrodermatitis enteropathica	
54. Factor H deficiency	AR	77. Anhidrotic ectodermal dysplasia	
55. Factor D deficiency	AR	78. Papillon-Lefèvre syndrome	
56. Properdin deficiency	XL	HEREDITARY METABOLIC DEFECTS	
G. Immunodeficiency Associated with or Secondary to Other Diseases		79. Transcobalamin 2 deficiency	
CHROMOSOMAL INSTABILITY OR DEFECTIVE REPAIR		80. Methylmalonic acidemia	
57. Bloom syndrome		81. Type 1 hereditary orotic aciduria	
58. Fanconi anemia		82. Biotin-dependent carboxylase deficiency	
59. ICF syndrome		83. Mannosidosis	
60. Nijmegen breakage syndrome		84. Glycogen storage disease, type 1b	
61. Seckel syndrome		85. Chédiak-Higashi syndrome	
62. Xeroderma pigmentosum		HYPERCATABOLISM OF IMMUNOGLOBULIN	
CHROMOSOMAL DEFECTS		86. Familial hypercatabolism	
63. Down syndrome		87. Intestinal lymphangiectasia	
64. Turner syndrome		**H. Other Immunodeficiencies**	
65. Chromosome 18 rings and deletions		78. Hyper-IgE syndrome	
SKELETAL ABNORMALITIES		89. Chronic mucocutaneous candidiasis	
66. Short-limbed skeletal dysplasia		90. Chronic mucocutaneous candidiasis with polyendocrinopathy (APECED)	AR
67. Cartilage-hair hypoplasia		91. Hereditary or congenital hyposplenia or asplenia	
IMMUNODEFICIENCY WITH GENERALIZED GROWTH RETARDATION		92. Ivemark syndrome	
68. Schimke immuno-osseous dysplasia		93. IPEX syndrome	XL
69. Immunodeficiency with absent thumbs		94. Ectodermal dysplasia (NEMO defect)	XL
70. Dubowitz syndrome			

AD = autosomal dominant; ADA = adenosine deaminase; AID = activation-induced cytidine deaminase; AR = autosomal recessive; capsace = cysteinyl; aspartate = specific proteinase; FLICE = Fas-associating protein with death domain-like IL-1-converting enzyme; G6PD = glucose 6-phosphate dehydrogenase; ICF = immunodeficiency, centromeric instability, facial anomalies; IFN = interferon; Ig = immunoglobulin; IL = interleukin; IPEX = immune dysregulation, polyendocrinopathy, enteropathy; MHC = major histocompatibility complex; NEMO = IKK-gamma; SCID = severe combined immunodeficiency; TAP-2 = transporter associated with antigen presentation; XL = X-linked.
Modified from report of an IUIS Scientific Committee. Primary immunodeficiency diseases: Clin Exp Immunol 118(suppl 1):1–28, 1999; and Chapel et al. Primary immunodeficiency diseases: an update. Clin Exp Immunol 132:9–15, 2003.

Classification

The immune system is conveniently divisible into the following distinct classifications:

B-lymphocyte (antibody) system
T-lymphocyte (cellular immune) system
Phagocytic (polymorphonuclear and mononuclear) system
Complement (opsonic) system

This division provides the usual and clinically convenient way to classify the primary immunodeficiencies. Many illnesses have deficiencies of two or more of the systems, particularly combined antibody and cellular (T-cell) deficiencies.

Secondary Immunodeficiency

Primary immunodeficiencies must be differentiated from secondary immunodeficiencies. Secondary immunodeficiencies are those disorders that, as a result of another illness, age, injury, or treatment, result in increased susceptibility to infection (Table 12-3). These disorders are very common and, in total, affect many more people than do the primary immunodeficiencies. Indeed, almost all serious illnesses are associated with some impairment of one or more components of the immune system.

Whereas antibody defects are the most common abnormality in primary immunodeficiency, cellular (T-cell) defects are the most common defect in the secondary immunodeficiencies. Examples of important secondary immunodeficiencies, as outlined in Part III, include infancy, human immunodeficiency virus (HIV) infection (acquired immune deficiency syndrome [AIDS]), primary malnutrition, and immunosuppressive treatment.

Distribution

The approximate division of the types of primary immunodeficiencies is shown in Figure 12-1. This figure

TABLE 12-3 · FACTORS ASSOCIATED WITH SECONDARY IMMUNODEFICIENCY

Premature and Newborn

Hereditary and Metabolic Diseases
Chromosomal abnormalities (Down syndrome, others)
Uremia
Diabetes mellitus
Malnutrition
Vitamin and mineral deficiencies
Protein-losing enteropathies
Nephrotic syndrome
Myotonic dystrophy
Sickle cell disease

Immunosuppressive Agents
Radiation
Immunosuppressive drugs
Corticosteroids
Antilymphocyte or antithymocyte globulin
Anti-B- or T-cell monoclonal antibodies

Infectious Diseases
Congenital rubella
Viral exanthems (e.g., measles, varicella)
HIV infection, AIDS
Cytomegalovirus
Infectious mononucleosis
Bacterial infections
Mycobacterial, fungal, or parasitic disease

Infiltrative and Hematologic Diseases
Histiocytosis
Sarcoidosis
Hodgkin's disease and lymphoma
Leukemia
Myeloma
Agranulocytosis and aplastic anemia
Lymphoma in immunocompromised transplant recipients

Surgery and Trauma
Burns
Splenectomy
Anesthesia
Head injury
Hypothermia

Miscellaneous
Lupus erythematosus
Chronic active hepatitis
Alcoholic cirrhosis
Aging

AIDS = acquired immune deficiency syndrome; HIV = human immunodeficiency virus.

RELATIVE DISTRIBUTION OF THE PRIMARY IMMUNODEFICIENCIES

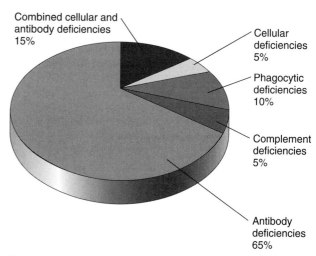

Figure 12-1 · Relative distribution of the primary immunodeficiencies.

reflects data from early registries (from Switzerland, Japan, Sweden, and Italy) summarized by Affentranger and colleagues (1993), from more recent registries as shown in Table 12-4, from the European Society of Immunodeficiency Registry, and from our own experience. It excludes asymptomatic selective IgA deficiency, and includes the hyper-IgE syndrome as a phagocytic disease because clinically it resembles this group of illnesses in terms of its infectious complications and management.

The antibody deficiencies constitute approximately 65% of all cases of primary immunodeficiencies and are covered in Chapter 13. They include disorders in which immunoregulatory T-cell abnormalities are present (e.g., the X-linked hyper-IgM [HIGM1] syndrome), but in which the major immune defect is poor antibody function.

A separate chapter (Chapter 14) is devoted to selective IgA deficiency because it is so common, heterogenous, and associated with many other conditions, and its management is distinct from the other antibody deficiencies.

Combined immunodeficiencies (antibody and T-cell deficiencies) compose the next largest group; they compose approximately 15% of the total primary immunodeficiencies. There are multiple disorders in this group and they are covered in Chapters 15 through 18. Many combined immunodeficiencies exhibit clinical features that constitute a distinct syndrome (e.g., ataxia-telangiectasia, WAS) or are associated with thymic hypoplasia or dysplasia.

Within the phenotypic syndrome of SCID, multiple genetic subtypes exist, and these are detailed in Chapter 15. A separate chapter is devoted to adenosine deaminase (ADA) deficiency (Chapter 16), because the metabolic defect is well established and replacement therapy (polyethylene glycol conjugated bovine ADA) has been used successfully in this disorder.

Pure cellular defects, without an antibody defect, are less common, and make up approximately 5% of the total. The two most common disorders in this group, DiGeorge anomaly and mucocutaneous candidiasis are covered in Chapter 17. Several other cellular immunodeficiency syndromes are also discussed in this chapter.

Phagocytic immunodeficiencies comprise approximately 10% of the total primary immunodeficiencies. These affect the polymorphonuclear phagocytic system and the mononuclear phagocytic (monocyte/macrophage) system, or both, and are discussed in Chapter 20.

Primary disorders of the complement system make up approximately 5% of immunodeficiencies and are covered in Chapter 21. These include hereditary angioneurotic edema caused by C1 esterase defects.

TABLE 12-4 · RELATIVE FREQUENCIES OF MAJOR PRIMARY IMMUNODEFICIENCIES* IN FOUR REGIONAL REGISTRIES

	Country/Region				
Disorder	Spain (Matamoros Flori et al., 1997)	Australia (Baumgart et al., 1997)	Latin America (Zelazko et al., 1998)	Norway (Stray-Pederson et al., 2000)	Total in four registries
	# (%)[†]	# (%)[†]	# (%)[†]	# (%)[†]	# (%)
Predominantly Antibody Defects					
X-linked agammaglobulinemia	49 (4.6)	41 (8.2)	109 (7.6)	15 (2.1)	214 (6.4)
Common variable immunodeficiency	213 (19.5)	137 (27.2)	154 (27.2)	117 (31.4)	614 (18.4)
Transient hypogammaglobulinemia of infancy	15 (1.4)	5 (1.0)	5 (1.0)	NR	80 (2.3)
Selective IgA deficiency	394 (36.9)	82 (16.8)	413 (16.8)	36 (9.2)	925 (27.5)
IgG subclass deficiency	60 (5.6)	50 (10.0)	45 (3.2)	10 (2.7)	165 (4.8)
Hyper-IgM syndrome	23 (2.1)	9 (1.8)	34 (2.4)	11 (3.0)	77 (2.3)
TOTAL	754 (70.5)	297 (59.0)	815 (57.1)	189 (50.8)	2082 (61.8)[‡]
Combined Antibody and T-Cell Defects					
Severe combined immunodeficiency	65 (6.1)	26 (5.2)	65 (4.6)	7 (1.8)	163 (4.8)
Wiskott-Aldrich syndrome	18 (1.7)	12 (2.4)	48 (3.4)	8 (2.2)	86 (2.5)
Ataxia-telangiectasia	29 (2.7)	10 (2.0)	149 (10.4)	17 (4.6)	205 (6.0)
TOTAL	112 (10.5)	48 (9.6)	262 (18.3)	32 (8.6)	454 (13.3)[‡]
Predominantly T-Cell Defects					
Chronic mucocutaneous candidiasis	32 (3.0)	8 (1.6)	48 (3.4)	23 (6.2)	111 (3.2)
DiGeorge anomaly	19 (1.8)	16 (3.2)	18 (1.3)	8 (2.2)	61 (1.8)
TOTAL	51 (4.8)	24 (4.8)	66 (4.7)	31 (8.4)	172 (5.1)[‡]
Phagocytic Defects					
Chronic granulomatous disease	32 (3.0)	12 (3.0)	64 (4.5)	4 (1.1)	115 (3.4)
Hyper-IgE syndrome	18 (1.7)	NR	43 (3.0)	1 (0.3)	68 (2.0)
TOTAL	50 (4.7)	12 (3.0)	107 (7.5)	5 (1.4)	183 (5.4)[‡]
Complement Defects					
C1 esterase deficiency	NR	32 (6.4)	12 (0.8)	67 (18.0)	111 (3.0)
Other complement deficiencies	NR	5 (1.0)	16 (1.2)	11 (3.))	32 (1.0)
TOTAL	65 (6.1)	37 (7.4)	28 (2.0)	78 (21.0)	145 (4.0)[‡]
TOTAL CASES REPORTED	1069	500	1428	372	3369 (89.6)

*The 15 disorders listed account for 90% of the 3369 total cases reported to the four registries.
†Percent in each registry.
‡Percent in combined registries.

Two unique groups of lymphocyte disorders are also covered in this section. These include the chromosomal breakage syndromes (Chapter 18) and the apoptosis syndrome associated with autoimmunity (Chapter 19).

Since 1952 more than 15,000 cases of primary immunodeficiency have been reported in the medical literature and to national and international registries. Many more remain undiagnosed or unreported.

Recognition of these disorders is increasing because of the wider availability of immunologic laboratory tests, the increasing ability of physicians to recognize the disorders, and the description of new syndromes heretofore unrecognized. Since the last edition of this book (1996), several new primary immunodeficiencies have been delineated (e.g., leukocyte mycobacterial defects, autosomal recessive forms of hyper-IgM syndrome), and many others have been subdivided into new biochemical or genetic variants (e.g., SCID).

Prevalence and Incidence

The prevalence of primary immunodeficiency was first estimated to be approximately one case per 100,000 population, based on a 1969 report of the Medical Research Council Working Party from the United Kingdom. Because this report did not include cases of cellular immunodeficiency and used strict criteria for diagnosis (an IgG level less than 200 mg/dl), this is a minimal figure.

Immunodeficiency Registries

Recent studies from registries in Switzerland (518 cases in a population of 7,000,000) (Affentranger et al., 1993) and Norway (372 patients in a population of 4,450,000) (Stray-Pederson et al., 2000) suggest that the prevalence is closer to 1 per 10,000, excluding asymptomatic IgA deficiency (which occurs at a frequency of 20 to 40 per 10,000).

Because of incomplete reporting to the registries, the true prevalence of symptomatic immunodeficiency is probably considerably higher, at least 1 per 5000 (.02%). Many of these additional cases are of late onset, and less severe.

The U.S. Immune Deficiency Foundation (IDF) (Immune Deficiency Foundation, 1999) conducted a combined physician–patient survey, and estimated that there were approximately 50,000 cases in the United States, making the prevalence of 1:5000 a reasonable estimate. Approximately 40% of reported cases were the genetically defined syndromes (e.g., XLA, CGD, SCID, DiGeorge anomaly), most of which are recognized before age 10. The other 60% were genetically ill-defined syndromes, most of which are diagnosed after childhood (e.g., CVID—34%, IgG subclass deficiencies—24%, IgA deficiency—17%). In this survey, there were more females (52%) and patients older than age 18 (62%).

The incidence of some specific disorders in the Norwegian Registry (Stray-Pedersen et al., 2000) include XLA (4.2 per 100,000), SCID (8.3 per 100,000), ataxia-telangiectasia (6.7 per 100,000), and WAS (10.4 per 100,000). We estimate that genetic testing at birth would identify approximately 1 per 10,000 infants, approximately half of the immunodeficiencies eventually diagnosed.

Overall Incidence

The overall 1:10,000 incidence of genetically defined primary immunodeficiency is one-fourth that of cystic fibrosis (1:2500), one-half that of congenital hypothyroidism (1:5000), and somewhat more common than phenylketonuria (1:14,000). Regional differences based on differing populations and environmental factors affect the relative incidence of each disorder. This can be appreciated by comparison of the immunodeficiency registries of four countries (see Table 12-4).

According to these figures, there are approximately 400 new cases of primary immunodeficiency in infants born each year in the United States (4.0 million live births). Such calculations are of particular value when the frequency of undiagnosed immunodeficiency in patients receiving potentially fatal live virus vaccines is determined, when the need for bone marrow transplant facilities is calculated, or when the need for intravenous Ig administration is estimated. Regarding the latter, approximately 70% of all immunodeficient patients are receiving Ig therapy.

Immunodeficiency Among Inpatients and Outpatients

Among hospitalized patients, the frequency of immunodeficiency is considerably higher. Hobbs (1966) noted that 138 of 6000 patients (2.3%) admitted to a general hospital in the United Kingdom demonstrated total gamma-globulin levels lower than 400 mg/dl. Only 20 of 6000 (0.3%) had a primary immunodeficiency. The remaining patients had hypogammaglobulinemia of immaturity (20 patients) or secondary hypogammaglobulinemia (98 patients). Other secondary immunodeficiencies, mostly those affecting cellular immunity, are also common among hospitalized patients.

In the outpatient setting, patients with less severe immunodeficiency syndromes are identified. Palma-Carlos and Palma-Carlos (1991) identified 37 primary immunodeficiencies in 5100 outpatients (0.74%) followed in an allergy and clinical immunology clinic, including 27 patients with selective IgA deficiency.

Age and Sex

The age of onset of symptoms, based on the time of diagnosis, can be estimated from British studies (Medical Research Council Working Party, 1969), Japanese studies (Hayakawa et al., 1981), and the Swiss Registry (Ryser et al., 1988). The age of onset varies from syndrome to syndrome. In these early studies, approximately 40% of cases were diagnosed in the first year, another 40% by age 5 years, another 15% by age 16, and only 5% in adulthood. In earlier registries only 10% of the registered cases were adults, and the diagnosis was established before age 16 in most of these cases.

Current registries contain many more adults (60%) than children, and many of the cases were diagnosed after age 18, (Immune Deficiency Foundation, 1999; Stray-Pedersen et al., 2000). Adult patients have a high frequency of CVID and IgG subclass deficiency.

Registry data indicate that the male/female ratios vary from 1.4:1 to 2:1, presumably because of the large number of X-linked disorders. However, even CVID is slightly more common in males (Affentranger et al., 1993; Baumgart et al., 1997; Stray-Pedersen et al., 2000). In the physician–patient IDF survey (1999), 52% were female, most of whom were adults.

There is a family history of a similar deficiency in approximately 25% of patients with immunodeficiency. This is more common in affected males (33%) than in females (5.5%). These differences are largely accounted for by the many boys with X-linked immunodeficiencies with early-onset disease.

ETIOLOGY

Immunodeficiencies can be classified as either primary immunodeficiencies, caused by a single gene defect (e.g., XLA caused by mutations of Btk) or genetic susceptibility (e.g., CVID), or as secondary immunodeficiencies caused by some other primary disorder such as prolonged protein malnutrition, chronic infection with lymphotropic viruses (e.g., HIV infection) or immunosuppressive therapy (e.g., ritixumab) (Table 12-5).

In recent years, the genetic basis of more than 100 primary immunodeficiencies has been identified, and their mode of inheritance identified as X-linked recessive, autosomal recessive, or autosomal dominant (Table 12-6). Some disorders are caused by mutations of genes required for the development of a functionally mature cell lineage (e.g., Btk for B-cell development)

TABLE 12-5 · PATHOGENESIS OF IMMUNODEFICIENCY AND EXAMPLES

Genetic Defects
Single-gene defects expressed in multiple tissues (e.g., ataxia-telangiectasia; adenosine deaminase deficiency)
Single-gene defects specific to the immune system (e.g., tyrosine kinase defect in X-linked agammaglobulinemia; ε chain of TCR abnormality)
Multifactorial disorders with genetic susceptibility (e.g., common variable immunodeficiency)

Drugs or Toxins
Immunosuppressives (e.g., corticosteroids, cyclosporine)
Anticonvulsants (e.g., phenytoin [Dilantin])

Nutritional and Metabolic Disorders
Malnutrition (e.g., kwashiorkor)
Protein-losing enteropathy (e.g., intestinal lymphangiectasia)
Vitamin deficiency (e.g., biotin or transcobalamin II deficiency)
Mineral deficiency (e.g., zinc deficiency in acrodermatitis enteropathica)

Infection
Transient immunodeficiency (e.g., varicella, rubeola)
Permanent immunodeficiency (e.g., HIV infection, congenital rubella)

Chromosome Abnormalities
DiGeorge anomaly (e.g., deletion of 22q11)
Selective IgA deficiency (e.g., trisomy 18)

HIV = human immunodeficiency virus; IG = immunoglobulin; TCR = T-cell receptor.

TABLE 12-6 · CHROMOSOME LOCATIONS OF ABNORMAL GENES OF PRIMARY IMMUNODEFICIENCIES

Disorder	Gene Symbol	Gene Location
XL Disorders		
XL chronic granulomatous disease	gp91phox	Xp26
XL SCID	IL2R	Xp13
XL lymphoproliferative syndrome	SAP/SH2D1A	Xq25
Wiskott-Aldrich syndrome	WASP	Xp11.22
XL agammaglobulinemia	BTK	Xq21.3
XL hyper-IgM syndrome	CD40L	Xq27
Ectodermal dysplasia with NEMO mutation	NEMO	
Properdin deficiency	PFC	Xp11
IPEX syndrome	FOXP3	Xp11.23 – Xp13.3
AR Disorders		
AR chronic granulomatous disease	p22-phox	16q24
	p47-phox	7q11.23
	p67-phox	1q25
Janus kinase 3 deficiency—SCID	JAK3	19p13.1
RAG-1 deficiency—SCID	RAG-1	11p13
RAG-2 deficiency—SCID	RAG-2	11p13
Athabascan—SCID	ARTEMIS	10p
ZAP 70 deficiency—SCID	ZAP70	Sq12
Adenosine deaminase deficiency	ADA	20q13
Purine nucleoside phosphorylase deficiency	PNP	14q13
MHC class II deficiency	CIITA	16p13
	RFX-5	1q21
	RFXAP	13q
MHC class I deficiency	TAP2	6q21.3
AR agammaglobulinemia		
μ Heavy chain deficiency	IGHM	14q32
λ5 Surrogate light chain deficiency	IGLL1	22q11.22
Igα deficiency	mb-1	1q13.2
BLNK deficiency	BLNK	10q23.22
CD40 deficiency	CD40	20q12–q13.2
AID deficiency	AID	
APECED	AIRE	21q22.3
Chédiak-Higashi syndrome	CHS1	1q42-q43
LAD-1	CD18	21q22.3
Ataxia-telangiectasia	ATM	11q22.3
Nijmegen-breakage syndrome	NBS	8q21
AD Disorders		
ALPS	FAS(AP01)	21q22–q23
WHIM syndrome	CXCR4	2q21

AD = autosomal dominant; AID = activation-induced cytidine deaminase; ALPS = autoimmune lymphoproliferative syndrome; APECED = autoimmune polyendocrinopathy, candidiasis, ectodermal dystrophy; AR = autosomal recessive; BLNK = ball linker protein; Ig = immunoglobulin; IPEX = immune dysregulation, polyendocrinopathy, enteropathy, XL; LAD = leukocyte adhesion defect; MHC = major histocompatibility complex; NEMO = IKK-gamma; SCID = severe combined immunodeficiency; WHIM = warts, hypogammaglobulinemia, infections, myelokathexis; XL = X-linked.

(see Table 12-5). Others are caused by mutations of genes required for the development and function of multiple cell lineages derived from a single precursor (e.g., the common γ-chain for T, B, and natural killer [NK] cells). In a third group of disorders, the mutated gene is expressed in multiple tissues resulting in a complex multisystem disorder including immunodeficiency (e.g., ataxia-telangiectasia, ADA deficiency).

Classification of primary immunodeficiency disorders is further complicated by the fact that a specific clinical and laboratory phenotype may be the result of mutations of more than one gene, sometimes with different patterns of inheritance. For example, mutations of the common γ-chain cause X-linked SCID and mutations of JAK-3 cause autosomal recessive SCID, and both present as T⁻B⁺NK⁻ SCID (see Chapter 15). Conversely, mutations of the same gene may result in strikingly different clinical phenotypes depending on the nature and location of the mutation. As an example, RAG-1/RAG-2 mutations generally result in T⁻B⁻NK⁺ SCID (see Chapter 15); however, if the mutation is less severe, (e.g., missense mutations that allow expression of mutated protein), the resulting phenotype may result in Omenn's syndrome (T⁺B⁻NK⁺) with a classic erythematous, itchy rash, elevated serum IgE, and eosinophilia (Villa et al., 2001) (see Chapter 15).

In the "premolecular era" primary immunodeficiencies were classified as to whether they affected antibody production (B cells), cellular immunity (T cells), phagocytic function (neutrophils and monocytes), or complement activation. Such a system is useful clinically, but from a mechanistic standpoint it is invalid because many immunodeficiencies do not easily fit into such a scheme. This classification does not consider new concepts of molecular immunology.

For example, the most prominent feature of X-linked HIGM1 syndrome, originally called *dysgammaglobulinemia*, is a pronounced antibody deficiency; however, molecular evaluation of this syndrome revealed that the responsible gene encodes the CD40 ligand expressed by activated CD4⁺ T cells (Allen et al., 1993), and such patients have subtle defects in T-cell immunity (see Chapter 13).

Another approach is to classify immunodeficiencies according to functional defects of cellular immunity—for example, grouping together disorders caused by genes coding for deoxyribonucleic acid (DNA)-binding proteins, genes involved in defects of DNA repair/DNA rearrangement, genes coding for lymphocyte receptor or cytoplasmic signaling molecules, or genes resulting in defects of cell adhesion. This approach has led to a better understanding of lymphocyte development, gene activation, and identification of several genes responsible for specific immunodeficiencies. Thus a shift from a descriptive to the molecular approach has resulted in precise diagnosis, carrier identification, prenatal diagnosis, accurate genetic counseling, and better therapies, including gene therapy.

Molecular studies also have shown that several genetic defects can result in the same clinical phenotype. For example, more than half a dozen independent genes, if mutated, result in an SCID phenotype (see Chapter 15). Mutations of four individual genes result in CGD with both X-linked or autosomal recessive modes of inheritance (see Chapter 20).

Single Gene Defects of the Immune System

To date, more than 100 genes are known to cause primary immunodeficiency diseases. The most common disorders and their genes are listed in Table 12-5. A large proportion are X-linked, many are autosomal recessive, and a few are autosomal dominant. The large number of genes that, if mutated, are associated with immunodeficiency attests to the complexity of the immune system. Genes involved in the maturation of lymphocyte subsets, such as Btk, ZAP70, RAG-1 and RAG-2, and Artemis are responsible for characteristic immune cytopenias and the resulting immune defects.

The importance of effective DNA repair is demonstrated by the complex pathology observed in ataxia-telangiectasia and Nijmegen-breakage syndrome (see Chapter 18). Examples of defective cell signaling include X-linked and autosomal recessive HIGM1 syndromes caused by mutations of genes involved in CD40 signaling (see Chapter 13). Antigen presentation is defective in patients with major histocompatibility complex (MHC) class II deficiency, leading to defects in both B and T lymphocytes (see Chapter 15).

Mutations of genes involved in the regulation of the immune response, including one required for lymphocyte apoptosis (e.g., Fas), causes autoimmune lymphoproliferative syndrome (ALPS) (see Chapter 19). Mutations of the AIRES gene encoding a DNA-binding protein required for self-recognition cause the autoimmune polyendocrinopathy-candidiasis-ectodermal dystrophy (APECED) syndrome (see Chapter 17). Mutations of a gene encoding another DNA-binding protein that is crucial for the generation of regulatory T cells cause the polyendocrinopathy, enteropathy, X-linked (IPEX) syndrome (see Chapter 17).

Metabolic defects resulting in primary immunodeficiency include the enzymes ADA and purine nucleoside phosphorylase (PNP) (see Chapter 16), biotinidase deficiency (Hurvitz et al., 1989), biotin-dependent carboxylase deficiency (Cowan et al., 1979), and transcobalamin II deficiency (Kaikov et al., 1991) (see Chapters 13 and 17).

Many of the genes involved in immune deficiency affect specific biochemical or cellular functions. For examples, failure to synthesize a complement component results in failure of complement activation, abnormalities of superoxide production cause defective granulocyte bactericidal activity in CGD, and defects in variable-diversity-joining (VDJ) rearrangement (caused by mutations of RAG-1/RAG-2 or Artemis genes) result in failure to generate T- and B-cell receptors with resultant combined immunodeficiency (Moshous et al., 2001; Schwarz et al., 1991). Defects in cytokine production or expression of cytokine receptors have a profound effect on the development and function of both B and T lymphocytes.

The importance of cell migration and cell adhesion for cell trafficking and cell interaction is exemplified by the immune deficiency associated with leukocyte adhesion defect type 1 (LAD-1), caused by mutations of CD18 (see Chapter 20).

Multigene Defects of the Immune System

Several primary immunodeficiencies do not follow a single pattern of inheritance, but are clearly influenced by genetic factors. A study of patients with CVID and their families has revealed an increased incidence of selective IgA deficiency and other immune disorders in some kinships (Cunningham-Rundles, 1989) (see Chapters 13 and 14). Studies of families with multiple affected members presenting with either CVID or selective IgA deficiency demonstrated the presence of certain characteristic "complotypes" of human leukocyte antigen (HLA) class I, II, and III antigens. These complotypes may function as susceptibility genes or, alternatively, they may be linked to a gene or genes not yet discovered that directly effect immune competence (Olerup et al., 1990; Schaffer et al., 1989).

Not every member of these families who inherits a particular complotype associated with risk develops an immunodeficiency, suggesting that additional genetic or environmental factors must be present to trigger the immune defect.

Other disorders that may occur in more than one member of a family, but not according to a consistent pattern of inheritance, are mucocutaneous candidiasis (Herrod, 1990) and some forms of hyper-IgE syndrome. Some immune disorders have a dominant inheritance with various penetrant; examples are ALPS and the DiGeorge syndrome. It is interesting to speculate that other susceptibility genes, perhaps with different polymorphisms, play a role in the manifestation of clinical symptoms.

Drugs, Toxins, and Nutrient Deficiency

Certain immunodeficiencies may result from exposure to a toxin or drug. The ingestion of phenytoin (Dilantin) or one of several other anticonvulsant drugs can be associated with selective IgA deficiency or hypogammaglobulinemia (Ishizaka et al., 1992; Ruff et al., 1987) (see Chapter 13). Maternal alcohol consumption during pregnancy has been associated with some cases of DiGeorge anomaly (Ammann et al., 1982b) (see Chapter 17); indeed, in most children with fetal alcohol syndrome, T-cell function is depressed (Johnson et al., 1981).

A lack of vitamins, minerals, calories, or protein may adversely affect the immune system with resultant immune deficiency (see Chapter 23). Zinc deficiency has been associated with acrodermatitis enteropathica,

which in turn has been associated with combined immunodeficiency (see Chapters 23 and 24). Vitamin B$_{12}$ deficiency, as a result of transcobalamin II deficiency, may lead to hypogammaglobulinemia (Kaikov et al., 1991) (see Chapters 13 and 24). Severe protein-calorie malnutrition leads to a profound but reversible T-cell immunodeficiency. Intrauterine malnutrition secondary to placental insufficiency may result in permanent cellular immunodeficiency (Chandra, 1975) (see Chapter 23).

Treatment with the tumor necrosis factor (TNF)-α receptor etenercept or with a monoclonal antibody to TNF-α increases susceptibility to intracellular bacteria (e.g., mycobacteria). Anti-CD20 monoclonal antibody therapy designed to eliminate B cells results in severe and prolonged antibody deficiency. Other drugs causing immunodeficiency are discussed in Chapters 13 and 27.

Infection

Infectious agents can cause or exacerbate immunodeficiency (see Chapters 28 and 29). HIV targets CD4+ T cells and macrophages, resulting in cellular immune deficiency and opportunistic infections. Congenital rubella infection is associated with a variety of immunodeficiency syndromes, including IgA deficiency and an HIGM syndrome. Both congenital rubella and HIV infection can result in permanent immunodeficiency. Infection with other microorganisms, including varicella, Epstein-Barr virus (EBV), and rubeola, can cause a transient increased susceptibility to infection.

Chromosomal Abnormalities

Chromosomal abnormalities are noted in several well described immunodeficiencies. Deletions in the long arm of chromosome 22 and other deletions and translocations are seen in a high proportion of patients with the DiGeorge anomaly (Driscoll et al., 1992; Greenberg et al., 1986) (see Chapter 17). Defects in chromosome 18 are sometimes associated with IgA deficiency (see Chapter 14). Chromosomal breakage syndromes, including ataxia-telangiectasia and Nijmegen-breakage syndrome, are associated with hypogammaglobulinemia and T-cell abnormalities (Taalman et al., 1989) (see Chapter 18).

CLINICAL GENETICS

Genetic Counseling

Because most primary immunodeficiencies are caused by single or multiple gene defects, comprehensive care for an affected child should include genetic counseling, not only for the child's parents, but also for siblings and the extended family. It may be helpful to refer the family to a genetic counselor who has experience in providing complex information in an unbiased and easily understood manner. However, it is also important to confirm the diagnosis using the most specific and accurate technology possible. Genetic counseling based on an incorrect diagnosis can be devastating.

Shortly after the patient is diagnosed as having a particular primary immunodeficiency, the pattern of inheritance should be described to the family and the potential for carrier detection and prenatal diagnosis discussed. The patient's siblings should be screened to ensure that they do not have the same disorder. In families with X-linked or autosomal dominant disorders, it is wise to discuss genetic risks again when the patient or the siblings reach reproductive age.

Genetic counseling issues vary, depending on the mode of inheritance of the immunodeficiency. In families who carry an autosomal recessive gene defect (see Table 12-6), such as ADA deficiency, ataxia-telangiectasia, or LAD-1, the major concern is prenatal diagnosis for the parents' future children. All of the autosomal recessive immunodeficiencies are sufficiently rare that one would not expect the patient or the patient's siblings to be at risk of having affected children. Although it is often possible to determine which family members are heterozygous for the autosomal recessive disorders, it is usually not clinically important. The issues are different in families with X-linked immunodeficiencies. Because the sisters, cousins, and aunts of boys with X-linked immunodeficiencies are at risk of having affected children, carrier detection as well as prenatal diagnosis is a concern for these families.

In other immunodeficiencies that follow less clearly defined patterns of inheritance, genetic issues should also be addressed. DiGeorge anomaly is associated with a high incidence of chromosomal defects, particularly partial monosomy of chromosome 22 (Driscoll et al., 1992) (see Chapter 17). Most cases are sporadic, but in occasional families one of the parents carries a balanced translocation or another silent defect. Thus it is important to screen all patients with the DiGeorge anomaly for chromosomal defects. If abnormalities are found, the parents and siblings should be studied.

Hyper-IgE syndrome can follow both autosomal recessive and autosomal dominant patterns of inheritance (Grimbacher et al., 1999), making it difficult to provide genetic counseling for affected families with these disorders (see Chapter 17).

Family members of patients with CVID and selective IgA deficiency have an increased risk of antibody deficiencies and autoimmune disorders, although data are insufficient to document the exact risk.

Approximately 25% to 35% of patients seen in an immunodeficiency clinic have abnormalities of the immune system that do not fall into any well-described syndrome. These patients may have disorders that are secondary to in utero infection or a toxic exposure, or they may have genetic disorders not yet identified The parents of these children probably have a risk of having another similarly affected child, although the risk is probably less than 25%.

Prenatal Diagnosis

A variety of approaches can be used to provide prenatal diagnosis (Table 12-7). Fetal blood obtained by periumbilical blood sampling can be analyzed by flow cytometry, and those disorders with a characteristic peripheral blood lymphocyte profile (e.g., T^-B^-, or $T^-B^+NK^-$ in severe combined immune deficiency or absence of B cells in XLA). For some disorders, for example, ADA deficiency, the enzymatic activity of the gene product in amniocytes or chorionic villous samples can be measured. This technique can be performed early in pregnancy and does not require the exact identification of the mutation of the affected gene in a particular family.

DNA-based assays using polymerase chain reaction (PCR) have become the procedure of choice for many immunodeficiencies (Rose, 1991). If the family is known to carry a specific mutation of a specific gene, this portion of the gene can be amplified, sequenced, and the results interpreted accurately.

Linkage analysis, used before genes were identified and mutations could be determined, which requires the availability of DNA from a large number of members of the family, is now used only in rare situations (Puck et al., 1990).

Carrier Detection

Most of the techniques described for prenatal diagnosis can be used to identify carriers. DNA-based assays,

---

TABLE 12-7 · TECHNIQUES USED IN PRENATAL DIAGNOSIS

Approaches	Indication (Example)
Immunologic studies on fetal blood	The defective gene is not known, but the disorder has a characteristic phenotype (severe combined immunodeficiency with no T or B cells).
Functional assay to measure the activity of the gene product in fetal blood or tissue	Assays are available to assess directly the function of the defective gene (adenosine deaminase activity in chorionic villus samples).
Mutation detection	The defective gene has been identified, and the mutation in the family at risk is known (e.g., C to T base pair substitution in codon 520 of Btk, the defective gene in X-linked agammaglobulinemia).
Linkage analysis	The defective gene has been mapped to a specific site on a single chromosome, and sufficient family members are available to identify haplotypes carrying the mutation (X-linked lymphoproliferative syndrome when DNA is available on the proband).

DNA = deoxyribonucleic acid.

including mutation analysis and linkage studies, are the most reliable. Carrier detection is particularly important for X-linked disorders. Each of the X-linked disorders of the immune system listed in Table 12-6 has been mapped to a specific site on the X chromosome and the responsible genes cloned and sequenced. If the mutation in a given family with X-linked immunodeficiency is known, sequence analysis of genomic DNA can be used to identify carrier females. In rare cases, it is possible to use linkage analysis to achieve carrier detection.

However, as with other X-linked disorders that are lethal prior to reproductive age, approximately one third of affected males are the result of new mutations. For this reason and the small family sizes, more than 50% of patients with X-linked disorders have a negative family history. If a new mutation has occurred, it may have started in the ovum that gave rise to the patient, or, more often, the mutation occurred in the sperm of the maternal grandfather.

Thus, to determine if the patient's sisters and other family members are carriers, the patient's mother and maternal grandmother must be tested. If the mutation occurred during cell division of the maternal egg, a certain proportion of the mother's eggs may have the mutated X-chromosome, but her somatic cells are normal. This situation is called *gonadal mosaicism* and creates a difficult problem for genetic counseling. Gonadal mosaicism is confirmed if the mother has borne more than one affected boy but has only wild-type gene product in her somatic cells.

In X-linked CGD and in properdin deficiency, the assays used to detect carriers are the same as those used to diagnose an affected patient. Neutrophils from carriers of CGD are usually intermediate in their ability to produce superoxide radicals when compared with those from controls and from affected patients (see Chapter 20). Carriers of properdin deficiency have approximately half the normal serum concentration of properdin (Sjoholm et al., 1988) (see Chapter 21). Approximately half of the neutrophils from carrier females for X-linked CGD are able to reduce nitroblue tetrazolium (NBT) or undergo an "oxidative burst" in the rhodamine flow cytometry assay.

In contrast, carrier females of XLA have B cells that are entirely normal and carrier females of XL-SCID and WAS have normal immune systems. This is due to the fact that the cell lineages primarily affected by the gene defect (i.e., B cells in XLA, T and B cells in XL-SCID, and all hematopoietic cell lineages in WAS) use exclusively the nonmutated X chromosome as the active chromosome (Conley, 1992).

This phenomenon, termed *nonrandom X-inactivation*, is based on the fact that cells expressing the X chromosome with the mutant gene are at a disadvantage in cell proliferation or differentiation compared with cells expressing the normal X chromosome. As a result, the majority of cells of that lineage are derived from precursors that have the normal X chromosome as the active X.

Several techniques have been used to analyze patterns of X chromosome inactivation. The most frequently used takes advantage of the fact that the active and inactive X chromosomes vary in methylation. Using a PCR technique and certain "housekeeping genes," for example, the androgen receptor gene, the inactive X chromosome can be identified by demonstrating increased methylation (Allen et al., 1994).

CLINICAL FEATURES

A variety of clinical presentations may prompt the suspicion of a primary immunodeficiency (Table 12-8). These include an increased susceptibility to infection, the presence of autoimmune or inflammatory disorders, or the presence of the features of a specific syndrome, a part of which is immunodeficiency.

Increased Susceptibility to Infection

The most common clinical presentation of immunodeficiency is an increased susceptibility to infection. This includes (1) recurrent infections, (2) increased severity or duration of infections, (3) unexpected or severe com-

TABLE 12-8 · CLINICAL FEATURES IN IMMUNODEFICIENCY

Usually Present
Recurrent upper respiratory infections
Severe bacterial infections
Persistent infections with incomplete or no response to therapy

Often Present
Failure to thrive or growth retardation
Paucity of lymph nodes and tonsils
Infection with an unusual organism
Skin lesions (e.g., rash, seborrhea, pyoderma, necrotic abscesses [noma], alopecia, eczema, telangiectasia, severe warts)
Recalcitrant thrush
Clubbing
Diarrhea and malabsorption
Persistent sinusitis, mastoiditis
Recurrent bronchitis, pneumonia
Autoimmune disorders
Hematologic abnormalities (e.g., aplastic anemia, hemolytic anemia, neutropenia, thrombocytopenia)

Occasionally Present
Weight loss, fevers
Chronic conjunctivitis
Periodontitis
Lymphadenopathy
Hepatosplenomegaly
Severe viral disease
Arthralgia or arthritis
Chronic encephalitis
Recurrent meningitis
Pyoderma gangrenosa
Sclerosing cholangitis
Chronic hepatitis (viral or autoimmune)
Adverse reaction to vaccines
Bronchiectasis
Urinary tract infection
Delayed umbilical cord detachment (>30 days)
Chronic stomatitis
Granulomas
Lymphoid malignancies

plications of infections, or (4) infections with unusual organisms, such as opportunistic organisms of low virulence. A poster distributed by the Jeffrey Modell Foundation and the American Red Cross for parents and physicians with early warning features is displayed in Figure 12-2.

In most patients, there is an increased frequency of infections plus one or more of the other characteristics listed previously. However, in some patients, their first infection may be of such severity, be associated with an unusual complication, or be caused by an unusual organism, that it gives rise to a suspicion of an immunodeficiency disease. For example, if the patient's first infection is *Pneumocystis carinii* pneumonia (PCP), there should be a strong suspicion of an immunodeficiency.

Most immunodeficient patients present with recurrent or chronic respiratory infections. However, infectious diarrhea and blood-borne infections, such as sepsis, meningitis, osteomyelitis, or septic arthritis, are not uncommon. Although one severe infection may

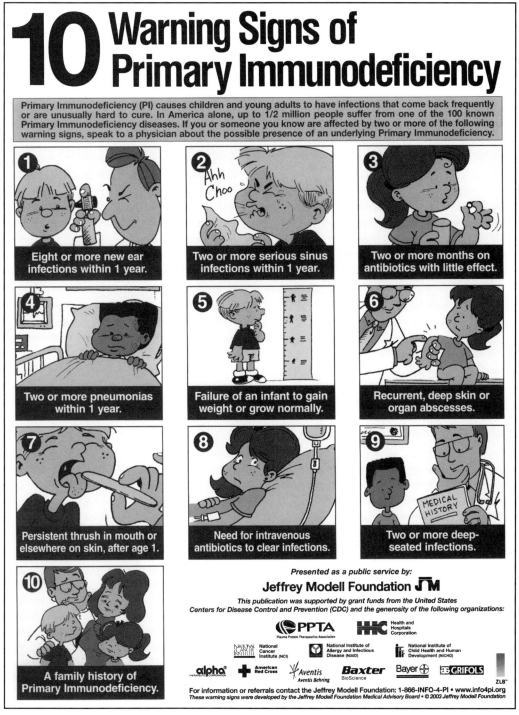

Figure 12-2 · Poster of the Modell Foundation detailing the 10 warning signs of primary immunodeficiency. (Courtesy of the Jeffrey Modell Foundation, New York.)

occur in a normal child, a second should alert the physician to possible immunodeficiency.

In immunodeficient patients, repeated respiratory infections may lead to chronic sinusitis, otitis media, mastoiditis, and bronchiectasis. Indeed, many hypogammaglobulinemic adults present initially with early-onset bronchiectasis. Other clinical features of immunodeficiency are shown in Table 12-8.

Respiratory Infection

Many immunocompetent children experience six to eight respiratory infections per year, and this number is increased with exposure to older siblings or other children at nursery school. In the immunologically normal child, the respiratory infections are usually mild, without fever, and last only a few days. Further, the normal child recovers completely between infections. Thus the presence of recurrent episodes of uncomplicated upper respiratory infections (URIs) is not necessarily a sign of immunodeficiency.

When respiratory infections occur repeatedly as the sole infectious manifestation, allergy must also be suspected. Allergic disorders, in contrast to immunodeficiency, are characterized by (1) absence of fever; (2) clear nonpurulent discharge; (3) prior history of colic, food intolerance, eczema, or other allergic symptoms; (4) a positive family history of allergy; (5) a characteristic seasonal or exposure pattern; (6) a poor response to antibiotics; and (7) a good response to antihistamines or bronchodilators.

Gastrointestinal Manifestations

Gastrointestinal (GI) infections also occur commonly in primary immunodeficiency and may be manifest as chronic diarrhea or emesis. These can be severe enough and protracted enough to lead to malabsorption and failure to thrive. Patients with severe cellular immunodeficiency are particularly likely to have chronic diarrhea. Liver disease and cholangitis are not uncommon. Indeed, 8 of 56 patients with sclerosing cholangitis had primary immunodeficiency (Debray et al., 1994).

Although failure to thrive was common as a presenting sign in many immunodeficiencies, it is now less common, presumably because of earlier diagnosis and improved therapy of the GI infections. Although the initial descriptions of several immunodeficiencies included poor weight gain and short stature, nowadays many immunodeficient children appear normal in the early months or years of life.

Types of Infection

The kind of infection often provides a clue as to which component of the immune system is deficient. In *antibody immunodeficiencies,* the infecting organisms are usually encapsulated pyogenic bacteria, such as *Streptococcus pneumoniae* and *Haemophilus influenzae,* organisms for which antibody-mediated opsonization is an important host defense mechanism. Most viral infections are tolerated well with the notable exception of enteroviruses, such as ECHOvirus, coxsackie, and poliovirus, because antibody-mediated viral neutralization is critical in preventing dissemination.

In *cellular (T-lymphocyte) immunodeficiencies,* the organisms responsible for infection usually are gram-negative bacteria, intracellular bacterial pathogens (e.g., mycobacteria), viruses, fungi, or protozoa. Thus patients with T-cell defects can present with mucocutaneous or systemic candidiasis, herpes virus infections, or *PCP.*

Patients with *complement deficiencies,* particularly deficiencies of the terminal components, are unduly susceptible to systemic *Neisserial* infections, such as meningococcemia and meningococcal meningitis, because complement-mediated bactericidal activity is critical in host defense against these gram-negative bacteria.

Patients with *phagocytic defects,* such as CGD, usually have infections caused by catalase-producing bacteria (e.g., *Staphylococci* and *Burkholderia*) or fungi (e.g., *Aspergillus, Nocardia,* and *Cryptococcus*).

Autoimmune and Inflammatory Disorders

Patients with primary immunodeficiencies can present with or develop a variety of autoimmune, rheumatic, or inflammatory disorders.

These are most common in patients with partial T-cell deficiencies, with or without concurrent defects in B-cell function. Paradoxically, even patients with some degree of hypogammaglobulinemia can produce autoantibodies and develop autoimmune disease. For example, patients with either selective IgA deficiency or CVID not uncommonly develop immune thrombocytopenic purpura (ITP) or autoimmune hemolytic anemia (Cunningham-Rundles and Bodian, 1999). Myasthenia gravis is a common feature of Good's syndrome, an immunodeficiency associated with thymomas. Systemic lupus erythematosus (SLE), rheumatoid arthritis, and juvenile rheumatoid arthritis all may occur in either selective IgA deficiency or CVID.

Inflammatory bowel disease (IBD) is not uncommon in primary immunodeficiency, particularly in patients with CVID (Cunningham-Rundles and Bodian, 1999). Finally, a granulomatous disorder that resembles sarcoidosis occurs in approximately 10% of patients with CVID (Fasano et al., 1996).

Patients with complement deficiencies, especially those with deficiencies of C1, C4, C2, or C3, often develop a lupus-like syndrome with prominent cutaneous manifestations (Figueroa and Densen, 1991). Although the mechanisms by which complement-deficient patients develop the lupus-like syndrome are unclear, they may relate to the role of C3 and other components that activate C3 (i.e., C1, C4, and C2) in the clearance and processing of circulating immune complexes and apoptotic cells.

Patients with either the autosomal recessive or X-linked forms of CGD may also develop discoid or SLE (Winkelstein et al., 2000). Interestingly, discoid lupus is also relatively common in the female carriers of the X-linked recessive form of CGD. In fact, it is more common in female carriers than in affected males.

In rare instances, an infection in an immunodeficient host can masquerade as a rheumatic disorder. In XLA, chronic enteroviral infection can cause a syndrome resembling dermatomyositis (Bardelas et al., 1977), and mycoplasma infection can resemble rheumatoid arthritis (Franz et al., 1997).

History

The patient's history is often of help in the diagnosis of a primary immunodeficiency.

The birth history and neonatal course should be explored for any maternal infections that could lead to immunodeficiency in the infant, such as congenital rubella or cytomegalovirus (CMV) infections. In addition, birth weight and length can provide insight into congenital infections or act as a baseline for assessing poor growth in infancy.

The nature and severity of past infectious diseases should be detailed because they may provide insight into the ability of the child to resist infection. In addition, the rash of a viral exanthem or contact dermatitis (poison ivy or oak) suggests intact cellular immunity.

Current and past medications should be recorded. IgA deficiency or CVID may be associated with certain drugs (e.g., phenytoin, gold salts [see Chapter 13]).

The past history should be explored for earlier surgery. In some instances the kind of surgery may provide insight into the severity of the infection (e.g., tympanoplasty and/or the placement of pressure equalizing [PE] tubes, drainage of an abscess). In other instances, the surgery may produce a secondary immunodeficiency (e.g., splenectomy, thymectomy) or create a physical finding that may be misconstrued as a sign of a primary immunodeficiency disease (e.g., tonsillectomy may be misconstrued as congenital absence of tonsils). The histology of the removed organs is sometimes valuable in establishing a retrospective diagnosis.

Prior blood transfusion; antibiotic or gamma globulin therapy (and their apparent clinical benefit); and adverse reactions to blood, plasma, or gamma globulin injections should all be noted. A history of marked clinical benefit from small doses of gamma globulin can usually be attributed to a placebo effect.

The immunization history is crucial when evaluating antibody or T-cell responses to antigens in vaccines, such as tetanus and diphtheria toxoids, Haemophilus influenzae type b vaccine, and pneumococcal polysaccharide or pneumococcal-conjugate vaccines. In addition, live virus vaccines, or exposure to a recently immunized individual, may cause progressive disease in a profoundly immunodeficient child.

Family History

The family history is important in assessing patients for possible immunodeficiency because many immunodeficiencies are inherited as single-gene defects. A relevant family history is of interest after clinical symptoms have developed, and may suggest a diagnosis before clinical symptoms appear. Only 25% of XLA patients born into families with a previously affected member had a diagnosis made before the onset of clinical symptoms (Lederman and Winkelstein, 1985).

The family history should also be explored for other affected family members with primary immunodeficiency and for family members with an increased susceptibility to infection, early deaths, or multiple hospitalizations. Other clinical manifestations not related to infection, such as bleeding from thrombocytopenia in WAS or lymphoreticular malignancy in CVID should be noted.

The family's racial, religious, or national background is relevant because some immunodeficiencies are more common in certain ethnic groups. For example, ataxia-telangiectasia is more common in the Amish, C3 deficiency is more common in South African blacks, and cartilage hair hypoplasia is more common in Finland. A history of consanguinity should also be sought.

Physical Examination

The physical findings in immunodeficient subjects may provide information as to their general health status, the presence of infection, autoimmune or inflammatory disease, or characteristic syndromic features.

General health status is assessed by growth charts, developmental milestones, and signs of weight loss or failure to thrive. If infections have been chronic and severe, muscle mass may be diminished, and the fat deposits of the buttocks may be atrophied. Pallor as a reflection of anemia is also helpful. Excoriation around the anus suggests chronic diarrhea.

Characteristic physical features are uncommon, but the complete absence of lymph nodes and tonsils in a child with frequent infections is very suggestive of immunodeficiency.

Physical features of infection may suggest which component of the immune system is defective. For example, candidal infections of the skin, severe warts, and molluscum contagiosum suggest a T-cell defect. Candidiasis of the mucous membranes, roof of the mouth, tongue, or corners of the mouth is also common in T-cell deficiency. Diffuse ulceration of the mucous membranes and necrotizing lesions of the tongue or mucous membranes (noma) are seen in severe T-cell deficiencies (Rotbart et al., 1986). Conjunctivitis is more characteristic of antibody defects. Periodontitis and dental decay are seen in neutropenia and granulocytic functional disorders such as the LADs.

Some physical findings are common to many types of immunodeficiency. Scarred or perforated tympanic membranes, sometimes with draining ears, indicate recurrent otitis or mastoiditis. The nostrils are often excoriated and crusted, indicative of a purulent nasal discharge. Cutaneous granulomas, pyodermas, or non-healing wounds are sometimes present. A deep cough or chest rattle with rales and digital clubbing suggests chronic lung disease. Occasionally the lymph nodes, liver, and spleen are enlarged.

Physical findings relating to inflammatory or autoimmune disease may include joint swelling, limitation of joint motion, and subcutaneous nodules. Other physical findings relating to autoimmune diseases may include the rashes of rheumatoid arthritis and lupus, vitiligo, or alopecia.

Some physical findings are characteristic of a specific immunodeficiency syndrome. Examples include ataxia-telangiectasia and developmental delay in ataxia-telangiectasia, atopic dermatitis in WAS, infected eczema in the hyper-IgE syndrome, dwarfism in cartilage hair hypoplasia, and oculocutaneous albinism in Chédiak-Higashi syndrome.

Clinical Syndromes

Certain clinical patterns among the primary immunodeficiencies are sufficiently characteristic to suggest the diagnosis to the astute clinician (Table 12-9). These are based on age of onset, type of infection, sex, and other characteristic clinical findings. For example, in a 1-year-old boy with recurrent pneumococcal infections since the age of 6 months whose tonsils are absent and who has no palpable lymph nodes, a diagnosis of XLA is suggested. For a definitive diagnosis in all instances, laboratory tests are required.

Diagnostic Criteria

Exact diagnosis rests on a combination of clinical and laboratory features. Conley and associates (1999) have developed criteria for 10 of the more common primary immunodeficiency syndromes, classifying them into definitive, probable, and possible diagnoses.

LABORATORY DIAGNOSIS

Because the clinical findings in immunodeficiency are rarely distinctive, the diagnosis must be established by appropriate laboratory procedures. In this section, the initial screening and advanced tests for the evaluation of each group of immunodeficiencies are outlined. These are summarized in Tables 12-10 and 12-11.

General Laboratory Tests

As with other ill patients, certain nonspecific laboratory tests are often indicated, including a complete blood cell (CBC) count, erythrocyte sedimentation rate or C-reactive protein (CRP), urinalysis, tuberculin test, and chest and sinus x-ray examinations. Specific laboratory tests are sometimes indicated to exclude cystic fibrosis (sweat test or genetic test), malabsorption (fecal fat, xylose tolerance test), malnutrition (protein, vitamin, and albumin levels), and allergy (skin tests or radioallergosorbent tests, nasal smear for eosinophils).

Chronic diarrhea may be accompanied by electrolyte imbalance. Autoantibodies (antinuclear antibodies, thyroid antibodies, direct and indirect Coombs' testing,

---

TABLE 12-9 · CHARACTERISTIC CLINICAL PATTERNS IN SOME PRIMARY IMMUNODEFICIENCIES

Features	Diagnosis
In Newborns and Young Infants (0 to 6 Months)	
Hypocalcemia, heart disease, unusual facies	DiGeorge anomaly
Delayed umbilical cord detachment, leukocytosis, recurrent infections	Leukocyte adhesion defect
Diarrhea, pneumonia, thrush, failure to thrive	Severe combined immunodeficiency
Maculopapular rash, alopecia, lymphadenopathy	Severe combined immunodeficiency with graft-versus-host disease
Bloody stools, draining ears, eczema	Wiskott-Aldrich syndrome
Mouth ulcers, neutropenia, recurrent infections	XL-Hyper IgM syndrome
In Infancy and Young Children (6 Months to 5 Years)	
Severe progressive infectious mononucleosis	X-linked lymphoproliferative syndrome
Paralytic disease following oral poliovirus immunization	X-linked agammaglobulinemia
Recurrent cutaneous and systemic staphylococcal infections, coarse features	Hyper-IgE syndrome
Persistent thrush, nail dystrophy, endocrinopathies	Chronic mucocutaneous candidiasis
Short stature, fine hair, severe varicella	Cartilage hair hypoplasia with short-limbed dwarfism
Oculocutaneous albinism, recurrent infection	Chédiak-Higashi syndrome
Lymphadenopathy, dermatitis, pneumonia, osteomyelitis	Chronic granulomatous disease
In Older Children (Older Than 5 Years) and Adults	
Progressive dermatomyositis with chronic enterovirus encephalitis	X-linked agammaglobulinemia
Sinopulmonary infections, neurologic deterioration, telangiectasia	Ataxia-telangiectasia
Recurrent neisserial meningitis	C6, C7, or C8 deficiency
Sinopulmonary infections, malabsorption, splenomegaly, autoimmunity	Common variable immunodeficiency
Candidiasis with raw egg ingestion	Biotin-dependent cocarboxylase deficiency

rheumatoid factor) may be present. Liver enlargement is an indication for obtaining liver function tests and tests for viral hepatitis (e.g., hepatitis B surface antigen [HBsAg]; CMV culture, PCR and antibody; HIV antibody or PCR tests; hepatitis C virus [HCV] antibody or PCR tests) and EBV antibody or PCR tests.

TABLE 12-10 · INITIAL SCREENING TESTS FOR IMMUNODEFICIENCY

Blood Cell Count
Hemoglobin, white blood cell count, lymphocyte morphology, differential count, platelet estimation or count

Quantitative Immunoglobulins
IgG, IgM, IgA, and IgE levels

Antibody Responses to Previous Vaccines
Tetanus, diphtheria, *Haemophilus influenzae* titers (for IgG function)

Classical Complement Pathway Assessment
Total hemolytic complement (CH_{50})

Infection Evaluation
Erythrocyte sedimentation rate or C-reactive protein, appropriate cultures, appropriate roentgenograms

Ig = immunoglobulin.

Special cultures, PCR analysis, or stains for specific organisms may be necessary in certain situations. Of particular importance are *Pneumocystis carinii* and CMV in the lung; *Giardia lamblia*, rotavirus, cryptosporidia, and poliovirus (particularly in recently vaccinated patients given live attenuated poliovirus) in the stool (Lopez et al., 1974); CMV in the urine, GI tract, or blood; and EBV in the blood.

Some rare nonimmunologic disorders should be excluded in certain clinical situations. Absence of the spleen should be suspected if a patient has repeated episodes of sepsis and bizarre red blood cell (RBC) forms or Howell-Jolly bodies on peripheral smear. Asplenia is confirmed by ultrasonography.

Immobile cilia may be present in some patients with sinusitis and bronchiectasis, owing to a lack of dynein arms within the cilia (Afzelius, 1976). Sperm motility is also decreased in these patients and can be used to diagnose the defect. This deficiency may be present in patients with Kartagener's syndrome. Complete absence of nasal cilia has also been reported (Welch et al., 1984).

Certain laboratory findings should suggest specific immunodeficiencies. These include an elevated level of

TABLE 12-11 · LABORATORY TESTS IN IMMUNODEFICIENCY

Screening Tests	Advanced Tests	Research/Special Tests
B-Cell Deficiency		
IgG, IgM, IgA levels	B-cell enumeration (CD 19 or CD20)	Advanced B-cell phenotyping
Isoagglutinin titers	IgG subclass levels	Biopsies (e.g., lymphnodes)
Ab response to vaccine antigens (e.g., tetanus, diphtheria, rubeola, *Haemophilus influenzae*)	IgD and IgE levels	Ab responses to special antigens (e.g., ϕX, KLH)
	Natural Ab titers (e.g., anti–streptolysin O, *Escherichia coli*)	In vivo Ig-survival
	Ab responses to new vaccines (e.g., typhoid, pneumococcal vaccines)	Secretory Ig levels
	Lateral pharyngeal x-ray study for adenoidal tissue	In vitro Ig synthesis
		Cell activation analysis
		Mutation analysis
T-Cell Deficiency		
Lymphocyte count and morphology	T-cell subset enumeration (CD3, CD4, CD8)	Advanced flow cytometry
Chest x-ray examination for thymic size*	Proliferative responses to mitogens, antigens, allogeneic cells	Cytokine and cytokine receptor analysis
Delayed skin tests (e.g., *Trichophyton*, mumps, *Candida*, tetanus toxoid, multitest panel)	HLA typing	Cytotoxic assays (e.g. NK, CTL).
	Chromosome analysis	Enzyme assays (e.g., ADA, PNP)
		Thymic imaging and function
		T-cell receptor analysis
		T-cell activation studies
		Apoptosis studies
		Biopsies
		Mutation analysis
Phagocytic Deficiency		
WBC count, morphology	Dihydrorhodamine reduction	Adhesion molecule assays (e.g., CD11b/CD18, selectin ligand)
NBT dye test	WBC turnover	Rebuck skin window
IgE level	Special morphology	Deformability, adherence, and aggregation
	Random mobility and chemotaxis	Oxidative metabolism
	Phagocytosis assays	Enzyme assays (e.g., MPO, G6PD, NADPH oxidase)
	Bactericidal assays	Mutation analysis
Complement Deficiency		
CH_{50} activity	Opsonic assays	Alternative pathway activity
C3 level	Component assays	Functional assays (e.g., chemotactic factor, immune adherence)
C4 level	Activation assays (e.g., C3a, C4a, C4d, C5a)	C allotype analysis

*In infants only.

Ab = Antibody; ADA = adenosine deaminase; ADCC = antibody-dependent cellular cytotoxicity; C = complement; CH = hemolytic complement; CTL = cytotoxic T lymphocyte; DR = class II histocompatibility antigen; G6PD = glucose-6-phosphate dehydrogenase; HLA = human leukocyte antigen; IFN = interferon; Ig = immunoglobulin; KLH = keyhole limpet hemocyanin; MIF = migration inhibition factor; MPO = myeloperoxidase; NADPH = nicotinamide adenine dinucleotide phosphate; NBT = nitroblue tetrazolium; NK = natural killer; PNP = purine nucleoside phosphorylase; WBC = white blood cell; ϕX = phage antigen.

α-2-fetoprotein, present in ataxia-telangiectasia (Waldmann and McIntire, 1972), presence of megaloblastic anemia in infancy (transcobalamin II deficiency), abnormal chromosome 18 or 22 (associated with IgA deficiency and the DiGeorge anomaly, respectively), increased chromosomal breakage (ataxia-telangiectasia), inability to grow chromosomes for karyotyping (SCID with lack of proliferation to phytohemagglutinin [PHA]), and situs inversus on chest x-ray examination (Kartagener's syndrome).

Initial Screening Tests

The initial screening evaluation for suspected immunodeficiency includes a CBC count; quantitation of serum IgG, IgM, and IgA levels; assessment of antibody function; measurement of total hemolytic complement (CH_{50}); and an infection evaluation (see Table 12-10). This and other advanced tests are depicted in a poster distributed by the Modell foundation (Fig. 12-3).

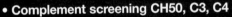

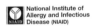
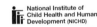

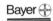

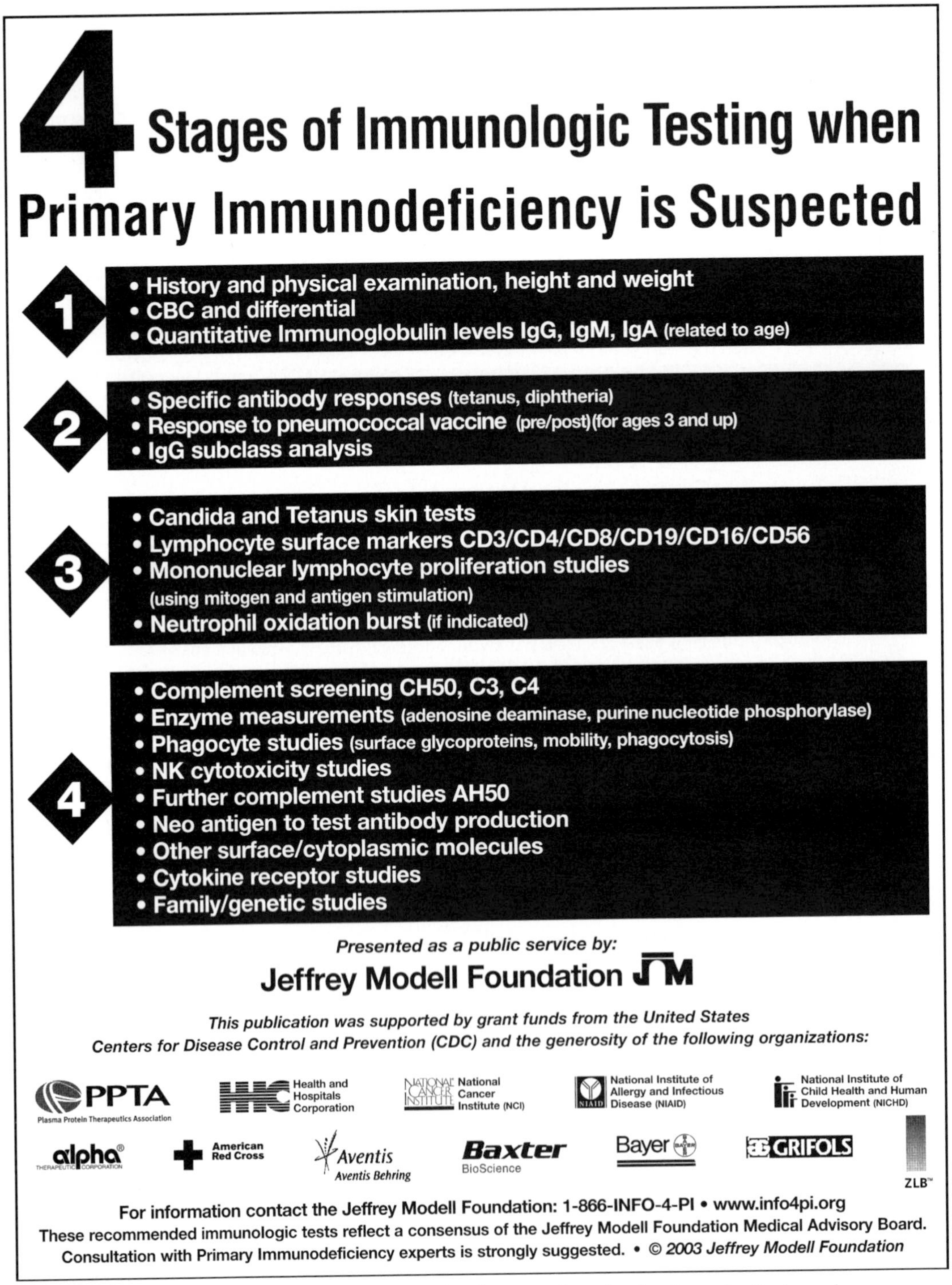

Figure 12-3· Poster of the Modell Foundation detailing procedures for the diagnosis of primary immunodeficiency. (Courtesy of the Jeffrey Modell Foundation, New York.)

Complete Blood Cell Count

The complete blood cell count, including hemoglobin level, leukocyte count, differential count, platelet enumeration, and examination of the blood smear, establishes the presence of anemia, thrombocytopenia, leukopenia, or leukocytosis; the latter, with a shift to the left, suggests the presence of acute or chronic infection. The total lymphocyte count should be calculated (WBC × percent lymphocytes); the normal lymphocyte count is 2000 to 6000 cells/µl (see Table 12-16). Lymphopenia is suggested if the lymphocyte count is less than 2000 cells/µl and is present if the count is less than 1500 cells/µl. When lymphopenia is noted, several counts over several weeks are indicated.

Persistent lymphopenia, generally associated with a paucity of small lymphocytes on the peripheral smear, is present in many cellular immunodeficiencies. By contrast, large lymphocytes with pale cytoplasm, reminiscent of monocytes rather than darkly stained small lymphocytes, are often present.

Lymphopenia in a newborn or an infant (less than 2500 cells/µl) is a special cause for concern because babies normally have high levels of total lymphocytes. A diagnosis of SCID should be suspected in all infants with a low lymphocyte count.

The peripheral smear should also be examined for the presence of Howell-Jolly bodies and other unusual RBC forms; these are characteristic features of asplenia. The granulocytes may also disclose morphologic abnormalities, such as the giant vacuoles of the Chédiak-Higashi syndrome (Blume et al., 1968) or the bilobed or kidney-shaped nuclei of the secondary granule deficiency syndrome (Strauss et al., 1974).

Thrombocytopenia is a feature of a few immunodeficiency syndromes, associated with autoantibodies to platelets (see Chapter 39). The platelet size is characteristically diminished in patients with WAS (see Chapter 17).

Immunoglobulin Assays

Quantitative determination of serum IgG, IgM, IgA, and IgE levels should be performed; IgD levels are not part of the initial screening. Levels of IgG, IgM, and IgA are usually performed by nephelometry, but radial immunodiffusion kits are also available. IgE assays require radioimmunoassay.

Quantitative Ig assays are recommended, inasmuch as immunoelectrophoresis or plasma electrophoresis do not provide exact information about the levels of individual Igs. A gamma globulin level by plasma electrophoresis lower than 600 mg/dl should be further studied by quantitative Ig assays.

The Ig levels must be interpreted with care because of marked alterations with each age (Stiehm and Fudenberg, 1966b). All infants aged 3 to 6 months are hypogammaglobulinemic if adult normal values are used. Therefore comparison of each Ig value with its age-matched control is essential (Tables 12-12 and 12-13).

Premature infants have particularly low levels of Igs in the first year of life. Ballow and colleagues (1986) have published values for premature infants and young children at various birth weights and ages, and these are presented in Table 12-14.

An Ig level within two standard deviations (SDs) of the mean for age is considered normal. In older children and adults, a total Ig level higher than 600 mg/dl with normal screening antibody tests excludes antibody deficiency. By contrast, a total Ig (IgG + IgM + IgA) lower than 400 mg/dl or an IgG globulin level lower than 200 mg/dl usually indicates antibody immunodeficiency. Total Ig levels of 400 to 600 mg/dl and IgG levels of 200 to 400 mg/dl are nondiagnostic and must be correlated with functional antibody tests.

Antibody Function Tests

Antibodies to tetanus, diphtheria, and *Haemophilus influenzae* B are useful functional tests recommended for

---

TABLE 12-12 · LEVELS OF IMMUNOGLOBULINS IN SERA OF NORMAL SUBJECTS BY AGE*

	IgG		IgM		IgA		Total Immunoglobulin	
Age	mg/dl	% of Adult Level	mg/dl	% of Adult Level	mg/dl	% of Adult Level	mg/dl	% of Adult Level
Newborn	1031 ± 200[†]	89 ± 17	11 ± 5	1.1 ± 5	2 ± 3	1 ± 2	1044 ± 201	67 ± 13
1–3 mo	430 ± 119	37 ± 10	30 ± 11	30 ± 11	21 ± 13	11 ± 7	481 ± 127	31 ± 9
4–6 mo	427 ± 186	37 ± 16	43 ± 17	43 ± 17	28 ± 18	14 ± 9	498 ± 204	32 ± 13
7–12 mo	661 ± 219	58 ± 19	54 ± 23	55 ± 23	37 ± 18	19 ± 9	752 ± 242	48 ± 15
13–24 mo	762 ± 209	66 ± 18	58 ± 23	59 ± 23	50 ± 24	25 ± 12	870 ± 258	56 ± 16
25–36 mo	892 ± 183	77 ± 16	61 ± 19	62 ± 19	71 ± 37	36 ± 19	1024 ± 205	65 ± 14
3–5 yr	929 ± 228	80 ± 20	56 ± 18	57 ± 18	93 ± 27	47 ± 14	1078 ± 245	69 ± 17
6–8 yr	923 ± 256	20 ± 22	65 ± 25	66 ± 25	124 ± 45	62 ± 23	1112 ± 293	71 ± 20
9–11 yr	1124 ± 235	97 ± 20	79 ± 33	80 ± 33	131 ± 60	66 ± 30	1334 ± 254	85 ± 17
12–16 yr	946 ± 124	82 ± 11	59 ± 20	60 ± 20	148 ± 63	74 ± 32	1153 ± 169	74 ± 12
Adults	1158 ± 305	100 ± 26	99 ± 27	100 ± 27	200 ± 61	100 ± 31	1457 ± 353	100 ± 24

*The values were divided from measurements made in 296 healthy children and 30 adults. Levels were determined by the radial diffusion technique using specific rabbit antisera to human immunoglobulins.
[†]One standard deviation.
From Stiehm ER, Fudenberg HH. Serum levels of immune globulins in health and disease. A survey. Pediatrics 37:715, 1966.

TABLE 12-13 · SERUM IgE LEVELS IN 425 WHITE SUBJECTS BY AGE GROUPS

Age (yr)	N	Natural Log Mean	Natural Log SD	Antilog Mean (IU/ml)	Antilog Mean + 1 SD (IU/ml)	Antilog Mean + 2 SD (IU/ml)
1–2	29	2.98	1.18	20	64	208
3–5	31	3.55	1.23	35	119	405
6–15	45	3.92	1.09	51	150	446
16–20	59	3.63	1.18	38	123	401
21–30	114	3.29	1.32	27	100	376
31–40	38	3.53	1.19	34	113	372
Over 40	109	3.52	1.21	34	114	382
Total	425	3.47	1.21	32	108	386

IU = international unit; N = number; SD = standard deviation.
From Wittig HJ, Belloit J, DeFillippi I, Royal G. Age-related serum immunoglobulin E levels in healthy subjects and in patients with allergic disease. J Allergy Clin Immunol 66:305–313, 1980.

the initial screening. These are valid only if the patient has previously been immunized to these antigens. These tests are available at many hospital laboratories or reference laboratories. Negative (nonprotective) titers, despite a positive immunization history, suggest functional antibody deficiency. These are usually IgG antibodies and thus test IgG function.

Total Hemolytic Complement Activity

Most complement component defects can be identified by a low CH_{50}; this test assesses the ability of the patient's serum to lyse antibody-coated sheep erythrocytes by the classical complement pathway. Values must be compared with standards used in the laboratory. The blood for this procedure must get to the laboratory

without delay because heat and time can diminish the complement levels in vitro.

Infection Evaluation

Patients with immunodeficiency often have chronic infection. The erythrocyte sedimentation rate or CRP is usually elevated in proportion to the severity of the chronic infection. The condition should be investigated by appropriate x-ray examinations and cultures of the suspected sites.

If these screening tests are all normal, immunodeficiency is usually excluded and the patient can be assured that IVIG or other long-term therapy is not indicated. However, if the screening tests are positive, if chronic infection is documented but unexplained, or if

TABLE 12-14 · LEVELS OF PLASMA IMMUNOGLOBULINS IN VERY SMALL PREMATURE INFANTS (<1500 g) DURING THE FIRST 10 MONTHS OF LIFE

	Premature infants 25 to 28 weeks' gestation				Premature infants 29 to 32 weeks' gestation			
Age (mo)	N	IgG* (mg/dl)	IgM* (mg/dl)	IgA* (mg/dl)	Age (mo)	N	IgG* (mg/dl)	IgM* (mg/dl)	IgA* (mg/dl)
0.25	18	251 (114–552)[†]	7.6 (1.3–43.3)	1.2 (0.07–20.8)	0.25	42	368 (186–728)[†]	9.1 (2.1–39.4)	0.6 (0.04–1.0)
0.5	14	202 (91–446)	14.1 (3.5–56.1)	3.1 (0.09–10.7)	0.5	35	275 (119–637)	13.9 (4.7–41)	0.9 (0.01–7.5)
1.0	10	158 (57–437)	12.7 (3.0–53.3)	4.5 (0.65–30.9)	1.0	26	209 (97–452)	14.4 (6.3–33)	1.9 (0.3–12.0)
1.5	14	134 (59–307)	16.2 (4.4–59.2)	4.3 (0.9–20.9)	1.5	22	156 (69–352)	15.4 (5.5–43.2)	2.2 (0.7–6.5)
2.0	12	89 (58–136)	16.0 (5.3–48.9)	4.1 (1.5–11.1)	2.0	11	123 (64–237)	15.2 (4.9–46.7)	3.0 (1.1–8.3)
3	13	60 (23–156)	13.8 (5.3–36.1)	3.0 (0.6–15.6)	3	14	104 (41–268)	16.3 (7.1–37.2)	3.6 (0.8–15.4)
4	10	82 (32–210)	22.2 (11.2–43.9)	6.8 (1.0–47.8)	4	21	128 (39–425)	26.5 (7.7–91.2)	9.8 (2.5–39.3)
6	11	159 (56–455)	41.3 (8.3–205)	9.7 (3.0–31.2)	6	21	179 (51–634)	29.3 (10.5–81.5)	12.3 (2.7–57.1)
8–10	6	273 (94–794)	41.8 (31.1–56.1)	9.5 (0.9–98.6)	8–10	16	280 (140–561)	34.7 (17–70.8)	20.9 (8.3–53)

*Geometric mean.
[†]The normal ranges in parentheses were determined by taking the antilog of (mean logarithm ± 2 standard deviations of the logarithms).
Data from Ballow M, Cater KL, Rowe JC, Goetz C, Desbonnet C. Development of the immune system in very low birth weight (less than 1500 g) premature infants: concentrations of plasma immunoglobulins and patients of infection. Pediatr Res 20:899–904, 1986, with permission.

the history is unusually suggestive for immunodeficiency, advanced tests are indicated (see Table 12-11).

Tests for Antibody Deficiencies

Initial Tests

Ig levels and functional antibody tests are part of the screening evaluation for immunodeficiency (see Table 12-10); in the antibody immunodeficiencies, one or more test results is abnormal. If the Ig levels are very low (total less than 100 mg/dl), a diagnosis of antibody immunodeficiency is established and further tests are done only to assess the degree of antibody impairment and the involvement of other components of the immune system.

B-Cell Enumeration

B cells are the precursors of the antibody-producing plasma cells and are characterized by the presence of one or more classes of surface membrane Ig (sIg) and certain B cell–related surface antigens, such as CD19, CD20, and CD21 (Tables 12-15 and 12-16).

B-cell enumeration is indicated when Igs are very low or absent; it is rarely indicated in the presence of normal or elevated Igs except to look for unusual surface Ig isotype distribution or density, which is characteristic of some antibody deficiencies.

B cells are usually measured by automated immunofluorescence (flow cytometry) (see T-Cell Enumeration, later) with an antibody to either the CD19 or CD20 B-cell surface antigen. This assay is often performed in conjunction with CD3, CD4, and CD8 T-cell enumeration. B cells make up 10% to 20% of the total lymphocytes but vary with age (see Table 12-16).

Alternatively, B cells can be assessed by measuring surface membrane Ig using immunofluorescence and a polyvalent antihuman Ig antisera with specificity for all Ig subclasses and κ and λ chains (World Health Organization [WHO]/International Agency for Research on Cancer [IARC] Technical Report, 1974). B cells with specificity for μ or δ chain or both are most common.

Pre-B cells are usually enumerated on a bone marrow aspirate with fluorescein-labeled antibodies to heavy chains. Pre-B cells are lymphocytes without surface membrane Ig but with small quantities of cytoplasmic μ heavy chains. Most pre-B cells are also CD10+.

B cells are very low (less than 1%) in XLA and in some forms of SCID, and are slightly reduced (2% to 6%) in transient hypogammaglobulinemia of infancy. In most antibody immunodeficiencies, B cells are present in normal quantities, indicating that the defect is one of differentiation rather than a lack of the precursor cells.

B-cell enumeration is of particular value in infant boys in whom XLA is suspected; the absence of B cells favors this diagnosis, and their presence favors a diagnosis of transient hypogammaglobulinemia, common

variable immunodeficiency, or an HIGM syndrome (see Chapter 13).

Abnormal distribution of SIG, such as the presence of several isotypes or selective increase or decrease of one isotype, may provide some diagnostic information in selective Ig deficiency (e.g., IgA deficiency, HIGM syndrome) or in B-cell malignancies.

IgG Subclass Levels

Selective deficiency of one of the four subclasses of IgG may occur in antibody deficiency (Schur et al., 1970) (see Chapter 13). The relative contributions of IgG1, IgG2, IgG3, and IgG4 to the total IgG are 70%, 20%, 7%, and 3%, respectively (see Chapter 4). Specific antisera for quantitative measurements are available; normal levels of IgG subclasses for age are presented in Table 12-17. Several reference laboratories offer these assays, but reproductivity and standardization are less than optimal.

Such measurements are indicated when IgG levels are normal or near-normal, but when functional antibody deficiency is present (Yount et al., 1970). IgG subclasses should also be measured in patients with selective IgA deficiency who exhibit increased susceptibility to infection. Many IgA-deficient patients have IgG2 subclass deficiency (Oxelius et al., 1981). Some patients with chronic lung disease have been reported with IgG4 subclass deficiency (Heiner et al., 1983), but isolated IgG4 deficiency also occurs in normal subjects.

A reasonable guideline for diagnosis of subclass deficiency is a value less than two SDs below the mean for age or an IgG1 less than 250 mg/dl, an IgG2 less than 50 mg/dl, and an IgG3 less than 25 mg/dl. An isolated IgG4 deficiency is not usually clinically significant. IgG subclass deficiencies are discussed in detail in Chapter 13.

IgD and IgE Levels

Determinations of IgD and IgE levels are indicated in the complete evaluation of suspected antibody immunodeficiency. IgD levels are determined by radial immunodiffusion, radioimmunoassay, or enzyme-linked immunosorbent assay (ELISA). IgE levels, because they are so low, are usually performed by radioimmunoassay or ELISA. Commercial kits are available. Table 12-13 provides normal levels of IgE at different ages.

Abnormalities of IgD and IgE levels, both high and low values, are not uncommon in incomplete antibody deficiency syndromes. IgE levels often parallel IgA levels, and IgD levels often parallel IgM levels.

Isolated deficiencies of IgD and IgE (see Chapter 13) are rare and of minimal significance. When other Ig levels are extremely low, levels of IgD and IgE are often low (Buckley and Fiscus, 1975). In partial cellular immunodeficiencies (e.g., Nezelof syndrome, WAS, DiGeorge anomaly), moderately elevated levels of IgE are commonly noted. In certain immunodeficiencies (e.g., hyper-IgE syndrome, Omenn's syndrome), IgE levels are markedly elevated (see Chapters 15 and 17).

TABLE 12-15 · PRINCIPAL CELL SURFACE ANTIGENS (CLUSTER DESIGNATIONS) USED TO IDENTIFY CELLS OF THE HUMAN IMMUNE SYSTEM

Cluster Designation	Predominant Reactivity	Names of Monoclonal Antibody Clones	Other Cellular Reactivity
Hematopoietic Stem Cells			
CD34	Progenitor cells	My10, B1-3C5	
All Leukocytes			
CD45	Tyrosine phosphatase	Anti-HLe-1	
CD43	Leukosialin	Leu-22	
T Cells			
Immature T Cells			
CD1a	Corticothymocytes	Leu-6, OKT6	Pre-B, dendritic cells
CD38	Immature cells	Leu-17, OKT10	Pre-B, plasma, NK, B subset
Pan-T Cells			
CD2	Sheep erythrocyte, LFA-3 receptor	Leu-5, OKT11, CT-2	NK subset
CD3	T-cell receptor complex	Leu-4, OKT3	
CD5	Mature T cells	Leu-1, OKT1, T101	B subset
CD7	Immature T cells	3A1, Leu-9	NK
CD28	Receptor for CD80 and CD86	Leu-28	Act B, Act T
Subsets of T Cells			
CD4	Helper/inducer T cells	Leu-3, OKT4	Mono
CD8	Cytotoxic/suppressor T cells	Leu-2, OKT8	NK subset
CD45RA	Naïve CD4 T cells (Suppressor/Inducer)	2H4, Leu18	CD8, B, NK
CD-62L	L-selectin, naïve cells	Leu8	CD8, Mono, B, NK, PMNs
CD45RO	Memory CD4 T cells (Helper/Inducer)	UCHL	CD4, Mono/Mφ, PMN
Activated T Cells			
CD25	IL-2α receptor	Tac	B subset
CD38	Immature cells	Leu 17, OKT10	Pre-B, plasma, NK, B subset
CD71	Transferrin receptor	OKT9	Act B, Mono
—*	HLA-DR (class II MHC)		B, Mono
CD69		Leu23	Act B, Act NK, Mono/Mφ
CD95	Fas ligand	APO-1	Act B, NK
CD154	Ligand for CD40	TRAP-1	Platelets, Mono/Mφ
B Cells			
Exclusive B-Cell Markers			
CD19	Pan-B cell	Leu-12, B4	
CD20	Pan-B cell	Leu-16, B1	
CD21	CR2, EBV receptor	B2	
CD22	Pan-B cell	Leu-14	
CD40	Ligand for CD154		
Nonexclusive B-Cell Markers			
CD35	CR1, C3b receptor		Mono, RBC, PMN
—*	HLA-DR (class II MHC)		Mono, Act T
—*	HLA-DP (class II MHC)		Mono, Act T
—*	HLA-DQ (class II MHC)		Mono, Act T
Monocytes			
CD11b	CR3, C3bi receptor	Leu-15, OKM1, Mac-1, Mo-1	NK, PMN, T subset
CD11c	CR4 receptor	Leu-M5	NK, T subset
CD14	Monocytes	Leu-M3, Mo-2	
Natural Killer Cells			
CD16	FcγRIll	Leu-11	Mono, PMN
CD11b	CR3, C3bi receptor	Leu-15, OKM1, Mac-1, Mo-1	Mono, PMN, T subset
CD56	N-CAM	Leu-19, NKH-1	T subset
CD57	Large granular lymphocytes	Leu-7, HNK-1	T subset

*No CD assigned.

Act = activated; CD = cluster designation; CR = complement receptor; EBV = Epstein-Barr virus; FcR = Fc receptor; LFA = leukocyte function associated antigen; MHC = major histocompatibility complex; Mono = monocytes; Mφ = macrophages; N-CAM = neural cell adhesion molecule; NK = natural killer; PMN = polymorphonuclear leukocytes. Other CD antigens are described in the Appendix.

TABLE 12-16 · NORMAL HUMAN BLOOD LYMPHOCYTE SUBPOPULATIONS AT VARIOUS AGES

Subpopulations	Age Groups						
	Cord Blood	2–3 Months	4–8 Months	12–23 Months	2–5 Years	7–17 Years	Adult
Total Lymphocytes							
Median cells/ul (%)	5400 (41%)	5680 (66%)	5990 (64%)	5160 (59%)	4060 (50%)	2400 (40%)	2100 (32%)
Confidence intervals	4200 (35%) to 6900 (47%)*	2920 (55%) to 8840 (78%)	3610 (45%) to 8840 (79%)	2180 (44%) to 8270 (72%)	2400 (38%) to 5810 (64%)	2000 (36%) to 2700 (43%)*	1600 (28%) to 2400 (39%)*
CD3 T Cells							
Median cells/ul (%)	3100 (55%)	4030 (72%)	4270 (71%)	3300 (66%)	3040 (72%)	1800 (70%)	1600 (73%)
Confidence intervals	2400 (49%) to 3700 (62%)*	2070 (55%) to 6540 (78%)	2280 (45%) to 6450 (79%)	1460 (53%) to 5440 (81%)	1610 (62%) to 4230 (80%)	1400 (66%) to 2000 (76%)*	960 (61%) to 2600 (84%)*
CD4 T Cells							
Median cells/ul (%)	1900 (35%)	2830 (52%)	2950 (49%)	2070 (43%)	1800 (42%)	800 (37%)	940 (46%)
Confidence intervals	1500 (28%) to 2400 (42%)*	1460 (41%) to 5116 (64%)	1690 (36%) to 4600 (61%)	1020 (31%) to 3600 (54%)	900 (35%) to 2860 (51%)	700 (33%) to 1100 (41%)*	540 (32%) to 1660 (60%)*
CD8 T Cells							
Median cells/ul (%)	1500 (29%)	1410 (25%)	1450 (24%)	1320 (25%)	1180 (30%)	800 (30%)	520 (27%)
Confidence intervals	1200 (26%) to 2000 (33%)*	650 (16%) to 2450 (35%)	720 (16%) to 2490 (34%)	570 (16%) to 2230 (38%)	630 (22%) to 1910 (38%)	600 (27%) to 900 (35%)*	270 (13%) to 930 (40%)*
B Cells (CD19 or CD20)†							
Median cells/ul (%)	1000 (20%)†	900 (23%)	900 (23%)	900 (23%)	900 (24%)	400 (16%)†	246 (13%)†
Confidence intervals	200 (14%) to 1500 (23%)*	500 (19%) to 1500 (31%)	500 (19%) to 1500 (31%)	500 (19%) to 1500 (31%)	700 (21%) to 1300 (28%)	300 (12%) to 500 (22%)*	122 (10%) to 632 (31%)
CD4:CD8 Ratio							
Median	1.2	2.2	2.1	1.6	1.4	1.3	1.7
Confidence intervals	0.8 to 1.8	1.3 to 3.5	1.2 to 3.5	1.0 to 3.0	1.0 to 2.1	1.1 to 1.4	0.9 to 4.5

Confidence intervals given are the 5th to 95th percentiles except where indicated (*); these are the 25th to 75th percentiles. B cells use the CD20 antigen except where indicated (†); these use the CD19 antigen. The lymphocyte % is the percentage of total leukocytes. The CD3, CD4, CD8, and B cell (CD19 or CD20) % is the percentage of total lymphocytes.
Combined data from Erkellor-Yuksel FM, et al. J Pediatr 120:216–222, 1992 (cord blood, 7–17 yrs; B cells); Denny T, et al. JAMA 267:1484–1488, 1992 (2–3 mo to 5 yr); Fahey JL, cited in Giorgi JV et al. In Rose NR, et al. Manual of Clinical Laboratory Immunology, 4th ed. Washington, D.C., American Society for Microbiology, 1992, pp 174–181 (adults).
Each subgroup contains at least 22 healthy subjects.

TABLE 12-17 · LEVELS OF IgG SUBCLASSES IN SERA OF NORMAL SUBJECTS BY AGE[*]

Age (yr)	No. of Subjects	IgG	IgG1	IgG2	IgG3	IgG4[†]
0–1	22	420[‡] (250–690)	340 (190–620)	59 (30–140)	39 (9–62)	19 (6–63)
1–2	42	470 (270–810)	410 (230–710)	68 (30–170)	34 (11–98)	13 (4–43)
2–3	36	540 (300–980)	480 (280–830)	98 (40–240)	28 (6–130)	18 (3–120)
3–4	52	600 (400–910)	530 (350–790)	120 (50–260)	30 (9–98)	32 (5–180)
4–6	31	660 (440–1000)	540 (360–810)	140 (60–310)	39 (9–160)	39 (9–160)
6–8	24	890 (560–1400)	560 (280–1120)	150 (30–630)	48 (40–250)	81 (11–620)
8–10	21	1000 (530–1900)	690 (280–1740)	210 (80–550)	85 (22–320)	42 (10–170)
10–13	33	910 (500–1660)	590 (270–1290)	240 (110–550)	58 (13–250)	60 (7–530)
13–16	19	910 (580–1450)	540 (280–1020)	210 (60–790)	58 (14–240)	60 (11–330)

[*]Levels were determined by radial diffusion using monospecific antisera.
[†]IgG4 levels appear to be absent in 10% of individuals.
[‡]Geometric means are presented for each Ig at every age. The normal bounds, given in parentheses, are obtained by taking the mean logarithm.
±2 Standard deviations of the logarithms and then take the antilogs of the results.
Data from Schur PH, Rosen F, Norman ME. Immunoglobulin subclasses in normal children. Pediatr Res 13:181–183, 1979.

The hyper-IgD syndrome, a rare disorder with elevated levels of IgD (IgD higher than 150 IU/ml [more than 20 mg/dl]) characterized by periodic bouts of fever, lymphadenitis, and occasional bouts of arthritis, has been described; recurrent infection was not seen (Drenth et al., 1994; Haraldson et al., 1992; Van der Meer et al., 1984) (see Chapter 36).

In allergic and parasitic disorders, IgE levels are markedly elevated. IgE levels higher than 50 IU/ml before age 1 year, higher than 100 IU/ml before age 2 years, or higher than 400 IU/ml after age 3 years are considered elevated (Wittig et al., 1980).

Natural Antibody Levels

The function of the antibody system can be assessed by measuring the antibody response to ubiquitous and injected antigens.

The saline isoagglutinin (anti-A, anti-B, or both) titers to measure IgM globulin function are sometimes performed. In most immunologically normal individuals older than 6 months of age (with the exception of those of blood group AB), titers are at least 1:8 to A1 and B cells, respectively. These titers are available in hospital blood banks, because the method is identical to that used to identify low titer O blood for exchange transfusion. Isoagglutinins are selectively deficient in older children with WAS; these patients often have low IgM globulin levels (Stiehm and McIntosh, 1967). Soothill (1962) showed correlation between serum IgM globulin levels and the isoagglutinin titers in normal subjects.

Other natural antibodies include the heterophile titer (antibody to sheep erythrocytes) and the streptolysin O titer. Nearly all normal individuals have antibodies at low titers (more than 1:10) to these antigens because of their widespread presence in food, inhaled particles, and the respiratory flora. Other natural antibodies that can be assayed are those to *Escherichia coli* (Webster et al., 1974) or endotoxin (Gupta and Reed, 1968).

Specific Antibody Responses

If the patient has not been immunized with diphtheria or tetanus toxoids, immunization with these agents (two or three injections), followed by antibody titers within 3 to 4 weeks after the last injection, is the preferred test for antibody function. The antibody response to tetanus toxoid is particularly valuable because delayed cutaneous hypersensitivity and in vitro proliferative responses to tetanus antigen can also be assessed following vaccine, thus providing information on T-cell responsiveness (Borut et al., 1980). ELISAs to tetanus antibodies that measure both IgG and IgM responses are available.

The antibody response to *Haemophilus influenzae* type B vaccine is also of value. The newer conjugate vaccines produce a good antibody response even in infants younger than 1 year of age. Titers to tetanus, diphtheria, and *Haemophilus influenzae* are often used together in the immunized infant for the initial antibody screening.

The antibody response to pneumococcal or meningococcal polysaccharide vaccines can also be used, particularly in subjects in whom the antibody response to polysaccharides is suspect (e.g., WAS, IgG2 subclass deficiency). The weak responses of normal infants to these antigens limit this procedure to children older than age 2 years.

The antibody response to typhoid vaccine has also been used to assess antibody function. The antibody response to the H and O antigens measures IgG and

IgM globulin function, respectively. Serum is obtained before and 3 weeks after three subcutaneous injections of 0.5 ml of typhoid vaccine (at 1- to 2-week intervals). Agglutinin titers to both antigens higher than 1:40 are normal; lower titers indicate poor antibody responses.

The antibody response to viral antigens can also be assessed. Rubeola, rubella, or varicella-zoster titers following measles, rubella, or varicella vaccinations, or following natural chickenpox infection are used. Antibody to hepatitis B virus following administration of vaccine is also of value.

Poliomyelitis titers following vaccination are less valuable in our experience because of low postimmunization titers even in normal subjects. As noted elsewhere, use of live virus vaccines to test for immunodeficiency is contraindicated because of the risk of disseminated infection.

RESPONSE TO ΦX-174 PHAGE ANTIGEN

Other antigens used to assess antibody responses include special antigens such as keyhole-limpet hemocyanin (KLH), and particularly bacteriophage ΦX-174. If screening tests suggest a primary or secondary antibody deficiency or if the patient is receiving IVIG infusions, intravenous immunization with bacteriophage ΦX-174, a T-cell dependent neoantigen, can be done. The antibody assay, phage neutralization, is sensitive, quantitative, and reproducible. ΦX-174 has a large molecular weight (MW) of 6×10^6 and thus is retained intravascularly until cleared from the circulation immunologically within 3 to 4 days after administration.

After phage clearance, neutralizing antibody activity develops in the serum of normal individuals. The primary response peaks at 2 weeks and consists predominantly of IgM antibody. The secondary response to a repeat immunization is brisk, peaks at 1 week, declines slowly, and consists of equal proportions of IgG and IgM antibody. A third immunization results in a further increase of the antibody titer and consists exclusively of IgG. Thus there are characteristic quantitative and qualitative differences between the primary, secondary, and tertiary responses to this antigen.

In the immunologically normal individual, the following components of the immune response to bacteriophage ΦX-174 can be distinguished:

1. Antigen clearance
2. The primary IgM response
3. The secondary response demonstrating amplification, immunologic memory, and limited isotype switch
4. The tertiary response characterized by amplification, a complete switch from IgM to IgG, and persistent immunologic memory

The generation of memory cells and the process of isotype switching is T-cell dependent. The early IgG antibody produced by normal subjects following the secondary immunization is of the IgG3 and IgG1 subclasses, later followed by the appearance of other IgG subclass antibodies. The persisting antibody after multiple immunizations is of the IgG1 class (Pyun et al., 1989).

Theoretically, six types of quantitatively and qualitatively abnormal immune responses to immunization with bacteriophage ΦX-174 are possible (Fig. 12-4). Examples of all such aberrant responses, following ΦX immunization, have been observed (Wedgwood et al., 1975) (Table 12-18).

1. Patients in whom the antigen is not cleared in a normal fashion and who produce no antibody (type 0)
2. Patients with normal (accelerated) antigen clearance, but absent antibody activity (type I)
3. Patients with normal antigen clearance, followed by production of small amounts of IgM antibody without immunologic memory (type II)
4. Patients with normal antigen clearance, antibody formation limited to IgM, some immunologic memory and limited amplification (type III)
5. Patients with normal antigen clearance, low antibody titers, immunologic memory and production of some, but limited IgG antibody (type IV)
6. Patients with normal antigen clearance and low antibody production consisting predominantly of IgG, intact memory and amplification, suggesting a qualitatively normal but quantitatively depressed response (type V)

Because ΦX-174 is a T-cell–dependent antigen, abnormal antibody responses may be observed in patients with a prototypic B-cell defect (e.g., XLA), a T-cell defect (e.g., patients with HIGM1 with CD40 ligand mutations) or both.

Approximately half of XLA patients have a prolonged phage clearance of up to 5 weeks, demonstrating no ability to make antibodies to bacteriophage. However, approximately half of XLA patients clear phage normally and some can produce small amounts of IgM and, occasionally, IgG antibody (see Table 12-18). Patients with XL-SCID clear phage normally, but their overall response is minute and only of the IgM class type 2 response. Of 44 patients with an SCID phenotype, 5 (2 boys, 3 girls) were unable to clear phage normally and failed to produce detectable antibodies to phage (type 0 response). Three of those are suspect to have RAG-1 or RAG-2 deficiency and two were members of the Navajo tribe, presumably with Abthascan SCID and Artemis mutations.

Patients with X-linked HIGM1 resulting from mutations of CD40 ligand (HIGM1) have normal phage clearance and a type II response. Patients with CVID clear phage normally, but some produce only IgM antibody, whereas others can isotype switch to various degrees (type III to V responses). Patients with classic WAS have a type II response, whereas those with X-linked thrombocytopenia have a type IV or V response.

Lateral Pharyngeal X-Ray Examination

A lateral radiograph of the pharynx that shows a marked decrease in adenoidal tissues is indicative of poor lymphoid development and immunodeficiency (Baker et al., 1962). This finding was first described in

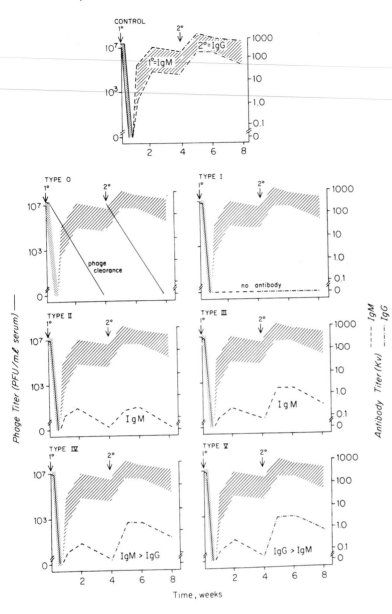

Figure 12-4 · Types of immune responses to bacteriophage φX-174 in patients with X-linked agammaglobulinemia. The phage injections, given at time 0 (1°) and at 4 weeks (2°), are indicated by a downward arrow (↓). Normal phage clearance is accomplished within 3 to 4 days after primary immunization (*stippled area*). Patients with prolonged phage clearance (*solid line*) are assigned to the type 0 category. All other types have normal clearance of phage. Range of antibody titers observed in a control population is shown by the hatched area (1° = primary antibody response, 2° = secondary antibody response). Patients classified as types 0 and I do not produce antibody to phage; those classified as type II make small amounts of IgM antibody without expressing immunologic memory. Patients classified as types III to V demonstrate immunologic memory but have either a qualitative (types III and IV with no or reduced amounts of IgG antibody) or a quantitative (type V) deficiency of antibody response. Of 50 X-linked agammaglobulinemic patients immunized with φX-174, 25 had a type 0 response, 4 had a type I response, 9 had a type II response, 6 had a type III response, and 6 had a type IV response.

WAS; it is also present in other antibody and cellular immunodeficiencies. By contrast, many immunologically normal children with recurrent upper respiratory tract infections have enlarged adenoids.

Biopsies

Biopsies are occasionally of value in patients with antibody immunodeficiencies if the diagnosis is equivocal; they are rarely necessary and entail some risk of infection at the biopsy site. A biopsy specimen should be obtained after local antigenic stimulation. A diphtheria-pertussis-tetanus or typhoid immunization is given in the anterior thigh, and an inguinal lymph node is obtained from the same side 5 to 7 days later. Lymph nodes are examined to assess the thymus-dependent paracortical areas, the medullary plasma cells, and the cortical germinal centers. Immunofluorescent studies

using antibodies to T- and B-cell surface antigens can identify the exact cells present in the biopsy.

Nodes from patients with antibody immunodeficiencies show a paucity of plasma cells, a diminished number of primary lymphoid follicles, a thin cortex, absence of germinal centers, and cellular disorganization. An increased number of histiocytes and other reticuloendothelial elements may be present. Biopsy results are especially valuable in immunodeficient patients with lymphadenopathy to exclude reticuloendothelial malignancy. In HIGM1 syndrome and WAS, the cervical lymph nodes are characteristically large with abundant plasma cells; however, the overall architecture is abnormal.

Biopsies of the enlarged lymph nodes of patients with CVID may identify granulomas or lymphoreticular malignancies.

The rectal mucosa is the preferred biopsy site for some investigators (Davis et al., 1971). A decreased

zation (a positive MLC). A positive stimulation index in an MLC and in an antigen-stimulated culture is usually 3 to 20, considerably less than the response to a mitogen.

Because the response to a specific antigen requires prior sensitization, it indicates cellular immunodeficiency only when prior contact with the antigen has been established. For example, a failure of response to *Candida* antigen in a patient with widespread mucocutaneous candidiasis indicates a T-cell defect to this antigen.

Superantigens can also be used to assess lymphocyte proliferation. Superantigens are bacterial products (e.g., staphylococcal toxins) that stimulate a large fraction of T cells without prior sensitization (Takei et al., 1993).

INHIBITORS

Because serum factors may modulate the response to mitogens or antigens, a decreased proliferative response may be further studied by culturing the washed lymphocytes in the presence of normal serum. If this improves the response and if the addition of the patient's serum depresses the response of normally responsive lymphocytes, an inhibitor is present. This inhibition can be specific to one or a few related antigens, or nonspecific. Specific inhibitors are usually antibodies to the antigens; they have been observed in miliary tuberculosis, atypical measles, and mucocutaneous candidiasis.

Nonspecific inhibitors include antibodies directed against lymphocytes; they may occur in SLE, pregnancy, and multitransfused blood recipients. Nonspecific inhibitors, poorly characterized but nonantibody in nature, are seen in uremia, certain malignancies, leprosy, hepatitis, and ataxia-telangiectasia.

OTHER LYMPHOPROLIFERATION ASSAYS

Techniques for using whole blood to measure mitogen responsiveness have been developed, but are considerably less sensitive (Fletcher et al., 1987). Techniques that assess lymphocyte reactivity by flow cytometry measure the appearance of activation antigens (e.g., IL-2 receptor [CD25] or CD69), or the presence of intracellular ATP (Sottang et al., 2000) are also available. The production of specific cytokines following lymphocyte activation (ELISPOT assays) (see later text) also indicates lymphocyte responsiveness.

HLA Typing

HLA typing is of value to identify potential stem cell transplant donors; siblings and parents are HLA typed along with the patient. An MLC between individuals of the same HLA type can confirm the existence of HLA identity between the patient and the donor (see Chapter 43).

HLA typing can also be used to detect chimerism. Certain infants with profound T-cell deficiencies may have lymphoid chimerism as a result of engraftment of maternal cells in utero or engraftment from a blood or plasma transfusion (Kadowaki et al., 1965; Parkman et al., 1974). In some infants, there is evidence of graft-versus-host disease (GVHD) with alopecia, rash, diar-

rhea, hepatitis, and GI disturbances, but in most the engraftment is silent.

The presence of more than two HLA antigens at any one locus or HLA antigens not present in either parent usually indicates engraftment with a second population of cells, either from the mother or from a blood donor. A few instances of multiple weak HLA antigens not caused by chimerism have been reported in SCID (Terasaki et al., 1972). Some patients with SCID have no class I or class II antigens, characteristic of the MHC deficiencies (bare lymphocyte syndrome) (de la Salle et al., 1994; Klein et al., 1993; Touraine and Betuel, 1983; Touraine et al., 1978) (see Chapter 15).

Karyotype analysis or DNA studies can also be used to identify chimerism or engraftment (Conley et al., 1984).

Chromosome Analysis

Chromosome analysis is of value in the diagnosis of certain immunodeficiencies, notably the DiGeorge anomaly and the chromosomal breakage syndromes (see Chapters 17 and 18). Chimerism may also be diagnosed by the simultaneous presence of XX and XY cell lines in routine chromosome counts of peripheral blood. In some instances, lymphocytes for chromosome analysis do not proliferate to the PHA used to induce mitosis: In such instances, SCID should be suspected.

Advanced Flow Cytometric Analysis

Identification of subtle T-cell abnormalities not discernible by the basic CD3, CD4, and CD8 panel may be achieved using monoclonal antibodies for other T-cell antigens, in three- or four-color flow cytometry analysis. These advanced panels may permit diagnosis of several T-cell defects, and provide a means to follow the course of the illness and response to treatment, including immune reconstitution.

An assessment of naïve and memory CD4 and CD8 cells is used to determine the immune system's ability to respond to neoantigens. CD45RA is a marker for naïve T cells that are able to respond to neoantigens, and thus an indirect assessment of thymic function. Naïve T cells also express high levels of the adhesion molecule L-selectin (CD62L) (Campbell and Butcher, 2000) The numbers of naïve T cells increase following stem cell or thymic transplantation in SCID, complete DiGeorge syndrome, or after potent antiviral therapy in HIV patients (Markert et al., 1997, McCune et al., 2000).

CD45RO is a marker for memory T cells; the proportion of memory to naïve cells increases with advancing age and immunologic maturity. CD45RO and CD45RA are usually mutually exclusive, so cells that are CD45RO$^-$ are naïve cells and CD45RA$^-$ cells are memory cells. The majority (more than 90%) of T cells of normal newborns are naïve cells, whereas normal adults have approximately half naïve and half memory T cells.

Activation markers such as CD25 (IL-2 receptor α chain) and HLA-D related are of value in identifying defects of CD3 activation; CD25 absence on activated T cells can be used in the diagnosis of XL-SCID and absence of DR on B cells or activated T cells is characteristic of the major histocompatibility class II deficiency (see Chapter 15). By contrast, activated T cells in the circulation may indicate immune activation such as is present in Omenn syndrome.

Other monoclonal antibody assays are of value in the diagnosis of several T-cell disorders such as CD7 deficiency, WAS (absent WASP protein on platelets) and HIGM1 (absent CD154 on activated T cells or platelets).

Flow cytometry can also be used to assess the function of granulocytes, to measure apoptosis, and to characterize the TCR, as described elsewhere in this chapter. Advanced flow techniques are also available to assess signal transduction, T-cell proliferation, T-cell cytotoxicity, and intracellular cytokine production.

Cytokine Assays

Elevations of some cytokines can be detected transiently in the blood after therapeutic administration, during the acute phase of an illness, or in certain chronic infections. They can also be elevated in body fluids, such as joint fluid or cerebrospinal fluid (CSF). Because of their low MW, they usually have very brief half lives in the circulation and thus they are usually measured in cultures of the patient's stimulated cells or occasionally in body fluids such as joint fluid or CSF. Alternatively, cellular ribonucleic acid (RNA) for a specific cytokine can be assessed in the lysate of unstimulated or stimulated cells.

The most common cytokine assays used clinically are IL-1, IL-2, TNF-α, and IFN-γ (Table 12-20). Biologic, ELISA, and radioimmunoassays are available using commercially available kits. Alternatively, reference laboratories can perform the assays.

Production of IL-2 is decreased in many T-cell immunodeficiencies, including HIV (Prince et al., 1984). A small number of children with SCID have a specific defect in IL-2 production (Weinberg and Parkman, 1990). A primary defect in the production of IFN-gamma has also been reported in a few children (Lipinski et al., 1980). IL-1 and TNF-α levels are increased in HIV and the CSF of several central nervous

system disorders (e.g., meningitis) (Arditi et al., 1991; Saez-Llorens et al., 1990).

The cytokine profile has been used to define Th1 and Th2 responses in various diseases, particularly AIDS and allergic states. Th1 responses are characterized by IL-2, IFN-γ, and IL-12 secretion, and are associated with a cellular (T-cell) immune response, whereas Th2 responses are characterized by IL-4, IL-5, IL-6, and IL-10 secretion with enhanced antibody responses (including IgE) and suppression of Th1 responses (see Chapter 2).

ELISPOT ASSAYS

To assess antigen-specific cytokine production by individual cells, an ELISPOT test can be used (Power et al., 1999). In this procedure antigen-activated lymphocytes are cultured in semisolid agar and the cytokines secreted by an individual cell are assessed using a monoclonal antibody and an ELISA assay; this creates a spot where a single cell has synthesized a specific cytokine. This permits an estimation of the number of cells synthesizing a specific cytokine in question (usually IFN-γ) following antigen activation. ELISPOT assays can also be used to measure Ig or antibody synthesis in single cells.

OTHER CYTOKINE ASSAYS

Flow cytometry can be used to measure the levels of intracellular cytokines produced after antigen or mitogen stimulation. Other methods are used to assess specific cytokine RNA production, including PCR assays and simultaneous quantitative analysis of multiple cytokines (cytokine microarray technology).

CYTOKINE RECEPTOR AND SOLUBLE CYTOKINE RECEPTOR ASSAYS

Several immunodeficiencies result from deficiency or structural defects of cytokine receptors such as IL-2 receptor common gamma chain in XL-SCID, IFN-γ–receptor defect in leukocyte mycobactericidal defect or CD40 ligand defect (CD156) in HIGM1 syndrome. Specific antibodies to some of these receptors are available so that flow cytometry can be performed on resting or activated cells to diagnose the defect.

Soluble cytokine receptor assays are available, including soluble IL-2 receptor, soluble TNF-α receptor, soluble CD4, soluble CD8, soluble CD23, soluble Fc receptor (FcR), and soluble intracellular adhesion mole-

---

TABLE 12-20 · CYTOKINES USED IN CLINICAL IMMUNOLOGY

Cytokine	Principal Cell Source	Principal Action	Comment
IL-1	MΦ, other cells	Stimulates T cells, augments inflammation, fever	↑ in inflammatory diseases, infections
IL-2	T, NK	T and B growth factor; LAK, NK stimulant	↓ in T cell IDD, HIV
IL-4	T	B-cell, IgE stimulant	↑ in hyper-IgE
IL-5	T	B-cell, eosinophil, IgA stimulant	↑ in eosinophilia
IL-6	Multiple cells	B-cell stimulant	↑ in HIV, Castleman's disease
TNF-α	T	Augments inflammation, tumoricidal	↑ in inflammatory diseases
IFN-α	Leukocytes	Antiviral	↓ in hepatitis, cancer
IFN-β	Fibroblasts	Antiviral	↓ in hepatitis, cancer
IFN-γ	T, NK	Antiviral, immune enhancer	↓ in IFN-IDD

IDD = immunodeficiency disease; IFN = interferon; Ig = immunoglobulin; IL = interleukin; LAK = lymphokine-activated killer cells; MΦ = macrophage; NK = natural killer; TNF = tumor necrosis factor.

TABLE 12-21 · TYPES OF CYTOTOXIC REACTIONS

Types	Cell	Activating or Enhancing Agent	Specificity
Natural killer (NK)	NK (CD16, CD56)	Interferon	Nonspecific
Antibody-dependent cellular cytotoxicity	NK, M/MΦ, granulocyte	IgG antibody on target surface	Specificity dependent on antibody
Cytotoxic T cell	T	Viral or tumor antigens, haptens	Specific, HLA-restricted
Cell-mediated lympholysis	T	Alloantigens	Specific, HLA-restricted
Lymphokine-activated	NK. T. M/MΦ	IL-2	Nonspecific
Lectin-dependent	NK, T, M/MΦ	Mitogens	Nonspecific

HLA = human leukocyte antigen; Ig = immunoglobulin; IL = interleukin; NK = natural killer; M/MΦ = monocyte/macrophage.

cule type 1 (CD54). Assays of serum, plasma, body fluids (e.g., CSF, joint fluid), or supernatants of activated lymphocytes can be done by ELISA or radioimmunoassay.

Alterations are present in a variety of inflammatory/autoimmune diseases and in GVHD. Because these factors are regulators of the immune system, alterations in many immunodeficiencies may be expected. For example, Jyonouchi and co-workers (1991) found normal levels of soluble FcεRII in the serum of patients with CVID, but elevated levels in the serum of patients with ectodermal dysplasia.

Natural cytokine inhibitors (e.g., IL-1 receptor antagonist), pharmacologic (e.g., anti–TNF-α monoclonal antibodies), and acquired antibodies following cytokine treatment (IFN-γ antibodies) can neutralize the effects of cytokines. Specialized assays are available for assessment of these inhibitors.

Because of the increased availability of these assays, cytokine abnormalities in various immunodeficiencies may be further identified.

Cytotoxic Assays

Determining the ability of a mononuclear cell to lyse a target is a valuable assay of lymphocyte function. In most of these assays, a target cell is isotopically labeled (e.g., with ^{51}Cr), and the amount of radioactivity released after exposure to the effector cell is used as a measure of cell lysis. Several types of cytotoxicity have been identified (Table 12-21) based on the effector cell involved, the type of target cell lysed, and the participation of soluble factors (e.g., antibodies, interferons, interleukins).

NATURAL KILLER ASSAYS

NK cells are non-T, non-B, large granular lymphocytes that lyse tumor or viral-infected target cells without presensitization. These cells are identified by the CD16 and CD56 antigens in the basic flow panel. NK function is measured by lysis of the K562 tumor cell line (Table 12-22).

NK deficiency is present in some patients with SCID (see Chapter 15), AIDS (see Chapter 29), Chédiak-Higashi syndrome (see Chapter 20), LAD-1 (see Chapter 20), X-linked lymphoproliferative syndrome (see Chapter 17), lymphohistiocytosis syndromes (see Chapter 26), Griscelli syndrome (see Chapters 17 and 20), and primary NK deficiency (see Chapter 17).

ANTIBODY-DEPENDENT CYTOTOXICITY

Antibody-dependent cellular cytotoxicity (ADCC) involves lysis of an antibody-coated target cell. The nonspecific effector cell is often termed a *killer cell*, although the cell has an NK phenotype. The specificity of the cytotoxic reaction comes from the antibody coat.

Sanel and Buckley (1978), using antibody-coated human lymphocytes as targets, noted profound ADCC defects in XLA and combined immunodeficiency; using human lymphocytes or chicken or human erythrocytes as targets, they noted less severe ADCC defects in CVID and HIGM1. Albrecht and Hong (1976) noted decreased cytotoxicity toward antibody-coated human erythrocytes in primary monocyte defects. Patients with LAD-1 also exhibit low ADCC (and NK) because their effector cells do not adhere to the target cells.

TABLE 12-22 · AGE-RELATED CHANGES IN NATURAL KILLER CELLS AND NATURAL KILLER LYTIC ACTIVITY

Age	N	Phenotypic Markers						K562 Lysis*	
		CD16		CD56		CD57			
		%	Cells/ul	%	Cells/ul	%	Cells/ul	N	%
Birth	11	13.8 ± 4.3	709 ± 316	9.1 ± 4.3	481 ± 198	1.2 ± 0.7	60 ± 40	26	15 ± 6
1–5 mo	6	12.7 ± 4.6	790 ± 352	10.6 ± 5.4	627 ± 308	1.4 ± 0.8	80 ± 40	7	36 ± 12
6–12 mo	7	12.5 ± 4.9	714 ± 300	12.2 ± 6.0	676 ± 295	1.7 ± 1.5	120 ± 110	12	42 ± 9
1–4 yr	8	12.9 ± 4.6	573 ± 264	13.1 ± 5.6	586 ± 310	2.6 ± 1.9	120 ± 90	23	41 ± 8
5–8 yr	6	14.4 ± 5.2	418 ± 134	15.0 ± 6.7	431 ± 181	12.5 ± 6.7	360 ± 170	13	40 ± 8
9–13 yr	7	15.2 ± 4.2	408 ± 196	16.5 ± 5.9	438 ± 181	15.8 ± 6.9	410 ± 190	19	38 ± 8
Adult	12	15.5 ± 5.4	318 ± 191	16.4 ± 6.5	343 ± 214	20.5 ± 5.5	400 ± 150	42	38 ± 8

Values are means ± 1 standard deviation.
*Percent specific lysis of K562 tumor cells using a 20:1 target/effector ratio and a 4-hour chromium release assay.
Data derived from Yabuhara A, Kawai H, Komiyama A. Development of natural killer cytotoxicity during childhood: marked increases in number of natural killer cells with adequate cytotoxic abilities during infancy to early childhood. Pediatr Res 28:316–322, 1990.

T-CELL CYTOTOXICITY

Antigen-specific, HLA-restricted cytotoxic T-cell reactions (cytoxic T cells [CTLs]), generally assess CD8+ T cells with an alpha/beta TCR, using target cells that share class I HLA determinants with the effector cell and express the antigen of interest. A common target cell is an autologous B-cell line that has been infected with a specific virus or with a virus vector containing a specific antigenic peptide.

The T cells are often stimulated with the antigen prior to the assay because resting CTLs are rarely detectable. CTLs are deficient in primary cellular immunodeficiencies (e.g., SCID and ataxia-telangiectasia), in severe viral infection (e.g., advanced AIDS), and in the newborn. Because of the complexity of these assays, CTL assays are not done routinely in the diagnosis of immunodeficiency.

HLA-nonrestrictive cytotoxic reactions of T cells can also be assessed and include lectin-dependent cytotoxicity (Lubens et al., 1982) and lymphokine-activated cytotoxicity (Grimm and Rosenberg, 1984). These nonspecific cytotoxic reactions tend to be decreased in newborns, in patients with cellular immunodeficiencies, and in patients following bone marrow ablative procedures. T cells with a gamma/delta TCR also participate in these reactions.

USE OF TETRAMERS

A new way to measure CTLs uses tetramers, antigenic peptides attached to specific MHC molecules and conjugated to a fluorochrome. Flow cytometry is used to assess the binding of antigen-specific, HLA-restricted T-cell populations to the tetramer. The identity of the T cell (e.g., CD8 or CD4, CD45RO or CD45RA) and its activation status can be determined simultaneously with monoclonal antibodies tagged with a different fluorochrome. This very sensitive method may become the preferred way to identify the numbers and specificity of individual cytotoxic cells (Moris et al., 2001).

Enzyme Assays

When combined immunodeficiency is suspected, assays should be performed for ADA and PNP, inasmuch as absence of these enzymes identifies variants of autosomal recessive combined immunodeficiency (Giblett et al., 1975; Meuwissen et al., 1975). ADA catalyzes the conversion of adenosine to inosine, and PNP catalyzes the conversion of inosine to hypoxanthine. Their absence may lead to intracellular accumulation of adenosine, inosine, deoxyadenosine, and deoxyinosine, which exert an immunosuppressive action (see Chapter 16). Radiologic abnormalities of the ribs and long bones may be seen in patients with this type of enzymatic deficiency.

ADA and PNP are best measured on hemolyzed erythrocytes (Scott et al., 1974). Heterozygotes have half-normal levels. Intrauterine diagnosis of ADA deficiency has been accomplished by showing decreased levels in cultured amniotic fluid cells (Hirschhorn et al., 1975). A complete discussion is presented in Chapter 16.

Several infants with deficiency of biotin-dependent carboxylase have been noted to have T-cell immunodeficiency, primarily manifested by mild mucocutaneous candidiasis (Cowan et al., 1979). Biotin is necessary for the catabolism of isoleucine and leucine; its absence causes organic aciduria with alopecia and central nervous system abnormalities (see Chapter 17).

Thymic Functional Assays

THYMIC HORMONE ASSAYS

Several factors from thymic epithelial cells with biologic activity have been isolated, including thymulin, thymosin, thymopoietin, and facteur thymique serique (FTS) (Hadden, 1993). Radioimmunoassays for thymosin and bioassays for FTS and thymopoietin have been reported but are not generally available (Goldstein et al., 1966; Incefy et al., 1977).

Thymic hormone levels are typically high at birth and early childhood, decreasing slowly with age. Thymic hormones are absent or greatly depressed in combined immunodeficiency and the DiGeorge anomaly (Lewis et al., 1977). Thymic hormone assays have been replaced to a large extent by assays of thymic output or thymic size, as outlined in the following text.

THYMIC IMAGING

Thymic imaging can be done by CT or MRI scanning of the thymus, providing additional information not obtained by ordinary chest x-ray examination (Han et al., 2001; Mendelson, 2001). Such procedures have been used in HIV to measure restoration of thymic function following antiretroviral therapy (Smith et al., 2000).

T-CELL REARRANGMENT EXCISION CIRCLES

Assessment of recent thymic emigrant (RTE) cells offers another way to assess thymic function. This is done by measuring the levels of T-cell rearrangement excision circles (TRECs) in peripheral blood T cells. TRECs are nonreplicating episomal DNA byproducts (containing a signal joint sequence) of the final step of TCR rearrangement that are present in newly emigrated thymic CD4 and CD8 T cells. Because they are not replicated during cell division, there is a progressive dilution of these cells with clonal expansion.

TRECs can be assessed using quantitative PCR (Douek et al., 1998). Levels in newborns are higher than in adults, and patients with acquired (e.g., HIV) or congenital defects in T-cell function have diminished levels of TRECs in proportion to the severity of the thymic dysfunction.

The TREC levels in all or specific lymphocyte subpopulations can be measured and compared with normal levels or levels prior to specific treatment. Serial TREC analyses have been used to indicate restoration of thymic function in combined immunodeficiency or DiGeorge syndrome following stem cell (Patel et al., 2000) or thymic transplantation (Markert et al., 1999, 2003) or in advanced HIV after retroviral therapy (Douek et al., 2000).

T-Cell Receptor Analysis

Analysis of the TCR is of value in the diagnosis of certain T-cell deficiencies, particularly those in which CD3 cells are present but proliferative responses are abnormal or in patients with increased numbers of double positive (CD4+,CD8+ cells) or double negative (CD4−,CD8−) CD3 cells on flow cytometry.

The TCR consists of the antigen-binding variant portion (the alpha/beta or gamma/delta heterodimer) and CD3, the signal transduction invariant portion. The latter is composed of four proteins, organized into three dimers, the gamma/epsilon and delta/epsilon heterodimers and the zeta/zeta dimer. (The gamma and delta segments of the invariant portion are structurally distinct from the gamma and delta segments of the variant portion).

ALPHA/BETA AND GAMMA/DELTA TCRs

Most circulating T cells originate in the thymus and have alpha/beta TCRs, but a small percentage (<5%), contain the gamma/delta heterodimer. The percentage of alpha/beta and gamma/delta TCRs can be examined using flow cytometry and monoclonal antibodies that recognize these chains.

Gamma/delta T cells mature outside of the thymus, and are usually CD4−,CD8− double negative cells. They are found normally in the tissues of the GI tract and may be present in increased numbers in the circulation in autoimmunity, certain infections, and some forms of immunodeficiency (De Libero, 1997; Fisch et al., 1999).

ANALYSIS OF THE CD3 COMPLEX

The invariant (CD3) portion of the TCR can be studied by advanced flow cytometry, noting low expression of CD3 on CD4 and CD8 cells (Kappes et al., 1995).

Confirmation of a CD3 defect requires mutation analysis of the CD3 complex using T-cell RNA and PCR amplification of each component using specific primers. These amplified DNA segments can undergo sequence analysis (Kappes et al., 1995). Abnormalities of the CD3 gamma chain (Arnaiz-Villena et al., 1992), delta chain (Dadi et al., 2003), epsilon chain (Soudais et al., 1993), and zeta chain (Alarcon et al., 1988) in patients with immunodeficiencies have been identified (see Chapter 15).

TCR Vβ REPERTOIRE ANALYSIS

Another way to study the TCR is to characterize the alpha/beta heterodimer repertoire. This is done by assessing the distribution of the approximately 26 different Vβ chains. In normal subjects each Vβ segment is used in approximately 1% to 9% (mean 4%) of the circulating T cells. Immunologic immaturity with diminished use of certain segments may lead to a skewed distribution. Alternatively, expansion of certain T-cell clones evoked by malignancy or repeated exposure to a specific antigen or superantigen may result in expansion (greater than threefold from the mean) of T cells of one or more Vβ segments and a skewed repertoire (Wahlstrom et al., 2001).

Two principal ways to measure Vβ usage include (1) flow cytometry using monoclonal antibodies to unique Vβ chains and (2) PCR amplification and quantitation using specific primers to these unique gene segments (Kharbanda et al., 2003). (Similar studies can be done for the Vα segments but are less commonly used).

Such methods have been used to determine the development of the T-cell repertoire following transplants, to search for clonal expansion in malignancy (e.g., lymphoma), and to characterize antigen-stimulated expansion in autoimmunity (e.g., scleroderma), infection (e.g., HIV), or organ rejection. Refined analyses can identify the repertoire in selected T-cell subpopulations such as CD4 or CD8 cells.

TCR REARRANGEMENTS

A final way to examine the TCR is to look for TCR rearrangements in isolated T-cell subpopulations (Pan et al., 2001) as a way to identify clonality (suggesting malignancy) or to identify the origin of a particular population of T cells (e.g., maternal or infant). This can be done either by Southern blot analysis or by PCR. Such rearrangements have been noted in patients with Omenn syndrome (Brooks et al., 1999).

T-Cell Activation Analysis

A complete analysis of certain T-cell immunodeficiencies requires assessment of T-cell activation, including the integrity of the TCR and the signal transduction pathway (Nel, 2002). Defects in T-cell activation or the TCR have been reported in a few patients with T-cell immunodeficiencies (Alarcon et al., 1988; Arpaia et al., 1994; Le Deist et al., 1995; Rijkers et al., 1991) (see Chapter 15). Such patients may have normal numbers of T cells and variable susceptibility to infection but poor proliferative responses to mitogens, antigens, or anti-CD3 monoclonal antibody (Stiehm, 1993).

T-cell activation includes antigen processing and presentation, an intact TCR, participation by CD45 phosphatase, inositol phospholipid turnover, translocation of protein kinase C (PKC) from cytosol to the plasma membrane, and activation of several protein tyrosine kinases (PTKs) (see Chapter 2). The PKC and PTK pathways are linked insofar as phospholipase C, which initiates phospholipid turnover, requires tyrosine phosphorylation for its activation. Phospholipase C converts phosphatidylinositol 4,5-diphosphate to inositol 1,4, 5-triphosphate (IP3), and diacylglycerol (DG). IP3 leads to intracellular Ca^{2+} mobilization, and DG activates phosphokinase C.

These alterations open the Ca^{2+} channels and this in turn activates IL-2 gene expression in conjunction with a nuclear factor of activated T cells. Finally, IL-2 receptor expression occurs. IL-2 gene transcription also requires the participation of several proto-oncogenes (e.g., C-Fos, C-Jun), a tyrosine protein kinase, and TCR ζ-chain phosphorylation.

Assessment of activation uses various stimulants or inhibitors, such as phorbol myristate acetate (PMA), ionophores, and anti-CD3 antibody, which stimulate or bypass certain pathways. Following these steps, IL-2 production, IL-2 receptor expression, intracellular calcium, biochemical events (enzyme levels, cyclic adenosine monophosphate levels), and specific DNA and RNA assays for various components (e.g., ζ-chains of CD3, IL-2, PTK) are performed. Such assays are available in only a few research laboratories.

Alternate activation pathways may also exist. For example, activation of CD43 (sialophorin) by anti-CD43 antibody occurs and can be abnormal in WAS. CD28 activation by anti-CD28 antibody can also be assessed; this is an important co-receptor for cellular growth versus tolerance or apoptosis. Nel (2002) and Nel and Slaughter (2002) have reviewed T-cell activation.

Apoptosis Assays

The assessment of apoptosis in lymphocytes is of value in selected immunodeficiencies. Spontaneous "programmed cell death" occurs normally after a lymphocyte performs its duties of cell activation and effector function. Elimination of these cells maintains immune homeostasis by limiting lymphocyte accumulation and self reactivity. Apoptotic cells have characteristic morphologic features of shrinkage, and disappearance of microvilli, with segmental cleavage of its DNA.

An important signal for apoptosis is ligation of the Fas surface antigen (CD95) by another cell expressing a Fas ligand or self-expression of Fas ligand, both of which results in cell suicide. This is done by activation of cytoplasmic proteases (caspases), which results in the characteristic structural abnormalities. TNF can also trigger apoptosis. An illness termed ALPS is associated with inherited mutations of the Fas gene (Rieux-Laucat et al., 1995) (see Chapter 19).

Assessment of Fas (CD95) on T cells can be done by flow cytometry, but is rarely diagnostic. Increased expression of CD95 is associated with increased apoptosis, as has been described in Blackfan-Diamond syndrome (Dror and Freedman, 2001). Diminished expression of CD95 may occur in homozygous ALPS.

Flow cytometry can be used to assess apoptosis using dyes that bind to fragmented DNA (e.g., 7-aminoactinomycin, propidium iodide) (Schmidt et al., 1994). Alternatively, expanded T-cell lines can be activated with anti-Fas or anti-CD3 monoclonal antibodies and the number or cells viable after incubation can be assessed (Puck and Sneller, 1997). Diminished cell death suggest defective apoptosis.

Increased apoptosis may lead to T-cell depletion such as in AIDS, whereas decreased apoptosis results in lymphoproliferation and autoimmunity (see Chapter 19).

Biopsies

Biopsies may also be helpful in the exact diagnosis of cellular immunodeficiency. Bone marrow and lymph node biopsies were discussed earlier. A lymph node biopsy is of value in cellular immunodeficiency if the laboratory evaluation is equivocal or if malignancy is a concern. However, there is some risk of infection, particularly if a specimen is obtained in the groin area.

The lymph node architecture of patients with cellular immunodeficiency shows considerable disorganization without a clear demarcation between cortical and medullary areas. Germinal centers are absent, and the lymphoid follicles are rudimentary. Lymphoid and plasma cells may be entirely absent if there is a combined B-cell and T-cell defect. Stromal cells, monocytes, and histiocytes predominate. Criteria for morphologic assessment of lymph nodes have been published (Cottier et al., 1972). Immunohistologic study to identify T and B subsets within the lymph nodes may help to identify the immunopathogenesis of the disorder.

A thymic biopsy can also provide useful diagnostic and therapeutic information in special cases. This type of biopsy should be performed by someone with special skills in the procedure. There is not complete correlation between thymic morphology and functional capacity (Borzy et al., 1979b). Autopsies of children with suspected immunodeficiency should always include a histologic examination of the thymus gland, lymph nodes, and lymphatic tissue of the GI system.

Intestinal biopsy can provide valuable information in the presence of a protein-losing enteropathy and may aid in establishing an exact diagnosis, such as intestinal lymphangiectasia or infiltrative disorder. Organisms such as *Cryptosporidia* and *Giardia* can also be identified.

A skin biopsy is sometimes of value in immunodeficiency when GVHD is suspected or when histiocytosis-X or another dermatosis must be excluded.

Mutation Analysis

Many of the cellular immunodeficiencies, particularly the various types of combined immunodeficiencies, have specific genetic mutations that can be identified by DNA analysis of leukocytes, skin, fibroblasts, or mucosal scrapings (see Chapter 15). A cell line using EBV-transformed lymphocytes is an ideal source of large amounts of DNA. Classification of the mutation in specific syndromes may permit genotype-phenotype correlation (see Chapter 12).

Tests for Phagocytic Deficiencies

Screening Tests

The screening tests for a phagocytic (granulocytic and monocytic) disorder include the total WBC count, the differential count, and the morphologic appearance of the granulocytes and monocytes. Other tests, such as the NBT dye reduction test (see Table 12-11) should be performed if there are clinical findings such as the presence of skin or mucous membrane infections, abscesses, or prominent adenopathy.

An absolute neutrophil count consistently lower than 2000 cells/μl or higher than 12,000 cells/μl is abnormal. The presence of chronic neutropenia may indicate a primary leukocyte disorder such as cyclic neutropenia, congenital neutropenia, or glycogen storage disease type 1B (see Chapters 20 and 39). Neutropenia may also be a component of a primary immunodeficiency disease (Cham et al., 2002) such as X-linked HIGM syndrome (Levy et al., 1997), CVID (see Chapter 13), and some complement deficiencies (see Chapter 21).

Conversely, patients with LAD-1 have a persistent neutrophilia, usually 20,000 to 40,000 cells/μl, even when free of infection. This reflects the fact that their neutrophils are unable to adhere to vascular endothelium and thus the neutrophils that normally are part of the marginating pool are in the circulation and result in the increased WBC and absolute neutrophil count.

Morphologic assessment of phagocytic cells may provide important clues to the presence of a phagocytic disorder. For example, the phagocytic cells of patients with Chédiak-Higashi syndrome contain characteristic giant vacuoles (Blum et al., 1968), whereas the phagocytic cells of patients with secondary granule deficiency contain bilobed or kidney shaped nuclei (Strauss et al., 1974).

Advanced tests of neutrophil function are indicated if quantitative abnormalities have been excluded, and morphologic abnormalities are not present

Nitroblue-Tetrazolium Test

The NBT test is the most common assay used to diagnose CGD (Segal et al., 2000). The NBT test is based on the fact that during phagocytosis, normal granulocytes and monocytes increase their oxidative metabolism, through nicotinamide adenine dinucleotide phosphate (NADPH) oxidase, and generate microbicidal reactive oxygen species such as superoxide, hydrogen peroxide, and hydroxyl anions. In contrast, CGD phagocytes have decreased or absent ability to generate reactive oxygen species. When the colorless dye, NBT, is added to normal phagocytozing leukocytes, the reactive oxygen species reduces the NBT creating purple formazan.

The leukocytes of patients with CGD or leukocyte glucose-6-phosphate dehydrogenase (G6PD) deficiency cannot reduce NBT in the normal fashion; this inability to reduce NBT is correlated with their inability to generate superoxide and hydrogen peroxide and kill certain microorganisms (see Chapter 20).

A number of procedures use NBT to diagnose CGD. The simplest NBT screening test is a histochemical slide test in which leukocytes are allowed to adhere to endotoxin-coated glass slides and incubated with NBT; the percentage of granulocytes containing blue-purple formazan granules is estimated microscopically (Ochs and Igo, 1973). In normal subjects, the percentage of NBT-positive granulocytes is more than 90%; patients with CGD usually have less than 1%. Female carriers of X-linked CGD have two populations of cells: one able to reduce NBT and another not.

In another NBT test, peripheral leukocytes are incubated with NBT and latex particles, the latter to stimulate phagocytosis. The reduction of the NBT is then assessed by examining the leukocytes for the presence of bluish-purple granules of reduced formazan in the leukocytes (Johnston, 1969). This assay is also able to identify carrier of X-linked CGD.

A quantitative NBT dye reduction test is also available (Baehner and Nathan, 1968). Leukocytes are incubated with and without latex particles in the presence of NBT dye. After 15 minutes, the reaction is stopped and the reduced NBT is assessed spectrophotometrically. The difference in optical density between the resting (no latex particles) and phagocytizing cells is calculated. Normal value is 0.233 ± 0.103; CGD patients range from 0.034 to 0.045, and carriers have intermediate values.

In some cases of CGD, particularly patients with the autosomal recessive forms of the disease, there may be low levels of oxidants produced and the presence of blue-purple formazan positive cells over time (Segal et al., 2000). Thus, in the face of a highly characteristic clinical picture and a negative NBT test for CGD (e.g., dye reduction), advanced testing of phagocytic oxidase function should be undertaken.

Dihydrorhodamine Reduction

Another assay of phagocytic oxidase activity in CGD uses dihydrorhodamine 123 (DHR) and flow cytometry (Jirapaongsananuruk et al., 2003; Vowells et al., 1996). DHR is added to stimulated white cells and its reduction by newly generated hydrogen peroxide forms a fluorescent compound rhodamine 123, which is assessed in each cell by flow cytometry. Not only is this assay capable of diagnosing CGD, but because of the increased sensitivity obtained by assessing the activity of each cell, it is able to provide provisional evidence for the genetic form of the disease (Jirapaongsananuruk et al., 2003; Vowells et al., 1996).

Most patients with the X-linked form of the CGD (e.g., gp91 [phox] defect) have no cells capable of reducing the dye, whereas patients with the most common autosomal recessive form (e.g., p47[phox] defect) have a few cells capable of dye reduction.

The carrier state of CGD can often be identified by this procedure and will have an average of 50% of cells capable of reducing the dye. Because of the increased availability of flow cytometry, and its simplicity and sensitivity, it now is the best diagnostic tool for CGD diagnosis.

Other Tests of Leukocyte Oxidative Activity

CHEMILUMINESCENCE

Allen and associates (1972) showed that during phagocytosis, human neutrophils produce chemiluminescence (chemically produced light). During phagocytosis, normal neutrophils and monocytes produce free oxygen radicals that react with oxidizable substrates on microbes, such as unsaturated lipids, nucleic acids, and peptides, to form unstable intermediates. When these intermediates return to their ground state, light energy measurable as chemiluminescence is released (Allen et al., 1972).

A direct correlation between chemiluminescence and intracellular bacterial killing was suggested when Stjernholm and colleagues (1973) demonstrated that granulocytes from patients with CGD produced no chemiluminescence during phagocytosis of opsonized bacteria. Because chemiluminescence is readily measured with a beta-scintillation spectrophotometer or a chemiluminometer, it has become a valuable assay of oxidative metabolism during phagocytosis and an aid in the diagnosis of CGD (Johnston et al., 1975a). It is also a sensitive and reliable way to diagnose the CGD carrier state (Mills et al., 1978). It should be noted that an increased chemiluminescent response to soluble stimuli (e.g., PMA) but a reduced one to particulate stimuli (e.g., zymosan) is characteristic of LAD-1 (see Chapter 20) (Anderson et al., 1984).

QUANTITATIVE IODINATION

Pincus and Klebanoff (1971) have used leukocyte iodination to assess microbicidal activity. In this reaction, inorganic iodide is fixed to bacteria (or a yeast particle) by myeloperoxidase in the presence of hydrogen peroxide generated by the hexose monophosphate shunt. Because of the failure of peroxide production, this reaction is defective in CGD. The assay employs radioactive inorganic iodide, isolated leukocytes, zymosan or bacteria, and serum; it can be used to detect CGD, CGD heterozygotes, or myeloperoxidase deficiency.

METABOLIC ASSAYS

Ingestion of organisms by phagocytes and intracellular killing is accompanied by a number of metabolic changes. Assays of glucose metabolism, oxygen consumption, NADPH oxidase activity, hexose monophosphate shunt activation, superoxide, singlet oxygen, and hydrogen peroxide production in phagocytizing leukocytes are deficient in CGD leukocytes (Hohn and Lehrer, 1975; Holmes et al., 1967; Johnston et al., 1975a).

Leukocyte Bactericidal Assays

The most definitive test for a functional defect of granulocytes is the quantitative bacterial killing assay developed by Quie and associates (1967). Peripheral blood leukocytes are isolated and suspended in a medium containing normal serum (as an opsonic source) and living bacteria (usually *Staphylococcus aureus*, *Escherichia coli*, or *Serratia marcescens*). During incubation, aliquots are removed at different times from the leukocyte-serum-bacteria mixture. Each aliquot is centrifuged so that the leukocytes (and any phagocytized bacteria) are in the cell button and free bacteria are in the supernatant. Both the cell button and the supernatant are then assayed for viable bacteria. Thus this test measures serum opsonic activity, phagocytosis (ingestion), and intracellular bactericidal activity.

Leukocytes from a normal subject usually phagocytize and kill more than 90% of the bacteria within 120 minutes. Leukocytes from a patient with CGD usually kill less than 50% of the bacteria in this period; further, in CGD the viable bacteria are within the leukocyte, indicating that phagocytosis has occurred but that intracellular killing is deficient. In a phagocytic (ingestion) defect, killing is deficient, but the viable bacteria remain in the supernatant fluid. An opsonic defect can also be identified with this assay by using normal cells and the test serum as an opsonic source.

Alternatively, a whole blood assay can also be used to assess intracellular bactericidal activity in CGD as long as bacteria resistant to the bactericidal activity of serum complement is used (e.g., staphylococci) (Keusch et al., 1975).

Chemotaxis and Random Mobility

Defects of mobility may be associated with lack of pus formation at the site of infection; conversely, the presence of pus provides some clinical evidence that leukocyte number, mobility, and chemotactic factor production are intact.

Random mobility and chemotaxis assays are usually performed on granulocytes, but purified monocytes and eosinophils can also be studied. There are two general types of assays used, the Boyden chamber technique and the agarose-gel plate technique. In the Boyden procedure (Boyden, 1962) a double chamber is used. Granulocytes are placed in the upper chamber, separated by Millipore filters from a chemotactic stimulus placed in the lower chamber.

The usual chemotactic stimulus is human serum to which endotoxin, zymosan, or antigen-antibody complexes have been added; these stimuli activate complement and cleave C5 and thereby generate the low-molecular-weight peptide C5a, which is a strong chemotactic stimulus. Other chemotactic substances employed are particle-activated plasma (through release of kallikrein and plasminogen activator), bacterial formulated peptides, or lymphocyte-derived chemotactic factor from antigen-activated lymphocytes.

Performing the assay in the absence of chemotactic stimuli assesses random mobility. The number of cells migrating toward a chemotactic stimulus is assessed by microscopy of the lower side of the filter. Alternatively, Cr^{51} radiolabeled cells can be used and the radioactivity in the lower filter can be assessed as an indicator of the number of migrating cells (Gallin et al., 1973).

Random mobility and chemotaxis can also be assessed by migration of the cells under agarose gel. In this assay, cell suspensions are placed in one well and a second well in close proximity is filled with a chemotactic factor (Nelson et al., 1975). The distance that the cells migrate under the gel from their origin in one well toward the chemotactic gradient emanating from the second well represents their chemotactic ability. Chemotactic values must be compared with normal age-matched controls run simultaneously in the same assay.

REBUCK SKIN WINDOW

The Rebuck skin window has been used in the past to assess the morphology and in vivo motility of cells in the inflammatory response (Rebuck and Crowley, 1955), but is rarely used today. The skin is abraded superficially with a scalpel blade over an area of 4 mm², and cover slips are placed over the site; the cover slips are changed at 30-minute intervals for the first few hours and at longer intervals up to 24 hours. The leukocytes migrate to the abrasion and adhere to the slides, which are stained and analyzed. An initial influx of polymorphonuclear granulocytes should occur within 2 hours; these cells should be replaced by mononuclear cells within 12 hours.

Deformability, Adherence, and Aggregation

When random mobility or chemotaxis is abnormal, advanced tests to identify the basis for the movement defect are available. These include assays of deformability (Miller, 1975), adherence (MacGregor et al., 1974), or aggregation (Hammerschmidt et al., 1980). If findings are abnormal, tests for spreading, chemotactic orientation, and membrane fluidity can be undertaken (Anderson et al., 1984).

Phagocytosis (Ingestion) Assays

Phagocytosis is assessed by the ability of granulocytes or other phagocytic cells to recognize and ingest particles, such as bacteria. Particles that are opsonized with antibody or complement are engulfed much easier than those that are not, primarily because phagocytes have Fc and complement receptors that interact with the opsonic ligand. More phagocytic defects are the result of opsonic defects rather than intrinsic abnormalities of the leukocyte phagocytosis.

In phagocytic assays, the patient's leukocytes are incubated with particles (polystyrene beads, paraffin-oil particles, erythrocytes) or bacteria in the presence of an opsonic source such as serum. After incubation, ingestion is assessed by microscopy (polystyrene beads or bacteria) (Miller and Nilsson, 1970), spectrophotometry (paraffin-oil particles) (Stossel, 1973), metabolic changes (Johnston et al., 1975a) or scintillation counting (radiolabeled bacteria) (Keusch et al., 1972).

Because ingestion must precede killing, a phagocytic defect is indirectly excluded if leukocyte microbial killing is present.

White Blood Cell Turnover

In neutropenic states, particularly when the bone marrow shows myeloid precursors, serial WBC counts should be done to determine the presence of cyclic neutropenia. Then the peripheral WBC response to the administration of corticosteroids, epinephrine, or endotoxin can be tested (Cline et al., 1976). The response to corticosteroid measures bone marrow reserve, whereas the response to epinephrine and endotoxin assesses the marginating pool (Metcalf et al., 1986). If increased leukocyte destruction is suggested by an active marrow, the presence of leukocyte antibodies should be sought (Lalezari and Bernard, 1966).

Special Morphology

Whereas ordinary light microscopy has the capability of detecting certain intrinsic disorders of granulocytes (such as bilobed nuclei and the giant vacuoles of Chédiak-Higashi syndrome), phase and electron microscopy are able to detect defects in granule formation, spreading, pseudopod formation, and mobility as seen in specific granule deficiency or LAD-1 (Anderson et al., 1984). Staining of granulocytes by histochemical techniques is used to demonstrate alkaline phosphatase, myeloperoxidase, and esterase activities. Absence of these enzymes should be followed by quantitative assays for each enzyme. Bone marrow aspiration can be done to assess the morphology of the granulocyte precursors, to exclude other hematopoietic disorders, and to obtain a culture for unusual organisms.

Adhesion Molecule Assays

Assays for adhesion molecules are performed when a leukocyte defect is suspected (see Chapter 20). Deficiencies of these glycoproteins on the granulocyte surface are best assessed by flow cytometry using specific monoclonal antibodies. In LAD-1 there is a deficiency of both CD11b (CR3; Mac-1) and CD18, the alpha and beta chains, respectively, of leakocyte function-associated antigen-1 (LFA-1). In LAD-2 an anti-sialyl-Lewis X monoclonal antibody can be used to identify a defect in the selectin ligand (see Chapter 20). The degree of deficiency of the LFA-1 molecule can be used to identify mild and severe phenotypes and heterozygotes of LAD-1. Leukocyte activation by ionophore prior to flow cytometry can greatly enhance the expression of these glycoproteins to magnify the differences between healthy subjects and patients (Todd et al., 1988) (see Chapter 20).

Enzyme Assays

Enzyme defects associated with defective granulocyte function include NADPH oxidase deficiency, myeloperoxidase deficiency, alkaline phosphatase deficiency, and G6PD deficiency. When CGD is suspected, certain laboratories can identify the exact enzymatic defect leading to the NADPH oxidase deficiency by immunoassay (Curnutte, 1993). When CGD has been excluded, the other enzyme defects should be sought. In myeloperoxidase deficiency, killing is abnormal, leukocyte iodination is abnormal, and hydrogen peroxide is normal (Klebanoff and Pincus, 1971). Specific diagnosis depends on demonstrating lack of myeloperoxidase activity (Lehrer and Cline, 1969).

A complete lack of leukocyte G6PD has been described in a patient in whom the neutrophils failed to kill staphylococci (Cooper et al., 1972). There was also deficient generation of hydrogen peroxide, and the case clinically resembled CGD. Most patients with erythrocyte G6PD deficiency have sufficient G6PD levels in their leukocytes for normal microbicidal activity.

A deficiency of glutathione peroxidase has been noted in some patients (Holmes et al., 1970) with an autosomal recessive form of CGD (DeChatelet et al., 1976).

Immunoglobulin E Levels

Elevated levels of IgE (see Table 12-13 for normal standards) are seen in several phagocytic deficiency syndromes, particularly those with chemotactic defects (see Chapter 20).

Mutation Analysis

For those phagocytic defects with defined genetic defects (e.g., the four types of CGD), mutation analysis can provide an exact molecular diagnosis.

Tests for Complement Immunodeficiencies

Screening Tests

The screening tests used to assess the complement system depend on the kind of disorders suspected. Genetically determined deficiencies of individual components that present with an increased susceptibility to infection or rheumatic diseases are best screened for by measurements of serum total hemolytic complement.

The measurement of serum total hemolytic complement is an excellent screening tool for genetically determined deficiencies of the classical pathway and the terminal components (C1 through C9) because marked deficiencies of any of these components all have markedly reduced levels of total hemolytic complement levels with one exception, that of deficiency of C9 (see Chapter 21). Because some complement-mediated hemolysis can occur in the absence of C9, levels of serum hemolytic complement are only reduced to between one third and one half of the normal level in these patients.

Total hemolytic complement is assessed by the hemolysis of antibody sensitized sheep erythrocytes by test serum (Gewurz and Suyehira, 1976). In most instances, the end point is that dilution of serum that yields 50% hemolysis, hence CH_{50}, although there are other end points used. There is a wide range of normal values (from 20 to 100 CH_{50} units), depending on the cells and antibody used, so that normal levels must be established by each laboratory. In addition, because some components of complement lose activity relatively rapidly at room temperature, if the blood or serum is not kept on ice or if the serum is not frozen, the sample may yield a false low value. It should be noted that decreases in the concentrations of individual components of up to 50% may not be identified in this test.

C3 and C4 levels can be measured immunochemically by radial immunodiffusion or nephelometry. Although very low or absent levels of C3 or C4 can indicate a genetically determined deficiency of one of these components, deficiencies of either of these two components are very rare and are suggested by markedly reduced levels of total hemolytic complement (e.g., CH_{50}).

Complement Component Assays

Assays of individual components of complement are usually performed when there is a suspicion of genetically determined deficiency (e.g., when a screening test for total hemolytic activity is markedly reduced). Complement components can be assayed either by functional assays or by immunochemical assays. Functional assays of individual complement components are performed by incubating the test serum with antibody-sensitized erythrocytes and a reagent containing all of the components of the classical pathway necessary for hemolysis except for the component for which the assay is designed to measure (Alper and Rosen, 1975). The hemolysis achieved then depends on the functional activity of individual component that is only present in the test serum.

Alternatively, complement component levels can be measured by immunoassays, such as radial immunodiffusion or nephelometry, using antisera to C1q, C1r, C1s, C2, C3, C4, C5, C6, C7, C8, B, P, and D. Patients with deficiencies of each of these components have been described (see Chapter 21). Functional and immunoassays for are also available for C1 inactivator and are of value in the diagnosis of hereditary angioneurotic edema.

A determination of which components are reduced may provide insight into which complement pathway is activated. Classical pathway activation is generally associated with extremely low levels of C1, C4, C2, and C3, and C5, and to a lesser extent C6, C7, C8, and C9. By contrast, alternative pathway activation is associated with normal levels of C1, C4, and C2, but with low levels of C3.

Alternative Pathway Assays

Functional activity of the alternative pathway can be assessed by antibody-independent hemolysis of rabbit erythrocytes (Platts-Mills and Ishizaka, 1974; Polhill et al., 1975). This assay depends on the fact that unsensitized rabbit erythrocytes are potent activators of the human alternative pathway. Thus hemolysis of rabbit erythrocytes by serum is mediated by the alternative pathway and the terminal complement components C5 through C9. Therefore patients with deficiencies of components of the alternative pathway or deficiencies of C5 through C9 have reduced hemolytic activity in this assay. Radial diffusion agar kits using rabbit erythrocytes are available for screening alternative pathway activity.

Complement Allotypes and Isotypes

Several proteins of the complement system are polymorphic. These polymorphisms generally are expressed as changes in the electrophoretic mobility of the protein. These assays are often performed on family members of individuals with a genetically determined deficiency of an individual component to determine whether they are heterozygous for the deficiency.

The fourth component of complement is unique in that it is encoded by two genes, C4A and C4B, which are closely linked within the MHC on chromosome 6. Not only are the two isotypes of C4 highly polymorphic, but deficiencies of one or the other are quite common and can be detected by electrophoresis in gel. Deficiencies of C4A are associated with a variety of autoimmune disorders, such as diabetes and lupus, whereas deficiencies of C4B are associated with an increased susceptibility to blood-borne infections, such as sepsis and meningitis (see Chapter 21).

Complement Activation Assays

Complement activation may occur in a number of clinical situations, but with only slight or transient decreases in complement levels. Complement activation is suggested by the presence of complement cleavage products, particularly of C3, C4, and C5. In the case of the larger cleavage products, such as C3b or C3bi, these are distinguishable from the native molecule by alterations of their immunoelectrophoretic mobility or by the appearance of low-molecular-weight breakdown products on crossed electrophoresis. In the case of the smaller cleavage products such as C3a, C4a, and C5a, immunoassays are available for their detection. Because the smaller cleavage products are of low MW and disappear rapidly from the circulation, they are present only during an ongoing or very recent event.

Complement Functional Assays

Other assays that assess the biologic functions of the complement system include serum chemotactic activity, serum opsonic activity, and serum bactericidal activity. Although other serum components can contribute to these activities, as usually performed, these assays generally reflect the integrity of the complement system. Because these tests depend on biologic assays, they are usually performed in specialized laboratories.

SERUM CHEMOTACTIC ACTIVITY

Serum chemotactic activity is assessed by activating the patient's serum complement with endotoxin, antigen-antibody complexes, or zymosan, using normal granulocytes or monocytes as the chemotaxing cells (Miller, 1975). A comparison with a normal serum and a known deficient serum must be performed. Chemotactic factor generation from serum depends on the formation of C5a, and thus is abnormal in C5 deficiency (Johnston and Stroud, 1977) or deficiencies of components necessary for the activation of C5, such as C1, C4, C2, or C3.

SERUM OPSONIC ACTIVITY

Serum opsonic activity is assessed by incubating a particle, such as bacteria, in the patient's serum and determining the rate, or degree, of ingestion of the opsonized particle by phagocytic cells such as polymorphonuclear leukocytes. The rate or degree of ingestion is determined

in a variety of ways, including microscopic assessment, the use of radioactive bacteria, and the assessment of metabolic changes associated with ingestion (Johnston et al., 1969).

SERUM BACTERICIDAL ACTIVITY

Serum bactericidal activity is assessed by incubating the patient's serum with gram-negative bacteria that are sensitive to the bactericidal activity of complement and measuring the survival of the bacteria (Skarnes and Watson, 1956).

TREATMENT

Prevention

Prevention of immunodeficiency is limited to averting certain viral infections that cause immunodeficiency, genetic counseling, and in utero prenatal diagnosis with interruption of pregnancy. However, a maximum effort in all these areas would have minimal effect on the prevalence of congenital immunodeficiencies. Nevertheless, rubella vaccination programs have resulted in the disappearance of immunodeficiency secondary to congenital rubella. Prevention of HIV infections would decrease the incidence of AIDS. Genetic counseling is of value only when the genetic pattern is established.

Patients with a personal or family history of hereditary immunodeficiency should be counseled as to the risks of occurrence in their offspring, as described earlier. Prenatal diagnosis is available for many illnesses if early treatment or therapeutic abortion are possibilities.

Ig and complement levels should be obtained in the immediate family of patients with antibody or complement deficiencies to determine a familial pattern. In disorders in which procedures are available for heterozygosity testing (e.g., LAD-1, CGD), the parents, siblings, and children of the affected subject can be tested. If other family members have suggestive histories, they should also be studied. Newborn siblings of an affected patient are followed carefully from birth for manifestations of a similar disorder.

Neonatal Management

If a previous sibling has had combined immunodeficiency and the mother is again pregnant and about to deliver, prior planning is imperative. Cesarean section may be considered if a difficult labor is anticipated; however, it is not routinely indicated.

Long-term cord blood storage should also be considered to be used as a source of stem cells for gene therapy, or if the infant is unaffected, for use as stem cells for a future affected sibling. This requires the availability of a cord blood bank facility for processing, freezing, and storing the cord blood sample.

At birth, blood should be obtained for blood count, Ig assays, B-cell and T-cell enumeration, PHA stimulation, and HLA typing to detect chimerism. The newborn infant with suspected immunodeficiency should be placed in a sterile isolator and maintained on reverse isolation until his or her immunologic status is clarified. A chest x-ray examination for thymic size should be done as soon as possible.

Newborns with combined immunodeficiency should remain in a protective environment with reverse isolation or in an isolator with food and liquid sterilized until definitive therapy is completed. Irradiated and CMV-negative blood products should be used.

GI sterilization (with nonabsorbable antibiotics) and *Pneumocystis carinii* prophylaxis (with trimethoprim-sulfamethoxazole) should be considered for patients suspected of combined immunodeficiency.

General Treatment

Patients with most primary immunodeficiency diseases require comprehensive pediatric care to manage their infections and rheumatologic and inflammatory conditions, to maintain their general health and nutrition, and to prevent emotional problems related to their illness.

Although no special dietary limitations are necessary, every effort should be made to provide a well-rounded, nutritious diet. In some instances, GI infections or IBD may preclude normal feeding and parenteral nutrition may be necessary.

Patients with immunodeficiencies should be protected from unnecessary exposure to infection as much as possible. Toward that end, they should be kept away from individuals with obvious respiratory or other infections as much as possible. Bottled water should be used if the local supply is suspect. Day care is associated with considerable infectious exposure, so it may not be appropriate for some severely deficient children.

In some situations, as may occur with chicken pox, immune deficient patients should also be kept away from individuals who are at risk for incubating an infection. Following chicken pox exposure in T-cell and antibody-deficient children, varicella-zoster Ig (VZIG) or acyclovir prophylaxis is indicated. For the antibody-deficient child with normal T-cell immunity receiving regular IVIG, VZIG is generally unnecessary, inasmuch as IVIG contains antibody to varicella-zoster virus, and chickenpox, even if not prevented, is attenuated by the IVIG infusions.

Any chronic infection, such as mastoiditis, sinusitis, bronchitis, and bronchiectasis, should be managed as in other patients. Long-term chronic antibiotic therapy may be of value in some patients who have a recurrent infection such as sinusitis or bronchitis shortly after finishing a course of antibiotics (Sweinberg et al., 1991).

In patients with recurrent pulmonary infections, pulmonary function tests should be performed at regular intervals. Those with chronic pulmonary disease should have a home treatment plan of physiotherapy and inhalation therapy similar to that used in cystic fibrosis.

As with patients with other chronic medical conditions, the parents, other family members, and friends should make every effort to avoid or prevent the occurrence of any concurrent emotional problems that may result from the primary immunodeficiency disease. The child should be encouraged to be outdoors, to play with other children in small groups, and to attend nursery and regular school. The aim is to teach such children to live in a near-normal fashion with their disease, in much the same way as the diabetic child.

Vigorous exercise, including team sports, should be strongly encouraged. Special attention must be directed such problems as hearing loss, the need for tutors to make up for school absences, financial help for the family, and access to support groups.

Precautions

Blood Products

Patients with suspected or proven T-cell immunodeficiencies should not be given routine blood or blood components that could contain viable lymphocytes because of the possibility of a graft-versus-host reaction. If transfusion is necessary, the blood should be irradiated prior to administration. The authors use 2500 rad, but higher and lower doses have been used (Strauss et al., 1993).

Because of the risks of CMV infection from blood products, it is advisable to use CMV-negative donors.

Surgery

The same indications for surgery that are applied to normal hosts apply to patients with primary immunodeficiency diseases. However, splenectomy should only be performed when there is a clear indication (e.g., severe hemolytic anemia or thrombocytopenia) and no reasonable alternative medical therapy is available. Antibiotics before and after surgery should be considered.

Corticosteroids and Other Immunosuppressive Drugs

Corticosteroids (and other immunosuppressive drugs) are occasionally necessary in patients with immunodeficiency for such problems as asthma, lymphoid interstitial pneumonia, obstructive GI or genitourinary tract lesions of CGD, hemolytic anemic, anaphylactic reactions, eczema, or graft-versus-host reactions. Short-term courses are usually well tolerated; long-term use has the hazard of additional immunosuppression with depressed lymphocyte counts and lowered Ig levels. Lymphoproliferative responses and preexisting humoral antibodies are usually maintained. *Pneumocystis carinii* prophylaxis should be considered.

We have used inhaled corticosteroids in children with CGD without complications and topical steroids for the eczema of WAS and the hyper-IgE syndrome without complications.

Immunizations

Patients with primary immunodeficiencies may contract a vaccine-related infection from live attenuated vaccines (smallpox, poliomyelitis, measles, mumps, rubella, varicella, and BCG). In general, all live attenuated vaccines should be avoided in severe antibody or cellular immunodeficiencies (American Academy of Pediatrics, 2000). However, the risk varies, depending on the component of the immune system that is deficient. For example, when smallpox vaccine was routine before 1970, many patients with SCID or other T-cell deficiencies developed fatal disseminated vaccinia infections after immunization; in fact, in some patients, the vaccinia infection was a clue to the diagnosis of the immunodeficiency.

Similarly, vaccine-associated paralytic poliomyelitis is a recognized complication of oral poliomyelitis immunization in patients with either B-cell or combined B- and T-cell immunodeficiency. In recent years the only polio infections in the western hemisphere have been vaccine-related and most of these have occurred in immunodeficient patients. It is for this reason that the current immunization schedule in the United States is limited to the killed, inactivated polio vaccine.

Live measles vaccine has also caused severe disease in patients with T-cell or combined deficiencies. Attenuated live varicella vaccine has not been reported to cause clinical disease in patients with primary immunodeficiency, but this may be due to the fact that it is given after age 2, by which time most patients with severe T-cell deficiencies have been diagnosed.

Finally, BCG has caused a disseminated infection in children with T-cell defects such as SCID, but also in children with CGD.

Live viral vaccines can be given to patients with selective IgA deficiency, phagocytic and complement immunodeficiencies, and to children fully reconstituted following stem cell transplantation 2 years after the procedure.

Yearly influenza vaccination is also recommended for immunodeficient children who can make an antibody response and for their immediate family members and other household residents.

Antibiotics

Antibiotics are lifesaving in the treatment of the infectious episodes of patients with immunodeficiency. Before their availability, most patients with immunodeficiencies probably succumbed early in life from infection. The choice and dosage of antibiotics for specific infections are identical to those used in normal subjects. However, because these patients may succumb rapidly to infection, antibiotic therapy for suspected infections should be initiated earlier than in other patients. Throat, blood, and other culture specimens deemed appropriate are obtained prior to therapy; these are especially important if the infection does not respond promptly to the initial antibiotic chosen.

If an infection does not respond to antibiotics, fungal, mycobacterial, viral, or protozoal *(P. carinii)* infection should be considered. Because certain of these infections can be treated only with special drugs (e.g., pentamidine or trimethoprim-sulfamethoxazole [TMP/SMX] for *P. carinii* infection, ribavirin for parainfluenza infection, and so on), an exact microbiologic diagnosis is essential.

Pneumocystis carinii Prophylaxis

P. carinii pneumonia (PCP) prophylaxis is recommended for children with significant primary and secondary cellular (T-cell) immunodeficiencies. The older guidelines for children with HIV infection can be followed (Centers for Disease Control and Prevention, 1991). Prophylaxis is recommended for infants younger than 12 months of age with a CD4 count less than 1500 cells/μl, for young children aged 12 to 23 months with a CD4 count less than 750 cells/μl, for children 2 to 5 years with a CD4 count less than 500 cells/μl, and for children older than 5 years of age and adults with a CD4 count less than 200 cells/μl. In addition, any patient with a CD4 count less than 25% of the total lymphocytes or a past history of PCP is a candidate for prophylaxis.

Prophylaxis usually consists of TMP/SMX—160 mg/M^2/day of the TMP and 750 mg/M^2/day of SMX given orally in divided doses twice per day three times per week, with frequent checks of the WBC count. Alternative drugs for PCP prophylaxis include pentamidine, atovaquone, and dapsone.

Continuous Antibiotics

Continuous prophylactic antibiotics often are of benefit in immunodeficiencies. They are especially useful in disorders characterized by rapid overwhelming infections (e.g., in WAS), in antibody immunodeficiencies when recurrent infections occur despite optimal Ig therapy, and in phagocytic disorders in which no other form of therapy is available. In these instances, penicillin, ampicillin, or dicloxacillin given orally, 0.5 to 1.0 g/day in divided doses, is recommended. If diarrhea or vomiting results, lower doses or other drugs are used.

If the patient is not neutropenic, TMP/SMX given daily at a half therapeutic dose is often well tolerated. Another well tolerated regimen is azithromycin given at full therapeutic doses for 3 consecutive days, followed by 11 days without drug, restarting on day 15 for 3 days, and so on. With severe refractory infections, full therapeutic oral doses can be used, and the antibiotics switched empirically every 2 months in an attempt to avoid resistance.

The continuous use of antibiotics in the antibody immunodeficiencies is not an adequate substitute for Ig therapy but can be used if patients refuse Ig on religious grounds. In CGD, the continuous use of sulfisoxazole or TMP/SMX is indicated not only because of its antimicrobial activity but because it may increase the bactericidal activity of the phagocytes (Johnston et al., 1975b). In CGD, continuous itraconazole is proven to decrease the risk of fungal infection (Gallin et al., 2003).

Some patients have chronic respiratory or other bacterial infection, despite optimal use of IVIG; they are candidates for prophylactic antibiotic therapy.

Antibiotics with Dental or Surgical Procedures

Antibiotics should be given prophylactically with each dental or surgical procedure. Amoxicillin and gentamicin can be give intravenously 1 hour before and 8 and 18 hours after major surgery, or 3 days of oral broad-spectrum antibiotics can be used for less serious procedures (e.g., dental prophylaxis).

Antivirals

Antiviral therapy can be used effectively in some immunodeficiencies. Exposure to influenza or early symptomatic influenza infection can be managed with amantadine, ranitidine, or the neuraminidase inhibitors zanamivir and oseltamivir (the latter is not approved for children). Severe herpes simplex, chicken pox, or herpes zoster can be treated with acyclovir. Ribavirin aerosols have been used in the treatment of respiratory syncytial virus (RSV) and parainfluenza viral infections in SCID (McIntosh et al., 1984).

VZIG or ganciclovir can be used in the incubation period to modify or prevent chickenpox (Asano et al., 1993). Pleconaril may be of value in enteroviral infection (Rotbart and Webster, 2001). Topical cidofovir has been used successfully in severe molluscum contagiosum (Davies et al., 1999).

Human Immune Globulin

Indications

Most severe antibody immunodeficiencies are treated successfully with repeated injections or infusions of human immune globulin (Table 12-23). This treatment allows many patients to be symptom-free, similar to the well-controlled diabetic on insulin therapy. Others given Ig remain chronically ill or undergo a progressive downhill course; often these patients have other immunologic or hematologic deficits. Ig is not of value in the treatment of cellular, phagocytic, or complement immunodeficiencies, but is of value (although not curative) in combined antibody and cellular immunodeficiencies.

Two forms of human immune serum globulin are available: 16% intramuscular Ig and IVIG. Currently, most antibody-deficient patients receive IVIG intravenously, although the 16% product is used extensively in Europe by subcutaneous infusions. A few patients continue to receive 16% IG by periodic intramuscular injections.

Immunoglobulin for Intramuscular or Subcutaneous Use

PHARMACOLOGY

Immune serum globulin (IG or ISG) is prepared by alcohol fractionation of pooled human sera by Cohn alcohol fractionation (thus deriving its alternative name of Cohn fraction II). An additional viral inactivation step such as solvent/deterrent or pasteurization is then performed. These procedures remove most other serum proteins and live viruses (e.g., hepatitis B virus, HIV), thus providing a sterile product for intramuscular or subcutaneous injection. IG is reconstituted as a sterile 16.5% solution (165 mg/ml) with thimerosal or one that is preservative free. IG contains a wide spectrum of antibodies to viral and bacterial antigens because it is derived from plasma pools derived from multiple (more than 10,000) donors.

TABLE 12-23 · SOME IMMUNODEFICIENCIES IN WHICH INTRAVENOUS IMMUNOGLOBULIN MAY BE OF BENEFIT

Antibody Deficiencies
Congenital agammaglobulinemias
Common variable immunodeficiency
Immunodeficiencies with hyper-IgM
Transient hypogammaglobulinemia of infancy (sometimes)
IgG subclass deficiency ± IgA deficiency (sometimes)
Antibody deficiency with normal immunoglobulins

Combined Deficiencies
Severe combined immunodeficiencies (all types)
Wiskott-Aldrich syndrome
Ataxia-telangiectasia
Short-limbed dwarfism
X-linked lymphoproliferative syndrome

Secondary Immunodeficiencies
Malignancies with antibody deficiencies; multiple myeloma, chronic lymphocytic leukemia, other cancers
Protein-losing enteropathy with hypogammaglobulinemia
Nephrotic syndrome with hypogammaglobulinemia
Pediatric acquired immunodeficiency syndrome
Intensive care patients: trauma/surgery/shock
Post-transplantation period
Post–bone marrow transplantation
Burns
Prematurity

Ig = immunoglobulin.

IG is more than 95% IgG globulin, but trace quantities of IgM and IgA globulins and other serum proteins are present. The IgM and IgA globulins are therapeutically insignificant because of their rapid half-lives (approximately 7 days) and their low concentrations in IG preparations. IG contains multiple IgG allotypes (Gm and Km types).

IG is approved only for intramuscular or subcutaneous use, and intravenous injection of IG is generally contraindicated. It aggregates in vitro to large-molecular-weight complexes (9.5 to 40 Svedberg units) that are strongly anticomplementary. These aggregates are probably responsible for the occasional systemic reactions to IG. The incidence of these reactions is increased if the recipient has received gamma globulin previously or if IG is given intravenously. Agammaglobulinemic boys with affected male relatives (suggesting X-linked inheritance) may experience a lower incidence of reactions (Medical Research Council Working Party, 1969). Small intradermal injections of IG are not of value (except as a placebo), and they are also contraindicated.

INTRAMUSCULAR IMMUNOGLOBULIN INJECTIONS

The recommended dose of IG for antibody immunodeficiency is 100 mg/kg per month, approximately equivalent to 0.7 ml/kg/month of the 16% (160 mg/ml) product. A double or triple dose is given at the onset of therapy, often over a 3- to 5-day period. The maximum dose should not exceed 20 or 30 ml/week. Few studies of the optimal dose are available; however, the Medical Research Council Working Party (1969) found that 25 mg/kg/week (100 mg/kg/month) was equivalent therapeutically to 50 mg/kg/week but that 10 mg/kg/week was inadequate.

The IG should be given at multiple sites to avoid giving more than 5 ml at any one site (10 ml in a large adult). The buttocks are the preferred sites, but the anterior thighs can also be used. Tenderness, sterile abscesses, fibrosis, and sciatic nerve injury may result from these injections. The danger of sciatic nerve injury is especially great in a small, malnourished infant with inadequate muscle and fat in the gluteal regions. IG injections should not be given to patients with thrombocytopenia because of the risk of hematoma and infection.

The injections are initially given at monthly intervals. If the patient continues to have infection or if a characteristic symptom recurs at the end of the injection period (such as cough, conjunctivitis, diarrhea, arthralgia, or purulent nasal discharge), the interval between doses is decreased to 3 or 2 weeks. Older patients often report that they can tell when the IgG level is low and when they need another injection. During acute infections, gamma globulin catabolism increases, so extra injections of IG are given. Many adults needing large doses (e.g., 40 ml/month) prefer to get weekly injections of 10 ml.

Because high levels of IgG cannot be maintained, serial Ig assays are not valuable in assessing the effectiveness of treatment. The maximum increase of the serum IgG level after a standard IG injection varies from patient to patient and from dose to dose because of different rates of absorption, local proteolysis at the injection site, and distribution within the tissues. An intramuscular injection of 100 mg/kg of IG usually raises the IgG serum level by 100 to 125 mg/dl after 2 to 4 days (Liese et al., 1992; Stiehm et al., 1966). Thus a recent IG injection usually does not obscure the diagnosis of hypogammaglobulinemia.

Because of the discomfort of these injections and the limited amount of IG that can be given, intramuscular IG is rarely used nowadays.

Subcutaneous Immunoglobulin Infusions

As an alternative to intramuscular injections or IVIG infusions, 10% to 16% IG can be given to immunodeficient patients by slow (0.05 to 0.20 ml/kg/hour) subcutaneous infusions (Berger et al., 1980). The usual maintenance dose is 100 mg/kg/week, preceded by several consecutive days of therapy as a loading dose. These infusions are given using a tiny needle into the abdominal wall or thigh using a battery-operated pump over several hours. These injections are well tolerated, often preferred by the patient over IVIG, and enable the patient to receive equivalent amounts of IgG as that given by IVIG infusions, with similar blood IgG levels.

The incidence of side effects with slow subcutaneous infusions is less than with IVIG infusions. These infusions can readily be done at home, with considerable savings in infusion costs. Subcutaneous infusions are the preferred route in many European countries (Gardulf et al., 1991; Waniewski et al., 1993). Rapid infusion (less than 1 hour) can be achieved by using several pumps and several infusion sites (Gardulf et al., 1991; Gardulf et al., 1995).

This route is especially attractive for individuals who have poor venous access or side reactions (including aseptic meningitis and anaphylaxis) to IVIG. Stiehm and colleagues (1998) have used 10% IVIG subcutaneously because preservative-free 16% IG has not been available in the United States. This route has been used safely during pregnancy and in children.

REACTIONS TO IMMUNOGLOBULIN

Although IG is one of the safest biologic products available, rare anaphylactic reactions to intramuscular injections have been reported, particularly in patients requiring repeat injections (Ellis and Henney, 1969). The Medical Research Council Working Party (1969) noted such reactions in 33 of 175 patients (19%) treated over a 10-year period. In all, there were 85 reactions to about 40,000 injections; in eight patients, the injections were stopped because of these adverse effects, and one death was recorded. Such reactions occurred at all stages of treatment and were unrelated to any particular lot number of gamma globulin or to its measured anticomplementary activity. The symptoms include anxiety, nausea, vomiting, malaise, flushing, facial swelling, cyanosis, and loss of consciousness. Immediate treatment with epinephrine and antihistamines is indicated.

Individuals who experience such reactions should be evaluated before a repeat injection. Skin testing, using several lots of IG, should be done (Ellis and Henney, 1969). A skin test that is positive for an old but not a new lot of IG may indicate a particular idiosyncratic reaction to a particular unit. Under these circumstances, incremental doses of IG from a new lot are recommended. In other patients, IgE antibodies to IgG develop, resulting in positive immediate skin tests. In others, no cause of the reactions can be found. Some of these patients tolerate repeated small doses of IG, particularly if they are premedicated with a nonsteroidal antiinflammatory drug, diphenhydramine, or corticosteroids.

A few patients have developed IgG or IgE antibodies to the IgA present in minute quantities in the IG; these IgA antibodies can be detected by serologic means in several laboratories. IVIG with low IgA content or IgA-deficient plasma can be used under these circumstances (Burks et al., 1986).

Immunologically normal patients given gamma globulin (or plasma) may develop antibodies to a genetic gamma globulin type different from their own (usually anti-Gm antibodies). These are clinically insignificant. Allen and Kunkel (1966) found anti-Gm antibodies in 17 of 24 thalassemic children given repeated blood transfusions. Stiehm and Fudenberg (1965) noted anti-Gm antibodies in normal children given single gamma globulin injections and in hypogammaglobulinemic children given repeated gamma globulin injections. In patients with severe antibody immunodeficiency, such antibodies do not develop. One plasma transfusion reaction was attributed to a Gm/anti-Gm interaction (Fudenberg and Fudenberg, 1964).

Patients with antibodies to IgA may have a reaction to gamma globulin as a result of the trace quantities of IgA in IG or IVIG (Vyas et al., 1968). However, some patients with combined IgA and IgG2 deficiency with anti-IgA antibodies tolerate treatment with IVIG, particularly IVIG with low levels of IgA (Bjorkander et al., 1987).

Administration of IG may inhibit the endogenous synthesis of Ig. Premature infants given IG monthly in the first year of life had lower IgG levels at 1 year of age than albumin-treated controls (Amer et al., 1963). In X-linked HIGM syndrome, intramuscular IgG results in diminution of IgM levels, suggesting inhibition of endogenous IgM synthesis (Stiehm and Fudenberg, 1966a). In some patients with transient hypogammaglobulinemia given IG from early infancy, persistently depressed IgG levels may return to normal when IG or IVIG is discontinued.

Late side effects with IG injections are uncommon; in a few patients, fibrosis of the buttocks or localized subcutaneous atrophy develops at the site of repeated injections. Repeat injections of IG may result in high levels of mercury because of the thimerosal preservative. Although acrodynia developed in one patient as a result of such therapy (Matheson et al., 1980), most patients remain asymptomatic.

Intravenous Immunoglobulin

PHARMACOLOGY

Intravenous administration of IVIG is the usual way to provide IgG to patients with primary and secondary immunodeficiencies (Table 12-23). IVIG is also used extensively in autoimmune and inflammatory conditions and occasionally in the management of infectious diseases.

There are several advantages to the administration of Ig by the intravenous route, including the following:

1. Ease of administering large doses
2. More rapid action
3. No loss in the tissues from proteolysis
4. Avoidance of painful intramuscular injections

Although 16% IG has been used intravenously (Barandun et al., 1962), severe reactions are common, and thus its intravenous use is usually contraindicated (although HBIG is often given intravenously in liver transplant recipients).

IVIG is prepared from Cohn fraction II that is further treated to eliminate high-molecular-weight complexes and their resultant anticomplementary activity. Methods to accomplish this are the following:

1. Physical removal of aggregates by ultracentrifugation or gel filtration
2. Treatment with proteolytic enzymes
3. Treatment with chemicals that reduce sulfhydryl bonds, followed by alkylation of the free disulfide bonds
4. Incubation at low pH

Although physical removal of aggregates is impractical, the other methods have been used with considerable success. In addition to these methods, a final viral inactivation step is added such as solvent/detergent treatment or pasteurization. Donors and the final product are tested for several viral pathogens such as hepatitis B and C and HIV.

The first IVIG licensed in the United States was a reduced (dithiothreitol) and alkylated (iodoacetamide) product formulated as a 5% solution in 10% maltose (Gamimune, Cutter Laboratories). This is no longer available because it was low in IgG3 and IgG4 subclasses. The second licensed IVIG (1984) was an acidified, pepsin-treated powder reconstituted to a 3% or 6% solution in 5% or 10% sucrose (Sandoglobulin, Sandoz Laboratories). Several other IVIGs are now available in the United States and throughout the world. For patients with anti-IgA antibodies, Gammagard-SD or Polygam-SD are the preparations of choice because they have the lowest levels of IgA (Apfelzweig et al., 1987).

All of these preparations offer acceptable serum half-lives (18 to 25 days), contain all IgG subclasses, have minimal anticomplementary activity, have a good and diverse antibody content, and are negative for HBsAg, HCV, and HIV.

Although each of the products differ slightly, they are generally therapeutically equivalent, and are usually selected on the basis of cost and convenience. There are minor IgA and IgG subclass differences (Stiehm, 1997), and they have varying antibody titers to specific pathogens. The latter is clinically significant if the IVIG is used in the treatment of a specific infection, in which a high titer to a less common pathogen (e.g., a specific enterovirus) is needed. Premixed liquids have the advantage of convenience because the reconstitution step is not required; however, most must be kept refrigerated, unlike the lyophilized powders.

DOSE OF IVIG IN IMMUNODEFICIENCY

Early studies with IVIG preparations indicate that they were as effective in preventing serious infections in antibody-deficient subjects as equivalent doses of intramuscular Ig, usually 100 mg/kg/month (Ammann et al., 1982a). Subsequent studies have indicated that higher-dose IVIG (400 to 600 mg/kg/month) given at 3- or 4-week intervals is clinically superior in terms of lessened infections, lessened need for antibiotics, and improved pulmonary function than the earlier recommended doses of 100 to 200 mg/kg/month (Bernatowska et al., 1987; Liese et al., 1992; Ochs et al., 1984).

Sufficient IVIG must be given to increase the trough IgG level at least 400 mg/dl above the preinfusion IgG level or over 500 mg/dl. This generally requires a dose of 400 to 600 mg/kg/month given every 3 to 4 weeks. After an IVIG infusion, the IgG level will immediately increase 250 mg/dl for every 100 mg/kg infused and increase the trough level (after 3 to 4 weeks) 100 mg/dl for every 100 mg/kg IVIG infused (Ochs et al., 1984). At the start of therapy, several additional doses are often given. With continued IVIG infusions, the trough level increases slowly over a 6-month period as the interstitial spaces become saturated with Ig.

These large doses are not necessary for all antibody-deficient subjects because of the increased expense, lack of proven efficacy, and variation of metabolism among different patients (Schiff et al., 1984; Schiff and Rudd, 1986).

Some authors recommend even higher doses. Eijkhout and colleagues (2001) found that doubling the IVIG dose to 600 mg/kg/month in adults and 800 mg/kg/month in children significantly decreased the number and duration of infections The mean IgG levels increased from 650 mg/dl to 940 mg/kg.

Some patients with severe disease do not improve with even very high doses or more frequent infusions of IVIG because of permanent tissue damage or deep-seated chronic infection.

ADMINISTRATION OF IVIG

IVIG is usually given in a clinic or in a physician office by individuals trained to administer and monitor the patient during the infusion (Stiehm, 1997). Emergency resuscitation drugs and equipment should be available. Large centers often have an infusion center with specially trained personnel, special chairs for the patient, and television/VCR/DVD modules to amuse children during their infusion.

The infusion usually takes several hours. The initial rate is 0.01 ml/kg/minute and this can be doubled at 20 to 30 minute intervals to the maximal rate of 0.08 ml/kg/minute (4.0 mg/kg/hour of a 5% product) if there are no side effects. Rates above 5 mg/kg/hour are not recommended. If the patient develops a minor reaction (headache or chills), the infusion is slowed, and medication administered as noted in the following text. For severe reactions, the infusions are stopped.

Premedication is used for individuals with a prior history of reactions. Acetaminophen (15 mg/kg) and diphenhydramine (Benadryl) (1 mg/kg) are given 30 minutes orally before the infusion. Hydrocortisone (6 mg/kg) can be given intravenously 1 hour before the infusion if a severe reaction is anticipated based on prior infusions. Repeat doses of the oral medication are often given after 4 hours. For individuals with delayed or persistent reactions, nonsteroidal antiinflammatory drugs such as naproxen (Naprosyn) can be used for 48 to 72 hours after the infusion.

Up to 15% of patients experience minor reactions such as headache or nausea. These can be minimized by slowing the rate or giving the previously noted medications. Occasionally switching to a different product (generally one available as a solution) may alleviate the reactions.

HOME ADMINISTRATION

IVIG can be given at home by a home-care service, by the parents, or by another adult. Home infusion is much more convenient, with considerable cost and time savings (Daly et al., 1991; Kobayashi et al., 1990). This also gives the patients (or parents) a feeling that they are in charge of their own (or their child's) health. The initial infusions should be given in the hospital or clinic; if the outcome is uneventful, the infusions can be administered at home subsequently.

Home infusions are not recommended for patients with difficult venous access or those with significant side effects from the infusions. Home infusions should never be administered without a responsible adult present. The patient should be under continued supervision, including periodic examination by a physician.

ADVERSE REACTIONS TO IVIG

Adverse reactions to IVIG are unusual, usually preventable, and easily treated. The pain of needle insertion can be minimized by applying eutectic mixture of local anesthetics cream, a local anesthetic, to the infusion site an hour before the infusion. The most common adverse reactions to IVIG are nonanaphylactic reactions, occurring in approximately 5% of infusions, usually in the first 30 minutes of administration and consisting of backache, abdominal pain, headache, chills, fever, and mild nausea.

Most reactions can be minimized by pretreatment with aspirin or diphenhydramine (or occasionally steroids) and treated by slowing the infusion. True anaphylactic reactions are extremely rare. Some of these reactions may be due to the presence of anti-IgA antibodies in the patient reacting with trace amounts of IgA present in the preparations.

Long-term side effects of IVIG are unusual (see Chapter 4). Several cases of aseptic meningitis have been noted shortly after the administration of IVIG; although most are in patients with autoimmune or inflammatory diseases given high dose IVIG, a few cases have occurred in patients with antibody deficiencies (Rao et al., 1992; Stiehm et al., 1998).

Several cases of transient or permanent renal insufficiency have been noted, mostly with high-dose therapy with an IVIG product containing sucrose (Barton et al., 1987; Miller et al., 1992; Schifferli et al., 1991). Thrombosis has been described in a few patients (Comenzo et al., 1992; Woodruff et al., 1986).

Other serious side effects include pulmonary insufficiency (Rault et al., 1991); and hemolytic anemia, Coombs' positivity, or both (Copeland et al., 1986; Moscow et al., 1987).

Hepatitis C

Hepatitis C has been noted following infusions of experimental lots of IVIG (Lever et al., 1984; Ochs et al., 1985; Trepo et al., 1986) and following infusions of Gammagard and Polygam, both made by the same manufacturer (Baxter Labs) (Centers for Disease Control, 1994; Yap et al., 1994; Yu et al., 1995).

This epidemic occurred after testing of donors for hepatitis C antibodies was instituted by the Food and Drug Administration and exclusion of these donors. Thus the immune globulin had no hepatitis C antibodies to neutralize the hepatitis C from donors who were in the window period; that is, donors who were viremic for hepatitis C but had not yet developed antibody, and thus were missed by antibody testing.

Viral inactivation methods (solvent-detergent treatment or pasteurization) as well as PCR assay for virus have now been instituted and no new cases of hepatitis C transmission through IVIG have been observed since 1994.

Bjoro and colleagues (1994) reported that hepatitis C in immune-deficient patients was often associated with severe and sometimes fatal outcome, and was resistant to IFN treatment. More recent studies indicate that the outlook is not as grave. High dose IFN therapy was effective in clearing the virus in more than 50% of the patients followed by Chapel and associates (2001). Razvi and co-workers (2001) reported that approximately one fourth of immunodeficient patients cleared their infection with or without IFN.

Risk of Prion (Mad Cow) and HIV Infection from IVIG

There is the potential risk of prion disease and HIV transmission by immune globulin. Donors are excluded if they have lived in the United Kingdom or Europe for 6 months after 1980, because of the potential risk of transmission of new variant (mad cow) Jacob-Creutzfeldt disease. There is no proven blood test for this illness. There are no cases known to be transmitted by blood product infusions, although Ziegner and colleagues (2002) reported a series of immunodeficient patients with progressive neurodegeneration exposed to IVIG preparations, but none had proven prion disease.

No cases of AIDS or HIV transmission have been reported as a result of immune globulin treatment. Indeed, the virus has been shown to be inactivated by the fractionation process.

SPECIAL USES OF IVIG IN IMMUNODEFICIENCY

Infections

During infections or prolonged fever, IgG catabolism increases, and consumption of antibody to the offending microorganism is consumed. Thus it is prudent to give extra IVIG infusions during severe infections so as to maintain IgG levels. In severe diarrhea, IgG may be lost in the stool and extra doses of IVIG should be considered. In refractory severe infections in immunodeficient subjects, particularly if neutropenia is present, high-dose IVIG therapy in addition to antimicrobial agents may be effective.

ENTEROVIRUS ENCEPHALITIS AND POLYMYOSITIS

Chronic meningocephalitis and polymyositis resulting from ECHOvirus or coxsackievirus characteristically occur in patients with XLA, and less commonly CVID or X-linked HIGM syndrome (Crennan et al., 1986; Cunningham et al., 1999; Lederman and Winkelstein, 1985; Quartier et al., 2000; Schmugge et al., 1999). Treatment with high doses of IVIG at frequent intervals may modify the severity of infection and improve survival (Mease et al., 1981). When possible, the IVIG should be tested for antibody to the patient's viral strain, and a product used that contains good titers to the virus.

A review of published reports indicated that 8 of 11 patients treated with IVIG survived, compared with only 2 of 10 patients given intramuscular IG or immune plasma and 0 of 4 patients who received no treatment (Stiehm, 1996). Two patients who received intraventricular Ig as well as IVIG showed resolution of CSF pleocytosis with eradication of the ECHOvirus from the CSF. However, most other patients, including two others given intraventricular Ig, have had a chronic fluctuating course with persistent CSF pleocytosis and positive CSF cultures.

A preliminary trial of the antiviral drug pleconaril was partially successful (Rotbart and Webster, 2001). With the use of enteroviral PCR, early diagnosis and therapeutic monitoring may make future trials of new antiviral agents more definitive (Chesky et al., 2000).

RESPIRATORY SYNCYTIAL VIRUS INFECTIONS

RSV infections present a major risk to immunodeficient subjects younger than age 2, particularly those who were born prematurely, who have profound deficiency, and who have chronic lung or heart disease. Such children are candidates for RSV prophylaxis with RSV-IVIG (RespiGam) a hyperimmune immune globulin enriched in RSV antibodies. This can be substituted for the regular IVIG infusions, but the prophylactic dose is 750 mg/kg/month, a dose not tolerated at a single infusions by all infants. In such instances we give 400 mg/kg of RSV-IVIG every 2 weeks.

Alternatively the anti-RSV monoclonal antibody palivizumab Synagis can be given monthly intramuscularly at a dose of 15 mg/kg in addition to regular IVIG. All patients receiving stem cell transplants who are younger than age 3 are candidates for RSV prophylaxis during the RSV season.

OTHER RESPIRATORY VIRAL INFECTIONS

In patients with severe T- or B-cell immunodeficiency, severe respiratory viral infections may develop, particularly in infants younger than age 2 with chronic lung or heart disease. IVIG preparations contain antibodies to several common respiratory tract pathogens, including adenovirus, influenza, and parainfluenza, and may be of value in management of these diseases (Stiehm et al., 1986).

Adenovirus pneumonia has occurred in immunodeficient children lacking neutralizing antibody to adenovirus, and one child recovered after receiving intramuscular IG. IVIG controls but does not eradicate these viral infections unless the patient's immunity is restored with a stem cell transplant.

PARVOVIRUS B19 INFECTION

Parvovirus B19 infection causes aplastic anemia in immunodeficient and immunocompromised subjects. Kurtzman and colleagues (1989) reported cure of pure RBC aplasia caused by parvovirus in a 24-year-old man. After intensive IVIG therapy, the virus disappeared permanently from the marrow and peripheral blood. The IVIG treatments were then discontinued without relapse. Others have reported similar experiences (Young et al., 1966).

Oral Immunoglobulin

Human IG has been used orally in immunodeficiency to diminish or abolish the shedding of rotavirus, poliovirus, or coxsackievirus (Losonsky et al., 1985). It has also been used in *Cryptosporidium* infection (Borowitz and Saulsbury, 1991). A recommended dose is 150 mg/kg/day in divided doses given at 4- to 6-hour intervals using a preservative-free IVIG preparation.

Hypercatabolic States

IVIG can be used to study the metabolism of IgG in hypogammaglobulinemic patients suspected of GI or urinary tract loss or hypercatabolism. A large dose of IVIG (2 g/kg) is given to raise the IgG levels acutely, and then serial IgG levels are studied to determine the rate of disappearance from the circulation. Patients with primary hypogammaglobulinemia have a normal or increased IgG half-life (greater than 20 days), whereas patients with loss or hypercatabolism have a shortened IgG half-life (less than 15 days).

Autoimmune Diseases

Patients with immunodeficiency may develop immunoregulatory disorders such as autoimmune hemolytic anemia, ITP, or vasculitis that may benefit from large-

dose IVIG. They can be treated with the larger doses of IVIG recommended for these disorders (see Chapter 4).

Pregnancy

IVIG has been used in pregnancy with safety and efficacy for immunodeficiency, thrombocytopenic purpura, and threatened abortion. The profound transient hypogammaglobulinemia of the infant born to a mother with agammaglobulinemia can be prevented by large doses of IVIG during late pregnancy; however, IVIG can also be given to the infant at birth. A few of these children have done well without IG therapy (Kobayashi et al., 1980).

IVIG IN SECONDARY IMMUNODEFICIENCIES

Some patients with secondary immunodeficiencies have low Ig levels, poor antibody responses to antigenic challenge, and low levels of natural antibodies. This may result from loss of Ig, loss of immune cells, or the toxic effect of therapy or infection on the immune system. Table 12-23 includes those diseases and conditions in which secondary antibody immunodeficiency can occur.

Laboratory criteria that support the use of IVIG include (1) significant hypogammaglobulinemia (serum IgG less than 200 mg/dl or total Ig level [IgG + IgM + IgA] less than 400 mg/dl), (2) absent or low natural antibodies, (3) absent or poor response to antigenic challenge (e.g., tetanus, pneumococcal vaccines), and (4) lack of an antibody response to the infecting organism (Stiehm, 1991).

Hematologic/Oncologic Diseases

Antibody deficiencies can occur with multiple myeloma, chronic lymphocytic leukemia, lymphomas, and advanced cancer. A double-blind multicenter study concluded that the prophylactic infusion of 400 mg/kg of IVIG every 3 weeks reduced the incidence of bacterial infections in patients with chronic lymphocytic leukemia (Cooperative Group for the Study of Immunoglobulin in Chronic Lymphocytic Leukemia, 1988). The treatment group had fewer infections with *Streptococcus pneumoniae* and *Haemophilus influenzae*, but there was no difference in infections resulting from other gram-negative bacteria or fungal or viral infections. This beneficial effect was confirmed in a subsequent study (Gamm et al., 1994). IVIG has also been shown to reduce the incidence of infections in patients with multiple myeloma (Chapel et al., 1994) and in patients with lung cancer receiving chemotherapy (Schmidt et al., 1994).

Protein-Losing Enteropathy and Nephrotic Syndrome

Some pediatric patients develop antibody deficiency associated with massive proteinuria (nephrosis) or diarrhea (protein-losing enteropathy) because of accelerated IgG catabolism. Most of these patients have minimal trouble with recurrent infection, probably because antibody synthesis is intact and probably accelerated; however, if the IgG loss greatly exceeds the synthetic capacity, symptomatic severe hypogammaglobulinemia may result. IVIG can be used diagnostically in such cases; a large intravenous infusion, followed by serial measurements of serum IgG levels, can document an accelerated IgG half-life (i.e., less than 10 days).

These patients are candidates for IVIG therapy if they have recurrent infections and very low IgG levels (e.g., less than 200 mg/dl). Large and repeated doses are necessary. Occasionally, antibody infusions help control the severe diarrhea of protein-losing enteropathy (Cannon et al., 1982). Subcutaneous IG has been used in this situation because its delayed release into the serum may result in higher IgG levels than an equivalent IVIG dose (Stiehm et al., 1998).

Trauma, Shock, and Surgery

Patients undergoing severe stress associated with trauma or extensive surgery have profound exposure and susceptibility to infection and a spectrum of immune deficiencies, including cutaneous anergy, leukocyte dysfunction, hypogammaglobulinemia, and transiently impaired antibody synthesis (Glinz et al., 1985; Munster, 1984; Wilson et al., 1989). Bowel stasis and hypotension may promote gram-negative sepsis or endotoxemia with development of severe and often irreversible shock.

Studies by Ziegler and associates (1982) and Baumgartner and associates (1985) suggested that when antisera to a mutant J5 *Escherichia coli* endotoxin with antilipid A activity was used in bacteremic or surgical intensive care unit (ICU) patients, the incidence and severity of severe shock could be reduced. However, Calandra and colleagues (1988), using a human IVIG to J5 *E. coli* in 71 patients with gram-negative infections and shock, could not confirm their results. They gave a single infusion of 200 mg/kg; a control group got a similar dose of regular IVIG. There was no difference in mortality, onset of time to shock, or complications.

Just and coworkers (1986) used regular IVIG and antibiotics in 50 ICU patients suspected of infection and compared their outcome with 54 control patients who received antibiotics alone. Although there was no difference in survival, there was a trend to indicate that the IVIG-antibiotic group had a shortened ICU stay, a shorter period during which respirator therapy was necessary, improved renal function, and a favorable effect on infection (i.e., infections were a less likely cause of death in these patients).

A multicenter study of 352 postsurgical patients confirmed the observation that standard IVIG (400 mg/kg at weekly intervals) reduced the incidence of infections and shortened the stay in the ICU compared with placebo or hyperimmune core-lipopolysaccharide immune globulin-treated patients (Intravenous Immunoglobulin Collaborative Study Group, 1991).

Werdan (1999) has reviewed the use of IVIG in sepsis and suggests that there may be specific subgroups that may benefit (e.g., postoperative sepsis, septic shock with endotoxinemia, and sepsis with neutropenia). Studies of IVIG in patients with trauma requiring surgery (deSimone et al., 1988; Douzinas et al., 2000; Glinz et al., 1985) and in head trauma patients (Wilson et al., 1989) have shown questionable efficacy.

Monoclonal antibodies to endotoxin have been tested in clinical trials of septic shock patients, but none were of proven efficacy (National Committee for the Evaluation of Centoxin, 1994; Wheeler and Bernard, 1999; Ziegler et al., 1991). In summary, there are no compelling data to suggest that antibody, either polyclonal or monoclonal, is of benefit in the acutely ill patient with shock.

Prematurity

All premature infants have low levels of maternally derived IgG at birth and most develop IgG levels approaching 100 mg/dl in the first months of life (Ballow et al., 1986) (see Table 12-14). These IgG levels may be further depressed by pulmonary disease (with transudation into the lung), stress (with increased IgG catabolism), and multiple blood drawing (Ruderman et al., 1988). In addition, their sluggish antibody responses; their concurrent IgM and IgA deficiency; and their immature complement, phagocytic, and T-cell systems make them extraordinarily susceptible to infection (see Chapter 22).

Attempts to decrease infections in premature infants with periodic IG injections date from the 1960s. Four controlled studies were performed, enrolling a total of 363 infants using IG doses from 80 mg/kg to 240 mg/kg/month during their stay in the nursery (two studies), for 4 months, and for 1 year (Amer et al., 1963; Conway et al., 1987; Diamond et al., 1966; Steen 1960). In two of these studies there was a slight decrease in the number and severity of infections, but no difference in survival. These mixed results suggest that Ig at the doses employed was not of value in prophylaxis of infection.

In the last decade, the increasing survival of very tiny premature infants and the availability of IVIG reawakened interest in use of antibody to prevent infections in the premature infant. In general, IVIG is well tolerated with minimal adverse effects in doses up to 1 g/kg/day.

A meta-analysis of 12 controlled, prospective, randomized, placebo-controlled prevention studies, (representing 4180 infants) was done by Jenson and Pollock (1997; 1998). These studies differed as to entry criteria, dose, and brand of IVIG. All infants weighed less than 2000 g, started IVIG therapy within the first week of life, received doses of at least 400 mg/kg/month, and used culture-proven sepsis. Five studies showed a significant benefit if IVIG, one showed a higher incidence in the control group, and six studies showed no difference. Overall, there were 345 cases of sepsis in 2136 IVIG-treated infants (16%) versus 408 cases in 2044 control infants (20.0%) (P = .02), a modest but statistically significant difference. A Cochrane review meta-analysis of 15 studies, including 5054 infants, also found a 3% to 4% reduction in serious infections without a difference in mortality (Ohlsson and Lacy, 2001).

Shamim and associates (1991) gave IVIG for 6 months to 15 of 30 matched premature infants with severe bronchopulmonary dysplasia, maintaining their IgG levels over 400 mg/dl, whereas the untreated infants had levels less than 200 mg/dl. The number of infections, notably pneumonia, were significantly reduced in the IVIG group (5 episodes of pneumonia and 4 other infections) compared with 15 episodes of pneumonia and 12 other infections in the control group.

Thus the evidence to date supports the National Institutes of Health Consensus Statement (1990), which concluded that IVIG should not be given routinely to infants of low birth weight, but may be of value in selected premature infants at high risk for infection.

IVIG is recommended for premature infants with a history of serious infections with underlying lung disease: Most such infants will have hypogammaglobulinemic and should be regarded as having transient hypogammaglobulinemia of infancy (see Chapters 13 and 22). Such infants need RSV prophylaxis also.

Post-transplantation

Conditioning regimens to eliminate or reduce the host's hematopoietic and immune systems during transplantation (stem cell and solid organ) render these patients extremely susceptible to infection (Tutscha, 1986).

The use of IVIG to prevent these infections, particularly sepsis, pneumonia, or GI infections have met with limited success (Copelon and Tutschka, 1986; Graham-Pole et al., 1988; Sullivan, 1987, 1989; Sullivan et al., 1990), with the exception of preventing complications from CMV infection (discussed in the next section).

One report demonstrated some benefit from infusions of IVIG in a controlled trial on 382 bone marrow recipients (Sullivan, 1989). The study patients received 500 mg/kg of IVIG weekly for 90 days, then monthly for 1 year, with a resultant decrease in the number of infections, number of platelet transfusions, and the incidence of GVHD. A review from the same group of investigators concluded that IVIG has shown benefit on reducing septicemia, interstitial pneumonia, fatal CMV disease, acute GVHD, and transplant-related mortality in adult recipients of related marrow transplants (Sullivan et al., 1990).

Thus IVIG has been recommended for allogeneic marrow transplant recipients (Keller et al., 1993; Rowe et al., 1994) but not for autologous transplantation (Guglielmo et al., 1994; Wolff et al., 1993).

Burns

Bacterial sepsis, particularly *Pseudomonas* and *Escherichia coli* sepsis, is the leading cause of death in the 300,000 patients hospitalized annually in the United States for burns (Munster, 1984, 1986). These patients develop hypogammaglobulinemia as a result of protein loss in proportion to the severity of the burn. High-dose IVIG prolonged survival in experimentally burned mice infected with *Pseudomonas,* and preliminary studies of hyperimmune Ig and plasma in human burn patients were encouraging, but proof of efficacy is lacking (Kefalides et al., 1962; Pollack, 1983; Shirani et al., 1984).

HIV Infection

There is considerable rationale for the use of IVIG in patients with advanced HIV disease (particularly children), including their increased susceptibility to common bacterial and viral infections; poor primary antibody responses to vaccine antigens despite hypergammaglobulinemia; and, in children, a limited antibody spectrum to common bacterial pathogens.

Although the central immune defect in AIDS is a loss of Th (CD4) numbers and function, the polyclonal B-cell activation and defective T-cell helper function results in a significant B-cell deficiency (Bernstein et al., 1985; Ochs, 1987). Thus, in children with pediatric AIDS, bacterial infections are more common than opportunistic infections. AIDS patients may also develop immune-mediated thrombocytopenic purpura and viral diseases (e.g., RSV, parainfluenza, CMV) amenable to IVIG therapy.

After preliminary uncontrolled studies suggested a benefit of IVIG in children with advanced HIV infection (Calvelli and Rubinstein, 1986; Siegel and Oleske, 1986), two large multicenter controlled studies undertaken by the National Institutes of Health (NIH)-supported Pediatric AIDS Clinical Trial Group determined the efficacy of IVIG in decreasing infections and improving survival in AIDS patients.

The first study of 372 children received 400 mg/kg of IVIG every 4 weeks or an albumin control for 2 years (Intravenous Immune Globulin Study Group, 1991). Of all children in the IVIG-treated group, 30% had serious infections as compared with 42% of the children in the placebo group. Less ill children (those with CD4 lymphocyte counts greater than 200 cells/mm^3) benefitted in particular from IVIG. Children in this category had fewer serious infections, were hospitalized less than the placebo group, and their CD4 counts dropped less rapidly than the placebo group. The mortality in both groups, however, was identical. The children with CD4 counts less than 200 cells/mm^3 (i.e., those with severely impaired immunity) who were given IVIG had no significant decrease in infections, days of hospitalization, or mortality as compared to their counterparts in the placebo group.

The authors concluded that IVIG significantly reduced the risk of serious infections in some children with symptomatic HIV infection, primarily those with CD4 counts between 200 and 500 CD4 cells/mm^3. In a follow-up study, the placebo group was allowed to cross over to receive IVIG with a drop in the rate of serious infection and hospitalizations (Mofenson et al., 1994).

In a second trial of IVIG in which all of the children received zidovudine, there again was a significant decrease in serious bacterial infections, but this benefit was limited to children who did not receive TMP/SMX prophylaxis for PCP (Spector et al., 1994). A consensus of an HIV working group was that HIV-infected children with significant hypogammaglobulinemia or documented poor antibody formation may be candidates for IVIG therapy (Working Group on Antiretroviral Therapy, 1993). We also use IVIG in HIV-infected children whose recurrent infections are not controlled by antibiotics or who have chronic nonspecific diarrhea with failure to thrive.

In addition to preventing serious bacterial infections, IVIG given to children with HIV reduced the number of nonserious bacterial infections (by 60% for ear infections, 13% for skin infections, and 10% for other URIs) and viral infections by approximately one third in both trials (Mofenson and Moye, 1992; Mofenson et al., 1992, 1994; Spector et al., 1994).

IVIG in large doses (0.5 to 1.0 g/kg for 3 to 5 days) has been shown to be effective in reducing infection in HIV-infected adults (Kiehl et al., 1996) and HIV-related thrombocytopenia (Bussel and Himi, 1988; Kurtzberg et al., 1987).

Regular IVIG infusions also improved left ventricular function in HIV-infected children with dilated cardiac myopathy (Lipshultz et al., 1995).

IVIG IN IMMUNOREGULATORY DISORDERS

High-dose IVIG has immunosuppressive and antiinflammatory effects that make it a valuable agent in the treatment of several autoimmune or inflammatory disorders. These may occur in patients with both primary and secondary immunodeficiencies. The mechanisms, indications, and doses of IVIG are discussed in Chapter 4.

Plasma

Periodic plasma infusions have been used to administer IgG, IgM, and IgA by the intravenous route to patients with antibody immunodeficiencies (Buckley, 1972; Stiehm et al., 1966). In addition to supplying large quantities of undenatured immune globulin, plasma supplies complement components and other proteins of possible importance in combating infection. Cannon and co-workers (1982) described two infants with diarrhea, malabsorption, and hypoproteinemia who were initially diagnosed as having SCID and who recovered with intensive plasma. Plasma can be used in complement component deficiencies to provide the missing factor.

Because plasma therapy may transmit hepatitis, CMV, or HIV, such treatment is rarely used today. If done, the plasma from a single hepatitis-free, CMV, and HIV antibody-negative donor, usually a relative, is recommended. This is collected by plasmapheresis, aliquoted in plasma bags, and frozen before use; freezing destroys lymphocytes that may cause GVHD. A minor crossmatch of the donor plasma with the patient's RBCs must be negative.

The usual dose of plasma is 20 ml/kg, which contains approximately 200 mg/kg of IgG, 40 mg/kg of IgA, and 20 mg/kg of IgM. Larger doses may be given if this dose is ineffective; in these instances, large quantities of plasma can be obtained from the recipient by plasmapheresis.

Leukocyte Transfusions

In patients with phagocytic immunodeficiencies, notably CGD, granulocytes from a normal donor may permit resolution of an infection not responsive to antibiotic therapy (Fanconi et al., 1985; Raubitschek et al., 1973). Although compatible leukocytes of the same HLA type are not imperative, they result in fewer reactions and have a longer half-life within the recipient. The separated granulocytes must be given within 3 to 4 hours of procurement, and repeated courses of therapy are generally necessary (Boggs, 1974). The donor is often given granulocyte colony stimulating factor (GCSF) prior to donation to increase the peripheral blood count and increase the yield.

Immediate side effects include chills, fevers, and anaphylactoid reactions. Late effects include pulmonary infiltrates. Amphotericin may aggravate the latter, and special care must be used when amphotericin is used concomitantly. Diminished effectiveness of the granulocytes may occur as a result of the development of HLA or granulocyte antibodies. A recent review is available (Hubel et al., 2001).

In patients with cellular immunodeficiencies, donor granulocytes should be irradiated to remove the risk of GVHD from contaminating lymphocytes. Granulocyte infusions can also transmit viral hepatitis, CMV, and HIV. CMV antibody-negative donors are recommended for a CMV antibody-negative recipient.

Pharmacologic Agents

Certain drugs have been used in an attempt to alter the basic immunologic defect in a few immunodeficiency syndromes.

Vitamin C enhances the chemotaxis of normal granulocytes, probably by increasing the intracellular levels of cyclic 3',5'-guanosine monophosphate, and improves the in vitro bactericidal capacity of the granulocytes from patients with Chédiak-Higashi syndrome (see Chapter 20). Accordingly, high-dose vitamin C may benefit certain patients with this syndrome (Boxer et al., 1976; Gallin et al., 1979; Weening et al., 1981). Vitamin B_{12} is beneficial in the treatment of the immunodeficiency of transcobalamin II deficiency (see Chapter 13).

Antihistamines may also enhance phagocytic chemotaxis under some circumstances. Hill and Quie (1974) found that patients with elevated IgE levels exhibit defective chemotaxis secondary to high levels of intracellular histamine, which in turn affects immune function.

Cimetidine, an antihistamine with primarily histamine 2–blocking activity that is widely used in peptic ulcer disease, diminishes suppressor-cell activity and enhances delayed cutaneous hypersensitivity in immunologically normal subjects (Avella et al., 1978). One patient with CVID had increased Ig synthesis following its use (White and Ballow, 1985).

Levamisole, an antihelminthic agent that enhances cutaneous reactivity by nonspecifically stimulating T lymphocytes and macrophages, has been used in immunodeficient subjects. Despite some restoration of immune function (Lieberman and Hsu, 1976), no clinical benefit has been observed in patients with WAS or mucocutaneous candidiasis. Some reports suggest therapeutic benefit of levamisole in the hyper-IgE syndrome by enhancing chemotaxis (DeCree et al., 1974; Wright et al., 1970); its efficacy is unproven.

Thalidomide was originally used as a sedative and antinausea drug, but was withdrawn from the market because of its teratogenicity. It has been revived because of its immunomodulating properties by opposing the effect of TNF and other immunosuppressive properties. It has been used with some benefit in aphthous ulcers (in HIV and Behçet's syndrome, in erythema nodosum, in leprosy, and in chronic GVHD (Moraes and Russo, 2001; Paterson et al., 1995; Vogelsang et al., 1992).

Immunomodulating Agents

Several agents that stimulate the immune system nonspecifically are available, but their value in primary immunodeficiency is limited at best. These include microbial products (BCG and other bacterial or fungal extracts), thymus-derived T-cell stimulants, thyromimetic drugs, muramyl peptides, lipid A analogs, isoprinosine, tuftsin, herbal remedies, and IFN inducers (e.g., Ampligen) (Hadden, 1993). Several are licensed in other countries, and clinical trials in cancer, HIV, and recurrent infections are under way. None shows proven clinical benefit in primary immunodeficiency.

BLyS, an agent that activates B cells, looks promising in animal experiments and is under clinical trials in some forms of antibody deficiency with B cells (see Chapter 3).

Thymic Hormones

The thymic epithelium synthesizes a number of soluble factors that regulate and differentiate T lymphocytes. These include thymosin, FTS, and thymopoietin. These can be assayed by biologic or immunoassays.

Thymosin, a 28–amino acid peptide extracted from bovine thymus, has been the most widely used therapeutically. Wara and Ammann (1976) treated 17 patients with cellular immunodeficiency with thymosin injections. No responses were noted in combined immunodeficiency and ataxia-telangiectasia, but some clinical benefit and restoration of immunologic function in vitro was noted in some patients with WAS, Nezelof syndrome, and DiGeorge syndrome.

Another thymic polypeptide in clinical use in some countries is thymic pentapeptide, a polypeptide that includes the active site (amino acids 32 to 36) of the intact thymopoietin molecule. Aiuti and colleagues (1983) have reported some clinical benefit in the DiGeorge and Nezelof syndromes. Therapeutic benefits in immunodeficiency for synthetic FTS (Bordigoni et al., 1982) and thymostimuline (Aiuti et al., 1984) have been reported.

Transfer Factor

Transfer factor (TF) is a dialyzable extract of immune leukocytes that is used to transfer cellular immunity from a skin-test–positive donor to a skin-test–negative recipient (Lawrence, 1969). It is often referred to as *dialyzable leukocyte extract*. Concomitantly, there may be the acquisition of proliferative responses and mediator production to a specific antigen. TF is a low-molecular-weight (1110–1600) nucleopeptide that is heterogeneous in column chromatography. Its exact mechanism of action is uncertain. It is nonantigenic and can be lyophilized and stored for years.

TF has been used in a variety of immunodeficiencies with very limited success. In some cases of WAS treated with TF, there has been some clinical benefit, as evidenced by decreased infection and eczema and lessening of the thrombocytopenia for up to 6 months (Spitler et al., 1972) (see Chapter 7). Repeated injections were necessary when skin tests became negative.

Some patients with mucocutaneous candidiasis have benefited, particularly when concomitant antifungal therapy is given to reduce the antigenic load (Schulkind et al., 1972). Several patients with combined deficiency have been given TF in conjunction with fetal thymus transplantation with engraftment of T cells from the fetal thymus (Ammann et al., 1973; Rachelefsky et al., 1975). In general, TF therapy is of dubious value in cellular immunodeficiency or any other disorder.

Enzyme Replacement

In many children with combined immunodeficiency with ADA deficiency, partial restoration of immune function and clinical improvement with erythrocyte transfusions containing adequate amounts of ADA have occurred (Polmar et al., 1976) (see Chapter 16). Other ADA-deficient children have not shown clinical benefit from transfusions (Schmalsteig et al., 1978).

Hershfield and associates (1987) first reported that the weekly intramuscular injection of bovine ADA conjugated with polyethylene glycol resulted in correction of the metabolic abnormalities, clinical improvement, and increased T cells in two children with ADA-deficient combined immunodeficiency. Since then, more than 100 patients have been treated with PEG-ADA (Hershfield, 1995) (see Chapter 16).

Cytokines

Cytokine therapy has been used successfully in selected primary immunodeficiencies. The best example is the use of IFN-γ in patients with CGD (Gallin, 1991) (see Chapter 20). IFN-γ is given weekly subcutaneously enhanced respiratory burst activity in some of these patients and nonoxidative bactericidal activity with a 72% reduction in infections in a double-blind placebo-controlled study. IFN-γ has also been used in the hyper-IgE syndrome, glycogen storage disease type 1b (McCawley et al., 1993), NK immunodeficiency (Lipinski et al., 1980), and some forms of mycobactericidal defect with partial IFN-γ deficiency (Jouanguy et al., 1997) (see Chapter 17).

GCSF has been used successfully in the treatment of congenital neutropenia (Kostmann's syndrome), cyclic neutropenia, glycogen storage disease-Ib, and other primary immunodeficiencies with neutropenia (e.g., X-linked HIGM syndrome) (Bonilla et al., 1989).

De Ugarte and associates (2002) successfully used local applications of granulocyte macrophage colony stimulating factor to promote wound healing in patients with phagocytic deficiencies, including one patient with a leukocyte adhesion defect.

IL-2 therapy may benefit children with SCID who have selective IL-2 deficiency (Paganelli et al., 1983; Weinberg and Parkman, 1990). IL-2 conjugated to polyethylene glycol given weekly intramuscularly has been used in patients with CVID (Cunningham-Rundles et al., 1994, 2001). There was some enhancement of in vitro lymphoproliferative responses and antibody responses to a neoantigen, but no clear clinical benefit.

Soluble cytokine receptors and monoclonal antibodies to cytokines or their receptors are being tested for their immunosuppressive, inflammatory, or antitumor effects. There are two reports of improvement of cutaneous granulomas in CVID with the use of the anti-TNF receptor antagonist (Liebhaber et al., 2002; Smith et al., 2001).

Fetal Organ Transplants

Liver

The fetal liver is a source of stem cells and can reconstitute lethally irradiated mice. Keightley and co-workers (1975) and Buckley and associates (1976b) reported successful reconstitution in combined immunodeficiency using large numbers of fresh liver cells from fetuses of less than 10 weeks' gestation. Another successful reconstitution used both fetal liver and thymus (Ackeret et al., 1976). Graft-versus-host reactions and chimerism have been observed in some cases. Fetal liver transplantation is no longer done because of the good results with haploidentical T-cell–depleted marrow and the incomplete nature of the immune reconstitution.

Thymus

Fetal thymus transplantation (into either the subcutaneous tissue or the peritoneum) from a fetus of less than 16 weeks' gestation restored cellular immunity to several patients with DiGeorge anomaly (August et al., 1970; Cleveland et al., 1968), combined immunodeficiency (Rachelefsky et al., 1975), and Nezelof syndrome (Ammann et al., 1973; Shearer et al., 1978). In the DiGeorge anomaly, fetal thymus brings about rapid reconstitution (within days), which appears to be permanent, and lymphoid chimerism is absent; the mechanism in this syndrome appears to result from the presence of an inducer that activates the patient's own thymic precursor cells (Wara and Ammann, 1976).

In combined immunodeficiency, including the Nezelof syndrome, fetal thymus transplantation resulted in slow reconstitution of T-cell immunity, mild graft-versus-host manifestations, and lymphoid chimerism derived from the implanted thymocytes. TF has been given concurrently with fetal thymus; its contribution is not clear. The timing and temporary reconstitution distinguishes this effect from the reconstitution in DiGeorge anomaly.

Fetal thymic tissue is difficult to obtain; intact fetuses are available only after hysterectomies, prostaglandin-induced abortions, or at laparotomy for the removal of an unruptured tubal pregnancy. Thus the popularity of this procedure has waned.

Cultured Thymic Tissue Transplants

Thymic epithelial transplantations were first used in combined immunodeficiency by Hong and co-workers (1976). Thymic fragments removed from normal infants undergoing heart surgery are held for several weeks in tissue culture, during which time most of the lymphoid cells die while the epithelial elements persist. The cultured thymic tissue was implanted intraperitoneally or intramuscularly.

After this procedure, increased Ig levels, antibody production, and restoration of T-cell numbers and proliferative responses associated with mild to moderate clinical improvement were noted. The incomplete nature of the immunologic reconstitution, the occurrence of lymphomas in 3 (of 30) patients given thymic epithelial transplants, and the availability of haploidentical transplants reduced the enthusiasm for this procedure in SCID (Borzy et al., 1979a).

Markert and associates (1997, 1999, 2003) have used cultured thymic tissue to treat several patients with complete DiGeorge syndrome. Thymic tissue, not necessarily HLA matched, is obtained from infants undergoing heart surgery from age 2 to 35 days. The thymus is sliced and cultured and then implanted surgically into the quadriceps muscle. Rapid restoration of immunity was identified by the development of lymphoproliferative responses, the appearance of CD4 and CD8 cells, and the presence of newly released thymic emigrant T cells with T-cell excision circles and the CD45RA phenotype characteristic of newly emerged thymic cells. Seven of twelve patients are doing well; six have antigen-specific T-cell responses (Markert et al., 2003).

Stem Cell Transplants

HLA-Matched Transplants

Stem cell transplantation from an HLA-identical, MLC, nonreactive (i.e., HLA-D identical) sibling is the treatment of choice for patients with all forms of combined immunodeficiency and WAS. It has also been used successfully in patients with reticular dysgenesis (Levinsky and Tiedeman, 1983), CGD (Rappeport et al., 1982), LAD-1 (Le Deist et al., 1989), Chédiak-Higashi syndrome (Virelizier et al., 1982), Omenn's syndrome (Fischer et al.,

1994), complete DiGeorge anomaly (Goldsobel et al., 1987), X-linked lymphoproliferative disorder (Williams et al., 1993; Vowels et al., 1993), and several other immunodeficiencies (see Chapter 43).

Most of these transplants have used bone marrow cells aspirated from an anesthetized donor. Alternatively, peripheral white blood cells can be obtained by leukapheresis and enriched for CD34 stem cells for infusion. There have been a few transplants of cord blood using an HLA identical newborn (HLA typed in utero) to treat a sibling with a severe T-cell deficiency.

More than 1000 infants with SCID and many others have been restored to health since the initial bone marrow transplants in 1968 (Bach et al., 1968; Gatti et al., 1968) (see Chapters 15 and 43). Dramatic and permanent (up to 30 years) restoration of both cellular and antibody functions may occur, with firm evidence of engraftment. Graft-versus-host reactions vary in severity, and some patients have succumbed from infection during this period. The graft-versus-host reaction is usually self-limited, and following its disappearance, the child is usually restored to a state of good health. Some patients have chronic graft-versus-host reactions with persistent dermatitis, hepatitis, or diarrhea.

Because each sibling of the patient has only a 1-in-4 chance of being HLA-identical, most patients will not have an HLA matched donor (see Chapter 43). When a sibling donor is not available, parents and relatives should be examined for HLA identity.

Stem cell transplantation for immunodeficiency is available in many major medical centers. If transplantation is contemplated, the parents and all siblings should be HLA-A and HLA-B typed, and if any are identical to the patient, an MLC is warranted. All MLC-identical matches should be confirmed by repeat testing. After testing the donor for viral diseases including HIV and hepatitis B and C, he or she is usually hospitalized at the time of transplantation for marrow obtained under anesthesia. It is enumerated, filtered, and injected intravenously (Thomas and Storb, 1970).

No immunosuppression is necessary if there is a complete lack of cellular immunity. *Pneumocystis carinii* prophylaxis is used before and throughout the procedure. If the donor is CMV antibody-positive, the recipient should receive prophylactic antiviral treatment.

In patients with intact or slightly decreased T-cell immunodeficiency, WAS, or SCID with some degree of cellular immunity (as indicated by positive lymphoproliferative responses such as a positive MLC reaction to an unrelated donor), immunosuppression before transplantation is necessary to ensure T-cell engraftment. In the WAS, immunosuppression is necessary to ensure hematopoietic engraftment and correction of the platelet defect.

One regimen is oral busulfan (3 to 4 mg/kg/day) for 4 days, and intravenous cyclophosphamide (50 mg/kg/day) for 4 days, followed by transplantation on day 10. After the transplant, cyclosporine is usually given to suppress a graft-versus-host reaction. Antithymocyte globulin and corticosteroids are also sometimes used (see Chapter 43).

Haploidentical Transplants

When an HLA-identical donor is unavailable for a patient with SCID, a haploidentical, T cell–depleted stem cell transplantation (half-matched) can be undertaken. In this procedure, mature T cells are removed from the donor marrow before infusion; the less mature T cells then reconstitute the patient without the occurrence of life-threatening GVHD.

Two techniques are used for T-cell depletion: (1) removal by agglutination with soybean lectin and (2) lysis of T cells with monoclonal anti–T-cell antibody plus complement. The former has been used in more than 1000 cases (Buckley et al., 1986, 1999; Cowan et al., 1985; Friedrich et al., 1985; O'Reilly et al., 1983), the latter method in more than 100 cases (Reinherz et al., 1982; Parkman, 1986; Fischer et al., 1994) with little or no GVHD and a 60% to 80% survival.

Immunosuppression is sometimes used to ensure T-cell engraftment. B-cell engraftment with antibody function is not always achieved, and graft-versus-host responses may still occur. Despite these limitations, this technique has been associated with many impressive successes and has replaced fetal liver or cultured thymic epithelial transplants for the SCID patient without a matched donor.

In Utero HLA Haploidentical Transplants

A few patients with SCID have been given haploidentical parental marrow in utero with at least four successes (Flake and Zanjani, 1997). This may allow easier engraftment without the need for immunosuppression.

Matched Unrelated Transplants

An alternative to a T-depleted haploidentical bone marrow transplant is an unrelated HLA, phenotypically identical, and (usually) MLC-identical nonrelated donor, usually identified through the National Marrow Donor Program. This has been used with success in children with SCID, the Chédiak-Higashi syndrome, and WAS (Filipovich et al., 1992; Lenarsky et al., 1993). Powerful immunosuppressives before and after the procedure are necessary, because the marrow is not T-depleted.

Cord Blood Transplants

A matched HLA-identical cord blood transplant is rarely available, but in utero HLA typing was used to identify a match for a child with WAS (Ochs, 2003, personal communication). With increasing use of cord blood banks, a matched sibling cord blood could be used.

Unrelated umbilical cord cells from one of the cord blood banks can also be used as an alternative to a haploidentical transplantation or a matched unrelated marrow transplant from the bone marrow transplant registry. Cord bloods matched in at least three of six HLA loci without T-cell depletion have been used successfully in several primary immunodeficiencies, including SCID, HIGM1 syndrome, WAS, and X-linked lymphoproliferative syndrome (Ziegner et al., 2001). In the latter disease, cord cells may be preferable because they are EBV negative.

Gene Therapy

Successful gene therapy necessitates identification and cloning of the gene lacking or abnormal in the disorder under question, such as ADA deficiency, X-linked SCID, one or more of the genetic variants CGD, and LAD-1. The isolated gene is inserted into peripheral leukocytes or bone marrow stem cells using a viral vector. The cells are then infused back into the patient and the patient is monitored for clinical improvement, immunologic restoration, and gene expression.

The first attempts were in patients with the ADA form of combined immunodeficiency in 1990 (Blaese, 1993) (see Chapter 16). Although prolonged survival of the gene-corrected T cells were identified, the patients continued to receive polyethylene glycol adenosine deaminase and clinical benefit was unproven. Aiuti and co-workers (2003) have reported successful gene therapy in ADA deficiency with discontinuation of enzyme replacement therapy.

Casazzana-Colvo (2000) succeeded in showing clearcut clinical benefit in gene therapy for X-linked SCID (IL-2 receptor gamma chain defect). Most infants so treated have restored immune systems and are off of IVIG replacement therapy. However, the occurrence of lymphoproliferative disease in two of the infants has led to interruption of further trials (see Chapter 15).

Gene therapy may be anticipated for other primary immunodeficiencies in which the gene defect has been identified such as other forms of combined immunodeficiency (see Chapter 15), XLA, and the HIGM1.

PROGNOSIS

The short-term prognosis depends on the severity of the infectious complications. The long-term prognosis is determined by the nature of the defect. Patients with cellular and combined immunodeficiencies usually have the poorest prognosis unless successful transplantation is achieved. Although acute infectious episodes can be controlled with antibiotics, chronic tissue damage, such as necrotizing colitis or bronchiectasis, may not be prevented.

The registry data suggest that patients are living longer inasmuch as half of the patients are adults. Further successfully transplanted patients with serious life-threatening illnesses are now disease free or markedly improved.

In the past, Gabrielson and associates (1969) estimated that one third of their patients died prematurely from infectious complications. Among patients with antibody immunodeficiency studied by the Medical Research Council Working Party (1969), the overall mortality was 29% (51 of 176 patients) and 14% died within 6 months of diagnosis. All 11 patients with combined immunodeficiency succumbed rapidly. The mortality for infants younger than 1 year of age was 45%, compared with 11% for older patients. Among eight patients older than age 2 years who stopped receiving gamma globulin therapy, five died shortly thereafter. The outlook for long-term survival is considerably better nowadays.

Cunningham-Rundles (1989) reported an overall mortality rate of 22% in 103 patients with CVID followed over a 13-year period. Males died at an earlier age (28.9 years) than females (55.4 years).

COMPLICATIONS

Complications other than bacterial infections include arthritis, amyloidosis, chronic hepatitis, sclerosing cholangitis, chronic lung disease, malignancy, and psychosocial problems. If live vaccines are given, systemic BCG infection, vaccinia gangrenosa, paralytic poliomyelitis, or giant cell (measles) pneumonia may develop in these patients.

There is a high incidence of lymphoreticular malignancy in certain primary immunodeficiencies, notably ataxia-telangiectasia, WAS, and CVID (see Chapter 39). Indeed, malignancy is the second leading cause of death after infections in immunodeficiency (see Chapter 39). Occasionally, the onset of immunodeficiency and malignancy is simultaneous; usually, however, the immunodeficiency precedes the malignancy by several years.

RECOVERY

An occasional adult may spontaneously recover the ability to synthesize antibody. In 3 (of 176) adult females in the Medical Research Council Working Party (1969) study, antibody function returned.

Hirschhorn and associates (1994) reported a young adult who had combined immunodeficiency resulting from ADA deficiency diagnosed at age 2 who spontaneously recovered because of somatic mosaicism and proliferation of a spontaneously appearing cell line with normal ADA activity.

A 36-year-old man with common variable hypogammaglobulinemia (CVID) diagnosed at age 24 showed normalization of antibody responsiveness and Ig levels following acquisition of HIV infection at age 30 (Wright et al., 1987). Another CVID patient with HIV recovered IgG and IgM production and antibody function but not IgA production (Jolles et al., 2001). Two other cases have been reported (Morell et al., 1986, Webster et al., 1989).

Several patients with selective IgA deficiency may undergo spontaneous cure; most of these have low but measurable IgA and are children younger than 5 years (Blum et al., 1982). In general, the primary immunodeficiencies are lifelong, incurable, and associated with a guarded prognosis for extended life.

REGISTRIES AND DATABASES

There are several registries for immune-deficient patients, including ones that are country- or region-wide (e.g., European Society for Immunodeficiency, The Latin American Registry) as well as disease-specific registries for XLA, HIGM1 syndrome, CGD, and other specific diseases. Some of these detail the specific types of mutations in individual patients. There also is a registry for malignancies in primary immunodeficiency. These registries are useful in genetic studies, prognostic studies and epidemiologic studies. They also allow access to special studies and therapies. Mutation databases for various immunodeficiencies are described by Vihinen and colleagues (1999).

Several professional organizations have a special interest in immunodeficiency, including the US Clinical Immunology Society, the European Society for Immunodeficiency, and the Pan American Society for Immunodeficiency.

SUPPORT ORGANIZATIONS

Two organizations are active for patients with primary immunodeficiency in the United States. These are the parent-based IDF, Courthouse Square, 3565 Ellicott Drive, Unit B2, Ellicott City, MD 21043 (1-800-296-4433); and the Jeffrey Modell Foundation, 43 W. 47th Street, New York, 10036 (1-800-JEFF-844). Similar organizations are available in Europe (Table 12-24).

The IDF has regional chapters in many areas and offers free publications for physicians, nurses, and patients (including children) on immunodeficiency. Both foundations sponsor parent support groups, research meetings, and physician fellowships. The IDF also provides scholarships for patients and helps with insurance and access to care issues.

FINANCIAL IMPLICATIONS

Among the patients surveyed by the IDF (1999), 52% had been hospitalized at some time; 25% were hospitalized in the last year. Of these patients, 58% had current physical limitations (30% moderate or severe), 60% had difficulty with insurance coverage, and 40% used savings for medical expenses.

These data indicate that primary immunodeficiency are not confined to pediatric populations, are more common than previously ascertained, and are a significant physical and financial burden to patients and their families. The need for expensive drugs, notably IVIG, antibiotics, and cytokines are a significant cost to the health care system.

R E F E R E N C E S

Ackeret C, Pluss HJ, Hitzig WH. Hereditary severe combined immunodeficiency and adenosine deaminase deficiency. Pediatr Res 10:67–70, 1976.

Affentranger P, Morell A, Spath P, Seger R. Registry of primary immunodeficiencies in Switzerland. Immunodeficiency 4:193–195, 1993.

Afzelius BA. A human syndrome caused by immobile cilia. Science 193:31–319, 1976.

Aiuti F, Businco L, Fiorilli M, Galli E, Quinti I, Rossi P, Seminara R, Goldstein G. Thymopoietin pentapeptide treatment of primary immunodeficiencies. Lancet 1:551–554, 1983.

Aiuti F, Sirianni MC, Fiorilli M, Paganelli R, Stella A, Turbessi G. A placebo-controlled trial of thymic hormone treatment of recurrent herpes simplex labialis infection in immunodeficient host: Results after a 1-year follow-up. Clin Immunol Immunopathol 30:11–18, 1984.

Aiuti A, Vai S, Mortellaro A, Casorati G, Ficara F, Andolfi G, Ferrari G, Tabucchi A, Carlucci F, Ochs HD, Notarangelo LD, Roncarolo MG, Bordignon C. Immune reconstitution in ADA-SCID after PBL gene therapy and discontinuation of enzyme replacement. Nat Med 8:423–5, 2002.

Alarcon B, Regueiro JR, Arnaiz-Villena A, Terhorst C. Familial defect in the surface expression of the T-cell receptor-CD3 complex. N Engl J Med 319:1203–1208, 1988.

Albrecht RM, Hong R. Basic and clinical consideration of the monocyte-macrophage system in man. J Pediatr 88:751–765, 1976.

Allen JC, Kunkel HG. Antibodies against gamma-globulin after repeated blood transfusions in man. J Clin Invest 45:29–39, 1966.

Allen RC, Armitage RJ, Conley ME, Rosenblatt H, Jenkins NA, Copeland NG, Bedell MA, Edelhoff S, Disteche CM, Simoneaux DK, Fanslow WC, Belmont JW, Spriggs MK. CD40 Ligand gene defects responsible for X-linked hyper-IgM syndrome. Science 259:990–993, 1993.

Allen RC, Nachtman RC, Rosenblatt HM, Belmont JW. Application of carrier testing to genetic counseling for X-linked agammaglobulinemia. Am J Hum Genet 54:25–35, 1994.

Allen RC, Stjernholm RL, Steele RH. Evidence for the generation of an electronic excitation state in human polymorphonuclear leukocytes and its participation in bactericidal activity. Biochem Biophys Res Comm 47:679–684, 1972.

Alper CA, Rosen FS. Complement in laboratory medicine. In Vyas GN, Stites DP, Brecher G, eds. Laboratory Diagnosis of Immunologic Disorders. New York, Grune & Stratton, 1975, pp 47–68.

TABLE 12-24 · ADDRESSES AND WEB SITES FOR IMMUNODEFICIENCY SUPPORT GROUPS

TABLE 12-24 · ADDRESSES AND WEB SITES FOR IMMUNODEFICIENCY SUPPORT GROUPS

International Patient Organisation for Primary Immunodeficiencies—General Secretary: Mr. Keith Gray, PIA, 12 Caxton Way, London, UK

National Immune Deficiency Foundation, 25 W. Chesapeake Avenue, Suite 206, Towson, MD 21204; USA telephone 1-800-296-4433

Jeffrey Modell Foundation, 43 W. 47th Street, New York, NY 10036 www.info4pi.org; telephone 1-866-INFO-4-PI

Primary Immunodeficiency Association, PiA, 12 Caxton Way, London, UK

Ataxia-Telangiectasia Children's Project, 6685 S. Military Tr., Deerfield Beach, FL 33442 USA www.atcp.org

National Organization for Rare Disorders, PO Box 8922, New Fairfield, CT 06812-8923 USA www.rarediseases.org

Amer J, Ott E, Ibbott FA, O'Brien D, Kempe H. The effect of monthly gamma-globulin administration on morbidity and mortality from infection in premature infants during the first year of life. Pediatrics 32:4–9, 1963.

American Academy of Pediatrics. Immunization in special clinical circumstances. In Pickering LK, ed. 2000 Red Book Report of the Committee on Infectious Diseases, ed 25. Elk Grove Village, IL, American Academy of Pediatrics, 2000, pp 54-61.

Ammann AJ, Wara DW, Salmon S, Perkins HL. Thymus transplantation: permanent reconstitution of cellular immunity in a patient with sex-linked combined immunodeficiency. N Engl J Med 289:5–9, 1973.

Ammann AJ, Ashman RF, Buckley RH, Hardie WR, Krantman HJ, Nelson J, Ochs H, Stiehm ER, Tiller T, Wara DW, Wedgwood R. Use of intravenous gamma globulin in antibody immunodeficiency. Results of a multicenter controlled trial. Clin Immunol Immunopathol 22:60–67, 1982a.

Ammann AJ, Wara DW, Cowan MJ, Barrett DJ, Stiehm ER. The DiGeorge syndrome and the fetal alcohol syndrome. Am J Dis Child 136:906–908, 1982b.

Anderson DC, Schmalstieg FC, Arnaout MA, Kohl S, Tosi MF, Dapa N, Buffone GJ, Hughes BJ, Brinkley BR, Dickey WD, Abramson JS, Springer T, Boxer LA, Hollers JM, Smith CW. Abnormalities of polymorphonuclear leukocyte function associated with a heritable deficiency of high molecular weight surface glycoproteins (GP138): common relationship to diminished cell adherence. J Clin Invest 74:536–551, 1984.

Anderson WF. Prospects of human gene therapy. Science 226:401–409, 1984.

Apfelzweig R, Piszkiewicz D, Hooper JA. Immunoglobulin A concentrations in commercial immune globulins. J Clin Immunol 7:46–50, 1987.

Arditi M, Kabat W, Togev BS, Yogev R. Serum tumor necrosis factor alpha, interleukin 1-beta, p24 antigen concentrations and CD4+ cells at various stages of human immunodeficiency virus 1 infection in children. Pediatr Infect Dis J 10:450–455, 1991.

Arnaiz-Villena A, Timon M, Corell A, Perez-Aciego P, Martin-Villa JM, Regueiro JR. Primary immunodeficiency caused by mutations in the gene encoding the CD3-γ subunit of the T-lymphocyte receptor. N Engl J Med 327:529–533, 1992.

Arpaia E, Sharar M, Dadi H, Cohen A, Roifman CM. Defective T-cell receptor signaling and CD8+ thymic selection in humans lacking Zap-70 kinase. Cell 76:947–958, 1994.

Asano Y, Yoshikawa T, Suga S, Kobayashi I, Nakashima T, Yazaki T, Ozaki T, Yamada A, Imanishi J. Postexposure prophylaxis of varicella in family contact by oral acyclovir. Pediatrics 92:219–222, 1993.

August CS, Levey RH, Berkel AI, Rosen FS. Establishment of immunological competence in a child with congenital thymic aplasia by a graft of fetal thymus. Lancet 1:1080–1083, 1970.

Avella J, Madsen JE, Binder HJ, Askenase PW. Effect of histamine H2-receptor antagonists on delayed hypersensitivity. Lancet 1:624–626, 1978.

Bach FH, Albertini RJ, Anderson JL, Joo P, Bortin MM. Bone-marrow transplantation in a patient with the Wiskott-Aldrich syndrome. Lancet 2:1364-1366, 1968.

Baehner RL, Nathan DG. Quantitative nitroblue tetrazolium test in chronic granulomatous disease. N Engl J Med 278:971–980, 1968.

Baker DH, Parmer EA, Wolff JA. Roentgen manifestation of the Aldrich syndrome. Am J Roentgenol 88:458–465, 1962.

Ballow M, Cater KL, Rowe JC, Goetz C, Desbonnet C. Development of the immune system in very low birth weight (less than 1500 g) premature infants: concentrations of plasma immunoglobulins and patterns of infections. Pediatr Res 20:899–904, 1986.

Barandun S, Kistler P, Jeunet F, Isliker H. Intravenous administration of human γ-globulin. Vox Sang 7:157–174, 1962.

Bardelas JA, Winkelstein, JA, Seto, DSY, Tsai T, Rogol AD. Fatal ECHO 24 infection in a patient with hypogammaglobulinemia: relationship to dermatomyositis-like syndrome. J Pediatr 90:396–401, 1977.

Barton JC, Herrera GA, Galla JH, Bertoli LF, Work J, Koopman WJ. Acute cryoglobulinemic renal failure after intravenous infusion of gamma globulin. Am J Med 82:624–629, 1987.

Baumgart KW, Britton WJ, Kemp A, French M, Roberton D. The spectrum of primary immunodeficiency disorders in Australia. J Allergy Clin Immunol 100:415–23, 1997.

Baumgartner JD, Glauser MP, McCutchan JA, Ziegler EJ, van Melle G, Klauber MR, Vogt M, Muehlen E, Luethy R, Chiolero R. Prevention of gram negative-shock and death in surgical patients by antibody to endotoxin core glycolipid. Lancet 2:59–63, 1985.

Berendes H, Bridges RA, Good RA. A fatal granulomatous disease of childhood: the clinical study of a new syndrome. Minn Med 40:309–312, 1957.

Berger M, Cupps TR, Fauci A. Immunoglobulin replacement therapy by slow subcutaneous infusion. Ann Intern Med 93:55–56, 1980.

Bernatowska E, Madalinski K, Janowicz W, Weremowicz R, Gutkowski P, Wolf HM, Eibl MM. Results of a prospective controlled two-dose crossover study with intravenous immunoglobulin and comparison (retrospective) with plasma treatment. Clin Immunol Immunopath 43:153–162, 1987.

Bernstein LJ, Krieger BZ, Novic B, Sicklick MJ, Runinstien A. Bacterial infections in acquired immunodeficiency syndrome of children. Pediatr Infect Dis 4:472–475, 1985.

Bjorkander J, Hammarstrom L, Smith CIE, Buckley RH, Cunningham-Rundles C, Hanson LA. Immunoglobulin prophylaxis in patients with antibody deficiency syndromes and anti-IgA antibodies. J Clin Immunol 7:8–15, 1987.

Bjoro K, Froland SS, Yun Z, Samdal HH, Haaland T. Hepatitis C infection in patients with contaminated immune globulin. N Engl J Med 331 :1607–1611, 1994.

Blaese RM. Development of gene therapy for immunodeficiency: adenosine deaminase deficiency. Pediatr Res 33(suppl):S49–S55, 1993.

Blum PM, Hong R, Stiehm ER. Spontaneous recovery of selective IgA deficiency: additional case report and a review. Clin Pediatr 21:77–80, 1982.

Blume RS, Beanett JM, Yankee RA, Wolff SM. Defective granulocyte regulation in the Chédiak-Higashi syndrome. N Engl J Med 279:1009–1015, 1968.

Boggs DP. Transfusions of neutrophils as prevention or treatment of infection in patients with neutropenia. N Engl J Med 290:1055–1062, 1974.

Bonilla MA, Gillio AP, Ruggeiro M, Kernan NA, Brochstein JA, Abboud M, Fumagalli L, Vincent M, Gabrilove JL, Welte K, Souza LM, O'Reilly RJ. Effects of recombinant human granulocyte colony-stimulating factor on neutropenia in patients with congenital agranulocytosis. N Engl J Med 320:1574–1580, 1989.

Bordigoni P, Faure G, Bene MC, Dardenne M, Bach JF, Duheille J. Improvement of cellular immunity and IgA production in immunodeficient children after treatment with synthetic serum thymic factor (FTS). Lancet 2:293–297, 1982.

Borowitz SM, Saulsbury FT. Treatment of chronic cryptosporidial infection with orally administered human serum immune globulin. J Pediatr 119:593–595, 1991.

Borut TC, Ank BJ, Gard SE, Stiehm ER. Tetanus toxoid skin test in children: correlation with in vitro lymphocyte stimulation and monocyte chemotaxis. J Pediatr 97:567–573, 1980.

Borzy MS, Hong R, Horowitz SD, Gilbert E, Kaufman D, DeMendonca W, Oxelius VA, Dictor M, Pachman L. Fatal lymphoma after transplantation of cultured thymus in children with combined immunodeficiency disease. N Engl J Med 301:565–568, 1979a.

Borzy MS, Schulte-Wissermann H, Gilbert E, Horowitz SD, Pellett J, Hong R. Thymic morphology in immunodeficiency diseases: results of thymic biopsies. Clin Immunol Immunopathol 12:31–51, 1979b.

Boxer LA, Watanabe AM, Rister M, Besch HR Jr, Allen J, Baehner RL. Correction of leukocyte function in Chédiak-Higashi syndrome by ascorbate. N Engl J Med 293:1041–1045, 1976.

Boyden S. The chemotactic effect of mixtures of antibody and antigen on polymorphonuclear leukocytes. J Exp Med 115:453–466, 1962.

Brandtzaeg P, Fjellanger I, Gjeruldsen ST. Immunoglobulin M: local synthesis and selective secretion in patients with immunoglobulin A deficiency. Science 160:789–791, 1968.

Brooks EG, Filipovich AH, Padgett JW, Mamlock R, Goldblum RM. T-cell receptor analysis in Omenn's syndrome: evidence for defects in gene rearrangement and assembly. Blood, 93:242–250, 1999.

Bruton OC. Agammaglobulinemia. Pediatrics 9:722–728, 1952.

Buckley RH. Plasma therapy in immunodeficiency diseases. Am J Dis Child 124:376–381, 1972.

Buckley RH, Fiscus SA. Serum IgD and IgE concentrations in immunodeficiency diseases. J Clin Invest 55:157–65, 1975.

Buckley RH, Gilbertsen RB, Schiff RI, Ferreira E, Sanal SO, Waldmann TA. Heterogeneity of lymphocyte subpopulations in severe combined immunodeficiency. J Clin Invest 58:130–136, 1976a.

Buckley RH, Whisnant JK, Schiff RI, Gilbertsen RB, Huang AT, Platt MS. Correction of severe combined immunodeficiency by fetal liver cells. N Engl J Med 294:1076–1082, 1976b.

Buckley RH, Schiff SE, Sampson HA, Schiff RI, Markert ML, Knutsen AP, Hershfield MS, Huang AT, Mickey GH, Ward FE. Development of immunity in human severe primary T cell deficiency following haploidentical bone marrow stem cell transplantation. J Immunol 136:2398–2407, 1986.

Buckley RH, Schiff SE, Schiff RI, Markert L, Williams LW, Roberts JL, Myers LA, Ward FE. Hematopoietic stem cell transplantation for the treatment of severe combined immunodeficiency. N Engl J Med 340:508–516, 1999.

Burks AW, Sampson HA, Buckley RH. Anaphylactic reactions after gamma globulin administration in patients with hypogammaglobulinemia. N Engl J Med 314:56–564, 1986.

Bussel JB, Himi JS. Isolated thrombocytopenia in patients infected with HIV: treatment with intravenous gammaglobulin. Am J Hematol 28:79–84, 1988.

Calandra T, Glauser MP, Schellekens J, Verhoef J. Treatment of gram negative septic shock with human IgG antibody to *Escherichia coli* J5: a prospective, double blind, randomized trial. J Infect Dis 158:312–319, 1988.

Calvelli TA, Rubinstein A. Intravenous gamma globulin in infant acquired immunodeficiency syndrome. Pediatr Infect Dis 5:S207–S210, 1986.

Campbell JJ, Butcher EC. Chemokines in tissue-specific and microenvironment-specific lymphocyte homing. Curr Opin Immunol 12:336–41, 2000.

Cannon RA, Blum PM, Ament ME, Byrne WJ, Soderberg-Warner M, Seeger RC, Saxon AE, Stiehm ER. Reversal of enterocolitis-associated combined immunodeficiency by plasma therapy. J Pediatr 101:711–717, 1982.

Cavazzana-Calvo M, Hacein-Bey S, de Saint Basile G, Gross F, Yvon E, Nusbaum P, Selz F, Hue C, Certain S, Casonova JL, Bousso P, LeDeist F, Fischer A. Gene therapy of human severe combined immunodeficiency (SCID-X) disease. Science 288:669–672, 2000.

Centers for Disease Control. Guidelines for prophylaxis against *Pneumocystis carinii* pneumonia for children infected with human immunodeficiency virus. MMWR 40:1–11, 1991.

Centers for Disease Control. Outbreak of hepatitis C associated with intravenous immunoglobulin administration—United States, Oct 1993–June 1994. MMWR 43:505–509, 1994.

Cham B, Bonilla MA, Winkelstein JA. Neutropenia associated with primary immunodeficiency diseases. Semin Hematol 39:107–113, 2002.

Chandra RK. Fetal malnutrition and postnatal immunocompetence. Am J Dis Child 129:450–454, 1975.

Chapel HM, Lee M, Hargreaves R, Pamphilon DH, Prentice AG. Randomized trial of intravenous immunoglobulin as prophylaxis against infection in plateau-phase multiple myeloma. Lancet 343:1059–1063, 1994.

Chapel H, Christie J, Peach V, Chapman R. Five year follow-up of patients with primary antibody deficiencies following an outbreak of acute hepatitis C. Clin Immunol 99:320–324, 2001

Chapel H, Geha R, Rosen F; IUIS PID (Primary Immunodeficiencies) Classification committee. Primary immunodeficiency diseases: an update. Clin Exp Immunol 132:9–15, 2003.

Chesky M, Scalco R, Failace L, Read S, Jobim LF. Polymerase chain reaction for the laboratory diagnosis of aseptic meningitis and encephalitis. Arq-Neuropsiquiatr 58:836–42, 2000.

Cleveland WW, Fogel BJ, Brown WT, Kay HEM. Foetal thymic transplant in a case of DiGeorge's syndrome. Lancet 2:1211–1214, 1968.

Cline MJ, Opelz G, Saxon A, Fahey JL, Golde DW. Autoimmune panleukopenia. N Engl J Med 295:1489–1493, 1976.

Comenzo RL, Malachowski ME, Meissner HC, Fulton DR, Berkman EM. Immune hemolysis, disseminated intravascular coagulation, and serum sickness after large doses of immune globulin given intravenously for Kawasaki disease. J Pediatr 120:926–928, 1992.

Conley ME. Molecular approaches to analysis of X-linked immunodeficiencies. Annu Rev Immunol 10:215–238, 1992.

Conley ME, Notarangelo LD, Etzioni A. Diagnostic criteria for primary immunodeficiencies. Clin Immunol 93:190–197, 1999.

Conley ME, Nowell PC, Henle G, Douglas SD. XX T cells and XY B cells in two patients with severe combined immune deficiency. Clin Immunol Immunopathol 31:87–95, 1984.

Conley ME, Park CL, Douglas SD. Childhood variable immunodeficiency with autoimmune disease. J Pediatr 108:915-922, 1986.

Conway SP, Gillies DRN, Docherty A. Neonatal infection in premature infants and use of human immunoglobulin. Arch Dis Child 62:1252–1256, 1987.

Cooper MR, DeChatelet LD, LaVia MF, McCall CE, Spurr CL, Baehner RL. Complete deficiency of leukocyte glucose-6-phosphate dehydrogenase with defective bactericidal activity. J Clin Invest 51:769–778, 1972.

Cooperative Group for the Study of Immunoglobulin in Chronic Lymphocytic Leukemia: Intravenous immunoglobulin for the prevention of infection in chronic lymphocytic leukemia. N Engl J Med 319:902–907, 1988.

Copeland EA, Strohm PL, Kennedy MS, Tutschka PJ. Hemolysis following intravenous immune globulin therapy. Transfusion 26:410–412, 1986.

Copelon EA, Tutschka PJ. Immunoglobulin in bone marrow transplantation. In Morell A and Nydegger UE, eds. Clinical Use of Intravenous Immunoglobulins. New York Academic Press, 1986, pp 117–121

Cottier H, Turk J, Sobin L. Propositions en vue de standardiser la description histologique du ganglion lymphatique humain dans ses rapports avec la fonction immunologique. Bull WHO 47:409–417, 1972.

Cowan MJ, Wara DW, Packman S, Ammann AJ. Multiple biotin-dependent carboxylase deficiencies associated with defects in T cell and B cell immunity. Lancet 2:117–119, 1979.

Cowan MJ, Wara DW, Weintrub PS, Pabst H, Ammann AJ. Haploidentical bone marrow transplantation for severe combined immunodeficiency disease using soybean agglutinin-negative, T-depleted marrow cells. J Clin Immunol 5:370–376, 1985.

Crennan JM, Van Scoy RE, McKenna CH, Smith TF. Echovirus polymyositis in patients with hypogammaglobulinemia: failure of high dose intravenous gammaglobulin therapy and review of the literature. Am J Med 81:35–42, 1986.

Cunningham CK, Bonville CA, Ochs, HD, Seyama K, John PA, Rotbart HA, Weiner LB. Enterovirus meningoencephalitis as a complication of X-linked hyper-IgM syndrome. J Pediatr 134:584–588, 1999.

Cunningham-Rundles C. Clinical and immunologic analyses of 103 patients with common variable immunodeficiency. J Clin Immunol 9:22–33, 1989.

Cunningham-Rundles C, Bodian C. Common variable immunodeficiency: clinical and immunologic features of 248 patients. Clin Immunol 92:34–48, 1999.

Cunningham-Rundles C, Bodian C, Ochs HD, Martin S, Reiter-Wong M, Zhao Z. Long-term low-dose IL-2 enhances immune function in common variable immunodeficiency. Clin Immunol 100:181–190, 2001.

Cunningham-Rundles C, Kazbay K, Hassett J, Zhou Z, Mayer L. Enhanced humoral immunity in common variable immunodeficiency after long-term treatment with polyethylene glycol-conjugated interleukin-2. N Engl J Med 331:918–921, 1994.

Curnutte JT. Chronic granulomatous disease: the solving of a clinical riddle at the molecular level. Clin Immunol Immunopathol 67:S2–S15, 1993.

Dadi HK, Simon AJ, Roifman CM. Effect of CD3δ deficiency on maturation of α/β and γ/δ T-cell lineages in severe combined immunodeficiency. N Engl J Med 349:1821–1828, 2003.

Daly PB, Evans JH, Kobayashi RH, Kobayashi AL, Ochs HD, Fischer SH, Pirofsky B, Sprouse C. Home-based immunoglobulin infusion therapy: quality of life and patient health perceptions. Ann Allergy 67:504–510, 1991.

Davies EG, Thrasher A, Lacey K, Harper J. Topical cidofovir for severe molluscum cantagiosum. Lancet 353:2042, 1999.

Davis SD, Schaller J, Wedgwood RJ. Antibody deficiency syndromes. In Kagan BM, Stiehm ER, eds. Immunologic Incompetence. Chicago, Year Book Medical Publishers, 1971, pp 179–189.

Debray D, Pariente D, Urvoas E, Hadchouel M, Bernard O. Sclerosing cholangitis in children. J Pediatr 124:49–56, 1994.

DeChatelet LP, Shirley PS, McPhail LC. Normal leukocyte glutathione peroxidase activity in patients with chronic granulomatous disease. J Pediatr 89:598–600, 1976.

DeCree J, Verhaegen H, DeCock W, Vanheule R, Brugmans J, Schuermans V. Impaired neutrophil phagocytosis. Lancet 2:294–295, 1974.

de la Salle H, Hanau D, Fricker D, Urlacher A, Kelly A, Salamero J, Powis SH, Donato L, Bausinger H, Laforet M, Jeras M, Spehner D, Bieber T, Falkenrodt A, Cazenave JP, Trowsdale J, Tongio MM. Homozygous human TAP peptide transporter mutation in HLA class 1 deficiency. Science 265:237–241, 1994.

De Libero. Sentinel function of broadly reactive human gamma delta T cells. Immunol Today 18:22–6, 1997.

DeSimone C, Delogu G, Corbetta G. Intravenous immunoglobulins in association with antibiotics: a therapeutic trial in septic intensive care unit patients. Crit Care Med 16:23–26, 1988.

De Ugarte DA, Roberts RL, Lerdluedeeporn P, Stiehm ER, Atkinson JB. Treatment of chronic wounds by local delivery of granulocyte-macrophage colony-stimulating factor in patients with neutrophil dysfunction. Pediatr Surg Int 18:517–20, 2002.

Diamond EF, Purugganan HB, Choi HJ. Effect of prophylactic administration on infection morbidity in premature infants. Illinois Med J 130:668–670, 1966.

Douek DC, Koup RA, McFarland RD, Sullivan JL, Luzuriaga K. Effect of HIV on thymic function before and after antiretroviral therapy in children. J Infect Dis181:1479–1482, 2000.

Douek DC, McFarland RD, Keiser PH, Gage EA, Massey JM, Haynes BF, Polis MA, Haase AT, Feinberg MB, Sullivan JL, Jamieson BD, Zack JA, Picker LJ, Koup RA. Changes in thymic function with age during the treatment of HIV infection. Nature 396:690–695, 1998.

Douzinas EE, Pitaridis MT, Louris G, Andrianakis I, Katsouyanni K, Karmpaliotis D, Economidou J, Syfras D, Roussos C. Prevention of infection in multiple trauma patients by high-dose intravenous immunoglobulins. Crit Care Med 28:8–15, 2000.

Drenth JPH, Haagsma CJ, van der Meer JWM, the International Hyper-IgD Study Group. Hyperimmunoglobulinemia D and periodic fever syndrome: the clinical spectrum in a series of 50 patients. Medicine 73:133–144, 1994.

Driscoll DA, Budarf ML, Emanuel BS. A genetic etiology for DiGeorge syndrome: consistent deletions and microdeletions of 22q11. Am J Hum Genet 50:924–933, 1992.

Dror Y, Freedman MH. Schwachman-Diamond syndrome marrow cells show increased apoptosis through the Fas pathway. Blood 97:3011–3016, 2001.

Durandy A, Schiff C, Bonnefoy JY, Forveille M, Rousset F, Mazzei G, Milili M, Fischer A. Induction by anti-CD40 antibody or soluble CD40 ligand and cytokines of IgG, IgA, and IgE production by B cells from patients with X-linked hyper-IgM syndrome. Eur J Immunol 23:2294–2299, 1993

Eijkhout HW, van Der Meer JW, Kallenberg CG, Weening RS, van Dissel JT, Sanders LA, Strengers PF, Nienhuis H, Schellekens PT; Inter-University Working Party for the Study of Immune Deficiencies. The effect of two different dosages of intravenous immunoglobulin on the incidence of recurrent infections in patients with primary hypogammaglobuinemia: a randomized, double-blind, multicenter crossover trial. Ann Intern Med 135:165–74, 2001.

Ellis EF, Henney CS. Adverse reactions following administration of human gammaglobulin. J Allergy 43:45–54, 1969.

Fanconi S, Seger R, Gmür J, Willi U, Schaer G, Spiess H, Otto R, Hitzig WH. Surgery and granulocyte transfusions for life-threatening infections in chronic granulomatous disease. Helv Paediatr Acta 40:277–284, 1985.

Fasano MB, Sullivan KE, Sarpong SB, Wood RA, Jones SM, Johns CH, Lederman HM, Bydowsky MH, Greene JM, Winkelstein JA. Sarcoidosis and common variable immunodeficiency. Medicine 75:251–259, 1996.

Figueroa JE, Densen P. Infectious diseases associated with complement deficiencies. Clin Microbiol Rev 4:359–395, 1991.

Filipovich AH, Shapiro RS, Ramsay NKC, Kim T, Blazar B, Kersey J, McGlave P. Unrelated donor bone marrow transplantation for correction of lethal congenital immunodeficiencies. Blood 80:270–276, 1992.

Fisch P, Millner M, Muller SM, Wahn U, Friedrich W, Renz H. Expansion of _ T cells in an infant with severe combined immunodeficiency syndrome after disseminated BCG infection and bone marrow transplantation. J Allergy Clin Immunol 103:1218–1219, 1999.

Fischer A, Landais P, Friedrich W, Gerritsen B, Fasth A, Porta F, Vellodi A, Benkerrou M, Jais JP, Cavazzana-Calvo M, Souillet G, Bordigoni P, Morgan G, VanDijken P, Vossen J, Locateli F, di Bartolomeo P. Bone marrow transplantation (BMT) in Europe for primary immunodeficiencies other than severe combined immunodeficiency: a report from the European group for BMT and the European group for immunodeficiency. Blood 83:1144–1154, 1994.

Flake AW, Zanjani ED. In utero hematopoietic stem cell transplantation: a status report. JAMA 278:932–937, 1997.

Fletcher MA, Baron GC, Ashman MR, Fischl MA, Kimas NG. Use of whole blood methods in assessment of immune parameters in immunodeficiency states. Diagn Clin Immunol 5:69–81, 1987.

Franz A, Webster AD, Furr PM, Taylor-Robinson D. Mycoplasmal arthritis in patients with primary immunoglobulin deficiency: clinical outcome in 18 patients. Br J Rheumatol 36:551–668, 1997.

Friedrich W, Goldman SF, Ebell W, Blutters-Sawatzki R, Gaedicke G, Raghavachar A, Peter HH, Belohradsky B, Kreth W, Kubanek B, Kleihauer E. Severe combined immunodeficiency: treatment by bone marrow transplantation in 15 infants using HLA-haploidentical donors. Eur J Pediatr 144:125–130, 1985.

Fudenberg HH, Fudenberg BR. Antibody to hereditary human gamma-globulin (Gm) factor resulting from maternal-fetal incompatibility. Science 145:170, 1964.

Gabrielson AE, Cooper MD, Peterson RDA, Good RA. The primary immunologic deficiency diseases. In Meischer PA, Muller-Eberhard HJ, eds. Textbook of Immunopathology, vol 2. New York, Grune & Stratton, 1969, pp 385–405.

Gallin JI. Interferon-γ in the treatment of the chronic granulomatous diseases of childhood. Clin Immunol Immunopath 61:S100–S105, 1991.

Gallin JI, Clark RA, Kimball HR. Granulocyte chemotaxis: an improved in vitro assay employing 51Cr-labeled granulocytes. J Immunol 110:233–240, 1973.

Gallin JI, Elin RJ, Hubert RT, Fauci AS, Kaliner MA, Wolff SM. Efficacy of ascorbic acid in Chédiak-Higashi syndrome (CHS). Studies in humans and mice. Blood 53:226–234, 1979.

Gallin JI, Alling DW, Malech HL, Wesley R, Koziol D, Marciano B, Eisenstein EM, Turner ML, DeCarlo ES, Starling JM, Holland SM. Itraconazole to prevent fungal infections in chronic granulomatous disease. N Engl J Med 348:2416–22, 2003.

Gamm H, Huber Ch, Chapel H, Lee M, Ries F, Dicato MA. Intravenous immune globulin in chronic lymphocytic leukemia. Clin Exp Immunol 97(suppl):17–20, 1994.

Gardulf A, Anderson V, Bjorkander J, Ericson D, Froland SS, Gustafson R, Hammarstrom L, Jacobsen MB, Jonsson E, Moller G, Nystrom T, Soeberg V, Smith CIE. Subcutaneous immunoglobulin replacement in patients with primary antibody deficiencies: safety and costs. Lancet 345:365–369, 1995.

Gardulf A, Hammarström L, Smith CIE. Home treatment of hypogammaglobulinemia with subcutaneous gammaglobulin by rapid infusion. Lancet 338:162-166, 1991.

Gatti RA, Meuwissen HJ, Allen HD, Hong R, Good RA. Immunological reconstitution of sex-linked lymphopenic immunological deficiency. Lancet 2:1366–1369, 1968.

Gewurz H, Suyehira LA. Complement. In Rose NR, Friedman H, eds. Manual of Clinical Immunology. Washington, DC, American Society of Microbiology, 1976, pp 36–47.

Giblett ER, Ammann AJ, Wara DW, Sandman R, Diamond LK. Nucleoside-phosphorylase deficiency in a child with severely defective T-cell immunity and normal B-cell immunity. Lancet 1:1010–1014, 1975.

Glanzmann E, Riniker P. Essentielle lymphocytophthise. Ein neues Krankheitsbild aus der Sauglings-pathologie. Ann Paediatr (Basel) 175:1–32, 1950.

Glinz W, Grob PVJ, Nydegger UE, Ricklin T, Stamm F, Stoffel D, Lasance A. Polyvalent immunoglobulins for prophylaxis of bacterial infections in patients following multiple trauma. Intensive Care Med 11:288–294, 1985.

Goldsobel AB, Haas A, Stiehm ER. Bone marrow transplantation in DiGeorge syndrome. J Pediatr 111:40–44, 1987.

Goldstein AL, Slater FD, White A. Preparation, assay, and partial purification of a thymic lymphocytopoietic factor (thymosin). Proc Natl Acad Sci USA 56:1010–1017, 1966.

Gordon EH, Krause A, Kinney JL, Stiehm ER, Klaustermeyer WB. Delayed cutaneous hypersensitivity in normals: choice of antigens and comparison to in vitro assays of cell-mediated immunity. J Allergy Clin Immunol 72:487–494, 1983.

Graham-Pole J, Camitta B, Casper J, Elfenbein G, Gross S, Herzig R, Koch P, Mahoney D, Marcus R, Munoz L, et al. Intravenous immunoglobulin may lessen all forms of infection in patients receiving allogeneic bone marrow transplantation for acute lymphoblastic leukemia: a Pediatric Oncology Group study. Bone Marrow Transplant 3:559–566, 1988.

Greenberg F, Valdes C, Rosenblatt HM, Kirkland JL, Ledbetter DH. Hypoparathyroidism and T cell immune defect in a patient with 10p deletion syndrome. J Pediatr 109:489–492, 1986.

Grimbacher B, Holland SM, Gallin JI, Greenberg F, Hill SC, Malech HL, Miller JA, O'Connell AC, Puck JM. Hyper-IgE syndrome with recurrent infections–an autosomal dominant multisymptom disorder. N Engl J Med 340:692–702, 1999.

Grimm EA, Rosenberg SA. The human lymphokine-activated killer cell phenomenon. In Pick E, Landy M, eds. Lymphokines, vol 19. New York, Academic Press, 1984, pp 279–311.

Guglielmo BJ, Wong-Beringer A, Linker CA. Immune globulin therapy in allogeneic bone marrow transplant: a critical review. Bone Marrow Transplant 13:499–510, 1994.

Gupta JD, Reed CE. Natural antibodies to Salmonella enteritidis endotoxin in maternal and cord sera and in patients with immunologic deficiency diseases. Int Arch Allergy 34:324–330, 1968.

Hadden JW. Immunostimulants. Immunol Today 14:275–280, 1993.

Hammerschmidt PE, Bowers TK, Kammi-Kepfe CJ, Jacob HS, Craddock PR. Granulocyte aggregometry: a sensitive technique for the detection of C5a and complement activation. Blood 55:898–902, 1980.

Han BK, Suh YL, Yoon HK. Thymic ultrasound. I. Intrathymic anatomy in infants, Pediatr Radiol 31:474–479, 2001.

Haraldson A, Weemaes CMR, De Boer AW, Bakkeren JAJM, Stoelinga GBA. Immunological studies in the hyper-immunoglobulin D syndrome. J Clin Immunol 12:424–428, 1992.

Hayakawa H, Iwata T, Yata J, Kobayashi N. Primary immunodeficiency syndrome in Japan. I. Overview of a nationwide survey on primary immunodeficiency syndrome. J Clin Immunol 1:31–39, 1981.

Heiner DC, Myers AS, Beck CS. Deficiency of IgG4: disorder associated with frequent infections and bronchiectasis which may be familial. Clin Rev Allergy 1:259–266, 1983.

Herrod HG. Chronic mucocutaneous candidiasis in childhood and complications of non-Candida infection: a report of the Pediatric Immunodeficiency Collaborative Study Group. J Pediatr 116:377–382, 1990.

Hershfield MS. PED-ADA replacement therapy or adenosine deaminase deficiency: an update after 8.5 years. Clin Immunol Immunopath 76:S228–S232, 1995.

Hershfield MS, Buckley RH, Greenberg ML, Melton AL, Schiff R, Hatem C, Kurtzberg J, Markert ML, Kobayashi RH, Kobayashi AL, Abuchowski A. Treatment of adenosine deaminase deficiency with polyethylene glycol-modified adenosine deaminase. N Engl J Med 316:589–596, 1987.

Hill HR, Quie PG. Raised serum-IgE levels and defective neutrophil chemotaxis in three children with eczema and recurrent bacterial infections. Lancet 1:183–187, 1974.

Hirschhorn R, Beratis N, Rosen FS, Parkman R, Stern R, Polmar S. Adenosine-deaminase deficiency in a child diagnosed prenatally. Lancet 1:73–75, 1975.

Hirschhorn R, Yang DR, Israni A, Huie M, Ownby DR. Somatic mosaicism for a newly identified splice-site mutation in a patient with adenosine deaminase-deficient immunodeficiency and spontaneous clinical recovery. Am J Hum Genet 55:59–68, 1994.

Hitzig WH, Biro A, Bosch H, Huser HJ. Agammaglobulinamie und Almphozytose mit Schwund des lymphatischen Gewebes. Helv Paediatr Acta 13:551–585, 1958.

Hobbs JR. Disturbances of the immunoglobulins. Sci Basis Med Annu Rev 106–127, 1966.

Hohn DC, Lehrer RI. NADPH oxidase deficiency in X-linked chronic granulomatous disease. J Clin Invest 55:707–713, 1975.

Holmes B, Park BH, Malawista SE, Quie PG, Nelson DL, Good RA. Chronic granulomatous disease in females. A deficiency of leukocyte glutathione peroxidase. N Engl J Med 283:217–221, 1970.

Hong R, Santosham M, Schulte-Wisserman H, Horowitz S, Hsu SH, Winkelstein JA. Reconstitution of B and T lymphocyte function in severe combined immunodeficiency disease following transplantation with thymic epithelium. Lancet 2:1270–1272, 1976.

Hubel K, Dale DC, Liles WC. Granulocyte transfusion therapy: update on potential clinical applications. Curr Opin Hematol 8:161–4, 2001.

Hurvitz H, Ginat-Israeli T, Elpeleg ON, Klar A, Amir N. Biotinidase deficiency associated with severe combined immunodeficiency. Lancet 2:228–229, 1989.

Immune Deficiency Foundation. Primary immune deficiency diseases in America: the first national survey of patients and specialists. Immune Deficiency Foundation, Towson, MD, 1999, pp 1–17.

Incefy G, Dardenne M, Pahwa S, Grimes E, Pahwa PN, Smithwick E, O'Reilly R, Good RA. Thymic activity in severe combined immunodeficiency diseases. Proc Natl Acad Sci USA 74:1250–1253, 1977.

International Chronic Granulomatous Disease Cooperative Study Group. A controlled trial of interferon gamma to prevent infection in chronic granulomatous disease. N Engl J Med 324:509–16, 1991.

Intravenous Immunoglobulin Collaborative Study Group: Prophylactic intravenous administration of standard immune globulin as compared with core-lipopolysaccharide immune globulin in patients at high risk of postsurgical infection. N Engl J Med 327:234–240, 1991.

Intravenous Immunoglobulin Study Group: Intravenous immune globulin for the prevention of bacterial infections in children with symptomatic human immunodeficiency virus infection. N Engl J Med 325:73–80, 1991.

Ishizaka A, Nakanishi M, Kasahara E, Mizutani K, Sakiyama Y, Matsumoto S. Phenytoin-induced IgG2 and IgG4 deficiencies in a patient with epilepsy. Acta Paediatr 81:646–648, 1992.

Jenson, HB, Pollock BH. Meta-analyses of the effectiveness of intravenous immune globulin for prevention and treatment of neonatal sepsis. Pediatrics 99:E2, 1997.

Jenson HB, Pollock BH. The role of intravenous immunoglobulin for the prevention and treatment of neonatal sepsis. Sem Perinatol 22:50–63, 1998.

Jirapaongsananuruk O, Malech HL, Kuhns DB, Niemela JE, Brown MR, Anderson-Cohen M, Fleisher TA. Diagnostic paradigm for evaluation of male patients with chronic granulomatous disease, based on the dihydrorhodamine 123 assay. J Allergy Clin Immunol 111:374—9, 2003.

Johnson S, Knight R, Marmer DJ, Steele RW. Immune deficiency in fetal alcohol syndrome. Pediatr Res 15:908–911, 1981.

Johnston RB Jr. Screening test for the diagnosis of chronic granulomatous disease. Pediatrics 43:122–124, 1969.

Johnston RB Jr, Keele BB Jr, Misra HP, Lehmeyer JE, Webb LE, Baehner RL, Rajagopalan, KV. The role of superoxide anion generation in phagocyte bactericidal activity. Studies with normal and chronic granulomatous disease leukocytes. J Clin Invest 55:1357–1372, 1975a.

Johnston RB Jr, Klemperer MR, Alper CA, Rosen FS. The enhancement of bacterial phagocytosis by serum. The role of complement components and two cofactors. J Exp Med 129:1275–1283, 1969.

Johnston RB Jr, Stroud RM. Complement and host defense against infection. J Pediatr 90:169–179, 1977.

Johnston RB Jr, Wilfert CM, Buckley RH, Webb LS, DeChatelet LR, McCall CE. Enhanced bactericidal activity of phagocytes from patients with chronic granulomatous disease in the presence of sulphisoxazole. Lancet 1:824–827, 1975b.

Jolles S, Tyrer M, Johnson M, Webster D. Long term recovery of IgG and IgM production during HIV infection in a patient with common variable immunodeficiency (CVID). J Clin Pathol 54:713–5, 2001.

Jouanguy E, Lamhamedi-Cherradi S, Altare F, Fondaneche MC, Tuerlinckx D, Blanche S, Emile JF, Gaillard JL, Schrieber R, Levin M, Fischer A, Hivroz C, Casanova JL. Partial interferon-γ receptor 1 deficiency in a child with tuberculoid bacillus Calmette-Guerin infection and a sibling with clinical tuberculosis. J Clin Invest 100:2658–2664, 1997.

Just HM, Voge W, Metzger M, et al. Treatment of intensive care unit patients with severe nosocomial infections. In Morell A, Nydegger UE, eds. Clinical use of intravenous immunoglobulins. New York, Academic Press, 1986, pp 346–352.

Jyonouchi H, Voss RM, Krishna S, Urval K, Sjahli H, Welty PB, Good RA. Soluble FcγR II levels in normal children and patients with immunodeficiency diseases. J Clin Immunol Allergy 87:965–970, 1991.

Kadowaki J, Zuelzer WW, Brough AJ, Thompson RI, Wooley PV Jr, Gruber D. XX/XY lymphoid chimaerism in congenital immunological deficiency syndrome with thymic alymphoplasia. Lancet 2:1152–1155, 1965.

Kaikov Y, Wadsworth LD, Hall CA, Rogers PCJ. Transcobalamin II deficiency: case report and review of the literature. Eur J Pediatr 150:841–843, 1991.

Kappes DJ, Alarcon B, Regueiro JR. T lymphocyte receptor deficiencies. Curr Opin Immunol 7:441–7, 1995.

Kefalides NA, Arana JA, Bazan A, et al. Role of infection in mortality from severe burns. Evaluation of plasma, gamma globulin, albumin, and saline solution therapy in a group of Peruvian children. N Engl J Med 267:317–323, 1962.

Keightley RG, Lawton AR, Cooper MD. Successful fetal liver transplantation in a child with severe combined immunodeficiency. Lancet 2:850–853, 1975.

Keller T, McGrath K, Newland A, Gatenby P, Cobcroft R, Gibson J. Indications for use of intravenous immunoglobulin. Recommendations of the Australasian Society of Blood Transfusion consensus symposium. Med J Aust 159:204–206, 1993.

Keusch GT, Douglas SD, Mildvan D, Hirschman SZ. 14C-glucose oxidation in whole blood: a clinical assay for phagocyte dysfunction. Infect Immun 5:414–415, 1972.

Keusch GT, Douglas SD, Ugurbil K. Intracellular bactericidal activity of leukocytes in whole blood for the diagnosis of chronic granulomatous disease of childhood. J Infect Dis 131:584–7, 1975.

Kharbanda M, McCloskey TW, Pahwa R, Sun M, Phhwa S. Alteration in T-cell receptor Vbeta repertoire of CD4 and CD8 T lymphocytes in human immunodeficiency virus-infected children. Clin Diagn Immunol 10:53–58, 2003.

Kiehl MG, Stoll R, Broder M, Mueller C, Foerster EC, Domschke W. A controlled trial of intravenous immune globulin for the prevention of serious infections in adults with advanced human immunodeficiency virus infection. Arch Intern Med 156:2545–2550, 1996.

Klebanoff SJ, Pincus SH. Hydrogen peroxide utilization in myeloperoxidase-deficient leukocytes: a possible microbicidal control mechanism. J Clin Invest 50:2226–2129, 1971.

Klein C, Lisowska-Grospierre B, Le Deist F, Fischer A, Griscelli C. Major histocompatibility complex class II deficiency. Clinical manifestations, immunologic features and outcome. J Pediatr 123:921–928, 1993.

Klemperer MR, Woodworth HC, Rosen FS, Austen KF. Hereditary deficiency of the second component of human complement: transmission as an autosomal codominant trait (abstract). J Lab Clin Med 66:886, 1965.

Kobayashi RH, Hyman CJ, Stiehm ER. Immunologic maturation in an infant born to a mother with agammaglobulinemia. Am J Dis Child 134:942–944, 1980.

Kobayashi RH, Kobayashi AD, Lee N, Fischer S, Ochs HD. Home self-administration of intravenous immunoglobulin therapy in children. Pediatrics 85:705–709, 1990.

Kurtzberg J, Friedman HS, Kinney TR, Chaffee S, Stine K, Falletta JM, Weinhold KJ. Management of human immunodeficiency virus-associated thrombocytopenia with intravenous gamma globulin. Am J Pediatr Hematol Oncol 9:299–301, 1987.

Kurtzman G, Frickhofen N, Kimball J, Jenkins DW, Nienhuis AW, Young NS. Pure red-cell aplasia of 10 years duration due to persistent parvovirus B19 infection and its cure with immunoglobulin therapy. N Engl J Med 321:519–521, 1989.

Lalezari P, Bernard GE. An isologous antigen-antibody reaction with human neutrophils related to neonatal neutropenia. J Clin Invest 45:1741–1750, 1966.

Lawrence HW. Transfer factor. Adv Immunol 11:195–266, 1969.

Lederman HM, Winkelstein JA. X-linked agammaglobulinemia: an analysis of 96 patients. Medicine 64:145–146, 1985.

Le Deist F, Blanche S, Keable H, Caud C, Pham J, Descamp-Latscha B, Wahn V, Griscelli C, Fischer A. Successful HLA nonidentical bone marrow transplantation in three patients with the leukocyte adhesion deficiency. Blood 74:512–516, 1989.

Le Deist F, Hivroz C, Partiseti M, Thomas C, Buc HA, Oleastro M, Belohradsky B, Choquet D, Fischer A. A primary T-cell immunodeficiency associated with defective transmembrane calcium flux. Blood 85:1053–1062, 1995.

Lehrer RI, Cline MJ. Leukocyte myeloperoxidase deficiency and disseminated candidiasis. The role of myeloperoxidase in resistance to Candida infection. J Clin Invest 48:1478–1488, 1969.

Lenarsky C, Weinberg K, Kohn DB, Parkman R. Unrelated donor BMT for Wiskott-Aldrich syndrome. Bone Marrow Transplant 12:145–147, 1993.

Lever AM, Webster ADB, Brown D, Thomas HC. Non-A, non-B hepatitis occurring in agammaglobulinaemic patients after intravenous immunoglobulin. Lancet 2:1062–1064, 1984.

Levinsky RJ, Tiedeman K. Successful bone marrow transplantation for reticular dysgenesis. Lancet 1:671–673, 1983.

Levy J, Espanol-Boren T, Thomas C, Fischer A, Tovo P, Bordigoni P, Resnick I, Fasth A, Baer M, Gomex L, Sanders EA, Tabone MD, Plantaz D, Etzioni A, Monafo V, Abinun M, Hammarstrom L, Abrabamsen T, Jones A, Finn A, Klemola T, DeVries E, Sanal O, Peitzch MC, Notarangelo LD. Clinical spectrum of X-linked hyper-IgM syndrome. J Pediatr 131:47–54, 1997.

Lewis V, Twomey JJ, Goldstein G, O'Reilly R, Smithwick E, Pahwa R, Pahwa S, Good RA, Schulte-Wisserman H, Horowitz S, Hong R, Jones J, Sieber O, Kirkpatrick C, Polmar S, Bealmear P. Circulating thymic hormone activity in congenital immunodeficiency. Lancet 2:471–475, 1977.

Lieberman R, Hsu M. Levamisole-mediated restoration of cellular immunity in peripheral blood lymphocytes of patients with immunodeficiency diseases. Clin Immunol Immunopathol 5:142–146, 1976.

Liebhaber M, Dyer Z, Stiehm ER, Roberts RC. Improvement in granulomatous lesions in a patient with common variable immunodeficiency during treatment with the TNF antagonist. Etanercept (Enbrel) J All Clin Immunol 109:S204–S205, 2002.

Liese JG, Wintergerst U, Tympner KD, Belohradsky B. High-vs. low-dose immunoglobulin therapy in the long-term treatment of X-linked agammaglobulinemia. Am J Dis Child 146:335–339, 1992.

Lipinski M, Virelizier JL, Tursz T, Griscelli C. Natural killer and killer cell activities in patients with primary immunodeficiencies or defects in immune interferon production. Eur J Immunol 10:246–249, 1980.

Lipshultz SE, Orav EJ, Sanders SP, Colan SD. Immunoglobulins and left ventricular structure and function in pediatric HIV infection. Circulation 92:2220–2225, 1995.

Lopez C, Biggar WD, Park BH, Good RA. Nonparalytic poliovirus infections in patients with severe combined immunodeficiency disease. J Pediatr 84:497–502, 1974.

Losonsky GA, Johnson JP, Winkelstein JA, Yolken RH. Oral administration of human serum immunoglobulin in immunodeficient patients with viral gastroenteritis. J Clin Invest 76:2362–2367, 1985.

Lubens RG, Gard SE, Soderberg-Warner M, Stiehm ER. Lectin-dependent T lymphocyte and natural killer cytotoxic deficiencies in human newborns. Cell Immunol 74:40–53, 1982.

MacGregor RR, Spagnuolo PJ, Lentnek AL. Inhibition of granulocyte adherence by ethanol, prednisone, and aspirin, measured with an assay system. N Engl J Med 291:642–646, 1974.

Markert ML, Boeck A, Hale LP, Kloster AL, McLaughlin TM, Batchvarova MN, Douek DC, Koup RA, Kostyu DD, Ward FE, Rice HE, Mahaffey SM, Schiff SE, Buckley RH, Haynes BF. Thymus transplantation in complete DiGeorge syndrome. N Engl J Med 341:1180–1189, 1999.

Markert ML, Kostyu DD, Ward FE, McLaughlin TM, Watson TJ, Buckley RH, Schiff SE, Ungerleider RM, Gaynor JW, Oldham KT, Mahaffey SM, Ballow M, Driscoll DA, Hale LP, Haynes BF. Successful formation of a chimeric human thymus allograft following transplantation of cultured postnatal human thymus. J Immunol 158:998–1005, 1997.

Markert ML, Sarzotti M, Ozaki DA, Sempowski GD, Rhein ME, Hale LP, Le Derst F, Alexieff MJ, Li J, Hauser ER, Haynes BF, Rice HE, Skinner MA, Mahaffey SM, Jaggers J, Stein LD, Mill MR. Thymus transplantation in complete DiGeorge syndrome: immunologic and safety evaluations in 12 patients. Blood 102:1121–1130, 2003.

Matamoros Flori N, Mila Llambi J, Espanol Boren T, Raga Borja S, Fontan Casariego G. Primary immunodeficiency syndrome in Spain: first report of the National Registry in Children and Adults. J Clin Immunol 17:333–9, 1997.

Matheson DS, Clarkson TW, Gelfand EW. Mercury toxicity (acrodynia) induced by long-term injection of gamma globulin. J Pediatr 97:153–155, 1980.

McCawley LJ, Korchak HM, Cutilli JR, Stanley CA, Baker L, Douglas SD, Kilpatrick L. Interferon-γ corrects the respiratory burst defect in vitro in monocyte-derived macrophages from glycogen storage disease type 1b patients. Pediatr Res 34:265–269, 1993.

McCune JM, Hanley MB, Cesar D, Halvorsen R, Hoh R, Schmidt D, Wieder E, Deeks S, Siler S, Neese R, Hellerstein M. Factors influencing T-cell turnover in HIV-1 seropositive patients. J Clin Invest 105:R1–8, 2000.

McIntosh K, Kurachek SC, Cairns LM, Burns JC, Goodspeed B. Treatment of respiratory viral infection in an immunodeficient infant with ribavirin aerosol. Am J Dis Child 138:305–308, 1984.

Mease PJ, Ochs HD, Wedgwood RJ. Successful treatment of Echovirus meningoencephalitis and myositis-fasciitis with intravenous immune globulin therapy in a patient with X-linked agammaglobulinemia. N Engl J Med 304:1278–1281, 1981.

Medical Research Council Working Party. Hypogammaglobulinemia in the United Kingdom. Lancet 1:163–169, 1969.

Mendelson DS. Imaging of the thymus. Chest Surg Clin N Am 11:269–293, 2001.

Metcalf JA, Gallin JI, Nauseet WM, Root RK. Laboratory Manual of Neutrophil Function. New York, Raven Press, 1986.

Meuwissen HJ, Pollara B, Pickering RJ. Combined immunodeficiency disease associated with adenosine deaminase deficiency. J Pediatr 86:169–181, 1975.

Miller FW, Leitman SF, Plotz PH. High-dose intravenous immune globulin and acute renal failure. N Engl J Med 327:1032–1033, 1992.

Miller ME. Pathology of chemotaxis and random mobility. Semin Hematol 12:59–82, 1975.

Miller ME, Nilsson UR. A familial deficiency of the phagocytosis-enhancing activity of serum related to a dysfunction of the fifth component of complement. N Engl J Med 282:354–358, 1970.

Mills EL, Rholl K, Quie PG. Chemiluminescence, a rapid sensitive method for detection of patients with chronic granulomatous disease (abstract). Pediatr Res 12:454, 1978.

Mofenson LM, Moye J, Bethel J, Hirschhorn R, Jordan C, Nugent R. Prophylactic intravenous immunoglobulin in HIV-infected children with CD4+ counts of .20 × 10⁹/L or more: effects on viral, opportunistic, and bacterial infections. JAMA 268:483–488, 1992.

Mofenson LM, Moye J, Korelitz J, Bethel J, Hirschhorn R, Nugent R. Crossover of placebo patients to intravenous immunoglobulin confirms efficacy for prophylaxis of bacterial infections and reduction of hospitalizations in human immunodeficiency virus-infected children. Pediatr Infect Dis J 13:477–484, 1994.

Mofenson LM, Moye J Jr. Intravenous immune globulin for the prevention of infections in children with symptomatic human immunodeficiency virus infection. Pediatr Res 33:S80–S89, 1992.

Moraes M, Russo G. Thalidomide and its dermatologic uses. Am J Med Sci 321:321–326, 2001.

Morell A, Baradun S, Locher G. HTLV-III seroconversion in a homosexual patient with common variable immunodeficiency. N Engl J Med 315:456–7, 1986.

Moris A, Teichgraber V, Gauthier L, Buhring HJ, Rammensee HG. Cutting edge: characterization of allorestricted and peptide-selective alloreactive T cells using HLA-tetramer selection. J Immunol 166:4818–4821, 2001.

Moscow JA, Casper AJ, Kodis C, Fricke WA. Positive direct antiglobulin test results after intravenous immune globulin administration. Transfusion 27:248–249, 1987.

Moshous D, Callebaut I, de Chasseval R, Corneo B, Cavazzana-Calvo M, Le Deist F, Tezcan I, Sanal O, Bertrand Y, Philippe N, Fischer A, de Villartay JP. Artemis, a novel DNA double-strand break repair/V(D)J recombination protein, is mutated in human severe combined immune deficiency. Cell 105:177–186, 2001.

Munster AM. Immunologic response of trauma and burns. Am J Med 7:142–145, 1984.

Munster AM. Infections in burns. In Morell A, Nydegger UE, eds. Clinical Use of Intravenous Immunoglobulins. New York, Academic Press, 1986, pp 339–344.

National Committee for the Evaluation of Centoxin. The French National Registry of HA-1A (Centoxin) in septic shock. A cohort study of 600 patients. Arch Intern Med 154:2484–2491, 1994.

National Institutes of Health Consensus Development Conference: Diseases, doses, recommendations for intravenous immunoglobulin. HLB Newsletter. Nat Inst Heart Lung Blood Dis 6:73–78, 1990.

Nel AR. T-cell activation through the antigen receptor. Part 1. Signaling components, signaling pathways, and signal integration at the T-cell antigen receptor synapse. J Allergy Clin Immunol 109:758–777, 2002.

Nel AE, Slaughter N. T-cell activation through the antigen receptor Part 2. Role of signaling cascade in T-cell differentiation, anergy immune senescence and development of immunotherapy. J Allergy Clin Immunol 109:901–915, 2002.

Nelson RD, Quie PG, Simmons RL. Chemotaxis under agarose: a new and simple method for measuring chemotaxis and spontaneous migration of human polymorphonuclear leukocytes and monocytes. J Immunol 115:1650–1656, 1975.

Ochs HD: Intravenous immunoglobulin in the treatment and prevention of acute infections in pediatric acquired immunodeficiency syndrome patients. Pediatr Infect Dis 6:509–511, 1987.

Ochs HD, Fischer SH, Virant FS, Lee ML, Kingdon HS, Wedgwood RJ. Non-A, non-B hepatitis and intravenous immunoglobulin. Lancet 1:404–405, 1985.

Ochs HD, Fischer SH, Wedgwood RJ, Wara DW, Cowan MJ, Ammann AJ, Saxon A, Budinger MD, Alfred RU, Rousell RH. Comparison of high-dose and low-dose intravenous immunoglobulin therapy in patients with primary immunodeficiency diseases. Am J Med 76:78–82, 1984.

Ochs HD, Igo RP. The NBT slide test: a simple screening method for detecting chronic granulomatous disease and female carriers. J Pediatr 83:77–82, 1973.

Ohlsson A, Lacy JB. Intravenous immunoglobulin for preventing infection in preterm and/or low birth-weight infants (Cochrane Review). The Cochrane Library, Oxford. Issue 1, 2001.

Olerup O, Smith CIE, Hammarström L. Different amino acids at position 57 of the HLA-DQβ chain associated with susceptibility and resistance to IgA deficiency. Nature 347:289–290, 1990.

Oppenheim JJ, Blaese RM, Waldmann TA. Defective-lymphocyte transformation and delayed hypersensitivity in Wiskott-Aldrich syndrome. J Immunol 104:835–844, 1970.

O'Reilly RJ, Kapoor N, Kirkpatrick D, Cunningham-Rundles S, Pollack MS, Dupont B, Hodes MZ, Good RA, Reisner Y. Transplantation for severe combined immunodeficiency using histoincompatible parental marrow fractionated by soybean agglutinin and sheep red blood cells: experience in six consecutive cases. Transplant Proc 15:1431–1435, 1983.

Oxelius V, Laurell A, Lindquist B, Golebiowska H, Axelsson U, Bjorkander J, Hanson LA. IgG subclasses in selective IgA deficiency: importance of IgG2-IgA deficiency. N Engl J Med 304:1476–1478, 1981.

Paganelli R, Aiuti F, Beverley PC, Levinsky RJ. Impaired production of interleukins in patients with cell-mediated immunodeficiencies. Clin Exp Immunol 51:338–344, 1983.

Palma-Carlos AG, Palma-Carlos ML. Incidence of primary and acquired immunodeficiencies in an outpatient population. In Chapel HM, Levinsky RJ, Webster ADB, eds. Progress in Immune Deficiency, ed 3. London Royal Society of Medicine Services, International Congress and Symposium Series No. 173, 1991, pp 100–101.

Pan L, Cesarman E, Knowles DM. Antigen receptor genes: structure, function, and genetic analysis of their rearrangements. In Knowles DM, ed. Neoplastic Hematopathology, ed 2, Lippincott, Philadelphia, 2001, pp 307–328.

Parkman R. Antibody-treated bone marrow transplantation for patients with severe combined immune deficiency. Clin Immunol Immunopathol 40:142–146, 1986.

Parkman R, Mosier D, Umansky I, Cochran W, Carpenter CB, Rosen FS. Graft-versus-host disease after intrauterine and exchange transfusions for hemolytic disease of the newborn. N Engl J Med 290:359–363, 1974.

Patel DD, Gooding ME, Parrott RE, Curtis KM, Haynes BF, Buckley RH. Thymic function after hematopoietic stem-cell transplantation for the treatment of severe combined immunodeficiency. New Engl J Med 341:1325–1332, 2000.

Paterson DL, Georghiou PR, Allworth AM, Kemp RJ. Thalidomide as treatment of refractory aphthous ulceration related to human immunodeficiency virus infection. Clin Inf Dis 20:250–254, 1995.

Pincus SH, Klebanoff SJ. Quantitative leukocyte iodination. N Engl J Med 284:744–750, 1971.

Platts-Mills TAE, Ishizaka K. Activation of the alternate pathway of human complement by rabbit cells. J Immunol 113:348–358, 1974.

Polhill RB Jr, Pruitt KM, Johnston RB Jr. Assessment of alternate complement pathway activity in a continuously monitored hemolytic system (abstract). Fed Proc 34:982, 1975.

Pollack M. Antibody activity against Pseudomonas aeruginosa in immune globulins prepared for intravenous use in humans. J Infect Dis 147:1090–1098, 1983.

Polmar SH, Stern RC, Schwartz AL, Wetzler EM, Chase PA, Hirschhorn R. Enzyme replacement therapy for adenosine deaminase deficiency and severe combined immunodeficiency. N Engl J Med 295:1337–1343, 1976.

Power CA, Grand CL, Ismail N, Peters NC, Yurkowski DP, Bretscher PA. A valid ELISPOT assay for enumeration of ex vivo, antigen-specific, IFN-gamma producing cells. J Immunol Methods 227:99–107, 1999.

Prince HE, Kermani-Arab V, Fahey JL. Depressed interleukin-2-receptor expression in acquired immune deficiency and lymphadenopathy syndromes. J Immunol 133:1313–1317, 1984.

Puck JM, Krauss CM, Puck SM, Buckley RH, Conley ME. Prenatal test for X-linked severe combined immunodeficiency by analysis of maternal X-chromosome inactivation and linkage analysis. N Engl J Med 322:1063–1066, 1990.

Puck JM, Sneller MC. ALPS: an autoimmune human lymphroliferative syndrome associated with abnormal lymphocyte apoptosis. Sem Immunol 9:77–84, 1997

Pyun KH, Ochs HD, Wedgwood RJ, Yang XQ, Heller SR, Reimer CB. Human antibody responses to bacteriophage φX174: sequential induction of IgM and IgG subclass antibody. Clin Immunol Immunopathol 51:252–63, 1989.

Quartier P, Foray S, Casanova JL, Hau-Rainsard I, Blanche S, Fischer A. Enteroviral meningoencephalitis in X-linked agammaglobulinemia: intensive immunoglobulin therapy and sequential viral detection in cerebrospinal fluid by polymerase chain reaction. Pediatr Infect Dis J 119:1106–1108, 2000.

Quie PG, White JG, Holmes B, Good RA. In vitro bactericidal capacity of human polymorphonuclear leukocytes: diminished activity in chronic granulomatous disease of childhood. J Clin Invest 46:668–679, 1967.

Rachelefsky GS, Stiehm ER, Ammann AJ, Cederbaum SD, Opelz G, Terasaki PI. T-cell reconstitution by thymus transplantation and transfer factor in severe combined immunodeficiency. Pediatrics 54:114–118, 1975.

Rao SP, Teitlebaum J, Miller ST. Intravenous immune globulin and aseptic meningitis. Am J Dis Child 146:147, 1992.

Rappeport JM, Newburger PE, Goldblum RM, Goldman AS, Nathan DG, Parkman R. Allogeneic bone marrow transplantation for chronic granulomatous disease. J Pediatr 101:952–955, 1982.

Raubitschek AA, Levin AS, Stites DP, Shaw EB, Fudenberg HH. Normal granulocyte infusion therapy for aspergillosis in chronic granulomatous disease. Pediatrics 51:230–233, 1973.

Rault R, Piraino B, Johnston JR, Oral A. Pulmonary and renal toxicity of intravenous immunoglobulin. Clin Nephrol 26:83–86, 1991.

Razvi S, Schneider L, Jonas MM, Cunningham-Rundles, C. Outcome of intravenous immunoglobulin transmitted hepatitis C virus (HCV) in primary immunodeficiency. Clin Immunol 101:284–288, 2001.

Rebuck JW, Crowley JH. A method of studying leukocytic functions in vivo. Ann NY Acad Sci 59:757–805, 1955.

Reinherz EL, Geha R, Rappeport JM, Wilson M, Penta AC, Hussey RE, Fitzgerald KA, Daley JR, Levine J, Rosen FS, Schlossman SF. Reconstitution after transplantation with T lymphocyte–depleted HLA haplotype–mismatched bone marrow for severe combined immunodeficiency. Proc Natl Acad Sci USA 79:6047–6051, 1982.

Rieux-Laucat F, Le Deist F, Hivroz C, Roberts IA, Debatin KM, Fischer A, de Villartay JP. Mutations in Fas associated with human lymphoproliferative syndrome and autoimmunity. Science 268:1347–1349, 1995.

Rijkers GT, Scharenberg JGM, Van Dongen JJM, Neijens HJ, Zegers BJ. Abnormal signal transduction in a patient with severe combined immunodeficiency disease. Pediatr Res 29:306–309, 1991.

Rose EA. Applications of the polymerase chain reaction to genome analysis. FASEB J 5:46–54, 1991.

Rotbart HA, Levin MJ, Jones JF, Hayward AR, Allan J, McLane MF, Essex M. Noma in children with severe combined immunodeficiency. J Pediatr 109:596–600, 1986.

Rotbart HA, Webster AD. Treatment of potentially life-threatening enterovirus infections with pleconaril. Clin Infect Dis 32:228–235, 2001.

Rowe JM, Ciobanu N, Ascensao J, Stadtmauer EA, Weiner RS, Schenkein DP, McGlave P, Lazarus HM. Recommended guidelines for the management of autologous and allogeneic bone marrow transplantation. Ann Intern Med 120:143–158, 1994.

Ruderman JW, Peter JB, Gall RC, Stewart ME, Pomerance JJ, Stiehm ER. Prevention of hypogammaglobulinemia of prematurity with intravenous immune globulin. J Perinatol 10:150–155, 1988.

Ruff ME, Pincus LG, Sampson HA. Phenytoin-induced IgA depression. Am J Dis Child 141:858–861, 1987.

Ryser O, Morell A, Hitzig WH. Primary immunodeficiencies in Switzerland: first report of the national registry in adults and children. J Clin Immunol 8:479–485, 1988.

Saez-Llorens X, Ramilo O, Mustafa MM, Mertsola J, McCracken GH. Molecular pathophysiology of bacterial meningitis: current concepts and therapeutic implications. J Pediatr 116:671–684, 1990.

Sanel SO, Buckley RH. Antibody-dependent cellular cytotoxicity in primary immunodeficiency diseases and with normal leukocyte subpopulations. J Clin Invest 61:1–10, 1978.

Sanford JP, Favour CB, Tribeman MS. Absence of serum gamma globulins in an adult. N Engl J Med 250:1027–1029, 1954.

Saxon A, Giorgi JV, Sherr EH, Kagan JM. Failure of B cells in common variable immunodeficiency to transit from proliferation to differentiation is associated with altered B cell surface–molecule display. J Allergy Clin Immunol 84:44–53, 1989.

Schaffer FM, Palermos J, Zhu ZB, Barger BO, Cooper MD, Volanakis JE. Individuals with IgA deficiency and common variable immunodeficiency share polymorphisms of major histocompatibility complex class III genes. Proc Natl Acad Sci USA 86:8015–8019, 1989.

Schiff RI, Rudd C. Alterations in the half-life and clearance of IgG during therapy with intravenous gamma globulin in 16 patients with severe primary humoral immunodeficiency. J Clin Immunol 6:256–264, 1986.

Schiff RI, Rudd C, Johnson R, Buckley RH. Use of a new chemically modified intravenous IgG preparation in severe primary humoral immunodeficiency: clinical efficacy and attempts to individualize dosage. Clin Immunol Immunopathol 31:13–23, 1984.

Schifferli J, Favre H, Nydegger U, Leski M, Imbach P, Davies K. High-dose intravenous IgG treatment and renal function. Lancet 337:457–458, 1991.

Schmalsteig FC, Mills GC, Nelson JA, May LT, Goldman AS, Goldblum RM. Limited effect of erythrocyte and plasma infusions in adenosine deaminase deficiency. J Pediatr 93:597–603, 1978.

Schmidt I, Uittenbogaart CH, Keld B, Giorgi JV. A rapid method for measuring apoptosis and dual-color immunofluorescence by single laser flow cytometry. J Immunol Methods 170:145–157, 1994.

Schmugge M, Lauener R, Seger RA, Gungor T, Bossart W. Chronic enteroviral meningo-encephalitis in X-linked agammaglobulinaemia: favourable response to anti-enteroviral treatment. Eur J Pediatr 158:1010–1011, 1999.

Schulkind ML, Adler WM, Altemeier WA, Ayoub EM. Transfer factor in the treatment of a case of chronic mucocutaneous moniliasis. Cell Immunol 3:606–615, 1972.

Schur PH, Borel H, Gelfand EW, Alper CA, Rosen FS. Gamma-G globulin deficiencies in patients with recurrent pyogenic infections. N Engl J Med 283:631–634, 1970.

Schwarz K, Hansen-Hagge TE, Knobloch C, Friedrich W, Kleihauer E, Bartram CR. Severe combined immunodeficiency (SCID) in man: B cell-negative (B–) SCID patients exhibit an irregular recombination pattern at the JH locus. J Exp Med 174:1039–1048, 1991.

Scott CR, Chen SH, Giblett ER. Detection of the carrier state in combined immunodeficiency associated with adenosine deaminase deficiency. J Clin Invest 53:1194–1196, 1974.

Seeger RC, Robins RA, Stevens RH, Klein RB, Waldman DJ, Zeltzer PM, Kessler SW. Severe combined immunodeficiency with B lymphocytes: in vitro correction of defective immunoglobulin production by addition of normal T lymphocytes. Clin Exp Immunol 26:1–10, 1976.

Segal BH, Leto TL, Gallin JI, Malech HL, Holland SM. Genetic, biochemical and clinical features of chronic granulomatous disease. Medicine 79:170–200, 2000.

Shamim M, Giacola GP, West K. The use of intravenous immunoglobulin (IVIG) to prevent infection in bronchopulmonary dysplasia: report of a pilot study. J Perinatol 40:239–244, 1991.

Shearer WT, Wedner HJ, Strominger DB, Kissane J, Hong R. Successful transplantation of the thymus in Nezelof's syndrome. Pediatrics 61:619–624, 1978.

Shirani KZ, Vaughan GM, McManus AT, et al. Replacement therapy with modified immunoglobulin G in burn patients: preliminary kinetic studies. Am J Med 76:175–180, 1984.

Siegel FP, Oleske J. Management of the acquired immune deficiency syndrome: is there a role for immune globulins? In Morell A, Nydegger UE, eds. Clinical Use of Intravenous Immunoglobulins. New York, Academic Press, 1986, pp 373–384.

Sjoholm AG, Kuijper EJ, Tijssen CC, Jansz A, Bo P, Spanjaard L, Zanen HC. Dysfunctional properdin in a Dutch family with meningococcal disease. N Engl J Med 319:33–37, 1988.

Skarnes RC, Watson DW. Characterization of leukin: an antibacterial factor from leukocytes active against gram-positive pathogens. J Exp Med 104:829–845, 1956.

Smith KJ, Skelton H. Common variable immunodeficiency treated with a recombinant human IgG, tumour necrosis factor-alpha receptor fusion protein. Br J Dermatol 144:597–600, 2001.

Smith KY. Thymic size and lymphocyte restoration in HIV-infected patients following 48 weeks of therapy with Zidovudine, lamivudine, and ritonavir. Infect Dis 18I:141, 2000.

Soothill JF. The concentration of gamma-macroglobulin in the serum of patients with hypogammaglobulinemia. Clin Sci 23:2–35, 1962.

Sottong PR, Rosebrock JA, Britz JA, Kramer TR. Measurement of T-lymphocyte responses in whole-blood cultures using newly synthesized DNA and ATP. Clin Diagn Lab Immunol 7:307–311, 2000.

Soudais C, de Villartay JP, Le Deist F, Fischer A, Lisowska-Grospierre B. Independent mutations of the human CD3-epsilon gene resulting in a T cell receptor/CD3 complex immunodeficiency. Nat Genet 3:77–81, 1993.

South MA, Warwick WJ, Wollheim FA, Good RA. The IgA system. III. IgA levels in the serum and saliva of pediatric patients: evidence for a local immunological system. J Pediatr 71:645–653, 1967.

Spector SA, Gelber RD, McGrath N, Wara D, Barzilai A, Abrams E, Bryson YJ, Dankner WM, Livingston RA, Connor EM. A controlled trial of intravenous immune globulin for the prevention of serious bacterial infections in children receiving zidovudine for advanced human immunodeficiency virus infection. N Engl J Med 331:1181–1187, 1994.

Spitler LE, Levin AS, Stites DP, Fudenberg HH, Pirofsky B, August CS, Stiehm ER, Hitzig WH, Gatti RA. The Wiskott-Aldrich syndrome: results of transfer factor therapy. J Clin Invest 51:3216–3224, 1972.

Steen JA. Gamma globulin in preventing infections in prematures. Arch Pediatr 77:291–294, 1960.

Stiehm ER. Human intravenous immunoglobulin in primary and secondary antibody deficiencies. Pediatr Infect Dis 16:696–707, 1997.

Stiehm ER. New and old immunodeficiencies. Pediatr Res 33(suppl):S2–S8, 1993.

Stiehm ER. Use of immunoglobulins in secondary immunodeficiencies. In Imbach P, ed. Immunotherapy with intravenous immunoglobulins. London, Academic Press, 1991, pp 115–126

Stiehm ER. Passive immunization. In Feigen RW, Cherry JD, eds. Textbook of Pediatric Infectious Diseases, 4th ed. Philadelphia: W B Saunders Co, pp 2769-2802, 1996.

Stiehm ER, Casillas AM, Finkelstein JZ, Gallagher KET, Groncy PM, Kobayashi RH, Oleske JM, Roberts RL, Sandbert ET, Wakim ME. Slow subcutaneous human intravenous immunoglobulin in the treatment of antibody immunodeficiency: use of an old method with a new product. J Allergy Clin Immunol 101:848–849, 1998.

Stiehm ER, Chin TW, Haas A, Peerless AG. Infectious complications of the primary immunodeficiencies. Clin Immunol Immunopathol 40:69–86, 1986.

Stiehm ER, Fudenberg HH. Antibodies to gamma-globulin in infants and children exposed to isologous gamma-globulin. Pediatrics 35:229–235, 1965.

Stiehm ER, Fudenberg HH. Clinical and immunologic features of dysgammaglobulinemia type I: report of a case diagnosed in the first year of life. Am J Med 40:805–815, 1966a.

Stiehm ER, Fudenberg HH. Serum levels of immune globulins in health and disease: a survey. Pediatrics 37:715–727, 1966b.

Stiehm ER, McIntosh RM. Wiskott-Aldrich syndrome: review and report of a large family. Clin Exp Immunol 2:179–189, 1967.

Stiehm ER, Vaerman JP, Fudenberg HH. Plasma infusions in immunologic deficiency states: metabolic and therapeutic studies. Blood 28:918–938, 1966.

Stjernholm RL, Allan RC, Steele RH, Waring WW, Harris JA. Impaired chemiluminescence during phagocytosis or opsonized bacteria. Infect Immun 7:313–314, 1973.

Stossel TP. Evaluation of opsonic and leukocyte function with a spectrophotometric test in patients with infection and with phagocytic disorders. Blood 42:121–130, 1973.

Strauss RG, Bove KE, Jones JF, Mauer AM, Fulginiti VA. An anomaly of neutrophil morphology with impaired function. N Engl J Med 290:478–484, 1974.

Strauss RG, Levy GJ, Sotelo-Avila C, Albanese MA, Hume H, Schloz L, Blazina JB, Werner A, Barrasso C, Blanchette V, Warkentin PI, Pepkowitz S, Mauer AM, Hines D. National survey of neonatal transfusion practices: II. Blood component therapy. Pediatrics 91:530–536, 1993.

Stray-Pedersen A, Abrahamsen TG, Froland SS. Primary immunodeficiency diseases in Norway. J Clin Immunol 20:477–85, 2000.

Sullivan KM. Immunoglobulin therapy in bone marrow transplantation. Am J Med 83(suppl 4A):34–35, 1987.

Sullivan KM. Intravenous immune globulin prophylaxis in recipients of a marrow transplant. J Allergy Clin Immunol 84:632–639, 1989.

Sullivan KM, Kopecky KJ, Jocom J, Fisher L, Buckner CD, Meyers JD, Counts GW, Bowden RA, Peterson FB, Witherspoon RP, et al. Immunomodulatory and antimicrobial efficacy of intravenous immunoglobulin in bone marrow transplantation. N Engl J Med 323:705–712, 1990.

Sweinberg SK, Wodell RA, Grodofsky MP, Greene JM, Conley ME. Retrospective analysis of the incidence of pulmonary disease in hypogammaglobulinemia. J Allergy Clin Immunol 88:96–104, 1991.

Syllaba L, Henner K. Contribution a l'independance de l'athetose double idiopathique et congenitale: atteinte familiale, syndrome dystrophique, signe du reseau vasculaire conjonctival, integrite psychique. Rev Neurol (Paris) 1:541–562, 1926.

Taalman RD,, Hustinx TWJ, Weemaes CM, Seemanova E, Schmidt A, Passarge E, Scheres JM. Further delineation of the Nijmegen breakage syndrome. Am J Med Genet 32:425–431, 1989.

Takei S, Arora YK, Walker SM. Intravenous immunoglobulin contains specific antibodies inhibitory to activation of T cells by staphylococcal superantigens. J Clin Invest 91:602–607, 1993.

Terasaki PI, Miyajima R, Sengar DPS, Stiehm ER. Extraneous lymphocytic HLA antigens in severe combined immunodeficiency disease. Transplantation 13:250–255, 1972.

Thomas ED, Storb R. Technique for human marrow grafting. Blood 36:507–515, 1970.

Thorpe ES, Handley HE. Chronic tetany and chronic mycelial stomatitis in a child aged four and one-half years. Am J Dis Child 38:328-338, 1929.Todd RF III, Fegen DR. The CD11/CD18 leukocyte glycoprotein deficiency. Hematol Oncol Clin North Am 4:13–31, 1988.

Touraine J-L, Betuel H. The bare lymphocyte syndrome: immunodeficiency resulting from the lack of expression of HLA antigens. Birth Defects Orig Artic Ser 19:83–85, 1983.

Touraine J-L, Betuel H, Souillet G, Jeune M. Combined immunodeficiency disease associated with absence of cell-surface HLA-A and -B antigens. J Pediatr 93:47–51, 1978.

Trepo C, Hantz O, Vitvitski L. Non-A, non-B hepatitis after intravenous gammaglobulin. Lancet 1:322, 1986.

Tutscha PJ. Diminishing morbidity and mortality of bone marrow transplantation. Vox Sang 51(suppl 2):87–94, 1986.

Van der Meer JWM, Vossen JM, Radl J, Van Nieuwkoop JA, Meijer CJLM, Lobatto S, Van Furth R. Hyperimmunoglobulinemia D and periodic fever: a new syndrome. Lancet 1:1087–1090, 1984.

Vihinen M, Lehvaslaiho, H, Cotton RGH. Immunodeficiency mutation databases. In Ochs HD, Smith CIE, Puck JM, eds. Primary Immunodeficiency Disease: A Molecular and Genetic Approach. Oxford University Press, New York, 1999, pp 443–447.

Villa A, Vezzoni P, Sobacci C, Notarangelo L, Bozzi F, Abinin M, Abrahamsen TG, Aekwright PD, Baniyash M, Brooks EG, Conley ME, Cortes P, Duse M, Fasth A, Filipovich AM, Infante AJ, Jones A, Mazzolari E, Muller SM, Pasic S, Rechavi G, Sacco MG, Santagata S, Schroeder ML, Seger R, Strina D, Ugazio A, Väliaho J, Vihinen M, Volger LB, Ochs HD, Vezzoni P, Friedrich W, Schwarz K. V(D)J recombination defects in lymphocytes: a severe immunodeficiency with a spectrum of clinical presentations due to Rag mutations. Blood. 97:81–88, 2001.

Virelizier JL, Lagrue A, Durandy A, Arenzana F, Oury C, Griscelli C. Reversal of natural killer defect in a patient with Chédiak-Higashi syndrome after bone-marrow transplantation. N Engl J Med 306:1055–1056, 1982.

Vogelsang GB, Farmer ER, Hess AD, Altamonte V, Beschorner WE, Jabs DA, Corio RL, Levin LS, Colvin OM, Wingard JR, Santos GW. Thalidomide for the treatment of chronic graft-versus-host disease. New Engl J Med 326:1055–1058, 1992.

Vowells SJ, Fleisher TA, Sekhsaria S, Alling DW, Maguire TE, Malech HL. Genotype-dependent variability in flow cytometric evaluation of reduced nicotinamide adenine dinucleotide phosphate oxidase function in patients with chronic granulomatous disease. J Pediatr 128:104–7, 1996.

Vowels MR, Lam-Poo-Tang R, Berdoukas V, Ford D, Thierry D, Purtilo D, Gluckman E. Correction of X-linked lymphoproliferative disease by transplantation of cord-blood stem cells. N Engl J Med 22:1623–1625, 1993.

Vyas GH, Perkins HA, Fudenberg HH. Anaphylactoid transfusion reaction associated with anti-IgA. Lancet 2:312–315, 1968.

Wahlstrom J, Gigliotti D, Roquet A, Wigzell H, Eklaund A, Grunewald, J. T cell receptor Vbeta expression in patients with allergic asthma before and after repeated low-dose allergen inhalation. Clin Immunol 100:31–39, 2001.

Waldmann TA, Broder S, Blaese RM, Durin M, Blackman M, Strober W. Role of suppressor T cells in pathogenesis of common variable hypogammaglobulinaemia. Lancet 2:609–613, 1974.

Waldmann TA, McIntire KR. Serum alpha-fetoprotein levels in patients with ataxia-telangiectasia. Lancet 2:1112–1115, 1972.

Waldmann TA, Strober W. Metabolism of immunoglobulins. Prog Allergy 13:1–110, 1969.

Waniewski J, Gardulf A, Hammarstrom L. Bioavailability of γ-globulin after subcutaneous infusions in patients with common variable immunodeficiency. J Clin Immunol 14:90–97, 1993.

Wara DW, Ammann AJ. Thymic cells and humoral factors as therapeutic agents. Pediatrics 57:643–646, 1976.

Webster ADB, Efter T, Asherson GL. Escherichia coli antibody: a screening test for immunodeficiency. Br Med J 3:16–18, 1974.

Webster AD, Lever A, Spickett G, Beattie R, North M, Thorpe R. Recovery of antibody production after HIV infection in 'common' variable hypogammaglobulinaemia. Clin Exp Immunol 77:309–13, 1989.

Wedgwood RJ, Ochs HD, Davis SD. The recognition and classification of immunodefiecimcy diseases with bacteriophage φX174. In Bergsma D, ed. Immunodifiodity in Man and Animals. Birth Defects: Original Article Series, Vol XI, No. 1. Sunderland, Mass, Sinauer Associates, 1975, pp 331–338.

Weening RS, Schoorel EP, Roos D, van Schaik MLJ, Voetman AA, Bot AAM, Batenburg-Plenter AM, Willems CH, Zeijlemaker WP, Astaldi A. Effect of ascorbate on abnormal neutrophil, platelet, and lymphocyte function in a patient with the Chediak-Higashi syndrome. Blood 57:856–865, 1981.

Weinberg K, Parkman R. Severe combined immunodeficiency due to a specific defect in the production of IL-2. N Engl J Med 322:1718–1720, 1990.

Welch MJ, Stiehm ER, Dudley JP. Isolated absence of nasal cilia: a case report. Ann Allergy 52:32B34, 1984.

Werdan K. Supplemental immune globulins in sepsis. Clin Chem Lab Med 37:341–349, 1999.

Wheeler AP, Bernard GR. Treating patients with severe sepsis. N Engl J Med 340:207–214, 1999.

White WB, Ballow M. Modulation of suppressor-cell activity in cimetidine in patients with common variable hypogammaglobulinemia. N Engl J Med 312:198–202, 1985.

Williams LL, Rooney CM, Conley ME, Brenner MK, Krance RA, Heslop HE. Correction of Duncan's syndrome by allogeneic bone marrow transplantation. Lancet 342:587–588, 1993.

Wilson NW, Ochs HD, Peterson R, et al. Abnormal primary antibody responses in pediatric trauma patients. J Pediatr 115:424–427, 1989.

Winkelstein JA, Marino MC, Johnston RB Jr, Boyle J, Curnutte J, Gallin JI, Malech HL, Holland SM, Ochs H, Quie P, Buckley RH, Foster CB, Chanock SJ, Dickler H. Chronic granulomatous disease: report on a national registry of 368 patients. Medicine 79:155–169, 2000.

Wiskott A. Familiarer, angeborener Morbus Werihofii? Aschr Kinderheilk 68:212–216, 1937.

Wittig HJ, Belloit J, De Fillippi I, Royal G. Age-related serum immunoglobulin E levels in healthy subjects and in patients with allergic disease. J Allergy Clin Immunol 66:305–313, 1980.

Woodruff RK, Grigg AP, Firkin FC, Smith IL. Fatal thrombotic events during treatment of autoimmune thrombocytopenia with intravenous immunoglobulin in elderly patients. Lancet 2:217–218, 1986.

Working Group on Antiretroviral Therapy. National Pediatric HIV Resource Center. Antiretroviral therapy and medical management of the human immunovirus-infected child. Pediatr Inf Dis J 12:513–522, 1993.

World Health Organization/International Agency for Research on Cancer. Technical report. Identification enumeration and isolation of B and T lymphocytes from human peripheral blood. Scand J Immunol 3:521–532, 1974.

Wright DG, Kirkpatrick CH, Gallin JI. Effects of levamisole on normal and abnormal leukocyte locomotion. J Clin Invest 59:941–950, 1970.

Wright JJ, Birx DL, Wagner DK, Waldmann TA, Blaese RM, Fleisher T. Normalization of antibody responsiveness in a patient with common variable hypogammaglobulinemia and HIV infection. New Engl J Med 317:1516–1520, 1987.

Yap PL, McOmish F, Webster ADB, Hammarstrom L, Smith CIE, Bjorkander J, Ochs HD, Fischer SH, Quinti I, Simmonds P. Hepatitis C virus transmission by intravenous immunoglobulin. J Hepatol 21:455–460, 1994.

Young NS. Parvovirus infection and its treatment. Clin Exp Immunol 104(suppl 1):26–30, 1996.

Yount WJ, Hong R, Seligmann M, Good RA, Kunkel HG. Imbalances of gammaglobulin subgroups and gene defects in patients with primary hypogammaglobulinemia. J Clin Invest 49:1957–1966, 1970.

Yu MW, Mason BL, Guo ZP, Tankersley DL, Nedjar S, Mitchell FD, Biswas RM. Hepatitis C transmission associated with intravenous immunoglobulins. Lancet 345:1173–1174, 1995.

Zelazko M, Carneiro-Sampaio M, Cornejo de Luigi M, Garcia de Olarte D, Porras Madrigal O, Berron Perez R, Cabello A, Rostan MV, Sorenson, RU. Primary immunodeficiency diseases in latin America: first report from eight countries participating in the LAGID. Latin America Group for Primary Immunodeficiency Diseases. J Clin Immunol 18:161–6,1998.

Ziegler, EJ, Fisher CJ Jr, Sprung CL, Straube RC, Sadoff JC, Foulke GE, Wortel CH, Fink MP, Dellinger RP, Teng NN, et al. Treatment of gram negative bacteremia and septic shock with HA 1A human monoclonal antibody against endotoxin. N Engl J Med 324:429–436, 1991.

Ziegler EJ, McCutchan JA, Fierer J, Glauser MP, Sadoff JC, Douglas H, Braude AI. Treatment of gram negative bacteremia and shock with human antiserum to a mutant Escherichia coli. N Engl J Med 307:1225–1230, 1982.

Ziegner UH, Ochs HD, Schanen C, Feig SA, Seyama K, Futatani T, Gross T, Wakim M, Roberts RL, Rawlings DJ, Dovat S, Fraser JK, Stiehm ER. Unrelated umbilical cord stem cell transplantation for X-linked immunodeficiencies. J Pediatr 138:570–573, 2001.

Ziegner UH, Kobayashi RH, Cunningham-Rundles C, Espanol T, Fasth A, Huttenlocher A, Krogstad P, Marthinsen L, Notarangelo LD, Pasic S, Rieger CH, Rudge P, Sankar R, Shigeoka AO, Stiehm ER, Sullivan KE, Webster AD, Ochs HD. Progressive neurodegeneration in patients with primary immunodeficiency disease on IVIG treatment. Clin Immunol 102:19–24, 2002.

13 Antibody Deficiencies

Hans D. Ochs, E. Richard Stiehm, and Jerry A. Winkelstein

With contributions by Charlotte Cunningham-Rundles, Anne Durandy, Howard M. Lederman, Luigi D. Notarangelo, David J. Rawlings, and Chaim M. Roifman

OVERVIEW

Predominant antibody deficiencies are the most numerous of the primary immunodeficiencies. Selective immunoglobulin (Ig)A deficiency is particularly common and this is covered in Chapter 14. The antibody deficiencies can be grouped into three categories, all of which are covered in this chapter.

1. Profound antibody deficiencies (e.g., X-linked agammaglobulinemia [XLA] and related syndromes, common variable immunodeficiency, the hyper-IgM syndromes, antibody deficiency with normal immunoglobulins and immunodeficiency with thymoma). These patients generally need intravenous immune globulin (IVIG), and some patients, for example, those with X-linked hyper-IgM syndrome, may require transplantation.
2. Common but less severe antibody deficiencies (e.g., transient hypogammaglobulinemia of infancy, IgG subclass deficiency, and impaired polysaccharide responsiveness). IVIG is rarely used in these patients.
3. Unusual and usually less severe antibody deficiencies, including immuno-osseous syndromes, transcobalamin 2 deficiency, immunodeficiency with specific infections, drug-induced antibody deficiencies, and selective IgE and IgM deficiencies.

Antibody deficiencies are also present in the combined immunodeficiencies (see Chapters 15 and 16) as well as in several specific immunodeficiency syndromes (see Chapter 17). They are also present in a number of genetic syndromes (termed *syndromic immunodeficiencies;* see Chapter 24), and in secondary immunodeficiencies, such as malignancy, malnutrition, chemotherapy, splenic deficiency, protein loss, and acute stress (Part III of this book; see Chapters 22 through 30).

X-LINKED AGAMMAGLOBULINEMIA

Definition

XLA is the prototypic genetic primary humoral immunodeficiency characterized by a profound deficiency of all immunoglobulins, mature B cells and plasma cells, secondary to mutations in the Btk gene. Most patients have an early onset of bacterial infections. XLA has an incidence of approximately 1 in 100,000 to 200,000 and a prevalence of 1 in 10,000.

Historical Aspects

Colonel Ogden Bruton first identified the disease in 1952 by noting the complete absence of the gamma-globulin peak on an electrophoretic pattern of the serum of a boy with severe recurrent infections (Bruton, 1952). Treatment with gamma-globulin injections led to marked improvement. The clinical and laboratory features of this X-linked recessive disorder have been of major interest for a half century (Good, 1954; Janeway et al., 1953; Lederman and Winkelstein, 1985; Rosen et al., 1984). Its discovery initiated a search for other primary immunodeficiencies, which in turn has led to the delineation, classification, and management of nearly 100 primary immunodeficiencies discussed in this section.

In the early 1990s two independent groups identified the gene responsible for XLA (Tsukada et al., 1993; Vetrie et al., 1993). Both XLA and a related immunodeficiency in mice (X-linked immunodeficiency [xid]) result from the deficient function of a cytoplasmic tyrosine kinase now aptly named *Bruton's tyrosine kinase* (Btk) (Conley et al., 1994c; Ochs and Smith, 1996; Rawlings et al., 1993; Smith and Witte, 1999).

Pathogenesis

Defective Function of Btk in XLA

BTK, the XLA gene, maps to the mid-portion of the long arm of the X-chromosome at Xq21.2-22.2 (Guiloi et al., 1989; Kwan et al., 1986, 1990; Malcolm et al., 1987; Mensink et al., 1986; Parolini et al., 1993). Physical maps of this region were developed using yeast artificial chromosomes and pulse-field gel analysis (O'Reilly et al., 1992; Parolini et al., 1993). *BTK* mapped to within 100 kb of a probe defining the polymorphism most closely linked to XLA at DXS178. Reduced Btk mRNA, protein, and kinase activity was subsequently demonstrated in B-cell lines from XLA patients (Tsukada et al., 1993). In an independent study, YAC clones from the DXS178 locus were used to isolate a BTK complementary deoxyribonucleic acid (cDNA) and sequencing demonstrated alterations in the transcripts from XLA patients (Vetrie et al., 1993).

Five lines of evidence support the critical role for *BTK* in XLA. First, Btk is expressed in all stages of the B-lymphocyte lineage (except plasma cells), but not in T lymphocytes (Smith et al., 1994a; Tsukada et al., 1993). Second, *BTK* maps to the same chromosomal location as the XLA locus. Third, most patients with XLA have reduced levels of *BTK* messenger ribonucleic acid (mRNA) and/or reduced Btk protein and kinase activity in B-cell lines derived from their peripheral blood or bone marrow. Fourth, extensive mutational analysis demonstrates sequence alterations within each of the Btk protein subdomains in more than 500 independent families (Vihinen et al., 1998). Finally, these mutations segregate with the X-chromosome carrying the XLA allele among many pedigrees.

Btk Structure and Function

Btk is representative of the Tec family of nonreceptor tyrosine kinases (Mano, 1999; Rawlings and Witte, 1995; Smith et al., 2001) and is expressed at all stages of B-lineage development from CD34+ CD19+ pro-B cells to mature B cells but is down-regulated in plasma cells (de Weers et al., 1993; Smith et al., 1994a; Tsukada et al., 1993). Btk is also expressed in erythroid precursors, myeloid cells, mast cells, monocytes, megakaryocytes, and platelets. Btk expression is absent in T and natural killer (NK) cell lineages.

Similar to the Src tyrosine kinases, Btk contains classical Src homology (SH) type 1 catalytic, and SH2 and SH3 protein interaction domains (Bolen, 1993). These SH2 and SH3 domains bind tyrosine-phosphorylated proteins and polyproline motifs, respectively (Pawson, 1995). A critical role for each of these domains has been demonstrated in mutational studies in XLA patients. However, although several potential interacting proteins have been identified in vitro, the biologic consequences of these interactions remain unclear (Baba et al., 1999; Bunnell et al., 1996; Guinamard et al., 1997).

Most notably, Btk contains a unique amino-terminal region composed of three distinct subdomains, including from closest to the amino-terminal: a pleckstrin homology (PH) domain, a Drosophila RasGAP or "Btk motif," and a proline rich region (PRR). Together, these latter two domains have also been termed the Tec homology (TH) domain (Vihinen et al., 1994). The PH domain is the most distinctive feature of Btk. This module is present in many divergent proteins involved in signal transduction (Gibson et al., 1994; Lemmon et al., 1996) and the Btk PH domain crystal structure is similar to that of other signaling proteins (Hyvönen and Saraste, 1997). The Btk PH contains a positively charged ligand-binding pocket that specifically binds phosphatidylinositol lipids and modulates recruitment of Btk to the cell membrane. All of the "functional" PH domain mutations resulting in XLA map to this pocket.

The carboxyl-terminus of the PH domain contains a conserved α-helix that can modulate binding to the βγ subunits of heterotrimeric G proteins (Tsukada et al., 1994). The Btk motif is an approximately 25 amino acid domain that has been shown to facilitate interaction with Gα subunits of two families of heterotrimeric G proteins (Jiang et al., 1998). The Btk PRR binds SH3 domains from other proteins (Cheng et al., 1994) and also can form an intramolecular loop between the Btk PRR and SH3 domains that may regulate access to these domains and Btk kinase activity (Andreotti et al., 1997).

B-Cell Development and Function in XLA

The B cells in female obligate carriers of XLA exhibit nonrandom X-chromosome inactivation consistent with an autonomous B-lineage defect (Conley and Puck, 1988; Conley et al., 1986; Fearon et al., 1987). Early observations also suggested that the XLA defect interfered progressively at several points in B-lymphocyte development (Conley, 1985; Kinnon et al., 1993). Consistent with these predictions, biochemical and functional studies demonstrate that Btk is required for both pre–B-cell expansion, and for mature B-cell survival and activation (Fig. 13-1) (see Chapter 3). Signaling through the pre–B-cell receptor (pre-BCR)

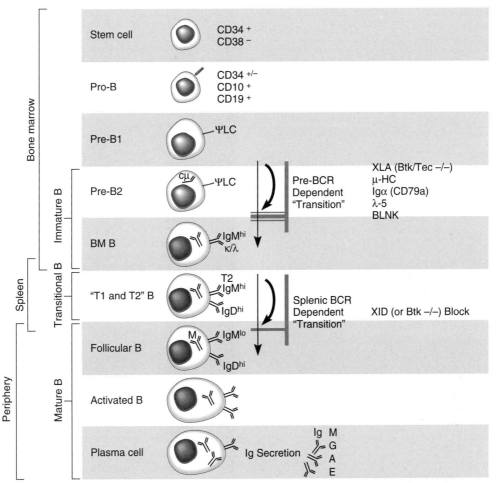

Figure 13-1 · **B-lineage developmental defects presenting with agammaglobulinemia and absent or markedly reduced peripheral B-cell numbers.** Schematic of bone marrow and peripheral B lineage development illustrating two key developmental transitions that require the signaling function of the pre–B-cell receptor (pre-BCR) and mature B-cell antigen receptor (BCR), respectively. In humans, deficient function of Btk leads to X-linked agammaglobulinemia (XLA) with developmental arrest at the pre-B transition (pre-B1 to pre-B2). Btk is also essential for the Transitional 2 to mature follicular B-cell transition mediated by signaling through the BCR. In mice, Btk deficiency alone leads to a defect at this later transition, whereas Btk/Tec doubly deficient mice exhibit a pre–B-cell developmental arrest nearly identical to XLA. Also shown are four additional genetic defects that lead to a defect in the human pre–B-cell developmental transition. Defects in additional components of the pre-BCR are likely to be responsible for other currently unidentified, rare cases of non-XLA. Ig, Immunoglobulin.

and B-cell antigen receptor (BCR), respectively, controls these developmental transitions. In Btk-deficient cells, these respective cell populations fail to proliferate and, instead, undergo apoptotic cell death.

Role of Btk in Pre–BCR-Dependent Signals

Pre-BCR cells are the major cycling B-lineage population; they are essential for generation of an adequate pool of B cells. Expression and signaling via the pre-BCR leads to immunoglobulin heavy chain allelic exclusion and pre–B-cell expansion (Karasuyama et al., 1996). B-lineage development is severely compromised when these events are disrupted.

The earliest and most severe consequence of the XLA defect occurs at the pre–B-cell transition. Early fluores-

cent microscopy studies demonstrated the presence of cytoplasmic μ^+ ($c\mu^+$) bone marrow B progenitors but markedly reduced numbers of surface IgM$^+$ B cells in XLA bone marrow. Consistent with an early developmental block, very few IgM$^+$ B cells were present in blood or lymphoid tissues (Aiuti et al., 1972; Bentwich and Kunkel, 1973; Cooper and Lawton, 1972; Geha et al., 1973; Pearl et al., 1978; Preud'Homme et al., 1973; Schiff et al., 1974; Siegal et al., 1971) and plasma cells; these cells were absent in marrow, lymph nodes, and the lamina propria of intestinal mucosa (Ament et al., 1973; Gitlin et al., 1959; Good, 1955). XLA bone marrow B-cell progenitors are predominantly pro-B cells that are $c\mu^-$, terminal deoxynucleotidyl transferase (TdT)$^+$ with very limited numbers of $c\mu^+$ pre-B lymphocytes. This limited pool of XLA pre-B cells has a reduced proliferative capacity (Campana et al., 1990).

Flow cytometric analysis (using an antibody to the surrogate light [ψLc] chain protein, VpreB, a key component of the pre-BCR) has provided a more precise resolution of the XLA developmental block (Nomura et al., 2000). XLA bone marrow progenitors exhibit a significantly increased percentage of pro-B (cμ$^-$ψLc^{++}) cells, and small (presumably noncycling) pre-B1a (cm^{lo} SL^{++}) cells. In contrast, there is a marked reduction in large (cycling) pre-B1a cells and all subsequent developmental stages, including pre-B1b (cμ^{lo}ψLc$^+$), pre-B2 (cμ^{lo}ψLc$^-$), and B cells (cμ^{hi}ψLc$^-$). Studies using a combination of several cell surface and intracellular markers (Noordzij et al., 2002) identified a similar developmental block at the pre-B1 (cμ$^-$) to pre-B2 (cμ$^+$) transition based on the schema of Ghia and colleagues (1996).

In most XLA patients the pro-B and pre-B1 compartment composes more than 80% of B-lineage cells in the marrow compared with less than 20% in normal individuals. In contrast, an XLA patient that expressed low levels of wild-type Btk exhibited no pre-B developmental block. This is consistent with the concept that a lower dosage of Btk is sufficient to rescue the pre-B versus the mature B-cell developmental transitions. Interestingly, XLA patients may also exhibit a partial developmental block at the pro-B to pre-B1 stage. This may reflect a potential role for Btk in signals mediated by a pro–B-cell receptor complex, as has been suggested in murine studies (Kouro et al., 2001).

Although markedly reduced in number, XLA B cells still exhibit clonally diverse μ heavy chain variable-diversity-joining (V-D-J) rearrangements (Anker et al., 1989; Mensink et al., 1986; Milili et al., 1993; Timmers et al., 1991). This suggests that Btk is not required prior to immunoglobulin rearrangement or pre-BCR expression but is essential for the pre–B-cell transition.

Studies of pre-BCR signaling provide a biochemical framework for understanding failure of pre-B clonal expansion in XLA. A fraction of the human pre-BCR is constitutively associated with detergent-insoluble membrane microdomains known as lipid rafts (Guo et al., 2000). Receptor engagement increases this association and promotes activation of src family kinases, Igα/β phosphorylation, and the generation of a signaling module or "signalosome" composed of tyrosine phosphorylated signaling molecules, including activated Btk. Formation of this signalosome is required for pre-BCR calcium signaling and probably for other pre-BCR–dependent signals. Failure to support these biochemical events likely explains the failed expansion and decreased survival of XLA pre-B cells.

Role of Btk in BCR-Dependent Signals

Mature B cells typically compose only 0.1% of circulating lymphocytes in XLA patients (Conley, 1985). The limited numbers of circulating B lymphocytes in XLA patients have an "immature" phenotype with relatively high expression of both surface IgM and the co-stimulatory molecule, CD38 (Conley, 1985; Golay and Webster, 1986; Leickley and Buckley, 1986a). This immature phenotype is consistent with the phenotype observed in Btk-deficient mice. This finding suggests that Btk is also required for mature B-lymphocyte function.

Disruption of BCR expression leads to mature B-cell death, suggesting that low-level BCR signaling is required for mature B cells' maintenance (Neuberger, 1997). BCR-dependent signaling determines the fate of both immature and mature B cells.

The phenotype in *xid* mice (or mice with targeted disruptions of the *btk* gene) is less severe than in XLA (Kerner et al., 1995; Khan et al., 1995; Scher, 1982; Wicker and Scher, 1986). *Xid* mice generate modestly (30% to 50%) reduced numbers of peripheral B cells, but exhibit altered splenic B-cell development. Immature, or transitional, splenic B cells can be divided into two distinct subsets: transitional 1 (T1) and transitional 2 (T2) cells that are located in distinct anatomic locations (Loder et al., 1999). *Xid* mice have normal numbers of T1 and T2 B cells but have a severe reduction in the number of follicular mature (M) B cells. This suggests that defects in BCR signaling in *xid* block B-cell development from T2 to the M follicular B-cell stage.

T2 immature B cells (in contrast to either T1, marginal zone, or B1 splenic B cells) comprise a unique developmental subset that mediates BCR-dependent, proliferative, pro-survival, and differentiation signals. These signals promote the generation and survival of mature, recirculating B cells (Petro et al., 2002; Su and Rawlings, 2002). *Xid* T2 cells fail to generate these signals and fail to differentiate into mature B cells in vitro. The loss of mature B cells is further accelerated in *Btk-/-CD40-/-* doubly deficient mice (Khan et al., 1997; Oka et al., 1996) and is partially rescued in *xid* animals overexpressing the antiapoptotic proteins Bcl-2 or Bcl$_{XL}$ (Solvason et al., 1998; Woodland et al., 1996).

These observations highlight the essential role for the BCR/Btk signalosome at the T2 stage (see Fig. 13-1). Notably, the difference in phenotype between Btk-deficient humans and mice is explained by partially redundant function of Tec, another Btk family kinase expressed in pre-B cells. Btk/Tec doubly deficient mice *(Btk-/-Tec-/-)* exhibit a block in B-lineage development essentially identical to human XLA (see Fig. 13-1) (Ellmeier et al., 2000).

Consistent with these findings, a major role for Btk in BCR-dependent signaling has been elucidated (Rawlings, 1999). Btk is activated in response to BCR engagement and promotes phosphorylation of at least two key regulatory residues in phospholipase C gamma (PLCγ). Activation of PLCg promotes generation of inositol-1,4,5-trisphosphate (IP3) and diacylglycerol (DAG). These key second messengers lead to intracellular calcium mobilization, and protein kinase C (PKC) activation, respectively. Depletion of calcium stores by peak IP3 levels leads to enhancement of store-operated calcium influx and maintenance of the Btk dependent, sustained calcium signal (Fig. 13-2) (Fluckiger et al., 1998; Rawlings, 1999).

Activation of protein kinase Cβ (PKCβ) is essential for activation of NF-κB and prosurvival signaling (Anderson

Pre-B cell or transitional 2 and mature splenic B cell

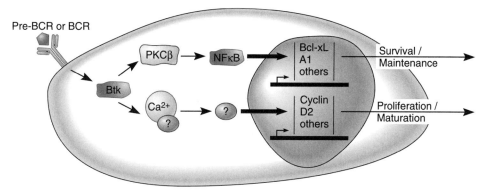

Figure 13-2 · Signaling function of Btk in bone marrow pre-B and splenic B cells. Btk is activated in response to pre-BCR or BCR engagement leading to increases in intracellular, sustained calcium signaling and protein kinase Cb (PKCb) activation. These events promote downstream transcriptional events that mediate protein kinase C (PKC)-dependent prosurvival signals and PKC-independent cell proliferation and maturation.

et al., 1996; Bajpai et al., 2000; Petro et al., 2000; Su et al., 2002). The amplitude and duration of calcium signals regulate proliferative responses and are a key determinant of the specific transcription program initiated following BCR activation (Berridge, 1993; Bootman and Berridge, 1995; Dolmetsch et al., 1997; Healy et al., 1997). Thus Btk-dependent signals modulate transcriptional events that determine the fate of splenic B cells (see Fig. 13-2).

Other Potential Btk Signaling Functions

Expression of Btk in non-B cells suggests that it participates in other lineage-dependent signaling events. Enhancement of Btk activity has been observed in multiple activation pathways in several cell lineages, including the B-cell co-stimulatory receptor, CD38 (Santos-Argumedo et al., 1998); the interleukin (IL)-5 (Kikuchi et al., 1995; Sato et al., 1994) and IL-6 receptors (Matsuda et al., 1995); the high affinity IgE receptor (FcεRI) on mast cells (Kawakami et al., 1994); G protein–coupled receptors via association with Gα12, Gαq, or Bg subunits (Jiang et al., 1998; Ma and Huang, 1998; Tsukada et al., 1994); and engagement of either the collagen receptor (glycoprotein VI and its associated Fc receptor gamma chain) (Quek et al., 1998); or the thrombin receptor (in association with alpha-IIb/beta-III integrins) in platelets (Laffargue et al., 1999). Additional receptors capable of activating other Btk/Tec kinase family members have been identified (Rawlings and Witte, 1994). The biologic relevance of these signaling pathways remains unclear. Defects in mast cell activation have been identified in Btk-deficient animal models. No clear evidence exists that functional defects in mast cells or other non-B cells contribute to the XLA phenotype. The relative specificity for Btk function in B cells is most likely explained by the redundant function of other Btk family kinases co-expressed in other cell lineages.

BTK Mutational Analysis and Clinical Phenotype

Identification of deficient function of Btk in XLA represented the first demonstration that mutation in a cytoplasmic tyrosine kinase could lead to a hereditary human disease. Extensive mutational analysis has demonstrated that alterations within each of the domains of Btk can result in XLA. These data have been the topic of several reviews and an international database cataloguing *BTK* mutations, designated *BTK*base, has been established (maintained at web address http://www.uta.fi/imt/bioinfo/BTKbase/) (Vihinen et al., 1995, 1998).

This resource lists more than 600 entries (including more than 500 unrelated families and more than 400 unique molecular events), including both published and directly submitted information. All major types of mutations, including missense, nonsense, insertions, and deletions, have been identified in XLA. All of these mutations, except those within the *BTK* promoter region, result in alterations in the *BTK* coding region or in the intron/exon splicing of *BTK* transcripts.

The genomic organization of *BTK* consists of 19 exons spanning approximately 37 kb in length (Hagemann et al., 1994; Ohta et al., 1994). Because of this relatively large genomic locus, rapid *BTK* mutational screening is best accomplished using either single-strand conformation polymorphism (SSCP) or reverse transcriptase-polymerase chain reaction (RT-PCR), screening of *BTK* exons, followed by direct gene sequencing to detect specific alterations. If mutations are not identified using these approaches and analysis of Btk protein or mRNA expression still suggests the diagnosis of XLA, then selected intronic screening may be required to identify the genetic abnormality. To date, this latter approach has been necessary in very few XLA patients.

BTK mutational analysis has identified mutations affecting every domain of the gene. Point mutations have been the most frequent defects identified, resulting in amino acid substitutions, premature stop codons, exon skipping resulting from splice junction mutations, and "non-start" from initiation codon mutations. With the exception of the SH3 domain (in which no missense mutations have been identified to date), the distribution of the mutations is approximately equal to the relative size of the individual domains.

The most frequently affected sites are CpG dinucleotides. Many of these missense mutations affect conserved, functionally significant residues. Molecular modeling of several of these residues supports their predicted effects on domain function. The most striking of these changes is the *xid* gene defect that alters a single residue (R28C) in the Btk PH domain (Rawlings et al., 1993; Thomas et al., 1993). This residue is also mutated in several XLA families, and has provided a major clue to the events controlling Btk activation.

Based on the crystal structure and binding studies, it is now clear that this residue lies directly within the Btk PH domain binding pocket. This change perturbs the recognition of PI(3,4,5)P3 and other phosphatidylinositol lipids, and may also block the interaction with protein ligands (Fukuda et al., 1996; Hyvönen and Saraste, 1997; Salim et al., 1996). Several TH domain mutations are predicted to affect Zn^{2+} binding, and those within the SH2 domain are predicted to alter phosphotyrosine ligand interactions. Similarly, mutations in the kinase domain affect functional and structural sites including the adenosine triphosphate (ATP) binding site.

Somewhat surprisingly, the location and type of mutation do not consistently correlate with the clinical phenotype of XLA. A number of families with a "leaky" or less severe disease phenotype have been described (e.g., with greater than 2% of normal B-cell numbers and/or higher levels of serum immunoglobulin) (Saffran et al., 1994; Zhu et al., 1994). However, significant disease variably exists even within the same family (Conley et al., 1994a; Wedgwood and Ochs, 1980), and patients presenting with typical XLA symptoms and clinical findings have been reported with mutations located within each of the Btk subdomains.

This phenotypic variation likely reflects multiple factors, including modifying alleles, infection history, and other events. The phenotypic differences in the human and murine Btk deficiency disorders (including variation in the severity of *xid* in different mouse strains) supports the importance of both modifier alleles and species-specific differences in B-lineage development.

Clinical Features

Because IgG is actively transported across the placenta, XLA patients have normal levels of serum IgG at birth and few, if any, symptoms. However, as the maternally derived IgG is catabolized, hypogammaglobulinemia and an increased susceptibility to infection develops. Thus most patients with XLA are asymptomatic in the first few months of life and begin to have recurrent infections between 4 and 12 months of age (Lederman

and Winkelstein, 1985). A significant number of patients, however, remain asymptomatic in the first year of life.

In a review of 96 XLA patients, nearly 20% experienced initial clinical symptoms after their first birthday and approximately 10% after 18 months of age (Lederman and Winkelstein, 1985). In another series of 44 patients, as many as 21% of patients first presented clinically as late as 3 to 5 years of age (Hermaszewski and Webster, 1993). There are also a number of reports of patients with onset of chronic infection recognized only in adulthood or misdiagnosed as common variable immunodeficiency (CVID) shown to have *BTK* mutations (Hashimoto et al., 1999; Kanegane et al., 2000; Kornfeld et al., 1997; Usui et al., 2001).

A retrospective review of 82 XLA patients suggests that the majority of patients experience chronic otitis media prior to definitive diagnosis and that attention to this history combined with physical signs of reduced lymphatic tissues might prompt more rapid diagnosis (Conley and Howard, 2002).

Bacterial Infections

Bacterial infections are the most common clinical manifestation of XLA, both before diagnosis and after IVIG therapy has been instituted (Hermaszewski and Webster, 1993; Lederman and Winkelstein, 1985; Liese et al., 1992). The infections are usually caused by pyogenic encapsulated bacteria including *Streptococcus pneumoniae*, *Haemophilus influenzae*, *Staphylococcus aureus*, and *Pseudomonas* species, organisms for which antibody is an important opsonin. These four organisms account for most of the cases of sepsis, pyogenic meningitis, and septic arthritis in patients with XLA (Kim et al., 2000; Lederman and Winkelstein, 1985; Zenone and Souilet, 1996).

Other bacterial species, such as *Salmonella* and *Campylobacter*, have also been described (Chusid et al., 1987; Hermaszewski and Webster, 1993; Lederman and Winkelstein, 1985; Van der Meer et al., 1986; Wyatt et al., 1977). Unusual chronic intravascular and intralymphatic infections secondary to *Flexispiral/Helicobacter*-related bacteria requiring prolonged antibiotics have also been reported (Cuccherini et al., 2000; Han et al., 2000; Weir et al., 1999).

The most common infection is chronic sinusitis. Indeed, this is present in nearly all patients and is very difficult to eradicate. Chronic sinusitis may lead to postnasal drip and a diminished gag reflex leading to chronic bronchitis, pneumonia, and even bronchiectasis.

Infections may be localized to the respiratory tract (e.g., otitis, sinusitis, pneumonia), skin (e.g., pyoderma), or gastrointestinal tract (e.g., diarrhea), or they may be systemic and blood-borne (e.g., sepsis, meningitis, septic arthritis). Although any single infection may be limited to one anatomic location, it usually occurs in multiple locations over time. For example, in a large multi-institutional series of patients with XLA, 74% of patients had infections of the upper respiratory tract (e.g., otitis, sinusitis) before diagnosis, but of these, more than two thirds also had infections of the lower respiratory tract (e.g., pneumonia, bronchiolitis) and/or gastrointestinal tract (Lederman and Winkelstein, 1985).

Although respiratory and gastrointestinal tract infections are most common, other infections also occur with regularity (Hermaszewski and Webster, 1993; Lederman and Winkelstein, 1985). Blood-borne systemic infections, such as sepsis, meningitis, osteomyelitis, and septic arthritis, each comprise approximately 5% to 15% of reported infections prior to IVIG therapy (Lederman and Winkelstein, 1985). When such infections do occur, they most often are secondary complications of infections in other sites. Gastroenteritis can be secondary to chronic infections with *Giardia lamblia* (LoGalbo et al., 1982; Ochs et al., 1972), rotavirus (Saulsbury et al., 1980), *Campylobacter* (Melamed et al., 1983), and other organisms.

Enteroviral Infections

Although resistance to viral infections is generally intact in XLA patients (Good and Zak, 1956; Janeway et al., 1953), there are some important exceptions. XLA patients are unusually susceptible to infections with enteroviruses, such as echovirus, coxsackievirus, and poliovirus (McKinney et al., 1987). These viruses usually cause primary infections in the gastrointestinal tract, with spread to the blood stream and secondary infection of the central nervous system (CNS) in some individuals. Antibody is important in neutralization of these viruses during their passage through the blood stream (Hammon et al., 1952). Transfer of immune B cells can rescue mice from chronic disease manifestations related to coxsackievirus B3 infection (Mena et al., 1999).

POLIOVIRUS

Several XLA patients have developed vaccine-related poliomyelitis after live attenuated (Sabin) poliovirus vaccine (Lederman and Winkelstein, 1985; Wright et al., 1977). Vaccine-related disease in these patients is usually characterized by a prolonged incubation period (often greater than 30 days), chronic CNS encephalomyelitis, a high mortality rate, and failure of the vaccine strain to revert to wild type virus (Wyatt, 1973).

ECHOVIRUS AND COXSACKIEVIRUS

Before the widespread use of high-dose IVIG, many XLA patients developed chronic and disseminated echovirus and coxsackievirus infections (Bardelas et al., 1977; McKinney et al., 1987; Wilfert et al., 1977). The infections involved several different organs (e.g., the CNS, skin, subcutaneous tissue, muscle, heart, and liver), leading to chronic meningoencephalitis (Wilfert et al., 1977), dermatomyositis (Bardelas et al., 1977; Gotoff et al., 1972) and hepatitis (Bardelas et al., 1977; Ziegler and Penny, 1975) (Fig. 13-3).

MENINGOENCEPHALITIS

Enterovirus meningoencephalitis is usually insidious in onset with slowly progressive neurologic symptoms,

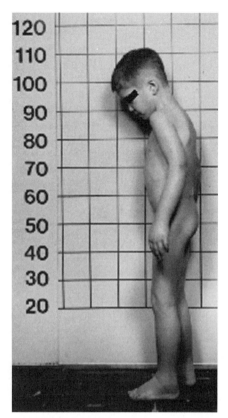

Figure 13-3· The patient is a 6-year-old boy with X-linked agammaglobulinemia and the dermatomyositis-like syndrome caused by disseminated echovirus 24 infection. Note the edema of the patient's extremities, especially the hands and feet, the gluteal wasting, and the flexion contractures of his arms and legs.

including emotional lability and personality changes, episodic confusional states, sensorineural hearing loss, retinal lesions, loss of cognitive function, lethargy, weakness, ataxia, and paresis. The clinical course is generally either a myelopathy progressing to encephalopathy or a pure encephalopathy (Rudge et al., 1996). In some patients, the onset is acute and manifested initially by fever, headache, and seizures.

Many patients have developed disease many years after their initial diagnosis and while receiving either intramuscular or IVIG. The course is often protracted, with some patients showing evidence of infection for 10 years despite treatment with high dose IVIG (McKinney et al., 1987; Mease et al., 1985; Rudge et al., 1996). Isolation of the virus from the cerebrospinal fluid (CSF) may be difficult or delayed until after symptoms and signs of CNS infection have progressed. Isolation of coxsackie A virus is especially difficult and may require inoculation of suckling mice (O'Neil et al., 1988). Newer diagnostic methods to identify viral genomic material by polymerase chain reaction (PCR) are useful in documenting infection (Leparc et al., 1994; Quartier et al., 2000; Rotbart et al., 1990; Webster et al., 1993). However, PCR analysis using conserved enteroviral nucleotide sequences still may not identify all cases of infection and nearly one half of reported cases lack an exact viral diagnosis.

In most cases, CSF findings are that of a viral meningoencephalitis with a mononuclear pleocytosis, elevated protein, and, occasionally, hypoglycorrhachia. Other patients have normal or near-normal CSF findings despite clinical evidence of encephalitis (Webster et al., 1993). Imaging studies are initially normal but eventually show progressive cortical and subcortical atrophy, periventricular changes, ventricular dilation, and hydrocephalus (Rudge et al., 1996). Brain autopsies typically demonstrate either end-stage encephalitis or leptomeningitis without vasculitis (Rudge et al., 1996).

The clinical picture is one of progressive decline associated with high mortality (McKinney et al., 1987; Rudge et al., 1996). Although several groups have described significant improvement following high-dose IVIG (including its intraventricular administration), the duration of these responses remains unclear (Erlendsson et al., 1985; Hadfield et al., 1985; Mease et al., 1981; Misbah et al., 1992), and many clinical failures have been reported. The higher serum IgG levels typically achieved with IVIG may provide protection against CNS enteroviral infection because the number of new cases is diminishing.

DERMATOMYOSITIS-LIKE SYNDROME

Patients with the *dermatomyositis-like syndrome* usually present with brawny edema of their extremities, an erythematous rash, and biopsy evidence of fasciitis and myositis (see Fig. 13-3). Biopsies show perivascular mononuclear infiltrates. Virus can be isolated from the skin, muscle, or liver (Bardelas et al., 1977; Junker and Dimmick, 1982; Mease et al., 1981; Ziegler and Penny, 1975). Most XLA patients with a dermatomyositis-like presentation ultimately develop encephalomyelitis.

Other Infections

Resistance to most other infections, presumed to depend on intact T-lymphocyte function (tuberculosis, histoplasmosis, varicella-zoster), appears to be intact. When these infections occur, they are no more serious than in normal patients. Although infection with *Pneumocystis carinii* has been observed in a few patients with XLA, it has usually occurred in patients who are also debilitated or otherwise compromised (Lederman and Winkelstein, 1985; Saulsbury et al., 1979). Fungal infections are also unusual but have been observed in a few patients, including one case report of cryptococcal empyema (Wahab et al., 1995). Interestingly, XLA patients lack Epstein-Barr virus (EBV)–specific cytotoxic T cells, suggesting that B cells are essential for acquisition of EBV infection (Faulkner et al., 1999).

HEPATITIS C

Several XLA patients developed hepatitis virus C (HVC) from contaminated IVIG in the early 1990s (see Chapter 4). Razvi and associates (2001) and Quinti and colleagues (2002) reported 9 and 11 patients respectively from U.S. and European centers. Approximately 10% to 30% of patients spontaneously cleared the HCV infection or remained asymptomatic, with the others exhibiting variable degree of hepatic dysfunction despite therapy. Hepatic failure was reported in one XLA patient co-infected with hepatitis B. This HCV risk has now been significantly reduced or eliminated by modified practices for screening and preparing IVIG.

Although 8 of 28 XLA patients reported by Morris and co-workers (1998) had passively acquired GB virus C RNA, there is no evidence that this was the cause of non-B non-C hepatitis (Morris et al., 1998). The capacity of XLA patients to generate normal CD4 T-cell responses to hepatitis B surface antigen (HBsAg) suggests that they may respond more favorably than CVID patients to acquired viral infections (Paroli et al., 2002; Plebani et al., 1997).

Arthritis

Up to 20% of XLA patients develop arthritis. Occasionally the arthritis is caused by pyogenic bacteria typical of septic arthritis (Hermaszewski and Webster, 1993; Lederman and Winkelstein, 1985). Usually the arthritis is not septic, but instead closely resembles juvenile chronic arthritis (Fu et al., 1999; Gitlin et al., 1959; Good and Rotstein, 1960; Good et al., 1957; Hansel et al., 1987; Janeway et al., 1956; McLaughlin et al., 1972). It characteristically affects the large joints with effusion, limited range of motion, and pain. Initially there is no joint destruction, and the erythrocyte sedimentation rate is normal. As expected, serologic tests for rheumatoid factor and antinuclear antibodies are negative.

The arthritis may improve when treatment with IVIG is initiated (with or without addition of nonsteroidal anti-inflammatory agents) or when the IVIG dose is increased, suggesting an infectious cause. In some cases the arthritis is associated with infection with enteroviruses or *Mycoplasma* (Ackerson et al., 1987; Frangogiannis and Cate, 1998; Franz et al., 1997; Hermaszewski and Webster, 1993). In seven XLA patients with chronic arthritis, *Ureaplasma* was cultured from the synovial fluid or biopsies in three patients; the remainder exhibited features consistent with previous or subsequent mycoplasma infection, including mycoplasma osteomyelitis in two individuals (Franz et al., 1997). Onset of disease was correlated with low IgG levels and the patients responded to IV antibiotics and IVIG therapy. With improved diagnostic tests for viruses and fastidious microorganisms, more infectious agents may be identified.

Gastrointestinal Disease

Chronic intestinal inflammation mimicking Crohn's disease has been reported in XLA patients (Abramowsky and Sorensen, 1988; Washington et al., 1996; Cellier et al., 2000). Its pathogenesis may reflect a failure of regulatory B-cell function (Mizoguchi et al., 2002), a response to chronic enteroviral infection (Cellier et al., 2000), or other events.

Gastroenteritis is not uncommon and may be associated with malabsorption. *Giardia lamblia* (LoGalbo et al., 1982; Ochs et al., 1972), *Campylobacter* species (Melamed et al., 1983), or rotavirus (Saulsbury et al., 1980) may be the causative agent.

Other Manifestations

Less common manifestations include neutropenia (see below), alopecia totalis (Ipp and Gelfand, 1976), glomerulonephritis (Avasthi et al., 1975), protein-losing enteropathy (Norman et al., 1975), malabsorption with disaccharidase deficiency (Dubois et al., 1970), and amyloidosis (Hermaszewski and Webster, 1993; Ziegler and Penny, 1975). Conjunctivitis is common in adults, and many note improvement with IVIG and its return as the IgG levels decrease toward the end of an infusion period.

Physical Examination

Abnormalities on physical examination directly related to XLA include markedly hypoplastic or absent tonsils, adenoids, and lymph nodes, tissues that are normally rich in B lymphocytes (Fig. 13-4). Other physical findings are usually secondary to specific infections such as chronic otitis, sinusitis, mastoiditis, or bronchiectasis. Growth delay and digital clubbing are not uncommon. However, patients treated before permanent structural damage has occurred appear normal (except for the paucity of lymphatic tissue) and their growth is age appropriate.

Laboratory Features

Immunoglobulins and Antibodies

XLA patients have markedly reduced levels of all classes of serum immunoglobulins (Lederman and Winkelstein, 1985; Rosen et al., 1984). IgG levels are generally below 100 mg/dl and in some cases may be nearly undetectable. Although markedly reduced in number, a few B cells are nearly always detectable in the blood.

Consistent with this, immunoglobulin production can be demonstrated in culture supernatants of peripheral blood lymphocytes (Cooperband et al., 1968; Levitt et al., 1984; Stites et al., 1971). Most patients have low but detectable levels of immunoglobulin of one or another isotypes in their serum (Lederman and Winkelstein, 1985; Rosen et al., 1984; Wedgwood and Ochs, 1980). In a rare XLA patient, the IgG level may be as high as 200 to 300 mg/dl. Serum levels of IgA, IgM, and IgE are also markedly reduced or undetectable.

XLA patients have low or undetectable antibody titers to ubiquitous antigens (e.g., isohemagglutinins, antistreptolysin, anti–*Escherichia coli*) and to previously administered vaccine antigens. Their antibody response to deliberate antigenic challenge with the usual childhood vaccines (e.g., tetanus, diphtheria, pertussis, and *H. influenzae* type b) or other immunogens (e.g., pneumococcal polysaccharide and typhoid vaccines) are markedly reduced or undetectable (Rosen et al., 1984).

When immunized with a potent neoantigen such as bacteriophage ϕX-174, 60% of XLA patients demonstrate an absolute inability to respond (Ching et al., 1966; Wedgwood et al., 1975). They did not clear phage from the blood in an accelerated manner and produce no detectable antibody. However, as many as 40% of patients with XLA clear phage from the blood in less than 1 week and produce small amounts of antigen-specific IgM antibody (see Fig. 12-4 and Table 12-18).

B Cells and Plasma Cells

Most XLA patients have few mature B lymphocytes (<2%) in their blood or tissues, as assessed by analysis of surface immunoglobulin or B-cell specific monoclonal

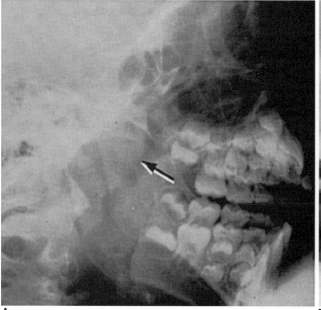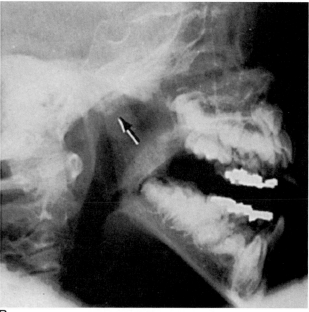

A   B

Figure 13-4· A. Lateral roentgenogram of the nasopharynx of a normal 10-year-old boy. Adenoidal tissue is present *(arrow)*. B. Lateral roentgenogram of the nasopharynx of a 10-year-old boy with X-linked agammaglobulinemia. Adenoidal tissue is absent *(arrow)*.

antibodies (such as anti-CD19, anti-CD20) (Aiuti et al., 1972; Bentwich and Kunkel, 1973; Cooper and Lawton, 1972; Geha et al., 1973; Preud'Homme et al., 1973; Schiff et al., 1974; Siegal et al., 1971). Advanced analysis of the sparse B-cell population shows a maturational arrest at the pre–B1 to pre–B2 stage and progressive decline in all subsequent developmental stages.

Because the diagnosis of XLA in the newborn period and in the first few months of life is obscured by the presence of passively acquired maternal IgG and the physiologically low IgA and IgM levels (Stiehm and Fudenberg, 1966b), the markedly reduced number of B cells enables an early diagnosis.

XLA patients also lack plasma cells in the bone marrow, the lamina propria of the rectal mucosa (Fig. 13-5), and lymph nodes (Ament et al., 1973; Gitlin et al., 1959; Good, 1955). Similarly, areas of lymph nodes typically rich in B lymphocytes and plasma cells, such as lymphoid follicles and germinal centers of lymph nodes, are markedly hypoplastic or absent.

Cellular Immunity

T-lymphocyte numbers and functions are normal. In vivo delayed cutaneous hypersensitivity skin tests to ubiquitous antigens (e.g., *Candida* species) or following antigenic sensitization (e.g., mumps, tetanus) are also normal.

Absolute NK-cell numbers have been reported to be reduced in XLA (Aspalter et al., 2000), that did not change in response to immunoglobulin therapy. Because Btk is not expressed in NK cells, the reason for these observations (also seen in patients with CVID) remains unclear, but may be relevant to the increased risk for malignancy in XLA.

Granulocytes (Neutropenia)

Significant neutropenia (Buckley and Rolands, 1973; Farrar et al., 1996; Hermaszewski and Webster, 1993; Lederman and Winkelstein, 1985; Plo et al., 1999) has been reported in approximately 10% to 25% of XLA patients. Neutropenia is nearly always associated with an acute illness (>90% of cases, including approximately 50% with sepsis). The duration is typically less than 1 week and resolves with antibiotic therapy. Neutropenia has not been reported with patients receiving IVIG. It is unclear whether there is a requirement for Btk for neutrophil function or development during stress.

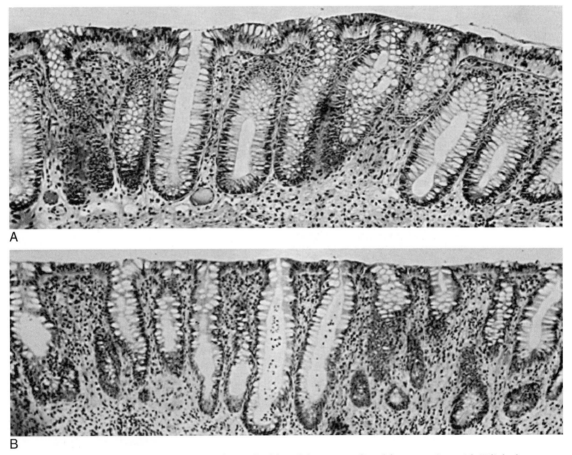

Figure 13-5· Rectal biopsy specimen from a healthy adult *(top panel)* and from a patient with X-linked agammaglobulinemia *(lower panel)*. Plasma cells are plentiful in the healthy adult (**A**) but are absent in the XLA patient (**B**). There are multiple polymorphonuclear leukocytes in the glands in the XLA patient. (×115.) (Courtesy of Dr. Marvin Ament.)

Btk Protein Expression

The B cells in female obligate XLA carriers exhibit non-random X-chromosome inactivation consistent with an autonomous B-lineage defect (Conley and Puck, 1988; Conley et al., 1986; Fearon et al., 1987). In normal females, B-cell progenitors comprise two nearly equal pools expressing either the active maternal, or the paternal X-chromosome, respectively. In contrast, female XLA carriers have a single predominant population expressing only the normal *BTK* allele (Conley and Puck, 1988; Conley et al., 1986; Fearon et al., 1987). Consistent with an intrinsic B-lineage defect, other cell populations that express Btk (including myeloid cells and platelet precursors) exhibit unbiased X-chromosome inactivation.

These observations pioneered the development of improved methods for the diagnosis of XLA (and XLA carrier status) using Btk-specific monoclonal antibodies. Using flow cytometric analysis of intracellular Btk expression in monocytes or platelets, 85% of hypogammaglobulinemic patients with reduced B-cell numbers (<1%) exhibit either absent or reduced Btk expression (Futatani et al., 1998, 2001; Kanegane et al., 2001; Tani et al., 2002). In addition, approximately 10% to 20% of patients with normal Btk expression exhibit missense mutations in *BTK*. This methodology is now the preferred initial diagnostic evaluation for patients with suspected XLA.

Diagnosis

Diagnostic criteria for XLA are based on the developmental, clinical, and genetic inheritance pattern of this disorder (Conley et al., 1999). These criteria are divided into three categories: definitive, probable, and possible (Table 13-1). These are designed to categorize individual patients based on the relative certainty of diagnosis, to assist in directing the diagnostic evaluation of affected individuals, and to facilitate clinical and molecular research.

Carrier Diagnosis

There are three major approaches for carrier detection in XLA: (1) analysis of an altered pattern of X-chromosome inactivation in carrier B lymphocytes, (2) analysis of closely linked X-chromosome genes (i.e., linkage analysis), and (3) mutational analysis of the *BTK* gene in those families with known mutations (Vorechovsky et al., 1993; Zhu et al., 1994).

The B cells of noncarrier females contain two populations, one in which the maternal X-chromosome is active and one in which the paternal X-chromosome is active. In contrast, the B lymphocytes of female XLA carriers contain only one population of B cells, that of the normal allele at the XLA locus.

Nonrandom X-chromosome inactivation in carriers can be identified by analysis of methylation patterns (Fearon et al., 1987), examination of somatic cell hybrids that have selectively retained the active X-chromosome (Conley and Puck, 1988), or by flow cytometric intracellular analysis of Btk expression in carrier monocytes or platelets. This latter approach is the current method of choice and identifies the majority of obligate carriers with the exception of those pedigrees with *BTK* missense mutations

TABLE 13-1 · CRITERIA FOR THE DIAGNOSIS OF X-LINKED AGAMMAGLOBULINEMIA

Definitive	Male patient with less than 2% CD19+ B cells and at least one of the following: 1. Mutation in *BTK* 2. Absent Btk mRNA on northern blot analysis of neutrophils or monocytes 3. Absent Btk protein in monocytes or platelets 4. Maternal cousins, uncles, or nephews with less than 2% CD19+ B cells
Probable	Male patient with less than 2% CD19+ B cells in whom all of the following are positive: 1. Onset of recurrent bacterial infection in the first 5 years of life 2. Serum IgG, IgM, and IgA more than 2 SDs below normal for age 3. Absent isohemagglutinins and/or poor response to vaccines 4. Other causes of hypogammaglobulinemia have been excluded (see later*)
Possible	Male patient with less than 2% CD19+ B cells in whom other causes of hypogammaglobulinemia have been excluded (see later*) and at least one of the following is positive: 1. Onset of recurrent bacterial infections in the first 5 years of life 2. Serum IgG, IgM, and IgA more than 2 SDs below normal for age 3. Absent isohemagglutinins
Spectrum of disease	Most patients with XLA develop recurrent bacterial infections, particularly otitis, sinusitis, and pneumonia in the first 2 years of life. The most common organisms are *Streptococcus pneumoniae* and *Haemophilus influenzae*. The serum IgG is usually less than 200 mg/dl (2 g/L) and the IgG and IgA are generally less than 20 mg/dl (0.2 g/L). Approximately 20% of patients present with a dramatic, overwhelming infection, often with neutropenia. Another 10%–15% have higher concentrations of serum immunoglobulin than expected or are not recognized to have immunodeficiency until after 5 years of age.
Differential diagnosis	I. Other causes of hypogammaglobulinemia described in this volume II. Alternative genetic causes for agammaglobulinemia with absent B cells 1. μ heavy chain deficiency 2. λ5 deficiency 3. Igα deficiency 4. BLNK deficiency

BLNK = B-cell linker protein; Ig = immunoglobulin; mRNA = messenger RNA; SD = standard deviation; XLA = X-linked agammaglobulinemia.
From Conley ME, Notarangelo LD, Etzioni A. Diagnostic criteria for primary immunodeficiencies. Representing PAGID (Pan-American Group for Immunodeficiency) and ESID (European Society for Immunodeficiencies). Clin Immunol 93:190–197, 1999.

leading to normal levels of protein expression, or very rare cases in which there is severe skewing toward the normal X chromosome. An advantage of X-chromosome inactivation analysis is that the mutation responsible for the XLA need not be known and a previously affected family member need not be available (Conley and Sweinberg, 1992; Winkelstein and Fearon, 1990).

Analysis of closely linked X-chromosome genes (i.e., linkage analysis) can also be used in cases in which a previously affected family member expresses a specific allele of a gene closely linked to *BTK*. A number of polymorphic loci (e.g., DXS178) that are closely linked to the XLA locus have been useful in carrier detection (Guioli et al., 1989; Kwan et al., 1986, 1990; Malcolm et al., 1987; Mensink et al., 1986; Parolini et al., 1993).

Prenatal Diagnosis

Prenatal diagnosis is possible by mutation analysis of Btk using amniotic fluid cells and/or enumeration and flow cytometric analysis of Btk expression in B lymphocytes of fetal cord blood. Prenatal diagnosis of an affected fetus has been performed using both techniques. These techniques have also been used to exclude the diagnosis in fetuses at risk (Journet et al., 1992; Kwan et al., 1994).

Treatment

Immunoglobulin Therapy

The primary goal of treating XLA patients is to replace immunoglobulin. Although intramuscular immunoglobulin was initially used, IVIG or subcutaneous immunoglobulin (SCIG) infusions are now used. IVIG has allowed XLA patients to achieve normal or near-normal serum IgG levels and has significantly improved their clinical course (Hermaszewski and Webster, 1993; Liese et al., 1992; Sweinberg et al., 1991). Liese and colleagues (1992) compared different doses of IVIG to intramuscular immunoglobulin and found that patients who received relatively high doses of IVIG (>400 mg/kg every 3 weeks) and maintained IgG trough levels at or near the lower limit of normal (>500 mg/dl) had significantly fewer hospitalizations and infections than patients who received lower doses of IVIG (<200 mg/kg every 3 weeks) or immunoglobulin. The effect of high-dose IVIG on the incidence of pneumonia, bacterial meningitis, and gastrointestinal infections was particularly evident when treatment was initiated early in life.

Slow SCIG infusions or more rapid SCIG administration are additional options that may improve patient compliance, decrease side effects, limit fluctuations in IgG levels, and result in lower cost (Gardulf et al., 1995; Hansen et al., 2002). Chapters 4 and 12 also discuss immunoglobulin therapy.

Several additional studies suggest that IgG trough levels at or near 500 mg/dl may not be sufficient to prevent chronic lung disease and chronic sinusitis in XLA (Kainulainen et al., 1999; Quartier et al., 1999; Roifman et al., 1987). Of 23 XLA patients who received higher dose IVIG (with median IgG trough levels of 700 mg/dl), 3 had obstructive lung disease, 6 had bronchiectasis, and 20 had chronic sinusitis. A recent survey of Italian XLA patients with similar trough IgG levels found that chronic lung disease developed in 80% of patients after 17 years of follow-up (Plebani et al., 2002). Thus the optimal immunoglobulin dosing regimen for XLA still remains incompletely defined.

Although IVIG therapy has been a major advance in the treatment of patients with XLA, it has some limitations. IVIG only replaces IgG and is unable to correct the defect in secretory antibody. In addition, the use of nonselected lots of IVIG does not provide high levels of specific antibody to all organisms, and the patients are still susceptible to a variety of infections.

Treatment of Enteroviral Infection

An important concern is the treatment of disseminated enteroviral infections (McKinney et al., 1987). Since the introduction of IVIG, the incidence of disseminated enteroviral infections has dropped dramatically, but it still may occur in some patients receiving IVIG (Misbah et al., 1992; Rotbart et al., 1990) or in children prior to a diagnosis. Most XLA patients with disseminated enteroviral infection have been treated with high-dose IVIG aimed at maintaining the IgG level greater than 1000 mg/dl. In some patients, selected lots of IVIG with high titers of antibody against the specific serotype of virus have been employed. In some instances, IVIG has also been given by the intraventricular route to deliver antibody to the site of CNS infection (Erlendsson et al., 1985).

These therapies have not proved uniformly successful. In some patients, relapses occurred (McKinney et al., 1987; Mease et al., 1985) despite temporary clinical improvement. In other patients, neurologic signs persisted (Ciliberti et al., 1994) or progressed despite high-dose IVIG given by both the IV and intraventricular routes (Johnson et al., 1985; McKinney et al., 1987; Webster et al., 1993), albeit more slowly than in untreated patients, indicating that IVIG therapy is not adequate in all cases of established infection.

Enterovirus encephalitis has been treated with a new antipicornaviral agent, pleconaril. In one patient with persistent symptoms despite high-dose IVIG, pleconaril therapy was associated with clinical improvement with rapid resolution of elevated cell counts, protein levels, and loss of PCR-detectable CSF enteroviral genome (Schmugge et al., 1999). In two other patients, very-high-dose IVIG (with IgG levels up to 8000 mg/dl) and pleconaril led to sustained clinical improvement and viral clearance by PCR analysis (Quartier et al., 2000).

Other Therapy and Vaccines

Prompt treatment of acute bacterial infections with antibiotics is mandatory (see Chapter 12). In patients with chronic sinusitis or chronic lung disease, long-term, broad-spectrum antibiotics are needed along with other supportive therapy such as inhaled steroids or bronchodilators, postural drainage, and even surgery. Antiviral therapy may be necessary for influenza or recurrent herpes infections.

Live viral vaccines are contraindicated because of the possibility of vaccine-related infections such as poliomyelitis (Hermaszewski and Webster, 1993; Lederman and Winkelstein, 1985; Wright et al., 1977; Wyatt, 1973). Killed vaccines may be useful for induction of T-cell immunity (Paroli et al., 2002; Plebani et al., 1997) as well to test for specific antibody or T-cell responses.

Gene Therapy

A strong selective pressure for survival of hematopoietic stem cells with wild-type (normal) BTK has been demonstrated by both nonrandom X-inactivation studies (described previously) and in competitive repopulation studies. Transplantation of mixtures of CBA/J (wild-type) and CBA/N (xid) bone marrow cells to lethally irradiated xid mice leads to the selective expansion and preferential survival of wild-type B lineage cells (Sprent and Bruce, 1984). Transfer of large numbers of normal marrow or fetal liver cells (10^7 cells/animal) into xid mice can restore their immune responses without conditioning (Quan et al., 1981; Quintans et al., 1979). Immune responses can also be restored in sublethally irradiated (200 to 400 cGy) mice with as few as 2.5×10^4 CBA/J marrow cells resulting in as few as 10% wild-type (normal) cells in the recipient's spleen (Rohrer and Conley, 1999). Thus gene therapy that results in even partial Btk reconstitution may be sufficient to restore B-cell function. Preclinical development of safe and efficient methods for BTK gene transfer is underway (Yu et al., 2000, 2002).

Complications and Prognosis

Before antibiotics and IVIG, few XLA patients survived past infancy or early childhood. Early diagnosis, regular IVIG therapy, and prompt use of antibiotics have increased their longevity dramatically. In a series of 44 XLA patients, age-related survival was significantly better in patients diagnosed and treated recently (Hermaszewski and Webster, 1993). Thus an increasing number of XLA patients are adults. Two follow-up studies in genetically defined XLA patients indicate that infectious and noninfectious morbidity remains high (Plebani et al., 2002; Van der Hilst et al., 2002). The mortality rates in XLA are also unclear but can be as high as 30% over approximately 10 years, even with current comprehensive care (Van der Hilst et al., 2002).

Long-term lung complications are more common in patients whose diagnosis has been delayed or in older patients who initially did not receive high-dose IVIG therapy. For example, in a series largely made up of patients who were diagnosed and treated before the introduction of IVIG, approximately 75% of the patients older than 20 years of age had chronic lung disease, either obstructive disease alone or combined obstructive and restrictive disease; and 5% to 10% had cor pulmonale (Lederman and Winkelstein, 1985). Even in patients treated with higher-dose IVIG therapy, the risk for chronic lung disease and chronic sinusitis is substantial (Plebani et al., 2002; Quartier et al., 1999).

Chronic otitis media and hearing loss may result in speech and learning disorders. Other complications include chronic disseminated enteroviral infection, vaccine-related poliomyelitis, and amyloidosis (Hermaszewski and Webster, 1993).

XLA patients may have an increased incidence of lymphoreticular malignancies (see Chapter 39). Estimates of the incidence of lymphoid malignancy in XLA range from 0.5% to 6% in various studies that may include some non-XLA patients (Frizzera et al., 1980; Hayakawa et al., 1986; Hermaszewski and Webster, 1993; Kinlen et al., 1985; Lederman, 1995; Lederman and Winkelstein, 1985; Luzi et al., 1991; Mueller and Pizzo, 1995; Page et al., 1963; Spector et al., 1978). In one series, lymphoreticular malignancies developed in 2 of 96 (2%) XLA patients (Lederman and Winkelstein, 1985). In another series, however, none of 44 patients with XLA had a malignancy (Hermaszewski and Webster, 1993).

Several case reports and a study from the Netherlands describe the early development of colorectal cancer in XLA patients (Adachi et al., 1992; Chisuwa et al., 1999; Kinlen et al., 1985; Van der Meer et al., 1993). If accurate, this risk is approximately 30-fold greater than that expected for age. The increased risk for colorectal cancer may be related to an absence of plasma or regulatory B cells in the gut (Mizoguchi et al., 2002), persistent asymptomatic inflammation, as suggested by the presence of multiple crypt abscesses and polymorphonuclear leukocyte infiltrates in the lamina propria (Ament et al., 1973), or other factors such as reduced levels of glutathione S-transferase in the colonic mucosa (Grubben et al., 2000).

Gastric adenocarcinoma has also been reported in XLA in association with chronic giardiasis and atrophic gastritis (Lavilla et al., 1993).

Huo and associates (1994) identified increased radiosensitivity in EBV-transformed B cells from XLA patients and proposed that Btk may play a role in signals regulating repair of radiation damage to deoxyribonucleic acid (DNA). This may increase their propensity to malignancy.

David J. Rawlings

X-LINKED HYPOGAMMAGLOBULINEMIA WITH GROWTH HORMONE DEFICIENCY

Definition

X-linked hypogammaglobulinemia with growth hormone deficiency is a rare familial disorder of short stature and hypogammaglobulinemia with absent B cells.

Historical Aspects

In 1980, Fleisher and colleagues reported a family in which the combination of hypogammaglobulinemia and growth hormone deficiency were inherited as an X-linked recessive disorder. Since that original report, three additional unrelated families have been identified (Conley et al., 1991; Monafo et al., 1991; Sitz et al., 1990), suggesting that X-linked hypogammaglobulinemia with growth hormone deficiency is a distinct clinical entity rather than the coincidental occurrence of two unrelated inherited disorders. Another report of growth hormone deficiency in a boy with immunodeficiency and increased IgM (Ohzeki et al., 1993) and the finding of isolated growth hormone deficiency and antibody deficiency in a girl with Mulibrey nanism (Haraldsson et al., 1993) support the alternative explanation of a nonspecific growth hormone deficiency that may develop in patients suffering from recurrent infections and an abnormal immune system.

Pathogenesis

The cause of X-linked hypogammaglobulinemia with growth hormone deficiency is unknown. Studies in two of the families using X-chromosome inactivation analysis of female carriers indicate that the immunologic defect is intrinsic to the B-lymphocyte lineage (Conley et al., 1991). Linkage analysis in two families indicated that the defect maps to a relatively large region of the X-chromosome (approximately 5%) that includes the BTK gene (Conley et al., 1991).

These findings have led to the suggestion that X-linked hypogammaglobulinemia with growth hormone deficiency is either an allelic variant of the more typical XLA, which in some fashion affects both B-lymphocyte development and growth hormone production, or is a small, contiguous gene deletion syndrome that includes both the gene for XLA and another closely linked gene involved in growth hormone production. In this regard, it is interesting to note that although the structural gene for growth hormone is located on the long arm of chromosome 17 (George et al., 1981), there is also an X-linked gene that controls growth hormone production (Najiar et al., 1990; Phillips and Vnencak-Jones, 1989).

Mapping and/or mutational analysis of BTK in several patients with this association has led to divergent results. Physical mapping in three patients excluded the possibility of a contiguous deletion of the BTK and an associated locus. Analysis of the patient originally described by Fleisher and co-workers in 1980 revealed normal BTK coding sequence and protein expression (Stewart et al., 1995). In contrast, analysis of two other cases revealed an insertion in BTK exon 6 (predicted to generate a premature stop codon) in one patient and two carrier females (Abo et al., 1998), and an intronic point mutation (predicted to alter splicing of the Btk kinase domain) in the second patient (Duriez et al., 1994). Neither of the latter studies confirmed the predicted change through an analysis of Btk protein expression.

Growth hormone studies in three sporadic and two familial cases suggest that the association of X-linked, B-cell immunodeficiency with "true" growth hormone deficiency is very rare (Buzi et al., 1994) and that most cases can be explained by delayed priming with testosterone resulting from delay in growth and puberty as described in other chronic diseases. Thus it is likely that this rare association represents a currently undefined, BTK-independent, X-linked disorder, leading to alterations in both B-cell development and growth hormone production.

Clinical Features

Patients with X-linked hypogammaglobulinemia with growth hormone deficiency presented with many of the same clinical features seen in typical XLA patients, including recurrent upper respiratory infections, pneumonia, sepsis, recurrent otitis media, conjunctivitis, dacryocystitis, and monarticular arthritis. Their growth hormone deficiency is manifested by short stature and delayed onset of puberty.

Laboratory Features

Most patients have marked hypogammaglobulinemia and absent B lymphocytes in the peripheral blood. However, one patient from the original kindred had normal levels of IgA and IgM and reduced but detectable (3%) numbers of B lymphocytes (Fleisher et al., 1980). Affected males do not respond to immunization with either protein or polysaccharide antigens. T-lymphocyte function is intact.

Growth hormone deficiency is manifested by retarded bone age and deficient growth hormone responses to insulin, arginine, and L-dopa (Conley et al., 1991; Monafo et al., 1991; Sitz et al., 1990). As expected, levels of circulating somatomedin are also reduced (Fleisher et al., 1980). Other tests of endocrine function, including cortisol responses to insulin-induced hypoglycemia and gonadal function, are normal (Fleisher et al., 1980).

Treatment

As with other antibody-deficient patients, IVIG is the mainstay of therapy. Growth retardation appears to respond appropriately to growth hormone injections.

Complications and Prognosis

Patients with X-linked hypogammaglobulinemia with growth hormone deficiency appear to have an excellent prognosis. In fact, many of the patients had not been identified as hypogammaglobulinemic until they were of school age or older (Conley et al., 1991; Fleisher et al., 1980; Monafo et al., 1991; Sitz et al., 1990), suggesting that the clinical expression of their immunodeficiency may be milder than typical XLA. However, in one member of the original kindred, chronic disseminated echovirus infection developed, manifested clinically as chronic meningoencephalitis and dermatomyositis (Wagner et al., 1989).

David J. Rawlings

AUTOSOMAL RECESSIVE AGAMMAGLOBULINEMIA

Definition

Autosomal recessive agammaglobulinemia is a profound antibody deficiency syndrome associated with absent or very low B cells, thus resembling XLA, but without characteristic *BTK* abnormalities. It occurs in either sex, may have an autosomal recessive pattern of inheritance, and is associated with several different genetic defects. A specific genetic defect has not yet been identified in more than 50% of the patients with these features.

Historical Aspects

Several groups reported female patients with absent B cells and hypogammaglobulinemia in the 1970s. Two of these reports also included partial phenotypic analysis of bone marrow progenitors demonstrating a very early blockade in bone marrow B lineage development. Mapping studies in several female agammaglobulinemic patients demonstrated no linkage with Xq22 (Conley and Sweinberg, 1992; Yel et al., 1996).

Based on these and related reports, it was predicted that approximately 5% to 10% of patients with agammaglobulinemia and B-cell deficiency are females. Because it is likely that a similar percentage of males with an XLA phenotype have normal Btk function, approximately 10% to 15% of all patients with B-cell negative, congenital agammaglobulinemia may have mutations in alternative gene products (Conley and Sweinberg, 1992; Conley et al., 1994c; Grunebaum, 2001; Minigeshi et al., 1999a; Yel et al., 1996).

Pathogenesis

B-lineage development is characterized by the sequential expression of a series of B-lineage–specific and ubiquitously expressed transcripts. Several key proteins are required for this development and have been identified primarily through gene targeting approaches in murine models (Cheng et al., 1995; Clayton et al., 2002; Fruman et al., 1999; Gong and Nussenzweig, 1996; Hashimoto et al., 2000; Jou et al., 2002; Jumaa et al., 1999; Kitamura et al., 1991, 1992; Okkenhaug et al., 2002; Pappu et al., 1999; Wang et al., 2000). These observations suggested that alternative genetic defects (in addition to *BTK* deficiency) might result in agammaglobulinemia.

Candidate gene abnormalities for these disorders include those coding for (1) B-lineage–specific transcription factors, (2) components of the pre-BCR, and (3) signaling molecules associated with the pre-BCR.

Recent studies have identified four autosomal recessive genetic disorders that result in early disruption of B-lineage development and congenital agammaglobulinemia. Conley and colleagues (1994a, 1994e; Minigeshi et al., 1998, 1999a, 1999b; Yel et al., 1996) have carried out most of these studies. Her group has used several approaches to delineate these defects, including (1) screening of candidate genetic loci using polymorphic short tandem repeats to identify potential genetic linkage, (2) genomic DNA screening using Southern blotting to detect large alterations such as deletion or duplications at these loci, and (3) SSCP analysis followed by direct gene sequencing to detect alterations in the coding sequence of candidate genes.

Mutations in μ Heavy-Chain Gene

Linkage analysis was initially performed in two families with autosomal recessive agammaglobulinemia (including two female and four male patients) using short tandem repeat sequences (Yel et al., 1996). Both families exhibited an inheritance pattern consistent with a defect at 14q32, the location of immunoglobulin heavy-chain genes. Southern blotting with a probe for the μ constant-region gene demonstrated deletion of the μ heavy chain in the affected children from one family. Because of parental consanguinity, both of these children inherited a common μ heavy-chain allele and were homozygous for the shared allele. This 75-kb deletion included all of the D and J region genes, the immunoglobulin enhancer, and the entire coding region of the μ constant-region.

Analysis of two additional unrelated patients (including one from the other family noted previously) showed no evidence of a deletion. SSCP identified altered exons in the fourth constant region of the μ heavy chain. In one individual with evidence for consanguinity, a single base substitution was identified that was predicted to lead to absent production of the membrane form of the μ heavy chain. In the second individual, a single base substitution led to replacement of a cysteine with glycine predicted to alter disulfide bonding, making the protein unstable. In this latter individual, the second μ heavy-chain allele was deleted. These combined mutations were predicted to lead to an absence of surface μ expression.

To date, μ heavy-chain disruption with autosomal recessive agammaglobulinemia has been identified in at least 21 members from 14 unrelated families (Lopez Granados et al., 2002; Meffre et al., 1996; Milili et al., 2002; Schiff et al., 2000). Together, the susceptibility of the μ heavy chain to potential mutations associated with immunoglobulin rearrangement, and the critical role for the μ heavy chain (in association with both the surrogate light chains, conventional light chains, and the immunoglobulin transducer complex including both Igα and Igβ) suggests that additional mutations in this protein are likely to be identified.

Mutations in the λ5/14.1 Gene IGLL1

The surrogate light chain components, VpreB and λ5/14.1, are likely candidates for target genes leading to autosomal recessive agammaglobulinemia, because they are required for normal B-lineage development as part of the pre-BCR complex. The VpreB and λ5 proteins assemble to produce a complex that is similar to the conventional λ light chain. The terminal portion of VpreB is homologous to the variable region of immunoglobulin and the carboxyl-terminal portion of λ5 is similar to the J and constant regions of the λ light chain. These proteins are noncovalently linked to one another and are covalently linked to the μ heavy chain via a cysteine in λ5.

Surrogate light chain is absolutely required for surface expression of the μ heavy chain in pre-B cells. These three proteins, expressed in association with the Igα and Igβ chains, form the pre-BCR. Expression of this receptor leads to pre–B-cell clonal survival and expansion and to subsequent conventional light-chain expression. This signal functionally permits the pre-BCR to test the integrity of the rearranged μ chain prior to initiating light-chain gene rearrangements.

Mutations have been identified in the λ5 gene (IGLL1) using SSCP analysis of genomic PCR products in a 5-year-old boy with sporadic agammaglobulinemia and absent B cells (Minegishi et al., 1998). These mutations resulted in a premature stop codon in the maternal allele and three base pair substitutions in the paternal allele. The latter change led to substitution of a leucine for proline at codon 142.

Analysis of this mutant protein expressed in fibroblasts suggested that this substitution resulted in improper protein folding with more rapid λ5 protein turnover and/or unstable association during formation of the pre-BCR. Interestingly, this missense mutation was also present in the λ5 pseudogene (16.1) suggesting that the mutant IGLL1 allele resulted from a gene conversion event (Minegishi et al., 1998).

Mutations in the Igα (B29; CD79A) Gene

The immunoreceptor tyrosine activation motif (ITAM)-containing proteins, Igα (CD79a) and Igβ (CD79b), form the transducer complex of the pre-BCR and the mature BCR and are encoded by the B29 and MB-1 genes, respectively. Hence, alterations in these genes are also predicted to lead to B-lineage immunodeficiency.

Consistent with this prediction, a defect in Igα was identified in a 2-year-old agammaglobulinemic female with absent B cells (Minegishi et al., 1999a). This patient was identified through SSCP screening of 25 agammaglobulinemia patients with normal BTK. Analysis of the Igα-coding exons identified an altered migration pattern in exon 3 of this patient. Genomic sequencing revealed a single base pair mutation leading to deletion of the transmembrane domain of Igα. Both parents were heterozygous for the identical mutation and no wild-type Igα transcripts were present in the patient's bone marrow, consistent with a homozygous defect.

Mutations in the B-Cell Adaptor Molecule BLNK

Engagement of the B-cell antigen receptor leads to the rapid tyrosine phosphorylation of the adapter protein BLNK (B-cell linker protein; also known as SLP-65; BASH) (see Chapter 3). Phosphorylated BLNK serves as a critical scaffold protein that nucleates the assembly of other signaling complexes, leading to increases in intracellular calcium and the activation of a cascade of MAP kinases. Targeted disruption of BLNK in mice results in a block in B-cell development in the pre–B-cell stage (Jumaa et al., 1999; Pappu et al., 1999). These observations suggested that autosomal recessive agammaglobulinemia might result from BLNK deficiency.

To test this hypothesis, the human BLNK gene was isolated and its genome structure determined (Minegishi et al., 1999a). SSCP primers amplifying each of the BLNK exons were used in analysis of 25 patients with agammaglobulinemia and normal BTK. This analysis revealed a homozygous alteration in the first exon of BLNK in one individual. Sequencing identified a homozygous splice defect predicted to alter processing of the BLNK message. Consistent with these findings, BLNK transcripts and protein expression were undetectable in marrow pro-B cells using RT-PCR and flow cytometric analysis.

Other Congenital Agammaglobulinemias

As noted, the genetic defect or defects responsible for approximately 50% of patients with absent B cells and congenital agammaglobulinemia and normal BTK remain undefined. These defects likely include additional components of the pre-BCR, as well as other genetic alterations such as transcriptional activators that might lead to either lymphoid-specific or more ubiquitous alterations in other tissues and organ systems. An example of the latter may include a recently described syndrome with agammaglobulinemia and absent B cells, intrauterine growth retardation, microcephaly, cerebellar hypoplasia, and progressive pancytopenia (Revy et al., 2000a).

B-Lineage Developmental Abnormalities

Development of both bone marrow and peripheral blood B-lymphocyte populations have been evaluated using flow cytometric analysis in each of the four forms of autosomal recessive agammaglobulinemia. As observed in XLA, patients with these disorders have normal numbers of CD34+ CD19+ pro-B cells, but have significantly reduced numbers of CD34− CD19+ pre-B cells (including large cycling pre-B cells) and all subsequent developmental stages. The λ5-deficient patient also had significantly reduced staining for cytoplasmic VpreB, consistent with an altered stability of the surrogate light chain. Together, these observations and the marked reduction in CD19+ CD34− pre-B cells in these disorders suggests a primary role for each of these gene products for the surface expression and the signaling function of the pre-BCR complex.

Comparing the peripheral B-cell numbers in XLA with the various forms of autosomal recessive agammaglobulinemia reveals several additional differences. CD19+ cells typically compose 0.1% of peripheral blood lymphocytes in both XLA- and λ5-deficient patients. In contrast, CD19+ cell are nearly undetectable (<0.01%) in patients with deficiencies in μ heavy chain, Igα, or BLNK. This suggests a more stringent requirement for the latter proteins in pre-BCR signaling.

Despite the slightly larger numbers of B cells in both Btk and λ-deficient patients, there are differences in the B-cell surface phenotype in these two disorders. Circulating B cells in the λ5-deficient patient exhibited relatively low IgM and CD38 surface expression. In contrast, XLA B cells have a more immature phenotype with increased expression of both surface IgM and CD38. This suggests that the mutant λ5 protein permits some level of pre-BCR function, leading to generation of a limited pool of relatively normal functioning mature B cells. In contrast, although Btk is not absolutely required for the generation of peripheral B cells, it is necessary for the survival and maturation of the peripheral B-cell pool.

Generation of a Pre–B-Cell Receptor Signaling Complex

As detailed previously, disruption of pre-BCR components (including μ, Igα, Igβ, or λ5) or their associated signaling molecules (including Syk, Btk, p85, and BLNK) results in partial or complete pre–B-cell developmental arrest in mice and humans. Studies of the signaling events initiated by pre-BCR engagement provide a biochemical framework for understanding immunodeficiencies leading to blockade at the pro– to pre–B-cell transition.

A fraction of the human pre-BCR is constitutively associated with detergent-insoluble membrane microdomains known as *lipid rafts* (Guo et al., 2000). Receptor engagement increases this association and promotes src family kinase activation; Igα/β phosphorylation; and the generation of a signaling module composed of tyrosine phosphorylated Syk, BLNK, Btk, PLCγ2 and additional signaling molecules. Formation of this molecule is required for pre-BCR calcium signaling.

These biochemical findings directly link these B-lineage signaling molecules to a functional role or roles in human pre-BCR signaling. The more severe phenotype associated with the human immunodeficiencies suggests that the pre-BCR signal is more stringent in humans than in mice.

These findings also suggest that mutations in other components of this signaling module (such as PLCγ2, PI-3-K isoforms, or others) may account for additional cases of agammaglobulinemia. The events necessary for successful μ heavy-chain rearrangement, pre-BCR expression, and pre-BCR signaling appear to be a critical bottleneck in human B-lineage development that can be disrupted at multiple levels and lead to a similar clinical phenotype.

Clinical Features

Most patients with autosomal recessive agammaglobulinemia have a disease phenotype very similar to that of X-linked agammaglobulinemia. However, patients with μ heavy chain alterations may have a more severe clinical phenotype (Lopez Granados et al., 2002). Although the numbers of patients described are small, they appear to present at an earlier mean age (11 months) than do XLA patients (32 months) (Yel et al., 1996). Notably, 7 of the 21 reported μ heavy chain deficient patients developed chronic enteroviral encephalitis versus a 10% frequency in XLA. One of these autosomal recessive patients died of chronic enteroviral encephalitis. The very small number of patients with either Igα, λ5, or BLNK deficiency had presentations similar to patients with XLA.

Laboratory Features and Diagnosis

In agammaglobulinemic males with an apparent X-linked inheritance pattern and severely decreased peripheral B lymphocytes, the diagnosis of XLA is extremely likely. However, because up to 50% of XLA cases are sporadic, methods for diagnosis of autosomal recessive agammaglobulinemia are required. A first step in males is to exclude Btk deficiency as outlined in the XLA section of this chapter. In males with normal *BTK* and in females additional testing is required, including screening of candidate genes using chromosomal localization in association with RT-PCR and/or SSCP analysis. Because these disorders are so rare, laboratories dedicated to this area of research must be consulted.

Treatment and Prognosis

The mainstay of therapy is immunoglobulin replacement as in XLA. Because of the small number of patients identified, it is not known whether these patients also have an increased risk for malignancies.

David J. Rawlings

COMMON VARIABLE IMMUNODEFICIENCY

Definition

CVID is a clinically heterogeneous disorder presenting at any age, characterized by recurrent bacterial infections, hypogammaglobulinemia, impaired antibody responses despite the presence of B cells, and normal or near-normal T-cell immunity (Cunningham-Rundles and Bodian, 1999; Hermaszewski and Webster, 1993; Janeway et al., 1953). Although this disorder was first recognized in 1953 (Janeway et al., 1953), its fundamental cause remains unknown.

The incidence of CVID lies between 1:25,000 and 1:66,000 (Hammarström et al., 2000). In most cases, the onset of symptoms appears after puberty, and the diagnosis is usually made in the second or third decade of life; however, approximately 25% are diagnosed prior to age 21. CVID is the most common form of severe antibody deficiency.

Pathogenesis

Because of the variability in age of onset and in the clinical and laboratory abnormalities, and an unpredictable genetic component (Schroeder et al., 1998; Vorechovsky et al., 2000), CVID is probably not caused by a single defect. Indeed, in spite of intensive investigation, a precise molecular defect resulting in most cases of CVID has not been identified.

Studies of T and B lymphocytes from patients with CVID, both in vitro and in vivo, have revealed a wide variety of abnormalities. Although most patients with CVID have normal numbers of mature B lymphocytes in the peripheral blood and lymphoid tissue, they have various defects in differentiation into immunoglobulin-secreting plasma cells. Specific defects identified are outlined in the following paragraphs.

B-Cell Defects

The main phenotype of CVID is the lack of immune globulin and antibody resulting from a variable block in B-cell differentiation (Bryant et al., 1990; Eisenstein et al., 1994; Saiki et al., 1982). Although most patients have normal numbers of B cells, a small proportion of CVID patients have low B-cell numbers (Farrant et al., 1994). A few male patients given the clinical diagnosis of CVID may actually have atypical XLA and should be studied for mutations of the Btk gene (Kanegane et al., 2000; Weston et al., 2001).

Defects in the expression of the B-cell co-receptors CD27 and CD134 ligand, important in promoting differentiation into plasma cells, have been demonstrated (Jacquot et al., 2001). In contrast to the mature memory B cells observed in normals, CVID B cells have the phenotypic characteristics of immature B lymphocytes, including the use of restricted V_H gene families and lack of somatic hypermutation (SHM) of variable heavy-chain genes (Bonhomme et al., 2000; Levy et al., 1998). Recent studies have demonstrated deficient numbers and activation of memory B cells (Brouet et al., 2000) and a severe deficiency of switched memory B cells (Agematsu et al., 2002; Warnatz et al., 2002).

A number of investigators have studied in vitro immunoglobulin synthesis in CVID (Nonoyama et al., 1993a). CVID B lymphocytes co-cultured with normal allogeneic T lymphocytes do not produce or secrete normal amounts of immunoglobulin. Conversely, T lymphocytes from many of these patients may support immunoglobulin production by normal B lymphocytes (Ashman et al., 1980). Purified CVID B lymphocytes activated by several stimuli identify several subgroups of patients: the B cells of one group fail to produce any immunoglobulin, a second group produces only IgM with little or no IgG, and a third group produces IgM and IgG in normal or near normal quantities (Bryant et al., 1990; Saiki et al., 1982).

CVID B cells usually produce immune globulin if stimulated by the polyclonal B-cell activator, the antisense oligomer to the rev gene of HIV-1 (Branda et al., 1996). It is not clear, however, whether the B-cell defects of CVID are permanent, or if under some circumstances the B cells could be induced to produce immunoglobulin. There are four CVID patients who have contacted human immunodeficiency virus (HIV) infection, and have had reconstitution of both immunoglobulin levels and antibody production (Jolles et al., 2001). The mechanism for this is unknown.

T-Cell Defects

Some CVID patients have associated T-cell defects. T-cell subsets are generally normal but many have lymphopenia. A subgroup of CVID patients (25% to 30%) have increased numbers of CD8+ lymphocytes, normal or decreased numbers of CD4+ lymphocytes, and a reduced CD4/CD8 ratio (Aukrust et al., 1994; Jaffe et al., 1993; Wright et al., 1990). A general lack of antigen-specific T cells is characteristic (Kondratenko et al., 1997) and a restricted T-cell receptor repertoire, with oligoclonal expansion of CD8+ T cells, may be present (Serrano et al., 2000). Many patients have decreased CD4+ CD45RA+ T cells suggesting a persistent activation of circulating naïve T cells with expansion of the CD45RO+ memory cell population or preferential homing of the CD45RA+ lymphocytes into chronically infected tissues (Baumert et al., 1992).

Many subjects with CVID have decreased proliferation of peripheral blood lymphocytes when stimulated in vitro with mitogens or antigens (Cunningham-Rundles and Bodian, 1999; Cunningham-Rundles et al., 1981; North et al., 1989; Reinherz et al., 1981). Proliferative defects are more common in older subjects. CVID T lymphocytes often have markedly decreased amounts of IL-specific mRNA and functional ILs, including IL-2 (Eisenstein et al., 1994; Kruger et al., 1984; Nonoyama et al., 1994), interferon (IFN)-γ, IL-2, IL-4, IL-5 (Pastorelli et al., 1989; Sneller and Strober, 1990), and IL-10 (Zhou et al., 1998).

Others have noted abnormalities of the T-cell receptor (TCR), resulting in defective T-cell activation following stimulation with anti-CD2 (Zielen et al., 1994), or anti-CD3 (Fischer et al., 1994, 1996), impaired intracellular tyrosine kinase expression following TCR ligation (Majolini et al., 1997), reduced ZAP-70 mobilization (Boncristiano et al., 2000), deficient CD28 co-signaling (DiRenzo et al., 2000), and accelerated T-cell death associated with increased expression of CD95 (DiRenzo et al., 2000; Iglesias et al., 1999).

Adhesion/Switching Defects

Perhaps contributing to their immune dysfunction, CVID patients have reduced expression of cell surface molecules involved in adhesion, including L-selectin (Zhang et al., 1996), attractin (Pozzi et al., 2001), and CD40 ligand (CD40L, CD154) (Farrington et al., 1994). CD40L, expressed by activated CD4+ lymphocytes, is of primary importance in B-cell proliferation, differentiation, and isotype switching. In a significant proportion of CVID patients, CD40L mRNA, as well as functional CD40L protein expression, is significantly depressed, suggesting inefficient signaling or defective activation (Farrington et al., 1994).

The fact that CVID B cells, when cultured in vitro in the presence of anti-CD40 and IL-4, undergo normal proliferation and synthesize normal quantities of IgE further supports the hypothesis that most patients with CVID have B lymphocytes capable of normal function (Nonoyama et al., 1993a; Saxon et al., 1992).

Four patterns of in vitro Ig isotype synthesis by CVID B cells can be observed. One third of CVID patients produced normal amounts of IgM, IgG, and IgA; 25% produced normal quantities of IgM and IgG, but no IgA. Of the remaining patients who did not synthesize IgG and IgA, the majority produced normal and/or decreased amounts of IgM (Nonoyama et al., 1993a).

Although the main characteristic of CVID is its profound antibody defects, several types of immune over-activation could contribute to some of the clinical pathology. In some subjects, especially those with splenomegaly and lymphadenopathy, there are increased levels of serum IL-4 and IL-6 (Adelman et al., 1990; Aukrust et al., 1994). Elevated IL-4 and IL-6 serum levels may be accompanied by elevated serum levels of neopterin and of soluble CD8 and by low numbers of both CD4+ T lymphocytes and CD19+ B lymphocytes.

Markers of oxidative stress, potentially caused by chronic inflammation, have been noted (Aukrust et al., 1994, 1997, 1999). Some subjects have increased cyclic adenosine monophosphate (cAMP)-dependent protein kinase A type 1 (PKA1) and elevated endogenous cAMP levels. Because PKA1 is an inhibitor of T-cell proliferation after antigen stimulation, this form of immune activation might result in defective T-cell function (Aukrust et al., 1999).

Monocyte/Macrophage Defects

Monocyte/macrophage defects have also been identified in CVID. The increased IL-6 concentration in blood and culture supernatants is mostly of monocyte origin (Adelman et al., 1990); in addition, a higher proportion of lipopolysaccharide (LPS)-stimulated circulating CD14-positive monocytes express intracellular IL-12 than monocytes from patients with XLA or normal subjects (Cambronero et al., 2000). This imbalance might skew the immune response away from antibody production and could explain the failure of CVID T cells to make antigen-specific memory cells.

Monocyte activation may also be involved in the pathogenesis of the chronic inflammatory and granulomatous complications that are present in some CVID patients (Aukrust et al., 1997; Mullighan et al., 1997, 1999).

Genetic Abnormalities

CVID is currently viewed as a heterogeneous group of disorders with an intrinsic B-cell defect or a B-cell dysfunction related to abnormal T cell–B cell interaction. In the majority of cases, there is no family history of a related or similar defect. However, in 10% to 20% of families, another member may have selective IgA deficiency, IgG deficiency, or much more rarely, CVID.

A large microsatellite linkage study of 101 multiple-case families with IgA deficiency and CVID demonstrated a susceptibility locus lying in the telomeric part of the major histocompatibility complex (MHC) class II region or the centromeric part of the MHC class III region on chromosome 6 (Schroeder et al., 1998; Vorechovsky et al., 2000). However, the issue is complicated by the observation that different regions of MHC haplotype exert different effects (de la Concha et al., 1999).

One polymorphism, the +448A polymorphism of the tumor necrosis factor (TNF)-α gene has been associated with a form of CVID in which granulomatous changes appear in many organs, especially the lungs (Mullighan et al., 1997, 1999).

In search of a genetic defect in CVID, Grimbacher and co-workers (2003) found that 4 of 32 CVID patients lacked the *inducible co-stimulator* (ICOS) expressed by activated T cells, because of a homozygous deletion in the *ICOS* gene. Loss of ICOS is associated with lack of T-cell help for late B-cell differentiation, class switching, and memory B-cell generation (Grimbacher et al., 2003).

Clinical Features

Most CVID patients present with recurrent sinopulmonary infections, most often bacterial pneumonia. Symptoms may first appear during childhood or, more often, after puberty. Physical examination may include features of otitis or sinusitis, acute or chronic lung disease, and weight loss. Clubbing suggests long-standing pulmonary disease. Some patients have lymphadenopathy and hepatosplenomegaly. Other patients may present with autoimmune manifestations such as hemolytic anemia, thrombocytopenia, arthritis, or gastrointestinal disease.

Although males and females are equally affected, there are clinical differences in the male and female CVID patients; a recent study of 248 subjects in New York City showed that the mean age at symptom onset was 23 for males and 28 for females. (Cunningham-Rundles and Bodian, 1999). The mean age at diagnosis was 29 for males and 33 for females (Fig. 13-6).

Approximately 27% of males were diagnosed prior to the age of 21, but only 14% of females were diagnosed before age 21. Among 248 patients with CVID, there were only 11 Hispanics and 4 African Americans; the remainder were Caucasians of European descent, suggesting either racial differences or lack of recognition in some ethnic groups.

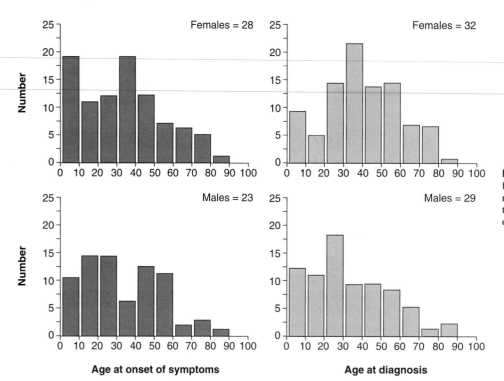

Figure 13-6· The ages of male and female common variable immunodeficiency patients at the onset of their symptoms and at their time of diagnosis.

Infections

In a study of CVID in the United Kingdom, 151 of 240 patients (63%) had one or more episodes of pneumonia prior to diagnosis, and 86 (36%) had sinusitis, otitis, and/or mastoiditis (Hermaszewski and Webster, 1993). In a U.S. study of 248 patients, 78% had experienced one or more episodes of pneumonia prior to diagnosis (Cunningham-Rundles and Bodian, 1999).

Bronchiectasis may develop if diagnosis and/or optimal therapy is delayed (Hermaszewski and Webster, 1993; Kainulainen et al., 1999; Martinez Garcia et al., 2001). In one series, 42 patients (18%) had already developed bronchiectasis at the time of diagnosis (Hermaszewski and Webster, 1993). In fact, unrecognized CVID cases may be identified in "chest" or pulmonary clinics; this finding emphasizes the necessity of evaluating all bronchiectasis patients for immunodeficiency.

The organisms most often involved in sinopulmonary infections are *H. influenzae, Streptococcus pneumoniae,* and staphylococci. In rare situations, infections may involve such unusual organisms as *Pneumocystis carinii, Mycobacterium* species, or fungi (Cunningham-Rundles and Bodian, 1999; Esolen et al., 1992; Sneller, 2001). Prolonged and persistent infection with *Mycoplasma pneumoniae* is not infrequent (Franz et al., 1997). Recurrent attacks of herpes simplex are sometimes observed, and herpes zoster may develop in up to 20% of CVID patients (Asherson et al., 1980).

HEPATITIS C

In the early 1990s a number of CVID patients became infected with hepatitis C through their IVIG infusions, apparently the result of changing the manufacturing process to exclude hepatitis C antibody-positive subjects from the donor pool. Several of these patients underwent spontaneous remission, others remained stable but infected, and others developed symptomatic hepatitis C, a few of which went on to death or liver transplantation (Chapel et al., 2001; Razvi et al., 2001). Thus patients who received IVIG during this period should be tested for hepatitis C, preferably by PCR.

Gastrointestinal Problems

Some CVID patients present with inflammatory bowel disease (Crohn's disease or ulcerative colitis) with characteristic pathology; more often, a morphologically atypical inflammatory gastrointestinal disease is found, resulting in diarrhea, malabsorption, and weight loss (Cunningham-Rundles and Bodian, 1999; Washington et al., 1996).

Gastrointestinal disease was present in 53 subjects of one group of 248 (21%) CVID patients (Cunningham-Rundles and Bodian, 1999). A chronic malabsorption syndrome with steatorrhea, folate and vitamin B$_{12}$ deficiency, lactose intolerance, generalized disaccharidase deficiency, protein-losing enteropathy, and abnormalities of villous architecture is seen frequently in CVID patients (Ament et al., 1973) (Fig. 13-7). *Giardia lamblia* or *Campylobacter* species may be found in some patients. Washington and colleagues (1996) examined the pathology of the gastrointestinal tract in CVID; 10 of 43 CVID subjects had one or more biopsies taken; the pathology ranged from mild to severe villous atrophy in those with malabsorption, to granulomatous infiltration or a pattern resembling graft-versus-host disease with a lymphocytic infiltrate in others. *Giardia* species was found in three subjects of this group, and a

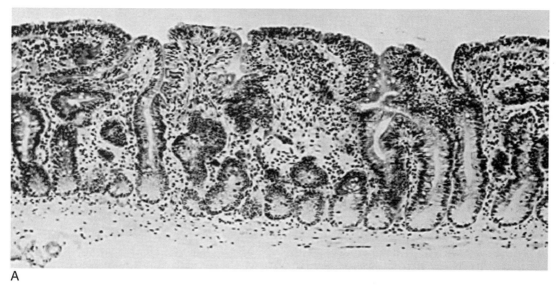

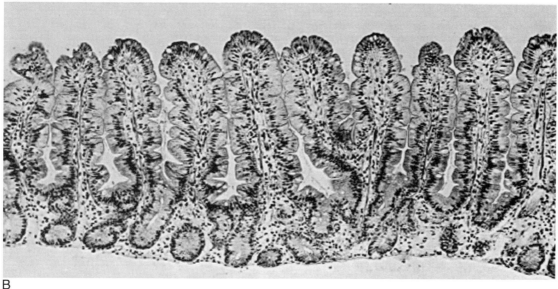

Figure 13-7· Intestinal biopsies in common variate immunodeficiency. **A.** Representative peroral biopsy specimen taken near the duodenojejunal junction of a patient with common variable immunodeficiency, gastrointestinal symptoms, and malabsorption caused by *Giardia lamblia* infestation. The villus architecture is markedly abnormal. (H and E, ×150.) **B.** Biopsy specimen taken 4 weeks after completion of treatment to eradicate giardiasis; the villus architecture is normal. (H and E, ×150.) (Courtesy of Dr. Marvin Ament.)

small bowel lymphoma in two subjects. Another agent of importance in CVID is *Helicobacter pylori;* Zullo and associates (1999) examined 34 dyspeptic CVID subjects and found *H. pylori* on gastric biopsy in 14 (41%).

Nodular lymphoid hyperplasia of the small bowel is frequently observed. Endoscopic examination reveals large lymphoid follicles with germinal centers within the lamina propria, causing protrusion of the overlying mucosa and nodular or polypoid appearance on radiographs (Washington et al., 1996). Plasma cells of the lamina propria are usually absent or markedly reduced.

Most patients with nodular lymphoid hyperplasia are asymptomatic unless they are infected with *G. lamblia;* eradication of the parasites improves symptomatology

but does not change the extent of nodular lymphoid hyperplasia. In addition to *G. lamblia* infection, patients with CVID are at risk for gastrointestinal infections with enteropathogens, including *Salmonella, Shigella, Campylobacter,* and perhaps rare organisms such as dysgonic fermenter-3 (DF-3), a gram-negative bacterium (Sneller et al., 1993).

Autoimmunity

Autoimmune disorders are more frequent in CVID patients and their relatives than in a normal control population: 20% to 25% of subjects with CVID at the time of diagnosis or later develop one or more autoimmune conditions (Asherson, 1980; Cunningham-Rundles and

Bodian, 1999; Hermaszewski and Webster, 1993; Sneller, 2001).

Disorders resembling rheumatoid arthritis, dermatomyositis, scleroderma, and systemic lupus erythematosus have been described in adult CVID patients. Autoimmune hemolytic anemia, immune thrombocytopenic purpura, autoimmune neutropenia, pernicious anemia, chronic active hepatitis, parotitis, alopecia, primary biliary cirrhosis, and Guillain-Barré syndrome have also been observed.

Polymorphisms of mannose binding lectin have been associated with autoimmunity in some patients (Mullighan et al., 2000).

Granulomata

In both adult and pediatric CVID patients, noncaseating granulomas of the lung, spleen, liver, skin, and other tissues may develop, a condition resembling sarcoidosis (Fasano et al., 1996; Mechanic et al., 1997). The cause is unknown, but granulomata are more common in subjects with T-cell defects, splenomegaly, and autoimmune disease; a role for tumor necrosis factor polymorphisms has been suggested (Mullighan et al., 1997, 1999).

Malignancy

There is an unusually high incidence of lymphoreticular and gastrointestinal malignancies in older CVID patients (Cunningham-Rundles and Bodian, 1999; Cunningham-Rundles et al., 1987; Sander et al., 1992). In comparison with normal populations, CVID subjects show an 8- to 13-fold increase in cancer in general and a 438-fold increase in lymphoma for females (Cunningham-Rundles et al., 1987). As with other congenital immunodeficiencies, the lymphomas in CVID tend to be extranodal in origin and of B-cell lineage. Unlike the nodular lymphoid hyperplasia found in other immunodeficiencies, which are often poorly differentiated, CVID lymphomas tend to be well differentiated, secrete immunoglobulins, and are mostly EBV-negative.

In one study, 19 lymphomas appeared in a group of 248 subjects; 14 of these patients were female (Cunningham-Rundles and Bodian, 1999). In five other cases, a low-grade B-cell lymphoma of mucosal-associated lymphoid tissue (MALT) type developed (Cunningham-Rundles et al., 2002). Three stomach cancers were noted in this patient group, and in another survey two stomach cancers were found among 240 CVID subjects (Hermaszewski and Webster, 1993).

Laboratory Features

Serum immunoglobulin levels are consistently depressed but are generally higher in CVID patients than in XLA patients. IgG levels rarely exceed 300 mg/dl but occasionally may reach 500 mg/dl. IgM and IgA levels are low or undetectable in most patients. Fluctuations in immunoglobulin levels do occur, however, and some IgA-deficient and IgG subclass deficient subjects may

develop CVID over time (Espanol et al., 1996; Johnson et al., 1997).

Isohemagglutinin titers and specific antibody levels are depressed or absent. For subjects with higher IgG levels (>450 mg/dl), verification of antibody deficiency (using a panel of antibodies postvaccine challenge) is important prior to starting immunoglobulin replacement. Following immunization with bacteriophage φX-174, all CVID patients studied have cleared antigen and the majority of patients produce neutralizing antibody. However, a large proportion of CVID patients exhibit low titers, abnormal amplification, and a depressed switch from IgM to IgG (Ochs et al., 1971; Wedgwood et al., 1975).

Lymphocyte subsets in the peripheral blood, as determined by surface markers, are normal in the majority of patients, including the presence of normal or only moderately decreased numbers of B lymphocytes. However, up to one third of patients with CVID have an abnormally low CD4/CD8 ratio (<1.0), primarily a result of a significant increase in CD8+ T lymphocytes and/or a reduced number of CD4+ T cells. The subset of CD8+ T cells, preferentially expressed by patients with splenomegaly and bronchiectasis, co-express human leukocyte antigen D-related (HLA-DR) and IL-2 receptor, suggesting in vivo activation (Wright et al., 1990).

The standard tests to assess T-cell function, including in vitro proliferation to mitogens, antigens, and allogeneic cells, are subnormal in up to 50% of CVID patients, with a small subgroup of patients having very low responses. In addition, as pointed out earlier, a number of investigators have demonstrated a decreased production of lymphokines and abnormally low expression of T-lymphocyte activation markers (e.g., CD40 ligand) in a subgroup of CVID patients (Farrington et al., 1994; Kruger et al., 1984; Pastorelli et al., 1989; Sneller and Strober, 1990).

In vitro assessment of B cells with techniques that eliminate the need of direct T-cell contact suggests that B cells from most CVID patients are normal or less mature, perhaps similar to cord blood B lymphocytes (Nonoyama et al., 1993a, 1995).

Diagnosis and Differential Diagnosis

The diagnosis of CVID depends on excluding other well-defined immunodeficiency syndromes, finding serum IgG and IgA and/or IgM levels that are substantially reduced, and finding that antibody responses are deficient. Most patients have IgG levels of 400 mg/dl or less and 70% have absent or very low levels of serum IgA. B lymphocytes are usually present, unlike the case in XLA.

A CVID diagnosis should not be made in children younger than the age of 2, because these cases may represent transient hypogammaglobulinemia of infancy (see elsewhere in this chapter). If a CVID diagnosis is made before the age of 5, it should be verified by retesting at later times. The diagnosis of CVID may also not apply to patients who develop lymphoma within 2 years of the diagnosis of hypogammaglobulinemia, because

Specific antibodies, when present, are of the IgM isotype, such as isohemagglutinins, (Benkerrou et al., 1990; Pascual-Salcedo et al., 1983). Following immunization with a T-cell–dependent antigen such as bacteriophage φX-174, HIGM1 patients have a low normal primary and a depressed secondary antibody response consisting of IgM only and either absent or markedly reduced amplification (Aruffo et al., 1993; Nonoyama et al., 1993a). CD40L/CD40 interaction is essential for memory B-cell generation and SHM. Consequently, the number of IgD⁻ CD27⁺ memory B cells is markedly diminished in HIGM1 (Agematsu et al., 1998). Moreover, somatic mutation of immunoglobulin variable genes is typically diminished (Chu et al., 1995; Razanajaona et al., 1996).

Because failure of terminal B-cell differentiation is due to a primary T-cell defect, B lymphocytes from HIGM1 patients in vitro switch normally to IgE production and can produce some IgG and IgA (Allen et al., 1993; Aruffo et al., 1993; Korthäuer et al., 1993).

The number and distribution of T-cell subsets is normal in HIGM1, although the proportion of CD45R0⁺ memory T cells is reduced (Jain et al., 1999). In vitro lymphoproliferative response to mitogens is normal, whereas the response to recall antigens is often defective (Ameratunga et al., 1997; Levy et al., 1997). Moreover, HIGM1 patients have a defective Th1 response, as shown by reduced secretion of interferon-γ and failure of antigen-presenting cells to synthesize IL-12 (Jain et al., 1999; Subauste et al., 1999).

Histologic examination of lymph nodes of HIGM1 patients disclose primary follicles, but germinal centers are typically absent (Facchetti et al., 1995) (Fig. 13-10).

HIGM1 patients frequently have hematologic abnormalities. More than 50% of patients have persistent or cyclic neutropenia (Benkerrou et al., 1990; Levy et al., 1997). Anemia is present in approximately 25%, commonly resulting from chronic infection (Levy et al., 1997), and rarely resulting from parvovirus B19-induced red cell aplasia. The latter has been the presenting feature in a group of HIGM1 patients with a mild phenotype (Seyama et al., 1998a).

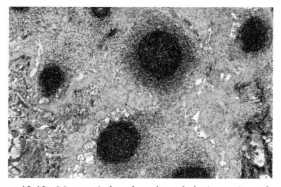

Figure 13-10 · **Mesenteric lymph node pathologic specimen from a patient with X-linked hyper-IgM syndrome type 1.** The lymph node contains primary follicles, but is devoid of germinal centers. (Courtesy Prof. F. Facchetti, Department of Pathology, University of Brescia, Italy.)

Diagnosis

The diagnosis of HIGM1 can be strongly suspected by demonstrating that in vitro–activated CD4⁺ T cells do not express CD40L (CD154), using a soluble form of the receptor for CD40L, a chimeric recombinant of CD40 termed *CD40-Ig*. Alternative tools, such as monoclonal or polyclonal antibodies to CD40L (CD154) may give false negative results, because they may recognize mutant forms of the protein (Callard et al., 1994; Seyama et al., 1998b).

In rare instances, the CD40-Ig construct may bind to mutant CD40L, although with reduced intensity (Seyama et al., 1998b). Reduced expression of CD40L has also been observed in the neonatal period (Brugnoni et al., 1994; Nonoyama et al., 1995) and in some patients with CVID (Farrington et al., 1994). Consequently, mutation analysis at the *CD40L (TNFSF5)* gene is ultimately required for final confirmation of HIGM1.

Molecular analysis is also the best approach for carrier detection, although immunologic assays, showing two populations of activated CD4⁺ T cells (only one of which expresses functional CD40L), can be used (Hollenbaugh et al., 1994b). Prenatal diagnosis of HIGM1 can also be done by mutation analysis on chorionic villus DNA (Villa et al., 1994).

Treatment and Prognosis

IVIG at dosages of 400 to 500 mg/kg/month (or more) is the most important way to reduce the frequency and severity of infections. IVIG may also reduce or normalize serum IgM levels (Benkerrou et al., 1990) and, in a minority of cases, increase the neutrophil count (Banatvala et al., 1994; Rieger et al., 1974).

Infants with HIGM1 are particularly susceptible to *Pneumocystis carinii* pneumonia and should receive prophylaxis with trimethoprim-sulfamethoxazole (Banatvala et al., 1994; Levy et al., 1997). Patients with persistent neutropenia may respond to granulocyte-colony stimulating factor (GCSF) injections (Banatvala et al., 1994).

Prevention of liver disease requires careful monitoring of liver and biliary tract function and structure (with ultrasound scanning and, in some cases, biopsies), and hygienic measures to avoid *Cryptosporidium* infection (i.e., use of boiled or filtered water). In some cases, malabsorption is a major complication, necessitating total parenteral nutrition (Benkerrou et al., 1990; Levy et al., 1997; Stiehm et al., 1986).

In spite of all these measures, the long-term prognosis of HIGM1 is guarded. According to data from the European HIGM1 registry, only 40% of the patients survive beyond 25 years of age (Levy et al., 1997). Severe infections early in life, and liver disease later on, are the major causes of death. Consequently, more aggressive treatment has been advocated. Liver transplantation has been attempted in patients with sclerosing cholangitis, but relapse is the rule (Levy et al., 1997).

Hematopoietic stem cell transplantation, particularly if performed early in life, from an human leukocyte antigen (HLA)-identical sibling, a matched unrelated donor, or umbilical cord blood may cure the disease (Bordigoni et al., 1998; Duplantier et al., 2001; Gennery et al., 2000; Kato et al., 1999; Kawai et al., 1999; Kutukculer et al., 2003; Scholl et al., 1998; Thomas et al., 1995; Ziegner et al., 2001) (see Chapter 43). Combined bone marrow and cadaveric orthotopic liver transplantation has been used successfully in one HIGM1 patient with severe liver disease (Hadzic et al., 2000).

Although gene therapy remains a possibility, several considerations make this problematic. Expression of CD40L is under tight regulatory control (Schubert et al., 1995), and experiments with CD40L$^{-/-}$ mice indicate that expression of CD40L under a constitutive promoter results in thymic T-lymphoproliferative disease (Brown et al., 1998). Similarly, transgenic mice with deregulated CD40L expression develop lymphoid proliferation that in some cases progresses into frank lymphomas (Sacco et al., 2000).

These considerations suggest the need for including autologous regulatory elements in CD40L gene transfer experiments, a goal that may be more easily achieved with use of lentiviral vectors (Barry et al., 2000). Another difficulty for HIGM1 gene therapy is the demonstration that mutant forms of CD40L may interact with wild-type molecules, and hence prevent membrane expression of functional CD40L trimers (Seyama et al., 1999; Su et al., 2001).

Luigi D. Notarangelo and Anne Durandy

AUTOSOMAL RECESSIVE HYPER-IgM SYNDROME TYPE 2 DUE TO AID DEFICIENCY (HIGM2)

Definition

Hyper-IgM type 2 (HIGM2) syndrome is an autosomal recessive immunodeficiency characterized by elevated IgM levels, decreased IgG and IgA immunoglobulins, lymphadenopathy, and normal cellular immunity, resulting from mutations in a gene encoding activation-induced cytidine deaminase (AID), an enzyme involved in isotype switching.

HIGM2 is much less common than HIGM1, and most patients are from consanguineous families.

Pathogenesis

Several investigators identified patients (including females) with the hyper-IgM syndrome who had susceptibility to bacterial, but not opportunistic, infections and an autosomal recessive pattern of inheritance (Callard et al., 1994; Conley et al., 1994b; Durandy et al., 1997). HIGM1 was excluded in these patients by finding normal T-cell expression of CD40L and a normal sequence of the CD40L gene (Durandy et al., 1997). Unlike HIGM1 patients, these patients have an intrinsic B-cell defect of class switch recombination (CSR) in the presence of CD40L agonists and appropriate interleukins.

Identification of the AID Gene

To identify the cause of the HIGM2, several candidate genes were studied. CD40 gene sequence and CD40 expression were normal (Durandy et al., 1997). Other molecules involved in CD40 signaling or activation of NF-κB activation were also normal (Cheng et al., 1995, 1996; Durandy et al., 1997; Hu et al., 1994; Ishida et al., 1996a, 1996b; Malinin et al., 1997; Rothe et al., 1996; Sato et al., 1995; Song et al., 1997). CD40 agonists could activate the patients' monocytes and dendritic cells (Revy et al., 1998), suggesting that the HIGM2 defect originates in the B cell, either as a B-cell–specific CD40-triggered event or in the CSR mechanism (Durandy et al., 1997).

Because analysis of family trees suggested an autosomal recessive pattern of inheritance, gene mapping of highly polymorphic markers in consanguineous families was performed. In all families, the disease co-segregated with the telomeric region of the short arm of chromosome 12 at region p13, with a multipoint logarithm of the odds (LOD) score of 10.45 (Revy et al., 2000b). Recombination analysis defined a 4.5 cM critical interval, in which a gene coding for a new molecule, the AID, had been recently localized (Muto et al., 2000).

Structure of the AID Gene

The AID gene was originally cloned in mice by subtractive hybridization using murine lymphoma CH12F3-2 B cells induced or not induced to undergo CSR in vitro. AID is expressed in B cells undergoing immunoglobulin CSR in vitro (after stimulation with soluble CD40-ligand or LPS plus appropriate cytokines) and in vivo (in germinal center B cells) (Muramatsu et al., 1999).

The human counterpart of murine AID has been cloned; it exhibits a strong homology (96%) with murine AID, especially in the cytidine deaminase domain (100%). Human AID is expressed in secondary lymphoid organs (spleen, lymph nodes and tonsils), in EBV-transformed B-cell lines, and in peripheral blood B cells induced to CSR by stimulation with soluble CD40-ligand and interleukins (IL-4 or IL-10) (Muto el al., 2000).

The human AID gene, located on chromosome 12p13, encompasses approximately 10 kb of genomic DNA and is organized in five exons and four intervening introns (Muto et al., 2000). Definition of the exon-intron boundaries allowed searching for mutations at the genomic level. As shown in Figure 13-11, deleterious mutations (deletions, premature stop codons, and missense mutations preferentially clustered in the cytidine deaminase domain) have been found in patients with HIGM2 (Minegishi et al., 2000; Revy et al., 2000a).

In contrast, none of the patients with sporadic forms of CD40L-positive HIGM tested had defects in AID sequence and/or AID expression, providing evidence for at least another form of HIGM, the transmission of which remains unclear (Minegishi et al., 2000).

Function of AID

The immunologic abnormalities of HIGM2 patients and AID-deficient mice resulting from AID deficiency suggests a critical role for AID in the terminal maturation of B cells, particularly CSR, SHM, and control of B-cell proliferation in germinal centers (Fig. 13-12).

The AID enzyme is structurally related (34% homology) to the apolipoprotein B (ApoB) RNA-editing enzyme APOBEC-1. RNA-editing is widely used to create new functional genes from the restricted genome in plants and protozoa (Scott et al., 1995; Simpson et al., 1995). A number of mammalian mRNAs are known to be edited, including ApoB mRNA by APOBEC-1. ApoB mRNA editing involves a site-specific C to U deamination of residue 2158, thus changing the CAA codon (that encodes for glutamine) into the UAA stop codon. ApoB100 and ApoB48 are translation products of the unedited and edited ApoB mRNA, respectively; these proteins have completely different functions and expression. APOBEC-1 requires an auxiliary factor (APOBEC-1 complementation factor [ACF]) for site-specific RNA editing of ApoB mRNA; this auxiliary factor is widely expressed, even in organs that do not express APOBEC-1 (Navaratnam et al., 1993; Teng et al., 1993; Yamanaka et al., 1994).

The open reading frame of the AID cDNA encodes a 198-residue protein with a molecular mass of approximately 24 kD. AID contains an active site for cytidine deamination, which is conserved in the large cytidine deaminase family. It also contains a leucine-rich region

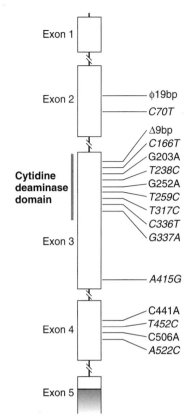

Figure 13-11 · Activation-induced cytidine deaminase gene mutations in patients with hyper-IgM syndrome type 2. Mutations in *italics* represent missense mutations; the remaining mutations lead to premature termination.

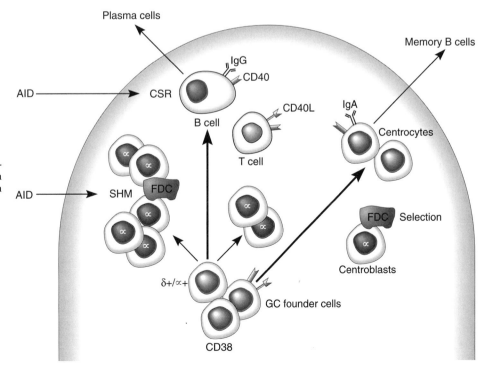

Figure 13-12 · Role of activation-induced cytidine deaminase (AID) in B-cell terminal differentiation within a germinal center.

located in the C terminus part of the protein, which is likely important for protein–protein interaction. Recombinant AID has been shown to exert an actual cytidine deaminase activity in vitro (Muramatsu et al., 2000).

Role of AID in Class Switch Recombination

The precise mechanisms responsible for CSR and SHM, although not completely understood, require germline transcription (Bottaro et al., 1994; Gu et al., 1993; Jung et al., 1993; Xu et al., 1993; Zhang et al., 1993), an efficient splicing machinery (Hein et al., 1998), and DNA double strand breaks (Bross et al., 2000; Papavasiliou et al., 2000; Wuerffel et al., 1997). Formation of RNA:DNA complexes with R-loop structure at the switch regions (Daniels and Lieber, 1995; Tian et al., 2000) has been described for CSR.

The role of DNA-protein kinase (DNA-PK) and the Ku70–Ku80 recombination complex in CSR has also been demonstrated (Casellas et al., 1998; Manis et al., 1998; Rolink et al., 1996), whereas DNA-PK has been shown to be dispensable for SHM (Bemark et al., 2000). It has been suggested that the DNA mismatch repair system (Cascalho et al., 1998; Wiesendanger et al., 1998), as well as newly described DNA polymerases (Pol i or Pol m) and UNG are specifically involved in SHM (Dominguez et al., 2000; Rada et al., 2002; Tissier et al., 2000).

As noted, the molecular mechanism for AID function is unclear. Considering its homology with the RNA-editing enzyme APOBEC-1, it has been hypothesized that AID acts by affecting a specific mRNA coding for a common substrate necessary for both CSR and SHM (e.g., a site-specific DNA double-strand break endonuclease). Another less likely hypothesis is that AID edits two different mRNAs, specific either for CSR or for SHM. Alternatively, there is strong evidence that AID functions as a DNA-editing enzyme (Rada et al., 2002).

Role of AID in Adenopathy

One explanation for the massive lymphadenopathy with giant germinal centers observed in HIGM2 is that, in the absence of functional AID, B cells are continuously triggered to proliferate by antigen (as they express the BCR normally), in the absence of successful immunoglobulin variable region gene SHM. However, a direct role of AID in regulating B-cell proliferation cannot be excluded.

Animal Models

Because no animal models of AID deficiency are available, AID-deficient mice have been generated by gene targeting. The gene encoding AID was disrupted in an embryonic stem (ES) cell line, and AID-disrupted ES cells were injected into RAG-2$^{-/-}$ 8-cell embryos, giving rise to chimeric animals in which all mature lymphocytes were derived from the injected ES cells.

The mouse phenotype is identical with that of HIGM2 patients, including defective CSR, defective SHM, and giant germinal center formation (Muramatsu et al., 2000).

Clinical Features

HIGM2 patients present during early childhood with recurrent bacterial sinorespiratory and gastrointestinal tract infections. Unlike HIGM1 patients (Levy et al., 1997; Facchetti et al., 1995) and HIGM3 patients (see later discussion), HIGM2 patients lack opportunistic infections (characteristic of T-cell abnormalities) and lymphoid hyperplasia, often leading to tonsillectomy or lymph node biopsy to rule out tumors (Table 13-2). Neutropenia is also absent.

Laboratory Features

HIGM2 patients have markedly diminished serum levels of IgG and IgA with normal or increased serum levels of IgM. IgG antibodies are not elicited by immunization, whereas IgM isoagglutinin titers are normal. Peripheral blood T-cell subsets are normal, as is in vitro T-cell proliferation to mitogens and antigens.

B Lymphocytes

Peripheral blood B cells in HIGM2 are normal in number, as is their expression of CD40 protein and their CD40 gene sequence. However, unlike CD19 B cells from age-matched controls that express either surface immunoglobulin (sIg)M or sIgD (and usually sIgG or sIgA), HIGM2 CD19 B cells express both sIgM and sIgD, suggesting a defect in CSR.

In vitro activation of HIGM2 B cells by soluble CD40L and IL-4, which induces IgE production in both normal and CD40L-deficient patients (Durandy et al., 1993), does not induce IgE synthesis in HIGM2 B cells. However, the same culture conditions did induce sterile intermediate transcripts, indicating that the first step of the CSR (the expression of the sterile transcripts) is normal (Durandy et al., 1997). Inability to undergo CSR is

TABLE 13-2 · CLINICAL MANIFESTATIONS IN HYPER-IgM SYNDROME TYPE 2

Clinical Manifestations	Frequency (%)
Recurrent infections affecting:	
· Upper respiratory tract	42
· Lower respiratory tract	58
· Digestive tract	27
· Urinary tract	6
· Central nervous system	25
Failure to thrive	10*
Arthritis	12
Lymphoid hyperplasia	
· Lymph nodes, tonsils	52
· Hepatosplenomegaly	6

*Observed only in pediatric series.

also observed in cultures stimulated with soluble CD40-L and IL-10.

CD27 has been identified as a marker for memory B cells, even in the IgM/IgD⁺ B-cell compartment (Klein et al., 1998). CD27 is expressed on a normal proportion (from 9% to 45%) and with the same intensity on AID-deficient B cells as in normal age-matched controls. In contrast, CD40L-deficient B cells lack CD27⁺ memory B cells (Agematsu et al., 1998).

Hypermutated B Cells

The frequency of SHM in the variable region of IgM expressed by CD19⁺/CD27⁺ B cells is significantly reduced in HIGM2 patients, ranging from 0% to 0.9% mutations per base pair (bp), as compared with 2.6% to 6.3% mutations per bp in age-matched controls. In some HIGM2 patients, all individual clones were completely devoid of mutation. The mutations in the V genes of normal B cells, unlike the rare mutations found in HIGM2 B cells, occurred in the major individual hotspots of mutations previously reported (Bonhomme et al., 2000; Levy et al., 1998) and reflects the process of antigenic selection. Thus HIGM2 patients not only lack CSR but also have defective SHM (Revy et al., 2000b).

Lymph Node Histology

Histologic sections of enlarged secondary lymphoid organs (tonsils, cervical lymph nodes) show marked follicular hyperplasia. Whereas the mantle zone and inter-follicular areas are normally present, germinal centers are 5 to 10 times larger than those from control reactive lymph nodes. Giant germinal centers contain a normal follicular dendritic cell network (DRC⁺), and CD38⁺, sIgM⁺, sIgD⁺, Ki67⁺ B cells. Strikingly, numerous germinal center B cells co-express sIgD. This contrasts with observations in normal reactive germinal centers, in which few IgD⁺ cells are found.

The phenotype and size of the germinal center B cells identify them as proliferating (Ki67⁺) germinal founder cells, prone to undergo SHM and selection (Lebecque et al., 1997). Occasional CD27⁺ B cells as well as IgM⁺ and IgD⁺ plasma cells are found in germinal centers and T-cell areas. Neither IgG nor IgA plasma cells are observed.

Thus secondary lymphoid organs from HIGM2 patients exhibit abnormal giant germinal centers, filled with IgM⁺/IgD⁺/CD38 proliferating germinal center founder cells (Revy et al., 2000b).

Diagnosis

Other causes of hyper-IgM must be ruled out. Normal expression of CD40L on activated T cells and normal CD40L gene sequence excludes HIGM1. Normal expression of CD40 on B cells excludes HIGM3. Congenital rubella with hyper-IgM must be considered; these patients have a T-cell activation defect leading to defective CD40L expression (Kawamura et al., 2000).

Rarely, ataxia-telangiectasia patients may develop hyper-IgM before neurologic features develop (Gatti et al., 1991). Definitive diagnosis of HIGM2 requires demonstration of a mutated AID gene (Minegishi et al., 2000; Revy et al., 2000b).

Treatment

Treatment includes regular infusions of IVIG (400 to 600 mg/kg every 3 to 4 weeks); this usually leads to a significant reduction in the severity and frequency of infection and may diminish or normalize the IgM levels. However, the lymphoid hyperplasia is not affected by IVIG.

Because HIGM2 is a pure B-cell defect, prophylaxis for *Pneumocystis carinii* or *Cryptosporidium* species is not necessary. Unlike XLA patients, severe enterovirus infections have not been reported, suggesting a protective role of IgM (even without SMH) as a first barrier against enteroviral and other viral infections.

Luigi D. Notarangelo and Anne Durandy

AUTOSOMAL RECESSIVE HYPER-IgM SYNDROME TYPE 3 DUE TO CD40 DEFICIENCY (HIGM3)

Definition

Hyper-IgM syndrome type 3 (HIGM3) is a rare autosomal recessive immunodeficiency with elevated IgM levels and decreased IgG and IgG antibody responses, associated with absence of CD40 antigen on the B lymphocytes.

Pathogenesis

Four patients from two unrelated families born to consanguineous parents have been described with HIGM3. All had most of the clinical and laboratory features of HIGM1, but had normal CD40L expression and gene sequence (Ferrari et al., 2001; Kutckculer et al., 2003). Their B cells were intrinsically unable to undergo immunoglobulin CSR when stimulated with anti-CD40 and cytokines in vitro.

These patients have a complete lack of CD40 expression on the surface of B lymphocytes and monocytes, allowing for the identification of HIGM3 (Ferrari et al., 2001). Like HIGM2, HIGM3 has an autosomal recessive pattern of inheritance, but clinically and immunologically it resembles HIGM1 (see Table 13-2).

The CD40 gene maps to chromosome 20q12-13.2. Characterization of its genomic structure has facilitated HIGM3 mutation analysis.

In the first HIGM3 family, of Italian origin, the affected patient was homozygous for a single nucleotide substitution in exon 5 of the CD40 gene, an exonic splicing enhancer. This prevented the correct splicing of the mRNA. The mature CD40 mRNA lacked exon 5, resulting in frameshift with complete absence of CD40 protein.

In the second family, of Arabic origin, two affected patients were homozygous for a missense mutation that affected a highly conserved cysteine residue, resulting in expression of a mutant CD40 protein that was retained in the cytoplasm and could not be expressed at the cell surface (Ferrari et al., 2001).

In the third family, of Turkish origin, the patient was homozygous for a mutation at the acceptor splice site of intron 3, resulting in incorrect splicing and the use of a cryptic splice site within exon 4 (Kutukculer et al., 2003).

Although the HIGM3 families shared autosomal recessive inheritance, based on the fact that CD40 is expressed as a homotrimer at the cell surface, it is possible that some patients with dominant-negative heterozygous mutations of the CD40 gene may present with clinical and immunologic features of HIGM3.

Clinical and Laboratory Features

The patients with HIGM3 described have a clinical phenotype resembling HIGM1. This includes early-onset interstitial pneumonia caused by *Pneumocystis carinii,* recurrent lower respiratory tract infections, and failure to thrive associated with severe hypogammaglobulinemia (Ferrari et al., 2001). One of the four HIGM3 patients also had neutropenia as seen in HIGM1. Because of this similarity, HIGM3 patients are probably at risk for *Cryptosporidium* infection. Severe liver disease has also been reported (Kutukculer et al., 2003).

HIGM3 patients have markedly reduced IgG and IgA serum levels, and normal to increased IgM. The numbers and distribution of T-cell subsets are normal, as are in vitro lymphoproliferative responses to mitogens and antigens. B lymphocytes are present in normal numbers, but lack membrane expression of CD40.

The proportion of IgD$^-$,CD27$^+$ B cells (e.g., isotype-switched memory B cells) is markedly decreased, as is the frequency of SHM in circulating B cells. These findings reflect defective maturation of humoral immune responses resulting from lack of CD40-mediated signaling in germinal center B cells. Indeed, when stimulated in vitro with CD40 agonists (CD40L, or anti-CD40 monoclonal antibody) and appropriate cytokines, HIGM3 B cells fail to undergo CSR (Ferrari et al., 2001).

CD40 is normally expressed on the surface of monocytes and of monocyte-derived dendritic cells (DCs). Not surprisingly, the differentiation and function of monocyte-derived DCs are defective in HIGM3 (Fontana et al., 2003). The probable lack of CD40 expression by activated endothelial and epithelial cells may affect their function and contribute to the severity of the clinical manifestations.

Treatment

Treatment of HIGM3 includes regular administration of IVIG, prompt and aggressive treatment of bacterial infections, and prophylactic use of co-trimoxazole to prevent *Pneumocystis carinii* pneumonia.

Hematopoietic stem cell transplantation (SCT) has been advocated in HIGM1 because of the poor long-term prognosis. Although the limited number of HIGM3 patients reported precludes analysis of the long-term outcome, SCT may be less effective in HIGM3 than in HIGM1, because it would restore CD40 expression only in hematopoietic cell types, but not on other CD40-expressing cell lineages. In contrast, CD40L is normally expressed only on T cells.

Luigi D. Notarangelo and Anne Durandy

OTHER AUTOSOMAL RECESSIVE HYPER-IgM SYNDROMES (HIGM4 AND UNG DEFICIENCY)

Hyper-IgM Syndrome Type 4 (HIGM4)

Definition

HIGM4 is a recently identified hyper-IgM syndrome described in 15 patients with a molecularly undefined defect clinically similar to HIGM2 (AID defect) but in which the defect is downstream from the action of AID (Imai et al., 2003a). Clinically, it resembles HIGM2, but with a slightly milder phenotype with some residual Ig synthesis.

Pathogenesis

B-cell CSR was intrinsically impaired in these patients, but SHM in the variable region of the Ig heavy-chain defect was similar to that in control lymphocytes. In vitro studies showed that the molecular defects for HIGM4 occur downstream of the AID activity and the *AID* gene was expressed normally; further AID-induced DNA double-strand breaks in the switch μ region of the Ig heavy-chain locus detected during CSR were similar to those of controls.

The authors conclude that HIGM4 is the consequence of a selective defect in a CSR-specific factor of the DNA repair machinery or in survival signals delivered to switched B cells (Imai et al., 2003a).

Clinical Features

A total of 15 patients from 14 families were identified with a hyper-IgM syndrome in which HIGM1, HIGM2, HIGM3, NEMO, and UNG defects were excluded by genetic analysis. They were from five countries, and one patient was born to a consanguineous family. Two of the patients were brothers; the others were sporadic. There were 11 males and 4 females. The mean age of diagnosis was 8.8 years, and the patients are now 2 to 32 years of age and receiving IVIG therapy.

Clinical features include recurrent respiratory infections and occasionally severe gastrointestinal infections, sepsis, lymphadenitis, and osteomyelitis. Similar to HIGM2, seven of the patients had lymphoid hyperplasia, but without the histologic pattern of HIGM2 nodes. Ten of the patients had elevated IgM, and most had low levels of IgG and IgA.

Hyper-IgM Syndrome Due to UNG Deficiency

Definition

HIGM with uracil-DNA glycosylane (UNG) deficiency is a newly described human disorder clinically resembling HIGM2 and HIGM4 (Imai et al., 2003b) and molecularly resembling UNG-deficient mice (Rada et al., 2002).

Pathogenesis

UNG-deficient mice have partially defective CSR and a biased pattern of SHM toward transition at dG–dC nucleotides (Rada et al., 2002). Imai and colleagues (2003b) showed that recessive mutations of the UNG gene in these patients was associated with profound impairment in CSR at a DNA precleavage step and a partial disturbance of the SHM pattern. Because UNG is normally expressed in activated B cells, they postulate that UNG is essential for normal CSR and SHM and that a defect in this enzyme leads to the observed HIGM defect.

Clinical Features

Three unrelated patients have been described, one 6-year-old child and two adults aged 27 and 40. The latter patient was born to first-cousin parents. All had recurrent respiratory infections since early childhood and lymphadenopathy, and in one adult, chronic epididymitis. The patients had increased serum IgM levels and profoundly decreased IgG and IgA levels. All are well controlled on IVIG therapy.

X-LINKED ANHIDROTIC ECTODERMAL DYSPLASIAS WITH IMMUNODEFICIENCY CAUSED BY MUTATIONS OF NEMO (EDA-ID AND OP-EDA-ID)

Definition

Anhidrotic (or hypohidrotic) ectodermal dysplasia (EDA) is a rare developmental syndrome with partial or complete absence of eccrine sweat glands, sparse hair growth, and abnormal dentition. Some EDA patients have an X-linked disorder associated with immunodeficiency (EDA-ID), characterized by frequent infections, low IgG levels, variably elevated IgM levels, and decreased antibody responses.

EDA-ID results from mutations in the IKK gamma gene coding for NEMO on the X chromosome; NEMO is a key regulatory subunit of the IκB kinase that regulates NF-κB nuclear signaling.

A subgroup of EDA-ID patients have a particularly severe immunodeficiency, with osteopetrosis and lymphedema (OL-EDA-ID) associated with more extensive

stop codon NEMO gene mutations. Some mothers of the OL-EDA-ID boys have had mild incontinentia pigmenti. Indeed, mutations in NEMO are also responsible for most cases of incontinentia pigmenti.

Pathogenesis

Mutations in the IKK-gamma (NEMO) gene have been identified in patients with EDA-ID. IKK-gamma is a regulatory component of a multiprotein kinase complex that phosphorylates and degrades IκB, an inhibitory molecule that mediates cytoplasmic retention of NF-κB (Israel et al., 2000). Members of the TNF cytokine family mediate activation of IKK-gamma, and consequently promote nuclear translocation of NF-κB, thereby inducing transcription of target genes.

Severe mutations of the IKK-gamma (NEMO) gene are lethal in males, and cause incontinentia pigmenti (an allelic form of ectodermal dysplasia) in females. In contrast, in four families with EDA-ID, the mutations were located in exon 10, affected the C-terminal region of the molecule, and were not always associated with severe infection. In lymphoblastoid B-cell lines from one family, expression of the mutant protein was documented by Western blotting (Zonana et al., 2000). Deletion of the C-terminus of IKK-gamma has been shown to markedly diminish, but not abolish, stimulation of NF-κB by Tax, the product of type 1 human leukemia virus (Harhaj and Sun, 1999). Therefore it is hypothesized that the mutations observed in EDA-ID also preserve partial functioning of the NF-κB pathway.

Clinical and Laboratory Features

Early reports suggested that patients with anhidrotic EDA may have an increased risk of viral and bacterial infections, and one case of miliary tuberculosis was reported (Frix and Bronson, 1986). Manifestations of EDA include facial dysmorphism, sparse hair, delayed eruption of teeth, conical teeth, and sweat gland abnormalities.

The association of EDA and significant immunodeficiency (EDA-ID) has been reported in several families with X-linked inheritance (Abinun et al., 1996; Conley et al., 1994b; Schweizer et al., 1999; Zonana et al., 2000). These males present with ectodermal dysplasia and increased susceptibility to bacterial infections of bones and soft tissues, pneumonia, sepsis, and meningitis.

A particularly severe phenotype associated with osteopetrosis and lymphedema (OP-ESD-ID) has been described in several families (Zonana et al., 2000), and in individual patients (Doffinger et al., 2001; Dupois-Girod et al., 2002). Most OP-EDA-ID children have died before age 3.

Immunologic investigations most often document reduced IgG serum levels, normal to increased IgM, and variable levels of serum IgA. Expression of CD40L by

CD4+ T cells upon in vitro activation with phorbol myristate acetate and ionomycin is normal. Stimulation of B cells with anti-CD40 monoclonal antibody and appropriate interleukins fails to induce immunoglobulin isotype switch, indicating an intrinsic B-cell defect (Conley et al., 1994b). Delayed or absent production of isohemagglutinins and an inability to form specific antibodies to polysaccharide antigens are other common features (Abinun et al., 1996; Schweizer et al., 1999).

Treatment and Prognosis

Treatment of patients with EDA-ID requires regular administration of IVIG, and careful surveillance for infectious episodes. In particular, care must be paid to early diagnosis and treatment of mycobacterial infections, to which patients with EDA-ID show increased susceptibility. Occurrence of mycobacterial infections, recurrent bacterial infections, and bronchiectasis compromise the long-term prognosis.

Luigi D. Notarangelo and Anne Durandy

IMMUNODEFICIENCY WITH THYMOMA (GOOD'S SYNDROME)

Definition

Immunodeficiency with thymoma, first described by Good in 1954, and thus sometimes referred to as *Good's syndrome,* is primarily a disorder of adults between ages 40 and 70. The immunodeficiency associated with thymoma may affect either B or T lymphocytes or both.

Few children have been described with immunodeficiency with thymoma, one an 8-year-old with combined cellular and humoral immunodeficiency (Watts and Kelly, 1990) and another a 15-year-old with a cellular immunodeficiency (Sicherer et al., 1998). The thymic tumors are predominantly of the spindle cell type and are rarely malignant.

Pathogenesis

The basis for the association between thymoma and immunodeficiency is unknown, but proposed mechanisms have included viral infection, autoantibodies (Jeunet and Good, 1968), and secretion of a substance by the thymoma that suppresses immunoglobulin synthesis (Goldstein and Mackay, 1969; Peterson et al., 1965).

There is some evidence that suppressor T cells generated in the thymoma interfere with B-cell maturation or function. Some patients with this syndrome have had excessive CD8+ suppressor cells that interfered with in vitro immunoglobulin synthesis by normal B cells (Hayward et al., 1982; Moretta et al., 1977).

Most patients with immunodeficiency and thymoma completely lack both pre-B cells in the bone marrow and B cells in the peripheral blood (Hayward et al., 1982; Pearl et al., 1978). However, the description of a thymoma patient with hypogammaglobulinemia and no evidence of suppressor T-cell activity and normal numbers of B cells (Brenner et al., 1984) suggests that more than one mechanism for its pathogenesis exists.

Histology

Thymomas associated with hypogammaglobulinemia cannot be distinguished histologically from other thymomas. Most thymomas arise from the anterior mediastinum and weigh up to 250 g; the maximum diameter is 4 to 20 cm. Two thirds of the tumors are encapsulated and benign, and one third are invasive (Gray and Gutowski, 1979). In a large series, 50% of the tumors consisted of round epithelial cells, 25% were of the spindle cell type, and 25% were of mixed type. Lymphocytes are present in most thymomas and are usually T cells. Functionally, they are similar to lymphocytes from a normal thymus (Lauriola et al., 1981; Musiani et al., 1982). The bone marrow lacks both pre-B lymphocytes and plasma cells, and lymph nodes and spleen are hypocellular with absence of germinal centers and decreased numbers of plasma cells.

Clinical Features

The incidence of hypogammaglobulinemia and/or cellular immunodeficiency in patients with thymoma is estimated to be between 4% and 12% (Gray and Gutowski, 1979; Otto, 1978; Souadjian et al., 1974; Waldmann et al., 1967). Conversely, the prevalence of thymoma in adult patients with hypogammaglobulinemia has been estimated at 4% (Van der Hilst et al., 2002). The thymoma and hypogammaglobulinemia are usually detected simultaneously, either during the initial investigation of hypogammaglobulinemia or when a mediastinal mass is detected on a chest film. Occasionally, the thymoma may be present for many years before symptoms of immune deficiency are noticed and hypogammaglobulinemia is diagnosed (Chapin, 1965; TeVelde et al., 1966). Removal of the thymoma does not affect the hypogammaglobulinemia. The onset of immunodeficiency may even occur several years after thymectomy (Lambie et al., 1957).

The infections associated with thymoma and immunodeficiency generally reflect the nature of the underlying immunodeficiency. Thus patients may have recurrent sinopulmonary infections with encapsulated bacteria, reflecting their hypogammaglobulinemia, or they may have opportunistic infections reflecting their T-cell deficiency (Tarr et al., 2001). The opportunistic infections have included invasive candidiasis (Gupta et al., 1985; Kirkpatrick and Windhorst, 1979), generalized cytomegalovirus infection (Bernadou et al., 1972; Gupta et al., 1985; Ide et al., 2000; Kauffman et al., 1979), cutaneous and systemic herpes simplex infection (Beck et al., 1981; Gupta et al., 1985), and *Pneumocystis carinii* pneumonia (TeVelde et al., 1966).

Anemia is frequently associated with the syndrome and may be due to pure red blood cell aplasia (Al-Mondhiry et al., 1971) or malabsorption of vitamin B_{12} (Jeandel et al., 1994). Muscle weakness caused by myasthenia gravis is a frequent complication (Gehrmann and Engstfeld, 1965). Other clinical findings associated with thymoma and immunodeficiency include thrombocytopenia (Peterson et al., 1965), neutropenia (Degos et al., 1982), arthritis (Webster, 1976), alopecia areata (Tan, 1974), and pemphigus vulgaris (Safai et al., 1978).

Laboratory Features

Every patient with a mediastinal mass should be studied for possible immunodeficiency. Typically, immunoglobulin levels of all isotypes are low, antibody responses to immunization with specific antigens are depressed, and in vitro immunoglobulin synthesis by peripheral blood lymphocytes is decreased because of the absence of functional B lymphocytes (Hayward et al., 1982; Litwin et al., 1979; Pearl et al., 1978) or the presence of CD8[+] suppressor lymphocytes (Hayward et al., 1982; Moretta et al., 1977). Most patients with thymoma and immunodeficiency also have abnormal T-cell function. Skin tests for delayed-type hypersensitivity are negative, in vitro lymphocyte responses to mitogens and specific antigens are often impaired, and the number of T cells is low, with an inverted CD4/CD8 ratio. Anemia, thrombocytopenia, neutropenia, and autoantibodies may also be present.

Treatment

To identify the nature of the tumor, the thymoma must be removed surgically. Removal of the thymoma does not correct the hypogammaglobulinemia, but it may improve the cellular immune defect. Symptoms of myasthenia gravis and other autoimmune diseases frequently improve after excision of the thymoma. Immunoglobulin therapy is effective in controlling recurrent bacterial infections and may alleviate chronic diarrhea (Conn and Quintiliani, 1966), but its effect on neutropenia or thrombocytopenia is unknown.

Prognosis

The prognosis of a benign thymoma by itself is excellent, with a 5-year survival of between 80% and 90% (Batata et al., 1974; Bernatz et al., 1973). However, the clinical course of patients with thymoma and immunodeficiency is less favorable. Immunologic deterioration is observed frequently, resulting in recurrent pulmonary infections that may progress to chronic lung disease and pulmonary insufficiency. Neutropenia, thrombocytopenia, and severe anemia are other serious complications. The nature of the tumor is of prognostic importance. If it is malignant, the clinical course is usually rapidly fatal.

TRANSIENT HYPOGAMMAGLOBULINEMIA OF INFANCY

Definition

Transient hypogammaglobulinemia of infancy (THI), first reported and named by Gitlin and Janeway in 1956, is defined as persistently low immunoglobulin levels in an infant beyond 6 months of age and in whom another immunodeficiency has been excluded. It is often asymptomatic and full recovery ensues. This disorder is also discussed in Chapter 22.

THI has been classically considered an accentuation and prolongation of the physiologic hypogammaglobulinemia of infancy that occurs during the first 3 to 6 months of life. Diagnostic criteria for THI are not well standardized. The World Health Organization in 1992 included both diminished IgG and IgA in defining the illness, whereas their latest report (Report of an International Union of Immunological Societies, 1999) states that one or more classes of Ig may be very low— "within an immunodeficient range."

Most authorities use a low IgG level as mandatory, whereas others have used low levels of other Ig isotypes, such as IgA (McGeady, 1987). However, the high frequency of selective IgA deficiency and the great variability of serum IgA in infants (Cunningham-Rundles, 1996) makes IgA levels an unreliable test for THI. In addition, most authors (Dalal et al., 1998; Dresser et al., 1989; Smolen et al., 1983) suggest that the level of Ig be less than two standard deviations (SDs) below the mean for age-matched controls.

We recommend that the definition of THI be based on an IgG level at least two SDs below the normal mean for age, with or without low levels of other Ig isotypes.

Incidence

The precise frequency of THI remains undetermined. There is no gender or racial difference or familial predilection. Ex-premature infants, because of their lower levels of transplacental IgG, may have a higher incidence, particularly in the youngest THI patients.

Tiller and Buckley (1978) reported that only 11 cases of THI were identified among more than 10,000 patients whose sera were sent for Ig measurements, suggesting that THI is not common. Dressler and associates (1989) supported this assumption by finding only 5 new cases in more than 8000 samples over a period of 11 years. Walker and colleagues (1994) reported 15 patients with proven THI and another 25 patients with possible THI among 2468 referrals over a 10-year period. This was an incidence of 23 or 61 per 10^6 live births, respectively. These figures most likely reflect selected patients with relatively severe symptomatic THI, rather than the true incidence of the disorder.

Indeed, a nationwide survey of primary immunodeficiency in Japan indicated that a substantial 18.5% of all patients were diagnosed with THI (Hayakawa et al., 1981). This disparity of the estimated THI incidence in various studies is best explained by the lack of strict diagnostic criteria and the lack of large-scale long-term studies.

Pathogenesis

Although THI has been recognized for years, and despite significant progress in understanding the molecular basis for other primary immunodeficiencies (PIDs), little is known about this entity. Several mechanisms have been proposed. Fudenberg and Fudenberg (1964) demonstrated that IgG (Gm) alloantigens present on human fetal but not on maternal IgGs can induce the synthesis of maternal IgG anti-Gm antibodies during pregnancy, and suggested that these alloantibodies cross the placenta and temporarily suppress fetal immunoglobulin production. However, a prospective study on this issue did not support this hypothesis (Hobbs and Davis, 1967).

Soothill (1968) identified THI in relatives of patients with a variety of PID disorders and suggested that THI is a manifestation of heterozygosity for other immunodeficiency diseases. Although this remains a possibility, confirmation is lacking.

Siegel and associates (1981) proposed that a defect in T-helper cell maturation might cause THI. This has not been confirmed by subsequent studies (Dalal et al., 1998; Dressler et al., 1989; Rieger et al., 1977).

Kowalczyk and co-workers (1997) have suggested cytokine abnormalities in the pathogenesis of THI by demonstrating enhanced production of TNF-α, TNF-β, and IL-10 but not IL-1, IL-4, and IL-6, in THI patients. Exogenous TNF-α and TNF-β inhibited IgG and IgA secretion in pokeweed mitogen-stimulated mononuclear cells. Normalization of the patient's IgG levels was associated with a decrease in TNF-α and TNF-β production, but IL-10 production remained unchanged. They concluded that TNF may be involved in the regulation of IgG and IgA production and the balance between TNF production (suppressing IgG synthesis), and IL-10 (inducing switching to IgG) is essential for the normal development of IgG-secreting B cells.

Clinical Features

Two distinct groups of infants with THI have been identified, based on the circumstances in which a diagnosis was obtained. The first group consisted of relatives of patients with other well defined immunodeficiency diseases. Most were healthy without recurrent infection, and diagnosis was made only because they were screened for immunoglobulin deficiency. These patients normalized their immunoglobulin levels and remained asymptomatic (Soothill, 1968). The second group was identified among infants screened for early onset of recurrent infection. The severity and type of infections varied from otitis media to bronchitis to life-threatening invasive infections, such as bacterial meningitis (Wilson et al., 1996).

The indication for immunologic evaluation in a long-term prospective study (Dalal et al., 1998) was recurrent upper respiratory infections, with or without ear infections, in 17 patients (49%). Of these, 8 (23%) also had at least one episode of pneumonia or sinusitis. Three (8%) presented with upper respiratory infection and recurrent gastroenteritis. Other illnesses included severe varicella (two infants), prolonged oral thrush (two infants), polio-like disease (one infant) and invasive infection (bacteremia with cellulitis and meningitis) (two infants).

In most series, atopic diseases have not been prominent (Dalal and Roifman, 2001; Tiller and Buckley, 1978). However, Fineman and colleagues (1979) described four THI infants with increased IgE levels and food allergy. Walker and associates (1994) found that 12 of 15 of their THI patients had either atopic disease or food allergy or intolerance.

A less frequent manifestation is hematologic abnormalities. Dalal and Roifman (2001) reported two patients with transient neutropenia and thrombocytopenia, one with persistent neutropenia (absolute neutrophils 0.5×10^9/L) and one who developed acute lymphoblastic leukemia (ALL). It is possible that the same immune dysregulation in this patient could be responsible for both the THI and the ALL.

Physical examination is generally normal except that tonsils and lymph nodes may be small. The presence of palpable lymph nodes, even small ones, excludes XLA. A thymus is usually visualized on chest x-ray examination.

Laboratory Features

Immunoglobulin levels are reduced, and by definition IgG levels are less than 2 SDs below the mean for age. For the 1-to 2-year-old, this means that the IgG is less than 400 mg/dl (see Chapter 12 for levels at various ages). IgM and IgA levels may also be reduced. IgE levels may be elevated and IgG subclasses are usually uniformly decreased.

Most THI patients have normal or near-normal antibody responses to tetanus and diphtheria vaccines, sometimes well before Ig levels normalize. They also have normal isohemagglutinin values for age (Rieger et al., 1977; Tiller and Buckley, 1978). In contrast, Cano and colleagues (1990) showed that 11 of 12 THI patients younger than 17 months did not make specific antibodies to a panel of respiratory viruses despite recurrent upper respiratory infections. Resolution of the THI was associated with the appearance of specific viral antibodies, even before the IgG levels normalized.

Dalal and Roifman (2001) reported that the ability to maintain protective levels of antibodies was as important as achieving an initial adequate response. Some of their patients (subsequently diagnosed with dysgammaglobulinemia) had a substantial but unsustained response to reimmunization even after the IgG levels normalized. This pattern of response is missed unless serial antibody determinations are performed over a period of years.

Lymphocyte subpopulations and lymphoproliferative assays to mitogens or specific antigens are generally normal.

Diagnosis

A diagnosis of THI cannot be made with confidence until after complete laboratory and clinical recovery. During this period, THI must be differentiated from other primary immunodeficiencies presenting in a similar manner such as XLA or early-onset CVID.

XLA can usually be differentiated from THI because of the severe deficiency of all immunoglobulin isotypes, the inability to produce specific antibodies, the absence of peripheral lymphoid tissue, and the absence or severe deficiency of circulating B lymphocytes. Furthermore, most XLA patients develop severe pyogenic infections starting in the first to second year of life (Buckley, 1992; Iseki and Heiner, 1993). Since the discovery that XLA is caused by BTK mutations (Vetrie et al., 1993), atypical XLA patients with milder phenotypes have been described, sometimes blurring the distinction between THI and XLA (Kornfield et al., 1995). Thus molecular testing of patients with persistent hypogammaglobulinemia for BTK mutations is recommended.

CVID is usually diagnosed in the second to third decade of life. CVID patients are usually unable to make specific antibodies, have variable immunoglobulin levels, and some impairment in cellular immunity (Buckley, 1992; Iseki and Heiner, 1993). Other types of humoral deficiencies such as the hyper-IgM syndromes (see elsewhere in this chapter) or X-linked lymphoproliferative disease (see Chapter 17) can occasionally be confused with THI.

Treatment

Most THI patients do not require IVIG treatment, particularly those in which antibody titers to one or more vaccine antigens are detected. Indeed, IVIG therapy may delay the onset of the patient's own immunoglobulin synthesis and delay complete recovery. Recurrent respiratory infections may be reduced in these children by removal from day care or continuous administration of prophylactic antibiotics. Pneumococcal vaccine should be given and the antibody response to it measured.

An occasional THI patient develops severe life-threatening infection such as meningitis, pneumonia, or recurrent cellulitis, or continues to have respiratory infections despite antibiotic therapy. Many of these patients have some degree of failure to thrive or gain weight and gastrointestinal problems. Under these circumstances, a trial of IVIG is indicated, usually for 6 to 12 months, at the usual therapeutic dose of 400 to 600 mg/kg every 3 to 4 weeks (Cano et al., 1990; Dalal et al., 1998; Wilson et al., 1996).

It is generally advisable to stop the IVIG infusions in the late spring or summer because there is less chance of getting a respiratory infection at that time. Immunizations are restarted after 3 months and immunoglobulin levels and antibody titers are followed serially.

Prognosis

Clinical recovery ensues by 9 to 15 months of age, but a rise to normal immunoglobulin levels may not occur until 2 to 4 years of age (Rosen and Janeway, 1966; Wilson et al., 1996); however, a few patients have persistent low IgG levels beyond infancy up to the age of 5 years (Benderly et al., 1986; McGeady, 1987; Tiller and Buckley, 1978).

In a prospective study, Dalal and co-workers (1998) and Dalal and Roifman (2001) followed the evolution of THI patients since infancy. All infants presented with recurrent infections. Clinical manifestations and specific antibody titers were recorded in 35 patients for 10 years. They identified three different patterns of illness.

The first and most common pattern was patients who experienced fewer infections as they grew older and eventually developed normal immunoglobulin and IgG subclass levels. Some of these patients initially had low levels of specific antibodies but responded normally to reimmunization and were able to sustain these titers. This process may span a decade and may include a transient phase whereby IgG subclasses may gradually normalize.

The second group consisted of patients who continued to suffer repeated infections and whose IgG levels remained low and who were unable to mount significant antibody titers despite reimmunization. These patients subsequently required permanent IVIG therapy. Such patients can be therefore classified as CVID despite the unusual presentation early in infancy.

The third pattern included patients who normalized their serum IgG levels but continued to experience significant infections. Upon reimmunization, they had a satisfactory but short-lived antibody response (declined within 6 to 12 months), despite obtaining normal IgG levels. This group of patients was classified as having dysgammaglobulinemia.

Although it is impossible to predict at presentation the pattern an individual patient will follow, invasive infections and low specific antibody levels at presentation appear to predict permanent antibody deficiency.

Chaim M. Roifman

IgG SUBCLASS DEFICIENCIES

Definition

Selective IgG subclass deficiency is defined as a deficiency of one or more IgG subclasses but normal or near normal total IgG concentrations (Herrod, 1993). The usual criterion of an IgG subclass deficiency is a level less than 2 SDs below the mean for age. Up to 20% of the population has an IgG subclass level for one or more subclasses.

Most IgG subclass-deficient subjects are asymptomatic, particularly those with an IgG4 deficiency (depending on the assay, as many as 10% to 20% of normals lack IgG4). Thus the aforementioned definition does not define a disease; instead, it defines a clinical laboratory finding.

A *clinically significant* IgG subclass deficiency occurs when the IgG subclass deficiency is associated with recurrent infection *and* a significant defect in antibody responsiveness. Most patients with an IgG1 subclass deficiency have panhypogammaglobulinemia (because IgG1 makes up 70% of the total IgG), and therefore these patients do not meet the definition of a selective IgG subclass deficiency.

IgG subclass deficiency is usually identified among individuals with recurrent upper respiratory infections or lung problems such as asthma, bronchitis, or bronchiectasis. IgG subclass deficiency may also occur as part of another primary immunodeficiency syndrome (e.g., selective IgA deficiency, impaired polysaccharide responsiveness, ataxia-telangiectasia, CVID, Wiskott-Aldrich syndrome) (Morell, 1994) or as part of a secondary antibody deficiency (e.g., HIV infection, cirrhosis). It has also been noted in a number of autoimmune disorders (e.g., immune thrombocytopenic purpura [ITP], lupus erythematosus) and as part of several miscellaneous syndromes.

Historical Aspects

Yount and colleagues (1970) reported immunoglobulin subclass imbalances in 13 patients with hypogammaglobulinemia. Schur and associates (1970) first reported IgG subclass deficiencies in three patients with progressive pulmonary infections. All had IgG1 and IgG2 deficiency; one had an IgG4 deficiency, and another an IgG3 deficiency. Because the total IgG level was low in two patients, they do not fit the current definition of a subclass deficiency.

In 1974, Oxelius and colleagues reported a mother and two children with recurrent infection and an IgG2 and IgG4 deficiency. In 1981, Oxelius and associates reported the frequent association of IgG2 and IgG4 deficiency with symptomatic selective IgA deficiency.

Morell and co-workers (1972), Schur and colleagues (1979), and Oxelius (1979) published normal levels of IgG subclass levels in infants and children at different ages, permitting definition of subnormal subclass levels.

Several reviews (Buckley, 2002; Herrod, 1993; Lawton, 1999; Morell, 1990; Shackleford, 1993) and a monograph (Levinsky, 1989) have been published detailing the clinical, laboratory, and therapeutic approaches to this disorder.

Pathogenesis

Each of the four IgG subclasses, defined by unique primary structures of the constant region of the heavy chain molecule (Grey et al., 1964; Terry and Fahey, 1964), have clear biologic and function differences (Ochs and Wedgwood, 1987; Shackleford, 1993) (see Chapters 3 and 4). For example, IgG1 and IgG3 bind C1 and can activate the classic pathway of complement. In contrast, IgG2 fixes C1 poorly and IgG4 does not fix C1 at all. IgG2 may not cross the placenta as well as other IgG subclasses (Hay et al., 1971). All IgG subclasses except IgG3 combine with staphylococcal protein A, a characteristic of the Fc portion of the molecule.

Differences in the regulation of IgG subclass expression is evident by the strikingly different levels in serum and characteristic differences in ontogeny. In infants, IgG1 and IgG3 levels increase quickly with age; IgG2 and IgG4 display a slower increase and reach adult levels at puberty (Fig. 13-13). The order of appearance of the IgG subclasses in children follows precisely the downstream order of the IgG heavy chain constant region gene segments on chromosome 14 (...γ3, γ1,...γ2, γ4) (Flanagan and Rabbitts, 1982). The half-life of IgG3 is 9 days, less than half that of the other subclasses. IgG3 and IgG4 are more susceptible to proteolytic digestion than the other subclasses.

IgG subclass restriction has been reported for antibodies against many bacterial and viral antigens. Antibody titers to pneumococcal polysaccharides correlate best with serum IgG2 concentrations (Siber et al., 1980). In adults antibody activity to polysaccharides is found predominantly in the IgG2 fraction (Freijd et al., 1984; Hammarström and Smith, 1986), whereas tetanus antibody is found predominantly in the IgG1 subclass (Stevens et al., 1983) and the high titer of antibody in patients with chronic schistosomiasis (Iskander et al., 1981) and filariasis (Ottesen et al., 1985) are limited to the IgG4 subclass. Following antigen exposure, a characteristic pattern of IgG subclass appearance has been observed. After the initial IgM response, IgG1 and

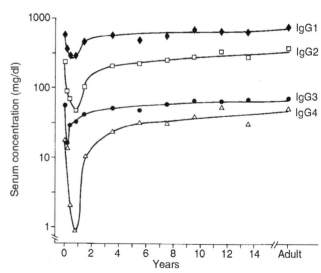

Figure 13-13· Serum immunoglobulin (Ig)G subclass levels in healthy infants and children. Time 0 represents the cord blood values. The means for each age group were obtained from data published by Oxelius. (Modified from Oxelius V-A. IgG subclass levels in infancy and childhood. Acta Paediatr Scand 68:23–27, 1979.)

IgG3 appear first, followed by IgG2 and IgG4 during the secondary immune response, in order of appearance that recapitulate ontogeny (Pyun et al., 1989).

The molecular mechanisms of IgG subclass deficiencies are not known, but may include DNA defects, transcriptional defects, mRNA translational defects or post-translational modification of the immunoglobulin molecule, or post-transcriptional abnormalities (Kavanaugh and Huston, 1989).

Because trace amounts of the IgG subclasses can be detected by sensitive methods in even severe subclass deficiencies, gene deletion is probably not common. Gene deletions have, however, been described in several patients: Lefranc and colleagues (1983) described a patient with IgG1, IgG2, IgG4, and IgA1 deficiency with a deletion of the heavy chain for Cγ1, Cγ2, Cγ4, and Cα1 genes. Migone and associates (1984) and Plebani and co-workers (1993) identified similar patients with gene deletions resulting in IgG2, IgG4, IgE, and IgA1 deficiencies; Smith and colleagues (1989) identified a familial IgG1 deficiency resulting from a homozygous deletion of the IgH Cγ1 gene.

Another possible cause of subclass deficiency is a regulatory defect in the initiation of DNA transcription, limited to certain gene segments. Heterologous gene deletions may also occur in 1% to 3% of the population, resulting in an IgG deficiency (Carbonara and Demarchi, 1986). The localization of the heavy chain genes may explain the frequent association of IgG1 and IgG3 deficiencies, Ig2 and IgG4 deficiencies, and combined IgA, IgG2, and IgG4 deficiencies.

A third possibility is the different use of variable chains coincident with defects in antibody specificities and affinities, thus explaining the heterogeneity of the antibody defects and the clinical severity.

IgG subclass levels can be influenced by a number of factors including placental passage, maturational age, Gm types, presence of infection, serum protein loss, or the use of drugs such as corticosteroids (Klaustermeyer et al., 1992). Individuals homozygous for the G3m(g) and G3m(b) allotypes may have selective IgG3 deficiency (Oxelius, 1993).

Clinical Features

Subclass deficiency should be suspected in patients who have recurrent respiratory infections, similar to patients with impaired polysaccharide responsiveness (see elsewhere in this chapter) or selective IgA deficiency (see Chapter 14). The usual respiratory infections are chronic otitis, sinusitis, or bronchitis, but occasionally may be more serious such as mastoiditis, pneumonia, or bronchiectasis. The offending bacteria are often those with a polysaccharide capsule such as pneumococci, *H. influenzae,* meningococci, and group B streptococci. Some patients present with refractory asthma triggered by respiratory infections.

Some patients are identified after laboratory testing discloses decreased antibody function, including poor polysaccharide antibody responses (see elsewhere in this

chapter). Some subclass-deficient patients are identified in patients with low normal IgG levels or selective IgA deficiency. Beck and Heiner (1981), Hill and colleagues (1998), and Klaustermeyer and associates (1992) have identified subclass deficiencies in patients with recurrent pulmonary infections. Moss and co-workers (1992) observed the frequent association of pulmonary infections with IgG4 deficiency and suggested that IgG4 is a marker for pulmonary infection. Bronchiectasis is also associated with selective IgG4 deficiency (Hill et al., 1998).

Many patients are found to have an IgG subclass deficiency who are not ill or have only mild respiratory symptoms. If their antibody function is intact, the subclass deficiency is probably not the cause of their problem. Most of these patients have low but not absent IgG1, IgG2, or IgG3 levels. IgG4 also may be absent in a significant percentage (i.e., 10% to 20%) of subjects, depending on the sensitivity of the assay. A clinically significant subclass deficiency necessitates an accompanying antibody deficiency with poor or absent response to vaccine antigens. Most of these latter patients have refractory respiratory infections.

The relative frequency of the subclass deficiencies are shown in Table 13-3. It can be noted that subclass deficiencies are often multiple and often associated with selective IgA deficiency. Although clinical features alone do not allow identification of which particular subclass is deficient, each subclass deficiency has some characteristic clinical features.

IgG1 Deficiency

IgG1 deficiency is usually associated with hypogammaglobulinemia because IgG1 makes up 70% of the total IgG, and if low, the total IgG level is low. Schur and colleagues (1970) and Page and associates (1988) described symptomatic IgG1 subclass deficiencies associated with

TABLE 13-3 · DISTRIBUTION OF DIAGNOSES IN 232 CHILDREN WITH AN IDENTIFIED IgG SUBCLASS AND/OR SELECTIVE IgA DEFICIENCY AND RECURRENT INFECTIONS

Phenotype	Percent of Cases
IgG4 deficiency (isolated)	23%
IgA deficiency (isolated)	21%
IgG3 deficiency (isolated)	12%
IgG1 deficiency (isolated)	11%
IgG2 deficiency (isolated)	10%
IgG2 and IgG4 deficiency	9%
IgA and IgG4 deficiency	4%
IgA and IgG3 deficiency	3%
IgA, IgG2, and IgG4 deficiency	3%
IgA and IgG2 deficiency	2%
IgA, IgG1, and IgG4 deficiency	2%

The deficiencies (either isolated or combined with another deficiency) involved immunoglobulin (Ig)G4 37%, IgA 35%, IgG2 26%, IgG3 15%, and IgG1 13%.
Data from Goldblatt D, Morgan G, Symour ND, et al. The clinical manifestations of IgG subclass deficiency. In Levinksy RJ, ed. IgG Subclass Deficiencies. London, Royal Society of Medicine Services, 1989, pp 19–25.

other subclass deficiencies and panhypogammaglobu-linemia. IgG1 deficiency is considerably more common in adults than children and is often associated with other subclass deficiencies (Söderström et al., 1989).

Usually the IgG1 level is low but not absent, although Smith and co-workers (1989) reported familial absence of IgG1 deficiency. Many of the pediatric IgG1-deficient patients are younger than 5 years of age and are recovering from transient hypogammaglobulinemia of infancy. Older patients with IgG1 deficiency may be developing CVID.

Beard and colleagues (1986) reported that 6 of 22 IgA-deficient children with recurrent infections had an associated IgG1 subclass deficiency. Most patients had low but not absent IgA. Total IgG levels were low to normal; antibody levels were not reported.

IgG2 Deficiency

After IgG4 deficiency, IgG2 deficiency is the most common subclass deficiency in children, and males are more commonly affected than females (Söderström et al., 1989). Nahm and colleagues (1990) noted subnormal IgG2 levels in 312 of 8015 (4%) of normal blood donors. In children, it is the subclass deficiency most often associated with recurrent infections (see Table 13-3).

Most symptomatic patients have recurrent or chronic respiratory infections, often with *H. influenzae* or pneumococci. Others may have allergy and asthma, and a rare child has severe infections, including meningitis (Bass et al., 1983; Ohga et al., 1995). O'Keefe and Finnegan (1993) reported IgG2 deficiency in many patients with obstructive lung disease, particularly in those with long duration of disease and receiving steroid therapy.

Because IgG2 contains most of the antibodies to polysaccharide antigens, a deficiency of IgG2 is often associated with impaired polysaccharide responsiveness (Geha, 1988; Insel and Anderson, 1986; Umetsu et al., 1985). Some of these children have permanent, but more commonly transient, defects in their ability to respond to polysaccharide antigens (Shackelford et al., 1986, 1990b, 1990b). However, among adults, Avanzini and colleagues (1994) could not correlate antibody responses to *H. influenzae* conjugate vaccines, IgG subclass deficiencies, and respiratory problems. IgG2 deficiency may be a marker for recurrent respiratory responses, rather than the cause of the problem (Shackelford et al., 1990a).

Association with IgA and Other IgG Subclass Deficiencies

IgG2 is often associated with another subclass deficiency or an IgA deficiency. Oxelius and associates (1981) found low or immeasurable levels of IgG2 in 7 of 37 IgA-deficient subjects, 6 of whom had an associated IgG4 deficiency. All of the patients had recurrent infections, unlike 11 IgA-deficient subjects without an IgG2 deficiency. Beard and co-workers (1986) found that 4 of 22 (18%) IgA deficient subjects had an IgG2 deficiency; another 9 had other subclass deficiencies.

Roberton and colleagues (1990) found that 17% of IgA-deficient children had an IgG2 deficiency (and 25% an IgG4 deficiency). By contrast, French and associates (1995) found an IgG2 deficiency in 5% of all their IgA deficient adults, and in 9% of IgA-deficient adults with severe recurrent infections.

IgG2 deficiency is often associated with an IgG4 deficiency or a combined IgA, IgG2, and IgG4 deficiency. French and co-workers (1995) found that among IgA-deficient subjects, the severity of infection was correlated with an associated IgG2 and or IgG4 deficiency. Plebani and colleagues (1993) report two children with undetectable IgA1, IgG2, IgG4, and IgE with mild sinusitis caused by a homozygous deletion of the IgA1-IgE genes.

Other Associations

Some patients with normal IgG2 levels (and other subclasses) have impaired polysaccharide responsiveness, including patients with the Wiskott-Aldrich syndrome (Nahm et al., 1986) (see Chapter 17). Conversely, many IgG2-deficient patients have intact polysaccharide antibody responsiveness and are asymptomatic (Nahm et al., 1990; Shackelford et al., 1990b).

Selective IgG2 deficiency has been associated with other immunodeficiencies, including ataxia-telangiectasia (Oxelius et al., 1982), C3 deficiencies (Jefferis and Kumararatre, 1990), and mucocutaneous candidiasis (Kalfa et al., 2003) and C2 deficiency. It has also been reported in lupus erythematosus, diabetes, and minimal change glomerulonephritis (Morell, 1990), growth hormone deficiency (Wilson et al., 1990), HIV infection (Parkin et al., 1989), Hodgkin's disease (Zenone et al., 1996), Wolf-Hirschhorn syndrome (Hanley-Lopez et al., 1998), IFN-γ deficiency (Inoue et al., 1995), familial enteropathy (Smith et al., 1994b), and following sulfasalazine therapy (with an IgA deficiency) (Leickley and Buckley, 1986b).

Kavanaugh and Huston (1990) reported an adult male with complete IgG2 deficiency who normalized his IgG2 following splenectomy. Soiffer and colleagues (1995) noted a slight decrease of IgG2 levels following IL-2 infusions.

IgG3 Deficiency

IgG3 deficiency is less common than IgG4 or IgG2 deficiency in children, it is often unassociated with another subclass deficiency (see Table 13-3). Oxelius and associates (1986) described IgG3 deficiency in 313 of 8580 (4.7%) patients with recurrent infections, half of whom had an isolated IgG3 deficiency. IgG3 deficiency is considerably more common in adults (Söderström et al., 1989).

IgG3 antibodies may be important in the response to respiratory viral infections as well as responses to *Moraxella catarrhalis* and *Streptococcus pyogenes* (Goldblatt et al., 1991; Hammarström et al., 1986; Walker et al., 1983). IgG3 has a short half-life and is the least resistant to proteolytic digestion. Armenaka and co-workers (1994) reported that some patients with low

IgG3 levels normalized their IgG3 following intensive antibiotic therapy, suggesting that consumption of IgG3 antibodies was occurring with infection.

Most symptomatic IgG3-deficient patients have an associated deficiency of another subclass. These patients have recurrent respiratory infection (Shackelford et al., 1993), including refractory sinusitis (Armanaka et al., 1994; Barlan et al., 1993; Shapiro et al., 1991) or asthma (Armanaka et al., 1994; Önes et al., 1998; Oxelius et al., 1986).

Familial IgG3 deficiency has been reported (Huston et al., 1989). Many family members were homozygous for the G3m(g) or G3m(b) allotypes (Oxelius et al., 1986). IgG3 deficiency has also been described in Friedreich's ataxia (Oxelius et al., 1986) and in patients with an elevated IgE and recurrent infections (often with an IgA or IgG4 deficiency) (Loh et al., 1990) and recurrent parotitis (Marsman and Sukhai, 1999).

IgG4 Deficiency

IgG4 deficiency is the most common subclass immunodeficiency. Using insensitive assays such as radial diffusion of immunoprecipitation in which levels less than 5 to 7 mg/dl are recorded as absent, up to 15% of normal children and 10% of adults may have an IgG4 deficiency (Buckley, 2002). Most are asymptomatic. In infants younger than 5 years, the incidence of IgG4 is even higher. Using more sensitive assays, such as ELISA or radioimmunoassay, IgG4 is detectable in nearly all sera, and a deficiency can be defined as a level less than 1 mg/dl (Beck and Heiner, 1981).

IgG4 makes up only 2% to 4% of the total IgG and has no known unique immunoglobulin function. The mean level in 94 adults was 22 mg/dl with a range of 5 to 96 mg/dl (±2 SDs) (Beck and Heiner, 1981). Schur and colleagues (1970) found a mean among 3- to 4-year-olds of 32 mg/dl, with a range of 5 to 180 mg/dl.

Although most IgG4-deficient patients are symptomatic, several groups have identified IgG4-deficient patients who have recurrent respiratory, particularly pulmonary, infection (Bartmann and Kleihauer, 1988; Beck and Heiner, 1981; Moss et al., 1992). Heiner and associates (1983) described a familial syndrome of IgG4 deficiency with bronchiectasis. Hill and co-workers (1998) found an IgG4 deficiency in 5% of patients with bronchiectasis while other subclass deficiencies were found in 1% of patients.

IgG4 deficiency may be a marker for susceptibility to respiratory infection, possibly associated with an enrichment of IgG4 in the secretions (Merrill et al., 1985; Moss et al., 1992). Most of these patients have normal antibody responses to vaccine antigens.

IgG4 deficiency is often associated with IgG2 deficiency, IgA deficiency, or combined IgG2-IgA deficiency, and many of these children have recurrent infections and poor antibody responses to polysaccharide antigens (French et al., 1995; Moss et al., 1992; Page et al., 1988). The contribution of the IgG4 deficiency to their infection proneness is not known.

IgG4 deficiency has been noted in Wiskott-Aldrich syndrome, IgM deficiency (Morrel, 1994) ataxia-telangiectasia (Oxelius, 1979), and mucocutaneous candidiasis (Bragger et al., 1989; Kalfa et al., 2003). Other disorders with IgG4 deficiency include Down syndrome (Annerén et al., 1992), immune thrombocytopenia, lupus erythematosus, and growth hormone deficiency (with IgG2 deficiency) (Jefferis and Kumararatne, 1990; Morell, 1994; Wilson et al., 1990).

Laboratory Features

IgG subclass determinations are not recommended in the initial evaluation of individuals with recurrent infection, because functional antibody studies identify patients requiring such tests; in the presence of normal antibody function, a subclass deficiency is not clinically significant. Some authorities question the value of subclass determination at any time (Buckley, 2002; Maguire et al., 2002).

We recommend IgG subclass determinations for patients with selective IgA deficiency, for patients with detectable immunoglobulins but selective antibody deficiencies, and for patients in which an early stage of CVID is suspected.

IgG subclass levels must be compared with age-matched controls, because levels increase with age, particularly in the first 2 years. Normal values for age are given in Table 12-17 in Chapter 12. For children ages 4 to 10, an IgG1 level less than 250 mg/dl, an IgG2 level less than 50 mg/dl, an IgG3 level less than 15 mg/dl, and an IgG4 level less than 1 mg/dl are considered abnormal. For subjects older than age 10, an IgG1 level less than 300 mg/dl, an IgG2 level less than 75 mg/dl, an IgG3 level less than 25 mg/dl, and an IgG4 level less than 1 mg/dl are abnormal. If radial diffusion is used to measure IgG4, levels between 1 mg/dl and 8 mg/dl are usually reported as nondetectable, thus increasing the frequency of the diagnosis of IgG4 deficiency.

To substantiate a *clinically significant* subclass deficiency, the response to protein and/or polysaccharide antigens must be deficient, as outlined in Chapter 12 and the section on impaired polysaccharide responsiveness in this chapter. The definition of a poor response to pneumococcal antigens is that used in the impaired polysaccharide responsive patients (i.e., failure to respond to a majority of the pneumococcal antigens following a pneumococcal polysaccharide vaccine, or failure to exhibit a twofold rise in titer to serotypes for which there are nonprotective levels). Most patients with an IgG4 deficiency are excluded by this criterion.

Pitfalls in the diagnosis of IgG subclass deficiency include discrepancies in the values reported by different laboratories and their normal ranges, the degree of sensitivity of the assays (particularly for IgG4 levels), the marked variability of levels with age, particularly in young children, and failure to perform specific antibody studies to identify a clinically significant deficiency. Because one or more IgG subclasses is depressed in transient hypogammaglobulinemia of infancy (THI), a subclass deficiency can rarely be diagnosed before age 4 (Lawton et al., 1999). Instead, these patients have THI.

Treatment

Asymptomatic individuals with one or more subclass deficiencies and normal antibody responses require no treatment. Because a tiny percentage of these patients (particularly those with IgG1, IgG2, or IgG3 deficiencies) may evolve into CVID, they should be followed periodically with repeat subclass levels and antibody titers.

Individuals with respiratory infections and an IgG subclass deficiency but with normal antibody function are not candidates for IVIG therapy; indeed, this is probably the most common reason for the misuse of IVIG treatment. Alternative treatments such as antibiotics, inhaled steroids, bronchodilators, and surgical procedures for obstructive lesions may be needed.

Individuals with severe recurrent respiratory infections and a subclass deficiency (sometimes with an associated IgA deficiency), as well as a documented antibody deficiency may benefit from IVIG therapy. This is particularly true for individuals who have deficient antibody responses to both protein and polysaccharide antigens. A failure of prolonged antibiotics, severe symptoms, and persistent radiographic abnormalities also favor the use of IVIG.

Under such circumstances, IVIG can be given as for other patients with primary antibody deficiency (e.g., 400 to 600 mg/kg every 3 to 4 weeks). This has reportedly been effective in reducing infection in several patients with subclass deficiencies (Chapel et al., 2000; Duncan et al., 1988; Silk and Geha, 1988). When the IVIG therapy is to be discontinued after several months of therapy, it should be stopped in the warmer months to avoid community respiratory viral infections (which will be blamed on cessation of the IVIG).

The child younger than age 5 with frequent, non–life-endangering respiratory infections and a subclass deficiency or impaired polysaccharide responsiveness is a special problem. Lawton (1999) points out that most infection-prone children attending preschool who are given IVIG will almost certainly have a decreased number of respiratory infections, and if a mild immunodeficiency has been diagnosed as the cause, this will emphatically affirm the diagnosis, and the parents will be reluctant to stop IVIG. Indeed, if stopped, the frequency of infection increases temporarily, and lessens the physician's credibility. Because many (most) of these patients outgrow their infection-proneness, judicious use of antibiotics, reassurance, and careful monitoring may avoid expensive and sometimes hazardous IVIG infusions that may cause delay in normal immunologic maturation.

Prognosis

Children younger than ages 6 to 8 usually outgrow their IgG subclass deficiency, but adults rarely do. Recovery is more common if the subclass is low but not absent. A rare patient may progress to CVID.

IMPAIRED POLYSACCHARIDE RESPONSIVENESS (SELECTIVE ANTIBODY DEFICIENCY)

Definition

Impaired polysaccharide responsiveness (IPR), also termed *selective antibody deficiency*, is characterized by recurrent bacterial respiratory infections, an absent or subnormal response to a majority of polysaccharide antigens, normal or elevated immunoglobulin and IgG subclass levels, and intact antibody responses to protein antigens in subjects older than age 2 years. This illness should not be confused with antibody deficiency with normal immunoglobulins (see Historical Aspects, following).

The usual respiratory infections in IPR are chronic otitis, sinusitis, or bronchitis, but occasionally may include more serious infections such as mastoiditis or pneumonia. The offending bacteria are those with a polysaccharide capsule such as pneumococci, *H. influenzae*, meningococci, and group B streptococci.

Because nearly all infants younger than 2 years old have a physiologic defect in response to polysaccharide antigens, patients with IPR are by definition older than age 2. Several other primary immunodeficiencies may have selective antibody deficiencies to polysaccharide antigens, including Wiskott-Aldrich syndrome (see Chapter 17), IgG subclass immunodeficiency (see elsewhere in this chapter), selective IgA deficiency (see Chapter 14), transient hypogammaglobulinemia of infancy (see elsewhere in this chapter), autoimmune lymphoproliferative syndrome (ALPS) (see Chapter 19), and DiGeorge syndrome (Gennery et al., 2002) (see Chapter 17), but because of their other immune defects, do not have IPR.

Many patients with secondary immunodeficiencies also have impaired polysaccharide antibody responses, including those with splenic deficiency (Molrine et al., 1999), lymphoma and leukemia (Siber et al., 1978; Spickermann et al., 1994), HIV (Ballet et al., 1987), advanced age (Fata et al., 1996), bone marrow transplants (Ambrosino et al., 1991), chronic lung disease (Ekdahl et al., 1997; Miravitlles et al., 1999), and those receiving immunosuppressive drugs (Gennery et al., 2001).

Historical Aspects

Several patients with antibody deficiency with normal immunoglobulins were reported prior to 1980 (Blecher et al., 1968; Rothbach et al., 1979; Saxon et al., 1980), but these children had a broad-spectrum antibody deficiency and severe infections, not unlike patients with CVID. Thus these patients did not have IPR.

In 1986, Granoff and colleagues (1986a) identified several children with invasive *H. influenzae* infection, despite *H. influenzae* capsular immunization. Of these, 14 of 26 (54%) had nonprotective titers to the polysaccharide capsular antigen, but only a few had an IgG subclass or tetanus antibody deficiency. Poor antibody responses to this capsular vaccine were also identified in Apache Native American (Siber et al., 1990) and Alaskan Eskimo children (Ward et al., 1990), two groups with increased susceptibility to *Haemophilus* infections.

In 1987, Ambrosino and colleagues reported a 30-year-old man with pneumococcal pneumonia who had recurrent otitis and bronchitis since age 7. The patient had normal immunoglobulin and IgG subclass levels, normal antibody responses to diphtheria and tetanus toxoids, and intact cellular immunity, but no response to capsular antigens of *H. influenzae, Neisseria meningitides* types A and C, and four types of pneumococci. Rijkers and associates (1987) reported five additional cases of IPR (one of whom had selective IgA deficiency) in children aged 3 to 11, and Gigliotti and co-workers (1988) reported a leukemic child with septic arthritis resulting from *S. pneumoniae* who had a selective inability to respond to pneumococcal and *H. influenzae* polysaccharides, but no other immunologic abnormalities.

Ambrosino and colleagues (1988) identified 26 children with recurrent infection and normal immunoglobulin levels, 20 of whom had diminished antibody responses to *H. influenzae* vaccine. Herrod and associates (1989) studied 51 children with recurrent respiratory infection and identified 10 (20%) who did not respond to *H. influenzae* capsular vaccine. Seven of eight of these children responded normally to the *H. influenzae* protein conjugate vaccine.

With the introduction of the *H. influenzae* conjugate vaccine, most patients with IPR have been identified by their deficient responses to the 23-valent pneumococcal polysaccharide vaccine. Several authors have reported substantial numbers of these patients (Epstein and Gruskay, 1995; Herrod et al., 1997; Sanders et al., 1993, 1995; Shapiro et al., 1991; Wolpert and Knutsen, 1998; Zora et al., 1993).

Pathogenesis

IPR is probably a heterogenous disorder with multiple causes. Normal infants have impaired polysaccharide responsiveness until 2 years of age (see Chapter 22). Older children with persistent transient hypogammaglobulinemia may have impaired polysaccharide responsiveness for several months beyond age 2 (see elsewhere in this chapter). Lucas and associates (1993) have found age-dependent alterations of the variable light (VL) chain utilization for *H. influenzae* antibodies of infants versus adults so that a defect or delay in V region usage could be implicated in IPR.

Genetic factors may play a role in certain populations or individuals unresponsive to polysaccharide antigens. Among Alaskan Eskimo children who exhibited poor responses to *H. influenzae* polysaccharide vaccine, there was no correlation between the extent of Eskimo her-

itage and immune responsiveness (Ward et al., 1990). In these and Apache Native American children, micronutrient deficiencies may play an important role (Siber et al., 1990). Granoff and co-workers (1986b) identified certain Gm and Km (IgG allotypes) types associated with enhanced or depressed antibody responses to *H. influenzae* capsular vaccine. They also found a poor response to this vaccine in 50% of siblings of patients who had *H. influenzae* meningitis (Granoff et al., 1983).

Ambrosino and colleagues (1987) postulated that IPR is due to a defect in the B-cell repertoire, similar to CBA/N mice who lack B cells expressing the Lyb5 marker and are unresponsive to polysaccharide antigens. In normal mice Lyb5+ B cells appear with maturity and the ability to respond to polysaccharide. They suggest that IPR may be due to a delay in the appearance or absence of the appropriate B-cell repertoire.

Timens and Poppema (1987) suggest that IPR is due to a deficiency of the marginal zone of the spleen where polysaccharide antigens are concentrated and where dendritic cells present antigen to marginal-zone B cells. This zone is absent in the spleen of the human fetus and newborn. They suggest that splenic marginal-zone B cells may be analogous to the murine Lyb5 B-cell subset responsible for antibody formation to polysaccharides.

Most polysaccharides are T-independent type 2 antigens, requiring limited T-cell help but not direct T-cell interactions (see Chapter 3). Thus a T-cell cytokine deficiency or maturational defect could result in IPR. However, most of these patients have no identifiable T-cell defect.

One adult male with IPR had few B cells and a BTK mutation characteristic of XLA (Wood et al., 2001). A final possibility is that IPR is an early stage of CVID. This consideration is more likely in older individuals who were well as infants.

Clinical Features

Approximately 60% of IPR patients are male. There is usually no familial pattern, but as noted previously, certain ethnic groups may be more susceptible to IPR. Thus the ethnicity of the patient should be explored for Native American or Eskimo heritage. A history of past illness or immunosuppressive medications should be sought. The vaccine record should be reviewed.

The usual age of onset is age 2 to 7, but older children and an occasional adult may be affected. Epstein and Gruskay (1995) found the mean age at diagnosis was 4.7 ± 1.2 years. Some, but not all, of these infants had THI.

Recurrent infections, including chronic sinusitis, purulent rhinitis, and otitis are most common, followed by bronchitis, pharyngitis, and pneumonia, both lobar or bronchial (Epstein and Gruskay, 1995; Wolpert and Knutsen, 1998). Less common are systemic infections such as sepsis or meningitis. Allergic disease, usually asthma or allergic rhinitis, is present in more than 50% of patients (Wolpert and Knutsesn, 1998), probably depending on referral patterns. Many of these patients have ear tubes, tonsillectomy and adenoidectomy, decreased hearing, and multiple courses of antibiotics.

The infections are not life threatening, but mastoiditis, draining ears, sleep disturbances, and recurrent bronchitis with wheezing are not uncommon. The overall clinical picture is similar to patients with IgG subclass deficiencies, selective IgA deficiency, and mild hypogammaglobulinemia.

On physical examination, pallor, a gaping mouth, and prominent cervical lymph nodes are often noted. The tonsils may be enlarged and there is evidence of sinusitis such as circles under the eyes, posterior pharyngeal cobblestoning, purulent nasal discharge, postnasal drip, and diminished gag reflex.

Laboratory Features and Diagnosis

The diagnosis is established by identifying deficient antibody responses to polysaccharide vaccine antigens (usually pneumococcal vaccine) after age 2, associated with a normal antibody responses to protein antigens and normal or elevated IgG, IgM, IgA, and IgG subclasses, including IgG2 subclass. A concomitant antibody deficiency to protein antigens excludes this diagnosis. Antibody responses to tetanus, diphtheria, and conjugated H. influenzae vaccines are usually normal. Normal complement levels, nitroblue tetrazolium (NBT) or rhodamine dye reduction tests, and T-cell subsets exclude other primary immunodeficiencies. Nasopharyngeal cultures positive for S. pneumoniae or H. influenzae provide supporting evidence for IPR, but are rarely done and rarely positive.

Controversy exists as to what degree of hyporesponsiveness to the 23-valent pneumococcal vaccine is necessary for diagnosis of IPR. Normal children ages 2 to 5 develop protective titers to half or more of the antigens in the vaccine, using a 12 serotype panel. Normal children aged 6 and older and normal adults respond to more than 70% of the serotypes (Sorensen et al., 1998b). Certain serotypes may be more antigenic (3, 7F, 8, and 9); whereas 12F and 18C are intermediate; and 1, 4, 6, 14, 19F, and 23F are poorly antigenic (Epstein and Gruskay, 1995; Zora et al., 1993). Antibody responses are assessed 1 month following vaccine administration.

Sorensen and colleagues (1998b) also use a fourfold rise in titer to a serotype to which there is a nonprotective initial titer as a positive response, thus excluding those serotypes in which an adequate titer is present prior to immunization. In children older than age 5 or who have had a prior pneumococcal vaccine, baseline antibody titers are recommended prior to immunization.

In some patients, the response to pneumococcal vaccine is transient so that protective titers are not maintained upon retesting in 6 months. Thus retesting should be done if symptoms persist, despite adequate initial antibody responses. In nonresponsive patients, repeat pneumococcal polysaccharide immunization does not usually result in a better response and thus is not recommended. However, it can be repeated after a year or so to determine whether the patient has outgrown the problem.

Immunization with another polysaccharide vaccine such as meningococcal vaccine can be done to confirm the diagnosis. However, Epstein and Gruskay (1995) report that the antibody response to meningococcal vaccine and H. influenzae vaccine was intact in most children who had a poor response to pneumococcal vaccine.

Immunization with the pneumococcal conjugate vaccine can also be given. An adequate antibody response is expected (Sorensen et al., 1998a) and may be therapeutically beneficial, but does not exclude the diagnosis of IPR.

Despite development of adequate response to the conjugate pneumococcal vaccine, many patients continue to have recurrent infections, indicating that this is not simply lack of an antibody response to selected antigens, but a global deficiency in response to some or all polysaccharide microbial antigens.

Treatment

Initial management is directed at treating the co-existing infection. Chronic sinusitis, otitis, and mastoiditis are treated with 6 weeks of antibiotics at full therapeutic doses to try to eradicate the infection. Radiographs or CT scans are needed to document improvement. Ancillary treatment with nasal steroids, bronchodilators, and inhaled steroids may be used concomitantly for nasal allergy, persistent sinusitis, or asthma. After control of pre-existing infection, a trial of prophylactic antibiotics is often of value, particularly during the respiratory infection season. A 6-month trial is usually necessary.

The patient should sleep alone if economically feasible. Removal from day care may be necessary. Other vaccines, including influenza vaccine, should be given to the patient and his or her family. Environmental allergy control measures should be instituted.

Patients with persistent or recurrent infections who fail antibiotic therapy may be candidates for IVIG, particularly if the infections are associated with school absenteeism, chronic disability, or recurrent invasive infection. Indeed, an experimental human hyperimmune polysaccharide immune globulin containing high antibody titers to H. influenzae, S. pneumoniae, and N. meningitides reduced serious pneumococcal and H. influenzae disease in high-risk infants (Santosham et al., 1987). It also reduced the number of cases of pneumococcal otitis media (Shurin et al., 1993).

Silk and colleagues (1990) documented decreased episodes of sinusitis, otitis, and pneumonia in several IPR children following IVIG therapy at doses of 300 to 400 mg/kg every 3 to 4 weeks. Wolpert and Knutson (1998) gave IVIG to 34 of 120 IPR patients for an aver-

males from 3 to 18 years were identified. All suffered severe infections, including pertussis, recurrent pneumoniae, hemorrhagic chickenpox, otitis media, sinusitis, and bronchitis. These patients collectively gave histories of immune thrombocytopenia, autoimmune encephalitis, juvenile rheumatoid arthritis, Crohn's-like disease, hypothyroidism, and vitiligo. IVIG therapy reduced, but did not eliminate, the sinus and pulmonary infections.

The skeletal changes in all patients involved exclusively the metaphyseal regions of long bones and mild to severe involvement of the spine. Irregularities to the superior and inferior end plates of the vertebral bodies, sclerotic metaphyseal bands with irregularities in the long bones (mainly proximal and distal humeri, femurs, distal radii ulnae, and tibiae) were noted.

The IgG level was elevated in two patients, the IgM was low in one, and the IgA was low in two. The antibody responses to tetanus, polio, and pneumococcal vaccines were nonprotective in all patients. All four had moderately low T cells with some reduction in T-cell function.

Their clinical presentation was similar to patients with a predominantly antibody deficiency, rather than a profound cell-mediated deficiency. The T-cell aberrations may have led to dysregulation of the immune system with predisposition to autoimmunity.

Combined Immunodeficiency with Short-Limbed Dwarfism and Ectodermal Dysplasia

Gatti and colleagues (1969) described two siblings, male and female, who presented with agammaglobulinemia, T-cell immunodeficiency, short-limbed dwarfism, and ectodermal dysplasia. Dysmorphic features included shortened upper and lower limbs, shortened and widened pelvis, short ribs, and cupping of the distal radii. Both had recurrent and overwhelming bacterial infections to which they eventually succumbed. One patient exhibited eczematoid skin changes and eventually lost all her hair. The male sibling had no hair or eyebrows.

Both children had decreased, but not absent, lymphoid tissue. Immunoglobulins were very low and the one sibling studied thoroughly had no isohemagglutinins, decreased phytohemagglutinin (PHA) proliferation, and cutaneous anergy. Both children had normal chromosomes.

Schimke Immuno-Osseous Dysplasia

Schimke immuno-osseous dysplasia is an autosomal recessive syndrome that includes short stature, renal failure, and immunodeficiency (Boerkoel et al., 2000) (see Chapter 24). Autoimmune hemolytic anemia, immune thrombocytopenia, hyperpigmented cutaneous lesions, and cerebral vascular attacks have also been observed. Skeletal abnormalities include flattened ovoid vertebrae, small and laterally displaced capital femoral epiphyses, and dysplastic hips. The epiphyses show a lack of columnization of endochondral bone and decreased cellularity of resting cartilage. Patients are normal neurologically and intellectually. Renal disease is typically a focal segmental glomerulosclerosis often resistant to treatment.

Defects of cell-mediated and humoral immunity may be present with moderate CD4 lymphocytopenia, reduced mitogenic responses, and antibody deficiency. Some of these patients develop overwhelming viral and opportunistic infections.

Roifman Syndrome: Antibody Deficiency, Growth Retardation, Spondyloepiphyseal Dysplasia, and Retinal Dystrophy

Roifman in 1997 described two brothers with a new syndrome of antibody deficiency, spondyloepiphyseal dysplasia, growth retardation, and retinal dystrophy in two brothers. Two additional patients have been described (Roifman, 1999).

All were males born between 35 and 37 weeks' gestation with intrauterine growth retardation (IUGR). Both initial patients had eczema and two had asthma. Infections included recurrent ear infections, pneumonias, sepsis, and recurrent herpes.

Dysmorphic features included long prominent eyelashes, down-slanting palpebral fissures, a long philtrum, and a thin upper lip. Clinodactyly of the fifth finger was present, as were short tapered fingers and toes, a simian crease, and hyperconvex nails. Hepatosplenomegaly was present. Hypogonadotrophic hypogonadism was described in an additional case (Robertson et al., 2000) and noncompaction of the myocardium was identified in one patient (Mandel et al., 2001). Motor milestones were delayed and linear growth was below the third percentile. Borderline to mild developmental delay was present.

Radiographs demonstrated irregular and wavy end plates of the epiphyseal areas of the vertebrae and flattening fragmentation and erosion of the femoral heads, femoral condyle, and tibia, as well as over-tubulous third and fourth metacarpals. Abnormalities of the retinal rod and cone system were present in two patients.

Most patients had a mild eosinophilia but a normal IgE. Serum immunoglobulins were normal or low and B cells were reduced. Antibody responses to vaccine antigens were markedly reduced. T-cell number and function were normal.

Chaim M. Roifman

κ AND λ CHAIN DEFICIENCIES

Deficiency of κ or λ immunoglobulin light chains has been reported in a few individuals with immunodeficiency. Bernier and associates (1972) described a child with recurrent respiratory infections and diarrhea who had a κ/λ ratio of 0.66 instead of the expected 1.5 to 2.1. She also had an IgA deficiency but normal IgG and some antibody function. Barundun and co-workers

(1976) reported two boys with hypogammaglobuline-mia, frequent infections, and pernicious anemia. One had a κ/λ ratio of 0.01 (κ chain deficiency) and the other a ratio of 6.0 (λ chain deficiency).

Zegers and colleagues (1976) also described a patient with complete absence of κ-type immunoglob-ulins, cystic fibrosis, and selective IgA deficiency. A sis-ter had a similar κ chain deficiency. Sequence analysis of the patient's constant κ chain region genes revealed two different point mutations, one in each allele, resulting in substitution of a single amino acid in each κ light chain molecule (Stavnezer-Nordren et al., 1985).

During normal B-cell development, an attempt is made to match a κ light chain (of which there are two allotypes) coded by genes on chromosome 2 to the heavy chain derived from gene rearrangement on chro-mosome 14. If this is unsuccessful, a λ light chain tran-script, coded by genes on chromosome 22, is tried and κ chain synthesis stops (Korsmeyer et al., 1981).

Diagnosis is made by assessing serum levels of κ and λ chains or by immunoelectrophoretic analysis of the patient's serum with antisera to κ and λ chains.

ANTIBODY DEFICIENCY WITH TRANSCOBALAMIN II DEFICIENCY

Hereditary transcobalamin II (TCII) deficiency is a rare autosomal recessive disorder (Hakami et al., 1971) caused by a mutation of the TCII gene located on chro-mosome 22 (Arwert et al., 1986). TCII is required for absorption of cobalamin from the bowel and transport to vitamin B_{12}-requiring tissues. Cobalamin is taken up by cells only when bound to TCII (Hall, 1981).

Typically patients with TCII deficiency present in the first few months of life with failure to thrive, diarrhea, mucous membrane ulcers, lethargy, irritability, delayed neurologic development, severe macrocytic anemia, and neutropenia.

Most patients have decreased serum IgG levels and a failure to respond to childhood vaccines (Hitzig and Kenny, 1975). In vitro and in vivo T-cell function is nor-mal (Hitzig et al., 1974; Kaikov et al., 1991). Following parenteral treatment with high-dose vitamin B_{12}, patients recover completely clinically, hematologically, and immunologically. Some patients remain symptom free on oral maintenance therapy with hydroxocobal-amin, 1 or 2 mg daily (Zeitlin et al., 1985).

Hitzig and colleagues (1974) noted that immuniza-tion attempts initially failed to induce specific anti-body production, but that the patients produced specific antibody as soon as vitamin B_{12} injections were begun without reimmunization. This suggested that antigen exposure initiated the differentiation of antigen-specific memory cells in the absence of vita-min B_{12} utilization, but B-cell function was compro-mised; this emphasizes the need for a continuous supply of vitamin B_{12} by rapidly replicating cells such as the intestinal mucosa and hematopoietic and lymphoid cells.

DRUG-INDUCED ANTIBODY DEFICIENCIES

Immunosuppressive agents including alkylating agents, purine antagonists, and other drugs that interfere with cell proliferation and DNA synthesis may have a pro-found effect on T-lymphocyte function with secondary suppression of antibody production. The abnormalities associated with these agents are usually reversible if treatment is discontinued (Table 13-5).

Corticosteroids

Glucocorticosteroids exert their primary effects on T lymphocytes and monocytes (Cupps and Fauci, 1982). Short-term use in immunologically normal adults causes small but probably unimportant decreases of serum IgG and IgA levels in many subjects (Butler and Rossen, 1973; Posey et al., 1978; Settipane et al., 1978). Long-term treatment with glucocorticosteroids may cause severe depression of IgG in a small percent-age of subjects, but the ability to produce specific anti-body to immunization is generally normal (Berger et al., 1978; Katz et al., 1988; Lack et al., 1996). However, prolonged high dose prednisone in neonates has resulted in hypogammaglobulinemia and antibody defi-ciency, requiring the use of IVIG (Lederman et al., 1989).

Anticonvulsants

Treatment with anticonvulsants, including phenytoin, carbamazepine, and valproic acid, has resulted in reduc-tions in one or more immunoglobulin classes or IgG subclasses (Basaran et al., 1994; Callenbach et al., 2003). The only clinically significant problems have been associated with phenytoin (Ruff et al., 1987; Seager et al., 1975; Sorrell et al., 1971). Selective IgA deficiency (IgA levels lower than 10 mg/dl) occurs in as many as 3% of subjects taking phenytoin, and panhy-pogammaglobulinemia has been reported in several cases (Guerra et al., 1986; Travin et al., 1989). In most,

TABLE 13-5 · PHARMACEUTICALS THAT MAY CAUSE HYPOGAMMAGLOBULINEMIA

Anticonvulsant Drugs
Phenytoin
Carbamazepine
Valproic acid

Anti-inflammatory Drugs
Glucocorticosteroids
Gold salts
Sulfasalazine
Antimalarials
Captopril
D-Penicillamine
Fenclofenac

Monoclonal Antibodies
Rituximab (anti-CD20)

but not all, subjects, the effects resolve when phenytoin is withdrawn (Gilhus and Aarli, 1981).

Phenytoin has also been associated with hypersensitivity reactions, manifesting as skin rash, fever, lymphadenopathy, nephritis, and other organ dysfunction (Haruda, 1979). This may be due to the accumulation of toxic arene oxide metabolites in individuals who have a genetically determined variation in drug detoxification (Shear and Spielberg, 1988).

Gold Salts

Gold salts used for rheumatoid arthritis cause moderate reductions of immunoglobulin (Lorber et al., 1978) and IgG subclass (Kiely et al., 2000) levels in a substantial number of patients, and a few develop selective IgA deficiency (Pelkonen et al., 1983). Up to 2% of patients treated with gold develop severe panhypogammaglobulinemia with defective antibody production, leading to severe infections (Snowden et al., 1996). There is no obvious relationship between the dose or duration of therapy and the severity of immunodeficiency. In most, but not all, cases, the immunosuppressive effects are reversible when therapy is stopped. For that reason, it is recommended that serum immunoglobulin levels be measured before gold therapy begins, after each 1000 ng, and if recurrent or severe bacterial infections occur. Severe panhypogammaglobulinemia or defects in specific antibody production are an indication to stop gold therapy and consider the use of IVIG or other prophylaxis against infection until immune reconstitution occurs.

Anti-inflammatory Drugs

A variety of other slow-acting anti-inflammatory drugs can lower serum immunoglobulin levels. Among patients treated for inflammatory joint disorders, sulfasalazine causes low serum IgM levels in 3%, selective IgA deficiency in 3%, and low IgG in 2% (Van Rossum et al., 2001). There also have been isolated reports of selective IgA deficiency associated with antimalarials (Pelkonen et al., 1983), captopril (Hammarström et al., 1991), D-penicillamine (Hjalmarson et al., 1977), sulphasalazine (Farr et al., 1991), and fenclofenac (Farr et al., 1985). None of the patients treated with these drugs developed chronic, severe, or unusual infections, and in most cases the immunoglobulin abnormalities resolved when drug therapy was discontinued.

Rituximab

Rituximab is a humanized anti-CD20 monoclonal antibody used to target B lymphocytes in lymphoma, posttransplant lymphoproliferative disease, and antibody-mediated autoimmune diseases. Therapy with rituximab usually occurs in combination with other immunosuppressive drugs, so it is difficult to precisely assess its effects on the immune system. However, transient hypogammaglobulinemia and an increased susceptibility to infection occur in many patients following rituximab therapy (Quartier et al., 2003; Sharma et al., 2000; Verschuuren et al., 2002), and in at least one case severe hypogammaglobulinemia has persisted for longer than 2 years after therapy stopped (Castagnola et al., 2003). Humoral immune function should be monitored in all patients receiving rituximab, and prophylactic IVIG therapy should be provided as necessary.

Howard M. Lederman

ANTIBODY DEFICIENCY WITH INFECTIOUS DISEASES

Most infections result in a vigorous antibody response and, if chronic, hypergammaglobulinemia (see Chapter 4). Nevertheless, several viral infections and possibly parasitic infections such as malaria (see Chapter 28) may impair immunity sufficiently that antibody responses are diminished. Viral diseases include measles, HIV, human T-cell leukemia virus-1 (HTLV-1), cytomegalovirus, and particularly EBV infection. Congenital infections, notably rubella, may even lead to hypogammaglobulinemia or a hyper-IgM syndrome.

Other severe acute infections resulting in transient T-cell dysfunction blunt the primary antibody responses to neoantigens without affecting pre-existing antibody levels.

Epstein-Barr Virus Infection

A group of healthy college students with EBV-associated acute infectious mononucleosis were studied for in vivo and in vitro antibody responses to φX-174 bacteriophage. Their antibody responses were depressed, and in vitro studies revealed the presence of suppressor T cells. These transient immune defects resolved with 6 to 8 weeks of onset of disease (Junker et al., 1968). The mechanisms by which EBV affects the immune system and develops persistence are discussed in Chapter 28. Boys with X-linked lymphoproliferative syndrome may develop profound antibody defects following EBV infections, including agammaglobulinemia (see Chapter 17).

Human Immunodeficiency Virus Infection

Although the principal immune defect in HIV infection is a profound defect in CD4 T-cell numbers and function, B-cell immunity is also affected (see Chapter 29). Depressed antibody responses to keyhole limpet hemocyanin (KLH) antigen and pneumococcal polysaccharide vaccine were observed in adult males with acquired immune deficiency syndrome (AIDS) (Ammann et al., 1984). Antibody responses to φX-174 bacteriophage were significantly depressed in pediatric AIDS patients (Bernstein et al., 1985) and in adults with HIV-related adenopathy (Ochs et al., 1988). Most of these patients have normal or elevated levels of immune globulins. The use of IVIG in reducing the severity and frequency of infection in pediatric HIV infection has been documented (Mofenson et al., 1992, 1993) (see Chapter 29).

Some infants with congenital HIV infection may develop profound hypogammaglobulinemia after 6 months of age, associated with absent antibody responses to vaccine antigens and HIV-antibody negativity.

Congenital Rubella

Although congenital rubella may be associated with hypogammaglobulinemia affecting all three major immunoglobulin isotypes (Hancock et al., 1968; Plotkin et al., 1966; Soothill et al., 1966), it is most often associated with a hyper-IgM immunoglobulin profile (e.g., elevated IgM, low IgG, and absent IgA) (Soothill et al., 1966). The immunoglobulin abnormalities may normalize when virus excretion diminishes or ceases (Michaels, 1969). Kawamura and colleagues (2000) described deficient expression of CD40L (CD154) that normalized following treatment with IVIG.

REFERENCES

Abinun M, Spickett G, Appleton AL, Flood T, Cant AJ. Anhidrotic ectodermal dysplasia associated with specific antibody deficiency. Eur J Pediatr 155:146–147, 1996.

Abo K, Nishio H, Lee MJ, Tsuzuki D, Takahashi T, Yoshida S, Nakajima T, Matsuo M, Sumino K. A novel single basepair insertion in exon 6 of the Bruton's tyrosine kinase (Btk) gene from a Japanese X-linked agammaglobulinemia patient with growth hormone insufficiency. Hum Mutat 11:336, 1998.

Abramowsky CR, Sorensen RU. Regional enteritis-like enteropathy in a patient with agammaglobulinemia: histologic and immunocytologic studies. Hum Pathol 19:483–486, 1988.

Ackerson BK, Raghunathan R, Keller MA, Bui RH, Phinney PR, Imagawa DT. Echovirus 11 arthritis in a patient with X-linked agammaglobulinemia. Pediatr Inf Dis J 6:485–8, 1987.

Adachi Y, Mori M, Kido A, Shimono R, Suehiro T, Sugimachi K. Multiple colorectal neoplasms in a young adult with hypogammaglobulinemia. Report of a case. Dis Colon Rectum 35:197–200, 1992.

Adelman DC, Matsuda T, Hirano T, Kishimoto T, Saxon A. Elevated serum interleukin-6 associated with a failure in B cell differentiation in common variable immunodeficiency. J Allergy Clin Immunol 86:512–521, 1990.

Agematsu K, Futatani T, Hokibara S, Kobayashi N, Takamoto M, Tsukada S, Suzuki H, Koyasu S, Miyawaki T, Sugane K, Komiyama A, Ochs HD. Absence of memory B cells in patients with common variable immunodeficiency. Clin Immunol 103:34–42, 2002.

Agematsu K, Nagumo H, Shinozaki K, Hokibara S, Yasui K, Terada K, Kawamura N, Yoba T, Nonoyama S, Ochs HD, Komiyama A. Absence of IgD–CD27+ memory B cell population in X-linked hyper-IgM syndrome. J Clin Invest 102:853–860, 1998.

Aiuti F, Lacava V, Fiorilli M. B lymphocytes in agammaglobulinaemia. Lancet 2:761, 1972.

Allen RC, Armitage RJ, Conley ME, Rosenblatt H, Jenkins NA, Copeland NG, Bedell MA, Edelhoff S, Disteche CM, Simoneaux DK, Fanslow WC, Belmont J, Spriggs MK. CD40 ligand gene defects responsible for X-linked hyper-IgM syndrome. Science 259:990–993, 1993.

Al-Mondhiry H, Zanjani ED, Spivack M, Zalusky R, Gordon AS. Pure red cell aplasia and thymoma: loss of serum inhibitor of erythropoiesis following thymectomy. Blood 38:576–582, 1971.

Ambrosino DM. Impaired polysaccharide responses in immunodeficient patients: relevance to bone marrow transplant patients. Bone Marrow Transplant 7(suppl 3):48–51, 1991.

Ambrosino DM, Siber GR, Chilmonczyk BA, Jernberg JB, Finberg RW. An immunodeficiency characterized by impaired antibody responses to polysaccharides. N Engl J Med 316:790–792, 1987.

Ambrosino DM, Umetsu DT, Siber GR, Howie G, Goularte TA, Michaels R, Martin P, Schur PH, Noyes J, Schiffman G, et al. Selective defect in the antibody response to Haemophilus influenzae type b in children with recurrent infections and normal serum IgG subclass levels. J Allergy Clin Immunol 81:1175–1180, 1988.

Ament ME, Ochs HD, Davis SD. Structure and function of the gastrointestinal tract in primary immunodeficiency syndromes. A study of 39 patients. Medicine 52:227–248, 1973.

Ameratunga R, Lederman HM, Sullivan KE, Ochs HD, Seyama K, French JK, Prestidge R, Marbrook J, Fanslow W, Winkelstein JA. Defective antigen-induced lymphocyte proliferation in the X-linked hyper-IgM syndrome. J Pediatr 131:147–150, 1997.

Ammann AJ, Schiffman G, Abrams D, Volberding P, Ziegler J, Conant M. B-cell immunodeficiency in acquired immune deficiency syndrome. JAMA 251:1447–1449, 1884.

Ammann AJ, Sutliff W, Millinichick E. Antibody-mediated immunodeficiency in short limbed dwarfism. J. Pediatr 84:200–203, 1974.

Anderson JS, Teutsch M, Dong Z, Wortis HH. An essential role for Bruton's tyrosine kinase in the regulation of B-cell apoptosis. Proc Natl Acad Sci USA 93:10966–10971, 1996.

Andreotti AH, Bunnell SC, Feng S, Berg LJ, Schreiber SL. Regulatory intramolecular association in a tyrosine kinase of the Tec family. Nature 385:93–97, 1997.

Anker R, Conley ME, Pollok BA. Clonal diversity in the B cell repertoire of patients with X-linked agammaglobulinemia. J Exp Med 169:2109–2119, 1989.

Anneren G, Magnusson CG, Lilja G, Nordvall SL. Abnormal serum IgG subclass pattern in children with Down's syndrome. Arch Dis Child 6:628–631, 1992.

Armenaka M, Grizzanti J, Rosenstreich DL. Serum immunoglobulins and IgG subclass levels in adults with chronic sinusitis: evidence for decreased IgG3 levels. Ann Allergy 72:507–514, 1994.

Aruffo A, Farrington M, Hollenbaugh D, Li X, Milatovich A, Nonoyama S, Bajorath J, Grosmaire L, Stenkamp R, Neubauer M, Roberts RL, Noelle RJ, Ledbetter JA, Francke U, Ochs HD. The CD40 ligand, gp39, is defective in activated T cells from patients with X-linked hyper-IgM syndrome. Cell 72:291–300, 1993.

Aruffo A, Hollenbaugh D, Wu LH, Ochs HD. The molecular basis of X-linked agammaglobulinemia, hyper-IgM syndrome, and severe combined immunodeficiency in humans. Curr Opin Hematol 1:12–18, 1994.

Arwert F, Porck HJ, Frater-Schroder M, Brahe C, Geurts van Kessel A, Westerveld A, Meera Khan P, Zang K, Frants RR, Kortbeek HT, et al. Assignment of human transcobalamin II (TCII) to chromosome 22 using somatic cell hybrids and monosomic meningioma cells. Hum Genet 74:378–381, 1986.

Asherson GL. Late onset hypogammaglobulinemia. In Asherson GL, Webster AD, eds. Diagnosis and Treatment of Immunodeficiency. Cambridge, Mass, Cambridge University Press, 1980, p 37.

Ashman RF, Saxon A, Stevens RH. Profile of multiple lymphocyte functional defects in acquired hypogrammaglobulinemia, derived from in vitro cell recombination analysis. J Allergy Clin Immunol 65:242–256, 1980.

Aspalter RM, Sewell WA, Dolman K, Farrant J, Webster AD. Deficiency in circulating natural killer (NK) cell subsets in common variable immunodeficiency and X-linked agammaglobulinemia. Clin Exp Immunol 121:506–514, 2000.

Aukrust P, Aandahl EM, Skalhegg BS, Nordoy I, Hansson V, Tasken K, Froland SS, Muller F. Increased activation of protein kinase A type I contributes to the T cell deficiency in common variable immunodeficiency. J Immunol 162:1178–1185, 1999.

Aukrust P, Berge RK, Muller F, Ueland PM, Svardal AM, Froland SS. Elevated plasma levels of reduced homocysteine in common variable immunodeficiency—a marker of enhanced oxidative stress. Eur J Clin Invest 27:723–730, 1997.

Aukrust P, Muller F, Froland SS. Elevated serum levels of interleukin-4 and interleukin-6 in patients with common variable immunodeficiency (CVI) are associated with chronic immune activation and low numbers of CD4+ lymphocytes. Clin Immunol Immunopathol 70:217–224, 1994.

Avanzini MA, Björkander J, Söderström, Söderström T, Schneerson R, Robbins JB, Hanson LA. Qualitative and quantitative analyses of the antibody response elicited by *Haemophilus influenzae* type b capsular polysaccharide-tetanus toxoid conjugates in adults with IgG subclass deficiencies and frequent infections. Clin Exp Immunol 96:54–58, 1994.

Avasthi PS, Avasthi P, Tung KS. Glomerulonephritis in agammaglobulinaemia. Br Med J 2:478, 1975.

Baba Y, Nonoyama S, Matsushita M, Yamadori T, Hashimoto S, Imai K, Arai S, Kunikata T, Kurimoto M, Kurosaki T, Ochs HD, Ji Y, Kishimoto T, Tsukada S. Involvement of Wiskott-Aldrich syndrome protein in B-cell cytoplasmic tyrosine kinase pathway. Blood 93:2003–2012, 1999.

Bajpai UD, Zhang K, Teutsch M, Sen R, Wortis HH. Bruton's tyrosine kinase links the B cell receptor to nuclear factor kappaB activation. J Exp Med 191:1735–1744, 2000.

Ballet J-J, Sulcebe G, Couderc L-J, Danon F, Rabian C, Lathrop M, Clauvel JP, Seligmann M. Impaired anti-pneumococcal antibody response in patients with AIDS-related persistent generalized lymphadenopathy. Clin Exp Immunol 68:479–487, 1987.

Banatvala N, Davies J, Kanariou M, Strobel S, Levinsky R, Morgan G. Hypogammaglobulinaemia associated with normal or increased IgM (the hyper IgM syndrome): a case series review. Arch Dis Child 71:150–152, 1994.

Barandun S, Morell A, Skvaril F, Oberdorfer A. Deficiency of kappa- or lambda-type immunoglobulins. Blood 47:79–89, 1976.

Barber TD, Barber MC, Cloutier TE, Timothy E, Friedman TB. PAX3 gene structure, alternative splicing and evolution. Gene 237:311–319, 1999.

Bardelas JA, Winkelstein JA, Seto DS, Tsai T, Rogol AD. Fatal ECHO 24 infection in a patient with hypogammaglobulinemia: relationship to dermatomyositis-like syndrome. J Pediatr 90:396–399, 1977.

Barkin RM, Bonis SL, Elghammer RM, Todd JK. Ludwig angina in children. J Pediatr 87:563–565, 1975.

Barlan IB, Geha RS, Schneider LC. Therapy for patients with recurrent infections and low serum IgG3 levels. J Allergy Clin Immunol 92:353–355, 1993.

Barry SC, Seppen J, Ramesh N, Foster JL, Seyama K, Ochs HD, Garcia JV, Osborne WRA. Lentiviral and murine retroviral transduction of T cells for expression of human CD40 ligand. Hum Gene Ther 11:323–332, 2000.

Barth WF, Asofsky R, Liddy TJ, Tanaka Y, Rowe DS, Fahey JL. An antibody deficiency syndrome: selective immunoglobulin deficiency with reduced synthesis of gamma and alpha immunoglobulin polypeptide chains. Am J Med 39:319–334, 1965.

Bartmann P, Kleihauer E. Undetectable IgG4 in immunoprecipitation: association with repeated infections in children? Eur J Pediatr 148:211–214, 1988.

Basaran N, Hincal F, Kansu E, Ciger A. Humoral and cellular immune parameters in untreated and phenytoin- or carbamazepine-treated epileptic patients. Int J Immunopharmacol 12:1071–1077, 1994.

Bass JL, Nuss R, Mehta KA, Morganelli P, Bennett L. Recurrent meningococcemia associated with IgG2-subclass deficiency. N Engl J Med 309:430, 1983.

Batata MA, Martini N, Huvos AG, Aguilar RI, Beattie EJ. Thymomas: clinicopathologic features, therapy, and prognosis. Cancer 34:389–396, 1974.

Baumert E, Wolff-Vorbeck G, Schlesier M, Peter HH. Immunophenotypical alterations in a subset of patients with common variable immunodeficiency (CVID). Clin Exp Immunol 90:25–30, 1992.

Beall GN, Ashman RF, Miller ME, Easwaran C, Raghunathan R, Louie J, Yoshikawa T. Hypogammaglobulinemia in mother and son. J Allergy Clin Immunol 65:471–481, 1980.

Beard LJ, Ferrante A, Oxelius V-A, Maxwell GM. IgG subclass deficiency in children with IgA deficiency presenting with recurrent or severe respiratory infections. Pediatr Res 20:937–942, 1986.

Beck CS, Heiner DC. Selective immunoglobulin G4 deficiency and recurrent infections of the respiratory tract. Am Rev Respir Dis 124:94–96, 1981.

Beck S, Slater D, Harrington CI. Fatal chronic cutaneous herpes simplex associated with thymoma and hypogammaglobulinaemia. Br J Dermatol 105:471–474, 1981.

Bemark M, Sale JE, Kim HJ, Berek C, Cosgrove RA, Neuberger MS. Somatic hypermutation in the absence of DNA-dependent protein kinase catalytic subunit (DNA-PK[cs]) or recombination-activating gene (RAG)1 activity. J Exp Med 192:1509–1514, 2000.

Benderly A, Pollack S, Etzioni A. Transient hypogammaglobulinemia of infancy with severe bacterial infections and persistent IgA deficiency. Isr J Med Sci 22:393–396, 1986.

Benkerrou M, Gougeon ML, Griscelli C, Fischer A. Hypogammaglobulinémie G et A avec hypergammaglobulinémie M: a propos de 12 observations. Arch Fr Pediatr 47:345–349, 1990.

Bentwich Z, Kunkel HG. Specific properties of human B and T lymphocytes and alterations in disease. Transplant Rev 16:29–50, 1973.

Berger W, Pollock J, Kiechel F, Danning M, Pearlman DS. Immunoglobulin levels in children with severe asthma. Ann Allergy 41:67–74, 1978.

Bernadou A, Devred C, Diebold J, Bilski-Pasquier G, Bousser J. Thymome fuso-cellulaire associe a une erythroblastopenie, une megacaryocytopenie et une maladie des inclusions cytomegaliques. Semin Hop Paris 48:3443–3449, 1972.

Bernatz PE, Khonsari S, Harrison EG Jr, Taylor WF. Thymoma: factors influencing prognosis. Surg Clin North Am 53:885–892, 1973.

Bernier GM, Gunderman JR, Ruymann FB. Kappa-chain deficiency Blood 40:795–805, 1972.

Bernstein LJ, Ochs HD, Wedgwood RJ, Rubinstein A. Defective humoral immunity in pediatric acquired immune deficiency syndrome. J Pediatr 107:352–357, 1985.

Berridge MJ. Inositol trisphosphate and calcium signalling. Nature 361:315–325, 1993.

Blecher TE, Soothill JF, Voyce MA, Walker WH. Antibody deficiency syndrome: a case with normal immunoglobulin levels. Clin Exp Immunol 3:47–56, 1968.

Boerkoel CF, O'Neill S, André JL, Benke PJ, Bogdanovíc R, Bulla M, Burguet A, Cockfield S, Cordeiro I, Ehrich JHH, Fründ S, Geary DF, Ieshima A, Illies F, Joseph MW, Kaitila I, Lama G, Leheup B, Ludman MD, McLeod DR, Medeira A, Milford DV, Örmälä T, Rener-Primec Z, Santava A, Santos HG, Schmidt B, Smith GC, Spranger J, Zupancic N, Weksberg R. Manifestations and treatment of Schimke immunoosseous dysplasia: 14 new cases and a review of the literature. Eur J Pediatr 159:1–7, 2000.

Bolen JB. Nonreceptor tyrosine protein kinases. Oncogene 8:2025–2031, 1993.

Boncristiano M, Majolini MB, D'Elios MM, Pacini S, Valensin S, Ulivieri C, Amedei A, Falini B, Del Prete G, Telford JL, Baldari CT. Defective recruitment and activation of ZAP-70 in common variable immunodeficiency patients with T cell defects. Eur J Immunol 30:2632–2638, 2000.

Bonhomme D, Hammarstrom L, Webster D, Chapel H, Hermine O, Le Deist F, Lepage E, Romeo PH, Levy Y. Impaired antibody affinity maturation process characterizes a subset of patients with common variable immunodeficiency. J Immunol 165:4725–4730, 2000.

Bootman MD, Berridge MJ. The elemental principles of calcium signaling. Cell 83:675–678, 1995.

Bordigoni P, Auburtin B, Carret AS, Schuhmacher A, Humbert JC, Le Deist F, Sommelet D. Bone marrow transplantation as treatment for X-linked immunodeficiency with hyper-IgM. Bone Marrow Transplant 22:1111–1114, 1998.

Bottaro A, Lansford R, Xu L, Zhang J, Rothman P, Alt FW. S region transcription per se promotes basal IgE class switch recombination but additional factors regulate the efficiency of the process. EMBO J 13:665–674, 1994.

Bragger C, Seger RA, Aeppli R, Halle F, Hitzig WH. IgG2/IgG4 subclass deficiency in a patient with chronic mucocutaneous candidiasis and bronchiectases. Eur J Pediatr 149:168–169, 1989.

Brahmi Z, Lazarus KH, Hodes ME, Baehner RL. Immunologic studies of three family members with the immunodeficiency with hyper-IgM syndrome. J Clin Immunol 3:127–134, 1983.

Branda RF, Moore AL, Hong R, McCormack JJ, Zon G, Cunningham-Rundles C. B-cell proliferation and differentiation in common variable immunodeficiency patients produced by an antisense oligomer to the rev gene of HIV-1. Clin Immunol Immunopathol 79:115–121, 1996.

Brenner MK, Reittie JGE, Chadda HR, Pollock A, Asherson GL. Thymoma and hypogammaglobulinaemia with and without T suppressor cells. Clin Exp Immunol 58:619–624, 1984.

Brilliant LB, Nakano JH, Kitamura T, Hodakevic LN, Bharucha PB. Occupationally acquired smallpox in an IgM deficient health worker. Bull World Health Organ 59:99–106, 1981.

Brooks EG, Schmalsteig FC, Wirt DR, Rosenblatt HM, Adkins LT, Lookingbill, DP, Rudoff HE, Rakusa TA, Goldman AS. A novel X-linked combined immunodeficiency disease. J Clin Invest 86:1623–16311, 1990.

Bross L, Fukita Y, McBlane F, Demolliere C, Rajewsky K, Jacobs H. DNA double-strand breaks in immunoglobulin genes undergoing somatic hypermutation. Immunity 13:589–597, 2000.

Brouet JC, Chedeville A, Fermand JP, Royer B. Study of the B cell memory compartment in common variable immunodeficiency. Eur J Immunol 30:2516–2520, 2000.

Brown MP, Topham DJ, Sangster MY, Zhao J, Flynn KJ, Surman SL, Woodland DL, Doherty PC, Farr AG, Pattengale PK, Brenner MK. Thymic lymphoproliferative disease after successful correction of CD40 ligand deficiency by gene transfer in mice. Nature Med 4:1253–1260, 1998.

Brugnoni D, Airò P, Graf D, Marconi M, Giliani S, Malacarne F, Cattaneo R, Ugazio AG, Albertini A, Kroczek RA, Notarangelo LD. Ineffective expression of CD40 ligand on cord blood T cells may contribute to poor immunoglobulin production in the newborn. Eur J Immunol 24:1919–1924, 1994.

Bruton OC. Agammaglobulinemia. Pediatrics 9:722–727, 1952.

Bryant A, Calver NC, Toubi E, Webster AD, Farrant J. Classification of patients with common variable immunodeficiency by B cell secretion of IgM and IgG in response to anti-IgM and interleukin-2. Clin Immunol Immunopathol 56:239–248, 1990.

Buckley RH. Immunoglobulin G subclass deficiency: fact or fancy? Current Allergy Asthma Reports 2:356–360, 2002.

Buckley RH. Immunodeficiency diseases. JAMA 268:2797–2806, 1992.

Buckley RH, Fiscus SA. Serum IgD and IgE concentrations in immunodeficiency diseases J. Clin Invest 55:157–165, 1975.

Buckley RH, Rowlands DTJ. Agammaglobulinemia, neutropenia, fever, and abdominal pain. J Allergy Clin Immunol 51:308–318, 1973.

Bunnell SC, Henry PA, Kolluri R, Kirchhausen T, Rickles RJ, Berg LJ. Identification of Itk/Tsk Src homology 3 domain ligands. J Biol Chem 271:25646–25656, 1996.

Burtin P. Un exemple d'agammaglobulinemie atypique (un cas de grande hypogammaglobulinemie avec augmentation de la β2-macroglobuline). Rev Franc Etud Clin et Biol 6:286–289, 1961.

Butler WT, Rossen RD. Effects of corticosteroids on immunity in man. I. Decreased serum IgG concentration caused by 3 or 5 days of high doses of methylprednisolone. J Clin Invest 52:2629–2640, 1973.

Buzi F, Notarangelo LD, Plebani A, Duse M, Parolini O, Monteleone M, Ugazio AG. X-linked agammaglobulinemia, growth hormone deficiency and delay of growth and puberty. Acta Paediatr 83:99–102, 1994.

Cain WA, Ammann AF, Hong R, Ishizaka K, Good RA. IgE deficiency associated with chronic sinopulmonary infection (abstract). J Clin Invest 48:12a, 1969.

Callard RE, Smith SH, Herbert J, Morgan G, Padayachee M, Lederman S, Chess L, Kroczek RA, Fanslow WC, Armitage RJ. CD40 ligand (CD40L) expression and B cell function in agammaglobulinemia with normal or elevated levels of IgM (HIM). Comparison of X-linked, autosomal recessive, and non-X-linked forms of the disease, and obligate carriers. J Immunol 153:3295–3306, 1994.

Callenbach PMC, Jol-Van Der Zijde CM, Geerts AT, Arts WFM, Van Donselaar CA, Peters AC, Stroink H, Brouwer OF, Van Tol MJ. Immunoglobulins in children with epilepsy: the Dutch study of epilepsy in childhood. Clin Exp Immunol 132:144–151, 2003.

Cambronero R, Sewell WA, North ME, Webster AD, Farrant J. Up-regulation of IL-12 in monocytes: a fundamental defect in common variable immunodeficiency. J Immunol 164:488–494, 2000.

Campana D, Farrant J, Inamdar N, Webster AD, Janossy G. Phenotypic features and proliferative activity of B cell progenitors in X-linked agammaglobulinemia. J Immunol 145:1675–1680, 1990.

Canalis E, McCarthy T, Centrella M. Growth factors and the regulation of bone remodeling. J Clin Inv 81:277–281, 1988.

Cano F, Mayo DR, Ballow M. Absent specific viral antibodies in patients with transient hypogammaglobulinemia of infancy. J Allergy Clin Immunol 85:510–513, 1990.

Carbonara AO, Demarchi M. Ig isotypes deficiency caused by gene deletions. Monogr Allergy 20:13–17, 1986.

Cascalho M, Wong J, Steinberg C, Wabl M. Mismatch repair co-opted by hypermutation. Science 279:1207–1210, 1998.

Casellas R, Nussenzweig A, Wuerffel R, Pelanda R, Reichlin A, Suh H, Qin XF, Besmer E, Kenter A, Rajewsky K, Nussenzweig MC. Ku80 is required for immunoglobulin isotype switching. EMBO J 17:2404–2411, 1998.

Cassidy JT, Nordby GL. Human serum immunoglobulin concentrations: prevalence of immunoglobulin deficiencies. J Allergy Clin Immunol 55:35–48, 1975.

Castagnola E, Dallorso S, Faraci M, Morreale G, Di Martino D, Cristina E, Scarso L, Lanino E. Long-lasting hypogammaglobulinemia following rituximab administration for Epstein-Barr virus-related post-transplant lymphoproliferative disease preemptive therapy. J Hematother Stem Cell Res 12:9–10, 2003.

Cellier C, Foray S, Hermine O. Regional enteritis associated with enterovirus in a patient with X-linked agammaglobulinemia. N Engl J Med 342:1611–1612, 2000.

Chakravarti VS, Borns P, Lobell J, Douglas SD. Chondroosseous dysplasia in severe combined immunodeficiency due to adenosine deaminase deficiency (chondroosseous dysplasia in ADA deficiency SCID). Pediatr Radiol 21:447–448, 1991.

Chapel HM, Christie JM, Peach V, Chapman RW. Five-year follow-up of patients with primary antibody deficiencies following an outbreak of acute hepatitis C. Clin Immunol 99:320–324, 2001.

Chapel HM, Spickett GP, Ericson D, Engl W, Eibl MM, Bjorkander J. The comparison of the efficacy and safety of intravenous versus subcutaneous immunoglobulin replacement therapy. J Clin Immunol 20:94–100, 2000.

Chapin MA. Benign thymoma, refractory anemia and hypogammaglobulinemia: case report. J Maine Med Assoc 56:83–87, 1965.

Cheng AM, Rowley B, Pao W, Hayday A, Bolen JB, Pawson T. Syk tyrosine kinase required for mouse viability and B-cell development. Nature 378:303–306, 1995.

Cheng G, Baltimore D. TANK, a co-inducer with TRAF2 of TNF- and CD40L-mediated NF-kappaB activation. Genes Dev 10:963–973, 1996.

Cheng G, Cleary AM, Ye ZS, Hong DI, Lederman S, Baltimore D. Involvement of CRAF1, a relative of TRAF, in CD40 signaling. Science 267:1494–1498, 1995.

Cheng G, Ye ZS, Baltimore D. Binding of Bruton's tyrosine kinase to Fyn, Lyn, or Hck through a Src homology 3 domain-mediated interaction. Proc Nat Acad Sci USA 91:8152–8155, 1994.

Ching YC, Davis SD, Wedgwood RJ. Antibody studies in hypogammaglobulinemia. J Clin Inv 45:1593–600, 1966.

Chisuwa H, Mori T, Fujimori K, Shigeno T, Maejima T. Colorectal cancer in a young adult with X-linked agammaglobulinemia (XLA). Report of a case. Nippon Shokakibyo Gakkai Zasshi 96:1392–1395, 1999.

Chu YW, Marin E, Fuleihan R, Ramesh N, Rosen FS, Geha RS, Insel RA. Somatic mutation of human immunoglobulin V genes in the X-linked hyperIgM syndrome. J Clin Invest 95:1389–1393, 1995.

Chusid MJ, Coleman CM, Dunne WM. Chronic asymptomatic *Campylobacter* bacteremia in a boy with X-linked hypogammaglobulinemia. Pediatr Inf Dis J 6:943–944, 1987.

Ciliberti MD, Zweiman B, Atkins PC, Levinson AI, Mittl RL, Phillips DM. Chronic enteroviral meningoencephalitis in X-linked agammaglobulinemia: prolonged survival with the use of intrathecal therapy. Immunol Allergy Prac 16:7–10, 1994.

Clayton E, Bardi G, Bell SE, Chantry D, Downes CP, Gray A, Humphries LA, Rawlings D, Reynolds H, Vigorito E, Turner M. A crucial role for the p110delta subunit of phosphatidylinositol 3-kinase in B cell development and activation. J Exp Med 196:753–763, 2002.

Conley ME. B cells in patients with X-linked agammaglobulinemia. J Immunol 134:3070–3074, 1985.

Conley ME, Brown P, Pickard AR, Buckley RH, Miller DS, Raskind WH, Singer JW, Fialkow PJ. Expression of the gene defect in X-linked agammaglobulinemia. N Engl J Med 315:564–567, 1986.

Conley ME, Burks AW, Herrod HG, Puck JM. Molecular analysis of X-linked agammaglobulinemia with growth hormone deficiency. J Pediatr 119:392–397, 1991.

Conley ME, Fitch-Hilgenberg ME, Cleveland JL, Parolini O, Rohrer J. Screening of genomic DNA to identify mutations in the gene for Bruton's tyrosine kinase. Hum Molecular Genetics 3:1751–1756, 1994a.

Conley ME, Howard V. Clinical findings leading to the diagnosis of X-linked agammaglobulinemia. J Pediatr 141:566–571, 2002.

Conley ME, Larche M, Bonagura VR, Lawton AR III, Buckley RH, Fu SM, Coustan-Smith E, Herrod HG, Campana D. Hyper IgM syndrome associated with defective CD40-mediated B cell activation. J Clin Invest 94:1404–1409, 1994b.

Conley ME, Notarangelo LD, Etzioni A. Diagnostic criteria for primary immunodeficiencies. Representing PAGID (Pan-American Group for Immunodeficiency) and ESID (European Society for Immunodeficiencies). Clin Immunol 93:190–197, 1999.

Conley ME, Parolini O, Rohrer J, Campana D. X-linked agammaglobulinemia: new approaches to old questions based on the identification of the defective gene. Immunol Rev 138:5–21, 1994c.

Conley ME, Puck JM. Carrier detection in typical and atypical X-linked agammaglobulinemia. J Pediatr 112:688–694, 1988.

Conley ME, Sweinberg S K. Females with a disorder phenotypically identical to X-linked agammaglobulinemia. J Clin Immunol 12:139–143, 1992.

Conn HO, Quintiliani R. Severe diarrhea controlled by gamma globulin in a patient with agammaglobulinemia, amyloidosis, and thymoma. Ann Intern Med 65:528–541, 1966.

Cooper MD, Lawton AR. Circulating B-cells in patients with immunodeficiency. Am J Path 69:513–528, 1972.

Cooperband SR, Rosen FS, Kibrick S. Studies on the in vitro behavior of agammaglobulinemic lymphocytes. J Clin Invest 47:836–847, 1968.

Cosyns M, Tsirkin S, Jones M, Flavell R, Kikutani H, Hayward AR. Requirement of CD40-CD40 ligand interaction for elimination of *Cryptosporidium parvum* from mice. Infect Immun 66:603–607, 1998.

Cuccherini B, Chua K, Gill V, Weir S, Wray B, Stewart D, Nelson D, Fuss I, Strober W. Bacteremia and skin/bone infections in two patients with X-linked agammaglobulinemia caused by an unusual organism related to *Flexispira/Helicobacter* species. Clin Immunol 97:121–129, 2000.

Cunningham CK, Bonville CA, Ochs HD, Seyama K, John PA, Rotbart HA, Weiner LB. Enteroviral meningoencephalitis as a complication of X-linked hyper IgM syndrome. J Pediatr 134:584–588, 1999.

Cunningham-Rundles C. Disorders of the IgA system. In Stiehm ER, ed. Immunologic Disorders in Infants and Children, ed 4. Philadelphia, WB Saunders, 1996, pp 423–442.

Cunningham-Rundles C, Bodian C. Common variable immunodeficiency: clinical and immunological features of 248 patients. Clin Immunol 92:34–48, 1999.

Cunningham-Rundles C, Bodian C, Ochs HD, Martin S, Reiter-Wong M, Zhuo Z. Long-term low-dose IL-2 enhances immune function in common variable immunodeficiency. Clin Immunol 100:181–190, 2001.

Cunningham-Rundles C, Cooper DL, Duffy TP, Strauchen J. Lymphomas of mucosal-associated lymphoid tissue in common variable immunodeficiency. Am J Hematol 69:171–178, 2002.

Cunningham-Rundles S, Cunningham-Rundles C, Siegal FP, Gupta S, Smithwick EM, Kosloff C, Good RA. Defective cellular immune response in vitro in common variable immunodeficiency. J Clin Immunol 1:65–72, 1981.

Cunningham-Rundles C, Siegal FP, Cunningham-Rundles S, Lieberman P. Incidence of cancer in 98 patients with common varied immunodeficiency. J Clin Immunol 7:294–299, 1987.

Cupps TR, Fauci AS. Corticosteroid-mediated immunoregulation in man. Immunol Rev 65:133–155, 1982.

Dalal I, Reid B, Nisbet-Brown E, Roifman CM. The outcome of patients with hypogammaglobulinemia in infancy and early childhood. J Pediatr 133:144–146, 1998.

Dalal I, Roifman CM. Hypogammaglobulinemia of infancy. Immunol Allergy Clin North Am 21:129–139, 2001.

Daniels GA, Lieber MR. RNA:DNA complex formation upon transcription of immunoglobulin switch regions: implications for the mechanism and regulation of class switch recombination. Nucleic Acids Res 25:5006–5011, 1995.

Davies CW, Juniper MC, Gray W, Gleeson FV, Chapel HM, Davies RJ. Lymphoid interstitial pneumonitis associated with common variable hypogammaglobulinaemia treated with cyclosporin A. Thorax 55:88–90, 2000.

de la Concha EG, Fernandez-Arquero M, Martinez A, Vidal F, Vigil P, Conejero L, Garcia-Rodriguez MC, Fontan G. HLA class II homozygosity confers susceptibility to common variable immunodeficiency (CVID). Clin Exp Immunol 116:516–520, 1999.

de la Concha EG, Garcia-Rodriquez MC, Zabay JM, Laso MT, Alonso R, Bootello A, Fontan G. Functional assessment of T and B lymphocytes in patients with selective IgM deficiency. Clin Exp Immunol 42:670–676, 1982.

Degos L, Faille A, Housset M, Boumsell L, Rabian C, Parames T. Syndrome of neutrophil agranulocytosis, hypogammaglobulinemia, and thymoma. Blood 60:968–972, 1982.

de Weers M, Verschuren MC, Kraakman ME, Mensink RG, Schuurman RK, vand Dongen JJ, Hendriks RW. The Bruton's tyrosine kinase gene is expressed throughout B cell differentiation, from early precursor B cell stages preceeding immunoglobulin gene rearrangement up to mature B cell stages. Eur J Immuno 23:3109–3114, 1993.

Di Renzo M, Zhou Z, George I, Becker K, Cunningham-Rundles C. Enhanced apoptosis of T cells in common variable immunodeficiency (CVID): role of defective CD28 co-stimulation. Clin Exp Immunol 120:503–511, 2000.

DiSanto JP, Bonnefoy JY, Gauchat JF, Fischer A, De Saint Basile G. CD40 ligand mutations in X-linked immunodeficiency with hyper IgM. Nature 361:541–543, 1993.

Doffinger R, Smahi A, Bessia C, Geissmann F, Feinberg J, Durandy A, Bodemer C, Kenwrick S, Dupuis-Girod S, Blanche S, Wood P, Rabia SH, Headon DJ, Overbeek PA, Le Deist F, Holland SM, Belani K, Kumararatne DS, Fischer A, Shapiro R, Conley ME, Reimund E, Kalhoff H, Abinun M, Munnich A, Israel A, Courtois G, Casanova JL. X-linked anhidrotic ectodermal dysplasia with immunodeficiency is caused by impaired NF-κB signaling. Nature Genetics 27:277–285, 2001.

Dolmetsch RE, Lewis RS, Goodnow CC, Healy JI. Differential activation of transcription factors induced by Ca2+ response amplitude and duration [see comments] [published erratum appears in Nature 1997 Jul 17;388]. Nature 386:855–858, 1997.

Dominguez O, Ruiz JF, Lain de Lera T, Garcia-Diaz M, Gonzalez MA, Kirchhoff T, Martinez-AC, Bernad A, Blanco L. DNA polymerase mu (Pol mu), homologous to TdT, could act as a DNA mutator in eukaryotic cells. EMBO J 19:1731–1742, 2000.

Dougall WC, Claccum M, Charrier K, Rohrbach K, Brasel K, De Smedt T, Daro E, Smith J, Tometsko ME, Maliszewski CR, Armstrong A, Shen V, Bain S, Cosman D, Anderson D, Morrissey PJ, Peschon JJ, Schuh J. RANK is essential for osteoclast and lymph node development. Genes Develop 13:2412–2424, 1999.

Dressler F, Peter HH, Muller W, Reiger CHL. Transient hypogammaglobulinemia of infancy: five new cases, review of the literature and redefinition. Acta Paediatr Scand 78:767–774, 1989.

Dubois RS, Roy CC, Fulginiti VA, Merrill DA, Murray RL. Disaccharidase deficiency in children with immunologic deficits. J Pediat 76:377–385, 1970.

Duncan JM, Herrod HG, Crawford LV. IgG subclass deficiency and recurrent respiratory tract disease in childhood. Ped Asthma Allergy Immunol 2:269–278, 1988.

Duplantier JE, Seyama K, Day NK, Hitchcock R, Nelson RP Jr, Ochs HD, Haraguchi S, Klemperer MR, Good RA. Immunologic reconstitution following bone marrow transplantation for X-linked hyper-IgM syndrome. Clin Immunol 98:313–318, 2001.

Durandy A, Hivroz C, Mazerolles F, Schiff C, Bernard F, Jouanguy E, Revy P, DiSanto JP, Gauchat JF, Bonnefoy JY, Casanova JL, Fischer A. Abnormal CD40-mediated activation pathway in B lymphocytes from patients with hyper-IgM syndrome and normal CD40 ligand expression. J. Immunol 158:2576–2584, 1997.

Durandy A, Schiff C, Bonnefoy JY, Forveille M, Rousset F, Mazzei G, Milili M, Fischer A. Induction by anti-CD40 antibody or soluble CD40 ligand and cytokines of IgG, IgA and IgE production by B cells from patients with X-linked hyper-IgM syndrome. Eur J Immunol 23:2294–2299, 1993.

Duriez B, Duquesnoy P, Dastot F, Bougneres P, Amselem S, Goossens M. An exon-skipping mutation in the btk gene of a patient with X-linked agammaglobulinemia and isolated growth hormone deficiency. FEBS Lett 346:165–170, 1994.

Dworzack DL, Murray CM, Hodges GR, Barnes WG. Community-acquired bacteremic Achromobacter xylosodicans type IIIa pneumonia in a patient with idiopathic IgM deficiency. Am J Clin Pathol 70:712–717, 1978.

Eisenstein EM, Chua K, Strober W. B-cell differentiation defects in common variable immunodeficiency are ameliorated after stimulation with anti-CD40 antibody and IL-10. J Immunol 152:5957–5968, 1994.

Ekdahl K, Braconier JH, Svanborg C. Immunoglobulin deficiencies and impaired immune response to polysaccharide antigens in adult patients with recurrent community-acquired pneumonia. Scand J Infect Dis 29:401–407, 1997.

Ellmeier W, Jung S, Sunshine MJ, Hatam F, Xu Y, Baltimore D, Mano H, Littman DR. Severe B cell deficiency in mice lacking the tec kinase family members Tec and Btk. J Exp Med 192:1611–1624, 2000.

Epstein MM, Gruskay F. Selective deficiency in pneumococcal antibody response in children with recurrent infections. Ann Allergy Asthma Immunol 75:125–131, 1995.

Erlendsson K, Swartz T, Dwyer JM. Successful reversal of echovirus encephalitis in X-linked hypogammaglobulinemia by intraventricular administration of immunoglobulin. N Engl J Med 312:351–353, 1985.

Esolen LM, Fasano MB, Flynn J, Burton A, Lederman HM. Pneumocystis carinii osteomyelitis in a patient with common variable immunodeficiency. N Engl J Med 326:999–1001, 1992.

Espanol T, Catala M, Hernandez M, Caragol I, Bertran JM. Development of a common variable immunodeficiency in IgA-deficient patients. Clin Immunol Immunopathol 80:333–335, 1996.

Facchetti F, Appiani C, Salvi L, Levy J, Notarangelo LD. Immunohistologic analysis of ineffective CD40-CD40 ligand interaction in lymphoid tissues from patients with X-linked immunodeficiency with hyper-IgM. J Immunol 154:6624–6633, 1995.

Farr M, Kitas GD, Tunn EJ, Bacon PA. Immunodeficiencies associated with sulphasalazine therapy in inflammatory arthritis. Br J Rheumatol 30:413–417, 1991.

Farr M, Struthers GR, Scott DGI, Bacon PA. Fenclofenac-induced selective IgA deficiency in rheumatoid arthritis. Br J Rheumatol 24:367–369, 1985.

Farrant J, Spickett G, Matamoros N, Copas D, Hernandez M, North M, Chapel H, Webster AD. Study of B and T cell phenotypes in blood from patients with common variable immunodeficiency (CVID). Immunodeficiency 5:159–169, 1994.

Farrar JE, Rohrer J, Conley ME. Neutropenia in X-linked agammaglobulinemia. Clin Immunol Immunopath 81:271–276, 1996.

Farrington M, Grosmaire LS, Nonoyama S, Fischer SH, Hollenbaugh D, Ledbetter JA, Noelle RJ, Aruffo A, Ochs HD. CD40 ligand expression is defective in a subset of patients with common variable immunodeficiency. Proc Natl Acad Sci USA 91:1099–1103, 1994.

Fasano MB, Sullivan KE, Sarpong SB, Wood RA, Jones SM, Johns CJ, Lederman HM, Bykowsky MJ, Greene JM, Winkelstein JA. Sarcoidosis and common variable immunodeficiency. Report of 8 cases and review of the literature. Medicine (Baltimore) 75:251–261, 1996.

Fata FT, Herzlich BC, Schiffman G, Ast AL. Impaired antibody responses to pneumococcal polysaccharide in elderly patients with low serum vitamin B_{12} levels. Ann Intern Med 124:299–304, 1996.

Faulk WP, Kiyasu WS, Cooper MD, Fudenberg HH. Deficiency of IgM. Pediatrics 47:399–404, 1971.

Faulkner GC, Burrows SR, Khanna R, Moss DJ, Bird AG, Crawford DH. X-Linked agammaglobulinemia patients are not infected with Epstein-Barr virus: implications for the biology of the virus. J Virol 73:1555–1564, 1999.

Fearon ER, Winkelstein JA, Civin CI, Pardoll DM, Vogelstein B. Carrier detection in X-linked agammaglobulinemia by analysis of X-chromosome inactivation. N Engl J Med 316:427–431, 1987.

Ferrari S, Giliani S, Insalaco A, Al-Ghonaium A, Soresina AR, Loubser M, Avanzini MA, Marconi M, Badolato R, Ugazio AG, Levy Y, Catalan N, Durandy A, Tbakhi A, Notarangelo LD, Plebani A. Mutations of CD40 gene cause an autosomal recessive form of immunodeficiency with hyper IgM. Proc Natl Acad Sci USA 98:12614–12619, 2001.

Fineman SM, Rosen FS, Geha RS. Transient hypogammaglobulinemia, elevated immunoglobulin E levels, and food allergy. J Allergy Clin Immunol 64:216–222, 1979.

Fischer MB, Hauber I, Eggenbauer H, Thon V, Vogel E, Schaffer E, Lokaj J, Litzman J, Wolf HM, Mannhalter JW, et al. A defect in the early phase of T-cell receptor-mediated T-cell activation in patients with common variable immunodeficiency. Blood 84:4234–4241, 1994.

Fischer MB, Wolf HM, Hauber I, Eggenbauer H, Thon V, Sasgary M, Eibl MM. Activation via the antigen receptor is impaired in T cells, but not in B cells from patients with common variable immunodeficiency. Eur J Immunol 26:231–237, 1996.

Flanagan JG, Rabbitts TH. Arrangement of human immunoglobulin heavy chain constant region genes implies evolutionary duplication of a segment containing gamma, epsilon, and alpha genes. Nature 300:709–713, 1982.

Fleisher TA, White RM, Broder S, Nissley SP, Blaese RM, Mulvihill JJ, Olive G, Waldmann TA. X-linked hypogammaglobulinemia and isolated growth hormone deficiency. N Engl J Med 302:1429–1434, 1980.

Fluckiger AC, Li Z, Kato RM, Wahl MI, Ochs HD, Longnecker R, Kinet JP, Witte ON, Scharenberg AM, Rawlings DJ. Btk/Tec kinases regulate sustained increases in intracellular Ca2+ following B-cell receptor activation. EMBO J 17:1973–1985, 1998.

Fontana S, Moratto D, Mangal S, De Francesco M, Vermi W, Ferrari S, Facchetti F, Kutukculer N, Fiorini C, Duse M, Das PK, Notarangelo LD, Plebani A, Badolato R. Functional defects of dendritic cells in CD40-deficient patients. Blood 102:4099–4106, 2003.

Frangogiannis NG, Cate TR. Endocarditis and Ureaplasma urealyticum osteomyelitis in a hypogammaglobulinemic patient. A case report and review of the literature. J Infect 37:181–184, 1998.

Franz A, Webster AD, Furr PM, Taylor-Robinson D. Mycoplasmal arthritis in patients with primary immunoglobulin deficiency: clinical features and outcome in 18 patients. Br J Rheumatol 36:661–668, 1997.

Freijd A, Hammarström L, Persson MAA, Smith CIE. Plasma antipneumococcal antibody activity of the IgG class and subclasses in otitis prone children. Clin Exp Immunol 565:233–238, 1984.

French MAH, Denis KA, Dawkins R, Peter JB. Severity of infectios in IgA deficiency: correlation with decreased serum antibodies to pneumococcal polysaccharides and decreased serum IgG2 and/or IgG4. Clin Exp Immunol 100:47–53, 1995.

Frix CD, Bronson DM. Acute miliary tuberculosis in a child with anhidrotic ectodermal dysplasia. Pediat Derm 3:464–467, 1986.

Frizzera G, Rosai J, Dehner LP, Spector BD, Kersey JH. Lymphoreticular disorders in primary immunodeficiencies: new findings based on an up-to-date histologic classification of 35 cases. Cancer 46:692–699, 1980.

Fruman DA, Snapper SB, Yballe CM, Davidson L, Yu JY, Alt FW, Cantley LC. Impaired B cell development and proliferation in absence of phosphoinositide 3-kinase p85alpha. Science 283:393–397, 1999.

Fu JL, Shyur SD, Lin HY, Lai YC. X-linked agammaglobulinemia presenting as juvenile chronic arthritis: report of one case. Chung-Hua Min Kuo Hsiao Erh Ko I Hsueh Hui Tsa Chih 40:280–283, 1999.

Fudenberg HH, Fudenberg BR. Antibody to hereditary human gammaglobulin (Gm) factor resulting from maternal-fetal incompatibility. Science 145:170, 1964.

Fukuda M, Kojima T, Kabayama H, Mikoshiba K. Mutation of the pleckstrin homology domain of Bruton's tyrosine kinase in immunodeficiency impaired inositol 1,3,4,5-tetrakisphosphate binding capacity. J Biol Chem 271:30303–30306, 1996.

Fuleihan R, Ramesh N, Loh R, Jabara H, Rosen FS, Chatila T, Fu SM, Stamenkovic I, Geha RS. Defective expression of the CD40 ligand in X chromosome-linked immunoglobulin deficiency with normal or elevated IgM. Proc Natl Acad Sci USA 90:2170–2173, 1993.

Futatani T, Miyawaki T, Tsukada S, Hashimoto S, Kunikata T, Arai S, Kurimoto M, Niida Y, Matsuoka H, Sakiyama Y, Iwata T, Tsuchiya S, Tatsuzawa O, Yoshizaki K, Kishimoto T. Deficient expression of Bruton's tyrosine kinase in monocytes from X-linked agammaglobulinemia as evaluated by a flow cytometric analysis and its clinical application to carrier detection. Blood 91:595–602, 1998.

Futatani T, Watanabe C, Baba Y, Tsukada S, Ochs HD. Bruton's tyrosine kinase is present in normal platelets and its absence identifies patients with X-linked agammaglobulinaemia and carrier females. Br J Haematol 114:141–149, 2001.

Gardulf A, Andersen V, Bjorkander J, Ericson D, Froland SS, Gustafson R, Hammarstrom L, Jacobsen MB, Jonsson E, Moller G, et al. Subcutaneous immunoglobulin replacement in patients with primary antibody deficiencies: safety and costs. Lancet 345:365–369, 1995.

Gatti RA, Boder E, Vinters HV, Sparkes RS, Norman A, Lange K. Ataxia-telangiectasia: an interdisciplinary approach to pathogenesis. Medicine (Baltimore) 70:99–117, 1991.

Gatti RA, Platt N, Pomerance HH, Hong R, Langer LO, Kay HEM, Good RA. Hereditary lymphopenic agammaglobulinemia associated with a distinctive form of short-limbed dwarfism and ectodermal dysplasia. J Pediatr 75:675–684, 1969.

Geha RS. IgG antibody response to polysaccharides in children with recurrent infections. Monogr Allergy 23:97–102, 1988.

Geha RS, Rosen FS, Merler E. Identification and characterization of subpopulations of lymphocytes in human peripheral blood after fractionation on discontinuous gradients of albumin. The cellular defect in X-linked agammaglobulinemia. J Clin Inv 52:1726–1734, 1973.

Gehrmann G, Engstfeld G. Thymoma and agammaglobulinemia. German Med Monthly 10:281–283, 1965.

Gennery AR, Barge D, O'Sullivan JJ, Flood TJ, Abinun M, Cant AJ. Antibody deficiency and autoimmunity in 22q11.2 deletion syndrome. Arch Dis Child 86:422–425, 2002.

Gennery AR, Cant AJ, Baldwin CI, Calvert JE. Characterization of the impaired antipneumococcal polysaccharide antibody production in immunosuppressed pediatric patients following cardiac transplantation. J Clin Immunol 21:43–50, 2001.

Gennery AR, Clark JE, Flood TJ, Abinun M, Cant A. T-cell-depleted bone marrow transplantation from allogeneic sibling for X-linked hyperimmunoglobulin M syndrome. J Pediatr 137:290, 2000.

George DL, Phillips JAD, Francke U, Seeburg PH. The genes for growth hormone and chorionic somatomammotropin are on the long arm of human chromosome 17 in region q21 to qter. Human Genetics 57:138–141, 1981.

Ghia P, ten Boekel E, Sanz E, de la Hera A, Rolink A, Melchers F. Ordering of human bone marrow B lymphocyte precursors by single-cell polymerase chain reaction analyses of the rearrangement status of the immunoglobulin H and L chain gene loci. J Exp Med 184:2217–2229, 1996.

Gibson TJ, Hyvonen M, Musacchio A, Saraste M, Birney E. PH domain: the first anniversary. Trends Biochem Sci 19:349–353, 1994.

Gigliotti F, Herrod HG, Kalwinsky DK, Insel RA. Immunodeficiency associated with recurrent infections and an isolated in vivo inability to respond to bacterial polysaccharides. Pediatr Infect Dis J 7:417–420, 1988.

Gilhus NE, Aarli JA. The reversibility of phenytoin-induced IgA deficiency. J Neurol 226:53–61, 1981.

Gilmour KC, Cranston T, Jones A, Davies EG, Goldblatt D, Thrasher A, Kinnon C, Nichols KE, Gaspar HB. Diagnosis of X-linked lymphoproliferative disease by analysis of SLAM-associated protein expression. Eur J Immunol 30:1691–1697, 2000.

Gitlin D, Janeway CA: Agammaglobulinemia: congenital, acquired and transient forms. Prog Hematol 1:318–329, 1956.

Gitlin D, Janeway CA, Apt L, Craig JM. Agammaglobulinemia., In Lawrence HS, ed. Cellular and Humoral Aspects of the Hypersensitivity States: A Symposium. New York, Hoeber-Harper, 1959, p 375–441.

Gleich GL, Averbeck AK, Swedlung HA. Measurement of IgE in normal and allergic serum by radioimmunoassay. J Lab Clin Med 77:690–698, 1971.

Golay JT, Webster AD. B cells in patients with X-linked and `common variable' hypogammaglobulinaemia. Clin Exp Immunol 65:100–104, 1986.

Goldblatt D, Turner MW, Levinsky RJ. Delayed maturation of antigen-specific IgG3: another variant of paediatric immunodeficiency? In Chapel HM, Levinsky RJ, Webster ADB, eds. Progress in Immune Deficiency III. Royal Society of Medicine Services International Congress Symposium Series 173:109–114, 1991.

Goldstein G, Mackay IR, eds. The Human Thymus. St. Louis, Warren H. Green, 1969, pp 194–227.

Gong S, Nussenzweig MC. Regulation of an early developmental checkpoint in the B cell pathway by Ig beta. Science 272:411–414, 1996.

Good RA. Agammaglobulinemia—a provocative experiment of nature. Bull Univ Minn Med Found 26:1–19, 1954.

Good RA. Studies on agammaglobulinemia: II. Failure of plasma cell formation in the bone marrow and lymph nodes of patients with agammaglobulinemia. J Lab Clin Med 46:167–181, 1955.

Good RA, Rotstein J. Rheumatoid arthritis and agammaglobulinemia. Bull Rheum Dis 10:203–206, 1960.

Good RA, Rotstein J, Mazzitello WF. The simultaneous occurrence of rheumatoid arthritis and agammaglobulinemia. J Lab Clin Med 49:343–357, 1957.

Good RA, Zak SJ. Disturbances in gamma globulin synthesis as "experiments of nature." Pediatrics 18:109–149, 1956.

Gotoff SP, Smith RD, Sugar O. Dermatomyositis with cerebral vasculitis in a patient with agammaglobulinemia. Am J Dis Child 123:53–56, 1972.

Graf D, Korthäuer U, Mages HW, Senger G, Kroczek R. Cloning of TRAP, a ligand for CD40 on human T cells. Eur J Immunol 22:3191–3194, 1992.

Granoff DM, Squires JE, Munson RS Jr, Suarez B. Siblings of patients with haemophilus meningitis have impaired anticapsular antibody responses to Haemophilus vaccine. J Pediatr 103:185–191, 1983.

Granoff DM, Shackelford PG, Suarez BK, Nahm MH, Cates KL, Murphy TV, Karasic R, Osterholm MT, Paudey JP, Daum MD, the Collaborative Group. Hemophilus influenzae type b disease in children vaccinated with type B polysaccharide vaccine. N Engl J Med 315:1584–1590, 1986a.

Granoff DM, Shackelford PG, Pandey JP, Boies EG. Antibody responses to Haemophilus influenzae type b polysaccharide vaccine in relation to Km(1) and G2m(23) immunoglobulin allotypes. J Infect Dis 154:257–264, 1986b.

Gray GF, Gutowski WT. Thymoma: a clinicopathologic study of 54 cases. Am J Surg Pathol 3:235–249, 1979.

Grey HM, Kunkel HG. H chain subgroups of myeloma proteins and normal 7S gamma-globulin. J Exp Med 120:253–266, 1964.

Grimbacher B, Hutloff A, Schlesier M, Glocker E, Warnatz K, Drager R, Eibel H, Fischer B, Schaffer AA, Mages HW, Kroczek RA, Peter HH. Homozygous loss of ICOS is associated with adult-onset common variable immunodeficiency. Nat Immunol 4:261–268, 2003.

Grubben MJ, van den Braak CC, Peters WH, van der Meer JW, Nagengast FM. Low levels of colonic glutathione S-transferase in patients with X-linked agammaglobulinaemia. Eur J Clin Invest 30:642–645, 2000.

Gruber HE. Bone and the immune system. Proc Soc Exp Biol Med 197:219–225, 1991.

Grunebaum E, Agammaglobulinemia caused by defects other than Btk. In Roifman CM, ed. Immunol Allergy Clin N Am 21:45–63, 2001.

Gu H, Zou YR, Rajewsky K. Independent control of immunoglobulin switch recombination at individual switch regions evidenced through Cre-loxP-mediated gene targeting. Cell 73:1155–1164, 1993.

Guerra IC, Fawcett WA IV, Redmon AH, Lawrence EC, Rosenbaltt HM, Shearer WT. Permanent intrinsic B cell immunodeficiency caused by phenytoin hypersensitivity. J Allergy Clin Immunol 77:603–608, 1986.

Guill MF, Brown DA, Ochs HD, Pyun KH, Moffitt JE. IgM deficiency: clinical spectrum and immunologic assessment. Ann Allergy 62:547–552, 1989.

Guinamard R, Fougereau M, Seckinger P. The SH3 domain of Bruton's tyrosine kinase interacts with Vav, Sam68 and EWS. Scand J Immunol 45:587–595, 1997.

Guioli S, Arveiler B, Bardoni B, Notarangelo LD, Panina P, Duse M, Ugazio A, Oberle I, de Saint Basile G, Mandel JL, et al. Close linkage of probe p212 (DXS178) to X-linked agammaglobulinemia. Hum Genet 84:19–21, 1989.

Guo B, Kato RM, Garcia-Lloret M, Wahl MI, Rawlings DJ. Engagement of the human pre-B cell receptor generates a lipid raft-dependent calcium signaling complex. Immunity 13:243–253, 2000.

Gupta S, Saverymuttu SH, Gibbs JSR, Evans DJ, Hodgson HJF. Watery diarrhea in a patient with myasthenia gravis, thymoma, and immunodeficiency. Am J Gastroenterol 80:877–881, 1985.

Hadfield MG, Seidlin M, Houff SA, Adair CF, Markowitz SM, Straus SE. Echovirus meningomyeloencephalitis with administration of intrathecal immunoglobulin. J Neuropathol Exp Neurol 44:520–529, 1985.

Hadzic N, Pagliuca A, Rela M, Portmann B, Jones A, Veys P, Heaton ND, Mufti GJ, Mieli-Vergani G. Correction of hyper-IgM syndrome after liver and bone marrow transplantation. N Engl J Med 342:320–324, 2000.

Hagemann TL, Chen Y, Rosen FS, Kwan SP. Genomic organization of the Btk gene and exon scanning for mutations in patients with X-linked agammaglobulinemia. Hum Molecul Gen 3:1743–1749, 1994.

Hakami N, Neiman PE, Canellos GP, Lazerson J. Neonatal megaloblastic anemia due to inherited transcobalamin II deficiency in two siblings. N Engl J Med 285:1163–1170, 1971.

Hall CA. Congenital disorders of vitamin B_{12} transport and their contribution to concept. II. Yale Biol Med 54:485–495, 1981.

Hammarström L, Smith CIE. IgG subclasses in bacterial infections. Monogr Allergy 19:122–133, 1986.

Hammarström L, Smith CI, Berg CI. Captopril-induced IgA deficiency. Lancet 337:436, 1991.

Hammarström L, Vorechovsky I, Webster D. Selective IgA deficiency (SIgAD) and common variable immunodeficiency (CVID). Clin Exp Immunol 120:225–231, 2000.

Hammon WM, Coriell LL, Stokes JJ. Evaluation of Red Cross gamma-globulin as a prophylactic agent for poliomyelitis. I. Plan of controlled field tests and results of 1951 pilot study in Utah. JAMA 150:739–749, 1952.

Han S, Schindel C, Genitsariotis R, Marker-Hermann E, Bhakdi S, Maeurer MJ. Identification of a unique Helicobacter species by 16S rRNA gene analysis in an abdominal abscess from a patient with X-linked hypogammaglobulinemia. J Clin Microbiol 38:2740–2742, 2000.

Hancock MP, Huntley CC, Sever JL. Congenital rubella syndrome with immunoglobulin disorder. J Pediatr 72:636–645, 1968.

Hanley-Lopez J, Estabrooks LL, Stiehm ER. Antibody deficiency in Wolf-Hirschhorn syndrome. J Pediatr 133:141–143, 1998.

Hansel TT, Haeney MR, Thompson RA. Primary hypogammaglobulinaemia and arthritis. Br Med J (Clin Res Ed) 295:174–175, 1987.

Hansen S, Gustafson R, Smith CI, Gardulf A. Express subcutaneous IgG infusions: decreased time of delivery with maintained safety. Clin Immunol 104:237–241, 2002.

Haraldsson A, van der Burgt CJ, Weemaes CM, Otten B, Bakkeren JA, Stoelinga GB. Antibody deficiency and isolated growth hormone deficiency in a girl with Mulibrey nanism. Eur J Pediatr 152:509–512, 1993.

Harhaj EW, Sun SC. IKKgamma serves as a docking subunit of the IkappaB kinase (IKK) and mediates interaction of IKK with the human T-cell leukemia virus Tax protein. J Biol Chem 274:22911–22914, 1999.

Haruda F. Phenytoin hypersensitivity: 38 cases. Neurology 29:1480–1485, 1979.

Hashimoto A, Takeda K, Inaba M, Sekimata M, Kaisho T, Ikehara S, Homma Y, Akira S, Kurosaki T. Cutting edge: essential role of phospholipase C-gamma 2 in B cell development and function. J Immunol 165:1738–1742, 2000.

Hashimoto S, Miyawaki T, Futatani T, Kanegane H, Usui K, Nukiwa T, Namiuchi S, Matsushita M, Yamadori T, Suemura M, Kishimoto T, Tsukada S. Atypical X-linked agammaglobulinemia diagnosed in three adults. Intern Med 38:722–725, 1999.

Hay FC, Hull MGR, Torriigiani G. The transfer of human IgG subclasses from mother to fetus. Clin Exp Immunol 9:355, 1971.

Hayakawa H, Iwata T, Yata J, Kobayashi N. Primary immunodeficiency syndrome in Japan. I. Overview of a nationwide survey on primary immunodeficiency syndrome. J Clin Immunol 1:3139, 1981.

Hayakawa H, Kobayashi N, Yata J. Primary immunodeficiency diseases and malignancy in Japan. Jpn J Cancer Res 77:74–79, 1986.

Hayward AR, Paolucci P, Webster ADB, Kohler P. Pre-B cell suppression by thymoma patient lymphocytes. Clin Exp Immunol 48:437–442, 1982.

Hayward AR, Levy J, Facchetti F, Notarangelo L, Ochs HD, Etzioni A, Bonnefoy J-Y, Cosyns M, Weinberg A. Cholangiopathy and tumors of the pancreas, liver, and biliary tree in boys with X-linked immunodeficiency with hyper-IgM. J Immunol 158:977–983, 1997.

Healy JI, Dolmetsch RE, Timmerman LA, Cyster JG, Thomas ML, Crabtree GR, Lewis RS, Goodnow CC. Different nuclear signals are activated by the B cell receptor during positive versus negative signaling. Immunity 6:419–428, 1997.

Hein K, Lorenz MG, Siebenkotten G, Petry K, Christine R, Radbruch A. Processing of switch transcripts is required for targeting of antibody class switch recombination. J Exp Med 188:2369–2374, 1998.

Heiner DC, Myers AS, Beck CS. Deficiency of IgG4: disorder associated with frequent infections and bronchiectasis that may be familiar. Clin Rev Allergy 1:259–266, 1983.

Hermaszewski RA, Webster AD. Primary hypogammaglobulinaemia: a survey of clinical manifestations and complications. Quart J Med 86:31–42, 1993.

Herrod HG. Follow-up of pediatric patients with recurrent infection and mild serologic immune abnormalities. Ann Allergy Asthma Immunol 79:460–464, 1997.

Herrod HG. Management of the patient with IgG subclass deficiency and/or selective antibody deficiency. Ann Allergy 70:3–7, 1993.

Herrod HG, Gross S, Insel R. Selective antibody deficiency to Haemophilus influenzae type b capsular polysaccharide vaccination in children with recurrent respiratory tract infection. J Clin Immunol 9:429–434, 1989.

Higuchi S, Awata H, Nunoi H, Tsuchiya H, Naore H, Igarashi H, Matsuda I. A family of selective immunodeficiency with normal immunoglobulins: possible autosomal dominant inheritance. Eur J Pediatr 153:328–332, 1994.

Hill SL, Mitchell JL, Burnett D, Stockley RA. IgG subclass in the serum and sputum from patients with bronchiectasis. Thorax 53:463–468, 1998.

Hitzig WH, Dohmann U, Pluss HJ, Vischer D. Hereditary transcobalamin II deficiency: clinical findings in a new family. J Pediatr 85:922–629, 1974.

Hitzig WH, Kenny AB. The role of vitamin B_{12} and its transport globulins in the production of antibodies. Clin Exp Immunol 20:105–111, 1975.

Hjalmarson O, Hanson LA, Nilssen LA. IgA deficiency during D-penicillamine treatment. Br Med J 1:549, 1977.

Hobbs JR, Davis JA. Serum gamma-G-globulin levels and gestational age in premature babies. Lancet 1:757–759, 1967.

Hobbs JR, Hepner GW. Deficiency of γM-globulin in coeliac disease. Lancet 1:217–219, 1968.

Hobbs JR, Milner RDG, Watt PJ. Gamma-M deficiency predisposing to meningococcal septicaemia. Br Med J 4:583–586, 1967.

Hollenbaugh D, Ochs HD, Noelle RJ, Ledbetter JA, Aruffo A. The role of CD40 and its ligand in the regulation of the immune response. Immunol Rev 138:23–37, 1994a.

Hollenbaugh D, Wu LH, Ochs HD, Nonoyama S, Grosmaire LS, Ledbetter JA, Noelle RJ, Hill H, Aruffo A. The random inactivation of the X chromosome carrying the defective gene responsible for X-linked hyper IgM syndrome (X-HIM) in female carriers of HIGM1. J Clin Invest 94:616–622, 1994b.

Hong R. The biologic significance of IgE in chronic respiratory infections. In Dayton DH Jr, Small PA Jr, Chanock RM, et al, eds. The Secretory Immunologic System. Washington DC, US Government Printing Office, 1971, pp 433–445.

Hu HM, O'Rourke K, Boguski MS, Dixit VM. A novel RING finger protein interacts with the cytoplasmic domain of CD40. J Biol Chem 269:30069–30072, 1994.

Huo YK, Wang Z, Hong JH, Chessa L, McBride WH, Perlman SL, Gatti RA. Radiosensitivity of ataxia-telangiectasia, X-linked agammaglobulinemia, and related syndromes using a modified colony survival assay. Cancer Res 54:2544–2547, 1994.

Huston DP, Kavanaugh AF, Andrew SL, Huston MM. Importance of IgG3 and IgG3 deficiency. Royal Society of Medicine Services International Congress and Symposium Series 143:43–51, 1989.

Hyvönen, M, Saraste M. Structure of the PH domain and Btk motif from Bruton's tyrosine kinase: molecular explanations for X-linked agammaglobulinaemia. EMBO J 16:3396–404, 1997.

Ide S, Koga T, Rikimaru T, Katsuki Y, Oisumi K. Good's syndrome presenting with cytomegalovirus pneumonia. Intern Med 39:1094–1096, 2000.

Iglesias J, Matamoros N, Raga S, Ferrer JM, Mila J. CD95 expression and function on lymphocyte subpopulations in common variable immunodeficiency (CVID); related to increased apoptosis. Clin Exp Immunol 117:138–146, 1999.

Imai K, Catalan N, Plebani A, Marodi L, Sanal O, Kumaki S, Nagendran V, Wood P, Glastre C, Sarrot-Reynauld F, Hermine O, Forveille M, Revy P, Fischer A, Durandy A. Hyper-IgM syndrome type 4 with a B lymphocyte-intrinsic selective deficiency in Ig class-switch recombination. J Clin Invest 112:136–142, 2003a.

Imai K, Slupphaug G, Lee WI, Revy P, Nonoyama S, Catalan N, Yel L, Forveille M, Kavli B, Krokan HE, Ochs HD, Fischer A, Durandy A. Human uracil-DNA glycosylase deficiency associated with profoundly impaired immunoglobulin class-switch recombination. Nat Immuno 4:1023–1028, 2003b.

Inoue R, Kondo N, Kobayashi Y, Fukutomi O, Orii T. IgG2 deficiency associated with defects in production of interferon-gamma; comparison with common variable immunodeficiency. Scand J Immunol 41:130–134, 1995.

Inoue T, Okumura Y, Shirama M, Ishibashi H, Kashiwagi S, Okubo H. Selective partial IgM deficiency: functional assessment of T and B lymphocytes in vitro. J Clin Immunol 6:130–135, 1986.

Insel RA, Anderson PW. Response to oligosaccharide-protein conjugate vaccine against Hemophilus influenzae b in two patients with IgG2 deficiency unresponsive to capsular polysaccharide vaccine. N Engl J Med 315:499–503, 1986.

Ipp MM, Gelfand EW. Antibody deficiency and alopecia. J Pediatr 89:728–731, 1976.

Iseki M, Heiner DC. Immunodeficiency disorders. Pediatr Rev 14:226–236, 1993.

Ishida TK, Mizushima SI, Azuma S, Kobayashi N, Tojo T, Suzuki K, Aizawa S, Watanabe T, Mosialos G, Kieff E, Yamamoto T, Inoue J. Identification of TRAF6, a novel tumor necrosis factor receptor-associated factor protein that mediates signaling from an amino-terminal domain of the CD40 cytoplasmic region. J Biol Chem 271:28745–28748, 1996a.

Ishida TK, Tojo T, Aoki T, Kobayashi N, Ohishi T, Watanabe T, Yamamoto T, Inoue J. TRAF5, a novel tumor necrosis factor receptor-associated factor family protein, mediates CD40 signaling. Proc Natl Acad Sci USA 93:9437–9442, 1996b.

Iskander R, Das PK, Aalberse RC. IgG4 antibodies in Egyptian patients with schistosemiasis. Int Arch Allergy Appl Immunol 66:200–207, 1981.

Israel A. The IKK complex: an integrator of all signals that activate NF-kappa B? Trends Cell Biol 10:129–133, 2000.

Israel-Asselain R, Burtin P, Chebat J. Un trouble biologique nuoveau: l'agammaglobulinémie avec beta2-macroglobulinémie (un cas). Bull Soc Med Hop Paris 76:519–523, 1960.

Jacquot S, Macon-Lemaitre L, Paris E, Kobata T, Tanaka Y, Morimoto C, Schlossman SF, Tron F. B cell co-receptors regulating T cell-dependent antibody production in common variable immunodeficiency: CD27 pathway defects identify subsets of severely immuno-compromised patients. Int Immunol 13:871–876, 2001.

Jaffe JS, Strober W, Sneller MC. Functional abnormalities of $CD8^+$ T cells define a unique subset of patients with common variable immunodeficiency. Blood 82:192–201, 1993.

Jain A, Atkinson TP, Lipsky PE, Slater JE, Nelson DL, Strober W. Defects of T-cell effector function and post-thymic maturation in X-linked hyper-IgM syndrome. J Clin Invest 103:1151–1158, 1999.

Janeway C A, Apt L, Gitlin D. Agammaglobulinemia. Trans Assoc Am Phys 66:200–202, 1953.

Janeway CA, Gitlin D, Craig JM, Grice DS. Collagen disease in patients with congenital agammaglobulinemia. Trans Assoc Am Phys 69:93–97, 1956.

Jeandel C, Gastin I, Blain H, Jouanny P, Laurain MC, Penin F, Saunier M, Nicolas JP, Guðant JL. Thymoma with immunodeficiency (Good's syndrome) associated with selective cobalamin malabsorption and benign IgM-6 gammopathy. J Intern Med 235:179–182, 1994.

Jefferis R, Kumararatne DS. Selective IgG subclass deficiency: quantification and clinical relevance. Clin Exp Immunol 81:357–367, 1990.

Jiang Y, Ma W, Wan Y, Kozasa T, Hattori S, Huang XY. The G protein G alpha12 stimulates Bruton's tyrosine kinase and a rasGAP through a conserved PH/BM domain. Nature 395:808–813, 1998.

Johnson PRJ, Edwards KM, Wright PF. Failure of intraventricular gamma globulin to eradicate echovirus encephalitis in a patient with X-linked agammaglobulinemia [letter]. N Engl J Med 313:1546–1547, 1985.

Johnson ML, Keeton LG, Zhu ZB, Volanakis JE, Cooper MD, Schroeder HW Jr. Age-related changes in serum immunoglobulins in patients with familial IgA deficiency and common variable immunodeficiency (CVID). Clin Exp Immunol 108:477–483, 1997.

Jolles S, Tyrer M, Johnson M, Webster D. Long term recovery of IgG and IgM production during HIV infection in a patient with common variable immunodeficiency (CVID). J Clin Pathol 54:713–715, 2001.

Jou ST, Carpino N, Takahashi Y, Piekorz R, Chao JR, Wang D, Ihle JN. Essential, nonredundant role for the phosphoinositide 3-kinase p110delta in signaling by the B-cell receptor complex. Mol Cell Biol 22:8580–8591, 2002.

Journet O, Durandy A, Doussau M, Le Deist F, Couvreur J, Griscelli C, Fischer A, de Saint-Basile G. Carrier detection and prenatal diagnosis of X-linked agammaglobulinemia. Am J Med Genet 43:885–887, 1992.

Juhlin I, Michaelson JG: A new syndrome characterized by absence of eosinophils and basophils. Lancet 1:1233–1235, 1977.

Jumaa H, Wollscheid B, Mitterer M, Wienands J, Reth M, Nielsen PJ. Abnormal development and function of B lymphocytes in mice deficient for the signaling adaptor protein SLP-65. Immunity 11:547–554, 1999.

Jung S, Rajewsky K, Radbruch A. Shut down of class switch recombination by deletion of a switch region control element. Science 259:984–987, 1993.

Junker AK, Dimmick JE. Progressive generalized edema in an 8-year-old boy with agammaglobulinemia. J Pediatr 101:147–153, 1982.

Junker AK, Ochs HD, Clark EA, Puterman ML, Wedgwood RJ. Transient immune deficiency in patients with acute Epstein-Barr virus infection. Clin Immunol Immunopath 40:436–446, 1968.

Kaikov Y, Wadsworth LD, Hall CA, Rogers PCJ. Transcobalamin II deficiency: case report and review of the literature. Eur J Pediatr 150:841–843, 1991.

Kainulainen L, Varpula M, Liippo K, Svedstrom E, Nikoskelainen J, Ruuskanen O. Pulmonary abnormalities in patients with primary hypogammaglobulinemia. J Allergy Clin Immunol 104:1031–1036, 1999.

Kalfa VC, Roberts RL, Stiehm ER. The syndrome of chronic mucocutaneous candidiasis with selective antibody deficiency. Ann Allergy Asthma Immunol 90:254–264, 2003.

Kamanaka MP, Yu T, Yasui K, Yoshida T, Kawabe T, Horii T, Kishimoto T, Kikutani H. Protective role of CD40 in *Leishmania major* infection at two distinct phases of cell-mediated immunity. Immunity 4:275–281, 1996.

Kanegane H, Futatani T, Wang Y, Nomura K, Shinozaki K, Matsukura H, Kubota T, Tsukada S, Miyawaki T. Clinical and mutational characteristics of X-linked agammaglobulinemia and its carrier identified by flow cytometric assessment combined with genetic analysis. J Allergy Clin Immunol 108:1012–1020, 2001.

Kanegane H, Tsukada S, Iwata T, Futatani T, Nomura K, Yamamoto J, Yoshida T, Agematsu K, Komiyama A, Miyawaki T. Detection of Bruton's tyrosine kinase mutations in hypogammaglobulinaemic males registered as common variable immunodeficiency (CVID) in the Japanese Immunodeficiency Registry. Clin Exp Immunol 120:512–517, 2000.

Karasuyama H, Rolink A, Melchers F. Surrogate light chain in B cell development. Adv Immunol 63:1–41, 1996.

Karpusas M, Hsu YM, Wang JH, Thompson J, Lederman S, Chess L, Thomas D. A crystal structure of an extracellular fragment of human CD40 ligand. Structure 3:1031–1039, 1995.

Karsh J, Watts CS, Osterland CK. Selective immunoglobulin M deficiency in an adult: assessment of immunoglobulin production by peripheral blood lymphocytes *in vitro*. Clin Immunol Immunopath 25:386–394, 1982.

Kato T, Tsuge I, Inaba J, Kato K, Matsuyama T, Kojima S. Successful bone marrow transplantation in a child with X-linked hyper-IgM syndrome. Bone Marrow Transplant 23:1081–1083, 1999.

Katz Y, Harbeck RJ, DeMichelle D, Mitchell B, Strunk RC. Steroid-treated asthmatic patients with low levels of IgG have a normal capacity to produce specific antibodies. Pediatr Asthma Allergy Immunol 2:309–316, 1988.

Kauffman CA, Linnemann CC Jr, Alvira MM. Cytomegalovirus encephalitis associated with thymoma and immunoglobulin deficiency. Am J Med 67:724–727, 1979.

Kavanaugh AF, Huston DP. Immunoglobulin G subclass deficiency. Insights in Allergy 4:1–7, 1989.

Kavanaugh AF, Huston DP. Variable expression of IgG2 deficiency. J Allergy Clin Immunol 86:4–10, 1990.

Kawabe T, Naka T, Yoshida K, Tanaka T, Fujiwara H, Suematsu S, Yoshida N, Kishimoto T, Kikutani H. The immune responses in CD40-deficient mice: impaired immunoglobulin class switching and germinal center formation. Immunity 1:167–178, 1994.

Kawai S, Sasahara Y, Minegishi M, Tsuchiya S, Fujie H, Ohashi Y, Kumaki S, Konno T. Immunological reconstitution by allogeneic bone marrow transplantation in a child with the X-linked hyper-IgM syndrome. Eur J Pediatr 158:394–397, 1999.

Kawakami Y, Yao L, Miura T, Tsukada S, Witte ON, Kawakami T. Tyrosine phosphorylation and activation of Bruton tyrosine kinase upon Fc epsilon RI cross-linking. Mol Cell Biol 14:5108–5113, 1994.

Kawamura N, Okamura A, Furuta H, Katow S, Yamada M, Kobayashi I, Okano M, Kobayashi K, Sakiyama Y. Improved dysgammaglobulinaemia in congenital rubella syndrome after immunoglobulin therapy: correlation with CD154 expression. Eur J Pediatr 159:764–766, 2000.

Kerner JD, Appleby MW, Mohr RN, Chien S, Rawlings DJ, Maliszewski CR, Witte ON, Perlmutter RM. Impaired expansion of mouse B cell progenitors lacking Btk. Immunity 3:301–312, 1995.

Khan WN, Alt FW, Gerstein RM, Malynn BA, Larsson I, Rathbun G, Davidson L, Muller S, Kantor AB, Herzenberg LA, et al. Defective B cell development and function in Btk-deficient mice. Immunity 3:283–299, 1995.

Khan WN, Nilsson A, Mizoguchi E, Castigli E, Forsell J, Bhan AK, Geha R, Sideras P, Alt FW. Impaired B cell maturation in mice lacking Bruton's tyrosine kinase (Btk) and CD40. International Immunology 9:395–405, 1997.

Kiely PDW, Helbert MR, Miles J, Oliveira DBG. Immunosuppressant effect of gold on IgG subclasses and IgE; evidence for sparing of Th2 responses. Clin Exp Immunol 120:369–374, 2000.

Kikuchi Y, Yasue T, Miyake K, Kimoto M, Takatsu K. CD38 ligation induces tyrosine phosphorylation of Bruton tyrosine kinase and enhanced expression of interleukin 5-receptor alpha chain: synergistic effects with interleukin 5. Proc Nat Acad Sci USA 92:11814–11818, 1995.

Kim DC, Cresswell A, Mitra A. Compartment syndrome in a patient with X-linked agammaglobulinaemia and ecthyma gangrenosum. Case report. Scand J Plast Reconstr Surg Hand Surg 34:87–89, 2000.

Kimura W, Tanigawa M, Nakahashi Y, Inoue M, Yamamura Y, Kato H, Sugino S, Kondo M. Selective IgM deficiency in a patient with Hashimoto's disease Intern Med 32:302–307, 1993.

Kinlen LJ, Webster AD, Bird AG, Haile R, Peto J, Soothill JF, Thompson RA. Prospective study of cancer in patients with hypogammaglobulinaemia. Lancet 1:263–266, 1985.

Kinnon C, Hinshelwood S, Levinsky RJ, Lovering RC. X-linked agammaglobulinaemia–gene cloning and future prospects. Immunol Today 14:554–558, 1993.

Kiratli HK, Akar Y. Multiple recurrent hordeola associated with selective IgM deficiency. J AAPOS 5:60–61, 2001.

Kirkpatrick CH, Windhorst DB. Mucocutaneous candidiasis and thymoma. Am J Med 66:939–945, 1979.

Kitamura D, Kudo A, Schaal S, Muller W, Melchers F, Rajewsky K. A critical role of lambda 5 protein in B cell development. Cell 69:823–831, 1992.

Kitamura D, Roes J, Kuhn R, Rajewsky K. A B cell-deficient mouse by targeted disruption of the membrane exon of the immunoglobulin mu chain gene. Nature 350:423–426, 1991.

Klausvermeyer WB, Gianos ME, Kurohara Ml, Dao HT, Heiner DC. IgG subclass deficiency associated with corticosteroids in obstructive lung disease. Chest 102:1137–1142, 1992.

Klein U, Rajewsky K, Küppers R. Human Immunoglobulin (Ig)M+IgD+ Peripheral blood B cells expressing the CD27 cell surface antigen carry somatically mutated variable region genes: CD27 as a general marker for somatically mutated (memory) B cells. J Exp Med 188:1679–1689, 1998.

Knutsen AP, Merten DF, Buckley RH. Colonic nodular lymphoid hyperplasia in a child with antibody deficiency and near-normal immunoglobulins. J Pediatr 98:420–423, 1981.

Kondratenko I, Amlot PL, Webster AD, Farrant J. Lack of specific antibody response in common variable immunodeficiency (CVID) associated with failure in production of antigen-specific memory T cells. MRC Immunodeficiency Group. Clin Exp Immunol 108:9–13, 1997.

Kornfeld SJ, Kratz J, Haire RN, Litman GW, Good RA. X-linked agammaglobulinemia presenting as transient hypogammaglobulinemia of infancy. J Allergy Clin Immunol 95:915–917, 1995.

Kornfeld SJ, Haire RN, Strong SJ, Brigino EN, Tang H, Sung SS, Fu SM, Litman GW. Extreme variation in X-linked agammaglobulinemia phenotype in a three-generation family. J Allergy Clin Immunol 100:702–706, 1997.

Korsmeyer SJ, Hieter PA, Ravetch J, Poplack DG, Waldmann TA, Leder P. Developmental hierarchy of immunoglobulin gene rearrangements in human leukemic pre B-cells Proc Natl Acad Sci USA 78:7096–7100, 1981.

Korthäuer U, Graf D, Mages HW, Brière F, Padayachee M, Malcolm S, Ugazio AG, Notarangelo LD, Levinsky RJ, Kroczek RA. Defective expression of T-cell CD40 ligand causes X-linked immunodeficiency with hyper IgM. Nature 361:539–543, 1993.

Kouro T, Nagata K, Takaki S, Nisitani S, Hirano M, Wahl MI, Witte ON, Karasuyama H, Takatsu K. Bruton's tyrosine kinase is required for signaling the CD79b-mediated pro-B to pre-B cell transition. Int Immunol 13:485–493, 2001.

Kowalczyk D, Mytar B, Zembala M. Cytokine production in transient hypogammaglobulinemia and isolated IgA deficiency. J Allergy Clin Immunol 100:556–562, 1997.

Krance SM, Amento EP, Goldring SR. Lymphocytes, monocytes and metabolic bone disease. In Cohn DV, Fujita T, Potts JT Jr, Talmage RV, eds. Endocrine Control of Bone and Calcium Metabolism. Amsterdam: Elsevier Science Publishers BV, 1984, pp 3–14.

Krantman HJ, Stiehm ER, Stevens RH, Saxon A, Seeger RC. Abnormal B cell differentiation and variable increased T cell suppression in immunodeficiency with hyper-IgM. Clin Exp Immunol 40:147–156, 1980.

Kruger G, Welte K, Ciobanu N, Cunningham-Rundles C, Ralph P, Venuta S, Feldman S, Koziner B, Wang CY, Moore MA, et al. Interleukin-2 correction of defective in vitro T-cell mitogenesis in patients with common varied immunodeficiency. J Clin Immunol 4:295–303, 1984.

Kutukculer N, Aksoylar S, Kansoy S, Cetingul N, Notarangelo ND. Outcome of hematopoietic stem cell transplantation in hyper-IgM syndrome caused by CD40 deficiency. J Pediatr 143:141–142, 2003.

Kwan SP, Kunkel L, Bruns G, Wedgwood RJ, Latt S, Rosen FS. Mapping of the X-linked agammaglobulinemia locus by use of restriction fragment-length polymorphism. J Clin Invest 77:649–652, 1986.

Kwan SP, Terwilliger J, Parmley R, Raghu G, Sandkuyl LA, Ott J, Ochs H, Wedgwood R, Rosen F. Identification of a closely linked DNA marker, DXS178, to further refine the X-linked agammaglobulinemia locus. Genomics 6:238–242, 1990.

Kwan SP, Walker AP, Hagemann T, Gupta S, Vayuvegula B, Ochs HD. A new RFLP marker, SP282, at the btk locus for genetic analysis in X-linked agammaglobulinaemia families. Prenat Diag 14:493–496, 1994.

Kyong CU, Virella G, Fudenberg HH, Darby CP. X-linked immunodeficiency with increased IgM: clinical, ethnic, and immunologic heterogeneity. Pediatr Res 12:1024–1026, 1978.

Lack G, Ochs HD, Gelfand EW. Humoral immunity in steroid-dependent children with asthma and hypogammaglobulinemia. J Pediatr 129:898–903, 1996.

Laffargue M, Ragab-Thomas JM, Ragab A, Tuech J, Missy K, Monnereau L, Blank U, Plantavid M, Payrastre B, Raynal P, Chap H. Phosphoinositide 3-kinase and integrin signalling are involved in activation of Bruton tyrosine kinase in thrombin-stimulated platelets. Febs Letters 443:66–70, 1999.

Lambie AT, Burrows BA, Sommers SC. Clinicopathologic conference: refractory anemia, agammaglobulinemia and mediastinal tumor. Am J Clin Pathol 27:444–452, 1957.

Lane P, Traunecker A, Hubele S, Inui S, Lanzavecchia A, Gray D. Activated human T cells express a ligand for the human B cell-associated antigen CD40 which participates in T cell-dependent activation of B lymphocytes. Eur J Immunol 22:2573–2578, 1992.

Lauriola L, Maggiano N, Marino M, Carbone A, Piantelli M, Musiani P. Human thymoma: immunologic characteristics of the lymphocytic component. Cancer 48:1992–1995, 1981.

Lavilla P, Gil A, Rodriguez MC, Dupla ML, Pintado V, Fontan G. X-linked agammaglobulinemia and gastric adenocarcinoma. Cancer 72:1528–1531, 1993.

Lawlor GR Jr, Ammann AJ, Wright WC, LaFranchi SH, Bilstrom D, Stiehm ER. The syndrome of cellular immunodeficiency with immunoglobulins J Pediatr 84:183–192, 1974.

Lawton AR. IgG subclass deficiency and the day-care generation. Pediatr Infect Dis J 18:462–466, 1999.

Lebecque S, de Bouteiller O, Arpin C, Banchereau J, Liu YJ. Germinal center founder cells display propensity for apoptosis before onset of somatic mutation. J Exp Med 185:563–571, 1997.

Lederman HM. Cancer in children with primary or secondary immunodeficiencies. J Pediatr 127:335, 1995.

Lederman HM, Metz SJ, Zuckerberg AL, Loughlin GM. Antibody deficiency complicating severe bronchopulmonary dysplasia. Pediatr Pulmonol 7:52–54, 1989.

Lederman HM, Winkelstein JA. X-linked agammaglobulinemia: an analysis of 96 patients. Medicine 64:145–156, 1985.

Lefranc G, Chaabani H, Loghem EV, et al. Simultaneous absence of the human IgG1, IgG2, IgG4, and IgA1 subclasses: immunological and immunogenetical considerations. Eur J Immunol 13:240–244, 1983.

Leickley FE, Buckley RH. Variability in B cell maturation and differentiation in X-linked agammaglobulinemia. Clin Exp Immunol 65:90–99, 1986a.

Leickley FE, Buckley RH. Development of IgA and IgG2 subclass deficiency after sulfasalazine therapy. J Pediatr 108:481–482, 1986b.

Lemmon MA, Ferguson KM, Schlessinger J. PH domains: diverse sequences with a common fold recruit signaling molecules to the cell surface. Cell 85:621–624, 1996.

Leparc I, Aymard M, Fuchs F. Acute, chronic and persistent enterovirus and poliovirus infections: detection of viral genome by seminested PCR amplification in culture-negative samples. Mol Cell Probes 8:487–495, 1994.

Levinsky RJ, ed. IgG subclass deficiencies. In Royal Society of Medicine Series London International Congress and Symposium Series 143:1–70, 1989.

Levitt D, Haber P, Rich K, Cooper MD. Hyper-IgM immunodeficiency: a primary dysfunction of B lymphocyte isotype switching. J Clin Invest 72:1650–1657, 1983.

Levitt D, Ochs H, Wedgwood RJ. Epstein-Barr virus-induced lymphoblastoid cell lines derived from the peripheral blood of patients with X-linked agammaglobulinemia can secrete IgM. J Clin Immunol 4:143–150, 1984.

Levy DA, Chen J. Healthy IgE-deficient person. N Engl J Med 283:541–542, 1970.

Levy J, Espanol-Boren T, Thomas C, Fischer A, Tovo P, Bordigoni P, Resnick I, Fasth A, Baer M, Gomez L, Sanders EA, Tabone MD, Plantaz D, Etzioni A, Monafo V, Abinun M, Hammarstrom L, Abrahamsen T, Jones A, Finn A, Klemola T, DeVries E, Sanal O, Peitsch MC, Notarangelo LD. Clinical spectrum of X-linked hyper-IgM syndrome. J Pediatr 131:47–54, 1997.

Levy Y, Gupta N, Le Deist F, Garcia C, Fischer A, Weill JC, Reynaud CA. Defect in IgV gene somatic hypermutation in common variable immuno-deficiency syndrome. Proc Natl Acad Sci USA 95:13135–13140, 1998.

Liese JG, Wintergerst U, Tympner KD, Belohradsky BH. High-vs low-dose immunoglobulin therapy in the long-term treatment of X-linked agammaglobulinemia. Am J Dis Child 146:335–339, 1992.

Litwin SD. Immunodeficiency with thymoma: failure to induce Ig production in immunodeficient lymphocytes cocultured with normal T cells. J Immunol 122:728–732, 1979.

Loder F, Mutschler B, Ray RJ, Paige CJ, Sideras P, Torres R, Lamers MC, Carsetti R. B cell development in the spleen takes place in discrete steps and is determined by the quality of B cell receptor-derived signals. J Exp Med 190:75–89, 1999.

LoGalbo PR, Sampson HA, Buckley RH. Symptomatic giardiasis in three patients with X-linked agammaglobulinemia. J Pediatr 101:78–80, 1982.

Loh RKS, Thong YH, Ferrante A. Immunoglobulin G subclass deficiency in children with high levels of immunoglobulin E and infection proneness. Int Arch Allergy Appl Immunol 93:285–288, 1990.

Lopez Granados E, Porpiglia AS, Hogan MB, Matamoros N, Krasovec S, Pignata C, Smith CI, Hammarstrom L, Bjorkander J, Belohradsky BH, Casariego GF, Garcia Rodriguez MC, Conley ME. Clinical and molecular analysis of patients with defects in micro heavy chain gene. J Clin Invest 110:1029–1035, 2002.

Lorber A, Simon T, Leeb J, Peter A, Wilcox S. Chrysotherapy: suppression of immunoglobulin synthesis. Arthritis Rheum 21:785–791, 1978.

Lucas AH, Azmi FH, Mink CM, Granoff DM. Age-dependent V region expression in the human antibody response to the *Haemophilus influenzae* type b polysaccharide. J Immunol 150:2056–2061, 1993.

Luzi G, Pesce AM, Rinaldi S. Primary immunodeficiencies in Italy. Data revised from the Italian Register of Immunodeficiencies—IRID (1977–1988). Allergol Immunopathol (Madr) 19:53–57, 1991.

Ma YC, Huang XY. Identification of the binding site for Gqalpha on its effector Bruton's tyrosine kinase. Proc Nat Acad Sci USA 95:12197–12201, 1998.

Maguire GA, Kamararatne DS, Joyce HJ. Are there any clinical indications for measuring IgG subclasses? Ann Clin Biochem 39:374–377, 2002.

Majolini MB, D'Elios MM, Boncristiano M, Galieni P, Del Prete G, Telford JL, Baldari CT. Uncoupling of T-cell antigen receptor and downstream protein tyrosine kinases in common variable immunodeficiency. Clin Immunol Immunopathol 84:98–102, 1997.

Makitie O, Kaitila I, Savilabti E. Deficiency of humoral immunity in cartilage-hair hypoplasia J Pediatr 137:487–492, 2000.

Malcolm S, de Saint Basile G, Arveiler B, Lau YL, Szabo P, Fischer A, Griscelli C, Debre B, Mandel JL, Callard RE, et al. Close linkage of random DNA fragments from Xq 21.3-22 to X-linked agammaglobulinaemia (XLA). Hum Genet 77:172–174, 1987.

Malinin NL, Boldin MP, Kovalenko AV, Wallach D. MAP3K-related kinase involved in NF-kappa B induction by TNF, CD95 and IL-1. Nature 385:540–544, 1997.

Mandel K, Grunebaum E, Benson L. Noncompaction of the myocardium associated with Roifman syndrome. Heart, Cardiol Young 11:227–230, 2001.

Manis JP, van der Stoep N, Tian M, Ferrini R, Davidson L, Bottaro A, Alt FW. Class switching in B cells lacking 3′ immunoglobulin heavy chain. J Exp Med 188:1421–1431, 1998.

Mano H. Tec family of protein-tyrosine kinases: an overview of their structure and function. Cytokine Growth Factor Rev 10:267–280, 1999.

Mansouri A, Hallonet M, Gruss P. Pax genes and their roles in cell differentiation and development. Current Opin Cell Biol 8:851–857, 1996.

Marsman WA, Sukhai RN. Recurrent parotitis and isolated IgG3 subclass deficiency. Eur J Pediatr 158:684, 1999.

Martinez Garcia MA, de Rojas MD, Nauffal Manzur MD, Munoz Pamplona MP, Compte Torrero L, Macian V, Perpina Tordera M. Respiratory disorders in common variable immunodeficiency. Respir Med 95:191–195, 2001.

Matsuda T, Takahashi-Tezuka M, Fukada T, Okuyama Y, Fujitani Y, Tsukada S, Mano H, Hirai H, Witte ON, Hirano T. Association and activation of Btk and Tec tyrosine kinases by gp130, a signal transducer of the interleukin-6 family of cytokines. Blood 85:627–633, 1995.

Matsushita S, Inoue T, Okubo H. A case of selective IgM deficiency: isotype-specific suppressor T lymphocytes. Jpn J Med 23:149–151, 1984.

Mayer L, Kwan SP, Thompson C, Ko HS, Chiorazzi N, Waldmann T, Rosen F. Evidence for a defect in "switch" T cells in patients with immunodeficiency and hyperimmunoglobulinemia M. N Engl J Med 314:409–418, 1986.

Mayumi M, Yamaoka K, Tsutsui T, Mizue H, Doi A, Matsuyama M, Ito S, Shinomiya K, Mikkawa H. Selective immunoglobulin M deficiency associated with disseminated molluscum contagiosum. Eur J Pediatr 145:99–103, 1986.

McGeady SJ. Transient hypogammaglobulinemia of infancy: need to reconsider name and definition. J Pediatr 110:47–50, 1987.

McKinney REJ, Katz SL, Wilfert CM. Chronic enteroviral meningoencephalitis in agammaglobulinemic patients. Rev Inf Dis 9:334–356, 1987.

McKusick VA, Eldridge R, Hostetler JA. Dwarfism in Amish. II. Cartilage-hair-hypoplasia. Bull Johns Hopkins Hosp 116:285–326, 1964.

McLaughlin JF, Schaller J, Wedgwood RJ. Arthritis and immunodeficiency. J Pediatr 81:801–803, 1972.

Mease PJ, Ochs HD, Wedgwood RJ. Successful treatment of echovirus meningoencephalitis and myositis-fasciitis with intravenous immune globulin therapy in a patient with X-linked agammaglobulinemia. N Engl J Med 304:1278–1281, 1981.

Mease PJ, Ochs HD, Corey L, Dragavon J, Wedgwood RJ. Echovirus encephalitis/myositis in X-linked agammaglobulinemia N Engl J Med 313:758, 1985.

Mechanic LJ, Dikman S, Cunningham-Rundles C. Granulomatous disease in common variable immunodeficiency. Ann Intern Med 127:613–617, 1997.

Meffre E, LeDeist F, de Saint-Basile G, Deville A, Fougereau M, Fischer A, Schiff C. A human non-XLA immunodeficiency disease characterized by blockage of B cell development at an early pro B cell stage. J Clin Invest 98:1519–1526, 1996.

Melamed I, Bujanover Y, Igra YS, Schwartz D, Zakuth V, Spirer Z. Campylobacter enteritis in normal and immunodeficient children. Am J Dis Child 137:752–753, 1983.

Mena I, Perry CM, Harkins S, Rodriguez F, Gebhard J, Whitton JL. The role of B lymphocytes in coxsackievirus B3 infection. Am J Path 155:1205–1215, 1999.

Mensink EJ, Thompson A, Schot JD, van de Greef WM, Sandkuyl LA, Schuurman RK. Mapping of a gene for X-linked agammaglobulinemia and evidence for genetic heterogeneity. Hum Genet 73:327–332, 1986.

Merrill WW, Naegel GP, Olchowski JJ, Reynolds HY. Immunoglobulin G subclass proteins in serum and lavage fluid of normal subjects. Am Rev Respir Dis 131:584–587, 1985.

Migone N, Oliviero S, Lange GE, Delacroix DL, Boschis D, Altruda F, Silengo L, DeMarchi M, Carbonara AO. Multiple gene deletions within the human immunoglobulin heavy-chain cluster. Proc Natl Acad Sci USA 81:5811–5815, 1984.

Milili M, Antunes H, Blanco-Betancourt C, Nogueiras A, Santos E, Vasconcelos J, Castro e Melo J, Schiff C. A new case of autosomal recessive agammaglobulinaemia with impaired pre-B cell differentiation due to a large deletion of the IGH locus. Eur J Pediatr 161:479–484, 2002.

Milili M, Le Deist F, de Saint-Basile G, Fischer A, Fougereau M, Schiff C. Bone marrow cells in X-linked agammaglobulinemia express pre-B-specific genes (lambda-like and V pre-B) and present immunoglobulin V-D-J gene usage strongly biased to a fetal-like repertoire. J Clin Invest 91:1616–1629, 1993.

Minegishi Y, Coustan-Smith E, Rapalus L, Ersoy F, Campana D, Conley ME. Mutations in Ig alpha (CD79a) result in a complete block in B-cell development. J Clin Inv 104:1115–1121, 1999a.

Minegishi Y, Coustan-Smith E, Wang YH, Cooper MD, Campana D, Conley ME. Mutations in the human lambda5/14.1 gene result in B cell deficiency and agammaglobulinemia. J Exp Med 187:71–77, 1998.

Minegishi Y, Lavoie A, Cunningham-Rundles C, Bedard PM, Hebert J, Cote L, Dan K, Sedlak D, Buckley RH, Fischer A, Durandy A, Conley ME. Mutations in activation-induced cytidine deaminase in patients with hyper IgM syndrome. Clin Immunol 97:203–210, 2000.

Minegishi Y, Rohrer J, Conley ME. Recent progress in the diagnosis and treatment of patients with defects in early B-cell development. Curr Opin Pediatr 11:528–532, 1999b.

Minegishi Y, Rohrer J, Coustan-Smith E, Lederman HM, Pappu R, Campana D, Chan AC, Conley ME. An essential role for BLNK in human B cell development. Science 286:1954–1957, 1999c.

Miravitlles M, De Gracia J, Rodrigo M-J, Cruz MJ, Vendrell M, Vidal R, Morell F. Specific antibody response against the 23-valent pneumococcal vaccine in patients with α1-antitrypsin deficiency with and without bronchiectasis. Chest 116:946–952, 1999.

Misbah SA, Spickett GP, Ryba PC, Hockaday JM, Kroll JS, Sherwood C, Kurtz JB, Moxon ER, Chapel HM. Chronic enteroviral meningoencephalitis in agammaglobulinemia: case report and literature review. J Clin Immunol 12:266–270, 1992.

Mitsuya H, Tomino S, Hisamitsu S, Kishimoto S. Evidence for the failure of IgA specific T helper activity in a patient with immunodeficiency with hyper IgM. J Clin Lab Immunol 2:337–342, 1979.

Mizoguchi A, Mizoguchi E, Takedatsu H, Blumberg RS, Bhan AK. Chronic intestinal inflammatory condition generates IL-10-producing regulatory B cell subset characterized by CD1d upregulation. Immunity 16:219–230, 2002.

Mofenson LM, Bethel J, Moye J Jr, Flyer P, Nugent R. Effect of intravenous immunoglobulin (IVIG) on CD4+ lymphocyte decline in HIV-infected children in a clinical trial of IVIG infection prophylaxis. J AIDS 6:1103–1113, 1993.

Mofenson LM, Moye J Jr, Bethel J, Hirschhorn R, Jordan C, Nugent R. Prophylactic intravenous immunoglobulin in HIV-infected children with CD4+ counts of 0.20 × 10⁹/L or more: effect on viral, opportunistic and bacterial infections: The National Institute of Child Health and Human Development Intravenous Immunoglobulin Clinical Trial Study Group. JAMA 268:483–488, 1992.

Molrine DC, Siber GR, Samra Y, Shevy DS, MacDonald K, Cieri R, Ambrosino DM. Normal IgG and impaired IgG responses to polysaccharide vaccines in asplenic patients. J Infect Dis 179:513–517, 1999.

Monafo V, Maghnie M, Terracciano L, Valtorta A, Massa M, Severi F. X-linked agammaglobulinemia and isolated growth hormone deficiency. Acta Paediatr Scand 80:563–566, 1991.

Monteil M, Hobbs J, Citron K. Selective immunodeficiency affecting staphylococcal response. Lancet 2:880–883, 1987.

Morell A. IgG subclass deficiency: a personal viewpoint. Pediatr Infect Dis J 9:S4–S8, 1990.

Morell A. Clinical relevance of IgG subclass deficiencies. Ann Biol Clin 52:49–52, 1994.

Morell A, Skvaril F, Hitzig WH, Barandun S. IgG subclasses: development of the serum concentrations in "normal" infants and children. J Pediatr 80:960–964, 1972.

Moretta L, Mingari MC, Webb SR, Pearl ER, Lydyard PM, Grossi CE, Lawton AR, Cooper MD. Imbalances in T cell subpopulations associated with immunodeficiency and autoimmune syndromes. Eur J Immunol 7:696–700, 1977.

Morra M, Silander O, Calpe S, Choi M, Oettgen H, Myers L, Etzioni A, Buckley R, Terhorst C. Alterations of the X-linked lymphoproliferative disease gene SH2D1A in common variable immunodeficiency syndrome. Blood 98:1321–1325, 2001.

Morris A, Webster AD, Brown D, Harrison TJ, Dusheiko G. GB virus C infection in patients with primary antibody deficiency. J Infect Dis 177:1719–1722, 1998.

Morrison AM, Nutt SL, Thevenin C, Rolink A, Busslinger M. Loss- and gain-of-function mutations reveal an important role of BSAP (Pax-5) at the start and end of B cell differentiation. Semin Immunol 10:133–142, 1998.

Moss RB, Carmack MA, Esrig S. Deficiency of IgG4 in children: association of isolated IgG4 deficiency with recurrent respiratory tract infection. J Pediatr 120:16–21, 1992.

Mueller BU, Pizzo PA. Cancer in children with primary or secondary immunodeficiencies. J Pediatr 126:1–10, 1995.

Mullighan CG, Fanning GC, Chapel HM, Welsh KI. TNF and lymphotoxin-alpha polymorphisms associated with common variable immunodeficiency: role in the pathogenesis of granulomatous disease. J Immunol 159:6236–6241, 1997.

Mullighan CG, Marshall SE, Bunce M, Welsh KI. Variation in immunoregulatory genes determines the clinical phenotype of common variable immunodeficiency. Genes Immun 1:137–148, 1999.

Mullighan CG, Marshall SE, Welsh I. Mannose binding lectin polymorphisms are associated with early age of disease onset and autoimmunity in common variable immunodeficiency. Scand J Immunol 51:111–122, 2000.

Muramatsu M, Kinoshita K, Fagarasan S, Yamada S, Shinkai Y, Honjo T. Class switch recombination and hypermutation require activation-induced cytidine deaminase (AID), a potential RNA editing enzyme. Cell 102:553–563, 2000.

Muramatsu M, Sankaranand VS, Anant S, Sugai M, Kinoshita K, Davidson NO, Honjo T. Specific expression of activation-induced cytidine deaminase (AID), a novel member of the RNA-editing deaminase family in germinal center B cells. J Biol Chem 274:18470–18476, 1999.

Musiani P, Lauriola L, Maggiano N, Tonali P, Piantelli M. Functional properties of human thymoma lymphocytes: role of subcellular factors in blastic activation. J Natl Cancer Inst 69:827–831, 1982.

Muto T, Muramatsu M, Taniwaki M, Kinoshita K, Honjo T. Isolation, tissue distribution, and chromosomal localization of the human activation-induced cytidine deaminase (AID) gene. Genomics 68:85–88, 2000.

Nahm MH, Blaese RM, Crain MJ, Briles DE. Patients with Wiskott-Aldrich syndrome have normal IgG2 levels. J Immunol 137:3484–3487, 1986.

Nahm MH, Macke K, Kwon OH, Madassery JV, Sherman LA, Scott MG. Immunologic and clinical status of blood donors with subnormal levels of IgG2. J Allergy Clin Immunol 85:769–777, 1990.

Najiar JL, Phillips JA, Manness KJ, Teague D, Summar ML, Lorenz RA. Some cases of non-classical growth hormone deficiency may be due to an X-linked disorder (abstract). 72nd Annual Meeting of the Endocrine Society. Atlanta GA, 1990.

Navaratnam N, Morrison JR, Bhattacharya S, Patel D, Funahashi T, Giannoni F, Teng BB, Davidson NO, Scott J. The p27 catalytic subunit of the apolipoprotein B mRNA editing enzyme is a cytidine deaminase. J Biol Chem 268:20709–20712, 1993.

Neuberger MS. Antigen receptor signaling gives lymphocytes a long life. Cell 90:971–973, 1997.

Nezelof C. Thymic dysplasia with normal immunoglobulins and immunologic deficiency: pure alymphocytosis. In Bergsma D, ed. Immunologic Deficiency Diseases in Man, Birth Defects Original Article Series. New York, The National Foundation, 1968, pp 1004–115.

Noelle RJ, Meenakshi R, Shepherd DM, Stamenkovic I, Ledbetter JA, Aruffo A. A 39-kDa protein on activated helper T cells binds CD40 and transduces the signal for cognate activation of B cells. Proc Natl Acad Sci USA 89:6550–6554, 1992.

Nomura K, Kanegane H, Karasuyama H, Tsukada S, Agematsu K, Murakami G, Sakazume S, Sako M, Tanaka R, Kuniya Y, Komeno T, Ishihara S, Hayashi K, Kishimoto T, Miyawaki T. Genetic defect in human X-linked agammaglobulinemia impedes a maturational evolution of pro-B cells into a later stage of pre-B cells in the B-cell differentiation pathway. Blood 96:610–617, 2000.

Nonoyama S, Farrington M, Ishida H, Howard M, Ochs HD. Activated B cells from patients with common variable immunodeficiency proliferate and synthesize immunoglobulin. J Clin Invest 92:1282–1287, 1993a.

Nonoyama S, Farrington ML, Ochs HD. Effect of IL-2 on immunoglobulin production by anti-CD40-activated human B cells: synergistic effect with IL-10 and antagonistic effect with IL-4. Clin Immunol Immunopathol 72:373–379, 1994.

Nonoyama S, Hollenbaugh D, Aruffo A, Ledbetter JA, Ochs HD. B cell activation via CD40 is required for specific antibody production by antigen-stimulated human B cells. J Exp Med 178:1097–1102, 1993b.

Nonoyama S, Penix LA, Edwards CP, Lewis DB, Ito S, Aruffo A, Wilson CB, Ochs HD. Diminished expression of CD40 ligand by activated neonatal T cells. J Clin Invest 95:66–75, 1995.

Noordzij JG, de Bruin-Versteeg S, Comans-Bitter WM, Hartwig NG, Hendriks RW, de Groot R, van Dongen JJ. Composition of precursor B-cell compartment in bone marrow from patients with X-linked agammaglobulinemia compared with healthy children. Pediatr Res 51:159–168, 2002.

Norman ME, Hansell JR, Holtzapple PG, Parks JS, Waldmann TA. Malabsorption and protein-losing enteropathy in a child with X-linked agammaglobulinemia. Clin Immunol Immunopath 4:157–164, 1975.

North ME, Spickett GP, Allsop J, Webster AD, Farrant J. Defective DNA synthesis by T cells in acquired 'common-variable' hypogammaglobulinaemia on stimulation with mitogens. Clin Exp Immunol 76:19–23, 1989.

Notarangelo LD, Duse M, Ugazio AG. Immunodeficiency with hyper-IgM (HIM). Immunodefic Rev 3:101–122, 1992.

Notarangelo LD, Hayward AR. X-linked immunodeficiency with hyper-IgM (XHIM). Clin Exp Immunol 120:399–405, 2000.

Notarangelo LD, Parolini O, Albertini A, Duse M, Mazzolari E, Plebani A, Camerino G, Ugazio AG. Analysis of X-chromosome inactivation in X-linked immunodeficiency with hyper-IgM (HIGM1): evidence for involvement of different hematopoietic cell lineages. Hum Genet 88:130–134, 1991.

Ochs HD, Ament ME, Davis SD. Giardiasis with malabsorption in X-linked agammaglobulinemia. N Engl J Med 287:341–342, 1972.

Ochs HD, Davis SD, Wedgwood RJ. Immunologic responses to bacteriophage φX-174 in immunodeficiency diseases. J Clin Invest 50:2559–2568, 1971.

Ochs HD, Junker AK, Collier AC, Virant FS, Handsfield HH, Wedgwood RJ. Abnormal antibody responses in patients with persistent generalized lymphadenopathy. J Clin Immunol 8:57–63 1988.

Ochs HD, Smith CI. X-linked agammaglobulinemia. A clinical and molecular analysis. Medicine 75:287–299, 1996.

Ochs HD, Wedgwood RJ. IgG subclass deficiencies. Ann Rev Med 38:325–340, 1987.

Ohga S, Okada K, Asahi T, Ueda K, Sakiyama Y, Matsumoto S. Recurrent pneumococcal meningitis in a patient with transient IgG subclass deficiency. Acta Pædiatr Jpn 37:196–200, 1995.

Ohno T, Inaba M, Kuribayashi K, Masuda T, Kanoh T, Uchino H. Selective IgM deficiency in adults: phenotypically and functionally altered profiles of peripheral blood lymphocytes. Clin Exp Immunol 68:630–637, 1987.

Ohta Y, Haire RN, Litman RT, Fu SM, Nelson RP, Kratz J, Kornfeld SJ, de la Morena M, Good RA, Litman GW. Genomic organization and structure of Bruton agammaglobulinemia tyrosine kinase: localization of mutations associated with varied clinical presentations and course in X chromosome-linked agammaglobulinemia. Proc Nat Acad Sci USA 91:9062–9066, 1994.

Ohtani I, Schukenecht HF. Temporal bone pathology in DiGeorge's syndrome. Ann Otol Rhinol Laryngol 93:220–224, 1984.

Ohzeki T, Hanaki K, Motozumi H, Ohtahara H, Hayashibara H, Harada Y, Okamoto H, Shiraki K, Tsuji Y, Emura H. Immunodeficiency with increased immunoglobulin M associated with growth hormone insufficiency. Acta Paediatr 82:620–623, 1993.

Oka Y, Rolink AG, Andersson J, Kamanaka M, Uchida J, Yasui T, Kishimoto T, Kikutani H, Melchers F. Profound reduction of mature B cell numbers, reactivities and serum Ig levels in mice which simultaneously carry the XID and CD40 deficiency genes. International Immunol 8:1675–1685, 1996.

O'Keeffe S, Finnegan P. IgG subclass deficiency. Chest 104:1940, 1993.

Okkenhaug K, Bilancio A, Farjot G, Priddle H, Sancho S, Peskett E, Pearce W, Meek SE, Salpekar A, Waterfield MD, Smith AJ, Vanhaesebroeck B. Impaired B and T cell antigen receptor signaling in p110delta PI 3-kinase mutant mice. Science 297:1031–1034, 2002.

O'Neil KM, Pallansch MA, Winkelstein JA, Lock TM, Modlin JF. Chronic group A coxsackievirus infection in agammaglobulinemia: demonstration of genomic variation of serotypically identical isolates persistently excreted by the same patient. J Inf Dis 157:183–186, 1988.

Önes Ü, Güler A, Salman N, Yalçin I. Low immunoglobulin G3 levels in wheezy children. Acte Pædiatr 87:368–370, 1998.

O'Reilly MA, Alterman LA, Malcolm S, Levinsky RJ, Kinnon C. Identification of CpG islands around the DXS178 locus in the region of the X-linked agammaglobulinaemia gene locus in Xq22. Hum Genet 90:275–278, 1992.

Ottesen EA, Skavaril F, Tripathy SP, Poindexter RW, Hussain R. Prominence of IgG4 in the IgG antibody response to human filariasis. J Immunol 134:2707–2711, 1985.

Otto HF. Klinisch-pathologische Studie zur Klassifikation und Prognose von 57 Thymustumoren: II. Prognostische Kriterien. Z Krebsforsch 91:103–115, 1978.

Oxelius VA. Quantitative and qualitative investigations of serum IgG subclasses in immunodeficiency diseases. Clin Exp Immunol 36:112–116, 1979.

Oxelius V-A. IgG subclass levels in infancy and childhood. Acta Pædiatr Scand 68:23–27, 1979.

Oxelius V-A. Chronic infections in a family with hereditary deficiency of IgG2 and IgG4. Clin Exp Immunol 17:19–27, 1974.

Oxelius V-A. Serum IgG and IgG subclass contents in different Gm phenotypes. Scand J Immunol 37:149–153, 1993.

Oxelius V-A, Berkel AI, Hanson LA. IgG2 deficiency in ataxia-telangiectasia. N Engl J Med 306:515–517, 1982.

Oxelius V-A, Hanson Lå, Björkander J, Jammarström L, Sjoholm A. IgG3 deficiency: common in obstructive lung disease. Monogr Allergy 20:106–115, 1986.

Oxelius V-A, Laurell A-B, Linquist B, Golebiowska H, Axelsson U, Bjorkander J, Hanson LA. IgG subclasses in selective IgA deficiency. N Engl J Med 304:1476–1477, 1981.

Ozawa T, Kondo N, Motoyoshi F, Kato Y, Orii T. Preferential damage to IgM production by ultraviolet B in the cells of patients with Bloom's syndrome. Scan J Immunol 38:225–232, 1993.

Padayachee M, Feighery C, Finn A, McKeown C, Levinsky RJ, Kinnon C, Malcolm S. Mapping of the X-linked form of hyper-IgM syndrome (HIGM1) to Xq26 by close linkage to HPRT. Genomics 14:551–553, 1992.

Page AR, Hansen AE, Good RA. Occurrence of leukemia and lymphoma in patients with agammaglobulinemia. Blood 21:197–206, 1963.

Page R, Friday G, Stillwagon P, Skoner D, Caliguiri L, Fireman P. Asthma and selective immunoglobulin subclass deficiency: improvement of asthma after immunoglobulin replacement therapy. J Pediatr 112:127–131, 1988.

Papavasiliou FN, Schatz DG. Cell-cycle-regulated DNA double-stranded breaks in somatic hypermutation of immunoglobulin genes. Nature 408:216–221, 2000.

Pappu R, Cheng AM, Li B, Gong Q, Chiu C, Griffin N, White M, Sleckman BP, Chan AC. Requirement for B cell linker protein (BLNK) in B cell development. Science 286:1949–1954, 1999.

Parkin JM. IgG2 subclass deficiency and pyogenic infection in patients with HIV-related disease. The clinical manifestations of IgG subclass deficiency. In Levinsky RJ, ed. IgG Subclass Deficiencies. Royal Society of Medicine, London, 1989, pp 37–39.

Paroli M, Accapezzato D, Francavilla V, Insalaco A, Plebani A, Balsano F, Barnaba V. Long-lasting memory-resting and memory-effector CD4+ T cells in human X-linked agammaglobulinemia. Blood 99:2131–2137, 2002.

Parolini O, Hejtmancik JF, Allen RC, Belmont JW, Lassiter GL, Henry MJ, Barker DF, Conley ME. Linkage analysis and physical mapping near the gene for X-linked agammaglobulinemia at Xq22. Genomics 15:342–349, 1993.

Pascual-Salcedo D, de la Concha EG, Garcia-Rodriguez MC, Zabay JM, Sainz T, Fontan G. Cellular basis of hyper IgM immunodeficiency. J Clin Lab Immunol 10:29–34, 1983.

Pastorelli G, Roncarolo MG, Touraine JL, Peronne G, Tovo PA, de Vries JE. Peripheral blood lymphocytes of patients with common variable immunodeficiency (CVI) produce reduced levels of interleukin-4, interleukin-2 and interferon-gamma, but proliferate normally upon activation by mitogens. Clin Exp Immunol 78:334–340, 1989.

Pawson T. Protein modules and signalling networks. Nature 373:573–580, 1995.

Pearl ER, Vogler LB, Okos AJ, Crist WM, Lawton AR III, Cooper MD. B lymphocyte precursors in human bone marrow: an analysis of normal individuals and patients with antibody deficiency states. J Immunol 120:1169–1175, 1978.

Pelkonen P, Savilhati E, Mäkelä A-L. Persistent and transient IgA deficiency in juvenile rheumatoid arthritis. Scand J Rheumatol 12:273–279, 1983.

Peterson RDA, Cooper MD, Good RA. The pathogenesis of immunologic deficiency diseases. Am J Med 38:579–604, 1965.

Petro JB, Gerstein RM, Lowe J, Carter RS, Shinners N, Khan WN. Transitional type 1 and 2 B lymphocyte subsets are differentially responsive to antigen receptor signaling. J Biol Chem 277:48009–48019, 2002.

Petro JB, Rahman SM, Ballard DW, Khan WN. Bruton's tyrosine kinase is required for activation of IkappaB kinase and nuclear factor kappaB in response to B cell receptor engagement. J Exp Med 191:1745–1754, 2000.

Phillips JAD, Vnencak-Jones CL. Genetics of growth hormone and its disorders. Adv Hum Genetics 18:305–363, 1989.

Plebani A, Fischer MB, Meini A, Duse M, Thon V, Eibl MM. T cell activity and cytokine production in X-linked agammaglobulinemia: implications for vaccination strategies. Int Arch Allergy Immunol 114:90–93, 1997.

Plebani A, Soresina A, Rondelli R, Amato GM, Azzari C, Cardinale F, Cazzola G, Consolini R, De Mattia D, Dell'Erba G, Duse M, Fiorini M, Martino S, Martire B, Masi M, Monafo V, Moschese V, Notarangelo LD, Orlandi P, Panei P, Pession A, Pietrogrande MC, Pignata C, Quinti I, Ragno V, Rossi P, Sciotto A, Stabile A.

Clinical, immunological, and molecular analysis in a large cohort of patients with X-linked agammaglobulinemia: an Italian multicenter study. Clin Immunol 104:221–230, 2002.

Plebani A, Ugazio AG, Meini A, Ruggeri L, Negrini A, Albertini A, Leibovitz M, Duse M, Bottaro A, Brusco R, et al. Extensive deletion of immunoglobulin heavy chain constant region genes in the absence of recurrent infections: when is IgG subclass deficiency clinically relevant? Clin Immunol Immunopathol 68:46–50, 1993.

Plo RF, Garcia RM, Ferreira CA, Fontan CG. Neutropenia as early manifestation of X-linked agammaglobulinemia. Report on 4 patients. Span An Esp Pediatr 51:235–240, 1999.

Plotkin SA, Klaus RM, Whitely JP. Hypogammaglobulinemia in an infant with congenital rubella syndrome: failure of l-adamantadine to stop virus excretion. J Pediatr 69:1085–1091, 1966.

Polmar SH, Waldmann TA, Balestra ST, Jost MC, Terry WD. Immunoglobulin E in immunologic deficiency diseases: I. Relation of IgE and IgA to respiratory tract disease in isolated IgE deficiency. J Clin Invest 51:326–330, 1972.

Posey WC, Nelson HS, Branch B, Pearlman DS. The effects of acute corticosteroid therapy for asthma on serum immunoglobulin levels. J Allergy Clin Immunol 62:340–348, 1978.

Pozzi N, Gaetaniello L, Martire B, De Mattia D, Balestrieri B, Cosentini E, Schlossman SF, Duke-Cohan JS, Pignata C. Defective surface expression of attractin on T cells in patients with common variable immunodeficiency (CVID). Clin Exp Immunol 123:99–104, 2001.

Preud'Homme JL, Griscelli C, Seligmann M. Immunoglobulins on the surface of lymphocytes in fifty patients with primary immunodeficiency diseases. Clin Immunol Immunopath 1:241–56, 1973.

Pyun KH, Ochs HD, Wedgwood RJ, Yang XQ, Heller SR, Reimer CB. Human antibody responses to bacteriophage φX-174: sequential induction of IgM and IgG subclass antibody. Clin Immunol Immunopathol 51:252–262, 1989.

Quan ZS, Dick RF, Regueiro B, Quintans J. B cell heterogeneity. II. Transplantation resistance in xid mice which affects the ontogeny of B cell subpopulations. Eur J Immunol 11:643–649, 1981.

Quartier P, Brethon B, Philippet P, Landman-Parker J, Le Deist F, Fischer A. Treatment of childhood autoimmune haemolytic anaemia with rituximab. Lancet 358:1511–1513, 2001.

Quartier P, Debre M, De Blic J, de Sauverzac R, Sayegh N, Jabado N, Haddad E, Blanche S, Casanova JL, Smith CI, Le Deist F, de Saint Basile G, Fischer A. Early and prolonged intravenous immunoglobulin replacement therapy in childhood agammaglobulinemia: a retrospective survey of 31 patients. J Pediatr 134:589–596, 1999.

Quartier P, Foray S, Casanova JL, Hau-Rainsard I, Blanche S, Fischer A. Enteroviral meningoencephalitis in X-linked agammaglobulinemia: intensive immunoglobulin therapy and sequential viral detection in cerebrospinal fluid by polymerase chain reaction. Pediatr Inf Dis J 19:1106–1108, 2000.

Quartier P, Tournilhac O, Archimbaud C, Lazaro L, Chaleteix C, Millet P, Peigue-Lafeuille H, Blanche S, Fischer A, Casanova JL, Travade P, Tardieu M. Enteroviral meningoencephalitis after anti-CD20 (rituximab) treatment. Clin Infect Dis 36:e47–e49, 2003.

Quek LS, Bolen J, Watson SP. A role for Bruton's tyrosine kinase (Btk) in platelet activation by collagen. Current Biol 8:1137–1140, 1998.

Quintans J, McKearn JP, Kaplan D. B cell heterogeneity. I. A study of B cell subpopulations involved in the reconstitution of an X-linked immune defect of B cell differentiation. J Immunol 122:1750–1756, 1979.

Quinti I, Pierdominici M, Marziali M, Giovannetti A, Donnanno S, Chapel H, Bjorkander J, Aiuti F. European surveillance of immunoglobulin safety—results of initial survey of 1243 patients with primary immunodeficiencies in 16 countries. Clin Immunol 104:231–236, 2002.

Rada C, Williams GT, Nilsen H, Barnes DE, Lindahl T, Neuberger MS. Immunoglobulin isotype switching is inhibited and somatic hypermutation perturbed in UNG-deficient mic. Curr Biol 12:1748–1755, 2002.

Rawlings DJ. Bruton's tyrosine kinase controls a sustained calcium signal essential for B lineage development and function. Clin Immunol 91:243–253, 1999.

Rawlings DJ, Saffran DC, Tsukada S, Largaespada DA, Grimaldi JC, Cohen L, Mohr RN, Bazan JF, Howard M, Copeland NG, et al. Mutation of unique region of Bruton's tyrosine kinase in immunodeficient XID mice. Science 261:358–361, 1993.

Rawlings DJ, Witte ON. Bruton's tyrosine kinase is a key regulator in B-cell development. Immunol Rev 138:105–119, 1994.

Rawlings DJ, Witte ON. The Btk subfamily of cytoplasmic tyrosine kinases: structure, regulation and function. Sem Immunol 7:237–246, 1995.

Razanajaona D, van Kooten C, Lebecque S, Bridon J-M, Ho S, Smith S, Callard R, Banchereau J, Brière F. Somatic mutations in human Ig variable genes correlate with a partially functional CD40-ligand in the X-linked hyper-IgM syndrome. J Immunol 157:1492–1498, 1996.

Raziuddin S, Assal HM, Teklu B. T cell malignancy in Richter's syndrome presenting as hyper IgM. Induction and characterization of a novel CD3+, CD4−, CD8+ T cell subset from phytohemagglutinin-stimulated patient's CD3+, CD4+, CD8+ leukemic T cells. Eur J Immunol 19:469–474, 1989.

Razvi S, Schneider L, Jonas MM, Cunningham-Rundles C. Outcome of intravenous immunoglobulin-transmitted hepatitis C virus infection in primary immunodeficiency. Clin Immunol 101:284–288, 2001.

Reinherz EL, Cooper MD, Schlossman SF, Rosen FS. Abnormalities of T cell maturation and regulation in human beings with immunodeficiency disorders. J Clin Invest 68:699–705, 1981.

Report of an International Union of Immunological Societies Scientific Committee: Primary immunodeficiency diseases. Clin Exp Immunol 118(suppl 1):1–28, 1999.

Revy P, Busslinger M, Tashiro K, Arenzana F, Pillet P, Fischer A, Durandy A. A syndrome involving intrauterine growth retardation, microcephaly, cerebellar hypoplasia, B lymphocyte deficiency, and progressive pancytopenia. Pediatrics 105:E39, 2000a.

Revy P, Geissmann F, Debre M, Fischer A, Durandy A. Normal CD40-mediated activation of monocytes and dendritic cells from patients with hyper-IgM syndrome due to a CD40 pathway defect in B cells. Eur J Immunol 28:3648–3654, 1998.

Revy P, Muto T, Levy Y, Geissmann F, Plebani A, Sanal O, Catalan N, Forveille M, Dufourcq-Lagelouse R, Gennery A, Tezcan I, Ersoy F, Kayserili H, Ugazio A, Brousse N, Muramatsu M, Notarangelo LD, Kinoshita K, Honjo T, Fischer A, Durandy A. Activation-induced cytidine deaminase (AID) deficiency causes the autosomal recessive form of the hyper-IgM syndrome (HIGM2). Cell 102:565–575, 2000b.

Ridanpaa M, van Eenennaam H, Pelin K, Chadwick R, Johnson C, Yuan B, van Venrooij W, Pruijn G, Salmela R, Rockas S, Makitie O, Kaitila I, de la Chapelle A. Mutations in the RNA component of RNase MRP cause a pleiotropic human disease cartilage-hair-hypoplasia. Cell 104:195–203, 2001.

Rieger CHL, Moohr JW, Rothberg RM, Todd JK. Correction of neutropenia associated with dysgammaglobulinemia. Pediatrics 54:508–511, 1974.

Rieger CHL, Nelson LA, Peri BA, Lustig JV, Newcomb RW. Transient hypogammaglobulinemia of infancy. J Pediatr 91:601–603, 1977.

Roberton DM, Colgan T, Ferrante A, Jones C, Mermelstein N, Sennhauser F. IgG subclass concentrations in absolute, partial and transient IgA deficiency in childhood. Pediatr Infect Dis J 9:S41–S45, 1990.

Robertson SP, Rodda C, Bankier A. Hypogonadotrophic hypogonadism in Roifman syndrome. Clin Genet 57:435–438, 2000.

Rohrer J, Conley ME. Correction of X-linked immunodeficient mice by competitive reconstitution with limiting numbers of normal bone marrow cells. Blood 94:3358–3365, 1999.

Roifman CM, Costa T. A novel syndrome including combined immunodeficiency, autoimmunity, and spondylometaphyseal dysplasia. Can J Allerg Clin Immunol 5:6–9, 2000.

Roifman CM. Immunological aspects of a novel immunodeficiency syndrome that includes antibody deficiency with normal immunoglobulins, spondyloepiphyseal dysplasia, growth and developmental delay, and retinal dystrophy. Can J Allergy Clin Imm 3:94–98, 1997.

Roifman CM. Antibody deficiency, growth retardation, spondyloepiphyseal dysplasia and retinal dystrophy: a novel syndrome. Clin Genet 55:103–109, 1999.

Roifman CM, Levison H, Gelfand EW. High-dose versus low-dose intravenous immunoglobulin in hypogammaglobulinaemia and chronic lung disease. Lancet 1:1075–1077, 1987.

Roifman CM, Melamed I. A novel syndrome of combined immunodeficiency, autoimmunity and spondylometaphyseal dysplasia. Clin Genet 63:1–9, 2003.

Rolink A, Melchers F, Andersson J. The SCID but not the RAG-2 gene product is required for S-mu-S epsilon heavy chain class switching. Immunity 4:319–330, 1996.

Rosen FS, Cooper MD, Wedgwood RJ. The primary immunodeficiencies (I). N Engl J Med 311:235–242, 1984.

Rosen FS, Janeway CA. The gamma globulins: III. The antibody deficiency syndromes. N Engl J Med 275:769–775, 1966.

Rosen FS, Kevy SV, Merler E, Janeway CA, Gitlin D. Recurrent bacterial infections and dysgammaglobulinemia: deficiency of 7S gammaglobulins in the presence of elevated 19S gammaglobulins. Pediatrics 28:182–195, 1961.

Ross IN, Thompson RA. Severe selective IgM deficiency. J Clin Path 29:773–777, 1976.

Rotbart HA. Diagnosis of enteroviral meningitis with the polymerase chain reaction. J Pediatr 117:85–89, 1990.

Rotbart HA, Webster AD. Treatment of potentially life-threatening enterovirus infections with pleconaril. Clin Infect Dis 32:228–235, 2001.

Rothbach CJ, Nagel J, Rabin B, Fireman PJ. Antibody deficiency with normal immunoglobulins. J Pediatr 94:250–253, 1979.

Rothe M, Xiong J, Shu HB, Williamson K, Goddard A, Goeddel DV. I-TRAF is a novel TRAF-interacting protein that regulates TRAF-mediated signal transduction. Proc Natl Acad Sci USA 93:8241–8246, 1996.

Rudge P, Webster AD, Revesz T, Warner T, Espanol T, Cunningham-Rundles C, Hyman N. Encephalomyelitis in primary hypogammaglobulinaemia. Brain 119:1–15, 1996.

Ruff ME, Pincus LG, Sampson HA. Phenytoin-induced IgA depression. Am J Dis Child 141:858–861, 1987.

Rump JA, Jahreis A, Schlesier M, Stecher S, Peter HH. A double-blind, placebo-controlled, crossover therapy study with natural human IL-2 (nhuIL-2) in combination with regular intravenous gammaglobulin (IVIG) infusions in 10 patients with common variable immunodeficiency (CVID). Clin Exp Immunol 110:167–173, 1997.

Sacco MG, Ungari M, Catò EM, Villa A, Strina D, Notarangelo LD, Jonkers J, Zecca L, Facchetti F, Vezzoni P. Lymphoid abnormalities in CD40 ligand transgenic mice suggest the need for tight regulation in gene therapy approaches to hyper immunoglobulin M (IgM) syndrome. Cancer Gene Ther 7:1299–1306, 2000.

Safai B, Gupta S, Good RA. Pemphigus vulgaris associated with a syndrome of immunodeficiency and thymoma: a case report. Clin Exp Dermatol 3:129–134, 1978.

Saffran DC, Parolini O, Fitch-Hilgenberg ME, Rawlings DJ, Afar DE, Witte ON, Conley ME. Brief report: a point mutation in the SH2 domain of Bruton's tyrosine kinase in atypical X-linked agammaglobulinemia. N Engl J Med 330:1488–1491, 1994.

Saiki O, Ralph P, Cunningham-Rundles C, Good RA. Three distinct stages of B-cell defects in common varied immunodeficiency. Proc Natl Acad Sci USA 79:6008–6012, 1982.

Salim K, Bottomley MJ, Querfurth E, Zvelebil MJ, Gout I, Scaife R, Margolis RL, Gigg R, Smith CI, Driscoll PC, Waterfield MD, Panayotou G. Distinct specificity in the recognition of phosphoinositides by the pleckstrin homology domains of dynamine and Bruton's tyrosine kinase. EMBO J 15:6241–6250, 1996.

Sander CA, Medeiros LJ, Weiss LM, Yano T, Sneller MC, Jaffe ES. Lymphoproliferative lesions in patients with common variable immunodeficiency syndrome. Am J Surg Pathol 16:1170–1182, 1992.

Sanders LAM, Rijkers GT, Kuis W, Tenbergen-Meekes AJ, de Graeff-Meeder BR, Hiemstra I, Zegers BJ. Defective antipneumococcal polysaccharide antibody response in children with recurrent respiratory tract infections. J Allergy Clin Immunol 91:110–119, 1993.

Sanders LAM, Rijkers GT, Tenbergen-Meekes A-M, Voorhorst-Ogink MM, Zegers BJ. Immunoglobulin isotype-specific antibody responses to pneumococcal polysaccharide vaccine in patients with recurrent bacterial respiratory tract infections. Pediatr Res 37:812–819, 1995.

Santos-Argumedo L, Lund FE, Heath AW, Solvason N, Wu WW, Grimaldi JC, Parkhouse RM, Howard M. CD38 unresponsiveness of xid B cells implicates Bruton's tyrosine kinase (btk) as a regular of CD38 induced signal transduction. International Immunol 7:163–170, 1998.

Santosham M, Reid R, Ambrosino DM, Wolff MC, Alemido-Hill J, Priehs C, Aspery KM, Garrett S, Croll L, Foster S, et al. Prevention of Haemophilus influenzae type b infections in high-risk infants treated with bacterial polysaccharide immune globulin. N Engl J Med 317:923–929, 1987.

Sato S, Katagiri T, Takaki S, Kikuchi Y, Hitoshi Y, Yonehara S, Tsukada S, Kitamura D, Watanabe T, Witte O, Takatsu K IL-5 receptor-mediated tyrosine phosphorylation of SH2/SH3-containing proteins and activation of Bruton's tyrosine and Janus 2 kinases. J Exp Med 180:2101–2111, 1994.

Sato T, Irie S, Reed JC. A novel member of the TRAF family of putative signal transducing proteins binds to the cytosolic domain of CD40. FEBS Lett 358:113–118, 1995.

Saulsbury FT, Bernstein MT, Winkelstein JA. Pneumocystis carinii pneumonia as the presenting infection in congenital hypogammaglobulinemia. J Pediatr 95:559–561, 1979.

Saulsbury FT, Winkelstein JA, Yolken RH. Chronic rotavirus infection in immunodeficiency. J Pediatr 97:61–65, 1980.

Saxon A, Keld B, Braun J, Dotson A, Sidell N. Long-term administration of 13-cis retinoic acid in common variable immunodeficiency: circulating interleukin-6 levels, B-cell surface molecule display, and in vitro and in vivo B-cell antibody production. Immunology 80:477–487, 1993.

Saxon A, Kobayashi RH, Stevens RH, Singer AD, Stiehm ER, Siegel SC. In vitro analysis of humoral immunity in antibody deficiency with normal immunoglobulins. Clin Immunol Immunopath 17:235–244, 1980.

Saxon A, Sidell N, Zhang K. B cells from subjects with CVI can be driven to Ig production in response to CD40 stimulation. Cell Immunol 144:169–181, 1992.

Scher I. The CBA/N mouse strain: an experimental model illustrating the influence of the X-chromosome on immunity. Adv Immunol 33:1–71, 1982.

Schiff C, Lemmers B, Deville A, Fougereau M, Meffre E. Autosomal primary immunodeficiencies affecting human bone marrow B-cell differentiation. Immunol Rev 178:91–98, 2000.

Schiff RI, Buckley RH, Gilbertsen RB, Metzgar RS. Membrane receptors and in vitro responsiveness of lymphocytes in human immunodeficiency. J Immunol 112:376–386, 1974.

Schimke RN, Bolano C, Kirkpatrick CH. Immunologic deficiency in the congenital rubella syndrome. Am J Dis Child 118:626–632, 1969.

Schmugge M, Lauener R, Bossart W, Seger RA, Gungor T. Chronic enteroviral meningo-encephalitis in X-linked agammaglobulinaemia: favourable response to anti-enteroviral treatment. Eur J Pediatr 158:10101011, 1999.

Schoettler JJ, Schleissner LA, Heiner DC. Familial IgE deficiency associated with with sinopulmonary disease. Chest 96:516–521, 1989.

Scholl PR, O'Gorman MR, Pachman LM, Haut P, Kletzel M. Correction of neutropenia and hypogammaglobulinemia in X-linked hyper-IgM syndrome by allogeneic bone marrow transplantation. Bone Marrow Transplant 22:1215–1218, 1998.

Schroeder HW Jr, Zhu ZB, March RE, Campbell RD, Berney SM, Nedospasov SA, Turetskaya RL, Atkinson TP, Go RC, Cooper MD, Volanakis JE. Susceptibility locus for IgA deficiency and common variable immunodeficiency in the HLA-DR3, -B8, -A1 haplotypes. MolMed 4:72–86, 1998.

Schubert LA, King G, Cront RQ, Lewis DB, Aruffo A, Hollenbaugh D. The human gp39 promoter. Two distinct nuclear factors of activated T cell protein-binding elements contribute independently to transcriptional activation. J Biol Chem 270:29624–29627, 1995.

Schur PH, Borel H, Gelfand EW, Alper CA, Rosen FS. Selective gamma-G globulin deficiencies in patients with recurrent pyogenic infections. N Engl J Med 283:631–634, 1970.

Schur PH, Rosen F, Norman ME. Immunoglobulin subclasses in normal children. Pediatr Res 13:181–183, 1979.

Schweizer P, Kalhoff H, Horneff G, Weahn V, Diekmann L. Polysaccharide specific humoral immunodeficiency in ectodermal dysplasia: case report of a boy with two affected brothers. Klin Pädiatr 211:459–461, 1999.

Scott J. A place in the world for RNA editing. Cell 81:833–836, 1995.

Seager J, Jamison DL, Wilson J, Hayward AR, Soothill JF. IgA deficiency, epilepsy, and phenytoin treatment. Lancet 2:632–635, 1975.

Serrano D, Becker K, Cunningham-Rundles C, Mayer L. Characterization of the T cell receptor repertoire in patients with common variable immunodeficiency: oligoclonal expansion of CD8(+) T cells. Clin Immunol 97:248–258, 2000.

Settipane GA, Pudupakkam RK, McGowan JH. Corticosteroid effect on immunoglobulins. J Allergy Clin Immunol 62:162–166, 1978.

Seyama K, Kobayashi R, Hasle H, Apter AJ, Rutledge JC, Rosen D, Ochs HD. Parvovirus B19-induced anemia as the presenting manifestation of X-linked hyper-IgM syndrome. J Infect Dis 178:318–324, 1998a.

Seyama K, Nonoyama S, Gangsaas I, Hollenbaugh D, Pabst HF, Aruffo A, Ochs HD. Mutations of the CD40 ligand gene and its effects on CD40 ligand expression in patients with X-linked hyper IgM syndrome. Blood 92:2421–2434, 1998b.

Seyama K, Osborne WRA, Ochs HD. CD40 ligand mutants responsible for X-linked hyper-IgM syndrome associate with wild-type CD40 ligand. J Biol Chem 274:11310–11320, 1999.

Shackelford PG. IgG subclasses: importance in pediatric practice. Pediatr Rev 14:291–296, 1993.

Shackelford PG, Granoff DM, Madassery JV, Scott MG, Nahm MH. Clinical and immunologic characteristics of healthy children with subnormal serum concentrations of IgG2. Pediatr Res 27:16–21, 1990a.

Shackelford PG, Granoff DM, Polmar SH, Scott MG, Goskowicz MC, Madassery JV, Nahm MH.. Subnormal serum concentrations of IgG2 in children with frequent infections associated with varied patterns of immunologic dysfunction. J Pediatr 116:529–538, 1990b.

Shackelford PG, Polmar SH, Mayus JL. Spectrum of IgG2 subclass deficiency in children with recurrent infections: prospective study. J Pediatr 108:647–653, 1986.

Shapiro GG, Virant FS, Furukawa CT, Pierson WE, Bierman CW. Immunologic defects in patients with refractory sinusitis. Pediatrics 87:311–316, 1991.

Sharma VR, Fleming DR, Slone SP. Pure red cell aplasia due to parvovirus B19 in a patient treatment with rituximab. Blood 96:1184–1186, 2000.

Shear NH, Spielberg SP. Anticonvulsant hypersensitivity syndrome. J Clin Invest 82:1826–1832, 1988.

Shovlin CL, Simmonds HA, Fairbanks LD, Deacock SJ, Hughes JM, Lechler RI, Webster AD, Sun XM, Webb JC, Soutar AK. Adult onset immunodeficiency caused by inherited adenosine deaminase deficiency. J Immunol 153:2331–2339, 1994.

Shurin PA, Rehmus JM, Johnson CE, et al. Bacterial polysaccharide immune globulin for prophylaxis of acute otitis media in high-risk children. J Pediatr 123:801–810, 1993.

Siber GR, Santosham M, Reid GR, Thompson C, Almeido-Hill J, Morell A, deLange G, Ketcham JK, Callahan EH. Impaired antibody response to Haemophilus influenzae type b polysaccharide and low IgG2 and IgG4 concentrations in Apache children. N Engl J Med 323:1387–1392, 1990.

Siber GR, Schur PH, Aisenberg AC, Weitzman SA, Schiffman G. Correlation between serum IgG2 concentrations and the antibody response to bacterial polysaccharide antigens. N Engl J Med 303:178–182, 1980.

Siber GR, Weitzman SA, Aisenberg AC, Weinstien HJ, Schiffman G. Impaired antibody response to pneumococcal vaccine after treatment for Hodgkin's disease. N Engl J Med 299:442–448, 1978.

Sicherer SH, Cabana MD, Perlman EJ, Lederman, HM, Matsakis RM, Winkelstein JA. Thymoma and cellular immunodeficiency in an adolescent. Pediatr Aller Immunol 9:49–52, 1998.

Siegal FP, Pernis B, Kunkel HG. Lymphocytes in human immunodeficiency states: a study of membrane-associated immunoglobulins. Eur J Immunol 1:482–486, 1971.

Siegel RL, Issekutz T, Schwaber J, Rosen FS, Geha RS. Deficiency of T helper cells in transient hypogammaglobulinemia of infancy. N Engl J Med 305:1307–1313, 1981.

Silk H, Geha RS. Asthma, recurrent infections and IgG2 deficiency. Ann Allergy 60:134–136, 1988.

Silk HJ, Ambrosino DM, Geha RS. Effect of intravenous gammaglobulin therapy in IgG2 deficient and IgG2 sufficient children with recurrent infections and poor response to immunization with Hemophilus influenzae type b capsular polysaccharide antigen. Ann Allergy 64:21–25, 1990.

Simpson L, Thiemann OH. Sense from Nonsense: RNA editing in mitochondria of kinetoplastic protozoa and slime molds. Cell 81:837–840, 1995.

Sitz KV, Burks AW, Williams LW, Kemp SF, Steele RW. Confirmation of X-linked hypogammaglobulinemia with isolated growth hormone deficiency as a disease entity. J Pediatr 116:292–294, 1990.

Smith C, Witte ON. X-linked agammaglobulinemia: a disease of Btk tyrosine kinase. In Smith CIE, Ochs HD, Puck JM, eds. Primary Immunodeficiency Diseases: A Molecular and Genetic Approach. New York, Oxford University Press, 1999 pp 263–284.

Smith CI, Baskin B, Humire-Greiff P, Zhou JN, Olsson PG, Maniar HS, Kjellen P, Lambris JD, Christensson B, Hammarstrom L, et al. Expression of Bruton's agammaglobulinemia tyrosine kinase gene, BTK, is selectively down-regulated in T lymphocytes and plasma cells. J Immunol 152:557–565, 1994a.

Smith CI, Islam TC, Mattsson PT, Mohamed AJ, Nore BF, Vihinen M. The Tec family of cytoplasmic tyrosine kinases: mammalian Btk, Bmx, Itk, Tec, Txk and homologs in other species. Bioessays 23:436–446, 2001.

Smith CIE, Hammarström L, Henter J-I, De Lange GG. Molecular and serologic analysis of IgG1 deficiency caused by new forms of the constant region of the Ig H chain gene deletions. J Immunol 142:4514–4519, 1989.

Smith JK, Krishnaswamy GH, Kykes, R, Reynods S, Berk SL. Clinical manifestations of IgE hypogammaglobulinemia. Ann Allergy Asthma Immunol 78:313–318, 1997.

Smith KJ, Skelton H. Common variable immunodeficiency treated with a recombinant human IgG, tumour necrosis factor-alpha receptor fusion protein. Br J Dermatol 144:597–600, 2001.

Smith LJ, Szymanski W, Foulston C, Jewell LD, Pabst HF. Familial enteropathy with villous edema and immunoglobulin G2 subclass deficiency. J Pediatr 125:541–548, 1994b.

Smolen P, Bland R, Heiligenstein EL, Dillard R, Abramson J. Antibody response to oral polio vaccine in premature infants. J Pediatr 103:917–919, 1983.

Sneller MC. Common variable immunodeficiency. Am J Med Sci 321:42–48, 2001.

Sneller MC, Strober W. Abnormalities of lymphokine gene expression in patients with common variable immunodeficiency. J Immunol 144:3762–3769, 1990.

Sneller MC, Strober W, Eisenstein E, Jaffe JS, Cunningham-Rundles C. NIH conference. New insights into common variable immunodeficiency. Ann Intern Med 118:720–730, 1993.

Snowden N, Dietch DM, Teh LS, Hilton RC, Haeney MR. Antibody deficiency associated with gold treatment: natural history and management in 22 patients. Ann Rheum Dis 55:616–621, 1996.

Söderström T, Söderström R, Avanzini A, Nilsson JE, Mattsby Baltzer I, Hamson LA. Determination of normal IgG subclass levels. In Levinsky RJ, ed. IgG Subclass Deficiencies. London, Royal Society of Medicine, 1989, pp 13–26.

Soiffer RJ, Murray C, Ritz J, Phillips N, Jacobsohn D, Chartier S, Ambrosino DM. Recombinant interleukin-2 infusions and decreased IgG2 subclass concentrations. Blood 85:925–928, 1995.

Solvason N, Wu WW, Kabra N, Lund-Johansen F, Roncarolo MG, Behrens TW, Grillot DA, Nunez G, Lees E, Howard M. Transgene expression of bcl-xL permits anti-immunoglobulin (Ig)-induced proliferation in xid B cells. J Exp Med 187:1081–1091, 1998.

Song HY, Regnier CH, Kirschning CJ, Goeddel DV, Rothe M. Tumor necrosis factor (TNF)-mediated kinase cascades: bifurcation of nuclear factor-kappaB and c-jun N-terminal kinase (JNK/SAPK) pathways at TNF receptor-associated factor 2. Proc Natl Acad Sci USA 94:9792–9796, 1997.

Soothill JF. Immunoglobulins in first-degree relatives of patients with hypogammaglobulinemia. Transient hypogammaglobulinaemia: a possible manifestation of heterozygosity. Lancet 1:1001–1003, 1968.

Soothill JF, Hayes K, Dudgeon JA. The immunoglobulins in congenital rubella. Lancet 1:1385–1388, 1966.

Sorensen RU, Leiva LE, Giangrosso PA, Butler B, Javier FC III, Sacerdote DM, Bradford N, Moore C. Response to a heptavalent conjugate Streptococcus pneumoniae vaccine in children with recurrent infections who are unresponsive to the polysaccharide vaccine. Pediatr Infect Dis J 17:685–691, 1998a.

Sorensen RU, Leiva LE, Javier FC III, Sacerdote DM, Bradford N, Butler B, Giangrosso PA, Moore C. Influence of age on the response to Streptococcus pneumoniae vaccine in patients with recurrent infections and normal immunoglobulin concentrations. J Allergy Clin Immunol 102:215–221, 1998b.

Sorrell TC, Forbes IJ, Burness FR, Rischbieth RH. Depression of immunological function in patients treated with phenytoin sodium (sodium diphenylhydantoin). Lancet 2:1233–1235, 1971.

Souadjian JV, Enriquez P, Silverstein MN, Pepin J-M. The spectrum of diseases associated with thymoma: coincidence or syndrome? Arch Int Med 134:374–379, 1974.

Spector BD, Perry GS, Kersey JH. Genetically determined immunodeficiency diseases (GDID) and malignancy: report from the immunodeficiency—cancer registry. Clinical Immunol Immunopath 11:12–29, 1978.

Spickermann D, Gause A, Pfreundschuh M, von Kalle A-K, Bohlen H, Diehl V. Impaired antibody levels to tetanus toxoid and pneumococcal polysaccharides in acute leukemias. Leukemia and Lymphoma 16:89–96, 1994.

Sprent J, Bruce J. Physiology of B cells in mice with X-linked immunodeficiency (xid). III. Disappearance of xid B cells in double bone marrow chimeras. J Exp Med 160:711–723, 1984.

Stavnezer-Nordgren J, Kekish O, Zegers BJM. Molecular defects in a human immunoglobulin kappa chain deficiency. Science 230:458–461, 1985.

Stevens R, Dicheck D, Keld B, Heiner D. IgG1 is the predominant subclass of in vivo and in vitro produced anti-tetanus toxoid antibodies and also serves as the membrane IgG molecule for delivering inhibitory signals to antitetanus toxoid antibody-producing B cells. J Clin Immunol 3:65–69, 1983.

Stewart DM, Notarangelo LD, Kurman CC, Staudt LM, Nelson DL. Molecular genetic analysis of X-linked hypogammaglobulinemia and isolated growth hormone deficiency. J Immunol 155:2770–2774, 1995.

Stiehm ER, Casillas AM, Finkelstein JZ, Gallagher KT, Groncy PM, Kobayashi RH, Oleske JM, Roberts RL, Sandberg ET, Wakim ME. Slow subcutaneous human intravenous immunoglobulin in the treatment of antibody immunodeficiency: use of an old method with a new product. J Allergy Clin Immunol 101:848–849, 1998.

Stiehm ER, Chin TW, Haas A, Peerless AG. Infectious complications of the primary immunodeficiencies. Clin Immunol Immunopathol 40:69–86, 1986.

Stiehm ER, Fudenberg HH. Clinical and immunologic features of dysgammaglobulinemia type I: report of a case diagnosed in the first year of life. Am J Med 40:805–815, 1966a.

Stiehm ER, Fudenberg HH. Serum levels of immune globulins in health and disease: a survey. Pediatrics 37:715–727, 1966b.

Stites DP, Levin AS, Austin KE, Fudenberg HH. Immunobiology of human lymphoid cell lines. I. Immunoglobulin biosynthesis in cultures from hypogammaglobulinemias and paraproteinemias. J Immunol 107:1376–1381, 1971.

Su L, Garber EA, Hsu Y-M. CD154 variant lacking tumor necrosis factor homologous domain inhibits cell surface expression of wild-type protein. J Biol Chem 276:1673–1676, 2001.

Su TT, Guo B, Kawakami Y, Sommer K, Chae K, Humphries LA, Kato RM, Kang S, Patrone L, Wall R, Teitell M, Leitges M, Kawakami T, Rawlings DJ. PKC-beta controls I kappa B kinase lipid raft recruitment and activation in response to BCR signaling. Nat Immunol 3:780–786, 2002.

Su TT, Rawlings DJ. Transitional B lymphocyte subsets operate as distinct checkpoints in murine splenic B cell development. J Immunol 168:2101–2110, 2002.

Subauste CS, Wessendarp M, Sorensen RU, Leiva LE. CD40-CD40 ligand interaction is central to cell-mediated immunity against Toxoplasma gondii: Patients with hyper-IgM syndrome have a defective type 1 immune response that can be restored by soluble CD40 ligand trimer. J Immunol 162:6690–6700, 1999.

Sweinberg SK, Wodell RA, Grodofsky MP, Greene JM, Conley ME. Retrospective analysis of the incidence of pulmonary disease in hypogammaglobulinemia. J Allergy Clin Immunol 88:96–104, 1991.

Takeuchi T, Nakagawa T, Maeda Y, Hirano S, Sasaki-Hayashi M, Makino S, Shimizu A. Functional defect of B lymphocytes in a patient with selective IgM deficiency associated with systemic lupus erythematosus Autoimmunity 34:115–122, 2001.

Tan RS-H. Thymoma, acquired hypogammaglobulinaemia, lichen planus, alopecia areata. Proc R Soc Med 67:196–198, 1974.

Tani SM, Wang Y, Kanegane H, Futatani T, Pinto J, Vilela MM, Miyawaki T. Identification of mutations of Bruton's tyrosine kinase gene (BTK) in Brazilian patients with X-linked agammaglobulinemia. Hum Mutat 20:235–236, 2002.

Tarr PE, Sneller MC, Mechanic LJ, Economides A, Eger CM, Strober W, Cunningham-Rundles C, Lucey DR. Infections in patients with immunodeficiency with thymoma (Good Syndrome). Report of 5 cases and review of the literature. Medicine 80:123–133, 2001.

Te Velde K, Huber J, Van der Slikke LB. Primary acquired hypogammaglobulinemia, myasthenia, and thymoma. Ann Intern Med 65:554–559, 1966.

Teng B, Burant CF, Davidson NO. Molecular cloning of an apolipoprotein B messenger RNA editing protein. Science 260:1816–1819, 1993.

Terry WD, Fahey JL. Subclasses of human gamma-2-globulin based on differences in the heavy polypeptide chains. Science 146:400–401, 1964.

Thomas C, de Saint Basile G, Le Deist F, Theophile D, Benkerrou M, Addad E, Blanche S, Fischer A. Correction of X-linked hyper-IgM syndrome by allogeneic bone marrow transplantation. N Engl J Med 333:426–429, 1995.

Thomas JD, Sideras P, Smith CI, Vorechovsky I, Chapman V, Paul WE. Colocalization of X-linked agammaglobulinemia and X-linked immunodeficiency genes. Science 261:355–358, 1993.

Thong YH, Maxwell GM, Primary selective deficiency of immunoglobulin M. Aust N Z J Med 8:436–438, 1978.

Tian M, Alt FW. RNA editing meets DNA shuffling. Nature 407:31–33, 2000.

Tiller TL, Buckley RH. Transient hypogammaglobulinemia of infancy: review of the literature, clinical and immunologic features of 11 new cases, and long-term follow-up. J Pediatr 92:347–353, 1978.

Timens W, Poppema S. Impaired immune response to polysaccharides. N Engl J Med 317:837–838, 1987.

Timmers E, Kenter M, Thompson A, Kraakman ME, Berman JE, Alt FW, Schuurman RK. Diversity of immunoglobulin heavy chain gene segment rearrangement in B lymphoblastoid cell lines from X-linked agammaglobulinemia patients. Eur J Immunol 21:2355–2363, 1991.

Tissier A, McDonald JP, Frank EG, Woodgate R. poliota, a remarkably error-prone human DNA polymerase. Genes Dev 14:1642–1650, 2000.

Travin M, Macris NT, Block JM, Schwimmer D. Reversible common variable immunodeficiency syndrome induced by phenytoin. Arch Intern Med 149:1421–1422, 1989.

Tsui HW, Siminovitch KA, de Souza L, Tsui FWL. Moth-eaten and viable moth-eaten mice have mutations in the haematopoietic cell phosphatase gene. Nature Gen 4:124–129, 1993.

Tsukada S, Saffran DC, Rawlings DJ, Parolini O, Allen RC, Klisak I, Sparkes RS, Kubagawa H, Mohandas T, Quan S, et al. Deficient expression of a B cell cytoplasmic tyrosine kinase in human X-linked agammaglobulinemia. Cell 72:279–290, 1993.

Tsukada S, Simon M, Witte O, Katz A. Binding of the beta gamma ?subunits of heterotrimeric G-proteins to the PH domain of Bruton's tyrosine kinase. Proc Natl Acad Sci USA 91:11256–11260, 1994.

Umetsu DT, Ambrosino DM, Quinti I, Siber GR, Geha RS. Recurrent sinopulmonary infections and impaired antibody response to bacterial capsular polysaccharide antigen in children with selective IgG subclass deficiency. N Engl J Med 313:1247–1251, 1985.

Usui K, Sasahara Y, Tazawa R, Hagiwara K, Tsukada S, Miyawaki T, Tsuchiya S, Nukiwa T. Recurrent pneumonia with mild hypogammaglobulinemia diagnosed as X-linked agammaglobulinemia in adults. Respir Res 2:188–192, 2001.

Van der Hilst JC, Smits BW, van der Meer JW. Hypogammaglobulinaemia: cumulative experience in 49 patients in a tertiary care institution. Neth J Med 60:140–147, 2002.

van der Meer JW, Mouton RP, Daha MR, Schuurman RK. Campylobacter jejuni bacteraemia as a cause of recurrent fever in a patient with hypogammaglobulinaemia. J Infection 12:235–239, 1986.

van der Meer JW, Weening RS, Schellekens PT, van Munster IP, Nagengast FM. Colorectal cancer in patients with X-linked agammaglobulinaemia. Lancet 341:1439–1440, 1993.

van Rossum MAJ, Fiselier TJW, Franssen MJAM, ten Cate R, et al. Effects of sulfasalazine treatment on serum immunoglobulin levels in children with juvenile chronic arthritis. Scand J Rheumatol 30:25–30, 2001.

Verschuuren EAM, Stevens SJC, van Imhoff GW, Middeldorp JM, de Boer C, Koeter G, The TH, van Der Bij W. Treatment of posttransplant lymphoproliferative disease with rituximab: the remission, the relapse, and the complication. Transplantation 73:100–104, 2002.

Vetrie D, Vorechovsk I, Sideras P, Holland J, Davies A, Flinter F, Hammarström L, Kinnon C, Levinsky R, Bobrow M, Smith CIE, Bentley DR. The gene involved in X-linked agammaglobulinemia is a member of the src family of protein-tyrosine kinases. Nature 361:226–233, 1993.

Vihinen M, Brandau O, Branden LJ, Kwan SP, Lappalainen I, Lester T, Noordzij JG, Ochs HD, Ollila J, Pienaar SM, Riikonen P, Saha BK, Smith CIE. BTKbase, mutation database for X-linked agammaglobulinemia (XLA). Nucleic Acids Res 26:242–247, 1998.

Vihinen M, Cooper MD, de Saint Basile G, Fischer A, Good RA, Hendriks RW, Kinnon C, Kwan SP, Litman GW, Notarangelo LD, et al. BTKbase: a database of XLA-causing mutations. International Study Group. Immunol Today 16:460–465, 1995.

Vihinen M, Nilsson L, Smith CI. Tec homology (TH) adjacent to the PH domain. FEBS Letters 350:263–265, 1994.

Villa A, Notarangelo LD, Di Santo JP, Macchi PP, Strina D, Frattini A, Lucchini F, Patrosso CM, Giliani S, Mantuano E, Agosti S, Nocera G, Kroczek RA, Fischer A, Ugazio AG, De Saint Basile G, Vezzoni P. Organization of the human CD40L gene: implications for molecular defects in X chromosome-linked hyper-IgM syndrome and prenatal diagnosis. Proc Natl Acad Sci USA 91:2110–2114, 1994.

Vogelzang NJ, Finlay JL, Pelletiere EV, Luskin AT, Di Camelli RF, Hong R. Clear cell sarcoma and selective IgM deficiency: a case report. Cancer 49:234–238, 1982.

Vorechovsky I, Cullen M, Carrington M, Hammarstrom L, Webster AD. Fine mapping of IGAD1 in IgA deficiency and common variable immunodeficiency: identification and characterization of haplotypes shared by affected members of 101 multiple-case families. J Immunol 164:4408–4416, 2000.

Vorechovsky I, Zhou JN, Hammarstrom L, Smith CI, Thomas D, Paul WE, Notarangelo LD, Bernatowska-Matuszkiewicz E. Absence of xid mutation in X-linked agammaglobulinaemia. Lancet 342:552, 1993.

Wagner DK, Marti GE, Jaffe ES, Straus SE, Nelson DL, Fleisher TA. Lymphocyte analysis in a patient with X-linked agammaglobulinemia and isolated growth hormone deficiency after development of echovirus dermatomyositis and meningoencephalitis. Inter Arch Allergy Appl Immunol 89:143–148, 1989.

Wahab JA, Hanifah MJ, Choo KE. Bruton's agammaglobulinaemia in a child presenting with cryptococcal empyema thoracis and periauricular pyogenic abscess. Singapore Med J 36:686–689, 1995.

Waldmann TA, Strober WS, Blaese MR, Strauss AJL. Thymoma, hypogammaglobulinemia and absence of eosinophils. J Clin Invest 46:1127–1128, 1967.

Walker AM, Kemp AS, Hill DJ, Shelton MJ. Features of transient hypogammaglobulinemia in infants screened for immunological abnormalities. Arch Dis Child 70:183–186, 1994.

Walker L, Johnson GD, MacLennan ICM. The IgG subclass responses of human lymphocytes to B cell activation. Immunology 50:269–272, 1983.

Wang D, Feng J, Wen R, Marine JC, Sangster MY, Parganas E, Hoffmeyer A, Jackson CW, Cleveland JL, Murray PJ, Ihle JN. Phospholipase Cgamma2 is essential in the functions of B cell and several Fc receptors. Immunity 13:25–35, 2000.

Ward J, Brenneman G, Letson GW, Heyward WL. Limited efficacy of a Hemophilus influenzae type b conjugate vaccine in Alaska native infants. N Engl J Med 323:1393–1401, 1990.

Warnatz K, Denz A, Drager R, Braun M, Groth C, Wolff-Vorbeck G, Eibel H, Schlesier M, Peter HH. Severe deficiency of switched memory B cells (CD27(+)IgM(−)IgD(−)) in subgroups of patients with common variable immunodeficiency: a new approach to classify a heterogeneous disease. Blood 99:1544–1551, 2002.

Washington K, Stenzel TT, Buckley RH, Gottfried MR. Gastrointestinal pathology in patients with common variable immunodeficiency and X-linked agammaglobulinemia. Am J Surg Pathol 20:1240–1252, 1996.

Watts RG, Kelly DR. Fatal varicella infection in a child associated with thymoma and immunodeficiency (Good's syndrome). Med Pediatr Oncol 18:246–251, 1990.

Webster ADB. Thymoma, polyarthropathy and hypogammaglobulinaemia. Proc Roy Soc Med 69:58–59, 1976.

Webster AD, Rotbart HA, Warner T, Rudge P, Hyman N. Diagnosis of enterovirus brain disease in hypogammaglobulinemic patients by polymerase chain reaction. Clin Inf Dis 17:657–661, 1993.

Wedgwood RJ, Ochs HD. Variability in the expression of X-linked agammaglobulinemia: the co-existence of classic X-LA (Bruton type) and "common variable immunodeficiency" in the same families. In Seligmann M, ed. Primary Immunodeficiencies. Horth, Holland, Biomedical Press, Elsevier, 1980, p 69–78.

Wedgwood RJ, Ochs HD, Davis SD. The recognition and classification of immunodeficiency diseases with bacteriophage ϕX-174. Birth Defects Original Article Series 11:331–338, 1975.

Weir S, Cuccherini B, Whitney AM, Ray ML, MacGregor JP, Steigerwalt A, Daneshvar MI, Weyant R, Wray B, Steele J, Strober W, Gill VJ. Recurrent bacteremia caused by a Flexispira-like organism in a patient with X-linked (Bruton's) agammaglobulinemia. J Clin Microbiol 37:2439–2445, 1999.

Weston SA, Prasad ML, Mullighan CG, Chapel H, Benson EM. Assessment of male CVID patients for mutations in the Btk gene: how many have been misdiagnosed? Clin Exp Immunol 124:465–469, 2001.

Wicker LS, Scher I. X-linked immune deficiency (xid) of CBA/N mice. Curr Top Microbiol Immunol 124:87–101, 1986.

Wiesendanger M, Scharff MD, Edelmann W. Somatic hypermutation, transcription, and DNA mismatch repair. Cell 94:415–418, 1998.

Wiley JA, Harmsen AG. CD40 ligand is required for resolution of Pneumocystis pneumonia in mice. J Immunol 155:3525–3529, 1995.

Wilfert CM, Buckley RH, Mohanakumar T, Griffith JF, Katz SL, Whisnant JK, Eggleston PA, Moore M, Treadwell E, Oxman MN, Rosen FS. Persistent and fatal central-nervous-system ECHOvirus infections in patients with agammaglobulinemia. N Engl J Med 296:1485–1489, 1977.

Wilson CB, Lewis DB, Penix LA. The physiologic immunodeficiency of immaturity. In Stiehm ER, ed. Immunologic Disorders in Infants and Children, ed 4, Philadelphia, WB Saunders, 1996, pp 253–295.

Wilson NW, Daaboul J, Bastian JF. Association of autoimmunity with IgG2 and IgG4 subclass deficiency in a growth hormone-deficient child. J Clin Immunol 10:330–334, 1990.

Winkelstein JA, Fearon E. Carrier detection of the X-linked primary immunodeficiency diseases using X-chromosome inactivation analysis. J Allergy Clin Immunol 85:1090–10907, 1990.

Wolpert J, Knutsen AP. Natural history of selective antibody deficiency to bacterial polysaccharide antigens in children. Pediatr Asthma, Allergy Immunol 12:183–191, 1998.

Wood P, Mayne A, Joyce H, Smith CI, Granoff DM, Kumararatne DS. A mutation in Bruton's tyrosine kinase as a cause of selective anti-polysaccharide antibody deficiency. J Pediatr 139:148–151, 2001.

Woodland RT, Schmidt MR, Korsmeyer SJ, Gravel KA. Regulation of B cell survival in xid mice by the proto-oncogene bcl-2. J Immunol 156:2143–2154, 1996.

World Health Organization Scientific Group. Primary immunodeficiency diseases. Immunodef Rev 3:195–236, 1992.

Wright JJ, Wagner DK, Blaese RM, Hagengruber C, Waldmann TA, Fleisher TA. Characterization of common variable immunodeficiency: identification of a subset of patients with distinctive immunophenotypic and clinical features. Blood 76:2046–2051, 1990.

Wright PF, Hatch MH, Kasselberg AG, Lowry SP, Wadlington WB, Karzon DT. Vaccine-associated poliomyelitis in a child with sex-linked agammaglobulinemia. J Pediatr 91:408–412, 1977.

Wuerffel RA, Du J, Thompson RJ, Kenter AL. Ig Sgamma3 DNA-specific double strand breaks are induced in mitogen-activated B cells and are implicated in switch recombination. J Immunol 159:4139–4144, 1997.

Wyatt HV. Poliomyelitis in hypogammaglobulinemics. J Inf Dis 128:802–806, 1973.

Wyatt RA, Younoszai K, Anuras S, Myers MG. Campylobacter fetus septicemia and hepatitis in a child with agammaglobulinemia. J Pediatr 91:441–442, 1977.

Xu J, Foy TM, Laman JD, Elliott EA, Dunn JJ, Waldschmidt TJ, Elsemore J, Noelle RJ, Flavell RA. Mice deficient for the CD40 ligand. Immunity 1:423–431, 1994.

Xu L, Gorham B, Li SC, Bottaro A, Alt FW, Rothman P. Replacement of germ-line epsilon promoter by gene targeting alters control of immunoglobulin heavy chain class switching. Proc Natl Acad Sci USA 90:3705–3709, 1993.

Yamanaka S, Poksay KS, Balestra ME, Zeng GQ, Innerarity TL. Cloning and mutagenesis of the rabbit ApoB mRNA editing protein. A zinc motif is essential for catalytic activity, and noncatalytic auxiliary factor(s) of the editing complex are widely distributed. J Biol Chem 269:21725–21734, 1994.

Yamasaki T. Selective IgM deficiency: functional assessment of peripheral blood lymphocytes in vitro. Intern Med 31:866–870, 1992.

Yel L, Minegishi Y, Coustan-Smith E, Buckley RH, Trubel H, Pachman LM, Kitchingman GR, Campana D, Rohrer J, Conley ME. Mutations in the mu heavy-chain gene in patients with agammaglobulinemia. N Engl J Med 335:1486–1493, 1996.

Yocum MW, Strong DM, Chusid MJ, Lakin JD. Selective immunoglobulin M (IgM) deficiency in two immunodeficient adults with recurrent staphylococcal pyoderma. Am J Med 60:486–493, 1976.

Yount WJ, Hong R, Seligmann M, Good RA, Kunkel HG. Imbalances of gamma globulin subgroups and gene defects in patients with primary hypogammaglobulinemia. J Clin Invest 49:1957–1966, 1970.

Yu PW, Tabuchi RS, Dang VK, Lansigan E, Hernandez R, Witte ON, Rawlings DJ. Correction of X-linked immunodeficiency by retroviral mediated transfer of Bruton's tyrosine kinase. Blood 96:210a, 2000.

Yu PW, Tabuchi RS, Kato RM, Chae K, Dang VK, Lansigan E, Hernandez R, Witte ON, Rawlings DJ. Reconstitution of Bruton's tyrosine kinase function in murine models of X-linked agammaglobulinemia (Abstract). Molecular Therapy 5:S22–S23, 2002.

Zegers BJM, Maertzdorf WJ, van Loghem E. Mul NAJ, Stoop JW, van der Laag J, Vossen JJ, Ballieux RE. Kappa-chain deficiency: an immunoglobulin disorder. N Engl J Med 294:1026–1030, 1976.

Zenone T, Souquet PJ, Cunningham-Rundles C, Bernard JP. Hodgkin's disease associated with IgA and IgG subclass deficiency. J Intern Med 240:99–102, 1996.

Zenone T, Souillet G. X-linked agammaglobulinemia presenting as Pseudomonas aeruginosa septicemia. Scand J Infect Dis 28:417–418, 1996.

Zhang J, Bottaro A, Li S, Stewart V, Alt FW. A selective defect in IgG2b switching as a result of targeted mutation of the I gamma 2b promoter and exon. EMBO J 12:3529–3537, 1993.

Zhang JG, Morgan L, Spickett GP. L-selectin in patients with common variable immunodeficiency (CVID): a comparative study with normal individuals. Clin Exp Immunol 104:275–279, 1996.

Zhou Z, Huang R, Danon M, Mayer L, Cunningham-Rundles C. IL-10 production in common variable immunodeficiency. Clin Immunol Immunopathol 86:298–304, 1998.

Zhu Q, Zhang M, Rawlings DJ, Vihinen M, Hagemann T, Saffran DC, Kwan SP, Nilsson L, Smith CI, Witte ON, et al. Deletion within the Src homology domain 3 of Bruton's tyrosine kinase resulting in X-linked agammaglobulinemia (XLA). J Exp Med 180:461–470, 1994.

Ziegler JB, Penny R. Fatal ECHO 30 virus infection and amyloidosis in X-linked hypogammaglobulinemia. Clin Immunol Immunopath 3:347–352, 1975.

Ziegner UHM, Ochs HD, Schanen C, Feig SA, Seyama K, Futatani T, Gross T, Wakim M, Roberts RL, Rawlings DJ, Dovat S, Fraser JK, Stiehm ER. Unrelated umbilical cord stem cell transplantation for X-linked immunodeficiencies. J Pediatr 138:570–573, 2001.

Zielen S, Dengler TJ, Bauscher P, Meuer SC. Defective CD2 T cell pathway activation in common variable immunodeficiency (CVID). Clin Exp Immunol 96:253–259, 1994.

Zonana J, Elder ME, Schneider LC, Orlow SJ, Moss C, Golabi M, Shapira SK, Farndon PA, Wara DW, Emmal SA, Ferguson BM. A novel X-linked disorder of immune deficiency and hypohidrotic ectodermal dysplasia is allelic to incontinentia pigmenti and due to mutations in IKK-gamma (NEMO). Am J Hum Genet 67:1555–1562, 2000.

Zora JA, Silk HJ, Tinkelman DG. Evaluation of postimmunization pneumococcal titers in children with recurrent infections and normal levels of immunoglobulin. Ann Allergy 70:283–288, 1993.

Zullo A, Romiti A, Rinaldi V, Vecchione A, Tomao S, Aiuti F, Frati L, Luzi G. Gastric pathology in patients with common variable immunodeficiency. Gut 45:77–81, 1999.

proteases (Plaut, 1983). IgA2 exists in two allotypic (genetic) variants, IgA2m(1) and IgA2m(2) (Van Loghem et al., 1973) (see Selective IgA Subclass Deficiency), which differ in the points of attachment between heavy and light chains.

IgA1 is the predominant subclass in serum, and IgA2 is the predominant subclass in secretions. Serum IgA (both IgA1 and IgA2) is monomeric (containing two heavy chains and two light chains). Secretory IgA is dimeric (i.e., two IgA monomers) and is joined by the J chain and the 80-kD secretory component (Fig. 14-1B, C) (see Chapter 9).

FUNCTION OF IgA

IgA is the most prevalent immunoglobulin in exocrine secretions and represents the predominant class of antibodies produced by plasma cells of the sinopulmonary, gastrointestinal, and genitourinary tracts (Mestecky and McGhee, 1987; Tomasi and Bienenstock, 1968). External antigens contacting the mucosa of these organs stimulate the secretion of IgA antibodies. Secretory IgA combines with antigen at these surfaces to prevent mucosal penetration and exclude foreign antigens from entering the body. Secretory IgA antibodies can neutralize viruses, bind toxins, agglutinate bacteria, prevent bacteria from binding to epithelial cells, and bind to various food antigens. Thus IgA is important in preventing infectious agents from penetrating mucosal surfaces (Arnold et al., 1977; Hanson, 1983; Mestecky and McGhee, 1987; Tomasi and Bienenstock, 1968). Table 14-1 summarizes some of the known binding activities of secretory IgA.

Other roles for IgA in mucosal immunity have also been identified. Dimeric IgA secreted by plasma cells is selectively transported to the intestinal or organ lumen through the epithelial cell by the polymeric immunoglobulin receptor in a process called *transcytosis*. Cleavage of this receptor releases the secretory component, and the secretory IgA portion is discharged into the mucosal gland lumen. Dimeric IgA transiting through epithelial cells in this way may impede the replication of intracellular viruses (Mazanec et al., 1992). IgA can also complex with antigens that have penetrated the lamina propria and transport them across epithelial cells to facilitate antigen exclusion (Kaetzel et al., 1991).

Although secretory IgA has many known functions, the role of serum IgA is less certain. Plasma cells producing serum IgA are located predominantly in the bone marrow and, to a lesser extent, in the spleen (Mestecky and McGhee, 1987). The role of the abundant serum IgA antibodies to microbial and food antigens in the systemic immune response is uncertain (Mestecky and McGhee, 1987). One clue to understanding the function of serum IgA may be the presence of receptors for the Fc portion of IgA on monocytes and granulocytes (Kerr, 1990; Monteiro et al., 1990). This receptor (FcRα), a glycosylated protein of 50 to 70 kD, can bind IgA1 or IgA2 monomers or even secretory IgA. Receptor-bound IgA antibodies can activate both granulocytes and monocytes and may initiate phagocytosis of bacteria and fungi. The FcRα receptor may play a role in the catabolism of IgA antibodies and in the clearance of IgA immune complexes from the circulation. Because IgA in the serum does not fix complement by the classical pathway, although it can do so by the alternative pathway (Kerr, 1990; Russell and Mansa, 1989), it has been suggested that IgA acts as a "discrete housekeeper," in which foreign antigens are bound by IgA into complexes and removed by the phagocytic system, but with little or no resultant inflammation (Conley and Delacroix, 1987).

Another biologic function is suggested by a biochemical feature of serum IgA, the presence of free cysteine residues located near the tip of the carboxy terminus of the Fc portion. These cysteines can complex IgA to other serum proteins, principally albumin, α-1-antitrypsin, and the heterogeneously charged (HC) protein. Both the heterogeneously charged protein and α-antitrypsin are leukocyte inhibitors. Thus these complexes, as well as other IgA complexes, may inhibit neutrophil chemotaxis and exert a subtle immune control mechanism (Kerr, 1990). Other proteins binding to serum IgA include fibronectin and lactoferrin (Kerr, 1990).

SELECTIVE IgA DEFICIENCY

Frequency of IgA Deficiency

Serum IgA deficiency was first described in children with ataxia-telangiectasia (Thieffry et al., 1961), but soon IgA deficiency was identified in other patients and even in normal subjects (West et al., 1962). Following this report, many investigators studied the frequency of IgA deficiency in various populations. Its prevalence has ranged from 1 in 223 to 1 in 1000 in community

TABLE 14-1 · SPECIFIC SECRETORY IgA ANTIBODY REACTIVITY IN HUMAN COLOSTRUM AND MILK

Bacteria	Coxsackievirus
Escherichia coli O, K antigens, enterotoxin	Respiratory syncytial virus
Salmonella	Cytomegalovirus
Shigella	Influenza A virus
Vibrio cholerae	Arboviruses—Semliki forest,
Bacteroides fragilis	Ross river, Japanese B, dengue
Streptococcus mutans, other *Streptococcus* species	Parainfluenza, rhinovirus
Bordetella pertussis	**Fungi**
Clostridium diphtheriae, Clostridium tetani	*Candida albicans*
Neisseria gonorrhoeae	**Protozoa**
Campylobacter	*Giardia*
Viruses	**Other**
Rotavirus	Milk proteins
Poliovirus 1, 2, 3	Soy lectin
Echovirus	Peanut lectin
	Wheat gluten, gliadin

Modified from Cunningham-Rundles C. IgA deficiency. Immunol Allergy Clin North Am 8:435–450, 1988.

populations from different countries (Bachmann, 1965; Cassidy and Nordby, 1975; Grundbacher, 1972) and from 1 in 400 to 1 in 3000 among healthy blood donors (Frommel et al., 1973; Koistinen, 1975; Natvig et al., 1971; Periera et al., 1997). These varying results may be the result of population differences, with the Finns having the highest frequency of IgA deficiency.

One difference in these studies is the serum IgA level used to establish the diagnosis of IgA deficiency. Some authors use 10 mg/dl or lower (Buckley and Dees, 1969); others use a level of 5 mg/dl or lower, as suggested by Hong and Ammann (1989). We define selective IgA deficiency as a level of less than 7 mg/dl because many commercial laboratories have this value as the lowest detectable limit under the conditions employed.

Some studies have investigated the prevalence of IgA deficiency in predominantly male blood donors or in Rh-negative women. Although there are no apparent gender differences in the occurrence of IgA deficiency in healthy persons (Bachmann, 1965; Koistinen, 1975), male IgA-deficient individuals appear more prevalent in hospitalized groups (Buckley, 1975). Buckley (1975) also suggested that IgA deficiency may be less common in blacks than in whites. A correlated observation is that IgA deficiency is much less prevalent in Japanese blood donors than in white donors (Kanoh et al., 1986); similarly, the incidence in Malaysians is low (Yadav and Iyngkaran, 1979).

IgA deficiency may occasionally be familial (see Patterns of Inheritance), and several studies have noted a higher frequency of mother-to-child inheritance of IgA deficiency than of father-to-child inheritance (Koistinen, 1976; Oen et al., 1982). Investigating 101 families in which IgA deficiency and common variable immunodeficiency were present in more than one individual, 30 affected children had affected fathers, whereas 118 affected children had normal fathers. In contrast, 75 affected children were born to affected mothers, and 95 affected children were born to unaffected mothers (Vorechovsky et al., 2000). One explanation is the potential transplacental passage of anti-IgA antibodies, which could result in IgA deficiency in the infant. Petty and colleagues (1985) studied 27 offspring of IgA-deficient mothers; 12 had IgA levels more than 1 standard deviation (SD) below normal, and 7 had levels more than 2 SDs below normal. Of the 7 with the lowest IgA levels, 5 had mothers with anti-IgA antibodies during gestation.

In vitro studies indicate that heterologous antihuman IgA can suppress mitogen-induced IgA synthesis by human B lymphocytes and that human anti-IgA suppresses the development of human IgA plaque-forming cells (Hammarstrom et al., 1983; Warrington et al., 1982). In one study, two IgA-deficient mothers with circulating anti-IgA antibodies gave birth to four children with IgA deficiency (De Laat et al., 1991). In three of these children, anti-IgA antibodies developed before puberty. In all four, in vitro studies showed an IgA B-cell defect combined with excess IgA-specific T suppressor function. These data suggest a means whereby IgA deficiency might be perpetuated among a population with a high prevalence of IgA deficiency.

Another hypothesis suggests that the maternal major histocompatibility complex (MHC) tissue type influences the occurrence of IgA deficiency in the offspring (Vorechovsky et al., 2000).

IgA Deficiency in Healthy Subjects

Because secretory IgA is important in protecting mucous surfaces, it is of course a mystery why most IgA-deficient subjects remain healthy. For example, an early report described IgA deficiency in two healthy young physicians (Rockey et al., 1964). This lack of disease in IgA deficiency has been attributed to a compensatory increase in IgM in the secretions (Brandtzaeg et al., 1986). In IgA-deficient individuals, there may be an increase in secretory IgM (IgM attached to secretory component) in the saliva and other intestinal fluids and in IgM-bearing plasma cells in the gastrointestinal mucosa. Similarly, the colostrum of IgA-deficient subjects has been shown to contain abundant amounts of IgM (Barros et al., 1985). The saliva of IgA-deficient individuals contains biologically active IgM antibody, such as secretory IgM to *Streptococcus mutans* (Arnold et al., 1977).

Although secretory IgM is functionally active, it may not confer mucosal protection equivalent to that of secretory IgA. Indeed, IgA-deficient blood donors harbor poliovirus longer after oral vaccination than do normal subjects (Savilahti et al., 1988). Additionally, secretory IgA is subject to rapid degradation in the intestinal lumen (Richman and Brown, 1977). Norhagen and associates (1989) have questioned the view that IgM can compensate for IgA deficiency in the secretions, and they could not relate salivary IgM levels to health or frequency of illness in 63 IgA-deficient subjects. Conversely, Mellander and colleagues (1986) found that infections are more common in IgA-deficient individuals with low or absent secretory IgM.

Nilssen and co-workers (1993) have shown that oral cholera–vaccinated, IgA-deficient individuals preferentially activate intestinal IgG-producing cells rather than IgM (Nilssen et al., 1993). The response to this vaccination (which in normal subjects produces a predominantly IgA response) was not significantly different from healthy, asymptomatic IgA-deficient individuals. Another reason some IgA-deficient individuals might remain healthy is that secretory IgA is produced in normal amounts. Up to 3% of IgA-deficient individuals have normal levels of secretory IgA (Ammann and Hong, 1971b; Hazenberg et al., 1968; Swanson et al., 1968) and possess normal numbers of IgA-bearing plasma cells in the intestine.

In any case, IgA deficiency in healthy adults appears to be a stable defect over many years of follow-up (Koistenen, 1996).

IgA Deficiency in Specific Disorders

Despite the fact that most IgA-deficient subjects are not ill, IgA deficiency has been associated with an astonishing number of specific disorders (Ammann and Hong, 1970, 1971b; Burks and Steele, 1986; Cunningham-Rundles, 1990; Hanson, 1983; Schaffer et al., 1991; Strober and Sneller, 1991). A partial list is given in Table 14-2.

IgA Deficiency and Sinopulmonary Infections

Recurrent sinopulmonary infections are the most common illnesses associated with selective IgA deficiency. Indeed, these infections often represent the reason why immunoglobulin levels are first obtained and the diagnosis established. The frequency of these infections in IgA-deficient subjects varies considerably. Most infections are caused by minor bacterial pathogens or, in the absence of exact bacteriologic diagnosis, various viral agents. Sinopulmonary infections are more likely to occur in IgA-deficient individuals who have IgG2 subclass deficiency, but they also occur in IgA-deficient individuals without a second known defect (see Chapter 13).

One group found that infections may be more common in IgA-deficient individuals with low or absent levels of secretory IgM (Mellander et al., 1986), although another group, studying a larger group of IgA-deficient subjects, did not find salivary IgM levels to be increased in healthy subjects or depressed in frequently infected individuals (Norhagen et al., 1989). Brandtzaeg and colleagues (1986) have suggested that some IgA-deficient patients with frequent infections have increased IgD B cells, rather than increased IgM B cells in the nasal mucosa. Selected polymorphisms of mannan-binding lectin, which in theory could predispose IgA-deficient individuals to infections, were not found

correlated with increased number of illnesses in IgA deficiency (Aittoniemi et al., 1999).

There are several reports of chronic serious lung disease in selective IgA deficiency, including sarcoidosis, recurrent pneumonia, chronic obstructive lung disease, chronic bronchitis, bronchiectasis (Burks and Steele, 1986; Hong and Ammann, 1989; Sharma and Chandor, 1972; Webb and Condemi, 1974), and pulmonary hemosiderosis (Kreiger and Brough, 1967). As noted, those with combined IgA and IgG2 deficiency are more likely to have severe chronic respiratory infections (Bjorkander et al., 1985).

IgA Deficiency and Allergy

IgA deficiency has long been associated with the development of allergy. Even in blood bank donors in whom IgA deficiency was discovered accidentally, allergy is more common (20%) than in healthy blood donors (10%) (Kaufman and Hobbs, 1970). IgE levels are often increased in IgA deficiency (Kanok et al., 1978). The most common allergic disorders in IgA-deficient individuals are allergic conjunctivitis, rhinitis, urticaria, atopic eczema, and bronchial asthma (Ammann and Hong, 1971b; Burks and Steele, 1986; Plebani et al., 1987). Many clinicians believe that IgA-deficient subjects with asthma have more refractory disease; perhaps their susceptibility to secondary respiratory infections aggravates the associated inflammation. Food allergy may be more common in IgA-deficient patients. In one study a reduced IgA response to luminal antigens and a lack of IgM compensation were noted in the mucosa of atopic children (Sloper et al., 1981); delayed development of IgA in the intestinal tract of infants and young children has also been associated with atopy (Taylor et al., 1973).

IgA Deficiency and Gastrointestinal Tract Disorders

Patients with IgA deficiency have an increased frequency of gastrointestinal diseases (Table 14-3). The best known association is infection with *Giardia lamblia*. Presumably the lack of secretory IgA permits the

TABLE 14-2 · CONDITIONS ASSOCIATED WITH SELECTIVE IgA DEFICIENCY

Allergic disorders (Ammann and Hong, 1971b; Buckley, 1975; Burgio et al., 1980; Burks and Steele, 1986; Kanok et al., 1978)
Recurrent infections (Ammann and Hong, 1971b; Burgio el al., 1980; Burks and Steele, 1986; Schaffer et al., 1991)
Familial history of hypogammaglobulinemia (Vorechovsky et al., 1995, 2000; Wolheim et al., 1964)
Malignancy (Ammann and Hong, 1971b; Cunningham-Rundles et al., 1980; Kersey et al., 1988)
Chronic *Candida* granuloma (Claman et al., 1966)
Mental retardation and seizures (Fontana et al., 1976; Haddow et al., 1970)
Congenital sensory neuropathy (Haddow et al., 1970)
Chronic nephritis (French et al., 1987)
α_1-Antitrypsin deficiency (Casterline et al., 1978)
Familial chronic lung disease (Webb and Condemi, 1974)
Cystic fibrosis (Ammann and Hong, 1971b)
Endocrinopathy (Francois et al., 1967; Liblau and Bach, 1992; Schaffer et al., 1991)
Sarcoidosis (Claman et al., 1966; Sharma and Chandor, 1972)
Pernicious anemia (Odgers and Wangel, 1968)
Epilepsy (Fontana et al., 1976; Joubert et al., 1977)
Gastrointestinal disease (see Table 14-3)
Autoimmune disease (see Table 14-4)
Chromosomal abnormalities (see Table 14-5)

TABLE 14-3 · GASTROINTESTINAL DISEASES ASSOCIATED WITH IgA DEFICIENCY

Giardiasis	Regional enteritis
Nonspecific gastroenteritis	Total villous atrophy in the presence
Allergic disorders	of antiepithelial cell antibody
Malabsorption	Achlorhydria
Celiac disease	Henoch-Schönlein syndrome
Pancreatic insufficiency	Cholelithiasis
Nodular hepatitis	Gastrointestinal lymphoma
Primary biliary cirrhosis	Adenocarcinoma of stomach
Pernicious anemia	Nodular lymphoid hyperplasia
Lactose intolerance	
Ulcerative colitis	

attachment and proliferation of these protozoa on the intestinal epithelium (Zinneman and Kaplan, 1975). If giardiasis occurs in IgA deficiency, malabsorption resulting from flattened villi, often accompanied by nodular lymphoid hyperplasia, may develop. Diagnosis warrants multiple stool analyses and an examination of the duodenal fluid. Relapses after treatment with metronidazole or quinacrine hydrochloride are fairly common.

Nodular lymphoid hyperplasia and malabsorption also occur in IgA deficiency, but malabsorption can be present without nodular lymphoid hyperplasia (Jacobson and De Shazo, 1979). Severe diarrhea in association with IgA deficiency and lymphoid hyperplasia or malabsorption may be difficult to treat. Dramatic improvement has been reported after infusions of fresh plasma (Gryboski et al., 1967). Lactose intolerance appears to be increased in patients with IgA deficiency (Dubois et al., 1970).

Patients with celiac disease have a high incidence of IgA deficiency; approximately 1 of every 200 patients with celiac disease has IgA deficiency (Crabbé and Heremans, 1966; Crabbé and Heremans, 1967; Hanson, 1983; Savilahti et al., 1984). Such patients will lack the characteristic IgA antiendomycelial antibody used in diagnosis of celiac disease (Prince et al., 2000). In a recent review, Heneghan and colleagues (1997) found that of 604 subjects with celiac sprue, 14 had IgA deficiency (2.3%); response to a gluten-free diet for these subjects was similar to those without this deficiency. This association is unique because gluten enteropathy is not associated with other primary immunodeficiencies. It is possible that there is increased absorption of wheat antigens because of the absence of secretory IgA. Indeed, secretory IgA can bind to wheat gluten and gliadin. Intestinal biopsy specimens of patients with co-existing IgA deficiency and celiac disease are similar to those of patients with celiac disease alone, and their responses to a gluten-free diet are also similar (Klemola, 1988).

Associations between IgA deficiency and other autoimmune intestinal diseases have included chronic hepatitis (Benbassat et al., 1973), biliary cirrhosis (James et al., 1986), and pernicious anemia (Odgers and Wangel, 1968). In these cases, autoantibodies to the relevant target organ are not uncommon. It is less clear whether the anti–basement membrane antibodies found in the sera of IgA-deficient individuals play a role in tissue damage; however, in one study 3 of 31 patients with IgA deficiency and celiac disease had such an antibody (Ammann and Hong, 1971c). In another case a serum antibody to the gastrointestinal epithelial cells was associated with total villous atrophy and malabsorption (McCarthy et al., 1978).

Ulcerative colitis and regional enteritis are also associated with IgA deficiency; again, their therapeutic response is similar to that of non–IgA-deficient patients. One report described an IgA-deficient patient who had both ulcerative colitis and gluten-sensitive enteropathy (Falchuk and Falchuk, 1975).

Food allergy may be a common clinical feature of IgA deficiency. This may represent another example of abnormal antigen processing at the mucosal surface. There may be an increase in infantile atopy in IgA infants with delayed IgA maturation (Taylor et al., 1973). Similarly, another study showed a reduced IgA response and a lack of IgM compensation in the intestinal mucosa of atopic children (Sloper et al., 1981).

A syndrome of malabsorption, IgA deficiency, diabetes mellitus, and a common human leukocyte antigen (HLA) haplotype (HLA-B8 and DRw3) was reported in 3 persons in a kindred of 43 individuals (Van Thiel et al., 1977). Although some of these family members were healthy, others had multiple medical problems, including Graves' disease, vitiligo, rheumatic fever, multiple sclerosis, and hypocomplementemia. Henoch-Schönlein purpura has been described in IgA deficiency (Martini et al., 1985). Cholelithiasis has been described in several children with selective IgA deficiency (Danon et al., 1983).

Gastrointestinal Pathology

Several studies on the pathology and immunology of the gastrointestinal tract in IgA deficiency have been conducted. The main immunologic difference between the IgA-deficient and the normal intestinal tract is the substitution of IgM-secreting plasma cells for IgA-secreting cells (Klemola, 1988; McClelland et al., 1979; Plebani et al., 1983), even though there are some IgA-bearing B cells in the peripheral blood of IgA-deficient subjects (Scotta et al., 1982). This is evident in both healthy and IgA-deficient subjects. When nodular lymphoid hyperplasia develops, the nodules contain a proliferation of IgM plasma cells.

Another gastrointestinal abnormality in IgA deficiency involves the increase of intraepithelial lymphocytes in the intestinal tract. The lamina propria of the normal intestinal mucosa contains many T lymphocytes, but IgA-deficient individuals have an increased number of these cells. In both healthy and IgA-deficient subjects, these cells express CD8, the T-suppressor phenotype. These CD8 cells may limit local antibody production, cytokine secretion, or both. In agreement with this, there are increased CD8 cells in the epithelium following gluten challenge of both IgA-deficient and non–IgA-deficient celiac patients (Klemola, 1988). This implies that a sensitizing antigen stimulates the appearance of suppressor T lymphocytes.

Nonimmunologic abnormalities of the mucosal architecture may also be present. In one study, goblet numbers were significantly related to cell-mediated immunity in the nasal mucosa in IgA deficiency (Karlsson et al., 1985), but in another report they were not present in increased amounts in the intestinal tract (KIemola, 1988).

Ultrastructural abnormalities of the gastrointestinal surface epithelium have been reported in IgA deficiency, including areas of missing glycocalyx and enterocytes with "frayed" microvilli (Giorgi et al., 1986). These abnormalities were found in the absence of associated disease and were thought characteristic of "normal" IgA-deficient individuals. The lesions described may permit increased absorption of antigens from the intestinal lumen, even in the presence of compensatory mechanisms. IgA-deficient patients fed polyethylene glycol polymers have an abnormally large urinary excretion of high-molecular-weight polymers, indicating excess gastrointestinal absorption of high-molecular-weight substances (Cunningham-Rundles et al., 1988). Because polyethylene glycol is immunologically inert, this supports the hypothesis that structural gastrointestinal lesions are present in IgA deficiency.

IgA Deficiency and the Nervous System

Early reported cases indicated a connection between selective IgA deficiency and mental retardation (Haddow et al., 1970; West et al., 1962). IgA deficiency also occurs in patients with ataxia-telangiectasia (Aguilar et al., 1968) and myasthenia gravis (Liblau et al., 1992). The relationship of IgA deficiency to neurologic disease is complicated by the fact that anticonvulsant therapy can, for unknown reasons, reduce serum IgA levels. Hydantoin (Dilantin) has been implicated most often (Ruff et al., 1987; Sorrell et al., 1971), but sodium valproate can also reduce the serum IgA level (Joubert et al., 1977). In persons with epilepsy treated with hydantoin who were found to be IgA deficient, the most prevalent HLA haplotypes were HLA-A1, HLA-A2, and HLA-B8 (Shakir et al., 1978). Serum IgA levels, however, are also sometimes low in untreated epileptic patients. Autoantibodies to muscle and brain nicotinic acetylcholine receptors were found in three subjects with epilepsy with IgA deficiency (Fontana et al., 1976, 1978).

IgA Deficiency and Autoimmune Diseases

A number of autoimmune diseases have been associated with selective IgA deficiency. Based on various reviews (Ammann and Hong, 1970, 1971b; Bluestone et al., 1970; Cunningham-Rundles et al., 1981; Hong and Ammann, 1989; Itescu, 1996; Liblau and Bach, 1992; Price et al., 1999; Rankin and Isenberg, 1997; Sandler and Zlotnick, 1976; Schaffer et al., 1991; Sleasman, 1996; Smith et al., 1978; Strober and Sneller, 1991), autoimmunity may represent the most common association with IgA deficiency (Table 14-4). The most common of these conditions are juvenile rheumatoid arthritis, adult rheumatoid arthritis, and systemic lupus erythematosus, but they also include endocrine disease, vitiligo, hemolytic anemia, idiopathic thrombocytopenic purpura, and neurologic diseases. Davies and colleagues (2001) have identified four children with IgA deficiency, polyarticular arthritis, and monoallelic deletion at 22q11, the DiGeorge region chromosomal site.

The sera of IgA-deficient subjects often contain autoantibodies, even in the absence of autoimmune illness. Antibodies against thyroglobulin, red blood cells, thyroid

TABLE 14-4 · AUTOIMMUNE DISEASES ASSOCIATED WITH IgA DEFICIENCY

Rheumatoid arthritis (Bluestone et al., 1970; Cassidy et al., 1971; Davies et al., 2001; Johns et al., 1978; Mbuyi et al., 1983)
Systemic lupus erythematosus (Ammann and Hong, 1970; Rankin and Isenberg, 1997; Smith et al., 1970)
Thyroiditis (Ammann and Hong, 1970, 1971b)
Still's disease (Bluestone et al., 1970; Cassidy et al., 1973)
Transfusion reactions (Vyas and Fudenberg, 1969; Vyas et al., 1968)
Pernicious anemia (Odgers and Wangel, 1968)
Pulmonary hemosiderosis (Ammann and Hong, 1970, 1971b; Krieger and Brough, 1967)
Myasthenia gravis (Liblau et al., 1992)
Vitiligo (Torrelo et al., 1992)
Dermatomyositis (Cassidy et al., 1969b)
Coombs' positive hemolytic anemia (Sandler and Zlotnick, 1976)
Idiopathic Addison's disease (Francois et al., 1967)
Henoch-Schönlein syndrome (Martini et al., 1985)
Cerebral vasculitis (Ammann and Hong, 1970)
Idiopathic thrombocytopenic purpura (Ozsoylu et al., 1988)
Regional enteritis (Claman et al., 1970)
Ulcerative colitis (Claman et al., 1970)
Diabetes mellitus (Price et al., 1999; Smith et al., 1978)
21-Hydroxylase deficiency (Cobain et al., 1985)
Primary biliary cirrhosis (James et al., 1986)

microsomal antigens, basement membrane, smooth muscle cells, pancreatic cells, nuclear proteins, cardiolipin, human collagen, and adrenal cells have been identified (Ablin, 1972; Ammann and Hong, 1970, 1971b; Cunningham-Rundles et al., 1981; Pascual-Salcedo et al., 1988; Sandler and Zlotnick, 1976; Silver et al., 1973; Torrelo et al., 1992; Wells et al., 1973). Cunningham-Rundles and colleagues (1981) found that IgA-deficient patients with high titers of antibodies to cow's milk are also more likely to have other autoantibodies. They suggested that IgA-deficient subjects with anti–food antibodies have enhanced gastrointestinal antigen absorption and that food-derived antigens could cross-react with internal self-antigens. The sera of IgA-deficient individuals may contain antibodies to a bovine mucoprotein of the fat globule membrane formed by the mammary gland (Butler and Oskvig, 1974). Sera with high levels of immune complexes may potentially stimulate autoantibody production and even autoimmune disease (Ammann and Hong, 1970; Cassidy et al., 1971; Cunningham-Rundles et al., 1981; Kornstadt and Nordhagen, 1974) (see Milk Antibodies).

Anti-IgA Antibodies

A significant proportion of IgA-deficient individuals have anti-IgA antibodies in their serum. Although blood or blood products given to IgA-deficient individuals with high titers of anti-IgA antibodies can lead to severe, even fatal, transfusion reactions, such reactions are actually quite rare. Hospitalized patients, some of whom are certain to be IgA deficient, are not screened for anti-IgA antibodies prior to blood transfusions. The actual incidence of anti-IgA–mediated blood infusion reactions, due to anti-IgA antibodies, has been estimated as 1.3 per million units of blood or blood products infused (Laschinger et al., 1984).

Anti-IgA antibodies can be directed to IgA1 (most commonly), IgA2, or the allotypic variants A2m(1) or A2m(2). These antibodies occur with a reported frequency of 9.6% to 44% in IgA-deficient subjects (Björkander et al., 1987; Koistinen et al., 1977). Anti-IgA antibodies are more common in IgA-deficient individuals with undetectable IgA but may occasionally occur when the IgA level is 10 mg/dl or higher. Ferreira and associates (1988) found that 39% of their IgA-deficient patients had anti-IgA antibodies; 22% of those in the antibody-positive group had IgA levels between 1.1 and 5 mg/dl, and the remaining 78% had IgA levels lower than 1.1 mg/dl.

Anti-IgA antibodies are usually of the IgG1 class, are more closely associated with the presence of HLA-DR3 (Hammarstrom et al., 1983), and are more common in IgA-deficient subjects who are also IgG2-deficient (Cunningham-Rundles et al., 1993; Ferreira et al., 1988). Anti-IgA antibodies may be of the IgE isotype, leading to true anaphylactic reactions (Burks et al., 1986); however, the actual incidence of such antibodies is unknown, and some studies have not found them (Björkander et al., 1987). Others have concluded that they are not likely to be important because direct skin-prick testing with IgA in a patient with IgE-anti-IgA and a prior reaction to immunoglobulin was negative (Nadorp et al., 1973.) Because IgA-deficient and IgG2-deficient individuals often have poor but not absent antibody responses and may require immunoglobulin treatment (Oxelius et al., 1981), they may be at particular risk for infusion reactions during immunoglobulin treatment.

IgA-Related Infusion Reactions

In the past, most IgA-related infusion reactions occurred following blood transfusions (Leikola and Vyas, 1971; Vyas and Fudenberg, 1969; Vyas et al., 1968); with the increased use of IVIG, however, more reactions now result from IVIG infusions. IVIGs contain varying amounts of IgA, but IgA-depleted preparations are available and are usually well tolerated, even in patients with high titers of anti-IgA antibodies (Cunningham-Rundles et al., 1993).

IgA Deficiency and Malignancy

Carcinoma (particularly adenocarcinoma of the stomach) and lymphoma (usually of B-cell origin) are also associated with IgA deficiency (Kersey et al., 1988). Often the lymphomas are extranodal and involve the jejunum. Whether nodular lymphoid hyperplasia leads to lymphoma is not known. In general, IgA deficiency is more common than expected in cancer patients; in one cancer hospital, 12 of 4210 patients had selective IgA deficiency, an incidence of 1 in 342 (0.3%). One patient had gastric cancer and another had primary hepatoma (Cunningham-Rundles et al., 1980). Ten other cancers did not involve the gastrointestinal tract.

Other reported cancers in selective IgA deficiency include carcinoma of the stomach and colon, ovarian cancer, lymphosarcoma, melanoma, and thymoma (Kersey et al., 1988). One case of multiple neoplasms in an adolescent IgA-deficient child involving the thymus, scalp, hand, eyes, colon, and brain has been reported. This child had an IgA-deficient sibling who died of lymphosarcoma (Hamoudi et al., 1974).

Transient IgA Deficiency

Although IgA deficiency is generally a permanent condition (Koskinen et al., 1994), occasionally a spontaneous remission occurs (Blum et al., 1982). Petty and co-workers (1973) gave fresh-frozen plasma repeatedly to an IgA-deficient child with rheumatoid arthritis, resulting in permanent normalization of the serum IgA level. In a few such instances of transient IgA deficiency with recovery, the original IgA level was lower than 5 mg/dl; in most such cases, however, the IgA level is between 5 and 30 mg/dl (i.e., partial IgA deficiency) (Plebani et al., 1986). In this cohort of IgA-deficient subjects, half of those who had partial deficiency underwent spontaneous resolution, whereas none with an IgA level lower than 5 mg/dl experienced spontaneous recovery (Plebani et al., 1986). Resolution of IgA deficiency is much more common in children under 5 years of age (Joller et al., 1981), presumably the result of a delayed maturation of the IgA system.

Acquired IgA Deficiency

IgA deficiency many follow drug therapy or viral infection. Penicillamine (Proesman et al., 1976), sulfasalazine (Leickly and Buckley, 1986), hydantoin (Fontana et al., 1976; Seager et al., 1975), cyclosporine (Murphy et al., 1993), gold (Johns et al., 1978), fenclofenac (Farr et al., 1985), sodium valproate (Joubert et al., 1977), and captopril can produce a usually reversible IgA deficiency (Hammarstrom et al., 1991). On the other hand, congenital rubella and Epstein-Barr virus infections may result in persistent IgA deficiency (Soothill et al., 1966). A unique case of acquired IgA deficiency was reported by Hammarstrom and colleagues (1985c), who noted that an IgA-deficient bone marrow transplant donor transferred the deficiency to the recipient, who previously had normal IgA levels.

Partial IgA Deficiency

Many patients have a serum IgA level lower than expected for age (i.e., less than 2 SDs from the mean, but above 5 mg/dl), a condition that can be considered "partial" IgA deficiency. This is more common in children, presumably because of the immaturity of the IgA system. As noted earlier, such patients are more likely to undergo spontaneous remission than patients with an

IgA level lower than 5 mg/dl. Many patients with partial IgA deficiency have normal levels of salivary IgA and are usually healthy. Partial IgA deficiency can be the result of deletions of genes controlling either the α1 or α2 chains, a condition termed selective IgA1 (or IgA2) subclass deficiency.

Selective IgA Subclass Deficiency

In rare cases, IgA1 or IgA2 deficiency has been identified as a result of gene deletions on chromosome 14. Sometimes the α1 gene is deleted along with other heavy-chain genes (Olsson et al., 1991). The first case of selective IgA subclass deficiency was identified in an inbred Tunisian Berber family. The propositus was a healthy, 75-year-old woman with absent serum IgA1, IgG1, IgG2, and IgG4; increased IgG3, IgA2, and IgM; and normal IgE. The gene deletions included three IgG subclass genes, γ1, γ2, and γ4, the pseudo-ε and α genes (Lefranc et al., 1982). Two brothers and one sister of the propositus were apparently heterozygous for this defect. Presumably, the good health of the index case was due to increased serum IgG3 and IgM levels and the presence of IgA2.

A similar, unrelated Tunisian family was described by Lefranc and colleagues (1983). In this family a 45-year-old Tunisian man whose only medical condition was a chronic cough had deleted genes for IgG1, IgG2, IgG4, and IgA1. Two other family members had two different chromosomal deletions, one a small deletion of the α1 gene and the other a larger deletion involving the γ1, γ2, γ4, and α1 genes. Migone and associates (1984) and Carbonara and Demarchi (1986) reported additional families in whom similar deletions were found. Deletion of the α2 gene occurs less commonly than deletions involving α1 genes, but in one case the α2 gene was deleted in conjunction with the pseudo-ε, γ2, γ4, and ε genes (Bottaro et al., 1989).

From these studies, it appears that there may be instability of a region of chromosome 14, with a potential "hot" recombination region being present between the γ2 and the switch α2 loci (Chaabani et al., 1985; Migone et al., 1984). Presumably, because of the location of this hot spot, no individuals have been both IgA1 deficient and IgA2 deficient on a genetic basis.

To ascertain the occurrence of such heavy-chain gene deletions, Carbonara and Demarchi (1986) studied 5000 normal Italian blood donors and found two subjects who lacked IgG2, IgG4, IgE, and IgA1. Although gene deletion is probably a rare cause of IgA1 deficiency, the data suggest that if the frequency of homozygous deletions were as high as that identified by this study (1 in 5000), the actual gene frequency might be of the order of 1 in 70.

Selective absence of IgA2 has been reported in a mother and daughter (Van Loghem et al., 1983). The mother had a low level of IgA1 and antibodies to IgA2, and the daughter had a normal IgA1 level. Both had normal IgG subclass levels. The molecular defect in this case is not known.

Pathogenesis

T-cell abnormalities have often been sought in IgA deficiency because a T-cell regulatory abnormality is an attractive hypothesis. In athymic or thymectomized animals, T cells are involved in B-cell differentiation into IgA-secreting plasma cells (McGhee et al., 1989). Neonatal thymectomy leads to IgA deficiency (Benveniste et al., 1969; Perey et al., 1970). The thymically impaired nude mouse is IgA deficient (Pritchard et al., 1973). A reversible T-cell influence might explain why IgA deficiency can resolve spontaneously after exposure to certain drugs. Despite these reasons for suspecting a T-cell defect in IgA deficiency, few IgA-deficient patients seem to have identifiable defects using current analytical methods.

IgA deficiency is associated with certain MHC haplotypes (see IgA Deficiency and the MHC). This suggests that the inheritance of a certain gene in the MHC area of chromosome 6 confers susceptibility to IgA deficiency. A gene of this sort may potentially activate IgA B-cell maturation.

Molecular analyses have demonstrated some errors of switch (S) μ to S α rearrangements in peripheral B cells from IgA-deficient subjects. Two types of defects, low expression of both secreted and membrane forms of productive constant (C) α messenger RNA (mRNA) in IgA-switched B cells and impaired IgA switching, were characterized in IgA-deficient subjects homozygous for the MHC haplotype (HLA-B8, HLA-SC01, HLA-DR3). This could reflect a blockade in post-IgA switch differentiation of B cells (Wang et al., 1999).

Animal Models

In addition to the IgA-deficient nude mouse, there are a few other animal models of IgA deficiency. Transgenic IgA−/− knockout mice have been generated by targeting the entire IgA switch region and the 5′ half of the constant region (Harriman et al., 1999; Mbawuike et al., 1999). A second, more indirect mouse model emphasizes the role of transforming growth factor-β (TGF-β1) in isotype switch and secretion of IgA, because the TGF-β1 knockout is partially IgA deficient (Van Glinkel et al., 1999) and the TGF-β1R knockout has impaired mucosal IgA responses (Cazac and Roes, 2000).

Similarly, mice with a deletion of the α chain of the interleukin-5 (IL-5) receptor (IL-5Rα−/−) have reduced levels of IgA in mucosal secretions as compared with wild-type mice, but the levels of IgA in serum are not reduced (Hiroi et al., 1999). IL-5 is important for the development of IgA B cells in the intestine (and perhaps elsewhere), and disruption of the IL-5 receptor reduces mucosal antibody responses. In another mouse model, the tumor necrosis factor and lymphotoxin-α (a double knockout, TNF/LT-α−/−) knockout, have only low numbers of total IgA-producing cells, no Peyer's patches, and no mucosal IgA (Koni et al., 1997). Mice lacking exon 2 of the polymeric Ig receptor (pIgR) have very reduced secretory IgA levels, whereas serum IgA is markedly increased (Shimada et al., 1999).

Genetics

Patterns of Inheritance

In most cases, IgA deficiency appears to be inherited in a sporadic fashion. Many familial cases, however, have been described (Ashman et al., 1992; Fudenberg et al., 1962; Huntley and Koistinen, 1976; Oen et al., 1982; Schaffer et al., 1989; Stephenson, 1968; Vorchovsky et al., 1999a, 2000). Modes of inheritance include autosomal recessive (Koistinen, 1976; Van Loghem, 1974), multifactorial (Buckley, 1975; Grundbacher, 1972), and autosomal dominant with variable (Stocker et al., 1968) or incomplete expression (Cleland and Bell, 1978).

How often are relatives of IgA-deficient subjects also IgA deficient? Oen and colleagues (1982) studied relatives of 60 IgA-deficient donors. In 48 families, no additional IgA-deficient members were discovered. In 21 of these families, all first-degree relatives of at least two consecutive generations were studied. For the remaining 12 families, IgA deficiency was found in three generations in one family, in two generations in six families, and in one generation in five families. Thus among first-degree relatives of affected blood donors, the prevalence of IgA deficiency was 7.5%, a 38-fold increase over that of unrelated donors. As noted earlier, IgA deficiency is more common in the children of IgA-deficient women than in the offspring of IgA-deficient men (Petty et al., 1985; Vorchovsky et al., 2000).

IgA deficiency is also relatively common in family members of patients with common variable immunodeficiency (CVID). Several families have shown IgA deficiency in the first generation, hypogammaglobulinemia in the second generation, and IgA deficiency in the third generation (Ashman et al., 1992; Hammarstrom et al., 2000; Vorchovsky et al., 2000; Wollheim et al., 1964). This suggests that IgA deficiency and CVID are genetically related diseases (see Chapter 13).

Cytogenetics

IgA deficiency has been reported in children with chromosomal abnormalities, particularly those involving chromosome 18 (Table 14-5). Ring chromosome 18 and deletion of the short or long arm of chromosome 18 have been described. These patients have other congenital defects, such as facial, ear, and hand abnormalities; growth retardation; muscular hypotonia; and mental retardation. The 18q– syndrome (long-arm deletion) is a predictable syndrome of mental retardation, short stature, hypotonia, and facial and hand abnormalities (Werteleki and Gerald, 1971; Wilson et al., 1979). To discern which area of the long arm leads to these abnormalities when deleted, Wilson and associates (1979) studied patients with overlapping areas of deletions. The consistently deleted band was 18q21.3, but only two of these patients were IgA deficient. About half of patients with the 18p– syndrome and ring chromosome 18 are IgA-deficient (Lewkonia et al., 1980). How these abnormalities lead to IgA deficiency is not understood; no particular area of chromosome 18 is consistently abnormal or deleted. A search for linkage to chromosome 18 in 83 families in whom IgA deficiency and/or common variable immunodeficiency had been identified, using 17 marker loci, did not reveal linkage of the defect to any marker (Vorchovsky et al., 1999b).

IgA deficiency occurs in other chromosome abnormalities, including a Turner's syndrome variant with an Xq isochromosome (Silver et al., 1973); IgE deficiency

---

TABLE 14-5 · CHROMOSOME ABNORMALITIES IN SELECTIVE IgA DEFICIENCY

Chromosome or Syndrome Involved	Associated Features	Reference
Chromosome 18		
18p–	Retardation and multiple anomalies	Ruvalcaba and Thuline (1969)
18p–	Multiple anomalies	Ogata et al. (1977)
18p–	Growth hormone deficiency	Leisti et al. (1973)
18q–	Multiple anomalies	Feingold et al. (1969)
18q–	Cleft palate, mental and growth retardation	Lewkonia et al. (1980)
18q–	Hypothyroidism	Faed et al. (1972)
18q–	—	Steward et al. (1970)
18q22	—	Wilson et al. (1979)
18q+ mosaic	Retardation, multiple dysmorphic features	Lewkonia et al. (1980)
Ring 18	Multiple dysmorphic features, retardation	Finley et al. (1968)
Ring 18/18p	Short stature, hypotonia, facial abnormalities	Taalman et al. (1987)
Ring 18, trisomy 21	—	Burgio et al. (1980)
17–18p–, 21–22q	Two primary cancers	Goh et al. (1976)
Ring 22	Microcephaly; large, low-set ears; epicanthal fold; syndactyly of toes; unstable gait; mental retardation	Taalman et al. (1987)
Turner's syndrome	Changes of Turner's syndrome	Silver et al. (1973)
Xq isochromosome	—	Choudat et al. (1979)
Branched chromosomes 1, 9, and 16 (lymphocytes only)	IgE deficiency, recurrent pulmonary infections; neurologic degeneration	Tiepolo et al. (1979)
Polymorphic chromosome changes	—	Munoz-López et al. (1977)
Klinefelter's syndrome	Changes of Klinefelter's syndrome	Tsung and Ajlouni (1978)
Karyotype instability with multiple 7/14 and 7/7 rearrangements	Microcephaly, growth retardation	Hustinx et al. (1979)
22q11 deletion syndrome	DiGeorge anomaly, velocardiofacial syndrome	Davies et al. (2001)

with multibranched chromosomes 1, 9, and 16 (Tiepolo et al., 1979); and Klinefelter's syndrome (Tsung and Ajlouni, 1978). IgA deficiency has been associated with the rare 20-nail dystrophy (Leong et al., 1982) and with α_1-antitrypsin deficiency (Casterline et al., 1978; Ostergaard, 1982). This latter association is of interest because α_1-antitrypsin is encoded near the α chain of IgA on chromosome 14 (Cox et al., 1982).

Most IgA-deficient individuals without physical or mental deficiencies, however, have no chromosome abnormalities. Herrmann and associates (1982) found no chromosome abnormalities in 70 IgA-deficient blood donors and in 10 symptomatic IgA-deficient patients. Taalman and co-workers (1987) reported that 2 of 17 of the IgA-deficient children studied had chromosome abnormalities, but both children had pronounced physical and mental abnormalities.

IgA Deficiency and the MHC

An association between IgA deficiency and certain HLA types of the MHC has been reported (Table 14-6). In diabetes mellitus and concomitant IgA deficiency, HLA-B8 frequency was significantly increased (Lakhanpal et al., 1988; Van Thiel et al., 1977). Juvenile-onset diabetes mellitus itself, however, is associated with HLA-B8 (and HLA-DR3), and therefore a relationship between HLA-B8 and IgA deficiency may be secondary to this disease association. Similarly, there is an increased frequency of HLA-A1 and HLA-B8 in patients with autoimmune disorders and IgA deficiency (Ambrus et al., 1977), but again, this may result from the HLA-B8–autoimmunity association. In one study of IgA-deficient patients with recurrent upper respiratory tract infections, no association with HLA-B8 was found (Seignalet et al., 1978). In a group of IgA-deficient patients with epilepsy, an association with HLA-A2 was identified (Fontana et al., 1978).

Hammarstrom and Smith (1983) studied 21 unrelated healthy IgA-deficient Swedish blood donors and noted a significant increase in HLA-A1 ($P < .05$), HLA-B8 ($P < .01$), and HLA-DR3 ($P < .001$). In a study of 23,782 healthy U.S. blood donors, 67 IgA-deficient individuals were identified; HLA typing in 36 indicated a significant association with HLA-A1, HLA-29, HLA-B8, and HLA-B14 (Strothman et al., 1986).

Wilton and colleagues (1985) studied HLA types in 17 individuals from 13 Australian families with complete or partial IgA deficiency (IgA levels < 30 mg/dl). They also studied DR antigens and the complement components C4A, C4B, and Bf. Their report noted an increased frequency of HLA-A1, HLA-B8, and HLA-DR3; in addition, of the 29 independent haplotypes

observed in the IgA-deficient subjects, 22 included deletions, duplications, or a defective C4 or 21-hydroxylase locus. The investigators suggested that there may be a gene regulating serum IgA concentration in the MHC region of chromosome 6 and that associations with three main extended haplotypes explained most previously reported HLA-IgA deficiency associations (see Table 14-6). A survey of 150 other individuals with at least one of these haplotypes revealed only two who were IgA-deficient, which suggested recessive inheritance, with penetrance determined by another factor not linked to the MHC (Wilton et al., 1985). The HLA-B14, HLA-C4A2, HLA-C4B1/2, BfS haplotype (which also carries a C4B duplication) is itself associated with 21-hydroxylase and IgA deficiencies (Cobain et al., 1985).

Others have investigated the connection between the MHC haplotype (HLA-B8, HLA-SC01, HLA-DR3) and selective IgA deficiency. The prevalence of individual immunoglobulin deficiencies in blood donors with this haplotype ranges from 13% to 37%, significantly higher than rates in noncarriers or general controls. There is an increased frequency of IgA and IgG4 deficiency only in homozygotes (13.3% and 30%, respectively) as compared with heterozygotes (1.7% and 3.4%) or noncarriers (1.6% each), suggesting recessive expression (Alper et al., 2000).

Other genes in the region of the MHC have been investigated in IgA deficiency such as TNF polymorphisms (de la Concha et al., 2000). The MHC class III genes encoding complement components C2, C4A, and C4B and 21-hydroxylase have also been studied in patients with IgA deficiency or CVI. Twelve of 19 patients with CVI (63%) and 9 of 16 with IgA deficiency (56%) had rare C2, C4A, or 21-hydroxylase A deletions, compared with 5 of 34 (14%) in healthy individuals (Schaffer et al., 1989, 1991). Olerup and associates (1990, 1992) implicated the amino acid at codon 57 of the HLA-DQB1 gene in susceptibility to IgA deficiency. The putative protective allele had aspartic acid at position 57, whereas the susceptibility allele had an alanine or valine at this position. Despite these findings, several pairs of discordant twins have been reported, with only one of each set having IgA deficiency (Huntley and Stephenson, 1968; Lewkonia et al., 1976).

Laboratory Findings

Milk Antibodies

A common feature of IgA deficiency is the occurrence of increased levels of serum antibodies to cow's milk

---

TABLE 14-6 · HISTOCOMPATIBILITY SUPRATYPES WITH IgA DEFICIENCY

Class I		Class III			Class II	
A1 Cw7	B8	C4AQO	C4B1	Bfs	DR3	
	Bw65(14)	C4A2	C4B1/s	Bfs	DR1	DQW1
	Bw57(17)	C4A6	C4B1	Bfs	—	

Data from Wilton et al., 1985; Schaffer et al., 1991; Olerup et al., 1992; Vorechovsky et al., 1995; Vorechovsky et al., 1999b; Vorechovsky et al., 2000; Wang et al., 1999.

proteins and other proteins of bovine origin (cow, sheep, and goat) (Ammann and Hong, 1971a; Buckley and Dees, 1969; Huntley et al., 1971; Lopez and Hyslop, 1968). When these antibodies are in high titer, they can be visualized by the double-diffusion procedure in agar gels and are known as milk precipitins (Fig. 14-2) (Buckley and Dees, 1969). Up to 50% of IgA-deficient individuals have precipitins to cow's milk (Cunningham-Rundles et al., 1978, 1979a; Tomasi and Katz, 1971). The antibody appears to be directed against bovine IgM, a component of cow's milk (Tomasi and Katz, 1971). Most IgA-deficient individuals have IgG1 and IgG4 antibodies directed to ovalbumin and β-lactoglobulin and IgG1, IgG2, IgG3, and IgG4 (IgG1 > IgG2 > IgG3 > IgG4) antibodies to casein, bovine IgM, and gliadin, a component of wheat gluten (Husby et al., 1992).

The presence in IgA-deficient serum of large amounts of IgG milk antibodies directed to bovine IgM, and that cross-react with sheep and goat IgM, can cause confusion when such sera are examined for IgA deficiency if the IgA antiserum used is produced in these species. A false-positive result in radial immunodiffusion or in nephelometry can occur, leading to the interpretation of normal or increased IgA levels (Ammann and Hong, 1971a; Leikola and Vyas, 1971). This problem is not entirely solved by switching to rabbit antiserum because the sera of IgA-deficient subjects may contain antibodies directed to rabbit IgM (Truedsson et al., 1982).

Immune Complexes

In IgA-deficient patients, the gastrointestinal tract is sufficiently leaky so that circulating immune complexes develop in the patient's serum 15 to 60 minutes after drinking a glass of milk (Fig. 14-3) (Cunningham-Rundles et al., 1978, 1979a, 1979b). The antigens identified in these immune complexes are bovine milk protein antigens (Cunningham-Rundles, 1981). These immune complexes are apparently benign because renal disease, vasculitis, and arthritis are not common in IgA deficiency. Arthralgia, autoimmune disease, and neurologic disease, however, are common in IgA-deficient patients and are associated with high titers of immune complexes (Cunningham-Rundles et al., 1981).

Other Humoral Abnormalities

Other immunologic abnormalities in some IgA-deficient subjects include increased levels of serum IgG, IgM, or IgE (but not IgD) (Ammann and Hong, 1971b; Buckley and Fiscus, 1975; Plebani et al., 1983). Other patients exhibit low-molecular-weight serum IgM (monomeric IgM instead of pentameric IgM) (Kwitko et al., 1982),

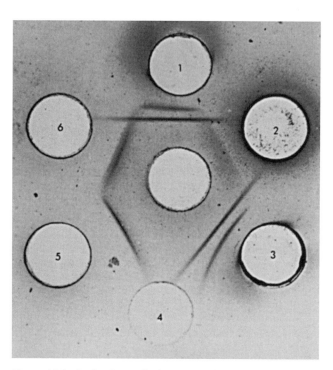

Figure 14-2 · Antibovine antibody examined by precipitation in agar wells. Wells 1 and 3 contain cow's milk, well 2 contains goat serum, well 4 contains horse serum, well 5 contains sheep serum, and well 6 contains selective IgA deficiency. A precipitin line indicating identity is shown between cow, sheep, and goat sera and cow's milk but not with horse serum. An additional precipitin line is seen with cow's milk, which is not present in cow, sheep, or goat serum.

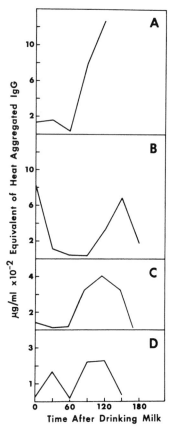

Figure 14-3 · Immune complexes in IgA deficiency. Four IgA-deficient subjects *(A–D)* were given 100 ml of cow's milk to drink. Before and at 30-minute intervals after milk ingestion, the amount of circulating immune complex was measured in the serum using the Raji cell radioimmunoassay. (Adapted from Cunningham-Rundles C et al. Bovine antigens and the formation of circulating immune complexes in selective IgA deficiency. J Clin Invest. 64:270–272, 1979. Copyright permission of The American Society for Clinical Investigation.)

increased J-chain–positive IgG B cells following stimulation with pokeweed mitogen (Yasuda et al., 1981), and a common cross-reactive idiotype on certain antibodies (Cunningham-Rundles and Feng, 1988). An associated IgA2 deficiency or IgG2 and IgG4 deficiency may occur (Oxelius et al., 1981). The frequency of the IgA-IgG2 dual deficiency may differ in ethnic groups; Oxelius and co-workers (1981) found that 7 out of 37 (19%) IgA-deficient Swedish patients were IgG2-deficient, whereas Cunningham-Rundles and colleagues (1983), using the same methods, found that 3 out of 39 (8%) IgA-deficient U.S. patients were IgG2 deficient.

IgA B Cells

A fundamental defect in IgA deficiency is the failure of IgA-bearing B lymphocytes to mature into IgA-secreting plasma cells. A cardinal feature is a paucity of IgA-bearing gastrointestinal plasma cells (Crabbé and Heremans, 1967) and the substitution of IgM- or IgG-bearing plasma cells instead, which are activated on antigen challenge (Nilssen et al., 1993). There are decreased (but not absent) numbers of IgA-bearing B cells in the peripheral circulation (Lawton et al., 1972), which bear an immature phenotype—that is, IgA-bearing B cells that are also positive for IgM and IgD (Conley and Cooper, 1981). The α heavy-chain genes and their switch regions have no known abnormalities (Hammarstrom et al., 1985a). The failure of terminal B-cell differentiation has been attributed to the following:

1. Inadequate or defective T-helper cells (King et al., 1979)
2. IgA-specific T-cell suppressors (Atwater and Tomasi, 1978; Waldmann et al., 1976)
3. An intrinsic B-cell defect (Cassidy et al., 1979; Inoue et al., 1984)
4. The presence of maternal anti-IgA antibodies that suppress fetal IgA development (Petty et al., 1985)
5. Impaired switching at a molecular level (Islam et al., 1994; Wang et al., 1999)
6. Inheritance of susceptibility factor on the sixth chromosome (Vorchovsky et al., 1999a; Wilton et al., 1985)
7. Cytokine skewing: defects in IL-5 or TGF-β secretion or receptor abnormalities (Cazac and Roes, 2000; Lio et al., 1998; Van Ginkel et al., 1999)

T-Cell Abnormalities

Other than the T-cell regulatory abnormalities postulated, T-cell effector function generally appears to be normal in IgA deficiency. Natural killer cells are normal (Stannegard et al., 1983). Inconsistent cellular abnormalities that have been reported include reduced B-cell expression of IgA Fc receptors (Adachi et al., 1983), low serum thymic factor (Iwata et al., 1981), decreased lymphoproliferative responses to phytohemagglutinin on limiting dilution (Cowan et al., 1980), and reduced interferon-γ production following phytohemagglutinin stimulation (Epstein and Ammann, 1974). Levitt and Cooper (1981) studied in vitro plasma cell differentiation in a family in whom three members were IgA deficient. Two healthy IgA-deficient family members had subtle cellular abnormalities of B and T lymphocytes, whereas lymphocytes of the symptomatic IgA-deficient child had decreased in vitro production of all immunoglobulin classes. Following clinical improvement and plasma infusions from her healthy, nonimmunodeficient father, the child's in vitro lymphocyte culture results became similar to those of her healthy IgA-deficient brother and sister. These data suggest that the mechanisms for IgA deficiency in a given family are inherited.

Pathology

The pathologic findings in selective IgA deficiency are dependent on the associated diseases. IgA-deficient patients with malabsorption have blunting of villi on jejunal biopsy as in celiac disease. In the few patients studied, lymph node specimens reveal normal follicle formation and intact thymic-dependent and thymic-independent areas (Hobbs, 1968). Intestinal biopsy usually reveals abundant plasma cells, mostly secreting IgM (Ammann and Hong, 1971c; Crabbé et al., 1965). A small number of IgA-containing plasma cells (usually IgA2) may be found (Andre et al., 1978). A few autopsy reports are available. Kreiger and Brough (1967) reported an unusual case with pulmonary hemosiderosis, bronchiectasis, and portal fibrosis of the liver. Detailed information was not given on the thymus, although the gland was present. Generalized hypertrophy of the lymph nodes was present, along with loss of normal architecture and diminution of the follicles.

Evaluation of the Patient with IgA Deficiency

When IgA deficiency is identified in a healthy person with no significant medical history, no further evaluation is needed. Usually, quantitative immunoglobulins have been ordered because a significant clinical problem has emerged. In these cases, especially when significant infections have been present, IgG subclass levels should be performed. A combined IgA-IgG2 subclass-deficient patient may have a normal IgG levels because of an elevation of other IgG subclasses; such individuals may have a history of serious or even life-threatening illness. Many of these patients may not respond to vaccination with pneumococcal polysaccharides. For these patients, IVIG is sometimes indicated, but anti-IgA antibodies are common in these patients. Thus assays for anti-IgA antibodies should be completed prior to IVIG therapy; if antibodies are present, IVIG should be given with trepidation, along with medication and under close supervision. An IgA-depleted IVIG preparation, such as Gammagard-SD or Polygam-SD, should be used (Cunningham-Rundles et al., 1993; Ferreira et al., 1988).

The antibody responses to polysaccharide antigen (pneumococcal or meningococcal vaccine) are assessed by obtaining a baseline serum titer, immunizing, and obtaining a postvaccination serum titer 1 month later. The paired sera should be tested simultaneously to enhance this reliability. Children under 2 years of age have poor responses to polysaccharide vaccines; therefore testing before age 2 is not done. Some IgA-deficient patients have persistent allergic symptoms. An allergic evaluation, including skin and or radioallergosorbent testing, may be indicated.

IgA deficiency can be induced by various drugs (see Acquired IgA Deficiency). In IgA-deficient patients taking such a drug, a substitute drug (e.g., phenobarbital for phenytoin) can be given for 3 to 6 months and the IgA level redrawn; sometimes the IgA deficiency will disappear.

Serum immunoglobulin levels on family members to ascertain the inheritance pattern, although of scientific interest, are not usually indicated unless a family member has symptoms. Similarly, HLA typing in patients or their families, except for research purposes, is not indicated unless a family member has symptoms. IgA-deficient patients with certain HLA types are not more likely to have specific medical problems.

Quantitation of IgA1 and IgA2 levels in the partially IgA-deficient patient is difficult and expensive and not especially informative. In one report, IgA-deficient children (ages 3 to 10 years) had variable IgA1 and IgA2 levels, with both subclasses present in all children (Conley et al., 1983). Although there is an association between IgA deficiency and autoimmune disease, the likelihood of an autoimmune disease developing in an individual IgA-deficient patient is probably low. Thus extensive screening for autoantibodies is not indicated in the asymptomatic IgA-deficient patient. Whether anti-IgA antibodies should be determined in all IgA-deficient patients is debatable. Although IgA antibodies can produce serious anaphylactic reactions if blood or blood products (including IVIG) are infused, the likelihood of such a reaction is low. Tests for anti-IgA antibodies are not widely available but can be done in several commercial laboratories.

Treatment of IgA Deficiency

There is no specific treatment for IgA deficiency because there are no drugs that activate IgA-producing B cells. Theoretically, an infusion of serum IgA or IgA containing plasma can correct the serum IgA deficiency, but there is limited transfer of infused IgA into the secretions (Butler et al., 1967; Stiehm et al., 1966). Nonetheless, there have been claims of the successful use of IgA-rich immunoglobulin preparations given intravenously (Blatrix et al., 1977) or orally (Eibl et al., 1988). Intermittent or continuous prophylactic antibiotics may be helpful in patients with recurrent respiratory tract infections, particularly those with chronic asthma, bronchitis, or sinusitis.

For the IgA-deficient individual with concomitant IgG2 subclass deficiency, or impaired antibody responses to bacterial or vaccine antigens, immunoglobulin replacement may be warranted, especially when lung damage is present or recurrent infections are prominent. IVIG in the usual therapeutic doses (300 to 400 mg/kg body weight, every 3 to 4 weeks) is indicated, using a product low in IgA (e.g., Gammagard-SD) to decrease the risk of sensitization. Subcutaneous infusions of immunoglobulin can also be used safely under these circumstances (Sundin et al., 1998).

Associated diseases in IgA deficiency are treated conventionally using standard therapies, and the results in most are the same as in nonimmunodeficient patients. For example, patients with systemic lupus erythematosus and selective IgA deficiency respond favorably to immunosuppressive treatment. An insufficient number of cases of selective IgA deficiency with associated diseases have been observed to predict their long-term prognosis. IgA-deficient asthmatic patients appear to be more resistant to standard antiasthma therapy, possibly because of their propensity to develop superimposed infections.

Transfusions with blood containing IgA may sensitize the selective IgA-deficient patient or may cause an anaphylactic reaction in a sensitized patient with anti-IgA antibodies (Vyas et al., 1968). Thus sensitized patients with selective IgA deficiency who require blood transfusions should be given blood from an IgA-deficient donor or saline-washed erythrocytes. The use of autologous erythrocytes, drawn prior to elective surgery, is also indicated. IgA-deficient patients, particularly those with anti-IgA antibodies, should wear a medical alert bracelet cautioning about blood, gamma globulin, or plasma infusions.

Lactose intolerance is not uncommon in IgA deficiency, and milk should be avoided in lactose-intolerant, IgA-deficient patients. IgA-deficient subjects with milk precipitins are not instructed to avoid milk, because there is no clear association with disease. In one child who was given a bone marrow transplant for severe combined immunodeficiency, chronic graft-versus-host disease and IgA deficiency developed. His serum had high levels of circulating immune complexes containing milk protein, and bovine casein was detected in his skin. Exclusion of milk from the diet resulted in a precipitous drop of serum immune complex levels with clinical improvement (Cunningham-Rundles et al., 1981).

Prognosis

Selective IgA deficiency is the mildest form of permanent primary immunodeficiency. On long-term follow-up studies of blood donors found to be IgA deficient, the defect is permanent (Koskinen et al., 1994). In most cases the prognosis is good, although there are some differences in overall health on long-term follow-up. Of 215 healthy blood donors with IgA deficiency who were followed after a median interval of 19 years, 80% of the group and 50% of the controls had experienced various infections, drug allergy, or autoimmune or atopic disease (Koskinen, 1996). Of these, respiratory infections and autoimmune diseases were more common in IgA-deficient subjects than in controls. When IgA deficiency is associated with another illness, the prognosis is that of the illness (e.g., lupus erythematosus, juvenile rheumatoid arthritis). Insufficient data are available to determine whether early onset of associated disease is correlated with increased morbidity or mortality. Selective IgA deficiency in an apparently healthy child, however, should not generate complacency.

A reasonable initial search and a periodic review for diseases associated with selective IgA deficiency (see Tables 14-2, 14-3, and 14-4) should be carried out. As noted, a few patients with selective IgA deficiency, particularly young children with low but detectable levels of IgA, may recover spontaneously, although this is unusual (Blum et al., 1982; Petty et al., 1973). A few individuals with IgA deficiency may go on to develop common variable immunodeficiency (Espanol et al., 1996). In one study, 2 subjects out of 215 IgA-deficient blood donors studied over a long interval were subsequently found to have reduced levels of IgG, as well as IgA (Koskinen, 1996).

REFERENCES

Ablin RJ. Anti-tissue IgG antibodies and deficiency of IgA. Vox Sang 23:371–375, 1972.

Adachi M, Yodoi J, Masuda T, Takatsuki K, Uchino H. Altered expression of lymphocyte Fc alpha receptor in selective IgA deficiency and IgA nephropathy. J Immunol 131:1246–1251, 1983.

Aguilar MM, Kamoshita S, Landing BH, Border E, Sedgwick RP. Pathological observations in ataxia-telangiectasia: report of five cases. J Neuropathol Exp Neurol 27:659–676, 1968.

Alper CA, Marcus-Bagley D, Awdeh Z, Kruskall MS, Eisenbarth GS, Brink SJ, Katz AJ, Stein R, Bing DH, Yunis EJ, Schur PH Prospective analysis suggests susceptibility genes for deficiencies of IgA and several other immunoglobulins on the HLA-B8, SC01, DR3 conserved extended haplotype. Tissue Antigens 56:207–216, 2000.

Ambrus M, Hernadi E, Bajtai G. Prevalence of HLA-A1 and HLA-B8 antigens in selective IgA deficiency. Clin Immunol Immunopathol 7:311–314, 1977.

Ammann AJ, Hong R. Anti-antisera antibody as a cause of double precipitin rings in immunoglobulin quantitation and its relation to milk precipitins. J Immunol 106:567–569, 1971a.

Ammann AJ, Hong R. Selective IgA deficiency and autoimmunity. Clin Exp Immunol 7:833–838, 1970.

Ammann AJ, Hong R. Selective IgA deficiency: presentation of 30 cases and a review of the literature. Medicine 60:223–236, 1971b.

Ammann AJ, Hong R. Unique antibody to basement membrane in patients with selective IgA deficiency and celiac disease. Lancet 1:1264–1267, 1971c.

Andre C, Andre F, Fargier MC. Distribution of IgA1 and IgA2 plasma cells in various normal human tissues and in the jejunum of plasma IgA deficient patients. Clin Exp Immunol 33:327–331, 1978.

Arnold RR, Cole MF, Prince S, McGhee J. Secretory IgM antibodies to *Streptococcus mutans* in subjects with selective IgA deficiency. Clin Immunol Immunopathol 8:475–486, 1977.

Ashman RF, Schaffer FM, Kemp JD, Yokoyama WM, Zhu ZB, Cooper MD, Volanakis JE. Genetic and immunologic analysis of a family containing five patients with common variable immune deficiency or selective IgA deficiency. J Clin Immunol 12:406–414, 1992.

Atwater JS, Tomasi TB. Suppressor cells and IgA deficiency. Clin Immunol Immunopathol 9:379–382, 1978.

Bachmann R. Studies on the serum gamma A-globulin level. III. The frequency of A-gamma-A-globulinemia. Scand J Clin Lab Invest 17:316–320, 1965.

Barros MD, Porto MHO, Leser PG, Greemach AS, Carniero-Sampaio MMS. Study of colostrum of a patient with selective IgA deficiency. Allergol Immunopathol (Madr) 13:331–334, 1985.

Benbassat J, Keren L, Zlotnic A. Hepatitis in selective IgA deficiency. Br Med J 4:762–763, 1973.

Benveniste J, Lespinats G, Salomon JC. Study of immunoglobulins in axenic mice thymectomized at birth. Proc Soc Exp Biol Med 130:936–940, 1969.

Bjørkander J, Bake B, Oxelius VA, Hanson LÅ. Impaired lung function in patients with IgA deficiency and low levels of IgG2 or IgG3. N Engl J Med 313:720–724, 1985.

Bjørkander J, Hammarström L, Smith CI, Buckley RH, Cunningham-Rundles C, Hanson LA. Immunoglobulin prophylaxis in patients with antibody deficiency syndromes and anti-IgA antibodies. J Clin Immunol 7:8–15, 1987.

Blatrix C, Thebault J, Steinbuch M. Properties of and information about a new preparation of immunoglobulins (IgGAM) enriched in IgA and IgM. Rev. Fr. Transfus Immunohematol, 20:419–426, 1977.

Bluestone R, Goldberg LS, Katz RM, Marchesano JM, Calabro JJ. Juvenile rheumatoid arthritis: a serologic survey of 200 consecutive patients. J Pediatr 77:98–102, 1970.

Blum PM, Stiehm ER, Hong R. Spontaneous recovery of selective IgA deficiency: additional case report and review. Clin Pediatr 21:77–80, 1982.

Bottaro A, de Marchi M, de Lange GG, Carbonara AO. Human Ig markers. Exp Clin Immunogenet 6:55–59, 1989.

Brandtzaeg P. Presence of J chains in human immunocytes containing various immunoglobulin classes. Nature 252:418–420, 1974.

Brandtzaeg P. Two types of IgA immunocytes in man. Nature New Biol 243:142–143, 1973.

Brandtzaeg P, Karlsson G, Hansson G, Petruson B, Bjørkander J, Hanson LÅ. The clinical condition of IgA-deficient patients is related to the proportion of IgD- and IgM-producing cells in their nasal mucosa. Clin Exp Immunol 67:626–636, 1986.

Buckley RH. Clinical and immunologic features of selective IgA deficiency. Birth Defects 11:134–141, 1975.

Buckley RH, Dees SC. Correlation of milk precipitins with IgA deficiency. N Engl J Med 281:465–469, 1969.

Buckley RH, Fiscus SA. Serum IgD and IgE concentrations in immunodeficiency diseases. J Clin Invest 55:157–161, 1975.

Burgio GR, Duse M, Monafo V, Ascione A, Nespoli L. Selective IgA deficiency: clinical and immunological evaluation of 50 pediatric patients. J Pediatr 133:101–106, 1980.

Burks AW, Sampson HA, Buckley RH. Anaphylactic reactions after gammaglobulin administration in patients with hypogammaglobulinemia. Detection of IgE antibodies to IgA. N Eng J Med, 314:560–564, 1986.

Burks AW Jr, Steele RW. Selective IgA deficiency. Ann Allergy 57: 3-13, 1986.

Butler JE, Oskvig R. Cancer, autoimmunity and IgA deficiency, related by a common antigen-antibody system. Nature 249:830–833, 1974.

Butler WT, Rosen R, Waldmann TA. The mechanism of appearance of immunoglobulin A in nasal secretion in man. J Clin Invest 46:1883–1887, 1967.

Carbonara AO, Demarchi M. Ig isotype deficiency caused by gene deletions. Monogr Allergy 20:13–17, 1986.

Cassidy JT, Burt A, Petty R, Sullivan D. Selective IgA deficiency and autoimmunity [letter]. N Engl J Med 284:985, 1971.

Cassidy JT, Nordby GL. Human serum immunoglobulin concentrations: prevalence of immunoglobulin deficiencies. J Allergy Clin Immunol 55:35–48, 1975.

Cassidy JT, Oldham G, Platts-Mills TAE. Functional assessment of a B cell defect in patients with selective IgA deficiency. Clin Exp Immunol 35:296–299, 1979.

Cassidy JT, Petty RE, Sullivan DB. Abnormalities in the distribution of serum immunoglobulin concentration in juvenile rheumatoid arthritis. Clin Invest 52:1931–1936, 1973.

Casterline CL, Evans R, Battista VC, Talamo RC. IgA deficiency and Pi ZZ anti-trypsin deficiency. Chest 73:885–886, 1978.

Cazac BB, Roes J TGF-beta receptor controls B cell responsiveness and induction of IgA *in vivo*. Immunity 13:443–451, 2000.

Chaabani H, Bech-Hansen TN, Cox DW. A multigene deletion within the immunoglobulin heavy chain region. Am J Hum Genet 37:1164–1171, 1985.

Chodirker WB, Tomasi TB. Gammaglobulins: quantitative relationships in human serum and nonvascular fluids. Science 142:1080–1081, 1963.

Claman HN, Hartley TF, Merrill D. Hypogammaglobulinemia, primary and secondary: immunoglobulin levels (gamma-G, gamma-A, gamma-M) in one hundred and twenty-five patients. J Allergy 38:215–225, 1966.

Choudat D, Taillemite JL, Hirsch-Marie H, Choubrac P, Lebas FX. Relation between Xq isochromosome and serum immunoglobulin A deficiency. Nouv Presse Med 30:2419–2422, 1979.

Claman HN, Merrill DA, Peakman D, Robinson A. Isolated severe gamma-A deficiency: immunoglobulin levels, clinical disorders, and chromosome studies. J Lab Clin Med 75:307–315, 1970.

Cleland LG, Bell DA. The occurrence of systemic lupus erythematosus in two kindreds in association with selective IgA deficiency. J Rheumatol 5:288–293, 1978.

Cobain TJ, Stuckey MS, McCluskey J, Wilton A, Gedeon A, Garlepp MJ, Christiansen FT, Dawkins RL. The coexistence of IgA deficiency and 21-hydroxylase deficiency marked by specific supra types. Ann N Y Acad Sci 458:76–84, 1985.

Conley ME, Arbetter A, Douglas SD. Serum levels of IgA1 and IgA2 in children and in patients with IgA deficiency. Mol Immunol 20:977–981, 1983.

Conley ME, Cooper MD. Immature IgA B cells in IgA-deficient patients. N Engl J Med 305:495–497, 1981.

Conley ME, Delacroix DL. Intravascular and mucosal immunoglobulin A: two separate but related systems of immune defence? Ann Intern Med 106:892–899, 1987.

Cowan MJ, Fujiwara P, Ammann AJ. Cellular immune defect in selective IgA deficiency using a microculture method for PHA stimulation and limiting dilution. Clin Immunol Immunopathol 17:595–605, 1980.

Cox DW, Markovic VD, Teshima IE. Genes for immunoglobulin heavy chains and for alpha-1-antitrypsin are localized to specific regions of chromosome 14q. Nature 297:428–430, 1982.

Crabbé PA, Carbonara AO, Heremans JF. The normal human intestinal mucosa as a major source of plasma cells containing gamma-A immunoglobulin. Lab Invest 14:235–248, 1965.

Crabbé PA, Heremans JF. Lack of gamma A-immunoglobulin in serum of patients with steatorrhea. Gut 7:119–125, 1966.

Crabbé PA, Heremans JF. Selective IgA deficiency with steatorrhea. A new syndrome. Am J Med 42:319–326, 1967.

Cunningham-Rundles C. IgA deficiency. Immunol Allergy Clin North Am 8:435–440, 1988.

Cunningham-Rundles C. Genetic aspects of immunoglobulin A deficiency. Adv Hum Genet 19:234–265, 1990.

Cunningham-Rundles C. The identification of antigens in circulating immune complexes by an enzyme-linked immunosorbent assay: detection of bovine κ-casein IgG complexes in human sera. Eur J Immunol 11:504–509, 1981.

Cunningham-Rundles C, Brandeis WE, Good RA, Day NK. Bovine antigens and the formation of circulating immune complexes in selective IgA deficiency. J Clin Invest 64:270–272, 1979a.

Cunningham-Rundles C, Brandeis W, Good RA, Day NK. Milk precipitins, circulating immune complexes and IgA deficiency. Proc Natl Acad Sci U S A 75:3387–3389, 1978.

Cunningham-Rundles C, Brandeis WE, Pudifin DJ, Day NK, Good RA. Autoimmunity in selective IgA deficiency: relationship to anti-bovine protein antibodies, circulating immune complexes and clinical disease. Clin Exp Immunol 45:299–304, 1981.

Cunningham-Rundles C, Brandeis WE, Safai B, O'Reilly R, Day NK, Good RA. Selective IgA deficiency and circulating immune complexes containing bovine proteins in a child with chronic graft vs. host disease. Am J Med 67:883–889, 1979b.

Cunningham-Rundles C, Feng ZK. Analysis of a common inheritable idiotype in IgA-deficient sera using monoclonal antibodies. J Immunol 140:3880–3886, 1988.

Cunningham-Rundles C, Magnusson KE, Lindblad BS. Abnormal gastrointestinal absorption of polyethylene glycol in common variable immunodeficiency [abstract]. Clin Res 36:65, 1988.

Cunningham-Rundles C, Oxelius VA, Good RA. IgG2 and IgG3 subclass deficiencies in selective IgA deficiency in the United States. Birth Defects 19:173–176, 1983.

Cunningham-Rundles C, Pudifin DJ, Armstrong D, Good RA. Selective IgA deficiency and neoplasia. Vox Sang 38:61–67, 1980.

Cunningham-Rundles C, Zhou Z, Mankarious S, Courter S. Long-term use of IgA-depleted intravenous immunoglobulin in immunodeficient subjects with anti-IgA antibodies. J Clin Immunol 13:272–278, 1993.

Danon YL, Dinari G, Garty BZ, Horodniceanu C, Nitzan M, Grunebaum M. Cholelithiasis in children with immunoglobulin A deficiency: a new gastroenterologic syndrome. J Pediatr Gastroenterol Nutr 2:663–666, 1983.

Davies K, Stiehm ER, Woo P, Murray KJ. Juvenile idiopathic polyarticular arthritis and IgA deficiency in the 22q11 deletion syndrome. J. Rheumat. 28:2326–2334, 2001.

De Graeff PA, The TH, Van Munster PJ, Out TA, Vossen JM, Zegers BJM. The primary immune response in patients with selective IgA deficiency. Clin Exp Immunol 54:778–784, 1983.

De Laat PCJ, Weemaes CMR, Bakkeren JAJM, Van den Brandt FCA, Van Lith TGPM, De Graaf R, Van Munster PJJ, Stoelinga GBA. Familial selective IgA deficiency with circulating anti-IgA antibodies: a distinct group of patients? Clin Immunol Immunopathol 58:92–101, 1991.

De la Concha EG, Fernandez-Arquero M, Vigil P, Lazaro F, Ferreira A, Garcia-Rodriguez MC, Fontan G. Tumor necrosis factor genomic polymorphism in Spanish IgA deficiency patients. Tissue Antigens 55:359–363, 2000.

Dubois RS, Roy CC, Fulginiti VA, Merrill DA, Murray RL. Disaccharidase deficiency in children with immunologic deficits. J Pediatr 76:377–385, 1970.

Epstein LB, Ammann AJ. Evaluation of T lymphocyte effector function in immunodeficiency diseases: abnormalities in mitogen-stimulated interferon in patients with selective IgA deficiency. J Immunol 112:617–622, 1974.

Espanol T, Catala M, Hernandez M, Caragol I, Bertran JM. Development of a common variable immunodeficiency in IgA-deficient patients. Clin Immunol Immunopathol 80:333-335, 1996.

Faed MJ, Whyle R, Patterson CR, McCathic M, Robertson J. Deletion of the long arm of chromosome 18 (46, XX, 18q⁻) associated with absence of IgA and hypothyroidism in an adult. J Med Genet 9:102–105, 1972.

Falchuk KR, Falchuk ZM. Selective immunoglobulin A deficiency, ulcerative colitis and gluten-sensitive enteropathy : a unique association. Gastroenterology 69:503–506, 1975.

Fallgreen-Gebauer E, Gebauer W, Bastian A, Kratzin HD, Eiffert H, Zimmermann B, Karas M, Hilschmann N.The covalent linkage of secretory component to IgA. Structure of sIgA. Biol Chem Hoppe Seyler 374:1023–1028, 1993.

Farr M, Struthers GR, Scott DGI, Bacon PA. Fendofenac-induced selective IgA deficiency in rheumatoid arthritis. J Rheumatol 24:367–369, 1985.

Ferreira A, Garcia-Rodriguez MC, Lopez-Trascasa M, Pascual-Salcedo D, Fontan G. Anti-IgA antibodies in selective IgA deficiency and in primary immunodeficient patients treated with gammaglobulin. Clin Immunol Immunopathol 47:199–207, 1988.

Finley SC, Finley WH, Uchida IA, Noto TA, Roddam RF. IgA absence associated with ring-18 chromosome. Lancet 1:1095–1096, 1968.

Fontana A, Grob PJ, Sauter R, Joller H. IgA deficiency, epilepsy and hydantoin medication. Lancet 2:228, 1976.

Fontana A, Joller H, Skvaril F, Grob P. Immunological abnormalities and HLA antigen frequencies in IgA-deficient patients with epilepsy. J Neurol Neurosurg Psychiatry 41:593–597, 1978.

Francois R, Rosenberg D, Bertrand J, Manuel Y. Adrenal insufficiency and immunological deficiency. Apropos of a case. Minerva Pedatr. 31;19:584–589, 1967.

French MA, Shortland JR, Coward RA, Brown CB. Glomerulonephritis and IgA deficiency. Clin Nephrol. 27:199–205, 1987.

Frommel D, Moullec J, Lambin P, Fine JM. Selective IgA deficiency: frequency among 15,200 French blood donors. Vox Sang 25:513–518, 1973.

Fudenberg H, German JL, Kunkel HG. The occurrence of rheumatoid factor and other abnormalities in families of patients with agammaglobulinemia. Arthritis Rheum 5:565–588, 1962.

Giorgi PL, Catassi C, Sbarbati A, Bearzi I, Cinti S. Ultrastructural findings in the jejunal mucosa of children with IgA deficiency. J Pediatr Gastroenterol Nutr 5:892–898, 1986.

Goh KO, Reddy MM, Webb DR. Cancer in a familial IgA deficiency patient: abnormal chromosomes and B lymphocytes. Oncology. 33:237–240, 1976.

Grabar P, Williams CA. Methode permettant d'etude conjugee des proprietes electrophoretique et immunochemiques d'un milange de protein: application au serum sanguin. Biochem Biophys Acta 10:193–194, 1953.

Grundbacher FJ. Genetic aspects of selective immunoglobulin A deficiency. J Med Genet 9:344–347, 1972.

Gugler E, Von Muralt G. Uber immunoelectrophoretische untersuchurgen an Frauenmilchproteinen. Schweiz Med Wochenschr 89:925–929, 1959.

Gryboski JD, Self TW, Clemett A, Herskovic T. Selective IgA deficiency and intestinal nodular lymphoid hyperplasia correction of diarrhea with antibiotics and plasma. Pediatrics 42:833–837, 1967.

Haddow JE, Shapiro SR, Gall DG. Congenital sensory neuropathy in siblings. Pediatrics 45:651–655, 1970.

Hammarstrom L, Carlsson B, Smith CIE, Wallin J, Wieslander L. Detection of IgA heavy chain constant region genes in IgA deficient donors: evidence against gene deletions. Clin Exp Immunol 60:661–664, 1985a.

Hammarstrom L, Persson MAA, Smith CIE. Anti-IgA in selective IgA deficiency. In vitro effects and Ig subclass patterns of human anti-IgA. Scand J Immunol 18:509–513, 1983.

Hammarstrom L, Persson MAA, Smith CIE. Immunoglobulin subclass distribution of human anti-carbohydrate antibodies: aberrant pattern in IgA-deficient donors. Immunology 54:821–826, 1985b.

Hammarstrom L, Ringden O, Lonngvist B, Smith CIE, Wiebe T. Transfer of IgA deficiency to a bone marrow grafted patient with aplastic anemia. Lancet 1:778–781, 1985c.

Hammarstrom L, Smith CI, Berg CI. Captopril-induced IgA deficiency. Lancet 1:436, 1991.

Hammarstrom L, Smith CIE. HLA-A, B, C, and DR antigens in immunoglobulin A deficiency. Tissue Antigens 21:75–79, 1983.

Hammarstrom L, Vorechovsky I, Webster D. Selective IgA deficiency (SIgAD) and common variable immunodeficiency (CVID). Clin Exp Immunol 120:225–231, 2000.

Hamoudi AB, Ertel I, Newton WA Jr, Reiner CB, Clatworthy HW Jr. Multiple neoplasms in an adolescent child associated with IgA deficiency. Canter, 33:1134–1144, 1974.

Hanson LÅ. Comparative analysis of human milk and blood plasma by means of diffusion in gel methods. Experientia 15:473–474, 1959.

Hanson LÅ. Comparative immunological studies of immunoglobulins of human milk and serum. Int Arch Allergy Appl Immunol 18:241–267, 1961.

Hanson LÅ. Selective IgA-deficiency. In Chandra RK, ed. Primary and Secondary Immunodeficiency Disorders. New York, Churchill Livingstone, 1983, pp 62–84.

Hanson LÅ, Brandtzaeg. Immunology Today. 14:416–417, 1993.

Harriman GR, Bogue M, Rogers P, Finegold M, Pacheco S, Bradley A, Zhang Y, Mbawuike IN. Targeted deletion of the IgA constant region in mice leads to IgA deficiency with alterations in expression of other Ig isotypes. J Immunol 162:2521–2529, 1999.

Hazenberg BP, Hoedemaeker PJ, Nieuwenhuis P, Mandema E. Source of IgA in jejunal secretions. In Peeters H, ed. Protides of the Biological Fluids: Proceedings of the Sixteenth Colloquium. Oxford, UK, Pergamon Press, 1968, pp 491–497.

Heneghan MA, Stevens FM, Cryan EM, Warner RH, McCarthy CF. Celiac sprue and immunodeficiency states: a 25-year review. J Clin Gastroenterol 25:421–425, 1997

Heremans JF. Immunoglobulin A. In Sela M, ed. The Antigens, vol 2. London, Academic Press, 1974, pp 365–522.

Herrmann RP, Chipper L, Bell S. Chromosome studies in healthy blood donors with IgA deficiency. Clin Genet 22:231–233, 1982.

Hiroi T, Yanagita M, Iijima H, Iwatani K, Yoshida T, Takatsu K, Kiyono H. Deficiency of IL-5 receptor alpha-chain selectively influences the development of the common mucosal immune system independent IgA-producing B-1 cell in mucosa-associated tissues. J Immunol 162:821–8, 1999

Hong R, Ammann RJ. Disorders of the IgA system. In Stiehm ER, ed. Immunologic Disorders of Infants and Children, ed 3. Philadelphia, WB Saunders, 1989, pp 329–342.

Huntley CC, Robbins JB, Lyerly AD, Buckley RH. Characterization of precipitating antibodies to ruminant serum and milk proteins in humans with selective IgA deficiency. N Engl J Med 284:7–10, 1971.

Huntley CC, Stephenson RL. IgA deficiency: family studies. N C Med J 29:326–335, 1968.

Husby S, Oxelius VA, Svehag SE. IgG subclass antibodies to dietary antigens in IgA deficiency: quantitation and correlation with serum IgG subclass levels. Clin Immunol Immunopathol 62:83–90, 1992.

Hustinx TWJ, Scheres JMJC, Weemaes CMR, Ter Haar BGA, Janssen AH. Karyotype instability with multiple 7/14 and 7/7 rearrangements. Hum Genet 49:199–208, 1979.

Inoue T, Okubo H, Kudo J, Ikuta T, Hachimine K, Shibata R, Yoshinari D, Fukada K, Ranase T. Selective IgA deficiency: analysis of Ig production in vitro. J Clin Immunol 4:235–241, 1984.

Islam KB, Baskin B, Nilsson L, Hammarstrom L, Sideras P, Smith CI. Molecular analysis of IgA deficiency. Evidence for impaired switching to IgA. J Immunol 152:1442–1452,1994.

Itescu S. Adult immunodeficiency and rheumatic disease. Rheum Dis Clin North Am 22:53–73, 1996.

Iwata T, Incefy GS, Cunningham-Rundles S, Cunningham-Rundles C, Smithwick E, Geller N, O'Reilly R, Good RA. Circulating thymic hormone activity in patients with primary and secondary immunodeficiency diseases. Am J Med 71:385–394, 1981.

Jacobson KW, De Shazo RD. Selective immunoglobulin A deficiency associated with nodular lymphoid hyperplasia. J Allergy Clin Immunol 64:516–521, 1979.

James SP, Jones EA, Schafer DF, Hoofnagle JH, Varma RR, Strober W. Selective immunoglobulin A deficiency associated with primary biliary cirrhosis in a family with liver disease. Gastroenterology 90:283–288, 1986.

Johns P, Felix-Davies DD, Hawkins CF, Macintosh P, Shadford MF, Stanworth DR, Thompson RA, Williamson N. IgA deficiency in patients with rheumatoid arthritis with D-penicillamine or gold [abstract]. Ann Rheum Dis 37:289, 1978.

Joller PW, Buehler AK, Hitzig WH. Transitory and persistent IgA deficiency: reevaluation of 19 pediatric patients once found to be IgA deficient. J Clin Lab Immunol 6:97–101, 1981.

Joubert PH, Aucamp AK, Potgieter GM, Verster F. Epilepsy and IgA deficiency: the effect of sodium valproate. South Afr Med J 52:642–644, 1977.

Kaetzel CS, Robinson JK, Chintalacharuvu KR, Vaerman JP, Lamm ME. The polymeric immunoglobulin receptor (secretory component) mediates transport of immune complexes across epithelial cells: a local defense function for IgA. Proc Natl Acad Sci U S A 88:8796–8800, 1991.

Kanoh T, Mizumoto T, Yasuda N, Koya M, Ohno Y, Uchino H, Yoshimura K, Ohkubo Y, Yamaguchi H. Selective IgA deficiency in Japanese blood donors: frequency and statistical analysis. Vox Sang 50:81–86, 1986.

Kanok JM, Steinberg P, Cassidy JT, Petty RE, Bayne NK. Serum IgE levels in patients with selective IgA deficiency. Ann Allergy 41:220–228, 1978.

Karlsson G, Hansson HA, Petruson B, Björkander J, Hanson LA. Goblet cell number in the nasal mucosa relates to cell-mediated immunity in patients with antibody deficiency syndromes. Int Arch Allergy Appl Immunol. 78:86–91, 1985.

Kaufman HS, Hobbs JR. Immunoglobulin deficiencies in an atopic population. Lancet 2:1061–1063, 1970.

Kerr MA. The structure and function of human IgA. J Biochem 271:285–296, 1990.

Kersey JH, Shapiro RS, Filipovich AH. Relationship of immunodeficiency to lymphoid malignancy. Pediatr Infect Dis J 7 (Suppl):S10–S12, 1988.

King MA, Wells JV, Nelson DS. IgA synthesis by peripheral blood mononuclear cells from normal and selectively IgA-deficient subjects. Clin Exp Immunol 38:306–310, 1979.

Klemola T. Immunohistochemical findings in the intestine of IgA-deficient persons. J Pediatr Gastroenterol Nutr 7:537–543, 1988.

Koistinen J. Familial clustering of selective IgA deficiency. Vox Sang 30:181–190, 1976.

Koistinen J. Selective IgA deficiency in blood donors. Vox Sang 29:192–202, 1975.

Koistinen J, Cardenas RM, Fudenberg HH. Anti-IgA antibodies of limited specificity in healthy IgA-deficient subjects. J Immunogenet 4:295–299, 1977.

Koni PA, Sacca R, Lawton P, Browning JL, Ruddle NH, Falvell RA. Distinct roles in lymphoid organogenesis for lymphotoxins and β revealed in lymphotoxin β-deficient mice. Immunity 6:491–495, 1997.

Kornstadt L, Nordhagen R. Immune deficiency and autoimmunity. Int Arch Allergy Appl Immunol 47:942–945, 1974.

Koskinen S, Tolo H, Hirvonen M, Koistinen J. Long-term persistence of selective IgA deficiency in healthy adults. J Clin Immunol 14:116–119,1994.

Krieger I, Brough JA. Gamma-A deficiency and hypochromic anemia due to defective iron mobilization. N Engl J Med 269:886–894, 1967.

Kwitko AO, Roberts-Thomas PJ, Shearman DJC. Low molecular weight IgM in selective IgA deficiency. Clin Exp Immunol 50:198–202, 1982.

Lakhanpal S, O'Duffy JD, Homburg HA, Moore SB. Evidence for linkage of IgA deficiency with the major histocompatibility complex. Mayo Clin Proc 63:461–465, 1988.

Laschinger C, Sheppard FA, Naylor DH. Anti-IgA-mediated transfusion reactions in Canada. Can Med Assoc J 130:141–144, 1984.

Lawton AR, Royal SA, Self KS, Cooper MD. IgA determinants on B lymphocytes in patients with deficiency of circulating IgA. J Lab Clin Med 80:26–33, 1972.

Lefranc MP, Lefranc G, Rabbits TM. Inherited deletion of immunoglobulin heavy chain region genes in normal human individuals. Nature 300:760–762, 1982.

Lefranc MP, Lefranc G, De Lange G, Out TA, Van Denbroek PJ, Van Nieuwkoop J, Radl J, Helal AM, Chabaani H, Van Loghem E, Rabbits TH. Instability of the human immunoglobulin heavy chain constant region locus indicated by different inherited chromosomal deletions. Mol Biol Med 1:207–217, 1983.

Leickley FE, Buckley RH. Development of IgA and IgG2 subclass deficiency after sulfasalazine therapy. J Pediatr 108:481–482, 1986.

Leikola J, Vyas GN. Human antibodies to ruminant IgM concealing the absence of IgA in man. J Lab Clin Med 77:629–638, 1971.

Leisti J, Leisti S, Perheentupa J, Savilahti E, Aula P. Absence of IgA and growth hormone deficiency associated with a short arm deletion of chromosome 18. Arch Dis Child 48:320–322, 1973.

Leong AB, Gange RW, O'Connor RD. Twenty nail dystrophy associated with selective IgA deficiency. J Pediatr 100:418–419, 1982.

Levitt D, Cooper MD. Immunoregulatory defects in a family with selective IgA deficiency. J Pediatr 98:52–58, 1981.

Lewkonia RM, Gairdner D, Doe WF. IgA deficiency in one of identical twins. Br Med J 1:311–313, 1976.

Lewkonia RM, Lin CC, Haslam RHA. Selective IgA deficiency with 18q+ and 18q− karyotypic anomalies. J Med Genet 17:453–456, 1980.

Liblau RS, Bach JF. Selective IgA deficiency and autoimmunity. Int Arch Allergy Immunol. 99:16–27, 1992.

Lio D, D'Anna C, Leone F, Curro MF, Candore G, Caruso C. Hypothesis: interleukin-5 production impairment can be a key point in the pathogenesis of the MHC-linked selective IgA deficiency. Autoimmunity 27:185–188, 1998.

Lopez M, Hyslop E. Precipitating antibody to bovidae serum proteins in dysgammaglobulinemic sera [abstract]. Fed Proc 27:684, 1968.

Nagao AT, Mai FH, Pereira AB, Carneiro-Sampaio MM. Measurement of salivary, urinary and fecal secretory IgA levels in children with partial or total IgA deficiency. J Investig Allergol Clin Immunol. 4:234–237, 1994

McCarthy DM, Katz SI, Gazzel L, Waldmann TA, Nelson DL, Strober W. Selective IgA deficiency associated with total villous atrophy of the small intestine and an organ-specific anti-epithelial cell antibody. J Immunol 120:932–938, 1978.

McClelland DBL, Shearman DJ, Van Furth R. Synthesis of immunoglobulin and secretory components by gastrointestinal mucosa in patients with hypogammaglobulinemia or IgA deficiency. Clin Exp Immunol 25:103–109, 1979.

McGhee JR, Mestecky J, Elson CO, Kiyono H. Regulation of IgA synthesis and immune response by T cells and interleukins. J Clin Immunol 9:175–199, 1989.

Martini A, Raveli A, Notarangelo LD, Burgio VL, Plebani A. Henoch-Schönlein syndrome and selective IgA deficiency. Arch Dis Child 60:160–162, 1985.

Mazanec MB, Kaetzel CS, Lamm ME, Fletcher D, Nedrud JG. Intracellular neutralization of virus by immunoglobulin A antibodies. Proc Natl Acad Sci U S A 89:6901–6905, 1992.

Mbawuike IN, Pacheco S, Acuna CL, Switzer KC, Zhang Y, Harriman GR. Mucosal immunity to influenza without IgA: an IgA knockout mouse model. J Immunol 162:2530–2537, 1999.

Mbuyi JM, Dequeker J, Francx L. IgA deficiency and drug induced IgA deficiency in rheumatoid arthritis. J Rheumatol 10:829–831, 1983.

Mellander L, Björkander J, Carlson B, Hanson LA. Secretory antibodies in IgA-deficient and immunosuppressed individuals. J Clin Immunol 6:284–291, 1986.

Mestecky J, McGhee JR. Immunoglobulin A (IgA): molecular and cellular interactions involved in IgA biosynthesis and immune response. Adv Immunol 40:153–245, 1987.

Migone N, Olivero S, De Lange G, Delacroix DL, Altruda F, Silengo L, Demarchi M, Carbona AO. Multiple gene deletions within the human immunoglobulin heavy chain cluster. Proc Natl Acad Sci USA 81:5811–5815, 1984.

Monteiro RC, Kubagawa H, Cooper MD. Cellular distribution, regulation, and biochemical nature of an Fc alpha receptor in humans. J Exp Med 171:597–613, 1990.

Mostov KE, Deitcher DL. Polymeric immunoglobulin receptor expressed in MDCK cells transcytoses IgA. Cell 46:613–621, 1986.

Mostov KE, Friedlander M, Blobel G. The receptor for transepithelial transport of IgA and IgM contains multiple immunoglobulin-like domains. Nature 308:37–43, 1984.

Munoz-Lopez F, Ballesta Martinez F, Martin Mateos MA. Selective IgA deficiency. Immunologic and cytogenetic studies. Allergol Immunopathol (Madr) 5:671–676, 1977.

Murphy EA, Morris AJ, Walker E, Lee FD, Sturrock RD. Cyclosporine A induced colitis and acquired selective IgA deficiency in a patient with juvenile chronic arthritis. J Rheumatol 20:1397–1398, 1993.

Nadorp JH, Voss M, Buys Wc, Van Munster PJ, Van Tongeren JH, Aalberse RC, Van Longhem E. The significance of the presence of anti-IgA antibodies in individuals with an IgA deficiency. Eur J Clin Invest. 3:317–323, 1973.

Natvig JB, Harboe M, Fausa O, Tveit A. Family studies in individuals with selective absence of gamma-A-globulin. Clin Exp Immunol 8:229–236, 1971.

Nilssen DE, Friman V, Theman K, Björkander J, Kilarder A, Holmgren J, Hanson LÅ, Brandtzaeg P. B cell activation in duodenal mucosa after oral cholera vaccination in IgA-deficient subjects with or without IgG subclass deficiency. Scand J Immunol 38:201–208, 1993.

Norhagen GE, Enaptrom PE, Hammerstrom L, Soder PO, Smith CIE. Immunoglobulin levels in saliva in individuals with selective IgA deficiency. Compensatory IgM secretion and its correlation with HLA and susceptibility to infections. J Clin Immunol 9:279–286, 1989.

Odgers RJ, Wangel AG. Abnormalities in IgA-containing mononuclear cells in the gastric lesions of pernicious anemia. Lancet 2:844–849, 1968.

Oen K, Petty RE, Schroeder ML. Immunoglobulin A deficiency in genetic studies. Tissue Antigens 19:174–182, 1982.

Ogata K, Iinuma K, Kamimura K, Morinaga R, Kato J. A case report of a presumptive +i(18p) associated with serum IgA deficiency. Clin Genet 11:184–188, 1977.

Olerup O, Smith CIE, Björkander J, Hammarström L. Shared HLA class II-associated genetic susceptibility and resistance, related to the HLA-DQB1 gene, in IgA deficiency and common variable immunodeficiency. Proc Natl Acad Sci U S A 89:10653–10657, 1992.

Olerup O, Smith CIE, Hammarström L. Different amino acids at position 57 of the HLA-DQ-beta chain associated with susceptibility and resistance to IgA deficiency. Nature 347:289–290, 1990.

Olsson PG, Hofker MH, Walter MA, Smith S, Hammarström L, Smith CIE, Cox DW. Ig H chain variable and C region genes in common variable immunodeficiency. J Immunol 147:2540–2546, 1991.

Ostergaard PA. Combined IgA and alpha-1-antitrypsin deficiency in a boy with severe respiratory tract infections and asthma. Eur J Pediatr 138:83–85, 1982.

Oxelius VA, Laurell AB, Linquist B, Golebiowska H, Axelsson U, Björkander J, Hanson LÅ. IgG subclasses in selective IgA deficiency. N Engl J Med 304:1476–1477, 1981.

Ozsoylu S. Karabent A, Irken G. Selective IgA deficiency in childhood ITP. Eur J Haematol 41:95, 1988.

Pascual-Salcedo D, Rodriguez MCG, Trascasa ML, Fontana G. Anti cardiolipin antibodies in patients with primary immunodeficiency disease. Ann Rheum Dis 47:410–413, 1988.

Pereira LF, Sapina AM, Arroyo J, Vinuelas J, Bardaji RM, Prieto L. Prevalence of selective IgA deficiency in Spain: more than we thought [abstract]. Blood 90:893, 1997.

Perey DYE, Frommel D, Hong R, Good RA. The mammalian homologue of the avian bursa of Fabricius. Lab Invest 22:212–227, 1970.

Petty RE, Cassidy JT, Sullivan DB. Reversal of selective IgA deficiency in a child with juvenile rheumatoid arthritis after plasma transfusions. Pediatrics 51:44–48, 1973.

Petty RE, Sherry DD, Johannson J. Anti-IgA antibodies in pregnancy. N Engl J Med 313:1620–1625, 1985.

Plaut AG. The IgA1 proteases of pathogenic bacteria. Ann Rev Microbiol 37:603–622, 1983.

Plebani A, Mira E, Mevio E, Monafo V, Notarangelo LD, Avanzini A, Ugazio AG. IgM and IgD concentrations in the serum and secretions of children with selective IgA deficiency. Clin Exp Immunol 53:689–696, 1983.

Plebani A, Monafo V, Ugazio AG, Monti MA, Avanzini P, Massimi P, Burgio GR. Comparison of the frequency of atopic disease in children with severe and partial IgA deficiency. Int Arch Allergy Appl Immunol 82:485–486, 1987.

Plebani A, Ugazio AG, Monafo V, Burgio GR. Clinical heterogeneity and reversibility of selective immunoglobulin A deficiency in 80 children. Lancet 1:829–831, 1986.

Price P, Witt C, Allcock R, Sayer D, Garlepp M, Kok CC, French M, Mallal S, Christiansen F. The genetic basis for the association of the 8.1 ancestral haplotype (A1, B8, DR3) with multiple immunopathological diseases. Immunol Rev 167:257–274, 1999.

Prince HE, Norman GL, Binder WL. Immunoglobulin A (IgA) deficiency and alternative celiac disease-associated antibodies in sera submitted to a reference laboratory for endomysial IgA testing. Clin Diagn Lab Immunol 7:192:6, 2000.

Pritchard H, Riddaway J, Micklem HS. Immune response in congenitally thymus-less mice: II. Quantitative studies of serum immunoglobulins, the antibody response to sheep red blood cells and the effectiveness of thymus allografting. Clin Exp Immunol 13:125–138, 1973.

Proesman W, Jaeken J, Eeckels R. D-Penicillamine-induced IgA deficiency in Wilson's disease. Lancet 1:804–805, 1976.

Rankin EC, Isenberg DA. IgA deficiency and SLE: prevalence in a clinic population and a review of the literature. Lupus 6:390–394, 1997.

Richman LK, Brown WR. Immunochemical characterization of IgM in intestinal fluids. J Immunol 199:1515–1521, 1977.

Rockey JH, Hanson LÅ, Heremans JF, Kunkel HG. Beta-2A-agammaglobulinemia in two healthy men. J Lab Clin Med 63:205–212, 1964.

Ruff ME, Pincus LG, Sampson HA. Phenytoin-induced IgA depression. Am J Dis Child 141:858–859, 1987.

Ruvalcaba RHA, Thuline HC. IgA absence associated with short arm deletion of chromosome no. 18. J Pediatr 74:964–965, 1969.

Sandler SC, Zlotnick A. IgA deficiency and autoimmune hemolytic disease. Arch Intern Med 136:93–94, 1976.

Savilahti E, Eskola J, Koskimies S. IgA deficiency in coeliac disease. In Griscelli C, Vossen J, eds. Progress in Immunodeficiency Research and Therapy. Amsterdam, Elsevier Science, 1984, pp 257–259.

Savilahti E, Klemola T, Carlsson B, Mellander L, Stenvile M, Hovi T. Inadequacy of mucosal IgM antibodies in selective IgA deficiency: excretion of attenuated polio viruses is prolonged. J Clin Immunol 8:89–94, 1988.

Schaffer FM, Palermos J, Zhou ZB, Barger BO, Cooper MD, Volanakis JE. Individuals with IgA deficiency and common variable immunodeficiency share polymorphisms of major histocompatibility complex class III genes. Proc Natl Acad Sci USA 86:8015–8019, 1989.

Schaffer FM, Monteiro RC, Volanakis JE, Cooper MD. IgA deficiency. Immunodefic Rev 3:15–44, 1991.

Scotta MS, Maggiore G, DeGiacomo C, Martini A, Burgio VL, Ugazio AG. IgA-containing plasma cells in the intestinal mucosa of children with selective IgA deficiency. J Clin Lab Immunol 9:173–175, 1982.

Seager J, Jamison DL, Wilson J, Hayward AR, Soothill JF. IgA deficiency, epilepsy and phenytoin treatment. Lancet 2:632–635, 1975.

Seignalet J, Michael FB, Guendon R, Thomas R, Robinet-Levy M, Lapinski H. HLA et dificit en IgA. Rev Fr Transfus Immunohematol 21:753–761, 1978.

Shakir RA, Behan PO, Dick H, Lambie DG. Metabolism of immunoglobulin A, lymphocyte function, and histocompatibility antigens in patients on anticonvulsants. J Neurol Neurosurg Psychiatry 41:307–311, 1978.

Sharma OP, Chandor SM. IgA deficiency in sarcoidosis. Am Rev Respir Dis 106:600–603, 1972.

Shimada S, Kawaguchi-MiyashitaM, Kushiro A, Sato T, Nanno M, Sako T, Matsuoka Y, Sudo K, Tagawa Y, Iwakura Y, Ohwaki M Generation of polymeric receptor-deficient mouse with marked reduction of secretory IgA. J Immunol 163:5367–5373, 1999.

Silver HKB, Shuster J, Gold P, Hawkins D, Freedman SO. Endocrinopathy and IgA deficiency. Clin Immunol Immunopathol 1:212–219, 1973.

Sleasman, JW The association between immunodeficiency and the development of autoimmune disease. Adv Dent Res 10:57–61, 1996.

Sloper KS, Brook CGD, Kingston D, Pearson JR, Shiner M. Eczema and atopy in early childhood: low IgA plasma cell counts in the jejunal mucosa. Arch Dis Child 56:939–943, 1981.

Smith WI, Rabin BS, Huelimantel A, Van Thiel DH, Drash A. Immunopathology of juvenile-onset diabetes mellitus I: IgA deficiency and juvenile diabetes. Diabetes 27:1092–1099, 1978.

Soothill JF, Hayes K, Dudgeon JA. The immunoglobulins in congenital rubella. Lancet 2:1385–1388, 1966.

Sorrell TC, Forbes IJ, Burness FR, Rischbieth RHC. Depression of immunological function in patients treated with phenytoin sodium (sodium diphenylhydantoin). Lancet 2:1233–1235, 1971.

Stannegard O, Björkander J, Hanson LÅ, Hermodsson S. Natural killer cells in common variable immunodeficiency and selective IgA deficiency. Clin Immunol Immunopathol 25:325–334, 1983.

Stewart JM, Go S, Ellis E, Robinson A. Absent IgA and deletions of chromosome 18. J Med Genet 7:11–19, 1970.

Stiehm ER, Vaerman J-P, Fudenberg HH. Plasma infusions in immunologic deficiency states: metabolic and therapeutic studies. Blood 28:918–937, 1966.

Stobo JD, Tomasi TB. A low molecular weight immunoglobulin antigenically related to 19S IgM. J Clin Invest 46:1329–1337, 1967.

Stocker F, Ammann P, Rossi E. Selective gamma-A-globulin deficiency, with dominant autosomal inheritance in a Swiss family. Arch Dis Child 43:585–588, 1968.

Strober W, Sneller MC. IgA deficiency. Ann Allergy 66:363–375, 1991.

Strothman R, White MB, Testin J, Chen SN, Ball MS. HLA and IgA deficiency in blood donors. Hum Immunol 16:289–294, 1986.

Sundin U, Nava S, Hammarstrom L Induction of unresponsiveness against IgA in IgA-deficient patients on subcutaneous immunoglobulin infusion therapy. Clin Exp Immunol 112:341–346, 1998.

Swanson V, Dyce B, Citron P, Roulea C, Feinstein D, Haverback BJ. Absence of IgA in serum with presence of IgA-containing cells in the intestinal tract [abstract]. Clin Res 16:119, 1968.

Taalman RDFM, Weemaes CMR, Hustinx TWJ, Scheres JMJC, Clement JME, Stoelinga GBA. Chromosome studies in IgA-deficient patients. Clin Genet 32:81–87, 1987.

Taylor B, Norman AP, Orgel HA, Stokes CR, Turner MW, Soothill JF. Transient IgA deficiency and pathogenesis of infantile atopy. Lancet 2:111–113, 1973.

Thieffry S, Arthuis M, Aicardi J, Lyon G. L'ataxie-telangiectasie (7 observations personnelles). Rev Neurol (Paris) 105:390–405, 1961.

Tiepolo L, Maraschio P, Gimeli G, Cuoco C, Gargani GF, Romano C. Multibranched chromosomes 1, 9, and 16 in a patient with combined IgA and IgE deficiency. Hum Genet 51:127–137, 1979.

Tomasi TB. The discovery of secretory IgA and the mucosal immune system. Immunol Today 13:416–418, 1992.

Tomasi TB, Bienenstock J. Secretory immunoglobulins. Adv Immunol 9:1–96, 1968.

Tomasi TB Jr, Katz L. Human antibodies against bovine immunoglobulin M in IgA-deficient sera. Clin Exp Immunol 9:3–10, 1971.

Torrelo A, Espana A, Balsa J, Ledo A. Vitiligo and polyglandular autoimmune syndrome with selective IgA deficiency. Int J Dermatol 31:343–344, 1992.

Truedsson L, Axelsson U, Laurell AB. Frequent occurrence of anti-rabbit IgM in IgA deficiency. Acta Pathol Microbiol Scand 90:315–316, 1982.

Tsung SH, Ajlouni K. Immune competence in patients with Klinefelter syndrome. Am J Med Sci 275:311–317, 1978.

Van Ginkel FW, Wahl SM, Kearney JF, Kweon MN, Fujihashi K, Burrows PD, Kiyono H, McGhee JR. Partial IgA-deficiency with increased Th2-type cytokines in TGF-beta 1 knockout mice J Immunol 163:1951–1957, 1999.

Van Loghem E. Familial occurrence of isolated IgA deficiency associated with antibodies to IgA: evidence against a structural gene defect. Eur J Immunol 4:57–61, 1974.

Van Loghem E, Wang AC, Shuster J. A new genetic marker of human immunoglobulin determined by an allele at the alpha 2 locus. Vox Sang 24:481–490, 1973.

Van Loghem E, Zegers BJM, Bast EJE, Kater L. Selective deficiency of immunoglobulin A2. J Clin Invest 72:1918–1923, 1983.

Van Thiel DH, Smith WI, Rabin BS, Fisher SE, Lester R. A syndrome of immunoglobulin A deficiency, diabetes mellitus, malabsorption, and a common HLA haplotype: immunologic and genetic studies of forty-three family members. Ann Intern Med 86:10–19, 1977.

Victoria CG, Smith PG, Vaughan JP, Nobre LC, Lombardi C, Teixeira AMB, Fuchs SMC, Moreira LB, Gigante LP, Barros FC. Evidence for protection by breast-feeding against infant deaths from infectious diseases in Brazil. Lancet 2:319–322, 1987.

Vorechovsky I, Blennow E, Nordenskjold M, Webster AD, Hammarstrom L. A putative susceptibility locus on chromosome 18 is not a major contributor to human selective IgA deficiency: evidence from meiotic mapping of 83 multiple-case families. J Immunol 163:2236–2242, 1999a.

Vorechovsky I, Cullen M, Carrington M, Hammarstrom L, Webster AD. Fine mapping of IGAD1 in IgA deficiency and common variable immunodeficiency: identification and characterization of haplotypes shared by affected members of 101 multiple-case families. J Immunol 164:4408–4416, 2000.

Vorechovsky I, Webster AD, Plebani A, Hammarstrom L. Genetic linkage of IgA deficiency to the major histocompatibility complex: evidence for allele segregation distortion, parent-of-origin penetrance differences, and the role of anti-IgA antibodies in disease predisposition. Am J Hum Genet 64:1096–1109, 1999b.

Vorechovsky I, Zetterquist H, Paganelli R, Koskinen S, Webster AD, Bjorkander J, Smith CI, Hammarstrom L. Family and linkage study of selective IgA deficiency and common variable immunodeficiency. Clin Immunol Immunopathol 77:185–192, 1995.

Vyas GN, Fudenberg HH. Immunogenetic study of Am(1), the first allotype of human IgA. Clin Res 17:469, 1969.

Vyas GN, Perkins HA, Fudenberg HH. Anaphylactoid transfusion reactions associated with anti-IgA. Lancet 2:312–315, 1968.

Waldmann TA, Broder S, Krakauer R, Durm M, Meade B, Goldman C. Defect in IgA secretion and in IgA-specific suppressor cells in patients with selective IgA deficiency. Trans Assoc Am Physicians 89:219–224, 1976.

Wang Z, Yunis D, Irigoyen M, Kitchens B, Bottaro A, Alt FW, Alper CA. Discordance between IgA switching at the DNA level and IgA expression at the mRNA level in IgA-deficient patients. Clin Immunol 91:263–270, 1999.

Webb RD, Condemi JJ. Selective immunoglobulin A deficiency and chronic obstructive lung disease: a family study. Ann Intern Med 80:618–621, 1974.

Wells JV, Michaeli D, Fudenberg HH. Antibodies to human collagen in subjects with selective IgA deficiency. Clin Exp Immunol 13:203–208, 1973.

Werteleki W, Gerald PS. Clinical chromosomal studies of the 18q syndrome. J Pediatr 78:44–51, 1971.

Wilson MG, Towner JW, Forsman L, Siris E. Syndromes associated with the deletion of the long arm of chromosome 18. Am J Med Genet 8:155–174, 1979.

Wilton AN, Cobain TJ, Dawkins RL. Family studies of IgA deficiency. Immunogenetics 21:333–342, 1985.

Wollheim FA, Belfrage S, Coster C, Lindholm H. Primary "acquired" hypogammaglobulinemia: clinical and genetic aspects of nine cases. Acta Med Scand 176:18–23, 1964.

Yadav M, Iyngkaran N. Low incidence of selective IgA deficiency in normal Malaysians. Med J Malaysia 34:145–148, 1979.

Yasuda N, Kanoh T, Uchino H. J chain synthesis in lymphocytes from patients with selective IgA deficiency. Clin Exp Immunol 46:142–148, 1981.

Zinneman HH, Kaplan AP. The association of giardiasis with reduced intestinal secretory immunoglobulin A. Dig Dis Sci 125:207–213, 1975.

C H A P T E R

15

Combined Immunodeficiencies

Alain Fischer and Luigi D. Notarangelo

With contributions by Fabio Candotti, Jean-Pierre de Villartay, Barbara Grospierre, and Allesandro Plebani

INTRODUCTION

Combined immunodeficiencies (CIDs) are a heterogeneous group of disorders characterized by defects in T-cell development and/or function, variably associated with abnormal development of other lymphocyte lineages (i.e., B or natural killer [NK] lymphocytes) (Table 15-1) (Buckley, 2002; Fischer, 2000; World Health Organization Scientific Group Report, 1999).

Incidence and Distribution

The overall frequency of these disorders is estimated to be 1 in 50,000 to 100,000 live births. Among CID, the forms with the most severe T-cell depletion are termed *severe combined immune deficiencies* (SCIDs). The approximate division of the various types of SCID is shown in Table 15-2. Apart from X-linked hyper-IgM (see Chapter 13), SCID associated with purine enzyme defects (see Chapter 16) and some other immunodeficiency syndromes in which severe CIDs may occur (e.g.,

TABLE 15-1 · CHARACTERISTIC FEATURES OF THE COMBINED IMMUNE DEFICIENCIES

Disease	Gene	Inheritance	Circulating Lymphocytes			Associated Findings
			T	B	NK	
1. B⁻ SCID						
a. Reticular dysgenesis	?	AR	↓↓	↓↓	↓↓	
b. RAG deficiency, T⁻B⁻ SCID	*RAG-1, RAG-2*	AR	↓↓	↓↓	N	
c. Omenn syndrome	*RAG-1, RAG-2*	AR	↓/N	↓↓	N/↑	Erythroderma, eosinophilia
d. Radiation sensitive T⁻B⁻ SCID	*Artemis*	AR	↓↓	↓↓	N	
2. T⁻B⁺ SCID						
a. X-linked SCID	*IL-2Rγ*	XL	↓↓	N/↑	↓↓	
b. Jak3 deficiency	*JAK3*	AR	↓↓	N/↑	↓↓	
c. IL-7Rα-deficiency	*IL-7Rα*	AR	↓↓	N/↑	N	
3. Purine metabolism deficiency						
a. Adenosine deaminase deficiency	*ADA*	AR	↓↓	↓	↓	
b. Nucleoside phosphorylase deficiency	*PNP*	AR	↓↓	↓/N	↓/N	
4. ZAP-70 deficiency	*ZAP70*	AR	(↓↓ CD8)	N	N	
5. CD25 deficiency	*IL-2Rα*	AR	↓	N	N	Lymphoproliferation, autoimmunity
6. CD3 deficiency						
a. CD3γ deficiency	*CD3γ*	AR	N (↓ CD3)	N	N	
b. CD3δ deficiency	*CD3δ*	AR	↓↓	N	N	
c. CD3ε deficiency	*CD3ε*	AR	N (↓ CD3)	N	N	
7. CD45 deficiency	*CD45*	AR	↓↓	N/↑	↓	
8. T-cell activation defects	?	AR	N	N	N	In some cases: myopathy
9. Multiple cytokine defects	?	AR (?)	N	N	N	
10. Human nude phenotype	*WHN*	AR	↓↓	N	N	Alopecia
11. TAP deficiency (MHC class I deficiency)	*TAP 1, TAP 2*	AR	↓ (↓↓ CD8)	N	N	Skin ulcers, lung disease
12. MHC class II deficiency	*CIITA, RFXANK, RFX5, RFXAP*	AR	↓ (↓↓ CD4)	N	N	
13. X-linked hyper-IgM syndrome	*TNFSF5*	XL	N	N	N	
14. ID with multiple intestinal atresias	?	AR (?)	↓	↓	N	Intestinal atresia

AR = autosomal recessive; ID = immunodeficiency; MHC = major histocompatibility complex; SCID = severe combined immunodeficiency; XL = X-linked.

TABLE 15-2 · RELATIVE FREQUENCY OF THE GENETIC FORMS OF SEVERE COMBINED IMMUNODEFICIENCY AND THEIR CHROMOSOMAL LOCI

Genetic Form of SCID	Gene	Locus	Estimated Frequency (%)
Reticular dysgenesis	?	?	<1
Adenosine deaminase deficiency	ADA	20q13.2-q13.11	~8
X-linked SCID	γc	Xq13.1-q13.3	50
AR T⁻B⁺NK⁻ SCID	JAK 3	19p13.1	10
T⁻B⁻ SCID	RAG-1/RAG-2	11p13	10
	Artemis	10p	10
T⁻B⁺NK⁺ SCID	Il-7Rα	—	10
T⁻B⁺NK⁺ SCID	CD45 (PTPRC)	1q31-32	<1
T⁻ SCID	?	?	~2

AR = autosomal recessive; SCID = severe combined immunodeficiency.

complete DiGeorge syndrome, cartilage hair hypoplasia; see Chapter 17). The other forms of CID presented in Table 15-1 are discussed in this chapter.

The molecular defects in many cases of SCID have not yet been identified. This heterogenous group makes up fewer than 10% of the cases; in some of them an autosomal recessive mode of inheritance has been documented. Molecular analysis of known causes of SCID should be attempted in each case. In those in which no known defect is identified, it is particularly important to establish cell lines to facilitate future investigations. Management, including stem cell transplantation, is identical to that for known causes of SCID.

Common Clinical Features

Clinically the CIDs are characterized by early-onset severe infections (chronic diarrhea, interstitial pneumonia, persistent candidiasis), usually leading to growth failure (Buckley et al., 1997; Stephan et al., 1993). Oral candidiasis occurs spontaneously even without the use of antibiotics, and can lead to swallowing difficulties if it extends to the esophagus. Opportunistic organisms, such as *Pneumocystis carinii* and *Aspergillus* species, or viruses (adenovirus, cytomegalovirus, respiratory syncytial virus) are a common cause of infection in CID.

Vaccination with bacillus Calmette-Guerin (BCG) may lead to uncontrolled dissemination, and is often fatal. In the past many patients developed progressive vaccinia following smallpox vaccination. Progressive central nervous system (CNS) poliovirus infection can occur secondary to oral polio vaccination or exposure to a recently immunized individual.

Graft-versus-host disease (GVHD) resulting from transplacental passage of alloreactive maternal T lymphocytes is not uncommon among SCID infants (Fischer, 2000). Although usually asymptomatic, the maternal cells may occasionally cause skin rashes, increased liver enzymes, eosinophilia, and pancytopenia. In contrast, transfusion of unirradiated blood products invariably causes overwhelming proliferation of alloreactive T lymphocytes, with rapidly fatal GVHD (Stephan et al., 1993).

Other features in some SCID patients include chronic hepatitis or sclerosing cholangitis (Thomas et al., 1974).

Chronic encephalopathy is not uncommon; for example, it was present in 11 of 24 autopsy cases reviewed by Dayan in 1971. In one case Jamestown-Canyon (JC) virus with progressive multifocal leukoencephalopathy was observed (ZuRhein et al., 1978).

Cutaneous lesions include recurrent warts or molluscum contagiosum, severe eczema, sparse hair or complete alopecia, seborrheic dermatitis, and cellulitis. Noma of the mucous membrane is noted in some forms of SCID.

Cause

Over the last 10 years, major advances in molecular immunology and genetics have unraveled the molecular basis of many forms of CID (see Table 15-1). The chromosome location of the defects is shown in Table 15-2. This has resulted in improved diagnosis (including prenatal diagnosis) and the introduction of novel forms of treatment, including gene therapy.

Treatment and Prognosis

The natural course of CID is severe, with most patients dying within the first years of life unless treated properly. Use of intravenous immunoglobulin (IVIG), prophylactic cotrimoxazole (to prevent *Pneumocystis carinii* pneumonia), aggressive treatment of infectious episodes, and use of irradiated (25 Gy) blood products may at best prolong survival. In contrast, allogeneic bone marrow transplantation (BMT) or other stem cell transplantation often results in permanent cure, with a recent survival rate of more than 90% if a human leukocyte antigen (HLA)-identical family donor is available (Buckley et al., 1999; Fischer et al., 1990). Excellent results (up to 78% survival) have also been obtained with haploidentical BMT (Buckley et al., 1999).

The discovery of many gene defects and advances in gene transfer technology have advanced the potential efficacy of gene therapy, a strategy that has recently proven effective in the most common form of SCID (i.e., X-linked SCID) (Cavazzana-Calvo et al., 2000). It is expected that additional forms of SCID can be successfully treated by this approach in the future.

X-LINKED SCID CAUSED BY γc DEFICIENCY

Definition

X-linked SCID (XL-SCID) is an X-linked inherited immunodeficiency characterized by the absent development of both mature T and NK lymphocytes and absent immunoglobulin synthesis, despite the presence of B cells, leading to the early onset of severe infections. It is caused by mutations in the interleukin (IL)-2 receptor common gamma chain (IL-2Rγc, γc) encoding a gene located on the long arm of the X chromosome. XL-SCID accounts for approximately half of the cases of SCID, thus explaining the male predominance of all affected SCID patients (see Table 15-2). Its estimated incidence is 1:150,000 to 1:200,000 live births.

Historical Aspects

SCID was recognized in the early 1950s and included both X-linked and autosomal recessive forms of SCID. The first successful BMT was performed in 1968 in a patient with XL-SCID (Gatti et al., 1968). Partial B-cell function in XL-SCID was described in the 1970s (Griscelli et al., 1978). The advent of genetic tools led to mapping of the XL-SCID locus to Xq13 (de Saint Basile et al., 1985; Puck et al., 1993). In 1993 it was recognized that mutations of the γc gene, cloned a year earlier (Takeshita et al., 1992), were associated with XL-SCID (Noguchi et al., 1993).

Pathogenesis

T-Cell Differentiation

In XL-SCID patients, mature T cells are absent not only in the peripheral blood but also in peripheral lymphoid tissues. The thymus lacks corticomedullary differentiation, lymphoid precursors are scarce, and Hassall's corpuscles are not present. These findings indicate that there is an early block in T-cell differentiation.

XL-SCID is curable by allogeneic BMT, indicating that the defect is intrinsic to the lymphoid lineage (Buckley et al., 1999). Studies of X-chromosome inactivation in obligate carriers have shown a skewed pattern in T and NK cells, as well as in B cells, whereas a random pattern was usually detected in other hematopoietic cell lineages (Conley et al., 1988; Wengler et al., 1993). The XL-SCID gene product is therefore expressed and involved in the maturation of the T-, B-, and NK-cell lineages.

Identification of the XL-SCID Gene Defect

The XL-SCID locus was mapped to Xq12-13.1 by de Saint Basile and colleagues in 1985. It was then recognized that the γc gene encoding for the common γ chain of the IL-2 receptor was localized to the same region, and mutations of the γc gene were found in XL-SCID patients (Noguchi et al., 1993; Puck et al., 1993). A direct causal relationship between γc mutations and XL-SCID has been demonstrated convincingly: All patients with XL-SCID exhibit γc gene mutations (Puck, 1996). In vitro gene transfer of γc into these patients' Epstein-Barr virus (EBV)-transformed B cells and marrow cells corrects expression of their high-affinity IL-2 receptor deficiency and T/NK-cell differentiation block, respectively (Candotti et al., 1996; Cavazzana-Calvo et al., 1996; Hacein-Bey-Abina et al., 1996; Taylor et al., 1996b).

Canine X-linked SCID is also associated with a mutation in the γc gene (Henthorn et al., 1994), and γc(−) mice exhibit a similar although not entirely identical phenotype (Cao et al., 1995; DiSanto et al., 1995a).

Function of the γc Chain

The common γc receptor belongs to the hematopoietic cytokine receptor family, characterized by four conserved cysteines and the repeated tryptophan, serine (WS) motif (Takeshita et al., 1992). The γc-chain is constitutively expressed by T, B, and NK cells, as well as myeloid cells and erythroblasts (Leonard et al., 1994). γc, together with the IL-2Rα and IL-2Rβ subunits, generates the high-affinity receptor for IL-2, which plays a major role in signal transduction through activation of its associated tyrosine kinase Jak-3 (Leonard et al., 1994).

Because XL-SCID is lethal, a 30% rate for new mutations is expected for each generation, accounting for the variety of mutations found to date. It is remarkable that many single amino acid substitutions in the extracellular domain are sufficient to abrogate T- and NK-cell differentiation. Some affect conserved cysteines and the WS motif, the structure of which is likely to be required for the overall configuration of the molecule (Puck et al., 1993).

The common γc receptor is not only a member of the IL-2 receptor but also of the IL-4, IL-7, IL-9, IL-15, and IL-21 receptors (Dumoutier et al., 2000; Malek et al., 1999), augmenting in each case the affinity of the receptor for the particular cytokine and participating in signal transduction. The XL-SCID phenotype appears therefore to be the complex association of defects in all six cytokine/receptor systems.

Role of IL-7

Studies of mutant mice generated by homologous recombination have underscored the role of IL-7 in T-cell differentiation. The T-cell phenotype of γc(−) mice is virtually identical to IL-7(−) and IL-7Rα(−) mice (Peschon et al., 1994; von Freeden-Jeffry et al., 1995). These data strongly argue for a major role of IL-7 in inducing survival and proliferation of early T-cell progenitors in the thymus (Akashi et al., 1997; DiSanto et al., 1995b; Maraskovsky et al., 1997). This conclusion is confirmed by the finding of a block in T-cell development in two patients with IL-7Rα deficiencies (Puel et al., 1998) (see later discussion). Furthermore, γδ T cells are completely lacking in γc(−) mice.

NK-Cell Deficiency

The NK-cell deficiency observed in XL-SCID is likely to be the consequence of defective IL-15-induced signaling, because IL-15 (in combination with stem cell factor [SCF]) can trigger CD56+ NK-cell generation from CD34+ marrow progenitors (Mrozek et al., 1996). Following γc gene transfer into XL-SCID patients' marrow cells, the differentiation of functional NK cells (CD56+) was observed in the presence of SCF and IL-15 (Cavazzana-Calvo et al., 1996).

B-Cell Function

In vitro, XL-SCID B cells produce IgE in the presence of IL-4 and a CD40-mediated signal (Matthews et al., 1995). However, XL-SCID EBV-transformed B cells do not activate Jak-3 and signal transducers and activators of transcription (STAT)6 in the presence of IL-4 (Izuhara et al., 1996). These results can be explained by the presence of a γc-independent IL-4 receptor able to transduce at least some signals after IL-4 binding. As expected, IL-2 and IL-15 do not induce an immunoglobulin switch in XL-SCID B cells, in contrast to their effects on normal B cells (Matthews et al., 1995). Whereas V(D)J elements of immunoglobulin genes rearrange normally in XL-SCID B cells, most of the JH elements are in germ-line configuration, probably reflecting a lack of T-cell help (Minegishi et al., 1994).

Clinical Features

Patients with XL-SCID usually present during the first months of life with oral candidiasis (thrush), persistent diarrhea with failure to thrive, and/or interstitial pneumonia often caused by *Pneumocystis carinii*. Occasionally, other intracellular organisms such as listeria or legionella can cause devastating disease, as can viruses, especially those of the herpes group or respiratory syncytial virus. In rare cases, EBV infection can lead to uncontrolled B-cell proliferation. Live attenuated vaccines are another cause of severe clinical manifestations. BCG vaccination may lead to disseminated, often lethal infection (Buckley et al., 1997; Stephan et al., 1993).

The presence of maternal T cells (see later discussion) can be associated with an exanthematous rash, skin exfoliation, eosinophilia, and mildly elevated liver enzymes.

Diagnosis

The diagnosis of XL-SCID should be suspected in male infants with severe lymphopenia, a finding present in more than 90% of these patients. Low T-cell counts associated with low numbers of NK cells and normal or, more often, elevated B cells are typically observed. On chest x-ray examination, no thymic shadow can be seen. Mitogen-induced lymphocyte proliferation is low, whereas serum immunoglobulin levels reflect the presence of maternal IgG immunoglobulin, with low serum IgM and IgA levels.

Occurrence of this phenotype in a boy is suggestive of XL-SCID. A family history of X-linked inheritance is found in approximately 50% of cases. The diagnosis should be confirmed by molecular testing.

Absence of the γc molecule on the surface of lymphocytes or monocytes by immunofluorescence may be difficult to interpret because the level of γc expression by normal cells is low. It is therefore important to perform the immunofluorescence procedure in an experienced laboratory. Furthermore, the presence of maternal T cells (in most cases between 50 to 5000/µl), which express normal levels of γc, can falsely exclude the diagnosis. The analysis of γc expression by monocytes (γc expression by B cells is very low) is the best technique to screen for XL-SCID. However, some patients' lymphocytes and monocytes express mutated γc protein in normal quantity, and only mutation analysis of the γc gene confirms the diagnosis of XL-SCID.

Atypical cases of XL-SCID include forms with progressive loss of T-cell number and function, leading to death during childhood (Brooks et al., 1990; de Saint-Basile et al., 1992). These atypical phenotypes may be due to splice-site or missense mutations that result in the expression of lower amounts of γc protein with a conserved binding for IL-2, or to γc gene mutations that reduce interaction with Jak-3, and thus impair T-cell activation (DiSanto et al., 1994; Russell et al., 1994; Schmalstieg et al., 1995). Finally, some missense mutations of the γc gene may result in the expression of normal amounts of protein with reduced IL-2 (or IL-7) binding (Kumaki et al., 1999; Sharfe et al., 1997).

A unique patient, in whom a reverse mutation occurred in an early T-cell progenitor, developed substantial amounts of circulating T cells (that lasted for years) that expressed normal amounts of γc protein. In these T cells, as a result of the reverse mutation, sequence of the γc gene was normal; in contrast, B cells had a mutated γc gene, resulting in lack of surface protein expression (Stephan et al., 1996).

Although in all of these cases the atypical phenotype was the direct consequence of the specific genetic defects, in other cases the mechanisms underlying clinical and phenotypic heterogeneity of XL-SCID remain poorly understood, as in a patient who had near-normal numbers of T cells in spite of a γc gene deletion encompassing most of the cytoplasmic tail of the protein (Morelon et al., 1996).

Differential Diagnosis

If a high T-cell count caused by maternal T-cell engraftment argues against a diagnosis of SCID, but the clinical manifestations are typical enough, a systematic search for the maternal origin of the circulating T cells should be performed.

Other forms of SCID may present with a similar phenotype but with autosomal recessive inheritance, as in the case of Jak-3 deficiency (see later discussion). Although IL-7Rα deficiency and nonmolecularly defined SCID can present with low T- and high B-cell counts, they generally have detectable NK cells in blood.

Complete DiGeorge syndrome, by definition, is associated with the absence of peripheral blood T cells, whereas B cells are usually normal or high. A correct differential diagnosis between XL-SCID and DiGeorge syndrome is important, because the two entities require different treatments. Associated clinical features, the presence of NK cells, and the demonstration of hemizygous interstitial deletion of chromosome 22q11 or a chromosome 10 abnormality support the diagnosis of DiGeorge syndrome (see Chapter 17).

About 2% to 5% of XL-SCID patients present with a low B-cell count (Buckley et al., 1997). In these cases, the diagnosis of autosomal recessive SCID associated with abnormal V(D)J recombination resulting from recombinase activating gene *(RAG) RAG-1* or *RAG-2* deficiency or to an *Artemis* gene defect (see later discussion) should be considered. Only the detection of a deleterious γc gene mutation, inherited from a carrier mother in two thirds of cases (the others being new mutations), ascertains the diagnosis of XL-SCID.

Prenatal Diagnosis and Carrier Detection

Carrier females can be detected either by studying the profile of X-chromosome inactivation in lymphocytes, which is highly skewed, or, preferably, by mutation detection. Male fetuses at risk can be screened by mutation analysis of the γc gene using deoxyribonucleic acid (DNA) obtained from chorionic villous biopsy performed at weeks 8 to 10 of pregnancy.

Treatment

If untreated, the prognosis of XL-SCID is poor and most affected boys die by age 1 year. Treatment of bacterial, viral, and fungal infections; IVIG, and cotrimoxazole prophylaxis for *P. carinii* can at best marginally prolong survival. Other obligatory measures include irradiation of blood products to avoid fatal GVHD and avoidance of live vaccines such as BCG.

Stem Cell Transplantation

The standard treatment for XL-SCID is allogeneic BMT (or other stem cell transplantation) as first described in 1968 (Gatti et al., 1968) (see Chapter 43). The BMT procedure for SCID patients requires neither myeloablation nor immunosuppression to achieve lymphoid engraftment, and usually results in split chimerism, because only T cells (+/– NK cells) are of donor origin. HLA-identical BMT is characterized by rapid T-cell reconstitution following expansion of the donor memory T-cell pool (Buckley et al., 1999; Fischer et al., 1990). Newly generated T cells can be detected 3 to 4 months after BMT, the minimal time interval required for efficient development of T cells in the host thymus (Buckley et al., 1999; Fischer et al., 1990). In recent years, the probability of success has reached more than 90% when an HLA-matched donor is available.

Since the early 1980s SCID patients lacking an HLA identical donor have been treated with haploidentical stem cell transplantation, usually from a parent. Elimination of T cells from the marrow inoculum to minimize GVHD was the key to success (Reisner et al., 1983). A recent survey showed that, in the absence of GVHD, survival can reach 78% (Buckley et al., 1999). Myeloablation is not a prerequisite (Buckley et al., 1999, 2000; Fischer et al., 1990).

Cord blood, matched unrelated bone marrow, or peripheral blood mobilized CD34 cells from suitable donors can also be used as a source of stem cells. Fully or partially matched cord blood cells are given without T-cell depletion (Knutsen and Wall, 2000).

An important shortcoming of BMT in SCID is the frequent persistence of B-cell deficiency with hypogammaglobulinemia. Most patients in whom donor B cells engraft acquire a repertoire of functional B cells (White et al., 2000). In contrast, the majority of patients with host B cells do not produce normal amounts of immunoglobulins and specific antibodies, making long-term treatment with IVIG necessary.

In Utero Stem Cell Transplantation

In utero stem cell transplantation following prenatal diagnosis is another option. Two reports have demonstrated that intrauterine injection of parental CD34+ cells can lead to normal T-cell development without harmful effects (Flake et al., 1996; Wengler et al., 1996). However, the advantage of this therapeutic procedure is decreased risk of GVHD and rapid and more complete immune reconstitution must be established, considering the risk, although small, associated with intrauterine puncture and the high likelihood of a cure accomplished by BMT in the neonatal period (Buckley et al., 1999).

Gene Therapy

Because of the invariably lethal outcome of XL-SCID unless treated by BMT—which may result in complications or incomplete immune reconstitution—gene therapy was considered an alternative treatment as soon as the γc gene was discovered. Selective advantage of transduced patient's cells was expected, because functional γc expression provides survival, growth, and differentiation signals to lymphocyte progenitors. The observation of reverse mutations of the γc gene (Stephan et al., 1996) provided further encouragement for a successful gene therapy approach.

Following γc gene transfer into CD34+ cells using an MFG vector, we achieved correction of the T- and NK-cell immunodeficiency in 9 of 11 patients with γc deficiency (Cavazzana-Calvo et al., 2000; Hacein-Bey-Abina et al., 2002). In nine of them, ex vivo gene transfer into hematopoietic progenitors led to the development of normal T-cell counts, which readily expressed the γc protein, the product of the transgene. They also recognize and react to microbial antigens, including vaccines. Therefore these nine patients were able to live in a normal environment in a normal fashion without the need for IVIG.

These results provide proof of the principle that gene therapy can work. They demonstrate that a selective survival advantage provided by the gene occurs, leading to immune reconstitution and clinical benefit.

However, two of the nine infants (ages 1 and 3 months) who successfully underwent gene therapy developed a clonal T-lymphocyte lymphoproliferation akin to T-cell leukemia 30 and 34 months following gene therapy, characterized by a marked increase in CD3 cells, anemia, and splenomegaly (Hacein-Bey-Abina et al., 2003).

The CD3 cells showed an expansion of a γδ TCR clone in one patient and an expansion of three αβ TCR clones in the other. The former received a matched unrelated marrow transplant and the latter received chemotherapy. Both are alive and well.

Analysis of the clones disclosed that the retrovirus vector integration occurred in proximity to the LMO-2 proto-oncogene promoter, leading to aberrant transcription and expression of LMO-2. LMO-2 is a transcription factor required for normal hematopoiesis.

Possible contributing factors include chicken pox in one patient prior to the clonal expansion, the young age of the patients, a large dose of transfected autologous cells, a probable expanded pool of target precursor cells, and the presence of immunodeficiency leading to selection and expansion of transduced cells.

Alain Fischer

AUTOSOMAL RECESSIVE SCID CAUSED BY Jak3 DEFICIENCY

Definition

Patients with autosomal recessive SCID resulting from Jak3 deficiency resemble patients with XL-SCID because both have a virtual absence of T cells and NK cells, but have normal or elevated numbers of nonfunctional B cells (e.g., a T⁻B⁺NK⁻ SCID) (Notarangelo and Candotti, 2000). Although a relatively low number of Jak3-deficient subjects have been diagnosed worldwide, it is an important cause of autosomal recessive SCID in the United States (Buckley, 2000), and its prevalence in Europe appears even higher (Ihle, 1996).

Historical Aspects

Jak3 deficiency was first suspected as a cause of SCID after XL-SCID patients were identified whose mutations of the γc receptor resulted in impaired interaction between γc and Jak3 (Russell et al., 1994). Several patients with autosomal recessive T⁻B⁺NK⁺ SCID with mutations of Jak3 were subsequently described (Bozzi et al., 1998; Buckley et al., 1997; Candotti et al., 1997; Macchi et al., 1995; Russell et al., 1995; Schumacher et al., 2000), thus confirming that Jak3 deficiency is a distinct entity with clinical features virtually indistinguishable from XL-SCID.

Pathogenesis

Jak3 is a member of the *Janus associated* family of protein tyrosine *k*inases and plays a crucial role in hematopoietic cytokine signaling (Leonard and O'Shea,

1998). Jak3 is the only enzyme associated with the common γ chain of multiple cytokine receptors (the molecule mutated in XL-SCID) and mediates the downstream signaling of crucial cytokines such as IL-2, IL-4, IL-7, IL-9, IL-15, and IL-21 (Fig. 15-1). In particular, binding of the cytokine to the specific γc-containing receptor results in dimerization of the cytokine receptor chains, and activation and cross-phosphorylation of the Jak1 and Jak3 kinases associated with the intracytoplasmic tails of the cytokine receptor.

The Jak kinases also phosphorylate tyrosine residues of the cytokine receptor chains, thus generating docking sites for SH2 domain-containing STAT proteins (Leonard and O'Shea, 1998). STATs are in turn phosphorylated by the Jaks; this allows dimerization of the STATs that then translocate to the nucleus where they bind to promoter sequences of cytokine-inducible genes mediating their transcription (Ihle, 1996).

The Jak3 protein is organized into seven Janus homology (JH) domains, the most C-terminal of which (JH1) mediates kinase activity. Molecular analysis of patients with Jak3 deficiency has demonstrated that mutations can occur throughout the *Jak3* gene (Fig. 15-2) with apparent clustering in the regions coding for the JH2 and JH3 domains of the Jak3 protein (Notarangelo and Candotti, 2000). EBV-transformed B-cell lines from Jak3-deficient patients have provided unique biologic tools to study the effects of these mutations on the expression and function of the Jak3 protein.

Lack of expression of Jak3 leads to profound impairment of signaling through all cytokine receptors using γc, thus duplicating the abnormalities caused by mutations of γc in XL-SCID patients (Candotti et al., 1997; Russell et al., 1995; Taylor et al., 1997). Although in a number of cases residual expression of the mutant protein was demonstrated, Jak3 function was found to be profoundly affected (Bozzi et al., 1998; Candotti et al., 1997; Notarangelo and Candotti, 2000), thus providing important clues as to the Jak3 structure/function relationship. In particular, mutations in the JH2 pseudokinase domain were shown to directly interfere

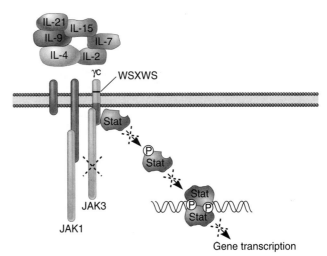

Figure 15-1 · Diagram describing the interaction of Jak3 with cytokine receptors and its role in the Jak/STAT signal transduction cascade.

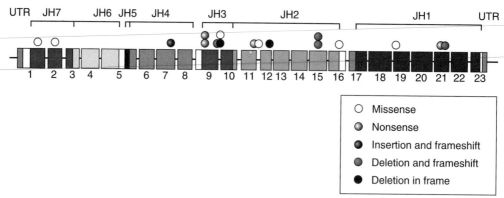

Figure 15-2 · Schematic representation of the *JAK3* open reading frame with position and type of 17 mutations identified in 11 Jak3-deficient families. The 23 Jak3 exons are represented by numbered boxes, and their specific contribution to the seven Jak homology (JH) domains is highlighted. UTR = untranslated region.

with the kinase activity of Jak3 (Chen et al., 2000), whereas mutations of the JH7 N-terminal domain abrogated Jak3 binding to γc (Cacalano et al., 1999).

In both instances downstream cytokine signaling events are impaired, thus providing a biochemical basis for this immunodeficiency (Cacalano et al., 1999; Chen et al., 2000). A mutation database for Jak3 deficiency has been organized, and is accessible at http://www.bioinfo/JAK3base/ (Vihinen et al., 2000).

Classic mouse genetics experiments have corroborated the critical role of Jak3 in lymphocyte development through the generation of knockout mice that also showed profound immune deficiency with lack of CD8+ T lymphocytes and NK cells. In contrast to the human illness, Jak3-knockout animals may develop a substantial number of CD4+ T cells (which, however, are phenotypically and functionally abnormal), and negligible numbers of B cells whose development seems blocked at the pro–B-cell stage (Nosaka et al., 1995; Park et al., 1995; Thomis and Berg, 1997; Thomis et al., 1995). The reasons for the differences in phenotype between Jak3-deficient mice and humans are not clear; however, the importance of IL-7 for B lymphopoiesis in mice, but not in humans, may explain these B-cell development differences (Thomis et al., 1995).

Clinical and Laboratory Features

Jak3-deficient patients present in the first few months of life with clinical features of SCID, including chronic diarrhea and failure to thrive, severe respiratory and/or generalized infections from opportunistic pathogens, or signs of graft-versus-host reaction from transplacentally acquired maternal T cells. Jak3-deficient patients may or may not be lymphopenic, but generally present with low to undetectable numbers of T cells and NK cells, whereas absolute B-cell counts are normal or increased (T–B+NK– SCID). Lymphocytes fail to proliferate to mitogenic stimulation and serum immune globulins are usually low or undetectable.

Because of the clinical and immunologic similarities of XL-SCID, Jak3 deficiency, and IL-7 receptor α chain deficiency, all three should be included in the differential diagnosis of patients with T–B+ SCID. The definitive diagnosis of Jak3 deficiency is established by Western blot analysis for Jak3 expression in the patients' fresh lymphocytes or lymphoid cell lines and/or demonstration of *JAK3* gene mutations. Because Jak3 deficiency may be present in the presence of significant numbers of circulating, although poorly functioning, T cells (Brugnoni et al., 1998), screening for Jak3 expression and/or mutations should be considered in all undefined cases of SCID, especially those presenting with a high proportion of peripheral B lymphocytes.

Availability of the structure of the human *JAK3* gene allows prenatal diagnosis based on DNA analysis of chorionic villus biopsies (Schumacher et al., 1999).

Treatment

The treatment of choice for Jak3 deficiency is allogeneic BMT, often life-saving for these patients. Although information is available for only a few BMTs in patients with molecularly defined Jak3 deficiency, reconstitution of normal T-cell numbers and function has been reported after both HLA-identical and haploidentical BMTs. Similar to other forms of T–B+ SCID, partially matched BMTs are less likely to result in complete restoration of the B-cell compartment compared with transplantation with HLA-matched donors (Buckley et al., 1999; Notarangelo and Candotti, 2000). Competition between host and donor B-cell progenitors may be responsible for the persistence of host-derived, nonfunctional B lymphocytes in Jak3-deficient patients.

Gene therapy is being investigated for Jak3-deficient patients. Because of the clinical and biochemical similarities between Jak3 deficiency and XL-SCID, genetic correction and engraftment of autologous hematopoietic stem cell should be possible in Jak3-deficient patients similar to the results in XL-SCID patients (Cavazzama-Calvo et al., 2000).

Preclinical experiments in *JAK3* knockout mice have demonstrated that retroviral-mediated *JAK3* gene transfer into hematopoietic stem cells is safe and leads to reconstitution of lymphoid development and specific immunity in treated mice (Bunting et al., 1998,

1999), thus supporting the use of similar strategies for humans.

Prognosis

Similar to other forms of SCID, Jak3 deficiency is a pediatric emergency and affected patients do not survive beyond infancy without reconstitution by allogeneic BMT. The results of BMTs performed in 14 Jak3-deficient patients showed excellent rates of engraftment and survival (Buckley et al., 1999; Notarangelo and Candotti, 2000), comparable to the results in other T⁻B⁺ SCID patients (Buckley et al., 1999; Fischer et al., 1990; Haddad et al., 1998).

The absence of host NK cells in Jak3-deficient and other T⁻B⁺ SCID patients is likely to reduce the occurrence of graft failures (Haddad et al., 1998). In contrast to the uniform reconstitution of T-cell immunity observed in all reported cases of Jak3 deficiency treated with BMT, 4 out of 12 Jak3-deficient patients who underwent haploidentical BMT had incomplete B-cell reconstitution and thus continued to need IVIG therapy. As noted, B-cell deficiency post-BMT is not unique to Jak3-deficient patients, but is common to many T⁻B⁺ SCID patients receiving haploidentical transplants (Buckley et al., 1999; Hadda et al., 1998). This may cause significant late morbidity in these patients.

Fabio Candotti and Luigi Notarangelo

AUTOSOMAL RECESSIVE SCID CAUSED BY IL-7Rα DEFICIENCY

Definition

IL-7 receptor-α deficiency results in an autosomal recessive form of SCID characterized by selective absence of T-lymphocyte development. So far, six cases in three families have been reported or mentioned (Buckley, 2000; Puel and Leonard, 2000; Puel et al., 1998; Roifman et al., 2000). B lymphocytes and NK lymphocytes are present in normal numbers, and B-cell counts can be elevated. It accounts for about 10% of the total SCID patients.

Pathogenesis

IL-7 is produced by stromal cells in bone marrow and in the thymus. The IL-7 receptor consists of two subunits, the γc chain shared with the IL-2, IL-4, IL-9, IL-15, and IL-21 receptors (see XL-SCID) and the α chain specific for IL-7R. IL-7Rα −/− mice exhibit a block in T-cell development at the TCR⁻CD4⁻CD8⁻CD44⁻CD25⁺ stage although some mature peripheral T cells can be detected (Peschon et al., 1994). The IL-7 receptor is expressed by lymphoid precursor cells, including a fraction of marrow CD34⁺ cells. IL-7 provides survival and proliferative signals to IL-7R⁺ cells.

Two patients with typical T⁻B⁺NK⁺ SCID were first reported with mutations in the *IL-7Rα* gene located on chromosome 5p13 (Puel et al., 1998). In one patient, the IL-7Rα messenger ribonucleic acid (mRNA) level was reduced and undetectable in the second. In the former, two heterozygous mutations (a splice function acceptor mutation and a nonsense mutation leading to a premature stop codon) were found. The latter patient had a homozygous donor splice site mutation. In both cases no functional IL-7R protein was made.

Three related patients were recently reported with a missense mutation at position 132, resulting in an IL-7Rα chain that was normally expressed but bound IL-7 poorly (Roifman et al., 2000). The phenotype of these three cases was similar to other IL-7Rα-deficient patients (i.e., T⁻B⁺NK⁺).

Clinical Features

The clinical presentation of all IL-7Rα-deficient patients is that of typical SCID, presenting with infections and lymph node hypoplasia during the first 4 months of age.

The diagnosis of IL-7Rα deficiency should be considered in patients with low T-cell counts and normal or elevated NK- and B-cell counts who do not have γc or Jak3 mutations. The identification of an *IL-7Rα* gene mutation confirms the diagnosis. IL-7Rα deficiency accounts for 1% to 2% of SCID patients.

DiGeorge syndrome can present with the same immunologic phenotype, but in most cases, associated features such as cardiac defects, hypoparathyroidism, and micrognathism distinguish DiGeorge syndrome from SCID. The demonstration of chromosome 22 or 10 hemizygous interstitial deletions distinguishes DiGeorge syndrome patients from SCID patients.

Treatment

Similar to other forms of SCID, supportive care (see previous discussion) should be provided. Allogeneic stem cell transplantation is the treatment of choice and may be curative. It is unclear, based on the low number of cases, whether haploidentical stem cell transplantation requires conditioning to prevent NK-cell mediated graft rejection. IL-7Rα deficiency is also a good candidate disease for gene therapy because *IL-7Rα* gene expression, similar to γc, should provide a growth advantage for transduced lymphoid precursors.

Alain Fischer

AUTOSOMAL RECESSIVE SCID CAUSED BY *RAG-1* OR *RAG-2* DEFICIENCIES

Definition

Autosomal recessive SCID associated with recombinase activating gene (RAG) abnormalities have the typical clinical features of SCID but lack both T and B cells but not NK cells. This T⁻B⁻NK⁺ phenotype composes approximately 20% of SCID patients. RAG-deficient patients have mutations in *RAG-1* or *RAG-2* genes leading to impaired V(D)J recombinational activity.

Another group of patients with defective recombinase activation have increased radiosensitivity and are termed *radiation-sensitive SCID* or *Athabascan SCID* associated with an *Artemis* gene defect. A third group of patients with defective recombinase activation have *Omenn syndrome* (OS) with distinct clinical features that differentiates them from other defective recombinase activation. These latter two forms are discussed subsequently.

Pathogenesis

B and T lymphocytes recognize foreign antigens through specialized receptors: the Ig and the T-cell receptor (TCR), respectively. Their highly polymorphic antigen-recognition regions are composed of variable (V), diversity (D), and joining (J) gene segments that undergo somatic rearrangement prior to their expression, a mechanism known as *V(D)J recombination* (Tonegawa, 1983).

V(D)J recombination occurs in three steps. RAG-1 and RAG-2 proteins initiate the rearrangement process through the recognition of recombination signal sequences (RSS) and the introduction of a DNA double-strand break (dsb) (Oettinger, 1990; Schatz et al., 1989). The next step is the recognition and signaling of the DNA damage to the DNA repair machinery and, finally, repair of the DNA.

The recognition that SCID mice (Bosma et al., 1983) have a general DNA repair defect with increased sensitivity to ionizing radiation or other agents causing DNA dsb suggested a link between V(D)J recombination and DNA dsb repair (Biedermann, 1991; Fulop, 1990; Hendrickson, 1991). The Ku70, Ku80, and the DNA-dependent protein kinase catalytic subunit (DNA-PKcs) complex was identified as a DNA damage sensor (Jackson and Jeggo, 1995). Cells from SCID mice lack DNA-PKcs activity owing to a mutation in the *DNA-PKcs* encoding gene; this compromises V(D)J recombination and results in an early arrest of T- and B-cell development (Blunt et al., 1996; Danska et al., 1996).

Additional proteins (XRCC4 and DNA ligase IV) mediate the final step of DNA repair through nonhomologous end joining. The crucial role of both the V(D)J recombination and the DNA repair machinery in lymphoid development is illustrated by the fact that all the animal models (either natural, such as murine and equine SCID, or those generated through homologous recombination) with defects in any of these proteins have a profound and early arrest in B- and T-cell maturation.

Schwarz and colleagues (1991) and Abe and associates (1994) identified defects in V(D)J recombination in some patients with T⁻B⁻ SCID. These patients can be further divided in two groups according to the response of their cells to ionizing radiation. Patients in group 1 are defective in the early phases of V(D)J recombination, carry mutations in either the *RAG-1* or *RAG-2* genes, and do not exhibit an increased radiosensitivity

(Notarangelo et al., 1999). Patients in group 2 have increased radiosensitivity to ionizing radiation, affecting both bone marrow cells and primary skin fibroblasts, suggesting a defect in the later phases of V(D)J recombination (Cavazzana-Calvo et al., 1993).

RAG-1 and RAG-2 are the lymphoid restricted factors of the V(D)J recombinase. They were identified through their capacity to accomplish V(D)J recombination of extrachromosomal substrates in fibroblasts, non-lymphoid cells normally devoid of V(D)J recombination activity. They initiate the recombination process through the recognition of RSSs that flank all Ig and TCR genes.

Their critical role during lymphoid development was documented through targeting experiments in mice (Mombaerts et al., 1992; Shinkai et al., 1992). RAG-1–/– and RAG-2–/– mice are devoid of both mature B and T cells owing to a defect in the V(D)J recombination process. In view of the similarity between RAG-1/RAG-2 knock-out mice and the human T⁻B⁻SCID phenotype, Schwarz and co-workers (1996) successfully identified mutations of either the *RAG-1* or *RAG-2* gene in a group of patients with this condition.

The identification of disease-causing mutations of the RAG proteins is of particular interest for the understanding of structure-function relationship. For RAG-2, a three-dimensional model has been proposed consisting of a β-propeller like structure, a motif known as the Kelch motif (Callebaut and Mornon, 1998), which is involved in protein–protein interactions. Interestingly, several mutations of the *RAG-2* gene were localized in the region of this putative β-propeller structure thought to represent the region of interaction with RAG-1 (Corneo et al., 2000). A review of RAG-1/RAG-2 mutations has been published (Villa et al., 2001), demonstrating that characteristic phenotypes correlate with certain genotypes, including OS.

Clinical Features

The clinical presentation of RAG-deficient T⁻B⁻ SCID includes severe respiratory infections (often sustained by opportunistic pathogens), chronic diarrhea, failure to thrive, persistent candidiasis, and eczematoid dermatitis. Transplacental passage and persistence of maternal T lymphocytes is common and may occasionally lead to clinical manifestations of GVHD. Although these features are usually mild, transfusion of unirradiated blood products results in dramatic, most often fatal, GVHD. Vaccination with live attenuated viruses or BCG may also lead to disseminated infection.

The immunologic phenotype is characterized by severe lymphopenia, with virtual absence of T and B lymphocytes, unless maternal T-cell engraftment has occurred; almost all circulating lymphocytes are NK cells. After the decline of maternally transferred immunoglobulins, profound hypogammaglobulinemia becomes apparent, and antibody production is not elicited following immunization.

Treatment

As for other forms of SCID, supportive therapy includes antibiotics, nutritional support, and IVIG. Definitive treatment is BMT.

Jean-Pierre de Villartay

AUTOSOMAL RECESSIVE SCID CAUSED BY A DEFECT OF THE *ARTEMIS* GENE (RADIATION-SENSITIVE SCID, ATHABASCAN SCID)

Definition

These patients have a T$^-$B$^-$NK$^+$ phenotype, and are characterized by increased cellular radiosensitivity, suggesting a general DNA repair defect (Nicolas et al., 1998). Mutations in *RAG-1* and *RAG-2* genes affecting DNA repair have been excluded by linkage analysis (Li et al., 1998), but recent studies have identified a point mutation in a gene termed *Artemis* located on chromosome 10p13.

A high incidence of SCID was reported in the Navajo and Apache American Indian tribes by Murphy and colleagues in 1980. These individuals are from the Athabascan linguistic group who migrated to the southwest United States from Asia via the Behring Strait, Alaska, and Canada between 700 and 1300 AD (Li et al., 2002). The incidence of Athabascan SCID is as high as 1 in 2000 in these groups (Hu et al., 1988; Jones et al., 1991; Murphy et al., 1980).

Pathogenesis

The lack of B and T lymphocytes and the increased radiosensitivity of RS-SCID cells is reminiscent of SCID mice, who have a general DNA repair defect. Indeed, V(D)J recombination assays in fibroblasts from radiosensitive (RS)-SCID patients confirmed the absence of coding-joint formation, whereas signal joints were formed normally (Nicolas et al., 1998). Abnormal V(D)J junctions of IgH genes were also demonstrated ex vivo in bone marrow cells from radiation-sensitive RS-SCID patients (Schwarz et al., 1991).

SCID Mice Model

RS-SCID patients are not the human homologue of SCID mice for several reasons. First, a direct defect in DNA-repair was not demonstrated by pulse-field gel electrophoresis following irradiation, whereas a distinctive defect in the kinetics of DNA repair is characteristic of murine SCID cells (Nicolas et al., 1996). Second, unlike SCID mice, RS-SCID patients' fibroblast extracts demonstrate a normal Ku70-80/DNA-PKcs complex with normal kinase activity (Nicolas et al., 1998). Finally murine SCID cells have a mutation in the DNA-

PKcs encoding gene, which was ultimately ruled out by genetic means in several consanguineous RS-SCID families (Nicolas et al., 1998).

Interestingly, cells from RS-SCID patients have no defect in cell cycle progression checkpoints (our unpublished observations). In particular, the G0/G1 arrest following irradiation was normal in these cells, whereas it is generally impaired in other human immune deficiency disorders associated with DNA-repair defects (e.g., ataxia-telangiectasia–like or Nijmegen-breakage syndromes [Petrini, 2000]).

A causal role for other known genes involved in V(D)J recombination/DNA repair has also been excluded by means of genetic linkage analysis.

Mapping and Cloning of Artemis

Genome-wide analysis revealed that in the Athabascan SCID and RS-SCID, the gene involved was located on the short arm of human chromosome 10 (Li et al., 1998; Moshous et al., 2000). The gene responsible for RS-SCID, eventually identified by positional cloning, is named *Artemis*. It is broadly expressed, and encodes a 78-kD protein with homology to β-lactamases (Moshous et al., 2001).

Artemis is composed of 14 exons, and a variety of mutations have been identified in patients with RS-SCID. Interestingly, nearly all the mutations described are functionally null, and are represented by intragenic deletions, frameshift, and nonsense mutations. Transfection of wild-type *Artemis* complementary DNA (cDNA) into fibroblasts from patients with RS-SCID has led to complementation of the V(D)J recombination defect, further demonstrating the crucial role of *Artemis* mutations in RS-SCID (Moshous et al., 2001). Although all cases with RS-SCID appear to be due to *Artemis* gene mutations, it is unclear whether leaky mutations in this gene may cause a subtler and less severe immune deficiency. In any case, identification of the molecular basis for RS-SCID has now made early prenatal diagnosis feasible.

Function of Artemis

In spite of successful cloning of the Artemis gene, the function of the encoded protein is still poorly defined. Recent evidence suggests that Artemis protein forms a complex with DNA-PKcs, and is in fact a substrate for DNA-PKcs kinase activity (Ma et al., 2002). It has been hypothesized that Artemis plays a role in opening of the DNA hairpin that is formed following the DNA dsb introduced by RAG activity.

Clinical Features

Similar to other infants with SCID, RS-SCID patients present early in life with serious infections, failure to thrive, and profound lymphopenia. T and B cells are very low but NK cells are abundant and function normally. A thymus shadow is absent on chest x-ray examination and engraftment of maternal cells is not uncommon.

A characteristic clinical feature of Athabascan SCID is the frequent appearance of noma-like ulcers of the oral mucosa or genitalia. This occurred in 12 of 18 infants; cultures and histologic studies revealed no unique abnormalities. Successful transplantation led to resolution of the lesions (Kwong et al., 1999; O'Marcaigh et al., 2001; Rotbart et al., 1986).

Treatment

Supportive care (antibiotics, IVIG, nutritional support) is used prior to bone marrow or stem cell transplantation. For patients who have an HLA-identical donor, the outcome is excellent for complete reconstitution. For patients who are not transplanted, the survival is less than patients with T⁻B⁺ SCID (35% survived at a median period of 52 months, compared with 60% survival with a median of 57 months [Bertrand et al., 1999]). Following parental haploidentical transplantation, there is a higher risk of failure and a delay in reconstitution compared with T⁻B⁺ recipients. Conditioning with busulfan and cyclophosphamide may be necessary to ensure B-cell engraftment (O'Marcaigh et al., 2001).

Jean-Pierre de Villartay

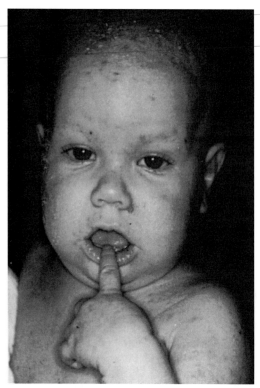

Figure 15-3 · An infant with Omenn syndrome. Note the scaly dermatitis and alopecia.

OMENN SYNDROME
Definition

OS is an autosomal recessive severe combined immune deficiency characterized by the early onset of a prominent generalized papular skin eruption or scaly exudative erythrodermia, enlarged lymph nodes, hepatosplenomegaly, severe respiratory infections and/or diarrhea, failure to thrive, hypoproteinemia with edema, and eosinophilia (Fig. 15-3). The latter is so prominent that OS is sometimes termed CID *with eosinophilia.*

The clinical picture may mimic histiocytosis X of the Letterer-Siwe type or GVHD, and may be occasionally seen in SCID infants with transplacental passage of alloreactive maternal T cells. Although the latter condition is also referred to as Omenn-like syndrome, the term OS is reserved for cases in which presence of alloreactive T cells has been ruled out.

Historical Aspects

In 1965 Omenn reported a large family with 12 infants affected with this disorder. Paucity of lymphoid tissue, associated with an increase of stromal cells and eosinophils was observed at autopsy. Immunologic studies performed in vitro and in vivo confirmed a combined immunodeficiency in such patients (Cederbaum et al., 1974; Ochs et al., 1974).

Pathogenesis

The pathogenesis of OS long remained a mystery. However, the demonstration of oligoclonal, activated T cells in OS infants, and the simultaneous occurrence of OS and of T⁻B⁻ SCID in two siblings (de Saint Basile et al., 1991) suggested that it may be genetically related to T⁻B⁻ SCID, and likely reflected defective T- and B-lymphocyte differentiation. This hypothesis was proven when mutations in the *RAG-1* and *RAG-2* genes, which play a critical role in V(D)J rearrangement (Notarangelo et al., 2001), were identified in OS patients (Villa et al., 1998).

Because the disease has an autosomal recessive pattern of inheritance, each patient carries at least one mutant allele that allows for partial RAG protein expression and function (Fig. 15-4) (Noordzij et al., 2000; Santagata et al., 2000; Villa et al., 2001, 1998; Wada et al., 2000). This results in a leaky V(D)J rearrangement defect, and permits some intrathymic T-cell differentiation, with generation of oligoclonal T cells that undergo peripheral expansion, possibly in response to autoantigens (Rieux-Laucat et al., 1998; Signorini et al., 1999).

Clinical and Laboratory Features

Patients with OS develop generalized erythyroderma and desquamation shortly after birth that is somewhat responsive to local steroid ointment. They later develop the characteristic infections of other SCID patients but in addition

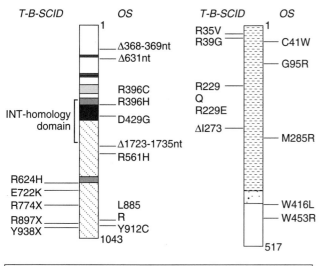

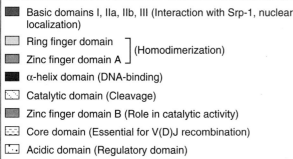

Basic domains I, IIa, IIb, III (Interaction with Srp-1, nuclear localization)

Ring finger domain ⎤
Zinc finger domain A ⎦ (Homodimerization)

α-helix domain (DNA-binding)

Catalytic domain (Cleavage)

Zinc finger domain B (Role in catalytic activity)

Core domain (Essential for V(D)J recombination)

Acidic domain (Regulatory domain)

Figure 15-4 · Schematic representation of the *RAG 1* (L) and *RAG 2* (R) genes indicating the known domains of each gene. Mutations that result in classic T⁻B⁻ SCID are shown on the left side and those associated with Omenn syndrome (OS) are shown on the right side of each gene cartoon.

have lymphadenopathy and hepatosplenomegaly. The skin lesions look like a graft-versus-host reaction, but lymphoid cells with foreign HLA antigens are not found in the skin or the blood. Other laboratory features include a marked eosinophilia, an elevated IgE level, but low levels of other immunoglobulins (Brugnoni et al., 1997).

Leukocytosis caused by the marked eosinophilia is a common finding. In contrast, lymphopenia is rare. Circulating T cells are usually normal to increased (Villa et al., 2001). The CD4/CD8 ratio is often unbalanced, but varies from patient to patient (Brugnoni et al., 1997). In one patient, a selective expansion of TCR αβ⁺ CD4⁻ CD8⁻ cells was observed (Wirt et al., 1989), possibly reflecting down-modulation of co-receptor molecules as an attempt to overcome in vivo T-cell activation.

A characteristic finding in OS is the coexpression of activation and/or memory markers (DR, CD45R0, CD25, CD95, CD30) on T lymphocytes (Brugnoni et al., 1997; Villa et al., 1999). This subset of T cells predominantly secretes Th2-type cytokines, such as IL-4 and IL-5 (Chilosi et al., 1996a; Schandené et al., 1993), which may contribute to the hypereosinophilia and elevated IgE levels (Ochs et al., 1974).

Analysis of in vitro lymphocyte function has yielded variable results; most often, proliferative responses to mitogens and antigens are markedly diminished, possi-

bly reflecting increased activation-induced cell death (Brugnoni et al., 1997). B lymphocytes are usually absent from the peripheral blood and lymphoid tissues (Martin et al., 1995) with hypogammaglobulinemia except for the notable exception of the elevated IgE levels (Ochs et al., 1974).

Histologic evaluation of lymph nodes demonstrates abnormal architecture, with depletion of lymphoid cells, and an increased proportion of interdigitating reticulum cells, eosinophils, and histiocytes (Fig. 15-5); the lymphoid component is predominantly composed of activated T lymphocytes (Chilosi et al., 1996b; Martin et al., 1995). Lymphoid depletion and lack of corticomedullary demarcation are observed in the thymus (Cederbaum et al., 1974; Signorini et al., 1999).

Diagnosis and Treatment

The diagnosis of OS is based on the typical clinical and laboratory features listed previously. However, GVHD resulting from engraftment of maternal T cells or of lymphocytes from unirradiated blood transfusions must be ruled out. Genetic analysis at *RAG-1* and *RAG-2* loci demonstrates specific mutations in the vast majority of OS patients, and serves as a basis for prenatal diagnosis based on analysis of chorionic villus DNA (Villa et al., 2000).

Some patients present with a milder phenotype, consisting of some, but not all, of the clinical features of OS. This condition, also referred to as *atypical OS,* or *leaky SCID,* shares with typical OS the molecular basis (i.e., mutations of the *RAG* genes that allow for residual protein expression and function) (Villa et al., 2001). Unless treated by BMT or other stem cell transplantation procedures, OS is invariably fatal within the first months of life. Use of interferon-γ (IFN-γ) may counteract the predominance of Th2-type T cells and improve the clinical status before BMT (Schandené et al., 1993). We have observed significant improvement of the skin manifestations with topical and systemic steroids and cyclosporine. Total parenteral nutrition is often required

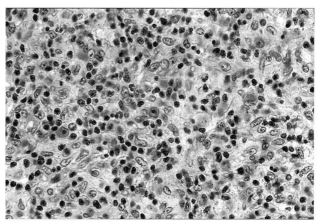

Figure 15-5 · Lymph node pathology of Omenn syndrome. Polymorphic cell infiltrate in the lymph node from a patient with Omenn syndrome.

for the chronic diarrhea. Use of antibiotics and IVIG is mandatory to prevent infections.

BMT using an HLA-matched sibling or unrelated donor, or a haploidentical family donor, represents the optimal treatment and leads to permanent cure in most cases (Fischer et al., 1994; Gomez et al., 1995; Junker et al., 1989).

Luigi D. Notarangelo

MAJOR HISTOCOMPATIBILITY COMPLEX (MHC) CLASS I DEFICIENCY (BARE LYMPHOCYTE SYNDROME TYPE I, TAP DEFICIENCY)

Definition

Major histocompatibility complex (MHC) class I deficiency is a less severe autosomal recessive combined immunodeficiency associated with mutations of the genes encoding for the *t*ransporter associated with *a*ntigen *p*resentation (TAP), a complex essential for HLA class I expression. It is also called bare lymphocyte syndrome type I (BLS I).

Historical Features

First described by Touraine and colleagues in 1978 in a child with severe combined immunodeficiency, MHC class I deficiency was termed BLS because of the absence of HLA antigens on the lymphocytes. Shortly thereafter, the same immunologic defect was observed in two other patients who presented with similar severe clinical features (Schuurman et al., 1979).

Since then, several other patients with MHC class I deficiency but a less severe clinical phenotype have been reported (de la Salle et al., 1994, 1998; Donato et al., 1995; Gadola et al., 2000; Maeda et al., 1985; Moins-Teisserenc et al., 1999; Payne et al., 1983; Plebani et al., 1996; Sugiyama et al., 1986; Teisserenc et al., 1997; Watanabe et al., 1987). Defective expression of HLA class I molecules has been found also in an apparently healthy subject (Payne et al., 1983).

Because the first reported patients with HLA class I deficiency had severe disease, similar to that observed in patients with HLA class II deficiency, there is doubt that HLA class I deficiency is a distinct entity. In the case reported by Touraine and colleagues (1978) a diagnosis of HLA class II deficiency associated with low expression of class I molecules was subsequently recognized (Sabatier et al., 1996). It has also been suggested that the cases reported by Schuurman were also HLA class II deficiencies (Griscelli et al., 1989).

The subsequent reports of patients with selective reduction of HLA class I, but normal expression of HLA class II, have confirmed that defective expression of HLA class I molecules is a distinct genetic disorder. This has been confirmed by the identification of patients with mutations of the genes encoding for TAP, a complex essential for expression of HLA class I molecules (de la Salle et al., 1994, 1999; Furukawa et al., 1999a; Moins-Teisserenc et al., 1999).

Pathogenesis

HLA class I molecules are polymorphic cell surface glycoproteins that play an essential role in presenting antigenic peptides to cytotoxic T lymphocytes and in modulating the activity of NK cells that bear HLA class I-binding receptors (Braud et al., 1998; Colonna, 1997; Pamer and Cresswell, 1998). HLA class I molecules are composed of a polymorphic heavy chain, encoded by HLA-A, HLA-B, and HLA-C genes, associated with β_2-microglobulin (β2M).

The assembly of HLA class I molecules occurs in the lumen of the endoplasmic reticulum (ER), where they are retained through interaction with several proteins (calnexin, calreticulin, Erp57, and tapasin), and where they are loaded with peptides derived from the degradation of intracellular organisms (Hughes and Cresswell, 1998; Sadasivan et al., 1996; Williams, 1995). These peptides, derived from cytosolic proteasome-mediated proteolysis, are transported into the ER via the TAP complex (Momburg and Hammerling, 1998).

TAP consists of two structurally related subunits (TAP 1 and TAP 2) that interact to form a functional peptide transporter system. In the ER lumen, TAP-transported peptides bind to newly synthesized HLA class I/β2M complexes. Binding of the peptide to the HLA class I/β2M complex results in its stabilization and transport to the cell surface. Studies with mutant mammalian cell lines have shown that both TAP 1 and TAP 2 are required for peptide binding to TAP and for peptide translocation into the ER (Androlewicz et al., 1994; Kelly et al., 1992).

Defects in either protein result in impaired peptide-HLA class I/β2M complex formation, with the result that the peptide-unloaded HLA class I/β2M complex is unstable and rapidly dissociates (Heemels and Ploegh, 1995). Hence, any defect that impairs the translocation of peptides into the ER (i.e., TAP 1 or TAP 2 deficiencies) results in reduced surface expression of HLA class I.

Clinical Features

Twelve well-documented cases of MHC I deficiency with normal expression of class II molecules have been reported (Table 15-3). Nine of these patients, from seven unrelated families, had a demonstrated TAP defect (Gadola et al., 2000); four had a TAP 2 defect (de la Salle et al., 1994; Moins-Teisserenc et al., 1999), and five had a TAP 1 defect (de la Salle et al., 1999; Furukawa et al., 1999a).

With the exception of 2 patients, one with aplastic anemia and the other apparently healthy (both with an unidentified molecular defect) (Payne et al., 1983), the

TABLE 15-3 · CHARACTERISTICS OF TWELVE PATIENTS WITH HLA CLASS I DEFICIENCY

Sex	Age	Clinical Features	HLA Class I	HLA Class II	Diagnosis	Reference
M	9 yr	Aplastic anemia	Reduced	Present	HLA class I def.	Payne et al., 1983
F	6 yr	Apparently healthy	Reduced	Present	HLA class I def.	Sullivan et al., 1985
F	33 yr	Sinobronchial disease, polyposis, skin lesions	Reduced	Present	TAP 1 defect	Maeda et al., 1985; de la Salle et al., 1999; Furukawa et al., 1999a, 1999b; Watanabe et al., 1987
M	41 yr	Recurrent sinopulmonary infections, bronchiectasis	Reduced	Present	HLA class I def.	Sugiyama et al., 1986; de la Salle et al., 1994
F	15 yr	Recurrent sinobronchial infections, polyposis, bronchiectasis	Reduced	Present	TAP 2 defect	Donato et al., 1995; Zimmer et al., 1998, 1999
M	8 yr	Recurrent sinopulmonary infections, polyposis, bronchiectasis, chronic otitis	Reduced	Present	TAP 2 defect	Zimmer et al., 1998, 1999
M	16 yr	Recurrent sinopulmonary infections, polyposis, bronchiectasis, skin ulcers	Reduced	Present	TAP 1 defect	de la Salle et al., 1999; Plebani et al., 1996
F	36 yr	Recurrent sinopulmonary infections, polyposis, bronchiectasis, skin ulcers, retinal vasculitis	Reduced	Present	TAP 2 defect	Moins-Teisserenc et al., 1999; Teisserenc et al., 1997
F	Unknown	Recurrent sinopulmonary infections, bronchiectasis, skin ulcers	Reduced	Present	TAP 1 defect	Moins-Teisserenc et al., 1999
F	Unknown	Recurrent sinobronchial infections, skin ulcers	Reduced	Present	TAP 2 defect	Moins-Teisserenc et al., 1999
F	Unknown	Recurrent sinopulmonary infections, bronchiectasis, skin ulcers	Reduced	Present	TAP 1 defect	Moins-Teisserenc et al., 1999
F	Unknown	Skin lesions, mutilating lesions in the midface	Reduced	Present	TAP 1 defect	Moins-Teisserenc et al., 1999

Two additional adult male brothers with reduced expression of HLA class I molecules due to TAP 2 mutations have been reported, one asymptomatic and one with late-onset granulomatous skin lesions (de la Salle et al., 2002). Another patient with an HLA class I defect has been described due to a tapasin deficiency. Tapasin links TAP to the heavy chain (Yabe et al., 2002).

other 10 patients with selective MHC I deficiency suffered from sinopulmonary infections (including chronic sinusitis and recurrent bronchitis and pneumonia) and/or granulomatous skin lesions (see Table 15-3). Bronchiectasis (more often during the second and third decades of life) and polyposis were common. *Haemophilus influenzae*, *Streptococcus pneumoniae*, *Staphylococcus aureus*, *Klebsiella*, and *Pseudomonas aeruginosa* were the predominant pathogens involved in sinopulmonary infections.

Skin lesions were present in seven patients. More common in adulthood, they were predominantly located on the legs (Fig. 15-6) and the midface. The lesions started as small expanding pustules and eventually evolved into ulcers that healed very slowly leading to muscle contractures and organ mutilation, such as nose scarring as a result of cartilage destruction (Moins-Teisserenc et al., 1999; Plebani et al., 1996).

Histologic analysis of the lesions showed an inflammatory pattern variably described as necrobiosis lipoidica, or necrotizing granulomatosis, with infiltration of blood vessels resembling Wegener's granulomatosis (Moins-Teisserenc et al., 1999; Plebani et al., 1996; Watanabe et al., 1987). No pathogens were cultured, and the lesions were unresponsive to antibiotic or immunosuppressive therapy. One patient developed retinal vasculitis (Moins-Teisserenc et al., 1999), and another had associated congenital albinism (Donato et al., 1995).

Laboratory Features

The effects of HLA class I deficiency on humoral and T-cell immunity have not been fully investigated in all patients, and this may partly explain the heterogeneity of the immune abnormalities reported. Defects of humoral immunity, when present, were mild. Immunoglobulin levels were normal in five out of seven patients studied (Donato et al., 1995; Payne et al., 1983; Sugiyama et al., 1986); one patient had low serum IgM (Maeda et al., 1985), and another had an IgG2 and IgG4 deficiency (Plebani et al., 1996). Complement levels and antibody responses against viral and bacterial antigens were also normal (Donato et al., 1995; Maeda et al., 1985; Plebani et al., 1996; Sugiyama et al., 1986).

No consistent T-cell defects have been observed. Delayed skin tests performed on three patients were normal to one or more of the antigens tested (Maeda et al., 1985; Plebani et al., 1996; Sugiyama et al., 1986). Two patients had normal in vitro lymphoproliferation

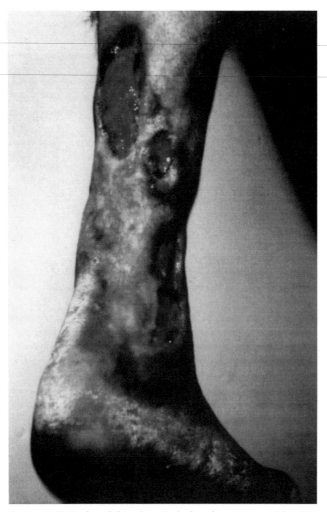

Figure 15-6· Profound skin ulcers in the leg of one patient with MHC class I (TAP 1) deficiency.

to alloantigens (de la Salle et al., 1994). Mitogen-induced lymphoproliferation was normal in two of three patients (Maeda et al., 1985; Plebani et al., 1996; Sugiyama et al., 1986).

T-cell subsets were normal in two of five patients (Maeda et al., 1985; Sugiyama et al., 1986); a progressive decrease of CD3+, CD4+, and CD8+ T-cell subsets occurred in one patient (Plebani et al., 1996); and two patients had a selective decrease of CD8 cells, with an expansion of γδ CD8 cells (de la Salle et al., 1994; Donato et al., 1995).

NK cells in three patients were present in normal numbers and expressed normal levels of inhibitory and activating NK receptors; they were unable to lyse HLA class I K562 cells, kill autologous lymphoblastoid B-cell lines (B-LCs), or exhibit LAK activity against class I deficient target cells following incubation with IL-2, IL-12, and IL-15 (de la Salle et al., 1994; Furukawa et al., 1999b; Zimmer et al., 1999). Interestingly, the cytotoxicity of activated NK cells from TAP-deficient patients to autologous B-LCs was

significantly greater than that of normal NK cells (Zimmer et al., 1998).

Because the immune defects in these patients are mild and inconsistent, their characteristic respiratory symptoms and the skin lesions cannot be readily explained. Instead, we speculate that an autoreactive mechanism may initiate or contribute to the damage to target organs (i.e., lung and skin), such as their increased NK-cell cytotoxic activity to autologous cells.

Cytokines such as IFN-γ that upregulate HLA class I expression protect normal but not TAP-deficient fibroblasts from lysis by activated autologous NK cells (Zimmer et al., 1999). IFN-γ protects several types of target cells (including fibroblasts) from NK-mediated lysis by increasing their expression of HLA class I molecules. Similar results have been observed using endothelial cells as target cells (Ayalon et al., 1998). In TAP-deficient patients, NK-cell activation (resulting from an inflammatory or infectious episode) cannot be counteracted by a sufficient increase in HLA class I expression and may lead to an exaggerated autoimmune process that initiates or contributes to the lung and skin lesions.

Diagnosis

HLA class I deficiency should be suspected in patients presenting with recurrent sinopulmonary infections and/or granulomatous skin lesions. The diagnosis is based on the demonstration of low expression of HLA class I molecules on peripheral blood mononuclear cells (PBMCs) using serologic HLA class I typing or flow cytometry following staining of PBMCs with the anti-HLA class I monomorphic monoclonal antibody W6/32 (Fig. 15-7). If, after activation of PBMCs, the expression of HLA class I molecules remains low, a TAP defect is likely.

Differential diagnoses to consider include other primary immunodeficiencies, cystic fibrosis, and systemic diseases that present with necrotizing granulomatous skin lesions and chronic inflammation of the upper respiratory tract (i.e., Wegener's granulomatosis and lethal midline granulomatosis).

Treatment and Prognosis

The major objectives of management are early recognition and aggressive treatment of respiratory infections to prevent the development of bronchiectasis. Treatment of respiratory tract infections in TAP-deficient patients is similar to that recommended in cystic fibrosis, including prompt and aggressive use of antibiotics and chest physiotherapy. Bacteriologic analysis of the sputum helps guide antimicrobial therapy.

Chronic pansinusitis with or without polyposis is a frequent complaint of TAP-deficient patients. Neither medical treatment with systemic antibiotics and topi-

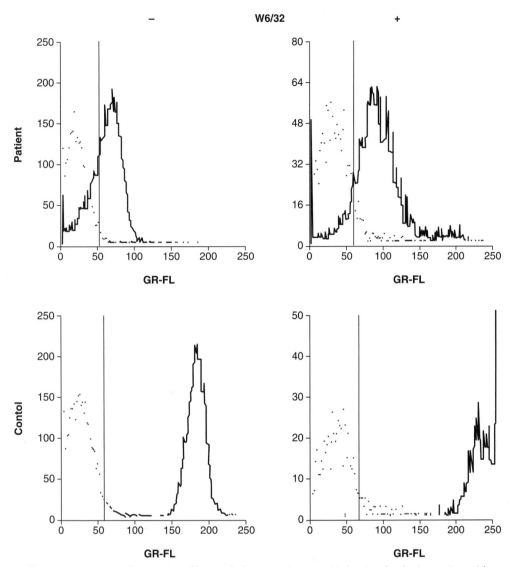

W6/32

Figure 15-7· Pattern of expression of human leukocyte antigen (HLA) class I molecules in a patient with HLA class I deficiency (TAP 1 defect) before (−) and after (+) incubation of a peripheral blood mononuclear blood mononuclear cell (PBMC) with recombinant interferon-γ. The cytometric analysis has been performed with the monoclonal antibody W6/32 that recognizes a nonpolymorphic epitope of major histocompatibility complex (MHC) class I molecules. There is no increase in expression of MHC in the patient unlike that in the control.

cal steroids nor surgical intervention is of convincing benefit.

The treatment of the skin lesions is equally unsatisfactory. Ulcer-cleansing procedures may be effective in avoiding bacterial colonization (Gadola et al., 2000), but immunosuppressive (steroids in combination with cyclophosphamide, methotrexate, azathioprine, or cyclosporine) or immunomodulatory therapy (IFN-α or IFN-γ) is not recommended because progression of both skin lesions and pulmonary disease has been reported (Gadola et al., 2000). It is unknown whether solid organ (lung) transplantation and BMT would be beneficial.

Allesandro Plebani

MHC CLASS II DEFICIENCY (BARE LYMPHOCYTE SYNDROME TYPE II)

Definition

MHC class II deficiency is an autosomal recessive primary immunodeficiency caused by the absence of MHC class II expression on the surface of cells normally expressing HLA class II molecules. The disease was identified in 1979 and is also referred to as the bare lymphocyte syndrome type II (BLS II), whereas MHC class I deficiency, first reported in 1978, is called BLS type I. Clinically there are severe defects in both cellular and humoral immune responses with extreme susceptibility to viral, bacterial, fungal, and protozoan infections, primarily of the respiratory and gastrointestinal tract. This leads to severe malabsorption with failure to thrive and death in early childhood.

Pathogenesis

Early molecular studies of MHC class II deficiency indicated that the genes encoding class II MHC are not directly affected. Instead, the defect lies in transcription factors that control MHC class II gene expression. BLS II thus became the first disease known to be caused by defective or absent transcription factors.

The genetic heterogeneity of MHC II expression defect was demonstrated by means of somatic fusion experiments. Four complementation groups A, B, C, and D have been identified (Table 15-4). Patient-derived cell lines with class II MHC transcription defects provide a unique way to identify the transcription factors controlling MHC II expression and the molecular mechanism underlying the disease.

MHC Class II Expression

MHC class II molecules are heterodimeric transmembrane molecules composed of α and β chains; they play a crucial role in presentation of exogenous antigens to CD4+ T cells, leading to helper T-cell activation required for the initiation and maintenance of immune responses (Chapman, 1998; McDevitt, 1998). These molecules are critical for numerous aspects of immune function, including antibody production, T-cell–mediated immunity, T-cell selection, tolerance induction, and the inflammatory response.

MHC class II molecules are expressed on the surface of B cells, dendritic cells, macrophages, thymic epithelia, and activated T cells. The non–antigen-presenting cells can be induced to express MHC class II by IFN-γ. In addition to a narrow tissue specificity, MHC II expression varies during development and differentiation. Thus the primary basis for the immunodeficiency resides in the inability of T cells to recognize antigens in the context of self-MHC II molecules expressed by antigen-presenting cells (APCs) (Bradley et al., 1997). In addition, defects in lymphocyte differentiation and function contribute to the defects in cellular and humoral immunity.

The expression of MHC II genes is essentially controlled at the transcription level. The genes encoding the three human MHC II isotypes (HLA-DR, HLA-DQ, and HLA-DP) and the *DMA* and *DMB* genes implicated in antigen presentation are coordinately expressed (Trowsdale, 1993). These genes contain conserved cis-acting elements in their proximal promoters: the W, X1, X2, and Y boxes. The binding of specific transcription factors allows the expression of the different HLA isotypes and DM molecules co-regulated in APCs. The RFX, X2BP, and NF-Y complexes bind respectively X, X2, and Y boxes. RFX is expressed ubiquitously and is a heteromeric complex consisting of three subunits: RFX5 (p75) (Steimle et al., 1995), RFXAP (p36) (Durand et al., 1997), and either RFXANK (p33) (Masternak et al., 1998) or RFX-B (Nagarajan et al., 1999).

MHC II Mutations

In MHC class II deficiency, mutations in either *RFX or CIITA* genes have been found. Mutations of the *RFX-ANK/RFX-B* gene were found in the complementation group B (Masternak et al., 1998; Nagarajan et al., 1999; Wiszniewski et al., 2000), of RFX5 in group C (Steimle et al., 1995; Villard et al., 1997b), and of RFXAP in group D (Fondaneche et al., 1998; Villard et al., 1997a). The defect of either of these proteins leads to the absence of the RFX complex with non-occupancy of the MHC class II promoter, as shown by DNAase protection assays and in vivo footprint experiments (Reith et al., 1999). This indicates that binding of NF-Y and X2BP to box Y and X2 is dependent on the RFX complex showing cooperative binding of these transcription factors.

TABLE 15-4 · PHENOTYPIC, BIOCHEMICAL, AND MOLECULAR DEFECTS OF MHC II DEFICIENCY PATIENTS AND REGULATORY MUTANTS FROM COMPLEMENTATION GROUPS A TO D MHC II DEFICIENCY COMPLEMENTATION GROUPS

	Wild Type	A	B	C	D
Prototypical patients/cell lines		BLS-2	BLS-1	SJO	DA, ABI
Number of unrelated families		8	32*	5	7
In vitro mutants		RJ 2.5.5	None	None	6.1.6
Ethnic origin		Spanish, Italian, Pakistani	Maghreb, Italian, Turkish	Turkish, American	Druze, Kabyl Turkish
MHC II expression	+	—	—	—	—
MHC II promotor activity	+	—	—	—	—
Binding of RFX	+	+	—	—	—
DNA-ase hypersensitive sites	+	+	—	—	—
Promoter occupancy in vivo	+	+	—	—	—

*22/32 group B patients share the same mutation, the 752delG-25. In one patient (B25) each RFXANK allele bears different mutations. The number of the defined RFXANK mutations is therefore 11.

CIITA Mutations

Although all of these promoter-bound factors are required for MHC class II expression, they are not sufficient. Group A cells express the X and Y binding proteins but fail to transcribe MHC class II. The class II transactivator, CIITA, is also required (Steimle et al., 1993). CIITA does not bind DNA but interacts with factors on the MHC class II promoter, as well as with the general transcriptional machinery, to activate transcription through its acidic activation domain (Fig. 15-8) (Harton and Ting, 2000).

CIITA expression correlates directly with MHC class II expression and is regulated by IFN-γ (Otten et al., 1998; Steimle et al., 1994). Thus CIITA functions as a molecular switch for MHC class II gene regulation. Mutations in the gene encoding CIITA are responsible for the MHC class II deficiency in patients belonging to group A. CIITA –/– mice have been generated (Chang et al., 1996) and exhibit a phenotype similar to that observed in BLS patients.

Other Mutations

CIITA, RFXANK/B, RFX5, and RFXAP genes were studied in 52 MHC-II-deficient patients. A prevalence of RFXANK/B defects (32 out of 52) is due to a founder effect for one of the RFXANK mutations: the 752delG-25 was detected in 22 patients, all from North African families with a high degree of consanguinity (Wiszniewski et al., 2000). Three recurrent mutations were also detected in the RFXAP gene (Fondaneche et al., 1998). In most patients, mutations in all four genes result in truncated product and lead to protein degradation. In two CIITA-deficient patients with a prolonged survival, a missense mutation was detected, which may explain their "leaky" phenotype (Quann et al., 1999; and see later discussion).

Molecular studies of BLS II cells confirm that the expression of all genes involved in antigen presentation are controlled by a common transcriptional mechanism. In DR-transfected BLS II cell lines, each of the molecular defects that silence MHC II transcription also results in a defective APC phenotype, providing strong evidence for co-regulation of all HLA D genes (Bradley et al., 1997). Because of the essential function of MHC class II, it is not surprising that their absence results in profound immunodeficiency.

Clinical Features

More than 80 cases of BLS II have been identified, mostly but not exclusively in patients originating from the Mediterranean area. Infections occur early (mean age of onset 4.8 months) and include gastrointestinal, upper and lower respiratory, and urinary tract infections and septicemia (Klein et al., 1993).

Most patients have severe diarrhea, malabsorption, and stunted growth. Acute diarrhea may develop during the first year of life and progress to protracted diarrhea after 2 years of life. Histologic examination of intestinal mucosa reveals variable degrees of villous atrophy. The most frequently isolated bacteria include *Staphylococcus, Streptococcus, Escherichia coli, Campylobacter, Proteus, Pseudomonas, Salmonella,* and *Shigella.* In some patients *Cryptosporidium parvum* and *Giardia intestinalis* were isolated in feces. All patients had *Candida* digestive tract colonization.

Hepatic abnormalities are frequent, with 50% of patients having hepatomegaly and elevated transaminase levels. Sclerosing cholangitis resulting from *C. parvum* is often observed.

Recurrent lower respiratory tract infections are observed in most patients and upper respiratory infections are common. The infectious agents identified include *Pneumocystis carinii,* bacteria (*Staphylococcus, Streptococcus, H. influenzae, Proteus, Pseudomonas*) and viruses (cytomegalovirus [CMV], respiratory syncytial virus [RSV], adenovirus).

Neurologic manifestations are caused by viral infections of the CNS (herpes simplex virus [HSV], enteroviruses [including poliovirus]). Three children developed paralytic polio, including one patient who died of polioencephalitis following oral poliovirus vaccination. Three patients presented with chronic lymphocytic meningitis caused by adenovirus, echovirus, and herpes virus, respectively.

A few patients developed autoimmune hemolytic anemia requiring steroid therapy or splenectomy. Three other patients had neutropenia.

The clinical course is characterized by progression of infectious complications, ultimately resulting in death. Among the 9 nontransplanted children in the largest complementation group, B, the mean age at the time of death was 7 years (range 16 months to 17 years). However, it has recently been recognized that a few patients survive to adulthood with only mild symptoms. The reasons for the variable outcome are not fully understood and do not necessarily reflect residual expression of MHC class II molecules.

MHC CLASS II DEFICIENCY COMPLEMENTATION GROUPS

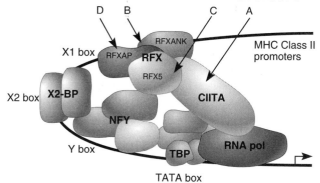

Figure 15-8·Binding of transcription factors to the major histocompatibility complex (MHC) class II promoter. Mutations in these transcription factors account for the various complementation groups A to D identified in MHC class II deficiency.

Laboratory Features

The hallmark of MHC class II deficiency is the lack of detectable HLA-DR, HLA-DQ, and HLA-DP molecules on the surface of all cells that constitutively express HLA class II (B cells, monocytes, dendritic cells) and of IFN-γ-activated cells (e.g., T cells, fibroblasts). HLA-DM molecule expression is also defective. MHC class I expression varies from markedly reduced to normal and can vary with time in a given patient. MHC class I expression can be corrected by incubation with IFN-γ. Although total T-cell numbers are preserved, CD4+ T-cell counts are decreased. This is often associated with a relative or absolute increase in CD8+ T cells, resulting in a reversed CD4/CD8 ratio. The remaining CD4+ T cells that reach the circulation appear to be phenotypically and functionally normal (see later discussion).

However, all MHC class II–deficient patients are unable to mount T-cell–mediated immune responses to antigens, as assessed by delayed hypersensitivity skin tests. This abnormality correlates with lack of T-cell responses in vitro to antigens to which the patients had been exposed. Their lymphocytes have a decreased capacity to stimulate HLA-nonidentical lymphocytes in mixed leukocyte culture. Humoral immunity is severely impaired with a variable degree of hypogammaglobulinemia and profoundly defective antibody production. In lymph nodes, follicle development is poor and germinal centers are absent. Virtually no plasma cells are found in tissues and bone marrow (Klein et al., 1993; Reith et al., 1999).

The reduced CD4 T cells are presumably a consequence of defective MHC class II expression in the thymus, similar to MHC class II(–) mice (Chang et al., 1996). However, MHC class II expression, although at low concentration, has been detected postmortem on medullary cells of thymuses from these children and, more importantly, from aborted MHC class II deficient fetuses. This observation suggests leakiness of the defect (although leakiness in the periphery is uncommon) or the presence of an alternative regulatory pattern of MHC class II gene transcription in thymic cells and may account for partially preserved T-cell differentiation and a capacity for self and nonself discrimination.

Vβ element use by TCRs of residual CD4+ T cells was found to be normal (Rieux-Leucat et al., 1993). This indicates that either residual MHC class II expression in the thymus is sufficient for normal repertoire building or that Vβ element use frequency is independent of selection events.

The immunologic abnormalities show considerable variability from one patient to another; this variability does not correlate with the genetic heterogeneity of the disease.

Diagnosis

Early diagnosis of BLS II is critical because it increases the success of BMT (see later discussion). A diagnosis of BLS II should be considered in all young children with recurrent respiratory tract infections, diarrhea, and failure to thrive, especially those born from consanguineous parents. The diagnosis is based on the absence of HLA class II molecules on the surface of B cells, monocytes, dendritic cells, or IFN-γ activated cells (T cells, fibroblasts).

The most sensitive technique to identify HLA class II molecules is flow cytometric analysis of blood lymphocytes using monoclonal antibodies reactive with nonpolymorphic regions of human MHC class II antigens. Decreased CD4+ T-cell counts, absence of in vitro proliferation to antigens confirmed by negative delayed cutaneous hypersensitivity skin tests, hypogammaglobulinemia, and profoundly defective antibody production complete the diagnosis of MHC II deficiency.

Molecular diagnosis by a direct sequencing of the affected gene is now possible in families with RFXANK-, RFX5-, and RFXAP-deficient patients, allowing early postnatal or prenatal diagnosis. A high prevalence of the 752delG-25 mutation in the *RFXANK* gene makes it possible to search for this mutation in siblings of affected patients and also to molecularly screened potential patients born to consanguineous parents of North African origin. For CIITA defects, the situation is more complex, not only because of the large size of the *CIITA* gene (50 Kb) and transcript but also because CIITA expression is tightly regulated by four distinct promoters.

Treatment and Prognosis

Despite antibiotics, IVIG, and parenteral nutrition, affected patients die of progressive organ dysfunction, generally between the ages of 5 and 18 years (Klein et al., 1993; Reith et al., 1997). Thus without BMT, the prognosis is poor (Klein et al., 1995). There is no difference in the prognosis for patients belonging to different complementation groups.

The leaky phenotype present in atypical patients of group A and B may be associated with a better outcome. Even in those cases, a clear genotype and phenotype correlation is difficult to establish. Among 22 North African patients, bearing the same mutation of the RFXANK, one 21-year-old patient is almost asymptomatic with only IVIG therapy.

BMT or other stem cell transplantation is the only cure for MHC class II deficiency. However, in a recent review, only 8 of 21 patients have been cured by the procedure (Klein at al., 1995). The outcome was much better in patients transplanted before the age of 2 years, probably because viral burden and organ dysfunction were less severe. The availability of an HLA-identical sibling further increases the rate of success.

Because all the genes affected in MHC II deficiency are now identified, gene therapy becomes a potential alternative to BMT. The proof of principle was demonstrated by the successful transfer of CIITA into cells from a MHC class II–deficient patient (Bradley et al., 1997).

Barbara Grospierre

AUTOSOMAL RECESSIVE SCID CAUSED BY A ZETA CHAIN–ASSOCIATED PROTEIN 70 (ZAP-70) DEFECT

Definition

ZAP-70 defect is a rare autosomal recessive form of SCID, characterized by early onset of infection, a lack of CD8+ T cells, and normal numbers of functionally deficient CD4+ T cells. It is due to mutations of the gene on chromosome 2q12 encoding ZAP-70, a non-src family protein tyrosine kinase necessary for T-cell signaling.

Historical Aspects

The original patient with ZAP-70 defect was a member of a Mennonite family who presented with *P. carinii* pneumonia, chronic diarrhea, failure to thrive, and persistent oral thrush and who had a selective absence of circulating CD8+ T cells (Roifman et al., 1989). Additional cases with a similar clinical phenotype were reported during the following years (Monafo et al., 1992). In 1994, two groups demonstrated that the failure to generate CD8+ T cells was due to mutations of the *ZAP-70* tyrosine kinase gene (Arpaia et al., 1994; Chan et al., 1994; Elder et al., 1994).

Since the original description, a total of 12 patients belonging to eight families with ZAP-70 deficiency have been reported. Most are Mennonites. Immunologic and molecular data have been collected in a database (ZAP70base), accessible at http://www.uta.fi/imt/bioinfo/ZAP70base/.

Pathogenesis

ZAP-70 is an intracellular tyrosine kinase, recruited to the CD3/T-cell receptor (TCR) and required for T-cell activation following TCR engagement. TCR-mediated stimulation results in activation of p56lck, which mediates tyrosine-phosphorylation of immunoreceptor tyrosine-based activation motifs (ITAMs) in the CD3-γ, δ and ϵ chains and in the TCR ζ chains (Iwashima et al., 1994).

Role of ZAP-70 in Signaling

The ZAP-70 tandem SH2 domains cooperatively form the binding pocket for one of the ITAMs phosphotyrosine residues, allowing recruitment of the ZAP-70 tyrosine kinase to the receptor complex (Gauen et al., 1994; Hatada et al., 1995). This results in phosphorylation of ZAP-70 itself by Src-family protein tyrosine kinases at specific tyrosine residues, resulting in increased catalytic activity (Chan et al., 1995; van Oers et al., 1996). Activated ZAP-70 can then phosphorylate the *linker of activated T cells* (LAT) and the Src homology 2 domain–containing 76-kD leukocyte protein (SLP-76), allowing recruitment and activation of other critical signaling molecules, such as phospholipase Cγ1 (PLCγ1) and Vav (van Leeuwen and Samelson, 1999).

These reactions are required for mobilization of intracellular free calcium ($[Ca^{2+}]_i$) and activation of the phosphatidylinositol-3-kinase and the Ras/MAP kinase pathways and ultimately culminate in T-cell activation and initiation of T-cell-specific responses (Qian and Weiss, 1997; van Leeuwen and Samelson, 1999).

Defective expression and/or function of ZAP-70 results in impaired T-cell development affecting T-cell activation and function. ZAP-70 is expressed during the early stages of thymocyte development. Syk, another tyrosine kinase, is also involved in signaling through the pre-TCR (Chu et al., 1999).

Murine ZAP-70 Defects

In murine T-cell development, Syk expression is rapidly downregulated, making CD4+CD8+ double positive (DP) thymocytes fully dependent on ZAP-70 for signaling via the TCR and for positive and negative selection. In contrast, human DP thymocytes continue to express Syk at relatively high levels, which may partially compensate for ZAP-70 deficiency during positive selection (Gelfand et al., 1995). Moreover, because Lck is preferentially associated with CD4 rather than with CD8 in DP thymocytes, signal transduction in human ZAP-70-deficient thymocytes may reach an appropriate threshold for CD4 but not CD8 lineage selection.

This hypothesis explains the differences observed in humans and mice with ZAP-70 defects: although ZAP-70–deficient mice lack both CD4+ and CD8+ circulating T cells (Negishi et al., 1995), normal numbers of circulating CD4 T cells have consistently been reported in patients with ZAP-70 deficiency. Furthermore, the thymus from Zap-70–deficient mice is devoid of single positive (SP) T cells, whereas CD4+ but not CD8+ SP cells are found in the thymic medulla of patients with ZAP-70 deficiency. Although Syk may partially compensate for ZAP-70 deficiency during human thymic development, ZAP-70 is critical for peripheral T-cell activation. Consequently, peripheral CD4+ T cells of patients with ZAP-70 deficiency have profoundly impaired TCR signaling.

ZAP-70 Gene Defects

Most *ZAP-70* gene defects identified to date prevent protein expression and are concentrated in a region that is critical for stability and enzymatic activity. These mutations include a 9-nucleotide insertion (resulting in the introduction of three amino acids after codon 541) (Arpaia et al., 1994; Chan et al., 1994), a deletion of 13 nucleotides resulting in frameshift and premature termination at codon 538 (Elder et al., 1994), and two missense mutations, S518R (Chan et al., 1994) and A507V (Noraz et al., 2000).

One patient was a compound heterozygote for two mutations (P80Q, M572L) that resulted in the production of a temperature-sensitive mutant, which was not expressed at 37°C (Matsuda et al., 1999). Recently, a ZAP-70 defect (R465C) that selectively affects kinase activity, without preventing protein expression, has been reported (Elder et al., 2001). An identical mutation is responsible for murine SCID in the ST mouse (Wiest et al., 1997).

Clinical Features

With one exception (Katamura et al., 1999), all patients with ZAP-70 defects have presented early in life with typical clinical features of SCID: severe pulmonary infections, generally resulting from opportunistic pathogens (*P. carinii* or viruses); chronic diarrhea; failure to thrive; persistent candidiasis; and oral ulcers. However, unlike those with other forms of SCID, patients with ZAP-70 defects have palpable lymph nodes and a normal thymic shadow (Roifman, 1995).

The unique patient reported by Katamura and associates (1999) did not suffer from respiratory infections or diarrhea but presented at birth with exudative skin lesions resulting from an accumulation of activated, memory, and presumably self-reactive CD4+ T cells. This patient was a compound heterozygote with two mutations that resulted in the production of a temperature-sensitive mutant that rapidly degraded at 37°C but was expressed and activated in self-reactive T cells in the skin, where the temperature is lower (Matsuda et al., 1999)

Laboratory Features

The distinctive laboratory feature of ZAP-70 deficiency is a selective absence of circulating CD8+ T cells, associated with an inability of peripheral lymphocytes to respond to activation signals (phytohemagglutinin, anti-CD3 monoclonal antibodies, allogeneic cells) that require integrity of membrane-proximal signal transduction. Thus, in vitro proliferation, intracellular calcium mobilization, IL-2 production, and IL-2 receptor expression are markedly depressed (Arpaia et al., 1994; Chan et al., 1994; Elder et al., 1994; Gelfand et al., 1995). In contrast, stimulation with phorbol esters and ionomycin results in normal lymphocyte proliferative responses. T-cell proliferation in response to TCR signaling, observed on rare occasions, is associated with the expression of high levels of Syk in the proliferating CD4+ T cells (Noraz et al., 2000).

Thymic biopsies reveal the presence of DP thymocytes in the cortex, whereas CD4+ SP thymocytes are only found in the medulla, compatible with a defect in positive selection of CD8+ T cells. As expected, TCR-mediated signaling is preserved in thymocytes, in keeping with the subsidiary role played by Syk in the thymus (Gelfand et al., 1995).

Serum immunoglobulins may be normal (Katamura et al., 1999; Monafo et al., 1992; Roifman et al.,

1989) or low (Elder et al., 1996, 2001; Gelfand et al., 1995), and antigen-specific antibody production is equally variable (Mazer et al., 1997; Roifman et al., 1989).

Treatment and Prognosis

ZAP-70 deficiency, like all forms of SCID, is ultimately fatal, unless treated by BMT or stem cell transplantation. Of four patients reported to have undergone BMT from an HLA-matched family donor, matched unrelated donor, or haploidentical donor, three have been cured (Elder et al., 2001; Mazer et al., 1997; Monafo et al., 1992). Isolation in a protected environment, antimicrobial prophylaxis, and IVIG are required before BMT.

Retroviral-mediated insertion of the *ZAP-70* gene into ZAP-70–deficient CD4+ cells in vitro has resulted in reconstitution of signaling, with a selective growth advantage of transduced cells (Steinberg et al., 2000; Taylor et al., 1996), indicating the potential for gene therapy.

Alain Fischer

SCID CAUSED BY AN IL-2 RECEPTOR-α (CD25) DEFICIENCY

Definition

IL-2 receptor alpha (IL-2Rα) deficiency has been described in a single patient who presented with a profound T-cell immunodeficiency associated with diffuse lymphocyte infiltrates and absence of expression of the alpha chain of the IL-2 receptor (Roifman et al., 2000).

Pathogenesis

The patient's lymphocytes lacked IL-2Rα (CD25) expression, but the IL-2Rβ chain was present at normal concentrations. A homozygous mutation of 4 bp was identified in the *IL-2Rα* gene, resulting in a translational frameshift and defective IL-2 signaling of mature T cells and accounting for the severe functional T-cell deficiency that was observed. This also indicates that T-cell development can occur in humans as in mice in the absence of IL-2 signaling.

The lymphoproliferative syndrome is not as easy to explain. IL-2Rα–/– mice develop inflammatory bowel disease (Willerford et al., 1995), which may represent an organ-limited manifestation of the general lymphoproliferation observed in this child. Van Parijs and Abbas (1998) proposed that IL-2 primes lymphocytes for fas-mediated apoptosis, accounting for the similarity between CD25 deficiency and the autoimmune lymphoproliferative syndrome caused by Fas deficiency (see Chapter 19).

Clinical Features

The patient presented early in life with severe viral infections (CMV, adenovirus), recurrent bacterial and fungal infections (*Candida* esophagitis), and chronic diarrhea. The patient had mild lymphopenia with a reduced CD4+ T-cell count, poor T-cell proliferation to mitogens that was not corrected by IL-2, and low IgA serum levels. A thymic biopsy revealed an abnormal corticomedullary separation. The patient also exhibited manifestations of lymphoproliferation (i.e., lymph node enlargement, hepatosplenomegaly, and lung infiltrates). These abnormalities responded to steroids and cyclosporine. The patient was successfully treated by allogeneic BMT.

AUTOSOMAL RECESSIVE SCID CAUSED BY CD45 DEFICIENCY

Definition

CD45 deficiency, resulting from mutations in the *CD45 tyrosine phosphatase* gene (Kung et al., 2000), is not unexpected because CD45-deficient mice also exhibit a profound immunodeficiency (Kishihara et al., 1993). CD45 is the common hematopoietic cell-specific transmembrane protein that plays a major role in regulating src kinases involved in T- and B-cell antigen receptor-triggered signaling.

Pathogenesis

The complete absence of CD45 membrane expression was the result of a large deletion of the CD45 maternal allele and a splice site mutation leading to aberrant splicing in the second allele.

Clinical Features

The first affected child was a 2-month-old infant who presented with the clinical picture of SCID and low CD4 numbers but normal numbers of B cells (Kung et al., 2000). There was complete absence of TCR αβ+ T cells, whereas γδ+ T cells were detected. NK cells were reduced but not absent. A second case of CD45 deficiency has been recently reported (Tchilian et al., 2001). CD45 deficiency should therefore be considered in patients with T⁻B⁺NK⁺ SCID who have none of the molecular defects more commonly associated with this form of SCID.

AUTOSOMAL RECESSIVE SCID CAUSED BY p56 lck DEFICIENCY

Definition

Autosomal recessive SCID may be due to a defect of p56 lck, an intracellular protein tyrosine kinase that is critically involved in TCR-mediated signaling. Its N-terminal region associates with the cytoplasmic tail of the CD4 and CD8 co-receptors (Chow and Veillette, 1995), thus bringing lck in close proximity with the TCR.

Pathogenesis

The lck contributes to tyrosine phosphorylation of the ITAMs of the TCR complex (Iwashima et al., 1994; van Oers et al., 1996). In mice, targeting of the *lck* gene (Molina et al., 1992) or expression of a dominant negative *lck* transgene (Levin et al., 1993) results in a severe T-cell developmental defect, with profound thymic atrophy, a dramatic reduction in the number of DP thymocytes, and only few circulating mature T cells.

In the affected infant, a marked reduction in the level of p56 lck and an alternatively spliced lck transcript, lacking the exon 7 coding domain, were demonstrated. The molecular basis for this abnormal finding is unclear. The milder immunologic phenotype observed in the patient compared with gene-targeted mice may be explained by residual, although low, expression of lck.

Clinical Features

One infant with a putative lck defect has been reported (Goldman et al., 1998). The patient presented with chronic diarrhea and failure to thrive at 1 month of age and developed *Enterobacter cloacae* sepsis, CMV infection, and persistent oral candidiasis.

Laboratory investigation disclosed panhypogammaglobulinemia, lymphopenia with a low proportion (9% to 22%) of CD4+ T cells, and a progressive decline in T-cell proliferation to mitogens and anti-CD3 monoclonal antibody. CD8+ T cells, when activated with anti-CD3, failed to express the activation marker CD69, whereas activation with phorbol esters and ionomycin resulted in normal CD69 expression, indicating a TCR signaling defect proximal to protein kinase C activation. B cells and NK cells were present making this a T⁺B⁺NK⁺ SCID.

The clinical course of the infant was typical for SCID, and the infant ultimately required BMT, which resulted in a complete cure.

RETICULAR DYSGENESIS

Definition

Reticular dysgenesis is a rare form of SCID associated with a block in myeloid differentiation with severe deficiencies of granulocyte precursors in the bone marrow. Autosomal recessive inheritance is presumed but not strictly proven, because of the rarity of the syndrome. It was first described in 1959 by DeVall and Seyneheve in male twins.

Pathogenesis

It is not clear whether some forms of SCID with neutropenia truly represent a unique syndrome or whether a block in hematopoiesis may be secondary to persistent viral infections. The molecular basis of the syndrome is unknown, but a hematopoietic origin is probable because it is curable by BMT (Levinsky and Teideman, 1983). The association of SCID with cyclic neutropenia has been described in an infant who was cured by BMT (Junker et al., 1991).

Clinical Features

Reticular dysgenesis manifests within the first days of life with failure to thrive, vomiting, diarrhea, or localized infection. The course is rapidly progressive, and most patients die by the 90th day of life.

The outstanding laboratory finding in all cases is the marked leukopenia (no cells in two patients, 200 to 600 cells/µl in the third, and 1200 to 1800 cells/µl in the fourth, and less than 4000 cells/µl in others (Hong, 1966). Immunoglobulin levels reflect transplacental passage. Autopsy studies show typical findings of SCID with a dysplastic thymus without Hassall's corpuscles. Granulocyte precursors were absent in the marrow but megakaryocytes and erythroid precursors were present. Erythrophagocytosis was present in two cases (De Vaal and Seynhaeve, 1959; Ownby et al., 1976).

Treatment

BMT from an HLA-identical sibling was curative (Levinsky and Tiedeman, 1983). Several haploidentical transplants have been recorded (Bertrand et al., 2002; Haas et al., 1986; Stephan et al., 1993). Bertrand and colleagues (2002) performed haploidentical stem cell transplants in 10 RD patients. The three patients with full lymphoid and myeloid engraftment needed intensive conditioning. Granulocyte transfusions may also be helpful; these should be irradiated to prevent GVHD.

T-CELL IMMUNODEFICIENCY

Definition

T-cell immunodeficiency describes a heterogeneous group of patients who have repeated infections starting in late infancy or childhood and peripheral T cells that are moderately reduced in number and function. Antibody function is usually reduced, immunoglobulin levels are variable, and autoimmunity is not uncommon. Onset of infection is usually delayed until early childhood. This clinical disorder is at least as frequent as that of typical SCID and is often associated with distinct syndromes that are neither fully recognized nor molecularly characterized (see Chapter 24).

The condition in patients who have this clinical pattern and who have significant levels of some immunoglobulins, usually with poor antibody function, has been termed cellular immunodeficiency with immunoglobulins or *Nezelof syndrome* (Nezelof et al., 1968).

Pathogenesis

The pathogenesis of T-cell deficiency is not clear and may occasionally result from gene mutations similar to those of SCID but with a less severe phenotype. Its heterogeneity suggests multiple genetic defects. Thymic dysplasia on postmortem may be present in severe cases (Nezelof, 1968).

The mechanisms leading to autoimmunity are also unclear. Abnormal T-cell activation causing impaired Fas ligand expression may lead to reduced fas-mediated lymphocyte apoptosis. Defective IL-2 production or IL-2R expression (see later discussion) may impair the sensitivity of T lymphocytes to fas-triggered cell death. These abnormalities may favor persistence and activation of autoimmune T- and B-cell clones. Alternatively, the negative selection process during T- and B-cell ontogeny may be impaired, resulting in the development of autoimmune clones. Finally, a deficiency in T regulatory cells producing immunosuppressive cytokines, such as IL-10 and TGF-β, may contribute to this phenomenon.

Clinical Features

Patients with T-cell immunodeficiency usually do not develop life-threatening infections during the first years of life but then develop a variety of complications that are directly or indirectly caused by the T-cell immunodeficiency, including infections, autoimmunity, allergy, and cancer. A number of patients have distinct genetic syndromes as detailed in Chapter 24.

In a survey of 25 patients with T-cell immunodeficiency, recurrent infections occurred in all and were the first clinical manifestation in 22 cases (Berthet et al., 1994). Respiratory tract infections, often leading to bronchiectasis, and recurrent or protracted diarrhea were the most frequent manifestations. Cutaneous and/or mucosal candidiasis and central nervous system infection of bacterial or viral origin were common. These complications may lead to failure to thrive, often necessitating parenteral nutrition. In two thirds of the patients, repeated and/or severe viral infections are reported, often caused by the herpesviruses. Severe recalcitrant warts are not uncommon.

Autoimmunity is a frequent complication of T-cell immunodeficiency, occurring in at least 50% of the patients during childhood or early adulthood. It is usually manifested by blood cell autoantibodies with Coombs'-positive hemolytic anemia, thrombocytopenia, or neutropenia. Autoimmune hepatitis and vasculitis of the brain and kidney have been observed. Because autoimmunity is often severe with a tendency to relapse, aggressive immunosuppression may be required, which can accentuate the immunodeficiency.

Patients with T-cell deficiency and immunoglobulins (Nezelof phenotype) may have somewhat milder courses, despite chronic diarrhea and recurrent pneumonia. Six patients reported by Lawlor and co-workers (1974) had variable patterns of serum immunoglobulins: only one had normal levels of all immunoglobulin, but she had poor antibody responses to keyhole limpet cyanin and pneumococcal polysaccharide vaccine. The lymphoproliferative response was reduced to phytohemagluttinin (PHA) but normal to allogeneic cells. All patients had functional antibody deficiency.

Allergic manifestations, including urticaria, eczema, and asthma, are common (48% in our series), and elevated serum IgE is a frequent finding. Malignancies, especially lymphomas, are often the cause of death in these patients.

Diagnosis

The diagnosis of T-cell immunodeficiency is usually suggested by the occurrence of repeated infections associated with allergic and autoimmune manifestations. The presence of mild T-cell lymphocytopenia and abnormal T-cell function (as assessed by in vivo skin tests and in vitro proliferative responses to vaccine antigens) in the absence of an acquired cause supports this diagnosis. Hypergammaglobulinemia involving one or more isotypes is not uncommon. However, hypogammaglobulinemia and abnormal antibody production in vivo are more common. HIV infection must be excluded.

Treatment and Prognosis

Despite prophylactic antibiotics, antifungals, and IVIG, the long-term outcome is generally poor, with a mean survival of 5 to 10 years. Causes of death include organ failure caused by poor nutritional status, uncontrolled infection by various organisms, and malignancy. Allogeneic BMT or other stem cell transplantation is therefore indicated at an early age, before chronic symptoms develop. Knutsen and Wall (2000) reported successful cord blood transplantation in two of three of these patients.

Alain Fischer

DEFECTIVE EXPRESSION OF THE T-CELL RECEPTOR-CD3 COMPLEX

Definition

The TCR is a structure complexed with CD3 to provide antigen specificity of the immune response. The TCR consists of four polypeptide chains, gamma, delta, epsilon, and zeta. Mutations of the genes for these chains lead to abnormal or absent expression of the TCR and a moderate to severe immune deficiency. Seven patients from four families with low CD3/TCR complex expression have been described. Two patients are from Spain, one is from Turkey, one is from France, and three are Mennonites from Canada.

Pathogenesis

Mutations affecting the CD3/TCR complex were identified in all cases. In the Spanish and Turkish patients, mutations were found in the gene encoding the gamma chain of the TCR. The Turkish patient, whose parents were first cousins, was homozygous for a nonsense mutation, and the Spanish patients were compound heterozygotes, with one mutation affecting the translation initiation codon and the other affecting a splice site. Interestingly, absence of CD3γ protein only reduced (50% of controls) but did not abolish TCR/CD3 expression (Perez-Aciego et al., 1991). Because CD8 T cells were reduced, they may interact with CD3γ in the antigen recognition unit.

In the French patient, the reduction of CD3/TCR expression resulted from two independent mutations (a splice site and a nonsense mutation) of the gene encoding the CD3 epsilon chain (Soudais et al., 1993; Thoenes et al., 1992).

The Canadian patients, two boys and a girl, all of whom are cousins, have a deficiency of the TCR delta chain because of a stop codon mutation of the extracellular domain of the CD3δ protein in thymocytes, preventing γ/δ assembly and transport to the periphery (Dadi et al., 2003).

These observations suggest that these CD3 abnormalities have variable phenotypic consequences depending on the deficient subunit and on the residual expression of the defective subunit.

Clinical Features

The clinical manifestations are variable. One of two siblings in a Spanish family had a severe phenotype, whereas the other had no symptoms (Alarcon et al., 1988). The former developed failure to thrive, protracted diarrhea, autoimmune hemolytic anemia, and fatal pneumonia at 32 months of age. His lymphocytes had poor proliferative responses and no cytotoxic function, but antibody function was normal. The asymptomatic sibling had few CD3-expressing cells and an IgG2 subclass deficiency.

In two other unrelated cases, one of French and one of Turkish origin, an immunodeficiency was suspected because of recurrent pneumonia and otitis media early in childhood. The infectious episodes responded well to prophylactic antibiotics and IVIG (Le Deist et al., 1991; Van Tol et al., 1997). In the three Canadian patients, manifestations of SCID occurred in the first months of life, leading to death in two infants with severe viral infection. The third infant was successfully transplanted at age 3 months (Dadi et al., 2003).

Laboratory Features

In the first four reported TCR-CD3 defects, lymphocyte counts were within the normal range. The most common laboratory finding was the defective expression (10% to 50% of normal) of the CD3/TCR complex on T lymphocytes. The proportion of CD8+ T lymphocytes was low in two patients, whereas the others had a mild depletion of CD4+ T lymphocytes. In all cases, anti-CD3 monoclonal antibody-induced T-cell activation was defective as determined by lymphoproliferation, CD25 expression, and intracellular calcium increase. Antigen-induced proliferation was either low or normal, depending on the antigens tested. B-cell function was variable: antibody responses to protein vaccines were normal or marginally decreased. In contrast, antibody responses to polysaccharide were defective.

In infants with CD3δ deficiency, there was a profound deficiency of CD3, CD4, but B cells and NK cells were normal or increased—for example, a T−B+NK+ phenotype. Immunoglobulins were low but detectable. A thymic shadow was present. There was a complete absence of γ/δ TCR cells in the periphery (Dadi et al., 2003).

Treatment

IVIG is indicated if there is a significant antibody deficiency. Stem cell transplantation is indicated for patients with profound T-cell deficiency.

Alain Fischer

OTHER PHENOTYPES WITH SCID AND T-CELL IMMUNODEFICIENCIES

T-Cell Transduction Defects

Patients with T-cell transduction defects have a severe T-cell or combined immunodeficiency because their T lymphocytes cannot be activated in response to antigen and therefore cannot undergo expansion.

The clinical manifestations include severe diarrhea and CMV pneumonia (Gehrz et al., 1980; Le Deist et al., 1995). Lymphocyte counts and subpopulations are usually within the normal range. Antigen-, lectin-, and anti-CD3 antibody-induced lymphocyte proliferation is absent or low. However, mitogens that bypass membrane receptors, such as phorbol ester and calcium ionophore, can induce T-lymphocyte proliferation. Serum Ig levels are either within normal range or elevated, but the heterogeneity of immunoglobulins is restricted. Antibody responses are impaired in most cases.

The mechanisms of these T-cell activation defects are not clear. In three cases, TCR-mediated calcium influx was found to be abolished despite normal calcium release from intracellular stores (Le Deist et al., 1995).

This failure was also observed in all of the hematopoietic cells tested, including platelets and polymorphonuclear cells, and in fibroblasts. Importantly, in these cases immune deficiency was associated with myopathy, suggesting that a ubiquitous calcium channel is involved in this immunodeficiency.

Cytokine Deficiencies

T-cell immunodeficiency may result from abnormal cytokine production, particularly IL-2, but sometimes other cytokine defects are present. Three patients have been reported with this form of immunodeficiency. Clinical features include opportunistic and viral infections, chronic diarrhea, failure to thrive, and erythrodermia. Blood lymphocyte counts are normal, as are the phenotype and distribution of T lymphocytes. Hypogammaglobulinemia was present. A common feature is poor mitogen-induced T-lymphocyte proliferation restored by exogenous IL-2. This T-cell dysfunction was associated with hypogammaglobulinemia in one of the patients (Chatila et al., 1990).

These immunodeficiencies are due to a defect in lymphokine production of IL-2, which in one case also involved other lymphokines (IL-4, IL-5, IFN-γ) production defects. In all cases, the defect resulted from failure of IL-2 gene transcription after T-cell activation, even though early steps of T-cell activation are normal (Chatila et al., 1990; DiSanto et al., 1990; Weinberg and Parkman, 1990). The precise molecular defects have not been identified. In the multilymphokine defect, abnormal binding of transcription complex NF-AT to the enhancer region of the IL-2 gene was identified by transfection of a reporter gene (Castigli et al., 1993). However, because the molecular definition of the NF-AT complex is unknown, the basis of this disorder has yet to be elucidated.

In other cases, the IL-2 defect may result either from a mutation in regulatory sequences of the IL-2 gene interfering with binding of regulatory proteins or from an abnormality in a regulatory protein. Although IL-2 may play a role in intrathymic T-cell development, it is interesting to note that normal T-cell differentiation can occur in the absence of IL-2 production.

One patient with a SCID phenotype was treated successfully with IL-2 (Pahwa et al., 1989).

Human Nude Phenotype

In one Italian kindred, a severe T-cell immunodeficiency was associated with complete alopecia and was termed human nude phenotype (WHN) (Frank et al., 1999). This phenotype is highly reminiscent of nude mice and led to the finding of mutations in the human equivalent of the winged–helix-nude (whn) gene mutated in the murine counterpart (Frank et al., 1999). The whn gene encodes a transcription factor expressed in epithelial cells in the skin and the thymus. Mutations of this gene leads to a defective thymic microenvironment and impaired T-cell development. Thus BMT may not permanently cure the disorder unless mature T cells are also injected, as is necessary for patients with complete DiGeorge syndrome.

Autosomal Recessive SCID with Multiple Intestinal Atresias

SCID associated with multiple gastrointestinal atresia has been observed in two kindreds, with absence of T cells and very low cell counts (Moreno et al., 1990; Walker et al., 1993). Inheritance is presumed to be autosomal recessive. The molecular mechanism underlying the intestinal abnormalities is unknown.

Alain Fischer

REFERENCES

Abe T, Tsuge I, Kamachi Y, Torii S, Utsumi K, Akahori Y, Ichihara Y, Kurosawa Y, Matsuoka H. Evidence for defects in V(D)J rearrangements in patients with severe combined immunodeficiency. J Immunol 152:5502–5513, 1994.

Akashi K, Kondo M, von Freeden-Jeffry U, Murray R, Weissman IL. Bcl-2 rescues T lymphopoiesis in interleukin-7 receptor-deficient mice. Cell 89:1033–1041, 1997.

Alarcon B, Regueiro JR, Arnaiz-Villena A, Terhorst C. Familial defect in the surface expression of the T-cell receptor-CD3 complex. N Engl J Med 319:1203–1208, 1988.

Androlewicz MJ, Ormann B, van-Endert P, Spies T, Cresswell P. Characteristics of peptide and major histocompatibility complex class I/β2-microglobulin binding to the transporters associated with antigen processing TAP1 and TAP2. Proc Natl Acad Sci USA 91:12716–12720, 1994.

Arpaia E, Shahar M, Dadi H, Cohan A, Roifman C. Defective T cell receptor signaling and CD8+ thymic selection in humans lacking Zap-70 kinase. Cell 76:947–958, 1994.

Ayalon O, Hughes EA, Cresswell P, Lee J, O'Donnell L, Pardi R, Bender JR. Induction of transporter associated with antigen processing by interferon γ confers endothelial cell cytoprotection against natural killer-mediated cytolysis. Proc Natl Acad Sci USA 95:2435–2440, 1998.

Berthet F, Le Deist F, Duliege A, Griscelli C, Fischer A. Clinical consequences and treatment of primary immunodeficiency syndromes characterized by functional T and B lymphocyte anomalies (combined immune deficiency). Pediatrics 93:265–270, 1994.

Bertand Y, Landais P, Friedrich W, Gerritsen B, Morgan G, Fasth A, Cavazzana-Calvo M, Porta F, Cant A, Espanol T, Muller S, Veys P, Vossen J, Haddad E, Fischer A. Influence of severe combined immunodeficiency phenotype on the outcome of HLS non-identical, T-cell-depleted bone marrow transplantation: a retrospective European survey from the European group for bone marrow transplantation and the European society for immunodeficiency. J Pediatr 134:740–748, 1999.

Bertrand Y, Muller SM, Casanova JL, Morgan G, Fischer A, Friedrich W. Reticular dysgenesis: HLS non-identical bone marrow transplants in a series of 10 patients. Bone Marrow Transplant 29:759–762, 2002.

Biedermann KA, Sum JR, Giaccia AJ, Tosto LM, Brown JM. SCID mutation in mice confers hypersensitivity to ionizing radiation and a deficiency in DNA double-strand break repair. Proc Natl Acad Sci USA 88:1394–1397, 1991.

Blunt T, Gell D, Fox M, Taccioli GE, Lehmann AR, Jackson SP, Jeggo PA Identification of a nonsense mutation in the carboxyl-terminal region of DNA-dependent protein kinase catalytic subunit in the SCID mouse. Proc Natl Acad Sci USA 93:10285–10290, 1996.

Bosma GC, Custer RP, Bosma MJ. A severe combined immunodeficiency mutation in the mouse. Nature 301:527–530, 1983.

Bozzi F, Lefranc G, Villa A, Badolato R, Schumacher RF, Khalil G, Loiselet J, Bresciani S, O'Shea JJ, Vezzoni P, Notarangelo LD, Candotti F. Molecular and biochemical characterization of JAK3 deficiency in a patient with severe combined immunodeficiency over 20 years after bone marrow transplantation: implications for treatment. Br J Haematol 102:1363–1366, 1998.

Bradley MB, Fernandez JM, Ungers G, Diaz-Barrientos T, Steimle V, Mach B, O'Reilly R, Lee JS. Correction of defective expression in MHC class II deficiency (bare lymphocyte syndrome) cells by retroviral transduction of CIITA. J Immunol 159:1086–1095, 1997.

Braud VM, Alian DSJ, O'Callaghan CA, Soderstrom K, D'Andrea A, Ogg GS, Lazetic S, Young NT, Bell JI, Phillips JH, Lanier LL, Mc Michael AJ. HLA-E binds to natural killer cell receptors CD94/NKG2A, B and C. Nature 391:795–799, 1998.

Brooks EG, Schmalstieg FC, Wirt DP, Rosenblatt HM, Adkins LT, Lookingbill DP, Rudloff HE, Rakusan TA, Goldman AS. A novel X-linked combined immunodeficiency disease. J Clin Invest 86:1623–1631, 1990.

Brugnoni D, Airò P, Facchetti F, Blanzuoli L, Ugazio AG, Cattaneo R, Notarangelo LD. In vitro cell death of activated lymphocytes in Omenn's syndrome. Eur J Immunol 27:2765–2773, 1997.

Brugnoni D, Notarangelo LD, Sottini A, Airò P, Pennacchio M, Mazzolari E, Signorini S, Candotti F, Villa A, Mella P, Vezzoni P, Cattaneo R, Ugazio AG, Imberti L. Development of autologous, oligoclonal, poorly functioning T lymphocytes in a patient with autosomal recessive severe combined immunodeficiency due to defects of the Jak3 tyrosine kinase. Blood 91:949–955, 1998.

Buckley RH. Primary immunodeficiency diseases due to defects in lymphocytes. N Engl J Med 343:1313–1324, 2000.

Buckley PH. Primary cellular immunodeficiencies. J Allergy Clin Immunol 109:747–757, 2002.

Buckley RH, Schiff RI, Schiff SE, Markert ML, Williams LW, Harville TO, Roberts JL, Puck JM. Human severe combined immunodeficiency: genetic, phenotypic, and functional diversity in one hundred eight infants. J Pediatr 130:378–387, 1997.

Buckley RH, Schiff SE, Schiff RI, Markert L, Williams LW, Roberts JL, Myers L A, Ward FE. Hematopoietic stem-cell transplantation for the treatment of severe combined immunodeficiency. N Engl J Med 340:508–516, 1999.

Bunting KD, Flynn KJ, Riberdy JM, Doherty PC, Sorrentino BP. Virus-specific immunity after gene therapy in a murine model of severe combined immunodeficiency. Proc Natl Acad Sci USA 96:232–237, 1999.

Bunting KD, Sangster MY, Ihle JN, Sorrentino BP. Restoration of lymphocyte function in Janus kinase 3-deficient mice by retroviral-mediated gene transfer. Nat Med 4:58–64, 1998.

Cacalano NA, Migone TS, Bazan F, Hanson EP, Chen M, Candotti F, O'Shea JJ, Johnston JA. Autosomal SCID caused by a point mutation in the N-terminus of Jak3: mapping of the Jak3-receptor interaction domain. EMBO J 18:1549–1558, 1999.

Callebaut I, Mornon JP. The V(D)J recombination activating protein RAG2 consists of a six-bladed propeller and a PHD fingerlike domain, as revealed by sequence analysis. Cell Mol Life Sci 54:880–891, 1998.

Candotti F, Johnston, JA, Puck JM, Sugamura K, O'Shea JJ, Blaese RM. Retroviral-mediated gene correction for X-linked severe combined immunodeficiency. Blood 87:3097–3102, 1996.

Candotti F, Oakes SA, Johnston JA, Giliani S, Schumacher RF, Mella P, Fiorini M, Ugazio AG, Badolato R, Notarangelo LD, Bozzi F, Macchi P, Strina D, Vezzoni P, Blaese RM, O'Shea JJ, Villa A. Structural and functional basis for JAK3-deficient severe combined immunodeficiency. Blood 90:3996–4003, 1997.

Cao X, Shores EW, Hu-Li J, Anver MR, Kelsall BL, Russell SM, Drago J, Noguchi M, Grinberg A, Bloom ET. Defective lymphoid development in mice lacking expression of the common cytokine receptor gamma chain. Immunity 2:223–228, 1995.

Castigli E, Pahwa R, Good RA, Geha RS, Chatila TA. Molecular basis of a multiple lymphokine deficiency in a patient with severe combined immunodeficiency. Proc Natl Acad Sci USA 90:4728–4732, 1993.

Cavazzana-Calvo M, Hacein-Bey S, de Saint Basile G, De Coene C, Selz F, Le Deist F, Fischer A. Role of interleukin-2 (IL-2), IL-7, and IL-15 in natural killer cell differentiation from cord blood hematopoietic progenitor cells and from gamma c transduced severe combined immunodeficiency X1 bone marrow cells. Blood 88:3901–3909, 1996.

Cavazzana-Calvo M, Hacein-Bey S, de Saint Basile G, Gross F, Yvon E, Nusbaum P, Selz F, Hue C, Certain S, Casanova JL, Bousso P, Deist FL, Fischer A. Gene therapy of human severe combined immunodeficiency (SCID)-X1 disease. Science 288:669–672, 2000.

Cavazzana-Calvo M, Le Deist F, de Saint Basile G, Papadopoulo D, de Villartay JP, Fischer A. Increased radiosensitivity of granulocyte macrophage colony-forming units and skin fibroblasts in human autosomal recessive severe combined immunodeficiency. J Clin Invest 91:1214–1218, 1993.

Cederbaum SD, Niwayama G, Stiehm ER, Neerhout RC, Ammann AJ, Berman W Jr. Combined immunodeficiency presenting as the Letterer-Siwe syndrome. J Pediatr 85:466–471, 1974.

Chan AC, Dalton M, Johnson R, Kong G-h, Wang T, Thoma R, Kurosaki T. Activation of ZAP-70 kinase activity by phosphorylation of tyrosine 493 is required for lymphocyte antigen receptor function. EMBO J 14:2499–2508, 1995.

Chan AC, Kadlecek TA, Elder ME, Filipovich AH, Kuo W-L, Iwashima M, Parslow T, Weiss A. ZAP-70 deficiency in an autosomal recessive form of severe combined immunodeficiency. Science 264:1599–1601, 1994.

Chang C-H, Guerder S, Hong S-C, van Ewijk W, Flavell RA. Mice lacking the MHC class II transactivator (CIITA) show tissue-specific impairment of MHC class II expression. Immunity 4:167–178, 1996.

Chapman H.A Endosomal proteolysis and MHC class II function. Curr Opin Immunol 10:93–102, 1998.

Chatila T, Castigli E, Pahwa R, Pahwa S, Chirmule N, Oyaizu N, Good RA, Geha RS. Primary combined immunodeficiency resulting from defective transcription of multiple T-cell lymphokine genes. Proc Natl Acad Sci USA 87:10033–10037, 1990.

Chen M, Cheng A, Candotti F, Zhou Y J, Hymel A, Fasth A, Notarangelo LD, O'Shea JJ. Complex effects of naturally occurring mutations in the JAK3 pseudokinase domain: evidence for interactions between the kinase and pseudokinase domains. Mol Cell Biol 20:947–956, 2000.

Chilosi M, Facchetti F, Notarangelo LD, Romagnani S, Del Prete G, Almerigogna F, De Carli M, Pizzolo G. CD30 cell expression and abnormal soluble CD30 serum accumulation in Omenn's syndrome: evidence for a T helper 2-mediated condition. Eur J Immunol 26:329–334, 1996a.

Chilosi M, Pizzolo G, Facchetti F, Notarangelo LD, Romagnani S, Del Prete G, Almerigogna F, De Carli M. The pathology of Omenn's syndrome. Am J Surg Pathol 20:773–774, 1996b.

Chow LML, Veillette A. The Src and Csk families of tyrosine protein, kinases in hemopoietic cells. Semin Immunol 7:207–226, 1995.

Chu DH, van Oers NSC, Malissen M, Harris J, Elder M, Weiss A. Pre-T cell receptor signals are responsible for the down-regulation of Syk protein tyrosine kinase expression. J Immunol 163:2610–2620, 1999.

Colonna M. Specificity and function of immunoglobulin superfamily of NK cell inhibitory and stimulatory receptors. Immunol Rev 155:127–133, 1997.

Conley ME, Lavoie A, Briggs C, Brown P, Guerra C, Puck JM. Nonrandom X chromosome inactivation in B cells from carriers of X chromosome-linked severe combined immunodeficiency. Proc Natl Acad Sci USA 85:3090–3094, 1988.

Corneo B, Moshous D, Callebaut I, de Chasseval R, Fischer A, de Villartay JP. Three-dimensional clustering of human RAG2 gene mutations in severe combined immune deficiency. J Biol Chem. 275:12672–12675, 2000.

Dadi HK, Simon AJ, Roifman CM. Effect of CD3δ deficiency on maturation of α/β and γ/δ T-cell lineages in severe combined immunodeficiency. N Engl J Med 349:1821–1828, 2003.

Danska JS, Holland DP, Mariathasan S, Williams KM, Guidos CJ. Biochemical and genetic defects in the DNA-dependent protein kinase in murine SCID lymphocytes. Mol Cell Biol 16:5507–5517, 1996.

Dayan AD. Chronic encephalitis in children with sever immunodeficiency. Acta Neuropathol (Berl) 19:234–241. 1971.

de la Salle H, Donato L, Zimmer J, Plebani A, Hanau D, Bonneville M, Tongio MM. HLA class I deficiencies. In Ochs HD, Smith CEI, Puck JM, eds. Primary Immunodeficiency Diseases: A Molecular and Genetic Approach. New York, Oxford University Press, 1998, pp 181–188.

de la Salle H, Hanau D, Fricker D, Urlacher A, Kelly A, Salamero J, Powis SH, Donato L, Bausinger H, Laforet M, Jeras M, Spehner D, Bieber T, Falkenrodt A, Cazenave JP, Trowsdale J, Tongio MM. Homozygous human TAP peptide transporter mutation in HLA class I deficiency. Science 265:237–240, 1994.

de la Salle H, Saulquin X, Mansour I, Klayme S, Fricker D, Zimmer J, Cazenave JP, Hanau D, Benneville M, Houssaint E, Lefranc G, Naman R. Asymptomatic deficiency in the peptide transported associated to antigen processing (TAP). Clin Exp Immunol 128:525–531, 2002.

de la Salle H, Zimmer J, Fricker D, Angenieux C, Cazenave JP, Okubo M, Maeda A, Plebani A, Tongio MM, Dormay A, Hanau D. HLA class I deficiencies due to mutations in subunit 1 of the peptide transporter TAP1. J Clin Invest 103:R9–R13, 1999.

de Saint Basile G, Fischer A, Dautzenberg MD, Durandy A, Le Deist F, Angles-Cano E, Griscelli C. Enhanced plasminogen-activator production by leukocytes in the human and murine Chediak-Higashi syndrome. Blood 65:1275–1281, 1985.

de Saint-Basile G, Le Deist F, Caniglia M, Lebranchu Y, Griscelli C, Fischer A. Genetic study of a new X-linked recessive immunodeficiency syndrome. J Clin Invest 89:861–866, 1992.

de Saint Basile G, Le Deist F, de Villartay J-P, Cerf-Bensussan N, Journet O, Brousse N, Griscelli C, Fischer A. Restricted heterogeneity of T lymphocytes in combined immunodeficiency with hypereosinophilia (Omenn's syndrome). J Clin Invest 87:1352–1359, 1991.

De Vaal O, Seyneheve V. Reticular dysgenesis. Lancet 2:1123–1125, 1959.

DiSanto JP, Keever CA, Small TN, Nicols GL, O'Reilly RJ, Flomenberg N. Absence of interleukin 2 production in a severe combined immunodeficiency disease syndrome with T cells. J Exp Med 171:1697–1704, 1990.

DiSanto JP, Muller W, Guy-Grand D, Fischer A, Rajewsky K. Lymphoid development in mice with a targeted deletion of the interleukin 2 receptor gamma chain. Proc Natl Acad Sci USA 92:377–381, 1995a.

DiSanto JP, Kuhn R, Muller W. Common cytokine receptor gamma chain (gamma c)-dependent cytokines: understanding in vivo functions by gene targeting. Immunol Rev 148:19–34, 1995b.

DiSanto JP, Rieux-Laucat F, Dautry-Varsat A, Fischer A, de Saint Basile G. Defective human interleukin 2 receptor gamma chain in an atypical X chromosome-linked severe combined immunodeficiency with peripheral T cells. Proc Natl Acad Sci USA 91:9466–9470, 1994.

Donato L, de la Salle H, Hanau D, Tongio MM, Oswald M, Vandevenne A, Gelsert J. Association of HLA class I antigen deficiency related to a TAP 2 gene mutation with familial bronchiectasis. J Pediatr 127:895–900, 1995.

Dumoutier L, Van Roost E, Colau D, Renauld JC. Human interleukin-10-related T cell-derived inducible factor: molecular cloning and functional characterization as an hepatocyte-stimulating factor. Proc Natl Acad Sci USA 97:10144–10149, 2000.

Durand B, Sperisen P, Emery P, Barras E, Zufferey M, Mach B, Reith W. RFXAP, a novel subunit of the RFX DNA binding complex is mutated in MHC class II deficiency. EMBO J 16:1045–1055, 1997.

Elder ME. Severe combined immunodeficiency due to a defect in the tyrosine kinase ZAP-70. Pediatr Res 39:743–748, 1996.

Elder ME, Lin D, Clever J, Chan AC, Hope TJ, Weiss A, Parslow TG. Human severe combined immunodeficiency due to a defect in ZAP-70, a T cell tyrosine kinase. Science 264:1596–1599, 1994.

Elder ME, Skoda-Smith S, Kadlecek T, Wang F, Wu J, Weiss A. Distinct T cell development consequences in humans and mice expressing identical mutations in the DLAARN motif of ZAP-70. J Immunol 166:656–661, 2001.

Fischer A. Thirty years of bone marrow transplantation for severe combined immunodeficiency. N Engl J Med 340:559–561, 1999.

Fischer A. Severe combined immunodeficiencies (SCID). Clin Exp Immunol 122:143–149, 2000.

Fischer A, Landais P, Friedrich W, Gerritsen B, Fasth A, Porta F, Vellodi A, Benkerrou M, Jais JP, Cavazzana-Calvo M. Bone marrow transplantation (BMT) in Europe for primary immunodeficiencies other than severe combined immunodeficiency: a report from the European Group for BMT and the European Group for Immunodeficiency. Blood 83:1149–1154, 1994.

Fischer A, Landais P, Friedrich W, Morgan G, Gerritsen B, Fasth A, Porta F, Griscelli C, Goldman SF, Levinsky R, Vossen J. European experience of bone-marrow transplantation for severe combined immunodeficiency. Lancet 336:850–854, 1990.

Flake AW, Roncarolo MG, Puck JM, Almeida-Porada G, Evans MI, Johnson MP, Abella EM, Harrison DD, Zanjani ED. Treatment of X-linked severe combined immunodeficiency by in utero transplantation of paternal bone marrow. N Engl J Med 335:1806–1810, 1996.

Fondaneche MC, Villard J, Wiszniewski W, Etzioni A, Le Deist F, Peijnenburg A, Casanova J-L, Reith W, Mach B, Fischer A, Lisowska-Grospierre B. Genetic and molecular definition of complementation group D in MHC class II deficiency. Hum Mol Gen 7:879–885, 1998.

Frank J, Pignata C, Panteleyev AA, Prowse DM, Baden H, Weiner L, Gaetaniello L, Ahmad W, Pozzi N, Cserhalmi-Friedman PB, Aita VM, Uyttendaele H, Gordon D, Ott J, Brissette JL, Christiano AM Exposing the human nude phenotype. Nature 398:473–474, 1999.

Fulop GM, Phillips RA. The SCID mutation in mice causes a general defect in DNA repair. Nature 347:479–482, 1990.

Furukawa H, Murata S, Yabe T, Shimbara N, Keicho N, Kashiwase K, Watanabe K, Ishikawa Y, Akaza T, Tadokoro K, Tohma S, Inoue T, Tokunaga K, Yamamoto K, Tanaka K, Juji T. Splice acceptor site mutation of the transporter associated with antigen processing-1 gene in human bare lymphocyte syndrome. J Clin Invest 103:649–652, 1999a.

Furukawa H, Yabe T, Watanabe K, Miyamoto R, Miki A, Akaza T, Tadokoro K, Tohma S, Inoue T, Yamamoto K, Juji T. Tolerance of NK and LAK activity for HLA class I-deficient targets in a TAP1-deficient patient (bare lymphocyte syndrome type I). Hum Immunol 60:32–40, 1999b.

Gadola SD, Mois-Teisserenc HT, Trowsdale J, Gross WL, Cerundolo V. TAP deficiency syndrome. Clin Exp Immunol 121:173–178, 2000.

Gatti RA, Meuwissen HJ, Allen HD, Hong R, Good RA. Immunological reconstitution of sex-linked lymphopenic immunological deficiency. Lancet 2:1366–1369, 1968.

Gauen LK, Zhu Y, Letourneur F, Hu Q, Bolen JB, Matis LA, Klausner RD, Shaw AS. Interactions of p59fyn and ZAP-70 with T-cell receptor activations motifs: defining the nature of a signalling motif. Mol Cell Biol 14:3729–3741, 1994.

Gehrz RC, McAuliffe JJ, Linner KM, Kersey JH. Defective membrane function in a patient with severe combined immunodeficiency disease. Clin Ep Immunol 39:344–348, 1980.

Gelfand EW, Weinberg K, Mazer BD, Kadlecek TA, Weiss A. Absence of ZAP-70 prevents signaling through the antigen receptor on peripheral blood T cells but not on thymocytes. J Exp Med 182:1057–1066, 1995.

Goldman FD, Ballas ZK, Schutte BC, Kemp J, Hollenback C, Noraz N, Taylor N. Defective expression of p56lck in an infant with severe combined immunodeficiency. J Clin Invest 102:421–429, 1998.

Gomez L, Le Deist F, Blanche S, Cavazzana-Calvo M, Griscelli C, Fischer A. Treatment of Omenn syndrome by bone marrow transplantation. J Pediatr 127:76-81, 1995.

Griscelli C, Durandy A, Virelizier JL, Ballet JJ, Daguillard F. Selective defect of precursor T cells associated with apparently normal B lymphocytes in severe combined immunodeficiency disease. J Pediatr 93:404–411, 1978.

Griscelli C, Lisowska-Grospierre B, Mach B. Combined immunodeficiency with defective expression in MHC class II genes. Immunodefic Rev 1:135–153, 1989.

Haas A, Wells J, Chin T, Stiehm ER, Successful treatment of reticular dysgenesis with haploidentical bone marrow transplantation. Clin Res 34:127, 1986.

Hacein-Bey-Abina S, Le Deist F, Carlier F, Bouneaud C, Hue C, De Villartay JP, Thrasher AJ, Wulffraat N, Sorensen R, Dupuis-Girod S, Fischer A, Davies EG, Kuis W, Leiva L, Cavazzana-Calvo M. Sustained correction of X-linked severe combined immunodeficiency by ex vivo gene therapy. N Engl J Med 346:1185–1193, 2002.

Hacein-Bey-Abina S, Von Kalle C, Schmidt M, McCormack MP, Wulffraat N, Lebouch P, Lim A, Osborne CS, Pawliuk R, Morillon E, Sorensen R, Forster A, Fraser P, Cohen JI, de Saint Basile G, Alexander I, Wintergerst U, Frebourg T, Aurias A, Stoppa-Lyonnet D, Romana S, Radford-Weiss I, Gross F, Valensi F, Delabesse E, Macintyre E, Sigaux F, Soulier J, Leiva LE, Wissler M, Prinz C, Rabbitts TH, Le Deist F, Fischer A, Cavazzana-Calvo M. LMO2-associated clonal T cell proliferation in two patients after gene therapy for SCID-X1. Science 302:415–419, 2003.

Haddad E, Landais P, Friedrich W, Gerritsen B, Cavazzana-Calvo M, Morgan G, Bertrand Y, Fasth A, Porta F, Cant A, Espanol T, Muller S, Veys P, Vossen J, Fischer A. Long-term immune reconstitution and outcome after HLA-nonidentical T-cell-depleted bone marrow transplantation for severe combined immunodeficiency: a European retrospective study of 116 patients. Blood 91:3646–3653, 1998.

Harton JA, Ting JP-Y. Class II transactivator: mastering the art of MHC complex expression. Mol Cell Biol 20:6185–6194, 2000.

Hatada MH, Lu X, Laird ER, Green J, Morgenstern JP, Lou M, Marr CS, Phillips TB, Ram MK, Theriault K, Zoller MJ, Karas JL. Molecular basis for interaction of the protein tyrosine kinase ZAP-70 with the T-cell receptor. Nature 377:32–38, 1995.

Heemels MT, Ploegh H. Generation, translocation, and presentation of MHC class I restricted peptides. Annu Rev Biochem 64:463–491, 1995.

Hendrickson EA, Qin XQ, Bump EA, Schatz DG, Oettinger M, Weaver DT. A link between double-strand break related repair and V(D)J recombination: the SCID mutation. Proc Natl Acad Sci USA 88:4061–4065, 1991.

Henthorn PS, Somberg RL, Fimiani VM, Puck JM, Patterson DF, Felsburg PJ. IL-2R gamma gene microdeletion demonstrates that canine X-linked severe combined immunodeficiency is a homologue of the human disease. Genomics 23:69–74, 1994.

Hong R. Disorders of the T-cell system. In Stiehm ER, ed. Immunologic Disorders in Infants and Children, ed 4, Philadelphia, WB Saunders, 1996, pp 339–408.

Hu DC, Gahagan S, Wara DW, Hayward A, Cowan MJ. Congenital severe combined immunodeficiency disease (SCID) in American Indians. Pediatr Res 24:239–244, 1988.

Hughes EA, Cresswell P. The thiol oxidoreductase ERp75 is a component of the MHC class I peptide-loading complex. Curr Biol 8:709–712, 1998.

Ihle JN. STATs: signal transducers and activators of transcription. Cell 84:331–334, 1996.

Iwashima M, Irving B, van Oers NSC, Chan AC, Weiss A. The sequential interaction of the T cell antigen receptor with two distinct cytoplasmic protein tyrosine kinases. Science 263:1136–1139, 1994.

Izuhara K, Heike T, Otsuka T, Yamaoka K, Mayumi M, Imamura T, Niho Y, Harada N. Signal transduction pathway of interleukin-4 and interleukin-13 in human B cells derived from X-linked severe combined immunodeficiency patients. J Biol Chem 271:619–622, 1996.

Jackson SP, Jeggo PA. DNA double-strand break repair and V(D)J recombination: involvement of DNA-PK. Trends Biochem Sci 20:412–415, 1995.

Jones J, Ritenbaugh C, Spence A, Hayward A. Severe combined immunodeficiency among the Navajo: characterization of phenotypes, epidemiology and population genetics. Hum Biol 63:669–682, 1991.

Junker AK, Chan KW, Massing BG. Clinical and immune recovery from Omenn syndrome after bone marrow transplantation. J Pediatr 114:596–600, 1988.

Junker AK, Poon MC, Hoar DI, Rogers PC. Severe combined immune deficiency presenting with cyclic hematopoiesis. J Clin Immunol 11:369–377, 1991.

Kaiser J. Seeking the cause of induced leukemias in X-SCID Science 299:495, 2003.

Katamura K, Tai G, Tachibana T, Yamabe H, Ohmori K, Mayumi M, Matsuda S, Koyasu S, Furusho K. Existence of activated and memory CD4+ T cells in peripheral blood and their skin infiltration in CD8 deficiency. Clin Exp Immunol 115:124–130, 1999.

Kelly A, Powis SH, Kerr LA, Mockridge I, Elliott T, Bastin J, Uchanska-Ziegler B, Ziegler A, Trowsdale J, Townsend A. Assembly and function of the two ABC transporter proteins encoded in the human major histocompatibility complex. Nature 355:641–644, 1992.

Kishihara K, Penninger J, Wallace VA, Kundig TM, Kawai K, Wakeham A, Timms E, Pfeffer K, Ohashi PS, Thomas ML. Normal B lymphocyte development but impaired T cell maturation in CD45-exon6 protein tyrosine phosphatase-deficient mice. Cell 74:143–156, 1993.

Klein C, Cavazzana-Calvo M, Le Deist F, Jabado N, Benkerrou N, Blanche S, Lisowska-Grospierre B, Griscelli C, Fischer A. Bone marrow transplantation in major histocompatibility complex class II deficiency: a single-center study of 19 patients. Blood 85:580–558, 1995.

Klein C, Lisowska-Grospierre B, LeDeist F, Fischer A, Griscelli C. Major histocompatibility complex class II deficiency: clinical manifestations, immunologic features, and outcome. J Pediatr 123:921–929, 1993.

Knutsen AP, Wall DA. Umbilical cord blood transplantation in severe T-cell immunodeficiency disorders: two-year experience. J. Clin Immunol. 20:466–476, 2000.

Kumaki S, Ishii N, Minegishi M, Tsuchiya S, Cosman D, Sugamura K, Konno T. Functional role of interleukin-4 (IL-4) and IL-7 in the development of X-linked severe combined immunodeficiency. Blood 93:607–612, 1999.

Kung C, Pingel JT, Heikinheimo M, Klemola T, Varkila K, Yoo LI, Vuopala K, Poyhonen M, Uhari M, Rogers M, Speck SH, Chatila T, Thomas ML. Mutations in the tyrosine phosphatase CD45 gene in a child with severe combined immunodeficiency disease. Nat Med 6:343–345, 2000.

Kwong PC, O'Marcaigh AS, Howard R, Cowan MJ, Frieden IJ. Oral and genital ulceration: a unique presentation of immunodeficiency in Athabascan-speaking American Indian children with severe combined immunodeficiency. Arch Dermatol 135:927–931, 1999.

Lawlor GR Jr, Ammann AJ, Wright WC, LaFranchi SH, Bilstrom D, Stiehm ER. The syndrome of cellular immunodeficiency with immunoglobulins. J Pediatr 84:183–192, 1974.

Le Deist F, Hivroz C, Partiseti M, Thomas C, Buc HA, Oleastro M, Belohradsky B, Choquet D, Fischer A. A primary T-cell immunodeficiency associated with defective transmembrane calcium influx. Blood 85:1053–1062, 1995.

Le Deist F, Thoenes G, Corado J, Lisowska-Grospierre B, Fischer A. Immunodeficiency with low expression of the T cell receptor/CD3 complex. Effect on T lymphocyte activation. Eur J Immunol 21:1641–1647, 1991.

Leonard WJ, O'Shea JJ. Jaks and STATs: biological implications. Annu Rev Immunol 16:293–322, 1998.

Leonard WJ, Noguchi M, Russell SM, McBride OW. The molecular basis of X-linked severe combined immunodeficiency: the role of the interleukin-2 receptor gamma chain as a common gamma chain, gamma c. Immunol Rev 138:61–86, 1994.

Levin SD, Anderson SJ, Forbush KA, Perlmutter RM. A dominant-negative transgene defines a role for p56lck in thymopoiesis. EMBO J 12:1671–1680, 1993.

Levinsky RJ, Tiedeman K. Successful bone-marrow transplantation for reticular dysgenesis. Lancet 1:671–673, 1983.

Li L, Drayna D, Hu D, Hayward A, Gahagan S, Pabst H, Cowan MJ. The gene for severe combined immunodeficiency disease in Athabascan-speaking Native Americans is located on chromosome 10p. Am J Hum Genet 62:136–144, 1998.

Li L, Moshous D, Zhou Y, Wang J, Xie G, Salido E, Hu D, de Villartay JP, Cowan MJ. A founder mutation in Artemis, an SNM1-like protein, causes SCID in Athabascan-speaking Native Americans. J Immunol. 168:6323–6329, 2002.

Ma Y, Pannicke U, Schwarz K, Lieber MR. Hairpin opening and overhang processing by an Artemis/DNA-dependent protein kinase complex in nonhomologous end joining and V(D)J recombination. Cell 108:781–794, 2002.

Macchi P, Villa A, Giliani S, Sacco MG, Frattini A, Porta F, Ugazio AG, Johnston JA, Candotti F, O'Shea JJ, Vezzoni P, Notarangelo LD. Mutations of Jak-3 gene in patients with autosomal severe combined immune deficiency (SCID). Nature 377:65–68, 1995.

Maeda H, Hirata R, Chen RF, Suzaki H, Kudoh S, Tohyama H. Defective expression of HLA class I antigens: a case of the bare lymphocyte syndrome without immunodeficiency. Immunogenetics 21:549–558, 1985.

Malek TR, Porter BO, He YW. Multiple gamma c-dependent cytokines regulate T-cell development. Immunol Today 20:71–76, 1999.

Maraskovsky E, O'Reilly LA, Teepe M, Corcoran LM, Peschon JJ, Strasser A. Bcl-2 can rescue T lymphocyte development in interleukin-7 receptor-deficient mice but not in mutant rag-1–/– mice. Cell 89:1011–1019, 1997.

Martin JV, Willoughby PB, Giusti V, Price G, Cerezo L. The lymph node pathology of Omenn's syndrome. Am J Surg Pathol 19:1082–1087, 1995.

Masternak K, Barras E, Zufferey M, Conrad B, Corthals G, Aebersold R, Sanchez JC, Hochstrasser DF, Mach B, Reith W. A gene encoding a novel RFX-associated transactivator is mutated in the majority of MHC class II deficiency patients. Nat Genet 20:273–277, 1998.

Matsuda S, Suzuki-Fujimoto T, Minowa A, Ueno H, Katamura K, Koyasu S. Temperature-sensitive ZAP-70 mutants degrading through a proteasome-independent pathway. J Biol Chem 274:34515–34518, 1999.

Matthews DJ, Clark PA, Herbert J, Morgan G, Armitage RJ, Kinnon C, Minty A, Grabstein KH, Caput D, Ferrara P. Function of the interleukin-2 (IL-2) receptor gamma-chain in biologic responses of X-linked severe combined immunodeficient B cells to IL-2, IL-4, IL-13, and IL-15. Blood 85:38–42, 1995.

Mazer B, Harbeck RJ, Franklin R, Schwinzer R, Kubo R, Hayward A, Gelfand EW. Phenotypic features of selective T cell deficiency characterized by absence of CD8+ T lymphocytes and undetectable mRNA for ZAP-70 kinase. Clin Immunol Immunopathol 84:129–136, 1997.

McDevitt HO. The role of MHC class II molecules in susceptibility and resistance to autoimmunity. Curr Opin Immunol 10:677–681, 1998.

Minegishi Y, Okawa H, Sugamura K, Yata J. Preferential utilization of the immature JH segment and absence of somatic mutation in the CDR3 junction of the Ig H chain gene in three X-linked severe combined immunodeficiency patients. Int Immunol 6:1709–1716,1994.

Moins-Teisserenc HT, Gadola SD, Cella M, Dunbar PR, Exley A, Blake N, Baycal C, Lambert J, Bigliardi P, Willemsen M, Jones M, Buechner S, Colonna M, Gross WL, Cerundolo V. Association of a syndrome resembling Wegener's granulomatosis with low surface expression of HLA class-I molecules. Lancet 354:1598–1603, 1999.

Molina TJ, Kishihara K, Siderovski DP, van Ewijk W, Narendran A, Timms E, Wakeham A, Paige CJ, Hartmann K-U, Veillette A, Davidson D, Mak TW. Profound block in thymocyte development in mice lacking p56lck. Nature 357:161–164, 1992.

Mombaerts P, Iacomini J, Johnson RS, Herrup K, Tonegawa S, Papaionnou VE. RAG-1 deficient mice have no mature B and T lymphocytes. Cell 68:869–877, 1992.

Momburg F, Hammerling G. Generation and TAP-mediated transport of peptides for major histocompatibility complex class I molecules. Adv Immunol 68:191–256, 1998.

Monafo WJ, Polmar SH, Neudorf S, Mather A, Filipovich AH. A hereditary immunodeficiency characterized by CD8+ T lymphocyte deficiency and impaired lymphocyte activation. Clin Exp Immunol 90:390–393, 1992.

Morelon E, Dautry-Varsat A, Le Deist F, Hacein-Bay S, Fischer A, de Saint Basile G. T-lymphocyte differentiation and proliferation in the absence of the cytoplasmic tail of the common cytokine receptor gamma c chain in a severe combined immune deficiency X1 patient. Blood 88:1708–1717, 1996.

Moreno LA, Gottrand F, Turck D, Manouvrier-Hanu S, Mazingue F, Morisot C, Le Deist F, Ricour C, Nihoul-Fekete C, Debeugny P. Severe combined immunodeficiency syndrome associated with autosomal recessive familial multiple gastrointestinal atresias: study of a family. Am J Med Genet 37:143–146, 1990.

Moshous D, Callebaut I, de Chasseval R, Corneo B, Cavazzana-Calvo M, Le Deist F, Tezcan I, Sanal O, Bertrand Y, Philippe N, Fischer A, de Villartay J-P. Artemis, a novel DNA double-strand break repair/V(D)J recombination protein, is mutated in human severe combined immune deficiency. Cell 105:177–186, 2001.

Moshous D, Li L, de Chasseval R, Philippe N, Jabado N, Cowan MJ, Fischer A, de Villartay JP. A new gene involved in DNA double-strand break repair and V(D)J recombination is located on human chromosome 10p. Hum Mol Genet 9:583–588, 2000.

Mrozek E, Anderson P, Caligiuri MA. Role of interleukin-15 in the development of human CD56$^+$ natural killer cells from CD34$^+$ hematopoietic progenitor cells. Blood 87:2632–2640, 1996.

Murphy S, Hayward A, Troup G, Devor EJ, Coons T. Gene enrichment in an American Indian population: an excess of severe combined immunodeficiency disease. Lancet 2:502–505, 1980.

Nagarajan UM, Louis-Plence P, DeSandro A, Nilsen R, Bushey A, Boss JM. RFX-B is the gene responsible for the most common cause of the bare lymphocyte syndrome, an MHC class II immunodeficiency (erratum, 10:399). Immunity 10:153–162, 1999.

Negishi I, Motoyama N, Nakayama K, Nakayama K, Senju S, Hatakeyama S, Zhang Q, Chan AC, Loh DY. Essential role for ZAP-70 in both positive and negative selection of thymocytes. Nature 376:435–438, 1995.

Nezelof C. Thymic dysplasia with normal immunoglobulins and immunologic deficiency: pure alymphocytosis. In Bergsma D, ed. Immunologic Deficiency in Man. Birth Defects, vol 4 (Original Article Series). New York, The National Foundation, 1968, pp 104–115.

Nicolas N, Finnie NJ, Cavazzana-Calvo M, Papadopoulo D, Le Deist F, Fischer A, Jackson SP, de Villartay JP. Lack of detectable defect in DNA double-strand break repair and DNA-dependant protein kinase activity in radiosensitive human severe combined immunodeficiency fibroblasts. Eur J Immunol 26:1118–1122, 1996.

Nicolas N, Moshous D, Papadopoulo D, Cavazzana-Calvo M, de Chasseval R, le Deist F, Fischer A, de Villartay JP. A human SCID condition with increased sensitivity to ionizing radiations and impaired V(D)J rearrangements defines a new DNA recombination/repair deficiency. J Exp Med 188:627–634, 1998.

Noguchi M, Yi H, Rosenblatt HM, Filipovich AH, Adelstein S, Modi WS, McBride OW, Leonard WJ. Interleukin-2 receptor gamma chain mutation results in X-linked severe combined immunodeficiency in humans. Cell 73:147–157, 1993.

Noordzij JG, Verkaik NS, Hartwig NG, de Groot R, van Gent DC, van Dongen JJM. N-terminal truncated human RAG1 proteins can direct T-cell receptor but not immunoglobulin gene rearrangements. Blood 96:203–209, 2000.

Noraz N, Schwarz K, Steinberg M, Dardalhon V, Rebouissou C, Hipskind R, Friedrich W, Yssel H, Bacon K, Taylor N. Alternative antigen receptor (TCR) signaling in T cells derived from ZAP-70–deficient patients expressing high levels of Syk. J Biol Chem 275:15832–15838, 2000.

Nosaka T, van Deursen JM, Tripp RA, Thierfelder WE, Witthuhn BA, McMickle AP, Doherty PC, Grosveld GC, Ihle JN. Defective lymphoid development in mice lacking Jak3. Science 270:800–802, 1995.

Notarangelo LD, Candotti F. JAK3-deficient severe combined immunodeficiency. Immunol Allergy Clin N Am 20:97–111, 2000.

Notarangelo LD, Santagata S, Villa A. Rearrangement-activating (RAG) enzymes of lymphocytes. Curr Opin Hematol 8:41–46, 2001.

Notarangelo LD, Villa A, Schwarz K. RAG and RAG defects. Curr Opin Immunol 11:435–442, 1999.

Ochs HD, Davis SD, Mickelson E, Lerner KG, Wedgwood RJ. Combined immunodeficiency and reticuloendotheliosis with eosinophilia. J Pediatr 85:463–465, 1974.

Oettinger MA, Schatz DG, Gorka C, Baltimore D. RAG-1 and RAG-2, adjacent genes that synergistically activate V(D)J recombination. Science 248:1517–1523, 1990.

O'Marcaigh AS, DeSantes K, Hu D, Pabst H, Horn B, Li L, Cowan MJ. Bone marrow transplantation for T-B-severe combined immunodeficiency disease in Athabascan-speaking native Americans. Bone Marrow Transplant 27:703–709, 2001.

Omenn GS. Familial reticuloendotheliosis with eosinophilia. N Engl J Med 273:427–432, 1965.

Otten LA, Steimle V, Bontron S, Mach B. Quantitative control of MHC class II expression by the transactivator CIITA. Eur J Immunol 28:473–478, 1998.

Ownby DR, Pizzo S, Blackmon L, Gall SA, Buckley RH. Severe combined immunodeficiency with leukopenia (reticular dysgenesis) in siblings: immunologic and histopathologic findings. J Pediatr 89:382–387, 1976.

Pahwa R, Chatila T, Pahwa S, Paradise C, Day NK, Geha R, Schwartz SA, Slade H. Oyaizu N, Good RA. Recombinant interleukin-2 therapy in severe combined immunodeficiency disease. Proc Natl Acad Sci USA 86:5069–5073, 1989.

Pamer E, Cresswell P. Mechanisms of MHC class I-restricted antigen processing. Annu Rev Immunol 16:323–358, 1998.

Park SY, Saijo K, Takahashi T, Osawa M, Arase H, Hirayama N, Miyake K, Nakauchi H, Shirasawa T, Saito T. Developmental defects of lymphoid cells in Jak3 kinase-deficient mice. Immunity 3:771–782, 1995.

Payne R, Brodsky F, Peterlin BM, Young LM. Bare lymphocytes without immunodeficiency. Hum Immunol 6:219–227, 1983.

Perez-Aciego P, Alarcon B, Arnaiz-Villena A, Terhorst C, Timon M, Segurado OG, Regueiro JR. Expression and function of a variant T cell receptor complex lacking CD3-gamma. J Exp Med 174:319–326, 1991.

Peschon JJ, Morrissey PJ, Grabstein KH, Ramsdell FJ, Maraskovsky E, Gliniak BC, Park LS, Ziegler SF, Williams DE, Ware CB. Early lymphocyte expansion is severely impaired in interleukin 7 receptor-deficient mice. J Exp Med 180:1955–1960, 1994.

Petrini JH. The Mre11 complex and ATM: collaborating to navigate S phase. Curr Opin Cell Biol 12:293–296, 2000.

Plebani A, Monafo V, Cattaneo R, Carella G, Brugnoni D, Facchetti F, Battocchio S, Meini A, Notarangelo LD, Duse M, Ugazio AG. Defective expression of HLA class I and CD1a molecules in a boy with Marfan-like phenotype and deep skin ulcers. J Am Acad Dermatol 35:814–818, 1996.

Puck JM. IL2RGbase: a database of gamma c-chain defects causing human X-SCID. Immunol Today 17:507–511, 1996.

Puck JM, Deschenes SM, Porter JC, Dutra AS, Brown CJ, Willard HF, Henthorn PS. The interleukin-2 receptor gamma chain maps to Xq13.1 and is mutated in X-linked severe combined immunodeficiency, SCIDX1. Hum Mol Genet 2:1099–1104, 1993.

Puel A, Leonard WJ. Mutations in the gene for the IL-7 receptor result in T-B+NK+ severe combined immunodeficiency disease. Curr Opin Immunol 12:468–473, 2000.

Puel A, Ziegler SF, Buckley RH, Leonard WJ. Defective IL-7R expression in T-B+NK+ severe combined immunodeficiency. Nat Genet 20:394–397, 1998.

Quann V, Towey M, Sacks S, Kelly AP. Absence of MHC class II gene expression in a patient with a single amino acid substitution in class II transactivator protein CIITA. Immunogenetics 49:957–963, 1999.

Qian D, Weiss A. T cell antigen receptor signal transduction. Curr Opin Cell Biol 9:205–212, 1997.

Reisner Y, Kapoor N, Kirkpatrick D, Pollack MS, Cunningham-Rundles S, Dupont B, Hodes MZ, Good RA, O'Reilly RJ. Transplantation for severe combined immunodeficiency with HLA-A,B,D,DR incompatible parental marrow cells fractionated by soybean agglutinin and sheep red blood cells. Blood 61:341–348, 1983.

Reith W, Steimle V, Lisowska-Grospierre B, Fischer A, Mach B. Molecular basis of major histocompatibility complex class II deficiency. In Ochs HD, Smith CIE, Puck JM, eds. Primary

Immunodeficiency Diseases: A Molecular and Genetic Approach. Oxford University Press, New York, 1999, pp 167–180.

Rieux-Laucat F, Bahadoran P, Brousse N, Selz F, Fischer A, Le Deist F, de Villartay JP. Highly restricted human T cell repertoire in peripheral blood and tissue-infiltrating lymphocytes in Omenn's syndrome. J Clin Invest 102:312–321, 1998.

Rieux-Leucat F, Le Deist F, Selz F, Fischer A, de Villartay J-P. Normal T cell receptor Vb usage in a primary immunodeficiency associated with HLA class II deficiency. Eur J Immunol 23:929–934, 1993.

Roifman CM. A mutation in ZAP-70 protein tyrosine kinase results in a selective immunodeficiency. J Clin Immunol 15:52S–62S, 1995.

Roifman CM, Hummel D, Martinez-Valdez H, Thorner P, Doherty PJ, Pan S, Cohen F, Cohen A. Depletion of CD8+ cells in human thymic medulla results in selective immune deficiency. J Exp Med 170:2177–2182, 1989.

Roifman CM, Zhang J, Chitayat D, Sharfe N. A partial deficiency of interleukin-7R alpha is sufficient to abrogate T-cell development and cause severe combined immunodeficiency. Blood 96:2803–2807, 2000.

Rotbart HA, Levin MJ, Jones JF, Hayward AR, Allan J, McLane MF, Essex M. Noma in children with severe combined immunodeficiency. J Pediatr 109:596–600, 1986.

Russell SM, Johnston JA, Noguchi M, Kawamura M, Bacon CM, Friedmann M,0 Berg M, McVicar DW, Witthuhn BA, Silvennoinen O, Goldman AS, Schmalsteig FC, Ihle JN, O'Shea JJ, Leonard WJ. Interaction of IL-2R beta and gamma c chains with Jak1 and Jak3: implications for XSCID and XCID. Science 266:1042–1045, 1994.

Russell SM, Tayebi N, Nakajima H, Riedy MC, Roberts JL, Aman MJ, Migone TS, Noguchi M, Markert ML, Buckley RH, O'Shea JJ, Leonard WJ. Mutation of Jak3 in a patient with SCID: essential role of Jak3 in lymphoid development. Science 270:797–800, 1995.

Sabatier C, Gimenez C, Calin-Laurens V, Rabourdin-Combe C, Touraine JL. Type III lymphocyte syndrome: lack of HLA class II gene expression and reduction in HLA class I gene expression. C R Acad Sci Paris, Sciences de la vie/Life Science 319:789–798, 1996.

Sadasivan B, Lehner PJ, Ortmann B, Spies T, Cresswell P. Roles for calreticulin and a novel glycoprotein, tapasin, in the interaction of MHC class molecules with TAP. Immunity 5:103–114, 1996.

Santagata S, Gomez CA, Sobacchi C, Bozzi F, Abinun M, Pasic S, Cortes P, Vezzoni P, Villa A. N-terminal RAG1 frameshift mutations in Omenn's syndrome: internal methionine usage leads to partial V(D)J recombination activity and reveals a fundamental role in vivo for the N-terminal domains. Proc Natl Acad Sci USA 97:14572–14577, 2000.

Schandené L, Ferster A, Mascart-Lemone F, Crusiaux A, Gérard C, Marchant A, Lybin M, Velu T, Sariban E, Goldman M. T helper type 2-like cells and therapeutic effects of interferon-γ in combined immunodeficiency with hypereosinophilia (Omenn's syndrome). Eur J Immunol 23:56–60, 1993.

Schatz DG, Oettiger MA, Baltimore D. The V(D)J recombination activating gene, RAG-1. Cell 59:1035–1048, 1989.

Schmalstieg FC, Leonard WJ, Noguchi M, Berg M, Rudloff HE, Denney RM, Dave SK, Brooks EG, Goldman AS. Missense mutation in exon 7 of the common gamma chain gene causes a moderate form of X-linked combined immunodeficiency. J Clin Invest 95:1169–1173, 1995.

Schumacher RF, Mella P, Badolato R, Fiorini M, Savoldi G, Giliani S, Villa A, Candotti F, Tampalini A, O'Shea JJ, Notarangelo LD Complete genomic organization of the human JAK3 gene and mutation analysis in severe combined immunodeficiency by single-strand conformation polymorphism. Hum Genet 106:73–79, 2000.

Schumacher RF, Mella P, Lalatta F, Fiorini M, Giliani S, Villa A, Candotti F, Notarangelo LD. Prenatal diagnosis of JAK3 deficient SCID. Prenat Diagn 19:653–656, 1999.

Schuurman RKB, Van Rood JJ, Vossen JM, Schellekens PTA, Feltkamp-Vroom TM, Doyer E, Gmelig-Meyling F, Visser HKA. Failure of lymphocyte-membrane HLA-A and -B expression in two siblings with combined immunodeficiency. Clin Immunol Immunopathol 14:418–434, 1979.

Schwarz K, Gauss GH, Ludwig L, Pannicke U, Li Z, Lindner D, Friedrich W, Seger RA, Hansen-Hagge TE, Desiderio S, Lieber MR, Bartram CR. RAG mutations in human B cell-negative SCID. Science 274:97–99, 1996.

Schwarz K, Hansen-Hagge TE, Knobloch C, Friedrich W, Kleihauer E and Bartram CR. Severe combined immunodeficiency (SCID) in man: B cell negative (B⁻) SCID patients exhibit an irregular recombination pattern at the Jh locus. J Exp Med 174:1039–1048, 1991.

Sharfe N, Shahar M, Roifman CM. An interleukin-2 receptor gamma chain mutation with normal thymus morphology. J Clin Invest 100:3036–3043, 1997.

Shinkai Y, Rathbun G, Lam KP, Oltz EM, Stewart V, Mendelsohn M, Charron J, Datta M, Young F, Stall AM, Alt FW. RAG-2 deficient mice lack mature lymphocytes owing to inability to initiate V(D)J rearrangement. Cell 68:855–867,1992.

Signorini S, Imberti L, Pirovano S, Villa A, Facchetti F, Ungari M, Bozzi F, Albertini A, Ugazio AG, Vezzoni P, Notarangelo LD. Intrathymic restriction and peripheral expansion of the T-cell repertoire in Omenn syndrome. Blood 94:3468–3478, 1999.

Soudais C, de Villartay JP, Le Deist F, Fischer A, Lisowska-Grospierre B. Independent mutations of the human CD3-epsilon gene resulting in a T cell receptor/CD3 complex immunodeficiency. Nat Genet 3:77–81, 1993.

Steimle V, Durand B, Barras E, Zufferey M, Hadam MR, Mach B, Reith W. A novel DNA-binding regulatory factor is mutated in primary MHC class II deficiency (bare lymphocyte syndrome). Genes Dev 9:1021–1032, 1995.

Steimle V, Otten LA, Zufferey M, Mach B. Complementation cloning of an MHC class II transactivator mutated in hereditary MHC class II deficiency (or bare lymphocyte syndrome). Cell 75:135–146, 1993.

Steimle V, Siegrist CA, Mottet A, Lisowska-Grospierre B, Mach B. Regulation of MHC class II expression by interferon-gamma mediated by the transactivator gene CIITA. Science 265:106–109, 1994.

Steinberg M, Swainson L, Schwarz K, Boyer M, Friedrich W, Yssel H, Taylor N. Retrovirus-mediated transduction of primary ZAP-70–deficient human T cells results in the selective growth advantage of gene-corrected cells: implications for gene therapy. Gene Ther 7:1392–1400, 2000.

Stephan JL, Vlekova V, Le Deist F, Blanche S, Donadieu J, De Saint-Basile G, Durandy A, Griscelli C, Fischer A. Severe combined immunodeficiency: a retrospective single-center study of clinical presentation and outcome in 117 patients. J Pediatr 123:921–928, 1993.

Stephan V, Wahn V, Le Deist F, Dirksen U, Broker B, Muller-Fleckenstein I, Horneff G, Schroten H, Fischer A, de Saint Basile G. Atypical X-linked severe combined immunodeficiency due to possible spontaneous reversion of the genetic defect in T cells. N Engl J Med 335:1563–1567, 1996.

Sugiyama Y, Maeda H, Okumura K, Takaku F. Progressive sinobronchiectasis associated with the "bare lymphocyte syndrome" in an adult. Chest 89:398–401, 1986.

Sullivan KE, Stobo JD, Peterlin BM. Molecular analysis of the bare lymphocyte syndrome. J Clin Invest 76:75–79, 1985.

Takeshita T, Asao H, Ohtani K, Ishii N, Kumaki S, Tanaka N, Munakata H, Nakamura M, Sugamura K. Cloning of the gamma chain of the human IL-2 receptor. Science 257:379–382, 1992.Taylor N, Bacon KB, Smith S, Jahn T, Kadlecek TA, Uribe L, Kohn DB, Gelfand EW, Weiss A, Weinberg K. Reconstitution of T cell receptor signaling in ZAP-70–deficient cells by retroviral transduction of the ZAP-70 gene. J Exp Med 184:2031–2036, 1996a.

Taylor N, Uribe L, Smith S, Jahn T, Kohn DB, Weinberg K. Correction of interleukin-2 receptor function in X-SCID lymphoblastoid cells by retrovirally mediated transfer of the gamma-c gene. Blood 87:3103–3107, 1996b.

Taylor N, Candotti F, Smith S, Oakes SA, Jahn T, Isakov J, Puck JM, O'Shea JJ, Weinberg K, Johnston JA. Interleukin-4 signaling in B lymphocytes from patients with X-linked severe combined immunodeficiency. J Biol Chem 272:7314–7319, 1997.

Tchilian EZ, Wallace DL, Wells RS, Flower DR, Morgan G, Beverley PC. A deletion in the gene encoding the CD45 antigen in a patient with SCID. J Immunol 166:1308–1313, 2001.

ATP, which may be less than half normal and below the level of dATP (Hershfield and Mitchell, 2001; Simmonds et al., 1979, 1982a). ATP depletion is due to increased catabolism induced by the buildup of dATP (Bagnara and Hershfield, 1982; Bontemps and Van den Berghe, 1989). Erythrocytes of patients with ADA deficiency also show greatly reduced activity, usually to less than 5% of normal, of the enzyme S-adenosylhomocysteine hydrolase (AdoHcyase). This is due to the "suicidelike" inactivation of AdoHcyase by dAdo (Hershfield, 1979; Hershfield et al., 1979).

In nonerythroid cells, dAdo and dGuo are substrates for deoxycytidine kinase (dCK), an enzyme expressed at particularly high levels in cytoplasm and nuclei of immature lymphoid cells (Hatzis et al., 1998; Johansson et al., 1997). Mitochondria possess a dGuo kinase (Johansson and Karlsson, 1996; Park and Ives, 1988). Because erythrocytes lack dCK and mitochondria, PNP deficiency results in only a slight accumulation of dGTP in red cells. However, GTP is decreased to about 10% of normal as a result of impaired guanine production and the absence of de novo purine nucleotide synthesis in erythrocytes (Cohen et al., 1978a; Simmonds et al., 1982b, 1987).

Effects of ADA and PNP Deficiency on Lymphoid Tissue

ADA and PNP are not essential for growth of lymphoblastoid cell lines, but their absence greatly potentiates the toxicity of exogenous Ado, dAdo, and dGuo. Several toxic biochemical effects of these ADA and PNP substrates have been identified (Fig. 16-2) (reviewed in Hershfield and Mitchell, 2001). Most were first identified in vitro, but many have also been observed in vivo in red cells from ADA-deficient patients or in lymphoblasts from patients with T-cell leukemia undergoing treatment with the ADA inhibitor deoxycoformycin (Hershfield et al., 1983, 1984).

One factor that may account for relatively selective immunodeficiency is that in vivo, dAdo and dGuo, the more toxic ADA and PNP substrates, arise largely from DNA breakdown. Thus they are generated at high levels by physiologic processes that operate in lymphoid organs: negative selection in thymus, activation-induced apoptosis in lymph nodes, and dissolution of nuclei of erythroid progenitors in marrow. The resulting nuclear debris is degraded by resident macrophages, which, in the absence of ADA or PNP, secrete dAdo or dGuo as products of DNA degradation (Chan, 1978, 1979; Smith and Henderson, 1982; Thompson et al., 2000) (Fig. 16-3).

These nucleosides can then enter viable lymphoid cells via the nucleoside transporter and exert toxic effects. High deoxynucleoside kinase and low deoxynucleotidase activity in lymphoid cells (particularly in T lymphoblasts) favors "trapping" of dAdo and dGuo as nucleotides, resulting in the accumulation of dATP and dGTP to toxic levels (Carson et al., 1978, 1979; Osborne, 1986).

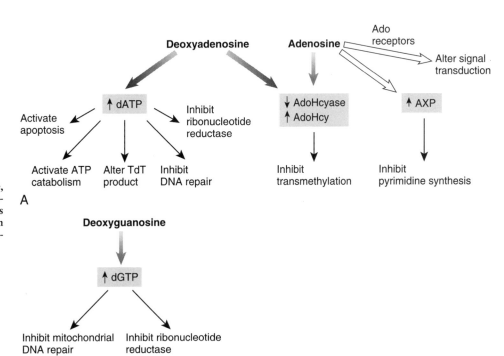

Figure 16-2· Actions of adenosine, deoxyadenosine, and deoxyguanosine that have been considered as causes of immunodeficiency in ADA deficiency (A) and PNP deficiency (B).

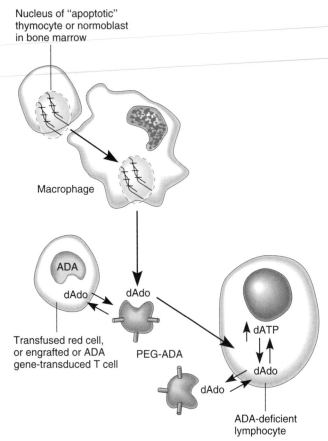

Nucleus of "apoptotic" thymocyte or normoblast in bone marrow

Macrophage

ADA

dAdo

Transfused red cell, or engrafted or ADA gene-transduced T cell

dAdo

PEG-ADA

dAdo

dAdo

↑ dATP

dAdo

ADA-deficient lymphocyte

Figure 16-3· Source of dAdo in ADA deficiency, and the basis for correction of dAdo-induced intracellular dATP accumulation during treatment. (From Hershfield MS, Chaffee S. PEG-enzyme replacement therapy for adenosine deaminase deficiency. In Desnick RJ, ed. Treatment of Genetic Diseases. New York, Churchill Livingstone, 1991, pp 169–182.)

Murine Models of ADA and PNP Deficiency

Studies in ADA- and PNP-deficient mice have confirmed many of the biochemical effects shown in Fig. 16-2. These animal models have permitted detailed studies of nonhematopoietic tissues, which are not possible in human patients. Perhaps because of differences in purine metabolism and development, mouse models only partially reproduce the human phenotypes.

The first ADA knockout mice to be developed died at birth, showing extensive hepatocyte degeneration, lung atelectasis, and small intestinal cell death; however, lymphoid development was normal, unlike newborn ADA-deficient humans (Blackburn et al., 2000b; Migchielsen et al., 1995; Wakamiya et al., 1995). Perinatal death of ADA knockout mice could be prevented by selectively expressing an ADA transgene in placenta (Blackburn et al., 1997). The "placentally rescued" ADA knockout mice died at 3 weeks of age of respiratory failure, associated with airway thickening and an increase in lung macrophages and eosinophils. T- and B-cell lymphopenia and ribcage abnormalities also appeared before death.

Enzyme replacement with PEG-ADA prevented lung pathology and permitted survival; higher doses of PEG-ADA were needed to prevent the lymphopenia (Blackburn et al., 2000a). The expression of a number of genes in lung tissue of ADA-deficient mice was significantly changed by treatment with PEG-ADA (Banerjee et al., 2002).

PNP deficiency in mice causes a progressive, predominantly cellular immune defect. The severity of the defect is related to the degree of enzyme deficiency and is milder in strains with missense mutations (Snyder et al., 1997) than in PNP knockout mice (Arpaia et al., 2000).

Specific Pathogenic Mechanisms

ADA and PNP substrates and their metabolites have a number of potentially toxic effects. Together these may cause lymphopenia and immune dysfunction by inhibiting proliferation and inducing apoptosis, by interfering with the generation of antigen receptor diversity, or by otherwise disrupting lymphocyte differentiation and function. Some actions may also contribute to nonimmunologic pathology.

Inhibition of Ribonucleoside Diphosphate Reductase

The cytotoxicity of dAdo is due largely, and of dGuo entirely, to the expansion of dATP and dGTP pools (Carson et al., 1978, 1979; Hershfield et al., 1982; Ullman et al., 1978, 1979). In dividing cells, the four deoxyribonucleoside triphosphates (dNTP) are produced coordinately at rates just sufficient to support ongoing DNA synthesis. Balanced production of dNTP is due to precise end-product control of the key enzyme ribonucleoside diphosphate (NDP) reductase, which converts ADP, GDP, CDP, and UDP to the corresponding 2′-deoxyNDP. dATP is a general allosteric inhibitor of NDP reductase. Thus dATP pool expansion (via dAdo salvage) inhibits the reduction of GDP, UDP, and CDP. In PNP deficiency, dGTP accumulation (from dGuo) selectively blocks CDP and UDP reduction. The resulting depletion of DNA precursors would block the rapid proliferation of immature thymocytes essential to production of the T-cell repertoire.

Induction of Apoptosis

Thymocytes and T lymphoblasts treated with dAdo and dGuo undergo apoptosis (Benveniste and Cohen, 1995; Gao et al., 1995; Kizaki et al., 1988). dAdo also induced apoptosis in nondividing mature T cells (Seto et al., 1985). The ADA inhibitor deoxycoformycin caused a p53-dependent depletion of $CD4^+CD8^+$ double-positive thymocytes in mice (Benveniste and Cohen, 1995), and it blocked the transition of double-negative to double-positive cells in murine fetal thymic organ cultures (Thompson et al., 2000).

dATP has been found to participate directly in activating aspartate-directed proteases (caspases) that mediate apoptosis. dATP has been shown to induce the release of cytochrome c from isolated mitochondria (Yang and Cortopassi, 1998; Yang et al., 1997). dATP also forms a complex with cytoplasmic cytochrome c, apoptosis-activating factor 1 (Apaf-1), and pro-caspase 9 in assembling an "apoptosome," which initiates a caspase cascade (Li et al., 1997, 1996; Purring-Koch and McLendon, 2000). The ability of dATP accumulation to inhibit DNA replication and repair, and to deplete ATP pools, could also promote apoptosis by inducing p53 expression and by destabilizing mitochondria.

Thymocytes from PNP knockout mice showed increased apoptosis in vivo and increased sensitivity to gamma irradiation in vitro (Arpaia et al., 2000). It was postulated that dGuo kinase-mediated intramitochondrial dGTP accumulation might inhibit mitochondrial DNA repair, leading to organelle injury that triggers apoptosis. dGTP-induced mitochondrial injury might also account for neurologic abnormalities often associated with PNP deficiency (Arpaia et al., 2000). Alternatively, PNP deficiency might cause neurologic injury by impairing the salvage of the PNP products hypoxanthine and guanine. This is metabolically equivalent to the salvage defect caused by HPRT deficiency (Lesch-Nyhan syndrome), in which neurologic dysfunction is a major feature.

Altered N-region Composition

Terminal deoxynucleotidyl transferase (TdT), a template-independent DNA polymerase expressed in thymocytes and B-lymphocyte progenitors, inserts nucleotides into N regions of immunoglobulin and T-cell receptor genes at sites of V(D)J recombination (Gilfillan et al., 1993; Komori et al., 1993). It has been suggested that dATP pool expansion might increase the insertion of dAMP residues by TdT (Coleman et al., 1978). Evidence of this effect has been obtained in a cell culture system and in Epstein-Barr virus (EBV) B-cell lines established from ADA-deficient patients (Gangi-Peterson et al., 1999).

Inhibition of Methylation

S-adenosylmethionine–dependent methylation has been implicated in many cellular processes, including gene expression. For normal methylation to occur, S-adenosylhomocysteine (AdoHcy), an inhibitory product of all methylation reactions, must be metabolized to Ado and homocysteine by AdoHcy hydrolase. In ADA deficiency, Ado accumulation inhibits and dAdo irreversibly inactivates AdoHcyase (Hershfield, 1979; Hershfield et al., 1979; Kredich and Martin, 1977). AdoHcyase inactivation, AdoHcy accumulation, and reduced nucleic acid methylation accompanied the lymphocytotoxic effects of Ado and dAdo in vitro and in vivo (Hershfield and Kredich, 1980; Hershfield et al., 1983, 1984; Kredich and Hershfield, 1979). Purine analogs that selectively inhibit AdoHcyase are toxic to lymphoblasts, interfere with thymocyte differentiation, and cause immunosuppression in mice (Benveniste et al., 1995; Greenberg et al., 1989; Wolos et al., 1993a, 1993b).

An 85% to more than 95% reduction in AdoHcyase activity was observed in tissues of ADA knockout mice, resulting in significant AdoHcy accumulation in liver (Migchielsen et al., 1995). This effect was postulated to contribute to hepatocyte degeneration in these mice and to metabolic hepatitis in some ADA-deficient patients (Bollinger et al., 1996).

Adenosine-Mediated Effects

Ado exerts many physiologic effects through G-protein–coupled plasma membrane Ado receptors (subtypes A1, A2a, A2b, A3), which are linked to various effectors, including adenylyl cyclase, ion channels, and phospholipases C and A2 (Olah and Stiles, 1998). Various in vitro effects of Ado on lymphoid cells have been postulated to contribute to immunodeficiency (Apasov and Sitkovsky, 1999; Apasov et al., 1997; Birch et al., 1982; Dong et al., 1996; Franco et al., 1998; Resta et al., 1997). Increased Ado signaling has also been implicated in causing pulmonary injury in ADA knockout mice (Blackburn et al., 2000a, 2000b; Zhong et al., 2001). However, no obvious clinical correlates of well-known pharmacologic effects of Ado on smooth muscle tone, heart rate, lipolysis, neurotransmitter release, mast cell degranulation, or platelet aggregation have been observed in ADA-deficient patients (i.e., more often than in other forms of SCID).

Loss of "ecto-ADA" bound to CD26-dipeptidyl peptidase IV has been implicated in the pathogenesis of immune dysfunction via postulated effects on signal transduction by extracellular Ado (Dong et al., 1996; Franco et al., 1998; Kameoka et al., 1993; Morimoto and Schlossman, 1998). It has also been proposed that ADA binding per se (unrelated to catalytic activity) might be crucial to a co-stimulatory function of CD26 essential to lymphocyte development or activation (Franco et al., 1998; Martin et al., 1995). Ado receptors and the co-stimulatory function of CD26 are conserved in humans and mice, but murine CD26 does not bind ADA (Dinjens et al., 1989b; Schrader et al., 1990). Neither CD26 knockout mice nor a CD26-deficient strain of rats are immune deficient (Erickson et al., 1992; Marguet et al., 2000; Tsuji et al., 1992). Also, a healthy human adult with partial ADA deficiency has been identified, whose only expressed ADA protein has a mutation (R142Q) that markedly impairs the binding of ADA to CD26 (Richard et al., 2000).

CLINICAL FEATURES

ADA Deficiency

The clinical presentation of typical ADA-deficient patients is similar to that in other forms of SCID (Hirschhorn, 1979a, 1979b) (see Chapter 15). The average age at diagnosis is 3 to 4 months (Arredondo-Vega et al., 1998; Stephan et al., 1993). Some distinguishing features of ADA-deficient SCID are noteworthy. Among 225 SCID patients treated at transplant centers in Paris,

France, and Durham, North Carolina, the 32 with ADA deficiency had the lowest lymphocyte counts, averaging less than 500/µl, with depletion of T, B, and natural killer (NK) cells (Buckley et al., 1997; Stephan et al., 1993). ADA-deficient patients were among the most seriously ill, often presenting by 1 month of age with life-threatening interstitial pneumonitis; they were also more likely to die before transplantation (Stephan et al., 1993). In contrast to other forms of SCID, maternal lymphoid engraftment was not observed with ADA deficiency (Buckley et al., 1997; Stephan et al., 1993).

Major physical findings are related to the absence of lymphoid tissues, infections, and failure to thrive. In addition, the underlying purine metabolic disorder may cause skeletal, hepatic, or neurologic abnormalities that are more variable in severity and penetrance. Prominent costochondral junctions ("rachitic rosary") and radiographic skeletal abnormalities (cupping and flaring of rib ends, pelvic dysplasia, platyspondyly) are found in up to half of ADA-deficient patients and appear to be due to a growth abnormality of chondrocytes (Cederbaum et al., 1976; Wolfson and Cross, 1975) (Fig. 16-4). These resolve after marrow transplantation (Bluetters-Sawatzki et al., 1989; Hirschhorn et al., 1979b) and have not been noted in patients receiving enzyme replacement therapy. Similar skeletal abnormalities may occur in patients who are not ADA deficient, so they do not play a major role in diagnosis.

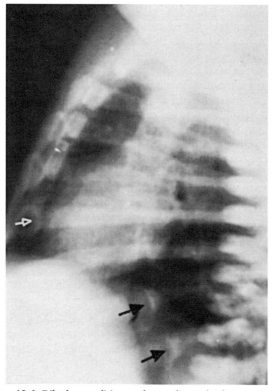

Figure 16-4· Rib abnormalities on chest radiograph of a patient with ADA deficiency.

Nonimmunologic Features

Transaminasemia is often present at diagnosis. Findings in one patient, who presented at age 2 months with persistent neonatal jaundice, suggested a metabolic hepatitis similar to that in newborn ADA knockout mice. An extensive evaluation excluded infection and GVHD (Bollinger et al., 1996). ADA replacement therapy led to resolution of the hepatitis, concomitant with normalization of erythrocyte dAXP but before recovery of T-cell function. In several other patients, interruption of ADA replacement therapy has been associated with a significant rise in serum transaminases (Kohn et al., 1998).

In addition to effects of viral encephalitis or hypoxia associated with pneumonia or mechanical ventilation, various neurologic abnormalities of uncertain etiology have been reported in patients with ADA deficiency, including spasticity, head lag, movement disorders, nystagmus, inability to focus, and sensorineural deafness (Hirschhorn et al., 1980a; Polmar et al., 1976; Tanaka et al., 1996; Tezcan et al., 1995). Neurologic improvement following red cell transfusion has been reported (Hirschhorn et al., 1980a; Tezcan et al., 1995). Developmental delay without evidence of central nervous system infection was found in 6 of 16 ADA-deficient patients, a higher frequency than was found in 100 patients with other forms of SCID (Stephan et al., 1993). Concerns have been raised that ADA deficiency might be associated with abnormal neuropsychologic development (Rogers et al., 2001).

Pathologic Findings

In autopsy specimens, the thymus is often hypoplastic, without corticomedullary demarcation; lymphocytes are absent, and fully developed Hassall bodies cannot be identified. Few or no lymphocytes are found in lymph nodes and spleen (Hirschhorn, 1979a; Ratech et al., 1989). Thymic tissue obtained from an affected fetus at 18 weeks' gestation showed similar findings (Linch et al., 1984). In some cases, areas of differentiated thymic epithelium and Hassall bodies are seen, and in one case thymic architecture and cellularity were normal when a biopsy was performed on the patient at 6 months of age (Schmalstieg et al., 1983).

Cartilaginous growth plate abnormalities, apparently due to metabolic effects of ADA deficiency, correspond to rib and radiographic abnormalities (Cederbaum et al., 1976; Ratech et al., 1985). Mesangial sclerosis in renal glomeruli and adrenal cortical sclerosis were noted in a review of autopsy material from eight patients; severe bridging portal fibrosis was found in livers of two of the three patients who lived beyond infancy (Ratech et al., 1985).

Delayed-Onset ADA Deficiency

A more variable delayed-onset presentation has characterized a number of patients diagnosed at 1 to 8 years of age (Arredondo-Vega et al., 2002; Cohen et al., 1979; Geffner et al., 1986; Giblett et al., 1972; Hirschhorn,

1979a; Hirschhorn et al., 1993; Levy et al., 1988; Notarangelo et al., 1992; Santisteban et al., 1993; Umetsu et al., 1994). Some were well for their first few years; others experienced frequent bouts of otitis, sinus and upper respiratory infections, pneumonia, or diarrhea by 6 to 18 months, but often these did not involve opportunistic organisms or require hospitalization and growth was not seriously impaired. Lymphocyte counts and immunoglobulin levels were less profoundly decreased than in SCID, and diagnoses such as asthma, allergy, or cystic fibrosis were considered. Eventually a life-threatening infection or the chronic consequences of recurrent infection focused attention on signs of underlying combined immunodeficiency.

Adult-Onset ADA Deficiency

Four patients from three families have been reported with a late- or adult-onset phenotype (Ozsahin et al., 1997; Santisteban et al., 1993; Shovlin et al., 1993). All had developed chronic consequences of immunodeficiency before ADA deficiency was suspected. For example, a 15-year-old was evaluated for enzyme deficiency after he developed *Pneumocystis carinii* pneumonia; the diagnosis had been considered unlikely when he had been treated for pneumonia 3 years earlier. At that time he was lymphopenic but had significant mitogenic responses and antibody titers to *Haemophilus influenzae* (Santisteban et al., 1993).

Two sisters in their mid-thirties had been treated for progressive pulmonary insufficiency and recurrent warts for more than a decade before lymphopenia was recognized and prompted a search for an underlying etiology (Shovlin et al., 1993, 1994). A fourth patient with recurrent pneumonia was diagnosed at age 39 (Ozsahin et al., 1997). As a child she had frequent infections, recurrent hepatitis, and persistent lymphopenia; immune deficiency was diagnosed at age 5 years (ADA deficiency was unknown at the time). She did relatively well in her teens and twenties but in her thirties developed chronic hepatobiliary disease, asthma with elevated serum immunoglobulin E (IgE), and tuberculosis. She died at age 40 of JC virus leukoencephalopathy.

All these women had given birth to healthy children (not ADA deficient). This is of interest because treating pregnant mice with an ADA inhibitor is embryotoxic (Knudsen et al., 1988, 1989) and because maternal portions of the placenta possess high ADA activity.

Several patients with delayed and late or adult onset have shown signs of immune dysregulation, including allergy, atopic dermatitis, asthma, eosinophilia, elevated IgE, IgG subclass deficiency, and autoimmunity (immune cytopenias, thyroid insufficiency, type I diabetes). Bronchiolitis obliterans and other pulmonary findings suggesting hypersensitivity have led to prolonged treatment of some patients with glucocorticoids and cyclophosphamide (Ozsahin et al., 1997; Shovlin et al., 1993). Had the significance of persistent lymphopenia and combined immune deficiency been appreciated, diagnosis might have been made and specific treatment initiated years earlier. No cases of unsuspected ADA or PNP deficiency were found among 44 patients who had been diagnosed with common variable immunodeficiency (Fleischman et al., 1998).

Phenotypic Variability

Phenotypic heterogeneity can occur within a family, usually when awareness of one affected child leads to diagnosis and treatment of subsequent affected siblings at birth, before clinical onset. However, one of Giblett's original patients was well until age 2 years, whereas her younger sibling had pneumonia at 9 months and was diagnosed with immunodeficiency at 14 months (Cohen et al., 1979; Giblett et al., 1972; Hong et al., 1970). In another family (Arredondo-Vega et al., 1994; Umetsu et al., 1994), the proband had persistent diarrhea, respiratory infections, and failure to thrive from age 4 months and was diagnosed at 9 months during evaluation of *Pseudomonas* sepsis and *P. carinii* pneumonia. Her 39-month-old "healthy" sister (normal growth, uncomplicated varicella at 12 months) was then tested and found to be ADA deficient. Lymphopenia had been found at 1 year of age, but at diagnosis some cellular and humoral immune function was still present. Clinical and immunologic deterioration eventually prompted enzyme replacement therapy.

PNP Deficiency

A serum uric acid of less than 1 mg/dl in association with T lymphopenia, recurrent infections, and often with neurologic findings and autoimmunity should raise suspicion of PNP deficiency. The full clinical spectrum may not be known because fewer than 50 PNP-deficient patients have been reported.

Thirty-three cases have been reviewed (Markert, 1991). Patients have presented at 4 months to 6 years, with recurrent otitis, pharyngitis, sinus infection, pneumonia, disseminated varicella, diarrhea, and urinary tract infections (Ammann, 1979). Bacterial pathogens and opportunistic organisms have been involved, but viral infections have been especially common, including cytomegalovirus, parainfluenza type 3, herpes, EBV, and ECHOvirus meningoencephalitis. Immunizations have usually been uncomplicated, but fatal generalized vaccinia has occurred (Virelizier et al., 1978). Although PNP deficiency was initially thought to affect cellular immunity selectively, the clinical profile of many cases indicates an associated humoral defect.

Neurologic Features

Neurologic abnormalities, sometimes diagnosed as cerebral palsy, have been reported in more than half of PNP-deficient children; these abnormalities include spastic diplegia or tetraparesis, delayed motor development, ataxia, tremor, hypertonia or hypotonia, behavioral difficulties, and mental retardation (Broome et al., 1996; Carpenter et al., 1996; Markert, 1991; Markert et al., 1987; Rich et al., 1979; Simmonds et al., 1987;

Stoop et al., 1977; Watson et al., 1981). Five children had a syndrome of dysequilibrium (difficulty in maintaining posture associated with hypotonia and spastic diplegia) and defective cellular immunity; PNP deficiency was found in the three children who were tested (Graham-Poole et al., 1975; Hagberg et al., 1970; Soutar and Day, 1991). Stroke occurred in one 13-year-old patient (Tam and Leshner, 1995). Neurologic impairment has preceded clinical immune deficiency in a number of patients.

Autoimmune Manifestations

Autoimmune disorders are also common; hemolytic anemia (seven cases), idiopathic thrombocytopenic purpura, and autoimmune neutropenia have been reported, as have single cases of systemic lupus erythematosus and central nervous system vasculitis (Carapella-De Luca et al., 1978; Markert, 1991; Markert et al., 1987; Rich et al., 1979). These disorders may reflect B-lymphocyte hyperactivity resulting from a loss of T-cell regulation. B-cell lymphomas, in one case associated with EBV infection, also occur and have been ascribed to primary T-cell dysfunction (Pannicke et al., 1996; Watson et al., 1981).

Physical and Laboratory Findings

Physical findings are related to recurrent infections and neurologic abnormalities; mild hepatomegaly and splenomegaly may occur. The thymus is absent on chest radiographs, and tonsils are small or absent. The total lymphocyte count is often less than 500/µl. T-cell counts have decreased over time in several patients, although fluctuations and occasional spontaneous increases may occur (Markert, 1991; Markert et al., 1987). In vitro T-cell responses to mitogens and allogeneic cells are reduced but may also fluctuate (Rijksen et al., 1987; Stoop et al., 1977). The number of B lymphocytes has been normal in most cases.

B-cell function may be normal, but dysregulation is often indicated by findings such as elevated immunoglobulins, monoclonal gammopathy, and specific autoantibodies. Among 33 patients, 9 had defective B-cell function, such as low antibody titers or immunoglobulin levels (Markert, 1991). Abnormal responses to immunization with the T-cell–dependent antigen bacteriophage φX-174 have been observed (Osborne and Ochs, 1999). Thus PNP deficiency should be considered a cause of combined immunodeficiency.

Molecular Basis for the Relationship between Genotype and Phenotype in ADA Deficiency

ADA and PNP deficiency are genetically heterogeneous (reviewed by Hershfield and Mitchell, 2001; Hirschhorn, 1999; and Osborne and Ochs, 1999). Among 67 reported ADA mutations there were 41 missense, 12 splicing, 9 deletion, and 5 nonsense mutations. Polymorphisms that do not affect enzymatic activity have also been identified (Hirschhorn et al., 1994a; Valerio et al., 1984). Ten different PNP mutations have been reported to date (6 missense, 2 deletion, 2 splicing).

Many ADA point mutations arise from codons that contain the hypermutable CpG dinucleotide. In an analysis of 50 nonsibling patients, 2 ADA mutations (R211H, G216R) each accounted for 11% and 13% of their 100 chromosomes; a few others (L107P, R156H, A329V, 955del5) accounted for 5% to 7% each (Arredondo-Vega et al., 1998). About half of all mutant alleles are "private," occurring in single families, and most patients are heteroallelic, having inherited two different mutant ADA alleles. Homozygosity for one allele is often associated with consanguinity or, in some cases, a specific geographic origin.

A few ADA missense mutations alter active site residues that directly contact substrate (E217K) or coordinate with the essential zinc ion (H15D, H17P). Almost all missense mutations from immunodeficient patients result in a labile ADA protein, so that immunologically detectable ADA is reduced or absent in patient cells or cell lines and when the cloned complementary DNA (cDNA) is expressed in *Escherichia coli* (Arredondo-Vega et al., 1998; Wiginton and Hutton, 1982).

Certain mutations found in patients with milder phenotypes were not found in those with the more common SCID phenotype (Hirschhorn et al., 1990; Santisteban et al., 1993). This observation, as well as the correlation between erythrocyte dAXP level and clinical severity, suggested that allele combinations providing more than some critical level of functional ADA might confer a milder phenotype.

To assess this more precisely, we have quantified ADA activity expressed by more than 30 missense mutant ADA cDNAs in an *E. coli* strain lacking the bacterial ADA gene (Ariga et al., 2001a; Arredondo-Vega et al., 1998, 2002). The mutants from immunodeficient patients expressed 0.001% to 0.6% of the activity expressed with normal (wild-type) human ADA cDNA. By contrast, those from five healthy individuals with partial ADA deficiency expressed from 1% to 28% of normal ADA activity.

Allele Ranking System

Based on the expression of ADA alleles in *E. coli*, we have developed a ranking system for analyzing the relationship of genotype to phenotype. The sample tested included 52 patients who possessed 43 different genotypes derived from 42 different mutant ADA alleles (Arredondo-Vega et al., 1998). Alleles were grouped according to their effect on expressed ADA activity: deletion and nonsense mutations were designated 0, and missense mutations were distributed among groups I to IV according to increasing activity expressed in *E. coli* (Table 16-1).

Of 31 SCID patients, 28 had genotypes 0/0, 0/I, or I/I, which expressed 0.05% or less of wild-type ADA activity, whereas genotypes from 19 of 21 patients with less

TABLE 16-1 · ADA ALLELES GROUPED BY ADA ACTIVITY EXPRESSED IN *E. COLI* SØ3834

Allele Group	Mutations	Expressed ADA Activity (% Wild Type*)
0	Deletions, nonsense	Inactive
I	H15D, G74V, G74D, A83D, R101L, R101Q, R101W, P104L, L107P, G140E, R149W, R156C, R211H, G216R, E217K, R235Q, S291L, A329V, E337del	0.015 ± 0.02 (0.001 to ~0.07)
II	V129M, R156H, V177M, A179D, Q199P, R253P	0.11 ± 0.04 (~0.06 to 0.2)
III	G74C, P126Q, R211C	0.42 ± 0.19 (0.3 to 0.6)
IV	R142Q, R149Q, A215T, G239S, M310T	8.3 ± 11.3 (1.0 to 28)
Spl	Splice-site mutations	Variable

*Mean ± standard deviation (SD; range); ADA alleles are grouped as defined in Arredondo-Vega, et al., 1998. Alleles with missense mutations in groups I to IV had increasing ADA activity (as shown) when expressed in *E. coli* SØ3834, which has a deletion of the bacterial ADA gene. Patients with genotypes consisting only of alleles from groups 0 or I were very likely to have SCID, whereas those with at least one allele from groups II or III were likely to have a milder delayed-onset or late- or adult-onset phenotype, respectively. Individuals who possessed one group IV allele were healthy and had partial ADA deficiency. Modified from Arredondo-Vega, et al. Am J Hum Genet 63:1049–1059, 1998; with additional data from Ariga T, et al. Molecular basis for paradoxical carriers of adenosine deaminase (ADA) deficiency that show extremely low levels of ADA activity in peripheral blood cells without immunodeficiency. J Immunol 166:1698–1702, 2001.

severe phenotypes expressed greater activity due to at least one allele from groups II to IV. Among the patients studied, there was an inverse correlation between total expressed ADA activity and erythrocyte dAXP content (Fig. 16-5).

Splice-site mutations have been associated with relatively mild or variable phenotypes, because normal splicing may not be disrupted completely, particularly with mutations that activate cryptic splice sites but leave the normal splice site intact. The amount of "leakiness" can vary among individuals carrying the same splicing allele, including siblings (Arredondo-Vega et al., 1994; Santisteban et al., 1993).

Mosaicism

As in some other genetic diseases, mosaicism for revertant somatic cells can moderate the effect of inherited genotype on phenotype. This is exemplified by two

ADA-deficient patients who presented with immunodeficiency as children and then had spontaneous clinical remissions (Hirschhorn et al., 1994b, 1996). B-cell lines derived from each patient possessed both a mutant and a wild-type ADA allele; in one case the latter arose by reversion of an inherited mutation (Hirschhorn et al., 1996). A similar phenomenon has been reported in a patient with X-linked SCID (Stephan et al., 1996).

An unusual mechanism of reversion has been found in a common progenitor of T and B cells in the older of two ADA-deficient siblings (Arredondo-Vega et al., 2002). Both patients had inherited two copies of an ADA allele with a point mutation in the last splice site of the gene. Nonlymphoid cells from the older patient, who was 16 years old at diagnosis, were homozygous for this mutation, but one mutant ADA allele in his T cells and a B-cell line had acquired a "second-site" deletion that suppressed the effects of the splice-site mutation, resulting in expression of 75% of normal ADA activity. Erythrocyte dAXP levels in the mosaic patient were much lower than in his more severely immunodeficient sibling (Arredondo-Vega et al., 2002).

These intriguing cases provide in vivo evidence that rare ADA-expressing lymphoid cells have a proliferative or survival advantage, an effect that may prove important in gene therapy (discussed later). To be of clinical benefit, mosaicism may have to be relatively extensive. This is indicated by findings in several patients whose T cells or T-cell lines expressed high ADA activity but in whom immunodeficiency was severe (Ariga et al., 2001b; Arredondo-Vega et al., 1990). Mosaicism in these cases may have occurred in a lymphoid clone at a later stage of differentiation, rather than in a stem cell or early progenitor, or selection may not have operated for a sufficiently long period to result in improved immune function.

LABORATORY DIAGNOSIS

The evaluation of infants suspected of having severe combined immunodeficiency is presented in Chapters 12 and 15. The following discussion focuses on ADA and PNP deficiency.

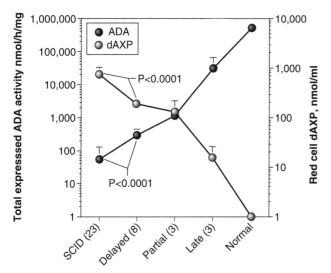

Figure 16-5 · Relationship of total ADA activity expressed by both patient alleles in *E. coli* SØ3834, erythrocyte dAXP content, and clinical phenotype. (Adapted from Arredondo-Vega FX, et al. Adenosine deaminase deficiency: genotype-phenotype correlations based on expressed activity of 29 mutant alleles. Am J Hum Genet 63:1049–1059, 1998.)

Enzyme Activity in Erythrocytes

ADA and PNP deficiency are usually diagnosed by finding less than 1% of normal catalytic activity in hemolysates prepared from fresh or frozen packed erythrocytes, using spectrophotometric or more sensitive radiochemical assays (Hershfield and Mitchell, 2001). We use a thin layer chromatographic method to measure the conversion of $[^{14}C]$Ado to Ino or of $[^{14}C]$Ino to hypoxanthine for ADA and PNP, respectively (Arredondo-Vega et al., 1990). Because of overlap with activity found in about 10% of normal individuals, erythrocyte ADA activity is not always reliable for carrier identification.

Measuring plasma ADA activity is not reliable for diagnosing ADA deficiency. ADA activity in plasma is much lower than in blood cells and is partly due to an aminohydrolase with low affinity for Ado and dAdo, and which is insensitive to specific ADA inhibitors. The inhibitor-resistant aminohydrolase activity has been termed ADA_2 to distinguish it from ADA_1, the ADA gene product (Daddona and Kelley, 1981; Muraoka et al., 1990).

When rapid sample delivery or shipment of frozen material is complicated, we have also measured enzyme activity and metabolite levels eluted from dried blood spots (Arredondo-Vega et al., 2002). These are prepared by applying fresh heparin or EDTA anticoagulated whole blood onto Guthrie filter paper cards (as used in newborn screening); air-dried filters are stable at room temperature. We have used this method to identify more than a dozen ADA or PNP-deficient patients from Asia, the Middle East, and South America. Diagnosis based on analyzing purine metabolites by mass spectrometry is being developed (Ito et al., 2000).

Analysis of Metabolites in Erythrocytes, Plasma, and Urine

When patients have been transfused prior to testing, measuring ADA and PNP substrates in plasma or urine, or their metabolites in red cells, may suggest the diagnosis. Because dAXP are normally almost undetectable in mature red cells, finding any appreciable dATP (dAXP) strongly suggests ADA deficiency, even when erythrocytes have appreciable ADA activity due to transfusion. By contrast with transfused SCID patients, obligate ADA heterozygotes with half-normal ADA activity show no elevation in erythrocyte dAXP. The diagnosis can be established definitively by assaying ADA and PNP activity in blood mononuclear cells or in fibroblasts.

Prenatal Diagnosis

For practical purposes, ADA or PNP genotyping can be used for diagnosis or carrier detection only if previous studies have identified the mutant alleles in the family. Prenatal diagnosis is usually based on finding low or absent enzyme activity in cultured amniocytes or chorionic villus fibroblasts (Aitken et al., 1980, 1986; Dooley et al., 1987; Hirschhorn, 1979c; Hirschhorn et al., 1975; Ziegler et al., 1981). In our experience with more than 20 pregnant patients at risk for ADA deficiency, results of enzyme assay have been unequivocal and have been confirmed by postnatal enzyme assay or by genotype analysis.

dATP is elevated in red cells of ADA-deficient fetuses at 16 to 17 weeks' gestation and in cord blood at birth (Hirschhorn et al., 1980b; Kohn et al., 1995; Linch et al., 1984; Morgan et al., 1987). Red-cell dAXP increases substantially during the week after birth (Hershfield and Mitchell, 2001).

Relationship of Metabolic and Clinical Phenotypes

Because of low ADA expression and lack of protein turnover in red cells, and the instability of mutant proteins, the level of ADA activity in erythrocytes does not distinguish patients with SCID from those with milder phenotypes or from most healthy individuals with partial deficiency. ADA activity is appreciable in peripheral blood lymphocytes (PBL) from those with partial deficiency. It is difficult to obtain sufficient PBL for analysis from immunodeficient patients, but ADA activity in lymphoid cell lines derived from patients has usually been reported as less than 1% to 2% of normal.

In contrast to red-cell ADA activity, there is a good correlation between clinical severity and the level of dATP (or dAXP) in erythrocytes, which reflects total systemic capacity to eliminate dAdo. dAXP normally comprise less than 2 nmol/ml of packed red blood cells (RBCs) but are elevated to about 300 to 2000 nmol/ml in patients with SCID, 30 to 300 nmol/ml in those with delayed or late onset, and less than 30 nmol/ml in individuals with partial deficiency (Ariga et al., 2001a; Arredondo-Vega et al., 1998; Borkowsky et al., 1980; Cohen et al., 1978b; Daddona et al., 1983; Hirschhorn et al., 1979a; Morgan et al., 1987; Santisteban et al., 1993, 1995).

Because of this correlation between metabolic and clinical phenotype, there is potentially prognostic value in measuring red-cell dAXP in newly diagnosed patients (if they have not been transfused). Monitoring red-cell dAXP levels can also be useful for assessing enzyme replacement therapy, the stability of engraftment after stem cell/marrow transplantation, and the systemic metabolic efficacy of gene therapy (discussed later).

TREATMENT

Overview

Newly diagnosed ADA-deficient patients require the same supportive care as do patients with SCID due to other causes (see Chapter 15). For patients with an HLA-identical sibling, bone marrow or blood stem cell transplantation (BMT/SCT) is usually the treatment of choice. This section focuses on alternative therapies for those patients who do not have such a donor, namely BMT/SCT from HLA-haploidentical or matched unrelated donors; enzyme replacement with PEG-ADA; and somatic cell gene therapy, which is still experimental (Fig. 16-6). Experience with SCT using closely matched heterologous umbilical cord blood for ADA and PNP deficiency is limited, and in utero therapy (transplantation, enzyme replacement, or gene transduction) has not, to the author's knowledge, yet been attempted in these patients.

In deciding on therapy, many factors must be considered, often in a brief time frame: clinical status, distance from a transplant center, cost, the judgment and experience of physicians consulted, and parents' expectations and assessment of risks and benefit. The latter may reflect outcome for a previous affected child, as well as information and advice from families of other children with SCID (often obtained via the Internet). Physicians must be prepared to provide or quickly obtain accurate and objective information about all approaches to treatment.

Stem Cell Transplantation

The general topic of BMT/SCT for SCID, including potential complications and delayed recovery of B-cell function, is covered in Chapter 43. However, the experience with ADA-deficient patients warrants separate consideration.

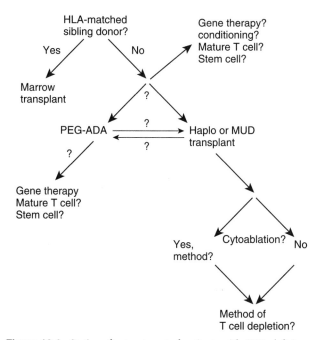

Figure 16-6 · Options for treatment of patients with ADA deficiency. (Adapted from Hershfield MS, Chaffee S. PEG-enzyme replacement therapy for adenosine deaminase deficiency. In Desnick RJ, ed. Treatment of Genetic Diseases. New York, Churchill Livingstone, 1991, pp 169–182.)

Several transplant centers in North America and Europe have noted more frequent graft failure in patients with ADA deficiency (O'Reilly et al., 1989; Porta and Friedrich, 1998). It has been speculated that ADA-deficient patients may possess T cells capable of graft rejection. However, such cells have not been identified. It is also possible that donor stem cells or their lymphoid progeny may be sensitive to the toxic metabolic environment or that metabolic injury to host microenvironment limits donor lymphoid engraftment.

Because of frequent graft failure, some have concluded that ADA-deficient patients require cytoreductive conditioning prior to HLA-haploidentical BMT (Bluetters-Sawatzki et al., 1989; Cowan et al., 1988; Moen et al., 1987; O'Reilly et al., 1989; Porta and Friedrich, 1998; Silber et al., 1987). Others feel that such conditioning may be unnecessary and is poorly tolerated (Buckley et al., 1999). ADA-deficient patients may be at an increased risk of transplant-associated morbidity due to systemic effects of their underlying disorder. It has been suggested that subclinical metabolic hepatitis due to effects of ADA substrates might exacerbate the effects of conditioning agents that are metabolized in liver or are hepatotoxic (Bollinger et al., 1996).

Because they account for only 15% of SCID patients, relatively few ADA-deficient patients have been treated at any single transplant center. Nevertheless, the view that ADA-deficient patients fare poorly is supported. For example, in summaries of the long-term experience of centers in Paris and San Francisco, combined overall survival was 57% for 74 SCID patients who received haploidentical BMT, but all 8 ADA-deficient patients who underwent this procedure died (Dror et al., 1993; Stephan et al., 1993). In a review of the combined European experience with haploidentical BMT, 82 of 167 (49%) non–ADA-deficient SCID patients were alive after 6 years, compared with 8 of 20 (40%) ADA-deficient patients (Haddad et al., 1998). The majority of these patients had undergone cytoablative conditioning.

Among 77 SCID patients who received unconditioned haploidentical BMT at Duke University Medical Center over roughly the same period, survival was 78% (Buckley et al., 1999). Among the ADA-deficient patients in this series, seven of nine who had received haploidentical BMT were alive. However, one of the survivors had twice failed to engraft and had been treated for 12 years with PEG-ADA (Buckley et al., 1999; Hershfield et al., 1987). Of eight additional ADA-deficient patients who have undergone unconditioned haploidentical BMT at Duke University Medical Center since this report, two died in the peritransplant period and six are now being treated with PEG-ADA or have entered a clinical trial of experimental gene therapy.

Erythrocyte Metabolite Levels Reflect Extent/Stability of Engraftment

After successful BMT, dAXP levels in red cells decline (Chen et al., 1978; Hirschhorn et al., 1981; Ochs et al., 1992; Rubocki et al., 2001). Erythrocyte dAXP may normalize after HLA-identical BMT, when erythroid and lymphoid engraftment have occurred (Hershfield and Mitchell, 2001; Ochs et al., 1992; Rubocki et al., 2001).

Following unconditioned haploidentical BMT, when chimerism is limited to T cells, the fall in dAXP content of host (ADA-deficient) erythrocytes is due to the uptake and deamination of dAdo by donor-derived (ADA-expressing) lymphocytes (see Fig. 16-3). Because circulating T cells are exclusively donor derived in these patients, it appears that engrafted T cells, although themselves resistant to ADA substrates, provide insufficient systemic ADA activity to protect endogenous host thymocytes, and possibly some other tissues, from metabolic toxicity.

We have monitored erythrocyte dAXP serially in a number of patients before and after unconditioned haploidentical BMT (unpublished). Long-term engraftment has been associated with a fall in red-cell dAXP to a new level, which, although still abnormal, is relatively stable over a period of many months or years. In contrast, primary failure to engraft is not associated with a significant decline in red-cell dAXP, and transient engraftment is associated with an initial decline by 3 to 4 months after transplant, followed later by an increase in dAXP to near pretreatment levels (unpublished data).

BMT for Patients with PNP Deficiency

Published experience with BMT for PNP deficiency is limited to 11 patients (Baguette et al., 2002; Broome et al., 1996; Carpenter et al., 1996; Classen et al., 2001; Fischer et al., 1994; Markert, 1991). HLA-identical sibling BMT has been successful in four patients. One patient who failed a first T-cell–depleted haploidentical BMT engrafted following a second BMT performed after more intensive conditioning (Fischer et al., 1994). The remaining PNP-deficient patients who underwent BMT have died from infection, graft failure, and graft-versus-host disease (GVHD).

At our institution, a 3-year-old patient recently underwent transplantation with partially matched stem cells from unrelated cord blood. He has done well clinically, and after 12 months, engrafted PBL showed normal PNP activity and immune function (Kurtzberg J, Myers L, unpublished).

Enzyme Replacement with PEG-ADA

The toxic compounds that accumulate in ADA and PNP deficiency (dATP, dGTP, AdoHcy) cross cell membranes poorly, but they are metabolized to ADA and PNP substrates that rapidly equilibrate with plasma via the nucleoside transporter. Thus maintaining sufficient levels of circulating "ectopic" ADA or PNP, either in plasma or in a population of cells, can normalize metabolite levels in enzyme-deficient cells (see Fig. 16-3). This was first demonstrated in ADA-deficient patients transfused with normal red cells (Cohen et al., 1978b; Polmar et al., 1976).

Prior to the era of T-cell–depleted haploidentical BMT, chronic transfusion was used as a replacement therapy for ADA and a few PNP-deficient patients. Immune function and clinical status improved in some ADA-deficient patients, but the response was usually transient (Davies et al., 1982; Hirschhorn et al., 1980a; Hutton et al., 1981; Polmar, 1979; Ziegler et al., 1980). This approach was abandoned after the introduction of PEG-ADA (Hershfield et al., 1987).

Pharmacology of PEG-ADA

PEG-ADA consists of highly purified bovine ADA decorated with multiple strands of monomethoxy-polyethylene glycol (PEG) of average molecular weight 5000. Covalently bound PEG is intended to prevent proteolysis and uptake by cells and to prolong circulating life and reduce immunogenicity (Davis et al., 1981). On a volume basis, the clinical preparation (Adagen, manufactured by Enzon, Inc.) has approximately 1800 times the ADA activity of packed erythrocytes; 3 ml contains the ADA equivalent of about 10^{12} T lymphocytes.

PEG-ADA is not taken up appreciably by blood cells. After intramuscular (IM) injection, plasma ADA activity peaks in 24 to 48 hours, then declines with a half-life of from 3 to more than 6 days. Clearance can be more rapid in some newly diagnosed SCID patients (Weinberg et al., 1993). Treatment of SCID patients is usually initiated with twice weekly IM injections, each of 30 U/kg (60 U/kg/week), based on ideal body weight (i.e., fiftieth percentile for the patient's age). At this schedule, preinjection plasma ADA activity ranges from 50 to 150 μmol/h/ml (normal is <0.4), or about 4 to 10 times normal total blood ADA activity. At a maintenance dose of 15 to 30 U/kg once a week, trough plasma ADA activity ranges from 20 to 60 μmol/h/ml.

Summary of Results

The lack of toxicity of free PEG and PEG-ADA in animals, and the potential for achieving much higher circulating ADA activity than is possible by transfusion, led to the first clinical test of PEG-ADA in two SCID patients who had failed unconditioned haploidentical BMT and had responded poorly to transfusion therapy (Hershfield et al., 1987). In the 16.5 years after it was introduced, 119 patients were treated with PEG-ADA (probably comparable to the numbers of ADA-deficient patients who underwent non–HLA-identical BMT over the same period). This slow accrual of 4 to 10 patients per year at widely dispersed locations in 15 countries, and the lack of dependence on specialized treatment centers (unlike BMT and gene therapy), has favored reports of single or a few cases, rather than large series (Bollinger et al., 1996; Bory et al., 1990; Chun et al., 1993; Girault et al., 1992; Hershfield, 1995; Hershfield et al., 1987, 1993; Hirschhorn et al., 1993; Levy et al., 1988; Notarangelo et al., 1992; Rosen and Bhan, 1998; Umetsu et al., 1994; Walcott et al., 1994; Weinberg et al., 1993).

The summary presented in this section is drawn from this published experience and from unpublished information gained from monitoring the metabolic and antibody responses to PEG-ADA by the author's laboratory (supported by a grant from the manufacturer). Physicians who have cared for patients and monitored their immunologic function have provided information on clinical status.

By 4 to 8 weeks of treatment at doses of 15 to 60 U/kg/week, erythrocyte dAXP falls to 2 to 10 nmol/ml packed RBC or less (normal = 2); erythrocyte AdoHcyase activity also normalizes (Fig. 16-7A). This metabolic state, which is achieved in virtually all patients treated for longer than 2 months, is similar to that of healthy individuals with partial ADA deficiency.

As metabolic correction proceeds, general clinical status improves; this may be evident even before immune reconstitution (Rosen and Bhan, 1998). Infections are usually controlled and weight gain often resumes in the first 1 to 3 months of treatment. By 6 months, opportunistic infections cease and the frequency and duration of respiratory infections and diarrhea have decreased. Maintaining clinical benefit requires continuous treatment with PEG-ADA. Any sustained fall in trough (preinjection) plasma ADA activity to below about 10 µmol/h/ml has been associated with an increase in erythrocyte dAXP and a decline in lymphocyte counts and function (Chaffee et al., 1992; Chun et al., 1993; Kohn et al., 1998).

Some SCID patients have developed marked but transient thrombocytosis, without clinical consequence, within 2 to 3 weeks of starting PEG-ADA (Marwaha et al., 2000; and unpublished). This has also been noted after initiation of erythrocyte transfusion therapy (Hirschhorn et al., 1992). B-cell counts also often increase within the first month of PEG-ADA therapy, in contrast to the much slower and more limited recovery of B cells following BMT/SCT (Fig. 16-7B).

T-cell counts and response to mitogens may not improve for 6 to 12 weeks (see Fig 16-7B). This time course, and the evolution of T-cell antigen expression, suggests maturation from an intrathymic progenitor (Weinberg et al., 1993). Lymphocyte counts may decrease

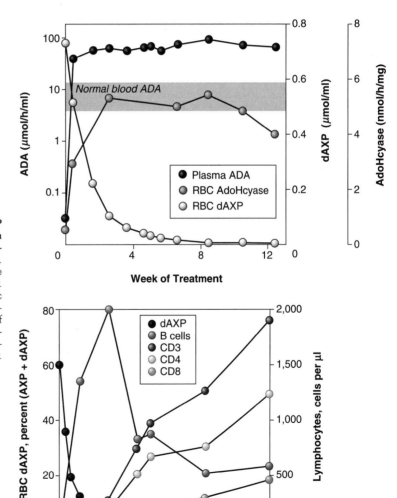

Figure 16-7· A. Plasma ADA activity and levels of dAXP and AdoHcyase activity in erythrocytes of a patient with ADA-deficient SCID during the first 3 months of treatment with PEG-ADA. (From Hershfield MS, Mitchell BS. Immunodeficiency diseases caused by adenosine deaminase deficiency and purine nucleoside phosphorylase deficiency. In Scriver CR, Beaudet AL, Sly WS, Valle D, eds. The Metabolic and Molecular Bases of Inherited Disease. New York, McGraw-Hill, 2001, pp 2585–2625.) **B.** Time course of appearance of circulating T and B lymphocytes in a patient with ADA-deficient SCID. (Adapted from Bollinger ME, et al. Hepatic dysfunction as a complication of adenosine deaminase deficiency. N Engl J Med 334:1367–1371, 1996.)

after the first year of treatment, and on long-term therapy most patients remain lymphopenic, with the response to mitogens fluctuating between 30% and more than 90% of normal controls. About 20% of SCID patients, including some patients who have been treated for more than 10 years with PEG-ADA, have shown little improvement in circulating T-cell counts and in vitro lymphocyte function.

Most patients tested have developed lymphocyte responses to some recall antigens, as well as normal immunoglobulin, isohemagglutinin, and specific antibody levels. The response to immunization with bacteriophage φX-174 suggests that humoral immunity may be more effectively reconstituted in patients who respond to PEG-ADA than in ADA-deficient patients with stable engraftment after BMT (Ochs et al., 1992). Approximately half of patients in the United States now receiving PEG-ADA have discontinued IVIG.

Antibodies to PEG-ADA

No toxic or allergic reactions to PEG-ADA have been reported. IgG antibody to bovine ADA-specific epitopes became detectable by enzyme-linked immunosorbent assay (ELISA), usually between 3 and 8 months of therapy, in 10 of the first 17 patients, who had been treated 1 to 5.5 years when studied (Chaffee et al., 1992). Plasma ADA activity had remained stable in 8 of the 10 anti-ADA–positive patients, but 2 patients developed enhanced enzyme clearance, associated with neutralizing antibody directed at the ADA active site. In one of these patients, tolerance was induced (Chaffee et al., 1992; Chun et al., 1993); in the other, twice-weekly injections have maintained a therapeutic level of plasma ADA activity (both have now been treated for more than 12 years).

Ongoing monitoring by ELISA indicates that 75% to 80% of patients develop detectable anti-ADA antibody on long-term therapy, and about 10% of patients show enhanced enzyme clearance (Hershfield, 1997; and unpublished). Because of this, it is advisable to monitor plasma ADA activity (and erythrocyte dATP or dAXP, if possible) every 1 to 2 months during the first 12 to 18 months of treatment and two to four times per year thereafter.

Immune Dysregulation

Transient thrombocytopenia or hemolytic anemia has occurred early in treatment with PEG-ADA in a few patients. In one case, hemolysis unresponsive to prednisone and azathioprine developed after 1 month of PEG-ADA therapy; the patient died of sepsis without recovering immune function. Hemolytic anemia, as well as neutralizing antibody to PEG-ADA, have occurred in three patients. In one of these patients with a delayed onset, hemolysis was present at diagnosis and recurred, along with anti-ADA antibody, following catheter sepsis after 6 months of PEG-ADA therapy. Catheter sepsis was also implicated in initiating hemolysis in a second patient. The third developed anti-ADA antibody after

2.5 years on PEG-ADA, and hemolytic anemia may have resulted from the ensuing loss of immune function. All three died, of infections or hepatic failure, following BMT performed after discontinuing PEG-ADA.

Lymphoproliferative disorders have occurred in two patients. In one case, pulmonary nodules, possibly EBV related, were discovered after 8 years on PEG-ADA. The nodules remained stable in size but failed to regress after rituximab therapy. PEG-ADA was discontinued after 10 years, and a matched unrelated BMT was performed. The patient died of a viral illness a month after the procedure. In the second patient, Hodgkin's lymphoma (EBV positive) developed after 13 years on PEG-ADA (an ADA-deficient sibling of this patient died of lymphoma in early childhood following haploidentical BMT [Hirschhorn et al., 1992]). This patient died at 16 years of age following a recurrence of lymphoma after an attempted cord blood stem cell transplant.

Long-Term Results of PEG-ADA Therapy

From April 1986 to September 2002, 119 ADA-deficient patients worldwide were treated with PEG-ADA (excluding 5 who received PEG-ADA for less than 1 month before undergoing BMT). Of these, 85 (71%) had SCID (64 diagnosed at 6 months of age or younger, 21 at 6 to 12 months); 34 patients (29%) had delayed or late onset and were diagnosed at age 1 to 34 years. Survival for all patients (including those who underwent BMT/SCT after discontinuing PEG-ADA) during this 16.5-year period was 75% (89 of 119); survival was 74% for the SCID patients (63 of 85).

Among the 89 survivors, 76 (85%) are still receiving PEG-ADA: 21 had been treated for 10 to 15 years, 19 for 5 to 9.9 years, 21 for 2 to 4.9 years, and 15 for less than 2 years. Of the remainder, 11 had undergone successful BMT (discussed later), and 2 late-onset patients discontinued treatment after 5 years.

Eighteen patients (15%) died while receiving PEG-ADA. Of these, 12 died within the first 6 months of treatment (8 in the first month), and 6 died after 2 to 15 years. Four of the 6 late deaths occurred after 5 to 15 years of therapy, due to progression to an end stage of chronic lung disease present at the time PEG-ADA therapy was initiated at 3, 4, 10, and 33 years of age. One patient died of infection after 6 years; she had severe central nervous system (CNS) and motor dysfunction when treatment was begun at age 2 years. One death after 2 years was due to hepatoblastoma that was probably present at the time of diagnosis.

PEG-ADA Prior to Transplantation

Twenty-four patients (20% of all PEG-ADA–treated patients) have discontinued PEG-ADA to undergo BMT (15 after 2 to 13 months, 7 after 1.4 to 5 years, and 2 after 10 years of therapy). In several patients in whom it was monitored, endogenous immune function deteriorated to baseline 4 to 6 weeks after the last PEG-ADA injection, coincident with the disappearance of plasma ADA activity and a sharp rise in erythrocyte dAXP. The transplants were performed 2 weeks to 3 months after the last dose of PEG-ADA. All 19 patients with non–HLA-identical sibling donors received some form of preconditioning.

For 18 of the 24 transplanted patients, PEG-ADA was intended as an interim therapy, to be used until clinical status had improved and a suitable donor could be identified. These patients were treated with PEG-ADA for 2 to 60 (mean = 14) months, and they were 3 to 63 (mean = 18.8) months of age when PEG-ADA was electively discontinued prior to transplant. Two of the patients in this group had developed neutralizing antibodies to PEG-ADA; in both cases the transplant was successful.

In the other six patients, all of whom died within a year of transplant, BMT was performed for medical problems that developed or had progressed during treatment with PEG-ADA. As mentioned earlier, three of these patients had developed refractory hemolytic anemia and neutralizing antibody to PEG-ADA, and two others had developed lymphoma, possibly EBV associated. The sixth patient had undergone unconditioned haploidentical BMT at birth (following prenatal diagnosis), which was complicated by pancytopenia thought to be due to GVHD. PEG-ADA was initiated at age 15 months. Pancytopenia persisted, and a second, conditioned haploidentical BMT was performed 20 months later.

Survival for patients undergoing transplant was 46% for the entire group (11 of 24), or 61% (11 of 18) among those who underwent BMT by initial intent. The 11 successful transplants include 3 of 4 with HLA-identical sibling donors, 3 of 9 with matched unrelated donors, and 5 of 10 with HLA-haploidentical donors. All the deaths occurred within a year after BMT and were related to infection, GVHD, or complications of the conditioning regimen.

Enzyme Replacement for PNP Deficiency

Four PNP-deficient patients have been treated by red cell transfusion. No improvement was noted in two patients (Gelfand et al., 1978; Sandman et al., 1977), and transient improvement in T-cell counts and response to mitogens was seen in the other two (Rich et al., 1980; Zegers et al., 1979). Transfusion brought about a marked decrease in urinary excretion of PNP substrates and an increase in plasma and urinary urate (Rich et al., 1980).

The development of PEG-PNP for treating PNP deficiency is a reasonable goal. Purified mammalian PNP appears to be too unstable at 37° to be used for therapy, but a PEG-PNP with prolonged circulating life and reduced immunogenicity in mice has been prepared from a genetically engineered variant of the stable PNP enzyme from E. coli (Hershfield et al., 1991). Treating PNP knockout mice with this PEG-PNP corrected metabolic abnormalities and prolonged life (Arpaia et al.,

2000). Unfortunately, manufacturing this material for use in an exceedingly small patient population poses great practical problems.

Gene Therapy

In the mid-1980s, when retroviral vectors for transducing hematopoietic cells and ADA cDNA made gene therapy for ADA deficiency plausible, the disorder seemed ideal for early human trials. At the time, the only options for treating patients who lacked an HLA-identical sibling, chronic red cell transfusion and haploidentical BMT, had significant morbidity and high rates of failure. It was anticipated that achieving relatively low ADA expression might be of benefit because individuals with partial ADA deficiency are healthy and because gene-corrected lymphoid cells should have a survival advantage.

Preclinical Studies

In preclinical studies, low abundance and other factors hindered efficient transduction of stem cells, the ideal target for gene therapy of SCID (Halene and Kohn, 2000). Conditions used successfully in mice did not work well in nonhuman primates (Kantoff et al., 1987; Van Beusechem et al., 1992) or with cultured human marrow (Bordignon et al., 1989; Cournoyer et al., 1991; Hughes et al., 1989; Nolta and Kohn, 1990). This experience, and the intervening development of PEG-ADA, led to a proposal to target mature T cells, rather than stem cells (Blaese, 1993). It was felt that the life span of ADA-deficient T cells might be prolonged by transducing normal ADA cDNA and that repeated cycles of transduction might over time stabilize the T-cell repertoire generated by PEG-ADA therapy.

Early Clinical Trials, 1990–1993

The T-cell approach was initiated in 1990 at the National Institutes of Health in two patients with relatively mild phenotypes. Other trials soon followed in the United States, Europe, and Japan, targeting stem cell–enriched populations of immunoselected CD34+ cells. In all cases, T cells or CD34+ cells from patients were placed in culture, induced to divide with anti-CD3 antibody, and then treated ex vivo with a retroviral vector carrying the normal human ADA cDNA. After a further period of expansion in interleukin-2 (IL-2) supplemented medium, the cells were reinfused, without preselection for ADA expression. Some patients received single treatments (Hoogerbrugge et al., 1996; Kohn et al., 1995); others underwent multiple cycles (up to a dozen) of ex vivo transduction, expansion, and reinfusion over a period of 1 to 2 years (Blaese et al., 1995; Bordignon et al., 1995; Onodera et al., 1998). Transduction efficiency (percentage of vector-containing infused cells), vector persistence, and ADA expression in circulating lymphoid cells were the major objective end points.

Results of Early Clinical Trials

The 5 early trials involved 11 PEG-ADA–treated patients, whose ages ranged from newborn, in the case of 3 patients diagnosed prenatally and treated at birth, to 9.5 years. These patients had varying degrees of lymphopenia and immune dysfunction, but all were clinically well and stable when they began gene therapy. They were all still receiving PEG-ADA at the time reports were prepared, 1 to 4 years after the last infusion of transduced cells (Blaese et al., 1995; Bordignon et al., 1995; Hoogerbrugge et al., 1996; Kohn et al., 1995, 1998; Onodera et al., 1998).

Results varied considerably among patients in the same trial, as well as among patients in the different trials. In patients whose stem cells were targeted, there was little evidence of ADA gene transfer, although in some cases the vector persisted in myeloid and lymphoid lineages for several years (Hoogerbrugge et al., 1996; Kohn et al., 1995, 1998). With mature T-cell targeting, ADA activity in circulating T cells increased to as much as 25% of normal in some patients but was essentially undetectable in others (Blaese et al., 1995; Bordignon et al., 1995; Onodera et al., 1998).

Concomitant treatment with PEG-ADA has precluded evaluation of clinical benefit in early gene therapy trials (Halene and Kohn, 2000; Orkin and Motulsky, 1995; Parkman et al., 2000). Nevertheless, increased lymphocyte counts and changes in immune function observed in some patients were taken as evidence of successful gene therapy (Blaese et al., 1995; Bordignon et al., 1995; Onodera et al., 1998). However, these changes began early in treatment, when transduction efficiency was 10% or less, and even when gene transfer and ADA expression were minimal, as in the second of the two NIH patients (Blaese et al., 1995). In one "successful" case, a progressive reversal of the CD4:CD8 ratio was associated with preferential proliferation of CD8[+] T cells during ex vivo gene transduction (Kawamura et al., 1998; Onodera et al., 1998). Marked increases in eosinophil count and serum IgE, which also began after the second infusion of treated T cells, were attributed to ADA gene transfer, even though more than 90% of the infused, IL-2–activated T cells were untransduced. No ADA gene therapy trial has evaluated the immunomodulatory effects of repeated infusions of mock-transduced, activated autologous T cells.

Influence of PEG-ADA on Gene Therapy Trials

It has been hoped that low transduction efficiency might be compensated for by a selection over time for ADA-expressing lymphoid cells, as has apparently led to clinical improvement in some mosaic patients (see Mosaicism). Concomitant enzyme replacement could blunt this selection. Indeed, the abundance of revertant T cells decreased when some mosaic patients began PEG-ADA therapy (Ariga et al., 2001b; Arredondo-Vega et al., 2002). Conversely, an increase in ADA-expressing T cells has followed interruption of PEG-ADA therapy in two gene therapy patients (Aiuti et al., 2002b; Kohn et al., 1998).

In the first case, PEG-ADA was withheld at 4 years of age in a patient who had received stem cell–targeted autologous CD34[+] umbilical cord cells at birth and in whom the ADA vector persisted in 1% to 10% of T cells (Kohn et al., 1998). In the second case, PEG-ADA was withdrawn over 6 months and then was withheld for 7 months; during this period, this patient also received 11 rounds of T-cell–targeted gene therapy (Aiuti et al., 2002b). In both patients a marked increase in the percentage of vector-positive T cells, as well as a rise in erythrocyte dAXP to pretreatment levels, occurred several weeks after discontinuing PEG-ADA, when plasma PEG-ADA activity returned to baseline. Clinical deterioration necessitated resumption of PEG-ADA therapy after 6 weeks in the first patient. The second patient did well clinically, but she developed pseudotumor cerebri, with papilledema and increased intracranial pressure, 6 months after discontinuing PEG-ADA. At present, both these patients are again receiving PEG-ADA.

In these two patients the increase in ADA-expressing T cells after withdrawal of PEG-ADA probably reflected not only selective growth of transduced T cells but also the metabolic death of ADA-deficient T cells that had been maintained during PEG-ADA therapy. The marked rise in erythrocyte dAXP in both patients indicates that the transduced T cells provided much less systemic ADA activity than was provided by PEG-ADA. There is concern that failure to effectively eliminate ADA substrates systemically may be harmful over time to some nonlymphoid organs.

Recent Success with Stem Cell Gene Therapy

Since the initial trials, retroviral vector design and transduction protocols have improved (Halene and Kohn, 2000; Parkman et al., 2000). New trials began in 2000 after reports from France of successful stem cell–targeted gene therapy for X-linked SCID (Cavazzana-Calvo et al., 2000; Hacein-Bey-Abina et al., 2002). Correction of SCID by stem cell gene therapy has now been reported in two ADA-deficient SCID patients treated in Italy (Aiuti et al., 2002a). These children, 7 months and 2.5 years of age, had not received PEG-ADA. Each was preconditioned with busulfan (2 mg/kg on days −3 and −2) before receiving a single infusion of 8.6 or 0.9×10^6 transduced autologous CD34[+] cells per kilogram.

Following treatment, T cells appeared in blood in about 90 days. NK cells increased in both patients, but B-cell counts increased only in the younger of the two. PBL had increased to 2000/μl at a 14-month follow-up in the younger patient and to 400/μl at 12 months in the older; in both cases, PBL showed significant responses to mitogens and recall antigens. Virtually 100% of circulating T cells contained vector and had normal ADA activity; lower percentages of ADA-expressing cells were found in granulocytic, erythroid, and megakaryocytic lineages. Erythrocyte dAXP normalized in the younger patient, reflecting significant erythroid transduction. Red-cell dAXP decreased in the older patient, but remained significantly elevated above normal. It would appear that recovery of immune function and normalization of metabolic abnormalities may vary among gene therapy patients.

Both these patients have done well clinically, and IVIG has been discontinued in the younger patient. The strikingly better results compared with earlier attempts can probably be attributed primarily to improved efficiency of transducing stem cells, with preservation of the capacity for multilineage differentiation. Lack of concomitant treatment with PEG-ADA may also have increased selection for transduced cells. The role of non-myeloablative conditioning is uncertain.

A Cautionary Note

The quasi-random chromosomal integration of retroviral vectors in stem cells poses two potential adverse complications: unstable expression of the transduced gene and insertional mutagenesis of critical genes (including oncogenes). Long-term monitoring of immune function and ADA expression in patients will be necessary to evaluate the possibility of ADA gene silencing.

Concerns about mutagenesis are no longer theoretical. Of 11 patients with X-linked SCID treated by stem cell–targeted gene therapy, 2 have developed a leukemia-like clonal T-cell expansion, apparently initiated by insertion of the retroviral vector into an oncogene (Check, 2002; see Chapter 15). Too few patients have undergone stem cell gene therapy to estimate the magnitude of the risk from insertional mutagenesis. Direct analysis of sites of retroviral vector integration in lymphoid and possibly other hematopoietic cells may be advisable in patients undergoing gene therapy for ADA deficiency.

PROGNOSIS

The outlook for children diagnosed with ADA deficiency today should be optimistic if specific therapy can be instituted before devastating consequences of SCID have occurred, which may be fatal or cause permanent neurologic or pulmonary injury. For those patients with an HLA-identical sibling, the chance of cure is great. For the majority, a choice must be made among very different alternatives (see Fig. 16-6).

BMT/SCT from a nonsibling donor offers a possible cure but has substantial and often unpredictable risks. After more than two decades, expert opinion remains divided about the need for preconditioning patients with ADA deficiency. Should BMT/SCT fail, enzyme replacement can be instituted. However, its efficacy may be diminished by effects of prior ablative conditioning on endogenous lymphopoiesis or by post-transplant clinical deterioration.

Systemic ADA replacement has the advantage of rapidly correcting the underlying metabolic cause of immunodeficiency and other pathology due to enzyme deficiency. PEG-ADA provides effective management with little risk, but it is not curative and about 10% of patients may develop neutralizing antibody. As an orphan drug for a rare disease, PEG-ADA is very expensive, although the cost is comparable to that for Gaucher disease or hemophilia A, more prevalent disorders for which parenteral replacement therapy is standard.

Because of cost, and because it is not curative, PEG-ADA has been used semiselectively, in many cases to treat patients who were considered poor candidates for BMT/SCT. The level of specific immune function restored is variable and in most cases partial. However, over the past 16 years, overall survival with PEG-ADA therapy has been better than has been reported by most centers for ADA-deficient SCID patients treated by BMT/SCT using HLA-haploidentical or matched unrelated donors.

Treating with PEG-ADA does not preclude subsequent BMT/SCT. However, the decision to discontinue PEG-ADA in favor of a transplant (or gene therapy) in a child who has responded well is difficult. Experience to date suggests that the success rate and complications of a preconditioned BMT/SCT performed after a period of PEG-ADA therapy will be about the same as when performed as initial therapy.

Recent results of gene therapy in a few ADA-deficient patients have been promising, but gene therapy is still experimental and not widely available. The potential complications are of concern, and because several different protocols have been pursued simultaneously, choosing the best technique is still uncertain.

R E F E R E N C E S

Abbott CA, McCaughan GW, Levy MT, Church WB, Gorell MD. Binding to human dipeptidyl peptidase IV by adenosine deaminase and antibodies that inhibit ligand binding involves overlapping, discontinuous sites on a predicted B propellor domain. Eur J Biochem 266:798–810, 1999.

Aitken DA, Gilmore DH, Frew CA, Ferguson-Smith ME, Carty MJ, Chatfield WR. Early prenatal investigation of a pregnancy at risk of adenosine deaminase deficiency using chorionic villi. J Med Genet 23:52–54, 1986.

Aitken DA, Kleijer WJ, Niermeijer MF, Herbschleb-Voogt E, Galjaard H. Prenatal detection of a probable heterozygote for ADA deficiency and severe combined immunodeficiency disease using a microradioassay. Clin Genet 17:293–298, 1980.

Aiuti A, Slavin S, Aker M, Ficara F, Deola S, Mortellaro A, Morecki S, Andolfi G, Tabucchi A, Carlucci F, Marinello E, Cattaneo F, Vai S, Servida P, Miniero R, Roncarolo MG, Bordignon C. Correction of ADA-SCID by stem cell gene therapy combined with nonmyeloablative conditioning. Science 296:2410–2413, 2002a.

Aiuti A, Vai S, Mortellaro A, Casorati G, Ficara F, Andolfi G, Ferrari G, Tabucchi A, Carlucci F, Ochs HD, Notarangelo LD, Roncarolo MG, Bordignon C. Immune reconstitution in ADA-SCID after PBL gene therapy and discontinuation of enzyme replacement. Nat Med 8:423–425, 2002b.

Ammann AJ. Immunologic aberrations in purine nucleoside phosphorylase deficiencies. In Elliot K, Whelan J, eds. Enzyme Defects and Immune Dysfunction, Ciba Foundation Symposium 68. New York, Exerpta Medica, 1979, pp 55–69.

Apasov SG, Koshiba M, Chused TM, Sitkovsky MV. Effects of extracellular ATP and adenosine on different thymocyte subsets:

possible role of ATP-gated channels and G protein–coupled purinergic receptor. J Immunol 158:5095–5105, 1997.

Apasov SG, Sitkovsky MV. The extracellular versus intracellular mechanisms of inhibition of TCR-triggered activation in thymocytes by adenosine under conditions of inhibited adenosine deaminase. Int Immunol 11:179–189, 1999.

Ariga T, Oda N, Santisteban I, Arredondo-Vega FX, Shioda M, Ueno H, Terada K, Kobayashi K, Hershfield MS, Sakiyama Y. Molecular basis for paradoxical carriers of adenosine deaminase (ADA) deficiency that show extremely low levels of ADA activity in peripheral blood cells without immunodeficiency. J Immunol 166:1698–1702, 2001a.

Ariga T, Oda N, Yamaguchi K, Kawamura K, Kikuta H, Taniuchi S, Kobayashi Y, Terada K, Ikeda H, Hershfield MS, Kobayashi K, Sakiyama Y. T cell lines from 2 patients with adenosine deaminase (ADA) deficiency showed the restoration of ADA activity resulted from the reversion of an inherited mutation. Blood 97:2896–2899, 2001b.

Aronow B, Lattier D, Silbiger R, Dusing M, Hutton J, Jones G, Stock J, McNeish J, Potter S, Witte D. Evidence for a complex regulatory array in the first intron of the human adenosine deaminase gene. Genes Dev 3:1384–1400, 1989.

Aronow BJ, Silbiger RN, Dusing MR, Stock JL, Yager KL, Potter S, Hutton JJ, Wiginton DA. Functional analysis of the human adenosine deaminase gene thymic regulatory region and its ability to generate position-independent transgene expression. Mol Cell Biol 12:4170–4185, 1992.

Arpaia E, Benveniste P, Di Cristofano A, Gu Y, Dalal I, Kelly S, Hershfield M, Pandolfi PP, Roifman CM, Cohen A. Mitochondrial basis for immune deficiency: evidence from purine nucleoside phosphorylase-deficient mice. J Exp Med 191:2197–2207, 2000.

Arredondo-Vega FX, Kurtzberg J, Chaffee S, Santisteban I, Reisner E, Povey MS, Hershfield MS. Paradoxical expression of adenosine deaminase in T cells cultured from a patient with adenosine deaminase deficiency and combined immunodeficiency. J Clin Invest 86:444–452, 1990.

Arredondo-Vega FX, Santisteban I, Fuhrer H, Tuchschmid P, Jochum W, Aguzzi A, Lederman HM, Fleischman A, Winkelstein JA, Seger RA, Hershfield MS. Adenosine deaminase deficiency in adults. Blood 89:2849–2855, 1997.

Arredondo-Vega FX, Santisteban I, Kelly S, Schlossman C, Umetsu D, Hershfield MS. Correct splicing despite a G>A mutation at the invariant first nucleotide of a 5′ splice site: a possible basis for disparate clinical phenotypes in siblings with adenosine deaminase (ADA) deficiency. Am J Hum Genet 54:820–830, 1994.

Arredondo-Vega FX, Santisteban I, Daniels S, Toutain S, Hershfield MS. Adenosine deaminase deficiency: genotype-phenotype correlations based on expressed activity of 29 mutant alleles. Am J Hum Genet 63:1049–1059, 1998.

Arredondo-Vega FX, Santisteban I, Richard E, Bali P, Koleilat M, Loubser M, Al-Ghonaium A, Al-Helali M, Hershfield MS. Adenosine deaminase deficiency with mosaicism for a "second-site suppressor" of a splicing mutation: decline in revertant T lymphocytes during enzyme replacement therapy. Blood 99:1005–1013, 2002.

Bagnara AS, Hershfield MS. Mechanism of deoxyadenosine-induced catabolism of adenine ribonucleotides in adenosine deaminase-inhibited human T lymphoblastoid cells. Proc Natl Acad Sci USA 79:2673–2677, 1982.

Baguette C, Vermylen C, Brichard B, Louis J, Dahan K, Vincent MF, Cornu G. Persistent developmental delay despite successful bone marrow transplantation for purine nucleoside phosphoylase deficiency. J Pediatr Hematol Oncol 24:69–71, 2002.

Banerjee SK, Young HW, Volmer JB, Blackburn MR. Gene expression profiling in inflammatory airway disease associated with elevated adenosine. Am J Physiol Lung Cell Mol Physiol 282:L169–L182, 2002.

Benveniste P, Cohen A. p53 expression is required for thymocyte apoptosis induced by adenosine deaminase deficiency. Proc Natl Acad Sci USA 92:8373–8377, 1995.

Benveniste P, Zhu W, Cohen A. Interference with thymocyte differentiation by an inhibitor of S-adenosylhomocysteine hydrolase. J Immunol 155:536–544, 1995.

Birch RE, Rosenthal AK, Polmar SH. Pharmacologic modification of immunoregulatory T-lymphocytes II. Modulation of T-lymphocyte cell surface characteristics. Clin Exp Immunol 48:231–238, 1982.

Blackburn MR, Aldrich M, Volmer JB, Chen W, Zhong H, Kelly S, Hershfield M, Datta SK, Kellems RE. The use of enzyme therapy to regulate the metabolic and phenotypic consequences of adenosine deaminase deficiency in mice: differential impact on pulmonary and immunologic abnormalities. J Biol Chem 275:32114–32121, 2000a.

Blackburn MR, Knudsen TB, Kellems RE. Genetically engineered mice demonstrate that adenosine deaminase is essential for early postimplantation development. Development 124:3089–3097, 1997.

Blackburn MR, Volmer JB, Thrasher JL, Zhong H, Crosby JR, Lee JJ, Kellems RE. Metabolic consequences of adenosine deaminase deficiency in mice are associated with defects in alveogenesis, pulmonary inflammation, and airway obstruction. J Exp Med 192:159–170, 2000b.

Blaese RM. Development of gene therapy for immunodeficiency: adenosine deaminase deficiency. Pediatr Res 33 (Suppl):S49–S55, 1993.

Blaese RM, Culver KW, Miller AD, Carter CS, Fleisher T, Clerici M, Shearer G, Chang L, Chiang Y, Tolstoshev P, Greenblatt JJ, Rosenberg SA, Klein H, Berger M, Mullen CA, Ramsey WJ, Muul L, Morgan RA, Anderson WF. T lymphocyte–directed gene therapy for ADA-SCID: initial trial results after 4 years. Science 270:475–480, 1995.

Bluetters-Sawatzki R, Friedrich W, Ebell W, Vetter U, Stoess H, Goldmann SF, Kleihauer E. HLA-haploidentical bone marrow transplantation in three infants with adenosine deaminase deficiency: stable immunologic reconstitution and reversal of skeletal abnormalities. Eur J Pediatr 149:104–109, 1989.

Bollinger ME, Arredondo-Vega FX, Santisteban I, Schwarz K, Hershfield MS, Lederman HM. Hepatic dysfunction as a complication of adenosine deaminase deficiency. N Engl J Med 334:1367–1371, 1996.

Bontemps F, Van den Berghe G. Mechanism of ATP catabolism induced by deoxyadenosine and other nucleosides in adenosine deaminase-inhibited human erythrocytes. Adv Exp Med Biol 253B:267–274, 1989.

Bordignon C, Notarangelo L, Nobili N, Ferrari G, Casorati G, Panina P, Mazzolari E, Maggioni D, Rossi C, Servida P, Ugazio AG, Mavilio F. Gene therapy in peripheral blood lymphocytes and bone marrow for ADA-immunodeficient patients. Science 270:470–475, 1995.

Bordignon C, Yu SF, Smith CA, Hantzopoulos P, Ungers GE, Keever CA, O'Reilly RJ, Gilboa E. Retroviral vector-mediated high-efficiency expression of adenosine deaminase (ADA) in hematopoietic long-term cultures of ADA-deficient marrow cells. Proc Natl Acad Sci USA 86:6748–6752, 1989.

Borkowsky W, Gershon AA, Shenkman L, Hirschhorn R. Adenosine deaminase deficiency without immunodeficiency: clinical and metabolic studies. Pediatr Res 14:885–889, 1980.

Bory C, Boulieu R, Souillet G, Chantin C, Rolland MO, Mathieu M, Hershfield MS. Comparison of red cell transfusion and polyethylene glycol–modified adenosine deaminase therapy in an adenosine deaminase–deficient child. Pediatr Res 28:127–130, 1990.

Broome CB, Graham ML, Saulsbury FT, Hershfield MS, Buckley RH. Correction of purine nucleoside phosphorylase deficiency by transplantation of allogeneic bone marrow from a sibling. J Pediatr 128:373–376, 1996.

Buckley RH, Schiff RI, Schiff SE, Markert ML, Williams LW, Harville TO, Roberts JL, Puck JP. Human severe combined immunodeficiency: genetic, phenotypic, and functional diversity in one hundred eight infants. J Pediatr 130:378–387, 1997.

Buckley RH, Schiff SE, Schiff RI, Markert ML, Williams LW, Roberts JL, Myers LA, Ward FE. Hematopoietic stem-cell transplantation for the treatment of severe combined immunodeficiency. N Engl J Med 340:508–516, 1999.

Carapella-De Luca E, Aiuti F, Lacarelli P, Bruni L, Baroni CD, Imperato C, Roos D, Astaldi A. A patient with nucleoside phosphorylase deficiency, selective T-cell deficiency, and autoimmune hemolytic anemia. J Pediatr 93:1000–1003, 1978.

Carpenter PA, Ziegler JB, Vowels MR. Late diagnosis and correction of purine nucleoside phosphorylase deficiency with allogeneic bone marrow transplantation. Bone Marrow Transplant 17:121–124, 1996.

Carson DA, Kaye J, Matsumoto S, Seegmiller JE, Thompson L. Biochemical basis for the enhanced toxicity of deoxyribonucleosides toward malignant human T cell lines. Proc Natl Acad Sci USA 76:2430–2433, 1979.

Carson DA, Kaye J, Seegmiller JE. Differential sensitivity of human leukemic T cell lines and B cell lines to growth inhibition by deoxyadenosine. J Immunol 121:1726–1731, 1978.

Cavazzana-Calvo M, Hacein-Bey S, de Saint Basile G, Gross F, Yvon E, Nusbaum P, Selz F, Hue C, Certain S, Casanova JL, Bousso P, Deist FL, Fischer A. Gene therapy of human severe combined immunodeficiency (SCID)-X1 disease. Science 288:669–672, 2000.

Cederbaum SD, Kaitila I, Rimoin DL, Stiehm ER. The chondro-osseous dysplasia of adenosine deaminase deficiency with severe combined immunodeficiency. J Pediatr 89:737–742, 1976.

Chaffee S, Mary A, Stiehm ER, Girault D, Fischer A, Hershfield MS. IgG antibody response to polyethylene glycol–modified adenosine deaminase (PEG-ADA) in patients with adenosine deaminase deficiency. J Clin Invest 89:1643–1651, 1992.

Chan TS. Deoxyguanosine toxicity on lymphoid cells as a cause for immunosuppression in purine nucleoside phosphorylase deficiency. Cell 14:523–530, 1978.

Chan TS. Purine excretion by mouse peritoneal macrophages lacking adenosine deaminase activity. Proc Natl Acad Sci USA 76:925–929, 1979.

Chechik BE, Schrader WP, Minowada J. An immunomorphologic study of adenosine deaminase distribution in human thymus tissue, normal lymphocytes, and hematopoietic cell lines. J Immunol 126:1003–1007, 1981.

Chechik BE, Schrader WP, Perets A, Fernandes B. Immunohistochemical localization of adenosine deaminase distribution in human benign extrathymic lymphoid tissues and B-cell lymphomas. Cancer 53:70–78, 1984.

Check E. Gene therapy: a tragic setback. Nature 420:116–118, 2002

Chen SH, Ochs HD, Scott CR, Giblett ER, Tingle AJ. Adenosine deaminase deficiency. Disappearance of adenine deoxynucleotides from a patient's erythrocytes after successful marrow transplantation. J Clin Invest 62:1386–1389, 1978.

Chun JD, Lee N, Kobayashi RH, Chaffee S, Hershfield MS, Stiehm ER. Suppression of an antibody to adenosine deaminase (ADA) in an ADA deficient severe combined immunodeficiency patient receiving polyethylene glycol modified adenosine deaminase (PEG-ADA). Ann Allergy 70:462–466, 1993.

Classen CF, Schulz AS, Sigl-Kraetzig M, Hoggmann GF, Simmonds HA, Fairbanks L, Debatin KM, Friedrich W. Successful HLA-identical bone marrow transplantation in a patient with PNP deficiency using busulfan and fludarabine for conditioning. Bone Marrow Transplant 28:93–96, 2001.

Cohen A, Doyle D, Martin DW, Jr, Ammann AJ. Abnormal purine metabolism and purine overproduction in a patient deficient in purine nucleoside phosphorylase. N Engl J Med 295:1449–1454, 1976.

Cohen A, Gudas LJ, Ammann AJ, Staal GEJ, Martin DW, Jr. Deoxyguanosine triphosphate as a possible toxic metabolite in the immunodeficiency associated with purine nucleoside phosphorylase deficiency. J Clin Invest 61:1405–1409, 1978a.

Cohen A, Hirschhorn R, Horowitz SD, Rubinstein A, Polmar SH, Hong R, Martin DW, Jr. Deoxyadenosine triphosphate as a potentially toxic metabolite in adenosine deaminase deficiency. Proc Natl Acad Sci USA 75:472–475, 1978b.

Cohen F, Cejka J, Chang CH, Brough AJ, Rowe BJ, Gaines PJ. Adenosine deaminase deficiency and immunodeficiency. In Pollara B, Pickering RJ, Meuwissen HJ, Porter IH, eds. Inborn Errors of Specific Immunity. New York, Academic Press, 1979, pp 401–424.

Coleman MS, Donofrio J, Hutton JJ, Hahn L, Daoud A, Lampkin B, Dyminski J. Identification and quantitation of adenine deoxynucleotides in erythrocytes of a patient with adenosine deaminase deficiency and severe combined immunodeficiency. J Biol Chem 253:1619–1626, 1978.

Cournoyer D, Scarpa M, Mitani K, Moore KA, Markowitz D, Bank A, Belmont JW, Caskey CT. Gene transfer of adenosine deaminase into primitive human hematopoietic progenitor cells. Hum Gene Ther 2:203–213, 1991.

Cowan MJ, Shannon KM, Wara DM, Ammann AJ. Rejection of bone marrow transplant and resistance of alloantigen reactive cells to in vivo deoxyadenosine in adenosine deaminase deficiency. Clin Immunol Immunopathol 49:242–250, 1988.

Daddona PE, Kelley WN. Characterization of an aminohydrolase distinct from adenosine deaminase in cultured human lymphocytes. Biochim Biophys Acta 658:280–290, 1981.

Daddona PE, Mitchell BS, Meuwissen HJ, Davidson BL, Wilson JM, Koller CA. Adenosine deaminase deficiency with normal immune function. J Clin Invest 72:483–492, 1983.

Davies EG, Levinsky RJ, Webster DR, Simmonds HA, Perrett D. Effect of red cell transfusions, thymic hormone and deoxycytidine in severe combined immunodeficiency due to adenosine deaminase deficiency. Clin Exp Immunol 50:303–310, 1982.

Davis S, Abuchowski A, Park YK, Davis FF. Alteration of the circulating life and antigenic properties of bovine adenosine deaminase in mice by attachment of polyethylene glycol. Clin Exp Immunol 46:649–652, 1981

Dinjens WN, Ten Kate J, Van der Linden E, Wijnen JT, Khan PM, Bosman FT. Distribution of adenosine deaminase complexing protein (ADCP) in human tissues. J Histochem Cytochem 37:1869–1875, 1989a.

Dinjens WN, Ten Kate J, Wijnen JT, Van der Linden EP, Beek CJ, Lenders MH, Khan PM, Bosman FT. Distribution of adenosine deaminase–complexing protein in murine tissues. J Biol Chem 264:19215–19220, 1989b.

Dong RP, Kameoka J, Hegen M, Tanaka T, Xu Y, Schlossman SF, Morimoto C. Characterization of adenosine deaminase binding to human CD26 on T cells and its biologic role in immune response. J Immunol 156:1349–1355, 1996.

Dong RP, Tachibana K, Hegen M, Munakata Y, Cho D, Schlossman SF, Morimoto C. Determination of adenosine deaminase binding domain on CD26 and its immunoregulatory effect on T cell activation. J Immunol 159:6070–6076, 1997.

Dooley T, Fairbanks LD, Simmonds HA, Rodeck CH, Nicolaides KH, Soothill PW, Stewart P, Morgan G, Levinsky RJ. First trimester diagnosis of adenosine deaminase deficiency. Prenat Diagn 7:561–565, 1987.

Dror Y, Gallagher R, Wara DW, Colombe BW, Merino A, Benkerrou M, Cowan MJ. Immune reconstitution in severe combined immunodeficiency disease after lectin-treated, T-cell–depleted haplocompatible bone marrow transplantation. Blood 81:2021–2030, 1993.

Dusing MR, Wiginton DA. Sp1 is essential for both enhancer-mediated and basal activation of the TATA-less human adenosine deaminase promoter. Nucl Acids Res 22:669–677, 1994.

Ealick SE, Rule SA, Carter DC, Greenhough TJ, Babu YS, Cook WJ, Habash J, Helliwell JR, Stoeckler JD, Parks RE, Jr, Chen S-F, Bugg CE. Three dimensional structure of human erythrocytic purine nucleoside phosphorylase at 3.2 å resolution. J Biol Chem 265:1812–1820, 1990.

Erickson RH, Suzuki Y, Sedlmayer A, Kim YS. Biosynthesis and degradation of altered immature forms of intestinal dipeptidyl peptidase IV in a rat strain lacking the enzyme. J Biol Chem 267:21623–21629, 1992.

Fischer A, Landais P, Friedrich W, Gerritsen B, Fasth A, Porta F, Vellodi A, Benkerrou M, Jais JP, Cavazzana-Calvo M, Souillet G, Bordigoni P, Morgan G, Van Dijken P, Vossen J, Locatelli F, di Bartolomeo P. Bone marrow transplantation (BMT) in Europe for primary immunodeficiencies other than severe combined immunodeficiency: a report from the European Group for BMT and the European Group for Immunodeficiency. Blood 83:1149–1154, 1994.

Fleischman A, Hershfield MS, Toutain S, Lederman HM, Sullivan KE, Fasano MB, Greene J, Winkelstein JA. Adenosine deaminase deficiency and purine nucleoside phosphorylase deficiency in common variable immunodeficiency. Clin Diagn Lab Immunol 5:399–400, 1998.

Franco R, Valenzuela A, Lluis C, Blanco J. Enzymatic and extraenzymatic role of ecto-adenosine deaminase in lymphocytes. Immunol Rev 161:27–42, 1998.

Gangi-Peterson L, Sorscher DH, Reynolds JW, Kepler TB, Mitchell BS. Nucleotide pool imbalance and adenosine deaminase deficiency induce alterations of N-region insertions during V(D)J recombination. J Clin Invest 103:833–841, 1999.

Gao X, Knudsen TB, Ibrahim MM, Haldar S. Bcl-2 relieves deoxyadenylate stress and suppresses apoptosis in pre-B leukemia cells. Cell Death Diff 2:69–78, 1995.

Geffner ME, Stiehm ER, Stephure D, Cowan MJ. Probable autoimmune thyroid disease and combined immunodeficiency disease. Am J Dis Child 140:1194–1196, 1986.

Gelfand EW, Dosch HM, Biggar WD, Fox IH. Partial purine nucleoside phosphorylase deficiency Studies of lymphocyte function. J Clin Invest 61:1071–1080, 1978.

George DL, Francke U. Gene dose effect: regional mapping of human nucleoside phosphorylase on chromosome 14. Science 194:851–852, 1976.

Giblett ER. ADA and PNP deficiencies: how it all began. Ann NY Acad Sci 451:1–8, 1985.

Giblett ER, Ammann AJ, Wara DW, Sandman R, Diamond LK. Nucleoside-phosphorylase deficiency in a child with severely defective T-cell immunity and normal B-cell immunity. Lancet 1:1010–1013, 1975.

Giblett ER, Anderson JE, Cohen F, Pollara B, Meuwissen HJ. Adenosine deaminase deficiency in two patients with severely impaired cellular immunity. Lancet 2:1067–1069, 1972.

Gilfillan S, Dierich A, Lemeur M, Benoist C, Mathis D. Mice lacking TdT: Mature animals with an immature lymphocyte repertoire. Science 261:1175–1178, 1993.

Girault D, Le Deist F, Debré M, Pérignon JL, Herbelin C, Griscelli C, Scudiery D, Hershfield M, Fischer A. Traitement du deficit en adenosine desaminase par l'adenosine desaminase couplee au polyethylene glycol (PEG-ADA). Arch Franç Pediatrie 49:339–343, 1992.

Graham-Poole J, Gibson AAM, Stephenson JBP. Familial dysequilibrium-diplegia with T lymphocyte deficiency. Arch Dis Child 50:927–932, 1975.

Greenberg ML, Chaffee S, Hershfield MS. Basis for resistance to 3-deazaaristeromycin, an inhibitor of S-adenosylhomocysteine hydrolase, in human B-lymphoblasts. J Biol Chem 264:795–803, 1989.

Hacein-Bey-Abina S, Le Deist F, Carlier F, Bouneaud C, Hue C, De Villartay JP, Thrasher AJ, Wulffraat N, Sorensen R, Dupuis-Girod S, Fischer A, Davies EG, Kuis W, Leiva L, Cavazzana-Calvo M. Sustained correction of X-linked severe combined immunodeficiency by ex vivo gene therapy. N Engl J Med 346:1185–1193, 2002.

Haddad E, Landais P, Friedrich W, Gerritsen B, Cavazzana-Calvo M, Morgan G, Bertrand Y, Fasth A, Porta F, Cant A, Espanol T, Muller S, Veys P, Vossen J, Fischer A. Long-term immune reconstitution and outcome after HLA-nonidentical T-cell–depleted bone marrow transplantation for severe combined immunodeficiency: A European retrospective study of 116 patients. Blood 91:3646–3653, 1998.

Hagberg B, Hansson O, Liden S, Nilsson K. Familial ataxic diplegia with deficient cellular immunity. Acta Pediatr Scand 59:545–546, 1970.

Halene S, Kohn DB. Gene therapy using hematopoietic stem cells: Sisyphus approaches the crest. Hum Gene Ther 11:1259–1267, 2000.

Hatzis P, Al-Madhoon AS, Jullig M, Petrakis TG, Eriksson S, Talianidis I. The intracellular localization of deoxycytidine kinase. J Biol Chem 273:30239–30243, 1998.

Hershfield MS. Apparent suicide inactivation of human lymphoblast S-adenosylhomocysteine hydrolase by 2'-deoxyadenosine and adenine arabinoside. A basis for direct toxic effects of analogs of adenosine. J Biol Chem 254:22–25, 1979.

Hershfield MS. Biochemistry and immunology of poly(ethylene glycol)–modified adenosine deaminase (PEG-ADA). In Harris JM, Zalipsky S eds. Poly(ethylene glycol) Chemistry and Biological Applications. Washington, DC, ACS, 1997, pp 145–154.

Hershfield MS. PEG-ADA replacement therapy for adenosine deaminase deficiency: an update after 8.5 years. Clin Immunol Immunopathol 76:S228–S232, 1995.

Hershfield MS, Buckley RH, Greenberg ML, Melton AL, Schiff R, Hatem C, Kurtzberg J, Markert ML, Kobayashi RH, Kobayashi AL, Abuchowski A. Treatment of adenosine deaminase deficiency with polyethylene glycol–modified adenosine deaminase. N Engl J Med 316:589–596, 1987.

Hershfield MS, Chaffee S. PEG-enzyme replacement therapy for adenosine deaminase deficiency. In Desnick RJ, ed. Treatment of Genetic Diseases. New York, Churchill Livingstone, 1991, pp 169–182.

Hershfield MS, Chaffee S, Koro-Johnson L, Mary A, Smith AA, Short SA. Use of site directed mutagenesis to enhance the epitope shielding effect of covalent modification of proteins with polyethylene glycol. Proc Natl Acad Sci USA 88:7185–7189, 1991.

Hershfield MS, Chaffee S, Sorensen RU. Enzyme replacement therapy with polyethylene glycol–adenosine deaminase in adenosine deaminase deficiency: overview and case reports of three patients, including two now receiving gene therapy. Pediatr Res 33 (Suppl):S42–S48, 1993.

Hershfield MS, Fetter JE, Small WC, Bagnara AS, Williams SR, Ullman B, Martin DW, Jr, Wasson DB, Carson DA. Effects of mutational loss of adenosine kinase and deoxycytidine kinase on deoxyATP accumulation and deoxyadenosine toxicity in cultured CEM cells. J Biol Chem 257:6380–6386, 1982.

Hershfield MH, Kredich NM. Resistance of an adenosine kinase–deficient human lymphoblastoid cell line to effects of deoxyadenosine on growth, S-adenosylhomocysteine hydrolase inactivation, and dATP accumulation. Proc Natl Acad Sci USA 77:4292–4296, 1980.

Hershfield MS, Kredich NM, Koller CA, Mitchell BS, Kurtzberg J, Kinney TR, Falletta JM. S-Adenosylhomocysteine catabolism and basis for acquired resistance during treatment of T-cell acute lymphoblastic leukemia with 2'-deoxycoformycin alone and in combination with 9-ß-D-arabinofuranosyladenine. Cancer Res 43:3451–3458, 1983.

Hershfield MS, Kredich NM, Ownby DR, Ownby H, Buckley R. In vivo inactivation of erythrocyte S-adenosylhomocysteine hydrolase by 2'-deoxyadenosine in adenosine deaminase-deficient patients. J Clin Invest 63:807–811, 1979.

Hershfield MS, Kurtzberg J, Moore JO, Whang Peng J, Haynes BF. Conversion of a stem cell leukemia from T-lymphoid to a myeloid phenotype by the adenosine deaminase inhibitor 2'-deoxycoformycin. Proc Natl Acad Sci USA 81:253–257, 1984.

Hershfield MS, Mitchell BS. Immunodeficiency diseases caused by adenosine deaminase deficiency and purine nucleoside phosphorylase deficiency. In Scriver CR, Beaudet AL, Sly WS, Valle D, eds. The Metabolic and Molecular Bases of Inherited Disease. New York, McGraw-Hill, 2001, pp 2585–2625.

Hirschhorn R. Clinical delineation of adenosine deaminase deficiency. In Elliot K, Whelan J, eds. Enzyme Defects and Immune Dysfunction, Ciba Foundation Symposium 68. New York, Excerpta Medica, 1979a, pp 35–54.

Hirschhorn R. Immunodeficiency disease due to deficiency of adenosine deaminase. In Ochs HD, Smith CIE, Puck JM, eds. Primary Immunodeficiency Diseases: A Molecular and Genetic Approach. New York, Oxford University Press, 1999, pp 121–139.

Hirschhorn R. Incidence and prenatal detection of adenosine deaminase deficiency and purine nucleoside phosphorylase deficiency. In Pollara B, Pickering RJ, Meuwissen HJ, Porter IH, eds. Inborn Errors of Specific Immunity. New York, Academic Press, 1979b, pp 5–12.

Hirschhorn R. Prenatal diagnosis and heterozygote detection in adenosine deaminase deficiency. In Guttler F, Seakins JWT, Harkness RA, eds. Inborn Errors of Immunity and Phagocytosis. Lancaster, Mass, MTP Press, 1979c, pp 121–128.

Hirschhorn R, Beratis N, Rosen FS, Parkman R, Stern R, Polmar S. Adenosine-deaminase deficiency in a child diagnosed prenatally. Lancet 1:73–75, 1975.

Hirschhorn R, Nicknam MN, Eng F, Yang DR, Borkowsky W. Novel deletion and a new missense mutation (Glu 217 Lys) at the catalytic site in two adenosine deaminase alleles of a patient with neonatal onset adenosine deaminase severe combined immunodeficiency. J Immunol 149:3107–3112, 1992.

Hirschhorn R, Papageorgiou PS, Kesarwala HH, Taft LT. Amelioration of neurologic abnormalities after "enzyme replacement" in adenosine deaminase deficiency. N Engl J Med 303:377–380, 1980a.

Hirschhorn R, Roegner-Maniscalco V, Kuritsky L, Rosen FS. Bone marrow transplantation only partially restores purine metabolites to normal in adenosine deaminase–deficient patients. J Clin Invest 68:1387–1393, 1981.

Hirschhorn R, Roegner V, Jenkins T, Seaman C, Piomelli S, Borkowsky W. Erythrocyte adenosine deaminase deficiency without immunodeficiency. Evidence for an unstable mutant enzyme. J Clin Invest 64:1130–1139, 1979a.

Hirschhorn R, Roegner V, Rubinstein A, Papageorgiou P. Plasma deoxyadenosine, adenosine, and erythrocyte deoxyATP are elevated at birth in an adenosine deaminase–deficient child. J Clin Invest 65:768–771, 1980b.

Hirschhorn R, Tzall S, Ellenbogen A. Hot spot mutations in adenosine deaminase deficiency. Proc Natl Acad Sci USA 87:6171–6175, 1990.

Hirschhorn R, Vawter GF, Kirkpatrick JA, Jr., Rosen FS. Adenosine deaminase deficiency: frequency and comparative pathology in autosomally recessive severe combined immunodeficiency. Clin Immunol Immunopathol 14:107–120, 1979b.

Hirschhorn R, Yang DR, Israni A. An Asp8Asn substitution in the adenosine deaminase (ADA) genetic polymorphism (ADA 2 allozyme): occurrence on different chromosomal backgrounds and apparent intragenic crossover. Ann Hum Genet 58:1–9, 1994a.

Hirschhorn R, Yang DR, Insel RA, Ballow M. Severe combined immunodeficiency of reduced severity due to homozygosity for an adenosine deaminase missense mutation (Arg253Pro). Cell Immunol 152:383–393, 1993.

Hirschhorn R, Yang DR, Israni A, Huie ML, Ownby DR. Somatic mosaicism for a newly identified splice-site mutation in a patient with adenosine deaminase–deficient immunodeficiency and spontaneous clinical recovery. Am J Hum Genet 55:59–68, 1994b.

Hirschhorn R, Yang DR, Puck JM, Huie ML, Jiang C-K, Kurlandsky LE. Spontaneous reversion to normal of an inherited mutation in a patient with adenosine deaminase deficiency. Nat Genet 13:290–295, 1996.

Hong R, Gatti R, Rathbun JC, Good RA. Thymic hypoplasia and thyroid dysfunction. N Engl J Med 282:470–474, 1970.

Hoogerbrugge PM, van Beusechem VW, Fischer A, Debree M, le Deist F, Perignon JL, Morgan G, Gaspar B, Fairbanks LD, Skeoch CH, Moseley A, Harvey M, Levinsky RJ, Valerio D. Bone marrow gene transfer in three patients with adenosine deaminase deficiency. Gene Ther 3:179–183, 1996.

Hughes PDF, Eaves CJ, Hogge DE, Humphries RK. High-efficiency gene transfer to human hematopoietic cells maintained in long-term marrow culture. Blood 74:1915–1922, 1989.

Hutton JJ, Wiginton DA, Coleman MS, Fuller SA, Limouze S, Lampkin BC. Biochemical and functional abnormalities in lymphocytes from an adenosine deaminase deficient patient during enzyme replacement therapy. J Clin Invest 68:413–421, 1981.

Ito T, van Kuilenburg AB, Bootsma AH, Haasnoot AJ, van Cruchten A, Wada Y, Van Gennip AH. Rapid screening of high-risk patients for disorders of purine and pyrimidine metabolism using HPLC-electrospray tandem mass spectrometry of liquid urine or urine-soaked filter paper strips. Clin Chem 46:445–452, 2000.

Johansson M, Brismar S, Karlsson A. Human deoxycytidine kinase is located in the cell nucleus. Proc Natl Acad Sci USA 94:11941–11945, 1997.

Johansson M, Karlsson A. Cloning and expression of human deoxyguanosine kinase cDNA. Proc Natl Acad Sci USA 93:7258–7262, 1996.

Jonsson JJ, Williams SR, McIvor RS. Sequence and functional characterization of the human purine nucleoside phosphorylase promoter. Nucl Acids Res 19:5015–5020, 1991.

Jonsson JJ, Converse A, McIvor RS. An enhancer in the first intron of the human purine nucleoside phosphorylase-encoding gene. Gene 140:187–193, 1994.

Kameoka J, Tanaka T, Nojima Y, Schlossman S, Morimoto C. Direct association of adenosine deaminase with a T cell activation antigen, CD26. Science 261:466–469, 1993.

Kantoff PW, Gillio A, McLachlin JR, Bordignon C, Eglitis MA, Kernan NA, Moen RC, Kohn DB, Yu SF, Karson E, Karlsson S, Zwiebel JA, Gilboa E, Blaese RM, Nienhuis A, O'reilly RJ, Anderson WF. Expression of human adenosine deaminase in non-human primates after retroviral mediated gene transfer. J Exp Med 166:219–234, 1987.

Kawamura N, Ariga T, Ohtsu M, Yamada M, Tame A, Furuta H, Kobayashi I, Okano M, Yanagihara Y, Sakiyama Y. Elevation of serum IgE level and peripheral eosinophil count during T lymphocyte–directed gene therapy for ADA deficiency: implication of Tc2-like cells after gene transduction procedure. Immunol Lett 64:49–53, 1998.

Kizaki H, Shimada H, Ohsaka F, Sakurada T. Adenosine, deoxyadenosine, and deoxyguanosine induce DNA cleavage in mouse thymocytes. J Immunol 141:1652–1657, 1988.

Knudsen TB, Gray MK, Church JK, Blackburn MR, Airhart MJ, Kellems RE, Skalko RG. Early postimplantation embryolethality in mice following in utero inhibition of adenosine deaminase with 2'-deoxycoformycin. Teratol 40:615–626, 1989.

Knudsen TB, Green JD, Airhart MJ, Higley HR, Chinsky JM, Kellems RD. Developmental expression of adenosine deaminase in placental tissues of the early postimplantation mouse embryo and uterine stroma. Biol Reprod 39:937–951, 1988.

Kohn DB, Hershfield MS, Carbonaro D, Shigeoka A, Brooks J, Smogorzewska EM, Barsky LW, Chan R, Burroto F, Annett G, Nolta JA, Crooks GM, Kapoor N, Elder M, Wara D, Bowen T, Madsden E, Snyder FF, Bastian J, Muul L, Blaese RM, Weinberg KI, Parkman R. Selective accumulation of T lymphocytes containing a normal ADA gene four years after transplantation of transduced autologous umbilical cord blood CD34+ cells in ADA-deficient SCID neonates. Nat Med 4:775–780, 1998.

Kohn DB, Weinberg KI, Nolta JA, Heiss LN, Lenarsky C, Crooks GM, Hanley ME, Annett G, Brooks JS, El-Khoureiy A, Lawrence K, Wells S, Shaw K, Moen RC, Bastian J, Williams-Herman D, Elder M, Wara D, Bowen T, Hershfield MS, Mullen CA, Blaese RM, Parkman R. Engraftment of gene-modified umbilical cord blood cells in neonates with adenosine deaminase deficiency. Nat Med 1:1017–1023, 1995.

Komori T, Okada A, Stewart V, Alt FW. Lack of N regions in antigen receptor variable region genes of TdT-deficient lymphocytes. Science 261:1171–1175, 1993.

Kredich NM, Hershfield MS. S-Adenosylhomocysteine toxicity in normal and adenosine kinase–deficient lymphoblasts of human origin. Proc Natl Acad Sci USA 76:2450–2454, 1979.

Kredich NM, Martin DW, Jr. Role of S-adenosylhomocysteine in adenosine-mediated toxicity in cultured mouse T-lymphoma cells. Cell 12:931–938, 1977.

Levy Y, Hershfield MS, Fernandez-Mejia C, Polmar SH, Scudiery D, Berger M, Sorensen RU. Adenosine deaminase deficiency with late onset of recurrent infections: Response to treatment with polyethylene glycol–modified adenosine deaminase (PEG-ADA). J Pediatr 113:312–317, 1988.

Li P, Nijhawan D, Budihardjo I, Srinivasula SM, Ahmad M, Alnemri ES, Wang X. Cytochrome c and dATP-dependent formation of Apaf-1/caspase-9 complex initiates an apoptotic protease cascade. Cell 91:479–489, 1997.

Linch DC, Levinski RJ, Rodeck CH, Maclennan KA, Simmonds HA. Prenatal diagnosis of three cases of severe combined immunodeficiency severe T cell deficiency—during the first half of gestation in fetuses with adenosine deaminase deficiency. Clin Exp Immunol 56:223–232, 1984.

Liu X, Kim CN, Yang J, Jemmerson R, Wang X. Induction of apoptotic program in cell-free extracts: requirement for dATP and cytochrome c. Cell 86:147–157, 1996.

Ma DDF, Sylwestrowicz TA, Granger S, Massaia M, Franks R, Janossy G, Hoffbrand AV. Distribution of terminal deoxynucleotidyl transferase and purine degradative and synthetic enzymes in subpopulations of human thymocytes. J Immunol 129:1430–1435, 1982.

Marguet D, Baggio L, Kobayashi T, Bernard AM, Pierres M, Nielsen PF, Ribel U, Watanabe T, Drucker DJ, Wagtmann N. Enhanced insulin secretion and improved glucose tolerance in mice lacking CD26. Proc Natl Acad Sci USA 97:6874–6879, 2000.

Markert ML. Purine nucleoside phosphorylase deficiency. Immunodef Rev 3:45–81, 1991.

Markert ML, Hershfield MS, Schiff RI, Buckley RH. Adenosine deaminase and purine nucleoside phosphorylase deficiencies: evaluation of therapeutic interventions in eight patients. J Clin Immunol 7:389–399, 1987.

Martin M, Huguet J, Centelles JJ, Franco R. Expression of ecto-adenosine deaminase and CD26 in human T cells triggered by the TCR-CD3 complex. J Immunol 155:4630–4643, 1995.

Marwaha VR, Italia DH, Esper F, Hostoffer RW. Extreme thrombocytosis in response to PEG-ADA: early therapeutic and risk indicator. Clin Pediatr (Phila) 39:183–186, 2000.

Migchielsen AA, Breuer ML, van Roon MA, te Riele H, Zurcher C, Ossendorp F, Toutain S, Hershfield MS, Berns A, Valerio D. Adenosine deaminase–deficient mice die perinatally and exhibit liver-cell degeneration, atelectasis and small intestinal cell death. Nat Genet 10:279–287, 1995.

Moen RC, Horowitz SD, Sondel PM, Borcherding WR, Trigg ME, Billing R, Hong R. Immunologic reconstitution after haploidentical bone marrow transplantation for immune deficiency disorders: treatment of bone marrow cells with monoclonal antibody CT-2 and complement. Blood 70:664–669, 1987.

Morgan C, Levinsky RJ, Hugh JK, Fairbanks LD, Morris GS, Simmonds HA. Heterogeneity of biochemical, clinical and immunological parameters in severe combined immunodeficiency due to adenosine deaminase deficiency. Clin Exp Immunol 70:491–499, 1987.

Morimoto C, Schlossman SF. The structure and function of CD26 in the T-cell immune response. Immunologic Rev 161:55–70, 1998.

Morrison ME, Vijayasaradhi S, Engelstein D, Albino AP, Houghton AN. A marker for neoplastic progression of human melanocytes is a cell surface ectopeptidase. J Exp Med 177:1135–1143, 1993.

Muraoka T, Katsuramaki T, Shiraishi H, Yokoyama MM. Automated enzymatic measurement of adenosine deaminase isoenzyme activities in serum. Anal Biochem 187:268–272, 1990.

Nolta JA, Kohn DB. Comparison of the effects of growth factors on retroviral vector-mediated gene transfer and the proliferative status of human hematopoietic progenitor cells. Hum Gene Ther 1:257–268, 1990.

Notarangelo LD, Stoppoloni G, Toraldo R, Mazzolari E, Coletta A, Airo P, Bordignon C, Ugazio AG. Insulin-dependent diabetes mellitus and severe atopic dermatitis in a child with adenosine deaminase deficiency. Eur J Pediatr 151:811–814, 1992.

Ochs HD, Buckley RH, Kobayashi RH, Kobayashi AL, Sorensen RU, Douglas SD, Hamilton BL, Hershfield.M.S. Antibody responses to bacteriophage (φX-174 in patients with adenosine deaminase deficiency. Blood 80:1163–1171, 1992.

Olah ME, Stiles GL. Adenosine receptor–mediated signal transduction. In Pelleg A, Belardinelli L, eds. Effects of Extracellular Adenosine and ATP on Cardiomyocytes. Austin, Tex, R. G. Landes, 1998, pp 1–31.

Onodera M, Ariga T, Kawamura N, Kobayashi I, Ohtsu M, Yamada M, Tame A, Furuta H, Okano M, Matsumoto S, Kotani H, McGarrity GJ, Blaese RM, Sakiyama Y. Successful peripheral T-lymphocyte–directed gene transfer for a patient with severe combined immune deficiency caused by adenosine deaminase deficiency. Blood 91:30–36, 1998.

O'Reilly RJ, Keever CA, Small TN, Brochstein J. The use of HLA–non-identical T-cell–depleted marrow for transplants for correction of severe combined immunodeficiency disease. Immunodef Rev 1:273–309, 1989.

Orkin S, Motulsky A. Report and recommendations of the panel to assess the NIH investment in research on gene therapy: http://www.nih.gov/news/panelrep.html. Accessed 1995.

Osborne WR. Human red cell purine nucleoside phosphorylase. Purification by biospecific affinity chromatography and physical properties. J Biol Chem 255:7089–7092, 1980.

Osborne WRA. Nucleoside kinases in T and B lymphoblasts distinguished by autoradiography. Proc Natl Acad Sci USA 83:4030–4034, 1986.

Osborne WRA, Ochs HD. Immunodeficiency disease due to deficiency of purine nucleoside phosphorylase. In Ochs HD, Smith CIE, Puck JM, eds. Primary Immunodeficiency Diseases: A Molecular and Genetic Approach. New York, Oxford University Press, 1999, pp 140–145.

Ozsahin H, Arredondo-Vega FX, Santisteban I, Fuhrer H, Tuchschmid P, Jochum W, Aguzzi A, Lederman HM, Fleischman A, Winkelstein JA, Seger RA, Hershfield MS. Adenosine deaminase deficiency in adults. Blood 89:2849–2855, 1997.

Pannicke U, Tuchschmid P, Friedrich W, Bartram CR, Schwarz K. Two novel missense and frameshift mutations in exons 5 and 6 of the purine nucleoside phosphorylase (PNP) gene in a severe combined immunodeficiency (SCID) patient. Hum Genet 1996:706–709, 1996.

Park I, Ives DH. Properties of a highly purified mitochondrial deoxyguanosine kinase. Arch Biochem Biophys 266:51–60, 1988.

Parkman R, Weinberg K, Crooks G, Nolta J, Kapoor N, Kohn D. Gene therapy for adenosine deaminase deficiency. Annu Rev Med 51:33–47, 2000.

Polmar SH. Enzyme replacement and other biochemical approaches to the therapy of adenosine deaminase deficiency. In Elliot K, Whelan J, eds. Enzyme Defects and Immune Dysfunction. Ciba Foundation Symposium. New York, Excerpta Medica, 1979, pp 213–230.

Polmar SH, Stern RC, Schwartz AL, Wetzler EM, Chase PA, Hirschhorn R. Enzyme replacement therapy for adenosine deaminase deficiency and severe combined immunodeficiency. N Engl J Med 295:1337–1343, 1976.

Porta F, Friedrich W. Bone marrow transplantation in congenital immunodeficiency diseases. Bone Marrow Transplant 21 (Suppl) 2:S21–S23, 1998.

Purring-Koch C, McLendon G. Cytochrome c binding to apaf-1: the effects of dATP and ionic strength. Proc Natl Acad Sci USA 97:11928–11931, 2000.

Ratech H, Greco MA, Gallo G, Rimoin DL, Kamino H, Hirschhorn R. Pathologic findings in adenosine deaminase–deficient severe combined immunodeficiency. Am J Pathol 120:157–169, 1985.

Ratech H, Hirschhorn R, Greco MA. Pathologic findings in adenosine deaminase deficient–severe combined immunodeficiency. II. Thymus, spleen, lymph node, and gastrointestinal tract lymphoid tissue alterations. Am J Pathol 135:1145–1156, 1989.

Resta R, Hooker SW, Laurent AB, Jamshedur Rahman SM, Franklin M, Knudsen TB, Nadon NL, Thompson LF. Insights into thymic purine metabolism and adenosine deaminase deficiency revealed by transgenic mice overexpressing ecto-5′-nucleotidase (CD73). J Clin Invest 99:676–683, 1997.

Ricciuti F, Ruddle FH. Assignment of nucleoside phosphorylase to D-14 and localization of X-linked loci in man by somatic cell genetics. Nature 241:180–182, 1973.

Rich KC, Arnold WJ, Palella T, Fox IH. Cellular immune deficiency with autoimmune hemolytic anemia in purine nucleoside phosphorylase deficiency. Am J Med 67:172–176, 1979.

Rich KC, Richman CM, Mejias E, Daddona PA. Immunoreconstitution by peripheral blood leukocytes in adenosine deaminase–deficient severe combined immunodeficiency. J Clin Invest 66:389–395, 1980.

Richard E, Alam SM, Arredondo-Vega FX, Patel DD, Hershfield MS. Clustered charged amino acids of human adenosine deaminase comprise a functional epitope for binding the adenosine deaminase complexing protein CD26/Dipeptidyl peptidase IV. J Biol Chem 277:19720–19726, 2002.

Richard E, Arredondo-Vega FX, Santisteban I, Kelly SJ, Patel DD, Hershfield MS. The binding site of human adenosine deaminase for CD26/dipeptidyl peptidase IV: The Arg142Gln mutation impairs binding to CD26 but does not cause immune deficiency. J Exp Med 192:1223–1235, 2000.

Rijksen G, Kuis W, Wadman SK, Spaapen L, Duran M, Voorbrood BS, Staal G, Stoop JW, Zegers B. A new case of purine nucleoside phosphorylase deficiency: enzymologic, clinical and immunologic characteristics. Pediatr Res 21:137–141, 1987.

Rogers MH, Lwin R, Fairbanks L, Gerritsen B, Gaspar HB. Cognitive and behavioral abnormalities in adenosine deaminase deficient severe combined immunodeficiency. J Pediatr 139:44–50, 2001.

Rosen FS, Bhan AK. Weekly Clinicopathological Exercises: Case 18-1998: A 54-day-old premature girl with respiratory distress and persistent pulmonary infiltrates. N Engl J Med 338:1752–1758, 1998.

Rubocki RJ, Parsa JR, Hershfield MS, Sanger WG, Pirruccello SJ, Santisteban I, Gordon BG, Strandjord SE, Warkentin PI, Coccia PF. Full hematopoietic engraftment after allogeneic bone marrow transplantation without cytoreduction in a child with severe combined immunodeficiency. Blood 97:809–811, 2001.

Sandman R, Ammann AJ, Grose C, Wara DW. Cellular immunodeficiency associated with nucleoside phosphorylase deficiency. Clin Immunol Immunopathol 8:247–253, 1977.

Santisteban I, Arredondo-Vega FX, Kelly S, Loubser M, Meydan N, Roifman C, Howell PL, Bowen T, Weinberg KI, Schroeder ML, Hershfield MS. Three new adenosine deaminase mutations that define a splicing enhancer and cause severe and partial phenotypes: implications for evolution of a CpG hotspot and expression of a transduced ADA cDNA. Hum Mol Genet 4:2081–2087, 1995.

Santisteban I, Arredondo-Vega FX, Kelly S, Mary A, Fischer A, Hummell DS, Lawton A, Sorensen RU, Stiehm ER, Uribe L, Weinberg K, Hershfield MS. Novel splicing, missense, and deletion mutations in 7 adenosine deaminase–deficient patients with late/delayed onset of combined immunodeficiency disease. Contribution of genotype to phenotype. J Clin Invest 92:2291–2302, 1993.

Schmalstieg FC, Mills GC, Tsuda H, Goldman AS. Severe combined immunodeficiency in a child with a healthy adenosine deaminase deficient mother. Pediatr Res 17:935–940, 1983.

Schrader WP, West CA, Miczek AD, Norton EK. Characterization of the adenosine deaminase–adenosine deaminase complexing protein binding reaction. J Biol Chem 265:19312–19318, 1990.

Seto S, Carrera CJ, Kubota M, Wasson DB, Carson DA. Mechanism of deoxyadenosine and 2-chlorodeoxyadenosine toxicity to nondividing human lymphocytes. J Clin Invest 75:377–383, 1985.

Shovlin CL, Hughes JMB, Simmonds HA, Fairbanks L, Deacock S, Lechler R, Roberts I, Webster ADB. Adult presentation of adenosine deaminase deficiency. Lancet 341:1471, 1993.

Shovlin CL, Simmonds HA, Fairbanks LD, Deacock SJ, Hughes JM, Lechler RI, Webster AD, Sun XM, Webb JC, Soutar AK. Adult onset immunodeficiency caused by inherited adenosine deaminase deficiency. J Immunol 153:2331–2339, 1994.

Silber GM, Winkelstein JA, Moen RC, Horowitz SD, Trigg M, Hong R. Reconstitution of T-and B-cell function after T-lymphocyte–depleted haploidentical bone marrow transplantation in severe combined immunodeficiency due to adenosine deaminase deficiency. Clin Immunol Immunopathol 44:317–320, 1987.

Simmonds HA, Fairbanks LD, Morris GS, Morgan G, Watson AR, Timms P, Singh B. Central nervous system dysfunction and erythrocyte guanosine triphosphate depletion in purine nucleoside phosphorylase deficiency. Arch Dis Child 62:385–391, 1987.

Simmonds HA, Levinsky RJ, Perrett D, Webster DR. Reciprocal relationship between erythrocyte ATP and deoxy-ATP levels in inherited ADA deficiency. Biochem Pharmacol 31:947–951, 1982a.

Simmonds HA, Sahota A, Potter CF, Cameron JS, Wadman SK. Purine metabolism and immunodeficiency. Urinary purine excretion as a diagnostic screening test in adenosine deaminase and purine nucleoside phosphorylase deficiency. Clin Sci Mol Med 54:579–584, 1978.

Simmonds HA, Sahota A, Potter CF, Perrett D, Hugh-Jones K, Watson JG. Purine metabolism in adenosine deaminase deficiency. In Elliot K, Whelan J, eds. Enzyme Defects and Immune Dysfunction, Ciba Foundation Symposium. New York, Excerpta Medica, 1979, pp 255–262.

Simmonds HA, Watson AR, Webster DR, Sahota A, Perrett D. GTP depletion and other erythrocyte abnormalities in inherited PNP deficiency. Biochem Pharmacol 31:941–946, 1982b.

Smith CM, Henderson JF. Deoxyadenosine triphosphate accumulation in erythrocytes of deoxycoformycin-treated mice. Biochem Pharmacol 31:1545–1551, 1982.

Snyder FF, Jenuth JP, Mably ER, Mangat RK. Point mutations at the purine nucleoside phosphorylase locus impair thymocyte differentiation in the mouse. Proc Natl Acad Sci USA 94:2522–2527, 1997.

Soutar RL, Day RE. Dysequilibrium/ataxic diplegia with immunodeficiency. Arch Dis Child 66:982–983, 1991.

Stephan JL, Vlekova V, Le Deist F, Blanche S, Donadieu J, De Saint-Basile G, Durandy A, Griscelli C, Fischer A. Severe combined immunodeficiency: a retrospective single center study of clinical presentation and outcome in 117 patients. J Pediatr 123:564–572, 1993.

Stephan JL, Wahn V, Le Deist F, Dirksen U, Broker B, Muller-Fleckenstein I, Horneff G, Schroten H, Fischer A, De Saint Basile G. Atypical X-linked severe combined immunodeficiency due to possible spontaneous reversion of the genetic defect in T cells. N Engl J Med 335:1563–1567, 1996.

Stoeckler JE, Agarwal RP, Agarwal KC, Schmid K, Parks RE, Jr. Purine nucleoside phosphorylase from human erythrocytes. Physiochemical properties of the crystalline enzyme. Biochemistry 17:278–283, 1978.

Stoop JW, Zegers BJM, Hendrickx GFM, Siegenbeek Van Heukelom LH, Staal GEJ, De Bree PK, Wadman SK, Ballieux RE. Purine nucleoside phosphorylase deficiency associated with selective cellular immunodeficiency. N Engl J Med 296:651–655, 1977.

Tam DA, Jr., Leshner RT. Stroke in purine nucleoside phosphorylase deficiency. Pediatr Neurol 12:146–148, 1995.

Tanaka C, Hara T, Suzaki I, Maegaki Y, Takeshita K. Sensorineural deafness in siblings with adenosine deaminase deficiency. Brain Devel 18:304–306, 1996.

Tezcan L, Ersoy F, Caglar M, Sanal O, Kotiloglu E, Aysun S. A case of adenosine deaminase–negative severe combined immunodeficiency with neurological abnormalities. Turk J Pediatr 37:383–389, 1995.

Thompson LF, Van De Wiele CJ, Laurent AB, Hooker SW, Vaughan JG, Jiang H, Khare K, Kellems RE, Blackburn MR, Hershfield MS, Resta R. Metabolites from apoptotic thymocytes inhibit thymopoiesis in adenosine deaminase–deficient fetal thymic organ cultures. J Clin Invest 106:1149–1157, 2000.

Tsuji E, Misumi Y, Fujiwara T, Takami N, Ogata S, Ikehara Y. An active-site mutation (Gly633>Arg) of dipeptidyl peptidase IV causes its retention and rapid degradation in the endoplasmic reticulum. Biochemistry 31:11921–11927, 1992.

Ullman B, Gudas LJ, Clift SM, Martin DW, Jr. Isolation and characterization of purine-nucleoside phosphorylase–deficient T-lymphoma cells and secondary mutants with altered ribonucleotide reductase. Genetic model for immunodeficiency disease. Proc Natl Acad Sci USA 76:1074–1078, 1979.

Ullman B, Gudas LJ, Cohen A, Martin DW, Jr. Deoxyadenosine metabolism and cytotoxicity in cultured mouse T lymphoma cells: a model for immunodeficiency disease. Cell 14:365–375, 1978.

Umetsu DT, Schlossman CM, Ochs HD, Hershfield MS. Heterogeneity of phenotype in two siblings with adenosine deaminase deficiency. J Allergy Clin Immunol 93:543–550, 1994.

Valerio D, Duyvesteyn MGC, van Ormondt H, Meera Khan P, van der Eb AJ. Adenosine deaminase (ADA) deficiency in cells derived from humans with severe combined immunodeficiency disease is due to an aberration of the ADA protein. Nucl Acids Res 12:1015–1024, 1984.

Van Beusechem VW, Kukler A, Heidt PJ, Valerio D. Long-term expression of human adenosine deaminase in rhesus monkeys transplanted with retrovirus-infected bone-marrow cells. Proc Natl Acad Sci USA 89:7640–7644, 1992.

Virelizier JL, Hamet M, Ballet JJ, Reinert P, Griscelli C. Impaired defense against vaccinia in a child with T-lymphocyte deficiency associated with inosine phosphorylase defect. J Pediatr 92:358–362, 1978.

Wakamiya M, Blackburn MR, Jurecic R, McArthur MJ, Geske RS, Cartwright J, Jr., Mitani K, Vaishnav S, Belmont JW, Kellems RE, Finegold MJ, Montgomery CA, Jr., Bradley A, Caskey CT. Disruption of the adenosine deaminase gene causes hepatocellular impairment and perinatal lethality in mice. Proc Natl Acad Sci USA 92:3673–3677, 1995.

Walcott DW, Linehan T, Hilman BC, Hershfield MS, El Dahr J. Failure to thrive, cough and oral candidiasis in a three month old male. Ann Allergy 72:408–414, 1994.

Watson AR, Evans DK, Marsden HB, Miller V, Rogers PA. Purine nucleoside phosphorylase deficiency associated with a fatal lymphoproliferative disorder. Arch Dis Child 56:563–565, 1981.

Weinberg K, Hershfield MS, Bastian J, Kohn D, Sender L, Parkman R, Lenarsky C. T lymphocyte ontogeny in adenosine deaminase deficient severe combined immune deficiency following treatment with polyethylene glycol modified adenosine deaminase. J Clin Invest 92:596–602, 1993.

Wiginton DA, Hutton JJ. Immunoreactive protein in adenosine deaminase deficient human lymphoblast cell lines. J Biol Chem 257:3211–3217, 1982.

Wiginton DA, Kaplan DJ, States JC, Akeson AL, Perme CM, Bilyk IJ, Vaughn AJ, Lattier DL, Hutton JJ. Complete sequence and structure of the gene for human adenosine deaminase. Biochemistry 25:8234–8244, 1986.

Williams SR, Goddard JM, Martin DW, Jr. Human purine nucleoside phosphorylase cDNA sequence and genomic clone characterization. Nucl Acids Res 12:5779–5787, 1984.

Wilson DK, Rudolph FB, Quiocho FA. Atomic structure of adenosine deaminase complexed with a transition-state analog: understanding catalysis and immunodeficiency mutations. Science 252:1278–1284, 1991.

Witte DP, Wiginton DA, Hutton JJ, Aronow BJ. Coordinate developmental regulation of purine catabolic enzyme expression in gastrointestinal and postimplantation reproductive tracts. J Cell Biol 115:179–190, 1991.

Wolfson JJ, Cross VF. The radiographic findings in 49 patients with combined immunodeficiency. In Pollara B, Pickering RJ, Meuwissen HJ, Porter IH, eds. Combined Immunodeficiency Disease and Adenosine Deaminase Deficiency: A Molecular Defect. New York, Academic Press, 1975, pp 255–277.

Wolos JA, Frondorf KA, Davis GF, Jarvi ET, McCarthy JR, Bowlin TL. Selective inhibition of T cell activation by an inhibitor of S-adenosyl-L-homocysteine hydrolase. J Immunol 150:3264–3273, 1993a.

Wolos JA, Frondorf KA, Esser RE. Immunosuppression mediated by an inhibitor of S-adenosyl-L-homocysteine hydrolase. J Immunol 151:526–534, 1993b.

Yang J, Liu X, Bhalla K, Kim CN, Ibrado AM, Cai J, Peng T-I, Jones DP, Wang X. Prevention of apoptosis by Bcl-2: release of cytochrome c from mitochondria blocked. Science 275:1129–1132, 1997.

Yang JC, Cortopassi GA. dATP causes specific release of cytochrome C from mitochondria. Biochem Biophys Res Comm 250:454–457, 1998.

Zannis V, Doyle D, Martin DW, Jr. Purification and characterization of human erythrocyte purine nucleoside phosphorylase and its subunits. J Biol Chem 253:504–510, 1978.

Zegers BJM, Stoop JW, Staal GEJ, Wadman SK. An approach to the restoration of T cell function in a purine nucleoside phosphorylase deficient patient. In Elliot K, Whelan J, eds. Enzyme Defects and Immune Dysfunction. New York, Excerpta Medica, 1979, pp 231–247.

Zhong H, Chunn JL, Volmer JB, Fozard JR, Blackburn MR. Adenosine-mediated mast cell degranulation in adenosine deaminase-deficient mice. J Pharmacol Exp Ther 298:433–440, 2001

Ziegler JB, Lee CL, Van der Weyden MB, Bagnara AS, Beveridge J. Severe combined immunodeficiency and adenosine deaminase deficiency failure of enzyme replacement therapy. Arch Dis Child 55:452–457, 1980.

Ziegler JB, Van der Weyden MB, Lee CH, Daniel A. Prenatal diagnosis for adenosine deaminase deficiency. J Med Genet 18:154–156, 1981.

C H A P T E R

17

Other Well-Defined Immunodeficiency Syndromes

Hans D. Ochs, David L. Nelson, and E. Richard Stiehm

With contributions by Rebecca H. Buckley, Genevieve de Saint-Basile, Eleonora Gambineri, Maria Ines Garcia Lloret, Anna Virginia Gulino, Charles H. Kirkpatrick, Steven M. Holland, Karin Nielsen, Luigi D. Notarangelo, Sergio D. Rosenzweig, John L. Sullivan, Kathleen E. Sullivan, and Troy R. Torgerson

OVERVIEW

This chapter discusses 14 familiar and not-so-familiar immunodeficiencies that have a striking heterogeneity in their clinical, laboratory, and genetic features. Four are primarily T-cell defects (DiGeorge syndrome, chronic mucocutaneous candidiasis, CD4 lymphocytopenia, OKT4 epitope deficiency), three are combined B- and T-cell defects (Wiskott-Aldrich syndrome, X-linked lymphoproliferative syndrome, cartilage-hair hypoplasia), three involve the natural killer (NK)/interferon/IL-12 system (Griscelli syndrome, IFN-γ/IL-12 receptor defects, NK-cell deficiency), one is a metabolic/nutritional defect (biotin-responsive immunodeficiency), and three defy ready categorization (hyper-IgE, WHIM, and IPEX syndromes). All modes of inheritance are represented but some have no clear hereditary pattern (NK-cell deficiency, idiopathic CD4 lymphocytopenia, most forms of chronic mucocutaneous candidiasis).

WISKOTT-ALDRICH SYNDROME (AND X-LINKED THROMBOCYTOPENIA)

Definition

The Wiskott-Aldrich syndrome (WAS) is an X-linked recessive disorder associated with microplatelet thrombocytopenia, eczema, recurrent infections, and an increased risk of autoimmunity and lymphoreticular neoplasia (Aldrich et al., 1954; Sullivan et al., 1994; Wiskott, 1937). In 1994, Derry and colleagues used positional cloning to identify the WASP gene (WAS protein) responsible for the disorder at Xp11.23.

Mutations of the WASP gene not only cause WAS but also cause X-linked thrombocytopenia (XLT), a milder form of the disease characterized by thrombocytopenia and small platelets but without the other clinical findings associated with the classic WAS phenotype (Derry et al., 1995; Villa et al., 1995; Zhu et al., 1995).

The identification of the WASP gene has provided an effective tool to confirm the diagnosis of WAS/XLT, to identify carrier females, and to facilitate prenatal diagnosis. WASP contains well-defined domains with unique functions suggesting a critical role of this complex protein in signal transduction and cytoskeletal reorganization (Machesky and Insall, 1998; Notarangelo and Ochs, 2003).

Historical Aspects

In 1937 Wiskott described three brothers with congenital thrombocytopenia, bloody diarrhea, eczema, and recurrent infections—one of the first immunodeficiency syndromes described. Seventeen years later, Aldrich and co-workers (1954) reported a large family with multiple affected males, demonstrating X-linked inheritance.

Following these clinical reports, the immunologic abnormalities characteristic of WAS were recognized, including progressive lymphopenia, absence of delayed-type hypersensitivity, and abnormal antibody production (Blaese et al., 1968; Cooper et al., 1968; Ochs et al., 1980). In addition to the consistent microplatelet thrombocytopenia, many functional and morphologic abnormalities of WAS platelets were recognized (Gröttum et al., 1969; Kuramoto et al., 1970; Ochs et al., 1980; Semple et al., 1997). An increased incidence of malignancies in WAS was observed as early as 1961 (Cotelingam at al., 1985; Kildeberg 1961; Sullivan et al., 1994; ten Bensel et al., 1966).

The WASP gene was mapped to the short arm of the X chromosome within the region of Xp11.23 (Kwan et al., 1991, 1995) and identified by positional cloning (Derry et al., 1994). Bone marrow transplantation (BMT) for WAS was first performed in 1968 (Bach et al., 1968) and is now the treatment of choice (Filipovich et al., 2001; Parkman et al., 1978).

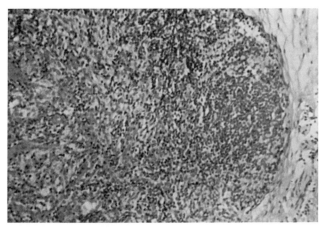

Figure 17-3· A lymph node biopsy from a 4-year-old patient with the Wiskott-Aldrich syndrome. There is moderated depletion of lymphoid cells in the thymic-dependent and thymic-independent areas and a lack of follicular formation.

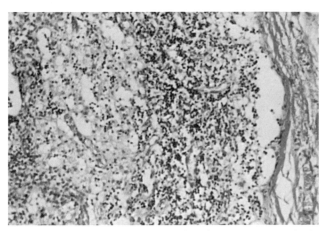

Figure 17-4· Lymph node biopsy taken from a patient with the Wiskott-Aldrich syndrome. He is the older brother (age 8 years) of the patient illustrated in Figure 17-3. There is a greater degree of lymphoid depletion and no evidence of follicular formation.

Diagnosis

Considering the wide spectrum of the clinical presentation, the diagnosis of WAS or XLT should be considered in any male with congenital or early-onset (or even transient) thrombocytopenia and small platelets, especially if other male relatives have been affected. A history of, or the presence of, mild or severe eczema supports the diagnosis.

Infections and immunologic abnormalities are characteristic of WAS but may be absent or mild in patients with the XLT phenotype. Autoimmune diseases and malignancies may develop in patients with WAS or less often in patients with XLT.

A presumptive diagnosis of WAS/XLT is based on congenital thrombocytopenia and small platelets (mean platelet volume <5.0 fl in most patients) in a male patient.

Flow cytometric analysis of lymphocytes for decreased or absent levels of WASP protein or RNA is a new but as yet commercially unavailable way to diagnose WAS/XLP. The gold standard, however, is to identify a mutation of the *WASP* gene.

Clinical Genetics

Mutation Analysis

The identification of the gene responsible for WAS/XLT has provided a definite tool to confirm the diagnosis in affected males, to identify carrier females, and to perform prenatal diagnosis. Techniques to sequence mRNA and/or genomic DNA of the *WASP* gene and to quantitate WASP by Western blot or flow cytometry are available in specialized laboratories. Knowing the quantity and size of mutated WAS protein expressed in cells from affected patients is of diagnostic value.

Of the 155 unrelated families studied at the University of Washington, Seattle, 79 had single base-pair (bp) substitutions within the coding region, resulting in 56 missense and 23 nonsense mutations (Fig. 17-5). Thirty mutations were caused by deletions and 13 by insertions, all but 2 resulting in frame shift. An additional 26 mutations affected a splice site. In seven families the mutation was complex.

Although mutations are found throughout the entire *WASP* gene and involve all 12 exons, the distribution of the independent mutations is skewed toward the N-terminal. The PH/WH1 domain, which includes exons 1, 2, and part of exon 3, comprises approximately 22% of the total amino acids but contains 45% of all mutations. This region also has an excess of substitutional events with 66% of missense/nonsense mutations located in exons 1 to 3. In contrast, exons 8 to 12, which encode more than 50% of the amino acids, contain only 26% of the mutations, which consist predominately of insertions and deletions resulting in frame shift or splice site mutations.

In the 155 unrelated families studied in a single center, 95 unique mutations were observed. A total of 24 mutations occurred more than once, representing 60 events. Five mutations were present in five or more families affecting a total of 38 families. Two of these hot spots (R211X and IVS8+1g–>n) are associated with classical WAS, and three (T45M, R86C/G/H/L, and IVS6+5g–>a) are associated with XLT.

Carrier Detection and Prenatal Diagnosis

X-inactivation studies in WAS carrier females have shown that the normal X chromosome is preferentially used as the active X chromosome in all hematopoietic cell lineages, including CD34+ cells (Wengler et al., 1995). One exception is in families with a very mild form of XLT in which X chromosome inactivation may be random (Inoue et al., 2002; Lutskiy et al., 2002; Zhu et al., 2002). If the WASP mutation is known in a given family, carrier females can be identified by mutation analysis. Similarly, prenatal diagnosis of a male fetus at risk for WAS/XLT can be accomplished by DNA analysis using chorionic villous sam-

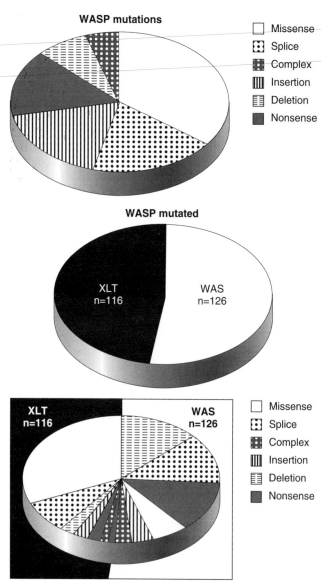

Figure 17-5 · **A.** Mutations of Wiskott-Aldrich syndrome protein (WASP) observed in a large cohort of Wiskott-Aldrich Syndrome (WAS)/X-linked thrombocytopenia (XLT) patients. **B.** The number of patients with XLT and WAS, respectively. **C.** Typical mutations observed in XLT patients and in WAS patients, respectively.

pling, or cultured amniocytes as the DNA source (Giliani et al., 1999).

Scoring System for WAS/XLT

A scoring system, presented in Table 17-1, postulates that patients with WAS or XLT have in common thrombocytopenia and small-sized platelets and that most affected males develop some form of immunodeficiency, although to a different degree (Zhu et al., 1997). The extent of eczema may be difficult to assess. Lack of a history of eczema or the presence of mild transient eczema that responds well to treatment, indicated by (+) in Table 17-1, and mild infrequent infections not resulting in sequelae indicated as (+) are consistent with XLT (score 1 or 2).

Treatment-resistant, moderate to severe eczema and recurrent infections despite optimal therapy are characteristic for classic WAS and are scored as moderate (score of 3) or severe (score of 4). If a patient, independent of his score, develops autoimmune disease or lymphoma, his original score (1 to 4) is changed to a score of 5.

Using these criteria, we and others (Lemahieu et al., 1999; Remold-O'Donnell et al., 1997; Zhu et al., 1997) observed a strong phenotype/genotype correlation, whereas others did not (Schindelhauer et al., 1996). Patients with missense mutations located within exons 1, 2, and 3 usually have mild disease. Other mutations observed in patients with mild disease include splice anomalies resulting in multiple splicing products.

As a rule, mutations associated with a mild phenotype have in common the expression of a normal-sized or truncated mutated protein, usually in decreased quantity. Mutations resulting in the absence of protein (e.g., nonsense mutations, out of frame insertions and deletions, and most splice site mutations) are associated with the classic WAS phenotype (Lemahieu et al., 1999; Remold-O'Donnell et al., 1997; Zhu et al., 1997).

Treatment

General Treatment

Improved nutrition, improved antimicrobial therapy, and prophylactic use of IVIG have markedly prolonged the life expectancy of WAS patients. Hematopoietic stem cell transplantation, especially if performed during infancy and childhood, has been highly successful in curing this lethal disease.

Early diagnosis is imperative for effective prophylaxis and treatment. Any infection requires an extensive evaluation for a bacterial, viral, or fungal cause followed by effective antimicrobial therapy. Because of the abnormal antibody responses to protein and polysaccharide antigens, patients with the classic WAS phenotype are candidates for prophylactic IVIG at full therapeutic doses. The dose of IVIG may be increased during infections that aggravate their already accelerated IgG catabolism. Continuous antibiotic therapy should be considered if infections are occurring despite IVIG therapy. PCP prophylaxis with trimethoprim-sulfamethoxazole should be used during the first 2 to 4 years of life.

Killed vaccines can be given, including pneumococcal polysaccharide-protein conjugate vaccines, but their response should be determined. Live-virus vaccines should not be used. Varicella-zoster immune globulin or acyclovir are indicated on exposure to chickenpox. Antivirals are used for herpes infections and for varicella. Bottled water can be used to prevent infectious diarrhea.

Eczema, if severe, requires aggressive therapy including local steroid and short-term systemic use of steroids. Cutaneous infection is common and necessitates local or systemic antibiotics. Lymphadenopathy is a feature of infected eczema. Whether the newly approved tacrolimus ointment (Protopic 0.03%) or primecrolimus cream (Elidel 1%) will be effective in the treatment of WAS-associated eczema remains to be seen. If

TABLE 17-1 · SCORING SYSTEM* TO DEFINE THE PHENOTYPES OF WASP MUTATIONS

	IXLT	XLT		WAS Classic			XLN
Score	<1	1	2	3	4	5	0
Thrombocytopenia	(+)	+	+	+	+	+	—
Small platelets	+	+	+	+	+	+	—
Eczema	—	—	(+)	+	++	(+)/+/++	—
Immunodeficiency	—	–/(+)	(+)	+	+	(+)/+	—
Infections	—	—	(+)	+	+/++	(+)/+/++	—
Autoimmunity and/or malignancy	—	—	—	—	—	+	—
Congenital neutropenia	—	—	—	—	—	—	+

*Scoring system:
  –/(+) absent or mild
  (+) mild, transient eczema or mild, infrequent infections, not resulting in sequelae
  + persistent but therapy-responsive eczema and recurrent infections requiring antibodies
  ++ eczema that is difficult to control and severe, life-threatening infections
Because patients with XLT may develop autoimmune disorders or lymphoma, although at a lower rate than those with classic WAS, a progression from a score of 1 or 2 to a score of 5 is possible for XLT.
IXLT = intermittent X-linked thrombocytopenia; WAS = Wiskott-Aldrich syndrome; WASP = Wiskott-Aldrich syndrome protein; XLN = X-linked neutropenia; XLT = X-linked thrombocytopenia.

food allergies are a problem, an appropriate restricted diet is indicated.

Platelet transfusions should be avoided unless the bleeding is serious; central nervous system (CNS) hemorrhages require immediate platelet transfusions. Blood products should be irradiated and cytomegalovirus (CMV) negative.

Aspirin, which interferes with platelet function, is contraindicated. Splenectomy, recommended by some for XLT patients, effectively stops the bleeding tendency by bringing the number of circulating platelets close to normal but will increase the risk of septicemia.

WAS and XLT patients who have undergone splenectomy require life-long prophylactic antibiotic therapy. Data collected at the National Institute of Health support the clinical experience that splenectomy does not affect the development of autoimmune diseases and malignancies (Blaese, personal communication, 2003).

High-dose IVIG and systemic steroids are indicated in the treatment of autoimmune complications. Immunosuppressive therapy, however, may cause reactivation of viruses or increase the risk for fungal infections.

TRANSPLANTATION

Hematopoietic stem cell transplantation, using bone marrow or cord blood and immunosuppression, is the only curative therapy available for WAS patients (Filipovich et al., 2001) (see Chapter 43). The most widely used conditioning regimen includes cyclophosphamide, busulfan, and anti-thymocyte globulin. Fully matched siblings are preferred donors, resulting in highly successful BMT even in older patients.

Matched unrelated donors can be used successfully in young boys with WAS; after the age of 5 to 8 years, the success rate of matched unrelated donor transplants decreases and unrelated donors are not recommended in older children (Filipovich et al., 2001).

Cord blood stem cells, fully or partially matched, are excellent alternatives for boys with WAS who weigh less than 25 kg, if a fully matched bone marrow donor is not available.

The use of haploidentical BMT has been disappointing (Brochstein et al., 1991; Hong, 1996; Ozsahin et al., 1996).

GENE THERAPY

Gene therapy for WAS is being explored. After transduction of WAS T cells with a retroviral vector expressing the WASP gene, the transformed T cells showed levels of WASP expression similar to those found in cells from normal individuals and, more importantly, became functionally normal (Wada et al., 2002). In a mouse model, WASP-deficient hematopoietic stem cells transduced with WASP-expressing retroviruses were transferred into lethally irradiated, RAG-2 deficient recipient mice. The gene-corrected cells developed into mature B and T cells. T-cell signaling was rescued, and the colitis associated with the transfer of WASP-deficient stem cells was prevented or ameliorated (Klein et al., 2002; Wada et al., 2002).

These in vivo experiments provide proof of principle that the WAS-associated T-cell signaling defect can be improved following transplantation of retrovirally transduced hematopoietic stem cells. In addition, the observation that several WAS patients spontaneously underwent in vivo reversions of an inherited mutation of the WASP gene in lymphocytes (Ariga et al., 2001; Wada et al., 2001) supports the hypothesis that in this syndrome genetically corrected stem cells have an in vivo advantage to develop into T cells, which is a prerequisite for successful gene therapy.

It is of interest that one patient with such a reversion had a typical WAS phenotype as a child but improved in his mid-20s, whereas all his affected relatives had classical WAS (Wada et al., 2001).

Prognosis

The life expectancy of infants with WAS born in the 1960s was less than 3 years (Cooper et al., 1968). Ten years later, the average age was 11 years (Sullivan et al., 1994), and many WAS patients now live past 20 years of age. However, the incidence of malignancies, most often B-cell lymphomas, increases substantially during the third decade of life in patients with classic WAS, and the causes of death have remained similar over the years: infections (44%), bleeding (23%), and malignancies (26%) (Hong, 1996). Patients undergoing successful BMT are cured from infections, bleeding, and autoimmune disease and seem not to develop excessive rates of malignancies.

X-LINKED LYMPHOPROLIFERATIVE SYNDROME

Definition

X-linked lymphoproliferative syndrome (XLP) is an X-linked primary immunodeficiency characterized by life-threatening vulnerability to EBV infection; EBV infection results in uncontrolled proliferation of B lymphocytes and cytotoxic T lymphocytes leading to fulminant infectious mononucleosis (IM); B-cell lymphomas; immunodeficiency; or, less commonly, aplastic anemia, necrotizing lymphoid vasculitis, and lymphoid granulomatosis. XLP is generally fatal by age 40 (Sullivan, 1999).

Historical Aspects

Thirty-five years ago Purtilo and Vawter performed an autopsy on an 8-year-old boy who died following IM (Purtilo et al., 1991). The death of the third male sibling in this family following a bout of IM led to the seminal publication in 1975 that described an X-linked progressive combined variable immunodeficiency termed Duncan's disease, now referred to as XLP (Purtilo et al., 1975).

Since its original description, more than 89 families with 309 affected males have been reported to the XLP registry, established in 1979 by Purtilo and colleagues (Hamilton and Purtilo, 1979; Seemayer et al., 1995; Sumegi et al., 2000).

In 1987, Skare and associates demonstrated that the XLP gene was located on the Xq24-27 interval of the long arm of the X chromosome; in 1989, they localized the gene to a region near DX572 and DXS37 (Skare et al., 1989). Also in 1989, Wyandt and colleagues reported an interstitial deletion in Xq25 in a male with XLP, localizing the gene to the Xq25 region of the X chromosome. In 1998, the XLP gene (SH2D1A) was cloned and its gene product identified as a small signal transduction protein (Coffey et al., 1998; Nichols et al., 1998; Sayos et al., 1998a).

Pathogenesis

There is some controversy as to whether the immune system of an individual with XLP is totally normal before EBV infection because most patients have normal numbers and function of T, B, and NK cells including proliferative responses to mitogens and antigens, a normal mixed leukocyte reaction, normal NK-cell activity; and normal antibody responses to vaccine antigens (Sullivan et al., 1983). However, some patients before EBV infection have subtle humoral deficiencies, and a few have severe infections (Grierson et al., 1991).

Response to EBV Infection

EBV is the trigger for the phenotypic expression of XLP in most individuals. Why EBV? EBV is a ubiquitous herpesvirus that infects most individuals beginning in early childhood. EBV is the only member of the herpesvirus family known to trigger the XLP phenotype. Individuals with XLP have normal responses to other viral infections including varicella zoster virus (VZV) and rubeola, viruses that are known to cause life-threatening infections in other T-cell immunodeficient patients (Hamilton et al., 1980; Purtilo et al., 1975; Sullivan et al., 1983).

The hallmark of acute EBV infection is a florid CD8 T-lymphocyte response to EBV-transformed B cells. Up to 10% of the total B cells may be EBV-infected and transformed during acute EBV infection. The vigorous EBV-specific cytotoxic CD8 response results in most circulating CD8 T cells becoming activated effector T cells (which accounts for the atypical lymphocytosis). Studies using major histocompatability complex (MHC) class I tetramer staining have confirmed that these CD8 T cells are EBV-specific and recognize lytic and latent EBV epitopes that can lyse EBV-transformed autologous B cells (Catalina et al., 2001). XLP patients with acute EBV infection have normal EBV antibody responses and CD8 T-lymphocyte responses, mimicking those of normals with acute EBV-induced IM.

The effector function of XLP CD8 T lymphocytes has not been extensively studied, but we demonstrated that, during acute EBV infection, cytotoxic T cells that recognize and kill autologous EBV-transformed B-lymphoblastoid cell lines are present in the peripheral blood (Sullivan et al., 1983). In addition, two laboratories have reported that males with XLP surviving EBV have MHC class I–restricted EBV-specific memory T-cell responses (Harada et al., 1982; Rousset et al., 1986).

Discovery and Function of the XLP Gene

In 1997 an international XLP consortium was formed to identify the XLP gene, and in 1998 Coffey and colleagues identified a gene encoding a polypeptide of 128 amino acid residues containing a single SH2 domain. The gene was designated SH2D1A for SH2 domain–containing gene 1A.

At the same time Sayos and co-workers (1998a, 1998b) reported the serendipitous discovery of the XLP gene when they identified a novel protein that binds to a signaling lymphocyte-activation molecule (SLAM), a type-1 transmembrane protein present on the surface of T and B cells. This novel protein, which they named SLAM-associated protein (SAP), was found to be encoded by a gene that mapped to a location on the murine X chromosome syntonous to the human Xq25 region. Subsequent studies showed that the SAP gene was identical to *SH2D1A*.

Work carried out simultaneously with that of Coffey and co-workers (1998), and Sayos and colleagues (1998a, 1998b) by Nichols and co-workers (1998) identified the XLP gene as a previously identified DSHP gene (with an unknown function). DSHP was also shown to be identical to *SH2D1A*.

Expression and Function of SH2D1A

Each of the three laboratories reporting the discovery of *SH2D1A* found messenger RNA (mRNA) expression in the thymus with lesser amounts expressed in the spleen, lymph nodes, peripheral blood, small intestine, lungs, and liver. T-cell populations including CD4 and CD8 cells, either isolated or in the tissues, also expressed SH2D1A mRNA, with activated cells expressing the largest amounts. Coffey and colleagues (1998) found SH2D1A expression in B lymphocytes and Nichols and co-workers (1998) reported mRNA expression in B cells by in situ hybridization.

Sayos and colleagues (1998b) on the other hand, failed to find SH2D1A mRNA expression in B cells of the normal mouse and reported that CD3 epsilon-null mice lacking T cells failed to express SH2D1A mRNA. All groups found that EBV-transformed B-lymphoblastoid cell lines did not express mRNA, whereas T-cell lines all showed mRNA expression. Nichols and co-workers (1998) demonstrated SH2D1A mRNA expression in both B- and T-cell lymphomas and in Hodgkin's disease.

The SH2D1A protein is one of the two known polypeptides (the other being EAT-2) (Thompson et al., 1996) that function as adaptor-like molecules and interact through their SH2 region with members of the SLAM family of immune receptors (Veillette and Latour, 2003).

The SH2D1A protein binds to at least three members of the SLAM family (Table 17-2). It has been hypothesized that the SH2 domain interacts with tyrosine phosphorylated molecules and that the COOH-terminal tail may play an important role in recruitment of downstream effector molecules in the signal transduction cascade. The interaction of SH2D1A with SLAM results in decreased interferon-γ (IFN-γ) production by activated T cells (Castro et al., 1999; Cocks et al., 1995), and the

SH2D1A-dependent stimulation of the 2B4 or NTB-A results in the triggering of NK-cell cytotoxicity (Sayos et al., 2000; Shlapatska et al., 2001; Tangye et al., 2000).

Sayos and colleagues (1998a, 1998b) hypothesized that the absence of SH2D1A in XLP results in defective helper and cytotoxic T-cell function and the inability of the immune system to completely eliminate EBV-infected B cells. Studies in SH2D1A-deficient mice have demonstrated exaggerated CD8 T-cell responses and excess IFN-γ production following infection with the Armstrong strain of lymphocytic choriomeningitis virus (Wu et al., 2001). Normal CD8 T-cell mediated cytotoxicity and NK-cell function was observed in SH2D1A-deficient mice before infection. These data are consistent with the observations made in patients with XLP.

Mutations in SH2D1A

In the largest study reported to date, Sumegi and co-workers (2000) found 28 different mutations in 34 XLP families. Table 17-3 lists the types of mutations observed. Deletions resulting in absence of the SH2D1A proteins were observed in 13 families, nonsense and missense mutations in 9 families each, and splice site mutation in 3 families. Each of the missense mutations altered critical amino acid residues in the SH2 domain of SH2D1A protein such as the substitution of a threonine for the arginine at position 32 of the SH2D1A protein found in patient 4 described by Coffey and colleagues (1998). All SH2 domains require this interior arginine residue to engage the phosphate group of the phosphotyrosine during protein-protein interactions. There is no correlation observed between genotype and phenotype or outcome.

Immunopathogenesis: A Role for Apoptosis?

Several points must be addressed by any hypothesis put forth to explain the pathogenesis of XLP. These include the following:

1. Most XLP patients have relatively normal immune systems before EBV infection and are able to mount normal immune responses to other viruses that require intact T-cell responses (Sullivan et al., 1983).

TABLE 17-2 · SLAM FAMILY OF IMMUNE CELL RECEPTORS THAT INTERACT WITH SH2D1A PROTEIN

Receptor	Tissue Expression	Function
SLAM	T cells, B cells, dendritic cells	Regulation of TCR-induced IFN-γ production
2B4	NK, CD8 T cells	Activation of NK-cell–mediated cytotoxicity
NTB-A	T, B, NK cells	Activation of NK-cell–mediated cytotoxicity

IFN = interferon; NK = natural killer; SLAM = signaling lymphocyte-activation molecule; TCR = T-cell receptor.

TABLE 17-3 · SPECTRUM OF SH2D1A GENE MUTATIONS REPORTED IN INDIVIDUALS WITH X-LINKED LYMPHOPROLIFERATIVE SYNDROME

Mutation	Number of Families (Individuals)	Predicated Effect
Deletion	13 (51)	No SH2D1A protein (5) Truncated SH2D1A protein (8)
Nonsense	9 (48)	Truncated SH2D1A protein (9) [6 ARG 55 stop]
Missense	9 (55)	Residue change at highly conserved sites in SH2 domain
Splice site	3 (16)	Truncated SH2D1A protein

2. Rare XLP patients develop a malignancy (usually a B-cell malignancy) before EBV infection (Seemayer et al., 1995).
3. Most XLP patients mount normal EBV-specific humoral and cell-mediated immune responses during the acute phase of their EBV infection (Harada et al., 1982; Rousset et al., 1986; Sullivan et al., 1983).

With these points in mind, we hypothesized in 1983 that control of the T-cell response initiated by EBV-infected B lymphocytes is the fundamental defect in XLP (Sullivan et al., 1983). In 1999, we modified this hypothesis to focus on the apoptosis pathway, which plays a central role in downregulating effector T-cell responses (Sullivan, 1999).

If SH2D1A plays a key role in initiating apoptosis in CD8 T cells, its absence would result in an exaggerated or abnormally prolonged cytotoxic T-cell response to EBV-infected B lymphocytes. Damage to the liver and the immune system would result from cytotoxic cytokines released by the proliferating CD8 T cells.

If SH2D1A plays an important role in a subpopulation of B lymphocytes, defective apoptosis may also result in the emergence of B-cell lymphomas following EBV infection. The rare occurrence of these lymphomas before EBV infection could be explained by a defect in an apoptosis pathway. A defect in a cell-type specific apoptosis pathway would explain the normal immune system before EBV infection and the ability of XLP patients to mount normal EBV-specific T- and B-cell responses.

Clinical Features

EBV-Uninfected Patients

Although most patients with XLP are asymptomatic before EBV infection, many have subtle immunologic abnormalities, notably hypogammaglobulinemia. Rare cases of severe infection including Neisserial meningitis, measles pneumonitis, and disseminated vaccinia have been described before EBV infection (Grierson et al., 1991).

Acute EBV Infection

Typical IM is the most common presenting feature, associated with fever, lymphadenopathy, hepatosplenomegaly,

pancytopenia, and hepatitis. The registry reports that 58% of the patients had severe progressive fatal IM (Hamilton et al., 1980; Seemayer et al., 1995).

Following EBV infection, several phenotypes may occur as presented in Table 17-4. These differ in frequency and prognosis with IM having the worst prognosis and immunodeficiency the best. Within the same kindred, different phenotypes can develop and indeed single patients may develop one or more clinical phenotypes during the course of the disease. Overall the outlook is unfavorable for prolonged survival.

Fulminant Infectious Mononucleosis

The most devastating form of XLP is fulminant IM, associated with uncontrolled EBV replication within B cells and polyclonal T-cell activation. The mean age of onset is age 5 years, but this may occur as early as 5 months of age. Classic features of acute IM are initially present including lymphocytosis, atypical lymphocytes, heterophile antibodies, and the appearance of other EBV antibodies (Purtilo et al., 1977; Sullivan et al., 1983).

The IM proceeds rapidly to hepatitis with liver failure, thrombocytopenia, coagulopathy, and encephalopathy. Bone marrow hypoplasia, myocarditis, and interstitial nephritis may develop. Virus-associated hemophagocytic syndrome (VACS) with hyperlipidemia, lymphadenopathy, macrophage activation, and widespread parenchymal infiltration of histiocytes containing erythrocytes and nuclear debris may develop.

The major cause of death in fulminant IM is liver failure secondary to widespread hepatic necrosis (Schuster and Kreth, 1999; Sullivan and and Woda, 1989; Weisenburger and Purtilo, 1986). Most die within 1 month of the onset of EBV infection. Examination of hepatic tissue reveals periportal infiltration of CD8 T lymphocytes.

Immunodeficiency

This phenotype usually occurs after EBV exposure but, as noted, may be present before EBV infection. About 30% of patients have this pattern. The median age of onset is 9 years. The immunodeficiency may be global, affecting T-, B-, or NK-cell function and is thought to be secondary to the widespread necrosis seen throughout the lymphoreticular system during acute EBV infection (Sullivan et al., 1983).

The most frequent manifestation of immunodeficiency is hypogammaglobulinemia with low IgG and IgG subclass levels, low IgA levels, low or normal IgM levels, and variable antibody deficiencies. Some patients may have elevated IgM and IgA levels. T-cell numbers may be normal, or there may be inversion of the CD4:CD8 ratio. T-cell and NK-cell function may be normal or low (Schuster and Kreth, 1999; Sullivan et al., 1983; Sullivan and Woda, 1989). These T-cell defects generally are not profound enough to result in the clinical picture of severe combined immunodeficiency (SCID).

With IVIG therapy, many of these children do well for many years, and this phenotype has the best prognosis. Some of these patients are misdiagnosed as having

TABLE 17-4 · PHENOTYPES EXPRESSED IN X-LINKED LYMPHOPROLIFERATIVE DISEASE COMPILED FROM THE X-LINKED LYMPHOPROLIFERATIVE SYNDROME REGISTRY

Phenotype	Frequency	Mortality
Life-threatening EBV infection	58%	96%
Immunodeficiency	31%	45%
Lymphoproliferative disorders	30%	69%
Aplastic anemia	3%	50%
Vasculitis, lymphomatoid granulomatosis	3%	61%

EBV = Epstein-Barr virus.

another primary immunodeficiency such as common variable immunodeficiency or a hyper-IgM syndrome.

Lymphoproliferative Disorders

About one third of patients with XLP develop lymphomas or other tumors. XLP has the highest incidence of malignancy of all the primary immunodeficiency syndromes (see Chapter 39). These patients have a risk of lymphoma 200-fold that of the general population (Grierson and Purtilo, 1987). The lymphomas are usually extranodal and most often affect the ileocecal region, but they can also occur in the CNS, liver, or kidney. As noted previously, they may occur before EBV infection.

Most of the lymphomas are non-Hodgkin's lymphomas of the Burkitt's type (53%), but Hodgkin's disease, other B-cell lymphomas, and T-cell lymphomas may occur. Some of these tumors appear before EBV infection, and some tumors following EBV infection have no EBV genome expression. The clinicopathologic features are similar to other lymphomas in terms of their histology, clonality, gene rearrangements, and response to therapy. Different histologic patterns may occur among lymphomas in the same kindred (Donhuijsen-Ant et al., 1988). Some lymphoproliferative patients develop other manifestations of XLP such as aplastic anemia or immunodeficiency following or during their treatment.

Aplastic Anemia

Aplastic anemia occurs in about 3% of XLP cases and is distinct from the marrow depletion associated with fulminant IM. It may consist of pancytopenia or pure red cell aplasia and is sometimes associated with other manifestation of XLP such as hypogammaglobulinemia or persistent hepatitis.

Lymphoid Vasculitis and Lymphomatoid Granulomatosis

An occasional patient may develop lymphoid vasculitis with arterial wall destruction and aneurysmal dilatation. Some have developed primary T-cell pulmonary lymphomatoid granulomatosis before EBV infection, and others have developed CNS granulomas (Purtilo et al., 1991).

Laboratory Features

As noted previously, some affected males have subtle immunologic defects before EBV infection. Usually these are not associated with symptoms, but some may be severe enough to cause serious infection. Grierson and colleagues (1991) identified variable deficiencies of IgG, IgG1 or IgG3, in all 13 patients studied before EBV infections. Some patients had elevated IgA and IgM levels. Seven were receiving IVIG.

Purtilo and co-workers (1989) described a failure of switching from IgM to IgG antibody following challenge with the neoantigen bacteriophage φX-174; this

was used as a diagnostic test before molecular identification of the gene.

During the initial EBV infection the characteristic laboratory features of IM are present and often exaggerated, including leukocytosis, atypical lymphocytosis, thrombocytopenia, and bone marrow hyperplasia. Liver abnormalities are common and progressive, often leading to coagulopathy with liver failure. Evidence of EBV infection is indicated by the presence of heterophile antibodies, other EBV antibodies, and positive tests for EBV genome in the blood or tissues. Activated T cells are present; these are usually cytotoxic CD8 cells, resulting in the atypical lymphocytosis.

The bone marrow, although initially hyperplastic, may become infiltrated with lymphoid and plasma cells. Necrosis and histiocytic hemophagocytosis may also be present.

Following EBV infection, a variety of immunologic abnormalities may develop including cutaneous anergy, an elevated CD8 count with a reversed CD4:CD8 ratio, and decreased lymphoproliferative responses to mitogens and antigens (Lindstren et al., 1982; Sullivan and Woda, 1989). Hypogammaglobulinemia may develop with diminished antibody responses and decreased in vitro immunoglobulin synthesis (Lai et al., 1987; Yasuda et al., 1991).

There may be diminished IFN-γ synthesis following activation of mononuclear cells (MNCs) with autologous T-cell lines (Yasuda et al., 1991), unlike the normal or increased IFN-γ synthesis during EBV infection (Sullivan, 1983). Sullivan and co-workers (1980) described a progressive loss of NK cytotoxicity, in part corrected by incubation with interferon.

Following EBV infection, EBV-specific antibody titers to EBNA are usually decreased or absent, and VCA antibodies are variable. Some patients with severe antibody defects have no EBV antibodies. Most patients have normal immune responses to other herpesvirus infections.

Definitive diagnosis of EBV infection is established by identifying EBV DNA within the blood or tissues using polymerase chain reaction (PCR) techniques.

Pathologic finding of patients succumbing with XLP include infiltration of proliferating lymphocytes, histiocytes, and plasma cells in the liver, spleen, and lymph nodes and thymic atrophy, in addition to the characteristic features of the phenotypic pattern of illness. As noted, some of the lymphomas identified are of T-cell origin.

Carrier females may have subtle immunoglobulin abnormalities (Grierson and Purtilo, 1987; Sakamoto et al., 1982) including an elevated serologic response to EBV. Grierson and Purtilo (1987) reported a high frequency of elevated levels of VCA antibodies, IgA and IgM VCA antibodies; EA antibodies were also noted. These serologic abnormalities are not reliable tests to identify the carrier state.

Diagnosis

The discovery of the *SH2D1A* gene now makes definitive diagnosis by mutation analysis of XLP possible in suspected patients, carriers, and uninfected siblings. Diagnostic criteria are listed in Table 17-5.

Before identification of the gene, the diagnosis was based on a combination of a family history, characteristic clinical and laboratory features, and indirect genotype analysis, using alleles of flanking markers at the XLP locus (Schuster et al., 1994).

Differential diagnosis of a boy suspected of XLP includes sporadic fatal IM (Mroczek et al., 1987); familial non-X linked severe EBV infection (Fleisher et al., 1982); and other primary immunodeficiencies such as X-linked agammaglobulinemia, common variable immunodeficiency, one of the hyper-IgM syndromes, and Fas deficiency (Schuster and Kreth, 1998). Antibody-deficient males without a molecular diagnosis should be screened for a *SH2D1A* mutation.

Treatment

Prevention of EBV Infection

Although the use of IVIG in asymptomatic EBV-seronegative patients in an attempt to prevent EBV infection is not reliably protective (Okano et al., 1990; Purtilo et al., 1991; Seemayer et al., 1995), we have used high-dose IVIG (600 mg/kg/month) in six males with XLP seronegative for EBV. All have remained EBV-uninfected as determined by EBV-PCR for up to 15 years after initiating therapy. Prophylactic antiviral therapy (e.g., acyclovir) is of unproven value in preventing EBV infection (Purtilo et al., 1991).

Treatment of Acute EBV Infection

During the initial EBV infection with severe IM, high-dose IVIG or acyclovir is ineffective. Therapy should be directed at elimination of both activated T cells and EBV-transformed B lymphocytes. The use of recently developed monoclonal antibodies against T cells (CAMPATH) and B cells (Campath and Rituxin) has not been reported, but their use in this setting may be warranted.

Etoposide to diminish macrophage activation and immunosuppressive agents (e.g., cyclosporine) to decrease cytotoxic activity may be of value in patients with a hemophagocytic syndrome or an aplastic crisis (Migliorati et al., 1994; Seemayer et al., 1995).

Other Therapy

The sequelae of EBV infection such as immunodeficiency, lymphoma, or aplastic anemia are treated as in other non-XLP afflicted patients. IVIG and other supportive care are used for patients with antibody deficiency. Many of these latter patients do well for prolonged periods on this therapy.

The lymphomas can often be brought into prolonged remission with standard chemotherapy or radiotherapy, but eventual relapse is the rule.

Transplantation

The only curative therapy is hematopoietic stem cell transplantation. Gross and colleagues (1996) reported on seven XLP patients who received human leukocyte antigen (HLA)-identical stem cell transplants with pretransplant immunosuppression. All seven of the patients were post-EBV and had one or more sequelae including lymphoproliferative disease (four patients), immunodeficiency (four patients), or fulminant IM (one patient). Six of the donors were siblings (including one umbilical cord blood), and one was an unrelated matched donor. All of the patients engrafted; six had acute graft-versus-host disease (GVHD); none had chronic GVHD. Four are alive and well 3 years after transplant. All but the cord blood infant donor were from EBV-seropositive donors. In the recipients, younger age and lack of infections were associated with a better prognosis.

Ziegner and co-workers (2001) used unrelated partially matched cord blood to transplant two boys with XLP before EBV infection; they point out that cord blood might be preferable to matched unrelated donors because cord blood is generally EBV negative.

Prognosis

As noted in Table 17-4, there is a very high mortality, particularly in those with fulminant IM. Seemayer and colleagues (1995) reported that 70% of patients die before age 10, and only two patients in the registry have survived beyond age 40. These grim statistics point out the importance of early diagnosis and stem cell transplantation.

John L. Sullivan

. . . .

TABLE 17-5 · X-LINKED LYMPHOPROLIFERATIVE SYNDROME (XLP) DIAGNOSTIC CRITERIA

Definitive Diagnosis of XLP

Male patient with lymphoma/Hodgkin's disease, fatal EBV infection, immunodeficiency, aplastic anemia, or lymphohistiocytic disorder and at least one of the following: (1) mutations in SH2D1A, (2) absent SH2D1A RNA on Northern blot analysis of lymphocytes, and (3) absent SH2D1A protein in lymphocytes.

Probable Diagnosis of XLP

Male patient experiencing death, lymphoma/Hodgkin's disease, immunodeficiency, aplastic anemia, or lymphohistiocytic disorder following acute EBV infection and maternal cousins, uncles, or nephews with a history of similar diagnoses following acute EBV infection.

XLP Phenotype

Male patient experiencing death, lymphoma/Hodgkin's disease, immunodeficiency disorder, aplastic anemia or lymphohistiocytic disorder following acute EBV infection and who have normal expression of SH2D1A.

EBV = Epstein-Barr virus.

X-LINKED IMMUNE DYSREGULATION WITH POLYENDOCRINOPATHY SYNDROME (IPEX SYNDROME)

Definition

Immune dysregulation, polyendocrinopathy, enteropathy, X-linked (IPEX) syndrome is an X-linked recessive disorder associated with mutations in the *FOXP3* gene at Xp11.23 and characterized by overwhelming, systemic autoimmunity resulting from a defect in immune system regulation. Affected males typically present during the first year of life with diarrhea (enteropathy), eczematous rash, endocrine disease (diabetes or thyroid disease), and other autoimmune phenomena (Torgerson and Ochs, 2002; Wildin et al., 2002).

Historical Aspects

IPEX was initially described in 1982 in a large family with 19 clinically affected males in a five-generation pedigree (Powell et al., 1982). Many of the patients had the characteristic triad of enteropathy, dermatitis, and endocrine abnormalities and some had other autoimmune phenomena including hemolytic anemia and collagen-vascular disease. Most of the affected patients died before the age of 3 of either metabolic or infectious causes (Powell et al., 1982).

Interestingly, 33 years before this initial description of IPEX, a spontaneously occurring mutant mouse strain called *Scurfy* was identified, which has many phenotypic similarities to IPEX including enteropathy with runting, dermatitis, X-linked inheritance, and early lethality (Russell et al., 1959). An indication that the human and mouse diseases were related came from linkage analysis, which pinpointed the responsible locus of the mutated gene in each to the pericentromeric region of the X chromosome (Xp11.23 to Xq21.1) (Ferguson et al., 2000; Means et al., 2000).

Because the gene encoding the WASP also lies within this region, IPEX was originally thought to be a WAS variant. However, the sequence of the *WASP* gene was found to be normal in IPEX patients and carrier females (Bennett et al., 2000; Ferguson et al., 2000).

Subsequent cloning of *Foxp3*, the causative gene in the *Scurfy* mouse (Brunkow et al., 2001), and the association of the human IPEX syndrome with mutations in *FOXP3*, the human orthologue of the mouse gene, verified that these two syndromes are indeed homologous (Bennett et al., 2001b; Chatila et al., 2000; Wildin et al., 2001).

Pathogenesis

Scurfy Mouse Model

Much of what is known about the pathogenesis of IPEX has been derived from observations on the *Scurfy* mouse model but is yet to be specifically confirmed in humans.

Affected *Scurfy* males typically appear sick in the second week of life and most die by age 3 weeks from an overwhelming autoimmune syndrome. Adoptive transfer experiments have demonstrated that CD4[+] T cells from an affected *Scurfy* male can transfer the disease to a lymphopenic mouse, thereby confirming that these are the effector cells that drive the process (Blair et al., 1994; Godfrey et al., 1994).

The CD4[+] *Scurfy* T cells are able to cause disease because they lack regulation by CD4[+]CD25[+] regulatory T cells, a lymphocyte subset absent in *Scurfy* mice (Fontenot et al., 2003; Hori et al., 2003; Khattri et al., 2003). This subset of regulatory cells typically makes up 5% to 10% of the normal CD4[+] T-cell population and plays an important role in maintaining peripheral immune tolerance by suppressing growth and proliferation of other activated cells (reviewed by Francois Bach, 2003).

Foxp3 has recently been shown to play a crucial role in the development and function of CD4[+]CD25[+] regulatory T cells and that animals lacking Foxp3 also lack these cells (Fontenot et al., 2003; Khattri et al., 2003). Absence of their regulatory activity allows other cells to take on an activated phenotype and respond in an uncontrolled fashion to both foreign and self-antigens. Thus as the disease progresses in *Scurfy* mice, there is a marked increase in Mac1[+] (monocytic) cells and a decrease in B220[+] cells within the spleen and lymph nodes.

These changes are accompanied by an increase in the proportion of CD4[+] T cells that express activation-related cell-surface markers including CD25, CD69, and CD40L. In addition, B220[+] cells show increased expression of B7.1 (CD80) and B7.2 (CD86) costimulatory molecules (Clark et al., 1999). Despite this activation, *Scurfy* T cells maintain their requirement for a second signal when they are activated through the T-cell receptor but are hyperresponsive to stimulation, producing large amounts of granulocyte-macrophage colony-stimulating factor (GM-CSF) (>1000-fold higher than wild-type CD4[+] T cells) and a number of other cytokines including IL-2, IL-4, IL-5, IL-6, IL-7, IL-10, IFN-γ, and tumor necrosis factor-α (TNF-α) (Clark et al., 1999).

Interestingly, this hyperresponsiveness is resistant to suppression by cyclosporine, genistein, or herbamycin A, which are potent inhibitors of key signaling molecules required for T-cell activation (Clark et al., 1999). Despite this hyperresponsiveness, the T cells do not consistently show an activated phenotype based on cell surface markers.

FOXP3 Gene

The *FOXP3* gene is located at Xp11.23 and consists of 11 translated exons that encode a protein of 431 amino acids in humans and 429 amino acids in mice. The two proteins have 86% sequence identity. The gene is expressed primarily in lymphoid tissues (thymus, spleen, and lymph nodes), particularly in CD4[+]CD25[+] regulatory T cells. It is expressed at low levels in CD4[+]CD25[-] cells and not significantly expressed in CD8[+] cells (Brunkow et al., 2001; Hori et al., 2003).

The mutation present in the *Scurfy* mouse is a two-bp insertion leading to a frame shift and loss of the entire forkhead domain (Brunkow et al., 2001). To date, 17 different *FOXP3* mutations in approximately 20 families have been identified (Gambineri et al., 2003). The majority of these are missense mutations within the C-terminal forkhead DNA-binding domain, but there are also mutations affecting the leucine zipper and N-terminal proline-rich domain, suggesting their importance for FOXP3 function (Gambineri et al., 2002). Two other mutations, one within an intron-exon splice junction and one in the first polyadenylation signal of the gene, tend to lead to a somewhat milder, late onset form of the disease (Bennett et al., 2001a).

Not all patients with the IPEX phenotype have *FOXP3* mutations. In a cohort of 27 affected males from 24 families, only 60% had an identifiable mutation. Another 10% who lacked mutations were found to have low mRNA expression levels (Gambineri et al., 2003). These data suggest that defects in other genes or gene products may generate a similar phenotype.

FOXP3 Protein

The FOXP3 protein has several interesting structural features including a proline-rich domain at the N-terminus, a zinc finger and leucine zipper (both conserved structural motifs involved in protein–protein interactions) in the central portion, and a forkhead DNA-binding domain at the C-terminus from which it derives its name (forkhead box) (Torgerson and Ochs, 2002). There is a putative nuclear localization signal at the C-terminal portion of the forkhead domain. Proteins bearing forkhead DNA-binding motifs comprise a large family of related molecules that play diverse roles in enhancing or suppressing transcription from specific binding sites, and several members of this protein family are involved in patterning and development (Gajiwala and Burley, 2000).

Clinical Features

As noted, the clinical triad among most patients with mutations of *FOXP3* is enteropathy, dermatitis, and endocrinopathy. Enteropathy with failure to thrive is present in virtually every case and usually presents in early infancy with watery diarrhea that may at times contain mucus and blood. Villous atrophy is the most common finding at biopsy, and some patients have been misdiagnosed as having inflammatory bowel disease.

Dermatitis is also described in virtually every case of IPEX and is most commonly eczematous in nature. Endocrinopathy is present in most but not all patients. Early-onset insulin-dependent diabetes mellitus is the most common endocrinopathy, but thyroid disease, either hypothyroidism or hyperthyroidism, is also common (Wildin et al., 2002).

In addition to the clinical triad, most patients have other autoimmune phenomena including Coombs'-positive hemolytic anemia, immune thrombocytopenia, autoimmune neutropenia, lymphadenopathy, splenomegaly, tubular nephropathy, or alopecia (Di Rocco and Marta, 1996; Ferguson et al., 2000; Hattevig et al., 1982; Jonas et al., 1991; Peake et al., 1996; Powell et al., 1982; Satake et al., 1993).

In most cases, affected males develop symptoms early in infancy, and most die within the first 2 years of life of either metabolic derangements or sepsis, which occurs in some patients before the initiation of immunosuppressive therapy (Kobayashi et al., 2001; Levy-Lahad and Wildin, 2001; Powell et al., 1982).

It is unclear whether IPEX patients have increased susceptibility to infection as a result of 2 years genetic defect or whether this is secondary to other clinical features such as decreased barrier function of the skin and gut or to immunosuppressive therapy. In a series of 27 patients with an IPEX phenotype, half had serious infections, including sepsis, meningitis, pneumonia, and osteomyelitis, many occurring before the initiation of immunosuppressive therapy. The most common pathogens were *Staphylococcus*, CMV, and *Candida* (Gambineri et al., 2003).

Heterozygous female carriers of *FOXP3* mutations appear to be healthy, although one female carrier was shown to have an expression level of *FOXP3* mRNA that is intermediate between the low level of expression by her affected son and that of a normal patient (Bennett et al., 2001a). X-chromosome inactivation analysis performed on one carrier female demonstrated that both normal and mutated *FOXP3* alleles are equally expressed in circulating T lymphocytes (Tommasini et al., 2002).

Laboratory Features

The laboratory findings in patients with IPEX syndrome are strikingly normal given the dramatic clinical phenotype. Anemia and thrombocytopenia resulting from autoantibodies may be present. Other than intermittent eosinophilia, circulating leukocyte counts and T- and B-cell subsets tend to remain normal (Ferguson et al., 2000; Peake et al., 1996; Powell et al., 1982; Wildin et al., 2002). Patients with IPEX have normal neutrophil function and normal complement levels.

The most consistent finding is a markedly elevated IgE level with normal IgG, IgM, and IgA levels. The patients are able to make protective antibody responses to immunizations, but, in some patients, immunization has been reported to precipitate a clinical crisis (Powell et al., 1982).

Over time, affected males typically generate a variety of autoantibodies to multiple targets including thyroid, islet cells, small bowel mucosa, erythrocytes, and platelets. Autoantibodies to a novel 75-kD gut and kidney-specific antigen, AIE-75, have been described in IPEX patients (Kobayashi et al., 1998).

Cultured peripheral blood MNCs from IPEX patients show increased response to activation with excess production of the Th2 cytokines IL-4, IL-5, IL-10, and IL-13 and decreased production of the Th1 cytokine IFN-γ (Chatila et al., 2000).

Caution must be exercised regarding the immune responses of IPEX patients because most are on immunosuppressive drugs at the time of diagnosis.

Treatment

Immunosuppressive agents that target T-cell activation such as cyclosporine and FK-506, either alone or in combination with steroids, are the most effective treatment (Di Rocco and Marta, 1996; Kobayashi et al., 1995). None of these drugs seems to maintain long-term remission, and many patients have ultimately failed therapy because of toxicity or infection.

Hematopoietic stem cell transplantation is the only cure for the IPEX syndrome, and some patients have achieved a complete remission following BMT despite the presence of achieving only 20% to 30% of donor T cells (Baud et al., 2001). The success of transplantation may be dependent on its performance before irreversible damage to target organs such as pancreas and thyroid.

The patient reported by Baud and colleagues (2001) had complete symptomatic remission during his conditioning regimen that consisted of anti–T-lymphocyte globulin, busulfan, and cyclophosphamide, raising the possibility that cytotoxic or biologic agents that target T cells may be effective in patients who have failed other therapies.

Prognosis

In general, the prognosis of IPEX is poor. Untreated, most patients die within the first 2 years of life. Patients with unusual mutations such as those affecting mRNA splicing or polyadenylation may make a small amount of normal messenger RNA and thereby have a relatively milder phenotype; however, even these patients do poorly, with most dying by the third decade of life (Bennett et al., 2001a; Powell et al., 1982).

Treatment with potent immunosuppressive agents targeting T cells are of some benefit short-term, but because of their toxicity and the increased susceptibility to infection, they generally do not result in long-term amelioration of symptoms.

BMT provides the possibility of cure; however, its risks are substantial and it must be performed before permanent organ damage ensues.

Troy R. Torgerson and Eleonora Gambineri

DIGEORGE SYNDROME AND CHROMOSOME 22q11.2 DELETION SYNDROME

Definition

DiGeorge syndrome (DGS) is classically defined as a congenital T-cell immunodeficiency characterized by a conotruncal cardiac anomaly, hypocalcemic tetany, unusual facies, and a hypoplastic thymus gland. Pathologically, in addition to the absence or hypoplasia of the thymus, there are parathyroid gland, aortic arch, and cardiac defects. Many, but not all, patients with DGS have a heterozygous deletion of chromosome 22q11.2.

When all patients with the deletion are considered, the clinical spectrum includes many children without the typical DiGeorge phenotype, and the spectrum of immunodeficiency ranges from a profound SCID to a completely normal immune system. In this chapter, patients with the deletion and patients with the clinical picture of DGS who do not have the deletion both are discussed.

Nomenclature

The phenotype of DGS may be seen in patients with isotretinoid fetopathy, maternal diabetes, fetal alcohol syndrome, Zellweger syndrome, CHARGE association, Opitz G/BBB syndrome, and a variety of other conditions (Greenberg, 1993). Some of these patients have the characteristic deletion and some do not. The most common cause of the syndrome is a hemizygous deletion of 22q11.2 (Adachi et al., 1998; de la Chapell et al., 1981; Kelley et al., 1982). This deletion is one of the most common chromosomal abnormalities known with a frequency in the general population of approximately 1:4000 (Devriendt et al., 1998; Goodship et al., 1998).

In DGS cases with the deletion, it is most appropriate to use the terminology of *DiGeorge syndrome with chromosome 22q11.2 deletion*. Not all patients with the 22q11.2 deletion have the clinical picture of DGS. Most patients with the deletion do not have the characteristic triad of conotruncal cardiac anomaly, hypocalcemia, and a hypoplastic thymus gland. They are often said to have *velocardiofacial (Shprintzen) syndrome* or *conotruncal anomaly face syndrome*, or their phenotypic features may be so mild that they do not carry a syndromic diagnosis.

Sometimes these patients are collectively called the *CATCH 22 syndrome* (for *c*ardiac defects, *t*hymic hypoplasia, *c*left palate, *h*ypocalcemia and chromosome 22 abnormalities); this mnemonic is best avoided, particularly when referring to individual patients. These patients are probably best served by stating that they have chromosome 22q11.2 deletion syndrome. For the unusual patients who have DGS but do not have the deletion, it is best to state that they have DGS without the chromosome 22q11.2 deletion.

The immunodeficiency has been characterized as either complete or partial. This categorization was based on the level of immunologic function. The distinction between the two categories was imprecise, and it is now better appreciated that there is a continuum of immunologic function in patients with the deletion. Nevertheless, the term *complete DiGeorge syndrome* continues to be used to designate those patients with profound cellular deficiency who require reconstitution.

Historical Aspects

In 1965, Dr. Angelo DiGeorge described congenital absence of the thymus gland associated with congenital hypoparathyroidism in four patients, one of which had absent T-cell immunity, normal immunoglobulin levels, and deficient antibody production (Lischner and DiGeorge, 1969).

This combination had been described by LH Harrington in 1829 and David Lobdell in 1959, but the recognition that these organs had a common developmental origin was not appreciated. Impaired neural crest cell migration into the third and fourth pharyngeal arches during the fourth week of embryonic development is believed to underlie many of the observed defects (Bockman and Kirby, 1985; Kirby and Bockman 1984).

In the early 1980s, the association of DGS with chromosome 22 defects was first described (de la Chapelle et al., 1981; Kelley et al., 1982). Later studies confirmed that 90% to 95% of patients with the clinical picture of DGS had monosomic submicroscopic deletions of chromosome 22q11.2 (Carey et al., 1992; Emanuel et al., 1992, 2003).

Several candidate genes within this region have been identified, and, using knockout mice, three genes, *TBX1, Crkol,* and *UFDIL,* have been implicated in the phenotype of DGS. To date no point mutations or single gene deletions have been identified in humans (Lindsay et al., 2001).

With the recognition that the profound immunologic defect present in some patients may be due to deficient thymic function, two early successful fetal thymus transplants were recorded (August et al., 1968; Cleveland et al., 1968). Hematopoietic stem cell transplantation from an HLA-identical sibling was first used with success in 1987 (Goldsobel et al., 1987). Most recently non-HLA matched cultured neonatal thymic tissue has been used successfully (Markert et al., 1997a, 1999, 2003).

Pathogenesis

Immunopathogenesis

Originally the T-cell defect was considered to result from the small thymic mass. However, small morphologically normal undescended thymi were found at autopsy in patients dying of causes unrelated to immune deficiency. This finding, associated with the observation that the T-cell deficiency was sometimes partial or transient, suggests that a small gland required time to grow to generate normal T-cell function. Bastian and co-workers (1989) reviewed 18 patients with DGS. All patients had cardiac surgery or were examined at autopsy or during cardiac surgery. In only three patients was the thymus present in the mediastinum. Additional studies confirmed that small thymic rests are found in the neck.

Hong (1996) postulated that there is a failure of descent in most cases of partial or incomplete DGS and that the undescended thymi reside in sites such as the tongue, thyroid, and middle ear where they cannot be clinically noticeable but are able to provide competent T-cell function. Thus he believes that an absent thymus gland results in the complete DGS.

Chromosomal Abnormalities

Following identification that most patients with DGS had a 22q11 deletion, it was shown that these deletions were mediated by low copy number repeats and typically encompass the same 2.5-Mb region (Edelman et al., 1999). Within this region are approximately 25 genes whose functions have been largely characterized.

Mice heterozygous for the *TBX1* gene (Jerome and Papaioannou, 2001; Lindsay et al., 2001; Merscher et al., 2001) have aortic arch anomalies but no other characteristics of DGS. Mice homozygous for the deletion die near birth but display hypoplasia of the thymus and parathyroid glands and cleft palate (Jerome and Papaioannou, 2001). TBX1 is a T-box transcription factor that may require specific concentrations for its effect. Thymic hypoplasia was revealed on different genetic backgrounds, suggesting some phenotypic variability in this syndrome may be due to partial compensation by other genes.

A second candidate gene, *Crkol,* is implicated in the development of aortic arch, thymus, and craniofacial structures (Guris et al., 2001). It is required for the development of neural crest cells in this region. A heterozygous deletion of *Crkol* in mice has no phenotypic abnormalities, whereas mice homozygous for the deletion die *in utero* of multiple congenital anomalies including aortic arch anomalies, thymic hypoplasia, and facial anomalies.

A third gene, *UFD1L,* is expressed in the relevant tissues and plays a role in the degradation of ubiquitinated proteins (Yamagishi et al., 1999). Mice homozygous for a deletion of this gene have aortic arch anomalies; however, heterozygous mice have a normal phenotype (Lindsay et al., 1999).

These studies suggest that there are differences in the manner in which mice and humans manifest different genetic defects or that multiple gene effects may be required for the full phenotypic expression of DGS. Importantly, when the whole region of murine chromosome 16 (which is syntenic with the human chromosome 22q11.2 region) was deleted, the heterozygous mice had only a cardiac phenotype (Lindsay et al., 1999, 2001). This would suggest that differences in the phenotype relate more to species differences than additive genetic effects.

Nevertheless, confirmation of a single gene effect in humans will require demonstration of a point mutation in the relevant gene replicating the full phenotype of DGS. To date, no point mutations or single gene deletions have been identified in humans (Lindsay et al., 2001).

The basis for the syndrome without the characteristic deletion is often unknown. Some patients will have a known exposure to toxins such as isotretinoin or maternal alcohol ingestion. There is also a small subset who have deletions of chromosome 10p13-14 (Greenberg et al., 1986; Schuffenhauer et al., 1998). These deletions are different from the chromosome 22q11.2 deletions in that they vary from patient to patient (Daw et al., 1996).

Two regions determine different phenotypic features with deletion of 10p13-14 causing hypoparathyroidism, cardiac anomalies, and immune deficiency. Deletion of the telomeric 10p14-10pter results in deafness, renal anomalies, and hypoparathyroidism. This syndrome is often termed the hypoparathyroidism, deafness, renal anomaly (HDR) syndrome and is due to deletion or mutation of the GATA3 gene (Van Esch et al., 2000).

When the phenotypic features of the patients with the 10p deletion are compared with those of the patients with the chromosome 22q11.2 deletion, the only difference is an increased association with deafness in the patients with the 10p deletion (Van Esch et al., 1999).

The chromosome 10p deletions are thought to cause the DGS phenotype in approximately 2% of the cases

and may be detected through the use of 10p FISH analyses. One center performs both the chromosome 22q11.2 and 10p FISH simultaneously (Berend et al., 2000).

Clinical Features

Infants

The original descriptions of children with DGS ascertained only the most severely affected infants (Barrett et al., 1981; Conley et al., 1979; DiGeorge, 1968; Lischner and Huff, 1975; Muller et al., 1988). These children were recognized by characteristic facial features including hypertelorism; downturning eyes; low-set, posteriorly rotated, prominent ears with notched pinnae and reduced helix formation; and micrognathia (Fig. 17-6). A short philtrum of the upper lip, a bifid uvula, a high arched palate, submucosal cleft palate, and nasal speech were often described. Other features included tapered fingers; esophageal atresia; imperforate

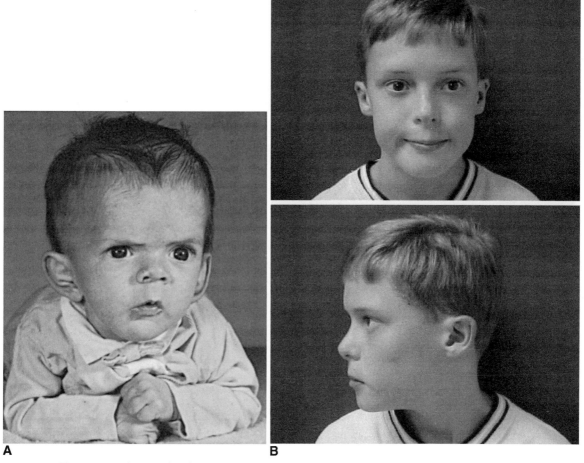

A **B**

Figure 17-6 · Photographs of patients with the DiGeorge syndrome. **A.** Infant with DiGeorge syndrome has the typical hypertelorism, antimongoloid slant of the eyes, ear malformation, and peculiar mouth. **B.** Older child with DiGeorge syndrome depicts characteristic facial features, which become more subtle with age. Relatively consistent features are hooded eyelids, a bulbous nose tip, a broad nasal bridge, posteriorly rotated ears, simple ear helices, and micrognathia. This child has posteriorly rotated ears with simple helices, slightly hooded eyelids, and a slightly bulbous nose tip.

anus; and urinary tract abnormalities, particularly hydronephrosis (Conley et al., 1979). Borderline microcephalia, delayed development, and learning problems are also noted.

Tetany secondary to hypocalcemia occurs in a subset of patients in the first 24 to 48 hours of life. Serum calcium levels are low, the phosphorus level is elevated, and parathyroid hormone is absent or very low.

The early studies emphasized the multiple congenital anomalies present and observed that infections were common and were a frequent contributor to death. The mortality rate in the three earliest studies ranged from 69% to 96%. In the 1988 study by Muller and colleagues, after technical advances in cardiac surgery became available, the mortality rate had decreased to 8%.

DGS patients with severely impaired immunologic function (so-called complete DGS) regardless of whether they have or do not have the characteristic deletion are susceptible to the same types of infections and complications as patients with SCID (see Chapter 15). For example, GVHD, severe adenoviral disease, disseminated CMV, disseminated parainfluenza, extraintestinal or prolonged rotaviral infections, and B-cell lymphomas have been described (Beard et al., 1980; Brouard et al., 1985; Deerojanawong et al., 1997; Gilger et al., 1992; Ocejo-Vinyals et al., 2000; Ramos et al., 1999; Sato et al., 1999; Tuvia et al., 1988; Washington et al., 1993, 1994; Wintergerst et al., 1989; Wood et al., 1988).

These patients require thymic tissue transplantation or fully matched sibling hematopoietic stem cell transplantation for survival. Even with appropriate treatment, mortality rates are high when the T-cell defect is severe.

Recent studies of patients with a 22q11.2 deletion suggest that mortality is rare and infrequently due to infection. A study of 558 patients with the characteristic deletion found an 8% mortality rate (Ryan et al., 1997). Most of the patients who died did so within the first 6 months of life, and most deaths were due to cardiac disease. In this same series, severe immunodeficiency was found in only two patients, suggesting that this feared phenotype has a frequency of approximately 0.3%. An American study of 250 patients with the deletion found a mortality rate of 5% with none of the patients having complete absence of T cells (McDonald-McGinn et al., 1999). Most patients had a mild to moderate T-cell defect.

Thus most patients with the deletion are modestly immunocompromised and do not develop opportunistic infections or life-threatening infections. Viral infections are often prolonged, and abnormal palatal anatomy leads to an increased susceptibility to upper airway bacterial infections. The combination of impaired T cells and abnormal palatal anatomy is associated with a high frequency of otitis media and sinusitis. Many have impaired polysaccharide responsiveness (Gennery et al., 2002) (see Chapter 12).

Kornfeld and colleagues (2000) compared the clinical picture in 13 patients with the characteristic deletion with three patients who had DGS without the deletion. Both groups of infants had frequent otitis media and sinusitis and both groups had comparable T-cell production and function.

Older Children and Adults

There are few studies of older children with DGS or chromosome 22q11.2 deletion syndrome. Jawad and co-workers (2001) found that adults and children older than 9 years often continue to have infections. Only 40% of patients with the deletion who were older than 9 years were thought to be as healthy as others their age. Approximately one fourth to one third of the patients had either recurrent sinusitis or otitis media, and 4% to 7% had recurrent lower airway infections. Interestingly, there was no correlation of recurrent infections with immunologic status, suggesting that infections have more to do with anatomic and functional airway problems than defects in host defense.

Autoimmune Disease and Malignancy

Cellular immunodeficiencies are commonly associated with an increased risk of autoimmune disease and an increased susceptibility to malignancies, particularly B-cell lymphomas (Elenitoba-Johnson and Jaffe, 1997) (see Chapter 39). This also appears to be true for patients with DGS or chromosome 22q11.2 deletion syndrome. The B-cell lymphomas tend to occur in patients with profound T-cell defects although this is not universally the case (Hong et al., 2001; Ramos et al., 1999; Sato et al., 1999).

The autoimmune disease does not correlate with severe T-cell dysfunction and includes a range of pediatric autoimmune diseases. Autoimmune cytopenias and juvenile rheumatoid arthritis appear to be the most common and may occur 20 to 100 times more frequently than in the general population (Davies et al., 2001; DePiero et al., 1997; Duke et al., 2000; Gennery et al., 2002; Jawad et al., 2001; Levy et al., 1996; Pinchas-Hamiel et al., 1994; Rasmussen et al., 1996; Verloes et al., 1998). The juvenile rheumatoid arthritis is often polyarticular and may be difficult to manage (Davies et al., 2001). Autoimmune thyroid disease and other autoimmune processes have also been described. It is likely that the T-cell defect acts synergistically with other predisposing factors to cause autoimmune disease (Ham Pong et al., 1985; Jawad et al., 2001; Kawamura et al., 2000).

Other Clinical Features

Patients with DGS or with a chromosome 22q11.2 deletion have complex medical needs and benefit from coordinated subspecialty care (Hopkin et al., 2000).

Because the immunodeficiency does not correlate with other phenotypic features, it is important to perform surveillance for other manifestations of the disease that could affect the child's life (Sullivan et al., 1998b). The dysmorphic facial features may be subtle and failure to recognize them may lead to delay in diagnosis (see Fig. 17-6). The cardiac defect occurs in 75% to 90% of patients with the deletion and is often the most critical issue in early infancy (Table 17-6) (McDonald-McGinn et al., 1999; Ryan et al., 1997).

Hypocalcemia is seen in 50% to 60% and is most common in infancy (McDonald-McGinn et al., 1999; Ryan et al., 1997). It is thought that hyperplasia of the parathyroids can compensate for its impaired development; however, late-onset hypocalcemia has been described, and it is often precipitated by stress.

Approximately 10% of patients have cleft palate but nearly one third have velopharyngeal incompetence, which contributes to their upper airway infections, feeding difficulties, speech delay, and speech characteristics.

As the patients age, the emphasis usually shifts to developmental and social issues. Language delay is exceedingly common, and only 9% of patients have normal expressive language early in life (Rommel et al., 1999; Scherer et al., 1999). The remaining patients are equally divided between mildly delayed in expressive language and severely delayed. Nonverbal learning disabilities are common in school-aged children, and testing typically reveals a discordance between verbal abilities and performance (Wang et al., 2000b). Therefore children have a delay in acquisition of speech but most ultimately have normal language. Many have special school needs, but most are able to attend regular school.

Teens and adults have an increased predisposition to behavioral and psychiatric problems (Ryan et al., 1997; Sugama et al., 1999; Usiskin et al., 1999; Wang et al., 2000b).

Only a minority of DGS patients with the characteristic chromosome deletions have the syndromic triad of cardiac disease, hypocalcemia, and immunodeficiency, and even among them there is a wide range of involvement. This has raised the question of when to perform chromosome 22q11.2 deletion fluorescent in situ hybridization (FISH) analysis. Patients with neonatal hypocalcemia and certain types of cardiac disease are quite likely to have the deletion, whereas patients with isolated behavioral problems are less likely (Table 17-7). One strategy to stratify risk for chromosome 22q11.2 deletion uses a combination of phenotypic features (Tobias et al., 1999).

Many clinics perform FISH analysis of parents of patients with DGS who have a deletion. Identification of an affected parent has implications for future pregnancies because 50% of the children will be affected. Genetic counseling is warranted in those cases.

Laboratory Features

Initial Tests

An infant suspected of having DGS should have an immediate cardiac evaluation, calcium and phosphorus levels, and a parathyroid hormone assay. Imaging of the thymus can confirm an absent thymic shadow but does not always correlate with immunologic function (see Chapter 12). A complete blood count (CBC) may indicate profound lymphopenia in complete DGS.

TABLE 17-6 · CLINICAL FINDINGS IN PATIENTS WITH CHROMOSOME 22q11.2 DELETION SYNDROME

Cardiac anomalies	49%–83%
Tetralogy of Fallot	17%–22%
Interrupted aortic arch	14%–15%
Ventriculoseptal defect	13%–14%
Truncus arteriosus	7%–9%
Hypocalcemia	17%–60%
Growth hormone deficiency	4%
Palatal anomalies	69%–100%
Cleft palate	9%–11%
Submucous cleft palate	5%–16%
Velopharyngeal insufficiency	27%–32%
Bifid uvula	5%
Renal anomalies	36%–37%
Absent/dysplastic	17%
Obstruction	10%
Reflux	4%
Ophthalmologic abnormalities	7%–70%
Tortuous retinal vessels	58%
Posterior embryotoxon (anterior segment dysgenesis)	69%
Neurologic	8%
Cerebral atrophy	1%
Cerebellar hypoplasia	0.4%
Dental: delayed eruption, enamel hypoplasia	2.5%
Skeletal abnormalities	17%–19%
Vertebral anomalies	19%
Lower extremity anomalies	15%
Speech delay	79%–84%
Developmental delay in infancy	75%
Developmental delay in childhood	45%
Behavior/psychiatric problems	9%–50%
Attention deficit hyperactivity disorder	25%
Schizophrenia	6%–30%

From Shprintzen et al., 1992; Motzkin et al., 1993; Ryan et al., 1997; Swillen et al., 1997; Yan et al., 1998; Gerdes et al., 1999; McDonald-McGinn et al., 1999; Moss et al., 1999; Vantrappen et al., 1999; Weller et al., 1999; Wang et al., 2000b.

TABLE 17-7 · FREQUENCY OF CHROMOSOME 22q11.2 DELETION IN PATIENTS WITH DIFFERENT CLINICAL FINDINGS IN DiGEORGE SYNDROME

Phenotypic Feature	Frequency of Chromosome 22q11.2 Deletion
Any cardiac lesion	1.1%
Interrupted aortic arch	50%–60%
Pulmonary atresia	33%–44%
Aberrant subclavian	25%
Truncus arteriosus	20%
Tetralogy of Fallot	11%–17%
Velopharyngeal insufficiency following adenoidectomy	64%
Isolated velopharyngeal insufficiency	37.5%
Neonatal hypocalcemia	71%
Schizophrenia	0.3%–6.4%

From Webber et al., 1996; Adachi et al., 1998; Goldmuntz et al., 1998; Rauch et al., 1998; Yan et al., 1998; Borgmann et al., 1999; Frohn-Mulder et al., 1999; Lu et al., 1999; Sugama et al., 1999; Swillen et al., 1999; Loffredo et al., 2000; Maeda et al., 2000; Perkins et al., 2000.

FISH studies for chromosome 22q11 deletion should be done as discussed previously, and, if negative, a karyotype examination for other chromosomal abnormalities is recommended. A 10p13-14 FISH study should also be considered if there is clinical evidence of DGS but a negative 22q11 FISH study.

In older children with possible 22q11.2 deletion syndrome, endocrine studies for parathyroid, growth hormone, and thyroid abnormalities should be considered. Selective patients may benefit from feeding and swallowing studies; radiologic examinations for infection; speech and language assessment; and renal, psychiatric, and orthopedic evaluation.

Cellular Immunity

When interpreting immunologic studies in DGS it must be remembered that normal T-cell counts decline rapidly in the first year of life and decline slowly during the next few years. T-cell counts in many patients with DGS or a chromosome 22q11.2 deletion rise slightly in the first year and then decline more slowly than in children without the deletion (Jawad et al., 2001). Thus the T-cell counts in these patients approach normal as they age because of a slight increase in their counts and the expected decline in normal children (Junker and Driscoll, 1995).

T-cell numbers and lymphoproliferative responses in young DGS patients range from normal to completely absent (Barrett et al., 1981; Bastian et al., 1989; Lischner and Huff, 1975; Muller et al., 1988, 1989). Several authors report that the patients with profound T-cell deficiencies were unlikely to improve, whereas less severely affected infants typically regain immunologic function (Barrett et al., 1981; Bastian et al., 1989; Markert et al., 1998; Muller et al., 1988).

Patients with the chromosome 22q11.2 deletion have a broad range of T-cell counts and proliferative responses. Mean CD3 counts (± standard deviation [SD]) from patients with the deletion were 1977 ± 1106 cells/mm^3 at 0 to 6 months of age, 1913 ± 914 cells/mm^3 at 6 to 38 months of age, 1537 ± 650 cells/mm^3 at 38 to 109 months of age, and 1188 ± 482 cells/mm^3 at older than 109 months. Mean CD4 counts from patients with the deletion are 1383 ± 839 cells/mm^3 at 0 to 6 months of age, 1333 ± 672 cells/mm^3 at 6 to 38 months of age, 953 ± 432 cells/mm^3 at 38 to 109 months of age, and 687 ± 302 cells/mm^3 at older than 109 months (Jawad et al., 2001).

Approximately 10% of infants with the chromosome 22q11.2 deletion who are younger than 1 year have a CD4 count less than 500 cells/mm^3; 2.5% of infants have a CD4 count less than 200 cells/mm^3. Slightly more than 2% of children with the deletion who are older than 1 year have a CD4 count less than 200 cells/mm^3 (Jawad et al., 2001). Patients with slight decreases in T-cell numbers have normal defenses against pathogens.

T-cell proliferative responses to mitogens are usually normal, except in those with profound immunodeficiency. These severely affected patients also have abnormalities in their T-cell repertoire (Collard et al., 1999; Pierdominici et al., 2000). T-cell receptor excision circles (TRECs), as a measure of newly emigrated thymic cells, are diminished in proportion to the degree of T-cell deficiency (Haynes et al., 2000). In contrast to the diminished T-cell numbers in patients with the deletion, the fraction, number, and function of NK cells are normal or increased (Muller et al., 1988, 1989).

Humoral Immunity

B-cell numbers are normal or increased (Muller et al., 1988, 1989). DGS patients with frequent infections have a B-cell repertoire intermediate between those of controls and patients with profound immunodeficiency, consistent with limitation of T-cell help (Haire et al., 1993). Immunoglobulin levels are usually normal although subtle immunoglobulin abnormalities are often noted. Hypogammaglobulinemia present in the first year of life usually resolves, and hypergammaglobulinemia may occur after age 5.

Although most DGS patients have normal antibody function and antibody avidity (Junker and Driscoll, 1995), some patients have functional antibody defects (Etzioni and Pollack, 1989; Jawad et al., 2001; Mayuni et al., 1989; Miranda et al., 1983; Schubert and Moss, 1992; Smith et al., 1998). Gennery and co-workers (2002) noted that 22q11.2 deletion patients with recurrent sinopulmonary infections had frequent immunoglobulin abnormalities, particularly impaired antibody responses to pneumococcal polysaccharide vaccine.

Selective IgA deficiency may occur in up to 10% of patients with DGS with a deletion, and the deficiency seems to be particularly common in DGS with autoimmune problems including arthritis (Davies et al., 2001; Smith et al., 1998). Autoimmune antibodies such as red cell autoantibodies, antinuclear antibodies, and thyroid antibodies are not uncommon, particularly in DGS patients with T-cell defects with limited somatic mutations. Gennery and colleagues (2002) noted that 10 of 30 patients had autoimmune phenomena, and 6 were symptomatic.

Diagnosis

A positive FISH test for a chromosome 22q11.2 deletion or a 10p deletion establishes the diagnosis. For patients without a deletion and no known exposures to fetal toxins, the diagnosis is based on the clinical phenotype. Generally, a combination of a conotruncal cardiac anomaly, hypocalcemia, hypoplastic thymus, and characteristic facial features are used as diagnostic criteria. A recent attempt to codify the diagnosis of DGS has revealed how difficult it is to develop such a system without leaving many patients uncategorized or with an uncertain diagnosis (Conley et al., 1999).

Treatment

Newborn Management

Once the diagnosis is established, coordinated subspecialty management should be initiated. The nonimmunologic features often require medical management immediately after birth. Cardiac repair and calcium supplementation are often the most urgent needs in the first few days of life. Asymptomatic infants should have an echocardiogram to ensure that anomalous vasculature is not present. A renal ultrasound is indicated because of the high frequency of renal anomalies. Feeding and swallowing problems should be managed according to the child's individual needs (Eicher et al., 2000). Palatal defects, reflux, and motility issues must be investigated and treated.

The infant with DGS suspected of having an immunodeficiency should be placed in isolation with precautions against the use of unirradiated or CMV-positive blood products. If T cells are absent, observation for a few weeks to determine if T cells will appear is warranted (Markert et al., 1998) while a search for an HLA-identical donor is sought or transfer to a center for transplantation is planned. IVIG and PCP prophylaxis is indicated just as in a patient with SCID.

Management of Older Children

Children with markedly diminished CD4 T cells should be given PCP prophylaxis although PCP has not been reported in these patients. Live viral vaccines should be withheld if the child has impaired T-cell function, an inability to produce functional antibodies, or markedly diminished peripheral blood T-cell counts. In the presence of antibody responses to killed vaccines, normal proliferative responses to mitogens and recall antigens, and a CD8 T-cell count of more than 300 cells/mm^3 at 1 year of age, we have given live virus vaccines without sequelae.

For patients who have not received varicella vaccine and are exposed to varicella, varicella-zoster immune globulin or acyclovir prophylaxis is indicated. When the hypogammaglobulinemia is severe and/or is accompanied by a defect in antibody function, IVIG is warranted. For patients with selective IgA deficiency and recurrent infection, a trial of prophylactic antibiotics can be given.

Toddler-aged DGS patients benefit from early intervention, particularly those with decreased language skills and developmental delay (Gerdes et al., 1999). Hearing defects should be suspected, particularly in those with speech delay and a 10p deletion. Velopharyngeal insufficiency should be suspected and when present requires surgical repair. Recurrent otitis is common, and tympanic tube placement may be of value (Ford et al., 2000). Brain imaging should be considered for those with developmental delay. Growth should be monitored because growth hormone deficiency is present in approximately 4% of patients with a 22q11.2 deletion (Weinzimer et al., 1998). Hypothyroidism may also contribute to growth failure.

Most older children with the characteristic deletion or with syndromically defined DGS have a mild to moderate T-cell defect. No outcome studies evaluating different managements have been performed.

Immune Reconstitution

The rationale for bone marrow or peripheral blood lymphocyte transplantation in DGS is to provide mature T cells rather than hematopoietic stem cells (Bensoussan et al., 2002). These latter cells, lacking thymic tissue, are unable to mature appropriately. Only sibling-matched transplants are attempted in this setting. Bone marrow and peripheral blood T-cell transplantation has an excellent record of success and results in nearly immediate appearance of functional T cells (Bensoussan et al., 2002; Borzy et al., 1989; Bowers et al., 1998; Goldsobel et al., 1987). There are theoretical concerns regarding the durability of the transplanted T cells; however, some recipients are now teenagers and are doing well.

The use of whole fetal thymus was first described by Cleveland and co-workers in 1968. Several years later, trials of fetal thymic tissue implantation to support T-cell development were done (Mayumi et al., 1989; Thong et al., 1978). This strategy had some success, but difficulties in obtaining fetal tissue limited its application in the United States.

Recently, postnatal thymic tissue obtained from another infant during cardiac surgery has been implanted to support T-cell development. The thymic tissue is cultured to ensure that mature T cells capable of causing GVHD have been eliminated (Markert et al., 1997b). Thin slices of the cultured thymus are implanted in the quadriceps muscle. Although partial HLA matching is desirable, it is not necessary (Markert et al., 1997a, 1999). Functional T cells appear approximately 3 to 4 months posttransplantation, and the T-cell repertoire posttransplant appears to be normal, suggesting that the graft is capable of supporting normal T-cell development (Davis et al., 1997).

Markert and colleagues (2003) have reported their results on 12 patients with the complete DiGeorge syndrome, 11 of whom had T-cell counts less than 50/mm^3. Of 12, 7 have survived; 6 of these have developed antigen-specific lymphoproliferative responses and 3 have intact B-cell function. Markert and colleagues conclude that thymic transplantation is efficacious, is well tolerated, and should be considered as treatment for the complete DiGeorge syndrome.

Prognosis

The patient of Cleveland and colleagues (1968) remained free of infections for many years after the thymus transplantation, as have the children who received allogeneic bone marrow or peripheral blood. The long-range outlook is more dependent on the cardiac defect, the degree of hypoparathyroidism, and the child's emotional and intellectual development than on the immune status because the latter is rarely life-limiting.

Most older children and adults with DGS lead full and active lives. A small number have behavioral or psychiatric problems, and a very small proportion are unable to attend regular school or hold a job. By this age, most of their medical issues have been addressed. Isolated cases of latent hypoparathyroidism have occurred in this group, but this is uncommon (Sykes et al., 1997).

Kathleen E. Sullivan

CHRONIC MUCOCUTANEOUS CANDIDIASIS

Definition

Chronic mucocutaneous candidiasis (CMC) refers to a group of immunodeficiencies characterized by persistent or recurrent infections of the skin, nails, and mucous membranes caused by organisms of the genus *Candida*; in most cases, the infecting species is *Candida albicans*. The immunodeficiency is usually a selective cellular defect to *Candida* and a few related organisms. There are seven clinical CMC subgroups, defined by the extent and location of the infections; the molecular defects; and associated disorders including endocrinopathies, thymomas, autoimmune disorders, and interstitial keratitis (Table 17-8).

Patients with CMC rarely develop *Candida* sepsis or candidiasis of parenchymal organs. The *Candida* infection usually responds to adequate treatment with antifungal drugs, but candidiasis of the mucous membranes, skin, and nails recurs soon after the antifungal therapy is stopped. Long-term remissions have been observed in patients who have received treatments that restored cell-mediated immunity against *Candida*.

Historical Aspects

The first reported case of CMC is attributed to Thorpe and Handley (1929), who described a 4½-year-old child with hypoparathyroidism and chronic oral candidiasis. This is the earliest report of an immunodeficiency.

Additional reports during the 1950s and 1960s confirmed the association of superficial candidiasis with childhood-onset endocrinopathies; some recorded that

TABLE 17-8 · CLINICAL SYNDROMES OF MUCOCUTANEOUS CANDIDIASIS

· Chronic oral candidiasis
  · Iron deficiency
  · HIV infection
  · Denture stomatitis
  · Inhaled corticosteroid use
· Familial chronic mucocutaneous candidiasis
· Autoimmune polyendocrinopathy-candidiasis-ectodermal dystrophy (APECED)
· Chronic localized candidiasis
· Chronic mucocutaneous candidiasis with thymoma
· Candidiasis with chronic keratitis
· Candidiasis with the hyper-IgE syndrome

multiple members of a sibship could be affected (Blizzard and Gibbs, 1968; Craig et al., 1955; Hung et al., 1963; Louria et al., 1967; Whitaker et al., 1956).

Pathogenesis

Immune Defects

Evidence for an immunologic basis of CMC was derived from observations of patients with DGS (August et al., 1968, 1970; Cleveland et al., 1968) or one of the syndromes of SCID (Hong, 1996). *Candida* infections in these immunodeficient patients were recurrent, widespread, and difficult to treat.

Chilgren and co-workers (1967) reported seven patients, aged 6 months to 14 years, who had chronic candidiasis, four of whom had endocrinopathies. Three did not express delayed-type hypersensitivity responses to *Candida* antigen and two lacked IgA *Candida* antibodies in their parotid fluids. In 1970, Kirkpatrick and colleagues described three patients with absent delayed hypersensitivity and lymphoproliferative responses to *Candida* antigen but intact responses to other antigens.

During the 1970s, in vitro tests of cell-mediated immunity were used to further define the immunologic defect in CMC. Kirkpatrick and co-workers (1971a) described patients whose lymphocytes failed to secrete macrophage migration inhibitory factor (MIF) on stimulation with *Candida* extracts; this finding was confirmed by Lehner and colleagues (1972) and Valdimarsson and co-workers (1973). Lehner and colleagues (1972) also noted that CMC lymphocytes could not be activated by *Candida* extracts to express cytolytic activity against chicken erythrocytes.

These studies have led to the classification of CMC as a T-cell immunodeficiency. However, CMC patients have a range of immunologic defects that predispose them to chronic candidiasis. The most profound defects are found in those patients who develop CMC during infancy and early childhood (Kirkpatrick and Sohnle, 1981) and in those with extensive candidiasis (Lehner et al., 1972).

CYTOKINE ABNORMALITIES

Murine models of systemic *Candida* infections correlate survival to the cytokine profiles of the host. The general rule is that mice with vigorous Th1 responses are resistant to systemic candidal infections, whereas mice with predominantly Th2 responses are susceptible. (Spaccapelo et al., 1997). A role for IL-4 in susceptibility also seems clear; treatment of mice with anti-IL-4 or with soluble IL-4 receptor produces a survival rate of more than 90% in mice with otherwise lethal infections (Puccetti et al., 1994). However, in humans with CMC no clear Th1 or Th2 predominance has been identified.

IMMUNOREGULATORY ABNORMALITIES

Stobo and co-workers (1976) studied 14 patients with cutaneous or systemic fungal infections, two of whom had CMC; they found that fresh T lymphocytes from some patients suppressed the proliferative responses of autologous precultured T cells, thus suggesting an immunoregulatory (suppressor) defect. Arulanantham and colleagues (1979), using a different suppressor cell assay, studied three children with the candidiasis-polyendocrinopathy-ectodermal dysplasia (APECED) syndrome, their parents, and three siblings; they found that two of the patients and one normal sibling had subnormal suppressor cell activity.

Thus suppressive factors may contribute to the immunologic abnormalities in some patients with recurrent candidiasis. Jorizzo and co-workers (1980) reversed the immunologic abnormalities and achieved clinical benefit in members of a family with CMC by treatment with cimetidine. Witkin and colleagues (1986) concluded that prostaglandin E_2 was an endogenous immunosuppressant in patients with chronic vaginal candidiasis and corrected the subnormal lymphoproliferative response to *Candida* antigen by adding cyclooxygenase inhibitors to the cultures.

Role of the Organism

C. albicans virulence factors may play a contributing pathogenetic role. Cassone and co-workers (1987) studied women with candidal vaginitis and compared the protease activity of their organisms with those from women who were asymptomatic carriers. The isolates from symptomatic women had significantly more proteolytic activity than isolates from the asymptomatic subjects, suggesting that the *Candida*-secreted protease may be a virulence factor.

Differential expression of secreted aspartyl proteinase genes has been observed between asymptomatic carriers and patients with oral candidiasis (Naglik et al., 1999; Schaller et al., 1998). The recently described Ash 1 protein is also a factor that is required for full expression of virulence of *C. albicans* in mice (Inglis and Johnson, 2002).

C. albicans expresses a protein that is antigenically and structurally related to β_2 integrins such as the CD11b/CD18 complex present on human neutrophils, monocytes, and macrophages, which is important for their adhesion to endothelial surfaces (Calderone and Braun, 1991; Gustafson et al., 1991). Expression of this integrin-like molecule is upregulated at 37°C and by the presence of glucose, an observation that may be relevant to the frequent *Candida* infections in patients with diabetes mellitus.

INT 1p is a recently described protein of *C. albicans* that is similar to integrins in vertebrates. Mutant organisms with altered INT 1 have decreased growth of hyphae, decreased adherence to epithelium, and decreased virulence for mice (Gale et al., 1998).

Iron is an essential nutrient for the pathogenicity of *C. albicans*. Ramanan and Wang (2000) described two iron permease genes in *C. albicans* (*CaFTR1* and *CaFTR2*) that code for proteins that have iron-binding domains. *CaFRT1* was expressed when iron-limiting conditions were studied. *CaFTR1*-negative mutants lacked virulence in mice.

AIRE Gene in APECED

In one clinical variant of CMC, the autosomal recessive polyendocrinopathy-candidiasis-ectodermal dysplasia (APECED) syndrome, the mutated gene has been identified.

Aaltonen and colleagues (1993) reported that DNA analyses on 15 family members with APECED did not disclose linkage to genes for T-cell receptors, immunoglobulin heavy chains, the delta chain of CD3, or the alpha chain of CD8. They had previously reported that they were unable to identify linkage to any HLA-DR groups (Ahonen et al., 1988).

In 1997, two groups simultaneously reported mapping the APECED gene to chromosome 21 (Finnish-German APECED Consortium, 1997; Nagamine et al., 1997). The gene, designated *AIRE* (auto-immune regulator) encodes a protein containing two zinc-finger (PHD-finger) motifs, a proline-rich region, and three LXXLL motifs. The mutations that were identified in the initial reports were arginine → stop codon (R257X) and a missense mutation that was the result of substitution of lysine by glutamic acid (K83E).

The murine *AIRE* gene has also been identified and cloned (Shi et al., 1999; Wang et al., 1999), which has allowed production of mice with gene knockout mutations. The gene product, AIRE, is a transcriptional regulator expressed in the medullary epithelial cells of the thymus, the spleen, bone marrow, lymph nodes, and other cells and tissues. Knockout mice (*AIRE* −/−) had normal thymi, spleens, thyroid glands, pancreases, and ovaries, but some of the mice had atrophic adrenal glands (Ramsey et al., 2002).

Autoantibodies were found against liver, testes, pancreas, and adrenals in some but not all *AIRE* −/− knockout mice. The pancreatic antibodies were directed against the exocrine pancreas in all but one animal rather than against the islet cells or glutamic decarboxylase as is usually found in humans with *AIRE* mutations. T-lymphocyte proliferative responses were studied with lymph node cells from mice that were immunized with hen egg lysozyme, and supranormal responses were observed.

Anderson and associates (2002) proposed that one function of the AIRE protein was to regulate expression of ectopic antigens such as insulin, thyrotropin, retinal S antigen, and myelin basic protein present on thymic medullary epithelial cells. The model was based on the observation that thymocytes with receptors that potentially recognize self-antigens were removed or silenced in the thymus by interaction with thymic medullary epithelial cells.

In the absence of the AIRE protein, these potentially autoreactive cells would not encounter the ectopic antigens and would not be "edited out" of the thymic populations. The thymic medullary epithelial cells from the *AIRE* knockout mice had diminished expression of transcripts for the suspected ectopic genes, and a greater frequency of lymphocytic infiltrates in tissues such as the salivary glands, ovary, stomach, and retina. They also had autoantibodies against many of these tissues. Thus there is a plausible relationship of the AIRE gene product to a predisposition to autoimmunity, but the cause of the immune deficiency remains undefined.

Clinical Features

CMC patients can be divided into seven quite diverse clinical syndromes (see Table 17-8).

Chronic Oral Candidiasis

Patients with chronic oral candidiasis have recurrent candidiasis of the buccal mucosa and tongue and usually have perlèche. Isolated tongue coating without buccal mucosal involvement is usually not due to *Candida*. The white patches on the mucous membranes are easily removed with a tongue blade. Microscopic examination of scrapings suspended in potassium hydroxide reveals a dense network of pseudohyphae, epithelial cells, inflammatory cells, and debris.

These patients usually do not have esophageal candidiasis, and the skin and nails are not involved. The disorder is common in middle-aged and elderly females and, in some instances, is accompanied by iron deficiency (Higgs and Wells, 1972; Wells et al., 1972). It has been suggested that an abnormality in iron metabolism was fundamental to the predisposition to candidiasis, but in our experience, iron therapy is ineffective for this form of candidiasis.

Recurrent oral candidiasis is common in patients with human immunodeficiency virus (HIV) infections. Four clinical forms of oral candidiasis in HIV-infected patients have been described (Greenspan and Greenspan, 1996). These include (1) typical pseudomembranous candidiasis described previously; (2) erythematous candidiasis presenting as smooth depapillated areas on the palate and dorsum of the tongue; (3) hyperplastic candidiasis, which differs from pseudomembranous candidiasis in that the white patches are firmly attached to the underlying mucosa; and (4) angular cheilitis (see Chapter 29).

Other important clinical considerations in patients with chronic or recurrent oral candidiasis are dentures that may reduce bathing of oral mucous membranes with saliva; inhaled glucocorticoids that apparently suppress mucosal immunity; and other medications such as antibiotics, systemic steroids, and immunosuppressive agents.

Familial Chronic Mucocutaneous Candidiasis

Wells and associates (1972) have described familial CMC. These patients have chronic and recurrent oral candidiasis. Cutaneous and ungual candidiasis is less common, and endocrinopathies were not present. Males and females were equally represented, and most patients had oral candidiasis by the age of 2 years. Of the eight pedigrees reported, consanguinity was established in four and suspected in another two.

Autoimmune Polyendocrinopathy-Candidiasis-Ectodermal Dystrophy

APECED most likely affected the patient described by Thorpe and Handley (1929). Its first manifestation is usually recurrent oral candidiasis and diaper dermatitis. With time, the lesions spread and involve the scalp, extremities, nails, and sometimes other skin sites (see Figs. 17-7 and 17-8). The candidiasis can range from mild to severe. In most instances T-cell proliferative responses to antigens, especially *Candida*, are subnormal. Siblings often have candidiasis and one or more endocrinopathies. The inheritance pattern is autosomal recessive.

Ahonen and co-workers (1990) reported the frequency of 11 accompanying disorders in 68 patients from 54 families: hypothyroidism, adrenal failure, gonadal failure, insulin-dependent diabetes mellitus, gastric parietal cell failure, hypoparathyroidism, keratopathy, vitiligo, alopecia, autoimmune hepatitis, and intestinal malabsorption (Table 17-9). Forty-seven percent of the patients had four or five of the associated disorders. The most common endocrinopathies were hypoparathyroidism (79% of patients), hypoadrenalism (72%), and ovarian failure (60%). Sixty percent of the patients had two or more endocrinopathies.

The endocrinopathies may not appear during childhood or adolescence. In some of our patients (numbering more than 100), hypoadrenalism and hypothyroidism did not appear until the fourth and fifth decades. For this reason, we recommend annual evaluation of endocrine function in patients with CMC. Even more frequent evaluations may be appropriate in patients with one endocrinopathy or in patients who have siblings with APECED.

The clinical observation of an autosomal-recessive inheritance led to the identification of the *AIRE* gene. Approximately 45 mutations occur throughout its coding region (Kumar et al., 2002; Vogel et al., 2002). Certain mutations are more frequent in different populations (Table 17-10), but attempts to correlate specific

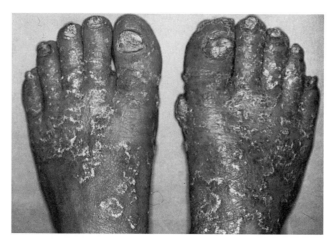

Figure 17-7· Candidiasis of the skin and toenails of a patient with the autoimmune polyendocrinopathy-candidiasis-ectodermal dystrophy (APECED) syndrome.

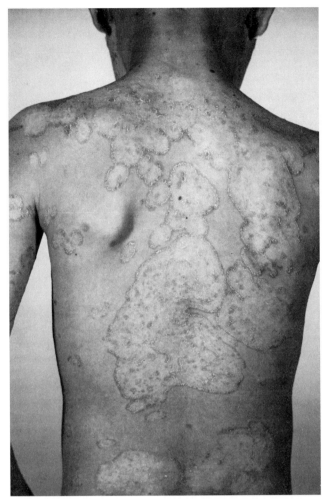

Figure 17-8 · Chronic mucocutaneous candidiasis of the skin of a patient with autoimmune polyendocrinopathy-candidiasis-ectodermal dystrophy (APECED) syndrome. Note the well-demarcated lesions with raised borders. Histologic studies show hyphal forms of *Candida albicans* in the lesional tissues but not in the fields of normal skin.

TABLE 17-9 · DISORDERS THAT ACCOMPANY MUCOCUTANEOUS CANDIDIASIS

Disorder	Ahonen et al., 1990 (% with disorder)	Kirkpatrick and Sohnle, 1981 (% with disorder)
Alopecia	29	15
Vitiligo	13	6
Keratoconjunctivitis	35	9
Enamel dysplasia	77	66
Autoimmune hepatitis	12	6
Malabsorption	18	13
Nail dystrophy	52	Not given

Ahonen and colleagues (1990) described 68 patients, each of whom had autoimmune polyendocrinopathy-candidiasis-ectodermal dystrophy (APECED). Kirkpatrick and Sohnle (1981) reported 58 patients with all forms of chronic mucocutaneous candidiasis. The percentages presented in this table used a denominator of 53, which includes only patients who developed candidiasis before age 15 years.

TABLE 17-10 · *AIRE* GENE MUTATIONS IN PATIENTS WITH APECED

Population	Most Common Mutation (% of cases)	Reference
Finnish	R257X (90)	Finnish-German APECED Consortium, 1997
Swedish	R257X (65)	Halonen et al., 2002
Iranian Jew	Y85C (100)	Vogel et al., 2002
Sardinian	R139X (90)	Rosatelli et al., 1998
South Italian	W78R (75)	Meloni et al., 2002
Norwegian	1094–1106 del (55)	Myhre et al., 2001
British	1094–1106 del (71)	Pearce et al., 1998
North American	1094–1106 del (30–50)	Vogel et al., 2002

APECED = autoimmune polyendocrinopathy-candidiasis-ectodermal dystrophy.

mutations with the phenotypic expression have not been successful (Anderson, 2002; Meloni et al., 2002; Vogel et al., 2002).

However, Halonen and co-workers (2002) reported that the prevalence of mucocutaneous candidiasis was greater in patients with the R257X mutation (the most common mutation in the Finnish population) than in patients with other mutations. They also noted that Iranian Jews, who have a different mutation (Y85C), had lesser prevalences of candidiasis (18%) and Addison's disease (22%). In addition, siblings within a pedigree may have different endocrinopathies, different nonendocrine disorders such as alopecia and vitiligo, and different severity of candidiasis even when they have the same *AIRE* gene mutation (Kogawa et al., 2002).

Chronic Localized Candidiasis (Candida Granuloma)

Chronic localized candidiasis has also been called *Candida granuloma* because the cutaneous lesions may present as thick and tightly adherent crusts on the scalp,

face, and hands (Fig. 17-9). Some patients have cutaneous horn formation (Kirkpatrick and Sohnle, 1981; Lehner, 1964). The cutaneous lesions show marked hyperkeratosis with acanthosis, and the underlying skin is infiltrated with lymphocytes, plasma cells, and rare giant cells. Most patients also have oral candidiasis. The disorder usually presents during early childhood (<5 years), and males and females are equally affected. There is no known genetic basis for this form of candidiasis.

Chronic Mucocutaneous Candidiasis with Thymoma

CMC with thymoma should be suspected when patients develop mucous membrane and cutaneous candidiasis during adult years. The youngest reported case is age 35 years (Kirkpatrick and Windhorst, 1979). The patients do not develop endocrinopathies, but they may develop other thymoma-associated disorders such as aplastic anemia, myasthenia gravis, or hypogammaglobulinemia (see Chapter 13).

It is not clear whether thymomas develop before or after the candidiasis because the chest imaging studies

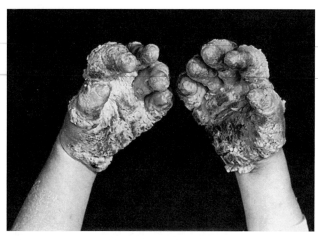

Figure 17-9· An example of the extraordinary hyperkeratosis that characterizes localized mucocutaneous candidiasis.

are usually not done until after the appearance of candidiasis. Malignant and benign thymomas have been reported. Removal of the thymic tumor usually does not result in resolution of the candidiasis.

Candidiasis with Keratitis

The original description of candidiasis with chronic keratitis was made by Okamato and co-workers (1977). Their patient developed photophobia by age 2 years and keratoconjunctivitis, alopecia, and oral and vaginal candidiasis by age 5 years. She was legally blind as a teenager. She had two daughters with keratoconjunctivitis and alopecia. One daughter had angular cheilitis, and the other had candidal diaper dermatitis. The proband's father was blind and may have had a similar disorder. The authors concluded that an AD form of inheritance was present.

Keratopathy was found in 24 of the 68 patients reported by Ahonen and colleagues (1990). It was accompanied by hypoparathyroidism in 22 patients, but 32 of 44 patients without keratopathy also had hypoparathyroidism ($P = .13$). There was a possible association of keratopathy with hypoadrenalism ($P = .048$) in these patients, but no familial cases were mentioned. We have seen alopecia, chronic candidiasis, and keratopathy in two Turkish siblings.

Candidiasis with the Hyper-IgE Syndrome

The hyper-IgE syndrome was described first as "Job's syndrome" in two patients with recurrent "cold" abscesses caused by *Staphylococcus aureus* (Davis et al., 1966; see section in this chapter). Grimbacher and co-workers (1999a) described 30 cases, and 25 of these (83%) had chronic candidiasis of the mucous membranes and nails. They concluded that the disorder was transmitted as a single locus AD trait with variable expressivity.

Associated Disorders

Patients with CMC are often susceptible to other infectious diseases and to disorders of other organ systems (see Table 17-9).

INFECTIOUS DISORDERS

Chipps and associates (1979) noted that CMC patients are susceptible to bacterial and viral infections of the skin and respiratory system. In some cases, the patients developed chronic bronchitis or bronchiectasis, sinusitis, and otitis media. In our review of 58 patients, 26 had significant non-candidal infections (Kirkpatrick and Sohnle, 1981). Herrod and colleagues (1990) reported the experience with non-candidal infections in 43 patients at eight medical centers. Thirty-five patients (81%) had significant infections with a variety of agents that included bacteria, viruses, other fungi, and parasites. Sepsis was common. Seven patients had died, and in each case an infectious disease was the direct cause of death.

Kalfa and associates (2003) suggested that the combination of respiratory infections, selective antibody defects, and IgG2 and IgG4 subclass deficiencies (and sometimes IgA deficiency) represents a distinct phenotype among CMC patients.

Infections with dermatophytes coexist in approximately 20% of patients with CMC (Shama and Kirkpatrick, 1980). These infections may not be appreciated unless cultures are performed or potassium hydroxide preparations are done. There are instances in which failure to recognize a dermatophyte infection has led to the incorrect diagnosis of resistant candidiasis.

VITILIGO, ALOPECIA, AND ENAMEL DYSPLASIA

In addition to their cosmetic challenge, vitiligo and alopecia may indicate the coexistence of an endocrinopathy. Dysplasia of the dental enamel is also common in patients with chronic candidiasis (see Table 17-9). It was present in 77% of the evaluable patients reported by Ahonen and colleagues (1990) and in 66% of our patients (Kirkpatrick and Sohnle, 1981). The mechanism is unknown, but it does not seem to be related to periodontal disease or to metabolic disorders such as hypoparathyroidism.

MALABSORPTION AND HEPATITIS

Although uncommon, intestinal malabsorption may be a cause of annoying symptoms and the basis for chronic iron deficiency. Patients with parietal cell atrophy may become deficient in Vitamin B_{12}.

Little is known about the cause of hepatitis in candidiasis patients except that it seems to be associated with circulating immune complexes. Hepatitis can lead to liver failure and death. The *AIRE*-knockout mice reported by Anderson and colleagues (2002) had autoantibodies against gastric parietal cells and lymphocytic infiltrates in the liver.

AUTOIMMUNE DISORDERS

In addition to the autoimmune endocrinopathies that accompany some CMC syndromes, other autoimmune disorders are also noted. The most common is autoimmune hemolytic anemia, present in 4 of 43 patients described by Herrod (1990) and Oyefara and co-workers (1994). Others include immune thrombocytopenic purpura, autoimmune neutropenia, pernicious anemia, chronic active hepatitis, and juvenile rheumatoid arthritis.

Disorders of other organ systems have been described, but they are infrequent and it is not certain if these events are incidental or components of the syndrome of CMC.

NEOPLASMS

Neoplastic diseases have been described in seven CMC patients. In six, the tumors involved the buccal cavity, and, in one, the esophagus was involved (Kirkpatrick and Hay, unpublished dissertation). Thymomas have been mentioned previously. In a review of 27 patients with candidiasis and thymoma, 11 of the tumors were malignant and 9 were benign; details of the other seven thymomas were not reported (Kirkpatrick and Windhorst, 1979).

Laboratory Features

Serum Inhibitors

An interesting observation is that the serum of some CMC patients suppresses proliferation of patient T cells and normal T cells. The inhibitory factor appears to be a product of *Candida,* rather than an antibody or a product that is released from host cells in response to *Candida* (Fischer et al., 1978). The same inhibitory effect was observed when *Candida* mannan was added to the lymphocyte cultures. The inhibitory activity was not found in the IgG fraction of the inhibitory serum. Subsequently, Lee and co-workers (1986) removed the inhibitory factor from serum with a polyvalent anti-*Candida* serum. In addition, antifungal treatment that improves clinical candidiasis is associated with loss of the inhibitory activity (Kirkpatrick and Smith, 1974).

Cellular Immunity

Lymphopenia is occasionally present. Lymphocyte subsets are generally normal. The exception is the CMC patient with a profound T-cell defect such as in HIV infection or immunodeficiency with thymoma (see Chapter 13). These patients have a broad-based T-cell defect, unlike the narrow T-cell defect characteristic of CMC.

Delayed cutaneous hypersensitivity tests to *Candida* antigen are usually negative. Generalized cutaneous anergy involving several antigens may also be present in some patients (see Chapter 12).

Lymphoproliferative responses to mitogens are usually intact. The response to *Candida* antigen is usually absent, particularly in patients who have anergy to *Candida*. Responses to other antigens to which the patient has been exposed to or immunized with are usually normal.

Cytokine production by CMC lymphocytes is generally impaired when activated by *Candida* antigen. CMC lymphocytes, when activated nonspecifically with phorbol myristate acetate (PMA) or phytohemagglutinin (PHA), also may show reductions of transcripts for IL-2, IL-3, IL-4, and IFN-γ (de la Morena et al., 1995). TNF-α mRNA may be increased.

Lilic and associates (1996) examined Th1- and Th2-dependent cytokine responses to *Candida* antigens in 10 patients with childhood-onset CMC but could find no clear-cut predominance of Th1 versus Th2 cytokines. There is little correlation between the cytokine profile and the clinical or other immunologic features.

Patterns of T-Cell Abnormalities

Several distinct patterns of T-cell abnormalities have emerged (Table 17-11).

COMPLETE ANERGY WITH LYMPHOPENIA

Patients with complete anergy have T-cell lymphopenia and poor lymphocyte proliferation to *Candida* and other antigens and to mitogens such as PHA (see Table 17-11). Their T cells do not secrete cytokines when they are stimulated with antigens or mitogens, and the patients are anergic to a panel of antigens that evoke delayed-type hypersensitivity.

COMPLETE ANERGY WITH SUBNORMAL T-CELL RESPONSES TO CANDIDA

Other patients have less marked immunologic defects. They have normal numbers of circulating T cells and normal distributions of T-cell subsets. Their T cells have normal proliferative responses to mitogens but do not respond to *Candida* antigens (Kirkpatrick et al., 1970). Production of cytokines such as macrophage MIF in response to *Candida* is subnormal or absent, but mitogens usually produce normal responses (Kirkpatrick et al., 1971a). This profile is usually seen in children who develop candidiasis by age 3 years. Most patients are also anergic.

COMPLETE ANERGY WITH DEFICIENT CYTOKINE PRODUCTION

In a third group of patients, the T cells proliferate normally to antigens and mitogens (Kirkpatrick and Sohnle, 1981). Mitogenic activation stimulates MIF production, but antigens do not. These patients are also anergic. About 20% of CMC patients have this immunologic profile.

ANERGY TO CANDIDA WITH DEFICIENT T-CELL RESPONSES TO CANDIDA

Another group of CMC patients has an immune deficiency that is limited to *Candida* antigens. They have normal T-cell proliferation and MIF production in response to mitogens and antigens such as tetanus toxoid, mumps antigen, and streptococcal antigens, but their cells do not secrete MIF in response to *Candida*. These patients do not express delayed-type hypersensitivity to *Candida* but may respond to skin tests with other antigens (Kirkpatrick and Sohnle, 1981).

TABLE 17-11 · PATTERNS OF CELL-MEDIATED IMMUNE ABNORMALITIES IN PATIENTS WITH CHRONIC MUCOCUTANEOUS CANDIDIASIS

			Lymphocyte Transformation		Cytokine Production	
Groups	DTH *(Candida)*	T-Cell Number	*Candida*	Mitogen	*Candida*	Mitogen
1	Anergy*	Few	SN	SN	SN	SN
2	Anergy	N	SN	N	SN	N
3	Anergy	N	N	N	SN	N
4	Negative**	N	SN	N	SN	N
5	Negative	N	N	N	SN	N
6	Negative	N	N	N	N	N

*No response to any antigen. **No response to Candida antigen.
DTH = delayed-type hypersensitivity; N = normal response; SN = subnormal or absent.

ANERGY TO CANDIDA WITH DEFICIENT CYTOKINE PRODUCTION TO CANDIDA

Patients in this group have normal numbers of T cells and normal responses to mitogens. Their T cells proliferate in response to *Candida* but do not secrete cytokines.

NO IDENTIFIABLE ABNORMALITY

A small number of CMC patients have no deficiency revealed by current assays. This is a group that deserves special study.

Humoral Immunity

Most CMC patients have normal serum immunoglobulins, high titers of antibodies against *C. albicans*, and normal responses to vaccines. However, many CMC patients have recurrent respiratory infections resulting from bacteria and viruses and may develop pyoderma and more severe infections. These patients need a thorough evaluation of their antibody responses.

Bentur and associates (1991) reported four CMC patients who had chronic pulmonary disease and repeated bacterial infections. None of the patients expressed cell-mediated immunity to *Candida*. Each patient had normal serum values for IgG, IgA, and IgM, but all four had subnormal values for IgG2 and IgG4 and subnormal antibody responses to immunization. Two of our CMC patients with endocrinopathy progressed to panhypogammaglobulinemia.

Kalfa and co-workers (2003) summarized nine CMC patients with recurrent respiratory infections and selective antibody deficiency to pneumococcal polysaccharide vaccine (including the four reported by Bentur et al., 1991). IgG2 deficiency was present in all nine patients, IgG4 deficiency was present in eight patients, and IgA deficiency was present in three patients.

Thus although the *Candida* infections are the most striking clinical features of CMC, many patients have antibody deficiencies that make them susceptible to infections with other organisms.

Granulocyte Function

Several groups have reported abnormalities of neutrophil function. Five of our patients had deficient chemotactic responses of neutrophils and monocytes to endotoxin-activated serum (Kirkpatrick and Sohnle, 1981). All of these patients had pyogenic infections of the skin, respiratory system, or both, and three of the patients had the hyper-IgE syndrome.

Djawari and associates (1978) reported five CMC patients including three from the same family who had abnormal neutrophil chemotactic responses. A mother and daughter with CMC reported by Van Scoy and colleagues (1975) had impaired chemotaxis and the hyper-IgE syndrome. These patients all had repeated infections with pyogenic organisms.

Snyderman and co-workers (1973) reported a CMC patient with abnormal monocyte chemotaxis. Yamazaki and colleagues (1984) reported defective monocyte chemotaxis both in vivo and in vitro in two siblings with chronic candidiasis. Although neutrophils constitute one mechanism of defense against *Candida* and other filamentous fungi, most CMC patients have normal phagocytic cell function, arguing against a major pathogenetic role.

Abnormal antigen presentation was apparently caused by a defect in macrophage function in a patient reported by Twomey and associates (1975). This patient had multiple abnormalities, including a thymoma and aplastic anemia. Impaired monocyte antibody-dependent cellular cytotoxicity has been found in a few patients (Rosenblatt et al., 1979).

Complement Function

The complement system may contribute to the cutaneous inflammation in CMC. Carbohydrates of *C. albicans* can activate the complement system through the alternative pathway and produce chemotactic cleavage fragments (Sohnle et al., 1976a). Deposits of C3 are present in the dermal-epidermal junctions of lesional skin of CMC patients (Sohnle et al., 1976b) and in the skin of guinea pigs with experimental cutaneous candidiasis (Sohnle and Kirkpatrick, 1976). C5-deficient mice have delayed recovery of experimental cutaneous candidiasis (Wilson and Sohnle, 1988). Despite these findings, complement abnormalities are uncommon in CMC (Drew, 1973).

Treatment

CMC patients are complex because they have multiple problems in addition to their candidal infection. Their endocrine problems, their associated autoimmune problems, and their propensity to viral and bacterial infections must be considered. The two approaches to their candidal infection include immune reconstitution and antifungal therapy. Very rarely surgical removal of an infected nail is performed before start of therapy.

Immune Reconstitution

Before the availability of absorbable oral antifungal drugs, there was considerable effort to treat CMC with immunologic procedures to correct the cell-mediated defects and restore immune competence. A few cases were successful.

Transplantation of thymic tissue in DGS led to clearance of the oral and cutaneous candidiasis (Cleveland et al., 1968). Benefits of thymus transplantation in CMC patients were also recorded (Ammann and Hong, 1989; Ballow and Hyman, 1977; Kirkpatrick et al., 1974; Levy et al., 1971).

Infusions of peripheral blood leukocytes from donors with intact cell-mediated immune responses to *Candida* transferred their immunity to CMC patients and resulted in clinical remission (Kirkpatrick et al., 1971b; Valdimarsson et al., 1972). One patient who received paternal leukocytes had a complete remission that lasted 8 months. He then lost delayed-type hypersensitivity to *Candida* and relapsed shortly thereafter. A second patient received leukocytes from an HLA-matched sibling and remained in remission for at least 17 months.

Aplastic anemia is an uncommon complication of CMC (Deeg et al., 1986; Twomey et al., 1975). A patient reported by Deeg and associates (1986) developed extensive mucous membrane candidiasis during the first year of life. At age 7 she developed aplastic anemia and underwent BMT from an HLA-identical sister. Three years later she could express cell-mediated immunity to *Candida*, was free of candidiasis, and no longer required antifungal therapy.

TRANSFER FACTORS

Candida-specific transfer factors have been used for immune reconstitution in CMC. Transfer factors are small proteins (MW = 5000) extracted from lymphocytes that transfer cell-mediated immunity from immune donors to nonimmune recipients (Rozzo and Kirkpatrick, 1992). This activity is antigen specific. Preliminary experiments showed that transfer factors were active in CMC patients and could correct the immune deficiency (Kirkpatrick et al., 1972). Using potent transfer factors from donors with strong delayed hypersensitivity reactions to *Candida*, immunologic reconstitution and clinical responses have been recorded (Kirkpatrick and Greenberg, 1979; Littman et al., 1978; Masi et al., 1996).

Transfer factors are not approved for clinical use, in part because their molecular structure and mechanisms of action are not fully known (Kirkpatrick, 2000). The acquired immunodeficiency syndrome (AIDS) epidemic has raised serious concerns about the safety of blood products. In addition, a number of highly effective, orally absorbed antifungal drugs have become available, rendering immune reconstitution unneeded (Como and Dismukes, 1994).

Antifungal Drugs

Mycostatin suspension (for oral candidiasis), ointment (for cutaneous candidiasis), or suppositories (for vaginal candidiasis) is often used initially. Because Mycostatin is not absorbed, it is very safe but usually of limited efficacy in CMC.

Ointments, troches, vaginal creams, or suppositories containing clotrimazole, terconazole, and tioconazole are of more benefit. With the possible exception of ciclopirox, topical preparations are usually not effective for nail candidiasis (Gupta et al., 2000). Because these agents do not correct the immune defect, relapses are common if treatment is interrupted.

Oral systemic antifungal drugs have been available since the early 1980s and are the mainstay of CMC therapy. Most owe their antifungal activity to inhibition of synthesis of ergosterol, the main sterol in fungal cell membranes. The dosage schedules for the most widely used drugs are shown in Table 17-12.

Ketoconazole was the first oral antifungal evaluated in CMC patients (Petersen et al., 1980). Improvement in oral candidiasis was noted in 7 ± 1 days (range 4 to 10 days), cutaneous candidiasis in 18 ± 4 days (range 10 to 29 days), and ungual candidiasis in 83 ± 20 days (range 16 to 131 days).

Continuous antifungal treatment is usually necessary, and liver function must be monitored at regular (3 to

TABLE 17-12 · ORAL ANTI-FUNGAL DRUGS FOR THE TREATMENT OF MUCOCUTANEOUS CANDIDIASIS

Class	Drug	Pediatric Dosage	Adult Dosage
Imidazole	Ketoconazole (Nizoral)	3.3–6.6 mg/kg/day	200–400 mg/kg/day
	Clotrimazole (Mycelex)	Not established	10 mg 3–5 times/day
Triazole	Fluconazole (Diflucan)	3–6 mg/kg/day	200 mg on first day, then 100 mg daily
	Itraconazole (Sporanox)*	5 mg/kg/day	200–400 mg/day
Allylamine	Terbinafine (Lamisil)*	Not established	250 mg/kg/day
Echinocandins	Caspofungin (Cancidas)	Not established	70 mg on first day, then 50 mg daily

*Not indicated for candidiasis.

6 months) intervals. Ketoconazole and itraconazole are not well absorbed if there is insufficient acid in the stomach, an important consideration for patients using antacids, H$_2$-blockers, and other medications. In such instances patients can dissolve the tablets in 0.2-N hydrochloric acid and take the medication through a straw to avoid contact of their teeth with the acid.

Because each of these drugs inhibits the cytochrome P450 system, their use may alter the catabolism of many other drugs including coumadin, immunosuppressive drugs such as tacrolimus and cyclosporine, antimycobacterial drugs such as rifampin, anti-HIV protease inhibitors, and certain cholesterol-lowering drugs.

Fluconazole and itraconazole are available as suspensions for pediatric patients. Clotrimazole (Mycelex) is available as a troche for oral candidiasis. Because 40% to 50% of primary isolates of *C. albicans* isolates are resistant to flucytosine, there is little use for this drug in CMC.

It is rarely necessary to use intravenous antifungal drugs such as amphotericin. Only in severe cases of esophageal candidiasis or systemic *Candida* infection is intravenous use indicated.

Additional antifungal drugs are under development. One group of compounds, the echinocandins, caspofungin and micafungin, have a novel mechanism of action: inhibition of synthesis of beta (1,3)-D-glucan, a component of the fungal cell wall. These drugs are active against organisms resistant to azole and polyene antifungal drugs. In a clinical trial of patients with invasive infections with various species of *Candida,* caspofungin given intravenously was equal to or superior to amphotericin B (Mora-Duarte et al., 2002). Dosage in pediatric patients has not been established, but one 13-year-old with chronic granulomatous disease has been treated with a first-day dose of 1.4 mg/kg and then 1.0 mg/kg daily (Sallman et al., 2003).

Prognosis

Factors that decrease survival of CMC patients include failure to recognize the extent of the immune deficiency, failure to recognize life-threatening endocrinopathies such as hypoadrenalism or hypoparathyroidism, and failure to consider thymoma. Patients with recurrent respiratory infections must be evaluated for defective antibody production or neutrophil function. Early recognition of these deficiencies will allow treatment to prevent structural airway changes and chronic pulmonary disease.

Although most endocrinopathies become evident during the first or second decade, some CMC patients may not show clinically significant endocrine failure until adulthood. An example is a 25-year-old man with candidiasis and hypoparathyroidism who boasted of his suntan during the winter; the diagnostic studies revealed adrenal insufficiency. It seems reasonable to conduct annual studies of endocrine function in such patients and any other members of the family who have mucocutaneous candidiasis. Thymoma should be considered in any person with an onset of candidiasis during adulthood. Early demise can also occur as a result of severe autoimmunity, notably autoimmune hepatis. With adequate care, most CMC patients have a good prognosis for a normal life and life span.

Charles H. Kirkpatrick

BIOTIN-RESPONSIVE IMMUNODEFICIENCIES: MULTIPLE COCARBOXYLASE DEFICIENCIES AND BIOTIN DEFICIENCY

Definition

Biotin-responsive immunodeficiency is due to genetic defects in one of the four human cocarboxylases for which biotin is a coenzyme or to a deficiency of biotin resulting from its lack in the diet or to excessive ingestion of egg white containing the biotin-binding protein avidin. The clinical features are highly variable, and the immunodeficiency is usually manifested by candidiasis; however, more severe infections may also be present. Other clinical manifestations include metabolic acidosis, neurologic abnormalities, dermatitis, and alopecia.

Two forms of cocarboxylase deficiency occur: a holocarboxylase synthetase deficiency (early-onset [neonatal] multiple cocarboxylase deficiency) and biotinidase deficiency (late-onset [juvenile] multiple cocarboxylase deficiency). Both are inherited as autosomal recessive traits.

Children with multiple carboxylase deficiencies usually present in early infancy or early childhood with severe acidosis, neurologic abnormalities, chronic dermatitis, alopecia, *Candida* infection, and systemic infection with bacteria and viruses. All manifestations of the disease respond to treatment with biotin.

Historical Aspects

Biotin-dependent multiple carboxylase deficiency was initially described as a biochemical disorder associated with severe acidosis in infancy (Packman et al., 1981; Roth, 1976). The infantile early-onset form was often associated with bacterial infections, including bacteremia and pneumonia. The delayed form of the disease usually occurs after the first year of life and was often associated with dermatitis, mucocutaneous candidiasis, alopecia, and keratoconjunctivitis (Charles et al., 1979; Cowan et al., 1979; Theone et al., 1979). A specific immunodeficiency was recognized in 1979 (Cowan et al., 1979).

Pathogenesis

A variety of carboxylation reactions require biotin as an essential coenzyme. These reactions involve nucleic acid, fatty acid, carbohydrate, and branched-chain amino acid metabolism. Patients with early-onset disease have been described with deficiencies of propionyl-

CoA carboxylase, B-methylcrotonyl-CoA carboxylase, and pyruvate carboxylase, all of which are biotin dependent, suggesting an abnormality in biotin transport or intracellular metabolism (Saunders et al., 1979).

Patients with late-onset disease associated with biotinidase defects cannot recycle endogenous biotin or release dietary protein-bound biotin, thus affecting cocarboxylase activity throughout the body and particularly in the brain.

In some patients, a nutritional deficiency of biotin may occur, resulting in identical clinical and laboratory abnormalities. Nutritional biotin deficiency has been reported under two circumstances: (1) omission of biotin from total parenteral nutrition or (2) the inclusion of large amounts of raw egg whites (avidin) in the diet (Baugh et al., 1968; Sweetman et al., 1979).

Experimental evidence suggests that biotin regulates immunologic function and, when deficient, is responsible for abnormal antibody formation, decreased T-cell cytotoxicity, and increased susceptibility to infection. Because biotin-dependent carboxylases are responsible for the metabolism of carbohydrates, amino acids, fatty acids, and purines, immunologic function is probably adversely affected by a deficiency in one or more of these pathways. Although large amounts of organic acids accumulate in the urine of these patients, a toxic metabolite for T cells has not been identified.

Clinical Features

Infants with the early-onset form of multiple carboxylase deficiency present with severe acidosis, bacterial infections, bacteremia, and pneumonia. In the late-onset form, chronic dermatitis, which may surround the eyes, is usually present. Alopecia is prominent. *Candida* infection of the involved skin and mucous membranes is a common finding. Progressive ataxia and dementia become prominent. The late-onset variety is characterized by a gradual onset and frequent episodes of remission.

Untreated, both forms of biotin-dependent multiple carboxylase deficiency are fatal. Patients may succumb to acute viral infections, develop acute bacterial infections, or have fatal reactions following immunization with live virus vaccines.

Laboratory Features

Detailed immunologic evaluations have been performed in only a few patients. Usually, delayed hypersensitivity skin test responses to *Candida* antigen are absent (Cowan et al., 1979). One patient had selective IgA deficiency and abnormal antibody responses to pneumococcal polysaccharide immunization. SCID with biotinidase deficiency has been described in a 7-month-old girl; a BMT and biotin therapy led to immunologic recovery but neurologic damage persisted (Ginat-Israeli et al., 1993).

If T-cell studies are performed by standard laboratory techniques using culture medium supplemented with biotin, a specific immunologic defect may not be detected. T-cell functional studies should be performed in a culture medium without supplemental biotin.

Other laboratory abnormalities reflect the metabolic effects of multiple carboxylase deficiencies and including organic aciduria, ketonuria, lactic acidosis, hypoglycemia, hyperglycinuria, hyperphosphatemia, and hyperammonemia. At autopsy, neuropathologic examination of the brain reveals atrophy and disappearance of the Purkinje layer of the cerebellum (Sander et al., 1980).

A diagnosis of multiple carboxylase deficiency can be established by demonstrating lactic acidosis and elevation of specific organic acids in the plasma or urine. The diagnosis is confirmed by demonstrating the enzyme deficiency in cultured leukocytes or fibroblasts. This method may also be used to establish an intrauterine diagnosis using cultured amniotic fluid cells.

Biotinidase deficiency is now diagnosed in some newborn genetic screening programs.

Treatment

Biotin is the therapy of choice. Biotin is administered orally in a dose ranging from 1 to 40 mg/day. Following treatment, neurologic, dermatologic, and immunologic abnormalities are corrected. Biotin must be administered on a continuous basis for an indefinite period of time. Biotin administered to a pregnant woman carrying an affected infant resulted in metabolic correction of the defect at the time of birth. Treatment was temporarily discontinued to confirm the diagnosis and immediately restarted on a long-term basis.

CARTILAGE-HAIR HYPOPLASIA

Definition

Cartilage-hair hypoplasia (CHH) is an autosomal recessive predominantly T-cell deficiency associated with metaphyseal chondrodysplasia, a form of short-limbed dwarfism. It is also termed metaphyseal chondrodysplasia, McKusick type, OMIM 250250. Sometimes erroneously referred to as chondrodystrophic or achondroplastic dwarfism, CHH is clearly distinct from true achondroplasia (OMIM 100800) on clinical and genetic grounds. Genetic penetrance, however, appears reduced when dwarfism is used as the phenotype for ascertainment. Short-limbed dwarfism is sometimes associated with other forms of immunodeficiency without the distinctive hair abnormalities of CHH (see Chapters 13 and 24).

Historical Aspects

McKusick (1964) first noted unusual susceptibility to varicella among Amish children with dwarfism in an Amish community in eastern Pennsylvania. He named this syndrome CHH (McKusick, 1964, 1965).

Davis (1966) and Alexander and Dunbar (1967) also reported patients with immunodeficiency and short-limbed dwarfism. Fulginiti and associates (1968) reported a patient with achondroplasia who developed progressive vaccinia and a predominant T-cell deficiency. Lux and co-workers (1970) and Hong and colleagues (1972) reported non-Amish CHH patients with T-cell deficiencies. Ammann and associates (1974) reported two siblings with short-limbed dwarfism who had a predominant antibody deficiency. CHH patients have been identified throughout the United States and among Dutch, Polish, French, Danish, Algerian, Italian, Spanish, Mexican, and Finnish populations (Makitie and Kaitila, 1993).

The incidence of CHH in Finland is 1:23,000 live births (three new patients per year; carrier rate of 1:76). In the Amish, the incidence is 1:1340 and a carrier rate as high as 1:19 (Ridanpaa et al., 2001).

Pathogenesis

The RNAase RNP (RMRP) Gene

The responsible gene for CHH has been mapped to 9p21-p12 (Sulisalo et al., 1993) and recently isolated (Ridanpaa et Al., 2001) and shown to be the gene encoding an RNAase RMRP protein. This gene had been cloned previously (Topper et al., 1990) and mapped to 9p21-p12 (Hsieh et al., 1990). RMRP is a ribonucleoprotein present in the nucleus and mitochondria of vertebrates implicated in the metabolism of RNA primers at the origins of DNA replication in mitochondria. The RNA component of this ribonucleoprotein is a nuclear gene, which may play a role in nuclear DNA replication (Tollervey and Kiss, 1997).

RNAase MRP also plays a role in ribosomal RNA production when 18S, 5.8S, and 25/28S ribosomal RNAs are generated by this enzyme from a large common precursor RNA. In yeast, RNAase MRP associates with at least three protein subunits Pop1p, Pop3p, and Pop 4p, each of which is required for stability of function of the enzyme. In humans RNAase associates with hPop1, hPop4, Rpp30, and Rpp38.

The RNA component and all the protein partners are required for cell growth but not viability (Tollervey and Kiss, 1997). This observation is in accord with the generalized defect in cell growth observed in T cells, B cells, and fibroblasts (Juvonen et al., 1995; Polmar and Pierce, 1986) and could thus explain part of the features of CHH.

RMRP Mutations

The mutations in CHH are of two types. The first are insertions or duplications between 6 and 30 nucleotides long, which are located between the TATA box and the transcription initiation site. These mutations interfere with the transcription of the RMPR gene and are considered null mutations.

The second type are single nucleotide substitutions or other mutations involving at most two nucleotides, which are located at highly conserved regions of the gene and result in "leaky" expression of the gene: this may in part may explain the variable phenotype observed in CHH (McKusick et al., 1965).

Among 70 CHH patients examined to date, 55 have mutations in both alleles of the RMRP gene (Ridanpaa et Al., 2001). In none of the patients with leaky mutations has the mutated protein failed to interact with hPop1, hPop4, Rpp30, and Rpp38. Additional protein partners have been suggested for RNAase MRP (Tollervey and Kiss, 1997), which could provide a better understanding of the condition.

The identification of the gene responsible for CHH should allow the determination of its relationship to other cases of dwarfism associated with immunodeficiency (Ammann et al., 1974; Castriota-Scanderberg et al., 1997; Corder et al., 1995; Davis, 1966; Fulginiti et al., 1967; Gatti et al., 1969; Lecora et al., 1995; MacDermot et al., 1991; Scanderberg et al., 1997; Schimke et al., 1974; Shokeir, 1978) (see Chapters 13 and 24).

Clinical Features

Morphologic Features

Birth weight is generally normal, but dwarfism is apparent at birth because of the reduced crown-to-heel measurement and abnormally short extremities. In early infancy the skin forms redundant folds around the neck and extremities (Gatti et al., 1969) (Fig. 17-10).

The dwarfism is of the short-limbed variety resembling achondroplasia; however, the head size is normal. The short stature is due to disproportionate shortening

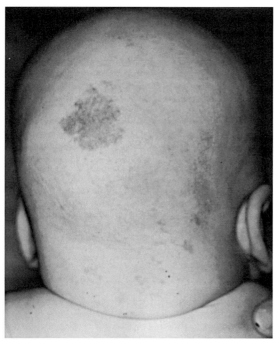

Figure 17-10 · Redundant skin folds in the neck of an infant with short-limbed dwarfism.

of the extremities. The hands are short and pudgy with short fingernails. The joints are loose, but there is limitation of elbow extension and a peculiar sternal defect (McKusick et al., 1964) The feet are often flat with weight bearing.

The hair of the scalp, eyebrows, and eyelashes is silky white or yellow in color, is very sparse and fine, and lacks a central pigmented core (Fig. 17-11). Body hair is similarly affected and along with the head hair, darkens with increasing age. Some patients appear bald; others rarely need haircuts because of hair breakage.

In females, breast development, menses, and sexual function are normal. Sexual development in males is also normal. Marriages of two affected individuals have produced families in which all children are affected and must be delivered by Caesarian section. Intelligence is normal. Adult height varies between 40 and 60 inches.

Infections

Most CHH patients have only a limited susceptibility to infection and thus live normal lives. Only 31% of 108 Finnish patients had increased susceptibility to infection (Mackitie et al., 1992). Varicella is the most common severe infection; two CHH children died of varicella at 6 and 9 year of age and five almost succumbed (Lux et al., 1970; McKusick et al., 1964). Vaccinia and poliovirus infections also are potentially lethal (Fulginiti et al., 1972; Hong et al., 1972; Saulsbury et al., 1975).

The occasional patient with short-limbed dwarfism (with or without CHH) and a SCID will have a broad susceptibility to overwhelming infection (Alexander and Dunbar, 1967; Davis, 1966; Gatti et al., 1969). These patients may succumb to overwhelming infection in infancy, and are susceptible to GVHD and *P. carinii* infection. CHH is a very rare cause of SCID; among 108 SCID patients in a large U.S. series, only one case of CHH was identified (Buckley et al., 1997).

Other Clinical Features

Anemia and neutropenia are common. GI manifestations including malabsorption, celiac disease, and aganglionic megacolon (Hirschsprung's disease) have been described (McKusick et al., 1994).

An increased incidence of cancer, particularly leukemia and lymphoma (Hodgkin's and non-Hodgkin's) has been described in CHH (Francomano et al., 1983; Makitie et al., 1999). BMT corrects the immunodeficiency but not the chondrodysplasia (Berthet et al., 1996).

Laboratory Features

In a large Finnish study, anemia and/or macrocytosis during childhood occurred in 86% of patients, lymphopenia in 62%, and neutropenia in 24% (Junoven et al., 1995; Makitie et al., 1993). The anemia is macrocytic and refractory to therapy. One child developed red blood cell aplasia (Lux et al., 1970). The anemia significantly correlated with growth failure and immunodeficiency and is thought to reflect a generalized defect in cellular proliferation (Makitie et al., 1992; Polmar and Pierce, 1986). Reduced colony formation of hematopoietic progenitors in vitro has been reported (Juvonen et al., 1995).

Immunologic Features

The immunodeficiency is variable. The major T-cell abnormalities include lymphopenia, reduced delayed-type hypersensitivity including allograft rejection, and reduced lymphoproliferative responses (Lux et al., 1970). Maktie and colleagues (1998) reported that 52% of their patients had reduced total T-cell numbers, 57% had reduced CD4 counts, 32% had a reduced CD4/CD8 ratio, and 40% had increased NK cells. B cells were normal. In the same series, proliferative responses were diminished to concanavalin A (Con A) in 69%, to PHA in 69%, and to pokeweed mitogen (PWM) in 83%. Others report similar findings (Polmar and Pierce et al., 1986; Thorjak et al., 1981; Van der Burgt et al., 1991). Immunoglobulin levels and antibody function are generally normal (Lux et al., 1970), although a few patients have antibody deficiency of varying severity.

Skeletal Features

Ultrasonography for prenatal diagnosis has revealed normal bone development at 14 weeks gestation but by 17 weeks there is significant shortening and bowing of the femur (Dungan et al., 1996).

Radiographic findings performed before epiphyseal closure reveal normal ossification centers with scalloping, irregular sclerosis, and cystic changes of the widened metaphyses of most bones (Fig. 17-12). All the tubular bones of the extremities are involved with this process, as are the ribs. Abnormalities of the sternum have also been reported. The skull is normal.

Histopathologically there is a relative paucity of cartilage cells and a failure of the cells to line up in orderly columns. Ossification appears normal with normal numbers of osteoblasts and osteoclasts. There appears

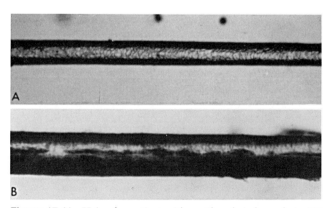

Figure 17-11 · Hair of a patient with cartilage-hair hypoplasia (A) compared with sample from the normal parent (B). The affected hair lacks the central pigment core, and the diameter is smaller.

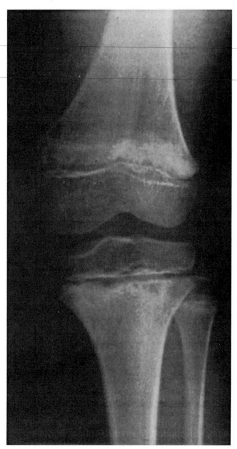

Figure 17-12 · X-ray film of the tibia in a child with short-limbed dwarfism. The irregular sclerosis, cystic changes, and scalloped appearance are apparent.

to be inadequate cartilage for bone deposition (McKusick et al., 1965).

Treatment

Immunoglobulin therapy is indicated if a significant antibody defect is present. Varicella vaccine should be given if the patient has near normal T-cell function and adequate antibody function; the antibody response following vaccine should be measured. Varicella-zoster immune globulin and antiviral drugs can be used for prevention (for the exposed seronegative patient) and treatment of varicella.

For CHH patients with profound T-cell defects, the same precautions are necessary as for patients with combined immunodeficiency (see Chapters 12 and 15). BMT for CHH patients with SCID is curative but will not affect the morphologic features or dwarfism (Berthet et al., 1966) (see Chapter 43).

Prognosis

The prognosis is better for CHH patients than for most T-cell deficiencies because their susceptibility to infection is less. For those with combined immunodeficiency,

the prognosis for long life is poor unless immunologic reconstitution is achieved.

IDIOPATHIC CD4+ LYMPHOCYTOPENIA

Definition

Idiopathic CD4+ lymphocytopenia (ICL) is a clinically heterogeneous syndrome defined as persistent depletion of peripheral blood CD4+ T lymphocytes less than 300 cells/mm^3 or less than 20% of the total lymphocytes in the absence of HIV infection or other known causes of immunodeficiency (CDC, 1992; Smith et al., 1993).

ICL was first recognized during the early years of the AIDS epidemic when an occasional patient was identified with profound CD4 T lymphocytopenia but without evidence of HIV infection. Concurrent CD8 lymphocytopenia was present in a few of these patients, whereas many others had abnormal immunoglobulin levels. Many of these patients had risk factors for HIV infection.

Clinical manifestations are heterogeneous; some patients have opportunistic infections typical of HIV-infected individuals with advanced disease, some have other conditions, and some are asymptomatic. In some patients complete or partial reversal of the CD4 lymphocytopenia occurs. An extensive search for a viral cause through serologic, culture, and PCR testing has been negative (Ho et al., 1993).

Pathogenesis

Epidemiology

In the initial CDC investigation, the prevalence of ICL was 0.0002%. Among 47 ICL patients, age, gender, ethnicity, and risk factors for HIV infection varied. Approximately 40% had engaged in high-risk sexual behavior or had a history of blood or blood product exposure. However, investigation of close contacts, sexual partners, children, and their blood donors provided no evidence of transmissibility (Smith et al., 1993).

Following the initial CDC report, a retrospective investigation of more than 1200 HIV-seronegative drug users in New York followed for more than 8 years identified only four patients who fulfilled the CDC case definition (Des Jarlais et al., 1993). Given the possibility that an unknown retrovirus was responsible for ICL, blood donor screening by assessing CD4 cell numbers was suggested. In a pilot study of approximately 2000 blood donors, 0.25% of HIV-seronegative individuals were found to have transient CD4 lymphocytopenia associated with temporary illnesses. Because no true cases of ICL were identified, CD4 cell count donor screening was deemed costly and unfeasible (Busch et al., 1994).

An investigation of more than 300 HIV-seronegative hemophiliac men and their sexual partners demonstrated that 2.3% of patients and 0.6% of their partners met the ICL case definition although three patients recovered spontaneously (O'Brien et al., 1995). When compared with hemophiliac ICL-negative controls, a history of liver disease and splenomegaly was more prevalent among the ICL patients. The presence of hepatitis C antibodies was nearly universal in both groups.

Role of Infection

Despite the high prevalence of ICL among intravenous drug users and hemophiliacs, no infectious agent has been identified such as HIV-1, HIV-2, HTLV-1, and HTLV-2 (Ho et al., 1993; Spira et al., 1993). Garry and colleagues (1996) demonstrated a cytopathic effect (CPE) on tissue culture of one ICL patient's peripheral blood mononuclear cells (PBMCs) with a lymphoblastoid cell line and identified A-type retroviral particles. In this study, sera from 8 of 13 ICL patients reacted by Western immunoblotting with these retroviral particles, and control sera remained negative. In addition, sera from 8 of 14 ICL patients were positive for antinuclear antibodies.

Mechanism of CD4 Lymphocytopenia

The mechanism of CD4 cell loss in ICL is due to spontaneous and accelerated CD4+ cell apoptosis (Laurence et al., 1996). Apoptosis may be associated with enhanced expression of Fas and Fas ligand. Patients with stable physiologic CD4 cell lymphopenia without opportunistic infections did not demonstrate accelerated apoptosis. Roger and associates (1999) demonstrated that a patient with ICL and disseminated *Mycobacterium xenopi* infection had overexpression of Fas/CD95c and spontaneous and Fas-induced apoptosis.

Alpha/beta and gamma/delta T-cell repertoires of ICL patients are highly restricted (Signorini et al., 2000). Biochemical defects of the CD3-TCR transduction pathway have been demonstrated in ICL patients (Hubert et al., 1999), possibly resulting from an abnormality of tyrosine kinase activity p56(Lck) (Hubert et al., 2000).

A 9-year-old child with ICL had reduced CD45RA (naïve T-cell phenotype) expression, enhanced CD45RO (memory T-cell phenotype) expression, and an increase in gamma/delta TCR-bearing T cells. Accelerated apoptosis was noted only in the CD45RO+ cell subsets, suggesting disturbed thymic T-cell maturation (Fruhwirth et al., 2001).

Clinical Features

Most of the originally reported ICL patients were adults; however, the condition has subsequently been described in a small number of children and adolescents (Fruhwirth et al., 2001; Lobato et al., 1995; Menon et al., 1998). ICL's gender, age, and geographic distribution are much wider than that of HIV infection. ICL has also been reported in the elderly (Kaiser and Morley, 1994; Matsuyama et al., 1998). The clinical manifestations that accompany ICL are variable.

Mycobacterial Infections

ICL patients may have opportunistic infections or other conditions or may be completely asymptomatic despite continuously low CD4 cell subsets. Tuberculosis is particularly common in ICL. In a study from West Africa, 14% of patients with advanced disseminated tuberculosis presented with CD4 cell subsets lower than 300 cells/mm³ in the absence of HIV infection (Kony et al., 2000).

The profound lymphocytopenia may result from the disseminated tuberculosis (Pilheu et al., 1997; Zaharatos et al., 2001), rather than the tuberculosis a result of the lymphocytopenia. Indeed, low numbers of CD4 and CD8 subsets in HIV-seronegative patients with severe pulmonary tuberculosis may serve as a surrogate for adverse clinical outcomes (Pilheu et al., 1997). ICL has also been identified in patients with atypical mycobacteria infections (Anzalone et al., 1996; Schantz et al., 2000).

Other Infections

ICL has been identified in several patients with opportunistic infections, including skin, musculoskeletal, CNS, and disseminated infections with *Cryptococcus* species (Kumlin et al., 1997; Menon et al., 1998; Nunez et al., 1999; Santos et al., 2002; Watanabe et al., 2000; Zanelli et al., 2001). Aspergillosis, toxoplasmosis, and histoplasmosis have also been reported (Nakahira et al., 2002; Tassinari et al., 1996) as has PCP (Ho et al., 1993; Sinicco et al., 1996).

Human papillomavirus (HPV) infections are not uncommon in ICL, particularly infections with HPV types 2, 3, and 18. Clinical manifestations included chronic pruritic papules, skin warts, alopecia areata, and Bowen's disease (Gubinelli et al., 2002; Hayashi et al., 1997; Manchado-Lopez et al., 1999; Paolini et al., 1996; Purnell et al., 2001; Stetson et al., 2002; Wakeel et al., 1994).

Other viral infections in ICL include hepatitis C (O'Brien et al., 1995), varicella-zoster (Warnatz et al., 2000), EBV (Shimano et al., 1997), CMV (Longo et al., 1999), JC virus, and polyoma viruses (the latter two in association with progressive multifocal leukoencephalopathy [PML]) (Haider et al., 2000; Iwase et al., 1998).

Sepsis-like illnesses with unusual pathogens such as *Fusobacterium nucleatum* and *Salmonella typhimurium* have been described in ICL (Burg et al., 1994; Etienne et al., 2001). Asymptomatic ICL has also been reported (Cascio et al., 1998).

Malignancies

Neoplastic disorders have been described in ICL, similar to those described in advanced HIV patients and other chronically immunocompromised patients with posttransplant lymphoproliferative disorder (PTLD). Lymphomas are not uncommon in ICL, including non-Hodgkin's lymphoma (Campbell et al., 2001; Hanamura et al., 1997; Longo et al., 1999), leptomeningeal lymphoma (Busse and Cunningham-Rundles, 2002), intravascular cerebral lymphomas (Guilloton et al., 1999), and EBV-related

Burkitt's lymphomas (Shimano et al., 1997). Viral-mediated malignancies such as Kaposi sarcoma of the digestive tract (Ben Rejeb et al., 2001) and cutaneous neoplasias such as vulval carcinoma (Rijnders et al., 1996) or epidermoid carcinomas (Michel et al., 1996) have been described.

Autoimmune Disorders

ICL has been associated with several autoimmune diseases, including Sjögren's syndrome (Kirtava et al., 1995), polyarteritis/vasculitis (Bordin et al., 1996), autoimmune skin disease including psoriasis (Hardman et al., 1997), erosive lichen of the scalp (Brudy et al., 1997), autoimmune vitiligo (Yamauchi et al., 2002), Behcet's-like syndrome (Venzor et al., 1997), and allergic conditions such as atopic dermatitis (Goodrich et al., 1993). Associations with sarcoidosis (Sinicco et al., 1996) and idiopathic bronchiolitis obliterans (Pohl, 1996) have also been described. Kirtava and associates (1995) showed that 6 of 115 Swedish patients with primary Sjögren's syndrome had ICL, and one progressed to lymphoma. Studies for a retrovirus were negative.

Laboratory Features

The diagnosis of ICL is based on persistently low numbers of CD4 cells on at least two separate analyses. Other immunologic or infectious disorders that would explain the CD4 deficiency must also be excluded, as should OKT4 epitope deficiency (OED) (discussed elsewhere in this chapter), particularly if there is a complete absence of CD4 cells.

In some patients there is an increased percentage of CD8 cells but not in their absolute numbers in conjunction with normal or slightly low levels of immunoglobulins. Lymphoproliferative responses to mitogens and antigens may be depressed (Spira et al., 1993). In four patients with ICL and opportunistic infections, only one patient had progressive decline of CD4 T cells, whereas all had significantly reduced CD8 T-cells, NK cells, and B cells (Duncan et al., 1993). In most cases of ICL, the CD4 cells stabilize at a low level rather than progress to zero as in HIV infection.

Treatment

There is no standard treatment for ICL except for management of the associated conditions. IL-2 was used successfully in ICL patients with relapsing herpes zoster infections (Warnatz et al., 2000) and in patients with interstitial nephritis (Wilhelm et al., 2001). Polyethylene glycol-conjugated IL-2 (PEG-IL-2) was used with success in an ICL patient with mycobacterial disease (Cunningham-Rundles et al., 1999). One ICL patient received an allogeneic BMT with restoration of CD4 T lymphocyte counts (Petersen et al., 1996).

Karin Nielsen

OKT4 EPITOPE DEFICIENCY

Definition

OED is a laboratory phenomenon in which there is an apparent absence of CD4 cells because the subject's CD4 antigen is not recognized by one of the anti-CD4 monoclonal antibodies (OKT4) often used to enumerate CD4 cells by flow cytometry. CD4 antigen is readily identified with other anti-CD4 monoclonal antibodies. Most subjects have normal CD4 cells and function.

Pathogenesis

CD4 is a surface molecule of T cells that binds to class II major histocompatibility complex (MHC) molecules (see Chapter 2). In so doing, it augments the ability of T cells to respond to antigen peptides carried in the class II MHC molecule cleft of antigen-presenting cells. Different epitopes (e.g., antigenic sites) of CD4 are distinguished by the monoclonal antibodies OKT4 and Leu-3a.

In 1981, Bach and colleagues described patients whose CD4[+] cells did not react with the anti-CD4 monoclonal antibody (MoAb) OKT4 but did bind to the anti-CD4 MoAb Leu-3a. Subsequently, numerous individuals with OED have been reported (Aozasa et al., 1985; Fukuda et al., 1984; Gill et al., 1985; Levinson et al., 1985; Sato el al., 1984; Stohl et al., 1985).

The CD4 epitope recognized by MoAb leu-3a is the HIV receptor, serving as a portal of entry into the T lymphocyte and macrophage. The epitope recognized by OKT4 is not required for HIV entry (Hoxie et al., 1986); indeed HIV infection has been identified in patients with OED (Khuong et al., 1994).

Clinical and Laboratory Features

Most patients with OED are asymptomatic and are able to resist infectious agents that are susceptible to T-cell control. Autoimmune problems such as Graves' disease and systemic lupus erythematosus have been reported (Fukuda et al., 1984; Stohl et al., 1985). An OED patient with thymoma, hypogammaglobulinemia, and red blood cell aplasia was reported by Levinson and co-workers (1985).

The T cells of OED patients respond to mitogens, and delayed hypersensitivity skin tests are normal. A slight defect in T-helper function support of immunoglobulin production may be present (Aozasa et al., 1985; Fukuda et al., 1984; Levinson et al., 1985; Sato et al., 1984; Stohl et al., 1985). Thus most, if not all, of the physiologic functions of CD4 are unaffected by OED.

The disorder is inherited as an autosomal codominant trait. Homozygotes lack completely OKT4[+] cells. Heterozygotes show normal numbers of OKT4[+] cells, but they express this antigen at approximately 50% of the density of normal persons (Aozasa et al., 1985; Takenaka et al., 1993). The trait is more common in blacks (8.3%) but rare in whites and Japanese (<1%) (Aozasa et al., 1985; Takenaka et al., 1993).

OED is important to recognize so that the subject is not labeled as having a severe T-cell deficiency. No treatment is indicated.

THE HYPER-IgE SYNDROME

Definition

The hyper-IgE syndrome, sometimes termed *Job's syndrome,* is a primary immunodeficiency characterized by recurrent infections, particularly staphylococcal infections; coarse facial features; skeletal abnormalities; and markedly elevated serum IgE levels (Buckley et al., 1972; Buckley, 2001). In some families it is inherited as an AD trait with incomplete penetrance.

Hyper-IgE patients have a lifelong history of severe recurrent staphylococcal abscesses involving the skin, lungs, joints, and other sites. In addition, there is a unique tendency to form persistent pneumatoceles following staphylococcal pneumonias. Although there usually is a history of pruritic dermatitis, the rash does not have the typical distribution of atopic dermatitis, and respiratory allergies are usually absent.

Historical Aspects

The first two patients with the hyper-IgE syndrome, both with the characteristic coarse features, were reported by Buckley and co-workers in 1972. In 1966, two girls with red hair, fair skin, and hyperextensible joints with cold, nontender, cutaneous abscesses had been described; IgE levels were not reported (Davis et al., 1966). The authors called the condition *Job's syndrome* after the biblical Job who was smitten with boils. ("So went Satan forth from the presence of the Lord, and smote Job with sore boils from the sole of his foot unto his crown" Job 2:7) Serum IgE concentrations were later found to be elevated in these and other similar patients (Hill et al., 1974).

Since 1972, we have evaluated more than 40 additional hyper-IgE patients (Buckley, 2001; Claassen et al., 1991; Sheerin and Buckley, 1991). Many other patients with this syndrome have also been reported from other centers (Blum et al., 1977; Chamlin et al., 2002; Church et al., 1976; Clark et al., 1973; Donabedian and Gallin, 1983; Geha and Leung, 1983; Grimbacher et al., 1999a; Hill et al., 1974; Soderberg-Warner et al., 1983; VanScoy et al., 1975; Weston et al., 1977).

Pathogenesis

Neither the precise host defect nor the fundamental biology underlying this condition has been found. The combination of an elevated serum IgE and osteoporosis is also a feature of IL-4 transgenic mice, suggesting one possible mechanism for their co-existence (Lewis et al., 1993). Such mice also have abnormalities in thymic selection (Lewis et al., 1991).

Genetics

Fourteen instances of familial occurrence of the hyper-IgE syndrome were noted among the 40 patients evaluated by Buckley (2001), and there are several additional familial reports (Blum et al., 1977; Van Scoy et al., 1975). The fact that both males and females were affected, as were members of succeeding generations, suggested an AD inheritance with incomplete penetrance (Buckley, 2001; Grimbacher et al., 1999a). In some patients of Turkish origin, there appears to be an autosomal recessive form of inheritance. There are also many sporadic cases.

The defect in some patients with an apparent AD inheritance has been mapped to chromosome 4 (Grimbacher et al., 1999b), but other cases could not be mapped to this chromosome. A candidate gene has not yet been identified (Grimbacher et al., 1999b). It is likely that genome research will soon identify the faulty gene (or genes) responsible for this syndrome.

IgE Regulation

Because of the apparent abnormal regulation of IgE synthesis in these patients, a regulatory T-cell defect has been sought. Using a reproducible system for studying IgE synthesis in vitro (Claassen et al., 1990), B cells from hyper-IgE patients were found to be paradoxically relatively refractory to stimulation with IL-4 (Fig. 17-13), suggesting that they may have already been stimulated with excessive endogenous IL-4 in vivo (Claassen et al., 1991). It has been difficult to prove, however, that patients with the hyper-IgE syndrome produce excessive IL-4, in part because IL-4 is difficult to measure as a result of its short half-life.

Cytokine Abnormalities

Del Prete and colleagues (1989) found that the precursor frequency of T cells of patients with the hyper-IgE syndrome able to produce IFN-γ and TNF-α is markedly decreased when compared with controls but that the precursor frequency of T cells producing IL-4 is normal. This was associated with decreased T-cell IFN-γ and TNF-α production following in vitro mitogen stimulation. Paganelli and co-workers (1991) reported that there were severely reduced or undetectable IFN-γ in the supernatants of mononuclear cells (MNCs) but that the precursor frequency of IL-4–producing T cells was normal. By contrast, neither Vercelli and associates (1990) nor we found deficient IFN-γ production by T cells in their patients with the hyper-IgE syndrome.

Borges and associates (2000) found less production of IFN-γ by the MNCs of hyper-IgE patients when activated by *S. aureus* than cells from normal subjects, and IL-12 augmentation of IFN-γ release was also less than in normal controls. Using flow cytometry, radioimmunoassays,

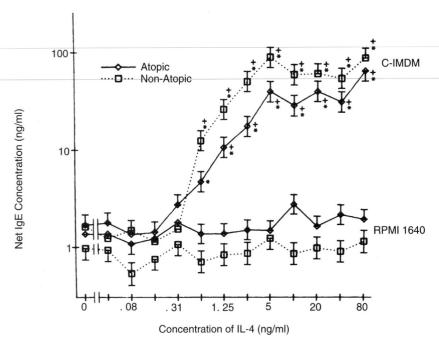

Figure 17-13 · Group mean net IgE concentrations in rhIL-4–stimulated mononuclear cell (MNC) cultures were lower in the donors with hyper-IgE (*N* = 9) than in the nonatopic (*N* = 9) and the atopic (*N* = 9) donors. Unfractionated MNCs were left unstimulated or were stimulated on day 0 with concentrations of IL-4 from 0.04 to 80 ng/ml. Net IgE concentrations were determined after 18 days of culture; +, IgE concentrations in rhIL-4–stimulated cultures were significantly greater compared to those of unstimulated cultures within a given donor group (*P* < .0042). *Significantly greater amounts of IgE were present in cultures of nonatopic and atopic MNCs, as compared with concentrations present in cultures of MNCs of donors with hyper-IgE undergoing the same treatment (*P* < .0013). Data are geometric means ± standard error of the mean (SEM). (From Claassen JL, Levine AD, Schiff SE, Buckley RH. Mononuclear cells from patients with the hyper IgE syndrome produce little IgE when stimulated with recombinant interleukin 4 in vitro. J Allergy Clin Immunol 88:713–721, 1991, with permission.)

and gene array analyses to assess cytokine and chemokine production, Chehimi and co-workers (2001) noted that hyper-IgE patients express more IL-12, whereas ENA-78, MCP-3, and cotaxin were deficient.

These mixed results indicate that there is as yet no clearly defined T-cell abnormality in the hyper-IgE syndrome. If such a deficiency is found, it is likely to be one of Th1 cells or cytokines. However, abnormal IgE regulation does not explain the infection susceptibility of these patients, because equally high levels of IgE are found in many patients with atopic dermatitis without susceptibility to abscess formation (Fiser and Buckley, 1979; Sampson and Buckley, 1981).

Clinical Features

The hyper-IgE syndrome is a rare disorder, and it must be emphasized that these are not merely individuals with atopic eczema with repeated superficial cutaneous infections. In our review of 40 patients with the hyper-IgE syndrome (Buckley et al., 2001) from a wide geographic area, the age range was from 1 to 44 years at the time of initial evaluation; two thirds were male and 30% were African American (Table 17-13). Dermatitis was present in nearly all, but wheezing was uncommon. IgE levels ranged from 320 IU/ml in an infant girl to 130,000 IU/ml in a 22-year-old female.

Infections

Hyper-IgE patients invariably have recurrent, severe bouts of furunculosis and pneumonia secondary to *S. aureus* starting in early infancy, some from day 1 of life. In most patients, persistent pneumatoceles developed as a result of recurrent pneumonias (Merten et al.,

TABLE 17-13 · CLINICAL FEATURES OF 40 PATIENTS WITH THE HYPER-IgE SYNDROME

1. Severe infections of the skin and lower respiratory tract from infancy. All have had furunculosis and staphylococcal pneumonia, and more than half have had persistent pneumatoceles; 11 have required lung surgery. Most have also had infections of ears, sinuses, eyes, and oral mucosa. Fewer have had infections of joints, viscera, or blood.
2. *Staphylococcus aureus*, coagulase-positive, has caused infections in all. *Candida albicans, Haemophilus influenzae,* pneumococci, and group A streptococci isolated in from 25% to 50%, miscellaneous gram-negative rods and other fungi in some.
3. Pruritic dermatitis chronically or (more often) in past, little or no respiratory allergy. Rash is *not* typical atopic eczema.
4. Both sexes affected (males 26; females 14); 28 were white, 12 were black.
5. Familial occurrence in 14/40 patients in 8 families; IgE normal in nonaffected relatives. Pattern in families suggests autosomal dominant trait with incomplete penetrance. No increased frequency of any HLA-A or HLA-B locus antigens.

From Buckley, 2001, with permission.

1979) (Fig. 17-14). Of our 40 patients, 11 required thoracic surgery because of giant persistent chronically infected pneumatoceles; 2 underwent complete pneumonectomies, 9 had lobectomies for lung abscesses, 1 had an empyema, and 1 had an anterior mediastinal *Candida* granuloma. The hyper-IgE syndrome may present with a clinical picture of CMC (see the section on CMC).

As shown in Table 17-14, all patients were plagued by infections with *S. aureus,* but some also had recurrent *H. influenzae,* pneumococcal, group A streptococcal, gram-negative, and fungal infections. The sites of infection are listed in Table 17-15. Infections of the skin and lungs predominated, but the ears, eyes, oral

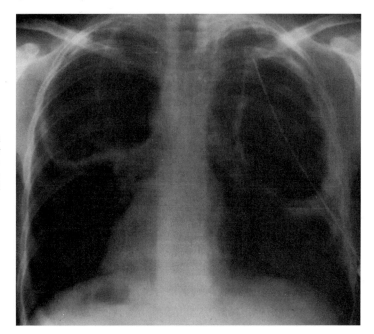

Figure 17-14 · Chest roentgenogram of 12-year-old boy with the hyper-IgE syndrome. Giant pneumatoceles were present for more than 1 year. A putrid abscess caused by *Enterobacter cloacae* led to chest tube insertion on the right. The left cyst necessitated emergency excision because of massive hemoptysis and was found to contain an aspergilloma.

TABLE 17-14 · ORGANISMS ASSOCIATED WITH INFECTION IN 40 PATIENTS WITH THE HYPER-IgE SYNDROME

Organisms	Number of Patients Infected
Staphylococcus aureus, coagulase positive	40/40
Candida albicans	20/40
Miscellaneous gram-negative organisms	11/40
Haemophilus influenzae	9/40
Pneumococci	9/40
Streptococci, group A	4/40
Aspergillus species	4/40
Trichophyton species	2/40
Cryptococcus neoformans	1/40
Pneumocystis carinii	1/40
Mycoplasma hominis	1/40

From Buckley, 2001, with permission.

TABLE 17-15 · SITES OF INFECTION IN 40 PATIENTS WITH THE HYPER-IgE SYNDROME

Sites of Infection	Number of Patients Affected
Skin	39/40
Abscesses	39/40
Deep cellulitis	3/40
Lung	39/40
Pneumatoceles	24/40
Resection of lobes	9/40
Total pneumonectomy	2/40
Ears	30/40
Mastoidectomy	2/40
Oral mucosa	20/40
Sinuses	18/40
Eyes	15/40
Viscera	10/40
Joints	6/40
Blood	4/40

From Buckley, 2001, with permission.

mucosa, sinuses, joints, blood, and even viscera were also involved. A peculiar tendency of the abscesses to localize about the scalp, face, and neck was observed in infants and younger children. Sites that were not foci of infections included the urinary and GI tracts and the bones (except for mastoids). Cryptococcal meningitis was observed in three patients, but bacterial meningitis was not seen.

Patients with the hyper-IgE syndrome and chronic granulomatous disease (CGD) (see Chapter 20) share a susceptibility to abscess formation but differ in several respects. Unlike CGD patients, hyper-IgE patients may have infections with catalase-negative organisms such as streptococci and pneumococci. Furthermore, although CGD patients may also have staphylococcal pneumonias, they rarely have persistent pneumatoceles as occur in hyper-IgE patients (Chamlin et al., 2002; Merten et al.,

1979). Finally, unlike CGD patients, hyper-IgE patients rarely have osteomyelitis, urinary tract infections or obstruction, diarrhea, or GI obstruction.

Although abscesses in our hyper-IgE patients have been tender and warm, many patients, despite having large deep-seated abscesses, had minimal systemic toxicity. The cold abscesses described in the original Job's syndrome patients (Davis et al., 1966) are unusual.

Dermatitis

All but 1 of our 40 patients had either a pruritic dermatitis at the time of evaluation or, more often, a history of such a dermatitis earlier in life. Although the lesions resembled those of an eczematoid dermatitis, the distribution and characteristics of the lesions are not typical of atopic eczema. A papulopustular eruption on the face and scalp in the first year of life has been noted by us and others (Chamlin et al., 2002).

Allergy

None of our patients had allergic rhinitis, and only three were noted to wheeze; even in these patients, it was not a prominent symptom. Two patients without a history of wheezing were given methacholine inhalation challenges without a significant drop in pulmonary function. Thus there was minimal evidence of respiratory allergy in these patients. None had evidence of parasitic infestation. Several patients were growth retarded, mainly those with chronic lower respiratory tract infection.

Facies

Coarse facial features were noted by Buckley (1972) in the first two patients. This has been a consistent feature of most patients with this syndrome (Buckley, 2001) (Figs. 17-15 and 17-16). Hyper-IgE syndrome patients look very different from their unaffected family members.

Distinctive facial characteristics were also pointed out by Grimbacher and his associates (Grimbacher et al., 1999a) (Table 17-16). Among their findings were a prominent forehead, deep-set eyes, a broad nasal bridge, a wide fleshy nasal tip, mild prognathism, facial asymmetry, and hemihypertrophy. The mean nasal interalar distance in these patients was above the 98th percentile ($P < .001$). These findings were present in all patients by age 16 years (Grimbacher et al., 1999a).

Bone and Teeth Abnormalities

An interesting previously unreported observation by Grimbacher and colleagues (1999a) was that 72% of their patients had a failure or delayed shedding of primary teeth, because of lack of root resorption. However, only 77% of their patients had the clinical diagnostic criteria of abscesses, pneumonias with pneumatoceles, and elevated IgE. Because there is no distinctive laboratory test for this condition, it is unclear whether all of these patients had the hyper-IgE syndrome.

A high incidence of scoliosis and hyperextensible joints has been noted. Osteopenia is also present in most patients with the hyper-IgE syndrome, many of whom have recurrent fractures (Chamlin et al., 2002;

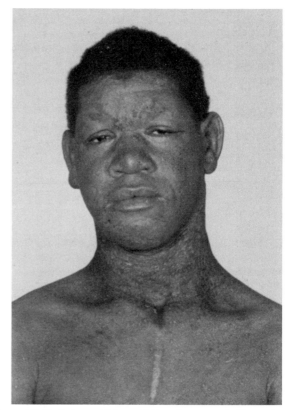

Figure 17-16· Patient with hyper-IgE syndrome, again illustrating the coarse facial features. Scar over upper chest is from excision of a *Candida* granuloma of the mediastinum.

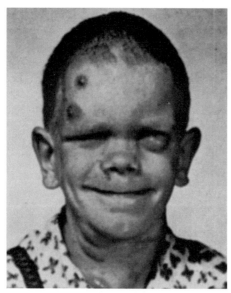

Figure 17-15· Patient with hyper-IgE syndrome showing multiple abscesses of the face and neck and coarse facial features. (From Buckley RH, Wray BB, Belmaker EZ. Extreme hyperimmunoglobulinemia E and undue susceptibility to infection. Pediatrics 49:59–70, 1972, with permission.)

TABLE 17-16· NONIMMUNOLOGIC FEATURES OF 30 PATIENTS WITH THE HYPER-IgE SYNDROME

Failure or delayed shedding of the primary teeth owing to lack of root resorption: 72%
Recurrent fractures resulting from minor trauma: 57%
Hyperextensible joints: 68%
Scoliosis: 76%
Facial asymmetry: hemihypertrophy, prominent forehead, deep-set eyes, broad nasal bridge, wide fleshy nasal tip, and mild prognathism. Present in all by age 16 years.

Modified from Grimbacher et al, 1999a.

Grimbacher et al., 1999a; Kirchner et al., 1985). This problem, which is not correlated with the patient's state of activity or accompanied by abnormalities in calcium or phosphorus metabolism, was so severe in one of our patients that collapse of most vertebral bodies occurred (Buckley et al., 1972). Leung and co-workers (1988b) noted that monocytes from hyper-IgE patients were activated to resorb bone in response to the spontaneous release of prostaglandin E_2 (PGE_2).

Laboratory Features

Hematologic Studies

Blood and sputum eosinophilia has been a consistent finding in the hyper-IgE syndrome (Buckley, 2001; Buckley et al., 1972; Chamlin et al., 2002). Peripheral eosinophilia as high as 55% to 60% has occurred in some infants. Both the percentage and the absolute number of eosinophils usually exceeds that present in most atopic patients. Total white blood cell (WBC) counts range from normal to markedly elevated (50,000 to 60,000/mm^3), but none of our patients were neutropenic or lymphopenic. Anemia is often present in those with chronic lower respiratory infections but is not present when infection is controlled.

Humoral Immunity

Serum IgE concentrations are exceedingly high, ranging from 3 to 82 times the upper limit of normal (Table 17-17). Serum IgE concentrations were normal in all first-degree relatives of nine patients studied by us.

The three major classes of immunoglobulins are elevated in some but not all patients. Josephs and Buckley (1979) noted that serum IgD levels were elevated in most patients, with a geometric mean of 94 IU/ml (confidence interval [CI] 6 to 1495 IU/ml), compared with normals (geometric mean of 14 IU/ml; CI 0.5 to 340 IU/ml; $P < .00001$).

Poor recall antibody responses to diphtheria and tetanus were noted in the first two hyper-IgE syndrome patients reported, who also failed to respond to the neoantigen keyhole limpet hemocyanin (KLH) (Buckley et al., 1972). To ascertain whether an antibody deficiency could account for their infection susceptibility, Sheerin and Buckley (1991) evaluated 11 additional patients for responses to bacteriophage φX-174, diphtheria and tetanus toxoids, pneumococcal polysaccharide (Pneumovax), and H. influenzae (HIB) vaccines. Three of nine patients immunized with φX-174 had normal primary and secondary antibody responses, five had accelerated declines in their titers (after initially normal primary antibody responses) and lower than normal secondary antibody responses, and two did not show normal switching from IgM to IgG antibody production (see Table 17-17).

Only 1 of 10 had a normal response to diphtheria toxoid, and postimmunization anti-tetanus titers were abnormally low in 5 of the 10 patients tested. Postimmunization antibody levels to H. influenzae polyribose phosphate were protective in seven of eight patients. Postimmunization titers to pneumococci were nonprotective to at least one of the serotypes 7, 9, or 14; however, all patients responded with protective antibody titers to type 3 (Table 17-18). There was no correlation between polysaccharide antibody responses and serum IgG2 levels. Leung and colleagues (1998a) also found deficient polysaccharide antibody responses to techoic acid of S. aureus and capsular polysaccharide of H. influenzae in nine hyper-IgE patients.

This heterogeneity suggests that antibody deficiency may contribute to the infection susceptibility of some but not all hyper-IgE patients. Dreskin and colleagues (1985) found normal S. aureus IgG, elevated IgM, and diminished IgA antibodies in 10 hyper-IgE patients. The titer of IgA anti–S. aureus present correlated inversely with the incidence of infection at mucosal surfaces and

---

TABLE 17-17 · MAJOR IMMUNOLOGIC FEATURES OF 40 PATIENTS WITH THE HYPER-IgE SYNDROME

1. Markedly elevated serum IgE levels; usually 2000 to 40,000 IU/ml; IgD also elevated in a majority; other immunoglobulins may be modestly low or elevated but are usually normal.
2. Positive immediate wheal and flare reactions to a variety of food, inhalant, bacterial, and fungal antigens.
3. Marked eosinophilia in blood, tissue, and sputum.
4. Impaired anamnestic (IgG) antibody responses and poor responses to neoantigens.
5. Depressed cell-mediated immunity to ubiquitous antigens **in vivo** in half and to specific antigens **in vitro** in a majority. Responses to mitogens are normal, as are percentages of CD4 and CD8 lymphocyte subpopulations.
6. Abnormal intrafamilial mixed leukocyte responses.
7. Decreased proportion of CD45RO-positive CD3$^+$ T cells.
8. Highly variable chemotactic abnormalities (not present in most).
9. Impaired IgE production in response to IL-4 in vitro.

From Buckley, 2001.

TABLE 17-18 · SUMMARY OF IgG CONCENTRATIONS AND POSTIMMUNIZATION ANTIBODY RESPONSES IN PATIENTS WITH THE HYPER-IgE SYNDROME

Immunologic Parameter	Number of Patients with Abnormal Value
Total IgG concentration	0/11 low
IgG1 concentration	0/11 low
IgG2 concentration	3/11 low
IgG3 concentration	2/11 low
IgG4 concentration	0/11 low
Diphtheria antibody titer	9/10 low
Tetanus antibody titer	5/10 low
Haemophilus influenzae antibody titer	1/8 nonprotective
Pneumococcus type 3 titer	0/9 nonprotective
Pneumococcus type 7 titer	3/9 nonprotective
Pneumococcus type 9 titer	2/9 nonprotective
Pneumococcus type 14 titer	4/9 nonprotective
Bacteriophage φX-174: primary	5/10 low
Bacteriophage φX-174: secondary	5/10 low
Bacteriophage φX-174: IgG antibody	2/10 low

From Sheerin and Buckley, 1991, with permission.

in adjacent lymph nodes, suggesting a role for a deficient IgA response in their infection susceptibility.

Serum antibodies to staphylococcal and *Candida* organisms were detected in the serum of one of the first two patients evaluated (Buckley et al., 1972). Schopfer and associates (1979) and Dreskin and co-workers (1985) reported high titers of IgE antibodies to *S. aureus* antigens in hyper-IgE syndrome patients and proposed that such antibodies may have a pathogenic role in their special susceptibility to staphylococci. However, similar antibodies were found in patients with eczema and other atopic diseases not susceptible to abscess formation (Motala et al., 1986; Walsh et al., 1981).

Moreover, Schmitt and Ballet (1983) and Berger and colleagues (1980) found high titers of IgE antibodies to tetanus and *Candida* antigens in patients with the hyper-IgE syndrome, suggesting that such antibodies are a consequence of their abnormal IgE regulation. IgE isolated from the serum of one of these patients contained both kappa and lambda chains, excluding the possibility that the IgE was monoclonal.

In keeping with their markedly elevated total serum IgE levels, these patients all had strongly positive immediate wheal and flare responses to a number of inhalant, food, and pollen allergens, as well as to *Candida*, staphylococcal, and other bacterial and fungal antigens (Buckley and Sampson, 1981).

Cellular Immunity

Although cutaneous anergy to ubiquitous antigens, such as *Candida* and streptokinase-streptodornase, was found in the first two patients described (Buckley et al., 1972), this was a feature in only 50% of other patients. Lymphocytes from hyper-IgE patients were reported by Geha and associates (1981) to be deficient in CD8+ T cells. However, others have reported normal numbers of CD3+, CD4+, and CD8+ lymphocytes and IgE-bearing B lymphocytes.

Buckley and associates (1991) found a deficiency of CD3+ T cells bearing the CD45RO isoform (memory T-cell phenotype) in all patients studied. In mice, Luqman and colleagues (1991) have shown this isoform to be present on Th1 but not on Th2 cells. These observations may be relevant to the abnormal anamnestic humoral and cellular responses and excess IgE production.

Lymphocyte responses in vitro to the mitogens PHA, Con A, and PWM are normal in most hyper-IgE patients. By contrast, lymphoproliferative responses to *C. albicans* and tetanus toxoid are absent or low. Because antigen-induced lymphoproliferation is primarily a T-cell response, mixed leukocyte culture (MLC) studies were conducted in nine patients (Buckley and Sampson, 1981). Six of nine patients' T lymphocytes did not respond in MLCs to MNCs from one or more genetically disparate family members.

By contrast, T lymphocytes from five of the six patients that were unresponsive in intrafamilial MLC reactions proliferated vigorously to the MNCs of unrelated subjects. HLA-A and HLA-B typing performed in nine patients and their first-degree relatives revealed no unusual antigens or antigen frequencies (Buckley and Sampson, 1981).

Chemotaxis

Defective polymorphonuclear (PMN) chemotaxis as reported in some hyper-IgE patients was suggested to be the basis for their infection susceptibility (Hill et al., 1974). These chemotactic abnormalities, however, are highly variable and infrequent. Rebuck skin window studies in the first two patients reported showed normal PMN influx (Buckley et al., 1972). Fluids from sites of infections contained numerous PMNs, and a brisk PMN leukocytosis occurs in the presence of infection.

Only three of nine patients studied repeatedly showed consistent depression of either PMN or mononuclear chemotaxis (one of each type and one with both) (Buckley and Sampson, 1981). In most patients with defective chemotaxis, repeat studies were normal. There has been no correlation of chemotactic defects with medications or the presence or absence of infection. The inconsistency of PMN chemotactic defects in this syndrome makes it highly unlikely that they are responsible for the extreme infectious susceptibility of these patients.

Complement and Phagocytic Function

Serum hemolytic complement activity has been normal in all patients tested. The first two patients reported had normal levels of all nine complement components (Buckley et al., 1972). Their sera were capable of generating C5a chemotactic factor normally.

PMN phagocytosis, metabolism, and killing have been normal in all patients studied. Because the clinical history in the hyper-IgE syndrome resembles that in chronic granulomatous disease (CGD), phagocytic functional studies are often among the first tests performed. The granulocytes have normal phagocytosis, bacterial killing, and oxidative metabolism; the latter demonstrated by normal nitroblue tetrazolium dye reduction, chemiluminescence, and flow cytometric respiratory burst assays.

Histologic Findings

Histologic sections of lymph nodes, spleen, and lung cysts obtained at surgery demonstrate tissue eosinophilia. This was particularly notable in the spleen of a boy who underwent splenectomy following trauma and in the wall of a giant lung cyst excised from another patient. The possibility exists that eosinophils or their products, such as eosinophil major basic protein, play a role in the observed tissue destruction leading to formation of pneumatoceles. Normal thymic architecture, including that of Hassall's corpuscles, was observed at the postmortem examination of one patient.

Treatment

Because the primary defect in the hyper-IgE syndrome is unknown, no definitive therapy is available. The most successful treatment is lifelong, continuous anti-staphylococcal antibiotic therapy to prevent staphylococcal infections (Buckley, 2001).

If pneumatoceles persist for more than 6 months, surgical excision should be considered because the cysts may enlarge and compress adjacent normal lung, become infected with other organisms, or predispose to fungus ball formation. Although cutaneous abscesses are unusual in patients receiving anti-staphylococcal antibiotics regularly, their occurrence may necessitate incision and drainage.

Although immunostimulants (e.g., transfer factor, levamisole) were used in some patients before their referral to our institution, none experienced any clinical benefit; deterioration sometimes occurred because of antibiotic discontinuance or delay of surgery. Levamisole was inferior to placebo in a controlled study in hyper-IgE patients (Donabedian et al., 1982).

Based on the observation by Coffman and Carty (1986) that IFN-γ inhibits murine IL-4–induced IgE synthesis and on confirmation of these findings in humans (Pene et al., 1988), King and colleagues (1989) administered recombinant human IFN-γ to five patients with the hyper-IgE syndrome in an open clinical trial in doses of 0.05 and 0.1 mg/m² three times weekly for 2 and 6 weeks, respectively. There was a decline in the serum IgE level in two of five patients on the higher dose. Although no adverse effects were noted, there was no obvious clinical benefit.

High-dose IVIG therapy in a few hyper-IgE patients has not been of marked benefit, although IgE levels decreased slightly during its administration (Wakim et al., 1998).

Prognosis

If the disorder is recognized early in life and the patient is maintained on chronic anti-staphylococcal antibiotic therapy, the prognosis is good. Many patients have reached adulthood, indicating that the defect is compatible with prolonged survival.

If the diagnosis is delayed, chronically infected giant pneumatoceles may develop and lung infections with agents other than staphylococci, such as *H. influenzae,* *Candida,* and *Aspergillus,* may occur. Putrid pyogenic secondary infections may develop within persistent pneumatoceles, and aspergilloma formation with severe hemoptysis may occur. The latter can lead to sudden death.

Hodgkin's disease developed at age 19 in one patient. In another patient, Burkitt's lymphoma developed at age 7 (Gorin et al., 1989); these are the only cases of malignancy reported in this syndrome.

Rebecca H. Buckley

WARTS, HYPOGAMMAGLOBULINEMIA, INFECTION, MYELOKATHEXIS (WHIM) SYNDROME

Definition

WHIM syndrome is a rare autosomal dominant immunodeficiency defined by the presence of *w*arts, *h*ypogammaglobulinemia, recurrent bacterial *i*nfections, and an unusual bone marrow condition termed *m*yelokathexis (reviewed by Gorlin et al., 2000). The latter refers to the failure of leukocytes to leave the marrow, resulting in hyperplasia and degeneration of mature myeloid cells. Despite this increased marrow reserve, there is profound chronic neutropenia. However, transient leukocytosis with neutrophilia can develop during acute systemic infections (O'Regan et al., 1977). This disorder is also discussed in Chapter 20.

Historical Aspects

Zuelzer and colleagues in 1964 (Krill et al., 1964; Zuelzer et al., 1964) reported the first cases of myelokathexis. They used a Greek compound word *myelo-kathexis* ("white blood cell–retention") to describe the marrow abnormalities and to suggest a pathogenic mechanism for the chronic neutropenia. There was no mention of warts or other immune defects. The occurrence of familial cases underscored its genetic basis, and, as new pedigrees were studied, an AD pattern of inheritance emerged (Christ et al., 1997; Gorlin et al., 2000; Hord et al., 1997; Mentzer et al., 1977; Wetzler et al., 1990).

The observation that myelokathexis is associated with hypogammaglobulinemia (Mentzer et al., 1977) and with susceptibility to human papillomavirus (HPV) infection (Wetzler et al., 1990) widened the spectrum of the disease. In 2002 two cases of EBV-related lymphoproliferative disease occurred in WHIM patients (Chae et al., 2002; Imashuku et al., 2002). The occurrence of hypogammaglobulinemia, HPV, and EBV vulnerability points to the definition of a new primary immunodeficiency.

Pathogenesis

The pathogenesis of WHIM initially focused on the hematologic features of the syndrome. Regulation of hematopoietic cell release, migration, and homing to the bone marrow relies on a complex interaction between adhesion molecules, chemokines, cytokines, proteolytic enzymes, stromal cells, and hematopoietic cells (Lapidot and Petit, 2002).

Two hypotheses for the pathogenesis of WHIM have been proposed: (1) defective release of mature granulocytes, caused by abnormal hematopoietic cytokine production and/or defects of leukocyte adhesion molecules (Mentzer et al., 1977; Wetzler et al., 1990; Zuelzer et al., 1964) or (2) accelerated apoptosis associated with the selective decrease in bcl-x expression affecting marrow myeloid cells (Aprikyan et al., 2000; Liles et al., 1995; Mackey et al., 2003; Taniuchi et al., 1999).

Gene Localization and Identification

Diaz's group, using linkage analysis, localized the WHIM gene to chromosome 2q21 and identified two nonsense mutations within the C-terminal of the chemokine receptor CXCR4 (Hernandez et al., 2003). CXCR4 is a co-receptor for HIV and the only receptor for CXC chemokine SDF-1 (stromal derived factor-1) (Nagasawa et al., 1998).

WHIM syndrome is the first human disorder caused by a chemokine signaling defect, and this discovery confirms the key role of CXCR4-SDF1 signaling in marrow homeostasis and leukocyte migration. All WHIM patients with mutations of CXCR4 (Gulino et al., unpublished; Hernandez et al., 2003) are heterozygous for nonsense mutations affecting its C-terminal cytoplasmic tail, resulting in the loss of 10, 17, or 19 amino acids.

Function of CXCR4

CXCR4 is the only receptor for the CXC chemokine SDF-1 (stromal-derived factor 1, or CXCL12). The engagement of SDF-1 and CSCR4 stimulates chemotaxis of progenitor and mature hematopoietic cells and is, at least in mice, essential for B-lymphocyte development and myelopoiesis (Ma et al., 1998; Nagasawa et al., 1998). In addition, CXCR signaling is essential for cardiac ventricular septum formation, vascularization of the GI tract, and development of cerebellar granule cell layer (Ma et al., 1998; Nagasawa et al., 1996). In human leukocytes, SDF1-CXCR4 interaction initiates cytoskeletal rearrangement and integrin-mediated adhesion and chemotaxis (Bleul et al., 1996).

Signaling via CXCR4, a G protein–coupled receptor, is associated with an increase of intracellular calcium ion levels. CXCR4 activation leads to the recruitment of multiple kinases including phosphoinositide-3 (PI-3) and downstream elements such as MAPKp38, ERK1/2, NFκB, and phospholipase C λ (Wang et al., 2000a). CXCR4-SDF1 binding also delivers both proapoptotic and antiapoptotic signals to the cell.

CXCR4 has been extensively studied because it acts as a co-receptor for the T-cell trophic HIV-1 (Berger et al., 1999). A role in inflammatory disease (e.g., rheumatoid arthritis) (Nanki et al., 2000) and cancer metastasis (Murphy, 2001) has also been proposed. Gonzalo and co-workers (2002) have shown that CXCR4 participates in the regulation of pulmonary inflammatory responses, possibly explaining the predisposition of some WHIM patients to bronchiectasis. Just how the mutation results in the other clinical and immunologic features of the disease is unexplained.

Apoptosis

Mature CD15+ bone marrow granulocytes have a high percentage of apoptotic nuclei as assessed by flow cytometry following propidium iodide and annexin V staining. Expression of the bcl-x antiapoptotic molecules is reduced but fas, fasL, and bcl-2 are normal (Aprikyan et al., 2000). This observation has led to the hypothesis that myelokathexis results from increased myeloid apoptosis (Aprikyan et al., 2000; Liles et al., 1995; Mackey et al., 2003; Taniuchi et al., 1999).

Clinical Features

WHIM patients present during early childhood with recurrent febrile bacterial infections, mostly affecting the respiratory tract including pneumonia, tonsillitis, otitis, and sinusitis (Gorlin et al., 2000). Bronchiectasis often develops during the third decade of life (Hord et al., 1997; Wetzler et al., 1990). Periodontitis is common and may result in premature tooth loss (Gorlin et al., 2000; Weston et al., 1991). Acute thrombophlebitis and omphalitis with abdominal wall cellulitis have been reported (Bohinjec, 1981; Weston et al., 1991).

The infections are caused by common pathogens (e.g., *H. influenzae*, *S. aureus*, *Proteus mirabilis*). Infections respond well to antibiotics, and only one fatality with septicemia and meningitis has been recorded (Wetzler et al., 1990).

Growth and development are normal, although one patient had dysmorphic features and skeletal abnormalities (Plebani et al., 1988).

Warts caused by HPV usually appear during the late teens but have been observed as early as 3 years of age (Hord et al., 1997). In 12 of 32 reported patients, warts were absent or not mentioned, which is possibly explained by phenotypic heterogeneity or short follow-up. When present, the warts are numerous and confluent. Most are on the hands (Fig. 17-17). Mucosal and

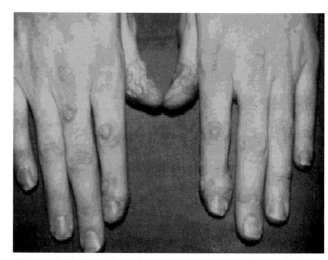

Figure 17-17· Extensive refractory cutaneous warts in a patient with the WHIM syndrome.

venereal warts may also occur, resulting in premalignant cervical papillomatosis and vulval condylomata acuminata (Gorlin et al., 2000; Wetzler et al., 1990). The oral mucosa can also be affected. HPV is detectable in the warts, and these are of the common serotypes. The warts respond poorly to treatment, including IVIG (Goddard et al., 1994).

Asthma, otitis with hearing loss, and chest infections are sometimes present. Bronchiectasis is not uncommon, particularly in the severely hypogammaglobulinemic patients; this may be aggravated by defective respiratory pathogen clearance because of the CXCR4 mutation (Gonzalo et al., 2000).

Cardiac defects have occurred in two patients, one with tetralogy of Fallot (authors' personal observation) and one with a ventricular septal defect with pulmonary artery atresia (Taniuchi et al., 1999), not unlike those described in the SDF1-knockout mice with abnormal B-cell lymphopoiesis and marrow myelopoiesis (Nagasawa et al., 1996).

Laboratory Features

Granulocytes

Neutropenia is severe with absolute neutrophil counts usually ranging between 100 and 500/mm^3. This may occur early in life and may be congenital. Lymphopenia with absolute lymphocyte counts less than 1500 cells/mm^3 is usually present. Thus the total WBC count is often less than 2500/mm^3.

Granulocyte morphology shows membrane blebbing, condensation of heterochromatin, and cell fragmentation suggesting apoptosis (Aprikyan et al., 2000). Granulocyte function is normal including chemotaxis, pus formation, phagocytosis, and bactericidal activity.

Bone Marrow

The bone marrow is normocellular or hypercellular with marked granulocyte hyperplasia. Granulocyte nuclei are highly condensed and often multilobulated with long, thin strands of chromatin separating the lobes. Vacuoles are small, multiple, and apparently empty. The karyotype is normal. The myeloid precursor cells and other marrow cells are normal.

Immunologic Findings

Moderate hypogammaglobulinemia, usually affecting IgG, is frequent but not always present. Antibody titers are usually present in low titers.

Lymphocyte subsets are normal except for moderately decreased B lymphocytes (Wetzler et al., 1990). Memory B cells (CD27$^+$, IgD$^-$) are markedly reduced. Lymphoproliferative responses are generally normal.

Endogenous levels of granulocyte colony-stimulating factor (G-CSF) were elevated in two patients studied by Hord and co-workers (1997), but GM-CSF levels were nondetectable.

Treatment

Daily G-CSF or monthly IVIG decreases their infectious episodes. There is a rapid response of the neutrophil count to G-CSF or GM-CSF (Arai et al., 2000; Bohinjec and Andoljsek, 1992; Cernelc et al., 2000; Ganser et al., 1989; Hord et al., 1997; Liles et al., 1995; Weston et al., 1991; Wetzler et al., 1992). In one case the IgG normalized following G-CSF treatment (Hord et al., 1997).

G-CSF may release proteinases (mainly leukocyte elastase [LE]) from primary granules of myeloid precursors, which cleaves the N-terminal of both SDF-1 and CXCR4, thus interrupting their interaction and permitting leukocyte release from the marrow (Petit et al., 2002; Valenzuela-Fernandez et al., 2002). Although long-term use of G-CSF or GM-CSF has not resulted in myelodysplastic changes, reversible marrow fibrosis was reported by Hess and colleagues (1992) in a 19-year-old girl after 110 days of GM-CSF treatment.

Vaccines, including live virus vaccines, have been given without sequelae.

Prognosis

Two early deaths among young adult WHIM patients have been reported, one resulting from EBV-driven lymphoproliferative syndrome (Imashuku et al., 2002) and one resulting from bacterial meningitis (Wetzler et al., 1990). One case of cutaneous B-cell lymphoma has also been reported (Chae et al., 2001).

Persistent warts on the hands and face have a severe cosmetic and psychologic effect. Malignant transformation of genital warts predisposes patients to cervical cancer.

Anna Virginia Gulino and Luigi D. Notarangelo

INTERFERON-γ/IL-12 PATHWAY DEFICIENCIES

Definition

IFN-γ and IL-12 pathway deficiencies are genetic immunodeficiencies characterized by undue susceptibility to mycobacterial and certain other infections associated with defects in the formation of or the response to IFN-γ and/or IL-12. These patients have no other associated antibody or cellular immunodeficiency.

Patients with defects in IFN-γR1 at chromosome 6q23-q24 (OMIM# 107470) IFN-γR2 at 21q22.1-q22.2 (OMIM# 147569), IL-12 receptor β1 at 19p13.1 (OMIM# 601604), IL-12p40 at 5q31.1-33.1 (OMIM# 161561), and STAT1 at 2q32.2-q32.3 (OMIM# 600555) have been recently identified because of their selective susceptibility to mycobacteria, *Salmonellae*, and some viral infections (reviewed in Casanova and Abel, 2002; Dorman and Holland, 2000).

Pathogenesis

The mononuclear phagocyte is a critical barrier both to pathogens and environmental organisms. Resistance to infection to the tuberculosis (TB) group of mycobacteria (*Mycobacterium tuberculosis, Mycobacterium bovis, Bacille Calmette-Guérin* [BCG], *Mycobacterium africanum,* and *Mycobacterium microti*) and to the nontuberculous mycobacteria (NTM) relies on the functional integrity of these cells. IFN-γ is critical and irreplaceable in this pathway.

Macrophage-engulfed mycobacteria stimulate the production of IL-12 (IL-12p70, a heterodimer of IL-12p40 and IL-12p35). IL-12 stimulates T cells and NK cells through its receptor (IL-12R, a heterodimer of IL-12Rβ1 and IL-12Rβ2) to produce IFN-γ. IFN-γ acts through its receptor (a heterodimer of IFN-γR1 and IFN-γR2) on macrophages to upregulate specific genes and activities. On phagocytes, IFN-γ increases production of TNF-α and further upregulates IL-12. IFN-γ also causes mycobacterial killing, but the mechanism is unknown.

IFN-γ binds to IFN-γR1, its ligand binding chain, leading to its dimerization. Following this event, two IFN-γR2 chains—the signal transducing chains—join the receptor complex. IFN-γR1 and IFN-γR2 are constitutively associated with their respective Janus kinases, Jak1 and Jak2. Mutual transphosphorylation of the Jaks leads to tyrosine phosphorylation of the intracellular domain of the IFN-γR1 at tyrosine 440.

This tyrosine is the docking site for the latent cytosolic signal transducer and activator of transcription-1 (STAT1). Jaks mediate STAT1 tyrosine 701 and serine 727 phosphorylation, leading to the homodimerization of two phospho-STAT1 (P-STAT1) molecules, which then translocate to the nucleus and upregulate the transcription of numerous IFN-γ regulated genes (reviewed in Bach et al., 1997; Casanova and Abel, 2002; Dorman and Holland, 2000) (Figs. 17-18 and 17-19).

Interferon-γ Receptor 1 (IFN-γR1) and Interferon-γ Receptor 2 (IFN-γR2) Deficiencies

Autosomal Recessive IFN-γR Deficiencies

Mutations in both IFN-γR chains have been identified and characterized. Autosomal recessive complete IFN-γR1–deficient or IFN-γR2–deficient patients tend to develop severe mycobacterial disease in infancy or childhood.

When BCG vaccine is administered, disseminated infection typically results. These patients fail to form well-circumscribed tuberculoid granulomata (Emile et al., 1997; Jouanguy et al., 1996). Although these genetic defects have been predominantly associated with mycobacteria and salmonella infection, the recognized phenotype has been expanded to include increased susceptibility to viruses such as CMV, respiratory syncytial

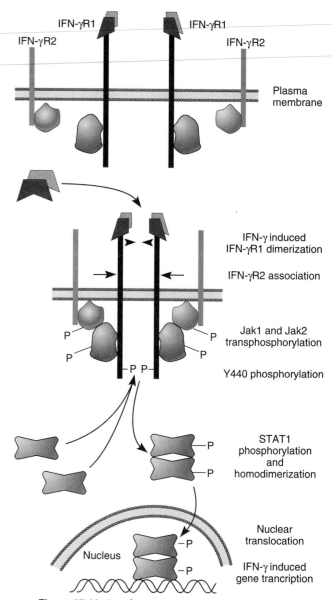

Figure 17-18 · Interferon-γ receptor stimulation pathway.

virus, varicella-zoster virus, and parainfluenza virus (Dorman et al., 1999), as well as the opportunistic pathogen *Listeria monocytogenes* (Roesler et al., 1999).

These autosomal recessive mutations of IFN-γR1 and IFN-γR2 have been mapped to the extracellular domains, where they usually lead to complete loss of protein expression (Casanova and Abel, 2002; Dorman and Holland, 2000). Another four-bp deletion mutational hotspot was recently described in IFN-γR1 in the extracellular domain (561del4). In contrast to the AD defect caused by mutations at 818, this extracellular defect leads to an autosomal recessive form of complete IFN-γR1 deficiency (Rosenzweig et al., 2001).

Rare partial defects in both IFN-γR1 and IFN-γR2, in which IFN-γ signal transduction is impaired by 2 to 3 logs but not abolished, have also been described (Doffinger et al., 2000; Jouanguy et al., 1997, 2000). These mutations are due to amino acid replacements in the extracellular domains.

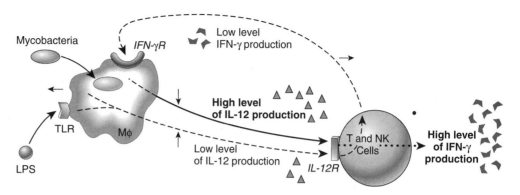

Figure 17-19 · Interferon-γ/
IL-12 induction pathway.

▲	IL-12
∨	Interferon-γ (IFN-γ)
LPS	Lipopolysaccharides
TLR	Toll-like receptor
Mφ	Macrophage
←	Macrophage stimulation after mycobacterial phagocytosis and/or through TLR stimulation
↓	Macrophage IL-12 production in response to IFN-γ
→	T-cell and NK-cell IFN-γ production in response to low amounts of IL-12
↑	Macrophage IL-12 production in response to mycobacterial engulfment and/or TLR stimulation
•	T-cell and NK-cell IFN-γ production in response to large amounts IL-12

Autosomal Dominant IFN-γR1 Deficiency

More common than the autosomal recessive IFN-γR deficiencies is the AD IFN-γR1 deficiency (Casanova and Abel, 2002; Dorman and Holland, 2000; Jouanguy et al., 1999). In this defect, the mutation is located in the intracellular domain, just beyond the transmembrane segment.

The most common AD mutation is a four-bp deletion (818del4) that leads to a frame shift and premature truncation of IFN-γR1, eliminating the Jak1 and STAT1 binding sites. In addition, the receptor recycling domain immediately C terminal to the Jak1 binding site is also removed. Loss of the receptor recycling domain severely impairs the normal removal and recycling of the receptor from the cell surface.

Therefore an overabundance of the extracellular domain of IFN-γR1 is displayed on the cell surface. The binding capacity of this truncated receptor is largely preserved, leading to sequestration of IFN-γ onto impotent receptors and the engagement of IFN-γR2 molecules. This AD mutation occurs relatively often, because of mispairing of DNA at a mutational hotspot around base 818 of IFN-γR1 (Jouanguy et al., 1999).

These patients tend to present later in childhood with circumscribed disease that is antibiotic responsive. Multifocal nontuberculous mycobacterial osteomyelitis and pulmonary nontuberculous mycobacterial infections are a frequent form of presentation among these patients.

Diagnosis

Diagnosis of IFN-γR1 or IFN-γR2 deficiency can be made by several means. STAT1 activation (detection of phosphorylated STAT1) following IFN-γ stimulation is only possible in the context of functional IFN-γ receptors (Fleisher et al., 1999). This provides a screening test for IFN-γR function that can be done in minutes on peripheral blood. In vitro TNF-α production by PBMC in response to LPS and IFN-γ is impaired in patients with IFN-γR1 or IFN-γR2 defects (Dorman and Holland, 2000; Holland et al., 1998; Newport, 1996). Overabundance of the IFN-γR1 on the cell surface (typically more than five times the normal level) suggests the AD form of IFN-γR1 deficiency and is easily detected by flow cytometry of unstimulated peripheral blood. Genetic analysis is necessary to definitively identify and characterize the genetic defect.

Treatment

Patients with the AD disorders are IFN-γ responsive, albeit at relatively higher doses, and are well controlled by a combination of antimycobacterials and IFN-γ. The duration of therapy should be prolonged, but the precise duration is undefined. However, they remain susceptible to recurrent mycobacterial infections throughout life, making ongoing antimycobacterial prophylaxis with macrolides the most appropriate course of long-term therapy. These patients are susceptible to other infections as well, including histoplasmosis and herpesviruses (Dorman and Holland, 2000).

Several patients with complete autosomal recessive IFN-γR deficiencies in Europe and the United States have had bone marrow transplants. Complications have included fatal GVHD, failure to clear infection, severe generalized granulomatous response, and gram-negative sepsis. It seems prudent to consider BMT only when the mycobacterial infection is under control. Even with infection control, whether there is a survival benefit to BMT in this disease remains to be determined.

It is important to note that BMT only replaces the hematopoietic compartment, whereas the IFN-γR is ubiquitously expressed on nucleated cells. Therefore the important contributions of the IFN-γR in infection control on somatic cells will remain uncorrected (Yap and Sher, 1999).

Autosomal Recessive IL-12 Receptor β1 Deficiency

Patients with disseminated nontuberculous mycobacterial and *Salmonella* infections in the setting of IL-12 unresponsiveness have been identified in Europe and Morocco with mutations in the IL-12 receptor β1 (IL-12Rβ1) (Altare et al., 1998a; Fieschi et al., 2003; de Jong et al., 1998). These patients develop severe, recurrent, disseminated *Salmonella* and nontuberculous mycobacterial infections or progressive BCG infection following vaccination. Granulomata are well contained and well organized. Delayed-type hypersensitivity is unaffected, as it is in IFN-γR deficiency as well.

These patients lack cell surface expression of IL-12Rβ1 on stimulated T and NK cells. As a result of defective IL-12R signaling, IFN-γ is poorly produced by T cells and NK cells. Verhagen and co-workers (2000) have shown that despite IL-12Rβ1 deficiency, T-cell clones from such patients can still be made to respond to IL-12, suggesting alternative pathways for IL-12 signaling.

The genetic defects are in the extracellular domains of the IL-12Rβ1 leading to premature stop codons. All reported patients with IL-12Rβ1 mutations have an autosomal recessive inheritance pattern. Heterozygous carriers are clinically healthy with normal IL-12 signaling and IFN-γ production. IFN-γ provides benefit in patients for whom antimycobacterials alone have been incompletely successful, because the IFN-γR remains intact and functional.

Autosomal Recessive IL-12p40 Deficiency

A patient with IL-12p40 (IL-12β) deficiency had disseminated BCG infection and *Salmonella enteritidis* sepsis (Altare et al., 1998b). This is a milder clinical phenotype than complete IFN-γR deficiency because residual IL-12–independent IFN-γ secretion pathways persist, as reflected in the patient's capacity to form organized granulomata. Interestingly, the patient's heterozygous father had had recurrent *Salmonella* infections earlier in life, suggesting a possible form of haploinsufficiency.

The mutation was a homozygous autosomal recessive deletion leading to loss of two exons of IL-12p40. Neither the IL-12p40 subunit nor the IL-12p70 heterodimer were detectable. The patient's lymphocytes secreted a reduced amount of IFN-γ, which could be corrected with recombinant IL-12 in vitro.

Picard and associates (2002) reviewed the clinical and laboratory data of 13 patients belonging to six different ethnic groups with IL-12p40 deficiency. The clinical outcome was surprisingly variable, ranging from patients who died early in life from nontuberculous mycobacterial infections to individuals in the second decade with only localized BCG. Two mutations (g.315_316insA and g.482+82_856-854del), related to different founder effects, were found in the two ethnic groups. Treatment with antibiotics and subcutaneous IFN-γ is typically successful.

STAT1 Deficiency

STAT1 is a critical molecule in the transduction of signal from both the IFN-γR and the IFN-α/βR. Following IFN-γ stimulation, STAT1 is phosphorylated and homodimerizes to form the gamma-activating-factor (GAF). In contrast, following IFN-α/β stimulation, STAT1 combines with STAT2 and the cytoplasmic protein p48 to form interferon-stimulated-gamma-factor-3 (ISGF3).

Dupuis and associates (2001) described two unrelated patients with the same heterozygous substitution (T2116C) in the coding sequence of STAT1, leading to the change of leucine 706 to serine (L706S). The first patient developed disseminated BCG after vaccination in childhood. Her affected daughter did not receive BCG vaccine and remains healthy. The American patient presented with disseminated *M. avium* infection in childhood. Despite antibody evidence of multiple viral exposures, there were no severe viral infections in these patients.

This mutation apparently interferes with the phosphorylation of STAT1 tyrosine 701. Phosphorylation of tyrosine 701 and serine 727 is critical for the integrity of IFN-triggered pathways. Hindrance of phosphorylation of serine 701 impedes STAT1 cytoplasmic dimerization and its subsequent nuclear translocation as GAF. Importantly, this AD mutation does not interfere with ISGF3 nuclear translocation. Therefore this mutation appears to selectively impair IFN-γ–mediated activity while sparing IFN-α/β–mediated activity. In contrast, autosomal recessive mutations in STAT1 causing complete loss of function lead to susceptibility to severe fatal mycobacterial and viral infections (Dupuis et al., 2003).

Steven M. Holland and Sergio D. Rosenzweig

NATURAL KILLER CELL DEFICIENCY

Definition

NK-cell deficiency is a rare primary immunodeficiency characterized by recurrent herpesvirus infections and a selective deficiency of NK-cell function and/or numbers.

In addition, several other primary immunodeficiencies have an NK defect in association with other immune defects.

Historical Aspects

In 1982 Fleisher and colleagues described a large family who had an NK-cell defect and increased susceptibility to severe EBV infection. Biron and colleagues (1989) described another early case of NK deficiency in a girl with severe varicella and CMV infections.

Since then several patients with impaired NK-cell responses have been reported, most displaying enhanced susceptibility to herpesvirus infections. Most have a selective deficiency of NK cells as assessed by flow cytometry and/or by diminished in vitro cytotoxicity. NK deficiency is also a component of several other secondary immunodeficiency syndromes.

Pathogenesis

NK cells are non-T, non-B lymphocytes that can lyse various target cells without prior sensitization or activation. NK cells make up 10% to 20% of the circulating lymphocytes. They belong to the innate immune system through their ability to lyse virus-infected and/or tumor cells, secrete cytokines, and serve as effector cells in antibody-dependent cellular cytotoxicity (ADCC) reactions (see Chapters 6 and 10). NK cells may also trigger innate immune responses by recognition of pathogen-derived receptors such as influenza hemagglutinins (Arnon et al., 2001; Mandelboim et al., 2001).

NK cells are large granular $CD3^-$ lymphocytes coexpressing CD56 (N-CAM) and CD16 ($Fc\gamma IIIa$). They are phenotypically and functionally heterogenous (Cooper et al., 2001). The majority (about 90%) are $CD56^{dim}CD16^{bright}$ cells that mediate cytotoxic functions and the rest (about 10%) are $CD56^{bright}CD16^{dim}$ cells that are responsible for cytokine production (Mandelboim et al., 1999).

Historically, the most compelling evidence of the role of NK cells in host defense comes from animal models in which NK cells have been depleted (Biron et al., 1999; Scharton and Scher, 1997). Their primary defect is impaired natural and ADCC reactions to viral-infected cells. Animals deficient in NK cells, human newborns with diminished NK function, and patients with primary immunodeficiencies that include an NK deficiency all have a propensity to recurrent viral infection (Orange, 2002; Scharton and Scher, 1997). The ADCC defect is probably less important than the NK defect because other cells with an Fc receptor (e.g., monocytes, B cells) can also perform in ADCC reactions.

Polymorphisms in $Fc\gamma IIIa$ (CD16), a low-affinity IgG receptor present on NK cells and phagocytes, has been associated with increased susceptibility to herpesvirus infections (de Vries et al., 1996; Jawahar et al., 1996) and, in one case, decreased NK-cell function. These individuals are homozygous for a mutation at position 230, resulting in a leucine → histidine substitution in the extracellular portion of the molecule that renders it unrecognizable by the B78.1 anti-CD16 monoclonal antibody (but not by other anti-CD16 antibodies). NK-cell numbers and in vitro cytotoxicity, including ADCC, was abnormal in one patient.

The molecular defects in other patients with selective NK deficiency have not been identified.

Clinical Features

Fleisher and colleagues (1982) reported a family with overwhelming susceptibility to EBV and bacterial infections. Three siblings from this family developed severe (two) or fatal (one) IM. Two of these patients but not their parents or an unaffected sibling with mild IM had deficiency of NK-cell activity that did not respond to interferon preincubation.

One of these patients, a 17-year-old girl, developed severe herpetic gingivostomatitis 1 year later and at age 27 developed intraepithelial neoplasia and condylomata (Starr et al., 1990). She also had recovered some NK cytotoxicity, suggesting that the EBV infection was responsible for the NK deficiency. This syndrome differs from XLP (see the section on XLP) inasmuch as the patients had bacterial infection, both sexes were affected, and one patient recovered completely.

Lopez and co-workers (1983) reported five patients with severe herpesvirus infections without a known cellular immunodeficiency whose NK cells had diminished lysis of herpes simplex virus (HSV)-1–infected fibroblasts, similar to that observed in five of six patients with WAS and in 70% of normal newborns.

Biron and associates (1989) reported an NK deficiency in a girl who was asymptomatic until she contracted disseminated varicella at age 13. She had been immunized with live virus varicella vaccine without incident. The varicella was complicated by pneumonia, leukopenia, and thrombocytopenia. She recovered with acyclovir but had severe scarring of the face and trunk. She also developed severe CMV pneumonia 4 years later.

Her T-cell subsets were normal, but $CD16^+/NKH-1^+$ cells were absent in the peripheral blood. NK cell cytotoxicity (spontaneous and cytokine-stimulated) against K562 tumor cells was undetectable as was the MNC-mediated ADCC reaction. However, in vitro T-cell responses and VZV antibody production were normal, indicating that other immune components were intact. She later developed aplastic anemia and died of complications of BMT.

Ballas and colleagues (1990) described a 23-year-old woman with recurrent HPV infection who had absent NK cells ($CD56^+/CD16^+/CD3^-$) and NK cytotoxicity but no other immune abnormalities. Komiyama and co-workers (1990) reported two brothers with an absolute NK-cell functional defect who were asymptomatic. One developed Hodgkin's disease 6 years after diagnosis.

Jawahar and associates (1996) reported a child with recurrent HSV stomatitis and whitlow who had depressed

NK cytotoxicity resulting from an FcRIII mutation. De Vries and colleagues (1996) described a 3-year-old boy with recurrent respiratory viral illness and protracted EBV and VZV infection with a similar FcRIII mutation. A younger brother, homozygous for the same mutation, had recurrent respiratory infection, food allergy, and eczema.

Wendland and co-workers (2000) described a 19-year-old man who was well until age 15, at which time he developed a marrow dysplastic syndrome, an *M. avium* infection, and fatal varicella infection. Immune abnormalities included absent NK (CD56$^+$) cells, absent NK cytotoxicity to K562 cells, normal T cells and in vitro T-cell responses, low B cells, mild hypogammaglobulinemia, monocytopenia, and cutaneous anergy.

In summary, the common feature of NK cell deficiency is an unusual susceptibility to acute and chronic herpes family viral infections, but other infections may also occur. Most patients come to medical attention in their teens or young adult years, but some have had infections since infancy. Family history is usually negative, but at least two pedigrees had other family members affected (Fleisher et al., 1982; Komiyama et al., 1990). Recurrent viral infections are common, but the patients are well between episodes. Malignancy has occurred in a few patients.

Natural Killer Cell Defects in Other Illnesses

Several other immunodeficiencies have NK defects as part of their immunologic defect. Patients with X-linked SCID (resulting from a γ-chain defect of the common cytokine receptor [γc]) and autosomal recessive SCID (resulting from a Jak3 defect, blocking signal transduction) have a profound NK deficiency (Buckley, 2000; see Chapter 15). These defects may result in an IL-15 deficiency, which is needed for NK-cell differentiation.

Gilmour and associates (2001) recently described a child with severe viral and fungal infections in whom the most prominent immunologic feature aside from a reduced number of T lymphocytes was the total absence of NK cells. PBMC expression of γc chain and Jak3 was comparable to controls, but there was a markedly reduced expression of the IL-2/IL-15β receptor subunit.

Patients with XLP have a progressive NK deficiency following acquisition of EBV infection (Parolini et al., 2000; see section on XLP). NK cell numbers and ADCC reactions are usually normal, and the impaired cytotoxicity appears restricted to that triggered by 2B4, an activating receptor present on NK and T cells (Garni et al., 1993). This molecule interacts with SAP (SLAM-associated protein or SH2D1A), the intracellular signaling molecule that is defective or absent in XLP (Sayos et al., 1998a).

Patients with X-linked agammaglobulinemia and common variable immunodeficiency (CVID) have been reported to have defects in NK and ADCC cytotoxicity (Bonagura et al., 1989; Koren et al., 1978; Sanal and Buckley, 1978) Aspalter and associates (2000) studied

NK-cell numbers in 55 CVID patients and found a 40% reduction in the total CD56$^+$/CD3$^-$ compared with controls; NK function was not studied.

One patient with X-linked hyper-IgM syndrome (HIGM1, Chapter 13) had a complete deficiency of CD56$^+$/CD16$^+$ cells (Ostenstad et al., 1997); other such patients have variable defects (Koren et al., 1978; Orange et al., 2002a). Because normal cells express CD40L, their absence in HIGM1 NK cells may prevent their activation by dendritic cells (Carbone et al., 1997).

Orange and co-workers (2002a) recently reported that intravenous administration of IL-2 partially restored in vivo NK-cell activity in a patient with a severe CMV infection and a NEMO mutation (see Chapter 13).

Immunodeficiency syndromes associated with defects in exocytosis of granule components may also have NK and cytotoxic T-cell defects (Russell and Ley, 2002). These include hemophagocytic lymphohistiocytosis (see Chapter 26), the Chédiak-Higashi syndrome (CHS) (see Chapter 20), and Griscelli syndrome (GS) (see section on this syndrome) (Abo et al., 1982; Perez et al., 1984; Roder et al., 1983; Sullivan et al., 1998).

Other primary immunodeficiencies with NK defects include leukocyte adhesion deficiency (LAD) (Kohl et al., 1984; Lau et al., 1991; Orange et al., 2001; see Chapter 20), CMC (Palma-Carlos, 2001; see section on CMC) and WAS (Orange 2002b; see section on WAS). The contribution of the NK-cell abnormality to immune dysfunction in these complex disorders remains unclear.

Secondary immunodeficiencies with NK-cell deficiency include the normal newborn, particularly the premature (see Chapter 22); severe malnutrition (see Chapter 23); HIV infection (see Chapter 29); and several hematologic and oncologic disorders (see Chapters 26 and 39).

Laboratory Features

Most patients have a selective deficiency of CD16/CD56 NK cells and a cytotoxic functional defect to K562 target cells. Normal levels of NK cells and function are shown in Chapter 12, Table 22. T- and B-cell function is usually normal. There may be failure of upregulation of NK-cell activity with such activators as IL-2 or various interferons. Advanced studies include FcRIII phenotyping, ADCC function, cytokine synthesis (e.g., IFN-γ, IL-2, etc.), and advanced analysis of NK-cell subsets by flow cytometry using different NK monoclonal antibodies.

Treatment and Prognosis

Treatment of infection and prophylactic use of antivirals may be indicated. IVIG reduced the frequency of infection in one patient reported by Jawahar and associates (1986). IL-2 partially restored in vivo NK cell activity in a patient with a NEMO mutation and a severe CMV infection (Orange et al., 2002a). The prognosis is dependent on the severity of the infection and the associated immune defects.

Maria Ines Garcia Lloret

GRISCELLI SYNDROME

Definition

GS (MIM 214450) is an autosomal recessive genetic disorder characterized by partial pigmentary dilution or albinism with silvery gray hair, frequent infections, cellular immunodeficiency, neurologic abnormalities, and early demise as a result of uncontrolled lymphocyte and macrophage activation, the so-called accelerated phase of the disorder. A defect of two closely linked genes, *MYO5A* and *RAB27A* on chromosome 15q21, is responsible for the two forms of the disease. This disorder is also discussed in Chapters 20 and 24.

Historical Aspects

GS was first described in two patients by Griscelli and associates in 1978. Since then, more than 60 cases have been described, mostly in patients of Turkish or Mediterranean heritage. (Chan et al., 1998; Gogus et al., 1995; Haraldsson et al., 1991; Harfi et al., 1992; Hurvitz et al., 1993; Klein et al., 1994; Ménasché et al., 2000; Pastural et al., 1997, 2000; Sanal et al., 2000, 2002; Schneider et al., 1990; Tezcan et al., 1999; Wagner et al., 1997). BMT was first performed in GS in 1990 (Schneider et al., 1990). The two genes responsible for the disorder were identified in the late 1990s by de Saint Basile and associates (Ménasché et al., 2000; Pastural et al., 1997). This group has recently reported genotype–phenotype correlations (2002).

Pathogenesis

Myosin-Va Gene Mutations

GS has some phenotypic resemblance to a murine mutant, the dilute mouse, which results from defects of myosin-Va (Mercer et al., 1991), an atypical myosin that acts as a molecular "motor" involved in transport of melanosomes and other cytoplasmic organelles (Titus, 1997). Genetic linkage to regions of the human genome homologous to the murine dilute region localized the GS gene to chromosome 15q21 in a region containing the myosin-Va *(MYO5A)* gene. Several GS patients had mutations in this gene, implicating defective myosin-Va protein in its pathogenesis. However, in other GS patients, myosin-Va is normally expressed, and *MYO5A* gene mutations are not detected.

RAB27A Gene Mutations

Further linkage analysis in GS families confirmed the original localization to 15q21, but fine haplotype analy-

sis suggested the existence of a second locus adjacent to the *MYO5A* gene (Pastural et al., 2000). The *RAB27A* gene, a member of the Rab GTPase family needed for vesicular transport and organelle dynamics, also localizes in this region. Mutations in *RAB27A* were detected in all GS patients who did not have an *MYO5A* mutation (Ménasché et al., 2000).

The ashen mutant mice are homologous to this form of GS, although this mutant does not develop an accelerated phase as occurs in GS (Wilson et al., 2000). Thus mutations in either *MYO5A* or *RAB27A* genes, separated by less than 1.6 cM at 15q21, can lead to GS.

Functional Defects

Myosin-Va is an unconventional myosin heavy chain implicated in intracellular vesicle transport that is particularly abundant in neurons and melanocytes. It has the expected structure for a member of this family, that is, a globular head domain containing the ATP- and actin-binding sites, a neck domain, the site of calmodulin (or light-chain) binding, and a tail domain, the cargo-binding domain. Myosin-Va acts as a dimer and moves cargo along actin filaments, allowing their capture and accumulation at the periphery of the cells. In addition, myosin-Va may be implicated in structural and functional cross-talk between the actin- and microtubule-based cytoskeleton. Figure 17-20 depicts its mechanism of action.

Myosin-Va binds to melanosomes in melanocytes (Wu et al., 1997) and to synaptic vesicles in nerve terminals (Prekeris and Terrian, 1997). Myosin-Va defects in dilute

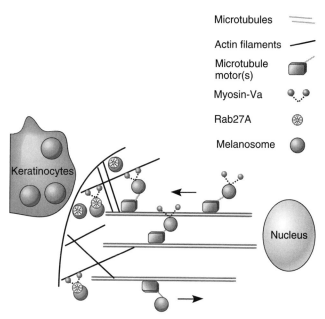

Figure 17-20· Model depicting the role of myosin-Va and Rab27A in intracellular melanosome transport. Myosin-Va serves to capture melanosomes delivered to the periphery of the cells via the centrifugal movement of microtubule motors, by mediating their interaction with F-actin. Rab27A participates in this capture probably by its interaction with myosin-Va. Defect of either myosin-Va or Rab27A leads to back movement and accumulation of the melanosomes in the center of the cells, preventing their delivery to adjacent keratinocytes.

mice result in the concentration of melanosomes in the center of the melanocytes, instead of in dendrites and dendritic tips of melanocytes. This defect impairs processing of presynaptic vesicles in the peripheral regions of the neurons and distribution of smooth endoplasmic reticulum in Purkinje cell neurons (Takagishi et al., 1996).

Rab27A is expressed in melanocytes, peripheral leukocytes, platelets, and many other cells and tissues but not in the brain (Chen et al., 1997). Each member of the Rab protein family has a characteristic intracellular distribution, suggesting a unique transport function. Similarly to myosin-Va, Rab27A co-localizes within melanosomes of melanocytes, resulting in the abnormal melanosome distribution observed in GS (Bahadoran et al., 2001). Rab27A is also necessary for cytotoxic granule exocytosis and intact T- and NK-cell cytotoxicity (Ménasché et al., 2000) (see Fig. 17-20).

Thus both myosin-Va and Rab27A anomalies lead to defective transport of melanosomes to surrounding keratinocytes, accounting for the pigmentary dilution characteristic of GS. Pigmentary dilution is identical in these two molecular defects. However, because of the presence of myosin-Va in brain tissue, only GS patients with the myosin-Va defect develop severe neurologic impairment in the absence of immunologic defects.

By contrast, defective Rab27A expression is always associated with abnormal lymphocyte cytotoxic activity, which can result in a lymphoproliferative syndrome similar to that present in familial hemophagocytic lymphohistiocytosis with perforin deficiency (Stepp et al., 1999). Neurologic problems in these patients during the accelerated phase are secondary to the widespread perivascular lymphohistiocytic infiltration.

Clinical Features

The two forms of GS are outlined in Table 17-19. Most patients are of Turkish and Mediterranean descent, many born to first-degree consanguineous parents. The age at diagnosis ranges from 1 month to 8 years with a mean of 17.5 months. Both genders are equally affected. Patients may present with the characteristic skin changes, the accelerated phase, or early onset of neuro-

logic features. Affected patients may have fevers or pneumonias before diagnosis, but recurrent respiratory infection are not reported.

Cutaneous Abnormalities

The most characteristic clinical feature of GS is cutaneous albinism and a silvery gray sheen to the hair (Klein et al., 1994; Ménasché et al., 2000). The latter is more obvious in patients with black hair, but it is also visible in light-haired patients. They generally have lighter hair than their unaffected family members. A few patients have only subtle pigmentary dilution of the skin and the retina. Hyperpigmentation in sun-exposed areas has also been noted. Hypopigmented spots in the retina have been described in some patients (Klein et al., 1994).

Accelerated Phase in RAB27A Mutation Patients

GS patients with the RAB27A mutation have anemia, neutropenia, and NK-cell deficiencies and will progress to the acute lymphophagocytic syndrome reflecting the accelerated phase. This may be triggered by a viral infection (e.g., EBV, hepatitis A, herpesvirus 6) or less commonly a bacterial infection (Klein et al., 1994; Wagner et al., 1997). Following remission, accelerated phase episodes recur with increasing severity. Twenty-three accelerated phase episodes, some self-limiting, were documented in one GS patient over a period of 7 years (Griscelli et al., 1978).

The accelerated phase, often the first manifestation of the disease, is characterized by high fever, jaundice, hepatosplenomegaly, lymphadenopathy, pancytopenia, and generalized lymphohistiocytic infiltrates of multiple organs including the CNS. This acute syndrome resembles that observed in the CHS (see Chapter 20), familial hemophagocytic lymphohistiocytosis (FHL) syndrome (see Chapter 26), VACS (Dufourcq-Lagelouse et al., 1999; see Chapter 26), and XLP syndrome (see the section on XLP).

Neurologic manifestations, caused by lymphocyte and macrophages activation within the CNS, may be the first sign of an accelerated phase (Chan et al., 1998;

TABLE 17-19 · COMPARISON OF THE TWO FORMS OF THE GRISCELLI SYNDROME

	Griscelli Syndrome 1	Griscelli Syndrome 2
Integument	Pigmentary dilution in skin and hair; Uneven distribution of large pigment granule in the hair shafts	
Immunologic	No immunologic symptoms	Defective natural killer and T-cell cytotoxicity Occurrence of accelerated phases
Neurologic	Severe, early, isolated, and static neurologic signs (hypotonia, absence of coordinated voluntary movements, psychomotor developmental delay)	Progressive neurologic signs secondary to cellular brain infiltration (seizures, hypertonic, ataxia, demyelination of the white matter), partly reversible
Curative treatment	—	Bone marrow transplantation
Chromosome localization	15q21	15q21
Molecular defect	Myosin-Va	Rab27A
Murine homologue	Dilute	Ashen
Related syndromes	Elejalde syndrome	PAID syndrome

PAID = partial albinism with immunodeficiency.

Hurvitz et al., 1993; Tezcan et al.,1999). Neurologic features include hyperreflexia, seizures, increased intracranial hypertension (vomiting, altered consciousness), hypertonia, nystagmus, and ataxia. Psychomotor development, usually normal at onset, may deteriorate; this may improve with remission although some changes may be irreversible.

Neurologic Features in MYO5A Mutation Patients

GS patients with *MYO5A* mutations may have severe neurologic abnormalities beginning at birth but without the occurrence of an accelerated phase. Neurologic features include hypotonia, absence of coordinated voluntary movements, and severe psychomotor developmental delay (Sanal et al., 2000). The CNS disorder is static or progressive but does not improve with time.

Laboratory Features

Hair and Skin Findings

The light microscopic examination and electron microscopic findings of the hair and skin are characteristic. Hair shafts have an uneven accumulation of large pigment granules, instead of the normal homogeneous distribution of small pigment granules. Fontana-stained silver sections of the skin show hyperpigmented melanocytes, contrasting to poorly pigmented adjacent keratinocytes, instead of the homogeneous distribution of melanin granules observed in melanocytes and surrounding keratinocytes in a normal epidermis.

Electron microscopy shows that the cytoplasm of melanocytes is filled with numerous mature stage IV melanosomes, predominantly around the nucleus but with normal dendritic processes (Chan et al., 1998; Griscelli et al., 1978; Klein et al., 1994; Takagishi et al., 1996). These findings are identical in both genetic groups of patients (e.g., myosin-Va or Rab27A defect).

Immunologic Findings

GS patients have normal numbers of T, B, and NK cells and normal neutrophil function, although decreased chemiluminescence and chemotactic responses have been reported in some patients (Klein et al., 1994). Immunoglobulin levels are usually normal. Delayed cutaneous hypersensitivity is decreased.

Patients with the Rab27A defect have a profound defect of T-cell mediated and NK-cell mediated cytotoxicity resulting in an inability to secrete cytotoxic granules and control activated cells throughout the body. A nonfunctional Rab27 protein is present in these patients and is the cause of accelerated phase onset (Ménasché et al., 2000; Stepp et al., 1999). Lymphoproliferative responses are preserved.

Other laboratory features of the accelerated phase include pancytopenia, hypertriglyceridemia, hypofibrinogenemia, cerebrospinal fluid pleocytosis, and the presence of activated macrophages and T lymphocytes, the latter mainly CD8 cells. These activated cells may infiltrate various organs to cause hemophagocytosis (Dufourcq-Lagelouse et al., 1999).

Patients with the myosin-Va defect have normal immunologic findings including normal cytotoxic activity. They do not develop an accelerated phase (Ménasché et al., 2000).

Central Nervous System Findings

Cranial computed tomography (CT) and magnetic resonance imaging (MRI) are different in the two groups of GS patients. Isolated congenital cerebellar atrophy was observed in a myosin-Va defect (Sanal et al., 2000). In the Rab27A defect, cerebellar hypodense areas, ventricular dilatation, or hyperdense areas compatible with inflammatory changes are observed. Generalized white matter changes and periventricular calcifications are also noted (Harfi et al., 1992; Hurvitz et al., 1993; Tezcan et al., 1999). Brain biopsy shows cerebral lymphohistiocytic infiltration, sometimes associated with erythrophagocytosis.

Diagnosis

GS must be considered in any child with decreased pigmentation accompanied by neurologic abnormalities or features of the accelerated phase (e.g., fever, hepatosplenomegaly, jaundice, or pancytopenia). Microscopic examination of the hair shaft provides strong support for the diagnosis of GS. The characteristic neurologic symptoms and decreased NK cytotoxicity also support the diagnosis. Confirmation is done by mutation analysis of the patient's DNA.

Prenatal Diagnosis

Prenatal diagnosis of GS was first accomplished by light microscopic examination of the hair shaft (Durandy et al., 1993). With identification of the GS genes, direct mutation-based carrier detection and prenatal diagnosis are now possible in families with defined *MYO5A* or *RAB27A* gene mutations. In addition, given the proximity of the two genes responsible for GS, polymorphic markers linked to the GS locus region in 15q21 can be used even if the precise mutation has not yet been identified in the family.

Differential Diagnosis

Several additional disorders that exhibit clinical similarities must be distinguished from GS.

Chediak-Higashi syndrome (CHS) is a disorder similar to GS involving variable hypopigmentation of the skin and the hair, frequent pyogenic infections, defective NK and T lymphocyte cytotoxicity, and an accelerated phase virtually identical to that of GS (Baetz et al., 1995; Beguez-Cesar, 1943; Blume and Wolff, 1972) (see Chapter 20). Light microscopic examination of the hair distinguishes these two disorders because in CHS the pigment clusters are smaller than in GS. The hallmark of CHS not present in GS is the presence of giant organelles (inclusion bodies) in virtually all granulated cells, including granulocytes, lymphocytes, monocytes, mast cells, melanocytes, Schwann cells, neurons, renal tubular epithelium, and fibroblasts.

Partial albinism with immunodeficiency (PAID syndrome) is similar to GS but is associated with progressive demyelination of the white matter of the brain (see Table 17-19). It has been described in eight Saudi Arabian kindred (Harfi et al., 1992). Genetic analysis in one of these families identified a *RAB27A* gene mutation, suggesting that PAID and GS are identical (de Saint Basile, unpublished data).

Elejalde syndrome (neuroectodermal melanolysosomal syndrome) has albinism resembling GS and an early onset of a severe CNS disorder but is without an accelerated phase (Elejalde et al., 1979) (see Table 17-19). This phenotype was present in four unrelated GS patients with myosin-Va defect, suggesting that Elejalde syndrome and this form of GS are allelic (Pastural et al., 2000; Sanal et al., 2000).

Familial hemophagocytic lymphohistiocytosis (see Chapter 26), XLP (see the section on XLP), and VACS (see Chapter 26) have accelerated phases identical to that in GS including diminished NK cytotoxicity (Dufourcq-Lagelouse et al., 1999). These disorders do not have partial albinism or hair abnormalities.

Treatment and Prognosis

Treatment for the accelerated phase includes supportive care, corticosteroids, and immunosuppressive drugs such as anti-thymocyte globulin (ATG), cyclosporine (CsA), or VP-16 eposide. Intrathecal methotrexate may be of value for the neurocerebral involvement (Gogus et al., 1995; Gurgey et al., 1994; Jabado et al., 1997; Klein et al., 1994; Tezcan et al., 1999). Chemotherapy of the accelerated phase is sometimes ineffective and rarely prevents relapses.

Allogeneic BMT for the Rab27A form of GS is the only curative treatment (Klein et al., 1994; Schneider et al., 1990). BMT corrects the cytotoxic defect and prevents reoccurrence of the accelerated phase. Even a low percentage of donor cells in the patient are enough to control the disease, probably because each cytotoxic cell may kill several targets. These findings indicate that successful transfer of a normal *RAB27A* gene, even to a small proportion of patient cells, may restore cytotoxic activity and control the disease.

In the myosin-Va form of GS, no specific treatment is available other than to control infection.

The prognosis for long-term survival in GS is poor. The Rab27A form is usually fatal within 1 to 4 years from the onset of the accelerated phase. The severe neurologic impairment and psychomotor delay do not improve with time.

Genevieve de Saint-Basile

REFERENCES

Aaltonen J, Komulainen J, Vikman A, Palotie A, Wadelius C, Perheentupa J, Peltonen L. Autoimmune polyglandular disease type I: exclusion map using amplifiable multiallelic markers in a microtiter well format. Eur J Hum Genet 1:164–171, 1993.

Abo T, Roder JC, Abo W, Cooper MD, Balch CM. Natural killer (HNK-1+) cells in Chediak-Higashi patients are present in normal numbers but are abnormal in function and morphology. J Clin Invest 170:193–197, 1982.

Adachi M, Tachibana K, Masuno M, Makita Y, Maesaka H, Okada T, Hizukuri K, Imaizumi K, Kuroki Y, Kurahashi H, Suwa S. Clinical characteristics of children with hypoparathyroidism due to 22q11.2 microdeletion. Eur J Pediatr 157:34–38, 1998.

Ahonen P, Koskimies S, Lokki ML, Tiilikainen A, Perheentupa J. The expression of autoimmune polyglandular disease type I appears associated with several HLA antigens, but not with HLA-DR. J Clin Endocrinol Metab 66:152–157, 1988.

Ahonen P, Myllärniemi S, Sipilä I, Perheentupa J. Clinical variation of autoimmune polyendocrinopathy-candidiasis-ectodermal dystrophy (APECED) in a series of 68 patients. N Engl J Med 322:1829–1836, 1990.

Aldrich RA, Steinberg AG, Campbell DC. Pedigree demonstrating a sex-linked recessive condition characterized by draining ears, eczematoid dermatitis and bloody diarrhea. Pediatrics 13:133–139, 1954.

Alexander WJ, Dunbar JS. Unusual bone changes in thmic alymphoplasia. Ann Radiol (Paris) 11:186–194, 1967.

Altare F, Durandy A, Lammas D, Emile JF, Lamhamedi S, Le Deist F, Drysdale P, Jouanguy E, Doffinger R, Bernaudin F, Jeppsson O, Gollob JA, Meinl E, Segal AW, Fischer A, Kumararatne D, Casanova JL. Impairment of mycobacterial immunity in human interleukin-12 receptor deficiency. Science 280:1432–1435, 1998a.

Altare F, Lammas D, Revy P, Jouanguy E, Doffinger R, Lamhamedi S, Drysdale P, Scheel-Toellner D, Girdlestone J, Darbyshire P, Wadhwa M, Dockrell H, Salmon M, Fischer A, Durandy A, Casanova JL, Kumararatne DS. Inherited interleukin 12 deficiency in a child with bacille Calmette-Guerin and *Salmonella enteritidis* disseminated infection. J Clin Invest 102:2035–2040, 1998b.

Ammann AJ, Hong R. Disorders of the T-cell system. In Stiehm ER, ed. Immunologic Disorders in Infants and Children, ed 3. Philadelphia, WB Saunders, 1989, pp 257–315.

Ammann, AJ, Sutliff, W. Millinchick E. Antibody mediated immunodeficiency in short limbed dwarfism. J Pediatr 84:200–203, 1974.

Anderson MS. Autoimmune endocrine disease. Curr Opin Immunol 14:760–764, 2002.

Anderson MS, Venanzi ES, Klein L, Chen Z, Berzins SP, Turley SJ, von Boehmer H, Bronson R, Dierich A, Benoist C, Mathis D. Projection of an immunological self-shadow within the thymus by the aire protein. Science 298:1395–1401, 2002.

Anzalone G, Cei M, Vizzaccaro A, Tramma B, Bisetti A. *M. Kansasii* pulmonary disease in idiopathic CD4+ T-lymphocytopenia. Eur Respir J 9:1754–6, 1996.

Aozasa M, Amino N, Iwatani Y, Tamaki H, Watanabe Y, Sato H, Hochito K, Umeda K, Gunji T, Yoshizawa T, Iyama S, Miya K. Familial OKT4 epitope deficiency: studies on antigen density and lymphocyte function. Clin Immunol Immunopathol 37:48–55, 1985.

Aprikyan AA, Liles WC, Park JR, Jonas M, Chi EY, Dale DC. Myelokathexis, a congenital disorder of severe neutropenia characterized by accelerated apoptosis and defective expression of bcl-x in neutrophil precursors. Blood 95:320–327, 2000.

Arai J, Wakiguchi H, Hisakawa H, Kubota H, Kurashige T. A variant of myelokathexis with hypogammaglobulinemia: lymphocytes as well as neutrophils may reverse in response to infections. Pediatr Hematol Oncol 17:171–176, 2000.

Ariga T, Kondoh T, Yamaguchi K, Yamada M, Sasaki S, Nelson DL, Ikeda H, Kobayashi K, Moriuchi H, Sakiyama Y. Spontaneous in vivo reversion of an inherited mutation in the Wiskott-Aldrich syndrome. J Immunol 166:5245–5249, 2001.

Arnon TI, Lev M, Katz G, Chernobrov Y, Porgador A, Mandelboim O. Recognition of viral hemagglutinins by NKp44 but not by NKp30. Eur J Immunol 31:2680–2689, 2001.

Arulanantham K, Dwyer JM, Genel M. Evidence for defective immunoregulation in the syndrome of familial candidiasis endocrinopathy. N Engl J Med 300:164–168, 1979.

Aspalter RM, Sewell WA, Dolman K, Farrant J, Webster AD. Deficiency in circulating natural killer (NK) cell subsets in common variable immunodeficiency and X-linked agammaglobulinaemia. Clin Exp Immunol 121:506–514, 2000.

Aspenstrom P, Lindberg U, Hall A. Two GTPases, Cdc42 and Rac, bind directly to a protein implicated in the immunodeficiency disorder Wiskott-Aldrich syndrome. Curr Biol 6:70–75, 1996.

August CS, Levey RH, Berkel AI, Rosen FS, Kay HEM. Establishment of immunological competence in a child with congenital thymic aplasia by a graft of fetal thymus. Lancet 1:1080–1083, 1970.

August CS, Rosen FS, Filler RM, Janeway CA, Markowski B, Kay HEM. Implantation of foetal thymus, restoring immunological competence in a patient with thymic aplasia (DiGeorge's syndrome). Lancet 2:1210-1211, 1968.

Baba Y, Nonoyama S, Matsushita M, Yamadori T, Hashimoto S, Imai K, Arai S, Kunikata T, Kurimoto M, Kurosaki T, Ochs HD, Yata J, Kishimoto T, Tsukada S. Involvement of Wiskott-Aldrich syndrome protein in B-cell cytoplasmic tyrosine kinase pathway. Blood 93:2003–2012, 1999.

Bach FH, Albertini RJ, Joo P, Anderson JL, Bortin MM. Bone-marrow transplantation in a patient with the Wiskott-Aldrich syndrome. Lancet 2:1364–1366, 1968.

Bach MA, Phan-Dinh-Tuy F, Bach JF, Wallach D, Biddison WE, Sharrow SO, Goldstein G, Kung PC. Unusual phenotypes of human inducer T cells as measured by OKT4 and related monoclonal antibodies. J Immunol 127:180, 1981, 1982.

Badolato R, Sozzani S, Malacarne F, Bresciani S, Fiorini M, Borsatti A, Albertini A, Mantovani A, Ugazio AG, Notarangelo LD. Monocytes from Wiskott-Aldrich patients display reduced chemotaxis and lack of cell polarization in response to monocyte chemoattractant protein-1 and formyl-methionyl-leucyl-phenylalanine. J Immunol 161:1026–1033, 1998.

Baetz K, Isaaz S, Griffiths GM. Loss of cytotoxic T lymphocyte function in Chediak-Higashi syndrome arise from a secretory defect that prevents lytic granule exocytosis. J Immunol 154:6122–6131, 1995.

Bahadoran P, Aberdam E, Mantoux F, Busca R, Bille K, Yalman N, De Saint Basile G, Casaroli R, Ortonne J-P, Ballotti R. Rab27A: a key to melanosome transport in human melanocytes. J Cell Biol 152:843–849, 2001.

Ballas ZK, Turner JM, Turner DA, Goetzman EA, Kemp JD. A patient with simultaneous absence of "classical" natural killer cells (CD3−, CD16+, and NKH1+) and expansion of CD3+, CD4−, CD8−, NKH1+ subset. J Allergy Clin Immunol 85:453–459, 1990.

Ballow M, Hyman LR. Combination immunotherapy in chronic mucocutaneous candidiasis. Synergism between transfer factor and fetal thymus tissue. Clin Immunol Immunopathol 8:504–512, 1977.

Barbosa MD, Nguyen QA, Tchernev VT, Aschley JA, Detter JC, Blaydes SM, Brandt SJ, Chotai D, Hodgman C, Solari RCE, Lovett M. Kingsmore SF. Identification of the homologous beige and Chediak-Higashi syndrome genes. Nature 382:262–265, 1996.

Barrat F, Auloge L, Pastural E, Dufourcq-Lagelouse, R, Vilmer E, Cant A, Weissenbach J, Le Paslier D, Fischer A, de Saint Basile G. Genetic and physical mapping of the Chédiak-Higashi syndrome on chromosome 1q42-43. Am J Hum Genet 59:625–632, 1996.

Barrett DJ, Ammann AJ, Wara DW, Cowan MJ, Fisher TJ, Stiehm ER. Clinical and immunologic spectrum of the DiGeorge syndrome. J Clin Lab Immunol 6:1–6, 1981.

Bastian J, Law S, Vogler L, Lawton A, Herrod H, Anderson S, Horowitz S, Hong R. Prediction of persistent immunodeficiency in the DiGeorge anomaly. J Pediatr 115:391–396, 1989.

Baud O, Goulet O, Canioni D, Le Deist F, Radford I, Rieu D, Dupuis-Girod S, Cerf-Bensussan N, Cavazzana-Calvo M, Brousse N, Fischer A, Casanova JL. Treatment of the immunedysregulation, polyendocrinopathy, enteropathy, X-linked syndrome (IPEX) by allogeneic bone marrow transplantation. N Engl J Med 344:1758–1762, 2001.

Baugh CM, Malone JH, Butterworth CE. Human biotin deficiency: a case history of biotin deficiency induced by raw egg white consumption in a cirrhotic patient. Am J Clin Nutr 21:173–182, 1968.

Beard LJ, Robertson EF, Thong YH. Para-influenza pneumonia in DiGeorge syndrome two years after thymic epithelial transplantation. Acta Paed Scand 69:403–406, 1980.

Beguez-Cesar A. Neutropenia cronica maligna familiar con granulaciones atipicas de los leucocitos. Sociedad Cubana de Pediatr Boletin 15:900–922, 1943.

Ben Rejeb A, Ebdelli N, Bouali MR, Goucha A, Bougrine F, Khediri F, Delsol G. Primary digestive tract Kaposi sarcoma with idiopathic CD4+ lymphocytopenia, HIV negative, HHV8 positive. Gastroenterol Clin Biol 25:707–710, 2001.

Bennett CL, Brunkow ME, Ramsdell F, O'Briant KC, Zhu Q, Fuleihan RL, Shigeoka AO, Ochs HD, Chance PF. A rare polyadenylation signal mutation of the FOXP3 gene (AAUAAA -> AAUGAA) leads to the IPEX syndrome. Immunogenetics 53:435–439, 2001a.

Bennett CL, Christie J, Ramsdell F, Brunkow ME, Ferguson PJ, Whitesell L, Kelly TE, Saulsbury FT, Chance PF, Ochs HD. The immune dysregulation, polyendocrinopathy, enteropathy, X-linked syndrome (IPEX) is caused by mutations of FOXP3. Nat Genet 27:20–21, 2001b.

Bensoussan D, Le Deist F, Latger-Cannard V, Gregoire MJ, Avinens O, Feugier P, Bourdon V, Andre-Botte C, Schmitt C, Jonveaux P, Eliaou JF, Stoltz JF, Bordigoni P. T-cell immune constitution after peripheral blood mononuclear cell transplantation in complete DiGeorge syndrome. Br J Haematol 117:899–906, 2002.

Bentur L, Nesbet-Brown E, Levinson H, Roifman CM. Lung disease associated with IgG subclass deficiency in chronic mucocutaneous candidiasis. J Pediatr 118:82–86, 1991.

Berend SA, Spikes AS, Kashork CD, Wu JM, Daw SC, Scambler PJ, Shaffer LG. Dual-probe fluorescence in situ hybridization assay for detecting deletions associated with VCFS/DiGeorge syndrome I and DiGeorge syndrome II loci. Am J Med Genet 91:313–317, 2000.

Berger EA, Murphy PM, Farber JM. Chemokine receptors as HIV-1 coreceptors: roles in viral entry, tropism, and disease. Annu Rev Immunol 17:657–700, 1999.

Berger M, Kirkpatrick CH, Goldsmith PK, Gallin JI. IgE antibodies to Staphylococcus aureus and Candida albicans in patients with the syndrome of hyperimmunoglobulin E and recurrent infections. J Immunol 125:2437–2443, 1980.

Berthet F, Siegrist CA, Lzsahin H, Tuchschmid P, Eich G, Superti-Furga A, Seger RA. Bone marrow transplantation in cartilage-hair hypoplasia: correction of the immunodeficiency but not of the chondrodysplasia. Eur J Pediatr 155:286–290, 1996.

Binks M, Jones GE, Brickell PM, Kinnon C, Katz DR, Thrasher AJ. Intrinsic dendritic cell abnormalities in Wiskott-Aldrich syndrome. Eur J Immunol 28:3259–3267, 1998.

Biron, A, Byron, KS, Sullivan, JL. Severe herpesvirus infections in an adolescent without natural killer cells. N Engl J Med 320:1731–1735, 1989.

Biron C, Nguyen KB, Pien GC, Cousens LP, Salazar-Mather T. Natural killer cells in antiviral defence: function and regulation by innate cytokines Annu Rev Immunol 17:189–220, 1999.

Blaese RM, Strober W, Brown RS, Waldmann TA. The Wiskott-Aldrich syndrome. A disorder with a possible defect in antigen processing or recognition. Lancet 1:1056–1061, 1968.

Blaese RM, Strober W, Levy AL, Waldmann TA. Hypercatabolism of IgG, IgA, IgM, and albumin in the Wiskott-Aldrich syndrome. A unique disorder of serum protein metabolism. J Clin Invest 50:2331–2338, 1971.

Blair PJ, Bultman SJ, Haas JC, Rouse BT, Wilkinson JE, Godfrey VL. CD4+CD8− T cells are the effector cells in disease pathogenesis in the scurfy (sf) mouse. J Immunol 153:3764–3774, 1994.

Bleul CC, Fuhlbrigge RC, Casasnovas JM, Aiuti A, Springer TA. A highly efficacious lymphocyte chemoattractant, stromal cell-derived factor 1 (SDF-1) J Exp Med 184:1101–1109, 1996.

Blizzard RM, Gibbs JH. Candidiasis: studies pertaining to its association with endocrinopathies and pernicious anemia. Pediatrics 42:231–237, 1968.

Blum R, Geller G, Fish LA. Recurrent severe staphylococcal infections, eczematoid rash, extreme elevations of IgE, eosinophilia, and divergent chemotactic responses in two generations. J Pediatr 90:607–609, 1977.

Blume R, Wolff S. The Chediak-Higashi syndrome: studies in four patients and a review of the literature. Medicine 51:247–280, 1972.

Bockman DE, Kirby ML. Neural crest interactions in the development of the immune system. J Immunol 135:766s–768s, 1985.

Bohinjec J, Andoljsek D. Neutrophil-releasing activity of recombinant human granulocyte-macrophage colony stimulating factor in myelokathexis. Br J Haematol 82:169–170, 1992.

Bohinjec J. Myelokathexis: chronic neutropenia with hyperplastic bone marrow and hypersegmented neutrophils in two siblings. Blut 42:191–196, 1981.

Bonagura VR, Cunningham-Rundles S, Edwards BL, Ilowite NT, Wedgwood JF, Valacer DJ. Common variable hypogammaglobulinemia, recurrent Pneumocystis carinii pneumonia on intravenous gamma-globulin therapy, and natural killer deficiency. Clin Immunol Immunopathol 51:216–231, 1989.

Bordin G, Ballare M, Paglino S, Ravanini P, Dulio D, Malosso MC, Boldorini R, Monteverde A. Idiopathic CD4+ lymphocytopenia and systemic vasculitis. J Intern Med 240:37–41, 1996.

Borges WG, Augustine NH, Hill HR. Defective interleukin-12/interferon-gamma pathway in patients with hyperimmunoglobulinemia E syndrome. J Pediatr 136:176–180, 2000.

Borgmann S, Luhmer I, Arslan-Kirchner M, Kallfelz HC, Schmidtke J. A search for chromosome 22q11.2 deletions in a series of 176 consecutively catheterized patients with congenital heart disease: no evidence for deletions in non-syndromic patients. Eur J Pediatr 158:958–963, 1999.

Borzy MS, Ridgway D, Noya FJ, Shearer WT. Successful bone marrow transplantation with split lymphoid chimerism in DiGeorge syndrome. J Clin Immunol 9:386–392, 1989.

Bowers DC, Lederman HM, Sicherer SH, Winkelstein JA, Chen AR. Immune constitution of complete DiGeorge anomaly by transplantation of unmobilised blood mononuclear cells. Lancet 352:1983–1984, 1998.

Brochstein JA, Gillio AP, Ruggiero M, Kernan NA, Emanuel D, Laver J, Small T, O'Reilly RJ. Marrow transplantation from human leukocyte antigen-identical or haploidentical donors for correction of Wiskott-Aldrich syndrome. J Pediatr 119:907–912, 1991.

Brouard J, Morin M, Borel B, Laloum D, Mandard JC, Duhamel JF, Venezia R. Syndrome de Di George complique d'une reaction du greffon contre l'hote. Arch Fr Pediatr 42:853–855, 1985.

Bruce RM, Blaese RM. Monoclonal gammopathy in the Wiskott-Aldrich syndrome. J Pediatr 85:204–207, 1974.

Brudy L, Janier M, Reboul D, Baviera E, Bonvalet D, Daniel F. Erosive lichen of the scalp. Ann Dermatol Venereol 124:703–706, 1997.

Brunkow ME, Jeffery EW, Hjerrild KA, Paeper B, Clark LB, Yasayko SA, Wilkinson JE, Galas D, Ziegler SF, Ramsdell F. Disruption of a new forkhead/winged-helix protein, scurfin, results in the fatal lymphoproliferative disorder of the scurfy mouse. Nat Genet 27:68–73, 2001.

Buckley RH. Primary immunodeficiency diseases due to defects in lymphocytes. N Engl J Med 343:1313–1324, 2000.

Buckley RH. The hyper-IgE syndrome. Clin Rev Allerg Immunol 20:139–154, 2001.

Buckley RH, Sampson HA. The Hyperimmunoglobulinemia E syndrome. In Clinical Immunology Update. New York, Elsevier North-Holland, 1981, pp 147–167.

Buckley RH, Schiff SE, Hayward AR. Reduced frequency of CD45RO+ T lymphocytes in blood of hyper IgE syndrome patients. J Allerg Clin Immunol 87:313a, 1991.

Buckley RH, Schiff RI, Schiff SE, Markert L, Williams LW, Harville TO, Roberts JL, Puck JM. Human severe combined immunodeficiency: genetic, phenotypic and functional diversity in one hundred eight infants. J Pediatr 130:378–387, 1997.

Buckley RH, Wray BB, Belmaker EZ. Extreme hyperimmunoglobulinemia E and undue susceptibility to infection. Pediatrics 49:59–70, 1972.

Burg S, Weber, W, Kucherer C. Idiopathic CD4 lymphocytopenia with lethal Salmonella typhimurium sepsis. Dtsch Med Wochenschr 119:956–958, 1994.

Busch MP, Valinsky JE, Paglieroni T, Prince HE, Crutcher GJ, Gjerset GF, Operskalski EA, Charlebois E, Bianco C, Holland PV, et al. Screening of blood donors for idiopathic CD4+ T-lymphocytopenia. Transfusion 34:192–197, 1994.

Busse PJ, Cunningham-Rundles C. Primary leptomeningeal lymphoma in a patient with concomitant CD4+ lymphocytopenia. Ann Allergy Asthma Immunol 88:339–342, 2002.

Calderone RA, Braun PC. Adherence and receptor relationships of Candida albicans. Microbiol Rev 55:1–20, 1991.

Campbell JK, Prince HM, Juneja SK, Seymour JF, Slavin M. Diffuse large cell lymphoma and t(8;22) (q24;q11) in a patient with idiopathic CD4+ T-lymphopenia. Leuk Lymphoma 41:421–423, 2001.

Canales ML, Mauer AM. Sex-linked hereditary thrombocytopenia as a variant of Wiskott-Aldrich syndrome. N Engl J Med 277:899–901, 1967.

Carbone E, Ruggiero G, Terrazzano G, Palomba C, Manzo C, Fontana S, Spits H, Karre K, Zappacosta S. A new mechanism of NK cell cytotoxicity activation: the CD40-CD40 ligand interaction. J Exp Med 185:2053–2060, 1997.

Carey AH, Kelly D, Halford S, Wadey R, Wilson D, Goodship J, Burn J, Paul T, Sharkey A, Dumanski J. Molecular genetic study of the frequency of monosomy 22q11 in DiGeorge syndrome. Am J Hum Genet 51:964–970, 1992.

Carlier MF, Ducruix A, Pantaloni D. Signalling to actin: the Cdc42-N-WASP-Arp2/3 connection. Chem Biol 6:R235–40, 1999.

Casanova JL, Abel L. Genetic dissection of immunity to mycobacteria: the human model. Annu Rev Immunol 20:581–620, 2002.

Cascio G, Massobrio AM, Cascio B, Anania A. Undefined CD4 lymphocytopenia without clinical complications. A report of two cases. Panminerva Med 40:69–71, 1998.

Cassone A, DeBernardis F, Mondello F, Ceddia T, Agatensi L. Evidence for a correlation between protease secretion and vulvovaginal candidiasis. J Infect Dis 156:777–783, 1987.

Castriota-Scanderberg A, Mingarelli R, Caramina G, Osimani P, Lachman RS, Rimoin DL, Wilcox WR, Dllapiccola B. Spondylo-mesomelic-acrodysplasia with joint dislocations and severe combined immunodeficiency: a newly recognized immuno-osseous dysplasia. J Med Genet 34:854–856, 1997.

Castro AG, Hauser TM, Cocks BG, Abrams J, Zurawski S, Churakova T, Zonin F, Robinson D, Tangye SG, Aversa G, Nichols KE, de Vries JE, Lanier LL, O'Garra A. Molecular and functional characterization of mouse signaling lymphocytic activation molecule (SLAM): differential expression and responsiveness in Th1 and Th2 cells. J Immunol 163:5860–5870, 1999.

Catalina MD, Sullivan JL, Bak KR, Luzuriaga K. Differential evolution and stability of epitope-specific CD8+ T-cell responses in EBV infection. J Immunol 167:4450–4457, 2001.

CDC. Unexplained CD4+ T-lymphocyte depletion in persons without evident HIV infection—United States. MMWR Morb Mortal Wkly Rep 41:541–545, 1992.

Cernelc P, Andoljsek D, Mlakar U, Pretnar J, Modic M, Zupan IP, Zver S. Effects of molgramostim, filgrastim and lenograstim in the treatment of myelokathexis. Pflugers Arch 440:R81–82, 2000.

Chae KM, Ertle JO, Tharp MD. B-cell lymphoma in a patient with WHIM syndrome. J Am Acad Dermatol 44:124–128, 2001.

Chamlin SL, McCalmont TH, Cunningham BB, Esterly NB, Lai CH, Mallory SB, Mancini AJ, Tamburro J, Frieden IJ. Cutaneous manifestations of hyper-IgE syndrome in infants and children. J Pediatr 141:572–575, 2002.

Chan L, Lapiere J, Chen M, Traczyk T, Mancini A, Paller A, Woodley D, Marinkovich M. Partial albinism with immunodeficiency: Griscelli syndrome: report of a case and review of the literature. J Am Acad Dermatol 38:295–300, 1998.

Charles BM, Hosking G, Green A, Pollitt R, Barlett K, Taitz LS. Biotin-responsive alopecia and developmental regression Lancet 2:118–120, 1979.

Chatila TA, Blaeser F, Ho N, Lederman HM, Voulgaropoulos C, Helms C, Bowcock AM. JM2, encoding a fork head-related protein, is mutated in X-linked autoimmunity-allergic dysregulation syndrome. J Clin Invest 106:R75–81, 2000.

Chehimi J, Elder M, Greene J, Noroski L, Stiehm ER, Winkelstein JA, Sullivan KE. Cytokine and chemokine dysregulation in hyper-IgE syndrome. Clin Immunol 100:49–56, 2001.

Chen D, Guo J, Miki T, Tachibana M. Gahl W. Molecular cloning and characterization of rab27a and rab27b, novel human rab proteins shared by melanocytes and platelets. Biochem Mol Med 60:7–37, 1997.

Chilgren RA, Quie PG, Meuwissen HJ, Hong R. Chronic mucocutaneous candidiasis, deficiency of delayed hypersensitivity, and selective local antibody defect. Lancet 2:688–693, 1967.

Chipps BE, Saulsbury FT, Hsu SH, Hughes WT, Winkelstein JA. Non-candidal infections in children with chronic mucocutaneous candidiasis. Johns Hopkins Med J 144:175–179, 1979.

Christ MJ, Dillon CA. Myelokathexis in a mother and infant: a second case suggesting dominant inheritance. Mil Med 162:827–828, 1997.

Church JA, Frenkel LD, Wright DG, Bellanti JA. T lymphocyte dysfunction, hyperimmunoglobulinemia E, recurrent bacterial infections, and defective neutrophil chemotaxis in a Negro child. J Pediatr 88:982–985, 1976.

Claassen JL, Levine AD, Buckley RH. A cell culture system that enhances mononuclear cell IgE synthesis induced by recombinant human interleukin-4. J Immunol Methods 126:213–222, 1990.

Claassen JL, Levine AD, Schiff SE, Buckley RH. Mononuclear cells from patients with the hyper IgE syndrome produce little IgE when stimulated with recombinant interleukin 4 in vitro. J Allergy Clin Immunol 88:713–721, 1991.

Clark LB, Appleby MW, Brunkow ME, Wilkinson JE, Ziegler SF, Ramsdell F. Cellular and molecular characterization of the scurfy mouse mutant. J Immunol 162:2546–2554, 1999.

Clark RA, Root RK, Kimball HR, Kirkpatrick CH. Defective neutrophil chemotaxis and cellular immunity in a child with recurrent infections. Ann Intern Med 78:515–519, 1973.

Cleveland WW, Fogel BJ, Brown WT, Kay HEM. Foetal thymic transplant in a case of DiGeorge's syndrome. Lancet 2:1211–1214, 1968.

Cocks BG, Chang CC, Carballido JM, Yssel H, de Vries JE, Aversa G. A novel receptor involved in T-cell activation. Nature 376:260-3, 1995.

Coffey AJ, Brooksbank RA, Brandau O, Oohashi T, Howell GR, Bye JM, Cahn AP, Durham J, Heath P, Wray P, Pavitt R, Wilkinson J, Leversha M, Huckle E, Shaw-Smith CJ, Dunham A, Rhodes S, Schuster V, Porta G, Yin L, Serafini P, Sylla B, Zollo M, Franco B, Bentley DR, et al. Host response to EBV infection in X-linked lymphoproliferative disease results from mutations in an SH2-domain encoding gene. Nat Genet 20:129–35, 1998.

Coffman RL, Carty J. A T cell activity that enhances polyclonal IgE production and its inhibition by interferon-γ. J Immunol 136:949–954, 1986.

Collard HR, Boeck A, Mc Laughlin TM, Watson TJ, Schiff SE, Hale LP, Markert ML. Possible extrathymic development of nonfunctional T cells in a patient with complete DiGeorge syndrome. Clin Immunol 91:156–162, 1999.

Como JA, Dismukes WE. Oral azole drugs as systemic antifungal therapy. N Engl J Med 330:263–272, 1994.

Conley ME, Beckwith JB, Mancer JF, Tenckhoff L. The spectrum of the DiGeorge syndrome. J Pediatr 94:883–890, 1979.

Conley ME, Notarangelo LD, Etzioni A. Diagnostic criteria for primary immunodeficiencies. Representing PAGID (Pan-American Group for Immunodeficiency) and ESID (European Society for Immunodeficiencies). Clin Immunol 93:190–197, 1999.

Conley ME, Wang WC, Parolini O, Shapiro DN, Campana D Siminovitch KA. Atypical Wiskott-Aldrich syndrome in a girl. Blood 80:1264–1269, 1992.

Cooper MA, Fehniger TA, Caligiuri MA. The biology of human natural killer-cell subsets. Trends Immunol 22:633–640, 2001.

Cooper MD, Chae HP, Lowman JT, Krivit W, Good RA. Wiskott-Aldrich syndrome. An immunologic deficiency disease involving the afferent limb of immunity. Am J Med 44:499–513, 1968.

Corder WT, Hummel M, Miller C. Wilson NW. Association of kyphomelic dysplasia with severe combined immunodeficiency Am J Med Genet 57:626–629,1995.

Cotelingam JD, Witebsky FG, Hsu SM, Blaese RM, Jaffe ES. Malignant lymphoma in patients with the Wiskott-Aldrich syndrome. Cancer Invest 3:515–522, 1985.

Cowan MJ, Wara D, Packman S, Ammann A, Yoshino M, Sweetman L, Nyhan W. Multiple biotin-dependent carboxylase deficiencies associated with defects in T-cell and B-cell immunity. Lancet 2:115–118, 1979.

Craig JM, Schiff LH, Boone JE. Chronic moniliasis associated with Addison's disease. Am J Dis Child 89:669–684, 1955.

Cunningham-Rundles C, Murray HW, Smith JP. Treatment of idiopathic CD4 T lymphocytopenia with IL-2. Clin Exp Immunol 116:322–5, 1999.

Davies, K, Stiehm ER, Woo P, Murray K. Juvenile idiopathic polyarticular arthritis and IgA deficiency in the 22q11 deletion syndrome, J Rheumatol 28:2326–2334, 2001.

Davis CM, McLaughlin TM, Watson TJ, Buckley RH, Schiff SE, Hale LP, Haynes BF, Markert ML. Normalization of the peripheral blood T cell receptor V beta repertoire after cultured postnatal human thymic transplantation in DiGeorge syndrome. J Clin Immunol 17:167–175, 1997.

Davis J. A case of Swiss type agammaglobulinemia and achondroplasia. BMJ 2:1371–1374, 1966.

Davis SD, Schaller J, Wedgwood RJ. Job's syndrome. Recurrent, "cold", staphylococcal abscesses. Lancet 2:1013–1015, 1966.

Daw SCM, Taylor C, Kraman M, Call K, Schuffenhauer S, Meitinger T, Lipson T, Goodship J, Scambler PJ. A common region of 10p deleted in DiGeorge and velocardiofacial syndromes. Nat Genet 13:458–460, 1996.

de Jong R, Altare F, Haagen IA, Elferink DG, Boer T, van Breda Vriesman PJ, Kabel PJ, Draaisma JM, van Dissel JT, Kroon FP, Casanova JL, Ottenhoff TH. Severe mycobacterial and Salmonella infections in interleukin-12 receptor-deficient patients. Science 280:1435–1438, 1998.

de la Chapelle A, Herva R, Koivisto M, Aula P. A deletion in chromosome 22 can cause DiGeorge syndrome. Hum Genet 57:253–256, 1981.

de la Morena M, James-Yarish M, Kirkpatrick CH, Good RA, Day NK. Studies of cytokine gene expression in patients with chronic mucocutaneous candidiasis. J Allergy Clin Immunol 95:234(abs), 1995.

de Vries E, Koene HR, Vossen JM, Gratama JW, von dem Borne AE, Waaijer JL, Haraldsson A, de Haas M, van Tol MJ. Identification of an unusual Fc gamma receptor IIIa (CD16) on natural killer cells in a patient with recurrent infections. Blood. 88:3022–3027, 1996.

Deeg HJ, Lum LG, Sanders J, Levy GJ, Sullivan KM, Beatty P, Thomas ED, Storb R. Severe aplastic anemia associated with chronic mucocutaneous candidiasis: immunologic and hematologic reconstitution after allogeneic bone marrow transplantation. Transplant 41:583–586, 1986.

Deerojanawong J, Chang AB, Eng PA, Robertson CF, Kemp AS. Pulmonary diseases in children with severe combined immune deficiency and DiGeorge syndrome. Pediatr Pulmonol 24:324–330, 1997.

Del Prete G, Tiri A, Maggi E, De Carli M, Macchia D, Parronchi P, Rossi ME, Pietrogrande MC, Ricci M, Romagnani S. Defective in vitro production of gamma interferon and tumor necrosis factor alpha by circulating T cells from patients with the hyper immunoglobulin E syndrome. J Clin Invest 84:1830–1835, 1989.

DePiero AD, Lourie EM, Berman BW, Robin NH, Zinn AB, Hostoffer RW. Recurrent immune cytopenias in two patients with DiGeorge/velocardiofacial syndorme. J Pediatr 131:484–486, 1997.

Derry JM, Kerns JA, Weinberg KI, Ochs HD, Volpini V, Estivill X, Walker AP, Francke U. WASP gene mutations in Wiskott-Aldrich syndrome and X-linked thrombocytopenia. Hum Mol Genet 4:1127–1135, 1995.

Derry JM, Ochs HD, Francke U. Isolation of a novel gene mutated in Wiskott-Aldrich syndrome. Cell 78:635–644, 1994.

Des Jarlais DC, Friedman SR, Marmor M, Mildvan D, Yancovitz S, Sotheran JL, Wenston J, Beatrice S. CD4 lymphocytopenia among injecting drug users in New York City. J Acquir Immune Defic Syndr 6:820–822, 1993.

Devriendt K, Fryns JP, Mortier G, van Thienen MN, Keymolen K. The annual incidence of DiGeorge/velocardiofacial syndrome. J Med Genet 35:789–790, 1998.

Devriendt K, Kim AS, Mathijs G, Frints SG, Schwartz M, Van Den Oord JJ, Verhoef GE, Boogaerts MA, Fryns JP, You D, Rosen MK, Vandenberghe P. Constitutively activating mutation in WASP causes X-linked severe congenital neutropenia. Nat Genet 27:313–317, 2001.

Di Rocco M, Marta R. X-linked immune dysregulation, neonatal insulin dependent diabetes, and intractable diarrhoea. Arch Dis Child 75:F144, 1996.

DiGeorge AM. A new concept of the cellular basis of immunology (discussion). J Pediatr 67:907–908, 1965.

DiGeorge AM. Congenital absence of the thymus and its immunological consequences: concurrance with congenital hypothyroidism. Birth Defects 4:116–121, 1968.

Djawari D, Bischoff T, Hornstein OP. Impairment of chemotactic activity of macrophages in chronic mucocutaneous candidiasis. Arch Derm Res 262:247–253, 1978.

Doffinger R, Jouanguy E, Dupuis S, Fondaneche MC, Stephan JL, Emile JF, Lamhamedi-Cherradi S, Altare F, Pallier A, Barcenas-Morales G, Meinl E, Krause C, Pestka S, Schreiber RD, Novelli F, Casanova JL. Partial interferon-gamma receptor signaling chain deficiency in a patient with bacille Calmette-Guerin and *Mycobacterium abscessus* infection. J Infect Dis 181:379–384, 2000.

Donabedian H, Alling DW, Gallin JI. Levamisole is inferior to placebo in the hyperimmunoglobulin E recurrent infection syndrome. N Engl J Med 307:290–292, 1982.

Donabedian H, Gallin JI. The hyperimmunoglobulin E recurrent-infection syndrome. A review of the NIH experience and the literature. Medicine 62:195–208, 1983.

Donhuijsen-Ant R, Abken H, Bornkamm G, et al. Fatal Hodgkin and non-Hodgkin lymphoma associated with persistent Epstein-Barr virus in four brothers. Ann Intern Med 103:946–952, 1988.

Dorman SE, Holland SM. Defects in the interferon gamma and IL-12 pathways. Cyto Growth Factor Rev 11:321–333, 2000.

Dorman SE, Uzel G, Roesler J, Bradley JS, Bastian J, Billman G, King S, Filie A, Schermerhorn J, Holland SM. Viral infections in interferon-gamma receptor deficiency. J Pediatr 135:640–643, 1999.

Dreskin SC, Goldsmith PK, Gallin JI. Immunoglobulins in the hyperimmunoglobulin E and recurrent infection syndrome. J Clin Invest 75:26–34, 1985.

Drew JH. Chronic mucocutaneous candidiasis with abnormal function of serum complement. Med J Aust 2:77–80, 1973.

Dufourcq-Lagelouse R, Pastural E, Barrat F, Feldmann J, Le Deist F, Fischer A. de Saint Basile G. Genetic basis of hemophagocytic lymphohistiocytosis syndrome. Int J Mol Med 4:127–133, 1999.

Duke SG, McGuirt WF Jr, Jewett T, Fasano MB. Velocardiofacial syndrome: incidence of immune cytopenias. Arch Otolaryngol Head Neck Surg 126:1141–1145, 2000.

Duncan RA, von Reyn CF, Alliegro GM, Toossi Z, Sugar AM, Levitz SM. Idiopathic CD4+ T-lymphocytopenia-four patients with opportunistic infections and no evidence of HIV infection. N Engl J Med 328:393–398, 1993.

Dungan JS, Emerson DS, Phillips OP. Shulman LP. Cartilage-hair hypoplasia syndrome: implications for prenatal diagnosis. Fetal Diagn Ther 11:398–401, 1996.

Dupuis S, Dargemont C, Fieschi C, Thomassin N, Rosenzweig S, Harris J, Holland SM, Schriber RD, Casanova JL. Impairment of mycobacterial but not viral immunity by a germline human STAT1 mutation. Science 293:300–303, 2001.

Dupuis S, Jouanguy E, Al-Hajjar S, Fieschi C, Al-Mohsen IZ, Al-Zumaah S, Yang K, Chapgier A, Eidenschenk C, Eid P, Al Ghonanium A, Tufenkeji H, Frayha H, Al-Gazlan S, Al-Rayes H, Schreiber RD, Gresser I, Casanova JL. Impaired response to interferon-alpha/beta and lethal viral disease in human STAT1 deficiency. Nat Genet 33:388–391, 2003.

Durandy A, Breton-Gorius J, Guy-Grand D, Dumez C, Griscelli C. Prenatal diagnosis of syndromes associating albinism and immune deficiencies (Chediak-Higashi syndrome and variant). Prenat Diagn 13:13–20, 1993.

Dustin ML, Cooper JA. The immunological synapse and the actin cytoskeleton: molecular hardware for T cell signaling. Nat Immunol 1:23–29, 2000.

Edelmann L, Pandita RK, Morrow BE. Low-copy repeats mediate the common 3-Mb deletion in patients with velo-cardio-facial syndrome. Am J Hum Genet 64:1076–1086, 1999.

Eicher PS, McDonald-McGinn DM, Fox CA, Driscoll DA, Emanuel BS, Zackai EH. Dysphagia in children with a 22q11.2 deletion: unusual pattern found on modified barium swallow. J Pediatr 137:158–164, 2000.

Elejalde BR, Holguin J, Valencia A, Gilbert EF, Molina J, Marin G, Arango LA. Mutations affecting pigmentation in man: I. neuroectodermal melanolysosomal disease Am J Med Genet 3:65–80, 1979.

Elenitoba-Johnson KS, Jaffe ES. Lymphoproliferative disorders associated with congenital immunodeficiencies. Semin Diagn Path 14:35–47, 1997.

Emanuel BS, Budarf ML, Selliger B, Goldmuntz E, Driscoll DA. Detection of microdeletions of 22q11.2 with fluorescence in situ hybridization (FISH): diagnosis of DiGeorge syndrome (DGS), velo-cardio-facial (VCF) syndrome, CHARGE association and conotruncal cardiac malformations. Am J Hum Genet 51(Suppl):A80, 1992.

Emile JF, Patey N, Altare F, Lamhamedi S, Jouanguy E, Boman F, Quillard J, Lecomte-Houcke M, Verola O, Mousnier JF, Dijoud F, Blanche S, Fischer A, Brousse N, Casanova JL. Correlation of granuloma structure with clinical outcome defines two types of idiopathic disseminated BCG infection. J Pathol 181:25–30, 1997.

Etienne M, Gueit I, Abboud P, Pons JL, Jacquot S, Caron F. Fusobacterium nucleatum hepatic abscess with pylephlebitis associated with idiopathic CD4(+) T lymphocytopenia. Clin Infect Dis 32:326–328, 2001.

Etzioni A, Pollack S. Hypogammaglobulinaemia in DiGeorge sequence Eur J Pediatr 149:143–144, 1989.

Evans DI, Holzel A. Immune deficiency state in a girl with eczema and low serum IgM. Possible female variant of Wiskott-Aldrich syndrome. Arch Dis Child 45:527–533, 1970.

Facchetti F, Blanzuoli L, Vermi W, Notarangelo LD, Giliani S, Fiorini M, Fasth A, Stewart D, Nelson DL. Defective actin polymerization in EBV-transformed B-cell lines from patients with the Wiskott-Aldrich syndrome. J Pathol 185:99–107, 1998.

Ferguson PJ, Blanton SH, Saulsbury FT, McDuffie MJ, Lemahieu V, Gastier JM, Francke U, Borowitz SM, Sutphen JL, Kelly TE. Manifestations and linkage analysis in X-linked autoimmunity-immunodeficiency syndrome. Am J Med Genet 90:390–397, 2000.

Fieschi C, Dupuis S, Catherinot E, Feinberg J, Bustamante J, Breiman A, Altare F, Baretto R, Le Deist F, Kayal S, Koch H, Richter D, Brezina M, Aksu G, Wood P, Al-Jumaah S, Raspall M, Da Silva Duarte AJ, Tuerlinckx D, Virelizier JL, Fischer A, Enright A, Bernhoft J, Cleary AM, Vermylen C, Rodriguez-Gallego C, Davies G, Blutters-Sawatzki R, Siegrist CA, Ehlayel MS, Novelli V, Haas WH, Levy J, Freihorst J, Al-Hajjar S, Nadal D, De Moraes Vasconcelos D, Jeppsson O, Kutukculer N, Frecerova K, Caragol I, Lammas D, Kumararatne DS, Abel L, Casanova JL. Low penetrance, broad resistance, and favorable outcome of interleukin 12 receptor β1 deficiency: medical and immunological implications. J Exp Med 197:527–535, 2003.

Filipovich AH, Stone JV, Tomany SC, Ireland M, Kollman C, Pelz CJ, Casper JT, Cowan MJ, Edwards JR, Fasth A, Gale RP, Junker A, Kamani NR, Loechelt BJ, Pietryga DW, Ringden O, Vowels M, Hegland J, Williams AV, Klein JP, Sobocinski KA, Rowlings PA, Horowitz MM. Impact of donor type on outcome of bone marrow transplantation for Wiskott-Aldrich syndrome: Collaborative Study of the International Bone Marrow Transplant Registry and the National Marrow Donor Program. Blood 97:1598–603, 2001.

Finnish-German APECED Consortium. An autoimmune disease, APECED, caused by mutations in a novel gene featuring two PHD-type zinc-finger mutations. Nat Genet 17:399–403, 1997.

Fischer A, Ballet J-J, Griscelli C. Specific inhibition in vitro *Candida*-induced lymphocyte proliferation by polysaccharide antigens present in the serum of patients with chronic mucocutaneous candidiasis. J Clin Invest 62:1005–1013, 1978.

Fiser PM, Buckley RH. Human IgE biosynthesis in vitro: studies with atopic and normal blood mononuclear cells and subpopulations. J Immunol 123:1788–1794, 1979.

Fleisher AT, Dorman SE, Anderson JA, Vail M, Brown MR, Holland SM. Detection of intracellular phosphorylated STAT-1 by flow cytometry. Clin Immunol 90:425–430, 1999.

Fleisher G, Starr S, Koven N, Kamiya H, Douglas SD, Henle W. A non X-linked syndrome with susceptibility to severe Epstein-Barr virus infections. J Pediatr 100:727–730, 1982.

Fontenot JD, Gavin MA, Rudensky AY. Foxp3 programs the development and function of CD4⁺CD25⁺ regulatory T cells. Nat Immunol 4:330–336, 2003.

Ford LC, Sulprizio SL, Rasgon BM. Otolaryngological manifestations of velocardiofacial syndrome: a retrospective review of 35 patients. Laryngoscope 110:362–367, 2000.

Francois Bach J. Regulatory T cells under scrutiny. Nat Rev Immunol 3:189–198, 2003.

Francomano CA, Trojak JE, McKusick VA. Cartilage-hair hypoplasia in the Amish: increased susceptibility to malignancy. Am J Hum Genet 35:89A, 1983.

Frohn-Mulder IM, Wesby Swaay E, Bouwhuis C, Van Hemel JO, Gerritsma E, Niermeyer MF, Hess J. Chromosome 22q11 deletions in patients with selected outflow tract malformations. Genet Counsel 10:35–41, 1999.

Fruhwirth M, Clodi K, Heitger A, Neu N. Lymphocyte diversity in a 9-year-old boy with idiopathic CD4⁺ T cell lymphocytopenia. Int Arch Allergy Immunol 125:80–85, 2001.

Fudenberg HH, Levin AS, Spitler LE, Wybran J, Byers V. The therapeutic uses of transfer factor. Hosp Pract 9:95–104, 1974.

Fukuda T, Matsunaga M, Kurata A, Mine M, Ikari N, Katamine S, Kanazawa H, Eguchi K, Nagataki S. Hereditary deficiency of OKT4-positive cells: studies for mode of inheritance and lymphocyte functions. Immunology 53:643–649, 1984.

Fulginiti VA, Hathaway. WE, Pearlman, DS, Kempe CH. Agammaglobulinemia and achondroplasia. BMJ 1:242, 1967.

Fulginiti VA, Kempke, GH, Hathaway WE, Pearlman DS, Sieber OF, Heller JJ, Joyner JJ, Robinson A. Progressive vaccinia in immunologically deficient individuals. In Bergsma D, Good RA, eds. Immunologic Deficiency Diseases in Man. National Foundation: Birth Defects. Baltimore, Williams and Wilkins, 1968 pp 129–151.

Gajiwala KS, Burley SK. Winged helix proteins. Curr Opin Struct Biol 10:110–116, 2000.

Gale CA, Bendel CM, McClellan M, Hauser M, Becker JM, Berman J, Hostetter MK. Linkage of adhesion, filamentous growth, and virulence in Candida albicans to a single gene, INT 1. Science 279:1355–1358, 1998.

Gallego MD, Santamaria M, Pena J, Molina IJ. Defective actin reorganization and polymerization of Wiskott-Aldrich T cells in response to CD3-mediated stimulation. Blood 90:3089–3097, 1997.

Gambineri E, Torgerson TR, Bennett CL, Amoroso A, Barker DF, Cunningham-Rundles C, Notarangelo L, Ronchetti R, Sakiyama Y, Ochs HD. Mutations of FOXP3 causing IPEX syndrome. Clin Immunol 103:S139–S140, 2002.

Gambineri E, Torgerson TR, Ochs HD. Immune dysregulation, polyendocrinopathy, enteropathy, and X-linked inheritance (IPEX), a syndrome of systemic autoimmunity caused by mutations of FOXP3, a critical regulator of T-cell homeostasis. Curr Opin Rheumatol 15:430–435, 2003.

Ganser A, Ottmann OG, Erdmann H, Schulz G, Hoelzer D. The effect of recombinant human granulocyte-macrophage colony-stimulating factor on neutropenia and related morbidity in chronic severe neutropenia. Ann Intern Med 111:887–892, 1989.

Garni-Wagner BA, Purohit A, Mathew PA, Bennett M, Kumar V. A novel function-associated molecule related to non-MHC-restricted cytotoxicity mediated by activated natural killer cells and T cells. J Immunol 151:60–70, 1993.

Garry RF, Fermin CD, Kohler PF, Markert ML, Luo H. Antibodies against retroviral proteins and nuclear antigens in a subset of idiopathic CD4⁺ T lymphocytopenia patients. AIDS Res Hum Retroviruses 12:931–940, 1996.

Gatti RA, Platt N, Pomerance HH, Hong R, Langer LO, Kay HE, Good RA. Hereditary lymphopenic agammaglobulinemia associated with a distinctive form of short-limbed dwarfism and ectodermal dysplasia. J Pediatr 75:6759–6784, 1969.

Geha RS, Leung DYM. Hyper-immunoglobulin E syndrome. Immunodefic Rev 1:155–172, 1989.

Geha RS, Reinherz E, Leung D, McKee JT, Schlossmann S, Rosen FS. Deficiency of suppressor T cells in the hyperimmunoglobulin E syndrome. J Clin Invest 68:783–791, 1981.

Gennery AR, Barge D, O'Sullivan JJ, Flood TJ, Abinun M, Cant AJ. Antibody deficiency and autoimmunity in 22q11.2 deletion syndrome. Arch Dis Child 86:422–425, 2002.

Gerdes M, Solot C, Wang PP, Moss E, LaRossa D, Randall P, Goldmuntz E, Clark BJ 3rd, Driscoll DA, Jawad A, Emanuel BS, McDonald-McGinn DM, Batshaw ML, Zackai EH. Cognitive and behavior profile of preschool children with chromosome 22q11.2 deletion. Am J Med Genet 85:127–133, 1999.

Gilger MA, Matson DO, Conner ME, Rosenblatt HM, Finegold MJ, Estes MK. Extraintestinal rotavirus infections in children with immunodeficiency. J Pediatr 120:912–917, 1992.

Giliani S, Fiorini M, Mella P, Candotti F, Schumacher RF, Wengler GS, Lalatta F, Fasth A, Badolato R, Ugazio AG, Albertini A, Notarangelo LD. Prenatal molecular diagnosis of Wiskott-Aldrich syndrome by direct mutation analysis. Prenat Diagn 19:36–40, 1999.

Gill JC, Maples J, Nikaein A, Kirchner P, Lockhard D, Snyder AJ, Montgomery RR, Casper JT. Inherited absence of OKT4 lymphocyte antigen in a chronically transfused patient with homozygous sickle cell disease. J. Pediatr 107:251–253, 1985.

Gilmour KC, Fujii H, Cranston T, Davies EG, Kinnon C, Gaspar HB. Defective expression of the interleukin-2/interleukin-15 receptor beta subunit leads to a natural killer cell-deficient form of severe combined immunodeficiency. Blood 98:877–879, 2001.

Ginat-Israeli T, Hurwitz H, Klar A, Blinder G, Branski D, Amir N. Deteriorating neurological and neuroradiological course in treated biotinidase deficiency. Neuropediatrics 24:103–106, 1993.

Goddard EA, Hughes EJ, Beatty DW. A case of immunodeficiency characterized by neutropenia, hypogammaglobulinaemia, recurrent infections and warts. Clin Lab Haematol 16:297–302, 1994.

Godfrey VL, Rouse BT, Wilkinson JE. Transplantation of T cell-mediated, lymphoreticular disease from the scurfy (sf) mouse. Am J Pathol 145:281–286, 1994.

Gogus S, Topcu M, Kucukali T, Akcoren Z, Berkel I, Ersoy F, Gunay M. Griscelli syndrome: report of three cases. Pediatr Pathol Lab Med 15:309–319, 1995.

Goldmuntz E, Clark BJ, Mitchell LE, Jawad AF, Cuneo BF, Reed L, McDonald-McGinn D, Chien P, Feuer J, Zackai EH, Emanuel BS, Driscoll DA. Frequency of 22q11 deletions in patients with conotruncal defects. J Am Coll Cardiol 32:492–498, 1998.

Goldsobel AB, Haas A, Stiehm ER. Bone marrow transplantation in DiGeorge syndrome. J Pediatr 111:40–44, 1987.

Gonzalo JA, Lloyd CM, Peled A, Delaney T, Coyle AJ, Gutierrez-Ramos JC. Critical involvement of the chemotactic axis CXCR4/stromal cell-derived factor-1 alpha in the inflammatory component of allergic airway disease. J Immunol 165:499–508, 2000.

Goodrich AL, Tigelaar RE, Watsky KL, Heald PW. Idiopathic CD4+ lymphocyte deficiency. Report of an unusual case associated with atopic dermatitis and allergic contact dermatitis and review of the literature. Arch Dermatol 129:876–878, 1993.

Goodship J, Cross I, LiLing J, Wren C. A population study of chromosome 22q11 deletions in infancy. Arch Dis Child 79:348–351, 1998.

Gorin LJ, Jeha SC, Sullivan MP, Rosenblatt HM, Shearer WT. Burkitt's lymphoma developing in a 7 year old boy with hyper IgE syndrome. J Allergy Clin Immunol 83:5–10, 1989.

Gorlin RJ, Gelb B, Diaz GA, Lofsness KG, Pittelkow MR, Fenyk JR Jr. WHIM syndrome, an autosomal dominant disorder: clinical, hematological, and molecular studies. Am J Med Genet 91:368–376, 2000.

Greenberg F. DiGeorge syndrome: an historical review of clinical and cytogenetic features. J Med Genetics 30:803–806, 1993.

Greenberg F, Valdes C, Rosenblatt HM, Kirkland JL, Ledbetter DH. Hypoparathyroidism and T cell immune defect in a patient with 10p deletion syndrome. J Pediatr 109:489–492, 1986.

Greenspan D, Greenspan JS. HIV-related oral disease. Lancet 348:729–733, 1996.

Greer WL, Kwong PC, Peacocke M, Ip P, Rubin LA, Siminovitch KA. X-chromosome inactivation in the Wiskott-Aldrich syndrome: a marker for detection of the carrier state and identification of cell lineages expressing the gene defect. Genomics 4:60–67, 1989.

Grierson H, Purtilo DT. Epstein-Barr virus infections in males with the X-linked lymphoproliferative syndrome. Ann Intern Med 106:538–545, 1987.

Grierson HL, Skare J, Hawk J, et al. Immunoglobulin class and subclass deficiencies prior to Epstein-Barr virus infection in males with X-linked lymphoproliferative disease. Am J Med Genet 40:294–297, 1991.

Grimbacher B, Holland SM, Gallin JI, Greenberg F, Hill SC, Malech HL, Miller JA, O'Connell AC, Puck JM. Hyper-IgE syndrome with recurrent infections–an autosomal dominant multisystem disorder. N Engl J Med 340:692–702, 1999a.

Grimbacher B, Schaffer AA, Holland SM, Davis J, Gallin JI, Malech HL, Atkinson TP, Belohradsky BH, Buckley RH, Cossu F, Espanol T, Garty BZ, Matamoros N, Myers LA, Nelson RP, Ochs HD, Renner ED, Wellinghausen N, Puck JM. Genetic linkage of hyper-IgE syndrome to chromosome 4. Am J Hum Genet 65:735–744, 1999b.

Griscelli C, Durandy A, Guy-Grand D, Daguillard F, Herzog C, Prunieras M. A syndrome associating partial albinism and immunodeficiency. Am J Med 65:691–702, 1978.

Gross TG, Filipovich AH, Conley ME, et al. Cure of X-linked lymphoproliferative disease (XLP) with allogeneic hematopoietic stem cell transplantation (HSCT): report from the XLP registry. Bone Marrow Transplant 17:741–744, 1996.

Grottum KA, Hovig T, Holmsen H, Abrahamsen AF, Jeremic M, Seip M. Wiskott-Aldrich syndrome: qualitative platelet defects and short platelet survival. Br J Haematol 17:373–388, 1969.

Gubinelli E, Posteraro P, Girolomoni G. Idiopathic CD4+ T lymphocytopenia associated with disseminated flat warts and alopecia areata. J Dermatol 29:653–656, 2002.

Guilloton L, Drouet A, Bernard P, Berbineau A, Berger F, Kopp N, Ribot C. Cerebral intravascular lymphoma during T CD4+ idiopathic lymphopenia syndrome Presse Med 28:1513–1515, 1999.

Gupta AK, Kleckman P, Baran R. Ciclopirox nail lacquer topical solution 8% in the treatment of toenail onychomycosis. J Am Acad Derm 43:S70–S80, 2000.

Gurgey A, Sayli T, Gunay M, Ersoy F, Kucukali T, Kale, G, Caglar M. High-dose methylprednisolone and VP-16 in treatment of Griscelli syndrome with central nervous system involvement. Am J Hematol 47:331–332, 1994.

Guris DL, Fantes J, Tara D, Druker BJ, Imamoto A. Mice lacking the homologue of the human 22q11.2 gene CRKL phenocopy neurocristopathies of DiGeorge syndrome. Nat Genet 27:293–298, 2001.

Gustafson KS, Vercellotti GM, Bendel CM, Hostetter MK. Molecular mimicry in Candida albicans. Role of an integrin analogue in adhesion of the yeast to human epithelium. J Clin Invest 87:1896–1902, 1991.

Haider S, Nafziger D, Gutierrez JA, Brar I, Mateo N, Fogle J. Progressive multifocal leukoencephalopathy and idiopathic CD4+ lymphocytopenia: a case report and review of reported cases. Clin Infect Dis 31:E20–22, 2000.

Haire RN, Buell RD, Litman RT, Ohta Y, Fu SM, Honjo T, Matsuda F, de la Morena M, Carro J, Good RA, Litman GW. Diversification, not use, of the immunoglobulin VH gene repertoire is restricted in DiGeorge syndrome. J Exp Med 178:825–834, 1993.

Halonen M, Eskelin P, Myhre AG, Perheentupa J, Husebye ES, Kämpe O, Rorsman F, Peltonen L, Ulmanen I, Partanen J. AIRE mutations and human leukocyte antigen genotypes as determinants of the autoimmune polyendocrinopathy-candidiasis-ectodermal dystrophy phenotype. J Clin Endocrinol Metab 87:2568–2574, 2002.

Ham Pong AJ, Cavallo A, Holman GH, Goldman AS. DiGeorge syndrome: long term survival complicated by Graves disease. J Pediatr 106:619–620, 1985.

Hamilton JK, Purtilo D. X-linked lymphoproliferative syndrome registry. JAMA 241:998–999, 1979.

Hamilton JK, Paquin LA, Sullivan JL, Maurer HS, Cruzi FG, Provisor AJ, Steuber CP, Hawkins E, Yawn D, Cornet JA, Clausen K, Finkelstein GZ, Landing B, Grunnet M, Purtilo DT. X-linked lymphoproliferative syndrome registry report. J Pediatr 96:669–673, 1980.

Hanamura I, Wakita A, Harada S, Tsuboi K, Komatsu H, Banno S, Iwaki O, Takeuchi G, Nitta M, Ueda R. Idiopathic CD4+ T-lymphocytopenia in a non-Hodgkin's lymphoma patient. Intern Med 36:643–646, 1997.

Harada S, Bechtold T, Seeley JK, Purtilo DT. Cell-mediated immunity to Epstein-Barr virus (EBV) and natural killer (NK)-cell activity in the X-linked lymphoproliferative syndrome. Int J Cancer 30:739–744, 1982.

Haraldsson A, Weemaes C, Bakkeren J, Happle, R. Griscelli disease with cerebral involvement Eur J Pediatr 150:419–422, 1991.

Hardman CM, Baker BS, Lortan J, Breuer J, Surentheran T, Powles A, Fry L. Active psoriasis and profound CD4+ lymphocytopenia. Br J Dermatol 136:930–932, 1997.

Harfi H, Brismar J, Hainau B, Sabbah R. Partial albinism, immunodeficiency, and progressive white matter disease: a new primary immunodeficiency. Allergy Proc 13:321–328, 1992.

Harrington LH. Absence of the thymus gland. London Med Gazette 3:314–320, 1829.

Hattevig G, Kjellman B, Fallstrom SP. Congenital permanent diabetes mellitus and celiac disease. J Pediatr 101:955–957, 1982.

Hayashi T, Hinoda Y, Takahashi T, Adachi M, Miura S, Izumi T, Kojima H, Yano S, Imai K. Idiopathic CD4+ T-lymphocytopenia with Bowen's disease. Intern Med 36:822–824, 1997.

Haynes BF, Market ML, Sempowski GD, Patel DD, Hale LP. The role of the thymus in immune reconstitution in aging, bone marrow transplantation, and HIV-1 infection. Annu Rev Immunol 18:529–560, 2000.

Hernandez PA, Gorlin RG, Lukens JN, Diaz GA. WHIM syndrome, a combined immunodeficiency disease, is caused by mutations in the HIV co-receptor gene CXCR4. Am J Hum Genet 69(Suppl):217abs, 2001.

Hernandez PA, Gorlin RJ, Lukens JN, Taniuchi S, Bohinjec J, Francois F, Klotman ME, Diaz GA. Mutations in the chemokine receptor gene CXCR4 are associated with WHIM syndrome, a combined immunodeficiency disease. Nat Genet 34:70–74, 2003.

Herrod HG. Chronic mucocutaneous candidiasis in childhood and complications of non-Candida infections: a report of the Pediatric Immunodeficiency Collaborative Study Group. J Pediatr 116:377–382, 1990.

Hess U, Ganser A, Schnurch HG, Seipelt G, Ottmann OG, Falk S, Schulz G, Hoelzer D. Myelokathexis treated with recombinant human granulocyte-macrophage colony-stimulating factor (rhGM-CSF). Br J Haematol 80:254–256, 1992.

Higgs JM, Wells RS. Chronic mucocutaneous candidiasis: associated abnormalities of iron metabolism. Br J Dermatol 86(Suppl 8):88–102, 1972.

Hill HR, Quie PG, Pabst HF, Ochs HD, Clark RA, Klebanoff SJ, Wedgwood RJ. Defect in neutrophil granulocyte chemotaxis in Job's syndrome of recurrent "cold" staphylococcal abscesses. Lancet 2:617–619, 1974.

Ho DD, Cao Y, Zhu T, Farthing C, Wang N, Gu G, Schooley RT, Daar ES. Idiopathic CD4+ T-lymphocytopenia—immunodeficiency without evidence of HIV infection. N Engl J Med 328:380–385, 1993.

Holland SM, Dorman SE, Kwon A, Pitha-Rowe IF, Frucht DM, Gerstberger SM, Noel GJ, Vesterhus P, Brown MR, Fleisher TA. Abnormal regulation of interferon-gamma, interleukin-12, and tumor necrosis factor-alpha in human interferon-gamma receptor 1 deficiency. J Infect Dis 178:1095–1104, 1998.

Hong R, Ammann AJ, Huang SW, Levy RI, Davenport G, Bach ML, Bach FH, Bortin MM, Kay HEM. Cartilage-hair hypoplasia: effect of thymus transplants. Clin Immunol Immunopathol 1:15–26, 1972.

Hong R, Shen V, Rooney C, Hughes DP, Smith C, Comoli P, Zhang L. Correction of DiGeorge anomaly with EBV-induced lymphoma by transplantation of organ-cultured thymus and Epstein-Barr-specific cytotoxic T lymphocytes. Clin Immunol 98:54–61, 2001.

Hong RT. Disorders of the T cell system. In Stiehm ER, ed. Immunologic Disorders in Infants and Children. Philadelphia, WB Saunders, 1996, pp 339–408.

Hopkin RJ, Schorry EK, Bofinger M, Saal HM. Increased need for medical interventions in infants with velocardiofacial (deletion 22q11) syndrome. J Pediatr 137:247–249, 2000.

Hord JD, Whitlock JA, Gay JC, Lukens JN. Clinical features of myelokathexis and treatment with hematopoietic cytokines: a case report of two patients and review of the literature. J Pediatr Hematol Oncol 19:443–448, 1997.

Hori S, Nomura T, Sakaguchi S. Control of regulatory T cell development by the transcription factor Foxp3. Science 299:1057–1061, 2003.

Hoxie JA, Flaherty LE, Haggarty BS, Rackowski JL. Infection of T4 lymphocytes by HTLV-III does not require expression of the OKT4 epitope. J Immunol 136:361–363, 1986.

Hsieh CL, Donlon TA, Darras, BT, Chang DD, Topper JN, Clayton DA, Francke U. The gene for the RNA component of the mitochondrial RNA-processing endoribonuclease is located on human chromosome 9p and on mouse chromosome 4. Genomics 6:540–544, 1990.

Hubert P, Bergeron F, Ferreira V, Seligmann M, Oksenhendler E, Debre P, Autran B. Defective p56Lck activity in T cells from an adult patient with idiopathic CD4+ lymphocytopenia. Int Immunol 12:449–457, 2000.

Hubert P, Bergeron F, Grenot P, Seligman M, Krivitzky A, Debre P, Autran B. Deficiency of the CD3-TCR signal pathway in three patients with idiopathic CD4+ lymphocytopenia. J Soc Biol 193:11–16, 1999.

Hung W, Migeon CJ, Parrott RH. A possible auto-immune basis for Addison's disease in three siblings, one with idiopathic hypoparathyroidism, pernicious anemia and superficial moniliasis. N Engl J Med 269:658–663, 1963.

Huntley CC, Dees SC. Eczema associated with thrombocytopenic purpura and purulent otitis media; report of five fatal cases. Pediatrics 19:351–361, 1957.

Hurvitz H, Gillis R, Klaus S, Gross-Kieselstein F, Okon E. A kindred with Griscelli disease: spectrum of neurological involvement Eur J Pediatr 152:402–405, 1993.

Imashuku S, Miyagawa A, Chiyonobu T, Ishida H, Yoshihara T, Teramura T, Kuriyama K, Imamura T, Hibi S, Morimoto A, Todo S. Epstein-Barr virus-associated T-lymphoproliferative disease with hemophagocytic syndrome, followed by fatal intestinal B lymphoma in a young adult female with WHIM syndrome. Warts, hypogammaglobulinemia, infections, and myelokathexis. Ann Hematol 81:470–473, 2002.

Inglis DO, Johnson AD. Ash 1 protein, an asymmetrically localized transcriptional regulator, controls filamentous growth and virulence of *Candida albicans*. Mol Cell Biol 22:8669–8680, 2002.

Inoue H, Kurosawa H, Nonoyama S, Imai K, Kumazaki H, Matsunaga T, Sato Y, Sugita K, Eguchi M. X-linked thrombocytopenia in a girl. Br J Haematol 118:1163–1165, 2002.

Iwase T, Ojika K, Katada E, Mitake S, Nakazawa H, Matsukawa N, Otsuka Y, Tsugu Y, Kanai H, Nakajima K. An unusual course of progressive multifocal leukoencephalopathy in a patient with idiopathic CD4+ T lymphocytopenia. J Neurol Neurosurg Psychiatry 64:788–791, 1998.

Jabado N, Degraeffmeeder ER, Cavazzana-Calvo M, Haddad E, Le Deist F, Benkerrou M, Dufourcq R, Caillat S, Blanche S, Fischer A. Treatment of familial hemophagocytic lymphohistiocytosis with bone marrow transplantation from HLA genetically nonidentical donors Blood 90, 4743–4748, 1997.

Jawad AF, McDonald-McGinn DM, Zackai E, Sullivan KE. Immunologic features of chromosome 22q11.2 deletion syndrome (DiGeorge syndrome/velocardiofacial syndrome). J Pediatr 139:715–723, 2001.

Jawahar S, Moody C, Chan M, Finberg R, Geha R, Chatila T. Natural killer (NK) cell deficiency associated with an epitope-deficient Fc receptor type IIIA (CD16-II). Clin Exp Immunol 103:408–413, 1996.

Jerome LA, Papaioannou VE. DiGeorge syndrome phenotype in mice mutant for the T-box gene, Tbx1. Nat Genet 27:286–291, 2001.

Jonas MM, Bell MD, Eidson MS, Koutouby R, Hensley GT. Congenital diabetes mellitus and fatal secretory diarrhea in two infants. J Pediatr Gastroenterol Nutr 13:415–425, 1991.

Jorizzo JJ, Sams WM, Jegasothy BV, Olansky AJ. Cimetidine as an immunomodulator: chronic mucocutaneous candidiasis as a model. Ann Intern Med 92:192–195, 1980.

Josephs SH, Buckley RH. Serum IgD concentrations in normal infants, children and adults and in patients with elevated serum IgE. J Pediatr 96: 417–420, 1979.

Jouanguy E, Altare F, Lamhanedi S, Revy P, Emile J-F, Newport M, Levin M, Blanche S, Seboun E, Fischer A, Casanova J-L. Interferon-γ receptor deficiency in an infant with fatal Bacille Calmette-Guerin infection. N Engl J Med 335:1956–1961, 1996.

Jouanguy E, Dupuis S, Pallier A, Doffinger R, Fondaneche MC, Fieschi C, Lamhamedi-Cherradi S, Altare F, Emile JF, Lutz P, Bordigoni P, Cokugras H, Akcakaya N, Landman-Parker J, Donnadieu J, Camcioglu Y, Casanova JL. In a novel form of IFN-gamma receptor 1 deficiency, cell surface receptors fail to bind IFN-gamma J Clin Invest 105:1429–1436, 2000.

Jouanguy E, Lamhamedi-Cherradi S, Altare F, Fondaneche MC, Tuerlinckx D, Blanche S, Emile JF, Gaillard JL, Schreiber R, Levin M, Fischer A, Hivroz C, Casanova JL. Partial interferon-gamma receptor 1 deficiency in a child with tuberculoid bacillus Calmette-Guerin infection and a sibling with clinical tuberculosis. J Clin Invest 100:2658–64, 1997.

Jouanguy E, Lamhamedi-Cherradi S, Lammas D, Dorman SE, Fondaneche MC, Dupuis S, Doffinger R, Altare F, Girdlestone J, Emile JF, Ducoulombier H, Edgar D, Clarke J, Oxelius VA, Brai M, Novelli V, Heyne K, Fischer A, Holland SM, Kumararatne DS, Schreiber RD, Casanova JL. A human IFN-γR1 small deletion hotspot associated with dominant susceptibility to mycobacterial infection. Nat Genet 21:370–378, 1999.

Junker AK, Driscoll DA. Humoral immunity in DiGeorge syndrome. J Pediatr 127:231–237, 1995.

Junoven E. Makitie O, Makipernaa A. Ruutu T, Kaitila I, Rajantie J. Defective in vitro colony formation of haematopoietic progenitors in patients with cartilage-hair hypoplasia and history of anaemia. Eur J Pediatr 154:30–34, 1995.

Kaiser FE, Morley JE. Idiopathic CD4+ T lymphopenia in older persons. J Am Geriatr Soc 42:1291–1294, 1994.

Kalfa V, Roberts RL, Stiehm ER. The syndrome of chronic mucocutaneous candidiasis with selective antibody deficiency. Ann Allergy Asthma Immunol 90:259–264, 2003.

Kawamura T, Nimura I, Hanafusa M, Fujikawa R, Okubo M, Egusa G, Amakido M. DiGeorge syndrome with Graves' disease: a case report. Endocrinol J 47:91–95, 2000.

Kelley RI, Zackai EH, Emanuel BS, Kistenmacher M, Greenberg F, Punnett HH. The association of the DiGeorge anomalad with partial monosomy of chromosome 22. J Pediatr 101:197–200, 1982.

Kenney D, Cairns L, Remold-O'Donnell E, Peterson J, Rosen FS, Parkman R. Morphological abnormalities in the lymphocytes of patients with the Wiskott-Aldrich syndrome. Blood 68:1329–32, 1986.

Khattri R, Cox T, Yasayko SA, Ramsdell F. An essential role for Scurfin in CD4+CD25+ T regulatory cells. Nat Immunol 4:337–342, 2003.

Khuong MA, Carage T, Komarover H, Mechali D. OKT4 epitope deficiency in patients infected with the human immunodeficiency virus: a cause of underestimation of the CD4 lymphocyte count. Clin Infect Dis 19:961–963, 1994.

Kildeberg P. The Aldrich syndrome: report of a case and discussion of pathogenesis. Pediatrics 27:362–369, 1961.

Kim AS, Kakalis LT, Abdul-Manan N, Liu GA, Rosen MK. Autoinhibition and activation mechanisms of the Wiskott-Aldrich syndrome protein. Nature 404:151–158, 2000.

King CL, Gallin JI, Malech HL, Abramson SL, Nutman TB. Regulation of immunoglobulin production in hyperimmunoglobulin E recurrent infection syndrome by interferon. Proc Natl Acad Sci USA 86:10085–10089, 1989.

Kirby ML, Bockman DE. Neural crest and normal development: a new perspective. Anat Rec 209:1–6, 1984.

Kirchner SG, Sivit CJ, Wright PF. Hyperimmunoglobulinemia E syndrome: association with osteoporosis and recurrent fractures. Radiology 156:362, 1985.

Kirkpatrick CH. Transfer factors: identification of conserved sequences in transfer factor molecules. Mol Med 6:332–341, 2000.

Kirkpatrick CH, Chandler JW Jr, Schimke RN. Chronic moniliasis with impaired delayed hypersensitivity. Clin Exp Immunol 6:375–386, 1970.

Kirkpatrick CH, Greenberg LE. Treatment of chronic mucocutaneous candidiasis with transfer factor. In Kahn A, Kirkpatrick CH, Hill NO, eds. Immune Regulators in Transfer Factor. New York, Academic Press, 1979, pp 547–562.

Kirkpatrick CH, Ottesen EA, Smith TK, Wells SA, Burdick JF. Reconstitution of defective cellular immunity with foetal thymus and dialysable transfer factor. Long-term studies in a patient with chronic mucocutaneous candidiasis. Clin Exp Immunol 23:414–448, 1974.

Kirkpatrick CH, Rich RR, Bennett JE. Chronic mucocutaneous candidiasis: model building in cellular immunity. Ann Intern Med 74:955–978, 1971a.

Kirkpatrick CH, Rich RR, Graw RG, Smith TK, Mickenberg ID, Rogentine GN. Treatment of chronic mucocutaneous moniliasis by immunologic reconstitution. Clin Exp Immunol 9:733–748, 1971b.

Kirkpatrick CH, Rich RR, Smith TK. Effect of transfer factor on lymphocyte function in anergic patients. J Clin Invest 51:2948–2958, 1972.

Kirkpatrick CH, Sohnle PG. Chronic mucocutaneous candidiasis. In Safai B, Good RA, eds. Immunodermatology. New York, Plenum Press, 1981, pp 495–514.

Kirkpatrick CH, Smith TK. Chronic mucocutaneous candidiasis: immunologic and antibiotic therapy. Ann Intern Med 80:310–320, 1974.

Kirkpatrick CH, Windhorst DB. Chronic mucocutaneous candidiasis and thymoma. Am J Med 66:939–945, 1979.

Kirtava Z, Blomberg J, Bredberg A, Henriksson G, Jacobsson L, Manthorpe R. CD4+ T-lymphocytopenia without HIV infection: increased prevalence among patients with primary Sjogren's syndrome. Clin Exp Rheumatol 13:609–616, 1995.

Klein C, Nguyen D, Liu CH, Mizoguchi A, Bhan AK, Miki H, Takenawa T, Rosen FS, Alt FW, Mulligan RC, Snapper SB. Gene therapy for Wiskott-Aldrich syndrome: rescue of T-cell signaling and amelioration of colitis upon transplantation of retrovirally transduced hematopoietic stem cells in mice. Blood 101:2159–2166, 2002.

Klein C, Philippe N, Le Deist F, Fraitag S, Prost C, Durandy A, Fischer A, Griscelli C. Partial albinism with immunodeficiency (Griscelli syndrome). J Pediatr 125:886–895, 1994.

Kobayashi I, Imamura K, Yamada M, Okano M, Yara A, Ikema S, Ishikawa N. A 75-kD autoantigen recognized by sera from patients with X-linked autoimmune enteropathy associated with nephropathy. Clin Exp Immunol 111:527–531, 1998.

Kobayashi I, Nakanishi M, Okano M, Sakiyama Y, Matsumoto S. Combination therapy with tacrolimus and betamethasone for a patient with X-linked auto-immune enteropathy. Eur J Pediatr 154:594–595, 1995.

Kobayashi I, Shiari R, Yamada M, Kawamura N, Okano M, Yara A, Iguchi A, Ishikawa N, Ariga T, Sakiyama Y, Ochs HD, Kobayashi K. Novel mutations of FOXP3 in two Japanese patients with immune dysregulation, polyendocrinopathy, enteropathy, X linked syndrome (IPEX). J Med Genet 38:874–876, 2001.

Kogawa K, Kudoh J, Nagafuchi S, Ohga S, Katsuta H, Ishibashi H, Harada M, Hara T, Shimizu N. Distinct clinical phenotype and immunoreactivity in Japanese siblings with autoimmune polyglandular syndrome type 1 (APS-1) associated with compound heterozygous novel AIRE gene mutations. Clin Immunol 103:277–283, 2002.

Kolluri R, Tolias KF, Carpenter CL, Rosen FS, Kirchhausen T. Direct interaction of the Wiskott-Aldrich syndrome protein with the GTPase Cdc42. Proc Natl Acad Sci USA 93:5615–5618, 1996.

Komiyama A, Kawai H, Yabuhara A, Yanagisawa M, Miyagawa Y, Ota M, Hasekura H, Akabane T. Natural killer cell immunodeficiency in siblings: defective killing in the absence or natural killer cytotoxic factor activity in natural killer and lymphokine-activated killer cytotoxicities. Pediatrics 85:323–330, 1990.

Kondoh T, Hayashi K, Matsumoto T, Yoshimoto M, Morio T, Yata J, Tsuji Y. Two sisters with clinical diagnosis of Wiskott-Aldrich syndrome: is the condition in the family autosomal recessive? Am J Med Genet 60:364–369, 1995.

Kony SJ, Hane AA, Larouze B, Samb A, Cissoko S, Sow PS, Sane M, Maynart M, Diouf G, Murray JF. Tuberculosis-associated severe CD4+ T-lymphocytopenia in HIV-seronegative patients from Dakar. SIDAK Research Group. J Infect 41:167–171, 2000.

Koren HS, Amos DB, Buckley RH. Natural killing in immunodeficient patients. J Immunol 120:796–799, 1978.

Kornfeld SJ, Zeffren B, Christodoulou CS, Day NK, Cawkwell G, Good RA. DiGeorge anomaly: a comparative study of the clinical and immunologic characteristics of patients positive and negative by fluorescence in situ hybridization. J Allergy Clin Immunol 105:983–987, 2000.

Kothakota S, Azuma T, Reinhard C, Klippel A, Tang J, Chu K, McGarry TJ, Kirschner MW, Koths K, Kwiatkowski DJ, Williams LT. Caspase-3-generated fragment of gelsolin: effector of morphological change in apoptosis. Science 278:294–298, 1997.

Krill CE, Dunlap Smith H, Mauer AM. Chronic idiopathic granulocytopenia. N Engl J Med 270:973–979, 1964.

Krivit W, Yunis E, White JG. Platelet survival studies in Aldrich syndrome. Pediatrics 37:339–341, 1966.

Kumar PG, Laloraya M, She JX. Population genetics and functions of the autoimmune regulator (AIRE). Endocrinol Metab Clin North Am 31:321–338, 2002.

Kumlin U, Elmqvist LG, Granlund M, Olsen B, Tarnvik A. CD4 lymphopenia in a patient with cryptococcal osteomyelitis. Scand J Infect Dis 29:205–206, 1997.

Kuramoto A, Steiner M, Baldini MG. Lack of platelet response to stimulation in the Wiskott-Aldrich syndrome. N Engl J Med 282:475–479, 1970.

Kwan SP, Hagemann TL, Blaese RM, Rosen FS. A high-resolution map of genes, microsatellite markers, and new dinucleotide repeats from UBE1 to the GATA locus in the region Xp11.23. Genomics 29:247–52, 1995.

Kwan SP, Lehner T, Hagemann T, Lu B, Blaese M, Ochs H, Wedgwood R, Ott J, Craig IW, Rosen FS. Localization of the gene for the Wiskott-Aldrich syndrome between two flanking markers, TIMP and DXS255, on Xp11.22-Xp11.3. Genomics 10:29–33, 1991.

Lai PK, Yasuda N, Purtilo DT. Immunoregulatory T cells in males vulnerable to Epstein-Barr virus with the X-linked lymphoproliferative syndrome. Am J Pediatr Hematol Oncol 9:179–182, 1987.

Lamarche N, Tapon N, Stowers L, Burbelo PD, Aspenstrom P, Bridges T, Chant J, Hall A. Rac and Cdc42 induce actin polymerization and G1 cell cycle progression independently of p65PAK and the JNK/SAPK MAP kinase cascade. Cell 87:519–29, 1996.

Lapidot T, Petit I. Current understanding of stem cell mobilization: the roles of chemokines, proteolytic enzymes, adhesion molecules, cytokines, and stromal cells. Exp Hematol 30:973–81, 2002.

Laurence J, Mitra D, Steiner M, Lynch DH, Siegal FP, Staiano-Coico L. Apoptotic depletion of CD4+ T cells in idiopathic CD4+ T lymphocytopenia. J Clin Invest 97:672–80, 1996.

Lecora M, Parenti G. Iaccarino E, Scarano G. Cucchiara S. Andria G. Immunological disorder and Hirschsprung disease in round femoral inferior epiphysis dysplasia. Clin Dysmorphol 4:130–135, 1995.

Lee WM, Holley HP, Stewart J, Galbraith GMP. Refractory esophageal candidiasis associated with a low molecular weight plasma inhibitor of T-lymphocyte function. Am J Med Sci 292:47–52, 1986.

Lehner T. Chronic candidiasis. Trans St Johns Hospital Derm Soc 50:8–21, 1964.

Lehner T, Wilton JMA, Ivanyi L. Immunodeficiencies in chronic mucocutaneous candidiasis. Immunology 22:775–787, 1972.

Lemahieu V, Gastier JM, Francke U. Novel mutations in the Wiskott-Aldrich syndrome protein gene and their effects on transcriptional, translational, and clinical phenotypes. Hum Mutat 14:54–66, 1999.

Lemmon MA, Ferguson KM, Schlessinger J. PH domains: diverse sequences with a common fold recruit signaling molecules to the cell surface. Cell 85:621–624, 1996.

Leung DYM, Ambrosino DM, Arbeit RD, Newton JL, Geha RS. Impaired antibody responses in the hyperimmunoglobulin E syndrome. J Allergy Clin Immunol 81:1082–1087, 1988a.

Leung DYM, Key L, Steinberg JJ, Young MD, Von Deck M, Wilkinson R, Geha RA. Increased in vitro bone resorption by monocytes in the hyperimmunoglobulin E syndrome. J Immunol 140:84–88, 1988b.

Leverrier Y, Lorenzi R, Blundell MP, Brickell P, Kinnon C, Ridley AJ, Thrasher AJ. The Wiskott-Aldrich syndrome protein is required for efficient phagocytosis of apoptotic cells. J Immunol 166:4831–4834, 2001.

Levinson AI, Hoxie JA, Kornstein MJ, Zembryki D, Matthews DM, Schreiber AD, Absence of the OKT4 epitope on blood T cells and thymus cells in a patient with thymoma, hypogammaglobulinemia, and red blood cell aplasia. J Allergy Clin Immunol 76:433–439, 1985.

Levy A, Michel G, Lemerrer M, Philip N. Idiopathic thrombocytopenia purpura in two mothers of children with DiGeorge syndrome sequence: a new component manifestation of CATCH 22? Am J Med Genet 69:356–359, 1996.

Levy RL, Huang SW, Bach ML, Bach FH, Hong R, Ammann AJ, Bortin M, Kay HEM. Thymic transplantation in a case of chronic mucocutaneous candidiasis. Lancet 2:898–900, 1971.

Levy-Lahad E, Wildin RS. Neonatal diabetes mellitus, enteropathy, thrombocytopenia, and endocrinopathy: Further evidence for an X-linked lethal syndrome. J Pediatr 138:577–580, 2001.

Lewis DB, Liggitt HD, Effmann EL, Motley ST, Teitelbaum SL, Jepsen KJ, Goldstein SA, Bonadio J, Carpenter J, Perlmutter RM. Osteoporosis induced in mice by overproduction of interleukin-4. Proc Nat Acad Sci U S A 90:11618–11622, 1993.

Lewis DB, Yu CC, Forbush KA, Carpenter J, Sato TA, Grossman A, Liggitt DH, Perlmutter RM. Interleukin-4 expressed in situ selectively alters thymocyte development. J Exp Med 173:89–100, 1991.

Liles WC, Park JR, Chi EY, Dale DC. Myelokathexis—a congenital form of neutropenia characterized by accelerated apoptosis and defective expression of Bclx in neutrophil precursors. Blood 86(Suppl):259abs, 1995.

Lilic D, Cant AJ, Abinun M, Calvert JE, Spickett GP. Chronic mucocutaneous candidiasis. I. Altered antigen-stimulated IL-2, IL-4, IL-6 and interferon-gamma (IFN-γ) production. Clin Exp Immunol 105:205–212, 1996.

Lin CY, Hsu HC. Acute immune complex mediated glomerulonephritis in a Chinese girl with Wiskott-Aldrich syndrome variant. Ann Allergy 53:74–8, 1984.

Linder S, Nelson D, Weiss M, Aepfelbacher M. Wiskott-Aldrich syndrome protein regulates podosomes in primary human macrophages. Proc Natl Acad Sci USA 96:9648–53, 1999.

Linder S, Wintegerst U, Bender-Gotze C, Schqarz K, Pannicke U, Aepfelbacher M. Macrophages of patients with X-linked thrombocytopenia display an attenuated Wiskott-Aldrich syndrome phenotype. Immunol Cell Biol 81:130–136, 2003.

Lindsay EA, Botta A, Jurecic V, Carattini-Rivera S, Cheah YC, Rosenblatt HM, Bradley A, Baldini A. Congenital heart disease in mice deficient for the DiGeorge syndrome region. Nature 401:379–383, 1999.

Lindsay EA, Vitelli F, Su H, Morishima M, Huynh T, Pramparo T, Jurecic V, Ogunrinu G, Sutherland HF, Scambler PJ, Bradley A, Baldini A. Tbx1 haploinsufficiency in the DiGeorge syndrome region causes aortic arch defects in mice. Nature 410:97–101, 2001.

Lindsten T, Seeley JK, Ballow M, et al. Immune deficiency in the X-linked lymphoproliferative syndrome. II. Immunoregulatory T cell defects. J Immunol 129:2536–2540, 1982.

Lischner HW, DiGeorge AM. Role of the thymus in humoral immunity. Lancet 2:1044–1049, 1969.

Lischner HW, Huff DS. T-cell deficiency in DiGeorge syndrome. Birth Defects Original Article Series 11:16–21, 1975.

Littman BH, Rocklin RE, Parkman R, David JR. Transfer factor treatment of chronic mucocutaneous candidiasis: requirement of donor reactivity to Candida antigen. Clin Immunol Immunopathol 9:97–110, 1978.

Litzman J, Jones A, Hann I, Chapel H, Strobel S, Morgan G. Intravenous immunoglobulin, splenectomy, and antibiotic prophylaxis in Wiskott-Aldrich syndrome. Arch Dis Child 75:436–439, 1996.

Lobato MN, Spira TJ, Rogers MF. CD4+ T lymphocytopenia in children: lack of evidence for a new acquired immunodeficiency syndrome agent. Pediatr Infect Dis J 14:527–535, 1995.

Lobdell DH. Congenital absence of the parathyroid gland. Arch Path 67:412–418, 1959.

Loffredo CA, Ferencz C, Wilson PD, Lurie IW. Interrupted aortic arch: an epidemiologic study. Teratology 61:368–375, 2000.

Longo F, Hebuterne X, Michiels JF, Maniere A, Caroli-Bosc FX, Rampal P. Multifocal MALT lymphoma and acute cytomegalovirus gastritis revealing CD4 lymphopenia without HIV infection. Gastroenterol Clin Biol 23:132–136, 1999.

Lopez C, Kirkpatrck D, Read SE, Fitzgerald PA, Pitt J, Pahwa S, Ching CY, Smithwick EM. Correlation between low natural killing of fibroblasts infected with herpes simplex virus type 1 and susceptibility to herpesvirus infections. J Infect Dis 147:1031–1035, 1983.

Lorenzi R, Brickell PM, Katz DR, Kinnon C, Thrasher AJ. Wiskott-Aldrich syndrome protein is necessary for efficient IgG-mediated phagocytosis. Blood 95:2943–2946, 2000.

Louria DB, Shannon D, Johnson G, Caroline L, Okas A, Taschdjian C. The susceptibility to moniliasis in children with endocrine hypofunction. Trans Assoc Am Physicians 80:236–248, 1967.

Lu JH, Chung MY, Hwang B, Chien HP. Prevalence and parental origin in tetralogy of Fallot associated with chromosome 22q11 microdeletion. Pediatrics 104:87–90, 1999.

Luqman M, Johnson P, Trowbridge I, Bottomly K. Differential expression of the alternatively spliced exons of murine CD45 in TH1 and TH2 cloned lines. Eur J Immunol 21:17–22, 1991.

Lutskiy MI, Sasahara Y, Kenney DM, Rosen FS, Remold-O'Donnell E. Wiskott-Aldrich syndrome in a female. Blood 100:2763–2768, 2002.

Luzzatto L, Martini G. X-linked Wiskott-Aldrich syndrome in a girl. N Engl J Med 338:1850–1851, 1998.

Lux, SE, Johnston, RB, August, CS, Say, B, Penchaszadeh, VB, Rosen, FS, McKusick, VA. Chronic neutropenia and abnormal cellular immunity in cartilage-hair hypoplasia. N Engl J Med 282:231–236, 1970.

Ma Q, Jones D, Borghesani PR, Segal RA, Nagasawa T, Kishimoto T, Bronson RT, Springer TA. Impaired B-lymphopoiesis, myelopoiesis, and derailed cerebellar neuron migration in CXCR4– and SDF-1-deficient mice. Proc Natl Acad Sci USA 95:9448–9453, 1998.

MacDermot, KD, Winter, R. NM, Wigglesworth, JS, Strobel, S. Short stature/short limb skeletal dysplasia with combined immunodeficiency and bowing of the femora: report of two patients and review. J Med Genet 28:10–17, 1991.

Machesky LM, Insall RH. Scar1 and the related Wiskott-Aldrich syndrome protein, WASP, regulate the actin cytoskeleton through the Arp2/3 complex. Curr Biol 8:1347–1356, 1998.

Mackey MC, Aprikyan AA, Dale DC. The rate of apoptosis in post mitotic neutrophil precursors of normal and neutropenic humans. Cell Prolif 36:27–34, 2003.

Maeda J, Yamagishi H, Matsuoka R, Ishihara J, Tokumura M, Fukushima H, Ueda H, Takahashi E, Yoshiba S, Kojima Y. Frequent association of 22q11.2 deletion with tetralogy of Fallot. Am J Med Genet 92:269–272, 2000.

Makitie O, Kaitila I. Cartilage-hair hypoplasia—clinical manifestations in 108 Finnish patients. Eur J Pediatr 152:211–217, 1993.

Makitie O, Kaitila I, Savilahti E. Susceptibility to infections and in vitro immune functions in cartilage-hair hypoplasia. Eur J Pediatr 157:816–820, 1998.

Makitie O, Pukkala E, Teppo L, Kailila I. Increased incidence of cancer in patients with cartilage-hair hypoplasia. J Pediatr 134:315–318, 1999.

Makitie O, Rajantie J, Kaitila I. Anaemia and macrocytosis—unrecognized features in cartilage-hair hypoplasia. Acta Paediatr 81:1026–1029, 1992.

Manchado-Lopez P, Ruiz de Morales JM, Ruiz Gonzalez I, Rodriguez Prieto MA. Cutaneous infections by papillomavirus, herpes zoster and Candida albicans as the only manifestation of idiopathic CD4+ T lymphocytopenia. Int J Dermatol 38:119–121, 1999.

Mandelboim O, Lieberman N, Lev M, Paul L, Arnon TI, Bushkin Y, Davis DM, Strominger JL, Yewdell JW, Porgador A. Recognition of haemagglutinins on virus-infected cells by NKp46 activates lysis by human NK cells. Nature 22:1055–1060, 2001.

Mandelboim O, Malik P, Davis DM, Jo CH, Boyson JE, Strominger JL. Human CD16 as a lysis receptor mediating direct natural killer cell cytotoxicity. Proc Natl Acad Sci U S A 96:5640–5644, 1999.

Markert ML, Boeck A, Hale LP, Kloster AL, McLaughlin TM, Batchvarova MN, Douek DC, Koup RA, Kostyu DD, Ward FE, Rice HE, Mahaffey SM, Schiff SE, Buckley RH, Haynes BF. Transplantation of thymus tissue in complete DiGeorge syndrome. N Engl J Med 341:1180–1189, 1999.

Markert ML, Hummell DS, Rosenblatt HM, Schiff SE, Harville TO, Williams LW, Schiff RI, Buckley RH. Complete DiGeorge syndrome: persistence of profound immunodeficiency. J Pediatr 132:15–21, 1998.

Markert ML, Kostyu DD, Ward FE, McLaughlin TM, Watson TJ, Buckley RH, Schiff SE, Ungerleider RM, Gaynor JW, Oldham KT, Mahaffey SM, Ballow M, Driscoll DA, Hale LP, Haynes BF. Successful formation of a chimeric human thymus allograft following transplantation of cultured postnatal human thymus. J Immunol 158:998–1005, 1997a.

Markert ML, Watson TJ, Kaplan I, Hale LP, Haynes BF. The human thymic microenvironment during organ culture. Clin Immunol Immunopathol 82:26–36, 1997b.

Markert ML, Sarzotti M, Ozaki DA, Sempowski GD, Rhein ME, Hale LP, Le Deist F, Alexieff MJ, Li J, Hauser ER, Haynes BF, Rice HE, Skinner MA, Mahaffey SM, Jaggers J, Stein LD, Mill MR. Thymus transplantation in complete DiGeorge syndrome: immunologic and safety evaluations in 12 patients. Blood 102:1121–1130, 2003.

Masi M, DeVinci C, Baricordi OR. Transfer factor in mucocutaneous candidiasis. Biotherapy 9:97–103, 1996.

Matsuyama W, Tsurukawa T, Iwami F, Wakimoto J, Mizoguchi A, Kawabata M, Osame M. Two cases of idiopathic CD4+ T-lymphocytopenia in elderly patients. Intern Med 37:891–895, 1998.

Mayumi M, Kimata H, Suehiro Y, Hosoi S, Ito S, Kuge Y, Shinomiya K, Mikawa H. DiGeorge syndrome with hypogammaglobulinemia: a patient with excess suppressor T cell activity treated with fetal thymus transplantation. Eur J Pediatr 148:143–144, 1989.

McDonald-McGinn DM, Kirschner R, Goldmuntz E, Sullivan K, Eicher P, Gerdes M, Moss E, Solot C, Wang P, Jacobs I, Handler S, Knightly C, Heher K, Wilson M, Ming JE, Grace K, Driscoll D, Pasquariello P, Randall P, Larossa D, Emanuel BS, Zackai EH. The Philadelphia story: the 22q11.2 deletion: report on 250 patients. Genet Counsel 10:11–24, 1999.

McKusick VA. Metaphyseal dysostosis and thin hair: A "new" recessively inherited syndrome? Lancet 1:832–833, 1964.

McKusick VA, Eldridge R, Hostetler JA, Ruangwit U, Egeland JA. Dwarfism in the Amish II. Cartilage-hair hypoplasia. Bull Johns Hopkins Hosp 116:285–326, 1965.

Means GD, Toy DY, Baum PR, Derry JM. A transcript map of a 2-Mb BAC contig in the proximal portion of the mouse X chromosome and regional mapping of the scurfy mutation. Genomics 65:213–223, 2000.

Melamed I, Gelfand EW. Microfilament assembly is involved in B-cell apoptosis. Cell Immunol 194:136–142, 1999.

Meloni A, Perniola R, Faa V, Corvaglia E, Cao A, Rosatelli MC. Delineation of the molecular defects in the AIRE gene in autoimmune polyendocrinopathy-candidiasis-ectodermal dystrophy patients from southern Italy. J Clin Endocrinol Metab 87:841–846, 2002.

Ménasché G, Pastural E, Feldmann J, Certain S, Ersoy F, Dupuis S, Wulffraat N, Bianci D, Fischer A, Le Deist, F de Saint Basile, G. Mutations in RAB27A cause Griscelli syndrome associated with hemophagocytic syndrome. Nat Genet 25:173–176, 2000.

Menon BS, Shuaib IL, Zamari M, Haq JA, Aiyar S, Noh LM. Idiopathic CD4+ T-lymphocytopenia in a child with disseminated cryptococcosis. Ann Trop Paediatr 18:45–48, 1998.

Mentzer WC Jr, Johnston RB, Jr, Baehner RL, Nathan DG. An unusual form of chronic neutropenia in a father and daughter with hypogammaglobulinaemia. Br J Haematol 36:313–22, 1977.

Mercer JA, Sepenack PK, Strobel MC, Copeland NG, Jenkins NA. Novel myosin heavy chain encoded by murine dilute coat colour locus. Nature 349:709–713, 1991.

Merscher S, Funke B, Epstein JA, Heyer J, Puech A, Lu MM, Xavier RJ, Demay MB, Russell RG, Factor S, Tokooya K, Jore BS, Lopez M, Pandita RK, Lia M, Carrion D, Xu H, Schorle H, Kobler JB, Scambler P, Wynshaw-Boris A, Skoultchi AI, Morrow BE, Kucherlapati R. TBX1 is responsible for cardiovascular defects in velo-cardio-facial/DiGeorge syndrome. Cell 104:619–629, 2001.

Merten DF, Buckley RH, Pratt PC, Effmann EL, Grossman H. The hyperimmunoglobulinemia E syndrome: radiographic observations. Radiology 132:71–78, 1979.

Michel JL, Perrot JL, Mitanne D, Boucheron S, Fond L, Cambazard F. Metastatic epidermoid carcinoma in idiopathic CD4+ T lymphocytopenia syndrome. Ann Dermatol Venereol 123:478–482, 1996.

Migliorati R, Castaldo A, Russo S. Treatment of EBV-induced lymphoproliferative disorder with epipodophyllotoxin VP16-213. Acta Pediatr 83:1322–1325, 1994.

Miki H, Miura K, Takenawa T. N-WASP, a novel actin-depolymerizing protein, regulates the cortical cytoskeletal rearrangement in a PIP2-dependent manner downstream of tyrosine kinases. EMBO J 15:5326–5335, 1996.

Miki H, Nonoyama S, Zhu Q, Aruffo A, Ochs HD, Takenawa T. Tyrosine kinase signaling regulates Wiskott-Aldrich syndrome protein function, which is essential for megakaryocyte differentiation. Cell Growth Differ 8:195–202, 1997.

Miranda JLG, Gomez AO, Ansedes HV, Torres NR, Espinosa CG, Cortabarria C, Salgado GS. Monosomy 22 with humoral immunodeficiency: is there an immunoglobulin chain deficit? J Med Genet 20:69–72, 1983.

Molina IJ, Kenney DM, Rosen FS, Remold-O'Donnell E. T cell lines characterize events in the pathogenesis of the Wiskott-Aldrich syndrome. J Exp Med 176:867–874, 1992.

Molina IJ, Sancho J, Terhorst C, Rosen FS, Remold-O'Donnell E. T cells of patients with the Wiskott-Aldrich syndrome have a restricted defect in proliferative responses. J Immunol 151:4383–4390, 1993.

Mora-Duarte J, Betts R, Rostein C, Colombo AL, Thompson-Moya L, Smietana J, Lupinacci R, Sable C, Kartsonis N, Perfect J, for the Caspofungin Invasive Candidiasis Study Group. Comparison of caspofungin and amphotericin B for invasive candidiasis. N Engl J Med 347:2020–2029, 2002.

Moss EM, Batshaw ML, Solot CB, Gerdes M, McDonald-McGinn DM, Driscoll DA, Emanuel BS, Zackai EH, Wang PP. Psychoeducational profile of the 22q11.2 microdeletion: a complex pattern. J Pediatr 134:193–198, 1999.

Motala C, Potter PC, Weinberg EG, Malherbe D, Hughes J. Anti-staphylococcus aureus specific IgE in atopic dermatitis. J Allergy Clin Immunol 78:583–589, 1986.

Motzkin B, Marion R, Goldberg R, Shprintzen R, Saenger P. Variable phenotypes in velocardiofacial syndrome with chromosomal deletion. J Pediatr 123:406–410, 1993.

Mroczek EC, Weisenburger DD, Grierson Hl, et al. Thymic lesions in fatal infectious mononucleosis. Clin Immunol Immunopathol 43:243–255, 1987.

Muller W, Peter HH, Kallfelz HC, Franz A, Rieger CH. The DiGeorge sequence. II. Immunologic findings in partial and complete forms of the disorder. Eur J Pediatr 149:96–103, 1989.

Muller W, Peter HH, Wilken M, Juppner H, Kallfelz HC, Krohn HP, Miller K, Rieger CH. The DiGeorge syndrome. I. Clinical evaluation and course of partial and complete forms of the syndrome. Eur J Pediatr 147:496–502, 1988.

Murphy PM. Chemokines and the molecular basis of cancer metastasis. N Engl J Med 345:833–5, 2001.

Myhre AG, Halonen M, Eskelin P, Ekwall O, Hedstrand H, Rorsman F, Kampe O, Husebye ES. Autoimmune polyendocrine syndrome type 1 (APS I) in Norway. Clin Endocrinol 54:211–217, 2001.

Nagamine K, Peterson P, Scott HS, Kodoh J, Minoshima S, Heino M, Krohn KJE, Lalioti MD, Mullis PE, Antonarakis SE, Kawaski K, Asakawa S, Ito F, Shimizu N. Positional cloning of the APECED gene. Nat Genet 17:393–398, 1997.

Nagasawa T, Hirota S, Tachibana K, Takakura N, Nishikawa S, Kitamura Y, Yoshida N, Kikutani H, Kishimoto T. Defects of B-cell lymphopoiesis and bone-marrow myelopoiesis in mice lacking the CXC chemokine PBSF/SDF-1. Nature 382:635–638, 1996.

Nagasawa T, Tachibana K, Kishimoto T. A novel CXC chemokine PBSF/SDF-1 and its receptor CXCR4: their functions in development, hematopoiesis and HIV infection. Semin Immunol 10:179–185, 1998.

Nagle, DL, Karim, AM, Woolf, EA, Holmgren, L, Bork, P, Misumi, DJ, McGrail, SH, Dussault, J, Perou, CM, Boissy, RE, Duyk, GM, Spritz, RA, Moore, KJ. Identification and mutation analysis of the complete gene for Chediak-Higashi syndrome. Nat Genet 14:307–311, 1996.

Naglik JR, Newport G, White TC, Fernandez-Naglik LL, Greenspan JS, Greenspan D, Sweet SP, Challacombe SJ, Agabain N. In vivo analysis of secreted aspartyl proteinase expression in human oral candidiasis. Infect Immun 67:2482–2490, 1999.

Nakahira M, Matsumoto S, Mukushita N, Nakatani H. Primary aspergillosis of the larynx associated with CD4+ T lymphocytopenia. J Laryngol Otol 116:304–306, 2002.

Nanki T, Hayashida K, El-Gabalawy HS, Suson S, Shi K, Girschick HJ, Yavuz S, Lipsky PE. Stromal cell-derived factor-1-CXC chemokine receptor 4 interactions play a central role in CD4+ T cell accumulation in rheumatoid arthritis synovium. J Immunol 165:6590–6598, 2000.

Newport M, Huxley CM, Huston S, Hawrylowicz C, Ostra BA, Williamson R, Levin M. A mutation in the interferon-γ receptor gene and susceptibility to mycobacterial infection. N Engl J Med 335:1941–1949, 1996.

Nichols KE, Harkin DP, Levitz S, Krainer M, Kolquist KA, Genovese C, Bernard A, Ferguson M, Zuo L, Snyder E, Buckler AJ, Wise C, Ashley J, Lovett M, Valentine MB, Look AT, Gerald W, Housman DE, Haber DA. Inactivating mutations in an SH2 domain-encoding gene in X-linked lymphoproliferative syndrome. Proc Natl Acad Sci U S A 95:13765–13770, 1998.

Notarangelo LD, Mazza C, Giliani S, D'Aria C, Gandellini F, Ravelli C, Locatelli MG, Nelson DL, Ochs HD. Missense mutations of the WASP gene cause intermittent X-linked thrombocytopenia. Blood 99:2268–2269, 2002.

Notarangelo LD, Ochs HD. Wiskott-Aldrich Syndrome: A model for defective actin reorganization, cell trafficking and synapse formation. Curr Opin Immunol 15:585–591, 2003.

Notarangelo LD, Parolini O, Faustini R, Porteri V, Albertini A, Ugazio AG. Presentation of Wiskott-Aldrich syndrome as isolated thrombocytopenia. Blood 77:1125–1126, 1991.

Nunez MJ, de Lis JM, Rodriguez JR, Allegue MJ, Viladrich A, Conde C, Santiago MP, Amigo MC. Disseminated encephalic cryptococcosis as a form of presentation of idiopathic T-CD4 lymphocytopenia. Rev Neurol 28:390–393, 1999.

O'Brien TR, Diamondstone L, Fried MW, Aledort LM, Eichinger S, Eyster ME, Hilgartner MW, White G, Di Bisceglie AM, Goedert JJ. Idiopathic CD4+ T-lymphocytopenia in HIV seronegative men with hemophilia and sex partners of HIV seropositive men. Multicenter Hemophilia Cohort Study. Am J Hematol 49:201–206, 1995.

Ocejo-Vinyals JG, Lozano MJ, Sanchez-Velasco P, Escribano de Diego J, Paz-Miguel JE, Leyva-Cobian F. An unusual concurrence of graft versus host disease caused by engraftment of maternal lymphocytes with DiGeorge anomaly. Arch Dis Child 83:165–169, 2000.

Ochs HD. The Wiskott-Aldrich syndrome. Clin Rev Allergy Immunol 20:61-86, 2001.

Ochs HD, Slichter SJ, Harker LA, Von Behrens WE, Clark RA, Wedgwood RJ. The Wiskott-Aldrich syndrome: studies of lymphocytes, granulocytes, and platelets. Blood 55:243–52, 1980.

Oda A, Ochs HD. Wiskott-Aldrich syndrome protein and platelets. Immunol Reviews 178:111–117, 2000.

Oda A, Ochs HD, Druker BJ, Ozaki K, Watanabe C, Handa M, Miyakawa Y, Ikeda Y. Collagen induces tyrosine phosphorylation of Wiskott-Aldrich syndrome protein in human platelets. Blood 92:1852–1858, 1998.

Okamato GA, Hall JG, Ochs H, Jackson C, Rodaway K, Chandler J. New syndrome of chronic mucocutaneous candidiasis. Birth Defects Original Article Series 13:117–125, 1977.

Okano M, Pirruccello SJ, Grierson HL, et al. Immunovirological studies of fatal infectious mononucleosis in a patient with X-linked lymphoproliferative syndrome treated with intravenous immunoglobulin and interferon-alpha. Clin Immunol Immunopathol 54:410–418, 1990.

Orange JS. Human natural killer cell deficiencies and susceptibility to infection. Microbes Infect 4:1545–1558, 2002.

Orange JS, Chehimi J, Ghavimi D, Campbell D, Sullivan KE. Decreased natural killer (NK) cell function in chronic NK cell lymphocytosis associated with decreased surface expression of CD11b. Clin Immunol 99:53–64, 2001.

Orange JS, Brodeur SR, Jain A, Bonilla FA, Schneider LC, Kretschmer R, Nurko S, Rasmussen WL, Kohler JR, Gellis SE, Ferguson BM, Strominger JL, Zonana J, Ramesh N, Ballas ZK, Geha RS. Deficient natural killer cell cytotoxicity in patients with IKK-gamma/NEMO mutations. J Clin Invest 109:1501–1509, 2002a.

Orange JS, Ramesh N, Remold-O'Donnell E, Sasahara Y, Koopman L, Byrne M, Bonilla FA, Rosen FS, Geha RS, Strominger JL. Wiskott-Aldrich syndrome protein is required for NK cell cytotoxicity and colocalizes with actin to NK cell-activating immunologic synapses. Proc Natl Acad Sci U S A 99:11351–6, 2002b.

O'Regan S, Newman AJ, Graham RC. `Myelokathexis'. Neutropenia with marrow hyperplasia. Am J Dis Child 131:655–8, 1977.

Ostenstad B, Giliani S, Mellbye OJ, Nilsen BR, Abrahamsen T. A boy with X-linked hyper-IgM syndrome and natural killer cell deficiency. Clin Exp Immunol 107:230–234, 1997.

Oyefara BI, Kim HC, Danziger RN, Carroll M, Greene JM, Douglas SD. Autoimmune hemolytic anemia in chronic mucocutaneous candidiasis. Clin Diagn Lab Immunol 1:38–43, 1994.

Ozsahin H, Le Deist F, Benkerrou M, Cavazzana-Calvo M, Gomez L, Griscelli C, Blanche S, Fischer A. Bone marrow transplantation in 26 patients with Wiskott-Aldrich syndrome from a single center. J Pediatr 129:238–44, 1996.

Packman S, Sweetman, L, Wall S. Biotin-responsive multiple carboxylase deficiency of infantile onset. J Pediatr 99:421–423, 1981.

Paganelli R, Scala E, Capobianchi MR, Fanales-Belasio E, D'Offizi G, Fiorilli M, Aiuti F. Selective deficiency of interferon-gamma production in the hyper IgE syndrome. Relationship to in vitro IgE synthesis. Clin Exp Immunol 84:28–33, 1991.

Palma-Carlos AG, Palma-Carlos ML. Chronic mucocutaneous candidiasis revisited. Allerg Immunol (Paris) 233:229–232, 2001.

Paolini R, D'Andrea E, Poletti A, Del Mistro A, Zerbinati P, Girolami A. B non-Hodgkin's lymphoma in a haemophilia patient with idiopathic CD4+ T-lymphocytopenia. Leuk Lymphoma 21:177–80, 1996.

Parkman R, Rappeport J, Geha R, Belli J, Cassady R, Levey R, Nathan DG, Rosen FS. Complete correction of the Wiskott-Aldrich syndrome by allogeneic bone-marrow transplantation. N Engl J Med 298:921–7, 1978.

Parolini O, Ressmann G, Haas OA, Pawlowsky J, Gadner H, Knapp W, Holter W. X-linked Wiskott-Aldrich syndrome in a girl. N Engl J Med 338:291–295. 1995.

Parolini S, Bottino C, Falco M, Augugliaro R, Giliani S, Franceschini R, Ochs HD, Wolf H, Bonnefoy JV, Biassoni R, Moretta L, Notarangelo L, Moretta A. X-linked lymphoproliferative disease: 2B4 molecules displaying inhibitory rather than activating function are responsible for the inability of natural killer cells to kill Epstein-Barr virus-infected cells. J Exp Med 192:337–346, 2000.

Pastural E, Barrat FJ, Dufourcq-Lagelouse R, Certain, S, Sanal O, Jabado N, Seger R, Griscelli C, Fischer A, de Saint Basile G. Griscelli disease maps to chromosome 15q21 and is associated with mutations in the myosin-Va gene. Nat Genet 16:289–292, 1997.

Pastural E, Ersoy F, Yalman N, Wulffraat N, Grillo E, Ozkinay F, Tezcan I, Gedikoglu G, Philippe N, Fischer A. and de Saint Basile, G. Two genes are responsible for Griscelli syndrome at the same 15q21 locus. Genomics 63, 299–306, 2000.

Peake JE, McCrossin RB, Byrne G, Shepherd R. X-linked immune dysregulation, neonatal insulin dependent diabetes, and intractable diarrhoea. Arch Dis Child 74:F195–199, 1996.

Pene J, Rousset F, Briere F, Chretien I, Bonnefoy J-Y, Spits H, Yokota T, Arai N, Arai K-I, Banchereau J, DeVries JE. IgE production by normal human lymphocytes is induced by interleukin 4 and suppressed by interferons and prostaglandin E2. Proc Nat Acad Sci U S A 85:6880–6884, 1988.

Perez N, Virelizier J, Arenzana-Seisdedos F, Fischer A, Griscelli C. Impaired natural killer activity in lymphohistiocytosis syndrome. J Pediatr 104:569–573, 1984

Perkins JA, Sie K, Gray S. Presence of 22q11 deletion in postadenoidectomy velopharyngeal insufficiency. Arch Otolaryngol Head Neck Surg 126:645–648, 2000.

Petersen EA, Alling DW, Kirkpatrick CH. Treatment of chronic mucocutaneous candidiasis with ketoconazole. A controlled clinical trial. Ann Intern Med 93:791–795, 1980.

Petersen EJ, Rozenberg-Arska M, Dekker AW, Clevers HC, Verdonck LF. Allogeneic bone marrow transplantation can restore CD4+ T-lymphocyte count and immune function in idiopathic CD4+ T-lymphocytopenia. Bone Marrow Transplant 18:813–815, 1996.

Petit I, Szyper-Kravitz M, Nagler A, Lahav M, Peled A, Habler L, Ponomaryov T, Taichman RS, Arenzana-Seisdedos F, Fujii N, Sandbank J, Zipori D, Lapidot T. G-CSF induces stem cell mobilization by decreasing bone marrow SDF-1 and up-regulating CXCR4. Nat Immunol 3:687–694, 2002.

Picard C, Fieschi C, Altare F, Al-Jumaah S, Al-Hajjar S, Feinberg J, Dupuis S, Soudais C, Al-Mohsen IZ, Genin E, Lammas D, Kumararatne D, Leclerc T, Rafii A, Frayha H, Murugasu B, Wah LB, Sinniah R, Loubser M, Okamoto E, Al-Ghonaium A, Tufunkeji H, Abel L, Casanova JL. Inherited interleukin-12 deficiency: IL-12β genotype and clinical phenotype of 13 patients from six kindreds. Am J Hum Genet 70:336–348, 2002.

Pierdominici M, Marziali M, Giovannetti A, Oliva A, Rosso R, Marino B, Digilio MC, Giannotti A, Novelli G, Dallapiccola B, Aiuti F, Pandolfi F. T cell receptor repertoire and function in patients with DiGeorge syndrome and velocardiofacial syndrome. Clin Exp Immunol 121:127–132, 2000.

Pilheu JA, De Salvo MC, Gonzalez J, Rey D, Elias MC, Ruppi MC. CD4+ T-lymphocytopenia in severe pulmonary tuberculosis without evidence of human immunodeficiency virus infection. Int J Tuberc Lung Dis 1:422–426, 1997.

Pinchas-Hamiel O, Engelberg S, Mandel M, Passwell JH. Immune hemolytic anemia, thrombocytopenia and liver disease in a patient with DiGeorge syndrome. Isr J Med Sci 30:530–532, 1994.

Plebani A, Cantu-Rajnoldi A, Collo G, Allavena P, Biolchini A, Pirelli A, Clerici Schoeller M, Masarone M. Myelokathexis associated with multiple congenital malformations: immunological study on phagocytic cells and lymphocytes. Eur J Haematol 40:12–17, 1988.

Pohl W. A patient with idiopathic bronchiolitis obliterans with organizing pneumonia and idiopathic CD4+ T-lymphocytopenia. Wien Klin Wochenschr 108:473–477, 1996.

Polmar SH, Pierce GF. Cartilage hair hypoplasia: immunological aspects and their clinical implications. Clin Immunol Immunopathol 40:87–93, 1986.

Powell BR, Buist NR, Stenzel P. An X-linked syndrome of diarrhea, polyendocrinopathy, and fatal infection in infancy. J Pediatr 100:731–737, 1982.

Prekeris R, Terrian D. Brain myosin V is a synaptic vesicle-associated motor protein: Evidence for a Ca2+-dependent interaction with the synaptobrevin-synaptophysin complex. J Cell Biol 137:1589–1601, 1997.

Puccetti P, Mencacci A, Cenci E, Spaccapelo R, Mosci P, Enssle K-H, Romani L, Bistoni F. Cure of murine candidiasis by recombinant soluble interleukin-4 receptor. J Infect Dis 169:1325–1331, 1994.

Purnell D, Ilchyshyn A, Jenkins D, Salim A, Seth R, Snead D. Isolated human papillomavirus 18-positive extragenital bowenoid papulosis and idiopathic CD4+ lymphocytopenia. Br J Dermatol 144:619–621, 2001.

Purtilo DT, Cassel CK, Yang JP, and Harper R. X-linked recessive progressive combined variable immunodeficiency (Duncan's disease). Lancet 1:935–40, 1975.

Purtilo DT, DeFlorio D Jr, Hutt LM, Bhawan J, Yang JP, Otto R, Edwards W. Variable phenotypic expression of an X-linked recessive lymphoproliferative syndrome. N Engl J Med 297:1077–1080, 1977.

Purtilo DT, Grierson HL, David JR, Okano M. The X-linked lymphoproliferative disease: from autopsy toward cloning the gene 1975-1990. Pediatr Pathol 11:685–710, 1991.

Purtilo DT, Grierson HL, Ochs H, Skare J. Detection of X-linked lymphoproliferative disease using molecular and immunovirologic markers Am J Med 87:421–424, 1989.

Radl J, Masopust J, Houstek J, Hrodek O. Paraproteinaemia and unusual dys-gamma-globulinaemia in a case of Wiskott-Aldrich syndrome. An immunochemical study. Arch Dis Child 42:608–614, 1967.

Ramanan R, Wang Y. A high-affinity iron permease essential for Candida albicans virulence. Science 288;1062–1064, 2000.

Ramesh N, Anton IM, Hartwig JH, Geha RS. WIP, a protein associated with Wiskott-Aldrich syndrome protein, induces actin polymerization and redistribution in lymphoid cells. Proc Natl Acad Sci USA 94:14671–14676, 1997.

Ramos JT, Lopez-Laso E, Ruiz-Contreras J, Giancaspro E, Madero S. B cell non-Hodgkin's lymphoma in a girl with the DiGeorge anomaly. Arch Dis Child 81:444–445, 1999.

Ramsey C, Winquist O, Puhakka L, Halonen M, Moro A, Kämpe O, Eskelin P, Pelto-Huikko M, Peltonen L. AIRE deficient mice develop multiple features of APECED phenotype and show altered immune response. Hum Mol Genet 11:397–409, 2002.

Rasmussen SA, Williams CA, Ayoub EM, Sleasman JW, Gray BA, Bent-Williams A, Stalker HJ, Zori RT. Juvenile rheumatoid arthritis in velo-cardio-facial syndrome: coincidence or unusual complication. Am J Med Genet 64:546–550, 1996

Rauch A, Hofbeck M, Leipold G, Klinge J, Trautmann U, Kirsch M, Singer H, Pfeiffer RA. Incidence and significance of 22q11.2 hemizygosity in patients with interrupted aortic arch. Am J Med Genet 78:322–331, 1998.

Rawlings SL, Crooks GM, Bockstoce D, Barsky LW, Parkman R, Weinberg KI. Spontaneous apoptosis in lymphocytes from patients with Wiskott-Aldrich syndrome: correlation of accelerated cell death and attenuated bcl-2 expression. Blood 94:3872–3882, 1999.

Reisinger D, Parkman R. Molecular heterogeneity of a lymphocyte glycoprotein in immunodeficient patients. J Clin Invest 79:595–599, 1987.

Remold-O'Donnell E, Cooley J, Shcherbina A, Hagemann TL, Kwan SP, Kenney DM, Rosen FS. Variable expression of WASP in B cell lines of Wiskott-Aldrich syndrome patients. J Immunol 158:4021–4025, 1997.

Rengan R, Ochs HD, Sweet LI, Keil ML, Gunning WT, Lachant NA, Boxer LA, Omann GM. Actin cytoskeletal function is spared, but apoptosis is increased, in WAS patient hematopoietic cells. Blood 95:1283–1292, 2000.

Ridanpaa M, van Eenennaam H, Pelin K, Chadwick R, Johnson C, Yuan B, vanVenrooij W, Pruijn G, Salmela R, Rockas S, Makitie O, Kaitila I, de la Chapelle A. Mutations in the RNA component of RNase MRP cause a pleiotropic human disease, cartilage-hair hypoplasia. Cell 104:195–203, 2001.

Rijnders RJ, van den Ende IE, Huikeshoven FJ. Suspected idiopathic CD4+ T-lymphocytopenia in a young patient with vulvar carcinoma stage IV. Gynecol Oncol 61:423–426, 1996.

Rivero-Lezcano OM, Marcilla A, Sameshima JH, Robbins KC. Wiskott-Aldrich syndrome protein physically associates with Nck through Src homology 3 domains. Mol Cell Biol 15:5725–5731, 1995.

Rocca B, Bellacosa A, De Cristofaro R, Neri G, Della Ventura M, Maggiano N, Rumi C, Landolfi R. Wiskott-Aldrich syndrome: report of an autosomal dominant variant. Blood 87:4538–4543, 1996.

Roder JC, Todd RF, Rubin P, Haliotis T, Helfand SL, Werkmeister J, Pross HF, Boxer LA, Schlossman SF, Fauci AS. The Chediak-Higashi gene in humans. III. Studies on the mechanisms of NK impairment. Clin Exp Immunol 51:359–68, 1983.

Roesler J, Kofink B, Wendisch J, Heyden S, Paul D, Friedrich W, Casanova JL, Leupold W, Gahr M, Rosen-Wolff A. Listeria monocytogenes and recurrent mycobacterial infections in a child with complete interferon-gamma-receptor (IFN-γR1) deficiency: mutational analysis and evaluation of therapeutic options. Exp Hematol 27:1368–1374, 1999.

Roger PM, Bernard-Pomier G, Counillon E, Breittmayer JP, Bernard A, Dellamonica P. Overexpression of Fas/CD95 and Fas-induced apoptosis in a patient with idiopathic CD4+ T lymphocytopenia. Clin Infect Dis 28:1012–1016, 1999.

Rohatgi R, Ma L, Miki H, Lopez M, Kirchhausen T, Takenawa T, Kirschner MW. The interaction between N-WASP and the Arp2/3 complex links Cdc42-dependent signals to actin assembly. Cell 97:221–231, 1999.

Root AW, Speicher CE. The triad of thrombocytopenia, eczema, and recurrent infections (Wiskott-Aldrich syndrome) associated with milk antibodies, giant-cell pneumonia, and cytomegalic inclusion disease. Pediatrics 31:444–454, 1963.

Rommel N, Vantrappen G, Swillen A, Devriendt K, Feenstra L, Fryns JP. Retrospective analysis of feeding and speech disorders in 50 patients with velo-cardio-facial syndrome. Genet Counsel 10:71–78, 1999.

Rosenblatt HR, Ladisch S, Albrecht RM, Lehrer RI, Fischer TJ, Hong R, Stiehm ER. Monocyte effector defects in chronic mucocutaneous candidiasis. Pediatr Res 13:454abs, 1979.

Rosenzweig S, Dorman SE, Roesler J, Palacios J, Zelazko M, Holland SM. 561del4 defines a novel deletion hotspot in the interferon gamma receptor 1 chain. Clin Immunol 102:25–27, 2002.

Roth K, Cohn R, Yandrasitz J, Preti G, Dodd P, Segal S. Beta-methylcrotonic aciduria associated with lactic acidosis. J Pediatr 88:229–235, 1976.

Rousset F, Souillet G, Roncarolo MG, Lamelin JP. Studies of EBV-lymphoid cell interactions in two patients with the X-linked lymphoproliferative syndrome: normal EBV-specific HLA-restricted cytotoxicity. Clin Exp Immunol 63:280–289, 1986.

Rozzo SJ, Kirkpatrick CH. Purification of transfer factors. Mol Immunol 29:167–182, 1992.

Rudolph MG, Bayer P, Abo A, Kuhlmann J, Vetter IR, Wittinghofer A. The Cdc42/Rac interactive binding region motif of the Wiskott Aldrich syndrome protein (WASP) is necessary but not sufficient for tight binding to Cdc42 and structure formation. J Biol Chem 273:18067–18076, 1998.

Russell JH, Ley TJ. Lymphocyte-mediated cytotoxicity. Annu Rev Immunol 20:323–370, 2002.

Russell WL, Russell LB, Gower JS. Exceptional inheritance of a sex-linked gene in the mouse explained on the basis that the X/O sex-chromosome constitution is female. Proc Natl Acad Sci U S A 45:554–560, 1959.

Ryan AK, Goodship JA, Wilson DI, Philip N, Levy A, Seidel H, Schuffenhauer S, Oechsler H, Belohradsky B, Prieur M, Aurias A, Raymond FL, Clayton-Smith J, Hatchwell E, McKeown C, Beemer FA, Dallapiccola B, Novelli G, Hurst JA, Ignatius J, Green AJ, Winter RM, Brueton L, Brondum-Nielson K, Stewart F, Van Essen T, Patton M, Paterson J, Scambler PJ. Spectrum of clinical features associated with interstitial chromosome 22q11 deletions: a European collaborative study. J Med Genet 34:798–804, 1997.

Sakamoto K, Seeley JK, Lindsten J, et al. Abnormal anti-Epstein Barr virus antibodies in carriers of the X-linked lymphoproliferative syndrome and in females at risk. J Immunol 128:904–907, 1982.

Sallmann S, Heilmann A, Heinke F, Kerkmann ML, Schuppler M, Hahn G, Gahr M, Rosen-Wolff A, Roesler J. Caspofungin therapy for aspergillus lung infection in a boy with chronic granulomatous disease. Pediatr Infect Dis 22:199–200, 2003.

Sampson HA, Buckley RH. Human IgE synthesis in vitro: a reassessment. J Immunol 127:829–834, 1981.

Sanal SO, Buckley RH. Antibody-dependent cellular cytotoxicity in primary immunodeficiency diseases and with normal leukocyte subpopulations. Importance of the type of target. J Clin Invest 61:1–10, 1978.

Sanal O, Yel L, Kucukali T, Gilbert-Barnes E, Tardieu M, Texcan I, Ersoy F, Metin A, de Saint Basile G. An allelic variant of Griscelli disease: presentation with severe hypotonia, mental-motor retardation, and hypopigmentation consistent with Elejalde syndrome (neuroectodermal melanolysosomal disorder) J Neurol 247:570–572, 2000.

Sanal O, Ersoy F, Tezcan I, Metin A, Yel L, Menasche G, Gurgey A, Berkel I, de Saint Basile G. Griscelli disease: genotype-phenotype correlation in an array of clinical heterogeneity. J Clin Immunol 22:237–243, 2002.

Sander JE, Malamud N, Cowan MJ, Packman S, Ammann AJ, Wara DW. Intermittent ataxia and immunodeficiency with multiple carboxylase deficiency: a biotin-responsive disorder. Ann Neurol 8:544–547, 1980.

Santos Gil I, Gonzalez-Ruano P, Sanz Sanz J. Idiopathic CD4+ lymphocytopenia associated with disseminated cryptococcosis. Rev Clin Esp 202:518–519, 2002.

Satake N, Nakanishi M, Okano M, Tomizawa K, Ishizaka A, Kojima K, Onodera M, Ariga T, Satake A, Sakiyama Y, et al. A Japanese family of X-linked auto-immune enteropathy with haemolytic anaemia and polyendocrinopathy. Eur J Pediatr 152:313–315, 1993.

Sato M, Hayashi Y, Yoshida H, Yanagawa T, Yura Y. A family with hereditary lack of T4+ inducer/helper T cell subsets in peripheral blood lymphocytes. J Immunol 132: 1071–1073, 1984

Sato T, Tatsuzawa O, Koike Y, Wada Y, Nagata M, Kobayashi S, Ishizawa A, Miyauchi J, Shimizu K. B-cell lymphoma associated with DiGeorge syndrome. Eur J Pediatr 158:609, 1999.

Saunders M, Sweetman L, Robinson B, Bolth K, Cohn R, Gravel RA. Multiple carboxylase deficiencies and complementation studies with proprionicacidemia in cultured fibroblasts. J Clin Invest 64:1695–1701, 1979.

Sayos J, Wu C, Morra M, Wang N, Zhang X, Allen D, van Schaik S, Notarangelo L, Geha R, Roncarolo MG, Oettgen H, De Vries JE, Aversa G, Terhorst C. The X-linked lymphoproliferative-disease gene product SAP regulates signals induced through the co-receptor SLAM. Nature 395:462–469, 1998a.

Sayos JC, Wu M, Morra N, et al. The X-linked lymphoproliferative-disease gene product SAP regulates signals induced through the co-receptor SLAM. Nature 395:462–469, 1998b.

Sayos J, Nguyen KB, Wu C, Stepp SE, Howie D, Schatzle JD, Kumar V, Biron, CA, Terhorst, C. Potential pathways for regulation of NK and T-cell responses: differential X-linked lymphoproliferative syndrome gene product SAP interactions with SLAM and 2B4. Int Immunol 12:1749–1757, 2000.

Schaller M, Schafer W, Korting HC, Hube B. Differential expression of secreted aspartyl proteinases in a model of human oral candidiasis and in patient samples from the oral cavity. Mol Microbiol 29:605–615, 1998.

Schantz V, Pedersen C, Homburg KM, Hansen ER. Mycobacterium avium complex infection in a patient with idiopathic CD4+ T-lymphocytopenia. Ugeskr Laeger 162:359–360, 2000.

Scharton-Kersten TM, Sher A. Role of natural killer cells in innate resistance to protozoan infections. Curr Opin Immunol 9:44–52, 1997.

Scherer NJ, D'Antonio LL, Kalbfleisch JH. Early speech and language development in children with velocardiofacial syndrome. Am J Med Genet 88:714–723, 1999.

Schimke, RN, Horton, WA, King, CR, Martin, NL. Chondroitin-6-sulfate, mucopolysaccharidosis in conjunction with lymphopenia, defective cellular immunity and nephrotic syndrome. Birth Defects 10:258–266, 1974.

Schindelhauer D, Weiss M, Hellebrand H, Golla A, Hergersberg M, Seger R, Belohradsky BH, Meindl A. Wiskott-Aldrich syndrome: no strict genotype-phenotype correlations but clustering of missense mutations in the amino-terminal part of the WASP gene product. Hum Genet 98:68–76, 1996.

Schmitt C, Ballet JJ. Serum IgE and IgG antibodies to tetanus toxoid and candidin in immunodeficient children with the hyper IgE syndrome. J Clin Immunol 3:178–183, 1983.

Schneider L, Berman R, Shea C, Perez-Atayde A, Weinstein H, Geha R. Bone marrow transplantation (BMT) for the syndrome of pigmentary dilution and lymphohistiocytosis (Griscelli's syndrome). J Clin Immunol 10, 146–53, 1990.

Schopfer K, Baerlocher K, Price P, Krech U, Quie PG, Douglas SD. Staphylococcal IgE antibodies, hyperimmunoglobulinemia E and Staphylococcus aureus infections. N Engl J Med 300:835–838, 1979.

Schubert MS, Moss RB. Selective polysaccharide antibody deficiency in familial DiGeorge syndrome. Ann Allergy 69:231–238, 1992.

Schuffenhauer S, Lichtner P, Peykar-Derakhshandeh P, Murken J, Haas OA, Back E, Wolff G, Zabel B, Barisic I, Rauch A, Borochowitz Z, Dallapiccola B, Ross M, Meitinger T. Deletion mapping on chromosome 10p and definition of a critical region for the second DiGeorge syndrome locus (DGS2). Eur J Hum Genet 6:213–225, 1998.

Schuster V, Kreth H. X-linked lymphoproliferative disease. In Smith C, Ochs HD, Puck JM, eds. Primary Immunodeficiency Diseases. Oxford, Oxford University Press, 1999, pp 222–232.

Schuster V, Seidenspinner S, Grimm T, et al. Molecular genetic haplotype segregation studies in three families with X-linked lymphoproliferative disease. Eur J Pediatr 153:432–437, 1994.

Seemayer TA, Gross TG, Egeler RM, Pirruccello SJ, Davis JR, Kelly CM, Okano M, Lanyi A, Sumegi J. X-linked lymphoproliferative disease: twenty-five years after the discovery. Pediatr Res 38:471–478, 1995.

Semple JW, Siminovitch KA, Mody M, Milev Y, Lazarus AH, Wright JF, Freedman J. Flow cytometric analysis of platelets from children with the Wiskott-Aldrich syndrome reveals defects in platelet development, activation and structure. Br J Haematol 97:747–754, 1997.

Shama SK, Kirkpatrick CH. Dermatophytosis in patients with chronic mucocutaneous candidiasis. J Am Acad Dermatol 2:285–294, 1980.

Sheerin KA, Buckley RH. Antibody responses to protein, polysaccharide, and φX-174 antigens in the hyperimmunoglobulinemia E (Hyper-IgE) syndrome. J Allergy Clin Immunol 87:803–811, 1991.

Shi JD, Wang CY, Marron MP, Ruan QG, Huang YQ, Detter JC, She JX. Chromosomal localization and complete genomic sequence of the murine autoimmune regulator gene (Aire). Autoimmunity 31:47–53, 1999.

Shimano S, Murata N, Tsuchiya J. Idiopathic CD4+ T-lymphocytopenia terminating in Burkitt's lymphoma. Rinsho Ketsueki 38:599–603, 1997.

Shlapatska LM, Mikhalap SV, Berdova AG, Zelensky OM, Yun TJ, Nichols KE, Clark EA, Sidorenko SP. CD150 association with either the SH2-containing inositol phosphatase or the SH2-containing protein tyrosine phosphatase is regulated by the adaptor protein SH2D1A. J Immunol 166:5480–5487, 2001.

Shokeir MHK. Short stature, absent thumbs, flat facies, anosmia and combined immune deficiency. Birth Defects 14:103–116, 1978.

Shprintzen RJ, Goldberg R, Golding-Kushner KJ, Marion RW. Late-onset psychosis in the velo-cardio-facial syndrome. Am J Med Genet 42:141–142, 1992.

Signorini S, Pirovano S, Fiorentini S, Stellini R, Bianchi V, Albertini A, Imberti L. Restriction of T-cell receptor repertoires in idiopathic CD4+ lymphocytopenia. Br J Haematol 110:434–447, 2000.

Siminovitch KA, Greer WL, Novogrodsky A, Axelsson B, Somani AK, Peacocke M. A diagnostic assay for the Wiskott-Aldrich syndrome and its variant forms. J Invest Med 43:159–169, 1995.

Sinicco A, Maiello A, Raiteri R, Sciandra M, Dassio G, Zamprogna C, Mecozzi B. Pneumocystis carinii in a patient with pulmonary sarcoidosis and idiopathic CD4+ T lymphocytopenia. Thorax 51:446–449: 1996.

Skare JC, Grierson HL, Sullivan JL, Nussbaum RL, Purtilo DT, Sylla BS, Lenoir GM, Reilly DS, White BN, Milunsky A. Linkage analysis of seven kindreds with the X-linked lymphoproliferative syndrome (XLP) confirms that the XLP locus is near DXS42 and DXS37. Hum Genet 82:354–358, 1989.

Skare JC, Milunsky A, Byron KS, Sullivan JL. Mapping the X-linked lymphoproliferative synrome. Proc Natl Acad Sci U S A 84:2015–2018, 1987.

Smith CA, Driscoll DA, Emanuel BS, McDonald-McGinn DM, Zackai EH, Sullivan KE. Increased prevalence of immunoglobulin A deficiency in patients with the chromosome 22q11.2 deletion syndrome (DiGeorge syndrome/velocardiofacial syndrome). Clin Diagn Lab Immunol 5:415–417, 1998.

Smith DK, Neal JJ, Holmberg SD. Unexplained opportunistic infections and CD4+ T-lymphocytopenia without HIV infection. An investigation of cases in the United States. The Centers for Disease Control Idiopathic CD4+ T-lymphocytopenia Task Force. N Engl J Med 328:373–379, 1993.

Snapper SB, Rosen FS. A family of WASPs. N Engl J Med 348:350–351, 2003.

Snyderman R, Altman LC, Frankel A, Blaese RM. Defective mononuclear leukocyte chemotaxis: a previously unrecognized immune dysfunction. Ann Intern Med 78:509–513, 1973.

Soderberg-Warner M, Rice-Mendoza CA, Mendoza GR, Stiehm ER. Neutrophil and T lymphocyte characteristics of two patients with the hyper IgE syndrome. Pediatr Res 17:820–824, 1983.

Sohnle PG, Frank MM, Kirkpatrick CH. Mechanisms involved in elimination of organisms from experimental cutaneous Candida albicans infections in guinea pigs. J Immunol 117:523–530, 1976a.

Sohnle PG, Frank MM, Kirkpatrick CH. Deposition of complement components in the cutaneous lesions of chronic mucocutaneous candidiasis. Clin Immunol Immunopathol 5:340–350, 1976b.

Sohnle PG, Kirkpatrick CH. Deposition of complement in the lesions of experimental cutaneous candidiasis in guinea pigs. J Cutan Path 3:232–238, 1976c.

Sole, D, Leser, PG, Soares, D, Naspitz, CK. Cartilage-hair hypoplasia syndrome: immunological evaluation of two cases. Rev Paul Med 111:314–319, 1993.

Spaccapelo R, Del Sero G, Mosci P, Bistoni F, Romani L. Early T cell unresponsiveness in mice with candidiasis and reversal by IL-2. Effect on T helper cell development. J Immunol 158:2294–2302, 1997.

Spira TJ, Jones BM, Nicholson JK, Lal RB, Rowe T, Mawle AC, Lauter CB, Shulman JA, Monson RA. Idiopathic CD4+ T-lymphocytopenia–an analysis of five patients with unexplained opportunistic infections. N Engl J Med 328:386–392, 1993.

Spritz RA. Genetic defects in Chediak-Higashi syndrome and the beige mouse. J Clin Immunol 18:97–105, 1998.

Starr SE, Hansen-Flaschen J, Miller D, Douglas SD, Perussia B. Reappearance of natural-killer-cell activity. N Engl J Med 322:133–134, 1990.

Stepp S, Dufourcq-Lagelouse R, Le Deist F, Bhawan S, Certain S, Mathew P, Henter J, Bennett M, Fischer A, de Saint Basile G, Kumar V. Perforin gene defects in familial hemophagocytic lymphohistiocytosis. Science 286:1957–1959, 1999.

Stetson CL, Rapini RP, Tyring SK, Kimbrough RC. CD4+ T lymphocytopenia with disseminated HPV. J Cutan Pathol 29:502–505, 2002.

Stobo JD, Paul S, Van Scoy RE, Hermans PE. Suppression of thymus-derived lymphocytes in fungal infection. J Clin Invest 57:319–328, 1976.

Stohl W, Crow MK, Kunkel HG. Systemic lupus erythematosus with deficiency of the T4 epitope on T helper/inducer cells. N Engl J Med 12:1671–1678, 1985.

Stormorken H, Hellum B, Egeland T, Abrahamsen TG, Hovig T. X-linked thrombocytopenia and thrombocytopathia: attenuated Wiskott-Aldrich syndrome. Functional and morphological studies of platelets and lymphocytes. Thromb Haemost 65:300–305, 1991.

Stowers L, Yelon D, Berg LJ, Chant J. Regulation of the polarization of T cells toward antigen-presenting cells by Ras-related GTPase CDC42. Proc Natl Acad Sci USA 92:5027–5031, 1995.

Sugama S, Namihira T, Matsuoka R, Taira N, Eto Y, Maekawa K. Psychiatric inpatients and chromosome deletions within 22q11.2. J Neuro Neurosurg Psychiatry 67:803–806, 1999.

Sulisalo T, Sistonen P, Hastbacka J, Wadelius C, Makitie O, de la Chapelle A, Kaitila I. Cartilage-hair hypoplasia gene assigned to chromosome 9 by linkage analysis. Nat Genet 3:338–341, 1993.

Sullivan JL. The abnormal gene in X-linked lymphoproliferative syndrome. Curr Opin Immunol 11:431–434, 1999.

Sullivan JL, Byron KS, Brewster FE, Baker SM, Ochs HD. X-linked lymphoproliferative syndrome: natural history of the immunodeficiency. J Clin Invest 71:1765–1778, 1983.

Sullivan JL, Byron KS, Brewster FE, Purtilo DT. Deficient natural killer cell activity in the X-linked lymphoproliferative syndrome. Science 210:543–545, 1980.

Sullivan KE, Delaat CA, Douglas SD, Filipovich, AH. Defective natural killer cell function in patients with hemophagocytic lymphohistiocytosis and in first degree relatives. Pediatr Res 44:465–468, 1998a.

Sullivan KE, Jawad AF, Randall P, Driscoll DA, Emanuel BS, McDonald-McGinn DM, Zackai EH. Lack of correlation between impaired T cell production, immunodeficiency and other phenotypic features in chromosome 22q11.2 deletions syndrome (DiGeorge syndrome/velocardiofacial syndrome). Clin Immunol Immunopathol 84:141–146, 1998b.

Sullivan KE, Mullen CA, Blaese RM Winkelstein JA. A multiinstitutional survey of the Wiskott-Aldrich syndrome. J Pediatr 125:876–885, 1994.

Sullivan JL, Woda BA. X-linked lymphoproliferative syndrome. Immunodefic Rev 1:325–347, 1989.

Sumegi J, Huang D, Lanyi A, Davis JD, Seemayer TA, Maeda A, Klein G, Seri M, Wakiguchi H, Purtilo DT, Gross TG. Correlation of mutations of the SH2D1A gene and Epstein-Barr virus infection with clinical phenotype and outcome in X-linked lymphoproliferative disease. Blood 96:3118–3125, 2000.

Sweetman L, Shur L, Nyhan WL, Deficiencies of proprionyl-CoA and 3-methylcrotonyl-CoA carboxylases in a patient with a dietary deficiency of biotin. Clin Res 27:118abs, 1979.

Swillen A, Devriendt K, Legius E, Eyskens B, Dumoulin M, Gewillig M, Fryns JP. Intelligence and psychosocial adjustment in velocardiofacial syndrome: a study of 37 children and adolescents with VCFS. J Med Genet 34:453–458, 1997.

Swillen A, Devriendt K, Legius E, Prinzie P, Vogels A, Ghesquiere P, Fryns JP. The behavioural phenotype in velo-cardio-facial syndrome (VCFS): from infancy to adolescence. Genet Counsel 10:79–88, 1999.

Sykes KS, Bachrach LK, Siegel-Bartelt J, Ipp M, Kooh SW, Cytrynbaum C. Velocardiofacial syndrome presenting as hypocalcemia in early adolescence. Arch Pediatr Adolesc Med 151:745–747, 1997.

Symons M, Derry JM, Karlak B, Jiang S, Lemahieu V, McCormick F, Francke U, Abo A. Wiskott-Aldrich syndrome protein, a novel effector for the GTPase CDC42Hs, is implicated in actin polymerization. Cell 84:723–734, 1996.

Takagishi Y, Oda S, Hayasaka S, Dekker Ohno, K, Shikata T, Inouye M, Yamamura H. The dilute-lethal (dl) gene attacks a Ca2+ store in the dendritic spine of Purkinje cells in mice Neurosci Lett 215:169–172, 1996.

Takenaka T, Kuribayashi K, Nakamine H, Yoshikawa F, Maeda J, Kishi S, Nakauchi H, Minatogawa Y, Kido R. Autosomal codominant inheritance and Japanese incidence of deficiency of OKT4 epitope with lack of reactivity resulting from conformational change. J Immunol 151:2864–2870, 1993.

Tangye SG, Phillips JH, Lanier LL, Nichols KE. Functional requirement for SAP in 2B4-mediated activation of human natural killer cells as revealed by the X-linked lymphoproliferative syndrome. J Immunol 165:2932–2936, 2000.

Taniuchi S, Yamamoto A, Fujiwara T, Hasui M, Tsuji S, Kobayashi Y. Dizygotic twin sisters with myelokathexis: mechanism of its neutropenia. Am J Hematol 62:106–111, 1999.

Tassinari P, Deibis L, Bianco N, Echeverria de Perez G. Lymphocyte subset diversity in idiopathic CD4+ T lymphocytopenia. Clin Diagn Lab Immunol 3:611–6613, 1996.

ten Bensel RW, Stadlan EM, Krivit W. The development of malignancy in the course of the Aldrich syndrome. J Pediatr 68:761–767, 1966.

Tezcan I, Sanal O, Ersoy F, Uckan D, Kilic S, Metin A, Cetin M, Akin R, Oner C, Tuncer A. Successful bone marrow transplantation in a case of Griscelli disease which presented in accelerated phase with neurological involvement. Bone Marrow Transplant 24:931–933, 1999.

Thompson AD, Braun BS, Arvand A, Stewart SD, May WA, Chen E, Korenberg J, Denny C. EAT-2 is a novel SH2 domain containing protein that is up regulated by Ewing's sarcoma EWS/FLI1 fusion gene. Oncogene 13:2649–2458, 1996.

Thong YH, Robertson EF, Rischbieth HG, Smith GF, Chetney K, Pollard AC. Successful restoration of immunity in the DiGeorge syndrome with fetal thymic epithelial transplant. Arch Dis Child 53:580–584, 1978.

Thorjak JE, Polmar SH, Winkelstein JA, Hsu S, Francomano C, Pierce GF, Scillian JJ, Gale AN, McKusick VA. Immunologic studies of cartilage hair hypoplasia in the Amish. John Hopkins Med J 148:157–164, 1981.

Thorpe ES, Handley HE. Chronic tetany and chronic mycelial stomatitis in a child aged four and one-half years. Am J Dis Child 38:228–338, 1929.

Thrasher AJ. WASP in immune-system organization and function. Nat Rev Immunol 2:635–646, 2002.

Thrasher AJ, Jones GE, Kinnon C, Brickell PM and Katz DR. Is Wiskott-Aldrich syndrome a cell trafficking disorder? Immunol Today 19:537–539, 1998.

Titus M. Myosins: myosin V—the multi-purpose transport motor. Curr Biol 7:R301–304, 1997.

Tobias ES, Morrison N, Whiteford ML, Tolmie JL. Towards earlier diagnosis of 22q11 deletions. Arch Dis Child 81:513–514, 1999.

Tollervey D, Kiss T. Function and synthesis of small nucleolar RNAs. Curr Opin Cell Biol 9:337–342, 1997.

Tommasini A, Ferrari S, Moratto D, Badolato R, Boniotto M, Pirulli D, Notarangelo LD, Andolina M. X-chromosome inactivation analysis in a female carrier of FOXP3 mutation. Clin Exp Immunol 130:127–130, 2002.

Topper JN, Clayton DA. Characterization of human MRP/Th RNA is an active endoribonuclease when assembled as RNP. Nucleic Acids Res 18:793–799, 1990.

Torgerson TR, Ochs HD. Immune dysregulation, polyendocrinopathy, enteropathy, X-linked syndrome: a model of immune dysregulation. Curr Opin Allergy Clin Immunol 2:481–487, 2002.

Tornai I, Kiss A, Laczko J. Wiskott-Aldrich syndrome in a heterozygous carrier woman. Eur J Haematol 42:501–502, 1989

Tuvia J, Weisselberg B, Shif I, Keren G. Aplastic anaemia complicating adenovirus infection in DiGeorge syndrome. Eur J Pediatr 147:643–644, 1988.

Twomey JJ, Waddell CC, Krantz S, O'Reilly R, L'Esperance P, Good RA. Chronic mucocutaneous candidiasis with macrophage dysfunction, a plasma inhibitor, and co-existent aplastic anemia. J Lab Clin Med 85:968–977, 1975.

Usiskin SI, Nicolson R, Krasnewich DM, Yan W, Lenane M, Wudarsky M, Hamburger SD, Rapoport JL. Velocardiofacial syndrome in childhood-onset schizophrenia. J Am Acad Child Adolesc Psych 38:1536–1543, 1999.

Valdimarsson H, Higgs JM, Wells RS, Yamamura M, Hobbs JR, Holt PJL. Immune abnormalities associated with chronic mucocutaneous candidiasis. Cell Immunol 6:348–361, 1973.

Valdimarsson H, Moss PD, Holt PJL, Hobbs JR. Treatment of chronic mucocutaneous candidiasis with leukocytes from HLA-compatible sibling. Lancet I:469–472, 1972.

Valenzuela-Fernandera A, Planchenault T, Baleux F, Staropoli I, Le-Barillec K, Leduc D, Delaunay T, Lazarini F, Virelizier JL, Chignard M, Pidard D, Arenzana-Seisdedos F. Leukocyte elastase negatively regulates Stromal cell-derived factor-1 (SDF-1)/CXCR4 binding and functions by amino-terminal processing of SDF-1 and CXCR4. J Biol Chem 277:15677–15689, 2002.

van der Burgt I, Haraldsson A, Oosterwijk JC, van Essen AJ, Weemaes KC, Hamel B. Cartilage hair hypoplasia, metaphyseal chondrodysplasia type McKusick: Description of seven patients and review of the literature. Am J Med Genet 41:371–380, 1991.

Van Esch H, Groenen P, Fryns JP, Van de Ven W, Devriendt K. The phenotypic spectrum of the 10p deletion syndrome versus the classical DiGeorge syndrome. Genet Counsel 10:59–65, 1999.

Van Esch H, Groenen P, Nesbitt MA, Schuffenhauer S, Lichtner P, Vanderlinden G, Harding B, Beetz R, Bilous RW, Holdaway I, Shaw NJ, Fryns J-P, Van de Ven W, Thakker RV, Devriendt K. GATA3 haplo-insufficiency causes human HDR syndrome. Nature 406:419–422, 2000.

Van Scoy RE, Hill HR, Ritts RE, Quie PG. Familial neutrophil chemotaxis defect, recurrent bacterial infections, mucocutaneous candidiasis, and hyperimmunoglobulinemia E. Ann Intern Med 82:776–781, 1975.

Vantrappen G, Devriendt K, Swillen A, Rommel N, Vogels A, Eyskens B, Gewillig M, Feenstra L, Fryns JP. Presenting symptoms and clinical features in 130 patients with the velo-cardio-facial syndrome. The Leuven experience. Genet Counsel 10:3–9, 1999.

Veillette A, Latour S. The SLAM family of immune-cell receptors. Curr Opin Immunol 15:277–285, 2003.

Venzor J, Hua Q, Bressler RB, Miranda CH, Huston DP. Behcet's-like syndrome associated with idiopathic CD4+ T-lymphocytopenia, opportunistic infections, and a large population of TCR alpha beta+ CD4- CD8- T cells. Am J Med Sci 313:236–238, 1997.

Vercelli D, Jabara HH, Cunningham-Rundles C, Abrams JS, Lewis DB, Meyer J, Schneider LC, Leung DYM, Geha RS. Regulation of immunoglobulin (Ig)E synthesis in the hyper IgE syndrome. J Clin Invest 85:1666–1671, 1990.

Verhagen CE, de Boer T, Smits H, Verreck FAW, Wierenga EA, Kurimoto M, Lammas A, Kumararatne D, Sanal O, Kroon F, van Dissel JT, Sinigaglia F, Ottenhoff THM. Residual type 1 immunity in patients genetically deficient for interleukin 12 β1 (IL-12β1): evidence for an IL-12Rβ1-independent pathway of IL-12 responsiveness in humans T cells. J Exp Med 192:517–528, 2000.

Verloes A, Curry C, Jamar M, Herens C, O'Lague P, Marks J, Sarda P, Blanchet P. Juvenile rheumatoid arthritis and del(22q11) syndrome: a non-random association. J Med Genet 35:943–947, 1998.

Villa A, Notarangelo L, Macchi P, Mantuano E, Cavagni G, Brugnoni D, Strina D, Patrosso MC, Ramenghi U, Sacco MG, et al. X-linked thrombocytopenia and Wiskott-Aldrich syndrome are allelic diseases with mutations in the WASP gene. Nat Genet 9:414–417, 1995.

Vogel A, Strassburg CP, Obermayer-Straub P, Brabant G, Manns MP. The genetic background of autoimmune polyendocrinopathy-candidiasis-ectodermal dystrophy and its autoimmune disease components. J Mol Med 80:201–211, 2002.

Wada T, Jagadeesh GJ, Nelson DL, Candotti F. Retrovirus-mediated WASP gene transfer corrects Wiskott-Aldrich syndrome T-cell dysfunction. Hum Gene Ther 13:1039–1046, 2002.

Wada T, Schurman SH, Otsu M, Garabedian EK, Ochs HD, Nelson DL, Candotti F. Somatic mosaicism in Wiskott–Aldrich syndrome suggests in vivo reversion by a DNA slippage mechanism. Proc Natl Acad Sci U S A 98:8697–8702, 2001.

Wagner M, Muller-Berghaus J, Schroeder RS, Luka J, Leyssens N, Schneider B, Krueger G. Human herpesvirus-6 (HHV-6)-associated necrotizing encephalitis in Griscelli's syndrome. J Med Virol 53:306–312, 1997.

Wakeel RA, Urbaniak SJ, Armstrong SS, Sewell HF, Herriot R, Kernohan N, White MI. Idiopathic CD4+ lymphocytopenia associated with chronic pruritic papules. Br J Dermatol 131:371–375, 1994.

Wakim M, Alazard M, Yajima A, Speights D, Saxon A, Stiehm ER. High dose intravenous immunoglobulin in atopic dermatitis and hyper-IgE syndrome. Ann Allergy Asthma Immunol 81:153–158, 1998.

Walsh GA, Richards KL, Douglas SD, Blumenthal MN. Immunoglobulin E anti-Staphylococcus aureus antibodies in atopic patients. J Clin Microbiol 13:1046–1048, 1981.

Wang CY, Shi JD, Davoodi-Semiromi A, She JX. Cloning of AIRE, the mouse homologue of the autoimmune regulator (AIRE) gene responsible for autoimmune polyglandular syndrome type 1. Genomics 55:322–326, 1999

Wang JF, Park IW, Groopman JE. Stromal cell-derived factor-1alpha stimulates tyrosine phosphorylation of multiple focal adhesion proteins and induces migration of hematopoietic progenitor cells: roles of phosphoinositide-3 kinase and protein kinase C. Blood 95:2505–2513, 2000a.

Wang PP, Woodin MF, Kreps-Falk R, Moss EM. Research on behavioral phenotypes: velocardiofacial syndrome (deletion 22q11.2). Develop Med Child Neurol 42:422–427, 2000b.

Warnatz K, Draeger R, Schlesier M, Peter HH. Successful IL-2 therapy for relapsing herpes zoster infection in a patient with idiopathic CD4+ T lymphocytopenia. Immunobiology 202:204–211, 2000.

Washington K, Gossage DL, Gottfried MR. Pathology of the liver in severe combined immunodeficiency and DiGeorge syndrome. Pediatr Path 13:485–504, 1993.

Washington K, Gossage DL, Gottfried MR. Pathology of the pancreas in severe combined immunodeficiency and DiGeorge syndrome: acute graft-versus-host disease and unusual viral infections. Hum Pathol 25:908–914, 1994.

Watanabe H, Inukai A, Doyu M, Sobue G. CNS cryptococcosis with idiopathic CD4+ T lymphocytopenia. Rinsho Shinkeigaku 40:249–253, 2000.

Webber SA, Hatchwell E, Barber JC, Daubeney PE, Crolla JA, Salmon AP, Keeton BR, Temple IK, Dennis NR. Importance of microdeletions of chromosomal region 22q11 as a cause of selected malformations of the ventricular outflow tracts and aortic arch: a three-year prospective study. J Pediatr 129:26–32, 1996.

Weinzimer SA, McDonald-McGinn DM, Driscoll DA, Emanuel BS, Zackai EH, Moshang T Jr. Growth hormone deficiency in patients with 22q11.2 deletion: expanding the phenotype. Pediatrics 101:929–932, 1998.

Weisenburger DD, Purtilo DT. Failure in immunological control of the virus infection: fatal infectious mononucleosis. In Epstein MA,

Achong BG, eds. Epstein-Barr Virus: Recent Advances. New York, John Wiley and Sons, 1986, pp 129–58.

Weller E, Weller R, Jawad A, Jessani N, Francisco-Solon E, Schecter J, Hoffman K, Hamarman S, Rowan A, Sanchez L. Psychiatric diagnoses in children with velocardiofacial syndrome. In American Academy of Child and Adolescent Psychiatry. Chicago, 1999.

Wells RS, Higgs JM, MacDonald A, Valdimarsson H, Holt PSL. Familial chronic mucocutaneous candidiasis. J Med Genet 9:302–310, 1972.

Wendland T, Herren S, Yawalkar N, Cerny A, Pichler WJ. Strong alpha/beta and gamma/delta TCR response in a patient with disseminated Mycobacterium avium infection and lack of NK cells and monocytopenia. Immunol Lett 72:75–82, 2000.

Wengler G, Gorlin JB, Williamson JM, Rosen FS, Bing DH. Nonrandom inactivation of the X chromosome in early lineage hematopoietic cells in carriers of Wiskott-Aldrich syndrome. Blood 85:2471–2477, 1995.

Weston B, Axtell RA, Todd RF, Vincent M, Balazovich KJ, Suchard SJ, Boxer LA. Clinical and biologic effects of granulocyte colony stimulating factor in the treatment of myelokathexis. J Pediatr 118:229–234, 1991.

Weston WL, Humbert JR, August CS, Harnett I, Mass MF, Dean PB, Hagan IM. A hyperimmunoglobulin E syndrome with normal chemotaxis in vitro and defective leukotaxis in vivo. J Allergy Clin Immunol 59:112–119, 1977.

Wetzler M, Talpaz M, Kellagher MJ, Gutterman JU, Kurzrock R. Myelokathexis: normalization of neutrophil counts and morphology by GM-CSF. JAMA 267:2179–2180, 1992.

Wetzler M, Talpaz M, Kleinerman ES, King A, Huh YO, Gutterman JU, Kurzrock R. A new familial immunodeficiency disorder characterized by severe neutropenia, a defective marrow release mechanism, and hypogammaglobulinemia. Am J Med 89:663–672, 1990.

Whitaker J, Landing BH, Esselborn VM, Williams RR. The syndrome of familial juvenile hypoadrenocorticism, hypothyroidism, and superficial moniliasis. J Clin Endocrinol 16:1374–1387, 1956.

Wildin RS, Ramsdell F, Peake J, Faravelli F, Casanova JL, Buist N, Levy-Lahad E, Mazzella M, Goulet O, Perroni L, Bricarelli FD, Byrne G, McEuen M, Proll S, Appleby M, Brunkow ME. X-linked neonatal diabetes mellitus, enteropathy and endocrinopathy syndrome is the human equivalent of mouse scurfy. Nat Genet 27:18–20, 2001.

Wildin RS, Smyk-Pearson S, Filipovich AH. Clinical and molecular features of the immunodysregulation, polyendocrinopathy, enteropathy, X linked (IPEX) syndrome. J Med Genet 39:537–545, 2002.

Wilhelm M, Weissinger F, Kunzmann V, Muller JG, Fahey JL. Idiopathic CD4+ T cell lymphocytopenia evolving to monoclonal immunoglobulins and progressive renal damage responsive to IL-2 therapy. Clin Immunol 99:298–304, 2001.

Wilson BD, Sohnle PG. Neutrophil accumulation and cutaneous responses in experimental cutaneous candidiasis of genetically complement-deficient mice. Clin Immunol Immunopathol 46:284–293, 1988.

Wilson, SM, Yip, R, Swing, DA, O'Sullivan, TN, Zhang, Y, Novak, EK, Swank, RT, Russell, LB, Copeland, NG, Jenkins, NA. A mutation in Rab27a causes the vesicle transport defects observed in ashen mice. Proc Natl Acad Sci U S A 97:7933–7938, 2000.

Wintergerst U, Meyer U, Remberger K, Belohradsky BH. Graft versus host reaction in an infant with DiGeorge syndrome. Monatsschrift Kinderheilkunde 137:345–347, 1989.

Wiskott A. Familiärer, angeborener Morbus Werlhofii? Monatsschr Kinderheilkd 68:212–216, 1937.

Witkin SS, Yu IR, Ledger WJ. A macrophage defect in women with recurrent Candida vaginitis and its reversal in vitro by prostaglandin inhibitors. Am J Obstet Gynecol 155:790–795, 1986.

Wolff JA, Bertucio M. A sex-linked genetic syndrome in a Negro family manifested by thrombocytopenia, eczema, bloody diarrhea, recurrent infection, anemia and epistaxis. Am J Dis Child 93:74, 1957.

Woolf Ja. Wiskott-Aldrich syndrome: clinical, immunologic, and pathologic observations. J Pediatr 70:221–232, 1967.

Wood DJ, David TJ, Chrystie IL, Totterdell B. Chronic enteric virus infection in two T-cell immunodeficient children. J Med Virol 24:435–444, 1988.

Wu C, Nguyen KB, Pien GC, Wang N, Gullo C, Howie D, Sosa MR, Edwards MJ, Borrow P, Satoskar AR, Sharpe AH, Biron CA, and Terhorst C. SAP controls T-cell responses to virus and terminal differentiation of TH2 cells. Nat Immunol 2:410–414, 2001.

Wu X, Bowers B, Wei Q, Kochner B, Hammer JA. Myosin V associates with melanosomes in mouse melanocytes: evidence that myosin V is an organelle motor J Cell Science 110:847–859, 1997.

Wyandt HE, Grierson HL, Sanger WG, Skare JC, Milunsky A, Purtilo DT. Chromosome deletion of Xq25 in an individual with X-linked lymphoproliferative disease. Am J Med Genet 33:426–430, 1989.

Yamada M, Ohtsu M, Kobayashi I, Kawamura N, Kobayashi K, Ariga T, Sakiyama Y, Nelson DL, Tsuruta S, Anakura M, Ishikawa N. Flow cytometric analysis of Wiskott-Aldrich syndrome (WAS) protein in lymphocytes from WAS patients and their familial carriers. Blood 93:756–757, 1999.

Yamagishi H, Garg V, Matsuoka R, Thomas T, Srivastava D. A molecular pathway revealing a genetic basis for human cardiac and craniofacial defects. Science 283:1158–1161, 1999.

Yamauchi PS, Nguyen NQ, Grimes PE. Idiopathic CD4+ T-cell lymphocytopenia associated with vitiligo. J Am Acad Dermatol 46:779–782, 2002.

Yamazaki M, Yasui K, Kawai H, Miyagawa Y, Komiyama A, Akabane T. A monocyte disorder in siblings with chronic candidiasis: a combined abnormality of monocyte mobility and phagocytosis killing ability. Am J Dis Child 138:192–196, 1984.

Yan W, Jacobsen LK, Krasnewich DM, Guan XY, Lenane MC, Paul SP, Dalwadi HN, Zhang H, Long RT, Kumra S, Martin BM, Scambler PJ, Trent JM, Sidransky E, Ginns EI, Rapoport JL. Chromosome 22q11.2 interstitial deletions among childhood-onset schizophrenics and "multidimensionally impaired". Am J Med Genet 81:41–43, 1998.

Yap GS, Sher A. Effector cells of both nonhematopoietic and hemopoietic origin are required for interferon (IFN)-gamma- and tumor necrosis factor (TNF)-alpha-dependent host resistance to the intracellular pathogen, *Toxoplasma gondii*. J Exp Med 189:1083–1092, 1999.

Yasuda N, Lai PK, Rogers J, Purtlo DT. Defective control of Epstein-Barr virus-infected B cell growth in patients with X-linked lymphoproliferative disease. Clin Exp Immunol 83:10–16, 1991.

Zaharatos GJ, Behr MA, Libman MD. Profound T-lymphocytopenia and cryptococcemia in a human immunodeficiency virus-seronegative patient with disseminated tuberculosis. Clin Infect Dis 33:E125–128, 2001.

Zanelli G, Sansoni A, Ricciardi B, Ciacci C, Cellesi C. Muscular-skeletal cryptococcosis in a patient with idiopathic CD4+ lymphopenia. Mycopathologia 149:137–139, 2001.

Zhu Q, Christie JR, Tyler EO, Watanabe M, Sibly B, Ochs HD. X-chromosome inactivation in symptomatic carrier females of X-linked thrombocytopenia. Clin Immunol 103:S129–130, 2002.

Zhu Q, Watanabe C, Liu T, Hollenbaugh D, Blaese RM, Kanner SB, Aruffo A, Ochs HD. Wiskott-Aldrich syndrome/X-linked thrombocytopenia: WASP gene mutations, protein expression, and phenotype. Blood 90:2680–2689, 1997.

Zhu Q, Zhang M, Blaese RM, Derry JM, Junker A, Francke U, Chen SH, Ochs HD. The Wiskott-Aldrich syndrome and X-linked congenital thrombocytopenia are caused by mutations of the same gene. Blood 86:3797–3804, 1995.

Zicha D, Allen WE, Brickell PM, Kinnon C, Dunn GA, Jones GE, Thrasher AJ. Chemotaxis of macrophages is abolished in the Wiskott-Aldrich syndrome. Br J Haematol 101:659–665, 1998.

Ziegner UH, Ochs HD, Schanen C, Feig SA, Seyama K, Futatani T, Gross T, Wakim M, Roberts RL, Rawlings DJ, Dovat S, Fraser JK, Stiehm ER. Unrelated umbilical cord stem cell transplantation for X-linked immunodeficiencies. J Pediatr 138:570–573, 2001.

Zuelzer WW. Myelokathexis—a new form of chronic granulocytopenia: report of a case. N Engl J Med 270:699–704, 1964.

CHAPTER

18

Chromosomal Breakage Syndromes Associated with Immunodeficiency

Martin F. Lavin and Howard M. Lederman

INTRODUCTION

Chromosomal breakage syndromes represent a number of human genetic disorders characterized by genome instability, detected in the basal state (spontaneously)

580

or in response to DNA-damaging agents (Table 18-1). These syndromes show defects in the recognition and/or repair of damage to DNA inflicted by different agents. In most cases the genome instability is accompanied by a predisposition to develop cancer.

This chapter focuses on a subgroup of chromosomal breakage syndromes that have an associated immunodeficiency. Each of these syndromes has a distinct clinical phenotype and a distinct pattern of chromosome aberrations. These syndromes include ataxia-telangiectasia (A-T), A-T–like disorder (ATLD), Nijmegen breakage syndrome (NBS), Bloom syndrome (BS), immunodeficiency/centromeric instability/facial anomalies syndrome (ICF), and Fanconi's anemia (FA). These disorders are also discussed in Chapter 24.

Although these syndromes are defined by specific characteristics, it is evident that they overlap in some features that can be explained by interactions between their protein products and/or common signaling pathways.

ATAXIA-TELANGIECTASIA

Ataxia-telangiectasia is an autosomal recessive disorder causing progressive neurodegeneration, immunodeficiency, cutaneous abnormalities (including telangiectasia), predisposition to malignancy, and premature aging.

Historical Aspects

Several reports of patients with ataxia and telangiectasia were published early in the twentieth century (Louis-Bar, 1941; Syllaba and Henner, 1926), but A-T was not recognized as a distinct disease until two groups published reports of children with a familial syndrome of progressive cerebellar ataxia, oculocutaneous telangiectasia, and frequent pulmonary infections (Biemond, 1957; Boder and Sedgwick, 1957).

Soon thereafter it was recognized that patients had a marked tendency to develop lymphoreticular malignancies (Boder and Sedgwick, 1963) and had a variable degree of humoral immune deficiency, as well as thymic hypoplasia (Peterson et al., 1964). On the basis of

TABLE 18-1 · CHARACTERISTICS OF CHROMOSOMAL BREAKAGE SYNDROMES

Syndrome	Immunodeficiency	Cancer Predisposition
Ataxia-telangiectasia	+	+
Ataxia-telangiectasia–like disorder	+	?
Bloom syndrome	+	+
Nijmegen breakage syndrome	+	+
Fanconi's anemia	±	+
Immunodeficiency/centromeric instability/facial anomalies syndrome	+	−
Cockayne syndrome	−	−
Trichothiodystrophy	−	−
Xeroderma pigmentosa	−	+
DNA ligase I deficiency	+	?

segregation analysis in 64 affected families, autosomal recessive inheritance was predicted (Tadjoedin and Fraser, 1965). The prevalence of A-T in the population has been estimated to be as high as 1 in 40,000 live births.

Pathogenesis

Genetics

The A-T locus was mapped by Gatti and colleagues (1988) to 11q 22-23. Combined genetic and molecular analyses provided detailed physical maps of the region and a high-density array of genetic markers (Lange et al., 1995), leading to the identification of the ataxia-telangiectasia mutated gene, *ATM* (Savitsky et al., 1995a).

The identification of a single gene for A-T, for which no alternative transcripts in the coding sequence were identified, questioned the earlier description of several separate complementation groups for this syndrome (Lange et al., 1993). The existence of separate complementation groups has still not been satisfactorily explained, but it seems likely that a limitation of the complementation assays may account for this observation.

The ATM gene is large, occupying 150 kb of genomic DNA, containing 66 exons, and encoding a 13-kb transcript (Savitsky et al., 1995b; Uziel et al., 1996). The open reading frame (complementary DNA [cDNA], 9.168 kb) predicts a 350-kD protein composed of 3056 amino acids, but the actual size is closer to 370 kD, at least in part due to phosphorylation of the protein (Chen and Lee, 1996). The N-terminal region of *ATM* has homology for yeast DNA repair/cell cycle checkpoint genes such as RAD3 and MEC1; the C-terminal region has phosphoinositol 3-kinase homology. There are no apparent "hot spots" for *ATM* mutations, but mutation sites span the entire open reading frame (for a catalog of mutations, see http://www.vmresearch.org/atm.htm).

Mutation analysis, using the protein truncation test, restriction endonuclease fingerprinting, single-strand conformation polymorphism, and conformation sensitive gel electrophoresis, has revealed that 70% of *ATM* mutations are predicted to give rise to a truncated protein (Byrd et al., 1996; Gilad et al., 1996; Telatar et al., 1996; Wright et al., 1996). Failure to detect ATM protein by immunoblotting in these cases suggests that truncated proteins are very unstable (Brown et al., 1997; Keegan et al., 1996; Lakin et al., 1996; Watters et al., 1997). In support of this, an unstable ATM arises from a truncating mutation that leads to the loss of only 10 amino acids from the C-terminal end of the protein (Gilad et al., 1998). In addition, missense mutations in the kinase domain of the protein also destabilize the protein. Short in-frame deletions are observed, with 7636del9 perhaps the most common mutation, enriched in the British/Irish population.

These patients have detectable levels of intracellular ATM, but no detectable levels of catalytic activity in the ATM protein and a typical A-T phenotype. A near full-length ATM protein is detected in A-T cells carrying this mutation (Watters et al., 1997), and a mouse homozygous for this knock-in mutation has been produced that differs significantly in its phenotype from ATM$^{-/-}$ mice (Spring et al., 2001).

Cellular and Molecular Biology

A comprehensive list of biochemical and cellular abnormalities in A-T is discussed in Lavin and Shiloh (1997). Of these, the cellular response to ionizing radiation is best described. The first indication of hypersensitivity to radiation in A-T was reported as an unexpectedly severe adverse response to radiotherapy for lymphoid malignancy (Gotoff et al., 1967; Morgan et al., 1968). Cellular sensitivity became evident from reduced survival and increased levels of chromosome aberrations after radiation exposure in vitro (Higurashi and Cohen, 1973; Taylor et al., 1975).

Intermediate sensitivity to radiation was subsequently demonstrated in A-T heterozygotes (Chen et al., 1978; Swift et al., 1991). It is still not firmly established why A-T cells are hypersensitive to radiation, but failure to repair 10% of double-strand breaks in DNA or inappropriate repair of some of these lesions could account for this sensitivity (Cornforth and Bedford, 1985; Foray et al., 1997).

It appears likely that ATM is a sensor of double-strand breaks in DNA and transduces this information to enzymes involved in the repair of DNA damage and in cell cycle checkpoint control (Fig. 18-1). Other proteins involved in double-strand break recognition and repair include DNA-dependent protein kinase (DNA-PK) and

DNA Double-Strand Break (dsbs) Damage Response

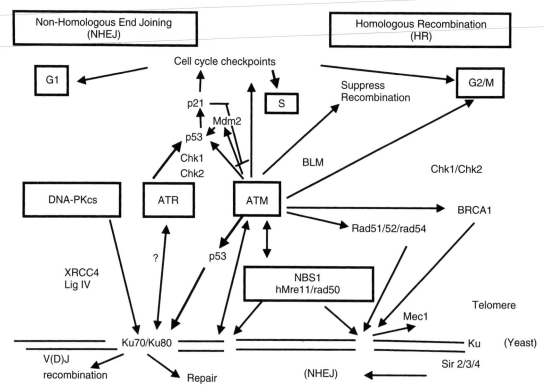

Figure 18-1 · **ATM and other proteins that regulate cell cycle progression and repair of double-strand DNA breaks.** ATM is at the center of a complicated pathway to detect double-strand DNA breaks. Activated ATM directly phosphorylates p53 (serine 15), Chk2 (threonine 68), MDM2 (serine 395), and NBS1 (serine 343). Chk2 subsequently phosphorylates p53 (serine 20), inhibiting the binding of p53 to MDM2 and thereby increasing the concentration of free p53 protein. This transcriptionally induces p21, which leads to cell cycle arrest in G1 phase. The phosphorylation of NBS1 causes S-phase cell cycle arrest. NBS1 exists in a complex with hMre11, rad 50, and BRCA1. These proteins become associated with double-strand DNA breaks in the early stages of cellular response.

NBS1, the product of the gene defective in Nijmegen breakage syndrome. DNA-PKcs, the catalytic subunit of DNA-PK, is one of a family of proteins that share a phosphoinositol 3-kinase domain and are involved in the cellular response to DNA damage and cell cycle control (Lavin et al., 1995). ATM is also a member of this family.

Mutations in DNA-PKcs give rise to the *scid* phenotype in mice, characterized by radiosensitivity, chromosomal instability, and combined immunodeficiency, features that are shared with A-T (Biedermann et al., 1991; Lieber et al., 1988). DNA-PKcs is recruited to double-strand breaks in DNA by the Ku proteins, KU70 and KU80, leading to its activation to phosphorylate substrates involved in DNA repair (Gottlieb and Jackson, 1994). In the absence of DNA-PK, the majority of double-strand breaks in DNA remain unrepaired, whereas this figure is only 10% in A-T cells.

Overlap between the DNA damage recognition pathways for ATM and DNA-PK is indicated by recent data describing negative regulatory control of c-Abl on DNA-PK in an ATM-dependent mechanism (Shangary et al., 2000). As is discussed later, overlap also exists between ATM and NBS1 in the recognition of breaks in

DNA, because ATM phosphorylates NBS1 in response to DNA damage and deficiency in this step contributes to radiosensitivity.

What distinguishes the functions of ATM and DNA-PK is that only ATM is capable of signaling DNA damage to cell cycle checkpoints. These checkpoints were first described in yeast and are activated to delay the passage of cells through the various phases of the cell cycle, ensuring that episodic DNA damage or DNA replication interruptions are repaired to maintain the integrity of the genome. In yeast, mutations in these checkpoints lead to uncontrolled passage through the cell cycle, spontaneous loss of chromosomes, and hypersensitivity to ionizing radiation (Al-Khodairy and Carr, 1992; Weinert and Hartwell, 1990).

In A-T, defective cell cycle checkpoint control impairs the usual inhibition of DNA synthesis after cells are exposed to ionizing radiation (Houldsworth and Lavin, 1980; Painter and Young, 1980). A-T cells are defective in both the G1/S and G2/M checkpoints after irradiation (Beamish and Lavin, 1994; Nagasawa and Little, 1983).

The involvement of ATM in checkpoint control is best described for the G1/S transition. In response to radiation, the activation/stabilization of p53 is defective (Kastan et al., 1992; Khanna and Lavin, 1993), the induction of p21/WAF1 is impaired, and there is a failure to inhibit cyclinE-cdk2 kinase in A-T cells (Beamish et al., 1996; Canman et al., 1994; Dulic et al., 1994; Khanna et al., 1995). Activation of this pathway by ATM appears to be by direct interaction with p53, because these two proteins co-immunoprecipitate (Watters et al., 1997) and they have been shown to interact in vitro (Khanna et al., 1998). Radiation-induced phosphorylation of p53 on serine 15, which may contribute to transcriptional activation of p53 (Chehab et al., 2000), is defective in A-T cells and ATM plays a direct role in phosphorylating this site (Banin et al., 1998; Canman et al., 1998; Khanna et al., 1998).

ATM-dependent phosphorylation of p53 on serine 20 contributes to the stabilization of p53 by reducing interaction with MDM2, which targets p53 for proteosome degradation. This phosphorylation is mediated through the cell cycle checkpoint protein kinase Chk2 (Hirao et al., 2000). A third modification to p53, dephosphorylation of serine 376, has also been reported to be ATM-dependent (Waterman et al., 1998).

In summary, ATM plays both direct and indirect roles in controlling the radiation signal transduction pathway operating through p53 and its downstream effector molecules. Inefficient operation of this pathway in A-T cells accounts for the defective G1/S checkpoint.

A-T cells are also defective in controlling the G2/M checkpoint, but the molecular basis of this defect is less clear. Rapid phosphorylation of Chk2 in response to DNA damage is ATM dependent, and this is associated with Chk2 activation and inhibition of cdc25C and consequently inhibition of cdc2 cyclin B kinase and G2 delay. ATM phosphorylates Chk2 directly on threonine 68 (Ahn et al., 2000; Matsuoka et al., 2000); this alteration is biologically significant in that mutation at the site causes radiosensitivity.

Radiation Signal Transduction

ATM is a member of the phosphatidylinositol 3-kinase (P13K) family of proteins (Keith and Schreiber, 1995; Lavin et al., 1995), which are involved in the cellular response to DNA damage and cell cycle control. These include ATM, ATR (A-T and rad3-like) DNA-PK, FRAP, and RAFT1 from mammalian cells; Tel1p, Mec1p, and Rad3p from yeast; and mei-41 from Drosophila (Lavin and Shiloh, 1999).

Although ATM is related to P13K through its C-terminal domain, it appears not to be a lipid kinase but rather a protein kinase. This kinase activity can be determined in vivo using an antibody against serine 15 of p53 to detect phosphorylation or in vitro by incubating a substrate such as p53 with immunoprecipitated ATM in the presence of ^{32}P-ATP (adenosine triphosphate).

It is evident that a basal level of ATM kinase activity exists in untreated cell extracts and this increases twofold to fourfold when the cells are exposed to radiation or radiomimetic agents (Banin et al., 1998; Canman et al., 1998). It appears likely that ATM recognizes double-strand breaks in DNA and is activated as a consequence to phosphorylate a number of key substrates associated with DNA damage recognition and cell cycle control. The mechanism of activation of ATM kinase by DNA damage remains undescribed but may involve a post-translational modification such as phosphorylation.

Once activated, ATM phosphorylates key substrates such as p53 to contribute to its transcriptional activation in inducing p21/WAF1 to bring about G1 delay as described earlier. ATM also phosphorylates Chk2 to in turn phosphorylate p53 on serine 20 to stabilize the protein. To add to the complexity of control of the G1/S checkpoint, ATM phosphorylates MDM2, which could alter its ability to bind to and destabilize p53, and may also phosphorylate p53BP1, which regulates p53. Thus ATM is capable of attenuating a specific signaling pathway at four levels of control, presumably to ensure fine regulation.

Recent evidence suggests that ATM phosphorylates BRCA1 in response to radiation damage and that mutations in the phosphorylation sites cause a failure to rescue radiation sensitivity in a BRCA1-deficient cell line (Cortez et al., 1999; Gatei et al., 2000). ATR has also been shown to phosphorylate BRCA1 at several sites, some of which overlap with those for ATM phosphorylation (Chen, 2000). Phosphorylated BRCA1 complexes with rad51 to carry out homologous recombinational repair of DNA double-strand breaks (Sharan et al., 1997). Mutations in BRCA1 lead to defects in cell proliferation, sensitivity to DNA-damaging agents, and genome instability (Scully et al., 1997). It is particularly intriguing that mutations in BRCA1 cause a predisposition to breast cancer (Wooster et al., 1995) and that A-T carriers may be predisposed to the same cancer.

Considerable overlap exists in the phenotype of A-T and NBS with respect to radiosensitivity and defective repair of breaks in DNA (Shiloh, 1997). Accordingly, it was expected that the products of the genes involved might overlap in their roles of recognizing breaks in DNA. The product of the gene mutated in NBS, NBS1, was subsequently shown to be a substrate for ATM kinase (Gatei et al., 2000; Lim et al., 2000; Zhao et al., 2000). Phosphorylation of NBS1 in response to radiation damage was defective in A-T cells, and the site of phosphorylation was shown to be physiologically significant for the correction of radiosensitivity. This is discussed further, later in the chapter.

Clinical Manifestations

Neurologic

Ataxia is the earliest clinical manifestation of A-T (Crawford, 1998; Crawford et al., 2000; Sedgwick and Boder, 1991). Most children appear healthy at birth and attain age-appropriate early gross and fine motor skills. They begin walking at a normal age but are slow to develop fluidity of gait and are wobbly beyond the usual period of a few months after a toddler learns to walk. The instability of gait has several unusual features. Children with A-T walk on an unusually narrow base, whereas most cerebellar disorders lead to widened stance. Although children with A-T weave and wobble, they fall and sustain significant injuries less often than one might expect. The children prefer to walk quickly or run because momentum appears to be helpful. Characteristically, an individual with A-T has difficulty holding the head and trunk still when sitting or standing, but Romberg's sign is negative—that is, the difficulty is not increased when the eyes are closed.

Although gross motor function remains abnormal, it is often relatively stable until the age of 3 to 7 years. In fact, many patients appear to improve slowly over this period, presumably because superimposed maturation of other parts of the brain compensate for A-T–induced abnormalities. The diagnosis of A-T may be quite difficult at this stage unless there is a high index of suspicion, and the majority of children are misdiagnosed with cerebral palsy (Cabana et al., 1998).

By approximately age 7 years, children demonstrate deterioration of gross and fine motor skills or oculocutaneous telangiectasia and the diagnosis of cerebral palsy is reconsidered. Thereafter there is slow but relentless progression of neurologic abnormalities. By the second decade of life, most patients are confined to wheelchairs and ambulation without assistance is impossible.

Eye movements are abnormal, even in young children. A-T patients have difficulty moving their eyes and heads in smooth, coordinated pursuit of a moving object (Baloh et al., 1978; Lewis et al., 1999; Smith and Cogan, 1959). There is a delay in initiating eye movement, and the eyes move in a series of small jumps rather than in a single smooth motion. As the head moves to track a slowly moving object, the eyes are often left behind.

Most patients never develop normal speech, but as with gross and fine motor skills, deterioration is often not noted until after the age of 5 to 8 years. There is a characteristic delay in initiation of speech, and the speech is typically slow, with inappropriate emphasis placed on single words or syllables. Progressive difficulty with chewing and swallowing develops over time (Lefton-Greif et al., 2000). In young children, drooling is the major manifestation. As they get older and neurologic disease progresses, most children have problems chewing and require a long time to finish a meal. Coughing, particularly when drinking thin liquids, is common. In the second decade of life, lack of cough response and silent aspiration become prominent and patients experience significant decreases in weight for height.

Other prominent neurologic abnormalities include choreiform movements of the hands and feet, intention and essential tremor, and myoclonus (Boder and Sedgwick, 1957; Louis-Bar, 1941; Syllaba and Henner, 1926). Finally, there is a mixed sensorimotor length-dependent neuropathy, which manifests itself by the loss of ankle and knee deep-tendon reflexes as patients age (Gardner and Goodman, 1969).

Cutaneous

The most prominent cutaneous finding is the presence of telangiectasia. These typically first appear between the ages of 3 and 6 years (Boder, 1985). Telangiectasia are observed as bright red horizontal torturous streaks across the bulbar conjunctivae (Fig. 18-2) but also occur on the pinnae and other sun-exposed areas of the face and neck. These telangiectasia are of venous origin and are thought to occur as progeric changes. It has been proposed that A-T cells are in a constant state of oxidative stress (Barlow et al., 1999; Watters et al., 1999). Under those circumstances, ischemic changes due to oxidative stress in endothelial cells could lead to dilation of blood vessels giving rise to telangiectasia. In keeping with this hypothesis, it is well established that exposure of normal tissues to therapeutic doses of ionizing radiation produces oxidative stress and gives rise to telangiectasia (Bentzen and Overgaard, 1991).

It is perhaps unfortunate that this disease is named ataxia-telangiectasia because the delayed appearance of telangiectasia often results in delayed diagnosis (Cabana et al., 1998) (Fig. 18-3). It is also worth noting that telangiectasia occur in most but not all patients with A-T. At least some of the patients who lack telangiectasia but have other clinical and laboratory manifestations of A-T have a related disease, ATLD, caused by a mutation of hMRE11 (discussed later).

Other progeric changes, including premature graying of hair, atrophic thinning of the skin on hands and feet, and progressive areas of hypopigmentation and hyperpigmentation, are common (Reed et al., 1966). Over time a significant number of A-T patients develop problems with chronic and recurrent cutaneous warts and noninfectious cutaneous granulomas of unknown etiology (Drolet et al., 1997; Paller et al., 1991).

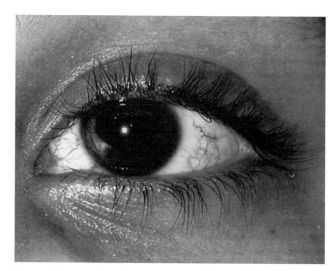

Figure 18-2 · Ocular telangiectasia in a patient with ataxia-telangiectasia. These large, tortuous, dilated blood vessels on the bulbar conjunctivae are typical findings in patients with A-T.

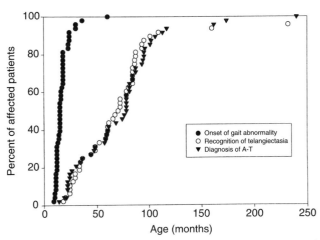

Figure 18-3 · Relationship among onset of ataxia, recognition of telangiectasia, and diagnosis of A-T. (Adapted from Cabana MD et al. Consequences of the delayed diagnosis of ataxia-telangiectasia. Pediatrics 102:98–100, 1998.)

Infection

Ataxia-telangiectasia is a primary immunodeficiency syndrome, but this characteristic is highly variable compared with the neurodegeneration. The incidence of infection, notably of the upper and lower respiratory tracts, varies from chronic sinopulmonary infections to levels of the same order as observed in unaffected siblings (McFarlin et al., 1972). Many patients do not develop difficulties with infections until the late stages of the disease, but historically, bacterial pneumonia and chronic lung disease have been a major cause of death (Sedgwick and Boder, 1991).

Infections outside the respiratory tract are generally not increased in frequency, and opportunistic infections rarely occur. For example, there are no published reports of fatal varicella or severe problems with herpes simplex virus, and only one report of a complication from a live viral vaccine (Pohl et al., 1992). Despite the common use of broad-spectrum antibiotics for respiratory tract infections, mucosal or cutaneous infections with *Candida* are unusual. Chronic and recurrent warts are the only opportunistic infection encountered with any regularity.

The lack of well-characterized cohorts of patients with longitudinal follow-up has made it difficult to determine the reasons for the predisposition to sinopulmonary infections. In some patients, infections are the result of antibody deficiency. However, swallowing dysfunction with aspiration, which becomes more severe as patients age (Lefton-Greif et al., 2000), may be as important as immunodeficiency in predisposing to lung infection.

Cancer

By most estimates, the lifetime prevalence of cancer in A-T patients is 10% to 30% (Spector et al., 1982) and cancer is the second most common cause of death (Boder and Sedgwick, 1963; Morrell et al., 1986; Taylor et al., 1996). This incidence is 60 to 184 times greater than expected for an age-matched population. Approximately 40% of cancers are non-Hodgkin's lymphomas, 25% are leukemias, 25% are assorted solid tumors, and 10% are Hodgkin's lymphomas (Hecht and Hecht, 1990; Spector et al., 1982). Of interest, most leukemias and lymphomas are of T-cell origin (Taylor et al., 1996), a pattern that is similar to that observed in A-T knockout mice (Barlow et al., 1996; Xu et al., 1996) but is remarkably different from the B-cell predominance of lymphoreticular malignancies in children without A-T. The solid tumors in A-T patients include adenocarcinoma, dysgerminoma, gonadoblastoma, and medulloblastoma.

The range and frequency of tumors (Hecht and Hecht, 1990) are probably best explained by genome instability arising from defective recognition and repair of double-strand DNA breaks, as well as defective cell cycle checkpoints. Genome instability is manifested as chromosomal aberrations, including translocations and inversions, especially involving chromosomes 7 and 14, with breakpoints traced to the T-cell receptor and immunoglobulin genes. Translocations involving chromosomes 12 and 14 are also observed, and in one case such an abnormal clone expanded to 80% of the lymphocyte population before the patient died of infection (Hecht et al., 1973).

The risk for cancer among heterozygotes is controversial. Swift and colleagues (1987, 1991; Athma et al., 1996) reported a 3.8-fold increased risk for breast cancer among A-T heterozygotes, particularly women older than age 60, compared with controls. These studies have been criticized because the incidence of breast cancer in the control population was unexpectedly low. However, several other epidemiologic studies also support an increased risk in A-T heterozygotes (Janin et al., 1999; Olsen et al., 2001). Fitzgerald and associates (1997) and others have performed tests for truncating ATM mutations in breast tumors occurring among the general population but have not found an increased incidence of A-T heterozygotes.

A unifying hypothesis proposes that the risk for breast cancer is greatest for heterozygotes with ATM missense mutations and that these are more difficult to detect in the general population (Gatti et al., 1999). Definitive studies have not yet been performed to resolve this issue. It is currently recommended that female obligate carriers scrupulously adhere to a schedule of monthly self-exams and routine mammography.

Because ATM plays a key role in DNA damage recognition and because the tumor types observed in A-T patients occur in the general population, it was expected that ATM might function as a tumor suppressor gene. Indeed, support for this hypothesis exists in that ATM mutations and impaired expression of ATM protein have been reported in T-cell prolymphocytic leukemia (Vorechovsky et al., 1997), B-cell chronic lymphocytic leukemia (Bullrich et al., 1999; Stankovic et al., 1999), and mantle cell lymphoma (Schaffner et al., 2000; Stankovic et al., 1999; Stoppa-Lyonnet et al., 1998; Yuille and Coignet, 1998).

Growth/Endocrine Problems

Many patients with A-T have somatic growth retardation. It is not known whether this is a direct effect of the ATM mutation or a nutritional consequence of abnormal swallow function. Problems with delayed or absent development of secondary sex characteristics are common. These include symptoms of irregular menstrual periods and amenorrhea due to ovarian dysgenesis in females (Miller and Chatten, 1967) and testicular atrophy in males. It is not known if A-T patients are capable of reproduction. Other endocrine abnormalities include diabetes mellitus, sometimes due to insulin resistance (Schalch et al., 1970); abnormalities of the anterior pituitary; and deficient growth hormone responses.

Survival

Most patients with A-T die in the second or third decade of life, though some individuals have survived longer. Historically, approximately half the patients have died from complications of chronic pulmonary disease and the other half from cancer. Rarely, patients have died from an infection at an extrapulmonary site or the sudden development of increased intracranial pressure associated with a central nervous system proliferation of telangiectasia.

Diagnosis and Differential Diagnosis

The diagnosis of A-T is relatively easy once the characteristic neurodegeneration and ocular telangiectasia have developed. In such cases the diagnosis can usually be confirmed by finding an elevated serum α-fetoprotein level. For this purpose, it should be remembered that α-fetoprotein levels in all children, with or without A-T, are elevated for the first 6 months of life when compared with the normal adult range. It is much more of a challenge to make the diagnosis in young children without progressive ataxia, in the minority of children who never develop telangiectasia, or in those children with atypical or mild phenotypes.

The identification of the ATM gene should theoretically facilitate diagnosis in such cases, but because the gene is so large and there are no mutational hot spots, mutational analysis has not been practical for clinical screening. Other confirmatory laboratory test results include absence of the ATM protein on Western blot, increased frequency of chromosomal breaks before and after exposure to x-irradiation, radioresistant DNA synthesis, and decreased colony survival after x-irradiation. None of these methods is 100% specific or 100% sensitive, and clinical correlation is essential.

A number of other disorders must be considered in the differential diagnosis. Chromosomal breakage and immunodeficiency may be features of Nijmegen breakage syndrome and Bloom syndrome, among others. At an age before telangiectasia or progressive neurologic dysfunction is present, cerebral palsy, structural abnormalities of the cerebellum, encephalitis or postencephalitis syndrome, brain tumor, and glycogen storage disease must be considered. Careful clinical follow-up and measurement of α-fetoprotein levels are the most useful tests for the majority of patients.

Laboratory Findings

The most consistent and characteristic laboratory abnormality is an elevation of the serum α-fetoprotein level in children older than age 8 months (Waldmann and McIntire, 1972). The level does not necessarily rise over time, and it does not correlate with severity of disease, presence of liver disease, or malignancy. Other causes for elevated α-fetoprotein levels in childhood include hepatitis, hereditary tyrosinemia, hepatoblastoma, and an asymptomatic autosomal recessive disorder of hereditary persistence of α-fetoprotein (Schefer et al., 1998). Each of these disorders can be easily excluded on the basis of associated physical or laboratory findings.

A wide range of laboratory abnormalities involving both humoral and cell-mediated immunity are present in individuals with A-T. However, it should be stressed that despite the high frequency of laboratory abnormalities, there is a striking lack of opportunistic infections and the risk for infection has never been closely correlated with any single or group of laboratory abnormalities (Nowak-Wegrzyn et al., 2004).

Absence or marked reductions of IgA (Ammann et al., 1969; Peterson et al., 1966; Waldmann et al., 1983), IgG2 and other IgG subclasses (Oxelius et al., 1982; Rivat-Peran et al., 1981; Sanal et al., 1999), and IgE (Ammann et al., 1969; Polmar et al., 1972; Waldmann et al., 1983) are the most commonly reported abnormalities of humoral immunity and each has been reported in as many as two thirds of patients.

Antibody responses to protein and polysaccharide vaccines vary from normal to markedly reduced (Berkel, 1986; Peterson et al., 1966; Roifman and Gelfand, 1985; Sanal et al., 1999; Sedgwick and Boder, 1972; Waldmann 1982). Deficiencies of antibody production have been ascribed to lack of T-cell helper function, overactivity of T-cell suppressor function, and intrinsic defects of B lymphocytes, but there is no consistent explanation.

Hypergammaglobulinemia, elevated levels of low-molecular-weight IgM, and oligoclonal or monoclonal gammopathy occur in as many as 8% of patients (Sadighi-Akha et al., 1999; Stobo and Tomasi, 1967). There is no apparent correlation between the presence of gammopathy and a particular T-lymphocyte subset profile, patient age, or emergence of neoplastic disease.

Throughout life, most A-T patients are moderately lymphopenic, with a prominent reduction in T lymphocytes (Waldmann 1982), a relative deficiency of total CD4 cells (Fiorilli et al., 1983; Lahat et al., 1988) and naïve CD4/CD45RA cells (Paganelli et al., 1992), and a relative increase in γ/δ-T cells (Carbonari et al., 1990). In all reports, the most consistent finding is the variability of immunodeficiency from patient to patient.

T-cell function is variably depressed, as measured by delayed-type hypersensitivity tests (Epstein et al., 1966; Ersoy et al., 1991; Kiran et al., 1974; Peterson et al., 1966; Roifman and Gelfand, 1985), in vitro lymphoproliferative responses to antigens and mitogens (Boutin et al., 1987; Fiorelli et al., 1983; Oppenheim et al., 1966; Paganelli et al., 1992; Rigas et al., 1970; Roifman and Gelfand, 1985), and skin homograft rejection (Epstein et al., 1966; Peterson et al., 1966).

In the vast majority of A-T patients, immunodeficiency is not progressive (Nowak-Wegrzyn et al., 2004). However, there have been several case reports of progressive lymphopenia, decreases in serum IgA, and increases in serum IgM (Ammann et al., 1969; Cawley and Schenken 1970).

Spontaneous cytogenetic abnormalities, including chromatid gaps, chromosomal breakage, translocations, rearrangements, and inversions, are observed in lymphocytes from the majority of patients (Taylor et al., 1981). The frequency of these abnormalities is greatly increased following in vitro exposure to radiographs and radiomimetic agents. Similarly, patient lymphoblasts have increased sensitivity to ionizing radiation when assessed in a colony survival assay (Huo et al., 1994).

The chromosomal damage is not random but tends to occur on chromosomes 7 and 14 within the immunoglobulin and T-cell receptor gene loci (Aurias et al., 1980; Kojis et al., 1991), pointing to a role for the ATM protein in recognition and processing of DNA double-strand breaks during the ontogeny of T and B cells (Taylor et al., 1976). Intrachromosomal recombination rates are elevated in A-T cells (Meyn, 1993), but no gross abnormality in signal and coding joint formation is evident during V(D)J recombination (Hsieh et al., 1993).

The immune defects recorded in A-T patients—thymus hypoplasia, defective T-cell–dependent immunity, and defective T-cell differentiation—are also observed in ATM gene-disrupted mice (Barlow et al., 1996; Xu et al., 1996; Elson et al., 1996). Introduction of a functional TCR transgene into $ATM^{-/-}$ mice rescued defective T-cell differentiation from the double-positive to the single-positive stage and partially rescued thymus hypoplasia (Chao et al., 2000). Because there were only slightly fewer T cells in $ATM^{-/-}$ TCR^+ compared with $ATM^{+/+}$ TCR^+, it has been suggested that lymphoid cells are functionally normal in $ATM^{-/-}$ mice and that the apparent developmental defect is secondary to defective thymocyte expansion. Nevertheless, given the marked thymic hypoplasia in A-T, it seems likely that developmental abnormalities contribute significantly to the defective cellular immunity.

Pathology

The most striking features of A-T occur in the cerebellum, where diffuse cortical degeneration primarily reflects progressive loss of Purkinje and granular cells (Boder, 1985; Sedgwick and Boder, 1991). In older patients the neurologic deterioration may extend to the dentate and olivary nuclei of the cerebellar cortex and outside the cerebellum to the substantia nigra, oculomotor nuclei, and dorsal root and sympathetic motor neurons (Sedgwick and Boder 1991). The presence of small numbers of ectopic Purkinje cells has led to speculation about a prenatal developmental defect in A-T. This is supported by data showing high levels of ATM expression in the fetal mouse brain (Herzog and McKinnon, 1998). Autopsies of occasional adults with A-T have shown prominent blood vessels or telangiectases within brain (Agamanolis and Greenstein, 1979; Amromin et al., 1979), but hemorrhage is rare (Terplan and Krauss, 1969).

Immunopathologic examination of A-T cases shows a variable degree of lymphoid hypoplasia (Aguilar et al., 1968; Peterson et al., 1964, 1966). However, interpretation is complicated by the fact that most material comes from autopsies of older individuals with lymphoreticular neoplasms, malnutrition, or a long history of corticosteroid therapy. The most instructive data come from a study of thymus and lymph node biopsies of young and relatively healthy A-T patients (Peterson, 1966). The thymus has normal lobules but is composed almost entirely of epithelial and stromal cells, with few lymphocytes and no Hassall's corpuscles. The appearance resembles the epithelial fetal thymus prior to its differentiation into a lymphoid organ. The findings of thymic atrophy, lymphoid depletion, and absence of Hassall's corpuscles are confirmed at autopsy of most A-T patients.

Inguinal lymph nodes, dissected 4 days after a regional injection of typhoid and diphtheria vaccines, show greater variability. The majority of nodes have normal general architecture, with germinal centers but depletion of cells from surrounding T-lymphocyte areas. A minority of patients lack germinal centers and plasma cells.

Treatment

At present, no therapy is known to slow or prevent neurologic deterioration, and care for patients with A-T is supportive. Immune function should be carefully evaluated. As in other disorders, hypogammaglobulinemia with antibody deficiency should be treated with immune globulin replacement. Individuals with recurrent lower respiratory tract infections should be assessed for swallowing dysfunction and aspiration. Corrective therapies include addition of thickeners to thin liquids and placement of a gastrostomy tube for feeding in some cases.

ATAXIA-TELANGIECTASIA–LIKE DISORDER

An A-T–like disorder has been described in four patients who presented with many but not all of the features of A-T. This disorder was subsequently found to be the result of mutations in hMRE11, a protein involved with

ATM in double-strand DNA break repair. There are still insufficient data to completely describe the clinical syndrome.

The reported patients with hMRE11 have progressive ataxia without telangiectasia (Hernandez et al., 1993; Klein et al., 1996). The progression of neurodegeneration in these patients was slow in comparison to that observed in the majority of A-T patients. For example, all were still ambulatory in their late teens and early twenties. However, in other respects they had characteristic neurologic features of A-T, including ataxic gait, abnormal eye movements, dysarthria, choreiform movements, intention tremor, and absent ankle reflexes. No ocular or cutaneous telangiectases were noted.

The laboratory findings also had some but not all of the characteristics of A-T. Peripheral blood lymphocytes had an increased level of spontaneous chromosome abnormalities and a large increase in chromatid-type damage after in vitro exposure to x-ray irradiation. Cultured skin fibroblasts showed decreased colony survival after exposure to gamma rays. However, in contrast to the findings in A-T patients, the levels of α-fetoprotein and immunoglobulins in the serum were normal.

At the time that the first kindred was described, the *ATM* gene had been mapped to chromosome 11q22-23 but not further identified. Haplotype analysis of ATLD patients found no linkage to this chromosomal location (Hernandez et al., 1993). The lack of ATM mutations was subsequently confirmed by restriction endonuclease fingerprinting, direct sequencing of selected parts of the cDNA, and detection of normal ATM protein levels on Western blots. Subsequent studies identified Nbs1 (mutated in Nijmegen breakage syndrome), hMre11, and hRad50 as members of a protein complex involved in recognition and repair of double-strand DNA breaks.

The presence of each of these proteins was therefore examined in the ATLD patients (Stewart et al., 1999). The patients of one kindred had complete absence of full-length hMre11 on Western blot, with a truncated protein observed in one of the patients. These cells also displayed a decrease in the levels of hRad50 and Nbs1 compared with normal controls. In the parents, hMre11 levels were reduced compared with normal control cells. In the second kindred, reduced levels of hMre11, hRad50, and Nbs1 proteins were observed in the patients and their mother, though their father had normal levels. Because levels of hMre11 were reduced in both kindreds, the sequence of the hMre11 gene was determined and mutations were identified in both kindreds (Pitts et al., 2001; Stewart et al., 1999).

The genetic locus for hMre11 is located on 11q21, and the locus for ATM is located on 11q23, so only detailed linkage analysis can separate ATLD from A-T. Mutation analysis will probably be required to distinguish the two disorders. Based on the relative size of the coding sequences of the two genes, it has been estimated that as many as 5% of A-T cases may, in fact, be due to mutations of hMre11. Until such studies are performed, it is not possible to know if the lack of oculocutaneous telangiectasia will reliably identify patients with hMre11. Similarly, genotype/phenotype correlations are needed before concluding that hMre11 mutations cause a milder form of neurodegeneration.

BLOOM SYNDROME

Bloom syndrome (BS) is an autosomal recessive chromosome instability syndrome characterized by short stature and predisposition to the early development of a variety of cancers (German, 1993; German and Ellis, 1996). Other variable features include sun-sensitive facial erythema, infertility, and immunodeficiency.

Although the syndrome is distinct from A-T, some of the characteristics overlap, including genome instability, aberrant DNA replication with extended S phase of the cell cycle, cancer predisposition, and propensity to develop diabetes (Ellis et al., 1995). Chromosomal interchanges represented by sister chromatid exchange (SCE) and those between chromosomes at homologous sites, manifested as quadraradials or telomeric associates, are characteristic of Bloom syndrome cells (Kuhn and Therman, 1986).

This syndrome is most common in people of Ashkenazi Jewish descent, among whom approximately 1% are carriers (Ellis et al., 1994). BS is grouped with other hereditary disorders manifesting age-related phenotypes. The protein products defective in these syndromes have in common seven conserved helicase motifs (Nakura et al., 2000).

Pathogenesis

Genetics

A high parental consanguinity rate among non-Ashkenazi families with BS allowed for homozygosity mapping to localize the gene defective in this syndrome (Ellis et al., 1994). Of the patients examined whose parents were related, 96% were homozygous for a polymorphic tetranucleotide repeat in the proto-oncogene FES, well in excess of that expected, indicating that the *BLM* gene is tightly linked to FES at 15q 26.1. Ironically the hypermutability of BS cells provided an important approach to more precisely mapping the *BLM* gene.

Ellis and associates (1995) observed that in some BS patients a minority of blood lymphocytes had normal SCE rates. Using lymphoblastoid cells from those low-SCE lymphocytes, they showed that polymorphic loci distal to the gene on 15q became homozygous, whereas markers proximal to the gene remained heterozygous.

These observations suggested that these low-SCE lymphocytes arose by recombination in patients who had inherited alleles from their parents that were mutated in different sites and thus had a functionally wild-type gene. The power of this approach was only limited by the density of polymorphic markers in the vicinity of the gene. A shift from heterozygosity to homozygosity was observed between the polymorphic loci D15S1108 and D15S127, a 250-kb region. A candidate for *BLM* was detected by direct selection of cDNA derived from this region (Ellis et al., 1995). Mutation analysis in BS patients revealed the presence of premature nonsense codons and missense mutations in this cDNA sequence. The size of the cDNA was 4437 nucleotides and coded for a 1417–amino acid peptide with homology to the RecQ family of helicases.

BLM is most closely related to the yeast proteins Rqhlp and Sgs1p (Kusano et al., 1999). Indeed, *BLM* has been demonstrated to suppress premature aging and increased homologous recombination caused by the *sgs1* mutation (Heo et al., 1999). Other human genes in the RecQ family include RECQ4, mutated in Rothmund Thomson syndrome (Lindor et al., 2000); RECQ3 (WRN), mutated in Werner's syndrome (Yu et al., 1996); and RECQL/RecQ1 and RECQ5, for which no syndromes have yet been identified. Stable transfection of BS cells with normal *BLM cDNA* restores the nuclear staining for BLM and reduces the mean number of SCEs (Neff et al., 1999).

On the other hand, *BLM cDNA* with missense mutations failed to reduce SCEs and did not localize in the nucleus in a normal pattern. Three-dimensional modeling of BLM helicase predicts that the I841T mutation is likely to weaken DNA binding, whereas other mutations, such as C891R, interfere with ATP binding (Rong et al., 2000). Furthermore, single amino acid substitutions found in BS patients abolish both the ATPase and helicase activities of BLM, pointing to the importance of these activities in the maintenance of genome integrity (Bahr et al., 1998).

Cellular and Molecular Biology

BLM was initially shown to be a nuclear protein found in three distinct nuclear locations—nuclear bodies that also contain the promyelocytic leukemia protein (PML), the adapter proteins Daxx and Sp100; the nucleolus; and a subset of telomeres (Ishov et al., 1999; Neff et al., 1999; Yankiwski et al., 2000). BLM is found only in PML bodies in G1-phase fibroblasts but co-localizes with WRN to the nucleolus during S phase (Dutertre et al., 2000).

BLM is also capable of co-localizing with a subset of telomeric clusters from within the PML bodies, suggesting that BLM may have a role in maintaining telomeric structure and function as part of the DNA surveillance mechanism (Yankiwski et al., 2000). Isolation of protein complexes using antibodies developed against the breast cancer susceptibility gene product, BRCA1, revealed the presence of BLM and other proteins involved in DNA repair and processing (Wang et al., 2000).

BLM was shown to be associated with diffuse nucleoplasmic patches and discrete foci, and BRCA1 co-localized primarily to the foci. Exposure of cells to hydroxyurea or ionizing radiation enhanced the co-localization of BLM and BRCA1 and caused a redistribution of BLM into nuclear foci (Wang et al., 2000). The BLM protein also co-localizes with the single-strand DNA-binding protein RPA within discrete foci during the late zygonema and early pachynema phases of meiotic prophase (Moens et al., 2000; Walpita et al.,

1999). Brosh and co-workers (2000) then demonstrated a functional interaction between these two proteins by showing that RPA stimulates the unwinding activity of BLM on short partial-duplex DNA substrate. These data suggest that BLM and RPA function together to unwind DNA duplexes during recombination repair and replication.

Exposure of BS cells to ultraviolet (UV) radiation and alkylating agents leads to a further elevation of SCE (Krepinsky et al., 1980; Kurihara et al., 1987). However, sensitivity to ionizing radiation has been demonstrated only with some BS lines (Aurias et al., 1985). A small but reproducible escape from radiation-induced G2/M delay could account for increased radiosensitivity (Ababou et al., 2000). This is a characteristic that BS cells share with A-T cells, in which all cell cycle checkpoints are defective and cells are hypersensitive to radiation. Further overlap between these syndromes is evident from the recent observation that radiation-induced phosphorylation of BLM is ATM dependent (Ababou et al., 2000). The presence of BLM, ATM, and BRCA1 in the same multiprotein complex is consistent with a common role in the G2/M checkpoint (Wang et al., 2000).

Because BLM contained consensus motifs conserved in DNA and RNA helicases, it suggested that BLM would be capable of unwinding DNA. Indeed, overexpression of BLM in *Saccharomyces cerevisiae* revealed DNA-dependent ATPase and 3'5' DNA helicase activities (Karow et al., 1997; Neff et al., 1999). Although the exact role of BLM remains unknown, the findings that point mutations in the helicase domain cause BS and lead to genome instability suggest that the helicase activity of BLM suppresses inappropriate recombination (Bahr et al., 1998).

There is also evidence that BLM plays a role in DNA replication. Immunodepletion of the *Xenopus laevis* homolog of BLM from an egg extract inhibited the replication of DNA in reconstituted nuclei, and this was restored with recombinant BLM protein (Liao et al., 2000). In chicken B-lymphocyte DT40 cells, BLM$^{-/-}$ mutants had phenotypic characteristics similar to BS cells (Wang et al., 2000). Generation of BLM$^{-/-}$ Rad54$^{-/-}$ cells led to an almost complete abolition of enhanced targeted integration and reduction in SCE, indicating that homologous recombination gives rise to the abnormal structures. Thus BLM appears to function to reduce DNA double-strand breaks during DNA replication.

Karow and colleagues (2000) have proposed a model in which BLM functions as an antirecombinase at blocked replication forks. In that model, Holliday junctions are formed by connecting of newly synthesized DNA strands at stalled replication forks; these structures are resolved by BLM. In BS cells, reverse branch migration is inefficient, giving rise to double-strand breaks and abnormal recombinants.

Separation of the strands of duplex DNA by RECQ helicases leads to torsional stress, which is resolved by the topoisomerases, enzymes essential for DNA replication and chromosome segregation (Wang, 1998).

Top3 mutants in *S. cerevisiae* display slow growth and genome instability, characteristics that are suppressed in *Sgs1* (the BLM homologue) top3 double mutants (Gangloff et al., 1994). It seems likely that Sgs1p gives rise to a deleterious topologic substrate that Top3 resolves. Physical interaction between these proteins was subsequently demonstrated (Watt et al., 1995).

A similar interaction was revealed between BLM and topoisomerase III (Johnson et al., 2000; Wu et al., 2000). These two proteins co-localize to PML bodies, are co-immunoprecipitates, and interact directly (Wu et al., 2000). Interaction between BLM and topoisomerases suggests that these proteins are intimately involved in maintaining the integrity of genomic DNA.

Clinical Manifestations

The major physical feature of Bloom syndrome is small stature with relatively normal body proportions. For this reason, Bloom syndrome may be mistaken for certain forms of dwarfism (German, 1999). Other clinical features may or may not be present and vary in severity. A characteristic keel-shaped face with a slightly small dolichocephalic cranium, malar hypoplasia, nasal prominence, small mandible, protuberant ears, and absence of upper lateral incisors are common.

Individuals are sun sensitive and develop erythematous lesions on exposed regions of the face. The erythema may appear as a faint blush on the cheeks, but in extreme cases it may manifest as a bright red disfiguring lesion (German, 1993).

Other abnormalities include the development of well-demarcated patchy areas of hypopigmentation and hyperpigmentation especially on the trunk, male and female infertility, restricted intellectual ability, and a predisposition to develop late-onset non–insulin-dependent diabetes mellitus. Problems with vomiting and diarrhea leading to life-threatening dehydration are common in infancy. The largest registry of Bloom syndrome patients has reported an increased incidence of otitis media and pneumonia. Chronic lung disease develops in 1 of 20 patients and is the second-leading cause of death (German, 1997, 1999). Approximately one in eight BS patients develops diabetes mellitus, with a mean age of 25 years (German, 1999).

Patients with Bloom syndrome have a remarkable predisposition to the early development of cancer (German, 1997). Approximately 50% of patients will develop cancer by age 25, and it is striking that many will have two or more primary malignancies. Cancers of virtually all types and at all locations have been reported. In the first two decades of life, the predominant types are leukemia and non-Hodgkin's lymphoma. Later in life, many carcinomas are common, especially those of the colon, skin, and breast.

Though immunodeficiency could account for some of the cancers seen in this syndrome, it is likely that genomic instability accounts for the majority of malignancies. For the most part, heterozygous carriers of the defective BLM gene do not exhibit any of the phenotype, but cytologic evidence of chromosomal damage in spermatozoa has been reported (Martin et al., 1994).

Laboratory Findings

Evidence of immunodeficiency has been reported in many Bloom syndrome patients, but it is highly variable and usually not severe (Etzioni et al., 1989; Hutteroth et al., 1975; Taniguchi et al., 1982; Van Kerckhove et al., 1988; Weemaes et al., 1979). The majority of patients have decreased levels of one or more serum immunoglobulin classes (IgM, IgA, and, less commonly, IgG) and decreased in vitro production of immunoglobulin, though the majority have normal antibody responses to vaccines.

Absolute lymphocyte counts and percentages of CD4 and CD8 T lymphocytes, B cells, and natural killer (NK) cells are typically normal. Most patients have normal in vitro lymphoproliferative responses to T-cell mitogens such as phytohemagglutinin A (PHA), but some have diminished responses to a T-cell–dependent B-cell mitogen such as pokeweed mitogen. As in A-T, the presence of laboratory evidence of immunodeficiency is not highly predictive of risk for infection. Other factors leading to the development of chronic lung disease have not been identified.

Diagnosis

The diagnosis of BS is based on the characteristic features of small but well-proportioned body size and a sun-sensitive, erythematous skin lesion affecting the butterfly area of the face. When the facial lesion is absent, BS may go unrecognized or the affected child may be misdiagnosed.

Once suspected on clinical grounds, the diagnosis is confirmed by finding excessive numbers of SCEs on a standard karyotype. Approximately 1% of PHA-stimulated T lymphocytes in metaphase display a characteristic quadriradial, composed of two homologous chromosomes with opposite arms of the figure of equal length and the centromeres positioned opposite one another. Cultured lymphoblasts and fibroblasts also exhibit increased chromosomal instability, with an abnormally large number of chromatid gaps and breaks, as well as structurally rearranged chromosomes.

Treatment

Efforts should be made to protect the face from the sun. Replacement of IgG is indicated if there is significant hypogammaglobulinemia and deficiency of antibody production. Gastrostomy tube feedings may be useful for providing nutrition and hydration, though the long-term benefits of this approach have not been proven. Infections should be promptly diagnosed and treated, with particular attention to prevention of life-threatening dehydration. Finally, patients and their families should be informed about the high risk for development of cancer, so that appropriate surveillance can be performed. Once diagnosed, doses of cancer chemotherapeutic agents may need to be adjusted because of the underlying tendency for chromosomal breakage and recombination.

NIJMEGEN BREAKAGE SYNDROME

Nijmegen breakage syndrome (NBS) is an autosomal recessive disorder characterized by chromosomal instability and radiosensitivity, immunodeficiency, short stature, microcephaly, a "bird-like" face, and a predisposition to malignancy (Weemaes et al., 1994).

This disease shares many characteristics with A-T and ATLD but can be distinguished from A-T by the fact that there is no neurodegeneration but rather microcephaly with mild to moderate mental retardation. Telangiectases are absent, and serum α-fetoprotein levels are normal.

Pathogenesis

Genetics

NBS was initially classified as a variant of A-T (A-TV) because of the overlap in cytogenetic characteristics (Jaspers et al., 1988). At that time A-T had been classified into four different complementation groups (Chen et al., 1984; Jaspers and Bootsma, 1982). Because of the overlapping cellular characteristics but distinct clinical presentation, NBS was called A-TV; it was further subdivided into A-TV1 and A-TV2 because of genetic heterogeneity (Jaspers et al., 1988; Wegner et al., 1988).

This heterogeneity was questioned after more recent studies (Saar et al., 1997). In total, 70 patients have been identified in the A-TV disorder (Wegner et al., 1999). Genotyping of six of these A-TV families, employing five microsatellite markers in the region of the A-T gene, 11q22-23, failed to find evidence of linkage and indicated that A-TV was not allelic to A-T (Green et al., 1995, Stumm et al., 1995). This was further confirmed by an inability of chromosome 11 to complement the A-TV phenotype (Komatsu et al., 1996), and Stumm and colleagues (1997) reported noncomplementation in A-T/A-TV cell hybrids.

A whole-genome screen in 14 families localized the NBS gene to a 1cM interval on chromosome 8q21 (Saar et al., 1997), and the use of microcell-mediated chromosome transfer, followed by complementation assays based on the correction of radiosensitivity, localized NBS to 8q21-24 (Matsuura et al., 1997).

Cerosaletti and co-workers (1998) generated a radiation-hybrid map of markers at 8q21, and examination of disease haplotypes segregating in different pedigrees revealed recombination events that placed the gene between the markers D8S1757 and D8S270. A common founder haplotype was present in 15 of 18 disease chromosomes from 9 of 11 NBS families.

The NBS gene was identified independently by three groups in 1998 employing different strategies. Varon

and colleagues (1998) used positional cloning to identify a gene, *nibrin*, mutated in patients with NBS. A truncating 5-bp deletion (657del5) was identified in the majority of patients. The protein encoded by *nibrin* contained a forkhead-associated (FHA) domain and a breast cancer carboxy-terminal (BRCT) domain, both previously found in other DNA-damage responsive cell cycle checkpoint proteins.

Matsuura and associates (1998) also used positional cloning to isolate the NBS gene, NBS1, from an 800-kb candidate region and detected the same 5-bp deletion in 13 individuals. On the other hand, Carney and colleagues (1998) used the reverse genetic approach, relying on protein sequence of a putative subunit (p95) of the Mre11/Rad50 complex. They showed that the locus encoding p95 mapped to 8q21.3, a region reported to contain the NBS gene (Saar et al., 1997), and were unable to detect p95 protein in extracts from NBS patients.

The NBS1/nibrin/p95 protein, hereafter referred to as NBS1, is a 754–amino acid polypeptide containing FHA and BRCT domains, which provides the potential for phosphorylation and protein–protein interactions, respectively.

Cellular and Molecular Biology

As indicated earlier, NBS overlaps with A-T in a number of characteristics, including chromosomal instability, radiosensitivity, and cancer predisposition (Shiloh, 1997). Chromosome rearrangements, as in the case of A-T, occur on chromosomes 7 and 14 and involve T-cell receptor and immunoglobulin gene sites (Aurius et al., 1980). The frequency of these rearrangements is twofold to threefold higher than in A-T lymphocytes (Van der Burgt et al., 1996). Chromatid and chromosome breaks, acentric fragments, marker chromosomes, and nonspecific exchanges are also found in NBS lymphocytes and fibroblasts (Weemaes et al., 1994). Telomeric fusions resulting in dicentric chromosomes are also seen, again in common with A-T cells (Pandita et al., 1995; Wegner et al., 1999).

Hypersensitivity of lymphocytes and fibroblasts to ionizing radiation and bleomycin is seen in chromosomal breakage assays (Green et al., 1995; Taalman et al., 1989; Wegner et al., 1999). Decrease in colony formation has also been used to reveal radiosensitivity (Jaspers et al., 1988; Taalman et al., 1983). Similar to A-T cells, radioresistant DNA synthesis, indicative of a defect in the S-phase checkpoint, is characteristic of NBS cells (Taalman et al., 1989).

Until recently the basis of this radiosensitivity has remained unresolved. Girard and associates (2000), employing pulse-field gel electrophoresis, showed that a small but significantly increased fraction of unreformed DNA double-strand breaks remained in NBS cells up to 24 hours after irradiation. The fraction is somewhat less than that observed in irradiated A-T cells, but the overall pattern of repair is similar (Foray et al., 1997). Increased chromosome breaks in noncycling NBS cells were also observed. Thus these unreformed breaks or their conversion to chromosome breaks could account for the radiosensitivity in NBS.

In addition to this cell cycle S-phase checkpoint defect, NBS cells accumulate in G2/M at 24 hours after irradiation at levels intermediate between those of control and A-T cells (Beamish and Lavin, 1994; Seyschab et al., 1992). A defective radiation-induced p53 response has also been reported for NBS cells (Jongmans et al., 1997; Sullivan et al., 1997; Yamazaki et al., 1998). In all cases the kinetics of induction of p53 revealed a slower or reduced response in NBS reminiscent of that seen in A-T. However, unlike that described for A-T, this has not been unequivocally associated with a defective G1/S checkpoint in NBS (Jongmans et al., 1997; Yamazaki et al., 1998).

As pointed out earlier, NBS1 is part of a complex with Mre11 and Rad50 (Carney et al., 1998). In *S. cerevisiae*, mutations in Mre11 and Rad50 cause radiosensitivity and defective meiosis (Ajimura et al., 1993). The third protein Xrs-2p forms a complex with Mre11/Rad50 in *S. cerevisiae* and, although not homologous to NBS1, appears to be functionally related. The Mre11/Rad50/Xrs2 complex is primarily involved in facilitating homologous recombination (Bressan et al., 1999) but also plays a role in nonhomologous end joining (NHEJ) (Haber, 2000). Mre11 and Rad50 are essential for survival in mice, presumably because of an essential role in homologous recombination (Luo et al., 1999; Xiao and Weaver, 1997).

As described earlier, the S-phase checkpoint is deficient in both NBS and A-T cells, indicating that they are linked in this pathway. Two pieces of evidence support this. First, ATM phosphorylates NBS1 in response to ionizing radiation exposure, which is required as part of the response to DNA damage (Gatei et al., 2000; Lim et al., 2000; Wu et al., 2000; Zhao et al., 2000). This phosphorylation does not affect the integrity of the Mre11 complex.

Second, mutations in hMre11 give rise to ATLD, emphasizing the functional cross-talk between ATM and the Mre11 complex. The recent localization of the Mre11 complex to sites of V(D)J recombination–induced double-strand breaks in immature thymocytes supports a role for this complex in both DNA damage recognition and other cellular processes involving recombination (Chen et al., 2000).

Previous data demonstrate that the Mre11 complex localizes rapidly to double-strand breaks in damaged DNA (Nelms et al., 1998). Because ATM phosphorylates NBS1 over the same time course, it is likely that this modification facilitates the role of the Mre11 complex in the repair process for double-strand breaks.

Clinical Manifestations

NBS was first described by Weemaes and colleagues (1981) in Nijmegen, Netherlands, with most of the patients coming from Eastern Europe, notably Poland and Czechoslovakia. Persons with the disease display a distinct pattern of malformations.

Virtually all patients have severe microcephaly, present at birth in 75% of cases, accompanied by mild to moderate mental retardation. Autopsy studies (Van De Kaa et al., 1994) and cranial magnetic resonance imaging (MRI) (Bekiesinska-Figatowska et al., 2000) have attributed this problem to stunted brain growth, with particularly severe effects on the frontal lobes and corpus callosum. The cerebellum appears to be normal.

There are abnormal facies with a sloping forehead, receding mandible, prominent mid-face, long nose, and upward slant of the palpebral fissures (Fig. 18-4). Other malformations occur in as many as 50% of patients. These include clinodactyly and syndactyly, atresia/stenosis along the gastrointestinal tract, ovarian dysgenesis, hydronephrosis, and hip dysplasia. Many patients develop café au lait spots and depigmented skin lesions, and hypergonadotropic hypogonadism is common in affected males.

Cancer is the leading cause of death for NBS patients, with a mean age of cancer-related death of only 9.2 years. The majority are lymphomas of all types, but there have been single case reports of glioma, rhabdomyosarcoma, and medulloblastoma. Although heterozygotes appear to be normal in other respects, an increased susceptibility to malignancy has been reported in at least one series (Seemanova, 1990).

Many patients suffer from recurrent upper and lower respiratory tract infections, and chronic lung disease with bronchiectasis is the second leading cause of death (The International Nijmegen Breakage Syndrome Study Group [TINBSSG], 2000; Seemanova et al., 1985). There are no published reports of opportunistic infections, but evidence of more generalized immune dysfunction exists, with patients exhibiting autoimmune (immune thrombocytopenia and hemolytic anemia) and chronic inflammatory (childhood sarcoidosis) disorders at much higher than expected rates.

Laboratory Findings

Immunodeficiency is common in NBS patients (Chrzanowska et al., 1995; Seemanova et al., 1985; TINBSSG, 2000). One third of patients are agammaglobulinemic. As many as 60% of the others have absent or low levels of one or more immunoglobulin classes or IgG subclasses, but no published reports document the extent or severity of antibody deficiency in these patients. The majority of patients are lymphopenic, with relatively similar diminution of CD4 and CD8 cells and reduced in vitro proliferative responses to mitogens.

The characteristic laboratory abnormality in NBS is chromosome instability. Cultured T lymphocytes show an extremely low mitotic index, making cytogenetic analysis difficult, but structural chromosomal aberrations are present in 10% to 35% of metaphases (Taalmon et al., 1989). Most of the rearrangements occur in chromosomes 7 and 14 at the locations of immunoglobulin and T-cell receptor genes. In a longitudinal study of a single patient over a 24-year period, the percentage of cells with rearrangements in chromosomes 7 or 14 increased to as high as 32%, and 35% of cells were characterized by other structural abnormali-

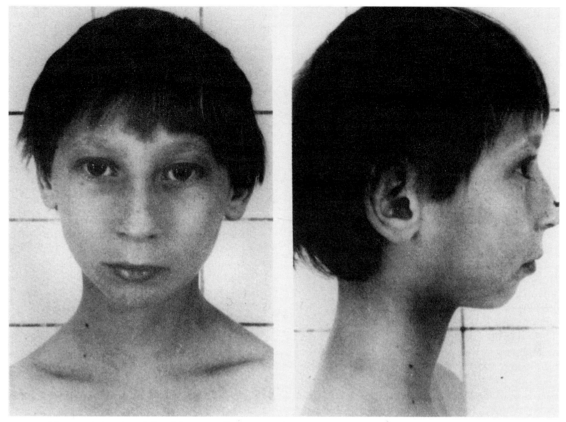

Figure 18-4 · Typical facial features of microcephaly, prominent nose, and mandibular hypoplasia in a child with Nijmegen breakage syndrome. (From Van der Burgt I, et al. Nijmegen breakage syndrome. J Med Genet 33:153–156, 1996.)

ties in the chromosomes (Weemaes et al., 1994). Hypersensitivity to x-rays has been documented in both lymphocytes and fibroblasts from NBS patients, with the extent of sensitivity comparable to that observed in A-T patients (Taalman et al., 1983). α-Fetoprotein levels are normal in NBS patients.

Pathology

At autopsy, the thymus is small and devoid of Hassall's corpuscles, suggesting dysplasia (Van De Kaa et al., 1994). Lymph nodes have normal architecture, but lymphoid follicles are small and germinal centers are reduced in number.

Diagnosis and Differential Diagnosis

The most prominent feature of NBS is severe microcephaly. Though the differential diagnosis of microcephaly is extensive, the relatively mild retardation and characteristic facies should point to the diagnosis. α-fetoprotein levels are normal.

The most useful laboratory test for confirmation is demonstration of chromosomal rearrangements typically involving chromosomes 7 and 14, and chromosomal hypersensitivity to x-irradiation. The 657del5 mutation

(Varon et al., 2000) is present in approximately 90% of cases in the United States, simplifying the task of genetic confirmation in many cases.

Treatment

As with A-T, there is no specific treatment for NBS. Subjects should be evaluated for immunodeficiency and treated as appropriate. Parents and caregivers should be counseled about the presenting signs of lymphoma and other malignancies.

FANCONI'S ANEMIA

The autosomal recessive disorder Fanconi's anemia (FA) features progressive pancytopenia in association with diverse congenital abnormalities (Alter and Young, 1993). The heterozygote frequency has been estimated at 1 in 200 (Swift, 1976).

This syndrome is included among the chromosomal instability syndromes because of high levels of spontaneous chromosomal breaks and a hypersensitivity to DNA crosslinking agents such as mitomycin C. These agents cause enhanced G2 phase delay in the cell cycle, chromosomal instability, and cell death in FA cells (D'Andrea and Grompe, 1997).

This is a heterogeneous disorder represented by eight genetic complementation groups (A–H), for which only some of the genes have been cloned and the products characterized. Mice deficient in complementation group A exhibit hypogonadism and impaired fertility. Because of the similar clinical and cellular phenotypes among the different FA complementation groups, it seems likely that their protein products cooperate in common cellular pathways.

Pathogenesis

Genetics

Somatic cell fusion studies were employed to identify up to eight distinct complementation groups among FA patients, FA-A through FA-H (Joenje et al., 1997). Complementation was assigned on the basis of correction of chromosomal breakage in hybrid cells taken from the different groups. However, it seems likely that the sole patient in FA-H belongs to FA-A (Joenje et al., 2000). This degree of heterogeneity predicted that mutation detection in this syndrome would be tedious.

Delineation of pathways involved also proved to be difficult because of the novelty of the genes initially identified (FA-A to FA-C) (D'Andrea, 1996). The heterogeneity seen at the clinical level obviously reflects the genetic heterogeneity evident from complementation and genetic studies. Again this syndrome is different from the other chromosome fragility syndromes, A-T, BS, and NBS, in which a single gene is involved (Carney et al., 1998; Ellis et al., 1995; Savitsky et al., 1995a).

A total of seven FA genes have been identified and given the names FANCA through FANCG. Because FA could be complemented in cell hybrids, Strathdee and colleagues (1992b) used transfection with a cDNA library prepared in an Epstein-Barr virus (EBV)–based vector (pREP4) to functionally complement and thus identify the cDNA for FANCC. This gene was subsequently localized to chromosome 9q22.3 (Strathdee et al., 1992a).

The predicted protein sequence did not contain any motifs common to other known proteins. Ten to 15 percent of FA patients in Western countries carry a mutation at this gene IVS4+4 A→T, a splice mutation in intron 4, found predominantly in Ashkenazi Jews (Whitney et al., 1993). Ashkenazi Jewish patients homozygous for this mutation have a severe phenotype compared with other FA patients. Ethnic background may have an influence on this, because a Japanese patient homozygous for IVS4 did not display a severe form of the disease (Futaki et al., 2000).

Using a panel of FA-A families, based on complementation analysis, Pronk and colleagues (1995) employed linkage analysis to localize FANCA to chromosome 16q24.3. Functional complementation similar to that used to clone FANCC was also successful in the isolation of a 5.5-kb cDNA corresponding to the FANCA gene. The predicted protein was 162 kD, containing two overlapping bipartite nuclear localization signals and a partial leucine zipper sequence suggestive of a nuclear protein (Lo Ten Foe et al., 1996). Somatic mosaicism due to reversion of a pathogenic allele to wild type was described previously for BS (Ellis et al., 1995).

Functional correction of a pathogenic microdeletion, microinsertion, and missense mutation in homozygous FA patients due to compensatory secondary sequence alterations in cis have also been described (Waisfisz et al., 1999a). Compensation for both FANCA and FANCC alleles was determined by complementation of hypersensitivity to crosslinking agents with cDNAs from EBV lines established from these patients.

Saar and colleagues (1998) mapped an additional FA gene to chromosome 9p, which was subsequently identified as FANCG (De Winter et al., 1998). The same approach of functional complementation with a cDNA library, as used to identify FANCA and FANCC, was employed to identify FANCG. De Winter and co-workers (1998) identified this gene as XRCC9, a human gene previously identified by its ability to correct chromosomal instability in Chinese hamster ovary (CHO) cells (Liu et al., 1997). This gene maps to chromosome 9p13, and loss of heterozygosity (LOH) is seen in 50% of small-cell lung cancer samples in this region. Thus it is a candidate tumor suppressor gene functioning to prevent genome instability.

Complementation cloning was also employed to clone the cDNA encoding FANCF from FA-F lymphoblasts (De Winter et al., 2000). This cDNA encodes a 374–amino acid novel protein containing a region of homology with the prokaryotic RNA-binding protein ROM (Predki et al., 1995) and has been localized more recently to a 200-kb region on chromosome 3p25.3, using noncomplemented microcell transfer (Hejna et al., 2000). Thus it is possible that FANCF may bind RNA or DNA as part of its function.

Homozygosity mapping and genetic linkage analysis was used to localize the FANCE gene to chromosome 6p21-22 (Waisfisz et al., 1999b), and complementation cloning was recently used to identify the FANCE gene that encodes a 536–amino acid protein containing two putative nuclear localization signals (De Winter et al., 2000). The gene for FANCD was initially mapped to chromosome 3p22-26 by microcell-mediated chromosome transfer (Whitney et al., 1995).

Cellular and Molecular Biology

Fibroblasts from patients with FA have decreased growth rates and increased generation times (Weksberg et al., 1979). Plating efficiencies for FA cells were found to be approximately 35% of those for control fibroblasts. When fibroblasts and lymphoblast cells were exposed to the crosslinking agent mitomycin C and D_{10} values (dose required to reduce survival to 10%), determined, FA cells were 3- to 27-fold more sensitive than controls.

Sensitivity to crosslinks in DNA was further substantiated using combined psoralen and long wavelength UV treatment (Weksberg et al., 1979). On the other hand, equitoxicity with control cells was observed when

FA-C cells were exposed to monofunctional alkylating agents (ethyl methane sulfonate and N-methyl-N1-nitro-N-nitrosoguanidine) or to actinomycin D. However, sensitivity is not confined to crosslinking agents because both peripheral blood lymphocytes and fibroblasts from three FA patients were approximately twofold more sensitive to the induction of chromatid-type aberrations after irradiation in the G1 phase of the cell cycle (Bigelow et al., 1979).

The increased aberration yields were not due to a prolonged G1 phase. It is not known what complementation groups were represented by these patients. The enhanced sensitivity of these FA cells to ionizing radiation is intermediate between that of control and A-T cells (Chen et al., 1978). In this respect it is of considerable interest because, similar to that for A-T cells, there is evidence for defective double-strand break repair in FA cells. Escarceller and associates (1997) established a host cell end-joining assay to analyze the fate of restriction enzyme–introduced breaks in plasmid DNA when transiently replicated in control FA-B and FA-D lymphoblasts (Escarceller et al., 1997). No difference in plasmid survival was observed, but the fidelity of end joining was significantly reduced in the FA cells. In an earlier study, increased mis-rejoining was also observed in one FA cell line, apparently due to complex mutations (Runger et al., 1993).

Other evidence in support of a defect in rejoining of breaks has been provided by Smith and colleagues (1998), who showed that an increased frequency of aberrant rearrangements is associated with V(D)J coding joint formation. This is consistent with excessive degradation of DNA ends and a defect in the fidelity of rejoining specific DNA breaks. A similar defect has been described in A-T cells transfected with restriction enzyme–cleaved plasmids (Cox et al., 1986).

To date, five of the seven likely genes that constitute the FA syndrome have been cloned and characterized. Even though FANCC was identified as early as 1992, little is known about the individual or combined functions of the FA gene products compared with the other chromosome breakage syndromes. This can be accounted to some extent by the findings that A-T, BS, and NBS are single-gene defects and FA has as many as seven gene products.

In the case of FANCC protein, it is primarily localized to the cytoplasm, maximally expressed in M phase (Yamashita et al., 1994), and interacts with a number of proteins, including FANCA, FANCG, cdc2, GRP94 (chaperone), NADPH cytochrome P450 reductase, and FAZF, a transcriptional repressor (Garcia-Higuera and D'Andrea, 1999; Hoatlin et al., 1999; Hoshino et al., 1998; Kruyt et al., 1998). FANCA and FANCC proteins form both cytoplasmic and nuclear complexes but do not interact directly (Kupfer et al., 1997).

FANCG/XRCC9 is also a component of this nuclear complex and is required for the interaction of FANCA and FANCC (Garcia-Higuera et al., 1999). The amino terminus of FANCA is required for FANCG binding, for FANCC binding, and for functional activity of the complex, and a carboxy terminal domain of FANCG is required for its function and the recruitment of FANCC to the complex (Kuang et al., 2000). It is also evident that the stability of the FANCA/FANCC/FANCG complex is enhanced by the individual components (Garcia-Higuera et al., 1999).

The protein products of the other FA complementation groups contribute to assembly, stabilization, and nuclear transport of the FA complex. Identification of other FA protein products in this complex, together with a description of biologic activities for these proteins, will assist in understanding the role of this complex in the fidelity of rejoining of double-strand breaks in DNA and maintenance of chromosome stability.

Clinical Manifestations

Patients with Fanconi's anemia most often present with short stature and abnormalities of skin pigmentation, such as café au lait spots, large hyperpigmented patches with diffuse boundaries, and smaller hypopigmented patches (Giampietro et al., 1993).

Approximately half the patients will have other congenital abnormalities. The most striking of these is bilateral absence or hypoplasia of thumbs and radii, but a variety of genitourinary (hypoplastic, aplastic or ectopic kidneys), gastrointestinal (atresia of esophagus, duodenum, jejunum, or imperforate anus), skeletal (spina bifida, rib hypoplasia, hip dysplasia or dislocation), and craniofacial (microcephaly and elfin features) malformations occur as well (De Kerviler et al., 2000). However, 20% to 40% of patients do not have significant malformations. Because there is so much variability in phenotypic expression, the diagnosis of Fanconi's anemia should be made only after confirmatory laboratory tests.

Symptomatic hematologic problems usually are not apparent until after the age of 2 years, but progressive pancytopenia usually ensues. More than 80% of patients will eventually develop aplastic pancytopenia.

There is also a significant predisposition to the development of cancer, with almost 10% of patients developing acute leukemia, predominantly of the myeloid lineage, at a mean age of 14 years (Auerbach and Allen, 1991). An additional 5% develop a myelodysplastic syndrome with cytogenetically detected clonal abnormalities (Alter, 1996). Among older patients, a variety of nonhematologic malignancies have been reported. These include hepatocellular carcinoma of the liver; squamous cell carcinomas of the oropharynx, esophagus, and vulva; and brain tumors. This pattern is clearly distinguishable from that observed in other chromosome breakage diseases.

The major factor predisposing Fanconi's anemia patients to develop infection is acquired neutropenia. Only a handful of cases report defined deficiencies of lymphoid function. One report exists of selective IgA deficiency of no obvious significance (Standen et al., 1989). One other patient had reduced in vitro lymphocyte proliferation and a clinical history of oral candidiasis and Pneumocystis carinii pneumonia, but these problems occurred only after oral corticosteroids had been used for treatment of pancytopenia (Pedersen et al., 1977).

Laboratory Findings

Macrocytic anemia and elevated levels of fetal hemoglobin are often the first manifestations of FA, occurring prior to the onset of pancytopenia.

However, the characteristic laboratory abnormality is excessive chromosomal breakage after exposure of lymphocytes, fibroblasts, or amniocytes to low concentrations of DNA crosslinking agents such as mitomycin C and diepoxybutane (German, 1969). Sensitivity to other agents including reactive oxygen intermediates and ionizing radiation has been described (Bigelow et al., 1979; Korkina et al., 1992).

As observed in A-T, serum α-fetoprotein (AFP) levels are elevated in FA but generally remain stable over a period of 4 years (Cassinat et al., 2000). AFP levels may be of diagnostic benefit in patients with limited numbers of physical features of FA.

Treatment

The aplastic pancytopenia typical of FA is managed transiently by treatment with cytokines such as granulocyte colony-stimulating factor (G-CSF) or granulocyte-macrophage colony-stimulating factor (GM-CSF), but bone marrow transplant using a histocompatible donor represents the most successful approach to treating the disease (De Medeiros et al., 1999; Kohli-Kumar et al., 1994).

IMMUNODEFICIENCY/CENTROMERIC INSTABILITY/FACIAL ANOMALIES SYNDROME

Approximately 20 patients with immunodeficiency/centromeric instability/facial anomalies (ICF) syndrome have been described with facial dysmorphism (hypertelorism, flat nasal bridge, epicanthal folds, and micrognathia), developmental delay, and mental retardation associated with centromere instability of chromosomes 1, 9, and 16 (Brown et al., 1995, Franceschini et al., 1995; Smeets et al., 1994).

Cultured lymphocytes show a characteristic pattern of chromosome breakage and recombination, with the formation of multibranched chromosomal configurations (Fig. 18-5). Chromosome 1 is affected in 60% of cultured cells, chromosome 9 in 27%, and chromosome 16 in 22% (Valkova et al., 1987). Of interest, a similar degree of chromosomal damage was not seen in fibroblasts. Karyotypic abnormalities are not increased by exposure to any known physical or chemical agents (Smeets et al., 1994); thus some do not characterize ICF syndrome as a chromosomal breakage disorder.

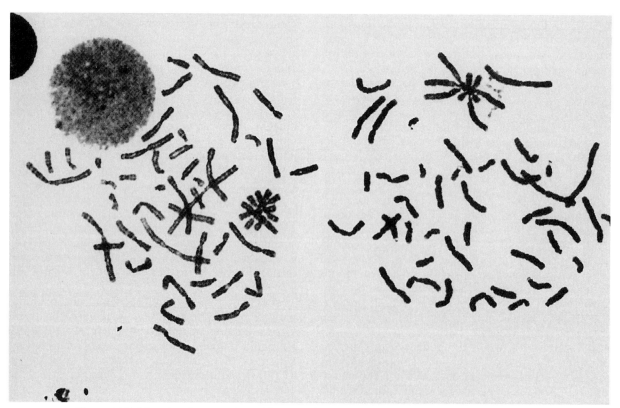

Figure 18-5· **Metaphase from a patient with ICF syndrome.** The association between the homologues of chromosome 16 with duplication of long and short arms gives a starburst effect. (From Brown DC, et al. ICF syndrome [immunodeficiency, centromeric instability and facial anomalies]: investigation of heterochromatin abnormalities and review of clinical outcome. Hum Genet 96:411–416, 1995.)

DNA samples from three consanguineous families were used to localize the ICF gene to chromosomal region 20q11-q13 (Wijmenga et al., 1998). Analysis of candidate genes led to the identification of mutations in a DNA methyltransferase gene DNMT3B (Okano et al., 1999; Xu et al., 1999). Under normal circumstances, this gene is responsible for methylation of cytosine residues in classical satellites 2 and 3 at juxtameric regions of chromosomes 1, 9, and 16. Findings in these patients indicate that cytosine methylation is required for the stabilization of these chromosomal regions. In the absence of methylation, the regions are greatly elongated and prone to breakage and rejoining.

Immunodeficiency has been reported in virtually every patient with ICF. Most children have significantly decreased levels of one or more immunoglobulin classes and reduced numbers of B lymphocytes; in many cases there is severe panhypogammaglobulinemia (Franceschini et al., 1995; Fryns et al., 1981; Howard et al., 1985; Hulton, 1978; Tiepolo et al., 1979). Of those studied in more detail, the majority have diminished or absent antibody responses to prior immunization and infection.

Many patients have reduced numbers of T lymphocytes but are able to mount responses to delayed-type hypersensitivity skin tests and have normal or near normal in vitro proliferation to T-cell mitogens (Franceschini et al., 1995; Fryns et al., 1981; Howard et al., 1985; Hulton, 1978).

Nevertheless, the broad range of reported organisms, including pyogenic bacteria, *Candida,* and cytomegalovirus, suggests dysfunction of both humoral and cell-mediated immune function. Almost all patients in these studies have problems with recurrent infections of the lungs and gastrointestinal tract, and infection was the cause of death in 5 of the 16 reported children. There is no apparent predisposition to skin lesions or neoplasia.

This disorder is also discussed in Chapter 24.

CHROMOSOMAL BREAKAGE SYNDROMES NOT CLEARLY ASSOCIATED WITH IMMUNODEFICIENCY

There are other syndromes with defects in the recognition or repair of DNA damage in which immunodeficiency does not occur or plays an uncertain role (Gennery et al., 2000). Three autosomal recessive syndromes of defective nucleotide excision repair have been described—*trichothiodystrophy, Cockayne syndrome,* and *xeroderma pigmentosa.* Each causes extreme sensitivity to sunlight. Neither trichothiodystrophy (Itin and Pittelkow, 1990) nor Cockayne syndrome (Nancy and Berry, 1992) has been associated with increased susceptibility to cancer or infection, and immunologic defects have not been described.

Patients with xeroderma pigmentosa have a 1000-fold increase in the prevalence of sunlight-induced skin cancers, but not other cancers. In a review of 830 previously published cases (Kraemer et al., 1987), only 10 were reported to have frequent infections. Unfortunately, neither the nature of infections nor information about the immunologic competence of each of these patients was reported.

Two patients with xeroderma pigmentosa had hypogammaglobulinemia. One had recurrent pneumonias and *Giardia* infection (Wysenbeek et al., 1980); the other had recurrent staphylococcal infections of the eyelids and conjunctivae, as well as hidradenitis suppurativa (Stenson, 1982). Four of four tested xeroderma pigmentosa patients were anergic to a panel of delayed-type hypersensitivity skin tests, and one of them subsequently died of varicella encephalitis (Dupuy and Lafforet, 1974). Neither anergy nor severe problems with infection have otherwise been reported among xeroderma pigmentosa patients, and there has never been a systematic study of immune function in a large number of such individuals.

A single patient with deficiency of DNA ligase I, a DNA repair enzyme, has been described (Barnes et al., 1992; Webster et al., 1992). She had retarded growth; skin hypersensitivity to sunlight; and immunodeficiency, including low serum IgG and absent IgA, impaired antibody responses to vaccines, and failure of peripheral blood lymphocytes to proliferate in response to mitogens. The patient died of pneumonia at age 19 years, after an illness characterized by hepatosplenomegaly with lymphocytic infiltration of the portal tracts suggestive of lymphoma.

REFERENCES

Ababou M, Dutertre S, Lécluse, Onclercq R, Chatton B, Amor-Guéret A. ATM-dependent phosphorylation and accumulation of endogenous BLM protein in response to ionizing radiation. Oncogene 19:5955–5963, 2000.

Agamanolis DP, Greenstein JI. Ataxia-telangiectasia. Report of a case with Lewy bodies and vascular abnormalities within cerebral tissue. J Neuropathol Exp Neurol 38:475–489, 1979.

Aguilar MJ, Kamoshita S, Landing BH, Boder E, Sedgwick RP. Pathological observations in ataxia-telangiectasia. A report of five cases. J Neuropathol Exp Neurol 27:659–676, 1968.

Ahn JY, Schwarz JK, Piwnica-Worms H, Canman CE. Threonine 68 phosphorylation by ataxia-telangiectasia mutated is required for efficient activation of Chk2 in response to ionizing radiation. Cancer Res 60:5934–5936, 2000.

Ajimura M, Leem SH, Ogawa H. Identification of new genes required for meiotic recombination in *Saccharomyces cerevisiae.* Genetics 133:51–66, 1993.

Al-Khodairy F, Carr AM. DNA repair mutants defining G2 checkpointpathways in *Schizosaccharomyces pombe.* EMBO J 11:1343–50, 1992.

Alter BP. Fanconi's anemia and malignancies. Am J Hematol 53:99–110, 1996.

Alter BP, Young NS. The bone marrow failure syndrome. In Nathan DG, Oski FA, eds. Hematology of Infancy and Childhood, ed 4, vol 1. Philadelphia, WB Saunders, 1993, p 216.

Ammann AJ, Good RA, Bier D, Fudenberg HH. Long-term plasma infusions in a patient with ataxia-telangiectasia and deficient IgA and IgE. Pediatrics 44:672–676, 1969.

Amromin GD, Boder E, Teplitz R. Ataxia-telangiectasia with a 32 year survival. A clinicopathologic report. J Neuropathol Exp Neurol 38:621–643, 1979.

Athma P, Rappaport R, Swift M. Molecular genotyping shows that ataxia-telangiectasia heterozygotes are predisposed to breast cancer. Cancer Genet Cytogenet 92:130–134, 1996.

Auerbach AD, Allen RG. Leukemia and preleukemia in Fanconi anemia patients. A review of the literature and report of the

International Fanconi Anemia Registry. Cancer Genet Cytogenet 51:1–12, 1991.

Aurias A, Antoine JL, Assathiany R, Odievre M, Dutrillaux B. Radiation sensitivity of Bloom's syndrome lymphocytes during S and G2 phases. Cancer Genet Cytogenet 16:131–136, 1985.

Aurias AB, Dutrillaux DB, Lejeune J. High frequencies of inversions and translocations of chromosomes 7 and 14 in ataxia-telangiectasaia. Mutat Res 69:369–374, 1980.

Bahr A, De Graeve F, Kedinger C, Chatton B. Point mutations causing Bloom's syndrome abolish ATPase and DNA helicase activities of the BLM protein. Oncogene 17:2565–2571, 1998.

Baloh RW, Yee RD, Boder E. Eye movements in ataxia-telangiectasia. Neurology 28:1099–1104, 1978.

Banin S, Moyal L, Shieh S, Taya Y, Anderson CW, Chessa I, Smorodinsky NI, Prives C, Reiss Y, Shiloh Y, Ziv Y. Enhanced phosphorylation of p53 by ATM in response to DNA damage. Science 281:1674–1677, 1998.

Barlow C, Dennery PA, Shigenaga MK, Smith MA, Morrow JD, Roberts LJ 2nd, Wynshaw-Boris A, Levine RL. Loss of the ataxia-telangiectasia gene product causes oxidative damage in target organs. Proc Natl Acad Sci USA 96:9915–9919, 1999.

Barlow C, Hirotsune S, Paylor R, Liyanage M, Eckhaus M, Collins F, Shiloh Y, Crawley JN, Ried T, Tagle D, Wynshaw-Boris A. ATM-deficient mice: a paradigm of ataxia telangiectasia. Cell 86:159–171, 1996.

Barnes DE, Tomkinson AE, Lehmann AR, Webster ADB, Lindahl T. Mutations in the DNA ligase I gene of an individual with immunodeficiencies and cellular hypersensitivity to DNA damaging agents. Cell 69:495–503, 1992.

Beamish H, Lavin MF. Radiosensitivity in ataxia-telangiectasia: anomalies in radiation-induced cell cycle delay. Int J Radiat Biol 65:175–184, 1994.

Beamish H, Williams R, Chen P, Khanna KK, Hobson K, Watters D, Shiloh Y, Lavin M. Rapamycin resistance in ataxia telangiectasia. Oncogene 13:963–970, 1996.

Bekiesinska-Figatowska M, Chrzanowska KH, Sikorska J, Walecki J, Krajewska-Walasek M, Jóźwiak S, Kleijer WJ. Cranial MRI in the Nijmegen breakage syndrome. Neuroradiology 42:43–47, 2000.

Bentzen SM, Overgaard M. Relationship between early and late normal-tissue injury after postmastectomy radiotherapy. Radiother Oncol 20:159–165, 1991.

Berkel AI. Studies of IgG subclasses in ataxia-telangiectasia patients. Monogr Allergy 20:100–105, 1986.

Biedermann KA, Sun JR, Giaccia AJ, Tosto LM, Brown JM. Scid mutation in mice confers hypersensitivity to ionizing radiation and a deficiency in DNA double-strand break repair. Proc Natl Acad Sci USA 88:1394–1397, 1991.

Biemond A. A Palaeocerebellar atrophy with extrapyramidal manifestations in association with bronchiectasia and telangiectasia of the conjunctiva bulbi as a familial syndrome. In Van Bogaert L, Radermecker J, eds. Proceeding of the First International Congress of Neurological Sciences, Brussels, July 1957. London, Pergamon Press, 1957, p 206.

Bigelow SB, Rary JM, Bender MA. G2 chromosomal radiosensitivity in Fanconi's anemia. Mutat Res 63:189–199, 1979.

Boder E. Ataxia-telangiectasia: an overview. Kroc Found Ser 19:1–63, 1985.

Boder E, Sedgwick RP. Ataxia-telangiectasia: A review of 101 cases. In Walsh G, ed. Little Club Clinics in Developmental Medicine, no 8. London, Heinemann Medical Books, 1963, pp 110–118.

Boder E, Sedgwick RP. Ataxia-telangiectasia. A familial syndrome of progressive cerebellar ataxia, oculocutaneous telangiectasia and frequent pulmonary infection. A preliminary report on 7 children, an autopsy, and a case history. Univ So Calif Med Bull 9:15–28, 1957.

Boutin B, Wagner DK, Nelson DL. Analysis of CD3 antigen expression in patients with ataxia-telangiectasia. Clin Exp Immunol 68:320–330, 1987.

Bressan DA, Baxter BK, Petrini JH. The Mre11-Rad50-Xrs2 protein complex facilitates homologous recombination-based double-strand break repair in Saccharomyces cerevisiae. Mol Cell Biol 19:7681–7687, 1999.

Brosh RM Jr, Li JL, Kenny MK, Karow JK, Cooper MP, Kureekattil RP, Hickson ID, Bohr VA. Replication protein A physically interacts with the Bloom's syndrome protein and stimulates its helicase activity. J Biol Chem 275:23500–23508, 2000.

Brown DC, Grace E, Sumner AT, Edmunds AT, Ellis PM. ICF syndrome (immunodeficiency, centromeric instability and facial anomalies): investigation of heterochromatin abnormalities and review of clinical outcome. Hum Genet 96:411–416, 1995.

Brown KD, Ziv Y, Sadanandan SN, Chessa L, Collins FS, Shiloh Y, Tagle, DA. The ataxia-telangiectasia gene product, a constitutively expressed nuclear that is not up-regulated following genome damage. Proc Natl Acad Sci USA 94:1840–1845, 1977.

Bullrich F, Rasio D, Kitada S, Starostik P, Kipps T, Keating M, Albitar M, Reed JC, Croce CM. ATM mutations in B-cell chronic lymphocytic leukemia. Cancer Res 59:24–27, 1999.

Byrd PJ, Cooper PR, Stankovic T, Kullar HS, Watts GD, Robinson PJ, Taylor MR. A gene transcribed from the bidirectional ATM promoter coding for a serine rich protein: amino acid sequence, structure and expression studies. Hum Mol Genet 5:1785–1791, 1996.

Cabana MD, Crawford TO, Winkelstein JA, Christensen JR, Lederman HM. Consequences of the delayed diagnosis of ataxia-telangiectasia. Pediatrics 102:98–100, 1998.

Canman CE, Lim DS, Cimprich KA, Taya Y, Tamai K, Sakaguchi K, Appella E, Kastan MB, Siliciano JD. Activation of the ATM kinase by ionizing radiation and phosphorylation of p53. Science 281:1677–1679, 1998.

Canman CE, Radany EH, Parsels LA, Davis MA, Lawrence TS, Maybaum M. WAF1/CIP1 is induced in p53-mediated G1 arrest and apoptosis. Cancer Res 54:1169–1174, 1994.

Carbonari M, Cherchi M, Paganelli R, Giannini G, Galli E, Gaetano C, Papetti C, Fiorilli M. Relative increase of T cells expressing the gamma/delta rather than the alpha/beta receptor in ataxia-telangiectasia. N Engl J Med 322:73–76, 1990.

Carney JP, Maser RS, Olivares H, Davis EM, Le Beau M, Yates JR 3rd, Hays L, Morgan WF, Petrini JH. The hMre11/hRad50 protein complex and Nijmegen breakage syndrome: linkage of double-strand break repair to the cellular DNA damage response. Cell 93:477–486, 1998.

Cassinat B, Guardiola P, Chevret S, Schlageter M-H, Toubert M-E, Rain J-D, Gluckman E. Constitutive elevation of serum alpha-fetoprotein in Fanconi anemia. Blood 96:859–863, 2000.

Cawley LP, Schenken, JR. Monoclonal hypergammaglobulinemia of the gamma M type in a nine-year girl with ataxia-telangiectasia. Am J Clin Pathol 54:790–801, 1970.

Cerosaletti KM, Lange E, Strngham HM, Weemaes CM, Smeets D, Solder B, Belohradsky BH, Taylor AM, Karnes P, Elliott A, Komatsu K, Gatti RA, Boehnke M, Concannon P. Fine localization of the Nijmegen breakage syndrome gene to 8q21: evidence for a common founder haplotype. Am J Hum Genet 63:125–134, 1998.

Chao C, Yang EM, Xu Y. Rescue of defective T cell development and function in Atm−/− mice by a functional TCR alpha beta transgene. J Immunol 164:345–349, 2000.

Chehab NH, Malikzay A, Appel M, Halazonetis TD. Chk2/hCds1 functions as a DNA damage checkpoint in G(1) by stablizing p53. Genes Dev 14:278–288, 2000.

Chen G, Lee EYHP. The product of the ATM gene is a 370 kDa nuclear phosphoprotein. J Biol Chem 271:33693–33697, 1996.

Chen J. Ataxia-telangiectasia-related protein is involved in the phosphorylation of BRCA1 following deoxyribonucleic acid damage. Cancer Res 60:5037–5039, 2000.

Chen P, Imray FP, Kidson C. Gene dosage and complementation analysis of ataxia-telangiectasia lymphoblastoid cell lines assayed by induced chromosome aberrations. Mutat Res 129:165–172, 1984.

Chen PC, Lavin MF, Kidson C, Moss D. Identification of ataxia-telangiectasia heterozygotes, a cancer prone population. Nature 274:484–486, 1978.

Chrzanowska KH, Kleijer WJ, Krajewska-Walasek M, Bialecka M, Gutkowska A, Goryluk-Kozakiewicz B, Michalkiewicz J, Stachowski J, Gregorek H, Lysón-Wojciechowska G, Janowicz W, Jóźwiak S. Eleven Polish patients with microcephaly, immunodeficiency, and chromosomal instability: the Nijmegen breakage syndrome. Am J Med Genet 57:462–471, 1995.

Cornforth MW, Bedford JS. On the nature of a defect in cells from individuals with ataxia-telangiectasia. Science 227:1589–1591, 1985.

Cortez D, Wang Y, Qin J, Elledge SJ. Requirement of ATM-dependent phosphorylation of brca1 in the DNA damage response to double-strand breaks. Science 286:1162–1166, 1999.

Cox R, Debenham PG, Masson WK, Webb MB. Ataxia-telangiectasia: a human mutation giving high-frequency misrepair double-stranded scissions. Mol Biol Med 3:229–244, 1986.

Crawford TO. Ataxia-telangiectasia. Semin Pediatr Neurol 5:287–294, 1998.

Crawford TO, Mandir AS, Lefton-Greif MA, Goodman SN, Goodman BK, Sengul H, Lederman HM. Quantitative neurologic assessment of ataxia-telangiectasia. Neurol 54:1505–1509, 2000.

D'Andrea AD. Fanconi anaemia forges a novel pathway. Nat Genet 14:240–242, 1996.

D'Andrea AD, Grompe M. Molecular biology of Fanconi anemia: implications for diagnosis and therapy. Blood 90:1725–1736, 1997.

De Kerviler E, Guermazi A, Zagdanski A-M, Gluckman E, Friga J. The clinical and radiological features of Fanconi's anemia. Clin Radiol 55:340–345, 2000.

De Medeiros CR, Zanis-Neto J, Pasquini R. Bone marrow transplantation for patients with Fanconi anemia: reduced doses of cyclophosphamide without irradiation as conditioning. Bone Marrow Transplant 24:849–852, 1999.

De Winter JP, Leveille F, Van Berkel CG, Rooimans MA, Van der Weel L, Steltenpool J, Demuth I, Morgan NV, Alon N, Bosnoyan-Collins L, Lightfoot J, Leegwater PA, Waisfisz Q, Komatsu K, Arwert F, Pronk JC, Mathew CG, Digweed M, Buchwald M. Joenje H. Isolation of cDNA representing the Fanconi anemia complementation group E gene. Am J Hum Genet 67:1306–1308, 2000.

De Winter JP, Waisfisz O, Rooimans MA, Van Berkel CG, Bosnoyan-Collins L, Alon N, Carreau M, Bender O, Demuth I, Schindler D, Pronk JC, Arwert F, Hoehn H, Digweed M, Buchwald M, Joenje H. The Fanconi anaemia group G gene FANCG is identical with XRCC9. Nat Genet 20:281–283, 1998.

Drolet BA, Drolet B, Zvulunov A, Jacobsen R, Troy J, Esterly NB. Cutaneous granulomas as a presenting sign in ataxia-telangiectasia. Dermatology 194:273–275, 1997.

Dulic V, Kaufmann WK, Wilson SJ, Tisty TD, Lees E, Harper JW, Elledge SJ, Reed SI. p53-dependent inhibition of cyclin-dependent kinase activities in human fibroblasts during radiation-induced G1 arrest. Cell 76:1013–1023, 1994.

Dupey JM, Lafforet A. A defect of cellular immunity in xeroderma pigmentosum. Clin Immunol Immunopathol 3:52–58, 1974.

Dutertre S, Ababou M, Onclercq R, Delic J, Chatton B, Jaulin C, Amor-Gueret M. Cell cycle regulation of the endogenous wild type Bloom's syndrome DNA helicase. Oncogene 19:2731–2738, 2000.

Ellis NA, Groden J, Ye TZ, Straughen J, Lennon DJ, Ciocci S, Proytcheva M, German J. The Bloom's syndrome gene product is homologous to RecQ helicases. Cell 83:655–666, 1995.

Ellis NA, Roe AM, Kozloski J, Proytcheva M, Falk C, German J. Linkage disequilibrium between the FES, D15S127, and BLM loci in Ashkenazi Jews with Bloom syndrome. Am J Human Genet 55:453–460, 1994.

Epstein WL, Fudenberg HH, Reed WB, Boder E, Sedgwick RP. Immunologic studies in ataxia-telangiectasia. I. Delayed hypersensitivity and serum immune globulin levels in probands and first-degree relatives. Int Arch Allergy Appl Immunol 30:15–29, 1966.

Ersoy F, Berkel AI, Sanal O, Oktay H. Twenty-year follow-up of 160 patients with ataxia-telangiectasia. Turk J Pediatr 33:205–215, 1991.

Escarceller M, Rousset S, Moustacchi E, Papadopoulo D. The fidelity of double strand breaks processing is impaired in complement groups B and D of Fanconi anemia, a genetic instability syndrome. Somat Cell Mol Genet 23:401–411, 1997.

Etzioni A, Lahat N, Benderly A, Katz R, Pollack S. Humoral and cellular immune dysfunction in a patient with Bloom's syndrome and recurrent infections. J Clin Lab Immunol 28:151–154, 1989.

Fiorilli M, Businco L, Pandolfi P, Paganelli R, Russo G, Aiuti F. Heterogeneity of immunological abnormalities in ataxia-telangiectasia. J Clin Immunol 3:135–141, 1983.

FitzGerald MG, Bean JM, Hegde SR, Unsal H, MacDonald DJ, Harkin DP, Finkelstein DM, Isselbacher KJ, Haber DA. Heterozygous ATM mutations do not contribute to early onset of breast cancer. Nat Genetics 15:307–310, 1997.

Foray N, Priestley A, Alsbeih G, Badie C, Capulas EP, Arlett CF, Malaise EP. Hypersensitivity of ataxia telangiectasia fibroblasts to ionizing radiation is associated with a repair deficiency of DNA double-strand breaks. Int J Radiat Biol 72:271–283, 1997.

Franceschini P, Martino S, Ciocchini M, Ciuti E, Vardeu MP, Guala A, Signorile F, Camerano P, Franceschini D, Tovo PA. Variability of clinical and immunological phenotype in immunodeficiency-centromeric instability-facial anomalies syndrome. Report of two new patients and review of the literature. Eur J Pediatr 154:840–846, 1995.

Fryns JP, Azou M, Jaeken J, Eggermont E, Pedersen JC, Van den Berghe H. Centromeric instability of chromosomes 1, 9, and 16 associated with combined immunodeficiency. Hum Genet 57:108–110, 1981.

Futaki M, Yamashita T, Yagasaki H, Toda T, Yabe M, Kato S, Asano S, Nakahata T. The IVS4+4 A to T mutation of the Fanconi anemia gene FANCC is not associated with a severe phenoype in Japanese patients. Blood 95:1493–1498, 2000.

Gangloff S, McDonald JP, Bendixen C, Arthur L, Rothstein R. The yeast type I topoisomerase Top3 interacts with Sgs1, a DNA helicase homolog: a potential eukaryotic reverse gyrase. Mol Cell Biol 14:8391–8398, 1994.

Garcia-Higuera I, D'Andrea AD. Regulated binding of the Fanconi anemia proteins, FANCA and FANCC. Blood 93:1430–1432, 1999.

Garcia-Higuera I, Kuang Y, Naf D, Wasik J, D'Andrea AD. Fanconi anemia proteins FANCA, FANCC, and FANCG/XRCC9 interact in a functional nuclear complex. Mol Cell Biol 19:4866–4873, 1999.

Gardner MB, Goodman WN. Ataxia-telangiectasia. Electron microscopic study of a nerve biopsy. Bull Los Angeles Neurol Soc 34:23–28, 1969.

Gatei M, Scott SP, Filippovitch I, Soronika N, Lavin MF, Weber B, Khanna KK. Role for ATM in DNA damage-induced phosphorylation of BRCA1. Cancer Res 60:3299–3304, 2000.

Gatti RA, Berkel I, Boder E, Bradedt G, Charmley P, Concannon P, Ersoy F, Foroud T, Jaspers NG, Lange K, et al. Localization of an ataxia-telangiectasia gene to chromosome 11q22-23. Nature 336:577–580, 1988.

Gatti RA, Tward A, Concannon P. Cancer risk in ATM heterozygotes: a model of phenotypic and mechanistic differences between missense and truncating mutations. Molec Genet Metab 68:419–423, 1999.

Gennery AR, Cant AJ, Jeggo PA. Immunodeficiency associated with DNA repair defects. Clin Exp Immunol 121:1–7, 2000.

German J. Bloom's syndrome. I. Genetical and clinical observations in the first twenty-seven patients. Am J Hum Genet 21:196–227, 1969.

German J. Bloom's syndrome. XX. The first 100 cancers. Cancer Genet Cytogenet 93:100–106, 1997.

German J. Bloom syndrome: a mendelian prototype of somatic mutational disease. Medicine (Baltimore) 72:393–406, 1993.

German J. The immunodeficiency of Bloom syndrome. In Ochs HD, Smith CIE, Puck JM, eds. Primary Immunodeficiency Diseases: A Molecular and Genetic Approach. New York, Oxford University Press, 1999, pp 335–338.

German J, Ellis NA. Molecular genetics of Bloom's syndrome. Hum Mol Genet 5:1457–1463, 1996.

Giampietro PF, Adler-Brecher B, Verlander PC, Pavlakis SG, Davis JG, Auerbach AD. The need for more accurate and timely diagnosis in Fanconi anemia: a report from the International Fanconi Anemia Registry. Pediatrics 91:1116–1120, 1993.

Gilad S, Chessa L, Khosravi R, Russell P, Galanty P, Piane M, Gatti RA, Jorgensen TJ, Shiloh Y, Bar-Shira A. Genotype-phenotype relationships in ataxia-teleangiectasia and variants. Am J Humn Genet 62:551–561, 1998.

Gilad S, Khosravi R, Shkedy D, Uziel T, Ziv Y, Savitsky K, Rotman G, Smith S, Chessa L, Jorgensen TJ, Harnik R, Frydman M, Sanal O,

Portnoi S, Goldwicz Z, Jaspers NG, Gatti RA, Lenoir G, Lavin MF, Tatsumi K, Wegner RD, Shiloh Y, Bar-Shira A. Predominance of null mutations in ataxia-telangiectasia. Hum Mol Genet 5:433–439, 1996.

Girard PM, Foray N. Stumm M, Waugh A, Riballo E, Maser RS. Radiosensitivity in Nijmegen breakage syndrome cells is attributable to a repair defect and not cell cycle checkpoint defects. Cancer Res 60:4881–4888, 2000.

Gotoff SP, Amirmokri E, Liebner EJ. Ataxia-telangiectasia. Neoplasia, untoward response to x-irradiation, and tuberous sclerosis. Am J Dis Child 114:617–625, 1967.

Gottlieb TM, Jackson SP. Protein kinases and DNA damage. Trends Biochem Sci 19:500–503, 1994.

Green AJ, Yates JRW, Taylor AMR, Biggs P, McGuire GM, McConville CM, Billing CJ, Barnes ND. Severe microcephaly with normal intellectual development: the Nijmegen breakage syndrome. Arch Dis Child 73:431–434, 1995.

Haber JE. Partners and pathways: repairing a double-strand break. Trends Genet 16:259–264, 2000.

Hecht F, Hecht BK. Cancer in ataxia-telangiectasia patients. Cancer Genet Cytogenet 46:9–19, 1990.

Hecht F, McCaw BK, Koler RD. Ataxia-telangiectasia—clonal growth of translocation lymphocytes. N Engl J Med 289:286–291, 1973.

Hejna JA, Timmers CD, Reifsteck C, Bruun DA, Lucas LW, Jakobs PM, Toth-Fejel S, Unsworth N, Clemens SL, Garcia DK, Naylor SL, Thayer MJ, Olson SB, Grompe M, Mose RE. Localization of the Fanconi anemia complementation group D to a 200-Kb region on chromosome 3p25.3. Am J Hum Genet 66:1540–1551, 2000.

Heo SJ, Tatebayashi K, Ohsugi I, Shimamoto A, Furuichi Y, Ikeda H. Bloom's syndrome gene suppresses premature ageing caused by Sgs1deficiency in yeast. Genes Cells 4:619–625, 1999.

Hernandez D, McConville CM, Stacey W, Woods CG, Brown MM, Shutt P, Rysiecki G, Taylor AMR. A family showing no evidence of linkage between the ataxia-telangiectasia gene and chromosome 11q22-23. J Med Genet 30:135–140, 1993.

Herzog KH, Chong MJ, Kapsetaki M, Morgan JI, McKinnon PJ. Requirement for ATM in ionizing radiation-induced cell death in the developing central nervous system. Science 280:1089–1091, 1998.

Higurashi M, Cohen PE. In vitro chromosomal radiosensitivity in "chromosomal breakage syndromes." Cancer 32:380–383, 1973.

Hirao A, Kong YY, Matsuoka S, Wakeham A, Ruland J, Yoshida H, Liu D, Elledge SJ, Mak TW. DNA damage-induced activation of p53 by the checkpoint kinase Chk2. Science 287:1824–1827, 2000.

Hoatlin ME, Zhi Y, Ball H, Silvey K, Melnick A, Stone S, Arai S, Hawe N, Owen G, Zelent A, Licht JD. A novel BTB/POZ transcriptional repressor protein interacts with the Fanconi anemia group C protein and PLZF. Blood 94:3737–3747, 1999.

Hoshino T, Wang J, Devetten MP, Iwata N, Kajigaya S, Wise RJ, Liu JM, Youssoufian H. Molecular chaperone GRP94 binds to the Fanconi anemia group C protein and regulates its intracellular expression. Blood 91:4379–4386, 1998.

Houldsworth J, Lavin MF. Effect of ionizing radiation on DNA synthesis in ataxia-telganiectasia cells. Nucleic Acids Res 8:3709–3720, 1980.

Howard PJ, Lewis IJ, Harris F, Walker S. Centromeric instability of chromosomes 1 and 16 with variable immune deficiency: a new syndrome. Clin Genet 27:501–505, 1985.

Hsieh CL, Arlett CF, Lieber MR. V(D)J recombination in ataxia telangiectasia, Bloom's syndrome, and a DNA ligase-I-associated immunodeficiency disorder. J Biol Chem 268:20105–20109, 1993.

Hulton M. Selective somatic pairing and fragility at 1q12 in a boy with common variable immunodeficiency. Clin Genet 14:294, 1978.

Huo YK, Wang Z, Hong JH, Chessa L, McBride WH, Perlman SL et al. Radiosensitivity of ataxia-telangiectasia, X-linked agammaglobulinemia, and related syndromes using a modified colony survival assay. Cancer Res 54:2544–2547, 1994.

Hütteroth TH, Litwin SD, German J. Abnormal immune responses of Bloom's syndrome lymphocytes in vitro. J Clin Invest 56:1–7, 1975.

Ishov AM, Sotnikov AG, Negorev D, Vladimirova OV, Neff N, Kamitani T, Yeh ET, Strauss Jf 3rd, Maul GG. PML is critical for ND10 formation and recruits the PML-interacting protein daxx to this nuclear structure when modified by SUMO-1. J Cell Biol 147:221–234, 1999.

Itin PH, Pittelkow MR. Trichothiodystrophy: Review of sulfur-deficient brittle hair syndromes and association with the ectodermal dysplasias. J Am Acad Dermatol 22:705–717, 1990.

Janin N, Andrieu N, Ossian K, Laugé A, Croquette M-F, Griscelli C, Debré M, Bressac-de-Paillerets B, Aurias A, Stoppa-Lyonnet D. Breast cancer risk in ataxia-telangiectasia (AT) heterozygotes: haplotype study in French AT families. Br J Cancer 80:1042–1045, 1999.

Jaspers NG, Bootsma D. Genetic complementation analysis of ataxia-telangiectasia by somatic cell fusion. IARC Sci Publ 39:127–136, 1982.

Jaspers NG, Gatti RA, Baan C, Linssen PC, Bootsma D. Genetic complementation analysis of ataxia-telangiectasia and Nijmegen breakage syndrome: a survey of 50 patients. Cytogenet Cell Genet 49:259–263, 1988.

Joenje H, Levitus M, Waisfisz Q, D'Andrea A, Garcia-Higuera I, Pearson T, Van Berkel CG, Rooimans MA, Morgan N, Mathew CG, Arwert F. Complementation analysis in Fanconi anemia: assignment of the reference FA-H patient to group A. Am J Hum Genet 67:759–762, 2000.

Joenje H, Oostra AB, Wijker M, Di Summa FM, Van Berkel CG, Rooimans MA, Ebell W, Van Weel M, Pronk JC, Buchwald M, Arwert F. Evidence for at least eight Fanconi anemia genes. Am J Hum Genet 61:940–944, 1997.

Johnson FB, Lombard DB, Neff NF, Mastrangelo MA, Dewolf W, Ellis NA, Marciniak RA, Yin Y, Jaenisch R, Guarente L. Association of the Bloom syndrome protein with topoisomerase III alpha in somatic and meiotic cells. Cancer Res 60:1162–1167, 2000.

Jongmans W, Vuillaume M, Chrzanowska K, Smeets D, Sperling K, Hall J. Nijmegen breakage syndrome cells fail to induce the p53-mediated DNA response following exposure to ionizing radiation. Mol Cell Biol 17:5016–5022, 1997.

Karow JK, Chakraverty RK, Hickson ID. The Bloom's Syndrome gene product is a 3′–5′ DNA helicase. J Biol Chem 272:30611–30614, 1997.

Karow JK, Constantinou A, Li JL, West SC, Hickson ID. The Bloom's syndrome gene product promotes branch migration of holliday junctions. Proc Natl Acad Sci USA 97:6504–6508, 2000.

Kastan MB, Zhan O, el-Deiry WS, Carrier F, Jacks T, Walsh WV, Plunkett BS, Vogelstein B, Fornace AJ Jr. A mammalian cell cycle checkpoint pathway utilizing p53 and GADD45 is defective in ataxia-telangiectasia. Cell 71:587–597, 1992.

Keith CT, Schreiber SL. PIK-related kinases: DNA repair, recombination, and cell cycle checkpoint. Science 270:50–51, 1995.

Keegan KS, Holtzman DA, Plug AW, Christenson ER, Brainerd EE, Flaggs G, Bentley NJ, Taylor EM, Meyn MS, Moss SB, Carr AM, Ashley T, Hoekstra MF. The Atr and Atm protein kinases associate with different sites along meiotic pairing chromosomes. Genes Dev 10:2423–2437, 1996.

Khanna KK, Beamish H, Yan Y, Hobson K, Williams R, Dunn I, Lavin MF. Nature of G1/S cell cycle checkpoint defect in ataxia-telangiectasia. Oncogene 11:609–618, 1995.

Khanna KK, Keating KE, Kozlov S, Scott S, Gatei M, Hobson K, Taya Y, Gabrielli B, Chan D, Lees-Miller SP, Lavin MF. ATM associates with and phosphorylates p53: mapping the region of interaction. Nat Genet 20:398–400, 1998.

Khanna KK, Lavin MF. Ionizing radiation and UV induction of p53 protein by different pathways ataxia-telangiectasia cells. Oncogene 8:3307–3312, 1993.

Kiran O, Yalaz K, Taysi K, Say B. Immunological studies in ataxia-telangiectasia. Clin Genet 5:40–45, 1974.

Klein C, Wenning GK, Quinn NP, Marsden CD. Ataxia without telangiectasia masquerading as benign hereditary chorea. Movement Dis 2:217–220, 1996.

Kohli-Kumar M, Morris C, DeLaat C, Sambrano J, Masterson M, Mueller R, Shahidi NT, Yanik G, Desanes K, Friedman DJ, Auerbach AD, Harris RE. Bone marrow transplantation in

Fanconi anemia using matched sibling donors. Blood 84:2050–2054, 1994.

Kojis TL, Gatti RA, Sparkes RS. The cytogenetics of ataxia-telangiectasia. Cancer Genet Cytogenet 56:143–156, 1991.

Komatsu K, Matsuura S, Tauchi H, Endo S, Kodama S, Smeets D, Weemaes C, Oshimura M. The gene for Nijmegen breakage syndrome (V2) is not located on chromosome 11. Am J Hum Genet 58:885–888, 1996.

Korkina LG, Durnev AD, Suslova TB, Cheremisina ZP, Daugel-Dauge NO, Afanas'ev IB. Oxygen radical-mediated mutagenic effect of asbestos on human lymphoctye suppression by oxygen radical scavengers. Mutat Res 265:245–253, 1992.

Kraemer KH, Lee MM, Scotto J. Xeroderma pigmentosum: Cutaneous, ocular and neurologic abnormalities in 830 published cases. Arch Dermatol 123:241–250, 1987.

Krepinsky AB, Rainbow AJ, Heddle JA. Studies on the ultraviolet light sensitivity of Bloom's syndrome fibroblasts. Mutat Res 69:357–368, 1980.

Kruyt FAE, Hoshino T, Liu JM, Joseph P, Jaiswal AK, Youssoufian H. Abnormal microsomal detoxification implicated in Fanconi anemia group C by interaction of the FAC protein with NADPH cytochrome P450 reductase. Blood 92:3050–3056, 1998.

Kuang Y, Garcia-Higuera I, Moran A, Mondoux M, Digweed M, D'Andrea AD. Carboxy terminal region of the Fanconi anemia protein, FANCG/XRCC9 required for functional activity. Blood 96:1625–1632, 2000.

Kuhn EM, Therman E. Cytogenetics of Bloom's syndrome. Cancer Genet Cytogenet 22:1–18, 1986.

Kupfer GM, Naf D, Suliman A, Pulsipher M, D'Andrea AD. The Fanconi anemia proteins, FAA and FAC, interact to form a nuclear complex. Nat Genet 17:487–490, 1997.

Kurihara T, Tatsumi K, Takahashi H, Inoue M. Sister-chromatid exchanges induced by ultraviolet light in Bloom's syndrome fibroblasts. Mutat Res 183:197–202, 1987.

Kusano K, Berres ME, Engels WR. Evolution of the RECQ family of helicases: A drosophila homolog, Dmblm is similar to the human bloom syndrome gene. Genetics 151:1027–1039, 1999.

Lahat N, Zelnik N, Froom P, Kinarty A, Etzioni A. Impaired autologous mixed lymphocyte reaction (AMLR) in patients with ataxia-telangiectasia and their family members. Clin Exp Immunol 74:32–35, 1988.

Lakin ND, Weber P, Stankovic T, Rottinghaus ST, Taylor AM, Jackson SP. Analysis of the ATM protein in wild-type and ataxia telangiectasia cells. Oncogene 13:2707–2716, 1996.

Lange E, Borresen AL, Chen X, Chessa L, Chiplunkar S, Concannon P, Dandekar S, Gerken S, Lange K, Liang T. Localization of an ataxia-telangiectasia gene to an approximately 500-kb interval on chromosome 11q23.1: linkage analysis of 176 families by an international consortium. Am J Hum Genet 57:112–119, 1995.

Lange E, Gatti RA, Sobel E, Concannon P, Lange K. How many ataxia-telangiectasia genes? In Gatti, RA, Painter RB, eds. Ataxia-telangiectasia. NATO ASJ Series. Berlin, Springer-Verlag, 1993, pp 37–54.

Lavin MF, Khanna KK, Beamish H, Spring K, Watters D, Shiloh Y. Relationship of the ataxia-telangiectasia protein ATM to phosphoinositide 3-kinase. Trends Biochem Sci 20:382–383, 1995.

Lavin MF, Shiloh Y. Ataxia-telangiectasia. In Primary Immunodeficiency Diseases: A Molecular and Genetic Approach. New York, Oxford University Press, pp 306–323, 1999.

Lavin MF, Shiloh Y. The genetic defect in ataxia-telangiectasia. Annu Rev Immunol 15:177–202, 1997.

Lefton-Greif MA, Crawford TO, Winkelstein JA, Loughlin GM, Koerner CB, Zaburak M, Lederman HM. Oropharyngeal dysphagia and aspiration in patients with ataxia-telangiectasia. J Pediatr 136:225–231, 2000.

Lewis RF, Lederman HM, Crawford TO. Ocular motor abnormalities in ataxia-telangiectasia. Ann Neurol 46:287–295, 1999.

Liao S, Graham J, Yan H. The function of Xenopus Bloom's syndrome protein homolog (xBLM) in replication. Genes Dev 14:2570–2575, 2000.

Lieber MR, Hesse JE, Lewis S, Bosma GC, Rosenberg N, Mizuuchi K, Bosma MJ, Gellert M. The defect in murine severe combined immune deficiency; joining of signal sequences but not coding segments in V(D)J recombination. Cell 55:7–16, 1988.

Lim DS, Kim ST, Xu B, Maser RS, Lin J, Petrini JH, Kastan MB. ATM phosphorylates p95/nbs1 in an S-phase checkpoint pathway. Nature 404:613–617, 2000.

Lindor NM, Furuichi Y, Kitao S, Shimamoto A, Arndt C, Jalal S. Rothmund-Thomson syndrome due to RECQ4 helicase mutations: report and clinical and molecular comparisons with Bloom syndrome and Werner syndrome. A J Med Genet 90:223–228, 2000.

Liu JM, Young NS, Walsh CE, Cottler-Fox M, Carter C, Dunbar C, Barrett AJ, Emmons R. Retroviral mediated gene transfer of the Fanconi anemia complementation group C gene to hematopoietic progenitors of group C patients. Hum Gene Ther 8:1715–1730, 1997.

Lo Ten Foe JR, Rooimans MA, Bosnoyan-Collins L, Alon N, Wijker M, Parker L, Lightfoot J, Carreau M, Callen DF, Savoia A, Cheng NC, Van Berkel CG, Strunk MH, Gille JJ, Pals G, Kruyt FA, Pronk JC, Arwert F, Buchwald M, Joenje H. Expression cloning of a cDNA for the major Fanconi anaemia gene, FAA. Nat Genet 14:320–323, 1996.

Louis-Bar D. Sur un syndrome progressif comprenant des télangiectasies capillaries cutanées et conjunctivales symétriques, à disposition naevode et de troubles cérébelleux. Confin Neurol (Basel) 4:32–42, 1941.

Luo G, Yao MS, Bender CF, Mills M, Bladl AR, Bradley A, Petrini JH. Disruption of mRad50 causes embryonic stem cell lethality, abnormal embryonic development, and sensitivity to ionizing radiation. Proc Natl Acad Sci USA 96:7376–7381, 1999.

McFarlin DE, Strober W, Waldmann TA. Ataxia-telangiectasia. Medicine (Baltimore) 51:281–314, 1972.

Martin RH, Rademaker A, German J. Chromosomal breakage in human spermatozoa, a heterozygous effect of the Bloom syndrome mutation. Am J Hum Genet 55:1242–1246, 1994.

Matsuoka S, Rotman G, Ogawa A, Shiloh Y, Tamai K, Elledge SJ. Ataxia telangiectasia-mutated phosphorylates Chk2 in vivo and in vitro. Proc Natl Acad Sci USA 97:10389–10394, 2000.

Matsuura S, Tauchi H, Nakamura A, Kondo N, Sakamoto S, Endo S, Smeets D, Solder B, Belohradsky BH, Der Kaloustian VM, Oshimura M, Isomura M, Nakamura Y, Komatsu K. Positional cloning of the gene for Nijmegen breakage syndrome. Nat Genet 19:179–181, 1998.

Matsuura S, Weemaes C, Smeets D, Takami H, Kondo N, Sakamoto S, Yano N, Nakamura A, Tauchi H, Endo S, Oshimura M, Komatsu K. Genetic mapping using microcell-mediated chromosome transfer suggests a locus for Nijmegen breakage syndrome at chromosome 8q21-24. Am J Hum Genet 60:1487–1494, 1997.

Meyn MS. High spontaneous intrachromosomal recombination rates in ataxia-telangiectasia. Science 260:1327–1330, 1993.

Miller ME, Chatten J. Ovarian changes in ataxia-telangiectasia. Acta Paediatr Scand. 56:559–561, 1967.

Moens PB, Freire R, Tarsounas M, Spyropoulos B, Jackson SP. Expression and nuclear localization of BLM, a chromosome stability protein mutated in Bloom's syndrome, suggest a role in recombination during meiotic prophase. J Cell Sci 113:663–672, 2000.

Morgan JL, Holcomb TM, Morrissey RW. Radiation reaction in ataxia-telangiectasia. Am J Dis Child 116:557–558, 1968.

Morrell D, Cromartie E, Swift M. Mortality and cancer incidence in 263 patients with ataxia-telangiectasia. J Natl Cancer Inst 77:89–92, 1986.

Nagasawa H, Little JB. Suppression of cytotoxic effect of mitomycin-C by superoxide dismutase in Fanconi's anemia and dyskeratosis congenita fibroblasts. Carcinogenesis 4:795–799, 1983.

Nakura J, Ye L, Morishima A, Kohara K, Miki T. Helicases and aging. Cell Mol Life Sci 57:716–730, 2000.

Nance MA, Berry SA. Cockayne syndrome: Review of 140 cases. Am J Med Genet 42:68–84, 1992.

Neff NF, Ellis NA, Ye TZ, Noonan J, Huang K, Sanz M, Proytcheva M. The DNA helicase activity of BLM is necessary for the correction of the genomic instability of Bloom syndrome cells. Mol Bio Cell 10:665–676, 1999.

Nelms BE, Maser RS, MacKay JF, Lagally MG, Petrini JH. In situ visualization of DNA double-strand break repair in human fibroblasts. Science 280:590–592, 1998.

Nowak-Wegrzyn A, Crawford TO, Winkelstein JA, Carson KA, Lederman HM. Immunodeficiency and infections in ataxia-telangiectasia. J Pediatr 2004 (in press).

Okano M, Bell DW, Haber DA, Li E. DNA methyl-transferases Dnmt3a and Dnmt3b are essential for de novo methylation and mammalian development. Cell 99:247–257, 1999.

Olsen JH, Hahnemann M, Børresen-Dale A-L, Brondum-Nielsen K, Hammarstrom L, Kleinerman R, Kääriäinen H, Lönnqvist T, Sankila R, Seersholm N, Tretli S, Yuen J, Boice JD Jr., Tucker M. Cancer in patients with ataxia-telangiectasia and in their relatives in the Nordic countries. J Natl Cancer Inst 93:121–127, 2001.

Oppenheim JJ, Barlow M, Waldmann TA, Block JB. Imparied in vitro lymphocyte transformation in patients with ataxia-telangiectasia. Br Med J 2:330–333, 1966.

Oxelius VA, Berkel AI, Hanson LA. IgG2 deficiency in ataxia-telangiectasia. N Engl J Med 306:515–517, 1982.

Paganelli R, Scala E, Scarselli E, Ortolani C, Cossarizza A, Carmini D et al. Selective deficiency of CD4⁺/CD45RA⁺ lymphocytes in patients with ataxia-telangiectasia. J Clin Immunol 12:84–91, 1992.

Painter RB, Young BR. Radiosensitivity in ataxia-telangiectasia: a new explanation. Proc Natl Acad Sci USA 77:7315–7317, 1980.

Paller AS, Massey RB, Curtis MA, Pelachyk JM, Dombrowski HC, Leickly FE, Swift M. Cutaneous granulomatous lesions in patients with ataxia-telangiectasia. J Pediatr 119:917–922, 1991.

Pandita TK, Pathak S, Geard CR. Chromosome end associations, telomeres and telomerase activity in ataxia telangiectasia cells. Cytogenet Cell Genet 71:86–93, 1995.

Pedersen FK, Hertz H, Lundsteen C, Platz P, Thomsen M. Indication of primary immune deficiency in Fanconi's anemia. Acta Paediatr Scand 66:745–751, 1977.

Peterson RD, Cooper MD, Good RA. Lymphoid tissue abnormalities associated with ataxia-telangiectasia. Am J Med 41:342–359, 1966.

Peterson RD, Kelly WD, Good RA. Ataxia-telangiectasia: Its association with a defective thymus, immunological-deficiency disease, and malignancy. Lancet 1:1189–1193, 1964.

Pitts SA, Kullar HS, Stankovic T, Stewart GS, Last JIK, Bedenham T, Armstrong SJ, Piane M, Chessa L, Taylor AMR, Byrd PJ. hMRE11: genomic structure and a null mutation, identified in a transcript protected from nonsense-mediated mRNA decay. Human Molec Genet 10:1155–1162, 2001.

Pohl KR, Farley JD, Jan JE, Junker AK. Ataxia-telangiectasia in a child with vaccine-associated paralytic poliomyelitis. J Pediatr 121:405–407, 1992.

Polmar SH, Waldmann TA, Balestra ST, Jost MC, Terry WD. Immunoglobulin E in immunologic deficiency diseases. I. Relation of IgE and IgA to respiratory tract disease in isolated IgE deficiency, IgA deficiency, and ataxia-telangiectasia. J Clin Invest 51:326–330, 1972.

Predki PF, Nayak LM, Gottlieb MB, Regan L. Dissecting RNA-protein interactions: RNA-RNA recognition by Rop. Cell 80:41–50, 1995.

Pronk JC, Gibson RA, Savoia A, Wijker M, Morgan NV, Melchionda S, Ford D, Temtamy S, Ortega JJ, Jansen S. Localization of the Fanconi anaemia complementation group A gene to chromosome 16q24.3. Nat Genet 11:338–340, 1995.

Reed WB, Epstein WL, Boder E, Sedgwick R. Cutaneous manifestations of ataxia-telangiectasia. JAMA 195:746–753, 1966.

Rigas DA, Tisdale VV, Hecht F. Transformation of blood lymphocytes in ataxia-telangiectasia. Dose and time response to phytohemagglutinin. Int Arch Allergy Appl Immunol 39:221–233, 1970.

Rivat-Peran L, Buriot D, Salier JP, Rivat C, Dumitresco SM, Griscelli C. Immunoglobulins in ataxia-telangiectasia: evidence for IgG4 and IgA2 subclass deficiencies. Clin Immunol Immunopathol 20:99–110, 1981.

Roifman CM, Gelfand EW. Heterogeneity of the immunological deficiency in ataxia-telangiectasia: absence of a clinical-pathological correlation. Kroc Found Ser 19:273–285, 1985.

Rong SB, Valiaho J, Vihinen M. Structural basis of Bloom syndrome (BS) causing mutations in the BLM helicase domain. Mol Med 6:155–164, 2000.

Runger TM, Sobotta P, Dekant B, Moller K, Bauer C, Kraemer KH. In-vivo assessment of DNA ligation efficiency and fidelity in cells from patients with Fanconi's anemia and other cancer-prone hereditary disorders. Toxicol Lett 67:309–324, 1993.

Saar K, Chrzanowska KH, Stumm M, Jung M, Nurnberg G, Wienker TF, Seemanova E, Wegner RD, Reis A, Sperling K. The gene for the ataxia-telangiectasia variant, Nijmegen breakage syndrome maps to a 1-cM interval on chromosome 8q21. Am J Hum Genet 60:605–610, 1997.

Saar K, Schindler D, Wegner RD, Reis A, Wienker TF, Hoehn H, Joenje H, Sperling K, Digweed M. Localisation of a Fanconi anaemia gene to chromosome 9p. Eur J Hum Genet 6:501–508, 1998.

Sadighi-Akha AA, Humphrey RL, Winkelstein JA, Loeb DM, Lederman HM. Oligo-/monoclonal gammopathy and hypergammaglobulinemia in ataxia-telangiectasia. A study of 90 patients. Medicine (Baltimore) 78:370–381, 1999.

Sanal O, Ersoy F, Yel L, Tezcan I, Metin A, Ozyurek H, Gariboglu S, Fikrig S, Berkel AI, Rijkers GT, Zegers BJ. Impaired IgG antibody production to pneumococcal polysaccharides in patients with ataxia-telangiectasia. J Clin Immunol 19:326–334, 1999.

Savitsky K, Bar-Shira A, Gilad S, Rotman G, Ziv Y, Vanagaite L, Tagle DA, Smith S, Uziel T, Sfez S, Ashkenazi M, Pecker I, Frydman M, Harnik R, Patanjali SR, Simmons A, Clines GA, Sartiel A, Gatti RA, Chessa L, Sanal O, Lavin MF, Jaspers NGJ, Taylor AMR, Arlett CF, Miki T, Weissman SM, Lovett M, Collins FS, Shiloh Y. A single ataxia-telangiectasia gene with a product similar to Pl-3 kinase. Science 268:1749–1753, 1995a.

Savitsky K, Sfez S, Tagle DA, Ziv Y, Sartiel A, Collins FS, Shiloh Y, Rotman G. The complete sequence of the coding region of the ATM gene reveals simple to cell cycle regulators in different species. Hum Mol Genet 4:2025–2032, 1995b.

Schaffner C, Idler I, Stilgenbauer S, Döhner H, Lichter P. Mantle cell lymphoma is characterized by inactivation of the ATM gene. Proc Natl Acad Sci USA 97:2773–2778, 2000.

Schalch DS, McFarlin DE, Barlow MH. An unusual form of diabetes mellitus in ataxia telangiectasia. N Engl J Med 282:1396–1402, 1970.

Schefer H, Mattmann S, Joss RA. Hereditary persistence of alpha-fetoprotein. Case report and review of the literature. Ann Oncol 9:667–672, 1998.

Scully R, Chen J, Ochs RL, Keegan K, Hoekstra M, Feunteun J, Livingston DM. Dynamic changes of BRCA1 subnuclear location and phosphorylation state are initiated by DNA damage. Cell 90:425–435, 1997.

Sedgwick RP, Boder E. Ataxia-telangiectasia. In De Jong JMBV, ed. Handbook of Clinical Neurology, vol 16. Hereditary Neuropathies and Spinocerebellar Atrophies. Amsterdam, Elsevier, 1991, pp 347–423.

Sedgwick RP, Boder E. Ataxia-telangiectasia. In Vinken PJ, Bruyn GW, eds. Handbook of Clinical Neurology, vol 14. Amsterdam, North Holland Publishers, 1972, pp 267–339.

Seemanová E. An increased risk for malignant neoplasms in heterozygotes for a syndrome of microcephaly, normal intelligence, growth retardation, remarkable facies, immunodeficiency and chromosomal instability. Mutat Res 238:321–324, 1990.

Seemanová E. Passarge E, Beneškova D, Houštěk J, Kasal P, Ševčiková M. Familial microcephaly with normal intelligence, immunodeficiency, and risk for lymphoreticular malignancies: a new autosomal recessive disorder. Am J Med Genet 20:639–648, 1985.

Seyschab H, Schindler D, Friedl R, Barbi G, Boltshauser E, Fryns JP, Hanefeld F, Korinthenberg R, Krageloh-Mann I, Scheres JM. Simultaneous measurement, using flow cytometry, of radiosensitivity and defective mitogen response in ataxia-telangiectasia and related syndromes. Eur J Pediatr 151:756–760, 1992.

Shangary S, Brown KD, Adamson AW, Edmonson S, Ng B, Pandita TK, Yalowich J, Taccioli GE, Baskaran R. Regulation of DNA-dependent protein kinase activity by ionizing radiation-activated abl kinase is an ATM-dependent process. J Biol Chem 275:30163–30168, 2000.

Sharan SK, Morimatsu M, Albrecht U, Lim DS, Regel E, Dinh C, Sands A, Eichele G, Hasty P, Bradley A. Embryonic lethality and radiation hypersensitivity mediated by Rad51 in mice lacking Brca2. Nature 386:804–810, 1997.

Shiloh Y. Ataxia-telangiectasia and the Nijmegen breakage syndrome: related disorders but genes apart. Annu Rev Genet 31:635–662, 1997.

Smeets DFCM, Moog U, Weemaes CMR, Vaes-Peeters G, Merkx GFM, Niehof JP, Hamers G. ICF syndrome: a new case and review of the literature. Hum Genet 94:240–246, 1994.

Smith J, Andrau JC, Kallenbach S, Laquerbe A, Doven N, Papadopoulo D. Abnormal rearrangements associated with V(D)J recombination in Fanconi anemia. J Mol Biol 281:815–825, 1998.

Smith JL, Cogan DG. Ataxia-telangiectasia. Arch Opthal 62:364–369, 1959.

Spector BD, Filipovich AH, Perry GS III, Kersey JH. Epidemiology of cancer in ataxia-telangiectasia. In Bridges BA, Harnden DG, eds. Ataxia-telangiectasia: A Cellular and Molecular Link Between Cancer, Neuropathology, and Immune Deficiency. New York, Wiley, 1982, pp 103–138.

Spring K, Cross S, Li C, Watters D, Ben-Senior L, Waring P, Ahangari F, Lu SL, Chen P, Misko I, Paterson C, Kay G, Smorodinsky NI, Shiloh Y, Lavin MF. ATM knock-in mice harbouring an in-frame deletion corresponding to the human ATM 7636del9 common mutation exhibit a variant phenotype. Cancer Res 61:4561–4568, 2001.

Standen GR, Hughes IA, Geddes AD, Jones BM, Wardrop CAJ. Myelodysplastic syndrome with trisomy 8 in an adolescent with Fanconi anaemia and selective IgA deficiency. Am J Hematol 31:280–283, 1989.

Stankovic T, Weber P, Stewart G, Bedenham T, Murray J, Byrd PJ, Moss PA, Taylor AM. Inactivation of ataxia-telangiectasia mutated gene in B-cell chronic lymphocytic leukaemia. Lancet 353:26–29, 1999.

Stenson S. Ocular findings in xeroderma pigmentosum: Report of two cases. Ann Ophthalmol 14:580–585, 1982.

Stewart GS, Maser RS, Stankovic T, Bressan DA, Kaplan MI, Jaspers NGJ, Raams A, Byrd PJ, Petrin JHJ, Taylor AMR. The DNA double-strand break repair gene hMRE11 is mutated in individuals with an ataxia-telangiectasia-like disorder. Cell 99:577–587, 1999.

Stobo JD, Tomasi TB Jr. A low molecular weight immunoglobulin antigenically related to 19S IgM. J Clin Invest 46:1329–1337, 1967.

Stoppa-Lyonnet D, Soulier J, Lauge A, Dastot H, Garand R, Sigaux F, Stern MH. Inactivation of the ATM gene in T-cell prolymphocytic leukemias. Blood 91:3920–3926, 1998.

Strathdee CA, Duncan AM, Buchwald M. Evidence for at least four Fanconi anaemia genes including FACC on chromosome 9. Nat Genet 1:196–198, 1992a.

Strathdee CA, Gavish H, Shannon WR, Buchwald M. Cloning of cDNAs for Fanconi's anaemia by functional complementation. Nature 356:763–767, 1992b.

Stumm M, Gatti RA, Reis A, Udar N, Chrzanowska K, Seemanova E, Sperling K, Wegner RD. The ataxia-telangiectasia-variant genes 1 and 2 are distinct from the ataxia-telangiectasia gene on chromosome 11q23.1. Am J Human Genet 57:960–962, 1995.

Stumm M, Sperling K, Wegner RD. Noncomplementation of radiation-induced chromosome aberrations in ataxia-telangiectasia/ataxia-telangiectasia-variant heterodikaryons. Am J Hum Genet 60:1246–1251, 1997.

Sullivan, KE, Veksler E, Lederman H, Lees-Miller SP. Cell cycle checkpoints and DNA repair in Nijmegen breakage syndrome. Clin Immunol Immunopathol 82:43–48, 1997.

Swift M. Malignant disease in heterozygous carriers. Birth Defects Orig Artic Ser 12:133–144, 1976.

Swift M, Morrell D, Massey RB, Chase CL. Incidence of cancer in 161 families affected by ataxia-telangiectasia. N Engl J Med 325:1831–1836, 1991.

Swift M, Reitnauer J, Morrell D, Chase CL. Breast and other cancers in families with ataxia-telangiectasia. N Engl J Med 316:1289–1294, 1987.

Syllaba L, Henner K. Contribution à l'indépendence de l'athétose double idiopathique et congénitale. Atteinte familiale, syndrome dystrophique, signe du reséau vasculaire conjonctival, intégrité psychique. Rev Neurol 1:541–562, 1926.

Taalman RDFM, Hustinx TWJ, Weemaes CMR, Seemanová E, Schmidt A, Passarge E, Scheres JMJC. Further delineation of the Nijmegen breakage syndrome. Am J Med Genet 32:425–431, 1989.

Taalman RDFM, Jaspers NGJ, Scheres JMJC, de Wit J, Hustinx TWJ. Hypersensitivity to ionizing radiation, in vitro, in a new chromosomal breakage disorder, the Nijmegen breakage syndrome. Mutat Res 112:23–32, 1983.

Tadjoedin MK, Fraser FC. Heredity of ataxia-telangiectasia (Louis-Bar syndrome). Am J Dis Child 110:64–68, 1965.

Taniguchi N, Mukai M, Nagaoki T, Mayawaki T, Moriya N, Takahashi H, Kondo N. Impaired B-cell differentiation and T-cell regulatory function in four patients with Bloom's syndrome. Clin Immunol Immunopathol 22:247–258, 1982.

Taylor AM, Harnden DG, Arlett CF, Harcourt SA, Lehmann AR, Stevens S, Bridges BA. Ataxia-telangiectasia: a human mutation with abnormal radiation sensitivity. Nature 258:427–429, 1975.

Taylor AM, Metcalfe JR, Oxford JM, Harnden DG. Is chromatid-type damage in ataxia-telangiectasia after irradiation at G0 a consequence of defective repair? Nature 260:441–443, 1976.

Taylor AM, Metcalfe JA, Thick J, Mak YF. Leukemia and lymphoma in ataxia telangiectasia. Blood 87:423–438, 1996.

Taylor AM, Oxford JM, Metcalfe JA. Spontaneous cytogenetic abnormalities in lymphocytes from thirteen patients with ataxia telangiectasia. Int J Cancer 27:311–319, 1981.

Telatar M, Wang Z, Udar W, Liang T, Concannon P, Bernatowska-Matuscklewicz E, Lavin MF, Sholoh Y, Good RA, Gatti RA. Ataxia-telangiectasia: mutations in ATM cDNA detected by protein-truncation screening. Am J Hum Genet 59:40–44, 1996.

Terplan KL, Krauss RF. Histopathologic brain changes in association with ataxia-telangiectasia. Neurology 19:446–454, 1969.

The International Nijmegen Breakage Syndrome Study Group. Nijmegen breakage syndrome. Arch Dis Child 82:400–406, 2000.

Tiepolo L, Maraschio P, Gimelli G, Cuoco C, Gargani GF, Romano C. Mulltibranched chromosomes 1,9, and 16 in a patient with combined IgA and IgE deficiency. Hum Genet 51:127–137.

Uziel T, Savitsky K, Platzer M, Ziv Y, Helbitz H, Nehls M, Boehm T, Rosenthal A, Shiloh Y, Rotman G. Genomic organization of the ATM Gene. Genomics 33:317–320, 1996.

Valkova G, Ghenev E, Tzancheva M. Centromeric instability of chromosomes 1,9 and 16 with variable immune deficiency. Support of a new syndrome. Clin Genet 31:119–124, 1987.

Van de Kaa CA, Weemaes CMR, Wesseling P, Schaafsma HE, Haraldsson A. Postmortem findings in the Nijmegen breakage syndrome. Pediatr Pathol 14:787–796, 1994.

Van der Burgt I, Chrzanowska KH, Smeets D, Weemaes C. Nijmegen breakage syndrome. J Med Genet 33:153–156, 1996.

Van Kerckhove CW, Ceuppens JL, Vanderschueren-Lodeweyckx M, Eggermont E, Vertessen S, Stevens EA. Bloom's syndrome. Clinical features and immunologic abnormalities of four patients. Am J Dis Child 142:1087–1093, 1988.

Varon R, Seemanova E, Chrzanowska K, Hnateyko O, Piekutowska-Abramczuk D, Krajewska-Walasek M, Sykut-Cegielska J, Sperling K, Reis A. Clinical ascertainment of Nijmegen breakage syndrome (NBS) and prevalence of the major mutation, 657del5, in three Slav populations. Eur J Hum Genet 8:900–902, 2000.

Varon R, Vissinga C, Platzer M, Cerosaletti KM, Chrzanowska KH, Saar K, Beckmann G, Seemanova E, Cooper PR, Nowak NJ, Stumm M, Weemaes CM, Gatti RA, Wilson RK, Digweed M, Rosenthal A, Sperling K, Concannon P, Reis A. Nibrin, a novel DNA double-strand break repair protein, is mutated in Nijmegen breakage syndrome. Cell 93:467–476, 1998.

Vorechovsky I, Luo L, Dyer MJ, Catovsky D, Amlot PL, Yaxley JC et al. Clustering of missense mutations in the ataxia-telangiectasia gene in a sporadic T-cell leukaemia. Nat Genet 17:96–99, 1997.

Waisfisz Q, Morgan NV, Savino M, De Winter JP, Van Berkel CG, Hoatlin ME, Ianzano L, Gibson RA, Arwert F, Savoia A, Mathew CG, Pronk JC, Joenje H. Spontaneous functional correction of homozygous Fanconi anaemia alleles reveals novel mechanistic basis for reverse mosaicism. Nat Genet 22:379–383, 1999a.

Waisfisz Q, Saar K, Morgan NV, Altay C, Leegwater PA, De Winter JP, Komatsu K, Evans GR, Wegner RD, Reis A, Joenje H, Arwert F, Mathew CG, Pronk JC, Digweed M. The Fanconi anemia group E gene, FANCE, maps to chromosome 6p. Am J Hum Genet 64:1400–1405, 1999b.

Waldmann TA. Immunological abnormalities in ataxia-telangiectasia. In Bridges BA, Harnden DG, eds. Ataxia-telangiectasia: A Cellular and Molecular Link Between Cancer Neuropathology and Immune Deficiency. New York, Wiley, 1982, pp 37–51.

Waldmann TA, Broder S, Goldman CK, Frost K, Korsmeyer SJ, Medici MA. Disorders of B cells and helper T cells in the pathogenesis of the immunoglobulin deficiency of patients with ataxia telangiectasia. J Clin Invest 71:282–295, 1983.

Waldmann TA, McIntire KR. Serum alpha-fetoprotein levels in patients with ataxia-telangiectasia. Lancet 1112–1115, 1972.

Walpita D, Plug AW, Neff NF, German J, Ashley T. Bloom's syndrome protein, BLM, colocalizes with replication protein A in meiotic prophase nuclei of mammalian spermatocytes. Proc Natl Acad Sci USA 96:5622–5627, 1999.

Wang JC. Moving one DNA double helix through another by a type II DNA topoisomerase: the story of a simple molecular machine. Q Rev Biophys 31:107–144, 1998.

Wang Y, Cortex D, Yazdi P, Neff N, Elledge SJ, Qin J. BASC, a super complex of BRCA1-associated proteins involved in the recognition and repair of aberrant DNA structures. Genes Dev 14:927–939, 2000.

Waterman MJ, Stavridi ES, Waterman JL, Halazonetis TD. ATM-dependent activation of p53 involves dephosphorylation and association with 14-3-3 proteins. Nat Genet 19:175–178, 1998.

Watt PM, Louis EJ, Borts RH, Hickson ID. Sgs1: a eukaryotic homolog of E. coli RecQ that interacts with topoisomerase II in vivo and is required for faithful chromosome segregation. Cell 81:253–260, 1995.

Watters D, Kedar P, Spring K, Bjorkman J, Chen P, Gatei M, Birrell G, Garrone B, Srinivasa P, Craine DI, Lavin MF. Localization of a portion of extranuclear ATM to peroxisomes. J Biol Chem 274:34277–34282, 1999.

Watters D, Khanna KK, Beamish H, Birrell G, Spring K, Kedar P, Gatei M, Stenzel D, Hobson K, Kozlov S, Zhang N, Farrell A, Ramsay J, Gatti R, Lavin M. Cellular localisation of the ataxia-telangiectasia (ATM) gene product and discrimination between mutated and normal forms. Oncogene 14:1911–1921, 1997.

Webster ADB, Barnes DE, Arlett CF, Lehmann AR, Lindahl T. Growth retardation and immunodeficiency in a patient with mutations in the DNA ligase I gene. Lancet 339:1508–1509, 1992.

Weemaes CMR, Bakkeren JAJM, Ter Haar BGA, Hustinx TWJ, Van Munster PJJ. Immune responses in four patients with Bloom syndrome. Clin Immunol Immunopathol 12:12–19, 1979.

Weemaes CMR, Hustinx TWJ, Scheres JMJC, Van Munster PJJ, Bakkern JAJM, Taalman RDFM. A new chromosomal instability disorder: the Nijmegen breakage syndrome. Acta Paediatr Scand 70:557–564, 1981.

Weemaes CM, Smeets DF, Van der Burgt CJ. Nijmegen breakage syndrome: a progress report. Int J Radiat Biol 66:S185–S188, 1994.

Wegner RD, Chrzanowska K, Sperling K, Stumm M. Ataxia-telangiectasia variants (Nijmegen breakage syndrome). In Ochs HD, Smith CIE, Puck JM, eds. Primary Immunodeficiency Diseases: A Molecular and Genetic Approach. New York, Oxford University Press, pp 324–334, 1999.

Wegner RD, Metzger M, Hanefeld F, Jaspers NGJ, Baan C, Magdorf K, Kunze J, Sperling K. A new chromosomal instability disorder confirmed by complementation studies. Clin Genet 33:20–32, 1988.

Weinert TA, Hartwell LH. Characterization of RAD9 of Saccharomyces cerevisiae and evidence that function acts posttranslationally in cell cycle arrest after DNA damage. Mol Cell Biol 10:6554–6564, 1990.

Weksberg R, Buchwald M, Sargent P, Thompson MW, Siminovitch L. Specific cellular defects in patients with Fanconi anemia. J Cell Physiol 101:311–323, 1979.

Whitney MA, Saito H, Jakobs PM, Gibson RA, Moses RE, Grompe M. A common mutation in the FACC gene causes Fanconi anaemia in Ashkenazi Jews. Nat Genet 4:202–205, 1993.

Whitney M, Thayer M, Reifsteck C, Olson S, Smith L, Jakobs PM, Leach R, Naylor S, Joenje H, Grompe M. Microcell mediated chromosome transfer maps the Fanconi anaemia group gene to chromosome 3p. Nat Genet 11:341–343, 1995.

Wijmenga C, Van den Heuvel LP, Strengman E, Luyten JA, Van der Burgt IJ, De Groot R, Smeets DF, Draaisma JM, Van Dongen JJ, De Abreu RA, Pearson PL, Sandkuijl LA, Weemaes CM. Localization of the ICF syndrome to chromosome 20 by homozygosity mapping. Am J Hum Genet 63:803–809, 1998.

Wooster R, Bignell G, Lancaster J, Swift S, Seal S, Mangion J, Collins N, Gregory S, Gumbs C, Micklem G. Identification of the breast cancer susceptibility gene BRCA2. Nature 378:789–792, 1995.

Wright J, Teraoka S, Onengut S, Tolun A, Gatti RA, Ochs HD, Concannon P. A high frequency of distinct ATM gene mutations in ataxia-telangiectasia. Am J Hum Genet 59:839–846, 1996.

Wu X, Ranganathan V, Weisman DS, Heine WF, Ciccone DN, O'Neill TB, Crick KE, Pierce KA, Lane WS, Rathbun G, Livingstone DM, Weaver DT. ATM phosphorylation of Nijmegen breakage syndrome protein is required in a DNA damage response. Nature 405:477–482, 2000.

Wysenbeek AJ, Pick AI, Weiss H. Tumores rari et inusitati: Impaired humoral and cellula immunity in xeroderma pigmentosum. Clin Oncol 6:361–365, 1980.

Xiao Y, Weaver DT. Conditional gene targeted deletion by Cre recombinase demonstrates the requirement for the double-strand break repair Mre11 protein in murine embryonic stem cells. Nucleic Acids Res 25:2985–2991, 1997.

Xu G-L, Bestor TH, Bourchis D, Hsieh C-L, Tommerup N, Bugge M, Hulten M, Qu X, Russo JJ, Viegas-Pequignot E. Chromosome instability and immunodeficiency syndrome caused by mutations in a DNA methyltransferase gene. Nature 402:187–191, 1999.

Xu Y, Ashley T, Brainerd EE, Bronson RT, Meyn SM, Baltimore D. Targeted disruption of ATM leads to growth retardation, chromosomal fragmentation during meiosis, immune defects and thymic lymphoma. Genes Dev 10:2411–2422, 1996.

Yamazaki V, Wegner RD, Kirchgessner CU. Characterization of cell cycle checkpoint responses after ionizing radiation in Nijmegen breakage syndrome cells. Cancer Res 58:2316–2322, 1998.

Yamashita T, Barber DL, Zhu Y, Wu N, D'Andrea AD. The Fanconi anemia polypeptide FACC is localized to the cytoplasm. Proc Natl Acad Sci USA 91:6712–6716, 1994.

Yankiwski V, Marciniak RA, Guarente L, Neff NF. Nuclear structure in normal and Bloom syndrome cells. Proc Natl Acad Sci USA 97:5214–5219, 2000.

Yu CE, Oshima J, Fu YH, Wijsman EM, Hisama F, Alisch R, Matthews S, Nakura J, Miki T, Ouais S, Martin GM, Mulligan J, Schellenberg GD. Positional cloning of the Werner's syndrome gene. Science 272:258–262, 1996.

Yuille MA, Coignet LJ. The ataxia-telangiectasia gene in familial and sporadic cancer. Recent Results Cancer Res 154:156–173, 1998.

Zhao S, Weng YC, Yuan SS, Lin YT, Hsu HC, Lin SC, Gerbino E, Song MH, Zdzienicka MZ, Gatti RA, Shay JW, Ziv Y, Shiloh Y, Lee EY. Functional link between ataxia-telangiectasia and Nijmegen breakage syndrome gene products. Nature 405:473–477, 2000.

CHAPTER

19

Autoimmune Lymphoproliferative Syndrome

Jack J.H. Bleesing, Thomas A. Fleisher, and Jennifer M. Puck

DEFINITION

Autoimmune lymphoproliferative syndrome (ALPS; also known as *Canale-Smith syndrome* or *lymphoproliferative syndrome with autoimmunity*) is defined as a triad of the chronic accumulation of nonmalignant lymphoid cells, increased α/β double-negative (CD4⁻ and CD8⁻) T cells, and defective in vitro lymphocyte apoptosis. In patients meeting these criteria, autoantibodies in significant titer and/or overt autoimmunity are usually present at some point.

ALPS is a disorder of apoptosis. Lymphocyte homeostasis requires that lymphocyte expansion from immune responses be appropriately balanced by lymphocyte elimination or death. Lymphocytes are eliminated by a process called *apoptosis*, or *programmed cell death*. Multiple pathways, many of which use common intracellular molecules, induce apoptosis. With respect to T lymphocytes, both antigen-driven and passive pathways can induce apoptosis. A characteristic feature of the antigen-induced pathway is the expression of the cell surface receptor Fas, which upon interaction with its ligand, induces T-cell apoptosis without the need for RNA transcription or protein synthesis (Lenardo et al., 1999).

In most patients with ALPS, there is a defect in the gene encoding the cell surface molecule Fas, a 45-kD transmembrane glycoprotein and a member of the tumor necrosis factor receptor superfamily (TNFRSF) of genes; Fas is also known as CD95, TNFRSF6, and APO-1. Its specific binding protein in vivo is Fas ligand (FasL), a member of the TNF superfamily (TNFSF); FasL is also known as CD95L and TNFSF6. A few patients with ALPS have defects in the gene encoding FasL or other downstream proteins of the Fas pathway of apoptosis (Chun et al., 2002; Pan et al., 1999; Wang et al., 1999; Wu et al., 1996). Other patients with ALPS have molecular defects that remain to be identified.

Criteria used by the U.S. National Institutes of Health ALPS Group (subsequently referred to as *the NIH Group*) to identify patients with ALPS are presented in Table 19-1. Table 19-2 contains a classification of the different genotypes of ALPS. If mutations in *TNFRSF6*, *TNFSF6*, and the gene encoding *cystinyl-asp*artate-requiring-protein*ase* (caspase) 10 *(CASP10)* and the gene encoding capase 8 *(CASP8)* have been ruled out, a patient meeting the clinical criteria for ALPS is currently classified as having ALPS type III. If the evaluation has been limited to ruling out a mutation in *TNFRSF6*, the patient is regarded as having ALPS non–type Ia.

HISTORICAL ASPECTS

In 1967, Canale and Smith described a group of patients with a symptom-complex consisting of generalized lymphadenopathy; hepatosplenomegaly; absence of fever; increased γ-globulin; variable lymph node histologic changes including the proliferation of lymphoid cells; and findings suggestive of episodes of autoimmune anemia, thrombocytopenia, or serum sickness (or all three). The onset of these distinctive features could be traced to early infancy, and they exhibited a chronic course. A patient with a similar clinical picture was reported in the German-language literature by Kellerer and Mutz (1976).

In 1992, Sneller and colleagues reported further observations on two such patients who, in addition to autoimmune blood cytopenias and chronic massive lymphadenopathy and splenomegaly, had an increase in

TABLE 19-1 · ALPS DIAGNOSTIC CRITERIA

Required

Chronic accumulation of nonmalignant lymphoid cells

Defective Fas-mediated lymphocyte apoptosis in vitro

>1% TCR αβ+ CD4− CD8− T cells (αβ-DNT cells) in peripheral blood and/or the presence of DNT cells in histologic specimens

Usually Present

Autoantibodies and/or autoimmunity

Supporting

Mutations in *TNFRSF6* or in other genes encoding proteins in apoptosis pathways

Family history of ALPS

Lymphoma

ALPS = autoimmune lymphoproliferative syndrome; DNT = double-negative T (cells); TCR = T-cell receptor; *TNFRSF6* = tumor necrosis factor receptor superfamily 6.

TABLE 19-2 · ALPS CLASSIFICATION FOR INDIVIDUALS MEETING CRITERIA IN TABLE 19-1

ALPS Ia: mutation in *TNFRSF6* (Fas, APO-1)

ALPS Ib: mutation in *TNFSF6* (FasL)

ALPS II: mutation in *CASP10* (caspase 10) or *CASP8* (caspase 8)

ALPS III: undefined genetic cause

ALPS = autoimmune lymphoproliferative syndrome; caspase = cysteinyl aspartate–specific protease; *TNFRSF6* = tumor necrosis factor receptor superfamily 6.

peripheral blood T cells (CD3+) that expressed the α/β–T-cell receptor (α/β-TCR) but lacked co-expression of CD4 or CD8 on their surfaces. These T cells are referred to as *α/β-TCR–positive, CD4/CD8 double-negative T cells (α/β-DNT cells)* and constitute 1% or fewer of peripheral blood lymphocytes in healthy individuals. One human case of increased α/β-DNT cells had been noted in a patient with generalized, persistent lymphoproliferation and humoral immunodeficiency (Illum et al., 1991).

Sneller and colleagues (1992) recognized the important connection between the clinical findings from their patients and two disease models of lymphoproliferation and autoimmunity in mice, the spontaneously occurring *lpr* and *gld* mutations (Takahashi et al., 1994; Watanabe-Fukunaga et al., 1992). In addition to increased αβ-DNT cells, these mice exhibited adenopathy and autoimmune features, similar to the findings now considered typical for humans with ALPS. One of their original patients plus additional patients reported both by the NIH Group and French investigators had defective in vitro Fas-mediated lymphocyte apoptosis attributable to mutations in the Fas-encoding gene *(TNFRSF6)* (Fisher et al., 1995; Rieux-Laucat et al., 1995).

Since these reports, an increasing number of patients with Fas defects have been identified including some of the patients originally described by Canale and Smith (Drappa et al., 1996). In addition, a substantial number of patients with some or all of the typical features of ALPS have been found who lack mutations in *TNFRSF6*, including patients with mutations in the FasL gene (*TNFSF6*), mutations in *CASP10*, and presently unknown genetic defects (Dianzani et al., 1997; Pan et al., 1999; Sneller et al., 1997; Wang et al., 1999).

PATHOGENESIS

Apoptosis

Lymphocytes, like most human cells, have the capacity to activate a genetically determined suicide program. This program, with characteristic morphologic and bio-chemical changes, is referred to as *programmed cell death* or *apoptosis* (derived from the Greek word meaning "a falling off"). After a lymphocyte, responding to extracellular or intracellular signals (e.g., the withdrawal of growth factors or the engagement of specific cell surface receptors), has made the commitment to undergo apoptosis, an irreversible sequence of events is initiated. The lymphocyte membrane structure is altered and becomes leaky; the cytoplasm shrinks and condenses; and in the nucleus, nucleases are activated that sequentially degrade the chromosomal DNA, first into large (i.e., 50 to 300 kb) and then into small oligonucleosomal fragments. Dense chromatin condensation, nuclear fragmentation, and cytoplasmic bleb formation follow, and the cell undergoes fragmentation and disintegration.

The plasma membrane changes of apoptosis include translocation of phosphatidylserine to the outer membrane surface, but the membrane remains sufficiently intact to surround the fragmented apoptotic bodies. Subsequent phagocytosis of these bodies is a key aspect of apoptosis, in that this type of cell destruction does not lead to spillage of cytosolic contents; therefore, no inflammatory response is induced. In contrast, necrosis—another form of cell death that occurs in response to acute nonphysiologic cell injury—is associated with swelling and lysis of the cell, the release of cytoplasmic and nuclear contents, and potentially harmful inflammation (Hetts, 1998).

Fas-Mediated Apoptosis

The Fas-mediated apoptosis pathway is important in downregulating antigen-induced immune responses and thus represents a critical pathway in lymphocyte homeostasis. In addition, the Fas pathway is involved in the long-term maintenance of clonotypic diversity. Lymphocytes reactive to a wide range of "foreign invaders" are permitted to survive, but potentially autoreactive lymphocytes are eliminated by Fas-mediated apoptosis (Lenardo et al., 1999). Moreover, the interaction between Fas and FasL may provide a mechanism for maintaining immune-privileged sites, such as the eye and testis (Griffith et al., 1995).

Resting T cells normally express a low level of surface Fas, which is upregulated after an encounter with cognate antigen. During this initial phase of TCR-mediated

T-cell activation, the low level of Fas expression is insufficient to activate the Fas apoptotic pathway. After activation and a number of cell divisions, T cells express high levels of surface Fas and become sensitive to Fas-induced apoptosis. The ability of activated T cells to proliferate and initiate an immune response is highly dependent on the autocrine interaction between IL-2 and its receptor; thus, IL-2 is an important permissive factor for T-cell apoptosis (Lenardo et al., 1999).

Fas becomes engaged with FasL attached to the surfaces of cytotoxic or T-helper cells or with soluble FasL. The engagement of Fas and FasL requires that each becomes organized as a homotrimer (Fig. 19-1). The

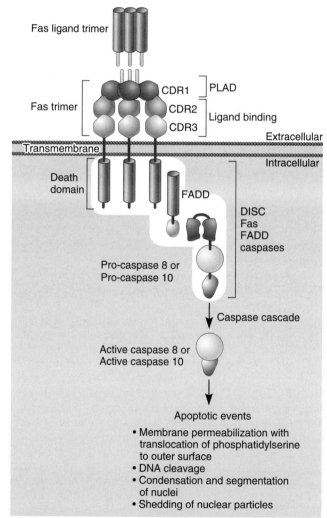

Figure 19-1 · The Fas-mediated apoptosis pathway. Apoptosis is initiated by trimerized Fas ligand binding to the ligand-binding domain of trimerized Fas (Fas cysteine-rich domains [CRD] 2 and 3). Fas is oligomerized into a trimer before FasL binding by its preligand assembly domain (PLAD [amino terminus and CRD1 domain]). Fas-FasL interaction initiates the recruitment of Fas-associated death domain (FADD) to the trimerized cytoplasmic death domains of Fas, which together with caspase 8 and 10 molecules (formed by autocleavage of pro-caspases), form the death-inducing signaling complex (DISC). Activation of the initiator caspases 8 and 10 leads to a lethal proteolytic cascade involving other effector caspases and ultimately causing cell death.

extracellular Fas-FasL interaction causes intracellular recruitment of the cytoplasmic adaptor protein FADD (*Fas-a*ssociated *d*eath *d*omain) to the trimerized cytoplasmic death domains of Fas. The cytosolic molecules pro-caspase 8 and pro-caspase 10 bind, through their death effector domains, to a similar death effector domain on the FADD. Together, Fas, FADD, and caspase molecules form the death-inducing signaling complex. Autoprocessing of pro-caspases 8 and 10 into their active caspase forms initiates a lethal proteolytic cascade, involving activation of other caspases that cleave specific substrates to generate the cytoskeletal and chromatin changes typical of apoptosis.

Transduction of a death signal can also be initiated by other, parallel induction mechanisms. For example, TNF and other similar molecules can, like FasL, engage other (trimerized) members of the TNFRSF, such as TNFR1, death receptor-3 (DR3), DR4 (TRAIL-R1), and DR5 (TRAIL-R2), that harbor cytoplasmic death domains (Lenardo et al., 1999). However, in mature lymphocytes, it appears that the Fas pathway is the dominant apoptotic pathway, with major physiologic roles in the removal of infected, malignant, superfluous, or self-reactive T cells. In addition, FasL-expressing T cells can also induce apoptosis and thus exert control over activated and autoreactive B cells expressing Fas, in addition to T cells.

TNFRSF6 Mutations

Fas is encoded by the gene *TNFRSF6*, located on chromosome 10q24.1. This gene contains 9 exons. The 5′ end contains a signal sequence that is cleaved off upon directing the protein to the cell membrane. Fas has three extracellular cysteine-rich domains (CRDs), a transmembrane domain, and an intracellular domain containing the site of the FADD-interacting death domain. In excess of 60 unique mutations, the majority of which affect the death domain, have been found in more than 70 unrelated families with ALPS.

With few exceptions, mutations involve changes, deletions, or additions of one or a small number of nucleotides, either in the coding regions or the splice sites of the gene (see the "Distribution of FAS [TNFRSF6] mutations" section of the online ALPS database [ALPSbase:http://www.nhgri.nih.gov/DIR/GMBB/ALPS]).

De novo mutations have been detected in a few families, but genetic analysis has revealed autosomal dominant inheritance in most families. The great majority of patients with ALPS studied to date carry a heterozygous mutation in the *TNFRSF6* gene. However, in three families, autosomal recessive ALPS has been associated with homozygous Fas mutations. In all three families, the carrier parents were first or second cousins and the affected children had mutations of both alleles of Fas giving rise to a complete absence of Fas, protein and severe lymphoproliferation and autoimmunity of prenatal or perinatal onset (Kasahara et al., 1998; Rieux-Laucat et al., 1995; van der Burg et al., 2000).

In vitro transfection studies have shown autosomal-dominant impairment of Fas-mediated apoptosis to be the consequence of a dominant-negative effect (Fisher et al., 1995). In these studies, mutant and wild-type Fas were co-expressed on the surface of a Fas-negative cell line to simulate the heterozygous defect present in lymphocytes of the patient with ALPS. The mutation-bearing Fas proteins interfered with apoptosis when co-expressed with normal Fas proteins to form chimeric trimers.

Clues to the actual mechanism of dominant-negative interference were provided by a series of patients who had ALPS with death domain mutations, in which it was shown that both localized and global disruptions of the death domain were associated with an inability to bind FADD and assemble the death-inducing signaling complex (Martin et al., 1999). The dominant-negative effect of mutant Fas chains in ALPS led to the recognition that functional Fas receptors oligomerize into trimeric complexes before binding to trimeric FasL. Indeed, Siegel and colleagues (2000) have demonstrated that the preassociation of Fas is mediated by the amino terminus and the CRD1 domains, now termed the *preligand assembly domain* (PLAD) (see Fig. 19-1).

Dominant interference by mutant Fas chains has been demonstrated for the great majority of ALPS-associated mutations (Jackson et al., 1999). However, the ALPS phenotype in homozygous and compound heterozygous (Kasahara et al., 1998) *TNFRSF6* mutations may be associated with the loss of function of Fas.

Phenotype/Genotype Relationships

Family studies of probands with ALPS caused by Fas mutation have contributed important information regarding the complex relationships among genotype, phenotype, and disease penetrance (Jackson et al., 1999; Rieux-Laucat et al., 1999; Vaishnaw et al., 1999). All mutation-bearing relatives have had defective in vitro Fas-mediated apoptosis, even if they lacked other ALPS features. Thus, interference with Fas-mediated apoptosis is inherited in an autosomal dominant fashion with full penetrance (Infante et al., 1998; Jackson et al., 1999).

In contrast to impaired apoptosis, clinical and immunologic manifestations have a highly variable expression, as demonstrated by Fas mutation–positive family members who lack some or even all of the clinical and laboratory features of ALPS (Infante et al., 1998; Jackson et al., 1999). As shown in the large kindred studied by Infante and colleagues (1998) (Fig. 19-2), of 11 individuals found carrying a death domain Fas mutation, all had impaired in vitro apoptosis, but only 8 had adenopathy or splenomegaly, 6 had elevated αβ-DNT cells, and 5 had autoantibodies or overt autoimmunity. Interestingly, two family members developed lymphoma, a recently recognized complication of ALPS (Straus et al., 2001).

The penetrance of ALPS features, other than impaired apoptosis, is significantly higher in families with intracellular mutations than in those with extracellular mutations (Jackson et al., 1999; Rieux-Laucat et al.,

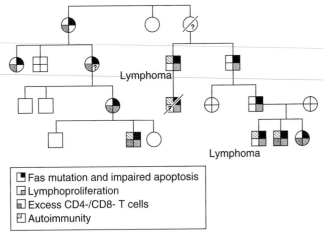

Figure 19-2 · Extended pedigree of a family with multiple individuals in four generations carrying a Fas death domain mutation. The features of autoimmune lymphoproliferative syndrome experienced by each person are shown. Squares = males; circles = females; slash = deceased; ? = not determined.

1999; Vaishnaw et al., 1999). In the study by Jackson and colleagues (1999), one or more features of ALPS (e.g., adenopathy, significant titers of autoantibodies, autoimmunity, and increased αβ-DNT cells) were present in 18% (3/17) of relatives with extracellular mutations versus 88% (38/43) of relatives with intracellular mutations. In addition, the penetrance of significant ALPS-related morbidity (i.e., splenomegaly requiring splenectomy, autoimmune disease requiring treatment, and lymphoma) was 0% (0/17) versus 44% (19/43) for relatives with extracellular versus intracellular mutations, respectively (Jackson et al., 1999).

The fact that there are many mutation-positive family members who lack clinical disease indicates that genetic or environmental factors, or both—in addition to Fas defects—are required for clinical ALPS to develop. Similar to *lpr* mice (discussed in the Animal Models of ALPS section), the genetic background may influence the penetrance of ALPS manifestations, in addition to the age of onset and the severity of these manifestations. Possible genetic modifiers include protective or deleterious changes in genes that interact directly with the Fas-FasL pathway, genes that exert influence on Fas-independent apoptosis pathways, and regulators of other aspects of lymphocyte function and survival.

The complex interplay among genotype, phenotype, and penetrance is also apparent in two families with the clinical features of ALPS, impaired in vitro apoptosis, and mutations in *CASP10* (Wang et al., 1999). In one proband, a dominant-negative heterozygous *CASP10* mutation caused defective Fas-mediated T-cell apoptosis and defective lymphocyte and dendritic cell apoptosis mediated through TNFRSF1 and TRAIL (TNFRSF4 [DR4] and TNFRSF5 [DR5]). In the other proband, defective apoptosis was associated with a homozygous *CASP10* mutation. Defective in vitro apoptosis was present in heterozygous family members of both probands. However, these relatives were not clinically affected, which is consistent with the concept that additional genetic or environmental factors, or both, are important.

CASP8 mutation has also been associated with a human autosomal recessive ALPS-related disease characterized by chronic adenopathy and impaired apoptosis; interestingly, affected patients had clinical signs of immunodeficiency, including recurrent sinopulmonary infections and recurrent herpes simplex (Chun et al., 2002; Puck and Zhu, 2003).

Animal Models of ALPS

Mouse strains originally used as models for lupus were found to have defects in Fas and FasL (Takahashi et al., 1994; Watanabe-Fukunaga et al., 1992). In contrast to humans with ALPS, these mutant mice have been studied primarily in the homozygous mutant state and their phenotypes are generally thought of as autosomal recessive. However, heterozygous littermates may, to a mild degree, develop increased lymph node and spleen weight, high immunoglobulin levels, and autoantibodies (Jachez et al., 1988).

Moreover, mild features of ALPS occurred in a recently developed transgenic mouse model carrying a dominant mutation in the death domain of murine Fas corresponding to a mutation in a patient with ALPS (Choi et al., 1999). In these transgenic mice expressing both mutated and endogenous wild-type Fas, a dominant-negative mechanism, similar to that of humans with ALPS, was demonstrated.

Experiments on mice with *lpr* mutations crossed into different mouse strains (e.g., C3H, MRL, and AKR) have revealed that the genetic background plays an important role in the age of onset and the severity of the murine phenotypes, especially the autoimmune manifestations (Choi et al., 2002; Kono and Theofilopoulos, 2000).

CLINICAL FEATURES

ALPS occurs in both sexes; however, in our patients with ALPS, there was a predominance among males. This sex skewing is in contrast to many autoimmune diseases in which females are more frequently affected. ALPS has been observed in diverse ethnic backgrounds, but currently there is no estimation of its incidence other than that the condition is rare. The range of clinical features of ALPS is shown in Table 19-3. The frequencies are estimated from published reports (Bleesing et al., 2000; Jackson and Puck, 1999) and unpublished data from the NIH Group.

Lymphoproliferation

All patients, by definition, must have either splenomegaly or lymphadenopathy, or both, for an extended period of time, and nearly half also have hepatomegaly. The manifestations of abnormal lymphocyte accumulation are

TABLE 19-3 · CLINICAL FINDINGS IN ALPS

Findings	Cases	Percentage*
Lymphoproliferation		
Proliferation of nonmalignant lymphoid cells	62/62	100
Lymphadenopathy	54/62	87
Splenomegaly (+/– hypersplenism)	56/62	90
Splenectomy	20/62	32
Hepatomegaly	28/62	45
Autoimmunity		
Autoimmune hemolytic anemia	33/62	53
Autoimmune thrombocytopenia	27/62	44
Autoimmune neutropenia	19/62	31
Glomerulonephritis	5/62	8
Autoimmune hepatitis	4/62	6
Guillain-Barré syndrome	3/62	5
Uveitis (+/– iridocyclitis)	3/62	5
Neoplasia (including benign tumors)†		
Lymphomas (Hodgkin's and non-Hodgkin's)	9	
Carcinomas (thyroid, breast, skin, tongue, and liver)	6	
Multiple neoplastic lesions (thyroid adenomas, breast adenomas, and gliomas)	1	
Other and Infrequent Findings		
Urticaria and other skin rashes	Common‡	
Vasculitis	1	
Panniculitis	1	
Arthritis and arthralgia	4	
Recurrent oral ulcers	1	
Aplastic anemia	1	
Pulmonary infiltrates	2	
Premature ovarian failure	1	
Hydrops fetalis	2	
Organic brain syndrome (mental status changes, seizures, and headaches)	1	

*Data are compiled from reported probands and from unpublished studies by the NIH ALPS Group.
†Reported cases in probands and their *TNFRSF6* mutation–positive relatives.
‡Present in most patients in the NIH Group; incidence not documented in many published reports.
ALPS = autoimmune lymphoproliferative syndrome; NIH = National Institutes of Health.

often present during the first year of life and are most pronounced before the fifth year. Cases of homozygous Fas mutation are rare; however, in these cases prenatal disease with lymphoproliferation is not rare. During infancy and childhood, the accumulation of lymphocytes is often massive, with distortion of normal anatomic relationships (Figs. 19-3 and 19-4), but it generally becomes less pronounced during adolescence and adulthood and may regress completely. The severity of lymphoproliferation also shows considerable variability among patients, including affected individuals in the same family.

Lymphadenopathy often involves (but is not limited to) the anterior and posterior cervical and axillary chains. At an examination, the lymph nodes are firm, nontender, nonsuppurative, and not attached to skin or underlying tissue. When considering the extensive differential diagnosis of lymphadenopathy in childhood, it is important to note that constitutional signs such as fever, weight loss, and night sweats are uncommon in ALPS. As reported by Canale and Smith (1967) and also

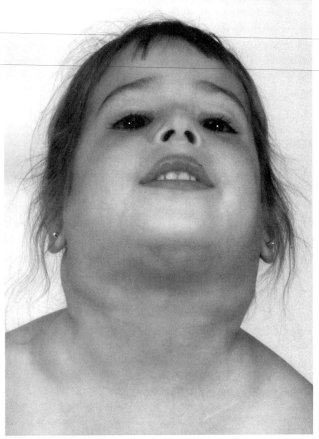

Figure 19-3 · A frontal view of anterior and posterior cervical adenopathy in a girl with autoimmune lymphoproliferative syndrome.

observed in the NIH cohort, during acute viral and bacterial infections, lymph node size may paradoxically undergo temporary regression (Sneller et al., 1992).

Isolated splenomegaly is uncommon when ALPS presents at an early age but may be the predominant

feature of ALPS lymphoproliferation during the course of the disease. Hypersplenism may cause or aggravate blood cytopenias, and the distinction between consumptive cytopenias and autoimmune cytopenia can be difficult. Approximately one third of the patients have undergone a splenectomy for hypersplenism, traumatic rupture, suspicion of malignancy, severe hemolysis, uncontrollable thrombocytopenia, or problems related to discomfort. The only premature death in the family illustrated in Figure 19-2 was in a boy who developed sepsis postsplenectomy despite receiving prophylactic antibiotics. Hepatomegaly is usually not associated with abnormalities of liver function, unless autoimmune hepatitis or viral hepatitis is present. Two patients with homozygous mutations in *TNFRSF6* were born with hydrops fetalis, and one of these patients plus another patient with a compound heterozygous mutation also developed pulmonary infiltrates.

Autoimmunity

Autoimmune features fall into two groups: autoimmunity involving blood cells and a group of other autoimmune manifestations (see Table 19-3) (Bleesing et al., 2000; Jackson and Puck, 1999). The identification of autoimmune cytopenia can be difficult in the presence of hypersplenism, but the degree of cytopenia, together with the level of compensation (e.g., reticulocytosis), is often greatest when associated with autoimmunity.

Almost all patients with ALPS develop at least one autoimmune manifestation, and many develop a combination of autoimmune features, most often thrombocytopenia and Coombs' positive autoimmune hemolytic anemia. There can be a delay between the lymphoproliferative phase of ALPS, which tends to occur early and regress in adolescence, and the development of autoimmunity.

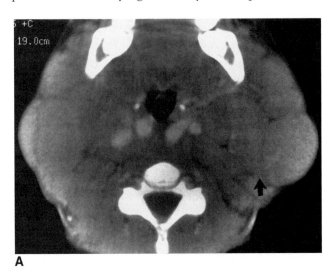
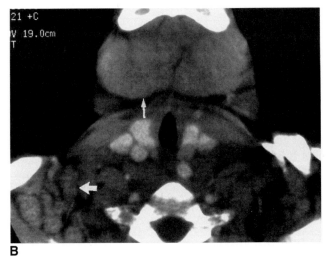

Figure 19-4 · Computed tomographs of the neck in a 4-year-old patient with autoimmune lymphoproliferative syndrome. A, An axial section at the level of the mandible depicts extensive cervical adenopathy *(arrow)*. B, An axial section at the base of the neck reveals extensive supraclavicular adenopathy *(large arrow)* and submental adenopathy *(small arrow)*. (Courtesy of Dr N.A. Avila, Diagnostic Radiology Department, Warren G. Magnuson Clinical Center, National Institutes of Health.)

As with other autoimmune diseases, autoimmunity in ALPS is often characterized by exacerbations and remissions. Autoimmune anemia and thrombocytopenia can present suddenly, with rapidly dropping hemoglobin levels or significant bleeding, each requiring interventions. The thrombocytopenia in ALPS contrasts with childhood immune thrombocytopenic purpura that rarely leads to bleeding, even though platelet levels may reach similarly low (i.e., <20,000/mm³) levels. Neutropenia in ALPS usually does not become severe enough to increase the risk for infections.

Uncommon autoimmune manifestations (see Table 19-3) include autoimmune hepatitis, uveitis, and Guillain-Barré syndrome. In contrast to findings in the MRL/lpr mouse, autoimmune glomerulonephritis has been observed in only a few patients with type Ia and in one patient with type Ib ALPS. Other manifestations that may or may not be autoimmune in nature are also listed in Table 19-3, with urticaria and other skin rashes being the most common (Bleesing et al., 2000; Jackson and Puck, 1999).

Malignancies

The abnormal survival of lymphocytes attributable to defective Fas-mediated apoptosis may sufficiently alter the balance between antiapoptotic and proapoptotic factors to allow malignant transformation of cells. In this context, Fas and other members of the Fas pathway play physiologic roles as tumor-suppressor genes (Peng et al., 1996). Now that many patients with ALPS and their families have been identified, it is clear that there is an increased risk of lymphomas associated with ALPS (Straus et al., 2001).

Individuals with inherited mutations in Fas have a significantly increased risk of Hodgkin's lymphoma (relative risk = 55) and non-Hodgkin's lymphoma (relative risk = 14). The following lymphoid malignancies have been reported in patients with ALPS and their mutation-positive family members: T-cell–rich B-cell lymphoma, Burkitt's lymphoma, atypical lymphoma, and Hodgkin's disease, nodular lymphocyte predominance type. Interestingly, the occurrence of both Hodgkin's lymphoma and non-Hodgkin's lymphoma in TNFRSF6 mutation–positive relatives within a single family has been observed twice (Peters et al., 1999; Straus et al., 2001). The majority of lymphoma cases have occurred in families with mutations affecting the death domain of Fas.

Thyroid cancer, hepatocellular carcinoma (with chronic hepatitis C), breast cancer, colon cancer, lung cancer, basal cell carcinoma of the skin, and squamous cell carcinoma of the tongue have been observed in patients with ALPS and their mutation-positive relatives; it is not clear whether inherited Fas mutations are associated with an increased risk for these nonlymphoid malignancies.

The role of the Fas gene and other apoptosis pathway genes as tumor suppressors is underscored by the recognition that somatic mutations in these genes have been identified in many lymphoid and nonlymphoid malignancies.

LABORATORY FEATURES

Hematologic Findings

Most patients with ALPS have lymphocytosis, often associated with atypical lymphocytes seen on a peripheral blood smear. The condition of patients taking immunosuppressives may revert from lymphocytosis to lymphopenia. An occasional patient with ALPS may have primary lymphopenia. Anemia (with or without hemolysis), iron deficiency, reticulocytosis, thrombocytopenia, and neutropenia may be present, depending on the severity of the autoimmune manifestations and hypersplenism. Many patients also have eosinophilia.

Splenectomy may normalize blood counts or may result in thrombocytosis, leukocytosis, and the presence of Howell-Jolly bodies. Postsplenectomy sepsis has occurred in multiple patients. Two patients with ALPS type Ia have been described with dyserythropoiesis, characterized by irregularities of the cytoplasm; multinucleated erythroblasts, dystrophic nuclei, and abnormal chromatin condensation on bone marrow smears; and a shortened erythrocyte half-life (Bader-Meunier et al., 2000).

Chemistry Profiles

Usually the chemistry profile is normal in patients with ALPS. Elevations of hepatic enzymes, conjugated bilirubin, and cholesterol, in addition to decreased albumin and clotting factors have been noted, with concomitant autoimmune or viral hepatitis (NIH Group, unpublished results; Pensati et al., 1997). Hyperlipidemia and proteinuria, both associated with glomerulonephritis, have been observed in a few patients with ALPS. An unexplained finding is elevated vitamin B_{12} levels in blood (NIH Group, unpublished results).

Immunologic Features

Immunologic findings in ALPS include alterations in lymphocyte phenotype and function (Table 19-4). An increase in αβ-DNT cells (Fig. 19-5A [I] and [II]) is a required element of the diagnosis of ALPS. The αβ-DNT cells are polyclonal and appear to be derived from proliferating cytotoxic T cells that have lost CD8 or CD4 expression after an antigen encounter (Table 19-5) (Bleesing et al., 2000). Like mice exhibiting mutations in lpr and gld, humans with ALPS have αβ-DNT cells that express the CD45RA isoform B220 (Fig. 19-5A [III]) (Bleesing et al., 2001; Cohen and Eisenberg, 1991). DNT cells respond poorly to in vitro stimulation, as assessed through lymphoproliferative

TABLE 19-4 · LABORATORY FINDINGS IN ALPS

Hematologic

Lymphocytosis or lymphopenia (primary or secondary to treatment)
Anemia (signs of hemolysis or iron deficiency on peripheral blood smear)
Dyserythropoiesis
Reticulocytosis
Thrombocytopenia
Neutropenia
Eosinophilia

Blood Chemical

Liver function abnormalities (in cases of autoimmune or viral hepatitis)
Proteinuria (in cases of glomerulonephritis)
Elevated vitamin B_{12} level

Immunologic

Expansion of α/β-DNT cells
Expansion of other lymphocyte subsets
γ/δ-DNT cells
CD8+ T Cells
CD8+/CD57+ T cells
HLA-DR+ T cells
B (CD5+) cells
Decrease in CD4+/CD25+ T cells
Decrease in CD27 expression ion B cells (associated with increased soluble CD27 levels in plasma/serum)
Elevated IL-10 levels in serum; increased IL-10 mRNA in DNT cells
Elevated IgG; IgA; IgM elevated, normal, or decreased; elevated IgE
Autoantibodies (most often positive: direct or indirect antiglobulin test, antiphospholipid antibody, antinuclear antibody, or rheumatoid factor)
Defective receptor-mediated lymphocyte apoptosis
Other reported findings (increased soluble CD25, CD30, and FasL; decreased soluble Fas; decreased in vitro lymphocyte function)

ALPS = autoimmune lymphoproliferative syndrome; DNT = double-negative T cells; FasL = Fas ligand.

and cytokine secretion assays (Fuss et al., 1997; Sneller et al., 1992).

T cells from patients with ALPS, including $\alpha\beta$-DNT cells, show increased expression of the activation marker HLA-DR (Fig. 19-5B [I]) but lack the α chain of the IL-2 receptor (CD25) (Fig. 19-5B [II]). This is because of a selective reduction in CD4+/CD25+, which may have regulatory properties and correlates with the severity of clinical ALPS (Fig. 19-5B [III]) (Bleesing et al., 2001). In addition to the expansion in $\alpha\beta$-DNT cells, there is typically an increase in DNT cells that express $\gamma\delta$-TcR and an increase in both CD8+ T cells that express CD57 (Fig. 19-5C [I]; see Table 19-5) and B cells, predominantly those expressing CD5 (Fig. 19-5C [II]).

Serum IgG levels are commonly increased in ALPS; IgA levels may also be increased, but IgM levels are often normal or decreased. Hypergammaglobulinemia is usually polyclonal, but a monoclonal component has been reported (Le Deist et al., 1996; Ströbel et al., 1999). Antibody responses to infection and protein antigen immunization are intact, but antibody responses to polysaccharide antigens, including pneumococcal and blood group antigens, may be reduced (Canale and Smith, 1967; Kellerer and Mutz, 1976; Peters et al., 1999). These observations and the lack of memory B cells with

CD2+, CD5+, CD27+/CD28+ and CD43+
CD45RA+/CD45RO−/B220+ (detected by rat antimouse monoclonal RA3-6B2)
CD57 increased*/CD16−, and CD56−
HLA-DR increased*/CD25−
CD62L reduced*
Perforin and CGP present†
Ki-67 present

*Relative to $\alpha\beta$-DNT cells from healthy control subjects.
†Marker detected in histologic specimens.
CGP = cytotoxic granule-associated protein; DNT = double-negative T cells.

the CD20+/CD27+ phenotype (Fig. 19-5C [III]) suggest that patients with ALPS have some degree of humoral immunodeficiency.

Autoantibodies in the majority of patients with ALPS are most often directed against erythrocytes, followed by antibodies to platelets and neutrophils, and, less frequently, rheumatoid factor, antinuclear antibodies, and antiphospholipid antibodies (Bleesing et al., 2000). Complement is usually normal, but one patient with a mutation of FasL had decreased CH50 and lupus erythematosus (Wu et al., 1996).

Cytokine abnormalities have been noted, the most striking of which is an elevation of serum IL-10. DNT cells of ALPS have high levels of IL-10 mRNA, and IL-10 is increased in DNT-containing lymph nodes. IL-10 is also produced by monocytes in patients in ALPS (Fuss et al., 1997; Lopatin et al., 2001). Other cytokine abnormalities, including increased in vitro IL-4 and IL-5, and decreased INF-γ and IL-12 production support a T-helper 2 cytokine pattern.

Apoptosis Assays

Functional in vitro assays of T-cell apoptosis must take into account that resting T cells that have not yet encountered antigen are resistant to Fas-induced apoptosis. T cells become Fas-sensitive after activation through the TCR (Lenardo et al., 1999). Lymphocyte apoptosis involves activating peripheral blood lymphocytes, usually with phytohemagglutinin, and expanding the T cells with growth factors such as IL-2. Apoptosis is subsequently induced by either restimulation of the TCR or by the addition of purified FasL or an antibody directed against Fas (mimicking FasL crosslinking) to test the Fas-FasL pathway. Apoptosis can be detected through the use of a variety of methods, including the assessment of viability with propidium iodide staining (Fisher et al., 1995; Jackson et al., 1999).

According to the NIH Group criteria, the demonstration of defective Fas-mediated apoptosis is a requirement for the diagnosis of ALPS (Fig. 19-6). Furthermore, relatives of patients with mutations in the TNFRSF6 gene have impaired Fas-mediated apoptosis in vitro; in contrast, almost all mutation-negative family members have normal Fas-induced apoptosis

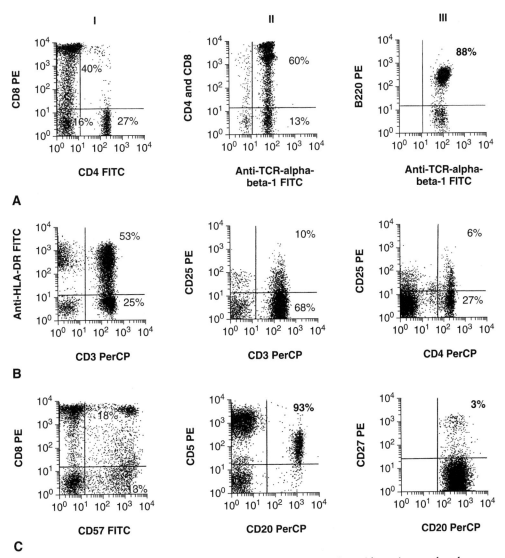

Figure 19-5 · Flow cytometric dot plot profiles from a representative patient with autoimmune lymphoproliferative syndrome. Dot plots in AI, AII, BIII, and CI represent percentages of total T cells; AIII represents T cells that are CD4-and CD8-negative (αβ double-negative T cells); BI, BII, and CII represent percentages of total lymphocytes; CIII represents a distribution gated on total B cells. *Numbers* denote percentages of gated cells present in each quadrant; *bold numbers* represent percentages of αβ double-negative T cells that are B220-positive (AIII) and B cells that express CD5 and CD27 (CII and CIII, respectively).

(Jackson et al., 1999; Rieux-Laucat et al., 1999). Similarly, mutation-positive relatives of ALPS probands with mutations in *CASP10* were found to have defective Fas-mediated apoptosis (Wang et al., 1999).

In addition to the apoptotic defect found in T cells, abnormal apoptosis has been demonstrated in B cells and Epstein-Barr virus–transformed B-cell lines. Other apoptosis pathways are intact in patients with ALPS, as shown through the results of in vitro assays demonstrating normal apoptosis induced by corticosteroids and antimetabolites (Bettinardi et al., 1997; Fisher et al., 1995). Increased spontaneous apoptosis of fresh lymphocytes held in vitro has also been described (Haas et al., 1998; Lopatin et al., 2001).

Histopathologic Features

Lymphoid tissues from patients with ALPS reveal histopathologic features distinct from other causes of lymph node and spleen enlargement. Paracortical hyperplasia of interfollicular areas and infiltration by proliferating DNT cells are the most consistent and notable findings in lymph nodes (Figs. 19-7 and 19-8). The extent of this infiltration correlates with disease severity (Le Deist et al., 1996; Lim et al., 1998). Splenic tissue shows lymphoid hyperplasia affecting the white pulp, with involvement of both T- and B-dependent zones. The splenic red pulp can be expanded secondary to autoimmune anemia and other autoimmune phenomena.

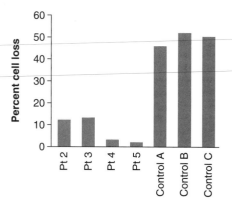

Figure 19-6 · The results of an apoptosis assay reveal cell loss (apoptosis) in cultures of cells activated with phytohemagglutinin (PHA), expanded in IL-2, and then restimulated with anti-CD3. Cells from patients with autoimmune lymphoproliferative syndrome (patients two through five) undergo significantly less cell death than cells from control subjects. Similar results would be obtained after exposing these cells to anti-Fas crosslinking antibody or to FasL instead of anti-CD3.

Phagocytosis of apoptotic lymphocytes by macrophages and histiocytes has been observed in the lymph nodes and the spleen (Le Deist et al., 1996), a finding in agreement with the results of normal in vitro apoptosis assays not involving the Fas pathway. Other features include prominent interfollicular vascularity, plasmacytosis, and abnormalities of the primary and secondary follicles, including follicular hyperplasia and progressive transformation of germinal centers (Fig. 19-7).

In contrast to lymphoproliferative disorders that develop after transplantation or are associated with primary immunodeficiencies, there has been no evidence of Epstein-Barr virus or other viral infections in histologic material from patients with ALPS.

The accumulation of nonmalignant lymphocytes in ALPS leaves the overall architecture of lymphoid tissues intact. The preservation of architecture, together with certain histopathologic features and the absence of T- or B-cell clonality, distinguish this disorder from lymphoid malignancies (Lim et al., 1998).

However, as previously noted, the apoptotic defect of ALPS is associated with a significantly increased risk of Hodgkin's and non-Hodgkin's lymphoma, which can be present with the typical features of ALPS, but usually not in the same lymph node. One patient with ALPS non–type Ia has been described who developed giant lymphadenopathy, with a loss of normal architecture and a massive monoclonal blastic B-cell population that underwent spontaneous remission (Ströbel et al., 1999).

Liver biopsy specimens have exhibited infiltration by DNT cells, extramedullary hematopoiesis in the presence of significant blood cytopenias, and, occasionally, signs of hepatitis with bile duct injury, intense inflammation, plasma cell infiltration, and evidence of micronodular cirrhosis (Lim et al., 1998; Pensati et al., 1997).

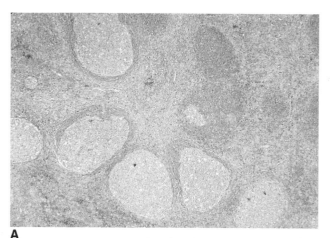

A

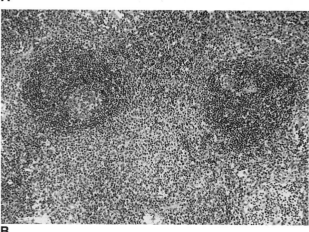

B

Figure 19-7 · Histopathologic features of autoimmune lymphoproliferative syndrome. **A.** The characteristic architecture of a lymph node biopsy specimen from a subject with autoimmune lymphoproliferative syndrome depicts progressively transformed germinal centers and a floridly hyperplastic germinal center. **B.** A higher-power view of the lymph node reveals follicular hyperplasia and marked paracortical expansion.

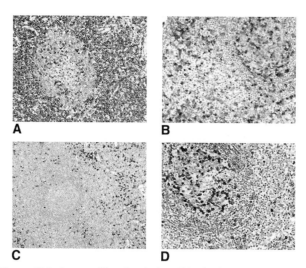

Figure 19-8 · Immunohistochemical results of a lymph node exhibiting autoimmune lymphoproliferative syndrome. CD3 (**A**) stains most paracortical T cells (the same cells seen in large numbers in **B**). These cells are largely negative for CD4 (**B**), CD8 (**C**), and CD45RO (**D**), corresponding to the immunophenotype of double-negative T cells in the peripheral blood of patients with autoimmune lymphoproliferative syndrome. Note that most of the T cells within germinal centers have the phenotype CD3+, CD4+, or CD45RO+, the same phenotype predominant in germinal centers from healthy subjects.

Bone marrow smears reveal increased erythroid hyperplasia during episodes of active hemolysis; an increase in megakaryocytes in response to autoimmune thrombocytopenia; and varying numbers of DNT cells, plasma cells, and eosinophils (Lim et al., 1998).

DIAGNOSIS

The diagnostic evaluation of ALPS is directed at identifying the required criteria (as outlined in Table 19-1), which combine clinical evidence of lymphoproliferation with immunophenotypic determination of αβ-DNT cells in peripheral blood and assessment of Fas-mediated apoptosis in vitro. Autoimmunity is not part of the required criteria, but it is almost always present at some stage in the disease.

In typical cases of ALPS, the diagnosis can be made without tissue biopsy specimens. However, in cases of an atypical presentation or if there is suspicion of malignancy, a histopathologic examination of enlarged lymph nodes, including a molecular analysis of clonality, is indicated. Documentation of a deleterious mutation in a Fas pathway gene confirms the diagnosis.

Differential diagnoses of ALPS include lupus erythematosus (see Chapter 35) and idiopathic autoimmune hemolytic anemia or thrombocytopenia (see Chapter 39); common variable immunodeficiency (see Chapter 13); and certain of the rare single-gene immunodeficiencies such as autosomal or X-linked hyper-IgM syndromes (see Chapter 13) or the immune dysregulation, polyendocrinopathy, X-linked (IPEX) syndrome (see Chapter 17). These disorders may present with autoimmunity and some degree of spleen or lymph node enlargement, but they are not characterized by increased numbers of αβ-DNT cells or apoptosis defects. Moreover, severe or opportunistic infections do not ordinarily occur in ALPS as they do in immunodeficiency diseases.

The first step in the classification of ALPS involves mutation detection (Jackson et al., 1999). Mutations causing frame shifts and protein truncation that affect the death domain can be predicted to be deleterious. However, to differentiate between pathogenic mutations and incidental polymorphisms, it is necessary to perform functional tests such as co-transfection assays to discern whether a mutation can be implicated as the cause of ALPS. To facilitate this important aspect of ALPS diagnosis/classification, submission of newly identified mutations to the ALPS mutation database (ALPSbase: http://www.nhgri.nih.gov/DIR/GMBB/ALPS) is recommended.

TREATMENT AND PROGNOSIS

Treatment of ALPS is directed primarily against clinically debilitating autoimmunity and malignancies. Lymphadenopathy and hepatosplenomegaly have been treated with corticosteroids and chemotherapeutic agents, but they generally reoccur after the cessation of such treatment (Sneller et al., 1997). Because of the side effects of these agents and the long-term risk of treatment-related malignancies, the presence of lymphadenopathy alone should not necessitate treatment. Hypersplenism is another frequent manifestation of ALPS; in the past, splenectomy was included among treatment options for hypersplenism.

The decision to remove an enlarged spleen can be difficult. Hypersplenism can contribute to blood cytopenias and complicate treatment, but splenectomy reduces the efficacy of anti-D therapy for thrombocytopenia (Scaradavou and Bussel, 1998), does not prevent subsequent autoimmune cytopenias, and introduces a lifelong additional risk of infection, which may be greater in ALPS than in other hypersplenic conditions because of the patients' decreased ability to make antipolysaccharide antibodies. Nevertheless, splenectomy is often necessary to control the blood cytopenias. Alternatives to conventional splenectomy have included partial splenectomy and (unsuccessful) splenic irradiation (Haas et al., 1998; Kellerer and Mutz, 1976; Peters et al., 1999).

Autoimmune thrombocytopenia responds somewhat less well to intravenous immunoglobulin than does typical childhood immune thrombocytopenic purpura (NIH Group, unpublished results). Thrombocytopenic episodes in ALPS do respond well to short courses of high-dose corticosteroids (e.g., prednisone, >1mg/kg per day). Autoimmune hemolytic anemia usually also responds well to short bursts of prednisone.

Occasionally, autoimmune manifestations require prolonged daily corticosteroids, intravenous immunoglobulin, and chemotherapeutic agents (e.g., cyclophosphamide, azathioprine, methotrexate, or chlorambucil) (Bleesing et al., 2000). Other treatments used in individual patients with varying results include cyclosporine, interferon-α (IFN-α), IL-2, recombinant granulocyte colony-stimulating factor for neutropenia, and antithymocyte globulin. Antimalarial drugs have shown some promise, particularly sulfadoxine-pyrimethamine (Fansidar) (van der Werff Ten Bosch et al., 2002).

Two patients with severe disease associated with homozygous mutations in the TNFRSF6 gene have been successfully treated by allogeneic bone marrow transplantation (Benkerrou et al., 1997; Sleight et al., 1998). Limited experience in the treatment of lymphomas in patients with ALPS suggests a normal response to standard chemotherapeutic agents (Infante et al., 1998; Peters et al., 1999, Straus et al., 2001).

Despite the often-impressive lymphadenopathy and splenomegaly, the prognosis with regard to lymphoproliferation is generally good and most patients demonstrate partial or complete regression of lymphadenopathy and splenomegaly over time. Autoimmune manifestations also tend to regress as children reach adolescence or adulthood, but autoimmune diseases have been noted to appear for the first time in adulthood (Jackson and Puck, 1999).

Further study will be needed to define the natural history of autoimmunity in ALPS. In addition, the increased risk of lymphoma offsets the generally favorable prognosis and mandates long-term follow-up of patients with ALPS and mutation-positive relatives.

ACKNOWLEDGMENT

We thank Christine Jackson, Elaine Jaffe, Janet Dale, and Stephen Straus for assistance in preparation of this chapter.

REFERENCES

Bader-Meunier B, Rieux-Laucat F, Croisille L, Yvart J, Mielot F, Dommergues JP, Ledeist F, Tchernia G. Dyserythropoiesis associated with a Fas-deficient condition in childhood. Br J Haematol 108:300–304, 2000.

Benkerrou M, Le Deist F, de Villartay JP, Caillat-Zucman S, Rieux-Laucat F, Jabado N, Cavazzana-Calvo M, Fischer A. Correction of Fas (CD95) deficiency by haploidentical bone marrow transplantation. Eur J Immunol 27:2043–2047, 1997.

Bettinardi A, Brugnoni D, Quiròs-Roldan E, Malagoli A, La Grutta S, Correra A, Notarangelo LD. Missense mutations in the Fas gene resulting in autoimmune lymphoproliferative syndrome: a molecular and immunological analysis. Blood 89:902–909, 1997.

Bleesing JJ, Brown MR, Straus SE, Dale JK, Siegel RM, Johnson M, Lenardo MJ, Puck JM, Fleisher TA. Immunophenotypic profiles in families with autoimmune lymphoproliferative syndrome. Blood 98:2466–2473, 2001.

Bleesing JJ, Straus SE, Fleisher TA. Autoimmune lymphoproliferative syndrome. A human disorder of abnormal lymphocyte survival. Pediatr Clin North Am 47:1291–1310, 2000.

Canale VC, Smith CH. Chronic lymphadenopathy simulating malignant lymphoma. J Pediatr 70:891–899, 1967.

Choi Y, Ramnath VR, Eaton AS, Chen A, Simon-Stoos K, Kleiner DE, Erikson J, Puck JM. Expression in transgenic mice of dominant interfering Fas mutations: a model for human autoimmune lymphoproliferative syndrome. Clin Immunol 93:34–45, 1999.

Choi Y, Simon-Stoos K, Puck JM. Hypo-active variant of IL-2 and associated decreased T cell activation contribute to impaired apoptosis in autoimmune prone MRL mice. Eur J Immunol. 32:677–685, 2002.

Cohen PL, Eisenberg RA. Lpr and gld: single gene models of systemic autoimmunity and lymphoproliferative disease. Annu Rev Immunol 9:243–269, 1991.

Chun HJ, Zheng L, Ahmad M, Wang J, Speirs CK, Siegel RM, Dale JK, Puck J, Davis J, Hall CG, Skoda-Smith S, Atkinson TP, Straus SE, Lenardo MJ. Pleiotropic defects in lymphocyte activation caused by caspase-8 mutations lead to human immunodeficiency. Nature 419:395–399, 2002.

Dianzani U, Bragardo M, DiFranco D, Alliaudi C, Scagni P, Buonfiglio D, Redoglia V, Bonissoni S, Correra A, Dianzani I, Ramenghi U. Deficiency of the Fas apoptosis pathway without Fas gene mutations in pediatric patients with autoimmunity/lymphoproliferation. Blood 89:2871–2879, 1997.

Drappa J, Vaishnaw AK, Sullivan KE, Chu JL, Elkon KB. Fas gene mutations in the Canale-Smith syndrome, an inherited lymphoproliferative disorder associated with autoimmunity. N Engl J Med 335:1643–1649, 1996.

Fisher GH, Rosenberg FJ, Straus SE, Dale JK, Middleton LA, Lin AY, Strober W, Lenardo MJ, Puck JM. Dominant interfering Fas gene mutations impair apoptosis in a human autoimmune lymphoproliferative syndrome. Cell 81:935–946, 1995.

Fuss IJ, Strober W, Dale JK, Fritz S, Pearlstein GR, Puck JM, Lenardo MJ, Straus SE. Characteristic T helper 2 T cell cytokine abnormalities in autoimmune lymphoproliferative syndrome, a syndrome marked by defective apoptosis and humoral autoimmunity. J Immunol 158:1912–1918, 1997.

Griffith TS, Brunner T, Fletcher SM, Green DR, Ferguson TA. Fas ligand–induced apoptosis as a mechanism of immune privilege. Science 270:1189–1192, 1995.

Haas JP, Grunke M, Frank C, Kolowos W, Dirnecker D, Leipold G, Hieronymus T, Lorenz HM, Herrmann M. Increased spontaneous apoptosis in double negative T cells of humans with fas/apo-1 mutation. Cell Death Differ 5:751–757, 1998.

Hetts SW. To die or not to die: an overview of apoptosis and its role in disease. JAMA 279:300–307, 1998.

Illum N, Ralfkiaer E, Pallesen G, Geisler C. Phenotypical and functional characterization of double-negative (CD4⁻ CD8⁻) alpha beta T-cell receptor positive cells from an immunodeficient patient. Scand J Immunol 34:635–645, 1991.

Infante AJ, Britton HA, DeNapoli T, Middelton LA, Lenardo MJ, Jackson CE, Wang J, Fleisher T, Straus SE, Puck JM. The clinical spectrum in a large kindred with autoimmune lymphoproliferative syndrome caused by a Fas mutation that impairs lymphocyte apoptosis. J Pediatr 133:629–633, 1998.

Jachez B, Montecino-Rodriguez E, Fonteneau P, Loor F. Partial expression of the lpr locus in the heterozygous state: presence of autoantibodies. Immunology 64:31–36, 1988.

Jachez B, Montecino-Rodriguez E, Pflumio F, Fonteneau P, Loor F. Lymphoid cell transfers between adult C57BL/6 mice differing at the lpr and/or nu locus. Humoral immunity phenotype of the chimeras. Immunology 68:169–174, 1989.

Jackson CE, Fischer RE, Hsu AP, Anderson SM, Choi Y, Wang J, Dale JK, Fleisher TA, Middelton LA, Sneller MC, Straus SE, Puck JM. Autoimmune lymphoproliferative syndrome with defective Fas: genotype influences penetrance. Am J Hum Genet 64:1002–1014, 1999.

Jackson CE, Puck JM. Autoimmune lymphoproliferative syndrome, a disorder of apoptosis. Curr Opin Pediatr 11:521–527, 1999.

Kasahara Y, Wada T, Niida Y, Yachie A, Seki H, Ishida Y, Sakai T, Koizumi F, Koizumi S, Miyawaki T, Taniguchi N. Novel Fas (CD95/APO-1) mutations in infants with a lymphoproliferative disorder. Int Immunol 10:195–202, 1998.

Kellerer K, Mutz I. Chronische pseudomaligne immunproliferation (Canale-Smith-Syndrom). Eur J Pediatr 121:203–213, 1976 (in German).

Kono DH, Theofilopoulos AN. Genetics of systemic autoimmunity in mouse models of lupus. Int Rev Immunol 19:367–387, 2000.

Le Deist F, Emile JF, Rieux-Laucat F, Benkerrou M, Roberts I, Brousse N, Fischer A. Clinical, immunological, and pathological consequences of Fas-deficient conditions. Lancet 348:719–723, 1996.

Lenardo M, Chan KM, Hornung F, McFarland H, Siegel R, Wang J, Zheng L. Mature T lymphocyte apoptosis—immune regulation in a dynamic and unpredictable antigenic environment. Annu Rev Immunol 17:221–253, 1999.

Lim MS, Straus SE, Dale JK, Fleisher TA, Stetler-Stevenson M, Strober W, Sneller MC, Puck JM, Lenardo MJ, Elenitoba-Johnson KS, Lin AY, Raffeld M, Jaffe ES. Pathological findings in human autoimmune lymphoproliferative syndrome. Am J Pathol 153:1541–1550, 1998.

Lopatin U, Yao X, Williams RK, Bleesing JJ, Dale JK, Wong D, Teruya-Feldstein J, Fritz S, Morrow MR, Fuss I, Sneller MC, Raffeld M, Fleisher TA, Puck JM, Strober W, Jaffe ES, Straus SE. Increases in circulating and lymphoid tissue interleukin-10 in autoimmune lymphoproliferative syndrome are associated with disease expression. Blood 97:3161–3170, 2001.

Martin DA, Zheng L, Siegel RM, Huang B, Fisher GH, Wang J, Jackson CE, Puck JM, Dale J, Straus SE, Peter ME, Krammer PH, Fesik S, Lenardo MJ. Defective CD95/APO-1/Fas signal complex formation in the human autoimmune lymphoproliferative syndrome, type Ia. Proc Natl Acad Sci USA 96:4552–4557, 1999.

Pan TQ, Atkinson TP, Makris CM, Cooper MD, MacDonald JM. ALPS (autoimmune lymphoproliferative syndrome) associated with a mutation in Fas-ligand [abstract 48], Fourteenth Annual Conference on Clinical Immunology and 5th International Symposium on Clinical Immunology. Washington DC, April 15-April 17, 1999.

Peng SL, Robert ME, Hayday AC, Craft J. A tumor-suppressor function for Fas (CD95) revealed in T cell–deficient mice. J Exp Med 184:1149–1154, 1996.

Pensati L, Costanzo A, Ianni A, Accapezzato D, Iorio R, Natoli G, Nisini R, Almerighi C, Balsano C, Vajro P, Vegnente A, Levrero M. Fas/APO1 mutations and autoimmune lymphoproliferative syndrome in a patient with type 2 autoimmune hepatitis. Gastroenterology 113:1384–1389, 1997.

Peters AM, Kohfink B, Martin H, Griesinger F, Wörmann B, Gahr M, Roesler J. Defective apoptosis due to a point mutation in the death domain of CD95 associated with autoimmune lymphoproliferative syndrome, T-cell lymphoma, and Hodgkin's disease. Exp Hematol 27:868–874, 1999.

Puck JM, Zhu S. Immune disorders caused by defects in the caspase cascade. Curr Allergy Asthma Rep 3:378–384, 2003.

Rieux-Laucat F, Blanchère S, Danielan S, De Villartay JP, Oleastro M, Solary E, Bader-Meunier B, Arkwright P, Pondaré C, Bernaudin F, Chapel H, Nielsen S, Berrah M, Fischer A, Le Deist F. Lymphoproliferative syndrome with autoimmunity: a possible genetic basis for dominant expression of the clinical manifestations. Blood 94:2575–2582, 1999.

Rieux-Laucat F, Le Deist F, Hivroz C, Roberts IA, Debatin KM, Fischer A, de Villartay JP. Mutations in Fas associated with human lymphoproliferative syndrome and autoimmunity. Science 268:1347–1349, 1995.

Scaradavou A, Bussel JB. Clinical experience with anti-D in the treatment of idiopathic thrombocytopenic purpura. Semin Hematol 35(1 Suppl 1):52–57, 1998.

Siegel RM, Frederiksen JK, Zacharias DA, Chan FK, Johnson M, Lynch D, Tsien RY, Lenardo MJ. Fas preassociation required for apoptosis signaling and dominant inhibition by pathogenic mutations. Science 288:2354–2357, 2000.

Sleight BJ, Prasad VS, DeLaat C, Steele P, Ballard E, Arceci RJ, Sidman CL. Correction of autoimmune lymphoproliferative syndrome by bone marrow transplantation. Bone Marrow Transplant 22:375–380, 1998.

Sneller MC, Straus SE, Jaffe ES, Jaffe JS, Fleisher TA, Stetler-Stevenson M, Strober W. A novel lymphoproliferative/autoimmune syndrome resembling murine lpr/gld disease. J Clin Invest 90:334–341, 1992.

Sneller MC, Wang J, Dale JK, Strober W, Middelton LA, Choi Y, Fleisher TA, Lim MS, Jaffe ES, Puck JM, Lenardo MJ, Straus SE. Clinical, immunologic, and genetic features of an autoimmune lymphoproliferative syndrome associated with abnormal lymphocyte apoptosis. Blood 89:1341–1348, 1997.

Straus SE, Jaffe ES, Puck JM, Dale JK, Elkon KB, Rosen-Wolff A, Peters AM, Sneller MC, Hallahan CW, Wang J, Fischer RE, Jackson CM, Lin AY, Baumler C, Siegert E, Marx A, Vaishnaw AK, Grodzicky T, Fleisher TA, Lenardo MJ. The development of

lymphomas in families with autoimmune lymphoproliferative syndrome with germline Fas mutations and defective lymphocyte apoptosis. Blood 98:194–200, 2001.

Ströbel P, Nanan R, Gattenlöhner S, Müller-Deubert S, Müller-Hermelink HK, Kreth HW, Marx A. Reversible monoclonal lymphadenopathy in autoimmune lymphoproliferative syndrome with functional FAS (CD95/APO-1) deficiency. Am J Surg Pathol 23:829–837, 1999.

Takahashi T, Tanaka M, Brannan CI, Jenkins NA, Copeland NG, Suda T, Nagata S. Generalized lymphoproliferative disease in mice, caused by a point mutation in the Fas ligand. Cell 76:969–976, 1994.

Vaishnaw AK, Orlinick JR, Chu JL, Krammer PH, Chao MV, Elkon KB. The molecular basis for apoptotic defects in patients with CD95 (Fas/Apo-1) mutations. J Clin Invest 103:355–363, 1999 [erratum in J Clin Invest 103:1099, 1999].

van der Burg M, de Groot R, Comans-Bitter WM, den Hollander JC, Hooijkaas H, Neijens HJ, Berger RM, Oranje AP, Langerak AW, van Dongen JJ. Autoimmune lymphoproliferative syndrome (ALPS) in a child from consanguineous parents: a dominant or recessive disease? Pediatr Res 47:336–343, 2000.

van der Werff Ten Bosch J, Schotte P, Ferster A, Azzi N, Boehler T, Laurey G, Arola M, Demanet C, Beyaert R, Thielemans K, Otten J. Reversion of autoimmune lymphoproliferative syndrome with an antimalarial drug: preliminary results of a clinical cohort study and molecular observations. Br J Haematol 117:176–188, 2002.

Wang J, Zheng L, Lobito A, Chan FK-M, Dale J, Sneller M, Yao X, Puck JM, Straus SE, Lenardo JM. Inherited human Caspase 10 mutations underlie defective lymphocyte and dendritic cell apoptosis in autoimmune lymphoproliferative syndrome type II. Cell 98:47–58, 1999.

Watanabe-Fukunaga R, Brannan CI, Copeland NG, Jenkins NA, Nagata S. Lymphoproliferative disorder in mice explained by defects in Fas antigen that mediates apoptosis. Nature 356:314–317, 1992.

Wu J, Wilson J, He J, Xiang L, Schur PH, Mountz JD. Fas ligand mutation in a patient with systemic lupus erythematosus and lymphoproliferative disease. J Clin Invest 98:1107–1113, 1996.

Phagocyte Disorders

Sergio D. Rosenzweig, Gülbû Uzel, and Steven M. Holland

INTRODUCTION

Phagocytes wear many hats and have many responsibilities in the healthy host. Although they are usually thought of as the uneducated grunts of the immune system, they have a dizzying array of responsibilities and activities. They are required to leave the bone marrow, circulate, if only briefly (7 hours for neutrophils, 2 to 4 days for monocytes), and then exit the circulation. Once out in the tissue, they must follow their "noses" to seek out intruders, using chemokines (interleuken-8 [IL-8]), bacterial products (N-formyl methionyl leucyl phenylalanine [fMLF]), and host factors (leukotriene B$_4$ [LTB4], platelet-activating factor [PAF]) for chemotactic guidance. Once they encounter a potential pathogen, they must recognize it by means of direct detection (binding to mannose and other motifs on bacteria and fungi), antibody-mediated detection (Fc receptors), or binding to deposited complement fragments.

Following these tasks comes the real reason for all the previous steps, as the neutrophil or monocyte tries to kill the intruder, using stored products in granules and the generation of toxic oxygen intermediates. In addition, throughout this period the phagocyte is producing its own cytokines and chemokines, calling in reinforcements. When the neutrophil has completed its work, ingested and perhaps killed its prey, it is ready to die; macrophages ingest their spent cousins and clean up the job. These steps are all done without the rearrangement of DNA by cells that are derived from the most ancient of immune systems. Their intrinsic importance is borne out with every neutropenic fever: Phagocytes are crucially important to our daily survival.

Phagocyte defects are still being discovered, and there are undoubtedly more to be identified. Although we have attained molecular knowledge of many of the classically described defects, we remain ignorant about some of the most basic aspects of pathophysiology and are still keen to sort out the mechanistic implications of the mutations found. These defects and mutations are especially important to identify, because they exist at the interface between microbes and the adaptive immune response. Further, these patients are quite difficult to manage. Each phagocyte defect has its own specific infection susceptibility and complications. Therefore treatment is not generic.

In this chapter we present a broad spectrum of the phagocyte disorders, including their molecular biology, clinical manifestations, and treatment. Table 20-1 lists the recognized defects and a brief summary of what is known about them. The generation of animal models of these defects has been highly informative. These models allow for experiments in pathophysiology and treatment that are not possible in humans. They also have been instrumental in the dissection of downstream pathways. Table 20-2 lists some of the most useful animal models of phagocyte defects for the interested reader. Interestingly, the animal and human models are not always identical, indicating subtle and still undiscovered differences in gene function between humans and other species.

TABLE 20-1 · GENETICALLY DEFINED PHAGOCYTE DEFECTS

Disease/MIM #	Gene Product Affected	Chromosomal Location	Inheritance Pattern	Functional Defect	Mutations
Chronic granulomatous disease (CGD) X-linked 306400	gp91^{phox}	Xp21.1	XR	Absent superoxide, granuloma formation	Deletions, point mutations
Autosomal recessive 233690	p22^{phox}	16q24	AR	Absent superoxide, granuloma formation	Deletions, point mutations
Autosomal recessive 233700	p47^{phox}	7q11.23	AR	Absent superoxide	GT deletion
Autosomal recessive 233710	p67^{phox}	1q25	AR	Absent superoxide	Deletions
Myeloperoxidase deficiency 254600	Myeloperoxidase, MPO	17q23.1	AR	*Candida* spp. infections, diabetes mellitus	Multiple
Glucose-6-phosphate dehydrogenase 305900	G6PDH	Xq28	XR	Anemia, infections	Multiple
Glutathione reductase deficiency	GR	8p21	AR	Hemolytic anemia; impaired respiratory burst	Unknown
Glutathione synthetase deficiency	GS	20q11.2	AR	Hemolytic anemia; 5-oxoprolinuria; recurrent bacterial infections	Multiple
Leukocyte adhesion deficiency type 1 116920	CD18	21q22.3	AR	Absent Mac-1, LFA-1, p150,95	Multiple
	CD11a (LFA-1) CD11b (Mo-1, Mac-1) CD11c (p150,95)	16p11–p13		Secondary to lack of CD18	None
Leukocyte adhesion deficiency type 2 or CDG IIc 266265	GDP-fucose transporter	11	AR	Absent CD15s, abnormal fucose metabolism, Bombay blood type	R147C T308R

Continued

TABLE 20-1 · PHAGOCYTE DEFECTS—cont'd

Disease/MIM #	Gene Product Affected	Chromosomal Location	Inheritance Pattern	Functional Defect	Mutations
Leukocyte adhesion deficiency with abnormal E-selection expression 131210	E-selectin (CD15s)	?	AR	Absent E-selectin, ineffective binding to endothelium	Unknown
Leukocyte adhesion deficiency due to Rac2 deficiency 602049	Rac2	22q12.3	AD	Inhibitory Rac2, abnormal binding, oxidative burst	D57N
Chédiak-Higashi syndrome 214500	Lysosomal transportation regulator, LYST or CHS1	1q42.1	AR	Giant granules, chemotactic defect NK-cell defect	Multiple
Griscelli syndrome 214450	Myosin-Va	15q21	AR	Partial albinism, absence of DTH, NK-cell defect	Multiple
603868	Ras-associated protein RAB27A	15q21	AR	Same as above	Multiple
606526	Melanophilin	2q37.3	AR	Partial albinism	Unknown
Kostmann's syndrome 202700	WASP (L270P)	Xp11.22	XL		
Cyclic neutropenia 162800	Neutrophil elastase (ELA2)	19p13.3	AD	Recurrent, severe neutropenia	Several
Myelokathexis/WHIM 193670	CRCR4	2q21	AD	Neutropenia, warts, hypogamma-globulinemia	Multiple
CD16 deficiency 146740	CD16 (FcγRIII)	1q23	AR	Absent CD16, abnormal ADCC, NK activity, isoimmune neutropenia	Unknown
Neutrophil-specific granule deficiency 245480	C/EBPε	14q11.2	AR	Myeloid transcription factor defect; absent specific granules, defensins	Deletions
Glycogen storage disease 16232220	Glu-6-phosphate transporter 1 (G6PT1)	11q3	AR	Lactic acidosis, neutropenia	Multiple
β-Actin deficiency 102630	β-Actin	7p22-p12	AD	Recurrent infections, neutrophil defects	G1174A substitution
Mannose-binding protein deficiency 154545	MBP	10q11.2-q21	AR	Recurrent bacterial infections, increased autoimmune phenomena	Multiple

AD = autosomal dominant; ADCC = antibody-dependent cell-mediated cytotoxicity; AR = autosomal recessive; DTH = delayed-type cell hypersensitivity; NK = natural killer; XR = X-linked recessive.

Defects of Oxidative Metabolism

CHRONIC GRANULOMATOUS DISEASE

Definition

Chronic granulomatous disease (CGD) is a genetically heterogeneous disease characterized by recurrent life-threatening infections with bacteria and fungi and dysregulated granuloma formation. CGD is caused by defects in the NADPH oxidase, the enzyme responsible for the phagocyte respiratory burst and the generation of phagocyte superoxide. There are four closely related genetic defects on different chromosomes that result in the phenotype.

The disease was first described by Janeway and colleagues (1954) and by Berendes and associates (1957) and Landing and Shirkey (1957) but was not well characterized until 1959 (Bridges et al., 1959). It was initially termed fatal granulomatous disease, but with early diagnosis and treatment, the prognosis no longer warrants this pessimistic name.

Pathogenesis

The functional NADPH oxidase is a six-protein complex. In the basal state, it exists as two components: as a membrane-bound complex embedded in the walls of secondary granules and as distinct cytosolic components (Segal et al., 2000). The granule membrane contains the heme and flavin binding cytochrome b_{558}, composed of a 91-kD glycosylated β chain (gp91^{phox}) and a 22-kD nonglycosylated α chain (p22^{phox}). The cytosolic components are p47^{phox}, p67^{phox}, p40^{phox}, and

TABLE 20-2 · ANIMAL MODELS OF PHAGOCYTIC IMMUNODEFICIENCIES

Disease	Animal Model (Spontaneous or Knockout)	References
CGD	*Cybb* knockout mice (X-linked CGD)	Pollock et al., 1995
	p47*phox* knockout mice (AR p47*phox* CGD)	Jackson et al., 1995
Chédiak-Higashi syndrome	Beige mouse	Gallin et al., 1974
Griscelli syndrome	Dilute mouse	Jenkins et al., 1981
Cyclic neutropenia/cyclic hematopoiesis	Canine cyclic neutropenia (Gray collie dog)	Chusid et al., 1975
	Neutrophil elastase knockout mice	Belaaouaj et al., 1998
Severe congenital neutropenia	*Gcsfr* knockout mice	Hermans et al., 1999
G6PDH deficiency	X-linked G6PDH deficient mice (*Mus musculus*)	Pretsch et al., 1981
Neutrophil-specific granule disease	CCAAT/enhancer binding protein-e (C/EBPε) knockout mice	Yamanaka et al., 1997
LAD-1	Bovine LAD (Holstein cattle)	Schuster et al., 1992
	Canine LAD (Irish setter)	Kijas et al., 1999
	CD18 mutant mice	Wilson et al., 1993
	CD18 knockout mice	Scharffetter-Kochanek et al., 1998
E-selectin deficiency/LAD-3	*Sele* knockout mice	Frenette et al., 1996
Rac2 deficiency/LAD-4	*Rac2* knockout mice	Roberts et al., 1999
IFN-γR1 deficiency	*IFN-γr1* knockout mice	Huang et al., 1993
IFN-γR2 deficiency	*IFN-γr2* knockout mice	Lu et al., 1998
IL-12R1 deficiency	*IL-12rβ1* knockout mice	Wu et al., 1997
IL-12p40 deficiency	*IL-12α* knockout mice	Magram et al., 1996
STAT1 mutations	*Stat1* knockout mice	Darnell et al., 1994

G6PDH = glucose-6-phosphate dehydrogenase; IFN-γR = interferon-γ receptor 1; LAD = leukocyte adhesion deficiency.

rac. All these components are necessary for the generation of superoxide except p40*phox*, which is thought to have a regulatory role (Fig. 20-1).

Genetic Heterogeneity

Four genes, with two different inheritance patterns, have been involved in CGD pathogenesis (Ariga et al., 1998; Rae et al., 1998; Roos, 1996; Roos et al., 1996) (Table 20-3):

1. CYBB (gp91*phox*, X-linked CGD; OMIM*306400) Xp21.1
2. CYBA (p22*phox*, AR-CGD; OMIM*233690) 16q24
3. NCF1 (p47*phox*, AR-CGD, OMIM*233700), 7q11.23
4. NCF2 (p67*phox*, AR-CGD; OMIM*233710), 1q25

The most common genotype, X-linked CGD, accounting for about 70% of U.S. cases, involves mutations in the β chain of the cytochrome b$_{558}$, CYBB, gp91*phox* (Winkelstein et al., 2000). Defects include those that result in absent gp91*phox* (X91^0), reduced amounts of hypofunctional protein (X91$^-$), or normal amounts of a nonfunctional protein (X91$^+$) (Segal et al., 2000). One corollary of X-linkage is lyonization in females. Heavy lyonization of the functional gene resulting in females with X-linked forms of CGD has been reported (Bolsher et al., 1981; Winkelstein et al., 2000).

Autosomal recessive CGD is caused by mutations of p22*phox*, the α chain of the cytochrome, and accounts for less than 5% of cases (Segal et al., 2000; Winkelstein et al., 2000). Failure to produce either member of the cytochrome heterodimer (gp91*phox* or p22*phox*) prevents significant expression of the other: Both subunits are required to stabilize each other within the membrane (Dinauer et al., 1990; Segal, 1987). In most of the p22*phox* defects, no flavocytochrome is present

(A22^0), but patients with normal expression of nonfunctional cytochrome b$_{558}$ due to a missense mutation in the p22*phox* gene (A22$^+$) have been described (Dinauer et al., 1991).

Autosomal recessive CGD caused by defects in p47*phox* is mainly due to failure of protein expression (A47^0) and accounts for about 25% of cases (Clark et al., 1989; Winkelstein et al., 2000). Most p47*phox*-deficient patients have at least one allele with a deletion of a GT couplet at the first intron-exon boundary, leading to improper splicing (Casimir et al., 1991). This common mutation is due to conversion with a highly homologous p47*phox* pseudogene (Roesler et al., 2000). There was a suggestion of autosomal dominant transmission in one family, but molecular analysis has confirmed only the recessive GT deletion (Gallin et al., 1983). The GT deletion allele is fairly common in the normal population, at around 1:2000 (Chanock, personal communication, 2000).

Autosomal recessive CGD caused by deficiency of p67*phox* has been documented in relatively few patients, typically without protein expression (A67^0), and accounts for less than 5% of cases (Segal et al., 2000; Winkelstein et al., 2000). Comprehensive reviews of mutations in CGD have been published (Roos, 1996; Roos et al., 1996).

Mechanisms of Defective Killing

After cell activation, the cytosolic components translocate to the cytochrome in the membrane, resulting in an active NADPH oxidase complex. The inability to generate superoxide in the CGD patient leads to a failure to make the downstream reactive oxygen species hydrogen peroxide and hydroxyl radical. This defect in turn manifests as defective microbial killing and recurrent infections with catalase-positive bacteria and fungi. The

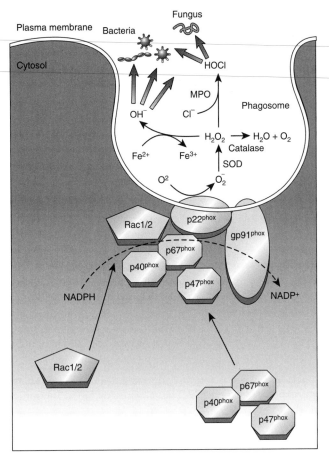

Figure 20-1 · NADPH oxidase components and activation. On activation of phagocytic cells, the three cytosolic components of the NADPH oxidase (p67^{phox}, p47^{phox}, and p40^{phox}), plus either Rac1 or Rac2, are translocated to the membrane of the phagocytic vacuole. The p47^{phox} subunit binds to the flavocytochrome$_{b558}$ component of the NADPH oxidase (gp91^{phox} plus p22^{phox}). The NADPH oxidase catalyses the formation of superoxide anion by transferring an electron to O_2, thereby forming superoxide. The unstable superoxide anion is converted to hydrogen peroxide, either spontaneously or by superoxide dismutase (SOD). Hydrogen peroxide can follow different metabolic pathways into more potent reactive oxidants (such as OH$^-$ or HOCl) or degradation to $H_2O + O_2 \cdot e^- =$ electron; $O^-_{2,} =$ superoxide anion; $H_2O_2 =$ hydrogen peroxide; MPO = myeloperoxidase; HOCl = hypochlorous acid; OH$^- =$ hydroxyl anion.

biochemical and functional dissection of the defect in CGD has led to an impressive body of information about the role of both oxidative and nonoxidative mechanisms in bacterial and fungal killing.

Quie and colleagues (1967) first noted normal phagocytosis associated with a defect in intracellular killing of bacteria in CGD. Baehner and Nathan (1968) developed a quantitative assay using nitroblue tetrazolium (NBT) to detect patients and carriers with CGD. This was modified and simplified by Ochs and Igo (1973) to essentially the NBT slide test that is used today.

In their elegant and classic paper, Klebanoff and White (1969) showed that CGD cells were able to halogenate bacteria that produced hydrogen peroxide but not killed organisms or those that produced catalase. This demonstrated that the defect in CGD cells was at the level of production of hydrogen peroxide and that distal mechanisms in the bactericidal pathway, most notably myeloperoxidase, were intact. This provided the pathophysiologic explanation for the clinical observation that patients with CGD are subject to infections almost exclusively with catalase-producing organisms. Organisms that produce and do not degrade hydrogen peroxide supply the substrate for the formation of hypohalous acid and therefore their own demise.

Other functional defects have been observed in CGD cells, including abnormal membrane potentials in response to phorbol myristate acetate (PMA) or fMLP stimulation, abnormal ADCC, and reduced tubulin tyrosinolation (Gallin and Buescher, 1983). Another corollary of an inability to form superoxide is the failure to oxidize NADPH. In this event, there is no mechanism to regenerate NADP$^+$, the terminal electron acceptor for the hexose monophosphate shunt (HMP). Therefore HMP activity is also defective in CGD cells.

Until recently, most evidence pointed at the metabolites of superoxide as the critical mediators of bacterial killing by themselves. However, Reeves and co-workers (2002) have recently shown that phagocyte production of reactive oxygen species is most critical for microbial killing through the activation of the primary granule proteins neutrophil elastase and cathepsin G inside the

TABLE 20-3 · CHRONIC GRANULOMATOUS DISEASE CLASSIFICATION

Component Affected	Gene Locus	Inheritance	Subtype Designation*	NBT (% Positive)	O$_2$ Production (% Normal)	Cytochrome b (% Normal)	Defect in Cell-Free System	Frequency (% of Cases)
gp91^{phox}	Xp21.1	XR	X91^0	0	0	0	Membrane	70
			X91$^-$	0–Weak	Low	Low	Membrane	
			X91$^+$	0–Weak	0	100	Membrane	
p22^{phox}	16q24	AR	A22^0	0	0	0	Membrane	<5
			A22$^+$	0	0	100	Membrane	
p47^{phox}	7q11.23	AR	A47^0	0	0–1	100	Cytosol	25
p67^{phox}	1q25	AR	A67^0	0	0–1	100	Cytosol	<5

*In this nomenclature, the letters indicate the inheritance mode and the superscript symbols indicate the following: 0 = undetectable, – diminished, + = normal as measured by immunoblot analysis.
AR = autosomal recessive; NBT = nitroblue tetrazolium; XR = X-linked recessive.
Modified from Roos D, Curnutte J: Chronic granulomatous disease. In Ochs H, Smith CIE, Puck J, eds. Primary Immunodeficiency Disorders. Oxford, UK, Oxford University Press, 1999.

phagocytic vacuole. This new paradigm for NADPH oxidase-mediated microbial killing suggests that the reactive oxidants are most critical as intracellular signaling molecules, leading to activation of other pathways, rather than exerting a microbicidal effect per se.

Clinical Features

Clinically, CGD is quite variable, ranging in time of presentation from infancy to late adulthood, with the majority of patients diagnosed as toddlers and young children. However, a significant number of patients are diagnosed in later childhood or adulthood (Winkelstein et al., 2000).

Bacterial Infections

The frequent sites of infection are lung (Fig. 20-2), skin, lymph nodes, and liver. Osteomyelitis, perianal abscesses, and gingivitis are also common (Segal et al., 2000; Winkelstein et al., 2000) (Table 20-4).

Pulmonary infections include recurrent pneumonia, hilar lymphadenopathy, empyema, and lung abscesses. Discrete reticulonodular densities may represent areas of granuloma. In certain patients, areas of bronchopneumonia may resolve into discrete areas of consolidation termed encapsulating pneumonia (Wolfson et al., 1968).

The microbiology of the infections of CGD is remarkable for its relative specificity (Table 20-5). The overwhelming majority of infections in CGD are due to only five organisms: *Staphylococcus aureus*, *Burkholderia (Pseudomonas) cepacia*, *Serratia marcescens*, *Nocardia*, and *Aspergillus*. In the preprophylaxis era, most lung, skin, and bone infections were staphylococcal. Now,

however, in the setting of trimethoprim/sulfamethoxazole prophylaxis, the frequency of bacterial infections in general and staphylococcal infections in particular are reduced. With current therapy, staphylococcal infections are essentially confined to the liver and lymph nodes (Winkelstein et al., 2000). Whereas the typical liver abscess in an immunologically normal patient involves enteric organisms and is liquid and easily drainable, the liver abscesses encountered in CGD are dense, caseous, and staphylococcal. This dense, undrainable abscess material is the reason that surgery is needed in almost all cases of CGD liver abscess (Lublin et al., 2002) (Fig. 20-3).

Infections with the gram-negative organisms listed earlier are most commonly pneumonia and cellulitis.

TABLE 20-4 · PREVALENCE OF INFECTION BY SITE IN 368 PATIENTS WITH CHRONIC GRANULOMATOUS DISEASE*

Type of Infection	Total (*n* = 368) No. (%)
Pneumonia	290 (79%)
Abscess	250 (68%)
Suppurative adenitis	194 (53%)
Osteomyelitis	90 (25%)
Bacteremia/fungemia	65 (18%)
Cellulitis	18 (5%)
Meningitis	15 (4%)
Other†	112 (30%)

*These data include patients on variable prophylactic regimens, if any, and are meant to portray the natural history of disease over the past 20 years.
†Includes impetigo, sinusitis, otitis media, septic arthritis, urinary tract infection/pyelonephritis, gingivitis/periodontitis, chorioretinitis, gastroenteritis, paronychia, conjunctivitis, hepatitis, epididymitis, empyema, epiglottitis, cardiac empyema, mastoiditis, and suppurative phlebitis.
Modified from Winkelstein JA et al. Chronic granulomatous disease. Report on a national registry of 368 patients. Medicine (Balt) 79:155–169, 2000.

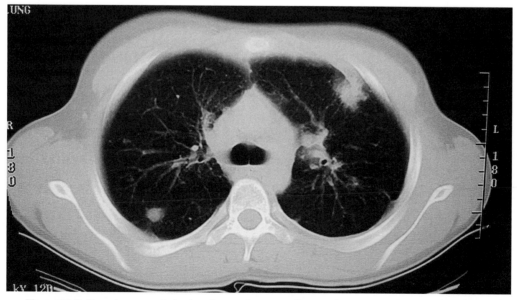

Figure 20-2 · Fungal pneumonia in chronic granulomatous disease. Chest computed tomography scan of a 17-year-old boy with X-linked CGD taken at a routine office visit. The patient was asymptomatic, had a normal erythrocyte sedimentation rate, and had no extrapulmonary involvement. A biopsy specimen grew *Paecilomyces lilacinus*. Treatment with amphotericin B was successful in clearing disease.

TABLE 20-5 · ISOLATION OF MICROORGANISMS BY TYPE OF INFECTION*

Type of Infection	Pneumonia (n = 290) No. (%)	Abscess (n = 250) Subcutaneous (n = 56) No. (%)	Liver (n = 98) No. (%)	Lung (n = 60) No. (%)	Perirectal (n = 57) No. (%)	Brain (n = 12) No. (%)	Suppurative Adenitis (n = 194) No. (%)	Osteomyelitis (n = 90) No. (%)	Bacteremia/ Fungemia (n = 65) No. (%)
Staphylococcus spp.	34 (12%)	42 (27%)	50 (50%)	5 (8%)	5 (9%)	1 (8%)	50 (26%)	5 (6%)	6 (9%)
Aspergillus spp.	120 (41%)	8 (5%)	3 (3%)	14 (23%)		7 (58%)		20 (22%)	8 (12%)
Burkholderia cepacia	24 (8%)			4 (7%)			4 (2%)	2 (2%)	
Nocardia spp.	21 (7%)	7 (5%)	3 (3%)	4 (7%)				3 (3%)	3 (5%)
Klebsiella spp.	7 (3%)	23 (15%)	5 (5%)		2 (2%)		10 (6%)	2 (2%)	4 (6%)
Serratia spp.	14 (5%)	6 (4%)	2 (2%)				18 (9%)	26 (29%)	7 (11%)
Candida spp.	5 (2%)						14 (7%)		
Mycobacteria spp.	12 (4%)								
Atypical mycobacteria	5 (2%)								
Pseudomonas spp.	7 (3%)								6 (9%)
Salmonella spp.									12 (18%)
Acinetobacter spp.							4 (2%)		3 (5%)
Escherichia coli					2 (2%)				
Enterobacteriaceae spp.	4 (1%)							2 (2%)	
Paecilomyces spp.								7 (8%)	
Streptococcus spp.			5 (5%)			1 (8%)			
Exophiala spp.									
Other	47 (17%)*	28 (18%)†	8 (8%)‡	9 (15%)§	5 (9%)**		16 (8%)††	5 (6%)‡‡	12 (18%)§§

*Include infections due to *Haemophilus parainfluenzae*, *Mycoplasma* spp., *Fusarium*, *Legionella* spp., respiratory syncytial virus, *Rhizopus*, *Acinetobacter*, *Enterobacter*, *Salmonella* spp., adenovirus, *Aerococcus*, *Exophiala*, *Moraxella*, *Streptomyces*, and *Chryseomonas*.
†Include infections due to *Escherichia coli*, *Pseudomonas*, *Enterococcus* spp., *Chromobacterium*, *Enterobacter*, *Nocardia*, *Salmonella*, *Acinetobacter*, *Diphtheroids*, *Exophiala*, *Fusarium*, *Microascus*, *Paecilomyces*, *Penicillium*, and *Providencia* spp.
‡Include infections due to *Coccidioidomycosis*, *Enterococcus*, *Klebsiella*, *Lactobacillus*, *Pediococcus*, *Peptostreptococcus*, *Pseudomonas*, and *Streptococcus milleri*.
§Include infections due to *Candida*, *Coccidioidomycosis*, *Fusobacterium*, *Klebsiella*, *Zygomycosis* (mucormycosis), *Mycobacterium tuberculosis*, *Paecilomyces*, and *Serratia* spp.
**Include infections due to *Edwardsiella*, *Enterococcus*, *Nocardia*, and *Proteus*.
††Include infections due to *B. cepacia*, *Pseudomonas* spp., *Acinetobacter*, *Aerococcus*, *Aspergillus*, *Bacillus subtilis*, *Enterobacter*, *Streptococcus*, and *Candida glabrata*.
‡‡Include infections due to *E. coli*, *Penicillium*, *Proteus*, and *Salmonella* spp.
§§Include infections due to *Arizona himanshi*, *Aspergillus*, *Enterobacter*, *Aerococcus*, *Corynebacterium*, *E. coli*, *Nocardia*, *Penicillium*, and *Rhodococcus*.
Modified from Winkelstein JA et al. Chronic granulomatous disease. Report on a national registry of 368 patients. Medicine (Baltimore) 79:155-169, 2000.
Columns do not sum to 100% because of culture negative or uncultured infections.

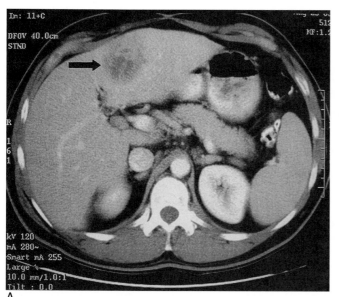
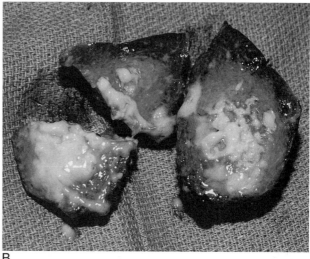

Figure 20-3 · Liver abscess in chronic granulomatous disease. **A.** This contrast computed tomography (CT) scan of the liver shows a large, complex, multiloculated mass *(arrow)* in a 30-year-old man with p47*phox*–deficient CGD. This liver abscess is typical of CGD in the paucity of liquefaction seen on the CT scan. **B.** The resected abscess is shown. Note that although the resected lesion has pus, it is not liquid but rather dense and interspersed in the hepatic parenchyma. This property makes catheter drainage of the lesions very difficult and almost always leads to open resection, as in this case.

Bacteremia is uncommon, but when it occurs it is usually due to *B. cepacia, S. marcescens,* or *Chromobacterium violaceum,* one of the gram-negative rods that inhabits soil and warm brackish water, such as that found in the southeastern United States. Bacterial and *Nocardia* infections in CGD tend to be symptomatic and associated with elevated erythrocyte sedimentation rates and may or may not be associated with elevated leukocyte counts (Dorman et al., 2002). However, normal laboratory values and a paucity of symptoms offer scant reassurance that a CGD patient is not significantly infected.

Fungal Infections

Aspergillus species and some of the rarer fungi such as *Exophiala dermatitidis* (Kenney et al., 1992) and *Paecilomyces* species (Williamson et al., 1992) are encountered in CGD. Fungal infections are now the leading cause of mortality in CGD (Winkelstein et al., 2000). Bony involvement by fungi typically occurs by direct extension from the lung. *Aspergillus nidulans* is an organism virtually exclusive in its occurrence in CGD. It causes a much higher rate of osteomyelitis than other fungi, and has a much higher rate of mortality than *Aspergillus fumigatus* or other fungi (Segal et al., 1998; Sponseller et al., 1991). Involvement of the vertebral bodies with fungi, typically by direct extension from the adjacent infected lung, is especially problematic. The rate of fungal infections in CGD is lower than that for bacterial infections and has apparently not changed in the setting of prophylactic antibiotics (Margolis et al., 1990).

Gastrointestinal and Genitourinary Tract Manifestations

The gastrointestinal and genitourinary tracts are often involved in CGD, sometimes as the site of the presenting complaint, sometimes asymptomatically (Figs. 20-4 and 20-5). Ament and Ochs (1973) described the clinical manifestations and laboratory and pathologic findings of gastrointestinal involvement in CGD. They noted frequent malabsorption, intrinsic factor–unresponsive vitamin B$_{12}$ deficiency, abundant lipid-laden pigmented histiocytes in small-bowel biopsy specimens, and pigmented histiocytes and granulomata in rectal biopsy specimens from both autosomal and X-linked patients. Esophageal, jejunal, ileal, cecal, rectal, and perirectal involvement with granulomas mimicking Crohn's disease have been described (Harris and Boles, 1973; Isaacs et al., 1985; Lindahl et al., 1984; Markowitz et al., 1982; Sty et al., 1979; Werlin et al., 1982).

Gastric outlet obstruction is an especially common manifestation and may be the initial presentation of CGD (Griscom et al., 1974; Johnson et al., 1975; Stopyrowa et al., 1989). Marciano and colleagues (2004) found 32% of 140 CGD patients had gastrointestinal involvement, with a marked preponderance among patients with X-linked CGD.

In a comprehensive review of the genitourinary manifestations of CGD, Walther and colleagues (1992) found that 38% of patients had some kind of urologic event. These included bladder granulomata, ureteral obstruction, and urinary tract infection. All patients with granulomata of the bladder or stricture of the

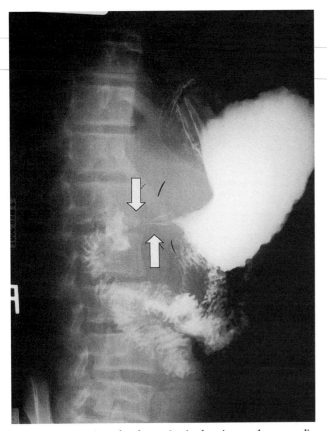

Figure 20-4 · Gastric outlet obstruction in chronic granulomatous disease. A 17-year-old boy with X-linked CGD had weight loss, nausea, and anorexia. Upper gastrointestinal series showed high-grade obstruction of the gastric outlet *(arrows)*. Upper endoscopy showed thickened folds without ulceration. Steroid therapy led to rapid resolution and return to normal food intake.

ureter had defects of the membrane component of the NADPH oxidase: eight had gp91^{phox} defects and one had a p22^{phox} defect. A previous report showed this same bias in favor of membrane component defects (Southwick and Van der Meer, 1988).

Steroid therapy in combination with antibiotics is quite effective and surprisingly well tolerated for resolution of obstructive lesions of both the gastrointestinal (GI)) and genitourinary (GU) tracts (see Fig. 20-4). Several reports and many anecdotes confirm the benefit of steroids given at about 1 mg/kg for a brief initial period and then tapered to a low dose on alternate days (Chin et al., 1987; Marciano et al., 2004; Narita et al., 1991; Quie and Belani, 1987; Southwick and Van der Meer, 1988). Prolonged low-dose maintenance is often necessary and is not associated with increased infections.

In the absence of NADPH oxidase, other host defense genes may be left with more discernible roles. Foster and co-workers (1998) examined assorted host defense genes in patients who have CGD and showed a striking influence of polymorphisms in myeloperoxidase and FcγRIII on the occurrence of gastrointestinal complications and an effect of polymorphisms in mannose-binding lectin on the development of autoimmune disorders.

Mucocutaneous Manifestations

Cutaneous inflammatory responses are often dysregulated in CGD. Patients with membrane component defects in particular may form exuberant granulomas and granulation tissue (Gallin and Buescher, 1983). This can manifest as wound dehiscence or delayed wound healing. Male CGD patients had abnormal persistence of neutrophils in Rebuck skin windows compared with female CGD patients and normal subjects. This suggested

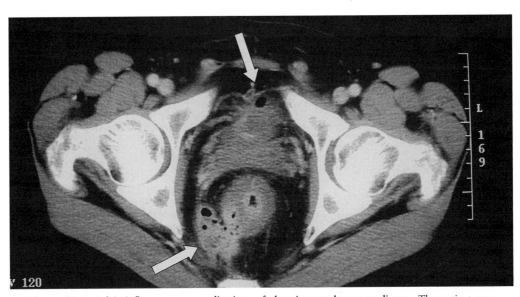

Figure 20-5 · Pelvic inflammatory complications of chronic granulomatous disease. The patient presented at age 17 with rectovesicle fistula thought to be Crohn's disease. Surgery and steroid therapy were initially successful, but the fistula recurred. The diagnosis of X-linked CGD was made (gp91$^+$). Extensive perirectal involvement is seen. The fistula has led to extensive bladder constriction and scarring. Arrows show air in the perirectal fat and bladder.

a defect in "turnoff" of the acute inflammatory response in CGD (Gallin and Buescher, 1983). Interestingly, this abnormal persistence of neutrophils was normalized in one patient who was receiving white blood cell transfusions simultaneously.

Blepharokeratoconjunctivitis, pannus formation, and stable chorioretinal scars have also been associated with CGD (Goldblatt et al., 1999; Palestine et al., 1983). The scars rarely involve the macula, but further study is needed to determine how often these lesions are sight threatening.

Growth Problems

Children with CGD tend to be short and small for their age, possibly in part due to chronic or recurrent infections or to some other aspect of defective oxidase function. However, children with CGD eventually tend to achieve the height predicted by their parents' heights. Bone age and chronologic age are most disparate in early childhood but achieve equivalence in late adolescence (Buescher and Gallin, 1984b). It is not uncommon for children with CGD to continue growing into their early 20s.

Clinical Features in Carriers of CGD

The X-linked carrier state for gp91^{phox} is not entirely silent. Lyonization of the X chromosome leads to two populations of phagocytes in carriers. One population has normal oxidase function and is detected as NBT-reducing or dihydrorhodamine oxidation (DHR)–oxidizing activity, whereas the other population, which has inactivated the normal X chromosome and has only the defective one functioning, is unable to produce superoxide. Therefore carriers give a characteristic mosaic pattern on oxidative testing.

Discoid lupus erythematosus–like lesions, aphthous ulcers, and photosensitive rashes have been seen in female relatives of gp91^{phox}-deficient patients, and screening of patients with discoid lupus erythematosus has detected unsuspected CGD carriers (Brandrup et al., 1981; Kragballe et al., 1981). The ease of determining which X chromosome is inactivated in a given phagocytic cell has been used to determine the presumed number of stem cells (exceeding 400) necessary to support human hematopoiesis (Buescher et al., 1985).

Characteristic infections are not usually seen in female carriers until the normal cells fall below 10% (Bolsher et al., 1991; Winkelstein et al., 2000). Several cases of extreme lyonization of the X chromosome carrying the functional X chromosome have been reported, leading to the rare appearance of X-linked CGD in females. This is due to skewed random inactivation in some cases, but it may be due to mutations in the gene controlling X chromosome inactivation, XIST, in others.

We have had an otherwise healthy highly lyonized X-linked carrier present with Serratia lymphadenitis as levels of her normal neutrophils fell below 10% (Malech and Holland, unpublished). Other investigators have noted progressive decline in the number of normal neutrophils in some lyonized X-linked carriers over time, leading to occurrence of CGD-type infections later in life (Lun et al., 2002).

Laboratory Features

There is usually only a mild to moderate leukocytosis with immature forms in the presence of infection with bacteria or Nocardia; fungal infections are typically relatively silent from the laboratory standpoint (Segal et al., 1998). The erythrocyte sedimentation rate and the C-reactive protein may be elevated. Immune globulins are generally elevated, and antibody titers are normal. Studies for T-cell immunity are also normal.

Kell Phenotype

The Kell blood antigens, expressed on white and red cells, are encoded at Xp21.2-1, right next to the X-CGD locus. Absence of Kell is referred to as the McLeod phenotype, named after the first identified case, Hugh McLeod (OMIM*314850). Therefore, in the event of X-CGD being caused by an interstitial deletion, there may also be deletion of the Kell locus, resulting in CGD with the McLeod phenotype (Marsh et al., 1975).

Because CGD patients may receive transfusions of granulocytes for the treatment of severe infections or of erythrocytes for blood loss, there is a potential transfusion hazard in X-CGD patients (Giblett et al., 1971). As a result of previous transfusions with Kell-positive erythrocytes, antibodies to Kell antigens may develop that cause transfusion reactions. Therefore Kell phenotyping should be done for all patients with X-CGD; if the patient is Kell negative, transfusion is best avoided or Kell-negative erythrocytes or granulocytes should be used.

Diagnosis

The index of suspicion of CGD should be raised by severe or recurrent infections in children, especially those involving pulmonary or hepatic parenchyma. Infections with unusual organisms such as B. cepacia, S. marcescens, C. violaceum, Nocardia, or Aspergillus species should always initiate a search for CGD in patients of any age without other predisposing factors. Granulomatous events such as gastrointestinal or genitourinary obstruction likewise are suggestive of the diagnosis.

The diagnosis of CGD is made by assays that rely on superoxide production. These include direct measurement of superoxide production, ferricytochrome c reduction, chemiluminescence, NBT reduction, or DHR. Currently, we prefer the lattermost assay because of its relative ease of use and its ability to distinguish X-linked from autosomal forms of CGD by flow cytometry (Vowells et al., 1995, 1996).

Several other conditions affect the phagocyte respiratory burst. Glucose-6-phosphate dehydrogenase (G6PD) deficiency may mimic certain aspects of neutrophil dysfunction of CGD, such as the decreased respiratory burst and increased susceptibility to bacterial infections (Roos et al., 1999). However, G6PD deficiency is most often associated with some degree of hemolytic anemia, whereas CGD is not. Diverse pathogens, including *Legionella pneumophila, Toxoplasma gondii, Chlamydia, Entamoeba histolytica,* and *Ehrlichia risticii,* have been shown to inhibit the respiratory burst in vitro. Recently, human granulocytic ehrlichiosis infection has been shown to depress the respiratory burst by down-regulating gp91^{phox} (Banerjee et al., 2000).

Immunoblot, flow cytometry, or molecular techniques can be used to determine the specific genotype. The history will usually suggest whether a patient has autosomal recessive or X-linked disease, based on sex, age of presentation, and severity. The subtype of CGD is important because autosomal CGD has a significantly better prognosis than X-linked disease (Winkelstein et al., 2000).

Treatment

Antimicrobial Prophylaxis

Advances in recent years have drastically altered the morbidity and mortality in patients with CGD. Prophylactic trimethoprim-sulfamethoxazole (TMP-SMX) reduced the frequency of major infections from about once every year to once every 3.5 years (Gallin et al., 1983). In addition, prophylactic TMP-SMX changes the type and site of serious infections in patients with CGD to fewer staphylococcal and skin infections (Forrest et al., 1988) without increasing the frequency of serious fungal infections (Margolis et al., 1990).

Although ketoconazole is ineffective at preventing aspergillus infection (Muoy et al., 1989), Cale and colleagues (2000) showed encouraging results with TMP-SMX and itraconazole prophylaxis in a cohort of 21 CGD patients followed at a single center; no invasive fungal infections and no deaths were registered in their group during 8 years. Itraconazole prophylaxis has now been shown to be highly effective and well tolerated in the prevention of fungal infection in CGD in a randomized prospective trial (100 mg daily for patients younger than 13 years or less than 50 kg; 200 mg daily for those 13 years or older or more than 50 kg) (Gallin et al., 2003). Therefore we routinely recommend itraconazole prophylaxis in all patients with CGD, regardless of age or previous fungal infections.

Interferon-γ Prophylaxis

Interferon-γ (IFN-γ) was unequivocally identified in 1983 as the lymphokine responsible for enhanced HMP activity and hydrogen peroxide generation in macrophages (Nathan et al., 1983). Ezekowitz and co-workers (1987) and Sechler and colleagues (1988) showed that IFN-γ could produce some of these same effects in vitro in cells from patients with an X-linked variant of CGD. When IFN-γ was administered to patients, Sechler and associates (1988) and Ezekowitz and co-workers (1988) found similar augmentation of bactericidal activity and superoxide production. In some patients this was concomitant with an increase in gp91^{phox} levels. The augmentation of superoxide production in neutrophils was demonstrable for several weeks, suggesting that IFN-γ was working at the progenitor cell level, as well as on more differentiated cells (Ezekowitz et al., 1990).

A large, multinational, multicenter, placebo-controlled study proved a marked clinical benefit for patients receiving IFN-γ. Recipients had 70% fewer and less severe infections than did placebo-treated patients. These benefits held true regardless of inheritance pattern of CGD, sex, or use of prophylactic antibiotics. Interestingly, no significant difference could be detected in terms of in vitro superoxide generation, bactericidal activity, or cytochrome b levels (International Chronic Granulomatous Disease Cooperative Study Group, 1991). Systemic IFN-γ did augment neutrophil activity against *Aspergillus conidia* in vitro (Rex et al., 1990).

Our current practice is to use prophylaxis with trimethoprim-sulfamethoxazole, itraconazole, and IFN-γ in all CGD patients.

Management of Infections

Treatment of infections in CGD must be extremely aggressive. Patients often fail to display symptoms commensurate with the extent of their disease and may present for care late in the course of infection. The erythrocyte sedimentation rate (ESR) is the most sensitive laboratory test to monitor the presence of ongoing infection: A newly elevated ESR should provoke active concern. Therapy for infections in CGD should be intravenous and prolonged, with more than one agent. The reduction in mortality and morbidity in recent years is attributable to the recognition, treatment, and prophylaxis of infections.

Microbiologic diagnosis is crucial: The differential diagnosis for any given process in these patients includes bacteria, fungi, and granulomatous processes. Transthoracic needle biopsy, bronchoscopy, and thoracotomy should be first-line diagnostic tests, not procedures considered after the failure of empirical therapy.

Hepatic abscesses are usually staphylococcal and require open excavation, débridement, and drainage (Lublin et al., 2002). Occasionally, percutaneous catheter placement has been successful in liver abscesses, but because of the dense consistency of these lesions it cannot be routinely recommended. Intralesional instillation of granulocytes has been used and may be helpful in particularly difficult cases (Lekstrom-Himes et al., 1994).

Granulocyte Transfusions

In severe infections, leukocyte transfusions are often used, although their efficacy is anecdotal. The principle is that the deficient product in CGD cells, superoxide, is highly diffusible, such that supplementation of defective cells with a few normal cells leads to complementation of the defective pathway and reconstituted bacterial and fungal killing (Ohno and Gallin, 1985). Therefore benefits accrue to granulocyte transfusions even though the overall number of peripheral blood leukocytes is not significantly altered. The number of infused granulocytes averages about 10^9 to 10^{10} per transfusion.

Buescher and Gallin (1982) showed transfused phagocyte penetration into and persistence in pulmonary secretions in a patient with *Nocardia* pneumonia. Using NBT reduction, they were able to detect transfused neutrophils in peripheral blood for up to 1 hour after transfusion, but they detected normal monocyte derived cells for up to 5 days in sputum. At 2 days after transfusion, half of the NBT-positive cells in sputum were monocytes. Emmendorffer and colleagues (1991) conducted a similar study in a boy with *Aspergillus* pneumonia using flow cytometric analysis for p22*phox* in peripheral blood and pulmonary secretions.

Although it is common practice to irradiate white blood cells before transfusion to prevent graft-versus-host disease (GVHD), this reduces the bactericidal activity and survivability of both neutrophils and monocytes in the transfused product (Buescher and Gallin, 1984a; Buescher and Gallin, 1987). Because CGD patients have no critical defect in lymphocytic immunity and there have been no reports of GVHD in recipients of unirradiated leukocytes who have CGD and irradiation of granulocytes may reduce efficacy, we do not recommend it.

Stem Cell Transplantation

Bone marrow or stem cell transplantation leading to stable chimerism was successfully performed in a patient with CGD in the 1980s (Kamani et al., 1988). The patient remained infection free despite having only 15% to 20% of his cells derived from the donor. Ozsahin and associates (1998) performed successful bone marrow transplantation on a child with CGD and active, refractory *Aspergillus* infection. Horwitz and colleagues (2001) reported low-intensity ablation (mini–bone marrow transplantation) from human leukocyte antigen (HLA)–identical siblings into 10 CGD patients. Success was greater in children than adults, but complications, including GVHD, rejection, and death, were significant.

Seger and colleagues (2002) reported 27 unmodified hemopoietic grafts in European CGD patients, some of whom had active infection. Most of these patients received HLA-matched transplants with T-cell–replete grafts following myeloablative conditioning. Survival and cure rates were 100% in those who received a transplant while well, but there were four deaths among the nine patients who received a transplant during active refractory infection. Myeloablative transplant regimens containing busulfan/cytoxan conditioning were by far the most successful. Transplantation during refractory infection may be lifesaving, but the risk is high.

Bhattacharya and colleagues (2003) reported successful umbilical cord stem cell transplantation for a child with CGD who had recurrent infections and persistent colitis. Preparation was with busulfan/cytoxan, and the transplant course was relatively uneventful. One year after the transplant, 92% of circulating neutrophils were of donor origin. The colitis resolved with transplantation, and the infections have ceased.

Del Guidice and co-workers (2003) reviewed the 24 published cases of HLA-identical sibling stem cell transplantations for CGD. They found 20 of 24 patients alive and disease free. Successful regimens typically included recipient preparation with busulfan/cytoxan and GVHD prophylaxis with cyclosporine-containing regimens.

Therefore, although there are potential benefits to reduced-intensity chemotherapeutic regimens for bone marrow ablation before transplantation for CGD, myeloablative approaches have proved reliably effective and successful in terms of engraftment and disease-free survival.

Gene Therapy

Clinical trials of p47*phox* gene therapy have shown marking of cells in the periphery for several months, but clinical benefit has not been shown, presumably due to the low numbers of corrected cells in the circulation (<0.01%) (Malech et al., 1997).

Prognosis

In a longitudinal analysis of 47 patients, Muoy and associates (1989) found an 8-year survival rate of 70.5% for children born before 1978 and 92.9% for those born later. More recently, Winkelstein and colleagues (2000) showed that mortality is about 5% per year for the X-linked form of the disease and 2% per year for the autosomal recessive varieties. The largest causes of mortality are *Aspergillus* pneumonia, followed by *B. cepacia* pneumonia or sepsis.

GLUCOSE-6-PHOSPHATE DEHYDROGENASE (G6PD) DEFICIENCY

Definition

G6PD deficiency, the most common enzymopathy in humans, affects 400 million persons worldwide. Its prevalence ranges from 0.1% in Japan and northern Europe to 62% in Kurdish Jews. G6PD maps to the long arm of the X chromosome, and its deficiency is inherited in an X-linked pattern (G6PD, Xq28; OMIM* 305900).

Hemolytic anemia, triggered by fava beans, drugs, infections or different oxidative challenges, is the most common clinical manifestation of G6PD deficiency, but when deficiency is severe, infection may result. A significant reduction in the risk of severe malaria has been associated with G6PD deficiency in males and in females heterozygous for G6PD deficiency (Ruwende et al., 1998).

Pathogenesis

G6PD is involved in NADPH generation through the hexose monophosphate pathway. As described earlier, NADPH is necessary for the respiratory burst and also for preventing erythrocyte oxidative damage (reviewed in Lazzotto, 1998).

A few patients with severe G6PD deficiency (less than 5% of normal enzyme activity) have had neutrophil respiratory burst impairment and severe infections. Neutrophil dysfunction in G6PD deficiency is less common than expected, probably because most of the affected patients have more than 20% of G6PD activity in neutrophils, which is sufficient to maintain the respiratory burst within the normal range.

Clinical Features

Recurrent bacterial pulmonary infections and a death due to *Chromobacterium violaceum* sepsis have been described (Mamlock et al., 1987; Roos et al., 1999; Vives Corrons et al., 1982). Through its compromise of the function of the NADPH oxidase by limiting the supply of NADPH, G6PD deficiency may somewhat resemble CGD (Ardati et al., 1997; Dinauer, 1998; Gray et al., 1972; Lazzotto, 1998; Mamlock et al., 1987; Roos et al., 1999; Vives Corrons et al., 1982).

Diagnosis is established by assessing G6PD activity in hemolysates or neutrophil homogenates; G6PD in neutrophils is significantly higher than that found in erythrocytes (Ardati et al., 1997; Dinauer, 1998).

Prevention includes avoidance of drugs such as primaquine, salicylates, sulfonamides, nitrofurans, phenacetin, and some vitamin K derivatives, as well as fava beans. Prompt treatment of infections is necessary.

MYELOPEROXIDASE DEFICIENCY

Definition

Myeloperoxidase (MPO) deficiency is an autosomal recessive trait with variable expressivity. It is the most common primary phagocyte disorder: 1 in 4000 individuals has complete MPO deficiency, and 1 in 2000 has a partial defect (MPO, 17q23.1; OMIM#254600) (Kitahara et al., 1981; Nauseef et al., 1983, 1988; Parry et al., 1981). Only a few patients are symptomatic, and most suffer from recurrent *Candida* infections.

Pathogenesis

Myeloperoxidase is synthesized in neutrophils and monocytes, packaged in the azurophilic granules, and released either into the phagosome or the extracellular space, where it catalyses the conversion of H_2O_2 to hypohalous acid. In neutrophils the halide is chloride and the product is bleach; in eosinophils the halide is bromine and the product is hypobromous acid. This reaction amplifies the presumed toxicity against bacteria and fungi of the reactive oxygen species generated during the respiratory burst.

Myeloperoxidase expression is affected by a promoter polymorphism in an SP1 transcription factor consensus binding site that confers higher (G allele) or lower (A allele) promoter activity (Piedrafita et al., 1996). Different genetic defects have been identified as causing MPO deficiency, but the R569W substitution is the most common (Kizaki et al., 1994; Nauseef, 1989; Nauseef et al., 1998).

Anti-MPO antibodies are associated with different autoimmune vasculitides (e.g., Wegener's granulomatosis and microscopic polyangiitis) (Kallenberg et al., 1998). MPO-derived oxidants have also been associated with atherosclerosis, where inflammation appears to play a critical role (Daugherty et al., 1994). Recently, MPO has been shown to have an impact on vascular tone through effects on nitric oxide (Eiserich et al., 2002). More recently, MPO has been recognized as a potent predictor of myocardial infarction, far exceeding the predictive value of C-reactive protein or troponins (Baldus et al., 2003).

Clinical Features

The vast majority of MPO-deficient patients are entirely asymptomatic: most of them are only found incidentally or through family screening (Laroccha et al., 1982). Of the MPO-deficient patients who have had associated clinical symptoms, infections due to different *Candida* strains have been the most common. Mucocutaneous, meningeal, and bone infections, as well as sepsis, have been described in MPO-deficient patients (Chiang et al., 2000; Ludviksson et al., 1993; Nauseef et al., 1988; Nguyen et al., 1997; Okuda et al., 1991; Weber et al., 1987). Diabetes mellitus appears to be a critical co-factor for *Candida* species infections in the context of MPO deficiency (Cech et al., 1979; Lehrer et al., 1969; Parry et al., 1981).

In vitro neutrophil function is affected in a variety of ways in MPO deficiency. The respiratory burst is prolonged, resulting in exaggerated amounts of superoxide production (Nauseef, 1990). Phagocytosis is normal to increased in MPO-deficient PMNs, whereas bactericidal activity is somewhat slower than normal (Nauseef, 1988). Candidacidal activity is markedly defective against the more pathogenic *Candida* species, such as *C. albicans*, *C. krusei*, and *C. tropicalis*. In contrast, candidacidal activity is preserved against the less pathogenic *C. parapsilosis* (Nauseef, 1988). The exaggerated respiratory burst, resulting in supranormal superoxide production, along with the presence of normal levels of eosinophil peroxidase and other oxidants, are possible explanations to the paucity of symptoms among these patients.

A secondary form of MPO deficiency has been described in patients with myelodysplastic syndromes, chronic myeloid leukemia, and the M2, M3, and M4 forms of acute myeloid leukemia (Bendix-Hansen et al., 1985, 1986; Nauseef, 1988). Aggressive treatment of infections, should they occur, is the recommended therapy in MPO deficiency. Also, diabetes should be diagnosed and controlled.

GLUTATHIONE PATHWAY ALTERATIONS: GLUTATHIONE REDUCTASE AND GLUTATHIONE SYNTHETASE DEFICIENCIES

The reduced form of glutathione (GSH) protects cells from the deleterious effects of reactive oxygen species produced during the respiratory burst and the metabolism of uric acid. Glutathione reductase (GR, 8p21.1) and glutathione synthetase (GS, 20q11.2) are involved in maintaining adequate intracellular levels of GSH (Dinauer et al., 1998). GR deficiency (OMIM*138300) and GS deficiencies (OMIM#266130 and #231900) are both extremely rare autosomal recessive inherited diseases associated with hemolysis after increased oxidant stress.

Most GS-deficient patients suffer from metabolic acidosis with increased 5-oxoproline levels, but only the most severely affected have recurrent bacterial infections. Impaired phagocytosis and intracellular bacterial killing has been reported in these patients (Boxer et al., 1979). In GR-deficient patients, premature termination of the respiratory burst has been described without an increased infection rate (Roos et al., 1979).

GR and GS deficiencies are diagnosed by measuring the respective enzymes in neutrophil, erythrocyte, or fibroblast homogenates. Vitamin E supplementation in GS-deficient patients has been associated with in vitro neutrophil functional improvement and reduced infection rates (Boxer et al., 1979; Ristoff et al., 2001).

Leukocyte Adhesion Deficiencies: General Considerations

For more than a century, leukocyte movement from the bloodstream toward inflamed sites has been recognized as critical in preventing and fighting infections.

Leukocyte adhesion to the endothelium, to other leukocytes, and to bacteria is critical in the ability of leukocytes to travel, communicate, inflame, and fight infection. Different families of adhesion molecules mediate these processes, critical among which are the integrins and selectins.

In this section we describe several different clinical and pathophysiologically defined phenotypes of leukocyte adhesion defects, impaired leukocyte movement, and severe infection (Table 20-6). Originally, leukocyte adhesion deficiency type 1 (LAD-1) was identified in children with defects in the β_2-integrins. Over the years, several new defects that affect leukocyte adhesion to the endothelium, thereby leading to recurrent hypoinflamed infections, have been identified.

Although these newer syndromes have appropriately been designated other leukocyte adhesion deficiencies because their underlying genetic defects have been worked out, more biochemically and genetically appropriate names have superseded the phenotypic ones. Thus leukocyte adhesion deficiency type 2 (LAD-2), a disease with impaired fucosylation leading to an abnormal sialyl-Lewis X, has been shown to be caused by a mutation in guanosine diphosphate (GDP)-fucose transporter-1, leading to a renaming of the syndrome as *congenital disorder of glycosylation IIc* (CDGIIc).

Therefore it is preferable to name syndromes as unique entities with names tied most closely to their specific defect, recognizing that renaming will be necessary when definitive genetic characterization takes place.

LEUKOCYTE ADHESION DEFICIENCY TYPE 1

Definition

LAD-1 is an autosomal recessive disorder caused by mutations in the common chain (CD18) of the β_2-integrin family (ITGB2, 21q22.3; OMIM#116920). LAD-1 patients usually present with recurrent severe infections, impaired pus formation, and impaired wound healing.

TABLE 20-6 · LEUKOCYTE ADHESION DEFICIENCY SYNDROMES

Leukocyte Adhesion Deficiency	Type 1 (LAD-1)	Type 2 (LAD-2 or CDGIIc)	E-selectin	Rac2	Rap-1
Affected gene	ITGB2 (21q22.3)	GDP-fucose transporter (chromosome 11)	Unknown	RAC2 (22q12.3-q13.2)	Unknown
Affected protein	β_2-Integrin common chain (CD18)	Fucosylated proteins (sialyl-Lewis X)	Endothelial E-selectin expression	Rac2	Rap-1, maybe β_2-integrin
Inheritance pattern	AR	AR	Unknown	AD	AR
Neutrophil function affected	Chemotaxis, tight adherence	Rolling, tethering	Rolling, tethering	Chemotaxis, superoxide production	Tight adhesion
Delayed umbilical cord separation	Yes (*severe phenotype* only)	No	Yes	Yes	No
Leukocytosis/ neutrophilia	Yes	Yes	No (mild neutropenia)	Yes	Yes (bleeding)

AD = autosomal dominant; AR = autosomal recessive.

Pathogenesis

Each of the β_2-integrins is a heterodimer composed of an α chain (CD11a, CD11b, or CD11c) noncovalently linked to a common β_2-subunit (CD18). The α-β heterodimers of the β_2-integrin family include CD11a/CD18 (lymphocyte function–associated antigen-1 [LFA-1]), CD11b/CD18 (macrophage antigen-1 [Mac-1] or complement receptor-3 [CR3]), and CD11c/CD18 (p150,95 or CR4) (Repo and Harlan, 1999). The CD18 gene, ITGB2, maps to chromosome 21q22.3, and its product is required for normal expression of the α-β heterodimers. Therefore defects in CD18 expression lead to either very low or no expression of CD11a, CD11b, and CD11c (Kishimoto et al., 1987; Springer et al., 1984). Mutations that result in failure to produce a functional β_2-subunit (point mutations, small insertions, deletions) cause LAD-1 (Kishimoto et al., 1989; Sligh et al., 1992). In the mid-1980s, LAD-1 clinical classifications were developed based on the degree of CD18 expression (Anderson and Springer, 1987; Anderson et al., 1985).

Clinical Features

Two relatively distinct clinical phenotypes of LAD-1 have been described. Patients with the severe phenotype (less than 1% of normal expression of CD18 on neutrophils) characteristically have delayed umbilical stump separation (more than 30 days); omphalitis; persistent leukocytosis (>15,000/µl) in the absence of overt active infection; and severe, destructive gingivitis with periodontitis and associated tooth loss and alveolar bone resorption (Anderson et al., 1985; Anderson and Springer, 1987; Fischer et al., 1988) (Fig. 20-6). Recurrent infections of the skin, upper and lower airways, bowel, and perirectal area are common and usually due to *S. aureus* or gram-negative bacilli. Infections tend to be necrotizing and may progress to ulceration

(Fig. 20-7). Typically, no pus is seen surrounding these lesions and there is an almost complete absence of neutrophil invasion on histopathology.

Aggressive medical management with antibiotics, neutrophil transfusions, and prompt surgery, when indicated, are required. Impaired healing of infectious, traumatic, or surgical wounds is also characteristic of LAD-1 patients. Scars tend to acquire a "cigarette-paper" appearance.

Patients with the moderate phenotype of LAD-1 (1% to 30% of normal expression of CD18 on neutrophils) tend to be diagnosed later in life. Normal umbilical separation and lower risk of life-threatening infections, along with longer life expectancy, are common (Anderson and Springer, 1987; Anderson et al., 1985; Fischer et al., 1988). However, leukocytosis, periodontal disease, and delayed wound healing are still the rule.

Although viral infections are not a major problem in LAD-1 patients in infancy, deaths due to viral infections have occurred in affected young adults (Anderson et al., 1985), presumably reflecting some specific antibody synthesis impairment due to poor cell–cell interaction.

Recently, patients with normal β_2-integrin expression but without functional activity were described (Hogg

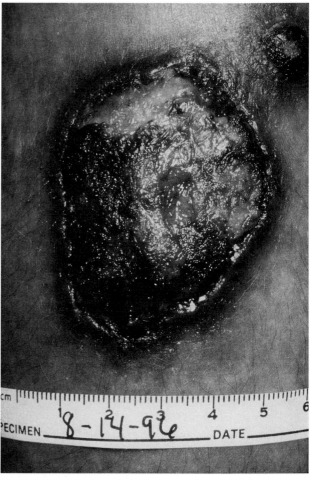

Figure 20-7 · Ulcerative skin lesion in a patient with LAD-1. No pus and poor inflammation are seen in the surrounding tissues.

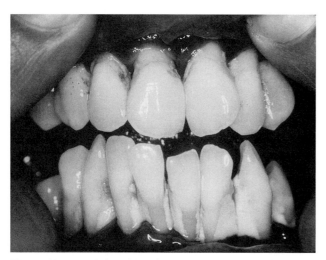

Figure 20-6 · Periodontal involvement in a patient with LAD-1. Gingivitis and gum recession are seen.

et al., 1999; Kuijpers et al., 1997). Therefore expression of CD18 alone is not sufficient to exclude the diagnosis of LAD-1: functional assays must be performed if the clinical suspicion is high. This consideration clearly makes the assignment of the labels *moderate* and *severe* complex, because surface expression alone cannot be a reliable indicator. So far, good quantitative techniques for this determination are not available in clinical laboratories.

Diagnosis

Flow cytometry analysis of LAD-1 blood samples shows significant reduction (moderate phenotype) or near absence (severe phenotype) of CD18 and its associated molecules CD11a, CD11b, and CD11c on neutrophils and other leukocytes.

LAD-1 patients have diminished neutrophil migration in vivo (Rebuck skin windows) and in vitro (Anderson and Springer, 1987; Anderson et al., 1985). Adherence of affected granulocytes to glass, plastic, nylon wool, and other LAD neutrophils is greatly reduced and does not improve after fMLF or phorbol myristate acetate (PMA) stimulation (Anderson and Springer, 1987; Anderson et al., 1985). Complement mediated phagocytosis is severely impaired due to absence of CD18/CD11b (CR3/Mac-1).

Nevertheless, immunoglobulin-G (IgG)–mediated phagocytosis is unaffected, as is NBT reduction, chemiluminescence, and primary and secondary granule release (Anderson and Springer, 1987; Anderson et al., 1985). Antibody-dependent cell-mediated cytotoxicity (ADCC) is diminished in LAD-1 patients and may contribute to the possible propensity to viral infection.

Treatment

Patients require early and aggressive treatment of infections with appropriate antibiotics. Bone marrow transplantation is the only definitive corrective treatment (Fischer et al., 1994; LeDiest et al., 1989; Thomas et al., 1995).

Preclinical gene therapy studies have been performed in LAD-1 (Bauer et al., 1998; Hibbs et al., 1990; Wilson et al., 1990), but as of yet there are no clinical benefits in humans.

LEUKOCYTE ADHESION DEFICIENCY TYPE 2

Definition

LAD-2 or congenital disorder of glycosylation type IIc (CDG-IIc) (OMIM#266265 and *605881) is a very rare autosomal recessive inherited disease of fucose metabolism. First described in 1992 by Etzioni and colleagues, LAD-2 is due to mutations in the GDP-fucose transporter gene on chromosome 11 (Lübke et al., 2001; Lühn

et al., 2001). LAD-2 is associated with lack of expression of different fucosylated molecules, leading to a complex phenotype, which includes neurologic and immunologic features.

Pathogenesis

The basic defect in LAD-2 is lack of fucosylation of various proteins, resulting in impaired expression of sialyl-Lewis X and other fucosylated proteins that function as ligands for the selectins (Etzioni et al., 1992; Frydman et al., 1992). Selectins are adhesive molecules expressed on the surface of activated endothelial cells that mediate the initial rolling of neutrophils and monocytes over the endothelium at sites of infection. Failure to adhere to selectins leads to impaired neutrophil adhesion to the endothelium, resulting in defective leukocyte migration to sites of infection.

In vitro evaluation of LAD-2 cells shows impaired random and chemoattractant-directed neutrophil migration, as well as defective neutrophil homotypic aggregation (Etzioni et al., 1994) and defective neutrophil adherence to IL-1β– or tumor necrosis factor-α (TNF-α)–stimulated endothelial cells (Phillips et al., 1995).

Clinical Features

The clinical phenotype of LAD-2 is one of increased infection susceptibility, leukocytosis, and poor pus formation. Severe mental retardation, short stature, distinctive facies, and the Bombay (hh) blood phenotype are also part of the syndrome. Infections, predominantly of the skin, lungs, and gums, resemble the "moderate phenotype" of LAD-1. However, unlike in those patients, the frequency and severity of infections tend to decline with age (Etzioni et al., 1998).

Marquart and colleagues (1999) used prolonged oral fucose treatment in LAD-2 and reported a significant reduction in infectious episodes and neutrophil baseline counts, as well as improved psychomotor capabilities. Using a different therapeutic scheme and fucose dose, Etzioni and Tonetti (2000) saw no changes in their two LAD-2 patients.

LEUKOCYTE ADHESION DEFICIENCY WITH ABNORMAL E-SELECTIN EXPRESSION

A female patient with deficient endothelial expression of E-selectin (OMIM*131210) was recently described by DeLisser and colleagues (1999). The patient had *Pseudomonas* omphalitis, recurrent ear and urinary tract infections, and severe soft tissue infections with impaired pus formation. She had a mild chronic neutropenia with appropriate leukocyte increases in response to infections or granulocyte-macrophage colony-stimulating factor (GM-CSF). The patient had two healthy half-sisters and a full sibling who died in utero due to a staphylococcal infection, thus leaving the inheritance pattern still unclear. No alterations in the E-selectin complementary DNA (cDNA) were detected, but circulating E-selectin levels were twice those of controls. So far, no specific neutrophil functional impairment has been found. Altogether, these data suggest a defect in E-selectin tethering or secretion.

LEUKOCYTE ADHESION DEFICIENCY DUE TO RAC2 DEFICIENCY

Ambruso and associates (2000) and Williams and co-workers (2000) reported a male patient with an autosomal dominant mutation in the Rho GTPase, RAC2 (RAC2, 22q12.13-q13.2; OMIM*602049). RAC2 comprises more than 96% of Rac in neutrophils, and is a member of the Rho family of GTPases critical to the regulation of the actin cytoskeleton and O^-_2 production. The patient had delayed umbilical cord separation, perirectal abscesses, a failure to heal surgical wounds, and an absence of pus in infected areas, accompanied by leukocytosis and neutrophilia.

Chemotaxis was impaired in response to fMLF, IL-8, and PMA; superoxide production was significantly reduced after fMLF stimulation but normal following PMA stimulation (Ambruso et al., 2000; Williams et al., 2000). In addition, the patient's neutrophils showed defective primary granule release (Ambruso et al., 2000) and impaired phagocytosis (Williams et al., 2000). These defects most likely reflect the necessity of Rac interaction with the actin cytoskeleton (chemotaxis) and with the NADPH oxidase (superoxide production).

Four months after a matched related bone marrow transplantation, the patient was thriving, with 100% donor cells in his bone marrow and normalized superoxide production in response to fMLF (Williams et al., 2000).

LEUKOCYTE ADHESION DEFICIENCY WITH IMPAIRED INTEGRIN REARRANGEMENT AND BLEEDING DIATHESIS

Alon and Etzioni (2003) described two Arab brothers with an apparently autosomal recessive disorder characterized by profound leukocytosis, recurrent infections, and platelet aggregation defects. The older brother died after bone marrow transplantation; the younger brother died at 1 week of life from sepsis. The cells from the older patient showed normal rolling along endothelial cultures but defective tethering and tight adhesion.

Because this defect involved both leukocyte and platelet functions and was distinct from the previous defects at biochemical and functional levels, it likely represented another mutation in an early myeloid response pathway. Kinashi and associates (2004) have

shown this defect to be associated with Rap-1 regulation, but its exact origins and mechanism, as well as the connection between the leukocyte and platelet dysfunctions, are incompletely understood. The authors have suggested that this syndrome of Rap-1 dysregulation be named LAD-III.

Immunodeficiencies Associated with Pigmentary Dilution

CHÉDIAK-HIGASHI SYNDROME

Definition

Chédiak-Higashi syndrome (CHS) is a rare, life-threatening autosomal recessive disease, clinically characterized by oculocutaneous albinism, frequent pyogenic infections, neurologic abnormalities, and a late lymphoma-like accelerated phase (Table 20-7).

Pathogenesis

In 1996 two groups identified mutations affecting a newly discovered gene, the lysosomal trafficking regulator gene, LYST or CHS1, that maps to chromosome 1q42.1-q42.2 (OMIM #214500) (Barbosa et al., 1996; Nagle et al., 1996). This gene is clearly involved in both endosomal trafficking and various aspects of surface molecule display, but the mechanism by which LYST works, and therefore the pathophysiology of CHS, is still elusive (Introne et al., 1999). A truncated LYST protein is the most common genetic defect found among CHS patients (Certain et al., 2000), but the complexity of this gene (more than 50 exons, 13.5-kb messenger RNA [mRNA], and 3801 amino acids), makes mutation analysis difficult.

Clinical Features

Oculocutaneous albinism, recurrent infections, neuropathy, and a late accelerated phase are the classical clinical features of CHS. Affected patients show hypopigmentation (pigmentary dilution) of the skin, iris, and hair, making CHS resemble other types of partial albinism (genetic abnormalities of melanin synthesis or distribution). Skin and ocular melanocytes show giant and aberrant melanosomes (macromelanosomes), with alterations in their maturation pathway. Inappropriate fusion of lysosomes with premelanosomes results in premature destruction and pigmentary dilution. Hair color is light brown to blonde, with a characteristic metallic silver-gray sheen. Under light microscopy, CHS hair shafts show pathognomonic small aggregates of clumped pigmentation (Fig. 20-8).

Frequent and recurrent pyogenic infections are characteristic, as is periodontitis. Neurologic involvement, affecting both the peripheral and central nervous systems, is also found. Progressive neuropathy of the lower

TABLE 20-7 · COMPARISON OF SYNDROMES WITH PARTIAL ALBINISM AND IMMUNODEFICIENCY

	Chédiak-Higashi Syndrome	Griscelli Syndrome
Affected gene(s)	CHS1/LYST (1q42.1-q42.2)	MYO5A (15q21) RAB27A (15q21) MLPH (2q37.3)
Affected protein	Lyst	Myosin-Va Rab27a Melanophilin
Inheritance pattern	Autosomal recessive	Autosomal recessive
Main immunologic disturbance	Neutropenia, deficient chemotaxis, impaired NK-cell activity	Impaired delayed-type hypersensitivity, impaired NK-cell activity
Giant intracellular granules	Yes	No
Accelerated phase	Yes	Yes for RAB27A mutations No for MYO5A mutations No for MLPH mutations

NK = natural killer.

limbs, cranial nerve palsies, seizures, mental retardation, and autonomic dysfunction are also reported (Lockman et al., 1967; Misra et al., 1991; Sung et al., 1969; Uyama et al., 1994).

Accelerated Phase

The phenomenon of the late accelerated phase of CHS is really a disease (accelerated phase) within a disease (CHS) and represents one of the principal causes of death in CHS. Fever, hepatosplenomegaly, lymphadenopathy, hematopoietic cytopenias, hypertriglyceridemia, hypofibrinogenemia, hemophagocytosis, and tissue lymphohistiocytic infiltration characterize the accelerated phase. The accelerated phase of CHS is clinically indistinguishable from other hemophagocytic syndromes, whether familial

or sporadic (Henter et al., 1991). Surface expression of CTLA-4, a molecule involved in T-cell response termination, is abnormal in CHS and may underlie the development of the accelerated phase (Barrat et al., 1999).

Laboratory Findings

Giant primary granules, products of the fusion of multiple primary granules, are found in neutrophils, eosinophils, and basophils in blood smears from CHS patients. In fact, enlarged cytoplasmic granules are found in all granule-containing cells, including lymphocytes, monocytes, histiocytes, mast cells, platelets, erythroid precursors, platelets, pancreatic cells, Schwann cells, neurons, renal tubular cells, and gastric mucosal

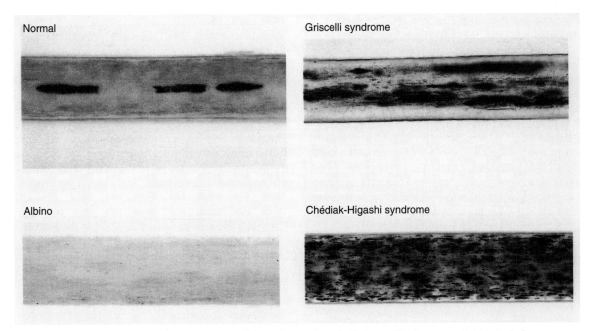

Figure 20-8 · Hair melanization. Normal hair: pigment is typically located in the cortex of the hair shaft; Griscelli syndrome: large clumps of pigment are distributed along the hair shaft; albinism: translucent hair with absent pigment; Chédiak-Higashi syndrome: small aggregates of melanin are irregularly distributed all along the hair shaft.

cells. Neutropenia is common (Blume et al., 1968), probably due to intramedullary destruction of neutrophils. The bone marrow is normocellular to hypercellular (Blume and Wolff, 1972), with poor response to stimuli of bone marrow granulocyte release (Blume et al., 1968). The normal granulocyte circulating half-life with elevated serum lysozyme levels indicate intramedullary destruction.

Functional defects have been described in different immune cells. Monocyte and neutrophil chemotaxis is diminished, possibly due to mechanical interference by the giant granules (Clawson et al., 1978). Rates of phagocytosis are normal or increased (Root et al., 1972; Wolff et al., 1972), but intracellular bacterial killing is delayed, probably due to lower-than-normal levels of some primary granule enzymes (Gallin et al., 1979; Stossel et al., 1972).

Natural killer (NK) cells are normal in number but show virtually absent cytotoxicity (Haliotis et al., 1980; Klein et al., 1980). Lymphocyte antibody-mediated cellular cytotoxicity (ADCC) is low, but neutrophil and monocyte ADCC is intact (Klein et al., 1980). Because T-cell cytotoxicity is dependent on the secretion of giant granule cytolytic proteins, it is probably impaired in CHS as a result of abnormal vesicle membrane fusion (Baetz et al., 1995). Elevated levels of $\gamma\delta$-T cells have been described in CHS patients (Holcombe et al., 1990). B-cell function is usually unaffected (Klein et al., 1980; Merino et al., 1983).

Prenatal diagnosis has been accomplished by the demonstration of large lysosomes in amniotic cells and chorionic villus cells (Diukman et al., 1992).

Treatment

Infections in CHS, as in other phagocytic immunodeficiencies, may be more extensive and severe than clinically apparent. Diagnosis and therapy should be directed at usual bacterial pathogens and should be at high doses for longer than normal periods. Neuropathies need early and careful attention from rehabilitation services.

Several regimens have been used to "brake" the accelerated phase. Etoposide (VP16), steroids, and intrathecal methotrexate comprise one of the more effective combinations (Bejaui et al., 1989). The accelerated phase usually recurs in a more aggressive and treatment-refractory form unless bone marrow transplantation is performed.

Promising results have been reported with related and unrelated HLA-matched bone marrow transplants (Haddad et al., 1995; Jabado et al., 1996; Liang et al., 2000).

GRISCELLI SYNDROME

Definition

Griscelli syndrome is a rare autosomal recessive disorder of partial albinism and immunodeficiency (see Chapter 17). It partially resembles CHS (silver-gray hair plus accelerated phase) but does not have neutropenia or giant intracellular granules (Griscelli et al., 1978) (see Table 20-7).

Pathogenesis

Griscelli syndrome (GS) has been associated with mutations in myosin-Va (MYO5A) on chromosome 15q21 (OMIM#214450 and *160777) (Pastural et al., 1997). Different allelic variants have also been described: Elejalde syndrome and partial albinism immunodeficiency (PAID) syndrome (Duran-McKinster et al., 1999; Harfi et al., 1992; Sanal et al., 2000; Spritz, 1999).

More recently, mutations in the GTP-binding protein RAB27A (OMIM*603868), a protein involved in regulating cytotoxic granule exocytosis, have been found in Griscelli syndrome patients who developed an accelerated phase (Menasche et al., 2000). Interestingly, RAB27A also maps to chromosome 15q21, very close to MYO5A. Moreover, one of the two originally described MYO5A mutations associated with Griscelli syndrome has turned out to be a relatively common polymorphism (Lambert et al., 2000; Pastural, 1999; Pastural et al., 1997).

These data suggest that two different genes, MYO5A and RAB27A, in the same region of the same chromosome may be responsible for a single disease. Whether these genes are equally contributory to cases of Griscelli syndrome, actually cause different diseases, or simply co-segregate remains to be definitively worked out. The *dilute* mouse is known to have a defect in MYO5A and is phenotypically similar to Griscelli syndrome, suggesting that this is at least one cause of GS (Jenkins et al., 1981; Mercer et al., 1991).

Menasche and colleagues (2003) reported mutations in human melanophilin (MLPH, 2q37.3) leading to defective interaction with Rab27a, resulting in yet another syndrome involving the same pathway as in Griscelli syndrome but clinically restricted to hypopigmentation.

Therefore mutations in three different genes, all involved in the process of intracellular trafficking, are involved in a common cutaneous phenotype. However, the neurologic involvement is limited to MYO5A mutations and the accelerated phase to those in Rab27a. These complex genotype/phenotype correlations should allow fine dissection of the role of these intracellular trafficking molecules in neuropathy and immune control of hemophagocytosis.

Clinical Features

Griscelli syndrome patients have characteristic silver-gray hair that under light microscopy shows big clumps of melanin, instead of the small aggregates seen in CHS (see Fig. 20-8). Viral and bacterial infections are frequent and are the most usual triggers for development of the accelerated phase. Late neurologic manifestations, such as seizures, dysmetria, ataxia, hemiparesis, nystagmus, and loss of developmental milestones, have been reported (Klein et al., 1994). The most constant immunologic abnormality in Griscelli syndrome is the absence of delayed-type hypersensitivity and impaired natural killer–cell activity (Klein et al., 1994). Hypogammaglobulinemia and neutrophil dysfunction have been described inconsistently.

As in CHS, early bone marrow transplantation is the only reliable way to prevent recurrences of the accelerated phase and early death in Griscelli syndrome (Baumeister et al., 2000; Klein et al., 1994).

Congenital Neutropenias

SEVERE CONGENITAL NEUTROPENIA (KOSTMANN'S SYNDROME, INFANTILE GENETIC AGRANULOCYTOSIS)

Definition

Severe congenital neutropenia (SCN) or Kostmann's syndrome (OMIM#202700) is composed of a heterogeneous group of disorders with variable inheritance patterns that share the following characteristics: (1) bone marrow granulocyte maturation arrest at the promyelocyte or myelocyte stage, (2) severe chronic neutropenia (<200 neutrophils/µl), and (3) increased susceptibility to acute myeloid leukemia.

Pathogenesis

In 1956 Kostmann described a Swedish kindred with severe congenital neutropenia inherited in an autosomal recessive pattern (Kostmann, 1956). Among patients with Kostmann's syndrome, single allele mutations in the granulocyte colony-stimulating factor (G-CSF) receptor gene (GCSFR, 1p35-p34.3) have been described and positively associated with the development of acute myeloid leukemia (Dong et al., 1995; Tidow et al 1997). However, not all patients with SCN or Kostmann's syndrome show mutations in the GCSFR gene, and causality was not conclusively established (Dong et al., 1994; Guba et al., 1993; Sandoval et al., 1993).

Dale and co-workers (2000) showed that 22 out of 25 patients with SCN had various heterozygous mutations in the gene encoding for neutrophil elastase 2 (ELA2, 19p13.3; OMIM*130130). Interestingly, mutations in this same gene are also responsible for cyclic neutropenia (Horwitz et al., 1999; see later discussion). Mutations that lead to cyclic neutropenia tend to be clustered around the enzymatically active site of ELA2, whereas mutations that lead to congenital neutropenia tend to be located on the opposite face of the three-dimensional structure of this protein (Dale et al., 2000). However, despite the growing knowledge of mutations leading to autosomal dominant and sporadic congenital neutropenia, the vast majority of which appears due to heterozygous mutations in ELA2, the autosomal recessive disease that Kostmann originally described does not

appear to be caused by mutations in this gene (Ancliff et al., 2001).

Recently, Devriendt and colleagues (2001) described a family with an X-linked form of severe congenital neutropenia (XLN) due to mutations in WASP, the gene that encodes the Wiskott-Aldrich syndrome protein (see Chapter 17). The mutations that produce Wiskott-Aldrich syndrome or X-linked thrombocytopenia lead to reduced WASP signaling due to reduced transcription or translation of WASP. In contrast, the WASP mutation leading to X-linked neutropenia, L270P, disrupts an autoinhibitory domain of WASP, creating a constitutively active protein.

Clinical Features

Despite the genetic heterogeneity, the clinical manifestations of these severe neutropenic disorders are rather homogeneous. Disease appears promptly after birth: 50% of affected infants are symptomatic before the first month of life, and 90% within 6 months. Omphalitis, upper and lower respiratory infections, and skin and liver abscesses are the most common infections.

Treatment is subcutaneous recombinant G-CSF (5 µg/kg/day; range 1 to 120 µg/kg, depending on patient response); this has dramatically changed the prognosis of these patients (Zeidler et al., 2000). Since the advent of recombinant G-CSF, the number of infections and hospital days in patients with SCN have been reduced and life expectancy has increased (Bonilla et al., 1989, 1994; Freedman, 1997).

CYCLIC NEUTROPENIA/CYCLIC HEMATOPOIESIS

Definition

Cyclic neutropenia/cyclic hematopoiesis (OMIM#162800 and *130130) is an autosomal dominant disease characterized by regular cyclic fluctuations in all hematopoietic lineages that are most remarkable among neutrophils (see Chapter 36). Neutrophil counts cycle at an average of 21 days (range 14 to 36 days), including periods of severe neutropenia (<200/µl) lasting from 3 to 10 days (Dale et al., 1988; Wright et al., 1981).

Pathogenesis

Different single-base substitutions in neutrophil elastase 2 (ELA2; 19p13.3), also known as leukocyte elastase or medullasin, have been identified in patients with cyclic neutropenia and their relatives (Horwitz et al., 1999). Neutrophil elastase has multiple disparate activities: It is involved in tissue destruction following its release from neutrophils migrating to sites of inflammation; it mediates tyrosyl-tRNA synthetase cleavage, yielding domains that induce neutrophil chemotaxis; it mediates the release of IL-8, a potent neutrophil chemoattractant, from endothelial cells; and it has direct activity against the outer membranes of gram-negative bacteria (Weinrauch et al., 2002); and it cleaves important growth factors, including G-CSF (El Ouriaghli et al., 2003).

Neutrophil elastase is inhibited by the serine protease inhibitor (serpin) α_1-antitrypsin. Disruption of this serpin-mediated neutralization has been proposed as a possible explanation for hematopoietic cycling, but the exact mechanism is still unclear (Horwitz et al.,1999). Interestingly, neutrophil elastase is a competitive ligand for the interaction of CD18/CD11a and ICAM1 (Cai and Wright, 1996). Therefore dysfunctional forms of elastase might alter the normal interactions of neutrophils or other leukocytes with the endothelium and each other.

Clinical Features

Most patients have clinical manifestations of neutropenia in early childhood. Oral ulcerations, gingivitis, lymphadenopathy, pharyngitis/tonsillitis, and skin lesions are the most commonly reported. Early loss of permanent teeth as a consequence of chronic gingivitis and periapical abscesses is common (Palmer et al., 1996).

Circulating monocytosis, eosinophilia, and reticulocytosis are found when neutrophils are at their nadir. Oscillations within the normal range in platelets are occasionally seen and tend to parallel neutrophil fluctuations (Wright et al., 1981). Bone marrow aspirates obtained during periods of neutropenia show maturation arrest at the myelocyte stage or, less commonly, hypoplasia (Souid et al., 1995).

G-CSF dramatically improves peripheral neutrophil counts and decreases morbidity in patients with cyclic neutropenia (Hammond et al., 1989; Palmer et al., 1996). Interestingly, infections and hospitalizations appear to naturally lessen with age (Palmer et al., 1996).

MYELOKATHEXIS/WHIM SYNDROME

Definition

Myelokathexis (from the Greek, meaning "retained in the bone marrow") is a congenital disorder associated with severe chronic neutropenia (see Chapter 17). Unlike other forms of congenital neutropenia, bone marrow aspirates from myelokathexis patients show myeloid hypercellularity with increased numbers of granulocytes at all stages of differentiation.

A significant number of patients with myelokathexis have warts, hypogammaglobulinemia, and infections, with different degrees of severity. The acronym WHIM (*w*arts, *h*ypogammaglobulinemia, *i*nfections, and *m*yelokathexis) has been proposed for this syndrome (OMIM*193670) (Wetzler et al., 1990). An autosomal dominant inheritance pattern has been shown to be due to mutations in the chemokine receptor CXCR4 (Gorlin et al., 2000; Hernandez et al., 2003).

Pathogenesis

Based on the morphology in bone marrow aspirates, Aprikyan and colleagues (2000) hypothesized that accelerated apoptosis of neutrophil precursors might account for the neutropenia. They demonstrated defective expression of *bcl-x*, an antiapoptotic product, in neutrophil precursors. This led to the hypothesis that myelokathexis/WHIM syndrome is caused by accelerated apoptosis of granulocytes due to depressed expression of *bcl-x* in bone marrow–derived granulocyte precursor cells. This hypothesis is supported by the fact that these abnormalities in *bcl-x* and apoptosis are partially corrected by in vivo administration of G-CSF (Aprikyan et al., 2000). However, the identification of CXCR4 as the responsible gene has opened a new line of investigation into the mechanisms by which neutrophils are retained in and traffic to the bone marrow (Martin et al., 2003).

Clinical Features

Recurrent sinopulmonary infections are common. During infectious episodes, neutrophils are typically increased over baseline. Neutrophil nuclei are hypersegmented with pyknotic nuclear lobes connected by thin chromatin filaments. Cytoplasmic vacuolation and heavy granulation are also common.

The presence of warts and hypogammaglobulinemia suggest a broader immunologic involvement affecting T and B cells. Neutrophil functional testing (chemotaxis, phagocytosis, bacterial lysis, and respiratory burst) has not shown any specific or characteristic abnormality. T-cell function, as evaluated by intradermal testing and in vitro lymphocyte proliferation in response to mitogens, has not shown any distinct abnormalities either.

Patients tend to have normal to moderately decreased levels of IgG, IgA, and IgM, but specific antibody production has been normal in evaluated cases (Arai et al., 2000; Wetzler et al., 1990). Interestingly, normalization of Ig levels has been observed during G-CSF or GM-CSF treatment (Hord et al., 1997; Wetzler et al., 1990).

Treatment

Steroids, subcutaneous epinephrine, intravenous endotoxin, and G-CSF and GM-CSF have all been shown to mobilize mature neutrophils from the bone marrow to the blood (Hord et al., 1997). Sustained therapy with G-CSF or GM-CSF has proved effective in rapidly increasing the number of neutrophils in the peripheral blood and decreasing the number of infections (Hord et al., 1997).

Immune-Mediated Neutropenias: Autoimmune and Alloimmune Neutropenia

Autoimmune neutropenia (AIN) is a rare disorder caused by peripheral destruction of neutrophils or their precursors. It can be caused by autoantibodies in a patient's serum or mediated by large granular lymphocytes (CD3+/CD8+/CD57+ T cells). Neutropenia is an isolated clinical entity in primary AIN and associated with another disease in secondary AIN.

Neonatal alloimmune neutropenia is caused by maternal sensitization to antigens present on neonatal neutrophils that differ from or are absent on their own neutrophils. These disorders are also discussed in Chapter 39.

PRIMARY AUTOIMMUNE NEUTROPENIA

Definition

Primary AIN is the most common cause of neutropenia in infancy and childhood (Bermomo, 1996; Bruin et al., 1999). The incidence has been reported at 1 in 100,000, with a slight predominance of females (Lyall et al., 1992).

Pathogenesis

Antineutrophil antibodies directed against different neutrophil antigens (NA) can be detected in almost all patients with primary AIN. Approximately one third of these antibodies are directed against NA1 or NA2, glycosylated isoforms of FcγRIII on neutrophils (Bux et al., 1998). Other antigens against which antibodies are directed are FcγRII (CD32), Mac-1 (CD11b/CD18), and C3b complement receptor (CR1, CD35) (Bux et al., 1998; Hartman and Wright, 1991).

The etiology of this disease remains unknown and is not usually associated with parvovirus B19 infection (Bux et al., 1998; Hartman et al., 1994; Murray and Morad, 1994).

Clinical Features

The majority of patients with primary AIN present with skin or upper respiratory tract infections, although some may have pneumonia, meningitis, or sepsis. AIN may be an asymptomatic incidental finding. Three percent of patients with AIN present with serious life-threatening infections, with clinical and bone marrow findings that mimic Kostmann's syndrome. In these patients, extensive destruction of neutrophils and band forms may cause a hypocellular marrow with maturation arrest at the myelocyte-metamyelocyte stage (Smith and Smith, 2001). The average age at diagnosis is for primary AIN is 8 months (Bux et al., 1998).

Laboratory Findings

Absolute neutrophil counts (ANC) usually vary between 0 and 1500/µl, with the majority of patients presenting with a neutrophil count greater than 500/µl. Despite low neutrophil counts, monocytosis is common. The ANC may transiently increase twofold to threefold during severe infection but return to neutropenic levels following resolution (Bruin et al., 1999; Bux et al., 1998). The bone marrow may be normal or hypercellular. Myeloid precursors reach at least the myelocyte/metamyelocyte stage before maturation arrest. Macrophages that have ingested neutrophils may be seen in the bone marrow, indicating the removal of sensitized cells in the marrow.

Detection of granulocyte-specific antibodies is the key to the diagnosis of primary AIN. In more than 70% of cases, granulocyte-specific antibodies were detected at the first determination. In some patients, detection of these autoantibodies may require repeat testing. Granulocyte immunofluorescence testing (GIFT) is a more sensitive method than granulocyte agglutination for detection of antigranulocyte antibodies. In addition to GIFT, neutrophil antigen typing should be performed (Bux et al., 1998).

Treatment and Prognosis

Symptomatic treatment with antibiotics for infections is usually sufficient. Prophylactic antibiotic treatment should be reserved for those with recurrent infections. Cotrimoxazole, ampicillin, and first-generation oral cephalosporins are the most commonly used agents.

Alternative treatment strategies for severe infections or in the setting of emergency surgical intervention include high-dose intravenous immunoglobulin (IVIG), corticosteroids, and G-CSF. In a recent report of 57 patients with primary AIN, serum G-CSF production was not increased, despite the low neutrophil count (Corbacioglu et al., 2000).

G-CSF is most effective in increasing the ANC (Bux et al., 1998; Smith and Smith, 2001). Most patients start treatment at 5 µg/kg/day subcutaneously. However, because the duration of neutrophil normalization is brief following G-CSF, maintenance should be based on response (one to three times weekly) (Smith and Smith, 2001). The ideal is to keep the peripheral neutrophil count greater than 1000/µl to prevent serious infection. In this clinical setting, the main side effects of G-CSF are malaise and mild bone pain. Osteopenia has not been reported in patients with primary AIN receiving G-CSF, as opposed to patients with severe congenital neutropenia (Smith and Smith, 2001).

The prognosis of primary AIN is very good because it is self-limited. Neutropenia remits spontaneously within 7 to 24 months in 95% of patients, preceded by disappearance of the autoantibodies from the circulation.

SECONDARY AUTOIMMUNE NEUTROPENIA

Secondary AIN may occur at any age but is more common in adults and has a more variable clinical course than primary AIN. Various systemic or autoimmune diseases, such as systemic lupus erythematosus (SLE), Hodgkin's disease, large granular lymphocyte (LGL) proliferation or LGL leukemia, Epstein-Barr virus (EBV), cytomegalovirus (CMV) (Soderberg et al., 1996), human immunodeficiency virus (HIV), and parvovirus B19 infections (Gautier et al., 1997) are often associated with secondary AIN.

Affected patients are at risk for developing other autoimmune problems. Antineutrophil antibodies typically have pan-FcγRIII specificity, rather than to the FcγRIII subunits, making the resulting neutropenia more severe. Anti-CD18/11b antibodies have been detected in a subset of patients with secondary AIN (Bruin et al., 1999). Secondary AIN responds best to therapy directed at the underlying cause (Bussel and Abboud, 1987).

ALLOIMMUNE NEONATAL NEUTROPENIA

First described by Lalezari and Bernard (1966), alloimmune neonatal neutropenia (ANN) is a different form of immune-mediated neutropenia. The pathophysiologic mechanisms for neonatal alloimmune neutropenia are similar to those that trigger hemolytic anemia due to Rh incompatibility: maternal sensitization to antigens present on the neutrophils of the neonates that differ from or are absent on maternal neutrophils.

ANN is caused by transplacental transfer of maternal antibodies against the FcγRIIIb isotypes NA1 and NA2, causing immune destruction of neonatal neutrophils (Dale, 1998). Several of the healthy mothers of affected infants did not express FcγRIIIb on their neutrophils, leading to the elaboration of antibodies against FcγRIIIb expressed on fetal neutrophils (Fromont et al., 1992; Huizinga et al., 1990; Stroncek et al., 1991). These complement-activating antineutrophil antibodies can be detected in 1 of 500 live births, making the potential incidence of ANN high.

ANN should be considered in the evaluation of all infants with neutropenia, with or without infection. Antibody-coated neutrophils in ANN are phagocytosed in the reticuloendothelial system (RES) and removed from the circulation, leaving the neonate neutropenic and prone to infections. Omphalitis, cellulitis, and pneumonia may be the presenting infections within the first 2 weeks of life. The diagnosis can be made by detection of neutrophil-specific alloantibodies in the maternal serum.

Parenteral antibiotics (even in the absence of other signs of sepsis) and G-CSF should be included in the initial management of ANN (Gilmore et al., 1994; Rodwell et al., 1996). Intravenous gamma globulin has not always been effective in reverting ANN (Gilmore et al., 1994). ANN tends to spontaneously improve with the waning of maternal antineutrophil antibody levels, but this process may take months.

Other Disorders Involving Phagocytic Cells

NEUTROPHIL-SPECIFIC GRANULE DEFICIENCY

Definition

Neutrophil-specific granule deficiency is a rare, heterogeneous, autosomal recessive disease characterized by the profound reduction or absence of neutrophil-specific granules and their contents and increased susceptibility to infection (OMIM#245480 and *600749) (Gallin et al., 1982; Strauss et al., 1974).

Pathogenesis

Homozygous, autosomal recessive, disabling mutations have been found by Lekstrom-Himes and colleagues (1999) and Gombart and associates (2001) in the C/EBPε gene of two affected patients. However, two subsequently examined cases did not have mutations in C/EBPε, suggesting that this is a genetically heterogeneous disease (Gombart and Koeffler, 2002; Lekstrom-Himes et al., unpublished observations). C/EBPε (14q11.2) is a member of the CCAAT/enhancer-binding protein family. It is a transcription factor that plays a critical role in myelopoiesis and cellular differentiation (Yamanaka et al., 1997).

Clinical Features

The cardinal features of the neutrophil-specific granule deficiency are paucity or absence of neutrophil-specific granules, predominantly bilobed neutrophil nuclei (pseudo–Pelger-Huët anomaly), and increased susceptibility to pyogenic infections, especially affecting the skin, ears, lungs, and lymph nodes (Ambruso et al., 1984; Breton-Gorius et al., 1980; Gallin et al., 1982; Komiyama et al., 1979). Associated abnormalities in the few patients reported include mononuclear eosinophils and absence of the primary granule protein, defensins. Hemostatic abnormalities were due to reduced levels of platelet-associated high-molecular-weight Von Willebrand factor, platelet fibrinogen, and fibronectin in one patient (Parker et al., 1992).

The diagnosis of specific granule deficiency rests on clinical suspicion bolstered by careful inspection of the peripheral smear. In some cases, eosinophils may not be detectable on routine smears (Gallin et al., 1982). Demonstration of absent or very low specific granule contents helps confirm the diagnosis. Electron microscopy shows absent peroxidase-negative granules in some patients and empty peroxidase-negative granules in others.

The specific granule protein lactoferrin is diminished or absent in these patients' neutrophils (Boxer et al., 1982; Gallin et al., 1982; Lomax et al., 1989). In contrast, lactoferrin protein was more abundant than normal in nasal secretions. Because there is only one lactoferrin gene, these data strongly suggested an underlying transcriptional factor defect (Lomax et al., 1989). NBT reduction and superoxide production are normal. In the patient studied by Strauss (1974), staphylococcal activity was reduced due to inadequate phagocytosis, whereas candidacidal activity was normal.

Treatment

Management of these patients is complicated by their impaired inflammatory response and impaired killing of some intracellular organisms. Gram-positive cocci are the most common offenders. As in other patients with defective inflammatory responses, clinical examination often understates the extent of infection. Aggressive diagnosis of infection, prolonged and intensive therapy, and early use of surgical excision and débridement are necessary.

GLYCOGEN STORAGE DISEASE TYPE 1b

Glycogen storage disease (GSD) type 1, or Von Gierke disease, is a recessively inherited disease characterized by the hepatic incapacity to convert glucose-6-phosphate to glucose. This process requires two different enzymes: glucose-6-phosphatase (17q21), which is deficient in GSD1a (OMIM*232200); and glucose-6-phosphate transporter 1 (G6PT1; 11q23; OMIM*602671), which is deficient in GSD1b (OMIM#232220). Both GSD1a and GSD1b present early in life with fasting hypoglycemia, seizures, lactic acidosis, hyperuricemia, hyperlipidemia, and hepatomegaly.

Only GSD1b, the defect in G6PT1, shows neutropenia and neutrophil dysfunction. Deficient chemotaxis (Anderson et al., 1981) and respiratory burst function (Kilpatrick et al., 1990) have been described. Different mutations affecting G6PT1 have been reported: G1184T and 1211delCT are the most prevalent in Caucasians, T521C in Japanese, and 338del7 and 1105insA in Pakistanis (Janacke et al., 2001).

Ambruso and colleagues (1985) showed that 15 of 21 GSD1b patients had moderate to severe infections that were mostly bacterial, affecting the ears, lungs, and skin. Oral and anal ulcers were also prevalent. These patients commonly develop an inflammatory bowel disease. Recently, Calderwood and associates (2001) reported significant objective and subjective improvements in infection-related morbidity in GSD1b patients receiving G-CSF therapy.

β-ACTIN DEFICIENCY

Several patients have been recognized with deficient actin polymerization leading to defective chemotaxis and recurrent infections (Boxer et al., 1974; Coates et al., 1991; Jung, 1991).

β-Actin is critical for the rapid reorganization of the phagocyte cytoskeleton. Nunoi and colleagues (1999) described a patient with a complex disorder and a heterozygous mutation in nonmuscle actin (β-actin) (OMIM*257150). The missense mutation found (G1174A) may act in a dominant-negative fashion.

The patient had a history of recurrent infections (otitis media, furunculosis, tuberculous pneumonia), photosensitivity, recurrent stomatitis, keratoconjunctivitis, polyarthralgia, and mental retardation. The patient's neutrophils had depressed chemotactic responses, reduced stimulated superoxide generation, and low fMLF-induced neutrophil membrane depolarization and repolarization. The patient also had hypergammaglobulinemia IgG, IgA, and IgE, as well as leukopenia, thrombocytopenia, and a positive rheumatoid factor.

The patient died from septicemia at the age of 15. The pathophysiologic link between the mutation found and the multiple clinical features is yet to be completely forged.

MANNOSE-BINDING PROTEIN ABNORMALITIES

The carbohydrate mannose is a natural constituent of the membranes of many microorganisms (viruses, bacteria, yeast, mycobacteria, and protozoa) but is not typically found in mammalian extracellular glycoproteins. There are at least two mannose-binding molecules involved in host defense: mannose-binding protein, a soluble factor synthesized as an acute-phase reactant, and macrophage-mannose receptor, expressed on macrophages and lymphatic endothelium (see Chapters 10 and 21).

Mannose-binding protein (MBP1; OMIM*154545, 10q11.2-q21) is a multimeric molecule. Once the mannose-binding protein complex has bound its target, it serves to activate complement and enhance phagocytosis through the C1q receptor (reviewed in Fraser et al., 1998). There are significant population-based polymorphisms, but their functional effect is still uncertain (Ezekowitz, 1998). Reports of increased susceptibility to Neisseria meningitidis infection (Bax et al., 1999), severe and unusual infections in adults (Summerfield et al., 1995), and differing infection rates and survival in patients with cystic fibrosis (Garred et al., 1999) suggest that under certain circumstances, mannose-binding protein polymorphisms may be important.

Koch and colleagues (2001) elegantly showed that polymorphisms in the mannose-binding protein promoter that lead to lower serum levels of MBP were linked to recurrent upper respiratory and ear infections in otherwise normal children in Greenland. Interestingly, the effect of these polymorphisms was only seen between the ages of 6 months and 2 years, the period during which maternal antibody protection wanes and endogenous antibody synthesis becomes established (see Chapter 21).

The macrophage-mannose receptor (MRC; OMIM* 153618, 10p13) is one of the best-characterized lectins. It binds glycoproteins, especially those with high mannose content (Linehan et al., 2000). Koziel and associates (1998) showed downregulation of the mannose receptor on the surface of alveolar macrophages in patients with *Pneumocystis carinii* and HIV infection with low CD4+ T lymphocytes.

SHWACHMAN-DIAMOND SYNDROME

Shwachman-Diamond syndrome (SDS; OMIM*260400) is a rare autosomal recessive disorder characterized by exocrine pancreatic insufficiency, metaphyseal dysostosis, short stature, and various immune disorders (Cipolli, 2001; Rothbaum et al., 2002) (see Chapters 24 and 39). The disease is caused by mutations in the Shwachman-Bodian-Diamond syndrome protein (SBDSP), in which characteristic mutations are found. The function of the gene is still under investigation (Boocock et al., 2003).

Intermittent neutropenia is present in almost all patients and is the most common immune manifestation. Cyclic or persistent neutropenia, anemia, and thrombocytopenia are also described (Cipolli, 2001; Dror and Freedman, 2002). Bone marrow findings do not always correlate with the level of cytopenia; bone marrow hypoplasia and fat infiltration are most common, but normal or even hypercellular aspirates have also been found (Dror and Freedman, 2002; Ginsberg et al., 1999; Smith et al., 1996). Neutrophils in SDS show impaired chemotaxis; neutrophil cytoskeletal dysfunction is probably involved (Dror and Freedman, 2002; Dror et al., 2001; Smith et al., 1996).

Recently, Dror and associates (2001) described other immune defects in a cohort of 11 SDS patients. Several quantitative and functional T- and B-cell abnormalities were detected, but NK lymphopenia was the most common.

Aside from pancreatic insufficiency and short stature, patients with SDS usually present with recurrent infections of the ears, sinuses, lungs, or bloodstream (Cipolli, 2001; Dror et al., 2002; Skapek et al., 1992; Smith et al., 1996).

G-CSF is effective in the management of neutropenia in SDS (Van der Sande and Hillen, 1996; Ventura et al., 1995). Concerns have been raised regarding the potential for G-CSF–induced myelodysplastic syndromes or acute myeloid leukemia in these patients. However, these conditions are part of the natural history of SDS, even in the absence of G-CSF treatment (Freedman and Alter, 2002).

Hematopoietic stem cell transplantation has been attempted for the most severe cases of hematologic dysfunction in SDS, such as severe aplasia, myelodysplastic syndromes, and acute myeloid leukemia. These patients have had high rates of acute complications and mortality after transplant (Hsu et al., 2002).

TRANSCOBALAMIN II DEFICIENCY

Transcobalamin II deficiency (OMIM*275350, 22q 11.2-qter) was first described by Hakami and co-workers (1971) in two siblings with the clinical manifestations of vitamin B_{12} deficiency but normal serum B_{12} levels. Transcobalamin II is the primary plasma transport protein for B_{12}, and its deficiency is inherited in an autosomal recessive manner. Megaloblastic anemia, neutropenia, leukopenia, thrombocytopenia, neurologic deficits, failure to thrive, diarrhea, and severe infections have been associated with this disease. Hypogammaglobulinemia, deficient antibody responses, and deficient neutrophil bacterial killing have also been reported (see Chapter 13).

Early and sustained treatment with hydroxycobalamin tends to reverse most of the manifestations, including the immunologic abnormalities (Hitzig et al., 1974, 1975; Seger et al., 1980).

PAPILLON-LEFÈBRE AND OTHER AGGRESSIVE PERIODONTITIS SYNDROMES

Papillon-Lefèbre syndrome (PLS; OMIM #245000) is an autosomal recessive disorder characterized by severe early-onset aggressive periodontitis (usually leading to dental loss) and palmoplantar hyperkeratosis. Mutations in cathepsin C (CTSC, 11q14) are responsible for PLS (Hart et al., 1999; Toomes et al., 1999). Cathepsin C is thought to be involved in protein degradation and proenzyme activation and is highly expressed in affected epithelial tissues such as palms, soles, and keratinized gingiva, as well as in PMN, macrophages, and their precursors. Impaired neutrophil chemotaxis, impaired spontaneous migration, and diminished phagocyte and intracellular killing have been described in PLS. All these factors may play a role in the periodontal disease (Firatli et al., 1996; Ghaffer et al., 1999).

Prepubertal periodontitis (PP) and *juvenile periodontitis* (JP) have recently been classified as forms of aggressive periodontitis syndromes (Eber and Wang, 2002). Following either a localized or generalized presentation, both syndromes share common characteristics: rapid alveolar bone loss, tooth mobility, and tooth loss. The generalized form of PP presents with acute gingival inflammation. Aggressive periodontitis syndromes are associated with bacterial plaque due to several specific microorganisms (e.g., *Actinobacillus actinomycetemcomitans*, *Prevotella intermedia*, *Porphyromonas gingivalis*, *Eikenella corrodens*, and *Fusobacterium nucleatum*), but discrete phagocyte disorders have been described as well (Eber and Wang, 2002).

Impaired neutrophil chemotaxis has been described in both PP and JP (Page et al., 1987; Van Dyke et al., 1990). When compared with control individuals, approximately half of JP patients showed lower numbers of phagocytes in the peripheral blood, as well as reduced PMN phagocytosis. Neither treatment of infections nor addition of normal serum to patient PMNs or patient serum to normal PMNs reproduced or corrected the phagocytosis defect, strongly suggesting a primary PMN phagocytic defect in these patients (Kimura et al., 1992).

TUFTSIN DEFICIENCY

Tuftsin is a tetrapeptide (Thr-Lys-Pro-Arg) originally described by Najjar and Nishioka in 1970 as a spleen-activated leukophilic fraction of IgG. After enzymatic cleavage by leukokininase on the neutrophil membrane, tuftsin enhances phagocytosis. Tuftsin deficiency (OMIM 191150) can be primary or secondary. Splenectomy, cirrhosis, long-term parenteral nutrition, and sickle cell anemia have been associated with secondary tuftsin deficiency (Constantopoulos et al., 1972, 1973; Spirer et al., 1980; Trevisani et al., 2002; Zoli et al., 1998). Tuftsin quantitation and functional testing are not widely available, making tuftsin deficiency difficult to diagnose. Constantopoulos (1983) reported five patients with congenital tuftsin deficiency who clinically improved after the administration of 1 to 2 g of intramuscular gamma globulin.

SECONDARY PHAGOCYTE DEFECTS

A variety of medical conditions are associated with increased risk of bacterial or fungal infections (Engelich et al., 2001). Diabetes mellitus (DM), burns, trauma, renal failure, and nutritional problems have been linked to secondary phagocyte functional disorders with increased infection susceptibility.

Reduced chemotaxis and impaired intracellular killing of bacteria have been described in diabetic patients (see Chapter 25). Data regarding adherence, phagocytosis, and oxidative burst have been more conflicting (Geerlings and Hoepelman, 1999; Rayfield et al., 1982). Excessive use of NADPH through the aldose reductase pathway in DM might lead to impaired respiratory burst activity and therefore impaired killing of microorganisms. Tight glucose control and treatment with aldose reductase inhibitors have improved phagocytosis and respiratory burst activity in some patients (Ihm et al., 1997; Tebbs et al., 1991). In a double-blind randomized placebo-controlled trial of G-CSF in diabetic foot infections, G-CSF–treated patients showed increased neutrophil superoxide production and a significantly better outcome (Gough et al., 1997).

Burn and trauma patients are also at increased risk of infections (see Chapter 30). Impaired neutrophil chemotaxis, phagocytosis, and intracellular bacterial killing have been described. Abnormalities of adherence and respiratory burst activity are less conclusive (Engelich et al., 2001; Krause et al., 1994; Moore et al., 1986; Rosenthal et al., 1986; Solomkin, 1990). Clinical trials using G-CSF, GM-CSF, and IFN-γ have not yielded definitive benefits (Cioffi et al., 1991; Dries, 1996; Polk et al., 1992).

Uremia has been linked to impaired phagocyte function and increased susceptibility to infection in end-stage renal failure (see Chapter 25). Impaired chemotaxis, phagocytosis, intracellular killing, and respiratory burst activity, as well as increased apoptosis, have been reported (Engelich et al., 2001; Haag-Weber and Horl, 1996; Jaber et al., 2001; Vanholder and Ringoir, 1993).

Elevated phagocyte intracellular calcium levels, iron overload, and uremic toxins have been associated with uremia-related phagocyte dysfunction (Haag-Weber et al., 1996). Therapy with calcium channel blockers or 1,25-vitamin D_3 has improved phagocyte function in patients with renal failure (Haag-Weber and Horl, 1996; Haag-Weber et al., 1993).

Cuprophane hemodialysis membranes, but not others, have been associated with overexpression of neutrophil adhesion molecules, pulmonary neutrophil sequestration, and transient neutropenia due to C5a generation (Skubitz et al., 1998).

Malnutrition is probably the most common cause of immunodeficiency worldwide (see Chapter 23). Phagocyte defects occur but are not as well characterized as lymphocyte defects in malnourished individuals. Chandra (1997) reported deficient phagocytosis and intracellular killing of bacteria in protein-energy malnutrition. Children with hemoglobin levels below 10 g/dl showed significant reduction on their bactericidal activity compared with those above 10 g/dl. Iron replacement alone reverted the anemia and the impaired intracellular killing of bacteria (Bashkaram et al., 1977; Srikantia et al., 1976). Zinc deficiency also impairs chemotaxis, phagocytosis, and NADPH oxidase activity (Chandra, 1999).

REFERENCES

Alon R, Etzioni A. LAD-III, a novel group of leukocyte integrin activation deficiencies. Trends Immunol 24:561–566, 2003.

Ambruso DR, Knall C, Abell AN, Panepinto J, Kurkchubasche A, Thurman G, Gonzalez-Aller C, Hiester A, deBoer M, Harbeck RJ, Oyer R, Johnson GL, Roos D. Human neutrophil immunodeficiency syndrome is associated with an inhibitory Rac2 mutation. Proc Natl Acad Sci USA 97:4654–4659, 2000.

Ambruso DR, McCabe ER, Anderson D, Beaudet A, Ballas LM, Brandt IK, Brown B, Coleman R, Dunger DB, Falleta JM, Friedman HS, Haymond MW, Keating JP, Kinney TR, Leonard JB, Mahoney DH, Matalon R, Roe TF, Simmons P, Slonim AE. Infectious and bleeding complications in patients with glycogenosis 1b. Am J Dis Child 139:691–697, 1985.

Ambruso DR, Sasada M, Nishiyama H, Kubo A, Komiyama A, Allen RH. Defective bactericidal activity and absence of specific granules in neutrophils from a patient with recurrent bacterial infections. J Clin Immunol 4:23–30, 1984.

Ament ME, Ochs HD. Gastrointestinal manifestations of chronic granulomatous disease. N Engl J Med 288:382–387, 1973.

Ancliff PJ, Gale RE, Liesner R, Hann IM, Linch DC. Mutations in the ELA2 gene encoding neutrophil elastase are present in most patients with sporadic severe congenital neutropenia but only in some patients with the familial form of the disease. Blood 98:2645–2650, 2001.

Anderson DC, Mace ML, Brinkley BR, Martin RR, Smith CW. Recurrent infection in glycogenosis type Ib: abnormal neutrophil motility related to impaired redistribution of adhesion sites. J Infect Dis 143:447–459, 1981.

Anderson DC, Schmalstieg FC, Finegold MJ, Hughes BJ, Rothlein R, Miller LJ, Kohl S, Tosi MF, Jacobs RL, Waldrop TC. The severe and moderate phenotypes of heritable Mac-1, LFA-1 deficiency: their quantitative definition and relation to leukocyte dysfunction and clinical features. J Infect Dis 152:668–689, 1985.

Anderson DC, Springer TA. Leukocyte adhesion deficiency: an inherited defect in the Mac-1, LFA-1, and P150,95 glycopotein. Annu Rev Med 38:175, 1987.

Aprikyan AAG, Conrad Liles W, Park JR, Jonas M, Chi EY, Dale DC. Myelokathexis, a congenital disorder of severe neutropenia characterized by accelerated apoptosis and defective expression of bcl-x in neutrophil precursors. Blood 95:320–327, 2000.

Arai J, Wakiguchi H, Hisakawa H, Kubota H, Kurashige T. A variant of myelokathexis with hypogammaglobulinemia: lymphocytes as well as neutrophils may reverse in response to infections. Ped Hematol Oncol 17:171–176, 2000.

Ardati KO, Bajakian KM, Tabbara KS. Effect of glucose-6-phosphate dehydrogenase deficiency on neutrophil function. Acta Hematol 97:211–215, 1997.

Ariga T, Furuta H, Cho K, Sakiyama Y. Genetic analysis of 13 families with X-linked chronic granulomatous disease reveals a low proportion of sporadic patients and a high proportion of sporadic carriers. Pediatr Res 44:85–92, 1998.

Bach E, Aguet M, Schriber R. The IFN-γ receptor: a paradigm for cytokine receptor signaling. Annu Rev Immunol 15:563–591, 1997.

Baehner RL, Nathan DG. Quantitative nitroblue tetrazolium test in chronic granulomatous disease. N Engl J Med 278:971–976, 1968.

Baetz K, Isaaz S, Griffiths GM. Loss of cytotoxic T lymphocyte function in Chédiak-Higashi syndrome arises from a secretory defect that prevents lytic granule exocytosis. J Immonol 154:6122–6131, 1995.

Baldus S, Heeschen C, Meinertz T, Zeiher AM, Eiserich JP, Munzel T, Simoons ML, Hamm CW, CAPTURE Investigators. Myeloperoxidase serum levels predict risk in patients with acute coronary syndromes. Circulation 108:1440–1445, 2003.

Banerjee R, Anguita J, Roos D, Fikrig E. Cutting edge: Infection by the agent of human granulocytic ehrlichiosis prevents the respiratory burst by down-regulating gp91phox. J Immunol 164:3946–3949, 2000.

Barbosa MD, Nguyen QA, Tchernev VT, Ashley JA, Detter JC, Blaydes SM, Brandt SJ, Chotai D, Hodgman C, Solari RC, Lovett M, Kingsmore SF. Identification of the homologous beige and Chédiak-Higashi syndrome genes. Nature 382:262–265, 1996.

Barrat FJ, Le Deist F, Benkerrou M, Bousso P, Feldmann J, Fischer A, de Saint Basile G. Defective CTLA-4 cycling pathway in Chédiak-Higashi syndrome: a possible mechanism for deregulation of T lymphocyte activation. Proc Natl Acad Sci USA 96:8645–8650, 1999.

Bauer TR, Schwartz BR, Conrad Liles W, Ochs HD, Hickstein DD. Retroviral-mediated gene transfer of the leukocyte integrin CD18 into peripheral blood CD34+ cells derived from a patient with leukocyte adhesion deficiency type 1. Blood 91:1520–1526, 1998.

Baumeister FA, Stachel D, Schuster F, Schmidt I, Schaller M, Wolff H, Weiss M, Belohradsky BH. Accelerated phase in partial albinism with immunodeficiency (Griscelli syndrome): genetics and stem cell transplantation in a 2-month-old girl. Eur J Pediatr 159:74–78, 2000.

Bax WA, Cluysenaer OJ, Bartelink AK, Aerts PC, Ezekowitz RA, Van Dijk H. Association of familial deficiency of mannose-binding lectin and meningococcal disease. Lancet 354:1094–1095, 1999.

Bejaoui M, Veber F, Girault D, Gaud C, Blanche S, Griscelli C, Fischer A. Phase acceleree de la maladie de Chédiak-Higashi. Arch Fr Pediatr 46:733, 1989.

Belaaouaj A, McCarthy R, Baumann M, Gao Z, Ley TJ, Abraham SN, Shapiro SD. Mice lacking neutrophil elastase reveal impaired host defense against gram negative bacterial sepsis. Nat Med 4:615–618, 1998.

Bendix-Hansen K, Kerndrup G. Myeloperoxidase-deficient polymorphonuclear leukocytes (V): relation to FAB classification and neutrophil alkaline phosphatase activity in primary myelodysplastic syndromes. Scand J Haematol 35:197, 1985.

Bendix-Hansen K, Kerndrup G, Pedersen B. Myeloperoxidase-deficient polymorphonuclear leukocytes (VI): relation to cytogenetic abnormalities in primary myelodysplastic syndromes. Scand J Haematol 36:3, 1986.

Berendes H, Bridges RA, Good RA. A fatal granulomatous disease of childhood: The clinical study of a new syndrome. Minn Med 40:309–312, 1957.

Bernard T, Gale RE, Evans JPM, Linch DC. Mutations of the granulocyte-colony stimulating factor receptor in patients with severe congenital neutropenia are not required for transformation to acute myeloid leukemia and may be a bystander phenomenon. Br J Hematol 101:141–149, 1998.

Bernini JC. Diagnosis and management of chronic neutropenia during childhood. Pediatr Clin North Am 43:773–792, 1996.

Bhaskaram C, Siva Prasad J, Krishnamachari KA. Anæmia and immune response. Lancet 1:1000, 1977.

Bhattacharya A, Slatter M, Curtis A, Chapman CE, Barge D, Jackson A, Flood TJ, Abinun M, Cant AJ, Gennery AR. Successful umbilical cord blood stem cell transplantation for chronic granulomatous disease. Bone Marrow Transplant 31:403–405, 2003.

Blume RS, Bennett JM, Yankee RA, Wolff SM. Defective granulocyte regulation in the Chédiak-Higashi syndrome. N Engl J Med 279:1009, 1968.

Blume RS, Wolff SM. The Chédiak-Higashi syndrome: Studies in four patients and a review of the literature. Medicine (Baltimore) 51:247, 1972.

Bolscher BG, de Boer M, de Klein A, Weening RS, Roos D. Point mutations in the B-subunit of cytochrome b558 leading to X-linked chronic granulomatous disease. Blood 77:2482–2487, 1991.

Bonilla MA, Dale D, Zeidler C, Last L, Reiter A, Ruggeiro M, Koci B, Hammond W, Gillio A. Long-term safety of treatment with recombinant human granulocyte colony-stimulating factor (r-metHuG-CSF) in patients with severe congenital neutropenias. Br J Hematol 88:723–730, 1994.

Bonilla MA, Gillio AP, Ruggeiro M, Kernan NA, Brochstein JA, Abboud M, Fumagalli L, Vincent M, Gabrilove, JL, Welte K. Effects of recombinant human granulocyte colony-stimulating factor on neutropenia in patients with congenital agranulocytosis. N Engl J Med 320:1574–1580, 1989.

Boocock GR, Morrison JA, Popovic M, Richards N, Ellis L, Durie PR, Rommens JM. Mutations in SBDS are associated with Shwachman-Diamond syndrome. Nat Genet 33:97–101, 2003.

Boxer LA, Coates TD, Haak RA, Wolach JB, Hoffstein S, Baehner RL. Lactoferrin deficiency associated with altered granulocyte function. N Engl J Med 307:404–410, 1982.

Boxer LA, Hedley-Whyte ET, Stossel TP. Neutrophil actin dysfunction and abnormal neutrophil behavior. N Engl J Med 291:1093–1099, 1974.

Boxer LA, Oliver JM, Spielberg SP, Allen JM, Schulman JD. Protection of granulocytes by vitamin E in glutathione synthetase deficiency. N Engl J Med 301:901–905, 1979.

Brandrup F, Koch C, Petri M, Schiodt M, Johansen KS. Discoid lupus erythematosus-like lesions and stomatitis in female carriers of X-linked chronic granulomatous disease. Br J Dermatol 104:495–505, 1981.

Breton-Gorius J, Mason DY, Buriot D, Vilde JL, Griscelli C. Lactoferrin deficiency as a consequence of a lack of specific granules in neutrophils from a patient with recurrent infections. Am J Pathol 99:413–428, 1980.

Bridges RA, Berendes H, Good RA. A fatal granulomatous disease of childhood. Am J Dis Child 97:387–408, 1959.

Bruin MC, Von dem Borne AE, Tamminga RY, Kleijer M, Buddelmeijer L, De Haas M: Neutrophil antibody specificity in different types of childhood autoimmune neutropenia. Blood 94:1797–1802, 1999.

Buescher ES, Alling DW, Gallin JI. Use of an X-linked human neutrophil marker to estimate timing of lyonization and size of the dividing stem cell pool. J Clin Invest 76:1581–1584, 1985.

Buescher ES, Gallin JI. Effects of storage and radiation on human neutrophil function in vitro. Inflammation 11:401–416, 1987.

Buescher ES, Gallin JI. Leukocyte transfusions in chronic granulomatous disease: persistence of transfused leukocytes in sputum. N Engl J Med 307:800–803, 1982.

Buescher ES, Gallin JI. Radiation effects on cultured human monocytes and on monocyte derived macrophages. Blood 63:1402–1407, 1984a.

Buescher ES, Gallin JI. Stature and weight in chronic granulomatous disease. J Pediatr 104:911–913, 1984b.

Bussel JB, Abboud MR: Autoimmune neutropenia of childhood. Crit Rev Oncol Hematol 7:37–51, 1987.

Bux J, Behrens G, Jaeger G, Welte K: Diagnosis and clinical course of autoimmune neutropenia in infancy: analysis of 240 cases. Blood 91:181–186, 1998.

Cai TQ, Wright SD. Human leukocyte elastase is an endogenous ligand for the integrin CR3 (CD11b/CD18, Mac-1, alpha M beta 2) and modulates polymorphonuclear leukocyte adhesion J Exp Med 184:1213–1223, 1996.

Calderwood S, Kilpatrick L, Douglas S, Freedman M, Smith-Whitly K, Rolland M, Kutzberg J. Recombinant human granulocyte colony-stimulating factor therapy for patients with neutropenia and/or neutrophil dysfunction secondary to glycogen storage disease 1b. Blood 97:376–382, 2001.

Cale CM, Jones AM, Goldblatt D. Follow-up of patients with chronic granulomatous disease diagnosed since 1990. Clin Exp Immunol 120:351–355, 2000.

Casimir CM, Bu-Ghaim HN, Rodaway AR, Bentley DL, Rowe P, Segal AW. Autosomal recessive chronic granulomatous disease caused by deletion at a dinucleotide repeat. Proc Natl Acad Sci USA 88:2753–2757, 1991.

Cech P, Stadler H, Widmann JJ, Rohner A, Miescher PA. Leukocyte myeloperoxidase deficiency and diabetes mellitus associated with Candida albicans liver abscess. Am J Med 66:149–153, 1979.

Certain S, Barrat F, Pastural E, Le Diest F, Goyo-Rivas J, Jabado N, Benkerrou M, Seger R, Vilmer E, Beullier G, Schwarz K, Fischer A, De Saint Basile G. Protein truncation test of LYST reveals heterogeneous mutations in patients with Chédiak-Higashi syndrome. Blood 95:979–983, 2000.

Chandra RK. Nutrition and immunology: from the clinic to cellular biology and back again. Proc Nutr Soc 58:681–683, 1999.

Chandra RK. Nutrition and the immune system: an introduction. Am J Clin Nutr 66:460S–463S, 1997.

Chiang AK, Chan GC, Ma SK, Ng YK, Ha SY, Lau YL. Disseminated fungal infection associated with myeloperoxidase deficiency in a premature neonate. Pediatr Infect Dis J 19:1027–1029, 2000.

Chin TW, Stiehm ER, Faloon J, Gallin J. Corticosteroids in treatment of obstructive lesions of chronic granulomatous disease. J Pediatr 111:349–352, 1987.

Chusid MJ, Bujak JS, Dale DC. Defective polymorphonuclear leukocyte metabolism in canine cyclic neutropenia. Blood 46:921–930, 1975.

Cioffi WG Jr, Burleson DG, Jordan BS, Becker WK, McManus WF, Mason AD Jr, et al. Effects of granulocyte-macrophage colony-stimulating factor in burn patients. Arch Surg 126:74–79, 1991.

Cipolli M. Shwachman-Diamond syndrome: clinical phenotypes. Pancreatology 1:543–548, 2001.

Clark RA, Malech HL, Gallin JI, Nunoi H, Volpp BD, Naussef WM, Curnutte JT. Genetic variants of chronic granulomatous disease: Prevalence of deficiencies of two cytosolic components of the NADPH oxidase system. N Engl J Med 321:647–652, 1989.

Clawson CC, White JG, Repine JE. The Chédiak-Higashi syndrome. Evidence that defective leukotaxis is primarily due to an impediment by giant granules. Am J Pathol 92:745, 1978.

Coates TD, Torkildson JC, Torres M, Church JA, Howard TH. An inherited defect of neutrophil motility and microfilamentous cytoskeleton associated with abnormalities in 47-Kd and 89-Kd proteins. Blood 78:1338–1346, 1991.

Constantopoulos A. Congenital tuftsin deficiency. Ann NY Acad Sci 419:214–219, 1983.

Constantopoulos A, Najjar VA, Smith JW. Tuftsin deficiency: a new syndrome with defective phagocytosis. J Pediatr 80:564–572, 1972.

Constantopoulos A, Najjar VA, Wish JB, Necheles TH, Stolbach LL. Defective phagocytosis due to tuftsin deficiency in splenoctomized subjects. Am J Dis Chil 125:663–665, 1973.

Corbacioglu S, Bux J, Konig A, Gabrilove JL, Welte K, Bussel JB. Serum granulocyte colony-stimulating factor levels are not increased in patients with autoimmune neutropenia of infancy. J Pediatr 137:96–99, 2000.

Dale DC: Immune and idiopathic neutropenia. Curr Opin Hematol 5:33–36, 1998.

Dale DC, Hammond WP. Cyclic neutropenia: a clinical review. Blood Rev 2:178–185, 1988.

Dale DC, Person RE, Bolyard AA, Aprikyan AG, Bos C, Bonilla MA, Boxer LA, Kannourakis G, Zeidler C, Welte K, Benson KF, Horwitz M. Mutations in the gene encoding neutrophils elastase in congenital and cyclic neutropenia. Blood 96:2317–2322, 2000.

Darnell JE Jr, Kerr IM, Starck GR. Jak-STAT pathways and transcriptional activation in response to IFNs and other extracellular signalling proteins. Science 264:1415–1421, 1994.

Daugherty A, Dunn JL, Rateri DL, Heinecke JW. Myeloperoxidase, a catalyst for lipoprotein oxidation, is expressed in human atherosclerotic lesions. J Clin Invest 94:437–444, 1994.

Del Giudice I, Iori AP, Mengarelli A, Testi AM, Romano A, Cerretti R, Macri F, Iacobini M, Arcese W. Allogeneic stem cell transplant from HLA-identical sibling for chronic granulomatous disease and review of the literature. Ann Hematol 82:189–192, 2003.

DeLisser HM, Christofidou-Solomidou M, Sun J, Nakada MT, Sullivan KE. Loss of endothelial surface expression of E-selectin in a patient with recurrent infections. Blood 94:884–894, 1999.

Devriendt K, Kim AS, Mathijs G, Frints SGM, Schwartz M, Van den Oord JJ, Verhoef EG, Boogaerts MA, Fryns J-P, You D, Rosen M, Vandenberghe P. Constitutively activating mutation in WASP causes X-linked severe congenital neutropenia. Nat Genet 27:313–317, 2001.

Dinauer M. The phagocyte system and disorders of granulopoiesis and granulocyte function. In Nathan DG, Oski FA. Hematology of Infancy and Childhood, ed 5, Philadelphia, WB Saunders, 1998, pp 889–967.

Dinauer MC, Pierce EA, Bruns GA, Curnutte JT, Orkin SH. Human neutrophil cytochrome b light chain (p22-phox). Gene structure, chromosomal location, and mutations in cytochrome negative autosomal recessive chronic granulomatous disease. J Clin Invest 86:1729–1737, 1990.

Dinauer MC, Pierce EA, Erickson RW, Muhlebach TJ, Messner H, Orkin SH, Seger RA, Curnutte JT. Point mutation in the cytoplasmic domain of the neutrophil p22-phox cytochrome b subunit is associated with nonfunctional NADPH oxidase and chronic granulomatous disease. Proc Natl Acad Sci USA 88:11231–11235, 1991.

Diukman R, Tanigawara S, Cowan MJ, Golbus, MS. Prenatal diagnosis of Chédiak-Higashi syndrome. Prenatal Diagnosis 12:677–665, 1968.

Dong F, Hoefsloot L, Schelen A, Broeders L, Meijer Y, Veerman A, Touw I, Lowenberg B. Identification of a nonsense mutation in the granulocyte-colony-stimulating factor receptor in severe congenital neutropenia. Proc Natl Acad Sci USA 91:4480–4484, 1994.

Dong F, Brynes R, Tidow N, Welte K, Lowenberg B, Touw I. Mutations in the gene for the granulocyte colony-stimulating-factor receptor in patients with acute myeloid leukemia preceded by severe congenital neutropenia. N Engl J Med 333:487–493, 1995.

Dorman SE, Guide SV, Conville PS, DeCarlo ES, Malech HL, Gallin JI, Witebsky FG, Holland SM. Nocardia infection in chronic granulomatous disease. Clin Infect Dis 35:390–394, 2002.

Dries DJ. Interferon gamma in trauma-related infections. Intensive Care Med 22 (Suppl 4):S462–S467, 1996

Dror Y, Freedman MH. Shwachman-Diamond syndrome. Br J Haematol 118:701–713, 2002.

Dror Y, Ginzberg H, Dalal I, Cherepanov V, Downey G, Durie P, et al. Immune function in patients with Shwachman-Diamond syndrome. Br J Haematol 114:712–717, 2001.

Duran-McKinster C, Rodriguez Jurado R, Riduara C, De la Luz Orozco-Covarrrubias MA, Tamayo L, Ruiz-Maldonado R. Elejalde syndrome: a melanolysosomal neurocutaneous syndrome. Arch Dermatol 135:182–186, 1999.

Eber OT-J, Wang H-L. Periodontal disease in the child and adolescent. J Clin Periodontol 29:400–410, 2002.

Eiserich JP, Baldus S, Brennan ML, Ma W, Zhang C, Tousson A, Castro L, Lusis AJ, Nauseef WM, White CR, Freeman BA. Myeloperoxidase, a leukocyte-derived vascular NO oxidase. Science 296:2391–2394, 2002.

El Ouriaghli F, Fujiwara H, Melenhorst JJ, Sconocchia G, Hensel N, Barrett AJ. Neutrophil elastase enzymatically antagonizes the in vitro action of G-CSF implication for the regulation of granulopoiesis. Blood 101:1752–1758, 2003.

Emmendorffer A, Lohmann-Matthes M-L, Roesler J. Kinetics of transfused neutrophils in peripheral blood and BAL fluid of a patient with variant X-linked chronic granulomatous disease. Eur J Haematol 47:246–252, 1991.

Engelich G, Wright DG, Hartshorn KL. Acquired disorders of phagocyte function complicating medical and surgical illness. CID 33:2040–2048, 2001.

Etzioni A. Adhesion molecule deficiencies and their clinical significance. Cell Adhesion Comm 2:257–260, 1994.

Etzioni A, Frydman M, Pollack S, Avidor I, Phillips ML, Paulson JC, Gershoni-Baruch R. Brief report: recurrent severe infections caused by a novel leukocyte adhesion deficiency. N Engl J Med 327:1789–1792, 1992.

Etzioni A, Gershoni-Baruch R, Pollack S, Shehadeh N. Leukocyte adhesion deficiency type II: long-term follow-up. J Allergy Clin Immunol 102:323–324, 1998.

Etzioni A, Tonetti M. Fucose supplementation in leukocyte adhesion deficiency type II [letter]. Blood 95:3641–3642, 2000.

Ezekowitz RA. Genetic heterogeneity of mannose-binding proteins: the Jekyll and Hyde of innate immunity? Am J Hum Genet 62:6–9, 1998.

Ezekowitz RAB, Dinauer MC, Jaffe HS, Orkin SH, Newburger PE. Partial correction of the phagocyte defect in patients with X-linked chronic granulomatous disease by subcutaneous interferon gamma. N Engl J Med 319:146–151, 1988.

Ezekowitz RAB, Orkin SH, Newburger PE. Recombinant interferon gamma augments phagocyte superoxide production and X-linked chronic granulomatous disease gene expression in X-linked variant chronic granulomatous disease. J Clin Invest 80:1009–1016, 1987.

Ezekowitz RAB, Sieff CA, Dinauer MC, Nathan DG, Orkin SH, Newburger PE. Restoration of phagocyte function by interferon gamma in X-linked chronic granulomatous disease occurs at the level of a progenitor cell. Blood 76:2443–2448, 1990.

Firatli E, Tuzun B, Efeoglu A. Papillon-Lefèbre syndrome. Analysis of neutrophil chemotaxis. J Periodontol 67:617–620, 1996.

Fischer A, Landais P, Friedrich W. Bone marrow transplantation (BMT) in Europe for primary immunodeficiencies other than severe combined immunodeficiency. Blood 83:1149–1154, 1994.

Fischer A, Lisowska-Grospierre B, Anderson DC, Springer TA. Leukocyte adhesion deficiency: molecular basis and functional consequences. Immunodefic Rev 1:39–54, 1988.

Forrest CB, Forehand JR, Axtell RA, Roberts RL, Johnston RB Jr. Clinical features and current management of chronic granulomatous disease. Hematol Oncol Clin North Am 2:253–266, 1988.

Foster CB, Lehrnbecher T, Mol F, Steinberg SM, Venzon DJ, Walsh TJ, Noack D, Rae J, Winkelstein JA, Curnutte JT, Chanock SJ. Host defense molecule polymorphisms influence the risk for immune-mediated complications in chronic granulomatous disease. J Clin Invest 102:2146–2155, 1998.

Fraser IP, Koziel H, Ezekowitz RA. The serum mannose-binding protein and the macrophage mannose receptor are pattern recognition molecules that link innate and adaptive immunity. Semin Immunol 10:363–372, 1998.

Freedman MH. Safety of long-term administration of granulocyte colony-stimulating factor for severe chronic neutropenia. Curr Opin Hematol 4:217–224, 1997.

Freedmann MH, Alter BP. Risk of myelodysplastic syndrome and acute myeloid leukemia in congenital neutropenias. Semin Hematol 39:128–133, 2002.

Frenette PS, Mayadas TN, Rayburn H, Hynes RO, Wagne DD. Susceptibility to infection and altered hematopoiesis in mice deficient in both P- and E-selectins. Cell 84:563–574, 1996.

Fromont P, Bettaieb A, Skouri H, Floch C, Poulet E, Duedari N, Bierling P. Frequency of the polymorphonuclear Fc-gamma receptor III deficiency in the French population and its involvement in the development of neonatal alloimmune neutropenia. Blood 79:2131–2134, 1992.

Frydman M, Etzioni A, Eidlitz-Markus T, Avidor I, Varsano Y, Shechter Y, Orlin JB, Gershoni-Baruch R. Ramban-Hasharon syndrome of psychomotor retardation, short stature, defective neutrophil motility and Bombay phenotype. Am J Med Genet 44:297–302, 1992.

Gallin JI, Alling DW, Malech HL, Wesley R, Koziol D, Marciano B, Eisenstein EM, Turner ML, DeCarlo ES, Starling JM, Holland SM. Itraconazole to prevent fungal infections in chronic granulomatous disease. N Engl J Med 348:2416–2422, 2003.

Gallin JI, Buescher ES. Abnormal regulation of inflammatory skin responses in male patients with chronic granulomatous disease. Inflammation 7:227–232, 1983.

Gallin JI, Buescher ES, Seligmann BE, Nath J, Gaither T, Katz P. NIH conference. Recent advances in chronic granulomatous disease. Ann Intern Med 99:657–674, 1983.

Gallin JI, Bujak JS, Patten E, Wolff SM. Granulocyte function in the Chédiak-Higashi syndrome of mice. Blood 43:201–206, 1974.

Gallin JI, Elin RJ, Hubert RT, Fauci AS, Kaliner MA, Wolff SM. Efficacy of ascorbic acid in Chédiak-Higashi syndrome (CHS): studies in humans and mice. Blood 53:226–234, 1979.

Gallin JI, Fletcher MP, Seligmann BE, Hoffstein S, Cehrs K, Mounessa N. Human neutrophil specific granule deficiency: a model to assess the role of the neutrophil specific granules in the evolution of the inflammatory response. Blood 59:1317–1329, 1982.

Garred P, Pressler T, Madsen HO, Frederiksen B, Svejgaard A, Hoiby N, Schwartz M, Koch C. Association of mannose-binding lectin gene heterogeneity with severity of lung disease and survival in cystic fibrosis. J Clin Invest 104:431–437, 1999.

Gautier E, Bourhis JH, Bayle C, Cartron J, Pico JL, Tchernia G. Parvovirus B19 associated neutropenia. Treatment with Rh G-CSF. Hematol Cell Ther 39:85–87, 1997.

Geerlings SE, Hoepelman AIM. Immune dysfunction in patients with diabetes mellitus (DM). FEMS Immunol Med Microbiol 26:259–265, 1999.

Ghaffer KA, Zahran FM, Fahmy HM, Brown RS. Papillon-Lefèbre syndrome: neutrophil function in 15 cases from 4 families in Egypt. Oral Surg Oral Med Oral Pathol Oral Radiol Endod 88:320–325, 1999.

Giblett ER, Klebanoff SJ, Pincus SH, Swanson J, Park BH, McCullough J. Kell phenotypes in chronic granulomatous disease: a potential transfusion hazard. Lancet 1:1235–1236, 1971.

Gilmore M, Stroncek D, Korones D. Treatment of alloimmune neonatal neutropenia with granulocyte colony-stimulating factor. J Pediatr 125:948–951, 1994.

Ginzberg H, Shin J, Ellis L, Morrison J, Ip W, Dror Y, Freedman M, Heitlinger LA, Belt MA, Corey M, Rommens JM, Durie PR. Shwachman syndrome: phenotypic manifestations of sibling sets and isolated cases in a large patient cohort are similar. J Pediatr 135:81–88, 1999.

Goldblatt D, Butcher J, Thrasher AJ, Russell-Eggitt I. Chorioretinal lesions in patients and carriers of chronic granulomatous disease. J Pediatr 134:780–783, 1999.

Gombart AF, Koeffler HP. Neutrophil specific granule deficiency and mutations in the gene encoding transcription factor C/EBP(epsilon). Curr Opin Hematol 9:36–42, 2002.

Gombart AF, Shiohara M, Kwok SH, Agematsu K, Komiyama A, Koeffler HP. Neutrophil-specific granule deficiency: homozygous recessive inheritance of a frameshift mutation in the gene encoding transcription factor CCAAT/enhancer binding protein—epsilon. Blood 97:2561–2567, 2001.

Goobie S, Popovic M, Morrison J, Ellis L, Ginzberg H, Boocock GR, Ehtesham N, Betard C, Brewer CG, Roslin NM, Hudson TJ, Morgan K, Fujiwara TM, Durie PR, Rommens JM. Shwachman-Diamond syndrome with exocrine pancreatic dysfunction and bone marrow failure maps to the centromeric region of chromosome 7. Am J Hum Genet 68:1048–1054, 2001.

Gorlin RJ, Gelg B, Diaz GA, Lofsness KG, Pittelkow MR, Fenyk JR. WHIM syndrome, an autosomal dominant disorder: clinical, hematological, and molecular studies. Am J Med Genet 91:368–376, 2000.

Gough A, Clapperton M, Rolando N, Foster AV, Philpott-Howard J, Edmonds ME. Randomised placebo-controlled trial of granulocyte-colony stimulating factor in diabetic foot infection. Lancet 350:855–859, 1997.

Gray GR, Klebanoff SJ, Stamatoyannopoulos G, Austin T, Naiman SC, Yoshida A, Kliman MR, Robinson GCF. Neutrophil dysfunction, chronic granulomatous disease, and non-spherocytic haemolytic anemia caused complete deficiency of glucose-6-phosphate dehydrogenase. Lancet 2:530–534, 1973.

Griscelli C, Durandy A, Guy-Grand D, Daguillard F, Herzog C, Prunerias M. A syndrome associating partial albinism and immunodeficiency. Am J Med 65:691–702, 1978.

Griscom NT, Kirkpatrick JA, Girdany BR, Berdon WE, Grand RJ, Mackie GG. Gastric antral narrowing in chronic granulomatous disease of childhood. Pediatrics 54:456–460, 1974.

Guba SC, Boxer LA, Emerson SG. G-CSF receptor transmembrane and intracytosolic structure in patients with congenital neutropenia. Blood (Suppl) 82:1:23a, 1993.

Haag-Weber M, Horl WH. Dysfunction of polymorphonuclear leukocytes in uremia. Semin Nephrol 16:192–201, 1996.

Haag-Weber M, Mai B, Horl WH. Normalization of enhanced neutrophil cytosolic free calcium of hemodialysis patients by 1,25-dihydroxyvitamin D3 or calcium channel blocker. Am J Nephrol 13:467–472, 1993.

Haddad E, LeDiest F, Blanche S, Benkerrou M, Rohorlich P, Vilmer E, Griscelli C, Fischer A. Treatment of Chédiak-Higashi syndrome by allogeneic bone marrow transplantation. Blood 85:3328–3333, 1995.

Hakami N, Neiman PE, Canellos GP, Lazerson J. Neonatal megaloblastic anemia due to inherited transcobalamin II deficiency in two siblings. N Engl J Med 285:1163–1170, 1971.

Haliotis T, Roder J, Klein M, Oraldo J, Fauci AS, Herberman RB. Chédiak-Higashi gene in humans. I. Impairment of natural-killer function. J Exp Med 151:1039–1048, 1980.

Hammond WP IV, Price TH, Souza LM, Dale DC. Treatment of cyclic neutropenia with granulocyte colony-stimulating factor. N Engl J Med 320:1306–1311, 1989.

Harfi HA, Brismar J, Hainau B, Sabbah R. Partial albinism, immunodeficiency, and progressive white matter disease: a new primary immunodeficiency. Allergy Proc 13:321–328, 1992.

Harris BH, Boles ET. Intestinal lesions in chronic granulomatous disease of childhood. J Pediatr Surg 8:955–956, 1973.

Hart TC, Hart PS, Bowden DW, Michalec MD, Callison SA, Walker SJ, et al. Mutations of the cathepsin c gene are responsible for Papillon-Lefèbre syndrome. J Med Genet 36:881–887, 1999.

Hartman KR, Brown KE, Green SW, Young NS. Lack of evidence for parvovirus B19 viraemia in children with chronic neutropenia [letter; comment]. Br J Haematol 88:895–896, 1994.

Hartman KR, Wright DG: Identification of autoantibodies specific for the neutrophil adhesion glycoproteins CD11b/CD18 in patients with autoimmune neutropenia. Blood 78:1096–1104, 1991.

Henter JI, Elinder G, Ost A. Diagnostic guidelines for hemophagocytic lymphohistiocytosis. Semin Oncol 18:29–33, 1991.

Hermans MH, Antonissen C, Ward AC, Mayen AE, Ploemacher RE, Touw IP. Sustained receptor activation and hyperproliferation in response to granulocyte colony-stimulating factor (G-CSF) in mice with severe congenital neutropenia/acute myeloid leukemia-derived mutation in the G-CSF receptor gene. J Exp Med 189:683–692, 1999.

Hernandez PA, Gorlin RJ, Lukens JN, Taniuchi S, Bohinjec J, Francoi F, Klotman ME, Diaz GA. Mutations in the chemokine receptor gene CXCR4 are associated with WHIM syndrome, a combined immunodeficiency disease. Nat Genet 34:70–74, 2003.

Hibbs ML, Wardlaw AJ, Stacker SA, Anderson DC, Lee A, Roberts TM, Springer TA. Transfection of cells from patients with leukocyte adhesion deficiency with an integrin beta subunit (CD18) restores lymphocyte function-associated antigen-1 expression and function. J Clin Invest 85:674–681, 1990.

Hitzig WH, Dohmann U, Pluss HJ, Vischer D. Hereditary transcobalamin II deficiency: clinical findings in a family. J Pediatr 85:622–628, 1974.

Hitzig WH, Kenny AB. The role of vitamin B12 and its transport globulins in the production of antibodies. Clin Exp Immunol 20:105–111, 1975.

Hogg N, Stewart MP, Scarth SL, Newton R, Shaw JM, Law SK, Klein N. A novel leukocyte adhesion deficiency caused by expressed but nonfunctional beta2 integrins Mac-1 and LFA-1 J Clin Invest 103:97–106, 1999.

Holcombe RF, van de Griend R, Ang SL, Bolhuis RL, Seidman JG. Gamma-delta T cells in Chédiak-Higashi syndrome. Acta Haematol (Basel) 83:193–197, 1990.

Hord JD, Whitlock JA, Gay JC, Lukens JN. Clinical features of myelokathexis and treatment with hematopoietic cytokines: a case report of two patients and review of the literature. J Pediatr Hematol Oncol 19:443–448, 1997.

Horwitz ME, Barrett AJ, Brown MR, Carter CS, Childs R, Gallin JI, Holland SM, Linton GF, Miller JA, Leitman SF, Read EJ, Malech HL. Treatment of chronic granulomatous disease with nonmyeloablative conditioning and T-cell-depleted hematopoietic allograft. N Engl J Med 344:881–888, 2001.

Horwitz M, Benson KF, Person RE, Aprikyan AG, Dale DC. Mutations in ELA2, encoding neutrophil elastase, define a 21-day biological clock in cyclic haematopoiesis. Nat Genet 23:433–436, 1999.

Hsu JW, Vogelsang G, Jones RJ, Brodsky RA. Bone marrow transplantation in Shwachman-Diamond syndrome. Bone Marrow Transplant 30:255–258, 2002.

Huang S, Hendricks W, Althage A, Hemmi S, Bluethmann H, Kamijo R, Vilcek J, Zinkernagel RM, Aguet M. Immune response in mice that lack the interferon-gamma receptor. Science 259:1742–1745, 1993.

Huizinga TW, Kuijpers RW, Kleijer M, Schulpen TW, Cuypers HT, Roos D, von dem Borne AE. Maternal genomic neutrophil FcRIII deficiency leading to neonatal isoimmune neutropenia. Blood 76:1927–1932, 1990.

Ihm SH, Yoo HJ, Park SW, Park CJ. Effect of tolrestat, an aldose reductase inhibitor, on neutrophil respiratory burst activity in diabetic patients. Metabolism 46:634–638, 1997.

International Chronic Granulomatous Disease Cooperative Study Group. A controlled trial of interferon gamma to prevent infection in chronic granulomatous disease. N Engl J Med 324:509–516, 1991.

Introne W, Boissy RE, Gahl WA. Clinical, molecular, and cell biological aspects of Chédiak-Higashi syndrome. Mol Genet Metab 68:283–303, 1999.

Isaacs D, Wright VM, Shaw DG, Raafat F, Walker-Smith JA. Chronic granulomatous disease mimicking Crohn's disease. J Pediatr Gastroenterol Nutr 4:498–501, 1985.

Jabado N, Le Diest F, Cant A, De Graeff-Meeders ER, Fasth A, Morgan G, Vellodi A, Hale G, Bujan W, Thomas C, Cavazzana-Calvo M, Widjenes J, Fischer A. Bone marrow transplantation from genetically HLA-nonidentical donors in children with fatal inherited disorders excluding severe combined immunodeficiencies: use of two monoclonal antibodies to prevent graft rejection. Pediatrics 98:420–428, 1996.

Jaber BL, Cendoroglo M, Balakrishnan VS, Perianayagam MC, King AJ, Pereira BJ. Apoptosis of leukocytes: basic concepts and implications in uremia. Kidney Int Suppl 78:S197–S205, 2001.

Jackson SH, Gallin JI, Holland SM. The p47phox mouse knock-out model of chronic granulomatous disease. J Exp Med 182:751–758, 1995.

Janecke AR, Mayatepek E, Utermann G. Minireview: molecular genetics of type 1 glycogen storage disease. Mol Genet Metab 73:117–125, 2001.

Janeway CA, Craig J, Davison M, Doroney W, Gitlin D, Sullivan JC. Hypergammaglobulinemia associated with severe, recurrent, and chronic non-specific infection. Am J Dis Child 88:388–392, 1954.

Jenkins NA, Copeland NG, Taylor BA, Lee BK. Dilute (d) coal colour mutation DBA/2J mice is associated with the site of integration of an ecotropic MuLV genome. Nature 293:370–374, 1981.

Johnson FE, Humbert JR, Kuzela DC, Todd JK, Lilly JR. Gastric outlet obstruction due to X-linked chronic granulomatous disease. Surgery 78:217–223, 1975.

Jung LK. Association of aberrant F-actin formation with defective leukocyte chemotaxis and recurrent pyoderma. Clin Immunol Immunopathol 61:41–54, 1991.

Kallenberg CG. Autoantibodies to myeloperoxidase: clinical and pathophysiological significance. J Mol Med 76:682–687, 1998.

Kamani N, August CS, Campbell DE, Hassan NF, Douglas SD. Marrow transplantation in chronic granulomatous disease: an update with 6 year follow-up. J Pediatr 113:697–700, 1988.

Kenney RT, Kwon-Chung KJ, Waytes AT, Melnick DA, Merino MJ, Gallin JI. Successful treatment of systemic Exophiala dermatitidis infection in a patient with chronic granulomatous disease. Clin Infect Dis 1:235–242, 1992.

Kilpatrick L, Garty BZ, Lundquist KF, Hunter K, Stanley CA, Baker L, Douglas SD, Korchak HM. Impaired metabolic function and signalling defects in phagocytic cells in glycogen storage disease 1b. J Clin Invest 86:196–202, 1990.

Kinashi T, Aker M, Sokolovsky-Eisenberg M, Grabovsky V, Tanaka C, Shamri R, Feigelson S, Etzioni A, Alon R. LAD-III, a leukocyte adhesion deficiency syndrome associated with defective Rap1 activation and impaired stabilization of integrin bonds. Blood 103:1033–1036, 2004.

Kimura S, Yonemura T, Hiraga T, Okada H. Flow cytometric evaluation of phagocytosis by peripheral blood polymorphonuclear leukocytes in human periodontal diseases. Arch Oral Biol 37:495–501, 1992.

Kishimoto TK, Hollander N, Roberts TM, Anderson DC, Springer TA. Heterogeneous mutations of the beta subunit common to the LFA-1, Mac-1 and p150,95 glycoproteins cause leukocyte adhesion deficiency. Cell 50:193–201, 1987.

Kishimoto TK, O'Connor K, Springer TA. Leukocyte adhesion deficiency: aberrant splicing of a conserved integrin sequence causes a moderate deficiency phenotype. J Biol Chem 264:3588–3596, 1989.

Kitahara M, Eyre HJ, Simonian Y, Atkin CL, Hasstedt SJ. Hereditary myeloperoxidase deficiency. Blood 57:888–893, 1981.

Kijas JM, Bauer TR, Gafvert S, Marklund S, Trowald-Wigh G, Johannisson A, Hedhammar A, Binns M, Juneja RK, Hickstein DD, Andersson L. A missense mutation in the beta-2 integrin gene (ITGB2) causes canine leukocyte adhesion deficiency. Genomics 61:101–107, 1999.

Kizaki M, Miller CW, Selsted ME, Koeffler HP. Myeloperoxidase (MPO) gene mutation in hereditary MPO deficiency. Blood 83:1935–1940, 1994.

Klebanoff SJ, White LR. Iodination defect in the leukocytes of a patient with chronic granulomatous disease of childhood. N Engl J Med 280:460, 1969.

Klein C, Phillipe N, LeDeist F, Fraitag S, Prost C, Durandy A, Fischer A, Griscelli C. Partial albinism with immunodeficiency (Griscelli syndrome). J Pediatr 125:886–895, 1994.

Klein M, Roder J, Haliotis T, Korec S, Jett JR, Herberman RB, Katz P, Fauci AS. Chédiak-Higashi gene in humans. II. The selectivity of the defect in natural killer and antibody-dependent cell-mediated cytotoxicity function. J Exp Med 151:1049–1058, 1980.

Koch A, Melbye M, Sorensen P, Homoe P, Madsen HO, Molbak K, Hansen LH, Hahn GW, Garred P. Acute respiratory tract infections and mannose-binding lectin insufficiency during early childhood. JAMA 285:1316–1321, 2001.

Komiyama A, Morosawa H, Hanamura K, Miyagawa Y, Akabane T. Abnormal neutrophil maturation in a neutrophil defect with morphologic abnormality and impaired function. J Pediatr 94:19–25, 1979.

Kostmann R. Infantile genetic agranulocytosis. Acta Paediatr Scand (Suppl) 45:1–178, 1956.

Koziel H, Eichbaum Q, Kruskal BA, Pinkston P, Rogers RA, Armstrong MY, Richards FF, Rose RM, Ezekowitz RA. Reduced binding and phagocytosis of Pneumocystis carinii by alveolar macrophages from persons infected with HIV-1 correlates with mannose receptor downregulation. J Clin Invest 102:1332–1344,1998.

Kragballe K, Borregaard N, Brandrup F, Koch C, Staehrjohansen K. Relation of monocyte and neutrophil oxidative metabolism to skin and oral lesions in carriers of chronic granulomatous disease. Clin Exp Immunol 43:390–398, 1981.

Krause PL, Woronick CL, Burke G, Slover N, Kosciol C, Kelly T, Spivack B, Maderazo EG. Depressed neutrophil chemotaxis in children suffering blunt trauma. Pediatrics 93:807–809, 1994.

Kuijpers TW, van Lier RAW, Hamann D, de Boer M, Thung LY, Weening RS, Verhoeven AJ, Roos D. Leukocyte adhesion deficiency type 1 (LAD/1)/variant. J Clin Invest 100:1725–1733, 1997.

Lalezari P, Bernard GE: An isologous antigen-antibody reaction with human neutrophiles, related to neonatal neutropenia. J Clin Invest 45:1741–1750, 1966.

Lambert J, Naeyaert JM, De Paepe A, Van Coster R, Ferster A, Song M, Messiaen L. Arg-cys substitution at codon 1246 of the human myosin Va gene is not associated with Griscelli syndrome. J Invest Dermatol 114:731–733, 2000.

Landing BH, Shirkey HS. A syndrome of recurrent infection and infiltration of viscera by pigmented lipid histiocytes. Pediatrics 20:431–408, 1957.

Larrocha C, Fernandez de Castro M, Fontan G, Viloria A, Fernandez-Chacon JL, Jimenez C. Hereditary myeloperoxidase deficiency: study of 12 cases. Scand J Haematol 29:389–397, 1982.

LeDiest F, Blanche S, Keable H, Descamps-Latscha B, Pham HT, Wahn V, Griscelli C, Fischer A. Successful HLA nonidentical bone marrow transplantation in three patients with leukocyte adhesion deficiency. Blood 74:512–518, 1989.

Lehrer RI, Cline MJ. Leukocyte myeloperoxidase deficiency and disseminated candidiasis: the role of myeloperoxidase in resistance to Candida infection. J Clin Invest 48:1478–1488, 1969.

Lekstrom-Himes JA, Dorman SE, Kopar P, Holland SM, Gallin JI. Neutrophil-specific granule deficiency results from a novel mutation with loss of function of the transcription factor CCAAT/enhancer binding protein epsilon. J Exp Med 189:1847–1852, 1999.

Lekstrom-Himes JA, Holland SM, DeCarlo ES, Miller J, Leitman SF, Chang R, Baker AR, Gallin JI. Treatment with intralesional granulocyte instillations and interferon-gamma for a patient with chronic granulomatous disease and multiple hepatic abscesses. Clin Infect Dis 19:770–773, 1994.

Lekstrom-Himes JA, Xanthopoulos KG. Biological role of the CCAAT/enhancer-binding protein family of transcription factors. J Biol Chem 273:28545–28548, 1998.

Liang JS, Lu MY, Tsai MJ, Lin DT, Lin KH. Bone marrow transplantation from HLA-matched unrelated donor for treatment of Chédiak-Higashi syndrome. J Formos Med Assoc 99:499–502, 2000.

Lieschke GJ, Grail D, Hodgson G, Metcalf D, Stanley E, Cheers C, Fowler KJ, Basu S, Zhan YF, Dunn AR. Mice lacking granulocyte colony-stimulating factor have chronic neutropenia, granulocyte and macrophage progenitor cell deficiency, and impaired neutrophil mobilization. Blood 84:1737–1746, 1994.

Lindahl JA, Williams FH, Newman SL. Small bowel obstruction in chronic granulomatous disease. J Pediatr Gastroenterol Nutr 3:637–640, 1984.

Linehan SA, Martinez-Pomares L, Gordon S. Macrophage lectins in host defense. Microbes and Infection 2:279–288, 2000.

Lockman LA, Kennedy WR, White JG. The Chédiak-Higashi syndrome: electrophysiological and electron microscopic observations on the peripheral neuropathy. J Pediatr 70:942–951, 1967.

Lomax KJ, Gallin JI, Rotrosen D, Raphael GD, Kaliner MA, Benz EJ Jr, Boxer LA, Malech HL. Selective defect in myeloid cell lactoferrin gene expression in neutrophil specific granule deficiency. J Clin Invest 83:514–519, 1989.

Lu B, Ebensperger C, Dembic Z, Wang Y, Kvatyuk M, Lu T, Coffman R, Petska S, Rothman P. Targeted disruption of the interferon-receptor 2 gene results in severe immune defects in mice. Proc Nat Acad Sci USA 95:8233–8238, 1998.

Lübke T, Marquardt T, Etzioni A, Hartmann E, Von Figura K, Körner C. Complementation cloning identifies CDG-IIc, a new type of congenital disorders of glycosylation, as a GDP-fucose transporter deficiency. Nat Genet 28:73–76, 2001.

Lublin M, Bartlett DL, Danforth DN, Kauffman H, Gallin JI, Malech HL, Shawker T, Choyke P, Kleiner DE, Schwartzentruber DJ, Chang R, DeCarlo ES, Holland SM. Hepatic abscess in patients with chronic granulomatous disease. Ann Surg 235:383–391, 2002.

Ludviksson BR, Thorarensen O, Gudnason T, Halldorsson S. Candida albicans meningitis in a child with myeloperoxidase deficiency. Pedritr Infect Dis J 12:162–164, 1993.

Lühn K, Wild MK, Eckhardt M, Gerardy-Schahn R, Vestweber D. The gene defective in leukocyte adhesion deficiency II encodes a putative GDP-fucose transporter. Nat Genet 28:69–72, 2001.

Lun A, Roesler J, Renz H. Unusual late onset of X-linked chronic granulomatous disease in an adult woman after unsuspicious childhood. Clin Chem 48:780–781, 2002.

Luzzatto L. Glucose-6-phosphate dehydrogenase deficiency and hemolytic anemia. In Nathan DG, Oski FA. Hematology of Infancy and Childhood, ed 5, Philadelphia, WB Saunders, 1998, Philadelphia, pp 704–726.

Lyall EG, Lucas GF, Eden OB. Autoimmune neutropenia of infancy. J Clin Pathol 45:431–434, 1992.

Magram J, Connaughton SE, Warrier WW, Carvajal DM, Wu CY, Ferrante J, Stewart C, Sarmiento U, Faherty DA, Gately MK. IL-12 deficient mice are defective in IFN-γ production and type 1 cytokine response. Immunity 4:471–481, 1996.

Malech HL, Maples PB, Whiting-Theobald N, Linton GF, Sekhsaria S, Vowells SJ, Li F, Miller JA, DeCarlo E, Holland SM, Leitman SF, Carter CS, Butz RE, Read EJ, Fleisher TA, Schneiderman RD, Van

Epps DE, Spratt SK, Maack CA, Rokovich JA, Cohen LK, Gallin JI. Prolonged production of NADPH oxidase-corrected granulocytes after gene therapy of chronic granulomatous disease. Proc Natl Acad Sci USA 94:12133–12138, 1997.

Mamlok RJ, Mamlok V, Mills GC, Daechner CW, Schmalstieg FC, Anderson DC. Glucose-6-phosphate dehydrogenase deficiency, neutrophil dysfunction and *Chromobacterium violaceum* sepsis. J Pediatr 111:852, 1987.

Marciano BE, Rosenzweig SD, Kleiner DE, Anderson VL, Darnell DN, Anaya-O'Brien S, Hilligoss DM, Malech HL, Gallin JI, Holland SM. Gastrointestinal involvement in chronic granulomatous disease. Pediatrics 2004 (in press).

Margolis DM, Melnick DA, Alling DW, Gallin JI. Trimethoprim-sulfamethoxazole prophylaxis in the management of chronic granulomatous disease. J Infect Dis 162:723–726, 1990.

Markowitz JF, Aranow E, Rausen AR, Silverberg M, Daum F. Progressive esophageal dysfunction in chronic granulomatous disease. J Pediatr Gastroenterol Nutr 1:145–149, 1982.

Marquardt T, Luhn K, Srikrishna G, Freeze HH, Harms E, Vestweber D. Correction of leukocyte adhesion deficiency type II with oral fucose. Blood 94:3976–3985, 1999.

Marsh WL, Uretsky, SC, Douglas SD. Antigens of the Kell blood group system on neutrophils and monocytes their relation to chronic granulomatous disease. J Pediatr 87:1117–1120, 1975.

Martin C, Burdon PC, Bridger G, Gutierrez-Ramos JC, Williams TJ, Rankin SM. Chemokines acting via CXCR2 and CXCR4 control the release of neutrophils from the bone marrow and their return following senscence. Immunity 19:583–593, 2003.

Menasche G, Ho CH, Sanal O, Feldmann J, Tezcan I, Ersoy F, Houdusse A, Fischer A, de Saint Basile G. Griscelli syndrome restricted to hypopigmentation results from melanophilin defect (gS3) or a MYO5A F-exon deletion (GS1). J Clin Invest 112:450–456, 2003.

Menasche G, Pastural E, Feldman J, Certain S, Ersoy F, Dupuis S, Wulffraat N, Bianchi D, Fischer A, Le Diest F, de Saint Basile G. Mutations in RAB27A cause Griscelli syndrome associated with hemophagocytic syndrome. Nat Genet 25:173–176, 2000.

Mercer JA, Separack PK, Srobel MC, Copeland NG, Jenkins NA. Novel myosin heavy chain encoded by murine *dilute* coat colour locus. Nature 349:709n713, 1991.

Merino F, Klein GO, Henle W, Ramirez-Duque P, Forsgren M, Amesty C. Elevated antibody titers to Epstein-Barr virus and low natural killer cell activity in patients with Chédiak-Higashi syndrome. Clin Immunol Immunopathol 27:326–339, 1983.

Misra VP, King RHM, Harding AE, Muddle JR, Thomas PK. Peripheral neuropathy in the Chédiak-Higashi syndrome. Acta Neuropathol 81:354–358, 1991.

Moore FD Jr, Davis C, Rodrick M, Mannick JA, Fearon DT. Neutrophil activation in thermal injury as assessed by increased expression of complement receptors. N Engl J Med 314:948–53, 1986.

Mouy R, Fischer A, Vilmer E, Seger R, Griscelli C. Incidence, severity and prevention of infections in chronic granulomatous disease. J Pediatr 114:555–560, 1989.

Murray JC, Morad AB. Childhood autoimmune neutropenia and human parvovirus B19 [letter]. Am J Hematol 47:336, 1994.

Nagle DL, Karim MA, Woolf EA, Holmgren L, Bork P, Misumi DJ, McGrail SH, Dussault BJ Jr, Perou CM, Boissy RE, Duyk GM, Spritz RA, Moore KJ. Identification and mutation analysis of the complete gene for Chédiak-Higashi syndrome. Nat Genet 14:307–311, 1996.

Najjar VA and Nishioka K. "Tuftsin": a natural phagocytosis stimulating peptide. Nature 228:672–673, 1970.

Narita M, Shibata M, Togashi T, Tomizawa K, Matsumoto S. Steroid therapy for bronchopneumonia in chronic granulomatous disease. Acta Pediatr Jpn Overseas Ed 33:181–5, 1991.

Nathan CF, Murray HW, Wiebe ME, Rubin BY. Identification of interferon gamma as the lymphokine that activates human macrophage oxidative metabolism and antimicrobial activity. J Exp Med 158:670–689, 1983.

Nauseef WM. Aberrant restriction endonuclease digests of DNA from subjects with hereditary myeloperoxidase deficiency. Blood 73:290–295, 1989.

Nauseef WM. Myeloperoxidase deficiency. Hematol Oncol Clin North Am 2:135–158, 1988.

Nauseef WM. Myeloperoxidase deficiency. Hematol Pathol 4:165–178, 1990.

Nauseef WM, Cogley M, Bock S, Petrides PE. Pattern of inheritance in hereditary myeloperoxidase deficiency associated with the R569W missense mutation. J Leuk Biol 63:264–269, 1998.

Nauseef WM, Root RK, Malech HL. Biochemical and immunologic analysis of hereditary myeloperoxidase deficiency. J Clin Invest 71:1297–1307, 1983.

Nguyen C, Katner HP. Myeloperoxidase deficiency manifesting as pustular candidal dermatitis. Clin Infect Dis 24:258–260, 1997.

Nunoi H, Yamazaki T, Tsuchiya H, Kato S, Malech HL, Matsuda I, Kanegasaki S. A heterozygous mutation of β-actin associated with neutrophil dysfunction and recurrent infection. Proc Natl Acad Sci USA 96:8693–8698, 1999.

Ochs HD, Igo RP. The NBT slide test: a simple screening method for detecting chronic granulomatous disease and female carriers. J Pediatr 83:77–82, 1973.

Ohno Y, Gallin JI. Diffusion of extracellular hydrogen peroxide into intracellular compartments of human neutrophils. Studies utilizing the inactivation of myeloperoxidase by hydrogen peroxide and azide. J Biol Chem 260:8438–8446, 1985.

Okuda T, Yasuoka T, Oka N. Myeloperoxidase deficiency as a predisposing factor for deep mucocutaneous candidiasis: a case report. J Oral Maxillofac Surg 49:183–186, 1991.

Ozsahin H, von Planta M, Muller I, Steinert HC, Nadal D, Lauener R, Tuchschmid P, Willi UV, Ozsahin M, Crompton NE, Seger RA. Successful treatment of invasive aspergillosis in chronic granulomatous disease by bone marrow transplantation, granulocyte colony-stimulating factor-mobilized granulocytes, and liposomal amphotericin-B. Blood 92:2719–2724, 1998.

Page RC, Beatty P, Waldrop TC. Molecular basis for the functional abnormality in neutrophils from patients with generalized prepuberal periodontitis. J Periodontal Res 22:182–183, 1987.

Palestine AG, Meyers SM, Fauci AS, Gallin JI. Ocular findings in patients with neutrophil dysfunction. Am J Ophthalmol 95:598–604, 1983.

Palmer SE, Stephens K, Dale DC. Genetics, phenotype, and natural history of autosomal dominant cyclic hematopoiesis. Am J Med Genet 66:413–422, 1996.

Parker RI, McKeown LP, Gallin JI, Gralnick HR. Absence of the largest platelet-von Willebrand multimers in a patient with lactoferrin deficiency and a bleeding tendency. Thromb Haemost 67:320–324, 1992.

Parry MF, Root RK, Metcalf JA, Delaney KK, Kaplow LS, Richar WJ. Myeloperoxidase deficiency: prevalence and clinical significance. Ann Intern Med 95:293–301, 1981.

Pastural E, Barrat FJ, Dufoureq-Lagelouse R, Certain S, Sanal O, Jabado N, Seger R, Griscelli C, Fischer A, de Saint Basile G. Griscelli disease maps to chromosome 15q21 and is associated with mutations in the myosin-Va gene. Nat Genet 16:289–292, 1997.

Phillips ML, Schwartz BR, Etzioni A, Bayer R, Ochs HD, Paulson JC. Neutrophil adhesion deficiency syndrome type 2. J Clin Invest 96:2898–2906, 1995.

Piedrafita FJ, Molander RB, Vansant G, Orlova EA, Pfahl M, Reynolds WF. An Alu element in the myeloperoxidase promoter contains a composite SP-1thyroid hormone–retinoic acid response element. J Biol Chem 271:14412–14420, 1996.

Polk HC Jr, Cheadle WG, Livingston DH, Rodriguez JL, Starko KM, Izu AE, et al. A randomized prospective clinical trial to determine the efficacy of interferon-gamma in severely injured patients. Am J Surg 163:191–196, 1992.

Pollock JD, Williams DA, Gifford MA, Li LL, Du X, Fisherman J, Orkin SH, Doerschuk CM, Dinauer MC. Mouse model of X-linked chronic granulomatous disease, an inherited defect in phagocyte superoxide production. Nat Genet 9:202–209, 1995.

Pretsch W, Charles DJ, Merkle S. X-linked glucose-6-phosphate dehydrogenase deficiency in Mus musculus. Biochem Genet 26:89–103, 1989.

Quie PG, Belani KK. Corticosteroids for chronic granulomatous disease. J Pediatr 111:393–3934, 1987.

Quie PG, White JG, Holmes B, Good RA. In vitro bactericidal capacity of human polymorphonuclear leukocytes: diminished activity in chronic granulomatous disease of childhood. J Clin Invest 46:668–679, 1967.

Rae J, Newburger PE, Dinauer MC, Noack D, Hopkins PJ, Kuruto R, Curnutte JT. X-Linked chronic granulomatous disease: mutations in the CYBB gene encoding the gp91-phox component of respiratory-burst oxidase. Am J Hum Genet 62:1320–1331, 1998.

Rayfield EJ, Ault MJ, Keusch GT, Brothers MJ, Nechemias C, Smith H. Infection and diabetes: the case for glucose control. Am J Med 72:439–450, 1982.

Reeves EP, Lu H, Jacobs HL, Messina CGM, Bolsover S, Gabella G, Potma EO, Warley A, Roes J, Segal AW. Killing activity of neutrophils is mediated through activation of proteases by K+ flux. Nature 416:291–297, 2002.

Repo H, Harlan JM. Mechanisms and consequences of phagocyte adhesion to endothelium. Ann Med 31:156–165, 1999.

Rex JH, Bennett JE, Gallin JI, Malech HL, Melnick DA. Normal and deficient neutrophils can cooperate to damage Aspergillus fumigatus hyphae. J Infect Dis 162:523–528, 1990.

Ristoff E, Mayatepek E, Larsson A. Long-term clinical outcome in patients with glutathione synthetase deficiency. J Pediatr 139:79–84, 2001.

Roberts AW, Kim C, Zhen L, Lowe JB, Kapur R, Petryniak B, Spaetti A, Pollock JD, Borneo JB, Bradford GB, Atkinson SJ, Dinauer MC, Williams DA. Deficiency of the hematopoietic cell-specific Rho family GTPase Rac2 is characterized by abnormalities in neutrophil function and host defense. Immunity 10:183–196, 1999.

Rodwell RL, Gray PH, Taylor KM, Minchinton R: Granulocyte colony stimulating factor treatment for alloimmune neonatal neutropenia. Arch Dis Child Fetal Neonatal Ed 75:F57–F58, 1996.

Roesler J, Curnutte JT, Rae J, Barrett D, Patino P, Chanock SJ, Goerlach A. Recombination events between the p47-phox gene and its highly homologous pseudogenes are the main cause of autosomal recessive chronic granulomatous disease. Blood 95:2150–2156, 2000.

Roos D. X-CGDbase: a database of X-CGD-causing mutations. Immunol Today 17:517–521, 1996.

Roos D, De Boer M, Kuribayashi F, Meischl C, Weening RS, Segal AW, Ahlin A, Nemet K, Hossle JP, Bernatowska-Matuszkiewicz E, Middleton-Price H. Mutations in the X-linked and autosomal recessive forms of chronic granulomatous disease. Blood 87:1663–1681, 1996.

Roos D, Van Zwieten R, Wijnen JT, Gomez-Gallego F, De Boer M, Stevens D, Pronk-Admiraal CJ, De Rijk T, Van Noorden CJ, Weening RS, Vulliamy TJ, Ploem JE, Mason PJ, Bautista JM, Khan PM, Beutler E. Molecular basis and enzymatic properties of glucose-6-phosphate dehydrogenase volendam, leading to chronic nonspherocytic anemia, granulocyte dysfunction, and increased susceptibility to infections. Blood 94:2955–2962, 1999.

Roos D, Weening RS, Voetman AA, van Schaik ML, Meehof LJ, Loos JA. Protection of phagocytic leukocytes by endogenous glutathione: studies in a family with glutathione reductase deficiency. Blood 53:851–866, 1979.

Root RK, Rosenthal AS, Balestra DJ. Abnormal bactericidal, metabolic, and lysosomal functions of Chédiak-Higashi syndrome leukocytes. J Clin Invest 51:649–665, 1972.

Rosenthal J, Thurman GW, Cusack N, Peterson VM, Malech HL, Ambruso DR. Neutrophils from patients after burn injury express a deficiency of the oxidase components p47-phox and p67-phox. Blood 88:4321–4329, 1996.

Rothbaum R, Perrault J, Vlachos A, Cipolli M, Blanche PA, Burroughs S, et al. Shwachman-Diamond syndrome: report from an international conference. J Pediatr 141:266–270, 2002.

Rowende C, Hill A. Glucose-6-phosphate dehydrogenase and malaria. J Mol Med 76:581–588, 1998.

Sanal O, Yel L, Kucukali T, Gilbert-Barnes E, Tardieu M, Tezcan I, Ersoy F, Metin A, de Saint Basile G. An allelic variant of Griscelli syndrome: presentation with severe hypotonia, mental retardation, and hypopigmentation consistent with Elejalde syndrome (neuroectodermal melanolysosomal disorder). J Neurol 247:570–572, 2000.

Sandoval C, Adams-Graves P, Parganas E, Wang W, Ihle JN. The cytoplasmic portion of the G-CSF receptor is normal in patients with Kostmann syndrome. Blood 82 (Suppl 1):185a, 1993.

Scharffetter-Kochanek K, Lu H, Norman K, Van Nood H, Munoz F, Grabbe S, McArthur M, Lorenzo I, Kaplan S, Ley K, Smith CW, Montgomery CA, Rich S, Beaudet A. Spontaneous skin ulceration and defective T cell function in CD18 null mice. J Exp Med 188:119–131, 1998.

Schuster DE, Kehrli ME, Ackerman MR, Gilbert RO. Identification and prevalence of a genetic defect that causes leukocyte adhesion deficiency in Holstein cattle. Proc Natl Acad Sci USA 89:9225–9229, 1992.

Sechler JM, Malech HL, White CJ, Gallin JI. Recombinant human interferon gamma reconstitutes defective phagocyte function in patients with chronic granulomatous disease of childhood. Proc Natl Acad Sci USA 85:4874–4878, 1988.

Segal AW. Absence of both cytochrome b-245 subunits from neutrophils in X-linked chronic granulomatous disease. Nature 326:88–91, 1987.

Segal BH, DeCarlo ES, Kwon-Chung KJ, Malech HL, Gallin JI, Holland SM. Aspergillus nidulans infection in chronic granulomatous disease. Medicine (Baltimore) 77:345–354, 1998.

Segal BH, Leto TL, Gallin JI, Malech HL, Holland SM. Genetic, biochemical, and clinical features of chronic granulomatous disease. Medicine (Baltimore) 79:170–200, 2000.

Seger RA, Gungor T, Belohradsky BH, Blanche S, Bordigoni P, Di Bartolomeo P, Flood T, Landais P, Muller S, Ozsahin H, Passwell JH, Porta F, Slavin S, Wulffraat N, Zintl F, Nagler A, Cant A, Fischer A. Treatment of chronic granulomatous disease with myeloablative conditioning and an unmodified hemopoietic allograft: a survey of the European experience, 1985–2000. Blood 100:4344–4350, 2002.

Seger R, Wildfeuer A, Frater-Schroeder M, Linnel J, Hitzig WH. Granulocyte dysfunction in transcobalamin II deficiency responding to leucovorin or hydroxycobalamin-plasma transfusion. J Inherit Metab Dis 3:3–9, 1980.

Skapek SX, Jones WS, Hoffman KM, Kuskie MR. Sinusitis and bacteremia caused by Flavobacterium meningosepticum in a sixteen-year-old with Shwachman-Diamond syndrome. Pediatr Infect Dis J 11:411–413, 1992.

Skubitz KM, Butterfield J, Ma K, Skubitz AP. Changes in neutrophil surface phenotype during hemodialysis. Inflammation 22:559–572, 1998.

Sligh JE, Hurwitz MY, Zhu C, Anderson DC, Beaudet AL. An initiation codon mutation in CD18 in association with the moderate phenotype of leukocyte adhesion deficiency. J Biol Chem 267:714–718, 1992.

Smith MA, Smith JG. The use of granulocyte colony-stimulating factor for treatment of autoimmune neutropenia. Curr Opin Hematol 8:165–169, 2001.

Smith OP, Hann IM, Chessells JM, Reeves BR, Milla P. Haematological abnormalities in Shwachman-Diamond syndrome. Br J Haematol 94:279–284, 1996.

Soderberg C, Sumitran-Karuppan S, Ljungman P, Moller E. CD13-specific autoimmunity in cytomegalovirus-infected immunocompromised patients. Transplantation 61:594–600, 1996.

Solomkin JS. Neutrophil disorders in burn injury: complement, cytokines, and organ injury. J Trauma 30:S80–S85, 1990.

Souid AK. Congenital cyclic neutropenia. Clin Pediatr (Phila) 34:151–155, 1995.

Southwick FS, Van der Meer JWM. Recurrent cystitis and bladder mass in two adults with chronic granulomatosis. Ann Intern Med 109:118–121, 1988.

Spirer Z, Weisman Y, Zakuth V, Fridkin M, Bogair N. Decreased serum tuftsin concentration in sickle cell disease. Arch Dis Child 55:566–567, 1980.

Sponseller PD, Malech HL, McCarthy EF Jr, Horowitz SF, Jaffe G, Gallin JI. Skeletal involvement in chronic granulomatous disease of childhood. J Bone Joint Surg Am 73:37–51, 1991.

Springer TA, Thompson NS, Miller LJ, Shmalstieg FC, Anderson DC. Inherited deficiency of the MAC-1, LFA-1, p150,95 glycoprotein family and its molecular basis. J Exp Med 160:1901–1918, 1984.

Spritz RA. Chédiak-Higashi syndrome. In Ochs HD, Smith CIE, Puck J, eds. Primary immunodeficiency diseases: a molecular and genetic approach. Oxford, UK, Oxford University Press, 1999, pp 389–396.

Srikantia SG, Bhaskaram C, Siva Prasad J, Krishnamachari KA. Anaemia and immune response. Lancet 1:1307–1309, 1976.

Stopyrowa J, Fyderek K, Sikorska B, Kowalczyk D, Zembala M. Chronic granulomatous disease of childhood: Gastric manifestation and response to salazosulfapyridine therapy. Eur J Pediatr 149:28–30, 1989.

Stossel TP, Root RK, Vaughan M. Phagocytosis in chronic granulomatous disease and Chédiak-Higashi syndrome. N Engl J Med 286:120–123, 1972.

Strauss RG, Bove KE, Jones JF, Mauer AM, Fulginiti VA. An anomaly of neutrophil morphology with impaired function. N Engl J Med 290:478–484, 1974.

Stroncek DF, Skubitz KM, Plachta LB, Shankar RA, Clay ME, Herman J, Fleit HB, McCullough J. Alloimmune neonatal neutropenia due to an antibody to the neutrophil Fc-gamma receptor III with maternal deficiency of CD16 antigen. Blood 77:1572–1580, 1991.

Sty JR, Chusid MJ, Babbit DP, Werlin SL. Involvement of the colon in chronic granulomatous disease of childhood. Radiology 132:618, 1979.

Summerfield JA, Ryder S, Sumiya M, Thursz M, Gorchein A, Monteil MA, Turner MW. Mannose binding protein gene mutations associated with unusual and severe infections in adults. Lancet 345:886–889, 1995.

Sung JH, Meyers JP, Stadlan EM, Cowen D, Wolf A. Neuropathological changes in Chédiak-Higashi syndrome. J Neuropathol Exp Neurol 28:86–118, 1969.

Tebbs ZSE, Gonzalez AM, Wilson RM. The role of aldose reductase inhibition in diabetic neutrophil phagocytosis and killing. Clin Exp Immunol 84:482–487, 1991.

Thomas C, Le Deist F, Cavazzana-Calvo M, Benkerrou M, Haddad E, Blanche S, Hartmann W, Friedrich W, Fischer A. Results of allogeneic bone marrow transplantation in patients with leukocyte adhesion deficiency. Blood 86:1629–1635, 1995.

Tidow N, Pilz C, Teichmann B, Muller-Brechlin A, Germanhausen M, Kasper B, Rauprich P, Sykora K-W. Clinical relevance of point mutations in the cytoplasmatic domain of the granulocyte-colony stimulating factor receptor gene in patients with severe congenital neutropenia. Blood 89:2369–2375, 1997.

Toomes C, James J, Wood AJ, Wu CL, McCormick D, Lench N, et al. Loss-of-function mutations in the cathepsin c gene result in periodontal disease and palmoplantar keratosis. Nat Genet 23:421–423, 1999.

Trevisani F, Castelli E, Foschi FG, Parazza M, Loggi E, Bertelli M, et al. Impaired tuftsin activity in cirrhosis: relationship with splenic function and clinical outcome. Gut 50:707–712, 2002.

Uyama E, Hirano T, Ito K, Nakashima H, Sugimoto M, Naito M, Uchino M, Ando M. Aduly Chédiak-Higashi syndrome presenting as Parkinsonism and dementia. Acta Neurol Scand 89:175–183, 1994.

Van Dyke TE, Warbington M, Gardner M, Offenbacher S. Neutrophil surface protein markers as indicators of defective chemotaxis in LJP. J Periodontol 61:180–184, 1990.

Van der Sande FM, Hillen HF. Correction of neutropenia following treatment with granulocyte colony-stimulating factor results in a decreased frequency of infections in Shwachman's syndrome. Neth J Med 48:92–95, 1996.

Vanholder R, Ringoir S. Infectious morbidity and defects in phagocytosis function in end-stage renal disease: a review. J Am Soc Nephrol 3:1541–1544, 1993.

Ventura A, Dragovich D, Luxardo P, Zanazzo G. Human granulocyte colony-stimulating factor (rHuG-CSF) for treatment of neutropenia in Shwachman syndrome. Haematologica 80:227–229, 1995.

Vives Corrons JL, Feliu E, Pujades MA, Cardellach F, Rozman C, Carreras A, Jou JM, Vallespi MT, Zauzu FJ. Severe glucose-6-phosphate dehydrogenase (G6PD) deficiency associated with chronic hemolytic anemia, granulocyte dysfunction and increase susceptibility to infections: description of a new molecular variant (G6PD barcelona). Blood 59:428, 1982.

Vowells SJ, Fleisher TA, Sekhsaria S, Alling DW, Maguire TE, Malech HL. Genotype-dependent variability in flow cytometric evaluation of reduced nicotinamide adenine dinucleotide phosphate oxidase function in patients with chronic granulomatous disease. J Pediatr 128:104–107, 1996.

Vowells SJ, Sekhsaria S, Malech HL, Shalit M, Fleisher TA. Flow cytometric analysis of the granulocyte respiratory burst: a comparison study of fluorescent probes. J Immunol Methods 178:89–97, 1995.

Walther MM, Malech HL, Berman A, Choyke P, Venzon DJ, Linehan WM, Gallin JI. The urologic manifestations of chronic granulomatous disease. J Urol 147:1314–1318, 1992.

Weber ML, Abela A, de Repentigny L, Garel L, Lapointe N. Myeloperoxidase deficiency with extensive candidal osteomyelitis of the base of the skull. Pediatrics 80:876–879, 1987.

Weinrauch Y, Drujan D, Shapiro SD, Weiss J, Zychlinsky A. Neutrophil elastase targets virulence factors of enterobacteria. Nature 417:91–94, 2002.

Werlin SL, Chusid MJ, Caya J, Oechler HW. Colitis in chronic granulomatous disease. Gastroenterology 82:328–331, 1982.

Wetzler M, Talpaz M, Kleinerman ES, King A, Huh YO, Gutterman JU, Kurzrock R. A new familial immunodeficiency disorder characterized by severe neutropenia, a defective marrow release mechanism and hypogammaglobulinemia. Am J Med 89:663–672, 1990.

Williams DA, Tao W, Yang F, Kim C, Gu Y, Mansfield P, Levine J, Petryniak B, Derrow C, Harris C, Jia B, Zheng Y, Ambruso D, Lowe J, Atkinson SJ, Dinauer M, Boxer L. Dominant negative mutation of the hematopoietic-specific Rho GTPase, Rac2, is associated with a human phagocyte immunodeficiency. Blood 96:1646–1654, 2000.

Williamson PR, Kwon-Chung KJ, Gallin JI. Successful treatment of *Paecilomyces varioti* infection in a patient with chronic granulomatous disease and a review of *Paecilomyces* species infections. *Clin Infect Dis* 5:1023–1026, 1992.

Wilson JM, Ping AJ, Krauss JC, Mayo-Bond L, Rogers CE, Anderson DC, Todd RF. Correction of CD18-deficient lymphocytes by retrovirus-mediated gene transfer. Science 248:1413–1416, 1990.

Wilson RW, Ballangtyne CM, Smith CW, Montgomery C, Bradley A, O'Brien WE, Beaudet AL. Gene targeting yields a CD18-mutant mouse for study of inflammation. J Immunol 151:1571–1578, 1993.

Winkelstein JA, Marino MC, Johnston RB Jr, Boyle J, Curnutte J, Gallin JI, Malech HL, Holland SM, Ochs HD, Quie P, Buckley RH, Foster CB, Chanock SJ, Dickler H. Chronic granulomatous disease. Report on a national registry of 368 patients. Medicine (Baltimore) 79:155–169, 2000.

Wolff SM, Dale DC, Clark RA, Root RK, Kimball HR. The Chédiak-Higashi syndrome: studies of host defense. Ann Intern Med 76:293–306, 1972.

Wright AH, Douglass WA, Taylor GM, Lau YL, Higginns D, Davis KA, Law SKA. Molecular characterization of leukocyte adhesion deficiency in six patients. Eur J Immunol 25:717–722, 1995.

Wright DG, Dale DC, Fauci AS, Wolff SM. Human cyclic neutropenia: clinical review and long-term follow-up of patients. Medicine (Baltimore) 60:1–13, 1981.

Wu CY, Ferrante J, Gately MK, Magram J. Characterization of IL-12 receptor beta1 chain (IL-12Rbeta1) deficient mice: IL-12Rbeta1 is an essential component of the functional mouse IL-12R. J Immunol 159:1658–1665, 1997.

Yamanaka R, Barlow C, Lekstrom-Himes J, Castilla LH, Liu PP, Eckhaus M, Decker T, Wynshaw-Boris A, Xanthopoulos KG. Impaired granulopoiesis, myelodysplasia, and early lethality in CCAAT/enhancer binding protein epsilon-deficient mice. Porc Natl Acad Sci USA 94:13187–13192, 1997.

Yamanaka R, Kim GD, Radomska HS, Lekstrom-Himes J, Smith LT, Antonson P, Tenen DG, Xanthopoulos KG. CCAAT/enhancer binding protein epsilon is preferentially up-regulated during granulocytic differentiation and its functional versatility is determined by alternative use of promoters and differential splicing. Proc Natl Acad Sci USA 94:6462–6467, 1994.

Ziedler C, Boxer L, Dale DC, Freedman MH, Kinsey S, Welte K. Management of Kostmann syndrome in the G-CSF era. Br J Hematol 109:490–495, 2000.

Zoli G, Corazza GR, Wood S, Bartoli R, Gasbarrini G, Farthing MJ. Impaired splenic function and tuftsin deficiency in patients with intestinal failure and long term intravenous nutrition. Gut 43:759–762, 1998.

C H A P T E R

21

Deficiencies of the Complement System

Kathleen E. Sullivan and Jerry A. Winkelstein

GENERAL CONSIDERATIONS

The complement system is composed of a series of plasma proteins and cellular receptors that play an important role in host defense, inflammation, immune complex clearance, induction of a normal humoral immune response, and clearance of apoptotic cells (see Chapter 7).

The first individual with a complement deficiency was described in 1960 (Silverstein, 1960). Since then, deficiencies of nearly all of the components of the complement system have been described. Most are inherited as autosomal recessive traits (Table 21-1); the only exceptions are C1 esterase inhibitor (C1 INH) deficiency, which is inherited as an autosomal dominant fashion, and properdin deficiency, which is inherited as an X-linked recessive fashion.

The clinical expressions of complement deficiencies include an increased susceptibility to infection, rheumatic disease, and angioedema (see Table 21-1). In addition, some patients with complement deficiencies are relatively asymptomatic and have been identified through family studies. In most instances, the nature of the clinical expression relates to the role of the deficient component in normal physiology and the pathophysiologic consequences of its absence. The pathophysiologic bases for two of the clinical expressions, infection and rheumatic diseases, are reasonably well understood.

Infections in Complement Deficiencies

An increased susceptibility to infection is a prominent clinical finding in some patients with complement deficiencies (Figueroa and Densen, 1991; Ross and Densen, 1984). Although studies in experimental animals have shown that complement contributes to the host's defense against a wide variety of bacteria, fungi, and viruses, clinical observations in complement-deficient humans indicates that their greatest susceptibility is to bacterial infections (Figueroa and Densen, 1991; Ross and Densen, 1984).

The kinds of bacteria that most commonly cause infection in a specific deficiency, however, reflect the biologic functions of the missing component. For example, C3 is an important opsonin in both the nonimmune and immune host (Johnston et al., 1969; Winkelstein et al., 1975). Therefore patients with a deficiency of C3, or with a deficiency of a component in the pathways necessary for the activation of C3, have an increased susceptibility to encapsulated bacteria for which opsonization is the primary host defense (e.g., the pneumococcus and *Haemophilus influenzae*).

This is reflected in two comprehensive reviews of complement-deficient patients, in which nearly 80% of the C3-deficient individuals had significant infections, 42% of the C1-deficient individuals had significant infections, 33% of the C4-deficient individuals had significant infections, and 50% of the C2-deficient individuals had significant infections (Figueroa and Densen, 1991; Ross and Densen, 1984).

TABLE 21-1 · HUMAN COMPLEMENT DEFICIENCY DISEASES

Component Deficient	Inheritance	Major Clinical Expression
Classical Pathway		
C1q	AR	Rheumatic disorders and pyogenic infections
C1r/s	AR	Rheumatic disorders
C4	AR	Rheumatic disorders and pyogenic infections
C2	AR	Rheumatic disorders and pyogenic infections
Alternative Pathway		
Factor D	AR	Meningococcal/pneumococcal sepsis
C3 and Terminal Components		
C3	AR	Pyogenic infections and rheumatic disorders
C5	AR	Meningococcal sepsis and meningitis
C6	AR	Meningococcal sepsis and meningitis
C7	AR	Meningococcal sepsis and meningitis
C8	AR	Meningococcal sepsis and meningitis
C9	AR	Meningococcal sepsis and meningitis
Control Proteins		
C1 inhibitor	AD	Angioedema
C4 binding protein		Behçet's disease and angioedema
Factor H	AR	Hemolytic uremic syndrome
Factor I	AR	Pyogenic infections
Properdin	XLR	Meningococcal sepsis and meningitis
Membrane/Receptor Proteins		
Decay-accelerating factor (CD55)	AR	Inab phenotype

AD = autosomal dominant; AR = autosomal recessive; XLR = X-linked recessive.

Patients with deficiencies of C1, C4, or C2 had a lower prevalence of infection, presumably because their alternative pathway is intact and able to activate C3. In vitro studies of serum opsonizing activity in C2- and C4-deficient patients have shown that they are able to generate serum opsonizing activity through the alternative pathway but more slowly and to a lesser degree than subjects with an intact classical pathway (Clark and Klebanoff, 1978; Repine et al., 1977).

The terminal components, C5 to C9, form the membrane attack complex and are therefore responsible for the bactericidal and bacteriolytic functions of complement. Patients with deficiencies of C5 to C9 can opsonize bacteria normally because they possess C3 and the components necessary for its activation. Thus these patients are not unduly susceptible to infection by bacteria for which opsonization is the primary host defense, such as the pneumococcus. These patients are, however, markedly susceptible to *Neisseria* species, because serum bactericidal activity is an important host defense against these organisms. Interestingly, although a variety of other gram-negative bacteria are susceptible to the bactericidal activity of the complement system in vitro, the increased susceptibility of patients with deficiencies of terminal components is limited to *Neisseria* (Figueroa and Densen, 1991; Ross and Densen, 1984).

Although blood-borne infections such as bacteremia, sepsis, and meningitis are the most common infections in patients with complement deficiencies (Figueroa and Densen, 1991; Ross and Densen, 1984), localized infections such as sinusitis and pneumonia have also been reported. Not only do patients with complement deficiencies have an increased frequency of infections, but the infections may also have features that differ from those in the normal population. For example, systemic blood-borne infections with *unencapsulated* bacteria are extremely rare in normal hosts. However, sepsis and meningitis caused by unencapsulated "avirulent" meningococci have occurred in complement-deficient individuals (Hummell et al., 1987; Kemp et al., 1985). Similarly, *Neisseria* infections caused by uncommon serotypes are more prevalent in complement-deficient patients (Figueroa and Densen, 1991; Platanoff et al., 1993; Ross and Densen, 1984). In addition, systemic meningococcal disease may have less morbidity and lower mortality in complement-deficient individuals (Figueroa and Densen, 1991; Platanoff et al., 1993; Ross and Densen, 1984).

Rheumatic Diseases in Complement Deficiencies

Patients with complement deficiencies also have a variety of clinical conditions that can best be characterized as rheumatic disorders (Figueroa and Densen, 1991; Ross and Densen, 1984). The pathophysiologic basis for this may relate to a number of different normal functions of the complement system. For example, the complement system has the potential to play a significant role in host defense against viral infections (Hirsch, 1982), and in some instances the rheumatic disorders seen in complement-deficient patients might be the consequence of an altered host response to recurrent or chronic viral infections. However, complement-deficient individuals do not appear to have an increased susceptibility to viral infections (Figueroa and Densen, 1991; Ross and Densen, 1984).

Second, the genes for three of the individual components of complement (C4, C2, and factor B) are located within the major histocompatibility complex (MHC) and are in linkage disequilibrium with specific human leukocyte antigen (HLA) haplotypes (Colten, 1986). Thus the rheumatic disorders seen in complement-deficient patients may be due in part to specific alleles of other genes within the MHC that influence immune function or antigen presentation, rather than to the deficiency in complement itself. However, it should also be noted that rheumatic diseases occur frequently in C3 deficiency, a component that is not linked to any other known genes influencing immune function.

Third, because the complement system is important in the generation and expression of an adequate antibody response (Dempsey et al., 1996; Ochs et al., 1983; O'Neill et al., 1988) and is required for tolerance (Prodeus et al., 1998), the rheumatic diseases seen in complement-deficient patients could result from disordered humoral immunity.

Role of Immune Complexes

One attractive hypothesis to explain the relationship between early complement component deficiencies and rheumatic diseases, such as lupus, has to do with the different roles of the complement system in the processing and clearance of immune complexes. A number of different mechanisms exist by which the complement system processes immune complexes. For example, the activation of C3 retards the precipitation of immune complexes from serum and helps solubilize them once they have formed (Miller and Nussenzweig, 1975; Schifferli et al., 1980).

In addition, primates possess the CR1 receptor for C3b on their erythrocytes (Fearon, 1980), and circulating immune complexes bearing C3b will fix to erythrocytes through these receptors (Cornacoff et al., 1983). The erythrocyte-bound immune complexes are then transported to the liver and spleen, where they are transferred to reticuloendothelial cells and the erythrocytes are returned to the circulation (Cornacoff et al., 1983). In this manner, erythrocytes serve to capture immune complexes, prevent their deposition in organs such as the kidney, and enhance their clearance by organs of the reticuloendothelial system.

For any given complement component deficiency, there is an excellent correlation between the patient's susceptibility to rheumatic diseases and the inability of the patient to process immune complexes normally. For example, the prevalence of rheumatic disorders is highest in those patients with deficiencies of the classical activating pathway (C1, C4, and C2) and of C3; approximately 80% of patients with C4 or C3 deficiency and slightly more than 30% of patients with C2 deficiency have had a rheumatic disorder (Figueroa and Densen, 1991; Ross and Densen, 1984).

In contrast, less than 10% of patients with deficiencies of terminal complement components have rheumatic disorders (Figueroa and Densen, 1991; Ross and Densen, 1984). As expected, serum from patients with genetically determined deficiencies of C1q, C4, C2, and C3 fails to prevent the precipitation of immune complexes as they are forming (Schifferli et al., 1980, 1985), has a reduced ability to resolubilize complexes once they have formed (Czop and Nussenzweig, 1976; Schifferli et al., 1985; Takahashi et al., 1978), and does not support the binding of preformed immune complexes to CR1 receptors on human erythrocytes (Paccaud et al., 1987).

In contrast, the sera of patients with deficiencies of terminal components (C5 to C9) are normal with respect to these activities. In addition, a C2-deficient individual has been shown to have markedly diminished binding of radiolabeled immune complexes to erythrocytes in vivo and impaired splenic uptake of the complexes, both of which normalized after C2 repletion, indicating a direct role of the complement deficiency in the faulty clearance of the immune complexes (Davies et al., 1993).

Role of Apoptotic Cells

Another hypothesis to explain the occurrence of rheumatic diseases in patients with deficiencies of early components of the classical pathway relates to their role, especially that of C1q, in the clearance of apoptotic cells (Botto et al., 1998; Navratil and Ahearn, 2000). As cells undergo apoptosis, intracellular constituents are reorganized and appear on the surface of the cell in blebs. Autoantigens targeted in patients with systemic lupus erythematosus (SLE), such as SSA and/or SSB, are often found on the surface in these blebs (Casciolo-Rosen et al., 1994), rendering a normally "invisible" antigen "visible." In addition, modification of proteins through cleavage or covalent binding may reveal cryptic epitopes.

Murine models support the importance of apoptotic body clearance in the prevention of lupus because defects in clearance mechanisms of apoptotic bodies, including absence of C1q, result in a murine disorder resembling lupus (Mohan, 2001). Although C2, C4, and C3 knockout mice do not have the same lupus-like phenotype as C1q knockout mice, it may be that additional background genes are required for the defect to become manifest. C3 and C4 also bind apoptotic cells, but it is not known whether they are required for clearance.

Types of Rheumatic Diseases in Complement Deficiencies

The rheumatic diseases seen in complement-deficient patients include SLE, discoid lupus, dermatomyositis, scleroderma, anaphylactoid purpura, vasculitis, and membranoproliferative glomerulonephritis (Figueroa and Densen, 1991; Ross and Densen, 1984). SLE is by far the most common rheumatic disease seen in patients with complement component deficiencies. There are some interesting and important differences between the rheumatic diseases seen in complement-deficient patients and their counterparts in non–complement-deficient individuals.

For example, the SLE seen in C2-deficient patients is frequently associated with photosensitive dermatitis. It is not uncommon for C2-deficient patients to have low (or absent) titers of antibodies to nuclear antigen and/or native DNA (Glass et al., 1976; Meyer et al., 1985; Provost et al., 1983). In contrast, the prevalence of anti-Ro antibodies in C2-deficient patients with lupus is much higher than in non–C2-deficient patients with lupus (Glass et al., 1976; Meyer et al., 1985; Provost et al., 1983). Patients deficient in C1 or C4 also have an earlier onset with prominent cutaneous manifestations but are more likely to have the usual array of autoantibodies and the classic end-organ effects of SLE such as cerebritis and nephritis (Bowness et al., 1994; Fredrikson et al., 1991; Walport et al., 1998; Welch et al., 1995).

Epidemiologic Studies of Complement Deficiency

There have been a number of studies performed to assess how often complement deficiencies occur within certain populations and to determine the utility of routine screening for these disorders.

Complement Defects in Specific Infections

A number of studies have examined the prevalence of complement deficiencies in patients with specific infections. Screening all patients with systemic blood-borne pneumococcal, streptococcal, or *H. influenzae* infections for complement deficiencies has not demonstrated significant rates of complement deficiency (Densen et al., 1990; Edkahl et al., 1995; Ernst et al., 1997; Rasmussen et al., 1987; Rowe et al., 1989).

The largest of these studies demonstrated only a single complement-deficient patient in 389 patients with bacteremia and/or meningitis caused by bacteria other than the meningococcus (Densen et al., 1990). The other studies found no evidence of complement deficiency in similar series ranging from 77 to 209 pediatric and/or adult patients with bacteremia or bacterial meningitis (Edkahl et al., 1995; Ernst et al., 1997; Rasmussen et al., 1987; Rowe et al., 1989).

Therefore screening of patients with a single episode of bacteremia or bacterial meningitis has not been recommended. However, a history of a blood-borne infection in a patient with autoimmune disease might warrant an evaluation for complement deficiency.

In contrast to the rarity of complement deficiencies in patients with blood-borne pneumococcal or *H. influenzae* infections, the frequency of complement deficiencies in sporadic cases of systemic meningococcal infections has been estimated to be as high as 15% (Ellison et al., 1983; Leggiadro et al., 1987; Merino et al., 1983; Platanov et al., 1993; Rasmussen et al., 1987). The prevalence is even greater in those patients who have had recurrent meningococcal disease (40%) (Nielsen et al., 1989b;

Platonov et al., 1993), a positive family history of meningococcal disease (10%) (Nielsen et al., 1989b), or an unusual serotype of the meningococcus (20% to 50%) (Fijen et al., 1989). Thus in the absence of an epidemic, it appears reasonable to screen any patient with a systemic meningococcal infection for a complement deficiency.

Complement Defects in Rheumatic Disorders

Relatively few studies have examined the frequency of complement deficiencies in rheumatic disorders. Genetically determined C2 deficiency is found in approximately 1:10,000 (0.01%) individuals in the general population (Ruddy, 1986; Sullivan et al., 1994). However, it is much more common in SLE populations with a prevalence of homozygous C2 deficiency between 0.4% and 2.0% (Glass et al., 1976; Hartung et al., 1989; Sullivan et al., 1994). C2 deficiency is associated with other rheumatic diseases as well (Figueroa and Densen, 1991; Ross and Densen, 1984), although there have been no studies documenting specific prevalence rates.

The most common complement deficiency associated with rheumatic disorders is a deficiency of one of the isotypes of C4. The fourth component of human complement is encoded by two closely linked genes, *C4A* and *C4B*, on the sixth chromosome (Carroll et al., 1984). The two isotypes of C4, C4A and C4B, are structurally very similar, but differences in a few amino acids are responsible for differences in certain specific antigenic determinants, electrophoretic mobility, and specific functional activity (Isenman and Young, 1984; Law et al., 1984) (see C4 deficiency in this chapter). Individuals who are homozygous deficient for one, but not the other, isotype are relatively common in the general population; approximately 1% of unselected individuals are C4A deficient and 3% are C4B deficient (Awdeh and Alper, 1978; O'Neill et al., 1978a).

A number of studies have shown that the prevalence of both homozygous and heterozygous C4A deficiency is increased in patients with lupus (Christiansen et al., 1983; DeJuan et al., 1993; Fiedler et al., 1983; Howard et al., 1986). Interestingly, some of the clinical features of lupus appear to be different in patients who are C4A deficient than in patients with lupus who are not (see C4 deficiency in this chapter).

It is difficult to know whether it is worthwhile to screen all patients with SLE for complement deficiencies. However, based on these studies, screening SLE patients, or patients with other rheumatic diseases, for complement deficiencies who have a positive family history of SLE, a history of recurrent infections, or atypical laboratory or clinical features appears to be reasonable.

Animal Models of Genetic Complement Deficiencies

For nearly 100 years, animal models of complement deficiency have been used to gain insight into the role of complement in normal physiology. The first naturally occurring animal with a genetically determined complement deficiency was described in 1919 and most probably had C3 deficiency (Moore, 1919). Subsequently, animals deficient in C4 (guinea pigs) (Ellman et al., 1970), C2 (guinea pigs) (Bottger et al., 1985), C3 (dogs) (Winkelstein et al., 1981), and C5 (mice) (Rosenberg and Tachibana, 1962) were discovered. Studies using these naturally occurring complement-deficient animals provided important information on the role of complement in host defense (Hammer et al., 1981; Hosea et al., 1980a; Winkelstein et al., 1975), inflammation (Hammer et al., 1981), modulation of antibody production (Ochs et al., 1983; O'Neil et al., 1988), rheumatic diseases (Bottger et al., 1986), and shock (Quezada et al., 1998).

Genetically engineered mice, so-called knockout mice, represent an opportunity to study the role of individual complement components in a variety of physiologic processes while controlling for any differences that might be attributable to differences in species. One of the more important contributions of knockout mice has been the insight that they have provided regarding the role of complement in antibody production (Fischer et al., 1996). The C3d cleavage product is an important co-stimulatory molecule for B cells (Dempsey et al., 1996). In the absence of C3, less antibody is made and the ability to sustain responsiveness is impaired. C3 knockout mice are more severely compromised than C4 knockout mice because the latter are capable of activating C3 through the alternative pathway and the mannose-binding lectin pathway.

Mice have a single gene product corresponding to the human CR1 and CR2 receptors. When this gene is knocked out, they also exhibit the defect in antibody production seen in C3 knockout mice (Ahearn et al., 1996; Molina et al., 1996). In addition, B1 B cells were decreased in one strain of CR1/2 knockout mice (Ahearn et al., 1996). The CR1/2 receptor associates with CD19 on the surface of B cells and acts as a co-stimulatory receptor. This receptor also appears to mediate antigen persistence on follicular dendritic cells that may account for the lack of persistence of antibody responses in complement-deficient mice (Fischer et al., 1998).

Knockout mice also provide insight into the role of complement in the genesis of rheumatic diseases, specifically lupus. Although a variety of rheumatic diseases are seen in patients with deficiencies of C1, C4, C2, and C3, the most striking association is with lupus (Walport et al., 1997). Furthermore, there is a gradient of association such that C1 and C4 deficiencies are most strongly associated with lupus, whereas C2 deficiency is only moderately associated with lupus and C3 deficiency even less so (Walport et al., 1997). Although defective immune complex clearance has been proposed as the basis for many of the rheumatic diseases seen in patients with deficiencies of C1, C4, C2, and C3 (such as their membranoproliferative glomerulonephritis), the basis for the graded association between C1, C4, C2, and C3 deficiency has not been elucidated.

The use of knockout mice has provided important insight; although knockouts for C1, C2, C3, and C4 have been examined for lupus, only the C1q knockout mice spontaneously develop a lupus-like syndrome (Botto et al., 1998). C4 deficiency accelerates lupus in the B6/lpr lupus model and may do so by affecting tolerance (Prodeus et al., 1998). The C1q knockout mice develop glomerulonephritis and their kidneys accumulate apoptotic bodies, suggesting that the C1q deficiency predisposes to autoimmune disease because it is required for clearance of apoptotic bodies (Botto et al., 1998). When apoptotic bodies accumulate, they allow access to cellular constituents normally hidden from the immune system such as nuclear proteins and DNA. Interestingly, mice deficient in factor B are resistant to autoimmune disease (Watanabe et al., 2000).

C1q DEFICIENCY

Pathogenesis

C1q is a member of the collectin family and is expressed primarily by liver, epithelial cells, and macrophages (Reid, 1985). The C1q complex is composed of 18 polypeptide chains. Three genes on the long arm of chromosome 1 encode highly homologous proteins known as C1qA, C1qB, and C1qC (Sellar et al., 1991), and one of each of the three C1q polypeptides combines to form the C1q subunit. Six subunits combine to form the intact C1q protein that is capable of binding the CH3 domain of IgM or the CH2 domain of IgG.

The primary role of C1q is to initiate activation of the classical pathway (Porter and Reid, 1978). Engagement of at least two subunits leads to activation of C1r and subsequently to activation of C1s, which in turn activates both C4 and C2. C1q has a number of other roles that it appears to directly mediate through its interaction with one or more C1q receptors. One of these is its ability to recognize apoptotic cells and target them for clearance (Botto et al., 1998; Korb and Ahearn, 1997; Mitchell et al., 1999; Taylor et al., 2000). C1q also regulates T-cell activation via specific T-cell C1q receptors (Chen et al., 1994) and activation of polymorphonuclear leukocytes via specific neutrophil C1q receptors (Jack et al., 1994).

Two significant features that are described in C1q deficiency for which the pathogenic basis is not understood are impaired natural killer cell activity (Toth et al., 1989) and defective interferon-γ production (Cutler et al., 1998). The former phenomenon has been described in humans and the latter in mice. Therefore deficiency of C1q not only affects one's ability to activate C3 and C5 to C9 through the classical pathway and generate those biologic activities related to C3 and C5 to C9, such as opsonization, chemotaxis, and bactericidal activity, but it also may affect the activation of immunologically relevant cells and the clearance of apoptotic cells.

As expected, affected individuals have markedly reduced total hemolytic complement (CH_{50}) activity and C1 functional activity. In some individuals there is an absence of C1q protein by immunochemical analysis,

whereas in others there is some immunoreactive C1q present in the serum but it is functionally deficient (i.e., they have a dysfunctional C1q protein).

Clinical Features

Only a limited number of patients with C1q deficiency have been identified (Figueroa and Densen, 1991; Ross and Densen, 1984). The deficiency is inherited as an autosomal recessive trait. C1q deficiency is associated with both SLE and recurrent infections (Bowness et al., 1994; Figueroa and Densen, 1991; Ross and Densen, 1984). C1q deficiency is the strongest known genetic risk factor for SLE. Approximately 40 patients with C1q deficiency have been described, and 93% have developed SLE (Berkel et al., 2000; Bowness et al., 1994). The reason C1q deficiency is a more potent risk factor for SLE than the other early complement component deficiencies may relate to its unique role in the clearance of apoptotic cells.

Although deficiencies of all of the early components of the classical pathway would be expected to impair immune complex clearance, C1q deficiency also impairs the ability to clear apoptotic cells, which in turn could result in the accumulation of, and immunologic exposure to, nuclear proteins (Botto et al., 1998; Korb and Ahearn, 1997; Mitchell et al., 1999; Taylor et al., 2000).

SLE seen in patients with C1q deficiency is usually more severe than in complement-sufficient individuals and the age of onset is usually prepubertal. Anti-nuclear antibodies are positive in most cases but are often of low titer. Anti-ds DNA antibodies are typically negative, although antibodies to extractable nuclear antigens are often positive (Walport et al., 1998). The cutaneous manifestations are typically prominent, and skin biopsies demonstrate IgG, IgM, and C3 deposition, as is characteristic of SLE (Berkel et al., 2000; Bowness et al., 1994; Petry et al., 1997). The presence of C3 suggests that in C1q deficiency complement activation through the alternative pathway plays a significant role in the immunopathogenesis of the cutaneous lesions.

Patients with C1q deficiency also have an increased frequency of infections with pyogenic organisms, reflecting their inability to activate the classical pathway and efficiently opsonize bacteria. Approximately 30% suffer from significant bacterial infections and 10% of the C1q-deficient patients have died of sepsis (Walport et al., 1998).

Molecular Genetics

There are multiple mutations occurring in each of the three genes responsible for C1q deficiency (Petry, 1998). A C to T mutation in exon 2 of C1qA is responsible for the high frequency of C1q deficiency in the Turkish population (Berkel et al., 2000; Petry et al., 1996). Outside of the Turkish population, the mutations are diverse. In most patients, C1q protein is not detectable, and the mutations are typically premature stop codons

(Berkel and Nakakuma, 1993; Leyva-Cobian et al., 1981; Loos and Colomb, 1993; Stone et al., 2000). Other patients produce small or dysfunctional C1q, which can neither bind to immunoglobulin heavy chains nor activate C1r (Chapius et al., 1982; Hannema et al., 1984; Reid and Thompson, 1983; Slingsby et al., 1996; Thompson et al., 1980). These patients typically exhibit missense mutations (Berkel et al., 2000; Petry et al., 1995).

C1r AND C1s DEFICIENCY

Pathogenesis

Like most other complement components, C1r and C1s are produced primarily in liver and macrophages (Kusumoto et al., 1988). The genes for C1r and C1s are closely linked on chromosome 12p13 and encode highly homologous serine proteases (Kusumoto et al., 1988). In addition to the serine protease domain, both proteins also include epidermal growth factor domains and homologous repeat domains. The C1 complex is composed of six C1q subunits and two molecules each of C1r and C1s. It is the C1s that activates both C4 and C2 by cleavage (Porter and Reid, 1978).

Patients have markedly reduced total hemolytic complement activity (CH_{50}) and C1 functional activity. Typically, C1r levels are markedly reduced (<1% of normal) and C1s levels are 20% to 50% of normal. However, three patients have been described in whom C1s was markedly reduced, whereas C1r levels were 50% of normal (Endo et al., 1999; Suzuki et al., 1992). The fact that absence of one protein results in diminution of the other suggests that neither monomer is stable in the absence of the other.

Clinical Features

Only a few individuals with combined C1r or C1s deficiency have been described (Chevailler et al., 1994; Ellison et al., 1987; Garty et al., 1987; Lee et al., 1978; Loos and Heinz, 1986). The deficiencies are inherited as autosomal recessive traits. The most common clinical presentations of C1r and C1s deficiency have been SLE or complex autoimmune processes, although bacterial infections and glomerulonephritis are also common in this patient population (Figueroa and Densen, 1991; Ross and Densen, 1984). One patient died of a virus-associated hemophagocytic syndrome (Endo et al., 1999).

Molecular Genetics

Three mutations have been found in C1s deficiency, a 4 base-pair (bp) deletion in exon 10, a nonsense mutation in exon 12, and a nonsense mutation in exon 12 (Dragon-Durey et al., 2001; Endo et al., 1999; Inoue et al., 1998). The mutations responsible for C1r deficiency have not been identified. However, 7 of the first 12 patients with C1r deficiency have been of Puerto Rican descent, suggesting they may be the descendants of a single individual who carried the mutation.

C2 DEFICIENCY

Pathogenesis

The C2 gene is similar in structure to the closely linked factor B gene, both of which are located within the MHC on chromosome 6 (Carroll et al., 1984; Ishikawa et al., 1990). Like C4, C2 is cleaved by C1s into two polypeptides of unequal size, the larger of which, C2a, can combine with C4b to create the bimolecular C3 cleaving enzyme of the classical pathway, C4b2a.

Like most of the other deficiencies of individual components of complement, C2 deficiency is inherited as an autosomal recessive trait. Individuals homozygous for C2 deficiency generally have less than 1% of the normal amount of C2 functional activity and undetectable C2 by standard immunochemical analysis (Ruddy et al., 1970).

Heterozygotes for C2 deficiency generally have C2 levels between 30% and 70% of the average values for normal individuals (Ruddy et al., 1970). The wide range of C2 levels in individuals who are heterozygous for C2 deficiency, and the fact that those levels may overlap the range of normal, makes identification of heterozygous status based on C2 levels alone difficult.

Complement-mediated serum activities, such as opsonization and chemotaxis, are present in patients with C2 deficiency, presumably because their alternative pathway is intact (Friend et al., 1975; Johnson FR et al., 1971; Sampson et al., 1982). However, these activities are not generated as quickly or to the same degree as in individuals with an intact classical pathway (Friend et al., 1975; Geibink et al., 1977; Johnston et al., 1969; Repine et al., 1977).

Clinical Features

Genetically determined C2 deficiency is the most common inherited complement deficiency, occurring in 1:10,000 whites (Ruddy, 1986; Sullivan et al., 1994). The clinical manifestations of C2 deficiency have varied and have included individuals who are clinically affected with either rheumatic diseases and/or an increased susceptibility to infection and asymptomatic individuals (Figueroa and Densen, 1991; Ross and Densen, 1984; Ruddy, 1986). Whether the patient expresses rheumatic diseases or an increased susceptibility to infection does not appear to be determined by linked MHC class I or class II genes (Johnson, 1992; Sullivan et al., 1994; Truedsson et al., 1993b).

Approximately 40% of C2-deficient individuals develop SLE or discoid lupus. The association of C2 deficiency with SLE is believed to be due to the compromise in immune complex clearance that results when C2 is deficient (Davies et al., 1993; Garred et al., 1990).

Normalization of serum complement by the administration of fresh frozen plasma has returned immune complex clearance to normal in C2-deficient patients (Davies et al., 1993). Some individuals have advocated the use of fresh frozen plasma for the treatment of SLE in complement-deficient patients (Steinsson et al., 1989).

Patients with C2 deficiency express many of the characteristic features of lupus, although severe nephritis, cerebritis, and aggressive arthritis are less common than in complement-sufficient SLE patients (Figueroa and Densen, 1991; Ross and Densen, 1984). Cutaneous lesions are common in C2-deficient patients with lupus and many have a characteristic annular photosensitive rash. Patients with C2 deficiency and SLE have a lower prevalence of anti-DNA antibodies than other SLE patients (Glass et al., 1976; Lipsker et al., 2000; Meyer et al., 1985; Provost et al., 1983), but their incidence of anti-Ro antibodies is higher (Lipsker et al., 2000; Meyer et al., 1985; Provost et al., 1983).

Other rheumatic disorders have also been described in C2 deficiency, including glomerulonephritis, inflammatory bowel disease, dermatomyositis, anaphylactoid purpura, and vasculitis (Friend et al., 1975; Gelfand et al., 1975; Kim et al., 1977; Leddy et al., 1975; Perlemuter et al., 1996; Ruddy, 1986).

Approximately 50% of C2-deficient patients have an increased susceptibility to bacterial infections. The infections are usually blood-borne and systemic (e.g., sepsis, meningitis, arthritis, and osteomyelitis), and caused by encapsulated organisms (e.g., pneumococcus, *H. influenzae,* and meningococcus) (Fasano et al., 1990; Figueroa and Densen, 1991; Hyatt et al., 1981; Newman et al., 1978; Ross and Densen, 1984; Ruddy, 1986).

It is unclear whether patients who are heterozygous for C2 deficiency have any clinical manifestations. An early study demonstrated an increased frequency of heterozygous C2 deficiency in SLE and juvenile rheumatoid arthritis (Glass et al., 1976). However, assignment of a given individual as heterozygous for C2 deficiency was based on serum levels of C2 and HLA haplotype. More recently, polymerase chain reaction (PCR) detection of the characteristic 28-bp deletion in ethnically and geographically matched SLE patients and controls found no increased frequency of C2 heterozygotes in SLE (Sullivan et al., 1994). However, a recent study suggested that heterozygous C2 deficiency in combination with C4 null alleles could be associated with an increased predisposition to SLE (Hartmann et al., 1997).

Molecular Genetics

The gene for C2 deficiency (C2*QO) is closely linked to genes of the MHC, and it is in linkage disequilibrium with specific alleles of the MHC (Awdeh et al., 1981; Day et al., 1975; Fu et al., 1975; Glass et al., 1976; Hauptmann et al., 1982; Rynes et al., 1982; Wolski et al., 1975). More than 95% of C2-deficient individuals are homozygous for a 28-bp deletion at the 3' end of

exon 6, which results in premature termination of transcription (Johnson et al., 1992; Sullivan et al., 1994; Truedsson et al., 1993a). The 28-bp deletion is associated with a conserved MHC haplotype consisting of HLA-B18, C2*QO, Bf*S, C4A*4, C4B*2, and DR*2 (Johnson et al., 1992; Sullivan et al., 1994; Truedsson et al., 1993a, 1993b). The gene frequency of this deletion has been found to be 0.005 to 0.007 in whites, which translates into a frequency of homozygous deficients of approximately 1:10,000 (Johnson et al., 1992; Sullivan et al., 1994; Truedsson et al., 1993b). In addition to the common 28-bp deletion, two different missense mutations have been identified that result in impaired secretion of mature C2 (Wetzel et al., 1996), and a 2-bp deletion has been found that results in a premature stop codon (Wang et al., 1998).

C3 DEFICIENCY

Pathogenesis

The human C3 gene consists of 41 exons spanning 42 kB (Vik et al., 1991) on chromosome 19 (Whitehead et al., 1982). Serum C3 is synthesized primarily in hepatocytes (Alper et al., 1969; Morris et al., 1982; Ramadori et al., 1985), although monocytes, fibroblasts, endothelium, and epithelial cells also produce C3 (Colten, 1992). Activation of C3, through either the classical pathway or alternative pathway, generates two cleavage products, C3a and C3b. The smaller product, C3a, possesses anaphylatoxic activity, and the larger product possesses opsonic activity. In addition, C3b is an important component of the C5 cleaving enzymes of the classical and alternative pathways and thus is integral to the generation of C5a-mediated anaphylatoxic and chemotactic activities and C5b- to C9-mediated cytolytic and bactericidal activities.

Affected individuals have severely depressed levels of serum C3 (<1% of normal) and markedly reduced total hemolytic activity (Singer et al., 1994). In some patients, a small amount of C3 antigen and function can be detected using highly sensitive techniques (Davis et al., 1977), whereas in others, no C3 protein is detected even when using extremely sensitive assays (Botto et al., 1990). Those serum functions either directly dependent on C3 or indirectly dependent on C3 because of its role in the activation of C5 to C9 are also markedly reduced. Serum opsonic, chemotactic, and bactericidal activities are either absent or markedly diminished in patients with C3 deficiency (Alper et al., 1976; Ballow et al., 1975; Botto et al., 1990; Davis et al., 1977; Hsieh et al., 1981; Osofsky et al., 1977; Pussell et al., 1980; Roord et al., 1983; Sano et al., 1981).

Clinical Features

Genetically determined C3 deficiency is inherited as an autosomal recessive trait (Figueroa and Densen, 1991; Ross and Densen, 1984; Singer et al., 1994). This genetic defect, although relatively rare, has been observed in many different ethnic groups throughout the world. An increased susceptibility to infection is the most common clinical finding in C3-deficient individuals (Figueroa and Densen, 1991; Ross and Densen, 1984; Singer et al., 1994). Infections have included pneumonia, bacteremia, meningitis, and osteomyelitis and are usually caused by encapsulated pyogenic bacteria, such as the pneumococcus, *H. influenzae,* and the meningococcus (Alper et al., 1972; Ballow et al., 1975; Botto et al., 1990; Davis et al., 1977; Figueroa and Densen, 1991; Grace et al., 1976; Hsieh et al., 1981; Roord et al., 1983; Ross and Densen, 1984; Sano et al., 1981; Singer et al., 1994). Patients tend to present early in life with recurrent severe infections.

Approximately 25% of C3-deficient patients develop rheumatic diseases (Figueroa and Densen, 1991; Ross and Densen, 1984; Singer et al., 1994). A number of patients have presented with a syndrome characterized by arthralgias and vasculitic skin rashes that resembles serum sickness and is frequently precipitated by an acute intercurrent illness (Osofsky et al., 1977; Roord et al., 1983). Some patients have developed a clinical picture consistent with SLE (Roord et al., 1983), although isolated glomerulonephritis is more common. Interestingly, although certain clinical features of lupus are present in some patients with C3 deficiency, as with some other complement-deficient patients, they may not have serologic evidence of lupus.

Renal disease has also been seen in C3-deficient patients (Berger et al., 1983; Borzy and Houghton, 1985; Pussell et al., 1980). Histologically, the lesions most closely resemble membranoproliferative glomerulonephritis with mesangial cell proliferation, an increased mesangial matrix, and electron-dense deposits in both the mesangium and the subendothelium of capillary loops (Berger et al., 1983; Borzy and Houghton, 1985).

Immunofluorescent studies have revealed all major immunoglobulin classes to be present but no C3. In some cases of renal disease, as well as in some of the cases of vasculitis or lupus in which there was no apparent renal disease, circulating immune complexes are found in the serum (Berger et al., 1983; Roord et al., 1983; Sano et al., 1981). The renal disease may reflect the role of C3 in immune complex clearance. For this reason, administration of fresh frozen plasma to replace C3 has been advocated as a treatment for the renal disease. However, evidence from C3-deficient dogs with membranoproliferative glomerulonephritis suggests that supplying C3 after the renal disease has occurred may make the glomerulonephritis worse (Cork et al., 1991).

Molecular Genetics

The molecular genetic defect in C3 deficiency has been identified in a limited number of patients. A single C3-deficient patient was found to have a mutation in the 5' donor splice site of intron 18, resulting in a premature stop codon (Botto et al., 1992). A second C3-deficient patient has a donor splice site mutation in intron 10 (Huang et al., 1994). In a third patient, a point mutation in exon 13 causes an amino acid change that blocks the maturation of intracellular pro-C3 to mature C3 (Singer et al., 1994). Finally, an Afrikaans-speaking patient was found to have an 800-bp deletion between two Alu repeats (Botto et al., 1990). This 800-bp deletion has been found with a relatively high gene frequency (0.0057) in the Afrikaans-speaking South African population (Botto et al., 1990).

C4 DEFICIENCY

Pathogenesis

The fourth component of complement is a three-chain disulfide-linked glycoprotein that is synthesized primarily in the liver. There are two loci for C4 within the MHC on chromosome 6 (O'Neill et al., 1978a). Although the products of the two loci (C4A and C4B) share functional, structural, and antigenic characteristics that identify them as C4, they differ with respect to other characteristics such as electrophoretic mobility (Awdeh and Alper, 1978), molecular weight of their alpha chain (Isenman and Young, 1984), specific epitopes (O'Neill et al., 1978b), and functional hemolytic activity (Isenman and Young, 1984; Law et al., 1984).

There are only four amino acid differences between the *C4A* and *C4B* genes (Yu et al., 1986). Activation of C4 by C1s results in the generation of a large molecular weight cleavage product C4b. The functional difference between the two isotypes relates to the different abilities of the C4b to transacylate with either hydroxyl or amino groups after activation. Nascent C4A is much more efficient than C4B in transacylating with amino groups of proteins, and nascent C4B is more efficient than C4A in transacylating with hydroxyl groups of carbohydrates (Isenman and Young, 1984; Law et al., 1984). Once activated, C4b can combine with the larger cleavage product of activated C2, C2a, to create the bimolecular C3-cleaving enzyme, C4b2a.

C4 deficiency is inherited in an autosomal recessive fashion. Patients with complete C4 deficiency (C4A*QO, C4B*QO) have severely depressed serum levels of both antigenic and functional C4 (<1%). Individuals who are heterozygous for C4 deficiency, at either or both C4 loci, as a group have serum C4 levels that generally reflect the number of active genes (Awdeh et al., 1981; Welch et al., 1985). However, assignment of a given individual as heterozygous for the deficiency is complicated by the fact that the range of C4 levels in normal individuals is quite wide and a deficiency of C4 at one or the other locus is relatively common (Awdeh and Alper, 1978; Hauptmann et al., 1988). Accordingly, assignment of an individual as heterozygous for the deficiency is usually based on kindred analysis using HLA linkage (Ochs et al., 1977), DNA Southern blot analysis (Schneider et al., 1986), or electrophoretic analysis of C4 allotypes in serum (Awdeh and Alper, 1978).

Patients with complete C4 deficiency have a markedly decreased ability to activate the classical pathway. Those serum activities that can be mediated via the alternative pathway, such as opsonic, chemotactic, and bactericidal activities, are present although usually reduced because of a lack of an intact classical pathway (Clark and Klebanoff, 1978; Mascart-Lemone et al., 1983).

Clinical Features

Complete deficiency of C4 is the result of being homozygous deficient at both the C4A and C4B locus (C4A*QO, C4B*QO) and is uncommon (Figueroa and Densen, 1991; Ross and Densen, 1984). The predominant clinical manifestation of complete C4 deficiency has been SLE (Figueroa and Densen, 1991; Hauptmann et al., 1988; Ross and Densen, 1984) (Fig. 21-1). The disease onset is usually early and cutaneous features, including photosensitive skin rash, Raynaud's phenomenon, and vasculitic ulcers, are common. Anti-DNA titers are sometimes absent as is also seen in C2-deficient patients with SLE.

Patients who have complete C4 deficiency also have an increased susceptibility to bacterial infections, probably as a consequence of impaired opsonization and possibly because of poor development of humoral immunity. Most deaths in C4-deficient patients are due to infection (Figueroa and Densen, 1991; Ross and Densen, 1984). As with many of the other complement deficiency diseases, there have also been a few asymptomatic C4-deficient patients ascertained as the result of family studies.

Although complete C4 deficiency is extremely rare, individuals who are homozygous deficient for either C4A or C4B are quite common (Awdeh and Alper, 1978; Hauptmann et al., 1988). For example, the frequency of the C4A*QO allele among whites has been estimated as between 13% and 14% and that of the C4B*QO allele as between 15% and 16%. The corre-

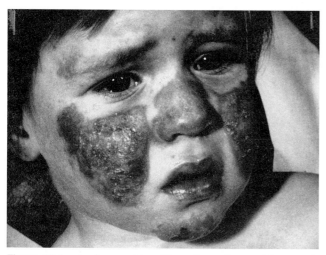

Figure 21-1 · A photosensitive skin rash consistent with systemic lupus erythematosus in a child with complete C4 deficiency. (Courtesy of Dr. Georges Hauptmann.)

sponding frequencies of homozygous null individuals at each locus would be just over 1% for C4A and just under 3% for C4B. Because of the differences in functional activity between C4A and C4B, individuals who are homozygous deficient in one or the other isotype might be predisposed to certain illnesses. For example, individuals with homozygous C4A deficiency lack the isotype that interacts most efficiently with proteins. They therefore might not be able to normally process protein-containing immune complexes and as a consequence might be at an increased risk for developing immune complex diseases such as SLE.

A number of studies have shown that the prevalence of homozygous C4A deficiency in SLE varies between 10% and 15%, a figure 10 to 15 times higher than the prevalence in the general population (Christiansen et al., 1983; Fiedler et al., 1983; Howard et al., 1986). The SLE patients with C4A deficiency appear to have a lower prevalence of anti-cardiolipin, anti-Ro, anti-dsDNA, and anti-Sm antibodies; less neurologic and renal disease; and more photosensitivity than other SLE patients (Petri et al., 1993; Welch et al., 1998).

C4A null alleles have also been associated with a variety of other autoimmune and immune complex disorders such as Henoch-Schönlein purpura, immune thrombocytopenic purpura, and celiac disease (Cahill et al., 1991; McLean et al., 1984; Nielsen et al., 1994).

Individuals with homozygous C4B deficiency lack the isotype that is most efficient in interacting with polysaccharides. They therefore may not be able to assemble the classical pathway C3 cleaving enzyme (C4b2a) and to deposit opsonically active C3b, on the polysaccharide capsules of pathogenic bacteria, thus predisposing them to blood-borne bacterial infections. There is an increased prevalence of homozygous C4B deficiency in children with bacteremia and bacterial meningitis (Biskoff et al., 1990; Rowe et al., 1989).

Molecular Genetics

C4A deficiency in whites is typically due to a large gene deletion and arises on the extended haplotype HLA-A1-Cw7-B8-C2C-BfS-C4AQ0-C4B1-DR3 (Kemp et al., 1987). In addition, a 2-bp insertion in exon 29 has been identified as the most common cause of non-expression of an intact C4A gene and is usually linked to HLA-B60-DR6 (Barba et al., 1993). Gene conversion can cause either C4A or C4B deficiency, and some C4B*Q0 alleles are the result of gene deletions (Braun et al., 1990).

C5 DEFICIENCY

Pathogenesis

C5 is transcribed from a single gene located on chromosome 9q34 and is produced primarily by hepatocytes, macrophages, alveolar epithelial cells, and lymphocytes (Carney et al., 1991; Haviland et al., 1991). When C5 is activated through either the classical or alternative pathway, two cleavage products, C5a and C5b, are generated. The smaller cleavage product C5a and its catabolite C5a (desArg) mediate their effects via a specific receptor CD88, which is expressed on cells of myeloid origin, lymphocytes, and bronchial epithelial cells (Floreani et al., 1998). Activation of this receptor is important in mediating neutrophil migration, T- and B-cell migration, and bronchial reactivity and can potentiate other inflammatory stimuli (Floreani et al., 1998; Nataf et al., 1999; Ottonello et al., 1999; Tsuji et al., 2000). C5a is the most potent endogenous neutrophil chemotactic factor (Fernandez et al., 1978). The larger cleavage product C5b initiates the formation of the membrane attack complex, which is responsible for the direct lysis of certain gram-negative bacteria such as *Neisseria*.

C5 deficiency is inherited as an autosomal recessive trait. Patients with C5 deficiency have nearly absent total hemolytic complement activity and very little C5 antigenic or functional activity in their serum. Serum chemotactic and bactericidal activities are severely compromised.

Clinical Features

C5 deficiency is not restricted to any particular geographic region or ethnicity. Although it occurs at a frequency of 1:10,000 in Japan (Fukumori et al., 1998), its frequency in other populations is not known (Figueroa and Densen, 1991; Ross and Densen 1984). The most common clinical manifestation of C5 deficiency has been an increased susceptibility to *Neisseria* infections (Figueroa and Densen, 1991; Ross and Densen 1984). A small number of C5-deficient patients have developed autoimmune disease (Figueroa and Densen, 1991; Ross and Densen, 1984; Schoonbrood et al., 1995).

Molecular Genetics

In three African-American patients, the mutations have been identified and are diverse (Wang et al., 1995); these same mutations have not been found in the four Caucasian C5-deficient patients who have been examined.

C6 DEFICIENCY

Pathogenesis

The genes for C6 and C7 lie 160 kb apart in a tail–tail orientation on chromosome 5p13 (Setien et al., 1993). C6 shares homology with C7, C8, and C9 and is a member of the channel-forming protein family (Chakravarti et al., 1989). The liver produces the majority of serum C6, but myeloid cells and fibroblasts also produce C6. C6 participates in the formation of the membrane attack complex and its highly complex structure suggests it evolved specifically to mediate pore formation (DiScipio et al., 1989).

C6 deficiency is inherited in an autosomal recessive fashion. Classic C6 deficiency is associated with a markedly low or absent CH_{50} and markedly reduced levels of C6 antigen and function. A condition designated as C6SD (for C6 subtotal deficiency) is characterized by 1% to 2% of the normal serum antigenic levels of C6 (Wurzner et al., 1995). The CH_{50} is diminished but detectable and antigenic C6 is present 1% to 2%. None of the C6SD patients has had recurrent infections (Orren et al., 1992). C6SD has also been seen in association with subtotal C7 deficiency (Fernie et al., 1996) and is the result of two independent mutations.

Clinical Features

C6 deficiency is one of the more common complement component deficiencies (Figueroa and Densen, 1991; Ross and Densen, 1984). In the United States, it is believed to occur with a frequency of 1:1600 (0.062%) in African Americans (Zhu et al., 2000). In contrast, its frequency among non-Caucasian individuals of the Western Cape province of South Africa is only 0.003% (Orren et al., 1987; Potter et al., 1990). Its prevalence in Japanese individuals is approximately 0.0027% (Inai et al., 1989). It is thought to be uncommon in whites.

C6 deficiency is most commonly associated with systemic blood-borne meningococcal infections (Figueroa and Densen, 1991; Ross and Densen et al., 1984). Disseminated gonococcal infections have also been described confirming the importance of an intact membrane attack complex in the defense against *Neisseria* organisms. Two cases of SLE and two cases of glomerulonephritis have been reported in C6-deficient patients. It is not known whether this represents a significant association or simply ascertainment bias, although there are no data to suggest that C6 deficiency in the rat predisposes to autoimmune disorders.

Molecular Genetics

The most common mutation leading to complete C6 deficiency in South Africa is a single-bp deletion at position 879 (Hobart et al., 1998). Importantly, there are multiple other mutations, and the mutations in the African population are somewhat different than those seen in the African-American population (Hobart et al., 1998; Zhu et al., 2000). Subtotal C6 deficiency is due to a loss of the splice donor site of intron 15 (Wurzner et al., 1995) and results in a truncated C6 that supports lytic activity to some degree.

C7 DEFICIENCY

Pathogenesis

The genes for C6, C7, and C9 are located on chromosome 5p12-14 (Setien et al., 1993). As a member of the membrane attack complex, C7 is a pore-forming protein whose structure, which is homologous to C6 and C8, suggests it evolved specifically to mediate pore formation (DiScipio et al., 1989). Although the tissue expression of C7 has not been investigated in detail, bone marrow–derived and hepatic synthesis of C7 has been studied in transplant recipients using protein polymorphisms (Naughton et al., 1996). Bone marrow transplant patients who received marrow from a donor with a different allotype were found to have 18% to 27% of their serum C7 made by the donor cells. This value increased during periods of inflammation, suggesting that C7 is an acute phase reactant. Conversely, liver transplant patients were shown to have approximately 60% of their serum C7 as liver derived.

C7 deficiency is inherited as an autosomal recessive trait. Patients with C7 deficiency have little if any detectable C7 antigen or function, and their CH_{50} and serum bactericidal activity are correspondingly diminished.

Clinical Features

More than 70 cases of C7 deficiency have been reported in the literature, and it has been found in diverse ethnic and racial groups (Figueroa and Densen, 1991; Ross and Densen, 1984). There may be an increased frequency in Moroccan Sephardic Jewish families, although true population studies have not been performed. *Neisseria* infections (predominantly meningococcal) have occurred in 60% of reported cases of C7-deficient individuals (Figueroa and Densen, 1991; Ross and Densen, 1984). A few patients have had SLE, rheumatoid arthritis, pyoderma gangrenosum, and scleroderma.

Molecular Genetics

The mutations causing C7 deficiency are diverse (Fernie and Hobart, 1998, 1999; Fernie et al., 1997; Horiuchi et al., 1999; Nishizaka et al., 1996; O'Hara et al., 1998), although founder mutations are seen in the Irish and the Moroccan Sephardic Jews (Fernie et al., 1997; O'Hara et al., 1998). A second type of C7 deficiency has been described in which the quantity of C7 is diminished and the protein exhibits an altered isoelectric point. This has also been seen in association with C6SD. This defect is due to a missense mutation in exon 11 that results in an arginine to serine change (Fernie et al., 1996).

C8 DEFICIENCY

Pathogenesis

C8 is composed of three polypeptide chains (α, β, γ) (Kolb et al., 1976). The α and γ chains are covalently joined to form one subunit (C8α,γ), which is joined to the other subunit, the β chain (C8β), by noncovalent bonds (Steckel et al., 1980). Each of the C8 polypeptides is encoded by separate genes (*C8A, C8B,* and *C8G*) (Howard et al., 1987; Kaufman et al., 1989; Rao et al., 1987; Rittner and Schneider, 1988). *C8A* and *C8B* map to chromosome 1p3.2 and *C8G* maps to 9q (Kaufman et al., 1989). The major site of synthesis of C8 is the liver (Ng and Sodetz, 1987).

Several variants of C8 deficiency have been recognized, and all are inherited as autosomal recessive traits. In one form of C8 deficiency, patients lack the C8β subunit, whereas in the other form, the α,γ subunit is deficient (Tedesco, 1986; Tedesco et al., 1983).

Two types of C8β deficiency have been identified thus far, one characterized by a complete absence of the C8β chain by both immunochemical and functional analysis and the other characterized by the presence of a dysfunctional protein (Tschopp et al., 1986; Tedesco, 1986; Warnick and Densen, 1991). In the case of C8β deficiency, C8 antigen can be detected in the serum of affected individuals because they possess the C8α,γ subunit, although the C8 lacks antigenic determinants present in the intact C8 molecule (Tedesco et al., 1980).

In the case of C8α,γ deficiency, analysis of serum from these patients using standard immunodiffusion techniques fails to detect any C8 antigen, even though they possess the C8β subunit (Jasin, 1977; Petersen et al., 1976). Patients with C8 deficiency have a marked reduction in serum bactericidal activity (Jasin, 1977; Nicholson and Lepow, 1979).

Clinical Features

The clinical presentation of C8 deficiency has been similar to the other deficiencies of terminal complement components (Figueroa and Densen, 1991; Ross and Densen, 1984; Tedesco, 1986). Systemic *Neisseria* infections, including meningococcemia, meningococcal meningitis, and disseminated gonococcal infections have predominated, but SLE has also rarely been seen.

Molecular Genetics

Deficiency of C8β is more common in whites, whereas C8α,γ deficiency is more common in African Americans; 86% of C8β null alleles are due to C-T transition in exon 9 producing a premature stop codon (Kaufmann et al., 1993; Kotnik et al., 1997; Saucedo et al., 1995), suggesting a founder effect. Three additional C-T transitions and two single-bp deletions causing premature stop codons have also been identified in C8β deficiency, implying that there are many different mutations occurring in the 14% of patients who do not carry the common mutation (Saucedo et al., 1995). The molecular basis of C8α,γ deficiency has been identified in three patients. In five of six null alleles, an intron mutation alters the splicing of exons 6 and 7 of C8A and creates a 10-bp insertion that generates a premature stop codon (Densen et al., 1996).

C9 DEFICIENCY

Pathogenesis

C9 is a 70-kD glycoprotein that has sequence homology to other members of the membrane attack complex (C8α, C8β, C6, and C7) and to perforin (Discipio et al., 1984; Stanley and Luzio, 1984; Stanley et al., 1985). The C9 gene 2.5 MB from the C6 and C7 genes on chromosome 5p13 (Abbott et al., 1989; Marazziti et al., 1987). C9 is produced primarily by the liver and is highly developmentally regulated; newborns produce substantially less than adults.

Like most of the other genetically determined deficiencies of complement, C9 deficiency is inherited as an autosomal recessive trait. Affected individuals usually have markedly reduced levels of C9, whether tested immunochemically or by functional analysis. In one patient, however, there were trace amounts of C9 antigen detectable in her serum and between 10% and 15% of the normal amount of C9 functional hemolytic activity (Harriman et al., 1981).

Because the hemolysis of sensitized erythrocytes can be mediated by a membrane attack complex composed of C5b-8 and is not therefore strictly dependent on C9 (Stolfi, 1968), patients with C9 deficiency have some total hemolytic complement activity, although it is usually between one third and one half of the lower limit of normal (Inai et al., 1979; Lint et al., 1980). Similarly, their sera possess some bactericidal activity, although the rate of killing is significantly reduced (Harriman et al., 1981).

Clinical Features

Only a few patients with C9 deficiency have been identified in individuals of European descent (Figueroa and Densen, 1991; Lint and Gewurz, 1986; Ross and Densen, 1984), but it appears to be the most common complement deficiency in Japan with a prevalence of 1:1000 (Horiuchi et al., 1998). Like patients with deficiencies of other terminal components, patients with C9 deficiency have an increased susceptibility to systemic meningococcal infections (Figueroa and Densen, 1991; Fine et al., 1983; Lint and Gewurz, 1986; Nagata et al., 1989; Ross and Densen, 1984). A few patients have presented with autoimmune disease, but the relationship of the autoimmune disease to C9 deficiency is unclear (Hironaka et al., 1993; Maruyama et al., 1995).

Molecular Genetics

The common mutation in Japanese patients is a nonsense mutation in exon 4 (Horiuchi et al., 1998). The molecular genetic basis for C9 deficiency has also been identified in one Swiss kindred. Two different point mutations in exon 2 and 4 resulted in premature stop codons (Witzel-Schlomp et al., 1997).

FACTOR D DEFICIENCY

Pathogenesis

Factor D was originally identified as adipsin, a molecule that is underexpressed in obesity (White et al., 1992). It has been mapped to chromosome 19 and is produced by adipocytes, myeloid cells, and hepatocytes (Barnum and Volanakis, 1985; Kitano and Kitamura, 2000). Factor D is a serine protease that cleaves a lysine-arginine bond in factor B and thereby participates in the activation of the alternative pathway (Lesavre et al., 1979). Factor D also plays a role in the stimulation of triglyceride synthesis in adipose tissue and acts as an inhibitor of neutrophil degranulation (Balke et al., 1995; Choy and Spiegelman, 1996).

Only nine patients with factor D deficiency have been identified, and each has had absent or very low levels of factor D and absent alternative pathway activity (Hiemstra et al., 1989; Kluin-Nelemans et al., 1984; Weiss et al., 1998). The deficiency appears to be inherited in an autosomal recessive fashion. The activity of the classical pathway was either normal or slightly below normal.

Clinical Features

Factor D deficiency is one of the more uncommon complement deficiencies (Biesma et al., 2001; Hiemstra et al., 1989; Kluin-Nelemans et al., 1984; Weiss et al., 1998). The true prevalence is not known, and, because alternative pathway assays are rarely performed, it is probably underdiagnosed. In this disorder, the CH_{50} is normal and the AH_{50} is extremely low or zero. In contrast to other alternative pathway deficiencies, the C3 level is normal. The patients with factor D deficiency all had significant infections and none have had autoimmune disease. All patients have presented in childhood with systemic *Neisseria* infections, pneumococcal infections, or sinopulmonary infections (Hiemstra et al., 1989; Kluin-Nelemans et al., 1984; Weiss et al., 1998). As is true for *Neisseria* infections in properdin-deficient patients, Factor D deficient patients may develop unusually severe disease, in contrast to patients with terminal component deficiencies who may have mild disease. Three asymptomatic individuals have also been identified.

Molecular Genetics

One kindred with five factor D–deficient individuals was found to carry a mutation causing a premature stop codon (Biesma et al., 2001).

FACTOR I DEFICIENCY

Pathogenesis

The gene for factor I is located on chromosome 4q (Goldberger et al., 1987). Factor I is synthesized in the liver, in mononuclear phagocytes, and in endothelial cells (Goldberger et al., 1984; Whaley, 1980). It is a serine protease that cleaves C3b to produce iC3b, an inactive cleavage product that cannot function in the C3 cleaving enzyme of the alternative pathway.

Factor I deficiency is inherited as an autosomal recessive trait. Patients with factor I deficiency have uncontrolled activation of C3 via the alternative pathway (Abramson et al., 1971; Alper et al., 1970a, 1970b; Zeigler et al., 1975). Because there is normally continuous low-grade generation of the alternative pathway C3 cleaving enzyme C3b, Bb, which is inhibited by factor I, in the absence of factor I there is no control imposed on the formation and expression of the alternative pathway C3 cleaving enzyme. As a result there is the continued cleavage and activation of C3 (Vyse et al., 1994; Wahn et al., 1981).

Patients with factor I deficiency therefore have a secondary consumption of native C3 with markedly reduced levels of both antigenic and functional C3 in their serum, most of which is in the form of the cleavage product C3b (Alper et al., 1970a). As expected, those serum activities that depend on C3, either directly or indirectly, such as bactericidal activity, opsonic activity, and chemotactic activity, are reduced in patients with factor I deficiency (Alper et al., 1970b).

Clinical Features

The most common clinical expression of factor I deficiency has been an increased susceptibility to infection (Figueroa and Densen, 1991; Ross and Densen, 1984; Solal-Celigny et al., 1982; Teisner et al., 1984; Thompson and Lachman, 1977; Vyse et al., 1994; Wahn et al., 1981). Like patients with C3 deficiency, factor I deficient patients have had infections caused by encapsulated pyogenic bacteria, such as the streptococcus, pneumococcus, meningococcus, and *H. influenzae*, organisms for which C3 is an important opsonic ligand. In addition to problems with infection, some patients have had elevated levels of circulating immune complexes (Solal-Celigny et al., 1982; Teisner et al., 1984). There has been one report of a transient illness resembling serum sickness and characterized by fever, rash, arthralgia, hematuria, and proteinuria (Solal-Celigny et al., 1984).

Molecular Genetics

The molecular genetic basis for factor I deficiency has been identified in only a few patients and is diverse (Vyse et al., 1996).

FACTOR H DEFICIENCY

Pathogenesis

The factor H gene maps to the regulator of complement activation (RCA) region of chromosome 1. It is composed of 20 homologous repeating units [short consensus repeats (SCRs)], which are also found in C4bp, DAF, MCP, CR1, and CR2 (Rodriques De Cordoba et al., 1985). It is synthesized in the liver (Skerka et al., 1992). Factor H is an inhibitor of the activation of the alternative pathway. It not only competes with factor B for binding to C3b in the assembly of the alternative pathway C3 convertase (Kazatchkine et al., 1979) but it also can displace Bb from the C3b, Bb complex once the C3 convertase has formed (Weiler et al., 1976). In addition, the rate of inactivation of C3b by factor I is markedly accelerated by factor H (Whaley and Ruddy, 1976).

In some cases of factor H deficiency, serum factor H has been undetectable (Brai et al., 1988; Nielsen et al., 1989a), whereas in most families Factor H has been detectable but reduced (Levy et al., 1986; Nielsen et al., 1989a). The levels of the alternative pathway components factor B and properdin are also reduced but not to the same degree as factor H. Similarly, serum levels of C3 are also reduced and the majority of the C3 that is present is in the form of an activation/cleavage product. Presumably, defective or absent factor H leads to continuous activation of the alternative pathway and the resultant depletion of C3 and other proteins of the alternative pathway, a situation comparable to factor I deficiency.

Clinical Features

Genetically determined factor H deficiency has been described in only a few families (Brai et al., 1988; Figueroa and Densen, 1991; Levy et al., 1986; Nielsen et al., 1989a; Ross and Densen, 1984; Sim et al., 1993; Thompson and Winterborn, 1981) and appears to be inherited as an autosomal recessive trait. The clinical manifestations of factor H deficiency have included glomerulonephritis, hemolytic uremic syndrome, SLE, and systemic meningococcal infections (Figueroa and Densen, 1991; Ross and Densen, 1984; Sim et al., 1993). The most common manifestation is familial hemolytic uremic syndrome or atypical (nondiarrheal) hemolytic uremic syndrome. In patients with factor H deficiency, the prognosis is poor, although twice-weekly infusions of fresh frozen plasma have prevented recurrences and renal failure (Landau et al., 2001). Some individuals with factor H deficiency have been ascertained because of family studies and have been asymptomatic (Thompson and Winterborn, 1981).

Molecular Genetics

One patient with factor H deficiency was found to be heterozygous for two missense mutations affecting conserved cysteine residues. This resulted in an inability to secrete the full-length protein (Ault et al., 1997). There are diverse point mutations affecting function (Neumann et al., 2003; Richards et al., 2001; Sanchez-Carral et al., 2002).

PROPERDIN DEFICIENCY

Pathogenesis

Properdin is the only gene of the complement system that is encoded on the X chromosome. Properdin is produced primarily by monocytes and T cells (Nolan et al., 1991; Wirthmueller et al., 1997). Properdin acts to stabilize the alternative pathway C3 and C5 convertases by extending the half-lives of the C3 and C5 converting enzymes and therefore enhancing the activity of the alternative pathway. It also plays a role in the efficient uptake of immune complexes through an undefined mechanism (Junker et al., 1998).

Properdin deficiency is inherited as X-linked recessive trait. It has been divided into three subtypes based on protein phenotypes. Type I properdin deficiency has no detectable properdin in the serum. Type II deficiency is associated with approximately 10% of the normal circulating properdin, and type III deficiency, identified in a single family, is associated with normal serum levels of properdin protein but absent function.

More than 70 properdin-deficient patients (Figueroa and Densen, 1991; Ross and Densen, 1984) have been described, and the classical finding is absent function of the alternative pathway. Similarly, serum bactericidal activity for some strains of the meningococcus is reduced in properdin-deficient serum. Patients with properdin deficiency have an intact classical pathway.

Clinical Features

Properdin deficiency appears to be one of the more common complement deficiencies, although prevalence figures are not available. Because its detection relies on the use of functional alternative pathway studies that are seldom obtained, it is likely that this disorder is underdiagnosed. Approximately 50% of the patients with properdin deficiency have had meningococcal disease (Figueroa and Densen, 1991; Ross and Densen, 1984). Interestingly, the mortality from meningococcal disease in patients with properdin deficiency is approximately 75% compared with the mortality of 3% in patients with terminal component deficiencies (Densen et al., 1987). Isolated cases of SLE and discoid lupus are also seen in properdin-deficient patients, and this could be due to ascertainment bias or through the role of properdin in the clearance of immune complexes (Junker et al., 1998).

Molecular Genetics

Mutations have been identified in some properdin-deficient patients and are diverse. The patients who produce no detectable properdin typically have early stop codons (Spath et al., 1999; Westberg et al., 1995), whereas the patients with type II deficiency have missense mutations or splicing defects (Westberg et al., 1995). The single kindred with dysfunctional properdin had a single-bp substitution that affected binding to C3 (Fredrikson et al., 1996).

C4 BINDING PROTEIN DEFICIENCY

Pathogenesis

The genes encoding the C4bp α and β chains are located on chromosome 1q32 and are arranged in tandem but are distinctly regulated (Arenzana et al., 1996). C4 binding protein (C4bp) is synthesized primarily by the liver and exists as three isoforms: α7β1, α7, α6β1. The major isoform is composed of seven 70-kD α chains (Sanchez-Corral et al., 1995) arrayed around a single 45-kD β chain. C4bp is one of the major regulators of the classical pathway. It acts by accelerating the decay of the classical pathway convertase and by aiding in the degradation of C4.

Only a single kindred with C4bp deficiency has been described (Trapp et al., 1987), and its mode of inheritance has not been determined. The family members with C4bp deficiency had approximately 25% of the normal antigenic levels of C4bp.

Clinical Features

The single known kindred with C4bp deficiency had two clinically well members who were deficient in C4bp and one C4bp-deficient member with a disorder described as atypical Behçet's disease (Trapp et al., 1987). The patient exhibited angioedema, central nervous system (CNS) changes, and oral ulcers with intermittent arthritis. The increased production of C3a and C5a might have led to angioedema through increased vascular permeability.

Molecular Genetics

The molecular genetic basis for C4bp deficiency has not been identified.

DECAY-ACCELERATING FACTOR DEFICIENCY

Pathogenesis

Decay-accelerating factor (DAF) is encoded on chromosome 1q32 (Lublin et al., 1987). It is a glycosyl phosphatidylinositol (GPI) anchored membrane protein found on erythrocytes, lymphocytes, granulocytes, endothelium, and epithelium. It inhibits the assembly of the classical and alternative pathway C3 converting enzymes (Nicholson-Weller et al., 1982). DAF functions primarily to protect cells from complement-mediated destruction (Mason et al., 1999; Sun et al., 1999);

however, it also plays a role in T-cell and macrophage activation (Hamann et al., 1999; Shenoy-Scaria et al., 1992; Tosello et al., 1998).

Inherited deficiency of DAF is uncommon. Because the Cromer blood group system is located on the DAF molecule (Lublin et al., 2000), patients with genetically determined DAF deficiency are negative for all Cromer antigens and possess the Inab phenotype (Telen and Green, 1989).

In addition to the inherited deficiency, an acquired deficiency also exists. Patients with the acquired deficiency have a clonal red cell population lacking GPI anchored proteins including CD59 and DAF and the clinical disorder paroxysmal nocturnal hemoglobinuria (PNH) (Takeda et al., 1993). Erythrocytes from patients with PNH have a positive Ham's test and increased susceptibility to complement mediated lysis.

Clinical Features

Surprisingly, DAF deficiency is not associated with spontaneous hemolysis (Shichishima et al., 1999). Hemolysis can be induced in vitro; however, deficiency of both CD59 and DAF is required to induce the characteristic clinical findings of PNH (Shichishima et al., 1999). Two patients with the Inab phenotype suffered from protein losing enteropathy that was of uncertain relationship to the DAF deficiency (Telen et al., 1989). It may have to do with the fact that DAF is a receptor for enteroviruses and *Escherichia coli*. Mutant forms of DAF may alter the pathologic response. The remainder of the individuals with the Inab phenotype have been well. No obvious T-cell dysfunction was noted in any of the patients. Therefore DAF deficiency may not have any clinical consequences.

Molecular Genetics

Various mutations in DAF have been identified (Lublin et al., 1994).

MANNOSE-BINDING LECTIN DEFICIENCY

Pathogenesis

Mannose-binding lectin (MBL) is a member of the collectin family and is encoded on chromosome 10 along with the three surfactant protein genes (Sastry et al., 1989) (see Chapter 10). C1q has a similar structure but does not contain the lectin domain, and thus C1q has no mannose-binding ability. MBL is composed of a trimer of which each polypeptide chain consists of a collagen-like region, cysteine repeats, and a lectin domain that interacts with various sugars. The predominant circulating form is a 600,000-kD multimer (Lipscombe et al., 1995). MBL binds N-acetylglucosamine and mannose more avidly than other sugars, and MBL binds both gram-positive and gram-negative bacteria. It has

also been shown to bind *Cryptococcus, Candida,* and several viruses.

One function of MBL is to provide a third activation arm of the complement cascade (Turner, 1996). The activation of C3 via this pathway does not involve the participation of immunoglobulin, thereby augmenting the alternative pathway early in infection before the development of protective antibody. MBL circulates with MBL-associated serine proteases (MASP1 and MASP 2), which are capable of activating C4 and C2 and therefore ultimately activating C3.

MBL deficiency is different than the other complement component deficiencies in that it is seldom, if ever, due to a null mutation. Instead, structural polymorphic variants destabilize the higher order structures and lead to loss of function (Lipscombe et al., 1995; Wallis and Cheng, 1999). Three relatively common structural variants are in codon 54 (known as structural allele *B*), codon 57 (known as structural allele *C*), and codon 52 (known as structural allele *D*). The wild-type is known as allele *A*. Collectively the structural variants are known as type *O*, and they have a combined allele frequency of approximately 20% in the Caucasian population (Babovic-Vuksanovic et al., 1999; Lipscombe et al., 1992; Madsen et al., 1995). Therefore MBL deficiency is the most common complement deficiency.

Inheritance of a single variant allele results in MBL serum levels of approximately 10%, although the functional level may be even lower (Madsen et al., 1995). Inheritance of two variant alleles results in nearly undetectable serum levels of MBL. These structural variants have been identified in all populations studied to date, although the frequency is different in different ethnicities. In addition to the structural polymorphisms, promoter polymorphisms are also seen with high frequency and these alter the production of MBL (Madsen et al., 1995). These promoter polymorphisms are typically referred to as H, L, X, Y, P, and Q. The low-producing promoter haplotype is LX and inheritance of LX and the wild-type structural allele results in approximately 10% of the normal serum level (Madsen et al., 1995). Other combinations are roughly additive in effect. The promoter polymorphisms are also found in all ethnicities.

Clinical Features

MBL deficiency was originally described in adults and children with recurrent and/or serious infections (Kakkanaiah et al., 1998; Sumiya et al., 1991; Summerfield et al., 1995). These infections included recurrent upper respiratory tract infections, abscesses, sepsis, and meningococcus. Similarly, the percent of children with meningitis who have MBL deficiency is higher than the percent of controls with MBL deficiency (Hibberd et al., 1999).

The odds ratio for any infection when an MBL variant is present is 2.4 among children (Summerfield et al., 1997), and there is a suggestion that the odds ratio would be higher for sepsis or severe infections. Finally, there is also some evidence that MBL deficiency plays a role in host defense against tuberculosis and influences the course of human immunodeficiency virus (HIV) (Bellamy, 2000; Garred et al., 1997; Hoal-Van Helden et al., 1999; Pastinen et al., 1998).

Other studies have shown that MBL deficiency accelerates the progression of rheumatoid arthritis and increases susceptibility to SLE (Davies et al., 1997; Garred et al., 1999; Graudal et al., 2000; Ip et al., 1998, 2000; Lau et al., 1996; Madsen et al., 1995; Senaldi et al., 1995; Sullivan et al., 1996).

MANAGEMENT OF GENETICALLY DETERMINED COMPLEMENT DEFICIENCIES

The management of complement deficiencies depends on the specific component that is deficient and its role in normal host defense and inflammation. Replacement of the specific component is usually not possible, with the notable exception of C1 esterase inhibitor deficiency. Therefore the management of complement deficiencies is usually limited to supportive care and relates to the clinical manifestations that are secondary to the specific deficiency.

Prevention of Infection

Infectious diseases are prominent clinical manifestations of nearly all the complement deficiency diseases, and two strategies have been attempted to reduce patients' susceptibility to infections and/or modify the clinical course of the infections.

One of these strategies is immunization against common bacterial pathogens such as the pneumococcus, *H. influenzae,* and the meningococcus. Unfortunately, there are important factors that may limit the utility of immunizations in these patients in preventing infections. For example, because of the role of complement in the development of a normal antibody response, when patients with C4 or C2 are immunized with neoantigens, such as φX-174, their primary response is limited and their secondary response delayed (Ochs et al., 1983). Other studies in patients with terminal component deficiencies have shown that, although initial responses to immunization to the meningococcus are normal, they have lower titers at distant time points (Andreoni et al., 1993; Biselli et al., 1993; Schlesinger at al., 1994, 2000).

Therefore it is possible that complement-deficient patients require more frequent immunization than a normal host (Fijen et al., 1998). One approach is to measure specific antibody titers and to re-immunize the patient when the titers fall below the protective range.

Another limitation to the use of immunizations in complement-deficient patients is that the vaccines may not include all of the serotypes to which complement-deficient patients are susceptible. For example, the new pneumococcal conjugate vaccine is limited to seven serotypes, and the meningococcal vaccine contains only serotypes A, C, Y, and W. These limitations may explain why a number of immunized patients with complement deficiencies have had *Neisseria* infections despite immunizations.

Another strategy in the prevention of infection is the use of prophylactic antibiotics. Because patients with complement deficiencies have a high risk for recurrent episodes of blood-borne infections and because immunizations may not afford them complete protection, some patients have been placed on antibiotic prophylaxis. However, any recommendation for antibiotic prophylaxis must be viewed in the context of the emergence of antibiotic resistance among bacteria.

Treatment of Rheumatic Diseases

Regardless of the rheumatologic disorder, it is most often treated with the same immunosuppressive agents and anti-inflammatory medications that one would use in a complement-sufficient patient.

One exception to this paradigm is the use of fresh frozen plasma in a series of patients with C2 deficiency and SLE in Iceland and Great Britain (Hudson-Peacock et al., 1997; Steinsson et al., 1989). There had been concerns that the provision of additional complement components would accelerate deposition of immune complexes in end organs and exacerbate the inflammation. This was not the case in the two patients for whom it has been attempted. In fact, nearly all clinical indicators improved on this regimen. Although it has only been used in a small number of patients, it is an attractive modality for those complement-deficient patients who are refractory to standard management or who have not done well on immunosuppression.

Immunosuppression would be predicted to exacerbate the defects in host defense associated with complement deficiency. There have been no formal studies to demonstrate that complement-deficient individuals do worse on immunosuppression than their complement-sufficient peers, but the potential for increased risk leads many caregivers to modify their immunosuppressive regimen.

HEREDITARY ANGIOEDEMA (C1 ESTERASE INHIBITOR DEFICIENCY/DEFECT)

Pathogenesis

C1 INH is encoded by a 17-kD gene on chromosome 11q (Bock, 1986 et al.; Carter et al., 1991; Davis et al., 1986). The liver is the major source of plasma C1 INH (Colten et al., 1972; Gitlin and Biasucci, 1969; Johnson AM et al., 1971; Morris et al., 1982), but mononuclear phagocytes and fibroblasts also synthesize and secrete C1 INH (Bensa et al., 1983). C1 INH is a glycoprotein that binds covalently to C1r and C1s leading to dissociation of the C1 macromolecular complex (Harpel and

Cooper, 1975) and inhibition of the enzymatic actions of C1r and C1s (Pensky et al., 1961).

There are two forms of genetically determined C1 INH deficiency and both are inherited as autosomal dominant traits (acquired forms of C1 INH deficiency are discussed later).

In the most common form (type I), accounting for approximately 85% of the patients, the serum of affected individuals is deficient in both C1 INH protein (5% to 30% of normal) and C1 INH functional activity (Cicardi et al., 1982; Donaldson and Evans, 1963; Frank et al., 1976; Rosen et al., 1971). In the other, less common form (type II), a dysfunctional protein is present in normal or elevated concentrations, but the functional activity of C1 INH is markedly reduced (Cicardi et al., 1982; Donaldson and Evans, 1963; Frank et al., 1976; Rosen et al., 1965).

In patients with type I C1 INH deficiency, the diagnosis can be established easily by demonstrating a decrease in serum C1 INH protein when assessed by immunochemical techniques. However, in patients with type II C1 INH deficiency, the diagnosis must rest on demonstrating a decrease in C1 INH functional activity. In either case, C4 levels or C2 levels are usually reduced below the lower limit of normal during attacks (Austen and Sheffer, 1965; Cicardi et al., 1982; Frank et al., 1976; Pickering et al., 1968) because of their uncontrolled cleavage by C1s. The level of C4 in serum is also reduced between attacks, making its measurement useful as a diagnostic clue (Frank et al., 1976; Pickering et al., 1968).

Several groups have examined the dysfunctional C1 INH molecules from different families and found that they not only differ from normal C1 INH but from each other with respect to their electrophoretic mobility, ability to bind C1s, and ability to inhibit both synthetic and natural substrates (Donaldson et al., 1985; Harpel et al., 1975; Rosen et al., 1965, 1971). The levels of normal C1 INH function in patients with either type of hereditary angioedema (HAE) are lower than one might expect in a hemizygote; 5% to 30% of normal in type I C1 INH deficiency and little or none in type II C1 INH deficiency. In addition, the immunochemical levels of the dysfunctional protein in the type II disorder are usually equivalent to normal, or higher than normal, rather than the expected 50% of normal.

In an attempt to explain these apparent discrepancies, metabolic studies using both normal and dysfunctional proteins have been performed in both normal and deficient subjects (Johnson AM et al., 1971; Quastel et al., 1983). These studies have been used to create a model to explain the low levels of C1 INH found in the type I disorder and the elevated levels of dysfunctional protein found in the type II disorder (Lachmann and Rosen, 1984).

It has been suggested that in the type I disorder, the markedly lowered levels of C1 INH are the result of both decreased synthesis and increased catabolism consequent to the complexing of the normal C1 INH with the activated enzymes that it normally inhibits. Similarly, it has been suggested that the low levels of normal C1 INH and elevated levels of dysfunctional C1 INH protein in the type II disorder are the result of decreased synthesis and increased catabolism of the normal C1 INH and, at least in some cases, decreased catabolism of the dysfunctional C1 INH consequent to its inability to complex with C1 and other enzymes.

The pathophysiologic mechanism(s) by which the absence of C1 INH activity leads to the angioedema characteristic of the disorder are still incompletely understood. C1 INH is the major inhibitor of kallikrein and factor XII (Curd et al., 1980; Donaldson and Rosen, 1964; Klemperer et al., 1968; Schapira et al., 1983; Schreiber et al., 1973). Diminished C1 INH leads to unregulated activation of kallikrein and the classical pathway after exposure to a mild trigger. Bradykinin and C2a appear to be the primary mediators of angioedema.

Clinical Features

Genetically determined deficiency of C1 INH is responsible for the clinical disorder termed HAE (Donaldson and Evans, 1963). The clinical symptoms of HAE are the result of submucosal or subcutaneous edema. The lesions are characterized by noninflammatory edema associated with capillary and venule dilation (Sheffer et al., 1971). The three most prominent areas of involvement are the skin, upper respiratory tract, and gastrointestinal tract (Cicardi et al., 1982; Donaldson and Rosen, 1966; Frank et al., 1976; Landerman, 1962). Although symptoms during attacks may relate to only one of these areas, they are not mutually exclusive and may be seen in combination.

Attacks involving the skin may involve an extremity, the face, or genitalia (Fig. 21-2). In some instances, there may be changes just preceding the edema such as mottling, a transient serpiginous erythema, or frank erythema marginatum. The edema usually expands centripetally from a single site and may vary in size from a few centimeters to involvement of a whole extremity. The lesions are pale rather than red, are usually not warm, and are characteristically nonpruritic. There may be, however, a feeling of tightness in the skin because of the accumulation of subcutaneous fluid. Attacks usually progress for 1 to 2 days and resolve over an additional 2 to 3 days.

Attacks involving the upper respiratory tract represent a serious threat to the patient with HAE. In one series, pharyngeal edema had occurred at least once in nearly two thirds of the patients (Frank et al., 1976). The patient may initially experience a "tightness" in the throat and swelling of the tongue, buccal mucosa, and oropharynx follows. In some instances laryngeal edema, accompanied by hoarseness and stridor occurs, progresses to respiratory obstruction and represents a life-threatening emergency. In a series from 20 years ago, tracheotomies had been performed in one out of every six patients with HAE (Frank et al., 1976).

The gastrointestinal tract can also be affected by HAE. Symptoms are probably related to edema of the bowel wall and may include anorexia, dull aching of

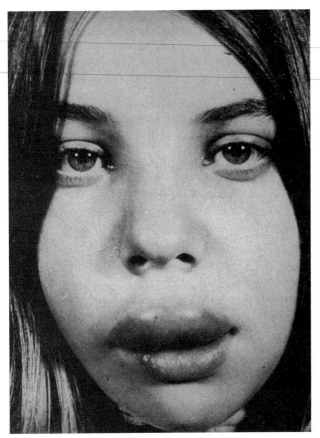

Figure 21-2 · Facial swelling in a child with C1 esterase deficiency during an attack of angioedema. (Courtesy of Dr. Fred Rosen.)

the abdomen, vomiting, and in some cases crampy abdominal pain. Abdominal symptoms can occur in the absence of concurrent cutaneous or pharyngeal involvement. In some instances, abdominal symptoms may be the only symptoms the patient has ever had, leading to difficulty in diagnosis.

The onset of symptoms referable to HAE occurs in more than half the patients before adolescence (Cicardi et al., 1982; Donaldson and Rosen, 1966; Frank et al., 1976), but in some patients, their first symptoms do not occur until they are well into adult life. Although in slightly more than half of the patients no specific events can be clearly identified as initiating attacks, anxiety and/or stress are frequently cited (Cicardi et al., 1982; Donaldson and Rosen, 1966; Frank et al., 1976). Dental extractions and tonsillectomy can initiate edema of the upper airway and cutaneous edema may follow trauma to an extremity. Some patients report attacks following the use of tight-fitting clothing or shoes, whereas others have related cold exposure to the onset of symptoms.

Molecular Genetics

The division of C1 INH deficiency into two categories based on the presence or absence of a dysfunctional protein has no correlation with clinical phenotype and only limited correlation with genotype because there are some examples of C1 INH mutations in which a dysfunctional protein is produced but is degraded so rapidly that it is not detectable in the serum (Agostoni and Cicardi, 1992; Davis et al., 1993).

Alu mediated deletions and duplications account for the most common C1 INH null genotypes (Davis et al., 1993; Stoppa-Lyonnet et al., 1991). The C1 INH gene contains a total of 17 Alu repetitive DNA elements and these are responsible for most of the gene rearrangements leading to C1 INH deficiency. A variety of single base changes and smaller deletions and duplications have also been identified (Davis et al., 1993).

Most patients with type II HAE deficiency have a mutation that interferes with the reactive center arginine residue. The other mutations identified in patients with a dysfunctional protein are usually found in the hinge region, thereby inactivating the C1 INH (Davis et al., 1993; Verpy et al., 1995). Several mutations just amino-terminal to the active site apparently generate changes in the stressed loop confirmation of the C1 INH serine protease inhibitor (SERPIN) (Davis et al., 1991; Levy et al., 1990; Skriver et al., 1991) and one located more distantly leads to an abnormal glycosylation signal (Parad et al., 1990).

Treatment

The therapy of HAE falls into three categories: (1) the long-term prophylaxis of attacks, (2) the short-term prophylaxis of attacks, and (3) the treatment of acute attacks.

In those patients who have had laryngeal obstruction or have suffered frequent and debilitating attacks that have interfered with work or other responsibilities, long-term prevention of attacks may be indicated. Impeded androgens such as danazol, stanozolol, and oxandrolone, which have attenuated androgenic potential, have been found to be useful in the long-term prophylaxis of HAE (Agostoni and Cicardi, 1992; Agostoni et al., 1993; Cicardi et al., 1991; Gelfand et al., 1976; Hosea et al., 1980c; Sheffer et al., 1987).

These impeded androgens increase serum concentrations of the normal C1 INH in these patients by increasing transcription of the wild-type C1 INH gene, whether they have the form of the disease characterized by low levels of C1 INH protein (type I) or the form characterized by a dysfunctional protein (type II) (Gadek et al., 1979; Gelfand et al., 1976).

Danazol is typically used at 50 to 600 mg per day, stanozolol is typically used at 1 to 10 mg per day, and oxandrolone is typically used at 2.5 to 25 mg per day in adults. It is possible to monitor C1 INH levels to titrate the effect of the medication. The goal is to bring the C1 INH functional level up to approximately 50% of normal although the dose of androgen should be specifically titrated to symptoms. Danazol therapy appears to be effective for extended periods of time, but because of dose-related adverse reactions (e.g., hirsutism, weight gain, abnormal liver function tests, microscopic hematuria, and altered libido), therapy must be closely monitored (Hosea et al., 1980c). Hepatic function and periodic ultrasound examinations of the liver should be performed. Attenuated androgens are usually not used in prepubertal children because of their side effects and should not be used in children with open epiphyses. However, children may safely receive intermittent treatment with attenuated androgens with little fear of premature closure of the epiphyses.

An alternative strategy for prophylaxis is to use antifibrinolytics (Agostoni et al., 1993). The mechanism of action is not completely understood; however, they act distally at the level of plasmin cleavage. Epsilon aminocaproic acid (EACA) was used initially as an antifibrinolytic agent. More recently, tranexamic acid has been used at doses of approximately 50 mg/kg/day. These are especially valuable in prepubertal children and patients who cannot tolerate attenuated androgens (Frank et al., 1972; Sheffer et al., 1972). Antifibrinolytics are not as effective as androgens; however, they can prevent a significant number of attacks.

Antifibrinolytics have been used occasionally as a therapy for an acute attack, but there seems to be little advantage of this approach.

In some instances, patients may need short-term prophylactic therapy, such as before elective surgery or oral surgery. There are a number of strategies used for short-term surgical prophylaxis. One option is to initiate therapy with attenuated androgens 1 week before surgery and continue its use for the first few days after surgery (Agostoni and Cicardi, 1992). Another option is the use of fresh frozen plasma. Although there is some controversy concerning the use of fresh frozen plasma during an acute attack, because the plasma not only supplies the missing C1 INH but also C1 enzyme and substrates such as C4 and C2, the use of plasma transfusions 12 hours before elective surgery has been shown to prevent morbidity from the procedure (Jaffe et al., 1975).

Perhaps the most effective strategy is to use purified C1 INH concentrate (Kunschak et al., 1998; Peled et al., 1997; Waytes et al., 1996). However, the use of purified C1 INH has not yet been approved in the United States. Antifibrinolytic therapy is not often used in this setting because of its comparatively weak action.

The management of an acute episode of angioedema requires a definition of the goals for each individual patient. Limited extremity swelling may require no intervention for some patients, whereas it may be disastrous for a pianist. Airway swelling or disabling abdominal pain almost always requires intervention. The most effective therapy is C1 INH concentrate given as an intravenous infusion that typically causes at least partial resolution of the swelling within 30 to 60 minutes (Kunschak et al., 1998; Waytes et al., 1996). However, until purified C1 esterase inhibitor is widely available, attenuated androgens are the most common specific treatment of an acute attack. Unfortunately, androgens do not begin to have an effect until 24 to 48 hours. The patients require careful monitoring during this time frame to ensure that the angioedema does not progress.

Epinephrine, corticosteroids, and antihistamines do not affect the angioedema in this disorder.

SECONDARY COMPLEMENT DEFICIENCIES

Secondary complement deficiencies are very common and can occasionally cause diagnostic confusion. Any pathologic process that results in activation of the complement cascade or interferes with the synthesis of complement can result in a secondary complement deficiency. In general, diminished, but not absent, levels of complement are usually due to consumption, whereas absent complement levels are usually due to inherited deficiencies.

In the following section, disorders associated with secondary deficiencies in complement are reviewed. In some cases, the hypocomplementemia is known to predispose to infection. In many cases, however, the relationship of the hypocomplementemia to susceptibility to infection has not been specifically studied and the risk must be inferred.

Systemic Lupus Erythematosus and Related Diseases

Circulating immune complexes are associated with a very large number of conditions, and they may be formed against both exogenous and endogenous antigens. Under normal physiologic conditions, immune complexes activate the classical pathway, depositing C3b on the complex. This results in binding of the immune complex to complement receptors and Fc receptors and clearance of the immune complex by the reticuloendothelial system. If production of immune complexes exceeds the clearance capacity of the reticuloendothelial system or there is a deficiency of complement, then clearance may be impaired and the immune complexes may be deposited in end organs such as the kidney. Once immune complexes are deposited in end organs, tissue destruction may occur.

SLE is a systemic disorder characterized by the presence of autoantibodies directed against common cellular constituents. Immune complexes are generated and deposited in end organs, leading to the classical pathologic changes in lupus. For example, immunoglobulin and C3 deposition in the skin is the basis for the lupus band test, and immunofluorescent labeling of C3 and IgG deposition in glomeruli are used as diagnostic indicators of the renal disease in lupus. Furthermore, activation and consumption of the complement cascade typically precedes clinical flare, suggesting that the exacerbations are driven by an increased production of immune complexes and/or activation of the classical pathway (Buyon et al., 1992; Davies et al., 1992; Lloyd and Schur, 1981; Swaak et al., 1986). The degree of hypocomplementemia, specifically levels of C3 and C4, generally reflects the degree of clinical activity (see Chapter 35).

Although complement activation as a result of the circulating immune complexes is particularly characteristic of lupus, it has also been described in rheumatoid arthritis, juvenile rheumatoid arthritis, Sjögren's syndrome, a variety of vasculitides, and mixed connective tissue disease. Hypocomplementemia as a result of immune complex formation is seen less frequently in inflammatory bowel disease, sarcoidosis, Behçet's syndrome, and myasthenia gravis.

Serum Sickness

Serum sickness is the consequence of immune complex formation in response to the administration of drugs (e.g., penicillin, cefaclor, and minocycline), foreign proteins (e.g., anti-thymocyte globulin, therapeutic monoclonal antibodies, or antivenoms), or in some instances infections (Hebert et al., 1991; Heckbert et al., 1990; Levenson et al., 1996; Parshuram and Phillips, 1998). When oral drugs are associated with serum sickness, it is believed that the drugs act as haptens.

In classic acute serum sickness, immune complexes are deposited in small vessels. Clinically, patients with serum sickness present with erythema between the fingers and toes, which spreads rapidly. The rash may become morbilliform or have an urticarial component. Resolution requires recognition and elimination of the cause. Severe cases may progress to renal involvement (Border and Noble, 1993), although rash, fever, and arthralgias/arthritis are the most common clinical findings. Immune complexes are present in the circulation early in the process. Most cases have significant hypocomplementemia, and when it occurs it is characterized by low CH_{50}, C3, and C4 (Bielory et al., 1986).

Sepsis

Acute bacterial sepsis, specifically gram-negative sepsis, may be associated with transient hypocomplementemia. Generally, the hypocomplementemia reflects activation of both the alternative and classical pathways and is characterized by low levels of C3, C4, and total hemolytic activity (CH_{50}) and the generation of the cleavage products C3a and C5a (Fearon et al., 1975; Fust et al., 1976; Sprung et al., 1986). The hypocomplementemia is most commonly found in patients who have some degree of cardiovascular compromise and is strongly correlated with the severity of the shock and morbidity.

Hypocomplementemic Urticarial Vasculitis

The hypocomplementemic urticarial vasculitis syndrome (HUVS) is an autoimmune disorder resulting from the production of antibodies directed against C1q (Wisnieski et al., 1995). The most common clinical features are urticaria, angioedema, and arthritis. Uveitis, glomerulonephritis, and obstructive lung disease have also been

described and are generally poor prognostic indicators. Anti-C1q antibodies are also seen in a subset of patients with SLE, and there can be some clinical overlap between the two disorders (Wisnieski and Jones, 1992); SLE patients with anti-C1q antibodies typically have more severe renal disease. C1q levels are markedly decreased as a result of the anti-C1q antibodies and the CH_{50} is consequently depressed. Other complement components, such as C4 and C3, may be normal when the disease is clinically inactive but moderately depressed when the disease is active (Sissons et al., 1974). When renal disease is seen in patients with hypocomplementemic urticarial vasculitis, it is immune complex mediated.

C3 Nephritic Factor

Antibodies to the C3 convertase C3b,Bb of the alternative pathway are termed C3 nephritic factors (Edwards et al., 1983). These IgG antibodies are directed against new epitopes on C3b that are exposed during the formation of the convertase. They act to stabilize the C3 converting enzyme, prolonging its half-life and thereby causing increased consumption of C3.

The term C3 nephritic factor arose because the most common phenotype associated with these antibodies is type II membranoproliferative glomerulonephritis. It also has been found in rare patients with lupus and in patients with partial lipodystrophy (Sissons et al., 1976; Walport et al., 1994). Not all C3 nephritic factors are identical, and some require properdin for full activity (Tanuma et al., 1990). C3 nephritic factors are sometimes classified according to whether they support fluid phase activation of C3 (type I) or not (type II). The specific type appears not to influence the clinical features. The development of C3 nephritic factor is acquired and is usually considered to be a sporadic occurrence, although one kindred with multiple affected members has been described (Power et al., 1990).

The age of onset of C3 nephritic factors ranges from early childhood through middle adulthood. The most common clinical features leading to diagnosis are the combination of glomerulonephritis and partial lipodystrophy. Patients typically report an acute onset and may describe an antecedent viral process (Sissons et al., 1976). C3 levels are characteristically low in these patients. Terminal components may be somewhat depressed, but the early components of the classical pathway are usually normal. As a result of the markedly depressed C3, the CH_{50} is low. The membranoproliferative glomerulonephritis is thought to be due to the immune complex effect of the C3 nephritic factor. The partial lipodystrophy is believed to result from activation of the complement cascade on adipocytes and their cytolysis.

The Newborn

A number of studies have examined levels of individual components of the complement system in normal, full-term infants (see Chapter 22). The levels of most components of either the classical or alternative pathways in full-term infants are 50% to 80% of adult levels (Johnston et al., 1979). However, both C8 and C9 seem to be more severely depressed with levels in full-term newborn infants as low as 28% and 10% of maternal levels (Adinolfi and Beck, 1975; Ballow et al., 1974).

The serum levels of individual components of complement in premature infants have also been studied. Significant levels of C4, C3, C7, C9, factor B, properdin, and C1 INH have been detected in fetal serum as early as the end of the first trimester or the beginning of the second trimester (Adinolfi, 1970, 1977; Adinolfi and Beck, 1975; Adinolfi and Gardner, 1967; Gitlin and Biasucci, 1969; Minta et al., 1976). There is a general tendency for levels of these components to increase with age, and their levels in premature infants generally correlate with gestational age (Adamkin et al., 1978; Adinolfi, 1970; Adinolfi and Beck, 1975; Fireman et al., 1969; Sawyer et al., 1971; Strunk et al., 1979).

In view of the fact that many of the individual components of complement are reduced in concentration in neonatal sera, it is not surprising that those serum activities that depend on the complement system, at least in part, are reduced as well. Thus serum opsonic and chemotactic activities are reduced in both full-term and premature infants (Dossett et al., 1969; Forman and Stiehm, 1969; Marodi et al., 1985; McCraken and Eichenwald, 1971). It has not always been possible to ascribe the deficient opsonizing or chemotactic activity found in the sera of newborn infants solely to a deficient complement system, because deficiencies in other humoral factors, such as IgM, important in the generation of these activities may contribute as well.

Nephrotic Syndrome

Children with the idiopathic nephrotic syndrome have an increased susceptibility to pneumococcal peritonitis and sepsis (Churg et al., 1970). Although they are susceptible at any point in their illness, they are at greatest risk when they are in relapse and spilling large amounts of protein, such as factor B, in their urine. Their serum opsonizing activity is reduced and when factor B is added back to their serum, the defect is corrected (McLean et al., 1977), suggesting that loss of factor B in the urine is responsible for their deficient opsonizing activity and thus may contribute to their increased susceptibility to infection.

Cirrhosis

Patients with cirrhosis have decreased serum concentrations of C3, C4, and total hemolytic activity (Ellison et al., 1990; Finlayson et al., 1972; Kourilsky et al., 1973; Potter et al., 1973, 1978). The presence of decreased levels of C3 and C4 correlate with the degree of liver decompensation and levels of serum proteins

synthesized in the liver, such as albumin and certain coagulation factors, suggesting that decreased hepatic synthesis is the basis for the decreased levels of C4 and C3. A number of studies have demonstrated a strong correlation between the low levels of C3 and a predisposition to spontaneous bacterial peritonitis and mortality in cirrhosis (Andreu et al., 1993; Homann et al., 1997; Mal et al., 1991; Runyon, 1988; Such et al., 1988).

Cardiopulmonary Bypass, Extracorporeal Membrane Oxygenation (ECMO), and Hemodialysis

A variety of therapeutic maneuvers, such as cardiopulmonary bypass, ECMO, and hemodialysis, may bring the patient's blood in contact with artificial surfaces or membranes. As a result there may be activation of the complement system and levels of individual components, such as C3, and of total hemolytic complement fall (Chenoweth et al., 1981; Jacob and Craddock, 1980). As a consequence of the activation of the complement system, the generation of biologically active cleavage products, such as C3a, C5a, also occurs. A number of studies have suggested that the generation of these anaphylatoxins are responsible for the generalized inflammatory response that follows cardiopulmonary bypass (postperfusion syndrome) and hemodialysis (pulmonary neutrophil sequestration) (Chenoweth et al., 1981; Hosea et al., 1980b; Jacob and Craddock, 1980; Till et al., 1982).

Malnutrition

Children with malnutrition, both kwashiorkor and marasmus, have decreased levels of serum total hemolytic complement activity and most of the individual components of complement, such as C3 and C5 (Sirisinha et al., 1973) (see Chapter 23). Dietary treatment of the malnutrition results in normalization of the complement levels. The degree of the decrease in complement components (e.g., C3) correlates strongly with serum albumin, suggesting that the decrease is due to poor synthetic function in the liver.

Acquired C1 Esterase Inhibitor Deficiency

Acquired C1 INH deficiency is due to antibodies to C1 INH (Agostoni and Cicardi, 1992; Gelfand et al., 1979; Oltvai et al., 1991). Many of the patients have an underlying lymphoproliferative process. The clinical presentation is similar to that of inherited C1 INH deficiency except that the age of onset is later, typically after the age of 30 years, and there is no family history. Certain laboratory features also allow the two disorders to be distinguished. In acquired C1 INH deficiency, C1q levels are low along with C4 and C2. C1 INH is produced appropriately; however, because of binding by the autoantibody, its turnover is rapid and its function is impaired (Melamed et al., 1986). Therefore these patients have very low levels of C1 INH antigen and function.

Therapy is typically directed at the lymphoproliferative process when applicable. Attenuated androgens have seldom been helpful, presumably because they are unable to compensate and correct such a large deficit (Agostoni and Cicardi, 1992). Fibrinolytics have demonstrated some clinical utility, and plasmapheresis has been used rarely (Donaldson et al., 1992). Purified C1 INH has also been used with some limited success, but very large doses are required to overcome the autoantibodies.

REFERENCES

Abbott C, West L, Povey S, Jeremiah S, Murad Z, Discipio R, Fey G. The gene for human complement component C9 mapped to chromosome 5 by polymerase chain reaction. Genomics 4:606–609, 1989.

Abramson N, Alper CA, Lachmann PJ, Rosen FS, Jandl JH. Deficiency of C3 inactivator in man. J Immunol 107:19–27, 1971.

Adamkin D, Stitzel A, Urmson J, Farnett ML, Post E, Spitzer R. Activity of the alternative pathway of complement in the newborn infant. J Pediatr 93:604–608, 1978.

Adinolfi M. Levels of two components of complement (C4 and C3) in human fetal and newborn sera. Develop Med Child Neurol 12:306–308, 1970.

Adinolfi M. Human complement: onset and site of synthesis during fetal life. Am J Dis Child 131:1015–1023, 1977.

Adinolfi M, Beck SE. Human complement C7 and C9 in fetal and newborn sera. Arch Dis Child 50:562–564, 1975.

Adinolfi M, Gardner B. Synthesis of B_1E and B_1C components of complement in human foetuses. Acta Paediatr Scand 56:450–454, 1967.

Agostoni A, Cicardi M. Hereditary and acquired C1-inhibitor deficiency: biological and clinical characteristics in 235 patients. Medicine 71:206–215, 1992.

Agostoni A, Cicardi M, Cugno M, Storti E. Clinical problems in the C1-inhibitor deficient patient. Behring Inst Mitt 93:306–312, 1993.

Ahearn JM, Fischer MB, Croix D, Goerg S, Ma M, Xia J, Zhou X, Howard RG, Rothstein TL, Carroll MC. Disruption of the Cr2 locus results in a reduction in B-1a cells and in an impaired B cell response to T-dependent antigens. Immunity 4:251–262, 1996.

Alper CA, Abramson N, Johnston RB Jr, Jandl JH, Rosen FS. Increased susceptibility to infection associated with abnormalities of complement-mediated functions and of the third component of complement (C3). N Engl J Med 282:350–354, 1970a.

Alper CA, Abramson N, Johnston RB, Jandl JH, Rosen FS. Studies in vivo and in vitro on an abnormality in the metabolism of C3 in a patient with increased susceptibility to infection. J Clin Invest 49:1975–1985, 1970b.

Alper CA, Colten HR, Gear JSS, Robson AR, Rosen FS. Homozygous human C3 deficiency: the role of C3 in antibody production, C1s-induced vasopermeability, and cobra venom–induced passive hemolysis. J Clin Invest 57:222–229, 1976.

Alper CA, Colten HR, Rosen FS, Robson AR, MacNab GM, Gear JSS. Homozygous deficiency of C3 in a patient with repeated infections. Lancet ii:1179–1181, 1972.

Alper CA, Johnson AM, Birtch AG, Moore RD. Human C3: evidence for the liver as the primary site of synthesis. Science 163:286–288, 1969.

Andreu M, Sola R, Sitges-Serra A, Alia C, Gallen M, Vila MC, Coll S, Oliver MI. Risk factors for spontaneous bacterial peritonitis in cirrhotic patients with ascites. Gastroenterology 104:1133–1138, 1993.

Andreoni J, Kayhty H, Densen P. Vaccination and the role of capsular polysaccharide antibody in prevention of recurrent meningococcal disease in late complement component-deficient individuals. J Infect Dis 168:227–231, 1993.

Arenzana N, Rodriguez de Cordoba S. Promoter region of the human gene coding for beta-chain of C4b binding protein. Hepatocyte nuclear factor-3 and nuclear factor-I/CTF transcription factors are required for efficient expression of C4BPB in HepG2 cells. J Immunol 156:168–175, 1996.

Ault BH, Schmidt BZ, Fowler NL, Kashtan CE, Ahmed AE, Vogt BA, Colten HR. Human factor H deficiency. Mutations in framework cysteine residues and block in H protein secretion and intracellular catabolism. J Biol Chem 272:25168–25175, 1997.

Austen KF, Sheffer AL. Detection of hereditary angioneurotic edema by demonstration of a reduction in the second component of human complement. N Engl J Med 272:649–654, 1965.

Awdeh ZL, Alper CA. Inherited structural polymorphism of the fourth component of human complement. Proc Natl Acad Sci USA 77:3576–3580, 1978.

Awdeh ZL, Ochs HD, Alper CA. Genetic analysis of C4 deficiency. J Clin Invest 67:260–263, 1981.

Awdeh ZL, Raum DD, Glass D, Agnello V, Schur PH, Johnston RB Jr, Gelfand EW, Ballow M, Yunis E, Alper CA. Complement-human histocompatibility antigen haplotypes in C2 deficiency. J Clin Invest 67:581–583, 1981.

Babovic-Vuksanovic D, Snow K, Ten RM. Mannose-binding lectin (MBL) deficiency. Variant alleles in a midwestern population of the United States. Ann Allergy Asthma Immunol 82:134–138, 141; quiz 142–143, 1999.

Ballow M, Fang F, Good RA, Day NK. Developmental aspects of complement components in the newborn. Clin Exp Immunol 18:257–266, 1974.

Ballow M, Shira JE, Harden L, Yang SY, Day NK. Complete absence of the third component of complement in man. J Clin Invest 56:703–710, 1975.

Balke N, Holtkamp U, Horl WH, Tschesche H. Inhibition of degranulation of human polymorphonuclear leukocytes by complement factor D. FEBS Lett 371:300–302, 1995.

Barnum SR, Volanakis JE. Biosynthesis of complement protein D by HepG2 cells: a comparison of D produced by HepG2 cells, U937 cells and blood monocytes. Eur J Immunol 15:1148–1151, 1985.

Barba G, Rittner C, Schneider PM. Genetics basis of human complement C4A deficiency. J Clin Invest 91:1681–1686, 1993.

Bellamy R. Identifying genetic susceptibility factors for tuberculosis in Africans: a combined approach using a candidate gene study and a genome-wide screen. Clin Sci (Colch) 98:245–250, 2000.

Bensa JC, Reboul A, Colomb MG. Biosynthesis in vitro of complement subcomponents C1q, C1s, and C1 inhibitor by resting and stimulated human monocytes. Biochem J 216:385–392, 1983.

Berger M, Balow JE, Wilson CB, Frank MM. Circulating immune complexes and glomerulonephritis in a patient with congenital absence of the third component of complement. N Engl J Med 308:1009–1012, 1983.

Berkel AI, Birben E, Oner C, Oner R, Loos M, Petry F. Molecular, genetic and epidemiologic studies on selective complete C1q deficiency in Turkey. Immunobiology 201:347–355, 2000.

Berkel AI, Nakakuma N. Studies of immune response in a patient with selective complete C1q deficiency. Turk J Pediatr 35:221–226, 1993.

Bielory L, Eascon P, Lawley TD, Nienhuis A, Frank MM, Yung NS. Serum sickness and hematopoietic recovery with antithymocyte globulin in bone marrow failure patients. Br J Haematol 63:729–736, 1986.

Biesma D, Hannema AJ, Van Velzen-Biad H, Mulder L, Van Zwieten R, Kluijt I, Roos D. A family with complement Factor D deficiency. J Clin Invest 108:233–240, 2001.

Biselli R, Casapollo I, D'Amelio R, Salvato S, Matricardi PM, Brai M. Antibody response to meningococcal polysaccharides A and C in patients with complement defects. Scand J Immunol 37:644–650. 1993.

Biskof NA, Welch TR, Beischel LS. C4B deficiency: a risk factor for bacteremia with encapsulated organisms. J Infect Dis 162:248–250, 1990.

Bock SC, Skriver K, Neilson E, Thogersen HC, Wiman B, Donaldson VH, Eddy RL, Muarinan J, Rodziejewska E, Huber R, Shows TB, Magnusson S. Human C1 inhibitor: primary structure, cDNA cloning and chromosomal localization. Biochem 25:4292–4301, 1986.

Border WA, Noble NA. From serum sickness to cytokines: advances in understanding the molecular pathogenesis of kidney disease [editorial]. Lab Invest 68:125–128, 1993.

Borzy MS, Houghton D. Mixed-pattern immune deposit glomerulonephritis in a child with inherited deficiency of the third component of complement. Am J Kid Dis 5:54–59, 1985.

Bottger EC, Hoffmann T, Hadding V, Bitter-Suermann D. Influence of genetically inherited complement deficiencies on humoral immune response in guinea pigs. J Immunol 135:4100–4107, 1985.

Bottger EC, Hoffmann T, Hadding U, Bitter-Suermann D. Guinea pigs with inherited deficiencies of complement components C2 or C4 have characteristics of immune complex disease. J Clin Invest 78:689–695, 1986.

Botto M, Dell'Agnola C, Bygrave AE, Thompson EM, Cook HT, Petry F, Loos M, Pandolfi PP, Walfport MJ. Homozygous C1q deficiency causes glomerulonephritis associated with multiple apoptotic bodies. Nat Genet 19:56–59, 1998.

Botto M, Fong KY, So AK, Barlow R, Routier R, Morley BJ, Walport MJ. Homozygous hereditary C3 deficiency due to a partial gene deletion. Proc Nat Acad Sci 89:4957–4961, 1992.

Botto M, Fong KY, So AK, Rudge A, Walport MJ. Molecular basis of hereditary C3 deficiency. J Clin Invest 86:1158–1163, 1990.

Bowness P, Davies KA, Norsworthy PJ, Athanassiou P, Taylor-Wiedeman J, Borysiewicz LK, Meyer PA, Walport MJ. Hereditary C1q deficiency and systemic lupus erythematosus. Q J Med 87:455–464, 1994.

Brai M, Misiano G, Maringhini S, Cutaja I, Hauptmann G. Combined homozygous factor H and heterozygous C2 deficiency in an Italian family. J Clin Immunol 8:50–56, 1988.

Braun L, Schneider PM, Giles CM, Bertrams J, Rittner C. Null alleles of human complement C4. Evidence for pseudogenes at the C4A locus and gene conversion at the C4B locus. J Exp Med 171:129–140, 1990.

Buyon JP, Tamerius J, Belmont HM, Abramson SB. Assessment of disease activity and impending flare in patients with systemic lupus erythematosus. Comparison of the use of complement split products and conventional measurements of complement. Arthritis Rheum 35:1028–1036, 1992.

Cahill J, Stevens FM, McCarthy CF. Complement C4 types in coeliacs and controls. Ir J Med Sci 160:168–169, 1991.

Carney DF, Haviland DL, Noack D, Wetsel RA, Vik DP, Tack BF. Structural aspects of the human C5 gene. J Biol Chem 266:18786–18791, 1991.

Carroll MC, Campbell RD, Bently DR, Porter RR. A molecular map of the human major histocompatibility complex class III region linking complement genes C4, C2, and factor B. Nature 307:237–240, 1984.

Carter PE, Duponchel C, Tosi M, Fothergill JE. Complete nucleotide sequence of the gene for human C1 inhibitor with an unusually high density of Alu elements. Eur J Biochem 197:301–308, 1991.

Casciola-Rosen LA, Anhalt G, Rosen A. Autoantigens targeted in systemic lupus erythematosus are clustered in two populations of surface structures on apoptotic keratinocytes. J Exp Med 179:1317–1330, 1994.

Chakravarti DN, Chakravarti B, Parra CA, Muller-Eberhard HJ. Structural homology of complement protein C6 with other channel-forming proteins of complement. Proc Nat Acad Sciences USA 86:2799–2803, 1989.

Chapius RM, Hauptmann G, Grosshans E, Isliker H. Structural and functional studies in C1q deficiency. J Immunol 129:1509–1515, 1982.

Chen A, Gaddipati S, Hong Y, Volkman DJ, Peerschke EI, Ghebrehiwet B. Human T cells express specific binding sites for C1q. Role in T cell activation and proliferation. J Immunol 153:1430–1440, 1994.

Chenoweth DE, Cooper SW, Hugli TE, Stewart RW, Blackstone EH, Kirklin JW. Complement activation during cardiopulmonary bypass. N Engl J Med 304:497–503, 1981.

Chevailler A, Drouet C, Ponard D, Alibeu C, Suraniti S, Carrere F, Renier G, Hurez P, Colomb MG. Non-coordinated biosynthesis of early complement components in a deficiency of complement proteins C1r and C1s. Scand J Immunol 40:383–388, 1994.

Choy LN, Spiegelman BM. Regulation of alternative pathway activation and C3a production by adipose cells. Obesity Res 4:521–532, 1996.

Christiansen FT, Dawkins RL, Uko G, McClusky J, Kay PH, Zilko PJ. Complement allotyping in SLE: association with C4A null. Aust N Z J Med 13:483–488, 1983.

Churg J, Habib RR, White RHR. Pathology of the nephrotic syndrome in children: a report of the International Study of Kidney Disease in Children. Lancet 1:1299–1302, 1970.

Cicardi M, Bergamaschini L, Cugno M, Hack E, Agostoni G, Agostoni A. Long-term treatment of hereditary angioedema with attenuated androgens: a survey of a 13-year experience. J Allergy Clin Immunol 87:768–773, 1991.

Cicardi M, Bergamaschini L, Marasini B, Boccassini G, Tucci A, Agostini A. Hereditary angioedema: an appraisal of 104 cases. Am J Med Sci 284:2–9, 1982.

Clark RA, Klebanoff SJ. Role of the classical and alternative complement pathways in chemotaxis and opsonization: studies of human serum deficient in C4. J Immunol 120:1102–1108, 1978.

Colten HR. Genetics and synthesis of components of the complement system. In Ross GD, ed. Immunobiology of the Complement System. New York, Academic Press, 1986, p 163.

Colten HR. Tissue specific regulation of inflammation. J Appl Physiol 72:1–7, 1992.

Cork LC, Morris JM, Olson JL, Krakowka S, Swift AJ, Winkelstein JA. Membranoproliferative glomerulonephritis in dogs with a genetically determined deficiency of the third component of complement. Clin Immunol Immunopathol 60:455–470, 1991.

Cornacoff JB, Hebert LA, Smead WL, Van Aman ME, Birmingham DJ, Waxman FJ. Primate erythrocyte-immune complex-clearing mechanism. J Clin Invest 71:236–247, 1983.

Curd JG, Progais LJ Jr, Cochrane CG. Detection of active kallikrein in induced blister fluids of hereditary angioedema patients. J Exp Med 152:742–747, 1980.

Cutler AJ, Botto M, van Essen D, Rivi R, Davies KA, Gray D, Walport MW. T-cell-dependent immune responses in C1q-deficient mice: defective interferon gamma production by antigen specific T cells. J Exp Med 187:1789–1797, 1998.

Czop J, Nussenzweig V. Studies on the mechanisms of solubilization of immune precipitates by serum. J Exp Med 143:615–630, 1976.

Davies EJ, The LS, Ordi-Ros J, Snowden N, Hillarby MD, Hajeer A, Donn R, Perez-Pemen P, Vilardell-Tarres M, Ollier WE. A dysfunctional allele of the mannose binding protein gene associates with systemic lupus erythematosus in a Spanish population. J Rheumatol 24:485–488, 1997.

Davies KA, Erlendsson K, Beynon HL, Peters AM, Steinsson K, Valdimarsson H, Walport MJ. Splenic uptake of immune complexes in man is complement dependent. J Immunol 151:3866–3873, 1993.

Davies KA, Peters M, Beynon HLC, Walport MJ. Immune complex processing in patients with systemic lupus erythematosus. J Clin Invest 90:2075–2083, 1992.

Davis AE, Aulak KS, Parad RB, Stecklein HP, Eldering E, Hack CG, Kramer J, Strunk RC, Rosen FS. Characterization and expression of C1 inhibitor non-reactive center mutations. Complem Inflamm 8:138abs, 1991.

Davis AE 3rd, Bissler JJ, Cicardi M. Mutations in the C1 inhibitor gene that result in hereditary angioneurotic edema. Behring Inst Mitt 93:313–320, 1993.

Davis AE III, Davis JS IV, Robson AR, Osofsky SG, Colten HR, Rosen FS, Alper CA. Homozygous C3 deficiency: detection of C3 by radioimmunoassay. Clin Immunol Immunopathol 8:543–550, 1977.

Davis AE, Whitehead AS, Harrison RA, Dauphinais A, Bruns GAP, Cicardi M, Rosen FS. Human inhibitor of the first component of complement, C1: characterization of cDNA clones and localization of the gene to chromosome 11. Proc Natl Acad Sci USA 83:3161–3165, 1986.

Day NK, L'esperance P, Good RA, Michael AF, Hansen JA, Dupont B, Jersild C. Hereditary C2 deficiency. Genetic studies and association with the HL-A system. J Exp Med 141:1464–1469, 1975.

DeJuan D, Martin-Villa JM, Gomez-Reino JJ, Vicario JL, Corell A, Martinez-Iaso J, Benmammar D, Arnaiz-Villena A. Differential contribution of C4 and HLA-DQ genes to systemic lupus erythematosus susceptibility. Hum Genet 91:579–584, 1993.

Dempsey PW, Allison MED, Akkaraju S, Goodnow CC, Fearon DT. C3d of complement as a molecular adjuvant: bridging innate and acquired immunity. Science 271:348–350, 1996.

Densen P, Ackerman L. The genetic basis of C8α-γ deficiency. Mol Immunol S1:68, 1996.

Densen P, Sanford M, Burke T, Densen E, Wintermeyer E. Prospective study of the prevalence of complement deficiency in meningitis. 30th Interscience Conference on Antimicrobial Agents and Chemotherapy, Abstract 320, 1990.

Densen P, Weiler JM, Griffs JM, Hoffmann LG. Familial properdin deficiency and fatal meningococcemia: correction of the bactericidal defect by vaccination. N Engl J Med 316:922–927, 1987.

DiScipio RG, Gehring MR, Podack ER, Kan CC, Hugli TE, Fey GH. Nucleotide sequence of human complement component C9. Proc Natl Acad Sci USA 81:7298–7302, 1984.

DiScipio RG, Hugli TE. The molecular architecture of human complement component C6. J Biol Chem 264:16197–16206, 1989.

Donaldson VH, Bernstein DI, Wagner CJ, Mitchell BH, Scinto J, Bernstein IL. Angioneurotic edema with acquired C1-inhibitor deficiency and autoantibody to C1-inhibitor: response to plasmapheresis and cytotoxic therapy. J Lab Clin Med 119:397–406, 1992.

Donaldson VH, Evans RR. A biochemical abnormality in hereditary angioneurotic edema. Absence of serum inhibitor of C1-esterase. Am J Med 35:37–43, 1963.

Donaldson VH, Harrison RA, Rosen FS, Being DH, Kindness G, Canar J, Wagner CJ, Awad S. Variability in purified dysfunctional C1-inhibitor proteins from patients with hereditary angioneurotic edema. Functional and analytical gel studies. J Clin Invest 75:124–132, 1985.

Donaldson VH, Rosen FS. Action of complement in hereditary angioneurotic edema: role of C1-esterase. J Clin Invest 43:2204–2208, 1964.

Donaldson VH, Rosen FS. Hereditary angioneurotic edema: a clinical survey. Pediatrics 37:1017–1027, 1966.

Dossett JH, Williams RC Jr, Quie PG. Studies on interaction of bacteria, serum factors and polymorphonuclear leukocytes in others and newborns. Pediatrics 44:49–57, 1969.

Dragon-Durey MA, Quartier P, Fremeaux-Bacchi V, Blouin J, de Barace C, Prieur A, Weiss L, Fridman WH. Molecular basis of selective C1s deficiency associated with multiple autoimmune diseases. J Immunol 166:7612–7616, 2001.

Edwards KM, Alford R, Gewurz H, Mold C. Recurrent bacterial infections associated with C3 nephritic factor and hypocomplementemia. N Engl J Med 308:1138–1141, 1983.

Edkahl K, Truedsson L, Sjoholm AG, Braconier JH. Complement analysis in adult patients with a history of bacteremic pneumococcal infections or recurrent pneumonia. Scand J Infect Dis 27:111–117, 1995.

Ellison RT III, Horsburgh R Jr, Curd J. Complement levels in patients with hepatic dysfunction. Dig Dis Sci 35:231–235. 1990.

Ellison RT, Kohler PH, Curd JG, Judson FN, Reller LB. Prevalence of congenital and acquired complement deficiency in patients with sporadic meningococcal disease. N Engl J Med 308:913–916, 1983.

Ellison RTD, Curd JG, Kohler PF, Reller LB, Judson FN. Underlying complement deficiency in patients with disseminated gonococcal infection. Sex Transm Dis 14:201–204, 1987.

Ellman L, Green I, Frank M. Genetically controlled deficiency of the fourth component of complement in the guinea pig. Science 170:74–75, 1970.

Endo Y, Kanno K, Takahashi M, Yamaguchi K, Kohno Y, Fujita T. Molecular basis of human complement C1s deficiency. J Immunol 162:2180–2183, 1999.

Ernst T, Spath PJ, Aebi C, Schaad UB, Bianchetti MG. Screening for complement deficiency in bacterial meningitis. Acta Paediatr 86:1009–1010, 1997.

Fasano MB, Hamosh A, Winkelstein JA. Recurrent systemic bacterial infections in homozygous C2 deficiency. Ped Allergy Immunol 1:46–49, 1990.

Fearon DT. Identification of the membrane glycoprotein that is the C3b receptor of the human erythrocyte, polymorphonuclear leukocyte, B lymphocyte and monocyte. J Exp Med 152:20–30, 1980.

Fearon DT, Ruddy S, Schur PH, McCabe WR. Activation of the properdin pathway of complement in patients with gram-negative bacteremia. N Engl J Med 292:937–940, 1975.

Fernandez HN, Henson PM, Otani A, Hugli TE. Chemotactic response to human C3a and C5a anaphylatoxins. I. Evaluation of C3a and C5a leukotaxis in vitro and under stimulated in vivo conditions. J Immunol 120:109–115, 1978.

Fernie BA, Hobart MJ. Complement C7 deficiency: seven further molecular defects and their associated marker haplotypes. Hum Genet 103:513–519. 1998.

Fernie BA, Hobart MJ. Five new polymorphisms in the complement C7 gene and their association with C7 deficiency. Exp Clin Immunogenet 16:150–161, 1999.

Fernie BA, Orren A, Sheehan G, Schlesinger M, Hobart MJ. Molecular bases of C7 deficiency. Three different defects. J Immunol 159:1019–1026, 1997.

Fernie BA, Wurzner R, Orren A, Morgan BP, Potter PC, Platonov AE. Molecular bases of combined subtotal deficiencies of C6 and C7: their effects in combination with other C6 and C7 deficiencies. J Immunol 157:3648–3657, 1996.

Fielder AHL, Walport MJ, Batchelor JR, Rynes RI, Black CM, Dodi IA, Hughes GRV. Family study of the major histocompatibility complex in patients with systemic lupus erythematosus: importance of null alleles of C4A and C4B in determining disease susceptibility. BMJ 286:425–428, 1983.

Figueroa JE, Densen P. Infectious diseases associated with complement deficiencies. Clin Microb Rev 4:359–395, 1991.

Fijen CA, Kuijper EJ, Hannema AJ, Sjohom AG, Van Putten JPM. Complement deficiencies in patients over ten years old with meningococcal disease due to uncommon serogroups. Lancet 2:585–588, 1989.

Fijen CA, Kuijper EJ, Drogari-Apiranthitou M, Van Leeuwen Y, Daha MR, Dankert J. Protection against meningococcal serogroup ACYW disease in complement-deficient individuals vaccinated with the tetravalent meningococcal capsular polysaccharide vaccine. Clin Exp Immunol 114:362–369, 1998.

Fine DP, Gewurz H, Griffis M, Lint TF. Meningococcal meningitis in a woman with inherited deficiency of the ninth component of complement. Clin Immunol Immunopathol 28:413–417, 1983.

Fireman P, Zuchowski DA, Taylor PM. Development of human complement system. J Immunol 103:25–31, 1969.

Finlayson NDC, Krohn K, Fauconnet MH, Anderson KE. Significance of serum complement levels in chronic liver disease. Gastroenterology 63:653–659, 1972.

Fischer MB, Goerg S, Shen L, Prodeus AP, Goodnaow CG, Kelsoe G, et al. Dependence of germinal center B cells on expression of CD21/CD35 for survival. Science 280:582–585, 1998.

Fischer MB, Ma M, Goerg S, Zhou X, Xia J, Finco O, et al. Regulation of the B cell response to T-dependent antigens by classical pathway complement. J Immunol 157:549–556, 1996.

Floreani A, Heires AJ, Welniak LA, Miller-Lindholm A, Clark-Pierce L, Rennard SI, Morgan EL, Sanderson SD. Expression of receptors for C5a anaphylatoxin (CD88) on human bronchial epithelial cells: enhancement of C5a-mediated release of IL-8 upon exposure to cigarette smoke. J Immunol 160:5073–5081, 1998.

Forman ML, Stiehm ER. Impaired opsonic activity but normal phagocytosis in low birth weight infants. N Engl J Med 281:926–931, 1969.

Frank MM, Gelfand JA, Atkinson JP. Hereditary angioedema: the clinical syndrome and its management. Ann Intern Med 84:580–593, 1976.

Frank MM, Sergent JS, Kane MA, Alling DW. Epsilon aminocaproic acid therapy of hereditary angioneurotic edema: a double blind study. N Engl J Med 286:808–812, 1972.

Fredrikson GN, Truedsson L, Sjoholm AG, Kjellman M. DNA analysis in a MHC heterozygous patients with complete C4 deficiency-homozygosity for C4 gene deletion and C4 pseudogene. Exp Clin Immunogen 8:29–35, 1991.

Fredrikson GN, Westberg J, Kuijper EJ, Tijssen CC, Sjoholm AG, Uhlen M, Truedsson L. Molecular genetic characterization of properdin deficiency type III: dysfunction due to a single point mutation in exon 9 of the structural gene causing a tyrosine to aspartic acid interchange. Mol Immunol 33(Suppl 1):1, 1996.

Friend P, Repine J, Kim Y, Clawson CC, Michael AF. Deficiency of the second component of complement (C2) with chronic vasculitis. Ann Intern Med 83:813–816, 1975.

Fu SM, Kunkel HG, Brusman HP, Allen FH Jr, Fotino M. Evidence for linkage between HL-A histocompatibility genes and those involved in the synthesis of the second component of complement. J Exp Med 140:1108–1111, 1975.

Fukumori Y, T Horiuchi. Terminal complement component deficiencies in Japan. Exp Clin Immunogenet 15:244–248, 1998.

Fust G, Petras GY, Ujhelyi E. Activation of the complement system during infections due to gram-negative bacteria. Clin Immunol Immunopathol 5:293–302, 1976.

Gadek JE, Hosea SW, Gelfand JA, Frank MM. Response of variant hereditary angioedema phenotypes to danazol therapy. J Clin Invest 64:280–286, 1979.

Garred P, Madsen HO, Balslev U, Hofmann B, Pedersen C, Gerstoft J, Svejgaard A. Susceptibility to HIV infection and progression of AIDS in relation to variant alleles of mannose-binding lectin. Lancet 349:236–240, 1997.

Garred P, Madsen HO, Halberg P, Petersen J, Kronborg G, Svejgaard A, Andersen V, Jacobsen S. Mannose-binding lectin polymorphisms and susceptibility to infection in systemic lupus erythematosus [see comments]. Arthritis Rheum 42:2145–2152, 1999.

Garred P, Mollnes TE, Thorsteinsson L, Erlendsson K, Steinsson K. Increased amounts of C4-containing immune complexes and inefficient activation of C3 and the terminal complement pathway in a patient with homozygous C2 deficiency and systemic lupus erythematosus. J Immunol 31:59–64, 1990.

Garty BZ, Conley ME, Douglas SD, Kolski GB. Recurrent infections and staphylococcal liver abscess in a child with C1r deficiency. J Allergy Clin Immunol 80:631–635, 1987.

Geibink GS, Verhoef J, Peterson PK, Quie PG. Opsonic requirements for phagocytosis of streptococcus pneumoniae types VI, XVIII, XXIII and XXV. Infect Immun 18:291–297, 1977.

Gelfand EW, Clarkson JE, Minta JO. Selective deficiency of the second component of complement in a patient with anaphylactoid purpura. Clin Immunol Immunopathol 4:269–276, 1975.

Gelfand JA, Boss GR, Conley CL, Reinhart R, Frank MM. Acquired C1 esterase inhibitor deficiency and angioedema: a review. Medicine 58:321–328, 1979.

Gelfand JA, Sherins RJ, Alling DW, Frank MM. Treatment of hereditary angioedema with danazol: reversal of clinical and biochemical abnormalities. N Engl J Med 295:1444–1448, 1976.

Gitlin D, Biasucci A. Development of gamma G, gamma A, gamma M, beta-1-C/beta-1-A, C1 esterase inhibitor, ceruloplasmin, transferrin, hemopexin, haptoglobin, fibrinogen, plasminogen, alpha₁ antitrypsin, orosomucoid, beta-lipoprotein, alpha₂ macroglobulin and prealbumin in the human conceptus. J Clin Invest 48:1433–1436, 1969.

Glass D, Raum D, Gibson D, Stillman JS, Schur PH. Inherited deficiency of the second component of complement. Rheumatic disease association. J Clin Invest 58:853–861, 1976.

Goldberger G, Arnaout MA, Aden D, Kay R, Rits M, Colten HR. Biosynthesis and postsynthetic processing of human C3b/C4b inactivator (factor I) in three hepatoma cell lines. J Biol Chem 259:6492–6497, 1984.

Goldberger G, Bruns GA, Rits M, Edge MD, Kwiatkowski DJ. Human complement factor I. Analysis of cDNA-derived primary structure and assignment of its gene to chromosome 4. J Biol Chem 262:10065–10071, 1987.

Grace HJ, Brereton-Stiles GG, Vos GH, Schonland M. A family with partial and total deficiency of complement C3. S Afr Med J 50:139–140, 1976.

Graudal NA, Madsen HO, Tarp U, Svejgaard A, Jurik G, Graudal HK, et al. The association of variant mannose-binding lectin genotypes with radiographic outcome in rheumatoid arthritis. Arthritis Rheum 43:515–521, 2000.

Hamann J, Wishaupt JO, van Lier RA, Smeets TJ, Breedveld FC, Tak PP. Expression of the activation antigen CD97 and its ligand

CD55 in rheumatoid synovial tissue. Arthritis Rheum 42:650–658, 1999.

Hammer CH, Gaither T, Frank MM. Complement deficiencies of laboratory animals. In Gershwin ME, Merchant B, eds. Immunologic Defects in Laboratory Animals. New York, Plenum Press, 1981.

Hannema AJ, Kluin-Nelemans JC, Hack E, Erenberg-Belmer AJM, Mallee C, Van Helden HPT. SLE-like syndromes and functional deficiency of C1q in members of a large family. Clin Exp Immunol 55:106–110, 1984.

Harpel PC, Cooper NR. Studies on human plasma C1 inactivator-enzyme interactions. I. Mechanisms of interactions with C1s, plasmin, and trypsin. J Clin Invest 55:593–604, 1975.

Harpel PC, Hugli TE, Cooper NR. Studies on human plasma C1 inactivator-enzyme interactions: II. Structural features of an abnormal C1 inactivator from a kindred with hereditary angioneurotic edema. J Clin Invest 55:605–611, 1975.

Harriman GR, Esser AF, Podack ER, Wunderlich AC, Braude AI, Lint TF, Curd JG. The role of C9 in complement-mediated killing of Neisseria. J Immunol 127:2386–2390, 1981.

Hartmann D, Fremeaux-Bacchi V, Weiss L, Meyer A, Blouin J, Haputmann G, Kazatchkine M, Uring-Lambert B. Combined heterozygous deficiency of the classical complement pathway proteins C2 and C4. J Clin Immunol 17:176–184, 1997.

Hartung K, Fontana A, Klar M, Krippner H, Jorgens K, Lang B, et al. Association of Class I, II, and III MHC geneproducts with systemic lupus erythematosus. Rheumatol Int 9:13–18, 1989.

Hauptmann G, Tappeiner G, Schifferli JA. Inherited deficiency of the fourth complement. Immunodef Rev 1:3–22, 1988.

Hauptmann G, Tongio MM, Goetz J, Mayer S, Fauchet R, Sobel A, Griscel C, Berthoux F, Rivat C, Rother U. Association of the C2-deficiency gene (C2*Q0) with the C4A*4, C4B*2 genes. J Immunogenet 9:127–132, 1982.

Haviland DL, Haviland JC, Fleischer DT, Wetsel RA. Structure of the murine fifth complement component (C5) gene. A large, highly interrupted gene with a variant donor splice site and organizational homology with the third and fourth complement component genes. J Biol Chem 266:11818–11825, 1991.

Hebert AA, Sigman ES, Levy ML. Serum sickness-like reactions from cefaclor in children. J Am Acad Dermatol 25:805–808, 1991.

Heckbert SR, Stryker WS, Coltin KL, Manson JE, Platt R. Serum sickness in children after antibiotic exposure: estimates of occurrence and morbidity in a health maintenance organization population. Am J Epidemiol 132:336–342, 1990.

Hibberd ML, Sumiya M, Summerfield JA, Booy R, Levin M. Association of variants of the gene for mannose-binding lectin with susceptibility to meningococcal disease. Meningococcal Research Group [see comments]. Lancet 353:1049–1053, 1999.

Hiemstra PS, Langeler E, Compier B, Keepers Y, Leijh PCJ, van den Barselaar MT, Overbosch D, Daha MR. Complete and partial deficiencies of complement factor D in a Dutch family. J Clin Invest 84:1957–1961, 1989.

Hironaka K, Makino H, Amano T, Ota Z. Immune complex glomerulonephritis in a pregnant woman with congenital C9 deficiency. Int Med 32:806–809, 1993.

Hirsch RL. The complement system: its importance in the host response to viral infection. Microbiol Rev 46:71–85, 1982.

Hoal-Van Helden EG, J Epstein, TC Victor, D Hon, LA Lewis, N Beyers, Zurakowski D, Ezekowtiz AB, Van Helden PD. Mannose-binding protein B allele confers protection against tuberculous meningitis. Pediatr Res 45:459–464, 1999.

Hobart MJ, Fernie BA, Fijen KA, Orren A. The molecular basis of C6 deficiency in the western Cape, South Africa. Hum Genet 103:506–512, 1998.

Homann C, Varming K, Hogasen K, Mollnes TE, Graudal N, Thomsen AC, Garred P. Acquired C3 deficiency in patients with alcoholic cirrhosis predisposes to infection and increased mortality. Gut 40:544–549, 1997.

Horiuchi T, Ferrer JM, Serra P, Matamoros N, Lopez-Trascasa M, Hashimura C, Niho Y. A novel nonsense mutation at Glu-631 in a Spanish family with complement component 7 deficiency. J Hum Genet 44:215–218, 1999.

Horiuchi T, Neshizaka H, Jojima T, Sawabe T, Niko Y, Schneider PM, Inaba S, Sakai K, Hayashi K, Hashimura C, Fukumori Y.

A nonsense mutation at Arg 95 is predominant in C9 deficiency in Japanese. J Immunol 160:1509–1513, 1998.

Hosea SW, Brown EJ, Frank MM. The critical role of complement in experimental pneumococcal sepsis. J Infect Dis 142:903–909, 1980a.

Hosea SW, Brown E, Hammer C, Frank M. Role of complement activation in a model of adult respiratory distress syndrome. J Clin Invest 66:375–382, 1980b.

Hosea SW, Santaella ML, Brown EJ, Berger M, Katusha K, Frank MM. Long-term therapy of hereditary angioedema with danazol. Ann Intern Med 93:809–812, 1980c.

Howard OM, Rao AG, Sodetz JM. cDNA and derived amino acid sequence of the beta subunit of human complement protein C8: Identification of a close structural and ancestral relationship to the alpha subunit and C9. Biochemistry 26:3565–3570, 1987.

Howard PF, Hochberg MC, Bias B, Arnett FC, Mclean RH. Relationship between C4 null genes, HLA-D region antigens, and genetic susceptibility to systemic lupus erythematosus in Caucasian and black Americans. Am J Med 81:187–192, 1986.

Hsieh K-H, Lin C-Y, Lee T-C. Complete absence of the third component of complement in a patient with repeated infections. Clin Immunol Immunopathol 20:305–312, 1981.

Huang JL, Lin CY. A hereditary C3 deficiency due to aberrant splicing of exon 10. Clin Immunol Immunopathol 73:267–273, 1994.

Hudson-Peacock MJ, Joseph SA, Cox J, Munro CS, Simpson NB. Systemic lupus erythematosus complicating complement type 2 deficiency: successful treatment with fresh frozen plasma. Br J Dermatol 136:388–392, 1997.

Hummel DS, Mocca LF, Frasch CE, Winkelstein JA, Jean-Baptiste HJJ, Canas JA, Leggiardro RJ. Meningitis caused by a nonencapsulated strain of Neisseria meningitidis in twin infants with a C6 deficiency. J Infect Dis 155:815–818, 1987.

Hyatt AC, Altenburger KM, Johnston RB Jr, Winkelstein JA. Increased susceptibility to severe pyogenic infections in patients with an inherited deficiency of the second component of complement. J Pediatr 98:417–419, 1981.

Inai S, Kitamura H, Hiramatsu S, Nagaki K. Deficiency of the ninth component of complement in man. J Clin Lab Immunol 2:85–87, 1979.

Inoue N, Saito T, Masuda R, Suzuki Y, Ohtomi M, Sakiyama H. Selective complement C1s deficiency caused by homozygous four-base deletion in the C1s gene. Hum Genet 103:415–418, 1998.

Ip WK, Chan SY, Lau CS, Lau YL. Association of systemic lupus erythematosus with promoter polymorphisms of the mannose-binding lectin gene. Arthritis Rheum 41:1663–1668, 1998.

Ip WK, Lau YL, Chan SY, Mok CC, Chan D, Tong KK, Lau CS. Mannose-binding lectin and rheumatoid arthritis in southern Chinese. Arthritis Rheum 43:1679–1687, 2000.

Isenman DE, Young JR. The molecular basis for the difference in immune hemolysis activity of the Chido and Rogers isotypes of human complement components C4. J Immunol 132:3019–3027, 1984.

Ishikawa N, Nonaka M, Wetsel RA, Colten HR. Murine complement C2 and factor B genomic and cDNA cloning reveals different mechanisms for multiple transcripts of C2 and B. J Biol Chem 265:19040–19046, 1990.

Jack RM, Lowenstein BA, Nicholson-Weller A. Regulation of C1q receptor expression on human polymorphonuclear leukocytes. J Immunol 153:262–269, 1994.

Jacob HS, Craddock PR, Hammerschmidt DE, Moldow CF. Complement-induced granulocyte aggregation, an unsuspected mechanism of disease. N Engl J Med 302:789–794, 1980.

Jaffe CJ, Atkinson JP, Gelfand JA, Frank MM. Hereditary angioedema: the use of fresh frozen plasma for prophylaxis in patients undergoing oral surgery. J Allergy Clin Immunol 55:386–393, 1975.

Jasin HE. Absence of the eighth component of complement in association with system lupus erythematosus-like disease. J Clin Invest 60:709–715, 1977.

Johnson AM, Alper CA, Rosen FS, Craig JM. Immunofluorescent hepatic localization of complement proteins: evidence for a biosynthetic defect in hereditary angioneurotic edema (HANE). J Clin Invest 50:50a, 1971.

Johnson CA, Densen P, Hurford R, Colten HR, Wetsel RA. Type I human complement C2 deficiency: a 28 basepair gene deletion causes skipping of exon 6 during RNA splicing. J Biol Chem 267:9347–9353, 1992.

Johnson FR, Agnello V, Williams RC Jr. Opsonic activity in human serum deficient in C2. J Immunol 109:141–145, 1971.

Johnston RB Jr, Altenburger KM, Atkinson AW Jr, Curry RH. Complement in the newborn infant. Pediatric 64:S781–786, 1979.

Johnston RB Jr, Klemperer MR, Alper CA, Rosen FS. The enhancement of bacterial phagocytosis by serum. The role of complement components and two co-factors. J Exp Med 129:1275–1290, 1969.

Junker A, Baatrup G, Svehag SE, Wang P, Holmstrom E, Sturfelt G, Sjoholm AG. Binding of properdin to solid-phase immune complexes: critical role of the classical activation pathway of complement. Scand J Immunol 47:481–486, 1998.

Kakkanaiah VN, Shen GQ, Ojo-Amaize EA, Peter JB. Association of low concentrations of serum mannose-binding protein with recurrent infections in adults. Clin Diag Lab Immunol 5:319–321, 1998.

Kaufman KM, Snider JV, Spurr NK, Schwartz CE, Sodety JM. Chromosomal assignments of genes encoding the α, β, γ subunits of human complement protein C8: identification of a close physical linkage between the α and β loci. Genomics 5:475–480, 1989.

Kaufmann T, Hansch G, Rittner C, Spath P, Tedesco F, Schneider PM. Genetic basis of human complement C8 beta deficiency. J Immunol 150:4943–4947, 1993.

Kazatchkine MD, Fearon DT, Austen KF. Human alternative complement pathway: membrane-associated sialic acid regulates the competition between B and B1H for cell-bound C3b. J Immunol 122:75–81, 1979.

Kemp AS, Vernon J, Muller-Eberhard HJ, Bau DCK. Complement C8 deficiency with recurrent meningococcemia. Aust Pediatr J 21:169–171, 1985.

Kemp ME, Atkinson JP, Skanes VM, Levine RP, Chaplin DD. Deletion of C4A genes in patients with systemic lupus erythematosus. Arthritis Rheum 30:1015–1022, 1987.

Kim Y, Friend PS, Dresner IG, Yunis EJ, Michael AF. Inherited deficiency of the second component of complement (C2) with membranoproliferative glomerulonephritis. Am J Med 62:765–771, 1977.

Kitano E, Kitamura H. Synthesis of factor D by normal human hepatocytes. Int Arch Allergy Immunol 122:299–302, 2000.

Klemperer MR, Donaldson VH, Rosen FS. Effect of C1 esterase on vascular permeability in man: studies in normal and complement-deficient individuals and in patients with hereditary angioneurotic edema. J Clin Invest 47:604–611, 1968.

Kluin-Nelemans H, van Velzen-Blad H, van Helden HPT, Daha MR. Functional deficiency of complement factor D in a monozygous twin. Clin Exp Immunol 58:724–730, 1984.

Kolb WP, Muller-Eberhard HJ. The membrane attack mechanism of complement. The three polypeptide chain structure of the eighth component (C8). J Exp Med 143:1131–1139, 1976.

Korb LC, Ahearn JM. C1q binds directly and specifically to surface blebs of apoptotic human keratinocytes. Complement deficiency and systemic lupus erythematosus revisited. J Immunol 158:4525–4528, 1997.

Kotnik V, Luznik-Bufon T, Schneider PM, Kirschfink M. Molecular, genetic and functional analysis of homozygous C8 β-chain deficiency in two siblings. Immunopharmacology 38:215–221, 1997.

Kourilsky O, Leroy C, Peltier AP. Complement and liver cell function in 53 patients with liver disease. Am J Med 55:783–790, 1973.

Kunschak M, Engl W, Maritsch F, Rosen FS, Edeer G, Zerlauth G, Schwarz HP. A randomized, controlled trial to study the efficacy and safety of C1 inhibitor concentrate in treating hereditary angioedema. Transfusion 38:540–549, 1998.

Kusumoto H, Hirasawa S, Salier JP, Hagen FS, Kurachi K. Human genes for complement components C1r and C1s in a close tail-to-tail arrangement. Proc Natl Acad Sci USA 85:7307–7311, 1988.

Lachmann PJ, Rosen FS. The catabolism of C1-Inhibitor and the pathogenesis of hereditary angio-edema. Acta Path Microbiol Immunol Scand 92:35–39, 1984.

Landau D, Shalev H, Levy-Finer G, Polonsky A, Segev Y, Katchko L. Familial hemolytic uremic syndrome associated with complement factor H deficiency. J Pediatr 138:412–417, 2001.

Landerman NS. Hereditary angioneurotic edema. I. Case reports and review of the literature. J Allergy 33:316–318, 1962.

Lassiter HA, Wilson JL, Feldhoff RC, Hoffpauir JM, Klueber KM. Supplemental complement component C9 enhances the capacity of neonatal serum to kill multiple isolates of pathogenic Escherichia coli. Pediatr Res 35:389–396, 1994.

Lau YL, Lau CS, Chan SY, Karlberg J, Turner MW. Mannose-binding protein in Chinese patients with systemic lupus erythematosus. Arthritis Rheum 39:706–708, 1996.

Law SK, Dodds AW, Porter RR. A comparison of the properties of two classes, C4A and C4B of the human complement components C4. EMBO J 3:1819–1823, 1984.

Leddy JP, Griggs RC, Klemperer MR, Frank MM. Hereditary complement (C2) deficiency with dermatomyositis. Am J Med 58:83–91, 1975.

Lee SL, Wallace SL, Barone R, Blum L, Chase PH. Familial deficiency of two subunits of the first component of complement: C1r and C1s associated with a lupus erythematosus-like disease. Arthritis Rheum 21:958–967, 1978.

Leggiadro RJ, Winkelstein JA. Prevalence of complement deficiencies in children with systemic meningococcal infections. Pediatr Infect Dis 6:75–79, 1987.

Lesavre PH, Hugli TE, Esser AF, Muller-Eberhard HJ. The alternative pathway C3/C5 convertase: chemical basis of factor B activation. J Immunol 123:529–534, 1979.

Levenson T, Masood D, Patterson R. Minocycline-induced serum sickness. Allergy Asthma Proc 17:79–81, 1996.

Levy M, Halbwachs-Mecarelli L, Gubler MC, Kohout G, Bensenouci A, Niaudet P, Hauptmann G, Lesavre P. H deficiency in two brothers with atypical dense intramembranous deposit disease. Kidney Int 30:949–956, 1986.

Levy NJ, Ramesh N, Cicardi M, Harrison RA, David AE. Type II hereditary angioneurotic edema that may result from a single nucleotide change in the codon for alanine-436 in the C1 inhibitor gene. Proc Natl Acad Sci USA 87:265–268, 1990.

Leyva-Cobian F, Moneo I, Mampaso R, Sanchez-Boyle M, Ecija JL. Familial C1q deficiency associated with renal and cutaneous disease. Clin Exp Immunol 44:173–176, 1981.

Lint TF, Gewurz H. Component deficiencies. The ninth component. Prog Allergy 39:307–310, 1986.

Lint TF, Zeitz HJ, Gewurz H. Inherited deficiency of the ninth component of complement in man. J Immunol 125:2252–2257, 1980.

Lipscombe RJ, Sumiya M, Hill AVS, Lau YL, Levinsky RJ, Summerfield JA, Turner MW. High frequencies in African and non-African populations of independent mutations in the mannose binding protein gene. Hum Mol Genet 1:709–715, 1992.

Lipscombe RJ, Sumiya M, Summerfield JA, Turner MW. Distinct physicochemical characteristics of human mannose binding protein expressed by individuals of different genotypes. Immunology 85:660–667, 1995.

Lipsker DM, Schreckenberg-Gilliot C, Uring-Lambert B, Meyer A, Hartmann D, Grosshans E, Hauptmann G. Lupus erythematosus associated with genetically determined deficiency of the second component of complement. Arch Dermatol 136:1508–1514, 2000.

Lloyd W, Schur PH. Immune complexes, complement, and anti-DNA in exacerbations of systemic lupus erythematosus (SLE). Medicine 60:208–217, 1981.

Loos M, Heinz HP. Component deficiencies. 1. The first component: C1q, C1r, C1s. Prog Allergy 39:212–231, 1986.

Loos M, Colomb M. C1, the first component of complement: structure-function-relationship of C1q and collectins (MBP, SP-A, SP-D, conglutinin), C1-esterases (C1r and C1s), and C1-inhibitor in health and disease. Behring Inst Mitt 1–5, 1993.

Lublin DM, Kompelli S, Storry JR, Reid ME. Molecular basis of Cromer blood group antigens. Transfusion 40:208–213, 2000.

Lublin DM, Lemons RS, LeBeau MM, Holers VM, Tykocinski ML, Medof ME, Atkinson JP. The gene encoding decay-accelerating factor (DAF) is located in the complement-regulatory locus on the long arm of chromosome 1. J Exp Med 165:1731–1736, 1987.

Lublin DM, Mallinson G, Poole J, Reid ME, Thompson S, Ferdman BR, Telen MJ, Anstee DJ, Tanner MJ. Molecular basis of reduced or absent expression of decay-accelerating factor in Cromer blood group phenotypes. Blood 84:1276–1282, 1994.

Madsen HO, Garred P, Thiel S, Kurtzhals JAL, Lamm LU, Ryder LP, Svejgaard A. Interplay between promoter and structural gene variants control basal serum level of mannan-binding protein. J Immunol 155:3013–3020, 1995.

Mal F, Pham Huu T, Bendahou M, Trinchet JC, Gardier M, Hakim J, Beaugrand M. Chemoattractant and opsonic activity in ascitic fluid. A study in 47 patients with cirrhosis or malignant peritonitis. J Hepatol 12:45–49, 1991.

Marazziti D, Eggersten G, Stanley KK, Fey G. Evolution of the cysteine-rich domains of C9. Complement 4:189–194, 1987.

Marodi L, Leijh PCJ, Braat A, Daha MR, VanFurth R. Opsonic activity of cord blood sera against various species of microorganisms. Pediatr Res 19:433–436, 1985.

Maruyama K, Arai H, Ogawa T, Hoshino M, Tomizawa S, Morikawa A. C9 deficiency in a patient with poststreptococcal glomerulonephritis. Pediatr Nephrol 9:746–748, 1995.

Mascart-Lemone F, Hauptmann G, Goetz J, Duchateau J, Delespesse G, Vray B, Dab I. Genetic deficiency of C4 presenting with recurrent infections and a SLE-like disease. Am J Med 75:295–304, 1983.

Mason JC, Yarwood H, Sugars K, Morgan BP, Davies KA, Haskard DO. Induction of decay-accelerating factor by cytokines or the membrane-attack complex protects vascular endothelial cells against complement deposition. Blood 94:1673–1682, 1999.

McCracken GH Jr, Eichenwald HF. Leukocyte function and the development of opsonic and complement activity in the neonate. Am J Dis Child 121:120–126, 1971.

McLean RH, Forsgren A, Bjorksten B, Kim Y, Quie PG, Michael AF. Decreased serum factor B concentration associated with decreased opsonization of Escherichia coli in the idiopathic nephrotic syndrome. Pediatr Res 11:910–916, 1977.

McLean RH, Wyatt RJ, Julian BA. Complement phenotypes in glomerulonephritis: increased frequency of homozygous null C4 phenotypes in IgA nephropathy and Henoch Schönlein purpura. Kid Int 26:855–860, 1984.

Melamed J, Alper CA, Cicardi M, Rosen FS. The metabolism of C1 inhibitor and C1q in patients with acquired C1-inhibitor deficiency. J Allergy Clin Immunol 77:322–326, 1986.

Merino J, Rodriguez-Valverde V, Lamelas JA. Prevalence of deficits of complement components in patients with recurrent meningococcal infections. J Infect Dis 148:331–336, 1983.

Meyer O, Hauptmann G, Tappeiner G, Ochs HD, Mascart-Lemone F. Genetic deficiency of C4, C2 or C1q and lupus syndromes. Association with anti-Ro (SS-A) antibodies. Clin Exp Immunol 62:678–684, 1985.

Miller GW, Nussenzweig V. A new complement function: solubilization of antigen-antibody aggregates. Proc Natl Acad Sci USA 72:418–422, 1975.

Minta JO, Jezyk PD, Lepow IH. Distribution and levels of properdin in human body fluids. Clin Immunol Immunopathol 5:84–90, 1976.

Mitchell DA, Taylor PR, Cook HT, Moss J, Bygrave AE, Walport MJ. Cutting edge: C1q protects against the development of glomerulonephritis independently of C3 activation. J Immunol 162:5676–5679, 1999.

Mohan C. Murine lupus genetics: lessons learned. Curr Opin Rheumatol 13:352–360, 2001.

Molina H, Holers VM, Li B, Fung Y, Mariathasan S, Goellner J, Strauss-Schoenberger J, Karr RW, Chaplin DD. Markedly impaired humoral immune response in mice deficient in complement receptors 1 and 2. Proc Natl Acad Sci USA 93:3357–3361, 1996.

Moore HD. Complementary and opsonic functions in their relation to immunity: a study of the serum of guinea pigs naturally deficient in complement. J Immunol 4:425–445, 1919.

Morris KM, Aden DP, Knowles BB, Colten HR. Complement biosynthesis by the human hepatoma-derived cell line, HepG2. J Clin Invest 70:906–913, 1982.

Nagata M, Hara T, Aoki T, Mizuno Y, Akeda H, Inaba S, Tsumoto K, Veda K. Inherited deficiency of the ninth component of complement: an increased risk of meningococcal meningitis. J Pediatr 114:260–264, 1989.

Nataf S, Davoust N, Ames RS, Barnum SR. Human T cells express the C5a receptor and are chemoattracted to C5a. J Immunol 162:4018–4023, 1999.

Naughton MA, Walport MJ, Wurzner R, Carter MJ, Alexander GJ, Goldman JM, Botto M. Organ-specific contribution to circulating C7 levels by the bone marrow and liver in humans. Eur J Immunol 26:2108–2112, 1996.

Navratil JS, Ahearn JM. Apoptosis and autoimmunity. Complement deficiency and systemic lupus erythematosus revisited. Curr Rheumatol Rep 2:32–38, 2000.

Newman SL, Vogler LB, Feigen RD, Johnston RB Jr. Recurrent septicemia associated with congenital deficiency of C2 and partial deficiency of factor B of the alternative pathway. N Engl J Med 299:290–292, 1978.

Neumann HP, Salzmann M, Bohnert-Iwan B, Mannuelian T, Skerka C, Lenk D, Bender BU, Cybulla M, Riegler P, Konigsrainer A, Never U, Bock A, Widmer U, Male DA, Franke G, Zipfel PF. Haemolytic uraemic syndrome and mutations of the factor H gene: a registry-based study of German speaking countries. J of Med Genetics 40:676–681, 2003.

Ng SC, Sodetz JM. Biosynthesis of C8 by hepatocytes: differential expression and intracellular association of the α-γ and β subunits. J Immunol 139:3021–3027, 1987.

Nicholson A, Lepow I. Host defense against Neisseria meningitidis requires a complement-dependent bactericidal activity. Science 205:298–299, 1979.

Nicholson-Weller A, Burge J, Fearon DT, Weller PF, Austen KF. Isolation of a human erythrocyte membrane glycoprotein with decay-accelerating activity for C3 convertases of the complement system. J Immunol 129:184–189, 1982.

Nielsen HE, Christensen KC, Koch C, Thomsen BS, Heegaard NHH, Tranum-Jensen J. Hereditary, complete deficiency of complement factor H associated with recurrent meningococcal disease. Scand J Immunol 30:711–718, 1989a.

Nielsen HE, Koch C, Magnussesn P, Lind I. Complement deficiencies in selected groups of patients with meningococcal disease. Scand J Infect Dis 21:389–396, 1989b.

Nielsen HE, Truedsson L, Donner M. Partial complement deficiencies in idiopathic thrombocytopenia of childhood. Acta Paediatr 83:749–753, 1994.

Nishizaka H, Horiuchi T, Zhu Z-B, Fukumori Y, Volanakis JE. Genetic bases of human complement C7 deficiency. J Immunol 157:4239–4243, 1996.

Nolan KF, Schwaeble W, Kaluz S, Dierich MP, Reid KBM. Molecular cloning of the cDNA coding for properdin, a positive regulator of the alternative pathway of human complement. Eur J Immunol 21:771–776, 1991.

Ochs HD, Rosenfeld SI, Thomas ED, Giblett ER, Alper CA, Dupont B, Schaller JG, Gilliland BC, Hansen JA, Wedgewood RJ. Linkage between the gene (or genes) controlling synthesis of the fourth component of complement and the major histocompatibility complex. N Engl J Med 296:470–475, 1977.

Ochs HD, Wedgewood RJ, Frank MM, Heller SR, Hosea SW. The role of complement in the induction of antibody responses. Clin Exp Immunol 53:208–216, 1983.

O'Hara AM, Fernie BA, Moran AP, Williams YE, Connaughton JJ, Orren A, et al. C7 deficiency in an Irish family: a deletion defect which is predominant in the Irish. Clin Exp Immunol 114:355–361, 1998.

Oltvai ZN, Wong EGG, Atkinson JP, Tung KSK. C1 inhibitor deficiency: molecular and immunologic basis of hereditary and acquired angioedema. Lab Invest 65:381–388, 1991.

O'Neil KM, Ochs HD, Heller SR, Cork LC, Morris JM, Winkelstein JA. Role of C3 in humoral immunity: defective antibody production in C3 deficient dogs. J Immunol 149:1939–1945, 1988.

O'Neill GJ, Yang SY, Dupont B. Two HLA-linked loci controlling the fourth component of human complement. Proc Natl Acad Sci U S A 75:5165–5169, 1978a.

O'Neill GJ, Yang SY, Tegoli J, Berger R, Dupont B. Chido and Rogers blood groups are distinct antigenic components of human complement C4. Nature 273:668–670, 1978b.

Orren A, Potter PC, Cooper RC, du Toit E. Deficiency of the sixth component of complement and susceptibility to Neisseria meningitidis infections: studies in 10 families and five isolated cases. Immunology 62:249–253, 1987.

Orren A, Wurzner R, Potter PC, Fernie BA, Coetzee S, Morgan BP, Lachmann PJ. Properties of a low molecular weight complement component C6 found in human subjects with subtotal C6 deficiency. Immunology 75:10–16, 1992.

Osofsky SG, Thompson BH, Lint TF, Gewurz H. Hereditary deficiency of the third component of complement in a child with fever, skin rash, and arthralgias: response to transfusion of whole blood. J Pediatr 90:180–186, 1977.

Ottonello L, Corcione A, Tortolina G, Airoldi I, Albesiano E, Favre A, D'Agostino R, Malavasi F, Pistoia V, Dallegri F. rC5a directs the in vitro migration of human memory and naive tonsillar B lymphocytes: implications for B cell trafficking in secondary lymphoid tissues. J Immunol 162:6510–6517, 1999.

Paccaud JP, Steiger G, Sjoholm AG, Spaeth PJ, Schifferli JA. Tetanus toxoid-anti-tetanus toxoid complexes: a potential model to study the complement transport system for immune complex in humans. Clin Exp Immunol 69:468–476, 1987.

Parad RB, Kramer J, Strunk RC, Rosen FS, Davis AE. Dysfunctional C1 inhibitor Ta: deletion of Lys-251 results in acquisition of an N-glycosylation site. Proc Natl Acad Sci U S A 87:6786–6790, 1990.

Parshuram CS, Phillips RJ. Retrospective review of antibiotic-associated serum sickness in children presenting to a paediatric emergency department. Med J Aust 169:116, 1998.

Pastinen T, Liitsola K, Niini P, Salminen M, Syvanen AC. Contribution of the CCR5 and MBL genes to susceptibility to HIV type 1 infection in the Finnish population. AIDS Res Hum Retroviruses 14:695–698, 1998.

Peled M, Ardekian L, Schnarch A, Laufer D. Preoperative prophylaxis for C1 esterase-inhibitor deficiency in patients undergoing oral surgery: a report of three cases. Quintessence Int 28:169–171, 1997.

Pensky J, Levy LR, Lepow IH. Partial purification of a serum inhibitor of C'1-esterase. J Biol Chem 236:1674–79, 1961.

Perlemuter G, Chassada S, Soubrane O, Degoy A, Lounal A, Barbet P, Legman P, Kahan A, Weiss L, Couturier D. Multifocal stenosing ulcerations of the small intestine revealing vasculitis associated with C2 deficiency. Gastroenterology 110:1628–1632, 1996.

Petersen BH, Graham JA, Brooks GF. Human deficiency of the eighth component of complement. The requirement of C8 for serum Neisseria gonorrhoeae bactericidal activity. J Clin Invest 57:283–290, 1976.

Petri M, Watson R, Winkelstein JA, McLean RH. Clinical expression of systemic lupus erythematosus in patients with C4A deficiency. Medicine 72:236–244, 1993.

Petry F. Molecular basis of hereditary C1q deficiency. Immunobiology 199:286–294, 1998.

Petry F, Berkel AI, Loos M. Repeated identification of a nonsense mutation in the C1qA-gene of deficient patients in South-East Europe. Mol Immunol 33(Suppl)1:9, 1996.

Petry F, Berkel AI, Loos M. Multiple identification of a particular type of hereditary C1q deficiency in the Turkish population: review of the cases and additional and functional analysis. Hum Genet 100:51–56, 1997.

Petry F, Le DT, Kirschfink M, Loos M. Non-sense and missense mutations in the structural genes of complement component C1q A and C chains are linked with two different types of complete selective C1q deficiencies. J Immunol 155:4734–4738, 1995.

Pickering RJ, Gewurz H, Kelly JR, Good RA. The complement system in hereditary angioneurotic oedema—a new perspective. Clin Exp Immunol 3:423–435, 1968.

Platonov AE, Beloborodov VB, Vershinina IV. Meningococcal disease in patients with late complement component deficiency: studies in the U.S.S.R. Medicine 72:374–392, 1993.

Porter RR, Reid KBM. The biochemistry of complement. Nature 275:699–704, 1978.

Potter BJ, Elias E, Fayers PM, Jones EA. Profiles of serum complement in patients with hepatobiliary diseases. Digestion 18:371–383, 1978.

Potter BJ, Trueman AM, Kones EA. Serum complement in chronic liver disease. Gut 14:451–456, 1973.

Potter PC, Frasch CE, van der Sande WJ, Cooper RC, Patel Y, Orren A. Prophylaxis against Neisseria meningitidis infections and antibody responses in patients with deficiency of the sixth component of complement. J Infect Dis 161:932–937, 1990.

Power DA, Ng YC, Simpson JG. Familial incidence of C3 nephritic factor, partial lipodystrophy and membranoproliferative glomerulonephritis. Q J Med 75:387–398, 1990.

Prodeus A, Goerg S, Shen L-M, Pozdnyakova OO, Chu L, Alicot E, Goodnow C, Carroll MC. A critical role for complement in maintenance of self-tolerance. Immunity 9:721–731, 1998.

Provost TT, Arnett FC, Reichlin M. Homozygous C2 deficiency, lupus erythematosus, and anti-Ro (SSA) antibodies. Arthritis Rheum 26:1279–1282, 1983.

Pussell BA, Bourke E, Nayef M, Morris S, Peters DK. Complement deficiency and nephritis: a report of a family. Lancet 675–677, 1980.

Quastel M, Harrison R, Cicardi M, Alper CA, Rosen FS. Behavior in vivo of normal and dysfunctional C1 inhibitor in normal subjects and patients with hereditary angioneurotic edema. J Clin Invest 83:1041–1046, 1983.

Quezada ZMN, Hoffman WD, Winkelstein JA, Yatsiv I, Koev TCA, Cork LC, Elin RJ, Eichacker PQ, Natanson C. The third component of complement protects against endotoxin-induced shock and multiple organ failure. J Exp Med 179:569–578, 1994.

Ramadori G, Tedesco F, Bitter-Buermann D, Meyer ZUM, Buschenfelde KH. Biosynthesis of the third (C3), eighth (C8), and ninth (C9) complement components by guinea pig hepatocyte primary cultures. Immunobiology 170:203–210, 1985.

Rao AG, Howard OM, Ng S, Whitehead AS, Colten HR, Sodetz JM. cDNA and derived amino acid sequence of the alpha subunit of human complement protein C8: evidence for the existence of separate alpha subunit mRNA. Biochemistry 26:3556–3564, 1987.

Rasmussen JM, Brandslund I, Teisner B, Isager H, Suehag S-E, Maarup L, Willumsen L, Ronne-Rasmussen JO, Permin H, Andersen PL. Screening for complement deficiencies in unselected patients with meningitis. Clin Exp Immunol 68:437–441, 1987.

Reid KBM. Molecular cloning and characterization of the complementary DNA and gene coding for the B-chain of subcomponent C1q of the human complement system. Biochem J 231:729–735, 1985.

Reid KBM, Thompson RA. Characterization of a non-functional form of C1q found in patients with a genetically linked deficiency of C1q activity. Mol Immunol 20:117–122, 1983.

Repine JE, Clawson CC, Friend PS. Influence of a deficiency of the second component of complement on the bactericidal activity of neutrophils in vitro. J Clin Invest 59:802–809, 1977.

Richards A, Buddles MR, Donne RL, Kaplan BS, Kirk E, Venning MC, Tielemans CL, Goodship JA, Goodship TH. Factor H mutations in hemolytic uremic syndrome cluster in exons 18–20, a domain important for host cell recognition. Am J of Human Genetics 68:485–490, 2001.

Rittner C, Schneider PM. Genetics and polymorphism of the complement components. In Rother K, Till GO, eds. The Complement System. Heidelberg, FRG, Springer-Verlag, Heidelberg, 1988, p 80.

Rodriquez de Cordoba S, Lublin DM, Rubinstein P, Atkinson JP. Human genes for 3 complement components that regulate the activation of C3 are tightly linked. J Exp Med 161:1189–1195, 1985.

Roord JJ, Daha M, Kuis W, Verbrugh HA, Verhoef J, Zegers BJM, Stoop JW. Inherited deficiency of the third component of complement associated with recurrent pyogenic infections, circulating immune complexes, and vasculitis in a Dutch family. Pediatrics 71:81–87, 1983.

Rosen FS, Alper CA, Pensky J, Klemperer MR, Donaldson VH. Genetically determined heterogeneity of the C1 esterase inhibitor in patients with hereditary angioneurotic edema. J Clin Invest 50:2143–2149, 1971.

Rosen FS, Charache P, Pensky J, Donaldson V. Hereditary angioneurotic edema: two genetic variants. Science 148:957–965, 1965.

Rosenberg LT, Tachibana DK. Activity of mouse complement. J Immunol 89:861–865, 1962.

Ross SC, Densen P. Complement deficiency states and infection: epidemiology, pathogenesis and consequences of Neisserial and other infections in an immune deficiency. Medicine 63:243–273, 1984.

Rowe PC, McLean RH, Wood RA, Leggiadro RJ, Winkelstein JA. Association of C4B deficiency with bacterial meningitis. J Infect Dis 160:448–451, 1989.

Ruddy S. Component deficiencies: the second component. Prog Allergy 39:250–266, 1986.

Ruddy S, Klemperer MR, Rosen FS, Austen KF, Kumate J. Hereditary deficiency of the second component of complement in man: correlation of C2 hemolytic activity with immunochemical measurements of C2 protein. Immunology 18:943–954, 1970.

Runyon BA. Patients with deficient ascitic fluid opsonic activity are predisposed to spontaneous bacterial peritonitis. Hepatology 8:632–635, 1988.

Rynes RI, Britten AF, Pickering RJ. Deficiency of the second component of complement association with the HLA haplotype A10, B18 in a normal population. Ann Rheum Dis 41:93–96, 1982.

Sampson HA, Walchner AM, Baker PJ. Recurrent pyogenic infections in individuals with absence of the second component of complement. J Clin Immunol 2:39–45, 1982.

Sanchez-Corral P, Criado-Garcia O, Rodriguez de Cordoba S. Isoforms of human C4b-binding protein. I. Molecular basis for the C4BP isoform pattern and its variations in human plasma. J Immunol 155:4030–4036, 1995.

Sanchez-Corral P, Perez-Caballero D, Huarte O, Simckes AM, Goicoechea E, Lopez-Trascasa M, de Cordoba, SR. Structural and functional characterization of factor H mutations associated with atypical hemolytic uremic syndrome. Am J of Human Genetics 71:1285–1295, 2002.

Sano Y, Nishimukai H, Kitamura H, Nagaki K, Inai S, Hamasaki Y, Maruyama I, Igata A. Hereditary deficiency of the third component of complement in two sisters with systemic lupus erythematosus-like symptoms. Arthritis Rheum 24:1255–1260, 1981.

Sastry K, Herman G, Day L, Deignan E, Bruns G, Morton CC, Ezekowitz RA. The human mannose-binding protein gene. J Exp Med 170:1175–1189, 1989.

Saucedo L, Ackermann L, Platonov AE, Gewurz A, Rakita RM, Densen P. Delineation of additional genetic basis for C8β deficiency. J Immunol 155:5022–5028, 1995.

Sawyer MK, Forman ML, Kuplic LS, Stiehm ER. Developmental aspects of the human complement system. Biol Neonate 19:148–162, 1971.

Schapira M, Silver LD, Scott CF, Schmaier AH, Prograis LJ, Curd JG, Colman RW. Prekallikrein activation and high-molecular-weight kininogen consumption in hereditary angioedema. N Engl J Med 308:1050–1053, 1983.

Schifferli JA, Bartolotti SR, Peters DK. Inhibition of immune precipitation by complement. Clin Exp Immunol 42:387–394, 1980.

Schifferli JA, Steiger G, Hauptmann G, Spaeth PJ, Sjoholm AG. Formation of soluble immune complexes by complement in sera of patients with various hypocomplementemic states. J Clin Invest 76:2127–2133, 1985.

Schlesinger M, Greenberg R, Levy J, Kayhty H, Levy R. Killing of meningococci by neutrophils: effect of vaccination on patients with complement deficiency. J Infect Dis 170:449–453, 1994.

Schlesinger M, Kayhty H, Levy R, Bibi C, Meydan N, Levy J. Phagocytic killing and antibody response during the first year after tetravalent meningococcal vaccine in complement-deficient and in normal individuals. J Clin Immunol 20:46–53, 2000.

Schneider PM, Carroll MC, Alper CA, Rittner C, Whitehead AS, Yunis EJ, Colten HR. Polymorphism of the human complement C4 and steroid 21-hydroxylase gene. Restriction fragment length polymorphisms revealing structural deletions, homoduplications and size variants. J Clin Invest 78:650–657, 1986.

Schoonbrood TH, Hannema A, Fijen CA, Markusse HM, Swaak AJ, Meri S. C5 deficiency in a patient with primary Sjögren's syndrome. J Rheumatol 22:1389–1390, 1995.

Schreiber AD, Kaplan AP, Austen KF. Inhibition by C1INH of Hageman factor fragment activation of coagulation, fibrinolysis, and kinin generation. J Clin Invest 52:1402–1409, 1973.

Sellar GC, Blake DJ, Reid KBM. Characterization and organization of the genes encoding the A-, B-, and C-chains of human complement subcomponent C1q. Biochem J 274:481–490, 1991.

Senaldi G, Davies ET, Peakman M, Vergani D, Lu J, Reid KBM. Frequency of mannose-binding protein deficiency in patients with systemic lupus erythematosus. Arthritis Rheum 38:1713–1714, 1995.

Setien F, Alvarez V, Coto E, DiScipio RG, Lopez-Larrea C. A physical map of the human complement component C6, C7, and C9 genes. Immunogenetics 38:341–344, 1993.

Sheffer AL, Austen KF, Rosen FS. Tranexamic acid therapy in hereditary angioneurotic edema. N Engl J Med 287:452–454, 1972.

Sheffer AL, Craig JM, Willims-Kretschmer K, Austen KF, Rosen FS. Histopathological and ultrastructural observations on tissues from patients with hereditary angioneurotic edema. J Allergy 47:292–297, 1971.

Sheffer AL, Fearon DT, Austen KF. Hereditary angioedema: a decade of management with stanozolol. J Allergy Clin Immunol 80:855–860, 1987.

Shenoy-Scaria AM, Kwong J, Fujita T, Olszowy MW, Shaw AS, Lublin DM. Signal transduction through decay-accelerating factor. J Immunol 149:3535–3541, 1992.

Shichishima T, Saitoh Y, Terasawa T, Noji H, Kai T, Maruyama Y. Complement sensitivity of erythrocytes in a patient with inherited complete deficiency of CD59 or with the Inab phenotype. Br J Haematol 104:303–306, 1999.

Silverstein AM. Essential hypocomplementemia: report of a case. Blood 16:1338–1345, 1960.

Sim RB, Kolble K, McAleer MA, Dominguez O, Dee VM. Genetics and deficiencies of the soluble regulatory proteins of the complement system. Int Rev Immunol 10:65–86, 1993.

Singer L, Colten HR, Wetsel RA. Complement C3 deficiency: human, animal, and experimental models. Pathobiology 62:14–28, 1994.

Sirisina S, Suskind R, Edelman R, Charupatana C, Olsen RE. Complement and C3-proactivator levels in children with protein-calorie malnutrition and effect of dietary treatment. Lancet i: 1016–1020, 1973.

Sissons JG, Peters DK, Williams DG, Boulton-Jones JM, Goldsmith HJ. Skin lesions, angio-oedema, and hypocomplementaemia. Lancet ii:1350–1352, 1974.

Sissons JP, West RJ, Fallows J, Williams DG, Boucher BJ, Amos N, Peters DK. The complement abnormalities of lipodystrophy. N Engl J Med 294:461–465, 1976.

Skerka C, Timmann C, Horstmann RD, Zipfel PE. Two additional human serum proteins structurally related to complement factor H. J Immunol 148:3313–3318, 1992.

Skriver K, Wikoff WR, Patston PA, Tausk F, Schapira M, Kaplan AP, Bock SC. Substrate properties of C1 inhibitor Ma (alanine 434-glutamic acid). General and structural evidence suggesting that the P12-region contains critical determinants of serine protease inhibitor/substrate status. J Biol Chem 266:9216–9221, 1991.

Slingsby JH, Norsworthy P, Pearce G, Vaishnaw AK, Issler H, Morley BJ, et al. Homozygous hereditary C1q deficiency and systemic lupus erythematosus. A new family and the molecular basis of C1q deficiency in three families. Arthritis Rheum 39:663–670, 1996.

Solal-Celigny P, Laviolette M, Hebert J, Atkins PC, Sirois M, Brun G, Lehner-Netsch G, Delage JM. C3b inactivator deficiency with immune complex manifestations. Clin Exp Immunol 47:197–205, 1982.

Spath PJ, Sjoholm AG, Fredrikson GN, Misiano G, Scherz R, Schaad UB, Uhring-Lambert B, Hauptmann G, Westberg J, Uhlen M, Wadelius C, Truedsson L. Properdin deficiency in a large Swiss family: identification of a stop codon in the properdin gene, and association of meningococcal disease with lack of the IgG2 allotype marker G2m(n). Clin Exp Immunol 118:278–284, 1999.

Sprung CL, Schultz DR, Marcial E, Caralis PV, Gelbard MA, Arnold PI, Long WM. Complement activation in septic shock patients. Crit Care Med 14:525–528, 1986.

Stanley KK, Kocher HP, Luzio JP, Jackson P, Tschopp J. The sequence and topology of human complement component C9. EMBO J 4:375–382, 1985.

Stanley KK, Luzio JP. Construction of a new family of high efficiency bacterial expression vectors: identification of cDNA clones for human liver proteins. EMBO J 3:1429–1434, 1984.

Steckel EW, York RG, Monahan JB, Sodety JM. The eighth component of human complement. Purification and physicochemical characterization of its unusual subunit structure. J Biol Chem 255:11997–12005, 1980.

Steinsson K, Erlandsson K, Valdimarsson H. Successful plasma infusion treatment of a patient with C2 deficiency and systemic lupus erythematosus: clinical experience over forty-five months. Arthritis Rheum 32:906–913, 1989.

Stolfi RL. Immune lytic transformation. A state of irreversible damage generated as a result of the reaction of the eighth component in the guinea pig complement system. J Immunol 100:46–54, 1968.

Stone NM, Williams A, Wilkinson JD, Bird G. Systemic lupus erythematosus with C1q deficiency. Br J Dermatol 142:521–524, 2000.

Stoppa-Lyonnet D, Duponchel C, Meo T, Laurent J, Carter PE, Arala-Chaves M, Cohen JH, Dewald G, Goetz J, Hauptmann G, Lagrue G, Lesavre P, Lopez-Trascasa M, Misiano G, Moraine C, Sobel A, Spath PJ, Tosi M. Recombinational biases in the rearranged C1-inhibitor genes of hereditary angioedema patients. Am J Hum Genet 49:1055–1062, 1991.

Strunk RC, Fenton LF, Gaines JA. Alternative pathway of complement activation in full term and premature infants. Pediatr Res 13:641–643, 1979.

Such J, Guarner C, Enriquez J, Rodriguez JL, Seres I, Vilardell F. Low C3 in cirrhotic ascites predisposes to spontaneous bacterial peritonitis. J Hepatol 6:80–84, 1988.

Sullivan KE, Petri M, McLean R, Schmeckpepper B, Winkelstein JA. Prevalence of a mutation which causes C2 deficiency in a population of patients with SLE. J Rheumatol 21:1128–1133, 1994.

Sullivan KE, Wooten C, Goldman D, Petri M. Mannose binding protein genetic polymorphisms in black patients with systemic lupus erythematosus. Arthritis Rheum 39:2046–2051, 1996.

Sumiya M, Super M, Tabona P, Levinsky RJ, Arai T, Turner MW, et al. Molecular basis of opsonic defect in immunodeficient children. Lancet 337:1569–1570, 1991.

Summerfield JA, Ryder S, Sumiya M, Thursz M, Gorchein A, Monteil MA, Turner MW. Mannose binding protein gene mutations associated with unusual and severe infections in adults. Lancet 345:886–889, 1995.

Summerfield JA, Sumiya M, Levin M, Turner MW. Association of mutations in mannose binding protein gene with childhood infection in consecutive hospital series [see comments]. Brit Med J 314:1229–1232, 1997.

Sun X, Funk CD, Deng C, Sahu A, Lambris JD, Song WC. Role of decay-accelerating factor in regulating complement activation on the erythrocyte surface as revealed by gene targeting. Proc Natl Acad Sci USA 96:628–633, 1999.

Suzuki Y, Ogura Y, Otsubo O, Akagi K, Fujita T. Selective deficiency of C1s associated with a systemic lupus erythematosus-like syndrome. Arthritis Rheum 35:576–579, 1992.

Swaak AJG, Groenwold J, Bronsveld W. Predictive value of complement profiles and anti-ds DNA in systemic lupus erythematosus. Ann Rheum Dis 45:359–366, 1986.

Takahashi M, Takahashi S, Brade V, Nussenzweig V. Requirements for solubilization of immune aggregates by complement. J Clin Invest 62:349–358, 1978.

Takeda J, Miyata T, Kawagoe K, Iida Y, Endo Y, Fujita T, Takahashi M, Kitani T, Kinoshita T. Deficiency of the GPI anchor caused by a somatic mutation of the PIG-A gene in paroxysmal nocturnal hemoglobinuria. Cell 73:703–711, 1993.

Tanuma Y, Ohi H, Hatano M. Two types of C3 nephritic factor: properdin-dependent C3NeF and properdin-independent C3NeF. Clin Immunol Immunopathol 56:226–238, 1990.

Taylor PR, Carugati A, Fadok VA, Cook HT, Andrews M, Carroll MC, Savill JS, Henson PM, Botto M, Walport MJ. A hierarchical role for classical pathway complement proteins in the clearance of apoptotic cells in vivo. J Exp Med 192:359–366, 2000.

Tedesco F. Component deficiencies. 8. The eighth component. Prog Allergy 39:295–306, 1986.

CD1b may be involved in the presentation of highly hydrophobic lipoglycan molecules of mycobacteria such as lipoarabinomannans, mycolic acid, and glucose monomycolate (Ernst et al., 1998; Porcelli et al., 1998).

CD1c presents mannosyl-β1-phosphodolichol, a mycobacterial-derived glycolipid to T cells (Moody et al., 2000). Fetal and neonatal B cells express higher levels of CD11c than adult B cells (Plebani, 1993), but the capacity of these cells to present antigens through CD1c is unknown.

CD1d appears to be specialized for the presentation of sphingolipids to NK T cells, but it is unclear whether these or similar molecules involved in physiological activation are typically derived from pathogens or from self-constituents (Matsuda and Kronenberg, 2001).

Dendritic Cells

Overview

Dendritic cells, the sentinels of the immune system, are bone marrow–derived cells that in their mature form display characteristic cytoplasmic protrusions. Dendritic cells in the circulation and tissues are heterogeneous on the basis of their surface phenotype and functional attributes, but the precursor–product relationship of these subsets with each other and with other cell types remains controversial (Banchereau et al., 2000; Liu, 2001a). Dendritic cells in the skin include Langerhans cells, which express CD1a and Birbeck granules but lack expression of factor XIIIa coagulation factor, and interstitial cells of the dermis, which conversely lack Birbeck granules but are factor XIIIa positive.

Skin dendritic cells and dendritic cells in the interstitial area of solid organs such as heart and kidney are highly effective in the uptake of antigen in soluble or particulate form (Mellman and Steinman, 2001). They express CD11c and ILT-1 (Banchereau et al., 2000; Cella et al., 1999) but are lineage negative (Lin⁻); that is, they lack expression of the markers characteristic of other cell lineages, such as T cells, B cells, NK cells, and granulocytes. In this chapter, these CD11c⁺Lin⁻ dendritic cells are collectively referred to as *myeloid dendritic cells* (Steinman and Inaba, 1999) or *DC1 cells* (Liu, 2001).

Dendritic Cells Type-1 (Myeloid)

DC1 cells have prominent cytoplasmic protrusions and express high levels of molecules involved in antigen presentation, including class I and class II MHC molecules. After exposure of immature DC1 cells to inflammatory stimuli, further antigen uptake is downregulated and maturation ensues in which these cells process and display previously internalized antigen. Concurrently, dendritic cells increase the surface expression of CC chemokine receptor 7 (CCR7) and decrease the expression of most other chemokine receptors. This results in the migration of these cells through lymphatics to T-cell–dependent areas of secondary lymphoid organs that express the CCR7 ligands, CCL19 and CCL21 (see Table 22-1 and Lanzavecchia and Salusto, 2001).

DC1 cell maturation and migration can be triggered by a variety of stimuli, including pathogen-derived products, such as peptides, cell walls, DNA, and lipopolysaccharide (LPS), that activate Toll-like receptors (TLRs) (Akira et al., 2001); by endogenous cytokines, such as IL-1, tumor necrosis factor-α (TNF-α), and granulocyte-macrophage colony-stimulating factor (GM-CSF) (see Tables 22-1 and 22-2); and by the engagement of CD40 on the dendritic cell surface by CD40 ligand (CD154), a molecule that is expressed at particularly high levels by activated CD4⁺ T cells.

Mature DC1 cells express high levels of molecules for T-cell co-stimulation, such as CD80 and CD86, and are highly efficient for presenting antigen and activating naïve T cells (Banchereau et al., 2000) (see Fig. 22-1 and Table 22-3). Dendritic cells may determine whether naïve CD4⁺ T cells differentiate into T-helper 1 (Th1; i.e., capable of producing IFN-γ but not IL-4, IL-5, or IL-13) or T-helper 2 (Th2; i.e., capable of producing IL-4, IL-5, or IL-13 but not IFN-γ) effector cell populations. For example, dendritic cell production of IL-12, a heterodimeric cytokine consisting of a p35 and a p40 chain, skews differentiation toward the Th1 pathway (Moser and Murphy, 2000).

Dendritic Cells Type II (Plasmacytoid)

DC2 cells and their immediate precursors, pre-DC2 cells, constitute a distinct dendritic cell lineage from DC1 cells. Human DC2 lineage cells are distinguished from DC1 cells by a characteristic surface phenotype of high levels of the IL-3 receptor (CD123), the expression of CD4, and a lack of CD11c and ILT1 (Cella et al., 1999). Pre-DC2 cells, also referred to as *plasmacytoid cells* or *lymphoid dendritic cells*, are found in secondary lymphoid organs in extrafollicular T-cell–dependent areas and the thymus. Some pre-DC2 cells are derived from a lymphoid, rather than a myeloid lineage precursor (Galy et al., 2000).

In contrast to immature DC1 cells, pre-DC2 cells express low levels of co-stimulatory molecules and have a limited capacity for antigen uptake and presentation (Cella et al., 1999). Pre-DC2 cells also differ from DC1 cells in their capacity to produce large amounts of type I interferon (IFN-α/β) and IL-12 in response to intact or inactivated DNA or RNA viruses or in response to DNA containing unmethylated CpG dinucleotide sequences (CpG DNA) (Bauer et al., 2001; Kadowaki et al., 2001b; Siegal et al., 1999).

Unmethylated CpG dinucleotide sequences, which are a constituent of DNA derived from sources other than the eukaryotic host (e.g., from bacteria) are an important pathogen-associated molecule. DC2 cells produce cytokines in response to CpG DNA, most likely after the recognition of CpG DNA by Toll-like receptor (TLR)-9, which is expressed at high concentrations (Kadowaki et al., 2001b). Murine studies have demonstrated that TLR-9 is absolutely required for leukocyte

TABLE 22-3 · PAIRS OF SURFACE MOLECULES INVOLVED IN THE INTERACTIONS BETWEEN T CELLS AND APCs

T-Cell Surface Molecule	T-Cell Distribution	Corresponding Ligand(s) on APCs	APC Distribution
CD2	Most T cells; higher on memory cells and lower on adult virgin and neonatal T cells	LFA-3 (CD58) and CD59	Leukocytes
CD4	Subset of αβ-T cells with predominantly helper activity	Class II MHC β chain	Dendritic cells, Mφ, B cells, and others
CD5	All T cells	CD72	B cells and Mφ
CD8	Subset of α/β-T cells with predominantly helper activity	Class I MHC heavy chain	Ubiquitous
LFA-1 (CD11a/CD18)	All T cells; higher on memory cells and lower on adult virgin and neonatal T cells	ICAM-1 (CD54), ICAM-2 (CD102), and ICAM-3 (CD50)	Leukocytes (ICAM-3 > ICAM-1 and ICAM-2) and endothelium (ICAM-1 and ICAM-2); most ICAM-1 expression requires activation
CD28	Most CD4 T cells; subset of CD8 T cells	CD80 (B7-1) CD86 (B7-2)	Dendritic cells, Mφ, and activated B cells
ICOS	Effector and memory T cells; not on resting naïve cells	B7-h (ICOS ligand)	B cells, Mφ, dendritic cells, and endothelial cells
CD45R0	High levels on memory cells and low levels on adult virgin and neonatal T cells	CD22 (?)	B cells
VLA-4 (CD49d/CD29)	All T cells; higher on memory cells and lower on adult virgin and neonatal T cells	VCAM-1 (CD106)	Activated or inflamed endothelium (increased by TNF, IL-1, and IL-4)
ICAM-1 (CD54)	All T cells; higher on memory cells, lower on adult virgin and neonatal T cells	LFA-1 (CD11a/CD18)	Leukocytes
CTLA-4 (CD152)	Activated T cells	CD80 and CD86	Dendritic cells, Mφ, and activated B cells
CD40 ligand (CD154)	Activated CD4 T cells; lower on neonatal CD4 T cells	CD40	Dendritic cells, Mφ, B cells, and thymic epithelial cells

APC = antigen-presenting cells; Mφ = mononuclear phagocytes; MHC = major histocompatibility complex; TNF = tumor necrosis factor.

responses to CpG DNA in vitro and in vivo (Kaisho and Akira, 2002).

Viruses trigger high levels of IFN-α/β secretion by pre-DC cells, but the mechanism remains unclear. This secretion results in a systemic antiviral state. Local exposure of secondary lymphoid tissue to IFN-α/β and IL-12 may also enhance local adaptive immune responses (Le Bon et al., 2001). The activation of pre-DC2 cells also results in their maturation, including acquisition of the cytoplasmic protrusions characteristic of dendritic cells and an increased capacity to present antigen to naïve T cells.

Ontogeny of DC1 and DC2 Cells

Epidermal Langerhans cells and dermal dendritic cells are found in fetal skin by 16 weeks' gestation (Drijkoningen et al., 1987), and immature DC1-type cells are found in the interstitium of solid organs by this age. Cells with the features of pre-DC2 are found in fetal lymph nodes between 19 and 21 days of gestation (Olweus et al., 1997); they have an immature phenotype and are not recent emigrants from inflamed tissues.

In the neonatal circulation, dendritic cells with a pre-DC2 surface phenotype (Lin⁻ HLA-DR^{mid}CD11c⁻CD33⁻ CD123^{high}) predominate in cord blood, constituting approximately 75% of the total Lin⁻ HLA-DR⁺ dendritic cells (Borras et al., 2001). The remaining 25% of dendritic cells have an HLA-DR^{high}CD11c⁺CD33⁺CD123^{low}

surface phenotype that is similar to that of circulating adult DC1 cells, except that CD83 expression is absent (Borras et al., 2001). The biological significance of the predominance of DC2 lineage cells in the neonatal circulation is uncertain, but this may reflect a high rate of colonization in the lymphoid tissue, which is undergoing rapid expansion at this age.

Ontogeny of Dendritic Cell Function

As discussed later, antigen-specific T-cell responses of the fetus and neonate are reduced or delayed compared with the responses of adults. These reduced or delayed responses may reflect limitations of neonatal dendritic cells. Results of rodent studies support a functional immaturity in neonatal dendritic cell function, inasmuch as dendritic cell recruitment into the rat lung after infectious challenge is markedly limited during the first several weeks of life (Nelson and Holt, 1995).

Most studies of dendritic cell function in the human neonate have focused on circulating cells; however, there are few studies on tissue dendritic cells. Cord blood dendritic cells isolated by cell fractionation and culture overnight in vitro were substantially less effective than adult cells in the activation of T-cell proliferation (Hunt et al., 1994; Petty and Hunt, 1998). This decreased activity was associated with reduced levels of expression of HLA-DR and the adhesion molecule, intercellular adhesion molecule (ICAM)-1 (see Table 22-3) (Hunt et al., 1994).

cules, such as CD40 ligand and Fas ligand. These have included decreases in anti-CD3 and CD28 monoclonal antibody–induced phosphorylation of CD3-ε and decreased phosphorylation and enzyme activity of the p56lck and zeta-associated protein of 70 kD (ZAP-70) tyrosine kinases and the extracellularly regulated kinase 2 (ERK2), c-jun N-terminal kinase (JNK), and p38 kinases (Sato et al., 1999). Researchers with a similar approach have found that anti-CD3 monoclonal antibody-stimulated neonatal T cells have reduced basal levels and the activation of phospholipase C isoenzymes (Miscia et al., 1999) and also display a generalized decrease in the overall level of tyrosine phosphorylation of intracellular proteins compared with unfractionated adult T cells (Ansart-Pirenne et al., 1999).

Whether these apparent deficiencies in proximal signal transduction events apply specifically to neonatal naïve T cells but not adult naïve T cells remains uncertain. This is plausible; our recent unpublished results suggest that some of these limitations in proximal signaling are intrinsic to the neonatal CD4+ T cell. We have observed that highly purified neonatal naïve CD4+ T cells have less of an increase in intracellular calcium after anti-CD3 monoclonal antibody crosslinkage than do identically treated adult naïve cells (Jullien et al., 2003).

Mechanisms for Decreased Cytokine mRNA Expression

Reduced IL-4 and IFN-γ mRNA expression by polyclonally activated neonatal CD4+ and CD8+ T cells compared with adult T cells is primarily attributable to reduced transcription of these cytokine genes (Lewis et al., 1991). These differences in cytokine mRNA expression occur for a variety of stimuli, including activation with ionomycin and phorbol ester, a pharmacologic stimulus that bypasses the early signal transduction events, as well as after engagement of the αβ-TCR/CD3 complex (Ehlers and Smith, 1991). IFN-γ and IL-4 are expressed mainly by memory/effector T-cell populations rather than by naïve T-cell populations (Lewis et al., 1988).

Thus the reduced expression of these cytokines by neonatal T cells after brief activation can be accounted for by the lack of memory/effector cells in the circulating neonatal T-cell population. The DNA of the IFN-γ genetic locus is methylated to a greater degree for neonatal and adult CD45RAhigh T cells than for adult CD45R0high T cells, potentially decreasing the accessibility of this gene to transcriptional activator proteins in these naïve T-cell populations and accounting for their limited capacity to transcribe this cytokine (Melvin et al., 1995). Recently, researchers studying neonatal CD4+ T cells also found that the DNA of the IFN-γ genetic locus is more highly methylated than adult cells at five of six CpG sites examined in the promoter and immediate downstream region (White et al., 2002). This hypermethylation could further decrease and delay the acquisition of an open chromatin configuration necessary for efficient IFN-γ gene expression by neonatal T cells compared with adult naïve T cells.

Decreased gene transcription is important in the reduced production of cytokines such as IFN-γ by neonatal T cells, but decreased mRNA stability may also play a role. For example, decreased IL-3 production by neonatal T cells appears to be mainly caused by reduced IL-3 mRNA stability rather than decreased gene transcription (Lee et al., 1993). The mechanism for this reduced mRNA stability remains unclear. Decreased mRNA stability has also been observed for other cytokines after the stimulation of cord blood mononuclear cells (Suen et al., 1998), but whether this also holds for purified neonatal T cells has not been addressed.

IFN-γ Production by Neonatal T Cells after Short-Term In Vitro Stimulation

In vitro studies have shown that as naïve T cells differentiate into effector cells, they acquire within days the capacity to produce IFN-γ and IL-4 on restimulation. The signals that are involved in determining whether T cells become producers of IFN-γ or IL-4 are discussed in more detail in the T-Helper 1 and T-Helper 2 Effector Generation In Vitro section. Our studies suggest that neonatal naïve CD4+ T cells have a decreased capacity to become IFN-γ–producing cells compared with adult naïve CD4+ T cells in response to short-term (i.e., 24 to 48 hours' duration) stimulation by allogeneic dendritic cells (Chen et al., 2001).

This decreased expression of IFN-γ by neonatal CD4+ T cells is likely attributable to several factors. First, neonatal CD4+ T cells are less effective than adult naïve cells at inducing the co-cultured dendritic cells to produce IL-12, a key cytokine for promoting IFN-γ production (Chen et al., 2001). Second, neonatal naïve CD4+ T cells have decreased expression of certain transcription factors that may play a role in the induction of IFN-γ gene expression, such as the NFATc2 protein (Kadereit et al., 1999; Kiani et al., 2001). Third, the greater methylation of DNA of the IFN-γ genetic locus in neonatal T cells may also contribute to the reduced, delayed acquisition of IFN-γ production after activation in vitro (White et al., 2002). Together, these mechanisms contribute to the delay in the appearance of IFN-γ production by antigen-specific CD4+ T cells after infection in the neonatal period (see Practical Aspects of T-Cell Function in the Fetus, Neonate, and Young Infant).

In contrast to the results with dendritic cell allostimulation, neonatal T cells, if polyclonally activated under conditions that favor repeated cell division (i.e., strong activation stimuli in common with the provision of exogenous IL-2), resemble antigenically naïve adult T cells in efficiently acquiring the characteristics of effector cells. These characteristics include a CD45RAlowCD45R0high surface phenotype, an enhanced ability to be activated by anti-CD2 or anti-CD3 monoclonal antibodies, and an increased capacity to produce cytokines (e.g., IL-4 and IFN-γ) (Clement, 1992; Ehlers and Smith, 1991; Hayward and Cosyns, 1994; Pirenne et al., 1992). This suggests that such approaches in vivo (e.g., IL-2 immunotherapy) might similarly enhance neonatal T-cell clonal expansion and differentiation.

Tumor Necrosis Factor Ligand Family Members

Role of CD40 Ligand

CD40 ligand (CD154) is a member of the TNF ligand family. CD40 ligand is expressed in high amounts on the surfaces of activated—but not resting—CD4$^+$ T cells and engages CD40, a molecule expressed by "professional" APCs, including dendritic cells and mononuclear phagocytes, and by B cells. The CD40 ligand/CD40 interaction is essential for many events in adaptive immunity, including the generation of memory CD4$^+$ T cells of the Th1 type (capable of producing IFN-γ but not IL-4), memory B cells, and immunoglobulin isotype switching (Schonbeck and Libby, 2001).

Durandy and colleagues (1995) reported that a substantial proportion of circulating fetal T cells between 19 and 31 weeks' gestation expressed CD40 ligand in vitro in response to polyclonal activation. Whether fetal T cells that can express CD40 ligand have a distinct surface phenotype, such as evidence of prior in vivo activation (Byrne et al., 1994) from those lacking this capacity, is unclear. In contrast, T cells from later gestational-age fetuses and from neonates have a much more limited capacity to produce CD40 ligand after activation with calcium ionophore and phorbol ester (Brugnoni et al., 1994; Durandy et al., 1995; Fuleihan et al., 1994; Nonoyama et al., 1995).

The expression of CD40 ligand by activated neonatal CD4$^+$ T cells remains reduced for at least 10 days postnatally but is almost equal to adult cells by 3 to 4 weeks after birth (Durandy et al., 1995; D. Lewis, unpublished observations). In most of these studies, activated neonatal T cells express markedly lower amounts of CD40 ligand surface protein and mRNA than either adult CD45RA^{high} or CD45R0^{high} CD4$^+$ T cells (Durandy et al., 1995; Fuleihan et al., 1994; Nonoyama et al., 1995). Thus decreased CD40 ligand expression may not be attributable to the lack of a memory/effector population in the neonatal T-cell compartment, but rather it may represent a true developmental limitation in cytokine production.

Decreased CD40 ligand production by neonatal T cells has also been documented in the mouse (Flamand et al., 1998), suggesting that it may be a feature of T cells that have recently emigrated from the thymus. Consistent with this idea, human CD4$^+$CD8$^-$ thymocytes, the immediate precursors of antigenically naïve CD4$^+$ T cells, also have a low capacity to express CD40 ligand (Fuleihan et al., 1995; Nonoyama et al., 1995). As for most other T-cell–derived cytokines, when neonatal T cells are activated in vitro into an effector T-cell population, they acquire a markedly increased capacity to produce CD40 ligand, which suggests that this reduction is not a fixed phenotype (Durandy et al., 1995; Nonoyama et al., 1995).

Given the importance of CD40 ligand in multiple aspects of the immune response (Schonbeck and Libby, 2001), limitations in CD40 ligand production could contribute to decreased antigen-specific immunity mediated by Th1 effector cells and B cells in the neonate. However, initial studies that reported a relative deficiency of CD40 ligand expression by neonatal T cells used calcium ionophore and phorbol ester stimulation, a combination that maximizes the production of most cytokines but may not accurately mimic physiologic T-cell activation. Neonatal CD4$^+$ T cells stimulated allogeneically can express some CD40 ligand and induce IL-12 production by dendritic cells (Ohshima and Delespesse, 1997). Reduced CD40 ligand surface expression by neonatal T cells after activation by a combination of anti-CD3 and anti-CD28 monoclonal antibodies has also been observed by some (Jullien et al., 2003; Sato et al., 1999), but not by others (Reen, 1998; Splawski et al., 1996).

One study found that CD40 ligand expression by neonatal T cells was similar to that of adult T cells after 5 days of allogeneic stimulation with irradiated adult monocyte-derived dendritic cells (Matthews et al., 2000). In contrast, Chen and colleagues (2001) found that CD40 ligand expression by purified neonatal naïve CD4$^+$ T cells was substantially less than in adult naïve CD4$^+$ T cells after 24 to 48 hours of stimulation. This reduced CD40 ligand production is accompanied by reduced IL-12 production (by monocyte-derived dendritic cells) and IFN-γ production (by naïve CD4$^+$ T cells). This suggests that CD40 ligand surface expression is at least initially more limited for neonatal T cells, but with continued priming in vitro, this can be overcome. As a consequence, the differentiation of these cells into Th1 effector cells by an IL-12–dependent process may be limited, at least during the early stages of T-cell differentiation.

Role of Other TNF Family Ligands

TNF-α and TRANCE (TNF-related activation-induced cytokine) are additional members of the TNF ligand family that are expressed on activated T cells. TNF-α and TRANCE expressed on the T-cell surface can stimulate the immune function of other cell types such as B cells and dendritic cells. A recent murine study also suggests that interaction of TRANCE with its specific receptor, RANK (receptor activator of nuclear factor-kappa B) may be important in the development of CD4$^+$CD25$^+$ regulatory T-cell function (Green et al., 2002). The capacity of activated neonatal T cells to express surface TNF-α and TRANCE is unknown.

Fas ligand (CD95L) is another member of the TNF ligand family and plays a key role in inducing apoptotic cell death on target cells that express Fas (CD95) on the surface. Fas ligand may trigger the apoptosis of any cell type that expresses Fas and, in so doing, eliminates intracellular pathogens, such as viruses; however, the key role of this interaction, at least in humans, appears to be to eliminate previously activated lymphocytes and prevent autoimmune disease. Thus Fas deficiency is associated with antibody-mediated autoimmunity rather than defects in viral clearance.

Neonatal T cells have decreased Fas ligand expression after anti-CD3 and CD28 monoclonal antibody stimulation in comparison with adult cells (Sato et al., 1999). Whether neonatal T cells have a decreased level of Fas expression compared with adult naïve T cells remains to be determined. Iwama and colleagues (2000) reported that circulating levels of Fas ligand are elevated in newborns, but the cellular source of this protein and its functional significance is unclear. The role of Fas/Fas ligand interactions in regulating apoptosis of neonatal T cells is discussed in the section "Neonatal T-Cell Apoptosis."

The activation of neonatal T cells with anti-CD3 monoclonal antibody and CD28 engagement by CD80 results in the induction of OX40, a member of the TNF receptor family (Ohshima et al., 1998). The engagement of OX40 on activated neonatal T cells skews effector T-cell development toward a Th2 profile (Ohshima et al., 1998). Whether adult naïve T cells express similar amounts of OX40 and have a similar outcome after OX40 engagement as neonatal T cells remains to be determined.

T-Cell Co-Stimulation and Anergy

Neonatal T cells produce IL-2 and proliferate as well as adult T cells in response to mouse APC expressing human CD80 or CD86 (B7-2) and to anti-CD3 monoclonal antibody, indicating that CD28-mediated signaling is intact (Cayabyab et al., 1994). This is also supported by the results of a study showing that anti-CD28 monoclonal antibody treatment of neonatal T cells markedly augments their ability to produce IL-2 and proliferate in response to anti-CD2 monoclonal antibody (Hassan et al., 1997).

Superantigens activate T cells by binding to a portion of the TCRβ chain outside of the peptide antigen recognition site, but they otherwise mimic activation by peptide/MHCs in most respects. Neonatal T cells differ from adult CD45RA^{high} T cells in their tendency to become anergic rather than competent for increased cytokine secretion after priming with bacterial superantigen bound to class II MHC–transfected murine fibroblasts (Takahashi et al., 1995). This is developmentally regulated because CD4$^+$CD8$^-$ thymocytes, the immediate precursors of antigenically naïve CD4$^+$ T cells, are also prone to anergy when treated under these conditions (Imanishi et al., 1998). Consistent with this anergic tendency, newborns with toxic shock syndrome–like exanthematous disease, in which Vβ_2-bearing T cells are markedly expanded in vivo by the superantigen toxic shock syndrome toxin-1 (TSST-1), have a greater fraction of anergic Vβ_2-bearing T cells than do adults with TSST-1–mediated disease (Takahashi et al., 2000).

Neonatal, but not adult, CD4$^+$ T cells primed by alloantigen, in the form of Epstein-Barr virus (EBV)–transformed human B cells, became nonresponsive to restimulation by alloantigen or by a combination of anti-CD3 and anti-CD28 monoclonal antibodies (Porcu et al., 1998; Risdon et al., 1995). Preliminary studies implicated a lack of ras signaling as the basis for this reduced responsiveness (Porcu et al., 1998). These results suggest that neonatal and, presumably, fetal T cells have a greater tendency to become anergic, particularly under conditions in which co-stimulation (e.g., through CD40, CD80, or CD86 on the APC) may be limited.

Recently, a CD28 homolog called ICOS has been identified that interacts with B7h, a B7 family molecule expressed on both APCs and nonhematopoietic cells (Sharpe and Freeman, 2002). ICOS is not expressed by naïve T cells but is detectable at the later stages of naïve T-cell activation and is constitutively expressed by established effector and memory T cells (Sharpe and Freeman, 2002). The results of murine studies initially indicated that the ICOS/B7h interaction is important for the activation of Th2 rather than Th1 effector cells, but recent investigations have also implicated ICOS co-stimulation in Th1-predominant immunopathosis (Rottman et al., 2001; Sporici et al., 2001). The expression of ICOS and B7h by neonatal cells has not been reported.

T-Helper 1 and T-Helper 2 Effector Generation In Vitro

Activated neonatal T cells can be differentiated in vitro into either Th1-like or Th2-like effector cells by incubation for several days to weeks with IL-12 and anti–IL-4 antibody or with IL-4 and anti–IL-12 antibody, respectively (Delespesse et al., 1998; Demeure et al., 1994; Rogge et al., 1997; Sornasse et al., 1996). Treatment of neonatal T cells with IL-4 and anti–IL-12 upregulates GATA-3 (Macaubas and Holt, 2001), which acts as a master transcription factor promoting Th2 effector generation. The findings of these studies indicate that neonatal T cells express functional receptors for IL-4 and IL-12, including the activation-induced IL-12 receptor β_2 subunit (Rogge et al., 1997). Mature single-positive (CD4$^+$CD8$^-$ or CD4$^-$CD8$^+$) fetal thymocytes obtained as early as 16 weeks' gestation can be also differentiated into either Th1 or Th2 effector cells by such cytokine treatment (Yamaguchi et al., 1999), indicating that the capacity to acquire a polarized cytokine profile is established relatively early in fetal life.

Purified neonatal CD45RA^{high} CD4$^+$ T cells proliferate substantially more in response to IL-4 than do analogous adult cells (Early and Reen, 1996), suggesting a way by which neonatal T cells might be more prone to become Th2 effectors. Studies by Delespesse and colleagues (1998) also suggest that neonatal and adult CD45RA^{high} CD4$^+$ T cells may differ in their tendency to become Th2-like effector cells under certain conditions in vitro; when these cells were primed by using a combination of anti-CD3 monoclonal antibody, a fibroblast cell line expressing low amounts of the CD80 co-stimulatory molecule, and exogenous IL-12, there was enhanced production of IL-4 by neonatal CD4+ T cells in comparison with adult cells. Moreover, this group found that the neonatal effector T cells generated had a substantially lower capacity to produce IFN-γ than adult cells and these differences persisted even when endogenous IL-4 was blocked with an anti–IL-4 receptor antibody (Bullens et al., 1999).

Chemokine Receptor Expression

The differential expression of chemokine receptors by T cells is important in their selective trafficking either to sites where naïve T cells may potentially encounter antigen for the first time, such as the spleen and lymph nodes, or to inflamed tissues for effector functions (Sallusto and Lanzavecchia, 2000). CCR7 expression by naïve T cells allows these cells to recirculate between the blood and uninflamed lymphoid organs, which constitutively express the two major ligands for CCR7: CCL19 and CCL21.

Naïve T cells in the adult express CCR1, CCR7, and CXCR4 on the cell surface and have low to undetectable levels of CCR5. Neonatal naïve T cells have a similar phenotype, except that they lack CCR1 surface expression and, unlike adult naïve T cells, they do not increase CXCR3 expression and decrease CCR7 expression after activation through anti-CD3 and CD28 monoclonal antibodies (Berkowitz et al., 1998; Sato et al., 2001). The CCR7 expressed on neonatal T cells is functional and mediates chemotaxis of these cells in response to SLC and ELC (Christopherson et al., 1999). These results suggest that activated neonatal T cells may be limited in their capacity to traffic to nonlymphoid tissue sites of inflammation and may preferentially recirculate between the blood and peripheral lymphoid organs.

Neonatal T cells can increase the surface expression of CCR5 by treatment with either mitogen or IL-2 (Mo et al., 1998). The observation that CCR5 is expressed by fetal mesenteric lymph node T cells during the second trimester of pregnancy (Kitchen and Zack, 1999) suggests that CCR5 can be upregulated in vivo by a mechanism that does not involve antigenic stimulation. CCR5 expression on CD4+ T cells also gradually increase after birth in parallel with the appearance of memory cells, suggesting that this process occurs in vivo as part of memory cell generation (Auewarakul et al., 2000).

Neonatal T cells also have the capacity to express chemokines characteristic of Th1 or Th2 effectors after differentiation in a polarized cytokine milieu (IL-12 and anti–IL-4 for Th1 and IL-4 and anti–IL-12 for Th2). The Th1 effectors generated in vitro tend to express CXCR3, CCR5, and CX3CR1, whereas Th2 effectors tend to express CCR4 and, to a lesser extent, CCR3 (Bonnechi et al., 1998; Fraticelli et al., 2001; Sallusto and Lanzavecchia, 2000). Studies of freshly isolated memory CD4+ T cells suggest that the expression of CXCR3 and of CCR4 may be more accurate predictors of cells with Th1 and Th2 cytokine profiles, respectively (Kim et al., 2001; Yamamoto et al., 2000).

Some (Sallusto and Lanzavecchia, 2000)—but not all (Kim et al., 2001)—studies suggest an intermediate step by which naïve T cells first acquire a memory cell (CD45RA^low CD45R0^high) surface phenotype but retain high levels of CCR7 expression and a limited capacity to produce cytokines. These intermediate cells, termed *central memory cells,* are thought to differentiate into CCR7^−/low memory/effector cells that have a more diverse repertoire of chemokine receptors and an increased capacity for cytokine production and, in the case of CD8+ T cells, for cell-mediated cytotoxicity (Sallusto and Lanzavecchia, 2000). Our preliminary results suggest that infants and young children accumulate a higher ratio of central memory to effector memory CD4+ T cells compared with adults (Tu and Lewis, unpublished results).

T-Cell–Mediated Cytotoxicity

T-cell–mediated cytotoxicity involves two major pathways of killing of cellular targets through either the secretion of perforin and granzymes or through the engagement of Fas by Fas ligand (Fig. 22-2). The recent and growing use of cord blood for hematopoietic cell transplantation and the finding that its use is associated with reduced graft-versus-host disease compared with adult bone marrow have led to great interest in the capacity of neonatal T cells to mediate cytotoxicity and potentiate graft rejection.

Early studies mostly used unfractionated mononuclear cells as a source of killer cells in a variety of non–antigen-specific assays, such as lectin-mediated cytotoxicity or redirected cytotoxicity with anti-CD3 monoclonal antibodies. Reduced cytotoxicity was observed with lectin-activated cord blood lymphocytes, particularly when purified T cells were used (Andersson et al., 1981; Campbell et al., 1974; Lubens et al., 1982).

T cells can also be sensitized in vitro for cytotoxicity by using allogeneic (MHC other than self) stimulator cells followed by testing for cytotoxic activity against allogeneic target cells. Using this approach, most researchers have found that neonatal T cells are moderately less effective than adult T cells as cytotoxic effector cells (Granberg and Hirvonen, 1980; Harris, 1995; Rayfield et al., 1980; Risdon et al., 1994a, 1994b). More substantial defects in T-cell–mediated cytotoxicity by neonatal T cells after allogeneic priming is observed when no exogenous cytokines are added, such as IL-2 (Barbey et al., 1998; Slavcev et al., 2002), suggesting that this decreased cytolytic activity may well be of physiologic significance in vivo.

Part of this deficiency reflects the absence of effector and memory CD8+ T cells, as identified by their expression of CD45R0 or their lack of CD27 and CD28 (Appay et al., 2002), or both, in that CD8+ effector and memory T cells kill more efficiently than antigenically naïve T cells after stimulation with lectin or anti-CD3 monoclonal antibody (de Jong et al., 1991) or after allogeneic sensitization (Akbar et al., 1991; Hamann et al., 1997; Mescher, 1995). Limited studies of virus-specific

Cytotoxic T Cell　　　　**Target Cell**

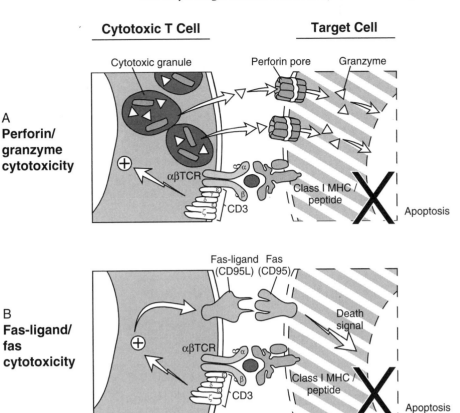

Figure 22-2 · Two major mechanisms of antigen-specific class I major histocompatibility (MHC)–restricted T-cell-mediated cytotoxicity. The engagement of αβ-T-cell receptors (TCRs) of CD8+ T cells by antigenic peptide bound to class I MHC on the target cell leads to T-cell activation and target cell death. A, Cytotoxicity may occur by the extracellular release of the contents of cytotoxic granules from the T cell, including perforins and granzymes. Perforins introduce pores by which granzymes can enter into the target cell, leading to the triggering of apoptosis and cell death. B, The activation of T cells results in their surface expression of Fas ligand (CD95L), which engages Fas (CD95) on the target cell, resulting in the delivery of death signal culminating in apoptosis. Both of these mechanisms are also used for killing by natural killer (NK) T cells and by NK cells.

T-cell–mediated cytotoxicity in the neonate and infant (discussed in the section "T-cell reactivity to postnatal infections and vaccines") also suggest that the capacity of the neonate to generate a functional T-cell effector population is reduced in comparison with that of adults for some viral pathogens but not others.

The mechanism for reduced neonatal T-cell–mediated cytotoxicity remains poorly understood. Two studies have found that only a low percentage of neonatal CD8+ T cells constitutively express perforin, whereas approximately 30% of adult CD8+ T cells contain this protein (Berthou et al., 1995; Kogawa et al., 2002). In contrast, another study found that approximately 30% of neonatal T cells expressed perforin, a frequency similar to that of adult T cells (Rukavina et al., 1998).

The capacity of fetal T cells to mediate cytotoxicity has not received as much scrutiny, despite its relevance to the development of fetal therapy with hematopoietic stem cells. CD8+ T cells bearing αβ-TCR can be cloned as polyclonal lines from human fetal liver by 16 weeks' gestation (Renda et al., 2000). These CD8+ T-cell lines have proliferative activity in response to allogeneic stimulation (Renda et al., 2000), but their reactivity toward HLAs and their cytolytic activity is not known. A recent study has found substantial numbers of circulating CMV-specific CD8+ T cells in CMV-infected fetuses that express perforin and IFN-γ (Marchant et al., 2003). This suggests that that the ability of the fetus to mount CD8+ T-cell responses to certain viruses may be intact.

Neonatal T-Cell Apoptosis

Effector T cells that are generated in vitro from naïve precursors are prone to apoptosis after their withdrawal from exogenous cytokines, such as IL-2, or with reactivation (e.g., by using anti-CD3 monoclonal antibody stimulation). IL-2 not only promotes the clonal expansion of T cells, but also makes effector T cells vulnerable to apoptosis after its withdrawal. This susceptibility of effector T cells to apoptosis compared with naïve T cells is attributable to the decreased expression of bcl-2 and the upregulation of Fas (CD95) and the p55 and p75 TNF receptors (Penninger and Kroemer, 1998).

Role of Fas and TNF Receptors

The engagement of Fas and TNF receptors by their cognate ligands of Fas ligand and TNF-α, respectively, results in the rapid induction of effector cell apoptosis. Effector B cells are similarly prone to the induction of apoptotic cell death by these pathways. Together, these observations account for the tendency of mice with genetic disruptions of either IL-2 or its specific receptor (CD25 [the IL-2 receptor α chain], the IL-2 receptor β chain, and the γc) to develop abnormal expansions of T-lymphocyte populations. In patients with Fas deficiency, abnormal accumulations of certain T-cell and B-cell populations are observed, along with the development of autoantibody-mediated hematologic disease.

Mononuclear cells from cord blood, including naïve CD4+ T cells, are more prone than those from the adult circulation to undergo spontaneous apoptosis during in vitro culture (El Ghalbzouri et al., 1999; Hassan and Reen, 1998, 2001; Soares et al., 1998; Tu et al., 2000). However, Fas expression is very low to undetectable on freshly isolated neonatal lymphocytes, including CD4[+] and CD8[+] T cells (Drenou et al., 1998; Kuntz et al., 2001; Potestio et al., 1999; Suda et al., 1997; Tu et al., 2000), a finding that is consistent with the restriction of Fas expression almost entirely to memory/effector cell populations (Potestio et al., 1999). This indicates that most spontaneous apoptosis of cord blood T cells is not mediated by Fas/Fas ligand interactions but other pathways.

Polyclonal activators such as anti-CD3 monoclonal antibody or PHA substantially increase Fas expression by neonatal T cells. However, activation-induced Fas expression by neonatal T cells is lower than that by adult cells (Aggarwal et al., 1997). Treatment of neonatal T cells with IFN-γ alone or with the combination of IL-2 and CD28 is effective in inducing neonatal T cells to express Fas and to become sensitive to apoptosis after Fas engagement (Suda et al., 1997). Neonatal T cells are initially more resistant than adult T cells to anti-CD3 monoclonal antibody-induced apoptosis and appear to be initially resistant to the TNF-α–mediated apoptosis, most likely because of decreased expression of the p55 TNF receptor, TNF receptor–associated death domain (TRADD) cytoplasmic protein, and caspase 3 enzyme involved in this process (Aggarwal et al., 2000).

However, primed neonatal T cells subsequently become more susceptible to apoptosis than adult cells after restimulation with anti-CD3 monoclonal antibody; nevertheless, they remain relatively resistant to Fas-induced apoptosis (Aggarwal et al., 1997). The increased apoptotic tendency after anti-CD3 monoclonal antibody stimulation is likely to be mediated by the p55 and p75 TNF receptors (Yang et al., 2001). These results suggest a mechanism by which the clonal expansion of neonatal T cells is limited after activation through the αβ-TCR/CD3 complex. They also suggest that exogenous cytokines (e.g., IL-2) could be used to counteract this apoptotic tendency, because IL-2 treatment in vitro blocks TNF receptor–mediated apoptosis of activated neonatal T cells (Yang et al., 2001).

The circulating levels of soluble Fas, soluble TNF, and soluble p55 TNF receptor increase in the first several days after birth (Malamitsi-Puchner et al., 2001). The apoptotic tendency of lymphocytes may be downregulated in the immediate postnatal period by these factors. These elevated levels may reflect increased surface expression at birth, an increased conversion to a shed form, or decreased clearance, or a combination of these possibilities.

Role of BCL-2 Family Members

The mechanisms responsible for neonatal naïve T cells to undergo increased apoptosis may be related to an abundance of members of the bcl-2 family. Neonatal T cells express a lower ratio of bcl-2 to *bax* mRNA and protein than do adult T cells, which may decrease protection from apoptosis (Aggarwal et al., 1997). This lower ratio has also been observed at the protein level

for neonatal naïve CD4[+] T cells (Hassan and Reen, 2001). Neonatal naïve T cells have a more marked decrease in the expression of bcl-2 and bcl-X$_L$ protein, which are both antiapoptotic, after 7 days in culture without exogenous cytokines (Soares et al., 1998). Treatment of neonatal naïve CD4[+] T cells with IL-7 can also block spontaneous apoptosis (Hassan and Reen, 1998; Soares et al., 1998; Webb et al., 1999) and is accompanied by increased expression of bcl-2 and bcl-X$_L$ (Hassan and Reen, 1998; Soares et al., 1998).

Role of Insulin-Like Growth Factor

This tendency for neonatal T cells to undergo apoptosis can also be blocked by incubation with insulin-like growth factor 1, but the mechanism whereby this occurs is unclear (Tu et al., 2000). The tendency of cord blood CD4[+] and CD8[+] T cells to undergo apoptosis after PHA stimulation and presumably after anti-CD3 monoclonal antibody stimulation, can be inhibited by incubation with insulin-like growth factor 1. In this context, insulin-like growth factor 1 may act by a mechanism that includes the inhibition of the upregulation of Fas surface expression (Tu et al., 2000), but the effect of this treatment on p55 and p75 TNF receptor expression has not been reported.

Role of MHC Engagement

Neonatal circulating mononuclear cells, most likely including T cells, are also more prone than adult mononuclear cells to undergo apoptosis after the engagement of class I MHC achieved by monoclonal antibody treatment (El Ghalbzouri et al., 1999), apparently by a mechanism independent of Fas/Fas ligand interactions. The physiologic importance of the spontaneous and class I MHC–induced apoptotic pathways for fetal lymphocytes is unclear. It is plausible that an increased tendency of fetal T lymphocytes to undergo apoptosis after the engagement of class I MHC might be a mechanism to maintain tolerance against noninherited maternal alloantigens.

Natural Killer T Cells

Definition

A small population of circulating human T cells expresses αβ-TCR—but not CD4 or CD8—and NKR-P1A, the human ortholog of the mouse NK1.1 protein. These features and others, such as CD56 and CD57 surface expression, in addition to a dependence on the cytokine IL-15 for their development (Ohteki et al., 1997), are characteristic of NK cells, a non-T-cell lymphocyte population. For this reason these cells are frequently referred to as *NK T cells* or *natural T cells*.

Similar to murine T cells expressing NK1.1, human NK T cells have a restricted repertoire of αβ-TCR (TCRα chains containing the Vα24JαQ segments in association with certain TCRβ chains containing Vβ11 segments) (Dellabona et al., 1994; Lantz and Bendelac,

1994; Porcelli et al., 1993) and mainly recognize antigens presented by the nonclassical MHC molecule CD1d rather than by class I or class II MHC molecules. These CD1d-restricted antigens that can be recognized by NK T cells include certain lipid molecules, such as α-galactosyl-ceramide (Kawano et al., 1999; Nieda et al., 2001), and certain hydrophobic peptides. NK T cells also have the ability to secrete high levels of IL-4 and IFN-γ and to express Fas ligand and TRAIL on their cell surfaces on primary stimulation, a capacity not observed with most antigenically naïve αβ-T cells (Godfrey et al., 2000; Nieda et al., 2001).

The physiologic role of NK T cells remains controversial. They may play a role in host defense against certain infections, but murine studies suggest that NK T cells are negative regulators of certain T-cell–mediated immune responses, particularly those involved in autoimmune disease (Wilson et al., 1998) and in graft-versus-host disease after hematopoietic cell transplantation (Zeng et al., 1999). The regulatory function of NK T cells in autoimmune disease may be relevant to humans in that if there is a lack of NK T cells, this may predispose one to the development of insulin-dependent diabetes mellitus (Bach, 2001).

Ontogeny of NK T Cells

Only small numbers of NK T cells (<1.0% of circulating T cells) are present in the neonatal circulation, but these subsequently increase with aging (Musha et al., 1998). This suggests that NK T cells may either undergo postnatal expansion (e.g., in relation to exposure to a ubiquitous antigen presented by CD1d molecules) or that their production by the thymus or at extrathymic sites occurs mainly postnatally. Neonatal NK T cells are similar to adult NK T cells in having a memory/effector–like cell surface phenotype, including the expression of CD25, the CD45R0 isoform, and a low level of expression of CD62L (L-selectin) (D'Andrea et al., 2000; van der Vliet et al., 2000). In the case of murine NK cells, many of these activation phenotypic features are found on NK T cells during intrathymic development, indicating that these are a result of differentiation rather than antigenic stimulation in the periphery before birth.

Neonatal NK T cells can be expanded in vitro by using a combination of anti-CD3 and CD28 monoclonal antibodies, PHA, IL-2, and IL-7 (Kadowaki et al., 2001a). Neonatal NK T cells have a similar surface phenotype to that of adult NK T cells, but they produce only limited amounts of IL-4 or IFN-γ on primary stimulation, indicating functional immaturity (D'Andrea et al., 2000). This decreased capacity may be attributable to mechanisms similar to those for the reduced IFN-γ production by neonatal CD4+ T cells, such as decreased levels of the NFATc2 transcription factor or increased methylation of the IFN-γ genetic locus.

Function of NK T Cells

After in vitro expansion, neonatal NK T cells produce higher levels of IL-4 and lower amounts of IFN-γ than

similarly treated adult NK T cells (Kadowaki et al., 2001a). The cytokine profile of neonatal NK T cells demonstrates greater plasticity than that of adult NK T cells; furthermore, the expansion and priming of neonatal NK T cells with either DC1-type or DC2-type dendritic cells—in conjunction with PHA, IL-2, and IL-7—result in an IL-4–predominant cytokine expression profile and an IFN-γ–predominant cytokine expression profile, respectively. In contrast, similarly treated adult NK T cells retain their ability to produce both cytokines (Kadowaki et al., 2001a), suggesting a loss of plasticity of NK T cells toward Th1 versus Th2 polarization after birth. Polarization of neonatal NK T cells toward IL-4 but not IFN-γ secretion might be potentially useful in the treatment of graft-versus-host disease and autoimmune diseases by adoptive transfer (Bach, 2001; Zeng et al., 1999).

The capacity of cytokine-derived neonatal NK T cells and those directly isolated from the infant to mediate cytotoxicity has not been reported. Neonatal CD56+ T cells constitutively express less perforin than do adult cells (Kogawa et al., 2002). Because the CD56+ T-cell population is highly enriched in NK T cells, NK T-cell cytotoxicity is probably limited at birth and gradually increases with age. Culturing of neonatal NK T cells in vitro for several weeks results in the acquisition of potent cytotoxic activity against a variety of tumor cell targets (Gansuvd et al., 2002), indicating that developmental limitations can be overcome after expansion and differentiation.

Gamma/delta–T Cells

Phenotype

γδ-T cells, which express a TCR heterodimer consisting of a γ chain and a δ chain in association with the CD3 complex proteins, are rarer than αβ-T cells in most tissues. A major exception is the intestinal epithelium, where they predominate (Kaufmann, 1996). Some γδ-TCRs can recognize conventional peptide antigens presented by MHC, but most directly recognize three-dimensional nonprotein or protein structures. The antigen-combining site of the γδ-TCR shares some structural features with that of immunoglobulin molecules (Li et al., 1998), which suggests that both γδ-TCR and immunoglobulin recognize three-dimensional structures rather than processed antigenic peptides bound to MHC molecules.

Human γδ-T cells expressing the Vγ2Vδ2 receptors can proliferate and secrete cytokines after the recognition of isopentenyl and prenyl phosphates derived from mycobacteria (Garcia et al., 1997; Tanaka et al., 1995) or of alkylamines derived from many species of bacteria, including important neonatal pathogens, such as *Listeria* and *Escherichia coli* (Bukowski et al., 1999; Feurle et al., 2002; Kabelitz, 1992; Kaufmann, 1996). Human γδ-T cells express NKG2D, which recognizes MICA (*MHC class I chain-related gene A*) (Bauer et al., 1999; Groh et al., 1998). This NKG2D/MICA interaction enhances the antigen-dependent effector function of Vγ2Vδ2 γδ-T cells (Das et al., 2001). Such enhancement in vivo may be a consequence of the induction of MICA on APCs by mycobacteria and other pathogens (Das et al., 2001).

Function

This in vitro activation of γδ-T cells is probably relevant in vivo because increased numbers are found in the skin lesions of patients with leprosy and in the blood of patients with malaria (Kabelitz, 1992; Kaufmann, 1996). Resident γδ-T cells of the murine skin can produce epithelial-specific growth factors that may help maintain epithelial integrity during stress (Witherden et al., 2000). The observation that MICA is expressed on heat-shock–stressed epithelial cells and, presumably, stressed or infected epithelium in vivo, is consistent with a similar role for human γδ-T cells.

γδ-T cells may also have important immunosurveillance function for malignancy, in that murine cutaneous γδ-T cells can kill skin carcinoma cells by a mechanism that involves the engagement of NKG2D by Rae-1 and H60, which have homology with human MICA (Girardi et al., 2001). The findings from murine studies also suggest that γδ-T cells may help decrease inflammatory responses to pathogens, such as *Listeria,* by killing activated macrophages by cell-mediated cytotoxicity (Egan and Carding, 2000).

Most activated γδ-T cells express high levels of perforins, serine esterases, and granulysin and are capable of cytotoxicity against tumor cells and other cell targets, such as infected cells (Dieli et al., 2001). γδ-T cells can also secrete a variety of cytokines in vitro, including TNF-α, IFN-γ, and IL-4 (Kabelitz, 1992; Kaufmann, 1996), as well as chemokines that may help recruit inflammatory cells to the tissues. Cytokine production can be potently activated by products from live bacteria, such as isobutylamine (Wang et al., 2001a) and by IFN-α/β or by agents that potently induce it, such as oligonucleotides containing unmethylated CpG motifs (Rothenfusser et al., 2001).

The results of murine studies suggest that these cells are critical for mucosal immunity. Mice lacking γδ cells have markedly decreased numbers of intestinal IgA plasma cells and decreased IgA production after oral immunization with foreign protein and adjuvant (Fujihashi et al., 1996). Murine γδ-T cells may also contribute to the defense of the host against intracellular pathogens, including herpes simplex virus (HSV), *Listeria,* and *Mycobacterium tuberculosis,* particularly if αβ-T-cell function is compromised (Ladel et al., 1995; 1996; Sciammas et al., 1997). Human Vγ2Vδ2 γδ-T cells after adoptive transfer into mice with genetically inherited severe-combined immunodeficiency (SCID) can mediate rapid and potent antibacterial activity against both gram-positive and gram-negative bacteria, with protection associated with the production of IFN-γ (Wang et al., 2001b).

Only approximately 2% to 5% of T-lineage cells of the thymus and peripheral blood express γδ-TCR in most individuals (Borst et al., 1991). Unlike most αβ-T cells, whose development requires an intact thymus, a significant portion of γδ-T cells can develop by a thymic-independent pathway, and normal numbers of γδ-T cells are found in cases of complete thymic aplasia (Borst et al., 1991). This may be explained, at least in part, by the differentiation of γδ-T cells directly from primitive lymphohematopoietic precursor cells found in clusters in the lamina propria of the small intestine, as has been demonstrated in the mouse (Saito et al., 1998).

Ontogeny of γδ-TCR Gene Rearrangements

The human TCRγ and TCRδ chain genes undergo a programmed rearrangement of dispersed segments analogous to that of the TCRβ and TCRα genes. However, most γδ-T cells lack surface expression of either CD4 or the CD8β chain, suggesting that they may not undergo the process of positive selection that is obligatory for αβ-T cells (Bigby et al., 1993). Unlike αβ-T cells, the development of γδ-T cells occurs normally in the absence of signaling through the pre-TCR complex (Saint-Ruf et al., 2000). Whether γδ-T cells undergo a negative selection process analogous to that of αβ-T cells is unclear (Chien et al., 1996).

Rearranged TCRδ genes are first expressed extrathymically in the liver and primitive gut between 6 and 9 weeks' gestation (McVay and Carding, 1999; McVay et al., 1998). Rearrangement of the human TCRγ and TCRδ genes in the fetal thymus begins shortly after its colonization with lymphoid cells, with TCRδ protein detectable by 9.5 weeks' gestation (Haynes and Heinly, 1995). Whether the differentiation of γδ-T cells occurs by a pathway that is largely or completely independent of that for αβ-thymocytes remains unclear (Burtrum et al., 1996; Robey and Fowlkes, 1998). γδ-T cells comprise approximately 10% of the circulating T-cell compartment at 16 weeks' gestation, a percentage that gradually declines to less than 3% by term (Bukowski et al., 1994; Peakman et al., 1992).

There is potential for the formation of a highly diverse γδ-TCR repertoire, but peripheral γδ-T cells use only a small number of V segments, which vary with age and with tissue location. These can be divided into two major groups: Vγ2Vδ2 cells and Vδ1 cells, in which a Vδ1-bearing TCRδ chain predominantly pairs with a TCRγ chain using a Vγ segment other than Vγ1.

Most γδ-thymocytes in the first trimester of fetal life express Vδ2 segments. This is followed by γδ-thymocytes that express Vδ1, which predominate at least through infancy in the thymus. Most circulating fetal and neonatal γδ-T cells are also Vδ1, with only approximately 10% bearing Vδ2 (Musha et al., 1998), and these Vδ1 cells are the predominant γδ-T-cell population of the small intestinal epithelium after birth. In contrast to the early gestation fetal thymus and the fetal and neonatal circulation, Vδ2 T cells predominate in the fetal liver and spleen early during the second trimester (Erbach et al., 1993; Wucherpfennig et al., 1993) and appear before γδ-thymocytes (Haynes and Heinly, 1995; Miyagawa et al., 1992), suggesting that they are produced extrathymically by the fetal liver.

TCR spectratyping results revealed that the TCRδ chains making use of either Vδ1 or Vδ2 segments are usually oligoclonal at birth (Beldjord et al., 1993; Shen et al., 1998). Because this oligoclonality is also characteristic of the adult γδ-T-cell repertoire, this is not attributable to postnatal clonal expansion, but it instead reflects an intrinsic feature of this cell lineage. By 6 months old, γδ-T cells bearing Vγ2Vδ2 segments become predominant and remain so during adulthood (Parker et al., 1990), most likely because of their preferential expansion in response to ubiquitous antigens such as endogenous bacterial flora (Bukowski et al., 1999).

Ontogeny of γδ-T-Cell Function

Neonatal γδ-T cells proliferate in vitro to mycobacterial lipid antigens (Tsuyuguchi et al., 1991), yet they express lower levels of serine esterases than do adult γδ-T cells, suggesting that they have less effective cytotoxic cells (Smith et al., 1990b). γδ-T-cell clones derived from cord blood also have a markedly reduced capacity to mediate cytotoxicity against tumor cell extracts (Bukowski et al., 1994). Because these neonatal clones also have lower CD45R0 surface expression than the adult clones, their reduced activity may reflect their antigenic naïveté.

In contrast to neonatal αβ-T cells, the activation and propagation of these cells in culture (e.g., with exogenous IL-2) does not enhance their function. The function of fetal liver γδ-T cells remains unclear, but one report suggests that they have cytotoxic reactivity against maternal class I MHC (Miyagawa et al., 1992) and thus may prevent engraftment of maternal T cells.

Practical Aspects of T-Cell Function in the Fetus, Neonate, and Young Infant

Delayed Cutaneous Hypersensitivity, Graft Rejection, and Graft-versus-Host Disease

Skin test reactivity to cell-free antigens assesses a form of DTH that requires the function of antigen-specific CD4+ T cells. Skin test reactivity to common antigens such as Candida, streptokinase-streptodornase, and tetanus toxoid is usually not detectable in neonates (Franz et al., 1976; Munoz and Limbert, 1977; Steele et al., 1976). This reflects a lack of antigen-specific sensitization because in vitro reactivity of these antigens is also absent. However, when leukocytes and, presumably, antigen-specific CD4+ T cells from sensitized adults are adoptively transferred to neonates, children, and adults, only neonates fail to respond to antigen-specific skin tests (Warwick et al., 1960).

As discussed later, this indicates that the neonate may be deficient in other components of the immune system required for DTH, such as monocyte or dendritic cell chemotaxis. Such deficiencies may account, at least in part, for diminished skin reactivity by the neonate after

specific sensitization or after intradermal injection with T-cell mitogens (Bonforte et al., 1972; Uhr et al., 1960). Diminished skin reactivity persists postnatally up to a year old (Kniker et al., 1985).

Nevertheless, neonates, including those born prematurely, are capable of rejecting foreign grafts (Fowler et al., 1960). Experiments on human-SCID mouse chimeras also suggest that second-trimester human fetal T cells are capable of becoming cytotoxic effector T cells in response to foreign antigens and in rejecting solid tissue allografts (Rouleau et al., 1996). Transplantation of fetal blood from one unaffected fraternal twin to another with β-thalassemia did not result in marrow engraftment, despite a sharing of similar MHC haplotypes; instead there was a postnatal recipient cytotoxic T-cell response against donor leukocytes (Orlandi et al., 1996). A T-cell response to alloantigens can also be detected in newborns after in utero irradiated red blood cell transfusions from unrelated donors; these neonates have a significantly greater percentage of CD45R0^high T cells than healthy control subjects (Vietor et al., 1997a, 1997b). Thus fetal T cells can mediate in vivo allogeneic responses, including graft rejection.

Another indication that neonatal T cells can mediate allogeneic responses is the fact that blood transfusions rarely induce graft-versus-host disease in the neonate. However, rare cases of persistence of donor lymphocytes and of graft-versus-host disease have developed after intrauterine transfusion in the last trimester and in transfused premature neonates (Berger and Dixon, 1989; Flidel et al., 1992; Naiman et al., 1969; Parkman et al., 1974). Because the infusion of fresh leukocytes induces partial tolerance to skin grafts (Fowler et al., 1960), tolerance for transfused lymphocytes might occur by a similar mechanism, predisposing the fetus or neonate to graft-versus-host disease.

Together, these observations suggest a partial immaturity in T-cell and inflammatory mechanisms required for DTH and for graft rejection.

T-Cell Reactivity to Environmental Antigens

Specific antigen reactivity can theoretically develop in the fetus by exposure to antigens transferred from the mother, by the transfer of specific cellular immunity from maternal lymphocytes, or by infection of the fetus itself (Field and Caspary, 1971). Several studies suggest that fetal T cells have become primed to environmental or dietary protein allergens as a result of maternal exposure and transfer of allergens to the fetus (Prescott et al., 1997; Szepfalusi et al., 1997; van Duren-Schmidt et al., 1997). A criticism of these studies is that the antigen-specific proliferation is low compared with the basal proliferation of cord blood mononuclear cells. In addition, many of these researchers used antigen extracts rather than defined recombinant proteins or peptides, and these may have nonspecific stimulatory effects.

Prenatal sensitization has been assessed in the incorporation of ³H-thymidine by cord blood mononuclear cells and in antigen-induced cytokine production, as determined by using either reverse transcriptase polymerase chain reaction for cytokine transcripts (IL-4, IL-5, IL-9, and IFN-γ), cell culture supernatant cytokine enzyme-linked immunosorbent assays (for IL-5, IL-10, and IL-13 [Miller et al., 2001; Prescott et al., 1998a, 1998b]), and a cell-based cytokine enzyme-linked immunosorbent assay (for IL-4 and IFN-γ [Devereux et al., 2000]). In some studies, the production of IL-10 in these cultures is high relative to the classic Th2 cytokines (IL-4, IL-5, IL-9, and IL-13). IFN-γ production was 100-fold higher than IL-4 production, a ratio that is still reduced compared with that of adult cells. This cytokine profile has been interpreted as a Th2-biased response or a regulatory T-cell (IL-10–dominant) response. Whether Th2 priming of fetal T cells to environmental antigens is a risk factor for the postnatal development of atopic disease remains controversial. Its frequent occurrence suggests that priming per se may be a normal outcome of fetal exposure to such antigens (Prescott et al., 1998b).

Prenatal priming of T cells by environmental allergens can be demonstrated as early as 20 weeks' gestation, on the basis of their proliferative responses to seasonal allergens (Szepfalusi et al., 2000). However, these responses are low and the cytokine profile was not reported. In one study, protein allergen-specific T-cell proliferation detected at birth was more common when allergen exposure occurred in the first or second trimester than in the third trimester (Van Duren-Schmidt et al., 1997). This could reflect decreased maternal-fetal transport of antigen during late pregnancy or an intrinsic capacity of early gestation and late-gestation fetal T cells to be primed.

Fetal T-Cell Sensitization to Maternally Administered Vaccines and Maternally Derived Antigens

In contrast to protein allergens, antigen-specific fetal T-cell priming to vaccines has not been documented (e.g., after maternal vaccination during the last trimester of pregnancy with tetanus toxoid or inactivated influenza A or influenza B virus [Englund et al., 1993]). This suggests that fetal sensitization to foreign proteins is inefficient, particularly when exposure is temporally limited. Whether this reflects inefficient maternal-fetal transfer of protein antigens or intrinsic limitations of the fetus for antigen presentation and T-cell priming is unclear. Even if fetal T cells could be primed, their immune response to maternally derived vaccine proteins would be expected to be decreased compared with the maternal response, because the antigen would enter the fetal circulation without accompanying activation of the innate response required for full T-cell activation.

However, fetal T-cell sensitization can occur from chronic infection of the mother with viruses or parasites: HIV peptide–specific IL-2 production by cord blood CD4[+] T cells can occur in uninfected infants born to HIV-infected mothers, indicating that fetal T-cell sensitization can occur (Kuhn et al., 2001). Parasite (schistosomal, filarial, and *Plasmodium*) antigen-specific cytokine production by peripheral blood lymphocytes, most likely of T-cell origin, was also detectable at birth in infants without congenital infection born to infected mothers (King et al., 2002; Malhotra et al., 1999). This T-cell immunity persisted for at least a year. Fetal exposure to parasitic antigens is also associated with decreased antigen-specific IFN-γ production during early infancy to other antigens, such as BCG vaccine given at birth (Malhotra et al., 1999). These results suggest that fetal exposure to parasitic antigens without infection can downregulate subsequent post-natal Th1 responses to unrelated antigens.

Maternal Transfer of T-Cell Immunity to the Fetus

There are many reports of cord blood lymphocyte proliferation or cytokine production in response to antigens that the fetus is presumed not to have encountered. These antigen responses have been attributed to passive transfer of T-cell immunity from the mother. For example, in studies in which the in vitro reactivity of lymphocytes was studied between birth and the first week of life, specific reactivity to tuberculin purified protein derivative (PPD) (Schlesinger and Covelli, 1977; Shiratsuchi and Tsuyuguchi, 1981), *Mycobacterium leprae* (Barnetson et al., 1976), measles (Gallagher et al., 1981), and rubella (Thong et al., 1974) was observed. However, infants with reactive lymphocytes were usually a minority (<20%) of those born to mothers without evidence of active infection, and the data were interpreted as evidence for the transfer of maternal cellular immunity (Leikin and Oppenheim, 1970; Thong et al., 1974). Responses are usually small and may represent laboratory artifacts rather than true sensitization. It is also important to consider that mycobacterial products, such as PPD or *M. leprae* extracts, can activate γδ-T cells in the absence of specific prior sensitization. Lipoglycan antigens bound to CD1 may mediate these responses.

In vitro reactivity of neonatal T cells to extracts of gram-negative bacteria or *Staphylococcus aureus* has also been reported (Brody et al., 1968; Ivanyi and Lehner, 1977; Rubin et al., 1981). However, some of these stimuli may act as mitogens or superantigens rather than as MHC-restricted peptide antigens. T cells, including those from the neonate, are effectively activated by superantigens of *S. aureus* and other bacteria (Garderet et al., 1998; Hayward and Cosyns, 1994).

Maternal-fetal transfer of leukocytes occurs, but their numbers in the fetus are very low (i.e., usually <0.1%) (Lo et al., 1996) and are unlikely to result in detectable antigen-specific cellular immunity. Thus reports of neonatal T-cell responses as a result of the transfer of maternal immunity should remain suspect unless the T-cell population is identified and its antigen specificity and MHC restriction is demonstrated.

T-Cell Response to Congenital Infection

Pathogen-specific T-cell proliferative responses and cytokine responses (IL-2 and IFN-γ) of infants and children who are congenitally infected (e.g., those with syphilis, CMV, varicella-zoster virus, or *Toxoplasma gondii*) are markedly decreased or absent compared with infants and children with postnatal infection (Buimovici-Klein and Cooper, 1985; Friedmann, 1977; McLeod et al., 1990; Paryani and Arvin, 1986; Pass et al., 1983; Starr et al., 1979). This is particularly true with first- or second-trimester infections. For severe infections of the first trimester, a direct deleterious effect on T-cell development may occur. However, T cells from infants and children with congenital toxoplasmosis retain the ability to respond to alloantigen, mitogen, and, in one case, tetanus toxoid (McLeod et al., 1990).

These reduced responses, which are mainly mediated by CD4$^+$ T cells, may be the result of antigen-specific unresponsiveness (e.g., anergy, deletion, or ignorance [the failure of the T cell to be initially activated by antigen]). As discussed earlier, it is unlikely that a decreased TCR repertoire limits these immune responses, particularly after the second trimester onward. Decreased responses do not occur to all pathogens, because, in one study, 10-year-old children congenitally infected with mumps had DTH reactions to mumps antigen, indicating the persistence of mumps-specific memory/effector T cells (Aase et al., 1972).

Congenital infection with viruses or *Toxoplasma* during the second and third trimesters may result in the appearance of CD45R0^{high} memory T cells and an inverse ratio of the number of circulating CD4$^+$ to CD8$^+$ T cells (Bruning et al., 1997; Hohlfeld et al., 1990; Thilaganathan et al., 1994). This suggests that fetal CD8$^+$ T cells are activated and expanded in response to serious infection. These alterations may also be present at birth and through early infancy (Hara et al., 1996; Michie and Harvey, 1994). Congenital CMV infection also results in detectable circulating levels of CMV-specific CD8$^+$ T cells in the neonate that are functional (Marchant et al., 2003).

T-cell Reactivity to Postnatal Infections and Vaccines

Postnatal infection with HSV results in antigen-specific proliferation and cytokine (IL-2 and IFN-γ) production by CD4$^+$ T cells. However, these responses are delayed compared with adults with primary HSV infection (Burchett et al., 1992; Sullender et al., 1987). Infants between 6 and 12 months old also have lower IL-2 production in response to tetanus toxoid than older children and adults (Clerici et al., 1993). This suggests that either antigen-specific memory CD4$^+$ T-cell generation or function is decreased during early infancy. Whether this reflects limitations in antigen processing, T-cell activation and co-stimulation, or proliferation and differentiation remains unclear.

In contrast to HSV infection, BCG vaccination at birth versus 2 months or 4 months old was equally effective in inducing T-cell proliferative and IFN-γ responses to PPD, secreted *M. tuberculosis* antigens, and an *M. tuberculosis* cellular extract (Marchant et al., 1999; Vekemans et al., 2001). The responses were robust not only at 2 months after immunization, but

also at 1 year old, and there was no skewing toward Th2 cytokine production (Marchant et al., 1999), even by PPD-specific CD4$^+$ T-cell clones (Vekemans et al., 2001). Thus early postnatal administration of BCG vaccine does not result in decreased vaccine-specific Th1 responses, tolerance, or Th2 skewing.

Early BCG vaccination may also influence antigen-specific responses to unrelated vaccine antigens. BCG given at birth increased Th1- and Th2-specific responses and antibody titers to hepatitis B surface antigen (HBsAg) given simultaneously (Ota et al., 2002). BCG at birth did not enhance the Th1 response to tetanus toxoid given at 2 months old but did increase the Th2 response (IL-13 production). It is likely that BCG vaccination may accelerate dendritic cell maturation so that these cells can augment either Th1 or Th2 responses.

In contrast to BCG, the T-cell–specific response to oral poliovirus vaccine (OPV), another live vaccine, suggests a decreased Th1 response. Neonates given OPV at birth, 1, 2, and 3 months of age have lower OPV-specific proliferation, IFN-γ production, and lower numbers of IFN-γ–positive cells than immunized (but not reimmunized) adults (Vekemans et al., 2002). In contrast, their antibody titers were higher than those of the adults.

Neonates and young infants are thought to have skewing toward a Th2 response, but this may be an oversimplification. For example, the tetanus toxoid–specific response after vaccination suggests that both Th1 (IFN-γ) and Th2 (IL-5 and IL-13) memory responses occur, particularly after the third vaccine dose at 6 months old (Rowe et al., 2001). The tetanus toxoid–specific Th1 response may transiently decrease by 1 year old, but Th2 responses are not affected (Rowe et al., 2001).

Antigen-Specific T-Cell–Mediated Cytotoxicity of the Fetus, Neonate, and Young Infant

There are few studies of antigen-specific cytotoxic T-cell responses in the fetus, neonate, or young infant. In congenital CMV infection, substantial numbers of CMV-specific CD8$^+$ T cells were detected in the circulation of the fetus or the neonate, and these appeared to have normal expression of cytolytic molecules and activation-induced cytokine production (Marchant et al., 2003). In congenital HIV-1 infection, an expansion of HIV-specific cytotoxic T cells was detected at birth, indicating that fetal T cells were activated by viral antigens (Luzuriaga et al., 1995). In another case of in utero HIV infection, HIV-specific T-cell–mediated cytotoxicity was detected at 4 months old and persisted for several years despite a high HIV viral load (Brander et al., 1999).

Cytotoxic responses to HIV in perinatally infected infants suggest that although CD8$^+$ T cells capable of mediating cytotoxicity have undergone clonal expansion in vivo as early as 4 months old (Buseyne et al., 1998), their cytotoxicity may be reduced and delayed in appearance compared with that of adults (Pikora et al., 1997). There is decreased HIV-specific CD8$^+$ T-cell production of IFN-γ by young infants with perinatal HIV infection (Scott et al., 2001) and an inability to generate HIV-specific cytotoxic T cells after highly active antiretroviral therapy (Luzuriaga et al., 2000).

HIV-1 infection may inhibit antigen-specific immunity by depleting circulating dendritic cells (Pacanowski et al., 2001), impairing antigen presentation (Stumptner-Cuvelette et al., 2001), decreasing thymic T-cell output (Nielsen et al., 2001), and promoting T-cell apoptosis (Badley et al., 2000). These suppressive effects of HIV-1 on cytotoxic responses may be relatively specific for HIV-1, in that HIV-infected infants who lack HIV-specific cytotoxic T cells may maintain cytolytic T cells against EBV and CMV (Luzuriaga et al., 2000; Scott et al., 2001). Some of the inhibitory effects of HIV-1 infection may also occur in HIV-exposed—but uninfected—infants born to HIV-infected mothers (Chougnet et al., 2000; Nielsen et al., 2001).

Respiratory syncytial virus–specific cytotoxicity is more pronounced and frequent in infants 6 to 24 months old than in younger infants (Chiba et al., 1989). The results of recent murine studies have indicated that respiratory syncytial virus infection suppresses CD8+ T-cell–mediated effector activity (IFN-γ production and cytolytic activity) and that only transient memory CD8+ T-cell responses occur after infection (Chang and Braciale, 2002).

Summary: Fetal and Neonatal T Cells

T-cell function in the fetus and neonate is impaired compared with that of adults. Diminished functions include T-cell–mediated cytotoxicity, T-cell participation in cutaneous DTH, and, as discussed in the next section, T-cell help for B-cell differentiation. Selective cytokine decreases by fetal and neonatal T cells, such as decreased IFN-γ, and surface expression of the TNF ligand family (notably CD40 ligand) may contribute to these deficits. The repertoire of αβ-T-cell receptors is probably adequate, except in early gestation.

After fetal or neonatal infection, the acquisition of T-cell antigen-specific responses is delayed, and this likely applies to fetal infection, particularly for CD4+ T-cell function. The findings of in vitro studies suggest that deficiencies of dendritic cell function and activation and differentiation of antigenically naïve T cells into memory/effector T cells may be contributory. The mother does not transfer T-cell–specific immunity to the fetus. T-cell sensitization may occur during fetal life to environmental allergens, but this must be confirmed.

DEVELOPMENT OF B CELLS AND IMMUNOGLOBULINS

Ontogeny of B-Cell Development and Immunoglobulin Isotype Expression

Antigen-specific humoral immunity is mediated by immunoglobulins produced by mature B cells and plasma cells (Fig. 22-3; see Chapters 3 and 4). Pre-B

cells are first detected in the human fetal liver and omentum by 8 weeks' gestation and in the fetal bone marrow by 13 weeks' gestation (Gathings et al., 1977; Solvason et al., 1992). Between 18 and 22 weeks' gestation, pro-B or pre-B cells can also be detected in the liver, lung, and kidney (Nunez et al., 1996). These fetal organs also express the SDF-1 chemokine (CXCL12), which serves as a critical chemoattractant for B-cell precursors expressing the CXCR4 chemokine receptor (Coulomb-L'Hermin et al., 1999). This raises the possibility that B-cell lymphopoiesis may occur in these organs in situ at this stage of fetal development.

By midgestation the bone marrow is the predominant site of pre-B–cell development (Nishimoto et al., 1991). B-cell lymphopoiesis occurs solely in the bone marrow after 30 weeks' gestation and for the remainder of life (Nunez et al., 1996). The neonatal circulation contains higher levels of CD34+CD38− progenitor cells that are capable of differentiating into B cells than the bone marrow compartment of children or adults (Arakawa-Hoyt et al., 1999). The concentration of B cells in the circulation is higher during the second and third

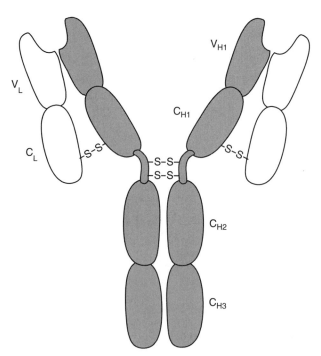

Figure 22-3 · The structure of an immunoglobulin molecule. The immunoglobulin molecule consists of two heavy chains *(dark shading)* and two light chains *(unshaded)* linked together by disulfide bonds. The amino-terminal region of the heavy and light chains contains variable heavy (V_H) and variable light (V_L) domains, respectively, that form the antigen-combining site. The remainder of the heavy and light chains consist of several constant heavy (C_H) domains and a single constant light (C_L) domain, respectively. For IgG, IgD, and IgA, the constant region C_{H3} domain of the heavy chain determines isotype or subclass specificity, which dictates the ability of the immunoglobulin to fix complement, bind to Fc receptors, and be actively transported from the mother to the fetus during gestation. IgM and IgE, which are not shown, are structurally similar except that they contain an additional C_{H4} domain conferring these properties and they lack a hinge region.

trimesters than at birth and further declines by adulthood (de Vries et al., 2000; Schultz et al., 2000).

Surface Immunoglobulin Expression

B cells expressing surface IgM are present by 10 weeks' gestation (Gathings et al., 1977). Unlike IgM+ adult B cells in the peripheral lymphoid organs, most of which also express surface IgD, fetal B cells at this stage express IgM without IgD (Gathings et al., 1977; Gupta et al., 1976). Such IgM+IgD- B cells are a transitory stage between pre-B cells and mature IgM+IgD+ B cells, and it is at this stage that the CD21 surface molecule is expressed.

Findings from murine studies have shown that antigenic exposure of IgM+IgD- B cells, including those found in the adult bone marrow, results in clonal anergy rather than activation (Metcalf and Klinman, 1976). The susceptibility of IgM+IgD- cells to clonal anergy maintains B-cell tolerance to soluble self-antigens present at high concentrations. Thus antigen exposure in utero may induce B-cell tolerance rather than an antibody response and may account for the observation that early congenital infection sometimes results in pathogen-specific defects in immunoglobulin production. In some cases, such as congenital mumps, these defects may occur despite normal T-cell responses, such as DTH (Aase et al., 1972), suggesting a direct inhibitory effect on antigen-specific B-cell function.

Between 8 and 11 weeks' gestation, transcripts for IgA and IgG can be detected in the liver (Baskin et al., 1998), followed shortly by the appearance of B cells bearing surface immunoglobulins of the IgA, IgG, and IgD isotypes. By 16 weeks' gestation, fetal bone marrow B cells expressing surface immunoglobulin of all heavy-chain isotypes are detectable (Dosch et al., 1989). The stimulus for isotype switching during fetal development remains unclear considering that, in the adult, isotype switching typically occurs in response to B-cell activation by foreign protein antigens. The frequency of B cells in tissues rapidly increases so that by 22 weeks' gestation, the proportion of B cells in the spleen, blood, and bone marrow is similar to that in the adult (Gathings et al., 1977; Gupta et al., 1976).

Neonatal B cells have increased surface levels of IgM compared with adult B cells; these differences persist for several years (Gagro et al., 2000; Macardle et al., 1997). In contrast to adult B cells bearing IgM plus IgD or IgG or IgA alone, neonatal B cells express IgG or IgA with IgM plus IgD (Gathings et al., 1977). This observation was based on the results of fluorescent microscopy with polyclonal antisera, but it has not been confirmed by multiparameter flow cytometry. In a flow cytometric study in which nonspecific binding was carefully excluded, neonatal B cells expressing surface IgG or IgA were below the limit of detectability (i.e., <1% of circulating B cells) (Wedgwood et al., 1997). True germinal centers in the spleen and lymph nodes are absent during fetal life but appear during the first months after postnatal antigenic stimulation (Zheng et al., 1996).

CD5 Expression and B-1 Cells

Another distinct feature of fetal and neonatal B cells is the high frequency of CD5 expression, indicating that they belong to the B-1 subset (Punnonen et al., 1992). More than 40% of B cells in the fetal spleen, omentum, and circulation at midgestation are CD5+ (Antin et al., 1986; Bhat et al., 1992; Kipps et al., 1990), but fewer are found in the fetal liver and bone marrow (Antin et al., 1986). CD5+ B cells are also frequent in the neonatal circulation (Hannet et al., 1992) and gradually decline with postnatal age (Bhat et al., 1992; Griffiths et al., 1984; Small et al., 1989). Like adult B-1 cells, the fetal and newborn B-1 cells tend to express IgM antibodies that are polyreactive, including reactivity with self-antigens such as DNA, compared with B-2 cells (Bhat et al., 1992; Chen et al., 1998; Kipps et al., 1990; Lydyard et al., 1990).

CD5+ B cells may help regulate the immune system in early ontogeny, including the induction of tolerance to self-antigens, yet they lack most surface markers characteristic of previously activated B cells (Bhat et al., 1992). The extent to which human CD5+ and CD5- B cells represent distinct lineages remains contentious. For example, activation through the use of a combination of antibody to IgM, the engagement of CD40, and exogenous IL-4 results in the loss of CD5 expression by both neonatal and adult CD5+ cells (Gagro et al., 2000), raising the possibility of a precursor-product relationship between CD5+ and CD5- B cells.

Natural IgM Antibodies

B-1 cells are the major source of the low amounts of circulating "natural" IgM present at birth produced in the absence of antigenic stimulation. Results of murine studies have defined a role for natural IgM: mice in which secretory, but not surface, IgM was eliminated by gene targeting had decreased primary responses to T-cell–dependent antigens (Ehrenstein et al., 1998) and an increased susceptibility to acute peritonitis from endogenous bacteria, apparently because of a lack of natural IgM antibodies with reactivity against phosphatidylcholine (Boes et al., 1998a).

Natural IgM antibodies are of low affinity, but they can activate complement, which may allow antigenically naïve B cells to become activated as a result of receiving of co-stimulation through CD21 (complement receptor 2). Natural IgM does not play a role in enhancing the response to polysaccharide antigens, at least in mice (Boes et al., 1998a, 1998b; Ehrenstein et al., 1998).

Development of the Immunoglobulin Repertoire

VDJ Segment Usage

The primary or preimmune immunoglobulin repertoire, consisting of all antibodies that can be expressed before an encounter with antigen, is determined by the number of different B-cell clones with distinct antigen specificity.

This preimmune immunoglobulin repertoire is limited during the initial stages of B-cell development in the fetus compared with that in the adult. In an early to midgestation human fetus, the set of V segments used to generate the heavy-chain gene is smaller than for the adult (Cuisinier et al., 1989; Schroeder et al., 1987). The V segments are scattered throughout the heavy-chain gene locus (Schutte et al., 1992). There are also differences in the usage of particular heavy-chain D and J segments between the first and second trimesters and term (Schroeder et al., 1998).

These developmental differences are genetically determined rather than the result of environmental influences. The evidence for this is that these differences occur in immature B-cell precursors lacking a surface pre–B-cell receptor complex (BCR); the pre-BCR complex contains a full-length immunoglobulin heavy chain, which could potentially respond to environmental influences.

By the third trimester, the V- and D-segment heavy-chain gene repertoire of peripheral B cells appears to be similar to that of the adult, but there may be overrepresentation of certain segments, such as DH7-27 (Zemlin et al., 2001). Certain heavy-chain V segments expressed by the adult repertoire are not found in the neonate (Mortari et al., 1992; Sanz, 1991), but it is unlikely that this limits the neonatal humoral immune response. Other V segments, such as VH3, are present at a greater frequency in the preimmune immunoglobulin repertoire (Mortari et al., 1992; Silverman et al., 1993). This increased representation may confer on antibody molecules an ability to bind protein A of *S. aureus*, thus providing some intrinsic immunity during the perinatal period.

Role of CDR3 Length and Terminal Deoxynucleotidyl Transferase (TdT)

The length of the heavy chain's third complementarity determining region (CDR3), which is formed at the junction of the V segment with the D and J segments, is shorter in the midgestation fetus than at birth (Raaphorst et al., 1992) or in adulthood, including in pre-B cells (Raaphorst et al., 1997). This is attributable in part, to decreased TdT, which is responsible for N-nucleotide additions. This decreased TdT expression is an intrinsic property of CD34+ precursor cells not yet committed to the B-cell lineage, because the in vitro differentiation of B-lineage cells from neonatal CD34+ cells results in lower amounts of TdT than are present in similar cells generated from adult CD34+ cells (Hirose et al., 2001).

Up to 25% of heavy-chain fetal CDR3 lack N-nucleotide additions, and in the remainder, the size of these additions is smaller than for neonatal or adult CDR3. The CDR3 is the most hypervariable portion of immunoglobulins, and a short CDR3 significantly reduces the diversity of the fetal immunoglobulin repertoire (Sanz, 1991). The CDR3 of the heavy-chain gene remains relatively short at the beginning of the third trimester and gradually increases in length until birth

(Cuisinier et al., 1990; Mortari, et al., 1993; Schroeder et al., 2001; Zemlin et al., 2001).

Because the CDR3 is at the center of the antigen-binding pocket of antibodies (Padlan, 1994), reduced CDR3 diversity could limit the efficiency of the antibody response. A complete lack of N-nucleotide additions would be predicted to result in antibodies with combining sites that are relatively flat and potentially inefficient at combining with antigen (Schroeder et al., 1998). However, the importance of shortened CDR3 alone in limiting antibody responses is doubtful, because gene knockout mice lacking TdT produce normal antibody responses after immunization or infection (Gilfillan et al., 1985). A combination of lack of TdT and limitations in V and D usage could limit the ability of the fetal B cells to recognize a full spectrum of foreign antigens, particularly before midgestation, but such a "hole in the repertoire" has not been documented.

Somatic Hypermutation

Raaphorst and colleagues (1992) and Mortari and co-workers (1992) found that most neonatal and fetal immunoglobulin heavy-chain gene variable regions appear not to have undergone somatic mutation; these researchers examined heavy-chain transcripts for IgM, an isotype in which somatic mutation is uncommon in the adult, except in IgM+IgD- memory cells (Nicholson et al., 1995; van Es et al., 1992). In contrast, somatic mutations are detectable in some neonatal B cells expressing IgG or IgA transcripts (Mortari et al., 1993). Among neonatal B cells that bear somatic mutations, the mutational frequency per length of DNA is similar to that of adult B cells. Together, these observations indicate that somatic hypermutation occurs normally by birth in the B-cell compartment.

B-Cell Surface Phenotype

In adults, CD10 expression ceases at the antigenically naïve B-cell stage. In contrast, most fetal bone marrow and spleen B cells express CD10 (LeBien et al., 1990; Punnonen et al., 1992). CD10+ B cells may constitute an immature transitional population but are functionally mature on the basis of their ability to undergo isotype switching. Small numbers of CD10+ B cells are found at birth and these gradually decline during infancy (Calado et al., 1999).

Increased expression of CD38 on neonatal B cells has also been observed (Gagro et al., 2000; Macardle et al., 1997). Unfractionated neonatal B cells, the majority of which are CD5+, and adult naïve B cells have similar levels of surface IgD, CD19, CD21, CD22, CD23, CD40, CD44, CD80, CD81, and CD86 (Elliott et al., 1999, 2000; Gagro et al., 2000; Macardle et al., 1997; Viemann et al., 2000), in addition to CCR6 (Kryzsiek et al., 2000). Rijkers and co-workers (1998) reported that neonatal B cells have reduced CD21 expression. Surface expression of the FcγRII receptor (CD32) is reduced on neonatal B cells (Jessup et al., 2001; Macardle et al., 1997). This FcγRII receptor binds to IgG molecules via their Fc moiety and contains a cytoplasmic ITIM domain characteristic of receptors with inhibitory function. Thus decreased expression of FcγRII by neonatal B cells may render them less subject to the inhibitory effect of antigen–antibody complexes.

Neonatal CD5⁻ B cells have reduced expression of several adhesion molecules, including CD11a, CD44, CD54 (ICAM-1), and CD62L (L-selectin) (Parra et al., 1996). A similar reduction is found in the CD5⁻ B cells of adult patients during the first 3 months after either autologous or heterologous hematopoietic cell transplantation, but this resolves by 14 months posttransplant (Parra et al., 1996).

Circulating neonatal B cells have lower levels of class II MHC than do adult splenic B cells and, unlike adult cells, an inability to increase intracellular calcium after the engagement of class II MHC by monoclonal antibodies (Garban et al., 1998). However, because neonatal B cells proliferate as well as or better than adult splenic B cells after class II engagement (Garban et al., 1998), these alterations in signaling appear unlikely to compromise neonatal B-cell function.

Cerutti and colleagues (1996) reported that circulating neonatal B cells, of which approximately 90% were of the B-1 subset, expressed CD28, which is typically found on T cells and not B cells. Neonatal B cells also expressed substantially more CD27 and CD80 than did adult spleen B cells, in which more than 95% of the cells were of the B-2 subset. Whether this unusual neonatal surface phenotype also applies to the adult B-1 subset was not determined. It is also unclear what role CD28 on B cells plays in the immune response in vivo. Nonetheless, the presence of CD80 and CD27, markers for adult memory B cells, suggests that some circulating neonatal B-1 cells have undergone activation in vivo.

T-Cell–Dependent Immunoglobulin Production and Isotype Switching

Early in vitro studies of neonatal immunoglobulin production made use of PWM, a polyclonal activator of both T and B cells. In this system, immunoglobulin production is low compared with that of adults and mixing experiments suggested that neonatal T cells acted as suppressors of immunoglobulin production by either adult or neonatal B cells. Further fractionation of the T-cell populations in this assay suggested that in the absence of memory/effector T cells, antigenically naïve (CD45RA^{high}CD45R0^{low}) CD4$^+$ T cells of either the neonate or the adult acted as suppressors of antibody production (Clement, 1992). Priming of neonatal or adult antigenically naïve CD4$^+$ T cells in vitro resulted in their acquisition of a CD45RA^{low}CD45R0^{high} phenotype and, concurrently, an ability to enhance rather than suppress PWM-induced immunoglobulin production (Clement, 1992). However, the relevance of this system to neonatal in vivo B-cell responses remains unclear, in part because of our limited under-standing of the cellular and molecular nature of T-cell suppression.

When B cells are activated by exogenous cytokines (e.g., IL-4, IL-10, or cytokine-containing supernatants from activated T cells) and a cellular source of CD40 ligand (e.g., CD40 ligand-expressing fibroblasts) or EBV infection, the neonatal B-cell production of IgM, IgG1, IgG2, IgG3, IgG4, and IgE is similar to that of adult antigenically naïve B cells (Banchereau et al., 1994; Gudmundsson et al., 1999; Nonoyama et al., 1995; Servet et al., 1996). Isotype switching occurs at the pre–B-cell stage, even during fetal ontogeny: isotype switching and IgE and IgG4 production occurs in fetal B and pre-B cells as early as 12 weeks' gestation (Punnonen et al., 1992, 1993, 1994, 1995).

Further support for the capacity of fetal and neonatal B cells to undergo isotype switching comes from several observations: IgA1 and IgA2 are produced in similar amounts by antigenically naïve fetal and adult B cells upon stimulation with anti-CD40 antibody and vasoactive intestinal peptide hormone. Fetal pre-B cells can also synthesize IgA under these conditions (Kimata et al., 1995). Finally, when human fetal or neonatal B and T cells develop in or are adoptively transferred into mice with genetic SCID, they are capable of isotype switching and immunoglobulin production if the appropriate T-cell–derived signals are present (Rouleau et al., 1996; Ueno et al., 1992; Vandekerckhove et al., 1993).

However, a few studies suggest that isotype switching and antibody production by fetal and neonatal B cells is limited compared with those of antigenically naïve (IgD$^+$) adult B cells. Durandy and co-workers (1995) found that IgM, IgG, and IgE production by fetal B cells at midgestation was substantially lower than that of neonatal or adult B cells, suggesting an intrinsic hyporesponsiveness to CD40 or cytokine receptor engagement, or both. Neonatal B cells produce substantially less IgA than do adult naïve B cells in the presence of adult T cells stimulated by a CD3 monoclonal antibody (as a source of CD40 ligand) and exogenous cytokines, such as IL-10 (Splawski et al., 1998). These limitations of fetal and neonatal isotype switching and antibody production probably reflect intrinsic limitations of B-cell function, particularly when T-cell help may be limited. This is not because of decreased activation or proliferation, because neonatal B cells proliferate normally in response to the engagement of CD40 or surface IgM (Gagro et al., 2000).

Neonatal T cells activated for a few hours and fixed provide less help for neonatal B-cell immunoglobulin production and isotype switching than do similarly treated adult T cells (Nonoyama et al., 1995). Because the help provided by these fixed T cells is probably CD40 ligand, its reduction or that of similar activation-induced molecules may limit fetal and neonatal B-cell immune responses. Decreased neonatal dendritic cell function may also contribute to diminished B-cell responses.

IgM and IgG synthesis is detected as early as 12 weeks in fetal organ cultures (Gitlin and Biasucci, 1969). Plasma cells secreting IgG and IgA are detectable at

718 / Secondary Immunodeficiencies

20 weeks' gestation (Gathings et al., 1981). In general, neonatal B cells can differentiate into IgM-secreting plasma cells as efficiently as adult cells and can undergo isotype switching after CD40 ligation. Splawski and Lipsky (1994) found that T-cell–dependent immunoglobulin production by neonatal CD5+ and CD5− B cells is more readily inhibited by agents that raise intracellular cyclic adenosine monophosphate, such as prostaglandin E2. The precise mechanism remains unclear.

Antibody Response to T-Cell–Dependent and T-Cell–Independent Antigens

Definitions of T-Dependent and T-Independent Antigens

The chronology of the response to different antigens differs depending on the need for cognate T-cell help (Table 22-4). On the basis of findings from murine studies, antigens can be divided into those dependent on a functional thymus and cognate help (direct cell–cell interactions) provided by mature αβ-T cells (T-dependent antigens) and those independent of T-cell help (T-independent antigens). The T-independent (TI) antigens can be further divided into TI type 1 or TI type II on the basis of their dependence on cytokines produced by T cells or other cell types.

Most proteins are T-dependent antigens requiring cognate T-cell–B-cell interaction for the production of antibodies (other than small amounts of IgM). The antibody response to T-dependent antigens is characterized by the generation of memory B cells with somatically mutated immunoglobulin and the potential for isotype switching.

TI type 1 antigens are those that bind to B cells and directly activate them in vitro to produce antibody without T cells or exogenous cytokines. In the human, one such TI type 1 antigen is fixed *Brucella abortus* bacteria.

TI type 2 antigens are mostly polysaccharides with multiple identical subunits, as well as certain proteins that contain multiple determinants of similar antigenic specificity. Responses to these antigens are enhanced in vitro and in vivo by a variety of cytokines, including IL-6, IL-12, IFN-γ, and GM-CSF (Ambrosino et al., 1990; Buchanan et al., 1998; Peeters et al., 1992; Snapper and Mond, 1996). NK cells, T cells, dendritic cells, or

macrophages may provide these cytokines. TI type 2 responses are also enhanced by bacterially derived LPS, lipoproteins, porin proteins, DNA, or CpG oligonucleotides (Chelvarajan et al., 1999; Snapper and Mond, 1996; Snapper et al., 1995). This enhancement probably occurs by the engagement of TLRs on B cells (Vos et al., 2000). The response to TI type 2 antigens is characterized by the lack of B-cell memory or somatic hypermutation and is largely restricted to the IgM and IgG2 isotypes (Rijkers et al., 1998).

Response to T-Dependent Antigens

The capacity of the neonate to respond to T-dependent antigens is well established at birth (see Table 22-4) and is only modestly reduced compared with the response of the adult. This modest reduction may be attributable to decreases in antigen presentation by dendritic cells, CD4+ T-cell activation and expansion into an effector population, CD4+ T-cell–B-cell interactions, dendritic cell–B-cell interactions, intrinsic B-cell signaling, or a combination of these factors. Another possibility is that T-dependent antigens preferentially upregulate CD22 on neonatal B cells, which increases the BCR signaling threshold and limits cell activation (Viemann et al., 2000).

Most researchers studying the neonatal immune response to T-dependent antigens have not evaluated antibody affinity, a reflection of somatic mutation, or isotype expression. Given the importance of CD40 ligand in both of these processes, the observation of reduced CD40 ligand expression by neonatal T cells (Brugnoni et al., 1994; Durandy et al., 1995; Fuleihan et al., 1994; Nonoyama et al., 1995) suggests a mechanism by which B-cell immune responses might be limited. Studies of CD40 ligand expression by antigen-specific T cells generated in response to vaccination and its correlation with reduced memory B-cell development, decreased isotype switching, and somatic hypermutation will be of interest.

Response to T-Independent TI Antigens

RESPONSE TO TI TYPE 1 ANTIGENS

Antibody production by human neonatal B cells to a TI type 1 antigen in vitro (*B. abortus*) is only modestly reduced (Golding et al., 1984) (see Table 22-4) and may

TABLE 22-4 · HIERARCHY OF ANTIBODY RESPONSIVENESS TO DIFFERENT ANTIGENS

Species	Type of Antigen	Examples of Antigen	Age at Onset of Antibody Response
Mouse	T-cell dependent	TNP-KLH	Birth
	T-cell independent type I	TNP–*Brucella abortus*	Birth
	T-cell independent type II	TNP-Ficoll	Delayed (2–3 wk old)
Human	T-cell dependent	Tetanus toxoid, HBsAg, *Haemophilus influenzae* conjugate vaccine, and bacteriophage φX-174	Birth
	T-cell independent type I	TNP–*Brucella abortus*	Birth
	T-cell-independent type II	Bacterial capsular polysaccharides (*H. influenzae* type b, *Neisseria meningitidis*, *Streptococcus pneumoniae*, and GBS)	Delayed (6–24 mo old)

GBS = group B streptococci; HBsAg = hepatitis B surface antigen; KLH = keyhole limpet hemocyanin; TNP = trinitrophenol.

reflect a decreased ability of antigen-activated B cells to proliferate rather than a decreased precursor frequency of antigen-specific clones (Golding et al., 1984). Human B cells (from both adults and neonates) are poorly responsive to high doses of LPS alone, a TI type 1 stimulus that is effective for murine B cells. However, low doses of LPS augment the response of human B cells to certain TI type 2–like stimuli (Snapper and Mond, 1996), suggesting that these cells express functional LPS receptors and signaling pathways.

RESPONSE TO TI TYPE 2 ANTIGENS

In humans and mice, the response to TI type 2 antigens is the last to appear chronologically (see Table 22-4). This helps account for the neonate's susceptibility to infection with encapsulated bacteria (e.g., group B streptococci [Edwards and Baker, 2001; Fink et al., 1962; Smith et al., 1964]) and the poor response to polysaccharide antigens, such as the unconjugated capsular polysaccharide of *Haemophilus influenzae* type b, meningococci, and pneumococci, until approximately 2 to 3 years old. Whether the decreased responses to TI type 2 antigens during early childhood reflect an intrinsic B-cell immaturity or decreased function of other cells such as APCs, or both, remains unclear.

One potential mechanism for these decreased responses may be due to decreased expression of CD21 by B cells. CD21 is expressed in association with CD19, the type 2 complement receptor, and serves to transduce B-cell activating signals when CD19 is engaged by C3 complement components; thus, a reduction in CD21 expression could limit B-cell activation. The incubation of human splenic tissue with pneumococcal polysaccharides and complement results in preferential binding of the polysaccharide and C3, presumably as a complex, to CD21$^+$ B cells in this area of the spleen (Peset-Llopis et al., 1996). Findings from in vitro studies of human splenic tissue suggest that TI type 2 antigens activate complement and bind C3, then localize to the marginal zone splenic B cells expressing type 2 complement receptors (Rijkers et al., 1998). This localization presumably induces polysaccharide-reactive B cells to proliferate in vivo.

Rijkers and colleagues (1998) and Griffioen and co-workers (1992) found lower CD21 expression on neonatal B cells than on adult B cells (Griffioen et al., 1992). Timens and colleagues (1987) found that the response to bacterial polysaccharides (at approximately 2 to 3 years old) correlates with the appearance of B cells expressing CD21 in the marginal zone region of the spleen. Although these observations argue for an intrinsic immaturity in B-cell responsiveness to TI type 2 antigens, decreased expression of CD21 by neonatal B cells has not been confirmed by others (Macardle et al., 1997). Moreover, animal experiments do not support decreased CD21 signaling as a plausible explanation for the severely decreased responses to polysaccharide antigens of the human neonate: mice genetically deficient in the type 2 complement receptor or CD21 have only a slight deficiency of their antibody response to polysaccharide antigens (Carroll, 1998; Tedder et al., 1997).

Human neonatal B cells have a marked decrease in CD22 expression after the engagement of IgM, a stimulus used to mimic a TI type 2 antigen (Viemann et al., 2000). This decreased expression of CD22, which acts as a negative regulator of B-cell activation, results in hyperresponsive neonatal B cells that are perhaps more prone to apoptosis. Thus the loss of activated B cells during the immune response due to decreased CD22 expression is another potential mechanism for the neonate's decreased antibody responses to TI type 2 antigens.

IN VITRO STUDIES MIMICKING TI TYPE 2 ANTIGEN RESPONSES

Dextran-conjugated anti-immunoglobulin monoclonal antibodies have been used to mimic the events in TI type II antibody responses in vitro (Snapper and Mond, 1996). Murine B cells treated in this manner proliferate but do not produce antibodies unless additional stimuli, such as NK cells, cytokines, or bacterial-derived products, are provided. Human neonatal B cells respond to this stimulus as well as do adult B cells, suggesting that the lack of the neonatal TI type 2 response is not attributable to an intrinsic limitation of B-cell function (Halista et al., 1998). However, dextran-conjugated anti-immunoglobulin monoclonal antibodies can potentially activate all B cells regardless of their particular surface immunoglobulin specificity. It is plausible that B cells reactive with polysaccharides or other TI type 2 antigens may be functionally distinct from other B cells and subject to selective developmental immaturity.

Murine neonatal B cells are able to proliferate in response to the TI type 2 antigen TNP-Ficoll or the polyclonal stimulus goat antimurine IgM, if CpG oligonucleotides containing unmethylated cytosine residues are present (Chelvarajan et al., 1999). These CpG oligonucleotides directly bind to TLR-9 (Kaisho and Akira, 2002) on the murine neonatal B cells. Murine neonatal B cells undergo apoptosis on engagement of surface IgM, and this is associated with increased levels of bcl-X$_S$, a proapoptotic member of the bcl-2 family. CpG oligonucleotides protect neonatal B cells from apoptosis, most likely by downregulating bcl-X$_S$. Whether CpG oligonucleotides "humanized" for interaction with human TLR-9 have a similar capacity to increase TI type 2 responses by B cells from neonates and young infants is not established.

Antibody Response of the Fetus to Maternal Immunization and Congenital Infection

Fetal Response to Immunization

Early studies by Silverstein and colleagues (1970) of the antibody response of fetal sheep and rhesus monkeys to immunization with foreign proteins were conceptually important in establishing two major features of the ontogeny of B-cell immune competence for T-cell–dependent antigens in larger mammals.

First, immune competence for T-cell–dependent antigens is established early during fetal ontogeny: primary immunization of fetal rhesus monkeys between 103 and 127 days' gestation (out of a total of 160 days) with sheep red blood cells, a T-cell–dependent antigen, results in the formation of sheep red blood cell–reactive B cells in the spleen; reimmunization 3 weeks later results in a rapid antibody response with IgG (Silverstein et al., 1970). In fetal sheep, the antibody response to bacteriophage φX-174 occurs as early as 40 days' postconception (Silverstein, 1977), and, again, isotype switching is evident during the fetal response. Together, this suggests that B-cell response to protein antigens, including isotype switching and probably memory cell generation, are functional during fetal life.

Second, these responses occur in a predictable, stepwise fashion for particular antigens. For example, in fetal sheep, the antibody response to keyhole limpet hemocyanin and lymphocytic choriomeningitis virus are first detectable at approximately 80 and 120 days' postconception (Silverstein, 1977), respectively. These differences in the responsiveness to particular antigens are not explained by limitations in the repertoires of surface immunoglobulins or αβ-TCRs, because it is known that a diverse repertoire is established early in ontogeny.

No correlation exists between the physical and chemical characteristics of particular antigens and their immunogenicity during ontogeny. For example, bacteriophage φX-174 and bacteriophage T-4 are both particulate antigens and would be expected to enter into antigen processing similarly. In fetal sheep, however, bacteriophage T-4 becomes immunogenic 60 days after that of φX-174. Baboons fetally immunized with HBsAg vaccine have a robust IgG antibody response without the development of tolerance because postnatal immunizations further increased the antibody titer (Watts et al., 1999).

Fetal Antibody Response to Maternal Immunization

Studies to determine whether the human fetus produces antibodies in response to maternal immunization have had variable results. In two studies, maternal immunization with tetanus toxoid during the third trimester but not earlier resulted in fetal immune responses, as shown by the presence of IgM tetanus antibodies at birth (Gill et al., 1983; Vanderbeeken et al., 1985). Infants with tetanus-specific antibodies at birth had enhanced secondary antibody responses after tetanus immunization, indicating that fetal antigen exposure was a priming, rather than a tolerizing, event (Gill et al., 1983). By contrast, Englund and co-workers (1993) were unable to demonstrate neonatal tetanus toxoid–specific IgM antibody or T-cell proliferation after maternal tetanus toxoid vaccination in the third trimester. Similarly, no fetal response to maternal immunization with inactivated trivalent influenza vaccine was noted (Englund et al., 1993). It is not known how reliably a fetal antibody response to maternal vaccination with polysaccharide-protein conjugate vaccines occurs.

Fetal Antibody Response to Intrauterine Infection

Specific antibody may be present at birth to intrauterine infection, including rubella virus, CMV, HSV, varicella-zoster virus, and T. gondii, and this often can be used to diagnose congenital infection. However, not all fetuses have an antibody response to intrauterine infection; specific IgM antibody was absent in 34% of infants with congenital rubella (Enders, 1985), in 19% to 33% of infants with congenital toxoplasmosis (Chumpitazi et al., 1995; Naot et al., 1981), and in 11% of infants with congenital CMV infection (Griffiths et al., 1982).

When congenital infection is severe during the first or second trimester, antibody production may be delayed until late childhood (Paryani and Arvin, 1986). This may reflect a lack of T-cell help, in that antigen-specific CD4+ T-cell responses are often reduced in parallel with B-cell responses.

Congenital toxoplasmosis may lead to detectable IgE and IgA anti-Toxoplasma antibodies at birth or during early infancy (Pinon et al., 1990). Similarly, filarial- and schistosome-specific IgE are present in the sera of most newborns after maternal filariasis or schistosomiasis (King et al., 1998). Thus T-cell–dependent isotype switching and immunoglobulin production occur during fetal life, at least for certain pathogens and antigens derived from maternal infection. With some infections, such as with T. gondii, non-IgM antibodies may be more sensitive than IgM antibodies for the diagnosis of congenital infection. However, in cases of congenital infection, the titers of these Toxoplasma-specific IgA and IgE-specific antibodies may be lower at 20 to 30 weeks' gestation than after birth (Decoster et al., 1992; Desmonts et al., 1985; Stepick-Biek et al., 1990), indicating that their production is delayed.

Antibody Response of the Neonate and Young Infant to Protein Antigens

The immunization of neonates usually elicits a protective response to protein antigens, including tetanus and diphtheria toxoids (Dengrove et al., 1986), OPV (Smolen et al., 1983), Salmonella flagellar antigen (Fink et al., 1962; Smith et al., 1964), bacteriophage φX-174 (Uhr et al., 1962), and HBsAg (hepatitis B vaccine) (West, 1989). However, the response to some vaccines may be less vigorous in the neonate than in older children or adults. This has occurred in the primary response to recombinant hepatitis B vaccine in term neonates lacking maternally derived HBsAg antibody, in comparison with unimmunized children and adults (Lee et al., 1995; West, 1989). The neonates' ultimate anti-HBsAg titers achieved after secondary and tertiary immunizations are similar to those of older children, indicating that neonatal immunization does not result in tolerance (West, 1989). If initial immunization is delayed until 1 month old, the antibody response to primary hepatitis B vaccination is increased and nearly equivalent to that of older children, suggesting that the developmental limitations responsible for reduced antibody responses are transient (Greenberg, 1993; West, 1989).

Similarly, 2-week-old infants immunized with a single dose of diphtheria or tetanus toxoid had delayed production of specific antibody compared with older infants; by 2 months of age, their response was similar to that of 6-month-old infants (Dancis et al., 1953), suggesting rapid maturation of T-dependent responses. The switch from IgM to IgG may also be delayed after neonatal vaccination for some (e.g., *Salmonella* H vaccine [Smith et al., 1964])—but not all—antigens (e.g., bacteriophage φX-174 [Uhr et al., 1962]). The immunization of infants of HIV-infected mothers with recombinant HIV-1 gp120 vaccine with MF59 adjuvant, beginning at birth, also results in high antibody titers, indicating that postnatal vaccination does not induce tolerance (McFarland et al., 2001).

Unlike what happens with other vaccines, newborns given whole-cell pertussis vaccination may not only have a poor initial antibody response, but their subsequent antibody response to certain antigenic components (e.g., lymphocyte-promoting toxin) may be less than in infants initially immunized at 1 month of age or older (Baraff et al., 1984; Peterson, 1951; Provenzano et al., 1965), suggesting partial tolerance. Whole-cell pertussis vaccine immunization of premature infants (i.e., those at 28 to 36 weeks' gestation) at 2 months of age elicited responses similar to that of 2-month-old term infants (Smolen et al., 1983). This suggests that the period in which the infant is prone to tolerance rather than immunity wanes rapidly and is relatively independent of gestational age.

This tendency for tolerance rather than immunity is highly antigen dependent, in that an inhibitory effect is not observed after the early administration of diphtheria or tetanus toxoid (Dengrove et al., 1986) or hepatitis B vaccine given within 48 hours of birth (West, 1989). OPV given at birth enhanced rather than inhibited the response to subsequent immunization, suggesting that the mucosal route does not produce tolerance (Schoub et al., 1988).

There may be other limitations in the antibody response to certain protein antigens. The antibody response to measles vaccine given at 6 months of age is significantly less than when given at 9 or 12 months of age, even when the inhibitory effect of maternal antibody is controlled for (Gans et al., 1998). This is not caused by a lack of measles-specific T cells, because measles antigen–specific T-cell proliferation and IL-12 and IFN-γ proliferation was similar in the three groups (Gans et al., 1998, 1999, 2001). Limitations in T-cell help, such as CD40 ligand production, or an intrinsic B-cell defect may be responsible.

Antibody Response of the Neonate to Polysaccharide and Polysaccharide-Protein Conjugates

In contrast to the response to protein antigens, the newborn's response to polysaccharide antigens is absent or severely blunted, as demonstrated by the inability to

mount an antibody response to *H. influenzae* type b unconjugated vaccine or to group B streptococci capsular antigens after infection. The response to some polysaccharide antigens can be demonstrated by 6 months old, but the response to vaccination with *H. influenzae* polysaccharides, *Neisseria meningitidis* type C, or to most pneumococcal polysaccharides is poor until approximately 18 to 24 months of age (Smith et al., 1973). This inability to respond to polysaccharides and other TI type 2 antigens is not clearly understood, but it appears not to be a lack of the appropriate antibody repertoire, at least for *H. influenzae* (Adderson et al., 1991).

The conjugation of *H. influenzae* capsular polysaccharide covalently to a protein carrier renders it immunogenic in infants as young as 2 months of age and an enhanced antibody response to unconjugated vaccine by 12 months of age. Because this is an age when the response to the unconjugated vaccine is usually poor, the conjugate vaccine has induced polysaccharide-specific B-cell memory (Granoff et al., 1993). Similarly, the administration of a single dose of *H. influenzae* type b polysaccharide–tetanus toxoid conjugate to term neonates as early as a few days of age may enhance the antibody response to unconjugated *H. influenzae* type b polysaccharide vaccine at 4 months of age (Eskola and Kayhty, 1998). However, this enhanced response is weak and does not occur when the neonate is primed with tetanus toxoid followed by immunization with conjugate vaccine at 2 months of age (Lieberman et al., 1995).

Coupling of the *H. influenzae* type b polysaccharide to a protein carrier converts a TI type 2 antigen to a T-dependent antigen with increased antibody avidity (Schlesinger and Granoff, 1992). This is presumably the result of T-dependent memory B-cell generation, which favors affinity maturation after somatic hypermutation. The early interactions between T cells and B cells in response to such carbohydrate-protein conjugate vaccines are summarized in Figure 22-4.

The conjugation of *H. influenzae* type b polysaccharide to tetanus or diphtheria toxoid does not change the repertoire of the antibodies produced from that of the free polysaccharide (Adderson et al., 1991; Granoff et al., 1993). The neonates' response to conjugate vaccines now mimics the response to other T-dependent antigens. Vaccination with protein conjugates of capsular polysaccharides of *Streptococcus pneumoniae* (types 4, 6B, 9V, 14, 18C, 19F, and 23F) (Anderson et al., 1996; Daum et al., 1997; Siber, 1994) and *N. meningitidis* (types A and C) (Fairley et al., 1996) is immunogenic in infants as young as 2 months of age and primes them for subsequent memory responses.

Antibody Response of the Premature Infant

Preterm neonates of 24 weeks' gestation or older produce antibody to protein antigens such as diphtheria toxoid, diphtheria-pertussis-tetanus vaccine, and oral

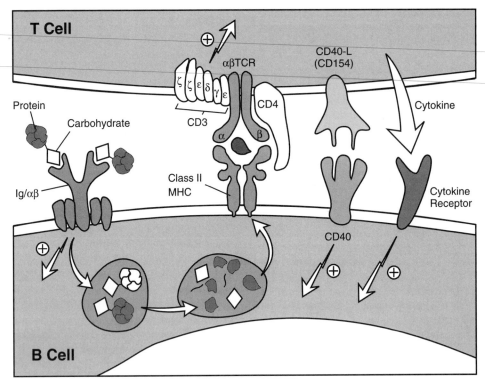

Figure 22-4 · **Interactions between B and T cells in the response to vaccines consisting of carbohydrate (e.g., bacterial capsular polysaccharide) covalently linked to protein carrier.** The carbohydrate moiety of the conjugate is bound by surface immunoglobulin (sIg) on B cells, resulting in the internalization of the conjugate. Peptides derived from the protein moiety of the conjugate are presented by class II major histocompatibility complex (MHC) on the B cell, resulting in the activation of the T cell and the expression of CD40 ligand (CD154). The engagement of CD40 on the B cell by CD40 ligand, in conjunction with cytokines secreted by the T cell, results in carbohydrate-specific B-cell proliferation, immunoglobulin isotype switching, secretion of antibody, and memory B-cell generation.

and inactivated poliovirus vaccines as well as do term neonates when administered at 2, 4, and 6 months of age (Adenyi-Jones et al., 1992; Bernbaum et al., 1985; Koblin et al., 1988; Smolen et al., 1983). The antibody responses of premature infants to multiple doses of hepatitis B vaccine, initially administered at birth, are clearly reduced compared with those of term infants (Lau et al., 1992). These titers are substantially increased if immunization of the premature infant is delayed until 5 weeks of age, indicating the importance of postnatal age rather than that of a particular body weight (Kim et al., 1997).

However, the antibody levels after three doses of *H. influenzae* type b capsular polysaccharide-tetanus conjugate vaccine are significantly lower in premature infants than in term infants when vaccination is begun at 2 months of age (Greenberg et al., 1994), particularly in premature infants with chronic lung disease (Washburn et al., 1993). Glucocorticoid treatment for chronic lung disease may decrease the antibody responses. As in term infants, the response of premature infants to polysaccharide antigens remains diminished during the first 2 years of life.

Placental Transport of Maternal IgG Antibody

IgG is the predominant immunoglobulin isotype at all ages (Stiehm and Fudenberg, 1966). Human IgG is composed of four different subclasses (IgG1, IgG2, IgG3, and IgG4) and is the only isotype that crosses the placenta (see Chapters 3 and 4). All subclasses, with the exception of IgG4, can activate the classic complement pathway. In adults, IgG1 is the predominant subclass (70%), whereas IgG2, IgG3, and IgG4 are approximately 20%, 7%, and 3% of the total, respectively (Lee et al., 1986).

The mechanism by which IgG is transferred to the fetus is only incompletely understood, but it depends on the recognition of maternal IgG through its Fc domain. Maternally derived placental syncytiotrophoblasts express surface type III Fc receptors for IgG, which are particularly abundant in the area in direct contact with the maternal circulation (Kameda et al., 1991), but other Fc receptors are important for internalizing maternal IgG for transport to the fetus (Landor, 1995), possibly by pinocytosis (Leach et al., 1996).

Role of FcRn

Once IgG is internalized by the trophoblast, the next step in transport involves the FcRn, an intracellular IgG receptor that is a unique β_2-microglobulin–associated nonpolymorphic member of the class I MHC family (Leach et al., 1996; Simister, 1998; Story et al., 1994) (see Chapter 3). FcRn lacks a functional peptide-binding groove and, instead, uses a different region of the molecule for binding IgG through its Fc domain. IgG bound to FcRn receptor undergoes transcytosis across the syncytiotrophoblast, followed by its release into the interstitium in the vicinity of endothelial cells surrounding fetal villous vessels (Story et al., 1994). How IgG is internalized and transported across the endothelium of fetal villous vessels is unclear, because these cells express only low or undetectable amounts of FcRn (Leach et al., 1996). In addition to the syncytiotrophoblast, FcRn is widely expressed by nonplacental tissues, where it binds to pinocytosed IgG and recycles it to the circulation. This recycling system accounts for the very long half-life of IgG. (FcRn is also discussed in Chapter 3.)

Maternal IgG and FcRn expression can be detected in placental syncytiotrophoblasts during the first trimester (Simister et al., 1998), but transport does not occur because circulating fetal concentrations of IgG remain below 100 mg/dl until approximately 17 weeks. The maternally derived placental cytotrophoblast, which is found between the syncytiotrophoblast and the fetal endothelium during the first trimester, may act as a barrier to IgG transport. This cytotrophoblast layer becomes discontinuous as the villous surface area expands during the second trimester (Simister et al., 1998).

Maternal IgG in the Fetus and Newborn

After 17 weeks' gestation, circulating IgG levels in the fetus rise steadily, reaching half of the term serum concentration by approximately 30 weeks and equaling that of the mother by approximately 33 weeks (Gusdon, 1969; Kohler and Farr, 1966). In some instances, fetal IgG concentrations may exceed those of the mother by twofold (Pitcher-Wilmott et al., 1980). This may reflect a locally increased IgG concentration within the syncytiotrophoblast before IgG release into the fetal interstitial space (Landor, 1995).

The fetus synthesizes little IgG so that the concentration in utero reflects almost solely maternally derived antibody (Fig. 22-5) (Martensson and Fudenberg, 1965). Accordingly, the degree of prematurity is reflected in proportionately lower neonatal IgG concentrations. There is a relatively low ratio of the IgG2 concentration in cord blood from term infants and particularly in preterm infants compared with maternal blood, whereas the fetal-to-maternal IgG ratio is usually near 1.0 for other subclasses (Hay et al., 1971; Malek et al., 1994; Oxelius and Svenningsen, 1994). The low IgG2 levels reflect the relatively low affinity of the type III Fc receptor for IgG2. IgM, IgA, IgD, and IgE do not cross the placenta. There is also no evidence for the transamniotic transfer of IgG to the fetus (Landor, 1995).

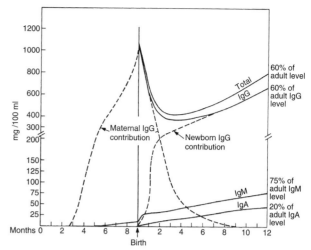

Figure 22-5 · Immunoglobulin (IgG, IgM, and IgA) levels in the fetus and infant in the first year of life. The IgG of the fetus and newborn infant is normally solely of maternal origin. The maternal IgG disappears by the age of 9 months, by which time endogenous synthesis of IgG by the infant is well established. The IgM and IgA of the neonate are entirely endogenously synthesized because maternal IgM and IgA do not cross the placenta.

By approximately 2 months of life, the amount of circulating IgG synthesized by the infant equals the amount derived from transplacental transfer; and by 10 to 12 months old, the IgG is nearly all derived from synthesis by the infant. As a consequence of the fall in passively derived IgG and the gradual increase in synthesis of IgG, values reach a nadir of approximately 400 mg/dl in term infants at 3 to 4 months old and rise thereafter (Table 22-5 and Fig. 22-5). The premature infant has lower IgG concentrations at birth. These reach a nadir at 3 months old, with mean IgG values of 82 and 104 mg/dl observed for infants born at 25 to 28 and at 29 to 32 weeks' gestation, respectively. Passive maternal antibody plays an important protective role, but it limits the value of IgG determinations in the diagnosis of immunodeficiency or infection in the young infant.

Function of Maternal Antibodies in the Newborn

The fetus receives IgG antibodies against antigens to which the mother has been exposed by infection or vaccination (Table 22-6). For example, in mothers immunized with *H. influenzae* type b capsular polyribosylphosphate-polysaccharide antigen at 34 to 36 weeks' gestation, antipolyribosylphosphate antibody is effectively transferred to the fetus. This results in protective neonatal antibody levels for approximately the first 4 months of life. However, if the maternal antibody levels are too low, it may protect the mother against infection without conferring protection to her infant. Furthermore, the mother can develop a rapid-recall antibody response upon infectious challenge, whereas the antigenically naïve infant will mount a slower primary antibody response.

TABLE 22-5 · LEVELS OF IMMUNOGLOBULINS IN SERA OF NORMAL SUBJECTS BY AGE*

Age	IgG mg/dl	IgG Percentage of Adult Level	IgM mg/dl	IgM Percentage of Adult Level	IgA mg/dl	IgA Percentage of Adult Level	Total Immunoglobulins mg/dl	Total Immunoglobulins Percentage of Adult Level
Newborn	1031 ± 200†	89 ± 17	11 ± 5	11 ± 5	2 ± 3	1 ± 2	1044 ± 201	67 ± 13
1–3 mo	430 ± 119	37 ± 10	30 ± 11	21 ± 13	11 ± 7	481 ± 127	31 ± 9	
4–6 mo	427 ± 186	37 ± 16	43 ± 17	43 ± 17	28 ± 18	14 ± 9	498 ± 204	32 ± 13
7–12 mo	661 ± 219	58 ± 19	54 ± 23	55 ± 23	37 ± 18	19 ± 9	752 ± 242	48 ± 15
13–24 mo	762 ± 209	66 ± 18	58 ± 23	59 ± 23	50 ± 24	25 ± 12	870 ± 258	56 ± 16
25–36 mo	892 ± 183	77 ± 16	61 ± 19	62 ± 19	71 ± 37	36 ± 19	1024 ± 205	65 ± 14
3–5 yr	929 ± 228	80 ± 20	56 ± 18	57 ± 18	93 ± 27	47 ± 14	1078 ± 245	69 ± 17
6–8 yr	923 ± 256	80 ± 22	65 ± 25	66 ± 25	124 ± 45	62 ± 23	1112 ± 293	71 ± 20
9–11 yr	1124 ± 235	97 ± 20	79 ± 33	80 ± 33	131 ± 60	66 ± 30	1334 ± 254	85 ±17
12–16 yr	946 ± 124	82 ± 11	59 ± 20	60 ± 20	148 ± 63	74 ± 32	1153 ± 169	74 ± 12
Adult	1158 ± 305	100 ± 26	99 ± 27	100 ± 27	200 ± 61	100 ± 31	1457 ± 353	100 ± 24

*The values were derived from measurements made for 296 normal children and 30 adults. Levels were determined by the radial diffusion technique using specific rabbit antisera to human immunoglobulins.
†One SD.
From Stiehm ER, Fudenberg HH. Serum levels of immune globulins in health and disease: a survey. Pediatrics 37:715, 1966.

TABLE 22-6 · PROPERTIES OF IgG SUBCLASSES

Subtype	Biologic Half-Life (Days)	Classical Pathway Complement Activation	Fc Receptor* Binding Type I	Fc Receptor* Binding Type II	Fc Receptor* Binding Type III	Placental Transfer†
IgG1	25	++	++	±	++	++
IgG2	23	+	±	+	±	+
IgG3	9	++	++	++	++	++
IgG4	25	‡	+	±	±	+

*Cells expressing FcγR: FcγRI—monocytes, macrophages, and IFN-γ–treated neutrophils; FcγRII—monocytes, macrophages, all granulocytes, and B cells; FcγRIII—some monocytes, macrophages, neutrophils, eosinophils, NK cells (rare T cells), and trophoblasts.
†See text.
‡Activates alternative pathway.
NK = natural killer.
From Lewis DB, Wilson CB. Developmental immunology and role of host defenses in neonatal susceptibility to infection. In Remington JS, Klein JO, eds. Infectious diseases of the fetus and newborn, ed 4. Philadelphia, WB Saunders, 1994.

Maternal antibodies are primarily IgM directed against gram-negative pathogens such as *E. coli* and *Salmonella* (Fink et al., 1962; Smith et al., 1964); however, the fetus will not receive them because IgM does not traverse the placenta. Further, premature infants may not receive sufficient amounts of IgG for protection, since the bulk of maternal IgG is transferred to the fetus after 34 weeks' gestation (Morell et al., 1986). This limited transfer to the premature infant accounts for their increased susceptibility to certain infections, such as varicella-zoster virus, compared with term infants (Linder et al., 2000).

Maternal Antibody Inhibition of Neonatal Antibody Responses

Maternal antibody may also inhibit the fetus or newborn from producing antibodies of the same specificity. This inhibition varies with the antigen, antigen dose, vaccine adjuvant, and the maternal antibody titer.

Maternal antibody markedly inhibits the response to measles and rubella vaccine, but not mumps vaccine (Sato et al., 1979); this is the reason for delaying measles-mumps-rubella vaccine until infants are at least 12 months old. One mechanism for this is the inhibition of viral replication necessary for an optimal antibody response to some live attenuated vaccines.

Maternal antibodies may also inhibit the neonatal response to nonreplicating vaccines such as whole-cell pertussis vaccine (Baraff et al., 1984), diphtheria toxoid (Vahlquist, 1949), *Salmonella* flagellar antigen (Smith et al., 1964), and inactivated poliovirus vaccine (Perkins et al., 1959). One possible inhibitory mechanism is that maternal IgG forms antigen–antibody complexes with the immunogen and blocks B-cell activation through the simultaneous engagement of the inhibitory FcγRII receptor by the IgG component of the complex and the surface immunoglobulin by immunogen. Another is that maternal antibody results in more rapid clearance of vaccine antigen and decreased immunogenicity.

For certain antibodies—such as anti-HBsAg—neither maternal antibodies nor hepatitis B immune globulin administration has a substantial inhibitory effect on the newborn's immune response to a hepatitis B vaccination.

Immunoglobulin Synthesis by the Fetus and Neonate

IgM

IgM is the only isotype other than IgG that binds and activates complement, requiring only a single IgM molecule for activation. IgM increases from a mean of 6 mg/dl in premature infants younger than 28 weeks' gestation to 11 mg/dl at term (Avrech et al., 1994; Cederqvist et al., 1978), which is approximately 8% of the maternal IgM level. This IgM is likely to be preimmune (i.e., not the result of a B-cell response to foreign antigens) and enriched for "natural" polyreactive antibodies produced by B-1 cells. The results of murine studies suggest that such natural IgM may fix complement and allow antigenically naïve B cells to efficiently activate complement receptor 2 (CD21) co-stimulation (Boes et al., 1998a, 1998b; Ehrenstein et al., 1998). Some of the neonatal IgM is monomeric and therefore nonfunctional, as opposed to its usual pentameric functional form (Allansmith et al., 1968; Perchalski et al., 1968).

Postnatal IgM concentrations rise rapidly for the first month and then more gradually thereafter, presumably in response to intestinal colonization and other antigenic stimuli (see Fig. 22-5). By 1 year old, values are approximately 60% of those in adults. The postnatal rise is similar in premature and term infants (Allansmith et al., 1968). Elevated (>20 mg/dl) IgM concentrations in cord blood suggest possible intrauterine infections (Alford et al., 1975), but many infants with congenital infections have normal cord blood IgM levels (Griffiths et al., 1982).

IgG

Passively derived maternal IgG is the source of virtually all the IgG subclasses detected in the normal fetus and neonate, and levels of these fall rapidly after birth. IgG synthesized by the neonate and that derived from the mother are approximately equal when the neonate reaches 2 months old. Because the IgG plasma half-life is approximately 21 days, by 10 to 12 months old, virtually all maternally derived IgG has been catabolized. As discussed earlier, maternal IgG may inhibit certain postnatal antibody responses by binding to FcγRII receptors and by rapidly clearing potential antigens. However, the slow onset of IgG synthesis in the neonate is predominantly an intrinsic limitation of the neonate, rather than maternal antibody; indeed, a similar pattern of IgG development was observed in a neonate born to a mother with untreated agammaglobulinemia (Kobayashi et al., 1980).

By 1 year, the total IgG concentration is approximately 60% that of adults. IgG3 and IgG1 subclasses reach adult concentrations by 8 years old, whereas IgG2 and IgG4 do so by 10 and 12 years old, respectively (Ochs and Wedgwood, 1987). The slow rise in IgG2 concentrations parallels the poor antibody response to bacterial polysaccharide antigens (e.g., *H. influenzae* type b polyribosylphosphate), which are predominantly IgG2 (Granoff et al., 1986).

Interestingly, the postpartum order in which adult levels of isotype expression are achieved closely parallels the order of the heavy-chain gene segments that encode these isotypes. Thus the postnatal regulation of isotype switching is mediated in part at the heavy-chain gene locus (i.e., its chromatin configuration may be developmentally regulated.

IgA

IgA is present in both sera and secretions, and this isotype is produced in the greatest amount per day in humans. IgA exists both as a monomer and as a dimer containing a covalently linked J chain. The J chain is not absolutely required for IgA dimerization, but it may play an important role in facilitating IgA secretion into the bile (Hendrickson et al., 1995) (see Chapter 9).

There are two subclasses of IgA. IgA1 makes up 90% of the IgA found in serum, whereas IgA2 makes up 60% of that found in secretions, indicating preferential localization of IgA2-secreting plasma cells near mucosal surfaces. IgA2 is also less susceptible to bacterial proteases, favoring its survival in the intestinal lumen. IgA does not cross the placenta, and its concentration in cord blood is usually 0.1 to 5.0 mg/dl, approximately 0.5% of the levels in maternal serum (Avrech et al., 1994). Concentrations are similar in term and premature neonates (Cederqvist et al., 1978), and both IgA1 and IgA2 are present.

At birth, the frequency of IgA1-bearing and IgA2-bearing B cells is equivalent. Subsequently, there is a preferential expansion of IgA1-bearing cells, presumably as a result of postnatal exposure to environmental antigens (Conley et al., 1980). The sera concentrations increase to 20% of those in adults by 1 year old and rise progressively through adolescence. Increased cord blood IgA concentrations are observed in some infants with congenital infection (Alford et al., 1975). Elevated IgA is common in young infants infected by vertical transmission with HIV. IgA has a relatively short half-life in plasma of approximately 5 days. Secretory IgA is present in substantial amounts in the saliva by 10 days after birth (Seidel et al., 2000).

IgD

IgD is detectable by means of sensitive techniques in sera from the cord blood of term and premature infants (Cederqvist et al., 1978; Josephs and Buckley, 1980). Mean sera levels at birth are approximately 0.05 mg/dl (Avrech et al., 1994) and increase during the first year of life. Circulating IgD has no clear functional role, but it may be elevated in certain disease states, such as hyper-IgD syndrome. The immune response of mice in which IgD expression has been eliminated by gene targeting appears to be normal. In contrast, surface IgD can replace surface IgM in B-cell function in the mouse. Together, these results suggest that the functions of IgM and IgD are largely redundant.

IgE

IgE synthesis by the fetus is detectable as early as 11 weeks' gestation, but levels in cord blood at birth are typically low, with a mean of approximately 0.5% of maternal levels (Avrech et al., 1994). These low levels of IgE are of fetal origin and are higher in infants born from a pregnancy of 40 to 42 weeks' gestation than those from a 37 to 39 weeks' gestation (Avrech et al., 1994). The rate of postnatal increase varies and is greater in infants predisposed to allergic disease or with greater environmental exposure to allergens (Bazaral et al., 1971). The level of IgE at birth appears to have limited predictive value regarding whether an individual will later develop atopic disease (Edenharter et al., 1998).

Summary

The neonate is partially protected from infection by passive maternal IgG antibody, predominantly transferred during the latter third of pregnancy. Fetal IgG concentrations are equal or higher than maternal concentrations after 34 weeks' gestation.

The inability of the neonate to produce antibodies in response to polysaccharides, particularly bacterial capsular polysaccharides, limits resistance to bacterial pathogens to which the mother has little or no IgG antibody. The basis for this defect remains unclear, but it may reflect an intrinsic limitation of B-cell function or a deficiency in the anatomic microenvironment required for B cells to become activated and differentiate into plasma cells.

By contrast, the neonatal IgM response to most protein antigens is intact and only slightly limited for IgG responses to certain vaccines. Nevertheless, there are clear differences between neonates and older infants in the magnitude of the antibody response to most protein neoantigens, but this rapidly resolves after birth. There is a limited antibody response of premature infants to immunization with protein antigens during the first month of life but not subsequently. Thus chronologic (i.e., postnatal) age is more of a determinant of antibody responses to T-dependent antigens than is gestational age.

Isotype expression by B cells after immunization with T-dependent antigens is limited by T-cell function, such as reduced CD40 ligand production, and intrinsic limitations of B-cell maturation and function. These limitations are exaggerated in the fetus.

DEVELOPMENT AND FUNCTION OF NATURAL KILLER CELLS

Definition

NK cells are large granular lymphocytes that have cytotoxic function and the ability to produce cytokines such as IFN-γ and chemokines such as CCL3 [macrophage inflammatory protein (MIP)-1α] and CCL4 (MIP-1β) (see Chapter 6). NK cells are critical for the early control of viral infections, particularly with herpesvirus infections, until peptide-specific cytolytic T lymphocytes (CTLs) can be generated approximately 5 to 7 days after the onset of infection. The elaboration of cytokines by NK cells may augment the development of cell-mediated immunity by Th1 effector cells and mononuclear phagocytes (Fig. 22-6). (NK cells are also discussed in Chapter 6.)

Mechanisms of Natural Killer Cell–Mediated Cytotoxicity

NK cells are functionally distinct from CTLs in their ability to lyse virally infected or tumor target cells in a non–MHC-restricted manner not requiring prior sensitization (Miller, 2001). Activation of NK cells for target cell lysis, termed *natural cytotoxicity*, in part involves the absence of the engagement of inhibitory receptors

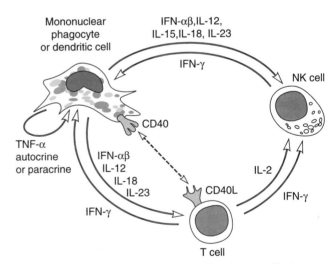

Figure 22-6 · Cytokines link innate and antigen-specific immune mechanisms against intracellular pathogens. The activation of T cells by antigen-presenting cells (APCs), such as mononuclear phagocytes or dendritic cells, results in the expression of CD40 ligand (CD154) and the secretion of cytokines, such as IL-2 and interferon gamma (IFN-γ). Mononuclear phagocytes are activated by IFN-γ and the engagement of CD40, with increased microbicidal activity. Mononuclear phagocytes produce tumor necrosis factor (TNF)-α, which enhances their microbicidal activity in a paracrine or autocrine manner. Mononuclear phagocytes and dendritic cells also secrete the cytokines IFN-α/β, IL-12, IL-15, IL-18, and IL-23. These cytokines promote T-helper 1 (Th1) effector cell differentiation and also natural killer (NK) cell activation. Activated NK cells in turn secrete IFN-γ, which further enhances mononuclear phagocyte activation and Th1 effector cell differentiation.

by self MHC class I alleles or HLA-E (Lanier, 1998) (Fig. 22-7). This contrasts with CTL cytotoxicity, in which foreign antigenic peptides bound to self MHC (MHC-restricted cytotoxicity) or self-peptides bound to foreign MHC (allogeneic cytotoxicity) are recognized.

Inhibitory and Activating Receptors

The two major groups of receptors that inhibit NK cells are the KIRs and CD94/NKG2A. The KIRs bind to portions of HLA-B and HLA-C molecules located outside of the peptide-binding groove, whereas CD94/NKG2A binds to HLA-E, a nonclassical and nonvariable MHC molecule that requires hydrophobic leader peptides from HLA-A, HLA-B, and HLA-C for its surface expression. These NK-cell receptors help counteract the ability of viruses, particularly herpesviruses and some adenoviruses, to decrease the surface expression of class I MHC molecules, thereby limiting CTL-mediated viral clearance. This negative regulation of natural cytotoxicity may also endow NK cells with the capacity to reject hematopoietic cell grafts from individuals lacking recipient MHC alleles even if they do not express foreign MHC alleles and to kill tumor cells that have reduced or absent class I MHC expression.

NK cells also express positive activating receptors such as 2B4 (CD244), NKG2D, NKp30, NKp44, NKp46, and NKR-P1A (CD161) (Boles et al., 1999; Lanier, 1998; 2001). The 2B4 receptor binds to CD48, a protein expressed by a variety of cell types that is upregulated by EBV infection of B cells. NKG2D binds to MICA and MICB, molecules that are class I MHC–like but not involved in peptide presentation and that are expressed at high levels by tumors and stressed cells. NKp44 and NKp46 can bind to the hemagglutinin protein of influenza virus, resulting in the lysis of cells expressing this viral protein (Arnon et al., 2001).

NK cells also express killer activating receptors, which are similar in structure and in binding specificity to KIRs, but have cytoplasmic domains that activate rather than inhibit the generation of signals for natural cytotoxicity (Lanier, 2001). CD94/NKG2C is also an activating receptor that has a similar specificity for HLA-E as the CD94/NKG2A inhibitory receptor. How NK-cell–mediated cytotoxicity can be appropriately regulated by inhibitory and activating receptors sharing the same ligand specificity remains unclear.

Antibody-Dependent Cellular Cytotoxicity

NK cells can also kill target cells that are coated with IgG antibodies, a process known as *antibody-dependent cellular cytotoxicity* (ADCC). ADCC requires the recognition

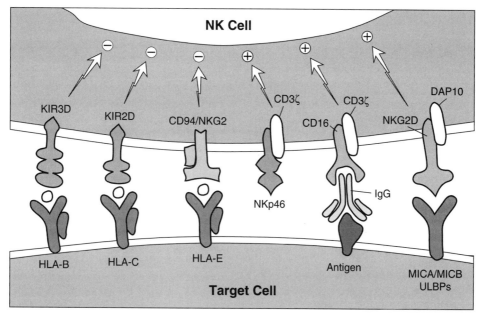

Figure 22-7 · **Positive and negative regulation of natural killer (NK)-cell cytotoxicity by receptor/ligand interactions, with only some of the known receptor ligand interactions shown.** NK-cell cytotoxicity is inhibited by the engagement of killer inhibitory receptors (KIRs) by class I major histocompatibility complex (MHC) molecules, such as HLA-B and HLA-C. In addition, NK cells are inhibited when the CD94/NKG2 complex, a member of the C-type lectin family, on the NK cell is engaged by HLA-E. HLA-E binds hydrophobic leader peptides derived from HLA-A, HLA-B, and HLA-C molecules and requires these for its surface expression. Thus HLA-E surface expression on a potential target cell indicates its overall production of conventional class I MHC molecules. These inhibitory influences on NK-cell cytotoxicity are overcome if viral infection of the target cell results in decreased class I MHC and HLA-E levels. NK-cell cytotoxicity is positively regulated by the engagement of NKp46, CD16—which is an Fc receptor for IgG—and NKG2D—which is a receptor for MICA, MICB, and UL16-binding proteins (ULBPs). These positive receptors are associated with CD3-ζ (CD16 and NKp46) or DAP-10 (NKG2D), which mediate intracellular activation signals.

of the target cell IgG by the NK-cell FcγRIIIB (CD16) receptor (Perussia, 1998). In contrast to natural cytotoxicity, in which perforin/granzyme–dependent mechanisms are predominant, ADCC uses both perforin/granzyme-dependent and Fas ligand–dependent cytotoxic mechanisms (Eischen et al., 1996).

NK-cell–mediated natural cytotoxicity and ADCC in vitro can be markedly increased by exposure to certain cytokines, such as IL-2 and IL-15, a mechanism that is probably important to optimal NK-cell function in vivo. NK-cell production of IFN-γ is induced by exposure to the cytokines IL-12 and IL-18.

Natural Killer–Cell Surface Phenotype

NK cells do not rearrange either the TCR or immunoglobulin genes and, as a consequence, lack surface expression of the TCRs or surface immunoglobulins, as well as their associated proteins, such as CD3, Ig-α, and Ig-β. Virtually all circulating adult human NK cells express NKp46, which appears to be NK cell specific (Sivori et al., 1997), and CD2, CD16, CD56, and NKR-P1A (Nakazawa et al., 1997; Phillips et al., 1992), which are not unique to the NK-cell lineage and are also found on populations of T cells or other cell types. Approximately 50% of adult NK cells express CD57 (Phillips et al., 1992), which, in conjunction with CD2 and CD56, is primarily involved in NK-cell adhesion to either target cells or endothelium. Adult NK cells include a distinct CD56^{high} population that is highly enriched in the capacity to produce cytokines compared with that of CD56^{low} cells (Cooper et al., 2001).

All NK cells also express cytoplasmic CD3-ζ and FcεR1γ, which are involved in the intracellular propagation of activation signals. Most or all NK cells express DAP-12, a CD3-like homolog with similar function, and DAP-10, which associates with NKG2D and propagates activation signals by activating the PI3 kinase (Lanier, 2001). NK cells are mainly produced in the bone marrow and are derived from a common T and NK precursor cell.

Ontogeny of Natural Killer Cells

The development of human NK cells precedes that of αβ-T cells during ontogeny, demonstrating their thymic independence. The fetal liver produces NK cells as early as 6 weeks' gestation; furthermore, they become increasingly abundant during the second trimester (Phillips et al., 1992). CD34$^+$CD38$^+$Lin$^-$ cells of the second trimester fetal liver give rise to NK-like cells rather than T-lineage cells after culture in vitro with the cytokines IL-7, IL-15, and Flt-3 ligand (Jaleco et al., 1997), suggesting that the fetal liver is the main site of development for NK cells rather than extrathymic T cells. In the murine fetal thymus, NK cells appear before αβ-thymocytes (Carlyle et al., 1998). A similar sequence of events applies to humans, but the immunologic importance of thymic-derived NK cells remains

unclear. The bone marrow is the major site for NK-cell production from late gestation onward.

The precise developmental sequence of NK-cell maturation in the bone marrow remains poorly understood. CD34$^+$Lin$^-$ cells expressing CD7 or CD38 are found in the adult bone marrow and the neonatal or adult circulation and appear to be enriched for NK-cell progenitors (Blom et al., 1998; Miller et al., 1994). In vitro treatment of these progenitor cells with cytokines or stromal cells, or both, results in the appearance of CD56$^+$ cells with NK-cell features, including natural cytotoxicity and CD94 surface expression (Carayol et al., 1998; Mrozek et al., 1996).

Findings from studies of in vitro cultures of single neonatal CD34$^+$Lin$^-$ blood cells suggest that during differentiation, the commitment to NK-cell lineage is made first, followed by the acquisition of inhibitory receptors (Miller and McCullar, 2001). CD34$^+$ cells with these or similar characteristics in the thymus can also differentiate into thymocytes or lymphoid dendritic cells, depending on the culture conditions, suggesting the existence of a common T/NK/lymphoid dendritic cell progenitor (Marquez et al., 1998).

IL-15 appears to be critical for directing less committed lymphocyte precursors into the NK-cell lineage (Miller and McCullar, 2001; Mingari et al., 1997) and for promoting the survival of mature NK cells (Carson et al., 1997). This is supported by murine studies in which IL-15 or its specific receptor components (the IL-15 receptor α chain, the IL-2 receptor β chain, and the γc chain) have been eliminated by selective gene targeting.

As in mice with SCID, NK cells and T cells are absent in humans with X-linked SCID, in whom there is a genetic deficiency of γc. The absence of IL-15–mediated signaling probably accounts for the absence of NK cells in γc chain deficiency in humans, rather than a lack of IL-7, because patients with deficiency of the IL-7 receptor α chain lack T cells but have normal numbers of NK cells (Puel et al., 1998).

Neonatal mononuclear cells produce less IL-15 than do adult cells after LPS stimulation (Qian et al., 1997). However, it is unlikely that this applies to IL-15–producing cells at major sites of NK-cell development, such as the fetal bone marrow and fetal liver, because NK cells are present in greatest numbers in the circulation during the second trimester of fetal development (Thilaganathan et al., 1993) and their number in the neonatal circulation (approximately 15% of total lymphocytes) is typically equal to or greater than that in adults (Phillips et al., 1992). These observations suggest that developing NK cells in the fetus and neonate have normal IL-15 responsiveness.

In contrast to adult NK cells, most fetal liver NK cells express the CD3-ε and CD3-δ components associated with the TCR and lack CD16 surface expression (Phillips et al., 1992): Virtually all fetal and neonatal NK cells lack the expression of CD57 (Kohl et al., 1999). The surface expression of CD16, CD18, CD44, and the KIR (p70 or NKB-1) by circulating neonatal and adult NK cells is similar (Kohl, 1999). However, the fraction of fetal and neonatal NK cells that express CD2 or CD56 is reduced by approximately 50% compared with that in the adult (Gaddy et al., 1995; Nakazawa et al., 1997; Phillips et al., 1992). Fetal NK cells, unlike adult NK cells, may express CD28, but it is unclear whether they respond to engagement by the B7 molecules CD80 and CD86, the ligands of CD28.

Neonatal Natural Killer-Cell–Mediated Cytotoxicity and Cytokine Production

The cytolytic function of NK cells increases progressively during fetal life to reach values approximately 50% (15% to 60% in various studies) of those in adult cells at term, as determined by means of assays with tumor cell targets, such as the K562 erythroleukemia cell line, and either unpurified (Baley and Schacter, 1985; Lubens et al., 1982; Nair et al., 1985; Seki et al., 1985; Tarkkanen and Saksela, 1982; Toivanen et al., 1981; Ueno et al., 1985) or NK-cell–enriched preparations (Kaplan et al., 1982; McDonald et al., 1992; Phillips et al., 1992; Tarkkanen and Saksela, 1982; Sancho et al., 1991; Seki et al., 1985). Reduced cytotoxic activity by neonatal NK cells has been observed by using cord blood from vaginal or cesarean section deliveries or peripheral blood obtained 2 to 4 days after birth (Georgeson et al., 2001). Full function is not achieved until at least 9 to 12 months old. Cytolytic function is also markedly reduced by bacterial sepsis in neonates (Georgeson et al., 2001). NK cells from the premature infant also have reduced cytotoxic function compared with those of the term neonate (Merrill et al., 1996; Phillips et al., 1992).

The reduced cytolytic activity appears to reflect primarily diminished postbinding cytotoxic activity and diminished recycling to kill multiple targets. This parallels the reduced number of CD56+ NK cells in the neonate and is consistent with the poor cytolytic activity of CD56- NK cells. When only CD56+ neonatal NK cells are studied, their cytolytic activity is usually similar to that of adult NK cells (Phillips et al., 1992; Sancho et al., 1991).

Role of Target Cells in NK-Cell Cytotoxicity

However, whether neonatal NK cells have decreased cytolytic activity compared with adult cells depends in part on the target cell used. For example, NK cells from term neonates were found to have similar cytotoxic activity to adult cells against non-K562 tumors. Decreased cytotoxic activity by neonatal NK cells in comparison with that of adult cells is also consistently observed with HSV-infected (Cicuttini et al., 1993; Phillips et al., 1992; Webb et al., 1994) and CMV-infected target cells (Harrison and Waner, 1985). In contrast, both neonatal and adult NK cells have equivalent cytotoxic activity against HIV-1–infected cells (Jenkins et al., 1993; Merrill et al., 1996).

These results suggest that ligands on the target cell or its intrinsic sensitivity to the induction of apoptosis may influence fetal and neonatal NK-cell function. The mechanisms of these pathogen-related differences remain unclear but may contribute to the severity of neonatal HSV infection. If neonatal NK-cell activity is reduced against enteroviruses, it may contribute to the severe outcome of this infection in the neonatal period.

Neonatal NK-Cell ADCC Activity

Paralleling the reduction in the natural cytotoxic activity of neonatal cells, the ADCC of neonatal mononuclear cells is approximately 50% that of adult mononuclear cells, including against HSV-infected targets (Merrill et al., 1996). In contrast to natural cytotoxicity, decreased ADCC mediated by purified neonatal NK cells appears to be caused in part by an adhesion defect in the presence of antibody (Kohl et al., 1999).

Cytokine Augmentation of NK Cytotoxicity

Similar to their effects on adult NK cells, cytokines such as IL-2, IL-12, IL-15, IFN-α, IFN-β, and IFN-γ can augment the cytolytic activity of neonatal NK cells within a few hours (Kohl, 1999; Lau et al., 1996; Nguyen et al., 1998a, 1998b). Consistent with the ability of IL-2 and IFN-γ to augment their cytolytic activity, neonatal NK cells have surface receptors for IL-2 and IFN-γ that are equal to or greater than those of adult NK cells (Han et al., 1995). However, neonatal NK cells are less responsive to activation by the combination of IL-12 and IL-15 than are adult NK cells, in terms of the induction of CD69 surface expression (Lin et al., 2000a, 2000b).

Circulating neonatal NK cells have increased natural cytotoxic activity and ADCC activity after incubation from 18 hours to 3 weeks with IL-2, IL-12, IL-15, IL-18, or combinations of these to generate lymphokine-activated killer (LAK) cells (Condiotti and Nagler, 1998; Condiotti et al., 2001; Gaddy and Broxmeyer, 1997; Gaddy et al., 1995; Harris, 1995; Keever et al., 1995; Lin et al., 2000a, 2000b; Merrill et al., 1996; Nguyen et al., 1998a, 1998b; Nomura et al., 2001; Umemoto et al., 1997; Webb et al., 1994). Neonatal LAK cells often have cytotoxic activity equivalent to that of adult LAK cells, suggesting that neonatal NK cells have a normal capacity to be primed by exogenous cytokines.

The generation of neonatal LAK cells from NK cells also increases their surface expression of CD56 because of the differentiation of CD56- NK cells into CD56+ LAK cells, rather than expansion from the pre-existing neonatal CD56+ NK population (Gaddy and Broxmeyer, 1997; Malygin and Timonen, 1993). This suggests that the neonatal CD56- NK-cell population is a phenotypically and functionally immature NK-cell subset that gives rise to a mature CD56+ population.

Mechanisms of Decreased Neonatal NK-Cell Cytotoxicity

The mechanisms responsible for decreased NK cytotoxicity in the neonate are undefined. Soluble class I MHC is present at a 10-fold greater concentration in cord serum than in adult serum, and this could contribute to decreased neonatal NK cytotoxicity by engaging KIRs (Webb et al., 1994). However, because exposure to levels of soluble class I MHC present in cord blood has only a modest inhibitory effect on NK cytotoxicity in vitro (Webb et al., 1994), this is unlikely to be a major factor. Cell-mediated suppression has also been proposed, yet this has not been shown in mixing experiments (Dominguez et al., 1998). Nor is decreased neonatal NK cytotoxicity attributable to decreased binding to target cells (Webb et al., 1994) or to decreased levels of intracellular perforin/granzyme B (Gaddy and Broxmeyer, 1997).

Treatment of neonatal NK cells, including the CD56 subset, with ionomycin and phorbol ester enhances natural cytotoxicity to levels present in adult NK cells (Gaddy and Broxmeyer, 1997). This increase is blocked by inhibitors of granule exocytosis, indicating that decreased release of granules containing perforin/granzyme may reduce neonatal NK cytotoxicity. Finally, decreased neonatal NK cytotoxicity is not determined at the level of HSCs or later precursor cells of the NK-cell lineage because donor-derived NK cells appear early after cord blood transplantation, with good cytotoxicity through the perforin/granzyme and Fas/Fas ligand cytotoxic pathways (Brahmi et al., 2001).

Cytokine Production by Neonatal NK Cells

Neonatal NK cells produce IFN-γ as effectively as adult NK cells in response to exogenous IL-2 and HSV (Hayward et al., 1986) or to polyclonal stimulation with ionomycin and phorbol ester (Krampera et al., 2000). IL-12–induced production of IFN-γ by neonatal mononuclear cells (most likely NK cells) may be reduced compared with that of adult cells (Lau et al., 1996; Lee et al., 1996). However, purified neonatal NK cells produce substantially more IFN-γ than adult NK cells after stimulation with the combination of IL-12 and IL-18 (Nomura et al., 2001). Fewer neonatal NK cells express TNF-α than do adult NK cells after ionomycin and phorbol ester stimulation (Krampera et al., 2000). The production of other cytokines by neonatal NK cells, particularly with physiologic stimuli, is not known.

NK-Cell Response to Congenital Infection

Congenital viral or *Toxoplasma* infection during the second trimester may increase the number of circulating NK cells (Thilaganathan et al., 1993). Elevated NK cells can persist until birth, accompanied by decreased NK-cell expression of the CD45RA isoform and increased expression of the CD45R0 isoform of the CD45 tyrosine phosphatase (Michie and Harvey, 1994). This CD45RA^{low}CD45R0^{high} phenotype suggests in vivo activation, similar to NK cells incubated in vitro with IL-2 or tumor cell targets (Braakman et al., 1991).

Summary

NK cells appear early during gestation and are present in normal numbers by mid- to late gestation; approximately 50% of these cells at birth are CD56⁻. This surface phenotype is a marker for NK-cell immaturity, but the relationship between CD56⁻ and CD56⁺ cells is unclear. Neonatal CD56⁻ NK cells have decreased cytotoxicity to several target cells, including virus-infected target cells, in comparison with the adult CD56⁺ phenotype. Neonatal NK-cell cytotoxicity can be augmented by incubation with cytokines in vitro, which suggests a potential immunotherapeutic strategy.

NEUTROPHILS OF THE FETUS AND NEONATE

Fetal and Neonatal Neutrophil Production and Release

Neutrophil precursors appear later than macrophage precursors and are first detected in the yolk sac and later in the liver and spleen (Christensen, 1989; Playfair et al., 1963) (see Chapter 5). Cells committed to the neutrophil lineage are detectable in the fetal bone marrow cavity by 10 to 11 weeks' gestation (Slayton et al., 1998), and mature neutrophils are detectable by 14 to 16 weeks' gestation. The numbers of circulating neutrophil precursors (GM–colony-forming units [GM-CFU]) are approximately 10- to 20-fold higher in the fetus and neonate than in adults; neonatal bone marrow also contains an abundance of neutrophil precursors (Christensen, 1989; Christensen and Rothstein, 1984; Ohls et al., 1995; Shapiro and Bassen, 1941).

The rate of proliferation of circulating neonatal neutrophil precursors is close to maximum (Ohls et al., 1995; Shapiro and Bassen, 1941), suggesting that further increases of GM-CFU in response to infection are limited. In contrast to the increased numbers of GM-CFU present in term newborns and adults, the midgestation human fetus has markedly fewer postmitotic neutrophils in the fetal liver and bone marrow (Laver et al., 1990). At this stage of gestation, neutrophils also constitute less than 10% of circulating leukocytes, rising to values of 50% to 60% at term.

Within hours of birth, the number of circulating neutrophils increase sharply in term and preterm neonates (Manroe et al., 1979). In healthy term neonates, the absolute neutrophil count 4 hours after birth ranges between 9.5 and 21.5 × 10³/μl (10th to 90th percentile), with an immature-to-mature neutrophil ratio of 0.05 to 0.27 (Schelonka et al., 1994). The absolute number of neutrophils normally peaks shortly thereafter, whereas the fraction of neutrophils that are immature (bands, metamyelocytes, and promyelocytes) remain at approximately 15% (Fig. 22-8). These values may be influenced by a number of factors, including sepsis.

Neutropenia and Leukemoid Reactions

Infants with sepsis may occasionally have normal or increased neutrophil counts, but many infants with sepsis or with other perinatal complications such as maternal hypertension, periventricular hemorrhage, and severe asphyxia have neutropenia. Severe or fatal sepsis is usually associated with persistent neutropenia, particularly in the premature infant (Christensen and Rothstein, 1980; Squire et al., 1979). Neutropenia may be associated with increased margination of circulating neutrophils, an early response to infection (Walker and Willemze, 1980). However, sustained neutropenia usually reflects depletion of the newborn's—particularly the premature newborn's—limited postmitotic neutrophil storage pool. Consistent with this, neonates with sepsis and neutropenia who have depleted neutrophil storage pools are more likely to die than are those with normal neutrophil storage pools (Christensen and Rothstein, 1980).

Leukemoid reactions are observed in approximately 1% of term neonates in the absence of infection or other definable cause. These reactions appear to be caused by increased marrow production of neutrophils. The mechanism for this is not clear, but in most cases these leukemoid reactions are not associated with increased G-CSF concentrations (Calhoun et al., 1996).

Effects of G-CSF and GM-CSF

G-CSF and, to a lesser extent, GM-CSF, are cytokines that promote neutrophil production, survival, and optimal function. G-CSF and its specific receptor are expressed within the bone marrow compartment by 6 weeks' gestation, approximately a month before committed neutrophil lineage cells are present (Slayton et al., 1998), consistent with a central role of G-CSF for fetal neutrophil formation. Circulating mononuclear cells and monocytes from midgestation fetuses and premature neonates produce less G-CSF and GM-CSF after in vitro stimulation than do cells from term neonates and adults. This decreased cytokine production also applies to the marrow microenvironment, in which nonhematopoietic cells, such as stromal cells, produce the bulk of these cytokines.

The circulating levels of G-CSF, which peak in the first hours after birth, are typically higher in premature infants than term neonates (Gessler et al., 1993; Ishiguro et al., 1996; Shimada et al., 1996; Wilimas et al., 1995). This suggests that G-CSF production in vivo is intact during midgestation. G-CSF levels rapidly decline in the neonatal period and subsequently decrease more slowly with age.

Whether levels of G-CSF in neonates correlate with their absolute neutrophil count remains controversial (Ishiguro et al., 1996). Circulating G-CSF levels tend to be elevated in infected mature and premature neonates (Gessler et al., 1993), but these overlap with levels in uninfected subjects (Kennon et al., 1996). Premature neonates with sepsis also have lower levels of G-CSF than do term neonates with sepsis (Weimann et al., 1998). Neutropenic neonates without sepsis do not have elevated G-CSF levels. Low levels of G-CSF may contribute to neutropenia in the premature infant with sepsis and other types of neonatal neutropenia (Schibler et al., 1993).

The most significant deficiency in phagocyte defenses of the neonate, particularly in premature infants, is their limited ability to accelerate neutrophil production in response to infection. This is mainly attributable to a limited neutrophil storage pool and a decreased ability to increase neutrophil production in response to infection, rather than to a deficiency of G-CSF. Nevertheless, trials of G-CSF and GM-CSF have been undertaken to ameliorate these deficits in neutrophil storage pools and production. These agents have not reduced the mortality from neonatal sepsis, but they may prevent later nosocomial infections and necrotizing enterocolitis (Miura et al., 2001), a complication that has been recalcitrant to many other therapies.

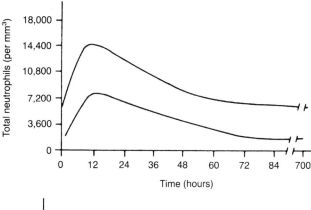

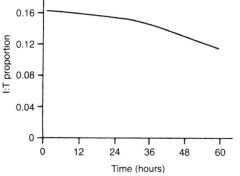

Figure 22-8 · Change in total number of neutrophils and in ratio of immature to total neutrophils (I:T proportion) in the neonate. The two lines of the upper panel bracket all valves obtained at each time point. (Adapted from Manroe BL, Weinberg AG, Rosenfeld CR, Browne R. The neonatal blood count in health and disease. I. Reference values for neutrophilic cells. J Pediatr 95:89–98, 1979.)

Assessment of Neonatal Neutrophil Function

Circulating neutrophils are poised for activation and entry into sites of infection or inflammation and for phagocytosis and killing of microbes. As a consequence, the in vitro measurement of their function is sensitive to a variety of influences, including anticoagulants, blood pH, the conditions used for cell isolation (e.g., dextran sedimentation and nonphysiologic temperature), and even in vivo exposure to low levels of anesthetics (e.g., lidocaine) systemically absorbed after local administration (Gasparoni et al., 1998). Neonatal neutrophils obtained at delivery may be activated, and this may influence certain assays. Many studies in which adult and neonatal neutrophil function are compared have not accounted for differences in cell maturity. Thus reported abnormalities of neonatal neutrophil function in vitro must be interpreted cautiously.

Adhesion of Neonatal Neutrophils

The capacity of neonatal neutrophils to exit from the blood into sites of infection and inflammation is reduced or delayed (Hill, 1987; Johnston, 1998) (see Chapter 5). The skin of the neonate often contains a large number of eosinophils in the early inflammatory response, and the transition from a neutrophilic to a mononuclear phagocytic response is delayed (Johnston, 1998). This diminished delivery of neutrophils to infected tissues may result from defects in adhesion or chemotaxis, or both.

The adhesion of neonatal neutrophils under resting conditions is normal or modestly impaired, whereas the adhesion of activated cells is deficient (Anderson et al., 1981, 1984). The adhesion of neonatal neutrophils to activated endothelium under conditions of flow mimicking those in capillaries or postcapillary venules is 40% to 45% that of adult neutrophils (Anderson et al., 1991; Smith et al., 1992). This may be attributable to the decreased expression of L-selectin (CD62L), a reduced ability to shed L-selectin from the surface, and decreased binding to P-selectin on the endothelium (CD62P) (Koenig, 1996; Rebuck, 1995). The decreased binding to P-selectin may reflect decreased expression of P-selectin glycoprotein ligand 1 (Tcharmtchi et al.,

2000), the major ligand for P-selectin on neutrophils. Moreover, Lorant and colleagues (1999) found reduced expression of P-selectin of mesenteric endothelial cells in premature infants compared with term neonates, a factor contributing to their decreased neutrophil influx.

Instead of decreased selectin expression by neonatal neutrophils, neonatal and adult neutrophils have similar basal surface levels of the heterodimeric β_2-integrins Mac-1 (CD11b/CD18) and LFA-1 (CD11a/CD18) (Abughali et al., 1994; Anderson et al., 1991; McEvoy et al., 1996; Smith et al., 1992), according to most studies. Activation-induced expression of Mac-1 from intracellular granule stores may be reduced in neonatal neutrophils, particularly in premature infants (Anderson et al., 1990), and this is associated with reduced adhesion to ICAM-1, the purified ligand for Mac-1, or to activated endothelium (Anderson et al., 1990). However, others have noted normal expression of Mac-1 and LFA-1 on both resting and stimulated neonatal neutrophils, surmising that the diminished expression in other studies was an artifact of the methods used to purify neutrophils (Adinolfi, 1988; Rebuck, 1995). Reddy and co-workers (1998) also found that reduced Mac-1 expression of activated neonatal neutrophils is almost entirely accounted for by an increase of immature neutrophils.

Chemotaxis of Neonatal Neutrophils

Chemotaxis of neonatal neutrophils in vitro is consistently less than that of adult neutrophils (Table 22-7) (Anderson et al., 1981; Hill, 1987; Klein et al., 1977; Merry et al., 1996; Pahwa, et al., 1977; Raghunathan et al., 1982; Tono-Oka et al., 1979). The chemotaxis of neonatal peripheral blood neutrophils seems to be more impaired than that of cord blood neutrophils (Pahwa et al., 1977). Neutrophil chemotaxis in premature infants is particularly impaired (Bektas et al., 1990; Carr et al., 1992; Kamran et al., 1993), especially in those with sepsis (Merry et al., 1996). Some researchers have found

TABLE 22-7 · CHEMOTAXIS OF NEONATAL GRANULOCYTES

Cell Source	Assay	Stimulus	% of Adult Response	Comment
Cord blood	3-µm Nucleopore filter	EAS	79	Normal random motility
Peripheral blood	Agarose	ZAS	27	Low until 2 yr old
Cord blood and peripheral blood	3-µm Nucleopore filter	EAS	53	Still low at 6 mo old; normal chemokinesis
Cord blood	Agarose	ZAS	≤30	More severe with lower concentrations of ZAS
Peripheral blood	5-µm cellulose filter and whole blood	ZAS	79	Ill neonates = 62%
Cord blood	Cellulose filter: 3, 5, or 8 µm	Casein	37–60	Normal random motility and normal chemokinesis
Cord blood	Agarose 3-µm cellulose	EAS	60–80 <15	Normal random motility
Peripheral blood	5-µm cellulose filter	ZAS	88	—
Peripheral blood	Cellulose filter	ZAS	~50	Equal to adult by 2 wk
Cord blood	Agarose	FMLP	70	Low until 1 yr old

EAS = endotoxin-activated serum; FMLP = N-foryml-methionine-leucine-phenylalanine peptide; ZAS = zymosan-activated serum.
Adapted from Lewis DB, Wilson CB. Developmental immunology and role of host defenses in neonatal susceptibility to infection. In Remington JS, Klein JO, eds. Infectious diseases of the fetus and newborn, ed 5. Philadelphia, WB Saunders, 2001.

that neonatal chemotaxis remains less than that of adult cells until at least 1 to 2 years old (Klein et al., 1977; Pahwa et al., 1977), whereas others (Carr et al., 1992) found more rapid maturation.

Neonatal neutrophils have a reduced response to chemotactic molecules including the bacterial peptide mimic, N-formyl-met-leu-phe (FMLP), leukotriene B$_4$, platelet-activating factor, IL-8, and zymosan-activated serum (Dos and Davidson, 1993; Merry et al., 1996; Tan and Davidson, 1995; Yasui et al., 1990). Most (Anderson et al., 1981; Sacchi and Hill, 1984; Strauss and Snyder, 1984), but not all (Nunoi et al., 1983), studies have found that the number and affinity of FMLP receptors are similar in adult and neonatal neutrophils, whereas receptors for C5a are reduced (Nybo et al., 1998).

Thus decreased chemotaxis to agents such as FMLP is attributable to limitations in events downstream of binding of the chemotaxin to its receptor, such as the generation of increased intracellular calcium, the generation of inositol phospholipid, and the alteration of cell membrane potential within the neutrophil (Sacchi and Hill, 1984; Santoro et al., 1995). However, not all responses to chemotactic factors are abnormal for neonatal neutrophils—for example, the upregulation of the type I complement receptor (CR1) is normal or at most slightly impaired (Bruce et al., 1987; Smith et al., 1990a), suggesting that postbinding signaling events are not globally impaired.

Neutrophil migration into the tissues may also be impaired by the reduced deformability of neonatal neutrophils, particularly immature forms (Anderson et al., 1984). This is because of the decreased capacity of the neonatal neutrophil to reorganize its cytoskeleton in response to stimulation, rather than decreases in tubulin, actin, or other cytoskeletal proteins (Hill, 1987; Merry et al., 1996; Raghunathan et al., 1982).

Chemotaxis by neonatal neutrophils is more impaired at low than at high concentrations of chemotactic factors (Boner et al., 1982). Therefore the decreased generation of chemotactic factors by neonatal serum (Boner et al., 1982; Pahwa et al., 1977) compounds the intrinsic deficits of neonatal neutrophils. However, the generation of all chemotactic agents is not impaired; for example, leukotriene B$_4$ production by neonatal neutrophils is similar to that of adult neutrophils (Kikawa et al., 1986).

Systemic treatment with G-CSF and GM-CSF increases the expression of CR3 (Mac1 or the C3bi receptor) on neonatal neutrophils (Goldman et al., 1998). In vitro exposure to IFN-γ and GM-CSF enhances chemotaxis of neonatal neutrophils (Cairo et al., 1989; Frenck et al., 1989; Hill et al., 1991). However, high concentrations of GM-CSF optimal for oxygen radical production may inhibit neonatal neutrophil chemotaxis (Cairo et al., 1989; Frenck et al., 1989). Cytokines do not completely normalize neonatal neutrophil chemotaxis when compared to adult neutrophils. Indomethacin, used clinically to close the ductus arteriosus in premature infants, impairs chemotaxis in both term and preterm neonates (Kamran et al., 1993).

Opsonization and Phagocytosis by Neonatal Neutrophils

Under optimal in vitro conditions, neutrophils from healthy term and preterm neonates bind and ingest gram-positive and gram-negative bacteria as well as or only slightly less efficiently than do adult neutrophils (Bektas et al., 1990; Harris et al., 1983; McCracken and Eichenwald, 1971). Opsonins, including IgG and complement, are reduced in the sera of preterm neonates. Thus bacterial phagocytosis by neutrophils from preterm neonates is reduced compared with term and adult neutrophils in whole blood assays (Falconer et al., 1995a, 1995b; Fujiwara et al., 1997).

This is primarily because of deficient opsonic activity rather than an intrinsic neutrophil defect (Fujiwara et al., 1997). The reduction of Fc receptors for IgG (e.g., FcγRIII, which is also known as CD16) and of receptors for complement (e.g., Mac-1, which is a receptor for the C3bi complement component and is also known as complement receptor 3) on premature neonatal neutrophils in comparison with neutrophils from term neonates and adults (Adinolfi et al., 1988; Bruce et al., 1987; Falconer et al., 1995a, 1995b; Payne and Fleit, 1996) may also contribute to reduced opsonization, but only modestly.

Neutrophils from term neonates also ingest bacteria less efficiently than those from adults at low concentrations of opsonins (Miller, 1979). The decreased opsonization of neonatal neutrophils is not attributable to decreased levels of opsonin receptors such as complement receptor 1 and Mac-1, which are similar in neutrophils from term neonates compared with adults (Falconer et al., 1995a, 1995b).

Neonatal neutrophil FcγRIII expression is similar to that of adult neutrophils in some studies (Carr and Davies, 1990; Falconer et al., 1995a, 1995b) and reduced in others (Maeda et al., 1996; Smith et al., 1990a). The decreased expression of FcγRIII by neutrophils from premature infants has also been reported (Carr and Davies, 1990). Because neutrophil FcγRIII surface expression is downregulated by exposure to activating cytokines (e.g., TNF-α and G-CSF) or during incipient apoptosis, decreased expression may not be an intrinsic property of neonatal neutrophils but rather a consequence of in vivo activation. As in the case of decreased neutrophil adhesion to activated endothelium, decreased activation-induced upregulation of Mac-1 β$_2$-integrin, the C3bi receptor, may also limit opsonic activity (Bruce et al., 1987; Jones et al., 1990; Qing et al., 1995; Smith et al., 1990a).

Microbicidal Activity of Neonatal Neutrophils

The killing of phagocytosed gram-positive and gram-negative bacteria and *Candida* by neutrophils from healthy neonates is similar to that of adult neutrophils (Dossett et al., 1969; McCracken and Eichenwald, 1971; Park et al., 1970). However, moderately decreased bactericidal activity has been noted against *Pseudomonas aeruginosa* (Cocchi and Marianelli, 1967), *S. aureus*

(Coen et al., 1969), and some (Becker et al., 1981; Stroobant et al., 1984)—but not all—strains of group B streptococci (Becker et al., 1981; Shigeoka et al., 1981). Defective neonatal neutrophil killing is more pronounced at high ratios of bacteria to neutrophils (Mills et al., 1979a).

Neutrophils from infected or stressed neonates, most of whom were premature and had sepsis, respiratory impairment, hyperbilirubinemia, premature rupture of membranes, and hypoglycemia, have clearly impaired microbicidal activity (Shigeoka et al., 1979; Wright et al., 1975), despite normal (Shigeoka et al., 1979) or only slightly decreased phagocytosis (Wright et al., 1975). Neutrophils from adults with similar illnesses may also have diminished microbicidal activity.

Neutrophils kill ingested microbes by oxygen-dependent (i.e., mediated by superoxide anion, peroxide, and hydroxyl radical), and oxygen-independent mechanisms (e.g., antimicrobial proteins and peptides). The generation of superoxide anion by neonatal (Ambruso et al., 1979; Shigeoka et al., 1981) and fetal (Newburger, 1982) neutrophils is similar to that by adult cells; however, Komatsu and co-workers (2001) noted reduced production in neutrophils from preterm neonates. Hydrogen peroxide generation by neutrophils from term and preterm neonates is also at least as efficient as that in adult cells (Fujiwara et al., 1997). In contrast, toxic hydroxyl radical generation and chemiluminescence, an index of oxygen radical production, may be decreased (Ambruso et al., 1979; Strauss et al., 1980; van Epps et al., 1978). The reduced generation of hydroxyl radicals may particularly contribute to impaired microbicidal activity for certain strains of group B streptococci (Stroobant et al., 1984; Wilson and Weaver, 1985).

Neonatal neutrophils have a reduced content of bactericidal permeability-increasing protein (Levy et al., 1999). Bactericidal permeability-increasing protein is stored in azurophilic granules. It binds to the lipid A portion of LPS with high affinity and directly kills gram-negative bacteria, in addition to acting as an opsonin (Iovine et al., 1997). This bactericidal permeability-increasing protein deficiency may particularly increase the susceptibility of the neonate to certain pathogens, such as the *E. coli* K1 strain.

Other azurophilic granule components, including defensin-1, lysozyme, and lactoferrin, are present in adult quantities (Levy et al., 1999). Yasui and colleagues (1988) found that newborn neutrophils had normal quantities of lysozyme and β-glucuronidase. However, activation-induced lactoferrin release by neonatal neutrophils may be reduced (Ambruso et al., 1984; Jones et al., 1990).

Cytokine Production by Neonatal Neutrophils

Neutrophils can synthesize cytokines, including IL-1, IL-8 (CXCL8), and TNF-α, which amplify inflammatory responses. Neonatal neutrophils have an increased capacity to produce IL-8, which binds to the CXCR1 and CXCR2 chemokine receptors, as compared with adult cells (Vancurova et al., 2001). This suggests a mechanism by which neutrophilic inflammation in neonates might be sustained, particularly in disorders such as chronic lung diseases of the newborn.

Summary

The most clearly defined deficiency of neonates' phagocytic defense is their diminished neutrophil storage pool. Neonatal neutrophils also have diminished adhesion to the endothelium and migration to sites of infection. Opsonic defects are present in the sera of premature infants. Phagocytic and killing defects are less pronounced, but they may contribute to decreased neutrophil function in situations in which opsonins or the local density of bacteria is high or the infant is stressed as a result of some other condition.

EOSINOPHILS OF THE FETUS AND NEONATE

In older children and adults, eosinophils normally represent only a few percent of circulating granulocytes and are increased in allergic disease, parasitic infection (particularly with metazoans), and in certain autoimmune and malignant diseases. By contrast, eosinophils in the fetus and neonate compose a sizable fraction of the total circulating granulocytes. At 18 to 30 weeks' gestation, granulocytes constitute approximately only 10% of the total circulating leukocytes, but eosinophils constitute 10% to 20% of the granulocytes (Forestier et al., 1986).

In preterm neonates, eosinophils are increased relative to term neonates, often reaching values of 1500 to 3000 cells/μl and constituting up to one third of the granulocytes in the first month after birth (Bhat and Scanlon, 1981). The number of eosinophils in inflammatory exudates is also increased in neonates, paralleling their greater numbers in the circulation (Smith et al., 1992).

Other neonatal conditions associated with eosinophilia include Rh disease, total parenteral nutrition, and blood transfusion (Bhat and Scanlon, 1981). In contrast to conditions such as allergic and parasitic diseases, eosinophilia in the neonate is not associated with increased circulating levels of IgE (Rothberg et al., 1983). The mechanisms or biologic significance of this eosinophilic tendency in the neonate is not known. Certain functional deficits of neonatal neutrophils, such as diminished L-selectin expression and leukocyte migration into tissues, have also been observed for neonatal eosinophils (Smith et al., 1992).

MONONUCLEAR PHAGOCYTES OF THE FETUS AND NEONATE

Production and Differentiation

Macrophages are detectable as early as 4 weeks of fetal life in the yolk sac and are found shortly thereafter in the liver and then in the bone marrow (Kelemen and Jaanossa, 1980) (see Chapter 6). The capacity of the fetus and the neonate to produce monocytes, as indicated by in vitro cultures of macrophage colonies of fetal liver, bone marrow, or blood is equal to or greater than that of adults (Ueno et al., 1981). The percent of monocytes in the blood in neonates is also equal to or greater than that in adults (Christensen, 1989; Weinberg et al., 1985).

The number of macrophages in various tissues of the human neonate is less well characterized. Limited data suggest that the human lung contains few macrophages until shortly before term (Alenghat and Esterly, 1984). The blood of premature neonates has increased numbers of damaged erythrocytes (e.g., Howell-Jolly bodies). These damaged cells are removed by splenic and perhaps liver macrophages (Kupffer's cells), so decreased macrophage number or function may exist in premature infants and during fetal life (Freedman et al., 1980).

Monocyte Migration and Delayed Cutaneous Hypersensitivity

The influx of monocytes into sites of inflammation and the subsequent inflammatory response is delayed and attenuated in neonates. After abrasion of adult skin, there is a rapid influx of neutrophils, but by 6 to 12 hours, mononuclear leukocytes become predominant (van Furth et al., 1979). This monocytic influx is delayed in term and preterm neonates, remaining below that seen in adult skin even after 24 hours (Table 22-8) (Bullock et al., 1969; Sheldon and Caldwell, 1963). This may be caused by diminished chemotaxis or decreased generation of chemotactic factors such as CC-chemokines (see Table 22-1). Monocyte chemotaxis, like that of polymorphonuclear leukocytes, is induced by a variety of chemotactic stimuli, including activated complement components, bacterial factors, leukotriene B_4, and certain chemokines, particularly those of the CC-chemokine family (see Table 22-1).

Most studies of cord blood monocytes have obtained similar amounts of chemotaxis in vitro compared with adult monocytes for a variety of chemotactic stimuli (Lewis and Wilson, 2001). However, in two studies of peripheral blood, neonatal monocyte chemotaxis was significantly less than that of adult monocytes (Klein et al., 1977; Raghunathan et al., 1982), and in one study it remained diminished until 6 to 10 years old (Klein et al., 1977). The mechanism for this reduced chemotaxis is unknown.

The expression of the β_2-integrin Mac-1 (CD11b/CD18) by resting and activated neonatal monocytes is either similar to (Adinolfi et al., 1988) or only slightly less than that of adult monocytes (Marwitz et al., 1988).

Delayed cutaneous hypersensitivity, which depends on an influx of monocytes and T lymphocytes into the site of antigen injection, is diminished in neonates (Fowler et al., 1960; Smith et al., 1997; Warwick et al., 1960), even when in vitro tests indicate T-cell sensitivity (e.g., antigen-specific cell proliferation). This suggests that a decreased influx of cells in vivo, including monocytes, contributes to this diminished response.

The capacity of fetal and neonatal mononuclear phagocytes to process and present antigen to T cells is discussed in the earlier section on antigen presentation.

Microbicidal Activity

Defense against Pyogenic Bacteria and Fungi

Neonatal monocytes ingest and kill *S. aureus*, *E. coli*, and group B streptococci as well as do adult monocytes (Becker et al., 1981; Hawes et al., 1980; Kretschmer et al., 1976; Orlowski et al., 1976; Weston et al., 1977), but the rate at which they ingest unopsonized latex particles is lower (Johnston, 1998; Schuit and Powell, 1980). Neonatal and adult monocytes have a similar capacity to produce microbicidal oxygen metabolites (Hawes et al., 1980; Speer et al., 1985). Neonatal monocytes also have comparable oxygen radical generation and microbicidal activity against staphylococci (Conley and Speert, 1991; Speer et al., 1988).

When cultured in vitro, neonatal and adult monocytes acquire many features of tissue-derived macrophages. These neonatal and adult monocyte-derived macrophages have a similar ability to phagocytose bacteria or other particles through receptors for mannose-fucose, IgG, complement, and opsonin-independent pathways. However, neonatal monocyte-derived macrophages are substantially less effective at killing ingested group B streptococci or *Candida albicans* than are adult cells and are relatively refractory to the enhancement of killing by treatment with IFN-γ (Marodi et al., 1994, 2000). In contrast, GM-CSF treatment can increase the microbicidal activity of neonatal monocyte-derived macrophages.

Because tissue macrophages are derived from monocytes, it might be assumed that neonatal tissue macrophages would be equally mature. However, local tissue conditions in neonates may differ and result in decreased tissue macrophage function. Indeed, neonatal macrophages from bronchial fluid were less effective at killing the yeast form of *Candida* than adult alveolar macrophages (D'Ambola et al., 1988). The results of similar studies of newborn and particularly premature

TABLE 22-8 · DELAYED MONOCYTE RESPONSE IN REBUCK SKIN WINDOWS IN HUMAN NEONATES AND ADULTS

Population	% Monocytes			
	2 hr	4 hr	6 hr	24 hr
Premature	4	13	18	30
Term <24 hr	4	9	13	20
Term 24–108 hr	2	7	11	19
Adult	5	21	38	76

From Lewis DB, Wilson CB. Developmental immunology and role of host defenses in neonatal susceptibility to infection. In Remington JS, Klein JO, eds. Infectious diseases of the fetus and newborn, ed 5. Philadelphia, WB Saunders, 2001.

newborn alveolar macrophages of monkeys, rabbits, and rats have revealed reduced phagocytic and microbicidal activity (Lewis and Wilson, 2001).

Defense against Intracellular Pathogens

Certain neonatal pathogens, including all viruses and some nonviral pathogens, require replication, including intracellular replication. Defense against obligatory or facultative intracellular pathogens is mediated by factors that (1) limit their entry into host cells, (2) inhibit their intracellular replication, (3) kill them intracellularly, or (4) destroy infected cells.

Neonatal monocytes can ingest and kill *Toxoplasma* and *Listeria* (Berman and Johnson, 1978; Wilson and Haas, 1984). Both cultured blood monocytes and placental macrophages from human neonates activated with IFN-γ kill or restrict the growth of these neonatal pathogens as well as adult cells. In contrast, IFN-γ treatment did not activate monocyte-derived macrophages from human neonates to kill *C. albicans* or to generate superoxide anion as effectively as it did for adult cells (Marodi et al., 1994).

Neonatal monocytes and monocyte-derived macrophages and fetal placental macrophages are not more permissive than adult cells of the replication of HSV (Mintz et al., 1980; Plaeger-Marshall et al., 1989). Monocytes and macrophages can also restrict viral replication by lysing infected cells both in the absence or presence of antibody. Neonatal monocytes may be slightly less cytotoxic for HSV-infected cells than adult cells in the absence of antibody, but equivalent to adult cells in the presence of antibody (Kohl, 1985).

Exogenous IFN-γ enhances resistance to *Listeria* and HSV infection for neonatal rodents, suggesting that a neonatal IFN-γ deficiency may be present and that treatment with IFN-γ (or other cytokines) might be beneficial in controlling intracellular infection. The role of IFN-γ was discussed earlier, in the section Neonatal T-Cell Function.

Cytokine and Inflammatory Mediator Production

CD14 and TLR-4 are components of a ligand-binding receptor for LPS of gram-negative bacteria. CD14 is also a component of other receptors, such as those recognizing the peptidoglycan of gram-positive bacteria. Ligation of CD14 by mononuclear phagocytes induces cytokine production (Guha and Mackman, 2001). Neonatal and adult monocytes express equivalent amounts of CD14 in most studies (Cohen et al., 1995; Kampalath et al., 1998), but Liu and colleagues (2001a) found a subtle decrease (Liu et al., 2001a). The neonatal expression of TLRs, including TLR-2, which is triggered by peptidoglycan and a variety of other bacterial products (Kaisho and Akira, 2002); TLR-3, which is triggered by double-stranded RNA (Alexopoulou et al., 2001); TLR-4, the LPS receptor; and TLR-9, which is triggered by DNA with unmethylated CpG dinu-

cleotides (Kaisho and Akira, 2002), is not known. There is a deficiency of cord blood for an as-yet uncharacterized plasma protein that facilitates the response of monocytes to LPS (Cohen et al., 1995).

Monocytes from term neonates stimulated with such agonists as LPS or IL-1 produce mediators that enhance neutrophil and monocyte production (e.g., G-CSF, GM-CSF, and M-CSF) or contribute to inflammation and acute-phase responses (e.g., IL-1, TNF-α, IL-6, IL-8, and leukotriene B_4) in amounts ranging from 25% to 75% of that produced by adult cells (see Table 22-2). In some studies, the production of G-CSF, IL-1, and IL-6 by neonatal monocytes is similar to that of adult cells (Bessler et al., 1999; Burchett et al., 1988; Chang et al., 1994; Cohen et al., 1995; English et al., 1992; Lee et al., 1996; Rowen et al., 1995; Sautois et al., 1997; Schibler et al., 1993). The neonatal monocyte production of IL-8 and IL-1α may even be greater than in adult cells (Hebra et al., 2001; Krampera et al., 2000) Thus any neonatal cytokine production defect is subtle. However, monocytes from premature neonates produce less TNF-α, IL-1β, and IL-6 in response to LPS than do term monocytes (Bessler et al., 1999).

Neonatal monocytes produce substantial amounts of TNF-α in response to heat-inactivated group B streptococci (Vallejo et al., 2000), but their IL-8 production is reduced compared with that of adult cells (Rowen et al., 1995). Neonatal mononuclear cells produce IL-12 and IFN-γ in response to group B streptococci, but in significantly lower amounts than with similarly treated adult cells (Joyner et al., 2000; Rowen et al., 1995).

Monocyte-derived and placental (tissue) macrophages from term neonates have reduced production of TNF-α compared with that of macrophages derived from peripheral blood monocytes of adults (Burchett et al., 1988). IFN-γ is also less effective in increasing TNF-α production by neonatal macrophages than by adult macrophages (Burchett et al., 1988). Deficient IFN-γ production by neonatal T cells may compound the deficit in TNF-α production. Indeed, neonatal rats have diminished resistance to *Listeria* infection associated with decreased IFN-γ and TNF-α production (Bortolussi et al., 1989, 1992).

The results of most studies suggest that neonatal monocytes have a modest deficiency in the production of proinflammatory cytokines, but this is balanced by reduced production of anti-inflammatory cytokines, such as IL-10 and transforming growth factor-beta (Chang et al., 1994; Chheda, 1996; Kotiranta-Ainamo et al., 1997). This may not apply to tissue macrophages, particularly in certain pathologic contexts. Alveolar macrophages from preterm neonates with respiratory distress syndrome produce less IL-10 in vivo relative to TNF-α than do alveolar macrophages from term neonates (Blahnik et al., 2001; Jones et al., 1996). This imbalance may predispose the prematurely born infant to the development of inflammatory lung disease.

Neonatal monocyte production of cytokines that enhance defenses against intracellular pathogens is reduced to a modest extent. IFN-α/β production by neonatal lymphocytes and monocytes is equivalent to that of adult cells for a variety of inducers, including

HSV and other viruses (Ray, 1970), but Cederblad and co-workers (1990) found that HSV-stimulated IFN production was diminished. The reason for these differing results is unclear. IL-12 and IL-15 production by mononuclear cells (presumably mainly by monocytes) from term neonates after stimulation with LPS was approximately 25% that of adult cells (Lee et al., 1996; Qian et al., 1997). In contrast, neonatal and adult blood mononuclear cells stimulated with *S. aureus* or meningococcal outer membrane proteins produce equivalent amounts of IL-12 (Lee et al., 1996; Perez-Melgosa et al., 2001; Qian et al., 1997; Scott et al., 1997).

Collectively, these results suggest a variable diminution in cytokine production by monocytes from neonates. However, Dembinski and colleagues (2002) used short-term whole blood assays, finding that LPS-stimulated cord blood produced substantially higher levels of IL-6 and IL-8 than does adult peripheral blood. These results likely reflect monocyte cytokine production, but indirect effects mediated by cytokines produced by NK cells and T cells may also contribute.

CD40 Expression by Neonatal Monocytes

Engagement of CD40 on monocytes by CD40 ligand of activated T cells induces proinflammatory cytokines (IL-1, TNF-α, and IL-12), prevents monocyte apoptosis, and promotes monocyte differentiation into dendritic cells in the absence of GM-CSF (Schonbeck and Libby, 2001). Because the expression of neonatal T-cell CD40 ligand may be diminished (see the Tumor Necrosis Factor Ligand Family Members section earlier), the activation of monocytes by CD40 ligand/CD40 interactions may be compromised. In addition, Sorg and co-workers (2001) reported that circulating neonatal monocytes obtained from cord blood express less CD40 than monocytes obtained from the peripheral blood of adults who have been treated with G-CSF before pheresis. This could further limit the monocyte activation by this pathway. However, this difference in CD40 expression needs to be confirmed by using cells from adults not treated with G-CSF, because this cytokine upregulates CD40 monocyte expression (Alderson et al., 1993). Moreover, others have reported that neonatal monocytes and adult monocytes express similar low levels of CD40 (Varis et al., 2001).

Chemokine Production

Using bioassays for total cytokines chemotactic for monocytes, Kretschmer and co-workers (1976) and Hawes and colleagues (1980) found no differences between adult and neonatal cells. This does not exclude decreased production of individual chemokines with particular stimuli. Indeed, cord blood mononuclear cells stimulated with mitogen generate 20% to 25% of the CC-chemokine MIP-1α (CCL3) produced by adult cells (Chang et al., 1994). To what extent this decreased

chemokine production is attributable to monocytes versus other cell types is not known.

Summary

Circulating monocytes from neonates are normal in number and similar to adult cells in their phagocytic and microbicidal activity. The diminished chemotactic activity of neonatal monocytes may delay or reduce their presence at sites of infection. Tissue macrophages from the neonates of certain animal species may have reduced phagocytosis and microbicidal activity, and this may also apply to humans. The capacity of mononuclear phagocytes to produce both proinflammatory and anti-inflammatory cytokines may be modestly reduced in term neonates and further reduced in preterm neonates. This neonatal cytokine deficiency may be compounded by the concomitant deficiency of IFN-γ production by neonatal T cells and NK cells, as well as their inability to respond fully to IFN-γ.

HUMORAL MEDIATORS OF INFLAMMATION AND OPSONIZATION

Introduction

Infection and inflammation induce or activate multiple mediators. Some of these are derived from components present in plasma, including complement components, mannan-binding lectin (MBL), fibronectin, coagulation factors, and components of the kinin system. Others, such as products of arachidonic acid metabolism (prostaglandins, platelet-activating factor, and leukotrienes), endorphins, amines (including histamine, catecholamines, and serotonin), and lysosomal enzymes, are produced and released from leukocytes, endothelial cells, and other cells. The production and interaction of these mediators are critical determinants of the outcome of infection (see Chapters 7 and 10).

Findings from experimental studies implicate certain of these mediators in the unfavorable response of the newborn animal to infection (Gibson et al., 1992; Hemming et al., 1984; O'Brien et al., 1985; Peevy et al., 1985) and suggest that therapy directed toward modulating their production would be beneficial. A better understanding of the relative role of these mediators in particular clinical situations such as septic shock will be required to develop therapies in which these mediators or their effects are modulated.

Complement

Complement Components and Activation

The complement system is composed of serum proteins that are activated in an orderly and sequential cascade (see Chapter 7). Interaction occurs along one of two pathways, the classic and the alternative pathway, that converge in a final common pathway in which C3b and terminal membrane attack complex are generated. The hepatocyte is the principal cell that synthesizes complement components, but mononuclear phagocytes can also synthesize complement proteins except those of the terminal membrane attack complex.

Activation of the classical pathway is initiated when antibodies capable of fixing complement to their Fc portion (IgM, IgG1, IgG2, and IgG3) complex with microbial or other antigens and bind C1. C1 is composed of three different proteins—C1q, C1r, and C1s—which are sequentially bound. Bound C1 then acts enzymatically on C4 and C2, components of which (C2a, C4b) are bound to the antigen. The C4b2a complex then acts on C3 to form C3b, which remains bound to the antigen, and C3a, which is released and serves as an inflammatory mediator.

MBL can also activate the classic complement pathway. In this case, two proteases specific for MBL are activated instead of C1r and C1s to initiate cleavage of C4 and C2. C-reactive protein, a host-derived acute-phase reactant that binds to C-type carbohydrate found in certain bacteria, particularly *S. pneumoniae,* may also substitute for antibody in the activation of the classic pathway.

Bound C3b, C4b, and C2a act together on C5 to release C5a. The larger C5b binds to a complex of the terminal complement components, C6, C7, C8, and C9. This C5b6789 complex, which is also known as the membrane attack complex, forms pores in cell membranes and causes cytolysis. The smaller fragment, C5a, serves as a chemoattractant and inflammatory mediator.

The alternative pathway is phylogenetically older and is constitutively active. Antibody is not required for its activation, but it can be facilitated by the $F(ab')_2$ portion of antibody. The continuous, but inefficient, interaction of factor B with factor D and C3 in the fluid phase generates low levels of C3b and Bb continuously. If C3b and Bb bind to a microorganism, they are effective in attracting and cleaving C3 to yield bound C3b. This interaction is facilitated by factor P (properdin) and inhibited by alternative pathway factors H and I.

Bacteria vary in their capacity to activate the alternative pathway, determined by their ability to bind C3b and to protect the complex of C3b and Bb from the inhibitory effects of factors H and I. Sialic acid, a component of several bacterial polysaccharide capsules, including those of group B streptococci and *E. coli* K1, favors factor H binding. Thus some virulent pathogens are protected from the alternative pathway by their capsules, and specific antibody is needed for their efficient opsonization. The classic pathway, by creating particle-bound C3b, also activates the alternative pathway, thus serving as an autocatalytic amplification mechanism. This may be particularly important when antibody is limited in amount or binding affinity.

Consequences of Complement Activation

A key consequence of complement activation is the binding of complement components to the microbial surface, which facilitates microbial killing or removal. C3b binds to CR1 receptors. C3b is also cleaved to C3bi, which binds to the CR3 receptor (Mac-1 or Cd11b/CD18) and CR4 receptor (CD11c/CD18). These C3bi receptors are β_2-integrin molecules, which are found on neutrophils, macrophages, and certain other cell types, and also play a role in cellular adhesion. Along with IgG antibody, which binds to Fc receptors on these phagocytes, C3b and C3bi promote ingestion (phagocytosis) of bacteria and fungi.

C3b is also a key component of the C5a convertase, which leads to the cleavage of C5, the release of C5a into the fluid phase, and the binding of C5b on the microbial surface. C5b acts to assemble the membrane attack complex, consisting of C5b and the terminal C6-C9 complement components. Once assembled, this complex lyses the cell to which it is bound. This mechanism is the principal defense mechanism against meningococci and gonococci. All gram-positive organisms and many gram-negative bacteria are resistant to complement lysis. As a result, the complement system may play a limited role in defense against common neonatal bacterial pathogens.

The C5a, and to a lesser extent, C3a, complement cleavage products that are released into the fluid phase cause vasodilation and increase vascular permeability. C5a is also a potent chemotactic factor for neutrophils, monocytes, and eosinophils. It stimulates these cells to degranulate, adhere to endothelium, and release leukotrienes, which themselves are potent mediators of inflammation.

Complement facilitates B-cell responses to T-cell–dependent antigens. C3d bound to antigen–antibody complexes (the antibody produced by initial B-cell response) may engage the B-cell C3d receptor (CD21), along with the BCR (surface immunoglobulin along with the associated Igα and Igβ chains involved in signal transduction), to amplify the antibody response. Mice genetically deficient in C3, C4, or the C3b and C3d complement receptors have diminished antibody responses to protein antigens.

Complement in the Fetus and Neonate

Little, if any, maternal complement is transferred to the fetus. Complement synthesis is detected in fetal tissues as early as 6 to 14 weeks' gestation, depending on the specific complement component and tissue examined (Ainbender et al., 1982; Gitlin and Biasucci, 1969).

Table 22-9 summarizes studies of the total hemolytic activity of the classic pathway (CH_{50}), alternative pathway (AH_{50}), and individual complement components in neonates. There is substantial individual variability such that some term neonates have individual complement components or CH_{50} or AH_{50} within the adult range. The hemolytic activity of the alternative pathway and

TABLE 22-9 · SUMMARY OF PUBLISHED
COMPLEMENT LEVELS IN NEONATES

Complement Component	Mean % of Adult Levels	
	Term Neonate*	Preterm Neonate*
CH_{50}	56–90 (4)	45–71 (3)
AP_{50}	49–65 (3)	40–51 (2)
C1q	65–90 (3)	—
C4	60–100 (4)	27–58 (2)
C2	76–100 (2)	42–91 (3)
C3	60–100 (5)	96 (1)
C5	75 (1)	—
C6	47 (1)	—
C7	67 (1)	—
C8	~20 (1)	—
C9	<20 (2)	—
B	35–59 (8)	36–50 (3)
P	33–71 (5)	13–65 (2)
H	61 (1)	—
C3bi	55 (1)	—

*Numbers in parentheses indicate the number of studies.
From Lewis DB, Wilson CB. Developmental immunology and role of host defenses in neonatal susceptibility to infection. In Remington JS, Klein JO, eds. Infectious diseases of the fetus and newborn, ed 4. Philadelphia, WB Saunders, 1994.

the levels of alternative pathway components (B and P) are more consistently decreased than those of the classic pathway.

There is also a marked neonatal deficiency of the terminal complement component C9 (Wolach et al., 1997), which is important for the lysis of certain gram-negative bacteria; furthermore, this deficiency correlates with poor killing of these organisms. The C9 deficiency of newborn sera is more important in the inefficient killing of E. coli K1 than is a deficiency of specific IgG antibodies (Lassiter et al., 1992). A functional deficiency of C3, which is deposited on microbes but not efficiently crosslinked, may also contribute to decreased opsonic activity (Zach and Hostetter, 1989).

Preterm infants have a more consistent decrease in both classic and alternative pathway hemolytic activity (Johnston et al., 1979) and levels of individual components such as C3 and C4 (Drossou et al., 1995) than do term infants. Mature but small-for-gestational-age neonates have CH_{50} and AH_{50} values similar to those of term neonates (Notarangelo et al., 1984). Component levels increase after birth and reach adult values between 6 and 18 months old (Davis et al., 1979).

Fibronectin

Fibronectin, a ubiquitous glycoprotein, exists in two forms: circulating and cellular (see Chapter 10). The liver synthesizes most of the plasma fibronectin, whereas fibroblasts, endothelial cells, and other cell types synthesize cellular fibronectin (Matsuura and Hakomori, 1985; Peters et al., 1986).

Fibronectin augments the initial neutrophil and monocyte adherence to endothelium as part of their migration from the blood to the tissues (Marino et al., 1985). Fibronectin also has opsonic properties in its binding to certain bacteria, including staphylococci and group B streptococci, but it is a less efficient opsonin than antibody or complement. Fibronectin may also have a direct phagocytosis-enhancing effect on monocytes and stimulated neutrophils (Pommier et al., 1984). Fibronectin fragments have chemotactic activity for mononuclear phagocytes (Norris et al., 1982). Fibronectin also activates TLR-4 (Okamura et al., 2001), with LPS-like effects on mononuclear phagocyte and dendritic cell activation.

Plasma fibronectin concentrations are low in neonates, particularly in premature infants (Barnard and Arthur, 1983; Drossou et al., 1995; Gerdes et al., 1983; Yoder et al., 1983). Levels may be further reduced in sepsis, birth asphyxia, and respiratory distress syndrome (Gerdes et al., 1983; Yoder et al., 1983). Plasma fibronectin concentrations approach the lower limit of adult normal limits by 1 year of age (McCafferty et al., 1983).

C-Reactive Protein

C-reactive protein (see Chapter 10) can activate the classical pathway when bound to certain gram-positive bacteria. It does not cross the placenta. Term and preterm neonates can produce this protein as well as can adults (Ainbender et al., 1982). Sera levels may be higher in healthy neonates than in healthy adults, and high levels can be used in the diagnosis of neonatal sepsis.

Mannan-Binding Lectin

With rare exceptions, glycoproteins containing terminal mannose sugars are not found on extracellular proteins in mammals, because these mannose residues are further modified in the endoplasmic reticulum before transport through the Golgi apparatus. In contrast, terminal mannose, fucose, glucose, and N-acetyl glucosamine are found on the surfaces of gram-positive and gram-negative bacteria, mycobacteria, yeast, and certain viruses and parasites (Epstein et al., 1996).

Tissue macrophages, but not neutrophils or monocytes, contain mannose-fucose receptors. These macrophages are activated for phagocytosis and killing by binding to microbial mannose-containing carbohydrate polymers. The liver synthesizes MBL (also referred to as *mannose-binding protein*), which is homologous to the tissue macrophage mannose-fucose receptor and which can bind to these organisms and serve as an opsonin for ingestion by neutrophils and circulating monocytes.

MBL is a calcium-dependent lectin that circulates as an 18-unit polymer composed of 3 to 6 identical homotrimeric structural units (see Chapter 10). It is homologous to C1q and thus can bind to C1q receptors on mononuclear phagocytes, facilitating the phagocytosis of microbes to which it is bound. MBL also activates the classical complement pathway and is an acute-phase protein, so that its plasma concentration increases in inflammation. The engagement of MBL is impeded by capsular polysaccharides of most virulent gram-negative pathogens.

Approximately 5% to 7% of the population is deficient in MBL because of a polymorphism in codon 54 (Lau et al., 1995; Super et al., 1989). Some individuals with MBL deficiency are more susceptible to infection, but most are not, suggesting that MBL plays an auxiliary—rather than a critical—role in host defense. The serum concentration of MBL of term neonates is similar to that in adults. Values in preterm neonates are approximately 50% less (Lau et al., 1995; Super et al., 1989), but no study links this reduction to their increased risk of infection (Lau et al., 1995).

Surfactant Apoproteins

Surfactant apoproteins A and D are members of the same collectin family to which MBL belongs (Lu, 1997) (see Chapter 10). They are synthesized by type II alveolar epithelial cells, Clara cells (nonciliated, nonmucous secretory cells of the airway), and certain extrapulmonary cell types (Epstein et al., 1996). Like MBL, surfactant apoprotein A binds to mannose-glucose polymers of gram-positive and gram-negative bacteria, *Mycobacteria,* and yeast. Mice made deficient in surfactant apoprotein A are much more susceptible to pulmonary infection with group B streptococci, *P. aeruginosa* (LeVine et al., 1997, 1998), and perhaps other microbes. These results raise the possibility that surfactant deficiency may be one factor in the greater risk of the preterm neonate for pulmonary infections. The biologic role of surfactant apoprotein D is uncertain.

Lipopolysaccharide-Binding Protein

The liver produces LPS-binding protein (LBP) constitutively and as an acute-phase protein. LBP facilitates the binding of LPS to the high-affinity CD14 receptor, which is expressed by mononuclear phagocytes and to a lesser extent by neutrophils (Wright, 1991) and presumably thereafter to TLR-4 (Akira et al., 2001). LPB and CD14 act together to lower by several orders of magnitude the concentration of LPS needed to prime or activate macrophages and the binding of gram-negative bacteria to these cells.

The level of LBP protein in neonates is not known. However, a deficiency of neonatal cord blood for an as-yet uncharacterized plasma protein that facilitates the response of monocytes to lipopolysaccharide has been reported (Cohen et al., 1995).

Serum Opsonic Activity

Serum opsonic activity reflects its ability to enhance phagocytosis (or phagocytosis and killing) of a particular organism or particle. Some organisms are effective activators of the alternative pathway, whereas others require antibody to activate complement. Thus depending on the organism or particle tested, opsonic activity reflects specific antibody, MBL, classic or alternative complement pathway hemolytic activity, or a combination of these factors. For this reason, it is not surprising that the efficiency with which neonatal sera opsonize varies greatly with the microbe tested.

For example, the opsonization of *S. aureus* is normal for neonatal sera in all studies, whereas the opsonization of some—but not all—strains of group B streptococci, *S. pneumoniae, E. coli,* and other gram-negative rods is decreased (Dossett et al., 1969; Geelen et al., 1990; Miller, 1979; Winkelstein et al., 1979). Neonatal sera are less able to opsonize organisms through antibody-independent complement activation (i.e., the activation of the alternative pathway and of the classic pathway by MBL) than strains that bind antibody and activate the classic complement pathway (Kobayashi and Usui, 1982; Marodi et al., 1985; Mills et al., 1979b). This difference is not attributable to a limitation in the ability of neonatal sera to activate the alternative pathway (Adamkin et al., 1978).

These findings, and the observation that neonatal sera are less effective in the opsonization of certain organisms (e.g., group B streptococci) through the CH_{50} in the absence of antibody (Eads et al., 1982), suggest a relative immaturity for the neonate of complement-dependent and antibody-independent opsonization. This deficiency is greater in sera from premature neonates and may be further impaired by the depletion of complement components in the presence of neonatal sepsis (Edwards and Baker, 2001).

Chemotactic Factor Generation

Complement activation also generates fluid-phase components with chemotactic activity for neutrophils and monocytes, most of which are derived from C5a. Sera from term neonates generate less chemotactic activity in vitro than adult sera, even in the presence of antigen–antibody complexes or pathogen plus specific antibody (Anderson et al., 1983; Miller, 1971; Pahwa et al., 1977). This most likely reflects a limitation of complement activation or the decreased generation of a chemotactic factor inactivator (Tannous et al., 1982). This reduced generation of chemotactic activity is even more striking in the sera of preterm neonates (Anderson et al., 1983). Because both term and preterm infants can generate substantial amounts of activated complement products in response to infection, C5a deficiency is not likely to be implicated in this abnormality (Zilow et al., 1997).

Summary

Compared with adults, neonates have moderately diminished AH_{50} activity, slightly diminished CH_{50} activity, and severely diminished activity of the terminal complement components, especially C9. Fibronectin and MBL concentrations are also reduced. These deficiencies correlate with diminished opsonic activity of neonatal sera, particularly when specific antibody levels are low or absent. The generation of complement-derived chemotactic activity is also moderately diminished.

These defects are greater in preterm than in term neonates. Preterm neonates may also have compromised lung defenses caused by reduced levels of surfactant apoprotein A.

These decreased functions, along with reduced phagocyte function, contribute to an attenuated inflammatory response and impaired bacterial clearance in neonates, particularly premature neonates.

REFERENCES

Aase JM, Noren GR, Reddy DV, St. Geme JW Jr. Mumps-virus infection in pregnant women and the immunologic response of their offspring. N Engl J Med 286:1379–1382, 1972.

Abughali N, Berger M, Tosi MF. Deficient total cell content of CR3 (CD11b) in neonatal neutrophils. Blood 83:1086–1092, 1994.

Adamkin D, Stitzel A, Urmson J, Farnett ML, Post E, Spitzer R. Activity of the alternative pathway of complement in the newborn infant. J Pediatr 93:604–608, 1978.

Adams EJ, Parham P. Species-specific evolution of MHC class I genes in the higher primates. Immunol Rev 183:41–64, 2001.

Adderson EE, Shackelford PG, Quinn A, Carroll WL. Restricted Ig H chain V gene usage in the human antibody response to *Haemophilus influenzae* type b capsular polysaccharide. J Immunol 147:1667–1674, 1991.

Adenyi-Jones SC, Faden H, Ferdon MB, Kwong MS, Ogra PL. Systemic and local immune responses to enhanced-potency inactivated poliovirus vaccine in premature and term infants. J Pediatr 120:686–689, 1992.

Adinolfi M, Cheetham M, Lee T, Rodin A. Ontogeny of human complement receptors CR1 and CR3: expression of these molecules on monocytes and neutrophils from maternal, newborn and fetal samples. Eur J Immunol 18:565–569, 1988.

Aggarwal S, Gollapudi S, Yel L, Gupta AS, Gupta S. TNF-alpha–induced apoptosis in neonatal lymphocytes: TNFRp55 expression and downstream pathways of apoptosis. Genes Immun 1:271–279, 2000.

Aggarwal S, Gupta A, Nagata S, Gupta S. Programmed cell death (apoptosis) in cord blood lymphocytes. J Clin Immunol 17:63–73, 1997.

Ainbender E, Cabatu EE, Guzman DM, Sweet AY. Serum C-reactive protein and problems of newborn infants. J Pediatr 101:438–440, 1982.

Aiuti A, Tavian M, Cipponi A, Ficara F, Zappone E, Hoxie J, Peault B, Bordignon C. Expression of CXCR4, the receptor for stromal cell-derived factor-1 on fetal and adult human lympho-hematopoietic progenitors. Eur J Immunol 29:1823–1831, 1999.

Akbar AN, Salmon M, Ivory K, Taki S, Pilling D, Janossy G. Human CD4+CD45R0+ and CD4+CD45RA+ T cells synergize in response to alloantigens. Eur J Immunol 21:2517–2522, 1991.

Akira S, Takeda K, Kaisho T. Toll-like receptors: critical proteins linking innate and acquired immunity. Nat Immunol 2:675–680, 2001.

Alderson MR, Armitage RJ, Tough TW, Strockbine L, Fanslow WC, Spriggs MK. CD40 expression by human monocytes: regulation by cytokines and activation of monocytes by the ligand for CD40. J Exp Med 178:669–674, 1993.

Alenghat E, Esterly JR. Alveolar macrophages in perinatal infants. Pediatrics 74:221–223, 1984.

Alexopoulou L, Holt AC, Medzhitov R, Flavell RA. Recognition of double-stranded RNA and activation of NF-kappa B by Toll-like receptor 3. Nature 413:732–738, 2001.

Alford CA Jr, Stagno S, Reynolds DW. Diagnosis of chronic perinatal infections. Am J Dis Child 129:455–463, 1975.

Allansmith M, McClellan BH, Butterworth M, Maloney JR. The development of immunoglobulin levels in man. J Pediatr 72:276–290, 1968.

Ambrosino DM, Delaney NR, Shamberger RC. Human polysaccharide-specific B cells are responsive to pokeweed mitogen and IL-6. J Immunol 144:1221–1226, 1990.

Ambruso DR, Altenburger KM, Johnston RB Jr. Defective oxidative metabolism in newborn neutrophils: discrepancy between superoxide anion and hydroxyl radical generation. Pediatrics 64:722–725, 1979.

Ambruso DR, Bentwood B, Henson PM, Johnston RB Jr. Oxidative metabolism of cord blood neutrophils: relationship to content and degranulation of cytoplasmic granules. Pediatr Res 18:1148–1153, 1984.

Anderson DC, Hughes BJ, Smith CW. Abnormal mobility of neonatal polymorphonuclear leukocytes. Relationship to impaired redistribution of surface adhesion sites by chemotactic factor or colchicine. J Clin Invest 68:863–874, 1981.

Anderson DC, Hughes BJ, Edwards MS, Buffone GJ, Baker CJ. Impaired chemotaxigenesis by type III group B streptococci in neonatal sera: relationship to diminished concentration of specific anticapsular antibody and abnormalities of serum complement. Pediatr Res 17:496–502, 1983.

Anderson DC, Hughes BJ, Wible LJ, Perry GJ, Smith CW, Brinkley BR. Impaired motility of neonatal PMN leukocytes: relationship to abnormalities of cell orientation and assembly of microtubules in chemotactic gradients. J Leukoc Biol 36:1–15, 1984.

Anderson DC, Rothlein R, Marlin SD, Krater SS, Smith CW. Impaired transendothelial migration by neonatal neutrophils: abnormalities of Mac-1 (CD11b/CD18)-dependent adherence reactions. Blood 76:2613–2621, 1990.

Anderson DC, Abbassi O, Kishimoto TK, Koenig JM, McIntire LV, Smith CW. Diminished lectin-, epidermal growth factor-, complement binding domain-cell adhesion molecule-1 on neonatal neutrophils underlies their impaired CD18-independent adhesion to endothelial cells in vitro. J Immunol 146:3372–3379, 1991.

Anderson EL, Kennedy DJ, Geldmacher KM, Donnelly J, Mendelman PM. Immunogenicity of heptavalent pneumococcal conjugate vaccine in infants. J Pediatr 128:649–653, 1996.

Andersson U, Bird AG, Britton BS, Palacios R. Humoral and cellular immunity in humans studied at the cell level from birth to two years of age. Immunol Rev 57:1–38, 1981.

Ansart-Pirenne H, Soulimani N, Tartour E, Blot P, Sterkers G. Defective IL2 gene expression in newborn is accompanied with impaired tyrosine-phosphorylation in T cells. Pediatr Res 45:409–413, 1999.

Antin JH, Emerson SG, Martin P, Gadol N, Ault KA. Leu-1+ (CD5+) B cells. A major lymphoid subpopulation in human fetal spleen: phenotypic and functional studies. J Immunol 136:505–510, 1986.

Appay V, Dunbar PR, Callan M, Klenerman P, Gillespie GM, Papagno L, Ogg GS, King A, Lechner F, Spina CA, Little S, Havlir DV, Richman DD, Gruener N, Pape G, Waters A, Easterbrook P, Salio M, Cerundolo V, McMichael AJ, Rowland-Jones SL. Memory CD8+ T cells vary in differentiation phenotype in different persistent virus infections. Nat Med 8:379–385, 2002.

Arakawa-Hoyt J, Dao MA, Thiemann F, Hao QL, Ertl DC, Weinberg KI, Crooks GM, Nolta JA. The number and generative capacity of human B lymphocyte progenitors, measured in vitro and in vivo, is higher in umbilical cord blood than in adult or pediatric bone marrow. Bone Marrow Transplant 24:1167–1176, 1999.

Arnon TI, Lev M, Katz G, Chernobrov Y, Porgador A, Mandelboim O. Recognition of viral hemagglutinins by NKp44 but not by NKp30. Eur J Immunol 31:2680–2689, 2001.

Arstila TP, Casrouge A, Baron V, Even J, Kanellopoulos J, Kourilsky P. A direct estimate of the human alpha/beta T cell receptor diversity. Science 286:958–961, 1999.

Asano S, Akaike Y, Muramatsu T, Mochizuki M, Tsuda T, Wakasa H. Immunohistologic detection of the primary follicle (PF) in human fetal and newborn lymph node anlages. Pathol Res Pract 189:921–927, 1993.

Asma GE, Van den Bergh RL, Vossen JM. Use of monoclonal antibodies in a study of the development of T lymphocytes in the human fetus. Clin Exp Immunol 53:429–436, 1983.

Auewarakul P, Sangsiriwut K, Pattanapanyasat K, Wasi C, Lee TH. Age-dependent expression of the HIV-1 coreceptor CCR5 on CD4+ lymphocytes in children. J Acquir Immune Defic Syndr 24:285–287, 2000.

Avrech OM, Samra Z, Lazarovich Z, Caspi E, Jacobovich A, Sompolinsky D. Efficacy of the placental barrier for immunoglobulins: correlations between maternal, paternal and fetal immunoglobulin levels. Int Arch Allergy Immunol 103:160–165, 1994.

Azuma M, Phillips JH, Lanier LL. CD28− T lymphocytes. Antigenic and functional properties. J Immunol 150:1147–1159, 1993a.

Azuma M, Cayabyab M, Phillips JH, Lanier LL. Requirements for CD28-dependent T cell–mediated cytotoxicity. J Immunol 150:2091–2101, 1993b.

Bach JF. Non-Th2 regulatory T-cell control of Th1 autoimmunity. Scand J Immunol 54:21–29, 2001.

Badley AD, Pilon AA, Landay A, Lynch DH. Mechanisms of HIV-associated lymphocyte apoptosis. Blood 96:2951–2964, 2000.

Baecher-Allan C, Brown JA, Freeman GJ, Hafler DA. CD4+CD25high regulatory cells in human peripheral blood. J Immunol 167:1245–1253, 2001.

Baley JE, Schacter BZ. Mechanisms of diminished natural killer cell activity in pregnant women and neonates. J Immunol 134:3042–3048, 1985.

Bancshereau J, Briere F, Liu YJ, Rousset F. Molecular control of B lymphocyte growth and differentiation. Stem Cells 12:278–288, 1994.

Bancshereau J, Briere F, Caux C, Davoust J, Lebecque S, Liu YJ, Pulendran B, Palucka K. Immunobiology of dendritic cells. Annu Rev Immunol 18:767–811, 2000.

Baraff LJ, Leake RD, Burstyn DG, Payne T, Cody CL, Manclark CR, St Geme JW Jr. Immunologic response to early and routine DTP immunization in infants. Pediatrics 73:37–42, 1984.

Barbey C, Irion O, Helg C, Chapuis B, Grand C, Chizzolini C, Jeannet M, Roosnek E. Characterisation of the cytotoxic alloresponse of cord blood. Bone Marrow Transplant 22:S26–S30, 1998.

Barnard DR, Arthur MM. Fibronectin (cold insoluble globulin) in the neonate. J Pediatr 102:453–455, 1983.

Barnetson RS, Bjune G, Duncan ME. Evidence for a soluble lymphocyte factor in the transplacental transmission of T-lymphocyte responses to Mycobacterium leprae. Nature 260:150–151, 1976.

Baroni CD, Valtieri M, Stoppacciaro A, Ruco LP, Uccini S, Ricci C. The human thymus in ageing: histologic involution paralleled by increased mitogen response and by enrichment of OKT3+ lymphocytes. Immunology 50:519–528, 1983.

Baskin B, Islam KB, Smith CI. Characterization of the CDR3 region of rearranged alpha heavy chain genes in human fetal liver. Clin Exp Immunol 112:44–47, 1998.

Bauer S, Groh V, Wu J, Steinle A, Phillips JH, Lanier LL, Spies T. Activation of NK cells and T cells by NKG2D, a receptor for stress-inducible MICA. Science 285:727–729, 1999.

Bauer M, Redecke V, Ellwart JW, Scherer B, Kremer JP, Wagner H, Lipford GB. Bacterial CpG-DNA triggers activation and maturation of human CD11c-, CD123+ dendritic cells. J Immunol 166:5000–5007, 2001.

Bazaral M, Orgel HA, Hamburger RN. IgE levels in normal infants and mothers and an inheritance hypothesis. J Immunol 107:794–801, 1971.

Becker ID, Robinson OM, Bazan TS, Lopez-Osuna M, Kretschmer RR. Bactericidal capacity of newborn phagocytes against group B beta-hemolytic streptococci. Infect Immun 34:535–539, 1981.

Beier KC, Hutloff A, Dittrich AM, Heuck C, Rauch A, Buchner K, Ludewig B, Ochs HD, Mages HW, Kroczek RA. Induction, binding specificity and function of human ICOS. Eur J Immunol 30:3707–3717, 2000.

Bektas S, Goetze B, Speer CP. Decreased adherence, chemotaxis and phagocytic activities of neutrophils from preterm neonates. Acta Paediatr Scand 79:1031–1038, 1990.

Beldjord K, Beldjord C, Macintyre E, Even P, Sigaux F. Peripheral selection of V delta 1+ cells with restricted T cell receptor delta gene junctional repertoire in the peripheral blood of healthy donors. J Exp Med 178:121–127, 1993.

Berger RS, Dixon SL. Fulminant transfusion-associated graft-versus-host disease in a premature infant. J Am Acad Dermatol 20:945–950, 1989.

Berkowitz RD, Beckerman KP, Schall TJ, McCune JM. CXCR4 and CCR5 expression delineates targets for HIV-1 disruption of T cell differentiation. J Immunol 161:3702–3710, 1998.

Berman JD, Johnson WD Jr. Monocyte function in human neonates. Infect Immun 19:898–902, 1978.

Bernbaum JC, Daft A, Anolik R, Samuelson J, Barkin R, Douglas S, Polin R. Response of preterm infants to diphtheria-tetanus-pertussis immunizations. J Pediatr 107:184–188, 1985.

Berthou C, Legros-Maida S, Souli'e A, Wargnier A, Guillet J, Rabian C, Gluckman E, Sasportes M. Cord blood T lymphocytes lack constitutive perforin expression in contrast to adult peripheral blood T lymphocytes. Blood 85:1540–1546, 1995.

Bessler H, Mendel C, Straussberg R, Gurary N, Aloni D, Sirota L. Effects of dexamethasone on IL-1beta, IL-6, and TNF-alpha production by mononuclear cells of newborns and adults. Biol Neonate 75:225–233, 1999.

Bhat AM, Scanlon JW. The pattern of eosinophilia in premature infants. A prospective study in premature infants using the absolute eosinophil count. J Pediatr 98:612, 1981.

Bhat NM, Kantor AB, Bieber MM, Stall AM, Herzenberg LA, Teng NN. The ontogeny and functional characteristics of human B-1 (CD5+ B) cells. Int Immunol 4:243–252, 1992.

Bigby M, Markowitz JS, Bleicher PA, Grusby MJ, Simha S, Siebrecht M, Wagner M, Nagler-Anderson C, Glimcher LH. Most gamma delta T cells develop normally in the absence of MHC class II molecules. J Immunol 151:4465–4475. 1993.

Blahnik MJ, Ramanathan R, Riley CR, Minoo P. Lipopolysaccharide-induced tumor necrosis factor-alpha and IL-10 production by lung macrophages from preterm and term neonates. Pediatr Res 50:726–731, 2001.

Blom B, Res PC, Spits H. T cell precursors in man and mice. Crit Rev Immunol 18:371–388, 1998.

Boes M, Prodeus AP, Schmidt T, Carroll MC, Chen J. A critical role of natural immunoglobulin M in immediate defense against systemic bacterial infection. J Exp Med 188:2381–2386, 1998.

Boes M, Esau C, Fischer MB, Schmidt T, Carroll M, Chen J. Enhanced B-1 cell development, but impaired IgG antibody responses in mice deficient in secreted IgM. J Immunol 160:4776–4787, 1998b.

Bofill M, Akbar AN, Salmon M, Robinson M, Burford G, Janossy G. Immature CD45RA(low)RO(low) T cells in the human cord blood. I. Antecedents of CD45RA+ unprimed T cells. J Immunol 152:5613–5623, 1994.

Boles KS, Nakajima H, Colonna M, Chuang SS, Stepp SE, Bennett M, Kumar V, Mathew PA. Molecular characterization of a novel human natural killer cell receptor homologous to mouse 2B4. Tissue Antigens 54:27–34, 1999.

Bonati A, Zanelli P, Ferrari S, Plebani A, Starcich B, Savi M, Neri TM. T-cell receptor beta-chain gene rearrangement and expression during human thymic ontogenesis. Blood 79:1472–1483, 1992.

Boner A, Zeligs BJ, Bellanti JA. Chemotactic responses of various differentiational stages of neutrophils from human cord and adult blood. Infect Immun 35:921–928, 1982.

Bonforte RJ, Topilsky M, Siltzbach LE, Glade PR. Phytohemagglutinin skin test: a possible in vivo measure of cell-mediated immunity. J Pediatr 81:775–780. 1972.

Bonecchi R, Bianchi G, Bordignon PP, D'Ambrosio D, Lang R, Borsatti A, Sozzani S, Allavena P, Gray PA, Mantovani A, Sinigaglia F. Differential expression of chemokine receptors and chemotactic responsiveness of type 1 T helper cells (Th1s) and Th2s. J Exp Med 187:129–134, 1998.

Borras FE, Matthews NC, Lowdell MW, Navarrete CV. Identification of both myeloid CD11c+ and lymphoid CD11c− dendritic cell subsets in cord blood. Br J Haematol 113:925–931, 2001.

Borst J, Vroom TM, Bos JD, van Dongen JJ. Tissue distribution and repertoire selection of human gamma delta T cells: comparison with the murine system. Curr Top Microbiol Immunol 173:41–46, 1991.

Bortolussi R, Issekutz T, Burbridge S, Schellekens H. Neonatal host defense mechanisms against Listeria monocytogenes infection: the role of lipopolysaccharides and interferons. Pediatr Res 25:311–315, 1989.

Bortolussi R, Rajaraman K, Serushago B. Role of tumor necrosis factor-alpha and interferon-gamma in newborn host defense against *Listeria monocytogenes* infection. Pediatr Res 32:460–464, 1992.

Braakman E, Sturm E, Vijverberg K, van Krimpen BA, Gratama JW, Bolhuis RL. Expression of CD45 isoforms by fresh and activated human gamma delta T lymphocytes and natural killer cells. Int Immunol 3:691–697, 1991.

Brahmi Z, Hommel-Berrey G, Smith F, Thomson B. NK cells recover early and mediate cytotoxicity via perforin/granzyme and Fas/FasL pathways in umbilical cord blood recipients. Hum Immunol 62:782–790, 2001.

Brander C, Goulder PJ, Luzuriaga K, Yang OO, Hartman KE, Jones NG, Walker BD, Kalams SA. Persistent HIV-1-specific CTL clonal expansion despite high viral burden post in utero HIV-1 infection. J Immunol 162:4796–4800, 1999.

Braud VM, Allan DS, Wilson D, McMichael AJ. TAP- and tapasin-dependent HLA-E surface expression correlates with the binding of an MHC class I leader peptide. Curr Biol 8:1–10, 1998.

Briken V, Moody DB, Porcelli SA. Diversification of CD1 proteins: sampling the lipid content of different cellular compartments. Semin Immunol 12:517–525, 2000.

Brody JI, Oski FA, Wallach EE. Neonatal lymphocyte reactivity as an indicator of intrauterine bacterial contact. Lancet 1:1396–1398, 1968.

Bruce MC, Baley JE, Medvik KA, Berger M. Impaired surface membrane expression of C3bi but not C3b receptors on neonatal neutrophils. Pediatr Res 21:306–311, 1987.

Brugnoni D, Airo P, Graf D, Marconi M, Lebowitz M, Plebani A, Giliani S, Malacarne F, Cattaneo R, Ugazio AG, et al. Ineffective expression of CD40 ligand on cord blood T cells may contribute to poor immunoglobulin production in the newborn. Eur J Immunol 24:1919–1924, 1994.

Bruning T, Daiminger A, Enders G. Diagnostic value of CD45RO expression on circulating T lymphocytes of fetuses and newborn infants with pre-, peri- or early post-natal infections. Clin Exp Immunol 107:306–311, 1997.

Buchanan RM, Arulanandam BP, Metzger DW. IL-12 enhances antibody responses to T-independent polysaccharide vaccines in the absence of T and NK cells. J Immunol 161:5525–5533, 1998.

Buimovici-Klein E, Cooper LZ. Cell-mediated immune response in rubella infections. Rev Infect Dis 7:S123–S128, 1985.

Bukowski JF, Morita CT, Brenner MB. Recognition and destruction of virus-infected cells by human gamma delta CTL. J Immunol 153:5133–5140, 1994.

Bukowski JF, Morita CT, Brenner MB. Human gamma delta T cells recognize alkylamines derived from microbes, edible plants, and tea: implications for innate immunity. Immunity 11:57–65, 1999.

Bullens DM, Rafiq K, Kasran A, Van Gool SW, Ceuppens JL. Naïve human T cells can be a source of IL-4 during primary immune responses. Clin Exp Immunol 118:384–391, 1999.

Bullock JD, Robertson AF, Bodenbender JG, Kontras SB, Miller CE. Inflammatory response in the neonate re-examined. Pediatrics 44:58–61, 1969.

Burchett SK, Weaver WM, Westall JA, Larsen A, Kronheim S, Wilson CB. Regulation of tumor necrosis factor/cachectin and IL-1 secretion in human mononuclear phagocytes. J Immunol 140:3473–3481, 1988.

Burchett SK, Corey L, Mohan KM, Westall J, Ashley R, Wilson CB. Diminished interferon-gamma and lymphocyte proliferation in neonatal and postpartum primary herpes simplex virus infection. J Infect Dis 165:813–818, 1992.

Burtrum DB, Kim S, Dudley EC, Hayday AC, Petrie HT. TCR gene recombination and alpha beta-gamma delta lineage divergence: productive TCR-beta rearrangement is neither exclusive nor preclusive of gamma delta cell development. J Immunol 157:4293–4296, 1996.

Buseyne F, Burgard M, Teglas JP, Bui E, Rouzioux C, Mayaux MJ, Blanche S, Riviere Y. Early HIV-specific cytotoxic T lymphocytes and disease progression in children born to HIV-infected mothers. AIDS Res Hum Retroviruses 14:1435–1444, 1998.

Byrne JA, Stankovic AK, Cooper MD. A novel subpopulation of primed T cells in the human fetus. J Immunol 152:3098–3106, 1994.

Cairo MS, van de Ven C, Toy C, Mauss D, Sender L. Recombinant human granulocyte-macrophage colony-stimulating factor primes neonatal granulocytes for enhanced oxidative metabolism and chemotaxis. Pediatr Res 26:395–399, 1989.

Calado RT, Garcia AB, Falcao RP. Age-related changes of immunophenotypically immature lymphocytes in normal human peripheral blood. Cytometry 38:133–137, 1999.

Calhoun DA, Kirk JF, Christensen RD. Incidence, significance, and kinetic mechanism responsible for leukemoid reactions in patients in the neonatal intensive care unit: a prospective evaluation. J Pediatr 129:403–409, 1996.

Campbell AC, Waller C, Wood J, Aynsley-Green A, Yu V. Lymphocyte subpopulations in the blood of newborn infants. Clin Exp Immunol 18:469–482, 1974.

Carayol G, Robin C, Bourhis JH, Bennaceur-Griscelli A, Chouaib S, Coulombel L, Caignard A. NK cells differentiated from bone marrow, cord blood and peripheral blood stem cells exhibit similar phenotype and functions. Eur J Immunol 28:1991–2002, 1998.

Carlyle JR, Michie AM, Cho SK, Zuniga-Pflucker JC. Natural killer cell development and function precede alpha beta T cell differentiation in mouse fetal thymic ontogeny. J Immunol 160:744–753, 1998.

Carr R, Davies JM. Abnormal FcRIII expression by neutrophils from very preterm neonates. Blood 76:607–611, 1990.

Carr R, Pumford D, Davies JM. Neutrophil chemotaxis and adhesion in preterm babies. Arch Dis Child 67:813–817, 1992.

Carroll MC. The role of complement and complement receptors in induction and regulation of immunity. Ann Rev Immunol 16:545–568, 1998.

Carson WE, Fehniger TA, Haldar S, Eckhert K, Lindemann MJ, Lai CF, Croce CM, Baumann H, Caligiuri MA. A potential role for interleukin-15 in the regulation of human natural killer cell survival. J Clin Invest 99:937–943, 1997.

Caux C, Massacrier C, Vanbervliet B, Barthelemy C, Liu YJ, Banchereau J. Interleukin 10 inhibits T cell alloreaction induced by human dendritic cells. Int Immunol 6:1177–1185, 1994.

Cayabyab M, Phillips JH, Lanier LL. CD40 preferentially costimulates activation of CD4+ T lymphocytes. J Immunol 152:1523–1531, 1994.

Cederblad B, Riesenfeld T, Alm GV. Deficient herpes simplex virus–induced interferon-alpha production by blood leukocytes of preterm and term newborn infants. Pediatr Res 27:7–10, 1990.

Cederqvist LL, Ewool LC, Litwin SD. The effect of fetal age, birth weight, and sex on cord blood immunoglobulin values. Am J Obstet Gynecol 131:520–525, 1978.

Cella M, Jarrossay D, Facchetti F, Alebardi O, Nakajima H, Lanzavecchia A, Colonna M. Plasmacytoid monocytes migrate to inflamed lymph nodes and produce large amounts of type I interferon. Nat Med 5:919–923, 1999.

Cella M, Facchetti F, Lanzavecchia A, Colonna M. Plasmacytoid dendritic cells activated by influenza virus and CD40L drive a potent TH1 polarization. Nat Immunol 1:305–310, 2000.

Cerutti A, Trentin L, Zambello R, Sancetta R, Milani A, Tassinari C, Adami F, Agostini C, Semenzato G. The CD5/CD72 receptor system is coexpressed with several functionally relevant counterstructures on human B cells and delivers a critical signaling activity. J Immunol 157:1854–1862, 1996.

Chalmers IM, Janossy G, Contreras M, Navarrete C. Intracellular cytokine profile of cord and adult blood lymphocytes. Blood 92:11–18, 1998.

Chang J, Braciale TJ. Respiratory syncytial virus infection suppresses lung CD8+ T-cell effector activity and peripheral CD8+ T-cell memory in the respiratory tract. Nat Med 8:54–60, 2002.

Chang M, Suen Y, Lee SM, Baly D, Buzby JS, Knoppel E, Wolpe S, Cairo MS. Transforming growth factor-beta 1, macrophage inflammatory protein-1 alpha, and interleukin-8 gene expression is lower in stimulated human neonatal compared with adult mononuclear cells. Blood 84:118–124, 1994.

Chatenoud L, Salomon B, Bluestone JA. Suppressor T cells—they're back and critical for regulation of autoimmunity! Immunol Rev 182:149–163, 2001.

Chelvarajan RL, Raithatha R, Venkataraman C, Kaul R, Han SS, Robertson DA, Bondada S. CpG oligodeoxynucleotides overcome the unresponsiveness of neonatal B cells to stimulation with the thymus-independent stimuli anti-IgM and TNP-Ficoll. Eur J Immunol 29:2808–2818, 1999.

Chen L, Jullien P, Stepick-Biek P, Lewis DB. Neonatal naïve CD4 T cells have a decreased capacity to express CD40-ligand (CD154) and to induce dendritic cell IL-12 production after allogeneic stimulation. Federation of Clinical Immunology Societies (FOCIS) Annual Meeting, Boston, MA, Abstract 309, pp 45, 2001.

Chen ZJ, Wheeler CJ, Shi W, Wu AJ, Yarboro CH, Gallagher M, Notkins AL. Polyreactive antigen-binding B cells are the predominant cell type in the newborn B cell repertoire. Eur J Immunol 28:989–994, 1998.

Chheda S, Palkowetz KH, Garofalo R, Rassin D, Goldman AS. Decreased interleukin-10 production by neonatal monocytes and T cells: relationship to decreased production and expression of tumor necrosis factor-alpha and its receptors. Pediatr Res 40:475–483, 1996.

Chiba Y, Higashidate Y, Suga K, Honjo K, Tsutsumi H, Ogra PL. Development of cell-mediated cytotoxic immunity to respiratory syncytial virus in human infants following naturally acquired infection. J Med Virol 28:133–139, 1989.

Chien YH, Jores R, Crowley MP. Recognition by gamma/delta T cells. Annu Rev Immunol 14:511–532, 1996.

Chilmonczyk BA, Levin MJ, McDuffy R, Hayward AR. Characterization of the human newborn response to herpesvirus antigen. J Immunol 134:4184–4188, 1985.

Chougnet C, Kovacs A, Baker R, Mueller BU, Luban NL, Liewehr DJ, Steinberg SM, Thomas EK, Shearer GM. Influence of human immunodeficiency virus-infected maternal environment on development of infant interleukin-12 production. J Infect Dis 181:1590–1597, 2000.

Christensen RD, Rothstein G. Exhaustion of mature marrow neutrophils in neonates with sepsis. J Pediatr 96:316–318, 1980.

Christensen RD, Rothstein G. Pre- and post-natal development of granulocytic stem cells in the rat. Pediatr Res 18:599–602, 1984.

Christensen RD. Hematopoiesis in the fetus and neonate. Pediatr Res 26:531–535, 1989.

Christopherson K II, Brahmi Z, Hromas R. Regulation of naïve fetal T-cell migration by the chemokines Exodus-2 and Exodus-3. Immunol Lett 69:269–273, 1999.

Chumpitazi BF, Boussaid A, Pelloux H, Racinet C, Bost M, Goullier-Fleuret A. Diagnosis of congenital toxoplasmosis by immunoblotting and relationship with other methods. J Clin Microbiol 33:1479–1485, 1995.

Cicuttini FM, Martin M, Petrie HT, Boyd AW. A novel population of natural killer progenitor cells isolated from human umbilical cord blood. J Immunol 151:29–37, 1993.

Cilio CM, Daws MR, Malashicheva A, Sentman CL, Holmberg D. Cytotoxic T lymphocyte antigen 4 is induced in the thymus upon in vivo activation and its blockade prevents anti-CD3-mediated depletion of thymocytes. J Exp Med 188:1239–1246, 1998.

Clement LT. Isoforms of the CD45 common leukocyte antigen family: markers for human T-cell differentiation. J Clin Immunol 12:1–10, 1992.

Clerici M, DePalma L, Roilides E, Baker R, Shearer GM. Analysis of T helper and antigen-presenting cell functions in cord blood and peripheral blood leukocytes from healthy children of different ages. J Clin Invest 91:2829–2836, 1993.

Cocchi P, Marianelli L. Phagocytosis and intracellular killing of Pseudomonas aeruginosa in premature infants. Helv Paediatr Acta 22:110–118, 1967.

Coen R, Grush O, Kauder E. Studies of bactericidal activity and metabolism of the leukocyte in full-term neonates. J Pediatr 75:400–406, 1969.

Cohen L, Haziot A, Shen DR, Lin XY, Sia C, Harper R, Silver J, Goyert SM. CD14-independent responses to LPS require a serum factor that is absent from neonates. J Immunol 155:5337–5342, 1995.

Condiotti R, Nagler A. Effect of interleukin-12 on antitumor activity of human umbilical cord blood and bone marrow cytotoxic cells. Exp Hematol 26:571–9, 1998.

Condiotti R, Zakai YB, Barak V, Nagler A. Ex vivo expansion of CD56+ cytotoxic cells from human umbilical cord blood. Exp Hematol 29:104–113, 2001.

Conley ME, Kearney JF, Lawton AR III, Cooper MD. Differentiation of human B cells expressing the IgA subclasses as demonstrated by monoclonal hybridoma antibodies. J Immunol 125:2311–2316, 1980.

Conley ME, Speert DP. Human neonatal monocyte-derived macrophages and neutrophils exhibit normal nonopsonic and opsonic receptor-mediated phagocytosis and superoxide anion production. Biol Neonate 60:361–366, 1991.

Cooper MA, Fehniger TA, Turner SC, Chen KS, Ghaheri BA, Ghayur T, Carson WE, Caligiuri MA. Human natural killer cells: a unique innate immunoregulatory role for the CD56(bright) subset. Blood 97:3146–3151, 2001.

Cossarizza A, Kahan M, Ortolani C, Franceschi C, Londei M. Preferential expression of V beta 6.7 domain on human peripheral CD4+ T cells. Implication for positive selection of T cells in man. Eur J Immunol 21:1571–1574, 1991.

Coulomb-L'Hermin A, Amara A, Schiff C, Durand-Gasselin I, Foussat A, Delaunay T, Chaouat G, Capron F, Ledee N, Galanaud P, Arenzana-Seisdedos F, Emilie D. Stromal cell-derived factor 1 (SDF-1) and antenatal human B cell lymphopoiesis: expression of SDF-1 by mesothelial cells and biliary ductal plate epithelial cells. Proc Natl Acad Sci USA 96:8585–8590, 1999.

Crow MK, Kunkel HG. Human dendritic cells: major stimulators of the autologous and allogeneic mixed leucocyte reactions. Clin Exp Immunol 49:338–346, 1982.

Cuisinier AM, Guigou V, Boubli L, Fougereau M, Tonnelle C. Preferential expression of VH5 and VH6 immunoglobulin genes in early human B-cell ontogeny. Scand J Immunol 30:493–497, 1989.

Cuisinier AM, Fumoux F, Moinier D, Boubli L, Guigou V, Milili M, Schiff C, Fougereau M, Tonnelle C. Rapid expansion of human immunoglobulin repertoire (VH, V kappa, V lambda) expressed in early fetal bone marrow. New Biol 2:689–699, 1990.

D'Andrea A, Lanier LL. Killer cell inhibitory receptor expression by T cells. Curr Top Microbiol Immunol 230:25–39, 1998.

D'Andrea A, Goux D, De Lalla C, Koezuka Y, Montagna D, Moretta A, Dellabona P, Casorati G, Abrignani S. Neonatal invariant Valpha24+ NK T lymphocytes are activated memory cells. Eur J Immunol 30:1544–1550, 2000.

D'Ambola JB, Sherman MP, Tashkin DP, Gong H Jr. Human and rabbit newborn lung macrophages have reduced anti-Candida activity. Pediatr Res 24:285–290, 1988.

Dancis J, Osborn JJ, Kunz HW. Studies of the immunology of the newborn infant. Pediatrics 12:151–156, 1953.

Dardalhon V, Jaleco S, Kinet S, Herpers B, Steinberg M, Ferrand C, Froger D, Leveau C, Tiberghien P, Charneau P, Noraz N, Taylor N. IL-7 differentially regulates cell cycle progression and HIV-1–based vector infection in neonatal and adult CD4+ T cells. Proc Natl Acad Sci U S A 98:9277–9282, 2001.

Das H, Groh V, Kuijl C, Sugita M, Morita CT, Spies T, Bukowski JF. MICA engagement by human Vgamma2Vdelta2 T cells enhances their antigen-dependent effector function. Immunity 15:83–93, 2001.

Daum RS, Hogerman D, Rennels MB, Bewley K, Malinoski F, Rothstein E, Reisinger K, Block S, Keyserling H, Steinhoff M. Infant immunization with pneumococcal CRM197 vaccines: effect of saccharide size on immunogenicity and interactions with simultaneously administered vaccines. J Infect Dis 176:445–455, 1997.

Davis CA, Vallota EH, Forristal J. Serum complement levels in infancy: age related changes. Pediatr Res 13:1043–1046, 1979.

Davis MM, Lyons DS, Altman JD, McHeyzer-Williams M, Hampl J, Boniface JJ, Chien Y. T cell receptor biochemistry, repertoire selection and general features of TCR and Ig structure. Ciba Found Symp 204:94–100, 1997.

de Jong R, Brouwer M, Miedema F, van Lier RA. Human CD8+ T lymphocytes can be divided into CD45RA+ and CD45RO+ cells with different requirements for activation and differentiation. J Immunol 146:2088–2094, 1991.

de Vries E, de Bruin-Versteeg S, Comans-Bitter WM, de Groot R, Hop WC, Boerma GJ, Lotgering FK, Sauer PJ, van Dongen JJ. Neonatal blood lymphocyte subpopulations: a different perspective when using absolute counts. Biol Neonate 77:230–235, 2000.

Decoster A, Darcy F, Caron A, Vinatier D, Houze de L'Aulnoit D, Vittu G, Niel G, Heyer F, Lecolier B, Delcroix M. Anti-P30 IgA antibodies as prenatal markers of congenital toxoplasma infection. Clin Exp Immunol 87:310–315, 1992.

Delespesse G, Yang LP, Ohshima Y, Demeure C, Shu U, Byun DG, Sarfati M. Maturation of human neonatal CD4+ and CD8+ T lymphocytes into Th1/Th2 effectors. Vaccine 16:1415–1419, 1998.

Dellabona P, Padovan E, Casorati G, Brockhaus M, Lanzavecchia A. An invariant V alpha 24-J alpha Q/V beta 11 T cell receptor is expressed in all individuals by clonally expanded CD4−8− T cells. J Exp Med 180:1171–1176, 1994.

Dembinski J, Behrendt D, Reinsberg J, Bartmann P. Endotoxin-stimulated production of IL-6 and IL-8 is increased in short-term cultures of whole blood from healthy term neonates. Cytokine 18:116–119, 2002.

Demeure CE, Wu CY, Shu U, SchneiderPV, Heusser C, Yssel H, Delespesse G. In vitro maturation of human neonatal CD4 T lymphocytes II. Cytokines present at priming modulate the development of lymphokine production. J Immunol 152:4775–4782, 1994.

Dengrove J, Lee EJ, Heiner DC, St. Geme JW Jr, Leake R, Baraff LJ, Ward JI. IgG and IgG subclass specific antibody responses to diphtheria and tetanus toxoids in newborns and infants given DTP immunization. Pediatr Res 20:735–739, 1986.

DerSimonian H, Band H, Brenner MB. Increased frequency of T cell receptor V alpha 12.1 expression on CD8+ T cells: evidence that V alpha participates in shaping the peripheral T cell repertoire. J Exp Med 174:639–648, 1991.

Desmonts G, Daffos F, Forestier F, Capella-Pavlovsky M, Thulliez P, Chartier M. Prenatal diagnosis of congenital toxoplasmosis. Lancet 1:500–504, 1985.

Devereux G, Hall AM, Barker RN. Measurement of T-helper cytokines secreted by cord blood mononuclear cells in response to allergens. J Immunol Methods 234:13–22, 2000.

Dieli F, Troye-Blomberg M, Farouk SE, Sirecil G, Salerno A. Biology of gamma/delta T cells in tuberculosis and malaria. Curr Mol Med 1:437–446, 2001.

Doherty PJ, Roifman CM, Pan SH, Cymerman U, Ho SW, Thompson E, Kamel-Reid S, Cohen A. Expression of the human T cell receptor V beta repertoire. Mol Immunol 28:607–612, 1991.

Dolganov G, Bort S, Lovett M, Burr J, Schubert L, Short D, McGurn M, Gibson C, Lewis DB. Coexpression of the interleukin-13 and interleukin-4 genes correlates with their physical linkage in the cytokine gene cluster on human chromosome 5q23-31. Blood 87:3316–3326, 1996.

Dominguez E, Madrigal JA, Layrisse Z, Cohen SB. Fetal natural killer cell function is suppressed. Immunology 94:109–114, 1998.

Dong C, Juedes AE, Temann UA, Shresta S, Allison JP, Ruddle NH, Flavell RA. ICOS co-stimulatory receptor is essential for T-cell activation and function. Nature 409:97–101, 2001.

Dos Santos C, Davidson D. Neutrophil chemotaxis to leukotriene B4 in vitro is decreased for the human neonate. Pediatr Res 33:242–246, 1993.

Dosch HM, Lam P, Hui MF, Hibi T. Concerted generation of Ig isotype diversity in human fetal bone marrow. J Immunol 143:2464–2469, 1989.

Dossett JH, Williams RC Jr, Quie PG. Studies on interaction of bacteria, serum factors and polymorphonuclear leukocytes in mothers and newborns. Pediatrics 44:49–57, 1969.

Douek D, McFarland R, Keiser P, Gage EA, Massey JM, Haynes BF, Polis MA, Haase AT, Feinberg MB, Sullivan JL, Jamieson BD, Zack JA, Picker LJ, Koup RA. Changes in thymic function with age and during the treatment of HIV infection. Nature 396:690–695, 1998.

Drenou B, Choqueux C, El Ghalbzouri A, Blancheteau V, Toubert A, Charron D, Mooney N. Characterisation of the roles of CD95 and CD95 ligand in cord blood. Bone Marrow Transplant 22:S44–S47, 1998.

Drijkoningen M, De Wolf-Peeters C, Van der Steen K, Moerman P, Desmet V. Epidermal Langerhans' cells and dermal dendritic cells in human fetal and neonatal skin: an immunohistochemical study. Pediatr Dermatol 4:11–17, 1987.

Drossou V, Kanakoudi F, Diamanti E, Tzimouli V, Konstantinidis T, Germenis A, Kremenopoulos G, Katsougiannopoulos V. Concentrations of main serum opsonins in early infancy. Arch Dis Child Fetal Neonatal Ed 72:F172–F175, 1995.

Durandy A, De Saint Basile G, Lisowska-Grospierre B, Gauchat JF, Forveille M, Kroczek RA, Bonnefoy JY, Fischer A. Undetectable CD40 ligand expression on T cells and low B cell responses to CD40 binding agonists in human newborns. J Immunol 154:1560–1568, 1995.

Eads ME, Levy NJ, Kasper DL, Baker CJ, Nicholson-Weller A. Antibody-independent activation of C1 by type Ia group B streptococci. J Infect Dis 146:665–672, 1982.

Early E, Reen D. Antigen-independent responsiveness to interleukin-4 demonstrates differential regulation of newborn human T cells. Eur J Immunol 26:2885–2889, 1996.

Edenharter G, Bergmann RL, Bergmann KE, Wahn V, Forster J, Zepp F, Wahn U. Cord blood-IgE as risk factor and predictor for atopic diseases. Clin Exp Allergy 28:671–678, 1998.

Edwards JA, Jones DB, Evans PR, Smith JL. Differential expression of HLA class II antigens on human fetal and adult lymphocytes and macrophages. Immunology 55:489–500, 1985.

Edwards MS, Baker CJ. Group B streptococcal infections. In Remington JS, Klein JO, eds. Infectious diseases of the fetus and newborn, 5th ed. Philadelphia, WB Saunders, 2001, pp 1091–1156.

Egan PJ, Carding SR. Downmodulation of the inflammatory response to bacterial infection by gamma/delta T cells cytotoxic for activated macrophages. J Exp Med 191:2145–2158, 2000.

Ehlers S, Smith KA. Differentiation of T cell lymphokine gene expression: the in vitro acquisition of T cell memory. J Exp Med 173:25–36, 1991.

Ehrenstein MR, O'Keefe TL, Davies SL, Neuberger MS. Targeted gene disruption reveals a role for natural secretory IgM in the maturation of the primary immune response. Proc Natl Acad Sci USA 95:10089–10093, 1998.

Eischen CM, Schilling JD, Lynch DH, Krammer PH, Leibson PJ. Fc receptor-induced expression of Fas ligand on activated NK cells facilitates cell-mediated cytotoxicity and subsequent autocrine NK cell apoptosis. J Immunol 156:2693–2699, 1996.

El Ghalbzouri A, Drenou B, Blancheteau V, Choqueux C, Fauchet R, Charron D, Mooney N. An in vitro model of allogeneic stimulation of cord blood: induction of Fas independent apoptosis. Hum Immunol 60:598–607, 1999.

Elliott SR, Macardle PJ, Roberton DM, Zola H. Expression of the costimulator molecules, CD80, CD86, CD28, and CD152 on lymphocytes from neonates and young children. Hum Immunol 60:1039–1048, 1999.

Elliott SR, Roberton DM, Zola H, Macardle PJ. Expression of the costimulator molecules, CD40 and CD154, on lymphocytes from neonates and young children. Hum Immunol 61:378–388, 2000.

Enders G. Serologic test combinations for safe detection of rubella infections. Rev Infect Dis 7:S113–S122, 1985.

English BK, Burchett SK, English JD, Ammann AJ, Wara DW, Wilson CB. Production of lymphotoxin and tumor necrosis factor by human neonatal mononuclear cells. Pediatr Res 24:717–722, 1988.

English BK, Hammond WP, Lewis DB, Brown CB, Wilson CB. Decreased granulocyte-macrophage colony-stimulating factor production by human neonatal blood mononuclear cells and T cells. Pediatr Res 31:211–216, 1992.

Englund JA, Mbawuike IN, Hammill H, Holleman MC, Baxter BD, Glezen WP. Maternal immunization with influenza or tetanus toxoid vaccine for passive antibody protection in young infants. J Infect Dis 168:647–656, 1993.

Epstein J, Eichbaum Q, Sheriff S, Ezekowitz RA. The collectins in innate immunity. Curr Opin Immunol 8:29–35, 1996.

Erbach GT, Semple JP, Osathanondh R, Kurnick JT. Phenotypic characteristics of lymphoid populations of middle gestation human fetal liver, spleen and thymus. J Reprod Immunol 25:81–88, 1993.

Ernst WA, Maher J, Cho S, Niazi KR, Chatterjee D, Moody DB, Besra GS, Watanabe Y, Jensen PE, Porcelli SA, Kronenberg M, Modlin RL. Molecular interaction of CD1b with lipoglycan antigens. Immunity 8:331–340, 1998.

Eskola J, Kayhty H. Early immunization with conjugate vaccines. Vaccine 16:1433–1438, 1998.

Fairley CK, Begg N, Borrow R, Fox AJ, Jones DM, Cartwright K. Conjugate meningococcal serogroup A and C vaccine: reactogenicity and immunogenicity in United Kingdom infants. J Infect Dis 174:1360–1363, 1996.

Falconer AE, Carr R, Edwards SW. Impaired neutrophil phagocytosis in preterm neonates: lack of correlation with expression of immunoglobulin or complement receptors. Biol Neonate 68:264–269, 1995a.

Falconer AE, Carr R, Edwards SW. Neutrophils from preterm neonates and adults show similar cell surface receptor expression: analysis using a whole blood assay. Biol Neonate 67:26–33, 1995b.

Farber DL. Differential TCR signaling and the generation of memory T cells. J Immunol 160:535–539, 1998.

Feurle J, Espinosa E, Eckstein S, Pont F, Kunzmann V, Fournie JJ, Herderich M, Wilhelm M. Escherichia coli produces phosphoantigens activating human gamma delta T cells. J Biol Chem 277:148–154, 2002.

Field EJ, Caspary EA. Is maternal lymphocyte sensitisation passed to the child? Lancet 2:337–342, 1971.

Fink CW, Miller WE, Dorward B, LoSpalluto J. The formation of macroglobulin antibodies II. Studies on neonatal infants and older children. J Clin Invest 41:1422–1428, 1962.

Flamand V, Donckier V, Demoor FX, Le Moine A, Matthys P, Vanderhaeghen ML, Tagawa Y, Iwakura Y, Billiau A, Abramowicz D, Goldman M. CD40 ligation prevents neonatal induction of transplantation tolerance. J Immunol 160:4666–4669, 1998.

Flidel O, Barak Y, Lifschitz-Mercer B, Frumkin A, Mogilner BM. Graft versus host disease in extremely low birth weight neonate. Pediatrics 89:689–690, 1992.

Forestier F, Daffos F, Galactaeros F, Bardakjian J, Rainaut M, Beuzard Y. Hematological values of 163 normal fetuses between 18 and 30 weeks of gestation. Pediatr Res 20:342–346, 1986.

Foster CA, Holbrook KA. Ontogeny of Langerhans cells in human embryonic and fetal skin: cell densities and phenotypic expression relative to epidermal growth. Am J Anat 184:157–164, 1989.

Fournel S, Aguerre-Girr M, Huc X, Lenfant F, Alam A, Toubert A, Bensussan A, Le Bouteiller P. Cutting edge: soluble HLA-G1 triggers CD95/CD95 ligand-mediated apoptosis in activated CD8+ cells by interacting with CD8. J Immunol 164:6100–6104, 2000.

Fowler R, Schubert WK, West CD. Acquired partial tolerance to homologous skin grafts in the human infant at birth. Ann NY Acad Sci 87:403–428, 1960.

Franz ML, Carella JA, Galant SP. Cutaneous delayed hypersensitivity in a healthy pediatric population: diagnostic value of diptheria-tetanus toxoids. J Pediatr 88:975–977, 1976.

Fraticelli P, Sironi M, Bianchi G, D'Ambrosio D, Albanesi C, Stoppacciaro A, Chieppa M, Allavena P, Ruco L, Girolomoni G, Sinigaglia F, Vecchi A, Mantovani A. Fractalkine (CX3CL1) as an amplification circuit of polarized Th1 responses. J Clin Invest 107:1173–1181, 2001.

Freedman RM, Johnston D, Mahoney MJ, Pearson HA. Development of splenic reticuloendothelial function in neonates. J Pediatr 96:466–468, 1980.

Frenck RW Jr, Buescher ES, Vadhan-Raj S. The effects of recombinant human granulocyte-macrophage colony stimulating factor on in vitro cord blood granulocyte function. Pediatr Res 26:43–48, 1989.

Frenkel L, Bryson YJ. Ontogeny of phytohemagglutinin-induced gamma interferon by leukocytes of healthy infants and children: evidence for decreased production in infants younger than 2 months of age. J Pediatr 111:97–100, 1987.

Friedmann PS. Cell-mediated immunological reactivity in neonates and infants with congenital syphilis. Clin Exp Immunol 30:271–276, 1977.

Fry TJ, Mackall CL. Interleukin-7: master regulator of peripheral T-cell homeostasis? Trends Immunol 22:564–571, 2001.

Fujihashi K, McGhee JR, Kweon MN, Cooper MD, Tonegawa S, Takahashi I, Hiroi T, Mestecky J, Kiyono H. Gamma/delta T cell-deficient mice have impaired mucosal immunoglobulin A responses. J Exp Med 183:1929–1935, 1996.

Fujiwara T, Kobayashi T, Takaya J, Taniuchi S, Kobayashi Y. Plasma effects on phagocytic activity and hydrogen peroxide production by polymorphonuclear leukocytes in neonates. Clin Immunol Immunopathol 85:67–72, 1997.

Fukui T, Katamura K, Abe N, Kiyomasu T, Iio J, Ueno H, Mayumi M, Furusho K. IL-7 induces proliferation, variable cytokine-producing ability and IL-2 responsiveness in naïve CD4+ T-cells from human cord blood. Immunol Lett 59:21–28, 1997.

Fuleihan R, Ahern D, Geha RS. Decreased expression of the ligand for CD40 in newborn lymphocytes. Eur J Immunol 24:1925–1928, 1994.

Fuleihan R, Ahern D, Geha RS. CD40 ligand expression is developmentally regulated in human thymocytes. Clin Immunol Immunopathol 76:52–58, 1995.

Gaddy J, Risdon G, Broxmeyer HE. Cord blood natural killer cells are functionally and phenotypically immature but readily respond to interleukin-2 and interleukin-12. J Interferon Cytokine Res 15:527–536, 1995.

Gaddy J, Broxmeyer HE. Cord blood CD16+56- cells with low lytic activity are possible precursors of mature natural killer cells. Cell Immunol 180:132–142, 1997.

Gagro A, McCloskey N, Challa A, Holder M, Grafton G, Pound JD, Gordon J. CD5-positive and CD5-negative human B cells converge to an indistinguishable population on signalling through B-cell receptors and CD40. Immunology 101:201–209, 2000.

Gallagher MR, Welliver R, Yamanaka T, Eisenberg B, Sun M, Ogra PL. Cell-mediated immune responsiveness to measles. Its occurrence as a result of naturally acquired or vaccine-induced infection and in infants of immune mothers. Am J Dis Child 135:48–51, 1981.

Galy A, Christopherson I, Ferlazzo G, Liu G, Spits H, Georgopoulos K. Distinct signals control the hematopoiesis of lymphoid-related dendritic cells. Blood 95:128–137, 2000.

Gans HA, Arvin AM, Galinus J, Logan L, DeHovitz R, Maldonado Y. Deficiency of the humoral immune response to measles vaccine in infants immunized at age 6 months. JAMA 280:527–532, 1998.

Gans HA, Maldonado Y, Yasukawa LL, Beeler J, Audet S, Rinki MM, DeHovitz R, Arvin AM. IL-12, IFN-gamma, and T cell proliferation to measles in immunized infants. J Immunol 162:5569–5575, 1999.

Gans H, Yasukawa L, Rinki M, DeHovitz R, Forghani B, Beeler J, Audet S, Maldonado Y, Arvin AM. Immune responses to measles and mumps vaccination of infants at 6, 9, and 12 months. J Infect Dis 184:817–826, 2001.

Gansuvd B, Hagihara M, Yu Y, Inoue H, Ueda Y, Tsuchiya T, Masui A, Ando K, Nakamura Y, Munkhtuvshin N, Kato S, Thomas JM, Hotta T. Human umbilical cord blood NK T cells kill tumors by multiple cytotoxic mechanisms. Hum Immunol 63:164–175, 2002.

Garban F, Ericson M, Roucard C, Rabian-Herzog C, Teisserenc H, Sauvanet E, Charron D, Mooney N. Detection of empty HLA class II molecules on cord blood B cells. Blood 87:3970–3976, 1996.

Garban F, Truman JP, Lord J, Draenou B, Plumas J, Jacob MC, Sotto JJ, Charron D, Mooney N. Signal transduction via human leucocyte antigen class II molecules distinguishes between cord blood, normal, and malignant adult B lymphocytes. Exp Hematol 26:874–884, 1998.

Garcia VE, Sieling PA, Gong J, Barnes PF, Uyemura K, Tanaka Y, Bloom BR, Morita CT, Modlin RL. Single-cell cytokine analysis of gamma delta T cell responses to nonpeptide mycobacterial antigens. J Immunol 159:1328–1335, 1997.

Garderet L, Dulphy N, Douay C, Chalumeau N, Schaeffer V, Zilber MT, Lim A, Even J, Mooney N, Gelin C, Gluckman E, Charron D, Toubert A. The umbilical cord blood alpha/beta T-cell repertoire: characteristics of a polyclonal and naïve but completely formed repertoire. Blood 91:340–346, 1998.

Gasparoni A, De Amici D, Ciardelli L, Autelli M, Regazzi-Bonora M, Bartoli A, Chirico G, Rondini G. Effect of lidocaine on neutrophil chemotaxis in newborn infants. J Clin Immunol 18:210–213, 1998.

Gathings WE, Lawton AR, Cooper MD. Immunofluorescent studies of the development of pre-B cells, B lymphocytes and immunoglobulin isotype diversity in humans. Eur J Immunol 7:804–810, 1977.

Lewis DB, Yu CC, Meyer J, English BK, Kahn SJ, Wilson CB. Cellular and molecular mechanisms for reduced interleukin 4 and interferon-gamma production by neonatal T cells. J Clin Invest 87:194–202, 1991.

Li H, Lebedeva MI, Llera AS, Fields BA, Brenner MB, Mariuzza RA. Structure of the Vdelta domain of a human gammadelta T-cell antigen receptor. Nature 391:502–506, 1998.

Lieberman JM, Greenberg DP, Wong VK, Partridge S, Chang SJ, Chiu CY, Ward JI. Effect of neonatal immunization with diphtheria and tetanus toxoids on antibody responses to Haemophilus influenzae type b conjugate vaccines. J Pediatr 126:198–205, 1995.

Lin SJ, Chao HC, Kuo ML. The effect of interleukin-12 and interleukin-15 on CD69 expression of T-lymphocytes and natural killer cells from umbilical cord blood. Biol Neonate 78:181–185, 2000a.

Lin SJ, Yang MH, Chao HC, Kuo ML, Huang JL. Effect of interleukin-15 and Flt3-ligand on natural killer cell expansion and activation: umbilical cord vs. adult peripheral blood mononuclear cells. Pediatr Allergy Immunol 11:168–174, 2000b.

Linder N, Waintraub I, Smetana Z, Barzilai A, Lubin D, Mendelson E, Sirota L. Placental transfer and decay of varicella-zoster virus antibodies in preterm infants. J Pediatr 137:85–89, 2000.

Liu YJ. Dendritic cell subsets and lineages, and their functions in innate and adaptive immunity. Cell 106:259–262, 2001.

Liu E, Tu W, Law HK, Lau YL. Decreased yield, phenotypic expression and function of immature monocyte-derived dendritic cells in cord blood. Br J Haematol 113:240–246, 2001a.

Liu K, Li Y, Prabhu V, Young L, Becker KG, Munson PJ, Weng NP. Augmentation in expression of activation-induced genes differentiates memory from naïve CD4+ T cells and is a molecular mechanism for enhanced cellular response of memory CD4+ T cells. J Immunol 166:7335–7344, 2001b.

Lo YM, Lo ES, Watson N, Noakes L, Sargent IL, Thilaganathan B, Wainscoat JS. Two-way cell traffic between mother and fetus: biologic and clinical implications. Blood 88:4390–4395, 1996.

Lorant DE, Li W, Tabatabaei N, Garver MK, Albertine KH. P-selectin expression by endothelial cells is decreased in neonatal rats and human premature infants. Blood 94:600–609, 1999.

Lorenzo ME, Ploegh HL, Tirabassi RS. Viral immune evasion strategies and the underlying cell biology. Semin Immunol 13:1–9, 2001.

Lu J. Collectins: collectors of microorganisms for the innate immune system. Bioessays 19:509–518, 1997.

Lubens RG, Gard SE, Soderberg-Warner M, Stiehm ER. Lectin-dependent T-lymphocyte and natural killer cytotoxic deficiencies in human newborns. Cell Immunol 74:40–53, 1982.

Luzuriaga K, Holmes D, Hereema A, Wong J, Panicali DL, Sullivan JL. HIV-1–specific cytotoxic T lymphocyte responses in the first year of life. J Immunol 154:433–443, 1995.

Luzuriaga K, McManus M, Catalina M, Mayack S, Sharkey M, Stevenson M, Sullivan JL. Early therapy of vertical human immunodeficiency virus type 1 (HIV-1) infection: control of viral replication and absence of persistent HIV-1-specific immune responses. J Virol 74:6984–6991, 2000.

Lydyard PM, Quartey-Papafio R, Broker B, Mackenzie L, Jouquan J, Blaschek MA, Steele J, Petrou M, Collins P, Isenberg D, et al. The antibody repertoire of early human B cells. I. High frequency of autoreactivity and polyreactivity. Scand J Immunol 31:33–43, 1990.

Lyons AB. Analysing cell division in vivo and in vitro using flow cytometric measurement of CFSE dye dilution. J Immunol Methods 243:147–154, 2000.

Macardle PJ, Weedon H, Fusco M, Nobbs S, Ridings J, Flego L, Roberton DM, Zola H. The antigen receptor complex on cord B lymphocytes. Immunology 90:376–382, 1997.

Macaubas C, Holt PG. Regulation of cytokine production in T-cell responses to inhalant allergen: GATA-3 expression distinguishes between Th1- and Th2-polarized immunity. Int Arch Allergy Immunol 124:176–179, 2001.

Mackall CL, Fleisher TA, Brown MR, Andrich MP, Chen CC, Feuerstein IM, Horowitz ME, Magrath IT, Shad AT, Steinberg SM, Wexler LH, Gress RE. Age, thymopoiesis, and CD4+ T-lymphocyte regeneration after intensive chemotherapy. N Engl J Med 332:143–149, 1995.

Maeda M, van Schie RC, Yuksel B, Greenough A, Fanger MW, Guyre PM, Lydyard PM. Differential expression of Fc receptors for IgG by monocytes and granulocytes from neonates and adults. Clin Exp Immunol 103:343–347, 1996.

Malamitsi-Puchner A, Sarandakou A, Tziotis J, Trikka P, Creatsas G. Evidence for a suppression of apoptosis in early postnatal life. Acta Obstet Gynecol Scand 80:994–997, 2001.

Malek A, Sager R, Schneider H. Maternal-fetal transport of immunoglobulin G and its subclasses during the third trimester of human pregnancy. Am J Reprod Immunol 32:8–14, 1994.

Malhotra I, Mungai P, Wamachi A, Kioko J, Ouma JH, Kazura JW, King CL. Helminth- and Bacillus Calmette-Guerin-induced immunity in children sensitized in utero to filariasis and schistosomiasis. J Immunol 162:6843–6848, 1999.

Malygin AM, Timonen T. Non-major histocompatibility complex-restricted killer cells in human cord blood: generation and cytotoxic activity in recombinant interleukin-2-supplemented cultures. Immunology 79:506–508, 1993.

Manroe BL, Weinberg AG, Rosenfeld CR, Browne R. The neonatal blood count in health and disease. I. Reference values for neutrophilic cells. J Pediatr 95:89–98, 1979.

Marchant A, Goetghebuer T, Ota MO, Wolfe I, Ceesay SJ, De Groote D, Corrah T, Bennett S, Wheeler J, Huygen K, Aaby P, McAdam KP, Newport MJ. Newborns develop a Th1-type immune response to Mycobacterium bovis bacillus Calmette-Guerin vaccination. J Immunol 163:2249–2255, 1999.

Marchant A, Appay V, van der Sande M, Dulphy N, Liesnard C, Kidd M, Kaye S, Ojuola O, Gillespie G, Cuero A, Cerundolo V, Callan M, McAdam K, Rowland-Jones S, Donner C, McMichael AJ, Whittle H. Mature CD8+ T lymphocyte response to viral infection during fetal life. J Clin Invest 111:1747–1755, 2003.

Marino JA, Pensky J, Culp LA, Spagnuolo PJ. Fibronectin mediates chemotactic factor-stimulated neutrophil substrate adhesion. J Lab Clin Med 105:725–730. 1985.

Marodi L, Leijh PC, Braat A, Daha MR, van Furth R. Opsonic activity of cord blood sera against various species of microorganism. Pediatr Res 19:433–436, 1985.

Marodi L, Káposzta R, Campbell DE, Polin RA, Csongor J, Johnston RB Jr. Candidacidal mechanisms in the human neonate. Impaired IFN-gamma activation of macrophages in newborn infants. J Immunol 153:5643–5649, 1994.

Marodi L, Kaposzta R, Nemes E. Survival of group B streptococcus type III in mononuclear phagocytes: differential regulation of bacterial killing in cord macrophages by human recombinant gamma interferon and granulocyte-macrophage colony-stimulating factor. Infect Immun 68:2167–2170, 2000.

Marquez C, Trigueros C, Franco JM, Ramiro AR, Carrasco YR, Lopez-Botet M, Toribio ML. Identification of a common developmental pathway for thymic natural killer cells and dendritic cells. Blood 91:2760–2771, 1998.

Marrack P, Bender J, Hildeman D, Jordan M, Mitchell T, Murakami M, Sakamoto A, Schaefer BC, Swanson B, Kappler J. Homeostasis of alpha beta TCR+ T cells. Nat Immunol 1:107–111, 2000.

Martensson L, Fudenberg HH. Gm genes and gamma G-globulin synthesis in the human fetus. J Immunol 94:514–520, 1965.

Marwitz PA, Van Arkel-Vigna E, Rijkers GT, Zegers BJ. Expression and modulation of cell surface determinants on human adult and neonatal monocytes. Clin Exp Immunol 72:260–266, 1988.

Matsuda JL, Kronenberg M. Presentation of self and microbial lipids by CD1 molecules. Curr Opin Immunol 13:19–25, 2001.

Matsuura H, Hakomori S. The oncofetal domain of fibronectin defined by monoclonal antibody FDC-6: its presence in fibronectins from fetal and tumor tissues and its absence in those from normal adult tissues and plasma. Proc Natl Acad Sci USA 82:6517–6521, 1985.

Matthews NC, Wadhwa M, Bird C, Borras FE, Navarrete CV. Sustained expression of CD154 (CD40L) and proinflammatory cytokine production by alloantigen-stimulated umbilical cord blood T cells. J Immunol 164:6206–6212, 2000.

McCafferty MH, Lepow M, Saba TM, Cho E, Meuwissen H, White J, Zuckerbrod SF. Normal fibronectin levels as a function of age in the pediatric population. Pediatr Res 17:482–485, 1983.

McCracken GH Jr, Eichenwald HF. Leukocyte function and the development of opsonic and complement activity in the neonate. Am J Dis Child 121:120–126, 1971.

McDonald T, Sneed J, Valenski WR, Dockter M, Cooke R, Herrod HG. Natural killer cell activity in very low birth weight infants. Pediatr Res 31:376–380, 1992.

McEvoy LT, Zakem-Cloud H, Tosi MF. Total cell content of CR3 (CD11b/CD18) and LFA-1 (CD11a/CD18) in neonatal neutrophils: relationship to gestational age. Blood 87:3929–3933, 1996.

McFarland EJ, Borkowsky W, Fenton T, Wara D, McNamara J, Samson P, Kang M, Mofenson L, Cunningham C, Duliege AM, Sinangil F, Spector SA, Jimenez E, Bryson Y, Burchett S, Frenkel LM, Yogev R, Gigliotti F, Luzuriaga K, Livingston RA. Human immunodeficiency virus type 1 (HIV-1) gp120-specific antibodies in neonates receiving an HIV-1 recombinant gp120 vaccine. J Infect Dis 184:1331–1335, 2001.

McFarland RD, Douek DC, Koup RA, Picker LJ. Identification of a human recent thymic emigrant phenotype. Proc Natl Acad Sci U S A 97:4215–4220, 2000.

McLeod R, Mack DG, Boyer K, Mets M, Roizen N, Swisher C, Patel D, Beckmann E, Vitullo D, Johnson D. Phenotypes and functions of lymphocytes in congenital toxoplasmosis. J Lab Clin Med 116:623–635, 1990.

McVay LD, Jaswal SS, Kennedy C, Hayday A, Carding SR. The generation of human gammadelta T cell repertoires during fetal development. J Immunol 160:5851–5860, 1998.

McVay LD, Carding SR. Generation of human gammadelta T-cell repertoires. Crit Rev Immunol 19:431–460, 1999.

Mehta-Damani A, Markowicz S, Engleman EG. Generation of antigen-specific CD4+ T cell lines from naïve precursors. Eur J Immunol 25:1206–1211, 1995.

Melian A, Beckman EM, Porcelli SA, Brenner MB. Antigen presentation by CD1 and MHC-encoded class I-like molecules. Curr Opin Immunol 8:82–88, 1996.

Mellman I, Steinman RM. Dendritic cells: specialized and regulated antigen processing machines. Cell 106:255–258, 2001.

Melvin AJ, McGurn ME, Bort SJ, Gibson C, Lewis DB. Hypomethylation of the interferon-gamma gene correlates with its expression by primary T-lineage cells. Eur J Immunol 25:426–430, 1995.

Merrill JD, Sigaroudinia M, Kohl S. Characterization of natural killer and antibody-dependent cellular cytotoxicity of preterm infants against human immunodeficiency virus-infected cells. Pediatr Res 40:498–503, 1996.

Merry C, Puri P, Reen DJ. Defective neutrophil actin polymerisation and chemotaxis in stressed newborns. J Pediatr Surg 31:481–485, 1996.

Mescher MF. Molecular interactions in the activation of effector and precursor cytotoxic T lymphocytes. Immunol Rev 146:177–210, 1995.

Metcalf ES, Klinman NR. In vitro tolerance induction of neonatal murine B cells. J Exp Med 143:1327–1340, 1976.

Michie C, Harvey D. Can expression of CD45RO, a T-cell surface molecule, be used to detect congenital infection? Lancet 343:1259–1260, 1994.

Miller JS, Alley KA, McGlave P. Differentiation of natural killer (NK) cells from human primitive marrow progenitors in a stroma-based long-term culture system: identification of a CD34+7+ NK progenitor. Blood 83:2594–2601, 1994.

Miller JS. The biology of natural killer cells in cancer, infection, and pregnancy. Exp Hematol 29:1157–1168, 2001.

Miller JS, McCullar V. Human natural killer cells with polyclonal lectin and immunoglobulin-like receptors develop from single hematopoietic stem cells with preferential expression of NKG2A and KIR2DL2/L3/S2. Blood 98:705–713, 2001.

Miller ME. Chemotactic function in the human neonate: humoral and cellular aspects. Pediatr Res 5:487–492, 1971.

Miller ME. Phagocyte function in the neonate: selected aspects. Pediatrics 64:709–712, 1979.

Miller RL, Chew GL, Bell CA, Biedermann SA, Aggarwal M, Kinney PL, Tsai WY, Whyatt RM, Perera FP, Ford JG. Prenatal exposure, maternal sensitization, and sensitization in utero to indoor allergens in an inner-city cohort. Am J Respir Crit Care Med 164:995–1001, 2001.

Mills EL, Thompson T, Bjorksten B, Filipovich D, Quie PG. The chemiluminescence response and bactericidal activity of polymorphonuclear neutrophils from newborns and their mothers. Pediatrics 63:429–434, 1979a.

Mills EL, Bjorksten B, Quie PG. Deficient alternative complement pathway activity in newborn sera. Pediatr Res 13:1341–1344, 1979b.

Mingari MC, Vitale C, Cantoni C, Bellomo R, Ponte M, Schiavetti F, Bertone S, Moretta A, Moretta L. Interleukin-15-induced maturation of human natural killer cells from early thymic precursors: selective expression of CD94/NKG2-A as the only HLA class I-specific inhibitory receptor. Eur J Immunol 27:1374–1380, 1997.

Mintz L, Drew WL, Hoo R, Finley TN. Age-dependent resistance of human alveolar macrophages to herpes simplex virus. Infect Immun 28:417–420, 1980.

Miscia S, Di Baldassarre A, Sabatino G, Bonvini E, Rana RA, Vitale M, Di Valerio V, Manzoli FA. Inefficient phospholipase C activation and reduced Lck expression characterize the signaling defect of umbilical cord T lymphocytes. J Immunol 163:2416–2424, 1999.

Miura E, Procianoy RS, Bittar C, Miura CS, Miura MS, Mello C, Christensen RD. A randomized, double-masked, placebo-controlled trial of recombinant granulocyte colony-stimulating factor administration to preterm infants with the clinical diagnosis of early-onset sepsis. Pediatrics 107:30–35, 2001.

Miyagawa Y, Matsuoka T, Baba A, Nakamura T, Tsuno T, Tamura A, Agematsu K, Yabuhara A, Uehara Y, Kawai H. Fetal liver T cell receptor gamma/delta+ T cells as cytotoxic T lymphocytes specific for maternal alloantigens. J Exp Med 176:1–7, 1992.

Mo H, Monard S, Pollack H, Ip J, Rochford G, Wu L, Hoxie J, Borkowsky W, Ho DD, Moore JP. Expression patterns of the HIV type 1 coreceptors CCR5 and CXCR4 on CD4+ T cells and monocytes from cord and adult blood. AIDS Res Hum Retroviruses 14:607–617, 1998.

Monteleone G, Pender SL, Wathen NC, MacDonald TT. Interferon-alpha drives T cell-mediated immunopathology in the intestine. Eur J Immunol 31:2247–2255, 2001.

Moody DB, Ulrichs T, Muhlecker W, Young DC, Gurcha SS, Grant E, Rosat JP, Brenner MB, Costello CE, Besra GS, Porcelli SA. CD1c-mediated T-cell recognition of isoprenoid glycolipids in Mycobacterium tuberculosis infection. Nature 404:884–888, 2000.

Morell A, Sidiropoulos D, Herrmann U, Christensen KK, Christensen P, Prellner K, Fey H, Skvaril F. IgG subclasses and antibodies to group B streptococci, pneumococci, and tetanus toxoid in preterm neonates after intravenous infusion of immunoglobulin to the mothers. Pediatr Res 20:933–936, 1986.

Mortari F, Newton JA, Wang JY, Schroeder HW Jr. The human cord blood antibody repertoire. Frequent usage of the VH7 gene family. Eur J Immunol 22:241–245, 1992.

Mortari F, Wang JY, Schroeder HW Jr. Human cord blood antibody repertoire. Mixed population of VH gene segments and CDR3 distribution in the expressed C alpha and C gamma repertoires. J Immunol 150:1348–1357, 1993.

Moser M, Murphy KM. Dendritic cell regulation of TH1-TH2 development. Nat Immunol 1:199–205, 2000.

Mrozek E, Anderson P, Caligiuri MA. Role of interleukin-15 in the development of human CD56+ natural killer cells from CD34+ hematopoietic progenitor cells. Blood 87:2632–2640, 1996.

Munoz AI, Limbert D. Skin reactivity to Candida and streptokinase-streptodornase antigens in normal pediatric subjects: influence of age and acute illness. J Pediatr 91:565–568, 1977.

Musha N, Yoshida Y, Sugahara S, Yamagiwa S, Koya T, Watanabe H, Hatakeyama K, Abo T. Expansion of CD56+ NK T and gamma delta T cells from cord blood of human neonates. Clin Exp Immunol 113:220–228, 1998.

Naiman JL, Punnett HH, Lischner HW, Destine ML, Arey JB. Possible graft-versus-host reaction after intrauterine transfusion for Rh erythroblastosis fetalis. N Engl J Med 281:697–701, 1969.

Nair MP, Schwartz SA, Menon M. Association of decreased natural and antibody-dependent cellular cytotoxicity and production of natural killer cytotoxic factor and interferon in neonates. Cell Immunol 94:159–171, 1985.

Nakazawa T, Agematsu K, Yabuhara A. Later development of Fas ligand-mediated cytotoxicity as compared with granule-mediated cytotoxicity during the maturation of natural killer cells. Immunology 92:180–187, 1997.

Naot Y, Desmonts G, Remington JS. IgM enzyme-linked immunosorbent assay test for the diagnosis of congenital Toxoplasma infection. J Pediatr 98:32–36, 1981.

Nel AE. T-cell activation through the antigen receptor. Part 1: signaling components, signaling pathways, and signal integration at the T-cell antigen receptor synapse. J Allergy Clin Immunol 109:758–770, 2002.

Nelson DJ, Holt PG. Defective regional immunity in the respiratory tract of neonates is attributable to hyporesponsiveness of local dendritic cells to activation signals. J Immunol 155:3517–3524, 1995.

Newburger PE. Superoxide generation by human fetal granulocytes. Pediatr Res 16:373–376, 1982.

Newman PJ. Switched at birth: a new family for PECAM-1. J Clin Invest 103:5–9, 1999.

Ng WF, Duggan PJ, Ponchel F, Matarese G, Lombardi G, Edwards AD, Isaacs JD, Lechler RI. Human CD4(+)CD25(+) cells: a naturally occurring population of regulatory T cells. Blood 98:2736–2744, 2001.

Nguyen QH, Roberts RL, Ank BJ, Lin SJ, Thomas EK, Stiehm ER. Interleukin (IL)-15 enhances antibody-dependent cellular cytotoxicity and natural killer activity in neonatal cells. Cell Immunol 185:83–92, 1998a.

Nguyen QH, Roberts RL, Ank BJ, Lin SJ, Lau CK, Stiehm ER. Enhancement of antibody-dependent cellular cytotoxicity of neonatal cells by interleukin-2 (IL-2) and IL-12. Clin Diagn Lab Immunol 5:98–104, 1998b.

Nicholson IC, Brisco MJ, Zola H. Memory B lymphocytes in human tonsil do not express surface IgD. J Immunol 154:1105–1113, 1995.

Nieda M, Nicol A, Koezuka Y, Kikuchi A, Lapteva N, Tanaka Y, Tokunaga K, Suzuki K, Kayagaki N, Yagita H, Hirai H, Juji T. TRAIL expression by activated human CD4(+)V alpha 24NKT cells induces in vitro and in vivo apoptosis of human acute myeloid leukemia cells. Blood 97:2067–2074, 2001.

Nielsen SD, Jeppesen DL, Kolte L, Clark DR, Sorensen TU, Dreves AM, Ersboll AK, Ryder LP, Valerius NH, Nielsen JO. Impaired progenitor cell function in HIV-negative infants of HIV-positive mothers results in decreased thymic output and low CD4 counts. Blood 98:398–404, 2001.

Nishimoto N, Kubagawa H, Ohno T, Gartland GL, Stankovic AK, Cooper MD. Normal pre-B cells express a receptor complex of mu heavy chains and surrogate light-chain proteins. Proc Natl Acad Sci U S A 88:6284–6288, 1991.

Nomura A, Takada H, Jin CH, Tanaka T, Ohga S, Hara T. Functional analyses of cord blood natural killer cells and T cells: a distinctive interleukin-18 response. Exp Hematol 29:1169–1176, 2001.

Nonoyama S, Penix LA, Edwards CP, Lewis DB, Ito S, Aruffo A, Wilson CB, Ochs HD. Diminished expression of CD40 ligand by activated neonatal T cells. J Clin Invest 95:66–75, 1995.

Norris DA, Clark RA, Swigart LM, Huff JC, Weston WL, Howell SE. Fibronectin fragment(s) are chemotactic for human peripheral blood monocytes. J Immunol 129:1612–1618, 1982.

Notarangelo LD, Chirico G, Chiara A, Colombo A, Rondini G, Plebani A, Martini A, Ugazio AG. Activity of classical and alternative pathways of complement in preterm and small for gestational age infants. Pediatr Res 18:281–285, 1984.

Nunes JA, Collette Y, Truneh A, Olive D, Cantrell DA. The role of p21ras in CD28 signal transduction: triggering of CD28 with antibodies, but not the ligand B7-1, activates p21ras. J Exp Med 180:1067–1076, 1994.

Nunez C, Nishimoto N, Gartland GL, Billips LG, Burrows PD, Kubagawa H, Cooper MD. B cells are generated throughout life in humans. J Immunol 156:866–872, 1996.

Nunoi H, Endo F, Chikazawa S, Namikawa T, Matsuda I. Chemotactic receptor of cord blood granulocytes to the synthesized chemotactic peptide N-formyl-methionyl-leucyl-phenylalanine. Pediatr Res 17:57–60, 1983.

Nybo M, Sorensen O, Leslie R, Wang P. Reduced expression of C5a receptors on neutrophils from cord blood. Arch Dis Child Fetal Neonatal Ed 78:129–132, 1998.

O'Brien WF, Golden SM, Bibro MC, Charkobardi PK, Davis SE, Hemming VG. Short-term responses in neonatal lambs after infusion of group B streptococcal extract. Obstet Gynecol 65:802–806, 1985.

O'Callaghan CA. Natural killer cell surveillance of intracellular antigen processing pathways mediated by recognition of HLA-E and Qa-1b by CD94/NKG2 receptors. Microbes Infect 2:371–80, 2000.

Ochs HD, Wedgwood RJ. IgG subclass deficiencies. Annu Rev Med 38:325–340, 1987.

Ohls RK, Li Y, Abdel-Mageed A, Buchanan G Jr, Mandell L, Christensen RD. Neutrophil pool sizes and granulocyte colony-stimulating factor production in human mid-trimester fetuses. Pediatr Res 37:806–811, 1995.

Ohshima Y, Delespesse G. T cell-derived IL-4 and dendritic cell-derived IL-12 regulate the lymphokine-producing phenotype of alloantigen-primed naïve human CD4 T cells. J Immunol 158:629–636, 1997.

Ohshima Y, Yang LP, Uchiyama T, Tanaka Y, Baum P, Sergerie M, Hermann P, Delespesse G. OX40 costimulation enhances interleukin-4 (IL-4) expression at priming and promotes the differentiation of naïve human CD4(+) T cells into high IL-4-producing effectors. Blood 92:3338–3345, 1998.

Ohteki T, Ho S, Suzuki H, Mak TW, Ohashi PS. Role for IL-15/IL-15 receptor beta-chain in natural killer 1.1+ T cell receptor-alpha beta+ cell development. J Immunol 159:5931–5935, 1997.

Okamura Y, Watari M, Jerud ES, Young DW, Ishizaka ST, Rose J, Chow JC, Strauss JF III. The extra domain A of fibronectin activates Toll-like receptor 4. J Biol Chem 276:10229–10233, 2001.

Olaussen RW, Farstad IN, Brandtzaeg P, Rugtveit J. Age-related changes in CCR9+ circulating lymphocytes: are CCR9+ naïve T cells recent thymic emigrants? Scand J Immunol 54:435–439, 2001.

Oliver AM, Thomson AW, Sewell HF, Abramovich DR. Major histocompatibility complex (MHC) class II antigen (HLA-DR, DQ, and DP) expression in human fetal endocrine organs and gut. Scand J Immunol 27:731–737, 1988.

Olweus J, BitMansour A, Warnke R, Thompson PA, Carballido J, Picker LJ, Lund-Johansen F. Dendritic cell ontogeny: a human dendritic cell lineage of myeloid origin. Proc Natl Acad Sci USA 94:12551–12556, 1997.

Orlandi F, Giambona A, Messana F, Marino M, Abate I, Calzolari R, Damiani F, Jakil C, Renda M, Dieli F, Buscemi F, Westgren M, Ringden O, Maggio A. Evidence of induced non-tolerance in HLA-identical twins with hemoglobinopathy after in utero fetal transplantation. Bone Marrow Transplant 18:637–639, 1996.

Orlowski JP, Sieger L, Anthony BF. Bactericidal capacity of monocytes of newborn infants. J Pediatr 89:797–801. 1976.

Ota MO, Vekemans J, Schlegel-Haueter SE, Fielding K, Sanneh M, Kidd M, Newport MJ, Aaby P, Whittle H, Lambert PH, McAdam KP, Siegrist CA, Marchant A. Influence of Mycobacterium bovis bacillus Calmette-Guérin on antibody and cytokine responses to human neonatal vaccination. J Immunol 168:919–925, 2002.

Oxelius VA, Svenningsen NW. IgG subclass concentrations in preterm neonates. Acta Paediatr Scand 73:626–630, 1984.

Pacanowski J, Kahi S, Baillet M, Lebon P, Deveau C, Goujard C, Meyer L, Oksenhendler E, Sinet M, Hosmalin A. Reduced blood CD123+ (lymphoid) and CD11c+ (myeloid) dendritic cell numbers in primary HIV-1 infection. Blood 98:3016–3021, 2001.

Padlan EA. Anatomy of the antibody molecule. Mol Immunol 31:169–217, 1994.

Pahal GS, Jauniaux E, Kinnon C, Thrasher AJ, Rodeck CH. Normal development of human fetal hematopoiesis between eight and seventeen weeks' gestation. Am J Obstet Gynecol 183:1029–1034, 2000.

Pahwa SG, Pahwa R, Grimes E, Smithwick E. Cellular and humoral components of monocyte and neutrophil chemotaxis in cord blood. Pediatr Res 11:677–680, 1977.

Park BH, Holmes B, Good RA. Metabolic activities in leukocytes of newborn infants. J Pediatr 76:237–241, 1970.

Parker CM, Groh V, Band H, Porcelli SA, Morita C, Fabbi M, Glass D, Strominger JL, Brenner MB. Evidence for extrathymic changes in the T-cell receptor gamma/delta repertoire. J Exp Med 171:1597–1612, 1990.

Parkman R, Mosier D, Umansky I, Cochran W, Carpenter CB, Rosen FS. Graft-versus-host disease after intrauterine and exchange transfusions for hemolytic disease of the newborn. N Engl J Med 290:359–363, 1974.

Parra C, Roldan E, Brieva JA. Deficient expression of adhesion molecules by human CD5⁻ B lymphocytes both after bone marrow transplantation and during normal ontogeny. Blood 88:1733 Parkman R, Mosier D, Umansky I, Cochran W, 1740, 1996.

Paryani SG, Arvin AM. Intrauterine infection with varicella-zoster virus after maternal varicella. N Engl J Med 314:1542–1546, 1986.

Pass RF, Stagno S, Britt WJ, Alford CA. Specific cell-mediated immunity and the natural history of congenital infection with cytomegalovirus. J Infect Dis 148:953–961, 1983.

Payne NR, Fleit HB. Extremely low birth weight infants have lower Fc gamma RIII (CD16) plasma levels and their PMN produce less Fc gamma RIII compared to adults. Biol Neonate 69:235–242, 1996.

Peakman M, Buggins AG, Nicolaides KH, Layton DM, Vergani D. Analysis of lymphocyte phenotypes in cord blood from early gestation fetuses. Clin Exp Immunol 90:345–350, 1992.

Peeters CC, Tenbergen-Meekes AM, Heijnen CJ, Poolman JT, Zegers JM, Rijkers GT. Interferon-gamma and interleukin-6 augment the human in vitro antibody response to the *Haemophilus influenzae* type b polysaccharide. J Infect Dis 165 Suppl 1:S161–S162, 1992.

Peevy KJ, Chartrand SA, Wiseman HJ, Boerth RC, Olson RD. Myocardial dysfunction in group B streptococcal shock. Pediatr Res 19:511–513, 1985.

Penninger JM, Kroemer G. Molecular and cellular mechanisms of T lymphocyte apoptosis. Adv Immunol 68:51–144, 1998.

Perchalski JE, Clem LW, Small PA Jr. 7S gamma-M immunoglobulins in normal human cord serum. Am J Med Sci 256:107–111, 1968.

Perez-Melgosa M, Ochs HD, Linsley PS, Laman JD, van Meurs M, Flavell RA, Ernst RK, Miller SI, Wilson CB. Carrier-mediated enhancement of cognate T cell help: the basis for enhanced immunogenicity of meningococcal outer membrane protein polysaccharide conjugate vaccine. Eur J Immunol 31:2373–2381, 2001.

Perkins FT, Yetto R, Gaisford W. Response of infants to a third dose of poliomyelitis vaccine given 10 to 12 months after primary immunization. Br Med J 1:680–682, 1959.

Perussia B. Fc receptors on natural killer cells. Curr Top Microbiol Immunol 230:63–88, 1998.

Peset Llopis MJ, Harms G, Hardonk MJ, Timens W. Human immune response to pneumococcal polysaccharides: complement-mediated localization preferentially on CD21-positive splenic marginal zone B cells and follicular dendritic cells. J Allergy Clin Immunol 97:1015–1024, 1996.

Peters JH, Ginsberg MH, Bohl BP, Sklar LA, Cochrane CG. Intravascular release of intact cellular fibronectin during oxidant-induced injury of the in vitro perfused rabbit lung. J Clin Invest 78:1596–1603, 1986.

Peterson JC. Immunization in the young infant. Response to combined vaccines: I-IV. Am J Dis Child 81:483–500, 1951.

Petty RE, Hunt DW. Neonatal dendritic cells. Vaccine 16:1378–1382, 1998.

Phillips JH, Hori T, Nagler A, Bhat N, Spits H, Lanier LL. Ontogeny of human natural killer (NK) cells: fetal NK cells mediate cytolytic function and express cytoplasmic CD3 epsilon,delta proteins. J Exp Med 175:1055–1066, 1992.

Pikora CA, Sullivan JL, Panicali D, Luzuriaga K. Early HIV-1 envelope-specific cytotoxic T lymphocyte responses in vertically infected infants. J Exp Med 185:1153–1161, 1997.

Pinon JM, Toubas D, Marx C, Mougeot G, Bonnin A, Bonhomme A, Villaume M, Foudrinier F, Lepan H. Detection of specific immunoglobulin E in patients with toxoplasmosis. J Clin Microbiol 28:1739–1743, 1990.

Pirenne H, Aujard Y, Eljaafari A, Bourillon A, Oury JF, Le-Gac S, Blot P, Sterkers G. Comparison of T cell functional changes during childhood with the ontogeny of CDw29 and CD45RA expression on CD4⁺ T cells. Pediatr Res 32:81–86, 1992.

Pitcher-Wilmott RW, Hindocha P, Wood CB. The placental transfer of IgG subclasses in human pregnancy. Clin Exp Immunol 41:303–308, 1980.

Pittard WB III, Miller K, Sorensen RU. Normal lymphocyte responses to mitogens in term and premature neonates following normal and abnormal intrauterine growth. Clin Immunol Immunopathol 30:178–187, 1984.

Plaeger-Marshall S, Ank BJ, Altenburger KM, Pizer LI, Johnston RB Jr, Stiehm ER. Replication of herpes simplex virus in blood monocytes and placental macrophages from human neonates. Pediatr Res 26:135–139, 1989.

Playfair JH, Wolfendale MR, Kay HE. The leucocytes of peripheral blood in the human foetus. Br J Haematol 9:336–344, 1963.

Plebani A, Proserpio AR, Guarneri D, Buscaglia M, Cattoretti G. B and T lymphocyte subsets in fetal and cord blood: age-related modulation of CD1c expression. Biol Neonate 63:1–7, 1993.

Poggi A, Demarest JF, Costa P, Biassoni R, Pella N, Pantaleo G, Mingari MC, Moretta L. Expression of a wide T cell receptor V beta repertoire in human T lymphocytes derived in vitro from embryonic liver cell precursors. Eur J Immunol 24:2258–2261, 1994.

Pommier CG, O'Shea J, Chused T, Yancey K, Frank MM, Takahashi T, Brown EJ. Studies on the fibronectin receptors of human peripheral blood leukocytes. Morphologic and functional characterization. J Exp Med 159:137–151, 1984.

Porcelli S, Yockey CE, Brenner MB, Balk SP. Analysis of T cell antigen receptor (TCR) expression by human peripheral blood CD4⁻8⁻ alpha/beta T cells demonstrates preferential use of several V beta genes and an invariant TCR alpha chain. J Exp Med 178:1–16, 1993.

Porcelli SA, Segelke BW, Sugita M, Wilson IA, Brenner MB. The CD1 family of lipid antigen-presenting molecules. Immunol Today 19:362–368, 1998.

Porcu P, Gaddy J, Broxmeyer HE. Alloantigen-induced unresponsiveness in cord blood T lymphocytes is associated with defective activation of Ras. Proc Natl Acad Sci USA 95:4538–4543, 1998.

Potestio M, Pawelec G, Di Lorenzo G, Candore G, D'Anna C, Gervasi F, Lio D, Tranchida G, Caruso C, Romano GC. Age-related changes in the expression of CD95 (APO1/FAS) on blood lymphocytes. Exp Gerontol 34:659–673, 1999.

Poulin JF, Viswanathan MN, Harris JM, Komanduri KV, Wieder E, Ringuette N, Jenkins M, McCune JM, Sekaly RP. Direct evidence for thymic function in adult humans. J Exp Med 190:479–486, 1999.

Prescott SL, Macaubas C, Yabuhara A, Venaille TJ, Holt BJ, Habre W, Loh R, Sly PD, Holt PG. Developing patterns of T cell memory to environmental allergens in the first two years of life. Int Arch Allergy Immunol 113:75–79, 1997.

Prescott SL, Macaubas C, Holt BJ, Smallacombe TB, Loh R, Sly PD, Holt PG. Transplacental priming of the human immune system to environmental allergens: universal skewing of initial T cell responses toward the Th2 cytokine profile. J Immunol 160:4730–4737, 1998a.

Prescott SL, Macaubas C, Smallacombe T, Holt BJ, Sly PD, Loh R, Holt PG. Reciprocal age-related patterns of allergen-specific T-cell immunity in normal vs. atopic infants. Clin Exp Allergy 28 Suppl 5:39–44, 1998b.

Provenzano RW, Wetterlow LH, Sullivan CL. Immunization and antibody response in the newborn infant. I. Pertussis inoculation within twenty-four hours of birth. N Engl J Med 273:959–965, 1965.

Puel A, Ziegler SF, Buckley RH, Leonard WJ. Defective IL7R expression in T(−)B(+)NK(+) severe combined immunodeficiency. Nat Genet 20:394–397, 1998.

Punnonen J, Aversa G, Vandekerckhove B, Roncarolo MG, de Vries JE. Induction of isotype switching and Ig production by CD5⁺ and CD10⁺ human fetal B cells. J Immunol 148:3398–3404, 1992.

Punnonen J, Aversa G, de Vries JE. Human pre-B cells differentiate into Ig-secreting plasma cells in the presence of interleukin-4 and activated CD4⁺ T cells or their membranes. Blood 82:2781–2789, 1993.

Punnonen J, de Vries JE. IL-13 induces proliferation, Ig isotype switching, and Ig synthesis by immature human fetal B cells. J Immunol 152:1094–1102, 1994.

Punnonen J, Cocks BG, de Vries JE. IL-4 induces germ-line IgE heavy chain gene transcription in human fetal pre-B cells.

Evidence for differential expression of functional IL-4 and IL-13 receptors during B cell ontogeny. J Immunol 155:4248–4254, 1995.

Qian JX, Lee SM, Suen Y, Knoppel E, van de Ven C, Cairo MS. Decreased interleukin-15 from activated cord versus adult peripheral blood mononuclear cells and the effect of interleukin-15 in upregulating antitumor immune activity and cytokine production in cord blood. Blood 90:3106–3117, 1997.

Qing G, Rajaraman K, Bortolussi R. Diminished priming of neonatal polymorphonuclear leukocytes by lipopolysaccharide is associated with reduced CD14 expression. Infect Immun 63:248–252, 1995.

Raaphorst FM, Timmers E, Kenter MJ, Van Tol MJ, Vossen JM, Schuurman RK. Restricted utilization of germ-line VH3 genes and short diverse third complementarity-determining regions (CDR3) in human fetal B lymphocyte immunoglobulin heavy chain rearrangements. Eur J Immunol 22:247–251, 1992.

Raaphorst FM, Kaijzel EL, Van Tol MJ, Vossen JM, van den Elsen PJ. Non-random employment of V beta 6 and J beta gene elements and conserved amino acid usage profiles in CDR3 regions of human fetal and adult TCR beta chain rearrangements. Int Immunol 6:1–9, 1994a.

Raaphorst FM, van Bergen J, van den Bergh RL, van der Keur M, de Krijger R, Bruining J, van Tol MJ, Vossen JM, van den Elsen PJ. Usage of TCRAV and TCRBV gene families in human fetal and adult TCR rearrangements. Immunogenetics 39:343–350, 1994b.

Raaphorst FM, Raman CS, Tami J, Fischbach M, Sanz I. Human Ig heavy chain CDR3 regions in adult bone marrow pre-B cells display an adult phenotype of diversity: evidence for structural selection of DH amino acid sequences. Int Immunol 9:1503–1515, 1997.

Raghunathan R, Miller ME, Everett S, Leake RD. Phagocyte chemotaxis in the perinatal period. J Clin Immunol 2:242–245, 1982.

Ramos SB, Garcia AB, Viana SR, Voltarelli JC, Falcao RP. Phenotypic and functional evaluation of natural killer cells in thymectomized children. Clin Immunol Immunopathol 81:277–281, 1996.

Randolph GJ, Beaulieu S, Lebecque S, Steinman RM, Muller WA. Differentiation of monocytes into dendritic cells in a model of transendothelial trafficking. Science 282:480–483, 1998.

Randolph GJ, Inaba K, Robbiani DF, Steinman RM, Muller WA. Differentiation of phagocytic monocytes into lymph node dendritic cells in vivo. Immunity 11:753–761, 1999.

Rao A, Avni O. Molecular aspects of T-cell differentiation. Br Med Bull 56:969–984, 2000.

Ray CG. The ontogeny of interferon production by human leukocytes. J Pediatr 76:94–98, 1970.

Rayfield LS, Brent L, Rodeck CH. Development of cell-mediated lympholysis in human foetal blood lymphocytes. Clin Exp Immunol 42:561–570, 1980.

Rebuck N, Gibson A, Finn A. Neutrophil adhesion molecules in term and premature infants: normal or enhanced leucocyte integrins but defective L-selectin expression and shedding. Clin Exp Immunol 101:183–189, 1995.

Reddy RK, Xia Y, Hanikyrova M, Ross GD. A mixed population of immature and mature leucocytes in umbilical cord blood results in a reduced expression and function of CR3 (CD11b/CD18). Clin Exp Immunol 114:462–467, 1998.

Reen DJ. Activation and functional capacity of human neonatal CD4 T-cells. Vaccine 16:1401–1408, 1998.

Renda MC, Fecarotta E, Dieli F, Markling L, Westgren M, Damiani G, Jakil C, Picciotto F, Maggio A. Evidence of alloreactive T lymphocytes in fetal liver: implications for fetal hematopoietic stem cell transplantation. Bone Marrow Transplant 25:135–141, 2000.

Ribeiro-do-Couto LM, Boeije LC, Kroon JS, Hooibrink B, Breur-Vriesendorp BS, Aarden LA, Boog CJ. High IL-13 production by human neonatal T cells: neonate immune system regulator? Eur J Immunol 31:3394–3402, 2001.

Rijkers GT, Sanders EA, Breukels MA, Zegers BJ. Infant B cell responses to polysaccharide determinants. Vaccine 16:1396–1400, 1998.

Risdon G, Gaddy J, Broxmeyer HE. Allogeneic responses of human umbilical cord blood. Blood Cells 20:566–570, 1994a.

Risdon G, Gaddy J, Stehman FB, Broxmeyer HE. Proliferative and cytotoxic responses of human cord blood T lymphocytes following allogeneic stimulation. Cell Immunol 154:14–24, 1994b.

Risdon G, Gaddy J, Horie M, Broxmeyer HE. Alloantigen priming induces a state of unresponsiveness in human umbilical cord blood T cells. Proc Natl Acad Sci USA 92:2413–2417, 1995.

Rissoan MC, Soumelis V, Kadowaki N, Grouard G, Briere F, de Waal Malefyt R, Liu YJ. Reciprocal control of T helper cell and dendritic cell differentiation. Science 283:1183–1186, 1999.

Riteau B, Menier C, Khalil-Daher I, Sedlik C, Dausset J, Rouas-Freiss N, Carosella ED. HLA-G inhibits the allogeneic proliferative response. J Reprod Immunol 43:203–211, 1999.

Robey E, Fowlkes BJ. The alpha beta versus gamma delta T-cell lineage choice. Curr Opin Immunol 10:181–187, 1998.

Rogge L, Barberis-Maino L, Biffi M, Passini N, Presky DH, Gubler U, Sinigaglia F. Selective expression of an interleukin-12 receptor component by human T helper 1 cells. J Exp Med 185:825–831, 1997.

Roncarolo MG, Bigler M, Ciuti E, Martino S, Tovo PA. Immune responses by cord blood cells. Blood Cells 20:573–585, 1994.

Rothberg AD, Cohn RJ, Argent AC, Sher R, Joffe M. Eosinophilia in premature neonates. Phase 2 of a biphasic granulopoietic response. S Afr Med J 64:539–541, 1983.

Rothenfusser S, Hornung V, Krug A, Towarowski A, Krieg AM, Endres S, Hartmann G. Distinct CpG oligonucleotide sequences activate human gamma delta T cells via interferon-alpha/-beta. Eur J Immunol 31:3525–3534, 2001.

Rottman JB, Smith T, Tonra JR, Ganley K, Bloom T, Silva R, Pierce B, Gutierrez-Ramos JC, Ozkaynak E, Coyle AJ. The costimulatory molecule ICOS plays an important role in the immunopathogenesis of EAE. Nat Immunol 2:605–611, 2001.

Rouas-Freiss N, Marchal RE, Kirszenbaum M, Dausset J, Carosella ED. The alpha1 domain of HLA-G1 and HLA-G2 inhibits cytotoxicity induced by natural killer cells: is HLA-G the public ligand for natural killer cell inhibitory receptors? Proc Natl Acad Sci USA 94:5249–5254, 1997.

Rouleau M, Namikawa R, Antonenko S, Carballido-Perrig N, Roncarolo MG. Antigen-specific cytotoxic T cells mediate human fetal pancreas allograft rejection in SCID-hu mice. J Immunol 157:5710–5720, 1996.

Rowe J, Macaubas C, Monger T, Holt BJ, Harvey J, Poolman JT, Loh R, Sly PD, Holt PG. Heterogeneity in diphtheria-tetanus-acellular pertussis vaccine-specific cellular immunity during infancy: relationship to variations in the kinetics of postnatal maturation of systemic th1 function. J Infect Dis 184:80–88, 2001.

Rowen JL, Smith CW, Edwards MS. Group B streptococci elicit leukotriene B4 and interleukin-8 from human monocytes: neonates exhibit a diminished response. J Infect Dis 172:420–426, 1995.

Rubin HR, Sorensen RU, Polmar SH. Lymphocyte responses of human neonates to bacterial antigens. Cell Immunol 57:307–315, 1981.

Rukavina D, Laskarin G, Rubesa G, Strbo N, Bedenicki I, Manestar D, Glavas M, Christmas SE, Podack ER. Age-related decline of perforin expression in human cytotoxic T lymphocytes and natural killer cells. Blood 92:2410–2420, 1998.

Sacchi F, Hill HR. Defective membrane potential changes in neutrophils from human neonates. J Exp Med 160:1247–1252, 1984.

Saint-Ruf C, Panigada M, Azogui O, Debey P, von Boehmer H, Grassi F. Different initiation of pre-TCR and gamma/deltaTCR signalling. Nature 406:524–527, 2000.

Saito H, Kanamori Y, Takemori T, Nariuchi H, Kubota E, Takahashi-Iwanaga H, Iwanaga T, Ishikawa H. Generation of intestinal T cells from progenitors residing in gut cryptopatches. Science 280:275–278, 1998.

Saito S, Morii T, Umekage H, Makita K, Nishikawa K, Narita N, Ichijo M, Morikawa H, Ishii N, Nakamura M, Sugamura K. Expression of the interleukin-2 receptor gamma chain on cord blood mononuclear cells. Blood 87:3344–3350, 1996.

Sakaguchi S, Sakaguchi N, Shimizu J, Yamazaki S, Sakihama T, Itoh M, Kuniyasu Y, Nomura T, Toda M, Takahashi T. Immunologic tolerance maintained by CD25+ CD4+ regulatory T cells: their common role in controlling autoimmunity, tumor immunity, and transplantation tolerance. Immunol Rev 182:18–32, 2001.

Sallusto F, Lanzavecchia A. Understanding dendritic cell and T-lymphocyte traffic through the analysis of chemokine receptor expression. Immunol Rev 177:134–140, 2000.

Salmon M, Kitas GD, Bacon PA. Production of lymphokine mRNA by CD45R+ and CD45R– helper T cells from human peripheral blood and by human CD4+ T cell clones. J Immunol 143:907–912, 1989.

Sancho L, de la Hera A, Casas J, Vaquer S, Martinez C, Alvarez-Mon M. Two different maturational stages of natural killer lymphocytes in human newborn infants. J Pediatr 119:446–454, 1991.

Sanders ME, Makgoba MW, June CH, Young HA, Shaw S. Enhanced responsiveness of human memory T cells to CD2 and CD3 receptor-mediated activation. Eur J Immunol 19:803–808, 1989.

Santoro P, Agosti V, Viggiano D, Palumbo A, Sarno T, Ciccimarra F. Impaired D-myo-inositol 1,4,5-triphosphate generation from cord blood polymorphonuclear leukocytes. Pediatr Res 38:564–567, 1995.

Sanz I. Multiple mechanisms participate in the generation of diversity of human H chain CDR3 regions. J Immunol 147:1720–1729, 1991.

Sato H, Albrecht P, Reynolds DW, Stagno S, Ennis FA. Transfer of measles, mumps, and rubella antibodies from mother to infant. Its effect on measles, mumps, and rubella immunization. Am J Dis Child 133:1240–1243, 1979.

Sato K, Nagayama H, Takahashi TA. Aberrant CD3- and CD28-mediated signaling events in cord blood T cells are associated with dysfunctional regulation of Fas ligand-mediated cytotoxicity. J Immunol 162:4464–4471, 1999.

Sato K, Kawasaki H, Nagayama H, Enomoto M, Morimoto C, Tadokoro K, Juji T, Takahashi T. Chemokine receptor expressions and responsiveness of cord blood T cells. J Immunol 166:1659–1666, 2001.

Sautois B, Fillet G, Beguin Y. Comparative cytokine production by in vitro stimulated mononucleated cells from cord blood and adult blood. Exp Hematol 25:103–108, 1997.

Schatt S, Holzgreve W, Hahn S. Stimulated cord blood lymphocytes have a low percentage of Th1 and Th2 cytokine secreting T cells although their activation is similar to adult controls. Immunol Lett 77:1–2, 2001.

Schelonka RL, Yoder BA, desJardins SE, Hall RB, Butler J. Peripheral leukocyte count and leukocyte indexes in healthy newborn term infants. J Pediatr 125:603–606, 1994.

Schelonka RL, Raaphorst FM, Infante D, Kraig E, Teale JM, Infante AJ. T cell receptor repertoire diversity and clonal expansion in human neonates. Pediatr Res 43:396–402, 1998.

Schibler KR, Liechty KW, White WL, Christensen RD. Production of granulocyte colony-stimulating factor in vitro by monocytes from preterm and term neonates. Blood 82:2478–2484, 1993.

Schlesinger JJ, Covelli HD. Evidence for transmission of lymphocyte responses to tuberculin by breast-feeding. Lancet 2:529–532, 1977.

Schlesinger Y, Granoff DM. Avidity and bactericidal activity of antibody elicited by different Haemophilus influenzae type b conjugate vaccines. The Vaccine Study Group. JAMA 267:1489–1494, 1992.

Schluns KS, Kieper WC, Jameson SC, Lefrancois L. Interleukin-7 mediates the homeostasis of naïve and memory CD8 T cells in vivo. Nat Immunol 1:426–432, 2000.

Schonbeck U, Libby P. The CD40/CD154 receptor/ligand dyad. Cell Mol Life Sci 58:4–43, 2001.

Schoub BD, Johnson S, McAnerney J, Gilbertson L, Klaassen KI, Reinach SG. Monovalent neonatal polio immunization—a strategy for the developing world. J Infect Dis 157:836–839, 1988.

Schroeder HW Jr, Hillson JL, Perlmutter RM. Early restriction of the human antibody repertoire. Science 238:791–793, 1987.

Schroeder HW Jr, Ippolito GC, Shiokawa S. Regulation of the antibody repertoire through control of HCDR3 diversity. Vaccine 16:1383–1390, 1998.

Schroeder HW Jr, Zhang L, Philips JB III. Slow, programmed maturation of the immunoglobulin HCDR3 repertoire during the third trimester of fetal life. Blood 98:2745–2751, 2001.

Schuit KE, Powell DA. Phagocytic dysfunction in monocytes of normal newborn infants. Pediatrics 65:501–504, 1980.

Schultz C, Reiss I, Bucsky P, Gopel W, Gembruch U, Ziesenitz S, Gortner L. Maturational changes of lymphocyte surface antigens in human blood: comparison between fetuses, neonates and adults. Biol Neonate 78:77–82, 2000.

Schutte ME, Ebeling SB, Akkermans-Koolhaas KE, Logtenberg T. Deletion mapping of Ig VH gene segments expressed in human CD5 B cell lines. JH proximity is not the sole determinant of the restricted fetal VH gene repertoire. J Immunol 149:3953–3960, 1992.

Sciammas R, Kodukula P, Tang Q, Hendricks RL, Bluestone JA. T cell receptor-gamma/delta cells protect mice from herpes simplex virus type 1-induced lethal encephalitis. J Exp Med 185:1969–1975, 1997.

Scott ME, Kubin M, Kohl S. High level interleukin-12 production, but diminished interferon-gamma production, by cord blood mononuclear cells. Pediatr Res 41:547–553, 1997.

Scott ZA, Chadwick EG, Gibson LL, Catalina MD, McManus MM, Yogev R, Palumbo P, Sullivan JL, Britto P, Gay H, Luzuriaga K. Infrequent detection of HIV-1-specific, but not cytomegalovirus-specific, CD8(+) T cell responses in young HIV-1-infected infants. J Immunol 167:7134–7140, 2001.

Seidel BM, Schulze B, Kiess W, Vogtmann C, Borte M. Determination of secretory IgA and albumin in saliva of newborn infants. Biol Neonate 78:186–190, 2000.

Seki H, Ueno Y, Taga K, Matsuda A, Miyawaki T, Taniguchi N. Mode of in vitro augmentation of natural killer cell activity by recombinant human interleukin 2: a comparative study of Leu-11+ and Leu-11– cell populations in cord blood and adult peripheral blood. J Immunol 135:2351–2356, 1985.

Servet-Delprat C, Bridon JM, Djossou O, Yahia SA, Banchereau J, Briere F. Delayed IgG2 humoral response in infants is not due to intrinsic T or B cell defects. Int Immunol 8:1495–1502, 1996.

Settmacher U, Volk HD, Jahn S, Neuhaus K, Kuhn F, von Baehr R. Characterization of human lymphocytes separated from fetal liver and spleen at different stages of ontogeny. Immunobiology 182:256–265, 1991.

Shapiro LM, Bassen F. Sternal marrow changes during the first week of life. Correlation with peripheral blood findings. Am J Med Sci 202:341–354, 1941.

Sharpe AH, Freeman GJ. The B7-CD28 superfamily. Nat Rev Immunol 2:116–126, 2002.

Sheldon WH, Caldwell JB. The mononuclear cell phase of inflammation in the newborn. Bull Johns Hopkins Hosp 112:258–269, 1963.

Shen J, Andrews DM, Pandolfi F, Boyle LA, Kersten CM, Blatman RN, Kurnick JT. Oligoclonality of Vdelta1 and Vdelta2 cells in human peripheral blood mononuclear cells: TCR selection is not altered by stimulation with gram-negative bacteria. J Immunol 160:3048–3055, 1998.

Shigeoka AO, Santos JI, Hill HR. Functional analysis of neutrophil granulocytes from healthy, infected, and stressed neonates. J Pediatr 95:454–460, 1979.

Shigeoka AO, Charette RP, Wyman ML, Hill HR. Defective oxidative metabolic responses of neutrophils from stressed neonates. J Pediatr 98:392–398, 1981.

Shimada M, Minato M, Takada M, Takahashi S, Harada K. Plasma concentration of granulocyte-colony-stimulating factor in neonates. 85:351–355, 1996.

Shiratsuchi H, Tsuyuguchi I. Tuberculin purified protein derivative-reactive T cells in cord blood lymphocytes. Infect Immun 33:651–657, 1981.

Siber GR. Pneumococcal disease: prospects for a new generation of vaccines. Science 265:1385–1387, 1994.

Siegal FP, Kadowaki N, Shodell M, Fitzgerald-Bocarsly PA, Shah K, Ho S, Antonenko S, Liu YJ. The nature of the principal type 1 interferon-producing cells in human blood. Science 284:1835–1837, 1999.

Silverman GJ, Sasano M, Wormsley SB. Age-associated changes in binding of human B lymphocytes to a VH3-restricted unconventional bacterial antigen. J Immunol 151:5840–5855, 1993.

Silverstein AM, Prendergast RA, Parshall CJ Jr. Cellular kinetics of the antibody response by the fetal rhesus monkey. J Immunol 104:269–271, 1970.

Silverstein A. Ontogeny of the immune response: a perspective. In Cooper MD, Dayton DH, eds. Development of host defenses. New York, NY, Raven Press, 1977, pp 1–10.

Simister NE. Human placental Fc receptors and the trapping of immune complexes. Vaccine 16:1451–1455, 1998.

Singh B, Read S, Asseman C, Malmstrom V, Mottet C, Stephens LA, Stepankova R, Tlaskalova H, Powrie F. Control of intestinal inflammation by regulatory T cells. Immunol Rev 182:190–200, 2001.

Sivori S, Vitale M, Morelli L, Sanseverino L, Augugliaro R, Bottino C, Moretta L, Moretta A. p46, a novel natural killer cell-specific surface molecule that mediates cell activation. J Exp Med 186:1129–1136, 1997.

Slavcev A, Striz I, Ivaskova E, Breur-Vriesendorp BS. Alloresponses of cord blood cells in primary mixed lymphocyte cultures. Hum Immunol 63:155–163, 2002.

Slayton WB, Li Y, Calhoun DA, Juul SE, Iturraspe J, Braylan RC, Christensen RD. The first-appearance of neutrophils in the human fetal bone marrow cavity. Early Hum Dev 53:129–144, 1998.

Small TN, Keever C, Collins N, Dupont B, O'Reilly RJ, Flomenberg N. Characterization of B cells in severe combined immunodeficiency disease. Hum Immunol 25:181–193, 1989.

Smith DH, Peter G, Ingram DL, Harding AL, Anderson P. Responses of children immunized with the capsular polysaccharide of *Hemophilus influenzae*, type b. Pediatrics 52:637–644, 1973.

Smith JB, Campbell DE, Ludomirsky A, Polin RA, Douglas SD, Garty BZ, Harris MC. Expression of the complement receptors CR1 and CR3 and the type III Fc gamma receptor on neutrophils from newborn infants and from fetuses with Rh disease. Pediatr Res 28:120–126, 1990a.

Smith JB, Kunjummen RD, Kishimoto TK, Anderson DC. Expression and regulation of L-selectin on eosinophils from human adults and neonates. Pediatr Res 32:465–471, 1992.

Smith MD, Worman C, Yuksel F, Yuksel B, Moretta L, Ciccone E, Grossi CE, Mackenzie L, Lydyard PM. T gamma delta-cell subsets in cord and adult blood. Scand J Immunol 32:491–496, 1990b.

Smith RT, Eitzman DV, Catlin ME, Wirtz EO, Miller BE. The development of the immune response. Pediatrics 33:163–183, 1964.

Smith S, Jacobs RF, Wilson CB. Immunobiology of childhood tuberculosis: a window on the ontogeny of cellular immunity. J Pediatr 131:16–26, 1997.

Smolen P, Bland R, Heiligenstein E, Lawless MR, Dillard R, Abramson J. Antibody response to oral polio vaccine in premature infants. J Pediatr 103:917–919, 1983.

Snapper CM, Rosas FR, Jin L, Wortham C, Kehry MR, Mond JJ. Bacterial lipoproteins may substitute for cytokines in the humoral immune response to T cell–independent type II antigens. J Immunol 155:5582–5589, 1995.

Snapper CM, Mond JJ. A model for induction of T cell–independent humoral immunity in response to polysaccharide antigens. J Immunol 157:2229–2233, 1996.

Soares MV, Borthwick NJ, Maini MK, Janossy G, Salmon M, Akbar AN. IL-7-dependent extrathymic expansion of CD45RA+ T cells enables preservation of a naïve repertoire. J Immunol 161:5909–5917, 1998.

Solvason N, Chen X, Shu F, Kearney JF. The fetal omentum in mice and humans. A site enriched for precursors of CD5 B cells early in development. Ann N Y Acad Sci 651:10–20, 1992.

Sorg RV, Kogler G, Wernet P. Functional competence of dendritic cells in human umbilical cord blood. Bone Marrow Transplant 22 (Suppl 1):S52–S54, 1998.

Sorg RV, Kogler G, Wernet P. Identification of cord blood dendritic cells as an immature CD11⁻ population. Blood 93:2302–2307, 1999.

Sorg RV, Andres S, Kogler G, Fischer J, Wernet P. Phenotypic and functional comparison of monocytes from cord blood and granulocyte colony-stimulating factor-mobilized apheresis products. Exp Hematol 29:1289–1294, 2001.

Sornasse T, Larenas PV, Davis KA, de Vries JE, Yssel H. Differentiation and stability of T helper 1 and 2 cells derived from naïve human neonatal CD4+ T cells, analyzed at the single-cell level. J Exp Med 184:473–483, 1996.

Speer CP, Ambruso DR, Grimsley J, Johnston RB Jr. Oxidative metabolism in cord blood monocytes and monocyte-derived macrophages. Infect Immun 50:919–921, 1985.

Speer CP, Gahr M, Wieland M, Eber S. Phagocytosis-associated functions in neonatal monocyte-derived macrophages. Pediatr Res 24:213–216, 1988.

Splawski JB, Jelinek DF, Lipsky PE. Delineation of the functional capacity of human neonatal lymphocytes. J Clin Invest 87:545–553, 1991.

Splawski JB, Lipsky PE. Cytokine regulation of immunoglobulin secretion by neonatal lymphocytes. J Clin Invest 88:967–977, 1991.

Splawski JB, Lipsky PE. Prostaglandin E2 inhibits T cell–dependent Ig secretion by neonatal but not adult lymphocytes. J Immunol 152:5259–5267, 1994.

Splawski JB, Nishioka J, Nishioka Y, Lipsky PE. CD40 ligand is expressed and functional on activated neonatal T cells. J Immunol 156:119–127, 1996.

Splawski, JB, Yamamoto, K, and Lipsky, PE. Deficient interleukin-10 production by neonatal T cells does not explain their ineffectiveness at promoting neonatal B cell differentiation. Eur J Immunol 28:4248–4256, 1998.

Sporici RA, Beswick RL, von Allmen C, Rumbley CA, Hayden-Ledbetter M, Ledbetter JA, Perrin PJ. ICOS ligand costimulation is required for T-cell encephalitogenicity. Clin Immunol 100:277–288, 2001.

Squire E, Favara B, Todd J. Diagnosis of neonatal bacterial infection: hematologic and pathologic findings in fatal and nonfatal cases. Pediatrics 64:60–64, 1979.

Starr SE, Tolpin MD, Friedman HM, Paucker K, Plotkin SA. Impaired cellular immunity to cytomegalovirus in congenitally infected children and their mothers. J Infect Dis 140:500–505, 1979.

Steele RW, Suttle DE, LeMaster PC, Patterson FD, Canales L. Screening for cell-mediated immunity in children. Am J Dis Child 130:1218–1221, 1976.

Steinman RM, Inaba K. Myeloid dendritic cells. J Leukoc Biol 66:205–208, 1999.

Stephens LA, Mottet C, Mason D, Powrie F. Human CD4(+)CD25(+) thymocytes and peripheral T cells have immune suppressive activity in vitro. Eur J Immunol 31:1247–1254, 2001.

Stepick-Biek P, Thulliez P, Araujo FG, Remington JS. IgA antibodies for diagnosis of acute congenital and acquired toxoplasmosis. J Infect Dis 162:270–273, 1990.

Stiehm ER, Fudenberg HH. Serum levels of immune globulins in health and disease: a survey. Pediatrics 37:715–727, 1966.

Story CM, Mikulska JE, Simister NE. A major histocompatibility complex class I–like Fc receptor cloned from human placenta: possible role in transfer of immunoglobulin G from mother to fetus. J Exp Med 180:2377–2381, 1994.

Strauss RG, Rosenberger TG, Wallace PD. Neutrophil chemiluminescence during the first month of life. Acta Haematol 63:326–329, 1980.

Strauss RG, Snyder EL. Chemotactic peptide binding by intact neutrophils from human neonates. Pediatr Res 18:63–66, 1984.

Stroobant J, Harris MC, Cody CS, Polin RA, Douglas SD. Diminished bactericidal capacity for group B *Streptococcus* in neutrophils from "stressed" and healthy neonates. Pediatr Res 18:634–637, 1984.

Stumptner-Cuvelette P, Morchoisne S, Dugast M, Le Gall S, Raposo G, Schwartz O, Benaroch P. HIV-1 Nef impairs MHC class II antigen presentation and surface expression. Proc Natl Acad Sci USA 98:12144–12149, 2001.

Suda T, Hashimoto H, Tanaka M, Ochi T, Nagata S. Membrane Fas ligand kills human peripheral blood T lymphocytes, and soluble Fas ligand blocks the killing. J Exp Med 186:1045–2050, 1997.

Suen Y, Lee SM, Qian J, van de Ven C, Cairo MS. Dysregulation of lymphokine production in the neonate and its impact on neonatal cell mediated immunity. Vaccine 16:1369–1377, 1998.

Sullender WM, Miller JL, Yasukawa LL, Bradley JS, Black SB, Yeager AS, Arvin A. Humoral and cell-mediated immunity in neonates with herpes simplex virus infection. J Infect Dis 155:28–37, 1987.

Super M, Thiel S, Lu J, Levinsky RJ, Turner MW. Association of low levels of mannan-binding protein with a common defect of opsonisation. Lancet 2:1236–1239, 1989.

Surh CD, Sprent J. Regulation of naïve and memory T-cell homeostasis. Microbes Infect 4:51–56, 2002.

Szepfalusi Z, Nentwich I, Gerstmayr M, Jost E, Todoran L, Gratzl R, Herkner K, Urbanek R. Prenatal allergen contact with milk proteins. Clin Exp Allergy 27:28–35, 1997.

Szepfalusi Z, Pichler J, Elsasser S, van Duren K, Ebner C, Bernaschek G, Urbanek R. Transplacental priming of the human immune system with environmental allergens can occur early in gestation. J Allergy Clin Immunol 106:530–536, 2000.

Taams LS, Smith J, Rustin MH, Salmon M, Poulter LW, Akbar AN. Human anergic/suppressive CD4(+)CD25(+) T cells: a highly differentiated and apoptosis-prone population. Eur J Immunol 31:1122–1131, 2001.

Takahashi N, Imanishi K, Nishida H, Uchiyama T. Evidence for immunologic immaturity of cord blood T cells. Cord blood T cells are susceptible to tolerance induction to in vitro stimulation with a superantigen. J Immunol 155:5213–5219, 1995.

Takahashi N, Kato H, Imanishi K, Miwa K, Yamanami S, Nishida H, Uchiyama T. Immunopathophysiological aspects of an emerging neonatal infectious disease induced by a bacterial superantigen. J Clin Invest 106:1409–1415, 2000.

Tan ND, Davidson D. Comparative differences and combined effects of interleukin-8, leukotriene B4, and platelet-activating factor on neutrophil chemotaxis of the newborn. Pediatr Res 38:11–16, 1995.

Tanaka Y, Morita CT, Nieves E, Brenner MB, Bloom BR. Natural and synthetic non-peptide antigens recognized by human gamma delta T cells. Nature 375:155–158, 1995.

Tannous R, Spitzer RE, Clarke WR, Goplerud CP, Cavendar-Zylich N. Decreased chemotactic activity in activated newborn plasma. J Lab Clin Med 99:331–341, 1982.

Tarkkanen J, Saksela E. Umbilical-cord-blood-derived suppressor cells of the human natural killer cell activity are inhibited by interferon. Scand J Immunol 15:149–157, 1982.

Tavian M, Robin C, Coulombel L, Peault B. The human embryo, but not its yolk sac, generates lympho-myeloid stem cells: mapping multipotent hematopoietic cell fate in intraembryonic mesoderm. Immunity 15:487–495, 2001.

Tcharmtchi MH, Smith CW, Mariscalco MM. Neonatal neutrophil interaction with P-selectin: contribution of P-selectin glycoprotein ligand-1 and sialic acid. J Leukoc Biol 67:73–80, 2000.

Tedder TF, Inaoki M, Sato S. The CD19-CD21 complex regulates signal transduction thresholds governing humoral immunity and autoimmunity. Immunity 6:107–118, 1997.

Thilaganathan B, Abbas A, Nicolaides KH. Fetal blood natural killer cells in human pregnancy. Fetal Diagn Ther 8:149–153, 1993.

Thilaganathan B, Carroll SG, Plachouras N, Makrydimas G, Nicolaides KH. Fetal immunological and haematological changes in intrauterine infection. Br J Obstet Gynaecol 101:418–421, 1994.

Thong YH, Hurtado RC, Rola-Pleszczynski M, Hensen SA, Vincent MM, Micheletti SA, Bellanti JA. Letter: Transplacental transmission of cell-mediated immunity. Lancet 1:1286–1287, 1974.

Timens W, Rozeboom T, Poppema S. Fetal and neonatal development of human spleen: an immunohistological study. Immunology 60:603–609, 1987.

Toivanen P, Uksila J, Leino A, Lassila O, Hirvonen T, Ruuskanen O. Development of mitogen responding T cells and natural killer cells in the human fetus. Immunol Rev 57:89–105, 1981.

Tono-Oka T, Nakayama M, Uehara H, Matsumoto S. Characteristics of impaired chemotactic function in cord blood leukocytes. Pediatr Res 13:148–151, 1979.

Trivedi HN, HayGlass KT, Gangur V, Allardice JG, Embree JE, Plummer FA. Analysis of neonatal T cell and antigen presenting cell functions. Hum Immunol 57:69–79, 1997.

Tsuyuguchi I, Kawasumi H, Ueta C, Yano I, Kishimoto S. Increase of T-cell receptor gamma/delta-bearing T cells in cord blood of newborn babies obtained by in vitro stimulation with mycobacterial cord factor. Infect Immun 59:3053–3059, 1991.

Tu W, Cheung PT, Lau YL. Insulin-like growth factor 1 promotes cord blood T cell maturation and inhibits its spontaneous and phytohemagglutinin-induced apoptosis through different mechanisms. J Immunol 165:1331–1336, 2000.

Ueno Y, Koizumi S, Yamagami M, Miura M, Taniguchi N. Characterization of hemopoietic stem cells (CFUc) in cord blood. Exp Hematol 9:716–722, 1981.

Ueno Y, Miyawaki T, Seki H, Matsuda A, Taga K, Sato H, Taniguchi N. Differential effects of recombinant human interferon-gamma and interleukin 2 on natural killer cell activity of peripheral blood in early human development. J Immunol 135:180–184, 1985.

Ueno Y, Ichihara T, Hasui M, Maruyama H, Miyawaki T, Taniguchi N, Komiyama A. T-cell-dependent production of IgG by human cord blood B cells in reconstituted SCID mice. Scand J Immunol 35:415–419, 1992.

Uhr JW, Dancis J, Neumann CG. Delayed-type hypersensitivity in premature neonatal humans. Nature 187:1130–1131, 1960.

Uhr JW, Dancis J, Franklin EC, Finkelstein MS, Lewis EW. The antibody response to bacteriophage in newborn premature infants. J Clin Invest 41:1509–1513, 1962.

Umemoto M, Azuma E, Hirayama M, Nagai M, Hiratake S, Qi J, Kumamoto T, Komada Y, Sakurai M. Two cytotoxic pathways of natural killer cells in human cord blood: implications in cord blood transplantation. Br J Haematol 98:1037–1040, 1997.

Vahlquist B. Response of infants to diphtheria immunization. Lancet 1:16–18, 1949.

Vallejo JG, Knuefermann P, Mann DL, Sivasubramanian N. Group B Streptococcus induces TNF-alpha gene expression and activation of the transcription factors NF-kappa B and activator protein-1 in human cord blood monocytes. J Immunol 165:419–425, 2000.

Vancurova I, Bellani P, Davidson D. Activation of nuclear factor-kappaB and its suppression by dexamethasone in polymorphonuclear leukocytes: newborn versus adult. Pediatr Res 49:257–262, 2001.

Vandekerckhove BA, Baccala R, Jones D, Kono DH, Theofilopoulos AN, Roncarolo MG. Thymic selection of the human T cell receptor V beta repertoire in SCID-hu mice. J Exp Med 176:1619–1624, 1992.

Vandekerckhove BA, Jones D, Punnonen J, Schols D, Lin HC, Duncan B, Bacchetta R, de Vries JE, Roncarolo MG. Human Ig production and isotype switching in severe combined immunodeficient-human mice. J Immunol 151:128–137, 1993.

van den Beemd R, Boor PP, van Lochem EG, Hop WC, Langerak AW, Wolvers-Tettero IL, Hooijkaas H, van Dongen JJ. Flow cytometric analysis of the Vbeta repertoire in healthy controls. Cytometry 40:336–345, 2000.

Vandenberghe P, Delabie J, de Boer M, de Wolf-Peeters C, Ceuppens JL. In situ expression of B7/BB1 on antigen-presenting cells and activated B cells: an immunohistochemical study. Int Immunol 5:317–321, 1993.

Vanderbeeken Y, Sarfati M, Bose R, Delespesse G. In utero immunization of the fetus to tetanus by maternal vaccination during pregnancy. Am J Reprod Immunol Microbiol 8:39–42, 1985.

van der Vliet HJ, Nishi N, de Gruijl TD, von Blomberg BM, van den Eertwegh AJ, Pinedo HM, Giaccone G, Scheper RJ. Human natural killer T cells acquire a memory-activated phenotype before birth. Blood 95:2440–2442, 2000.

Van Duren-Schmidt K, Pichler J, Ebner C, Bartmann P, Forster E, Urbanek R, Szepfalusi Z. Prenatal contact with inhalant allergens. Pediatr Res 41:128–131, 1997.

Van Epps DE, Goodwin JS, Murphy S. Age-dependent variations in polymorphonuclear leukocyte chemiluminescence. Infect Immun 22:57–61, 1978.

van Es JH, Meyling FH, Logtenberg T. High frequency of somatically mutated IgM molecules in the human adult blood B cell repertoire. Eur J Immunol 22:2761–2764, 1992.

van Furth R, Raeburn JA, van Zwet TL. Characteristics of human mononuclear phagocytes. Blood 54:485–500, 1979.

Varas A, Jimenez E, Sacedon R, Rodriguez-Mahou M, Maroto E, Zapata AG, Vicente A. Analysis of the human neonatal thymus: evidence for a transient thymic involution. J Immunol 164:6260–6267, 2000.

Varis I, Deneys V, Mazzon A, de Bruyere M, Cornu G, Brichard B. Expression of HLA-DR, CAM and co-stimulatory molecules on cord blood monocytes. Eur J Haematol 66:107–114, 2001.

Vekemans J, Amedei A, Ota MO, D'Elios MM, Goetghebuer T, Ismaili J, Newport MJ, Del Prete G, Goldman M, McAdam KP, Marchant A. Neonatal bacillus Calmette-Guerin vaccination induces adult-like IFN-gamma production by CD4+ T lymphocytes. Eur J Immunol 31:1531–1535, 2001.

Vekemans J, Ota MO, Wang EC, Kidd M, Borysiewicz LK, Whittle H, McAdam KP, Morgan G, Marchant A. T cell responses to vaccines in infants: defective IFN-gamma production after oral polio vaccination. Clin Exp Immunol 127:495–498, 2002.

Verhasselt B, Kerre T, Naessens E, Vanhecke D, De Smedt M, Vandekerckhove B, Plum J. Thymic repopulation by CD34(+) human cord blood cells after expansion in stroma-free culture. Blood 94:3644–3552, 1999.

Viemann D, Schlenke P, Hammers HJ, Kirchner H, Kruse A. Differential expression of the B cell-restricted molecule CD22 on neonatal B lymphocytes depending upon antigen stimulation. Eur J Immunol 30:550–559, 2000.

Vietor HE, Bolk J, Vreugdenhil GR, Kanhai HH, van den Elsen PJ, Brand A. Alterations in cord blood leukocyte subsets of patients with severe hemolytic disease after intrauterine transfusion therapy. J Pediatr 130:718–724, 1997a.

Vietor HE, Hawes GE, van den Oever C, van Beelen E, Kanhai HH, Brand A, van den Elsen PJ. Intrauterine transfusions affect fetal T-cell immunity. Blood 90:2492–2501, 1997b.

Vigano A, Esposito S, Arienti D, Zagliani A, Massironi E, Principi N, Clerici M. Differential development of type 1 and type 2 cytokines and beta-chemokines in the ontogeny of healthy newborns. Biol Neonate 75:1–8, 1999.

Vivien L, Benoist C, Mathis D. T lymphocytes need IL-7 but not IL-4 or IL-6 to survive in vivo. Int Immunol 13:763–768, 2001.

Vos Q, Lees A, Wu ZQ, Snapper CM, Mond JJ. B-cell activation by T-cell-independent type 2 antigens as an integral part of the humoral immune response to pathogenic microorganisms. Immunol Rev 176:154–170, 2000.

Walker RI, Willemze R. Neutrophil kinetics and the regulation of granulopoiesis. Rev Infect Dis 2:282–292, 1980.

Wang L, Das H, Kamath A, Bukowski JF. Human Vgamma2 Vdelta2 T cells produce IFN-gamma and TNF-alpha with an on/off/on cycling pattern in response to live bacterial products. J Immunol 167:6195–6201, 2001a.

Wang L, Kamath A, Das H, Li L, Bukowski JF. Antibacterial effect of human V gamma 2V delta 2 T cells in vivo. J Clin Invest 108:1349–1357, 2001b.

Warwick WJ, Good RA, Smith RT. Failure of passive transfer of delayed hypersensitivity in the newborn human infant. J Lab Clin Med 56:139–147, 1960.

Washburn LK, O'Shea TM, Gillis DC, Block SM, Abramson JS. Response to Haemophilus influenzae type b conjugate vaccine in chronically ill premature infants. J Pediatr 123:791–794, 1993.

Watts AM, Stanley JR, Shearer MH, Hefty PS, Kennedy RC. Fetal immunization of baboons induces a fetal-specific antibody response. Nat Med 5:427–430, 1999.

Webb BJ, Bochan MR, Montel A, Padilla LM, Brahmi Z. The lack of NK cytotoxicity associated with fresh HUCB may be due to the presence of soluble HLA in the serum. Cell Immunol 159:246–261, 1994.

Webb LM, Foxwell BM, Feldmann M. Putative role for interleukin-7 in the maintenance of the recirculating naïve CD4+ T-cell pool. Immunology 98:400–405, 1999.

Wedgwood JF, Weinberger BI, Hatam L, Palmer R. Umbilical cord blood lacks circulating B lymphocytes expressing surface IgG or IgA. Clin Immunol Immunopathol 84:276–282, 1997.

Weimann E, Rutkowski S, Reisbach G. G-CSF, GM-CSF and IL-6 levels in cord blood: diminished increase of G-CSF and IL-6 in preterms with perinatal infection compared to term neonates. J Perinat Med 26:211–218, 1998.

Weinberg AG, Rosenfeld CR, Manroe BL, Browne R. Neonatal blood cell count in health and disease. II. Values for lymphocytes, monocytes, and eosinophils. J Pediatr 106:462–466, 1985.

West DJ. Clinical experience with hepatitis B vaccines. Am J Infect Control 17:172–180, 1989.

Weston WL, Carson BS, Barkin RM, Slater GD, Dustin RD, Hecht SK. Monocyte-macrophage function in the newborn. Am J Dis Child 131:1241–1242, 1977.

White GP, Watt PM, Holt BJ, Holt PG. Differential patterns of methylation of the IFN-gamma promoter at CpG and non-CpG sites underlie differences in IFN-gamma gene expression between human neonatal and adult CD45RO- T cells. J Immunol 168:2820–2827, 2002.

Wilimas JA, Wall JE, Fairclough DL, Dancy R, Griffin C, Karanth S, Wang W, Evans WE. A longitudinal study of granulocyte colony-stimulating factor levels and neutrophil counts in newborn infants. J Pediatr Hematol Oncol 17:176–179, 1995.

Wilson CB, Haas JE. Cellular defenses against Toxoplasma gondii in newborns. J Clin Invest 73:1606–1616, 1984.

Wilson CB, Weaver WM. Comparative susceptibility of group B streptococci and Staphylococcus aureus to killing by oxygen metabolites. J Infect Dis 152:323–329, 1985.

Wilson CB, Westall J, Johnston L, Lewis DB, Dower SK, Alpert AR. Decreased production of interferon-gamma by human neonatal cells. Intrinsic and regulatory deficiencies. J Clin Invest 77:860–867, 1986.

Wilson M, Rosen FS, Schlossman SF, Reinherz EL. Ontogeny of human T and B lymphocytes during stressed and normal gestation: phenotypic analysis of umbilical cord lymphocytes from term and preterm infants. Clin Immunol Immunopathol 37:1–12, 1985.

Wilson SB, Kent SC, Patton KT, Orban T, Jackson RA, Exley M, Porcelli S, Schatz DA, Atkinson MA, Balk SP, Strominger JL, Hafler DA. Extreme Th1 bias of invariant Valpha24JalphaQ T cells in type 1 diabetes. Nature 391:177–181, 1998.

Winkelstein JA, Kurlandsky LE, Swift AJ. Defective activation of the third component of complement in the sera of newborn infants. Pediatr Res 13:1093–1096, 1979.

Witherden DA, Rieder SE, Boismenu R, Havran WL. A role for epithelial gamma delta T cells in tissue repair. Springer Semin Immunopathol 22:265–281, 2000.

Wolach B, Dolfin T, Regev R, Gilboa S, Schlesinger M. The development of the complement system after 28 weeks' gestation. Acta Paediatr 86:523–527, 1997.

Woodside DG, Long DA, McIntyre BW. Intracellular analysis of interleukin-2 induction provides direct evidence at the single cell level of differential coactivation requirements for CD45RA+ and CD45RO+ T cell subsets. J Interferon Cytokine Res 19:769–779, 1999.

Wright SD. Multiple receptors for endotoxin. Curr Opin Immunol 3:83–90, 1991.

Wright WC Jr, Ank BJ, Herbert J, Stiehm ER. Decreased bactericidal activity of leukocytes of stressed newborn infants. Pediatrics 56:579–584, 1975.

Wucherpfennig KW, Liao YJ, Prendergast M, Prendergast J, Hafler DA, Strominger JL. Human fetal liver gamma/delta T cells predominantly use unusual rearrangements of the T cell receptor delta and gamma loci expressed on both CD4+CD8- and CD4-CD8- gamma/delta T cells. J Exp Med 177:425–432, 1993.

Yamaguchi E, de Vries J, Yssel H. Differentiation of human single-positive fetal thymocytes in vitro into IL-4-and/or IFN-gamma-producing CD4+ and CD8+ T cells. Int Immunol 11:593–603, 1999.

Yamamoto J, Adachi Y, Onoue Y, Adachi YS, Okabe Y, Itazawa T, Toyoda M, Seki T, Morohashi M, Matsushima K, Miyawaki T. Differential expression of the chemokine receptors by the Th1- and Th2-type effector populations within circulating CD4+ T cells. J Leukoc Biol 68:568–574, 2000.

Yang Y, Chu W, Geraghty DE, Hunt JS. Expression of HLA-G in human mononuclear phagocytes and selective induction by IFN-gamma. J Immunol 156:4224–4231, 1996.

Yang YC, Hsu TY, Chen JY, Yang CS, Lin RH. Tumour necrosis factor-alpha-induced apoptosis in cord blood T lymphocytes: involvement of both tumour necrosis factor receptor types 1 and 2. Br J Haematol 115:435–441, 2001.

Yasui K, Masuda M, Matsuoka T, Yamazaki M, Komiyama A, Akabane T, Hasui M, Kobayashi Y, Murata K. Abnormal membrane fluidity as a cause of impaired functional dynamics of chemoattractant receptors on neonatal polymorphonuclear leukocytes: lack of modulation of the receptors by a membrane fluidizer. Pediatr Res 24:442–446, 1988.

Yasui K, Masuda M, Tsuno T, Matsuoka T, Komiyama A, Akabane T, Murata K. An increase in polymorphonuclear leucocyte chemotaxis accompanied by a change in the membrane fluidity with age during childhood. Clin Exp Immunol 81:156–159, 1990.

Yoder MC, Douglas SD, Gerdes J, Kline J, Polin RA. Plasma fibronectin in healthy newborn infants: respiratory distress syndrome and perinatal asphyxia. J Pediatr 102:777–780, 1983.

Zach TL, Hostetter MK. Biochemical abnormalities of the third component of complement in neonates. Pediatr Res 26:116–120, 1989.

Zemlin M, Bauer K, Hummel M, Pfeiffer S, Devers S, Zemlin C, Stein H, Versmold HT. The diversity of rearranged immunoglobulin heavy chain variable region genes in peripheral blood B cells of preterm infants is restricted by short third complementarity-determining regions but not by limited gene segment usage. Blood 97:1511–1513, 2001.

Zeng D, Lewis D, Dejbakhsh-Jones S, Lan F, Garcia-Ojeda M, Sibley R, Strober S. Bone marrow NK1.1(−) and NK1.1(+) T cells reciprocally regulate acute graft versus host disease. J Exp Med 189:1073–1081, 1999.

Zheng B, Kelsoe G, Han S. Somatic diversification of antibody responses. J Clin Immunol 16:1–11, 1996.

Zheng Z, Takahashi M, Narita M, Toba K, Liu A, Furukawa T, Koike T, Aizawa Y. Generation of dendritic cells from adherent cells of cord blood with granulocyte-macrophage colony-stimulating factor, interleukin-4, and tumor necrosis factor-alpha. J Hematother Stem Cell Res 9:453–464, 2000.

Zilow EP, Hauck W, Linderkamp O, Zilow G. Alternative pathway activation of the complement system in preterm infants with early onset infection. Pediatr Res 41:334–339, 1997.

CHAPTER

23 Immune Responses in Malnutrition

Susanna Cunningham-Rundles, David F. McNeeley, and Jintanat Ananworanich

MALNUTRITION, INFECTION, AND IMMUNODEFICIENCY

Malnutrition, an inadequacy of nutrients sufficient to interfere with normal physiologic function, is a major cause of immune deficiency, leading to serious and frequent infections in children (Adhikari et al., 1997; Cunningham-Rundles and Cervia, 1996a; Morris and Potter, 1997). The normal maturation of the immune system that occurs during development can be impaired by malnutrition during gestation, in the neonatal period, and during weaning (Hay, 1994; Insoft et al., 1996; Zuin and Principi, 1997). Even where food is available, poverty and ignorance can cause malnutrition. Infection due to poor sanitation, crowding, unsafe water, and contaminated foods often becomes chronic in the malnourished child. Chronic undernutrition leading to immune deficiency and exposure to endemic pathogens can then lead to a cycle of repetitive infections (Hirve and Ganatra, 1997; Scrimshaw and San Giovanni, 1997). Chronic infection imposes a metabolic burden that worsens malnutrition and prevents growth (Beisel, 1995; Peters et al., 1998).

The key interactions involved in this vicious cycle are depicted in Figure 23-1. Selective nutrient deficiencies of micronutrients, such as iron, zinc, or vitamin A, may occur even when food intake is adequate and may also cause specific immune deficiencies (Johnson et al., 1994; Kennedy and Goldberg, 1995; Rose et al., 1998). When combined with caloric deficiency, this leads to multiple clinical features, as shown in Table 23-1. Even when not lethal, nutritional deficiencies may have long-term adverse effects that persist after the nutritional defects are corrected. These include persistent T-cell defects (e.g., in zinc deficiency) and cognitive defects (e.g., in iron deficiency).

Overnutrition, an excess intake of calories relative to energy expenditure, leads to obesity and may also be associated with abnormalities of the immune system (Boeck et al., 1993); it is becoming increasingly common (Troiano et al., 1991). Eating disorders (bulimia and anorexia nervosa) also cause lymphocyte subset balance with reduced immune responses (Marcos et al., 1997a, 1997b).

The mechanisms by which nutrient deficiencies impair host defense may implicate cellular, humoral, and regulatory cytokine pathways (Lin et al., 1998; Rink and Kirchner, 2000; Savendall and Underwood, 1997; Wallace et al., 1997) and lead to specific dietary recommendations (Zeisel, 2000). This chapter discusses primary and secondary malnutrition, the impact of chronic infection, and the implications of these interactions for the development of host defense.

MALNUTRITION AND HOST DEFENSE

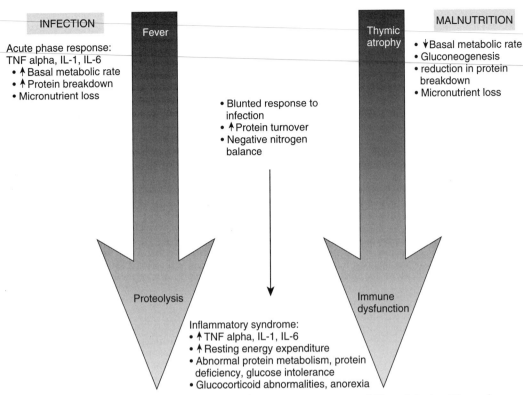

Figure 23-1 · Host defenses in malnutrition. Malnutrition increases susceptibility to infection. The resulting infection increases nutritional requirements and aggravates malnutrition. The worsening malnutrition aggravates the infection, which decreases the appetite and increases nutritional requirements. The growing child is especially vulnerable to this vicious cycle because of the immaturity of the immune system and increased nutritional requirements. IL = interleukin; TNF = tumor necrosis factor.

Etiology and Mechanisms

The mechanism by which malnutrition causes immune deficiency, whether from general food deprivation or specific micronutrient deficiencies (vitamin or trace element) are multiple and complicated by the presence, duration, and severity of infection (see Fig. 23-1). Specific nutrient defects can also be caused by genetic defects leading to zinc deficiency in acrodermatitis enteropathica (Moynahan, 1974; Sandstrom et al., 1994) or to defects of copper metabolism in Menkes and Wilson's disease (Menkes, 1999; Wilson et al., 2000).

Diets limited to grains or legumes can cause protein insufficiency and reduced immune responses. The effects of a single-grain diet such as maize may be related to metabolites of dietary constituents rather than to nutrient absence. For example, the high level of linoleic acid in maize in the absence of other polyunsaturated fatty acids may increase production of prostaglandin E_2 (PGE$_2$), leading to downregulation of T-helper 1 (Th1) cytokine production (Sammon, 1999). Some grains also contain large amounts of phytic acid, which impairs zinc intake.

Micronutrients in general have a crucial impact on immune response, both through antioxidant effects and through modulation of cytokine expression. Three antioxidant enzymes, the copper, zinc, and manganese superoxide dismutases, require trace metals for biologic activity. These reactions protect against oxidative damage caused by free radical formation.

Iron, copper, and zinc deficiencies are the most common trace element nutrient deficits in North America and are usually due to dietary insufficiency. Selenium deficiency, like that of iodine, affects those parts of the world with low levels in soil. Micronutrients are often deficient in patients with systemic illnesses and severe infections such as chronic viral infection.

Infections can be a direct cause of malnutrition (Schmidt, 1997). Cytokine production during the acute-phase response produces effects ranging from fever to septic shock with loss of lean tissue and body fat (Lin et al., 1998). Fever, cellular hypermetabolism, and various endocrine and metabolic changes eventually lead to increased catabolism and gluconeogenesis. These are accompanied by multiple effects on metals and minerals, such as fluxes of iron and zinc; losses of nitrogen, potassium, magnesium, phosphate, zinc, and vitamins; and retention of salt and water. Interleukin-1 (IL-1), IL-6, and tumor necrosis factor-α (TNF-α) are the key mediators implicated (Moldower and Lowry, 1993). IL-1 is also implicated in intestinal enteropathy (Mowat et al.,

TABLE 23-5 · CLINICAL AND IMMUNOLOGIC FEATURES OF MALNUTRITION SYNDROMES OF CHILDHOOD

Syndrome	Clinical Features of Malnutrition	Effects on Immune System
Intrauterine growth retardation	Low birth weight, small for gestational age, failure to thrive	Susceptibility to infection, T-cell abnormalities, skin test anergy
Failure to thrive	Growth failure, inability to gain weight, developmental delay, malabsorption, diarrhea	Frequent infections, deficient immune response
Short bowel syndrome	Severe fluid loss and electrolyte imbalance requiring initial parenteral and then enteral nutrition; PCM, zinc, vitamin D deficiency, poor growth, bony demineralization	Infections including nosocomial infections, bacterial overgrowth; parenteral nutrition may cause micronutrient deficiencies
Inflammatory bowel disease	Anorexia, diarrhea, gut blood and protein loss, malabsorption, impaired linear growth retarded bone development, delayed puberty	Chronic inflammatory response, increased macrophage inhibitory factor, antibodies to gut bacteria
Crohn's disease	Lactose intolerance if small bowel involvement, transmural inflammation, granuloma formation, genetic predisposition	T-cell–driven autoimmune disease, activated mucosal T cells
Ulcerative colitis	Hypercoagulability of blood, cow's milk intolerance, genetic predisposition	Antibodies to neutrophil cytoplasm, mucin
Malabsorption syndromes	Nausea, cramping, abdominal pain, diarrhea; lactase deficiency, sucrase-isomaltase deficiency, starch intolerance	Affects bacterial composition of the gut and thereby bacterial immune interaction.
Gluten-sensitive enteropathy (celiac disease)	Small intestinal damage, loss of absorptive villi, hyperplasia of crypts in response to gliadin, malabsorption, malnutrition, risk of malignancy	HLA-linked host response, IgA antibodies to gliadin, endomysium; autoantigen is tissue transglutaminase

HLA = human leukocyte antigen.

Intrauterine Growth Retardation

Intrauterine growth retardation (IUGR) can be caused by primary maternal malnutrition in developing countries but is usually attributed to placental insufficiency, congenital infection, maternal smoking, exposure to toxins, or a combination of factors (Pardi et al., 1997; Prada et al., 1998; Rondo et al., 1997; Strauss and Dietz, 1999). Maternal nutrient deficiencies linked to IUGR include calcium; vitamins A, B_1, and E; and folate (Jiang and Shao, 1994; Rondo and Tomkins, 2000). Low maternal weight in the second and third trimester is associated with IUGR (Strauss and Dietz, 1999). Increasing maternal protein and calories in the second and third trimester reduce the risk of IUGR (De Onis et al., 1998). Other studies have explored the use of zinc, folate, and magnesium in its prevention.

The low-birth-weight infant has significantly increased susceptibility to infection and reduced immune function compared with term infants, even when growth is appropriate for gestational age (AGA) and there is no evidence of infection (see Chapter 22). This leads to increased mortality, particularly when associated with congenital anomalies (Ashworth, 1998) Low-birth-weight infants have impaired cell-mediated immunity with diminished cytokine responses and reduced phagocyte function (Baltimore, 1998; Cunningham-Rundles and Nesin, 2000; Klein and Remington, 1995). Small-for-gestational-age (SGA) infants also have smaller thymic glands and deficient cytokine responses relative to the AGA infant (Nesin and Cunningham-Rundles, 2000).

Intrauterine growth retardation has also been linked to poor future health, including postnatal infections, sudden infant death syndrome, hypertension, ischemic heart disease, and diabetes (Hofman et al., 1997; Henriksen, 1999; Tenhola et al., 2000). A common feature for the latter may be insulin resistance. Children stunted in early childhood have higher salivary cortisol levels and an increased heart rate (Fernald et al., 1998).

Without specific postnatal support, catch-up growth is limited (Arifeen et al., 2000); however, addition of semi-essential nutrients such as dietary nucleotides may be beneficial (Yu, 1998). Sazawah and associates (2001) found that zinc supplementation given to SGA infants reduced their infectious mortality. Human growth hormone has been extensively used to correct growth impairment caused by IUGR, but with variable success (Chernausek et al., 1996).

Failure to Thrive

Failure to thrive (FTT), a major malnutrition syndrome, is often defined as weight (or weight for height) less than two standard deviations below the mean for sex and age. Alternatively, a child whose weight curve has crossed more than two percentile lines on the standard growth chart after a previous history of stable growth is also defined as having FFT. This definition reflects the fact that weight loss and growth failure are distinctly abnormal in childhood. Although FTT may be due to simple undernutrition, presence of organic illness such as malignancy, exposure to toxins, or congenital anomalies can be causative (Forchielli et al., 1999). Behavioral abnormalities and poor parenting may also result in growth failure (Wright and Birks, 2000).

A complete evaluation may reveal a genetic disorder such as Bloom's syndrome or Russell Silver syndrome (see Chapter 24), a psychosocial feeding disorder, an immune deficiency, a gastrointestinal disorder, or a combination of these factors. Immunologic screening tests are an important part of the diagnostic evaluation.

Short Bowel Syndrome

A shortened small intestine, termed short bowel syndrome, may be secondary to congenital atresia or surgical resection and commonly leads to severe nutritional problems (Horwitz et al., 1995; Vanderhoof, 1996; Weber, 1995). Malabsorption of fat-soluble vitamins, fats, and carbohydrates are common due to loss of absorptive area, digestive enzymes, and carrier proteins. Altered flux of water and electrolytes and changes in absorption due to loss of functional surface area may produce osmotic diarrhea and fluid loss.

Prolonged parenteral nutrition is usually necessary but often associated with impaired immune responses secondary to loss of antigenic stimuli (Bistrian, 1999; De Witt and Kudsk, 1999), caloric insufficiency, micronutrient insufficiency, and poor intestinal absorption (Rannem et al., 1996). Efforts to stimulate gastrointestinal cell growth with growth hormone or glutamine are promising (Byrne et al., 1995; Scolapio et al., 1997). Alterations in normal flora and microinfections of the gastrointestinal (GI) tract may cause motility abnormalities, provoking an inflammatory response necessitating the use of parenteral nutrition (Kaufman et al., 1997).

Inflammatory Bowel Disease

Ulcerative colitis (UC) and Crohn's disease, usually presenting in the second decade of life, are often associated with malnutrition and malabsorption (see Chapter 34). Whereas IgA is the major intestinal immunoglobulin in health, IgG predominates in the intestine of patients with inflammatory bowel disease, and its reactivity is against commensal bacterial cytoplasmic proteins, suggesting a possible abrogation of tolerance (Macpherson et al., 1996). Inflammatory cytokines have been implicated in the pathogenesis of UC (Murakami et al., 2001), possibly linked with gene polymorphism of the IL-1 receptor antagonist (Carter et al., 2001). Antibodies to neutrophil cytoplasmic antigens (ANCAs) and to mucin are often present in UC patients (Hayashi et al., 2001; Kossa et al., 1995). Immune responses to cow's milk antigens, either antibodies or cellular, are often present; these may reflect a generalized hyperreactivity rather than a specific response to a single antigen (Mishkin, 1997).

Crohn's disease is associated with increased numbers of circulating memory CD4+ T cells and activated mucosal T cells that have defective proliferative responses (Jacquot et al., 1996; Roman et al., 1996). Their mucosal T cells are balanced toward proliferation and away from apoptosis (Ina et al., 1999). An abnormal immune response toward endogenous bacteria may be causative (Duchmann et al., 1996). Clinical improvement may occur with restoration of normal bacterial flora (Malin et al., 1996). Infectious agents such as *Mycobacterium avium paratuberculosis* are suspected but unproved.

Poor nutrition is aggravated by inadequate dietary intake associated with altered taste and anorexia, in part related to partial zinc deficiency. Nutritional management includes elemental and hypoallergenic diets and, in severe cases, bowel rest with parenteral nutrition.

Food Intolerance and Gluten Sensitivity

Food intolerance includes food allergy (see Chapter 31), carbohydrate malabsorption, and gluten sensitivity (see Chapter 34). Carbohydrate malabsorption allows unabsorbed carbohydrate to undergo bacterial fermentation in the colon, producing gas and fluid. Lactose intolerance is the most common disorder. Maturational lactose deficiency may occur in premature infants, and congenital defects may occur with both early and late onset.

Gluten-sensitive enteropathy, or celiac disease, is a specific intolerance to the wheat gluten, gliadin, leading to villous flattening and, sometimes, severe malnutrition (Fasano and Catassi, 2001; Ferguson, 1995). Celiac disease, although genetically linked to human leukocyte antigen (HLA) class II DQ-A1 *0501 B1 *0201 (Goggins and Kelleher, 1994), may differ in clinical severity from silent to severe. Other genes must participate in disease expression, because even among celiac siblings risk is less than 40% (King and Ciclitira, 2000). Dermatitis herpetiformis (see Chapter 32), a blistering skin disease with cutaneous IgA deposition, shares the same genetic pattern but usually has no bowel symptoms, despite similar GI histologic changes (Hall et al., 2000).

Diagnosis of celiac disease has classically relied on intestinal biopsy following wheat gluten challenge. The intestinal mucosa can be normalized by a gluten-free diet, but changes in the intraepithelial lymphocytes, specifically increase in $\gamma\delta$-T-cell levels, persist (Camarero et al., 2000). The presence of serum IgA antibodies to gliadin and to endomysium, a structure of smooth muscle connective tissue, is used to diagnose celiac disease (Wahab et al., 2001). Gliadin is the substrate for tissue transglutaminase, which has been identified as a key target autoantigen (Dieterich et al., 1997). Antibodies to transglutaminase are now used diagnostically (Fasano and Catassi, 2001; Mc Pherson et al., 2001).

MALNUTRITION IN PEDIATRIC DISORDERS

Malnutrition is a common but not invariable complication of many pediatric conditions and leads to secondary immunodeficiency. These conditions are summarized in Table 23-6.

Cystic Fibrosis

Most children with cystic fibrosis (CF) eventually develop some degree of malnutrition as a result of malabsorption or chronic respiratory infection (see Chapter

TABLE 23-6 · CLINICAL AND IMMUNOLOGIC FEATURES OF SOME PEDIATRIC DISORDERS WITH MALNUTRITION-INDUCED IMMUNE DEFICIENCY

Disorder	Clinical Features of Malnutrition	Effects on Immune System
Cystic fibrosis	Pancreatic insufficiency, cirrhosis, neonatal meconium ileus, intestinal obstruction, esophagitis, hypoproteinemia, malabsorption, wasting, stunting	Hypergammaglobulinemia, elevated IgE infections
Liver diseases, hepatitis viruses, autoimmune hepatitis, Wilson's disease, iron overload (chronic transfusion), hereditary hemochromatosis	Increased energy expenditure and inefficient utilization, hypoglycemia/hyperglycemia, hypoalbuminemia, fat malabsorption, malabsorption of fat soluble vitamins, trace metal deficiency, anemia, wasting, stunting	Increased plasma TGF-β1, increased soluble adhesion molecules, decreased responses in vitro to mitogens and antigens, impaired skin test reactivity, increased IL-6
Chronic renal insufficiency	Growth decline, decrease in final height, muscle wasting, low serum albumin dehydration, sodium depletion, metabolic acidosis, PCM, anorexia	Increased loss of CD4 cells, immune activation, cytokine activation
HIV infection	Diarrhea; malabsorption; loss of micronutrients, especially vitamins A and E and selenium; anorexia; increased resting energy expenditure; wasting; stunting; delayed puberty	Progressive loss of CD4 cells, activation of the immune system; immune dysregulation
Diabetes mellitus	Type 1: insulin dependent, initially often presents with weight loss Type 2: non–insulin dependent, usually obese, hyperlipidemic	Type 1: autoimmune response antibodies to cow's milk, altered T cells, NK cells Type 2: obesity
Hyperlipidemia	Accelerated metabolism or diminished catabolism of lipoproteins; many genetic and non-genetic types Obesity, hypertriglyceridemia, hyperinsulinemia, and glucose intolerance common over time	Reduced CD4 cells, spontaneous TNF-α production
Chronic anemias	Deficiency of vitamins A, B$_6$, B$_{12}$, riboflavin, folic acid, iron, copper	Interferes with immune development and function
Cancer	Reduced intake, cancer cachexia, short stature, enteritis secondary to treatment	Immune deficiency associated with malignancy, treatment

TGF = transforming growth factor.

33). Genetic defects in the CF transmembrane conductance regulator have been identified, but genotype-phenotype correlations are weak, suggesting an important role for disease modifiers (Zielenski, 2000). Nor is there a good correlation between the severity of the pulmonary infection and the degree of intestinal involvement/nutritional status, also suggesting a role for other factors and stressing the need for nutritional supplementation in all patients. Malabsorption and increased energy expenditure may lead to hypoproteinemia, poor weight gain, and growth failure. Chronic pulmonary infections aggravate these problems (Burns et al., 2001; Tummler and Kiewitz, 1999); they are associated with an increase in inflammatory markers, such as soluble interleukin-2 receptor (sIL-2R) and eosinophilic cationic protein; the latter is a possible correlate of disease severity (Koller et al., 1996).

Recent studies suggest that intestinal inflammation may be a fundamental feature of CF (Smyth et al., 2000). Activation of IFN-γ production and a Th1 cytokine response have been associated with better lung function in CF, whereas reduced IFN-γ activity and an increased Th2 cytokine response were correlated with chronic *Pseudomonas aeruginosa* lung infection (Moser et al., 2000). A Th2 cytokine increase has also been observed in CF patients with aspergillosis (Skov et al., 1999). Infections are worsened by diminished immune responsiveness, possibly related to abnormal zinc turnover, reduced thymulin activity, and reduced IL-2 and NK activity (Mocchegiani, et al., 1995).

Nutritional therapy includes dietary supplements, increasing fat and protein absorption with oral pancreatic enzymes, providing supplemental fat-soluble vitamins such as vitamin K, and giving omega-3 long-chain polyunsaturated fatty acids such as docosahexanoic acid (DHA) (Winklhofer-Roob, 2000). Prevention of malnutrition is associated with improved linear growth (Farrell et al., 2001) and survival (Beker et al., 2001).

Liver Disease

Several liver disorders can affect growth, including metabolic disorders (galactosemia, glycogen storage disease), liver cancer, and hepatitis (infectious and autoimmune) (Protheroe, 1998; Ramaccioni et al., 2000) (see Chapter 34). Hepatocellular carcinoma has declined with hepatitis B vaccination (Chang et al., 2000) but may increase because of the increasing incidence of hepatitis C (Aizawa et al., 2000). Immune defects with liver disease may result from selective vitamin or trace element deficiency, as well as generalized malnutrition. Increased levels of transforming growth factor-β1 (TGF-β1) correlate with liver insufficiency (Flisiak and Prokopowitz, 2000; Tsai, et al., 1997), probably reflecting liver fibrogenesis. Increased levels of adhesion molecules such as E-selectin, ICAM-1, and LFA-3 (Cervello et al., 2000; Hoffman et al., 1996; Pirisi et al., 1997) are found in chronic liver disease, reflecting inflammation or infection. Risk factors for progressive liver disease following hepatitis C infection include HLA-DR5, HLA-DR4, and female gender (Czaja et al., 1998; Peano et al., 1994).

Renal Disease

Maternal protein insufficiency during pregnancy can lead to neonatal susceptibility to renal failure associated with fewer nephrons (Langley-Evans et al., 1999; Nwagwu et al., 2000). Conversely, a neonatal diet too rich in protein may cause metabolic acidosis, renal injury, and failure to thrive. Patients with acute renal disease have increased energy expenditure, nitrogen excretion, and caloric requirements. Chronic renal insufficiency leads to growth delay, in part a consequence of the uremia and in part secondary hyperparathyroidism. A low protein intake in the uremic infant retards growth more than excess protein. Growth failure is associated with increased morbidity and mortality (Norman et al., 2000; Wong et al., 2000) (see Chapter 25).

Dialysis also creates nutritional imbalance associated with hyperglycemia due to glucose in the dialysing solutions and protein loss. Peritoneal dialysis results in loss of micronutrients and carnitine, whereas peritoneal dialysis results in loss of amino acids (Swinford et al., 1996). Growth hormone has been successfully used to accelerate growth and increase body mineral mass in children with chronic renal insufficiency (Johnson et al., 2000).

Lipid Disorders

Lipid abnormalities include primary hyperlipidemias with hypercholesterolemia and secondary hyperlipidemias resulting from diabetes, nephrotic syndrome, hepatitis, lupus erythematosus, anorexia nervosa, and chronic steroid use. Many of the genes responsible for the hyperlipidemias have been identified, and of these, many present early in life. Children born SGA are at risk for higher levels in later life (Tenhola et al., 2000). Lowering dietary fat reduces body fat in hypercholesterolemic children (Tershakovec et al., 1998). Moreno and associates (1998) found that a low-fat diet reduced previously elevated T-cell subsets and triglycerides in children with hypercholesterolemia.

Low-fat diets may result in undernutrition. Diets deficient in essential fatty acids can result in anemia, growth retardation, and severe dermatitis.

Obesity

Obesity is a major nutritional problem with adverse effects on growth and immune function. Stunting can be associated with obesity (Popkin et al., 1996). The effect of genetic phenotype on predisposition to obesity is unsettled (Perusse and Bouchard, 2000). Adolescents with an increased body mass index (BMI) have increased CD8 T cells relative to CD4 T cells and increased TNF-α production (Boeck et al., 1993). Weight loss in obesity is associated with reduced immune function (Nieman et al., 1996). Although obesity is not associated with a major increase in susceptibility to infection, there is an increased risk for tumors, including renal cell, endometrial, and colonic adenocarcinomas and some forms of breast cancer (Carroll, 1998; Li and Mobarhan, 2000; Stoll, 2000; Weber et al., 2000).

Plasma levels of leptin, the fat-specific energy balance hormone, correlate with BMI; this increase may be associated with a loss of leptin sensitivity (Considine et al., 1996; Maffei et al., 1995). However, leptin increases the proinflammatory response (Loffreda et al., 1998), which may in turn stimulate leptin production. Leptin has been used to reverse the immunosuppressive effects of acute starvation by increasing Th1 and decreasing Th2 cytokines and promoting host defense in general (Loffreda et al., 1998; Lord et al., 1998).

Diabetes

Dietary modification can prevent the development of diabetes in diabetes-prone animals, by increasing insulin production in beta cells and downregulating glutamine oxidation in mesenteric lymph node cells (Scott et al., 2000). Cow's milk protein may trigger onset of type 1 diabetes in susceptible individuals (Vaarala, 1999) such as those with major histocompatibility complex (MHC) haplotype HLA B8-DR3-DQ2 (Harrison and Honeyman, 1999). Insulin in cow's milk may result in insulin antibodies in susceptible persons (Paronen et al., 2000).

Although type I diabetes continues to be far more common in children, type 2 diabetes is increasing because of childhood obesity (see Chapter 37). Loss-of-function mutations in the nuclear receptor peroxisome proliferator-activated receptor-γ (PPAR-γ) gene affects regulation of insulin resistance and blood pressure, whereas gain-of-function mutations are associated with obesity. A possible association between dietary fats and polymorphisms in PPAR-γ gene that affects fasting insulin and BMI has been suggested (Luan et al., 2001).

Anemia

Iron Deficiency Anemia

The usual cause of anemia is iron deficiency, resulting in a microcytic hypochromic anemia. Starvation, malabsorption, and infection may contribute to iron deficiency. A continuing controversy is whether the incidence or severity of infection is increased in the presence of iron deficiency or supplementation. Two large studies in Chile (Heresi et al., 1985) and India (Damadaran et al., 1979) found no difference in morbidity between children receiving iron supplements and a control group. In contrast, Cantwell (1972), studying children with severe iron deficiency, found a slight decrease in hospitalizations in an iron-treated group compared with controls.

Several studies have measured immunologic abnormalities in iron deficiency. B-cell immunity is generally intact. Serum immunoglobulins and salivary IgA are normal (Chandra and Saraya, 1975; MacDougall et al., 1975). Feng and associates (1994) noted subtle defects of pneumococcal polysaccharide antibody responses and IgG1 and IgG2 deficiencies in iron-deficient children.

Total hemolytic complement levels were reported as normal (Chandra and Saraya, 1975; MacDougall et al., 1975). One study noted a decrease in the total hemolytic complement when iron deficiency was severe (Jagaadeesan and Reddy, 1983).

Impaired bactericidal activity of neutrophils in iron-deficient patients is reversible after iron supplementation (Chandra, 1973; Walter et al., 1986; Yetgin et al., 1979). Conflicting evidence exists for a defect in phagocytic function as assessed by hexose monophosphate shunt activity and myeloperoxidase activity (Dhur et al., 1989).

Several studies have reported decreased T-cell numbers and impaired delayed cutaneous hypersensitivity consistent with impaired cell-mediated immunity (Chandra and Saraya, 1975; Krantman et al., 1982; MacDougall et al., 1975). Impaired lymphoproliferative response has been noted by several groups (Chandra and Saraya, 1975; Joynson et al., 1972; Scrimshaw and San Giovanni, 1997) but not by others (Kulapongs et al., 1974). One study found increased TNF-α and IL-1β production in response to lipopolysaccharide in vitro; this corrected with iron supplementation (Munoz et al., 1994).

There is a persistent concern that iron therapy may increase the severity of bacterial infection by providing an essential bacterial nutrient (Sussman, 1974). Use of parenteral iron as iron-dextran is now considered safe and effective but is contraindicated in the setting of acute infection (Burns et al., 1995).

Other Anemias

Vitamin A, pyridoxine, riboflavin, folic acid, and vitamin B_{12} deficiencies can cause a megaloblastic anemia. B_{12} deficiency may be a result of pernicious anemia, intestinal parasites, and transcobalamin defects. Vitamin B_{12}–deficient knockout mice have low levels of IgG, IgM, and C3; high levels of IgE; and a shift to a Th2 cytokine response (Funada et al., 2001).

Cancer

In general, children with cancer experience less malnutrition than do adults with cancer because leukemia, the most common childhood tumor, does not affect energy expenditure, and solid tumors affecting the digestive system are less common. In some children, loss of appetite and increased metabolic demands leads to cancer cachexia, in part mediated by cytokine activation, especially TNF-α and IL-6.

Chemotherapy can also lead to cachexia. Stem cell transplantation utilizing high-dose chemotherapy has major effects on gastrointestinal function and often results in significant nutrient imbalance. As noted in Chapter 27, these drugs and the radiation used can further decrease immune function. Loss of immune responsiveness as found in advanced neoplastic disease is associated with a poor prognosis (Heimdal et al., 1999; Lee et al., 1997; Melichar et al., 1996).

Eating Disorders

Anorexia nervosa is rarely associated with increased frequency or severity of infections. It is associated with both reduced immune responses and lymphocyte subsets, which persist even after weight gain occurs (Marcos et al., 1997a). These are probably mediated through the HPA axis, as suggested by peripheral resistance to glucocorticoids, hypercortisolism, low leptin levels, and altered secretion of leptin and cortisol (Herpetz et al., 1998).

Bulimia nervosa also leads to reduced lymphocyte subsets (Marcos et al., 1997b), even when body weight is maintained; this may be related to repetitive vomiting.

Parenteral Nutrition

Parenteral nutrition can reverse nutritional defects, but at the same time a lack of enteral intake has a suppressive effect on the mucosal immune system (Bistrian, 1999; De Witt and Kudsk, 1999). Lack of enteral dietary intake impairs mucosal IgA and secretory component production and decreases the number of IgA-containing cells and the level of IgG (Bengmark, 1999; Hulsewe et al., 1999). Thus the enteral route directly promotes mucosal growth (Heel et al., 1998).

Provision of glutamine, arginine, n-3 polyunsaturated fatty acids, and dietary nucleotides promotes GI immunity (Calder and Yaqoob, 1999). Catabolic stress increases the need for normally nonessential amino acids, specifically arginine and glutamine; these must be supplied to promote cellular proliferation in the gut, positive nitrogen balance, adequate T-cell production, and adequate host defense against infection. A glutamine deficiency reduces Th2 cytokine responses essential for gut immunity (Kew et al., 1999); supplementation leads to increased IL-4 and mucosal IgA production (Kudsk et al., 2000). Arginine has a similar function and modulates monocyte TNF-α production (Moinard et al., 1999).

MICRONUTRIENT DEFICIENCIES

Newborns require micronutrients such as iron, zinc, and selenium for normal growth. Premature infants, even if appropriate for gestational age, have higher requirements (Hay, 1996). They may develop selenium and zinc deficiencies, even when oral intake is adequate (Klinger et al., 1999; Obladen et al., 1998). Human milk normally provides adequate levels of zinc, along with milk antibodies and growth factors (Donnet-Hughes et al., 2000). However, some maternal milk may be deficient in zinc, resulting in a condition resembling *Acrodermatitis enteropathica* (Stevens and Lubitz, 1998).

Low dietary intake of antioxidants may increase susceptibility to gastritis and *H. pylori* infection (Nair et al., 2000). In mice, antioxidant supplements reduced gastric inflammation, lowered bacterial load, and shifted the Th1 response to a mixed Th1/Th2 response (Bennedsen, 1999). Micronutrients are often deficient in generalized infections (Schmidt, 1997), leading to reduced antioxidant effects and impaired cytokine secretion.

Iron, copper, and zinc deficiencies are the most common trace element deficiencies in North America. Selenium deficiency, like that of iodine, affects parts of the world with low levels in soil.

Iron Deficiency

Controversy about the value of iron supplementation in infections has continued over several decades because of the possibility that excess or inappropriate timing of iron repletion may promote bacterial growth by saturating iron receptors on antibacterial transferrin and lactoferrin (Weinberg, 1984). Part of the controversy stems from complex issues in assessing iron pools. Both iron and inflammatory cytokines increase hepatic secretion of ferritin, an acute-phase protein (Tran et al., 1997), so increases of serum ferritin, a commonly used index of iron overload, may be due to infection, rather than changes in iron status. Iron overload (e.g., from chronic transfusion) may increase susceptibility to some infections (Cunningham-Rundles et al., 2000a). Conversely, as noted, iron deficiency impairs T-cell responses and IL-2 production (Santos and Falcao, 1990; Tibault et al., 1993). Iron deficiency may aggravate chronic mucocutaneous candidiasis, and iron therapy may be beneficial (Cunningham-Rundles et al., 1990b) (see Chapter 17).

Zinc Deficiency

Zinc deficiency may occur in IgA deficiency, fetal alcohol syndrome, sickle cell disease, enteritis, celiac disease, and diarrhea. Zinc deficiency inhibits Th1 cytokine responses, thymic hormone activity, and lymphopoiesis (Fraker et al., 2000; Mocchegiani et al., 1999). *Acrodermatitis enteropathica,* a genetic defect in zinc absorption, presents in infancy as skin lesions (acute dermatitis or hyperkeratotic plaques), diarrhea, alopecia, and increased susceptibility to infection (Moynahan, 1974); it responds dramatically to zinc therapy (Neldner and Hambidge, 1975). Immune

defects include thymic atrophy, profound lymphopenia, cutaneous anergy, and low natural killer cell activity (Cook-Mills and Fraker, 1993; Kaplan et al., 1988; Keen and Gershwin, 1990).

Mild or marginal zinc deficiency, as present in chronic illnesses such as beta thalassemia and epidermolysis bullosa, may be associated with significant immune impairment (Cunningham-Rundles et al., 1990a). In severely malnourished infants, zinc-fortified formula improves linear growth, enhances delayed cutaneous hypersensitivity and lymphoproliferative responses, and increases salivary IgA (Schlesinger et al., 1992). In a large controlled study of diarrhea in Nepalese children, zinc but not vitamin A supplements significantly reduced the risk of prolonged diarrhea (Strand et al., 2002).

Because zinc competes with copper for gastrointestinal uptake, zinc supplements can induce copper deficiency with resultant neutropenia (Botash et al., 1992). In Menkes syndrome, a genetic defect of copper metabolism, death is often associated with intractable infections (Prohaska, 1993).

Selenium Deficiency

Selenoproteins are an important component of the antioxidant host defense system (Turner and Finch, 1991) and promote leukocyte adherence (Maddox, 1999). Selenium supplementation of volunteers increases lymphoproliferative responses and cytotoxic effector cell activity (Kiremidjian-Schumacher et al., 1994; Roy et al., 1994). Low selenium levels are correlated with deficient immune responses in children with HIV (Bologna et al., 1994); selenium supplements can enhance IL-2 production and improve T-helper function (Baum et al., 2000).

Vitamin A Deficiency

Vitamin A (retinol and it derivatives) deficiency has long been appreciated as a significant factor in the severity of infection including measles, rotavirus diarrhea, and HIV in the malnourished host (Bloch, 1924; Bloem et al., 1942; Malvy, 1999). Neonates have low stores of vitamin A largely because of poor placental transport, and children younger than 5 years are at greatest risk of vitamin A deficiency (Rumore et al., 1993). Pure vitamin A deficiency is uncommon; it is usually associated with other nutritional defects.

Many studies have indicated that vitamin A supplements reduce mortality in high-risk children. This has been observed in hospitalized patients and in community-based supplementation studies (Fawzi et al., 1993). The greatest reduction occurred in children younger than age 3 (Rahmathhullah et al., 1990). Stansfield and associates (1993), however, found an increased morbidity during a trial of megadose vitamin A supplementation; this study has been criticized for a low follow-up rate and for failure to assess the duration or severity of the morbidity (Semba and Hussey, 1993).

The role of vitamin A in measles has been explored in depth. Infections in general and measles in particular induce depression of vitamin A levels (Arrieta et al., 1992; Arroyave and Calcano, 1979). Treatment of severe measles with vitamin A dramatically improves morbidity and mortality (Hussey and Klein, 1990). Measles vaccine responsiveness was also increased in malnourished but not in healthy children (Bahl et al., 1999; Benn et al., 1997).

Peruvian children with low retinal levels have more severe diarrhea (Salzar-Lindo et al., 1993). Vitamin A supplements in Chinese children decreased diarrhea and respiratory disease (Lie et al., 1993).

Coutsoudis and associates (1992) found that vitamin A treatment corrects the infection-induced lymphopenia and increased the IgG measles antibody responses. Children with mild vitamin A deficiency given vitamin A had better IgG responses to tetanus vaccination (Semba et al., 1992, 1994). Rahman and colleagues (1977) found that vitamin A administration with each diphtheria-pertussis-tetanus (DPT) vaccine improved diphtheria but not tetanus titers among Bangladeshi infants.

Vitamin A deficiency may increase the risk of maternal-infant HIV transmission in women who are vitamin A deficient (Greenberg et al., 1997). Vitamin A given to HIV-infected children in conjunction with influenza vaccine diminished the HIV viremia that occurred following vaccination (Hanekorn et al., 2000) (see Chapter 29).

The mechanism by which vitamin A increases resistance to infection includes maintenance of the integrity of the skin and mucous membranes (Chandra, 1988; Olson, 1972). Deficiency leads to reduced antibody responses, impaired natural killer activity, and decreased interferon production (Arora and Ross, 1994; Bowman et al., 1990; Semba et al., 1992), whereas supplementation increases the humoral immune response in developing animals (Guzman and Caren, 1991). Vitamin A also promotes a Th2 cytokine response (Semba et al., 1993). Thus vitamin A deficiency leads to impaired T-cell responses to mitogens and antigens both in vivo and in vitro (Scrimshaw and San Giovanni, 1997). Semba and co-workers (1993) noted altered T subsets with lower CD4 naïve cells and higher CD8, CD45RO$^+$ memory cells in vitamin A deficiency; these were normalized with vitamin A supplements. Elderly subjects receiving vitamin A, C, and E supplements had increased CD4 cells and improved PHA lymphoproliferative responses (Penn et al., 1991).

Vitamin A may reduce the incidence of cancers, particularly those of epithelial origin (Hughes, 1999; Ziegler et al., 1986). In animal models, vitamin A enhances rejection of immunogenic tumors (Malkovsky et al., 1983), possibly through regulation of genes by retinoic acid (Petkovich, 1992).

Vitamin C and E Deficiencies

Plasma vitamin E levels correlate significantly with proliferative response of both T and B lymphocytes in vitro and with resistance to infection (Bendich, 1988). Vitamin E influences T-cell function by downmodulating PGE$_2$ (Meydani and Beharka, 1998). Parenteral nutrient formula inadequate vitamin E, and selenium may cause antioxidant deficiency and lipid peroxidation (Reimund et al., 2000).

Vitamin C supplementation leads to increased levels of the antioxidant plasma glutathione levels (Johnston et al., 1993) and inhibits T-cell apoptosis (Cambell et al., 1999). It has been used successfully to treat recurrent furunculosis in patients with deficient neutrophil function (Levy et al., 1996). Vitamin C may lower the incidence of colds associated with acute physical stress (Hemila et al., 1996), but there is no substantial evidence that megadoses decrease the severity or frequency of respiratory infection.

MALNUTRITION AND CHRONIC INFECTION

The acute-phase response to infection includes the formation and release of proinflammatory cytokines such as IL-1, IL-6, TNF, and IFN-γ. This may result in fever, malaise, myalgia, arthralgia, anorexia, nausea, vomiting, somnolence, weight loss, and negative nitrogen balance. The increased energy expenditure occurs at the same time that oral intake decreases and intestinal absorption of nutrients is impaired (Beisel, 2000).

HIV Infection

Malnutrition may occur during the asymptomatic phase of HIV infection in children (Cunningham-Rundles et al., 1997; Oleske et al., 1996; Wolf et al., 1995) (see Chapter 29). Before the availability of effective antiretroviral therapy, growth failure could be the presenting feature (Peters et al., 1998). Micronutrient impairment in HIV-infected children accentuates their immune deficiency and accelerates the course of their disease (Allavena et al., 1995; Baum et al., 1994; Cunningham-Rundles, 2000b; Sappy et al., 1994; Skurnick et al., 1996).

The anemia of HIV infection may be caused by iron deficiency, poor erythropoietin response, reduced number of red blood cell progenitors, or abnormalities of iron metabolism (Kreutzer and Rockstroh, 1997). As noted, iron deficiency can decrease T-cell responses, thus aggravating their immune defect (Omara and Blakely, 1994). Although iron deficiency secondary to malabsorption is common (Castaldo et al., 1996), iron overload also occurs frequently (Riera et al., 1994). Under these circumstances, iron chelation may inhibit HIV replication, possibly by decreasing the effect of HIV *tat* protein on nuclear factor κB (NF-κB) or inhibiting superoxide dismutase (Sappey et al., 1995; Shatrov et al., 1997).

The occurrence of oxidative stress in HIV infection causes increased lipid peroxidation (McCallan et al., 1995), which can be ameliorated with vitamin E and C supplements. These may also decrease viral load (Allard et al., 1998). HIV infection is sometimes associated with magnesium, zinc, and selenium deficiency, the latter two associated with a more rapid clinical course (Allavena et al., 1995; Baum et al., 1994, 2000; Sappy et al., 1994; Skurnick et al., 1996). The use of vitamin supplements was, not surprisingly, associated with higher levels of micronutrients, but almost one third of supplemented patients had reduced levels of at least one nutrient, including vitamins A, C, E, and B_{12} and carotenoids (Semba, 1999).

Trace elements such as zinc and selenium also decline in HIV disease as lipid peroxidase levels increase. Look and associates (1997) found a strong correlation between reduced selenium levels and CD4 cell count. Co-infection with hepatitis C virus is associated with further reduction in selenium levels. Baum and colleagues (1994) showed a correlation between very low selenium levels and morbidity.

Vitamin A deficiency may increase maternal-infant HIV transmission and increase its infectious mortality (Schwartz, 1994; Semba, 1997; West et al., 1999). Children congenitally exposed to HIV have low levels of vitamin A (Cunningham-Rundles et al., 1996b, 2002). Semba (1999a, 1999b) showed that vitamin A supplementation reduces morbidity and mortality to bacterial and viral infections, including HIV infection.

Parasitic Infections

The relationship among parasitic infection, malnutrition, and host immune response is complex because parasitic infections not only contribute to malnutrition and decrease host defenses, but they also are affected by host nutrition and immunity. Intestinal parasites may irritate the intestinal tract and cause pain, anorexia, flatulence, tenderness, loose stools, or diarrhea. Intestinal protozoa that damage the intestinal tract impair host nutrition directly as a result of inflammatory or noninflammatory diarrhea, resulting in the loss of nutrients and micronutrients (e.g., *Blastocystis hominis, Balantidium coli, Cryptosporidium* spp., *Dientamoeba fragilis, Entamoeba histolytica, Isospora belli, Cyclospora cayetanensis, Microsporidia* spp., *Giardia lamblia*).

The role of intestinal hookworms *(Necator americanus* and *Ancylostoma duodenale)* as the cause of anemia has been well documented (Stoltzfus, 2000). Blood loss occurs from the worms feeding on the intestinal mucosa and is directly proportional to the intensity of infection. Even a modest infection of *N. americanus* can result in blood loss that exceeds physiologic daily requirements. Minor infections of *A. duodenale* may cause severe anemia in an infant that is difficult to correct with iron supplementation alone. Severe infections with *Ascaris* may result in malabsorption, mild anemia, wasting, and poor growth. The worm metabolizes vitamin A, and severe infections may result in vitamin A deficiency.

Impairment of food absorption occurs from sheer parasite bulk and severe infection with intestinal helminths. The adverse effects of ascariasis on child growth and development can be reversed by periodic deworming (Latham et al., 1977, 1978; Stephenson et al., 1980). More elusive is the inter-relationship between parasite and host nutrition. An exception is schistosomiasis, long known to have serious nutritional consequences. Both urinary *(Schistosoma haematobium)* and intestinal *(Schistosoma mansoni* and other species) infections cause significant blood loss, malabsorption, protein loss, and anemia. Additional nutritional compromise results from the liver damage of advanced schistosomiasis.

The balance between the host's immune response and the parasite's strategies for survival is one that centers on host expulsion of the worms versus persistence of the worms and their products (Mecusen et al., 1999). The results are critical for both the production of host pathology and survival of parasite progeny. The protective effect of IL-4–dependent expulsion of intestinal nematodes involves regulation of TNF and operates by mechanisms other than degradation of the parasite's environment through immune enteropathy (Lawrence et al., 1998).

Zinc deficiency may impair the immune response to intestinal nematode infections (Scott and Koski, 2000). Further, the resultant zinc deficiency can cause diarrhea; thus oral zinc may be of therapeutic benefit. Zinc deficiency may predispose to giardiasis, but whether the parasite depletes body zinc levels is not known (Solomons, 2000).

In general, CD4 T cells are critical for host protection, IL-12 and IFN-γ inhibit protective immunity, and a Th2 cytokine response, particularly IL-4 with IgE production, favors protective immunity. Not all cytokines produced in response to gut nematode infections are protective (Findelman et al., 1997). The nutritional status of children is worsened by the parasitic infections, which in turn blunts the host response, as shown by studies on the IgE response against *Ascaris lumbricoides* (Hagel et al., 1995). Protein malnutrition may increase the survival of nematode parasites by decreasing gut-associated IL-4 (Th2 response) and increasing IFN-γ (Th1 response) (Ing et al., 2000).

Malaria

Malaria causes the most serious nutritional consequences of any major parasite (Stoltzfus, 2000). It causes hypochromic, microcytic anemia, but this is not associated with iron deficiency except in the case of hemoglobinuria of blackwater fever *(Plasmodium falciparum)*. Anemia also results from rapid hemolysis and in chronic malaria *(Plasmodium ovale, Plasmodium malariae, Plasmodium vivax)*. Erythroid recovery from malaria requires increased amounts of folate. The malaria parasite infects the placenta of pregnant women, compromising blood flow to the fetus and increasing the risk of low birth weight. Malaria is associated with PCM in the pregnant or lactating woman and in young children, as a result of increased caloric requirements, recurrent fever, and the acute-phase cytokine response. Clinical illness also causes vomiting and anorexia, which produce adverse nutritional consequences in an already fragile child or pregnant woman.

REFERENCES

Adhikari M, Pillay T, Pillay D. Tuberculosis in the newborn: an emerging disease. Pediatr Infect Dis J 16:1108–1112, 1997.

Aizawa Y, Shibamoto Y, Takagi I, Zeniya M, Toda G. Analysis of factors affecting the appearance of hepatocellular carcinoma in patients with chronic hepatitis C. A long term follow-up study after histologic diagnosis. Cancer 89:53–59, 2000.

Allard J, Aghdassi E, Chau J, Tam C, Kovacs C, Salit I, Walmsley S. Effects of vitamin E and C supplementation on oxidative stress and viral load in HIV-infected subjects. AIDS 12:1653–1659, 1998.

Allavena C, Dousset B, May T, Dubois F, Canton P, Belleville F. Relationship of trace element, immunological markers, and HIV-1 infection progression. Biol Trace Elem Res 47:133–138, 1995.

Arifeen SE, Black RE, Caulfield LE, Antelman G, Baqui AH, Nahar Q, Alamgir S, Mahmud H. Infant growth patterns in the slums of Dhaka in relation to birth weight, intrauterine growth retardation, and prematurity. Am J Clin Nutr 72:1010–1017, 2000.

Arora D, Ross A. Antibody response against tetanus toxoid is enhanced by lipopolysaccharide or tumor necrosis factor-alpha in vitamin A-sufficient and deficient rats. Am J Clin Nutr 59:922–928, 1994.

Arrieta AC, Zaleska M, Stutman HR, Marks MI. Vitamin A levels in children with measles in Long Beach, California. J. Pediatr 121:75–78, 1992.

Arroyave G, Calcano M. Descenso de los niveles sericos de retinol y su proteina de enlace (RBP) durante las infecciones. Arch Latinoam Nutr 29:233–260, 1979.

Ashworth A. Effects of intrauterine growth retardation on mortality and morbidity in infants and young children. Eur J Clin Nutr: 52:S34–S41, 1998.

Bahl R, Kumar R, Bhandari N, Kant S, Srivastava R, Bhan MK. Vitamin A administered with measles vaccine to nine-month-old infants does not reduce vaccine immunogenicity. J Nutr 129:1569–1573, 1999.

Baltimore R. Neonatal nosocomial infections. Sem Perinatol 22:25–32, 1998.

Batourina E, Gim S, Bello N, Shy M, Clagett-Dame M, Srinivas S, Costantini F, Mendelsohn C. Vitamin A controls epithelial/mesenchymal interactions through Ret expression. Nat Genet 27:74–78, 2001.

Baum M, Cassetti L, Bonvehi P, Shor-Posner G, Lu Y, Sauberlich H. Inadequate dietary intake and altered nutrition status in early HIV-1 infection. Nutrition 10:16–20, 1994.

Baum MK, Miguez-Burbano M, Campa A, Shor-Posner G. Selenium and interleukins in persons infected with human immunodeficiency virus type 1. J Infect Dis 182:S69–s73, 2000.

Beisel WR. Interactions between nutrition and infection. In Strickland GT, ed. Hunter's Tropical Medicine and Emerging Infectious Diseases, ed 8. Philadelphia, WB Saunders, 2000.

Beker LT, Russek-Cohen E, Fink RJ. Stature as a prognostic factor in cystic fibrosis survival. J Am Diet Assoc 101:438–442, 2001.

Bendich A. Antioxidant vitamins and immune responses. In Ranjit CK, ed. Nutrition and Immunology. New York, Alan R. Liss, 1988, pp 125–147.

Bengmark S. Gut microenvironment and immune function. Curr Opin Clin Nutr Metab Care 2:83–85, 1999.

Benn CS, Aaby P, Bale C, Olsen J, Michaelsen KF, George E, Whittle H. Randomized trial of effect of vitamin A supplementation on antibody response to measles vaccine in Guinea-Bissau, West Africa. Lancet 12:101–105, 1997.

Bennedsen M, Wang X, Willen R, Wadstrom T, Andersen LP. Treatment of H. pylori infected mice with antioxidant astaxanthin reduces gastric inflammation, bacterial load and modulates cytokine release by splenocytes. Immunol Lett 70:185–189, 1999.

Bern C, Zucker JR, Perkins BA, Otieno J, Oloo AJ, Yip R. Assessment of potential indicators for protein-energy malnutrition in the algorithm for integrated management of childhood illness. Bull World Health Org 75:87–96, 1997.

Bistrian BR. Enteral nutrition: just a fuel or an immunity enhancer? Minerva Anestesiol 65:471–474, 1999.

Blanchard RK, Cousins RJ. Regulation of intestinal gene expression by dietary zinc: induction of uroguanylin mRNA by zinc deficiency. J Nutr 130:1393S–1398S, 2000.

Bloem, MW, Wedel, M, Egger RJ, Speek AJ, Schrojver J, Saowakontha S, Schreurs WH. Mild Vitamin A deficiency and risk of respiratory tract diseases and diarrhea in preschool and school children in northeastern Thailand. Am J Epidemiol 131:332–339, 1992.

Boeck MA, Chen CX and Cunningham-Rundles S. Altered immune function in a morbidly obese pediatric population. Ann NY Acad Sci 699:252–256, 1993.

Bologna R, Indacochea F, Shor-Posner G, Mantero-Atienza E, Grazziutti M, Sotomayor MC, Fletcher MA, Cabrejos C, Scott GB, Baum MK. Selenium and immunity in HIV-1 infected pediatric patients. J Nutr Immunol 3:41–49, 1994.

Botash AS, Nasca J, Dubowy R, Weinberger HL, Oliphant M. Zinc-induced copper deficiency in an infant. Am J Dis Child 146:709–711, 1992.

Bowman TA, Goonewardene IM, Pasatiempo AM, Ross AC, and Taylor CE. Vitamin A deficiency decreases natural killer cell activity and interferon production in rats. J Nutr 120:1264–1273, 1990.

Brewster DR, Manary MJ, Menzies IS, Henry RL, O'Loughlin EV. Comparison of milk and maize based diets in kwashiorkor. Arch Dis Child 76:242–248, 1997.

Brown RE, Katz M. Failure of antibody production to yellow fever vaccine in children with kwashiorkor. Trop Geogr Med 18:125–128, 1966.

Brown RE, Katz M. Passive transfer of delayed hypersensitivity reaction to tuberculin in children with protein calorie malnutrition. J Pediatr 70:126–128, 1967.

Burns DL, Mascioli EA, Bistrian BR. Parenteral iron dextran therapy: a review. Nutrition 11:163–168, 1995.

Burns JL, Gibson RL, McNamara S, Yim D, Emerson J, Rosenfeld M, Hiatt P, McCoy K, Castile R, Smith AL, Ramsey BW. Longitudinal assessment of *Pseudomonas aeruginosa* in young children with cystic fibrosis. J Infect Dis 183:444–452, 2001.

Byrne TA, Persinger RL, Young LS, Ziegler TR, Wilmore DW. A new treatment for patients with short-bowel syndrome. Growth hormone, glutamine, and a modified diet. Ann Surg 222:243–254, discussion 254–255, 1995.

Cakir B, Yonem A, Guler S, Odabasi E, Demirbas B, Gursoy G, Aral Y. Relation of leptin and tumor necrosis factor alpha to body weight changes in patients with pulmonary tuberculosis. Horm Res 52:279–283, 1999.

Calder PC, Yaqoob P. Glutamine and the immune system. Amino Acids 17:227–241, 1999.

Camarero C, Eiras P, Asensio A, Leon F, Olivares F, Escobar R. Intraepithelial lymphocytes and coeliac disease: permanent changes in CD3-/CD7+ and T-cell receptor gamma delta subsets studied by flow cytometry. Acta Paediatr 89:285–290, 2000.

Campbell JD, Cole M, Bunditrutavorn B, Vella AT. Ascorbic acid is a potent inhibitor of various forms of T-cell apoptosis. Cell Immunol 25:194:1–5, 1999.

Cantwell RJ. Iron deficiency anemia of infancy: some clinical principles illustrated by the response of Maori infants to neonatal parenteral iron administration. Clin Pediatr 11:443–449, 1972.

Carroll K. Obesity as a risk factor for certain types of cancer. Lipids 33:1055–1059, 1998.

Carter MJ, Di Giovine FS, Jones S, Mee J, Camp NJ, Lobo AJ, Duff GW. Association of the interleukin 1 receptor antagonist gene with ulcerative colitis in Northern European Caucasians. Gut 48:461–467, 2001.

Castaldo A, Tarallo L, Palomba E, Albano F, Russo S, Zuin G, Buffardi F, Guarino A: Iron deficiency and intestinal malabsorption in HIV disease. J Pediatr Gastroenterol Nutr 22:359–363, 1996.

Cervello M, Virruso L, Lipani G, Giannitrapani L, Soresi M, Carroccio A, Gambino R, Sanfililippo R, Marasa L, Montalto G. Serum concentration of E-selectin in patients with chronic hepatitis, liver cirrhosis and hepatocellular carcinoma. J Cancer Res Clin Oncol 126:345–351, 2000.

Chandra, RK. Reduced bactericidal capacity of polymorphs in iron deficiency. Arch Dis Child 48:864–866, 1973.

Chandra, RK. Rosette-forming T lymphocytes and cell-mediated immunity in malnutrition. Br Med J 3:608–609, 1974.

Chandra, RK. Reduced secretory antibody response to live attenuated measles and poliovirus vaccines in malnourished children. Br. Med J 2:583–585, 1975.

Chandra, RK. Immunoglobulins and antibody response in malnutrition—a review. In Suskind R, ed. Malnutrition and the Immune Response. New York, Raven Press, 1977, pp 155–168.

Chandra, RK. Increased bacterial binding to respiratory epithelial cells in vitamin A deficiency. Br Med Journal 297:834–835, 1988.

Chandra, RK, Saraya AK. Impaired immunocompetence associated with iron deficiency. J Pediatr 86:899–902, 1975.

Chandra RK, Gupta S, Singh H. Inducer and suppressor T cell subsets in protein-energy malnutrition. Analysis by monoclonal antibodies. Nutr Res 2:21–26, 1982.

Chandra, RK, Chandra S, Gupta S. Antibody affinity and immune complexes after immunization with tetanus toxoid in protein-energy malnutrition. Am J Clin Nutr 40:131–134, 1984.

Chang MH, Shau WY, Chen CJ, Wu TC, Kong MS, Liang DC, Hsu HM, Chen HL, Hsu HY, Chen DS. Hepatitis B vaccination and hepatocellular carcinoma rates in boys and girls. JAMA 284:3040–3042, 2000.

Chernausek SD, Breen TJ, Frank GR. Linear growth in response to growth hormone treatment in children with short stature associated with intrauterine growth retardation: the National Cooperative Growth Study experience. J Pediatr 128:S22–S27, 1996.

Chevalier P, Sevilla R, Zalles L, Sejas E, Belmonte G, Parent G, Jambon B. Immuno-nutritional recovery of children with severe malnutrition Sante 6:201–208, 1996.

Chlebowski RT, Grosvenor MB, Bernhard NH, Morales LS, Bulcavage LM: Nutritional status, gastrointestinal dysfunction and survival in patients with AIDS [Comments]. Am J Gastroenterol 85:476, 1990.

Choudhary RP. Anthropometric indices and nutritional deficiency signs in preschool children of the Pahariya tribe of the Rajmahal Hills, Bihar. Anthropol Anz 59:61–71, 2001.

Cippitelli M, Santoni A. Vitamin D3: a transcriptional modulator of the interferon-gamma gene. Eur J Immunol 28:3017–3030, 1998.

Cohen S, Hansen JDL. Metabolism of albumin and gamma globulin in kwashiorkor. Clin Sci 23:351–359, 1962.

Considine R, Sinha M, Heiman M. Serum immunoreactive-leptin concentrations in normal-weight and obese humans. N Engl J Med 334:292–295, 1996.

Cook-Mills JM, Fraker PJ. The role of metals in the production of toxic oxygen metabolites by mononuclear phagocytes. In Cunningham-Rundles S, ed. Nutrient Modulation of the Immune Response. New York, Marcel Dekker, 1993, pp 127–140.

Coutsoudis A, Kiepiela P, Coovadia HM, Broughton M. Vitamin A supplementation enhances specific IgG antibody levels and total lymphocyte numbers while improving morbidity in measles. Pediatr Infect Dis J 11:203–209, 1992.

Cunningham-Rundles S. Analytical methods for evaluation of nutrient intervention. Nutr Rev S27–S37, 1998.

Cunningham-Rundles S. Issues in assessment of human immune function. In Military Strategies for Sustainment of Nutrition and Immune Function in the Field. Washington DC, Institute of Medicine National Academy of Sciences Press, 1999, pp 235–248.

Cunningham-Rundles S. Evaluation of Nutrient Interaction in Immune Function. In PC Calder, ed. Nutrition and Immune Function. Oxford, British Nutrition Society, 2002.

Cunningham-Rundles S, Bockman RS, Lin A, Giardina PV, Hilgartner MW, Caldwell-Brown D, Carter DM. Physiological and pharmacological effects of zinc on immune response. Ann NY Acad Sci 587:113–122, 1990a.

Cunningham-Rundles S, Cervia JS. Malnutrition and host defense. In Walker WA, Watkins JB, eds. Nutrition in Pediatrics: Basic Science and Clinical Application, ed 2. London, Marcel Dekker Europe, 1996a, 295–307.

Cunningham-Rundles S, Yeger-Arbitman R, Nachman SA, Kaul S, Fotino M. New variant of MHC Class II deficiency with

interleukin-2 abnormality. Clin Immunol Imunopathol 56:116–123, 1990b.

Cunningham-Rundles S, Kim S, Dnistrian A, Noroski L, Menendez-Botet C, Grassey C, Hinds G, Cervia J. Micronutrient and cytokine interaction in congenital pediatric HIV infection. J. Nutr 126:2674S–2679S, 1996b.

Cunningham-Rundles S, Noroski L, Cervia JS. Malnutrition as a cofactor in HIV disease. J Nutr Immunol 5:33–38, 1997.

Cunningham-Rundles S, Giardina P, Grady R, Califano C, McKenzie P, DeSousa M. Immune response in iron overload: implications for host defense. J Inf Dis 182:S115–S121, 2000a.

Cunningham-Rundles S, Nesin M. Bacterial infections in the Immunologically compromised host. In Nataro J, Blaser M, Cunningham-Rundles S, eds. Persistent Bacterial Infections. Washington, DC, American Society of Biology Press, 2000b, 145–164.

Cunningham-Rundles S. Nutrition and the mucosal immune system. Curr Opin Gastroenterol 17:171–176, 2001.

Cunningham-Rundles S, Ahrne S, Dnistrian A. Development of immunocompetence: role of micronutrients and microorganisms. Natr. Reviews 60:568–572, 2002.

Cunningham-Rundles S, McNeeley D. Malnutrition in the host defense. In Walker WA, Watkins JB, eds. Nutrition in Pediatrics, ed 3. Hamilton, Ontario, Canada, BC Decker, 2003, pp 367–385.

Czaja AJ, Dos Santos RM, Porto A, Santrach PJ, Moore SB. Immune phenotype of chronic liver disease. Dig Dis Sci 43:2149–2155, 1998.

Dale A, Thomas JE, Darboe MK, Coward WA, Harding M, Weaver LT. Helicobacter pylori infection, gastric acid secretion, and infant growth. Pediatr Gastroenterol Nutr 26:393–397, 1998.

Damodaran M, Naidu AN, Sarma KV. Anaemia and morbidity in rural preschool children. Indian J Med Res 69:448–456, 1979.

De Onis M, Villar J, Gulmezoglu M. Nutritional interventions to prevent intrauterine growth retardation: evidence from randomized controlled trials. Eur J Clin Nutr 52(Suppl 1):S83–S93, 1998.

Dhur A, Galan P, Hercberg S. Iron status, immune capacity and resistance to infections. Comp Biochem Physiol 94A:11–19, 1989.

Dieterich W, Ehnis T, Bauer M, Donner P, Volta U, Riecken EO, Schuppan D. Identification of tissue transglutaminase as the autoantigen of celiac disease. Nat Med 3:797–801, 1997.

Doherty DG, Norris S, Madrigal-Estebas L, McEntee G, Traynor O, Hegarty JE, O'Farrelly C. The human liver contains multiple populations of NK cells, T cells, and CD3+CD56+ natural T cells with distinct cytotoxic activities and Th1, Th2, and Th0 cytokine secretion patterns. J Immunol 163:2314–2321, 1999.

Doherty JF, Golden MH, Remick DG, Griffin GE. Production of interleukin-6 and tumor necrosis factor-alpha in vitro is reduced in whole blood of severely malnourished children. Clin Sci 86:347–351, 1994.

Donnet-Hughes A, Duc N, Serrant P, Vidal K, Schiffrin EJ: Bioactive molecules in milk and their role in health and disease: the role of transforming growth factor-beta. Immunol Cell Biol 78:74–79, 2000.

Douglas SD, Schopfer K. Phagocyte function in protein-calorie malnutrition. Clin Exp Immunol 17:121–128, 1974.

Dourov N. Thymic atrophy and immune deficiency in malnutrition. Curr Top Pathol 75:127–150, 1986.

Duchmann R, Schmitt E, Knolle P, Meyer zum Buschenfelde KH, Neurath M. Tolerance towards resident intestinal flora in mice is abrogated in experimental colitis and restored by treatment with interleukin-10 or antibodies to interleukin-12. Eur J Immunol 26:934–938, 1996.

Edelman R. Cutaneous hypersensitivity in protein-calorie malnutrition. Lancet 1:1244–1245, 1973.

el-Gamal Y, Aly RH, Hossny E, Afify E, el-Taliawy D. Response of Egyptian infants with protein calorie malnutrition to hepatitis B vaccination. J Trop Pediatr 42:144–145, 1996.

Elstad CA, Meadows GG, Aslakson CJ, Starkey JR. Evidence for nutrient modulation of tumor phenotype: impact of tyrosine and phenylalanine restriction. Adv Exp Med Biol 354:171–183, 1994.

Erickson KL, Medina EA, Hubbard NE. Micronutrients and innate immunity. J Infect Dis 182:S5–S10, 2000.

Faggioni R, Feingold KR, Grunfeld C. Leptin regulation of the immune response and the immunodeficiency of malnutrition. FASEB J 15:2565–2571, 2001.

Fantuzzi G, Faggioni R. Leptin in the regulation of immunity, inflammation, and hematopoiesis. J Leukoc Biol 68:437–446, 2000.

Farrell PM, Kosorok MR, Rock MJ, Laxova A, Zeng L, Lai HC, Hoffman G, Laessig RH, Splaingard ML. Early diagnosis of cystic fibrosis through neonatal screening prevents severe malnutrition and improves long-term growth. Pediatrics 107:1–13, 2001.

Fasano A, Catassi C. Current approaches to diagnosis and treatment of celiac disease: an evolving spectrum. Gastroenterology 120:636–651, 2001.

Fawzi WW, Chalmers TC, Herrera MG, Mosteller F. Vitamin A supplementation and child mortality. A meta-analysis. JAMA 269:898–903, 1993.

Ferguson A. Celiac disease research and clinical practice: maintaining momentum into the twenty-first century. Baillieres Clin Gastroenterol 9:395–412, 1995.

Ferguson AC, Lawlor GJ Jr, Neumann CG, Oh W, Stiehm ER. Decreased rosette-forming lymphocytes in malnutrition and intrauterine growth retardation. J Pediatr 85:717–723, 1974.

Fernald LC, Grantham-McGregor SM. Stress response in school-age children who have been growth retarded since early childhood. Am J Clin Nutr 68:691–8, 1998.

Findelman FD, Shea-Donohue T, Goldhill J, Sullivan CA, Morris SC, Madden KB, Gause WC, Urban JF Jr. Cytokine regulation of host defense against parasitic gastrointestinal nematodes: lessons from studies with rodent models. Ann Rev Immunol 15:505–533, 1997.

Flisiak R, Prokopowicz D. Transforming growth factor-beta1 as a surrogate marker of hepatic dysfunction in chronic liver diseases. Clin Chem Lab Med 38:1129–1131, 2000.

Forchielli ML, Paolucci G, Lo CW. Total parenteral nutrition and home parenteral nutrition: an effective combination to sustain malnourished children with cancer. Nutr Rev 57:15–20, 1999.

Fraker PJ, King LE, Laakko T, Vollmer TL. The dynamic link between the integrity of the immune system and zinc status. Nutrition 130:1399S–406S, 2000.

Freedman LP. Transcriptional targets of the vitamin D3 receptor-mediating cell cycle arrest and differentiation. J Nutr 129:581S–586S, 1999.

Funada U, Wada M, Kawata T, Mori K, Tamai H, Isshiki T, Onoda J, Tanaka N, Tadokoro T, Maekawa A. Vitamin B$_{12}$-deficiency affects immunoglobulin production and cytokine levels in mice. Int J Vitam Nutr Res 71:60–65, 2001.

Garcia VE, Uyemura K, Sieling PA, Ochoa MT, Morita CT, Okamura H, Kurimoto M, Rea TH, Modlin RL. IL-18 promotes type 1 cytokine production from NK cells and T cells in human intracellular infection. J Immunol 162:6114–6121, 1999.

Gautsch TA, Kandl SM, Donovan SM, Layman DK. Growth hormone promotes somatic and skeletal muscle growth recovery in rats following chronic protein-energy malnutrition. J Nutr 129:828–837, 1999.

Gernaat HB, Voorhoeve HW. A new classification of acute protein-energy malnutrition. J Trop Pediatr 46:97–106, 2000.

Goggins M, Kelleher D. Celiac disease and other nutrient related injuries to the gastrointestinal tract. Am J Gastroenterol 89:S2–S17, 1994.

Granot E, Binsztok M, Fraser D, Deckelbaum RJ, Weizman Z. Oxidative stress is not enhanced in non-malnourished infants with persistent diarrhea. J Trop Pediatr 47:284–27, 2001.

Greenberg BL, Semba RD, Vink PE, Farley, JJ, Sivapalasingam M, Steketee, RW, Thea DM, Schoenbaum EE. Vitamin A deficiency and maternal-infant transmissions of HIV in two metropolitan areas in the United States AIDS 11:325–32,1997.

Guzman JJ, Caren LD. Effects of prenatal and postnatal exposure to vitamin A on the development of the murine immune system. Life Sci 49:1455–1462, 1991.

Hagel I, Lynch NR, Di Prisco MC, Sanchez J, Perez M. Nutritional status and the IgE response against Ascaris lumbricoides in children from a tropical slum. Trans Royal Soc Trop Med Hyg 89:562–565, 1995.

Hall RP, Owen S, Smith A, Keough M, Bagheri B, Church P, Streilein R. TCR V beta expression in the small bowel of patients

with dermatitis herpetiformis and gluten-sensitive enteropathy. Limited expression in dermatitis herpetiformis and treated asymptomatic gluten sensitive enteropathy. Exp Dermatol 9:275–282, 2000.

Hanekom W, Yogev R, Heald L, Edwards K, Hussey G, Chadwick E. Effects of vitamin A therapy on serologic responses and viral load changes after influenza vaccination in children infected with the human immunodeficiency virus. J Pediatr 136:550–552, 2000.

Harland PSEG, Brown RE. Tuberculin sensitivity following BCG vaccination in undernourished children. East Afr Med J 42:233–238, 1965.

Harrison LC, Honeyman MC. Cow's milk and type 1 diabetes: the real debate is about mucosal immune function. Diabetes 48:1501–1507, 1999.

Hay WW Jr. Assessing the effect of disease on nutrition of the pre-term infant. Clin Biochem 29:399–417, 1996.

Hay WW Jr. Placental transport of nutrients to the fetus. Horm Res 42:215–222, 1994.

Hayashi T, Ishida T, Motoya S, Itoh F, Takahashi T, Hinoda Y, Imai K. Mucins and immune reactions to mucins in ulcerative colitis. Digestion 63(Suppl 1):28–31, 2001.

Heel KA, Kong SE, McCauley RD, Erber WN, Hall J. The effect of minimum luminal nutrition on mucosal cellularity and immunity of the gut. J Gastroenterol Hepatol 10:1015–1019, 1998.

Heimdal JH, Aarstad HJ, Klementsen B, Olofsson J. Peripheral blood mononuclear cell (PBMC) responsiveness in patients with head and neck cancer in relation to tumor stage and prognosis. Acta Otolaryngol 119:281–284, 1999.

Hemila H. Vitamin C and common cold incidence: a review of studies with subjects under heavy physical stress. Int J Sports Med 17:379–383, 1996.

Henriksen T. Foetal nutrition, foetal growth restriction and health later in life. Acta Paediatr Suppl 88:4–8, 1999.

Heresi G. Olivaress M, Pizzaro F, Cayazao M, Hertrampf E, Walter T, Stekel A. Effect of iron fortification on infant morbidity. In Proceeding of the Thirteenth International Congress of Nutrition, Brighton, England, 1985. London, Libbey, 1986, p 129.

Herpertz S, Wagner R, Albers N, Blum WF, Pelz B, Langkafel M, Kopp W, Henning A, Oberste-Berghaus C, Mann K, Senf W, Hebebrand J. Circadian plasma leptin levels in patients with anorexia nervosa: relation to insulin and cortisol. Horm Res 50:197–204, 1998.

Hill AD, Naama HA, Gallagher HJ, Shou J, Calvano SE, Daly JM. Glucocorticoids mediate macrophage dysfunction in protein calorie malnutrition. Surgery 118:130–136, discussion 136–137, 1995.

Hira S, Dupont H, Lanjewar D, Dholakia Y. Severe weight loss: the predominant clinical presentation of tuberculosis in patients with HIV infection in India. Natl Med J India 11:256–258, 1998.

Hirve S, Ganatra B. A prospective cohort study on the survival experience of under five children in rural western India. Indian Pediatr 34:995–1001, 1997.

Hoffmann JC, Bahr MJ, Tietge UJ, Braunstein J, Bayer B, Boker KH, Manns MP. Detection of a soluble form of the human adhesion receptor lymphocyte function-associated antigen-3 (LFA-3) in patients with chronic liver disease. J Hepatol 25:465–473, 1996.

Hofman PL, Cutfield WS, Robinson EM, Bergman RN, Menon RK, Sperling MA, Gluckman PD. Insulin resistance in short children with intrauterine growth retardation. J Clin Endocrinol Metab 82:402–406, 1997.

Horwitz JR, Lally KP, Cheu HW, Vazquez WD, Grosfeld JL, Ziegler MM. Complications after surgical intervention for necrotizing enterocolitis: a multicenter review. J Pediatr Surg 30:994–8, 1995.

Howard JK, Lord GM, Matarese G, Vendetti S, Ghatei MA, Ritter MA, Lechler RI, Bloom SR. Leptin protects mice from starvation-induced lymphoid atrophy and increases thymic cellularity in ob/ob mice. J Clin Invest 104:1051–1059, 1999.

Hubbard VS, Hubbard LR. Clinical assessment of nutritional status. In Walker WA and Watkins JB eds. Nutrition in Pediatrics: Basic Science and Clinical Applications, ed 2. Hamilton, Ontario, Canada, BC Decker, 1996, pp 14–17.

Hughes D. Effects of carotenoids on human immune function. Proc Nutr Soc 58:713–718, 1999.

Hulsewe KW, Van Acker BA, Von Meyenfeldt MF, Soeters PB: Nutritional depletion and dietary manipulation: effects on the immune response. World J Surg 23:536–544, 1999.

Hussey GD, Klein M. A randomized, controlled trial of vitamin A in children with severe measles. N Engl J Med 323:160–164, 1990.

Ina K, Itoh J, Fukushima K, Kusugami K, Yamaguchi T, Kyokane K, Imada A, Binion DG, Musso A, West GA, Dobrea GM, McCormick TS, Lapetina EG, Levine AD, Ottaway CA, Fiocchi C. Resistance of Crohn's disease T cells to multiple apoptotic signals is associated with a Bcl-2/Bax mucosal imbalance. J Immunol 163:1081–1090, 1999.

Ing R, Su Z, Scott ME, Koske KG. Suppressed T helper 2 immunity and prolonged survival of a nematode parasite in protein-malnourished mice. Proc Natl Acad Sci USA 97:7078–7083, 2000.

Insoft RM, Sanderson IR, Walker WA. Development of immune function in the intestine and its role in neonatal diseases. Pediatr Clin North Am 43:551–571, 1996.

Jacquot S, Modigliani R, Kuzniak I, Boumsell L, Bensussan A. Enhanced CD3 monoclonal antibody induced proliferation of colonic mucosal T lymphocytes in Crohn's disease patients free of corticosteroid or immunosuppressor treatment. Clin Immunol Immunopathol 79:20–24, 1996.

Jagadeesan V, Reddy V. Complement system in iron deficiency anemia. Experientia 39:146, 1983.

Jiang Y, Shao YF. Case-control study on intrauterine growth retardation and vitamin nutritional status in late pregnancy. Zhonghua Yu Fang Yi Xue Za Zhi 28:210–212, 1994.

Johnson RK, Guthrie H, Smiciklas-Wright H, Wang MQ. Characterizing nutrient intakes of children by sociodemographic factors. Public Health Rep 109:414–420, 1994.

Johnson VL, Wang J, Kaskel FJ, Pierson RN. Changes in body composition of children with chronic renal failure on growth hormone. Pediatr Nephrol 14:695–700, 2000.

Johnston CS, Meyer CG, Srlakshmi JC. Vitamin C elevates red blood cell glutathione in healthy adults. Am J Clin Nutr 58:103–105, 1993.

Joynson DH, Walker DM, Jacobs A, Dolby AE, Defect of cell-mediated immunity in patients with iron-deficiency anemia. Lancet 2:1058–1059, 1972.

Kahn E, Stein H, Zoutendyk A. Isohemagglutinins and immunity in malnutrition. Am J Clin Nutr 5:70–71, 1957.

Kaplan J, Highs JH, Prasad AS. Impaired interleukin-2 production in the elderly: association with mild zinc deficiency. J Trace Elements Exp Med 1:3–8, 1988.

Kaufman SS, Loseke CA, Lupo JV, Young RJ, Murray ND, Pinch LW, Vanderhoof JA. Influence of bacterial overgrowth and intestinal inflammation on duration of parenteral nutrition in children with short bowel syndrome. J Pediatr 131:356–361, 1997.

Keen CL, Gershwin ME. Zinc deficiency and immune function. Ann Rev Nutr 10:415–431, 1990.

Keet MP, Thom H. Serum immunoglobulins in kwashiorkor. Arch Dis Child 44:600–603, 1969.

Kennedy E, Goldberg J. What are American children eating? Implications for public policy. Nutr Rev 53:111–126, 1995.

Kew S, Wells SM, Yaqoob P, Wallace FA, Miles EA, Calder PC: Dietary glutamine enhances murine T-lymphocyte responsiveness. J Nutrition 129:1524–1531, 1999.

King AL, Ciclitira PJ. Celiac disease: strongly heritable, oligogenic, but genetically complex. Mol Genet Metab 71:70–75 2000.

King LE, Osati-Ashtiani F, Fraker PJ. Depletion of cells of the B lineage in the bone marrow of zinc-deficient mice. Immunology 85:69–73, 1995.

Kiremidjian-Schumacher L, Roy M, Wishe HI, Cohen MW, Stotzky G. Supplementation with selenium and human immune cell functions II: effect on cytotoxic lymphocytes and natural killer cells. Biol Trace Elem Res 41:115–127, 1994.

Klein J, Remington J. Current concepts of infections of the fetus and newborn infant. In Remington JS, Klein JO, eds. Infectious Diseases of the Fetus and Newborn Infant, ed 4. Philadelphia, WB Saunders, 1995, pp 11–13.

Klinger G, Shamir R, Singer P, Diamond EM, Josefsberg Z, Sirota L. Parenteral selenium supplementation in extremely low birth weight infants: inadequate dosage but no correlation with hypothyroidism. J Perinatol 19:568–572, 1999.

Koller DY, Gotz M, Wojnarowski C, Eichler I. Relationship between disease severity and inflammatory markers in cystic fibrosis. Arch Dis Child 75:498–501, 1996.

Kossa K, Coulthart A, Ives CT, Pusey CD, Hodgson HJ. Antigen specificity of circulating anti-neutrophil cytoplasmic antibodies in inflammatory bowel disease. Eur J Gastroenterol Hepatol 7:783–789, 1995.

Kotler DP, Tierney AR, Culpepper-Morgan JA, Wang J, Pierson RN Jr: Effect of home total parenteral nutrition on body composition in patients with acquired immunodeficiency syndrome. J Parenter Enteral Nutr 14:454–458, 1990.

Krantman HJ, Young SR, Ank BJ, O'Donnell CM, Rachelefsky GS, Stiehm ER. Immune function in pure iron deficiency. Am J Dis Child 136:840–844, 1982.

Kreutzer KA, Rockstroh JK. Pathogenesis and pathophysiology of anemia in HIV infection. Ann Hematol 75:179–187, 1997.

Kudsk KA, Wu Y, Fukatsu K, Zarzaur BL, Johnson CD, Wang R, Hanna MK. Glutamine-enriched total parenteral nutrition maintains intestinal interleukin-4 and mucosal immunoglobulin A levels. J Parenter Enteral Nutr 24:270–274, 2000.

Kulapongs P, Vithayasai V, Suskind R, Olson RE. Cell-mediated immunity and phagocytosis and killing function in children with severe iron-deficiency anaemia. Lancet 289–691, 1974.

Langley-Evans SC, Welham SJ, Jackson AA. Fetal exposure to a maternal low protein diet impairs nephrogenesis and promotes hypertension in the rat. Life Sci 64:965–974, 1999.

Latham LS. Nutritional and economic implications of Ascaris infection in Kenya: studies in experimental animals and pre-school children. Doctoral Thesis, Cornell University Graduate School, 1978.

Latham LS, Latham M, Basta SS. The nutritional and economic implications of Ascaris infection in Kenya. World Bank Staff Working Paper No. 271. Washington, DC, World Bank, 1977.

Lawrence CE, Patterson JC, Higgins LM, Mac Donald TT, Kennedy MW, Garside P. Il-4 regulated enteropathy in an intestinal nematode infection. Europ J Immunol 28:2672–2684, 1998.

Lee PP, Zeng D, McCaulay AE, Chen YF, Geiler C, Umetsu DT, Chao NJ. T helper 2-dominant anti-lymphoma immune response is associated with fatal outcome. Blood 90:1611–1617, 1997.

Leite-De-Moraes MC, Moreau G, Arnould A, Machavoine F, Garcia C, Papiernik M, Dy M. IL-4-producing NK T cells are biased towards IFN-gamma production by IL-12. Influence of the microenvironment on the functional capacities of NK T cells. Eur J Immunol 28:1507–1515, 1998.

Levy R, Shriker O, Porath A, Reisenberg K, Schlaeffer F. Vitamin C for the treatment of recurrent furunculosis in patients with impaired neutrophil functions. J Infect Dis 173:1502–1505, 1996.

Li SD, Mobarhan S. Association between body mass index and adenocarcinoma of the esophagus and gastric cardia. Nutr Rev 58:54–56, 2000.

Lie C, Ying C, Wang EL, Brun T, Geissler C. Impact of large-dose vitamin A supplementation on childhood diarrhea, respiratory disease and growth. Eur J Clin Nutr 47:88–96, 1993.

Lin E, Kotani JG, Lowry SF. Nutritional modulation of immunity and the inflammatory response. Nutrition 14:545–550, 1998.

Loffreda S, Yang SQ, Lin HZ, Karp CL, Brengman ML, Wang DJ, Klein AS, Bulkley GB, Bao C, Noble PW, Lane MD, Diehl AM. Leptin regulates proinflammatory immune response. FASEB J 12:57–65, 1998.

Look MP, Rockstroh JK, Rao GS, Kreuzer KA, Barton S, Lemoch H, Sudhop T, Hoch J, Stockinger K, Spengler U, Sauerbruch T. Serum selenium, plasma glutathione and erythrocyte glutathione peroxidase levels in asymptomatic versus symptomatic human immunodeficiency virus-1 infection. Eur J Clin Nutr 51:266–272, 1997.

Lord GM, Matarese G, Howard JK Baker RJ, Bloom SR, Lechler RI. Leptin modulates the T-cell immune response and reverses starvation-induced immunosuppression. Nature 394:897–901, 1998.

Luan J, Browne PO, Harding AH, Halsall DJ, O'Rahilly S, Chatterjee VK, Wareham NJ. Evidence for gene-nutrient interaction at the PPAR gamma locus. Diabetes 50:686–689, 2001.

MacDougall LG, Anderson R, McNab GM, Katz J. The immune response in iron-deficient children: impaired cellular defense mechanisms with altered humoral components. J Pediatr 86:833–843, 1975.

Macpherson A, Khoo UY, Forgacs I, Philpott-Howard J, Bjarnason I. Mucosal antibodies in inflammatory bowel disease are directed against intestinal bacteria. Gut 38:365–375, 1996.

Maddox JF, Aherne KM, Reddy CC, Sordillo LM. Increased neutrophil adherence and adhesion molecule mRNA expression in endothelial cells during selenium deficiency. J Leuk Biol 65:658–664, 1999.

Maffei M, Halaas J, Ravussin E. Leptin levels in human and rodent; measurement of plasma leptin and obRNA in obese and weight-reduced subjects. Nature Medicine 1:1155–1161, 1995.

Malin M, Suomalainen H, Saxelin M, Isolauri E. Promotion of IgA immune response in patients with Crohn's disease by oral bacteriotherapy with Lactobacillus GG. Ann Nutr Metab 40:137–45, 1996.

Malkovsky M, Edwards AJ, Hunt R. Palmer L, Medawar PB. T-cell-mediated enhancement of host-versus-graft reactivity in mice fed a diet enriched in vitamin A acetate. Nature 302:338–340, 1983.

Malvy, D. Micronutrients and topical viral infections: one aspect of pathogenic complexity in tropical medicine. Med Trop 59:442–448, 1999.

Manary MJ, Yarasheski KE, Hart CA, Broadhead RL. Plasma urea appearance rate is lower when children with kwashiorkor and infection are fed egg white-tryptophan rather than milk protein. J Nutr 130:183–188, 2000.

Marcos A, Varela P, Toro O, Lopez-Vidriero I, Nova E, Madruga D, Casas J, Morande G. Interactions between nutrition and immunity in anorexia nervosa: a 1-y follow-up study Am J Clin Nutr 66:485S–490S, 1997a.

Marcos A, Varela P, Toro O, Nova E, Lopez-Vidriero I, Morande G. Evaluation of nutritional status by immunologic assessment in bulimia nervosa: influence of body mass index and vomiting episodes. Am J Clin Nutr 66:491S–497S, 1997b.

McCallan DC, McNurlan MA, Milne E, Calder AG, Garlick PJ, Griffin GE Whole-body protein turnover from leucine kinetics and the response to nutrition in human immunodeficiency virus infection. Am J Clin Nutr, 61:818–826, 1995.

McMurray DN. Cell-mediated immunity in nutritional deficiency. Prog Food Nutr Sci 8:193–228, 1984.

McPherson RA. Commentary: advances in the laboratory diagnosis of celiac disease. J Clin Lab Anal 15:105–107, 2001.

Mecusen EN. Immunology of helminth infections, with reference to immunopathology. Veter Parasitology 84:259–273, 1999.

Melichar B, Jandik P, Krejsek J, Solichova D, Drahosova M, Skopec F, Mergancova J, Voboril Z. Mitogen-induced lymphocyte proliferation and systemic immune activation in cancer patients. Tumori 82:218–220, 1996.

Menkes JH. Menkes disease and Wilson disease: two sides of the same copper coin. Part II: Wilson disease. Eur J Paediatr Neurol 3:245–253, 1999.

Meydani SN, Beharka AA. Recent Developments in vitamin E and immune response. Nutr Rev 56:S49–S58, 1998.

Mishkin S. Dairy sensitivity, lactose malabsorption, and elimination diets in inflammatory bowel disease. Am J Clin Nutr 65:564–567, 1997.

MMWR. The role of BCG vaccine in the prevention and control of tuberculosis in the United States. A joint statement by the Advisory Council for the Elimination of Tuberculosis and the Advisory Committee on Immunization Practices. MMWR 45:1–18, 1996.

Mocchegiani E, Ciavattini A, Santarelli L, Tibaldi A, Muzzioli M, Bonazzi P, Giacconi R, Fabris N, Garzetti GG. Role of zinc and alpha2 macroglobulin on thymic endocrine activity and on peripheral immune efficiency (natural killer activity and interleukin-2) in cervical carcinoma. Br J Cancer 79:244–250, 1999.

Mocchegiani E, Provinciali M, Di Stefano G, Nobilini A, Caramia G, Santarelli L, Tibaldi A, Fabris N. Role of the low zinc bioavailability on cellular immune effectiveness in cystic fibrosis. Clin Immunol Immunopathol 75:214–224, 1995.

Moinard C, Chauveau B, Walrand S, Felgines C, Chassagne J, Caldefie F, Cynober LA, Vasson MP. Phagocyte functions in stressed rats: comparison of modulation by glutamine, arginine and ornithine 2-oxoglutarate. Clin Sci 97:59–65, 1999.

Moldawer LL and Lowry SF. Interactions between cytokine production and inflammation: implications for therapies aimed at modulating the host defense to infection. In Cunningham-Rundles S, ed. Nutrient Modulation of Immune Response. New York, Marcel Dekker, 1993, pp 511–522.

Moreno LA, Sarria A, Lazaro A, Lasierra MP, Larrad L, Bueno M. Lymphocyte T subset counts in children with hypercholesterolemia receiving dietary therapy. Ann Nutr Metab 42:261–265, 1998.

Morris JG Jr, Potter M. Emergence of new pathogens as a function of changes in host susceptibility. Emerg Infect Dis 3:435–440, 1997.

Moser C, Kjaergaard S, Pressler T, Kharazmi A, Koch C, Hoiby N. The immune response to chronic Pseudomonas aeruginosa lung infection in cystic fibrosis patients is predominantly of the Th2 type. Acta Path Microbiol Immunol Scand 108:329–335, 2000.

Mowat AM, Hutton AK, Garside P, Steel M. A role for interleukin-1 alpha in immunologically mediated intestinal pathology. Immunology 80:110–115, 1993.

Moynahan, EM. Acrodermatitis enteropathica. A lethal inherited human zinc deficiency disorder. Lancet 2:399–400, 1974.

Muga SJ, Grider A. Partial characterization of a human zinc-deficiency syndrome by differential display. Biol Trace Elem Res 68:1–12, 1999.

Munoz C, Olivares M, Schlesinger L, Lopez M, Letelier A. Increased in vitro tumor necrosis factor-alpha production in iron deficiency anemia. Eur Cytokine Netw 5:401–404, 1994.

Murakami H, Akbar SM, Matsui H, Onji M. Macrophage migration inhibitory factor in the sera and at the colonic mucosa in patients with ulcerative colitis: clinical implications and pathogenic significance. Eur J Clin Invest 31:337–343, 2001.

Nagao AT, Carneiro-Sampaio MM, Carlsson B, Hanson LA. Antibody titre and avidity in saliva and serum are not impaired in mildly to moderately undernourished children. J Trop Pediatr 41:153–157, 1995.

Nair S, Norkus EP, Hertan H, Pitchumoni CS. Micronutrient antioxidants in gastric mucosa and serum in patients with gastritis and gastric ulcer: does Helicobacter pylori infection affect the mucosal levels? J Clin Gastroenterol 30:381–385, 2000.

Najera O, Gonzalez C, Toledo G, Lopez L, Cortes E, Betencourt M, Ortiz R. CD45RA and CD45RO isoforms in infected malnourished and infected well-nourished children. Clin Exp Immunol 126:461–465, 2001.

Neldner KH, Hambidge KM. Zinc therapy of acrodermatitis enteropathica. N Engl J Med 292:879–882, 1975.

Nesin M, Cunningham-Rundles S. Cytokines and neonates. Am J Perinat 17:393–404, 2000.

Neumann CG, Lawlor CJ Jr, Stiehm ER, Swenseld ME, Newton C. Herbert J, Ammann AJ, Jacob M. Immunologic responses in malnourished children. Am J Clin Nutr 28:89–104, 1975.

Neumann CG, Harrison CG. Onset and evolution of stunting in infants and children—examples from the human nutrition collaborative research support program—Kenya and Egypt studies. Eur J Clin Nutr 48:S90–S102, 1994.

Nieman DC, Nehlsen-Cannarella SI, Henson DA, Butterworth DE, Fagoaga OR, Warren BJ, Rainwater MK. Immune response to obesity and moderate weight loss. Int J Obes Relat Metab Disord 20:353–360, 1996.

Norman LJ, Coleman JE, Macdonald IA, Tomsett AM, Watson AR. Nutrition and growth in relation to severity of renal disease in children. Pediatr Nephrol 15:259–265, 2000.

Nwagwu MO, Cook A, Langley-Evans SC. Evidence of progressive deterioration of renal function in rats exposed to a maternal low-protein diet in utero. Br J Nutr 83:79–85, 2000.

Obladen M, Loui A, Kampmann W, Renz H. Zinc deficiency in rapidly growing preterm infants. Acta Paediatr 87:685–691, 1998.

Oleske JM, Rothpletz-Puglia PM, Winter H. Historical perspectives on the evolution in understanding the importance of nutritional care in pediatric HIV infection. J Nutr 126:2616S–2619S, 1996.

Olson JA. The biological role of vitamin A in maintaining epithelial tissues. Isr J Med Sci 8:1170–1178, 1972.

Omara FO, Blakley BR. The effects of iron deficiency and iron overload on cell-mediated immunity in the mouse. Br J Nutr 72:899–909, 1994.

Ozkan H, Olgun N, Sasmaz E, Abacioglu H, Okuyan M, Cevik N. Nutrition, immunity and infections: T lymphocyte subpopulations in protein-energy malnutrition. J Trop Pediatr 39:257–260, 1993.

Pardi G, Marconi AM, Cetin I. Pathophysiology of intrauterine growth retardation: role of the placenta. Acta Paediatr Suppl 423:170–172, 1997.

Paronen J, Knip M, Savilahti E, Virtanen SM, Ilonen J, Akerblom HK, Vaarala O: Effect of cow's milk exposure and maternal type 1 diabetes on cellular and humoral immunization to dietary insulin in infants at genetic risk for type 1 diabetes. Finnish Trial to Reduce IDDM in the Genetically at Risk Study Group. Diabetes 49:1657–1665, 2000.

Peano G, Menardi G, Ponzetto A, Fenoglio LM. HLA-DR5 antigen. A genetic factor influencing the outcome of hepatitis C virus infection? Arch Intern Med 154:2733–2736, 1994.

Perusse L, Bouchard C. Gene-diet interactions in obesity. Am J Clin Nutr 721285S–1290S, 2000.

Peters VB, Rosh JR, Mugrditchian L, Birnbaum AH, Benkov KJ, Hodes DS, Le Leiko NS. Growth failure as the first expression of malnutrition in children with human immunodeficiency virus infection Mt Sinai J Med 65:1–4, 1998.

Petkovich M. Regulation of gene expression by vitamin A: the role of nuclear retinoic acid receptors. Annu Rev Nutr 12:443–471, 1992.

Pirisi M, Vitulli D, Falleti E, Fabris C, Soardo G, Del Forno M. Bardus P, Gonano F, Bartoli E. Increased soluble ICAM-1 concentration and impaired delayed-type hypersensitivity skin tests in patients with chronic liver disease. J Clin Pathol 50:50–53, 1997.

Popkin BM, Richards MK, Montiero CA. Stunting is associated with overweight in children of four nations that are undergoing the nutrition transition. J Nutr 126:3009–3016, 1996.

Prada JA, Tsang RC. Biological mechanisms of environmentally induced causes of intrauterine growth retardation. Eur J Clin Nutr 52:S21–S27.

Pretorius PJ, De Villiers LS, Antibody response in children with protein malnutrition. Am J Clin Nutr 10:379–383, 1962.

Prindull G, Ahmad M. The ontogeny of the gut mucosal immune system and the susceptibility to infections in infants of developing countries. Eur J Pediatr 152:786–792, 1993.

Probert L, Keiffer J, Corbella P, Cazlaris H, Patsavoudi E, Stephens S, Kaslaris E, Kioussis D, Kollias G: Wasting, ischemia, and lymphoid abnormalities in mice expressing T-cell-targeted human tumor necrosis factor transgenes. J Immunol 151:1894–1906, 1993.

Prohaska JR, Failla ML. Copper and immunity. In Klurfeld DM, ed. Nutrition and Immunology. New York, Plenum Press, 1993, pp 309–332.

Protheroe SM. Feeding the child with chronic liver disease. Nutrition 14:796–800, 1998.

Rahman MM, Mahalanabis D, Alvarez JO, Wahed MA, Islam MA, Habte D. Effect of early vitamin A supplementation on cell-mediated immunity in infants younger than 6 months. Am J Clin Nutr 65:144–148, 1997.

Rahman MM, Mahalanabis D, Hossain S, Wahed MA, Alvarez JO, Siber GR, Thompson C, Santosham M, Fuchs GJ. Simultaneous vitamin A administration at routine immunization contact enhances antibody response to diphtheria vaccine in infants younger than six months. J Nutr 129:2191–2195, 1999.

Rahmathullah L, Underwood BA, Thulasiraj RD, Milton RC, Ramaswamy K, Rahmathullah R, Babu G. Reduced mortality among children in southern India receiving a small weekly does of vitamin A. N Engl J Med 323:929–935, 1990.

Ramaccioni V, Soriano HE, Arumugam R, Klish WJ. Nutritional aspects of chronic liver disease and liver transplantation in children. J Pediatr Gastroenterol Nutr 30:361–367, 2000.

Rannem T, Hylander E, Ladefoged K, Staun M, Tjellesen L, Jarnum S. The metabolism of [75Se] selenite in patients with short bowel syndrome. JPEN J Parenter Enteral Nutr 20:412–416, 1996.

Reddy V, Raghuramulu N, Bhaskaram C. Secretory IgA in protein-calorie malnutrition. Arch Dis Child 51:871–874, 1976.

Redmond HP, Gallagher HJ, Shou J, Daly JM. Antigen presentation in protein-energy malnutrition. Cell Immunol 163:80–87, 1995.

Reimund JM, Arondel Y, Duclos B, Baumann R. Vitamins and trace elements in home parenteral nutrition patients. J Nutr Health Aging 4:13–18, 2000.

Riera A, Gimferrer E, Cadafalch J, Remacha A, Martin S: Prevalence of high serum and red cell ferritin levels in HIV-infected patients. Haematologica 79:165–167, 1994.

Rikimaru T, Taniguchi K, Yartey JE, Kennedy DO, Nkrumah FK Malvy, Humoral and cell-mediated immunity in malnourished children in Ghana. Eur J Clin Nutr 52:344–350, 1998.

Rink L, Kirchner H. Zinc-altered immune function and cytokine production. J Nutr 130:1407S–1411S, 2000.

Roman LI, Manzano L, De La Hera A, Abreu L, Rossi I, Alvarez-Mon M. Expanded CD4+CD45RO+ phenotype and defective proliferative response in T lymphocytes from patients with Crohn's disease. Gastroenterology 110:1008–1019, 1996.

Rondo PH, Abbott R, Rodrigues LC, Tomkins AM. The influence of maternal nutritional factors on intrauterine growth retardation in Brazil. Paediatr Perinat Epidemiol 11:152–166, 1997.

Rondo PH, Tomkins AM. Folate and intrauterine growth retardation. Ann Trop Paediatr 20:253–258, 2000.

Rose D, Habicht JP, Devaney B. Household participation in the Food Stamp and WIC programs increases the nutrient intakes of preschool children. J Nutr 128:548–555, 1998.

Rosen EU, Geefhuysen J, Ipp T. Immunoglobulin levels in protein calorie malnutrition. South Afr Med J 45:980–982, 1971.

Ross AC, Gardner EM. The function of vitamin A in cellular growth and differentiation, and its roles during pregnancy and lactation. Adv Exp Med Biol 352:187–200, 1994.

Roy M, Kiremidjian-Schumacher L, Wishe HI, Cohen MW, Stotzky G. Supplementation with selenium and human immune cell functions. Effect on lymphocyte proliferation and interleukin-2 receptor expression. Biol Trace Elem Res 46:103–114, 1994.

Rumore MM. Vitamin A as an immunomodulating agent. Clin Pharm 12:506–514, 1993.

Salimonu S, Ojo-Amaize, E, Williams AIO, Johnson AOK, Cooke AR, Adekunle FA, Alm GV, Wigzell H. Depressed natural killer cell activity in children with protein-calorie malnutrition Clin immunol Immunopath 24:1–7, 1982.

Salzar-Lindo E, Salazar M, Alvarez JO. Association of diarrhea and low serum retinol in Peruvian children. Am J Clin Nutr 58:110–113, 1993.

Sakamoto M, Fujisawa Y, Nishioka K Physiologic role of the complement system in host defense, disease, and malnutrition. Nutrition 14:391–398, 1998.

Sammon AM. Dietary linoleic acid, immune inhibition and disease. Postgrad Med J 75:129–132, 1999.

Sanderson IR, Naik S. Dietary regulation of intestinal gene expression. Annu Rev Nutr 20:311–338, 2000.

Sandstrom B, Cederblad A, Lindblad BS, Lonnerdal B. Acrodermatitis enteropathica, zinc metabolism, copper status, and immune function. Arch Pediatr Adolesc Med 148:980–985, 1994.

Santos PC, Falcao RP. Decreased lymphocyte subsets and K-cell activity in iron deficiency anemia. Acta Hematol 84:118–121, 1990.

Sappey C, Boelaert JR, Legrand-Poels S, Forceille C, Favier A, Piette J. Iron chelation decreases NF-kappa B and HIV type activation due to oxidative stress. AIDS Res Hum Retroviruses 11:1049–1061, 1995.

Sappy C, Leclercq P, Coudray C, Faure P, Micoud M, Favier A. Vitamins, trace elements and peroxide status in HIV seropositive patients: asymptomatic patients present a severe beta-carotene deficiency. Clin Chim Acta, 230:35–42, 1994.

Sauerwein RW, Mulder JA, Mulder L, Lowe B, Peshu N, Demacker PN, Van der Meer JW, Marsh K. Inflammatory mediators in children with protein-energy malnutrition. Am J Clin Nutr 65:1534–1339, 1997.

Savendahl L, Underwood LE. Decreased interleukin-2 production from cultured peripheral blood mononuclear cells in human acute starvation. J Clin Endocrinol Metab 82:1177–1180, 1997.

Schlesinger L, Stekel A. Impaired cellular immunity in marasmic infants. Am J Clin Nutr 27:615–620, 1974.

Schlesinger L, Arevalo M, Arredondo S, Diaz M, Lonnerdal B, Stekel A. Effect of a zinc-fortified formula on immunocompetence and growth of malnourished infants. Am J Clin Nutr 56:491–498, 1992.

Schmidt K. Interaction of antioxidative micronutrients with host defense mechanisms. A critical review Int J Vitam Nutr Res, 67:307–311, 1997.

Schnare M, Barton GM, Holt AC, Takeda K, Akira S, Medzhitov R. Toll-like receptors control activation of adaptive immune responses. Nat Immunol 2:947–950, 2001.

Schonland M. Depression of immunity in protein-calorie malnutrition: a post-mortem study. J Trop Pediatr Environ Child Health 18:217–224, 1972.

Schopfer K, Douglas SD. Neutrophil function in children with kwashiorkor. J Lab Clin Med 88:450–461, 1976b.

Schwartz RD, Miotti PG, Chiphangwi JD, Saah AJ, Canner JK, Dallabetta GA, Hoover DR. Maternal vitamin A deficiency and mother to child transmission of HIV-1. Lancet 343:1593–1596, 1994.

Scolapio JS, Camilleri M, Fleming CR, Oenning LV, Burton DD, Sebo TJ, Batts KP, Kelly DG. Effect of growth hormone, glutamine, and diet on adaptation in short-bowel syndrome: a randomized, controlled study. Gastroenterology 113:1074–1081, 1997.

Scott FW, Olivares E, Sener A, Malaisse WJ. Dietary effects on insulin and nutrient metabolism in mesenteric lymph node cells, splenocytes, and pancreatic islets of BB rats. Metabolism 49:1111–1117, 2000.

Scott ME, Koski KG. Zinc deficiency impairs immune responses against parasitic nematode infections at intestinal and systemic sites. J Nutr 130:1412S–20S, 2000.

Scrimshaw NS, Behar M. Protein malnutrition in young children. Science 133:2039–2047, 1961.

Scrimshaw NS, San Giovanni JP. Synergism of nutrition, infection, and immunity: an overview. Am J Clin Nutr 66:S464–S477, 1997.

Semba R. Overview of the potential role of vitamin A in mother-to-child transmission of HIV-1. Acta Pediatr Suppl 421:107–112, 1997.

Semba R. Vitamin A and immunity to viral, bacterial and protozoan infections. Proc Nutr Soc 58:719–27, 1999.

Semba R, Hussey G. Vitamin A supplementation and childhood morbidity. Lancet 342:1176, 1993.

Semba R, Tang A. Micronutrients and the pathogenesis of human immunodeficiency virus infection. Br J Nutr 81:181–189, 1999.

Semba RD, Muhilal, Scott AL, Natadisastra G, Wirasasmita S, Mele L, Ridwan E, West KP Jr, Sommer A. Depressed immune response to tetanus in children with vitamin A deficiency. J Nutr 122:101–107, 1992.

Semba RD, Muhilal, Ward BJ, Griffin DE, Scott AL, Natadisastra G, West KP Jr, Sommer A. Abnormal T-cell subset proportions in vitamin-A-deficient children. Lancet 341:5–8, 1993.

Semba RD, Muhilal, Scott AL, Natadisatra G, West KP Jr., Sommer A. Effect of vitamin A Supplementation on immunoglobulin G subclass responses to tetanus toxoid in children. Clin Diag Lab Immunol 1:172–175, 1994.

Seth V, Chandra RK. Opsonic activity, phagocytosis, and bactericidal capacity of polymorphs in undernutrition. Arch Dis Child 47:282–284, 1972.

Shamir R, Tershakovec AM, Gallagher PR, Liacouras CA, Hayman LL, Cortner JA. The influence of age and relative weight on the presentation of familial combined hyperlipidemia in childhood. Atherosclerosis 121:85–91, 1996.

Shatrov VA, Boelaert JR, Chouaib S, Droge W, Lehmann V. Iron chelation decreases human immunodeficiency virus-1 Tat potentiated tumor necrosis factor-induced NF-κB activation in Jurat cells. Eur Cytokine Netw 8:37–43, 1997.

Shrimpton R, Victora CG, de Onis M, Lima RC, Blossner M, Clugston G. Worldwide timing of growth faltering: implications for nutritional interventions. Pediatrics 107:E75, 2001.

Singla PN, Chand P, Kumar A, Kachhawaha JS. Serum magnesium levels in protein-energy malnutrition. J Trop Pediatr 44:117–119, 1998.

Sirisinha S, Edelman R, Suskind R, Charupatana C, Olson RE. Complement and C3-proactivator levels in children with protein-calorie malnutrition and effect of dietary treatment. Lancet 1:1016–1020, 1973.

Sirisinha S, Suskind R, Edelman R, Asvapaka C, Olson RE. Secretory and serum IgA in children with protein-calorie malnutrition. Pediatrics 55:166–170, 1975.

Skov M, Poulsen LK, Koch C. Increased antigen-specific Th-2 response in allergic bronchopulmonary aspergillosis (ABPA) in patients with cystic fibrosis. Pediatr Pulmonol 27:74–79, 1999.

Skurnick JH, Bogden JD, Baker H, Kemp FW, Sheffet A, Quattrone G, Louria DB. Micronutrient profiles in HIV-1 infected heterosexual adults. J Acquir Immune Defic Sndr Hum Retrovirol 12:75–83, 1996.

Smythe PM, Brereton Stiles GG, Grace HJ, Mafoyane A, Schonland M, Coovadia HM, Loening WE, Parent MA, Vos GH. Thymolymphatic deficiency and depression of cell-mediated immunity in protein-calorie malnutrition. Lancet 2:939–943, 1971.

Smythe RL, Croft NM, O'Hea U, Marshall TG, Ferguson A. Intestinal inflammation in cystic fibrosis. Arch Dis Child 82:394–399, 2000.

Soliman AT, El Zalabany MM, Salama M, Ansari BM. Serum leptin concentrations during severe protein-energy malnutrition: correlation with growth parameters and endocrine function. Metabolism 49:819–825, 2000.

Solomons NW. Zinc and other trace mineral deficiencies and excesses. In Strickland GT, ed. Hunter's Tropical Medicine and Emerging Infectious Diseases, ed 8. Philadelphia, WB Saunders, 2000, p 962.

Stansfield SK, Pierre Louis M, Lerebours G, Augustin A. Vitamin A supplementation and increased prevalence of childhood diarrhoea and acute respiratory infections. Lancet 342:578–582, 1993.

Stephenson LS. Crompton, DWT, Latham MC, Schulpen TWJ, Nesheim MC, Jansen AAJ. Relationship between Ascaris infection and growth of malnourished pre-schoolchildren in Kenya. Am J Clin Nutr 33:1165–1172, 1980.

Stevens J, Lubitz L. Symptomatic zinc deficiency in breast-fed term and premature infants. J Paediatr Child Health 34:97–100, 1998.

Stiehm ER. Humoral immunity in malnutrition. Fed Proc 39:3093–3097, 1980.

Stoll BA. Adiposity as a risk determinant for postmenopausal breast cancer. Int J Obes Relat Metab Disord 24:527–533, 2000.

Stoltzfus RJ. The impact of parasitic infections on nutrition. In Strickland GT, ed. Hunter's Tropical Medicine and Emerging Infectious Diseases, ed 8. Philadelphia, WB Saunders, 2000, pp 970–971.

Strand TA, Chandyo RK, Bahl R, Sharma PR, Adhikari RK, Bhandari N, Ulvik RJ, Molbak K, Bhan MK, Sommerfelt H. Effectiveness and efficacy of zinc for the treatment of acute diarrhea in young children. Pediatrics 109:898–903, 2002.

Strauss RS, Dietz WH. Low maternal weight gain in the second or third trimester increases the risk for intrauterine growth retardation. J Nutr 129:988–993, 1999.

Sullivan DA, Vaerman JP, Soo C. Influence of severe protein malnutrition on rat lacrimal, salivary and gastrointestinal immune expression during development, adulthood and aging. Immunology 78:308–317, 1993.

Sussman M. Iron and infection. In Jacobs A, Worwood M, eds. Biochemistry and Medicine. New York, Academic Press, 1974, pp 649–679.

Taylor CG, Giesbrecht JA. Dietary zinc deficiency and expression of T lymphocyte signal transduction proteins. Can J Physiol Pharmacol 78:823–838, 2000.

Tenhola S, Martikainen A, Rahiala E, Herrgard E, Halonen P, Voutilainen R. Serum lipid concentrations and growth characteristics in 12-year-old children born small for gestational age. Pediatr Res 48:623–628, 2000.

Tershakovec AM, Jawad AF, Stallings VA, Zemel BS, McKenzie JM, Stolley PD, Shannon BM. Growth of hypercholesterolemic children completing physician-initiated low-fat dietary intervention. J Pediatr 133:28–34, 1998.

Tibault H, Galan P, Selz F, Preziosi P, Olivier C, Badoual J, Hercberg S. The immune response in iron-deficient young children: effect of iron supplementation on cell-mediated immunity. Eur J Pediatr 152:120–124, 1993.

Touger-Decker R. Oral manifestations of nutrient deficiencies. Mt Sinai J Med 65:355–361, 1998.

Tran T, Eubanks S, Schaffer K, Zhou C, Linder M. Secretion of ferritin by rat hepatoma cells and its regulation by inflammatory cytokines and iron. Blood 90:4979, 1997.

Treem WR. New developments in the pathophysiology, clinical spectrum, and diagnosis of disorders of fatty acid oxidation. Curr Opin Pediatr 12:463–468, 2000.

Troiano RP, Flegal KM, Kuczmarski RJ, Campbell SM, Johnson CL. Overweight prevalence and trends for children and adolescents: the National Health and Nutrition Examination Surveys, 1963 to 1991. Arch Pediatr Adolesc Med 149:1085–1091, 1995.

Tsai JF, Jeng JE, Chuang LY, Chang WY, Tsai JH. Urinary transforming growth factor beta1 levels in hepatitis C virus-related chronic liver disease: correlation between high levels and severity of disease. Hepatology 25:1141–1146, 1997.

Tummler B, Kiewitz C. Cystic fibrosis: an inherited susceptibility to bacterial respiratory infections. Mol Med Today 5:351–358, 1999.

Turner RJ and Finch JM. Selenium and the immune response. Proc Nutr Soc 50:275–285, 1991.

Udani PM. BCG vaccination in India and tuberculosis in children: newer facets. Indian J Pediatr 5:451–462, 1994.

Vaarala O. Gut and the induction of immune tolerance in type-1 diabetes. Diabetes Metab Res Rev 15:353–361, 1999.

Vanderhoof JA. Short bowel syndrome in children and small intestinal transplantation. Pediatr Clin North Am 43:533–550, 1996.

Victora CG, Kirkwood BR, Ashworth A, Black RE, Rogers S, Sazawal S, Campbell H, Gove S. Potential interventions for the prevention of childhood pneumonia in developing countries: improving nutrition. Am J Clin Nutr 70:309–320, 1999.

Vint FW. Post-mortem findings in the natives of Kenya. East Afr Med J 13:332–340, 1937.

Wahab PJ, Crusius JB, Meijer JW, Mulder CJ. Gluten challenge in borderline gluten-sensitive enteropathy. Am J Gastroenterol 96:1464–1469, 2001.

Wallace JM, Ferguson SJ, Loane P, Kell M, Millar S, Gillmore WS. Cytokines in human breast milk. Br J Biomed Sci 54:85–87, 1997.

Walker AM, Garcia R, Pate P. Mata LJ, David JR. Transfer factor in the immune deficiency of protein-calorie malnutrition: a controlled study with 32 cases. Cell immunol 15:372–381, 1975.

Walter R. Arredondo S, Arevalo M, Stekel A. Effect of iron therapy on phagocytosis and bactericidal activity in neutrophils of iron-deficient infants. Am J Clin Nutr 44:877–882, 1986.

Wang YR, WU JY, Reaves SK, Lei KY. Enhanced expression of hepatic genes in copper-deficient rats detected by the messenger RNA differential display method. J Nutr 126:1772–1781, 1996.

Watzl B, Bub A, Brandstetter B, Rechkemmer G. Modulation of human T-lymphocyte functions by the consumption of carotenoid-rich vegetables. Br J Nutr 82:383–389, 1999.

Weber RV, Stein DE, Scholes J, Kral JG. Obesity potentiates AOM-induced colon cancer. Dig Dis Sci 45:890–895, 2000.

Weber TR. Enteral feeding increases sepsis in infants with short bowel syndrome. J Pediatr Surg 30:1086–1088, 1995.

Weinberg ED. Iron withholding: a defense against infection and neoplasia. Physiol Rev 64:65–102, 1984.

West K Jr, Katz J, Khatry S, Le Clerq S, Pradhan E, Shrestha S, Connor P, Dali S, Christian P, Pokhrel R. Sommer double blind, cluster randomized trial of low dose supplementation with vitamin A or beta carotene on morality related to pregnancy in Nepal. The NNIPS-2 Study Group. Br Med J 27:318:50–55, 1999.

Wilson DC, Phillips MJ, Cox DW, Roberts EA. Severe hepatic Wilson's disease in preschool-aged children. J Pediatr 137:719–722, 2000.

Winklhofer-Roob BM. Cystic fibrosis: nutritional status and micronutrients. Curr Opin Clin Nutr Metab Care 3:293–297, 2000.

Wolf BH, Ikeogu MO, Vos ET. Effect of nutritional and HIV status on bacteraemia in Zimbabwean Children who died at home. Eur J Pediatr 154:299–303, 1995.

Wong CS, Gipson DS, Gillen DL, Emerson S, Koepsell T, Sherrard DJ, Watkins SL, Stehman-Breen C. Anthropometric measures and risk of death in children with end-stage renal disease. Am J Kidney Dis 36:811–819, 2000.

Wright C, Birks E. Risk factors for failure to thrive: a population-based survey. Child Care Health Dev 26:5–16, 2000.

Yetgin S, Altay C, Ciliv G, Laleli Y. Myeloperoxidase activity and bactericidal function of PMN in iron deficiency. Acta Haematol 61:10–14, 1979.

Yu VY. The role of dietary nucleotides in neonatal and infant nutrition. Singapore Med J 39:145–150, 1998.

Zamboni G, Dufillot D, Antoniazzi F, Valentini R, Gendrel D, Tato L. Growth hormone-binding proteins and insulin-like growth factor-binding proteins in protein-energy malnutrition, before and after nutritional rehabilitation. Pediatr Res 39:410–414, 1996.

Zeisel SH. Is there a metabolic basis for dietary supplementation? Am J Clin Nutr 72:507S–511S, 2000.

Zhang W, Parentau H, Greenly RL, Metz CA, Aggarwal S, Wainer IW, Tracy TS. Effect of protein-calorie malnutrition on cytochromes P450 and glutathione S-transferase. Eur J Drug Metab Pharmacokinet 24:141–147, 1999.

Ziegler RG, Mason TJ, Stemhagen A, Hoover R. Schoenberg JB, Gridley G, Virgo PW, Fraumeni JF Jr. Carotenoid intake, vegetables, and the risk of lung cancer among white men in New Jersey. Am J Epidemiol 123:1080–1093, 1986.

Zielenski J. Genotype and phenotype in cystic fibrosis. Respiration 67:117–133, 2000.

Zuin G, Principi N. Trace elements and vitamins in immunomodulation in infancy and childhood. Eur J Cancer Prev 6:S69–S77, 1997.

C H A P T E R

24

Genetic Disorders, Including Syndromic Immunodeficiencies

Jeffrey E. Ming and John M. Graham, Jr.

SYNDROMIC IMMUNODEFICIENCIES—DEFINITION

Many immunodeficiency disorders have a genetic component, and numerous primary immunodeficiencies are now known to be due to single gene defects. In primary immunodeficiencies, the patient generally comes to medical attention because of manifestations resulting from defective immune function. Most have no phenotypic abnormalities except for immune deficiency. However, immune defects may also be associated with abnormalities in other organ systems, often as part of recognizable syndromes. We term these conditions *syndromic immunodeficiencies.*

In syndromic immunodeficiencies, the immune abnormalities are often identified after the syndrome has been diagnosed. The immunodeficiency may not represent the major clinical problem, and the immune defects may not be present in all cases. Several genetic disorders, such as Wiskott-Aldrich syndrome and ataxia-telangiectasia (AT), may fit into both primary and syndromic immunodeficiency categories. These conditions have both characteristic organ dysfunction and/or dysmorphology unrelated to the immune system and a consistent, well-defined immune deficiency.

Immunodeficiency may occur in combination with several diverse processes, including faulty embryogenesis, metabolic derangements, chromosomal abnormalities, or teratogenic disorders. Recognition of syndromes resulting from such processes, which can affect both the immune and other organ systems, may facilitate accurate diagnosis and management and yield information regarding genes critical for the development of the involved systems. This chapter delineates those immunodeficiencies that are associated with recognizable genetic syndromes. We provide an overview of the clinical manifestations and genetic aspects of each syndrome and delineate the specific associated immune defects. Many of the more common conditions are discussed in detail in other chapters and are presented here only briefly. In addition, we also consider two genetic hemoglobinopathies, sickle cell disease and thalassemia, because frequent infections are associated with both of these conditions.

The inheritance pattern of each condition and the chromosomal location of the disease-related genes, when known, are indicated in the tables. Mendelian Inheritance in Man (MIM) (OMIM, 2000) numbers are indicated within parentheses in the text.

SYNDROMES ASSOCIATED WITH GROWTH DEFICIENCY

Several immunodeficiency states are associated with growth deficiency (Tables 24-1 and 24-2). The growth deficiency may be due to a skeletal dysplasia, in which there is an abnormality of bone formation. Many skeletal dysplasias are associated with disproportionate short stature, in which the limbs and trunk are not proportional in relation to each other. Other forms of short stature are not associated with skeletal abnormalities. These forms usually show proportionate growth failure, in which case the overall height is small, but the various body parts are commensurate with one another.

Syndromes Associated with Skeletal Dysplasia

The disproportionate short stature that occurs with immunodeficiency often affects the limbs more than the trunk, resulting in short-limb skeletal dysplasia. Short-limb skeletal dysplasia has been reported in association with combined immunodeficiency, predominantly cellular defects, or with a primarily humoral defect.

Short-Limb Skeletal Dysplasia with Combined Immunodeficiency (MIM 200900)

The conditions in which short-limb skeletal dysplasia is associated with combined immunodeficiency are a heterogeneous group. Although some of these patients have adenosine deaminase (ADA) deficiency (see section on metabolic conditions), other patients have more severe bony changes affecting the metaphyses than is typically found in ADA deficiency. Several reports describe Omenn syndrome, a fatal disorder characterized by eosinophilia, skin eruptions, and reticuloendotheliosis, with short-limb skeletal dysplasia (Gatti et al., 1969; Gotoff et al., 1972; Schofer et al., 1991). Further discussion of Omenn syndrome may be found in the section on dermatologic disorders. A child with severe combined immunodeficiency (SCID), normal ADA and purine nucleoside phosphorylase activity, and short-limb skeletal dysplasia also developed a B-cell lymphoma (van den Berg et al., 1997).

MacDermot Syndrome

A patient with proximal shortening of the extremities, bowing of the femora, and increased skin folds had neutropenia and undetectable IgG2 and IgA (MacDermot et al., 1991). No mature B cells were detected, although normal numbers of immature B cells were present. CD4+ T-cell number and responses to phytohemagglutinin and alloantigen were decreased.

TABLE 24-1 · SYNDROMES ASSOCIATED WITH GROWTH DEFICIENCY: SKELETAL DYSPLASIAS

Name	Inheritance (Chromosome)	Associated Features	Immune Defect	Frequency of ID
1. Short limb skeletal dysplasia with combined immune deficiency	AR	Metaphyseal dysplasia, bowed femurs; may be seen with adenosine deaminase deficiency or Omenn syndrome	T, B	++++
2. MacDermot syndrome	?AR	Short limbs, bowed femora	T, B, Ph	++++ (1 case)
3. Kyphomelic dysplasia	AR	Short/bowed limbs, metaphyseal irregularities, 11 ribs	T, B	+
4. Spondylo-mesomelic-acrodysplasia	?	Meso/rhizomelia, hypoplastic vertebrae, brachydactyly	T, B	++++ (1 case)
5. Cartilage-hair hypoplasia	AR (9p13)	McKusick type metaphyseal dysplasia, mild leg bowing, fine/sparse hair	T, Ph	++++
6. Short limb skeletal dysplasia with humoral immune deficiency	?AR	Metaphyseal dysplasia, recurrent infection in male and female siblings		++++ (2 siblings)
7. Schimke immunoosseous dysplasia	AR	Spondyloepiphyseal dysplasia, progressive nephropathy, episodic lymphopenia, pigmentary skin changes	T	++++
8. Roifman syndrome	?XL	Spondyloepiphyseal dysplasia, retinal dystrophy	B	++++
9. Braegger syndrome	?	Prenatal growth deficiency, ischiadic hypoplasia, renal dysfunction, craniofacial anomalies, postaxial polydactyly, hypospadias	B	++++ (1 case)
10. Kenny-Caffey syndrome	AD, AR (1q42-q43)	Bone medullary stenosis, myopia, hypocalcemia; some have deletions of 22q11	T, Ph	++

Frequency of ID: +, less than 5% of reported cases with documented ID; ++, 5%–30%; +++, 30%–65%; ++++, >65%.
AD = autosomal dominant; AR = autosomal recessive; B = B-cell defect; ID = immunodeficiency; NK = NK-cell defect Ph = phagocyte defect; T = T-cell defect; XL = X linked.

Kyphomelic Dysplasia (MIM 211350)

Kyphomelic dysplasia is characterized by broad, short, and bent femora. The humeri, radii, and ulnae may also be affected and show flared and irregular metaphyses (Prasad et al., 2000). There may be mild platyspondyly. An affected male infant had severe T- and B-cell abnormalities and died from cytomegalovirus (CMV) pneumonia (Corder et al., 1995). Autosomal recessive inheritance has been suggested, although most reported patients are male.

Spondylo-Mesomelic-Acrodysplasia

A girl with spondylo-acrodysplasia, mild short-limb dwarfism, and joint dislocations had SCID (Castriota-Scanderbeg et al., 1997). She had greatly reduced T-cell number and very low IgG and IgA.

Cartilage-Hair Hypoplasia (MIM 250250)

Cartilage-hair hypoplasia (CHH), or metaphyseal chondrodysplasia, McKusick type, is an autosomal recessive disorder that was first described in the Amish population (McKusick et al., 1965) and has subsequently been reported in several ethnic groups. It is a recognized primary immunodeficiency (see Chapter 17). Affected individuals have short-limb dwarfism, metaphyseal chondrodysplasia, and fine sparse hair. Immunologic defects generally affect the cellular immune response (Makitie and Kaitila, 1993). Mutations in the gene encoding the endoribonuclease RNase mitochondrial RNA-processing endoribonuclease (MRP) were detected in affected patients (Ridanpaa et al., 2001). This nuclear gene (RMRP) encodes a structural RNA molecule. The molecule functions to cleave RNA in mitochondrial DNA synthesis and in nucleolar cleaving of pre-rRNA.

Short-Limb Skeletal Dysplasia with Humoral Immune Defect

A primary immunodeficiency with short-limb skeletal dysplasia was described in two siblings with metaphyseal dysostosis and low IgG, IgA, and IgM levels (Ammann et al., 1974). T-cell number, response to phytohemagglutinin, and delayed-type hypersensitivity tests were normal; however, T-cell proliferation to alloantigen was somewhat decreased.

TABLE 24-2 · SYNDROMES ASSOCIATED WITH GROWTH DEFICIENCY: PROPORTIONATE SHORT STATURE

Name	Inheritance (Chromosome)	Associated Features	Immune Defect	Frequency of ID
1. X-linked agamma-globulinemia with growth hormone deficiency	XL (Xq21-q22)	Hypogammaglobulinemia, isolated growth hormone deficiency	B	++++
2. Mulvihill-Smith syndrome	?AD	Prenatal growth deficiency, microcephaly, small face, premature aging, multiple nevi, mental retardation	T,B	++++
3. Mulibrey nanism	AR (17q22-q23)	Prenatal growth deficiency, muscle weakness, abnormal sella turcica, hepatomegaly, ocular fundi lesions	B	+
4. CHARGE association	?	Coloboma, heart defect, atresia choanae, retarded growth and development, genital hypoplasia, ear anomalies/deafness	T	++
5. Kabuki syndrome	?AD	Long palpebral fissures, prominent eyelashes, skeletal anomalies, congenital heart disease	B	+
6. Dubowitz syndrome	AR	Microcephaly, eczema, pre/postnatal growth deficiency	Ph	+
7. Rubinstein-Taybi syndrome	AD (16p13)	Broad thumbs and halluces, prominent nasal septum below ala nasi, cryptorchidism, mental retardation	T, Ph	+
8. Sutor syndrome	?	Hypogonadotropic hypogonadism, growth hormone deficiency	T, B, NK	++++ (1 case)
9. Shokeir syndrome	AR	Absent thumbs, anosmia, ichthyosiform dermatosis, congenital heart defect; 3 sibships	T, B, Ph	++++ (1 kindred)
10. Toriello syndrome	?AR	Prenatal growth deficiency, cataracts, microcephaly, enamel hypoplasia, mental retardation	B, Ph	++++ (1 kindred)
11. Stoll syndrome	?AR	Developmental delay, facial dysmorphism, congenital heart disease	Ph	++++ (3 siblings)
12. Hoffman syndrome	?	Postnatal growth retardation, triphalangeal thumbs, hypoplastic first metatarsals, microcephaly	B	++++ (1 case)

Frequency of ID: +, less than 5% of reported cases with documented ID; ++, 5%–30%; +++, 30%–65%; ++++, >65%.
AD = autosomal dominant; AR = autosomal recessive; B = B-cell defect; ID = immunodeficiency; NK = NK-cell defect; Ph = phagocyte defect; T = T-cell defect; XL = X linked.

Schimke Immunoosseous Dysplasia (MIM 242900)

The principal features of Schimke immunoosseous dysplasia, an autosomal recessive syndrome, are short stature with exaggerated lumbar lordosis, protruding abdomen, spondyloepiphyseal dysplasia, defective cellular immunity, and progressive renal failure (Boerkoel et al., 2000; Saraiva et al., 1999) (see Chapter 13). A broad and low nasal bridge with a bulbous nasal tip is characteristic, and hyperpigmented macules are commonly present. The vertebral bodies are usually ovoid, and the pelvis and proximal femora show dysplastic changes. Epiphyseal changes are most frequently present in the proximal femur. Proteinuria eventually develops in all patients, usually as a result of focal segmental glomerulosclerosis, and it often progresses to end-stage renal disease. Approximately 50% have an arteriopathy with cerebral infarcts and/or ischemia. Elevated thyroid-stimulating hormone level is present in approximately one half of patients, although T_3 and T_4 levels are generally normal. Nearly all patients have normal intellectual and neurologic development.

Mutations in the gene encoding the chromatin remodeling protein (SWI/SNF2-related matrix-associated, actin-dependent regulator of chromatin, subfamily a-like 1; *SMARCAL1*) have been detected in affected patients (Boerkoel et al., 2002). The protein participates in DNA-nucleosome restructuring that occurs during gene regulation and DNA replication and recombination.

Patients are prone to viral and bacterial infections, and all patients demonstrate T-cell deficiency with decreased CD4+ number (Ludman et al., 1993; Spranger et al., 1991). Mitogen-induced T-cell proliferation is impaired, and delayed-type hypersensitivity responses are absent. Lymphopenia is characteristic (94%) and is often associated with other hematologic abnormalities, including pancytopenia. The immunoglobulin levels are abnormal in two thirds, although the absolute B-cell (CD19+) counts were normal (Boerkoel et al., 2000).

Roifman Syndrome (MIM 300258)

Four boys from three families had a humoral immunodeficiency in association with growth restriction, spondyloepiphyseal dysplasia, impaired intelligence, and retinal dystrophy (Roifman, 1999) (see Chapter 13). They had low or absent antibody titers in response to infection, decreased isohemagglutinins, and decreased mitogenic response to *Staphylococcus aureus* Cowan A. T-cell number and function were normal. There was epiphyseal dysplasia of the hips and long bones and vertebral anomalies. Microcephaly, developmental delay, hypotonia, and eczema were present. Facial features included a long philtrum, narrow upturned nose, and thin upper lip. Another male patient with humoral immunodeficiency, spondyloepithelial dysplasia, and hypogonadotrophic hypogonadism was reported (Robertson et al., 2000). Because all reported patients have been male, the authors have suggested X-linked inheritance.

Braegger Syndrome (MIM 243340)

A boy of consanguineous parents had intrauterine growth deficiency, ischiadic hypoplasia, microcephaly, facial dysmorphism, renal dysfunction, cryptorchidism, postaxial polydactyly, cutaneous syndactyly, and conductive hearing loss (Braegger et al., 1991). He had multiple respiratory infections. IgG and IgM were decreased, and IgA, isohemagglutinins, and antidiphtheria antibodies were not detectable.

Kenny-Caffey Syndrome (MIM 127000, 244460)

Cortical thickening of long bones with medullary stenosis, growth deficiency, hypoparathyroidism, facial dysmorphism, and various ophthalmologic anomalies occur in Kenny-Caffey syndrome. Both autosomal recessive (type 1) and autosomal dominant (type 2) forms have been described. Neutropenia and abnormal T-cell function were noted in an affected 18-month-old girl (Bergada et al., 1988). Two siblings, who may have had the recessive form, had decreased T-cell numbers and impaired neutrophil phagocytosis (Sabry et al., 1998). Four affected siblings in a consanguineous kindred had a deletion of 22q11 (Sabry et al., 1998). However, other affected individuals do not have this deletion. The Sanjad-Sakati syndrome (MIM 241410), also termed the *hypoparathyroidism-retardation-dysmorphism (HRD) syndrome,* has significant clinical overlap. Both autosomal recessive Kenny-Caffey syndrome and Sanjad-Sakati syndrome have been mapped to chromosome 1q42-q43 (Diaz et al., 1999; Parvari et al., 1998), so these disorders may be allelic.

Syndromes Associated with Proportionate Short Stature

Growth Hormone Deficiency with X-Linked Agammaglobulinemia (MIM 307200)

Affected individuals have recurrent sinopulmonary infections, short stature, and decreased growth hormone levels without other endocrinologic abnormalities (Fleisher et al., 1980) (see Chapter 13). Both B-cell number and immunoglobulin levels are greatly decreased or absent,

consistent with X-linked agammaglobulinemia (XLA). T-cell number and function are normal. XLA/growth hormone deficiency (GHD) has been mapped at or near the XLA locus at Xq21-q22 (Conley et al., 1991). The growth hormone gene is located on chromosome 17. In two patients, a point mutation leading to premature termination of the protein has been detected in *BTK*, the gene associated with XLA (Abo et al., 1998; Duriez et al., 1994). Another patient did not have a mutation in the coding sequence of *BTK* (Stewart et al., 1995). Further studies will be needed to determine whether *BTK* is generally involved in XLA/GHD and whether XLA and XLA/GHD are distinct linked loci or allelic variations of a single locus or whether XLA/GHD usually results from a contiguous gene deletion.

Additional immune defects have been reported in association with isolated GHD, including combined immunodeficiency (Maghnie et al., 1992; Tang and Kemp, 1993), decreased natural killer (NK) activity (Kiess et al., 1988), and hypogammaglobulinemia (Ohzeki et al., 1993). However, most children with GHD do not display an increased susceptibility to infection (Church et al., 1989; Spadoni et al., 1991).

Mulvihill-Smith Syndrome (MIM 176690)

Mulvihill-Smith syndrome is characterized by prenatal and postnatal growth restriction, multiple pigmented nevi, microcephaly, reduced facial fat, genitourinary anomalies, and a high-pitched voice (de Silva et al., 1997; Mulvihill and Smith, 1975). Oligodontia, brachydactyly, mental retardation, and hearing loss have also been reported. Infectious complications are common, and the immune deficiency is often progressive. There can be impaired T-cell response to mitogen, decreased CD4 count, and/or low Ig levels (Bartsch et al., 1994; de Silva et al., 1997; Ohashi et al., 1993).

Mulibrey Nanism (MIM 253250)

Mulibrey nanism, an autosomal recessive condition, features prenatal-onset growth failure, muscular hypotonia, hepatomegaly, long and shallow sella turcica, retinal abnormalities, and constrictive pericarditis. Frequent infections have been noted. Low IgG (especially IgG2 and IgG4) and IgM were found in an affected patient who also had isolated GHD (Haraldsson et al., 1993). IgE was absent, and IgA and IgD were elevated. Specific antibody and isohemagglutinin titers were greatly diminished. Total B-cell number was low. T-cell numbers and function were normal. Mutations in the *MUL* gene have been identified (Avela et al., 2000). The MUL protein is a member of the RING-B-box-coiled-coil family of zinc-finger proteins.

CHARGE Association (MIM 214800)

The abnormalities that comprise the CHARGE association include coloboma, heart defects, atresia of the choanae, retardation of growth and development, genital hypoplasia, and ear anomalies and/or deafness (Fig. 24-1) (Pagon et al., 1981; Tellier et al., 1998). Other associated features include cranial nerve deficits resulting in swallowing deficits and facial palsy, renal anomalies, orofacial clefts, and tracheoesophageal fistula (Blake et al., 1998; Graham, 2001). Most cases are sporadic, and the disorder is thought to represent a new dominant mutation in most instances. The features are consistent with a developmental defect involving cephalic neural crest cells contributing to the third and fourth pharyngeal arches (Siebert et al., 1985). Of 21 patients with choanal atresia and/or ocular coloboma, 3 were found with DiGeorge sequence, although the presence of the 22q11 deletion was not assessed (Pagon et al., 1981). Five patients with CHARGE association who also showed DiGeorge sequence without a 22q11 deletion were described (de Lonlay-Debeney et al., 1997). A patient with malakoplakia of the colon, combined immunodeficiency with decreased CD4 count, coloboma, great vessel anomalies, and choanal atresia lacked detectable thymus tissue (Boudny et al., 2000). Overall, patients with CHARGE association do not have deletions of 22q11.

Kabuki Syndrome (MIM 147920)

Kabuki syndrome, a sporadic syndrome, features short stature, congenital heart disease, developmental delay, skeletal anomalies, and cleft palate (Niikawa et al., 1988; Schrander-Stumpel et al., 1994; Wilson, 1998). The distinctive facial features include long palpebral fissures with eversion of the lower lateral eyelid, promi-nent eyelashes, and abnormal ears (Fig. 24-2). Frequent infections occur in approximately 60% of patients (Chrzanowska et al., 1998). Patients with hypogamma-globulinemia, including decreased IgG and very low IgA, have been reported (Artigas et al., 1997; Chrzanowska et al., 1998; Hostoffer et al., 1996; Watanabe et al., 1994). Autoimmune hemolytic anemia and idiopathic thrombocytopenic purpura have also been reported (Ewart-Toland et al., 1998; Kawame et al., 1999; Watanabe et al., 1994) and may reflect the underlying immune dysfunction.

Dubowitz Syndrome (MIM 223370)

Dubowitz syndrome is an autosomal recessive condition characterized by prenatal and postnatal growth deficiency, mental retardation, microcephaly, sparse hair, eczema, and dysmorphic facies (ptosis, short palpebral fissures with lateral telecanthus, and dysplastic ears). Respiratory and gastrointestinal infections are common. Granulocytopenia resulting from bone marrow failure has been reported (Tsukahara and Opitz, 1996), and hyper-IgE syndrome was reported in one patient (Antoniades et al., 1996).

Rubinstein-Taybi Syndrome (MIM 180849)

Rubinstein-Taybi syndrome is characterized by broad thumbs and great toes, characteristic facial features, short stature, mental retardation, and cardiac abnormalities. There is an increased susceptibility to infec-

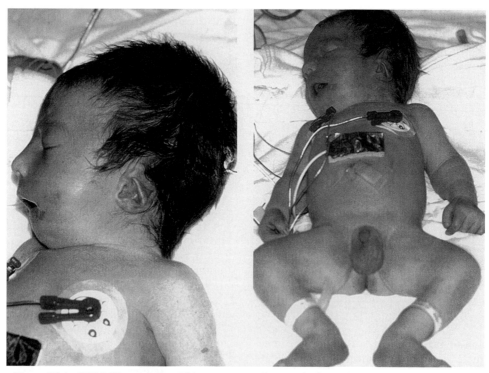

Figure 24-1 · CHARGE association. This neonate was born with choanal atresia, retinal colobomata, cleft palate, tetralogy of Fallot, absent thymus and parathyroid glands, and ears typical of CHARGE association.

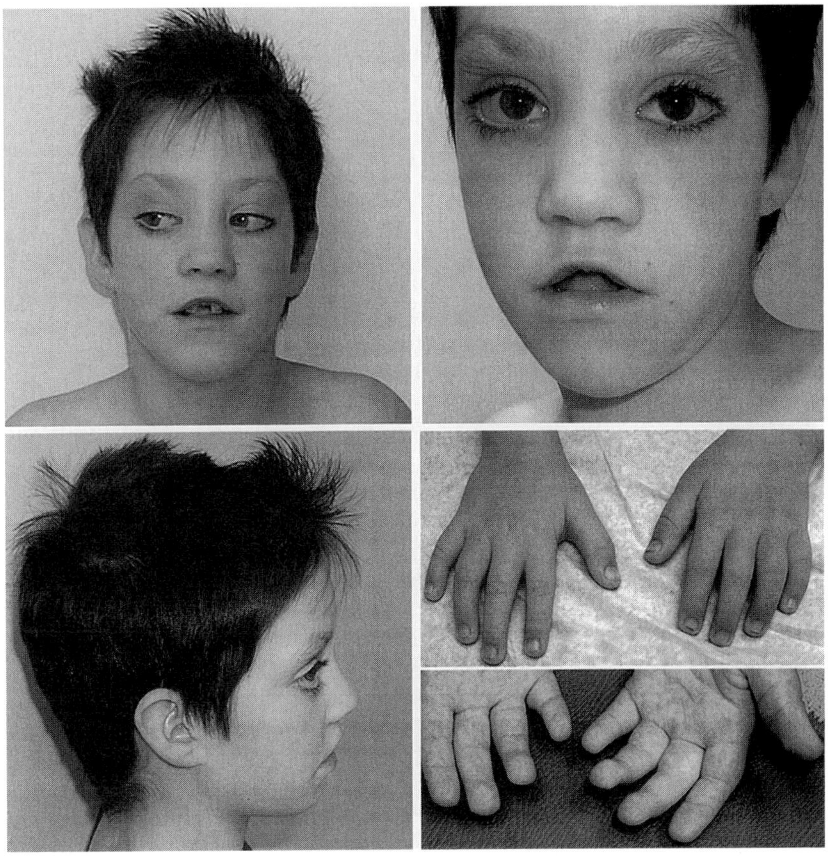

Figure 24-2 · Kabuki syndrome. This 9-year-old boy was the normal-sized product of a term delivery who experienced failure to thrive with multiple infections and developmental delay. He demonstrates typical features of Kabuki syndrome, including long palpebral fissures, medial eyebrow flare, trapezoidal philtrum, and persistent fetal fingertip pads.

tion. Thymic hypoplasia and defective T-cell function were reported in one patient (Kimura et al., 1993). Decreased T-cell number, impaired delayed-type hypersensitivity response (Rivas et al., 1980), lymphopenia, and poor response to pneumococcal vaccine (Villella et al., 2000) have been reported. Microdeletions and truncating mutations in the gene encoding CREB-binding protein (CBP) gene at 16p13.3 account for approximately 20% of the mutations in affected individuals (Petrij et al., 1995, 2000).

Sutor Syndrome

A woman with recurrent viral, fungal, and bacterial infections had hypogonadotropic hypogonadism and short stature with GHD (Sutor et al., 1998). She had low helper T cells, and antigen response and skin tests were defective. Hypogammaglobinemia, especially of IgG2 and IgG4, was noted, as were decreased NK-cell number and activity.

Shokeir Syndrome (MIM 274190)

Nine individuals from three sibships had absent thumbs, proportionate short stature, anosmia, and ichthyosiform dermatosis (Shokeir, 1978). One kindred showed cardiac defects. There was an increased susceptibility to infections, especially mucocutaneous candidiasis and varicella. Some individuals had decreased immunoglobulin levels, and decreased or absent IgA was the most

constant feature. Decreased T-cell response to phytohemagglutinin and neutropenia were present in all individuals studied. ADA and purine nucleoside phosphorylase levels were normal.

Toriello Syndrome (MIM 251190)

Two sisters with prenatal-onset growth deficiency, cataracts, microcephaly, mental retardation, enamel hypoplasia, and generalized delay of ossification were reported (Toriello et al., 1986). The older girl died of pneumonia at age 5 years. They had decreased IgM and IgG levels and neutropenia during infections.

Stoll Syndrome (MIM 601347)

Three siblings of first cousin parents had short stature, developmental delay, congenital heart disease, vesicoureteral reflux, and facial dysmorphism (prominent forehead, short philtrum, midface hypoplasia) (Stoll et al., 1994). All three siblings had bronchiectasis, which may have resulted from frequent severe pulmonary infections. Neutropenia was present.

Hoffman Syndrome

Hypogammaglobulinemia and absent B cells were noted in a girl with postnatal growth retardation, triphalangeal thumbs, and hypoplastic first metatarsals

(Hoffman et al., 2001). She also had microcephaly, micrognathia, and partial 4-5 syndactyly of the toes.

SYNDROMES ASSOCIATED WITH GASTROINTESTINAL DYSFUNCTION

Gastrointestinal abnormalities may lead to malnutrition and secondarily result in an immunodeficient state. However, in the syndromes described herein, the immunodeficiency precedes nutritional deprivation and thus is likely to be intrinsic to each condition (Table 24-3).

Familial Intestinal Polyatresia (MIM 243150)

The wide zone of distribution of the multiple atretic lesions found throughout the gastrointestinal tract in this condition distinguishes it from other types of intestinal atresia. SCID was described in three affected brothers (Moreno et al., 1990). They had panhypogammaglobulinemia and severely decreased T-cell number and function. ADA activity was normal. The recurrent infections were not secondary to the intestinal problems because they occurred early in life while the patients still had good nutritional status. Several other cases of multiple intestinal atresia associated with immune defects (Rothenberg et al., 1995; Snyder et al., 2000; Walker et al., 1993) have been described. In addition, two families with duodenal atresia and immunodeficiency have been reported (Moore et al., 1996), and this condition may be either a variant of familial intestinal polyatresia or a distinct entity with some clinical overlap.

Enteropathy with Villous Edema (MIM 600351)

Villous edema and recurrent episodes of acute severe secretory diarrhea were described in a Mennonite kindred (Smith et al., 1994). In the acute phase, massive protein and neutrophil loss occurs. During asympto-matic periods, jejunal villi are edematous, and breaks in the basement membrane are present, but without significant inflammatory infiltrate. During remission, IgG2 subclass deficiency was noted with normal IgA and B-cell levels. The abnormal mucosa and IgG2 deficiency may predispose these patients to bacterial overgrowth, infection, and resultant diarrhea.

Girault Syndrome

Severe infant diarrhea associated with low birth weight; dysmorphic features, including hypertelorism, prominent forehead, flat/broad nose, and wooly hair that came out in clumps; and immunodeficiency were reported in eight children (Girault et al., 1994). Jejunal biopsy showed villous atrophy, and no autoantibodies were detected. Severe infection, including sepsis, pneumonia, and CMV hepatitis, was typical. Skin tests were negative, and specific antibody response and isohemagglutinin titers were absent. A monoclonal IgA was detected in three children, without evidence of a lymphoproliferative disorder.

Dawson Syndrome (MIM 125890)

Severe secretory diarrhea with malabsorption of fat, vitamin B12, bile acids, and xylose was described in a male patient who also had four paternal relatives with histories of diarrhea (Dawson et al., 1979). Serum IgG, IgA, and IgM were all depressed. IgG synthesis rate was half the normal rate, whereas half-life and catabolic rate were normal. The albumin level was normal. In contrast to most individuals with common variable immunodeficiency, the patient had normal plasma cells in the intestinal mucosa.

Sclerosing Cholangitis with Immunodeficiency (MIM 242850)

Between 10% and 14% of children with sclerosing cholangitis have documented immunodeficiency, most

TABLE 24-3 · SYNDROMES ASSOCIATED WITH GASTROINTESTINAL DYSFUNCTION

Name	Inheritance	Associated Features	Immune Defect	Frequency of ID
1. Familial intestinal polyatresia	AR	Multiple atresias from pylorus to rectum	T, B	++
2. Enteropathy with villous edema	AD	Fulminant plasma-like stools, edematous jejunal villi; in Mennonites	B, Ph	+++
3. Girault syndrome	?	Diarrhea, villous atrophy, characteristic facies, abnormally easily removable hair	T, B	++++
4. Dawson syndrome	?	Diarrhea, malabsorption of fat, bile acids and xylose	B	++++ (1 case)
5. Sclerosing cholangitis with immunodeficiency	?AR	Intrahepatic sclerosing cholangitis, frequent infections	T, B	++

Frequency of ID: +, less than 5% of reported cases with documented ID; ++, 5%–30%; +++, 30%–65%; ++++, >65%.
AD = autosomal dominant; AR = autosomal recessive; B = B-cell defect; ID = immunodeficiency; NK = NK-cell defect; Ph = phagocyte defect; T = T-cell defect.

frequently involving both T and B cells (Debray et al., 1994; Sisto et al., 1987). Chronic infection of the biliary tract with organisms such as CMV or *Cryptosporidium* may lead to sclerosing cholangitis. Familial cases of sclerosing cholangitis with immune defects have been reported (Naveh et al., 1983; Record et al., 1973).

SYNDROMES ASSOCIATED WITH CUTANEOUS ABNORMALITIES

Although dermatologic symptoms such as dermatitis or skin infection often occur in immune-deficient patients, some immunodeficiency syndromes present with primarily cutaneous manifestations (Table 24-4). Some of these conditions present with alterations in pigmentation.

Griscelli Syndrome (MIM 214450)

An autosomal recessive syndrome of partial albinism, acute episodes of fever, neutropenia and thrombocytopenia, and lymphohistiocytosis have been described (Dufourcq-Lagelouse et al., 1999; Griscelli et al., 1978; Mancini et al., 1998) (see Chapters 17 and 20). Neurologic involvement may include seizures and neurodegenerative disease, possibly resulting from cerebral lymphohistiocytic infiltration (Hurvitz et al., 1993; Klein et al., 1994). Pigmentary dilution is due to accumulation of melanosomes in melanocytes, resulting in large clumps of pigment in hair shafts. The absence of giant granules and the histologic characteristics of the hypopigmentation differentiate this condition from Chédiak-Higashi. Most patients suffer from recurrent and severe fungal, viral, and bacterial infections. T-cell dysfunction, hypogammaglobulinemia, and neutropenia have been reported (Dufourcq-Lagelouse et al., 1999). Mutations in the *myosin VA* gene have been detected in affected patients (Pastural et al., 1997) with primarily neurologic symptoms. Mutations in a second gene on 15q21, *RAB27A,* were found in patients presenting primarily with the hemophagocytic syndrome resulting from uncontrolled T-lymphocyte and macrophage activation (Menasche et al., 2000). This gene encodes a GTP-binding protein of the Ras family.

TABLE 24-4 · SYNDROMES ASSOCIATED WITH CUTANEOUS ABNORMALITIES

Name	Inheritance (Chromosome)	Associated Features	Immune Defect	Frequency of ID
1. Griscelli syndrome	AR (15q21)	Partial albinism, frequent pyogenic infections, lymphohistiocytosis, episodic neutropenia/thrombocytopenia	T, B, NK, Ph	++++
2. Incontinentia pigmenti	XL (Xq28)	Erythematous vesiculobullous eruptions, CNS involvement, swirling macules of hyperpigmentation	T, B	+
3. Hypohydrotic/ anhidrotic ectodermal dysplasia	XL (Xq28)	Alopecia, hypo/anhidrosis, tooth anomalies	T, B	++
4. Dyskeratosis congenita	XL, AR, AD (Xq28)	Atrophy and pigmentation of skin, nail dystrophy, leukoplakia of oral mucosa	T, B, Ph	++
5. Acrodermatitis enteropathica	AR	Vesiculobullous dermatitis, alopecia, diarrhea; due to zinc deficiency	T, B, Ph	++
6. Netherton syndrome	AR (5q32)	Trichorrhexis invaginata (bamboo hair), ichthyosiform dermatitis, atopic diathesis	T, B	++
7. Papillon-Lefevre syndrome	AR (11q14)	Palmar/plantar hyperkeratosis, precocious periodontal disease	Ph	+
8. Pignata syndrome	AR (17q11-q12)	Congenital alopecia, nail dystrophy	T	++++ (2 siblings)
9. Onychotrichodys-plasia	AR	Dysplastic/hypoplastic nails, trichorrhexis	Ph	++++
10. Xeroderma pigmentosum	AR*	Photophobia, conjunctivitis, atrophic and pigmentary skin changes, skin tumors	T, NK	++
11. Kotzot syndrome	AR	Tyrosinase-positive oculocutaneous albinism, mental retardation, thrombocytopenia, microcephaly	Ph	++++ (2 siblings)
12. Navajo poikiloderma	?	Erythematous rash, telangiectasias, in Navajo population	Ph	++
13. Jung syndrome	?AD/XL	Pyoderma, folliculitis, atopic dermatitis, response to histamine-1 antagonist	T, B, Ph	++++ (1 kindred)
14. Neutrophil chemotactic defect	?AD	Congenital ichthyosis, recurrent skin infections, eczema	Ph	++++ (2 kindreds)
15. Davenport syndrome	?AR	White hair, muscle contractures, sensorineural hearing loss	Ph	++++ (1 kindred)
16. Ipp-Gelfand syndrome	?AR	Alopecia areata, pyogenic and respiratory infections	B	++++ (2 siblings)

*Multiple complementation groups suggest multiple genetic loci.
Frequency of ID: +, less than 5% of reported cases with documented ID; ++, 5%–30%; +++, 30%–65%; ++++, >65%.
AD = autosomal dominant; AR = autosomal recessive; B = B-cell defect; ID = immunodeficiency; NK = NK-cell defect; Ph = phagocyte defect; T = T-cell defect; XL = X linked.

Incontinentia Pigmenti (MIM 308310)

Linear erythematous vesiculobullous lesions shortly after birth that evolve into hyperpigmented swirling macules on the trunk and proximal extremities are typical findings for this X-linked dominant neurocutaneous disorder with fetal lethality in most affected males. Mental retardation, seizures, and ataxia can be associated features in some cases. Other findings include alopecia, ocular abnormalities, nail dystrophy, and malformed teeth. In a review of 77 cases, 13% had significant infection and 4 died of infectious causes (Diamantopoulos et al., 1985). No consistent immunologic abnormality has been detected, but decreased neutrophil chemotaxis and impaired proliferative response to phytohemagglutinin have been described in a few individuals (Jessen et al., 1978; Menni et al., 1990).

The gene encoding IKKγ, also termed *NEMO*, causes incontinentia pigmenti (Smahi et al., 2000) (see Chapter 13). The protein is involved in the regulation of phosphorylation and subsequent degradation of IκB, an inhibitor of nuclear factor-κB (NF-κB). NF-κB is involved in the regulation of expression of multiple genes. A variety of mutations in IKKγ have been detected, and approximately 80% of new mutations cause deletion of part of the gene. The deletion is mediated by directly repeated sequences within intron 3 and downstream of exon 10. Interestingly, mutations in this gene, which are presumably less disruptive, cause a form of ectodermal dysplasia associated with immune defects (see later discussion).

Hypohidrotic/Anhidrotic Ectodermal Dysplasia (MIM 300291)

Hypohidrotic/anhidrotic ectodermal dysplasia (HED) is marked by diminished or absent sweat glands, thin and sparse hair, and hypodontia (see Chapter 13). It is usually inherited in an X-linked recessive fashion, although autosomal recessive and dominant forms have been described. A subset of patients had been found to have immune defects (Abinun et al., 1996; Davis and Solomon, 1976). The most common defect involves hypogammaglobulinemia and may affect IgG and IgG2 levels (Doffinger et al., 2001; Zonana et al., 2000). Interestingly, the form with immune defects appears to be genetically distinct from those without immune defects. Four kindreds with X-linked HED and immune defects were found to have a mutation in exon 10 of the *NEMO* gene (Doffinger et al., 2001; Zonana et al., 2000). The mutations are predicted to affect the carboxy-terminal end of the protein, which may be involved in linking the IKK complex to upstream activators. Mutations in this gene have also been described in incontinentia pigmenti. Most cases of HED are caused by mutations in the gene encoding ectodysplasin (ED1) or its receptor (Kere et al., 1996; Monreal et al., 1998, 1999).

Interestingly, some patients with HED also have an X-linked hyper-IgM immunodeficiency (XHIM). Patients with isolated XHIM have a defect in the gene encoding the ligand for CD40 (Aruffo et al., 1993). However, patients with ectodermal dysplasia (ED) and XHIM have normal CD40L expression on T cells. Two patients with XHIM-ED and decreased IgG levels had a mutation in the *NEMO* gene in a predicted zinc-finger motif (Jain et al., 2001) (see Chapter 13).

Two male patients with anhidrotic ED, osteopetrosis, lymphedema, and immunodeficiency (MIM 300301) were born from mothers with mild incontinentia pigmenti (Doffinger et al., 2001). Both had multiple infections and died from infectious causes. The inflammatory response was poor, and isohemagglutinin titers and titers to *Pneumococcus* (despite documented infection) were decreased. Both patients had a mutation converting a stop codon to a tryptophan in *NEMO* (Doffinger et al., 2001). Thus four X-linked clinical conditions have been linked with different types of mutations in the *NEMO* gene.

Dyskeratosis Congenita (MIM 305000)

Dyskeratosis congenita is an X-linked disorder marked by reticulate skin pigmentation, nail dystrophy, leukoplakia of the oral mucosa, aplastic anemia, and an increased risk of malignancy. Progressive bone marrow failure develops in most patients and is the major cause of early mortality. Neutropenia occurs in approximately half of the patients (Dokal, 1996; Drachtman and Alter, 1992). Both humoral and cellular immune responses may be defective (Solder et al., 1998; Womer et al., 1983). Thymic aplasia was reported in two patients (Trowbridge et al., 1977). The gene causing dyskeratosis congenita (*DKC1*) codes for dyskerin, a protein predicted to function in the nucleolus in the formation of ribosomes (Heiss et al., 1998).

Acrodermatitis Enteropathica (MIM 201100)

Acrodermatitis enteropathica is an autosomal recessive disorder characterized by diarrhea, dermatitis, and alopecia arising in infancy and is due to inadequate zinc metabolism (see Chapters 23 and 34). Neurologic disturbances may occur. Severe infection with opportunistic pathogens occurs frequently, and recurrent infection occurs in 30% (Van Wouwe, 1989). Decreased response to phytohemagglutinin and abnormal delayed-type hypersensitivity skin response is typical (Oleske et al., 1979). Hypogammaglobulinemia and defective chemotaxis of neutrophils and monocytes are variably present (Van Wouwe, 1989; Weston et al., 1977). Both the clinical and immunologic abnormalities resolve after normalization of serum zinc levels.

Netherton Syndrome (MIM 256500)

The triad of trichorrhexis (brittle "bamboo" hair), ichthyosiform erythroderma, and atopic diathesis has been designated the Netherton syndrome, an autosomal recessive disorder. Recurrent infections occur in 28%, with skin involvement the most common site (Greene and Muller, 1985; Stryk et al., 1999). IgG abnormalities (both hypo-IgG and hyper-IgG) are present in 12% to 14%. Impairment of delayed-type hypersensitivity response, mitogen response, and neutrophil phagocytosis can occur. Increased IgE is found in 10% (Smith et al., 1995). Mutations in the gene SPINK5, which encodes a serine protease inhibitor, have been detected in affected patients (Chavanas et al., 2000).

Papillon-Lefevre Syndrome (MIM 245000)

Papillon-Lefevre syndrome is an autosomal recessive disorder associated with palmar-plantar hyperkeratosis and severe precocious periodontal disease leading to loss of both primary and permanent teeth (see Chapter 20). Approximately 17% of cases are associated with infections other than periodontal disease, most frequently furunculosis and pyoderma (Van Dyke et al., 1984). Neutrophil chemotaxis and random movement are both decreased. Mutations in the gene encoding cathepsin C (CTSC) have been demonstrated in several ethnic groups (Hart et al., 1999, 2000).

Pignata Syndrome (MIM 601705)

Two sisters with congenital alopecia, nail dystrophy, and T-cell dysfunction were reported (Pignata et al., 1996). Helper T-cell count was decreased with poor mitogen response. A homozygous mutation in the gene WHN, or winged-helix nude, was found in this kindred (Frank et al., 1999). Mutations in the mouse ortholog cause the nude phenotype of abnormal hair growth and thymus development (Nehls et al., 1994).

Onychotrichodysplasia with Neutropenia (MIM 258360)

Individuals with autosomal recessive dysplasia and hypoplasia of the nails and trichorrhexis have been reported (Cantu et al., 1975; Dallapiccola et al., 1994). Mild mental retardation has been reported in some patients and may be related to repeated infections. These patients had chronic and intermittent neutropenia leading to recurrent infections.

Xeroderma Pigmentosum (MIM 278700)

Xeroderma pigmentosum (XP) is characterized by sensitivity to sunlight with development of carcinoma at an early age, freckle-like lesions, photophobia, and poikiloderma. Neurologic complications are frequent, including progressive mental retardation, ataxia, microcephaly, and hearing loss. Seven distinct complementation groups (A to G) have been described (Cleaver, 1994). The protein products of these seven genes are believed to play roles in DNA repair in the process of nucleotide excision repair. Some form of immune alteration is found in 4% of patients, and only 1.2% show recurrent infection (Kraemer et al., 1987). The immune defects are variable. T-cell number may be decreased, because of decreased CD4 cells (Mariani et al., 1992; Wysenbeek et al., 1986), and delayed-type hypersensitivity response can be impaired (Dupuy and Lafforet, 1974). It remains to be determined if immunodeficiency is more prevalent in specific complementation groups. XP is also discussed in Chapter 18.

Kotzot Syndrome (MIM 203285)

A brother and sister of two related sets of consanguineous parents had tyrosinase-positive oculocutaneous albinism, intermittent thrombocytopenia, microcephaly, rough and projecting hair, and mild mental retardation (Kotzot et al., 1994). They had a protruding midface, thin upper lip, and nystagmus. Giant granules were not present. Bleeding time was prolonged with decreased factor XIII and antithrombin III. Neutropenia resulted in recurrent bacterial infections.

Navajo Poikiloderma (MIM 604173)

Navajo poikiloderma is characterized by a progressive erythematous rash, which begins in infancy, and the development of telangiectasias (Clericuzio et al., 1991). Neutropenia is variably present, and recurrent pneumonias have been described. All described patients have been Navajo.

Jung Syndrome (MIM 146840)

A father and son had recurrent pyoderma, folliculitis, herpetic corneal lesions, and atopic dermatitis (Jung et al., 1983). The child's grandfather had a similar history, and male-to-male transmission suggests autosomal dominant inheritance. T-cell responses to phytohemagglutinin, Candida, and tetanus toxoid were reduced. Pokeweed mitogen-induced immunoglobulin production was also decreased. IgE was increased. Phagocytic bactericidal activity was reduced, whereas chemotaxis and NBT reduction were normal. The immune abnormalities and clinical manifestations improved after treatment with the histamine-1 antagonist chlorpheniramine, and the abnormalities recurred after the agent was withdrawn.

Neutrophil Chemotactic Defect (MIM 162820)

Three children from two kindreds with congenital ichthyosis and recurrent infections with Trichophyton rubrum were reported (Miller et al., 1973). Chemotactic activity of neutrophils of both the patients and their fathers was defective. Bone marrow and peripheral blood neutrophil counts, phagocytosis, and bactericidal activity were normal. Immunoglobulin levels and phytohemagglutinin response were normal.

Davenport Syndrome

A boy, his mother, and his maternal grandmother had generalized hypopigmentation, white hair, a psoriasiform rash, muscle contractures, sensorineural hearing loss, and hyperkeratotic papillomata (Davenport et al., 1979). They had mucocutaneous candidiasis, and both granulocyte and monocyte chemotaxis were impaired.

Ipp-Gelfand Syndrome

Two siblings with alopecia areata arising at age 5 years, short stature, and recurrent pyogenic skin and respiratory infections were found to have mildly decreased levels of IgG and IgM (Ipp and Gelfand, 1976). Isohemagglutinin levels and antibody response to polio vaccine were low. An unrelated patient with congenital agammaglobulinemia also suffered from alopecia areata at age 12 years.

SYNDROMES ASSOCIATED WITH NEUROLOGIC DYSFUNCTION

Neurologic abnormalities ranging from structural abnormalities to epilepsy or ataxia have been reported in association with immunodeficiency (Table 24-5).

Myotonic Dystrophy (MIM 160900)

This autosomal dominant condition is a multisystem disorder characterized by difficulty in relaxing a contracted muscle. Muscle weakness and wasting, cataracts, hypogonadism, and cardiac conduction defects are also frequent manifestations. Cognitive function may deteriorate in adults. A severe congenital form of myotonic dystrophy has been described in which severe hypotonia, respiratory insufficiency, and feeding problems are present. This form is transmitted from the mother.

Most cases of myotonic dystrophy are due to a trinucleotide repeat expansion in the 3′ untranslated region of the *DMPK* gene, which encodes the dystrophia myotonica protein kinase (Brook et al., 1992; Fu et al., 1992; Mahadevan et al., 1992). In general, the size of the expansion correlates with the severity of the disease and the age of onset. Interestingly, a large family with features typical of myotonic dystrophy but who did not have the repeat expansion in the *DMPK* gene was described (Ranum et al., 1998). This family was found to have an

TABLE 24-5 · SYNDROMES ASSOCIATED WITH NEUROLOGIC DYSFUNCTION

Name	Inheritance (Chromosome)	Associated Features	Immune Defect	Frequency of ID
1. Myotonic dystrophy	AD (19q13, 3q)	Myotonia, muscle wasting, cataract, hypogonadism, cardiac arrhythmia; due to triplet repeat expansion	B	++
2. Ritscher-Schinzel syndrome	AR	Dandy-Walker-like malformation, atrio-ventricular canal defect, short stature; 2 sisters	B	++
3. Rambam-Hasharon syndrome	AR	Severe mental retardation, seizures, growth failure, abnormal facies	Ph	++++
4. Dionisi Vici syndrome	AR	Agenesis of corpus callosum, cleft lip, cutaneous hypopigmentation, bilateral cataracts; 2 brothers	T, B	++++
5. Høyeraal-Hreidarsson syndrome	XL (Xq28)	Cerebellar hypoplasia, absent corpus callosum, microcephaly, growth failure, pancytopenia	T, B, Ph	++++
6. Cohen syndrome	AR (8q22-q23)	Prominent central incisors, hypotonia, obesity	Ph	++
7. Microcephaly with immune defects	?AR/XL	Microcephaly, eczema, growth and developmental retardation, hypogonadism, epiphyseal dysplasia	B, Ph	++++ (2 siblings)
8. Mousa syndrome	AR	Spastic ataxia, congenital cataracts, macular corneal dystrophy	B	+++ (1 kindred)
9. Aguilar syndrome	?AR	Seizures, recurrent infection, conjunctival telangiectasias, mental retardation	B	++++ (1 kindred)
10. Adderson syndrome	?	Growth failure, intracranial calcifications, pancytopenia	B, Ph	++++ (2 cases)
11. Krawinkel syndrome	?	Lissencephaly, abnormal lymph nodes, spastic tetraplegia, transient arthritis, mental retardation	T, B, Ph	++++ (1 case)

Frequency of ID: +, less than 5% of reported cases with documented ID; ++, 5%–30%; +++, 30%–65%; ++++, >65%.
AD = autosomal dominant; AR = autosomal recessive; B = B-cell defect; ID = immunodeficiency; NK = NK-cell defect; Ph = phagocyte defect; T = T-cell defect; XL = X linked.

expansion in a CCTG repeat in intron one of the *ZNF9* gene (Liquori et al., 2001). The gene contains zinc-finger domains and is broadly expressed, with the highest levels of expression in the cardiac and skeletal muscles.

The most common immunologic abnormality in affected patients is a reduction in IgG level (Wochner et al., 1966). Other classes of immunoglobulin are generally normal, although decreased IgA and IgM levels have been noted. Increased repeat length correlates with decreased serum IgG level, decreased total lymphocyte count, and low T-cell number (Nakamura et al., 1996). Susceptibility to infection is generally not increased (Suzumura et al., 1986).

Ritscher-Schinzel Syndrome (MIM 220210)

Ritscher-Schinzel syndrome, an autosomal recessive syndrome, is also termed the 3C syndrome because of associated cerebellar abnormalities (including Dandy-Walker–like malformation and posterior fossa anomalies), craniofacial anomalies, and cardiac defects (atrioventricular septal defects) (Kosaki et al., 1997; Ritscher et al., 1987). One sister died after unsuccessful cardiac surgery. Immune abnormalities were demonstrated in the surviving sister (Lauener et al., 1989). Total IgG level was low, especially the IgG2 and IgG4 subclasses. Antibodies to polysaccharide antigens were not detected, but those to protein antigens were normal.

Rambam-Hasharon Syndrome (Leukocyte Adhesion Deficiency Type II) (MIM 266265)

Rambam-Hasharon syndrome, an autosomal recessive condition, is characterized by severe mental retardation, microcephaly, seizures, cortical atrophy, short stature, and abnormal facial features (see Chapter 20). The patients lack the red blood cell marker H, which is known as the Bombay blood phenotype. Despite an increased number of neutrophils, there are recurrent infections. Neutrophil motility is greatly decreased, with normal phagocytic activity (Frydman et al., 1992). The leukocyte defect is due to lack of CD15 on the surface of the neutrophils. This anomaly is also termed *leukocyte adhesion deficiency* (LAD) type II because it affects binding of the leukocytes to other cells. Both CD15 and erythrocyte substance H are fucosylated, and other fucosylated carbohydrates have defective synthesis (Price et al., 1994). The defect has been localized to the de novo pathway of GDP-fucose biosynthesis (Karsan et al., 1998).

Dionisi Vici Syndrome (MIM 242840)

An autosomal recessive syndrome of agenesis of the corpus callosum, bilateral cataracts, seizures, cleft lip/palate, cerebellar hypoplasia, and cutaneous hypopigmentation was initially described in two brothers (Dionisi

Vici et al., 1988). They suffered from recurrent respiratory infections and chronic mucocutaneous candidiasis, and both died from pneumonia. Persistent leukopenia was present in one of the brothers. Autopsy showed hypoplasia of the thymus and depletion of T-dependent areas of lymph nodes. CD4[+] T-cell number was decreased, and delayed-type hypersensitivity responses were absent. Serum IgG2 was selectively decreased. Four patients from three kindreds with agenesis of the corpus callosum, oculocutaneous albinism, and severe developmental delay also had recurrent viral, bacterial, and fungal infections (del Campo et al., 1999). The immunodeficiency was variable and included decreased T-cell number and response to mitogen.

Høyeraal-Hreidarsson Syndrome (MIM 300240)

X-linked cerebellar hypoplasia, psychomotor retardation, microcephaly, growth failure, and progressive pancytopenia have been reported in several affected males. Decreased IgG (Høyeraal et al., 1970) and death from candidal sepsis (Hreidarsson et al., 1988) have been described. Another patient with pancytopenia, severe T- and B-cell lymphopenia, hypogammaglobulinemia, and impaired lymphoproliferative responses to antigens died from *Aspergillus* sepsis (Berthet et al., 1994). Pancytopenia and SCID were described in two kindreds in which affected boys were found to have a missense mutation in the *DKC1* gene, which is associated with dyskeratosis congenita (Knight et al., 1999). Another affected patient with brittle scalp hair and nail dystrophy also had a missense mutation in the *DKC1* gene (Yaghmai et al., 2000).

Cohen Syndrome (MIM 216550)

Cohen syndrome features hypotonia, microcephaly, mental retardation, short stature, obesity, and characteristic facies with prominent upper central incisors. Neutropenia is mild to moderate, intermittent, and not generally associated with severe infection, although gingivitis, periodontitis, and cutaneous infections are common (Alaluusua et al., 1997; Kivitie-Kallio et al., 1997). Greatly increased neutrophil adhesive capability consistent with generalized neutrophil activation and granulocytopenia has been demonstrated (Olivieri et al., 1998).

Microcephaly with Immune Defects (MIM 251240)

Two brothers with microcephaly, facial dysmorphism, hypogonadism, scoliosis, hypoplastic patellae, postnatal growth retardation, and developmental delay suffered from recurrent respiratory infections and eczema (Say et al., 1986). Findings consistent with multiple epiphyseal dysplasia, scoliosis, and retinal pigmentation were noted during the teenage years (Carpenter et al., 2000). B-cell number and immunoglobulin levels were transiently decreased in early childhood. Subsequently, the patients displayed decreased IgG2 and/or IgG4 levels. Defective neutrophil chemotaxis was persistent.

Mousa Syndrome (MIM 271320)

Autosomal recessive spastic ataxia with cerebellar degeneration, cataracts, macular corneal dystrophy, and myopia were described in 22 individuals from a consanguineous Bedouin family (Mousa et al., 1986). Immunoglobulin levels were variably depressed in 12 individuals. Antithyroid antibodies were present in four persons. Recurrent infections were not a feature.

Aguilar Syndrome (MIM 226850)

Epilepsy, telangiectasia of palpebral conjunctivae, and mental retardation were reported in six of seven siblings in a Mexican family (Aguilar et al., 1978). The patients also had a long philtrum and anteverted nostrils. Five of six affected individuals had decreased serum IgA levels. There was no history of recurrent infection.

Adderson Syndrome

Two unrelated children had intracranial calcifications, growth failure, and acquired pancytopenia (Adderson et al., 2000). The patients also had developmental delay and one had hydrocephalus. They had greatly decreased immunoglobulin-bearing B-cell numbers and hypogammaglobulinemia.

Krawinkel Syndrome

A boy with lissencephaly, spastic tetraplegia, transient arthritis, and psychomotor retardation suffered from recurrent bacterial and mycotic infections (Krawinkel et al., 1989). Serum immunoglobulin levels were normal, but there was no specific antibody to tetanus toxoid. Initially, T-cell proliferation was reduced in response to phytohemagglutinin or allogeneic cells, and delayed-type hypersensitivity response was absent. No germinal centers were found on lymph node biopsy.

SYNDROMES ASSOCIATED WITH HEMATOLOGIC DYSFUNCTION

Some conditions with immunodeficiency may also feature hematologic abnormalities leading to bone marrow failure, neutropenia, anemia, and/or thrombocytopenia (Table 24-6). We also discuss in this section two important genetic causes of secondary immunodeficiency: sickle cell disease and β-thalassemia major.

TABLE 24-6 · SYNDROMES ASSOCIATED WITH HEMATOLOGIC DYSFUNCTION

Name	Inheritance (Chromosome)	Associated Features	Immune Defect	Frequency of ID
1. Sickle cell disease	AR (11p15)	Sickled erythrocytes, anemia, vascular occlusion; valine for glutamic acid substitution in β-hemoglobin	T, B	++
2. β-Thalassemia major	AR (11p15)	Hypochromic anemia, major form has severe anemia, requires transfusions	B	++
3. Wiskott-Aldrich syndrome	XL (Xp11)	Severe eczematous dermatitis, thrombocytopenia, bloody diarrhea, recurrent infection	T, B	++++
4. Chédiak-Higashi syndrome	AR (1q42)	Partial albinism, leukopenia, neuropathy, giant cytoplasmic granules in leukocytes	Ph, NK	++++
5. Omenn syndrome	AR (11p13)	Erythematous dermatitis, eosinophilia, lymphadenopathy, hemophagocytosis	T, B	++++
6. Shwachman syndrome	AR	Metaphyseal dysplasia, exocrine pancreatic insufficiency, cyclic neutropenia	B, Ph	++++
7. Pearson syndrome	Mito	Exocrine pancreatic deficiency, pancytopenia	Ph	++++
8. WHIM syndrome	AD	Warts, hypogammaglobulinemia, infection, myelokathexis	B, Ph	++++
9. IPEX syndrome	XL (Xp11)	Intractable diarrhea, polyendocrinopathy, neonatal diabetes mellitus, hemolytic anemia	T, B	++++
10. Transcobalamin II deficiency	AR (22q12-q13)	Transport protein for B12; severe megaloblastic anemia, leukopenia, thrombocytopenia	B	++
11. Glutathione synthetase deficiency	AR (20q11)	Hemolytic anemia, acidosis, neutropenia; decreased bactericidal activity, failure to assemble microtubules	Ph	+
12. Folic acid malabsorption (transport defect)	AR	Megaloblastic anemia, convulsions, movement disorder	T, B	++

Frequency of ID: +, less than 5% of reported cases with documented ID; ++, 5%–30%; +++, 30%–65%; ++++, >65%.
AD = autosomal dominant; AR = autosomal recessive; B = B-cell defect; ID = immunodeficiency; Mito = mitochondrial; NK = NK-cell defect; Ph = phagocyte defect; T = T-cell defect; XL = X linked.

Sickle Cell Disease (MIM 603903)

Sickle cell disease is the most common lethal autosomal recessive condition among African populations. It is caused by a point mutation leading to the amino acid substitution of valine for glutamic acid. Sickling disorders include sickle cell trait (heterozygous hemoglobin AS), sickle cell disease (SS), and compound heterozygotes with other ß globin chain variants such as hemoglobin C or D or ß-thalassemia. Individuals with sickle cell trait have a protective advantage against *Plasmodium falciparum* malaria. In certain regions of Africa, the frequency of HbS may be up to 24% at birth (Fleming et al., 1979). In the United States, the frequency of HbAS at birth is approximately 8%, with the expected incidence of sickle cell disease at 1 per 625 live births (Motulsky, 1973).

Infectious Susceptibility

There is an increased susceptibility to septicemia and meningitis (Overturf et al., 1977), including *Streptococcus pneumoniae*, *Escherichia coli*, *Haemophilus influenzae*, and *Salmonella*. Infection is a common reason for hospitalization and can result in sickle cell crises or death (Barrett-Connor, 1971). The relative risk of pneumococcal meningitis is more than 500-fold that of the general population (Barrett-Connor, 1971). The risk of infection in sickle cell disease variants, such as hemoglobin SC disease, is higher than in the normal population but considerably less than that present in individuals with homozygous sickle cell disease (Serjeant and Serjeant, 1993).

Septicemia with gram-negative enteric organisms is more common in the second decade (Overturf et al., 1977). *Salmonella* infections are a particularly important cause of osteomyelitis, which may result from infection of infarcted bone.

There is generally a good immune response to parvovirus B19, which can be associated with transient aplastic crisis. Patients with sickle cell disease do form antibodies and clear the virus, even if aplastic crisis has occurred (Rao et al., 1992).

Splenic Function

Patients with sickle cell disease often have progressive fibrosis and reduced size of the spleen. Splenic hypofunction may be due to sickling of the red blood cells, increased blood viscosity, vascular obstruction, infarction, and decreased blood flow (Usami et al., 1975). Splenic hypofunction may affect B-cell maturation. Assessment of splenic function can be made by counting of pitted erythrocytes or by clearance of autologous heat-damaged 99m-technicium–labeled erythrocytes from the circulation into the spleen (Zago and Bottura, 1983) (see Chapter 30).

Humoral Function

Total B-cell number is normal or increased (Wang et al., 1985). IgG levels may be increased (Ballas et al., 1980). IgM levels are often normal or may be decreased (Ballas et al., 1980; Boghossian et al., 1985). Many patients with sickle cell disease do not generate an adequate antibody response following immunization for *S. pneumoniae* or *H. influenzae* type b (Frank et al., 1988). Immunoglobulin synthesis in response to both mitogen and antigen may be decreased (Rautonen et al., 1992). B-cell proliferation was also decreased.

Cellular Function

The overall number of peripheral blood lymphocytes is generally increased, with a decreased percentage of T cells (Ballester et al., 1986). The absolute number of T cells is normal. CD4 helper T-cell proportion is either normal or may be decreased (Ades et al., 1980; Hernandez et al., 1980).

Complement

Defective serum opsonization activity has been noted (Bjornson et al., 1985; Winkelstein and Drachman, 1968). This was found to be due to reduction of opsonization by the alternative complement pathway (Johnston et al., 1973). It has been proposed that the decreased opsonization was due to consumption of some of the complement components, such as C3, by increased activation of the alternative pathway (Chudwin et al., 1985; Wilson, 1983). Alternatively, the defect may be due to decreased specific antibody levels (Bjornson and Lobel, 1987). However, other investigators have not found defects in complement activation (Bjornson et al., 1977; Boghossian et al., 1985).

Management

Early identification of patients with sickle cell disease through newborn screening has led to improved clinical management. Penicillin prophylaxis should be initiated by 2 months of age or at the time of diagnosis, if after 2 months, for patients with HbSS and sickle-ß-thalassemia disease (American Academy of Pediatrics, 2002). Because fetal hemoglobin synthesis generally stops after 4 months, it is important to start antibiotic prophylaxis before that time. A routine immunization schedule, including *H. influenzae* type b and hepatitis B immunization, should be followed. The American Academy of Pediatrics (2002) recommends that 7-valent pneumococcal conjugate vaccine be administered beginning at 2 months of age as per routine, and the 23-valent pneumococcal polysaccharide vaccine at 2 and 5 years of age. Influenza vaccine should be administered annually for children 6 months of age and older. The American Academy of Pediatrics also recommends that penicillin prophylaxis be continued at least until 5 years of age. After that time, the decision to continue penicillin prophylaxis should be based on the specific clinical history of the patient (Bjornson et al., 1996).

Thalassemia

β-Thalassemia major (MIM 141900) is characterized by a hypochromic anemia resulting from a defect in the β chain of hemoglobin. The major form requires transfusions of packed erythrocytes. Patients with β-thalassemia major and other severe forms of thalassemia have an increased risk of infection. Affected patients may require splenectomy for hypersplenism. Following splenectomy, the patients have an increased risk for pneumococcal sepsis. Thus penicillin prophylaxis and pneumococcal vaccine are indicated for these patients. Defects in the alternative pathway of complement have also been noted.

Other Hematologic Disorders

Wiskott-Aldrich Syndrome (MIM 301000)

Wiskott-Aldrich syndrome, a well-defined X-linked primary immunodeficiency disorder, is characterized by chronic eczema, thrombocytopenia (with small, defective platelets), and bloody diarrhea (see Chapter 17). Recurrent and life-threatening infections are a leading cause of death (Sullivan et al., 1994). Abnormal humoral immune responses are typical. The disease phenotype ranges from mostly thrombocytopenia to mild or severe forms of the disease (Villa et al., 1995). A novel gene expressed only in lymphocytic and megakaryocytic lineages, termed WAS, is mutated in Wiskott-Aldrich patients (Derry et al., 1994). Inactivating mutations in WAS have also been detected in isolated X-linked thrombocytopenia (Villa et al., 1995), whereas mutations resulting in constitutive activation have been detected in X-linked congenital neutropenia (Devriendt et al., 2001).

Chédiak-Higashi Syndrome (MIM 214500)

Chédiak-Higashi syndrome is a well-defined autosomal recessive primary immunodeficiency disorder that presents with recurrent bacterial infections (especially with S. aureus and streptococci), partial oculocutaneous albinism, prolonged bleeding time, nystagmus, and neuropathy (see Chapters 17 and 20). Most patients eventually develop a distinctive lymphoproliferative disorder characterized by generalized lymphohistiocytic infiltrates, which are difficult to treat. The defective gene, CHS1, may code for a protein involved in endosomal trafficking (Nagle et al., 1996).

Omenn Syndrome (MIM 267700)

Omenn disease is an autosomal recessive form of familial histiocytic reticulocytosis that presents with an erythematous skin rash, eosinophilia, reticulosis, hepatosplenomegaly, protracted diarrhea, alopecia, and lymphadenopathy (see Chapter 15). It has also been termed familial hemophagocytic lymphohistiocytosis. A characteristic SCID leads to failure to thrive, recurrent infection, and premature death. Although discussed previously in the context of short-limbed skeletal dysplasia, it most commonly occurs without associated skeletal anomalies. The immunologic derangements are quite variable and may include abnormal T-cell number and function and greatly elevated IgE. Mutations in genes encoding either of two lymphoid specific proteins, RAG-1 or RAG-2, cause SCID and Omenn syndrome (Villa et al., 1998). These two proteins interact and play a role in V(D)J recombination.

Shwachman Syndrome (MIM 260400)

Shwachman syndrome is autosomal recessive and presents with pancreatic insufficiency, neutropenia, and metaphyseal dysostosis resulting in short stature (see Chapter 20). The patients have a predisposition to hematologic malignancy. Neutropenia (which may be intermittent or cyclic) occurs in 88%, and leukopenia and/or pancytopenia may arise (Mack et al., 1996; Smith et al., 1996).

Pearson Syndrome (MIM 557000)

Pearson syndrome is a mitochondrial disorder that features exocrine pancreas dysfunction and bone marrow failure resulting in anemia, thrombocytopenia, and neutropenia. Mitochondrial DNA deletions have been detected (Rotig et al., 1991, 1995), and they are flanked by short repeats that may promote intramolecular recombinations, deletions, or duplications in human mitochondrial DNA. Surviving patients progress to clinical Kearns-Sayre syndrome, which shows the same mitochondrial DNA changes as in Pearson syndrome (Casademont et al., 1994; Poulton et al., 1994).

WHIM Syndrome (MIM 193670)

WHIM syndrome is a disorder consisting of multiple warts, hypogammaglobulinemia, infection, and myelokathexis (bone marrow retention of neutrophils) (Wetzler et al., 1990) (see Chapters 17 and 20). Neutrophil function is normal, but the count is reduced and they are hypersegmented. B-cell number and IgG and IgA levels were mildly decreased. Depressed T-cell number and diminished response to mitogen and skin tests have been noted. A three-generation pedigree was described with neutropenia, hypogammaglobulinemia, and warts (Gorlin et al., 2000).

IPEX Syndrome (MIM 304930)

The name of this condition—IPEX syndrome—is an acronym for immunodeficiency, polyendocrinopathy, and enteropathy, X-linked (see Chapter 17). It is generally lethal in infancy and is marked by intractable diarrhea with extensive villous atrophy, polyendocrinopathy (neonatal diabetes mellitus, autoimmune hypothyroidism), and hemolytic anemia (Peake et al., 1996;

Powell et al., 1982). Death is often secondary to infection or following immunization with live viral agents. IgE levels are greatly elevated, and there may be intermittent eosinophilia. Other features of immunodeficiency are variable. Mutations in the gene *FOXP3* have been identified in IPEX patients (Bennett et al., 2001; Wildin et al., 2001). FOXP3 is a member of the winged helix/forkhead transcription factor family. The mutant *FoxP3* mouse is termed the scurfy mouse and has many of the features of the human condition (Wildin et al., 2001). Mouse scurfy T cells are hyperresponsive to activation via the T-cell receptor and are less sensitive to cyclosporin A and inhibitors of tyrosine kinases (Clark et al., 1999).

Transcobalamin II Deficiency (MIM 275350)

Deficiency of transcobalamin II, the molecule responsible for intestinal absorption of cobalamin and transport to tissues, leads to severe megaloblastic anemia, failure to thrive, diarrhea, vomiting, and lethargy (see Chapter 13). Hypogammaglobulinemia (most frequently affecting IgG) (Hitzig et al., 1974; Kaikov et al., 1991) and failure to produce specific antibody to diphtheria or polio can occur. Although phagocytic killing is usually normal, a specific impairment of neutrophils against *S. aureus* has been reported (Seger et al., 1980). Clinical manifestations and immunologic abnormalities resolve after cobalamin supplementation.

Glutathione Synthetase Deficiency (MIM 266130)

Glutathione synthetase deficiency causes severe metabolic acidosis and hemolytic anemia. Glutathione eliminates hydrogen peroxide and protects the cell from oxidative damage. After particle ingestion by phagocytes, excess hydrogen peroxide accumulates, and bacterial killing is impaired (Spielberg et al., 1979). The neutrophils show normal phagocytosis and chemotaxis. Neutrophils fail to assemble microtubules during phagocytosis and damage to membranous structures subsequently occurs. The susceptibility to recurrent infection is relatively mild. Supplementation with the oxidant scavenger vitamin E can restore immunologic function (Boxer et al., 1979).

Folic Acid Malabsorption (MIM 229050)

Deficiency in intestinal folic acid absorption leads to megaloblastic anemia, ataxia, mental retardation, and seizures. Folic acid supplementation is corrective. Recurrent infections are an occasional feature. Humoral defects are variable and may include decreased IgM, IgG, and/or IgA (Corbeel et al., 1985; Malatack et al., 1999; Urbach et al., 1987). Cellular defects have included decreased response to phytohemagglutinin or to tetanus (Malatack et al., 1999; Urbach et al., 1987).

TABLE 24-7 · INBORN ERRORS OF METABOLISM ASSOCIATED WITH IMMUNODEFICIENCY

Name	Inheritance (Chromosome)	Associated Features	Immune Defect	Frequency of ID
1. Adenosine deaminase deficiency	AR (20q13)	Severe immunodeficiency, cupping and flaring of costochondral junctions	T, B	++++
2. Purine nucleoside phosphorylase deficiency	AR (14q13)	Severe immunodeficiency, neurological findings, hemolytic anemia	T	++++
3. 5'-nucleotidase elevation	?	Increased nucleotide catabolism, developmental delay, seizures, megaloblastic anemia, aggressive behavior	B	++++ (1 case)
4. Glycogen storage disease Ib/Ic	AR (11q23)	Hypoglycemia, glucose-6-phosphate transport defect	Ph	+++
5. Galactosemia	AR (9p13, 17q24)	Hepatomegaly, hypoglycemia, jaundice, feeding difficulties	Ph	+
6. Barth syndrome	XL (Xq28)	Endocardial fibroelastosis, myopathy, abnormal mitochondria, 3-methylglutaconicaciduria	Ph	++++
7. Methylmalonic aciduria	AR (6p21)	Acidosis, recurrent severe infection	T, B, Ph	+++
8. Propionic acidemia	AR (13q32)	Acidosis, vomiting, ketosis	B, Ph	+++
9. Isovaleric acidemia	AR (15q14-q15)	Acidosis, urinary odor of sweaty socks	Ph	++
10. Lysinuric protein intolerance	AR (14q11)	Dibasic aminoaciduria, hepatomegaly, failure to thrive	T, Ph, NK	+++
11. Orotic aciduria	AR (3q13)	Megaloblastic anemia, severe infection	T	++
12. Alpha-mannosidosis	AR (19cen-q12)	Hepatosplenomegaly, psychomotor retardation, dysostosis multiplex	T, B, Ph	++
13. Biotinidase deficiency	AR (3p25)	Alopecia, developmental delay, hypotonia, seizures; multiple carboxylase deficiency	T, B	+

Frequency of ID: +, less than 5% of reported cases with documented ID; ++, 5%–30%; +++, 30%–65%; ++++, >65%.
AR = autosomal recessive; B = B-cell defect; ID = immunodeficiency; NK = NK-cell defect; Ph = phagocyte defect; T = T-cell defect; XL = X linked.

INBORN ERRORS OF METABOLISM ASSOCIATED WITH IMMUNODEFICIENCY

Several metabolic defects are associated with immunodeficiency (Table 24-7). For most of these syndromes, it is unknown whether the immunologic deficit is due to block of a metabolic process important for immune function or whether the buildup of toxic metabolites adversely affects the cells. Alternatively, a nonspecific deleterious effect on cell proliferation would also affect immune cells. Most of the immunologic abnormalities appear to be secondary to the metabolic derangement, because correction of the metabolic defect usually results in normal immune function.

Adenosine Deaminase (ADA) Deficiency (MIM 102700)

ADA deficiency is a well-characterized metabolic defect associated with immunodeficiency and is the most common single genetic cause of autosomal recessive SCID (Hirschhorn, 1993) (see Chapter 16). The enzyme converts adenosine and deoxyadenosine to inosine and deoxyinosine, and their accumulation may lead to lymphocyte toxicity. The skeletal system is affected in a majority of patients, and manifestations include cupping and flaring of the costochondral junctions, platyspondylisis, thick growth arrest lines, and an abnormal bony pelvis.

Purine Nucleoside Phosphorylase (PNP) Deficiency (MIM 164050)

PNP is required for normal catabolism of purines. Enzyme substrates accumulate, principally affecting the immune and nervous systems. Cell-mediated immunity is defective. Abnormal motor development, including ataxia and spasticity, may occur (see Chapter 16). Patients may develop autoantibodies and autoimmune hemolytic anemia (Carapella-de Luca et al., 1978). Viral and fungal infections frequently arise. T-cell number and function are greatly decreased.

5′-Nucleotidase Elevation

A 3-year-old girl with recurrent sinusitis, developmental delay, seizures, megaloblastic anemia, ataxia, alopecia, and overly aggressive behavior was found to have increased catabolism of purine and pyrimidine nucleotides (Page et al., 1991). 5′-Nucleotidase activity was increased. Folic acid and B_{12} levels were normal. IgG level was low to borderline. It is unknown if the increased nucleotidase activity is primary or is in response to abnormal amounts of a nucleotide. Pyrimidine nucleotide supplementation resulted in improvement in clinical symptoms and behavior.

Glycogen Storage Disease (GSD) Ib/Ic (MIM 232220, 232240)

GSD Ib and Ic are marked by hypoglycemia and are due to a defect in the hepatic microsomal translocase for glucose-6-phosphate (see Chapter 20). Severe neutropenia was noted at some point in 87% of patients with GSD Ib (Visser et al., 2000) and is also frequently found in GSD Ic (Visser et al., 1998). Neutrophil function is variable, although random movement, chemotaxis, microbial killing, and respiratory burst are frequently diminished (Gitzelmann and Bosshard, 1993). Inflammatory bowel disease, oral lesions, and perianal abscesses occur with increased frequency and are most likely due to defective neutrophil function. Mutations in the glucose-6-phosphate translocase gene have been identified in both GSD Ib and Ic (Gerin et al., 1997; Veiga-da-Cunha et al., 1998).

Galactosemia (MIM 230400)

A defect in galactose-1-phosphate uridyl transferase results in galactosemia and presents with jaundice, hepatomegaly, cataracts, developmental delay, and feeding difficulties. It is part of the newborn screening panel in many states. The incidence in the United States is estimated at 1:50,000 (DeClue et al., 1991; Suzuki et al., 2001). These patients are at increased risk for fatal sepsis from *E. coli* in the neonatal period (Levy et al., 1977). Granulocyte chemotaxis is impaired, whereas bactericidal activity is usually normal. In vitro exposure of neutrophils to galactose also results in impaired function, especially in neonates (Kobayashi et al., 1983). Galactosemia may rarely be due to galactokinase deficiency. One affected individual suffered from recurrent bacterial infections and had deficiency of the complement component C2 and decreased neutrophil chemotaxis and bactericidal activity (Borzy et al., 1984).

Barth Syndrome (MIM 302060)

Barth syndrome, an X-linked condition, is characterized by short stature, cardiac and skeletal myopathy, endocardial fibroelastosis, and structural mitochondrial anomalies (Barth et al., 1999). Urinary 3-methylglutaconate and 3-methylglutarate are increased (Kelley et al., 1991). Neutropenia is often persistent and can lead to serious infections. The defective gene, *G4.5*, codes for a tafazzin and may play a role in acyltransferase activity (Barth et al., 1999; Bione et al., 1996).

Branched-Chain Amino Acidurias

Three diseases affecting branched-chain amino acid metabolism have been associated with leukopenia: *methylmalonic acidemia* (MMA) (MIM 251000), *propionic acidemia* (PA) (MIM 232000), and *isovaleric acidemia* (IVA) (MIM 243500). The conditions present with metabolic acidosis, lethargy, failure to thrive, and recurrent vomiting. Mental retardation generally occurs. These individuals are at increased risk for infection, which may precipitate episodes of acidosis. Leukopenia occurs in 60% of MMA patients (Matsui et al., 1983). The immune defect associated with MMA is variable, including neutropenia and pancytopenia; decreased B- and T-cell number; low IgG level; and impaired phagocyte chemotaxis (Church et al., 1984; Wong et al., 1992). Methylmalonic acid inhibits bone marrow stem cell growth in vitro (Inoue et al., 1981). Patients with PA may have neutropenia (Muller et al., 1980) or decreased IgG and IgM and B-cell number (Raby et al., 1994) during periods of metabolic acidosis. In IVA, neutropenia and pancytopenia can occur during periods of acidosis, and neonatal death from sepsis can result (Kelleher et al., 1980). The bone marrow contains large numbers of immature cells, suggesting an arrest of maturation.

Lysinuric Protein Intolerance (MIM 222700)

Lysinuric protein intolerance is marked by defective transport of the dibasic amino acids lysine, arginine, and ornithine in the intestine and renal tubules, leading to decreased levels of these substances in the blood, hyperammonemia, protein intolerance, and failure to thrive. Decreases in CD4 T-cell number (Dionisi-Vici et al., 1998), lymphopenia (Nagata et al., 1987), IgG subclass deficiency and poor humoral response to vaccination (Lukkarinen et al., 1999), and leukopenia with decreased leukocyte phagocytic activity (Yoshida et al., 1995) have been reported. Varicella infection may be severe (Lukkarinen et al., 1998). Intravenous immunoglobulin therapy has been used (Dionisi-Vici et al., 1998). Treatment of a 10-year-old boy with high-dose intravenous immunoglobulin (1 g/kg) resulted in improvement (but not normalization) of CD4 T-cell number and resolution of associated anemia and cutaneous lesions (Dionisi-Vici et al., 1998).

Orotic Aciduria (MIM 258900)

Orotic aciduria is an error of pyrimidine metabolism manifested by retarded growth and development and megaloblastic anemia unresponsive to vitamin B_{12} and folic acid. Musculoskeletal abnormalities, strabismus, and congenital heart disease can be associated. Several affected patients had lymphopenia and increased susceptibility to infection, including candidiasis, fatal varicella, and meningitis. Immune findings are variable and include low T-cell number, impaired delayed-type hypersensitivity response, reduced T-cell–mediated killing, and decreased IgG and IgA (Alvarado et al., 1988; Girot et al., 1983). Other patients have normal immune function (Becroft et al., 1984). The defective enzyme is uridine monophosphate synthase.

Alpha-Mannosidosis (MIM 248500)

Mannosidosis, a lysosomal storage disease, is characterized by psychomotor retardation, dysostosis multiplex, hepatosplenomegaly, and lenticular opacification. Mannose-rich oligosaccharides accumulate in neural and visceral tissues. Most patients have recurrent infections. Decreased serum IgG and impaired lymphoproliferation to phytohemagglutinin have been noted (Desnick et al., 1976). Defective chemotaxis, phagocytosis, and bactericidal killing occur, whereas nitro-blue tetrazolium reduction is normal. Accumulation of mannose-rich molecules may interfere with leukocyte plasma membrane-mediated processes. Pancytopenia was reported in association with antineutrophil antibodies (Press et al., 1983).

Biotinidase Deficiency (MIM 253260)

Biotinidase deficiency results in multiple carboxylase deficiency because biotin is a required cofactor for several carboxylases (see Chapter 17). Symptoms include lactic acidosis, hypotonia, developmental delay, seizures, dermatitis, and alopecia. Biotin supplementation corrects the defects. Two siblings with mucocutaneous candidiasis and keratoconjunctivitis had absent skin test responses (Cowan et al., 1979). One had decreased IgA and poor antibody formation to pneumococcal vaccine.

MISCELLANEOUS GENETIC SYNDROMES ASSOCIATED WITH IMMUNODEFICIENCY

The immunodeficiencies discussed in this section are associated with extraimmune features not addressed previously (Table 24-8).

Thymic-Renal-Anal-Lung Dysplasia (MIM 274265)

Three sisters with an absent or unilobed thymus, renal agenesis/dysgenesis, and prenatal growth failure were reported (Rudd et al., 1990). Cysts and dysplasia of the kidney were noted. No parathyroid tissue was identified. Two also had a unilobed lung (one with gut malrotation) and imperforate anus.

Hisama Syndrome

Three brothers with renal tubular dysgenesis, absent nipples, and nail anomalies were reported (Hisama et al., 1998). One had an absent thymus. Accessory spleens, a pulmonary lobation defect, and imperforate anus were also noted among the three siblings. All three died in the neonatal period.

TABLE 24-8 · MISCELLANEOUS GENETIC SYNDROMES ASSOCIATED WITH IMMUNODEFICIENCY

Name	Inheritance (Chromosome)	Associated Features	Immune Defect	Frequency of ID
1. Thymic-renal-anal-lung dysplasia	?AR	Hypoplastic thymus, renal dysgenesis, growth failure, unilobed lung, imperforate anus	T	++++ (3 sisters)
2. Hisama syndrome	?AR/XL	Renal tubular dysgenesis, absent nipples, nail anomalies	T	++++ (3 brothers)
3. Frenkel-Russe syndrome	?AR	Retinal telangiectasias, recurrent infections	T, B	++++ (2 siblings)
4. Asplenia syndrome	AR, ?XL	Asplenia, complex congenital heart disease, laterality defect	T	++
5. Lichtenstein syndrome	?	Osteoporosis, bony anomalies, lung cysts, neutropenia; monozygotic female twins	B, Ph	++++ (2 twins)
6. Hypercatabolic hypoproteinemia	AR	Chemical diabetes, shortened ulnae/bowed radii, hypogammaglobulinemia	B	++++ (2 siblings)
7. Schaller syndrome	?	Autoimmune hemolytic anemia, glomerulonephritis	B	++++ (1 kindred)
8. Turner-like phenotype with immunodeficiency	?	Anemia, neutropenia, webbed neck, short stature	B, Ph	++++ (1 case)

Frequency of ID: +, less than 5% of reported cases with documented ID; ++, 5%–30%; +++, 30%–65%; ++++, >65%.
AR = autosomal recessive; B = B-cell defect; ID = immunodeficiency; NK = NK-cell defect; Ph = phagocyte defect; T = T-cell defect; XL = X linked.

Frenkel-Russe Syndrome (MIM 267900)

A 13-year-old boy with retinal telangiectasias had meningitis and recurrent respiratory infections (Frenkel and Russe, 1967). IgG was decreased, and IgA and IgM were undetectable. Delayed-type hypersensitivity response was absent. Bone marrow aspirate showed no plasma cells. His sister had less extensive telangiectasias and showed impaired delayed-type hypersensitivity response.

Asplenia Syndrome (MIM 208530)

Asplenia may be accompanied by complex congenital heart disease and laterality defects affecting the position of thoracic and/or abdominal viscera (see Chapter 30). Severe bacterial infections often occur. In 13 children with asplenia, the average percentage of CD3 cells was decreased (54%, vs. 70% in controls with congenital heart disease), and the CD4/CD8 ratio was abnormal (1.1 vs. 1.9 in controls), largely resulting from decreased CD4 cell number (Wang and Hsieh, 1991). Proliferative responses to concanavalin A, phytohemagglutinin, and pokeweed mitogen were diminished. Immunoglobulin levels were normal.

Lichtenstein Syndrome (MIM 246550)

Monozygotic twins with facial anomalies (carp mouth, anteverted nostrils, synophrys), bony anomalies (osteoporosis of the long bones, failure of fusion of posterior spinal arches, subluxation of C1 on C2, spondylolysis of L5 on S1), and giant lung cysts were described (Lichtenstein, 1972). Neutrophil counts were frequently depressed, and the children suffered from recurrent infections. IgG and IgM levels were normal, and IgA

was deficient. Bone marrow was hypocellular with a decrease in myeloid precursors.

Hypercatabolic Hypoproteinemia (MIM 241600)

Two siblings of a first cousin marriage manifested hypoproteinemia, chemical diabetes, shortened ulnae, and bowed radii (Waldmann and Terry, 1990). Total circulating and body pools of IgG were less than 28% of normal, resulting from a fivefold increase in IgG catabolic rate, leading to decreased IgG survival. IgG synthetic rates were normal. Albumin levels were also reduced because of increased albumin catabolism. There was no evidence of anti-IgG autoantibodies, proteinuria, liver dysfunction, or gastrointestinal losses. One of the patients also had increased breakdown of IgA, but serum IgA level was normal because of an increased IgA synthetic rate.

Schaller Syndrome (MIM 247800)

A female infant with lymphopenia, autoimmune hemolytic anemia, and glomerulonephritis died from *Pneumocystis carinii* pneumonia (Schaller et al., 1966). Two siblings had also died of infection by 6 months of age. Specific antibody and isohemagglutinin titers were undetectable. Lymph nodes were hypoplastic, and the thymus lacked lymphoid elements and Hassall's corpuscles.

Turner-Like Phenotype

Immunodeficiency was found in a female patient with webbed neck and Turner-like phenotype with a normal karyotype (Feldman et al., 1976). The authors stated that the patient had features distinct from Noonan syndrome. The patient had recurrent hypoplastic anemia and intermittent neutropenia. Specific antibody production was decreased. B- and T-cell numbers, proliferative responses to mitogens and allogeneic cells, and delayed-type hypersensitivity response were normal.

WELL-RECOGNIZED SYNDROMES WITH IMMUNODEFICIENCY AS AN OCCASIONAL FEATURE

Immunodeficiency has been identified in a small number of patients in several well-established malformation syndromes (Table 24-9). Frequent sinopulmonary infections occur in many of the conditions, but whether this is due to anatomic and facial anomalies or to true immune defects is unclear. Generally, an increased susceptibility to serious infection is not a frequent feature in these syndromes, and immune status has been investigated in only a few patients. It is unclear if the rare reports of immunodeficiency are coincidental co-occurrences of two rare conditions or if immune defects actually do occur with some frequency in affected individuals. If immunologic studies were conducted on additional patients, the prevalence of detected immunodeficiency might increase. For some of the conditions,

normal immune status has been documented in some children. A contiguous gene deletion extending beyond the area necessary to produce the features of the syndrome could result in additional genetic defects, resulting in immunodeficiency.

Decreased T- and B-cell number has been described in *Schwartz-Jampel syndrome* (Mollica et al., 1979). Thymic hypoplasia and defective T-cell function has been noted in *Beckwith-Wiedemann syndrome* (Greene et al., 1973; Thorburn et al., 1970) and *Zellweger syndrome* (Hong et al., 1981). A hypoplastic thymus and reduced T cells in secondary lymphatic origin was described in a patient with the *ectrodactyly-ectodermal dysplasia-cleft lip/palate syndrome with urinary tract anomalies (EECUT)* (Frick et al., 1997). Impaired T-cell function has been described in *Menkes syndrome* (Pedroni et al., 1975) and *pseudoachondroplasia* (Kultursay et al., 1988). Hypogammaglobulinemia has been described in *Hallerman-Streiff syndrome* (Chandra et al., 1978). Monocyte dysfunction has been seen in *Smith-Lemli-Opitz syndrome* (Ostergaard et al., 1992). A combined immunodeficiency was present in *Hutchinson-Gilford syndrome* (Harjacek et al., 1990). Pancytopenia and hypogammaglobulinemia have been noted in *Seckel syndrome* (Lilleyman, 1984). Progressive diaphyseal dysplasia *(Engelmann syndrome)* is occasionally associated with leukopenia (Crisp and Brenton, 1982). Neutropenia was described in two cousins with

TABLE 24-9 · WELL-RECOGNIZED SYNDROMES WITH IMMUNODEFICIENCY AS AN OCCASIONAL FEATURE

Name	Inheritance (Chromosome)	Associated Features	Immune Defect	Frequency of ID
1. Schwartz-Jampel syndrome	AR (1p36-p34)	Myotonia, myopia, blepharophimosis, short stature, joint contractures	T, B	+
2. Beckwith-Wiedemann syndrome	AD (11p15)	Macroglossia, exomphalos, gigantism	T	+
3. Zellweger syndrome	AR (various)	Hypotonia, flat facies with high forehead, renal and hepatic anomalies	T	+
4. Ectrodactyly-ectodermal dysplasia-clefting syndrome	AD	Ectrodactyly, ectodermal dysplasia, cleft lip/palate, renal/genitourinary anomalies	T	+
5. Menkes syndrome	XL (Xq12-q13)	Kinky hair, seizures, progressive neurological deterioration; due to copper deficiency	T	+
6. Pseudoachondroplasia	AD (19p13)	Short-limb short stature, spondyloepiphyseal dysplasia, normal craniofacial appearance	T, B	+
7. Hallermann-Streiff syndrome	?AD	Thin pinched nose, congenital cataracts, hypotrichosis, microphthalmia	B	+
8. Smith-Lemli-Opitz syndrome	AR (11q12-q13)	Mental retardation, cryptorchidism, partial syndactyly of 2nd/3rd toes; defect in cholesterol metabolism	Ph	+
9. Hutchinson-Gilford syndrome	?AD	Postnatal growth deficiency, alopecia, atrophy of subcutaneous fat, atherosclerosis	T, B	+
10. Seckel syndrome	AR (3q22-q24)	Bird-like facies, microcephaly, mental retardation	Ph	+
11. Engelmann syndrome	AD	Progressive diaphyseal dysplasia, leg pain, weakness	Ph	+
12. Wolfram syndrome	AR (4p16)	Diabetes insipidus, diabetes mellitus, optic atrophy, deafness	Ph	+
13. Proteus syndrome	?AD	Overgrowth, hemihypertrophy, subcutaneous tumors	B	+
14. Cowden syndrome	AD (10q23)	Multiple hamartomas of skin, gastrointestinal tract, thyroid, breast	T	+

Frequency of ID: +, less than 5% of reported cases with documented ID; ++, 5%–30%; +++, 30%–65%; ++++, >65%.
AD = autosomal dominant; AR = autosomal recessive; B = B-cell defect; ID = immunodeficiency; NK = NK-cell defect; Ph = phagocyte defect; T = T-cell defect; XL = X linked.

Wolfram syndrome (Borgna-Pignatti et al., 1989). Hypogammaglobulinemia and lymphopenia were reported in a patient with *Proteus syndrome* (Hodge et al., 2000). Abnormal T-cell number and function and decreased NK activity have been reported in *Cowden syndrome* (Guerin et al., 1989; Ruschak et al., 1981; Starink et al., 1986).

SYNDROMES ASSOCIATED WITH CHROMOSOME INSTABILITY AND/OR DEFECTIVE DNA REPAIR

Syndromes associated with chromosome instability often have immune abnormalities, and the patient is at increased risk for malignancy (Table 24-10). Spontaneous and induced chromosome breakage is often increased, and defective DNA repair may play a role. These conditions are discussed in detail in Chapter 18 and are addressed here only briefly.

Bloom Syndrome (MIM 210900)

Bloom syndrome is an autosomal recessive condition characterized by low birth weight, proportionate short stature, skin rashes resulting from hypersensitivity to sunlight, malar hypoplasia, and telangiectatic erythema of the face (see Chapter 18). Risk of neoplasia, especially leukemia, is greatly increased. Sister chromatid exchanges occur at an increased frequency and can aid in the diagnosis. In this respect, Bloom syndrome differs from other chromosome breakage syndromes, which usually feature nonhomologous chromosome exchanges. The frequency of exchange is not increased in heterozygotes. There is an increased susceptibility to infection, and immunologic defects may involve the humoral and cellular responses (Kondo et al., 1992). The product of the *BLM* gene encodes a RecQ DNA helicase (Ellis

et al., 1995) and may interact with topoisomerases or other proteins involved in DNA repair (Ellis and German, 1996).

Fanconi Pancytopenia (MIM 227650)

Fanconi pancytopenia, an autosomal recessive syndrome, is associated with hyperpigmentation of the skin, café au lait spots, radial hypoplasia, and a characteristic facial appearance (microphthalmia, micrognathia, broad nasal base, and epicanthal folds) (see Chapter 18). Short stature, microcephaly, renal and genital anomalies, and mental retardation may also occur. Single chromatid breaks and gaps and multiradials of the nonhomologous type are present. Increased sensitivity to the clastogenic agent diepoxybutane is useful for diagnosis and prenatal detection, although heterozygotes are not reliably detected (Joenje et al., 1997). Neutropenia secondary to bone marrow failure occurs in more than 95% of patients. T- and B-cell function are generally normal.

Eight complementation groups (A to H) have been identified (Joenje et al., 1997). The genes for complementation groups A (Fanconi Anaemia/Breast Cancer Consortium, 1996; Lo Ten Foe et al., 1996) and C (Strathdee et al., 1992) have been isolated, and mutations in these two genes account for 72% of patients with Fanconi pancytopenia. These two gene products (FAA, FAC) bind to form a nuclear protein complex (Kupfer et al., 1997), although their exact function remains unknown.

Ataxia-Telangiectasia (MIM 208900)

AT is an autosomal recessive condition marked by progressive cerebellar ataxia, telangiectasias (especially of the conjunctiva), and chromosome instability (see

TABLE 24-10 · SYNDROMES ASSOCIATED WITH CHROMOSOMAL INSTABILITY AND/OR DEFECTIVE DNA REPAIR

Name	Inheritance (Chromosome)	Associated Features	Immune Defect	Frequency of ID
1. Bloom syndrome	AR (15q26)	Short stature, telangiectatic erythema of face, sensitivity to sunlight	T, B, NK	+++
2. DNA ligase I deficiency	?AR (19q13)	Short stature, sensitivity to sunlight	T, B	++++ (1 case)
3. Fanconi pancytopenia	AR*	Radial hypoplasia, hyperpigmentation, pancytopenia, short stature	Ph	++++
4. Ataxia-telangiectasia	AR (11q22)	Progressive cerebellar ataxia, telangiectasias (conjunctival), choreoathetosis	T, B	++++
5. Nijmegen breakage syndrome	AR (8q21)	Microcephaly, mental retardation, prenatal onset short stature, bird-like facies, café-au-lait spots, malignancy	T, B	++++
6. ICF syndrome (immunodeficiency-centromeric instability-facial anomalies)	AR (20q11)	Variable immune deficiency, mental retardation, chromosome instability, facial dysmorphism	T, B, NK	+++

*Multiple genetic loci.
Frequency of ID: +, less than 5% of reported cases with documented ID; ++, 5%–30%; +++, 30%–65%; ++++, >65%.
AR = autosomal recessive; B = B-cell defect; ID = immunodeficiency; NK = NK-cell defect; Ph = phagocyte defect; T = T-cell defect.

Chapter 18). Patients with AT are at increased risk for malignancy, especially leukemia and lymphoma. Elevated alpha-fetoprotein is a consistent finding. Most breaks occur at sites involved in the assembly of immunoglobulin and the T-cell receptor for antigen (chromosomes 2, 7, 14, 22) (Aurias and Dutrillaux, 1986). Most patients suffer from clinical immune deficiency, and a proportion of those individuals have severe infections (Woods and Taylor, 1992). A variety of immunologic defects have been reported, and very low levels of IgA and IgE are frequent aberrations. Impaired T-cell function may also occur.

The different complementation groups of AT were all found to be due to mutations in the gene *ATM* (Concannon and Gatti, 1997; Savitsky et al., 1995). Many of the mutations are due to defective splicing (Teraoka et al., 1999). ATM is involved in several signaling pathways (Brown et al., 1999). Interestingly, ATM can phosphorylate the protein product of the *NBS1* gene, which is implicated in Nijmegen breakage syndrome (NBS) (Gatei et al., 2000; Zhao et al., 2000).

Nijmegen Breakage Syndrome (MIM 251260)

Patients with the NBS have short stature, microcephaly, and bird-like facies (International NBS Study Group, 2000) (see Chapter 18). Mental retardation occurs in approximately half of the patients. The syndrome is similar to AT in that rearrangements of chromosomes 7 and 14, hypersensitivity to irradiation, and immunodeficiency are present.

However, the syndrome is distinct from AT because the patients do not generally display either ataxia or telangiectasias, alpha-fetoprotein is normal, and AT patients do not usually have dysmorphic features. There is a greatly increased risk of lymphoreticular malignancy, most often a lymphoma. The immunodeficiency, percentage of chromosome rearrangements, and frequency of malignancy are all higher than in AT. Affected individuals suffer from recurrent sinopulmonary infections including otitis media, sinusitis, mastoiditis, and pneumonia. Dysgammaglobulinemia and defects in T-cell function are present in most patients (International NBS Study Group, 2000).

The gene causing NBS has been termed *Nibrin* and the protein p95 (Matsuura et al., 1998; Varon et al., 1998). Approximately 90% of the patients have a specific five base-pair deletion at position 657 of *Nibrin* that results in premature truncation of the protein (Carney et al., 1998; Varon et al., 1998). Other identified mutations also result in premature truncation. The protein, named nibrin or p95, is a subunit of the hMRe11-hRad50 protein complex involved in double-stranded break repair (Carney et al., 1998).

Some individuals with bird-like facies, short stature, microcephaly, and mental retardation were diagnosed with Seckel syndrome and were subsequently found to have chromosomal fragility and hematologic abnormalities (Butler et al., 1987). These individuals may actu-ally have NBS. Because of the overlap in clinical appearance, NBS should be considered in an individual with features of Seckel syndrome and increased chromosomal breakage.

ICF Syndrome (MIM 242860)

ICF syndrome is an unusual condition composed of immunodeficiency, centromeric instability (involving chromosomes 1 and 16, often 9, rarely 2 and 10), and facial anomalies (Maraschio et al., 1988; Tiepolo et al., 1979). Mental retardation is frequent. Facial features include ocular hypertelorism, flat nasal bridge, and protrusion of the tongue. Deletions, breaks, interchanges between homologous and nonhomologous chromosomes, and multibranched configurations involving pericentric heterochromatin have been described.

The ICF syndrome differs from other chromosome instability syndromes in that no hypersensitivity to clastogenic agents has been demonstrated, so the condition should not be considered a chromosome breakage syndrome. Severe chronic sinopulmonary, gastrointestinal, and cutaneous infections occur. The immune defect may affect both immunoglobulin levels and T-cell number and function. Mutations in the gene encoding the DNA methyltransferase DNMT3B were identified (Okano et al., 1999; Xu et al., 1999).

DNA Ligase I Deficiency (MIM 126391)

A girl with growth retardation, sun sensitivity, conjunctival telangiectasias, and recurrent ear and pulmonary infections was described (Webster et al., 1992). IgA, IgG2, and IgG3 were decreased, and isohemagglutinins were not detectable. She later developed T-cell defects and died from pneumonia. Her fibroblasts were killed by unusually low doses of irradiation, and increased sister chromatid exchange was noted. Miscoding mutations in DNA ligase I, the enzyme involved in DNA replication of proliferating cells, were detected.

SYNDROMES ASSOCIATED WITH CHROMOSOMAL ABNORMALITIES OF NUMBER OR STRUCTURE

Several syndromes with known chromosome abnormalities are associated with immunodeficiency (Table 24-11).

Trisomy 21 (MIM 190685)

Down syndrome usually results from trisomy 21 and is associated with mental retardation, cardiac defects, gastrointestinal abnormalities, leukemia, and early-onset Alzheimer disease. Affected individuals can experience significant morbidity and mortality resulting from infections, especially respiratory infections (Ugazio et al., 1990). Although a number of immunologic abnormalities

TABLE 24-11 · SYNDROME ASSOCIATED WITH CHROMOSOMAL ABNORMALITIES OF NUMBER OR STRUCTURE

Name	Associated Features	Immune Defect	Frequency of ID
1. Trisomy 21 (Down syndrome)	Hypotonia, flat facies, upslanting palpebral fissures, mental retardation	T, B, Ph, NK	++
2. Deletion of long arm of chromosome 22 (22q11.2) (DiGeorge/velo-cardio-facial syndrome)	Aortic arch anomalies, hypocalcemia, thymic hypoplasia, cleft palate, facial dysmorphism	T	++++
3. Deletion of short arm of chromosome 10 (10p13-p14)	Hypoparathyroidism, DiGeorge anomaly; some with deafness, renal anomaly	T	++
4. Missing or abnormal X chromosome (XO, isoX, ring X; Turner syndrome)	Short stature, webbed neck, broad chest, ovarian dysgenesis, congenital lymphedema	T, B	++
5. Deletion of short arm of chromosome 4 (4p16) (Wolf-Hirschhorn syndrome)	Growth and developmental deficiency, "Greek helmet"-like facies, microcephaly, coloboma	B	+++
6. Deletion of short arm of chromosome 18	Mental and growth deficiency, microcephaly, ptosis	B	+
7. Deletion of long arm of chromosome 18	Midface hypoplasia, microcephaly, mental retardation, nystagmus	B	++

Frequency of ID: +, less than 5% of reported cases with documented ID; ++, 5%–30%; +++, 30%–65%; ++++, >65%.
B = B-cell defect; ID = immunodeficiency; NK = NK-cell defect; Ph = phagocyte defect; T = T-cell defect.

have been noted in individuals with Down syndrome, most do not have clear immune dysfunction. Decreased B-cell number and low specific antibody response have been reported (Lockitch et al., 1987; Ugazio et al., 1990). Increased IgG and decreased IgM levels may occur during late childhood and adolescence (Burgio et al., 1983). The thymus may be small with marked thymocyte depletion and an increased number of Hassall's corpuscles (Levin et al., 1979). Proliferation in response to phytohemagglutinin and alloantigens, delayed-type hypersensitivity response, and T-cell–mediated killing is variably reduced (Montagna et al., 1988; Ugazio et al., 1990). Total NK-cell number is increased, but the activity is decreased (Cossarizza et al., 1990; Montagna et al., 1988). Phagocyte number is normal, but chemotaxis and oxidative metabolism, and hence killing, is impaired (Barroeta et al., 1983). There is an increased incidence of autoimmune conditions (Cuadrado and Barrena, 1996). Some of the immunologic findings are similar to age-related changes in normal individuals and may reflect premature senescence of the immune system. Proliferation and interleukin-2 (IL-2) production in response to phytohemagglutinin were decreased in adult men with Down syndrome (Park et al., 2000).

Deletion of Chromosome 22q11.2 (MIM 188400)

The DiGeorge malformation sequence is due to defective development of the third and fourth pharyngeal pouches, resulting in thymic absence or hypoplasia, conotruncal cardiac defects, and parathyroid hypoplasia (with hypocalcemia) (see Chapter 17). Facial characteristics include hypoplastic mandible; short philtrum; short bulbous nose; and low-set, malformed, or posteriorly rotated ears (Fig. 24-3). Environmental

causes of DiGeorge sequence include exposure to retinoic acid (Lammer et al., 1985), maternal ethanol exposure (Ammann et al., 1982), and diabetic embryopathy (Gosseye et al., 1982; Wilson et al., 1993). Although the causes are diverse, the underlying cause of DiGeorge sequence is abnormal migration of neural crest cells (Bockman and Kirby, 1984), leading to a polytopic developmental field defect (Lammer and Opitz, 1986).

Deletions of chromosome 22q11 are found in at least 85% of cases of DiGeorge sequence. In addition, the same deletion is associated with velocardiofacial syndrome (*Shprintzen* syndrome, MIM 192430). Affected individuals have conotruncal heart defects, cleft palate, and a distinctive facies. There is great variability in the manifestations of the 22q11 deletion (McDonald-McGinn et al., 1999; Thomas and Graham, 1997). Microdeletions of 22q11 are the most frequent cytogenetic alterations in DiGeorge sequence, but other chromosome anomalies have also been identified, such as deletion 10p (Greenberg et al., 1988). Overall, 77% of patients with the 22q11 deletion have immunocompromise (Sullivan et al., 1998). The severity of the immunodeficiency does not correlate with any specific clinical feature, and immunodeficiency was not limited to those with "classic" DiGeorge sequence (Sullivan et al., 1998).

Most patients have similar overlapping deletions that span approximately 3 megabases (Shaikh et al., 2000), and there is marked variability even within patients with the same size deletion or within a single family. In addition, the size of the deletion does not correlate with the clinical phenotype. Recent findings have shed light on the role of certain genes located within the commonly deleted region on 22q11. Homozygous null mutant mice for the gene *Tbx1* were found to have several features consistent with DiGeorge sequence, includ-

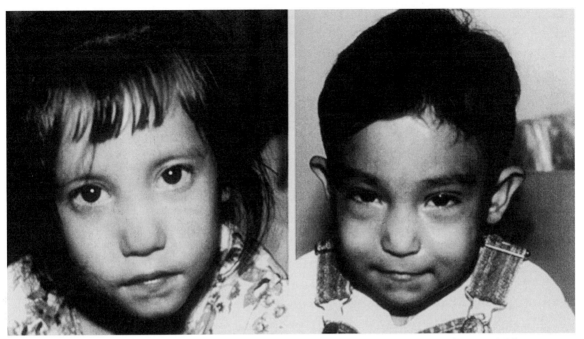

Figure 24-3· **Velocardiofacial syndrome.** These two children with velocardiofacial syndrome and deletion 22q11.2 demonstrate typical facial features with short palpebral fissures, squared-off nasal root with prominent bulbous tip, and small jaw with bifid uvula and velopharyngeal insufficiency.

ing conotruncal heart defects, thymic hypoplasia, and parathyroid defects (Jerome and Papaioannou, 2001; Lindsay et al., 2001; Merscher et al., 2001). In addition, a patient with a very small deletion of 22q11.2 involving the genes *UFD1L* and *CDC45L* and features of the DiGeorge anomaly was reported (Yamagishi et al., 1999). However, other patients with clinical features characteristic of the 22q11.2 deletion but who do not have a detectable deletion did not have mutations in these genes (Wadey et al., 1999). Future studies will determine more precisely the role of these genes in human DiGeorge anomaly.

Deletion of Chromosome 10p13-p14 (MIM)

Some patients diagnosed with DiGeorge anomaly or with hypoparathyroidism were found to have terminal deletions with breakpoints at 10p13-p14 (Daw et al., 1996; Greenberg et al., 1988). There is considerable variability in phenotype. The region has been narrowed to a 1-cM interval (Schuffenhauer et al., 1998). The 22q11 deletion is a much more frequent cause of DiGeorge syndrome than deletions involving 10p (Bartsch et al., 1999). Some of the patients with DiGeorge anomaly and a 10p deletion also have deafness and renal anomalies. These patients may have a 10p deletion that extends further in the telomeric direction beyond the DiGeorge syndrome critical region to include the *GATA3* gene (Lichtner et al., 2000), which is mutated in the syndrome of hypoparathyroidism, deafness, and renal dysplasia (Van Esch et al., 2000).

Partial Deletions of Chromosome 4p (Wolf-Hirschhorn Syndrome) (MIM 194190)

Patients with partial deletions of chromosome 4p have prenatal-onset growth deficiency, mental retardation, microcephaly, ocular hypertelorism, coloboma of the iris, and seizures (Fig. 24-4). There is some correlation between deletion size and clinical severity (Zollino et al., 2000). The critical region has been narrowed to 165 kb on 4p16.3 (Wright et al., 1997). Patients have frequent episodes of respiratory infections, due in part to recurrent aspiration, but antibody deficiencies are also common. Immune defects include common variable immunodeficiency, IgA and IgG2 subclass deficiency, IgA deficiency, and impaired polysaccharide responsiveness (Hanley-Lopez et al., 1998). T-cell immunity is normal. Immunodeficiency does not appear to correlate with deletion size, and all of these patients were deleted for the 4p16.3 critical region. This region likely contains a gene or genes critical for B-cell function.

Turner Syndrome

Patients with a missing or structurally abnormal X chromosome often present with short stature, shield chest, congenital lymphedema, and ovarian dysgenesis. The syndrome is associated with an increased risk for upper respiratory and ear infections, autoimmunity, and occasional neoplasia. In a review of 28 patients, decreased IgG was found in 50%, decreased IgM in 42%, decreased IgA in 10%, and increased IgA in 25%

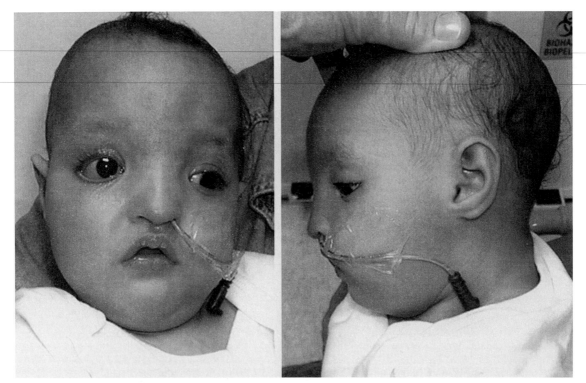

Figure 24-4 · Wolf-Hirschhorn syndrome. This 14-month-old boy with Wolf-Hirschhorn syndrome and a 4p15.2 deletion was born small for gestational age with an atrial septal defect, generalized clonic-tonic seizures, feeding problems with gastroesophageal reflux, postnatal failure to thrive, recurrent infections, and developmental delay.

(Lorini et al., 1983). Other occasional findings include decreased T-cell number with poor response to phytohemagglutinin and absent delayed-type hypersensitivity reactions (Cacciari et al., 1981; Donti et al., 1989) and common variable immunodeficiency (al-Attas et al., 1997; Robson and Potter, 1990). The X chromosome has an important role in immunoregulation. Several primary immunodeficiencies are X-linked. The relationship, if any, between the immune defects in Turner syndrome and the X-linked primary immunodeficiencies is unknown.

Partial Deletions of Chromosome 18

Deletion of the short arm of chromosome 18 (18p-) is marked by mental retardation, growth deficiency, and ptosis. Deletion of the long arm of chromosome 18 (18q-) is characterized by midface hypoplasia, conductive hearing loss, and mental retardation. Decreased or absent IgA has been found in 2 of 6 patients with ring 18, 5 of 15 with 18q-, and 2 of 5 with 18p- (Stewart et al., 1970; Wertelecki and Gerald, 1971) (see Chapter 14). Thus decreased IgA levels are found in some, but not all, individuals affected with structural chromosome 18 derangements. One patient with 18q- and IgA deficiency developed common variable immunodeficiency (Slyper and Pietryga, 1997). Individuals with 18p- also have an increased incidence of autoimmune diseases.

CONCLUSION

A variety of genetic syndromes are associated with immunodeficiency. The occurrence of immunodeficiency with other physical features could result from several underlying pathogenetic mechanisms. First, a mutation of a gene involved in the function, regulation, or development of both the involved systems could occur. Alteration of the activity or structure of such proteins could cause dysfunction in both the immune system and another organ system. Second, a gene critical in the development of one of the involved systems could be closely linked to a gene important for the immune system. A contiguous gene deletion would affect both genes. Third, insults at crucial times in embryologic development could affect more than one organ system if both were developing at that time. Fourth, abnormalities in bone or thymic development could cause improper development of immune cells by providing an inhospitable environment. Last, exposure to acidosis or toxic metabolites, as may be found in some inborn errors of metabolism, could affect function of the immune system.

Recognition of the association of immune defects with other organ system involvement is critical for optimal clinical care. For a child with a recognizable syndrome that is associated with immune deficiency, it is important to establish that the immune defect is present so that appropriate treatment can be undertaken. Alternatively, for a child with an immune defect and other anomalies, it is vital to determine whether the other malformations fit into a recognizable pattern. This will aid in giving accurate prognosis for the immune deficiency and other involved organ systems, including cognitive development. In addition, the diagnosis may have implications for other family members or for future pregnancies.

REFERENCES

Abinun M, Spickett G, Appleton AL, Flood T, Cant AJ. Anhidrotic ectodermal dysplasia associated with specific antibody deficiency. Eur J Pediatr 155:146–147, 1996.

Abo K, Nishio H, Lee MJ, Tsuzuki D, Takahashi T, Yoshida S, Nakajima T, Matsuo M, Sumino K. A novel single basepair insertion in exon 6 of the Bruton's tyrosine kinase (Btk) gene from a Japanese X-linked agammaglobulinemia patient with growth hormone insufficiency. Hum Mutat 11:336, 1998.

Adderson EE, Viskochil DH, Carey JC, Shigeoka AO, Christenson JC, Bohnsack JF, Hill HR. Growth failure, intracranial calcifications, acquired pancytopenia, and unusual humoral immunodeficiency: a genetic syndrome? Am J Med Genet 95:17–20, 2000.

Ades EW, Hinson A, Morgan SK. Immunological studies in sickle cell disease. I. Analysis of circulating T-lymphocyte subpopulations. Clin Immunol Immunopathol 17:459–462, 1980.

Aguilar L, Lisker R, Hernandez-Peniche J, Martinez-Villar C. A new syndrome characterized by mental retardation, epilepsy, palpebral conjunctival telangiectasias and IgA deficiency. Clin Genet 13:154–158, 1978.

al-Attas RA, Rahi AH, Ahmed el FE. Common variable immunodeficiency with CD4+ T lymphocytopenia and overproduction of soluble IL-2 receptor associated with Turner's syndrome and dorsal kyphoscoliosis. J Clin Pathol 50:876–879, 1997.

Alaluusua S, Kivitie-Kallio S, Wolf J, Haavio ML, Asikainen S, Pirinen S. Periodontal findings in Cohen syndrome with chronic neutropenia. J Periodontol 68:473–478, 1997.

Alvarado CS, Livingstone LR, Jones ME, Ravielle A, McKolanis J, Elsas LJ. Uridine-responsive hypogammaglobulinemia and congenital heart disease in a patient with hereditary orotic aciduria. J Pediatr 113:867–871, 1988.

American Academy of Pediatrics. Section on Hematology/Oncology, Committee on Genetics. Health supervision for children with sickle cell disease. American Academy of Pediatrics. Pediatrics 109:526–535, 2002.

Ammann AJ, Sutliff W, Millinchick E. Antibody-mediated immunodeficiency in short-limbed dwarfism. J Pediatr 84:200–203, 1974.

Ammann AJ, Wara DW, Cowan MJ, Barrett DJ, Stiehm ER. The DiGeorge syndrome and the fetal alcohol syndrome. Am J Dis Child 136:906–908, 1982.

Antoniades K, Hatzistilianou M, Pitsavas G, Agouridaki C, Athanassiadou F. Co-existence of Dubowitz and hyper-IgE syndromes: a case report. Eur J Pediatr 155:390–392, 1996.

Artigas M, Alcazar R, Bel J, Fernandez P, Javier G, Ortega E, Pintos G, Venderell T, Prats J. Kabuki syndrome and common variable immunodeficiency. Am J Hum Genet 61(Suppl):A91, 1997.

Aruffo A, Farrington M, Hollenbaugh D, Li X, Milatovich A, Nonoyama S, Bajorath J, Grosmaire LS, Stenkamp R, Neubauer M, et al. The CD40 ligand, gp39, is defective in activated T cells from patients with X-linked hyper-IgM syndrome. Cell 72:291–300, 1993.

Aurias A, Dutrillaux B. Probable involvement of immunoglobulin superfamily genes in most recurrent chromosomal rearrangements from ataxia telangiectasia. Hum Genet 72:210–214, 1986.

Avela K, Lipsanen-Nyman M, Idanheimo N, Seemanova E, Rosengren S, Makela TP, Perheentupa J, Chapelle A, Lehesjoki AE. Gene encoding a new RING-B-box-Coiled-coil protein is mutated in mulibrey nanism. Nat Genet 25:298–301, 2000.

Ballas SK, Burka ER, Lewis CN, Krasnow SH. Serum immunoglobulin levels in patients having sickle cell syndromes. Am J Clin Pathol 73:394–396, 1980.

Ballester OF, Abdallah JM, Prasad AS. Lymphocyte subpopulation abnormalities in sickle cell anemia: a distinctive pattern from that of AIDS. Am J Hematol 21:23–27, 1986.

Barrett-Connor E. Bacterial infection and sickle cell anemia. An analysis of 250 infections in 166 patients and a review of the literature. Medicine (Baltimore) 50:97–112, 1971.

Barroeta O, Nungaray L, Lopez-Osuna M, Armendares S, Salamanca F, Kretschmer RR. Defective monocyte chemotaxis in children with Down's syndrome. Pediatr Res 17:292–295, 1983.

Barth PG, Wanders RJ, Vreken P, Janssen EA, Lam J, Baas F. X-linked cardioskeletal myopathy and neutropenia (Barth syndrome) (MIM 302060). J Inherit Metab Dis 22:555–567, 1999.

Bartsch O, Tympner KD, Schwinger E, Gorlin RJ. Mulvihill-Smith syndrome: case report and review. J Med Genet 31:707–711, 1994.

Bartsch O, Wagner A, Hinkel GK, Lichtner P, Murken J, Schuffenhauer S. No evidence for chromosomal microdeletions at the second DiGeorge syndrome locus on 10p near D10S585. Am J Med Genet 83:425–426, 1999.

Becroft DM, Phillips LI, Webster DR, Wilson JD. Absence of immune deficiency in hereditary orotic aciduria. N Engl J Med 310:1333–1334, 1984.

Bennett CL, Christie J, Ramsdell F, Brunkow ME, Ferguson PJ, Whitesell L, Kelly TE, Saulsbury FT, Chance PF, Ochs HD. The immune dysregulation, polyendocrinopathy, enteropathy, X-linked syndrome (IPEX) is caused by mutations of FOXP3. Nat Genet 27:20–21, 2001.

Bergada I, Schiffrin A, Abu Srair H, Kaplan P, Dornan J, Goltzman D, Hendy GN. Kenny syndrome: description of additional abnormalities and molecular studies. Hum Genet 80:39–42, 1988.

Berthet F, Caduff R, Schaad UB, Roten H, Tuchschmid P, Boltshauser E, Seger RA. A syndrome of primary combined immunodeficiency with microcephaly, cerebellar hypoplasia, growth failure and progressive pancytopenia. Eur J Pediatr 153:333–338, 1994.

Bione S, D'Adamo P, Maestrini E, Gedeon AK, Bolhuis PA, Toniolo D. A novel X-linked gene, G4.5, is responsible for Barth syndrome. Nat Genet 12:385–389, 1996.

Bjornson AB, Falletta JM, Verter JI, Buchanan GR, Miller ST, Pegelow CH, Iyer RV, Johnstone HS, DeBaun MR, Wethers DL, Wang WC, Woods GM, Holbrook CT, Becton DL, Kinney TR, et al. Serotype-specific immunoglobulin G antibody responses to pneumococcal polysaccharide vaccine in children with sickle cell anemia: effects of continued penicillin prophylaxis. J Pediatr 129:828–835, 1996.

Bjornson AB, Gaston MH, Zellner CL. Decreased opsonization for Streptococcus pneumoniae in sickle cell disease: studies on selected complement components and immunoglobulins. J Pediatr 91:371–378, 1977.

Bjornson AB, Lobel JS. Direct evidence that decreased serum opsonization of Streptococcus pneumoniae via the alternative complement pathway in sickle cell disease is related to antibody deficiency. J Clin Invest 79:388–398, 1987.

Bjornson AB, Lobel JS, Harr KS. Relation between serum opsonic activity for Streptococcus pneumoniae and complement function in sickle cell disease. J Infect Dis 152:701–709, 1985.

Blake KD, Davenport SL, Hall BD, Hefner MA, Pagon RA, Williams MS, Lin AE, Graham JM. CHARGE association: an update and review for the primary pediatrician. Clin Pediatr (Phila) 37:159–173, 1998.

Bockman DE, Kirby ML. Dependence of thymus development on derivatives of the neural crest. Science 223:498–500, 1984.

Boerkoel CF, O'Neill S, Andre JL, Benke PJ, Bogdanovic R, Bulla M, Burguet A, Cockfield S, Cordeiro I, Ehrich JH, Frund S, Geary DF, Ieshima A, Illies F, Joseph MW, Kaitila I, Lama G, Leheup B, Ludman MD, McLeod DR, Medeira A, Milford DV, Ormala T, Rener-Primec Z, Weksberg R, et al. Manifestations and treatment of Schimke immuno-osseous dysplasia: 14 new cases and a review of the literature. Eur J Pediatr 159:1–7, 2000.

Boerkoel CF, Takashima H, John J, Yan J, Stankiewicz P, Rosenbarker L, Andre JL, Bogdanovic R, Burguet A, Cockfield S, Cordeiro I, Frund S, Illies F, Joseph M, Kaitila I, et al. Mutant chromatin remodeling protein SMARCAL1 causes Schimke immuno-osseous dysplasia. Nat Genet 30:215–220, 2002.

Boghossian SH, Wright G, Webster AD, Segal AW. Investigations of host defence in patients with sickle cell disease. Br J Haematol 59:523–531, 1985.

Borgna-Pignatti C, Marradi P, Pinelli L, Monetti N, Patrini C. Thiamine-responsive anemia in DIDMOAD syndrome. J Pediatr 114:405–410, 1989.

Borzy MS, Wolff L, Gewurz A, Buist NR, Lovrien E. Recurrent sepsis with deficiencies of C2 and galactokinase. Am J Dis Child 138:186–191, 1984.

Boudny P, Kurrer MO, Stamm B, Laeng RH. Malakoplakia of the colon in an infant with severe combined immunodeficiency (SCID) and CHARGE association. Pathol Res Pract 196:577–582, 2000.

Boxer LA, Oliver JM, Spielberg SP, Allen JM, Schulman JD. Protection of granulocytes by vitamin E in glutathione synthetase deficiency. N Engl J Med 301:901–905, 1979.

Braegger C, Bottani A, Halle F, Giedion A, Leumann E, Seger R, Willi U, Schinzel A. Unknown syndrome: ischiadic hypoplasia, renal dysfunction, immunodeficiency, and a pattern of minor congenital anomalies. J Med Genet 28:56–59, 1991.

Brook JD, McCurrach ME, Harley HG, Buckler AJ, Church D, Aburatani H, Hunter K, Stanton VP, Thirion JP, Hudson T, et al. Molecular basis of myotonic dystrophy: expansion of a trinucleotide (CTG) repeat at the 3′ end of a transcript encoding a protein kinase family member. Cell 68:799–808, 1992.

Brown KD, Barlow C, Wynshaw-Boris A. Multiple ATM-dependent pathways: an explanation for pleiotropy. Am J Hum Genet 64:46–50, 1999.

Burgio GR, Ugazio A, Nespoli L, Maccario R. Down syndrome: a model of immunodeficiency. Birth Defects Orig Artic Ser 19:325–327, 1983.

Butler MG, Hall BD, Maclean RN, Lozzio CB. Do some patients with Seckel syndrome have hematological problems and/or chromosome breakage? Am J Med Genet 27:645–649, 1987.

Cacciari E, Masi M, Fantini MP, Licastro F, Cicognani A, Pirazzoli P, Villa MP, Specchia F, Forabosco A, Franceschi C, Martoni L. Serum immunoglobulins and lymphocyte subpopulations derangement in Turner's syndrome. J Immunogenet 8:337–344, 1981.

Cantu JM, Arias J, Foncerrada M, Hernandez A, Podoswa G, Rostenberg I, Macotelaruiz E. Syndrome of onychotrichodysplasia with chronic neutropenia in an infant from consanguineous parents. Birth Defects Orig Artic Ser 11:63–66, 1975.

Carapella-de Luca E, Aiuti F, Lucarelli P, Bruni L, Baroni CD, Imperato C, Roos D, Astaldi A. A patient with nucleoside phosphorylase deficiency, selective T-cell deficiency, and autoimmune hemolytic anemia. J Pediatr 93:1000–1003, 1978.

Carney JP, Maser RS, Olivares H, Davis EM, Le Beau M, Yates JR, Hays L, Morgan WF, Petrini JH. The hMre11/hRad50 protein complex and Nijmegen breakage syndrome: linkage of double-strand break repair to the cellular DNA damage response. Cell 93:477–486, 1998.

Carpenter NJ, Berkel I, Say B. 'Novel' immunodeficiency syndrome may be a previously described entity. Clin Genet 57:90–92, 2000.

Casademont J, Barrientos A, Cardellach F, Rotig A, Grau JM, Montoya J, Beltran B, Cervantes F, Rozman C, Estivill X, et al. Multiple deletions of mtDNA in two brothers with sideroblastic anemia and mitochondrial myopathy and in their asymptomatic mother. Hum Mol Genet 3:1945–1949, 1994.

Castriota-Scanderbeg A, Mingarelli R, Caramia G, Osimani P, Lachman RS, Rimoin DL, Wilcox WR, Dallapiccola B. Spondylo-mesomelic-acrodysplasia with joint dislocations and severe combined immunodeficiency: a newly recognised immuno-osseous dysplasia. J Med Genet 34:854–856, 1997.

Chandra RK, Joglekar S, Antonio Z. Deficiency of humoral immunity and hypoparathyroidism associated with the Hallerman-Streiff syndrome. J Pediatr 93:892–893, 1978.

Chavanas S, Bodemer C, Rochat A, Hamel-Teillac D, Ali M, Irvine AD, Bonafe JL, Wilkinson J, Taieb A, Barrandon Y, Harper JI, de Prost Y, Hovnanian A. Mutations in SPINK5, encoding a serine protease inhibitor, cause Netherton syndrome. Nat Genet 25:141–142, 2000.

Chrzanowska KH, Krajewska-Walasek M, Kus J, Michalkiewicz J, Maziarka D, Wolski JK, Brecevic L, Madalinski K. Kabuki (Niikawa-Kuroki) syndrome associated with immunodeficiency. Clin Genet 53:308–312, 1998.

Chudwin DS, Korenblit AD, Kingzette M, Artrip S, Rao S. Increased activation of the alternative complement pathway in sickle cell disease. Clin Immunol Immunopathol 37:93–97, 1985.

Church JA, Costin G, Brooks J. Immune functions in children treated with biosynthetic growth hormone. J Pediatr 115:420–423, 1989.

Church JA, Koch R, Shaw KN, Nye CA, Donnell GN. Immune functions in methylmalonicaciduria. J Inherit Metab Dis 7:12–14, 1984.

Clark LB, Appleby MW, Brunkow ME, Wilkinson JE, Ziegler SF, Ramsdell F. Cellular and molecular characterization of the scurfy mouse mutant. J Immunol 162:2546–2554, 1999.

Cleaver JE. It was a very good year for DNA repair. Cell 76:1–4, 1994.

Clericuzio C, Hoyme HE, Aase JM. Immune deficient poikiloderma: a new genodermatosis. (Abstract). Am J Hum Genet 49:131, 1991.

Concannon P, Gatti RA. Diversity of ATM gene mutations detected in patients with ataxia-telangiectasia. Hum Mutat 10:100–107, 1997.

Conley ME, Burks AW, Herrod HG, Puck JM. Molecular analysis of X-linked agammaglobulinemia with growth hormone deficiency. J Pediatr 119:392–397, 1991.

Corbeel L, Van den Berghe G, Jaeken J, Van Tornout J, Eeckels R. Congenital folate malabsorption. Eur J Pediatr 143:284–290, 1985.

Corder WT, Hummel M, Miller C, Wilson NW. Association of kyphomelic dysplasia with severe combined immunodeficiency. Am J Med Genet 57:626–629, 1995.

Cossarizza A, Monti D, Montagnani G, Ortolani C, Masi M, Zannotti M, Franceschi C. Precocious aging of the immune system in Down syndrome: alteration of B lymphocytes, T-lymphocyte subsets, and cells with natural killer markers. Am J Med Genet Suppl 7:213–218, 1990.

Cowan MJ, Wara DW, Packman S, Ammann AJ, Yoshino M, Sweetman L, Nyhan W. Multiple biotin-dependent carboxylase deficiencies associated with defects in T-cell and B-cell immunity. Lancet 2:115–118, 1979.

Crisp AJ, Brenton DP. Engelmann's disease of bone–a systemic disorder? Ann Rheum Dis 41:183–188, 1982.

Cuadrado E, Barrena MJ. Immune dysfunction in Down's syndrome: primary immune deficiency or early senescence of the immune system? Clin Immunol Immunopathol 78:209–214, 1996.

Dallapiccola B, Mingarelli R, Obregon G. Onychotrichodysplasia and chronic neutropenia without mental retardation (ONS): a second case report. Clin Genet 45:200–202, 1994.

Davenport SL, Donlan MA, Dolan CR, Ochs HD. Dominant hearing loss, white hair, contractures, hyperkeratotic papillomata, and depressed chemotaxis. Birth Defects Orig Artic Ser 15:227–237, 1979.

Davis JR, Solomon LM. Cellular immunodeficiency in anhidrotic ectodermal dysplasia. Acta Derm Venereol 56:115–120, 1976.

Daw SC, Taylor C, Kraman M, Call K, Mao J, Schuffenhauer S, Meitinger T, Lipson T, Goodship J, Scambler P. A common region of 10p deleted in DiGeorge and velocardiofacial syndromes. Nat Genet 13:458–460, 1996.

Dawson J, Hodgson HJ, Pepys MB, Peters TJ, Chadwick VS. Immunodeficiency, malabsorption and secretory diarrhea. A new syndrome. Am J Med 67:540–546, 1979.

DeClue TJ, Malone JI, Tedesco TA. Florida newborn screening for galactosemia. J Fla Med Assoc 78:369–371, 1991.

de Lonlay-Debeney P, Cormier-Daire V, Amiel J, Abadie V, Odent S, Paupe A, Couderc S, Tellier AL, Bonnet D, Prieur M, Vekemans M, Munnich A, Lyonnet S. Features of DiGeorge syndrome and CHARGE association in five patients. J Med Genet 34:986–989, 1997.

de Silva DC, Wheatley DN, Herriot R, Brown T, Stevenson DA, Helms P, Dean JC. Mulvihill-Smith progeria-like syndrome: a further report with delineation of phenotype, immunologic deficits, and novel observation of fibroblast abnormalities. Am J Med Genet 69:56–64, 1997.

Debray D, Pariente D, Urvoas E, Hadchouel M, Bernard O. Sclerosing cholangitis in children. J Pediatr 124:49–56, 1994.

del Campo M, Hall BD, Aeby A, Nassogne MC, Verloes A, Roche C, Gonzalez C, Sanchez H, Garcia-Alix A, Cabanas F, Escudero RM, Hernandez R, Quero J. Albinism and agenesis of the corpus callosum with profound developmental delay: Vici syndrome, evidence for autosomal recessive inheritance. Am J Med Genet 85:479–485, 1999.

Derry JM, Ochs HD, Francke U. Isolation of a novel gene mutated in Wiskott-Aldrich syndrome. Cell 79:635–644, 1994.

Desnick RJ, Sharp HL, Grabowski GA, Brunning RD, Quie PG, Sung JH, Gorlin RJ, Ikonne JU. Mannosidosis: clinical, morphologic, immunologic, and biochemical studies. Pediatr Res 10:985–996, 1976.

Devriendt K, Kim AS, Mathijs G, Frints SG, Schwartz M, Van Den Oord JJ, Verhoef GE, Boogaerts MA, Fryns JP, You D, Rosen MK, Vandenberghe P. Constitutively activating mutation in WASP causes X-linked severe congenital neutropenia. Nat Genet 27:313–317, 2001.

Diamantopoulos N, Bergman I, Kaplan S. Actinomycosis meningitis in a girl with incontinentia pigmenti. Clin Pediatr (Phila) 24:651–654, 1985.

Diaz GA, Gelb BD, Ali F, Sakati N, Sanjad S, Meyer BF, Kambouris M. Sanjad-Sakati and autosomal recessive Kenny-Caffey syndromes are allelic: evidence for an ancestral founder mutation and locus refinement. Am J Med Genet 85:48–52, 1999.

Dionisi-Vici C, De Felice L, el Hachem M, Bottero S, Rizzo C, Paoloni A, Goffredo B, Sabetta G, Caniglia M. Intravenous immune globulin in lysinuric protein intolerance. J Inherit Metab Dis 21:95–102, 1998.

Dionisi-Vici C, Sabetta G, Gambarara M, Vigevano F, Bertini E, Boldrini R, Parisi SG, Quinti I, Aiuti F, Fiorilli M. Agenesis of the corpus callosum, combined immunodeficiency, bilateral cataract, and hypopigmentation in two brothers. Am J Med Genet 29:1–8, 1988.

Doffinger R, Smahi A, Bessia C, Geissmann F, Feinberg J, Durandy A, Bodemer C, Kenwrick S, Dupuis-Girod S, Blanche S, Wood P, Rabia SH, Headon DJ, Overbeek PA, Le Deist F, Holland SM, Belani K, Kumararatne DS, Fischer A, Shapiro R, Conley ME, Reimund E, Kalhoff H, Abinun M, Munnich A, Israel A, Courtois G, Casanova JL. X-linked anhidrotic ectodermal dysplasia with immunodeficiency is caused by impaired NF-kappaB signaling. Nat Genet 27:277–285, 2001.

Dokal I. Dyskeratosis congenita: an inherited bone marrow failure syndrome. Br J Haematol 92:775–779, 1996.

Donti E, Nicoletti I, Venti G, Filipponi P, Gerli R, Spinozzi F, Cernetti C, Rambotti P. X-ring Turner's syndrome with combined immunodeficiency and selective gonadotropin defect. J Endocrinol Invest 12:257–263, 1989.

Drachtman RA, Alter BP. Dyskeratosis congenita: clinical and genetic heterogeneity. Report of a new case and review of the literature. Am J Pediatr Hematol Oncol 14:297–304, 1992.

Dufourcq-Lagelouse R, Pastural E, Barrat FJ, Feldmann J, Le Deist F, Fischer A, De Saint Basile G. Genetic basis of hemophagocytic lymphohistiocytosis syndrome (Review). Int J Mol Med 4:127–133, 1999.

Dupuy JM, Lafforet D. A defect of cellular immunity in xeroderma pigmentosum. Clin Immunol Immunopathol 3:52–58, 1974.

Duriez B, Duquesnoy P, Dastot F, Bougneres P, Amselem S, Goossens M. An exon-skipping mutation in the btk gene of a patient with X-linked agammaglobulinemia and isolated growth hormone deficiency. FEBS Lett 346:165–170, 1994.

Ellis NA, German J. Molecular genetics of Bloom's syndrome. Hum Mol Genet 5(Spec No):1457–1463, 1996.

Ellis NA, Groden J, Ye TZ, Straughen J, Lennon DJ, Ciocci S, Proytcheva M, German J. The Bloom's syndrome gene product is homologous to RecQ helicases. Cell 83:655–666, 1995.

Ewart-Toland A, Enns GM, Cox VA, Mohan GC, Rosenthal P, Golabi M. Severe congenital anomalies requiring transplantation in children with Kabuki syndrome. Am J Med Genet 80:362–367, 1998.

Fanconi Anaemia/Breast Cancer Consortium. Positional cloning of the Fanconi anaemia group A gene. Nat Genet 14:324–328, 1996.

Feldman KW, Ochs HD, Price TH, Wedgwood RJ. Congenital stem cell dysfunction associated with Turner-like phenotype. J Pediatr 88:979–982, 1976.

Fleisher TA, White RM, Broder S, Nissley SP, Blaese RM, Mulvihill JJ, Olive G, Waldmann TA. X-linked hypogammaglobulinemia and isolated growth hormone deficiency. N Engl J Med 302:1429–1434, 1980.

Fleming AF, Storey J, Molineaux L, Iroko EA, Attai ED. Abnormal haemoglobins in the Sudan savanna of Nigeria. I. Prevalence of haemoglobins and relationships between sickle cell trait, malaria and survival. Ann Trop Med Parasitol 73:161–172, 1979.

Frank AL, Labotka RJ, Rao S, Frisone LR, McVerry PH, Samuelson JS, Maurer H, Yogev R. *Haemophilus influenzae* type b immunization of children with sickle cell diseases. Pediatrics 82:571–575, 1988.

Frank J, Pignata C, Panteleyev AA, Prowse DM, Baden H, Weiner L, Gaetaniello L, Ahmad W, Pozzi N, Cserhalmi-Friedman PB, Aita VM, Uyttendaele H, Gordon D, Ott J, Brissette JL, Christiano AM. Exposing the human nude phenotype. Nature 398:473–474, 1999.

Frenkel M, Russe HP. Retinal telangiectasia associated with hypogammaglobulinemia. Am J Ophthalmol 63:215–220, 1967.

Frick H, Munger DM, Fauchere JC, Stallmach T. Hypoplastic thymus and T-cell reduction in EECUT syndrome. Am J Med Genet 69:65–68, 1997.

Frydman M, Etzioni A, Eidlitz-Markus T, Avidor I, Varsano I, Shechter Y, Orlin JB, Gershoni-Baruch R. Rambam-Hasharon syndrome of psychomotor retardation, short stature, defective neutrophil motility, and Bombay phenotype. Am J Med Genet 44:297–302, 1992.

Fu YH, Pizzuti A, Fenwick RG Jr, King J, Rajnarayan S, Dunne PW, Dubel J, Nasser GA, Ashizawa T, de Jong P, et al. An unstable triplet repeat in a gene related to myotonic muscular dystrophy. Science 255:1256–1258, 1992.

Gatei M, Young D, Cerosaletti KM, Desai-Mehta A, Spring K, Kozlov S, Lavin MF, Gatti RA, Concannon P, Khanna K. ATM-dependent phosphorylation of nibrin in response to radiation exposure. Nat Genet 25:115–119, 2000.

Gatti RA, Platt N, Pomerance HH, Hong R, Langer LO, Kay HE, Good RA. Hereditary lymphopenic agammaglobulinemia associated with a distinctive form of short-limbed dwarfism and ectodermal dysplasia. J Pediatr 75:675–684, 1969.

Gerin I, Veiga-da-Cunha M, Achouri Y, Collet JF, Van Schaftingen E. Sequence of a putative glucose 6-phosphate translocase, mutated in glycogen storage disease type Ib. FEBS Lett 419:235–238, 1997.

Girault D, Goulet O, Le Deist F, Brousse N, Colomb V, Cesarini JP, de Potter S, Canioni D, Griscelli C, Fischer A, et al. Intractable infant diarrhea associated with phenotypic abnormalities and immunodeficiency. J Pediatr 125:36–42, 1994.

Girot R, Hamet M, Perignon JL, Guesnu M, Fox RM, Cartier P, Durandy A, Griscelli C. Cellular immune deficiency in two siblings with hereditary orotic aciduria. N Engl J Med 308:700–704, 1983.

Gitzelmann R, Bosshard NU. Defective neutrophil and monocyte functions in glycogen storage disease type Ib: a literature review. Eur J Pediatr 152 Suppl 1:S33–38, 1993.

Gorlin RJ, Gelb B, Diaz GA, Lofsness KG, Pittelkow MR, Fenyk JR. WHIM syndrome, an autosomal dominant disorder: clinical, hematological, and molecular studies. Am J Med Genet 91:368–376, 2000.

Gosseye S, Golaire MC, Verellen G, Van Lierde M, Claus D. Association of bilateral renal agenesis and Di George syndrome in an infant of a diabetic mother. Helv Paediatr Acta 37:471–474, 1982.

Gotoff SP, Esterly NB, Gottbrath E, Liebner EJ, Lajvardi SR. Granulomatous reaction in an infant with combined immunodeficiency disease and short-limbed dwarfism. J Pediatr 80:1010–1017, 1972.

Graham JM. A recognizable syndrome within CHARGE association: Hall-Hittner syndrome. Am J Med Genet 99:120–123, 2001.

Greenberg F, Elder FF, Haffner P, Northrup H, Ledbetter DH. Cytogenetic findings in a prospective series of patients with DiGeorge anomaly. Am J Hum Genet 43:605–611, 1988.

Greene RJ, Gilbert EF, Huang SW, Horowitz S, Levy RL, Herrmann JP, Hong R. Immunodeficiency associated with exomphalos-macroglossia-gigantism syndrome. J Pediatr 82:814–820, 1973.

Greene SL, Muller SA. Netherton's syndrome. Report of a case and review of the literature. J Am Acad Dermatol 13:329–337, 1985.

Griscelli C, Durandy A, Guy-Grand D, Daguillard F, Herzog C, Prunieras M. A syndrome associating partial albinism and immunodeficiency. Am J Med 65:691–702, 1978.

Guerin V, Bene MC, Judlin P, Beurey J, Landes P, Faure G. Cowden disease in a young girl: gynecologic and immunologic overview in a case and in the literature. Obstet Gynecol 73:890–892, 1989.

Hanley-Lopez J, Estabrooks LL, Stiehm ER. Antibody deficiency in Wolf-Hirschhorn syndrome. J Pediatr 133:141–143, 1998.

Haraldsson A, van der Burgt CJ, Weemaes CM, Otten B, Bakkeren JA, Stoelinga GB. Antibody deficiency and isolated growth hormone deficiency in a girl with Mulibrey nanism. Eur J Pediatr 152:509–512, 1993.

Harjacek M, Batinic D, Sarnavka V, Uzarevic B, Mardesic D, Marusic M. Immunological aspects of progeria (Hutchinson-Gilford syndrome) in a 15-month-old child. Eur J Pediatr 150:40–42, 1990.

Hart PS, Zhang Y, Firatli E, Uygur C, Lotfazar M, Michalec MD, Marks JJ, Lu X, Coates BJ, Seow WK, Marshall R, Williams D, Reed JB, Wright JT, Hart TC. Identification of cathepsin C mutations in ethnically diverse Papillon-Lefevre syndrome patients. J Med Genet 37:927–932, 2000.

Hart TC, Hart PS, Bowden DW, Michalec MD, Callison SA, Walker SJ, Zhang Y, Firatli E. Mutations of the cathepsin C gene are responsible for Papillon-Lefèvre syndrome. J Med Genet 36:881–887, 1999.

Heiss NS, Knight SW, Vulliamy TJ, Klauck SM, Wiemann S, Mason PJ, Poustka A, Dokal I. X-linked dyskeratosis congenita is caused by mutations in a highly conserved gene with putative nucleolar functions. Nat Genet 19:32–38, 1998.

Hernandez P, Cruz C, Santos MN, Ballester JM. Immunologic dysfunction in Sickle cell anaemia. Acta Haematol 63:156–161, 1980.

Hirschhorn R. Overview of biochemical abnormalities and molecular genetics of adenosine deaminase deficiency. Pediatr Res 33:S35–41, 1993.

Hisama FM, Reyes-Mugica M, Wargowski DS, Thompson KJ, Mahoney MJ. Renal tubular dysgenesis, absent nipples, and multiple malformations in three brothers: a new, lethal syndrome. Am J Med Genet 80:335–342, 1998.

Hitzig WH, Dohmann U, Pluss HJ, Vischer D. Hereditary transcobalamin II deficiency: clinical findings in a new family. J Pediatr 85:622–628, 1974.

Hodge D, Misbah SA, Mueller RF, Glass EJ, Chetcuti PA. Proteus syndrome and immunodeficiency. Arch Dis Child 82:234–235, 2000.

Hoffman HM, Bastian JF, Bird LM. Humoral immunodeficiency with facial dysmorphology and limb anomalies: a new syndrome. Clin Dysmorphol 10:1–8, 2001.

Hong R, Horowitz SD, Borzy MF, Gilbert EF, Arya S, McLeod N, Peterson RD. The cerebro-hepato-renal syndrome of Zellweger: similarity to and differentiation from the DiGeorge syndrome. Thymus 3:97–104, 1981.

Hostoffer RW, Bay CA, Wagner K, Venglarcik J 3rd, Sahara H, Omair E, Clark HT. Kabuki make-up syndrome associated with an acquired hypogammaglobulinemia and anti-IgA antibodies. Clin Pediatr 35:273–276, 1996.

Hoyeraal HM, Lamvik J, Moe PJ. Congenital hypoplastic thrombocytopenia and cerebral malformations in two brothers. Acta Paediatr Scand 59:185–191, 1970.

Hreidarsson S, Kristjansson K, Johannesson G, Johannsson JH. A syndrome of progressive pancytopenia with microcephaly, cerebellar hypoplasia and growth failure. Acta Paediatr Scand 77:773–775, 1988.

Hurvitz H, Gillis R, Klaus S, Klar A, Gross-Kieselstein F, Okon E. A kindred with Griscelli disease: spectrum of neurological involvement. Eur J Pediatr 152:402–405, 1993.

Inoue S, Krieger I, Sarnaik A, Ravindranath Y, Fracassa M, Ottenbreit MJ. Inhibition of bone marrow stem cell growth in vitro by methylmalonic acid: a mechanism for pancytopenia in a patient with methylmalonic acidemia. Pediatr Res 15:95–98, 1981.

International Nijmegen Breakage Syndrome Study Group. Nijmegen breakage syndrome. Arch Dis Child 82:400–406, 2000.

Ipp MM, Gelfand EW. Antibody deficiency and alopecia. J Pediatr 89:728–731, 1976.

Jain A, Ma CA, Liu S, Brown M, Cohen J, Strober W. Specific missense mutations in NEMO result in hyper-IgM syndrome with hypohydrotic ectodermal dysplasia. 2:223–228, 2001.

Jerome LA, Papaioannou VE. DiGeorge syndrome phenotype in mice mutant for the T-box gene, Tbx1. Nat Genet 27:286–291, 2001.

Jessen RT, Van Epps DE, Goodwin JS, Bowerman J. Incontinentia pigmenti. Evidence for both neutrophil and lymphocyte dysfunction. Arch Dermatol 114:1182–1186, 1978.

Joenje H, Oostra AB, Wijker M, di Summa FM, van Berkel CG, Rooimans MA, Ebell W, van Weel M, Pronk JC, Buchwald M, Arwert F. Evidence for at least eight Fanconi anemia genes. Am J Hum Genet 61:940–944, 1997.

Johnston RB Jr, Newman SL, Struth AG. An abnormality of the alternate pathway of complement activation in sickle-cell disease. N Engl J Med 288:803–808, 1973.

Jung LK, Engelhard D, Kapoor N, Pih K, Good RA. Pyoderma eczema and folliculitis with defective leucocyte and lymphocyte function: a new familial immunodeficiency disease responsive to a histamine-1 antagonist. Lancet 2:185–187, 1983.

Kaikov Y, Wadsworth LD, Hall CA, Rogers PC. Transcobalamin II deficiency: case report and review of the literature. Eur J Pediatr 150:841–843, 1991.

Karsan A, Cornejo CJ, Winn RK, Schwartz BR, Way W, Lannir N, Gershoni-Baruch R, Etzioni A, Ochs HD, Harlan JM. Leukocyte adhesion deficiency type II is a generalized defect of de novo GDP-fucose biosynthesis. Endothelial cell fucosylation is not required for neutrophil rolling on human nonlymphoid endothelium. J Clin Invest 101:2438–2445, 1998.

Kawame H, Hannibal MC, Hudgins L, Pagon RA. Phenotypic spectrum and management issues in Kabuki syndrome. J Pediatr 134:480–485, 1999.

Kelleher JF, Yudkoff M, Hutchinson R, August CS, Cohn RM. The pancytopenia of isovaleric acidemia. Pediatrics 65:1023–1027, 1980.

Kelley RI, Cheatham JP, Clark BJ, Nigro MA, Powell BR, Sherwood GW, Sladky JT, Swisher WP. X-linked dilated cardiomyopathy with neutropenia, growth retardation, and 3-methylglutaconic aciduria. J Pediatr 119:738–747, 1991.

Kere J, Srivastava AK, Montonen O, Zonana J, Thomas N, Ferguson B, Munoz F, Morgan D, Clarke A, Baybayan P, Chen EY, Ezer S, Saarialho-Kere U, de la Chapelle A, Schlessinger D. X-linked anhidrotic (hypohidrotic) ectodermal dysplasia is caused by mutation in a novel transmembrane protein. Nat Genet 13:409–416, 1996.

Kiess W, Malozowski S, Gelato M, Butenand O, Doerr H, Crisp B, Eisl E, Maluish A, Belohradsky BH. Lymphocyte subset distribution and natural killer activity in growth hormone deficiency before and during short-term treatment with growth hormone releasing hormone. Clin Immunol Immunopathol 48:85–94, 1988.

Kimura H, Ito Y, Koda Y, Hase Y. Rubinstein-Taybi syndrome with thymic hypoplasia. Am J Med Genet 46:293–296, 1993.

Kivitie-Kallio S, Rajantie J, Juvonen E, Norio R. Granulocytopenia in Cohen syndrome. Br J Haematol 98:308–311, 1997.

Klein C, Philippe N, Le Deist F, Fraitag S, Prost C, Durandy A, Fischer A, Griscelli C. Partial albinism with immunodeficiency (Griscelli syndrome). J Pediatr 125:886–895, 1994.

Knight SW, Heiss NS, Vulliamy TJ, Aalfs CM, McMahon C, Richmond P, Jones A, Hennekam RC, Poustka A, Mason PJ, Dokal I. Unexplained aplastic anaemia, immunodeficiency, and cerebellar hypoplasia (Hoyeraal-Hreidarsson syndrome) due to mutations in the dyskeratosis congenita gene, DKC1. Br J Haematol 107:335–339, 1999.

Kobayashi RH, Kettelhut BV, Kobayashi AL. Galactose inhibition of neonatal neutrophil function. Pediatr Infect Dis 2:442–445, 1983.

Kondo N, Motoyoshi F, Mori S, Kuwabara N, Orii T, German J. Long-term study of the immunodeficiency of Bloom's syndrome. Acta Paediatr 81:86–90, 1992.

Kosaki K, Curry CJ, Roeder E, Jones KL. Ritscher-Schinzel (3C) syndrome: documentation of the phenotype. Am J Med Genet 68:421–427, 1997.

Kotzot D, Richter K, Gierth-Fiebig K. Oculocutaneous albinism, immunodeficiency, hematological disorders, and minor anomalies: a new autosomal recessive syndrome? Am J Med Genet 50:224–227, 1994.

Kraemer KH, Lee MM, Scotto J. Xeroderma pigmentosum. Cutaneous, ocular, and neurologic abnormalities in 830 published cases. Arch Dermatol 123:241–250, 1987.

Krawinkel MB, Ernst M, Feller A, Flad HD, Mueller-Hermelink HK, Ulmer AJ, Schaub J. Lissencephaly, abnormal lymph nodes, and T-cell deficiency in one patient. Am J Med Genet 33:436–443, 1989.

Kultursay N, Taneli B, Cavusoglu A. Pseudoachondroplasia with immune deficiency. Pediatr Radiol 18:505–508, 1988.

Kupfer GM, Naf D, Suliman A, Pulsipher M, D'Andrea AD. The Fanconi anaemia proteins, FAA and FAC, interact to form a nuclear complex. Nat Genet 17:487–490, 1997.

Lammer EJ, Chen DT, Hoar RM, Agnish ND, Benke PJ, Braun JT, Curry CJ, Fernhoff PM, Grix AW, Lott IT, et al. Retinoic acid embryopathy. N Engl J Med 313:837–841, 1985.

Lammer EJ, Opitz JM. The DiGeorge anomaly as a developmental field defect. Am J Med Genet Suppl 2:113–127, 1986.

Lauener R, Seger R, Jorg W, Halle F, Aeppli R, Schinzel A. Immunodeficiency associated with Dandy-Walker-like malformation, congenital heart defect, and craniofacial abnormalities. Am J Med Genet 33:280–281, 1989.

Levin S, Schlesinger M, Handzel Z, Hahn T, Altman Y, Czernobilsky B, Boss J. Thymic deficiency in Down's syndrome. Pediatrics 63:80–87, 1979.

Levy HL, Sepe SJ, Shih VE, Vawter GF, Klein JO. Sepsis due to *Escherichia coli* in neonates with galactosemia. N Engl J Med 297:823–825, 1977.

Lichtenstein J. A 'new' syndrome with neutropenia, immunoglobulin deficiency, peculiar facies and bony anomalies. Birth Defects Orig Art Ser 8:178–190, 1972.

Lichtner P, Konig R, Hasegawa T, Van Esch H, Meitinger T, Schuffenhauer S. An HDR (hypoparathyroidism, deafness, renal dysplasia) syndrome locus maps distal to the DiGeorge syndrome region on 10p13/14. J Med Genet 37:33–37, 2000.

Liquori CL, Ricker K, Moseley ML, Jacobsen JF, Kress W, Naylor SL, Day JW, Ranum LP. Myotonic dystrophy type 2 caused by a CCTG expansion in intron 1 of ZNF9. Science 293:864–7, 2001.

Lilleyman JS. Constitutional hypoplastic anemia associated with familial "bird-headed" dwarfism (Seckel syndrome). Am J Pediatr Hematol Oncol 6:207–209, 1984.

Lindsay EA, Vitelli F, Su H, Morishima M, Huynh T, Pramparo T, Jurecic V, Ogunrinu G, Sutherland HF, Scambler PJ, Bradley A, Baldini A. Tbx1 haploinsufficieny in the DiGeorge syndrome region causes aortic arch defects in mice. Nature 410:97–101, 2001.

Lo Ten Foe JR, Rooimans MA, Bosnoyan-Collins L, Alon N, Wijker M, Parker L, Lightfoot J, Carreau M, Callen DF, Savoia A, Cheng NC, van Berkel CG, Strunk MH, Gille JJ, Pals G, Kruyt FA, Pronk JC, Arwert F, Buchwald M, Joenje H. Expression cloning of a cDNA for the major Fanconi anaemia gene, FAA. Nat Genet 14:320–323, 1996.

Lockitch G, Singh VK, Puterman ML, Godolphin WJ, Sheps S, Tingle AJ, Wong F, Quigley G. Age-related changes in humoral and cell-mediated immunity in Down syndrome children living at home. Pediatr Res 22:536–540, 1987.

Lorini R, Ugazio AG, Cammareri V, Larizza D, Castellazzi AM, Brugo MA, Severi F. Immunoglobulin levels, T-cell markers, mitogen responsiveness and thymic hormone activity in Turner's syndrome. Thymus 5:61–66, 1983.

Ludman MD, Cole DE, Crocker JF, Cohen MM. Schimke immuno-osseous dysplasia: case report and review. Am J Med Genet 47:793–796, 1993.

Lukkarinen M, Nanto-Salonen K, Ruuskanen O, Lauteala T, Sako S, Nuutinen M, Simell O. Varicella and varicella immunity in patients with lysinuric protein intolerance. J Inherit Metab Dis 21:103–111, 1998.

Lukkarinen M, Parto K, Ruuskanen O, Vainio O, Kayhty H, Olander RM, Simell O. B and T cell immunity in patients with lysinuric protein intolerance. Clin Exp Immunol 116:430–4, 1999.

MacDermot KD, Winter RM, Wigglesworth JS, Strobel S. Short stature/short limb skeletal dysplasia with severe combined immunodeficiency and bowing of the femora: report of two patients and review. J Med Genet 28:10–17, 1991.

Mack DR, Forstner GG, Wilschanski M, Freedman MH, Durie PR. Shwachman syndrome: exocrine pancreatic dysfunction and variable phenotypic expression. Gastroenterology 111:1593–1602, 1996.

Maghnie M, Monafo V, Marseglia GL, Valtorta A, Avanzini A, Moretta A, Balottin U, Touraine JL, Severi F. Immunodeficiency, growth hormone deficiency and central nervous system involvement in a girl. Thymus 20:69–76, 1992.

Mahadevan M, Tsilfidis C, Sabourin L, Shutler G, Amemiya C, Jansen G, Neville C, Narang M, Barcelo J, O'Hoy K, et al. Myotonic dystrophy mutation: an unstable CTG repeat in the 3' untranslated region of the gene. Science 255:1253–1255, 1992.

Makitie O, Kaitila I. Cartilage-hair hypoplasia–clinical manifestations in 108 Finnish patients. Eur J Pediatr 152:211–217, 1993.

Malatack JJ, Moran MM, Moughan B. Isolated congenital malabsorption of folic acid in a male infant: insights into treatment and mechanism of defect. Pediatrics 104:1133–1137, 1999.

Mancini AJ, Chan LS, Paller AS. Partial albinism with immunodeficiency: Griscelli syndrome: report of a case and review of the literature. J Am Acad Dermatol 38:295–300, 1998.

Maraschio P, Zuffardi O, Dalla Fior T, Tiepolo L. Immunodeficiency, centromeric heterochromatin instability of chromosomes 1, 9, and 16, and facial anomalies: the ICF syndrome. J Med Genet 25:173–180, 1988.

Mariani E, Facchini A, Honorati MC, Lalli E, Berardesca E, Ghetti P, Marinoni S, Nuzzo F, Astaldi Ricotti GC, Stefanini M. Immune defects in families and patients with xeroderma pigmentosum and trichothiodystrophy. Clin Exp Immunol 88:376–382, 1992.

Matsui SM, Mahoney MJ, Rosenberg LE. The natural history of the inherited methylmalonic acidemias. N Engl J Med 308:857–861, 1983.

Matsuura S, Tauchi H, Nakamura A, Kondo N, Sakamoto S, Endo S, Smeets D, Solder B, Belohradsky BH, Der Kaloustian VM, Oshimura M, Isomura M, Nakamura Y, Komatsu K. Positional cloning of the gene for Nijmegen breakage syndrome. Nat Genet 19:179–181, 1998.

McDonald-McGinn DM, Kirschner R, Goldmuntz E, Sullivan K, Eicher P, Gerdes M, Moss E, Solot C, Wang P, Jacobs I, Handler S, Knightly C, Heher K, Wilson M, Ming JE, Grace K, Driscoll D, Pasquariello P, Randall P, Larossa D, Emanuel BS, Zackai EH. The Philadelphia story: the 22q11.2 deletion: report on 250 patients. Genet Couns 10:11–24, 1999.

McKusick V, Eldridge R, Hostetler J, Egeland J, Ruangwit U. Dwarfism in the Amish: II. cartilage-hair hypoplasia. Bull Johns Hopkins Hosp 116:232–272, 1965.

Menasche G, Pastural E, Feldmann J, Certain S, Ersoy F, Dupuis S, Wulffraat N, Bianchi D, Fischer A, Le Deist F, de Saint Basile G. Mutations in RAB27A cause Griscelli syndrome associated with haemophagocytic syndrome. Nat Genet 25:173–176, 2000.

Menni S, Piccinno R, Biolchini A, Plebani A. Immunologic investigations in eight patients with incontinentia pigmenti. Pediatr Dermatol 7:275–277, 1990.

Merscher S, Funke B, Epstein JA, Heyer J, Puech A, Lu MM, Xavier RJ, Demay MB, Russell RG, Factor S, Tokooya K, Jore BS, Lopez M, Pandita RK, Lia M, Carrion D, Xu H, Schorle H, Kobler JB, Scambler P, Wynshaw-Boris A, Skoultchi AI, Morrow BE, Kucherlapati R. TBX1 is responsible for cardiovascular defects in velo-cardio-facial/DiGeorge syndrome. Cell 104:619–629, 2001.

Miller ME, Norman ME, Koblenzer PJ, Schonauer T. A new familial defect of neutrophil movement. J Lab Clin Med 82:1–8, 1973.

Mollica F, Messina A, Stivala F, Pavone L. Immuno-deficiency in Schwartz-Jampel syndrome. Acta Paediatr Scand 68:133–135, 1979.

Monreal AW, Ferguson BM, Headon DJ, Street SL, Overbeek PA, Zonana J. Mutations in the human homologue of mouse dl cause autosomal recessive and dominant hypohidrotic ectodermal dysplasia. Nat Genet 22:366–369, 1999.

Monreal AW, Zonana J, Ferguson B. Identification of a new splice form of the EDA1 gene permits detection of nearly all X-linked hypohidrotic ectodermal dysplasia mutations. Am J Hum Genet 63:380–389, 1998.

Montagna D, Maccario R, Ugazio AG, Nespoli L, Pedroni E, Faggiano P, Burgio GR. Cell-mediated cytotoxicity in Down syndrome: impairment of allogeneic mixed lymphocyte reaction, NK and NK-like activities. Eur J Pediatr 148:53–57, 1988.

Moore SW, de Jongh G, Bouic P, Brown RA, Kirsten G. Immune deficiency in familial duodenal atresia. J Pediatr Surg 31:1733–1735, 1996.

Moreno LA, Gottrand F, Turck D, Manouvrier-Hanu S, Mazingue F, Morisot C, Le Deist F, Ricour C, Nihoul-Fekete C, Debeugny P, et al. Severe combined immunodeficiency syndrome associated with autosomal recessive familial multiple gastrointestinal atresias: study of a family. Am J Med Genet 37:143–146, 1990.

Motulsky AG. Frequency of sickling disorders in U.S. blacks. N Engl J Med 288:31–33, 1973.

Mousa AR, Al-Din AS, Al-Nassar KE, Al-Rifai KM, Rudwan M, Sunba MS, Behbehani K. Autosomally inherited recessive spastic ataxia, macular corneal dystrophy, congenital cataracts, myopia and vertically oval temporally tilted discs. Report of a Bedouin family–a new syndrome. J Neurol Sci 76:105–121, 1986.

Muller S, Falkenberg N, Monch E, Jakobs C. Propionic acidaemia and immunodeficiency. Lancet 1:551–552, 1980.

Mulvihill JJ, Smith DW. Another disorder with prenatal shortness of stature and premature aging. Birth Defects Orig Artic Ser 11:368–370, 1975.

Nagata M, Suzuki M, Kawamura G, Kono S, Koda N, Yamaguchi S, Aoki K. Immunological abnormalities in a patient with lysinuric protein intolerance. Eur J Pediatr 146:427–428, 1987.

Nagle DL, Karim MA, Woolf EA, Holmgren L, Bork P, Misumi DJ, McGrail SH, Dussault BJ, Perou CM, Boissy RE, Duyk GM, Spritz RA, Moore KJ. Identification and mutation analysis of the complete gene for Chediak-Higashi syndrome. Nat Genet 14:307–311, 1996.

Nakamura A, Kojo T, Arahata K, Takeda S. Reduction of serum IgG level and peripheral T-cell counts are correlated with CTG repeat lengths in myotonic dystrophy patients. Neuromusc Disord 6:203–10, 1996.

Naveh Y, Mendelsohn H, Spira G, Auslaender L, Mandel H, Berant M. Primary sclerosing cholangitis associated with immunodeficiency. Am J Dis Child 137:114–117, 1983.

Nehls M, Pfeifer D, Schorpp M, Hedrich H, Boehm T. New member of the winged-helix protein family disrupted in mouse and rat nude mutations. Nature 372:103–107, 1994.

Niikawa N, Kuroki Y, Kajii T, Matsuura N, Ishikiriyama S, Tonoki H, Ishikawa N, Yamada Y, Fujita M, Umemoto H, et al. Kabuki make-up (Niikawa-Kuroki) syndrome: a study of 62 patients. Am J Med Genet 31:565–589, 1988.

Ohashi H, Tsukahara M, Murano I, Fujita K, Matsuura S, Fukushima Y, Kajii T. Premature aging and immunodeficiency: Mulvihill-Smith syndrome? Am J Med Genet 45:597–600, 1993.

Ohzeki T, Hanaki K, Motozumi H, Ohtahara H, Hayashibara H, Harada Y, Okamoto M, Shiraki K, Tsuji Y, Emura H. Immunodeficiency with increased immunoglobulin M associated with growth hormone insufficiency. Acta Paediatr 82:620–623, 1993.

Okano M, Bell DW, Haber DA, Li E. DNA methyltransferases Dnmt3a and Dnmt3b are essential for de novo methylation and mammalian development. Cell 99:247–257, 1999.

Oleske JM, Westphal ML, Shore S, Gorden D, Bogden JD, Nahmias A. Zinc therapy of depressed cellular immunity in acrodermatitis enteropathica. Its correction. Am J Dis Child 133:915–918, 1979.

Olivieri O, Lombardi S, Russo C, Corrocher R. Increased neutrophil adhesive capability in Cohen syndrome, an autosomal recessive disorder associated with granulocytopenia. Haematologica 83:778–782, 1998.

OMIM. Online Mendelian Inheritance in Man, OMIM (TM). McKusick-Nathans Institute for Genetic Medicine, Johns Hopkins University (Baltimore, MD) and National Center for Biotechnology Information, National Library of Medicine (Bethesda, MD), 2000. Available at http://www.ncbi.nlm.nih.gov/omim/.

Ostergaard GZ, Nielsen H, Friis B. Defective monocyte oxidative metabolism in a child with Smith-Lemli-Opitz syndrome. Eur J Pediatr 151:291–294, 1992.

Overturf GD, Powars D, Baraff LJ. Bacterial meningitis and septicemia in sickle cell disease. Am J Dis Child 131:784–787, 1977.

Page T, Nyhan WL, Yu AL, Yu J. A syndrome of megaloblastic anemia, immunodeficiency, and excessive nucleotide degradation. Adv Exp Med Biol 309B:345–348, 1991.

Pagon RA, Graham JM, Zonana J, Yong SL. Coloboma, congenital heart disease, and choanal atresia with multiple anomalies: CHARGE association. J Pediatr 99:223–227, 1981.

Park E, Alberti J, Mehta P, Dalton A, Sersen E, Schuller-Levis G. Partial impairment of immune functions in peripheral blood leukocytes from aged men with Down's syndrome. Clin Immunol 95:62–69, 2000.

Parvari R, Hershkovitz E, Kanis A, Gorodischer R, Shalitin S, Sheffield VC, Carmi R. Homozygosity and linkage-disequilibrium mapping of the syndrome of congenital hypoparathyroidism, growth and mental retardation, and dysmorphism to a 1-cM interval on chromosome 1q42-43. Am J Hum Genet 63:163–169, 1998.

Pastural E, Barrat FJ, Dufourcq-Lagelouse R, Certain S, Sanal O, Jabado N, Seger R, Griscelli C, Fischer A, de Saint Basile G. Griscelli disease maps to chromosome 15q21 and is associated with mutations in the myosin-Va gene. Nat Genet 16:289–292, 1997.

Peake JE, McCrossin RB, Byrne G, Shepherd R. X-linked immune dysregulation, neonatal insulin dependent diabetes, and intractable diarrhoea. Arch Dis Child Fetal Neonatal Ed 74:F195–199, 1996.

Pedroni E, Bianchi E, Ugazio AG, Burgio GR. Immunodeficiency and steely hair (Letter). Lancet 1:1303–1304, 1975.

Petrij F, Dauwerse HG, Blough RI, Giles RH, van der Smagt JJ, Wallerstein R, Maaswinkel-Mooy PD, van Karnebeek CD, van Ommen GJ, van Haeringen A, Rubinstein JH, Saal HM, Hennekam RC, Peters DJ, Breuning MH. Diagnostic analysis of the Rubinstein-Taybi syndrome: five cosmids should be used for microdeletion detection and low number of protein truncating mutations. J Med Genet 37:168–176, 2000.

Petrij F, Giles RH, Dauwerse HG, Saris JJ, Hennekam RC, Masuno M, Tommerup N, van Ommen GJ, Goodman RH, Peters DJ, et al. Rubinstein-Taybi syndrome caused by mutations in the transcriptional co-activator CBP. Nature 376:348–351, 1995.

Pignata C, Fiore M, Guzzetta V, Castaldo A, Sebastio G, Porta F, Guarino A. Congenital Alopecia and nail dystrophy associated with severe functional T-cell immunodeficiency in two sibs. Am J Med Genet 65:167–170, 1996.

Poulton J, Morten KJ, Weber K, Brown GK, Bindoff L. Are duplications of mitochondrial DNA characteristic of Kearns-Sayre syndrome? Hum Mol Genet 3:947–951, 1994.

Powell BR, Buist NR, Stenzel P. An X-linked syndrome of diarrhea, polyendocrinopathy, and fatal infection in infancy. J Pediatr 100:731–737, 1982.

Prasad C, Cramer BC, Pushpanathan C, Crowley MC, Ives EJ. Kyphomelic dysplasia: a rare form of semilethal skeletal dysplasia. Clin Genet 58:390–395, 2000.

Press OW, Fingert H, Lott IT, Dickersin CR. Pancytopenia in mannosidosis. Arch Intern Med 143:1266–1268, 1983.

Price TH, Ochs HD, Gershoni-Baruch R, Harlan JM, Etzioni A. In vivo neutrophil and lymphocyte function studies in a patient with leukocyte adhesion deficiency type II. Blood 84:1635–1639, 1994.

Raby RB, Ward JC, Herrod HG. Propionic acidaemia and immunodeficiency. J Inherit Metab Dis 17:250–251, 1994.

Ranum LP, Rasmussen PF, Benzow KA, Koob MD, Day JW. Genetic mapping of a second myotonic dystrophy locus. Nat Genet 19:196–198, 1998.

Rao SP, Miller ST, Cohen BJ. Transient aplastic crisis in patients with sickle cell disease. B19 parvovirus studies during a 7-year period. Am J Dis Child 146:1328–1330, 1992.

Rautonen N, Martin NL, Rautonen J, Rooks Y, Mentzer WC, Wara DW. Low number of antibody producing cells in patients with sickle cell anemia. Immunol Lett 34:207–211, 1992.

Record CO, Shilkin KB, Eddleston AL, Williams R. Intrahepatic sclerosing cholangitis associated with a familial immunodeficiency syndrome. Lancet 2:18–20, 1973.

Ridanpaa M, van Eenennaam H, Pelin K, Chadwick R, Johnson C, Yuan B, vanVenrooij W, Pruijn G, Salmela R, Rockas S, Makitie O, Kaitila I, de la Chapelle A. Mutations in the RNA component of RNase MRP cause a pleiotropic human disease, cartilage-hair hypoplasia. Cell 104:195–203, 2001.

Ritscher D, Schinzel A, Boltshauser E, Briner J, Arbenz U, Sigg P. Dandy-Walker(like) malformation, atrio-ventricular septal defect and a similar pattern of minor anomalies in 2 sisters: a new syndrome? Am J Med Genet 26:481–491, 1987.

Rivas F, Fragoso R, Ramos-Zepeda R, Vaca G, Hernandez A, Gonzalez-Quiroga G, Olivares N, Cantu JM. Deficient cell immunity and mild intermittent hyperaminoacidemia in a patient with the Rubinstein-Taybi Syndrome. Acta Paediatr Scand 69:123–125, 1980.

Robertson SP, Rodda C, Bankier A. Hypogonadotrophic hypogonadism in Roifman syndrome. Clin Genet 57:435–438, 2000.

Robson SC, Potter PC. Common variable immunodeficiency in association with Turner's syndrome. J Clin Lab Immunol 32:143–146, 1990.

Roifman CM. Antibody deficiency, growth retardation, spondyloepiphyseal dysplasia and retinal dystrophy: a novel syndrome. Clin Genet 55:103–109, 1999.

Rothenberg ME, White FV, Chilmonczyk B, Chatila T. A syndrome involving immunodeficiency and multiple intestinal atresias. Immunodeficiency 5:171–178, 1995.

Rotig A, Bourgeron T, Chretien D, Rustin P, Munnich A. Spectrum of mitochondrial DNA rearrangements in the Pearson marrow-pancreas syndrome. Hum Mol Genet 4:1327–1330, 1995.

Rotig A, Cormier V, Koll F, Mize CE, Saudubray JM, Veerman A, Pearson HA, Munnich A. Site-specific deletions of the mitochondrial genome in the Pearson marrow-pancreas syndrome. Genomics 10:502–504, 1991.

Rudd NL, Curry C, Chen KT, Capusten B, Trevenen CL. Thymic-renal-anal-lung dysplasia in sibs: a new autosomal recessive error of early morphogenesis. Am J Med Genet 37:401–405, 1990.

Ruschak PJ, Kauh YC, Luscombe HA. Cowden's disease associated with immunodeficiency. Arch Dermatol 117:573–575, 1981.

Sabry MA, Zaki M, Abul Hassan SJ, Ramadan DG, Abdel Rasool MA, al Awadi SA, al Saleh Q. Kenny-Caffey syndrome is part of the CATCH 22 haploinsufficiency cluster. J Med Genet 35:31–36, 1998.

Saraiva JM, Dinis A, Resende C, Faria E, Gomes C, Correia AJ, Gil J, da Fonseca N. Schimke immuno-osseous dysplasia: case report and review of 25 patients. J Med Genet 36:786–789, 1999.

Savitsky K, Sfez S, Tagle DA, Ziv Y, Sartiel A, Collins FS, Shiloh Y, Rotman G. The complete sequence of the coding region of the ATM gene reveals similarity to cell cycle regulators in different species. Hum Mol Genet 4:2025–2032, 1995.

Say B, Barber N, Miller GC, Grogg SE. Microcephaly, short stature, and developmental delay associated with a chemotactic defect and transient hypogammaglobulinaemia in two brothers. J Med Genet 23:355–359, 1986.

Schaller J, Davis SD, Ching YC, Lagunoff D, Williams CP, Wedgwood RJ. Hypergammaglobulinaemia, antibody deficiency, autoimmune haemolytic anaemia, and nephritis in an infant with a familial lymphopenic immune defect. Lancet 2:825–829, 1966.

Schofer O, Blaha I, Mannhardt W, Zepp F, Stallmach T, Spranger J. Omenn phenotype with short-limbed dwarfism. J Pediatr 118:86–89, 1991.

Schrander-Stumpel C, Meinecke P, Wilson G, Gillessen-Kaesbach G, Tinschert S, Konig R, Philip N, Rizzo R, Schrander J, Pfeiffer L, et al. The Kabuki (Niikawa-Kuroki) syndrome: further delineation of the phenotype in 29 non-Japanese patients. Eur J Pediatr 153:438–445, 1994.

Schuffenhauer S, Lichtner P, Peykar-Derakhshandeh P, Murken J, Haas OA, Back E, Wolff G, Zabel B, Barisic I, Rauch A, Borochowitz Z, Dallapiccola B, Ross M, Meitinger T. Deletion mapping on chromosome 10p and definition of a critical region for the second DiGeorge syndrome locus (DGS2). Eur J Hum Genet 6:213–225, 1998.

Seger R, Frater-Schroder M, Hitzig WH, Wildfeuer A, Linnell JC. Granulocyte dysfunction in transcobalamin II deficiency responding to leucovorin or hydroxocobalamin-plasma transfusion. J Inherit Metab Dis 3:3–9, 1980.

Serjeant GR, Serjeant BE. Management of sickle cell disease; lessons from the Jamaican Cohort Study. Blood Rev 7:137–145, 1993.

Shaikh TH, Kurahashi H, Saitta SC, O'Hare AM, Hu P, Roe BA, Driscoll DA, McDonald-McGinn DM, Zackai EH, Budarf ML, Emanuel BS. Chromosome 22-specific low copy repeats and the 22q11.2 deletion syndrome: genomic organization and deletion endpoint analysis. Hum Mol Genet 9:489–501, 2000.

Shokeir MH. Short stature, absent thumbs, flat facies, anosmia and combined immune deficiency (CID). Birth Defects Orig Artic Ser 14:103–116, 1978.

Siebert JR, Graham JM, MacDonald C. Pathologic features of the CHARGE association: support for involvement of the neural crest. Teratology 31:331–336, 1985.

Sisto A, Feldman P, Garel L, Seidman E, Brochu P, Morin CL, Weber AM, Roy CC. Primary sclerosing cholangitis in children: study of five cases and review of the literature. Pediatrics 80:918–923, 1987.

Slyper AH, Pietryga D. Conversion of selective IgA deficiency to common variable immunodeficiency in an adolescent female with 18q deletion syndrome. Eur J Pediatr 156:155–156, 1997.

Smahi A, Courtois G, Vabres P, Yamaoka S, Heuertz S, Munnich A, Israel A, Heiss NS, Klauck SM, Kioschis P, Wiemann S, Poustka A, Esposito T, Bardaro T, Gianfrancesco F, Ciccodicola A, D'Urso M, Woffendin H, Jakins T, Donnai D, Stewart H, Kenwrick SJ, Aradhya S, Yamagata T, Levy M, Lewis RA, Nelson DL. Genomic rearrangement in NEMO impairs NF-kappaB activation and is a cause of incontinentia pigmenti. The International Incontinentia Pigmenti (IP) Consortium. Nature 405:466–472, 2000.

Smith DL, Smith JG, Wong SW, deShazo RD. Netherton's syndrome: a syndrome of elevated IgE and characteristic skin and hair findings. J Allergy Clin Immunol 95:116–123, 1995.

Smith LJ, Szymanski W, Foulston C, Jewell LD, Pabst HF. Familial enteropathy with villous edema and immunoglobulin G2 subclass deficiency. J Pediatr 125:541–548, 1994.

Smith OP, Hann IM, Chessells JM, Reeves BR, Milla P. Haematological abnormalities in Shwachman-Diamond syndrome. Br J Haematol 94:279–284, 1996.

Snyder CL, Mancini ML, Kennedy AP, Amoury RA. Multiple gastrointestinal atresias with cystic dilatation of the biliary duct. Pediatr Surg Int 16:211–213, 2000.

Solder B, Weiss M, Jager A, Belohradsky BH. Dyskeratosis congenita: multisystemic disorder with special consideration of immunologic aspects. A review of the literature. Clin Pediatr 37:521–530, 1998.

Spadoni GL, Rossi P, Ragno W, Galli E, Cianfarani S, Galasso C, Boscherini B. Immune function in growth hormone-deficient children treated with biosynthetic growth hormone. Acta Paediatr Scand 80:75–79, 1991.

Spielberg SP, Boxer LA, Oliver JM, Allen JM, Schulman JD. Oxidative damage to neutrophils in glutathione synthetase deficiency. Br J Haematol 42:215–223, 1979.

Spranger J, Hinkel GK, Stoss H, Thoenes W, Wargowski D, Zepp F. Schimke immuno-osseous dysplasia: a newly recognized multisystem disease. J Pediatr 119:64–72, 1991.

Starink TM, van der Veen JP, Goldschmeding R. Decreased natural killer cell activity in Cowden's syndrome. J Am Acad Dermatol 15:294–296, 1986.

Stewart DM, Notarangelo LD, Kurman CC, Staudt LM, Nelson DL. Molecular genetic analysis of X-linked hypogammaglobulinemia and isolated growth hormone deficiency. J Immunol 155:2770–2774, 1995.

Stewart JM, Go S, Ellis E, Robinson A. Absent IgA and deletions of chromosome 18. J Med Genet 7:11–19, 1970.

Stoll C, Alembik Y, Lutz P. A syndrome of facial dysmorphia, birth defects, myelodysplasia and immunodeficiency in three sibs of consanguineous parents. Genet Couns 5:161–165, 1994.

Strathdee CA, Gavish H, Shannon WR, Buchwald M. Cloning of cDNAs for Fanconi's anaemia by functional complementation. Nature 358:434, 1992.

Stryk S, Siegfried EC, Knutsen AP. Selective antibody deficiency to bacterial polysaccharide antigens in patients with Netherton syndrome. Pediatr Dermatol 16:19–22, 1999.

Sullivan KE, Jawad AF, Randall P, Driscoll DA, Emanuel BS, McDonald-McGinn DM, Zackai EH. Lack of correlation between impaired T cell production, immunodeficiency, and other phenotypic features in chromosome 22q11.2 deletion syndromes. Clin Immunol Immunopathol 86:141–146, 1998.

Sullivan KE, Mullen CA, Blaese RM, Winkelstein JA. A multiinstitutional survey of the Wiskott-Aldrich syndrome. J Pediatr 125:876–885, 1994.

Sutor GC, Schuppert F, Schatzle C, Schmidt RE. Primary combined immunodeficiency, growth retardation, and disturbed sexual development: a novel syndrome of congenital impairment of the cellular immune system and the endocrine system. J Allergy Clin Immunol 102:327–328, 1998.

Suzuki M, West C, Beutler E. Large-scale molecular screening for galactosemia alleles in a pan-ethnic population. Hum Genet 109:210–215, 2001.

Suzumura A, Yamada H, Matsuoka Y, Sobue I. Immunoglobulin abnormalities in patients with myotonic dystrophy. Acta Neurol Scand 74:132–9, 1986.

Tang ML, Kemp AS. Growth hormone deficiency and combined immunodeficiency. Arch Dis Child 68:231–232, 1993.

Tellier AL, Cormier-Daire V, Abadie V, Amiel J, Sigaudy S, Bonnet D, de Lonlay-Debeney P, Morrisseau-Durand MP, Hubert P, Michel JL, Jan D, Dollfus H, Baumann C, Labrune P, Lacombe D, Philip N, LeMerrer M, Briard ML, Munnich A, Lyonnet S. CHARGE syndrome: report of 47 cases and review. Am J Med Genet 76:402–409, 1998.

Teraoka SN, Telatar M, Becker-Catania S, Liang T, Onengut S, Tolun A, Chessa L, Sanal O, Bernatowska E, Gatti RA, Concannon P. Splicing defects in the ataxia-telangiectasia gene, ATM: underlying mutations and consequences. Am J Hum Genet 64:1617–1631, 1999.

Thomas JA, Graham JM. Chromosomes 22q11 deletion syndrome: an update and review for the primary pediatrician. Clin Pediatr (Phila) 36:253–266, 1997.

Thorburn MJ, Wright ES, Miller CG, Smith-Read EH. Exomphalos-macroglossia-gigantism syndrome in Jamaican infants. Am J Dis Child 119:316–321, 1970.

Tiepolo L, Maraschio P, Gimelli G, Cuoco C, Gargani GF, Romano C. Multibranched chromosomes 1, 9, and 16 in a patient with combined IgA and IgE deficiency. Hum Genet 51:127–137, 1979.

Toriello HV, Horton WA, Oostendorp A, Waterman DF, Higgins JV. An apparently new syndrome of microcephalic primordial dwarfism and cataracts. Am J Med Genet 25:1–8, 1986.

Trowbridge AA, Sirinavin C, Linman JW. Dyskeratosis congenita: hematologic evaluation of a sibship and review of the literature. Am J Hematol 3:143–152, 1977.

Tsukahara M, Opitz JM. Dubowitz syndrome: review of 141 cases including 36 previously unreported patients. Am J Med Genet 63:277–289, 1996.

Ugazio AG, Maccario R, Notarangelo LD, Burgio GR. Immunology of Down syndrome: a review. Am J Med Genet Suppl 7:204–212, 1990.

Urbach J, Abrahamov A, Grossowicz N. Congenital isolated folic acid malabsorption. Arch Dis Child 62:78–80, 1987.

Usami S, Chien S, Bertles JF. Deformability of sickle cells as studied by microsieving. J Lab Clin Med 86:274–9, 1975.

van den Berg H, Wage K, Burggraaf JD, Peters M. Malignant B-cell lymphoma in an infant with severe combined immunodeficiency with short-limbed skeletal dysplasia. Acta Paediatr 86:778–780, 1997.

Van Dyke TE, Taubman MA, Ebersole JL, Haffajee AD, Socransky SS, Smith DJ, Genco RJ. The Papillon-Lefèvre syndrome: neutrophil dysfunction with severe periodontal disease. Clin Immunol Immunopathol 31:419–429, 1984.

Van Esch H, Groenen P, Nesbit MA, Schuffenhauer S, Lichtner P, Vanderlinden G, Harding B, Beetz R, Bilous RW, Holdaway I, Shaw NJ, Fryns JP, Van de Ven W, Thakker RV, Devriendt K. GATA3 haplo-insufficiency causes human HDR syndrome. Nature 406:419–422, 2000.

Van Wouwe JP. Clinical and laboratory diagnosis of acrodermatitis enteropathica. Eur J Pediatr 149:2–8, 1989.

Varon R, Vissinga C, Platzer M, Cerosaletti KM, Chrzanowska KH, Saar K, Beckmann G, Seemanova E, Cooper PR, Nowak NJ, Stumm M, Weemaes CM, Gatti RA, Wilson RK, Digweed M, Rosenthal A, Sperling K, Concannon P, Reis A. Nibrin, a novel DNA double-strand break repair protein, is mutated in Nijmegen breakage syndrome. Cell 93:467–476, 1998.

Veiga-da-Cunha M, Gerin I, Chen YT, de Barsy T, de Lonlay P, Dionisi-Vici C, Fenske CD, Lee PJ, Leonard JV, Maire I, McConkie-Rosell A, Schweitzer S, Vikkula M, Van Schaftingen E. A gene on chromosome 11q23 coding for a putative glucose-6-phosphate translocase is mutated in glycogen-storage disease types Ib and Ic. Am J Hum Genet 63:976–983, 1998.

Villa A, Notarangelo L, Macchi P, Mantuano E, Cavagni G, Brugnoni D, Strina D, Patrosso MC, Ramenghi U, Sacco MG, et al. X-linked thrombocytopenia and Wiskott-Aldrich syndrome are allelic diseases with mutations in the WASP gene. Nat Genet 9:414–417, 1995.

Villa A, Santagata S, Bozzi F, Giliani S, Frattini A, Imberti L, Gatta LB, Ochs HD, Schwarz K, Notarangelo LD, Vezzoni P, Spanopoulou E. Partial V(D)J recombination activity leads to Omenn syndrome. Cell 93:885–896, 1998.

Villella A, Bialostocky D, Lori E, Meyerson H, Hostoffer RW. Rubinstein-Taybi syndrome with humoral and cellular defects: a case report. Arch Dis Child 83:360–361, 2000.

Visser G, Herwig J, Rake JP, Niezen-Koning KE, Verhoeven AJ, Smit GP. Neutropenia and neutrophil dysfunction in glycogen storage disease type 1c. J Inherit Metab Dis 21:227–231, 1998.

Visser G, Rake JP, Fernandes J, Labrune P, Leonard JV, Moses S, Ullrich K, Smit GP. Neutropenia, neutrophil dysfunction, and inflammatory bowel disease in glycogen storage disease type Ib: results of the European Study on Glycogen Storage Disease type I. J Pediatr 137:187–191, 2000.

Wadey R, McKie J, Papapetrou C, Sutherland H, Lohman F, Osinga J, Frohn I, Hofstra R, Meijers C, Amati F, Conti E, Pizzuti A, Dallapiccola B, Novelli G, Scambler P. Mutations of UFD1L are not responsible for the majority of cases of DiGeorge syndrome/velocardiofacial syndrome without deletions within chromosome 22q11. Am J Hum Genet 65:247–249, 1999.

Waldmann TA, Terry WD. Familial hypercatabolic hypoproteinemia. A disorder of endogenous catabolism of albumin and immunoglobulin. J Clin Invest 86:2093–2098, 1990.

Walker MW, Lovell MA, Kelly TE, Golden W, Saulsbury FT. Multiple areas of intestinal atresia associated with immunodeficiency and posttransfusion graft-versus-host disease. J Pediatr 123:93–95, 1993.

Wang JK, Hsieh KH. Immunologic study of the asplenia syndrome. Pediatr Infect Dis J 10:819–822, 1991.

Wang W, Herrod H, Presbury G, Wilimas J. Lymphocyte phenotype and function in chronically transfused children with sickle cell disease. Am J Hematol 20:31–40, 1985.

Watanabe T, Miyakawa M, Satoh M, Abe T, Oda Y. Kabuki make-up syndrome associated with chronic idiopathic thrombocytopenic purpura. Acta Paediatr Japonica 36:727–729, 1994.

Webster AD, Barnes DE, Arlett CF, Lehmann AR, Lindahl T. Growth retardation and immunodeficiency in a patient with mutations in the DNA ligase I gene. Lancet 339:1508–1509, 1992.

Wertelecki W, Gerald PS. Clinical and chromosomal studies of the 18q-syndrome. J Pediatr 78:44–52, 1971.

Weston WL, Huff JC, Humbert JR, Hambidge KM, Neldner KH, Walravens PA. Zinc correction of defective chemotaxis in acrodermatitis enteropathica. Arch Dermatol 113:422–425, 1977.

Wetzler M, Talpaz M, Kleinerman ES, King A, Huh YO, Gutterman JU, Kurzrock R. A new familial immunodeficiency disorder characterized by severe neutropenia, a defective marrow release mechanism, and hypogammaglobulinemia. Am J Med 89:663–672, 1990.

Wildin RS, Ramsdell F, Peake J, Faravelli F, Casanova JL, Buist N, Levy-Lahad E, Mazzella M, Goulet O, Perroni L, Bricarelli FD, Byrne G, McEuen M, Proll S, Appleby M, Brunkow ME. X-linked neonatal diabetes mellitus, enteropathy and endocrinopathy syndrome is the human equivalent of mouse scurfy. Nat Genet 27:18–20, 2001.

Wilson GN. Thirteen cases of Niikawa-Kuroki syndrome: report and review with emphasis on medical complications and preventive management. Am J Med Genet 79:112–120, 1998.

Wilson TA, Blethen SL, Vallone A, Alenick DS, Nolan P, Katz A, Amorillo TP, Goldmuntz E, Emanuel BS, Driscoll DA. DiGeorge anomaly with renal agenesis in infants of mothers with diabetes. Am J Med Genet 47:1078–1082, 1993.

Wilson WA. Nature of complement deficiency in sickle cell disease. Arch Dis Child 58:236–237, 1983.

Winkelstein JA, Drachman RH. Deficiency of pneumococcal serum opsonizing activity in sickle-cell disease. N Engl J Med 279:459–466, 1968.

Wochner RD, Drews G, Strober W, Waldmann TA. Accelerated breakdown of immunoglobulin G (IgG) in myotonic dystrophy: a hereditary error of immunoglobulin catabolism. J Clin Invest 45:321–329, 1966.

Womer R, Clark JE, Wood P, Sabio H, Kelly TE. Dyskeratosis congenita: two examples of this multisystem disorder. Pediatrics 71:603–609, 1983.

Wong SN, Low LC, Lau YL, Nicholls J, Chan MY. Immunodeficiency in methylmalonic acidaemia. J Paediatr Child Health 28:180–183, 1992.

Woods CG, Taylor AM. Ataxia telangiectasia in the British Isles: the clinical and laboratory features of 70 affected individuals. Q J Med 82:169–179, 1992.

Wright TJ, Ricke DO, Denison K, Abmayr S, Cotter PD, Hirschhorn K, Keinanen M, McDonald-McGinn D, Somer M, Spinner N, Yang-Feng T, Zackai E, Altherr MR. A transcript map of the newly defined 165 kb Wolf-Hirschhorn syndrome critical region. Hum Mol Genet 6:317–324, 1997.

Wysenbeek AJ, Weiss H, Duczyminer-Kahana M, Grunwald MH, Pick AI. Immunologic alterations in xeroderma pigmentosum patients. Cancer 58:219–221, 1986.

Xu GL, Bestor TH, Bourc'his D, Hsieh CL, Tommerup N, Bugge M, Hulten M, Qu X, Russo JJ, Viegas-Pequignot E. Chromosome instability and immunodeficiency syndrome caused by mutations in a DNA methyltransferase gene. Nature 402:187–191, 1999.

Yaghmai R, Kimyai-Asadi A, Rostamiani K, Heiss NS, Poustka A, Eyaid W, Bodurtha J, Nousari HC, Hamosh A, Metzenberg A. Overlap of dyskeratosis congenita with the Hoyeraal-Hreidarsson syndrome. J Pediatr 136:390–393, 2000.

Yamagishi H, Garg V, Matsuoka R, Thomas T, Srivastava D. A molecular pathway revealing a genetic basis for human cardiac and craniofacial defects. Science 283:1158–1161, 1999.

Yoshida Y, Machigashira K, Suehara M, Arimura H, Moritoyo T, Nagamatsu K, Osame M. Immunological abnormality in patients with lysinuric protein intolerance. J Neurol Sci 134:178–182, 1995.

Zago MA, Bottura C. Splenic function in sickle-cell diseases. Clin Sci (Lond) 65:297–302, 1983.

Zhao S, Weng YC, Yuan SS, Lin YT, Hsu HC, Lin SC, Gerbino E, Song MH, Zdzienicka MZ, Gatti RA, Shay JW, Ziv Y, Shiloh Y, Lee EY. Functional link between ataxia-telangiectasia and Nijmegen breakage syndrome gene products. Nature 405:473–477, 2000.

Zollino M, Di Stefano C, Zampino G, Mastroiacovo P, Wright TJ, Sorge G, Selicorni A, Tenconi R, Zappala A, Battaglia A, Di Rocco M, Palka G, Pallotta R, Altherr MR, Neri G. Genotype-phenotype correlations and clinical diagnostic criteria in Wolf-Hirschhorn syndrome. Am J Med Genet 94:254–261, 2000.

Zonana J, Elder ME, Schneider LC, Orlow SJ, Moss C, Golabi M, Shapira SK, Farndon PA, Wara DW, Emmal SA, Ferguson BM. A novel X-linked disorder of immune deficiency and hypohidrotic ectodermal dysplasia is allelic to incontinentia pigmenti and due to mutations in IKK-gamma (NEMO). Am J Hum Genet 67:1555–1562, 2000.

25

Immune Deficiency in Metabolic Diseases

Jintanat Ananworanich and William T. Shearer

INTRODUCTION

A large majority of immune deficiency–related infections occur in patients with secondary immunodeficiency. Patients with certain metabolic disorders exhibit immune dysfunction resulting in predisposition to infection and autoimmunity. The main goal of management of metabolic disorder–related immune defects is not directed at the specific immune dysfunction but at the primary metabolic disorder, which is beyond the scope of this volume.

820

In this chapter we discuss the pathogenesis and nature of the immune defects associated with six disorders: nephrotic syndrome, inflammatory bowel disease, protein-losing enteropathy, diabetes mellitus, uremia and dialysis, and cirrhosis (Table 25-1). We also outline treatment directed at the associated immune defects. In three of the disorders, defects of innate immunity predominate, and in three others, defects of adaptive immunity predominate (Fig. 25-1). Other metabolic disorders of clear-cut genetic origin are covered in Chapter 24.

Each of the metabolic disorders described has diverse immune defects and clinical manifestations. The evaluation of such patients depends on the nature of the infection, the presence of associated autoimmunity, and the most likely immune dysfunction that occurs in that disorder. For instance, inflammatory bowel disease is associated with cell-mediated immune defects. Patients with uremia, patients on dialysis treatment, and patients with diabetes mellitus generally have phagocytic cell dysfunction, whereas patients with alcoholic cirrhosis may have complement deficiencies.

As in the primary immunodeficiencies, patients with T-cell dysfunction are predisposed to infections with intracellular organisms such as viruses, mycobacteria, and fungi. Patients with antibody (B-cell) defects have recurrent and invasive bacterial infections, including respiratory infections. Patients with phagocytic cell defects have severe fungal and bacterial infections, including abscesses and pyodermas. Patients with early-component complement (C2–C4) defects may have rheumatologic disorders and bacterial infections, whereas patients with late-component complement defects (C5–C9) have recurrent *Neisseria* infections.

NEPHROTIC SYNDROME

Predisposition to Infection

Nephrotic syndrome (NS) patients have a predisposition to infection, especially invasive pneumococcal disease (Janoff and Rubins, 1997) (see Chapter 38). Volhard and Fahr (1914) first reported pneumococcal peritonitis as a fatal complication of the nephrotic syndrome. Subsequently, other pneumococcal infections were noted in the nephrotic syndrome; this suggests a unique susceptibility not found in other patients with cavity was due to increased pressure in the lymphatic vessels.

Chylous ascites, sometimes occurring in association with peripheral lymphedema, has often been reported with hypoproteinemia (Rosen et al., 1962). Pomeranz and Waldmann (1963) demonstrated systemic lymphatic abnormalities by lymphangiography in four patients with intestinal lymphangiectasia, including one child with congenital chylous ascites.

Etiology

Protein-losing enteropathy can result from gastrointestinal anatomic defects, cardiac defects, autoimmunity, allergies, malignancies, and infections (see Table 25-2). *Helicobacter pylori* and CMV are among the infectious causes of intestinal protein loss (Nakase et al., 1998; Yoshikawa et al., 1999).

Protein loss occurs most commonly in patients with gastrointestinal surface abnormalities, such as regional enteritis, ulcerative colitis (Schwartz and Jarnum, 1959; Steinfeld et al., 1960), sprue (London et al., 1961; Parkins, 1960), and celiac disease (Rotem and Czerniak, 1964). Milk allergy has been incriminated as a cause of protein-losing enteropathy in infants (Waldmann et al., 1967). Edema, hypoalbuminemia, and hypogammaglobulinemia were associated with growth retardation, iron deficiency anemia, and eosinophilia. In three patients studied, significant improvement was noted on a milk-free diet and a return of symptoms when milk was reintroduced. Transient hypoproteinemia and edema have followed gastroenteritis in a few children (Degnan, 1957; Herskovic et al., 1968; Pitman et al., 1964; Waldmann et al., 1961).

Gastrointestinal protein loss also may occur as the result of lymphatic obstruction. The concurrent loss of lymphocytes into the intestinal tract and subsequent lymphopenia distinguish this mechanism of protein loss from the enteropathy caused by surface abnormalities. Direct obstruction of the intestinal lymphatics may occur in entities such as intestinal lymphangiectasia, neoplasia, and regional enteritis.

Intestinal lymphangiectasia is a congenital disorder with intestinal lymphatic obstruction and loss of lymph contents resulting in hypogammaglobulinemia and lymphopenia. Significant reduction of CD4$^+$CD45RA$^+$ (naïve) T cells has recently been documented (Fuss et al., 1998).

Allergic colitis is the most common cause of noninfective colitis in infancy. Low levels of IgA, IgG2, and IgG4, which have been documented in more than 50% of patients, may contribute to their higher prevalence of upper respiratory tract infections (Ojuawo et al., 1997).

Ménétrier's disease is characterized by hypertrophic gastritis, protein-losing enteropathy, hypoproteinemia, and edema. This disorder, when it occurs in children, is often a result of CMV infection (Ricci et al., 1996).

Familial enteropathy with villous edema and IgG2 subclass deficiency is an unusual syndrome of episodic life-threatening secretory diarrhea and characteristic histologic abnormalities of the jejunum. Almost all patients have IgG2 subclass deficiency, and half of these have subnormal total IgG levels. The immunoglobulin level is lowest during an acute diarrheal attack. Oral immune globulin therapy possibly alleviates symptoms. Despite low IgG2, upper respiratory tract infections are not problematic in these patients. The likely inheritance pattern is autosomal dominant with variable penetrance (Smith et al., 1994).

Indirect lymphatic obstruction occurs as the result of high venous pressure on lymphatic flow, as occurs in patients with congestive *heart failure*, especially in those with constrictive pericarditis. A few cases of constrictive pericarditis in children have been reported (Davidson et al., 1961; Nelson et al., 1975; Plauth et al., 1964). Patients with other causes of congestive heart failure, such as congenital heart disease and rheumatic fever, also may have excessive gastrointestinal protein losses (Waldmann, 1966).

Cardiac surgery can result in hypoproteinemia, elevated stool α_1-antitrypsin levels and lymphopenia but normal lymphoproliferative responses. This is thought to be from intestinal hemodynamic changes during the procedure (Koch et al., 1999).

Several *vasculitic* conditions, including systemic lupus erythematosus (SLE) (Pelletier et al., 1992), Henoch-Schönlein purpura (Kobayashi et al., 1991), and Churg-Strauss syndrome (Malaval et al., 1993), have been described as causes of gastrointestinal protein loss. Intestinal protein loss in SLE most likely occurs as the result of increased microvascular permeability (Perednia and Curosh, 1990).

Immunologic Defects

Lymphopenia has been reported in patients with intestinal lymphangiectasia and the protein-losing enteropathy of regional enteritis, Whipple's disease, and constrictive pericarditis (Strober et al., 1967). Normal lymphocyte counts are reported in protein-losing enteropathies associated with sprue, gluten enteropathy, allergic enteropathy, and variable agammaglobulinemia. The lymphopenic enteropathies are secondary to structural abnormalities of the lymphatic channels, such as intestinal lymphangiectasia (Strober et al., 1967; Weiden et al., 1972). Diminished skin test responses to purified protein derivative (PPD), mumps, *Trichophyton*, and *C. albicans*; negative reactions to dinitrochlorobenzene; and prolonged skin allograft retention were related to lymphopenia. Although immunoglobulin levels were depressed, the antibody responses were normal. Despite these defects, significant infections occurred in only two children younger than 10 years; furunculosis, pneumonia, and peritonitis associated with severe debilitation developed.

In a child with intestinal lymphangiectasia with lymphopenia and impaired cutaneous delayed hypersensitivity, the lymphoproliferative response to phytohemagglutinin (PHA) was normal, suggesting a quantitative defect of lymphocyte function (McGuigan et al., 1968).

Weiden and colleagues (1972) found impaired lympho-proliferative responses to mitogens, antigens, and allo-geneic cells in patients with intestinal lymphangiectasia. Lymphocytes from chylous effusions were normal, sug-gesting GI loss of recirculating long-lived lymphocytes.

Illustrative examples of gastrointestinal anomalies producing combined immunodeficiency were reported by Fawcett and associates (1986), who described severe B- and T-cell defects in two children originally thought to have food allergy. These children suffered from a mal-rotation of the small intestine and a cavernous heman-gioma of the mid-jejunum, respectively. Following surgical correction, there was gradual restoration of both B- and T-cell immunity (Fig. 25-2). In addition to normalizing serum IgG and mitogen reactivity, the num-ber of T lymphocytes and the inverted CD4/CD8 ratios became normal. These two cases emphasize the impor-tance of a careful immune evaluation in children with diarrhea when a food allergy is suspected.

Management

Irrespective of the etiology, intestinal protein loss invari-ably results in hypogammaglobulinemia. Nevertheless, the ability to produce functional antibodies is usually preserved and increased susceptibility to infections is uncommon. Use of intravenous immunoglobulin (IVIG) will raise the IgG level only transiently. Stiehm and col-leagues (1998) have used subcutaneous immunoglobu-lin at weekly intervals as a means to stabilize the IgG levels. However, correction of the primary defect and not intravenous immunoglobulin replacement will

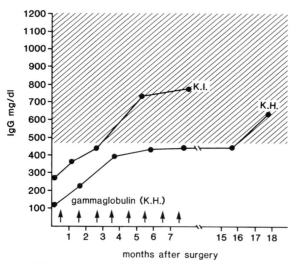

Figure 25-2 · Serum IgG concentrations in two patients with anatomic intestinal abnormalities corrected by surgery. Patient K. H. had a malrotation of the small bowel, and patient K. I. had a cav-ernous hemangioma of the mid-jejunum. Patient K. H. received intra-venous gamma globulin replacement therapy for several months until IgG levels were self-sustained. The shaded area represents the 95% confidence range for age-matched controls. (From Fawcett WA IV et al. Immunodeficiency secondary to structural intestinal defects. Malrotation of the small bowel and cavernous hemangioma of the jejunum. Am J Dis Child 140:169–172, 1986.)

reverse the low immunoglobulin levels (see Fig. 25-2). Live viral vaccine should not be administered in patients with significant antibody deficiency or T-cell defects. Blood products should be from CMV-negative donors and irradiated prior to use.

INFLAMMATORY BOWEL DISEASE

Etiology

The causes of inflammatory bowel disease (IBD), Crohn's disease (CD), and ulcerative colitis remain an enigma (see Chapter 34). Measles and mumps infections in early childhood may be associated with increased risk for IBD (Montgomery et al., 1999). A link between measles vaccination during infancy and subsequent development of CD has been suggested (Feeney et al., 1997; Thompson et al., 1995). The presence of her-pesvirus and Epstein-Barr virus (EBV) in affected gas-trointestinal mucosa suggest that a relationship between viral infection and IBD may exist (Ruther et al., 1998; Yanai et al., 1999). The lack of colitis in mice raised in a germ-free environment supports this notion. Furthermore, Th1 cells reactive with bacterial antigens from mice with colitis cause disease when transferred to immunodeficient hosts (Groux and Fiona, 1999).

Dysregulation of cell-mediated immune responses that can damage the gastrointestinal tract can be found in both humans and mice. A predominance of Th1 cells in Crohn's disease and Th2 cells in ulcerative colitis has been reported (McClane and Roombeau, 1999). IL-10 has been shown to have an immunoregulatory role in controlling gastrointestinal inflammation, and IL-10–deficient mice do not develop colitis. Following PHA stimulation, IL-2 production from peripheral blood mononuclear cells (PBMC) of ulcerative colitis patients was significantly increased, whereas their lam-ina propria mononuclear cells showed the reverse. By contrast, Crohn's patients had significant IL-2 produc-tion from these cells in response to PHA (Gurbindo et al., 1993). Adhesion molecules on colonic T cells from both diseases are different as well (Elewaut et al., 1998). These findings suggest unique immunopathogenetic mechanisms for each type of IBD.

Predisposition to Infection

Patients with ulcerative colitis have increased suscepti-bility to infection aggravated by their use of immuno-suppressive medications. Patients with IBD can have gastrointestinal infections from opportunistic organisms such as cytomegalovirus, which is not uncommon in refractory IBD disease (Ojanguren and Gassull, 1999; Rachima et al., 1998; Vega et al., 1999). Abscesses of abdominal and retroperitoneal cavities and osteomyelitis can occur as a result of fistulas and extravasation of enteric organisms (Murata et al., 1999). Life-threatening septic thrombophlebitis of the portal vein has been reported in Crohn's disease (Baddley et al., 1999).

Immunologic Defects

Impaired lymphoproliferation to PHA, anti-CD28, and anti-CD3 have been documented in IBD (Perez-Machado et al., 1999; Roman et al., 1996). Correction of abnormal LPRs can be accomplished with exogenous IL-2 and phorbol ester, suggesting a defect in the IL-2–dependent and early signaling pathway (Manzano et al., 1994). Depressed LPRs to several recall antigens are noted in Crohn's disease (D'Haens et al., 1994). Serum from patients with Crohn's disease inhibits the ability of normal PBMC to respond to mitogens (Iwao et al., 1992). The numbers of CD4+ T cells are typically normal, but the numbers of CD8+ T cells can be variable. Patients with IBD tend to have more activated cells, including CD3+ CD25+ (IL-2R) T cells and CD19+ CD78+ B cells (Senju et al., 1991).

Serum immunoglobulins are usually elevated, especially IgG1 in ulcerative colitis and IgG2 in Crohn's disease (Gouni-Berthold, et al., 1999; Gryboski and Buie, 1994). However, low IgG2 and high IgM has been reported in a patient with Crohn's disease (Korber et al., 1998). IgA level appears to correlate positively with disease activity in Crohn's disease and has an inverse relationship in ulcerative colitis activity (Philipsen et al., 1995). Decreased tetanus-specific antibody-producing B cells following in vivo immunization has been shown (Stevens et al., 1985).

Associated Autoimmune Disorders

Persons with IBD are at risk for other autoimmune diseases. Primary Sjögren's syndrome has been reported in a young man with ulcerative colitis and IgA deficiency; the latter has been associated with primary Sjögren's syndrome in the absence of ulcerative colitis (Steuer et al., 1996). In ulcerative colitis, antigliadin antibodies of both IgA and IgG types are found in one third of patients (Kull et al., 1999); however, the occurrence of celiac disease is not common. Celiac disease is especially rare in children with ulcerative colitis (Day and Abbott, 1999).

The presence of antineutrophil cytoplasmic antibodies has been documented in 41% to 73% and 2% to 14% of ulcerative colitis and Crohn's disease patients, respectively (Olives et al., 1997; Papo et al., 1996). The significance of these antibodies remains uncertain because they do not correlate with IBD activity (Frenzer et al., 1998). IgG and IgA anti-*Saccharomyces cerevisiae* antibodies (ASCA) have been used as serologic markers with a high specificity for Crohn's disease. ASCA are found in 50% to 80% of patients with Crohn's disease but only in less than 10% of ulcerative colitis patients and 5% of healthy control subjects (Nielsen et al., 2000).

Management

No specific immunization recommendations have been made for patients with IBD. However, patients who are on immunosuppressive medications should not receive live viral vaccine and blood products should be from CMV-negative donors and irradiated prior to use. The use of antibodies to intracellular adhesion molecule-1 (ICAM-1) and TNF-α (infliximab), and the use of recombinant IL-10 have been effective in some IBD patients (Heresbach et al., 1999). However, treatment with infliximab has been associated with reactivation of tuberculosis, warranting pretreatment screening for tuberculosis (Keane et al., 2001).

CIRRHOSIS

Predisposition to Infection

Patients with cirrhosis have a predisposition to infection, particularly bacterial infections. Bacteremia, spontaneous bacterial peritonitis, and urinary tract and respiratory tract infections are the most common (Navasa et al., 1999). Twenty percent of hospitalized patients with cirrhosis develop infection; of these, 39% and 32% have generalized infection and spontaneous bacterial peritonitis, respectively (Deschenes and Villeneuve, 1999). The risk of spontaneous bacterial peritonitis is higher in patients with low ascitic fluid protein levels (Guarner et al., 1999). Gram-negative bacterial infections are common in cirrhotic patients with gastrointestinal bleeding (Bernard et al., 1999).

Immunologic Defects

Impaired phagocytic, complement, and cell-mediated immune defects have been reported in patients with cirrhosis, similar to other patients with nutritional disorders. Frank protein-calorie malnutrition is not uncommon. Poor nutrition, increased protein catabolism, and increased fat oxidation are contributing factors. Alcohol ingestion further increases protein catabolism, placing these patients at greater risk for malnutrition-related immune dysfunction (Hirsch et al., 1999). Patients with alcoholic cirrhosis have low serum C3 and C4 levels that correlate with the severity of liver disease. Decreased C3 and defects of the alternative pathway are associated with a high incidence of infections and increased mortality (Homann et al., 1997). Defective neutrophil phagocytosis and chemotaxis have also been reported (Garcia-Gonzalez et al., 1993).

Cutaneous anergy is not uncommon. Impaired LPRs to PHA is documented in 60% of patients. However, there is normal LPR to phorbol esters, anti-CD2, CD3-TCR, CD28, and exogenous IL-2 and IL-4 (Giron-Gonzalez et al., 1994; Schirren et al., 1997; Vega Robledo et al., 1994).

Management

The use of quinolone antibiotics during gastrointestinal bleeding episodes results in a lower incidence of spontaneous bacterial peritonitis or bacteremia and a higher survival rate (Bernard et al., 1999). Prophylactic perioperative antibiotics for procedures such as transjugular intrahepatic portosystemic shunt reduces the incidence of bacterial infections (Gulberg et al., 1999). Granulocyte-macrophage colony-stimulating factor improves phagocytosis and chemotaxis in patients cirrhosis with and without peritonitis (Garcia-Gonzalez et al., 1993).

Typically, live viral vaccines and nonirradiated blood products can be given to cirrhotic patients. However, in cases with significant cell-mediated immune defects, avoidance of these measures may be indicated.

REFERENCES

Abrutyn E, Solomons NW, St Clair L, MacGregor RR, Root RK. Granulocyte function in patients with chronic renal failure: surface adherence, phagocytosis, and bactericidal activity in vitro. J Infect Dis 135:1–8, 1977.

Al-Bander HA, Martin VI, Kaysen GA. Plasma IgG pool is not defended from urinary loss in nephrotic syndrome. Am J Physiol 262:F333–F337, 1992.

Alexander RE. Routine prophylactic antibiotic use in diabetic dental patients. J Calif Dent Assoc 27:611–618, 1999.

Alexiewicz JM, Smogorzewski M, Fadda GZ, Massry SG. Impaired phagocytosis in dialysis patients: studies on mechanisms. Am J Nephrol 11:102–111, 1991.

American Academy of Pediatrics. Immunization in special clinical circumstances. In Pickering LK, ed. 2000 Red Book: Report of the Committee on Infectious Diseases, ed 25. Elk Grove Village, IL, American Academy of Pediatrics, 2000a, 56–62.

American Academy of Pediatrics. Hepatitis B. In Pickering LK, ed. 2000 Red Book: Report of the Committee on Infectious Diseases, ed 25. Elk Grove Village, IL, American Academy of Pediatrics, 2000b, 289–302.

Anderson DC, York TL, Rose G, Smith CW. Assessment of serum factor B, serum opsonins, granulocyte chemotaxis, and infection in nephrotic syndrome of children. J Infect Dis 140:1–11, 1979.

Arneil GC, Lam CN. Long-term assessment of steroid therapy in childhood nephrosis. Lancet 2:819–821, 1966.

Avanzini MA, Vitali L, d'Annunzio G, De Amici M, Strigazzi C, Alibrandi A, Lorini R. Enhancement of soluble CD23 serum levels and cell-surface CD23-expression in subjects at increased risk of type 1 diabetes mellitus and in diabetic patients. Diabet Med 15:320–326, 1998.

Baddley JW, Singh D, Correa P, Persich NJ. Crohn's disease presenting as septic thrombophlebitis of the portal vein (pylephlebitis): case report and review of the literature. Am J Gastroenterol 94:847–849, 1999.

Bagdade JD, Root RK, Bulger RJ. Impaired leukocyte function in patients with poorly controlled diabetes. Diabetes 23:9–15, 1974.

Bagdade JD. Infection in diabetes, predisposing factors. Postgrad Med 59:160–164, 1976.

Barandun S, Aebersold J, Bianchi R, Kluthe R, Muralt GV, Poretti G, Riva G. "Protein diarrhoe": Zugleich ein Beitrag zur Frage der sogenannten essentiellen Hypoproteinaimie. Schweiz Med Wschr 90:1458–1467, 1960.

Barth WF, Wochner RD, Waldmann TA, Fahey JL. Metabolism of human gamma macroglobulins. J Clin Invest 43:1036–1048, 1964.

Bernard B, Grange JD, Khac EN, Amiot X, Opolon P, Poynard T. Antibiotic prophylaxis for the prevention of bacterial infections in cirrhotic patients with gastrointestinal bleeding: a meta-analysis. Hepatology 29:1655–1661, 1999.

Black MM, De Chabon A. Reactivity of lymph nodes in azotaemic patients. Am J Clin Pathol 41:503–508, 1964.

Bloembergen WE, Port FK. Epidemiological perspective on infections in chronic dialysis patients. Adv Ren Replace Ther 3:201–207, 1996.

Bongiovanni AM, Wolman IJ. Plasma protein fractionation in pediatrics: a review of its present status. Am J Med Sci 218:700–714, 1949.

Bradley JR, Evans DB, Calne RY. Long-term survival in haemodialysis patients. Lancet 1:295–296, 1987.

Brayton RG, Stokes PE, Schwartz MS, Louria DB. Effect of alcohol and various diseases on leukocyte mobilization, phagocytosis and intracellular bacterial killing. N Engl J Med 282:123–128, 1970.

Bridges JM, Nelson SD, McGeown MG. Evaluation of lymphocyte transfer test in normal and uremic subjects. Lancet 1:581–584, 1964.

Bybee JD, Rogers DE. The phagocytic activity of polymorphonuclear leukocytes obtained from patients with diabetes mellitus. J Lab Clin Med 64:1–13, 1964.

Byron PR, Mallick NP, Taylor G. Immune potential in human uraemia. 1. Relationship of glomerular filtration rate to depression of immune potential. J Clin Pathol 29:765–769, 1976.

Carpenter CB, Glassock RJ, Gleason R, Corson JM, Merrill JP. The application of the normal lymphocyte transfer reaction to histocompatibility testing in man. J Clin Invest 45:1452–1466, 1966.

Chang HR, Bistrian B. The role of cytokines in the catabolic consequences of infection and injury. J Parenter Enter Nutr 22:156–166, 1998.

Citrin Y, Sterling K, Halsted JA. The mechanism of hypoproteinemia associated with giant hypertrophy of the gastric mucosa. N Engl J Med 257:906–912, 1957.

Cohen G, Haag-Weber M, Horl WH. Immune dysfunction in uremia. Kidney Int Suppl 62:S79–S82, 1997.

Cohen G, Rudnicki M, Horl WH. Isolation of modified ubiquitin as a neutrophil chemotaxis inhibitor from uremic patients. J Am Soc Nephrol 9:451–456, 1998.

Cortona L, Avanzini MA, Martinetti M, Lorini R. Transient IgG subclasses deficiencies in newly diagnosed diabetic children. Eur J Pediatr 151:179–182, 1992.

Couser WG. Pathogenesis of glomerular damage in glomerulonephritis. Nephrol Dial Transplant 13:10–15, 1998.

Curtis JR, Wing AJ, Coleman JC. Bacillus cereus bacteraemia: a complication of intermittent haemodialysis. Lancet 1:136–138, 1967.

Daichou Y, Kurushige S, Hashimoto S, Suzuki S. Characteristic cytokine products of Th1 and Th2 cells in hemodialysis patients. Nephron 83:237–245, 1999.

Dammin GJ, Couch NP, Murray JE. Prolonged survival of skin homografts in uremic patients. Ann NY Acad Sci 64:967–976, 1957.

Daniel V, Trautmann Y, Konrad M, Nayir A, Scharer K. T-lymphocytes populations, cytokines and other growth factors in serum and urine of children with idiopathic nephrotic syndrome. Clin Nephrol 47:289–297, 1997.

Davidson JD, Waldmann TA, Goodman DS, Gordon JRS. Protein-losing gastroenteropathy in congestive heart failure. Lancet 1:899–902, 1961.

Day AS, Abbott GD. Simultaneous presentation of coeliac disease and ulcerative colitis in a child. J Paediatr Child Health 35:204–206, 1999.

Degnan TJ. Idiopathic hypoproteinemia. J Pediatr 51:448–452, 1957.

Delamaire M, Maugendre D, Moreno M, Le Goff MC, Allannic H, Genetet B. Impaired leucocyte functions in diabetic patients. Diabet Med 14:29–34, 1997.

Descamps-Latscha B, Chatenoud L. T cells and B cells in chronic renal failure. Semin Nephrol 16:183–191, 1996.

Deschenes M, Villeneuve JP. Risk factors for the development of bacterial infections in hospitalized patients with cirrhosis. Am J Gastroenterol 94:2193–2197, 1999.

D'Haens G, Hiele M, Rutgeerts P, Geboes K, Ceuppens JL. Depressed T cell reactivity to recall antigens in Crohn's disease before and after surgical resection. Gut 35:1728–1733, 1994.

Dziatkowiak H, Kowalska M, Denys A. Phagocytic and bactericidal activity of granulocytes in diabetic children. Diabetes 31:1041–1043, 1982.

Elewaut D, De Keyser F, Cuvelier C, Lazarovits AI, Mielants H, Verbruggen G, Sas S, Devos M, Veys EM. Distinctive activated cellular subsets in colon from patients with Crohn's disease and ulcerative colitis. Scand J Gastroenterol 33:743–748, 1998.

el-Reshaid K, al-Mufti S, Johny KV, Sugathan TN. Comparison of two immunization schedules with recombinant hepatitis B vaccine and natural immunity acquired by hepatitis B infection in dialysis patient. Vaccine 12:223–234, 1994.

Estevez ME, Voyer LE, Craviotto RJ, Ballart IJ, Goicoa MA, Palacios F, Quadri B, Corti S, Wainstein RE, Sen L. Dysfunction of the monocyte-macrophage system in the idiopathic minimal change nephrotic syndrome. Acta Paediatr Scand 78:87–93, 1989.

Ewigs S, Torres A. Severe community-acquired pneumonia. Clin Chest Med 20:575–587, 1999.

Fabrizi F, Andrulli S, Bacchini G, Corti M, Locatelli F. Intradermal versus intramuscular hepatitis B re-vaccination in non-responsive chronic dialysis patients: a prospective randomized study with cost-effectiveness evaluation. Nephrol Dial Transplant 12:1204–1211, 1997.

Farid NR. Immunologic aspects of diabetes mellitus. In Chandra RK, ed. Nutrition in Immunology. New York, Alan R. Liss, 1988, 269–313.

Fawcett WA IV, Ferry GD, Gorin LJ, Rosenblatt HM, Brown BS, Shearer WT. Immunodeficiency secondary to structural intestinal defects: malrotation of the small bowel and cavernous hemangioma of the jejunum. Am J Dis Child 140:169–172, 1986.

Feeney M, Clegg A, Winwood P, Snook J. A case control study of measles vaccination and inflammatory bowel disease. Lancet 350:764–766, 1997.

Frenzer A, Fierz W, Rundler E, Hammer B, Binek J. Atypical, cytoplasmic and perinuclear anti-neutrophil cytoplasmic antibodies in patients with inflammatory bowel disease. Gastroenterol Hepatol 13:950–954, 1998.

Fuchshuber A, Khunemund O, Keuth B, Lutticken R, Michalk D, Querfeld U. Pneumococcal vaccine in children and young adults with chronic renal disease. Nephrol Dial Transplant 11:468–473, 1996.

Furth SL, Neu AM, Case BM, Lederman HM, Steinhoff M, Fivush B. Pneumococcal polysaccharide vaccine in children with chronic renal disease: a prospective study of antibody response and duration. J Pediatr 128:99–101, 1996.

Furnary AP, Zerr KJ, Grunkemeier GL, Starr A. Continuous intravenous insulin infusion reduces the incidence of deep sternal wound infection in diabetic patients after cardiac surgical procedures. Ann Thorac Surg 67:352–360, 1999.

Fuss IJ, Strober W, Cuccherini BA, Pearlstein GR, Bossuyt X, Brown M, Fleisher TA, Horgan K. Intestinal lymphagiectasia, a disease characterized by selective loss of naive CD45RA+ lymphocytes into gastrointestinal tract. Eur J Immunol 28:4275–4285, 1998.

Gallacher SJ, Thomson G, Fraser WD, Fisher BM, Gemmell CG, MacCuish AC. Neutrophil bactericidal function in diabetes mellitus: evidence for association with blood glucose control. Diabet Med 12:916–920, 1995.

Garcia-Gonzalez M, Boixeda D, Herrero D, Burgaleta C. Effect of granulocyte-macrophage colony-stimulating factor on leukocyte function in cirrhosis. Gastroenterology 105:527–531, 1993.

Garcia-Leoni ME, Martin-Scapa C, Rodeno P, Valderrabano F, Moreno S, Bouza E. High incidence of tuberculosis in renal patients. Eur J Clin Microbiol Infect Dis 9:283–285, 1990.

Gascon A, Orfao A, Lerma JL, Cindad J, Lopez A, Hernandez MD, Tabernero JM. Antigen phenotype and cytotoxic activity of natural killer cells in hemodialysis patients. Am J Kidney Dis 27:373–379, 1996.

Geerlings SE, Hoepelman AI. Immune dysfunction in patients with diabetes mellitus (DM). Federation of European Microbiological Societies (FEMS) Immunol Med Microbiol 26:259–265, 1999.

Giangiacomo J, Cleary TG, Cole BR, Hoffsten P, Robson AM. Serum immunoglobulins in the nephrotic syndrome: a possible cause of minimal-change nephrotic syndrome. N Engl J Med 293:8–12, 1975.

Giron-Gonzalez JA, Alvarez-Mon M, Menendez-Caro JL, Manzano L, Abreu L, Yebra M, Durantez-Martinez A. T lymphocytes from alcoholic cirrhosis patients show normal interleukin-2 production but a defective proliferative response to polyclonal mitogens. Am J Gastroenterol 89:767–773, 1994.

Goldblum SE, Reed WP. Host defenses and immunologic alterations associated with chronic hemodialysis. Ann Intern Med 93:597–613, 1980.

Gordon RS. Exudative enteropathy. Abnormal permeability of the gastrointestinal tract demonstrable with labelled polyvinylpyrolidone. Lancet 1:325–326, 1959.

Gorensek MJ, Lebel MH, Nelson JD. Peritonitis in children with nephrotic syndrome. Pediatrics 81:849–856, 1988.

Gouni-Berthold I, Baumeister B, Berthold HK, Schmidt C. Immunoglobulins and IgG subclasses in patients with inflammatory bowel disease. Hepatogastroenterol 46:1720–1723, 1999.

Groshong T, Mendelson L, Mendoza S, Bazaral M, Hamburger R, Tune B. Serum IgE in patients with minimal-change nephrotic syndrome. J Pediatr 83:767–771, 1973.

Groux H, Powrie F. Regulatory T cells and inflammatory bowel disease. Immunol Today 20:442–446, 1999.

Gryboski JD, Buie T. Immunoglobulin studies in children with inflammatory bowel disease. Ann Allergy 72:525–527, 1994.

Guarner C, Sola R, Soriano G, Andreu M, Novella MT, Vila MC, Sabat M, Coll S, Ortiz J, Gomez C, Balanzo J. Risk of a first community-acquired spontaneous bacterial peritonitis in cirrhotics with low ascitic fluid protein levels. Gastroenterol 117:414–419, 1999.

Gulberg V, Deibert P, Ochs A, Rossle M, Gerbes AL. Prevention of infectious complications after transjugular intrahepatic portosystemic shunt in cirrhotic patients with a single dose of ceftriaxone. Hepatogastroenterology 46:1126–1130, 1999.

Gurbindo C, Sabbah S, Menzes J, Justinich C, Marchand R, Seidman EG. Interleukin-2 production in pediatric inflammatory bowel disease: evidence for dissimilar mononuclear cell function in Crohn's disease and ulcerative colitis. J Pediatr Gastroenterol Nutr 17:247–254, 1993.

Haag-Weber M, Horl WH. The immune system in uremia and during its treatment. New Horiz 3:669–679, 1995.

Haag-Weber M, Horl WH. Dysfunction of polymorphonuclear leukocytes in uremia. Semin Nephrol 16:192-201, 1996.

Heresbach D, Semana G, Gosselin M, Bretagne MG. An immunomodulation strategy targeted towards immunocompetent cells or cytokines in inflammatory bowel diseases (IBD). Eur Cytokine Netw 10:7–15, 1999.

Herskovic T, Spiro HM, Gryboski JD. Acute transient gastrointestinal protein loss. Pediatrics 41:818–821, 1968.

Hill HR, Sauls HS, Dettloff JL, Quie PG. Impaired leukotactic responsiveness in patients with juvenile diabetes mellitus. Clin Immunol Immunopathol 2:395–403, 1974.

Hindman SH, Favero MS, Carson LA, Petersen NJ, Schonberger LB, Solano JT. Pyogenic reactions during haemodialysis caused by extramural endotoxin. Lancet 2:732–734, 1975.

Hirsch S, Maza M, Gattas V, Barrera G, Petermann M, Gotteland M, Munoz C, Lopez M, Bunout D. Nutritional support in alcoholic cirrhotic patients improves host defences. J Am Coll Nutr 18:434–441, 1999.

Hisano S, Miyazaki C, Hatae K, Kaku Y, Yamane I, Ueda K, Okamna S. Immune status of children on continuous ambulatory peritoneal dialysis. Pediatr Nephrol 6:179–181, 1992.

Hodes H (quoted by Janeway CA). In Metcoff J, ed. Proceedings of the Fourth Annual Conference on the Nephrotic Syndrome. New York, National Kidney Disease Foundation, 1952, 46.

Hodges R. In Metcoff J, ed. Proceedings of the Sixth Annual Conference on the Nephrotic Syndrome. Cleveland, National Kidney Disease Foundation, 1954, 265–271.

Homann C, Varming K, Hogasen K, Mollness TE, Graudal N, Thomsen AC, Garred P. Acquired C3 deficiency in patients with alcoholic cirrhosis predisposes to infection and increased mortality. Gut 40:544–549, 1997.

Hoy WE, Cestero RV, Freeman RB. Deficiency of T and B lymphocytes in uremic subjects and partial improvement with maintenance hemodialysis. Nephron 20:182–188, 1978.

Huber H, Pastner D, Dittrich P, Braunsteiner H. In vitro reactivity of human lymphocytes in uraemia—a comparison with the impairment of delayed hypersensitivity. Clin Exp Immunol 5:75–82, 1969.

Hulton SA, Shah V, Byrne MR, Morgan G, Barratt TM, Dillon MJ. Lymphocyte subpopulations, interleukin-2 and interleukin-2 receptor expression in childhood nephrotic syndrome. Pediatr Nephrol 8:135–139, 1994.

Hume DM, Merrill JP, Miller BS, Thorn GW. Experiences with renal homotransplantation in the human: report of nine cases. J Clin Invest 34:327–332, 1955.

Ingelfinger JR, Link DA, Davis AE, Grupe WE. Serum immunoglobulins in idiopathic minimal change nephrotic syndrome. N Engl J Med 294:50–51, 1976.

Iwao Y, Hibi T, Watanabe M, Takaishi H, Hosoda Y, Hayashi A, Ohara M, Ogata H, Aiso S, Toda K, et al. The mechanism of action of serum immunosuppressive factor in Crohn's disease: it blocks the growth of mitogen-stimulated lymphocytes in early G1 phase through an inhibition of transferrin receptor expression. J Clin Lab Immunol 38:15–27, 1992.

Jaber BL, Balakrishnan VS, Cendoroglo MN, Perianayagam MC, King AJ, Pereira BJG. Modulation of neutrophil apoptosis by uremic plasma during hemodialysis. Blood Purif 16:325–335, 1998.

Janoff EN, Rubins JB. Invasive pneumococcal disease in the immunocompromised host. Microb Drug Resist 3:215–232, 1997.

Jarnum S, Petersen VP. Protein-losing eneropathy. Lancet 1:417–421, 1961.

Johnston MF, Slavin RG. Mechanism of inhibition of adoptive transfer of tuberculin sensitivity in acute uremia. J Lab Clin Med 87:457–461, 1976.

Joshi N, Caputo GM, Weitekamp MR, Karchmer AW. Infections in patients with diabetes mellitus. N Engl J Med 341:1906–1912, 1999.

Kass EH. Hormones and host resistance to infection. Bacteriol Rev 24:177–195, 1960.

Keane J, Gershon S, Wise RP, Mirabile-Levens E, Kasznica J, Schwieterman WD, Siegel JN, Braun MM. Tuberculosis associated with infliximab, a tumor necrosis factor alpha-neutralizing agent. N Engl J Med 345:1098–1104, 2001.

Kelley VC, Ziegler MR, Doeden D, McQuarrie L. Labeled methionine as an indicator of protein formation in children with lipoid nephrosis. Proc Soc Exp Biol Med 75:153–155, 1950.

Kim MS, Stablein D, Harmon WE. Renal transplantation in children with congenital nephrotic syndrome: a report of the North American Pediatric Renal Transplant Cooperative Study (NAPRTCS). Pediatr Transplant 2:305–308, 1998.

Kirkpatrick CH, Wilson WEC, Talmage DW. Immunologic studies in human organ transplantation: I. Observation and characterization of suppressed cutaneous reactivity in uremia. J Exp Med 119:727–742, 1964.

Krensky AM, Ingelfinger JR, Grupe WE. Peritonitis in childhood nephrotic syndrome: 1970–1980. Am J Dis Child 136:732–736, 1982.

Kobayashi K, Manaka K, Ebihara Y, Funazu Y, Ueno M, Funazu K, Mizuno Y, Takeuchi M, Serizawa H, Miura S. A case of Schönlein-Henoch purpura complicated with protein-losing enteropathy and hyperamylasemia. Nippon Shokakibyo Gakkai Zasshi 88:2171–2176, 1991.

Koch A, Hofbeck M, Feistel H, Buheitel G, Singer H. Circumscribed intestinal protein loss with deficiency in CD4+ lymphocytes after the Fontan procedure. Eur J Pediatr 158:847–850, 1999.

Korber J, Kottgen E, Renz H. A case of Crohn's disease with increased CD8 T-cell activation and remission during therapy with intravenous immunoglobulin. Scand J Gastroenterol 33:1113–1117, 1998.

Kull K, Uibo O, Salupere R, Metskula K, Uibo R. High frequency of antigliadin antibodies and absence of antireticulin and antiendomysium antibodies in patients with ulcerative colitis. J Gastroenterol 34:61–65, 1999.

Kunin CM, Schwartz R, Yaffe S, Knapp J, Fellers FX, Janeway CA, Finland M. Antibody response to influenza virus vaccine in children with nephrosis: effect of cortisone. Pediatrics 23:54–62, 1959.

Kurz P, Kohler H, Meuer S, Hutteroth T, Meyer zum Buschenfelde KH. Impaired cellular immune response in chronic renal failure: evidence for a T cell defect. Kidney Int 29:1209–1214, 1986.

Lee HJ, Kang JH, Henrichsen J, Konradsen HB, Jang SH, Shin HY, Ahn HS, Choi Y, Hessel L, Nam SW. Immunogenicity and safety of a 23-valent pneumococcal polysaccharide vaccine in healthy children and in children at increased risk of pneumococcal infection. Vaccine 13:1533–1538, 1995.

Leutscher JA Jr, Deming QB. Treatment of nephrosis with cortisone. J Clin Invest 29:1576–1587, 1950.

Lewis SL, Van Epps DE. Neutrophil and monocyte alterations in chronic dialysis patients. Am J Kidney Dis 9:381–395, 1987.

Lewis SL. C5a receptors on neutrophils and monocytes from chronic dialysis patients. In Horl WH, Schollmeyer PJ, eds. New Aspects of Human Polymorphonuclear Leukocytes. New York, Plenum Press, 1991, 167–181.

Lin CY, Su SN. A chemotactic inhibitory factor in the minimal change nephrotic syndrome. Int J Pediatr Nephrol 7:191–196, 1986.

Li Volti S, Caruso-Nicoletti M, Biazzo F, Sciacca A, Mandara G, Mancuso M, Mollica F. Hyporesponsiveness to intradermal administration of hepatitis B vaccine in insulin dependent diabetes mellitus. Arch Dis Child 78:54–57, 1998.

London DR, Bamforth J, Creamer B. Steatorrhea presenting with gastrointestinal protein loss. Lancet 2:18–19, 1961.

Lorini R, Moretta A, Voltorta A, d'Annunzio G, Cortona L, Vitali L, Bozzola M, Severi F. Cytotoxicity activity in children with insulin-dependent diabetes mellitus. Diabetes Res Clin Pract 23:37–42, 1994.

Lorini R, d'Annunzio G, Montecucco C, Caporali R, Vitali L, Pessino P, Severi F. Anticardiolipin antibodies in children and adolescents with insulin-dependent diabetes mellitus. Eur J Pediatr 154:105–108, 1995.

Lorini R, d'Annunzio G, Vitali L, Scaramuzza A. IDDM and autoimmune thyroid disease in the pediatric age group. J Pediatr Endocrinol Metab 9:89–94, 1996.

Lorini R, Scaramuzza A, Vitali L, d'Annunzio G, Avanzini MA, De Giacomo C, Severi F. Clinical aspects of coeliac disease in children with insulin-dependent diabetes mellitus. J Pediatr Endocrinol Metab 9:101–111, 1996.

Lorini R, Alibrandi A, Ravelli A, d'Annunzio G, Castelnuovo P, Martini A. Wegener's granulomatosis presenting with life-threatening pulmonary hemorrhage in a boy with type 1 diabetes. Diabetes Care 22:1591–1592, 1999.

Lowrie EG, Lazarus JM, Mocelin AJ, Bailey GL, Hampers CL, Wilson RE, Merrill JP. Survival of patients undergoing chronic hemodialysis and renal transplantation. N Engl J Med 288:863–867, 1973.

MacLeod CM, Farr LE. Relation of the carrier state to pneumococcal peritonitis in young children with the nephrotic syndrome. Proc Soc Exp Biol Med 37:556–558, 1937.

Mailloux LU, Bellucci AG, Wilkes BM, Napolitano B, Mossey RT, Lesser M, Bluestone PA. Mortality in dialysis patients: analysis of the causes of death. Am J Kidney Dis 18:326–335, 1991.

Malaval T, Li V, Jang G, Martins-Ramos J, Mezin P, Fournet J, Hostein J. Churg-Strauss syndrome with rectal localization and exudative enteropathy. Gastroenterol Clin Biol 17:386–390, 1993.

Manzano L, Alvarez-Mon M, Vargas JA, Giron JA, Abreu L, Fernandez-Corugedo A, Roman LI, Albarran F, Durantez A. Deficient interleukin-2 dependent proliferation pathway in T lymphocytes from active and inactive ulcerative colitis patients. Gut 35:955–960, 1994.

Marseglia GL, Scaramuzza A, d'Annunzio G, Comolli G, Gatti M, Lorini R. Successful immune response to a recombinant hepatitis B vaccine in young patients with insulin-dependent diabetes mellitus. Diabet Med 13:630–633, 1996.

Matsumoto Y, Shinzato T, Amano I, Takai I, Kimura Y, Morita H, Miwa M, Nakane K, Yoshikai Y, Maeda K. Relationship between susceptibility to apoptosis and Fas expression in peripheral blood T cells from uremic patients: a possible mechanism for lymphopenia in chronic renal failure. Biochem Biophys Res Commun 215:98–105, 1995.

McClane SJ, Roombeau JL. Cytokines and inflammatory bowel disease: a review. JPEN 23:S20–24, 1999.

McGuigan JE, Purkerson ML, Trudeau WL, Peterson ML. Studies of the immunologic defects associated with intestinal lymphangiectasia, with some observations on dietary control of chylous ascites. Ann Intern Med 68:398–404, 1968.

McIntyre P, Craig JC. Prevention of serious bacterial infection in children with nephrotic syndrome. J Paediatr Child Health 34:314–317, 1998.

McMahon MM, Bistrian BR. Host defenses and susceptibility to infection in patients with diabetes mellitus. Infect Dis Clin North Am 9:1–9, 1995.

Memoli B, Marzano L, Bisesti V, Andreucci M, Guida B. Hemodialysis-related lymphomononuclear release of interleukin-12 in patients with end-stage renal disease. J Am Soc Nephrol 10:2171–2176, 1999.

Michael AF, McLean RH, Roy LP, Westberg NG, Hoyer JR, Fish AJ, Vernier RL. Immunologic aspects of the nephrotic syndrome. Kidney Int 3:105–115, 1973.

Miller ME, Baker L. Leukocyte function in juvenile diabetes mellitus: humoral and cellular aspects. J Pediatr 81:979–982, 1972.

Mishra OP, Garg R, Usha, Ali Z, Das BK. Immunoglobulins and circulating immune complexes in nephrotic syndrome. J Trop Pediatr 43:93–97, 1997.

Mishra OP, Agrawal S, Usha, Ali Z. Adenosine deaminase activity in protein-energy malnutrition. Acta Paediatr 87:1116–1119, 1998.

Montgomerie JZ, Kalmanson GM, Guze LB. Renal failure and infection. Medicine 47:1–32, 1968.

Montgomery SM, Morris DL, Pounder RE, Wakefield AJ. Paramyxovirus infections in childhood and subsequent inflammatory bowel disease. Gastroenterol 116:796–803, 1999.

Mowat AG, Baum J. Polymorphonuclear leucocyte chemotaxis in patients with bacterial infections. Br Med J 3:617–619, 1971.

Muchova J, Liptakova A, Orszaghova Z, Garaiora I, Tison P, Carsky J, Durackova J. Antioxidant systems in polymorphonuclear leucocytes of type 2 diabetes mellitus. Diabet Med 16:74–78, 1999.

Murata I, Satoh K, Yoshikawa I, Masumoto A, Sasaki e, Otsuki M. Recurrent subcutaneous abscess of the sternal region in ulcerative colitis. Am J Gastroenterol 94:844–845, 1999.

Nakase H, Itani T, Mimura J, Takeuchi R, Kawasaki T, Komori H, Hashimoto K, Chiba T. Transient protein-losing enteropathy associated with cytomegalovirus infection in a noncompromised host: a case report. Am J Gastroenterol 93:1005–1006, 1998.

Navasa M, Fernandez J, Rodes J. Bacterial infections in liver cirrhosis. Ital J Gastroenterol Hepatol 31:616–625, 1999.

Nelson DL, Blaese RM, Strober W, Bruce R, Waldmann TA. Constrictive pericarditis, intestinal lymphangiectasia, and reversible immunologic deficiency. J Pediatr 86:548–554, 1975.

Nielsen OH, Vainer B, Madsen SM, Seidelin JB, Heegaard NH. Established and emerging biological activity markers of inflammatory bowel disease. Am J Gastroenterol 95:359–367, 2000.

Ojanguren I, Gassull MA. Cytomegalovirus infection in patients with inflammatory bowel disease. Am J Gastroenterol 94:1053–1056, 1999.

Ojuawo A, St Louis D, Lindley KJ, Milla PJ. Non-infective colitis in infancy: evidence in favour of minor immunodeficiency in its pathogenesis. Arch Dis Child 76:345–348, 1997.

Olives JP, Breton A, Hugot JP, Oksman F, Johannet C, Ghisolfi J, Navarro J, Cezard JP. Antineutrophil cytoplasmic antibodies in children with inflammatory bowel disease: prevalence and diagnostic value. Pediatr Gastroenterol Nutr 25:142–148, 1997.

Pabico RC, Douglas RG, Betts RF, McKenna BA, Freeman RB. Influenza vaccination of patients with glomerular diseases: effects on creatinine clearance, urinary protein excretion, and antibody response. Ann Intern Med 81:171–177, 1974.

Papo M, Quer JC, Pastor RM, Garcia-Pardo G, Prats E Mirapeix E, Rodriguez R, Richart C. Antineutrophil cytoplasmic antibodies in relatives of patients with inflammatory bowel disease. Am J Gastroenterol 91:1512–1515, 1996.

Parkins RA. Protein-losing enteropathy in the sprue syndrome. Lancet 2:1366–1368, 1960.

Pelletier S, Ekert P, Landi B, Coutellier A, Bletry O, Herson S. Exudative enteropathy in disseminated lupus erythematosus. Ann Gastroenterol Hepatol 28:259–262, 1992.

Perednia DA, Curosh NA. Lupus-associated protein-losing enteropathy. Arch Intern Med 150:1806–1810, 1990.

Pereira BJ. Hepatitis C virus infection in dialysis: a continuing problem. Artif Organs 23:51–60, 1999.

Perez-Machado MA, Espinosa LM, De la Madrigal Ej, Abreu L, Lorente GM, Alvarez-Mon M. Impaired mitogenic response of peripheral blood T cells in ulcerative colitis is not due to apoptosis. Dig Dis Sci 44:2530–2537, 1999.

Philipsen EK, Bondesen S, Andersen J, Larsen S. Serum immunoglobulin G subclasses in patients with ulcerative colitis and Crohn's disease of different disease activities. Scand J Gastroenterol 30:50–53, 1995.

Pickering RJ, Herdman RC, Michael AF, Vernier RL, Gewurz H, Fish AJ, Good RA. Chronic glomerulonephritis associated with low serum complement activity (chronic hypocomplementemic glomerulonephritis). Medicine 49:207–226, 1970.

Pitman FE, Harris RC, Barker HG. Transient edema and hypoproteinemia. Am J Dis Child 108:189–197, 1964.

Plauth WH Jr, Waldmann TA, Wochner RD, Braunwald NS, Braunwald E. Protein-losing enteropathy secondary to constrictive pericarditis in childhood. Pediatrics 34:636–648, 1964.

Pomerantz M, Waldmann TA. Systemic lymphatic abnormalities associated with gastrointestinal protein loss secondary to intestinal lymphangiectasia. Gastroenterology 45:703–711, 1963.

Pozzilli P, Leslie RD. Infections and diabetes: mechanisms and prospects for prevention. Diabet Med 11:935–941, 1994.

Quie PG. Disorders of phagocyte function. Curr Probl Pediatr 2:3–53, 1972.

Quien RM, Kaiser BA, Deforest A, Polinsky MS, Fisher M, Baluarte HJ. Response to the varicella vaccine in children with nephrotic syndrome. J Pediatr 131:688–690, 1997.

Rachima C, Maoz E, Apter S. Cytomegalovirus infection associated with ulcerative colitis in immunocompetent individuals. Postgrad Med J 74:486–489, 1998.

Raska K Jr, Raskova J, Shea SM, Frankel RM, Wood RH, Lifter J, Ghobrial I, Eisinger RP, Homer L. T cell subsets and cellular immunity in end-stage renal disease. Am J Med 75:734–740, 1983.

Raskova J, Ghobrial I, Czerwinski DK, Shea SM, Eisinger RP, Raska K Jr. B-cell activation and immunoregulation in end-stage renal disease patients receiving hemodialysis. Arch Intern Med 147:89–93, 1987.

Rassias AJ, Marrin CA, Arruda J, Whalen PK, Beach M, Yeager MD. Insulin infusion improves neutrophil function in diabetic cardiac surgery patients. Anesth Analg 88:1011–1016, 1999.

Reddingius RE, Schroder CH, Daha MR, Monnens LA. The serum complement system in children on continuous ambulatory peritoneal dialysis. Perit Dial Int 13:214–218, 1993.

Reiss U, Wingen AM, Scharer K. Mortality trends in pediatric patients with chronic renal failure. Pediatr Nephrol 10:41–45, 1996.

Repine JE, Clawson CC, Goetz FC. Bactericidal function of neutrophils from patients with acute bacterial infections and from diabetics. J Infect Dis 142:869–875, 1980.

Ricci S, Bonucci A, Fabiani E, Catassi C, Carlucci A, Bearzi I, Giorgi PL. Protein-losing gastroenteropathy (Menetrier's disease) in childhood: a report of 3 cases. Pediatr Med Chir 18:269–273, 1996.

Roman LI, Manzano L, DeLaHera A, Abreu L, Rossi I, Alvarez-Mon M. Expanded CD4+CD45RO+ phenotype and defective proliferative response in T lymphocytes from patients with Crohn's disease. Gastroenterol 110:1008–1019, 1996.

Rosen FS, Smith DH, Earle JR, Janeway CA, Gitlin D. The etiology of hypoproteinemia in a patient with congenital chylous ascites. Pediatrics 30:696–706, 1962.

Rotem Y, Czerniak P. Gastrointestinal protein leakage in celiac disease as studied by labeled PVP. Am J Dis Child 107:58–66, 1964.

Rubin HM, Blau EB, Michaels RH. Hemophilus and pneumococcal peritonitis in children with the nephrotic syndrome. Pediatrics 56:598–601, 1975.

Ruther U, Nunnensiek C, Muller HA, Bader H, May U, Jipp P. Interferon alpha (IFN-alpha 2a) therapy for herpes virus-associated inflammatory bowel disease (ulcerative colitis and Crohn's disease). Hepatogastroenterol 45:692–699, 1998.

Sardegna KM, Beck AM, Strife CF. Evaluation of perioperative antibiotics at the time of dialysis catheter placement. Pediatr Nephrol 12:149–52, 1998.

Saxena KM, Crawford JD. The treatment of nephrosis. N Engl J Med 272:522–526, 1965.

Schirren CA, Jung MC, Zachoval R, Diepolder H, Hoffmann R, Riethmuller G, Pape GR. Analysis of T cell activation pathway in patients with liver cirrhosis, impaired delayed hypersensitivity and other T cell-dependent functions. Clin Exp Immunol 108:144–150, 1997.

Schwabe RF, Engelmann H, Hess S, Fricke H. Soluble CD40 in the serum of healthy donors, patients with chronic renal failure, haemodialysis and chronic ambulatory peritoneal dialysis (CAPD). Clin Exp Immunol 117:153–158, 1999.

Schwartz M, Jarnum S. Gastrointestinal protein loss in idiopathic (hypercatabolic) proteinemia. Lancet 1:327–328, 1959.

Senju M, Hulstaert F, Lowder J, Jewell DP. Flow cytometric analysis of peripheral blood lymphocytes in ulcerative colitis and Crohn's disease. Gut 32:779–783, 1991.

Sensi M, Pozzilli P, Gorsuch AN, Bottazzo GF, Cudworth AG. Increased killer cell activity in insulin-dependent (type 1) diabetes mellitus. Diabetologia 20:106–109, 1981.

Serlenga E, Garofalo AR, DePergola G, Ventura MT, Tortorella C, Antonaci S. Polymorphonuclear cell-mediated phagocytosis and superoxide anion release in insulin-dependent diabetes mellitus. Cytobios 74:189–195, 1993.

Smith LJ, Szymanski W, Foulston C, Jewell LD, Pabst HF. Familial enteropathy with villous edema and immunoglobulin G2 subclass deficiency. J Pediatr 125:541–548, 1994.

Steinfeld JL, Davidson JD, Gordon JRS, Greene FE. The mechanism of hypoproteinemia in patients with regional enteritis and ulcerative colitis. Am J Med 29:405–415, 1960.

Steuer A, McCrea DJ, Colaco CB. Primary Sjögren's syndrome, ulcerative colitis and selective IgA deficiency. Postgrad Med J 72:499–450, 1996.

Stevens CE, Alter HJ, Taylor PE, Zang EA, Harley EJ, Szmuness W. Hepatitis B vaccine in patients receiving hemodialysis: immunogenicity and efficacy. N Engl J Med 311:496–501, 1984.

Stevens R, Oliver M, Brogan M, Heiserodt J, Targan S. Defective generation of tetanus-specific antibody-producing B cells after in vivo immunization of Crohn's disease and ulcerative colitis patients. Gastroenterol 88:1860–1866, 1985.

Stiehm ER, Casillas AM, Finkelstein JZ, Gallagher KT, Groncy PM, Kobayashi RH, Oleske JM, Roberts RL, Sandberg ET, Wakim ME. Slow subcutaneous human intravenous immunoglobulin in the treatment of antibody immunodeficiency: use of an old method with a new product. J Allergy Clin Immunol 101:849–850, 1998.

Strober W, Wochner RD, Carbone PP, Waldmann TA. Intestinal lymphangiectasia: a protein-losing enteropathy with hypogammaglobulinemia, lymphocytopenia and impaired homograft rejection. J Clin Invest 46:1643–1656, 1967.

Sturgeon P, Brubaker C. Copper deficiency in infants: a syndrome characterized by hypocupremia, iron deficiency anemia, and hypoproteinemia. Am J Dis Child 92:254–265, 1956.

Such J, Runyon BA. Spontaneous bacterial peritonitis. Clin Infect Dis 27:669–674, 1998.

Sunder-Plassmann G, Patruta SI, Horl WH. Pathobiology of the role of iron in infection. Am J Kidney Dis 34:S25–S29, 1999.

Sunder-Plassmann G, Patrula SI, Horl WH. Pathobiology of the role of iron in infection. Am J Kidney Dis 34:S25–S29, 1999.

Suri A, Katz JD. Dissecting the role of CD4$^+$ T cells in autoimmune diabetes through the use of TCR transgenic mice. Immunol Rev 169:55–65, 1999.

Szmuness W, Prince AM, Grady GF, Mann MK, Levine RW, Friedman EA, Jacobs MJ, Josephson A, Ribot S, Shapiro FL, Stenzel KH, Suki WN, Vyas G. Hepatitis B infection. A point-prevalence study in 15 US hemodialysis centers. JAMA 227:901–906, 1974.

Tan JS, Anderson JL, Watanakunakorn C, Phair JP. Neutrophil dysfunction in diabetes mellitus. J Lab Clin Med 85:26–33, 1975.

Tielemans C, Gastaldello K, Husson C, Marchant A, Delville JP, Vanherweghem JL, Goldman M. Efficacy of oral immunotherapy on respiratory infections in hemodialysis patients: a double-blind, placebo-controlled study. Clin Nephrol 51:153–160, 1999.

Thompson NP, Montgomery SM, Pounder RE, Wakefield AJ. Is measles vaccination a risk factor for inflammatory bowel disease? Lancet 345:1071–1074, 1995.

Thomson GA, Fisher BM, Gemmell CG, MacCuish AC, Gallacher SJ. Attenuated neutrophil respiratory burst following acute hypoglycemia in diabetic patients and normal subjects. Acta Diabetol 34:253–256, 1997.

Tokars J, Alter MJ, Favero MS, Moyer LA, Miller E, Bland L. National surveillance of hemodialysis associated disease in the United States, 1992. American Society for Artificial Internal Organs (ASAIO) 40:1020–1031, 1994.

Turk S, Bozfakioglu S, Ecder ST, Karaman T, Gurel N, Erkoc R, Aysuna N, Turkman A, Bekiroglu N, Ark E. Effects of zinc supplementation on the immune system and on antibody response to multivalent influenza vaccine in hemodialysis patients. Int J Artif Organs 21:274–278, 1998.

Ulstrom RA, Smith NJ, Heimlich E. Transient dysproteinemia in infants: a new syndrome. Am J Dis Child 92:219–253, 1956.

Ulstrom RA, Smith NJ, Nakamura K, Heimlich E. Transient dysproteinemia in infants: II. Studies of protein metabolism using amino acid isotopes. Am J Dis Child 93:536–547, 1957.

Vega R, Bertran X, Menacho M, Domenech E, Moreno de Vega V, Hombrados M, Cabre E, Ojanguren I, Gassull MA. Cytomegalovirus infection in patients with inflammatory bowel disease. Am J Gastroenterol 94:1053–1056, 1999.

Vega Robledo GB, Guinzberg AL, Ramos Garcia C, Ortiz Oriz L. Patients with hepatic cirrhosis altered lymphocyte response to mitogens and its relation with plasmatic zinc, albumin and transferrin. Arch Med Res 25:5–9, 1994.

Volhard F, Fahr T. Die Brightsche Nierenkrankheit: Klinik, Pathologie und Atlas. Berlin, Springer, 1914.

Waldmann TA. Protein-losing enteropathy. Gastroenterology 50:422–443, 1966.

Waldmann TA, Schwab PJ. IgG (7S gamma globulin) metabolism in hypogammaglobulinemia: studies in patients with defective gamma globulin synthesis, gastrointestinal protein loss, or both. J Clin Invest 44:1523–1533, 1965.

Waldmann TA, Steinfeld JL, Dutcher TF, Davidson JD, Gordon RS Jr. The role of the gastrointestinal system in "idiopathic hypoproteinemia." Gastroenterology 41:197–207, 1961.

Waldmann TA, Wochner RD, Laster L, Gordon RS Jr. Allergic gastroenteropathy: a cause of excessive gastrointestinal protein loss. N Engl J Med 276:762–769, 1967.

Weiden PL, Blaese RM, Strober W, Block JB, Waldmann TA. Impaired lymphocyte transformation in intestinal lymphangiectasia: evidence for at least two functionally distinct lymphocyte populations in man. J Clin Invest 51:1319–1325, 1972.

Wilfert CM, Katz SL. Etiology of bacterial sepsis in nephrotic children 1963–1967. Pediatrics 42:840–843, 1968.

Wilson WEC, Kirkpatrick CH, Talmage DW. Suppression of immunologic responsiveness in uremia. Ann Intern Med 62:1–14, 1965.

Yan K, Nakahara K, Awa S, Nishibori Y, Nakajima N, kataoka S, Maeda M, Watanabe T, Matsushima S, Watanabe N. The increase of memory T cell subsets in children with idiopathic nephrotic syndrome. Nephron 79:274–278, 1998.

Yanai H, Shimizu N, Nagasaki S, Mitani N, Okita K. Epstein-Barr virus infection of the colon with inflammatory bowel disease. Am J Gastroenterol 94:1582–1586, 1999.

Yoshikawa I, Murata I, Tamura M, Kume K, Nakuno S, Otsuki M. A case of protein-losing gastropathy caused by acute Helicobacter pylori infection. Gastrointest Endosc 49:245–248, 1999.

Young AW Jr, Sweeney EW, David DS, Cheigh J, Hochgelerenl EL, Sakai S, Stenzel KH, Rubin AL. Dermatologic evaluation of pruritus in patients on hemodialysis. NY State J Med 73:2670–2674, 1973.

C H A P T E R

26

Proliferative and Histiocytic Disorders

Fabienne Dayer Pastore, Yves Pastore, Kenneth L. McClain, and William T. Shearer

INTRODUCTION

Alterations in immunologic function and increased susceptibility to infection may occur as a result of many systemic diseases, including proliferative and histiocytic disorders. These secondary forms of immunodeficiency are considerably more common than primary immunodeficiencies. Patients with secondary immunodeficiencies have an intact immune system but, during or following the primary disease, their host defenses become transiently or permanently impaired. This impairment can result in abnormalities of humoral and/or cellular immunity.

Mechanisms involved in the immune control of malignancies and the various immune defects described in selective malignancies, hematologic disorders, histiocytoses, and sarcoidosis are discussed in this chapter.

IMMUNE CONTROL OF MALIGNANCIES

Immune Escape of Tumor Cells

An important function of the immune system is to recognize and attack cells displaying foreign surface antigens, such as infectious pathogens, human leukocyte antigen (HLA)-incompatible cells or tissues, or mutated host cells presenting unique proteins. The growth of malignant cells implies a reduced or absent response of immune function. Several mechanisms of immune escape by neoplastic cells have been described.

Antigen-presenting cells (APCs), including monocytes, macrophages, dendritic cells, and histiocytes, play an essential role in presenting antigens, including tumor antigens, to the cellular immune system. These tumor peptides are presented in association with a major histocompatibility complex (MHC) class I molecule to CD8+

T cells and with a MHC class II molecule to CD4+ T cells (see Chapter 6).

Another necessary co-stimulator is the B7 (CD80) molecule expressed on the APC surface, which interacts with CD28 present on the T-cell surface. If complete recognition is made, CD8+ T cells can bind to and lyse the tumor cells. If an antigenic peptide associated with a MHC class II is recognized by CD4+ T cells, it will induce lymphokine production, which can stimulate CD8+ T cells, or the CD4+ cells can become cytotoxic (see Chapter 2).

Natural killer (NK) cells can be activated without the help of the MHC system (see Chapter 6). They attach to tumor cells and cause cell lysis by membrane-perforating molecules. Failure of this recognition system favors tumor growth. Various phenomena may lead to an ineffective cytotoxic cell response (Kavanaugh and Carbone, 1996) as discussed later (see Chapter 6).

Role of Major Histocompatibility Complex Class I Antigens

Downregulation or suppression of MHC class I expression on primary human tumors or metastases have been described (Cromme et al., 1994a; Lopez-Nevot et al., 1989; Zinkernagel and Doherty, 1979), leading to impaired immune recognition. This may result in loss of class I allospecificity (Kageshita et al., 1993) or a complete loss of MHC expression (Nouri et al., 1994). For normal surface expression, the processed antigenic peptides need the help of transporter associated with antigen presentation (TAP), a heterodimer protein that mediates their transport from the cytosol into the endoplasmic reticulum for association with the MHC class I molecules. A loss of MHC class I expression resulting from lack of TAP has been described in cervical carcinoma (Cromme et al., 1994b). Loss of CD80 that has been described in a mouse melanoma cell line K1735 (Townsend and Allison, 1993) led to decreased immune response in vivo despite the presence of MHC class I and class II molecules. After stimulation of the B7 receptor or after the CD80 gene was transfected by a B7-expression vector, cytotoxic cell killing was restored. Several solid tumors do not express B7 (Chen et al., 1993). When the B7 gene was transduced in tumors, T-cell immunity against the tumor was enhanced (Chen et al., 1994; Lee et al., 1996).

Role of the T-Cell Receptor

When an antigenic tumor peptide is presented in combination with MHC class I molecules, it must be recognized by the T-cell receptor (TCR) to induce a T-cell–mediated immunologic response. The CD3 zeta chain (CD3ζ) was completely absent in tumor-bearing mice (Mizoguchi et al., 1992), replaced by a protein similar to the Fcεγ chain. This change led to a decreased amount of CD3γ and loss of the Src family protein kinases, *fyn* and *lck*, and a functional defect in TCR-dependent phosphorylation. The peripheral blood T cells of some cancer patients show absence of CD3ζ and *fyn* proteins and defective T-cell activation (Loeffler et al., 1992). Another essential component of cytolysis is the presence of CD3δ, which is required for the surface expression of the TCRαβ molecule (Buferne et al., 1992).

Factors Secreted by Tumor Cells

Transforming growth factor-beta (TGF-β), a T-cell cytokine affecting cell differentiation and proliferation (Sporn et al., 1986), enhances growth of tumor cells (Kehrl et al., 1986). TGF-β reduces the DNA synthesis of concanavalin-activated lymphocytes by 60% to 80%. TGF-β may also deactivate macrophages (Tsunawaki et al., 1988); its presence in tumor tissue culture fluid inhibited the H_2O_2–induced respiratory burst, tumor necrosis factor-alpha (TNF-α) production, and MHC class II expression. These factors combined affect the ability of macrophages to kill tumor cells and the impairment of T-cell activation by decreasing the expression of processed antigens at the cell surface. TGF-β has different effects on the immune system, depending on its concentration (Wahl et al., 1988). At high concentration it has been shown that TGF-β inhibited interleukin (IL)-1 production and decreased the lymphocyte proliferation induced by mitogens, despite the presence of IL-2 and IL-2R.

TGF-β is present in more than 90% of primary human malignant astrocytomas and glioblastomas (Maxwell et al., 1992). A polyclonal anti–TGF-β neutralizing antibody increased T-cell cytotoxicity against autologous target cells. Preincubation of target cells with antisense oligonucleotides, which were used to inhibit transcription of the TGF-β gene, enhanced lymphocyte proliferation and autologous tumor cytotoxicity (Jachimczak et al., 1993). Another function of TGF-β that can affect tumor growth is decreased cytolytic activity of NK cells (Rook et al., 1986).

Soluble IL-2 receptor (sIL-2R) is often elevated in the serum of patients with cancer and may be used to determine the presence of a neoplasia (Zerler, 1991). Release of sIL-2R is a nonspecific marker of cellular immune regulation (Waldmann, 1986), and it increases in multiple myeloma or solid tumor metastases (Lissoni et al., 1990; Vacca et al., 1991). sIL-2R may be useful to follow tumor progression or regression in childhood solid tumor patients (Bodey et al., 1996) and as a prognostic factor (Bodey et al., 1996; Pui et al., 1987, 1988). Because sIL-2R binds IL-2 (Rubin et al., 1986), it interferes with IL-2–dependent immune function against tumor cells.

Complement-Inhibiting Factors

The complement system protects the host from invasive microorganisms and other antigen-bearing cells, including tumor cells. When activated, a membrane attack complex

(MAC) is formed and results in pore formation and cell lysis. Protection against uncontrolled activation is provided by regulatory proteins, either circulating or expressed on cell surfaces (Paraskevas, 1999). Tumor cells exposed to complement in the bloodstream during proliferation or metastasis release complement-inhibiting factors to avoid complement deposition and cell lysis.

Jurianz and co-workers (1999) have reviewed studies of complement regulatory proteins (soluble or membrane bound) that showed overexpression on malignant cells. Tumor cells also express proteases, which cleave complement components and inhibit the complement cascade (Jurianz et al., 1999).

Role of Adhesion Molecules

Adhesion molecules and their receptors are crucial for embryogenesis, cell growth, differentiation, and wound repair (Frenette and Wagner, 1996). Intercellular adhesion molecule-1 (ICAM-1, CD54), the ligand for lymphocyte function-associated antigen 1 (LFA-1), is essential not only for cell–cell and cell–tissue interactions but also for binding of cytolytic T cells and NK cells to their targets (Vanky et al., 1990). Circulating levels of ICAM-1 are elevated in many malignancies (Gruss et al., 1993; Harning et al., 1991; Tsujisaki et al., 1991) and may be secondary to cellular expression and tumor activity (Pizzolo et al., 1993). Circulating sICAM-1 may bind to LFA-1 on cytotoxic effector cells, thus inhibiting adhesion and cytotoxic reactions.

Downregulation of adhesion molecules on tumor cells may prevent formation of stable conjugates with cytotoxic T lymphocytes (CTL), thus evading CTL-mediated killing (Pandolfi et al., 1992).

Vascular cell adhesion molecule-1 (VCAM-1) is an endothelial adhesion molecule known to promote lymphocyte infiltration in inflamed tissues and presumably in tumors. Downregulation of VCAM-1 allows vascularized melanomas and carcinomas to avoid invasion by cytotoxic cells (Piali et al., 1995).

INTERACTION AMONG IMMUNODEFICIENCY, VIRAL INFECTION, AND MALIGNANCY

Individuals with primary or secondary immunodeficiencies are more susceptible to malignancy, presumably because of impaired immune surveillance. They are not at risk for all cancers but are particularly susceptible to lymphoproliferative disorders and selected epithelial tumors (Filipovich et al., 1994). Factors contributing to this increased risk may include endemic Epstein-Barr virus (EBV) infection, a predominance of Th2 over Th1 responses, and genetic defects that impair signaling between lymphoid cells.

EBV not only immortalizes B lymphocytes, it also contains genes inhibiting cell-mediated immunity. Following EBV infection in a normal host, cell-mediated immunity develops and causes the virus to become latent. In primary and secondary immunodeficiencies with impaired cell-mediated immunity EBV-immortalized B cells proliferate and, unchecked by regulatory stimuli, may undergo malignant transformation.

A predominance of type 2 cytokine production such as IL-4 and IL-10 stimulates B-cell activation and inhibits type 1 cytokine production and cellular immunity that inhibits EBV-transformed B cells. Patients with X-linked lymphoproliferative syndrome, Omenn syndrome, severe combined immunodeficiency (SCID), and Wiskott-Aldrich syndrome (WAS) and those receiving immunosuppressive agents for transplant procedures are particularly susceptible to lymphoproliferative disease (Mathur et al., 1994). Thus most tumors in primary immunodeficiencies are lymphomas, often related to EBV (Table 26-1) (see Chapter 39).

The incidence of cancers in primary immunodeficiency has increased with improved survival rates and represents the second most common cause of death (after infectious causes) (Mueller and Pizzo, 1995). The incidence of tumors has been reported to be between 13% and 25%, especially in WAS (Sullivan et al., 1994) (see Chapter 17), ataxia-telangiectasia (Morrell et al., 1986) (see Chapter 18), and common variable immunodeficiency (CVID) (Cunningham-Rundles and Bodian, 1999) (see Chapter 13).

Based on the international Immunodeficiency Cancer Registry (ICR) (Gatti and Good, 1971; Kersey et al., 1988), Hodgkin's disease (HD) represents approximately 10% of tumors arising in patients with primary immunodeficiencies, is often EBV positive, and occurs at a younger median age (before age 10). Their 5-year survival was 53% versus 86% in nonimmunodeficient patients (Robison et al., 1987).

The most common epithelial tumor in immunodeficient patients is gastric carcinoma. There is an association with immunoglobulin A (IgA) deficiency (see Chapter 14), CVID, and ataxia-telangiectasia. Chronic *Helicobacter*

. . . .
TABLE 26-1 · TUMORS OCCURRING IN PRIMARY IMMUNODEFICIENCIES

Lymphoma
Severe combined immunodeficiency (SCID)
  X-SCID*
  Omenn syndrome*
  Purine nucleoside phosphorylase (PNP) deficiency
Ataxia-telangiectasia
Wiskott-Aldrich syndrome*
X-linked lymphoproliferative syndrome (XLP)*
Chédiak-Higashi syndrome*
Hyper-IgE syndrome
Autoimmune lymphoproliferative syndrome (ALPS)
IgA deficiency*
Common variable immunodeficiency (CVID)*

Hodgkin's Disease
Hyper-IgM1 syndrome (CD40 ligand deficiency)

Biliary Tract Tumors
Hyper-IgM1 Syndrome

Gastric Carcinoma
IgA deficiency
CVID

---
*Frequently associated with Epstein-Barr virus (EBV).

pylori infection may be implicated by stimulating cytokines that promote epithelial and lymphoid proliferation. IgA antibodies may be important in the control of this infection. Other epithelial tumors associated with primary immunodeficiencies include skin, hepatic, and genitourinary tumors in ataxia-telangiectasia and biliary tree carcinomas in hyper-IgM1 syndrome (see Chapter 13).

In human immunodeficiency virus (HIV) infection, the incidence of lymphomas ranges from 4% to 10% (Knowles, 1997), and the use of multidrug therapies decreases this susceptibility (O'Connor and Scadden, 2000). EBV is implicated in 30% to 60% of these tumors. Central nervous system (CNS) tumors are not uncommon. Kaposi's sarcoma resulting from human herpes virus-8 (HHV-8) is associated with advanced stages of HIV infection (Goedert et al., 1998) (see Chapter 29).

IMMUNE DEFECTS IN LEUKEMIAS

Nonspecific Immunity

Leukopenia is the major but not the only cause of the increased susceptibility to infection in patients with acute leukemia. Leukocyte mobilization is markedly decreased (Senn and Jungi, 1975). Others have reported decreased neutrophil nitro-blue tetrazolium reduction both in relapse and remission (Humbert et al., 1976), reduced $H_2O_2^-$ and O_2^- production during induction, and decreased bactericidal activity (Lejeune et al., 1998). Both chemotactic and phagocytic activities of neutrophils are also impaired. Clearance of granulocytes from the circulation is normal in acute lymphoblastic leukemia (ALL) but is impaired in acute myelocytic leukemia. Reticuloendothelial phagocytic function is also impaired in some patients with acute leukemia (Groch et al., 1965).

B and T Lymphocytes and Cellular Immunity

Unlike lymphoma, patients with acute leukemia generally have normal antibody and cell-mediated immunity before intensive chemotherapy and/or before a terminal state. B and T cells are usually normal, but after chemotherapy there is progressive lymphopenia (Wehinger and Kartizky, 1977) affecting B-cell numbers more than T cells (Caver et al., 1998; Esber et al., 1976; Reid et al., 1977). Proliferation of T lymphocytes is attenuated at diagnosis and at the time of initiation of therapy (Abrahamsson et al., 1995) but had mainly been reported as normal later on during therapy (Borella and Webster, 1971; Nash et al., 1993).

Humoral Immunity

Immunoglobulin levels at diagnosis are usually normal, although hypergammaglobulinemia has been observed (Surico et al., 1999). During therapy, immunoglobulin levels and plasma cells decrease, affecting all isotypes (Abrahamsson and Mellander, 1997; Abrahamsson et al., 1995).

Antibody responses are normal at diagnosis but can be depressed by chemotherapy. Feldman and colleagues (1998) reported that measles and mumps seropositivity was greater than 90% in 39 previously healthy vaccinated children; after chemotherapy, the seropositivity for measles declined to 13%, for mumps to 18%, and for rubella to 21%.

Vaccine responsiveness during chemotherapy varies with the individual vaccine. Responses to booster immunization with tetanus and diphtheria are similar to those in healthy children, whereas the response to pneumococcal vaccine is suboptimal (Ridgway and Wolff, 1993). Only inactivated or toxoid vaccines should be used.

In sum, B- and T-cell function in leukemia is essentially normal at diagnosis, but phagocytic and chemotactic function of polymorphonuclear cells are diminished. During chemotherapy, patients usually develop progressive lymphopenia, particularly of B cells, and an associated decrease in immunoglobulin levels and antibody responses.

IMMUNE DEFECTS IN HODGKIN'S DISEASE

HD was the first lymphoma to be associated with abnormalities of the immune response. In some cases, the immunologic defects are related to the clinical stage of the disease and the histologic type (Lukes and Butler, 1966; Lukes et al., 1966). The four histologic expressions of HD are (1) lymphocyte predominance, (2) nodular sclerosis, (3) mixed cellularity, and (4) lymphocytic depletion. HD is clinically classified according to its anatomic distribution and systemic symptoms. Patients with lymphocytic depletion tend to be diagnosed at a more advanced stage compared with other histologic subtypes, and lymphocyte depletion is associated with a greater impairment of immunologic function and a poorer prognosis. Regardless of histologic type, HD must also be classified for clinical staging, as defined in Table 26-2. This clinical staging correlates with immunologic defects and ultimate prognosis.

Phagocytic Function

Leukocytosis is present in more than 50% of patients with HD, despite the presence of lymphopenia as the disease progresses (Aisenberg, 1965a). Both lymphopenia (lymphocyte count < 6/mm^3) and leukocytosis (white cell count ≥ 15,000/mm^3) at diagnosis were associated with a poor prognosis, in a large retrospective study on 4695 patients (Hasenclever and Diehl, 1998). Phagocytic function of the reticuloendothelial system, measured by the clearance of ^{125}I-labeled aggregated human serum albumin, is normal or enhanced (Sheagren et al., 1967). Physiologic granulocyte removal from circulation by the

TABLE 26-2 · CLINICAL STAGING OF HODGKIN'S DISEASE

Stage	Definition
Stage I	Involvement of single lymph node region (I) or nonlymphoid structure (I_E)
Stage II	Involvement of two or more lymph node regions on the same side of the diaphragm or localized involvement of an extralymphatic organ or site and one or more lymph node regions on the same side of the diaphragm
Stage III	Involvement of lymph node regions or structures on both sides of the diaphragm
Stage IV	Diffuse or disseminated involvement of one or more extralymphatic organs or tissues (e.g., bone marrow, bone, lung) with associated lymph node involvement

Suffix A: absence of systemic symptoms

Suffix B: presence of systemic symptoms such as fever > 38°C for 3 consecutive days, drenching night sweats, unexplained loss of 10% or more of body weight during the 6 months before admission

reticuloendothelial system is decreased in patients in stages III and IV, but neutrophil mobilization is normal (Senn and Jungi, 1975).

The bactericidal capacity of mononuclear phagocytes is normal in HD (Steigbigel et al., 1976). However, leukocyte chemotaxis is abnormal, apparently associated with excessive levels of chemotactic factor inactivator (Ward and Berenberg, 1974). Perez-Soler and co-workers (1985) found impaired superoxide production in monocytes from patients with active disease compared with patients in remission and normal controls.

B and T Lymphocytes

Reed-Sternberg cells are pathognomonic of HD. It is now clear that these cells arise from B lymphocytes (Staudt, 2000). For example, Cossman and associates (1999) compared gene expression of Hodgkin's and Reed-Sternberg cells with those derived from normal tissues and found that Reed-Sternberg cells from patients with nodular sclerosing and lymphocyte-predominant HD are derived from unusual B-cell lineage cells. Also, Foss and co-workers (1999) have found that the expression of a B-cell–specific transcription factor, B-cell–specific activator protein (BSAP), was present in Reed-Sternberg cells derived from 22 of 25 patients HD patients.

Lymphocyte depletion of lymphoid tissue is well recognized in HD (Lukes and Butler, 1966) and may be associated with peripheral leukopenia (Eltringham and Kaplan, 1973; Young et al., 1972). Although lymphopenia correlates with clinical stage, this by itself is not a prognostic factor (Ayoub et al., 1999). Historically, studies of B and T lymphocytes in HD show decreased percentages of T cells when using E rosette assays (Andersen, 1974; Bobrove et al., 1975)

but normal percentages when using specific anti–T-cell sera (Bobrove et al., 1975; Chin et al., 1973). In addition, reduced numbers of B cells occur and are associated with low T-cell levels (Bobrove et al., 1975).

Watanabe and colleagues (1997) showed a significant decrease in B cells, CD4 T cells, and CD8 T cells at diagnosis in adult patients. Whereas B lymphocytes recover quickly after therapy, T lymphocytes remain depressed for a prolonged period. This delayed recovery particularly affects naïve T lymphocytes, which may take several years to return to normal. This delayed recovery of the T lymphocytes in HD resembles the delayed recovery of naïve cells after treatment in HIV disease (Roederer et al., 1997).

Humoral Immunity

Serum immunoglobulins are usually normal in HD (Ultmann et al., 1966; Weitzman et al., 1977). Hypergammaglobulinemia or hypogammaglobulinemia occurs in about 10% of patients; the latter is associated with advanced disease. Patients with untreated HD may respond normally to polysaccharide and protein vaccines (Siber et al., 1981). However, this ability is lost during treatment and recovery of function depends on the vaccines as discussed subsequently.

Cellular Immunity

In Vivo Studies

Defects of cell-mediated immunity are common in patients with HD (Slivnick et al., 1990), demonstrated either with in vivo or by in vitro studies. As a result, patients with HD have increased incidence of infection, particularly with fungi, viruses (particularly herpes zoster and varicella), and tuberculosis (Casazza et al., 1966).

In earlier decades, when most adults were tuberculin positive, most HD patients had negative tuberculin results despite tuberculosis exposure or tuberculosis proven at autopsy. Schier and co-workers (1956) showed that tuberculin negativity was part of a generalized cutaneous anergy; in a control group, 71% responded to purified protein derivative of *Mycobacterium tuberculosis* (PPD), 90% to mumps, 92% to *Candida albicans,* and 66% to *Trichophyton;* in HD, the response rates to the same antigens were 23%, 14%, 19%, and 16%, respectively. Others have also noted anergy, even in patients who are asymptomatic or in good condition (Lamb et al., 1962; Sokal and Primikirios, 1961).

A consensus of several studies indicates that 12% to 25% of untreated patients with HD have complete anergy to six intradermal antigens (Slivnick et al., 1990). The anergic state is relative because increasing the concentration of the antigen increases the number of positive reactions. The tuberculin reaction in advanced HD may be delayed (Morganfeld and Bonchil, 1968); a negative reaction at 48 hours may become positive at 5 to 7 days. Conversion from tuberculin positivity to negativity occurs with the development of the disease, and reconversion to tuberculin positivity may occur with remission. Thus the anergy of HD occurs early even when the patient is asymptomatic or in good clinical condition; in contrast, anergy appears much later in patients with leukemia, carcinoma, or non Hodgkin's lymphoma.

To distinguish the anergic patients from those not exposed to antigen, Aisenberg (1962) attempted to sensitize patients with HD to dinitrochlorobenzene (DNCB). All 25 patients with active HD were anergic, whereas 12 patients with disease quiescent for more than 2 years became sensitized. Brown and colleagues (1967) were able to sensitize 35 of 50 patients to DNCB; the reactors tended to have localized disease and normal lymphocyte counts. Sokal and Aungst (1969) found that patients with advanced HD with positive tuberculin tests after bacillus Calmette-Guérin (BCG) vaccination had a longer survival than those who remained anergic.

In Vitro Studies

Hersh and Oppenhein (1965) reported decreased transformation of lymphocytes in response to phytohemagglutinin (PHA) in HD. Less transformation was seen in anergic patients than in those with positive skin tests. In three cases, plasma factors contributed to the impaired PHA response. Similar findings were reported by Trubovitz and colleagues (1966) and by Aisenberg (1965b). Brown and associates (1967) found that the PHA response in HD was related to clinical staging and histology. Jackson and co-workers (1970) also found a reduced lymphocyte response in patients with systemic symptoms and advanced disease; most patients with stage I disease showed a normal response.

Han and Sokal (1970) and Winkelstein and co-workers (1974) reported considerable variability of the in vitro lymphocyte response to PHA in active HD. Although the mean response was significantly lower than that of controls, half the patients had normal responses. A few patients in remission exhibited a diminished PHA response. Chemotherapy diminished the response in some cases. Patients with nodular sclerosing disease had normal PHA responses. In general, a diminished PHA response is correlated with advanced disease, systemic symptoms, lymphopenia, cutaneous anergy, and radiation therapy. Because PHA is such a strong lymphocyte stimulator, the response to it may remain positive even when the patient is nonreactive to weaker antigenic stimuli.

Gotoff and associates (1973) demonstrated impaired synthesis of a lymphokine, macrophage aggregation factor, by lymphocytes from patients with HD. Subnormal mixed leukocyte culture reactions of Hodgkin's lymphocytes suggest a relative excess of suppressor lymphocytes (Twoney et al., 1975).

Monocyte-related immunosuppression may be present in HD, resulting in an increased number of bacterial and fungal infections (Coker et al., 1983). Removal of glass-adherent cells from mononuclear cells of patients with HD resulted in increased PHA responsiveness (Sibbitt et al., 1978). Increased prostaglandin E_2 (PGE_2) production by monocytes from patients and reversal of their suppressive activity by indomethacin has been documented (Goodwin et al., 1977; Passwell et al., 1983).

Another cause of suppression includes circulating plasma factors. Pui and colleagues (1989) showed that increased serum soluble CD8 was associated with aggressive clinical disease and suggested that this correlated with regulatory T-cell activity.

Immune Surveillance

Examination of tissue samples from patients with HD classically reveals the presence of rare Hodgkin's and RS tumor cells within a large population of bystander cells, predominantly CD4+ cells. Despite the fact that RS cells are derived from B cells and resemble APCs, the surrounding immune cells are unable to clear the malignant cells, illustrating the principle of immune escape.

Several hypotheses have been raised to explain the pathophysiologic pathway to such escape. Poppema and Visser (1994) have shown that RS cells had a downregulation of the MHC class I molecules, therefore reducing the function of cytotoxic T lymphocytes. Bosshart and Jarrett (1998) have also shown that a subset of RS cells was deficient in MHC class II antigen presentation. Also, RS cells produce serum factors, such as TGF-β, that inhibit B and T lymphocytes (Slivnick et al., 1990). Finally, T lymphocytes might also show some abnormalities, such as a decreased expression of the TCR ζ chain (Roskrow et al., 1998). Future treatment may be directed at educating the immune system to recognize and eliminate the malignant Hodgkin's cells.

IMMUNE DEFECTS IN NON-HODGKIN'S LYMPHOMA

The lymphomas are the third most common childhood malignancy, accounting for approximately 10% of cancers in children. About two thirds of the lymphomas of childhood are non-Hodgkin's lymphoma (NHL), and the remainder are HD. The pattern of NHL seen in children differs significantly from that seen in adult patients. The three major histologic categories of NHL in children are lymphoblastic, small noncleaved cell or Burkitt's, and large cell lymphoma (Ries et al., 1994). Many lymphomas in children are of T-cell origin; in contrast, lymphomas in adults are usually B-cell derived (Shipp et al., 1997).

Immunoglobulin levels are decreased in NHL (Amlot and Green, 1979; Solanki et al., 1990), and antibody responses are usually impaired (Heath et al., 1964). The total number of lymphocytes is decreased in patients with NHL. T- and B-cell percentages are within normal limits, but because of the lymphopenia, the mean total numbers of T lymphocytes are decreased (Heier et al., 1977). Delayed hypersensitivity skin tests are depressed in NHL (Anderson et al., 1981; Gupta et al., 1980). The greatest impairment is found in diffuse lymphoma, particularly in those cases with histiocytic features (Jones et al., 1977). In vitro cell-mediated immunity measured by lymphocyte responses to PHA and concanavalin A (ConA) is also reduced (Heier et al., 1977; Hersh and Irvin, 1969). Leukocyte mobilization and granulocyte clearance rates are normal (Senn and Jungi, 1975).

CASTELMAN'S DISEASE: ANGIOFOLLICULAR LYMPH NODE HYPERPLASIA

Castelman's disease is a distinct lymphoproliferative disorder of unknown origin. Three histologic variants have been described: hyaline vascular, plasma cell, and mixed. Two different clinical types are localized or multicentric. The onset is generally in adolescence or early adulthood, rarely childhood (Perel, 1989). In the localized form, a single large mass or lymph node develops in the mediastinum or occasionally at other lymph node sites, exceptionally in extranodal sites. Multicentric disease is a systemic lymphoproliferative disorder with widespread lymphadenopathies, hepatosplenomegaly, fever, anemia, hypoalbuminemia, and polyclonal hypergammaglobulinemia, most often representing an increase in IgA and IgG (Frizzera et al., 1985; Maslovsky et al., 2000).

Lymphocyte subsets and function have been described in a few cases with contradictory results: normal numbers and function (Palacios et al., 1991) and predominance of CD4[+] T lymphocytes over CD8[+] T lymphocytes with absent lymphocyte proliferative response to PHA and ConA (Massey et al., 1991).

Some manifestations of Castelman's disease are due to excessive production of IL-6 that induces B-cell differentiation to immunoglobulin-producing cells and stimulates biosynthesis of acute phase proteins. Increased amounts of IL-6 are present in the germinal centers of B cells and in the plasma (Hsu et al., 1993; Yoshizaki et al., 1989). IL-6 levels correlate with extent of lymph node hyperplasia, hypergammaglobulinemia, increased level of acute phase proteins, and clinical manifestations.

Human herpesvirus 8 (HHV-8) DNA sequences have been detected in CD19 B lymphocytes of patients with localized Castelman's disease and in CD19 B lymphocytes and CD2 T lymphocytes in patients with multicentric Castelman's disease (Kikuta et al., 1997). HHV-8 has been shown to be present in lymph nodes from patients with multicentric Castelman's disease (Soulier et al., 1995), suggesting that HHV-8 has tropism for both B and T lymphocytes in Castelman's disease. HHV-8 may play a crucial role in producing IL-6 and in releasing angiogenic factors (Palestro et al., 1999).

Management of localized Castelman's disease can be achieved by surgery, with or without radiation therapy (Maslovsky et al., 2000; Weisenburger et al., 1979).

Treatment of multicentric Castelman's disease has used glucocorticoids, angiogenic factors, and chemotherapy. Clinical benefit has been achieved with a monoclonal antibody to IL-6 (Beck et al., 1994), humanized anti–IL-6 receptor antibody (Nishimoto et al., 2000), interferon-α (Maloisel et al., 2000; Tamayo et al., 1995), and other chemotherapeutic agents (Parez et al., 1999; Peterson and Frizzera, 1993); however, multicentric Castelman's disease has a poor long-term prognosis.

LYMPHOPROLIFERATIVE DISEASE IN TRANSPLANT RECIPIENTS

Transplantation of bone marrow or organs is lifesaving for some patients with congenital or acquired disorders such as malignancy. Potent immunosuppression must generally be used to achieve and maintain engraftment. Transplantation in both immunologically normal and immunologically deficient humans is accompanied by the frequent development of continually proliferating B lymphocytes that results in lymphoproliferative disease. The suppression of cell-mediated immunity necessary for successful transplantation also permits proliferation of transformed B lymphocytes.

Pathogenesis

With rare exceptions (Garcia et al., 1987), EBV infection is the causative agent of post-transplantation lymphoproliferative disease. The sequence of events has been reviewed (Ho et al., 1988; Malatack et al., 1991); EBV infects cells through a cell-specific complement receptor (CD21) on B cells. The normal immune response controls the infection by development of EBV-specific cytotoxic T cells directed against infected B cells (Klein, 1975). Without these cytotoxic T cells, the EBV-induced B-cell proliferation continues. Initial proliferation is polyclonal and can be reversed if the normal immune response is restored. A decreased dose of immunosuppressive drugs may allow sufficient restoration of the immune system to halt progression of the lymphoproliferation without compromising graft survival. Unimpeded progression of the disease may lead to a monoclonal malignant lymphoma that requires surgical excision, even if immune dysfunction can be reversed.

Three phases of lymphoproliferation have been described (Malatack et al., 1991). The first consists of a mononucleosis syndrome with benign polymorphous B-cell hyperplasia. The second is characterized by a polymorphic B-cell lymphoma with an illness similar to mononucleosis, but the tissues have the morphologic characteristics of a malignancy resembling large cell lymphoma. Associated clinical features can include pancreatitis, meningoencephalitis, and pneumonitis. Whether these symptoms are a direct result of EBV infection or from other opportunistic infection remains unresolved. The third phase is characterized by the development of extranodal tumors that are monoclonal and malignant. Chromosomal translocations in these tumors may occur; abnormalities in protooncogenes and tumor suppressor genes may also occur (Knowles et al., 1995).

Pathologic classification of these lymphoproliferative tumors emphasizes the progressive nature of the disease (Nalesnik et al., 1988). Polymorphic tumors consist of lymphoid cells in various stages of differentiation. Monomorphic tumors contain lymphocytes in the same stage of differentiation. Monomorphic lymphoid cells are further classified by clonality using immunocytochemical staining or genetic analysis of gene rearrangements. Polyclonal tumors have a nearly normal ratio of κ to λ light chains, whereas monoclonal tumors express a skewed ratio with either κ or λ light chains present in great excess.

Incidence

The incidence of lymphomas in immunosuppressed transplant patients is 1-fold higher than in the general population (Penn, 1981, 1998). After stem cell transplantation, the incidence of lymphoproliferative disorders ranges from less than 1% following unmanipulated matched sibling transplants to more than 30% following mismatched T-depleted transplants for immunodeficiencies (Gross et al., 1999). In practically all cases, the tumor arises within the first 6 months after transplant and is associated with EBV. Methods of marrow T-cell depletion that remove or inactivate B cells reduce the risk of lymphoproliferative disorders.

Immunocompetent subjects receiving organ transplants are also at risk for lymphoproliferative disorders because of the use of potent immunosuppressive agents. A multicenter study of 45,000 kidney transplant recipients found a 40-fold increase in NHL during the first post-transplant year (Opelz and Henderson, 1993; Penn, 2000). A similar risk occurs for heart and liver transplant recipients (Kelley et al., 2000; Krikorian et al., 1978; Okano et al., 1988). Rates can reach 25% after liver transplants, especially in EBV-negative pediatric recipients receiving a liver from an EBV-positive donor (Cox et al., 1995).

Treatment

Remissions of lymphoproliferative disorders have been reported using anti–B-cell monoclonal antibody therapies (Ifthikharuddin et al., 2000; Milpied et al., 2000), interferon-α for immune enhancement (Gaynor and Fisher, 1991), and donor lymphocyte infusions (Giralt and Kolb, 1996), especially in cases of polyclonal or anatomically limited disease. Infusion of cytotoxic T cells for the prevention and treatment of EBV-induced lymphoma in allogeneic transplant recipients has also been described (Rooney et al., 1998).

IMMUNE DEFECTS WITH CHEMOTHERAPY

Cancer chemotherapy with cytostatics and corticosteroids can result in marked immunosuppression. Mustafa and associates (1998) found that a majority of such patients showed a decrease in the absolute lymphocyte count at the end of therapy, irrespective of the type of malignancy (e.g., solid tumors, ALL, HD). Recovery occurred slowly, and a significant number show a decrease in $CD4^+$ counts 9 to 12 months after cessation of therapy with an abnormally low CD4/CD8 ratio. B-cell numbers were subnormal after cessation of therapy and returned to normal after approximately 1 month (Alanko et al., 1992; Mustafa et al., 1998).

Immunoglobulin levels are usually normal before initiation of chemotherapy in ALL and HD, but significant decrease in all immunoglobulin levels after therapy are seen. Recovery after cessation of therapy starts with restoration of IgG levels in 1 to 9 months, followed by IgA in 18 to 24 months. A profound depression of IgM levels, lasting several months or even years after completion of therapy, was seen in all tumor types (Abrahamsson et al., 1995; De Vaan et al., 1982). Normalization of serum immunoglobulins after ALL chemotherapy may take several years (Alanko et al., 1992; Layward et al., 1981).

Protective titers against tetanus, diphtheria, poliomyelitis, and sometimes pneumococcus in patients treated for leukemia and other malignancies such as Hodgkin's lymphoma are maintained. In contrast, antibodies to varicella, influenza, and hepatitis B (naturally acquired) or measles (acquired by vaccination) may decrease or disappear during chemotherapy (Ridgway and Wolff, 1993). The antibody response to initial or booster immunizations against tetanus and diphtheria are normal, but they are decreased for *Haemophilus influenzae* b, influenza virus, hepatitis B, and pneumococcus. General guidelines for immunization of patients with hematologic malignancies are described in Table 26-3 (Molrine and Ambrosino, 1996).

T-cell function, as measured by proliferative response to PHA, pokeweed mitogen (PWM), or ConA were decreased during chemotherapy (Lovat et al., 1993; Nash et al., 1993) but soon returned to normal in patients with ALL (Nash et al., 1993). Immune defects induced by radiotherapy and immune recovery are discussed in Chapter 27.

IMMUNE DEFECTS FOLLOWING STEM CELL TRANSPLANTATION

After bone marrow transplantation (BMT) or stem cell transplantation, hematopoietic reconstitution consists of two distinct phenomena—numerical recovery of hematopoietic cellular elements and recovery of cellular function. Hematologic recovery with reappearance of neutrophils and platelets occurs in 2 to 3 weeks (Bensinger et al., 21), but functional recovery of lymphoid cells occurs very gradually; full reconstitution may take a year or more (Guillaume et al., 1998). Mature B-cell numbers attain a normal plateau in 6 to 9 months. IgM production normalizes by 6 months, IgG by 12 months, and IgA by 2 years, reflecting a recapitulation of normal B-cell development (Pedrazzini et al., 1989) (see Chapter 43).

TABLE 26-3 · RECOMMENDATIONS FOR IMMUNIZATION OF PATIENTS WITH HEMATOLOGIC MALIGNANCIES

Vaccine	Chemotherapy	Hodgkin's Disease	BMT
DT or DPT*	Complete primary series during chemotherapy (C) Booster at 1 year after completion of chemotherapy	Not indicated	12 and 24 months
IPV	Complete primary series during chemotherapy (C) Booster at 1 year after completion of chemotherapy	Not indicated	12 and 24 months
Hib-conjugate	Complete primary series during chemotherapy (C) Booster at 1 year after completion of chemotherapy	Immunize before treatment and give booster immunization as early as 2 years after treatment	12 and 24 months
23-Valent pneumococcal	Recommended (A/C)	Immunize before treatment and give booster immunization as early as 2 years after treatment	12 and 24 months
Heptavalent pneumococcal conjugate (PCV7)	Recommended (C)	Recommended (C)	No recommendation†
4-valent meningococcal	Recommended (A/C)	Immunize before treatment and give booster immunization as early as 2 years after treatment	12 and 24 months
Influenza	Recommended (A/C)	Recommended	Recommended
MMR	Contraindicated (A/C)‡	Contraindicated	Recommended§
OPV	Contraindicated	Contraindicated	Contraindicated
Varicella	Contraindicated¶	Contraindicated¶	Contraindicated¶

*Pertussis vaccine is included if the child is younger than 7 years.
†Guidelines for preventing opportunistic infections among hematopoietic stem cell transplant recipients: recommendations of CDC, the Infectious Disease Society of America, and the American Society of Blood and Marrow Transplantation (MMWR 49:9, 2000).
‡May be considered in previously nonimmunized children with leukemia who are in remission and off therapy for at least 3 months.
§Contraindicated in BMT patients with graft-versus-host disease who are receiving immunosuppressors.
¶Prevention of varicella: updated recommendations of the Advisory Committee on Immunization Practices (ACIP). MMWR 48:1–5, 1999.
A/C = adults/children; BMT = bone marrow transplant; C = children; DT = diphtheria-tetanus toxoids; DPT = diphtheria-pertussis-tetanus; Hib-conjugate = *H. influenzae* type B-conjugate vaccine; IPV = inactivated polio vaccine; MMR = measles-mumps-rubella vaccine; OPV = oral polio vaccine.

CD3 total T-cell counts usually return to normal levels within 3 months (Sugita et al., 1994a), but low levels of CD4 cells may persist for a year or more. In contrast, the relative and absolute number of CD8 cells is restored more rapidly, leading to an inverted CD4/CD8 ratio for several months after BMT (Olsen et al., 1988; Sugita et al., 1994a).

Functional subsets of T cells include memory CD4⁺CD45RO⁺ that can respond to recall antigens, whereas naïve CD4⁺CD45RA⁺ are newly released cells from the thymus that can respond to neoantigens. CD4⁺CD4RA⁺ cells are profoundly decreased during the first 3 months following BMT but return to normal levels 1 to 2 years after BMT (Storek et al., 1995). The CD8⁺CD45RA⁺ (naïve cytotoxic T cells) subset normalizes during the first month after BMT. T-cell function measured by lymphoproliferation to mitogenic monoclonal antibodies to CD2 and CD3 alone or in the presence of IL-2, show decreased response shortly after BMT (Cayeux et al., 1989; Sugita et al., 1994b) with full restoration after 1 year (Sugita et al., 1994b).

NK cells are among the first cells to recover after BMT. NK-cell function reaches normal level within 1 month (Talmadge et al., 1996).

Antibodies to many common childhood vaccines, such as polio and tetanus, disappear after ablative therapy in autologous or allogeneic BMT, thus necessitating revaccination. Post-transplantation response to pneumococcal polysaccharide vaccine is poor early after transplant but a good response is obtained following

two booster doses of tetanus toxoid and *H. influenzae* b-conjugate vaccine after stable engraftment (Barra et al., 1992; Somani and Larson, 1995). General guidelines for immunization of patients with hematologic malignancies and patients after BMT are available (see Table 26-3) (Molrine and Ambrosino, 1996).

APLASTIC ANEMIA

Definition

Bone marrow failure affects one or more cellular elements. The term *aplastic anemia* should be reserved for illnesses in which pancytopenia develops, with decreased production of all hematologic cell types, with severe hypoplasia or aplasia of the marrow, and with exclusion of other causes (Scott et al., 1959). A congenital form of aplastic anemia, *Fanconi's anemia*, is discussed earlier (see Chapter 18).

Acquired forms of aplastic anemia may occur following certain infections, notably hepatitis, a history of autoimmune disease, and the previous use of various drugs (Baumelou et al., 1993; Williams, 1999) (Table 26-4).

No single cause of aplastic anemia has been identified (Appelbaum and Fefer, 1981). It may be a qualitative defect of a common stem cell population, a defective marrow environment, impaired production or effectiveness of hematopoietic growth factors, or immune suppression.

TABLE 26-4 · CLASSIFICATION OF APLASTIC ANEMIA

Acquired
Chemical and physical agents
Ionizing agents, benzene, certain drugs (chloramphenicol, anti-
  inflammatory drugs, antiepileptic drugs, gold)
Viral infections
  Hepatitis, EBV, HIV, parvovirus, dengue
Mycobacterial infections
Miscellaneous causes
  Diffuse eosinophilic fasciitis, pregnancy, sclerosis of the thyroid,
    Simmond disease
Idiopathic
Familial
Fanconi's anemia
Congenital dyskeratosis
Shwachman-Diamond syndrome
Reticular dysgenesis
Amegakaryocytic thrombocytopenia
Preleukemia, myelodysplasia, monosomy 7
Syndromes: Down, Dubowitz, Seckel
Putative hereditary defect in cellular uptake of folate

See Williams (1999) for details.
EBV = Epstein-Barr virus; HIV = human immunodeficiency virus.

Tsuda and Yamasaki (2000) have described an overproduction of type I cytokines in aplastic anemia that are
inhibitory to hematopoiesis.

Laboratory Findings

The predominant immunologic deficiency results
from the granulocytopenia. Monocytopenia has also
been noted in aplastic anemia (Twoney et al., 1973).
Foon and co-workers (1984), studying 16 patients
with hepatitis-associated aplastic anemia, documented
decreased circulating T cells, decreased mitogen reactivity of T cells, decreased response to skin-test
antigens, and low serum IgG and IgM levels. By contrast, Falcao and colleagues (1983) found normal
immunoglobulin levels, and Lum and associates (1987)
found normal T-cell proliferative responses. Decrease
in NK-cell activity has also been described (Porwit
et al., 1988).

Treatment

Management includes cessation of exposure to potentially noxious agents, blood and/or platelet transfusions, prevention of infections, immunosuppressive
therapy with high-dose methylprednisolone or antilymphocyte globulin, hematopoietic growth factors (i.e.,
granulocyte colony-stimulating factor [G-CSF]), and
BMT (Williams, 1999).

The prognosis of aplastic anemia is highly variable
depending on the severity of the disease and its response
to treatment. A recent study showed a 6-year survival of
93% in patients treated with BMT versus 70% in
patients treated with immunosuppression (Fouladi
et al., 2000).

AGRANULOCYTOSIS

Pathogenesis

Severe neutropenia (agranulocytosis) is associated with
marrow suppression induced by drugs or radiation therapy (Mauer and Krill, 1964). Neutropenia related to
increased cell destruction has been described in a variety of diseases, including cirrhosis with splenomegaly,
lupus erythematosus, megaloblastic anemia, viral infection, Felty syndrome, and other conditions (Bishop
et al., 1971; Mauer and Krill, 1964). Neutropenia is
present in the hyper-IgM1 syndrome (Levy et al., 1997)
and other cellular immunodeficiencies (Lux et al., 1970).

The risk of major bacterial infections is inversely proportional to the absolute granulocyte count. Children
with chronic neutropenia generally have infections
involving the skin, mucous membranes, and lungs, usually caused by *Staphylococcus aureus* or enteric organisms (Pincus et al., 1976). Cines and associates (1982)
noted a high incidence of underlying immunologic disturbances, such as immune thrombocytopenia and
autoimmune hemolytic anemia.

Treatment

Management of neutropenic states includes attempts to
reverse the primary defect and prevention and treatment
of infectious complications. Neutropenia has been corrected with plasma infusions (Pachman et al., 1975;
Rieger et al., 1974), leukocyte transfusions (Vallejos
et al., 1975), and BMT. A major advance has been the use
of cytokines that stimulate hematopoiesis. Recombinant
human granulocyte colony-stimulating factor (rhG-
CSF) and recombinant human granulocyte-macrophage
colony-stimulating factor (rhGM-CSF) are very effective especially in the neutropenias associated with
chemotherapy (Voss and Armitage, 1995).

Supportive therapeutic measures are directed at the
complications of the disease (Freireich et al., 1970).
Hemorrhage with thrombocytopenia is managed with
platelet transfusions. In leukopenia, acute leukemia,
and lymphomas, the granulocyte count often predicts
susceptibility to infection. Patients with fewer than 4
granulocytes/µl are at higher risk, and those with granulocyte counts of 4 to 8/µl are at moderate risk. Prompt
recognition of infection, with confirmation by appropriate cultures, is imperative.

In acute leukemia, in which more than 70% of the
febrile episodes are associated with infection, antimicrobial therapy should be started immediately after cultures are obtained. Selection of an antimicrobial agent
depends on the severity of the infection, the probable
location of the infection, or the prior response to antibiotics. Broad-spectrum antibiotics are used until the
organism is identified and sensitivity patterns are determined.

Many infections in patients with depressed resistance are endogenous and are almost impossible to prevent. Prophylactic antibiotics and/or antifungals are

sometimes used, but their long-term efficacy is uncertain. Transfusion of granulocytes in large numbers raises circulating blood levels for short periods of time (half-life of approximately 6 hours) and can be used for severe refractory infections. During remission of leukemia, there does not appear to be increased susceptibility to bacterial infection, and normal childhood activity should be maintained. Live viral vaccines are contraindicated in patients with leukemia and lymphomas and in those receiving immunosuppressive drugs or radiation therapy.

HISTIOCYTOSES

The histiocytoses are caused by nonmalignant proliferation of antigen-presenting dendritic cells and antigen-processing macrophages. In 1987, the Histiocyte Society grouped these disorders into three classes (Chu et al., 1987) (Table 26-5). Class I now represents Langerhans cell histiocytosis (LCH), which comprises disorders formerly termed *histiocytosis X* (Lichtenstein, 1953). Class II comprises hemophagocytic lymphohistiocytosis, juvenile xanthogranuloma, and reticulohistiocytoma. Finally, class III includes malignant histiocytic disorders, such as acute monocytic leukemia (FAB M5), malignant histiocytosis, and true histiocytic lymphoma. Each class has its own clinical picture and associated immunologic features.

Class I Histiocytosis: Langerhans Cell Histiocytosis

Lichtenstein (1953) was the first to group eosinophilic granuloma of bone, Hand-Schüller-Christian disease, and Letterer-Siwe disease under the term *histiocytosis X*. The lesion of histiocytosis X resulted from the proliferation and dissemination of abnormal histiocytic cells of the Langerhans cell system (Nezelof et al., 1973). Tissue analysis showed clonal proliferation of CD1a$^+$ cells or Langerhans-type dendritic cells (Willman and

McClain, 1998). The hypothesis that the clonal proliferation was driven by viral infection is not supported by DNA studies (for review, see Willman and McClain, 1998).

LCH can occur at any age, but more than 50% of cases are diagnosed between the ages 1 and 15 (Bhatia et al., 1997). The annual incidence has been estimated to be between 3 and 7 cases per million (Arceci, 1999). LCH can present as a restricted form, affecting one organ, or as an extensive disease, affecting many organs. Bone is often affected, in both restricted or extensive disease, and occurs in 80% to 1% of LCH patients (Arico and Egeler, 1998).

Clinical Features

Histopathology of LCH lesions reveals the presence of proliferating Langerhans cells mixed with macrophages and surrounded by T lymphocytes. The presence of proliferating Langerhans cells, using markers such as CD1 or S-1, is essential to the diagnosis of LCH (Schmitz and Favara, 1998). These cells produce an excessive amount of different cytokines, the so-called cytokine storm (Egeler et al., 1999). Increase in TNF-α, GM-CSF, and IL-1 has been documented in some patients with active disease. The increase in TNF-α production might contribute to features of the disease, including fever, bone lysis, hematologic abnormalities, and hepatic dysfunction. The proliferation of Langerhans cells is of clonal origin, whereas the surrounding T lymphocytes are polyclonal. The clonal proliferation of Langerhans cells raises the possibility that LCH is a neoplastic disease (Willman and McClain, 1998). Despite some immune defects, LCH does not result from a primary defect in the immune system.

Immunologic Features

Normal Langerhans cells are APCs and activators of T lymphocytes. Chu and Jaffe (1994) found that LCH cells were unable to stimulate T lymphocytes. Kragballe and colleagues (1981) found normal granulocyte function but decreased monocyte cytotoxicity. Tomooka and co-workers (1986) found decreased chemotactic response in 35 LCH patients and decreased chemiluminescence in 20 of the 35 patients. This decreased polymorphonuclear function might account for their increased susceptibility to bacterial infections (Tomooka et al., 1986).

In a study of 102 children, Lahey and associates (1985) found that 74% had an elevation in at least one immunoglobulin isotype and 15% had an elevation of all three immunoglobulins isotypes; hypogammaglobulinemia was rare. Leikin and colleagues (1973) found normal immunoglobulin levels, delayed cutaneous hypersensitivity reaction, and decreased in vitro lymphocyte responses to mitogens and allogeneic cells in six infants with Letterer-Siwe disease. Nesbit and associates (1981) found that one of eight patients had decreased lymphoproliferative responses to PHA, Con-A, and PWM; there was decreased response to the tetanus antigen in three of eight patients.

TABLE 26-5 · CLASSIFICATION OF HISTIOCYTOSIS

Class	Syndrome
I	Langerhans cell histiocytosis
II	Histiocytosis of mononuclear phagocytes (but not Langerhans cells)
	Hemophagocytic lymphohistiocytosis (familial or reactive—immune associated, virus associated, or malignancy associated)
	Sinus histiocytosis with massive lymphadenopathy (Rasai-Dorfman disease)
	Juvenile xanthogranuloma
	Reticulohistiocytoma
III	Malignant histiocytic disorders
	Acute monocytic leukemia (FAB M5)
	Malignant histiocytosis
	True histiocytic lymphoma

Modified from Chu T, D'Angio GJ, Favara BE, Ladisch S, Nesbit M, Pritchard J. Histiocytosis syndromes in children. Lancet 2:41–42, 1987.

Lymphopenia is not uncommon in histiocytosis, particularly in patients with multisystemic and advanced disease (Martin-Mateos et al., 1991). Both CD4 and CD8 cells are decreased, with an increase in the CD4/CD8 ratio in some patients (Shannon and Newton, 1986). Hosmalin and co-workers (1997) found a decrease in memory T lymphocytes (CD4[+]/CD45RO and CD8[+]/CD45RO) with a reciprocal increase of naïve cells (CD4[+]/CD45RA) in adults with LCH. These abnormalities disappeared in vitro when triggered by CD3 and CD28 molecules in the absence of APCs, hence demonstrating that there was no constitutive defect in the capacity of CD4[+] and CD8[+] T cells to convert from the CD45RO[-] to the CD45RO[+] isoform. They concluded that the lymphopenia and the lymphocyte subsets may result from an abnormal antigen activation rather than from a primary thymic defect.

Class II Histiocytosis: Hemophagocytic Syndromes

Farquhar and Claireaux (1952) described the cases of a brother and sister who presented with a sepsis-like syndrome: persistent fever, progressive pancytopenia, hepatosplenomegaly, and bruising beginning at 9 weeks of age. Autopsies revealed a lymphocytic and plasma cells infiltrate in the liver and a highly reactive marrow in the brother and a histiocytic proliferation of the spleen in the sister. This first report became the archetypical pathologic representation of the hemophagocytic syndrome. Since then, Risdall and associates (1979) described 19 patients with a similar syndrome but at an older age and without a familial history. Immunosuppressive treatment was given to 14, but 5 had no underlying disease; 15 patients had an active viral infection, which may have precipitated the development of the hemophagocytic syndrome.

This has led to the distinction between primary hemophagocytic syndrome or familial hemophagocytic syndrome (FHL), and secondary hemophagocytic syndrome such as virus-associated hemophagocytic syndrome (VAHS), infection-associated hemophagocytic syndrome (IAHS), and malignancy-associated hemophagocytic syndrome (MAHS). The distinction between primary and secondary syndromes is of etiologic significance, but the treatment in both is similar.

Primary Hemophagocytic Lymphohistiocytosis

The incidence of primary hemophagocytic lymphohistiocytosis (HLH) in children has been estimated to be 0.12 per 100,000 children per year in a Swedish study (Henter et al., 1991). The male to female ratio is 1:1. The disease has been reported from all continents and many ethnic groups. Although there is an increased incidence in certain ethnic groups, it is believed to be secondary to higher rates of consanguinity, because the disease is inherited in an autosomal recessive fashion (Henter et al., 1998). The onset of disease is usually

before age 1, but some cases have not appeared until the age of 8. Patients usually present with persistent high fever, hepatosplenomegaly, and in some cases, a rash. Laboratory findings include anemia, thrombocytopenia, neutropenia, hypertriglyceridemia, and hypofibrinogenemia (Favara, 1992).

Secondary Hemophagocytic Lymphohistiocytosis

The incidence of secondary HLH is not well defined, but Janka and associates (1998) found 219 cases reported in the literature from 1979 until 1995. The age of onset is older than the age of presentation with FHL; only 18% of patients were younger than 1 year and about half were younger than 3 years.

The clinical presentation is similar to that in FHL, with high fever, hepatosplenomegaly, and progressive pancytopenia. Laboratory findings include pancytopenia, elevated transaminases, low fibrinogen, disseminated intravascular coagulation, and high ferritin values.

Janka and colleagues (1998) identified a triggering infection in 163 of 219 cases. EBV infection was reported in 121 cases. Other viruses implicated include human herpesvirus 6, cytomegalovirus, adenovirus, parvovirus, and varicella-zoster virus. Bacterial infections were reported in 11 cases.

In both primary and secondary HLH, there is significant immune dysfunction. In both, there is a significant activation of macrophages, with presence of profound hemophagocytosis with vacuolated cytoplasm and large numbers of cells. Immunoglobulins show no consistent abnormalities (Egeler et al., 1996; McClain et al., 1988). Lymphopenia is frequent and often profound. Lymphocyte subset studies reveal a decrease in B lymphocytes in most patients. McClain and associates (1988) also found low numbers of T cells, with a relative decrease in suppressor cells. The CD4/CD8 ratio was also inverted in patients with EBV infection. Egeler and colleagues (1996), however, reported normal T-cell numbers and distribution. McClain and co-workers (1988) noted severely depressed lymphoproliferation to ConA, PHA, or PWM in five of nine HLH patients. Egeler and associates (1996) noted depressed cytotoxic T lymphocytes function in 11 of 12 patients.

NK-cell defects are common in HLH (Arceci, 1999). Arico and associates (1996) found impaired NK function in 36 of 37 patients. Although patients with familial HLH usually exhibit NK defects at diagnosis, patients with IAHS may have normal NK function and never completely lose NK function (Janka et al., 1998). Sullivan and colleagues (1998) studied the NK function in FHL patients and their first-degree relatives. Impaired NK function was present in all patients and at least one family member, implying that genetic defect in HLH may affect NK function to a degree insufficient to lead to disease progression, because no relative developed HLH.

At least two chromosomal loci have been implicated in HLH. Ohadi and co-workers (1999) analyzed four inbred FHL families and found a linkage at position 9q21.3-22.

Dufourcq-Lagelouse and associates (1999) analyzed 17 families with FHL and described linkage at position 10q21-22 in 10 families but not in the other 7, suggesting a genetic heterogeneity. Analysis of those markers in FHL led to the discovery of the gene encoding perforin, an important mediator in lymphocyte cytotoxicity (Stepp et al., 1999). However, the link between this defect and the clinical manifestations remains to be determined.

Class III Histiocytosis: Malignant Histiocytic Disorders

Class III histiocytosis includes malignant histiocytic disorders, such as acute monocytic leukemia, malignant histiocytosis, and true histiocytic lymphoma. The immune disorders associated with leukemic malignancies and lymphoma are described elsewhere in this chapter.

SARCOIDOSIS

Clinical Features

Sarcoidosis is a chronic, multisystem, granulomatous disorder that most often affects young adults. Although essentially all organs of the body may be affected, the lung is the most common organ involved and accounts for most morbidity and mortality (Thomas and Hunninghake, 1987). Although the cause of sarcoidosis is unknown, the host immune response clearly plays a major role in its pathogenesis. Sarcoidosis demonstrates a dichotomy of heightened immune activity at sites of disease activity and impaired responses elsewhere (Hunninghake et al., 1979). The diagnosis rests on the characteristic clinical and radiologic findings combined with histologic evidence of noncaseating epithelioid cell granulomas in more than one organ and exclusion of granulomas of known causes.

The course and prognosis depends on ethnicity, duration of the illness, site and extent of organ involvement, and activity of the granulomatous process. Sarcoidosis shows a predilection for adults younger than 40 years; the incidence peaks in adults between 20 to 29 years of age (Gordis, 1973). Most studies suggest a slightly higher rate among women and among Swedish, Danish, and African-American populations (Milman and Selroos, 1990; Rybicki et al., 1998). Sarcoidosis in children is uncommon, but Kendig (1974) found that the distribution of organs was the same as in adults; however, the prognosis is more favorable than in adults (James and Kendig, 1988).

Pathogenesis

Genetic Factors

Genetic factors may be implicated in sarcoidosis, as suggested by the predilection of African Americans to sarcoidosis. They are affected eight times more frequently and more severely than Caucasian Americans

(Johns et al., 1976). There are occasional familial cases (Buck, 1961). The genetic influence of MHC loci is suggested by studies that show an association of specific manifestations of sarcoidosis with particular MHC antigens. For example, erythema nodosum and arthritis are noted more commonly in patients with HLA-B8 (Guyatt et al., 1982; James and Neville, 1977), whereas uveitis is more common in those with HLA-B27 (Scharf and Zonis, 1980).

Environmental Factors

Possible etiologic factors for sarcoidosis are viruses, mycobacteria, and aberrant lymphokine expression. Mitchell and Rees (1969) reported the transfer of granulomatous reactions from human sarcoid tissue to mice. These results have been reproduced by some (Mitchell and Rees, 1976; Taub and Siltzbach, 1974) but not by others (Iwai and Takahashi, 1976). There are also reports of sarcoidosis in recipients of transplants from patients with sarcoidosis (Heyll et al., 1994).

Although viruses, particularly herpesviruses, have been suspect based on seroepidemiologic evidence (Byrne et al., 1973), conclusive support is lacking (Steplewski, 1976). Siltzbach (1976) suggested that the transfer experiments are also consistent with transmission by lymphokines. Mycobacterial infections have also received considerable attention.

Antibodies to mycobacteria are identified in the sera of 50% to 80% of patients (Chapman and Speight, 1964; Milman and Andersen, 1993). Antibodies were not present in the affected tissues nor were mycobacteria cultured. Mycobacterial DNA or ribosomal RNA in tissue specimens or bronchoalveolar lavage (BAL) cells from sarcoid patients have been identified (Mitchell et al., 1992; Saboor et al., 1992). These results must be interpreted with caution. Mycobacteria are difficult to cultivate, and cross-contamination may occur. The antibodies may result from the enhanced polyclonal synthesis of immunoglobulins against common antigens.

A further possibility is that both mycobacterial and viral infection may interact to produce sarcoidosis. James and Neville (1977) suggested that a virus-induced T-cell defect combined with an exposure to mycobacteria might result in sarcoidosis.

A role of environmental factors in the pathogenesis of sarcoidosis is suggested by the similar clinical and pathologic characteristics of berylliosis and sarcoidosis (Newman, 1995; Thomas and Hunninghake, 1987). Similar features have been noted with aluminum and zirconium exposure (De Vuyst et al., 1987; Skelton et al., 1993).

Immune Defects

Because sarcoidosis in children is relatively uncommon (Jasper and Denny, 1968; McGovern and Merritt, 1956; Pattischall and Kendig 1990; Waldman and Stiehm, 1977), most immunologic studies are in adult patients. Immune abnormalities include lymphocytic activation within the lungs (Hunninghake and Crystal, 1981) and depressed cellular immunity in peripheral blood lymphocytes (Pasquali et al., 1985). However, patients with sarcoidosis do not generally show an increased susceptibility to infection. Pascual and colleagues (1973) found elevated serum lysozyme levels in sarcoidosis that correlated with disease activity.

The serum angiotensin-converting enzyme (ACE) level is elevated in 60% of patients with sarcoidosis, but it also is elevated in many other disorders (Bascom and Johns, 1986). Activated macrophages are the likely source of lysozyme and ACE.

B and T Lymphocytes

The absolute number of circulating lymphocytes is usually decreased in patients with sarcoidosis (Hedfors et al., 1974; Ramachandar et al., 1975; Tannenbaum et al., 1976). Hedfors and co-workers (1974) report a modest but significant deficiency of T cells as measured by E rosettes, an observation confirmed in other laboratories (Kalden et al., 1976; Veien et al., 1976). Daniele and Rowlands (1976) have demonstrated antibodies to T lymphocytes in the sera of 9 of 15 sarcoid patients. Circulating B cells, as identified by surface membrane immunoglobulin, erythrocyte antibody (EA), or erythrocyte antibody and complement (EAC) rosettes, are normal (Hedfors, 1976; Kalden et al., 1976) or increased (Fernandez et al., 1976; Hedfors, 1975). Kataria and associates (1976) found increased numbers of B lymphocytes with surface membrane immunoglobulin but normal numbers of EAC rosette–forming lymphocytes. Increased subpopulations of CD8-positive cells have been described in sarcoidosis (Johnson et al., 1981; Semenzato et al., 1981), but there is an increase in CD4-helper T-cell function (Kataria and Glaus, 1978).

Humoral Immunity

Serum immunoglobulin levels are often normal in sarcoidosis, but IgG is increased in about half the patients (Blasi and Olivieri, 1974; James et al., 1975; Kataria et al., 1982). Other immunoglobulins abnormalities are not uncommon (Celikoglu et al., 1971). Buckley and associates (1966) reported significant elevations of IgA and IgG but not of IgM or C3 in 16 patients with active sarcoidosis. Low IgD levels (Buckley and Trayer, 1972) and high IgE levels (Bergmann et al., 1972) have been recorded. The variability does not consistently reflect disease activity or staging (James et al., 1975), but ethnicity may affect results, because IgA and IgG are reportedly higher in normal African Americans (Goldstein et al., 1969). Levels of secretory immunoglobulins in patients with pulmonary sarcoidosis are similar to those in other bronchopulmonary diseases (Blasi and Olivieri, 1974).

With the exception of the failure to form antibody to mycobacteriophage (Mankiewicz, 1967), patients with sarcoidosis generally exhibit normal or accentuated antibody responses. Carnes and Raffel (1949) reported that complement-fixing antibodies to mycobacterial antigens are comparable in patients with sarcoidosis and tuberculin-positive controls. Using the Middlebrook-Dubos test for antibody to mycobacteria, Flemming and colleagues (1951) found a normal response in patients with sarcoidosis. The antibody response to typhoid and pertussis vaccines (Sones and Israel, 1954) and tetanus toxoid (Greenwood et al., 1958) is essentially normal in sarcoidosis, except for a diminished primary response to tetanus toxoid. Quinn and associates (1955) reported normal titers of mumps antibody in patients with sarcoidosis. Sones and Israel (1954) found normal wheal-and-flare reaction to histamine and normal Prausnitz-Küstner reaction with serum of patient highly reactive to ragweed pollen.

High titers of antibody to EBV have been noted (Hedfors, 1975; Hirshaut et al., 1970), but the similar titers in acute and chronic sarcoidosis argues against EBV as the causative agent (James et al., 1975). Increased antibody titers to other members of the herpes group (Lebbe et al., 1999; Wahren et al., 1971) and other viruses (Byrne et al., 1973) have been recorded. The frequency of autoantibodies to gastric, thyroid, mitochondrial, and nucleic acid antigens were increased in one study (Veien et al., 1976) but normal in another (James et al., 1975).

Circulating immune complexes play an important role in some acute manifestations in sarcoidosis such as erythema nodosum or acute uveitis. Kataria and Holter (1997) reported the presence of immune complexes in 23% to 1% of sarcoid patients. A positive correlation with disease activity has been established (Daniele et al., 1978), and immune complexes tend to disappear with disease resolution.

Serum complement, reflecting an acute phase reaction, is increased in active sarcoidosis (Buckley et al., 1966), but CH_{50}, C2, and C4 levels are generally normal (Scheffer et al., 1971; Simececk et al., 1971).

Delayed Cutaneous Hypersensitivity

Decreased delayed cutaneous hypersensitivity to tuberculin was first observed in sarcoidosis by Jadassohn in 1914 and Schaumann in 1916, a period during which most adults tested had positive tuberculin reactions. These results have been confirmed with PPD, although the percentage of nonreactors has varied (Citron, 1957; Sones and Israel, 1954). In the pediatric age group, 14 of 86 patients had positive tuberculin test results (Jasper and Denny, 1968). Citron (1957) and Siltzbach (1969) have shown that increasing the test strength of tuberculin from 10 to 1 tuberculin units (TUs) significantly increased the number of reactors. The depressed delayed cutaneous hypersensitivity is an acquired defect, because conversion from positive to negative on acquiring sarcoidosis and a return of reactivity on remission have been observed (Israel and Sones, 1967; Nitter, 1953; Sommer, 1964).

Israel and Sones (1966, 1967) noted that tuberculin anergy persisted in most patients even during remission;

furthermore, only 1 of 12 patients given BCG remained tuberculin positive. With use of BCG vaccine that converted 95% of controls, a low degree of reactivity in patients with sarcoidosis was reported. Three patients who did not become tuberculin positive after receiving the BCG vaccine developed sarcoidosis shortly thereafter, suggesting that the immunologic defect might be causative.

Other data from a BCG and vole bacillus (*Mycobacterium microti*) vaccine study in Britain indicated no preceding impairment of delayed hypersensitivity in sarcoidosis. Sutherland and associates (1965) found that the incidence of intrathoracic sarcoidosis was similar in BCG-vaccinated subjects and tuberculin-negative or tuberculin-positive unvaccinated controls. They concluded that the occurrence of sarcoidosis (1.49 per 10,000) was not dependent on the level of previous tuberculin sensitivity; instead, tuberculin sensitivity is depressed in sarcoidosis during and shortly after the onset of the disease.

The loss of tuberculin reactivity is not absolute, because the addition of cortisone to the antigen and the use of depot tuberculin increase the number of reactors (Pyke and Scadding, 1952). Sarcoidosis patients also have decreased cutaneous hypersensitivity response to mumps, coccidioidin, *Trichophyton,* and pertussis (Friou, 1952; Sones and Israel, 1954). Epstein and Mayock (1957) found that sarcoid patients had normal contact sensitivity to the potent allergen pentadactyl catechol of poison ivy but a diminished response to the less potent chemical sensitizers DNCB and para-nitrosodimethyl aniline.

Skin allograft rejection was normal in five patients with sarcoidosis (Snyder, 1964). In this study, skin tests to PPD, histoplasmin, blastomycin, and coccioidin were negative, but all patients rejected their grafts by day 14. Lymphocytes from patients with sarcoidosis produce smaller graft-versus-host reactions in immunosuppressed rats (Topilsky et al., 1972).

Further insight into the immunologic defect in sarcoidosis comes from experiments on the transfer of delayed hypersensitivity reactions with leukocytes (Sones and Israel, 1954; Urbach et al., 1952) or transfer factor (Lawrence and Zweiman, 1968). In sarcoid patients who receive leukocytes from tuberculin-sensitive donors, a positive skin test result develops, excluding a cutaneous abnormality and suggesting that their defect is in their leukocyte. In five of seven sarcoid patients, transfer factor conferred a transient local immunity but systemic transfer was observed in only two of the five. Horsmanheimo and Virolainen (1976) reported transfer of systemic tuberculin sensitivity with transfer factor in six of eight sarcoid patients.

In Vitro Cell-Mediated Immunity

Hirschhorn and associates (1964) showed that peripheral blood leukocytes from sarcoid patients had an impaired response to PHA. Buckley and colleagues (1966) found a significantly decreased response to PHA in sick patients with sarcoidosis, whereas the lymphocytic response from patients in remission was normal. Impaired responses to PHA were reported by Siltzbach and co-workers (1971), Topilsky and associates (1972), and Kataria and colleagues (1973) but not by Girard and associates (1971), Fernandez and co-workers (1976), and Hedfors (1976). Similarly, impaired responses to ConA were reported by Hedfors (1976) but not by Girard and colleagues (1971). Hedfors (1975) and Horsmanheimo (1974) reported impaired lymphocyte response to PPD in some sarcoid patients, but other sarcoid patients with stage I disease or extrapulmonary manifestations had normal responses (Kalden et al., 1976). Belcher and colleagues (1974) and Mangi and associates (1974) demonstrated a serum inhibitor that reduced the in vitro response of normal lymphocytes to PHA, *Candida,* and mumps. Several investigators have reported increased thymidine incorporation by unstimulated lymphocytes. Fernandez and co-workers (1976) suggested that the increased spontaneous DNA synthesis might be due to replicating B cells.

Lymphoproliferative studies have been performed using Kveim suspension, a preparation of human sarcoid tissue. The active material of Kveim suspensions is unknown. Originally, Kveim preparations stimulated blast transformation of lymphocytes from patients with sarcoidosis (Hirschhorn et al., 1964; Schweiger and Mandi, 1967), but studies with thymidine incorporation were negative (Izumi et al., 1973; Siltzbach et al., 1971). However, Zweiman and Israel (1976) reported positive proliferative responses in 14 of 45 patients, but with some variation depending on the source of Kveim material. There was no correlation with in vivo Kveim reactivity, clinical stage, or lymphocyte response to other antigens in vitro. Inhibition of leukocyte migration with Kveim material has yielded conflicting results (Becker et al., 1972; Brostoff and Walker, 1971; Topilsky et al., 1972; Williams et al., 1972; Zweiman and Israel, 1976).

Immunoregulatory Defects

Hunninghake and Crystal (1981) demonstrated an imbalance of local immunoregulatory T lymphocytes in patients with active sarcoidosis (i.e., those with high-intensity alveolitis). Their findings demonstrated a relative excess of CD4 T-helper lymphocytes in BAL. Thus the CD4/CD8 ratio of lung cells was high (10.8:1 versus 1.8:1 for control) and the CD4$^+$ cell population was shown to spontaneously release interferon-γ (IFN-γ) and IL-2 and other cytokines (Konishi et al., 1988; Robinson et al., 1988). Furthermore, alveolar macrophages found in sarcoid lungs release a great number of different cytokines including TNF-α, IL-1, IL-12, IL-15, and growth factors (Agostini et al., 1996a; Baughman et al., 1990; Hunninghake, 1984; Kreipe et al., 1990; Moller et al., 1996).

The increased number of inflammatory cells in sarcoid tissues, especially CD4 memory cells, seems to be due to a cellular redistribution from the peripheral blood to the lung, mediated by chemoattractant cytokines such as IL-8, IL-15, IL-16, and regulated upon activation, normal T expressed and secreted (RANTES) (Agostini et al., 1996a; Agostini et al., 1996b; Taub et al., 1996) and an in situ proliferation (Muller-Quernheim et al., 1989) mainly mediated by IL-2. A large number of BAL lymphocytes from patients with sarcoidosis spontaneously release IL-2 and express a functional IL-2 receptor system (Agostini et al., 1996a; Saltini et al., 1986; Semenzato et al., 1984). Elevated levels of IFN-γ mRNA and the protein involved in the differentiation from Th0 cells into Th1 cells have been described (Moller et al., 1996). Thus a Th1-type T-cell response is probably responsible for the granuloma formation seen in sarcoidosis.

T cells also secrete factors that stimulate polyclonal activation of B cells, resulting in large amounts of immunoglobulin in fluid surrounding lung tissue. These imbalances of immunoregulatory subsets of lymphocytes in lung and blood may explain the excess production of immunoglobulins in the lung (Hunninghake et al., 1979; Lawrence et al., 1980) and the decreased antibody and immunoglobulin production of blood lymphocytes (Katz and Fauci, 1978; Lawrence et al., 1982). A role for suppressor monocytes in peripheral blood has also been demonstrated (Goodwin et al., 1979; Lawrence et al., 1982).

CONCLUSION

Some immune defects are common and characteristic of particular diseases. For example, in HD the defect in cell-mediated cytotoxicity is probably implicated in the disease pathogenesis. Patients with HD have downregulated MHC class I antigens, overexpression of TGF-β, and downregulation of certain adhesion molecules. Defects in NK cells are a hallmark of class II histiocytic disorders and are almost uniformly present at diagnosis. In contrast, immunologic impairment in leukemia is usually late and the consequence of chemotherapies. With a few exceptions, the immune dysfunction associated with these disorders usually disappears within a year after successful treatment.

R E F E R E N C E S

Abrahamsson J, Marky I, Mellander L. Immunoglobulin levels and lymphocyte response to mitogenic stimulation in children with malignant during treatment and follow-up. Acta Paediatr 84:177–182, 1995.

Abrahamsson J, Mellander L. Bone marrow immunoglobulin-secreting cells are not reduced in children with leukaemia as compared to children with solid tumors. Acta Pediatr 86:165–169, 1997.

Agostini C, Trentin L, Facco M, Sancetta R, Cerutti A, Tassinari C, Cimarosto L, Adami F, Cipriani A, Zambello R, Semenzato G. Role of IL-15, IL-2, and their receptors in the development of T cell alveolitis in pulmonary sarcoidosis. J Immunol 157:910–918, 1996a.

Agostini C, Zambello R, Sancetta R, Cerutti A, Milani A, Tassinari C, Facco M, Cipriani A, Trentin L, Semenzato G. Expression of tumor necrosis factor-receptor superfamily members by lung T lymphocytes in interstitial lung disease. Am J Respir Crit Care Med 153:1359–1367, 1996b.

Aisenberg AC. Studies on delayed hypersensitivity in Hodgkin's disease. J Clin Invest 41:1964–1970, 1962.

Aisenberg AC. Lymphopenia in Hodgkin's disease. J Clin Invest 251:1037–1042, 1965a.

Aisenberg AC. Quantitative estimation of the reactivity of normal and Hodgkin's disease lymphocytes with thymidine-2-C14. Nature 205:1233–1235, 1965b.

Alanko S, Pelliniemi TT, Salmi TT. Recovery of blood B-lymphocytes and serum immunoglobulins after chemotherapy for childhood acute lymphoblastic leukemia. Cancer 69:1481–1486, 1992.

Amlot PL, Green L. Serum immunoglobulins G, A, M, D and E concentrations in lymphomas. Br J Cancer 40:371–379, 1979.

Andersen E. Depletion of thymus-dependent lymphocytes in Hodgkin's disease. Scand J Haematol 12:263–269, 1974.

Anderson TC, Jones SE, Soehnlen BJ, Moon TE, Griffith K, Stanley P. Immunocompetence and malignant lymphoma: immunologic status before therapy. Cancer 48:2702–2709, 1981.

Appelbaum FR, Fefer A. The pathogenesis of aplastic anemia. Semin Hematol 18:24–257, 1981.

Arceci RJ. The histiocytosis: the fall of the Tower of Babel. Eur J Cancer 35:747–767, 1999.

Arico M, Egeler RM. Clinical aspects of Langerhans cell histiocytosis. Hematol Oncol Clin North Am 12:247–258, 1998.

Arico M, Janka G, Fischer A, Henter JI, Blanche S, Elinder G, Martinetti M, Rusca MP. Hemophagocytic lymphohistiocytosis. Report of 122 children from the international registry. FHL Study Group of the Histiocyte Society. Leukemia 10:197–203, 1996.

Ayoub JP, Palmer JL, Huh Y, Cabanillas F, Younes A. Therapeutic and prognostic implications of peripheral blood lymphopenia in patients with Hodgkin's disease. Leuk Lymphoma 34:519–527, 1999.

Barra A, Cordonnier C, Preziosi MP, Intrator L, Hessel L, Fritzell B, Preud'homme JL. Immunogenicity of Haemophilus influenzae type B conjugate vaccine in allogeneic bone marrow recipients. J Infect Dis 166:1021–1028, 1992.

Bascom R, Johns CJ. The natural history and management of sarcoidosis. Adv Intern Med 31:213–241, 1986.

Baughman RP, Strohofer SA, Buchsbaum J, Lower EE. Release of tumor necrosis factor by alveolar macrophages of patients with sarcoidosis. J Lab Clin Med 115:36–42, 1990.

Baumelou E, Guiguet M, Mary JY. Epidemiology of aplastic anemia in France: a case-control study. I. Medical history and medication use. The French Cooperative Group for Epidemiological Study of Aplastic Anemia. Blood 81:1471–1478, 1993.

Beck JT, Hsu SM, Widjenes J, Bataille R, Klein B, Vesole D, Hayden K, Jagannath S, Barlogie B. Brief report: alleviation of systemic manifestations of Castelman's disease by monoclonal anti-interleukin-6 antibody. N Engl J Med 330:602–605, 1994.

Becker FW, Krull P, Deicher H, Kalden JR. Leucocyte-migration test in sarcoidosis. Lancet 1:120–123, 1972.

Belcher RW, Carney JF, Nankervis GA. Effect of sera from patients with sarcoidosis on in vitro lymphocyte response. Int Arch Allergy Appl Immunol 46:183–190, 1974.

Bensinger WI, Martin PJ, Storer B, Clift R, Forman SJ, Negrin R, Kashyap A, Flowers MED, Lilleby K, Chauncey TR, Storb R, Appelbaum FR. Transplantation of bone marrow as compared with peripheral blood cells from HLA-identical relatives in patients with hematologic cancers. N Engl J Med 344:175–181, 21.

Bergmann KC, Zaumseil I, Lachmann B. IgE Konzentrationen im Serum von Patienten mit Sarkoidose und Lungertuberkulose. Dtsch Gesundheitsw 27:1774–1775, 1972.

Bhatia S, Nesbit ME Jr, Egeler RM, Buckley JD, Mertens A, Robison LL. Epidemiologic study of Langerhans cell histiocytosis in children. J Pediatr 130:774–784, 1997.

Bishop CR, Rothstein G, Ashenbrucker HE, Athens JW. Leukokinetic studies. XIV. Blood neutrophil kinetics in chronic, steady-state neutropenia. J Clin Invest 50:1678–1689, 1971.

Blasi A, Olivieri D. Immunoglobulins in serum and bronchial secretions in pulmonary sarcoidosis. In Proceedings of the Sixth International Conference on Sarcoidosis. Tokyo, Tokyo University Press, 1974, pp 204–207.

Bobrove AM, Fuks Z, Strober S, Kaplan HS. Quantitation of T and B lymphocytes and cellular immune function in Hodgkin's disease. Cancer 36:169–179, 1975.

Bodey B, Psenko V, Lipsey AL, Kaiser HE. Soluble interleukin-2 receptors in sera of children with primary malignant neoplasms. Anticancer Res 16:219–224, 1996.

Borella L, Webster RG. The immunosuppressive effects of long-term combination chemotherapy in children with acute leukemia in remission. Cancer Res 31:420–426, 1971.

Bosshart H, Jarrett RF. Deficient major histocompatibility complex class II antigen presentation in a subset of Hodgkin's disease tumor cells. Blood, 92:2252–2259, 1998.

Brostoff J, Walker JG. Leucocyte migration inhibition with Kveim antigen in Crohn's disease. Clin Exp Immunol 9:707–711, 1971.

Brown RS, Haynes HA, Foley HT, Godwin HA, Berard CW, Carbone PP. Hodgkin's disease. Immunologic, clinical, and histological features of 50 untreated patients. Ann Intern Med 67:291–302, 1967.

Buck AA. Epidemiologic investigations of sarcoidosis. IV. Discussion and summary. Am J Hyg 74:189–202, 1961.

Buckley CE, Nagaya H, Sieker HO. Altered immunologic activity in sarcoidosis. Ann Intern Med 64:508–520, 1966.

Buckley CE, Trayer HR. Serum IgD concentrations in sarcoidosis and tuberculosis. Clin Exp Immunol 10:257–265, 1972.

Buferne M, Luton F, Letourneur F, Hoeveler A, Couez D, Barad M, Malissen B, Schmitt-Verhulst AM, Boyer C. Role of CD3 delta in surface expression of the TCR/CD3 complex and in activation for killing analyzed with a CD3 delta-negative cytotoxic T lymphocyte variant. J Immunol 148:657–664, 1992.

Byrne EB, Evans AS, Fouts DW, Israel HL. A seroepidemiological study of Epstein-Barr virus and other viral antigens in sarcoidosis. Am J Epidemiol 97:355–363, 1973.

Carnes WH, Raffel S. A comparison of sarcoidosis and tuberculosis with respect to complement fixation with antigens derived from the tubercule bacillus. Bull Johns Hopkins Hosp 85:204–220, 1949.

Casazza AR, Duvall CP, Carbone PP. Infection in lymphoma. Histology, treatment, and duration in relation to incidence and survival. JAMA 197:710–716, 1966.

Caver TE, Slobod KS, Flynn PM, Behm FG, Hudson MM, Turner EV, Webster RG, Boyett JM, Tassie TL, Pui CH, Hurwitz JL. Profound abnormality of the B/T lymphocyte ratio during chemotherapy for pediatric acute lymphoblastic leukemia. Leukemia 12:619–622, 1998.

Cayeux S, Meuer S, Pezzuto A, Korling M, Haas R, Schulz R, Dorken B. T-cell ontogeny after autologous bone marrow transplantation: failure to synthetize interleukin-2 (IL-2) and lack of CD2-and CD3-mediated proliferation by both CD4+ and CD8+ cells even in the presence of exogenous IL-2. Blood 74:2270–2277, 1989.

Celikoglu S, Vieria LO, Siltzbach LE. Serum immunoglobulin levels in sarcoidosis. In Levinsky L, Macholda F, eds. Proceedings of the Fifth International Conference on Sarcoidosis. XIVth scientific conference of the faculty of Charles University, Prague, 1969. Prague, University Karlova, 1971, pp 168–170.

Chapman JS, Speight M. Further studies of mycobacterial antibodies in the sera of sarcoidosis patients. Acta Med Scand Suppl 425:61–67, 1964.

Chen L, Linsley PS, Hellstrom KE. Costimulation of T cells for tumor immunity. Immunol Today 14:483–486, 1993.

Chen L, McGowan P, Ashe S, Johnston J, Li Y, Hellstrom I, Hellstrom KE. Tumor immunogenicity determines the effect of B7 costimulation on T cell-mediated tumor immunity. J Exp Med 179:523–532, 1994.

Chin AH, Saiki JH, Trujillo JM, Williams RC Jr. Peripheral blood T- and B-lymphocytes in patients with lymphoma and acute leukemia. Clin Immunol Immunopathol 1:499–510, 1973.

Chu T, D'Angio GJ, Favara BE, Ladisch S, Nesbit M, Pritchard J. Histiocytosis syndromes in children. Lancet 2:41–42, 1987.

Chu T, Jaffe R. The normal Langerhans cell and the LCH cell. Br J Cancer Suppl 23:S4–10, 1994.

Cines DB, Passero F, Guerry D IV, Bina M, Dusak B, Schreiber AD. Granulocyte-associated IgG in neutropenic disorders. Blood 59:124–132, 1982.

Citron KM. Skin tests in sarcoidosis. Tubercle 38:33–41, 1957.

Coker DD, Morris DM, Coleman JJ, Schimpff SC, Wiernik PH, Elias EG. Infection among 210 patients with surgically staged Hodgkin's disease. Am J Med 75:97–109, 1983.

Cossman J, Annunziata CM, Barash S, Staudt L, Dillon P, He W-W, Ricciardi-Castagnoli P, Rosen CA, Carter KC. Reed-Sternberg cell genome expression supports a B cell lineage. Blood 94:411–416, 1999.

Cox KL, Lawrence-Miyasaki LS, Garcia-Kennedy R, Lennette ET, Martinez OM, Krams SM, Berquist WE, So SK, Esquivel CO. An increased incidence of Epstein-Barr virus infection and lymphoproliferative disorder in young children on FK506 after liver transplantation. Transplantation 59:524–529, 1995.

Cromme FV, Airey J, Heemels MT, Ploegh HL, Keating PJ, Stern PL, Meijer CJ, Walboomers JM. Loss of transporter protein, encoded by the TAP-1 gene, is highly correlated with loss of HLA expression in cervical carcinoma. J Exp Med 179:335–340, 1994a.

Cromme FV, van Bommel PF, Walboomers JM, Gallee MP, Stern PL, Kenemans P, Helmerhorst TJ, Stukart MJ, Meijer CJ. Differences in MHC and TAP-1 expression in cervical cancer lymph node metastases as compared with the primary tumors. Br J Cancer 69:1176–1181, 1994b.

Cunningham-Rundles C, Bodian C. Common variable immunodeficiency: clinical and immunological features of 248 patients. Clin Immunol 92:34–48, 1999.

Daniele RP, McMillan LJ, Dauber JH, Rossman MD. Immune complexes in sarcoidosis: a correlation with activity and duration of disease. Chest 74:261–264, 1978.

Daniele RP, Rowlands DT. Antibodies to T cells in sarcoidosis. Ann NY Acad Sci 278:88–1, 1976.

De Vaan GA, van Munster PJ, Bakkeren JA. Recovery of immune function after cessation of maintenance therapy in acute lymphoblastic leukemia (ALL) of childhood. Eur J Pediatr 139:113–117, 1982.

De Vuyst P, Dumortier L, Schandene L, Estenne M, Verherst A, Yernault JC. Sarcoidlike lung granulomatosis induced by aluminum dusts. Am Rev Respir Dis 135:493–497, 1987.

Dufourcq-Lagelouse R, Jabado N, Le Deist F, Stephan JL, Souillet G, Bruin M, Vilmer E, Schneider M, Janka G, Fischer A, de Saint Basile G. Linkage of familial hemophagocytic lymphohistiocytosis to 10q21-22 and evidence for heterogeneity. Am J Hum Genet 64:172–179, 1999.

Egeler RM, Favara BE, van Meurs M, Laman JD, Claassen E. Differential In situ cytokine profiles of Langerhans-like cells and T cells in Langerhans cell histiocytosis: abundant expression of cytokines relevant to disease and treatment. Blood 94:4195–4201, 1999.

Egeler RM, Shapiro R, Loechelt B, Filipovich A. Characteristic immune abnormalities in hemophagocytic lymphohistiocytosis. J Pediatr Hematol Oncol 18:340–345, 1996.

Eltringham JR, Kaplan HS. Impaired delayed-hypersensitivity responses in 154 patients with untreated Hodgkin's disease. Natl Cancer Inst Monogr 36:107–115, 1973.

Epstein WL, Mayock RL. Induction of allergic contact dermatitis in patients with sarcoidosis. Proc Soc Exp Biol Med 96:786–787, 1957.

Esber E, DiNicola W, Movassaghi N, Leikin S. T and B lymphocytes in leukemia therapy. Am J Hematol 1:211–218, 1976.

Falcao RP, Voltarelli JC, Bottura C. Some immunological studies in aplastic anemia. J Clin Lab Immunol 10:25–28, 1983.

Farquhar J, Clairveaux A. Familial haemophagocytic reticulosis. Arch Dis Child 27:519–525, 1952.

Favara BE. Hemophagocytic lymphohistiocytosis: a hemophagocytic syndrome. Semin Diagn Pathol 9:63–74, 1992.

Feldman S, Andrew M, Norris M, McIntyre B, Iyer R. Decline in rates of seropositivity for measles, mumps, and rubella antibodies among previously immunized children treated for acute leukemia. Clin Infect Dis 27:388–390, 1998.

Fernandez B, Press P, Girard JP. Distribution and function of T- and B-cell subpopulations in sarcoidosis. Ann NY Acad Sci 278:80–87, 1976.

Filipovich AH, Mathur A, Kamat D, Kersey JH, Shapiro RS. Lymphoproliferative disorders and other tumors complicating immunodeficiencies. Immunodeficiency 5:91–112, 1994.

Flemming JW, Runyon EH, Cummings MM. An evaluation of the hemagglutination test for tuberculosis. Am J Med 10:704–710, 1951.

Foon KA, Mitsayasu RT, Schroff RW, McIntyre RE, Champlin R, Gale RP. Immunologic defects in young male patients with hepatitis-associated aplastic anemia. Ann Intern Med 1:657–662, 1984.

Foss HD, Reusch R, Demel G, Lenz G, Anagnostopoulos I, Hummel M, Stein H. Frequent expression of the B-Cell-specific activator protein in Reed-Sternberg cells of classical Hodgkin's disease provides further evidence for its B-cell origin. Blood 94:3108–3113, 1999.

Fouladi M, Herman R, Rolland-Grinton M, Jones-Wallace D, Blanchette V, Calderwood S, Doyle J, Halperin D, Leaker M, Saunders EF, Zipursky A, Freedman MH. Improved survival in severe acquired aplastic anemia of childhood. Bone Marrow Transplant 26:1149–1156, 2000.

Freireich EJ, Bodey GP, DeJongh DS, Curtis JE, Hersh EM. Supportive therapeutic measures for patients under treatment for leukemia or lymphoma. In Leukemia-lymphoma. Chicago, Anderson Hospital, Year Book Medical Publishers, 1970, pp 275–284.

Frenette PS, Wagner DD. Adhesion molecules part I. N Engl J Med 334:1526–1529, 1996.

Friou GJ. A study of the cutaneous reactions to oidiomycin, trichophytin, and mumps skin test antigens in patients with sarcoidosis. Yale J Biol Med 24:533–539, 1952.

Frizzera G, Peterson BA, Bayrd ED, Goldman A. A systemic lymphoproliferative disorder with morphologic features of Castelman's disease: clinical findings and clinicopathologic correlations in 15 patients. J Clin Oncol 3:1202–1216, 1985.

Garcia CR, Brown NA, Schreck R, Stiehm ER, Hudnall SD. B-cell lymphoma in severe combined immunodeficiency not associated with the Epstein-Barr virus. Cancer 60:2941–2947, 1987.

Gatti RA, Good RA. Occurrence of malignancy in immunodeficiency diseases. A literature review. Cancer 28:89–98, 1971.

Gaynor ER, Fisher RI. Clinical trials of alpha-interferon in the treatment of non-Hodgkin's lymphoma. Semin Oncol 18:12–17, 1991.

Giralt SA, Kolb HJ. Donor lymphocyte infusions. Curr Opin Oncol 8:96–102, 1996.

Girard JP, Poupon MF, Press P. Culture of peripheral blood lymphocytes from sarcoidosis: response to mitogenic factor. Int Arch Allergy Appl Immunol 41:604–619, 1971.

Goedert JJ, Cote TR, Virgo P, Scoppa SM, Kingma DW, Gail MH, Jaffe ES, Biggar RJ. Spectrum of AIDS-associated malignant disorders. Lancet 351:1833–1839, 1998.

Goldstein RA, Israel HL, Rawnsley HM. Effect of race and stage of disease on the serum immunoglobulins in sarcoidosis. JAMA 208:1153–1155, 1969.

Goodwin JS, DeHoratius R, Israel H, Peake GT, Messner RP. Suppressor cell function in sarcoidosis. Ann Intern Med 90:169–173, 1979.

Goodwin JS, Messner RP, Bankhurst AD, Peake GT, Saiki JH, Williams RC Jr. Prostaglandin-producing suppressor cells in Hodgkin's disease. N Engl J Med 297:963–968, 1977.

Gordis L. Sarcoidosis: epidemiology of chronic lung diseases in children. Baltimore, John Hopkins University Press, 1973, pp 53–78.

Gotoff SP, Lolekha S, Lopata M, Kopp J, Kopp RL, Malecki TJ. The macrophage aggregation assay for cell-mediated immunity in many studies of patients with Hodgkin's disease and sarcoidosis. J Lab Clin Med 82:682–691, 1973.

Greenwood R, Smellie H, Barr M, Cunliffe AC. Circulating antibodies in sarcoidosis. BMJ 1:1388–1391, 1958.

Groch GS, Perillie PE, Finch SC. Reticuloendothelial phagocytic function in patients with leukemia and multiple myeloma. Blood 26:489–499, 1965.

Gross TG, Steinbuch M, DeFor T, Shapiro RS, McGlave P, Ramsay NK, Wagner JE, Filipovich AH. B cell lymphoproliferative disorders following hematopoietic stem cell transplantation: risk factors, treatment and outcome. Bone Marrow Transplant 23:251–258, 1999.

Gruss HJ, Dolken G, Brach MA, Mertelsmann R, Herrmann F. Serum levels of circulating ICAM-1 are increased in Hodgkin's disease. Leukemia 7:1245–1249, 1993.

Guillaume T, Rubinstein DB, Symann M. Immune reconstitution and immunotherapy after autologous hematopoietic stem cell transplantation. Blood 92:1471–1490, 1998.

Gupta S, Seth SK, Udupa KN, Sen PC, Rastogi BL. Delayed cutaneous hypersensitivity and blood lymphocyte count in advanced Hodgkin's and non-Hodgkin's lymphomas. Ann Chir Gynaecol 69:79–83, 1980.

Guyatt GH, Bensen WG, Stolmon LP, Fagnilli L, Singal DP. HLA-B8 and erythema nodosum. Can Med Assoc J 127:15–16, 1982.

Han T, Sokal JE. Lymphocyte response to phytohemagglutinin in Hodgkin's disease. Am J Med 48:728–734, 1970.

Harning R, Mainolfi E, Bystryn JC, Henn M, Merluzzi VJ, Rothlein R. Serum levels of circulating intercellular adhesion molecule 1 in human malignant melanoma. Cancer Res 51:53–55, 1991.

Hasenclever D, Diehl V. A prognostic score for advanced Hodgkin's disease. N Engl J Med 339:1506–1514, 1998.

Heath RB, Fairley GH, Malpas JS. Production of antibodies against viruses in leukemia and related diseases. Br J Haematol 10:365–370, 1964.

Hedfors E. Immunological aspects of sarcoidosis. Scan J Respir Dis 56:1–19, 1975.

Hedfors E. Characterization of peripheral blood lymphocytes in sarcoidosis. Ann NY Acad Sci 278:101–107, 1976.

Hedfors E, Holm G, Pettersson D. Lymphocyte subpopulations in sarcoidosis. Clin Exp Immunol 17:219–226, 1974.

Heier HE, Klepp R, Gundersen S, Godal T, Normann T. Blood B and T lymphocytes and in vitro cellular immune reactivity in untreated human malignant lymphomas and other malignant tumors. Scand J Haematol 18:137–148, 1977.

Henter JI, Arico M, Elinder G, Imashuku S, Janka G. Familial hemophagocytic lymphohistiocytosis. Primary hemophagocytic lympho-histiocytosis. Hematol Oncol Clin North Am 12:417–433, 1998.

Henter JI, Elinder G, Soder O, Ost A. Incidence in Sweden and clinical features of familial hemophagocytic lymphohistiocytosis. Acta Paediatr Scan 80:428–435, 1991.

Hersh EM, Irvin WS. Blastogenic responses of lymphocytes from patients with untreated and treated lymphomas. Lymphology 2:150–160, 1969.

Hersh EM, Oppenheim JJ. Impaired in vitro lymphocyte transformation in Hodgkin's disease. N Engl J Med 273:16–1012, 1965.

Heyll A, Meckenstock G, Aul C, Sohngen D, BorchardF, Hadding U, Modder U, Leschke M, Schneider W. Possible transmission of sarcoidosis via allogeneic bone marrow transplantation. Bone Marrow Transplant 14:161–164, 1994.

Hirschhorn K, Schreibman RR, Bach FH, Siltzbach LE. In vitro studies of lymphocytes from patients with sarcoidosis and lymphoproliferative diseases. Lancet 2:842–843, 1964.

Hirshaut Y, Glade P, Vieria BD, Ainbender E, Dvorak B, Siltzbach LE. Sarcoidosis, another disease associated with serologic evidence for herpes-like virus infection. N Engl J Med 283:502–506, 1970.

Ho M, Jaffe R, Miller G, Breinig MK, Dummer JS, Makowka L, Atchinson RW, Karrer F, Nalesnik MA, Starzl TE. The frequency of Epstein-Barr virus infection and associated lymphoproliferative syndrome after transplantation and its manifestations in children. Transplantation 45:719–727, 1988.

Horsmanheimo M. Lymphocyte transforming factor in sarcoidosis. Cell Immunol 10:338–343, 1974.

Horsmanheimo M, Virolainen M. Transfer of tuberculin sensitivity by transfer factor in sarcoidosis. Clin Immunol Immunopathol 6:231–237, 1976.

Hosmalin A, McIlroy D, Autran B, Ragot JP, Debre P, Herson S, Karmochkine M. Imbalanced "memory" T lymphocyte subsets and analysis of dendritic cell precursors in the peripheral blood of adult patients with Langerhans cell histiocytosis. Clin Exp Rheumatol 15:649–654, 1997.

Hsu SM, Waldron JA, Xie SS, Barlogie B. Expression of interleukin-6 in Castelman's disease. Hum Pathol 24:833–839, 1993.

Humbert JR, Hutter JJ Jr, Thoren CH, DeArmey PA. Decreased neutrophil bactericidal activity in acute leukemia of childhood. Cancer 37:2194–22, 1976.

Hunninghake GW. Release of interleukin-1 by alveolar macrophages of patients with active pulmonary sarcoidosis. Am Rev Respir Dis 129:569–572, 1984.

Hunninghake GW, Crystal RG. Pulmonary sarcoidosis: a disorder mediated by excess helper T-lymphocyte activity at sites of disease activity. N Engl J Med 305:429–434, 1981.

Hunninghake GW, Gadek JE, Kawanami O, Ferrans VJ, Crystal RG. Inflammatory and immune processes in the human lung in health and disease: evaluation by bronchoalveolar lavage. Am J Pathol 97:149–206, 1979.

Ifthikharuddin JJ, Mieles LA, Rosenblatt JD, Ryan CK, Sahasrabudhe DM. CD-20 expression in post-transplant lymphoproliferative disorders: treatment with rituximab. Am J Hematol 65:171–173, 2000.

Israel H, Sones M. A study of bacillus Calmette-Guerin vaccination and the Kveim reaction. Ann Intern Med 64:87–91, 1966.

Israel HL, Sones M. The tuberculin reaction in patients recovered from sarcoidosis. In Turiaf J, Chabot J, eds. La Sarcoidose. Paris, Masson, 1967, pp 295–298.

Iwai K, Takahashi S. Transmissibility of sarcoid-specific granulomas in the footpads of mice. Ann NY Acad Sci 278:249–259, 1976.

Izumi T, Nilsson BS, Ripe E. In vitro lymphocyte reactivity to different Kveim preparations in patients with sarcoidosis. Scand J Respir Dis 54:123–127, 1973.

Jachimczak P, Bogdahn U, Schneider J, Behl C, Meixensberger J, Apfel R, Dorries R, Schlingensiepen KH, Brysch W. The effect of transforming growth factor β_2-specific phosphorothioate-antisense oligodeoxynucleotides in reversing cellular immunosuppression in malignant glioma. J Neurosurg 78:944–951, 1993.

Jackson SM, Garrett JV, Craig AW. Lymphocyte transformation changes during the clinical course of Hodgkin's disease. Cancer 25:843–850, 1970.

Jadassohn J. Sietuberkulide. Arch Dermatol Syph 119:10–83, 1916.

James DG, Neville E, Walker A. Immunology of sarcoidosis. Am J Med 59:388–394, 1975.

James DG, Neville E. Pathobiology of sarcoidosis. Pathobiol Annu 7:31–61, 1977.

James DG, Kendig EL Jr. Childhood sarcoidosis. Sarcoidosis 5:57–59, 1988.

Janka G, Imashuku S, Elinder G, Schneider M, Henter JI. Infection- and malignancy-associated hemophagocytic syndromes. Secondary hemophagocytic lymphohistiocytosis. Hematol Oncol Clin North Am 12:435–444, 1998.

Jasper PL, Denny FW. Sarcoidosis in children. With special emphasis on the natural history and treatment. J Pediatr 73:499–512, 1968.

Johns CJ, Macgregor MI, Zachary JB, Ball WC. Extended experience in the long-term corticosteroid treatment of pulmonary sarcoidosis. Ann NY Acad Sci 278:722–731, 1976.

Johnson NM, Brostoff J, Hudspith BN, Boot JR, McNicol MW. T gamma cells in sarcoidosis: E rosetting monocytes suppress lymphocyte transformation. Clin Exp Immunol 43:491–496, 1981.

Jones SE, Griffith K, Dombrowski P, Gaines JA. Immunodeficiency in patients with non-Hodgkin's lymphomas. Blood 49:335–344, 1977.

Jurianz K, Ziegler S, Garcia-Schuler H, Kraus S, Bohana-Kashtan O, Fishelson Z, Kirschfink M. Complement resistance of tumor cells: basal and induced mechanisms. Mol Immunol 36:929–939, 1999.

Kageshita T, Wang Z, Calorini L, Yoshii A, Kimura T, Ono T, Gattoni-Celli S, Ferrone S. Selective loss of human leukocyte class I allospecificities and staining of melanoma cells by monoclonal antibodies recognizing monomorphic determinants of class I human leukocyte antigens. Cancer Res 53:3349–3354, 1993.

Kalden JR, Peter HH, Lohmann E, Schedel J, Diehl V, Vallee D. Estimation of T- and K-cell activity in the peripheral blood of sarcoidosis patients. Ann NY Acad Sci 278:52–68, 1976.

Kataria YP, Glaus KR. Phytohemagglutinin response of lymphocyte fractions isolated by velocity sedimentation and enhanced helper cell activity. Am Rev Respir Dis 117:519–526, 1978.

Kataria YP, Holter JF. Immunology of sarcoidosis. Clin Chest Med 18:719–739, 1997.

Kataria YP, LoBuglio AF, Bromberg PA, Hurtubise PE. Sarcoid lymphocytes: B- and T-cell quantitation. Ann NY Acad Sci 278:69–79, 1976.

Kataria YP, Sagone AL, LoBuglio AG, Bromberg PA. In vitro observations on sarcoid lymphocytes and their correlation with cutaneous anergy and clinical severity of disease. Am Rev Respir Dis 108:767–776, 1973.

Kataria YP, Shaw RA, Campbell PB. Sarcoidosis: an overview II. Clin Notes Respir Dis 20:1–16, 1982.

Katz P, Fauci AS. Inhibition of polyclonal B-cell activation by suppressor monocytes in patients with sarcoidosis. Clin Exp Immunol 32:554–562, 1978.

Kavanaugh DY, Carbone DP. Immunologic dysfunction in cancer. Hematol Oncol Clin North Am 10:927–951, 1996.

Kehrl JH, Wakefield LM, Roberts AB, Jakowlew S, Alvarez-Mon M, Derynck R, Sporn MB, Fauci AS. Production of transforming growth factor beta by human T lymphocytes and its potential role in the regulation of T cell growth. J Exp Med 163:1037–1050, 1986.

Kelley MP, Narula N, Loh E, Acker MA, Tomaszewski JE, DeNofrio D. Early post-transplant lymphoproliferative disease following heart transplantation in the absence of lymphocytolytic induction therapy. J Heart Lung Transplant 19:805–809, 2000.

Kendig EL Jr. The clinical picture of sarcoidosis in children. Pediatrics 54:289–292, 1974.

Kersey JH, Shapiro RS, Filipovich AH. Relationship of immunodeficiency to lymphoid malignancy. Pediatr Infect Dis J 7:S10–2, 1988.

Kikuta H, Itakura O, Taneichi K, Kohno M. Tropism of human herpesvirus 8 for peripheral blood lymphocytes in patients with Castelman's disease. Br J Haematol 99:790–793, 1997.

Klein G. The Epstein-Barr virus and neoplasia. N Engl J Med 293:1353–1357, 1975.

Knowles DM. Pathology and pathogenesis of non-Hodgkin's lymphomas associated with HIV infection. In Magrath T, ed. The non-Hodgkin's lymphomas. New York, Arnold, 1997, p 471.

Knowles DM, Cesarman E, Chadburn A, Frizzera G, Chen J, Rose EA, Michler RE. Correlative morphologic and molecular genetic analysis demonstrates three distinct categories of posttransplantation lymphoproliferative disorders. Blood 85:552–565, 1995.

Konishi K, Moller DR, Saltini C, Kirby M, Crystal RG. Spontaneous expression of the interleukin 2 receptor gene and presence of functional interleukin 2 receptors on T lymphocytes in the blood of individuals with active pulmonary sarcoidosis. J Clin Invest 82:775–781, 1988.

Kragballe K, Zachariae H, Herlin T, Jensen J. Histiocytosis X—an immune deficiency disease? Studies on antibody-dependent monocyte-mediated cytotoxicity. Br J Dermatol 105:13–18, 1981.

Kreipe H, Radzun HJ, Heidorn K, Barth J, Kiemle-Kallee J, Petermann W, Gerdes J, Parwaresch MR. Proliferation, macrophage colony-stimulating factor, and macrophage colony-stimulating factor-receptor expression of alveolar macrophages in active sarcoidosis. Lab Invest 62:697–703, 1990.

Krikorian JG, Anderson JL, Bieber CP, Penn I, Stinson EB. Maligant neoplasms following cardiac transplantation. JAMA 240:639–643, 1978.

Lahey ME, Heyn R, Ladisch S, Leikin S, Neerhout R, Newton W, Shore N, Smith B, Wara W, Hammond D. Hypergammaglobulinemia in histiocytosis X. J Pediatr 107:572–574, 1985.

Lamb D, Pilney F, Kelly WD, Good RA. A comparative study of the incidence of anergy in patients with carcinoma, leukemia, Hodgkin's disease and other lymphomas. J Immunol 89:555–558, 1962.

Lawrence EC, Martin RR, Blaese RM, Teague RB, Awe RJ, Wilson RK, Deaton WJ, Bloom K, Greenberg SD, Stevens PM. Increased bronchoalveolar lavage IgG-secreting cells in interstitial lung diseases. N Engl J Med 302:1186–1188, 1980.

Lawrence EC, Theodore BJ, Teague RB, Gottlieb MS. Defective immunoglobulin secretion in response to pokeweed mitogen in sarcoidosis. Clin Exp Immunol 49:96–104, 1982.

Lawrence EC, Zweiman B. Transfer factor deficiency response-a mechanism of anergy in Boeck's sarcoid. Trans Assoc Am Physicians 81:240–248, 1968.

Layward L, Levinsky RJ, Butler M. Long-term abnormalities in T and B lymphocyte function in children following treatment for acute lymphoblastic leukemia. Br J Haematol 49:251–258, 1981.

Lebbe C, Agbalika F, Flageul B, Pellet C, Rybojad M, Cordoliani F, Farge D, Vignon-Pennamen MD, Sheldon J, Morel P, Calvo F,

Schulz TF. No evidence for a role of human herpesvirus type 8 in sarcoidosis: molecular and serological analysis. Br J Dermatol 141:492–496, 1999.

Lee CT, Ciernik IF, Wu S, Tang DC, Chen HL, Truelson JM, Carbone DP. Increased immunogenicity of tumors bearing mutant p53 and P1A epitopes after transduction of B7-1 via recombinant adenovirus. Cancer Gene Ther 3:238–244, 1996.

Leikin S, Puruganan G, Frankel A, Steerman R, Chandra R. Immunologic parameters in histocytosis-X. Cancer 32:796–802, 1973.

Lejeune M, Ferster A, Cantinieaux B, Sariban E. Prolonged but reversible neutrophil dysfunctions differentially sensitive to granulocyte colony-stimulating factor in children with acute lymphoblastic leukaemia. Br J Haematol 102:1284–1291, 1998.

Levy J, Espanol-Boren T, Thomas C, Fischer A, Tovo P, Bordigoni P, Resnick I, Fasth A, Baer M, Gomez L, Sanders EA, Tabone MD, Plantaz D, Etzioni A, Monafo V, Abinun M, Hammarstrom L, Abramsen T, Jones A, Finn A, Klemola T, DeVries E, Sanal O, Peitsch MC, Notarangelo LD. Clinical spectrum of X-linked hyper-IgM syndrome. J Pediatr 131:47–54, 1997.

Lichtenstein L. Histiocytosis X: integration of eosinophilic granuloma of the bone, Letterer-Siwe disease and Schuller-Christian disease as related manifestations of a single nosologic entity. Arch Pathol 56:84–102, 1953.

Lissoni P, Barni S, Rovelli F, Viviani S, Maestroni GJ, Conti A, Tancini G. The biological significance of soluble interleukin-2 receptors in solid tumors. Eur J Cancer 26:33–36, 1990.

Loeffler CM, Smyth MJ, Longo DL, Kopp WC, Harvey LK, Tribble HR, Tase JE, Urba WJ, Leonard AS, Young HA, Ochoa AC. Immunoregulation in cancer bearing hosts. Down-regulation of gene expression and cytotoxic function in CD8+ T cells. J Immunol 149:949–956, 1992.

Lopez-Nevot MA, Esteban F, Ferron A, Gutierrez J, Oliva MR, Romero C, Huelin C, Ruiz-Cabello F, Garrido F. HLA class I gene expression on human primary tumors and autologous metastases: demonstration of selective losses of HLA antigens on colorectal, gastric and laryngeal carcinomas. Br J Cancer 59:221–226, 1989.

Lovat PE, Robinson JH, Windebank KP, Kernahan J, Watson JG. Serial study of T lymphocytes in childhood leukemia during remission. Pediatr Hematol Oncol 10:129–139, 1993.

Lukes RJ, Butler JJ. The pathology and nomenclature of Hodgkin's disease. Cancer Res 26:1063–1083, 1966.

Lukes RJ, Craver LF, Hall TC, Rappaport H, Ruben P. Report of the nomenclature committee. Cancer Res 26:1311, 1966.

Lum LG, Seigneuret MC, Doney KC, Storb R. In vitro immunoglobulin production, proliferation, and cell markers before and after antithymocyte globulin therapy in patients with aplastic anemia. Am J Hematol 26:1–15, 1987.

Lux SE, Johnston RB Jr, August CS, Say B, Penchszadeh VB, Rosen FS, McKusick VA. Chronic neutropenia and abnormal cellular immunity in cartilage-hair hypoplasia. N Engl J Med 282:231–236, 1970.

Malatack JF, Gartner JC Jr, Urbach AH, Zitelli BJ. Orthotopic liver transplantation, Epstein-Barr virus, cyclosporine, and lymphoproliferative disease: a growing concern. J Pediatr 118:667–675, 1991.

Maloisel F, Andres E, Campos F, Oprea C, Deslandres M, Randriamahazaka R, Kurtz JE, Koumarianou A, Dufour P. Is there a place for interferon-alpha in the treatment strategy of multicentric Castelman's disease. Rev Med Interne 21:435–438, 2000.

Mangi RJ, Dwyer JM, Kantor FS. The effect of plasma upon lymphocyte response in vitro: demonstration of a humoral inhibitor in patients with sarcoidosis. Clin Exp Immunol 18:519–528, 1974.

Mankiewicz E. Le role des mycobacteries lysogenes dans l'etiologie de la sarcoidose. In Turiaf J, Chabot J, eds. La Sarcoidose. Paris, Masson, 1967, pp 487–495.

Martin-Mateos MA, Munoz-Lopez F, Monferrer R, Cruz M. Immunological findings in 14 cases of Langerhans cells histiocytosis. J Investig Allergol Clin Immunol 1:308–314, 1991.

Maslovsky I, Uriev L, Lugassy G. The heterogeneity of Castelman disease: report of five cases and review of the literature. Am J Med Sci 320:292–295, 2000.

Massey GV, Kornstein MJ, Wahl D, Huang XL, McCrady CW, Carchman RA. Angiofollicular lymph node hyperplasia (Castelman's disease) in an adolescent female. Clinical and immunologic findings. Cancer 68:1365–1372, 1991.

Mathur A, Kamat DM, Filipovich AH, Steinbuch M, Shapiro RS. Immunoregulatory abnormalities in patients with EBV-associated B-cell lymphoproliferative disorders. Transplantation 57:1042–1045, 1994.

Mauer AM, Krill CE. A study of the mechanisms for granulocytopenia. Ann NY Acad Sci 113:13–18, 1964.

Maxwell M, Galanopoulos T, Neville-Golden J, Antoniades HN. Effect of the expression of transforming growth factor-beta 2 in primary human glioblastomas on immunosuppression and loss of immune surveillance. J Neurosurg 76:799–804, 1992.

McClain K, Gehrz R, Grierson H, Purtilo D, Filipovich A. Virus-associated histiocytic proliferations in children. Frequent association with Epstein-Barr virus and congenital or acquired immunodeficiencies. Am J Pediatr Hematol Oncol 10:196–205, 1988.

McGovern JP, Merritt DH. Sarcoidosis in childhood. Adv Pediatr 8:97–135, 1956.

Milman N, Andersen AB. Detection of antibodies in serum against M. tuberculosis using Western Blot technique: comparison between sarcoidosis patients and healthy subjects. Sarcoidosis 10:29–31, 1993.

Milman N, Selroos O. Pulmonary sarcoidosis in the Nordic countries 1950–1982. Epidemiology and clinical picture. Sarcoidosis 7:50–57, 1990.

Milpied N, Vasseur B, Parquet N, Garnier JL, Antoine C, Quartier P, Carret AS, Bouscary D, Faye A, Bourbigot B, Reguerre Y, Stoppa AM, Bourquard P, Hurault de Ligny B, Dubief F, Mathieu-Boue A, Leblond V. Humanized anti-CD20 monoclonal antibody (Rituximab) in post transplant B-lymphoproliferative disorder: a retrospective analysis of 32 patients. Ann Oncol 11:113–116, 2000.

Mitchell DN, Rees RJ. A transmissible agent from sarcoid tissue. Lancet 2:81–84, 1969.

Mitchell DN, Rees RJW. The nature and physical characteristics of a transmissible agent from human sarcoid tissue. Ann NY Acad Sci 278:233–248, 1976.

Mitchell IC, Turk JL, Mitchell DN. Detection of mycobacterial rRNA in sarcoidosis with liquid-phase hybridisation. Lancet 339:1015–1017, 1992.

Mizoguchi H, O'Shea JJ, Longo DL, Loeffler CM, McVicar DW, Ochoa AC. Alterations in signal transduction molecules in T lymphocytes from tumor-bearing mice. Science 258:1795–1798, 1992.

Moller DR, Forman JD, Liu MC, Noble PW, Greenlee BM, Vyas P, Holden DA, Forrester JM, Lazarus A, Wysocka M, Trinchieri G, Karp C. Enhanced expression of IL-12 associated with Th1 cytokine profiles in active pulmonary sarcoidosis. J Immunol 156:4952–4960, 1996.

Molrine DC, Ambrosino DM. Immunizations in immunocompromised cancer patients. Infect Med 13:259–280, 1996.

Morganfeld MD, Bonchil G. Tuberculin reactions in Hodgkin's disease. N Engl J Med 278:565, 1968.

Morrell D, Cromartie E, Swift M. Mortality and cancer in 263 patients with ataxia-telangiectasia. J Natl Cancer Inst 77:89–92, 1986.

Mueller BU, Pizzo PA. Cancer in children with primary and secondary immunodeficiencies. J Pediatr 126:1–10, 1995.

Muller-Quernheim J, Kronke M, Strausz J, Schykowski M, Ferlinz R. Interleukin-2 receptor gene expression by bronchoalveolar lavage lymphocytes in pulmonary sarcoidosis. Am Rev Respir Dis 140:82–88, 1989.

Mustafa MM, Buchana GR, Winick NJ, McCracken GH, Tkaczewsi I, Lipscomb M, Ansari Q, Agopian MS. Immune recovery in children with malignancy after cessation of chemotherapy. J Pediatr Hematol Oncol 20:451–457, 1998.

Nalesnik MA, Jaffe R, Starzl TE, Demetris AJ, Porter K, Burnham JA, Makowka L, Ho M, Locker J. The pathology of posttransplant lymphoproliferative disorders occurring in the setting of cyclosporine A-prednisone immunosuppression. Am J Pathol 133:173–192, 1988.

Nash KA, Mohammed G, Nandapalan N, Kernahan J, Scott R, Craft AW, Toms GL. T cell function in children with acute lymphoblastic leukaemia. Br J Haematol 83:419–427, 1993.

Nesbit ME Jr, O'Leary M, Dehner LP, Ramsay NK. The immune system and the histiocytosis syndromes. Am J Pediatr Hematol Oncol 3:141–149, 1981.

Newman LS. Beryllium disease and sarcoidosis: clinical and laboratory links. Sarcoidosis 12:7–19, 1995.

Nezelof C, Basset F, Rousseau MF. Histiocytosis X histogenetic arguments for a Langerhans cell origin. Biomedicine 18:365–371, 1973.

Nishimoto N, Sasai M, Shima Y, Nakagawa M, Matsumoto T, Shirai T, Kishimoto T, Yoshizaki K. Improvement in Castelman's disease by humanized anti-interleukin-6 receptor antibody therapy. Blood 95:56–61, 2000.

Nitter L. Changes in the chest roentgenogram in Boeck's sarcoid of the lungs. Acta Radiol 105(Suppl):7–202, 1953.

Nouri AM, Hussain RF, Oliver RT. The frequency of major histocompatibility complex antigen abnormalities in urological tumors and their correction by gene transfection or cytokine stimulation. Cancer Gene Ther 1:119–123, 1994.

O'Connor PG, Scadden DT. AIDS oncology. Infect Dis Clin North Am 14:945–965, 2000.

Ohadi M, Lalloz MR, Sham P, Zhao J, Dearlove AM, Shiach C, Kinsey S, Rhodes M, Layton DM. Localization of a gene for familial hemophagocytic lymphohistiocytosis at chromosome 9q21.3-22 by homozygosity mapping. Am J Hum Genet 64:165–171, 1999.

Okano M, Thiele GM, Davis JR, Grierson HL, Purtilo DT. Epstein-Barr virus and human diseases: recent advances in diagnosis. Clin Microbiol Rev 1:3–312, 1988.

Olsen GA, Gockerman JP, Bast RC Jr, Borowitz M, Peters WP. Altered immunologic reconstitution after standard-dose chemotherapy or high-dose chemotherapy with autologous bone marrow support. Transplantation 46:57–60, 1988.

Opelz G, Henderson R. Incidence of non-Hodgkin lymphoma in kidney and heart transplant recipients. Lancet 342:1514–1516, 1993.

Pachman LM, Schwartz AD, Barron R, Golde DW. Chronic neutropenia: response to plasma with high colony-stimulating activity. J Pediatr 87:713–719, 1975.

Palacios MF, Fondevilla CG, Fernandez J, Gonzalez NH. Circulating lymphocyte populations and B-cell differentiation in a young female with multicentric giant lymph node hyperplasia. Sangre 36:423–426, 1991.

Palestro G, Turrini F, Pagano M, Chiusa L. Castelman's disease. Adv Clin Path 3:11–22, 1999.

Pandolfi F, Trentin L, Boyle LA, Stamenkovic I, Byers HR, Colvin RB, Kurnick JT. Expression of cell adhesion molecules in human melanoma cell lines and their role in cytotoxicity mediated by tumor-infiltrating lymphocytes. Cancer 69:1165–1173, 1992.

Paraskevas F. Cell interactions in the immune response. In Lee GR, Foerster J, Lukens J, Paraskevas F, Greer JP, Rodgers GM, eds. Wintrobe's clinical hematology. Baltimore, Lippincott Williams and Wilkins, 1999, pp 584–595.

Parez N, Bader-Meunier B, Roy CC, Dommergues JP. Paediatric Castelman disease: report of seven cases and review of the literature. Eur J Pediatr 158:631–637, 1999.

Pascual RS, Gee JB, Finch SC. Usefulness of serum lysozyme measurement in diagnosis and evaluation of sarcoidosis. N Engl J Med 289:1074–1076, 1973.

Pasquali JL, Godin D, Urlacher A, Pelletier A, Pauli G, Storck D. Abnormalities of in vitro responses to polyclonal activation of peripheral blood lymphocytes in patients with active sarcoidosis. Eur J Clin Invest 15:82–88, 1985.

Passwell J, Levanon M, Davidsohn J, Ramot B. Monocyte PGE2 secretion in Hodgkin's disease and its relation to decreased cellular immunity. Clin Exp Immunol 51:61–68, 1983.

Pattischall EN, Kendig EL. Sarcoidosis. In Chernick V, ed. Kendig's disorders of the respiratory tract in children. Philadelphia, WB Saunders, 1990, pp 769–780.

Pedrazzini A, Freedman AS, Andersen J, Heflin L, Anderson K, Takvorian T, Canellos GP, Whitman J, Coral F, Ritz J, Nadler LM. Anti-B-cell monoclonal antibody-purged autologous bone marrow transplantation for B-cell non-Hodgkin's lymphoma: Phenotypic reconstitution and B-cell function. Blood 74:2203–2211, 1989.

Penn I. The price of immunotherapy. Curr Probl Surg 18:681–751, 1981.

Penn I. De novo malignancies in pediatric organ transplant recipients. Pediatr Transplant 2:56–63, 1998.

Penn I. Cancers in renal transplant recipients. Adv Ren Replace Ther 7:147–156, 2000.

Perel Y. Castelman's disease (angiofollicular hyperplasia) in children. Ann Pediatr 36:510–516, 1989.

Perez-Soler R, Lopez-Berestein G, Cabanillas F, McLaughlin P, Hersh EM. Superoxide anion (O_2^-) production by peripheral blood monocytes in Hodgkin's disease and malignant lymphoma. J Clin Oncol 3:641–645, 1985.

Peterson BA, Frizzera G. Multicentric Castelman's disease. Semin Oncol 20:636–647, 1993.

Piali L, Fichtel A, Terpe HJ, Imhof BA, Gisler RH. Endothelial vascular cell adhesion molecule 1 expression is suppressed by melanoma and carcinoma. J Exp Med 181:811–816, 1995.

Pincus SH, Boxer LA, Stossel TP. Chronic neutropenia in childhood: analysis of 16 cases and a review of the literature. Am J Med 61:849–861, 1976.

Pizzolo G, Vinante F, Nadali G, Ricetti MM, Morosato L, Marrocchella R, Vincenzi C, Semenzato G, Chilosi M. ICAM-1 tissue overexpression associated with increased serum levels of its soluble form in Hodgkin's disease. Br J Haematol 84:161–162, 1993.

Poppema S, Visser L. Absence of HLA class I expression by Reed-Sternberg cells. Am J Pathol 145:37–41, 1994.

Porwit A, Hast R, Stenke L, Wasserman J, Reizenstein P. Decreased blood natural killer cell activity and immunoglobulin synthesis in vitro in aplastic anemia. Acta Med Scand 224:391–397, 1988.

Pui CH, Ip SH, Iflah S, Behm FG, Grose BH, Dodge RK, Crist WM, Furman WL, Murphy SB, Rivera GK. Serum interleukin 2 receptor levels in childhood acute lymphoblastic leukemia. Blood 71:1135–1137, 1988.

Pui CH, Ip SH, Kung P, Dodge RK, Berard CW, Crist WM, Murphy SB. High serum interleukin-2 receptor levels are related to advanced disease and a poor outcome in childhood non-Hodgkin's lymphoma. Blood 70:624–628, 1987.

Pui CH, Ip SH, Thompson E, Dodge RK, Brown M, Wilimas J, Carrabis S, Kung P, Berard CW, Crist WM. Increased serum CD8 antigen level in childhood Hodgkin's disease relates to advanced stage and poor treatment outcome. Blood 73:209–213, 1989.

Pyke DA, Scadding JG. Effect of cortisone upon skin sensitivity to tuberculin in sarcoidosis. Br Med J 2:1126–1128, 1952.

Quinn EL, Bunch DC, Yagle EM. The mumps skin test and complement fixation test as a diagnostic aid in sarcoidosis. J Invest Dermatol 24:595–598, 1955.

Ramachandar K, Douglas SD, Siltzbach LE, Taub RN. Peripheral blood lymphocyte subpopulations in sarcoidosis. Cell Immunol 16:422–426, 1975.

Reid MM, Craft AW, Todd JA. Serial studies of numbers of circulating T and B lymphocytes in children with acute lymphoblastic leukaemia. Arch Dis Child 52:245–247, 1977.

Ridgway D, Wolff LJ. Active immunization of children with leukemia and other malignancies. Leuk Lymphoma 9:177–192, 1993.

Ries LA, Miller RW, Smith M. Cancer in children (ages 0–14 and ages 0–19). In Miller B, Ries LA, Hankey B, eds. SEER cancer statistics review 1973–1991. Bethesda: US Department of Health and Human Services, National Institutes of Health Publication #94-2789, 1994.

Risdall RJ, McKenna RW, Nesbit ME, Krivit W, Balfour HH Jr, Simmons RL, Brunning RD. Virus-associated hemophagocytic syndrome: a benign histiocytic proliferation distinct from malignant histiocytosis. Cancer 44:993–12, 1979.

Robinson RBW, McLemore TL, Crystal RG. Gamma interferon is spontaneously released by alveolary macrophages and lung T lymphocytes in patients with pulmonary sarcoidosis. J Clin Invest 75:1488–1505, 1988.

Robison LL, Stoker V, Frizzera G, Heinitz K, Meadows AT, Filipovich AH. Hodgkin's disease in pediatric patients with naturally occurring immunodeficiency. Am J Pediatr Hematol Oncol 9:189–192, 1987.

Roederer M, De Rosa SC, Watanabe N, Herzenberg LA. Dynamics of fine T-cell subsets during HIV disease and after thymic ablation by mediastinal irradiation. Semin Immunol 9:389–396, 1997.

Rook AH, Kehrl JH, Wakefield LM, Roberts AB, Sporn MB, Burlington DB, Lane HC, Fauci AS. Effects of transforming growth factor beta on the functions of natural killer cells: depressed cytolytic activity and blunting of interferon responsiveness. J Immunol 136:3916–3920, 1986.

Rooney CM, Smith CA, Ng CY, Loftin SK, Sixbey JW, Gan Y, Srivastava DK, Bowman LC, Krance RA, Brenner MK, Heslop HE. Infusion of cytotoxic T cells for the prevention and treatment of Epstein-Barr virus-induced lymphoma in allogeneic transplant recipients. Blood 92:1549–1555, 1998.

Roskrow MA, Suzuki N, Gan YJ, Sixbey JW, Ng CY, Kimbrough S, Hudson M, Brenner MK, Heslop HE, Rooney CM. Epstein-Barr virus (EBV)-specific cytotoxic T lymphocyte for the treatment of patients with EBV-positive relapsed Hodgkin's disease. Blood 91:2925–2934, 1998.

Rubin LA, Jay G, Nelson DL. The released interleukin-2 receptor binds interleukin-2 efficiently. J Immunol 137:3841–3844, 1986.

Rybicki RA, Maliarik MJ, Major M, Popovich J Jr, Iannuzzi MC. Epidemiology, demographics, and genetics of sarcoidosis. Semin Respir Infect 13:166–173, 1998.

Saboor SA, Johnson NM, McFadden J. Detection of mycobacterial DNA in sarcoidosis and tuberculosis with polymerase chain reaction. Lancet 339:1012–1015, 1992.

Saltini C, Spurzem JR, Lee JJ, Pinkston P, Crystal RG. Spontaneous release of interleukin 2 by lung T lymphocytes in active pulmonary sarcoidosis is primarily from the Leu3+DR+ T cell subset. J Clin Invest 77:1962–1970, 1986.

Scharf Y, Zonis S. Histocompatibility antigens (HLA) and uveitis. Surv Ophtalmol. 24:220–228, 1980.

Schaumann J. Étude sur le lupus pernio et ses rapports avec les sarcoides et la tuberculose. Ann Dermatol Syph (Paris) 6:357–373, 1916.

Scheffer AL, Ruddy S, Israel HL. Serum complement levels in sarcoidosis. In Levinsky L, Macholda F, eds. Proceedings of the Fifth International Conference on Sarcoidosis: XIVth scientific conference of the medical faculty of Charles University, Prague, 1969. Prague, University Karlova, 1971, pp 195–197.

Schier WW, Roth A, Ostroff G, Schrift MH. Hodgkin's disease and immunity. Am J Med 20:94–99, 1956.

Schmitz L, Favara BE. Nosology and pathology of Langerhans cell histiocytosis. Hematol Oncol Clin North Am 12:221–246, 1998.

Schweiger O, Mandi L. Effect of Kveim substance on the respiration of circulating leukocytes of patients suffering from pulmonary sarcoidosis or other lung disease. Am Rev Respir Dis 96:1064–1066, 1967.

Scott JL, Cartwright GE, Wintrobe MM. Acquired aplastic anemia. An analysis of thirty-nine cases and review of the pertinent literature. Medicine 38:119–172, 1959.

Semenzato G, Agostini C, Trentin L, Zambello R, Chilosi M, Cipriani A, Ossi E, Angi MR, Morittu L, Pizzolo G. Evidence of cells bearing interleukin-2 receptor at sites of disease activity in sarcoid patients. Clin Exp Immunol 57331–337, 1984.

Semenzato G, Pezzutto A, Agostini C, Gasparotto G, Cipriani A. Immunoregulation in sarcoidosis. Clin Immunol Immunopathol 19:416–427, 1981.

Senn HJ, Jungi WF. Neutrophil migration in health and disease. Semin Hematol 12:27–45, 1975.

Shannon BT, Newton WA. Suppressor-cell dysfunction in children with histiocytosis-X. J Clin Immunol 6:510–514, 1986.

Sheagren JN, Block JB, Wolff SM. Reticuloendothelial system phagocytic function in patients with Hodgkin's disease. J Clin Invest 46:855–862, 1967.

Shipp MA, Maugh PM, Harris NL. Non-Hodgkin's lymphomas. In DeVita VT Jr, Hellman S, Rosenberg SA, eds. Cancer: principles and practice of oncology. Philadelphia, Lippincott-Raven Publishers, 1997, pp 2165–2166.

Sibbitt WL Jr, Bankhurst AD, Williams RC Jr. Studies of cell subpopulations mediating mitogen hyporesponsiveness in patients with Hodgkin's disease. J Clin Invest 61:55–63, 1978.

Siber GR, Weitzman SA, Aisenberg AC. Antibody response of patients with Hodgkin's disease to protein and polysaccharide antigens. Rev Infect Dis 3(Suppl):144–159, 1981.

Siltzbach LE. Etiology of sarcoidosis. Practitioner 202:613–618, 1969.

Siltzbach LE. Discussion of sarcoidosis. Ann NY Acad Sci 278:247–248, 1976.

Siltzbach LE, Glade PR, Hurschaut Y, Viera LOBP, Celikoglu IS, Hirschhorn K. In vitro stimulation of peripheral lymphocytes in sarcoidosis. In Levinsky L, Macholda F, eds. Proceedings of the Fifth International Conference on Sarcoidosis: XIVth scientific conference of the medical faculty of Charles University, Prague, 1969. Prague, Universita Karlova, 1971, pp 217–224.

Simececk C, Zavagal V, Sach J, Kulich V. Serum proteins and serum complement in sarcoidosis. In Levinsky L, Macholda F, eds. Proceedings of the Fifth International Conference on Sarcoidosis: XIVth scientific conference of the medical faculty of Charles University, Prague, 1969. Prague, Universita Karlova, 1971, pp 188–194.

Skelton HGD, Smith KJ, Johnson FB, Cooper CR, Tyler WF, Lupton GP. Zirconium granuloma resulting from an aluminum zirconium complex: a previously unrecognized agent in the development of hypersensitivity granulomas. J Am Acad Dermatol 28:874–876, 1993.

Slivnick DJ, Ellis TM, Nawrocki JF, Fischer RI. The impact of Hodgkin's disease on the immune system. Sem Oncol 17:673–682, 1990.

Snyder GB. The fate of skin homografts in patients with sarcoidosis. Bull Johns Hopkins Hosp 115:81–91, 1964.

Sokal JE, Aungst CW. Response to BCG vaccination and survival in advanced Hodgkin's disease. Cancer 24:128–134, 1969.

Sokal JE, Primikirios N. The delayed skin test response in Hodgkin's disease and lymphosarcoma. Effect of disease activity. Cancer 14:597–607, 1961.

Solanki RL, Anand VK, Arora HL. Serum immunoglobulins in leukaemia and malignant lymphoma. J Indian Med Assoc 88:305–307, 1990.

Somani J, Larson RA. Reimmunization after allogeneic bone marrow transplantation. Am J Med 98:389–398, 1995.

Sommer E. Primary and secondary anergy to sarcoidosis. Acta Med Scand 425(Suppl):195–197, 1964.

Sones M, Israel HL. Altered immunologic reactions in sarcoidosis. Ann Intern Med 40:260–268, 1954.

Soulier J, Grollet L, Oksenhendler E, Cacoub P, Cazals-Hatem D, Babinet P, d'Agay MF, Clauvel JP, Raphael M, Degos L, Sigaux F. Kaposi's sarcoma-associated herpesvirus-like DNA sequences in multicentric Castelman's disease. Blood 86:1276–1280, 1995.

Sporn MB, Roberts AB, Wakefield LM, Assoian RK. Transforming growth factor-beta: biological function and chemical structure. Science 233:532–534,1986.

Staudt LM. The molecular and cellular origins of Hodgkin's disease. J Exp Med 191:207–212, 2000.

Steigbigel RT, Lambert LH Jr, Remington JS. Polymorphonuclear leukocyte, monocyte, and macrophage bactericidal function in patients with Hodgkin's disease. J Lab Clin Med 88:54–62, 1976.

Steplewski Z. The search for viruses in sarcoidosis. Ann NY Acad Sci 278:260–263, 1976.

Stepp SE, Dufourcq-Lagelouse, Le Deist F, Bhawan S, Certain S, Mathew PA, Henter JI, Bennett M, Fischer A, de Saint Basile G, Kumar V. Perforin gene defects in familial hemophagocytic lymphohistiocytosis. Science 286:1957–1959, 1999.

Storek J, Witherspoon RP, Storb R. T cell reconstitution after bone marrow transplantation in adult patients does not resemble T cell development in early life. Bone Marrow Transplant 16:413–425, 1995.

Sugita K, Nojima Y, Tachibana K, Soiffer RJ, Murray C, Schlossman SF, Ritz J, Morimoto C. Prolonged impairment of very late activating antigen-mediated T cell proliferation via the CD3 pathway after T cell-depleted allogeneic bone marrow transplantation. J Clin Invest 94:481–488, 1994a.

Sugita K, Soiffer RJ, Murray C, Schlossman SF, Ritz J, Morimoto C. The phenotype and reconstitution of immunoregulatory T cell subsets after T-cell-depleted allogenic and autologous bone marrow transplantation. Transplantation 57:1465–1473, 1994b.

Sullivan KE, Mullen CA, Blaese RM, Winkelstein JA. A multiinstitutional survey of the Wiskott-Aldrich syndrome. J Pediatr 125:876–885, 1994.

Sullivan KE, Delaat CA, Douglas SD, Filipovich AH. Defective natural killer cell function in patients with hemophagocytic lymphohistiocytosis and in first degree relatives. Pediatr Res 44:465–468, 1998.

Surico G, Muggeo P, Muggeo V, Lucarelli A, Novielli C, Conti V, Rigillo N. Polyclonal hypergammaglobulinemia at the onset of acute myeloid leukemia in children. Ann Hematol 78:445–448, 1999.

Sutherland I, Mitchell DN, D'Arcy Hart P. Incidence of intrathoracic sarcoidosis among young adults participating in a trial of tuberculosis vaccines. BMJ 2:497–503, 1965.

Talmadge JE, Reed EC, Kessinger A, Kuszynski CA, Perry GA, Gordy CL, Mills KC, Thomas ML, Pirruccello SJ, Letheby BA, Arneson MA, Jackson JD. Immunologic attributes of cytokine mobilized peripheral blood stem cells and recovery following transplantation. Bone Marrow Transplant 17:101–109, 1996.

Tamayo M, Gonzalez C, Majado MJ, Candel R, Ramos J. Long-term complete remission after interferon treatment in case of multicentric Castelman's disease. Am J Hematol 49:359–360, 1995.

Tannenbaum H, Pikus GS, Schur PH. Immunological characterization of subpopulations of mononuclear cells in tissue and peripheral blood from patients with sarcoidosis. Clin Immunol Immunopathol 5:133–141, 1976.

Taub DD, Anver M, Oppenheim JJ, Longo DL, Murphy WJ. T lymphocyte recruitment by interleukin-8 (IL-8). IL-8-induced degranulation of neutrophils releases potent chemoattractants for human T lymphocytes both in vitro and in vivo. J Clin Invest 97:1931–1941, 1996.

Taub RN, Siltzbach LE. Induction of granulomas in mice by injection of human sarcoid and ileitis homogenates. In Iwai K, Hosoda Y, eds. Proceedings of the sixth international conferences on Sarcoidosis. Tokyo, 1972. Baltimore, University Park Press, 1974, pp 20–21.

Thomas PD, Hunninghake GW. Current concepts of the pathogenesis of sarcoidosis. Am Rev Respir Dis 135:747–760, 1987.

Tomooka Y, Torisu M, Miyazaki S, Goya N. Immunological studies on histiocytosis X. I. Special reference to the chemotactic defect and the HLA antigen. J Clin Immunol 6:355–362, 1986.

Topilsky M, Siltzbach LE, Williams M, Glade PR. Lymphocyte response in sarcoidosis. Lancet 1:117–120, 1972.

Townsend SE, Allison JP. Tumor rejection after direct costimulation of CD8+ T cells by B7-transfected melanoma cells. Science 259:368–370, 1993.

Trubovitz S, Masek B, Del Rosario A. Lymphocyte response to phytohemagglutinin in Hodgkin's disease, lymphatic leukemia and lymphosarcoma. Cancer 19:2019–2023, 1966.

Tsuda H, Yamasaki H. Type I and type II T-cell profiles in aplastic anemia and refractory anemia. Am J Hematol 64:271–274, 2000.

Tsujisaki M, Imai K, Hirata H, Hanzawa Y, Masuya J, Nakano T, Sugiyama T, Matsui M, Hinoda Y, Yachi A. Detection of circulating intercellular adhesion molecule-1 antigen in malignant diseases. Clin Exp Immunol 85:3–8, 1991.

Tsunawaki S, Sporn M, Ding A, Nathan C. Deactivation of macrophages by transforming growth factor-beta. Nature 334:260–262, 1988.

Twoney JJ, Douglass CC, Morris SM. Inability of leukocytes to stimulate mixed leukocyte reactions. J Natl Cancer Inst 51:345–351, 1973.

Twoney JJ, Laughter AH, Farrow S, Douglass CC. Hodgkin's disease: an immunodepleting and immunosuppressive disorder. J Clin Invest 56:467–475, 1975.

Ultmann JE, Cunningham JK, Gellhorn A. The clinical picture of Hodgkin's disease. Cancer Res 26:1047–1062, 1966.

Urbach F, Sones M, Israel HL. Passive transfer of tuberculin sensitivity to patients with sarcoidosis. N Engl J Med 247:794–797, 1952.

Vacca A, Di Stefano R, Frassanito A, Iodice G, Dammacco F. A disturbance of the IL-2/IL-2 receptor system parallels the activity of multiple myeloma. Clin Exp Immunol 84:429–434, 1991.

Vallejos C, McCredie KB, Bodey GP, Hester JP, Freireich EJ. White blood cell transfusions for control of infections in neutropenic patients. Transfusion 15:28–33, 1975.

Vanky F, Wang P, Patarroyo M, Klein E. Expression of the adhesion molecule ICAM-1 and major histocompatibility complex class I antigens on human tumor cells is required for their interaction with autologous lymphocytes in vitro. Cancer Immunol Immunother 31:19–27, 1990.

Veien NK, Hardt F, Bendixen G, Ringsted J, Brodthagen H, Faber V, Genner J, Heckscher T, Svejgaard A, Freisleben S, Sorensen S, Wanstrup J, Wiik A. Immunological studies in sarcoidosis: a comparison of disease activity and various immunological parameters. Ann NY Acad Sci 278:47–51, 1976.

Voss JM, Armitage JO. Clinical applications of hematopoietic growth factors. J Clin Oncol 13:1023–1035, 1995.

Wahl SM, Hunt DA, Wong HL, Dougherty S, McCartney-Francis N, Wahl LM, Ellingsworth L, Schmidt JA, Hall G, Roberts AB. Transforming growth factor-beta is a potent immunosuppressive agent that inhibits IL-1-dependent lymphocyte proliferation. J Immunol 140:3026–3032, 1988.

Wahren B, Carlens E, Espmark A, Lundbeck H, Lofgren S, Madar E, Henle G, Henle W. Antibodies to various herpesvirus in sera from patients with sarcoidosis. J Natl Cancer Inst 47:747–755, 1971.

Waldman DJ, Stiehm ER. Cutaneous sarcoidosis of childhood. J Pediatr 91:271–273, 1977.

Waldmann TA. The structure, function, and expression of interleukin-2 receptors on normal and malignant lymphocytes. Science 232:727–732, 1986.

Ward PA, Berenberg JL. Defective regulation of inflammatory mediators in Hodgkin's disease. Supernormal levels of chemotactic-factor inactivator. N Engl J Med 290:76–80, 1974.

Watanabe N, De Rosa SC, Cmelak A, Hoppe R, Herzenberg LA, Roederer M. Long-term depletion of naïve T cells in patients treated for Hodgkin's disease. Blood; 90:3662–3672, 1997.

Wehinger H, Karitzky D. [T and B lymphocytes before, during, and after cytostatic therapy of acute lymphoblastic leukemia (ALL) in children. Klin Padiatr 189:234–241, 1977.

Weisenburger DD, DeGowin RL, Gibson P, Armitage JO. Remission of giant lymph node hyperplasia with anemia after radiotherapy. Cancer 44:457–462, 1979.

Weitzman SA, Aisenberg AC, Siber GR, Smith DH. Impaired humoral immunity in treated Hodgkin's disease. N Engl J Med 297:245–248, 1977.

Williams DM. Pancytopenia, aplastic anemia, and pure red cell aplasia. In Lee GR, Foerster J, Lukens J, Paraskevas F, Greer JP, Rodgers GM, eds. Wintrobe's clinical hematology. Baltimore, Lippincott Williams and Wilkins, 1999, pp 1451–1474.

Williams WJ, Pioli E, Jones DJ, Dighero M. The Kmif (Kveim-induced macrophage migration inhibition factor) test in sarcoidosis. J Clin Pathol 25:951–954, 1972.

Willman CL, McClain KL. An update on clonality, cytokines and viral etiology in Langerhans cell histiocytosis. Hematol Oncol Clin North Am 12:407–416, 1998.

Winkelstein JA, Mikulla JM, Sartiano GP, Ellis LD. Cellular immunity in Hodgkin's disease: comparison of cutaneous reactivity and lymphoproliferative responses to phytohemagglutinin. Cancer 34:549–553, 1974.

Yoshizaki K, Matsuda T, Nishimoto N, Kuritani T, Taeho L, Aozasa K, Nakahata T, Kawai H, Tagoh H, Komori T. Pathogenic significance of interleukin-6 (IL-6/BSF-2) in Castelman's disease. Blood 74:1360–1367, 1989.

Young RC, Corder MP, Haynes HA, DeVita VT. Delayed hypersensitivity in Hodgkin's disease. A study of 103 untreated patients. Am J Med 52:63–72, 1972.

Zerler B. The soluble interleukin-2 receptor as a marker for human neoplasia and immune status. Cancer Cells 3:471–479, 1991.

Zinkernagel RM, Doherty PC. MHC-restricted cytotoxic T cells: studies on the biological role of the polymorphic major transplantation antigens determining T-cell restriction-specificity, function, and responsiveness. Adv Immunol 27:51–177, 1979.

Zweiman B, Israel HL. Comparative in vitro reactivities of leukocytes from sarcoids and normals to different Kveim preparations. Ann NY Acad Sci 278:7–710, 1976.

Immunosuppression Induced by Therapeutic Agents and Environmental Conditions

Javier Chinen and William T. Shearer

Humans are exposed to multiple drugs and environmental conditions, some of which affect the immune system. In this chapter we summarize the significant effects of drugs and environmental agents on immunity.

Immunosuppressive agents may be classified as follows:
· *Chemical,* including drugs and chemotherapeutic agents
· *Biologic,* including immunoglobulins and interleukins
· *Physical,* including radiation and environmental conditions

These agents often affect the different components of the immune system, such as B-cell function, T-cell function, and phagocytic function, simultaneously. Complement function has rarely been evaluated; however, primary or secondary complement deficiencies are exceedingly uncommon.

DRUGS AND CHEMOTHERAPEUTIC AGENTS

Several anti-inflammatory drugs and cytotoxic drugs are used for transplant rejection, autoimmune disease, and chronic inflammatory conditions. Their mechanisms of action are mainly the inhibition of T-cell activation or proliferation (Fig. 27-1). Their use is commonly associated with an increased frequency of infections and neoplasias.

Cyclosporine, Tacrolimus, and Sirolimus

Cyclosporine is the prototype of a powerful class of drugs that confers immunosuppression by inhibiting intracellular signaling of T cells (Kahan, 1989). FK506 (Tacrolimus) and rapamycin (Sirolimus) are additional drugs within the same group (Gummert et al., 1999; Sigal and Dumont, 1992). These drugs differ from glucocorticoid and cytotoxic drugs by their immunologic specificity. Cyclosporine binds intracellularly to a protein known as cyclophilin, inhibiting its interaction with calcineurin, a calcium-calmodulin–dependent phosphatase. Inhibition of calcineurin results in suppression of interleukin-2 (IL-2) production because of the absence of activation signals for the IL-2 promoter (O'Keefe et al., 1992). This results in reversible inhibition of T-cell alloimmune and autoimmune responses (Fig. 27-2).

Cyclosporine has played a significant role in permitting successful organ transplantation; particularly, kidney, liver, heart, and lung transplantation (Gummert et al., 1999; Kahan, 1989). Several autoimmune conditions are ameliorated by cyclosporine, including uveitis, psoriasis, and insulin-dependent diabetes (Bougneres et al., 1988; Ellis et al., 1986; Nussenblatt et al., 1983). Because of its specificity, many infections seen in other immunosuppression regimens are avoided. Cyclosporine has reduced the incidence of acute viral, bacterial, and fungal infections in transplant recipients (Canadian Multicentre Transplant Study Group, 1986; Showstack et al., 1989). In vitro, cyclosporine inhibits T-cell activation and proliferation response to mitogens (Kuo et al., 1992; Zenke et al., 1993). Although cyclosporine usually spares B-cell function, antibody responses to some T-cell–independent antigens are inhibited (O'Garra et al., 1986). Macrophage function, including antigen presentation, phagocytosis, and cytotoxicity, is unaffected (Esa et al., 1988; Granelli-Piperno et al., 1988).

The most common adverse effects of cyclosporine are renal dysfunction and hypertension. Bone marrow

Calabrese L and Fleischer AB. Thalidomide: current and potential clinical applications. Am J Med 108:487–495, 2000.

Campbell AC, Hersey P, MacLennan IC, Kay HC, Pike MC. Immunosuppressive consequences of radiotherapy and chemotherapy in patients with acute lymphoblastic leukemia. Br Med J 2:385–388, 1973.

Canadian Multicentre Transplant Study Group. A randomized clinical trial of cyclosporine in cadaveric renal transplantation. Analysis at three years. N Engl J Med 314:1219–1225, 1986.

Champlin R, Ho W, Gale RP. Antithymocyte globulin treatment in patients with aplastic anemia: a prospective randomized trial. N Engl J Med 308:113–118, 1983.

Chan GL, Canafax DM, Johnson CA. The therapeutic use of azathioprine in renal transplantation. Pharmacotherapy 7:165–177, 1987.

Chatenoud L, Baudrihaye MF, Kreis H, Goldstin G, Schindler J. Bach JF. Human in vivo antigenic modulation induced by the anti T cell OKT3 monoclonal antibody. Eur J Immunol 12:979–982, 1982.

Choy EH, Panayi GS, Kingsley GH. Therapeutic monoclonal antibodies. Br J Rheumatol 34:707–715, 1995.

Claman HN. Corticosteroids and lymphoid cells. N Engl J Med 287:388–397, 1972.

Cockburn IT, Krupp P. The risk of neoplasm in patients treated with cyclosporine A. J Autoimmun 2:723–731, 1989.

Cogoli A. Effect of hypogravity on cells of the immune system. J Leuk Biol 54:259–268, 1993.

Corral LG, Haslett PA, Muller GW, Chen R, Wong LM, Ocampo CJ, Patterson RT, Stirling DI, Kaplan G. Differential cytokine modulation and T-cell activation by two distinct classes of thalidomide analogues that are potent inhibitors of TNF-alpha. J Immunol 163:380–386, 1999.

Cosimi AB, Colvin RB, Burton RC, Rubin RH, Goldstein G, Kung PC, Hansen WP, Delmonico FL, Russell PS. Use of monoclonal antibodies to T-cell subsets for immunologic monitoring and treatment in recipients of renal allografts. N Engl J Med 305:308–314, 1981.

Cosimi AB, Delmonico FL, Wright FK, Wee SL, Preffer FI, Jolliffee LK, Colvin RB. Prolonged survival of nonhuman primate renal allograft recipients treated with anti-CD4 monoclonal antibody. Surgery 108:406–413, 1990.

Cupps TR, Edgar LC, Thomas CA, Fauci AS. Multiple mechanisms of B cell immunoregulation in man after in vivo administration of corticosteroids. J Immunol 132:170–175, 1984.

Currey HL. A comparison of immunosuppressive and anti-inflammatory agents in the rat. Clin Exp Immunol 9:879–887, 1971.

Dale DC, Petersdorf RG. Corticosteroids and infectious diseases. Med Clin North Am 57:1277–1287, 1973.

Debol SM, Herron MJ, Nelson RD. Anti-inflammatory action of dapsone: inhibition of neutrophil adherence is associated with inhibition of chemoattractant-induced signal transduction. J Leuk Biol 62:827–836, 1997.

De La Rocque L, Campos MM, Olej B, Castilho F, Mediano IF, Rumjanek VM. Inhibition of human LAK-cell activity by the anti-depressant trifluoperazine. Immunopharmacology 29:1–10, 1995.

Dosch HM, Jason J, Gelfand EW. Transient antibody deficiency and abnormal T-suppressor cells induced by phenytoin. N Engl J Med 306:406–409, 1982.

Dresdale AR, Lutz S, Drost C, Levine TB, Fenn N, Paone G, del Busto R, Silverman NA. Prospective evaluation of malignant neoplasms in cardiac transplant recipients uniformly treated with prophylactic antilymphocyte globulin. J Thorac Cardiovas Surg 106:1202–1207, 1993.

Drobyski WR, Ul-Haq R, Majewski D, Chitambar CR. Modulation of in vitro and in vivo T-cell responses by transferrin-gallium and gallium nitrate. Blood 88:3056–3064, 1996.

Ebert RH, Barclay WR. Changes in connective tissue reaction induced by cortisone. Ann Intern Med 37:506–518, 1952.

Ellis CN, Gorsulowsky DC, Hamilton TA, Billings JK, Brown MD, Headington JT, Cooper KD, Baadsgaard O, Annesley TM, Turcotte JG Voorhees JJ. Cyclosporine improves psoriasis in a double blind study. JAMA 256:3110–3116, 1986.

Esa AH, Paxman DG, Noga SJ, Hess AD. Sensitivity of monocyte populations to cyclosporine. Arachidonate metabolism and in vitro antigen presentation. Transplant Proc 20:80–86, 1988.

Fauci AS, Dale DC. Alternate-day prednisone therapy and human lymphocyte subpopulations. J Clin Invest 55:22–32, 1975.

Fauci AS, Dale DC, Balow JE. Glucocorticosteroid therapy: mechanisms of action and clinical considerations. Ann Intern Med 84:304–315, 1976.

Feehally J, Beattie TJ, Brenchley PE, Coupes BM, Houston IB, Mallick NP, Wistlethwaite RJ. Modulation of immune function by cyclophosphamide in children with minimal change nephropathy. N Engl J Med 310:415–420, 1984.

Fernandez LP, Schlegel PG, Baker J, Chen Y, Chao NJ. Does thalidomide affect IL-2 response and production? Exp Hematol 23:978–985, 1995.

Fuks Z, Strober S, Bobrove AM, Sasazuki T, Mcmichael A, Kaplan HS. Long-term effects of radiation of T and B lymphocytes in peripheral blood of patients with Hodgkin's disease. J Clin Invest 58:803–814, 1976.

Gilhus NE, Aarli JA. The reversibility of phenytoin-induced IgA deficiency. J Neurol 226:53–61, 1981.

Goud SN. Effects of sublethal radiation on bone marrow cells: induction of apoptosis and inhibition of antibody formation. Toxicology 135:69–76, 1999.

Goutet M, Ban M, Binet S. Effects of nickel sulfate on pulmonary natural immunity in Wistar rats. Toxicology 145:15–26, 2000.

Granelli-Piperno A, Keane M, Steinman RM. Evidence that cyclosporine inhibits cell-mediated immunity primarily at the level of the T lymphocyte rather than the accessory cell. Transplantation 46:53S–60S, 1988.

Griem P, Takahashi K, Kalbacher H, Gleichmann E. The antirheumatic drug disodium aurothiomalate inhibits CD4$^+$ T cell recognition of peptides containing two or more cysteine residues. J Immunol 155:1575–1587, 1995.

Gronemeyer H. Control of transcription activation by steroid hormone receptors. FASEB J 6:2524–2529, 1992.

Guerra IC, Fawcett WA, Redmon AH, Lawrence EC, Rosenblatt HM, Shearer WT. Permanent intrinsic B cell immunodeficiency caused by phenytoin hypersensitivity. J Allergy Clin Immunol 77:603–607, 1986.

Gummert JF, Ikonen T, Morris RE. Newer immunosuppressive drugs: a review. J Am Soc Nephrol 10:1366–1380, 1999.

Hashemi BB, Penkala JE, Vens C, Huls H, Cubbage M, Sams CF. T cell activation responses are differentially regulated during clinorotation and in spaceflight. FASEB J 13:2071–2082, 1999.

Haynes BF, Fauci AS. The differential effect of in vivo hydrocortisone on the kinetics of subpopulations of human peripheral blood thymus-derived lymphocytes. J Clin Invest 61:703–707, 1978.

Hersh EM, Oppenheimer JJ. Impaired in vitro lymphocyte transformation in Hodgkin's disease. N Engl J Med 273:1006–1012, 1965.

Ishizaka A, Nakanishi M, Kasahara E, Mizutani K, Sakiyama Y, Matsumoto S. Phenytoin-induced IgG2 and IgG4 deficiencies in a patient with epilepsy. Acta Paediatr 81:646–648, 1992.

Jolivet J, Cowan KH, Curt GA, Cledennin NJ, Chabner BA. The pharmacology and clinical use of methotrexate. N Engl J Med 309:1094–1104, 1983.

Josephs SH, Rothman SJ, Buckley R. Phenytoin hypersensitivity. J Allergy Clin Immunol 66:166–172, 1980.

Judge TA, Tang A, Lurka LA. Immunosuppression through blockade of CD28:B7 mediated costimulatory signals. Immunol Res 15:38–49, 1996.

Kahan BD. Cyclosporine. N Engl J Med 321:1725–1738, 1989.

Kaplan HS, Hoppe RS, Strober S. Selective immunosuppressive effect of total lymphoid irradiation. In Chandra RK, ed. Primary and Secondary Immunodeficiency Disorders. New York, Churchill Livingstone, 1983, 272–279.

Kebudi R, Ayan I, Darendelile E, Agaoglu L, Piskin S, Bilge N. Immunologic status in children with brain tumor and the effects of therapy. J Neurooncol 24:219–227, 1995.

Kikuchi K, McCormick CI, Neuwelt EA. Immunosuppression by phenytoin: implication for altered immune competence in brain-tumor patients. J Neurosurg 61:1085–1090, 1984.

Kondo N, Kasahara K, Kameyama T, Suzuki Y, Shimokawa N, Tomatsu S, Nakashima Y, Hori Y, Yamagishi A, Ogawa T. Intravenous immunoglobulin suppress immunoglobulin production by suppressing Ca^{++} dependent signal transduction through Fc gamma receptors in B lymphocytes. Scand J Immunol 40:37–42, 1994.

Konstantinova IV, Rykova MP, Lesnyak AT, Antropova EA. Immune changes during long-duration missions. J Leukoc Biol 54:189–201, 1993.

Koo J. Phototherapy. Semin Dermatol 11:11–16, 1992.

Kotzin BL, Strober S, Engleman EG, Galin A, Hoppe RT, Kansan GS, Terrell CP, Kaplan HS. Treatment of intractable rheumatoid arthritis with total lymphoid irradiation. N Engl J Med 305:969–976, 1981.

Kovarsky J. Clinical pharmacology and toxicology of cyclophosphamide: emphasis on use in rheumatic disease. Semin Arthritis Rheum 12:359–372, 1983.

Kuo CJ, Chung J, Fiorentino DF, Flanagan WM, Blenis J, Crabtree GR. Rapamycin selectively inhibits interleukin-2 activation of p70S6 kinase. Nature 358:70–73, 1992.

Lacy CF, Armstrong LL, Godmar MP, Lane LL. Drug Information Handbook, ed 8. Lexi-Comp Editors, Hudson, Ohio, 2000.

Lall SB, Dan R. Role of corticosteroids in cadmium induced immunotoxicity. Drug Chem Toxicol 22:401–409, 1999.

Lance EM, Medawar PB, Taub RN. Antilymphocyte serum. Adv Immunol 17:1–92, 1973.

Lesnyak A, Sonnenfeld G, Avery L, Konstantinova I, Rykova M, Meshkov D, Orlova T. Effect of SLS-3 spaceflight on immune parameters of rats. J Appl Physiol 81:178–182, 1996.

Levy J, Zalkinder I, Kuperman O, Skibin A, Apte R, Bearman JE, Mielke PW, Tal A. Effect of prolonged use of inhaled steroids on the cellular immunity of children with asthma. J Allergy Clin Immunol 95:806–812, 1995.

Lew W, Oppenheim JJ, Matsushima K. Analysis of the suppression of IL-1 alpha and IL-1 beta production in human peripheral blood mononuclear adherent cells by a glucocorticoid hormone. J Immunol 140:1895–1902, 1988.

Linden GK and Wenstein GD. Psoriasis: current perspectives with an emphasis on treatment. Am J Med 107: 595–605, 1999.

Lo CJ, Cryer HG, Fu M, Lo FR. Regulation of macrophage eicosanoid generation is dependent of nuclear factor kappa B. J Trauma 45:19–23, 1998.

Luger TA, Schwarz T, Kalden H, Scholzen T, Schwarz A, Brzoska T. Role of epidermal derived alpha-melanocyte stimulating hormone in ultraviolet light mediated local immunosuppression. Ann N Y Acad Sci 885:209–216, 1999.

Lyn RY, Nahal A, Lee M, Menikoff H. Changes in nasal leukocytes and epithelial cells associated with topical beclomethasone treatment. Ann Allergy Asthma Immunol 84:618–622, 2000.

Mackall CL. T-cell immunodeficiency following cytotoxic antineoplastic therapy: a review. Stem Cells 18:10–18, 2000.

Macklis RM, Mauch PM, Burakoff SJ, Smith BR. Lymphoid irradiation results in long-term increases in natural killer cells in patients treated for Hodgkin's disease. Cancer 69:778–783, 1992.

MacLennan IC, Kay HE. Analysis of treatment in childhood leukemia. IV. The critical association between dose fractionation and immunosuppression induced by cranial irradiation. Cancer 41:108–111, 1978.

Maibach HI, Epstein WL. Immunologic responses of healthy volunteers receiving azathioprine (Imuran). Int Arch Allergy 27:102–109, 1965.

Malatack JF, Garner JC Jr, Urbach AH, Zitelli BJ. Orthotopic liver transplantation, Epstein-Barr virus, cyclosporine, and lymphoproliferative disease: a growing concern. J Pediatr 118:667–675, 1991.

Margaretten MC, Hincks JR, Warren RP, Coulombe RA. Effects of phenytoin and carbamazepine on human natural killer activity and genotoxicity in vitro. Toxicol Appl Pharmacol 87:10–17, 1987.

Martin PJ, Shulman HM, Schubach WH, Hansen JA, Fefer A, Miller G, Thomas ED. Fatal Epstein-Barr virus associated proliferation of donor B cells after treatment of acute graft-versus-host disease with a murine anti-T-cell antibody. Ann Intern Med 101:310–315, 1984.

Matthews DC, Appelbaum FR, Eary JF, Fisher DR, Durack LD, Bush SA, Hui TE, Martin PJ, Mitchell D, Press OW. Development of a marrow transplant regimen for acute leukemia using targeted hematopoietic irradiation delivered by ^{131}I-labeled anti-CD45 antibody, combined with cyclophosphamide and total body irradiation. Blood 85:1122–1131, 1995.

McCabe MJ, Singh KP, Reiners JJ. Lead intoxication impairs the generation of a delayed type hypersensitivity response. Toxicology 139:255–264, 1999.

McHugh SM, Rifkin IR, Deighton J, Wilson AB, Lachmann PJ, Lockwood CM, Ewan PW. The immunosuppressive drug thalidomide induces T-helper cell type 2 and concomitantly inhibits Th1 cytokine production in mitogen- and antigen-stimulated human peripheral blood mononuclear cell cultures. Clin Exp Immunol 99:160–167, 1995.

Meehan R, Duncan U, Neale L, Taylor G, Scott N, Ramsey K, Smith E, Rock P. Operation Everest II: alterations in the immune system at high altitudes. J Clin Immunol 8:397–406, 1988.

Mele TS, Halloran PF. The use of mycophenolate mofetil in transplant patients. Immunopharmacology 47:215–245, 2000.

Melli G, Mazzei D, Rugarli C, Ortolani C, Bazzi C. Blastosis during anti-lymphocyte globulin treatment. Lancet 2:975, 1968.

Moriera AL, Sampaio EP, Zmuidzinas A. Thalidomide exerts its inhibitory action on tumor necrosis factor alpha by enhancing mRNA degradation. J Exp Med 177:1675–1680, 1993.

Moszczynski P. Mercury compounds and the immune system: a review. Int J Occup Med Environ Health 10:247–258, 1997.

Nachbauer D, Herold M, Eibl B, Glass H, Schwaighofer H, Huber C, Gachter A, Pichl M, Niederweiser D. A comparative study of the in vitro immunomodulatory activity of human intact immunoglobulin, Fab and Fc fragments. Evidence of post-transcriptional IL-2 modulation. Immunology 90:212–218, 1997.

Najarian JS, Ferguson RM, Sutherland DE, Slavin S, Kim T, Kersey J, Simmons RS. Fractionated total lymphoid irradiation as preparative immunosuppression in high risk renal transplantation: clinical and immunological studies. Ann Surg 196:442–452, 1982.

Najarian JS, Simmons RL. The clinical use of antilymphocyte globulin. N Engl J Med 285:158–166, 1971.

Nussenblatt RB, Palestine AG, Chan CC. Cyclosporin A therapy in the treatment of intraocular inflammatory disease resistant to systemic corticosteroids and cytotoxic agents. Am J Ophthalmol 96:275–282, 1983.

O'Garra A, Warren DJ, Holman M, Popham AM, Sanderson CJ, Klaus GG. Effects of cyclosporine on responses of murine B cells to T cell-derived lymphokines. J Immunol 137:2220–2224, 1986.

O'Keefe SJ, Tamura J, Kincaid RL, Tocci MJ, O'Neill EA. FK-506- and CsA-sensitive activation of the interleukin-2 promoter by calcineurin. Nature 357:692–694, 1992.

Olszyna DP, Pajkrt D, Lauw FN, Van Deventer SJ, Van Der Poll T. Interleukin 10 inhibits the release of CC chemokines during human endotoxemia. J Infect Dis 181:613–620, 2000.

O'Malley BW. Steroid hormone action in eukaryotic cells. J Clin Invest 74:307–312, 1984.

Ooi BS, Kant KS, Hanenson IB, Pesce AJ, Pollak VE. Lymphocytotoxin in epileptic patients receiving phenytoin. Clin Exp Immunol 30:56–61, 1977.

Orosz CG, Wakely E, Sedmak DD, Bergese SD, Van Burskirk AM. Prolonged murine cardiac allograft acceptance: characteristics of persistent active alloimmunity after treatment with gallium nitrate versus anti-CD4 monoclonal antibody. Transplantation 63:1109–1117, 1997.

Page AR, Condie RM, Good RA. Suppression of plasma cell hepatitis with 6-mercaptopurine. Am J Med 36:200–214, 1964.

Pedersen BK, Kappel M, Klokker M, Nielsen HB, Secher NH. The immune system during exposure to extreme physiologic conditions. Int J Sports Med 15:S116–S121, 1994.

Perper RJ, Sanda M, Chinea G, Oronsky AL. Leukocyte chemotaxis in vivo. I. Description of a model of cell accumulation using adoptively transferred Cr-labeled cells. J Lab Clin Med 84:378–393, 1974.

Petrini B, Wasserman J, Rotstein S, Blomgren H. Radiotherapy and persistent reduction of peripheral T cells. J Clin Lab Immunol 11:159–160, 1983.

Pirofsky B, Beaulieu R, August A. Immunologic effects of anti-thymocyte antisera in human. In Seiler FR, Schwik HG, eds. ALG Therapy and Standardization Workshop. Marburg, Behringwerke AG, 1972, 237–242.

Pirsch JD, Miller J, Deierhoi MH, Vincenti F, Filo RS. A comparison of tacrolimus and cyclosporine for immunosuppression after cadaveric renal transplantation. FK506 Kidney Transplant Study Group. Transplantation 63:977–983, 1997.

Prasad NK, Papoff G, Zeuner A, Bonnin E, Kazatchkine MD, Ruberti G, Kaveri SV. Therapeutic preparations of normal polyspecific IgG induce apoptosis in human lymphocytes and monocytes: a novel mechanism of action of IVIG involving the Fas apoptotic pathway. J Immunol 161:3781–3790, 1998.

Radwansky E, Chakraborty A, Van Wart S, Huhn RD, Cutler DL, Affirme MB, Jusko WJ. Pharmacokinetics and leukocyte responses of recombinant interleukin-10. Pharm Res 15:1895–1901, 1998.

Reinherz EL, Geha R, Rappeport JM, Wilson M, Penta AC, Hussey RE, Fitzgerald KA, Daley JF, Levine H, Rosen FS, Schlossman SF. Reconstitution after transplantation with T-lymphocyte-depleted HLA, haplotype-mismatched bone marrow for severe combined immunodeficiency. Proc Natl Acad Sci U S A 79:6047–6051, 1982.

Revillard JP, Brochier J. Selective deficiency of cell-mediated immunity in humans treated with anti-lymphocyte globulins. Transplant Proc 3:725–729, 1971.

Rinehart JJ, Sagone AL, Balcerzak SP, Ackerman GA, LoBuglio AF. Effects of corticosteroid therapy on human monocyte function. N Engl J Med 292:236–241, 1975.

Roudebush RE, Berry PL, Layman NK, Butler LD, Bryant HU. Dissociation of immunosuppression by chlorpromazine and trifluoperazine from pharmacologic activities as dopamine antagonists. Int J Immunopharmacol 13:961–968, 1991.

Sands BE. Therapy of inflammatory bowel disease. Gastroenterology 118:S68–S82, 2000.

Santos GW, Owens AH, Sensenbrenner LL. Effects of selected cytotoxic agents on antibody production in man. Ann N Y Acad Sci 114:404–423, 1964.

Santos GW, Sensenbrenner LL, Burke PJ, Colvin M, Owens AH, Bias WB, Slavin RE. Marrow transplantation in man following cyclophosphamide. Transplant Proc 3:400–404, 1971.

Sanz-Guajardo D. Plasmapheresis in the treatment of glomerulonephritis: indications and complications. Am J Kidney Dis 36:liv–lvi, 2000.

Schneider KM. Plasmapheresis and immunoadsorption: different techniques and their current role in medical therapy. Kidney Int Suppl 64:S61–S65, 1998.

Schwartz RS. Immunosuppressive drugs. Prog Allergy 9:246–289, 1965.

Sharafuddin MG, Spanheimer RG, McClune GL. Phenytoin-induced agranulocytosis: a nonimmunologic idiosyncratic reaction? Acta Haematol 86:212–213, 1991.

Shearer WT, Finegold MJ, Guerra IC, Rosenblatt HM, Lewis DE, Pollack MS, Taber LH, Sumaya CV, Grumet FC, Cleary ML, Warnke R, Sklar J. Epstein-Barr virus associated B-cell proliferation of diverse clonal origins after bone marrow transplantation in a 12-year-old patient with severe combined immunodeficiency. N Engl J Med 312:1151–1159, 1985.

Shearer WT, Reuben JM, Mullington JM, Price NJ, Bang-Ning L, Smith EO, VanDongen HPA, Dinges DF. Soluble tumor necrosis factor-alpha receptor I and interleukin-6 plasma levels in humans subjected to the sleep deprivation model of space flight. J Allergy Clin Immunol 197:165–170, 2001.

Shepard RJ, Castellani JW, Shek PN. Immune deficits induced by strenuous exertion under adverse environmental conditions: manifestations and countermeasures. Crit Rev Immunol 18:545–568, 1998.

Showstack J, Katz P, Amend W, Bernstein L, Lipton H, O'Leary M, Bindman A, Salvatierra O. The effect of cyclosporine in the use of hospital resources for kidney transplantation. N Engl J Med 321:1086–1092, 1989.

Sigal NH, Dumont FJ. Cyclosporine A, FK-506, and rapamycin: pharmacologic probes of lymphocyte signal transduction. Annu Rev Immunol 10:519–560, 1992.

Silverman ED, Myones BL, Miller JJ. Lymphocyte subpopulation alterations induced by intravenous megadose pulse methylprednisolone. J Rheumatol 11:287–290, 1984.

Simmons RL, Moberg AW, Gewurz H, Soll R, Najarian JS. Immunosuppression by anti-human lymphocyte globulin: correlation of human and animal assay systems with clinical results. Transplant Proc 3:745–748, 1971.

Smialowicz RJ, Rogers RR, Riddle MM, Scott GA. Immunologic effects of nickel. Suppression of cellular and humoral immunity. Environ Res 33:413–427, 1984.

Sommerfeld G, Miller ES. Role of cytokines in immune changes induced by space flight. J Leuk Biol 54:253–258, 1993.

Sorrell TC, Forbes IJ. Depression of immune competence by phenytoin and carbamazepine. Studies in vivo and in vitro. Clin Exp Immunol 20:273–285, 1975.

Stangel M, Joly E, Scolding NJ, Compston DA. Normal polyclonal immunoglobulins inhibit microglial phagocytosis in vitro. J Neuroimmunol 106:137–144, 2000.

Starzl TE, Marchioro TL, Porter KA, Iwasaki Y, Cerilli GJ. The use of heterologous antilymphoid agents in canine renal and liver homotransplantation and in human renal homotransplantation. Surg Gynecol Obstet 124:301–308, 1967.

Starzl TE, Putnam CW, Halgrimson CG, Schroter GT, Martineau G, Launois B, Corman JL, Penn I, Booth AS, Groth CG, Porter KA. Cyclophosphamide and whole organ transplantation in human beings. Surg Gynecol Obstet 133:981–991, 1971.

Stevens JE, Willoughby DA. The antiinflammatory effect of some immunosuppressive agents. J Pathol 97:367–373, 1969.

Swanson MA, Schwartz RS. Immunosuppressive therapy: the relation between clinical response and immunologic competence. N Engl J Med 277:163–170, 1967.

Swinnen LJ, Costanzo-Nordin MR, Fisher SG, O'Sullivan EJ, Johnson MR, Heroux AL, Dizikes GJ, Pifarre R, Fisher RI. Increased incidence of lymphoproliferative disorder after immunosuppression with the monoclonal antibody OKT3 in cardiac-transplant recipients. N Engl J Med 323:1723–1728, 1990.

Taylor GR. Immune changes during short-duration mission. J Leuk Biol 54:202–208, 1993.

Thistlethwaite JR, Gaber AO, Haag BW, Aronson AJ, Broelsch CE, Stuart JK, Stuart FP. OKT3 treatment of steroid-resistant renal allograft rejection. Transplantation 43:176–184, 1987.

Toogood JH, White FA, Baskerville JC, Fraher LJ, Jennings B. Comparison of the antiasthmatic, oropharyngeal, and systemic glucocorticoid effects of budesonide administered through a pressurized aerosol plus spacer or the Turbohaler dry powder inhaler. J Allergy Clin Immunol 99:186–193, 1997.

Townes AS, Sowa JM, Shuman LE. Controlled trial of cyclophosphamide in rheumatoid arthritis. Arthritis Rheum 19:563–573, 1976.

Trentham DE, Belli JA, Anderson JA, Buckey JA, Goetzl EJ, David JR, Austen KF. Clinical and immunologic effect of fractionated total lymphoid irradiation in refractory rheumatoid arthritis. N Engl J Med 305:976–982, 1981.

Tuchinda M, Newcomb RW, DeVald BL. Effect of prednisone treatment on the human immune response to keyhole limpet hemocyanin. Int Arch Allergy Appl Immunol 42:533–544, 1972.

Turk JL, Poulter LW. Selective depletion of lymphoid tissue by cyclophosphamide. Clin Exp Immunol 10:285–296, 1972.

Uh S, Lee SM, Kim HT, Chung Y, Kim YH, Park C, Huh SJ, Lee HB. The effect of radiation therapy on immune function in patients with squamous cell lung carcinoma. Chest 105:132–137, 1994.

United Nations Scientific Committee on the effects of atomic radiation. Ionizing radiation: Sources and biological effects. New York, United Nations, 1972, 28–30.

Van Gelder T, Balk AH, Jonkman FA, Zietze R, Zondervan P. Hesse CJ, Vaesse LM, Mochtar B, Weimar W. A randomized trial comparing safety and efficacy of OKT3 and a monoclonal anti-interleukin-2 receptor antibody (BT563) in the prevention of acute rejection after heart transplantation. Transplantation 62:51–55, 1996.

Vermeer BJ, Hurks M. The clinical relevance of immunosuppression by UV irradiation. J Photochem Photobiol B 24:149–154, 1994.

Vernon-Roberts B. The Macrophage. Cambridge, UK, Cambridge University Press, 1972,92.

Vitetta ES, Thorpe PE, Uhr JW. Immunotoxins: magic bullets or misguided missiles? Immunol Today 14: 252–259, 1993.

Wang JY, Tsukayama DT, Wicklund BH, Gustilo RB. Inhibition of T and B cell proliferation by titanium, cobalt and chromium. J Biomed Mater Res 32:655–661, 1996.

Weston WL, Claman HN, Kruger GG. Site of action of cortisol in cellular immunity. J Immunol 110:880–883, 1973.

Wilson JW, Djukanovic R, Howarth PH, Holgate ST. Inhaled beclomethasone dipropionate downregulates airway lymphocyte activation in atopic asthma. Am J Respir Crit Care Med 149:86–90, 1994.

Woodle ES, Thistlethwaite JR, Jolliffe LK, Zilvin RA, Collins A, Adair JR, Bodmer M, Athwal D, Alegre ML, Bluestone JA. Humanized OKT3 antibodies: successful transfer of immune modulating properties and idiotype expression. J Immunol 148:2756–2763, 1992.

Young JW, Baggers J, Soergel SA. High Dose UVB irradiation alters human dendritic cell costimulatory activity but does not allow dendritic cells to tolerize T lymphocytes to alloantigen in vitro. Blood 81:2987–2997, 1993.

Zan-Bar I. Modulation of B and T cell subsets in mice treated with fractionated total lymphoid irradiation. II. Tolerance susceptibility of B cell subsets. Eur J Immunol 13:40–44, 1983.

Zenke G, Baumann G, Wengeer R, Hiestand P, Quesnieaux V, Andersen E, Schreier MH. Molecular mechanisms of immunosuppression by cyclosporins. Ann N Y Acad Sci 685:330–335, 1993.

CHAPTER

28 Immune Mechanisms in Infectious Disease

Katherine Luzuriaga and John L. Sullivan

Humans live in an environment rife with infectious agents. Whether infection occurs after exposure to an infectious agent depends on an intricate balance between the infectious agent and host defenses. The success of many pathogens depends on their ability to evade or counteract host defense mechanisms. This chapter reviews the mechanisms by which infectious agents subvert the host immune system to establish infection or develop persistent infection. Examples of how certain pathogens use these mechanisms are provided.

OVERVIEW OF HOST DEFENSE MECHANISMS

Remarkable progress in the past 30 years has led to delineation of the key effector mechanisms of the adaptive immune response (Hallman et al., 2001; Kimbrell and Beutler, 2001). Less is understood of the mechanisms of the innate immune response that precede the development of an adaptive immune response.

Components of the innate immune system signal the presence of microorganisms, prevent or limit the extent of an infection, and initiate an adaptive immune response. The effector mechanisms of the innate immune system include cells (e.g., epithelial, natural killer [NK], and phagocytic cells), and soluble factors (e.g., cytokines, chemokines, antimicrobial peptides, and complement components). These are discussed in detail in Chapter 10.

Innate Immunity

Three mechanisms are used by the innate immune system to distinguish self from nonself and thus facilitate the recognition of pathogens. As reviewed by Medzhitov and Janeway (2002), these include distinguishing "microbial nonself," "missing self," and "altered self."

The recognition of "microbial nonself" relies on specific receptor-ligand interactions between receptors of the innate immune system and molecular components of microbial cell surface membranes (e.g., lipopolysaccharides [LPSs] of gram-negative bacteria, peptidoglycans of gram-positive bacteria, and mannans of yeast). These components, known as *pathogen-associated molecular patterns,* are found on all microorganisms, regardless of their pathogenicity, but are not present on host cells. Their highly conserved and essential nature for the organism makes evolution of microbial resistance unlikely.

The pathogen-associated molecular pattern receptors on host cells, termed *pattern recognition receptors* (PRRs), are encoded in the germline (and thus passed from generation to generation) and, unlike cellular receptors of the adaptive immune response, are not clonal. Some PRRs are secreted and facilitate complement activation (e.g., mannose-binding protein) and pathogen phagocytosis. Other PRRs are present on mucosal epithelial cells or immune cells and facilitate pathogen internalization for microbial killing, antigen degradation, or antigen processing.

Toll-like receptors (TLRs) are type 1 membrane proteins that activate intracellular signaling pathways leading to nuclear NF-κB activation; this results in the secretion of cytokines or antimicrobial peptides. These antimicrobial peptides include cathelicidins (produced by leukocytes) and defensins (α-defensins are produced by blood granulocytes or intestinal Paneth cells; β-defensins are produced by specialized epithelial cells). The activation of TLRs on dendritic and other antigen-presenting cells also facilitates the initiation of adaptive immune responses by enhancing antigen presentation. For example, TLR-4 activation by LPS increases the expression of co-stimulatory molecules on the surfaces of dendritic cells (DCs). These co-stimulatory molecules, together with pathogen-derived peptides complexed to DC major histocompatibility complex (MHC) antigens, interact with ligands on naïve T cells to initiate an adaptive immune response.

The "missing self" surveillance system prevents the destruction of host cells by the host's own immune system. Constitutively expressed host cell molecules (Table 28-1) inhibit host–effector cell mechanisms. Pathogen cell surfaces lack these molecules and make them susceptible to host defense mechanisms such as complement-mediated damage, NK-cell lysis, or phagocytosis.

The "altered self" recognition system uses the induced expression of cell surface molecules (e.g., MHC–related chain A [MICA] and UL16-binding protein [ULBP]) on NK or CD8+ cells to enhance their ability to recognize infected or transformed cells. Recognition initiates enhanced NK- or cytolytic T-cell function and cytokine secretion.

Adaptive Immunity

The adaptive immune system generates pathogen-specific immune responses. These responses take days to weeks to develop. Immunologic memory, or the ability to respond to specific pathogens with increased speed and amplitude, is a hallmark of adaptive immunity. Immunologic memory requires the clonal expansion of antigen-specific T or B lymphocytes with unique receptors resulting from gene rearrangement.

DCs are an important bridge between innate and adaptive immunity (Rescigno and Borrow, 2001). DCs are found in the subepithelial layer of the skin and submucosa, usually in proximity to cells (e.g., intestinal M cells) that move antigens or microorganisms across the epithelial layer. DCs may sample the extraepithelial environment through their dendritic processes. Pathogen binding or phagocytosis leads to DC activation and their migration to secondary lymphoid organs, where antigen processing and interaction with naïve B or T cells initiates adaptive immune responses.

DCs and macrophages express cell surface receptors (including TLRs and lectins) that aid in the initial recognition of pathogens. Signaling through these receptors enhances the release of cytokine and other soluble factors, which further activate DCs for antigen processing and presentation, and initiates an adaptive immune response.

As outlined later, some pathogens exploit this sentinel function of DCs and macrophages to initiate and propagate infection.

LOCAL DEFENSE MECHANISMS

Because most infections begin at mucosal surfaces, intricate mucosal defense mechanisms have evolved to prevent pathogen entry (Hornef et al., 2002; Young et al., 2002). Epithelial cells form an anatomic barrier to pathogen entry. Other mechanisms maintain mucosal epithelial integrity or hinder pathogen replication and entry (Table 28-2). Mucosal injury may lead to infection through physical disruption of epithelial barriers and through functional disruption of mucosal defense systems.

Most epithelial surfaces are bathed in fluids that help to reduce the number of microorganisms. The low pH of some mucosal fluids (e.g., gastric juice and urine) renders the mucosal environment less conducive to microbial growth. The presence of peptides (e.g., defensins or cathelicidins) or antibodies in the mucosal fluid instigates antimicrobial activity. Promotion of motility minimizes contact time and reduces microbial adherence to the epithelial cells.

Developmental Defects of Local Immunity

Mucosal defense mechanisms are incompletely developed at birth, contributing to the newborn's susceptibility to certain pathogens (see Chapter 9). The reduced produc-

---

TABLE 28-1 · EXAMPLES OF CONSTITUTIVELY EXPRESSED CELL SURFACE MOLECULES THAT AID IN THE DISCRIMINATION OF "SELF" FROM "MISSING SELF"

Molecule	Host Cell Distribution	Mechanism of Action
MHC class I	All nucleated cells (except neurons)	MHC class I interaction with inhibitory receptors on NK cells blocks NK-cell lysis; downregulation of MHC I by infection or transformation targets cells for NK-cell lysis
CD46 and CD55	All nucleated cells	Inhibit formation and increase the decay of C3 convertases and activation of the alternative complement pathway
Sialic acid	Vertebrate cell surface glycoproteins and glycolipids	Presence of sialic acid inhibits formation of the C3 convertase and activation of the alternative complement pathway. Lack of sialic acids targets microbes or cells for phagocytosis
CD47	Erythrocytes	Ligation of SIRPα receptors on macrophages prevents phagocytosis; downregulation of CD47 targets cells for phagocytosis

MHC = major histocompatibility complex; NK = natural killer; SIRPα = signal regulatory protein.

TABLE 28-2 · EARLY HOST DEFENSE MECHANISMS

Stages	Barriers or Defense Mechanisms	Examples
Mucosal exposure and colonization	Epithelial integrity	Epithelial tight junctions (e.g., intestinal)
	Protective coating	Vernix caseosa (newborn skin) and mucin
	Secreted substances	Gastric acid, secretory antibodies, and antimicrobial peptides (e.g., cathelicidins and defensins)
	Motility	Ciliary movement (respiratory tract) and peristalsis (gastrointestinal tract)
Replication and dissemination	Submucosal macrophages and dendritic cells	Bind and phagocytose pathogens, initiating an inflammatory response and adaptive immunity
	Acute-phase reactants	Soluble pattern recognition receptors
	Complement	Opsonization, chemoattractants, and pore generation resulting in cell lysis
	NK cells	Direct lysis of altered cells

NK = natural killer.

tion of gastric acid renders infants more susceptible to enteric infections. Delayed closure of intestinal tight junctions facilitates microbial entry.

Delayed or abnormal development of components of the innate immune system may also increase the newborn's susceptibility to infection. Defensin secretion by intestinal Paneth's cells occurs as early as 25 weeks' gestation; Paneth's cell density increases during the third trimester (Salzman et al., 1998; Zasloff, 2003). TLR-2 and TLR-4 expression is decreased in the immature lung (Hallman et al., 2001). Surfactant protein SP-A, which has antimicrobial properties, is decreased in the newborn lung and may contribute to the susceptibility of premature infants to pulmonary infections (see Chapters 10 and 22).

Pathogen-Induced Defects of Local Immunity

Some pathogens subvert local defenses to initiate infection (Hornef et al., 2002). Biofilm formation by certain bacteria (e.g., *Pseudomonas aeruginosa* and *Staphylococcus epidermidis*) may impede mucosal clearance. Some bacteria (e.g., *Bordetella pertussis*) secrete toxins that paralyze respiratory mucosal ciliary clearance. Others (e.g., *Haemophilus influenzae*) degrade secretory immunoglobulins.

Pathogen entry requires breaching of the epithelial cell barrier. Some pathogenic bacteria contain factors (adhesins) that allow attachment to cell surfaces, thus preventing their mechanical removal. Pathogen binding to epithelial cells and epithelial cell infection (e.g., in measles) may facilitate penetrating the epithelial barrier. Epithelial tight junctions in the small intestine impede pathogen transfer; developmental delay in their closure may allow pathogen entry. Finally, pathogen-induced inflammation may disrupt the epithelial barrier and facilitate pathogen entry.

PATHOGEN SUBVERSION OF THE HOST IMMUNE SYSTEM

Pathogens may also create an environment favoring infection through direct immunosuppression of the host. Generalized immunosuppression is commonly present during the early stages of viral or parasitic infections. The precise mechanisms remain unclear, but the underlying mechanisms for the immunosuppression during measles virus (MV) and malarial infections have been delineated.

Role of Macrophages and Dendritic Cells

Once the epithelial barrier has been breached, establishment of infection requires that the pathogen reach cells able to replicate and disseminate it (Table 28-3). Antigen-presenting cells such as DCs or macrophages are abundant in submucosal tissues and are commonly exploited by pathogens for this purpose (Rescigno and Borrow, 2001).

TABLE 26-3 · CELLS OF THE IMMUNE SYSTEM THAT SERVE AS SUBSTRATES FOR INFECTION, AS VENUES FOR DISSEMINATION, OR AS SITES FOR THE PERSISTENCE OF PATHOGENS

Virus	Cell	Receptor
Human immunodeficiency virus	T cells and macrophages	CD4, CCR5, or CXCR3
	Dendritic cells	DC-SIGN
Epstein-Barr virus	B cells	CD21
Measles	Dendritic and T cells	CD46 and SLAM
Human herpesvirus 6		CD46

CCR5 = chemokine receptor 5; CXCR4 = chemokine receptor 4; DC-SIGN = dendritic cell–specific ICAM-3–grabbing nonintegrin; SLAM = signaling lymphocyte activation molecule.

Macrophages and DCs may serve as the initial site of replication for pathogens (e.g., dengue virus) or facilitate their transport to secondary lymphoid tissues. They may also facilitate infection of other susceptible cells. A calcium-dependent lectin known as DC-SIGN (*dendritic cell–specific ICAM-3–grabbing nonintegrin*; CD209) that is expressed on the surface of macrophages and some DCs and has high-affinity binding to carbohydrate domains on the surfaces of viruses such as human immunodeficiency virus (HIV) (Geijtenbeek et al., 2000), Ebola virus (Baribaud et al., 2002), hepatitis C virus (Pohlmann et al., 2003), or fungi Candida albicans (Cambi et al., 2003) was recently identified. Binding to permissive cells through this lectin may facilitate infection, and binding to nonpermissive cells may facilitate infection of nearby susceptible cells.

Pathogens may stimulate DCs or macrophages to secrete chemokines that recruit other cells that can become infected. In vitro studies demonstrate that the presence of HIV tat (Izmailova et al., 2003) and nef (Swingler et al., 1999) proteins in macrophages or DCs stimulates their synthesis of cytokines that attract monocytes and activated CD4 cells; the latter cells are the major producers of new viral particles (Griffin et al., 1994; Perelson, 2002). The cell-to-cell transfer of virus from DCs or macrophages to mobile CD4+ T cells is probably more efficient than cell-free viral transfer, minimizes exposure of the pathogen to immune surveillance, and provides a mechanism for HIV dissemination.

Measles-Induced Immune Suppression

Timing of Measles Immunosuppression

MV infections remain a major cause of morbidity and mortality in children worldwide. MV is an enveloped, single-strand RNA virus of the genus *Morbillivirus* and the family Paramyxoviridae. MV transmission occurs through direct nasopharyngeal mucosal contact or inhalation of aerosolized respiratory secretions of an infected individual.

In human and nonhuman primate studies, MV replication occurs in nasal, tracheal, bronchial, and pulmonary epithelial cells shortly after exposure (Griffin et al., 1994; Hilleman, 2001); cell-associated viremia (occurring primarily in monocytes) is commonly documented within a few days of exposure. Viral replication continues locally and within the reticuloendothelial system, resulting in secondary viremia 5 to 7 days after exposure.

Symptoms of measles develop 1 to 2 weeks after exposure and include fever, conjunctivitis, upper respiratory tract symptoms (e.g., coryza and cough), and a maculopapular rash. The resolution of symptoms coincides with the development of virus-specific antibodies and cell-mediated immunity, approximately 17 days to 3 weeks after exposure.

Most measles-related morbidity and mortality is attributable to secondary infection. Diarrhea and bacterial pneumonia are common sequelae and are thought to result from direct infection and disruption of the mucosal epithelial barriers. Generalized immunosuppression may also contribute to secondary infection. Lymphocytopenia is common during the viremic phases of MV infection and resolves as the rash appears. T-cell activation is observed during MV infection, but altered cell-mediated immunity also is commonly observed and may persist for weeks to months after the resolution of acute infection. Impaired delayed hypersensitivity reactions during MV infection have long been recognized. Decreased NK-cell function, increased lymphocyte apoptosis, impaired neutrophil function, and decreased lymphoproliferative responses have been documented in vitro, but MV-specific antibodies and CD8+ T-cell responses develop in vivo after infection.

Immunosuppression occurs after either natural MV infection or after attenuated MV vaccination. Killed virus is also immunosuppressive in vitro. These data suggest that direct interaction of viral particles with host cells may contribute to MV-induced immunosuppression.

MV Receptors

The MV envelope glycoprotein hemagglutinin (Benninger-Doring et al., 1999) interacts with host cell surface receptors to allow attachment; the fusion glycoprotein interacts with the cell membrane to allow entry of the viral genome. MV nucleoprotein binding to the Fcγ receptor on macrophages and DCs also occurs with resultant impaired activation of these cells (Marie et al., 2001).

Several cellular receptors have been implicated in MV pathogenesis. CD46, the first cellular receptor identified for MV (Dorig et al., 1993), is a 70-kD type 1 transmembrane glycoprotein expressed on all human cells except erythrocytes. CD46 has also been identified as a cellular receptor for human herpesvirus 6 and pathogenic *Neisseria* species. CD46 was initially identified as important in protecting human cells from complement lysis by serving as a co-factor for plasma serine protease factor I inactivation of C3b and C4b complement fragments. More recently, CD46 has also been shown to play an important role in adaptive immunity by modulating the threshold for T-cell activation (Marie et al., 2002).

Role of IL-12

The results of studies by Karp (1999) and Karp and colleagues (1996) have demonstrated that infection of monocytes and macrophages with laboratory strains of MV resulted in reduced IL-12 production in vitro. Decreased IL-12 production was observed despite the fact that relatively few monocytes were productively infected with MV. Decreased IL-2 production was also observed following exposure to inactivated viruses.

Monoclonal antibody-induced crosslinking of CD46 with dimerized C3b, its natural ligand, also decreased IL-12 production. Decreased in vivo IL-12 production by MV-infected macaques (Polack et al., 2002) and decreased in vitro IL-12 production by monocytes from

MV-infected patients (Atabani et al., 2001) have been observed. On the basis of these observations, a model for MV immunosuppression has been proposed in which the interaction of MV or complement-opsonized MV with CD46 leads to decreased IL-12 production. Because IL-12 stimulates IFN-γ production by T and NK cells, enhances NK-cell cytotoxicity, and is necessary for delayed cutaneous hypersensitivity responses, its deficiency may result in the other immune defects present in MV infection.

Role of Signaling Lymphocyte Activation Molecule

An additional cellular receptor for MV is the signaling lymphocyte activation molecule (SLAM) (Oldstone et al., 2002; Yanagi et al., 2002). All MV strains appear to use SLAM, whereas only MV grown in Vero cells appears to use CD46 as a receptor, suggesting that SLAM may be an important in vivo cellular receptor for MV. SLAM is constitutively expressed on CD45RO^{high} memory T cells, some B cells, and immature thymocytes, and it is upregulated on activated B and T cells. It is also present on activated monocytes and mature DCs, but not on resting monocytes or immature DCs. In ways that are not yet fully understood, MV infection of SLAM-expressing cells may also contribute to immunosuppression.

Malaria-Induced Immune Suppression

Malaria, an important global pathogen, is a common cause of childhood morbidity and mortality (Urban and Roberts, 2002; Wilson, 2003). Two thirds of the world's population is exposed annually to one or more of the four following *Plasmodium* species causing malaria: *Plasmodium falciparum*, *Plasmodium vivax*, *Plasmodium ovale*, and *Plasmodium malariae*. Infection with *P. falciparum* is associated with the most severe sequelae; an estimated 2 million children die from *P. falciparum* infection yearly.

Plasmodium Life Cycle

Sporozoites enter the host's bloodstream through the bite of the *Anopheles* mosquito. An initial round of asexual multiplication occurs in the liver, followed by the release of the merozoites, which invade erythrocytes. Within erythrocytes, the parasites undergo asexual multiplication (schizogeny) or sexual differentiation to produce gametocytes and then undergo mitosis and differentiation into merozoites. The subsequent rupture of the erythrocyte and release of the merozoites cause the fever and other symptoms of malaria. The *Plasmodium* life cycle is completed in the gastrointestinal tract of *Anopheles* mosquitoes after the ingestion of a blood meal.

Immune Defects in Malaria

During active *Plasmodium* infections, both concurrent infections (e.g., bacteremia) and impaired responses to childhood vaccines are frequently observed, suggesting a period of immune hyporesponsiveness. Recent studies (Urban and Roberts, 2002) have demonstrated that phagocytosis of infected erythrocytes impairs subsequent phagocytosis and generation of superoxide radicals. In vitro binding of infected red blood cells to macrophages and DCs through CD36 or CD51 diminishes the upregulation of MHC class II molecules, adhesion molecules, and co-stimulatory molecules (e.g., CD86); decreases the secretion of anti-inflammatory cytokines; and increases the secretion of proinflammatory cytokines (e.g., IL-10 and tumor necrosis factor-β).

Reduction of sporozoite replication in the liver is important for limiting subsequent parasitemia, and only low-level CD8$^+$ responses to liver-stage *Plasmodium* antigen develop during natural malarial infections (Urban and Roberts, 2003). Immunization with irradiated sporozoites was successful in preventing liver infection (Nussenzweig et al., 1969).

In a murine model of malaria, Ocana-Morgner and colleagues (2003) have demonstrated that *Plasmodium*-infected erythrocytes inhibit the generation of sporozoite-specific CD8$^+$ T-cell responses. Moreover, the transfer of DCs exposed to *Plasmodium*-infected erythrocytes suppressed IFN-γ production by circumsporozoite-specific CD8$^+$ T cells generated by immunization with irradiated sporozoites. In vitro studies demonstrated that the DCs exposed to *Plasmodium*-infected erythrocytes and then stimulated with LPS had decreased expression of MHC and co-stimulatory molecules, reduced IL-12 production, and increased IL-10 production.

Thus *Plasmodia* suppress the immune responses that limit their replication in the liver, enhancing the likelihood of malarial infection or reinfection. This suppression of cell-mediated immunity may also explain the impaired responses to childhood vaccines.

MECHANISMS OF VIRAL PERSISTENCE

Pathogens, particularly viruses, may subvert immune mechanisms to establish persistent infection. DNA viruses with large genomes, notably Epstein-Barr virus (EBV) or cytomegalovirus (CMV), code for immunomodulatory proteins that allow viral persistence.

Cytomegalovirus

CMV, a member of the Herpesviridae family, is an enveloped virus with a 230-kb linear double-stranded DNA genome that codes for more than 200 proteins (178 unique proteins). It is the largest virus to infect humans. CMV is spread by close or intimate (including sexual) contact with an infected individual, by blood products, organ transplantation, and vertically from mother to infant. CMV is the most common human congenital infection worldwide and a common cause of multiorgan disease in immunocompromised hosts.

Persistent CMV infection results from a dynamic interplay between viral evasion strategies and host immune responses. Vigorous CMV-specific immune responses develop during infection; nonetheless, numerous CMV immune evasion strategies have been identified (Reddehase, 2002).

Mechanisms of CMV Persistence

At least seven CMV gene products encode cytokine, chemokine, and chemokine receptor mimickers, thus constituting the largest group of viral homologs of host proteins (Murphy, 2001). For example, CMV encodes a viral IL-10 homolog, UL111A, that impairs host cellular immune responses by decreasing the secretion of proinflammatory cytokines. In vitro studies also demonstrate that a CMV-encoded G protein–coupled receptor, US28, binds to and thus reduces the concentration of the antiviral chemokine RANTES (regulated upon activation, normal T-cell expressed and secreted).

Other CMV-encoded proteins interfere with antigen processing and presentation. For example, proteins encoded by human CMV US11 and US2 mediate the translocation of newly synthesized HLA class I heavy chains from the endoplasmic reticulum to the cytosol for degradation, thus reducing cell surface HLA expression. The gP21 protein encoded by US6 blocks the transporter associated with antigen presentation–mediated translocation of peptides into the endoplasmic reticulum. Another CMV protein, UL18, binds to β_2-microglobulin and may serve as an HLA class I decoy by interacting with killer cell inhibitory receptors on NK cells.

Epstein-Barr Virus

EBV, also a member of the Herpesviridae family, is an enveloped virus with a 172-kb linear double-stranded DNA genome that codes for approximately 100 proteins. EBV has infected more than 90% of the world's population and is spread by contact with oropharyngeal secretions from a virus carrier. The tonsils appear to be the initial site of viral entry and replication. Primary EBV infection is usually asymptomatic or only mildly symptomatic in young children, but primary EBV infection in older children or adults may result in infectious mononucleosis.

The EBV genome is also detected in a variety of neoplasms, including Hodgkin's disease, Burkitt's lymphoma, and nasopharyngeal carcinoma. The role of EBV in their pathogenesis is not completely understood, yet EBV-associated lymphoproliferative disease is a common cause of morbidity in individuals undergoing transplantation or immunosuppressive therapy.

Persistent EBV infection also results from a dynamic interplay between viral evasion strategies and host immune responses (Thorley-Lawson, 2001). Acute EBV infection results in T-cell activation (Tomkinson et al., 1987, 1989a) and the development of high levels of EBV-specific CD4+ (Precopio et al., 2003) and CD8+ cells (Catalina et al., 2001; Tomkinson et al., 1989b).

Mechanisms of EBV Persistence

Recent studies have provided insight into how EBV persists despite these brisk immune responses. An EBV IL-10 homolog (BCRF1) has been identified that has potent immunosuppressive activity. EBV exploits normal B-cell differentiation to allow it to persist in a transcriptionally quiescent state in memory B cells and thus minimize immune recognition.

EBV infection of resting naïve B cells in the tonsillar mantle zone results in the generation of activated, proliferating B-cell blasts under the regulation of the transcription factor EBV nuclear antigen 2 (EBNA2). These EBV-infected B-cell blasts express many EBV proteins and are thus potentially subject to immune effector mechanisms, including lysis by EBV-specific CD8+ T cells.

However, some EBV-infected B-cell blasts escape immune surveillance and traffic to follicles where they form germinal centers, turn off EBNA2, and express a more restricted set of viral proteins: EBNA1, latent membrane protein 1 (LMP-1), and latent membrane protein 2 (LMP-2). Normally, the survival of germinal center B cells requires signals from antigen on antigen-presenting cells through the B-cell receptor and signals from CD40L on T-helper cells through CD40. EBV LMP-1, a functional homolog of CD40, and EBV LMP-2 protein, a functional homolog of the B-cell receptor, may mimic these signals. This allows survival of the EBV-infected B cells and their acquisition of a memory B-cell phenotype with limited EBV protein expression.

EBV-infected B cells leave the tonsil and enter the circulation as memory B cells with little transcriptional activity. These cells are highly mobile, long-lived, and invisible to the hosts' immune responses, allowing lifelong EBV persistence.

REFERENCES

Atabani SF, Byrnes AA, Jaye A, Kidd IM, Magnusen AF, Whittle H, Karp CL. Natural measles causes prolonged suppression of interleukin-12 production. J Infect Dis 184:1–9, 2001.

Baribaud F, Doms RW, Pohlmann S. The role of DC-SIGN and DC-SIGNR in HIV and Ebola virus infection: can potential therapeutics block virus transmission and dissemination? Expert Opin Ther Targets 6:423–431, 2002.

Benninger-Doring G, Pepperl S, Deml L, Modrow S, Wolf H, Jilg W. Frequency of CD8(+) T lymphocytes specific for lytic and latent antigens of Epstein-Barr virus in healthy virus carriers. Virology 264:289–297, 1999.

Cambi A, Gijzen K, de Vries JM, Torensma R, Joosten B, Adema GJ, Netea MG, Kullberg BJ, Romani L, Figdor CG. The C-type lectin DC-SIGN (CD209) is an antigen-uptake receptor for Candida albicans on dendritic cells. Eur J Immunol 33:532–538, 2003.

Catalina MD, Sullivan JL, Bak KR, Luzuriaga K. Differential evolution and stability of epitope-specific CD8(+) T cell responses in EBV infection. J Immunol 167:4450–4457, 2001 [erratum in: J Immunol 167:6045, 2001].

Dorig RE, Marcil A, Chopra A, Richardson CD. The human CD46 molecule is a receptor for measles virus (Edmonston strain). Cell 75:295–305, 1993.

Geijtenbeek TB, Kwon DS, Torensma R, van Vliet SJ, van Duijnhoven GC, Middel J, Cornelissen IL, Nottet HS, KewalRamani VN, Littman DR, Figdor CG, van Kooyk Y. DC-SIGN, a dendritic cell-specific HIV-1-binding protein that enhances trans-infection of T cells. Cell 100:587–597, 2000.

Griffin DE, Ward BJ, Esolen LM. Pathogenesis of measles virus infection: an hypothesis for altered immune responses. J Infect Dis 170 Suppl 1:S24–31, 1994.

Hallman M, Ramet M, Ezekowitz RA. Toll-like receptors as sensors of pathogens. Pediatr Res 50:315–321, 2001.

Hilleman MR. Current overview of the pathogenesis and prophylaxis of measles with focus on practical implications. Vaccine 20:651–665, 2001.

Hornef MW, Wick MJ, Rhen M, Normark S. Bacterial strategies for overcoming host innate and adaptive immune responses. Nat Immunol 3:1033–1040, 2002.

Izmailova E, Bertley FM, Huang Q, Makori N, Miller CJ, Young RA, Aldovini A. HIV-1 Tat reprograms immature dendritic cells to express chemoattractants for activated T cells and macrophages. Nat Med 9:191–197, 2003.

Karp CL. Measles: immunosuppression, interleukin-12, and complement receptors. Immunol Rev 168:91–101, 1999.

Karp CL, Wysocka M, Wahl LM, Ahearn JM, Cuomo PJ, Sherry B, Trinchieri G, Griffin DE. Mechanism of suppression of cell-mediated immunity by measles virus. Science 273:228–231, 1996 [erratum in: Science 275:1053, 1997].

Kimbrell DA, Beutler B. The evolution and genetics of innate immunity. Nat Rev Genet 2:256–267, 2001.

Marie JC, Astier AL, Rivailler P, Rabourdin-Combe C, Wild TF, Horvat B. Linking innate and acquired immunity: divergent role of CD46 cytoplasmic domains in T cell induced inflammation. Nat Immunol 3:659–666, 2002.

Marie JC, Kehren J, Trescol-Biemont MC, Evlashev A, Valentin H, Walzer T, Tedone R, Loveland B, Nicolas JF, Rabourdin-Combe C, Horvat B. Mechanism of measles virus-induced suppression of inflammatory immune responses. Immunity 14:69–79, 2001.

Medzhitov R, Janeway CA Jr. Decoding the patterns of self and nonself by the innate immune system. Science 296:298–300, 2002.

Murphy PM. Viral exploitation and subversion of the immune system through chemokine mimicry. Nat Immunol 2:116–122, 2001.

Nussenzweig RS, Vanderberg JP, Most H, Orton C. Specificity of protective immunity produced by x-irradiated *Plasmodium berghei* sporozoites. Nature 222:488–489, 1969.

Ocana-Morgner C, Mota MM, Rodriguez A. Malaria blood stage suppression of liver stage immunity by dendritic cells. J Exp Med 197:143–151, 2003.

Oldstone MB, Homann D, Lewicki H, Stevenson D. One, two, or three step: measles virus receptor dance. Virology 299:162–163, 2002.

Perelson AS. Modelling viral and immune system dynamics. Nat Rev Immunol 2:28–36, 2002.

Pohlmann S, Zhang J, Baribaud F, Chen Z, Leslie GJ, Lin G, Granelli-Piperno A, Doms RW, Rice CM, McKeating JA. Hepatitis C virus glycoproteins interact with DC-SIGN and DC-SIGNR. J Virol 77:4070–4080, 2003.

Polack FP, Hoffman SJ, Moss WJ, Griffin DE. Altered synthesis of interleukin-12 and type 1 and type 2 cytokines in rhesus macaques during measles and atypical measles. J Infect Dis 185:13–19, 2002.

Precopio ML, Sullivan JL, Willard C, Somasundaran M, Luzuriaga K. Differential kinetics and specificity of EBV-specific CD4+ and CD8+ T cells during primary infection. J Immunol 170:2590–2598, 2003.

Reddehase MJ. Antigens and immunoevasins: opponents in cytomegalovirus immune surveillance. Nat Rev Immunol 2:831–844, 2002.

Rescigno M, Borrow P. The host-pathogen interaction: new themes from dendritic cell biology. Cell 106:267–270, 2001.

Salzman NH, Polin RA, Harris MC, Ruchelli E, Hebra A, Zirin-Butler S, Jawad A, Martin Porter E, Bevins CL. Enteric defensin expression in necrotizing enterocolitis. Pediatr Res 44:20–26, 1998.

Swingler S, Mann A, Jacque J, Brichacek B, Sasseville VG, Williams K, Lackner AA, Janoff EN, Wang R, Fisher D, Stevenson M. HIV-1 Nef mediates lymphocyte chemotaxis and activation by infected macrophages. Nat Med 5:997–103, 1999.

Thorley-Lawson DA. Epstein-Barr virus: exploiting the immune system. Nat Rev Immunol 1:75–82, 2001.

Tomkinson BE, Brown MC, Ip SH, Carrabis S, Sullivan JL. Soluble CD8 during T cell activation. J Immunol 142:2230–2236, 1989a.

Tomkinson BE, Maziarz R, Sullivan JL. Characterization of the T cell-mediated cellular cytotoxicity during acute infectious mononucleosis. J Immunol 143:660–670, 1989b.

Tomkinson BE, Wagner DK, Nelson DL, Sullivan JL. Activated lymphocytes during acute Epstein-Barr virus infection. J Immunol 139:3802–3807, 1987.

Urban BC, Roberts DJ. Inhibition of T cell function during malaria: implications for immunology and vaccinology. J Exp Med 197:137–141, 2003.

Urban BC, Roberts DJ. Malaria, monocytes, macrophages and myeloid dendritic cells: sticking of infected erythrocytes switches off host cells. Curr Opin Immunol 14:458–465, 2002.

Wilson CM. *Plasmodium* species (malaria). In Long SS, Pickering LK, Prober CG, eds. Principles and practice of pediatric infectious diseases. New York, Churchill Livingstone, 2nd ed, 2003. pp. 1295–1301.

Yanagi Y, Ono N, Tatsuo H, Hashimoto K, Minagawa H. Measles virus receptor SLAM (CD150). Virology 299:155–161, 2002.

Young D, Hussell T, Dougan G. Chronic bacterial infections: living with unwanted guests. Nat Immunol 3:1026–1032, 2002.

Zasloff M. Vernix, the newborn, and innate defense. Pediatr Res 53:203–204, 2003.

CHAPTER

29

Pediatric Human Immunodeficiency Virus Infection

Arthur J. Ammann

INTRODUCTION

The first reports of an acquired immunodeficiency syndrome (AIDS) in children, possibly thought caused by a transmissible agent, appeared in 1982 (Ammann, 1983; Ammann et al., 1983a, 1983b; Centers for Disease Control and Prevention [CDC], 1982; Oleske et al., 1983; Rubinstein et al., 1983). Currently there are an estimated 4000 children aged younger than 13 years living with AIDS in the United States; of these, approximately 90% were infected perinatally (CDC, 1991b, 1993e, 2002b). As a result of antiretroviral treatment during pregnancy, the number of newly infected infants per year in the United States has declined from an estimated peak of approximately 1800 to fewer than 150 currently (CDC, 2002b).

Although treatment to prevent perinatal human immunodeficiency virus (HIV) transmission has dramatically altered the number of new pediatric infections in the United States, the number of infants born with HIV infection worldwide is estimated to be at least 1800 each day (UNAIDS/WHO, 2002). Importantly, the number of HIV-infected woman continues to increase both in the United States and globally, emphasizing the continued need for voluntary HIV counseling and testing (VCT) to prevent further escalation of HIV infection in infants. As a result of HIV-1 infection, obstetricians and pediatricians throughout the world are increasingly required to recognize and treat women and children infected with HIV at all stages of disease.

Unlike families of children with other life-threatening diseases, the parents of HIV-infected children are also frequently infected and ill and face discrimination rather than support from their communities. The care of HIV-infected children therefore involves a comprehensive, multidisciplinary approach. In developing countries in particular, the HIV/AIDS epidemic is contributing to a rapidly increasing epidemic of orphaned children (UNAIDS/WHO, 2002).

Although there are no cures for HIV at this time and no vaccine to prevent HIV, many advances are being made. This chapter provides an overview of the current state of understanding of the disease, clinical issues, and approaches to the management of HIV-1–infected children.

Detailed up-to-date information is also available on the Internet (http://www.womenchildrenhiv.org; http://www.GlobalStrategies.org; http://www.aidsinfo.nih.gov/guidelines/).

Elsevier, the publisher of this textbook, has kindly agreed to allow publication of this chapter on a CD-ROM titled "Women, Children, and HIV: Resources for Prevention and Treatment" and on the Internet at http://www.womenchildrenhiv.org. The chapter on the Internet site will be regularly updated, providing access to new information not currently incorporated in this chapter.

EPIDEMIOLOGY

Worldwide Epidemiology

Worldwide, more than 42 million people are estimated to be living with HIV/AIDS; 19.2 million are women, 17.4 million are men, and 3.2 million are children (UNAIDS/WHO, 2002). Fifty percent of the infected population is between the ages of 15 and 24 years. In 2002, for the first time since the beginning of the epidemic, the number of women with HIV/AIDS exceeded that of men. The implications of this shift are significant. As more women become infected, especially those of childbearing age, the number of HIV-infected children and orphans is likely to increase dramatically.

New HIV infections in 2002 were estimated to be 5 million, with 2.2 million new infections in men, 2 million new infections in women, and 800,000 new infections in children younger than 15 years. The number of AIDS deaths in 2002 was estimated to be 3.1 million, with 1.3 million deaths among men, 1.2 million deaths among women, and 610,000 deaths among children younger than 15 years. Since the beginning of the epidemic, approximately 20 million people have died from AIDS, including 4 million children (http://hivinsite.ucsf.edu). Seventy-five percent of individuals with HIV/AIDS reside in sub-Saharan Africa (http://www.cdc.gov/; UNAIDS/WHO, 2002; Quinn, 1994).

The spread of HIV-1 throughout the world has varied from region to region, but there are now no countries free of the virus. Emerging epidemics are observed in Central Europe and Asia. The number of HIV infections in India is expected to exceed that of any other country. China has reported a rapid increase in HIV infections related to migration, intravenous drug use, prostitution, and failure to adequately protect the blood supply (Ammann, 2000a; Kumar, 1999; Shan et al., 2002).

Worldwide, HIV seroprevalence varies considerably. The highest rates are observed in sub-Saharan Africa, especially in Botswana, South Africa, and Zimbabwe, which have rates as high as 30% to 40%. Outside of Africa, the highest seroprevalence is in Haiti and the Dominican Republic at between 3.5% and 7%, considerably less than that in sub-Saharan Africa (UNAIDS/WHO, 2002). However, even a low seroprevalence is not reassuring in countries such as India and China, where populations of more than 1 billion will push the total number of HIV infections to high levels (Ammann, 2000a, 2000b). AIDS is the leading cause of death in Africa and the fourth leading cause of death worldwide.

United States Epidemiology

In the United States, AIDS incidence increased rapidly throughout the 1980s and then peaked in the early 1990s at approximately 80,000 new cases per year. This was followed by a significant decline in 1996 that persisted until 1999 when the AIDS incidence began to level. An estimated 41,000 new AIDS cases were diagnosed in 1999 and 2000 (CDC, 2002b; Gayle, 2000; Gayle and Hill, 2001; http://hivinsite.ucsf.edu; Osmond, 2003). Subgroup analysis showed that the AIDS incidence declined most sharply among men who have sex with men (MSM) and injection drug users (IDUs). A decline in AIDS incidence to approximately 11,000 was observed during this time period in individuals who acquired HIV as a result of heterosexual contact. However, 25% of AIDS in the United States occurs in women, representing a 5% increase since 1988. African-American women represent 63% of AIDS cases in women although they represent only 13% of the U.S. population. Many women acquire HIV during adolescence.

AIDS prevalence has increased over time, with an estimated 700,000 individuals in the United States living with AIDS. Estimating the total number of individuals living with HIV and living with AIDS is somewhat problematic because there may be as many as 300,000 HIV-infected individuals who have never been tested and are thus unaware of their HIV status. Some epidemiologists put the total number living with HIV/AIDS at 700,000 to 900,000 (Osmond, 2003). Of these cases, 41% are black, 30% white, 20% Hispanic, 1% Asian/Pacific Islanders, and 1% American Indians/Alaska natives. The CDC estimates that of the 260,000 adults and adolescent males living with AIDS, 57% are MSM, 24% are IDUs, and 9% are exposed through heterosexual contact.

Of the estimated 70,000 adult and adolescent women living with AIDS, 57% were exposed through heterosexual contact and 39% through IDUs. An estimated 4000 children younger than 13 years are living with AIDS, most of whom were infected perinatally (CDC, 2002b). The number of AIDS deaths declined by a dramatic 47% in the United States in 1996. The decline was primarily associated with widespread use of highly active antiretroviral therapy (HAART) (CDC, 2002b, 2002e, 2002f).

In children, the incidence of AIDS began to decline in the mid-1990s and has continued to decline since then. AIDS mortality in 2000 was estimated to be less than 100 children. The recent declines in mortality in the United States are due to both the fewer number of newly infected infants (<150 per year) and the widespread use of HAART.

PATHOGENESIS

Current and future strategies for therapeutic intervention require a clear understanding of the pathogenesis of HIV-1 infection. Although it is likely that the viral life cycle is essentially the same in children and adults, viral replication and host cell susceptibility to infection may vary. Much remains to be learned regarding the influence of growth and cellular differentiation, which are an integral part of the pediatric host, on viral replication and pathogenesis. These influences may help explain some of the differences in the course of disease noted between adults and children.

Molecular and Cellular Biology

Considerations of molecular and cellular biology involve an understanding of viral structure, life cycle, cellular tropism, and regulation of gene expression.

HIV-1 Structure

HIV-1 is a member of the Lentivirinae subfamily of retroviruses. HIV most likely originated sometime in the latter half of the 20th century, evolving from the simian immunodeficiency virus (SIV) and crossing from chimpanzees into humans (Gao et al., 1999; Hahn et al., 2000; Korber et al., 1998). SIV has several variants and is found in multiple species of simian hosts.

Two major strains of HIV exist: HIV-1 and HIV-2. The latter is less common globally and less pathogenic, whereas HIV-1 major group M is the primary cause of AIDS worldwide (Korber et al., 1998; Weiss, 2001). Multiple subtypes of HIV-1 group M exist, classified as clades A to J. Each has a somewhat different geographic distribution although mixing of viral subtypes and recombinants exist simultaneously in many of the emerging epidemics (Korber et al., 1998). Clade B is the most common in the United States and Europe, whereas C is dominant in sub-Saharan Africa. As the epidemic continues to expand worldwide, mixtures of clades exist in many countries.

The distinguishing feature of all retroviruses is their ability to transcribe genetic material in a reverse direction (i.e., from RNA into DNA). The HIV-1 virion comprises a bullet-shaped, electron-dense nucleocapsid that contains the genomic RNA, surrounded by an envelope (Fig. 29-1) (Bryant and Ratner, 1992; Greene, 1991; Haseltine, 1991; Stevenson et al., 1992). The components of the virion are assigned numbers based on their molecular weights (in kilodaltons) and migration on Western blots. The genomic organization is illustrated in Figure 29-2. Nine genes control HIV replication (Emerman and Malim, 1998; Sleasman and Goodenow, 2003; Steffy and Wong-Staal, 1991; Trono, 1992, 1995).

The envelope gp120 consists of a highly glycosylated, lipid bilayer derived from the host cell plasma membrane during virus budding. The gp120 glycoprotein is anchored noncovalently to gp41, the transmembrane protein. A variety of additional host proteins, including class I and class II histocompatibility antigens, may be incorporated into the viral envelope as the virions bud (Gelderblom et al., 1987).

The core contains the duplex single-stranded RNA genome bound to nucleic acid–binding proteins p9 and p7. Surrounding this nucleoid core is the cylindric or bullet-shaped capsid formed by the p24 core antigen protein (Leis et al., 1988). Lining the inside of the

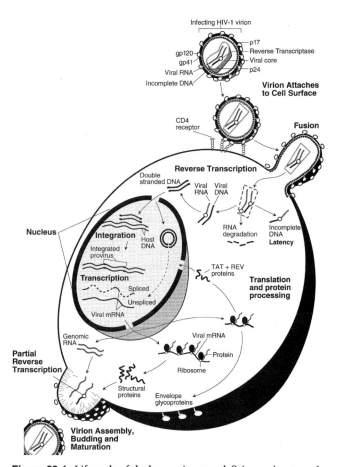

Figure 29-1 · Life cycle of the human immunodeficiency virus type 1.

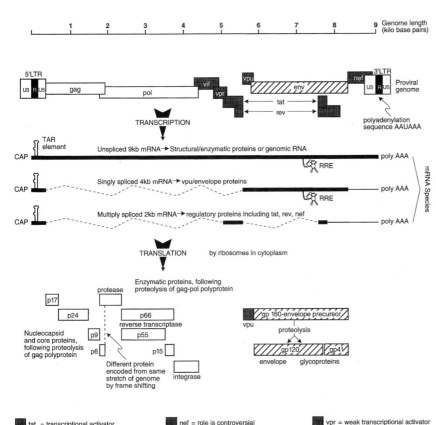

Figure 29-2 · Genomic organization of HIV-1, transcription of spliced (2- and 4-kb) and full-length (9-kb) messenger RNA species, and translation of structural, enzymatic, and regulatory proteins. RRE = rev responsive element; TAR = transactivation response element.

viral envelope with its amino terminal inserted into the membrane is the p17 matrix protein.

Within the virus, an inner core is surrounded by structural proteins containing enzymes and proteins required for viral replication, the viral genome consists of two identical linear copies of RNA (Emerman and Malim, 1998). The group-specific *antigen (gag)*, polymerase *(pol)*, and *env* genes, contained in the HIV-1 genome, are characteristic of all retroviruses. The *gag* gene encodes core structural proteins, and the *env* gene encodes the envelope glycoproteins gp120 and gp41 required for attachment of HIV to immune cells. The *pol* gene encodes for three viral enzymes, reverse transcriptase (RT), integrase, and protease. Two additional genes control viral replication. *Rev* facilitates gene transcriptions and *tat* is the major transactivator of the viral promoter within the long terminal repeats. Accessory genes that contribute to viral replication and include *nef, vpu, vpr,* and *vif* (Emerman and Malim, 1998; Sleasman and Goodenow, 2003; Steffy and Wong-Staal, 1991; Wyatt and Sodroski, 1998).

HIV-1 Life Cycle, Cellular Tropism, and Regulation of Gene Expression

VIRUS BINDING

As shown in Figure 29-1, the life cycle begins with the attachment of the virion to a target cell. The CD4 antigen of T lymphocytes and macrophages serves as the principal cell surface receptor for HIV-1 (Dalgleish et al., 1984; Gartner et al., 1986; Ho et al., 1986; Klatzmann et al., 1984). Several co-receptors are important alternate viral attachment and entry sites. CCR5 and CXCR4, chemokine receptors, determine HIV tropism R5 and X4, respectively (Garzino-Demo et al., 2000; Luster, 1998; O'Brien and Moore, 2000). CCR5 facilitates viral entry to macrophages and a subset of memory CD4 T cells, whereas CXCR4 facilitate viral entry into most CD4 T cells, some macrophages, monocyte cell lines, and transformed T cells.

Physiologically, the CD4 receptor stabilizes the interaction between major histocompatibility complex (MHC) class II molecules on an antigen-presenting cell and the T-cell receptor reactive with the MHC class II peptide complex. Binding of virions to the T cell involves the interaction of specific conformational domains of gp120 with the CD4 molecule (Lasky et al., 1987).

The binding affinity appears to vary among HIV isolates, with lower affinities observed for primary isolates than for laboratory-adapted viruses (Daar et al., 1990; Ivey-Hoyle et al., 1991). This may explain in part the disappointing results of clinical trials using soluble CD4 as a decoy to block viral binding to CD4 T cells and the poor neutralizing activity of its antibody, although other mechanisms are also implicated (Brighty et al., 1991).

Conformational alterations in the binding epitopes of gp120 are crucial determinants of the cellular tropism of HIV-1 variants (Cheng-Meyer et al., 1991; York-Higgins et al., 1990). Cordonnier and colleagues (1989) showed that a single amino acid substitution in a highly conserved domain of gp120 abrogated the ability of a cloned virus to infect monocytes, although it was still able to infect T-cell lines. Chesebro and associates (1992) defined critical amino acids in the third variable region (V3 loop) as determinants of macrophage tropism.

VIRAL ENTRY

Following binding to the target cell surface, the virus gains entry by simple fusion of the two membranes (Dimitrov et al., 1991; Stein et al., 1987). Alternatively, virus may be transmitted from an infected cell directly to an uninfected cell by fusion, a process that results in in vitro syncytia formation (Sodroski et al., 1986). Clinical isolates of HIV-1 vary in their ability to induce syncytia in donor peripheral blood mononuclear cells (PBMCs) (Tersmette et al., 1988). Syncytium-inducing (SI) variants tend to be recovered from patients later in the course of disease, whereas non–syncytium-inducing (NSI) isolates can be detected throughout HIV-1 infection.

REVERSE TRANSCRIPTION

Following fusion, the virion capsid is released into the host cell cytoplasm and uncoating occurs. Reverse transcription then proceeds in a complex series of steps involving the sequential creation of a partial, "strong stop" complementary DNA (cDNA) strand, degradation of the RNA component of the RNA–DNA duplex, and "jumping" of the cDNA from the 5′ to the 3′ end of the same or the second RNA strand to enable completion of the cDNA (Varmus and Swanstrom, 1991). The process is catalyzed by the *pol* gene product of HIV-1, RT (see Fig. 29-2).

Unlike cellular polymerases, HIV-1 RT is error-prone and lacks a "proofreading" mechanism. One base per 1.7 to 4.0 kb is estimated to be misincorporated (Bebenek et al., 1989; Hubner et al., 1992; Takeuchi et al., 1988). Because the genome is approximately 9 kb, this may produce several misincorporations per replication cycle and accounts for the rapid mutation rates observed in vivo. Some mutations may be lethal to the virus, but others may confer significant biologic advantage and result in selection of that strain or quasispecies within the host (Meyerhans et al., 1989).

Under different selection pressures of humoral and cellular responses and different antiretroviral therapies, this process may result in a heterogeneous population of viruses or "swarm" in infected individuals. The high mutation rate of HIV contributes to its ability to escape from immunologic and therapeutic control (Coffin, 1995; Richman, 1993). Drug escape mutants plague therapeutic control of infection and both cellular and antibody escape mutants prevent the development of lifelong immunity and successful vaccine development (Nabel, 2001; Wei et al., 2003; Wyatt and Sodroski, 1998).

PROVIRAL DNA

The double-stranded proviral DNA is translocated into the nucleus and integrated into the host chromosomal DNA by another *pol* gene-encoded enzyme, integrase. Integration depends on the state of activation of the host cell. In quiescent T lymphocytes, substantial amounts of unintegrated HIV DNA have been demonstrated that retained the capacity to integrate after in vitro activation of the cells (Stevenson et al., 1990).

The integrated proviral DNA functions like a host cell gene, providing a formidable obstacle to the eradication of HIV from infected individuals. Transcription is dependent initially on interactions between cellular transcription factors and the HIV promoter sequences in the 5′-LTR. Cellular transcription factors include the constitutively expressed Sp1 protein and the inducible nuclear factor kappa B, which normally regulates the expression of T-cell genes involved in cell growth following activation. NFκB can be induced by cytokines, such as tumor necrosis factor alpha (TNF-α), and interleukin-1 (IL-1) (Duh et al., 1989; Osborn et al., 1989), or by gene products of viruses, such as human T-cell leukemia virus type 1 (HTLV-1) and human herpesviruses such as herpes simplex virus (HSV) or human herpesvirus 6 (HHV-6) (Ensoli et al., 1989; Heng et al., 1994; Mosca et al., 1987; Siekevitz et al., 1987) and JC virus (Gendelman et al., 1986).

Other upstream regulatory sequences are being characterized that regulate LTR-driven gene expression in certain cells at different stages of differentiation (Zeichner et al., 1992). These may play an important role in the pathogenesis of perinatally acquired HIV disease.

The formation of a transcription complex on the 5-LTR initiates a low level of transcription of viral messenger RNA (mRNA) by the host enzyme RNA polymerase II (Fig. 29-3A and B). The early mRNA transcripts are multiply spliced, resulting in the synthesis of the HIV-1 regulatory proteins tat, rev, and nef. In studies of the kinetics of expression, these mRNAs can be detected within 8 to 12 hours of infection of cell lines in vitro (Klotman et al., 1991).

The tat protein is a potent transactivator, increasing transcription from the HIV LTR by as much as two orders of magnitude (Fisher et al., 1986). The protein binds to the transactivation response element (TAR) at the 5′ end of all HIV mRNAs (see Figs. 29-2 and 29-3B). It is thereby brought into close proximity with the transcription start site of the proviral DNA. In conjunction with the cellular proteins of the transcription complex, tat increases the rate of transcription initiation and allows elongation to take place (Laspia et al., 1989).

TRANSLATION

The resulting increased production of multiply spliced mRNA leads to higher levels of translation of the rev protein (see Fig. 29-3C). This also acts in the nucleus, binding to the rev response element (RRE), which is a segment of RNA in the env region, with a complex secondary structure. In the absence of rev, all mRNAs containing the RRE are held up in the nucleus to be spliced or degraded. Following binding with rev, export into the cytoplasm can occur, and production of structural and enzymatic proteins proceeds (see Fig. 29-3D) (Cullen and Greene, 1989).

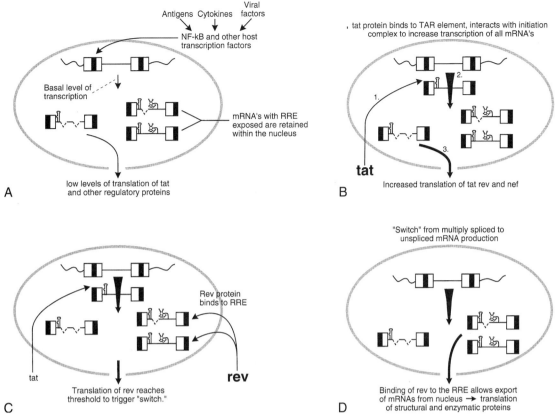

Figure 29-3· Function of tat and rev proteins in self-regulation of HIV-1 replication. **A.** Host-transcription factors, influenced by a variety of signals, bind to the 5'-LTR. A low level of transcription is initiated. The 9- and 4-kb mRNAs are retained in the nucleus because of the presence of the unbound rev response element (RRE). Only the multiply spliced 2-kb mRNA lacking an RRE can move out to the ribosomes in the cytoplasm, resulting in low levels of transcription of the regulatory proteins only. **B.** The tat protein is an extremely potent transactivator: 1, low concentrations of tat bind to the transactivation response element (TAR) element and interact with the initiation complex; 2, this results in increased transcription of all mRNAs; 3, at this stage, the 9- and 4-kb mRNAs are still retained in the nucleus and only the 2-kb messages can be exported, resulting selectively in increased translation of the regulatory proteins. **C.** The rev protein reaches a threshold concentration, binding in a multimeric fashion to the RRE and thereby enabling export of all mRNAs from the nucleus. **D.** As a result of rev binding, production of HIV-1 proteins is effectively switched from purely regulatory to all structural and enzymatic proteins also. Ovals = nuclear membrane; LTR = long terminal repeat; mRNA = messenger RNA; TAR = transactivation response element.

The roles of the auxiliary proteins are indicated in Figure 29-2 (Cullen and Greene, 1990). The precise function of the nef protein in HIV-1 is controversial, but it is required for the maintenance of high virus loads and clinical disease progression in rhesus monkeys with SIV infection (Kestler et al., 1991). In addition, down-regulation of CD4 receptor expression is a widely accepted role of the nef protein (Anderson et al., 1993; Inoue et al., 1993).

As depicted in Figure 29-2, the viral core structural proteins are encoded by the *gag* gene and the enzymatic proteins by the *pol* gene via a gag–pol fusion protein. The ribosomes slip back by one nucleotide (ribosomal frame shifting) during translation with 5% to 10% efficiency, thereby gaining access to the pol open reading frame (Jacks et al., 1988). This mechanism ensures that a much higher ratio of gag-to-pol proteins is produced. The polyproteins are modified post-translationally by the attachment of a myristyl group onto their shared amino terminal glycine. Myristoylation appears to be required for intracellular transport to the cell membrane (Bryant and Ratner, 1990).

During the final stages of virion assembly, the polyproteins are cleaved into functional proteins by the viral protease enzyme (Fitzgerald and Springer, 1991). Proteolysis of the gag proteins results in self-assembly of the virion nucleocapsid, with a predisposition for budding from the host cell.

Translation of the envelope precursor gp160 occurs in the rough endoplasmic reticulum. The protein is promptly glycosylated and is cleaved by cellular proteases in the Golgi complex into its components, gp120 and gp41, which are inserted across the host cytoplasmic membrane (Willey et al., 1988). Full-length genomic RNA is packaged into the assembling virion through interactions with a conserved zinc-finger sequence of the p9 gag protein (Gorelick et al., 1990). The host cell membrane, replete with gp120 anchored by gp41 and incidental host cell surface proteins, forms the viral envelope for the infectious, mature virion.

A new round of infection can now occur, either by direct interaction during budding of the envelope glycoproteins with a neighboring CD4 T cell or by the release of mature virions to infect distant cells.

Immunopathogenesis

Immunopathogenetic considerations include the course of the infection, mechanisms of CD4 depletion, interactions with cellular and humoral immune systems, and host genetic factors.

Initiation of HIV Infection

Immunopathologic studies in adults have revealed a common pattern of events following acute infection, although great individual variation has been noted (Fauci, 1993; Levy, 1993; Weiss, 1993). In children, there are many gaps in knowledge, but in broad terms a similar pattern is discernible. Acute infection by cell-associated or cell-free virus may occur parenterally (e.g., via a break in the integrity of the placental barrier) or across a mucosal surface (e.g., by ingestion of contaminated maternal blood during delivery, by breastfeeding, or by exposure of the rectal or vaginal mucosa to HIV-infected semen) (Fowler and Newell, 2002; Sato et al., 1992; Wofsy et al., 1986).

Infection occurs via CD4 receptors or chemokines on CD4+ T cell or monocytes or via an adhesion molecular complex on dendritic cells termed *dendritic cell–specific intercellular adhesion molecule–grabbing nonintegrin* (DC-SIGN) (Baribaud et al., 2001). Once the local cells are infected, they migrate throughout the lymphoid system and infect other cells by cell-to-cell contact.

Acute Viral Syndrome

Within 2 to 6 weeks after exposure, a rapid increase in viral reproduction occurs. An acute mononucleosis-like illness is experienced by 50% to 70% of adults (Quinn, 1997; Sleasman and Goodenow, 2003). Common signs and symptoms include fever, headache, fatigue, a variable rash, and lymphadenopathy. Many patients also experience pharyngitis along with myalgia and arthralgia, retro-orbital pain, weight loss, nausea, vomiting, diarrhea, night sweats, oral ulcers, and less commonly, ulceration of the genital tract or anus and oral candidiasis. Symptoms may last from a few days to a few weeks. Vanhems and associates (2003) found that a short incubation of fever, fatigue, and myalgias and a long duration of symptoms were associated with faster progression to disease. In their study, the incubation time to onset of acute symptoms varied from 17 to 35 days.

The equivalent clinical manifestations of primary infection are not as evident in infants. This may be due to the timing of perinatal transmission, differences in transmitted viral burden or phenotype, or immaturities

of the host immune response. In addition, infants of infected mothers generally have pre-existing (maternally derived) HIV-specific antibodies, unlike acute infection occurring outside the perinatal period, which may attenuate the acute syndrome.

The acute illness is associated with high levels of viremia and wide dissemination of the virus, particularly to lymphoid tissue but also to other organs, including the central nervous system (CNS). Plasma viremia, as high as 10^6 HIV RNA copies/ml, and p24 antigenemia occur (Daar et al., 1991; Niu et al., 1993). About 95% of plasma virus comes from newly infected CD4 T cells, with the remainder produced by macrophages and dendritic cells. High viral loads are sustained for prolonged periods of time in perinatally infected infants with only a gradual decline over the first 12 months of life (Palumbo et al., 1998; Shearer et al., 1997), and as a consequence virologic set points tend to be higher in children.

HIV-infected T cells that are cleared by cytotoxic T lymphocytes (CTLs) have a half-life of less than 20 hours. Free virus has a half-life of about 6 hours and is cleared by neutralizing antibody or by binding to new target cells (Ho, 1998). In adults, an abrupt drop in CD4 T-cell counts in the peripheral blood is observed (Daar et al., 1991). As many as 50% to 90% of new HIV infections may be transmitted during this time.

Latent Period

Within 1 to 2 weeks, antiviral cellular CTL and antibody immune responses develop and coincide with a dramatic decrease in circulating viral burden. Cytotoxic and noncytotoxic T cell and CD8 CTL responses appear before a neutralizing antibody response (Ariyoshi et al., 1992; Cooper et al., 1988; Safrit et al., 1993). Trapping of virus-antibody-complement immune complexes on the cytoplasmic processes of follicular dendritic cells (FDCs) in lymph nodes may contribute to the removal of virus from the circulation (Fox et al., 1991).

With the decrease in circulating virus, a partial recovery of CD4 T-cell counts is seen, although not usually back to preillness baseline levels. Studies have shown that the concentration of plasma virus at the end of the acute phase of infection (set point) correlates with the clinical course of disease; a high set point is associated with rapid disease progression (Mellors et al., 1995; Vergis and Mellors, 2000).

A clinically asymptomatic period follows primary infection, which may last for many years in adults. In children, there appears to be a subset with more rapid disease progression, and a second group that may follow a pattern of clinical latency, which is generally shorter than that seen in adult disease (Blanche et al., 1989, 1990; Byers et al., 1993; Scott et al., 1989; Tovo et al., 1992).

There may be no period of viral latency, and throughout the course of infection progressive destruction of CD4 T cells and of the FDC network in lymph nodes takes place (Michael et al., 1992; Pantaleo et al., 1993a; Vago et al., 1989). Figure 29-4 shows a section

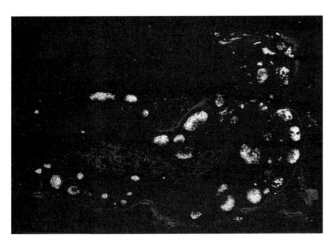

Figure 29-4 · In situ hybridization demonstrating large amounts of HIV-1 RNA in the germinal centers of a lymph node from a 3-year-old boy with well-preserved CD4+ count (36%; absolute count, 2695 cells/mm³). (×1.3 darkfield view using antisense probes that bind HIV-1 RNA. The gray reticulin stain reveals an orderly distribution of reticulin around the node, without extensive fibrosis in the tissue. The white grains represent hybridization signals using ³⁵S-labeled RNA antisense probes.) (Courtesy of Dr. Cecil Fox.)

of a lymph node from a relatively asymptomatic 2-year-old with a CD4 count of 2965 (36%). In situ hybridization of HIV-1 RNA reveals an abundance of virus localized to the germinal centers. Dual in situ and immunohistochemical staining reveals a pattern consistent with the attachment of immune complexed virions to the surface of the interlacing processes of the FDC.

The amount of virus in the lymphoid tissue may not be directly reflected by measurements of circulating viral burden or by the degree of immune impairment. The final breakdown of the germinal centers and FDC architecture and the profound impairment of HIV-specific host defenses result in a recurrence of high levels of viremia and depletion of virus trapped in lymphoid tissue.

A state of viral latency has been described in several reports in which CD4 T cells and other cells continue to harbor inactive virus (Butera and Folks, 1992; Ho, 1998; Levy, 1993). Under certain in vitro and in vivo conditions, this latent virus may be activated and new ways of virus replication may occur. At one time it was thought that with appropriate treatment, HIV could be eradicated, but the latent state of HIV and reservoirs of infected cells suggests that this will be extremely difficult to accomplish (Finzi et al., 1997; Ho, 1998). Latent HIV persists in resting memory CD4 T cells in a postintegrated form despite 1 to 2 years of combination antiretroviral therapy (ART) (Cohen, 1998; Ho, 1998; Wong et al., 1997).

CD4 Count and Viral Load in Infants and Children

In infants, the dynamics of viral replication and CD4 depletion are not well studied. CD4 T-cell counts in "normal" (i.e., uninfected) infants are much higher during the first 2 years of life, falling to adult levels by the time a child is 6 years of age (European Collaborative Study, 1992; McKinney and Wilfert, 1992; Raszka et al., 1994). HIV-infected infants have a progressive decline in CD4 T-cell number and percent and a loss in thymic volume and activity (Douek at al., 2000; Vigano et al., 1999).

A change in CD4 percentage may be a better marker of identifying disease progression in children than the CD4 count (Table 29-1). Although the use of the CD4 count and percent are good predictors of progression to disease and mortality, the combined use of CD4 counts and viral load are more predictive (Mofenson et al., 1997; Palumbo et al., 1998).

The percentage of CD4 T cells has been used to define the various grades of immunosuppression (see the section on CDC classification of HIV infection and AIDS in children younger than 13 years).

· Mild immunosuppression (>25%) correlates with either a lack of symptoms or mild symptomatology such as respiratory infections, lymphadenopathy, and splenomegaly.
· Moderate immunosuppression (15% to 24%) correlates with recurrent viral infections and systemic bacterial infections.
· Severe immunosuppression (<15%) correlates with high risk of opportunistic infection and life-threatening bacterial disease, neoplasms, and death (CDC, 2002c; http://www.aidsinfo.nih.gov/guidelines/).

Levels of HIV RNA in infants with more than 100,000 copies/ml are associated with high risk of disease progression and mortality, especially if the CD4 T-cell percentage is less than 15% (Tables 29-2 and 29-3). The baseline virologic data are also correlated with the risk for disease progression during long-term follow-up (Table 29-4).

TABLE 29-1 · ASSOCIATION OF BASELINE CD4 T-CELL PERCENTAGE WITH LONG-TERM RISK FOR DEATH IN HUMAN IMMUNODEFICIENCY VIRUS (HIV)-INFECTED CHILDREN BASELINE

CD4 Percentage	Number of Patients*	Number of Deaths[†]	Percent of Deaths
<5	33	32	97
5–9	29	22	76
10–14	30	13	43
15–19	41	18	44
20–24	52	13	23
25–29	49	15	31
30–34	48	5	10
≥35	92	30	33

*Includes 374 patients for whom baseline CD4+ T-cell percentage data were available.
[†]Mean follow-up: 5.1 years.
Data from Mofenson LM, Korelitz J, Meyer WA, et al. The relationship between serum human immunodeficiency virus type 1 (HIV-1) RNA level, CD4 lymphocyte percent, and long-term mortality risk in HIV-1-infected children. The National Institute of Child Health and Human Development Intravenous Immunoglobulin Clinical Trial. J Infect Dis 175:1029–1038, 1997.

TABLE 29-2 · ASSOCIATION OF BASELINE HUMAN IMMUNODEFICIENCY VIRUS (HIV) RNA COPY NUMBER AND CD4+ T-CELL PERCENTAGE WITH LONG-TERM RISK FOR DEATH IN HIV-INFECTED CHILDREN

Baseline HIV RNA[†] (copies/ml)	Baseline CD4+ T-cell Percentage	Number of Patients[‡]	Deaths* Number	Deaths* %
≤100,000				
	≥15	103	15	15
	<15	24	15	63
>100,000				
	≥15	89	32	36
	<15	36	29	81

*Mean follow-up: 5.1 years.
[†]Tested by NASBA assay (manufactured by Organon Teknika, Durham, North Carolina) on frozen stored serum.
[‡]Mean age: 3.4 years.
Data from Mofenson LM, Korelitz J, Meyer WA, et al. The relationship between serum human immunodeficiency virus type 1 (HIV-1) RNA level, CD4 lymphocyte percent, and long-term mortality risk in HIV-1-infected children. The National Institute of Child Health and Human Development Intravenous Immunoglobulin Clinical Trial. J Infect Dis 175:1029–1038, 1997.

TABLE 29-3 · ASSOCIATION OF BASELINE HUMAN IMMUNODEFICIENCY VIRUS (HIV) RNA COPY NUMBER WITH LONG-TERM RISK FOR DEATH IN HIV-INFECTED CHILDREN

Baseline (copies/ml)[†]	Number of Patients	Number of Deaths*	Percent of Deaths
Undetectable (i.e., ≤4,000)	25	6	24
4,001–50,000	69	19	28
50,001–100,000	33	5	15
100,001–500,000	72	29	40
500,001–1,000,000	20	8	40
>1,000,000	35	25	71
Total	254	92	36

*Mean follow-up: 5.1 years.
[†]Tested by NASBA assay (manufactured by Organon Teknika, Durham, North Carolina) on frozen stored serum.
*Mean age: 3.4 years.
Data from Mofenson LM, Korelitz J, Meyer WA, et al. The relationship between serum human immunodeficiency virus type 1 (HIV-1) RNA level, CD4 lymphocyte percent, and long-term mortality risk in HIV-1-infected children. The National Institute of Child Health and Human Development Intravenous Immunoglobulin Clinical Trial. J Infect Dis 175:1029–1038, 1997.

Mechanisms of CD4 T-Cell Depletion

HIV infection results in the progressive loss of CD4 T cells from the circulation and CD4 T-cell depletion from total body stores (McCune, 2001). The normal adult has about 2×10^{11} mature CD4 T cells, whereas HIV-infected individuals have approximately one half this number by the time that they reach a CD4 count of 200 cells/ml (Haase, 1999; Rosok et al., 1996). There is also a quantitative decrease in the proportion of peripheral quiescent naïve T cells and an increase in the proportion of memory effector cells (Gorochov et al., 1998).

The central event in the course of HIV disease is the development of functional abnormalities and progressive destruction of the CD4 T-cell population. Numerous

TABLE 29-4 · ASSOCIATION OF BASELINE HUMAN IMMUNODEFICIENCY VIRUS (HIV) RNA QUARTILE BY AGE AT ENTRY WITH RISK FOR DISEASE PROGRESSION OR DEATH DURING STUDY FOLLOW-UP AMONG HIV-INFECTED CHILDREN RECEIVING ANTIRETROVIRAL TREATMENT

Age at Entry	Baseline HIV RNA quartiles (copies/ml)*	Disease Progression or Death Number of Patients	Disease Progression or Death Number	Disease Progression or Death %
<30 months[†]				
	<1,000–150,000	79	9	11
	150,000–500,000	66	13	20
	500,000–1,700,000	76	29	38
	>1,700,000	18	42	52
≥30 months[‡]				
	<1,000–15,000	66	0	0
	15,001–50,000	54	7	13
	50,001–150,000	80	13	16
	>150,000	64	22	34

*Tested by NASBA assay (manufactured by Organon Teknika, Durham, North Carolina) on frozen stored serum.
[†]Mean age: 1.1 years.
[‡]Mean age: 7.3 years.
Data from Palumbo PE, Raskino C, Fiscus S, et al. Disease progression in HIV-infected infants and children: predictive value of quantitative plasma HIV RNA and CD4 lymphocyte count. The Pediatric AIDS Clinical Trial Group protocol. JAMA 279:756–761, 1998.

theories about how this occurs have been proposed, and it seems probable that both direct and indirect mechanisms are involved. Direct killing may occur because of the accumulation of unintegrated viral DNA, inhibition of cellular protein synthesis, or disruption during budding and release of virions (Garry, 1989). The demonstration of much higher levels of virus in PBMCs than were previously detectable support the role of direct cell killing in cytopathicity (Bagasra et al., 1992; Embretson et al., 1993; Patterson et al., 1993; Piatak et al., 1993b).

Numerous indirect mechanisms have also been postulated. Syncytia formation, in which infected cells fuse with neighboring uninfected CD4 T cells, can be demonstrated in vitro. This capability correlates with cytopathicity and with disease progression (see earlier section on life cycle) but has only rarely been observed in vivo (Lifson et al., 1986). The host's immune response may destroy virus-infected cells, principally by HIV-specific cytotoxic T cells and also by antibody-dependent cell-mediated cytotoxicity (ADCC) in conjunction with natural killer (NK) cells (Walker et al., 1987).

HIV may also trigger autoimmune destruction through the molecular mimicry of cellular antigens. For example, gp120 and gp41 glycoproteins share some structural homology with regions of the MHC class II molecules. Anti-HIV envelope antibodies may therefore cross-react with the patient's class II molecules. There are limited in vivo data supporting this finding (Golding et al., 1989). Such an alloreaction has been likened to a chronic graft-versus-host type disease (Habeshaw et al., 1992). However, a graft-versus-host mechanism is unlikely to be present in HIV infection (Ammann, 1993).

because some blood donors were in the "window" period during which time they were HIV infected but had not yet converted to antibody positivity (Busch and Satten, 1997).

With the initiation of DNA/RNA polymerase chain reaction (PCR) testing, the risk of transfusion-associated HIV decreased to about 1 out of every 800,000 to 1 million transfusions (Busch et al., 2003). Since the initiation of blood donor testing, heat treatment of factor VIII, and availability of recombinant factor VIII, there have been virtually no infants or children who have become HIV infected from blood products in the United States. However, use of untested blood products or contaminated needles continues to present a significant risk in developing countries (Shan et al., 2002).

SEXUAL TRANSMISSION

The risk of acquiring HIV from sexually activity is greatest among MSM practicing anal intercourse (0.8% to 5%) compared with vaginal intercourse (0.01% to 0.5%). Heterosexual transmission is the primary mode of acquiring HIV in developing countries. Intravenous drug abuse carries a risk of approximately 0.5% to 1%. Accidental inoculation from an HIV-infected donor carries a risk of 0.1% to 1.0% depending on the type of exposure (e.g., mucous membranes, hollow-bore needles, or devices that are inserted in arteries or veins) (Gerberding, 2003; Gray et al., 2001; Katz and Gerberding, 1997; Royce et al., 1997). A number of factors can increase the risk of donors transmitting HIV, including high viral load, low CD4 count, poor clinical status, associated diseases such as sexually transmitted diseases (STDs), amount of inoculum, lack of circumcision, advanced disease, and primary (recent) HIV infection.

HOME AND SCHOOL TRANSMISSION

Several large studies have confirmed the extremely low risk of transmission through casual contacts with household members (Friedland et al., 1986; Mann et al., 1986; Simonds and Chanock, 1993). There is one description of transmission from a child with AIDS to an unrelated 2-year-old in the same household. The authors concluded that the mode of transmission was an unrecognized exposure of the 2-year-old's mucous membranes or excoriated skin to blood from nosebleeds or a laceration of the child with AIDS (Fitzgibbon et al., 1993). A second report described transmission between siblings with hemophilia. The brothers could not recall sharing equipment for infusions of factor VIII, but the potential for a needle stick transmission in this setting is high (CDC, 1993b, 1993c). An earlier, brief report of suspected household transmission between young children, possibly by biting, was not supported by genotypic analysis (Wahn et al., 1986). Rogers and colleagues (1990) documented lack of HIV transmission in seven individuals known to have bitten HIV-infected children.

There have been no reports of transmission in out-of-home childcare settings or in school. Only one case of HIV transmission attributed to sports has been reported

worldwide to date (Torre et al., 1990). This involved a collision of heads during a soccer match, with copious bleeding from both players. Other modes of transmission for the person who became infected, however, could not be definitively excluded.

Transmission in Adolescents

Adolescents are at risk from unprotected sexual intercourse or the use of contaminated needles. The magnitude of this risk is underscored by the fact that 20% of people developing AIDS in the United States are aged 20 to 29 years. Given the prolonged incubation period, it is clear that a substantial proportion acquired their infection as teenagers (Gayle and D'Angelo, 1991).

Sexual Transmission to Young Children

Worldwide, sexual abuse and sex trafficking of children increases the risk of HIV infection even in very young children. Some studies place the number of children in forced prostitution as high as 10 million (Willis and Levy, 2002). The fairly widespread myth that having sex with a virgin can cure HIV infection has resulted in HIV-infected men seeking younger sexual partners (Willis and Levy, 2002). In some cases, children as young as 5 years have been raped. Young girls may command a premium as prostitutes, placing them at higher risk for HIV. Some young girls may associate with older men (sugar daddies), providing sex for income. In some countries, such as South Africa, Tanzania, and Zimbabwe, ratios of HIV-infected teenage girls to HIV-infected teenage boys may be as high as 6:1 (Ladner et al., 2002). This probably reflects the increased susceptibility of young girls to HIV and the fact that most of the older male sexual partners are HIV infected (Ladner et al., 2002).

Perinatal HIV Transmission

Perinatal transmission encompasses the transmission of virus from an infected mother to her child before delivery (prepartum), during delivery (intrapartum), or following delivery through breastfeeding (postpartum). In the literature on HIV, the term *perinatal* is used synonymously with *vertical,* to describe mother–infant transmission. In developed countries, in the absence of breastfeeding, perinatal HIV transmission accounts for virtually all new cases of HIV infection in children. A small proportion of children may be infected as the result of child sexual abuse (Gutman et al., 1991).

Factors Affecting Perinatal Transmission

Most infants born to infected mothers are uninfected. Published transmission rates in untreated mother–infant pairs varied from 13% in the European Collaborative Study to about 40% in Africa (Blanche et al., 1989; European Collaborative Study, 1991; Goedert et al., 1989; Gwinn et al., 1991; Hoff et al., 1988; Ryder et al., 1989). The reasons for such geographic variation have yet to be identified definitively. Higher levels of maternal viremia, lower CD4 counts, more advanced maternal disease, prolonged duration of ruptured membranes, chorioamnionitis, associated diseases, and whether an elective cesarean section has been performed have been associated with increased risk of transmission in some cohorts (Boue et al., 1990; Boyer et al., 1994; Cao et al., 1997; D'Arminio Monforte et al., 1991; International Perinatal Group, 1999; Ladner et al., 1998; Mofenson et al., 1999; Ryder et al., 1989; Tibaldi et al., 1993) but not in others (Papaevangelou et al., 1992; Tovo et al., 1991).

John and colleagues (2001) found increased transmission in Kenyan HIV-infected pregnant women associated with maternal viral RNA levels greater than 43,000 copies/ml, maternal cervical HIV-1 DNA, vaginal HIV-1 DNA, and cervical or vaginal ulcers. Breastfeeding and mastitis were associated with increased transmission overall, and mastitis and breast abscess were associated with late transmission occurring more than 2 months postpartum.

Mother–infant concordance at any HLA class I locus was a strong predictor of transmission (Polycarpou et al., 2002). Transmission was not associated with HLA class II concordance. Class I HLA concordance retained its importance after adjusting for maternal viral load, ART, duration of rupture of membranes, or histologic chorioamnionitis. HLA alleles, and in particular the HLA-1 concordance between maternal and neonatal HLA, may regulate the risk of perinatal HIV-1 transmission.

Most transmitting mothers in the United States are asymptomatic at delivery (Scott et al., 1985). Intrapartum events that increase fetal exposure to maternal blood, such as amniocentesis, placenta previa, abruptio placentae, fetal scalp monitoring, episiotomy, and second-degree tears, are associated with an increased risk of transmission (Boyer et al., 1994).

EFFECT OF VIRUS PHENOTYPE

Some selection of maternal viral quasispecies may occur, with preliminary evidence for preferential transmission of NSI variants and certain gp120 glycosylation motifs (Wolinsky et al., 1992; Zhu et al., 1993). In contrast, Lamers and colleagues (1994) found that sequences in samples obtained from two infants within 4 weeks of birth displayed greater genetic variation than maternal samples. The influence of viral genotype and phenotype is a focus of continued research. Viruses with a rapid-high replicative capacity do not appear to be transmitted more readily than those with a slow-low phenotype (Scarlatti et al., 1993).

MATERNAL FACTORS

The rate of disease progression in infants has been linked to the severity of disease in the mother at the time of delivery, but whether this is the result of a larger viral inoculum, earlier intrauterine transmission, or transmission of other pathogens that might influence disease progression is not clear (Blanche et al., 1994).

Maternal immune factors are equally controversial. High-titer antibodies to certain epitopes of gp120 of HIV-1 laboratory isolates were initially associated with lower transmission rates (Goedert et al., 1989), but this has not been confirmed in subsequent studies (Halsey et al., 1992). Preliminary data suggested that higher maternal neutralizing antibody titers to autologous HIV isolates might correlate with decreased transmission (Bryson et al., 1993b; Scarlatti et al., 1993). A phase III study of passive immunization of mothers (and of babies within 12 hours of birth) with human immune globulin containing high titers of antibody to HIV structural proteins (hyperimmune HIV immune globulin [HIVIG]) did not show any added benefit of HIVIG to existing ART (Stiehm et al., 1999). Furthermore, there is evidence that neither maternal CTLs nor neutralizing antibody will exert selective pressure on maternal HIV species that results in escape mutants that are transmitted to the infant (Goulder et al., 2001b, 2001c).

TWIN DISCORDANCE

Any theories regarding vertical transmission must explain the well-documented discordance of transmission from one pregnancy to the next and between twins. A multinational study of 100 sets of twins born to seropositive mothers demonstrated that transmission is more common to the first-born twin ($P = 0.004$) (Goedert et al., 1991). Fifty percent of vaginally delivered and 38% of cesarean section delivered first-born twins were infected, as opposed to 19% of second-born twins delivered by either route. Confounding variables, such as increased monitoring of the first twin with scalp electrodes, were excluded. The first-born twin has more prolonged exposure to cervical and vaginal secretions, which have been shown to harbor infectious virus (Pomerantz et al., 1988; Vogt et al., 1987).

BIRTH CANAL EXPOSURE

Intrapartum transmission is presumed to occur across the infant's mucous membranes, principally in the oropharynx and possibly in the esophagus and stomach. In support of this mechanism, four out of four healthy Rhesus monkeys inoculated orally at birth with cell-free SIV, equivalent to 5 ml of viremic plasma, became infected (Baba et al., 1994). Field studies, conducted to test whether cleansing of the birth canal during labor can reduce the risk of transmission, have not shown any benefit in preventing HIV transmission (Gailliard et al., 2001; Mandelbrot et al., 2002; Shey et al., 2002). Successful interventions to reduce perinatal infection, particularly in areas of the world where ART is not yet an option, are likely to require a more precise understanding of the mechanisms and timing of transmission.

In Utero Versus Intrapartum Transmission

With the advent of highly sensitive techniques for detecting virus in the peripheral circulation of the infant, it is possible to define the predominant time of transmission more accurately. A consensus opinion from the Pediatric Virology Committee of the AIDS Clinical Trials Group defined an infant infected in utero as one in whom virus could be cultured or HIV-1 genome detected by PCR from blood within 48 hours of birth (Bryson et al., 1992). A child infected intrapartum would have negative results within the first 48 hours, becoming positive from day 7 to day 90. Breastfed infants are excluded from this category. This is a reasonable working definition, although it does not exclude the possibility that infants are infected in utero but only develop detectable viremia postnatally as viral replication is upregulated following immune stimulation.

When the previous criteria are used, preliminary estimates indicate that in the absence of breastfeeding, 50% to 70% of transmission occurs around the time of delivery (Bertolli et al., 1996; Boyer et al., 1994). Perinatal HIV transmission is presumed to be a result of late viral transmission via the placenta during labor or acquisition of virus by vaginal delivery. Support for this concept comes from studies of cesarean section in which it has been shown that HIV transmission is significantly reduced following elective cesarean section (Duliege et al., 1995; International Perinatal HIV Group, 1999).

Timing of Transmission and Disease Progression

As mentioned, a bimodal pattern of disease progression has been observed in perinatally infected children (Blanche et al., 1989, 1990; Byers et al., 1993; Scott et al., 1989; Tovo et al., 1992). One explanation for this is that children infected in utero may have dissemination of virus to organs such as the thymus at a critical stage of development (Uittenbogaart et al., 1993). This may result in early and profound impairment of cellular and humoral immunity, with more rapid disease progression. Consistent with this are reports that infants who have detectable virus by culture, PCR, or p24 antigen levels within the first week of life are at increased risk for rapid disease progression (Bryson et al., 1993a; Burgard et al., 1992; Kalish et al., 1999; Krivine et al., 1992; Levine et al., 1993). Early reports of an embryopathy associated with HIV disease, suggesting first-trimester transmission, have not been confirmed (Iosub et al., 1987; Marion et al., 1986).

Breastfeeding Transmission

Despite several studies documenting the presence of HIV-1 in the breast milk of seropositive mothers, the additional risk of infection by this route rather than in utero or intrapartum appears to be around 15% to 20% (Davis, 1991; Dunn et al., 1992; Ruff et al., 1992; Thiry et al., 1985). The risk may be higher if the mother's primary infection occurs in the perinatal period, consistent with wide dissemination of virus and a lack of protective secretory IgA at the time of acute infection (Stiehm and Vink, 1991; Van De Perre et al., 1991). Ryder and colleagues (1991) did not find a statistically significant difference in infection rates of breastfed as opposed to bottle-fed infants in Zaire. This may be an exception in this setting; however, bottle-feeding was associated with a higher morbidity.

Increased risk of breastfeeding transmission is associated with prolonged breastfeeding, presence of mastitis, and recent HIV infection of the mother during or shortly after pregnancy (Dunn et al., 1992; Fowler and Newell, 2002; Leroy et al., 1998; Miotti et al., 1999; Van de Perre et al., 1991). Despite the risk of breastfeeding and HIV transmission, not breastfeeding is not an option in most developing countries because increased infant mortality may result. Mathematical modeling has demonstrated that the benefits of breastfeeding can outweigh the risks of transmission in countries in which safe water supplies and maintenance of sterility of bottle feeding equipment cannot be guaranteed (Lederman, 1992).

The World Health Organization (WHO) (UNAIDS/WHO, 1999) encourages breastfeeding in countries "where infectious diseases and malnutrition are the main causes of infant deaths and the infant mortality rate is high." In the United States, the United Kingdom, Europe, and other countries with relatively safe alternatives to breastfeeding, bottle-feeding is strongly encouraged (Brierley et al., 1988).

Some women who do not breastfeed may experience discrimination within the community because it is assumed that a mother who does not breastfeed is HIV infected. There is evidence that exclusive breastfeeding and early weaning may reduce the risk of acquiring HIV infection (Coutsoudis, 2000). A study from Nairobi suggested that breastfeeding by HIV-infected mothers may increase maternal mortality (Mbori-Ngacha et al., 2001). In areas where there are no sources of clean water, safe breast milk substitutes and societal discrimination makes this a difficult issue (Fowler and Newell, 2002).

Effect of Antiretroviral Therapy on Perinatal Transmission

In 1991, it was estimated that there would be 1800 new cases of HIV-infected children in the United States, based on projections of 6000 infected mothers delivering per year, with a transmission rate of 30% (Gwinn et al., 1991). The estimated number now is less than 100 HIV-infected infants each year (1800 occur each day in developing countries) as a result of early prenatal diagnosis, combination ART of pregnant women, and use of elective cesarean section. One study showed that women who have RNA virus of less than 1000 copies/ml viral loads have an HIV transmission rate of less than 1% (Ioannidis et al., 2001).

The impact of ART on HIV transmission in developing countries has been less significant. Combination ART is most often not available and too costly. Even abbreviated oral courses of monotherapy with zidovudine (AZT) can cost $40 to $50, exceeding most health care budgets. In 1999, a National Institutes of Health (NIH)-sponsored study in Uganda showed a 50%

reduction in HIV transmission using a single dose of nevirapine (NVP) given to the mother at the time of labor and delivery and a single dose to the infant (Guay et al., 1999). The beneficial effect of perinatal HIV transmission was observed even with continued breast-feeding.

Prevention of Perinatal HIV Transmission

A summary of studies to prevent HIV mother-to-child transmission (PMTCT) is presented in Table 29-5 and on the Internet (http://www.GlobalStrategies.org; http://www.womenchildrenhiv.org).

The first PMTCT study was a large double-blind, placebo-controlled, multicenter trial in the United States of AZT given to mothers during pregnancy and delivery and to their infants postnatally. Reported in 1994, the study demonstrated a highly significant reduction in transmission, from 25.5% to 8.3% (see later discussion on treatment) (CDC, 1994b; Connor et al., 1994). This was clearly of great importance for the management of women throughout the world who can be identified as infected early enough in pregnancy. It did not, however, clarify the issue of timing of transmission because treatment was started in the second trimester and extended throughout the perinatal period.

Subsequent studies, using abbreviated regimens of AZT alone or combinations of AZT and lamivudine (3TC), in the absence of breastfeeding with or without treatment of the infant, showed reductions of approximately 30% to 50% (Chaisilwattana et al., 2002; Dabis et al., 1999, 2001; Petra Study Team, 2002; Shaffer et al., 1999; Wiktor et al., 1999). In these abbreviated studies, AZT was given to the mother for the last 4 weeks of pregnancy and to the infant for 1 week.

An important study was completed in 1999 in Uganda demonstrating that a single dose of NVP given to the mother at the onset of labor and a single oral dose to the infant after birth could reduce perinatal HIV transmission by 50% (Guay et al., 1999). These effects persisted even with continued breastfeeding. These later studies support the concept that most HIV is transmitted during the perinatal period.

Use of Zidovudine (AZT)

AZT monotherapy as outlined later remains the mainstay of ART for PMTCT and continues to be used in developing countries either alone or with additional ART (see Table 29-5) (http://www.GlobalStrategies.org; http://www.womenchildrenhiv.org). The use of AZT in HIV-infected women during pregnancy, labor, and delivery and in nursing mothers and their infants during the first few weeks of life has been documented through several studies to significantly reduce mother-to-child transmission (CDC, 2002f; Connor et al., 1994).

The AZT regimen consists of antepartum administration of 100 mg of AZT orally, five times daily, initiated at 14 to 34 weeks' gestation and continued throughout

pregnancy. The intrapartum AZT dose is administered intravenously in a 1-hour initial infusion of 2 mg/kg body weight, followed by continuous infusion of 1 mg/kg body weight/hour and delivery. Postpartum, oral administration of AZT to the newborn infant is given for the first 6 weeks of life in the form of AZT syrup at 2 mg/kg body weight/dose every 6 hours, beginning at 8 to 12 hours after birth. If an infant cannot tolerate the oral medication, intravenous AZT is given at a dose of 1.5 mg/kg body weight every 6 hours.

The oral formulations of AZT include 100- and 300-mg tablets for women and a 10 mg/ml syrup for infants. The oral dosing regimens for women are as follows: 300 mg orally twice a day after the first trimester (14 weeks' gestation) until the onset of labor or 200 mg orally three times a day. If intravenous AZT is not available, oral administration of AZT may be given in a dose of 300 mg orally at the onset of labor and every 3 hours until delivery. If the mother did not receive antepartum AZT, then 600 mg of oral AZT should be administered at the onset of labor followed by 300 mg orally every 3 hours until delivery.

Treatment regimens that combine AZT with 3TC add the latter at a dose of 150 mg orally every 12 hours during the antepartum period and continue the dose during the intrapartum period. In breastfeeding populations in developing countries, AZT or AZT and 3TC, when available, should be continued in the mother. Although breastfeeding is not recommended in developed countries, there are few options available to mothers in developing countries despite the risk of breast milk transmission (Coutsoudis, 2000).

Maternal and infant side effects and toxicities possibly associated with AZT use have been evaluated for several years. The most frequently observed side effect is anemia. If anemia does occur in association with AZT in PMTCT trials, it is usually mild and resolves after discontinuation of the medication. There have been rare reports of liver toxicity in women receiving AZT, but this is usually when used for a long period beyond what is needed to prevent MTCT. Rare reports of mitochondrial toxicity have been reported in infants (see the section on toxicity of ART).

Use of Nevirapine (NVP)

Single-dose NVP is one of the most frequently used PMTCT regimens in developing countries because of its low cost, ease of use, and stability of drug at room temperatures (Marseille et al., 1999). The dose for the mother is 200 mg (one tablet) as a single dose at the onset of labor or at least 2 hours before a cesarean section. It is important to administer the NVP at the onset of labor and not during delivery because adequate levels of NVP may not be achieved in the mother for placental transfer to the infant if the dose is too close to the time of delivery. If more than 48 hours have elapsed since the dose of NVP and delivery has not yet occurred, a second dose of NVP should be administered.

In resource-poor settings, some health care professionals give a single capsule of NVP to the mother to

TABLE 29-5 · REGIMENS FOR PREVENTION OF HIV TRANSMISSION FROM MOTHERS TO INFANTS*

Regimen	Antepartum	Intrapartum	Postpartum	Infant	Efficacy/Results	References
U.S. (PACTG 076) ZDV only 2 arm, randomized, placebo-control (enrolled 1991–1993) Formula-feeding n = 477	Starting at 14–34 wk Arm 1: ZDV 100 mg 5 times/day Arm 2: Placebo	Arm 1: ZDV intravenous infusion Arm 2: Placebo	No ART	Arm 1: ZDV 2 mg/kg qid × 6 wk Arm 2: Placebo	At 18 mo, Tx 7.6% ZDV vs. 22.6% placebo, 68% efficacy ZDV resistance delivery—mother: no high-level, 3% low-level at delivery; at 6 wk, infant: none	Connor et al., 1994; Eastman et al., 1998; McSherry et al., 1999
Thailand (CDC) ZDV only 2 arm, randomized, placebo-control (enrolled 1996–1997) Formula-feeding n = 392	Starting at 36 wk Arm 1: ZDV 300 mg bid Arm 2: Placebo	Arm 1: ZDV 300 mg q3h Arm 2: Placebo	No ART	No ART	At 6 mo, Tx 9.4% ZDV vs. 18.9% placebo, 50% efficacy	Shaffer et al., 1999
Ivory Coast (CDC) ZDV only 2 arm, randomized, placebo-control (enrolled 1996–1998) Breastfeeding n = 280	Starting at 36 wk Arm 1: ZDV 300 mg bid Arm 2: Placebo (stopped 2/98)	Arm 1: ZDV 300 mg q3h Arm 2: Placebo (stopped 2/98)	No ART	No ART	At 3 mo, Tx 16.5% ZDV vs. 26.1% placebo, 37% efficacy. Pooled analysis from CDC and ANRS 049a trials: At 24 mo, Tx 22.5% ZDV vs. 30.2% placebo, 26% efficacy	Wiktor et al., 1999;
Ivory Coast, Burkina Faso (ANRS) ZDV only (DITRAME; ANRS 049a) 2 arm, randomized, placebo-control (enrolled 1995–1998) After trial completion, continued to enroll into an open-label ZDV regimen cohort Breastfeeding n = 400	Starting at 36–38 wk Arm 1: ZDV 300 mg bid Arm 2: Placebo (stopped 2/98)	Arm 1: ZDV 600 mg × 1 Arm 2: Placebo (stopped 2/98)	Arm 1: ZDV 300 mg bid × 1 wk Arm 2: Placebo (stopped 2/98)	No ART	At 6 mo, Tx 18.0% ZDV vs. 27.5% placebo, 38% efficacy. At 15 mo, Tx 21.5% ZDV vs. 30.6% placebo, 30% efficacy. At 24 mo (pooled analysis with CDC), Tx 22.5% ZDV vs. 30.2% placebo, 26% efficacy. 18 mo mortality: 17.6% ZDV vs. 22.1% placebo. Open-label ZDV cohort (n = 209), 15 mo Tx with ZDV regimen, 19.6%	Dabis et al., 1999, 2001

Continued

Regimen	Antepartum	Intrapartum	Postpartum	Infant	Efficacy/Results	References
South Africa, Uganda, Tanzania (PETRA) ZDV/3TC 4 arm, randomized, placebo-control (enrolled 1996–2000) Breastfeeding n = 1797	Starting at 36 wk Arm 1: ZDV 300 mg bid plus 3TC 150 mg bid Arm 2: Placebo Arm 3: Placebo Arm 4: Placebo (stopped 2/98)	Arm 1: ZDV 300 mg q3h plus 3TC 150 mg q12h Arm 2: ZDV 300 mg q3h plus 3TC 150 mg q12h Arm 3: ZDV 300 mg q3h plus 3TC 150 mg q12h Arm 4: Placebo (stopped 2/98)	Arm 1: ZDV 300 mg bid plus 3TC 150 mg bid × 7 day Arm 2: ZDV 300 mg bid plus 3TC 150 mg bid × 7 day Arm 3: Placebo Arm 4: Placebo (stopped 2/98)	Arm 1: ZDV 4 mg/kg bid plus 3TC 2 mg/kg bid × 7 day Arm 2: ZDV 4 mg/kg bid plus 3TC 2 mg/kg bid × 7 day Arm 3: Placebo Arm 4: Placebo (stopped 2/98)	At 6 wk, Tx: 5.7% AP/IP/PP (63% efficacy) 8.9% IP/PP (42% efficacy) 14.2% IP 15.3% placebo At 18 mo, Tx: 14.9% 20.0% IP 22.2% placebo	Petra Study Team, 2002
France (ANRS) ZDV/3TC (ANRS 075) Nonrandomized, open-label 1997–1998) Formula-feeding n = 445	Standard ZDV after 14 wk 3TC 150 mg bid added at 32 wk	Standard intravenous ZDV	Nonstudy ART	Standard ZDV × 6 wk 3TC 2 mg/kg bid × 6 wk	Tx 1.6% ZDV/3TC vs. 6.8% 1994–1997 historical, ZDV-alone control M184V mutation in 39% women (only if ≥4 wk 3TC)	Mandelbrot et al., 2001
Uganda (HIVNET 012) NVP vs. ZDV 2 arm, randomized; originally had third placebo arm, stopped 2/98 (enrolled 1997–99) Breastfeeding n = 626	Arm 1: No ARV Arm 2: No ARV Arm 3: No ARV	Arm 1: NVP 200 mg × 1 Arm 2: ZDV 300 mg q3h Arm 3: Placebo (stopped 2/98)	No ART	Arm 1: NVP 2 mg/kg × 1 at 48–72 hr Arm 2: ZDV 4 mg/kg bid × 7 day Arm 3: Placebo (stopped 2/98)	At 14–16 wk, Tx 13.1% NVP vs. 25.1% ZDV, 47% efficacy. At 18 mo, Tx 15.7% NVP vs. 25.8% ZDV, 41% efficacy. NVP resistance 6 wk PP: Mother (n = 271), 24% (not detected at 12–15 mo in those tested). Infant, 46% subtype D > A. At 18 mo, mortality in HIV-infected infants did not differ between arms, 38% NVP vs. 37% ZDV	Guay et al, 1999
South Africa (SAINT) NVP vs. ZDV/3TC 2 arm, randomized, comparative (enrolled 1999–2000) Breastfeeding (42%) and formula-feeding n = 1331	Arm 1: No ARV Arm 2: No ARV	Arm 1: NVP 200 mg × 1 Arm 2: ZDV 600 mg then 300 mg q3h plus 3TC 150 mg q12h	Arm 1: NVP 200 mg × 1 at 24–48 hr Arm 2: ZDV 300 mg bid plus 3TC 150 mg bid × 7 day	Arm 1: NVP 6 mg × 1 at 24–48 hr (>2kg) Arm 2: ZDV 12 mg bid plus 3TC 6 mg bid × 7 day (>2 kg)	At 8 wk, Tx 12.3% NVP vs. 9.3% ZDV/3TC (P = 0.11). NVP resistance 6 wk PP: mother, 67% (received 2 NVP doses; 20% persist at 12 mo) infant, 53%	

*Selected summarized regimens from Mofenson LM, Munderi P. Safety of antiretroviral prophylaxis of perinatal transmission for HIV-infected pregnant women and their infants. J Acquir Immune Defic Syndr 30:200–215, 2002 (http://www.womenchildrenhiv.org).

AP = antepartum; ART = antiretroviral therapy; ddI = didanosine; d4T = stavudine; IP = intrapartum; PP = postpartum; 3TC = lamivudine; Tx = transmission; ZDV = zidovudine.

keep with her and take as soon as labor begins. Under these circumstances, the NVP capsule should be kept in a safe location and away from light, and instructions should be given that the NVP should not to be used to treat HIV.

Her infant is given a single oral dose between 48 and 72 hours after birth to ensure an adequate NVP blood level. If the infant weighs 2000 g or more, 0.6 ml (6 mg) is given orally. For infants weighing less than 2000 g, the oral dose is 0.2 ml/kg (2 mg/kg).

If the mother and infant are to go home before 48 hours, then the infant NVP dose can be administered just before the mother and infant leave. If the mother received her NVP dose less than 2 hours before delivery, then the infant should be given a dose of NVP immediately after birth, followed by the usual infant postnatal dose as described later. In some resource-poor settings the NVP is given to the infant immediately after delivery. There are no efficacy studies to indicate that a 50% decrease in transmission is achieved with this dosing regimen. Therefore if this regimen is used, the infant's dose should be followed by a second dose at 5 to 7 days of age.

In the PMTCT trial of NVP in Uganda, breastfeeding was continued (Guay et al., 1999). Follow-up studies indicated that the beneficial effect of NVP in HIV prevention was still observed. However, if there is an option to safely formula-feed, the likelihood of the infant becoming infected with HIV is decreased.

In U.S., European, and African studies, this NVP regimen has not been associated with maternal or infant adverse effects. However, viral resistance to NVP has been observed in approximately 19% of women and 46% of their HIV-infected infants 6 to 8 weeks after single-dose NVP treatment (Eshleman et al., 2001). Furthermore, NVP and other non-nucleoside reverse transcriptase inhibitors (NNRTIs) are not active against HIV-2 and so should not be used to treat or prevent HIV-2 infection.

Combination Therapy during Pregnancy

A fundamental principle of ART during pregnancy is that ART of known benefit to the pregnant woman should not be withheld unless there are known adverse effects to her or to her infant or unless the adverse effects outweigh the potential benefits. Most of the treatment guidelines for pregnant women generally follow those of therapy in adolescents and adults (CDC 2002c; Cooper et al., 2002). This usually means that a combination of ART will be used consisting of two nucleoside analog RT inhibitors and a protease inhibitor (PI). Combination ART during pregnancy has reduced perinatal HIV transmission to less than 2% (http://www.womenchildrenhiv.org).

Cesarean Section

In one study, the use of cesarean sections in HIV-infected women was associated with an increase in endometritis, but it was not more severe than in non–HIV-infected women (Urbani et al., 2001). If a cesarean section is performed to decrease the risk of HIV transmission, it is recommended that it be performed at 38 weeks' gestation (Bartlett, 1999; Landesman et al., 1996).

Safety of ART in Pregnancy

Detailed and long-term studies of the safety of ART during pregnancy and for the infant are limited (Sperling et al., 1998). AZT has been used in pregnant women since the early 1990s as monotherapy and now is a necessary component of combination therapy. Safety data of combination ART in pregnant women are more limited. A Swiss report evaluated pregnancy and infant outcome. Eighty percent of the women develop anemia, nausea and vomiting, elevation of liver enzymes, or hyperglycemia (Lorenzi et al., 1998). A possible association with preterm births was noted. The European Collaborative Study (2003) and the Pediatric AIDS Clinical Trials Group 185 (Lambert et al., 2000) did not find an association of AZT use and preterm birth, low birth weight, or intrauterine growth retardation in infants born to HIV-infected versus uninfected mothers.

Additional safety issues related to the use of ART in pregnancy and infants is discussed in the section on antiretroviral safety and toxicity, but in general, no long-term safety issues have arisen (Culnane et al., 1999; Mofenson and Munderi, 2002).

Effectiveness of Prevention Trials

Aggressive prenatal HIV testing coupled with combination ART and cesarean section has further reduced HIV transmission to less than 2% in several clinical trials in the United States and Europe (European Collaborative Study, 1994, 1999; International Perinatal HIV Group, 1999; Ioannidis et al., 2001). As evidence accumulates that abbreviated courses of ART may prevent 50% or more of HIV infection of infants, there is increasing optimism that HIV infection of infants may be eradicated in the United States. Early diagnosis of HIV infection in women coupled with combination therapy during pregnancy, and in many instances cesarean section, has reduced the transmission rate to 1%. These results are associated with marked reductions in HIV RNA (Ioannidis et al., 2001).

Donation Programs for Prevention of Perinatal HIV Transmission

Donation programs that provide NVP free-of-charge to perinatal HIV prevention programs are available (http://www.GlobalStrategies.org/donations; http://www.axios-group.com/en/proj_donations.asp). NVP can also be purchased in developing countries at discounts, so the cost is less than $1 US for both doses. Rapid HIV testing (same day testing) ($1.85 to $2.50 per test) has contributed substantially to expanding perinatal HIV testing in resource-poor countries where prenatal care is limited. Rapid testing has the advantage of increasing knowledge of test results because the patient can be told the results before leaving the clinic.

CLINICAL CONSIDERATIONS

Key clinical issues include diagnosis of HIV, classification, comparison of HIV infection in adults and children, and complications of HIV infection. The significant differences between adults and children affect diagnosis, management, and prognosis of HIV-infected children.

Diagnosis

HIV Antibody Testing

The diagnosis of HIV infection is normally established in adults by serologic tests for HIV-specific IgG antibodies, which become detectable within 4 to 24 weeks of initial infection (Horsburgh et al., 1989). Without an antibody test it was difficult to distinguish AIDS from some forms of congenital immunodeficiency disorders early in the epidemic (Ammann et al., 1983a). Antibody assays subsequently allowed this distinction (Ammann et al., 1985; Newell et al., 1995).

Several licensed ELISAs are available, and the results can be confirmed with Western blot (Consortium for Retrovirus Serology Standardization, 1988). The Western blot provides a profile of antibody reactivity to multiple HIV-1 proteins. Antibodies to the envelope glycoproteins gp160, gp120, and gp41 tend to persist, whereas those to the gag proteins may be lost with advancing disease. This loss of reactivity has prognostic significance in children (Walter et al., 1990). A profound antibody deficiency may result in false-negative ELISA or Western blot tests (Rogers et al., 1991). Currently available tests detect HIV-1 and HIV-2.

For vertically infected infants or infants exposed to HIV perinatally, antibody-based tests are of no diagnostic value beyond confirming the serologic status of the mother. Almost 100% of infants of infected mothers acquire IgG antibodies to HIV transplacentally. These passively acquired antibodies gradually wane, with a median time to disappearance of 10 months; although up to 2% of uninfected infants have detectable antibodies at 18 months (Blanche et al., 1989; European Collaborative Study, 1991). Positive ELISA and Western blots are therefore only diagnostic of infection in children older than the age of 18 months.

Direct HIV Detection

The current approach to establishing the diagnosis in infants is to use tests that directly detect the virus or its components (Consensus Report, 1992; Husson et al., 1990; Rogers et al., 1991; Tudor-Williams, 1991). The four most widely accepted methods are (1) detection of proviral DNA from blood mononuclear cells by PCR, (2) detection of plasma viral RNA by PCR, (3) virus culture, and (4) detection of serum p24 antigen by ELISA.

PROVIRAL DNA PCR

PCR techniques have become standard for diagnosis of infants and for blood-product safety testing. Proviral

DNA extracted from PBMC or whole blood (including dried blood spots on filter papers) can be amplified (Cassol et al., 1992). By the use of a reverse transcription step before amplification (reverse transcriptase polymerase chain reaction [RT-PCR]), virion RNA from plasma or the various species of mRNA in cells or whole blood can be detected. For diagnostic purposes, the DNA PCR method is straightforward. PCR is more rapid than culture for diagnosis, is more accurate than p24, and provides a high degree of sensitivity and specificity, approaching 100% by 2 to 3 months of age (Consensus Report, 1992). Quality assurance procedures for rapidly detecting contamination and false-positive results in a PCR laboratory are mandatory. Careful selection of primers in highly conserved regions of the genome are important because genotypic variation can affect the efficiency of amplification (Candotti et al., 1991).

HIV RNA PCR

Reliable methods for quantitative plasma RNA PCR are now available (Mulder et al., 1994; Piatak et al., 1993a). RNA PCR methodology has now been standardized, especially for monitoring the antiviral response following treatment. Quantitative RNA tests are more widely available than are DNA PCR, have a quicker turnaround time, provide quantitation of viral load, and use less blood (Pavia, 2003). At the same time, an initial quantitative HIV RNA test can be used for diagnosis (Nesheim et al., 2003). In more than 90% of perinatally exposed infants, RNA PCR and DNA PCR are positive by day 14 after birth (Dunn et al., 1995). False-positive results may occur. A positive PCR test should always be confirmed by a second test. ART of the mother or infant does not interfere with test results (Connor et al., 1994).

HIV CULTURE

Virus can be cultured from plasma, PBMCs, whole blood, or body fluids in qualitative or quantitative assays (Alimenti et al., 1991, 1992; Coombs et al., 1989; Ho et al., 1989; Jackson et al., 1988). The requirement for Biosafety Level 2 or 3 facilities and the lengthy, labor-intensive nature of these assays makes them expensive and limits their availability. Culture of the virus is essential, however, if additional studies such as phenotypic assays and neutralizing antibody assay against autologous viral isolates are needed.

HIV p24 ANTIGEN

The sensitivity of p24 antigen detection has been considerably enhanced by the use of immune complex disruption and dissociation (ICD p24) techniques (Bollinger et al., 1992). Both in vivo and in vitro lysis of virions release p24 antigen, which is immediately complexed with antibody. Acid hydrolysis of such complexes frees the p24 antigen and allows it to bind with the test reagent. Results in the neonatal period were promising (Chandwani et al., 1993; Walter et al., 1993). In one study, however, 2 of 22 cord blood samples from seroreverting infants tested falsely positive just above the cutoff value. When a second serum sample was used, all 29 children evaluated in the first 3 weeks of life were correctly assigned (Miles et al., 1993). Despite the enhanced sensitivity of the p24 assays, the test has been largely replaced by RNA or DNA PCR, except in some resource-poor settings.

HIV-infected cells synthesizing p24 antigen can be detected by flow cytometry; fluorescent anti-p24 antibody probes that bind with intracellular p24 antigen in lymphocytes may be a potentially sensitive diagnostic technique (Connelly et al., 1992; Ohlsson-Wilhelm et al., 1990).

NEWBORN TESTING

Despite the sensitivity of culture, PCR, and to a marginally lesser extent, ICD p24 antigen assays, between 50% and 70% of children who subsequently prove to be infected have negative results in the first few days of life (Krivine et al., 1992). This suggests that peripartum transmission occurs with extremely low or absent initial circulating viral burden. The need for follow-up samples to confirm an initial positive result or establish a negative diagnosis is apparent.

In Vitro Antibody Synthesis

Several tests that demonstrate evidence of infection less directly have been developed. In vitro antibody production (IVAP) and enzyme-linked immunospot (Elispot) methodologies detect the presence of B cells that secrete HIV-specific antibodies in vitro (Nesheim et al., 1992; Pahwa et al., 1989). These methods have low sensitivity and specificity in the first 3 months of life and have not become widely used.

Detection of IgA-specific antibodies (which do not cross the placenta) was previously used, although they cannot usually be detected earlier than 2 months of age (Landesman et al., 1991; Martin et al., 1991). The assays in development are in ELISA format, are much less costly than PCR or culture, and may prove useful as an additional screening test.

Prenatal Diagnosis

Prenatal diagnosis has been attempted in a limited number of women, for example, those undergoing cordocentesis for clinical indications (Cullen et al., 1992). HIV has also been cultured from amniotic fluid (Mundy et al., 1987). Any invasive procedure in the prenatal period, however, runs the risk of carrying maternal blood to the infant and causing infections and thus are not recommended.

Rapid HIV Testing

The U.S. Food and Drug Administration (FDA) has approved several simple screening tests, designed for use in medical office, clinic, or home settings. OraSure detects HIV antibodies in the saliva and is 99.9% sensitive. A follow-up Western blot must be performed (Brodie and Sax, 1997; Gallo et al., 1997). A urine antibody test, manufactured by Calypte, is available in

some developing countries but not in the United States. A single-use diagnostic system (SUDS) to be used in medical offices or clinics or as a home-based test (Confide) is used for screening purposes only and requires confirmation by ELISA and Western blot (Martin and Keren, 2002).

Rapid HIV tests on blood samples have been available for many years in developing countries. They are not as accurate as an ELISA confirmed by Western blot or DNA or RNA PCR. However, the use of two or more rapid tests on a single blood sample increases the accuracy of the test to a degree comparable to ELISA and Western blot.

There are significant advantages to rapid HIV testing in which the result is available in less than 2 hours. Results can also be given to the patient on the same clinic visit increasing the opportunity for counseling. The tests are inexpensive in developing countries ($1.85 to $2.50). They need not be performed by highly trained technicians, thus increasing their availability and decreasing the cost. The (OraQuick) test recently approved by the FDA for use in the United States may expand HIV testing throughout the United States, especially for the estimated 200,000 HIV-infected individuals unaware of their infection (FDA, 2002).

Although rapid HIV tests are not of value for the diagnosis of infection in newborns exposed to HIV, they are a value in determining the HIV status of women who present late in labor, who have had no prenatal care, or who have no record of previous HIV testing. Under these circumstances, they provide guidance as to whether ART, such as NVP, should be used immediately for the mother and the infant.

Clinical and Laboratory Features of HIV Infection

Clinical and laboratory studies can suggest an HIV infection. A classification system (see later) for pediatric HIV disease has been developed (CDC, 1994a). The onset of category C symptoms, in association with a positive test for HIV, is considered diagnostic of AIDS, but category A symptoms have poor specificity (Mayers et al., 1991). Persistent oral candidiasis and parotitis were found to be highly discriminatory for HIV infection in the European Collaborative Study, whereas lymphadenopathy, hepatosplenomegaly, eczema, fever, rhinitis, otitis, and non–gram-negative pneumonias were not (European Collaborative Study, 1991).

A low CD4 count and percent, taking into account the age-dependent normal range, are suggestive but not diagnostic of HIV (CDC, 1992; Erkeller-Yuksel et al., 1992; McKinney and Wilfert, 1992). Hypergammaglobulinemia is a common finding by 3 months of age but is of poor predictive value, because many uninfected infants of infected mothers have high levels of passively acquired IgG (Kline et al., 1993). By 6 months of age, however, hypergammaglobulinemia was a useful indicator, present in 77% of infected infants and 3% of uninfected infants (European Collaborative Study, 1991). β_2-Microglobulin and neopterin levels, of interest early in the epidemic, are nonspecific indicators of infection (Chan et al., 1990; Ellaurie et al., 1992; Siller et al., 1993).

The 1994 CDC revised diagnostic classification system for children younger than 13 years (Table 29-6) considers a child younger than 18 months infected if either of the following are positive on two separate blood samples (excluding cord blood): (1) HIV virus culture, (2) HIV PCR, (3) HIV p24 antigen, and (4) diagnosis of AIDS based on the 1987 AIDS case definition. A child older than 18 months is considered HIV infected if the HIV antibody test is repeatedly reactive by ELISA assay and a confirmatory test is positive using the criteria listed previously for infants younger than 18 months.

HIV Seroreversion

A special category of seroreverter is an infant born to an HIV-infected mother who is not infected as evidenced by two or more antibody tests after 16 months of age or one negative test after 18 months of age and has no other laboratory evidence of HIV infection by the previously listed viral assays and has none of the clinical conditions listed in category C of the CDC classification system (severely symptomatic).

· ·
TABLE 29-6 · CDC 1994 REVISED DIAGNOSTIC CLASSIFICATION SYSTEM FOR HIV INFECTION IN CHILDREN YOUNGER THAN 13 YEARS OLD

Confirmed HIV Infection
1. In a child <18 months of age who is known to be HIV-seropositive or born to an HIV-infected mother with positive results by any of the following HIV detection tests on two separate samples (excluding cord blood):
   a. HIV virus culture
   b. HIV polymerase chain reaction (PCR)
   c. HIV antigen (p24) (FDA-licensed assay)
   d. Diagnosis of AIDS based on the 1987 AIDS case definition
2. In a child >18 months of age:
   a. HIV antibody-positive by repeatedly reactive EIA and confirmatory test
   b. Any of the criteria in (1) above

Exposed Infection Status (Prefix E)
1. A child who does not meet the criteria above but who is:
   a. HIV-seropositive by EIA and confirmatory test (<18 months old at the time of test)
   b. Born to an HIV-infected mother, infant's antibody status unknown

Seroreverter (SR)
1. A child born to an HIV-infected mother has seroreverted (SR) and is assumed uninfected when:
   a. He or she is documented HIV antibody-negative (two or more negative ELISA tests after 6 months of age) or one negative test after 18 months of age *and*
   b. Has no other laboratory evidence of infection (has not had two positive viral detections tests, described above) *and*
   c. Has not had any clinical condition listed in category C (see Table 29-7)

AIDS = acquired immunodeficiency syndrome; EIA = enzyme immunoassay; FDA = Food and Drug Administration; HIV = human immunodeficiency virus. From Centers for Disease Control and Prevention. Revised classification system for human immunodeficiency virus infection in children less than 13 years of age. MMWR Morb Mortal Wkly Rep 43:1–12, 1994a.

Differential Diagnosis

The differential diagnosis of HIV infection in symptomatic infants and children includes the primary combined immunodeficiency disorders, other congenital infections (e.g., toxoplasmosis, syphilis, parvovirus B19, listeriosis), and the extensive list of causes of failure to thrive. A careful history that includes maternal risk factors may suggest HIV exposure. Initial laboratory tests, including an immunoglobulin profile and lymphocyte subsets using age-adjusted standards, may indicate a cellular or humoral immune abnormality, but direct tests for the presence of HIV, as outlined earlier, should be done before an extensive workup for rare primary immunodeficiency diseases.

It should be noted that infants with severe combined immunodeficiency generally have absent or extremely low numbers of T cells (e.g., <100 cells/μl), which is rarely seen in HIV-infected infants (see Chapter 15).

Classification Systems

Classification systems have been developed for children 13 years old and younger, because there are significant differences between HIV infection in children and adults. The most widely used system is that first developed by the CDC in 1985, modified in 1987, and updated in 1994 (CDC, 1987, 1993a, 1994a). These systems have been used to obtain epidemiologic information and to track the epidemic.

Before the identification of the virus and a diagnostic test, the CDC classification systems provided a constellation of signs and symptoms that constituted the syndrome of acquired immunodeficiency. Once HIV was discovered as the cause of AIDS, a more precise classification system was developed.

The current classification for children is complex. Although useful for epidemiologic purposes, it is not useful for making treatment decisions in HIV-infected children because it does not include one of the most important laboratory features, the HIV viral load. It must also be recognized that many of the initial symptoms in HIV-infected patients are similar to those occurring in other children (e.g., recurrent respiratory tract infections, frequent episodes of diarrhea, thrush, anemia, leukopenia, lymphadenopathy). The severity and chronicity of these symptoms are used to suspect HIV and perform an HIV test that will establish a definitive diagnosis.

CDC Classification of HIV Infection and AIDS in Children Younger Than 13 Years

Under the 1994 classification system, HIV-infected children are classified into three mutually exclusive categories: (1) infection status (see Table 29-6), (2) clinical status (Table 29-7), and (3) immunologic status (Tables 29-8 and 29-9). It is immediately apparent that this classification system does not include the virologic

TABLE 29-7 · CDC 1994 REVISED CLASSIFICATION SYSTEM FOR HIV INFECTION IN CHILDREN YOUNGER THAN 13 YEARS OF AGE

Category N: No Symptoms

Child has no signs or symptoms that are believed to be the result of HIV infection and/or are indicative of immunologic deficits attributable to HIV infection, or has only one of the conditions listed in category A, below

Category A: Mildly Symptomatic

Two or more of the conditions listed below occurring in an HIV-infected or exposed child; conditions listed in categories B and C must not have occurred:

· Lymphadenopathy (>0.5 cm at more than two sites; bilateral = one site)
· Hepatomegaly
· Splenomegaly
· Dermatitis
· Parotitis
· Recurrent or persistent upper respiratory tract infections, including sinusitis or otitis media (four or more episodes in a 12-month period)

Category B: Moderately Symptomatic

Symptomatic conditions occurring in a child that are not included among conditions listed in clinical category C and that are attributed to HIV infection and/or are indicative of immunologic deficits attributable to HIV infection. Examples of conditions in clinical category B include, *but are not limited to:*

· Anemia, <8 g/dl, or neutropenia, <1000/mm³, or thrombocytopenia, <100,000/mm³ persisting for >30 days
· Bacterial meningitis, pneumonia, or sepsis (single episode)
· Candidiasis, oropharyngeal (thrush), persistent (>2 months) in children >6 months of age
· Cardiomyopathy
· Cytomegalovirus infection, with onset before 1 month of age
· Diarrhea, recurrent or chronic
· Hepatitis
· Herpes simplex virus stomatitis, recurrent (more than two episodes within 1 year)
· Herpes simplex virus, pneumonitis, or esophagitis with onset before 1 month of age
· Herpes zoster (shingles) involving at least two distinct episodes or more than one dermatome
· Leiomyosarcoma
· Lymphoid interstitial pneumonia (LIP) or pulmonary lymphoid hyperplasia complex (PLH)
· Nephropathy
· Nocardiosis
· Persistent fever >1 month
· Varicella, disseminated (complicated primary chickenpox)

Category C: Severely Symptomatic

Any condition listed in the 1987 surveillance case definition for AIDS, *with the exception of LIP.* The conditions in clinical category C are strongly associated with severe immunodeficiency, occur frequently in HIV-infected individuals, and cause serious morbidity or mortality:

· Serious bacterial infections, multiple or recurrent (any combination of at least two culture-proven infections within a 2-year period of the following types: septicemia, pneumonia, meningitis, bone or joint infection, or abscess of an internal organ or body cavity (excluding otitis media, superficial skin or mucosal abscesses, and indwelling catheter-related infections).
· Candidiasis, esophageal or pulmonary (bronchi, trachea, lungs)
· Coccidioidomycosis, disseminated (at site other than or in addition to lungs or cervical or hilar lymph nodes)
· Cryptococcosis extrapulmonary
· Cryptosporidiosis or isosporiasis with diarrhea persisting 1 month
· Cytomegalovirus disease with onset of symptoms at age >1 month (at a site other than liver, spleen, or nodes)
· Encephalopathy (at least one of the following progressive findings present for at least 2 months in the absence of a concurrent illness other than HIV infection that could explain the findings): (1) failure to attain or loss of developmental milestones or loss of intellectual ability verified by standard developmental scale or neuropsychologic tests; (2) impaired brain growth or acquired microcephaly or brain atrophy demonstrated by head circumference measurement or brain atrophy demonstrated by computerized tomography or magnetic resonance imaging (serial imaging is required for children <2 years of age); (3) acquired symmetric motor deficit manifested by two or more of the following with paresis, pathologic reflexes, ataxia, or gait disturbance
· Herpes simplex virus infection causing a mucocutaneous ulcer that persists longer than 1 month, or bronchitis, pneumonitis, or esophagitis for any duration affecting a child older than 1 month
· Histoplasmosis, disseminated (at site other than or in addition to lungs or cervical or hilar lymph nodes)
· Kaposi's sarcoma
· Lymphoma, primary in brain
· Lymphoma, small, noncleaved cell (Burkitt's), or immunoblastic or large-cell lymphoma of B-cell or unknown immunologic phenotype
· *Mycobacterium tuberculosis,* disseminated or extrapulmonary
· *Mycobacterium,* other species or unidentified species, disseminated or extrapulmonary
· *Mycobacterium avium* complex or *Mycobacterium kansasii,* disseminated (at site other than or in addition to lungs, skin, or cervical or hilar lymph nodes)
· *Pneumocystis carinii* pneumonia
· Progressive multifocal leukoencephalopathy
· Toxoplasmosis of the brain with onset at age >1 month
· Wasting syndrome in the absence of a concurrent illness other than HIV that could explain the following findings: (1) persistent weight loss >10% of baseline, (2) downward crossing of at least two of the following percentile lines on the weight-for-age chart (e.g., 95th, 75th, 50th, 25th, 5th) in a child >1 year, or (3) <5th percentile on weight-for-height chart on two consecutive measurements, >30 days apart PLUS (a) chronic diarrhea (i.e., at least two loose stools per day for >30 days) OR (b) documented fever (for >30 days, intermittent or constant)

AIDS = acquired immunodeficiency syndrome; HIV = human immunodeficiency syndrome.
From Centers for Disease Control and Prevention. Revised classification system for human immunodeficiency virus infection in children less than 13 years of age. MMWR Morb Mortal Wkly Rep 43:1–12, 1994a.

status other than whether the patient is HIV-infected (e.g., viral load considerations are omitted). (This is discussed subsequently under the treatment section.)

For purposes of the CDC classification system, once a child is classified in a specific category, the child cannot be reclassified in a less severe category even if the clinical or immunologic status improves. This again is in contrast to treatment approaches in which significant alterations in treatment may occur depending on the clinical, immunologic, or virologic status of the child.

Table 29-8 refers to the combined symptom and immunologic categories using the numbers 1, 2, and 3, which refer to increasing degrees of immunodeficiency (defined by age in Table 29-9). The letters N, A, B, and

TABLE 29-8 · CDC 1994 PEDIATRIC HUMAN IMMUNODEFICIENCY VIRUS (HIV) CLASSIFICATION

Immunologic Categories	Clinical Categories			
	N: No Signs/ Symptoms	A: Mild Signs/ Symptoms	B: Moderate Signs/ Symptoms	C: Severe Signs/ Symptoms
No evidence of immunosuppression	N1	A1	B1	C1
Evidence of moderate immunosuppression	N2	A2	B2	C2
Evidence of severe immunosuppression	N3	A3	B3	C3

Children whose HIV infection status is not confirmed are classified by using the above grade with a letter E (for perinatally exposed) placed before the appropriate classification code (e.g., EN2).
From Centers for Disease Control and Prevention. Revised classification system for human immunodeficiency virus infection in children less than 13 years of age. MMWR Morb Mortal Wkly Rep 43:1–12, 1994a.

TABLE 29-9 · CDC 1994 CD4 T-LYMPHOCYTE AND PERCENTAGE CATEGORIES FOR HIV-INFECTED CHILDREN YOUNGER THAN 13 YEARS OF AGE

Category	<12 Months		1–5 Years		6–12 Years	
	No./microliter	%	No./microliter	%	No./microliter	%
Category 1 No immunosuppression	>1500	>25	>1000	>25	>500	>25
Category 2 Moderate immunosuppression	750–1499	15–24	500–999	15–24	200–499	15–24
Category 3 Severe immunosuppression	<750	<15	<500	<15	<200	<15

From Centers for Disease Control and Prevention. Revised classification system for human immunodeficiency virus infection in children less than 13 years of age. MMWR Morb Mortal Wkly Rep 43:1–12, 1994a.

C refer to increasing degrees of clinical symptomatology beginning with N (no signs or symptoms) and progressing to C (severe symptomatology).

Three immunologic categories were devised for purposes of defining the degree of immunodeficiency. This was necessary because CD4 T-cell counts in infants are considerably higher than those in older children or adults; they decline with increasing age and do not reach adult levels until children are older than 12 years (Denny et al., 1992; Erkeller-Yuksel, et al., 1992; European Collaborative Study, 1992; Waeker et al., 1993). It is important to emphasize that CD4 counts do not reflect CD4 function, as evidenced by the fact that children may develop opportunistic infection at higher CD4 levels than adults do (Connor et al., 1991a; Kovacs et al., 1991). Included in Table 29-9 are both CD4 T-lymphocyte counts and the percentage of CD4 T lymphocytes. There is less variability in CD4 percentage values at different ages.

The clinical categories are outlined in Table 29-7. The signs and symptoms should be HIV related. For examples, hepatitis is ascribed to category B only when other causes of hepatitis, such as other viral infection or drug toxicity, have been excluded, and cytomegalovirus (CMV) infection is ascribed to HIV only when it occurs before 1 months of age.

Category C conditions include all those listed in the 1987 surveillance case definition for AIDS (see Table 29-7) except for lymphocytic interstitial pneumonitis (LIP). LIP is not associated with shortened survival (Blanche et al., 1990; Tovo et al., 1992). LIP and other category C conditions, however, are reportable to state and local health departments as AIDS. Common features of the conditions listed in category C are their severity and duration in HIV-infected individuals (e.g., candidia-sis of the esophagus or pulmonary tract, *Pneumocystis carinii* pneumonia [PCP]) and their rarity in other diseases other than in primary immunodeficiencies.

The CDC classification system requires systematic laboratory testing of children, both to establish the diagnosis and to assess immune function. Geographic variations in clinical manifestations of AIDS, such as severe diarrheal disease and measles in sub-Saharan Africa, may make this classification less useful in these settings.

WHO Classification

A clinical case definition for AIDS was published by the WHO (1986). Subsequent field evaluation demonstrated 90% specificity but only 35% sensitivity and positive predictive value (Lepage et al., 1989). Proposals for a revision have been proposed (Belec et al., 1992).

CDC Classification for Adolescents

For adolescents, the 1993 revised classification system should be used (CDC, 1993a). This includes an expansion of the surveillance case definition for AIDS to include all HIV-infected persons with CD4 counts lower than 200/mm³ or less than 14% and patients with pulmonary tuberculosis (TB), recurrent pneumonia, or invasive cervical cancer.

Comparison of HIV Infection in Adults and Children

The 1994 classification of clinical conditions for children with HIV contains much overlap with the current classification for adults and adolescents. A number of important differences, however, have become apparent. The most important difference is that disease progression may be more rapid in children. Disease progression has a bimodal distribution (see earlier), but the latency period is reduced compared with that of adults (Byers et al., 1993; Tovo et al., 1992).

In infants, the subtle initial symptoms must be distinguished from problems associated with prematurity, intrauterine drug exposure, or congenital infections other than HIV (Ammann, 1983, 1984; Ammann et al., 1984, 1985). It is unusual to detect a mononucleosis-like illness as described in adults with acute HIV infection. The incidence of encephalopathy is higher in children, ranging from 30% to 90% with advancing disease (European Collaborative Study, 1990). Failure to thrive, in particular the failure of normal linear growth, is considered a specific manifestation of pediatric HIV infection (McKinney et al., 1993; Working Group on Antiretroviral Therapy, 1993). Recurrent bacterial infections, particularly with polysaccharide-encapsulated bacteria, are more common, reflecting the immaturity of the humoral immune system. Toxoplasmosis and cryptococcosis are less common in children. LIP and chronic parotid swelling has been seen almost exclusively in the pediatric population. Malignancies are less common in children and Kaposi's sarcoma (KS) in particular is rare in children.

Pediatric Long-Term Survivors

Some children become long-term survivors even without therapy (Kline et al., 1995; Nielsen et al., 1997; Thorne et al., 2002). Attempts to ascertain whether long-term survival is associated with an immunologic factor(s) or specific viral variants have not been successful. It is more likely that host genetic factors may provide resistance to viral proliferation such as specific HLA types and mutations in chemokine receptors (see section on genetic factors).

Long-term surviving children are defined as those surviving 5 years or more following perinatal HIV infection with no or minimal ART. In 54 of 143 perinatally infected children meeting this definition, 27% had absolute CD4 counts greater than 500/ml and 40% had developed AIDS-defining conditions. Generalized lymphadenopathy, LIP, and recurrent bacterial infections were the most frequent clinical conditions (Nielsen et al., 1997). The long-term survivors who did not develop PCP had a median survival of 8.4 years. Long-term survival has also been associated with LIP in other series (Kline et al., 1995).

Long-term evaluation of a cohort of HIV-infected children in New York City indicated that the age of children in care increased from 3 years in 1989 to 1991 to 6 years in 1995 to 1998 (Abrams et al., 2001). AIDS-free survival increased significantly in severely immunosuppressed children, most likely related to the increased use of combined ART (66%) and the use of PCP prophylaxis (88%).

Another indication of improved long-term survival is the fact that perinatally infected girls are now surviving to reproductive age. The CDC has recently reported eight perinatally HIV-infected Puerto Rican teenagers who have given birth to uninfected infants (CDC, 2003).

COMPLICATIONS

Complications of pediatric HIV infection are of two major types: organ specific and infectious. Organ-specific complications include LIP, CNS problems, growth and endocrine dysfunction, nutritional and gastrointestinal problems, cardiac abnormalities, hematologic manifestations, and malignancies.

Lymphocytic Interstitial Pneumonitis

LIP is a chronic lung disorder of unknown cause that affects up to 40% to 50% of perinatally HIV-infected children (Connor et al., 1991b; Gonzalez et al., 2000). It is less common in older children and hemophiliacs. The disorder is characterized by a diffuse, interstitial, reticulonodular infiltrate on plain x-ray film (Fig. 29-5). If it is associated with larger nodules and hilar or mediastinal lymphadenopathy, it is referred to as pulmonary lymphoid hyperplasia (PLH), which appears to represent one end of the continuum of this process (Joshi et al., 1990). Clinically, there is a wide spectrum of severity, from an asymptomatic individual in whom LIP is a purely radiologic diagnosis to someone with severely compromised exercise tolerance and oxygen dependency.

A presumptive diagnosis may be made on the basis of suggestive x-ray changes that persist for months, are unresponsive to antimicrobial therapy, and are not the result of other specific infectious pathogens. PCP can co-exist with LIP, and any new onset of oxygen dependency should prompt an induced sputum examination

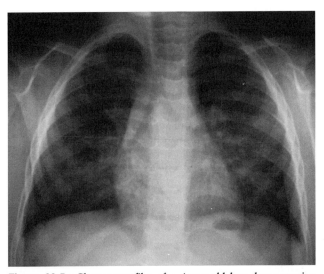

Figure 29-5 · Chest x-ray film of a 4-year-old boy demonstrating bilateral perihilar infiltrates of mild to moderate lymphoid interstitial pneumonitis (**LIP**). (Courtesy of Dr. Irwin Feuerstein.)

and consideration of bronchoscopy to look for pneumocysts or trophozoites.

Additional clinical findings include lymphadenopathy and salivary gland enlargement, the latter of which may be confused with chronic parotitis. Diffuse hypergammaglobulinemia with all immunoglobulin classes significantly elevated is a distinguishing laboratory characteristic. A definitive diagnosis of LIP is made by lung biopsy, although this is rarely necessary. Characteristic findings are a diffuse lymphoid infiltration of the alveolar septa and peribronchiolar areas, with varying degrees of lymphoid aggregation that may show organization into early germinal centers. Both Epstein-Barr virus (EBV) DNA and HIV RNA have been identified by in situ hybridization in biopsy specimens from children with LIP (Andiman et al., 1985; Joshi et al., 1987; Katz et al., 1992).

Interstitial lung disease may be a cytokine-mediated process, both in initiation and perpetuation, triggered by immune responses to HIV antigens, direct effects of HIV, or co-infection with pathogens such as EBV (Agostini at et al., 1996; Fishback and Koss, 1996). The reason why LIP is less frequently seen in adults is unclear. The fact that children may be experiencing a primary infection with EBV may be relevant. Other viral agents causing primary infections in childhood, such as HHV-6, may also play a role in the pathogenesis of LIP.

Children with LIP may experience long-term survival without ART (Kline et al., 1995; Nielsen et al., 1997). LIP may also remit spontaneously. Some children with LIP who have developed non-Hodgkin's lymphoma (NHL), particularly mucosa-associated lymphoid tumors, have been described (Gonzalez et al., 2000).

Treatment for LIP is only indicated in the presence of hypoxemia and shortness of breath. High-dose oral steroids are used for at least 6 weeks to suppress the lymphocytic proliferation. Symptoms frequently return on weaning steroids, and the lowest maintenance dosage must be sought for each individual.

Central Nervous System Abnormalities

Encephalopathy

HIV encephalopathy is rarely evident at birth but may present in infancy with such signs as delayed acquisition of a social smile, poor head control, or truncal hypotonia. Subsequently progressive motor abnormalities, such as spastic diplegia and oral motor dysfunction, become apparent (Belman, 1992; Civitello, 1991; European Collaborative Study, 1990; Sanchez-Ramon et al., 2002). Expressive language is usually more affected than is receptive language. The course varies from static (with acquisition of developmental milestones at a slower rate than normal) to progressive (with overt loss of previously acquired skills). Acquired microcephaly resulting from cerebral atrophy may be present. Seizures are unusual in the absence of other complications because HIV infection is predominately a disease of white matter (Civitello, 1991). Cerebrovascular

disease resulting in strokes can occur (Park et al., 1990). Giant aneurysms of the circle of Willis have also been described (Husson et al., 1992; Lang et al., 1992).

CNS problems occur frequently in symptomatic HIV-infected children; estimates vary from 31% to 89% (Belman, 1992; European Collaborative Study, 1990). Of 131 children followed at the National Cancer Institute until death, 86 (66%) had neurodevelopmental evidence of encephalopathy at some stage of their disease. Lower CD4 percentages, higher viral loads, and positive p24 antigen levels are significantly associated with the occurrence of CNS abnormalities (Cooper et al., 1998; Lindsey et al., 2000; Mitchell, 2001). Although a high viral load in infancy is predictive of encephalopathy, it is not predictive of age of onset (Cooper et al., 1998).

In a study of 1811 children followed in the Pediatric Spectrum of Disease Project, 23% had encephalopathy (Lobato et al., 1995). Milder neurologic dysfunction and developmental difficulties are more frequent. A similar percentage was found in a WITS Study in which 21% of the children developed encephalopathy (Cooper et al., 1998). Children with encephalopathy, in contrast to encephalopathic adults, more often have severe early-onset encephalopathy associated with less immunosuppression and prominent brain atrophy and motor abnormalities (Tardieu et al., 2000). In the first year of life, 10% of HIV-infected infants develop encephalopathy compared with an overall incidence of 0.3% in adults. After age 2 years about 1% of children developed encephalopathy, similar in frequency to that of adults.

Other Neurologic Problems

A high prevalence of behavioral problems exist among HIV-infected children. Neither HIV infection nor prenatal drug exposure has been identified as an underlying cause. The behavior disorders may be related to other biologic or environmental factors (Mellins et al., 2003).

Neurodevelopmental markers have been assessed as predictors of mortality. In 157 perinatally infected infants Llorente and co-workers (2003) noted that the Bayley scale of infant development independently predicted mortality after adjusting for treatment, clinical category, gestational age, plasma viral load, and CD4 percentage.

Mechanisms of CNS Damage

Only macrophage-tropic strains of HIV gain entry into the CNS, suggesting that HIV-infected peripheral blood macrophages are the "Trojan horses" that carry HIV across the blood–brain barrier (Levy, 1993). HIV can be identified in the microglia (CNS macrophages) and, to a lesser extent, in astrocytes.

Because neurons are not directly infected, several mechanisms for neuronal cell damage have been proposed. HIV proteins, in particular gp120 and possibly tat, may be toxic to neuroglial cells. In vivo support for this has been demonstrated in a transgenic mouse model, in which the expression of gp120 alone correlated with reactive astrocytosis, microglial activation and clustering, and neuronal dendritic vacuolization (Toggas et al., 1994).

Activated macrophages may produce toxic factors such as TNF, which has been implicated in demyelination (Epstein and Gendelman, 1993). Metabolic products, such as quinolinic acid, can mediate neuronal toxicity by binding to postsynaptic N-methyl-D-aspartate (NMDA) receptors, causing toxic calcium influx. One study in HIV-infected children has shown a significant relation between cerebrospinal fluid (CSF), quinolinic acid levels, and encephalopathy (Brouwers et al., 1993).

Nitric oxide, in conjunction with superoxide anion, is believed to be a mediator of neuronal damage following NMDA receptor stimulation (Dawson et al., 1993). Arachidonic acid metabolites, such as leukotrienes and prostaglandins, may also cause toxicity by different mechanisms (Epstein and Gendelman, 1993; Lipton, 1994).

CNS disease may progress more rapidly with CNS co-infection with other viruses or protozoal agents (Kovacs et al., 1999). Until the pathogenesis of CNS damage is better understood, reducing the virus burden using agents that penetrate the CNS is the most logical approach to intervention.

CNS Imaging

Computed tomography (CT) may demonstrate ventricular enlargement and cortical atrophy (Fig. 29-6) or cerebral calcification, which is seen particularly in the basal ganglia (Fig. 29-7) (DeCarli et al., 1993). DeCarli and colleagues (1993) found that calcification is a hallmark of vertically acquired HIV infection and is rare in children with transfusion-acquired disease, even if the transfusion was given in the neonatal period. Among children with vertically acquired disease, 33% had calcifications, and all were encephalopathic. Cerebral calcification may be a surrogate marker for intrauterine transmission.

Cerebellar atrophy was noted in 12% of scans from this series of symptomatic children. Abnormalities on CT scan were significantly associated with decline in neuropsychologic function and decline in CD4 percentages.

Magnetic resonance imaging (MRI) techniques are better than CT scans at delineating white matter abnormalities (Fig. 29-8) (Kauffman et al., 1992). Neuroimaging changes that may precede or follow clinical signs of neurologic involvement include calcifying microangiopathy on CT, white matter lesions and central atrophy on MRI, and lenticulostriate vessel echogenicity on cranial ultrasound (Mitchell, 2001).

Cerebrospinal Fluid Findings

Early reports suggested that PCR detection of HIV DNA of the CSF is a marker for CNS involvement in

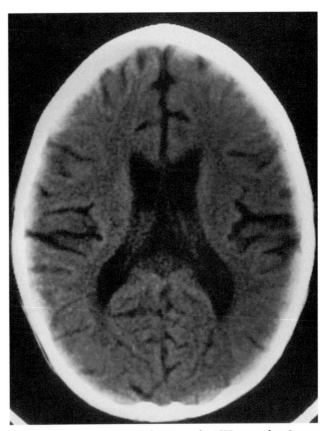

Figure 29-6 · Cranial computed tomography (CT) scan of an 8-year-old girl with perinatally acquired HIV-1 infection, demonstrating enlargement of the ventricles and widening of the sulci because of cerebral atrophy. This may be partially reversible with zidovudine therapy. (Courtesy of Dr. Nicholas Patronas.)

adults (Shaunak et al., 1990). A subsequent study, however, found that HIV-1 sequences could be amplified from CSF in 80% of patients, independent of clinical stage or neurologic symptoms (Chiodi et al., 1992). As a supplemental marker for HIV-related neurologic disease, CSF quinolinic acid determinations may be more useful than PCR.

Pathologic Features

Postmortem pathologic findings include cerebral atrophy, calcification, focal necrosis, gliosis, reactive astrocytosis, vascular lesions, and inflammatory infiltrates often containing multinucleated giant cells. Ultrastructural studies and in situ hybridization have demonstrated HIV within these giant cells (Epstein et al., 1988; Kure et al., 1991).

Treatment of CNS HIV Complications

ART may significantly improve CNS disease. However, saquinavir (SQV), nelfinavir (NFV), didanosine (ddI), and ddC have poor CNS penetration. Striking improvement in motor abnormalities, neurophysiologic functioning, and radiologic findings have been associated with AZT therapy, particularly when given by continuous infusion (Brouwers et al., 1990; Pizzo et al., 1988;

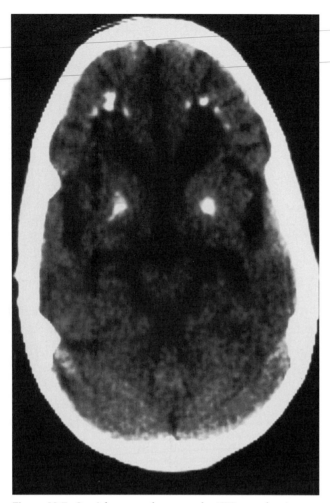

Figure 29-7 · Cranial computed tomography (CT) scan showing typical distribution of basal ganglia and frontal periventricular calcification. This is a hallmark of perinatally acquired HIV-1 infection (see text). Marked cerebral atrophy is also present. (Courtesy of Dr. Nicholas Patronas.)

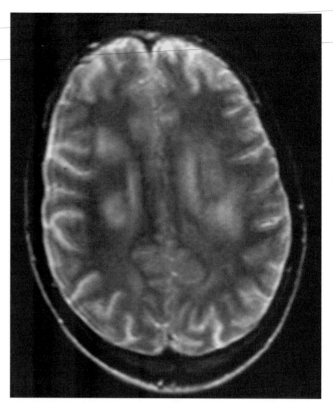

Figure 29-8 · Cranial magnetic resonance imaging (MRI) scan (T2-weighted image) demonstrating extensive periventricular white matter changes consistent with HIV-1 leukomalacia. Cytomegalovirus may cause a similar appearance but usually shows greater evidence of subependymal involvement. Periventricular multifocal leukomalacia, associated with JC virus infection, is usually subcortical initially, with finger-like projections to the surface of the gray matter, and may be more diffuse and patchy. (Courtesy of Dr. Nicholas Patronas.)

Raskino et al., 1999). Combination therapy with AZT and ddI was more effective than either drug alone (Raskino et al., 1999). HAART is more effective than nucleoside reverse transcriptase inhibitor (NRTI) combinations in the treatment of encephalopathic symptoms (Rosenfeldt et al., 2000).

Improvement has also been noted anecdotally with corticosteroid treatments (Stiehm et al., 1992). The rapidity with which steroids induce improvements in a subset of patients suggests that they may reverse some toxic effect on the CNS rather than inhibiting infection. Modulation of proinflammatory cytokines is a possible mechanism.

Growth and Endocrine Abnormalities

Growth Failure

Growth failure is a common finding in HIV-infected children, and its cause is multifactorial (Lindsey et al., 2000; Peters et al., 1998; Zeitler et al., 1999). In one retrospective analysis of 170 children born to infected

mothers, the 62 HIV-infected children had significantly decreased linear growth and weight gain by the age of 4 months compared with uninfected controls (McKinney et al., 1993). These decreases were proportional, so weight for height measurements were normal and the children did not appear wasted.

Growth failure is a specific marker of HIV disease progression (Brettler et al., 1990; Chiarelli et al., 1999, 2001; McKinney et al., 1991; Tovo et al., 1992). Proportionately decreased linear and ponderal growth is the most common abnormality in perinatally infected children and is usually accompanied by preferential decreases of fat-free or lean body mass.

There is no consistent information as to the primary cause of growth failure. Deficiency of micronutrients, including vitamin A, neuroendocrine abnormalities, abnormalities of thyroid, growth hormone, insulin-like growth factor-1 (IGF-1), and adrenal function, have been described. Gastrointestinal infection may result in malabsorption of proteins, fats, and carbohydrates, but it does not fully explain growth failure (Arpardi 2000). There is an association between growth failure and high levels of HIV replication (Arpardi et al., 2000). A meta-analysis of 15 large studies indicated that virologic markers were significant predictors of weight, growth and cognitive failure in children older than 1 year (Lindsey et al., 2003; Newell et al., 2003).

Growth failure may result from inadequate nutritional intake, caused by suppressed appetite, oropharyngeal pathology, or neurologic disease (see other topics). HIV enteropathy or bacterial overgrowth of the small intestine may result in malabsorption (Agostoni et al., 1998; Miller et al., 1991). The metabolic requirements of HIV-infected children may be increased, and wasting may result from cytokine dysregulation associated with immune activation (Grunfeld et al., 1992; Matsuyama et al., 1991).

Endocrine Abnormalities

Systematic studies of endocrine abnormalities at different stages of HIV disease are lacking. In one study of nine children with growth failure, there was one case of primary hypothyroidism, six cases of deficient nocturnal increase of thyroid-stimulating hormone (TSH), and one case of growth hormone deficiency (Laue et al., 1990). End-organ resistance may contribute to growth failure; in vitro resistance to growth hormone, IGF-1, and insulin has been demonstrated in erythroid progenitor cells from HIV-infected children (Geffner et al., 1990, 1993).

Among 124 children at various stages of HIV disease, Tudor-Williams and Pizzo (1996) reported an elevated TSH level in 35 (28%) of children. The prevalence increased as CD4 counts fell; 42% of children with less than 200 CD4 cells/mm^3 had an elevated TSH level. The thyroid-binding globulin level was frequently elevated (74% of 73 patients tested). These data suggest that compensated hypothyroidism is a frequent enough finding to merit annual testing of thyroxin and TSH in symptomatic children.

Endocrinologic factors were evaluated in 27 HIV-infected children before and after HAART (Van Rossum et al., 2003). Hypothyroidism and adrenal axis abnormalities were not associated with restoration of growth after HAART. However, the combination of any relatively high serum IGFBP-3 level and relatively low serum IGF-1 level suggested the presence of a growth hormone resistant state. Normalization of these values after HAART suggested restoration of normal sensitivity to growth hormone and recovery to an anabolic state.

Height, weight, and growth of children born to HIV-infected mothers in Europe were extensively analyzed prospectively from birth to approximately 10 years of age (Newell et al., 2003). HIV-infected children grew significantly slower than uninfected children and these differences increased with age. The growth patterns in asymptomatic-infected children were similar to those with mild or moderate symptoms. Severely ill children had poorer growth at all ages. A limited number of children who received combination ART had improved weight gain but a minimal effect on linear growth.

The beneficial effect of HAART on growth and development can be sustained for several years (Dreimane et al., 2001; Nadal et al., 1998). Height and weight are most favorably influenced in children whose therapy leads to a reduction of the viral load of at least 1.5 log or less than 500 copies/ml and an increase in the CD4 T-cell count (Buchacz et al., 2003; Steiner et al., 2001; Verweel et al., 2002).

HIV infection interferes with sexual maturation (de Martino et al., 2001). The onset of puberty was not related to clinical and immunologic status, antiretroviral treatment, weight for height, age at onset of severe disease, or degree of immune suppression.

Metabolic Abnormalities

An elevated serum anion gap and renal tubular acidosis occurring in some children with advanced HIV disease are associated with height and growth failure (Chakraborty et al., 2003). Prophylaxis with sulfur/sulfone-containing antibiotics may also cause renal tubular damage.

Zamboni and associates (2003) noted that low serum osteocalcin levels were an early indicator of altered bone metabolism in HIV-infected children. Children with severely compromised immune systems have bone loss as assessed by bone densitometry. Leonard and McComsey (2003) also noted osteopenia in HIV-infected children.

Nutritional and Gastrointestinal Complications

Nutritional deficiencies and wasting are common among HIV-infected children. They may result from reduced food intake, nutrient malabsorption, or metabolic alterations. Physical abnormalities such as painful lesions of the mouth, larynx, or esophagus may result in decreased food intake. *Candida albicans* and HSV are the most common causes of oropharyngeal pathology (Smith et al., 1993). Esophagitis that is minimally symptomatic, sometimes only detected by barium swallow, can lead to anorexia and weight loss.

The multiple HIV medications may lead to anorexia as a result of unpleasant taste, nausea, vomiting, diarrhea, or abdominal pain. Enteric infections with anorexia, diarrhea, or abdominal pain are not uncommon. *Cryptosporidia, Mycobacterium avium-intracellulare* (MAI), *Microsporidium, Salmonella,* and *Shigella* are particularly troublesome and should be excluded (Pickering and Cleary, 1991). HIV infection of enterochromaffin cells of the intestinal mucosa may result in abnormal motility, and cytokines released by macrophages in the lamina propria may promote secretory diarrhea (Babameto and Kotler, 1997; Matsuyama et al., 1991; Semba and Tang, 1999; Ulrich et al., 1989).

Disaccharide intolerance caused by lactase deficiency has been documented and may improve with dietary manipulation (Yolken et al., 1991). Malabsorption of fats and carbohydrates is common at all stages of HIV infection in both adults and children. This may affect the absorption and utilization of fat-soluble vitamins.

The metabolic abnormalities in HIV are multifactorial. Infection results in increased energy and protein requirements, inefficient utilization of nutrients, and loss of nutrients (Macallan, 1999). This may result from the HIV infection itself, the body's immune response, or decreased food intake. As carbohydrate stores are used, protein loss and muscle wasting occurs, leading to cachexia.

Specific Nutrient Deficiencies

Specific nutrient deficiencies have been evaluated in adults and children with HIV, often with inconsistent findings. Even when deficiencies are identified, supplementation does not always result in improved clinical outcome.

Selenium deficiency was documented in 61% of 23 children with wasting (Miller et al., 1993) and in 37% of 22 other symptomatic children (Mantero-Atienza et al., 1992). Low selenium and zinc levels have also been associated with a significantly higher risk of opportunistic infections and mortality, even with adjustment of baseline CD4 counts and other variables (Baum et al., 1997). Low zinc levels have been associated with HIV progression and increased mortality in intravenous drug users (Baum et al., 1997). In contrast, a high intake of zinc from diets and supplements was associated with decreased survival in HIV-infected men (Tang et al., 1996).

The administration of multivitamins, excluding vitamin A, resulted in significant improvement in CD3, CD4, and CD8 cell counts of women in Tanzania (Fawzi et al., 1998). Although low levels of vitamin A were associated with a higher risk of perinatal HIV transmission in Africa, controlled trials have not shown that vitamin A or other vitamin supplementation could decrease the rate of perinatal HIV transmission (Coutsoudis et al., 1999; Fawzi et al., 2000).

Micronutrient intake or micronutrient levels are not consistently correlated with disease progression (Abrams et al., 1993; Baum and Shor-Posner 1998; Baum et al., 1997; Duggan and Fawzi, 2001; Tang et al., 1993). Coutsoudis and associates (1995) reported that vitamin A supplementation reduced diarrheal morbidity in HIV-infected children by about 50%. Improved immune status was reported in other studies (Guarino et al., 2002; Hanekom et al., 2002).

Vitamin A supplementation reduced overall mortality by 63%, AIDS-related mortality by 68%, and diarrhea-associated mortality by 92% among HIV-infected Tanzanian children aged 6 months to 5 years (Fawzi et al., 1999).

Low serum B_{12} levels have been observed in HIV-infected individuals. Low B_{12} levels are associated with neurologic abnormalities, impaired cognition, decreased CD4 counts, and increased toxicity of antiretroviral drugs (Tang and Smit, 1998).

High baseline values of vitamin E have been associated with decreased HIV progression; supplementation with vitamin E and vitamin C decreased viral load (Allard et al., 1998; Tang and Smit, 1998).

A high intake of micronutrients is associated with slower HIV disease progression (Abrams et al., 1993; Tang et al., 1996). A higher baseline CD4 count is correlated with intake of riboflavin, thiamine, and niacin. Multivitamin use and vitamin E, riboflavin, vitamin C, thiamine, and vitamin A intake is inversely associated with disease progression. High intakes of niacin, vitamins B_1, B_2, and B_6 are associated with slower progression to AIDS and lower mortality.

Liver and Pancreatic Abnormalities

Fluctuating elevations of hepatic transaminases are a frequent finding and often a diagnostic challenge. Infectious causes, notably the hepatitis viruses and CMV, EBV, and MAI must be excluded. Cryptosporidial infection of the biliary tree is described in adults and in one child (Margulis et al., 1986). Drugs may be implicated, especially the rifamycins and antifungal azoles. Ceftriaxone and other antibiotics are implicated in biliary sludging (Zinberg et al., 1991). Indinavir (IDV) causes jaundice in children and adults.

Pancreatitis is an uncommon finding in children before the AIDS era. It can result from opportunistic infections, such as CMV, or more often a side effect of therapy, in particular as a dose-dependent toxicity of dideoxyinosine (ddI) or 3TC (Butler et al., 1993; Miller et al., 1992). The precise mechanism is not well understood (Underwood and Frye, 1993).

Therapy

Therapeutic interventions for growth failure must be individualized after a thorough diagnostic evaluation. In the absence of specific infections or endocrine complications, a combination of appetite stimulants, enteral supplements and, if necessary, parenteral feeding to counteract wasting can be used.

Hematologic Abnormalities

Anemia

All three hematopoietic cell lines can be affected by HIV infection, but direct HIV infection of marrow precursors is unusual (Molina et al., 1990; Scadden et al., 1989). HIV can infect human bone marrow stromal fibroblasts, an important source of trophic and inhibitory regulators of hematopoietic progenitors (Scadden et al., 1990). Disruption of the bone marrow microenvironment may explain some of the effects of HIV on hematopoiesis. Marrow aspirates or biopsies in HIV-infected children typically show maturational arrest of each cell line. The cell lines may be differentially affected. Dyserythropoiesis with megaloblastic changes and nucleated red blood cells, dysmegakaryopoiesis, and a shift to the left of myeloid precursors may be found.

The most common hematologic abnormality is anemia, which, depending on definition, stage of disease, and concomitant myelosuppressive drug exposure, is seen in up to 94% of HIV-infected children (Butler et al., 1991; Ellaurie et al., 1990; Folks et al., 1988; Northfelt et al., 1991; Pizzo et al., 1988; Stella et al., 1987). Severe anemia has been shown to be an indicator for disease progression in some series (Ellaurie et al., 1990; Tovo et al., 1992). The incidence of anemia increases with HIV severity (Northfelt et al., 1991).

AZT therapy is a common cause of anemia; it begins to appear 6 weeks after therapy with a fall in hemoglobin and a progressive increase in erythrocyte mean corpuscular volume (Richman et al., 1987). Recombinant human erythropoietin can be used to treat AZT-induced anemia (Eron et al., 1995). Drugs used for treatment or opportunistic infection prophylaxis may also cause anemia (Gordin et al., 1984; Kovacs et al., 1989; Real et al., 1986; Rios et al., 1985; Sattler et al., 1988). Dapsone may cause hemolytic anemia or generalized myelosuppression. Children with HIV-associated malignancy may develop anemia from the chemotherapy.

Infectious causes of anemia are common. *Mycobacterium avium* complex (MAC) can cause anemia, especially in its advanced stage. Parvovirus B19 can cause anemia in HIV and in other immunodeficiencies (Frickhofen et al., 1990; Northfelt et al., 1991; Mitchell et al., 1990). Parvovirus B19 can also result in pure red cell aplasia (Frickhofen et al., 1990; Parmentier et al., 1992). Autoimmune hemolytic anemia may occur in HIV, often associated with hypergammaglobulinemia (Murphy et al., 1987; Toy et al., 1985; Van der Lelie et al., 1987). Bone marrow infiltration with tuberculosis, histoplasmosis, and other infectious agents may result in generalized pancytopenia.

Neutropenia

Neutropenia (defined as an absolute neutrophil count below 500 or 1500 cells/μl) is common and is the major dose-limiting toxicity to AZT and other antiretroviral drugs. Ganciclovir for CMV and trimethoprim-sulfamethoxazole (TMP-SMX) for PCP are common causes of neutropenia. Side effects of therapy are the most common cause of neutropenia, but opportunistic infections with CMV and MAI may be implicated (Northfelt et al., 1991).

Defective neutrophil chemotaxis, killing, and phagocytosis have been reported (Ellis et al., 1988; Groopman et al., 1987; Murphy et al., 1988). Granulocytic stimulating factors (GM-CSF and granulocyte colony-stimulating factor [G-CSF]) have been used to treat granulocytopenia in adults; but few data are available in children (Groopman et al., 1987).

Thrombocytopenia

Thrombocytopenia may be the presenting complaint of HIV infection (Rigaud et al., 1992). It may result from direct effects of HIV, opportunistic infections of the marrow, autoimmune destruction, sequestration in the spleen, antiretroviral medication, or rarely, an artifact caused by platelet clumping in EDTA-anticoagulated samples. HIV immune complexes containing antibody to envelope glycoproteins may nonspecifically deposit on platelet membranes, causing their removal by the reticuloendothelial system (Karpatkin, 1989). Direct infection of megakaryocytes may be an additional etiology of thrombocytopenia.

Treatment of thrombocytopenia includes corticosteroids, intravenous immunoglobulin, Rho (D) immune globulin, cytotoxic agents, plasmapheresis, IFN-α, and splenectomy (Northfelt et al., 1991).

Coagulopathies

Several coagulopathies have been described in HIV infection. Vitamin K deficiency is not uncommon and easily corrected. Lupus anticoagulants may cause a prolongation of the activated partial thromboplastin time not corrected by the addition of normal plasma (Scadden et al., 1989). Disseminated intravascular coagulation complicating fulminant infections is rare in HIV-infected children.

Cardiac Abnormalities

HIV-infected children may develop a number of cardiovascular abnormalities, many of which are associated with poor survival (Harmon et al., 2002; Lipshultz et al., 1998, 2000a, 2000b, 2002; Starc et al., 1999a, 1999b; UNAIDS/WHO, 2002). These include persistent tachycardia, increased left ventricular mass, decreased left ventricular function, and abnormalities of cardiovascular structure and function on the fetal echocardiogram. An association between encephalopathy and cardiovascular morbidity has also been described (Lipshultz et al., 2002).

HIV-infected children who have baseline depressed left ventricular fractional shortening or contractibility; increased left ventricular dimension, thickness, mass, or wall stress; or increased heart rate or blood pressure have a higher mortality than HIV-infected children without these cardiac abnormalities. An increased risk of sudden infant death has also been reported (Harmon et al., 2002).

Malignancies

Many pediatric immunodeficiencies are associated with an increased risk malignancy (Groopman and Broder, 1989; Penn, 1988) (see Chapter 39). In adults with HIV, the risk of KS is estimated to be 20,000 times greater than in the general population, particularly among homosexual and bisexual men following sexual exposure (Beral et al., 1990). KS lesions regularly harbor DNA of human herpesvirus 8 (HHV-8) or KS-associated herpesvirus (KSHV); virus is found in the spindle cells of the tumor, most of which are latently infected. Latent infection by HHV-8 also occurs in B lymphocytes and is associated with several uncommon lymphoproliferative syndromes (Cesarman and Knowles, 1999; Chuck et al., 1996).

NHL is about 60 times more common in AIDS patients than in the general U.S. population (Beral et al.,

1991; Pluda et al., 1990a). In 1992, HIV-associated lymphomas were estimated to be 8% to 27% of approximately 36,000 of all newly diagnosed cases of lymphoma in the United States (Gail et al., 1991). Following aggressive treatment with antiretroviral agents and prophylaxis for opportunistic infections, the incidence of HIV-associated lymphomas has remained constant at about 1.6% per year (Moore et al., 1991).

Other malignancies associated with HIV include papilloma virus–associated malignancies such as anal carcinoma and invasive cervical cancer (Goedert, 2000).

In children, the exact incidence of malignancies is not known. Currently the number of HIV-infected children who ultimately develop a malignancy represents about 2% of the AIDS-defining events in the United States. This increases to about 3% in adolescents 13 to 19 years of age and to 9% in young adults 20 to 24 years of age (Mueller et al., 1999a, 1999b). The majority of these malignancies are NHL, divided equally between Burkitt's and immunoblastic NHL of the CNS and KS.

The Italian registry of 1331 HIV-infected children followed for a median time of 6.5 years identified 35 patients and 36 malignancies (Caselli et al., 2000; Serraino and Franceschi, 1996; Serraino et al., 1992). The cumulative incidence of HIV-associated malignancies was 4.2 per 1000 children per year among perinatally infected children. Overall, 393 children died at a median age of 3 years. Malignancies primarily occurred in symptomatic children with significant immunodeficiency although asymptomatic and immunologically competent children also developed malignancies.

The most common tumor (81%) was NHL, which involved the lymph nodes, parotid glands, and most commonly the CNS. The immunophenotype was characteristically of the B-cell lineage with detection of EBV genome in most cases. Other less common malignancies included splenic sarcoma, KS, acute lymphoblastic leukemia, Hodgkin's disease, leiomyoma, carcinoma of the vulva, and hepatoblastoma.

In the United States the cumulative number of children younger than the age of 13 years in whom a malignancy was the AIDS-defining illness was 99 (as of December 1993). This represented 2% of the total 5210 children with AIDS. Of these, 25 had KS, 39 had Burkitt's lymphoma (which is not normally associated with immunosuppression), 20 had an immunoblastic lymphoma, and 15 had a primary CNS lymphoma. Grouping the lymphomas together yields a 360-fold increased risk of observed to expected cases in the AIDS group from birth to 19 years old. In addition, an increased incidence of leiomyomas and leiomyosarcomas, not previously associated with immunodeficiency, was noted (Mueller, 1999a, 1999b; Mueller et al., 1992a).

Granovsky and associates (1998) retrospectively surveyed the Children's Cancer Group and the NCI for the types of cancer that occurred between July 1982 and February 1997 in HIV-infected children. They identified 64 children with malignancies, 58% of whom acquired HIV perinatally and 34% of whom acquired HIV through transfusion of blood products. The median age for cancer diagnosis was 13.4 years. Sixty-five percent of the malignancies were NHL, and seventy percent were leiomyosarcomas. Five children developed acute leukemia, three children had KS, two children had Hodgkin's disease, one child had vaginal carcinoma, and one child had neuroendocrine carcinoma. The median survival in NHL was 6 months, and in leiomyosarcoma the survival was 12 months.

The incidence of malignancy in HIV-infected children is likely to be significantly higher in developing countries with different tumor types represented (e.g., retinoblastoma, nasopharyngeal carcinoma, rhabdomyosarcomas) (Mueller, 1999a, 1999b). The most common malignancies include NHL, acute lymphoblastic leukemia, and KS (Athale et al., 1995; Chitsike and Siziya, 1998).

The diagnosis of NHL is often delayed in HIV-infected children because of similarities in the symptomatology between HIV infection and NHL. Differences in histology of NHL exist between HIV-infected and noninfected children. A more indolent anaplastic large-cell lymphoma is frequent in HIV-infected children, whereas small noncleaved tumors with the high-growth fraction are most common in uninfected children (Mueller et al., 1999a, 1999b). Most CNS lymphomas in HIV-infected children are high-grade tumors, primarily of B-cell origin and most often associated with EBV (Del Mistro et al., 1990; Epstein et al., 1988; Funkhouser et al., 1998; Shad and McGrath, 1997; Tirelli et al., 1995).

Hodgkin's disease occurs in an earlier age in HIV-infected children than in the general population (Tirelli et al., 1995). Both in adults and in children, Hodgkin's disease in HIV presents as an aggressive, lymphocytic-depleted tumor with mixed cellularity. In more than 78% of patients, there is evidence for latent EBV infection, and 80% of the tumors contain monoclonal EBV genomes (Tirelli et al., 1995). Mueller (1999a, 1999b) suggested that lymphoproliferative disorders represent a link between lymphocyte proliferation in HIV-infected children and malignancy.

Although smooth muscle tumors are rare in HIV-infected children, representing less than 2% of all cancers, an increased incidence of leiomyomas and leiomyosarcomas has been described (Granovsky et al., 1998). EBV has been demonstrated by in situ hybridization and PCR (Mueller, 1999a, 1999b).

The shorter life expectancy, along with concerns regarding additional immunosuppression and infectious complications, has prevented HIV-infected children from receiving adequate tumor chemotherapy. Studies from the Italian registry indicate that severe toxicity is uncommon in HIV-infected patients with malignancy, at least for NHL (Caselli et al., 2000). In general, however, the types of malignancies occurring in HIV-infected children respond poorly to treatment (Mueller, 1999a, 1999b).

Bacterial Infections

Infectious complications include recurrent bacterial, mycobacterial, viral, protozoal, and fungal infections. HIV-infected children are very susceptible to invasive bacterial infections compared with HIV-infected adults, prompting the CDC to add the category of invasive bacterial infections to the list of pediatric AIDS-defining illnesses (CDC, 1994a).

Recurrent and serious bacterial infections are a hallmark of the B-cell defect in HIV-infected children, which may occur even before evidence of a T-cell deficiency. Antibody deficiency alone, however, does not explain their marked susceptibility to infection; thus it is likely that defects in neutrophil function, functional asplenia, complement defects, and macrophage dysfunction contribute to this susceptibility (Krasinski et al., 1988).

If central venous catheter–associated infections are excluded, the most common bacterial pathogens are the polysaccharide-encapsulated organisms, particularly *Streptococcus pneumoniae* (Krasinski et al., 1988; Roilides et al., 1991b). Excluding otitis media, among 204 infectious episodes in 105 children reported by Roilides and colleagues (1991b), soft tissue infections were most frequent (34%), followed by bacteremias, pneumonia, and sinusitis. In other series the most common clinical syndromes resulting from bacterial infection were pneumonia, bacteremia, and urinary tract infection (Dankner et al., 2001). Less frequent are osteomyelitis, meningitis, abscesses, and septic arthritis. Sinusitis, adenitis, mastoiditis, and internal organ abscess sites occurred at frequencies less than 2%.

Severe bacterial infections may occur at a much higher CD4 count and percentage than that observed for susceptibility to PCP (Spector et al., 1994). Late-onset group B streptococcal disease may occur as late as 5 months of age (Di John et al., 1990).

An increasing incidence of *Pseudomonas* infections has been reported (Roilides et al., 1992). These were most commonly associated with central venous catheters, especially if a *Pseudomonas* species other than *Pseudomonas aeruginosa* was isolated. Only 4 of the 13 bacteremic children in this series were neutropenic. Of the catheter-related infections, 65% were cured without removal of the line.

Several case reports of *Bordetella pertussis* infection presenting in older children and adults with HIV infection despite complete prior immunizations have been reported (Adamson et al., 1989; Nordmann et al., 1992). Nasopharyngeal carriage may be prolonged, despite erythromycin therapy. This susceptibility may result from an impaired antibody response to bacterial toxoids as present in HIV-infected children (Borkowsky et al., 1992). Furthermore, intact cell-mediated immunity may be required to eliminate an intracellular phase of *B. pertussis* (Doebbeling et al., 1990).

The use of ART in children has dramatically decreased the morbidity and mortality from bacterial and opportunistic infections in the United States. However, both remain high in developing countries, with the combined adverse effects of immunodeficiency, malnutrition, crowding, contaminated water supply, and inadequate health care. In addition to the types of infections observed in developed countries, TB, CMV, and syphilis are common. Mortality rates may reach as much as 50% by 1 year of age in some developing countries. The deaths are primarily due to pulmonary infections, diarrhea, and malnutrition.

Mycobacterial Infections

Mycobacterial infections, particularly with MAI, are common in HIV-infected children and adults with advanced disease (CD4, <50 cells/mm^3) (Chaisson et al., 1998; Lewis et al., 1992; Nightingale et al., 1993). MAC consists of several related species that are ubiquitous in the environment. Typical presentation includes recurrent fevers, night sweats, abdominal pain and bloating, and weight loss. A diagnosis of systemic infection requires culture of the organisms from blood because stool and respiratory isolates may only represent colonization. However, in most prospectively studied adults with such colonization, bacteremia eventually develops (Chin et al., 1994). Two blood cultures can identify 98% of cases of MAC bacteremia.

Prophylaxis with either clarithromycin or azithromycin is recommended in patients with severe immunodeficiency. Although azithromycin combined with rifabutin is more effective it is not recommended routinely because of the increased risk of adverse effects and increased costs (CDC, 2002a, 2002c; http://www.aidsinfo.nih.gov/guidelines/).

Current therapy consists of initial treatment with clarithromycin plus ethambutol. Rifabutin may be added to this regimen, but the dose may require modification if other drugs are administered. Efficacy studies in adults with less than 75 CD4 cells/mm^3 indicate that rifabutin can halve the incidence of MAI infection during the course of treatment (Nightingale et al., 1993).

Mycobacterium tuberculosis is an emerging problem, especially in developing countries. The development of strains multiply resistant to isoniazid, rifampin, and other drugs in Miami and New York poses a serious threat to patients and their caregivers (Beck-Sague et al., 1992; Fischl et al., 1992; Khouri et al., 1992; Starke et al., 1992).

Diagnosis is confounded by anergy to purified protein derivative (PPD) in HIV-infected children. Gastric lavage was more sensitive than bronchoalveolar lavage (BAL) in one series of 20 children (Abadco and Steiner, 1992).

All HIV-infected children with a positive tuberculin skin test should receive a chest x-ray and clinical evaluation for TB. HIV-infected individuals with symptoms suggestive of TB should undergo prompt evaluation regardless of their skin test status (CDC, 2002a, 2002c; http://www.aidsinfo.nih.gov/guidelines/). HIV-infected individuals with a positive tuberculin skin test but no evidence of active TB or no history of treatment for active or latent TB should be treated as if they had latent TB.

Options for treatment include isoniazid, rifampin, or rifabutin or therapy with either rifampin and pyrazinamide or rifabutin and pyrazinamide (CDC, 1993d, 2002a, 2002c; Neu et al., 1999; http://www.aidsinfo.

nih.gov/guidelines/). Infants who are born to HIV-infected mothers should have a skin test for TB at or before 9 to 12 months of age. The infant should be retested at least once per year. HIV-infected children who live in households with skin test–positive individuals should be evaluated for TB. Children exposed to a person who has active TB should be given preventive therapy after the valuation for active TB has been performed regardless of their skin test results (CDC, 2002a, 2002c; Pape et al., 1993; http://www.aidsinfo.nih.gov/guidelines/).

Viral Infections

Varicella-Zoster

HIV-infected children are at substantially greater risk for serious morbidity and mortality from a wide variety of viral pathogens. Of the herpes group, primary varicella can be associated with visceral dissemination (Jura et al., 1989) and encephalitis (Silliman et al., 1993). Subsequent varicella-zoster virus (VZV) infection may recur with increasing frequency as the underlying immunodeficiency progresses, although it is seen at all stages of disease. Lesions may be atypical, with hyperkeratosis and increased pigmentation or hypopigmentation without obvious vesiculation (Leibovitz et al., 1992; Pahwa et al., 1988). They are usually painful. Chronic suppressive therapy with acyclovir, famciclovir, or foscarnet may be required, but the development of drug resistance is a problem (Jacobson et al., 1990; Pahwa et al., 1988; Zeichner and Read, 1999).

Herpes Simplex

Herpes simplex virus (HSV) has been associated with severe herpetic gingivostomatitis, esophagitis, and chronic labial infections (Hanson and Kaplan, 1990). Oral acyclovir may be useful for preventing frequent occurrences of severe mucocutaneous HSV infections (Working Group on Antiretroviral Therapy, 1993; Zeichner and Read, 1999) and for treatment of disseminated infection. For patients with acyclovir-resistant HSV infection, alternative therapies include foscarnet, valacyclovir, or famciclovir.

Cytomegalovirus

CMV may cause retinitis; pneumonitis; enterocolitis; hepatitis; and, more rarely, esophagitis, pancreatitis, or adrenal insufficiency (Hanson and Kaplan, 1990). Treatment options for CMV include ganciclovir, cidofovir, and foscarnet (Bueno et al., 2002; Butler et al., 1992; Zeichner and Read, 1999). Ganciclovir is more effective than acyclovir, but its tolerable profile is less optimal and it is associated with myelosuppression. Foscarnet and cidofovir are not associated with myelosuppression but have significant nephrotoxicity. Retinal implants with slow-release formulations of ganciclovir are used in adults with some promise. It may be possible to use this approach in children older than 6 years of age. HAART has dramatically decreased CMV and its complications.

Other Herpesviruses

EBV is implicated in the cause of LIP and a polyclonal lymphoproliferative disorder difficult to distinguish from lymphoma (see earlier section on malignancies).

Illnesses with HHV-6 and HHV-7 in this population are largely unknown, although seroepidemiologic studies suggest that most children seroconvert by age 2 or 3 years (Clark et al., 1993a; Pruksananonda et al., 1992). In vitro, individual CD4 T cells can be co-infected with HHV-6 and HIV, and HHV-6 transactivates the HIV LTR (Ensoli et al., 1989; Lusso and Gallo, 1994).

HHV-8 has similarities in DNA sequences to EBV. HHV-8 DNA sequences have been found in patients with KS. Studies in infants and children in Zambia indicate that in utero infection is possible but that transmission can also occur intrapartum or postpartum (Brayfield et al., 2003).

Hepatitis Viruses

Infection with hepatitis viruses A, B, and C may resultant in fulminant hepatitis, and hepatis B virus (HBV) and hepatitis C virus (HBC) can result in a chronic aggressive or frequently relapsing course (Bodsworth et al., 1991; Martin et al., 1989). Conflicting results have been reported on the frequency of perinatal HCV transmission (Dal Molin et al., 2002; Hershow et al., 1997), varying from no transmission to high rates. This may result from differing criteria to define perinatal infection, variation in the study population, or the length of follow-up. Cesarean section may reduce the risk of perinatal HCV infection (Steininger et al., 2003).

New treatments are available for hepatitis B and C. IFN-α for was approved for treatment of pediatric hepatitis B after it was shown to promote DNA negativity and HBeAg loss in a significant number of patients. Lamivudine efficacy trials demonstrated complete virologic responses in only 25% of patients after 1 year and a higher percentage of patients who had transaminase levels more than two times the upper limit of normal (Dikici et al., 2002; Jonas et al., 2002; Sokal, 2002). Combination therapy with IFN-α and lamivudine had a greater beneficial effect than IFN-α monotherapy, but at 6 months, both groups were similar (Dikici et al., 2002).

Nucleotide analogs such as adefovir dipoxivil (Preveon) are under evaluation in adults and children (Hadziyannis et al., 2003; Marcellin et al., 2003). Adults treated with 4 weeks of therapy demonstrated significant histologic, biologic, and biochemical improvement without serious side effects. There was no evidence of emergence of tenofovir-resistant HBV mutations. HCV infection in adults and children has been treated with IFN-α plus ribavirin (Wirth et al., 2002).

Other Viral Infections

Respiratory pathogens, particularly respiratory syncytial virus (RSV), parainfluenza III, and adenoviruses may cause severe and even fatal pneumonitis. They may also be shed for prolonged periods, creating a significant dilemma during hospitalization. PCP complicated by superinfection with any of these respiratory pathogens carries a poor prognosis.

Measles is associated with a high incidence of pneumonitis and occasionally encephalitis (Kaplan et al., 1992). The case fatality rate of measles pneumonitis is estimated to be between 33% and 45% in developing countries, although this may be an overestimate based on a series of hospitalized patients. The clinical presentation is frequently atypical, and rash is absent in about 30% of cases. Treatment options are limited, enhancing the need for widespread preventative vaccination in the community.

Protozoal and Fungal Infections

It is appropriate to discuss protozoal and fungal infections together, because one of the most significant opportunistic pathogens, *P. carinii*, has features of both groups. Morphologically, and in terms of treatment, *P. carinii* resembles a protozoon, but at a biochemical and molecular level it has features of a fungus (Masur, 1992). Invasive fungal infections with *Cryptococcus neoformans*, *Coccidioides immitis*, and *Histoplasma capsulatum* occur less frequently in the pediatric population than in adults but carry a similar high morbidity and mortality. Over the past 10 years, the therapeutic options for invasive fungal infections have widened with the introduction of the triazole compounds fluconazole and itraconazole and lipid formulations of amphotericin B.

Pneumocystis carinii *Infection*

CLINICAL FEATURES

Early in the HIV epidemic, *P. carinii* was noted to be a cause of pulmonary disease in young children with HIV despite high CD4 counts (Rubinstein et al., 1986). PCP was the AIDS indicator disease in 38% of 3471 reported pediatric AIDS cases through 1991. An early and frequently fatal peak is observed in infants around the age of 6 months who presumably experience their primary infection.

Scott and co-workers (1989) reported a median survival time of 1 month from the onset of PCP in a natural history study of HIV-infected children. The presenting features were tachypnea (88%), dyspnea (88%), cough (86%), and fever (79%) in the series of 27 cases reported by Connor and associates (1991a). The presentation may be insidious over weeks rather than acute. Hypoxemia is the hallmark of the disease. Radiologically, PCP can present as a spectrum with almost no infiltrates to frank consolidation.

DIAGNOSIS

The diagnosis can frequently be established by induced sputum analysis, but if this is negative and clinical suspicion is high, BAL is indicated (Ognibene et al., 1989). BAL is the diagnostic procedure of choice where the prevalence of *Pneumocystis* is low and where induced sputum analysis is difficult to obtain. Fiberoptic bronchoscopy with transbronchial biopsy has been used as the initial diagnostic procedure in patients with diffuse lung disease but carries a risk of pneumothorax (Mitchell et al., 1981). Open lung biopsy is rarely necessary but is the most sensitive means of establishing a diagnosis. PCR for *P. carinii* sequences is under research evaluation.

TREATMENT

Therapy should take into account which prophylactic regimen has failed. The drug of choice remains TMP-SMX, and only a documented serious allergic response (e.g., angioneurotic edema) should prompt alternative therapy. Based on data from adult studies, adjunctive steroids are used for any child with an arterial oxygen pressure lower than 70 mm Hg (National Institutes of Health/University of California Expert Panel, 1990).

Intravenous pentamidine may be used in patients who have broken through TMP-SMX prophylaxis, but careful monitoring for hypoglycemia, pancreatitis, and dysrhythmias is mandatory. Atovaquone is a hydroxynaphthoquinone with activity against both *P. carinii* and *Toxoplasma gondii* (see later). It can only be given orally, and the bioavailability of the initial tablet preparation is erratic. Absorption can be improved twofold to threefold if taken with fat-containing meals, which many individuals with advanced HIV disease cannot tolerate.

PROPHYLAXIS

Prophylaxis for PCP is a constantly evolving subject (CDC, 1991a, 1995, 2002a, 2002c). Prophylaxis may have benefits beyond prevention of PCP. Maldonado and associates (1998) showed that there is an overall delay in reaching AIDS-defining end points during the first 3 years of life, although there was a higher occurrence of encephalopathy as the AIDS-defining event.

HIV-infected adults and adolescents (including pregnant women and those on HAART) should receive chemoprophylaxis against PCP if they have a CD4 count less than 200 cells/mm^3 or a history of oropharyngeal candidiasis. Persons with a CD4 percentage less than 14% or a history of an AIDS-defining illness but who do not otherwise qualify should be considered for prophylaxis. When monitoring the CD4 count at least every 3 months is not possible, initiation of chemoprophylaxis at a CD4 count of less than 250 cells/mm^3 also should be considered.

TMP-SMX (Bactrim, Septra, Co-trimoxazole) is the recommended prophylactic agent (Table 29-10). In adults, one double-strength tablet per day is preferred (160 mg trimethoprim/800 mg sulfamethoxazole). However, one single-strength tablet per day is also effective and might be better tolerated. One double-strength tablet three times per week is also effective. One double-strength tablet per day confers cross-protection against toxoplasmosis and some common respiratory bacterial infections. Lower dosages of TMP-SMX also might confer such protection.

....

TABLE 29-10 · PROPHYLACTIC DRUGS FOR PCP IN ADULTS

Preferred Prophylaxis (Trimethoprim-Sulfamethoxazole) (TMP-SMX)

TMP-SMX 1 double strength (DS) tablet each day
TMP-SMX 1 single strength (SS) tablet each day
TMP-SMX 1 DS tablet orally three times per week

Alternate Prophylaxis

Dapsone, 50 mg orally twice each day or 100 mg orally once each day

Dapsone, 50 mg orally each day plus pyrimethamine 50 mg orally each day plus leucovorin 25 mg orally each week

Dapsone, 200 mg orally each day plus pyrimethamine 75 mg orally each day plus leucovorin 25 mg orally each week

Aerosolized pentamidine 300 mg via Respirgard II nebulizer once each month

Atovaquone 1500 mg orally once each day

PCP = *Pneumocystis carinii* pneumonia.

For patients with an adverse reaction that is not life threatening, TMP-SMX should be continued if clinically feasible; for those who have discontinued such therapy because of an adverse reaction, reinstitution of TMP-SMX should be strongly considered after the adverse event has resolved. Patients who have experienced adverse events, especially fever and rash, might better tolerate reintroduction of the drug with a gradual increase in dose (desensitization) as per published regimens or reintroduction of TMP-SMX at a reduced dose or frequency; up to 70% of patients can tolerate reinstitution of therapy.

If TMP-SMX cannot be tolerated, alternative prophylactic regimens include dapsone, dapsone plus pyrimethamine plus folinic acid (leucovorin), aerosolized pentamidine administered by the Respirgard nebulizer (Marquest, Englewood, Colorado), and atovaquone. Because dapsone causes hemolytic anemia in individuals with low levels of erythrocyte glucose-5-phosphate dehydrogenase, this should be assessed before its use. Atovaquone appears to be as effective as aerosolized pentamidine or dapsone but is substantially more expensive than the other regimens.

For patients seropositive for *T. gondii* who cannot tolerate TMP-SMX, recommended alternatives to TMP-SMX for prophylaxis against both PCP and toxoplasmosis include dapsone plus pyrimethamine or atovaquone with or without pyrimethamine. Regimens containing pyrimethamine must also include folinic acid (leucovorin).

The following regimens generally cannot be recommended as alternatives because data regarding their efficacy for PCP prophylaxis are insufficient for a firm recommendation: aerosolized pentamidine administered by other nebulization devices, intermittently administered parenteral pentamidine, oral pyrimethamine plus sulfadoxine, oral clindamycin plus primaquine, and intravenous trimetrexate. However, clinicians may consider using these agents in unusual situations in which the recommended agents cannot be administered.

DISCONTINUING PROPHYLAXIS IN ADULTS

Recommendations have been provided for the discontinuation of PCP prophylaxis (CDC, 2002a). Initial reports from three prospective observational studies, one retrospective review, and one randomized trial suggest that PCP prophylaxis in adults can be safely discontinued in patients responding to HAART who have a sustained increase in CD4 cells from less than 200 cells/mm³ to more than 200 cells/mm³.

Such reports have mostly included patients receiving primary prophylaxis (e.g., no prior episode of PCP) and PI-containing ART regimens. In these studies, median follow-up ranged from 6 to 12 months and the median CD4 T-lymphocyte count at the time prophylaxis was discontinued was greater than 300 cell/mm³. At the time PCP prophylaxis was discontinued, many patients had sustained suppression of HIV plasma RNA levels below detection limits.

Although optimal criteria for discontinuing PCP prophylaxis are still being assessed, providers may wish to discontinue prophylaxis when patients have sustained a CD4 cells more than 200 cells/mm³ for at least 3 to 6 months. Additional criteria might include sustained reduction in viral load for at least 3 to 6 months.

No data are available to guide recommendations for reinstituting primary prophylaxis. Pending the availability of such data, a reasonable approach would be to use the criteria for initiating prophylaxis. Adults and adolescents with a history of PCP should be given chemoprophylaxis (i.e., secondary prophylaxis or chronic maintenance therapy).

SECONDARY PROPHYLAXIS

Adult patients receiving secondary prophylaxis (e.g., prior episode of PCP) also appear to be a low risk for PCP when their CD4 cells have increased to more than 200 cells/mm³ on combination ART and have remained above this level for at least 3 months. Discontinuation of PCP prophylaxis (with continuation of effective ART) appears to be safe in such patients.

PROPHYLAXIS IN PREGNANCY AND THE NEONATAL PERIOD

Chemoprophylaxis for PCP should be administered to pregnant women as is done for other adults and adolescents. TMP-SMX is the recommended agent; dapsone is an alternative. However, caution should be used in providing TMP-SMX during pregnancy in women who may be nutritionally deprived because the drug may result in folic acid deficiency.

Because of concerns regarding the possible teratogenicity associated with drug exposure during the first trimester, providers may choose to withhold prophylaxis during the first trimester. In such cases, aerosolized pentamidine may be considered because of its lack of systemic absorption.

Discontinuing prophylaxis with TMP-SMX for 1 week after delivery may be considered in women who breastfeed to avoid jaundice in the infant.

Children born to HIV-infected mothers should start prophylaxis with TMP-SMX at 4 to 6 weeks of age

(Table 29-11). Prophylaxis can be discontinued when it is established that the infant is not HIV infected. HIV infection is excluded when two or more diagnostic tests are negative (i.e., HIV culture or HIV PCR). These are performed at 1 and 4 months of age or later. HIV can also be excluded in an asymptomatic infant when two or more HIV antibody tests are negative after 6 months of age.

HIV-infected children and children whose infection status remains unknown should continue prophylaxis for the first year of life. (See Table 29-12 for dosing.) The need for subsequent prophylaxis should be determined on the basis of age-specific CD4 T-lymphocyte count thresholds.

DISCONTINUING PROPHYLAXIS IN CHILDREN

The safety of discontinuing prophylaxis in HIV-infected children receiving HAART has not been studied. Children 1 to 2 years of age with CD4 cells less than $750/mm^3$ or CD4 percentage less than 15% or younger than 12 months should continue prophylaxis. Children with a history of PCP should receive lifelong chemoprophylaxis. Prophylaxis should be considered on a case-by-case basis for children who might otherwise be at risk for PCP, such as those with rapidly declining CD4 cells or children with category C status of HIV infection.

Toxoplasma gondii

Although there are several case reports of children with *T. gondii* infection, its prevalence is much lower in children than in adults (Miller and Remington, 1991). In adults, continuous pyrimethamine-sulfadiazine and folinic acid is recommended following treatment for active ocular or CNS toxoplasmosis (CDC, 2002a; Working Group on Antiretroviral Therapy, 1993; Zeichner and Read, 1999).

Candida albicans

C. albicans is the most common fungal infection in HIV. Recurrent oropharyngeal candidiasis was seen in 71%

TABLE 29-11 · RECOMMENDATIONS FOR PCP PROPHYLAXIS IN HIV EXPOSED INFANTS AND CHILDREN BY AGE AND INFECTION STATUS

Age and HIV Infection Status	PCP Prophylaxis
Birth to 4–6 weeks HIV exposed	None
4–6 weeks to 4 months HIV exposed	Prophylaxis
4–12 months	
HIV infected or indeterminate	Prophylaxis
HIV infection excluded	None
1–5 years HIV-infected	Prophylaxis if CD4 <500 cells/mm³ or <15% or history of PCP
>5 years HIV-infected	Prophylaxis if CD4 <200 cells/mm³ or <15% or history of PCP

PCP = *Pneumocystis carinii* pneumonia.

TABLE 29-12 · DRUG REGIMENS FOR PCP PROPHYLAXIS FOR CHILDREN 4 WEEKS OF AGE OR OLDER

Recommended Regimen

Oral suspension of TMX-SMX usually contains 40 mg of trimethoprim and 200 mg of sulfamethoxazole per teaspoon (5 ml)

Trimethoprim-sulfamethoxazole, 150 mg/m² per day of trimethoprim with 750 mg/m² per day of sulfamethoxazole administered orally in divided doses twice each day three times per week on consecutive days (e.g., Monday-Tuesday-Wednesday).

Acceptable Alternative TMX-SMX Dosage Schedules

150 mg/m² per day per day of trimethoprim with 750 mg/m² per day of sulfamethoxazole administered orally as a single daily dose three times per week on consecutive days (e.g., Monday-Tuesday-Wednesday).

150 mg/m² per day per day of trimethoprim with 750 mg/m² per day of sulfamethoxazole administered orally in divided doses twice a day and administered seven days per week.

150 mg/m² per day per day of trimethoprim with 750 mg/m² per day of sulfamethoxazole administered orally in divided doses twice a day and administered three times per week on alternate days (e.g., Monday-Wednesday-Friday).

Alternative Regimens If TMX-SMX Is Not Tolerated

Dapsone (children >1 month of age): 2 mg/kg (maximum 100 mg) administered orally once a day or 4 mg/kg (maximum 200 mg) orally every week. Because dapsone causes hemolytic anemia in individuals with low levels of the enzyme G6PD in their red blood cells, levels of this enzyme should be checked before using dapsone. In terms of side effects and survival, weekly dosing may be safer in children than daily dosing, but weekly dosing appears less effective in preventing PCP.

Aerosolized pentamidine (children 5 years of age or older) 300 mg administered via Respirgard II inhaler monthly.

Atovaquone (children 1–3 months of age and greater than 24 months of age): 30 mg/kg orally once a day (children 4–24 months of age) 45 mg/kg orally once a day.

If dapsone, aerosolized and pentamidine, and atovaquone are not tolerated, some clinicians use intravenous pentamidine (4 mg/kg) administered every 2 to 4 weeks.

PCP = *Pneumocystis carinii* pneumonia; TMX-SMX = trimethoprim-sulfamethoxazole.
Available at http://www.aidsinfo.nih.gov/guidelines/.

of 123 deceased patients followed at the NIH (Tudor-Williams and Pizzo, 1996). *Candida* esophagitis was diagnosed in 24%, usually on clinical and radiologic evidence. Disseminated candidiasis or fungemias are rare, except in patients with chronic indwelling intravenous devices (Walsh et al., 1993). *Torulopsis glabrata* and other candidal species may cause fungemia in association with such catheters.

For persistent or recurrent mucocutaneous candidiasis, chronic suppressive therapy is frequently required. Topical treatment with nystatin has limited efficacy for oropharyngeal candidiasis. Clotrimazole, ketoconazole, or fluconazole are alternatives (CDC, 2002a, 2002c; Zeichner and Read, 1999; http://www.aidsinfo.nih.gov/guidelines/). Esophageal and invasive infection require aggressive and often prolonged therapy with amphotericin or fluconazole. Alternative therapy includes ketoconazole or itraconazole (CDC, 2002a; Working Group on Antiretroviral Therapy, 1993; Zeichner and Read, 1999; http://www.aidsinfo.nih.gov/guidelines) (see Chapter 41).

Cryptococcus neoformans

C. neoformans is less prevalent in pediatric patients than in adults but can cause meningitis, with an insidious onset of malaise and altered mental status in older children (Ting et al., 1991). Chronic suppressive therapy with oral fluconazole is required following initial treatment with amphotericin B and 5-flucytosine (Working Group on Antiretroviral Therapy, 1993; Zeichner and Read, 1999). Studies in adults indicate that a combination of amphotericin B plus flucytosine results in fewer relapses then amphotericin B alone (Van der Horst et al., 1997).

Histoplasma capsulatum

Histoplasmosis presenting with fever, cough, pulmonary interstitial infiltrates, and sometimes dissemination to the CNS may occur, particularly in endemic areas of the Midwestern United States (Hanson and Kaplan, 1990). Treatment with amphotericin B or itraconazole is recommended. Pulmonary and sinus aspergillosis is an occasional complication that is seen in HIV-infected children, who usually have profound and persistent neutropenia (Walsh et al., 1993). Treatment consists of amphotericin B (Zeichner and Read, 1999).

Other Fungal and Protozoal Infections

Cryptosporidial infection may cause intractable diarrhea in some children, and there are few effective therapies (Curry et al., 1991). Complications include ascending infection of the biliary tree and pancreatitis. The role of *Isospora* and *Microsporidia* is not well documented in children, but *Giardia lamblia* can cause chronic diarrhea and malabsorption (CDC, 2002a; Smith et al., 1992).

LABORATORY FEATURES

CD4 Counts

The CD4 T-lymphocyte cell count (CD4 cells) and viral load, as determined by HIV RNA tests, have become the most reliable surrogate markers for following the course of HIV infection and making decisions regarding instituting therapy, changing therapy, discontinuing therapy, and instituting or discontinuing prophylactic antibiotics (Hughes et al., 1997).

An increase in CD4 cells coupled with a decrease in the viral load is indicative of a response to therapy and an improved prognosis (Kim et al., 2000; Marschner et al., 1998). In adults, CD4 T cells typically increase by more than 50 cells/ml 4 to 8 weeks after ART is started (Le Moing et al., 2002; Yamashita et al., 2001; Yeni et al., 2002). When the CD4 cells are more than $200/mm^3$ for 3 to 6 months, prophylaxis against certain opportunistic infections can often be stopped (CDC, 1995, 2002a). In children, changes in CD4 percentages of 5% should be viewed as significant (CDC, 2002c; http://www.aidsinfo.nih.gov/guidelines/).

RNA Viral Load

RNA tests are reliable to detection limits of 50 copies/ml. With repeated measurements, differences of 0.2 to 0.3 log_{10} (30% to 50%) are considered a significant change in viral load (Yeni et al., 2002). If ART is effective, a reduction of more than 90% is usually observed within 8 weeks of treatment. Failure to observe a decrease in viral load or an increase in viral load while on therapy suggests either inadequate combination therapy or pre-existing viral resistance.

In children, virologic response should be determined 4 weeks after therapy (CDC, 2002c; http://www.aidsinfo.nih.gov/guidelines/). The time to achieve a maximum response in children may vary because their baseline HIV RNA value may be significantly higher than that of adults (e.g., >1 million copies/ml), and a virologic response might not be observed until 12 or more weeks of therapy.

Sequential Measurements of CD4 Counts and Viral Load

Sequential measurements of CD4 cells and viral load are important to ascertain whether a continued beneficial effect of therapy exists. Changes in CD4 cells and HIV RNA levels are independent predicators of disease progression (CDC, 2002c; Yeni et al., 2002; http://www.aidsinfo.nih.gov/guidelines/; http://www.womenchildrenhiv.org; http://hivinsite.ucsf.edu).

Measurements of these variables are usually recommended at 4, 8 to 12, and 16 to 24 weeks following initiation of therapy. Once virologic control has been achieved (two sequential measurements below the level of detection; e.g., 50 copies/ml), measurements can be obtained every 8 to 12 weeks.

TREATMENT

Treatment for HIV is constantly evolving as understanding of the immunopathogenesis deepens and improved therapies are developed. Because current recommendations will likely be modified by the time this chapter appears, this discussion is limited to the broad principles of treatment and a review of selected published clinical studies. Drug doses and side effects are listed in Table 29-13. For detailed descriptions and information refer to "Guidelines for the Use of Antiretroviral Agents in Pediatric HIV Infection" (CDC, 2002c; http://www.aidsinfo.nih.gov/guidelines/; http://www.womenchildrenhiv.org; http://hivinsite.ucsf.edu).

Antiretroviral Therapy

The central role of the virus in the immunopathogenesis of HIV infection is becoming increasingly clear as more sensitive detection methods delineate the abundance of virus in the circulation and lymphoid organs at all

TABLE 29-13 · ANTIRETROVIRAL THERAPY DRUG DOSES AND TOXICITIES

Antiretroviral	Dose	Major Toxicities	Comments
Nucleoside Reverse Transcriptase Inhibitors	Neonatal is birth to <90 days of age		
Zidovudine (ZDV, AZT, Retrovir)	Oral 160 mg/m^2/dose every 8 hours Neonatal dose: 2 mg/kg every 6 hours IV 120 mg/m^2 every 6 hours or 20 mg/m^2/hour (continuous infusion) Adult: 200 mg 3 times a day or 300 mg twice daily	Neutropenia, anemia, nausea, headaches Rare: myopathy, myositis, lactic acidosis, hepatomegaly	Large volume of syrup not well tolerated in older children. Double dose for HIV encephalopathy.
Didanosine (ddI, dideoxyinosine, Videx)	90 to 150 mg/m^2 every 12 hours Neonatal: 50 mg/m^2/dose every 12 hours Enteric coated 125/200/250/400 mg capsules for older children Adult: 200 mg twice daily	Diarrhea and abdominal pain Rare: pancreatitis, peripheral neuropathy, lactic acidosis, hepatomegaly, steatosis	Constituted suspension stable for 30 days refrigerated. Ideally taken 1 hour before food or 2 hours after, but may be less important in children.
Stavudine (d4T, Zerit)	1 mg/kg/dose every 12 hours up to 30 kg 30–60 kg: 30 mg twice daily >60 kg: 40 mg twice daily Neonatal: unknown Adult: 40 mg twice daily	Headache, GI upset, skin rash, Rare: peripheral neuropathy and pancreatitis, hepatomegaly and steatosis	Large volume of suspension; capsules opened up well tolerated. Keep solution refrigerated. Stable for 30 days. Can give with food.
Lamivudine (3TC, Epivir)	3 mo–16 yr: 4 mg/kg/dose twice daily orally Maximum 150 mg bid Neonatal <30 days: 2 mg/kg/dose every 12 hours Adult: one tablet twice daily orally Combivir ZDV 300 mg + 3TC 150 mg per tablet	Headache, abdominal pain, rash Rare: pancreatitis, peripheral neuropathy, and neutropenia, abnormal liver function	Well tolerated. Can be given with food. Store solution at room temperature (use within 1 month of opening).
Abacavir (ABC, Ziagen)	3 mo–16 yr: 8 mg/kg/dose twice daily orally Maximum dose 300 mg twice daily Neonatal: no data, not approved Trizivir: ZDV 300 mg + 3TC 150 mg + ABC 300 mg per tablet Adult: 1 tablet twice daily orally	Up to 5% may develop hypersensitivity reaction, fever, malaise, mucositis, rash usually in first 6 weeks. Do not rechallenge with drug if hypersensitivity occurs	Syrup well tolerated or crush tablets. Must warn parents about hypersensitivity reaction.
Zalcitabine (ddC, dideoxycytidine, Hivid)	Adult: 0.75 mg 3 times per day Neonatal: 0.01 mg/kg/dose every 8 hours	Headache, GI upset, peripheral neuropathy; pancreatitis rare in children; hepatic toxicity; oral ulcers	Small tablets; syrup no longer available. No longer widely used in children.
Non-Nucleoside Reverse Transcriptase Inhibitors			
Nevirapine (NVP, Viramune)	2 mo–8 yr: initiate with 120–200 mg/m^2/dose once daily for 2 weeks then increase to 120–200 mg/m^2/dose every 12 hours if no rash occurs Neonatal: (still under evaluation) 120 mg/m^2/dose once daily for 2 weeks followed by 120 mg/m^2/dose every 12 hours for 2 weeks followed by 200 mg/m^2/dose every 12 hours Adult: 200 mg every 12 hours	Rash 10%–20% (can treat through), fever nausea, headache Rare: Stevens-Johnson; stop drug and monitor liver enzymes	Can be given with food. Few data on use with PI. Practice is to increase PI dose by about 30%. Induces cytochrome P450. Decreases concentrations of most protease inhibitors.
Efavirenz (EFV, DMP-266, Sustiva)	Daily single dose: 10–<15 kg: 200 mg; 15–<20 kg: 250 mg; 20–<25 kg: 300 mg; 25–<33 kg: 350 mg; 33–<40 kg 400 mg; >40 kg 600 mg Neonatal: no data Adult dose: 600 mg once daily	Rash (mild), CNS toxicity, somnolence, vivid dreams, abnormal thinking, confusion	Syrup available but with decreased bioavailability compared with tablets. Best given as bedtime dosing to reduce CNS side effects. Teratogenic in primates (avoid using in pregnancy).
Delavirdine (DLV, Rescriptor)	Pediatric and neonatal dose: unknown Adult dose: 600 mg twice daily or 400 mg 3 times a day orally	Headache, fatigue, rash, GI complaints	Dispersible tablets can be dissolved in water/Coke. No commercially available suspension. Rarely used.
Nucleotide Reverse Transcriptase Inhibitors			
Tenofovir (Viread)	Pediatric and neonatal dose: unknown Adult dose: 300 mg once daily		Approved for adults. Under evaluation in children.

Continued

TABLE 29-13 · ANTIRETROVIRAL THERAPY DRUG DOSES AND TOXICITIES—cont'd

Antiretroviral	Dose	Major Toxicities	Comments
Protease Inhibitors			
Indinavir (IDV, Crixivan)	Under evaluation 500 mg/m²/dose every 8 hours; lower doses in children with small body surface Neonatal: unknown Adult: 800 mg every 8 hours	Nausea, abdominal pain, hyperbilirubinemia (should not be used in neonates), renal stones, nephritis, hemolytic anemia, liver dysfunction, abnormal lipids Rare: diabetes, hemolytic anemia	Do not take with meals. Complex formula for syrup available. Advise fluid intake.
Ritonavir (RTV, Norvir)	Children >2 yr: 400 mg/m²/dose every 12 hours Start with 250 mg/m²/dose 12 hourly and increase over 5 days Neonatal: unknown Adult: 300 mg bid day 1; 400 mg bid day 2; 600 mg bid day 3	GI intolerance, headache, anorexia, increased liver enzymes, abnormal lipids Rare: hyperglycemia, hepatitis, diabetes, ketoacidosis	Take with food. Liquid tastes extremely bitter. Can help to take with peanut butter and follow with chocolate sauce or cheese. Note drug interactions. Syrup 80 mg/ml.
Saquinavir (SQV, Invirase) hard gel (Fortovase soft gel)	Children <16 yr: 50 mg/kg/dose every 8 hours (33 mg/kg every 8 hours when given with nelfinavir) Neonatal: unknown Adult: soft gel 1200 mg 3 times a day or 1600 twice daily	Rash, headache, GI complaints, abnormal lipids Rare: hyperglycemia, ketoacidosis, diabetes	Give with food. Sun photosensitivity.
Nelfinavir (NFV, Viracept)	Children: 20–30 mg/kg/dose 3 times a day Neonatal: under evaluation 40 mg/kg/dose every 12 hours Adult: 1250 twice daily or 750 mg 3 times a day	Mild/moderate diarrhea, vomiting, rash, abnormal lipids Rare: hyperglycemia, ketoacidosis, diabetes	Take with food. Crush tablets; powder available.
Lopinavir/ritonavir, (LPV, Kaletra)	Children: 230 mg/m² lopinavir/57.5 mg/m² ritonavir twice daily with food up to 400 mg lopinavir/100 mg ritonavir (when not using NVP or EFV) (higher dose when using NNRTI) Neonatal: unknown Adult: 533 mg lopinavir/133 mg ritonavir (4 capsules) twice daily	Rash, GI intolerance, abnormal lipids Rare: pancreatitis, hyperglycemia, ketoacidosis, diabetes, hepatitis	Liquid formulation: 80 mg lopinavir and 20 mg ritonavir per ml, bitter taste. Capsules large. Take with food. Drug interactions.
Amprenavir (APV, Agenerase)	<50 kg (4–12 years of age or 13–16 years of age): oral solution 22.5 mg/kg/dose twice daily or 17 mg/kg/dose 3 times a day Capsules 20 mg/kg/dose twice daily or 15 mg/kg/dose 3 times a day Not recommended for children <3 yr Neonatal: not recommended Adult: 1200 mg twice each day	GI, rash, abnormal lipids Rare: hyperglycemia, diabetes, hemolytic anemia	Large volume of syrup, bitter taste. Capsules either large size (200 mg) or need to take many small (50 mg). Pro-drug in development with improved bioavailability. Suspension contains polyethylene glycol: unsuitable for children <3 years.

CNS = central nervous system; GI = gastrointestinal; NNRTI = non-nucleoside reverse transcriptase inhibitor; PI = protease inhibitor.
Available at http://www.aidsinfo.nih.gov/guidelines/ CDC, 2002c; CDC 2002f http://www.aidsinfo.nih.gov/guidelines/; http://www.womenchildrenhiv.org; http://hivinsite.ucsf.edu.

stages of disease (Bagasra et al., 1992; Embretson et al., 1993; Pantaleo et al., 1993a; Piatak et al., 1993b). If antiretroviral agents were developed that could completely prevent viral replication, it would be rational to use these at the earliest possible stage of disease. In adults and adolescents, this would be at the time of acute infection, with the aim of reducing the initial burst of viremia and limiting the seeding of virus to the lymphoid organs, brain, and other sites. In infants, it would similarly be at the earliest stage of infection, which includes the perinatal period to diminish transmission or as soon as infection is confirmed postnatally.

The available agents cannot switch off viral replication completely, allowing subpopulations of virus to

evolve and mutate into potentially resistant or more pathogenic strains. Long-term therapy is necessary, requiring a balance between the potential benefits of early intervention and the side effects, cost, and selection of more resistant quasispecies associated with each drug. Table 29-13 lists the currently available ARTs.

Although many phase I and phase II studies have been performed in infants and children for pharmacokinetics and safety, fewer phase III efficacy trials have been conducted. Most antiretroviral combination approaches therefore rely on prior studies in adults. As new drugs become available, it is critical to assess their pharmacokinetics before they are used extensively in infants and children. Pediatric drugs usually require liquid formulations especially for infants, frequently delaying their availability. Efficacy studies are complicated by the need to evaluate multiple drug combinations, often in the context of pre-existing drug resistance.

Combination drug trials in pediatric patients have included the evaluation of stavudine (d4T), ddI, and IDV (Kline et al., 1999); AZT, ddI, and NVP (Luzuriaga et al., 1997); combinations of NNRTIs, NRTIs, and PIs (King et al., 2002, 2003; Krogstad et al., 1999, 2002; Starr et al., 1999; Staszewski et al., 1999). The addition of a PI to combination therapy in children increases the number of children achieving a virologic response by as much as 50% (Nachman et al., 2000; Wiznia et al., 2000).

These results have been achieved in trials of new drugs. Furthermore, adding a single new antiretroviral therapy to combination therapy is not an ideal approach to treatment (see later discussion). The use of combination therapy, including a PI, termed *HAART,* has significantly increased the survival of HIV-infected infants and children (de Martino et al., 2000).

Principles of Treatment

Initial ART therapy using monotherapy met with limited success. The inability of a single drug to significantly reduce viral load and the rapid emergence of resistance were two factors difficult to overcome until additional therapeutic agents became available. Dramatic slowing in disease progression, decrease of opportunistic infections, improved growth, better long-term survival, and restoration of immunity have followed the introduction of combination ART therapy, especially the introduction of HAART, which includes a PI (Clevenbergh et al., 2000; De Martino et al., 2000; Gavin and Yoger, 2002; Johnston et al., 2001; Mofenson and Munderi, 2002; Verweel et al., 2002).

Initiation of treatment should take into account the patient's clinical and immunologic status (Table 29-14). One difficult area is the initiation of treatment in the asymptomatic infant who acquired HIV perinatally. Reasons to begin treatment as early as possible include preservation of immune function, prevention of spread of virus to tissues and organs, prevention of destruction of immune cells, and prevention of dissemination and injury to the developing nervous system. In addition, infants begin HIV infection with higher viral loads than adults do and an immature immune system.

Therapeutic choice may be limited because some drugs are not approved for infants because of untested pharmacokinetics or unusual toxicities (CDC, 2002c; http://www.aidsinfo.nih.gov/guidelines/; http://www. womenchildrenhiv.org; http://hivinsite.ucsf.edu). Other factors to be considered include the ability of caregivers to administer complex drug regimens and recognize adverse treatment effects. Availability of appropriate laboratory studies is also important because therapeutic decisions are based on viral load assays, CD4 counts, and clinical response. In some circumstances viral resistance testing is essential (Baxter et al., 2000; Clevenbergh et al., 2000; Condra et al., 2000).

TABLE 29-14 · INDICATIONS FOR INITIATION OF ANTIRETROVIRAL THERAPY IN CHILDREN WITH HUMAN IMMUNODEFICIENCY VIRUS (HIV) INFECTION*

- Clinical symptoms associated with HIV infection (i.e. clinical categories A, B, or C in Table 29-7)
- Evidence of immune suppression, indicated by CD4 T-cell absolute number of percentage (i.e., immune category 2 or 3. Tables 29-8 and 29-9)
- Age <12 months, regardless of clinical, immunologic, or virologic status†
- For asymptomatic children aged ≥1 year with normal immune status, two options can be considered:
  Option 1: Initiate therapy regardless of age or symptom status
  Option 2: Defer treatment in situations in which the risk for clinical disease progression is low and other factors (i.e., concern for the durability of response, safety, and adherence) favor postponing treatment. In such cases, the health care provider should regularly monitor virologic, immunologic, and clinical status. Factors to be considered in deciding to initiate therapy include the following:
  - High or increasing HIV RNA copy number
  - Rapidly declining CD4 T-cell number or percentage to values approaching those indicative of moderate immune suppression (i.e., immune category 2, Tables 29-8 and 29-9)
  - Development of clinical symptoms

*Indications for initiation of antiretroviral therapy need to address issues of adherence. Postpubertal adolescents should follow the Guidelines for the Use of Antiretroviral Agents in Adults and Adolescents (available at http://www.aidsinfo.nih.gov/guidelines/).
†The Working Group recognizes that clinical trial data documenting therapeutic benefit from this approach are not currently available, and information on pharmacokinetics in infants younger than 3–6 months is limited. This recommendation is based on expert opinion. Issues associated with adherence should be fully assessed, discussed, and addressed with the HIV-infected infant's caregivers before the decision to initiate therapy is made.

TREATMENT OF ASYMPTOMATIC INFANTS

Initiation of ART to asymptomatic children before age 2 years, including primary infection in the neonatal period, may result in long-term suppression of viral replication and preservation of immune function (Luzuriaga et al., 2000). Because infants younger than 1 year have a higher risk for disease progression, HAART should be initiated in this group regardless of symptomatology or laboratory studies. The number of infants achieving HIV RNA levels below the limits of detection is lower than in older children and adults, possibly related to the high viral load at onset of therapy (Nachman et al., 2000).

TREATMENT OF SYMPTOMATIC CHILDREN

HAART is recommended for all symptomatic HIV-infected children (e.g., those children in clinical categories A, B, or C [see Table 29-7]) and/or children who have evidence of immunosuppression (e.g., those in immune categories 2 or 3 [see Table 29-9] regardless of the age or viral load). Additional factors to consider when initiating therapy include a high or increasing HIV RNA level, a rapidly decreasing CD4 count or percentage, or the development of clinical symptoms. The HIV RNA level at which treatment should be initiated has not been clearly demarcated. However, values of more than 100,000 copies/ml are associated with a high risk of mortality (CDC, 2002c; http://www.aidsinfo.nih.gov/guidelines/; http://www.womenchildrenhiv.org; http://hivinsite.ucsf.edu). Treatment of symptomatic HIV-infected children and adults slows the course of the disease (Englund et al., 1997; Katzenstein et al., 1996).

Choice of Antiretroviral Therapy

Monotherapy should not be used for the treatment of HIV-infected individuals. Theoretically, the initial choice of treatment for infants should be influenced by the treatment that the mother has received during pregnancy. However, data from several studies indicate that maternal ART is not associated with decreased effectiveness of therapy in infants (Eastman et al., 1998; McSherry et al., 1999; Stiehm et al., 1999). The goal of ART is to maximally suppress viral replication to undetectable levels for as long as possible while preserving and/or restoring immunologic function and minimizing drug toxicity.

Based on clinical trials it is strongly recommended that initial therapy consist of two NRTIs and a PI (Table 29-15) (CDC, 2002c). In adults, a PI-sparing regimen of efavirenz (EFV) in combination with AZT and 3TC was associated with a good virologic response (Staszewski et al., 1999). However, there are few clinical trials of this combination in children. Alternative combination therapies are listed in Table 29-15. The use of alternative regimens is determined by such factors as viral resistance, toxicity, and failure to respond. There are several ARTs that are not recommended for treatment, including monotherapy and the combination of certain NRTIs (see Table 29-15).

Changing Antiretroviral Therapy

Careful consideration must be given when changing therapy (Table 29-16). Indications for changing therapy include failure of the current regimen as evidenced by disease progression, virologic progression, immunologic deterioration; drug toxicity or intolerance; and new information that a particular drug regimen is superior to the current regimen. A single drug change within a regimen of treatment should not be done; instead a change should include new drugs to minimize development of resistance and maximize an optimal virologic response.

Although there are no definitive rules for when to change therapy, several situations may indicate that the change should be made. These include (1) less than a

---

TABLE 29-15 · RECOMMENDED ANTIRETROVIRAL REGIMENS FOR INITIAL THERAPY FOR HUMAN IMMUNODEFICIENCY VIRUS (HIV) INFECTION IN CHILDREN*

Strongly Recommended

Clinical trial evidence of clinical benefit and/or sustained suppression of HIV replication in adults and/or children.
- One highly active protease inhibitors (nelfinavir or ritonavir) plus two nucleoside analogue reverse transcriptase inhibitors
- Recommended dual nucleoside reverse transcriptase inhibitor (NRTI) combinations: the most data on use in children are available for the combinations or zidovudine (ZDV) and didanosine (ddI), ZDV and lamivudine (3TC), and stavudine (d4T) and ddI. More limited data are available for the combinations of d4T and 3TC and ZDV and dideoxycytosine (ddC)*
- For children who can swallow capsules: the non-nucleoside reverse transcriptase inhibitor (NNRTI) efavirenz (Sustiva)† plus two NRTIs, or efavirenz (Sustiva) plus nelfinavir and one NRTI.

Recommended as an Alternative

Clinical trial evidence of suppression of HIV replication, but (1) durability may be less in adults and/or children than with strongly recommended regimens or may not yet be defined, (2) evidence of efficacy may not outweigh potential adverse consequences (i.e., toxicity, drug interactions, cost, etc.), or (3) experience in infants and children is limited.
- NVP and two NRTIs
- Abacavir (ABC) in combination with ZDV and 3TC
- Lopinavir/ritonavir with two NRTIs or one NRTI and NNRTI‡
- Indinavir (IDV) or saquinavir (SQV) soft gel capsule with two NRTIs for children who can swallow capsules

Offered Only in Special Circumstances

Clinical trial evidence of either (1) virologic suppression that is less durable than for the strongly recommended or alternative regimens or (2) data are preliminary or inconclusive for use as initial therapy but may be reasonable offered in special circumstances.
- Two NRTIs
- Amprenavir (APV) in combination with two NRTIs or ABC

Not Recommended

Evidence against use because (1) overlapping toxicity may occur and/or (2) use may be virologically undesirable.
- Any monotherapy
- d4T and ZDV
- ddC* and ddI
- ddC* and d4T
- ddC* and 3TC

---

*ddC is not available commercially in a liquid preparation; however, a liquid formulation is available through a compassionate use program of the manufacturer [Hoffman-LaRoche Inc. (http://www.rocheusa.com), Nutley, New Jersey]. ZDV and ddC is a less preferred choice for use in combination with a PI.
†EFV is currently available only in capsule form, although a liquid formulation is available through an expanded access program of the manufacturer [Bristol-Myers Squibb Company (http://www.bms.com)]. There are currently no data on appropriate dosage of EFV in children younger than age 3 years.
‡CDC, 2002c; http://www.aidsinfo.nih.gov/guidelines/; http://www.womenchildrenhiv.org; http://hivinsite.ucsf.edu CDC, 2002c; http://www.aidsinfo.nih.gov/guidelines/; http://www.womenchildrenhiv.org; http://hivinsite.ucsf.edu). The data presented to the Food and Drug Administration for review during the drug approval process provided significant data on the pharmacokinetics and safety in children receiving lopinavir/ritonavir (Kaletra) for 24 weeks. The combination of lopinavir/ritonavir with either two NRTIs or one NRTI and an NNRTI may be moved up to the strongly recommended category as experience with this drug is gained by U.S. investigators.

TABLE 29-16 · CONSIDERATIONS FOR CHANGING ANTIRETROVIRAL THERAPY FOR HUMAN IMMUNODEFICIENCY VIRUS (HIV)-INFECTED CHILDREN*

Virologic Considerations
- Less than a minimally acceptable virologic response after 8 to 12 weeks of therapy. For children receiving antiretroviral therapy with two nucleoside reverse transcriptase inhibitors (NRTIs) and a protease inhibitor (PI), such a response is defined as a less than tenfold ($1.0 \log_{10}$) decrease from baseline HIV RNA levels. For children who are receiving less potent antiretroviral therapy (i.e., dual NRTI combinations), an insufficient response is defined as a less than fivefold ($0.7 \log_{10}$) decrease in HIV RNA levels from baseline.
- HIV RNA not suppressed to undetectable levels after 4 to 6 months of antiretroviral therapy.[†]
- Repeated detection of HIV RNA in children who initially responded to antiretroviral therapy with undetectable levels.[‡]
- A reproducible increase in HIV RNA copy number among children who have had a substantial HIV RNA response but still have low levels of detectable HIV RNA. Such an increase would warrant change in therapy if, after initiation of the therapeutic regimen, a greater than threefold ($0.5 \log_{10}$) increase in copy number for children aged >2 years and greater than fivefold ($0.7 \log_{10}$) increase is observed for children aged <2 years.

Immunologic Considerations*
- Change in immunologic classification (Table 29-9).
- For children with CD4+ cell percentages of <15% (i.e., those in immune category 3), a persistent decline of five percentiles or more in CD4 cell percentage (i.e., from 15% to 10%).
- A rapid and substantial decrease in absolute CD4+ T-cell count (i.e., >30% decline in <6 months).

Clinical Considerations
- Progressive neurodevelopmental deterioration.
- Growth failure defined as persistent decline in weight-growth velocity despite adequate nutritional support and without other explanation.
- Disease progression defined as advancement from one pediatric clinical category to another (i.e., from clinical category A to clinical category B).

*Available at http://www.aidsinfo.nih.gov/guidelines/
[†]At least two measurements (taken 1 week apart) should be performed before considering a change in therapy.
[‡]The initial HIV RNA level of the child at the start of therapy and the level achieved with therapy should be considered when contemplating potential drug changes. For example, an immediate change in therapy may not be warranted if there is a sustained 1.5 to 2.0 $\log_{10}$ decrease in HIV RNA copy number, even if RNA remains detectable at low levels.

tenfold ($1.0 \log_{10}$) decrease from baseline HIV RNA level after 12 weeks of therapy, (2) HIV RNA levels not suppressed to undetectable levels after 4 to 6 months of therapy, (3) repeated detection of HIV RNA in individuals who initially had undetectable levels in response to therapy, (4) a reproducible increase in HIV RNA in individuals who initially responded, (5) a change in the immune classification based on CD4 percentages, (6) a rapid and substantial decrease in the absolute CD4 count, (7) progressive neurodevelopmental deterioration, (8) growth failure, and (9) disease progression (CDC, 2002c; http://www.aidsinfo.nih.gov/guidelines/; http://www.womenchildrenhiv.org; http://hivinsite.ucsf.edu).

Viral Resistance

The chronic, persistent nature of HIV infection, with substantial virus replication at all stages and a naturally high mutation rate caused by the error-prone nature of the RT, results in the appearance of drug-resistant mutants under the selective pressure of prolonged treatment. Site-directed mutagenesis experiments with recombinant HIV clones have delineated the effect of specific mutations on viral resistance (St. Clair et al., 1991).

REVERSE TRANSCRIPTASE INHIBITOR RESISTANCE

Partial resistance to AZT is conferred by one to three virus mutations, whereas four to five mutations produce a highly AZT-resistant virus (Kellam et al., 1992). Relatively low-level resistance to ddI is conferred by the

amino acid substitution at codon 74 (St. Clair et al., 1991). In contrast, 1000-fold reduction in sensitivity to 3-TC is associated with the substitution at codon 184 (Tisdale et al., 1993). Through conformational changes adjacent to the nucleoside binding sites, certain mutations that confer resistance to one nucleoside analog (e.g., codon 74 to ddI or codon 181 to 3-TC) increase susceptibility to other nucleoside analogs (e.g., AZT) to which the virus has already developed resistance mutations (St. Clair et al., 1991; Tisdale et al., 1993).

The multiple mutations required to escape triple RT inhibitor combinations might result in nonviable viruses, the "convergent combination therapy" concept (Chow et al., 1993b). Subsequent reports demonstrated that HIV-1 was capable of developing multidrug-resistant variants in vitro, with growth kinetics similar to that of wild-type viruses (Chow et al., 1993a; Emini et al., 1993; Larder et al., 1993). It seems likely that such selection can occur in vivo also. Combination therapy, especially HAART, delays the development of resistance (Clevenbergh et al., 2000; Nikolic-Djokic et al., 2002).

Risk factors for the development of AZT resistance include low CD4 counts, an SI phenotype, and a high plasma viral load at initiation of therapy (Mayers et al., 1993; Newell et al., 2003; Richman, 1993; Richman et al., 1990). Drug resistance develops gradually, and mixtures of viruses with different resistance phenotypes may coexist. Proving that drug resistance causes disease progression is confounded by co-variables such as virus burden, SI phenotype, and impaired host defenses. Surrogate markers for disease progression worsen following the rapid emergence of resistance (Grant et al., 2002; Richman, 1992).

Two studies in children have demonstrated a highly significant relation between AZT resistance and disease progression (Ogino et al., 1993; Tudor-Williams et al., 1992). Ogino and colleagues (1993) documented improvement in growth following a change of retroviral therapy. This has been noted in additional studies in children and anecdotally in adults and supports the notion that drug resistance plays a role in disease progression (Newell et al., 2003).

VIRAL RESISTANCE IN PREGNANT WOMEN

Antiretroviral resistance mutations were evaluated in pregnant HIV-infected women and in the newborns in a prospective study between the years 1991 and 1997 by Palumbo and colleagues (2001). They studied 220 HIV-infected AZT-exposed pregnant women and 24 of their infected infants. AZT-associated mutations were detected in 17% of pregnant women and 8% of their newborns. The mutation pattern in the infant was not identical to the mother's pattern; furthermore, no association was found between perinatal transmission and the presence of AZT-resistant mutations.

A higher percentage of AZT resistance was found in infant viral isolates (20%) in a French Perinatal Cohort (Masquelier et al., 2002). Evidence of transmission of resistance virus from mothers to infants was observed in four cases.

VIRAL RESISTANCE DURING COMBINATION THERAPY

Eshleman and co-workers (2001) evaluated treatment-experienced children who were randomized into four treatment arms that included different combinations of d4T, lamivudine, NVP, NFV, and ritonavir. Some patients had previous treatment with NRTIs. NVP and lamivudine mutations were detected most frequently with virologic failure. NVP mutations were more common among children who had received three-drug versus four-drug NVP-containing regimens. Ritonavir and NFV mutations were detected at low rates.

NEVIRAPINE RESISTANCE IN THE PERINATAL PERIOD

A major advance in providing an effective, low-cost, and safe HIV prevention therapy for developing countries occurred with the report from Uganda that single doses of NVP prevented maternal–infant HIV transmission (PMTCT) in Uganda (Guay et al., 1999). In this study HIV transmission was reduced by 50%. Viral isolates after a single dose of NVP demonstrated a single point mutation in 19% of mothers and 46% of their infected infants. It was surprising to see resistance emerge after a single NVP dose. Follow-up studies showed that NVP resistance disappeared rapidly.

NVP-resistance mutations were also observed in a PACTG 316 study following single-dose NVP therapy for PMTCT. The most common mutation was K103N. In other studies, 5% of women had resistance mutations before the receipt of drug (Cunningham et al., 2002). Evaluation of viral resistance after 1 year indicated that all viruses had reverted to wild type (Nolan et al.,

2002). The risk of developing NVP resistance did not correlate with CD4 counts or HIV RNA at delivery.

Mullen and colleagues (2002) evaluated 26 children who had experienced virologic failure after combination ART. They found that at the time of treatment failure, 33% had resistance mutations in the protease gene and 90% in the RT gene. No resistance mutations were detected before treatment. Genotypic resistance was most frequently associated with lamivudine, followed by NVP and AZT.

Drug Resistance Testing

Both genotypic and phenotypic assays are used to test ART resistance (Clevenbergh et al., 2000; Condra et al., 2000). The assays are based on amplification procedures that can detect mutations in plasma samples with more than 1000 copies/ml of HIV RNA. HIV resistance assays are useful in guiding initial therapy and changing regimens but they are not entirely predictive. Resistance may not mean that an individual will fail to respond to a particular regimen containing that drug. Likewise, an individual may respond to combination therapy containing a drug to which some resistance is evident. Studies of resistance and response to therapy have not been performed in children.

Guidelines for the use of drug resistance testing have been published (Havlir et al., 2001; Hirsch et al., 1998, 2000). As expected, hundreds of mutations occur in response to ART. The significance of a single mutation in relation to response to therapy or loss of virologic control is uncertain in most instances. Randomized, prospective clinical trials have been performed using both genotypic and phenotypic assays. Although there are many limitations in the use of assays, including interpretation and expense, many consider viral resistance assays standard-of-care in the management of treatment failure (Hirsch et al., 2000). Resistance testing should be performed during the failing regimen because resistance may not be detected following withdrawal of ART. Resistance mutations may persist or re-emerge rapidly following reinstitution of therapy (Yeni et al., 2002).

Reverse Transcriptase Inhibitors

Antiretroviral agents are generally targeted to specific steps in the viral life cycle. Of these targets, the virus-encoded RT enzyme has been the most exploited to date. Because RT is an RNA-dependent and DNA-dependent DNA polymerase, it could be anticipated that nucleoside analogs might provide suitable substrates for the enzyme. Both purine (adenosine and guanosine and their precursor inosine) and pyrimidine (thymidine and cytidine) nucleoside analogs that have potent activity against a wide range of retroviruses have been identified.

Each drug requires intracellular anabolic phosphorylation by cellular kinases to form the active triphosphate. The rate of phosphorylation depends on the state of activation of the host cell; AZT is more efficiently phosphorylated in PHA-stimulated PBMC, as opposed to ddI and dideoxycytidine (ddC), which are metabolized to their triphosphate forms fivefold to 15-fold more efficiently in resting PBMCs (Gao et al., 1993). This is of possible relevance in the perinatal period, because neonates have a lower proportion of activated lymphocytes (Erkeller-Yuksel et al., 1992).

ZIDOVUDINE (ZDV, AZT, RETROVIR)

AZT prolongs the short-term survival of adults with advanced HIV-1 disease (Fischl et al., 1987) and delays the development of AIDS-defining conditions in symptomatic and asymptomatic adults with CD4 cells of less than 500 cells/mm^3 (Fischl et al., 1990; Graham et al., 1992; Volberding et al., 1990). Optimism from these initial studies, however, was tempered by data from the Veterans Affairs Cooperative Study and the European Concorde Study (Aboulker and Swart, 1993; Hamilton et al., 1992).

The most compelling evidence to date for the efficacy of AZT as an antiretroviral agent is provided by the ACTG 076 trial to diminish perinatal transmission (CDC, 1994b, 1994c; Connor et al., 1994). This was a placebo-controlled study of AZT given to mothers antepartum and intrapartum and to infants for 6 weeks after birth. At an analysis of 364 evaluable infants in February 1994, the estimated rate of transmission was 25.5% in the placebo recipients (*n* = 184) and 8.3% in the AZT-treated group (*n* = 180).

In children with symptomatic disease, uncontrolled clinical trials have demonstrated improvement in clinical, neurodevelopmental, and virologic parameters with AZT therapy (Brouwers et al., 1990; McKinney et al., 1990, 1991; Pizzo et al., 1988). Pharmacokinetic studies demonstrated good oral bioavailability (65%) and reasonable CSF levels (24% of serum levels) (Balis et al., 1989a, 1989b). The plasma half-life was only 1 hour in children older than 12 months but was considerably prolonged in neonates (14 hours after maternal ingestion in one study) (Chavanet et al., 1989; Watts et al., 1991).

The primary toxicities of AZT are anemia (30% to 40% of symptomatic children) and neutropenia. These may occur at any stage during treatment but are more frequent in children with more advanced disease. Dosage reduction (to no lower than 75 mg/m^2/dose) is indicated. Neutropenia may be ameliorated with G-CSF (Mueller et al., 1992b). Erythropoietin may be considered for transfusion-dependent anemia. Myopathy, myositis, liver toxicity, and lactic acidosis may occur. Additional toxicities of AZT and other ARTs are discussed in the section on antiretroviral toxicities. AZT monotherapy can no longer be recommended as initial therapy. AZT should not be co-administered with d4T.

DIDANOSINE (ddI, DIDEOXYINOSINE, VIDEX)

Didanosine has a longer plasma half-life than AZT, allowing 8- to 12-hour dosing. The oral bioavailability is highly variable (about 19%) and, because ddI is acid labile, the drug must be taken with antacid (Balis et al., 1992). Penetration of the blood–brain barrier is poor. Didanosine should not be co-administered with ddC.

ACTG study 116A compared ddI to AZT as first-line therapy for adults with advanced HIV disease. No difference in disease progression was found, but the survival trends favored AZT (relative risk 1.4) (Sande et al., 1993). Adults who had tolerated AZT for at least 16 weeks (median 14 months) reached study morbidity and mortality end points less frequently if they were switched to 500 mg/day of ddI rather than continuing on AZT (ACTG studies 116B/117) (Kahn et al., 1992).

In a randomized study of 312 adults with disease progression on AZT, switching to ddI was associated with fewer new AIDS-defining events or deaths after 2 years of follow-up (Spruance et al., 1994). The benefit was most apparent among those with a CD4 count above 100 cells/mm^3 at entry.

Studies of ddI in children were initiated concurrently with the adult studies. In the phase I/II trial, 43 children with symptomatic HIV-1 infection received escalating doses from 60 to 540 mg/m^2/day in three divided doses. Median CD4 counts increased from 218 to 327 cells/mm^3, and p24 antigen levels declined during the first 24 weeks (Butler et al., 1991). As in adults, bone marrow suppression was not observed, but pancreatitis was observed in two patients on higher doses ($\geq$360 mg/m^2/day), and peripheral atrophy of the retinal pigment epithelium occurred in three children.

In 1991, the data from this study contributed to the simultaneous licensing of ddI for adults and children, a historic event in the history of the FDA. The interim analysis of a large randomized trial (ACTG study 152) comparing ddI or AZT monotherapy with a combination of the two as first-line therapy for symptomatic children was terminated in February 1995, when the AZT monotherapy arm was found to be less active and more toxic than ddI monotherapy and/or the combination.

DIDEOXYCYTIDINE (ddC, ZALCITABINE, HIVID)

Dideoxycytidine is about 10 times more potent in vitro than AZT on a molar basis (Yarchoan et al., 1991). Despite the in vitro data, a study of 635 adults with CD4 cells less than 200/mm^3 (ACTG 114) demonstrated that both mortality and disease progression are significantly more frequent on ddC compared with AZT monotherapy (Remick et al., 1993). Moderate to severe peripheral neuropathy was observed in 23% of the ddC recipients versus 6% in the AZT group. In addition, oral ulcers and rash were common toxicities. Granulocytopenia (10%) and anemia (6%) occurred, although at a lower frequency than with AZT. Pancreatitis is an uncommon toxicity. Dideoxycytidine should not be co-administered with ddI, d4T, or 3TC.

Subsequently, ddI or ddC monotherapy has been compared in 467 adults who had disease progression or were intolerant to AZT (Abrams et al., 1994). The median CD4 count was lower than 50 cells/mm^3 at entry. After 16 months median follow-up, there were 100 deaths in the ddI arm and 88 in the ddC arm, yielding an adjusted relative risk of 0.63 in favor of ddC. Disease progression was not significantly different, and adverse events were common in both groups. It appears, however, that ddC is equivalent to ddI in this context. Two pediatric trials of ddC have been performed (PACTG 138, 190) (Bakshi et al., 1997; Spector et al., 1997). They were relatively few differences in relation to ZDV versus ddC efficacy and toxicity.

LAMIVUDINE (3TC, EPIVIR)

3TC is derived from cytosine. The drug is relatively well tolerated, and is frequently used in combination with other ARTs. PACTG 300 compared AZT and 3TC to ddI monotherapy. The combination of AZT and 3TC was superior to that of monotherapy. 3TC is an important component of combination therapy. 3TC should not be co-administered with ddC.

STAVUDINE (d4T, ZERIT)

Stavudine is a thymidine-derived nucleotide with efficacy similar to that of AZT. The pharmacokinetics of d4T is such that it can be given twice daily (Yarchoan et al., 1991; Yogev et al., 2002). Stavudine has been studied in children as monotherapy and in combination with ddI or 3TC demonstrating a good safety profile (Kline et al., 1996, 1999). It should not be co-administered with AZT or ddC, but it can be combined with PIs or NNRTIs.

ABACAVIR (ABC, ZIAGEN)

ABC is carbocyclic guanosine analog nucleoside with excellent antiviral activity. The pharmacokinetics are such that it can be administered every 12 hours. It is synergistic with other nucleosides but may also develop cross-resistance.

Approximately 5% of children and adults who receive ABC develop a potentially fatal hypersensitivity reaction consisting of fever, fatigue, malaise, nausea, vomiting, diarrhea, abdominal pain, and shortness of breath. The rash may not be present in all hypersensitivity reactions. Abnormal laboratory values include elevated liver enzymes, creatine phosphokinase (CPK), creatinine, and lymphopenia. Lactic acidosis with hepatomegaly and steatosis has been reported. Some of the reactions are fatal. Rarely, pancreatitis occurs along with elevated glucose, triglycerides, and liver enzymes.

Nucleotide Reverse Transcriptase Inhibitor

TENOFOVIR (VIREAD, TENOFOVIR, DISOPROXIL FUMARATE)

Tenofovir is a nucleotide RT inhibitor that has anti-HIV activity and antiviral activity against HSV and CMV. The drug has been approved for use in adults. Pediatric clinical trials are underway. An important potential use of this drug is for prevention of perinatal HIV transmission. Tenofovir does not have cross-resistance with NNRTIs, has a long duration of action, can be given orally, is safe in pharmacologic doses, crosses the placenta, and protects against SIV infection in a Rhesus macaque model of perinatal HIV transmission (Van Rompay et al., 2001). It is not yet approved for use in children.

Non-Nucleoside Reverse Transcriptase Inhibitors (Delavirdine, Efavirenz, Nevirapine)

Several structurally distinct groups of compounds that specifically inhibit HIV-1 RT at sites remote from the nucleoside binding domains have been identified. These include NVP (Viramune), delavirdine (DLV, Rescriptor), and EFV (Sustiva). All have high antiviral potency in vitro and have been shown to be synergistic with nucleoside analogs. They do not require intracellular metabolism and have low cellular toxicity. They are equally active against AZT-sensitive or AZT-resistant isolates. Their "Achilles heel" has been the rapid emergence of resistant HIV strains when they are given as single agents, both in vitro and in vivo (Richman, 1993). For this reason, they are used selectively in combination therapy and never as monotherapy except for the prevention of perinatal HIV transmission.

PACTG 180 evaluated NVP used in combination with AZT and ddI. It was also evaluated in PACTG 245, a study of advanced HIV disease in children (Luzuriaga et al., 1997). In the studies, NVP seemed to be a useful addition to combination therapy. The data in pediatrics for DLV and EFV are limited. NVP has been used primarily for the prevention of HIV transmission from mothers to infants (Mofenson and Monderi, 2002).

Protease Inhibitors

A variety of compounds have been designed containing nonhydrolyzable moieties that mimic the putative transition state of the protease-catalyzed reaction (Kageyama et al., 1993; Mimoto et al., 1991) or as symmetric inhibitors designed rationally on the basis of crystallographic resolution of the enzyme structure (Erickson et al., 1990; Roberts et al., 1990).

HIV PIs revolutionized combination therapy and resulted in the development of HAART, permitting significant control of viral replication, reconstitution of immunity, and delay in progression to AIDS-defining events (CDC, 2002c; Clevenbergh et al., 2000; Gavin and Yogev, 2002; Johnston et al., 2001; Mofenson and Monderi, 2002; http://www.aidsinfo.nih.gov/guidelines/; http://www.womenchildrenhiv.org; http://hivinsite.ucsf.edu).

PIs specifically inhibit HIV protease while not affecting host proteases. Pharmacologically, the PIs are difficult to manufacture, are not easily made into suspensions or water-based solutions, do not taste good, and interact with liver P450 cytochromes in a complex manner. The effects of PIs on P450 cytochrome isoforms are not consistent in relation to stimulation or inhibition of isoforms. Drug interactions with PIs and other antiretrovirals and non-antiretrovirals is significant, and pharmacologic interactions among drugs should be investigated when designing combination drug therapy, especially PIs.

RITONOVIR (RTV, NORVIR)

PACTG 338 evaluated the effect of a combination of AZT, 3TC, and RTV versus d4T and RTV versus

ZDV and 3TC. The RTV combinations suppressed viral load and enhanced CD4 counts to a greater extent than a combination of AZT and 3TC (CDC, 2002c; http://www.aidsinfo.nih.gov/guidelines/; http://www.womenchildrenhiv.org; http://hivinsite.ucsf.edu).

NELFINAVIR (NFV, VIRACEPT)

A phase I/II clinical trial in children demonstrated potent antiviral effects of NFV when used in combination with NRTIs, with many of the children reaching undetectable viral loads (Krogstad et al., 2002). Studies in adults demonstrate that NFV in combination with AZT and 3TC results in more than 80% of individuals reaching undetectable levels of virus.

INDINAVIR (IDV, CRIXIVAN)

Pediatric experience with IDV is limited. In adults the drug is effective when used in combination with other antiretrovirals. Significant side effects limit its use in pediatrics. IDV can cause jaundice and thus is contraindicated for use in newborns. Patients may also developed hematuria and flank pain associated with the formation of crystals and stones in the kidney.

SAQUINAVIR (SQV, INVIRASE, FORTASE) AND AMPRENAVIR (APV, AGENERASE)

Pediatric experience and data for these agents are limited.

Fusion Inhibitors

Enfuvirtide (Fuzeon, T-20) was the first fusion inhibitor to be approved by the FDA for adults and children older than 6 years. It functions by binding the region of the HIV envelope glycoprotein gp41, preventing viral fusion with the target cell membrane. The drug was evaluated in patients that have been highly experienced to NRTIs, NNRTIs, and protease inhibitors (CDC, 2002c; http://www.aidsinfo.nih.gov/guidelines/; http://www.women-childrenhiv.org; http://hivinsite.ucsf.edu). Efficacy was based on significantly greater decreases in viral load and increases in CD4 T-cell counts in the enfuvirtide group than in the control groups. The drug is administered by subcutaneous injection two times daily. Currently there are no data using enfuvirtide as initial therapy. The most common side effects were injection site reactions, insomnia, headache, dizziness, and nausea. Resistance results from one or more mutations in gp41.

New Antiretroviral Therapy

Currently there are 17 antiretroviral agents that have been approved by the FDA for treatment of HIV infection. The emergence of resistance to all categories of antiretroviral agents continues to spur pharmaceutical and academic research into developing drugs that are more potent, less frequently associated with resistance, and directed toward new targets of viral inhibition (Gulick, 2003). The newest category of drugs is related to entry inhibitors and integrase inhibitors.

Some new drugs include RT inhibitors such as emtricitabine, which has activity against both HIV and HBV.

Amdoxovir is also effective against HIV and HBV (Furman et al., 2001). DPC 083 is a new NNRTI that is a derivative of EFV (Gulick, 2003).

New PIs under evaluation include atazanavir and tipranavir with potent activity in vitro and with drug levels that are markedly increased by the co-administration of RTV (Gulick, 2003).

New entry inhibitor drugs are under evaluation. Their targets are prevention of viral binding to CD4 T cells and other cells. Pro 542 is an antibody-like fusion protein of CD4 and IgG2. SCH 351125 and SCH-C are chemokine receptor inhibitors. T-1249 is an HIV fusion inhibitor 100 times more active than enfuvirtide (Gulick, 2003).

Safety and Toxicity of Antiretroviral Therapy

Table 29-13 lists many common side effects of the antiretroviral drugs. In this section attention is given to side effects that are unique to ART and/or are most life threatening.

METABOLIC COMPLICATIONS

Metabolic complications of PIs include lipid abnormalities and lipodystrophy (Carr et al., 1998, 1999, 2003; Lo et al., 1998). It is most common in individuals taking PIs but is also found in individuals taking nucleoside analog RT inhibitors. The lipodystrophy syndrome consists of two main phenotypes—lipoatrophy (subcutaneous fat wasting) and central or visceral fat accumulation (Carr et al., 1998; Miller et al., 1998). The prevalence of lipodystrophy in self-reported adults is as high as 50% (Lichtenstein et al., 2001).

The prevalence of lipodystrophy in children ranged from 29% to 33% in a study using anthropometric measurements and in studies using dual-energy x-ray absorptiometry (DXA) (Arpadi et al., 2001; Jaquet et al., 2000). Vigano and associates (2003) studied a group of children during HAART using similar measurements, but in addition to body mass index, they performed MRIs. They found increasing numbers of children affected as the duration of therapy increased. DXA scans showed an increase in lean mass, peripheral fat loss, and central fat accumulation. Peripheral fat loss and intra-abdominal adipose tissue content were associated with duration of therapy and independent of immunologic stage of disease and immunologic response.

The disfiguring nature of lipodystrophy results in stigmatization and can interfere with adherence to therapy. The metabolic abnormalities associated with lipodystrophy include reduced high-density lipoprotein (HDL) cholesterol, hypercholesterolemia, hypertriglyceridemia, insulin resistance, type 2 diabetes, and lactic acidemia. They may contribute to the risk of cardiovascular disease (Arpadi et al., 2000; Hadigan et al., 2001; Leonard and McComsey, 2003; Martinez et al., 2001b). Similar metabolic complications have been observed in children (Leonard and McComsey, 2003).

Guidelines for management of the dyslipidemias have been published (Dube et al., 2003).

MITOCHONDRIAL DYSFUNCTION

Nucleoside analog drugs are associated with mitochondrial dysfunction by interfering with mitochondrial gamma DNA polymerase resulting in mitochondrial depletion and dysfunction (Brinkman et al., 1998; Martin et al., 1994). Clinical investigators in France reported suggestive mitochondrial dysfunction among eight HIV-uninfected infants who were exposed to NRTIs in the perinatal period (Blanche et al., 1999). Two deaths were reported in infants exposed to AZT and 3TC combination who developed neurologic abnormalities.

Because of the widespread use of AZT for PMTCT, several groups retrospectively analyzed infants treated with or exposed to AZT during pregnancy and infancy (Bulterys et al., 2000; Dominguez et al., 2000; Lindegren et al., 2000). None of these studies, evaluating several thousand AZT exposed and treated infants, found evidence of death as a result of mitochondrial dysfunction. The discrepancy between the results of the French study and the U.S. studies is not apparent. It is clear, however, that mitochondrial dysfunction and disease develops in HIV-infected children and adults who receive chronic ART.

Chronic compensated hyperlactatemia can occur during treatment, and rarely, compensated lactic acidosis with hepatomegaly and steatosis may occur (Brinkman et al., 1998; Cote et al., 2002). Severe lactic acidosis with or without pancreatitis has been reported in pregnancy or in postpartum women whose therapy included d4T and ddI in combination with other antiretroviral agents (CDC, 1994c, 2002f; http://www.aidsinfo.nih.gov/guidelines/).

OTHER METABOLIC ABNORMALITIES

Hepatotoxicity, defined as a threefold to fivefold increase in serum transaminases, has been reported in patients receiving ART (den Brinker et al., 2000). Among the NNRTIs, NVP has the greatest potential for causing clinical hepatitis and in some cases fatal liver failure (Martinez et al., 2001a). This may be part of a hypersensitivity syndrome accompanied by skin rash, fever, and eosinophilia.

Hyperglycemia, new onset diabetes mellitus, diabetic ketoacidosis, and exacerbation of pre-existing diabetes mellitus are associated with HAART and most strongly with PI use (Dube et al., 2003; Eastone and Decker, 1997). There are no data to assist in the decision to continue or discontinue ART in patients with new onset or pre-existing diabetes.

Avascular necrosis and decreased bone density are recognized metabolic complications of HIV infection and may be linked to HAART (Mora et al., 2001; Scribner et al., 2000). The disorder occurs in both adults and children (Legg-Calvé-Perthes disease). CT scanning or MRI can confirm the diagnosis in patients who complained of pain in an affected hip or in the spine. Asymptomatic disease may occur in approximately 5% of patients.

ART Safety in Pregnancy

All of the ARTs have been labeled either as FDA category B or C in relation to risk in pregnancy. Category B drugs are those in which animal reproduction studies fail to demonstrate the risk to the fetus, and adequate and well-controlled studies of pregnant women have not been conducted. Drugs included in category B are ddI, RTV, SQV, and NFV.

Category C drugs are those in which safety in human pregnancy has not been determined, animal studies are either positive for fetal risk or have not been conducted, and the drug should not be used unless the potential benefit outweighs the potential risk to the fetus. Most ARTs fall into this category and include AZT, ddC, d4T, 3TC, ABC, NVP, DLV, EFV, IDV, APV, and lopinavir. Animal teratogen studies have demonstrated abnormalities with AZT (near lethal doses), ddC, ABC, DLV, and EFV (CDC, 1994b, 1994c, 2002c, 2002f; http://www.aidsinfo.nih.gov/guidelines/; http://www.womenchildrenhiv.org).

Passive Immunotherapy with HIV Antibody

Passive immunotherapy using plasma from HIV-infected donors with high titers of anti-HIV antibodies provided no discernible clinical or laboratory benefit in a randomized study of 63 adults with advanced disease (Jacobson et al., 1993). Two other controlled studies showed some clinical promise (Levy et al., 1994; Vittecoq et al., 1995). A trial of HIVIG in symptomatic HIV-infected children showed no clinical or laboratory benefit (Stiehm et al., 2000). High concentrations of HIVIG were unable to prevent infection of monkeys with a chimeric HIV/SIV under conditions in which neutralizing monoclonal antibodies (MAbs) clearly worked (Mascola et al., 1999).

Enthusiasm for HIVIG as a way to interrupt mother–child transmission by treating the mother was diminished when it was shown that antibodies had a weak effect on viral load in established infection (Binley et al., 2000; Poignard et al., 1999). In a large multicenter study (ACTG 185) HIVIG added to AZT did not reduce the low rate of maternal-fetal transmission (Stiehm et al., 1999). In addition, the ease with which HIV-1 escapes from neutralizing antibody suggests that treatment of the mother could even be detrimental by selecting for antibody-resistant virus variants (Poignard et al., 1999).

Positive results were obtained in an animal model using polyclonal antibody as a method to prevent mother–child transmission (Van Rompay et al., 1998). In this model large doses of SIV immune globulin (SIVIG) provided partial protection of some newborn macaques against oral SIV challenge.

Intravenous Immunoglobulin

A double-blind study of 372 HIV-1 infected children compared human intravenous immune globulin (IVIG) (400 mg/kg) every 28 days with placebo (0.1% albumin), over a median length of follow-up of 17 months.

A reduction of bacterial infections and hospitalizations was observed for those children with CD4 counts greater than 200 cells/mm³ at entry (Lambert et al., 1997; Mofenson et al., 1992). Subsequent age-adjusted CD4 slope analysis demonstrated a slowing of CD4 count decline by 13.5 cells/month in the IVIG recipients (Mofenson et al., 1993).

The benefits, however, were not observed in children receiving TMP-SMX for PCP prophylaxis and were not found in another study of children with lower CD4 counts (Spector et al., 1994).

The consensus of the Working Group was that children with significant recurrent bacterial infections, hypogammaglobulinemia, or documented poor functional antibody development might be candidates for IVIG 400 mg/kg every 28 days (Working Group on Antiretroviral Therapy, 1993). Higher dosages may be useful in children with thrombocytopenia (0.5 to 1.0 g/kg/dose for 3 to 5 days).

Supportive Care

Caring for a child with HIV infection imposes a heavy burden for any caregiver. In the context of perinatal transmission, this is frequently compounded by illness in the parent, social isolation, and feelings of guilt. An effective multidisciplinary team needs to determine the major concerns for each caregiver. These may be emotional, financial, or legal (e.g., regarding schooling, inheritance, property). Caregivers may need more information about HIV, help informing the child or siblings about the diagnosis, advice about treatment for themselves, or help with substance abuse problems. Without addressing these issues, the child is unlikely to receive optimal care.

Ideally, a social worker and primary nurse should be assigned to each family. The team should also include psychologists, dietitians, clergy, teachers, occupational and physical therapists, and recreation therapists. Formal and informal group support should be provided for both children and their caregivers. Involvement of appropriate community-based supportive services, from early intervention programs to hospice services, may be required. Ideally, care for all infected and affected family members should be coordinated in one facility. This requires close collaboration among pediatricians, adult physicians, obstetricians-gynecologists, and their affiliated teams (Jansen and Ammann, 1994).

Medical supportive care includes teaching parents to be alert for subtle signs of new illness and to seek help promptly. Fevers need to be evaluated carefully, with early intervention for treatable bacterial or opportunistic infections. Creative and aggressive attention to pain management is important. Pain is frequently associated with procedures but also arises, for example, from infectious complications, side effects of drugs, or spasticity associated with CNS involvement.

Nutritional monitoring and dietary intervention should begin early, because malnutrition may aggravate immunodeficiency (Beisel et al., 1981) (see Chapter 23).

Iron, vitamin, and other micronutrient deficiencies should be considered. Providing sufficient calories and protein to maintain linear growth and weight gain is frequently difficult. A variety of calorically dense formulas and supplements should be available to find one that the child can tolerate. Dietary advice should be sensitive to the family's ethnic and cultural constraints.

Appetite stimulants, such as cyproheptadine (Periactin), dronabinol (Marinol), and megestrol acetate (Megace) are worth considering but rarely improve caloric intake more than 10% to 20%. If oral intake remains inadequate, tube feeding may be necessary. Gastrostomy sites may heal poorly and leak, however, and nasogastric tubes may exacerbate sinusitis and upper airway infection. Parenteral nutrition may therefore become necessary.

Pain Management

Despite the availability of new ART and prevention of disease progression and opportunistic infections, many children continued to suffer from acute and chronic pain. Chronic pain management is an integral part of treating advanced disease. Pain management in children with HIV infection should be carefully evaluated to avoid undertreatment (Boland, 2000; Gaughan et al., 2002; O'Hara and Czarneiecki, 1997).

Immunizations

The safety and effectiveness of vaccines in HIV-infected children is determined by the degree of immunosuppression. This varies considerably from patient to patient. In general, persons who are severely immunocompromised or in whom immune status is uncertain should not receive live vaccines, either viral or bacterial, because of the risk of vaccine-induced disease. Inactivated vaccines and immune globulins are safe in these situations, although the antibody response to the vaccine may be inadequate and the subject not protected (American Academy of Pediatrics, 2003).

Data on the use of currently available live-virus and bacterial vaccines in HIV-infected children are limited, but complications have been reported after bacille Calmette-Guérin (BCG) and measles immunizations.

Measles Vaccine

Because of reports of severe measles in symptomatic HIV-infected children, including fatalities, measles immunization (given as measles-mumps-rubella [MMR]) is recommended for HIV-infected children in most circumstances, including children who are symptomatic but are not severely immunocompromised and those who are asymptomatic. Vaccine should be given at 12 months of age to enhance the likelihood of an appropriate immune response. In a measles epidemic, vaccine should be given at an earlier age, such as at 6 to 9 months of age followed by the routinely recommended dose at 12 months of age (or 1 month after this initial dose). The second dose after the 12-month immunization may be administered as soon as 1 month (28 days) later in an attempt to induce seroconversion as early as possible.

Severely immunocompromised patients with HIV infection, as defined by low CD4 T-lymphocyte counts or low percentage of total circulating lymphocytes should not receive measles vaccine. MMR vaccine viruses are not transmitted so other children in the household may be immunized.

Varicella Vaccine

Varicella vaccine should be considered for asymptomatic or mildly symptomatic HIV-infected children with CD4 percentage of 25% or more. Because the vaccine strain of varicella has rarely been transmitted, household contacts of HIV-infected persons can be immunized. No precautions are needed after immunization of healthy children who do not develop a rash. Vaccine recipients who develop a rash should avoid direct contact with susceptible immunocompromised hosts for the duration of the rash.

BCG Vaccine

In the United States, BCG is contraindicated for HIV-infected patients. In areas of the world with a high incidence of TB, the WHO recommends giving BCG to HIV-infected children who are asymptomatic. Efficacy or adverse effects data are not available.

Other Vaccines

Children with asymptomatic or symptomatic HIV infection also should receive other routinely recommended childhood vaccines, including diphtheria, tetanus and adult pertussis vaccine (DTaP); inactivated polio vaccine (IPV); hepatitis B; and Haemophilus influenzae b (Hib) conjugate vaccines, according to recommended schedules (see Chapter 42). Annual influenza immunization of HIV-infected persons is recommended. Pneumococcal immunization is also recommended based on age and vaccine-specific recommendations.

Immunization of Asymptomatic At-Risk Infants

Routine or widespread screening to detect asymptomatic HIV-infected children before routine immunization is not recommended. Children without clinical manifestations of or known risk factors for HIV infection should be immunized in accordance with the recommendations for routine childhood immunization.

Vaccine Effect on Viral Load

Data are limited on the effect of routine immunizations on viral load in children. Some studies in adults have demonstrated transient increases of HIV RNA levels after immunization with influenza or pneumococcal vaccine, whereas other studies have shown no increase. No evidence indicates that this transient increase enhances progression of disease.

Vaccine Failure

Because the ability of HIV-infected children to respond to vaccine antigens is related to their degree of immunosuppression at the time of immunization, these children should be considered potentially susceptible to vaccine-preventable diseases, even after appropriate immunization, unless a recent serologic test demonstrates adequate antibody concentrations. Children with subtle antibody deficiencies have an intermediate degree of vaccine responsiveness and may require postimmunization antibody titers to confirm vaccine immunogenicity.

Passive Immunization

Passive immunization (or chemoprophylaxis) after exposure should be considered even if the child previously has received the recommended vaccines (see Chapters 41 and 42). Passive immunization is recommended for susceptible children with symptomatic HIV infection who are in contact with measles or varicella-zoster. Children receiving IVIG are considered susceptible if the last dose was given more than 2 weeks before exposure.

Children with a documented past history of varicella or recurrent zoster need not be treated with varicella-zoster immune globulin (VZIG). If a susceptible child is re-exposed more than 2 weeks after VZIG, however, another dose is recommended. The administration of VZIG may prolong the incubation period to 28 days, so clinic visits should be postponed for this period.

In urban areas where measles outbreaks are frequent, antibody responses in HIV-infected children should be checked after MMR vaccination. If the response has been poor, a second dose of MMR should be given. If the child fails to respond to a second dose, regular IVIG prophylaxis should be considered.

Detailed recommendations for active and passive immunization immunodeficient for infants and children are available and regularly updated from the CDC and the American Academy of Pediatrics and should be consulted regularly for immunization details (CDC, http://www.cdc.gov/; American Academy of Pediatrics, 2003).

HIV Vaccines

The continued escalation of the HIV epidemic worldwide, now reaching 5 million new HIV infections each year, coupled with increasing viral resistance to ART has made the need for an HIV vaccine even more imperative than when AIDS was first described in 1981 (Gottlieb et al., 1981).

Unlike many vaccines for other infectious diseases, HIV presents a formidable problem for vaccine development. The high mutation rate of HIV coupled with a high degree of envelop glycosylation, escape from CTL and neutralizing antibody, conformational changes in immunogenic epitopes, and existence of multiple viral clades (strains) contribute to difficulties in HIV vaccine development (Barouch and Letvin, 2002; Burton, 1997; Cohen, 1998; Goulder et al., 2001a, 2001b, 2001c; Korber et al., 1998; Letvin, 1998; Letvin and Walker, 2002; Nabel, 2001). Furthermore, the immunologic response to HIV infection and to vaccine antigens does not follow the immunologic pattern observed with other infectious agents. Most protein antigens elicit an initial IgM response followed by an IgG response along with CTL immunity. Following booster immunization, an amnestic response occurs with prolonged duration of IgG and CTL immunity. Polysaccharide antigens such as pneumococcal polysaccharide induced an immediate and prolonged IgG immunologic response. The immunologic response to HIV antigens follows neither of these patterns.

Potent CTL responses controlling HIV replication have been observed in acute HIV infection in humans and in animal models (Barouch et al., 2000; O'Connor et al., 2002; Schmitz et al., 1999). The presence of CTL and resistance to infection has been observed in a cohort of Nairobi prostitutes (Rowland-Jones et al., 1998). CTL alone, however, is unlikely to prevent or control HIV infection. Long-lived immunity can be provided by antibody, and protection in critical mucosal sites such as the gastrointestinal tract and vagina might be more important for HIV than other infectious agents (Burton, 1997; Nabel, 2001; Parren et al., 1997; Sattentau, 1996).

A significant number of antigens are being evaluated clinically as HIV vaccine candidates (reviewed in Nabel, 2001). HIV encodes for more than 12 gene products, one or more of which are targets for immune recognition. Because GP 120 binds to CD4 T lymphocytes, it is a common component of most vaccines. It elicits primarily neutralizing antibody; however, the antibody is poorly cross-reactive and of short duration. Gag proteins, on the other hand, elicit CTL responses.

The first multivalent envelope vaccine recently completed phase III clinical trials in the United States and Thailand, but initial results did not show a protective effect when compared with placebo (Watanabe, 2003).

DNA vaccines have been explored as alternatives to defined antigens as a mechanism of bypassing live-attenuated viral vaccines. Despite promising results in rodent models, DNA immunization has proven less effective in primates (Andre et al., 1998; Barouch et al., 2000). The basis for considering live-attenuated vaccines was the observation that naturally occurring HIV nef mutations were identified in patients who had slow disease progression (Learmont et al., 1999). However, unknown short-term and long-term risks of an attenuated HIV virus, which has the ability to become sequestered in the CNS, makes this an unlikely approach for vaccine development.

In an effort to enhance immune response to HIV antigens, a variety of viral vectors have been used in association with specific HIV antigens. These include replication defective forms of canarypox, fowlpox, modified vaccinia Ankara, and Sinibis and Venezuelan equine encephalitis virus alphaviruses (Nabel, 2001; Moss et al., 1996; Tartaglia et al., 1998). Significant safety concerns are associated with many of these viral constructs.

Adjuvants form the basis of enhancing the immune response to a variety of immunogens, and many adjuvants have a long safety record in their use in infants and children. Adjuvants include aluminum hydroxide, Freund's adjuvant, and a variety of polymers and lipopeptides (Cox and Coulter, 1997; Nabel, 2001). Despite the variety of adjuvants, tested along with a large number of HIV antigens, significant enhancement of immunity has not been achieved, attesting to the difficulties in developing an effective HIV vaccine.

SOCIAL AND LEGAL ISSUES

Orphans

The large number of HIV-infected women of childbearing age has resulted in a secondary epidemic of AIDS orphans (defined as a child who has lost one or both parents). In the United States, between the years 1980 and 1998, 51,000 women died of AIDS, leaving 97,000 offspring; 21,000 of these were HIV infected (Lee and Fleming, 2003).

Worldwide there are an estimated 13.2 million orphans 15 years or younger, with 6100 new orphans per day. Most (95%) of these orphans are in Africa. Before AIDS 2% of children in developing countries were orphans. With the HIV/AIDS epidemic this number increased to 7% and now is as high as 11% in some countries (Foster, 2002). Worldwide, infant and child mortality rates will increase as much as 30% above previously projected rates as a direct consequence of perinatal HIV infection (Quinn, 1994).

In a study from Malawi, mortality of children living with HIV-infected mothers was 27% in the first month, 46% in children younger than 5 years, and 49% in children younger than 10 years (Crampin et al., 2003). In contrast the mortality of children living with HIV-uninfected mothers was 11% in the first month, 16% in children younger than 5 years, and 17% in children younger than 10 years.

There is increasing concern about the fate of children orphaned by HIV. Their poor socioeconomic, educational, and legal status make them vulnerable to sexual, economic, and military exploitation. It is estimated that 1 million children enter the sex trade industry each year; many of them are children orphaned by HIV/AIDS (Bicego et al., 2003; Willis and Levy, 2002).

Confidentiality

The HIV-infected child encounters significant legal issues relating to confidentiality, access to medical care, adoption, inheritance, and property rights (especially in developing countries), and availability of FDA-approved therapy (Ammann, 1998; Boland, 2000). Disclosure of HIV status also presents significant psychosocial issues for school-aged children.

Prenatal Testing

The success of prenatal HIV testing in detecting early HIV infection of pregnant women has resulted in legislation in many states directed toward optimizing the availability of prenatal HIV testing. Recent reports indicate that widespread use of prenatal HIV testing and acceptance of testing by pregnant women is most effective when either mandatory or "opt-out" testing regimens are offered (CDC, 2002d, 2002e, 2002g). Mandatory testing is problematic, however, in that it may violate the confidentiality of the mother. Mandatory testing of newborns, although effective in determining HIV exposure of infants, does not enhance a diagnosis of HIV infection because antibody is positive in all HIV-exposed infants regardless of infection status. In addition, optimal prevention of HIV transmission from mothers to infants requires knowledge of HIV status during early pregnancy and delivery (Ammann, 1995).

Opt-out methods for prenatal testing resolve many of the issues related to mandatory testing. *Opt-out* refers to offering of HIV testing with the option of the mother refusing the HIV testing. Some states use voluntary offering, whereas others use mandatory offering with opt-out provisions. Opt-out and mandatory offering of HIV testing are both successful approaches to gaining acceptance for routine HIV testing. Regimens that use opt-in approaches (voluntary offering and acceptance) for HIV testing are less successful in gaining widespread acceptance of prenatal HIV testing (CDC, 2002d, 2002e, 2002g).

Newborn Infant Testing

Mandatory infant testing continues to capture a small number of HIV-exposed and/or infected infants in whom the mothers have not been tested during pregnancy (Cusick et al., 2003). Rapid HIV testing increases the likelihood of acceptance of prenatal HIV testing in developing countries (Malonza et al., 2003) and has recently been recommended by the U.S. Public Health Service for both prenatal and routine HIV testing in the United States to increase the acceptability and extent of HIV testing.

Failure to Test for HIV in Pregnant Women

Several lawsuits have been filed against physicians or obstetricians who failed to offer HIV testing to a pregnant woman in instances in which the infant was born HIV infected. The basis for these lawsuits is that failure to provide HIV testing did not provide the mother an opportunity to consider ART to prevent vertical HIV

transmission. In these cases, proof of high-risk behavior was not required. Pregnancy, by itself, was considered unprotected sex, and therefore a risk factor for HIV infection.

FUTURE CONSIDERATIONS

Treatment

Numerous refinements of existing ARTs in various combinations can be expected over the next few years. The role of new therapeutic strategies, particularly the use of immunomodulating therapies and gene therapy, are cause for optimism. Such advances depend on gaining increased insights into both viral pathogenesis and host defenses in this disease (Ammann, 1995).

Clinical Management

Validation of the new techniques for monitoring viral burden as surrogate markers for drug efficacy can perhaps enable more rapid identification of useful treatment strategies. Much work is being done to improve both the diagnostic and therapeutic options for the opportunistic infections associated with immunosuppressed hosts. Lessons learned from HIV-infected individuals may help in the care of children undergoing cancer chemotherapy and vice versa. Multidisciplinary approaches should continue to focus on ways to improve the quality of lives that may be extended by medical advances. More family-based care facilities can help in this regard.

Prevention of Maternal–Infant Transmission

The implementation of prevention of perinatal HIV transmission is of the highest priority for developing countries where as many as 300,000 to 500,000 infants' lives could be saved each year (Ammann, 2000a, 2000c). The results of the ACTG 076 study in 1994 provided the major impetus to develop less complicated but equally effective interventions that may be useful worldwide. The HIVNET 012 study in Uganda brought hope that perinatal HIV prevention could be initiated in even the poorest countries.

Targeted prevention such as PMTCT, however, can only be achieved if HIV-infected mothers can be identified prenatally. Success in this arena requires a concerted effort by health professionals, community organizations, and public health planners to train and educate in all possible areas—public health, educational institutions, governments, industry, and nongovernment organizations.

Prevention

Prevention efforts must incorporate all known methods to slow the HIV epidemic. Abstinence, monogamy, reduced sexual partners, delayed sexual intercourse, condoms, needle and syringe exchange, testing of blood donors, expansion of routine HIV testing, treatment of HIV-infected pregnant women and their infants, infant formula-feeding, and treatment of HIV infection are known to reduce HIV transmission and the seroincidence of infection in developed and developing countries (Ammann, 2000a, 2000b, 2000c).

REFERENCES

Abadco DL, Steiner P. Gastric lavage is better than bronchoalveolar lavage for isolation of *Mycobacterium tuberculosis* in childhood pulmonary tuberculosis. Pediatr Infect Dis J 11:735–738, 1992.

Aboulker JP, Swart AM. Preliminary analysis of the Concorde trial. Concorde Coordinating Committee (letter). Lancet 341:889–890, 1993.

Abrams B, Duncan D, Hertz-Picciotto I. A prospective study of dietary intake and acquired immune deficiency syndrome in HIV-seropositive homosexual men. J Acquir Immune Defic Syndr 6:949–958, 1993.

Abrams D, Goldman A, Launer C, Korvick J, Neaton J, Crane L, Grodesky M, Wakefield S, Muth K, Kornegay S, Cohn D, Harris A, Luskin-Hawk R, Markowitz N, Sampson J, Thompson M, Deyton L. A comparative trial of didanosine or zalcitabine after treatment with zidovudine in patients with human immunodeficiency virus infection. N Engl J Med 330:657–662, 1994.

Abrams EJ, Weedon J, Bertolli J, Bornschlegel K, Cervia J, Mendez H, Lambert G, Singh T, Thomas P. Aging cohort of perinatally human immunodeficiency virus-infected children in New York City. New York City Pediatric Surveillance of Disease Consortium. Pediatr Infect Dis J 20:511–517, 2001.

Adamson PC, Wu TC, Meade BD, Rubin M, Manclark CR, Pizzo PA. Pertussis in a previously immunized child with human immunodeficiency virus infection. J Pediatr 115:589–592, 1989.

Agostoni C, Zuccotti GV, Giovannini M, Decarlis S, Gianni ML, Piacentini E, D'Auria E, Riva E. Growth in the first two years of uninfected children born to HIV-1 seropositive mothers. Arch Dis Child 79:175–178, 1998.

Alimenti A, Luzuriaga K, Stechenberg B, Sullivan JL. Quantitation of human immunodeficiency virus in vertically infected infants and children. J Pediatr 119:225–229, 1991.

Alimenti A, O'Neill M, Sullivan JL, Luzuriaga K. Diagnosis of vertical human immunodeficiency virus type 1 by whole blood culture. J Infect Dis 166:1146–1148, 1992.

Allard JP, Aghdassi E, Chau J, Tam C, Koracs CM, Salit IE, Walmsley SL. Effects of vitamin E and C supplementation on oxidative stress and viral load in HIV-infected subjects. AIDS 12:1653–1659, 1998.

American Academy of Pediatrics. Active and passive immunization. In Pickering LK, ed. Red Book, 2003. Report of the Committee on Infectious Diseases. 26th ed. Elk Grove Village, IL: American Academy of Pediatrics: 2003:1–98.

Ammann AJ. Is there an acquired immune deficiency syndrome in infants and children? Pediatrics 72:430–432, 1983.

Ammann AJ. Etiology of AIDS. JAMA 252:1281–1282, 1984.

Ammann AJ. The acquired immunodeficiency syndrome in infants and children. Ann Intern Med 103:734–737, 1985.

Ammann AJ. Human immunodeficiency virus infections in infants and children. Adv Pediatr Infect Dis 3:91–109, 1988a.

Ammann AJ. Hypothesis: absence of graft-versus-host disease in AIDS is a consequence of HIV-1 infection of CD4+ T cells. J Acquir Immune Defic Syndr 6:1224–1227, 1993.

Ammann AJ. Human immunodeficiency virus infection/AIDS in children: the next decade. Pediatrics 93:930–935, 1994.

Ammann AJ. Unrestricted routine prenatal HIV testing: the standard of care. J Am Med Womens Assoc 50:83–84, 1995.

Ammann AJ. The need to resolve emerging ethical, legal and policy issues affecting children with serious and life threatening diseases. Childrens Legal Rights J 18:1–5, 1998.

Ammann AJ. HIV in China: an opportunity to halt an emerging epidemic. AIDS Patient Care STDS 14:109–112, 2000a.

Ammann AJ. Human immunodeficiency virus: an epidemic without precedent. Ann NY Acad Sci 918:3–8, 2000b.

Ammann AJ. Introduction to the Second Conference on Global Strategies for the Prevention of HIV Transmission from Mothers to Infants. Ann NY Acad Sci 918:1–2, 2000c.

Ammann AJ, Abrams D, Conant M, Chudwin D, Cowan M, Volberding P, Lewis B, Casavant C. Acquired immune dysfunction in homosexual men: immunologic profiles. Clin Immunol Immunopathol 27:315–325, 1983b.

Ammann AJ, Cowan MJ, Wara DW, Weintrub P, Dritz S, Goldman H, Perkins HA. Acquired immunodeficiency in an infant: possible transmission by means of blood products. Lancet 1:956–958, 1983a.

Ammann AJ, Schiffman G, Abrams D, Volberding P, Ziegler J, Conant M. B-cell immunodeficiency in acquired immune deficiency syndrome. JAMA 251:1447–1449, 1984a.

Ammann AJ, Wara DW, Cowan MJ. Pediatric acquired immunodeficiency syndrome. Ann NY Acad Sci 437:340–349, 1984b.

Anderson S, Shugars DC, Swanstrom R, Garcia JV. Nef from primary isolates of human immunodeficiency virus type 1 suppresses surface CD4 expression in human and mouse T cells. J Virol 67:4923–4931, 1993.

Andiman WA, Martin K, Rubinstein A, Pahwa S, Eastman R, Katz BZ, Pitt J, Miller G. Opportunistic lymphoproliferations associated with Epstein-Barr viral DNA in infants and children with AIDS. Lancet 2:1390–1393, 1985.

Andre S, Seed B, Eberle J, Schraut W, Bultmann A, Haas J. Increased immune response elicited by DNA vaccination with a synthetic gp120 sequence with optimized codon usage. J Virol 72:1497–1503, 1998.

Appay V, Nixon DF, Donahoe SM, Gillespie GM, Dong T, King A, Ogg GS, Spiegel HM, Conlon C, Spina CA, Havlir DV, Richman DD, Waters A, Easterbrook P, McMichael AJ, Rowland-Jones SL. HIV-specific CD8+ T cells produce antiviral cytokines but are impaired in cytolytic function. J Exp Med 192:63–75, 2000.

Ariyoshi K, Harwood E, Chiengsong-Popov R, Weber J. Is clearance of HIV-1 viraemia at seroconversion mediated by neutralising antibodies? Lancet 340:1257–1258, 1992.

Arpadi SM. Growth failure in children with HIV infection. J Acquir Immune Defic Syndr 25(Suppl 1):S37–42, 2000.

Arpadi SM, Cuff PA, Horlick M, Wang J, Kotler DP. Lipodystrophy in HIV-infected children is associated with high viral load and low CD4+-lymphocyte count and CD4+-lymphocyte percentage at baseline and use of protease inhibitors and stavudine. J Acquir Immune Defic Syndr 27:30–34, 2001.

Arpadi SM, Cuff PA, Kotler DP, Wang J, Bamji M, Lange M, Pierson RN, Matthews DE. Growth velocity, fat-free mass and energy intake are inversely related to viral load in HIV-infected children. J Nutr 130:2498–2502, 2000.

Athale UH, Patil PS, Chintu C, Elem B. Influence of HIV epidemic on the incidence of Kaposi's sarcoma in Zambian children. J Acquir Immune Defic Syndr Hum Retrovirol 8:96–100, 1995.

Baba T, Koch J, Mittler E, Greene M, Wyand M, Penninck D, Ruprecht R. Mucosal infection of neonatal Rhesus monkeys with cell-free SIV. AIDS Res Hum Retroviruses 10:351–357, 1994.

Babameto G, Kotler DP. Malnutrition in HIV infection. Gastroenterol Clin North Am 26:393–415, 1997.

Bagasra O, Hauptman SP, Lischner HW, Sachs M, Pomerantz RJ. Detection of human immunodeficiency virus type 1 provirus in mononuclear cells by in situ polymerase chain reaction. N Engl J Med 326:1385–1391, 1992.

Bakshi SS, Britto P, Capparelli E, Mofenson L, Fowler MG, Rasheed S, Schoenfeld D, Zimmer B, Frank Y, Yogev R, Jimenez E, Salgo M, Boone G, Pahwa SG. Evaluation of pharmacokinetics, safety, tolerance, and activity of combination of zalcitabine and zidovudine in stable, zidovudine-treated pediatric patients with human immunodeficiency virus infection. AIDS Clinical Trials Group Protocol 190 Team. J Infect Dis 175:1039–1050, 1997.

Balis FM, Pizzo PA, Butler KM, Hawkins ME, Brouwers P, Husson RN, Jacobsen F, Blaney SM, Gress J, Jarosinski P, Poplack DG. Clinical pharmacology of 2', 3'-dideoxyinosine in human immunodeficiency virus-infected children. J Infect Dis 165:99–104, 1992.

Balis FM, Pizzo PA, Eddy J, Wilfert C, McKinney R, Scott G, Murphy RF, Jarosinski PF, Falloon J, Poplack DG. Pharmacokinetics of zidovudine administered intravenously and orally in children with human immunodeficiency virus infection. J Pediatr 114:880–884, 1989a.

Balis FM, Pizzo PA, Murphy RF, Eddy J, Jarosinski PF, Falloon J, Broder S, Poplack DG. The pharmacokinetics of zidovudine administered by continuous infusion in children. Ann Intern Med 110:279–285, 1989b.

Banda NK, Bernier J, Kurahara DK, Kurrle R, Haigwood N, Sekaly RP, Finkel TH. Crosslinking CD4 by human immunodeficiency virus gp120 primes T cells for activation-induced apoptosis. J Exp Med 176:1099–1106, 1992.

Baribaud F, Pohlmann S, Doms RW. The role of DC-SIGN and DC-SIGNR in HIV and SIV attachment, infection, and transmission. Virology 286:1–6, 2001.

Barouch DH, Letvin NL. Viral evolution and challenges in the development of HIV vaccines. Vaccine 20(Suppl 4):A66–A68, 2002.

Barouch DH, Santra S, Schmitz JE, Kuroda MJ, Fu TM, Wagner W, Bilska M, Craiu A, Zheng XX, Krivulka GR, Beaudry K, Lifton MA, Nickerson CE, Trigona WL, Punt K, Freed DC, Guan L, Dubey S, Casimiro D, Simon A, Davies ME, Chastain M, Strom TB, Gelman RS, Montefiori DC, Lewis MG, Emini EA, Shiver JW, Letvin NL. Control of viremia and prevention of clinical AIDS in rhesus monkeys by cytokine-augmented DNA vaccination. Science 290:486–492, 2000.

Bartlett JG. ACOG committee opinion. "Scheduled cesarean delivery and the prevention of vertical transmission of HIV infection" [ACOG committee opinion #219, August 1999]. Hopkins HIV Rep 11:7, 1999.

Baum MK, Shor-Posner G. Micronutrient status in relationship to mortality in HIV-1 disease. Nutr Rev 56:S135–139, 1998.

Baum MK, Shor-Posner G, Lai S, Zhang G, Lai H, Fletcher MA, Sauberlich H, Page JB. High risk of HIV-related mortality is associated with selenium deficiency. J Acquir Immune Defic Syndr Hum Retrovirol 15:370–374, 1997.

Baxter JD, Mayers DL, Wentworth DN, Neaton JD, Hoover ML, Winters MA, Mannheimer SB, Thompson MA, Abrams DI, Brizz BJ, Ioannidis JP, Merigan TC. A randomized study of antiretroviral management based on plasma genotypic antiretroviral resistance testing in patients failing therapy. CPCRA 046 Study Team for the Terry Beirn Community Programs for Clinical Research on AIDS. AIDS 14:F83–93, 2000.

Bebenek K, Abbotts J, Roberts J, Wilson S, Kunkel T. Specificity and mechanism of error-prone replication by human immunodeficiency virus-1 reverse transcriptase. J Biol Chem 264:16948–16956, 1989.

Beck-Sague C, Dooley SW, Hutton MD, Otten J, Breeden A, Crawford JT, Pitchenik AE, Woodley C, Cauthen G, Jarvis WR. Hospital outbreak of multidrug-resistant Mycobacterium tuberculosis infections: factors in transmission to staff and HIV-infected patients. JAMA 268:1280–1286, 1992.

Beisel WR, Edelman R, Nauss K, Suskind RM. Single nutrient effects on immunological functions. JAMA 254:52–58, 1981.

Belec L, Mbopi Keou F, Georges A. A case for the revision of the WHO clinical definition for African AIDS. AIDS 6:880–881, 1992.

Belman AL. Acquired immunodeficiency syndrome and the child's central nervous system. Pediatr Clin North Am 39:691–714, 1992.

Beral V, Peterman TA, Berkelman RL, Jaffe HW. Kaposi's sarcoma among persons with AIDS: a sexually transmitted infection? Lancet 335:123–128, 1990.

Beral V, Peterman T, Berkelman R, Jaffe H. AIDS-associated non-Hodgkin's lymphoma. Lancet 337:805–809, 1991.

Berman PW, Matthews TJ, Riddle L, Champe M, Hobbs MR, Nakamura GR, Mercer J, Eastman DJ, Lucas C, Langlois AJ. Neutralization of multiple laboratory and clinical isolates of human immunodeficiency virus type 1 (HIV-1) by antisera raised against gp120 from the MN isolate of HIV-1. J Virol 66:4464–4469, 1992.

Bertolli J, St Louis ME, Simonds RJ, Nieburg P, Kamenga M, Brown C, Tarande M, Quinn T, Ou CY. Estimating the timing of mother-to-child transmission of human immunodeficiency virus in a breast-feeding population in Kinshasa, Zaire. J Infect Dis 174:722–726, 1996.

Bicego G, Rutstein S, Johnson K. Dimensions of the emerging orphan crisis in sub-Saharan Africa. Soc Sci Med 56:1235–1247, 2003.

Binley JM, Clas B, Gettie A, Vesanen M, Montefiori DC, Sawyer L, Booth J, Lewis M, Marx PA, Bonhoeffer S, Moore JP. Passive infusion of immune serum into simian immunodeficiency virus-infected rhesus macaques undergoing a rapid disease course has minimal effect on plasma viremia. Virology 270:237–249, 2000.

Blanche S, Mayaux MJ, Rouzioux C, Teglas JP, Firtion G, Monpoux F, Ciraru VN, Meier F, Tricoire J, Courpotin C, Vilmer E, Griscelli C, Delfraissy J-F, French Pediatric HIV Infection Study Group. Relation of the course of HIV infection in children to the severity of the disease in their mothers at delivery. N Engl J Med 330:308–312, 1994.

Blanche S, Rouzioux C, Guihard Moscato M-L, Veber F, Mayaux M-J, Jacomet C, Tricoire J, De Ville A, Vial M, Firtion G, De Crepy A, Douard D, Robin M, Courpotin C, Ciraru-Vigneron N, Le Deist F, Griscelli C. A prospective study of infants born to women seropositive for human immunodeficiency virus type 1. HIV Infection in Newborns French Collaborative Study Group. N Engl J Med 320:1643–1648, 1989.

Blanche S, Tardieu M, Duliege A-M, Rouzioux C, Le Deist F, Fukunaga K, Caniglia M, Jacomet C, Messiah A, Griscelli C. Longitudinal study of 94 symptomatic infants with perinatally acquired human immunodeficiency virus infection. Am J Dis Child 144:1210–1215, 1990.

Blanche S, Tardieu M, Rustin P, Slama A, Barret B, Firtion G, Ciraru-Vigneron N, Lacroix C, Rouzioux C, Mandelbrot L, Desguerre I, Rotig A, Mayaux MJ, Delfraissy JF. Persistent mitochondrial dysfunction and perinatal exposure to antiretroviral nucleoside analogues. Lancet 354:1084–1089, 1999.

Bodsworth NJ, Cooper DA, Donovan B. The influence of human immunodeficiency virus type 1 infection on the development of the hepatitis B virus carrier state. J Infect Dis 163:1138–1140, 1991.

Boland MG. Caring for the child and family with HIV disease. Pediatr Clin North Am 47:189–202, 2000.

Bollinger RC, Kline RL, Francis HL, Moss MW, Bartlett JG, Quinn TC. Acid dissociation increases the sensitivity of p24 antigen detection for the evaluation of antiviral therapy and disease progression in asymptomatic human immunodeficiency virus-infected persons. J Infect Dis 165:913–916, 1992.

Bonavida B, Katz J, Gottlieb M. Mechanism of defective NK cell activity in patients with acquired immunodeficiency syndrome (AIDS) and AIDS-related complex: I. defective trigger on NK cells for NKCF production by target cells, and partial restoration by IL 2. J Immunol 137:1157–1163, 1986.

Borkowsky W, Rigaud M, Krasinski K, Moore T, Lawrence R, Pollack H. Cell-mediated and humoral immune responses in children infected with human immunodeficiency virus during the first four years of life. J Pediatr 120:371–375, 1992.

Boyer P, Dillon M, Navaie M, Deveikis A, Keller M, O'Rourke S, Bryson Y. Factors predictive of maternal-fetal transmission of HIV-1. JAMA 271:1925–1930, 1994.

Brayfield BP, Phiri S, Kankasa C, Muyanga J, Mantina H, Kwenda G, West JT, Bhat G, Marx DB, Klaskala W, Mitchell CD, Wood C. Postnatal human herpesvirus 8 and human immunodeficiency virus type 1 infection in mothers and infants from Zambia. J Infect Dis 187:559–568, 2003.

Brettler DB, Forsberg A, Bolivar E, Brewster F, Sullivan J. Growth failure as a prognostic indicator for progression to acquired immunodeficiency syndrome in children with hemophilia. J Pediatr 117:584–588, 1990.

Brierley J, Roth C, Warwick C. Breast-feeding and HIV infection. Lancet 1:1346, 1988.

Brighty D, Rosenberg M, Chen I, Ivey-Hoyle M. Envelope proteins from clinical isolates of HIV-1 that are refractory to neutralization by soluble CD4 possess high affinity for the CD4 receptor. Proc Natl Acad Sci USA 88:7802–7805, 1991.

Brinkman K, ter Hofstede HJ, Burger DM, Smeitink JA, Koopmans PP. Adverse effects of reverse transcriptase inhibitors:

mitochondrial toxicity as common pathway. AIDS 12:1735–1744, 1998.

Brodie S, Sax P. Novel approaches to HIV antibody testing. AIDS Clin Care 9:1–5, 10, 1997.

Broliden K, Sievers E, Tovo PA, Moschese V, Scarlatti G, Broliden PA, Fundaro C, Rossi P. Antibody-dependent cellular cytotoxicity and neutralizing activity in sera of HIV-1-infected mothers and their children. Clin Exp Immunol 93:56–64, 1993.

Broliden PA, Makitalo B, Akerblom L, Rosen J, Broliden K, Utter G, Jondal M, Norrby E, Wahren B. Identification of amino acids in the V3 region of gp120 critical for virus neutralization by human HIV-1-specific antibodies. Immunology 73:371–376, 1991.

Brouwers P, Heyes MP, Moss HA, Wolters PL, Poplack DG, Markey SP, Pizzo PA. Quinolinic acid in the cerebrospinal fluid of children with symptomatic human immunodeficiency virus type 1 disease: relationships to clinical status and therapeutic response. J Infect Dis 168:1380–1386, 1993.

Brouwers P, Moss H, Wolters P, Eddy J, Balis F, Poplack DG, Pizzo PA. Effect of continuous-infusion zidovudine therapy on neuropsychologic functioning in children with symptomatic human immunodeficiency virus infection. J Pediatr 117:980–985, 1990.

Brunell P. Antibody in human immunodeficiency virus infection. Ann NY Acad Sci 693:9–13, 1993.

Bryant M, Ratner L. Myristoylation-dependent replication and assembly of human immunodeficiency virus I. Proc Natl Acad Sci USA 87:523–527, 1990.

Bryant M, Ratner L. Biology and molecular biology of human immunodeficiency virus. Pediatr Infect Dis J 11:390–400, 1992.

Bryson Y, Dillon M, Garratty E, Dickover R, Keller M, Deveikis A. The role of timing of HIV maternal-fetal transmission (in utero vs. intrapartum) and HIV phenotype on onset of symptoms in vertically infected infants. Int Conf AIDS 9:c10–c12, 1993a.

Bryson Y, Lehman D, Garratty E, Dickover R, Plaeger-Marshall S, O'Rourke S. The role of maternal autologous neutralizing antibody in prevention of maternal fetal HIV-1 transmission (abstract). J Cell Biochem S17E:95, 1993b.

Bryson Y, Luzuriaga K, Sullivan J, Wara D. Proposed definition for in utero versus intrapartum transmission of HIV-1. N Engl J Med 327:1246–1247, 1992.

Buchacz K, Rogol AD, Lindsey JC, Wilson CM, Hughes MD, Seage GR, 3rd, Oleske JM, Rogers AS. Delayed onset of pubertal development in children and adolescents with perinatally acquired HIV infection. J Acquir Immune Defic Syndr 33:56–65, 2003.

Bueno J, Ramil C, Green M. Current management strategies for the prevention and treatment of cytomegalovirus infection in pediatric transplant recipients. Paediatr Drugs 4:279–290, 2002.

Bulterys M, Nesheim S, Abrams EJ, Palumbo P, Farley J, Lampe M, Fowler MG. Lack of evidence of mitochondrial dysfunction in the offspring of HIV-infected women. Retrospective review of perinatal exposure to antiretroviral drugs in the Perinatal AIDS Collaborative Transmission Study. Ann NY Acad Sci 918:212–221, 2000.

Burgard M, Mayaux MJ, Blanche S, Ferroni A, Guihard MM, Allemon MC, Ciraru VN, Firtion G, Floch C, Guillot F, EL, Vial M, Griscelli C, Rouzioux C, HIV Infection in Newborns French Collaborative Study Group. The use of viral culture and p24 antigen testing to diagnose human immunodeficiency virus infection in neonates. N Engl J Med 327:1192–1197, 1992.

Burton DR. A vaccine for HIV type 1: the antibody perspective. Proc Natl Acad Sci USA 94:10018–10023, 1997.

Busch MP, Kleinman SH, Nemo GJ. Current and emerging infectious risks of blood transfusions. JAMA 289:959–962, 2003.

Busch MP, Satten GA. Time course of viremia and antibody seroconversion following human immunodeficiency virus exposure. Am J Med 102:117–124; discussion 125–116, 1997.

Buseyne F, Blanche S, Schmitt D, Griscelli C, Riviere Y. Detection of HIV-specific cell-mediated cytotoxicity in the peripheral blood from infected children. J Immunol 150:3569–3581, 1993.

Butera ST, Folks TM. Application of latent HIV-1 infected cellular models to therapeutic intervention. AIDS Res Hum Retroviruses 8:991–995, 1992.

Butler KM, De Smet MD, RNH, Mueller B, Manjunath K, Montrella K, Lovato G, Jarosinski P, Nussenblatt RB, Pizzo PA.

Treatment of aggressive cytomegalovirus retinitis with ganciclovir in combination with foscarnet in a child infected with human immunodeficiency virus. J Pediatr 120:483–486, 1992.

Butler KM, Husson RN, Balis FM, Brouwers P, Eddy J, El-Amin D, Gress J, Hawkins M, Jarosinski P, Moss H, Poplack D, Santacroce S, Venzon D, Wiener L, Wolters P, Pizzo PA. Dideoxyinosine in children with symptomatic human immunodeficiency virus infection. N Engl J Med 324:137–144, 1991.

Butler KM, Venzon D, Henry N, Husson RN, Mueller BU, Balis FM, Jacobsen F, Lewis LL, Pizzo PA. Pancreatitis in human immunodeficiency virus-infected children receiving dideoxyinosine. Pediatrics 91:747–751, 1993.

Byers B, Caldwell B, Oxtoby M. Pediatric Spectrum of Disease Project. Survival of children with perinatal HIV-infection: evidence for two distinct populations. Presented at the Ninth International Conference on AIDS, Berlin, 1993.

Cai Q, Huang XL, Rappocciolo G, Rinaldo CJ. Natural killer cell responses in homosexual men with early HIV infection. J AIDS 3:669–676, 1990.

Candotti D, Jung M, Kerouedan D, Rosenheim M, Gentilini M, M'Pele P, Huraux J. Genetic variability affects the detection of HIV by polymerase chain reaction. AIDS 5:1003–1007, 1991.

Cao Y, Krogstad P, Korber BT, Koup RA, Muldoon M, Macken C, Song JL, Jin Z, Zhao JQ, Clapp S, Chen IS, Ho DD, Ammann AJ. Maternal HIV-1 viral load and vertical transmission of infection: the Ariel Project for the prevention of HIV transmission from mother to infant. Nat Med 3:549–552, 1997.

Carr A, Emery S, Law M, Puls R, Lundgren JD, Powderly WG. An objective case definition of lipodystrophy in HIV-infected adults: a case-control study. Lancet 361:726–735, 2003.

Carr A, Samaras K, Chisholm DJ, Cooper DA. Pathogenesis of HIV-1-protease inhibitor-associated peripheral lipodystrophy, hyperlipidaemia, and insulin resistance. Lancet 351:1881–1883, 1998.

Carr A, Samaras K, Thorisdottir A, Kaufmann GR, Chisholm DJ, Cooper DA. Diagnosis, prediction, and natural course of HIV-1 protease-inhibitor-associated lipodystrophy, hyperlipidaemia, and diabetes mellitus: a cohort study. Lancet 353:2093–2099, 1999.

Carrington M, Nelson GW, Martin MP, Kissner T, Vlahov D, Goedert JJ, Kaslow R, Buchbinder S, Hoots K, O'Brien SJ. HLA and HIV-1: heterozygote advantage and B*35-Cw*04 disadvantage. Science 283:1748–1752, 1999.

Caselli D, Klersy C, de Martino M, Gabiano C, Galli L, Tovo PA, Arico M. Human immunodeficiency virus-related cancer in children: incidence and treatment outcome—report of the Italian Register. J Clin Oncol 18:3854–3861, 2000.

Cassol SA, Lapointe N, Salas T, Hankins C, Arella M, Fauvel M, Delage G, Boucher M, Samson J, Charest J. Diagnosis of vertical HIV-1 transmission using the polymerase chain reaction and dried blood spot specimens. J AIDS 5:113–119, 1992.

Cesarman E, Knowles DM. The role of Kaposi's sarcoma-associated herpesvinus (KSHV/HHV-8) in lymphoproliferative diseases. Semin Cancer Biol 9:165–174, 1999.

CDC [Centers for Disease Control and Prevention]. Unexplained immunodeficiency and opportunistic infections in infants—New York, New Jersey, California. MMWR Morb Mortal Wkly Rep 31:665–667, 1982.

CDC [Centers for Disease Control and Prevention]. Classification system for human immunodeficiency virus (HIV) infection in children under 13 years of age. MMWR Morb Mortal Wkly Rep 36:225–236, 1987.

CDC [Centers for Disease Control and Prevention]. Guidelines for prophylaxis against *Pneumocystis carinii* pneumonia for children with human immunodeficiency virus infection/exposure. MMWR Morb Mortal Wkly Rep 40:1–13, 1991a.

CDC [Centers for Disease Control and Prevention]. Mortality attributable to HIV infection/AIDS—United States, 1981–1990. MMWR Morb Mortal Wkly Rep 40:41–44, 1991b.

CDC [Centers for Disease Control and Prevention]. Guidelines for the performance of CD4+ T-cell determinations in persons with human immunodeficiency virus infection. MMWR Morb Mortal Wkly Rep 41:1–17, 1992.

CDC [Centers for Disease Control and Prevention]. 1993 revised classification system for HIV infection and expanded surveillance case definition for AIDS among adolescents and adults. MMWR Morb Mortal Wkly Rep 41:1–19, 1993a.

CDC [Centers for Disease Control and Prevention]. HIV transmission between two adolescent brothers with hemophilia. MMWR Morb Mortal Wkly Rep 42:948–951, 1993b.

CDC [Centers for Disease Control and Prevention]. HIV/AIDS Surveillance Rep 5:1–19, 1993c.

CDC [Centers for Disease Control and Prevention]. Initial therapy for tuberculosis in the era of multidrug resistance: recommendations of the Advisory Council for the Elimination of Tuberculosis. MMWR Morb Mortal Wkly Rep 42:1–8, 1993d.

CDC [Centers for Disease Control and Prevention]. Update: acquired immunodeficiency syndrome—United States, MMWR Morb Mortal Wkly Rep 42:547–557, 1993e.

CDC [Centers for Disease Control and Prevention]. Revised classification system for human immunodeficiency virus infection in children less than 13 years of age. MMWR Morb Mortal Wkly Rep 43:1–12, 1994a.

CDC [Centers for Disease Control and Prevention]. Zidovudine for the prevention of HIV transmission from mother to infant. MMWR Morb Mortal Wkly Rep 43:285–287, 1994b.

CDC [Centers for Disease Control and Prevention]. Recommendations of the U.S. Public Health Service Task Force on the use of zidovudine to reduce perinatal transmission of human immunodeficiency virus. MMWR Recomm Rep 43:1–20, 1994c.

CDC [Centers for Disease Control and Prevention]. Revised guidelines for prophylaxis against *Pneumocystis carinii* pneumonia for children infected with or perinatally exposed to human immunodeficiency virus. MMWR Morb Mortal Wkly Rep 44:1–11, 1995.

CDC. 2002 Guidelines for the prevention of opportunistic infections in persons infected with human immunodeficiency virus. U.S. Public Health Service (USPHS) and Infectious Diseases Society of America (IDSA). MMWR Recomm Rep 51:1–46, 2002a.

CDC [Centers for Disease Control and Prevention]. Diagnosis and reporting of HIV and AIDS in states with HIV/AIDS surveillance—United States, 1994–2000. MMWR Morb Mortal Wkly Rep 51:595–598, 2002b.

CDC [Centers for Disease Control and Prevention]. Guidelines for the use of antiretroviral agents in pediatric HIV infection. http://www.aidsinfo.nih.gov/guidelines, 2002c.

CDC [Centers for Disease Control and Prevention]. HIV testing among pregnant women—United States and Canada, 1998–2001. MMWR Morb Mortal Wkly Rep 51:1013–1016, 2002d.

CDC [Centers for Disease Control and Prevention]. Progress toward elimination of perinatal HIV infection—Michigan, 1993–2000. MMWR Morb Mortal Wkly Rep 51:93–97, 2002e.

CDC [Centers for Disease Control and Prevention]. U.S. Public Health Service Task Force recommendations for use of antiretroviral drugs in pregnant HIV-1 infected women for maternal health and interventions to reduce perinatal HIV-1 transmission in the United States. Morb Mortal Wkly Rep 51:1–61, 2002f.

CDC [Centers for Disease Control and Prevention]. HIV testing among pregnant women—United States and Canada, 1998–2001. JAMA 288:2679–2680, 2002g.

CDC [Centers for Disease Control and Prevention]. Pregnancy in perinatally HIV-infected adolescents and young adults—Puerto Rico, 2002. MMWR Morb Mortal Wkly Rep 52:149–151, 2003.

Chaisson RE. Gallant JE, Keruly JC, Moore RD. Impact of opportunistic disease on survival in patients with HIV infection. AIDS 12:29–33, 1998.

Chaisilwattana P, Chokephaibulkit K, Chalermchockcharoenkit A, Vanprapar N, Sirimai K, Chearskul S, Sutthent R, Oparktiattikul N. Short-course therapy with zidovudine plus lamivudine for prevention of mother-to-child transmission of human immunodeficiency virus type 1 in Thailand. Clin Infect Dis 35:1405–1413, 2002.

Chakraborty R, Uy CS, Oleske JM, Coen PG, McSherry GD. Persistent non-gastrointestinal metabolic acidosis in pediatric HIV-1 infection. Aids 17:673–677, 2003.

Chan MM, Campos JM, Josephs S, Rifai N. β₂-microglobulin and neopterin: predictive markers for human immunodeficiency virus type 1 infection in children? J Clin Microbiol 28:2215–2219, 1990.

Chandwani S, Moore T, Kaul A, Krasinski K, Borkowsky W. Early diagnosis of human immunodeficiency virus type 1-infected infants by plasma p24 antigen assay after immune complex disruption. Pediatr Infect Dis J 12:96–97, 1993.

Chanh T, Kennedy R, Kanda P. Synthetic peptides homologous to HIV transmembrane glycoprotein suppress normal human lymphocyte blastogenic response. Cell Immunol 111:77–86, 1988.

Chavanet P, Diquet B, Waldner A. Perinatal pharmacokinetics of zidovudine. N Engl J Med 321:1548–1549, 1989.

Chehimi J, Starr SE, Frank I, Rengaraju M, Jackson SJ, Llanes C, Kobayashi M, Perussia B, Young D, Nickbarg E. Natural killer (NK) cell stimulatory factor increases the cytotoxic activity of NK cells from both healthy donors and human immunodeficiency virus-infected patients. J Exp Med 175:789–796, 1992.

Chen YH, Xiao Y, Wu W, Zhao Y, Speth C, Dierich MP. The immunosuppressive peptide of HIV-1 gp41 like human type I interferons up-regulates MHC class I expression on H9 and U937 cells. Immunol Lett 59:93–97, 1997.

Cheng-Meyer C, Shiodo T, Levy J. Host range, replicative, and cytopathic properties of human immunodeficiency virus type 1 are determined by very few amino acid changes in Tat and gp120. J Virol 65:6931–6941, 1991.

Chesebro B, Wehrly K, Nishio J, Perryman S. Macrophage-tropic human immunodeficiency virus isolates from different patients exhibit unusual V3 envelope sequence homogeneity in comparison with T-cell-tropic isolates: definition of critical amino acids involved in cell tropism. J Virol 66:6547–6554, 1992.

Cheynier R, Langlade DP, Marescot MR, Blanche S, Blondin G, Wain HS, Griscelli C, Vilmer E, Plata F. Cytotoxic T lymphocyte responses in the peripheral blood of children born to human immunodeficiency virus-1-infected mothers. Eur J Immunol 22:2211–2217, 1992.

Chiarelli F, Galli L, Pomilio M, De Luca M, Verrotti A, De Martino M. Early detection and treatment of altered growth and puberty in children and adolescents with vertically-acquired HIV-1 infection: it's time to think about it. Int J Immunopathol Pharmacol 14:45–47, 2001.

Chiarelli F, Verrotti A, Galli L, Basciani F, de Martino M. Endocrine dysfunction in children with HIV-1 infection. J Pediatr Endocrinol Metab 12:17–26, 1999.

Chin DP, Hopewell PC, Yajko DM, Vittinghoff E, Horsburgh CJ, Hadley WK, Stone EN, Nassos PS, Ostroff SM, Jacobson MA. Mycobacterium avium complex in the respiratory or gastrointestinal tract and the risk of M. *avium* complex bacteremia in patients with human immunodeficiency virus infection. J Infect Dis 169:289–295, 1994.

Chiodi F, Keys B, Albert J, Hagberg L, Lundeberg J, Uhlen M, Fenyo EM, Norkrans G. Human immunodeficiency virus type 1 is present in the cerebrospinal fluid of a majority of infected individuals. J Clin Microbiol 30:1768–1771, 1992.

Chitsike I, Siziya S. Seroprevalence of human immunodeficiency virus type 1 infection in childhood malignancy in Zimbabwe. Cent Afr J Med 44:242–245, 1998.

Choi S, Lagakos SW, Schooley RT, Volberding PA. CD4+ lymphocytes are an incomplete surrogate marker for clinical progression in persons with asymptomatic HIV infection taking zidovudine. Ann Intern Med 118:674–680, 1993.

Chow YK, Hirsch MS, Kaplan JC, D'Aquila RT. HIV-1 error revealed (letter). Nature 364:679–793, 1993a.

Chow YK, Hirsch MS, Merrill DP, Bechtel LJ, Eron JJ, Kaplan JC, D'Aquila RT. Use of evolutionary limitations of HIV-1 multidrug resistance to optimize therapy [see erratum in Nature 364:679, 737, 1993]. Nature 361:650–654, 1993b.

Chuck S, Grant RM, Katongole-Mbidde E, Conant M, Ganem D. Frequent presence of a novel herpesvirus genome in lesions of human immunodeficiency virus-negative Kaposi's sarcoma. J Infect Dis 173:248–251, 1996.

Civitello L. Neurological complications of HIV infection in children. Pediatr Neurosurg 17:104–112, 1991.

Clark DA, Freeland ML, Mackie LK, Jarrett RF, Onions DE. Prevalence of antibody to human herpesvirus 7 by age (letter). J Infect Dis 168:251–252, 1993a.

Clement LT, Vink PE, Bradley GE. Novel immunoregulatory functions of phenotypically distinct subpopulations of CD4$^+$ cells in the human neonate. J Immunol 145:102–108, 1990.

Clerici M, Giorgi JV, Chou CC, Gudeman VK, Zack JA, Gupta P, Ho HN, Nishanian PG, Berzofsky JA, Shearer GM. Cell-mediated immune response to human immunodeficiency virus (HIV) type 1 in seronegative homosexual men with recent sexual exposure to HIV-1. J Infect Dis 165:1012–1019, 1992a.

Clerici M, Hakim F, Venzon D, Blatt S, Hendrix C, Wynn T, Shearer G. Changes in interleukin-2 and interleukin-4 production in asymptomatic, human immunodeficiency virus-seropositive individuals. J Clin Invest 91:759–765, 1993a.

Clerici M, Landay AL, Kessler HA, Phair JP, Venzon DJ, Hendrix CW, Lucey DR, Shearer GM. Reconstitution of long-term T helper cell function after zidovudine therapy in human immunodeficiency virus-infected patients. J Infect Dis 166:723–730, 1992b.

Clerici M, Lucey D, Berzofsky J, Pinto L, Wynn T, Blatt S, Dolan M, Hendrix C, Wolf S, Shearer G. Restoration of HIV-specific cell-mediated immune responses by interleukin-12 in vitro. Science 262:1721–1724, 1993b.

Clerici M, Lucey DR, Zajac RA, Boswell RN, Gebel HM, Takahashi H, Berzofsky JA, Shearer GM. Detection of cytotoxic T lymphocytes specific for synthetic peptides of gp160 in HIV-seropositive individuals. J Immunol 146:2214–2219, 1991.

Clerici M, Roilides E, Butler K, DePalma L, Venzon D, Shearer G, Pizzo P. Changes in T-helper function in human immunodeficiency virus-infected children during didanosine therapy as a measure of antiretroviral activity. Blood 80:2196–2202, 1992c.

Clerici M, Shearer G. A Th1-Th2 switch is a critical step in the etiology of HIV infection. Immunol Today 14:107–111, 1993.

Clerici M, Stocks N, Zajac R, Boswell R, Lucey D, Via C, Shearer G. Detection of three distinct patterns of T helper cell dysfunction in asymptomatic, human immunodeficiency virus-seropositive patients. J Clin Invest 84:1892–1899, 1989.

Clerici M, Yarchoan R, Blatt S, Hendrix CW, Ammann AJ, Broder S, Shearer GM. Effect of a recombinant CD4-IgG on in vitro T helper cell function: data from a phase I/II study of patients with AIDS. J Infect Dis 168:1012–1016, 1993c.

Clevenbergh P, Durant J, Halfon P, del Giudice P, Mondain V, Montagne N, Schapiro JM, Boucher CA, Dellamonica P. Persisting long-term benefit of genotype-guided treatment for HIV-infected patients failing HAART. The Viradapt Study: week 48 follow-up. Antivir Ther 5:65–70, 2000.

Cohen J. Apoptosis: physiological cell death. J Lab Clin Med 124:761–765, 1994.

Cohen J. Exploring how to get at—and eradicate—hidden HIV. Science 279:1854–1855, 1998.

Collins DP, Luebering BJ, Shaut DM. T-lymphocyte functionality assessed by analysis of cytokine receptor expression, intracellular cytokine expression, and femtomolar detection of cytokine secretion by quantitative flow cytometry. Cytometry 33:249–255, 1998.

Condra JH, Petropoulos CJ, Ziermann R, Schleif WA, Shivaprakash M, Emini EA. Drug resistance and predicted virologic responses to human immunodeficiency virus type 1 protease inhibitor therapy. J Infect Dis 182:758–765, 2000.

Connelly M, McSharry J, Rao P. A simple and rapid flow cytometric method for the detection of HIV infected cells and their immunophenotype. Presented at the International Conference on AIDS, Florence, Italy, 1992.

Connor E, Bagarazzi M, McSherry G, Holland B, Boland M, Denny T, Oleske J. Clinical and laboratory correlates of *Pneumocystis carinii* pneumonia in children infected with HIV. JAMA 265:1693–1697, 1991a.

Connor E, Marquis J, Oleske J. Lymphoid interstitial pneumonitis. In Pizzo PA, Wilfert CM, eds. The Challenge of HIV Infection in Infants, Children, and Adolescents. Baltimore, Williams and Wilkins, 1991b, pp 343–354.

Connor EM, Sperling RS, Gelber R, Kiselev P, Scott G, O'Sullivan MJ, VanDyke R, Bey M, Shearer W, Jacobson RL, Jimenez E, O'Neil E, Bazin B, Delfraissy JF, Culnane M, Coombs R, Elkins M, Moye J, Stratton P, Balsley J, for the Pediatric AIDS Clinical Trials Group Protocol 076 Study Group. Reduction of maternal-infant transmission of human immunodeficiency virus type I with zidovudine treatment. N Engl J Med 331:1173–1180, 1994.

Consensus Report. Early diagnosis of HIV infection in infants. J AIDS 5:1169–1178, 1992.

Consortium for Retrovirus Serology Standardization. Serological diagnosis of human immunodeficiency virus infection by Western blot testing. JAMA 260:674–679, 1988.

Coombs RW, Collier AC, Allain J-P, Nikora B, Leuther M, Gjerset GF, Corey L. Plasma viremia in human immunodeficiency virus infection. N Engl J Med 321:1626–1631, 1989.

Cooper DA, Tindall B, Wilson EJ, Imrie AA, Penny R. Characterization of T lymphocyte responses during primary infection with human immunodeficiency virus. J Infect Dis 157:889–896, 1988.

Cooper ER, Charurat M, Mofenson L, Hanson IC, Pitt J, Diaz C, Hayani K, Handelsman E, Smeriglio V, Hoff R, Blattner W. Combination antiretroviral strategies for the treatment of pregnant HIV-1-infected women and prevention of perinatal HIV-1 transmission. J Acquir Immune Defic Syndr 29:484–494, 2002.

Cooper ER, Hanson C, Diaz C, Mendez H, Abboud R, Nugent R, Pitt J, Rich K, Rodriguez EM, Smeriglio V. Encephalopathy and progression of human immunodeficiency virus disease in a cohort of children with perinatally acquired human immunodeficiency virus infection. Women and Infants Transmission Study Group. J Pediatr 132:808–812, 1998.

Cordonnier A, Montagnier L, Emerman M. Single amino-acid changes in HIV envelope affect viral tropism and receptor binding. Nature 340:571–574, 1989.

Cote HC, Brumme ZL, Craib KJ, Alexander CS, Wynhoven B, Ting L, Wong H, Harris M, Harrigan PR, O'Shaughnessy MV, Montaner JS. Changes in mitochondrial DNA as a marker of nucleoside toxicity in HIV-infected patients. N Engl J Med 346:811–820, 2002.

Coutsoudis A. Promotion of exclusive breastfeeding in the face of the HIV pandemic. Lancet 356:1620–1621, 2000.

Coutsoudis A, Bobat RA, Coovadia HM, Kuhn L, Tsai WY, Stein ZA. The effects of vitamin A supplementation on the morbidity of children born to HIV-infected women. Am J Public Health 85:1076–1081, 1995.

Coutsoudis A, Pillay K, Spooner E, Kuhn L, Coovadia HM. Randomized trial testing the effect of vitamin A supplementation on pregnancy outcomes and early mother-to-child HIV-1 transmission in Durban, South Africa. South African Vitamin A Study Group. AIDS 13:1517–1524, 1999.

Cox JC, Coulter AR. Adjuvants—a classification and review of their modes of action. Vaccine 15:248–256, 1997.

Crampin AC, Floyd S, Glynn JR, Madise N, Nyondo A, Khondowe MM, Njoka CL, Kanyongoloka H, Ngwira B, Zaba B, Fine PE. The long-term impact of HIV and orphanhood on the mortality and physical well-being of children in rural Malawi. AIDS 17:389–397, 2003.

Cullen B, Greene W. Regulatory pathways governing HIV-1 replication. Cell 58:423–426, 1989.

Cullen B, Greene W. Functions of the auxiliary gene products of the human immunodeficiency virus type 1. Virology 178:1–5, 1990.

Cullen M, Viscarello R, Paryani S, Sanchez-Ramos L. Prenatal diagnosis of HIV infection: the use of cordocentesis, polymerase chain reaction, and p24 antigen assay. Am J Obstet Gynecol 166:386, 1992.

Culnane M, Fowler M, Lee SS, McSherry G, Brady M, O'Donnell K, Mofenson L, Gortmaker SL, Shapiro DE, Scott G, Jimenez E, Moore EC, Diaz C, Flynn PM, Cunningham B, Oleske J. Lack of long-term effects of in utero exposure to zidovudine among uninfected children born to HIV-infected women. Pediatric AIDS Clinical Trials Group Protocol 219/076 Teams. JAMA 281:151–157, 1999.

Cunningham CK, Chaix ML, Rekacewicz C, Britto P, Rouzioux C, Gelber RD, Dorenbaum A, Delfraissy JF, Bazin B, Mofenson L, Sullivan JL. Development of resistance mutations in women receiving standard antiretroviral therapy who received intrapartum nevirapine to prevent perinatal human immunodeficiency virus type 1 transmission: a substudy of pediatric AIDS clinical trials group protocol 316. J Infect Dis 186:181–8, 2002.

Curry A, Turner AJ, Lucas S. Opportunistic infections in human immunodeficiency virus disease: review highlighting diagnostic and therapeutic aspects. J Clin Pathol 44:182–193, 1991.

Cusick W, Stewart J, Parry M, McLeod G, Rakos G, Sullivan C, Rodis J. State mandated prenatal human immunodeficiency virus screening at a large community hospital. Conn Med 67:7–10, 2003.

Daar E, Li X, Moudgil T, Ho D. High concentrations of recombinant soluble CD4 are required to neutralize primary human immunodeficiency virus type 1 isolates. Proc Natl Acad Sci USA 87:6574–6578, 1990.

Daar ES, Moudgil T, Meyer RD, Ho DD. Transient high levels of viremia in patients with primary human immunodeficiency virus type 1 infection. N Engl J Med 324:961–964, 1991.

Dabis F, Elenga N, Meda N, Leroy V, Viho I, Manigart O, Dequae-Merchadou L, Msellati P, Sombie I. 18-Month mortality and perinatal exposure to zidovudine in West Africa. Aids 15:771–779, 2001.

Dabis F, Msellati P, Meda N, Welffens-Ekra C, You B, Manigart O, Leroy V, Simonon A, Cartoux M, Combe P, Ouangre A, Ramon R, Ky-Zerbo O, Montcho C, Salamon R, Rouzioux C, Van de Perre P, Mandelbrot L. 6-month efficacy, tolerance, and acceptability of a short regimen of oral zidovudine to reduce vertical transmission of HIV in breastfed children in Cote d'Ivoire and Burkina Faso: a double-blind placebo-controlled multicentre trial. DITRAME Study Group. Diminution de la Transmission Mere-Enfant. Lancet 353:786–792, 1999.

Dalgleish A, Beverley P, Clapham P, Crawford D, Greaves M, Weiss R. The CD4 (T4) antigen is an essential component of the receptor for the AIDS virus. Nature 312:763–767, 1984.

D'Arminio Monforte A, Ravizza M, Muggiasca ML, Novati R, Bini T, Tornaghi R, Zuccotti GV, Cavalli G, Musicco M, Giovannini M. HIV-infected pregnant women: possible predictors of vertical transmission. Int Conf AIDS 7:1991.

Dal Molin G, D'Agaro P, Ansaldi F, Cianan G, Fertz C, Alberico S, Campello C. Mother-to-infant transmission of hepatitis C virus: rate of infection and assessment of viral load and IgM anti-HCV as risk factors. J Med Virol 67:137–142, 2002.

Dankner WM, Lindsey JC, Levin MJ. Correlates of opportunistic infections in children infected with the human immunodeficiency virus managed before highly active antiretroviral therapy. Pediatr Infect Dis J 20:40–8, 2001.

Davis MK. Human milk and HIV infection: epidemiologic and laboratory data. In Symposium on Immunology of Milk and the Neonate. New York, Plenum Press, 1991, pp 271–280.

Dawson VL, Dawson TM, Uhl GR, Snyder SH. Human immunodeficiency virus type 1 coat protein neurotoxicity mediated by nitric oxide in primary cortical cultures. Proc Natl Acad Sci USA 90:3256–3259, 1993.

de Martino M, Tovo PA, Balducci M, Galli L, Gabiano C, Rezza G, Pezzotti P. Reduction in mortality with availability of antiretroviral therapy for children with perinatal HIV-1 infection. Italian Register for HIV Infection in Children and the Italian National AIDS Registry. JAMA 284:190–197, 2000.

de Martino M, Tovo PA, Galli L, Gabiano C, Chiarelli F, Zappa M, Gattinara GC, Bassetti D, Giacomet V, Chiappini E, Duse M, Garetto S, Caselli D. Puberty in perinatal HIV-1 infection: a multicentre longitudinal study of 212 children. AIDS 15:1527–1534, 2001.

DeCarli C, Civitello LA, Brouwers P, Pizzo PA. The prevalence of computed tomographic abnormalities of the cerebrum in 100 consecutive children symptomatic with the human immune deficiency virus. Ann Neurol 34:198–205, 1993.

Del Mistro A, Laverda A, Calabrese F, De Martino M, Calabri G, Cogo P, Cocchi P, D'Andrea E, De Rossi A, Giaquinto C. Primary lymphoma of the central nervous system in two children with acquired immune deficiency syndrome. Am J Clin Pathol 94:722–728, 1990.

den Brinker M, Wit FW, Wertheim-van Dillen PM, Jurriaans S, Weel J, van Leeuwen R, Pakker NG, Reiss P, Danner SA, Weverling GJ, Lange JM. Hepatitis B and C virus co-infection and the risk of hepatotoxicity of high active antiretrovial therapy in HIV-1 infection. AIDS 14:2895–2902, 2000.

Denny T, Yogev R, Gelman R, Skuza C, Oleske J, Chadwick E, Cheng SC, Connor E. Lymphocyte subsets in healthy children during ht efirst 5 years of age. JAMA 267:1484–1488, 1992.

Di John D, Krasinski K, Lawrence R, Borkowsky W, Johnson JP, Schieken LS, Rennels MB. Very late onset of group B streptococcal disease in infants infected with the human immunodeficiency virus. Pediatr Infect Dis J 9:925–928, 1990.

Diamond D, Sleckman B, Gregory T, Lasky L, Greenstein J, Burakoff S. Inhibition of CD4+ T cell function by the HIV envelope protein, gp120. J Immunol 141:3715–3717, 1988.

Dikici B, Bosnak M, Bosnak V, Dagli A, Davutoglu M, Yagci RV, Haspolat K. Comparison of treatments of chronic hepatitis B in children with lamivudine and alpha-interferon combination and alpha-interferon alone. Pediatr Int 44:517–521, 2002.

Dimitrov D, Golding H, Blumenthal R. Initial steps in HIV-1 envelope glycoprotein mediated cell fusion monitored by a new assay based on redistribution of fluorescence markers. AIDS Res Hum Retroviruses 7:799–805, 1991.

Doebbeling BN, Feilmeier ML, Herwaldt LA. Pertussis in an adult man infected with the human immunodeficiency virus. J Infect Dis 161:1296–1298, 1990.

Dominguez K, Bertolli J, Fowler M, Peters V, Ortiz I, Melville S, Rakusan T, Frederick T, Hsu H, D'Almada P, Maldonado Y, Wilfert C. Lack of definitive severe mitochondrial signs and symptoms among deceased HIV-uninfected and HIV-indeterminate children < or = 5 years of age, Pediatric Spectrum of HIV Disease project (PSD), USA. Ann NY Acad Sci 918:236–246, 2000.

Douek DC, Koup RA, McFarland RD, Sullivan JL, Luzuriaga K. Effect of HIV on thymic function before and after antiretroviral therapy in children. J Infect Dis 181:1479–1482, 2000.

Dreimane D, Nielsen K, Deveikis A, Bryson YJ, Geffner ME. Effect of protease inhibitors combined with standard antiretroviral therapy on linear growth and weight gain in human immunodeficiency virus type 1-infected children. Pediatr Infect Dis J 20:315–316, 2001.

Dube MP. Disorders of glucose metabolism in patients infected with human immunodeficiency virus. Clin Infect Dis 31:1467–1475, 2000.

Dube MP, Stein JH, Aberg JA, Fichtenbaum CJ, Gerber JG, Tashima KT, Henry WK, Currier JS, Sprecher D, Glesby MJ. Adult AIDS Clinical Trial Group Cardiovascular Subcommittee; HIV Medical Association of the Infectious Disease Society of America. Guidelines for the evaluation and management of dyslipidemia in human immunodeficiency virus (HIV)-infected adults receiving antiretroviral therapy: recommendations of the HIV Medical Association of the Infectious Disease Society of America and the Adult AIDS Clinical Trials Group. Clin Infect Dis 37:613–627, 2003.

Dube M, Fenton M. Lipid abnormalities. Clin Infect Dis 36S2:S79–83, 2003.

Duggan C, Fawzi W. Micronutrients and child health: studies in international nutrition and HIV infection. Nutr Rev 59:358–369, 2001.

Duh E, Maury E, Folks T, Fauci A, Rabson A. Tumor necrosis factor alpha activates human immunodeficiency virus type 1 through induction of nuclear factor binding to the NF-kappa B sites in the long terminal repeat. Proc Natl Acad Sci USA 86:5974–5978, 1989.

Duliege AM, Amos CI, Felton S, Biggar RJ, Goedert JJ. Birth order, delivery route, and concordance in the transmission of human immunodeficiency virus type 1 from mothers to twins. International Registry of HIV-Exposed Twins. J Pediatr 126:625–632, 1995.

Dunn DT, Brandt CD, Krivine A, Cassol SA, Roques P, Borkowsky W, De Rossi A, Denamur E, Ehrnst A, Loveday C. The sensitivity of HIV-1 DNA polymerase chain reaction in the neonatal period and the relative contributions of intra-uterine and intra-partum transmission. AIDS 9:F7–11, 1995.

Dunn DT, Newell ML, Ades AE, Peckham CS. Risk of human immunodeficiency virus type 1 transmission through breastfeeding. Lancet 340:585–588, 1992.

Dybul M, Fauci AS, Bartlett JG, Kaplan JE, Pau AK. Guidelines for using antiretroviral agents among HIV-infected adults and adolescents. Recommendations of the Panel on Clinical Practices for Treatment of HIV. MMWR Recomm Rep 51:1–55, 2002.

Eastman PS, Shapiro DE, Coombs RW, Frenkel LM, McSherry GD, Britto P, Herman SA, Sperling RS. Maternal viral genotypic zidovudine resistance and infrequent failure of zidovudine therapy to prevent perinatal transmission of human immunodeficiency virus type 1 in pediatric AIDS Clinical Trials Group Protocol 076. J Infect Dis 177:557–564, 1998.

Eastone JA, Decker CF. New-onset diabetes mellitus associated with use of protease inhibitor. Ann Intern Med 127:948, 1997.

Economides A, Anisman D, Schmid I, Zack J, Hays E, Uittenbogaart C. Apoptosis in human HIV-1 infected thymocytes (abstract). J Cell Biochem S17E:62, 1993.

Ellaurie M, Burns ER, Rubinstein A. Hematologic manifestations in pediatric HIV infection: severe anemia as a prognostic factor. Am J Pediatr Hematol Oncol 12:449–453, 1990.

Ellaurie M, Calvelli T, Rubinstein A. Neopterin concentrations in pediatric human immunodeficiency virus infection as predictor of disease activity. Pediatr Infect Dis J 11:286–289, 1992.

Ellis M, Gupta S, Galant S, Hakim S, VandeVen C, Toy C, Cairo MS. Impaired neutrophil function in patients with AIDS or AIDS-related complex: a comprehensive evaluation. J Infect Dis 158:1268–1276, 1988.

Embretson J, Zupancic M, Ribas JL, Burke A, Racz P, Tenner RK, Haase AT. Massive covert infection of helper T lymphocytes and macrophages by HIV during the incubation period of AIDS. Nature 362:359–362, 1993.

Emerman M, Malim MH. HIV-1 regulatory/accessory genes: keys to unraveling viral and host cell biology. Science 280:1880–1884, 1998.

Emini EA, Graham DJ, Gotlib L, Condra JH, Byrnes VW, Schleif WA. HIV and multidrug resistance (letter). Nature 364:679, 1993.

Englund JA, Baker CJ, Raskino C, McKinney RE, Petrie B, Fowler MG, Pearson D, Gershon A, McSherry GD, Abrams EJ, Schliozberg J, Sullivan JL. Zidovudine, didanosine, or both as the initial treatment for symptomatic HIV-infected children. AIDS Clinical Trials Group (ACTG) Study 152 Team. N Engl J Med 336:1704–1712, 1997.

Ensoli B, Lusso P, Schachter F, Josephs S, Rappaport J, Negro F, Gallo R, Wong-Staal F. Human herpes virus-6 increases HIV-1 expression in co-infected T cells via nuclear factors binding to the HIV-1 enhancer. EMBO J 8:3019–3027, 1989.

Epstein LG, Gendelman HE. Human immunodeficiency virus type 1 infection of the nervous system: pathogenetic mechanisms. Ann Neurol 33:429–436, 1993.

Epstein LG, Sharer LR, Goudsmit J. Neurological and neuropathological features of human immunodeficiency virus infection in children. Ann Neurol 23(Suppl):S19–S23, 1988.

Erickson J, Neidhart DJ, VanDrie J, Kempf DJ, Wang XC, Norbeck DW, Plattner JJ, Rittenhouse JW, Turon M, Wideburg N. Design, activity, and 2.8 A crystal structure of a C2 symmetric inhibitor complexed to HIV-1 protease. Science 249:527–533, 1990.

Erkeller-Yuksel FM, Deneys V, Hannet I, Hulstaert F, Hamilton C, Mackinnon H, Turner Stokes L, Munhyeshuli V, Vanlangendonck F, De Bruyere M, Bach BA, Lydyard PM. Age-related changes in human blood lymphocyte subpopulations. J Pediatr 120:216–222, 1992.

Eron JJ, Benoit SL, Jemsek J, MacArthur RD, Santana J, Quinn JB, Kuritzkes DR, Fallon MA, Rubin M. Treatment with lamivudine, zidovudine, or both in HIV-positive patients with 200 to 500 CD4+ cells per cubic millimeter. North American HIV Working Party. N Engl J Med 333:1662–1669, 1995.

Eshleman SH, Krogstad P, Jackson JB, Wang YG, Lee S, Wei LJ, Cunningham M, Wantman M, Wiznia A, Johnson G, Nachman S, Palumbo P. Analysis of human immunodeficiency virus type 1 drug resistance in children receiving nucleoside analogue reverse-transcriptase inhibitors plus nevirapine, nelfinavir, or ritonavir (Pediatric AIDS Clinical Trials Group 377). J Infect Dis 183:1732–1738, 2001.

Fabio G, Scorza R, Lazzarin A, Marchini M, Zarantonello M, D'Arminio A, Marchisio P, Plebani A, Luzzati R, Costigliola P. HLA-associated susceptibility to HIV-1 infection. Clin Exp Immunol 87:20–23, 1992.

Fauci A. Multifactorial nature of human immunodeficiency virus disease: implications for therapy. Science 262:1011–1018, 1993.

Fawzi WW, Mbise RL, Hertzmark E, Fataki MR, Herrera MG, Ndossi G, Spiegelman D. A randomized trial of vitamin A supplements in relation to mortality among human immunodeficiency virus-infected and uninfected children in Tanzania. Pediatr Infect Dis J 18:127–133, 1999.

Fawzi WW, Msamanga G, Hunter D, Urassa E, Renjifo B, Mwakagile D, Hertzmark E, Coley J, Garland M, Kapiga S, Antelman G, Essex M, Spiegelman D. Randomized trial of vitamin supplements in relation to vertical transmission of HIV-1 in Tanzania. J Acquir Immune Defic Syndr 23(3): 246–254, 2000.

Fawzi WW, Msamanga GI, Spiegelman D, Urassa EJ, McGrath N, Mwakagile D, Antelman G, Mbise R, Herrera G, Kapiga S, Willett W, Hunter DJ. Randomised trial of effects of vitamin supplements on pregnancy outcomes and T cell counts in HIV-1-infected women in Tanzania. Lancet 351:1477–1482, 1998.

FDA [Food and Drug Administration]. FDA approves new rapid HIV test kit. FDA News, 2002. Available at www.fda.gov/bbs/topics/news/2002/new000852.

Finzi D, Hermankova M, Pierson T, Carruth LM, Buck C, Chaisson RE, Quinn TC, Chadwick K, Margolick J, Brookmeyer R, Gallant J, Markowitz M, Ho DD, Richman DD, Siliciano RF. Identification of a reservoir for HIV-1 in patients on highly active antiretroviral therapy. Science 278:1295–1300, 1997.

Fischl MA, Richman DD, Grieco MH, Gottlieb MS, Volberding PA, Laskin OL, Leedom JM, Groopman JE, Mildvan D, Schooley RT, Jackson GG, Durack DT, King D, Group TACW. The efficacy of azidothymidine (AZT) in the treatment of patients with AIDS and AIDS-related complex. N Engl J Med 317:185–191, 1987.

Fischl MA, Richman DD, Hansen N, Collier AC, Carey JT, Para MF, Hardy WD, Dolin R, Powderly WG, Allan JD, Wong B, Merigan TC, McAuliffe VJ, Hyslop NE, Rhame FS, Balfour HH, Spector SA, Volberding P, Pettinelli C, Anderson J, Group TACT. The safety and efficacy of zidovudine (AZT) in the treatment of subjects with mildly symptomatic human immunodeficiency virus type 1 (HIV) infection. Ann Intern Med 112:727–737, 1990.

Fischl MA, Uttamchandani RB, Daikos GL, Poblete RB, Moreno JN, Reyes RR, Boota AM, Thompson LM, Cleary TJ, Lai S. An outbreak of tuberculosis caused by multiple-drug-resistant tubercle bacilli among patients with HIV infection. Ann Intern Med 117:177–183, 1992.

Fishback N, Koss M. Update on lymphoid interstitial pneumonitis. Curr Opin Pulm Med 2:429–433, 1996.

Fisher A, Feinberg M, Josephs S, Harper M, Marsell L, Reyes G, Gonda M, Aldovini A, Debouk C, Gallo R, Wong-Staal F. The trans-activator gene of HTLV-III is essential for virus replication. Nature 320:367–371, 1986.

Fitzgerald P, Springer J. Structure and function of retroviral proteases. Annu Rev Biophys Chem 20:299–320, 1991.

Fitzgibbon J, Gaur S, Frenkel L, Laraque F, Edlin B, Dubin D. Transmission from one child to another of human immunodeficiency virus type 1 with a zidovudine-resistance mutation. N Engl J Med 329:1835–1841, 1993.

Folks TM, Kessler SW, Orenstein JM, Justement JS, Jaffe ES, Fauci AS. Infection and replication of HIV-1 in purified progenitor cells of normal human bone marrow. Science 242:919–922, 1988.

Foster G. Supporting community efforts to assist orphans in Africa. N Engl J Med 346:1907–1910, 2002.

Fowler MG, Newell ML. Breast-feeding and HIV-1 transmission in resource-limited settings. J Acquir Immune Defic Syndr 30:230–239, 2002.

Fox CH, Tenner-Racz K, Racz P, Firpo A, Pizzo PA, Fauci AS. Lymphoid germinal centers are reservoirs of human immunodeficiency virus type 1 RNA. J Infect Dis 164:1051–1057, 1991.

Frickhofen N, Abkowitz JL, Safford M, Berry JM, Antunez-de-Mayolo J, Astrow A, Cohen R, Halperin I, King L, Mintzer D, Cohen B, Young NS. Persistent B19 parvovirus infection in patients infected with human immunodeficiency virus type 1 (HIV-1): a treatable cause of anemia in AIDS. Ann Intern Med 113:926–933, 1990.

Friedland GH, Saltzman BR, Rogers MF, Kahl PA, Lesser ML, Mayers MM, Klein RS. Lack of transmission of HTLV-III/LAV infection to household contacts of patients with AIDS or AIDS-related complex with oral candidiasis. N Engl J Med 314:344–339, 1986.

Froebel KS, Doherty KV, Whitelaw JA, Hague RA, Mok JY, Bird AG. Increased expression of the CD45RO (memory) antigen on T cells in HIV-infected children. AIDS 5:97–99, 1991.

Funkhouser AW, Katzman PJ, Sickel JZ, Lambert JS. CD30-positive anaplastic large cell lymphoma (ALCL) of T-cell lineage in a 14-month-old infant with perinatally acquired HIV-1 infection. J Pediatr Hematol Oncol 20:556–559, 1998.

Furman PA, Jeffrey J, Kiefer LL, Feng JY, Anderson KS, Borroto-Esoda K, Hill E, Copeland WC, Chu CK, Sommadossi JP, Liberman I, Schinazi RF, Painter GR. Mechanism of action of 1-beta-D-2,6-diaminopurine dioxolane, a prodrug of the human immunodeficiency virus type 1 inhibitor 1-beta-D-dioxolane guanosine. Antimicrob Agents Chemother 45:158–165, 2001.

Gail MH, Pluda JM, Rabkin CS, Biggar RJ, Goedert JJ, Horm JW, Sondik EJ, Yarchoan R, Broder S. Projections of the incidence of non-Hodgkin's lymphoma related to acquired immunodeficiency syndrome. J Natl Cancer Inst 83:695–701, 1991.

Gaillard P, Mwanyumba F, Verhofstede C, Claeys P, Chohan V, Goetghebeur E, Mandaliya K, Ndinya-Achola J, Temmerman M. Vaginal lavage with chlorhexidine during labour to reduce mother-to-child HIV transmission: clinical trial in Mombasa, Kenya. AIDS 15:389–396, 2001.

Gallo D, George JR, Fitchen JH, Goldstein AS, Hindahl MS. Evaluation of a system using oral mucosal transudate for HIV-1 antibody screening and confirmatory testing. OraSure HIV Clinical Trials Group. JAMA 277:254–258, 1997.

Gao F, Bailes E, Robertson DL, Chen Y, Rodenburg CM, Michael SF, Cummins LB, Arthur LO, Peeters M, Shaw GM, Sharp PM, Hahn BH. Origin of HIV-1 in the chimpanzee Pan troglodytes. Nature 397:436–441, 1999.

Gao WY, Shirasaka T, Johns DG, Broder S, Mitsuya H. Differential phosphorylation of azidothymidine, dideoxycytidine, and dideoxyinosine in resting and activated peripheral blood mononuclear cells. J Clin Invest 91:2326–2333, 1993.

Garry R. Potential mechanisms for the cytopathic properties of HIV. AIDS 3:683–694, 1989.

Gartner S, Markovits P, Markovitz D, Kaplan M, Gallo R, Popovic M. The role of mononuclear phagocytes in HTLV-III/LAV infection. Science 233:215–219, 1986.

Garzino-Demo A, DeVico AL, Conant KE, Gallo RC. The role of chemokines in human immunodeficiency virus infection. Immunol Rev 177:79–87, 2000.

Gaughan DM, Hughes MD, Seage GR III, Selwyn PA, Carey VJ, Gortmaker SL, Oleske JM. The prevalence of pain in pediatric human immunodeficiency virus/acquired immunodeficiency syndrome as reported by participants in the Pediatric Late Outcomes Study (PACTG 219). Pediatrics 109:1144–1152, 2002.

Gavin PJ, Yogev R. The role of protease inhibitor therapy in children with HIV infection. Paediatr Drugs 4:581–607, 2002.

Gayle H. An overview of the global HIV/AIDS epidemic, with a focus on the United States. AIDS 14(Suppl 2):S8–17, 2000.

Gayle H, D'Angelo L. Epidemiology of acquired immunodeficiency syndrome and human immunodeficiency virus infection in adolescents. J Pediatr Infect Dis 10:322–328, 1991.

Gayle HD, Hill GL. Global impact of human immunodeficiency virus and AIDS. Clin Microbiol Rev 14:327–335, 2001.

Geffner ME, Bersch N, Lippe BM, Rosenfeld RG, Hintz RL, Golde DW. Growth hormone mediates the growth of T-lymphoblast cell lines via locally generated insulin-like growth factor-I. J Clin Endocrinol Metab 71:464–469, 1990.

Geffner ME, Yeh DY, Landaw EM, Scott ML, Stiehm ER, Bryson YJ, Israele V. In vitro insulin-like growth factor-I, growth hormone, and insulin resistance occurs in symptomatic human immunodeficiency virus-1-infected children. Pediatr Res 34:66–72, 1993.

Gelderblom H, Hausmann E, Ozel M, Pauli G, Koch M. Fine structure of human immunodeficiency virus (HIV) and immunolocalization of structural proteins. Virology 156:171–176, 1987.

Gendelman H, Phelps W, Feigenbaum L, Ostrove J, Adachi A, Howley P, Khoury G, Ginsberg H, Martin M. Trans-activation of

the human immunodeficiency virus long terminal repeat sequence by DNA viruses. Proc Natl Acad Sci USA 83:9759–9763, 1986.

Gerberding JL. Clinical practice. Occupational exposure to HIV in health care settings. N Engl J Med 348:826–833, 2003.

Goedert JJ. The epidemiology of acquired immunodeficiency syndrome malignancies. Semin Oncol 27:390–401, 2000.

Goedert JJ, Drummond JE, Minkoff HL, Stevens R, Blattner WA, Landesman SH, Mendez H, Robert-Guroff M, Holman S, Rubinstein A, Willoughby A. Mother-to-infant transmission of human immunodeficiency virus type 1: association with prematurity or low anti-gp120. Lancet 2:1351–1354, 1989.

Goedert JJ, Duliege A, Amos C, Felton S, Biggar R. The International Registry of HIV-exposed twins. High risk of HIV-1 infection for first-born twins. Lancet 338:1471–1475, 1991.

Golding H, Shearer G, Hillman K, Lucas P, Manischewitz J, Zajac R, Clerici M, Gress R, Boswell R, Golding B. Common epitope in human immunodeficiency virus (HIV) 1-gp41 and HLA class II elicits immunosuppressive autoantibodies capable of contributing to immune dysfunction in HIV I-infected individuals. J Clin Invest 83:1430–1435, 1989.

Gonzalez CE, Samakoses R, Boler AM, Hill S, Wood LV. Lymphoid interstitial pneumonitis in pediatric AIDS. Natural history of the disease. Ann NY Acad Sci 918:358–361, 2000.

Gordin FM, Simon GL, Wofsy CB, Mills J. Adverse reactions to trimethoprim-sulfamethoxazole in patients with the acquired immunodeficiency syndrome. Ann Intern Med 100:495–499, 1984.

Gorelick R, Nigida S, Bess J, Arthur L, Henderson L, Rein A. Noninfectious human immunodeficiency virus type 1 mutants deficient in genomic RNA. J Virol 64:3207–3211, 1990.

Gorochov G, Neumann AU, Kereveur A, Parizot C, Li T, Katlama C, Karmochkine M, Raguin G, Autran B, Debre P. Perturbation of CD4+ and CD8+ T-cell repertoires during progression to AIDS and regulation of the CD4+ repertoire during antiviral therapy. Nat Med 4:215–221, 1998.

Gottlieb MS, Schroff R, Schanker HM, Weisman JD, Fan PT, Wolf RA, Saxon A. Pneumocystis carinii pneumonia and mucosal candidiasis in previously healthy homosexual men: evidence of a new acquired cellular immunodeficiency. N Engl J Med 305:1425–1431, 1981.

Goulder PJ, Brander C, Tang Y, Tremblay C, Colbert RA, Addo MM, Rosenberg ES, Nguyen T, Allen R, Trocha A, Altfeld M, He S, Bunce M, Funkhouser R, Pelton SI, Burchett SK, McIntosh K, Korber BT, Walker BD. Evolution and transmission of stable CTL escape mutations in HIV infection. Nature 412:334–338, 2001a.

Goulder PJ, Jeena P, Tudor-Williams G, Burchett S. Paediatric HIV infection: correlates of protective immunity and global perspectives in prevention and management. Br Med Bull 58:89–108, 2001b.

Goulder PJ, Pasquier C, Holmes EC, Liang B, Tang Y, Izopet J, Saune K, Rosenberg ES, Burchett SK, McIntosh K, Barnardo M, Bunce M, Walker BD, Brander C, Phillips RE. Mother-to-child transmission of HIV infection and CTL escape through HLA-A2-SLYNTVATL epitope sequence variation. Immunol Lett 79:109–116, 2001c.

Graham NMH, Zeger SL, Park LP, Vermund SH, Detels R, Rinaldo CR, Phair JP. The effects on survival of early treatment of human immunodeficiency virus infection. N Engl J Med 326:1037–1042, 1992.

Granovsky MO, Mueller BU, Nicholson HS, Rosenberg PS, Rabkin CS. Cancer in human immunodeficiency virus-infected children: a case series from the Children's Cancer Group and the National Cancer Institute. J Clin Oncol 16:1729–1735, 1998.

Grant RM, Hecht FM, Warmerdam M, Liu L, Liegler T, Petropoulos CJ, Hellmann NS, Chesney M, Busch MP, Kahn JO. Time trends in primary HIV-1 drug resistance among recently infected persons. JAMA 288:181–188, 2002.

Gray L, Newell ML, Thorne C, Peckham C, Levy J. Fluctuations in symptoms in human immunodeficiency virus-infected children: the first 10 years of life. Pediatrics 108:116–122, 2001.

Greene WC. The molecular biology of human immunodeficiency virus type 1 infection. N Engl J Med 324:308–317, 1991.

Groopman JE, Broder S. Cancers in AIDS and other immunodeficiency states. In DeVita VT, Hilman S, Rosenberg S, eds. Cancer: Principles and Practice of Oncology. Philadelphia, JB Lippincott, 1989, pp 1953–1970.

Groopman JE, Mitsuyasu RT, DeLeo MJ, Oette DH, Golde DW. Effect of recombinant human granulocyte-macrophage colony-stimulating factor on myelopoiesis in the acquired immunodeficiency syndrome. N Engl J Med 317:593–598, 1987.

Groux H, Torpier G, Monte D, Mouton Y, Capron A, Ameisen J-C. Activation-induced death by apoptosis in CD4+ T cells from human immunodeficiency virus-infected asymptomatic individuals. J Exp Med 175:331–340, 1992.

Grunfeld C, Pang M, Shimuzu L, Shigenga JK, Jensen P, Feingold KR. Resting energy expenditure, caloric intake and short-term weight change in human immunodeficiency virus infection and the acquired immunodeficiency syndrome. Am J Clin Nutr 55:455–460, 1992.

Guarino A, Spagnuolo MI, Giacomet V, Canani RB, Bruzzese E, Giaquinto C, Roggero P, Plebani A, Gattinara GC. Effects of nutritional rehabilitation on intestinal function and on CD4 T-cell number in children with HIV. J Pediatr Gastroenterol Nutr 34:366–371, 2002.

Guay LA, Musoke P, Fleming T, Bagenda D, Allen M, Nakabiito C, Sherman J, Bakaki P, Ducar C, Deseyve M, Emel L, Mirochnick M, Fowler MG, Mofenson L, Miotti P, Dransfield K, Bray D, Mmiro F, Jackson JB. Intrapartum and neonatal single-dose nevirapine compared with zidovudine for prevention of mother-to-child transmission of HIV-1 in Kampala, Uganda: HIVNET 012 randomised trial. Lancet 354:795–802, 1999.

Gulick RM. New antiretroviral drugs. Clin Microbiol Infect 9:186–193, 2003.

Gutman LT, St. Claire KK, Weedy C, Herman-Giddens ME, Lane BA, Niemeyer JG, McKinney RE. Human immunodeficiency virus transmission by child sexual abuse. Am J Dis Child 145:137–141, 1991.

Gwinn M, Pappaioanou M, George J, Hannon W, Wasser S, Redus M, Hoff R, Grady G, Willoughby A, Novello A, Peterson L, Dondero T, Curran J. Prevalence of HIV infection in childbearing women in the United States: surveillance using newborn blood samples. JAMA 265:1704–1708, 1991.

Haase AT. Population biology of HIV-1 infection: viral and CD4+ T cell demographics and dynamics in lymphatic tissues. Annu Rev Immunol 17:625–656, 1999.

Habeshaw J, Hounsell E, Dalgleish A. Does the HIV envelope induce a chronic graft-versus-host-like disease? Immunol Today 13:207–210, 1992.

Hadigan C, Meigs JB, Corcoran C, Rietschel P, Piecuch S, Basgoz N, Davis B, Sax P, Stanley T, Wilson PW, D'Agostino RB, Grinspoon S. Metabolic abnormalities and cardiovascular disease risk factors in adults with human immunodeficiency virus infection and lipodystrophy. Clin Infect Dis 32:130–139, 2001.

Hadziyannis SJ, Tassopoulos NC, Heathcote EJ, Chang TT, Kitis G, Rizzetto M, Marcellin P, Lim SG, Goodman Z, Wulfsohn MS, Xiong S, Fry J, Brosgart CL. Adefovir dipivoxil for the treatment of hepatitis B e antigen-negative chronic hepatitis B. N Engl J Med 348:800–807, 2003.

Hahn BH, Shaw GM, De Cock KM, Sharp PM. AIDS as a zoonosis: scientific and public health implications. Science 287:607–614, 2000.

Halsey N, Markham R, Wahren B, Boulos R, Rossi P, Wigzell H. Lack of association between maternal antibodies to V3 loop peptides and maternal-infant transmission. J AIDS 5:153–157, 1992.

Hamilton JD, Hartigan PM, Simberkoff MS, Day PL, Diamond GR, Dickinson GM, Drusano GL, Egorin MJ, George WL, Gordin FM, Hawkes CA, Jensen PC, Klimas NG, Labriola AM, Lahart CJ, O'Brien WA, Oster CN, Weinhold KJ, Wray NP, Zolla-Pazner SB, the Veterans Affairs Cooperative Study Group on AIDS Treatment. A controlled trial of early versus late treatment with zidovudine in symptomatic human immunodeficiency virus infection: results of the Veterans Affairs Cooperative Study. N Engl J Med 326:437–443, 1992.

Hanekom WA, Yogev R, Heald LM, Edwards KM, Hussey GD, Chadwick EG. Effect of vitamin A therapy on serologic responses and viral load changes after influenza vaccination in children infected with the human immunodeficiency virus. J Pediatr 136:550–552, 2002.

Hanson I, Kaplan S. Opportunistic infections. Semin Pediatr Infect Dis 1:31–39, 1990.

Harmon WG, Dadlani GH, Fisher SD, Lipshultz SE. Myocardial and Pericardial Disease in HIV. Curr Treat Options Cardiovasc Med 4:497–509, 2002.

Haseltine W. Molecular biology of the human immunodeficiency virus type 1. FASEB J 5:2349–2360, 1991.

Havlir DV, Bassett R, Levitan D, Gilbert P, Tebas P, Collier AC, Hirsch MS, Ignacio C, Condra J, Gunthard HF, Richman DD, Wong JK. Prevalence and predictive value of intermittent viremia with combination HIV therapy. JAMA 286:171–179, 2001.

Heng MC, Heng SY, Allen SG. Co-infection and synergy of human immunodeficiency virus-1 and herpes simplex virus-1. Lancet 343:255–258, 1994.

Hersh BS, Popovici F, Jezek Z, Satten GA, Apetrei RC, Beldescu N, George JR, Shapiro CN, Gayle HD, Heymann DL. Risk factors for HIV infection among abandoned Romanian children. AIDS 7:1617–1624, 1993.

Hershow RC, Riester KA, Lew J, Quinn TC, Mofenson LM, Davenny K, Landesman S, Cotton D, Hanson IC, Hillyer GV, Tang HB, Thomas DL. Increased vertical transmission of human immunodeficiency virus from hepatitis C virus-coinfected mothers. Women and Infants Transmission Study. J Infect Dis 176:414–420, 1997.

Hirsch MS, Brun-Vezinet F, D'Aquila RT, Hammer SM, Johnson VA, Kuritzkes DR, Loveday C, Mellors JW, Clotet B, Conway B, Demeter LM, Vella S, Jacobsen DM, Richman DD. Antiretroviral drug resistance testing in adult HIV-1 infection: recommendations of an International AIDS Society-USA Panel. JAMA 283:2417–2426, 2000.

Hirsch MS, Conway B, D'Aquila RT, Johnson VA, Brun-Vezinet F, Clotet B, Demeter LM, Hammer SM, Jacobsen DM, Kuritzkes DR, Loveday C, Mellors JW, Vella S, Richman DD. Antiretroviral drug resistance testing in adults with HIV infection: implications for clinical management. International AIDS Society—USA Panel. JAMA 279:1984–1991, 1998.

Ho D, Rota T, Hirsch M. Infection of monocyte/macrophages by human T lymphotropic viruses type III. J Clin Invest 77:1712–1715, 1986.

Ho DD. Toward HIV eradication or remission: the tasks ahead. Science 280:1866–1867, 1998.

Ho DD, Moudgil T, Alam M. Quantitation of human immunodeficiency virus type 1 in the blood of infected persons. N Engl J Med 321:1621–1625, 1989.

Hoff R, Berardi VP, Weiblen BJ, Mahoney-Trout L, Mitchell ML, Grady GF. Seroprevalence of human immunodeficiency virus among childbearing women. Estimation by testing samples of blood from newborns. N Engl J Med 318:525–530, 1988.

Hoffenbach A, Langlade DP, Dadaglio G, Vilmer E, Michel F, Mayaud C, Autran B, Plata F. Unusually high frequencies of HIV-specific cytotoxic T lymphocytes in humans. J Immunol 142:452–462, 1989.

Homsy J, Tateno M, Levy J. Antibody-dependent enhancement of HIV infection. Lancet 1:1285–1286, 1988.

Horsburgh CJ, Ou CY, Jason J, Holmberg SD, Longini IJ, Schable C, Mayer KH, Lifson AR, Schochetman G, Ward JW. Duration of human immunodeficiency virus infection before detection of antibody. Lancet 2:637–640, 1989.

Hubner A, Kruhoffer M, Grosse F, Krauss G. Fidelity of human immunodeficiency virus type 1 reverse transcriptase in copying natural RNA. J Mol Biol 223:595–600, 1992.

Hughes MD, Johnson VA, Hirsch MS, Bremer JW, Elbeik T, Erice A, Kuritzkes DR, Scott WA, Spector SA, Basgoz N, Fischl MA, D'Aquila RT. Monitoring plasma HIV-1 RNA levels in addition to CD4+ lymphocyte count improves assessment of antiretroviral therapeutic response. ACTG 241 Protocol Virology Substudy Team. Ann Intern Med 126:929–938, 1997.

Husson RN, Comeau AM, Hoff R. Diagnosis of human immunodeficiency virus infection in infants and children. Pediatrics 86:1–10, 1990.

Husson RN, Saini R, Lewis LL, Butler KM, Patronas N, Pizzo PA. Cerebral artery aneurysms in children infected with human immunodeficiency virus. J Pediatr 121:927–930, 1992.

Imberti L, Sottini A, Bettinardi A, Puoti M, Primi D. Selective depletion of T cells that bear specific T cell receptor V-beta sequences. Science 254:860–862, 1991.

Inoue M, Koga Y, Djordjijevic D, Fukuma T, Reddy EP, Yokoyama MM, Sagawa K. Down-regulation of CD4 molecules by the expression of Nef: a quantitative analysis of CD4 antigens on the cell surfaces. Int Immunol 5:1067–1073, 1993.

Ioannidis JP, Abrams EJ, Ammann A, Bulterys M, Goedert JJ, Gray L, Korber BT, Mayaux MJ, Mofenson LM, Newell ML, Shapiro DE, Teglas JP, Wilfert CM. Perinatal transmission of human immunodeficiency virus type 1 by pregnant women with RNA virus loads <1000 copies/mL. J Infect Dis 183:539–545, 2001.

Iosub S, Bamji M, Stone RK, Gromisch DS, Wasserman E. More on human immunodeficiency virus embryopathy. Pediatrics 80:512–516, 1987.

Issel CJ, Horohov DW, Lea DF, Adams WJ, Hagius SD, McManus JM, Allison AC, Montelaro RC. Efficacy of inactivated whole-virus and subunit vaccines in preventing infection and disease caused by equine infectious anemia virus. J Virol 66:3398–3408, 1992.

Itescu S, Winchester R. Diffuse infiltrative lymphocytosis syndrome: a disorder occurring in human immunodeficiency virus-1 infection that may present as a sicca syndrome. Rheum Dis Clin North Am 18:683–697, 1992.

Ivey-Hoyle M, Culp J, Caikin M, Hellmig B, Matthews T. Envelope glycoproteins from biologically diverse isolates of human immunodeficiency viruses have widely different affinities for CD4. Proc Natl Acad Sci USA 88:7802–7805, 1991.

Jacks T, Power M, Masiarz F, Luciw P, Barr P, Varmus H. Characterization of ribosomal frameshifting in HIV-1 gag-pol expression. Nature 331:280–283, 1988.

Jackson J, Coombs R, Sannerud K, Rhame F, Balfour H. Rapid and sensitive viral culture method for human immunodeficiency virus type 1. J Clin Microbiol 26:1416–1418, 1988.

Jacobson JM, Colman N, Ostrow NA, Simson RW, Tomesch D, Marlin L, Rao M, Mills JL, Clemens J, Prince AM. Passive immunotherapy in the treatment of advanced human immunodeficiency virus infection [see published erratum appears in J Infect Dis 168:802, 1993]. J Infect Dis 168:298–305, 1993.

Jacobson MA, Berger TG, Fikrig S, Becherer P, Moohr JW, Stanat SC, Biron KK. Acyclovir-resistant varicella zoster virus infection after chronic oral acyclovir therapy in patients with the acquired immunodeficiency syndrome (AIDS). Ann Intern Med 112:187–191, 1990.

Jansen J, Ammann A. Priorities in psychosocial research in pediatric human immunodeficiency virus infection. Develop Behav Pediatr 15:S3–4, 1994.

Jaquet D, Levine M, Ortega-Rodriguez E, Faye A, Polak M, Vilmer E, Levy-Marchal C. Clinical and metabolic presentation of the lipodystrophic syndrome in HIV-infected children. AIDS 14:2123–2128, 2000.

Jenkinson E, Kingston R, Smith C, Williams G, Owen J. Antigen-induced apoptosis in developing T cells: a mechanism for negative selection of the T cell receptor repertoire. Eur J Immunol 19:2175–2177, 1989.

John GC, Nduati RW, Mbori-Ngacha DA, Richardson BA, Panteleeff D, Mwatha A, Overbaugh J, Bwayo J, Ndinya-Achola JO, Kreiss JK. Correlates of mother-to-child human immunodeficiency virus type 1 (HIV-1) transmission: association with maternal plasma HIV-1 RNA load, genital HIV-1 DNA shedding, and breast infections. J Infect Dis 183:206–212, 2001.

Johnston AM, Valentine ME, Ottinger J, Baydo R, Gryszowka V, Vavro C, Weinhold K, St Clair M, McKinney RE. Immune reconstitution in human immunodeficiency virus-infected children receiving highly active antiretroviral therapy: a cohort study. Pediatr Infect Dis J 20:941–946, 2001.

Jonas MM, Kelley DA, Mizerski J, Badia IB, Areias JA, Schwarz KB, Little NR, Greensmith MJ, Gardner SD, Bell MS, Sokal EM. Clinical trial of lamivudine in children with chronic hepatitis B. N Engl J Med 346:1706–1713, 2002.

Joshi VV, Kauffman S, Oleske JM, Fikrig S, Denny T, Gadol C, Lee E. Polyclonal polymorphic B-cell lymphoproliferative disorder with prominent pulmonary involvement in children with acquired immune deficiency syndrome. Cancer 59:1455–1462, 1987.

Joshi VV, Oleske JM. Pathologic appraisal of the thymus gland in acquired immunodeficiency syndrome in children. A study of four cases and a review of the literature. Arch Pathol Lab Med 109:142–146, 1985.

Joshi VV, Oleske JM, Connor EM. Morphologic findings in children with acquired immune deficiency syndrome: pathogenesis and clinical implications. In Childhood AIDS. Hemisphere Publishing, 1990, pp 155–165.

Jura E, Chadwick EG, Josephs SH, Steinberg SP, Yogev R, Gershon AA, Krasinski KM, Borkowsky W. Varicella-zoster virus infections in children infected with human immunodeficiency virus. Pediatr Infect Dis J 8:586–590, 1989.

Kageyama S, Mimoto T, Murakawa Y, Nomizu M, Ford HJ, Shirasaka T, Gulnik S, Erickson J, Takada K, Hayashi H. In vitro anti-human immunodeficiency virus (HIV) activities of transition state mimetic HIV protease inhibitors containing allophenylnorstatine. Antimicrob Agents Chemother 37:810–817, 1993.

Kahn JO, Lagakos SW, Richman DD, Cross A, Pettinelli C, Liou S-H, Brown M, Volberding PA, Crumpacker CS, Beall G, Sacks HS, Merigan TC, Beltangady M, Smaldone L, Dolin R, the NIAID AIDS Clinical Trials Group. A controlled trial comparing zidovudine with didanosine in human immunodeficiency virus infection. N Engl J Med 327:581–587, 1992.

Kalish LA, McIntosh K, Read JS, Diaz C, Landesman SH, Pitt J, Rich KC, Shearer WT, Davenny K, Lew JF. Evaluation of human immunodeficiency virus (HIV) type 1 load, CD4 T cell level, and clinical class as time-fixed and time-varying markers of disease progression in HIV-1-infected children. J Infect Dis 180:1514–1520, 1999.

Kaplan LJ, Daum RS, Smaron M, McCarthy CA. Severe measles in immunocompromised patients. JAMA 267:1237–1241, 1992.

Karpatkin S. Autoimmune thrombocytopenia and AIDS-related tyrombocytopenia. Curr Opin Immunol 2:625–632, 1989.

Kaslow RA, Carrington M, Apple R, Park L, Munoz A, Saah AJ, Goedert JJ, Winkler C, O'Brien SJ, Rinaldo C, Detels R, Blattner W, Phair J, Erlich H, Mann DL. Influence of combinations of human major histocompatibility complex genes on the course of HIV-1 infection. Nat Med 2:405–411, 1996.

Kaslow RA, Duquesnoy R, VanRaden M, Kingsley L, Marrari M, Friedman H, Su S, Saah AJ, Detels R, Phair J. A1, Cw7, B8, DR3 HLA antigen combination associated with rapid decline of T-helper lymphocytes in HIV-1 infection: a report from the Multicenter AIDS Cohort Study. Lancet 335:927–930, 1990.

Katz B, Berkman A, Shapiro E. Serologic evidence of active Epstein-Barr virus infection in Epstein-Barr virus-associated lymphoproliferative disorders of children with acquired immunodeficiency syndrome. J Pediatr 120:228–232, 1992.

Katz MH, Gerberding JL. Postexposure treatment of people exposed to the human immunodeficiency virus through sexual contact or injection-drug use. N Engl J Med 336:1097–1100, 1997.

Katzenstein DA, Hammer SM, Hughes MD, Gundacker H, Jackson JB, Fiscus S, Rasheed S, Elbeik T, Reichman R, Japour A, Merigan TC, Hirsch MS. The relation of virologic and immunologic markers to clinical outcomes after nucleoside therapy in HIV-infected adults with 200 to 500 CD4 T-cells per cubic millimeter. AIDS Clinical Trials Group Study 175 Virology Study Team. N Engl J Med 335:1091–1098, 1996.

Kauffman WM, Sivit CJ, Fitz CR, Rakusan TA, Herzog K, Chandra RS. CT and MR evaluation of intracranial involvement in pediatric HIV infection: a clinical-imaging correlation. Am J Neuroradiol 13:949–957, 1992.

Kellam P, Boucher CA, Larder BA. Fifth mutation in human immunodeficiency virus type 1 reverse transcriptase contributes to the development of high-level resistance to zidovudine. Proc Natl Acad Sci USA 89:1934–1938, 1992.

Kestler HW, Ringler DJ, Mori K, Panicali DL, Sehgal PK, Daniel MD, Desrosiers RC. Importance of the nef gene for maintenance of high virus loads and for the development of AIDS. Cell 65:651–662, 1991.

Khouri YF, Mastrucci MT, Hutto C, Mitchell CD, Scott GB. Mycobacterium tuberculosis in children with human immunodeficiency virus type 1 infection. Pediatr Infect Dis J 11:950–955, 1992.

Kim S, Hughes MD, Hammer SM, Jackson JB, DeGruttola V, Katzenstein DA. Both serum HIV type 1 RNA levels and CD4+ lymphocyte counts predict clinical outcome in HIV type 1-infected subjects with 200 to 500 CD4+ cells per cubic millimeter. AIDS Clinical Trials Group Study 175 Virology Study Team. AIDS Res Hum Retroviruses 16:645–653, 2000.

King JR, Acosta EP, Chadwick E, Yogev R, Crain M, Pass R, Kimberlin DW, Sturdevant MS, Aldrovandi GM. Evaluation of multiple drug therapy in human immunodeficiency virus-infected pediatric patients. Pediatr Infect Dis J 22:239–244, 2003.

King JR, Kimberlin DW, Aldrovandi GM, Acosta EP. Antiretroviral pharmacokinetics in the paediatric population: a review. Clin Pharmacokinet 41:1115–1133, 2002.

Klatzmann D, Champagne E, Chamaret S, Gruest J, Guetard D, Hercend T, Gluckman J-C, Montagnier L. T-lymphocyte T4 behaves as the receptor for human retrovirus LAV. Nature 312:767–768, 1984.

Kliks SC, Nisalak A, Brandt WE, Wahl L, Burke DS. Antibody-dependent enhancement of dengue virus growth in human monocytes as a risk factor for dengue hemorrhagic fever. Am J Trop Med Hyg 40:444–451, 1989.

Kline M, Hollinger F, Rosenblatt H, Bohannon B, Kozinetz C, Shearer W. Sensitivity, specificity and predictive value of physical examination, culture and other laboratory studies in the diagnosis during early infancy of vertically acquired human immunodeficiency virus infection. Pediatr Infect Dis J 12:33–36, 1993.

Kline MW, Fletcher CV, Federici ME, Harris AT, Evans KD, Rutkiewicz VL, Shearer WT, Dunkle LM. Combination therapy with stavudine and didanosine in children with advanced human immunodeficiency virus infection: pharmacokinetic properties, safety, and immunologic and virologic effects. Pediatrics 97:886–890, 1996.

Kline MW, Fletcher CV, Harris AT, Evans KD, Brundage RC, Remmel RP, Calles NR, Kirkpatrick SB, Simon C. A pilot study of combination therapy with indinavir, stavudine (d4T), and didanosine (ddI) in children infected with the human immunodeficiency virus. J Pediatr 132:543–546, 1998.

Kline MW, Paul ME, Bohannon B, Kozinetz CA, Shearer WT. Characteristics of children surviving to 5 years of age or older with vertically acquired HIV infection. Pediatr AIDS HIV Infect 6:350–353, 1995.

Kline MW, Van Dyke RB, Lindsey JC, Gwynne M, Culnane M, Diaz C, Yogev R, McKinney RE Jr, Abrams EJ, Mofenson LM. Combination therapy with stavudine (d4T) plus didanosine (ddI) in children with human immunodeficiency virus infection. The Pediatric AIDS Clinical Trials Group 327 Team. Pediatrics 103:e62, 1999.

Klotman ME, Kim S, Buchbinder A, DeRossi A, Baltimore D, Wong-Staal F. Kinetics of expression of multiply spliced RNA in early human immunodeficiency virus type 1 infection of lymphocytes and monocytes. Proc Natl Acad Sci USA 88:5011–5015, 1991.

Korber B, Theiler J, Wolinsky S. Limitations of a molecular clock applied to considerations of the origin of HIV-1. Science 280:1868–1871, 1998.

Kovacs A, Schluchter M, Easley K, Demmler G, Shearer W, La Russa P, Pitt J, Cooper E, Goldfarb J, Hodes D, Kattan M, McIntosh K. Cytomegalovirus infection and HIV-1 disease progression in infants born to HIV-1-infected women. Pediatric Pulmonary and Cardiovascular Complications of Vertically Transmitted HIV Infection Study Group. N Engl J Med 341:77–84, 1999.

Kovacs JA, Deyton L, Davey R, Falloon J, Zunich K, Lee D, Metcalf JA, Bigley JW, Sawyer LA, Zoon KC. Combined zidovudine and interferon-alpha therapy in patients with Kaposi sarcoma and the acquired immunodeficiency syndrome (AIDS). Ann Intern Med 111:280–287, 1989.

Kovacs A, Frederick T, Church J, Eller A, Oxtoby M, Mascola L. CD4 T-lymphocyte counts and Pneumocystis carinii pneumonia in pediatric HIV infection. JAMA 265:1698–1703, 1991.

Krasinski K, Borkowsky W, Bonk S, Lawrence R, Chandwani S. Bacterial infections in human immunodeficiency virusBinfected children. Pediatr Infect Dis J 7:323–328, 1988.

Krivine A, Firtion G, Cao L, Francoual C, Henrion R, Lebon P. HIV replication during the first weeks of life. Lancet 339:1187–1189, 1992.

Krogstad P, Lee S, Johnson G, Stanley K, McNamara J, Moye J, Jackson JB, Aguayo R, Dieudonne A, Khoury M, Mendez H, Nachman S, Wiznia A. Nucleoside-analogue reverse-transcriptase inhibitors plus nevirapine, nelfinavir, or ritonavir for pretreated children infected with human immunodeficiency virus type 1. Clin Infect Dis 34:991–1001, 2002.

Krogstad P, Wiznia A, Luzuriaga K, Dankner W, Nielsen K, Gersten M, Kerr B, Hendricks A, Boczany B, Rosenberg M, Jung D, Spector SA, Bryson Y. Treatment of human immunodeficiency virus 1-infected infants and children with the protease inhibitor nelfinavir mesylate. Clin Infect Dis 28:1109–1118, 1999.

Kumar S. India has the largest number of people infected with HIV. Lancet 353:48, 1999.

Kure K, Llena JF, Lyman WD, Soeiro R, Weidenheim KM, Hirano A, Dickson DW. Human immunodeficiency virusB1 infection of the nervous system: an autopsy study of 268 adult, pediatric, and fetal brains. Hum Pathol 22:700–710, 1991.

Ladner J, Cartoux M, Dauchet L, Van de Perre P, Czernichow P. Teenage African women and HIV-1 infection. Lancet 360:1889, 2002.

Ladner J, Leroy V, Hoffman P, Nyiraziraje M, De Clercq A, Van de Perre P, Dabis F. Chorioamnionitis and pregnancy outcome in HIV-infected African women. Pregnancy and HIV Study Group. J Acquir Immune Defic Syndr Hum Retrovirol 18:293–298, 1998.

Lambert JS, Mofenson LM, Fletcher CV, Moye J Jr, Stiehm ER, Meyer WA, 3rd, Nemo GJ, Mathieson BJ, Hirsch G, Sapan CV, Cummins LM, Jimenez E, O'Neill E, Kovacs A, Stek A. Safety and pharmacokinetics of hyperimmune anti-human immunodeficiency virus (HIV) immunoglobulin administered to HIV-infected pregnant women and their newborns. Pediatric AIDS Clinical Trials Group Protocol 185 Pharmacokinetic Study Group. J Infect Dis 175:283–291, 1997.

Lambert JS, Watts DH, Mofenson L, Stiehm ER, Harris DR, Bethel J, Whitehouse J, Jimenez E, Gandia J, Scott G, O'Sullivan MJ, Kovacs A, Stek A, Shearer WT, Hammill H, van Dyke R, Maupin R, Silio M, Fowler MG. Risk factors for preterm birth, low birth weight, and intrauterine growth retardation in infants born to HIV-infected pregnant women receiving zidovudine. Pediatric AIDS Clinical Trials Group 185 Team. AIDS 14:1389–1399, 2000.

Lamers SL, Sleasman JW, She JX, Barrie KA, Pomeroy SM, Barrett DJ, Goodenow MM. Persistence of multiple maternal genotypes of human immunodeficiency virus type I in infants infected by vertical transmission. J Clin Invest 93:380–390, 1994.

Landesman S, Weiblen B, Mendez H, Willoughby A, Goedert J, Rubinstein A, Minkoff H, Moroso G, Hoff R. Clinical utility of HIV-IgA immunoblot assay in the early diagnosis of perinatal HIV infection. JAMA 266:3443–3446, 1991.

Landesman SH, Kalish LA, Burns DN, Minkoff H, Fox HE, Zorrilla C, Garcia P, Fowler MG, Mofenson L, Tuomala R. Obstetrical factors and the transmission of human immunodeficiency virus type 1 from mother to child. The Women and Infants Transmission Study. N Engl J Med 334:1617–1623, 1996.

Lang C, Jacobi G, Kreuz W, Hacker H, Herrmmann G, Keul H-G, Thomas E. Rapid development of giant aneurysm at the base of the brain in an 8-year-old boy with perinatal HIV infection. Acta Histochem Suppl 42:S83–S90, 1992.

Larder BA, Kellam P, Kemp SD. Convergent combination therapy can select viable multidrug-resistant HIV-1 in vitro. Nature 365:451–453, 1993.

Lasky L, Nakamura G, Smith D, Fennie C, Shimasaki C, Patzer E, Berman P, Gregory T, Capon D. Delineation of a region of the human immunodeficiency virus type 1 gp120 glycoprotein critical for interaction with the CD4 receptor. Cell 50:975–985, 1987.

Laspia M, Rice A, Mathews M. HIV-1 tat protein increases transcriptional initiation and stabilizes elongation. Cell 59:283–292, 1989.

Laue L, Pizzo PA, Butler K, Cutler GB. Growth and neuroendocrine dysfunction in children with acquired immunodeficiency syndrome. J Pediatr 117:541–545, 1990.

Lee LM, Fleming PL. Estimated number of children left motherless by AIDS in the United States 1978–1998. J Acquir Immune Defic Syndr 34:231–236, 2003.

Le Moing V, Thiebaut R, Chene G, Leport C, Cailleton V, Michelet C, Fleury H, Herson S, Raffi F. Predictors of long-term increase in CD4(+) cell counts in human immunodeficiency virus-infected patients receiving a protease inhibitor-containing antiretroviral regimen. J Infect Dis 185:471–480, 2002.

Learmont JC, Geczy AF, Mills J, Ashton LJ, Raynes-Greenow CH, Garsia RJ, Dyer WB, McIntyre L, Oelrichs RB, Rhodes DI, Deacon NJ, Sullivan JS. Immunologic and virologic status after 14 to 18 years of infection with an attenuated strain of HIV-1. A report from the Sydney Blood Bank Cohort. N Engl J Med 340:1715–1722, 1999.

Lederman S. Estimating infant mortality from human immunodeficiency virus and other causes in breast-feeding and bottle-feeding populations. Pediatrics 89:290–296, 1992.

Leibovitz E, Kaul A, Rigaud M, Bebenroth D, Krasinski K, Borkowsky W. Chronic varicella zoster in a child infected with human immunodeficiency virus: case report and review of the literature. Cutis 49:27–31, 1992.

Leis J, Baltimore D, Bishop J, Coffin J, Fleissner E, Goff S, Oroszlan S, Robinson H, Skalka A, Temin H, Vogt V. Standardized and simplified nomenclature for proteins common to all retroviruses. J Virol 62:1808–1809, 1988.

Leonard EG, McComsey GA. Metabolic complications of antiretroviral therapy in children. Pediatr Infect Dis J 22:77–84, 2003.

Lepage P, van de Perre P, Dabis F, Commenges D, Orbinski J, Hitimana D, Bazubagira A, van Goethem C, Allen S, Butzler J. Evaluation and simplification of the World Health Organization clinical case definition for paediatric AIDS. AIDS 3:221–225, 1989.

Leroy V, Newell ML, Dabis F, Peckham C, Van de Perre P, Bulterys M, Kind C, Simonds RJ, Wiktor S, Msellati P. International multicentre pooled analysis of late postnatal mother-to-child transmission of HIV-1 infection. Ghent International Working Group on Mother-to-Child Transmission of HIV. Lancet 352:597–600, 1998.

Letvin NL. Progress in the development of an HIV-1 vaccine. Science 280:1875–1880, 1998.

Levin NL, Walker BD. Immunopathogenesis and immunotherapy in AIDS virus infections. Nat Med 9:861–866, 2003.

Levine M, Denamur E, Simon F, De Crepy A, Blot P, Vilmer. E. Conversion of HIV viral markers during the first months of life in HIV infected children born to seropositive mothers. Presented at the Ninth International Conference on AIDS, Berlin, June 6–11, 1993.

Levy J. Pathogenesis of human immunodeficiency virus infection. Microbiol Rev 57:183–289, 1993.

Levy J, Youvan Y, Lee ML, the Passive Hyperimmune Therapy Study Group. Passive hyperimmune plasma therapy in the treatment of acquired immunodeficiency syndrome: results of a 12-month multicenter double-blind controlled trial. Blood 84:2130–2135, 1994.

Lewis LL, Butler KM, Husson RN, Mueller BU, Fowler CL, Steinberg SM, Pizzo PA. Defining the population of human immunodeficiency virus-infected children at risk for Mycobacterium avium-intracellulare infection. J Pediatr 121:677–683, 1992.

Lichtenstein KA, Ward DJ, Moorman AC, Delaney KM, Young B, Palella FJ Jr, Rhodes PH, Wood KC, Holmberg SD. Clinical assessment of HIV-associated lipodystrophy in an ambulatory population. AIDS 15:1389–1398, 2001.

Lifson J, Reyes G, McGrath M, Stein B, Engleman E. AIDS retrovirus induced cytopathology: giant cell formation and involvement of CD4 antigen. Science 232:1123–1127, 1986.

Lindegren ML, Rhodes P, Gordon L, Fleming P. Drug safety during pregnancy and in infants. Lack of mortality related to mitochondrial dysfunction among perinatally HIV-exposed children in pediatric HIV surveillance. Ann NY Acad Sci 918:222–235, 2000.

Lindsey JC, Hughes MD, McKinney RE, Cowles MK, Englund JA, Baker CJ, Burchett SK, Kline MW, Kovacs A, Moye J. Treatment-mediated changes in human immunodeficiency virus (HIV) type 1 RNA and CD4 cell counts as predictors of weight growth failure, cognitive decline, and survival in HIV-infected children. J Infect Dis 182:1385–1393, 2000.

Lipshultz SE, Easley KA, Orav EJ, Kaplan S, Starc TJ, Bricker JT, Lai WW, Moodie DS, McIntosh K, Schluchter MD, Colan SD. Left ventricular structure and function in children infected with human immunodeficiency virus: the prospective P2C2 HIV Multicenter Study. Pediatric Pulmonary and Cardiac Complications of Vertically Transmitted HIV Infection (P2C2 HIV) Study Group. Circulation 97:1246–1256, 1998.

Lipshultz SE, Easley KA, Orav EJ, Kaplan S, Starc TJ, Bricker JT, Lai WW, Moodie DS, Sopko G, Colan SD. Cardiac dysfunction and mortality in HIV-infected children: The Prospective P2C2 HIV Multicenter Study. Pediatric Pulmonary and Cardiac Complications of Vertically Transmitted HIV Infection (P2C2 HIV) Study Group. Circulation 102:1542–1548, 2000a.

Lipshultz SE, Easley KA, Orav EJ, Kaplan S, Starc TJ, Bricker JT, Lai WW, Moodie DS, Sopko G, McIntosh K, Colan SD. Absence of cardiac toxicity of zidovudine in infants. Pediatric Pulmonary and Cardiac Complications of Vertically Transmitted HIV Infection Study Group. N Engl J Med 343:759–766, 2000b.

Lipshultz SE, Easley KA, Orav EJ, Kaplan S, Starc TJ, Bricker JT, Lai WW, Moodie DS, Sopko G, Schluchter MD, Colan SD. Cardiovascular status of infants and children of women infected with HIV-1 (P2C2 HIV): a cohort study. Lancet 360:368–373, 2002.

Lipton S. HIV displays its coat of arms. Nature 367:113–114, 1994.

Liu R, Paxton WA, Choe S, Ceradini D, Martin SR, Horuk R, MacDonald ME, Stuhlmann H, Koup RA, Landau NR. Homozygous defect in HIV-1 coreceptor accounts for resistance of some multiply-exposed individuals to HIV-1 infection. Cell 86:367–377, 1996.

Llorente A, Brouwers P, Charurat M, Magder L, Malee K, Mellins C, Ware J, Hittleman J, Mofenson L, Velez-Borras J, Adenyl-Jones S; Women and Infant Transmission Study Group. Early neurodevelopmental markers predictive of mortality in infants infected with HIV-1. Dev Med Child Neurol 45:76–84, 2003.

Lo JC, Mulligan K, Tai VW, Algren H, Schambelan M. "Buffalo hump" in men with HIV-1 infection. Lancet 351:867–870, 1998.

Lobato MN, Caldwell MB, Ng P, Oxtoby MJ. Encephalopathy in children with perinatally acquired human immunodeficiency virus infection. Pediatric Spectrum of Disease Clinical Consortium. J Pediatr 126:710–715, 1995.

Lorenzi P, Spicher VM, Laubereau B, Hirschel B, Kind C, Rudin C, Irion O, Kaiser L. Antiretroviral therapies in pregnancy: maternal, fetal and neonatal effects. Swiss HIV Cohort Study, the Swiss Collaborative HIV and Pregnancy Study, and the Swiss Neonatal HIV Study. AIDS 12:F241–247, 1998.

Lucey DR, Melcher GP, Hendrix CW, Zajac RA, Goetz DW, Butzin CA, Clerici M, Warner RD, Abbadessa S, Hall K, Shearer G. Human immunodeficiency virus infection in the US Air Force: seroconversions, clinical staging, and assessment of a T helper cell functional assay to predict change in CD4+ T cell counts. J Infect Dis 164:631–637, 1991.

Lusso P, Gallo R. Human herpesvirus 6 in AIDS. Lancet 343:555–556, 1994.

Luster AD. Chemokines—chemotactic cytokines that mediate inflammation. N Engl J Med 338:436–445, 1998.

Luzuriaga K, Bryson Y, Krogstad P, Robinson J, Stechenberg B, Lamson M, Cort S, Sullivan JL. Combination treatment with zidovudine, didanosine, and nevirapine in infants with human immunodeficiency virus type 1 infection. N Engl J Med 336:1343–1349, 1997.

Luzuriaga K, McManus M, Catalina M, Mayack S, Sharkey M, Stevenson M, Sullivan JL. Early therapy of vertical human immunodeficiency virus type 1 (HIV-1) infection: control of viral replication and absence of persistent HIV-1-specific immune responses. J Virol 74:6984–6991, 2000.

Luzuriaga K, McQuilken P, Alimenti A, Somasundaran M, Hesselton R, Sullivan JL. Early viremia and immune responses in

Robinson WJ, Montefiori DC, Mitchell WM. Antibody-dependent enhancement of human immunodeficiency virus type 1 infection. Lancet 1:790–794, 1988.

Rogers M, Ou C-Y, Kilbourne B, Schochetman G. Advances and problems in the diagnosis of human immunodeficiency virus infection in infants. Pediatr Infect Dis J 10:523–531, 1991.

Rogers M, White C, Sanders R, Schable C, Ksell T, Wasserman R, Bellanti J, Peters S, Wray B. Lack of transmission of human immunodeficiency virus from infected children to their household contacts. Pediatrics 85:210–214, 1990.

Roilides E, Butler KM, Husson RN, Mueller BU, Lewis LL, Pizzo PA. Pseudomonas infections in children with human immunodeficiency virus infection. Pediatr Infect Dis J 11:547–553, 1992.

Roilides E, Clerici M, DePalma L, Rubin M, Pizzo PA, Shearer GM. T helper cell responses in children infected with human immunodeficiency virus type 1. J Pediatr 118:724–730, 1991a.

Roilides E, Marshall D, Venzon D, Butler K, Husson R, Pizzo PA. Bacterial infections in human immunodeficiency virus type 1-infected children: the impact of central venous catheters and antiretroviral agents. Pediatr Infect Dis J 10:813–819, 1991b.

Roilides E, Mertins S, Eddy J, Walsh TJ, Pizzo PA, Rubin M. Impairment of neutrophil chemotactic and bactericidal function in children infected with human immunodeficiency virus type 1 and partial reversal after in vitro exposure to granulocyte-macrophage colony-stimulating factor. J Pediatr 117:531–540, 1990.

Rook AH, Masur H, Lane HC, Frederick W, Kasahara T, Macher AM, Djeu JY, Manischewitz JF, Jackson L, Fauci AS, Quinnan GJ. Interleukin-2 enhances the depressed natural killer and cytomegalovirus-specific cytotoxic activities of lymphocytes from patients with the acquired immune deficiency syndrome. J Clin Invest 72:398–403, 1983.

Rosenfeldt V, Valerius NH, Paerregaard A. Regression of HIV-associated progressive encephalopathy of childhood during HAART. Scand J Infect Dis 32:571–574, 2000.

Rosok BI, Bostad L, Voltersvik P, Bjerknes R, Olofsson J, Asjo B, Brinchmann JE. Reduced CD4 cell counts in blood do not reflect CD4 cell depletion in tonsillar tissue in asymptomatic HIV-1 infection. AIDS 10:F35–38, 1996.

Rousseau CM, Just JJ, Abrams EJ, Casabona J, Stein Z, King MC. CCR5del32 in perinatal HIV-1 infection. J Acquir Immune Defic Syndr Hum Retrovirol 16:239–242, 1997.

Rowland-Jones S, Nixon DF, Aldhous MC, Gotch F, Ariyoshi K, Hallam N, Kroll JS, Froebel K, McMichael A. HIV-specific cytotoxic T-cell activity in an HIV-exposed but uninfected infant. Lancet 341:860–861, 1993.

Rowland-Jones SL, Dong T, Fowke KR, Kimani J, Krausa P, Newell H, Blanchard T, Ariyoshi K, Oyugi J, Ngugi E, Bwayo J, MacDonald KS, McMichael AJ, Plummer FA. Cytotoxic T cell responses to multiple conserved HIV epitopes in HIV-resistant prostitutes in Nairobi. J Clin Invest 102:1758–1765, 1998.

Royce RA, Sena A, Cates W Jr, Cohen MS. Sexual transmission of HIV. N Engl J Med 336:1072–1078, 1997.

Rubinstein A, Morecki R, Silverman B, Charytan M, Krieger BZ, Andiman W, Ziprkowski MN, Goldman H. Pulmonary disease in children with acquired immune deficiency syndrome and AIDS-related complex. J Pediatr 108:498–503, 1986.

Rubinstein A, Sicklick M, Gupta A, Bernstein L, Klein N, Rubinstein E, Spigland I, Fruchter L, Litman N, Lee H, Hollander M. Acquired immunodeficiency with reversed T4/T8 ratios in infants born to promiscuous and drug-addicted mothers. JAMA 249:2350–2356, 1983.

Ruff AJ, Halsey NA, Coberly J, Boulos R. Breast-feeding and maternal-infant transmission of human immunodeficiency virus type 1. J Pediatr 121:325–329, 1992.

Ryder RW, Manzila T, Baende E, Kabagabo U, Behets F, Batter V, Paquot E, Binyingo E, Heyward WL. Evidence from Zaire that breast-feeding by HIV-1-seropositive mothers is not a major route for perinatal HIV-1 transmission but does decrease morbidity. AIDS 5:709–714, 1991.

Ryder RW, Nsa W, Hassig SE, Behets F, Rayfield M, Ekungola B, Nelson AM, Mulenda U, Francis H, Mwandagalirwa K, Davachi F, Rogers M, Nzilambi N, Greenberg A, Mann J, Quinn TC, Piot P, Curran JW. Perinatal transmission of the human

immunodeficiency virus type 1 to infants of seropositive women in Zaire. N Engl J Med 320:1637–1642, 1989.

Safrit J, Cao Y, Andrews C, Ho D, Koup R. Role of cytotoxic T lymphocytes in acute HIV-1 infection. Presented at the International Conference on AIDS, Berlin, June 6–11, 1993.

Sahmoud T, Laurian Y, Gazengel C, Sultan Y, Gautreau C, Costagliola D. Progression to AIDS in French haemophiliacs: association with HLA-B35. AIDS 7:497–500, 1993.

Sanchez-Ramon S, Canto-Nogues C, Munoz-Fernandez A. Reconstructing the course of HIV-1-associated progressive encephalopathy in children. Med Sci Monit 8:RA249–252, 2002.

Sande MA, Carpenter CC, Cobbs CG, Holmes KK, Sanford JP. Antiretroviral therapy for adult HIV-infected patients. Recommendations from a state-of-the-art conference. National Institute of Allergy and Infectious Diseases State-of-the-Art Panel on Anti-Retroviral Therapy for Adult HIV-Infected Patients. JAMA 270:2583–2589, 1993.

Sato H, Orenstein J, Dimitrov D, Martin M. Cell-to-cell spread of HIv-1 occurs within minutes and may not involved the participation of virus particles. Virology 186:712–724, 1992.

Sattentau QJ. Neutralization of HIV-1 by antibody. curr Opin Immunol 8:540–545, 1996.

Sattler FR, Cowan R, Nielsen DM, Ruskin J. Trimethoprim-sulfamethoxazole compared with pentamidine for treatment of Pneumocystis carinii pneumonia in the acquired immunodeficiency syndrome. A prospective, noncrossover study. Ann Intern Med 109:280–287, 1988.

Scadden DT, Zeira M, Woon A, Wang Z, Schieve L, Ikeuchi K, Lim B, Groopman JE. Human immunodeficiency virus infection of human bone marrow stromal fibroblasts. Blood 76:317–322, 1990.

Scadden DT, Zon LI, Groopman JE. Pathophysiology and management of HIV-associated hematologic disorders. Blood 74:1455–1463, 1989.

Scarlatti G, Leitner T, Hodara V, Halapi E, Rossi P, Albert J, Fenyo E. Neutralizing antibodies and viral characteristics in mother-to-child transmission of HIV-1. AIDS 7:S45–S48, 1993.

Schmitz JE, Kuroda MJ, Santra S, Sasseville VG, Simon MA, Lifton MA, Racz P, Tenner-Racz K, Dalesandro M, Scallon BJ, Ghrayeb J, Forman MA, Montefiori DC, Rieber EP, Letvin NL, Reimann KA. Control of viremia in simian immunodeficiency virus infection by CD8+ lymphocytes. Science 283:857–860, 1999.

Scott GB, Fischl MA, Klimas N, Fletcher MA, Dickinson GM, Levine RS, Parks WP. Mothers of infants with the acquired immunodeficiency syndrome. Evidence for both symptomatic and asymptomatic carriers. JAMA 253:363–366, 1985.

Scott GB, Hutto C, Makuch RW, Mastrucci MT, O'Connor T, Mitchell CD, Trapido EJ, Parks WP. Survival in children with perinatally acquired human immunodeficiency virus type 1 infection. N Engl J Med 321:1791–1796, 1989.

Scribner AN, Troia-Cancio PV, Cox BA, Marcantonio D, Hamid F, Keiser P, Levi M, Allen B, Murphy K, Jones RE, Skiest DJ. Osteonecrosis in HIV: a case-control study. J Acquir Immune Defic Syndr 25:19–25, 2000.

Semba RD, Tang AM. Micronutrients and the pathogenesis of human immunodeficiency virus infection. Br J Nutr 81:181–189, 1999.

Serraino D, Franceschi S. Kaposi's sarcoma and non-Hodgkin's lymphomas in children and adolescents with AIDS. AIDS 10:643–647, 1996.

Serraino D, Zaccarelli M, Franceschi S, Greco D. The epidemiology of AIDS-associated Kaposi's sarcoma in Italy. AIDS 6:1015–1019, 1992.

Shadduck PP, Weinberg JB, Haney AF, Bartlett JA, Langlois AJ, Bolognesi DP, Matthews TJ. Lack of enhancing effect of human anti-human immunodeficiency virus type 1 (HIV-1) antibody on HIV-1 infection of human blood monocytes and peritoneal macrophages. J Virol 65:4309–4316, 1991.

Shaffer N, Chuachoowong R, Mock PA, Bhadrakom C, Siriwasin W, Young NL, Chotpitayasunondh T, Chearskul S, Roongpisuthipong A, Chinayon P, Karon J, Mastro TD, Simonds RJ. Short-course zidovudine for perinatal HIV-1 transmission in Bangkok, Thailand: a randomised controlled trial. Bangkok Collaborative Perinatal HIV Transmission Study Group. Lancet 353:773–780, 1999.

Shan H, Wang JX, Ren FR, Zhang YZ, Zhao HY, Gao GJ, Ji Y, Ness PM. Blood banking in China. Lancet 360:1770–1775, 2002.

Shaunak S, Albright RE, Klotman ME, Henry SC, Bartlett JA, Hamilton JD. Amplification of HIV-1 provirus from cerebrospinal fluid and its correlation with neurologic disease. J Infect Dis 161:1068–1072, 1990.

Shearer G, Clerici M. Abnormalities of immune regulation in human immunodeficiency virus infection. Pediatr Res 33:S71–S74, 1993.

Shearer WT, Quinn TC, LaRussa P, Lew JF, Mofenson L, Almy S, Rich K, Handelsman E, Diaz C, Pagano M, Smeriglio V, Kalish LA. Viral load and disease progression in infants infected with human immunodeficiency virus type 1. Women and Infants Transmission Study Group. N Engl J Med 336:1337–1342, 1997.

Shey WI, Brocklehurst P, Sterne JA. Vaginal disinfection during labour for reducing the risk of mother-to-child transmission of HIV infection. Cochrane Database Syst Rev CD003651, 2002.

Siekevitz M, Josephs S, Dukovich M, Peffer N, Wong-Staal F, Greene W. Activation of the HIV-1 LTR by T cell mitogens and the transactivator protein of HTLV-1. Science 238:1575–1578, 1987.

Siller L, Martin N, Kostuchenko P, Beckett L, Rautonen J, Cheng S, Wara DW. Serum levels of soluble CD8, neopterin, beta 2-microglobulin and p24 antigen as indicators of disease progression in children with AIDS on zidovudine therapy. AIDS 7:369–373, 1993.

Silliman CC, Tedder D, Ogle JW, Simon J, Kleinschmidt D, Masters B, Manco JM, Levin MJ. Unsuspected varicella-zoster virus encephalitis in a child with acquired immunodeficiency syndrome. J Pediatr 123:418–422, 1993.

Simonds R, Chanock S. Medical issues related to caring for human immunodeficiency virus-infected children in and out of the home. Pediatr Infect Dis J 12:845–852, 1993.

Sirianni MC, Soddu S, Malorni W, Arancia G, Aiuti F. Mechanism of defective natural killer cell activity in patients with AIDS is associated with defective distribution of tubulin [see erratum in J Immunol 141:1709, 1988]. J Immunol 140:2565–2568, 1988.

Sleasman JW, Goodenow MM. 13. HIV-1 infection. J Allergy Clin Immunol 111:582–592, 2003.

Smith PD, Eisner MS, Manischewitz JF, Gill VJ, Masur H, Fox CF. Esophageal disease in AIDS is associated with pathologic processes rather than mucosal human immunodeficiency virus type 1. J Infect Dis 167:547–552, 1993.

Smith PD, Quinn TC, Strober W, Janoff EN, Masur H. Gastrointestinal infections in AIDS. Ann Intern Med 116:63–77, 1992.

Sodroski J, Goh W, Rosen C, Campbell K, Haseltine W. Role of the HTLV-III/LAV envelope in syncytium formation and cytopathicity. Nature 322:470–474, 1986.

Sokal E. Drug treatment of pediatric chronic hepatitis B. Paediatr Drugs 4:361–369, 2002.

Spector SA, Blanchard S. Wara DW, Oleske JM, McIntosh K, Hodes D, Dankner WM, Salgo M, McNamara J. Comparative trial of two dosages of zalcitabine in zidovudine-experienced children with advanced human immunodeficiency virus disease. Pediatric AIDS Clinical Trial Group. Pediatr Infec Dis J 16:623–626, 1997.

Spector SA, Gelber RD, McGrath N, Wara D, Barzilai A, Abrams E, Bryson YJ, Dankner WM, Livingston RA, Connor EM. A controlled trial of intravenous immune globulin for the prevention of serious bacterial infections in chldren receiving zidovudine for advanced human immunodeficiency virus infection. Pediatric AIDS Clincal Trials Group. N Engl J Med 331:1181–1187, 1994.

Sperling RS, Shapiro DE, McSherry GD, Britto P, Cunningham BE, Culnane M, Coombs RW, Scott G, Van Dyke RB, Shearer WT, Jimenez E, Diaz C, Harrison DD, Delfraissy JF. Safety of the maternal-infant zidovudine regimen utilized in the Pediatric AIDS Clinical Trial Group 076 Study. AIDS 12:1805–1813, 1998.

Spruance S, Pavia A, Peterson D, Berry A, Pollard R, Patterson T, Frank I, Remick S, Thompson M, MacArthur R, Morey G, Ramirez-Ronda C, Bernstein B, Sweet D, Crane L, Peterson E, Pachucki C, Green S, Brand J, Rios A, Dunkle L, Smaldone L. Didanosine compared with continuation of zidovudine in HIV-infected patients with signs of clinical deterioration while receiving zidovudine. Ann Intern Med 120:360–368, 1994.

St. Clair MH, Martin JL, Tudor-Williams G, Bach MC, Vavro CL, King DM, Kellam P, Kemp SD, Larder BA. Resistance to ddI and sensitivity to AZT induced by a mutation in HIV-1 reverse transcriptase. Science 253:1557–1559, 1991.

Starc TJ, Langston C, Goldfarb J, Colin AA, Cooper ER, Easley KA, Sunkle S, Schluchter MD. Unexpected non-HIV causes of death in children born to HIV-infected mothers. Pediatric Pulmonary and Cardiac Complications of Vertically Transmitted HIV Infection Study Group. Pediatrics 104:e6, 1999a.

Starc TJ, Lipshultz SE, Kaplan S, Easley KA, Bricker JT, Colan SD, Lai WW, Gersony WM, Sopko G, Moodie DS, Schluchter MD. Cardiac complications in children with human immunodeficiency virus infection. Pediatric Pulmonary and Cardiac Complications of Vertically Transmitted HIV Infection (P2C2 HIV) Study Group, National Heart, Lung, and Blood Institute. Pediatrics 104:e14, 1999b.

Starke JR, Jacobs RF, Jereb J. Resurgence of tuberculosis in children. J Pediatr 120:839–855, 1992.

Starr SE, Fletcher CV, Spector SA, Yong FH, Fenton T, Brundage RC, Manion D, Ruiz N, Gersten M, Becker M, McNamara J, Mofenson LM, Purdue L, Siminski S, Graham B, Kornhauser DM, Fiske W, Vincent C, Lischner HW, Dankner WM, Flynn PM. Combination therapy with efavirenz, nelfinavir, and nucleoside reverse-transcriptase inhibitors in children infected with human immunodeficiency virus type 1. Pediatric AIDS Clinical Trials Group 382 Team. N Engl J Med 341:1874–1881, 1999.

Staszewski S, Morales-Ramirez J, Tashima KT, Rachlis A, Skiest D, Stanford J, Stryker R, Johnson P, Labriola DF, Farina D, Manion DJ, Ruiz NM. Efavirenz plus zidovudine and lamivudine, efavirenz plus indinavir, and indinavir plus zidovudine and lamivudine in the treatment of HIV-1 infection in adults. Study 006 Team. N Engl J Med 341:1865–1873, 1999.

Steffy K, Wong-Staal F. Genetic regulation of human immunodeficiency virus. Microbiol Rev 55:193–205, 1991.

Steimer KS, Scandella CJ, Skiles PV, Haigwood NL. Neutralization of divergent HIV-1 isolates by conformation-dependent human antibodies to Gp120. Science 254:105–108, 1991.

Stein B, Gowda S, Lifson J, Penhallow R, Bensch K, Engleman E. pH-independent HIV entry into CD4-positive cells via virus envelope fusion to the plasma membrane. Cell 49:659–668, 1987.

Steiner F, Kind C, Aebi C, Wyler-Lazarevitch CA, Cheseaux JJ, Rudin C, Molinari L, Nadal D. Growth in human immunodeficiency virus type 1-infected children treated with protease inhibitors. Eur J Pediatr 160:611–616, 2001.

Steininger C, Kundi M, Jatzko G, Kiss H, Lischka A, Holzmann H. Increased risk of mother-to-infant transmission of hepatitis C virus by intrapartum infantile exposure to maternal blood. J Infect Dis 187:345–351, 2003.

Stella CC, Ganser A, Hoelzer D. Defective in vitro growth of the hemopoietic progenitor cells in the acquired immunodeficiency syndrome. J Clin Invest 80:286–293, 1987.

Stevenson M, Bukrinsky M, Haggerty S. HIV-1 replication and potential targets for intervention. AIDS Res Hum Retroviruses 8:107–117, 1992.

Stevenson M, Stanwick T, Dempsey M, Lamonica C. HIV-1 replication is controlled at the level of T cell activation and proviral integration. EMBO J 9:1551–1560, 1990.

Stiehm ER, Bryson YJ, Frenkel LM, Szelc CM, Gillespie S, Williams ME, Watkins ME. Prednisone improves human immunodeficiency virus encephalopathy in children. Pediatr Infect Dis J 11:49–50, 1992.

Stiehm ER, Fletcher, CV, Mofenson LM, Palumbo PE, Kang M, Fenton T, Sapan CV, Meyer WA, Shearer WT, Hawkins E, Fowler MG, Bouquin P, Purdue L, Sloand EM, Nemo GJ, Wara D, Bryson YJ, Starr SE, Petru A, Burchett S. Use of human immunodeficiency virus (HIV) human ihyperimmune immunoglobulin in HIV type-1 infected children (Pediatric AIDS clinical trials group protocol 273) J. Infect. Dis 181:548–54, 2000.

Stiehm ER, Lambert JS, Mofenson LM, Bethel J, Whitehouse J, Nugent R, Moye J Jr, Glenn Fowler M, Mathieson BJ, Reichelderfer P, Nemo GJ, Korelitz J, Meyer WA, 3rd, Sapan CV, Jimenez E, Gandia J, Scott G, O'Sullivan MJ, Kovacs A, Stek A, Shearer WT, Hammill H. Efficacy of zidovudine and human immunodeficiency virus (HIV) hyperimmune immunoglobulin for reducing perinatal HIV transmission from HIV-infected women asplenia described by Waldman and co-workers (1977). This is sometimes familial, with an autosomal recessive pattern of inheritance.

More often, it is part of a complex disorder termed *Ivemark syndrome,* also termed *asplenia syndrome,* which is characterized by splenic absence, hypoplasia, lobulation, polysplenia, or dextroposition in association with cardiac and visceral abnormalities (Ivemark, 1955). The common cardiac defects are transposition, pulmonary atresia or stenosis, and anomalous pulmonary venous return; dextrocardia is sometimes seen as well (Rose et al., 1975). The visceral abnormalities include lobulated lungs, isomerism of the liver, and gut malrotation. This occurs more commonly in males, and familial cases have been described (Cesko, 1997; Gillis et al., 1992). Most patients die in infancy because of cardiac disease, infection, or the congenital organ abnormalities.

Wang and Hseih (1991) noted decreased percentages of CD3 and CD4 cells, slightly diminished lymphoproliferative responses to mitogens, and slower clearance of antibody-coated autologous erythrocytes in 13 patients with asplenia syndrome. They suggest that these defects may contribute to their susceptibility to infection.

Britz-Cunningham and associates (1995) have described mutations in the *connexin43* gap junction gene in seven children with the visceroatrial heterotaxia of Ivemark syndrome. The gap junction protein promotes cell-to-cell communication within the developing heart, and disruption prevents tissues with similar functions to migrate properly.

Asplenia is a component of other genetic syndromes (Table 30-5). Familial asplenia is not uncommon and may be a subset of a developmental defect that includes polysplenia (Niikawa et al., 1983). Both autosomal dominant and autosomal recessive inheritance have been suggested (Gillis et al., 1992; Niikawa et al., 1983). Crawfurd (1978) described two siblings with asplenia, polycystic kidneys, and an enlarged cystic pancreas. Asplenia has also been reported in association with microgastria and limb reduction defects (Lueder et al., 1989). Stormorken and colleagues (1985) reported an association of bleeding tendency, extreme miosis, and asplenia in a six-generation family. Ades and colleagues (1991) reported two brothers with Smith-Fineman-Myers syndrome, one of whom had asplenia. Asplenia has also been associated with caudal deficiency (Fullana et al., 1986).

. . . .
TABLE 30-5 · SYNDROMES ASSOCIATED WITH CONGENITAL ASPLENIA

Asplenia with congenital heart disease (Ivemark syndrome)
Familial asplenia
Asplenia with cystic liver, kidney, and pancreas
Asplenia with microgastria and limb reduction defects
Thrombocytopenia, asplenia, and miosis (Stormorken's syndrome)
Distinctive facies, mental retardation, short stature, and cryptorchidism (Smith-Fineman-Myers syndrome)
Caudal deficiency and asplenia

Surgical Splenectomy

The spleen is removed surgically after trauma, lymphoid malignancies, and massive enlargement; less commonly, it may be removed for hemolytic anemia (particularly hereditary spherocytosis) and refractory immune thrombocytopenic purpura. Following trauma, nonoperative management of splenic injury has been introduced (Hebeler et al., 1982; Howman-Giles et al., 1978; Traub and Perry, 1982) and used successfully in 95% of cases (Touloukian, 1985). Other approaches to preservation of splenic tissue included splenorrhaphy, hemisplenectomy, and splenectomy with autotransplantation of splenic tissue (Martin, 1994; Morgenstern and Shapiro, 1979).

Functional Asplenia

The presence of a spleen that is functioning poorly also predisposes patients to infection and is present in a variety of conditions, including the newborn period, portal hypertension, autoimmune disease such as lupus erythematosus, infiltrative diseases, human immunodeficiency virus (HIV) infection, prolonged parenteral nutrition, and graft-versus-host disease.

The most common cause of clinical functional hyposplenism is homozygous sickle cell disease. Pearson and co-workers (1969) have shown that despite an enlarged spleen, splenic function decreases during the first 2 or 3 years of life, which can be reversed by transfusion of normal erythrocytes for the first 10 years (O'Brien et al., 1976; Pearson et al., 1969). Splenic function decreases with age at rates depending on the molecular nature of the sickle cell defect (Fig. 30-2). After several years, the spleen undergoes repeated infarctions and diminishes in size, a situation termed *autosplenectomy* (Pearson et al., 1979). Feder and Pearson (1999) advocated erythrocyte pit enumeration to discern the degree of splenic function. Patients with functional hyposplenism have the same susceptibility to infection as do patients who have undergone surgical splenectomy.

Management

Elective splenectomy for hereditary spherocytosis should be postponed beyond infancy (Diamond, 1969). If the patient is not adequately immunized, immunizations should be given several weeks before elective splenectomy. Medical therapy for illnesses such as immune thrombocytopenic purpura should be exhausted before splenectomy is performed.

As noted previously, following splenic injury, repair or partial splenectomy rather than complete spleen removal should be done when possible. Autotransplantation at the time of splenectomy can also be done. Successful autotransplantation does not restore the clearance function of the spleen, but it does improve the antibody responses to vaccine antigens.

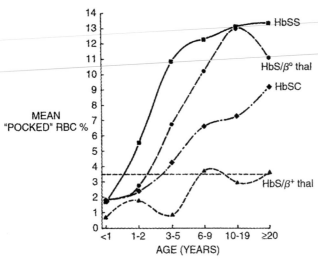

Figure 30-2· Developmental patterns of pocked red cells in different types of sickle hemoglobinopathies. Pocked red cells greater than 3.5% indicate functional hyposplenism. Nonvisualization of the spleen by technetium-99 metastable (^{99m}Tc) sulfur colloid scan correlated strongly with pocked red cells 3.5% or greater. (From Pearson, Gallagher, Chilcote, Sullivan, Wilimas, Espeland, Ritchey, and the Cooperative Study of Sickle Cell Disease. Developmental pattern of splenic dysfunction in sickle cell disorders. Pediatrics 76:392–397, 1985.)

Antibiotic Prophylaxis

Penicillin prophylaxis is indicated for all children after a splenectomy and for those with sickle cell disease at least up to age 5. Gaston and colleagues (1986) showed that such treatment reduced the incidence of bacterial sepsis in children with sickle cell disease by 84%. However, compliance is a problem in these patients (Buchanan et al., 1982).

The emergence of penicillin resistance to *S. pneumoniae* is another concern for patients who have undergone splenectomy and are taking penicillin prophylaxis. Nasopharyngeal colonization rates are generally around 10% to 12%; however, 33% to 62% of the colonizing strains are resistant to penicillin, and as many as 29% of the strains are resistant to high concentrations of penicillin (>2.0 fg/ml) (Norris et al., 1996; Steele et al., 1996).

Falletta and co-workers (1995) examined the consequences of discontinuing penicillin prophylaxis after 5 years of age in patients with sickle cell disease and thalassemia. Children received at least 2 years of penicillin prophylaxis before their fifth birthday and one dose of pneumococcal vaccine. No difference was noted in the rate of invasive pneumococcal infection among children receiving continued penicillin prophylaxis and those receiving placebo.

Although some physicians recommend prophylaxis until age 5, others suggest that prophylactic antibiotics be continued indefinitely, particularly for those with increased risk of infection. Prophylaxis is recommended for all children regardless of age for 1 year following splenectomy (American Academy of Pediatrics, 2000).

The Working Party of the British Committee for Standards in Hematology Clinical Hematology Task Force (1996) has recommended penicillin prophylaxis for these patients. Patients allergic to penicillin should be given erythromycin. Prophylactic antibiotics should be given at least until age 16, or indefinitely if there is impaired immune function. A supply of amoxicillin for immediate use at the first signs and symptoms of an infection should be available at home or when traveling. Patients should wear a Medic-Alert bracelet. Traveling patients should be warned about the dangers of malaria and babesiosis.

A patient with impaired splenic function who is suspected of having an infection needs urgent evaluation with appropriate cultures. In some cases, broad-spectrum antibiotics should be started empirically, even if the patient is taking prophylactic antibiotics (Brigden and Pattulio, 1999).

Vaccines

H. influenzae, pneumococcal, and meningococcal vaccines are particularly imperative for patients with asplenia (Chesney, 2001). These infants should receive the conjugated *H. influenzae* and 7-valent pneumococcal vaccines. Patients older than age 2 should also receive pneumococcal polysaccharide and the quadrivalent meningococcal vaccine. Boosters of these vaccines may be given every 5 years to maintain adequate antibody titers. Children older than age 2 who have received the 7-valent conjugated pneumococcal vaccine as infants should also receive the 23-valent polysaccharide vaccine. Similarly, older children with asplenia may benefit from both types of pneumococcal vaccines (American Academy of Pediatrics, 2000).

Other Precautions

In addition to receiving penicillin prophylaxis and immunization with the appropriate vaccines, patients who have undergone splenectomy must be educated about their enhanced susceptibility to bacterial infections. Despite the use of vaccines and penicillin prophylaxis, high rates of invasive pneumococcal infection still are observed (e.g., 3000 per 100,000 in some groups of children with sickle cell disease) (Overturf, 1999; Zarkowsky et al., 1986). The emerging resistance patterns of pneumococci may also dictate antibiotic choices and is an extremely important reason for immunization with pneumococcal vaccines.

SUMMARY

Secondary or acquired immune deficiencies are more common then the clinician realizes. It is surprising that much of the research done in several of these conditions dates back some 10 to 20 years. Clearly, more research is needed to understand the mechanisms by which the immune system is compromised in these conditions, as well as new approaches to prevention and therapy.

By contrast, there is much interest in the modulation of immune responses in exercise and stress, both physical and psychologic. Whether the stress of today's society can lead to an increased susceptibility to cancers by the "breakdown" of immune surveillance is debatable.

ACKNOWLEDGMENT

I thank Michele Bauer for her secretarial and editorial assistance in the preparation of this manuscript.

REFERENCES

Abraham E, Regan RF. The effects of hemorrhage and trauma on interleukin-2 production. Arch Surg 120:1341–1344, 1985.

Ades LC, Kerr B, Turner G, Wise G. Smith-Fineman-Myers syndrome in two brothers. Am J Med Genetics 40:467–470, 1991.

Akriotis V, Biggar WD. The effects of hypothermia on neutrophil function in vitro. Pediatr Res 19:1044–1047, 1985.

American Academy of Pediatrics. Immunization in special clinical circumstances. In Pickering LK, ed. 2000 Red Book: Report of the Committee on Infectious Diseases, ed 25. American Academy of Pediatrics, Elk Grove Village, IL, 2000, pp 54–81.

Ammann AJ, Addiego JD, Wara DW, Lubin BW, Smith B, Mentzer WC. Polyvalent pneumococcal-polysaccharide immunization of patients with sickle-cell anemia and patients with splenectomy. N Engl J Med 297:897–900, 1977.

Amsbaugh DF, Prescott B, Baker PJ. Effect of splenectomy on the expression of regulatory T cell activity. J Immunol 121:1483–1485, 1978.

Barlow Y. T lymphocytes and immunosuppression in the burned patient: a review. Burns 20:487–490, 1994.

Beilin B, Shavit Y, Hart J, Mordashov B, Cohn S, Nott I, Bessler H. Effects of anaesthesia based on large vs small doses of fentanyl on natural killer cell cytotoxicity in the perioperative period. Anesth Analg 82:492–497, 1996.

Bost KL. Hormone and neuropeptide receptors on mononuclear leukocytes. Prog Allergy 43:68–83, 1988.

Brigden ML, Pattulio AL. Prevention and management of overwhelming postsplenectomy infection—An update. Crit Care Med 27:836–842, 1999.

Britz-Cunningham SH, Shah MM, Zuppan CW, Fletcher WH. Mutation of the *connexin43* gap-junction gene in patients with heart malformations and defects of laterality. N Engl J Med 332:1323–1329, 1995.

Broberger O, Gyulai F, Hirschfeldt J. Splenectomy in childhood. Acta Paediatr 49:679–689, 1960.

Bruunsgaard H, Hartkopp A, Mohr T, Konradsen H, Heron I, Mordhorst CH, Pedersen BK. In vivo cell-mediated immunity and vaccination response following prolonged, intense exercise. Med Sci Sports Exerc 29:1176–1181, 1997.

Buchanan GR, Siegel JD, Smith SJ, DePasse DM. Oral penicillin prophylaxis in children with impaired splenic function: a study of compliance. Pediatrics 70:926–930, 1982.

Burke JF, Quinby WC, Bondoc CC. Primary excision and prompt grafting as routine therapy for the treatment of thermal burns in children. Surg Clin North Am 56:477–481, 1976.

Burleson DG, Mason AD, Pruitt BA. Lymphoid subpopulation changes after thermal injury and thermal injury with infection in an experimental model. Ann Surg 207:208–212, 1988.

Camus G, Deby-Dupont G, Duchateau J, Deby C, Princemail J, Lamy M. Are similar inflammatory factors involved in strenuous exercise and sepsis? Intens Care Med 20:602–610, 1994.

Cannon JG, Kluger MJ. Exercise enhances survival rate in mice-infected with *Salmonella typhimurium*. Exper Biol Med 175:518–521, 1984.

Carlisle HN, Saslaw S. Properdin levels in splenectomized persons. Proc Soc Exp Biol Med 102:150–154, 1959.

Cesko I, Hajdu J, Toth T, Marton T, Papp C, Papp Z. Ivemark syndrome with asplenia in siblings. J. Pediatr 130:822–824, 1997.

Chesney PJ. Asplenia. In Patrick C, ed. Clinical management of infections in immunocompromised infants and children. Lippincott Williams & Williams, Philadelphia, 2001, pp 307–326.

Chilcote RR, Baehner RL, Hammond D. Septicemia and meningitis in children splenectomized for Hodgkin's disease. N Engl J Med 295:798–800, 1976.

Christou NV, Meakins JL. Neutrophil function in surgical patients: Two inhibitors of granulocyte chemotaxis associated with sepsis. J Surg Res 26:355–364, 1979.

Christou NV, Meakins JL, Gordon J. The delayed hypersensitivity response and host resistance in surgical patients. Ann Surg 222:534–548, 1995.

Claret I, Morales L, Montaner A. Immunological studies in the postsplenectomy syndrome. J Pediatr Surg 10:59–64, 1975.

Coatney GR. Simian malarias in man: facts, implications, and predictions. Am J Trop Med Hygiene 17:147–155, 1968.

Corry JM, Polhill RB Jr, Edmonds SR, Johnston RB Jr. Activity of the alternative complement pathway after splenectomy: Comparison to activity in sickle cell disease and hypogammaglobulinemia. J Pediatr 95:964–969, 1979.

Crary B, Hauser SL, Borysenko M, Kutz I, Hoban C, Ault KA, Weiner HL, Benson H. Epinephrine induced changes in the distribution of lymphocyte subsets in peripheral blood of humans. J Immunol 131:1178–1181, 1983.

Crawfurd MD. Renal dysplasia and asplenia in two sibs. Clin Genetics 14:338–344, 1978.

De AK, Kodys KM, Pellegrini J, Yeh B, Furse RK, Bankey P, Miller-Graziano CL. Induction of global anergy rather than inhibitory Th2 lymphokines mediates post-trauma T cell immunodepression. Clin Immunol 96:52–66, 2000.

De AK, Kodys KM, Puyana JC, Fudem G, Pellegrini J, Miller-Graziano CL. Only a subset of trauma patients with depressed mitogen responses have true T cell dysfunctions. Clin Immunol Immunopathol 82:73–82, 1997.

Deitch EA, Xu D, Qi L. Different lymphocyte compartments respond differently to mitogenic stimulation after thermal injury. Ann Surg 211:72–77, 1990.

Devlin EG, Clark RSJ, Mirakhur RK. The effects of thiopentone and propofol on delayed hypersensitivity reactions. Anaesthesia 50:496–498, 1995.

Diamond LK. Splenectomy in childhood and the hazard of overwhelming infection. Pediatr 43:886–889, 1969.

Drew PA, Kiroff GK, Ferrant A, Cohen RC. Alterations in immunoglobulin synthesis by peripheral blood mononuclear cells from splenectomized patients with and without splenic regrowth. J Immunol 132:191–196, 1984.

Eraklis AJ, Filler RM. Splenectomy in childhood: a review of 1413 cases. J Pediatr Surg 7:382–388, 1972.

Falletta JM, Woods GM, Verter JI, Buchanan G, Pegelow C, Iyer S, Miller RS, Holbrook C, Kinney T, Vichinsky E. Discontinuing penicillin prophylaxis in children with sickle cell anemia: Prophylactic Penicillin Study II. J Pediatr 127:685–690, 1995.

Feder HM, Pearson HA. Assessment of splenic function in familial asplenia. N Engl J Med 341:210–211, 1999.

Ferry A, Weill B, Amiridis I, Laziry F, Rieu M. Splenic immunomodulation with swimming-induced stress in rats. Immunol Lett 29:261–264, 1991.

Fitzgerald L. Exercise and the immune system. Immunology Today 9:337–339, 1988.

Forward AD, Ashmore PG. Infection following splenectomy in infants and children. Can J Surg 3:229–233, 1960.

Fraser J, Nadau J, Robertson D, Wood JJ. Regulation of human leukocyte beta receptors by endogenous catecholamines: Relationship of leukocyte beta receptor density to the cardiac sensitivity to isoproterenol. J Clin Invest 67:1777–1784, 1981.

Frey MJ, Mancini D, Fischberg D, Wilson JR, Molinoff PB. Effect of exercise duration on density and coupling of beta-adrenergic receptors on human mononuclear cells. J Appl Physiol 66:1495–1500, 1989.

Fry RW, Morton AR, Keast D. Acute intensive interval training and T-lymphocyte function. Med Sci Sports Exerc 24:339–345, 1992.

Fullana A, Garcia-Frias E, Martinez-Frias ML, Razquin S, Quero J. Caudal deficiency and asplenia anomalies in sibs. Am J Med Genetics 2(Suppl.):23–29, 1986.

Gabriel H, Kindermann W. Adhesion molecules during immune response to exercise. Can J Physiol Pharmacol 76:512–523, 1998.

Gannon GA, Rhind SG, Shek PN, Shephard RJ. The majority of CD4+, but not CD8hi+, T cells mobilized to peripheral blood during exercise express a CD45 RO+ memory phenotype. Int J Sports Med 19:S213–S218, 1998.

Gaston MH, Verter JI, Woods G, Pegelow C, Kelleher J, Presbury G, Zarkowsky H, Vichinsky E, Iyer R, Lobel JS. Prophylaxis with oral penicillin in children with sickle cell anemia. A randomized trial. N Engl J Med 314:1593–1599, 1986.

Gatmaitan BG, Chason JL, Lerner AM. Augmentation of the virulence of murine coxsackie-virus B-3 myocardiopathy by exercise. J Exp Med 131:1121–1136, 1970.

Gillis J, Harvey J, Isaacs D, Freelander M, Wyeth B. Familial asplenia. Arch Dis Child 67:665–666, 1992.

Gleeson M, McDonald WA, Pyne DB, Clancy RL, Cripps AW, Francis JL, Fricker PA. Immune status and respiratory illness for elite swimmers during a 12-week training cycle. Int Sports Med 21:302–307, 2000.

Greif R, Akca O, Horn E, Kurz A, Sessler D. Supplemental perioperative oxygen to reduce the incidence of surgical wound infections. N Engl J Med 342:161–167, 2000.

Hansbrough JF, Zapata-Sirvent R, Peterson VM, Wang X, Bender E, Claman H, Boswick J. Characterization of the immunosuppressive effect of burned tissue in an animal model. J Surg Res 37:383–393, 1984.

Hebeler RF, Ward RE, Miller PW, Ben-Menachem Y. The management of splenic injury. J Trauma 22:492–495, 1982.

Heine J, Leuwer M, Scheinichen D. Flow cytometry evaluation of the in-vitro influence of four i.v. anaesthetics on respiratory burst of neutrophils. Br J Anaesth 77:387–392, 1996.

Hoffman-Goetz L, Pedersen BK. Exercise and the immune system: a model of stress response? Immunol Today 15:382–387, 1994.

Holdsworth RJ, Irving AD, Cuschieri A. Postsplenectomy sepsis and its mortality rate: actual versus perceived risks. Br J Surg 78:1031–1038, 1991.

Hopf H, Hunt T, West J. Wound tissue oxygen tension predicts the risk of wound infection in surgical patients. Arch Surg 132:997–1004, 1997.

Hosea SW, Brown EJ, Hamburger MI, Frank MM. Opsonic requirements for intravascular clearance after splenectomy. N Engl J Med 304:245–250, 1981a.

Hosea SW, Burch CG, Brown EJ, Berg RA, Frank MM. Impaired immune response of splenectomized patients to polyvalent pneumococcal vaccine. Lancet 1:804–807, 1981b.

Howman-Giles R, Gilday DL, Venugopal S, Shandling SB, Ash JM. Splenic trauma: Nonoperative management and long-term follow-up by scintiscan. J Pediatr Surg 13:121–126, 1978.

Ivemark BI. Implications of agenesis of the spleen on the pathogenesis of cono-truncus anomalies in childhood: analysis of the heart malformations of the splenic agenesis syndrome, with fourteen new cases. Acta Paediatr 44(Suppl. 104):1, 1955.

Johnson HM, Smith EM, Torres BA, Blalock JE. Regulation of the in vitro antibody response by neuroendocrine hormones. Proc Natl Acad Sci USA 79:4171–4174, 1982.

Jordan JR, Beneke R, Hutler M, Veith A, Haller H, Luft FC. Moderate exercise leads to decreased expression of β1 and β2 integrins on leukocytes. Eur J Appl Physiol 76:192–194, 1997.

Kaufmann SH. Heat shock proteins and the immune response. Immunol Today 11:129–136, 1990.

Keane RM, Birmingham W, Shatney CM, Winchurch RA, Munster AM. Prediction of sepsis in the multitraumatic patient by assays of lymphocyte responsiveness. Surg Gynecol Obstet 156:163–167, 1983.

Kelly JL, Lyons A, Soberg CC, Mannick JA, Lederer JA. Anti-interleukin-10 antibody restores burn-induced defects in T-cell function. Surgery 122:146–152, 1997.

King H, Shumacker H. Splenic studies: Susceptibility to infection after splenectomy performed in infancy. Ann Surg 136:239–242, 1952.

Kurokawa Y, Shinkai S, Torii J, Hino S, Shek PN. Exercise-induced changes in the expression of surface adhesion molecules on circulating granulocytes and lymphocyte subpopulations. Eur J Appl Physiol 71:245–252, 1995.

Landmann R. Beta-adrenergic receptors in human leukocyte subpopulations. Eur Clin Invest 22:30–36, 1992.

Lueder GT, Fitz-James A, Dowton SB. Congenital microgastria and hypoplastic upper limb anomalies. Am J Med Genet 32:368–370, 1989.

Mack VE, McCarter MD, Naama HA, Calvano SE, Daly JM. Dominance of T helper 2 type cytokines after severe injury. Arch Surg 131:1303–1308, 1996.

Maldonado MD, Venturoli A, Franco A, Nunez-Roldan A. Specific changes in peripheral blood lymphocyte phenotype from burn patients. Probable origin of the thermal injury-related lymphopenia. Burns 17:188–192, 1991.

Marshall GD, Agarwal SK, Lloyd C, Cohen L, Henninger EM, Morris GJ. Cytokine dysregulation in healthy medical students associated with exam stress. Brain Behav Immun 12:297–307, 1998.

Martin LW. Autologous splenic transplantation. Ann Surg 219:223, 1994.

McAnally HB, Cutter GR, Ruttenber AJ, Clarke D, Todd JK. Hypothermia as a risk factor for pediatric cardiothoracic surgical site infection. Pediatr Infect Dis J 20:459–461, 2001.

McFadzean AJS, Tsang KC. Antibody formation in cryptogenic splenomegaly: II. Response to antigen infected subcutaneously. Trans R Soc Trop Med Hyg 50:438–441, 1956.

Morgenstern L, Shapiro SJ. Techniques of splenic conservation. Arch Surg 114:449–454, 1979.

Morris DH, Bullock FD. The importance of the spleen in resistance to infection. Ann Surg 70:513–521, 1919.

Murray DR, Irwin M, Rearden CA, Ziegler M, Motulsky H, Maisel AS. Sympathetic and immune interactions during dynamic exercise. Mediation via a beta-2 adrenergic-dependent mechanism. Circulation 86:203–213, 1992.

Nakagawara M, Takeshigne K, Takamatsu J, Takahashi S, Roshitake K, Minakami S. Inhibition of superoxide production and Ca²⁺ mobilization in human neutrophils by halothane, enflurane and isoflurane. Anesthesiology 64:4–12, 1986.

Nieman DC. Exercise, infection, and immunity. Int Sports Med 15(Suppl. 3):S131–S141, 1994.

Nieman DC. Influence of carbohydrate on the immune response to intensive, prolonged exercise. Exercise Immunol Rev 4:64–76, 1998.

Nieman DC, Johanssen LM, Lee JW, Arabatzis K. Infectious episodes in runners before and after the Los Angeles Marathon. J Sports Med Phys Fitness 30:316–328, 1990a.

Nieman DC, Miller AR, Henson DA, Warren BJ, Gusewitch G, Johnson RL, Davis JM, Butterworth, DE, Nehlsen-Cannarella SL. Effects of high vs moderate-intensity exercise on natural killer cell activity. Med Sci Sports Exerc 25:1126–1134, 1993.

Nieman DC, Nehlsen-Cannarella SL, Fagoaga OR, Henson D, Utter A, Davis J, Williams F, Butterworth D. Influence of mode and carbohydrate on the granulocyte and monocyte response to intensive, prolonged exercise. J Appl Physiol 84:1252–1259, 1998.

Nieman DC, Nehlsen-Cannarella SL, Markoff PA, Balk-Lamberton AJ, Yang H, Chritton DB, Lee JW, Arabatzis K. The effects of moderate exercise training on natural killer cells and acute upper respiratory tract infections. Int Sports Med 11:467–473, 1990b.

Nieman DC, Pedersen BF. Exercise and immune function recent developments. Sports Med 27:73–80, 1999.

Niikawa N, Kohsaka S, Mizumoto M, Hamada I, Kajii T. Familial clustering of situs inversus totalis, and asplenia and polysplenia syndromes. Am J Med Genet 16:43–47, 1983.

Ninnemann JL, Condie JT, Davis SE, Crockett RA. Isolation of immunosuppressive serum components following thermal injury. J Trauma 22:837–844, 1982.

Norris CF, Mahannah SR, Smith-Whitley K, Ohene-Frempong K, McGowan KL. Pneumococcal colonization in children with sickle cell disease. J Pediatr 129:821–827, 1996.

O'Brien RT, McIntosh S, Aspnes GT, Pearson HA. Prospective studies of sickle-cell anemia in infancy. J Pediatr 89:205–210, 1976.

O'Mahony JB, Palder SB, Wood JJ, McIrvine A, Rodrick ML, Demling RH, Mannick JA. Depression of cellular immunity after multiple trauma in the absence of sepsis. J Trauma 24:869–875, 1984.

O'Sullivan ST, Lederer JA, Horgan AF, Chin DHL, Mannick JA, Rodrick ML. Major injury leads to predominance of the T helper-2 lymphocyte phenotype and diminished interleukin-12 production associated with decreased resistance to infection. Ann Surg 222:482–492, 1995.

Ostrowski K, Rohde T, Asp S, Schjerling P, Pedersen BK. Pro- and anti-inflammatory cytokine balance in strenuous exercise in humans. J Physiol 515:287–291, 1999.

Overturf GD. Infections and immunizations of children with sickle cell disease. Adv Pediatr Infect Dis 14:191–218, 1999.

Ozkan AN, Hoyt DB, Tomopkins S, Ninnemann JL, Sullivan JJ. Immunosuppressive effects of a trauma-induced suppressor active peptide. J Trauma 28:589–592, 1988.

Parry-Billings M, Budgett R, Koutedakis Y, Blomstrand E, Brooks S, Williams C, Calder PC, Pilling S, Baigrie R, Newsholme EA. Plasma amino acid concentrations in the overtraining syndrome: possible effects on the immune system. Med Science Sports Exerc 24:1353–1358, 1992.

Pearson HA, McIntosh S, Ritchey AK, Lobel JS, Rooks Y, Johnston D. Developmental aspects of splenic function in sickle cell disease. Blood 53:358–365, 1979.

Pearson HA, Spencer RP, Cornelius EA. Functional asplenia in sickle-cell anemia. N Engl J Med 281:923–926, 1969.

Pedersen BK, Ostrowski K, Rohde T, Bruunsgaard H. The cytokine response to strenuous exercise. Can J Physiol Pharmacol 76:505–511, 1998.

Pedersen BK, Tvede N, Klarlund K, Christensen LD, Hansen FR, Galbo H, Kharazmi A, Kalkjaer-Kristensen J. Indomethacin in vitro and in vivo abolishes post-exercise suppression of natural killer cell activity in peripheral blood. Int Sports Med 11:127–131, 1990.

Peters EM. Exercise and upper respiratory tract infections: a review. S Afr J Sports Med 11:9–14, 1996.

Rodrick ML, Wood JJ, Mahony JB, Davis CF, Moss NM, Blazar BA, Demling RH, Mannick JA. Defective IL-2 production in patients with severe burns and sepsis. Lymphokine Res 5(Suppl. 1):S75–S80, 1986.

Rohde T, MacLean D, Hartkopp A, Pedersen B. The immune system and serum glutamine during triathlon. Eur J Appl Physiol 74:428–434, 1996.

Rose V, Izukawa T, Moes CA. Syndromes of asplenia and polysplenia. A review of cardiac and non-cardiac malformations in 60 cases with special reference to diagnosis and prognosis. Br Heart J 37:840–852, 1975.

Rossano F, Tufano R, de L'Ero C, Servillo G, Baroni A, Tufano MA. Anaesthetic agents induce human mononuclear leukocytes to release cytokines. Immunopharmacol Immunotoxicol 14:439–450, 1992.

Roumen RM, Hendriks T, van der Ven-Jongekrijg Nieuwenhuijzen GA, Sauerwein RW, van der Meer JS, Goris RJ. Cytokine patterns in patients after vascular surgery, hemorrhagic shock, and severe blunt trauma. Ann Surg 218:769–776, 1993.

Saslaw S, Bouroncle BA, Wall RL, Doan CA. Studies on antibody response in splenectomized persons. N Engl J Med 261:120–125, 1959.

Schulkind ML, Ellis EE, Smith RT. Effect of antibody upon clearance of ^{125}I-labelled pneumococci by the spleen and liver. Pediatr Res 1:178–184, 1967.

Schumacher MJ. Serum immunoglobulin and transferrin levels after childhood splenectomy. Arch Dis Child 45:114–117, 1970.

Shephard RJ, Shek PN. Effects of exercise and training on natural killer cell counts and cytolytic activity: a meta-analysis. Sports Med 28:177–195, 1999.

Shinefield HR, Steinberg CR, Kaye D. Effect of splenectomy on the susceptibility of mice inoculated with *Diplococcus pneumoniae*. J Exp Med 123:777–794, 1966.

Singer D. Postsplenectomy sepsis. Perspect Pediatr Pathol 1:285–311, 1973.

Smith CH, Erlandson M, Schulman I, Stern G. Hazard of severe infections in splenectomized infants and children. Am J Med 22:390–404, 1957.

Sparkes BG. Influence of burn induced lipid-protein complex on IL-2 secretion by PBMC in vitro. Burns 17:128–135, 1991.

Sparkes BG, Monge G, Marshall SL, Peters WJ, Allgower M, Schoenenberger GA. Plasma levels of cutaneous burn toxin and lipid peroxides in thermal injury. Burns 16:118–122, 1990.

Steele RW, Warrier R, Unkel PJ, Foch BJ, Howes RF, Shah S, Williams K, Moore S, Jue SJ. Colonization with antibiotic-resistant *Streptococcus pneumoniae* in children with sickle cell disease. J Pediatr 128:531–535, 1996.

Steerenberg PA, Van-Aspersen IA, Van-Nieuw-Ameron-Gen A, Mold BA, Medema GJ. Salivary levels of immunoglobulin A in triathletes. Eur J Oral Sci 105:305–309, 1997.

Sternfeld B. Cancer and the protective effect of physical activity: the epidemiological evidence. Med Sci Sports Exerc 24:1195–1209, 1993.

Stormorken H, Sjaastad O, Langslet A, Sulg I, Egge K, Diderichsen J. A new syndrome: thrombocytopathia, muscle fatigue, asplenia, miosis, migraine, dyslexia and ichthyosis. Clin Genetics 28:367–374, 1985.

Sullivan JL, Ochs HD, Schiffman G, Hammerschlag MR, Miser J, Vichinsky E, Wedgwood RJ. Immune response after splenectomy. Lancet 1:178–181, 1978.

Sung Y, Akriotis V, Barker C, Calderwood S, Biggar WD. Susceptibility of human and porcine neutrophils to hypothermia in vitro. Pediatr Res 19:1044–1047, 1985.

Svoboda P, Kantorova I, Ochmann J. Dynamics of interleukin-1, -2, and -6 and tumor necrosis factor alpha in multiple trauma patients. J Trauma 36:336–340, 1994.

Teodorczyk-Injeyan JA, Sparkes BG, Mills GB, Falk RE, Peters WJ. Impairment of T cell activation in burn patients: A possible mechanism of thermal injury-induced immunosuppression. Clin Exp Immunol 65:570–581, 1986.

Teodorczyk-Injeyan JA, Sparkes BG, Mills GB, Falk RE, Peters WJ. Impaired expression of interleukin-2 receptor (IL-2R) in the immunosuppressed burned patient: Reversal by exogenous IL-2. J Trauma-Injury Infect Crit Care 27:180–187, 1987.

Tharp GD, Barnes MW. Reduction of saliva immunoglobulin levels by swim training. Eur J Appl Physiol 60:61–64, 1990.

Toft P, Svendsen P, Tonnesen E. Redistribution of lymphocytes after major surgical stress. Acta Anaesthesiol Scand 37:245–249, 1993.

Tomasi TB, Trudeau BV, Czerwinski D, Erredge S. Immune parameters in athletes before and after strenuous exercise. J Clin Immunol 2:173–178, 1982.

Touloukian RJ. Splenic preservation in children. World J Surg 9:214–221, 1985.

Traub AC, Perry JF Jr. Splenic preservation following splenic trauma. J Trauma 22:496–501, 1982.

Tvede NC, Heilmann C, Halkjaer-Kristensen J, Pedersen BK. Mechanisms of B-lymphocyte suppression induced by acute physical exercise. J Clin Lab Immunol 30:169–173, 1989a.

Tvede N, Kappel M, Halkjaer-Kristensen J, Galbo H, Pedersen BK. The effect of light, moderate and severe bicycle exercise on lymphocyte subsets, natural and lymphokine activated killer cells, lymphocyte proliferative response and interleukin-2 production. Int Sports Med 14:275–282, 1993.

Tvede N, Kappel M, Klarlund K, Duhn S, Halkjaer-Kristensen J, Kjaer M, Galbo H, Pedersen BK. Evidence that the effect of bicycle exercise on blood mononuclear cell proliferative responses and subsets is mediated by epinephrine. Int J Sports Med 15:100–104, 1994.

Tvede N, Pedersen BK, Hansen FR, Bendix T, Christensen LD, Galbo H, Halkjaer-Kristensen J. Effect of physical exercise on blood mononuclear cell subpopulations and in vitro proliferative responses. Scand J Immunol 29:383–389, 1989b.

Waldman JD, Rosenthal A, Smith AL, Shurin S, Nadas AS. Sepsis and congenital asplenia. J Pediatr 90:555–559, 1977.

Walker W. Splenectomy in childhood: A review in England and Wales, 1960–4. Br J Surg 63:36–43, 1976.

Wang JK, Hsieh KH. Immunologic study of the asplenia syndrome. Pediatr Infect Dis J 10:819–822, 1991.

Watson RS, Moriguchi S, Fackson JC, Werner L, Willmore JH, Freund BJ. Modification of cellular immune function in humans by endurance exercise training during β-adrenergic blockade with atenolol or propranolol. Med Sci Sports Exerc 18:95–100, 1986.

Weigent DA, Carr DJJ, Blalock JE. Bidirectional communication between the neuroendocrine and immune systems. Ann NY Acad Sci 579:17–27, 1990.

Wenisch C, Narzt E, Sessler DI, Parschalk B, Lenhardt R, Kurz A, Graninger W. Mild intraoperative hypothermia reduces production of reactive oxygen intermediates by polymorphonuclear leukocytes. Anesth Analg 82:810–816, 1996.

Western KA, Benson GD, Gleason NN, Healy GR, Schultz MG. Babesiosis in a Massachusetts resident. N Engl J Med 283:854–856, 1970.

Winkelstein JA, Lambert GH, Swift A. Pneumococcal serum opsonizing activity in splenectomized children. J Pediatr 87:430–433, 1975.

Working Party of the British Committee for Standards in Haematology Clinical Haematology Task Force. Guidelines for the prevention and treatment of infection in patients with an absent or dysfunctional spleen. Br Med J 312:430–434, 1996.

Xiao GX, Chopra RK, Adler W, Munster A, Winchurch RA. Altered expression of lymphocyte IL-2 receptors in burned patients. J Trauma 28:1669–1672, 1988.

Xu YX, Ayala A, Chaundry IH. Prolonged immunodepression after trauma and hemorrhagic shock. J Trauma 44:335–341, 1998.

Yeager MP, Colacchio T, Yu CT. Morphine inhibits spontaneous and cytokine enhanced natural killer cell cytotoxicity in volunteers. Anesthesiology 83:500–508, 1995.

Zarkowsky HS, Gallagher D, Gill FM, Wang WC, Falletta JM, Lande W, Levy PS, Verter JI, Wethers D. Bacteremia in sickle hemoglobinopathies. J Pediatr 109:579–585, 1986.

P A R T IV

Immunologic Aspects of Pediatric Illness

C H A P T E R

31 Allergic Diseases

Scott H. Sicherer and Hugh A. Sampson

DEFINITIONS

Clemens von Pirquet first coined the term *allergy* ("changed activity") and applied it to induced immune responses of either a protective nature, as illustrated by responses to vaccination, or a detrimental nature as he observed with serum sickness induced by horse serum. Over the years, however, the term has been linked to the latter hypersensitivity responses. Thus allergy may be defined as an adverse physiologic event resulting from an immunologically mediated response. This definition requires that the host experience a symptom or disease related to an antigen-induced immune response such as those derived from foods, medications, airborne biologic agents such as pollens or animal danders, and other foreign proteins. Defined as such, otherwise healthy persons may experience allergic responses from immune reactivity to foreign antigens that occur during reactions to mismatched blood transfusions, transplant rejection, and contact with poison ivy.

In contrast to allergy, *atopic diseases* are chronic disorders with a strong genetic predisposition that are classically attributed to immunoglobulin E (IgE)-mediated mechanisms. Coca and Cooke first coined the term *atopy* ("strange disease") in 1923 and suggested that atopic disorders included asthma, allergic rhinitis, and atopic dermatitis (AD). The current state of understanding suggests that food allergy should also be considered an atopic disorder. In addition, an expanded appreciation of the pathophysiologic basis of atopic disorders has disclosed that numerous immunologic pathways are involved. Indeed, the phenotypic manifestations of atopic disorders may, in some cases, not require IgE antibodies at all.

HISTORICAL CLASSIFICATION OF HYPERSENSITIVITY REACTIONS

In 1963, Gell and Coombs classified allergic reactions into four types. This classification is antiquated considering the current understanding of the complex interactions among multiple components of the immune system in any given reaction or atopic disease. However, this simple classification system still provides a helpful framework for understanding allergic responses.

Type I (anaphylactic reactions): These reactions generally occur within minutes of exposure to an environmental trigger and are mediated by allergen-specific IgE antibodies bound to the surface of effector cells such as mast cells. Interaction of the cell surface–bound IgE antibodies to allergen results in the activation of the mast cells and the release of a variety of mediators that cause physiologic responses such as vasodilation, pruritus, bronchoconstriction, and capillary leak. Examples of this type of allergy include drug-induced anaphylaxis, food-induced urticaria, allergic rhinitis, and asthma.

Type II (cytotoxic reactions): Antibodies of the IgG or IgM class that are directed to environmental antigens, or self-antigens in autoimmune disease, are responsible for mediating this type of reaction through direct binding of antibody to tissue that expresses the triggering antigen or has absorbed the antigen to its surface. Following antibody binding, local complement activation results in damage to the tissue. Examples include autoimmune hemolytic anemia, drug-induced leukopenia, and Goodpasture disease.

Type III (Arthus or immune complex reactions): Similar to type II reactions, IgG or IgM antibodies bind to extrinsic or self-antigens, but in this type of reaction antigen–antibody complexes of various sizes are formed. Although small complexes usually circulate harmlessly and large complexes are cleared by the reticuloendothelial system, intermediate-sized complexes may deposit in blood vessel walls and tissues. There the immune microprecipitates induce vascular and tissue damage through activation of complement, granulocytes, and platelets. Examples of this reaction include glomerulonephritis and serum sickness.

Type IV (cell-mediated reactions, delayed-type hypersensitivity): This hypersensitivity reaction does not involve antibody. Rather, antigen-specific T lymphocytes are activated by exposure to the relevant antigen and differentiate into cells capable of cytolysis or of secreting mediators that direct local inflammatory reactions, including the influx of effector cells such as macrophages or eosinophils. Examples include contact dermatitis from poison ivy, tuberculin skin reactions, and graft-versus-host disease.

BIOLOGIC BASIS OF IMMEDIATE, LATE PHASE, AND CHRONIC ALLERGIC RESPONSES

Allergen-specific IgE antibody is central to immediate, type I allergic reactions; however, acute responses following release of mast cell and basophil mediators are only one component of allergic inflammatory disease. Local IgE antibody–mediated reactions are linked to late-phase tissue responses characterized by the influx of eosinophils and neutrophils into the affected site 6 to 8 hours after the immediate response. By 48 hours, mononuclear cells predominate and the histologic picture is similar to that seen in type IV, cell-mediated reactions. Possibly an extension of the late-phase response, chronic allergic inflammation accounts for the symptoms observed in atopic diseases such as allergic asthma, rhinitis, and AD. A complex panoply of immune cells, soluble mediators, and surface molecules orchestrate these processes.

Immunoglobulin E Antibody

IgE antibody was identified independently by Ishizaka and Ishizaka (1967) and Johansson and Bennich (1967) as the skin-sensitizing (reaginic) protein central to type I hypersensitivity reactions. In nonallergic individuals, this 190-Kd immunoglobulin is present in low concentrations (<50 IU/ml), but elevated IgE is commonly associated with atopic disorders. IgE binds efficiently to high-affinity Fc receptors, FcεRI, on mast cells and basophils. The FcεRI is composed of an α, β, and γ chain. The α chain binds to the IgE, whereas the β and γ chains mediate signal transduction following the crosslinking of IgE antibodies by multivalent allergens (Hulett et al., 1994; Mallamaci et al., 1993; Sayers and Helm, 1999).

This series of events leads to changes in phospholipid and calcium metabolism and an energy-dependent secretion of pharmacologically active molecules that result in the observed reaction. Langerhans cells also bear FcεRI, and this may facilitate antigen presentation to T lymphocytes that direct allergic inflammation (Mudde et al., 1990). Low-affinity IgE receptors, CD23 (FcεRII), on monocytes, macrophages, and lymphocytes appear to play a role in regulation of IgE responses (Gustavsson et al., 2000).

Regulation of IgE Responses

For an IgM-bearing B cell to switch to an IgE isotype, two signals provided by T cells are needed following major histocompatibility complex (MHC) class II restricted antigen presentation. The first signal is provided by the cytokines interleukin (IL)-4 or IL-13 and stimulates transcription of the epsilon constant region. A second signal provided by the binding of CD40 ligand on the T cell to CD40 on the B cell triggers recombination events (Bacharier and Geha, 2000). Further augmentation of IgE synthesis results from the interaction of B cell CD80 with T cell CD28. Genetic studies have linked the phenotype of high IgE antibody to a region of chromosome 5q31 with the candidate genes IL-4 and IL-13 (Marsh et al., 1994), and there is also an association in families with asthma between elevated IgE and polymorphisms in the IL-4 promoter region (Rosenwasser et al., 1995).

Th1/Th2 Paradigm

CD4$^+$ T cells preferentially secrete particular profiles of cytokines that direct specific patterns of immune responses. T cells of the Th2 phenotype preferentially secrete the cytokines IL-4, IL-5, and IL-13, but not interferon-γ (IFN-γ) and thereby induce IgE synthesis and promote eosinophilic inflammation. Th1 cells are polarized to elaborate IFN-γ and not IL-4 or IL-5 and promote cell-mediated responses. Th0 cells produce both Th1 and Th2 cytokines and may become polarized depending on the subject's genetic background, co-stimulatory molecules activated during sensitization, and the characteristics of the antigen. For example, IL-12 produced by macrophages and dendritic cells may induce a Th1 response, whereas IL-4 promotes a Th2 response (Abehsira-Amar et al., 1992; Rissoan et al., 1999).

Regulatory Cytokines and Adhesion Molecules

In addition to the cytokines that direct IgE production, a number of cytokines are central to allergic inflammation because they promote eosinophilia. IL-5 plays a primary role in eosinophil activation and delay of apoptosis (Gleich et al., 2000), and IL-3 and granulocyte-macrophage colony-stimulating factor (GM-CSF) play a role in eosinophil activation. Eosinophils are attracted to sites of inflammation in part by chemokines such as regulated upon activation, normal T expressed and secreted (RANTES); eotaxin; and macrophage chemotactic proteins (MCP) MCP-2, MCP-3, and MCP-4. Expression of the chemokine receptor CCR3 by eosinophils is vital to these responses (Shahabuddin et al., 2000).

The initial immigration of eosinophils into sites of inflammation depends on a number of adhesion molecules. Initial low-affinity rolling on vascular endothelium is mediated by E and P selectins, whereas firm adhesion and diapedesis requires expression of the β$_2$ integrin VLA-4 (very late activation molecules-4) on the eosinophil that binds to vascular cell adhesion molecule-1 (VCAM-1) on the endothelium. These molecules are upregulated by several cytokines, including IL-1, IL-4,

IL-13, and tumor necrosis factor-alpha (TNF-α) (Bochner et al., 1991). These surface molecules and growth factors work together to maintain the eosinophilic inflammatory response.

Mast Cells and Basophils

Mast cells arise from CD34$^+$ pluripotential stem cells and migrate into tissues where they mature in the presence of stem cell factor and other locally produced cytokines (Metcalfe et al., 1997). A number of characteristics differentiate mast cells found primarily in skin, vascular walls, and other connective tissue sites (designated MC$_{tc}$) from those found primarily in mucosal sites such as the lung, nasal mucosa, and small intestinal mucosa (designated MC$_t$). MC$_{tc}$ demonstrate a lattice structure on electron microscopy and contain chymase, tryptase, and cathepsin G, whereas MC$_t$ are rich in scroll-appearing structures on electron microscopy and have tryptase but no chymase or cathepsin G.

In addition to the mediators mentioned previously, preformed mast cell mediators include histamine, heparin, and chondroitin sulfates A and E. Newly generated metabolites include leukotriene (LT) C$_4$, LT B$_4$, and prostaglandin (PG) D$_2$ and cytokines such as IL-4, IL-5, IL-6, IL-13, and TNF-α.

Basophils are derived from bone marrow promyelocytes, are fewer in number than mast cells, and remain primarily in the circulation. Although basophils share a number of mediators with mast cells (e.g., histamine, tryptase in small amounts, LTC$_4$, LTB$_4$, and a number of cytokines), they do not form heparin or PGD$_2$ and there are a number of differences in cell surface cytokine receptors, complement receptors, and other surface proteins (Bochner, 2000).

Eosinophils

The eosinophil is central to chronic allergic inflammation (Bochner, 2000; Rothenberg, 1998) and in immune responses to helminths. For purposes of regulation, target recognition, and effector functions, the eosinophil surface is studded with a variety of adhesion molecules, enzymes, and receptors for immunoglobulin, complement, cytokines, chemokines, LTs, and histamine.

Once recruited to sites of inflammation, the eosinophil may generate and release a large number of inflammatory mediators. Eosinophil-specific granules contain major basic protein (MBP) in a crystalloid core, whereas the matrix of granules contains eosinophil cationic protein, eosinophil peroxidase, and eosinophil-derived neurotoxin. MBP is active against helminths but also induces basophil histamine release and neutrophil superoxide release and can directly damage respiratory epithelial cells and promote bronchospasm. The matrix proteins are toxic to helminths and also affect coagulation and induce cell damage.

Eosinophils are also capable of producing a host of cytokines, arachidonic acid metabolites, reactive oxygen species, and enzymes such as collagenase and Charcot-Leyden crystal protein. The eosinophil's role in local tissue damage, especially in regard to airway epithelium, and its ability to sustain allergic inflammation distinguish it as the hallmark of allergic inflammation.

Chemical Mediators

A number of products released from cells participating in allergic inflammation result in physiologic events recognized as symptoms of classic allergic reactions. Histamine released from cytoplasmic granules in mast cells and basophils is particularly important in the type I hypersensitivity response. Histamine responses are mediated through H_1 receptors found on blood vessels and smooth muscle of the gut and lung. Stimulation of these receptors induces increased vascular permeability, pruritus, tachycardia, flushing, and bronchoconstriction.

However, histamine is also found in a variety of other cells and plays a role in neurotransmission, gastric acid secretion, and tissue growth and repair. Through stimulation of H_2 receptors in gastric mucosa, the heart, uterus, and central nervous system (CNS), there is induction of gastric acid, vasodilation, increased vascular permeability, uterine contractions, and increased bronchial mucus production. Activation of H_3 receptors in the CNS and gastrointestinal tract appears to inhibit the synthesis and release of histamine.

Oxidative metabolites of arachidonic acid also play a significant role in the allergic inflammatory response primarily through effects induced near their site of release. The lipoxygenase pathway is active in several cell populations, including mast cells, eosinophils, macrophages, and epithelial cells. Products of this pathway include LTs that induce neutrophil chemotaxis (LTB_4), bronchoconstriction, enhanced airway secretion, and increased vascular permeability (LTC_4, LTD_4, and LTE_4). The cyclo-oxygenase pathway is active in a broader variety of cells, and PGs induce bronchoconstriction (PGD_2 and PGF_2), bronchodilation, and microvessel dilation (PGE_2).

ALLERGENS

Molecular Characteristics of Allergens

An *allergen* may be defined as an antigen that (1) elicits a symptomatic allergic response, (2) elicits an allergic immune response (e.g., production of IgE antibody), or (3) binds specifically to IgE antibody. Although these three definitions overlap somewhat, they reflect the fact that an allergen does not always fulfill all three definitions. Some chemicals or proteins are "incomplete allergens," or *haptens* that are too small to elicit immune responses and must bind to larger proteins to act as allergens. Many drug allergies exemplify this phenomenon. Other allergens are "complete" and can elicit production of specific IgE and also elicit reactions on re-exposure. Still other antigens may be rare causes of primary sensitization but because of homologous struc-

tures to other allergens, may elicit reactions resulting from cross-reactivity.

The allergenicity of a protein is not dependent on specific structure but rather is dependent on a variety of characteristics, including stability, solubility, size, an ability to come in contact with immune cells, and failure to activate Th2 suppressive mechanisms (Aalberse, 2000). When one considers an airborne environmental or ingested food allergen, it must be appreciated that these single items actually represent a collection of proteins of potential allergenicity and that each protein has numerous potential sites (epitopes) to which immune responses may be directed.

Many of these epitopes involve presentation of amino acids dependent on the three-dimensional conformational structure of the protein, but linear (or sequential) epitopes may be more important in food allergens (Chatchatee et al., 2001). Digestion or alteration at mucosal sites may cause variation in the final configuration of the conformational epitope presented to the immune system but has much less of an effect on linear epitopes. A particular protein is considered a major allergen when more than 50% of allergic subjects are sensitized. Thus an allergenic substance such as peanut contains several major allergens.

Environmental Allergens

Environmental allergens are carried on airborne bioparticles from wind-pollinated plants, fungi, animal danders, insect emanations, and other biologic materials. Relevant particles are 2 to 60 μm in diameter. Particles less than 5 to 7 μm in diameter are capable of reaching terminal bronchioles, whereas larger particles are trapped in the upper airway. Pollen represents the major source of outdoor allergen. Pollens are the male genetic material for plant sexual reproduction and are composed of a variety of proteins to drive the fertilization process.

Plants that pollinate by wind dispersal are the most relevant to allergy because the proteins reach high concentrations and have access to the respiratory tract. In temperate regions, pollen seasons are traditionally grouped as trees (early spring), grasses (late spring), and weeds (fall) with characteristic seasons of dispersal. Specific flora and time of pollination vary by region.

Fungal spores and particles are responsible for both seasonal and perennial allergic symptoms and are both indoor and outdoor allergens. Although able to survive a variety of extremes in temperature and humidity, most fungal forms grow best on a moist substrate. *Alternaria* species are prevalent in dry, warm climates, whereas *Cladosporium* dominates temperate regions. Both are dispersed by wind as "dry spores." In contrast, slime spores such as *Fusarium* are dispersed during wet periods of rain and humidity.

Outdoor fungal particle levels peak seasonally, particularly in the midsummer in temperate regions, but this is variable. Fungal spore exposure may also increase in the spring when snow uncovers decaying vegetation and immediately after rain. Examples of common indoor fungi include *Penicillium, Aspergillus,* and *Cladosporium.* Fungal colonies may be visible as darkly stained growths on damp surfaces in basements and bathrooms. Sensitization and exposure to *Alternaria* has been associated with severe asthma (O'Hollaren et al., 1991).

In addition to fungi, indoor allergens are derived from dust mites, cockroaches, and animal danders. House dust mites, the most prominent of which are *Dermatophagoides pteronyssinus* and *Dermatophagoides farinae* are in the same phylogenetic family as scabies (Arlian et al., 2001). They are microscopic (approximately 0.3 mm in length) members of the spider family that feed on human skin scales and debris. They rely on ambient humidity for water and grow best at a relative humidity in excess of 75%. This degree of moisture may be achieved in, for example, a mattress, even when ambient humidity is lower. This requirement for humidity also results in a lower concentration of mites in surface dust. The optimal temperature for their growth is 18.3°C to 26.7°C. These requirements for growth explain why they are not as prevalent in cold, dry regions or at high altitudes. The major source of mite allergen is derived from fecal particles that are 10 to 35 μm in diameter. The fecal particles can become airborne with disturbance but settle rapidly.

Sensitization with continued exposure to cockroach has been linked to asthma in the inner city (Rosenstreich et al., 1997). Three main species of cockroach inhabit buildings: *Blattella germanica, Periplaneta americana,* and *Blattella orientalis. B. Germanica* is the most prevalent in crowded North American cities.

In suburban homes, furred pets are a common allergen. The major allergen responsible for cat allergy is *Fel d* 1, although reactivity to other proteins, including cat albumin, a serum protein, plays a role. All breeds, both long and short hair, produce *Fel d* 1 to varying extents and males produce more than females. The allergen is found in saliva and skin from sebaceous glands. The size of vectors that carry the allergen are generally less than 25 μm and 10% to 30% are smaller than 2.5 μm (Wood et al., 1993). Cat allergen is tenacious in that it has been detected on walls and fabrics and can remain for months after a cat is removed from the home (Wood et al., 1989).

The prevalence of sensitivity to dog allergen is about half of that seen with cat. The major dog allergen is *Can f* 1, which is detected on the coat and in saliva. The amount produced by different breeds varies, but all breeds produce the major allergen, so there is not a truly allergen-free breed. Breeds produce breed-specific allergens, but the clinical relevance of this is not well understood.

Other furred mammals, such as mice, rats, gerbils, rabbits, and hamsters, are potential sources of allergens in dwellings as pests or pets and also in laboratory research work.

Food Allergens

Allergic responses are directed primarily to water-soluble, heat- and acid-stable glycoproteins of molecular weights ranging from 10 to 70 kD. Although hypersensitivity reactions have been described to virtually all foods, it is remarkable that in infants and young children, about 90% of reactions are attributed to cow's milk, egg, peanut, soybean, wheat, tree nuts (e.g., walnut, hazel, Brazil nut), fish, and shellfish. In older children and adults, peanut, tree nuts, fish, and shellfish account for the majority of significant reactions. Generally, milder allergic reactions may be attributed to proteins of various classes that are homologous among particular plants or between pollens and ingested plant proteins. Many of these proteins are not stable to heating or digestive enzymes and are less likely to trigger systemic allergic responses.

The presence of cross-reacting protein does not equate with clinical allergy. For example, most individuals allergic to wheat tolerate other grains (Jones et al., 1995), and those allergic to peanuts (a legume) tolerate other beans (Bernhisel-Broadbent et al., 1989). Conversely, cow's milk allergic individuals may react to many mammalian milks such as goat's milk (Bellioni-Businco et al., 1999; Restani et al., 1999), and there is also a higher rate of clinical cross-reactivity among fish. Examples of common, well-characterized environmental and food allergens are shown in Table 31-1.

DIAGNOSTIC TESTS

Allergic disorders are diagnosed clinically. A careful history and physical examination are central to excluding alternative diagnoses, confirming that clinical symptoms are allergy-related, and identifying potential triggers. Laboratory evaluations are generally aimed at confirming clinical suspicions in the context of a thorough history and a solid understanding of the characteristics of environmental exposures. These elements require a history that elicits information concerning the seasonality of symptoms and/or relation of symptoms to particular exposures, the reproducibility of symptoms

TABLE 31-1 · REPRESENTATIVE ENVIRONMENTAL AND FOOD ALLERGENS

Common Name	Allergen	Function/Component
Ragweed	Amb a 1	
Birch	Bet v 1, Bet v 2 (profillin)	
Rye grass	Lol p 1	
Aspergillus	Asp f 1	
House dust mites	Der p 1, Der f 1	Cysteine protease
	Der p 3, Der f 3	Serine protease
Cat	Feld d 1	
Dog	Can f 1	
Mouse	Mus m 1	
Cockroach	Blag 1, Per a 1	
Chicken egg	Gal d 1	Ovomucoid
	Gal d 2	Ovalbumin
Codfish	Gad c 1	Parvalbumin
Shrimp	Pena 1	Tropomyosin
Peanut	Ara h 1	Vicilin (seed storage)
	Ara h 2	Conglutin (seed storage)
	Ara h 3	Conglycin (seed storage)

with exposures, the response to prior medications or avoidance, and the presence of associated atopic diseases. A number of modalities are available to confirm or refute particular triggers, but all tests have specific indications and limitations.

Immediate-Type Skin Tests to Detect Specific IgE Antibody

Skin testing with allergens is performed either by placing an extract on the skin and scratching through the extract and into the epidermis with a small needle, lancet, or other probe (prick/puncture) or by injecting the allergen intradermally. This methodology is based on the principle that allergen-specific IgE bound to skin mast cells is triggered to release mediators leading to a local wheal and flare response. Histamine and saline are placed as positive and negative controls, respectively. Patients must avoid antihistamines and drugs with antihistaminic properties for five half-lives of the drug before testing.

Extracts are commercially available, but most are not standardized; glycerinated forms are available for prick skin testing. Freshly made extracts of foods with labile proteins (a number of fresh fruits and vegetables) are needed for accurate assessment of these allergens. Reliable extracts are not available for many substances, particularly medications, because many of these are incomplete allergens and the structure of the relevant epitopes are unknown. Some substances directly cause mast cell release (narcotics) and cannot be used for skin testing.

Intradermal tests introduce a higher concentration of allergen and increase sensitivity and risk for a systemic reaction to the testing procedure (a rare event for skin testing in general). For most extracts, sensitivity of prick/puncture tests is very high, and increasing sensitivity by using intradermal tests may lead to an increase in clinically irrelevant (false-positive) tests. In particular, prick skin tests for foods carry a high false-positive rate for clinical symptoms (Sampson and McCaskill, 1985).

Studies comparing results of prick and intradermal skin tests to clinical reactions on exposure to Timothy grass (Nelson et al., 1996) and cat (Wood et al., 1999) revealed a poor correlation of reactivity to positive intradermal, compared with positive prick skin tests. The limitations of test interpretation underscores the need to select tests based on a careful clinical history. Negative skin tests are highly accurate to rule out IgE-mediated allergic reactions.

Serologic Tests for Specific IgE Antibody

Measurement of specific IgE antibody in the serum by immunoassay is widely available to a large variety of allergens. The classic radioallergosorbent test (RAST) is based on coupling allergen to an insoluble matrix, combining the tests serum with this reagent, and, following a wash step, detecting specific IgE by using radiolabeled anti-IgE antibody. A number of these assays are commercially available, although most are now based on fluorometric detection methods, and a variety of insoluble matrices are used. Results are expressed as counts, classes (e.g., class I to V or VI), or arbitrary units of concentration. The results generally correlate well with prick skin test results, but the RAST is usually less sensitive in comparison and more expensive. However, the RAST can be performed regardless of antihistamine use or widespread dermatitis that would preclude skin testing. Quantification of allergen-specific IgE antibodies, such as obtained with the CAP System FEIA (Yunginger et al., 2000) shows promise as an improved diagnostic strategy, especially in food allergy (Sampson and Ho, 1997).

Patch Tests

Contact dermatitis is a cell-mediated response to local application of allergen. Patch tests are a useful modality to identify causal allergens in this disorder. Tests are performed by applying the suspected agent to the surface of the skin under an occlusive dressing and leaving this in place for 24 hours. The test site is evaluated at the time of removal and 1 to 2 days later for evidence of inflammation that can be scored by severity. Controls are applied to compare for possible irritant reactions.

Patch test kits are commercially available for common contact allergens found in cosmetics, industrial chemicals, and topical medications. In contrast to classic patch tests for delayed-type hypersensitivity reactions to chemical sensitizers, patch testing with classic environmental allergens (e.g., dust mite) and food allergens is under investigation as a diagnostic modality for evaluating the role of these allergens in disorders such as AD. This so-called atopy patch test has shown some promising results in the evaluation of food allergy in infants with AD (Niggemann et al., 2000).

Other In Vitro Tests

The proliferative response of peripheral blood lymphocytes, secretion of relevant cytokines, or production of cytokine mRNA following in vitro stimulation with allergen has been used to characterize allergic sensitivity. However, direct relevance to clinical reactivity is debated. Allergen-induced basophil histamine release assays have been used to characterize IgE responses. These and other modalities are generally used in research studies because they are not of clear diagnostic value or are supplanted by other tests for clinical diagnosis. Assays using polyclonal or monoclonal antibodies to common environmental allergens have been used to evaluate exposure in the environment of atopic individuals in a variety of studies.

Provocation

Provocation studies are performed by exposing relevant allergens to their site of natural contact while monitoring for clinical reactivity. In research studies, the application of allergen to the eyes, nose, lung (by inhalation or bronchoscopy), gastrointestinal tract, and skin are routinely undertaken to characterize allergic responses.

For clinical purposes, the most common provocation tests are those performed to evaluate exposures for which other testing modalities are insufficient and for which continued avoidance for presumed reactivity is potentially detrimental: environmental exposure to occupational allergens and oral food challenges. Exposures to airborne occupational agents may be undertaken through exposure "on site" or with controlled experimental exposure with serial testing of pulmonary function.

Oral food challenges are performed by feeding gradually increasing amounts of the test food under physician supervision either in its natural form (open challenge) or hidden in another substance and given in a single blind or double-blind, placebo-controlled format. The use of blinding and placebos decreases false-positive interpretations of challenges. These challenges are selected when the results of the history and laboratory studies do not confirm a causal agent and also to monitor for tolerance.

Controversial and Unproven Testing Procedures

There are a host of tests that have been touted to be useful in the diagnosis of allergy (particularly food allergy) but have never been shown to be useful in blinded studies. These include measurement of IgG4 antibody, provocation-neutralization (drops placed under the tongue or injected to diagnose and treat various symptoms), cytotoxicity testing (cell death observed subjectively on a glass slide containing foods), and applied kinesiology (muscle strength testing), among other unproved methods (American Academy of Allergy and Immunology, 1986).

ALLERGEN AVOIDANCE THERAPY

Avoidance of identified allergic triggers and prophylactic avoidance of potential allergens are at the heart of therapy for allergic disorders. Allergen avoidance is not a simple task. Measures to avoid common environmental allergens are shown in Table 31-2. Understanding the characteristics of particular allergens is important to the design of effective environmental control measures. For example, dust mite allergens settle quickly, so air filtration does not reduce exposure. Cat allergen is tenacious, and meticulous cleaning after removal of the animal is needed to reduce the allergen load.

Environmental allergen avoidance is not without costs; patients are often loathe to part with family pets or remove carpets, and the placement of dust mite–proof bed covers and air filters carry expenses. However, decreased symptoms and reduced dependency on medications are an impetus to follow avoidance advice. Prophylactic avoidance of environmental allergens in children at high risk for atopic diseases may reduce the prevalence and severity of allergy (Hide et al., 1996).

Avoidance of food allergens is a complex undertaking with numerous pitfalls. Food allergens can be

TABLE 31-2 · AVOIDANCE STRATEGIES FOR MAJOR ENVIRONMENTAL ALLERGENS

Pollen
Keep windows closed
Use HEPA filters
Remove nearby sources
Limit outdoor activities in season

House Dust Mite
Remove reservoirs (stuffed animals, thick moisture-retaining cloth items)
Encase mattresses and pillows in impermeable covers
Hot water wash of bedclothes (>130°F)
Decrease humidity (<45%)

Fungi
Remove sources (wet papers, soiled carpet, visible mold)
Decrease humidity
Clean source areas with bleach solution

Animals
Remove pet
Reduce reservoirs (carpet, upholstery)
Seclude from patient (keep outside, out of bedroom)
Use HEPA filters

Cockroach
Use insecticides
Seal entry points (around pipes, cracks)
Remove breeding and feeding sites (food, moisture, accumulated trash)

HEPA = high-efficiency particle arresting.

passed via human breast milk, so lactating mothers, in addition to their affected children, may need dietary advice (Zeiger and Heller, 1995). Aside from obvious sources, small amounts of food protein may contaminate otherwise safe foods in the cooking and preparation process and in industrial processing because of factory line cross-contamination. Ingredient labels may contain technical terms such as casein rather than cow's milk, and patients must be educated about these issues as well.

MEDICATIONS FOR ALLERGIC DISEASE

Adrenergic Agents

The therapeutic effects of adrenergic agents rest on their ability to stimulate specific adrenergic receptors; nine types have been characterized. These receptors are transmembrane proteins coupled to G proteins for signal transduction. The relevant physiologic activity of α-adrenergic receptor activation in allergy is vasoconstriction, an important effect for local treatment of vascular congestion of the nose and for systemic treatment to support blood pressure in anaphylaxis.

Activation of β_1-adrenergic receptors results in increased heart rate and cardiac contractility, whereas activation of β_2-adrenergic receptors results in bronchodilation, relaxation of vascular smooth muscle, relaxation of uterine muscle, and stimulation of skeletal muscle. For evident reasons, β_2 receptors are a focus of research in asthma. Particular polymorphisms in the receptor are associated with asthma severity and response to β agonists (Israel et al., 2000). Continuous treatment with β agonists can lead to downregulation, but corticosteroid treatment reduces this effect (Mak et al., 1995).

Epinephrine is a catecholamine able to stimulate both α- and β-adrenergic receptors with the useful antiallergy properties of constricting blood vessels, decreasing edema, and inducing bronchodilation. Phenylephrine is primarily an α-adrenergic agonist and is useful as a vasoconstrictor to treat nasal congestion. Isoproterenol, by its highly β-adrenergic specific binding, provides bronchodilation without the α-adrenergic effects seen with epinephrine, but there is binding to both β_1 and β_2 receptors resulting in tachycardia as a side effect. Modification of catecholamines by substitutions at the N-alkyl position alters relative receptor specificity and modification of the 3,4-hydroxyl group results in resistance to digestive enzymes. Further structural modifications alter binding characteristics that prolong duration of action. Thus a number of specific β_2 agonists are available for asthma therapy that offer oral dosing, inhaled dosing, and prolonged action.

Short-acting, β_2-selective agents include albuterol and terbutaline. These agents produce bronchodilation with less cardiac stimulation than less selective agents such as metaproterenol and fenoterol. There is also evidence that β_2 agonists have benefits in addition to bronchodilation such as inhibition of mediator release from mast cells and eosinophils and increased mucociliary clearance (Barnes, 1999).

These agents are available in oral and parenteral formulations, but the inhaled route of administration by nebulization or from a metered dose inhaler is generally preferred for its profile of rapid onset with fewer side effects. Standard formulations of albuterol and other commercial adrenergics are an equal mixture of R and S isomers, but the R isomer (e.g., levalbuterol) is the active component, whereas its mirror-image enantiomer is either inactive or potentially deleterious.

New formulations with pure R isomer show promise in providing bronchodilation with fewer side effects and a better therapeutic profile (Gawchik et al., 1999; Nelson et al., 1998), but their exact place in therapy is evolving.

Salmeterol and formoterol are highly β_2 selective and have a long duration of action, up to 12 hours. Salmeterol has a delayed onset of action; thus, although it holds a place in chronic management of asthma, it is not a first-line treatment for acute exacerbations.

Methylxanthines

Theophylline and its derivative aminophylline are cyclic nucleotide phosphodiesterase (PDE) inhibitors. Although bronchodilation is a primary antiasthma benefit, the drug appears to have effects beyond PDE inhibition with evidence for improving mucociliary clearance, improving diaphragmatic contractility, and a variety of weak anti-inflammatory effects (Weinberger and Hendeles, 1996). Although theophylline inhibits early-phase methacholine-induced bronchoconstriction, it does not reduce allergen-induced increases in airway hyperreactivity. Sustained-release formulations may improve nocturnal asthma, but the drug has been shown to add little to the management of acute asthma and may actually increase side effects when used in this setting.

Theophylline remains an option for chronic treatment of persistent asthma, although other agents are generally preferred. Serum concentrations should be maintained between 5 and 15 μg/ml, which provides efficacy without undue risks for side effects from high serum concentrations. Above these concentrations there is a greater risk for side effects such as nausea, vomiting, palpitations, headache, seizures, and potentially, but very rarely, death. Metabolism of theophylline is primarily through the cytochrome P450 pathway, and thus numerous physiologic and pharmacologic interactions can result in alteration of serum levels.

Antihistamines

A variety of antihistamines are available for oral, parenteral, and topical use. The primary antiallergy effects are based on blockade of H_1 receptors, but additional efficacy may be related to inhibition of mediator release and direct anti-inflammatory effects. These medications reduce symptoms of pruritus, rhinorrhea, urticaria, and sneezing.

Chemical classes with examples of first-generation, sedating antihistamines include the alkylamines (chlorpheniramine, brompheniramine), piperazines (hydroxyzine), piperidines (cyproheptadine), ethanolamines (diphenhydramine, clemastine), ethylenediamines (tripelennamine), and phenothiazines (promethazine). These antihistamines cross the blood–brain barrier and impair concentration and induce sedation, although tachyphylaxis to these effects occurs to some degree. Many of these antihistamines also possess weak anticholinergic effects and may thus induce dry mouth, constipation, and difficulty in micturition. Cyproheptadine also blocks serotonin activity.

Newer second- and third-generation antihistamines (e.g., acrivastine, azelastine, cetirizine, fexofenadine, levocarbastine, desloratidine) are larger, lipophilic (reducing CNS penetration and sedation), and lack anticholinergic effects. Many of these compounds are metabolites of first-generation antihistamines. Time to onset, potency, duration of action, side effect profile, and route of metabolism vary slightly among these newer compounds. More than a dozen different preparations have come to market.

Several of the second-generation antihistamines were removed from the market because of their potential to prolong the cardiac Q-Tc interval and induce dysrhythmias such as torsades de pointes, particularly when given along with compounds that altered metabolism through the P450 CYP3A4 pathway.

Corticosteroids

The broad anti-inflammatory actions of adrenal glucocorticoids and their synthetic analogs make them indispensable treatment modalities for all allergic disorders. Oral, topical, inhaled, and parenteral forms of varying potency and duration of action are available.

Steroids act by binding to cytoplasmic receptors followed by translocation to the nucleus, where binding to specific glucocorticoid response elements triggers modification of gene transcription. Through a variety of mechanisms, steroids generally repress gene expression. This results in suppression of vital cytokines active in the allergic inflammatory process leading to apoptosis of eosinophils, failure to recruit inflammatory cells to target organs, and reduction in lymphocyte and macrophage activation. Steroids also increase responsiveness to β agonists, reduce the production and release of arachidonic acid metabolites, decrease mucus production, and decrease vascular permeability. Ultimately, steroids reduce chronic inflammation and late-phase responses to allergen.

Unfortunately, steroids also carry a substantial list of side effects; a major one for the pediatric patient is growth suppression. Additional problems include increased risk for infection, impaired wound healing, adrenal suppression, myopathy, osteoporosis, peptic ulcers, and hypertension among others.

The use of topical and inhaled preparations at the lowest effective dosage and oral steroids in bursts rather than for chronic treatment helps increase the benefit-to-risk ratio. New topical steroids with little systemic absorption are also improving the safety profile. Although use of inhaled steroids in children is associated with growth suppression, the use of newer inhaled steroid preparations does not usually result in decreased adult height (Agertoft et al., 2000; Childhood Asthma Management Program Research Group, 2000). Topical calcineurin inhibitors represent another alternative anti-inflammatory therapy for allergic disease.

Mast Cell Stabilizers

Cromolyn sodium and nedocromil sodium are chemically unique from other antiallergy medications. Both are generally considered mast cell stabilizers, although their anti-inflammatory effects are actually broader. Both drugs inhibit mediator release from mast cells, and nedocromil also inhibits eosinophil chemotaxis and mediator release. The mechanism of action for these drugs is not completely understood but may involve inhibition of calcium channel activation and alteration in chloride transport or inactivation of a mast cell protein involved in regulating cytoskeletal elements needed for degranulation (Theoharides et al., 2000).

The clinical efficacy observed with these medications for treatment of asthma is the result of improvements in pulmonary function and reduced airway hyperreactivity. They show efficacy in reducing both the acute and late phase responses to allergen (Cockcroft and Murdock, 1987) and also to physical triggers. Their safety profile is excellent, although cromolyn must be dosed four times each day and 12% of patients experience an unpleasant taste from nedocromil. Cromolyn also has been used topically for treatment of allergic rhinitis and is available in an oral form for treatment of the gastrointestinal manifestations of systemic mastocytosis. Other drugs with mast cell stabilizing properties are available, or becoming available, for topical treatment of allergic rhinitis and conjunctivitis.

Anticholinergics

Release of acetylcholine from parasympathetic nerves mediates a component of bronchial constriction through stimulation of muscarinic receptors. Increased glandular secretion is also involved in this process. Ipratropium is an anticholinergic agent that provides bronchodilation. Unlike atropine, it is not absorbed, thus systemic anticholinergic side effects are avoided. The medication is available in inhaled forms for treatment of severe acute exacerbations of asthma, as additional therapy to β agonists. It can be used in place of β agonists for patients with intolerance to these agents. A nasal spray is available for symptomatic treatment of rhinorrhea in nonallergic rhinitis, allergic rhinitis, and the common cold.

Leukotriene Antagonists

LT antagonists represent the first new treatment strategy for asthma in more than two decades. The agents work by blocking synthesis of these mediators (5-lipoxygenase and 5-lipoxygenase activating protein inhibitors) or as receptor antagonists. These medications inhibit bronchoconstriction and have anti-inflammatory effects. They reduce early- and late-phase bronchial responses to allergen and also are efficacious in asthma related to aspirin sensitivity and exercise (Drazen, 1998; Wenzel, 1998). They appear to work particularly well in a subset of patients with asthma, but as yet no distinguishing features to identify these patients are available. Side effects are agent dependent and include elevation of liver enzymes for some preparations. The role of these drugs in the treatment of chronic asthma, as monotherapy, or in combination regimens is evolving.

IMMUNOTHERAPY

Immunotherapy with Allergens

Immunotherapy is a form of immunomodulation that alters immune responses to the allergens being injected from an allergic, Th2 response toward a nonallergic, Th1 response. Gradually increasing amounts of allergen are injected, usually over a period of months. Observed alterations in immune responses to the allergen include an initial increase followed by a gradual decrease in allergen-specific IgE antibody, increases in allergen-specific IgG antibody, dampening of postseasonal rises in IgE, decreased CD4+ T-cell proliferation to antigen, and reduced late-phase skin responses (Creticos et al., 1996; Lack et al., 1997).

Clinically, most controlled trials have shown efficacy for treatment of perennial and seasonal allergic rhinitis and asthma (Abramson et al., 1995). Efficacy for insect sting anaphylaxis is particularly high, reducing the rate of repeat reactions from more than 50% to less than 2% (Hunt et al., 1978; Reisman and Livingston, 1992). Immunotherapeutic treatment of peanut allergy showed efficacy in some patients, but adverse side effects resulting from the injections in patients highly allergic to peanuts precluded general use of this therapy (Nelson et al., 1997).

A number of factors come into play in selecting candidates for allergen immunotherapy. The clinical history must indicate a potential relationship between symptoms and exposure, and evidence of IgE antibody to the allergen in question must be demonstrable. Furthermore, attempts at allergen avoidance and trial of medication should be undertaken (Dykewicz et al., 1998).

If symptoms are not reasonably controlled with these measures, immunotherapy should be considered. Selection of allergens is based on the history and laboratory results. Subcutaneous injections begin with very small doses and are administered in graduating doses with the final aim of achieving a dose of 6 to 12 µg of each allergen (Creticos, 1992). Maintenance doses are usually administered at 2- to 4-week intervals. Patients are screened to ensure that they are asymptomatic before injection and are observed for at least 30 minutes after treatment. Dosages are adjusted if side effects develop.

The adverse reaction rate is less than 4%, but deaths from anaphylaxis have been reported. Strict adherence to the precautions and observation period, availability of medications to reverse reactions, and care in avoiding dosing errors is crucial. In addition, immunotherapy is not given to patients in poor general health or who are on β-blockers or angiotensin-converting enzyme (ACE) inhibitors that may complicate the ability to treat reactions.

Desensitization Procedures

Unlike immunotherapy, desensitization therapy does not cause a specific alteration in the immune system. This procedure is typically undertaken for IgE-mediated drug hypersensitivity or for sensitivity to aspirin and other nonsteroidal anti-inflammatory medications (Joint Task Force on Practice Parameters, 1999). It involves the administration of gradually increasing amounts of the agent over relatively short periods, usually within a day or several days. This procedure also has been used for cell-mediated drug reactions but is contraindicated for Stevens-Johnson syndrome or toxic epidermal necrolysis.

The mechanism by which one is able to avoid severe reactions with this procedure is not known, but it is hypothesized to represent a very gradual and controlled subclinical reaction that leaves the immune system in a refractory state as long as allergen exposure continues uninterrupted. Because there is no change in the immune response, the procedure must be repeated on future courses once the medication is discontinued. The risk to the procedure appears to be less when using the oral rather than parenteral route. This procedure is generally conducted under direct medical supervision in a controlled setting.

Immunomodulatory Therapies under Development

Administration of standard allergens by the nasal or oral route has been investigated with some promising results. Alteration of allergen in a variety of ways to bypass activation of IgE and to promote nonallergic immune responses (Th1 responses and tolerance) has been a theme in novel therapeutic approaches. Several methodologies have demonstrated at least partial success and include aggregation or polymerization of allergen, use of peptides expressing primarily T-cell epitopes, overlapping peptides, and engineered proteins with site-directed mutations in IgE-binding epitopes.

Another approach involves administration of immunostimulatory DNA sequences covalently linked to allergens. These immunostimulatory sequences consist of a central nonmethylated CG dinucleotide flanked by less highly conserved sequences and are termed CpG motifs. These sequences stimulate Th1 responses and sterically hinder IgE binding, thereby reducing mast cell activation during administration. Other methodologies for specific immunotherapy include administration of plasmid DNA encoding the relevant allergen. Endogenous production of this allergen potentially leads to nonallergic immune responses.

Administration of Th1-promoting cytokines or agents that block Th2-promoting cytokines are also under investigation. Anti-IgE antibody has emerged as a useful allergen-nonspecific treatment whose exact place in allergy therapy is evolving. Ultimately, combinations of these modalities may prove effective.

ASTHMA

The 1997 expert panel report of the National Asthma Education Program (National Institutes of Health, 1997) defined asthma with an emphasis on several key aspects. Foremost, asthma is recognized as a chronic inflammatory disorder of the airways. In susceptible individuals, this inflammation results in symptoms due to widespread, variable, and at least partially reversible, airflow obstruction. It is also recognized that the inflammation causes an increase in bronchial hyperresponsiveness (BHR) to numerous stimuli and that prolonged inflammation may lead to sub-basement membrane fibrosis that contributes to persistent lung abnormalities. This expanded definition highlights the crucial need to address the inflammatory component of this atopic disease.

Epidemiology

The prevalence of childhood asthma appears to be increasing worldwide (Beasley et al., 2000). In the United States, 6.9% of children have asthma with non-white, urban poor at particular risk. Asthma is the leading cause for childhood hospitalizations and accounts for 10 million missed school days annually with an indirect cost alone of more than $1 billion.

The course of childhood asthma was elucidated in a prospective epidemiologic study of 826 children followed beyond age 6 years; 51.5% never wheezed, 19.9% had transient wheezing with respiratory infections before age 3 years, 13.7% continued to wheeze following symptoms while younger than 3 years, and 15% had no asthma in the first 3 years but did by age 6 (Martinez et al., 1995). Although early, transient wheezing was associated with diminished lung mechanics and exposure to tobacco smoke, persistent wheezing was associated with elevated IgE and a maternal history of asthma.

The genetic influence on asthma appears strong, and genome-wide screens in several populations have shown evidence for linkage to multiple regions on 16 different chromosomes (Howard et al., 2000). Candidate genes with evidence for linkage include those genes encoding cytokines; chemokines; HLA molecules; and T-cell, cytokine, glucocorticoid, and β_2-adrenergic receptors. Regions showing linkage to increased bronchial hyperreactivity also generally show linkage to elevated IgE (Postma et al., 1995).

In addition to complex gene–gene interactions, various environmental factors, including respiratory infections, diet, prematurity, air pollution, tobacco smoke, and environmental allergens, and their interactions are also important factors.

Pathogenesis

Typical histologic features of asthmatic lungs include tissue infiltration with eosinophils, mast cells, lymphocytes, macrophages, and plasma cells with tissue edema, vascular congestion, mucus secretion, and smooth muscle hypertrophy. Thickening below the basement membrane may also be observed. The cytokine profile in allergic asthma is typical of the Th2 profile with increased IL-4 and IL-5 but not IFN-γ (Ying et al., 1995). In sudden-onset asphyxiating asthma, a neutrophilic infiltration has been observed at autopsy (Carroll et al., 1996).

The relationship of airway inflammation to the characteristic BHR and airflow obstruction that characterize asthma is complex. BHR is increased in asthma to small doses of inhaled methacholine or histamine or to stimuli such as cold, dry air; hypertonic saline; or exercise. Measures of airway inflammation generally correlate with the degree of BHR, and treatment of inflammation ameliorates the degree of reactivity, but the relationship is complex and incomplete. A variety of stimuli, including allergen challenge and physical stimuli, can result in acute bronchoconstriction from contraction of airway smooth muscle via release of mediators or neurogenic mechanisms. Chronic obstruction results from airway edema, mucus plugging and, over longer periods of chronic inflammation, from airway remodeling.

Clinical Manifestations

The underlying genetic and pathophysiologic features of asthma translate into characteristic clinical features. The disease is more likely to develop in individuals with an atopic family history and personal development of other atopic disorders (Bergmann et al., 1998). Airway constriction and obstruction result in recurrent wheezing, coughing, sputum production, and chest tightness. Diurnal variation in endogenous steroid production results in symptom variation with increase of symptoms at night.

Triggers that increase inflammation such as viral infection and allergen exposure may lead to exacerbation of symptoms or increase the risk of exacerbation to other triggers. Additional triggers include irritants such as smoke or weather changes, physical triggers such as exercise, and neurologic triggers such as excitement.

Diagnosis

The diagnosis of asthma is a clinical exercise predicated on identifying episodic symptoms of airflow obstruction that are at least partially reversible and excluding alternative diagnoses. The history and physical examination are therefore pivotal in the diagnosis. The history should address the symptoms, pattern of symptoms and typical exacerbations, triggers, previous response to therapy, family and personal health history aimed at asthma and atopic disorders, and environmental exposures. In addition to establishing that symptoms are consistent with asthma, questions are directed toward assessing the severity and frequency of exacerbations and their impact on daily activities.

The physical examination is aimed at identifying and quantifying asthma symptoms such as wheezing, use of accessory muscles, chest hyperexpansion, prolonged exhalation, pulsus paradoxus, and signs of hypoxemia. In addition, supporting evidence of an atopic disposition, such as rhinorrhea or AD, are sought.

In severe exacerbations, additional tests such as arterial blood gases and pulse oximetry may become warranted. Although the diagnosis may be reached with no laboratory tests, ancillary testing can be helpful in assessing the severity of asthma, confirming the diagnosis, excluding other disorders, and identifying triggers.

Spirometry performed before and after administration of a bronchodilator is especially useful in this regard and is suggested for children able to cooperate. Typical findings in asthma include reduction from normal in the forced expiratory volume in the first second of forceful expiration (FEV$_1$), midexpiratory flow (FEF$_{25-75}$), and peak flow rates (PFR). Air trapping in the lung leads to increased residual volume, functional residual capacity, and total lung capacity. Spirometry results in patients with asthma should improve acutely with bronchodilator therapy and may be followed over the long term to monitor responses to anti-inflammatory therapies.

The differential diagnosis of asthma includes numerous disorders as listed in Table 31-3. In some cases,

TABLE 31-3 · DIFFERENTIAL DIAGNOSIS OF ASTHMA

Upper airway disease
  Allergic rhinitis/sinusitis
Obstruction of large airways
  Foreign body
  Vocal cord dysfunction
  Vascular ring/laryngeal webs
  Laryngotracheomalacia, tracheal stenosis
  Enlarged lymph nodes
  Tumor
Obstruction of small airways
  Viral bronchiolitis
  Cystic fibrosis
  Bronchopulmonary dysplasia
  Heart disease
Other causes
  Other causes of recurrent cough
  Aspiration

Adapted from National Institutes of Health, 1997.

specific studies may be needed to exclude these alternative diagnoses, including radiographs, bronchoprovocation with methacholine, evaluation for gastroesophageal reflux, and others. Peak flow monitoring with a portable device may be helpful in long-term management but not for diagnosis. Allergy testing is indicated to identify potential agents either triggering exacerbations or contributing to perennial symptoms in any patient but especially for those with persistent asthma on daily medications.

Management

The primary goals of asthma management are to prevent chronic symptoms, maintain normal or near-normal pulmonary function, maintain normal activity levels, prevent recurrent exacerbations and minimize emergency department visits and hospitalizations, provide optimal pharmacotherapy with minimal side effects, and meet patient and family expectations of and satisfaction with asthma care (National Institutes of Health, 1997). Treatment is based on control of environmental factors that contribute to asthma and on pharmacotherapy.

Environmental factors that contribute to asthma should be addressed; these factors include inhalant allergens, occupational exposures, and irritants. Avoidance measures should be undertaken as appropriate and consideration given for allergen immunotherapy. Additional factors associated with asthma that, if treated, may lead to amelioration of symptoms include treatment of rhinitis and sinusitis, gastrointestinal reflux, aspirin sensitivity, and medications that may trigger asthma or cough such as β-blockers and ACE inhibitors. Annual influenza vaccination is recommended to avoid this potent trigger.

Pharmacologic therapy of chronic asthma is directed not only toward symptom relief but, more important, toward reduction of inflammation in patients with persistent symptoms. A stepwise approach has been suggested that begins by delineating patients into one of four categories by history of symptoms and lung function (Table 31-4) and then suggests medication regimens based on these categories as shown in Table 31-5. Frequent reassessment and monitoring with objective assessments of lung function are central features of therapy. In addition, it is imperative that techniques of administration of medications be reviewed.

For cough-variant asthma, in which chronic cough follows typical asthma triggers but wheezing is not appreciated, trials of therapy with anti-inflammatory medication and monitoring of lung function are recommended. Treatment of exercise-induced asthma is based on reducing baseline inflammation and asthma symptoms. For residual exercise-induced bronchospasm, pre-exercise warm-up and use of β agonists, cromolyn, or nedocromil are helpful.

The treatment of acute exacerbations of asthma begins with patient education concerning signs of deterioration of asthma control. Written action plans should be established that detail what measures the patient should take if symptoms become more severe or frequent. Management of acute exacerbations of asthma may require medical intervention in the emergency room or

TABLE 31-4 · CLASSIFICATION OF ASTHMA BY SEVERITY IN CHILDREN OLDER THAN 5 YEARS

Category	Symptoms	Nighttime Symptoms	Lung Function
Severe, persistent	Continual symptoms Limited physical activity Frequent exacerbations	Frequent	FEV_1 or PEF ≤60% predicted; PEF variability >30%
Moderate, persistent	Daily Requires daily β agonist Exacerbations affect activity ≥2 exacerbations/week, may last days	>1/week	FEV_1 or PEF 60%–80% predicted; PEF variability >30%
Mild, persistent	Symptoms >2 times/week but <1/day Exacerbations may affect activity	>2/month	FEV_1 or PEF ≥80% predicted; PEF variability 20%–30%
Mild, intermittent	Symptoms ≤2 times/week Normal PEF between exacerbations Brief exacerbations (hours to days)	≤2/month	FEV_1 or PEF ≥80% predicted; PEF variability <20%

Any one of the features of severity is sufficient to warrant inclusion in that category and patients are categorized by their most severe symptom.
FEV_1 = forced expiratory volume at 1 second; PEF = peak expiratory flow.

TABLE 31-5 · MANAGEMENT OF ASTHMA BY SEVERITY IN CHILDREN OLDER THAN 5 YEARS

Severity	Medications
Severe, persistent	High-dose inhaled corticosteroid and Long-acting β_2 agonist or theophylline and Oral steroid
Moderate, persistent	Medium-dose inhaled corticosteroid or Low-medium or medium-high dose inhaled corticosteroid with long-acting β_2 agonist or theophylline
Mild, persistent	Low-dose inhaled corticosteroid or cromolyn or nedocromil or (alternative, not preferred) sustained-release theophylline or leukotriene antagonist
Mild, intermittent	No daily medication needed

Short-acting β_2 agonists are used for quick relief medication for symptoms. Treatments plans are reviewed every 1 to 6 months. Oral steroids may be needed for rescue at any step. Education on asthma management is key at any severity level. Dosing equivalents for children of beclomethasone dipropionate are low dose, 84 to 336 μg; medium dose, 336 to 672 μg; and high dose, >672 μg/day.

inpatient hospital setting when patients with moderate to severe symptoms fail to respond to treatments at home.

The treatment of asthma in the emergency setting entails a continuous process of evaluation, treatment, and re-evaluation. In general, when exacerbations are severe, treatment with oxygen to maintain blood saturation higher than 90% and repeated administration of aerosolized short-acting β agonist (every 20 minutes for 1 hour) and an anticholinergic agent are given. Corticosteroids are added for treatment during significant exacerbations. If there is good response to therapy, the patient may continue with hourly, aerosolized bronchodilators for several hours and continue therapy at home, weaning therapy as symptoms improve.

Severe or moderate exacerbations with incomplete or poor response to therapy may require hospitalization for further treatment. With increasingly severe symptoms and/or partial pressures of CO_2 greater than 41 mm Hg, observation in an intensive care setting is warranted. Intubation and mechanical ventilation are used for impending or actual respiratory arrest. For patients undergoing mechanical ventilation, barotrauma is a risk and allowance for hypercapnia, rather than use of high-pressure settings, is suggested. Treatment with chest physical therapy, mucolytics, or sedation is not generally recommended, and hydration should aim for appropriate corrections of dehydration and maintenance of hydration.

ALLERGIC RHINITIS AND CONJUNCTIVITIS

Epidemiology

Allergic rhinitis is an IgE-mediated response to environmental allergens that results in symptoms of nasal congestion, rhinorrhea, pruritus, and sneezing. Symptoms may be seasonal ("hayfever") in response to pollens, perennial in response to year-long exposure to indoor environmental allergens, or a combination (perennial with seasonal exacerbations). Once the inflammation is established, nonspecific irritant triggers such as cold air and pollutants may also induce symptoms.

The disorder is reported by 9.1% of children younger than 18 years (Nathan et al., 1997). Risk factors for physician-diagnosed allergic rhinitis include maternal history of atopy, personal history of asthma, and elevated IgE antibody (Wright et al., 1994). There is a strong association with asthma and increased bronchial hyperreactivity.

Pathogenesis

The pathophysiology of allergic rhinitis is that of the immediate, late-phase, and chronic allergic inflammatory responses and mirrors that are seen in asthma. Nasonasal cholinergic reflexes are responsible for orchestrating contralateral secretion from ipsilateral allergen stimulation (Cruz et al., 1992). Neuropeptides such as substance P, calcitonin gene–related peptide (CGRP), and vasoactive intestinal polypeptide (VIP) are released and induce secretion, vasodilation, and increased airway resistance. Late-phase and chronic inflammation is characterized by infiltration with eosinophils.

Clinical Manifestations

Patients typically experience symptoms reflecting the neurogenic and inflammatory mechanisms with sneezing, rhinorrhea, pruritus, and congestion. Patients may develop "allergic shiners," darkened lower eyelids from vascular congestion, but this is not pathognomonic for allergic rhinitis. The pruritus leads to rubbing and eventually patients find the most efficient manner to relieve this discomfort is either a lateral rubbing with the index finger or a long swipe of the nares from finger to lower palm termed the "allergic salute." Repetitive rubbing in this manner may lead to a horizontal crease on the nasal bridge. There also may be a component of oral pruritus.

Symptoms may escalate later in the pollen season because of the priming effect of repeated allergen exposure leading to increased clinical sensitivity to equivalent doses of allergen. Associated symptoms of ocular pruritus, tearing, and erythema are termed allergic conjunctivitis; this must be differentiated from vernal conjunctivitis, keratoconjunctivitis, and other forms of ocular allergy that are more likely to threaten vision (Bielory, 2000).

Diagnosis

There is no single diagnostic test for allergic rhinitis; thus, like asthma, the diagnosis rests on the history, physical examination, and consideration of alternative diagnoses. The history should be directed toward the typical symptoms with particular attention paid to a family history of atopy, seasonality of symptoms, and environmental triggers.

The physical examination may reveal pale, boggy turbinates with bluish or hyperemic mucosa. Secretions are typically prominent. Although nasal polyps are associated with allergic rhinitis in adults, this finding in children should prompt an evaluation for cystic fibrosis.

Prick skin tests and RAST tests can be used to identify and verify the role of specific environmental allergens. Food allergy is rarely a cause of isolated respiratory symptoms.

In children, the challenge is often to differentiate allergic rhinitis from frequent upper respiratory infections. The latter typically has less prominent pruritus and sneezing, and positive tests for specific IgE antibody to suspected environmental triggers are expected primarily in the former. In addition, smears of nasal discharge in allergic rhinitis should reveal eosinophils.

However, nasal eosinophilia and perennial symptoms exacerbated by irritants defines the disorder of *non-allergic rhinitis with eosinophilia* (NARES) that may mimic allergic rhinitis. In NARES, IgE to specific allergens is absent. Another disorder that may masquerade as allergic rhinitis is vasomotor rhinitis. In this disorder, there is no eosinophilia, and symptoms are provoked by nonallergen triggers such as strong odors, cold air, and spicy foods.

Additional diagnostic possibilities to consider in children with nasal symptoms are cerebrospinal fluid (CSF) leak, foreign bodies, and anatomic causes of congestion (adenoidal hypertrophy, choanal atresia, tumor, and others).

Management

Treatment of allergic rhinitis is predicated on the identification and elimination of environmental allergens and reduction of exposure to irritants such as tobacco smoke. Oral and topical formulations of antihistamines and decongestants provide symptom relief, but topical decongestants that act by vasoconstriction must be used sparingly to avoid rebound symptoms and dependence (rhinitis medicamentosum). Topical cromolyn and steroids reduce inflammation and can bring significant relief.

When symptoms are recalcitrant to medical and environmental measures, or if these therapies induce side effects, immunotherapy may be considered and is highly effective. Sinusitis is a potential complication and may require antibiotic therapy or, in some cases, surgical intervention.

ATOPIC DERMATITIS

Epidemiology

AD (eczema) generally begins in early infancy and is characterized by extreme pruritus, a chronically relapsing course, and distinctive distribution (Hanifin and Rajka, 1980). More than 10% of children are affected (Laughter et al., 2000; Williams et al., 1999). AD is typically the first manifestation of atopic disease, with approximately 80% going on to develop asthma or allergic rhinitis; many lose their AD only to experience the onset of respiratory allergy (see Chapter 32).

Pathogenesis

Acute skin lesions of AD are described as spongiotic, with epidermal hyperplasia and ballooning of the keratinocytes secondary to intracellular edema. Mast cell and basophil numbers are normal, and eosinophils are rare; however, eosinophil degranulation products are present. In chronic skin lesions, the epidermis has moderate to marked hyperplasia, with elongation of the rete ridges and prominent hyperkeratosis. Spongiosis is variable, and the number of mast cells and Langerhans cells are significantly increased.

Numerous cellular and molecular studies of AD emphasize an allergic inflammatory process underlying this disorder (Leung, 2000). Approximately 85% of patients with AD have elevated serum IgE levels, and eosinophilia is common.

The pattern of cytokine expression found in lymphocytes infiltrating skin lesions in AD has been studied using in situ hybridization and reflects an allergic milieu. Infiltrating T lymphocytes in acute AD lesions express predominantly the Th2 cytokines, IL-4, IL-5, and IL-13, whereas T cells in chronic lesions express predominantly IL-5 and IL-13 with expression also of IL-12 and IFN-γ (Hamid et al., 1994; Hamid et al., 1996). This is in contrast to classic type IV cellular responses, such as purified protein derivative (PPD) or rhus dermatitis (poison ivy), in which cells express primarily mRNA for IFN-γ and IL-2 but not IL-4 and IL-5.

Overt superinfection with *Staphylococcus aureus* and colonization by this microorganism are common, and the exotoxins secreted by these organisms play a pathologic role in maintaining the inflammatory response. Ultimately, the disorder reflects the result of complex relationships among allergic inflammation, tissue injury and repair, allergen triggers, exposure to irritants, microbial toxin exposure, neurologic responses, and even psychologic factors.

Clinical Manifestations

The acute rash of AD is typically an erythematous, papulovesicular eruption, often with weeping and crusting, that is more commonly seen in early life. It typically progresses to a subacute form marked by erythema and scaling papules and, in older patients, to a chronic form characterized by thickened, lichenified skin and fibrous papules. The distribution of the rash varies with age, involving the cheeks and extensor surfaces of the arms and legs in infancy; the flexor surfaces in the young child; and flexor surfaces, hands, and feet in the teenage patient and young adult. Scratching of pruritic skin is a central factor in maintaining and triggering inflammation and skin damage.

Triggers of rash and pruritus include irritants (wool, residual soap, sweat, emotional upset) and allergens (foods and environmental). Postinflammatory hyperpigmentation and hypopigmentation and uneven tanning gives the skin a variegated appearance. Xerosis and hand and foot dermatitis are common. Involvement of the eyelids may lead to infraorbital folds termed *Dennie-Morgan lines*. Hyperlinearity of the palms may result from lichenification. Curiously, the nose is spared.

Diagnosis

Diagnosis is based on the characteristic rash, its distribution, and chronicity in the context of a personal or family history of atopy. Skin tests are often positive and total serum IgE elevated. Positive skin tests do not necessarily correlate with clinical reactions, particularly to foods.

The rash must be differentiated from similar exanthems such as seborrheic dermatitis (usually on the scalp and ears with a yellow scale and little pruritus) and contact dermatitis (that can be triggered by numerous allergens and may look similar to AD, but the distribution often reflects the inciting agent). Eczematous rashes are also a feature of other disorders such as zinc deficiency, hyper-IgE syndrome, Wiskott-Aldrich syndrome, and so forth.

Management

Medical treatment is generally aimed at skin hydration, which can be achieved by soaking baths or wet wraps followed immediately by liberal application of moisturizers (Leung et al., 1997). Topical anti-inflammatory ointments such as steroids and calcineurin inhibitors reduce skin inflammation; sedating antihistamines given near bedtime help reduce itching and promote sleep. Topical or oral antibiotics reduce skin infection and inflammation and allow healing.

Identification and elimination of food and environmental allergens is key in the overall management but can be a very tricky procedure in this disorder that has so many triggers (Sicherer and Sampson, 1999). Allergen immunotherapy is generally not indicated.

AD may remit over time, but for some the rash persists indefinitely. Physical and psychologic scarring is a serious issue. Complications of AD include eye damage (keratoconus, cataracts) and potentially severe skin infection with viruses (molluscum, herpes) and with fungi.

FOOD ALLERGY

Epidemiology

A number of adverse reactions can be attributed to food, but only those based on immune responses can be considered food allergies. About 6% of infants and young children experience true food allergies, and egg, cow's milk, soy, wheat, peanut, nuts from trees (e.g., walnut, cashew, Brazil nut), and seafood account for most of the significant food allergies (Bock, 1987). Epidemiologic studies on large cohorts of unselected newborns indicate that 2.5% have cow's milk allergy. Allergy to peanut affects 1 in 150 children in the United States (Sicherer et al., 1999). The foods responsible for allergic reactions vary somewhat by local feeding patterns.

Food allergy is the most common cause of severe, anaphylactic reactions occurring outside of the hospital setting, affects 37% of children with AD, is responsible for 20% of acute urticarial episodes, and affects 6% of children with asthma.

Pathogenesis

There are many adverse reactions to foods that occur from nonimmunologic mechanisms such as from toxins or pharmacologic agents in foods or from intolerance caused by failure to digest particular sugars or fats in foods. In contrast, food allergies represent a specific immune response, either IgE antibody–mediated or cell-mediated, to the proteins in foods (Sampson, 1999a).

IgE-mediated reactions are typically of sudden onset resulting from release of mediators such as histamine from mast cells in target organs. Subacute or chronic disorders may be caused by continued exposure to the food protein to which IgE antibody has been formed, resulting in chronic inflammation in target sites, or may be the result of T-cell–mediated responses.

Most of the chronic or subacute food allergic responses involve the gastrointestinal tract. Particular target organs such as the skin, lung, and gastrointestinal tract may be affected either from systemic distribution of ingested allergen, targeting of T cells to particular organs, or from specific target organ hyperreactivity.

Clinical Manifestations

IgE-mediated reactions may affect the skin with hives, urticaria, angioedema, or flaring of AD. The lung is affected with bronchoconstriction and mucus production and the upper airway with laryngeal edema and rhinitis. Gastrointestinal symptoms include abdominal pain, nausea, vomiting, and diarrhea. In severe anaphylactic reactions, the cardiovascular system is involved with hypotension and cardiac failure. Severe respiratory and cardiovascular symptoms can be fatal.

Peanuts, tree nuts, and seafood account for most of the fatal or near fatal reactions, and teenagers with known food allergy and underlying asthma appear to be at significantly increased risk (Sampson et al., 1992). In food-associated *exercise-induced anaphylaxis*, reactions to particular foods, such as wheat or celery, occur only when ingestion is followed by exercise.

Cell-mediated reactions are primarily manifested as gastrointestinal disorders that may result in failure to thrive; however, there are examples of skin (dermatitis herpetiformis) and pulmonary (Heiner's syndrome) reactions to foods that are also not IgE mediated (Sampson, 1999b). Gastrointestinal reactions span from mild proctocolitis, with the only symptom being blood and mucus in stools; to enteropathy with malabsorption; to enterocolitis with severe vomiting, diarrhea, and progression to dehydration and occasionally shock.

Gastroesophageal reflux and colic have been shown to be symptoms of cow's milk allergy for a subset of infants. Eosinophilic gastroenteropathy, a severe eosinophilic inflammation in the esophagus and other segments of the intestinal tract, is also associated with food allergy in a subset of children but has both IgE- and non–IgE-mediated pathophysiologies.

Diagnosis

For acute IgE-mediated reactions with isolated foods, the diagnosis usually can be secured through a careful history and demonstration of the relevant IgE antibodies by prick skin test or RAST. For chronic disorders, the diagnosis is much more difficult because the false-positive rate of tests for food-specific IgE antibody is roughly 50%. When specific concentrations of antibody are highly elevated, the chance of true reactivity is higher (Sampson and Ho, 1997).

In chronic IgE-mediated disorders such as AD, demonstration of cause and effect with food allergy depends, in many cases, on responses to elimination of potentially causal foods and readministration under physician supervision (oral food challenges). In a subset of patients with AD, tests for IgE antibody may be negative but tests for delayed-type hypersensitivity with allergy patch testing for foods may be positive and have been reported to correlate with symptoms (Niggemann et al., 2000). Unfortunately, there are no reliable in vitro tests for non–IgE-mediated gastrointestinal disorders; thus the diagnosis is predicated on elimination and challenge.

Management

The primary treatment of food allergy is the strict elimination of the responsible food(s). Small traces of the responsible food protein can trigger reactions in sensitive children. Consequently, careful reading of ingredient labels and an appreciation for cross-contamination in processing, meal preparation, and in restaurants must be taught. A dietitian can provide assistance in suggesting substitutions to maintain a balanced diet.

For children with a history of or at risk for anaphylaxis, self-administered epinephrine should be prescribed, and the circumstances requiring and technique of administering should be periodically reviewed. Approximately 80% of children outgrow allergy to milk, egg, wheat, and soy by their third birthday, so re-evaluation is a critical component of management. Although a small minority of children outgrow allergies to peanut, nuts, and seafood, most have these for life.

In infants at high risk for allergy (biparental or parental and sibling atopy), prophylactic measures to prevent allergies have been suggested. These include breastfeeding (with consideration for maternal restriction of highly allergenic foods, e.g., peanuts); delayed introduction of solid foods until 6 months; and avoidance of cow's milk to age 1, egg to age 2, and peanut, nuts, and seafood to age 3 years (Committee on Nutrition, American Academy of Pediatrics, 2000).

ANAPHYLAXIS

Anaphylaxis refers to a rapid, systemic response caused by IgE-mediated release of immune mediators. Although the definition does not specify severity, these reactions can be fatal. A retrospective, population-based study of anaphylaxis in Minnesota found the annual incidence rate to be 21 per 100,000 person-years (Yocum et al., 1999).

Signs and symptoms affect the skin and gastrointestinal, respiratory, and cardiovascular systems and include pruritus; flushing; urticaria; angioedema; nasal congestion, pruritus, and rhinorrhea; cough; wheeze; dysphonia; laryngeal edema; vomiting, diarrhea; abdominal pain; syncope; dysrhythmias; and a sense of impending doom. Symptoms usually occur within minutes of exposure but are sometimes delayed, usually not beyond 2 hours. Biphasic responses with recurrence of symptoms within hours and protracted anaphylaxis lasting for days have been documented.

When similar symptoms are caused by non–immune-mediated release of mediators, the term *anaphylactoid* is used.

Common causes of anaphylactic and anaphylactoid reactions are shown in Table 31-6. When reactions that may represent anaphylaxis are being evaluated, alternative diagnoses may include vasovagal syncope, carcinoid, scombroid fish poisoning, mastocytosis, hereditary angioedema, and other causes of cardiovascular or respiratory compromise. When the history indicates possible triggers, testing for IgE antibody can often assist in confirming the diagnosis. In some cases, a combination of factors is responsible (food-associated, exercise-induced anaphylaxis). Assessment of risk factors may

---

TABLE 31-6 · REPRESENTATIVE CAUSES OF ANAPHYLAXIS AND ANAPHYLACTOID REACTIONS

Anaphylaxis
Foods
Drugs
Vaccines
Insect stings
Latex
Allergen extracts and immunotherapy
Insulin
Protamine
Exercise
Seminal fluid
Idiopathic

Anaphylactoid
ASA/NSAIDs
Radiocontrast dye

ASA = aspirin; NSAIDs = nonsteroidal anti-inflammatory drugs.

help pinpoint a diagnosis. For example, health care workers and children who have undergone multiple surgeries are at increased risk for latex allergy.

The treatment of acute anaphylaxis is based on early recognition of the typical signs and symptoms; rapid assessment of the airway and cardiopulmonary status; and prompt administration of epinephrine and appropriate supportive measures such as CPR, oxygen, vasopressors, intravenous fluids, and respiratory support (Joint Task Force on Practice Parameters, 1998). Additional treatments include antihistamines (H_1 and H_2 blockers), corticosteroids, and continued assessment for late-phase responses.

Long-term management requires careful searches for triggers and education about avoidance, signs and symptoms of anaphylaxis, and placement of an emergency plan including self-injectable epinephrine.

STINGING INSECT ALLERGY

Stinging insects, rather than insects that bite such as mosquitoes, are responsible for anaphylactic reactions because they inject venom that can elicit immune responses. Three families of stinging insects (order Hymenoptera) are responsible for these reactions: Apids (honeybee and bumblebee), Vespids (yellow jacket, yellow and white-faced hornets, and paper wasp), and Formicids (fire and harvester ants). The Vespid venoms cross-react as do the Apid venoms, but there is little cross-reactivity among the other insects.

IgE-mediated reactions to venom result in a variety of symptoms typically seen with anaphylaxis to a variety of agents. Local skin reactions of pain, erythema, and edema or even large local reactions that may involve large contiguous areas may also occur. Large numbers of stings may induce toxic reactions from large doses of venom vasoactive amines.

Stings can also induce non-IgE immune responses such as serum-sickness reactions or Guillain-Barré syndrome. Differentiation of the type of reaction is important because non–IgE-mediated and local reactions are not associated with significantly increased risks for severe reactions from future stings.

Increased risks for systemic reactions on future stings in subjects with documented venom-specific IgE antibody are greatest for adults who experienced systemic symptoms or children with systemic symptoms involving more than urticaria (Portnoy et al., 1999). In these individuals, venom immunotherapy should be considered because treatment can reduce the risk of systemic reactions from approximately 60% to 2% at a maintenance dose of 100 μg (Hunt et al., 1978; Reisman and Livingston, 1992).

Immunotherapy efficacy and spontaneous resolution of allergy usually permit discontinuation of immunotherapy after 3 to 5 years in patients with a history of mild to moderate reactions, whereas those with severe reactions may need to be maintained on treatment indefinitely (Portnoy et al., 1999). In any case, suggestions to reduce exposure risks (e.g., wearing long pants, avoiding areas of infestation) and instructions on the use of self-injectable epinephrine should be provided.

DRUG ALLERGY

Adverse reactions to medications occur on an immunologic and nonimmunologic basis with the latter accounting for most of the observed ill effects (some of which are common, expected side effects, whereas others are idiosyncratic) (Table 31-7). Immune-mediated reactions include all four types of hypersensitivity reactions. A special category of "pseudoallergic" or anaphylactoid reactions are those that are due to release of immunologic mediators in a nonspecific manner as can occur in reactions to narcotics and radiocontrast media that cause histamine release. Reactions to components of vaccines are also observed. Examples include reactions to egg protein in influenza and yellow fever vaccines and to gelatin in a number of vaccines.

The evaluation of drug hypersensitivity takes into account the historical information concerning potential agents, time course, type of symptoms, and a priori knowledge about the actions of particular drugs and their likelihood of triggering allergic responses. Consideration is also given for other causes of the adverse reactions (rash induced by the underlying illness rather than the treatment).

Immediate treatment of severe allergic reactions caused by type I hypersensitivity mirrors that for treatment of anaphylaxis from other causes. Immune-mediated reactions typically require withdrawal of the medication, choosing an alternative medication, and symptomatic treatments that may include antihistamines and corticosteroids. In some cases of mild reactions, "treating-through" may be attempted when the benefits outweigh the risks.

Mild maculopapular eruptions occurring late in the course of treatment with penicillins, especially in the context of an underlying viral infection, are not generally predictive of increased risks for severe reactions on

---

TABLE 31-7 · CATEGORIES OF ADVERSE DRUG REACTIONS

Predictable, nonimmune adverse reactions
   Overdosage (vomiting from theophylline toxicity)
   Side effects (tachycardia from albuterol)
   Drug–drug interactions (theophylline toxicity with erythromycin)
Unpredictable, immune
   IgE-mediated (anaphylaxis from PCN)
   Non–IgE-mediated
      Type II hypersensitivity (hemolysis from PCN)
      Type III hypersensitivity (serum sickness from sulfonamides)
      Type IV hypersensitivity (late-onset morbilliform eruptions from PCN)
Unpredictable, nonimmune
   Pseudoallergic, anaphylactoid ("red man" from vancomycin)
   Idiosyncratic (ASA, NSAID sensitivity)
   Intolerance

ASA = aspirin; NSAID = nonsteroidal anti-inflammatory drug; PCN = penicillin.

future courses of the antibiotic. In contrast, reactions such as Stevens-Johnson syndrome and toxic epidermal necrolysis are contraindications to future treatment with the causative drug or related compound.

For persons with anaphylactoid reactions to radiocontrast media, low-ionic radiocontrast formulations and premedication with corticosteroids and antihistamines should be used before radiocontrast media have been administered to circumvent a reaction (Greenberger and Patterson, 1991).

Unfortunately, skin tests are of limited value in the diagnosis of drug allergy because the cause of immune reactivity is most often not mediated by IgE. Even if reactions are IgE mediated, methods are not standardized for most drugs except penicillin and uncharacterized metabolites may be responsible for reactions.

The clinician must consider the suspected pathophysiology of reactions when deciding to perform skin tests and in interpreting the results. Although positive skin tests to appropriate concentrations of the drug in question may indicate a risk for type 1 reactions, a negative test cannot rule out the possibility.

For IgE-mediated reactions, when alternative agents are unavailable, desensitization procedures can be performed. Desensitization protocols have also been used with some success for mild, non–IgE-mediated reactions to aspirin, allopurinol, and sulfa medications.

Only a small percentage of individuals with a history of penicillin allergy experience reactions to cephalosporins, and specific protocols to evaluate this possibility have been suggested (Joint Task Force on Practice Parameters, 1999).

URTICARIA AND ANGIOEDEMA

Urticaria is characterized by pruritic, raised, erythematous wheals (localized edema) that blanch with pressure. Lesions may coalesce and may have surrounding areas of erythema. Individual lesions typically resolve within 24 hours, leaving no residual scarring, unlike vasculitis (Greaves, 1995).

Chronic urticaria, by definition, is frequent episodes of urticaria that persist beyond 6 weeks. Although acute urticaria is a common disorder affecting 10% to 20% of individuals at some time in their life and is often attributable to a particular exposure, chronic urticaria is uncommon and underlying causes are most often not identifiable.

Angioedema, a similar process to urticaria occurring in deeper skin layers, often accompanies urticaria. Cholinergic urticaria is characterized by small pinpoint wheals surrounded by large areas of erythema and is most commonly triggered by exercise, heat, sweating, and emotional factors.

Acute urticaria may result from histamine release following the interaction of allergen with IgE antibodies on the surface of mast cells but may also occur from elaboration of mediators triggered by other immune responses such as immune complexes (urticarial vasculitis) or nonimmune mechanisms as in physical urticaria.

Chronic urticaria may be attributed to an autoimmune response in about half of patients (Ferrer et al., 1998). In these patients, an IgG autoantibody is directed to the α subunit of the high-affinity IgE receptor.

There are a number of physical urticarias. Cold-induced urticaria comes in several forms, some acquired and others inherited. Acquired cold-induced urticaria generally presents as isolated urticaria at the skin site where temperature is lowered (rather than the absolute temperature of exposure). However, anaphylactic reactions have occurred when large areas are cooled, as can occur with swimming. Reactions may occur in association with production of cold-dependent autoantibodies. Systemic cold urticaria is distinct in that the site of exposure may not wheal, but systemic anaphylaxis can ensue. Dominantly inherited forms include an immediate form with macules, fever, and arthralgia and a delayed form with deep-seated edema hours after local exposure.

Episodic angioedema without urticaria may represent C1 esterase inhibitor deficiency, which is discussed in Chapter 21. Trauma (dermatographism), heat, vibration, sweating, and even water exposure are additional physical causes of urticaria.

The history is particularly important in identifying allergic and physical triggers. Directed laboratory tests such as skin prick tests for allergen can confirm clinical suspicions. Physical urticaria can be evaluated, for example, by applying ice to the skin and observing for wheal formation following removal in some forms of cold-induced urticaria and by scratching the skin in dermatographism.

Searching for underlying causes or associations in chronic urticaria such as infection, autoimmune disorders (thyroid disease), neoplasia, or vasculitic syndromes may be warranted as indicated by the history and physical examination. These ancillary tests may include stool for parasites, erythrocyte sedimentation rate (ESR), complete blood count (CBC), urinalysis, testing for cold agglutinins, cryoglobulins, and skin biopsy, among others.

Identification and avoidance of the allergen and pharmacologic and physical triggers is a major step in therapy. Unfortunately, such triggers are usually not identified in chronic urticaria; thus medical therapy remains the primary route for relief. The mainstay of therapy is an H_1 antihistamine, but recalcitrant urticaria may respond to the addition of H_2 antihistamines. Cyproheptadine has particular efficacy in cold-induced urticaria. Epinephrine for self-injection should be available for those at risk of systemic reactions. Systemic steroids at the lowest dosage possible to control symptoms are needed in some cases.

The natural course of chronic urticaria is that there is not progression to anaphylaxis and that symptoms usually remit over several years.

SERUM SICKNESS

Serum sickness is primarily a type III hypersensitivity response to foreign proteins from a variety of sources. Although classically described as a response to horse antisera, the most common triggers now include medications, but other triggers include infections and vaccines. Immune complexes are deposited in various organs, particularly the kidney, skin, and joints, and activation of inflammatory mediators ensues. Responses may develop days to weeks following exposure with symptoms such as skin rashes, adenopathy, arthralgia, fever, peripheral neuritis, and angioedema. Supporting laboratory evidence includes leukocytosis or leukopenia, eosinophilia, and abnormal urinary sediment. Treatment begins with withdrawal and avoidance of the offending agent and includes supportive care, antihistamines for skin rashes, and, in some cases, corticosteroids.

CONCLUSION

Allergy and atopic disorders are increasing in prevalence, and as a group represent the most common immunologic disorders in children. Although in some ways these disorders represent an overactive immune response, they may be more appropriately considered the result of immune dysregulation. The immune disorder is due to a genetic predisposition to mount a Th2-biased immune response. As such, the clinician must be aware that the symptoms and the underlying pathophysiology overlap those of autoimmune and immunodeficiency diseases. For example, the clinician must differentiate AD from the dermatitis of hyper-IgE syndrome and Wiskott-Aldrich syndrome and differentiate urticarial exanthemas from vasculitis.

Similarly, the atopic child may suffer from increased infections as a result of blunted Th1 responses (children with AD have impaired type IV hypersensitivity responses of the skin and are susceptible to cutaneous viral infections) or impaired nonspecific immune defenses resulting from anatomic compromise (pneumonia in a child with asthma or sinusitis in a rhinitis patient). Advances attributed to the Human Genome Project and improved molecular biologic techniques are improving the ability to diagnose and treat these disorders.

R E F E R E N C E S

Aalberse RC. Structural biology of allergens. J Allergy Clin Immunol 106:228–238, 2000.

Abehsira-Amar O, Gibert M, Joliy M, Theze J, Jankovic DL. IL-4 plays a dominant role in the differential development of Th0 into Th1 and Th2 cells. J Immunol 148:3820–3829, 1992.

Abramson MJ, Puy RM, Weiner JM. Is allergen immunotherapy effective in asthma? A meta-analysis of randomized controlled trials. Am J Respir Crit Care Med 151:969–974, 1995.

Agertoft L, Pedersen S. Effect of long-term treatment with inhaled budesonide on adult height in children with asthma. N Engl J Med 343:1064–1069, 2000.

American Academy of Allergy and Immunology. Unproven procedures for diagnosis and treatment of allergic and immunologic diseases. J Allergy Clin Immunol 78:275–277, 1986.

Arlian LG, Platts-Mills TA. The biology of dust mites and the remediation of mite allergens in allergic disease. J Allergy Clin Immunol 107:406–413, 2001.

Bacharier LB, Geha RS Molecular mechanisms of IgE regulation. J Allergy Clin Immunol 105:S547–S58, 2000.

Barnes PJ. Effect of beta-agonists on inflammatory cells. J Allergy Clin Immunol 104:S10–S17, 1999.

Beasley R, Crane J, Lai CK, Pearce N. Prevalence and etiology of asthma. J Allergy Clin Immunol 105:S466–S472, 2000.

Bellioni-Businco B, Paganelli R, Lucenti P, Giampietro PG, Perborn H, Businco. Allergenicity of goat's milk in children with cow's milk allergy. J Allergy Clin Immunol 103:1191–1194, 1999.

Bergmann RL, Edenharter G, Bergmann KE, Forster J, Bauer CP, Wahn V, Zepp F, Wahn U. Atopic dermatitis in early infancy predicts allergic airway disease at 5 years. Clin Exp Allergy 28:965–970, 1998.

Bernhisel-Broadbent J, Sampson HA. Cross-allergenicity in the legume botanical family in children with food hypersensitivity. J Allergy Clin Immunol 83:435–440, 1989.

Bielory L. Allergic and immunologic disorders of the eye. Part II: ocular allergy. J Allergy Clin Immunol 106:1019–1032, 2000.

Bochner BS. Systemic activation of basophils and eosinophils: markers and consequences. J Allergy Clin Immunol 106:S292–302, 2000.

Bochner BS, Luscinskas FW, Gimbrone MA Jr, Newman W, Sterbinsky SA, Derse-Anthony CP, Klunk D, Schleimer RP. Adhesion of human basophils, eosinophils, and neutrophils to interleukin 1-activated human vascular endothelial cells: contributions of endothelial cell adhesion molecules. J Exp Med 173:1553–1557, 1991.

Bock SA. Prospective appraisal of complaints of adverse reactions to foods in children during the first 3 years of life. Pediatrics 79:683–688, 1987.

Carroll N, Carello S, Cooke C, James A. Airway structure and inflammatory cells in fatal attacks of asthma. Eur Respir J 9:709–715, 1996.

Childhood Asthma Management Program Research Group. Long-term effects of budesonide or nedocromil in children with asthma. N Engl J Med 343:1054–1063, 2000.

Cockcroft DW, Murdock KY. Comparative effects of inhaled salbutamol, sodium cromoglycate, and beclomethasone dipropionate on allergen-induced early asthmatic responses, late asthmatic responses, and increased bronchial responsiveness to histamine. J Allergy Clin Immunol 79:734–740, 1987.

Committee on Nutrition. American Academy of Pediatrics. Hypoallergenic infant formulas. Pediatrics 106:346–349, 2000.

Chatchatee P, Järvinen K-M, Bardina L, Beyer K, Sampson HA. Identification of IgE- and IgG-binding epitopes on α_{s1}-casein: differences in patients with persistent and transient cow's milk allergy. J Allergy Clin Immunol, 107:379–383, 2001.

Creticos PS. Immunotherapy with allergens. JAMA 268:2834–2839, 1992.

Creticos PS, Reed CE, Norman PS, Khoury J, Adkinson NF Jr, Buncher CR, Busse WW, Bush RK, Gadde J, Li JT, et al. Ragweed immunotherapy in adult asthma. N Engl J Med 334:501–506, 1996.

Cruz AA, Togias AG, Lichtenstein LM, Kagey-Sobotka A, Proud D, Naclerio RM. Local application of atropine attenuates the upper airway reaction to cold, dry air. Am Rev Respir Dis 146:340–346, 1992.

Drazen J. Clinical pharmacology of leukotriene receptor antagonists and 5-lipoxygenase inhibitors. Am J Respir Crit Care Med 157:S233–S237, 1998.

Dykewicz MS, Fineman S, Skoner DP, Nicklas R, Lee R, Blessing-Moore J, Li JT, Bernstein IL, Berger W, Spector S, Schuller D. Diagnosis and management of rhinitis: complete guidelines of the Joint Task Force on Practice Parameters in Allergy, Asthma and Immunology. American Academy of Allergy, Asthma, and Immunology. Ann Allergy Asthma Immunol 81:478–518, 1998.

Ferrer M, Kinet JP, Kaplan AP. Comparative studies of functional and binding assays for IgG anti-Fc(epsilon)RIalpha (alpha-subunit) in chronic urticaria. J Allergy Clin Immunol 101:672–676, 1998.

Gawchik SM, Saccar CL, Noonan M, Reasner DS, DeGraw SS. The safety and efficacy of nebulized levalbuterol compared with racemic albuterol and placebo in the treatment of asthma in pediatric patients. J Allergy Clin Immunol 103:615–621, 1999.

Gleich GJ. Mechanisms of eosinophil-associated inflammation. J Allergy Clin Immunol 105:651–663, 2000.

Greaves MW. Chronic urticaria. N Engl J Med 332:1767–1772, 1995.

Greenberger PA, Patterson R. The prevention of immediate generalized reactions to radiocontrast media in high-risk patients. J Allergy Clin Immunol 87:867–872, 1991.

Gustavsson S, Wernersson S, Heyman B. Restoration of the antibody response to IgE/antigen complexes in CD23-deficient mice by CD23+ spleen or bone marrow cells. J Immunol 164:3990–3995, 2000.

Hamid Q, Boguniewicz M, Leung DY. Differential in situ cytokine gene expression in acute versus chronic atopic dermatitis. J Clin Invest 94:870–876, 1994.

Hamid Q, Naseer T, Minshall EM, Song YL, Boguniewicz M, Leung DY. In vivo expression of IL-12 and IL-13 in atopic dermatitis. J Allergy Clin Immunol 98:225–231, 1996.

Hanifin JM, Rajka L. Diagnostic features of atopic dermatitis. Acta Dermatol Venereol 92(Suppl):44–47, 1980.

Hide DW, Matthews S, Tariq S, Arshad SH. Allergen avoidance in infancy and allergy at 4 years of age. Allergy 51:89–93, 1996.

Howard TD, Meyers DA, Bleecker ER. Mapping susceptibility genes for asthma and allergy. J Allergy Clin Immunol 105:S477–S481, 2000.

Hulett MD, Hogarth PM. Molecular basis of Fc receptor function. Adv Immunol 57:1–127, 1994.

Hunt KJ, Valentine MD, Sobotka AK, Benton AW, Amodio FJ, Lichtenstein LM. A controlled trial of immunotherapy in insect hypersensitivity. N Engl J Med 299:157–161, 1978.

Ishizaka K, Ishizaka I. Identification of IgE antibodies as a carrier of reaginic activity J Immunol 99:1187–1198, 1967.

Israel E, Drazen JM, Liggett SB, Boushey HA, Cherniack RM, Chinchilli VM, Cooper DM, Fahy JV, Fish JE, Ford JG, Kraft M, Kunselman S, Lazarus SC, Lemanske RF, Martin RJ, McLean DE, Peters SP, Silverman EK, Sorkness CA, Szefler SJ, Weiss ST, Yandava CN. The effect of polymorphisms of the beta(2)-adrenergic receptor on the response to regular use of albuterol in asthma. Am J Respir Crit Care Med 162:75–80, 2000.

Johansson SGO and Bennich H. Immunologic studies of an atypical (myeloma) immunoglobulin. Immunology 13:381–394, 1967.

Joint Task Force on Practice Parameters, American Academy of Allergy, Asthma and Immunology, American College of Allergy, Asthma and Immunology, and the Joint Council of Allergy, Asthma and Immunology. The diagnosis and management of anaphylaxis. J Allergy Clin Immunol 101:S465–528, 1998.

Joint Task Force on Practice Parameters, the American Academy of Allergy, Asthma and Immunology, the American Academy of Allergy, Asthma and Immunology, and the Joint Council of Allergy, Asthma and Immunology. Executive summary of disease management of drug hypersensitivity: a practice parameter. Ann Allergy Asthma Immunol 83:665–700, 1999.

Jones SM, Magnolfi CF, Cooke SK, Sampson HA. Immunologic cross-reactivity among cereal grains and grasses in children with food hypersensitivity. J Allergy Clin Immunol 96:341–351, 1995.

Lack G, Nelson HS, Amran D, Oshiba A, Jung T, Bradley KL, Giclas PC, Gelfand EW. Rush immunotherapy results in allergen-specific alterations in lymphocyte function and interferon-gamma production in CD4+ T cells. J Allergy Clin Immunol 99:530–538, 1997.

Laughter D, Istvan JA, Tofte SJ, Hanifin JM. The prevalence of atopic dermatitis in Oregon schoolchildren. J Am Acad Dermatol 43:649–655, 2000.

Leung DY. Atopic dermatitis: new insights and opportunities for therapeutic intervention. J Allergy Clin Immunol 105:860–876, 2000.

Leung DY, Hanifin JM, Charlesworth EN, Li JT, Bernstein IL, Berger WE, Blessing-Moore J, Fineman S, Lee FE, Nicklas RA, Spector SL. Joint Task Force on Practice Parameters, representing the American Academy of Allergy, Asthma and Immunology, the American College of Allergy, Asthma and Immunology, and the Joint Council of Allergy, Asthma and Immunology. Work Group on Atopic Dermatitis. Disease management of atopic dermatitis: a practice parameter. Ann Allergy Asthma Immunol 79:197–211, 1997.

Mak JC, Nishikawa M, Shirasaki H, Miyayasu K, Barnes PJ. Protective effects of a glucocorticoid on downregulation of pulmonary beta 2-adrenergic receptors in vivo. J Clin Invest 96:99–106, 1995.

Mallamaci MA, Chizzonite R, Griffin M, Nettleton M, Hakimi J, Tsien WH, Kochan JP. Identification of sites on the human Fc epsilon RI alpha subunit which are involved in binding human and rat IgE. J Biol Chem 268:22076–22083, 1993.

Marsh DG, Neely JD, Breazeale DR, Ghosh B, Freidhoff LR, Ehrlich-Kautzky E, Schou C, Krishnaswamy G, Beaty TH. Linkage analysis of IL4 and other chromosome 5q31.1 markers and total serum immunoglobulin E concentrations. Science 264:1152–1156, 1994.

Martinez FD, Wright AL, Taussig LM, Holberg CJ, Halonen M, Morgan WJ. Asthma and wheezing in the first six years of life. The Group Health Medical Associates. N Engl J Med 332:133–138, 1995.

Metcalfe DD, Baram D, Mekori YA. Mast cells. Physiol Rev 77:1033–1079, 1997.

Mudde GC, Van Reijsen FC, Boland GJ, de Gast GC, Bruijnzeel PL, Bruijnzeel-Koomen CA. Allergen presentation by epidermal Langerhans' cells from patients with atopic dermatitis is mediated by IgE. Immunology 69:335–341, 1990.

Nathan RA, Meltzer EO, Selner JC, Storms W. Prevalence of allergic rhinitis in the United States. J Allergy Clin Immunol 99:S808–S814, 1997.

National Institutes of Health, National Heart, Lung, and Blood Institute. Expert panel Report 2: guidelines for the diagnosis and management of asthma, NIH Publication No. 97-4051, 1997.

Nelson HS, Bensch G, Pleskow WW, DiSantostefano R, DeGraw S, Reasner DS, Rollins TE, Rubin PD. Improved bronchodilation with levalbuterol compared with racemic albuterol in patients with asthma. J Allergy Clin Immunol 102:943–952, 1998.

Nelson HS, Lahr J, Rule R, Bock A, Leung D. Treatment of anaphylactic sensitivity to peanuts by immunotherapy with injections of aqueous peanut extract. J Allergy Clin Immunol 99:744–751, 1997.

Nelson HS, Oppenheimer J, Buchmeier A, Kordash TR, Freshwater LL. An assessment of the role of intradermal skin testing in the diagnosis of clinically relevant allergy to timothy grass. J Allergy Clin Immunol 97:1193–1201, 1996.

Niggemann B, Reibel S, Wahn U. The atopy patch test (APT)—a useful tool for the diagnosis of food allergy in children with atopic dermatitis. Allergy 55:281–285, 2000.

O'Hollaren MT, Yunginger JW, Offord KP, Somers MJ, O'Connell EJ, Ballard DJ, Sachs MI. Exposure to an aeroallergen as a possible precipitating factor in respiratory arrest in young patients with asthma. N Engl J Med 324:359–363, 1991.

Portnoy JM, Moffitt JE, Golden DB, Bernstein WE, Dykewicz MS, Fineman SM, Lee RE, Li JT, Nicklas RA, Schuller DE, Spector SL. Stinging insect hypersensitivity: a practice parameter. The Joint Force on Practice Parameters, the American Academy of Allergy, Asthma and Immunology, the American College of Allergy, Asthma and Immunology, and the Joint Council of Allergy, Asthma and Immunology. J Allergy Clin Immunol 103:963–980, 1999.

Postma DS, Bleecker ER, Amelung PJ, Holroyd KJ, Xu J, Panhuysen CI, Meyers DA, Levitt RC. Genetic susceptibility to asthma—bronchial hyperresponsiveness coinherited with a major gene for atopy. N Engl J Med 333:894–900, 1995.

Reisman RE, Livingston A. Venom immunotherapy: 10 years of experience with administration of single venoms and 50 micrograms maintenance doses. J Allergy Clin Immunol 89:1189–1195, 1992.

Restani P, Gaiaschi A, Plebani A, Beretta B, Cavagni G, Fiocchi A, Poiesi C, Velona T, Ugazio AG, Galli CL. Cross-reactivity between milk proteins from different animal species. Clin Exp Allergy 29:997–1004, 1999.

Rissoan MC, Soumelis V, Kadowaki N, Grouard G, Briere F, de Waal Malefyt R, Liu YJ. Reciprocal control of T helper cell and dendritic cell differentiation. Science 19;283:1183–1186, 1999.

Rosenstreich DL, Eggleston P, Kattan M, Baker D, Slavin RG, Gergen P, Mitchell H, McNiff-Mortimer K, Lynn H, Ownby D, Malveaux F. The role of cockroach allergy and exposure to cockroach allergen in causing morbidity among inner-city children with asthma. N Engl J Med 336:1356–1363, 1997.

Rosenwasser LJ, Klemm DJ, Dresback JK, Inamura H, Mascali JJ, Klinnert M, Borish L. Promoter polymorphisms in the chromosome 5 gene cluster in asthma and atopy. Clin Exp Allergy Suppl 2:74–78, 1995.

Rothenberg ME. Eosinophilia. N Engl J Med 338:1592–1600, 1998.

Sampson HA. Food allergy. Part 1: immunopathogenesis and clinical disorders. J Allergy Clin Immunol 103:717–728, 1999.

Sampson HA. Food allergy. Part 2: diagnosis and management. J Allergy Clin Immunol 103:981–989, 1999.

Sampson HA, Ho DG. Relationship between food-specific IgE concentrations and the risk of positive food challenges in children and adolescents. J Allergy Clin Immunol 100:444–451, 1997.

Sampson HA, McCaskill CC. Food hypersensitivity and atopic dermatitis: evaluation of 113 patients. J Pediatr 107:669–675, 1985.

Sampson HA, Mendelson L, Rosen JP. Fatal and near-fatal anaphylactic reactions to food in children and adolescents. N Engl J Med 327:380–384, 1992.

Sayers I, Helm BA. The structural basis of human IgE-Fc receptor interactions. Clin Exp Allergy 29:585–594, 1999.

Shahabuddin S, Ponath P, Schleimer RP. Migration of eosinophils across endothelial cell monolayers: interactions among IL-5, endothelial-activating cytokines, and C-C chemokines. J Immunol 164:3847–3854, 2000.

Sicherer SH, Muñoz-Furlong A, Burks AW, Sampson HA. Prevalence of peanut and tree nut allergy in the US determined by a random digit dial telephone survey. J Allergy Clin Immunol 103:559–562, 1999.

Sicherer SH, Sampson HA. Food hypersensitivity and atopic dermatitis: pathophysiology, epidemiology, diagnosis, and management. J Allergy Clin Immunol 104:114–122, 1999.

Theoharides TC, Wang L, Pang X, Letourneau R, Culm KE, Basu S, Wang Y, Correia I. Cloning and cellular localization of the rat mast cell 78-kDa protein phosphorylated in response to the mast cell "stabilizer" cromolyn. J Pharmacol Exp Ther 294:810–821, 2000.

Weinberger M, Hendeles L. Theophylline in asthma. N Engl J Med 334:1380–1388, 1996.

Wenzel SE. Antileukotriene drugs in the management of asthma. JAMA 280:2068–2069, 1998.

Williams H, Robertson C, Stewart A, Ait-Khaled N, Anabwani G, Anderson R, Asher I, Beasley R, Bjorksten B, Burr M, Clayton T, Crane J, Ellwood P, Keil U, Lai C, Mallol J, Martinez F, Mitchell E, Montefort S, Pearce N, Shah J, Sibbald B, Strachan D, von Mutius E, Weiland SK. Worldwide variations in the prevalence of symptoms of atopic eczema in the International Study of Asthma and Allergies in Childhood. J Allergy Clin Immunol 103:125–138, 1999.

Wood RA, Chapman MD, Adkinson NF Jr, Eggleston PA. The effect of cat removal on allergen content in household-dust samples. J Allergy Clin Immunol 83:730–734, 1989.

Wood RA, Laheri AN, Eggleston PA. The aerodynamic characteristics of cat allergen. Clin Exp Allergy 23:733–739, 1993.

Wood RA, Phipatanakul W, Hamilton RG, Eggleston PA. A comparison of skin prick tests, intradermal skin tests, and RASTs in the diagnosis of cat allergy. J Allergy Clin Immunol 103:773–779, 1999.

Wright AL, Holberg CJ, Martinez FD, Halonen M, Morgan W, Taussig LM. Epidemiology of physician-diagnosed allergic rhinitis in childhood. Pediatrics 94:895–901, 1994.

Ying S, Durham SR, Corrigan CJ, Hamid Q, Kay AB. Phenotype of cells expressing mRNA for TH2-type (interleukin 4 and interleukin 5) and TH1-type (interleukin 2 and interferon gamma) cytokines in bronchoalveolar lavage and bronchial biopsies from atopic asthmatic and normal control subjects. Am J Respir Cell Mol Biol 12:477–487, 1995.

Yocum MW, Butterfield JH, Klein JS, Volcheck GW, Schroeder DR, Silverstein MD. Epidemiology of anaphylaxis in Olmsted County: a population-based study. J Allergy Clin Immunol 104:452–456, 1999.

Yunginger JW, Ahlstedt S, Eggleston PA, Homburger HA, Nelson HS, Ownby DR, Platts-Mills TA, Sampson HA, Sicherer SH, Weinstein AM, Williams PB, Wood RA, Zeiger RS. Quantitative IgE antibody assays in allergic diseases. J Allergy Clin Immunol 105:1077–1084, 2000.

Zeiger RS, Heller S. The development and prediction of atopy in high-risk children: follow-up at age seven years in a prospective randomized study of combined maternal and infant food allergen avoidance. J Allergy Clin Immunol 95:1179–1190, 1995.

C H A P T E R

32 Dermatologic Disorders

Lynne H. Morrison and Jon M. Hanifin

INTRODUCTION

The entities discussed in this chapter are diverse and include the following:

1. Autoimmune disorders such as immunologically mediated blistering skin diseases and lupus erythematosus (LE)

2. Reactive erythemas, which are cutaneous reactions secondary to a variety of antigenic stimuli
3. Figurate erythemas such as erythema multiforme (EM), a morphologically defined group of reactive lesions with an annular appearance
4. Henoch-Schönlein purpura (HSP)
5. Immune-associated eczemas, including atopic dermatitis (AD) and allergic contact dermatitis

The skin manifestations of primary immunodeficiency diseases are discussed in chapters dealing with those disorders.

Although cutaneous lupus is discussed here, skin manifestations of other collagen-vascular diseases are covered in Chapter 35. By far, the most common of the diseases covered in this chapter is AD. HSP and EM minor are fairly common but are not seen with the frequency of AD, and the remaining diseases are considered uncommon to rare.

Because of the diversity of this group of skin disorders, there are no unifying historical or laboratory features that suggest a diagnosis of an immunologically mediated disease. The diagnosis often rests on recognition of the individual morphologic features of the various dermatoses and the histologic findings. In the immunologically mediated blistering skin diseases, immunohistology is essential in establishing a correct diagnosis.

Again, because of the wide range of entities considered here, the therapies vary widely and can range from simple observation in neonatal lupus with only skin findings or mild HSP to systemic corticosteroids in bullous diseases.

In general, many of the diseases discussed here are cutaneous reactions to an inciting allergen, and identification and elimination of the allergen are of prime importance. This consideration applies to allergic contact dermatitis, reactive erythemas such as EM, figurate erythemas, and HSP. Avoidance of exacerbating environmental agents is of great importance in managing AD.

Therapeutic control of the skin eruption often involves but is not limited to topical corticosteroids. Therapy for psoriasis includes ultraviolet light, topical corticosteroids, tar, topical calcipotriol, and anthralin. Systemic therapy is generally required for the bullous diseases. Both dermatitis herpetiformis (DH) and linear immunoglobulin A (IgA)/bullous dermatosis are treated with dapsone, and pemphigus and bullous pemphigoid (BP) are most often treated with systemic corticosteroids. Dapsone and tetracycline (in appropriately aged children) are alternatives to corticosteroids in BP.

IMMUNOBULLOUS DISEASES

Dermatitis Herpetiformis

DH is an intensely pruritic, chronic, papulovesicular eruption with a characteristic distribution involving extensor surfaces. Histologically, it is characterized by subepidermal blister formation with infiltration of neutrophils in the papillary tips. Because the clinical and histologic findings can overlap those of other immunologically mediated blistering diseases, direct immunofluorescence (IF) studies of perilesional skin are most reliable for diagnosing DH (McCord and Hall, 1993; Zone, 1991). The characteristic direct IF features of DH demonstrate granular deposition of IgA in the papillary tips or continuously beneath the basement membrane zone.

The disease usually occurs between the third and fifth decades, but cases of juvenile DH have been reported. The exact prevalence in the pediatric age group is hard to determine, because the disease was confused with linear IgA/bullous dermatosis (LABD) until direct IF studies were routinely performed in these patients. Some authors consider juvenile DH to be rare.

History

The initial description of DH is generally attributed to Dr. Louis Duhring in 1884. Over the next 80 years, the clinical description was refined, the histopathologic features were described, systemic ingestion of iodide was found to exacerbate the eruption, and a favorable response to sulfapyridine was noted. An association with gluten-sensitive enteropathy was first described by Marks and colleagues in 1966, and gluten sensitivity is now thought to play a role in its pathogenesis.

In 1971, Cormane and Gianetti recognized the presence of immunoglobulins in the skin, suggesting an immune pathogenesis. Since then, the granular deposition of IgA in the papillary tips has become the diagnostic hallmark of DH and a focus of investigation. A strong association with human leukocyte antigen (HLA)-B8, HLA-DR3, and HLA-DQ2 was recognized in the mid-1970s, indicating a genetic basis for DH immune disorder (McCord and Hall, 1993).

Clinical Features

DH in children occurs most often between 2 and 7 years of age. The cutaneous eruption in children is similar to that in adults, with red papules or papulovesicles and an intense burning or stinging itch that leads to rapid excoriation of lesions. The lesions are often grouped and distributed symmetrically over extensor areas including elbows, knees, buttocks, upper back, posterior neck, and scalp (Fig. 32-1). Small hemorrhagic papules and vesicles of the palms and soles are present in most patients (Rabinowitz and Esterly, 1993). Mucous membrane involvement rarely occurs.

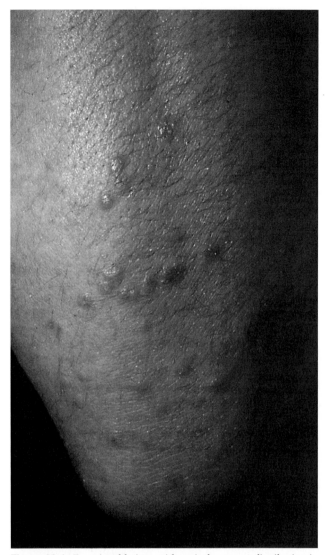

Figure 32-1 · Excoriated lesions with typical extensor distribution in a patient with dermatitis herpetiformis. Although the primary lesions are vesicopapules, the patient may present with excoriated lesions because of the intense pruritus.

Gluten-sensitive enteropathy has been found in 75% to 90% of children with DH (Rabinowitz and Esterly, 1993; Zone, 1991). Signs of malabsorption are not usually present in children with the disease, but some may have chronic diarrhea and anemia. A gluten-free diet can induce remission of both the gastrointestinal and cutaneous lesions.

Pathogenesis

The strong association between gluten ingestion and the skin eruptions suggests an as yet obscure pathogenic relationship with the intestinal abnormality. Gluten may act as an antigen that stimulates circulating or local IgA antibodies, which bind to the skin as cross-reacting antibodies or as immune complexes. Alternatively, a gluten-induced intestinal defect may allow passage of other dietary antigens that initiate the development of circulating IgA antibodies, which subsequently bind to the skin (Zone, 1991, 1993).

Diagnosis

Clinical and routine histologic features overlap those of other immunologically mediated vesicobullous dermatoses such as LABD, BP, or epidermolysis bullosa acquisita (EBA). Accurate diagnosis necessitates direct IF studies of biopsy specimens, which show granular deposition of IgA in dermal papillary tips (Fig. 32-2). The biopsy specimen for IF must be from perilesional skin of typically affected areas.

Treatment and Prognosis

Institution of a gluten-free diet can lead to complete control of skin disease and reversal of intestinal abnormalities. This treatment requires strict adherence and

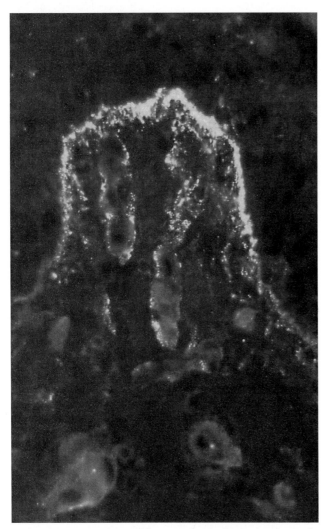

Figure 32-2 · Direct immunofluorescence of a biopsy specimen of a patient with dermatitis herpetiformis showing the characteristic granular deposition of IgA in the dermal papillary tips.

patience, because 1 to 2 years of a gluten-free diet may be necessary to obtain control (Rabinowitz and Esterly, 1993; Zone, 1991).

Alternatively, dapsone at a dosage of 1.5 to 2 mg/kg/day is effective and usually controls the symptoms and eruption within a few days of beginning therapy (Rabinowitz and Esterly, 1993). A combination of dapsone and a gluten-free diet may be used with either a decrease or discontinuance of the dapsone as the dietary regimen takes effect. Side effects of dapsone include dose-related hemolytic anemia; methemoglobinemia; and rare idiosyncratic effects, including agranulocytosis, neuropathy, and toxic hepatitis.

Typically, DH in adults is lifelong, with treatment-free remissions occurring in less than 1% of patients. Although the long-term prognosis for children is not clear, it is best to consider juvenile DH a lifelong disease.

Linear IgA/Bullous Dermatosis of Childhood

LABD, also known as *chronic bullous disease of childhood*, is a blistering cutaneous eruption that usually presents in preschool children. It is self-limited but lasts several years. The characteristic finding is the linear deposition of IgA along the basement membrane by IF studies of perilesional skin (Marsden, 1990). The exact incidence and prevalence of LABD are unknown because of its rarity. Cases are reported in both black and white children, and the frequency is the same in females and males.

History

LABD was initially considered a variant of DH because of shared histologic features. However, it has now been clearly differentiated from the latter, based on the linear IgA deposition in IF studies, absence of gluten-sensitive enteropathy, and HLA typing differences (McCord and Hall, 1993; Smith and Zone, 1993).

Clinical Features

Patients have large, tense bullae, either clear or hemorrhagic. These can arise on either normal skin or preexisting urticarial lesions. Sites of predilection are the lower abdomen, genital area, buttocks, face, and scalp. Other characteristic features include clustering of blisters and annular configurations of blisters encircling a crusted healing lesion, referred to as a "crown of jewels" or "rosette" (McCord and Hall, 1993; Rabinowitz and Esterly, 1993). The eruption may be mildly to markedly pruritic (Fig. 32-3).

Mucous membrane involvement is relatively common, in contrast to the situation in DH. Oral and ocular lesions are noted in a significant number of patients, and conjunctival scarring has been identified. Patients do not have an associated gluten-sensitive enteropathy, in contrast to those with childhood DH. Some, but not

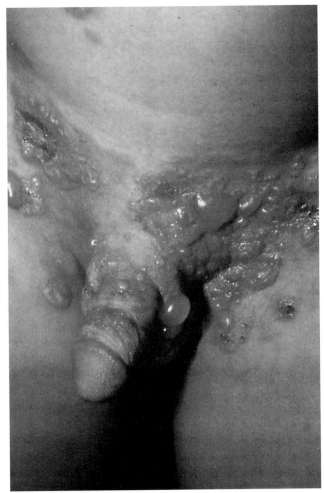

Figure 32-3· Tense blisters with an annular configuration in a patient with linear IgA/bullous dermatosis.

when mucous membrane changes predominate, the disease can resemble cicatricial pemphigoid. Histologic study shows a subepidermal blister with a neutrophilic infiltrate, often indistinguishable from DH. Direct IF studies are diagnostic and the most reliable means of establishing a diagnosis (Marsden, 1990; Rabinowitz and Esterly, 1993; Smith and Zone, 1993). The characteristic finding is linear deposition of IgA along the basement membrane zone of perilesional skin. In addition, a circulating IgA anti-basement membrane zone antibody is present in 31% to 72% of patients.

Treatment and Prognosis

Patients usually respond to dapsone at dosages of 1.5 to 2.0 mg/kg/day. If improvement is not satisfactory, the addition of either sulfapyridine or small amounts of systemic corticosteroids may be helpful. Topical steroids are generally ineffective. Topical antipruritics or systemic antihistamines may provide symptomatic relief. LABD is a self-limited disease, usually resolving after 2 to 3 years.

Pemphigus Vulgaris

Three other rare immunobullous diseases of adults are occasionally seen in children. The first of these is pemphigus vulgaris (PV), a serious chronic, intraepidermal bullous dermatosis with autoantibodies directed against antigens on the surface of epidermal cells. It affects both the mucosa and skin, producing flaccid blisters that may be limited in extent or generalized with large areas of denuded skin.

Patients with active PV typically have a positive Nikolsky sign (i.e., generation of a blister by displacement of perilesional skin by friction). Patients with widespread disease are subject to fluid and electrolyte imbalances, are susceptible to cutaneous and systemic infection, and often require inpatient management. The presentation in children does not differ significantly from that in adults; however, diagnosis in children has been delayed for months to years because the index of suspicion is low for pemphigus in a young child. PV should be included in the differential diagnosis in children with chronic mucous membrane erosions.

Biopsy specimens of oral or cutaneous bullae or erosions characteristically show suprabasilar acantholysis, a diagnostic pathologic finding in pemphigus. Direct IF shows deposition of both IgG and C3 in the epidermal intercellular spaces. Furthermore, circulating autoantibodies are detected in most patients.

Management of PV depends on the degree of severity. Mild localized lesions may respond to topical corticosteroids; however, more severe disease necessitates the use of systemic corticosteroids. Intravenous immune globulin has also been reported to be effective, possibly by downregulating production of interleukin (IL)-1α and IL-1β and enhancing production of interleukin-1 receptor antagonist (IL-1Ra) (Bhol et al., 2001).

all, studies suggest that there may be an increased frequency of HLA-B8 in these patients, but there is no increased frequency of HLA-DR3 and HLA-DQ2 as there is in DH (McCord and Hall, 1993; Rabinowitz and Esterly, 1993).

Pathogenesis

LABD is thought to be an autoimmune process mediated by IgA autoantibodies directed against a basement membrane antigen of skin. Immunoelectron microscopy reveals two patterns of IgA deposition: one with immunoglobulin deposition in the sublamina densa and the other with deposition of immunoglobulin within the lamina lucida (Rabinowitz and Esterly, 1993; Smith and Zone, 1993). There are no clinical differences related to the two immunoelectron microscopic findings.

Diagnosis

Clinically, LABD has a heterogeneous presentation and may be confused with other immunologically mediated blistering skin diseases such as BP or DH. Occasionally,

Bullous Pemphigoid

BP is an autoimmune bullous disorder characterized by tense subepidermal blisters typically occurring in elderly patients. Childhood cases are rare, but BP has been reported in infants 2 months of age. Most childhood cases occur before 8 years of age. BP is manifest as tense blisters arising either on an urticarial base or on normal skin. The blisters heal without scarring. Clinical features of the disease are similar in adults and children. Mucous membrane lesions are more common in children. Lesions of the palms and soles may occur in children younger than 1 year (Rabinowitz and Esterly, 1993).

Histologically, subepidermal blister formation with a dermal inflammatory infiltrate heavily mixed with eosinophils is seen. Direct IF shows linear deposition of IgG and C3 on the basement membrane. As with pemphigus, systemic corticosteroids are often necessary. Sulfones, such as dapsone and sulfapyridine, are alternatives. Sporadic reports of benefit from treatment of both pemphigus and pemphigoid with intravenous immunoglobulin (IVIG) suggest that this may provide adjunctive steroid-sparing value in various autoimmune blistering diseases (Beckers et al., 1995).

Epidermolysis Bullosa Acquisita

EBA is another subepidermal blistering disease that usually occurs in adults. However, several well-documented cases in children have been reported (Rabinowitz and Esterly, 1993). Cases beginning in children as young as 3 months have been noted.

EBA, like pemphigus and BP, is an autoimmune disorder mediated by antibodies to type VII collagen. The cutaneous eruption classically presents as noninflammatory blistering with skin fragility. The blisters and erosions, which are usually localized to acral and extensor surfaces, heal with atrophic scarring and milia. Nail dystrophy and scarring alopecia may also occur. The similarity of EBA to inherited epidermolysis bullosa accounts for its name.

Affected children, like affected adults, have, on routine histologic examination, subepidermal blister formation with a dermal inflammatory infiltrate significantly mixed with neutrophils. Direct IF shows linear deposition of IgG along the basement membrane, as found in BP; indirect IF (on salt split-skin substrates) can help differentiate the two diseases.

EBA in adults is generally refractory to therapy. In contrast, the childhood disease responds fairly well to the combination of prednisone and dapsone (Rabinowitz and Esterly, 1993). The long-term prognosis is uncertain.

LUPUS ERYTHEMATOSUS

Cutaneous Lupus Erythematosus

The cutaneous manifestations of LE include (1) acute cutaneous lupus; (2) chronic cutaneous lupus, also referred to as discoid LE (DLE); (3) subacute cutaneous LE; and (4) neonatal LE (Rothfield, 1993). Acute cutaneous lupus is similar in adults and children and is associated with active systemic lupus. The systemic manifestations usually overshadow the cutaneous changes. The most characteristic feature is the facial butterfly erythema; however, similar changes may extend to the upper extremities and trunk. These changes are typically transient and improve as the systemic disease is brought under control (see Chapter 35).

The most common form of chronic cutaneous LE is DLE. Other variants include lupus panniculitis and hypertrophic DLE. The cutaneous findings in children and adults are similar (Hurwitz, 1981). Red papules and plaques with scaling and prominent follicular hyperkeratosis occur. The lesions expand and heal with central scarring and pigmentary change and, when present in the scalp, can lead to permanent alopecia. They are mostly distributed over the face, scalp, and ears. DLE can be confused with polymorphous light eruption, lymphocytic infiltrate of Jessner, rosacea, sarcoid, granuloma faciale, and lichen planus. A skin biopsy is helpful in establishing the diagnosis.

Chronic cutaneous lupus can occur as an isolated manifestation of LE or as one feature of the systemic disease. Only 5% of adults with discoid lupus develop systemic disease, whereas in children there is a greater tendency for systemic involvement (George and Tunnessen, 1993). Other features unique to childhood DLE are lack of female preponderance and lower incidence of photosensitivity.

Subacute cutaneous LE is a recently recognized entity that presents as either papulosquamous or annular lesions with a prominent photodistribution (Lee, 1993). The lesions, in contrast to those in discoid lupus, do not scar. Most patients with subacute cutaneous lupus have relatively mild systemic involvement, and the skin disease is the greatest problem.

Neonatal Lupus Erythematosus

Neonatal LE is an uncommon autoimmune disease occurring in the neonatal period in which the major findings are nonscarring skin lesions and congenital heart block (see Chapter 35). Mothers of infants with neonatal lupus usually have anti-Ro/SS-A autoantibodies that cross the placenta into the infant and contribute to the pathogenesis of the disease (Watson and Provost, 1987). This disorder is also discussed in Chapter 35.

History

McCuistion and Schoch (1954) first reported LE in a newborn and hypothesized that a maternal factor passing transplacentally caused the eruption. In the early 1980s, Weston and colleagues (1982) identified the anti-Ro/SS-A autoantibody as a serologic marker of neonatal LE. Subsequently, it was recognized that many infants with congenital heart block had anti-Ro/SS-A autoantibodies.

Clinical Manifestations

About half of the infants with neonatal LE have cutaneous lesions and half have congenital heart block, but rarely do the two occur together. Liver disease and thrombocytopenia with petechiae or purpura are uncommon features. Liver disease and thrombocytopenia are generally not present at birth but develop a few weeks after birth and resolve within a few more weeks.

The cutaneous lesions are scaling, erythematous plaques and patches that lack the follicular plugging of DLE. They resolve without scarring or atrophy but may show residual hypopigmentation. The lesions are most often distributed over the face and scalp, particularly in periorbital and forehead areas, and are commonly exacerbated by sunlight. Less often, they occur in photoprotected areas such as the diaper area. Lesions are transient, typically appearing several weeks after birth or less often at birth, and resolve by 6 months of age (McCuistion and Schoch, 1954). Postinflammatory hypopigmentation may take months to resolve, and occasionally, persistent telangiectasias have been observed.

Complete heart block in neonatal LE begins during gestation as early as the 16th week (Lee, 1993; Watson and Provost, 1987). Although other cardiac problems are not usually present, patent ductus arteriosus has been reported in a few cases. Suspicion of heart block might arise during a routine obstetric examination with detection of a slow fetal heart rate. Diagnosis of heart block can be confirmed by fetal ultrasonography. The heart block is due to fibrosis and calcification of the conduction system that involves the atrioventricular node and also affects the sinoatrial node in some cases. Because the pathologic change is fibrosis, the heart block is generally permanent.

Pathogenesis

Several observations support the hypothesis that anti-Ro/SS-A autoantibodies are involved in the pathogenesis of neonatal LE (Lee, 1993). First, these autoantibodies are regularly present in the serum of mothers of babies with neonatal lupus. Second, these IgG autoantibodies can pass through the placenta and into the child's serum. Third, the infant's skin lesions begin to resolve as the maternal autoantibodies diminish and disappear. Furthermore, IgG antibodies have been shown to be present in neonatal lupus lesions. Particulate deposits of IgG have been demonstrated in the epidermis in skin lesions and in the conduction system in myocardium of affected cardiac tissue. A similar pattern was demonstrated in human skin grafted to immunodeficient mice after passive transfer of both sera from mothers of infants with neonatal lupus and purified Ro autoantibodies, suggesting that the particulate deposits of IgG are due to anti-Ro/SS-A autoantibodies.

It is not clear why some infants develop skin disease and others present only with cardiac disease. The antibody specificities in these two groups are not significantly different. Genetic factors may play a role in the disease. The mothers of infants with neonatal lupus

have an increased incidence of HLA-B8 and HLA-DR3 antigens. Sex steroids may be important because cutaneous lesions of neonatal LE are three times more common in female than in male infants. Of interest, there is no sexual predilection for the heart block.

Sun exposure may potentiate or initiate the skin lesions but is not essential because they occur in photoprotected areas and at birth.

Diagnosis

Clinical findings, serologic findings, skin biopsy results, and cardiac evaluation are all important in establishing a diagnosis of neonatal LE. If a diagnosis of neonatal lupus is suspected, the sera of mother and infant should be evaluated for autoantibodies. In about 95% of the cases, anti-Ro/SS-A autoantibodies are detected (Lee, 1993; Watson and Provost, 1987). Anti-La/SS-B antibodies are also present in many patients. A few patients with only anti-U_1-RNP autoantibodies have been reported. Characteristic clinical findings in association with the presence of either anti-Ro/SS-A, anti-La/SS-B, or anti-U_1-RNP antibodies strongly suggest the diagnosis of neonatal LE.

A skin biopsy showing vacuolar changes along the epidermal junction with sparse lymphohistiocytic infiltrate can confirm the diagnosis. IF studies show particulate deposition of IgG in epidermal cells.

During gestation, a slow heart rate may be detected on routine obstetric examination and confirmed by ultrasonography and postnatal electrocardiography. Blood and liver tests should also be done.

Treatment and Prognosis

Management of skin disease includes protection from and avoidance of sun exposure and nonfluorinated low-potency topical steroids. Because the skin changes are transient and nonscarring, more aggressive treatment is not indicated.

Treatment of cardiac disease may not be necessary but, if indicated, consists of pacemaker implantation. Systemic steroids can be considered when heart failure ensues.

The skin lesions generally heal by 6 months of age without scarring or atrophy, although persistent telangiectasias have been noted in some patients. Pigmentary change may take months to resolve.

Despite a markedly decreased heart rate, about half the infants with heart block related to neonatal LE do not need treatment and the other half require pacemaker placement. A small number fail to respond to pacemaker placement, presumably because of myocardial disease.

Children with congenital heart block who survive infancy generally have a good prognosis regardless of organ system involvement. Rarely, some children develop cardiac rhythm disturbances or congestive heart failure during later childhood. The long-term outlook is unknown, but there are occasional reports of connective tissue disease arising in adulthood.

About half the mothers of infants with neonatal lupus are asymptomatic at the time of delivery. However, at 5 years after delivery, 86% of the mothers had either symptoms of Sjögren's disease (Lee, 1993) or a diagnosis of systemic LE (SLE) or subacute cutaneous LE.

REACTIVE ERYTHEMAS

The reactive erythemas are a diverse group of cutaneous immunologic disorders representing varied host reactions to various antigenic stimuli. In some cases, the different patterns may occur together or occur at different times in the chronology of the process, suggesting that some of these conditions have similar causes or pathogenic mechanisms. Many of the disorders are associated with urticaria. Also, although certain of the reactive erythemas are associated with certain drugs (e.g., EM with sulfonamides), specific inflammatory diseases (e.g., erythema marginatum with rheumatic fever), or infections (e.g., erythema chronicum migrans with Lyme disease), virtually any of the reaction patterns may be triggered by any antigen.

Erythema Multiforme and Stevens-Johnson Syndrome

EM is an acute, self-limited mucocutaneous eruption, occurring as a cutaneous response to a variety of triggering agents. The disease is usefully classified into two forms: EM minor and EM major (e.g., the Stevens-Johnson syndrome) (Huff, 1991). EM minor affects primarily cutaneous surfaces, especially acral areas, with limited mucous membrane involvement. EM major is the more severe form, with evolution of lesions to bullae, extensive mucosal erosions, and marked constitutional symptoms.

History

Although the cutaneous eruptions of EM have been recognized for centuries, von Hebra in 1866 first used the term and recognized the multiform rash as it evolved from papules to target lesions. Subsequently, patients with severe mucosal involvement and skin changes similar to those of EM minor were reported by Stevens and Johnson in 1922. This is now considered a more severe variant of EM and is commonly referred to as the *Stevens-Johnson syndrome*.

Clinical Manifestations

EM minor most often occurs in young adults, but approximately 20% of cases occur in children, usually in preteen or adolescent patients. The disease is rare in infants. The course and evolution of lesions in children are similar to those in adults. EM minor is relatively common, slightly more frequent in males, and without a racial predilection. Recurrent episodes are common,

occurring in about half of cases. Seasonal outbreaks are common (Huff, 1993).

Stevens-Johnson syndrome is much less common than EM minor. One survey of hospitalized patients found an annual incidence of 1 to 10 cases per million. In contrast to EM minor, EM major occurs at any age but is more likely to occur in the pediatric population, particularly in the second decade (Huff, 1993).

A clinical prodrome is absent in most patients with EM minor. The primary lesions begin as red macules, which rapidly evolve into papules that may itch or burn. These may extend to form small plaques that clear centrally to produce annular lesions. The plaques may develop central duskiness surrounded by concentric zones of red to pink, producing the target or iris lesion, the hallmark of EM. Lesions are typically distributed symmetrically and most prominently over the distal extremities. In EM minor, the mucosal changes are limited to the mouth and present as discrete erosions with erythematous borders, often accompanied by cervical lymphadenopathy (Fritsch and Elias, 1993; Huff, 1993).

EM major is commonly preceded by fever, headache, and malaise. Mucous membrane and skin lesions begin abruptly, and cutaneous lesions may initially resemble those of EM minor but evolve quickly into large areas of tender erythema and blisters. The blisters usually break, leaving extensive, denuded, tender erosions involving from 10% to 90% of the body surface. Mucosal involvement is generally severe and usually involves at least two sites. Most patients have oral, mucosal, lip, and eye lesions. Mucosal changes include bullae that rupture to leave painful erosions, swelling, and hemorrhagic crusting. Ocular lesions are painful and manifest as erythema, erosions, and purulent conjunctivitis (Fritsch and Elias, 1993; Huff, 1993).

Pathogenesis

For years, it has been postulated that EM is a hypersensitivity reaction to a variety of precipitating factors. The association between preceding herpes simplex virus (HSV) infection and EM is well established, and HSV infection is probably the most common precipitating cause of EM minor (Huff, 1993). The HSV-associated reaction typically occurs between 3 and 21 days after an episode of HSV infection and often recurs. Other factors associated with outbreaks of EM include infectious mononucleosis, tuberculosis, histoplasmosis, coccidioidomycosis, *Yersinia* infections, vaccinia, and x-ray therapy.

Immunocytochemical studies indicate that the dermal infiltrate in EM consists primarily of T lymphocytes, with both helper and suppressor subsets present. Keratinocytes may express class II histocompatibility antigens, which they do not do constitutively. This suggests that lymphocyte-produced interferon-γ (IFN-γ) has activated the keratinocytes. This information, together with the finding of HSV antigens and nucleic acids in keratinocytes of the lesions, suggests that a cellular immune response to HSV antigens within the epidermis is responsible for the final lesion production in EM.

The best-documented precipitating factors of the Stevens-Johnson syndrome are drugs, mycoplasmal infections, and HSV infections (Fritsch and Elias, 1993). Drugs commonly involved include sulfonamides, anticonvulsants, and nonsteroidal anti-inflammatory agents. Similar to the hypothesis put forth for EM minor, it has been proposed that an antigen from either a drug or an infectious agent localizes at the mucocutaneous site of the eruption and a cell-mediated immune response causes the tissue damage.

Diagnosis

Proposed criteria for the diagnosis of EM minor (Huff, 1993) include the following:

· A self-limited illness not lasting more than 4 weeks
· Fixed discrete lesions lasting at least 7 days
· Some lesions with characteristic features of target lesions
· Minimal or no mucosal involvement
· Compatible histology

Atypical urticaria is most often confused with EM, but urticaria is much more transient and is histologically distinct.

Stevens-Johnson syndrome with severe mucous membrane involvement can resemble other immunologically mediated blistering diseases such as PV, BP, and paraneoplastic pemphigus. Direct IF studies of biopsy specimens are important in differentiating these conditions.

There is overlap between EM major and toxic epidermal necrolysis (TEN) (see later discussion); some believe that the latter is a more severe form of EM major. Acute severe graft-versus-host disease can also resemble Stevens-Johnson syndrome. History and routine histology can usually distinguish these two entities.

Treatment

Episodes of EM minor can be so mild that only symptomatic treatment is necessary. It is important to identify and eliminate potential precipitating factors. In recurrent cases secondary to HSV infection, prophylactic acyclovir prevents most episodes of recurrent HSV and EM (Huff, 1993). There is no good evidence that systemic steroids are of value in treating this condition.

EM major can be associated with severe complications, including sepsis, fluid and electrolyte imbalances, and pneumonia. Consideration of care in a burn unit is appropriate for those having large denuded areas of the skin. Cultures of skin erosions, mouth, blood, and sputum are important, as is meticulous fluid and electrolyte balance monitoring. Ophthalmologic consultation should be sought promptly to help manage ocular complications.

It is essential to discontinue any potential causative medications or treat underlying infections. Although some authors have suggested early use of systemic corticosteroids while new lesions are still evolving, there

have been no controlled studies of systemic steroids in the treatment of Stevens-Johnson syndrome (Eichenfield and Honig, 1991). Meticulous wound care, careful fluid and electrolyte therapy, good ophthalmologic care, and avoidance of systemic corticosteroids can lead to good outcomes (Prendiville et al., 1989). The use of systemic corticosteroids in patients with extensive skin erosions can increase the risk of infection and prolong the hospital stay.

Reports during the past decade have described the use of IVIG for treatment of Stevens-Johnson syndrome (Amato et al., 1992; Moudgil et al., 1995) and the dramatic demonstration of therapeutic benefit of IVIG for TEN (Viard et al., 1998) has led to increasing use of this modality (Brett et al., 2001; Morici et al., 2000).

Prognosis

EM minor typically has a course of 1 to 4 weeks and resolves without sequelae. About half the patients have recurrent episodes, often associated with HSV infections. EM major has a more prolonged course, lasting 3 to 4 weeks. Mucosal erosions may heal with scarring, including ocular scarring. Scarring can lead to esophageal and anal strictures and vaginal or urethral stenosis. Skin lesions usually heal without sequelae; however, permanent loss of nails may occur.

Toxic Epidermal Necrolysis

TEN defies precise categorization but at times may resemble Stevens-Johnson syndrome, both morphologically and in clinical course. TEN, or *Lyell's syndrome,* is an abrupt onset, often overwhelming condition in which the epidermis separates from the dermis in sheets. The net effect is similar to a second-degree burn, and similarly, the condition is often fatal. TEN is generally found to be drug-induced, in contrast to the scalded skin syndrome, which is related to staphylococcal toxins similar to those in the toxic shock syndrome. Although the ultimate appearance of TEN is similar to scalded skin, the condition often begins as a dusky, deep erythema. Epidermal detachment follows quickly and histology shows full epidermal necrolysis.

Studies in the past decade indicated that this was the result of apoptotic keratinocyte death (Paul et al., 1996; Roujeau and Stern, 1994). One mechanism for apoptosis is activation of the cell surface death receptor, Fas (CD95). Viard and co-workers demonstrated high levels of soluble Fas ligand in the serum of TEN patients (Viard et al., 1998). They then showed that keratinocytes from TEN patients expressed large amounts of Fas ligand, which was lytic for Fas-sensitive cells, and that the lytic reaction was inhibited by blocking antibodies. They then used treatment with IVIG and showed rapid reversal of the necrolysis and clinical healing in patients with TEN (Viard et al., 1998). They suggest that treatment with IVIG in doses from 0.2 to 0.75 g/kg body weight may be the treatment of choice for these patients, in whom no other form of therapy has previously been available other than supportive care in a burn unit.

Erythema Annulare Centrifugum

Figurative Erythemas

The figurate erythemas are a poorly defined, descriptive group of erythematous lesions caused by reaction to unknown antigens that have in common a lymphocytic inflammatory infiltrate around vessels in the upper and middle dermis. Most of the lesions are annular (but occasionally irregular or gyrate), multiple, chronic, and remitting. As with chronic urticaria, a cause is seldom identified, but patients should be assessed for an antigenic source for the reactive lesions. Infections, drugs, autoimmune diseases, and malignancies have all been associated with cases of figurate erythemas.

Erythema annulare centrifugum is the most common of the figurate erythemas. The appearance can vary considerably depending on the acuteness and intensity of the process, the depth of blood vessels affected, and the degree of involvement of the epidermis. The lesions range from the initial and transient pink indurated papules to annules with central clearing and often a trailing collarette of scale. This latter appearance can resemble that of tinea, which is easily ruled out with potassium hydroxide (KOH) examination. The rings are multiple, sometimes generalized, sometimes clustered over only one area. Erythema annulare centrifugum may appear at any age, including the newborn period (Fried et al., 1957). Lesions are usually chronic or recurring and may continue for years. They can be quite dynamic, enlarging over days to weeks and then fading while others appear. Itching is variable but is seldom severe.

The cause is obscure, but reactions to fungal infections are probably the most common associations. The immunologic nature of these lesions can occasionally be demonstrated when intradermal trichophytin antigen reproduces the process, resulting in an enlarging annular lesion that can continue for weeks (Champion, 1992). *Candida* infections, ingestion of blue cheese, carcinomas, lymphomas, drugs, and a variety of bacterial and viral infections have been reported in association with erythema annulare centrifugum (Troy and Goetz, 1991).

In addition to dermatophytosis, the differential diagnosis includes granuloma annulare, mycosis fungoides, sarcoid, LE, and leprosy.

Management is aimed primarily at eliminating the suspected antigen. Topical corticosteroids can reduce the inflammation of the superficial and scaly lesions. Prednisone controls the process but is rarely justified for such benign and minimally symptomatic lesions.

Erythema Marginatum

Erythema marginatum, classically associated with rheumatic fever, consists of superficial, macular, or urticarial erythemas in rings or ring segments that may coalesce into a polycyclic or reticular pattern (see Chapter 35). Typically, lesions are evanescent, appearing for a few hours in the afternoon, expanding rapidly, clearing centrally, and then fading, although some may last 2 to 3 days. Erythema marginatum occurs in 10% to 18% of patients with rheumatic fever and is considered specific (it is part of the Jones criteria) for rheumatic fever, although we have seen morphologically similar lesions associated with hepatitis B.

Erythema Chronicum Migrans

This annular erythema centered on the tick bite inoculation of *Borrelia burgdorferi* can be the cutaneous prodrome to Lyme disease (see Chapter 35). It differs from erythema annulare centrifugum because it is usually solitary and retains a central papulation at the bite site. Lesions usually occur on the extremities or trunk 4 to 20 days after the bite (Schachner and Hansen, 1988) and usually persist for 1 to 2 months. Treatment with penicillin, tetracycline, or amoxicillin may prevent the later development of Lyme disease, although the value of prophylaxis remains controversial (Shapiro et al., 1992).

HENOCH-SCHÖNLEIN PURPURA

HSP (also termed *anaphylactoid purpura* or *Henoch-Schönlein vasculitis*) is an illness affecting the skin, joints, gastrointestinal tract, kidneys, and in rare instances, central nervous system and other organs subject to hemorrhage (Allen et al., 1960; Hall, 1991; Jones and Callen, 1991). The condition can occur at any age but is more common in children, usually between 2 and 12 years of age. Symptoms typically appear suddenly and subside over 3 to 4 weeks, although they may recur in about 50% of patients and rarely persist or recur for years. Reflecting its diverse clinical manifestations, this disorder is also discussed in Chapters 33, 34, 35, and 38.

Clinical Features

The cutaneous manifestation of HSP is purpuric, usually palpable and symmetrical lesions arrayed over the buttocks and lower extremities. Lesions can appear in any site, and the earliest may be urticarial or petechial, evolving within hours to the typical palpable purpura. These gradually darken, flatten, and fade, usually within 2 weeks, leaving transient brownish pigmentation. Although skin lesions appear at some point in 100% of patients, the presenting complaint is cutaneous in only about 60%, and skin lesions may occur weeks after arthritic or gastrointestinal symptoms. In other cases, purpuric eruptions may be the only manifestation. In some patients, soft tissue swelling may occur over the head, extremities, or scrotum and may be quite painful. This edema is more common in younger children and is distinct from the joint manifestations that occur in up to 85% of children. The latter are limited to arthralgias and sometimes periarticular swelling. True inflammatory arthritis is uncommon, is self-limited, and leaves no joint damage.

Gastrointestinal symptoms occur in 70% to 95% of patients and include abdominal pain and vomiting (Jones and Callen, 1991). Evidence of gastrointestinal hemorrhage ranging from guaiac-positive stools to melena is seen in about 70% of cases. Occasional severe and even fatal manifestations such as hemorrhage and intussusception occur. It is important to consider HSP in any case of unexplained abdominal pain. Of the patients reported by Allen and colleagues (1960), 15% had severe pain before the development of purpura and many required laparotomy.

Renal disease occurs in about 30% of children (Crumb, 1976), usually in the first month (see Chapter 38). This is usually transient microscopic hematuria or proteinuria, but glomerulonephritis and renal failure occur. Of the 131 children studied by Allen and colleagues (1960), 6 developed severe renal disease and 2 died. In addition, 40% of those with acute renal disease had late renal findings not present initially. Thus all patients with HSP should have periodic urinalysis for 2 years after onset.

Pathology

Skin biopsy specimens show changes typical of leukocytoclastic vasculitis with perivascular neutrophilic infiltrate, erythrocyte extravasation, and nuclear debris. In some cases, epidermal necrosis and bulla formation are seen. Renal histopathology is highly variable, ranging from mild glomerular changes to proliferative glomerulonephritis. Immunopathologic studies first identified the presence of mesangial IgA deposits in more than 90% of renal biopsy specimens (Counahan and Cameron, 1977). This led to the demonstration of perivascular IgA deposits in 75% to 100% of lesional skin biopsy specimens and even in a high proportion of normal skin specimens from patients with HSP (Jones and Callen, 1991). These findings, along with the similarity of skin biopsy features to those of the Arthus reaction, have suggested that HSP is caused by deposition of circulating IgA immune complexes.

Treatment

Most cases of HSP resolve spontaneously. Systemic corticosteroids may improve joint and gastrointestinal symptoms but do not appear to affect the skin or renal disease. No controlled studies of corticosteroid therapy, other immunosuppressive agents, or plasmapheresis are available. Aspirin should be avoided because it may increase gastrointestinal hemorrhage.

ATOPIC DERMATITIS

Definition

AD (eczema) is a chronic inflammatory disease characterized by erythema, papulation, and intense itching, often accompanied by excoriations, lichenification, weeping, and crusting (see Chapter 31). It usually begins in infancy, and 95% of cases begin within the first 5 years of age. The disorder is extremely common, and the incidence has increased from 3% in 1950 to an estimated 7% to 17% of infants more recently (Laughter et al., 2000). The disease appears to affect all races, although Asians may have the greatest susceptibility.

This multifactorial condition may not appear while individuals live in rural or underdeveloped areas but may become manifest when the genetically susceptible person moves to an urban local (Shultz Larsen and Hanifin, 2002). Environmental pollution, psychologic stress, and excess exposure to antigens may exacerbate the disease in susceptible individuals. AD is also associated with asthma, and persons with AD often have methacholine-reactive airways, which suggests a predisposition to asthma (Barker et al., 1991).

The natural course of AD is one of gradual improvement. Complete clearing occurs in approximately 40% of patients observed over periods from 15 to 25 years (Musgrove and Morgan, 1976), but children with severe AD often have persistent disease.

Pathogenesis

AD and other atopic conditions, including IgE reactivity to specific antigens, are transferred by bone marrow transplantation; this provides strong evidence for a basic defect in hematopoietic cells rather than in the skin (Agosti et al., 1988). Conversely, transplantation of normal marrow corrects the AD of the Wiskott-Aldrich syndrome (Saurat, 1985). A genetic basis for AD is well established, based on the strong familial association and the high concordance rate in monozygotic twins (Schultz Larsen et al., 1986). The mode of inheritance is not consistent and may display autosomal dominant, autosomal recessive, and multifactorial inheritance patterns.

Gene mapping studies have led to identification of positive loci for AD at chromosome positions 3q21, 1p22, and 19p13 (Lee et al., 2000). Interestingly, a variety of other inflammatory or autoimmune diseases, including asthma, psoriasis, Crohn's disease, celiac disease, SLE, rheumatoid arthritis, type 1 diabetes, and multiple sclerosis, have been mapped to loci within 10 cM of the three identified in AD (Becker and Barnes, 2001). These findings suggest the possibility that different inflammatory diseases may share common defective immune regulatory pathways. HLA associations have shown no consistent patterns.

Two other generalizations can be made about AD: (1) patients have abnormal immune responses, and

(2) they have a number of pharmacophysiologic abnormalities (Hanifin, 1986). Immunologic abnormalities include IgE overproduction and altered cell-mediated immune responses. Serum IgE levels are elevated in 80% of patients with AD, but it is important to recognize the crucial 20% exception; the latter patients have normal serum IgE levels, negative radioallergosorbent tests (RASTs) and skin tests, and no asthma or allergic rhinoconjunctivitis (Hanifin and Lobitz, 1977). Thus IgE reactivity may simply be an epiphenomenon without true pathogenic importance.

Similar caution may avoid overinterpreting the high IL-4 production in AD (Chan et al., 1993). This cytokine, produced by type 2 T-helper cells (Th2 cells), is an important regulator of IgE synthesis and may well contribute to the excessive IgE production in atopic conditions. Th2 cells also produce IL-5, which regulates eosinophils, an important component of the inflammatory infiltrate in AD (Leiferman et al., 1985). In addition to Th2 cells and eosinophils, abnormal control of cytokine production and perhaps IgE synthesis may originate with atopic monocytes. These cells have abnormal cyclic nucleotide metabolism because of elevated phosphodiesterase (PDE) hydrolysis of cyclic adenosine monophosphate (cAMP), providing a functional state that encourages hyperresponsiveness of multiple cell types (Hanifin and Chan, 1995).

Likewise, studies have shown increased antigen-presenting capabilities of epidermal Langerhans cells (Maurer and Stingl, 1995), which, along with atopic monocytes, express high-affinity FcRI receptors. Thus the elevated IgE may enhance cellular immune responses to environmental antigens such as dust mites, animal proteins, pollens, and foods.

A consequence of inflammatory activity in the skin is breakdown in the function of the stratum corneum barrier. Trautmann and associates (2000) demonstrated that spongiosis in both atopic and allergic contact dermatitis results from keratinocyte apoptosis induced by T-cell–liberated Fas ligand. The resulting barrier defect allows for ingress of antigens, which stimulate 100- to 1000-fold greater IgE production than antigens introduced via mucosal routes. This suggests that the reason for the very high levels of IgE reactivity in AD may be secondary to inadequate stratum corneum protection. These perceptions also indicate the need for rapid effective therapy of eczematous skin at the earliest possible age.

Clinical Features

Pruritus is the cardinal symptom of AD. Many have paraphrased Jacqet's dictum that "atopic dermatitis is the itch that rashes rather than the rash that itches" (Rajka, 1989), although in reality erythematous inflammation closely precedes the itching. Erythema, edema, papulation, and induration are the primary clinical features of acute AD. It is also characterized by repeated episodes of flaring, sometimes several times a day or sometimes once or twice a month.

The secondary clinical features include dryness, scaling, excoriation, weeping, and lichenification. All are caused by the inflammation and itching, resulting from intractable, involuntary scratching, rubbing, and slapping of the skin throughout the day and night. Individuals with pigmented skin such as blacks and Asians also present with perifollicular accentuation, giving the skin a pebbled appearance; they also tend to have more severely lichenified skin in areas of rubbing. On some occasions, urticarial-type lesions accompany the flares, but patients with atopy and AD have no increased tendency toward acute or chronic urticaria.

Many pigmentary effects of inflammation occur in patients with AD. These include postinflammatory hypopigmentation (i.e., pityriasis alba) or hyperpigmentation, sometimes reticulated or sometimes patchy and persistent. Occasionally, vitiliginous depigmentation also develops. Patients often refer to these pigmentary defects as "scars," but parents should be reassured that AD essentially never leads to true scarring.

Dry, cracked skin is a nearly universal finding in patients with AD; the only exceptions occur in tropical or other humid locales (Hanifin and Rajka, 1980; Rajka, 1989; Uehara and Miyauchi, 1984). In pure AD, without associated ichthyosis vulgaris, the dryness and scaling are simply manifestations of preceding inflammation. Ichthyosis is seen often in patients with AD and is best appreciated by finding the polygonal "fish scale" skin markings along with dryness and roughness over the anterior tibial areas (Rajka, 1989).

The fine, papular, keratotic lesions over the posterior arms, called *keratosis pilaris,* along with palmar hyperlinearity, are typical manifestations of ichthyosis vulgaris, although they are too often considered hallmarks of AD (Hanifin and Rajka, 1980). The relationship between ichthyosis vulgaris and AD is probably functional rather than genetic. The genetic susceptibility to atopy, combined with the defective stratum corneum barrier of ichthyosis, primes the inflammation of AD.

Dryness and scaling over the scalp are typical of AD, but the more greasy scale of seborrheic dermatitis (i.e., cradle cap) can also be a presenting feature, along with periauricular fissures and chapped lips (cheilitis). Hand eczema is a commonly associated condition in AD, even in childhood. Foot eczematoid dermatitis is often called *atopic foot, winter foot,* or *juvenile plantar dermatosis* (Fig. 32-4). By recognizing this entity one can avoid unnecessary treatment and diagnostic procedures based on misdiagnoses such as contact allergy or athlete's foot.

AD can affect any body region, but it is important to recognize that the diaper area is usually spared (Fig. 32-5) because the moisture maintains a soft, pliable stratum corneum barrier. Atopic infants are not impervious to diaper dermatitis, however. A large study comparing atopic and normal infants found a slightly increased incidence of diaper dermatitis in the former (Seymour et al., 1987).

Cutaneous infection is a frequent concomitant of AD. Staphylococcal infections are the most common, but patients may develop HSV, warts, and molluscum contagiosum (Hanifin and Lobitz, 1977). The increased susceptibility to infection is due to a mild immune deficit in

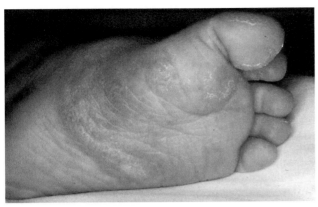

Figure 32-4· Juvenile plantar dermatosis, one of many manifestations of atopic dermatitis that may affect the foot.

the skin, heavy colonization with *Staphylococcus aureus,* and chronic excoriation. The colonization is lower in infants than in older patients (Seymour et al., 1987); the prevalence increases with age.

A practical management approach is to assume that infants and children with flaring or crusted or weeping lesions are infected and are best treated with systemic antibiotics. Such children usually have enlarged regional lymph nodes. Staphylococcal lesions in AD tend to be superficial and usually arise on the extremities or around the head and neck. These are important distinctions from the findings in hyper-IgE syndrome or other immunodeficiency syndromes, in which the patients typically have furuncles and other deep infections. Patients with AD have good resistance to sepsis and other invasive bacterial infections.

Treatment

Therapy of AD begins with prompt attention to the dry skin and the constant need for barrier protection through use of moisturizers. Good management also necessitates recognition and reduction of exacerbating

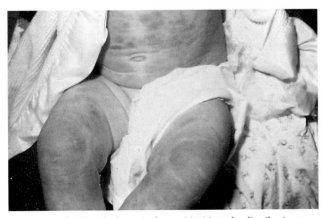

Figure 32-5· Lichenified atopic dermatitis. Note the distribution over the extensor surfaces and sparing of the well-hydrated diaper area.

factors. These "trigger" factors include infection, emotional stress, sweating or overheating, and allergens. Allergen avoidance is overemphasized and of questionable import for most eczematous children. The search for an allergen should not distract from basic management measures such as the use of moisturizing agents, antibiotics, and topical corticosteroids (Hanifin and Tofte, 1999).

Children and parents should be educated early about the need for immediate application of emollients after bathing. With that simple requisite, daily baths do no harm and in fact reduce infection and enhance corticosteroid effects. Topical steroids, usually triamcinolone 0.1% cream or ointment, should be applied twice daily to inflamed or flaring areas at the same time as emollients are used on noninflamed skin areas. When inflammation is controlled, topical steroids should be tapered to twice weekly to prevent steroid skin atrophy, although 1% hydrocortisone can be used more often.

If the eczema cannot be controlled with safe, intermittent topical corticosteroids, the newly introduced topical calcineurin inhibitors (IVIG, tacrolimus, pimecrolimus) should be used. These agents have shown excellent efficacy and they appear to be safe, even in studies of 1 to 4 years' duration (Kang et al., 2001). For children whose dermatitis cannot be controlled with topical agents, systemic medications such as cyclosporin A, methotrexate, IFN-γ, or IVIG should be considered (Sidbury and Hanifin, 2000). Oral antibiotics, usually cephalosporin, should be used for 5 days and repeated immediately whenever flaring associated with infection recurs.

When the child does not respond to this regimen or continues to have flares, allergen avoidance measures should be considered. Unfortunately, allergen identification is imprecise. Careful history and a 1-week restriction of the most suspect foods, including the high-probability foods (eggs, dairy products, peanuts, soy, wheat, and fish) (Sampson and McCaskill, 1985), while optimizing therapy may provide stability; then one food can be added back each day (if there has been no history of anaphylaxis).

If this approach does not induce remission, allergy tests are indicated, but the parents should be cautioned that a positive RAST or skin test will show false-positive results up to 80% of the time (Sampson and Albergo, 1984) and do not prove that the allergens causing the positive skin test cause the disease. Foods that trigger serious reactions usually are recognized by parents and then avoided, obviating the need for medical help. Double-blind challenge tests in highly selected patients indicate that temporary itching and rash can develop (Sampson and McCaskill, 1985), but such challenges are more likely to be urticarial rather than eczematous.

Food-induced eczema is extremely rare and represents less than 1% of the cases. The physician should be alert for the occasional undetected food allergy but never at the expense of proper general skin therapy or good nutrition.

ALLERGIC CONTACT DERMATITIS

Clinical Features

Allergic contact dermatitis is relatively uncommon in childhood, although not because of lack of sensitizing capability. Infants can be sensitized to the *Rhus* pentadecacatechol antigen even in the newborn period (Epstein, 1961). This highly antigenic moiety of poison ivy and poison oak (*Toxicodendron* species) plants is probably the most common cause of allergic contact dermatitis in both children and adults (see Chapter 31).

The acute form of allergic contact dermatitis presents as erythematous papulation or vesiculation with oozing. Those with *Toxicodendron rhus* dermatitis often have linear streaks of vesiculation. The dermatitis is usually in areas of contact with plants; however, because it can be spread by pets, shoelaces, and clothing, the eruption may affect any body surface.

The chronic form of allergic contact dermatitis is indolent with mild erythema, scaling, and induration, usually well marginated but occasionally diffuse. This subacute or chronic dermatitis occurs as a result of repeated exposure to weaker chemical allergens and may be indistinguishable from AD. Typically, the cause of the dermatitis is evident and avoidance clears up the problem. However, when contact allergy is suspected but the allergen is unknown, patch testing with common contact allergens is necessary to make a diagnosis.

Pathogenesis

The immunologic basis for allergic contact dermatitis has been well delineated through experimental studies in animals. Allergic contact dermatitis involves a sensitization and an elicitation phase. The antigens are low-molecular-weight haptens that conjugate with proteins. These haptens have the ability to penetrate the epidermis and form strong covalent bonds with proteins. Lipid solubility of haptens also enhances sensitization capacity because it leads to better skin penetration.

The hapten–protein carrier complex is processed by Langerhans cells or other antigen-presenting cells (APCs) in the skin. The antigen-bearing Langerhans cells migrate into the dermis and initiate T-lymphocyte sensitization, either locally or in draining lymph nodes (Tron and Sauder, 1991). The sensitization process generally takes 9 to 21 days, but with very strong antigens, reactions can occur within 5 days. The elicitation phase occurs in 24 to 48 hours, hence the usual 48-hour duration for patch testing. Histologic features of allergic contact dermatitis are the same as those of any other form of eczema.

Diagnosis

The types of allergen exposure are infinite. A typical list of compounds tested, based on the most probable allergens encountered in North America, has been developed by the North American Contact Dermatitis Group and is shown in Table 32-1. In children, topically applied medications and skin care preparations may be the most common cause of contact allergy. These include benzocaine and other "caine" derivatives, neomycin, preservatives (e.g., parabens, ethylenediamine, thimerosal), fragrances, and balsam of Peru. Rubbers and glues, especially in footwear, are other common sensitizers. Nickel is a common sensitizing antigen because of its presence in earrings and other body-piercing jewelry in our society.

Patch testing involves the application of the suspected antigen to the skin of the back in a nonirritating form for 48 hours. Any adhesive plaster can be used, but most dermatologists now apply antigens under small aluminum disks called *Finn chambers* held in place with paper tape. Two readings are recommended, the first at 48 hours and the second 4 to 7 days after the application. Clearly positive reactions are easy to discern, but reactions are often ambiguous because of irritation or flaring of surrounding inflamed skin ("angry back" syndrome). If positive reactions are found, patients should be advised about the many cross-reacting substances present in the environment.

Treatment

Treatment consists of anti-inflammatory agents, usually medium-potency corticosteroid creams such as 0.1% triamcinolone, although this and 1% hydrocortisone cream are generally inadequate for controlling severe acute allergic contact dermatitis. In such cases, high-potency corticosteroids such as betamethasone propionate may be necessary. For severe widespread contact dermatitis, such as that in patients exposed to poison ivy or oak, systemic corticosteroids are required.

TABLE 32-1 · NORTH AMERICAN CONTACT DERMATITIS GROUP STANDARD ALLERGENS

1. Benzocaine 5% petrolatum
2. Mercaptobenzothiazole 1% petrolatum
3. Colophony 20% petrolatum
4. *p*-Phenylenediamine 1% petrolatum
5. Imidazolidinyl urea 2% aqueous
6. Cinnamic aldehyde 1% petrolatum
7. Lanolin alcohol 30% petrolatum
8. Carba mix 3% petrolatum
9. Neomycin sulfate 20% petrolatum
10. Thiuram mix 1% petrolatum
11. Formaldehyde 1% aqueous
12. Ethylenediamine dihydrochloride 1% petrolatum
13. Epoxy resin 1% petrolatum
14. Quaternium-15 2% petrolatum
15. *p-tert*-Butylphenol formaldehyde resin 1% petrolatum
16. Mercapto mix 1% petrolatum
17. Black rubber mix 0.6% petrolatum
18. Potassium dichromate 0.25% petrolatum
19. Balsam of Peru 25% petrolatum
20. Nickel sulfate 2.5% petrolatum

Data from Hermal, Inc., Delmar, New York.

Because reactions can last up to 3 weeks, a course of systemic corticosteroids tapering over a 2-week period may be necessary. Prednisone at 1 mg/kg/day in a single or twice-daily dose may be used for younger children. In adolescents and adults, a prednisone dosage of 1 to 2 mg/kg (e.g., 60 to 80 mg/day) is required to interrupt the severe inflammatory reaction. Pre-prepared steroid dose packs usually have an inadequate supply to cover the necessary duration of treatment. A simplified plan for a teenager might be prednisone at 60 mg/day for 7 days, followed by 30 mg/day for 7 days. For patients with severe dermatitis, wet dressings or cool baths may provide considerable relief.

Patients and parents must be educated about the need to wash all clothing and about other possible sources of exposure, including family pets, immediately when poison oak dermatitis is recognized. For prevention in patients repeatedly exposed to poison ivy or oak, Stokogard cream, which inactivates the antigen (Orchard et al., 1986), can be used; it is available at industrial supply retailers. If the skin is rinsed with water immediately after contact with the offending plants, the reaction can usually be averted. Encouraging avoidance through education, using pictures of the offending plants, is often helpful.

PSORIASIS

Psoriasis is a papulosquamous inflammatory disease, rare in childhood but common in adults at any age. Girls are affected more often than boys (Esterly and Kever, 1978), and a family history is noted in about 50% of cases. The pathogenesis of psoriasis is unknown; for years, faulty control of proliferating epidermal cells was suspected. More recently, immunologic aberration as the cause of psoriasis has been suggested (Cooper, 1990; Krueger, 1989). Langerhans cells and other APCs in the epidermis present stimulatory antigens (e.g., microbial products) in association with HLA-DR to specific T-cell receptors on the lymphocytes. Lymphokine production then leads to recruitment of increased numbers of APCs and increased T-cell activation. The lymphokines also stimulate epidermal proliferation and inflammation. Cyclosporine, methotrexate, and ultraviolet light may act on T cells, APCs, or keratinocytes to inhibit the inflammatory process.

Clinical Features

There are two general forms of psoriasis in children. The classic form appears over typical locations of elbows, knees, scalp, and presacrum. Slowly evolving erythematous papules coalesce into well-demarcated plaques overlain by white or silvery scale. Nail pitting and onycholysis are common.

The second form is eruptive, guttate psoriasis, which can appear explosively with profuse, small, round or oval lesions over the face, trunk, and proximal extremities. This may follow a streptococcal or other infection but can also be triggered by sunburn or systemic corticosteroid withdrawal. Guttate psoriasis may be of short duration, receding with resolution of infection. Alternatively, patients may progress to erythroderma or pustular psoriasis, necessitating hospitalization.

Infantile psoriasis may occur with the subtle onset of lesions in skin folds and periauricular and diaper areas and may be indistinguishable from seborrheic dermatitis. Psoriasis of the diaper region may also be confused with candidiasis or eczematous diaper dermatitis.

Treatment

Therapy for psoriasis varies, depending on the clinical form, location, extent, and intensity of inflammation. Topical corticosteroids are generally the first line of therapy, but for classic, plaque-type lesions the thickened epidermis may prevent adequate drug penetration, necessitating medium- to high-potency agents or the use of occlusive dressings. A reasonable first-line therapeutic agent is triamcinolone 0.1% ointment applied after the bath once or twice daily for 2 weeks. Prolonged use leads to atrophy, so careful monitoring is necessary.

Cessation of corticosteroid therapy usually leads to prompt rebound of psoriatic inflammation. Thus topical corticosteroid therapy should be combined with stabilizers such as tar preparations (e.g., 1% to 5% crude coal tar ointment, 5% to 15% liquor carbonis detergens [LCD]) or ultraviolet light therapy. With seborrheiform psoriasis or inverse psoriasis (affecting mainly folds and genitals), hydrocortisone 1% cream or ointment is safe and usually effective. Use of tar preparations in these areas can lead to worsening of inflammation. For the scalp, tar shampoos are quite helpful, and if necessary, twice-daily application of a low- to medium-potency corticosteroid solution is indicated.

Biologic agents have been used with promising results and minimal toxicity in severe psoriasis in adults. These target TNF-α (e.g., etanercept, infliximab) or memory T cells (efalizumab and alefacept) (Weinberg, 2003).

In guttate psoriasis, streptococcal infection should be treated with penicillin. Baths and topical corticosteroids are used initially. If the eruption becomes chronic or progresses, systemic therapy or methotrexate may be indicated.

CUTANEOUS MANIFESTATIONS OF PRIMARY IMMUNODEFICIENCIES

Various skin abnormalities have been described in children with a variety of immunodeficiency syndromes. Other than the thrombocytopenic purpura of Wiskott-Aldrich syndrome and mucocutaneous candidiasis, these are nonspecific (see Chapters 12 and 17). They include pyodermas, oral candidiasis, viral exanthems, and AD (Buckley et al., 1972; Hanifin and Lobitz, 1977). Typical AD occurs in Wiskott-Aldrich syndrome (Saurat, 1985) and in X-linked agammaglobulinemia (Peterson et al., 1962), and atypical eczematous lesions occur in other conditions (Hanifin, 1991; Hanifin and Rajka, 1980). Patients with hyperimmunoglobulinemia

E syndrome have coarse facial lesions, furuncles, and intertriginous lesions but seldom have AD (Peterson et al., 1962) (see Chapter 17).

R E F E R E N C E S

Agosti JM, Sprenger JD, Lum LG, Witherspoon RP, Fisher LD, Storb R, Henderson WR Jr. Transfer of allergen-specific IgE-mediated hypersensitivity with allogeneic bone marrow transplantation. N Engl J Med 319:1623–1628, 1988.

Allen DM, Diamond LK, Howell DA. Anaphylactoid purpura in children (Schönlein-Henoch syndrome). Am J Dis Child 99:833–853, 1960.

Amato GM, Travia A, Ziino O. The use of intravenous high-dose immunoglobulins (IVIG) in a case of Stevens-Johnson syndrome. Pediatr Med Chir 14:555–556, 1992.

Barker AF, Hirshman CA, D'Silva R, Hanifin JM. Airway responsiveness in atopic dermatitis. J Allergy Clin Immunol 87:780–783, 1991.

Becker KG, Barnes KC. Underlying disease specificity of genetic loci in atopic dermatitis. J Invest Dermatol 117:1325–1327, 2001.

Beckers RCY, Brand A, VerMeer BJ, Boom BW. Adjuvant high-dose intravenous gammaglobulin in the treatment of pemphigus and bullous pemphigoid: experience in six patients. Br J Dermatol 113:289–293, 1995.

Bhol KC, Desai S, Colon JE, Ahmed AR. Pemphigus vulgaris: the role of IL-1 and IL-1 receptor antagonist in pathogenesis and effects of intravenous immunoglobulin on their production. Clin Immunol 100:172–180, 2001.

Brett AS, Philips D, Lynn AW. Intravenous immunoglobulin therapy for Stevens-Johnson syndrome. South Med J 94:342–343, 2001.

Buckley RH, Ray BB, Belmaker EZ. Extreme hyperimmunoglobulinemia-E and undue susceptibility to infection. Pediatrics 49:59–70, 1972.

Champion RH. Disorders of blood vessels. In Champion RH, Burton JL, Ebling FJG, eds. Rook/Wilkinson/Ebling textbook of dermatology, 5th ed. Oxford, Blackwell Scientific Publications, 1992, pp 1839–1840.

Chan SC, Li S-H, Hanifin JM. Increased interleukin 4 production by atopic mononuclear leukocytes correlates with increased cyclic AMP-phosphodiesterase activity and is reversible by phosphodiesterase inhibition. J Invest Dermatol 100:681–684, 1993.

Cooper KD. Psoriasis: leukocytes and cytokines. Dermatol Clin 8:737–745, 1990.

Cormane RH, Gianetti A. IgA in various dermatoses: immunofluorescence studies. Br J Dermatol 84:523–533, 1971.

Counahan R, Cameron JS. Henoch-Schönlein nephritis. Contrib Nephrol 76:143–165, 1977.

Crumb CK. Renal involvement in Schönlein-Henoch syndrome. In Suki WN, ed. In The kidney in systemic disease. New York, John Wiley and Sons, 1976, pp 43–55.

Eichenfield L, Honig P. Blistering disorders in childhood. Pediatr Clin North Am 38:959–976, 1991.

Epstein WL. Contact-type delayed hypersensitivity in infants and children: induction of Rhus sensitivity. Pediatrics 27:51–53, 1961.

Esterly NB, Kever E. Maculopapular eruptions. In Weinberg S, Hoekelman RA, eds. Pediatric dermatology for the primary care practitioner. New York, McGraw-Hill, 1978, pp 30–38.

Fried R, Schonberg IL, Litt JZ. Erythema annulare centrifugum (Darier) in a newborn infant. J Pediatr 50:66–67, 1957.

Fritsch P, Elias P. Erythema multiforme and toxic epidermal necrolysis. In Wolff K, Freedberg I, Austen K, eds. Dermatology in general medicine, 4th ed. New York, McGraw-Hill, 1993, pp 585–600.

George P, Tunnessen W. Childhood discoid lupus erythematosus. Arch Dermatol 129:613–617, 1993.

Hall RP III. Henoch-Schönlein purpura. In Jordon RE, ed. Immunologic diseases of the skin. East Norwalk, CT, Appleton & Lange, 1991, p 451.

Hanifin JM. Pharmacophysiology of atopic dermatitis. Clin Rev Allergy 4:43–65, 1986.

Hanifin JM. Atopic dermatitis in infants and children: pediatric dermatology. Pediatr Clin North Am 38:763–789, 1991.

Hanifin JM, Chan SC. Monocyte phosphodiesteraae abnormalties and dysregulation of lymphocyte function in atopic dermatitis. J Invest Dermatol 105(Suppl):84S–88S, 1995.

Hanifin JM, Lobitz WC. Newer concepts of atopic dermatitis. Arch Dermatol 113:663–670, 1977.

Hanifin JM, Rajka G. Diagnostic features of atopic dermatitis. Acta Derm Venereol (Stockh) 92(Suppl):44–47, 1980.

Hanifin JM, Tofte SJ. Update on therapy of atopic dermatitis. J Allergy Clin Immunol 104 (4 Pt 2):S123–S125, 1999.

Huff CV. Erythema multiforme. In Provost TT, Weston WL, eds. Bullous diseases. St. Louis, Mosby-Year Book, 1993, pp 213–256.

Huff JC. Erythema multiforme. In Jordon RE, ed. Immunologic diseases of the skin. East Norwalk, CT, Appleton & Lange, 1991, pp 463–475.

Hurwitz S. The skin and systemic disease. In Clinical pediatric dermatology. Philadelphia, WB Saunders, 1981, pp 411–413.

Jones EM, Callen JP. Collagen vascular diseases of childhood. Pediatr Clin North Am 38:1033–1038, 1991.

Kang S, Lucky AW, Pariser D, Lawrence I, Hanifin JM, Tacrolimus Ointment Study Groups. Long-term safety and efficacy of tacrolimus ointment for the treatment of atopic dermatitis in children. J Am Acad Dermatol 44:S58–S64, 2001.

Krueger GG. A perspective on psoriasis as an aberration in skin modified to expression by the inflammatory/repair system. In Norris DA, ed. Immune mechanisms in cutaneous disease. New York, Marcel Dekker, 1989, pp 425–445.

Laughter D, Istvan J, Tofte S, Hanifin J. The prevalence of atopic dermatitis in Oregon schoolchildren. J Am Acad Dermatol 43:649–655, 2000.

Lee L. Neonatal lupus erythematosus. J Invest Dermatol 100:9S–13S, 1993.

Lee YA, Wahn U, Kehrt R, Tarani L, Businco L, Gustafsson D, Andersson F, Oranje AP, Wolkerstorfer A, v Berg A, Hoffmann U, Kuster W, Wienker T, Ruschendorf F, Reis A. Major susceptibility locus for atopic dermatitis maps to chromosome 3q21. Nat Genet 26:470–473, 2000.

Leiferman KM, Ackerman SJ, Sampson HA, Haugen H, Venenci PY, Gleich GJ. Dermal deposition of eosinophil-granule major basic protein in atopic dermatitis. N Engl J Med 313:282–285, 1985.

Marks J, Shuster S, Watson AJ. Small bowel changes in dermatitis herpetiformis. Lancet 2:1280–1282, 1966.

Marsden RA. Linear IgA disease of childhood. In Wojnarowska F, Briggaman R, eds. Management of blistering diseases. London, Chapman & Hall Medical, 1990, pp 119–126.

Maurer D, Stingl G. Immunoglobulin E-binding structures on antigen-presenting cells present in skin and blood. J Invest Dermatol 104:707–710, 1995.

McCord M, Hall R. IgA-mediated autoimmune blistering diseases. In Fine J-D, ed. Topics in clinical dermatology: bullous diseases. New York, Igaku-Shoin, 1993, pp 97–120.

McCuistion CH, Schoch EP. Possible discoid lupus erythematosus in a newborn infant; report of a case with subsequent development of acute systemic lupus erythematosus in the mother. Arch Dermatol 70:782–785, 1954.

Morici MV, Galen WK, Shetty AK, Lebouef RP, Gouri TP, Cowan GS, Gedalia A. Intravenous immunoglobulin therapy for children with Stevens-Johnson syndrome. J Rheumatol 27:2494–2497, 2000.

Moudgil A, Porat S, Brunnel P, Jordan SC. Treatment of Stevens-Johnson syndrome with pooled human intravenous immune globulin. Clin Pediatr (Phila) 34:48–51, 1995.

Musgrove K, Morgan JK. Infantile eczema. Br J Dermatol 95:365–372, 1976.

Orchard S, Fellman JH, Storrs FJ. Poison ivy/oak dermatitis. Arch Dermatol 122:783–789, 1986.

Paul C, Wolkenstein P, Adle H, Wechsler J, Garchon HJ, Revuz J, Roujeau JC. Apoptosis as a mechanism of keratinocyte death in toxic epidermal necrolysis. Br J Dermatol 134:710–714, 1996.

Peterson RDA, Page AR, Good RA. Wheal and erythema allergy in patients with agammaglobulinemia. J Allergy Clin Immunol 33:406–411, 1962.

Prendiville J, Hebert A, Greenwald M, Esterly N. Management of Stevens-Johnson syndrome and toxic epidermolysis in children. J Pediatr 115:881–887, 1989.

B. cepacia make infection-control measures to prevent spread an important aspect of patient care in CF. In addition, because of diminished survival after lung transplantation, reluctance has developed in some transplantation centers to provide lungs to *B. cepacia*–infected patients (Warner, 1999).

Allergic Bronchopulmonary Aspergillosis in Cystic Fibrosis

ABPA is commonly seen in those with CF (Henry et al., 2000; Mastella et al., 2000; Skov et al., 2000). The colonization rates for *Aspergillus fumigatus* have been reported to be as high as 57% (Nelson et al., 1979) and 66% (Geller et al., 1999). A significant minority of these patients (5% to 11%) develop ABPA (vs. 1% to 2% of those with asthma) (Henry et al., 2000).

Hypersensitivity reactions to *Aspergillus* species are characterized by the stimulation of IgE and IgG specific for *A. fumigatus* (Skov et al., 1999a; Taccetti et al., 2000), the generation of proteolytic enzymes causing local immunosuppression, and the inhibition of phagocytosis, in addition to epithelial cell detachment (Mastella et al., 2000). The diagnosis of ABPA depends on clinical and immunologic evidence of disease, as discussed later.

The clinical features of these patients overlap significantly with those of patients without ABPA and include wheezing, decreasing pulmonary function, cough, hemoptysis, pneumothorax, and bronchiectasis. In one large epidemiologic study of 12,477 patients, ABPA was found to be associated with (1) age greater than 6 years; (2) 10% lower lung function; (3) lung colonization with *P. aeruginosa, S. maltophilia, Candida albicans,* and *B. cepacia*; (4) the continuous use of antibiotics; (5) the more frequent use of respiratory therapies such as bronchodilators and inhaled steroids; and (6) oral steroids (Mastella et al., 2000).

The treatment of patients with CF identified as having ABPA includes steroid and antifungal therapy; furthermore, screening total IgE levels may be appropriate to identify patients at risk (Nepomuceno et al., 1999). Fatal invasive aspergillosis lung disease has also been reported in CF (Brown et al., 1999).

Host Defenses

Host defense mechanisms in CF have been studied extensively (Moss and Lewiston, 1984; Piedra and Ogra, 1986; Schiotz, 1981; Talamo and Schwartz, 1984). Before the identification of the CFTR product of the CF gene, a primary immune defect was an attractive hypothesis, given the multiple organ system involvement in this disorder. However, no unique defect in the host defense system has been found to explain all the manifestations of disease. Many of the immunologic findings have been discrepant (Table 33-4).

Because the CFTR protein is expressed by cells of nonepithelial origin, such as fibroblasts, macrophages, and neutrophils (Yoshimura et al., 1991), the possibility

TABLE 33-4 · HOST DEFENSE MECHANISMS IN CYSTIC-FIBROSIS

B-Cell Function
Normal to increased number of circulating B cells
Normal to increased serum levels of IgG and IgA
Increased serum levels of precipitins to bacterial species
Increased number of IgA- and IgG-producing cells in bronchial mucosa and bronchial lymph glands
Increased levels of salivary IgA
Increased jejunal production of IgA (prenatally and postnatally)
Decreased levels of secretory IgA in sputum
Decreased affinity binding of sputum antibodies
Serum and sputum precipitins to *Pseudomonas aeruginosa* and *Staphylococcus aureus*
CF serum depresses phagocytosis of *P. aeruginosa* (but not of *S. aureus*) by rabbit alveolar macrophages (? defect in IgA opsonic function)
Immune complexes in serum and sputum
Immunoglobulins found in complexes in lungs and pancreas
Increased frequency of ANA
Increased levels of IgE (? increased incidence of allergy)
High serum precipitin and IgE levels to *Aspergillus fumigatus*

T-Cell Function
Normal to increased number of circulating T cells
Normal skin test reactivity
Normal and abnormal lymphocyte transformation
Abnormal lymphocyte response to *P. aeruginosa* (but not to *S. aureus*)

Complement
Normal to increased C3 levels
Transient depressions of C3, C4, and CH_{50} with viral infections
Found in immune complexes in lungs and pancreas
Normal and abnormal alternative pathways
Normal bacterial activation of terminal complement components

Neutrophil Function
Normal to low opsonins
Normal phagocytic and bactericidal activity against *P. aeruginosa*
Increased leukotaxis (related to activity of lung infection)
Increased NBT test (related to activity of lung infection)
Inhibition of leukocyte migration when exposed to certain antigens (lung, pancreas, *A. fumigatus*, and *P. aeruginosa*)

Other Host Defense Mechanisms
Depressed tracheal mucociliary transport rates
Sodium reabsorption inhibitory factor
Normal to elevated serum protease inhibitors (e.g., α_1-antitrypsin)
Decreased lung antiproteases (especially in advanced disease)
Normal levels of secretory piece

ANA = antinuclear antibody; NBT = nitroblue tetrazolium.

of a primary functional defect of certain immune cells must be considered. Immune dysfunction, most of which is attributable to secondary effects, is discussed here. In the future, careful analysis of specific activation and effector pathways may reveal subtle functional abnormalities in immune cell lines (Sorensen et al., 1991).

Immunoglobulins

Serum immunoglobulin levels, especially IgG and IgA, are usually elevated (Moss and Lewiston, 1980; Pritcher-Wilmot et al., 1982; Schwartz, 1966), and may be correlated with *P. aeruginosa* pulmonary involvement (Moss and Lewiston, 1980; Smith, 1997); moreover, they may play a protective role against sepsis. However, a subset of patients with CF who are younger than 10 years of age and who have milder lung disease has been found to have low levels of IgG (Matthews et al., 1980). A 5-year follow-up study of these patients demonstrated that they had better lung function, fewer hospitalizations, and less colonization with *P. aeruginosa* (Wheeler et al., 1984). With immune responses to mucosal injury and to the secretory products of *P. aeruginosa* (e.g., exotoxin A, phospholipase C, proteases, and other exotoxins), immune complexes are formed in the bronchial lumen that in turn perpetuate the acute inflammation (Smith, 1997).

Hemagglutination-inhibiting antibody responses to influenza vaccine have been reported to be normal (Feery et al., 1979). The bronchial mucosae in patients with CF contain an increased number of IgA-producing cells (Martinez-Tello et al., 1968). Free secretory component of IgA can be found in the sera of one third of patients with CF (Wallwork and MacFarlane, 1976), and this finding has led to the proposal that a defect in the synthesis of IgA may be the cause of increased allergic symptoms in some patients (Hodson, 1980). The increase in immunoglobulin levels and the number of immunocompetent cells most likely reflects the continuous antigenic stimulation by bacterial organisms in the tracheobronchial tree.

Salivary IgA levels have been reported to be elevated (Gugler et al., 1968; Wallwork et al., 1974) or normal (South et al., 1967). Elevated IgA levels were found in the meconium of neonates with CF (Rule et al., 1971), and because IgA is not normally produced in large quantities before birth, these authors suggested that this finding may be unique to CF and may have etiologic significance. However, Falchuk and Taussig (1973) demonstrated that IgA production by the jejunal mucosa is inversely related to the degree of pancreatic insufficiency. Patients with hereditary pancreatitis and pancreatic insufficiency also had increased jejunal IgA production. Most likely, the increased IgA found in CF meconium is a result of local noninfectious antigenic stimulus and probably represents a secondary manifestation.

An elevated IgE level is a common finding not clearly correlated with the presence of atopy (Moss and Lewiston, 1980; Tobin et al., 1980). This observation suggests that IgE may provide a screening tool for identifying patients at risk for ABPA (Nepomuceno et al., 1999).

Pseudomonal Antibodies

The BAL fluid from patients with CF who have chronic *P. aeruginosa* infection contains higher levels of IgG, IgA, IgE, and C3c than those from healthy individuals and from patients with chronic bronchitis who have *P. aeruginosa* infection. The elastolytic activity in the BAL fluid of these patients with CF is reported to be strikingly elevated, whereas α_1-antitrypsin antigenic levels were normal (Fick et al., 1984).

The chronic colonization of the respiratory tract by *S. aureus* and *P. aeruginosa* produces high levels of precipitating antibody to these organisms in the serum. Most of the *Pseudomonas*-specific precipitins are IgG and IgA (Høiby and Hertz, 1979, 1981), but *Pseudomonas*-specific IgE antibodies have been reported (Pathial et al., 1992; Shen et al., 1981). Precipitating antibodies against *Escherichia coli* and *Bacteroides fragilis* are also elevated in patients with CF; however, unlike the situation with *Pseudomonas* precipitins, their presence or titers do not correlate with the severity of clinical disease (Høiby and Hertz, 1979).

Certain *Pseudomonas* exoprotein–specific antibodies have been shown not only to correlate with the severity of disease, but to rise significantly during active pulmonary infection (exacerbation) and fall with antibiotic treatment (Granstrom et al., 1984). Antibodies to *Pseudomonas* mucoid exopolysaccharide (Speert et al., 1984) and exoproteins, such as exotoxin A and phospholipase C, can easily enable the identification of a patient with chronic *Pseudomonas* colonization (Smith, 1997).

Monitoring levels of exoprotein antibody has been proposed as a potentially useful objective guide to the treatment of patients with CF (Granstrom et al., 1984). By keeping IgG titers against *P. aeruginosa* in the control range with the use of early and frequent anti-*Pseudomonas* antibiotic therapy, Brett and co-workers (1992) were able to limit sputum conversion to positive for *P. aeruginosa* and improve lung function. The presence of not just large numbers, but also a wide variety of antipseudomonal antibodies, may explain why immunization attempts with *Pseudomonas* vaccine have not been beneficial in preventing pulmonary exacerbations in CF (Pennington et al., 1975; Wood et al., 1983).

CF sputum has been shown to contain precipitins to *S. aureus*, *P. aeruginosa*, and *H. influenzae* (Clarke, 1976; Schiller and Millard, 1983; Schiotz and Høiby, 1975 and 1979; Schiotz et al., 1979b, 1980; Wallwork et al., 1974). These antibodies are of the IgG and IgA classes and may cross-react with bacteria of the gut and pharyngeal flora, raising the possibility that they are not induced by chronic pulmonary infection alone (Schiotz, 1981). Specific IgA antibody titers may be higher in sputum than in serum, suggesting local production (Schiotz and Høiby, 1979).

The presence of antibodies to specific *Pseudomonas* toxic products has been linked to lung colonization in patients with CF (Hollsing et al., 1987; Jagger et al., 1982; Koch and Høiby, 1993). The presence of these antibodies may explain the conversion of sputum isolates to mucoid strains that express fewer proteinases than their nonmucoid counterparts (Storey et al., 1992) and would therefore be less vulnerable to opsonization. Attempts to link the *P. aeruginosa* toxic products exotoxin A (*tox* A) and elastase B (*las* B) to isolate types from patients with CF through the use of mRNA transcript and transcript product accumulation have met with limited success (Storey et al., 1992). This method may, however, be used to more clearly elucidate the pattern of lung injury caused by specific *Pseudomonas* toxic products in colonized patients.

The precise function of antibodies found in CF sputum or BAL fluid is unknown. IgA is thought to inhibit the attachment of bacteria to mucosal cells, and IgG may act as an opsonin (Schiotz, 1981). However, the presence of large amounts of antibody does not necessarily imply normal function. Indeed, the functional ability of IgG antibodies to act as opsonins has been shown to be impaired in patients with CF (Fick et al., 1981). Fick and colleagues (1984) found that BAL fluid from patients with CF contained as little as 18% intact IgG and that the level of IgG cleavage fragments correlated with impairment of opsonizing ability. This opsonizing defect could be duplicated by using proteolytically produced IgG peptide fragments and could be corrected by adding intact IgG to CF BAL fluid specimens. Furthermore, it has been demonstrated that elastase cleaves IgG at the Fc region, thus rendering it ineffective in opsonization (Davis, 1991; Greenberger, 1997).

Moss and co-workers (1986) described a 30-fold increase in *P. aeruginosa* serotype-specific lipopolysaccharide IgG antibodies and the elevation of IgG subclass antibodies in colonized patients with CF compared with uncolonized patients and healthy control subjects. Elevated levels of IgG antibodies in these patients with CF were associated with an isotypic shift in the distribution of IgG subclasses. This shift in IgG subclasses has been substantiated by several investigators who have shown that IgG subclass IgG2 or IgG4, or both, against *P. aeruginosa* are increased in the sera of patients with CF (Fick et al., 1986; Moss et al., 1986; Shryock et al., 1986). Because alveolar macrophages have surface receptors that bind primarily IgG1 and IgG3 antibodies, the excessive production of IgG2 and IgG4 may create a ligand-receptor mismatch for opsonized *P. aeruginosa* (Sorensen et al., 1991).

In colonized patients, serum opsonic capacity for phagocytosis of *P. aeruginosa* was significantly impaired and was correlated with elevated levels of IgG4 subclass antibodies and high concentrations of functional antibody (Moss et al., 1986). Because a major defense mechanism against *Pseudomonas* is provided by IgG *Pseudomonas* antibodies and macrophages with appropriate surface Fc receptors, the proteolytic destruction of IgG antibodies or the presence of antibody isotypes that may inhibit efficient macrophage uptake of *Pseudomonas* organisms is significant (Davis, 1991; Greenberger, 1997). Thus, despite the large numbers of anti-*Pseudomonas* precipitins in sera and respiratory tract secretions, their functional role is ill-defined and protection of the lungs in patients with CF has not been convincingly demonstrated.

Cellular Immunity

Elevated numbers of B and T lymphocytes but a normal ratio of B to T cells in patients with CF was reported by Høiby and Mathiesen in 1974. It is, however, generally thought that cell-mediated immunity—including lymphocyte numbers and migration, leukocyte migration, and delayed hypersensitivity—is normal in patients with CF (Sorensen et al., 1991). One report established a correlation among deteriorating nutritional status, T-helper cell number, and blas-

togenic responses to mitogens (Smith et al., 1987). If the presence of an abnormal chloride channel in B lymphocytes (Chen et al., 1989) can be confirmed, it may be possible to study the effects of this defect on cellular function. Lymphocytes from patients with CF produce less 3′,5′-cyclic monophosphate than normal lymphocytes in response to isoproterenol (Davis et al., 1983); have increased mitochondrial Ca^{2+} compared with normal cells (Waller et al., 1984); and produce less IL-10 in response to concanavalin A (conA) stimulation (Moss et al., 1995). These findings suggest that CF lymphocytes may have abnormalities that could affect their protective capacity in vivo (Sorensen et al., 1991).

Lymphoproliferative studies (Wallwork et al., 1974) have yielded normal results, but Gibbons and colleagues (1976) demonstrated the inhibition of leukocyte migration of CF cells to the lungs and pancreas, in addition to *A. fumigatus* and *P. aeruginosa* antigens. This inhibition is related to disease severity and is reversed by corticosteroids. Lymphocyte reactivity to *Pseudomonas* has been shown to be impaired in patients with CF (Sorensen et al., 1977, 1978, 1979, 1981a, 1981b, and 1983), as has reactivity to *Klebsiella pneumoniae, Serratia marcescens,* and *Proteus mirabilis* (Sorensen et al., 1979). This impaired lymphocyte proliferative response to *Pseudomonas* could not be corrected by incubation of lymphocytes in non-CF serum and could not be induced in non-CF lymphocytes by incubation in CF serum (Sorensen et al., 1981b). The cellular mechanisms to explain this defect in reactivity to *Pseudomonas* have yet to be established (Sorensen et al., 1991). It may be reversible with antibiotic treatment in some patients (Sorensen et al., 1981a).

Alveolar Macrophages

Alveolar macrophages from patients with CF are morphologically normal and phagocytize *Pseudomonas* in normal serum (Thomassen et al., 1980). However, sera from patients with CF depresses the phagocytosis of *P. aeruginosa*—but not *S. aureus*—by isolated rabbit and human alveolar macrophages (Biggar et al., 1971; Boxerbaum et al., 1973; Davis, 1991; Fick et al., 1984; Thomassen et al., 1980). In one study, the defect was less in concentrated serum (Biggar et al., 1971), whereas in another, the defect was accentuated by increasing the serum concentration (Boxerbaum et al., 1973). In the study by Thomassen and co-workers (1980), phagocytosis by both CF and normal alveolar macrophages was markedly inhibited by CF serum. Suggested explanations include lymphokines, nonopsonizing or blocking antibodies (Høiby and Olling, 1977; Thomassen et al., 1979), and a defect in IgA opsonic function specific for *Pseudomonas* (Biggar et al., 1971).

Opsonin-mediated macrophage phagocytosis and intracellular killing of *Pseudomonas* are markedly impaired in the presence of IgG opsonins derived from CF sera (Fick et al., 1981) or respiratory fluids (Fick et al., 1984). In the 1984 study, Fick and colleagues found that this impairment was related to the proteolytic fragmentation of IgG opsonins and further showed, as mentioned previously, that abnormal overrepresentation of IgG2 and IgG4 subclasses to *P. aeruginosa* may prevent normal opsonization of this bacterium by macrophages that primarily bind IgG1 and IgG3 (Fick et al., 1986). These observations are most likely attributable to elastase, which cleaves IgG at the Fc region and impairs opsonization, as discussed earlier (Davis, 1991).

Increased monocyte oxidase activity with increased superoxide production by macrophages from both patients with CF and carriers has led to speculation that CF gene carriers may have a selective advantage for intracellular microbe killing (Regelmann et al., 1991). In contrast, as mentioned earlier, the presence of increased macrophage-derived oxidants may make the CF lung extracellular matrix more susceptible to protease degradation (Bowden, 1984; Crystal, 1991; Willoughby and Willoughby, 1984). Thomassen and co-workers (1980), on the basis of the results of morphologic studies showing no difference between the appearance of alveolar macrophages from infected patients with CF and uninfected healthy subjects, suggested an in vivo inhibition of macrophage function.

In contrast, polymorphonuclear neutrophils from the same CF group were obviously engaged in phagocytic activity, unlike polymorphonuclear neutrophils from uninfected control subjects. As a potential source of the neutrophil chemoattractant, IL-8, the macrophage may provide an important signal for neutrophil recruitment into the lung and may help explain the elevation of this cytokine in the BAL fluid of patients with CF (Dai et al., 1994).

Neutrophil Function

Neutrophils are the principal effector cells causing damaging inflammation in the lung with CF (Bedrossian et al., 1976; Conese and Assael, 2001). Neutrophil function has been shown to be both normal (Biggar et al., 1971; Boxerbaum et al., 1973) and depressed (Holland et al., 1981) in the presence of CF serum. Granulocyte chemiluminescence, a measure of oxidative metabolism, has been used to study granulocyte function in CF. Graft and colleagues (1982) found that the peak response was normal in patients with CF but that a more rapid time of onset correlated with the severity of lung disease. They concluded that the granulocytes of patients with CF seem to be "primed" in their response to a phagocytic stimulus. In the same study, neutrophil concentration and the release of β-glucuronidase were found to be similar in control subjects and patients with CF, suggesting normal degranulation.

By contrast, granulocytes from patients with CF have reduced superoxide degeneration (Waller et al., 1984), decreased chemiluminescence, and decreased lysosomal ß-glucuronidase release in response to *N*-formylmethionyl-leucyl-phenylalanine (Kemp et al., 1986). The functional implications of these findings are not yet clear.

Leukotaxis and nitroblue tetrazolium dye reduction by CF neutrophils have been reported to be normal (Church et al., 1979, 1980) or above normal (Hill et al., 1974), probably owing to the presence of active pulmonary infection. Random neutrophil migration was normal. The nitroblue tetrazolium test has been used to search for active bacterial infections in patients with CF (Sullivan et al., 1973), but this test does not always enable the distinction of bacterial from viral infection (Berry and Brewster, 1977; Sieber et al., 1976).

Neutrophil recruitment in the CF lung is an area of intense interest. The epithelial cell in patients with CF is a poor source of IL-10, an immunosuppressive cytokine. Without IL-10 inhibition the proinflammatory cytokines IL-1, IL-8, and TNF are found in high concentrations in the airway (Conese and Assael, 2001). Recent observations have indicated that protein overload in the endoplasmic reticulum may lead to calcium release and activation of the transcription factor NFκB, which in turn stimulates IL-8 production (Jaffe and Bush, 2001). This inflammatory pathway has been shown to be activated by endoplasmic reticulum overload of mutant CFTR (DiMango et al., 1998).

Neutrophil recruitment into the lung is thought to occur through cytokine signaling (e.g., through epithelial and possibly macrophage-derived IL-8). In fact, BAL fluid concentrations of IL-8 are correlated strongly with disease severity (Dai et al., 1994). Other observers have found elevated IL-8 levels and neutrophil numbers in the BAL fluid of 4-week-old infants with CF, even before infection is evident (Khan et al., 1995).

Under the influence of the potent activator and chemoattractant macrophage-derived IL-1, neutrophils produce free radicals, leukotriene B$_4$, and proteolytic enzymes. Another indication that neutrophils are highly activated in the lungs of patients with CF is the local inactivation of endogenous α_1-proteinase inhibitor by neutrophil elastase (Birrer et al., 1994; Goldstein and Döring, 1986). Together with oxidative damage, this mechanism is thought to be one of the primary causes of CF lung injury (Döring et al., 1988; Greenberger, 1997).

Complement

McFarlane and co-workers (1975) found deposits of immunoglobulins (i.e., IgG, IgA, and IgM) and complement (i.e., Clq, C3, and C4) in the lungs and gastrointestinal tracts of patients with CF. In addition, 18 of 40 patients had low serum C3 levels. Other studies, however, have demonstrated elevated levels of C3 (Holzhauer et al., 1976; Lieberman, 1975; Polley and Bearn, 1974). Strunk and co-workers (1977) have shown that C3 and C4 levels are depressed in patients with CF (but not in healthy children) during documented viral illnesses; these levels return to normal after recovery from the viral illness. The alternative complement pathway was not abnormal in this study or in the one by Lyrene and colleagues (1977), but it was abnormal in the study by Polley and Bearn (1974).

12% to 95% eosinophils (Marchand et al., 1998). The etiology and immunopathogenesis of this disorder are unknown, but the presence of major basic protein (MBP) in lung tissue and pleural fluid suggests that eosinophilic granule constituents may lead to lung damage in this disease (Grantham et al., 1986). A type I mechanism has been suggested but remains unproven (McCarthy and Pepys, 1973; Schatz et al., 1981).

Steroids are of benefit in treating acute episodes (Rogers et al., 1975), but the disease may worsen when steroids are tapered. Recurrence after long periods of remission is not uncommon (Marchand et al., 1998; Schatz et al., 1981), but the prolongation of therapy for 6 months reduces the frequency of relapse (Jederlinic et al., 1988).

Drug Reactions

Many drugs can produce PIE syndrome, and the acute nitrofurantoin reaction is characteristic. Beginning within 10 days of the onset of treatment with nitrofurantoin, the patient experiences fever, dyspnea, and cough. Cyanosis and bibasilar crackles are often present, and the chest x-ray usually depicts basilar infiltrates and, at times, pleural effusions (Schatz et al., 1981; Weller, 1984). The lung pathologic state is characterized by histiocytic and eosinophilic alveolar infiltration, sometimes with vasculitis, interstitial inflammation, and granuloma formation. Type IV immunologic reactivity is thought to be the mechanism of injury, but antibodies against nitrofurantoin have been found (Schatz et al., 1981). A pulmonary syndrome including tissue eosinophilia has been reported in patients with β-thalassemia major receiving intravenous deferoxamine therapy (Freedman et al., 1990).

Other drugs reported to cause the PIE syndrome are listed in Table 33-6. Unfortunately, a pattern of interstitial eosinophilia with features of usual interstitial pneumonia (UIP) may develop, suggesting progression to fibrosis and chronic disease (Smith, 1990). This occurs more commonly with nitrofurantoin or gold salts, whereas the pattern of acute eosinophilic pneumonia is more typical of reactions to antibiotics. Treatment consists mainly of withdrawal of the offending drug and steroid therapy in severe cases (Schatz et al., 1981). The use of steroids in this setting is controversial (Carroll and Sterni, 1999).

Hypereosinophilic Syndrome

Hypereosinophilic syndrome is a disease of middle-aged men and is discussed only briefly here. It has been reported in children (Chusid et al., 1975; Simon et al., 1999; Wynants et al., 2000). The diagnosis is made when there is marked eosinophilia (>1500 cells/mm³) for more than 6 months, organ infiltration, and no other cause of the eosinophilia (Chusid et al., 1975; Fauci et al., 1982). Fever, diarrhea, edema, cough, cardiac murmurs, hepatomegaly, splenomegaly, arthral-

TABLE 33-6 · DRUGS ASSOCIATED WITH EOSINOPHILIA AND PULMONARY INFILTRATES

Nitrofurantoin
Penicillin
Sulfonamides
Imipramine
Mephenesin
Aspirin
Methylphenidate
Carbamazepine
Chloroquine
Gold salts
Captopril
Beclomethasone
Tetracycline
Cromolyn
Para-aminosalicylic acid
Aminosalicylic acid
Methotrexate
Chlorpropamide
Chlorpromazine

Data from Schatz M, Wasserman S, Patterson R. Eosinophils and immunologic lung disease. Med Clin North Am 65:1055–1071, 1981 and Smith GJ. The histopathology of pulmonary reactions to drugs. Clin Chest Med 11:95–117, 1990.

gias, and abdominal pain are common. Restrictive cardiomyopathy occurs and is a major source of morbidity and mortality. There is also nervous system and skin involvement. Histologically, the disease is characterized by the infiltration of mature eosinophils in many organs, and the immunopathogenesis may be linked, at least in some patients, to clonal populations of T cells expressing IL-5 (Fauci et al., 1982; Schatz et al., 1981; Simon et al., 1999). The response to treatment—which includes steroids or cytotoxic agents, or both—is variable (Carroll and Sterni, 1999). A history of recent travel to a tropical country has been the focus of one recent study (Wynants et al., 2000).

Tropical Eosinophilia (Parasitic Infestation)

The life cycles of several helminthic parasites are characterized by transpulmonary migration of larvae. The result may be blood eosinophilia, reversible obstructive airways disease, and transient infiltration in the lungs. Infestation with parasites such as *Ascaris,* hookworm, or *Strongyloides* can create this clinical picture; in fact, *Ascaris* infestation was probably the etiology in many of Löffler's original patients (Weller, 1984). Other parasites that may cause eosinophilia are listed in the review article by Schatz and co-workers (1982).

Tropical eosinophilia is a distinct PIE syndrome caused by infestation with filarial organisms of the genera *Brugia* and *Wuchereria*. It is most commonly found in men in the third and fourth decades of life and is characterized by a dry cough, dyspnea, wheezing (often worse at night), weight loss, and fatigue (Cooray and Ismail, 1999; Neva and Ottesen, 1978). The chest radiograph may appear normal or show linear markings and hilar prominence

(98%). Diffuse, finely nodular infiltrates and consolidation are also seen, usually with ill-defined margins and subsegmental distribution. Restrictive abnormalities are found during pulmonary function testing, but these are superimposed on an obstructive pattern in 30% of patients (Lopez and Salvaggio, 1991; Schatz et al., 1981). Intense eosinophilia (>2000 cells/mm^3), elevated total IgE (>1000 IU/ml), and high titers of antifilarial complement-fixing antibodies in the absence of circulating microfilaria characterize the laboratory findings.

Granulomas may develop, and microfilariae can be seen in the lesions. The disease is usually confined to the lungs without peripheral tissue invasion. Type I, III, and IV immune mechanisms are thought to be operative in this form of PIE syndrome (Schatz et al., 1981). Treatment consists of diethylcarbamazine for 2 weeks, and the prognosis is favorable (Cooray and Ismail, 1999).

Churg-Strauss Syndrome (Pulmonary Vasculitis)

Vasculitis was a category in the original Crofton classification, yet eosinophilia is characteristic of only one vasculitis syndrome: allergic granulomatous angiitis, or Churg-Strauss syndrome (Weller, 1984). It remains a rare cause of systemic vasculitis in children (Louthrenoo et al., 1999). Churg-Strauss syndrome has been considered a variant of polyarteritis nodosa (Wolfe and Hunninghake, 1991) but has unique features that distinguish it from polyarteritis nodosa (Guillevin et al., 1999). Asthma, peripheral eosinophilia (>10%), the involvement of various types and sizes of pulmonary vessels, intravascular and extravascular granuloma formation, and eosinophilic tissue infiltration with paranasal sinusitis and mononeuritis multiplex characterize this disease.

Laboratory findings often include elevated erythrocyte sedimentation rates (present in >80% of patients) and antineutrophil cytoplasmic antibodies (present in 47%). Thin-section CT of the lung may show changes, including patchy, ground-glass opacities with a predilection for the lower lobes; centrilobular nodules; lobar hyperinflation; bronchial wall thickening; and increased vascular caliber (Choi et al., 2000). Polyarteritis nodosa, by contrast, is characterized by occasional asthma and peripheral eosinophilia, neutrophilic cellular infiltrates, the involvement of small and medium arteries, and the absence of extravascular granuloma formation (Lopez and Salvaggio, 1991).

The treatment for Churg-Strauss syndrome involves high-dose corticosteroids and cytotoxic agents (cyclophosphamide or azathioprine or both) and plasma exchange when necessary (Guillevin et al., 1999). Intravenous immunoglobulin has been reported to be of benefit (Hamilos et al., 1991). Type I, III, and IV reactions may be involved in producing the lung changes seen with vasculitis (Cohen and Ottesen, 1983; Lopez and Salvaggio, 1991) and collagen-vascular disease. Such findings from the histologic evaluation are not typical of Churg-Strauss syndrome (Guillevin et al., 1999) and are usually minor features of the diseases listed in Table 33-7.

Allergic Bronchopulmonary Aspergillosis

Aspergillus lung disease occurs in a variety of forms that can be divided into three major groups: (1) invasive, (2) noninvasive (e.g., aspergilloma and suppurative aspergillosis), and (3) *Aspergillus hypersensitivity* syndromes, such as extrinsic asthma, extrinsic allergic alveolitis, and ABPA (Pennington, 1980, 1988).

Invasive aspergillosis is rare in children. A variant form, pseudomembranous necrotizing bronchial aspergillosis, has been reported in a 15-year-old boy with HIV (Pervez et al., 1985). *Aspergillus* may trigger bronchospasm in the sensitized patient with extrinsic asthma, but fever and lung infiltration are not common. By contrast, ABPA, which usually occurs in those with atopy or asthma (or as aforementioned in patients with CF), is a distinct clinical entity with lung infiltration, fever, and bronchiectasis. When *Aspergillus* is excluded as a trigger in extrinsic asthma, the other forms of

TABLE 33-7 · IMMUNOLOGIC CHARACTERISTICS OF CERTAIN IMMUNOLOGIC LUNG DISORDERS

Disease Category	Eosino-philia	Precipitins	Autoanti-bodies	Elevated IgE	Skin Tests Immediate	Skin Tests Arthus	Lung Immunofluorescence* IgG	Lung Immunofluorescence* IgM	Lung Immunofluorescence* IgA	Lung Immunofluorescence* Complement
PIE[†]	‡	§	‖	†	‖	‖	‖	‖	‖	‖
EAA	§	†	‖	§	§	†	§	‖	‖	§
ABPA	†	†	‖	†	†	†	‖	‖	‖	‖
Vasculitides[¶]	†	‖	†	‖	‖	‖	§	§	§	§
CFA	§	‖	†	‖	‖	‖	§	§	‖	§

* = Immunofluorescence in capillary and/or bronchial walls.
† = When not associated with one of the vasculitides or ABPA.
‡ = Usually, but not always, associated with the disease.
§ = Occasionally associated, but not a characteristic feature.
‖ = Rarely or never associated with the disease.
¶ = Includes systemic lupus erythematosus and rheumatoid arthritis.
ABPA = allergic bronchopulmonary aspergillosis; CFA = cryptogenic fibrosing alveolitis; EAA = extrinsic allergic alveolitis; PIE = pulmonary infiltrates with eosinophilia.

Aspergillus lung disease are not found to occur more frequently in persons with asthma (Pennington, 1980).

ABPA is an allergic bronchopulmonary mycosis characterized by reactive airways disease, *Aspergillus* skin reactivity (immediate), pulmonary infiltration, increased serum IgE, blood eosinophilia, *Aspergillus* precipitating antibodies, increased IgG/IgE-*Aspergillus* antigen complexes, and proximal bronchiectasis (Detjen et al., 1991; Greenberger, 1984, 2002; Longbottom, 1983; McCarthy and Pepys, 1971a, 1971b) (see Table 33-7).

Historically, ABPA is more commonly diagnosed in England than in the United States, with pediatric cases being less common overall (Slavin et al., 1970; Wang et al., 1979a). The disease has been reported in several infants younger than 2 years old (Imbeau et al., 1977; Katz and Kniker, 1973; Kiefer et al., 1986), and the diagnosis is often delayed, sometimes for years. ABPA may be diagnosed in patients with CF, persons with intermittent or persistent asthma, those with previously diagnosed bronchiectasis, and in patients with neutrophil disorders such as hyperimmunoglobulin E syndrome and chronic granulomatous disease. Some patients with ABPA may have a normal chest radiograph. The disease may occur at any time in a patient with asthma, and those with ABPA are more likely to have a history of food and drug allergies (Greenberger, 2002).

Clinical Manifestations

In the asthmatic patient with ABPA, there is a marked increase in wheezing, cough, peripheral eosinophilia, fever, pleuritic chest pain, and sputum production. The sputum contains tenacious, firm, spindle-shaped yellow-brown mucous plugs. The chest radiograph depicts nodular lesions ranging in size from 1.0 cm to entire lobar involvement. Atelectasis and pneumonia-type lesions are migratory, usually resolving within 6 weeks, only to recur later in different lung segments. With numerous recurrences, a characteristic bronchiectasis involving the central airways may develop and any lobe may be involved. This is in contrast to other causes of bronchiectasis, which usually involve the more distal airways (Greenberger, 2002; Pepys and Simon, 1973).

The alveoli are filled with eosinophils and mononuclear cells, and the alveolar septa are engorged with mast cells, fibroblasts, and edematous fluid. Polypoid masses of granulation tissue may protrude into the bronchioles. Some patients with ABPA may develop bronchocentric granulomatosis or bronchial mucoid impaction resulting in distal bronchiolitis obliterans (Bosken et al., 1988). Fungal hyphae are present in the bronchial mucus and the organism can be easily cultured from this source, but bronchial wall invasion is not seen. A lung biopsy will reveal characteristic changes but is not necessary for diagnosis. The most advanced form of disease has pulmonary fibrotic changes with very severe obstructive and restrictive changes seen on lung function testing. Pleural disease can be seen with adhesions to the lung (Greenberger, 2002).

Laboratory Findings

Laboratory findings in patients with ABPA have been extensively investigated and are summarized briefly here. *Aspergillus* antigen or mixes should produce an immediate positive reaction upon skin prick or intradermal testing. High levels of specific IgE and/or IgG precipitins to *Aspergillus* antigens can be found in at least 90% of patients (Patterson and Roberts, 1974; Hart et al., 1976; Pauwels et al., 1976). The IgA level is also elevated in serum, whereas IgM and complement levels are normal. The serum IgE level is almost always elevated in ABPA and rises sharply during exacerbations. Elevated levels of IgG and IgE antibodies directed against *A. fumigatus* (IgG-Af and IgE-Af) are found in the sera of affected patients, but the markedly elevated IgE level is usually nonspecific and not directed against *Aspergillus* (Detjen et al., 1991). IgE levels decrease with effective therapy and can be used as a sensitive marker of treatment efficacy (Ricketti et al., 1984).

T and B cells are present in normal numbers in stable patients, but a growing body of literature suggests that CD4+ T-cell activation is involved (Greenberger, 2002). Basophils from patients with ABPA have been demonstrated to have markedly increased histamine release in response to *Aspergillus* antigens when compared with those from persons with asthma who are mold-sensitive (Ricketti et al., 1983). Immunoglobulins are increased in BAL fluid, and concentrations suggest increased local production of IgE and IgA, but not IgG (Greenberger, 2002; Kauffman et al., 1984). Peripheral blood eosinophilia is common in untreated patients but may be suppressed or absent with steroid treatment. Sputum cultures may be positive but are not diagnostic. Expectorated mucous plugs reveal mycelium, eosinophils, fibrin, Charcot-Leyden crystals (lysophospholipase), and Curschmann's spirals and are culture-positive for *A. fumigatus*. Sputum cultures for the organism become negative when the chest radiograph normalizes (Greenberger and Patterson, 1987).

Radiographs of those with ABPA reveal unilateral or bilateral consolidation, perihilar infiltrates, and signs of secretion-occluded distal bronchi ("gloved-finger" and "toothpaste" shadows). These findings characteristically involve the middle and upper lung fields. Tramline shadows represent edematous bronchial walls, and permanent changes may be seen where proximal bronchiectasis and fibrosis exist. The typical finding of proximal bronchiectasis is best defined by using CT (Neeld et al., 1990; Shah et al., 1992; Vlahakis and Aksamit, 2001).

Pathogenesis

Type I, III, and IV immune reactions appear to be involved in the development of various manifestations of ABPA; in fact, evidence suggests that a type I reaction is necessary for the type III reaction to occur (Cochrane, 1971; Ottesen, 1976). Dual skin reactions can easily be demonstrated in the patient with ABPA by both skin testing and inhalation challenges. In both types of challenges, an immediate type I reaction is usually followed 4 to 6 hours later by a delayed Arthus (type III) reaction. In nonatopic individuals, only a type III reaction occurs. Granuloma formation and infiltrates of mononuclear cells in the lung suggest that type IV reactions are involved. Furthermore, some patients have lymphocytes that undergo blastogenesis after exposure to *Aspergillus* antigen (Forman et al., 1978; Turner et al., 1972).

Eosinophilic inflammation is induced through the activation of a T-helper 2 CD4+ lymphocyte response. The cytokines produced lead to the release of degradative proteins. MBP from eosinophils may promote fungal growth (Latgé, 1999; Slavin et al., 1988; Vlahakis and Aksamit, 2001). Immune complex activation of eosinophils to produce leukotriene C_4 has been suggested in the pathogenesis (Cromwell et al., 1988). Damage may also occur from proteolytic enzymes produced by the *Aspergillus* organisms (Greenberger, 1984).

After a mucous plug is expectorated, the radiographic infiltrates may resolve spontaneously or may remain for months if not medically treated. Resolution of infiltrates is accelerated by steroid treatment (Greenberger, 1984). It has been noted that the locations of the bronchiectatic lesions and the radiographic infiltrates coincide (Scadding, 1967).

Diagnosis

The diagnosis of ABPA may be difficult. Many patients, such as those with CF (Schwartz et al., 1970), may be colonized with *A. fumigatus* without active disease. Furthermore, sputum cultures are positive in only 35% to 65% of all symptomatic patients with ABPA and thus may not be helpful in confirming the diagnosis. Presensitized persons without ABPA may have serum precipitins and positive skin test results (Hart et al., 1976). A patient with asthma may have an elevated IgE level, positive skin test results, wheezing, peripheral blood eosinophilia, and precipitating antibodies to *Aspergillus* and still not have ABPA. The diagnosis is based on a constellation of findings, including a clinical syndrome such as asthma or CF and supportive laboratory.

Brownish mucous plugs are suggestive as are positive sputum cultures for *A. fumigatus*. Immediate cutaneous reactivity to *Aspergillus* antigen is seen at the site of the skin prick or intradermal injection. Blood tests include peripheral eosinophilia (>1000/mm³), elevated IgE levels (>1000 IU/ml), precipitating antibodies to *Aspergillus,* and elevated serum IgE and IgG levels specific to *Aspergillus* antigens. Radiographs show infiltrates, fixed or transient, and may demonstrate proximal bronchiectasis. Vlahakis and Aksamit (2001) have advocated the use of total serum IgE levels, together with *Aspergillus*-specific IgG and IgE, to establish the diagnosis in any patient with suggestive clinical or laboratory findings. This approach may allow early diagnosis and prevent missing patients who are not acutely ill at the time of evaluation. *Aspergillus*-specific IgE and IgG have been used to diagnosis ABPA in a 20-month-old child (Kiefer et al., 1986).

Pulmonary function tests may reveal severe restrictive or irreversible obstructive airways disease, or both. Acute exacerbations are accompanied by a reduction in lung volumes and diffusing capacity. During remission, pulmonary function may return to normal, even in the face of bronchiectatic changes, making such measurements an insensitive indicator of early changes of ABPA (Detjen et al., 1991).

Treatment

Spontaneous remissions may occur, yet the treatment of choice is prednisone. Radiographic lesions usually begin resolving by 2 weeks, and a reduction in total serum IgE level occurs at 4 to 8 weeks (Greenberger, 1984). In fact, it is recommended that failure to achieve a 35% reduction in total serum IgE level after 2 months of corticosteroid therapy should alert the physician to the possibility of noncompliance with medications or an incorrect diagnosis (Ricketti et al., 1984). Specific treatment recommendations are published elsewhere (Detjen et al., 1991; Ricketti et al., 1984; Wang et al., 1979b). Other forms of therapy, such as antifungal agents, inhaled steroids, and disodium cromoglycate, have not been as effective as prednisone (Greenberger, 1984).

The use of several inhaled antifungal drugs has been attempted with mixed and usually disappointing results (Hostetler et al., 1992). The poor response to specific antifungal therapy reflects the immunologic nature of this disorder. The oral antifungal agent itraconazole has proved an effective adjunct to steroid therapy. This drug may help by decreasing the antigenic load presented to the airways (Denning et al., 1991; Hostetler et al., 1992), through its antifungal action or possibly through slowing steroid clearance by the liver and adding potency to the primary treatment drug (Greenberger, 2002). Experience thus far suggests that treatment with steroids is effective in preventing progression to pulmonary fibrosis (Detjen et al., 1991).

Pathogenesis of Eosinophilia

The role of eosinophils in PIE syndrome disorders has not been fully elucidated. However, the many enzymes and cationic polypeptides contained in eosinophilic granules have putative functions that may be of major significance in the development of PIE syndromes (Lopez and Salvaggio, 1991). These include the following:

1. Major basic protein (MBP) represents 95% of core granule proteins. MBP mediates eosinophil adhesion and activates mast cells (type I immune reaction).
2. Eosinophil cationic protein is found in the granule matrix and alters Hageman factor function, enhances plasmin activity, is helminthicidal, is neurotoxic, and activates mast cells (type I immune reaction).
3. Eosinophil-derived neurotoxin and eosinophilic protein X may be identical polypeptides and are centrally neurotoxic.

4. Eosinophil peroxidase, a granule matrix enzyme, is microbicidal and activates mast cells (type I immune reaction).
5. Charcot-Leyden crystal protein is a plasma membrane–derived enzyme that inactivates lysophospholipids.
6. Phospholipase D is found in eosinophilic granules and inactivates platelet-activating factor.
7. Histaminase, also found in granules, inactivates histamine.

Activated eosinophils are hypodense and are found in the BAL fluid of patients with PIE syndromes (Chihara et al., 1988). Hypodense eosinophils exhibit enhanced antibody-mediated cytotoxicity against certain parasites, increased ligand-initiated chemotactic activity, enhanced ionophore-induced generation of leukotriene C_4, increased glucose and O_2 consumption, and enhanced expression of low-affinity IgE receptors and other surface receptors (Lopez and Salvaggio, 1991). Eosinophil chemotactic activity is maximal in the lung and is influenced by numerous chemoattractants, such as eosinophil chemotactic factor of anaphylaxis, histamine, platelet-activating factor, and leukotriene B_4.

Eosinophils are also capable of downregulating hypersensitivity reactions through the prostaglandin E_2–induced suppression of mast cell–mediator release, ingestion of mast cell granules, inactivation of histamine by histaminase, and heparin binding by MBP. Despite the obvious beneficial effects on host protection, the presence of these inflammatory cells and their associated mediators may lead to the hypereosinophilic state.

Neutrophil-derived eosinophil chemotactic factor of anaphylaxis-like peptides are implicated in cell-mediated (type IV) reactions (Fantone and Ward, 1983). Eosinophils generate superoxide and hydroxyl radicals, prostaglandin E_2 and leukotriene C_4, and several hydroxyeicosatetraneoic acid metabolites (Lopez and Salvaggio, 1991). Complement components C3a, C5, C5a, and C567 (a trimolecular complex) are known to assist in the development of eosinophilic states and are important in type II and III reactions (Fantone and Ward, 1983; Ottesen, 1976). Eosinophils alone or in concert with mast cells and macrophages are capable of participating actively in host defenses, promote processes that injure host tissue, and may involve all four immune mechanisms in the development of the hypereosinophilic states.

HYPERSENSITIVITY PNEUMONITIS (EXTRINSIC ALLERGIC ALVEOLITIS)

A number of pulmonary disorders produced by an immunologic reaction to inhaled organic dusts (high molecular weight) and inorganic substances (low molecular weight) have been grouped together under the term *hypersensitivity pneumonitis* (HP) or extrinsic allergic alveolitis (Table 33-8) (Schuyler and Salvaggio, 1984; Wild and Lopez, 2001). Patients may have recurrent acute respiratory distress, but these disorders are easily separable from asthma in that (1) they occur in both those without atopy and with allergies; (2) they are not usually associated with IgE (i.e., they are not type I

TABLE 33-8 · ETIOLOGIC AGENTS IN HYPERSENSITIVITY PNEUMONITIS*

Disease	Exposure	Antigen
Farmer's lung disease	Moldy hay	*Micropolyspora faeni* *Thermoactinomyces vulgaris Aspergillus* sp.
Bagassosis	Moldy pressed sugarcane (bagasse)	Thermophilic actinomycetes: *Thermoactinomyces sacchari* and *T. vulgaris*
Suberosis	Moldy cork	*Penicillium* sp.
Maple bark disease	Contaminated maple logs	*Cryptostroma corticale*
Sequoiosis	Contaminated wood dust	*Graphium* sp. and *Pullularia* sp.

Humidifier lung disease	Contaminated humidifiers, air conditioners, and dehumidifiers	Thermophilic actinomycetes:
		Thermoactinomyces candidus, T. vulgaris,
		    Penicillium sp., *Cephalosporium* sp., and
		    Amoebae

Familial hypersensitivity pneumonitis	Contaminated wood dust in walls	*Bacillus subtilis*
Thatched roof disease	Dried grasses and leaves	*Saccharomonospora viridis*
Cephalosporium hypersensitivity pneumonitis	Contaminated basement (sewage)	*Cephalosporium* sp.
Sauna taker's disease	Sauna water	*Pullularia* sp.
Japanese summer-type hypersensitivity pneumonitis	Contaminated home and environment	*Trichosporon* sp.: *T. asahii* and *T. mucoides*
Paprika splitter's lung	Paprika dust	*Mucor stolonifer*
Pigeon breeder's disease	Pigeon droppings	Altered pigeon serum (probably IgA)
Duck fever	Duck feathers	Duck proteins
Wheat weevil disease (miller's lung)	Wheat flour weevils	*Sitophilus granarius*
TDI hypersensitivity	TDI	Altered proteins
TMA hypersensitivity	TMA	Altered proteins
MDI hypersensitivity	Diphenylmethane diisocyanate	Altered proteins
Epoxy resin lung	Heated epoxy resin	Phthalic anhydride

*Agents that have been reported to or might produce disease in children.
TDI = Toluene diisocyanate; TMA = trimetallic anhydride; MDI = metered dose inhaler.
Modified from Wild LG, Lopez M. Hypersensitivity pneumonitis: a comprehensive review. J Investig Allergol Clin Immunol 11:3–15, 2001.

reactions); (3) they involve the terminal airways and lung parenchyma, in addition to larger bronchioles and bronchi; and (4) bronchospasm is not a characteristic feature.

The importance of exposure to organic dusts in producing lung disease was described by Ramazzini in 1713 (Schlueter, 1974), but it was nearly 200 years later before investigators demonstrated the relationship of hay and maple bark exposure to the development of pulmonary symptoms. In the 1960s, bird antigens were reported to be causally related to pulmonary disease (Reed et al., 1965).

Pathogenesis

It has been repeatedly demonstrated that the inhalation of various organic materials is the cause of acute and chronic lung disorders in susceptible individuals, yet the immunologic mechanisms underlying the lung damage are still not precisely defined (Table 33-7). Small dust particles (i.e., those <5 μm) can penetrate to the distal airways and alveoli, where they may initiate a complex immunologic reaction. In susceptible individuals, the initial event occurring after acute exposure to antigen inhalation is transient neutrophil alveolitis, which reverts within 1 week to the well-known pattern of lymphocyte predominance found in patients with chronic HP (Fournier et al., 1985). Lung biopsy, usually performed in patients with subacute or chronic disease, reveals interstitial infiltration with lymphocytes, macrophages, and plasma cells. There is often interstitial fibrosis with granulomas containing foam cells (i.e., alveolar macrophages with lipid inclusion bodies). Bronchi are inflamed and may be obstructed.

Localized vascular inflammation may be seen, but generalized pulmonary vasculitis does not occur (Schuyler and Salvaggio, 1984). Biopsy specimens may contain antibody, antigen, complement components, and nodular ("lumpy") deposits of proteinaceous material along alveolar capillary basement membranes (Ghose et al., 1974; McCombs, 1972; Pepys, 1973; Wenzel et al., 1971), but evidence for classic immune complex–mediated lung injury is lacking (Calvanico et al., 1984; Fink, 1984; Salvaggio and deShazo, 1986).

The presence of mononuclear cell infiltrates and noncaseating granuloma formation suggests an important role for cell-mediated immunity in the pathogenesis of HP. Lymphocytes from the peripheral blood of symptomatic patients respond to tests of in vitro cell-mediated immunity, such as antigen-induced blastogenesis and lymphokine release (Fink, 1984, 1992; Hansen and Penny, 1974; Moore et al., 1974; Purtilo et al., 1975; Schuyler et al., 1978). Bronchial and circulating lymphocytes can produce macrophage inhibitory factor (Caldwell et al., 1973), and suppressor cell function may be abnormal (Fink, 1984).

BAL fluid from patients with chronic HP contains approximately 65% lymphocytes, most of which are T cells (helper–to-suppressor cell ratios of <1) (Leatherman et al., 1984b; Salvaggio and deShazo,

1986; Semenzato, 1991). This inversion of the CD4:CD8 ratio persists in farm workers with continued exposure to sensitizing antigen but reverts to normal after 6 months in those removed from antigen exposure. The presence of very late activation antigen-1 on CD8+ T cells from the BAL fluid of those with HP suggests that CD8+ cells are an activated homing population in these patients. Very late activation antigen-1 may be involved in cell–cell interactions and may contribute to cytotoxicity. Strong experimental evidence exists that granuloma formation is associated with the presence of T-helper cells and that granulomas resolve under the influence of suppressor/cytotoxic T cells and natural killer cells (Semenzato, 1991). Yamasaki and colleagues (1999) demonstrated increases in BAL fluid concentrations of CD4+ and CD8+ cells, producing increased levels of TNF-α, increased high-affinity receptor for IL-12, and decreased IL-10 production. In an animal model of HP, interferon-γ is needed for the development of disease and is induced by IL-12 (Gudmundsson and Hunninghake, 1997).

Taken together with the finding of activated macrophages in the BAL fluid of these patients, activation or dampening of suppressor cells by macrophages may be important in the pathogenesis of HP (Fink, 1992; Guzman et al., 1992). Alveolar infiltrates of lymphocytes and macrophages with granuloma formation is characteristic of delayed hypersensitivity reactions (Wild and Lopez, 2001). Thus current evidence is suggestive of a type IV immunologic mechanism, likely involving genetically determined immunoregulatory abnormalities. This is not conclusive, however, because some of these findings may occur by nonimmunologic mechanisms in response to inhaled particles.

A type III immune mechanism is suggested by the presence of high levels of precipitating antibodies (IgG, IgM, and IgA classes) (Faux et al., 1971) to the offending antigen (Patterson et al., 1976), the latent period after exposure, and the occasional presence of antibody in bronchial walls. The Arthus reaction to skin tests is also suggestive. However, the pathologic state of the lung is inconsistent with a type III mechanism, and when susceptible individuals are made symptomatic by inhalation challenge, serum complement levels are not usually lowered. The presence of precipitins and complement-fixing antibodies in asymptomatic individuals suggests an immune response to exposure and not disease. Positive rheumatoid factors and Monospot test results have been reported. Autoantibodies are not present.

The immediate wheal-flare skin testing reaction seen in 80% of patients with pigeon breeder's disease may be mediated by IgG4 subclass short-latent sensitizing antibody (Fink, 1984). Data to support a role for a type I immune mechanism are lacking, because IgE levels are normal and specific IgE antibody has not been found in symptomatic patients. Type II immune reactions are apparently not involved in the pathogenesis of HP. Fink (1984) has pointed out that several nonspecific mechanisms of lung injury may be of pathogenic importance. A variety of potentially potent inflammatory agents

arteries (Wiener-Kronish et al., 1981). Positive granular staining for IgG, C3, and Clq in the blood vessels of the lungs and patchy interstitial fibrosis have been demonstrated, but clear evidence of immune complex deposition (i.e., a type III reaction) is lacking (Wiener-Kronish et al., 1981). Selective IgA deficiency may be associated with childhood MCTD (Sanders et al., 1973).

Children with MCTD and lung involvement usually respond well to corticosteroid therapy (Fraga et al., 1978; Sanders et al., 1973; Singsen et al., 1977); however, the response is variable and the addition of cytotoxic agents has been used to prevent the severe and rapidly progressive lung disease seen in adults (Weiner-Kronish et al., 1981).

Scleroderma

Not clinically apparent, scleroderma in most children manifests as mild pulmonary function abnormalities, such as impaired diffusing capacity, decreasing lung volumes, and decreased alveolar-capillary permeability (Falcini et al., 1992) (see Chapter 35). Pleural effusion occurs infrequently (Dabich et al., 1974; Silver and Miller, 1990). Vasculitis with progression to pulmonary hypertension has been reported in children (Wagener, 1999). High-resolution CT demonstrates pulmonary disease in up to 90% of children with scleroderma and is much more sensitive than conventional radiographs (Seely et al., 1998).

Dermatomyositis and Polymyositis

Diffuse interstitial fibrosis occurs in approximately 5% of patients with DM and polymyositis and is characterized by chronic nonproductive cough and shortness of breath (Hunninghake and Fauci, 1979; see Chapter 35). Neuromuscular involvement of the pharyngeal and respiratory muscles often results in a weak and ineffective cough, aspiration pneumonia, and respiratory failure caused by muscle weakness (Bitnum et al., 1964). DM may be associated with rapidly progressive, life-threatening interstitial pneumonia (Park and Nyhan, 1975) and with spontaneous pneumothorax (Singsen et al., 1978). A recently described serum test for the mucinous protein KL-6 shows strong correlation with ILD in DM in a small series of children (Kobayashi et al., 2001).

Sjögren's Syndrome

Sjögren's syndrome, a chronic inflammatory condition characterized by dry mucous membranes, including the mouth, eyes, and tracheobronchial tree, occurs with a wide variety of rheumatic diseases and has been reported in children (Fraga et al., 1978; Sanders et al., 1973; see Chapter 35). Pleuropulmonary manifestations are common and include pleurisy and effusion, interstitial fibrosis, desiccation of the tracheobronchial tree, and lymphoid interstitial disease. Desiccation of the respiratory tract apparently results in cough, chronic bronchitis, atelectasis, and pneumonia (Hunninghake and Fauci, 1979). Low CD4:CD8 ratios from BAL fluid in advanced disease are suggestive of alveolitis and thus may be correlated with decreased pulmonary function (Dalavanga et al., 1991), but this association has not been strong and deserves further study. The major antigens are thought to be cell nuclei, altered γ-globulin, salivary duct cells, and thyroid antigens. ANAs and rheumatoid factor are found in Sjögren's syndrome, as are salivary duct and thyroid microsomal antibodies (Turner-Warwick, 1984). Some patients respond to corticosteroid therapy (Hunninghake and Fauci, 1979). Sjögren's syndrome is often associated with other collagen-vascular diseases (Wagener, 1999).

Ankylosing Spondylitis

Ankylosing spondylitis is a chronic inflammatory disease that typically begins between the ages of 15 and 30 and results in a progressive limitation of spinal mobility (see Chapter 35). Upper lobe fibrobullous disease and chest wall restriction are the two major types of respiratory involvement. The chest wall restriction often fixes the thorax at high lung volumes, and functional impairment is usually minimal. Typical pulmonary function changes include a reduced vital capacity and total lung volume with normal lung compliance (Feltelius et al., 1986). Cavities manifesting fibrobullous disease may become secondarily infected with mycobacteria or fungi, which can result in massive hemoptysis. Clinically evident disease is rare in the absence of infection (Wiedeman and Matthay, 1989). The cause of fibrobullous disease is unknown (Hunninghake and Fauci, 1979).

Henoch-Schönlein Purpura (Anaphylactoid Purpura)

Henoch-Schönlein purpura or syndrome, thought to be IgA immune complex mediated, is a necrotizing vasculitis that occurs predominantly in prepubertal children and occasionally involves the lungs with diffuse alveolitis or pneumonia (see Chapters 32, 34, 35, and 38). Typical clinical features include a purpuric rash on the lower extremities, abdominal pain, and joint symptoms. Renal involvement is associated with glomerular IgA deposits. One patient with fatal Henoch-Schönlein purpura pulmonary involvement had extensive deposition of IgA along the alveolar septa, with smaller amounts of IgG and fibrinogen (Kathuria and Cheifec, 1982). The mildly decreased lung diffusion capacity seen in these individuals typically returns to normal as the disease resolves (Cazzato et al., 1999; Chaussain et al., 1992). The rare complication of pulmonary hemorrhage carries a high mortality rate, but survival is possible with aggressive supportive care (Olson et al., 1992; Vats et al., 1999).

Pulmonary Manifestations of Gastrointestinal and Liver Disease

Chronic active hepatitis and primary biliary cirrhosis may be associated with pulmonary manifestations, which are thought to be produced by immunologic mechanisms (see Chapter 34). These patients have alveolitis with or without pleural effusion, alveolar wall thickening, honeycombing, increased pulmonary lymphoid tissue, and complement and immunoglobulin deposits in the lung. Rheumatoid factor and antinuclear, mitochondrial, and smooth muscle autoantibodies are often present (Turner-Warwick, 1974, 1984). Alveolitis and bronchiectasis are associated with ulcerative colitis and colonic mucosal antibodies. A similar mechanism may be involved in the alveolitis and granuloma formation seen in some persons with celiac disease (Turner-Warwick, 1984).

Lung diffusion abnormalities in patients with inflammatory bowel disease signaled the presence of interstitial involvement, even in the absence of clinical symptoms, in more than 50% of patients in one large series (Kuzela et al., 1999). Bronchiolitis obliterans with granulomatous disease has been reported complicating Crohn's disease in a pediatric patient and was not attributable to medication toxicity (Bentur et al., 2000). In fact, the resolution of ILD has been demonstrated with effective therapy for inflammatory bowel disease in children (Mazer et al., 1993).

Rheumatic Fever

Numerous reports have established that rheumatic pneumonitis (RP) is a distinct clinical manifestation of acute rheumatic fever, separate from congestive heart failure, acute bacterial pneumonia, or other collagen-vascular diseases (de la Fuente et al., 2001; Serlin et al., 1975; see Chapter 35). Over the past several decades only a few reports of RP have appeared in the literature (Ephrem, 1990). RP occurs in approximately 10% to 15% of patients and may precede other manifestations of acute rheumatic fever, but it is usually associated with active carditis. Patients with pneumonitis usually have extensive and progressive pulmonary symptoms, with crackles and friction rubs.

Chest radiographs show increased lung markings extending from the hila to the midlung. These infiltrates are often migratory, and in some survivors, a chronic interstitial pneumonia develops. Pleurisy with pleural effusions has also been associated with RP. At autopsy, the alveoli contain exudate and there is considerable hemorrhage and necrosis of parenchyma and bronchiolar mucosa. The evidence for arteritis (vasculitis) is usually present. The streptococcal antigen is thought to be responsible for RP, producing a type III immune reaction.

These patients are usually unresponsive to steroid therapy, and in some, the pulmonary manifestations worsen with steroid therapy. Nonetheless, successful therapy with corticosteroids has been reported (de la Fuente et al., 2001). The symptoms improve as other manifestations of acute rheumatic fever improve. However, the prognosis for RP is generally poor, with high rates of mortality reported.

Wegener's Granulomatosis

Wegener's granulomatosis is characterized by (1) the development of necrotizing, granulomatous vasculitis of small vessels, primarily of the upper and lower respiratory tract; (2) focal glomerulonephritis; and (3) disseminated vasculitis (Fauci, 1976; Faul and Kuschner, 2001). It is primarily a disease of adults, but it does occur in childhood (Hansen et al., 1983; Rottem et al., 1993; see Chapter 35). Ninety-four percent of adult patients have lung disease with pulmonary infiltrates, sinusitis, fever, otitis, cough, rhinitis, and hemoptysis being the usual signs and symptoms (Fauci et al., 1983). The complications of subglottic stenosis and nasal deformity are more common in pediatric patients (Rottem et al., 1993).

Chest radiographs demonstrate solitary or multiple nodular densities, which are usually bilateral and may be cavitated. CT may aid in identifying cavitary and opacified lesions in the lung (Cordier et al., 1990; Wagener, 1999). Pleural effusions, atelectasis, and hilar adenopathy are common (Fauci and Wolff, 1973; Landman and Burgener, 1974), as are macroscopic findings of inflammation, stenosis, and hemorrhage at the time of bronchoscopy (Cordier et al., 1990).

Both immune complexes and granulomas have been demonstrated in the glomerular lesions, suggesting that Wegener's granulomatosis may be caused by both type III and type IV immune reactions (Fauci, 1976). However, at least one case of Wegener's granulomatosis was reported in which vascular lymphoid infiltrates consisted predominantly of T cells and monocytes and IgG, IgM, IgA, and C3 were not found in the pulmonary alveoli, septa, or vessels (Gephardt et al., 1983). Diagnosis has been facilitated by the demonstration of antineutrophil cytoplasmic antibodies in as many as 88% of patients with this disorder (Rottem et al., 1993; Specks et al., 1989).

In the recent past, the prognosis for persons with Wegener's granulomatosis was extremely grave, with a mean survival of 12.5 months for those treated with steroids. Long-term remissions can now be induced and maintained with a combination of prednisone and cytotoxic drugs, such as cyclophosphamide or azathioprine. The treatment of this challenging disorder has been extensively reviewed by Regan and colleagues (2001). After aggressive management to induce remission, a less toxic maintenance schedule should be followed. Serious infections occur in up to 50% of patients during therapy. Therefore a switch to alternate-day glucocorticoids should take place as soon as possible; the use of antibiotic prophylaxis for Pneumocystis carinii is now considered essential. Relapse occurs in 38% of children within 5 years of remission (Rottem et al., 1993). Rising antineutrophil cytoplasmic antibody titers may precede relapses and may be a valuable monitoring tool in the management of these patients (Day and Savage, 2001; Specks et al., 1989).

DRUG-INDUCED HYPERSENSITIVITY LUNG DISEASE

Many drugs are suspected of producing a hypersensitivity reaction in the lung (Table 33-10), but there is meager evidence to confirm that the reaction is truly immunologic. In the majority of individuals, circulating antibodies or sensitized lymphocytes cannot be found. The diagnosis of drug-induced hypersensitivity lung disease often lacks objectivity and is usually made on the basis of the following:

1. The reaction observed is not a known pharmacologic effect.
2. The onset of the reaction occurred after a latent period of 7 to 10 days (reactions may occur sooner if the patient has already been exposed to the same drug or to similar antigenic determinants).
3. The reaction recurred after exposure to the same drug (Rosenow, 1976). Hypersensitivity reactions must be distinguished from other adverse reactions, such as overdosage, side effects, secondary effects, drug interactions, intolerance, and idiosyncrasy (Rosenow, 1972).

As many as 25% of all drug-induced diseases may be attributable to hypersensitivity, and many of these illnesses involve the lung. Most drugs have a low molecular mass, and, to be antigenic, they must bind proteins. In the lung, these antigens may produce pulmonary edema (increased vascular permeability), bronchospasm, mucous hypersecretion, cellular infiltrates, granulomas,

TABLE 33-10 · DRUGS THAT MAY PRODUCE HYPERSENSITIVITY LUNG DISEASES

Nitrofurantoin
Sulfonamides
Penicillin
Busulfan
Cyclophosphamide
Methotrexate
Bleomycin
Procarbazine
Melphalan
Heroin/Methadone
Propoxyphene
Pituitary snuff
Methysergide
Hexamethonium
Blood
Drugs that induce systemic lupus erythematosus*
Hydrochlorothiazide
Chlordiazepoxide

*See Table 33-11.
Modified from Rosenow EC III. Drug-induced hypersensitivity disease of the lung. In Kirkpatrick CH, Reynolds HY, eds. Immunologic and Infectious Reactions in the Lung. New York, Marcel Dekker, 1976, pp 261–287.

neoplastic changes, and fibrosis (Alvarado et al., 1978; Sostman et al., 1977). Leukocytosis, eosinophilia, and elevated IgE levels have been reported (Clayton and Schidlow, 1999). BAL fluid reveals a predominance of lymphocytes, the majority of which are T-suppressor cells. A tissue evaluation reveals eosinophilic infiltration but no evidence of vasculitis. Occasionally, fibrotic changes may be progressive with resultant restrictive lung disease (Evans et al., 1987).

All four types of immunologic mechanisms may be involved (not necessarily simultaneously) in producing these pulmonary changes. Conversely, some drugs such as penicillin may, depending on the circumstances, produce all four types of reactions. Type I reactions are thought to be caused by procainamide, hormones, and antitoxins; type II, by quinidine; type III, by penicillin, sulfa drugs, and p-aminosalicylic acid; and type IV, by topical exposure with such drugs as penicillin (Rosenow, 1976).

Certain drugs (e.g., nitrofurantoin) may produce acute pulmonary disorders (bronchospasm, eosinophilia, and pleural effusions) and chronic disease (interstitial lung changes with fibrosis). The immunologic mechanisms underlying these responses may be different. Nitrofurantoin pulmonary toxicity in children has been reported since the drug was introduced in 1953 (Broughton and Wilson, 1986; Coraggio et al., 1989).

A large number of drugs (Table 33-11) are implicated in inducing illnesses resembling SLE. The disease produced by these drugs differs from SLE in that there is less involvement of the skin and kidneys, more involvement of the lungs, and no depression of serum complement, but antibodies to DNA and other cellular elements are found. Drugs such as pituitary snuff may cause extrinsic allergic alveolitis with measurable serum antibodies to an extract of the snuff.

The treatment of these drug-induced disorders consists of discontinuation and future avoidance of the drug and other drugs with similar antigenic structure. Corticosteroids may hasten recovery in some persons, and the response may be one of dramatic improvement (Clayton and Schidlow, 1999).

CHRONIC INTERSTITIAL LUNG DISEASE

Cryptogenic Fibrosing Alveolitis (Idiopathic Pulmonary Fibrosis)

Chronic ILD is rare in childhood. The largest study series to date reports 48 patients and spans a 12-year period (Fan et al., 1992). A group of such disorders with no association to known causes of interstitial disease has been classified as CFA, or idiopathic pulmonary fibrosis. Hamman and Rich (1944) first described an entity of acute, rapidly progressive interstitial pneumonia in adult patients who usually died within months. Bradley (1956) first described this disorder in children, and numerous patients have been reported since (Fan et al., 1992; Hewitt et al., 1977).

TABLE 33-11 · DRUGS THAT CAN INDUCE SYSTEMIC LUPUS ERYTHEMATOSUS

Antiarrhythmic drugs
  Practolol
  Procainamide
  Quinidine
Antibiotics
  Griseofulvin
  Nitrofurantoin
  Penicillin
  Sulfonamides
  Tetracycline
Anticonvulsant drugs
  Carbamazepine
  Diphenylhydantoin (phenytoin)
  Ethosuximide
  Mephenytoin
  Phenylethylacetylurea
  Primidone
  Trimethadione
Antihypertensive drugs
  Guanoxan
  Hydralazine
  Levodopa
  Methyldopa
  Reserpine
Antituberculous drugs
  Isoniazid
  Para-aminosalicylic acid
  Streptomycin
Phenothiazines
  Chlorpromazine
  Levomepromazine
  Perazine
  Perphenazine
  Promethazine
  Thioridazine
Miscellaneous
  Amoproxan
  Anthiolimine
  D-penicillamine
  Digitalis
  Gold
  Methysergide
  Methylthiouracil
  Oral contraceptives
  Oxyphenistatin
  Phenylbutazone
  Propylthiouracil
  Thiazides

Modified from Ginsburg WW. Drug-induced systemic lupus erythematosus. Semin Respir Med 2:51–58, 1980.

Several entities, which collectively comprise the CFA disorders, may constitute a spectrum of disease with varying pathologic features (Crystal et al., 1976; Redding and Fan, 1999). These include UIP and DIP. LIP is histologically distinct from UIP and DIP but shares many clinical similarities. LIP appears to be almost as prevalent as DIP and UIP (Fan et al., 1992; Diaz and Bowman, 1990). Despite the obvious reference to the interstitium in the nomenclature of these disorders, it should be remembered that alveolitis is an essential feature and that veins, arteries, and airways may also be involved (Cherniack et al., 1991; Crystal et al., 1981).

Although idiopathic by designation, all of these disorders have been seen in association with systemic disease. CFA has been seen with SLE and scleroderma and LIP with a variety of immune disorders (e.g., myasthenia gravis and agammaglobulinemia). Familial patterns of ILD expression have occurred (Farrell et al., 1986; Hewitt et al., 1977); for example, in one family, six affected siblings all carried the immunoglobulin allotype Glm(1), suggesting transmission by a dominantly inherited gene on chromosome 14 (Musk et al., 1986).

The histopathologic subclassification into UIP, DIP, and LIP is given here. Some researchers argue that DIP and UIP represent different stages of the same disease, with UIP being the more advanced (Crystal et al., 1976; Patchefsky et al., 1973; Reynolds, 1986).

Usual Interstitial Pneumonia

Usual interstitial pneumonia (UIP) refers to the disorder originally described by Hamman and Rich, also known as *idiopathic pulmonary fibrosis* or *Hamman-Rich syndrome*. Pathologically, it is characterized by patchy areas of inflammation at varying degrees of ongoing injury and repair adjacent to normal areas of lung ("honeycomb lung"). Interstitial edema and alveolar hyaline membrane formation accompany interstitial infiltration by monocytes and lymphocytes. Alveolar wall necrosis and organization result in the obliteration of air spaces. Peribronchial fibrous tissue with inflammatory cells is seen, and the walls of the muscular pulmonary arteries are thickened—but without vasculitis (Redding and Fan, 1999).

Desquamative Interstitial Pneumonia

In 1965, Liebow and co-workers originally described desquamative interstitial pneumonia (DIP) as an entity distinct from UIP. Since then, it has been described in a number of infants and children (Bhagwat et al., 1970; Buchta et al., 1970; Howatt et al., 1973; Leahy et al., 1985; Rosenow et al., 1970; Schneider et al., 1967). Familial forms, affecting an infant as young as 6 weeks old, have been described (Farrell et al., 1986; Nogee et al., 2001). In DIP, there is minimal necrosis of alveolar septa and honeycombing is much less common.

It is defined histologically by a diffuse, but uniform, pattern of type II alveolar cell hyperplasia, septal hypertrophy, abundant intra-alveolar macrophages, and the interstitial accumulation of lymphocytes and plasma cells. Histiocytes and eosinophils may also be present. There is little fibrosis despite widespread inflammation. Patients with a diagnosis of DIP can, however, have progression of their disease to fatal pulmonary fibrosis (Carrington et al., 1978) and a histologic state consistent with UIP (Nogee et al., 2001).

Lymphocytic Interstitial Pneumonia

Lymphocytic interstitial pneumonia (LIP) is characterized by sheets of mature lymphocytes within the interstitium and alveolar spaces and along lymphatic pathways. Plasma cells and macrophages are seen in lesser numbers. Noncaseating granulomas occur with mononuclear and giant cell micronodules having lymphoid germinal centers. No tissue necrosis is seen in the airways, and the lung vessels and lymph nodes are spared. Like UIP and DIP, the progression of this disease to life-threatening fibrosis has also been described, and familial LIP has been reported (O'Brodovich et al., 1980). LIP is a feature of disease in many children with HIV infection and is discussed later in this chapter with pulmonary manifestations of HIV infection (Kornstein et al., 1986) and in Chapter 29.

Clinical Manifestations

The clinical, radiographic, and physiologic findings are similar in all three conditions and are discussed collectively as ILD. The primary symptom is dyspnea, which may be associated with a nonproductive, chronic cough, chest pain, anorexia, weight loss, fatigue, and eventual cor pulmonale and heart failure. Late inspiratory crackles (sometimes known as "Velcro crackles") are usually heard, but bronchospasm with wheezing is a less common finding (Hewitt et al., 1977; Olson et al., 1990). Clubbing occurs earlier than in the course of extrinsic allergic alveolitis. Hypoxia and subsequent cyanosis are almost always present.

Chest radiographic abnormalities may lag behind clinical manifestations; in fact, extensive lung histologic changes and dyspnea can be present despite a normal chest radiograph (Epler et al., 1978; Renzi and Lopez-Majano, 1976). Radiographs may demonstrate one of five patterns: ground glass, reticular, nodular, reticulonodular, or honeycomb pattern (Redding and Fan, 1999). Diffuse reticulonodular markings may sometimes obliterate the vascular markings, and hilar adenopathy may be present. Conventional radiographs correlate poorly with disease severity, but high-resolution CT has been shown to be a sensitive method of detecting and describing diseases in these patients (Müller and Ostrow, 1991).

Pulmonary function tests reveal a pattern of lung restriction with decreased lung volumes and decreased compliance. Also seen is an increased physiologic dead space and the preservation of flow rates, dictated by large airway function (i.e., specific conductance at functional residual capacity [FRC] may be increased) (Kerem et al., 1990b; Zapletal et al., 1985). Decreases in flow rates influenced by small airways have been described in some (Ostrow and Cherniack, 1973)—but not all—persons (Schofield et al., 1976; Zapletal et al., 1985). Hyperventilation and hypoxia, the latter mainly caused by ventilation-perfusion abnormalities and not diffusion (alveolar-capillary block) problems, are common. Increased epithelial permeability may explain the plasma extravasation, which contributes to hypoxia (Cherniack et al., 1991). Young infants with ILD may have hyperinflation of the chest, suggesting small airways obstruction and air trapping.

Diagnosis

The differential diagnosis of ILD includes connective tissue disorders, sarcoidosis, granulomatous disease, pulmonary hemorrhage syndromes, radiation injury, vasculitis, alveolar proteinosis, histiocytosis, extrinsic allergic alveolitis, and *Mycoplasma pneumoniae* and viral infections. The diagnosis is made by exclusion of other entities and almost always requires an open-lung biopsy. Supporting evidence is provided by serologic, physiologic, radiographic, and BAL findings. High-resolution CT scans may be able to demonstrate fibrotic changes and elucidate the nonhomogeneous distribution of lesions seen in ILD, thus aiding in site selection for biopsy (Cherniack et al., 1991; Koh and Hansell, 2000; Redding and Fan, 1999). The gallium scan is more commonly used to correlate disease severity in adults.

BAL fluid analysis may someday be a useful diagnostic aid in pediatric patients with ILD, but at this time limited studies exist to define cellularity in control subjects, and standardization in technique is lacking (Redding and Fan, 1999). In contrast with extrinsic allergic alveolitis (increased lymphocytes, absent neutrophils), BAL fluid from patients with CFA may contain an increased proportion of neutrophils and normal proportions of lymphocytes and lymphocyte subpopulations are typical (Crystal et al., 1981). Eosinophil percentages in BAL fluid are higher in those with CFA than in control subjects, are not usually accompanied by peripheral eosinophilia, and have been associated with a poor prognosis (Cherniack et al., 1991; Haslam et al., 1980; Rudd et al., 1981). Analysis of BAL immune and inflammatory proteins is generally not helpful, but patients with CFA may have increased levels of free collagenase (Crystal et al., 1981) and fibronectin (Morgan et al., 1984) in BAL fluid.

Pathogenesis

The cause of ILD is obscure. Toxic agents, collagen-vascular diseases, familial predisposition, and pneumoconioses have all been proposed. A viral cause was originally proposed by Hamman and Rich (1944). Electron microscopic studies have demonstrated viral-like inclusion bodies in lung tissue (Kawai et al., 1976; O'Shea and Yardley, 1970), and many children with CFA had a previous upper respiratory tract infection, presumably of viral origin.

The general pathogenetic sequence is similar for all of the ILDs and can be divided into several stages. First, a stimulus (unknown in the CFA disorders) results in immune-mediated alveolitis characterized by the presence of effector cells (neutrophils, alveolar macrophages, and eosinophils) capable of damaging alveolar structures. Then, persistence of the alveolitis results in chronic, continuous damage; the derangement of alveolar structures; and, eventually, the irreversible loss of functional alveolar-capillary units (end-stage). These concepts are well supported by the following observations (Cherniack et al., 1991; Crystal et al., 1981):

1. Serial histologic evaluation has revealed that alveolitis precedes derangement.
2. Alveolitis without structural derangement is present in early ILD.
3. Alveolitis is the predecessor of structural alterations in experimental models.
4. Activated effector cells present are clearly capable of causing alveolar derangement.

Patients with CFA have a macrophage-neutrophil type of alveolitis in which macrophages predominate and neutrophils are chronically present. When properly stained, neutrophils are seen associated with interstitial connective tissue and parenchymal lung cells. B lymphocytes, albeit present in normal numbers, are secreting immunoglobulin, and macrophages are in an activated state (Cherniack et al., 1991; Hunninghake and Moseley, 1984).

Lung mononuclear cells are stimulated by an unknown antigen(s) to produce immunoglobulins, resulting in local immune complex production (Hunninghake and Moseley, 1984). Alveolar macrophages respond by producing chemotactic factors that cause influx of neutrophils from the circulation into lung tissues. A study by Carré and associates (1991) correlates the expression of alveolar macrophage IL-8 mRNA with the number of neutrophils per milliliter of BAL fluid and with disease severity. Once present, neutrophils are stimulated to release their array of potent mediators of destruction, including reactive oxygen species and collagenase.

The result is injury to alveolar, capillary, and interstitial structures. Involvement of the interstitium can then lead to bronchiolitis, bronchiolectasis, and pulmonary vascular injury. Peripheral airway obstruction and pulmonary hypertension follows in a significant percentage of patients (Hewitt et al., 1977; Stillwell et al., 1980; Zapletal et al., 1985).

In individuals with CFA, alveolar macrophages secrete fibronectin and a potent fibroblast growth factor that induces cell division; the latter sets the stage for cell division and is a chemoattractant for lung fibroblasts, in addition to being 1000 times more powerful than serum fibronectin. Thus collagen is constantly destroyed and replaced, and the stage is set for structural alveolar derangement (fibrosis). Ultrastructural and immunohistochemical analysis of myofibroblasts suggests active contraction, analogous to wound contraction, which may contribute to the distorted lung architecture (Kuhn and McDonald, 1991).

The antigens and immunoglobulin specificities are not known, but immunoglobulins may be directed against alveolar components as a result of injury (Hunninghake and Moseley, 1984). Autoantibodies to specific antigens have been identified but seem to have very private speci-

ficities, making general conclusions about their role in pathogenesis difficult (Robinson et al., 2001). Some patients with CFA exhibit cell-mediated immune responses specific for type I collagen. There is ample evidence that immune complexes are produced locally in lung tissue and that circulating immune complexes are not of etiologic significance. Continuous production of antigen or abnormal suppressor T-cell function has been proposed, but the actual mechanisms responsible for maintaining the unremitting immune response are unknown (Morgan et al., 1984; Redding and Fan, 1999).

Treatment and Prognosis

In CFA, a hypothesis linking levels of neutrophils in BAL fluid with a prognosis has been made (Crystal et al., 1981). This has been more clearly defined by Rudd and colleagues (1981). Patients with increased lymphocytes tended to have a better response to corticosteroids and a good prognosis. Increased neutrophils or eosinophils in BAL fluid were associated with a poor response to treatment, and progressive deterioration was likely in those with increased proportions of eosinophils. CFA has been classified as either high-intensity (>10% neutrophils in BAL fluid) or low-intensity (>10% neutrophils in BAL fluid) and has been evaluated longitudinally. Patients with low-intensity alveolitis had less deterioration of pulmonary function with time, thus providing additional support for the link between prognosis and the intensity of the alveolitis (Crystal et al., 1981).

Patients classified as having UIP and LIP generally have a poor response to therapy and an unfavorable prognosis: 55% survive for 5 years and 28% for 10 years from disease onset. Those with DIP, who often respond well to steroid treatment, have a more favorable prognosis (95% survive for 5 years, and 70% survive for 10 years) (Carrington et al., 1978). The survival pattern for children may be slightly better than for adults (Hewitt et al., 1977), but the differences in survival among pathologic type are not as distinct in children as in adults. Disease of early onset (<1 year) and familial forms of CFA have less chance of long-term survival.

Ultimately, the morbidity and mortality in patients with CFA are caused by irreversibly damaged, nonfunctional alveolar-capillary units. The main principle of therapy is therefore to arrest or suppress the alveolitis before permanent damage occurs. Because alveolitis is so closely linked to prognosis, the use of gallium scans or BAL to stage the activity or intensity of the alveolitis has been recommended (Crystal et al., 1981). However, the use of these techniques in routine clinical practice is still controversial (Cherniack et al., 1991; Morgan et al., 1984; Redding and Fan, 1999; Turner-Warwick and Haslam, 1986).

Treatment consists of the use of anti-inflammatory agents and supportive care for children diagnosed with ILD. Children do not experience spontaneous remission, as has been reported in adults. Corticosteroids have been used extensively to slow the progression of disease (Brown and Turner-Warwick, 1971; Carrington et al., 1978; Weese et al., 1975). Newer treatment regimens initially consist of prednisone, followed by long-term maintenance with anti-inflammatory drugs. Patients who do not respond to steroid treatment may benefit from azathioprine, penicillamine, vincristine, chlorambucil, cyclophosphamide (alone or with corticosteroids), or colchicine (Crystal et al., 1981; Peters et al., 1993; Turner-Warwick and Haslam, 1986).

Treatment of children should be initiated with prednisone at 2 mg/kg/day or more for 6 to 8 weeks. Tapering to lesser doses should be done cautiously, with the eventual goal to be that of alternate-day steroids. Numerous anecdotes of a positive response to chloroquine or hydroxychloroquine have been described in children, and these have become the treatment drugs of choice when prednisone alone is ineffective (Leahy et al., 1985; Springer et al., 1987; Waters et al., 1991). Hydroxychloroquine has less associated retinopathy (Maksymowych and Russel, 1987).

Clinical improvement is marked by a reduction in symptoms and may be accompanied by improved lung function and radiographic appearance (Hewitt et al., 1977; Stillwell et al., 1980). Chest physiotherapy, bronchodilators, and other nonspecific measures are often used in the management of ILD in children. Antibiotics are useful in treating secondary infections, and long-term oxygen therapy may improve the quality of life in those with hypoxemia and slow the progression to pulmonary hypertension.

PULMONARY HEMOSIDEROSIS

PH results when recurrent pulmonary hemorrhage produces a progressive accumulation of iron (hemosiderin) in the lungs. Certain cardiac and collagen-vascular diseases secondarily produce PH. However, in a number of disorders, PH is a primary feature of the disease and may have an immunologic basis; the disorders can be classified as follows:

1. Idiopathic pulmonary fibrosis
2. Pulmonary hemosclerosis from sensitivity to cow's milk
   a. Without upper airway obstruction
   b. With upper airway obstruction
3. Pulmonary hemosiderosis with glomerulonephritis (Goodpasture's syndrome)

Idiopathic Pulmonary Hemosiderosis

IPH, also known as *isolated primary pulmonary hemosiderosis*, is the result of diffuse alveolar hemorrhage with accumulation of hemosiderin in lung tissue. It occurs in the absence of an apparent cause (e.g., coagulopathy, hemodynamic abnormalities, or infection) or associated systemic disease (Kiper et al., 1999; Leatherman, 1991; Leatherman et al., 1984a). IPH is a disease of young children, usually between 1 and 10 years of age, occurring equally in boys and girls, often with a long delay between the onset of symptoms and diagnosis (Chryssanthopoulos et al., 1983; Kjellman et al., 1984). The strong association of pulmonary hemorrhage with systemic vasculitis has led many authors to propose an immunologic mechanism (Le Clainche et al., 2000). No specific genetic pattern of disease has been observed and most cases occur sporadically, but there are several reports of familial IPH (Beckerman et al., 1979).

Clinical Findings

Hemoptysis, cough, tachypnea, malaise, weight loss, and iron deficiency anemia characterize IPH. During an acute hemorrhage, there may be abdominal pain, tachycardia, and leukocytosis, findings compatible with a diagnosis of pneumonia. After episodes of acute hemorrhage, reticulocytosis and elevated serum bilirubin may be found. IPH is sometimes subclinical because some patients have minimal symptoms and demonstrate only a mild anemia. Hemolysis is not a feature of IPH, and Coombs' tests are usually negative (Leatherman et al., 1984a). Eosinophilia and hepatosplenomegaly are present in approximately 20% of patients; clubbing is not unusual. Radiographic abnormalities of the chest range from reticular and interstitial patterns to extensive infiltrates with segmental or lobar involvement. Chronic disease produces interstitial fibrosis with a reticulonodular radiographic picture; acute hemorrhage often results in transient infiltrates, which may be unilateral. There may be symptom-radiographic dissociation, in that radiographic abnormalities of the chest may precede or lag behind clinical symptoms.

Diagnosis

The diagnosis is made by a history of recurrent pulmonary hemorrhages (hemoptysis or transient infiltrates), the presence of iron deficiency anemia, and the finding of hemosiderin-laden macrophages in sputum or early morning gastric aspirates. The presence of hemosiderin-filled macrophages is a universal finding in the BAL fluid from these individuals (Saeed et al., 1999). A lung biopsy is not always required for diagnosis; moreover, apparently stable patients have rapidly decompensated after lung biopsy (Repetto et al., 1967; Soergel and Sommers, 1962).

Laboratory Findings

Pulmonary function abnormalities in IPH range from normal to either a restrictive or obstructive pattern (Allue et al., 1973; Beckerman et al., 1979; Le Clainche et al., 2000; Repetto et al., 1967). The examination of lung tissue by means of light microscopy reveals alveolar epithelial hyperplasia with shedding of cells, hemosiderin-laden macrophages in alveoli, erythrocytes in alveoli and the interstitium, and the degeneration of elastic fibers (fibrosis). Vasculitis, alveolar septal necrosis, and granuloma formation are usually absent; their presence suggests that the hemosiderosis is secondary to some other process (e.g., collagen-vascular disease).

Electron microscopy has demonstrated intact alveolar-capillary basement membranes (Dolan et al., 1975; Gonzalez-Crussi et al., 1976), breaks in the basement membranes (Donald et al., 1975; Hyatt et al., 1972), thickened basement membranes with reduplication (Gonzalez-Crussi et al., 1976), and the absence of immune complexes or protein deposits in the subendothelial areas (Dolan et al., 1975; Hyatt et al., 1972). In a recent study of 13 patients, 4 demonstrated fibrosis at the time of lung biopsy, all had evidence of recurrent hemorrhage, and none had evidence of vasculitis or other pathology (Saeed et al., 1999).

Pathogenesis

An immunologic basis for IPH is frequently postulated, yet no consistent defect has been found. However, an immune basis is suggested by several observations:

1. The IgA level is elevated in more than half of patients.
2. IPH and celiac sprue have occurred in the same individuals.
3. The alveolar hemorrhage of IPH is similar to that of several immune disorders.
4. Immunosuppressive agents are beneficial in some people (Leatherman et al., 1984a; Saeed et al., 1999).

Serum IgA elevation is not accompanied by increased salivary IgA production (Valassi-Adam et al., 1975). Other serum immunoglobulins are normal. No immunofluorescence to IgG, IgM, IgA, and C3, and no immune complexes have been found in lung tissue with IPH (Dolan et al., 1975; Donald et al., 1975; Irwin et al., 1974). Serum autoantibodies to lung tissue are not detectable (Hyatt et al., 1972).

Treatment

Because of variability in the clinical course, it has been difficult to assess the various forms of therapy. Splenectomy does not appear to be of benefit (Soergel and Sommers, 1962). Steroids are helpful in the treatment of acute hemorrhage (Soergel and Sommers, 1962); immunosuppressive agents (Byrd and Gracey, 1973) and plasmapheresis (Leatherman et al., 1984a) have apparently been beneficial in a small number of patients. The use of prednisone has been used to prevent recurrent hemoptysis, and combined therapy with hydroxychloroquine and azathioprine is reported (Saeed et al., 1999). One anecdotal report exists of successful treatment with long-term inhaled corticosteroids alone after stabilization with systemic steroids (Tutor and Eid, 1995). Deferoxamine may be helpful in mobilizing the excessive iron sequestered in the lung. Patients should be asked to abstain from milk products (in the presence or absence of serum milk precipitins, discussed later); some with IPH demonstrate considerable improvement while abstaining from milk and experience recurrence of symptoms when challenged with cow's milk.

Prognosis

The prognosis for patients with IPH is variable. Many individuals succumb within the first 2 years after the onset of manifestations, but others may have a spontaneous remission of variable duration. The rarity of adult patients with IPH suggests that older patients either die or go into a near-permanent remission as they approach adult life. Males and females are equally represented at the time of presentation, yet Chryssanthopoulos and co-workers (1983) have reported that females tend to survive longer: the male-to-female ratio is 1:2 among survivors. In addition, they found that younger age at the time of onset carries a poor prognosis; severity of disease at the time of onset does not dictate outcome; and the current therapeutic modalities do not appear to affect long-term prognosis. A more recent report detailing the outcome of 17 patients indicates 5-year survivals of 86% (Saeed et al., 1999).

Pulmonary Hemosiderosis from Sensitivity to Cow's Milk (Heiner Syndrome)

Heiner and colleagues (1962) described a disorder similar to IPH in infants who had serum precipitins to cow's milk and positive immediate skin test results to cow's milk proteins. These children (some of whom were as young as 13 to 14 days old) also had eosinophilia, growth retardation, recurrent otitis media, chronic rhinitis, gastrointestinal symptoms (diarrhea and vomiting), and gastrointestinal bleeding; notably, eczema was not a frequent finding. The pulmonary and gastrointestinal manifestations subsided with the withdrawal of milk products and recurred when milk was reintroduced. A few patients without milk precipitins also appear to improve when cow's milk is removed, raising the question of what role—if any—these precipitins play in the pathogenesis of the bleeding.

Boat and colleagues (1975) described PH occurring in early infancy with associated eosinophilia; serum precipitins to milk proteins; high IgE levels; normal IgG, IgM, and IgA levels; immediate and delayed skin reactions to milk antigens; chronic nasal discharge; diarrhea with gastrointestinal bleeding; and enlarged adenoids, producing upper airway obstruction and cor pulmonale. This syndrome occurred only in black children of both sexes. The syndrome described by Heiner and co-workers (1962) also occurred more frequently in black children. A unique immunologic mechanism causing milk-induced PH was not found in a later study by the same group (Stafford et al., 1977), but it was observed that, when milk was withdrawn, the IgE levels and milk precipitin titers dropped markedly in some infants. Pulmonary and gastrointestinal bleeding subsided, and nasal symptoms improved.

An association has been reported between the administration of cow's milk protein and the elevation of blood and BAL levels of histamine and eosinophil cationic protein in a newborn with PH (Torres et al.,

1996). The upper and lower respiratory tract disease produced by sensitivity to cow's milk seems to be mediated by both type I (high IgE levels) and type III (milk precipitins) immunologic reactions. The immediate and Arthus-type skin responses tend to confirm this hypothesis. Therapy consists of the withdrawal of milk products and, when needed, adenoidectomy.

Pulmonary Hemosiderosis with Glomerulonephritis (Goodpasture's Syndrome)

Goodpasture's syndrome generally refers to the combination of diffuse alveolar hemorrhage and glomerulonephritis resulting from anti–basement membrane (ABM) antibody disease (see Chapter 38). It is primarily a disease of adolescents and young adults, but a few cases have been reported in childhood (O'Connell et al., 1964; Rees, 1984). The strong male predominance seen in older series was not found by Rees (1984).

Clinical Manifestations

Hemoptysis, anemia, exertional dyspnea, and microscopic hematuria are common findings at the time of presentation (Leatherman et al., 1984a). Azotemia is present in approximately 55% of patients at diagnosis, and, as with IPH, there is often a considerable delay between the onset of symptoms and the correct diagnosis (Leatherman et al., 1984a).

Pathogenesis

Historically, Goodpasture's syndrome was thought to typify a type II (cytotoxic) immunologic reaction in the kidneys and lungs. Circulating anti–glomerular basement membrane antibody is present in the sera of most patients. The renal lesions demonstrate linear immunofluorescence along the basement membranes to IgA, IgG, IgM, and C3 (Donald et al., 1975), findings characteristic of a type II reaction. In the lungs, linear deposits of IgG, IgM, and C3 have been found along alveolar septa (Beirne et al., 1968; Poskitt, 1970; Sturgill and Westervelt, 1965); others have not seen such deposits in the lungs (Donald et al., 1975). A case of glomerulonephritis and alveolar hemorrhage with linear deposits of IgA in the lungs and kidneys has been reported (Border et al., 1979). Histologically, the pulmonary findings are diffuse alveolar hemorrhage and hemosiderin-laden macrophages. Recurrent hemorrhage may result in fibrosis. Severe inflammation is unusual, and neither alveolar septal necrosis nor vasculitis is found (Leatherman et al., 1984b).

ROLE OF ANTI–BASEMENT MEMBRANE ANTIBODIES

The pathogenesis of the lung involvement is unclear. ABM antibody is specific for only a few basement membranes, including those of the renal tubule, glomerulus, alveolus, and choroid plexus. It is possible that an autoimmune process in one organ may produce antibodies that cross-react with similar basement membranes in other organs (Leatherman, 1991). The antigenic component to which the Goodpasture's antibody binds is the α3(IV) chain of type IV collagen (Gunwar et al., 1991). ABM glomerulonephritis may occur without lung disease in 20% to 40% of individuals, but ABM antibody lung disease rarely occurs without renal involvement (Rees, 1984). Difficulties with the concept that high levels of circulating ABM antibody are solely responsible for the lung disease include the following:

1. New episodes of hemorrhage and their severity do not correlate with serum levels of ABM antibody.
2. ABM antibody (in animal experiments) does not appear to bind to alveolar basement membrane in vivo.
3. Most patients with ABM glomerulonephritis without lung involvement have levels of circulating antibody comparable to those with lung disease.
4. Human ABM antibody injected into sheep causes glomerulonephritis but not lung disease (Leatherman et al., 1984a).
5. Alveolar capillaries are usually not permeable to molecules the size of IgG (Rees, 1984).

It is logical, then, to postulate that lung involvement in Goodpasture's syndrome is precipitated by some insult that increases pulmonary capillary permeability, thus allowing circulating antibody to reach the alveolar basement membrane, setting the stage for lung injury (Rees, 1984).

ROLE OF OTHER FACTORS

Duncan and colleagues (1965) suggested that viruses may be implicated, either by sharing antigens with lung and kidney basement membranes or by altering lung and kidney antigens. Viruses may also be implicated by increasing pulmonary capillary permeability; indeed, approximately 50% of patients describe an upper respiratory tract infection immediately before presentation (Leatherman, 1991; Rees, 1984).

Similarly, smoking may be linked to the lung involvement in Goodpasture's syndrome. Donaghy and Rees (1983) studied 51 patients with ABM glomerulonephritis; only 2 of 10 nonsmokers had lung involvement, whereas all smokers had lung and renal disease.

Goodpasture's syndrome is strongly linked to the histocompatibility antigen HLA-DR2, and more severe glomerulonephritis occurs in association with HLA-B7 (Rees, 1984). Thus the expression of injury in this disorder appears to depend on a complex interrelationship among genetic, immunologic, and environmental influences.

GOODPASTURE VARIANTS

Several adults (Beirne et al., 1973; Lewis et al., 1973) and children (Loughlin et al., 1978; van der Ent et al., 1995) show pathologic evidence suggesting that a variant of Goodpasture's syndrome is produced by a type III immunologic process. In these persons, there was no demonstrable circulating ABM antibody; the deposits in the kidney along the basement membrane were granular ("lumpy-bumpy"), suggestive of circulating immune complexes that are cleared by the kidney; and an immunofluorescent study of the lungs revealed no immunoglobulin or complement (Loughlin et al., 1978).

Diagnosis

The identification of ABM antibody in the sera of patients may be performed with high specificity and sensitivity by radioimmunoassay, enzyme-linked immunosorbent assay, and indirect immunofluorescence (least sensitive). The hallmark of this disease is the linear staining of IgG along glomerular basement membrane in renal biopsy specimens. Biopsy and staining should be performed unless strongly contraindicated (Leatherman, 1991).

Treatment and Prognosis

The prognosis is generally poor, with death resulting from massive pulmonary hemorrhage (20%) or renal failure (75%). Plasma exchange and immunosuppressive agents (prednisone and cyclophosphamide, with or without azathioprine) are the currently recommended therapies; however, large comparative clinical trials are needed (Leatherman, 1991; Rees, 1984). The results with steroids are less clear. High-dose methylprednisolone has been successfully used to treat alveolar hemorrhage associated with ABM disease, but not the renal involvement (Briggs et al., 1979). Some clinicians believe that alveolar hemorrhage is better controlled with a combination of plasma exchange and steroids.

Renal transplantation should be postponed until ABM antibodies have disappeared, because the recurrence of glomerular lesions may be noted in up to 30% of renal allografts (Garrick and Neilson, 1988). Nephrectomy, once thought to diminish pulmonary involvement, no longer has a place in the management of Goodpasture's syndrome (Leatherman et al., 1984a).

PULMONARY MANIFESTATIONS OF HUMAN IMMUNODEFICIENCY VIRUS INFECTION

Pulmonary complications occur in two thirds of children infected with HIV and constitute the most frequent cause of death (Cunningham et al., 1991; Hauger, 1991; see Chapter 29). Infectious complications include both opportunistic organisms such as *P. carinii* and *Cryptococcus neoformans* and *Pneumococcus, Salmonella, and Enterococcus* (Bye, 1996). The immunopathogenesis of HIV infection is discussed in detail in Chapter 29. Several unique problems related to the respiratory tract deserve mention here.

Lymphocytic Interstitial Pneumonia

LIP is the most common respiratory complication of pediatric HIV infection. HIV-associated LIP usually occurs in children older than 20 months of age and is common with perinatally acquired disease (i.e., the incidence is 30% to 50%) (Sharland et al., 1997). The clinical presentation varies but typically has an indolent onset without fever. A predominance of rales is heard on auscultation, together with low serum lactate dehydrogenase levels and mild hypoxia with digital clubbing. Pulmonary function changes are typified by a decrease in lung compliance and expiratory flows. Chest radiographs may depict a diffuse reticular or reticulonodular pattern with widening of the mediastinum and hilum (Cunningham et al., 1991; Oldam et al., 1989). Patchy alveolar infiltrates and bronchiectasis have been described (Amorosa et al., 1992).

LIP occurs more often in children with relatively high CD4+ lymphocytes than in those with *P. carinii* infection. Lung biopsy specimens demonstrate diffuse interstitial thickening with occasional nodules. When nodules predominate, the pathogenic picture is referred to as *pulmonary lymphoid hyperplasia* or the *LIP–pulmonary lymphoid hyperplasia complex* (Bye, 1996). Benign, small, noncleaved lymphocytes and plasma cells are found in the alveolar septa, interlobular septa, and subpleural and peribronchial lymph channels. Whereas the pleura, blood vessels, and bronchi are often spared, cellular aggregates may be found around small arteries and distal airways, and pulmonary fibrosis may develop (Oldam et al., 1989; Pitt, 1991).

Bronchiectasis is seen to develop in some with LIP, but the etiology of these changes may be related to infection rather than to the lymphoid aggregates themselves (Bye, 1996; Sheikh et al., 1997). Characteristic findings of LIP are seen on thin-section CT scans and may be helpful in detecting early disease or differentiating this from other causes of respiratory compromise in those infected with HIV (Ambrosino et al., 1995; Becciolini et al., 2001).

Immunophenotypic studies have identified both B- and T-lymphocyte infiltrates (Barbera et al., 1992). CD8+ T-cell clones expressing very late activation antigen-4 bind preferentially to pulmonary vessels expressing high levels of vascular cell adhesion molecule-1. The vascular cell adhesion molecule-1/very late activation adhesion pathway may be responsible for the accumulation of T cells in alveolar septae (Brodie et al., 1999).

The Epstein-Barr virus has been implicated as a synergist in the development of LIP and may act by stimulating B-lymphocyte proliferation (Barbera et al., 1992; Katz et al., 1992). Because zidovudine leads to a positive clinical response in some patients, HIV itself may be a direct causative agent of pulmonary changes (Pitt, 1991). The alveolar macrophage has also been implicated in the pathogenesis of LIP (Semenzato et al., 1991). BAL may be useful in excluding opportunistic infection and may thereby help confirm the diagnosis of LIP. Marked BAL fluid lymphocytosis is seen, but cellular differentials and noncellular components of fluid cannot be accurately related to disease severity or disease progression (de Blic et al., 1989; Midulla et al., 2001).

Treatment consists of supportive care, which may include bronchodilators and supplemental oxygen. Prednisone, human immunoglobulin, and zidovudine have been used in the treatment of LIP, but responses have been variable, and some of these agents lack proof of efficacy by clinical trials (Pitt, 1991). Systemic steroids are typically reserved for those with significant hypoxia (Bye, 1996).

The presence of LIP may represent a period in the natural course of HIV infection when the host's immunoproliferative responses are still somewhat intact. This may precede the period of vulnerability to opportunistic infection. The median age of survival in HIV-infected children who initially present with LIP is 72 months. LIP may be clinically suspected in the child with chronic interstitial pneumonia, lymphocytosis, hypergammaglobulinemia, and lymphadenopathy or parotid enlargement, but a definitive diagnosis is dependent on a lung biopsy.

Other Interstitial Disorders

Other interstitial diseases have been reported in the child with HIV infection but are less frequent (Joshi and Oleske, 1986; Kornstein et al., 1986). DIP differs from LIP in that the normal pulmonary architecture is preserved. The intra-alveolar proliferation of macrophages and cuboidal metaplasia of alveolar type II cells are found on biopsy specimens. Nonspecific chronic interstitial pneumonia only rarely occurs as a complication of HIV infection in children and involves bronchiolar destruction with peribronchiolar interstitial infiltration of lymphocytes, plasma cells, and macrophages. Diagnosis is made at biopsy. Treatment of these entities is the same as for LIP in the child infected with HIV.

Malignancies

Immunoblastic sarcoma has been reported in the lung of a child with HIV infection, with tumor nodules penetrating the bronchial walls and surrounding pleura (Zimmerman et al., 1987). Kaposi's sarcoma is not found in the lungs of children with HIV despite its fairly frequent occurrence in other tissues (Rogers et al., 1987).

Infections

Opportunistic infections are frequent complications in children with HIV infection and are discussed in detail elsewhere (Hauger, 1991; Murray and Mills, 1990; see also Chapters 29 and 41). *P. carinii* infection is also discussed in Chapter 41. Pulmonary infection is typically found in the child whose helper (CD4+) lymphocytes are low ($<400/mm^3$), the helper/suppressor (CD4:CD8) ratio is less than 1.0, and the total lymphocyte count is less than $1500/mm^3$ (Inselman, 1990). BAL fluid typically exhibits increased total lymphocyte numbers, predominantly CD8+ cells, and a low CD4:CD8 ratio. Increases in IgA and IgG levels are found, and the total number of macrophages is low. Clinical disease with

opportunistic infection typically has a more acute onset than interstitial pneumonia. However, differentiation by clinical or radiographic means is often difficult and histologic or microbiologic differentiation is often required.

BRONCHIAL CASTS

Bronchial casts or "plastic bronchitis" is a rare disorder in pediatric patients. Airway obstruction and asphyxiation can occur, with deaths in children reported (Languepin et al., 1999; Seear et al., 1997). The first review on the subject by Bettman (1902) describes the presence of fibrinous casts in the airway and attributes the first reported case to Galen (AD 131-200).

A distinction can be made between two primary types of bronchial cast on the basis of the composition and underlying disease process. Inflammatory casts are composed primarily of fibrin, with a dense eosinophilic infiltrate both in the casts and the surrounding interstitium of the lung. This disorder occurs where underlying bronchopulmonary disease leads to excessive mucous production, such as that seen with asthma, ABPA, CF, tuberculosis, or recent acute pulmonary infection. Acellular casts are characterized by mucin-containing bronchial impaction with little or no inflammatory infiltration.

This disorder is primarily associated with congenital cyanotic heart disease in which palliative procedures have provided increased pulmonary blood flow. An epithelial response to increased pulmonary venous pressure is one proposed mechanism for excessive mucin production in these patients (Seear et al., 1997). Acellular casts have also been described in those with lymphatic drainage abnormalities, and the expectoration of chylous casts has been reported (Nair and Kurtz, 1996; Wetherill et al., 1990; Wiggins et al., 1989). Bronchial cast formation has also been found in individuals manifesting elevated systemic venous pressures and disrupted lymphatic circulation after the surgical treatment of congenital heart disease (Languepin et al., 1999). These patients were also found to have significant acquired immunodeficiency states with severe lymphopenia and low IgG or IgG subclass levels.

The initial treatment of bronchial casts has been directed toward the management of the respiratory distress with support measures, including mechanical ventilation and bronchoscopic removal of casts from the airway. The successful use of aerosolized tissue plasminogen activator has been reported (Costello et al., 2002). Treatment of the underlying disorder is imperative to eliminate the excessive production of mucus in the airway. Patients with inflammatory cast disorders may benefit from the use of systemic and inhaled corticosteroids, antibiotics, bronchodilators, and mucolytics.

The successful management of acellular casts depends on the improvement of underlying cardiac dysfunction, the reduction of central venous pressures, and, in some, the correction of pulmonary lymphatic drainage problems (Languepin et al., 1999; McMahon et al., 2001; Nair and Kurtz, 1996; Seear et al., 1997). In the absence of available treatment, patients with acellular casts have a poor prognosis for survival.

CHYLOTHORAX

Chylothorax describes the accumulation of chyle in the pleural space and is caused by disruption of the thoracic duct or one of its major divisions. The origin of this disorder ranges from tumors (Valentine and Raffin, 1992) to trauma (MacFarlane and Holman, 1972), both surgical and nonsurgical, and to miscellaneous causes (Postma and Keyser, 1997; van Straaten et al., 1993). Chylothorax is seen in children and is the most common cause of pleural effusion in the neonate (de Beer and Janssen, 2000; van Straaten et al., 1993). In newborns, it is found more commonly with congenital duct defects rather than as a result of birth trauma. Chyle is composed of triglycerides, and its turbidity is attributed to its chylomicrons.

The egress of chyle into the pleural space may result in metabolic disturbances, malnutrition, and immunodeficiency states. The diagnosis is made by testing pleural fluid for the presence of triglycerides and chylomicrons (with Sudan III or IV staining). If triglycerides exceed 110 mg/dl, the diagnosis is essentially assured (Staats et al., 1980). Chylous effusions may be bloody (26%), yellow/turbid (10%), have a characteristic "milky" appearance (47%), or rarely be serosanguinous in appearance (de Beer and Janssen, 2000).

The initial management of chylothorax is medical and includes careful monitoring of patient weight, serum albumin, total protein, and absolute lymphocyte counts. Electrolyte monitoring is also important, and chest tube drainage minimizes problems with loss of lung volume. Dietary measures include the use of medium-chain triglycerides, which are directly absorbed into the portal system and minimize thoracic duct flow. If ductal flow requires even more suppression, total parenteral nutrition may be necessary. Somatostatin has been described as an adjunct to total parenteral nutrition in reducing thoracic ductal flow (Ullibarri et al., 1990).

Lymphopenia secondary to pleural loss, together with other metabolic disturbances, make surgical therapy of chylothorax necessary in medical treatment failures (de Beer and Janssen, 2000). Chemical pleurodesis has been successful in a variety of situations and may include the use of talc, tetracycline, or bleomycin (Aoki et al., 1996; Mares and Mathur, 1998). Thoracic ductal ligation, when necessary, can be performed thoracoscopically or at thoracotomy. Pleuroperitoneal shunting may avoid nutritional and immunologic consequences (Cummings et al., 1992), and parietal pleurectomy has been advocated if no chylous leak is found (Browse et al., 1997).

LUNG TRANSPLANTATION

Lung transplantation provides a final hope for long-term survival in a growing number of pediatric patients with end-stage pulmonary disease (see Chapter 43).

The disorders for which lung transplantation has been performed include pulmonary fibrosis, obliterative bronchiolitis, emphysema, pulmonary hypertension, bronchopulmonary dysplasia, pulmonary vein stenosis, surfactant protein–B deficiency, and cystic fibrosis (Gaynor et al., 1998; Hamvas et al., 1997; Warner, 1999). The most common condition for which lung transplantation has been performed in children is CF; more than 50 living-donor lobar transplants have been performed in this group (Warner, 1999; Yankaskas and Mallory, 1998). The relative contraindications for lung transplantation include psychosocial problems, other serious organ system disease, and ventilator dependency. The growth of transplant center activity has been inhibited by a serious shortage of donor organs.

The survival rates after lung transplantation in children, as reported by Sweet and colleagues (1997), are 69%, 67%, and 60% at 12, 24, and 48 months, respectively. Their data suggest little difference in survival between children younger than 3 years old at transplantation and those undergoing transplantation later in childhood. In fact, infants may be less likely to reject their donor graft than older children and do not develop bronchiolitis obliterans (Huddleston and Mendeloff, 2001; Sweet et al., 1997).

ABO blood group compatibility, body size, cytomegalovirus (CMV) serologic status, and HLA compatibility are considered in donor and recipient evaluations (Lau et al., 2000; Warner, 1999; Wisser et al., 1996). HLA incompatibilities may be through expanded immunosuppressive treatment regimens (van den Berg et al., 2001). Careful management of the donor lung during harvesting and transfer is essential; donor cooling with cardiopulmonary bypass has allowed ischemia times up to 5 hours (Heritier et al., 1992). Infections, bronchiolitis obliterans, and the complications of immunosuppressive therapy pose many serious challenges to the long-term success of lung transplantation in children (Gaynor et al., 1998).

Survival after the transplantation of thoracic organs improved dramatically after introduction of cyclosporine (Borell and Kiss, 1991). Still the mainstay of suppression for allograft rejection, its blood level must be carefully monitored to prevent toxicity. Potential complications include nephrotoxicity, hyperkalemia, hepatotoxicity, gingival hyperplasia, hirsutism, hypertension, and convulsions (Heritier et al., 1992). Cyclosporine is lipophilic, and gastrointestinal absorption is impaired in CF patients. A newer microemulsion form of cyclosporine has helped in overcoming this problem to some extent (Girault et al., 1995).

Additional immunosuppression is achieved with azathioprine. In the perioperative period, methylprednisolone, antithymocyte globulin, and anti–T-cell monoclonal antibodies are used to ensure graft survival (Gaynor et al., 1998). OKT3 (murine monoclonal anti-CD3 antibody) and polyclonal antithymocyte globulin are used during induction therapy but are associated with posttransplant lymphoproliferative disease and viral illness with CMV, respiratory syncytial virus, and adenovirus.

Tacrolimus (FK506) is an attractive alternative to cyclosporine in some pediatric patients because of its more favorable toxicity profile, but anemia, renal toxicity, and chronic diarrhea do occur. The side effects of corticosteroids are poorly tolerated in children and include hypertension, growth retardation, osteoporosis, and diabetes mellitus. Attempts are usually made to withdraw this drug during the establishment of maintenance immunosuppressive therapy. Immunosuppressive agents function through interaction with intracellular binding proteins known as *immunophilins*. The formation of these complexes blocks the calcium-dependent signal transduction pathway, which is initiated by the activation of T-cell receptors. The inactivation of T cells prevents the initiation of graft rejection (Briffa and Morris, 1997).

Acute pulmonary rejection is common and manifests as increasing breathlessness, cough, low-grade fever, and crackles or wheezes. Successful monitoring for rejection includes a high index of suspicion and the use of pulmonary function tests, in addition to the aggressive use of bronchoscopy for bronchoalveolar lavage and transbronchial biopsy (Warner, 1999). Transbronchial biopsy remains the definitive test for detecting rejection in the transplanted organ (Whitehead et al., 1992) and is used in the surveillance of treatment of acute episodes of rejection (Aboyoun et al., 2001). Histologic testing reveals dense perivascular cuffing by mononuclear cells (Higgenbottam et al., 1988). Less invasive methods of detecting early rejection episodes are under investigation (Sedivá et al., 2001).

Treatment of acute rejection involves intensified immunosuppression with increased doses of cyclosporine and high-dose prednisone and the use, in some cases, of antithymocyte globulin and T-cell receptor antibodies (Gaynor et al., 1998). Early death caused by acute rejection is rare (10%).

Bronchiolitis obliterans is an inflammatory and proliferative injury to the small airways of the donor lung and may be rapidly progressive. The etiology is felt to be chronic rejection, but viral infection, airway ischemia, and airway denervation have also been suggested (Boucek et al., 1997).

Infectious complications account for up to 25% of deaths in the first 90 days after transplantation. Bacterial pneumonias are usually responsive to appropriate antibiotics. In addition, patients are at risk for fungal and parasitic infections such as *P. carinii* and toxoplasmosis. Viral infections pose a serious risk for individuals with transplants. CMV pneumonia occurs in up to 25% of patients, and is especially common in CMV-negative recipients of CMV-positive organs. Treatment consists of ganciclovir and CMV hyperimmune globulin (Hutter et al., 1989). Primary herpesvirus infections occur in up to 10% of patients and are treated with acyclovir. Epstein-Barr virus infections are less frequent but are associated with the development of posttransplant lymphoproliferative syndrome (Harwood et al., 1999).

Organisms found in the respiratory tract of CF patients may cause posttransplant complications and include *B. cepacia*, *P. aeruginosa* resistant to multiple drugs, *Aspergillus* species, and nontuberculous mycobacterium. Special consideration must be made in the management of these patients to prevent complications of invasive disease during immunosuppression after transplantation (Yankaskas and Mallory, 1998).

Lung transplantation requires that the patient and family exchange a life-ending condition for what is hoped will be a life-prolonging procedure that includes significant health risks (Stubblefield and Murray, 2000). Fortunately, our experience in this field has led to significant improvements in survival and in quality of life for many lung recipients. The experience is one that requires significant commitment and the careful selection of patients.

The psychological demands on the patient—even after the sometimes agonizing wait for a donor organ—are extreme. The transplantation experience has been described as an "awesome, demanding and stressful journey" (Suszycki, 1988). The needs of these patients and their families are unique and extreme, and a highly developed multidisciplinary team is necessary.

ACKNOWLEDGMENT

I am deeply indebted to Karen L. Keller, MLS, and Dena Fracolli Hanson, MLS, AHIP, of the Edwin G. Schwartz Health Sciences Library at Cook Children's Medical Center for their support and guidance.

REFERENCES

Aboyoun CL, Tamm M, Chhajed PN, Hopkins P, Malouf MA, Rainer S, Glanville AR. Diagnostic value of follow-up transbronchial lung biopsy after lung rejection. Am J Respir Crit Care Med 164:460–463, 2001.

Aitken ML, Fiel SB, Stern RC. Cystic fibrosis: respiratory manifestations. In Taussig LM, Landau LI, eds. Pediatric respiratory medicine. St. Louis, Mosby, 1999, pp 1009–1032.

Allen DH, Williams GV, Woolcock AJ. Bird breeder's hypersensitivity pneumonitis: progress studies of lung function after cessation of exposure to the provoking antigen. Am Rev Respir Dis 114:555–566, 1976.

Allen JN, Davis WB. Eosinophilic lung diseases. Am J Respir Crit Care Med 150:1423–1438, 1994.

Allue X, Wise MB, Beaudry PH. Pulmonary function studies in idiopathic pulmonary hemosiderosis in children. Am Rev Respir Dis 107:410–415, 1973.

Alton E, Geddes D. Cystic fibrosis clinical trials. Adv Drug Deliv Rev 30:205–217, 1998.

Alvarado CS, Boat TF, Newman AJ. Late-onset pulmonary fibrosis and chest deformity in two children treated with cyclophosphamide. J Pediatr 92:443–446, 1978.

Ambrosino MM, Roche KJ, Genieser NB, Kaul A, Lawrence RM. Application of thin-section low-dose chest CT (TSCT) in the management of pediatric AIDS. Pediatr Radiol 25:393–400, 1995.

Amorosa JK, Miller RW, Laraya-Cuasay L, Gaur S, Marone R, Frenkel L, Nosher JL. Bronchiectasis in children with lymphocytic interstitial pneumonia and acquired immune deficiency syndrome. Plain film and CT observations. Pediatr Radiol 22:603–607, 1992.

Aoki M, Kato F, Saito H, Mimatsu K, Iwata H. Successful treatment of chylothorax by bleomycin for Gorham's disease. Clin Orthop 330:193–197, 1996.

Asherson RA, Oakley CM. Pulmonary hypertension and systemic lupus erythematosus. J Rheumatol 13:1–5, 1986.

Asherson RA, Cervera R. Review: antiphospholipid antibodies and the lung. J Rheumatol 22:62–66, 1995.

Athreya BH, Doughty RA, Bookspan M, Schumacher HR, Sewell EM, Chatten J. Pulmonary manifestations of juvenile rheumatoid arthritis. A report of eight cases and review. Clin Chest Med 1:361–374, 1980.

Auerbach HS, Kirkpatrick JA, Williams M, Colten HR. Alternate-day prednisone reduces morbidity and improves pulmonary function in cystic fibrosis. Lancet 2:686–688, 1985.

Barbera JA, Hayashi S, Hegele RG, Hogg JC. Detection of Epstein-Barr virus in lymphocytic interstitial pneumonia by in situ hybridization. Am Rev Respir Dis 145:940–946, 1992.

Bardana EJ, Sobti KL, Cianciulli FD, Noonan MJ. *Aspergillus* antibody in patients with cystic fibrosis. Am J Dis Child 129:1164–1167, 1975.

Beckerman RC, Taussig LM, Pinnas JL. Familial idiopathic pulmonary hemosiderosis. Am J Dis Child 133:609–611, 1979.

Becciolini V, Gudinchet F, Cheseaux JJ, Schnyder P. Lymphocytic interstitial pneumonia in children with AIDS: high-resolution CT findings. Eur Radiol 11:1015–1020, 2001.

Bedrossian CW, Greenberg SD, Singer DB, Hansen JJ, Rosenberg HS. The lung in cystic fibrosis. A quantitative study including the prevalence of pathologic findings among different age groups. Hum Pathol 7:195–204, 1976.

Beirne GJ, Kopp WL, Zimmerman SW. Goodpasture syndrome. Dissociation from antibodies to glomerular basement membrane. Arch Intern Med 132:261–263, 1973.

Beirne GJ, Octaviano GN, Kopp WL, Burns RO. Immunohistology of the lung in Goodpasture's syndrome. Ann Intern Med 69:1207–1212, 1968.

Bennett WD, Olivier KN, Zeman KL, Hohneker KW, Boucher RC, Knowles MR. Effect of uridine 5′-triphosphate plus amiloride on mucociliary clearance in adult cystic fibrosis. Am J Respir Crit Care Med 153:1796–1801, 1996.

Bentur L, McKlusky I, Levison H, Roifman CM. Advanced lung disease in a patient with cystic fibrosis and hypogammaglobulinemia: response to intravenous immune globulin therapy. J Pediatr 117:741–743, 1990.

Bentur L, Lachter J, Koren I, Ben-Izhak O, Lavy A, Bentur Y, Rosenthal E. Severe pulmonary disease in association with Crohn's disease in a 13-year-old girl. Pediatr Pulmonol 29:151–154, 2000.

Berdischewsky M, Pollack M, Young LS, Chia D, Osher AB, Barnett EV. Circulating immune complexes in cystic fibrosis. Pediatr Res 14:830–833, 1980.

Berrill WT, van Rood JJ. HLA-DW6 and avian hypersensitivity. Lancet 2:248–249, 1977.

Berry DH, Brewster MA. Granulocyte NADH oxidase in cystic fibrosis. Ann Allergy 38:316–319, 1977.

Bettman M. Report of a case of fibrinous bronchiolitis, with a review of all cases in the literature. Am J Med Sci 123:304–329, 1902.

Bhagwat AG, Wentworth P, Conen PE. Observations on the relationship of desquamative interstitial pneumonia and pulmonary alveolar proteinosis in childhood: a pathologic and experimental study. Chest 58:326–332, 1970.

Bienenstock J. The lung as an immunologic organ. Annu Rev Med 35:49–62, 1984.

Biggar WD, Holmes B, Good RA. Opsonic defect in patients with cystic fibrosis of the pancreas. Proc Natl Acad Sci U S A 68:1716–1719, 1971.

Bigger B, Coutelle C. Perspectives on gene therapy for cystic fibrosis airway disease. BioDrugs 15:615–634, 2001.

Birrer P, McElvaney NG, Rudeberg A, Sommer CW, Liechti-Gallati S, Kraemer R, Hubbard R, Crystal RG. Protease-antiprotease imbalance in the lungs of children with cystic fibrosis. Am J Respir Crit Care Med 150:207–213, 1994.

Bitnum S, Daeschner CW Jr, Travis LB, Dodge WF, Hopps HC. Dermatomyositis. J Pediatr 64:101–131, 1964.

Boat TF, Polmar SH, Whitman V, Kleinerman JI, Stern RC, Doershuk CF. Hyperreactivity to cow milk in young children with pulmonary hemosiderosis and cor pulmonale secondary to nasopharyngeal obstruction. J Pediatr 87:23–29, 1975.

Boat TF, Welsh MJ, Beaudet AL. Cystic fibrosis. In Beaudet AL, Sly WS, Valle D, eds. Metabolic basis of inherited disease. New York, McGraw-Hill, 1989, pp 2649–2680.

Border WA, Baehler RW, Bhathena D, Glassock RJ. IgA antibasement membrane nephritis with pulmonary hemorrhage. Ann Intern Med 91:21–25, 1979.

Borell JF, Kiss ZL. The discovery and development of cyclosporine (Sandimmune). Transplant Proc 23:1867–1874, 1991.

Bosken CH, Myers JL, Greenberger PA, Katzenstein AL. Pathologic features of allergic bronchopulmonary aspergillosis. Am J Surg Pathol 12:216–222, 1988.

Boucek MM, Novick RJ, Bennett LE, Fiol B, Keck BM, Hosenpud JD. The Registry of the International Society of Heart and Lung Transplantation: first official pediatric report—1997. J Heart Lung Transplant 16:1189–1206, 1997.

Boucher RC. Pathogenesis of cystic fibrosis airways disease. Trans Am Clin Climatol Assoc 112:99–107, 2001.

Bowden DH. The alveolar macrophage. Environ Health Perspect 55:327–341, 1984.

Boxerbaum B, Kagumba A, Matthews LW. Selective inhibition of phagocytic activity of rabbit alveolar macrophages by cystic fibrosis serum. Am Rev Respir Dis 108:777–783, 1973.

Bradley CA III. Diffuse interstitial fibrosis of the lungs in children. J Pediatr 48:442–450, 1956.

Brett MM, Simmonds EJ, Ghoneim AT, Littlewood JM. The value of serum IgG titres against *Pseudomonas aeruginosa* in the management of early pseudomonal infection in cystic fibrosis. Arch Dis Child 67:1086–1088, 1992.

Briffa N, Morris RE. New immunosuppressive regimens in lung transplatation. Eur Respir J 10:2630–2637, 1997.

Briggs WA, Johnson JP, Teichman S, Yeager HC, Wilson CB. Antiglomerular basement membrane antibody–mediated glomerulonephritis and Goodpasture's syndrome. Medicine (Baltimore) 58:348–361, 1979.

Brodie SJ, de la Rosa C, Howe JG, Crouch J, Travis WD, Diem K. Pediatric AIDS-associated lymphocytic interstitial pneumonia and pulmonary arterio-occlusive disease: role of VCAM-1/VLA-4 adhesion pathway and human herpesvirus. Am J Pathol 154:1453–1464, 1999.

Broughton RA, Wilson HD. Nitrofurantoin pulmonary toxicity in a child. Pediatr Infect Dis 5:466–469, 1986.

Brown CH, Turner-Warwick M. The treatment of cryptogenic fibrosing alveolitis with immunosuppressant drugs. Q J Med 40:289–302, 1971.

Brown K, Rosenthal M, Bush A. Fatal invasive aspergillosis in an addolescent with cystic fibrosis. Pediatr Pulmonol 27:130–133, 1999.

Browse NL, Allen DR, Wilson NM. Management of chylothorax. Br J Surg 84:1711–1716, 1997.

Buchta RM, Park S, Giammona ST. Desquamative interstitial pneumonia in a 7-week-old infant. Am J Dis Child 120:341–343, 1970.

Buescher ES, Winkelstein JA. The ability of bacteria to activate the terminal complement components in serum of patients with cystic fibrosis. J Pediatr 93:530–531, 1978.

Bye MR. HIV in children. Clin Chest Med 17:787–796, 1996.

Byrd RB, Gracey DR. Immunosuppressive treatment of idiopathic pulmonary hemosiderosis. JAMA 226:458–459, 1973.

Caeiro F, Michielson FM, Bernstein R, Hughes GR, Ansell BM. Systemic lupus erythematosus in childhood. Ann Rheum Dis 40:325–331, 1981.

Caldwell JR, Pearce DE, Spencer C, Leder R, Waldman RH. Immunologic mechanisms in hypersensitivity pneumonitis. I. Evidence for cell-mediated immunity and complement fixation in pigeon breeders' disease. J Allergy Clin Immunol 52:225–230, 1973.

Calvanico NJ, Fink JN, Keller RH. Hypersensitivity pneumonitis. In Bienenstock J, ed. Immunology of the lung and upper respiratory tract. New York, McGraw-Hill, 1984, pp 365–385.

Campbell PW III, Phillips JA III, Krishnamani MR, Maness KJ, Hazinski TA. Cystic fibrosis: relationship between clinical status and F508 deletion. J Pediatr 118:239–241, 1991.

Carette S. Cardiopulmonary manifestations of systemic lupus erythematosous. Rheum Dis Clin North Am 14:135–147, 1988.

Carré PC, Mortenson RL, King TE Jr, Noble PW, Sable CL, Riches WD. Increased expression of interleukin-8 gene by alveolar macrophages in idiopathic pulmonary fibrosis. A potential mechanism for the recruitment and activation of neutrophils in lung fibrosis. J Clin Invest 88:1802–1810, 1991.

Carrington CB, Addington WW, Goff AM, Madoff IM, Marks A, Schwaber JR, Gaensler EA. Chronic eosinophilic pneumonia. N Engl J Med 280:787–798, 1969.

Carrington CB, Gaensler EA, Coutu RE, FitzGerald MX, Gupta RG. Natural history and treated course of usual and desquamative interstitial pneumonia. N Engl J Med 298:801–809, 1978.

Carroll JL, Sterni LM. Eosinophilic lung disorders and hypersensitivity pneumonitis. In Taussig LM, Landau LI, eds. Pediatric respiratory medicine. St. Louis, Mosby, 1999, pp 804–811.

Carswell F, Oliver J, Silverman M. Allergy in cystic fibrosis. Clin Exp Immunol 35:141–146, 1979.

Cazzato S, Bernardi F, Cinti C, Tassinari D, Canzi A, Bergamaschi R, Corsini I, Capecchi V, Cacciari E. Pulmonary function abnormalities in children with Henoch-Schönlein purpura. Eur Respir J 13:597–601, 1999.

Chandra S, Jones HE. Pigeon fancier's lung in children. Arch Dis Child 47:716–718, 1972.

Chaussain M, de Boissieu D, Kalifa G, Epelbaum S, Niaudet P, Badoual J, Gendrel D. Impairment of lung diffusion capacity in Schönlein-Henoch purpura. J Pediatr 121:12–16, 1992.

Chen JH, Schulman H, Gardner P. A cAMP-regulated chloride channel in lymphocytes that is affected in cystic fibrosis. Science 243:657–660, 1989.

Cheng K, Smyth RL, Govan JR, Doherty C, Winstanley C, Denning N, Heaf DP, van Saene H, Hart CA. Spread of a-lactam–resistant Pseudomonas aeruginosa in a cystic fibrosis clinic. Lancet 348:639–642, 1996.

Cheng SH, Gregory RJ, Marshall J, Paul S, Souza DW, White GA, O'Riordan CR, Smith AE. Defective intracellular transport and processing of CFTR is the molecular basis of most cystic fibrosis. Cell 63:827–834, 1990.

Cherniack RM, Crystal RG, Kalica AR. NHLBI Workshop summary. Current concepts in idiopathic pulmonary fibrosis: a road map for the future. Am Rev Respir Dis 143:680–683, 1991.

Chihara J, Kino T, Nakajima S. Observation of eosinophil chemotactic activity in sera and bronchoalveolar lavage fluid in patients with eosinophilic pneumonia. Nihon Kyobu Shikkan Gakkai Zasshi 26:714–719, 1988.

Chillon M, Casals T, Mercier B, Bassas L, Lissens W, Silber S, Romey MC, Ruiz-Romero J, Verlingue C, Claustres M, et al. Mutations in the cystic fibrosis gene in patients with congenital absence of the vas deferens. N Engl J Med 332:1475–1480, 1995.

Chiron C, Gaultier C, Boule M, Grimfeld A, Girard F. Lung function in children with hypersensitivity pneumonitis. Eur J Respir Dis 65:79–91, 1984.

Choi YH, Im JG, Han BK, Kim JH, Lee KY, Myoung NH. Thoracic manifestation of Churg-Strauss syndrome: radiologic and clinical findings. Chest 117:117–124, 2000.

Chryssanthopoulos C, Cassimos C, Panagiotidou C. Prognostic criteria in idiopathic pulmonary hemosiderosis in children. Eur J Pediatr 140:123–125, 1983.

Church JA, Jordan SC, Keens TG, Wang CI. Circulating immune complexes in patients with cystic fibrosis. Chest 80:405–411, 1981.

Church JA, Keens TG, Wang CI. Neutrophil and monocyte chemotaxis in acutely infected patients with cystic fibrosis. Ann Allergy 45:217–219, 1980.

Church JA, Keens TG, Wang CI, O'Neal M, Richards W. Normal neutrophil and monocyte chemotaxis in patients with cystic fibrosis. J Pediatr 95:2724, 1979.

Chusid MJ, Dale DC, West BC, Wolff SM. The hypereosinophilic syndrome: analysis of fourteen cases with review of the literature. Medicine (Baltimore) 54:1–27, 1975.

Citro LA, Gordon ME, Miller WT. Eosinophilic lung disease (or how to slice P.I.E.). AJR Am J Roentgenol Radium Ther Nucl Med 117:787–797, 1973.

Clarke CW. Aspects of serum and sputum antibody in chronic airways obstruction. Thorax 31:702–707, 1976.

Clarke LL, Grubb BR, Gabriel SE, Smithies O, Koller BH, Boucher RC. Defective epithelial chloride transport in a gene-targeted mouse model of cystic fibrosis. Science 257:1125–1128, 1992.

Clarke SW, Pavia D. Mucociliary clearance. In Crystal RG, West JB, et al., eds. The lung scientific foundations. New York, Raven Press, 1991, pp 1845–1859.

Clayton RG, Schidlow DV. Drug-induced pulmonary disease. In Taussig LM, Landau LI, eds. Pediatric respiratory medicine. St. Louis, Mosby, 1999, pp 457–461.

Cochrane CG. Mechanisms involved in the deposition of immune complexes in tissues. J Exp Med 134:75–89, 1971.

Cohen SG, Ottesen EA. The eosinophil, eosinophilia, and eosinophil-related disorders. In Middleton E Jr, Reed CE, Ellis EF, eds. Allergy: principles and practice. 2nd ed. St. Louis, Mosby, 1983, pp 701–769.

Cohn JA, Friedman KJ, Noone PG, Knowles MR, Silverman LM, Jowell PS. Relation between mutations of the cystic fibrosis gene and idiopathic pancreatitis. N Engl J Med 339:653–658, 1998.

Collins FS. Cystic fibrosis: molecular biology and therapeutic implications. Science 256:774–779, 1992.

Conese M, Assael BM. Bacterial infections and inflammation in the lungs of cystic fibrosis patients. Pediatr Infect Dis J 20:207–213, 2001.

Coombs RR, Gell PG. The classification of allergic reactions underlying disease. In Gell PGH, Coombs RRA, eds. Clinical aspects of immunology. 2nd ed. Oxford, Blackwell, 1968, pp 317–337.

Cooray JH, Ismail MM. Re-examination of the diagnositc criteria of tropical pulmonary eosinophilia. Respir Med 93:655–659, 1999.

Coraggio MJ, Gross TP, Roscelli JD. Nitrofurantoin toxicity in children. Pediatr Infect Dis J 8:163–166, 1989.

Cordier JF, Valeyre D, Guillevin L, Loire R, Brechot JM. Pulmonary Wegener's granulomatosis. A clinical and imaging study of 77 cases. Chest 97:906–912, 1990.

Costello JM, Steinhorn D, McColley S, Gerber ME, Kumar SP. Treatment of plastic bronchitis in a Fontan patient with tissue plasminogen activator: a case report and review of the literature (electronic article). Pediatrics 109:e67, 2002.

Crofton JW, Livingstone JL, Oswald NC, Roberts AT. Pulmonary eosinophilia. Thorax 7:1–35, 1952.

Cromwell O, Moqbel R, Fitzharris P, Kurlak L, Harvey C, Walsh GM, Shaw RJ, Kay AB. Leukotriene C4 generation from human eosinophils stimulated with IgG-Aspergillus fumigatus antigen immune complexes. J Allergy Clin Immunol 82:535–543, 1988.

Crystal RG. Alveolar macrophages. In Crystal RG, Barnes PJ, Cherniak NS, Werbel ER, West JB, eds. The lung: scientific foundations. New York, Raven Press, 1991, pp 527–538.

Crystal RG, Fulmer JD, Roberts WC, Moss ML, Reynolds HY. Idiopathic pulmonary fibrosis. Clinical, histologic, radiographic, physiologic, scintigraphic, cytologic, and biochemical aspects. Ann Intern Med 85:769–788, 1976.

Crystal RG, Gadek JE, Ferrans VJ, Fulmer JD, Line BR, Hunninghake GW. Interstitial lung disease: current concepts of pathogenesis, staging and therapy. Am J Med 70:542–568, 1981.

Crystal RG, McElvaney NG, Rosenfeld MA, Chu CS, Mastrangeli A, Hay JG, Brody SL, Jaffe HA, Eissa NT, Danel C. Administration of an adenovirus containing the human CFTR cDNA to the respiratory tract of individuals with cystic fibrosis. Nat Genet 8:42–51, 1994.

Cummings SP, Wyatt DA, Baker JW, Flanagan TL, Spotnitz WD, Rodgers BM, Kron IL, Tribble CG. Successful treatment of postoperative chylothorax using external pleuroperitoneal shunt. Ann Thorac Surg 54:276–278, 1992.

Cunningham AS, Fink JN, Schlueter DP. Childhood hypersensitivity pneumonitis due to dove antigens. Pediatrics 58:436–442, 1976.

Cunningham SJ, Crain EF, Bernstein LJ. Evaluating the HIV-infected child with pulmonary signs and symptoms. Pediatr Emerg Care 7:32–37, 1991.

Cupps TR, Fauci AS. The vasculitides. Major Probl Intern Med 21:1–211, 1981.

Cystic Fibrosis Genetic Analysis Consortium. Worldwide survey of the delta F508 mutation—report from the cystic fibrosis genetic analysis consortium. Am J Hum Genet 47:354–359, 1990.

Dabich L, Sullivan DB, Cassidy JT. Scleroderma in the child. J Pediatr 85:770–775, 1974.

Dai Y, Dean TP, Church MK, Warner JO, Shute JK. Desensitisation of neutrophil responses by systemic interleukin 8 in cystic fibrosis. Thorax 49:867–871, 1994.

Dalavanga YA, Constantopoulos SH, Galanopoulou V, Zerva L, Moutsopoulos HM. Alveolitis correlates with clinical pulmonary involvement in primary Sjögren's syndrome. Chest 99:1394–1397, 1991.

Daniele RP, Whiteside TL, Rowlands DT. Cells and secretory products of the immune system. In Daniele RP, ed. Immunology and immunologic diseases of the lung. Boston, Mass., Blackwell Scientific Publications, 1988, pp 3–19.

Davies JC, Stern M, Dewar A, Caplen NJ, Munkonge FM, Pitt T, Sorgi F, Huang L, Bush A, Geddes DM, Alton EW. CFTR gene transfer reduces the binding of Pseudomonas aeruginosa to cystic fibrosis respiratory epithelium. Am J Respir Cell Mol Biol 16:657–663, 1997.

Davis PB, Dieckman L, Boat TF, Stern RC, Doershuk CF. Beta adrenergic receptors in lymphocytes and granulocytes from patients with cystic fibrosis. J Clin Invest 71:1787–1795, 1983.

Davis PB, di Sant'Agnese PA. Diagnosis and treatment of cystic fibrosis. An update. Chest 85:802–809, 1984.

Davis PB. Cystic fibrosis from bench to bedside. N Engl J Med 325:575–577, 1991.

Day C, Savage C. Primary systemic vasculitis. Minerva Med 92:349–363, 2001.

de Beer HG, Mol MJ, Janssen JP. Chylothorax. Neth J Med 56:25–31, 2000.

de Blic J, Blanche S, Danel C, Le Bourgeois M, Caniglia M, Scheinmann P. Bronchoalveolar lavage in HIV infected patients with interstitial pneumonitis. Arch Dis Child 64:1246–1250, 1989.

DeHoratius RJ, Abruzzo JL, Williams RC Jr. Immunofluorescent and immunologic studies of rheumatoid lung. Arch Intern Med 129:441–446, 1972.

Dejaegher P, Derveaux L, Dubois P, Demedts M. Eosinophilic pneumonia without radiographic pulmonary infiltrates. Chest 84:637–638, 1983.

de Jongste JC, Neijens HJ, Duiverman EJ, Bogaard JM, Kerrebijn KF. Respiratory tract disease in systemic lupus erythematosus. Arch Dis Child 61:478–483, 1986.

de la Fuente J, Nodar A, Sopena B, Martinez CA, Fernandez A. Rheumatic pneumonia. Ann Rheum Dis 60:990–991, 2001.

Delgado EA, Malleson PN, Pirie GE, Petty RE. The pulmonary manifestations of childhood onset systemic lupus erythematosus. Semin Arthritis Rheum 19:285–293, 1990.

Denning DW, Van Wye JE, Lewiston NJ, Stevens DA. Adjunctive therapy of allergic bronchopulmonary aspergillosis with itraconazole. Chest 100:813–819, 1991.

Desnoyers MR, Bernstein S, Cooper AG, Kopelman RI. Pulmonary hemorrhage in lupus erythematosus without evidence of an immunologic cause. Arch Intern Med 144:1398–1400, 1984.

Detjen PF, Greenberger PA, Patterson R. Allergic bronchopulmonary aspergillosis. In Lynch JP, DeRemee RA, eds. Immunologically mediated pulmonary diseases. Philadelphia, Lippincott, 1991, pp 378–398.

Diaz RP, Bowman CM. Childhood interstitial lung disease. Semin Respir Med 11:253–268, 1990.

DiMango E, Ratner AJ, Bryan R, Tabibi S, Prince A. Activation of NF-κB by adherent Pseudomonas aeruginosa in normal and cystic fibrosis respiratory epithelial cells. J Clin Invest 101:2598–2605, 1998.

Dinwiddie R. Pathogenesis of lung disease in cystic fibrosis. Respiration 67:3–8, 2000.

di Sant'Agnese PA, Darling RC, Perea GA, Shea E. Abnormal electrolyte composition of sweat in cystic fibrosis of the pancreas. Pediatrics 12:549–563, 1963.

Disis ML, McDonald TL, Colombo JL, Kobayashi R, Angle CR, Murray S. Circulating immune complexes in cystic fibrosis and their correlation to clinical parameters. Pediatr Res 20:385–390, 1986.

Dolan CJ Jr, Srodes CH, Duffy FD. Idiopathic pulmonary hemosiderosis. Electron microscopic, immunofluorescent, and iron kinetic studies. Chest 68:577–580, 1975.

Doll NJ, Salvaggio JE. Pulmonary manifestations of the collagen-vascular disease. Semin Respir Med 5:273–281, 1984.

Donaghy M, Rees AJ. Cigarette smoking and lung hemorrhage in glomerulonephritis caused by autoantibodies to glomerular basement membrane. Lancet 2:1390–1393, 1983.

Donald KJ, Edwards RL, McEvoy JD. Alveolar capillary basement membrane lesions in Goodpasture's syndrome and idiopathic pulmonary hemosiderosis. Am J Med 59:642–649, 1975.

Donati MA, Guenette G, Auerbach H. Prospective controlled study of home and hospital therapy of cystic fibrosis pulmonary disease. J Pediatr 111:28–33, 1987.

Döring G, Albus A, Høiby N. Immunologic aspects of cystic fibrosis. Chest 94:109S–115S, 1988.

Douar AM, Adebakin S, Themis M, Pavirani A, Cook T, Coutelle C. Foetal gene delivery in mice by intra-amniotic administration of retroviral producer cells and adenovirus. Gene Ther 4:883–890, 1997.

Doull IJM. Recent advances in cystic fibrosis. Arch Dis Child 85:62–66, 2001.

Duan D, Yue Y, Yan Z, McCray PB Jr, Engelhardt JF. Polarity influences the efficiency of recombinant adenoassociated virus infection in differentiated airway epithelia. Hum Gene Ther 9:2761–2776, 1998.

Duncan DA, Drummond KN, Michael AF, Vernier RL. Pulmonary hemorrhage and glomerulonephritis. Report of six cases and study of the renal lesion by the fluorescent antibody technique and electron microscopy. Ann Intern Med 62:920–938, 1965.

Eisenberg H. The interstitial lung diseases associated with the collagen-vascular disorders. Clin Chest Med 3:565–578, 1982.

Eisenberg H, Dubois EL, Sherwin RP, Balchum OJ. Diffuse interstitial lung disease in systemic lupus erythematosus. Ann Intern Med 79:37–45, 1973.

Elborn JS, Shale DJ, Britton JR. Cystic fibrosis: current survival and population estimates to the year 2000. Thorax 46:881–885, 1991.

Emrie P, Fisher JH. Genetic basis of cystic fibrosis. Semin Respir Med 7:359–361, 1986.

Ephrem D. Rheumatic pneumonia in a 10-year-old Ethiopian child. East Afr Med J 67:740–742, 1990.

Epler GR, McLoud TC, Gaensler EA, Mikus JP, Carrington CB. Normal chest roentgenograms in chronic diffuse infiltrative lung disease. N Engl J Med 298:934–939, 1978.

Evans RB, Ettensohn DB, Fawaz-Estrup F, Lally EV, Kaplan SR. Gold lung: recent developments in pathogenesis, diagnosis, and therapy. Semin Arthritis Rheum 16:196–205, 1987.

Falchuk ZM, Taussig LM. IgA synthesis by jejunal biopsies from patients with cystic fibrosis and hereditary pancreatitis. Pediatrics 51:49–54, 1973.

Falcini F, Pignone A, Matucci-Cerinic M, Camiciottoli G, Taccetti G, Trapani S, Zammarchi E, Lombardi A, Bartolozzi G, Cagnoni M. Clinical utility of non invasive methods in the evaluation of scleroderma lung in pediatric age. Scand J Rheumatol 21:82–84, 1992.

Falk M, Kelstrup M, Andersen JB, Kinoshita T, Falk P, Stovring S, Gothgen I. Improving the ketchup bottle method with positive expiratory pressure, PEP, in cystic fibrosis. Eur J Respir Dis 65:423–432, 1984.

Fan LL, Mullen AL, Brugman SM, Inscore SC, Parks DP, White CW. Clinical spectrum of chronic interstitial lung disease in children. J Pediatr 121:867–872, 1992.

Fantone JC, Ward PA. Chemotactic mechanisms in the lung. In Newball HH, eds. Immunopharmacology of the lung. New York, Marcel Dekker, 1983, pp 243–272.

Farhood H, Serbina N, Huang L. The role of dioleoyl phophatidylethanolamine in cationic liposome mediated gene transfer. Biochem Biophys Acta 1235:289–295, 1995.

Farrell PM, Gilbert EF, Zimmerman JJ, Warner TF, Saari TN. Familial lung disease associated with proliferation and desquamation of type II pneumocytes. Am J Dis Child 140:262–266, 1986.

Farrell PM, Kosorok MR, Laxova A, Shen G, Koscik RE, Bruns WT, Splaingard M, Mischler EH. Nutritional benefits of neonatal screening for cystic fibrosis. Wisconsin Cystic Fibrosis Neonatal Screening Study Group. N Engl J Med 337:963–969, 1997.

Farrell PM, Kosorok MR, Rock MJ, Laxova A, Zeng L, Lai HC, Hoffman G, Laessig RH, Splaingard ML. Early diagnosis of cystic fibrosis through neonatal screening prevents severe malnutrition and improves long-term growth. Wisconsin Cystic Fibrosis Neonatal Screening Study Group. Pediatrics 107:1–13, 2001.

Fauci A. Pulmonary vasculitis. In Kirkpatrick CH, Reynolds HY, eds. Immunologic and infectious reactions in the lung. New York, Marcel Dekker, 1976, pp 243–257.

Fauci AS, Wolff SM. Wegener's granulomatosis: studies in eighteen patients and a review of the literature. Medicine (Baltimore) 52:535–561, 1973.

Fauci AS, Harley JB, Roberts WC, Ferrans VJ, Gralnick HR, Bjornson BH. NIH conference. The idiopathic hypereosinophilic syndrome. Clinical, pathophysiologic, and therapeutic considerations. Ann Intern Med 97:78–92, 1982.

Fauci AS, Haynes BF, Katz P, Wolff SM. Wegener's granulomatosis: prospective clinical and therapeutic experience with 85 patients for 21 years. Ann Intern Med 98:76–85, 1983.

Faul JL, Kuschner WG. Wegener's granulomatosis and the Churg-Strauss syndrome. Clin Rev Allergy Immunol 21:17–26, 2001.

Faux JA, Wide L, Hargreave FE, Longbottom JL, Pepys J. Immunological aspects of respiratory allergy in budgerigar (Melopsittacus undulatus) fanciers. Clin Allergy 1:149–158, 1971.

Feery BJ, Phelan PD, Gallichio HA, Hampson AW. Antibody responses to influenza virus vaccine in patients with cystic fibrosis. Aust Paediatr J 15:181–182, 1979.

Feltelius N, Hedenstrom H, Hillerdal G, Hallgren R. Pulmonary involvement in ankylosing spondylitis. Ann Rheum Dis 45:736–740, 1986.

Fick RB Jr, Naegel GP, Matthay RA, Reynolds HY. Cystic fibrosis Pseudomonas opsonins. Inhibitory nature in an in vitro phagocytic assay. J Clin Invest 68:899–914, 1981.

Fick RB Jr, Naegel GP, Squier SU, Wood RE, Gee JB, Reynolds HY. Proteins of the cystic fibrosis respiratory tract. Fragmented immunoglobulin G opsonic antibody causing defective opsonophagocytosis. J Clin Invest 74:236–248, 1984.

Fick RB Jr, Olchowski J, Squier SU, Merrill WW, Reynolds HY. Immunoglobulin-G subclasses in cystic fibrosis. IgG2 response to Pseudomonas aeruginosa lipopolysaccharide. Am Rev Respir Dis 133:418–422, 1986.

Fink JN. Hypersensitivity pneumonitis. J Allergy Clin Immunol 74:1–10, 1984.

Fink JN. Clinical features of hypersensitivity pneumonitis. Chest 89(Suppl.):193S–195S, 1986.

Fink JN. Hypersensitivity pneumonitis. Clin Chest Med 13:303–309, 1992.

Flotte TR, Laube BL. Gene therapy in cystic fibrosis. Chest 120(Suppl.):124S–131S, 2001.

Flume PA, Egan TM, Paradowski LJ, Detterbeck FC, Thompson JT, Yankaskas JR. Infectious complications of lung transplantation. Impact of cystic fibrosis. Am J Respir Crit Care Med 149:1601–1607, 1994.

Forman SR, Fink JN, Moore VL, Wang J, Patterson R. Humoral and cellular immune responses in Aspergillus fumigatus pulmonary disease. J Allergy Clin Immunol 62:131–136, 1978.

Fournier E, Tonnel AB, Gosset PH, Wallaert B, Ameisen JC, Voisin C. Early neutrophil alveolitis after antigen inhalation in hypersensitivity pneumonitis. Chest 88:563–566, 1985.

Fraga A, Gudino J, Ramos-Niembro F, Aiarcon-Segovia D. Mixed connective tissue disease in childhood. Relationship Sjogren's syndrome. Am J Dis Child 132:263–265, 1978.

Frank ST, Weg JG, Harkleroad LE, Fitch RF. Pulmonary dysfunction in rheumatoid disease. Chest 63:27–34, 1973.

Fraser RG, Paré JA. Extrinsic allergic alveolitis. Semin Roentgenol 10:31–42, 1975.

Freedman MH, Grisaru D, Olivieri N, MacLusky I, Thorner PS. Pulmonary syndrome in patients with thalassemia major receiving intravenous deferoxamine infusions. Am J Dis Child 144:565–569, 1990.

Fuchs HJ, Borowitz DS, Christiansen DH, Morris EM, Nash ML, Ramsey BW, Rosenstein BJ, Smith AL, Wohl ME. Effect of aerosolized recombinant human DNase on exacerbations of respiratory symptoms and on pulmonary function in patients with cystic fibrosis. The Pulmozyme Study Group. N Engl J Med 331:637–642, 1994.

Fujimura J, Murakami Y, Tsuda A, Chiba T, Migita M, Fukunaga Y. A neonate with Löffler syndrome. J Perinatol 21:207–208, 2001.

Fulmer JD, Kaltreider HB. The pulmonary vasculitides. Chest 82:615–624, 1982.

Gadek JE, Fells GA, Zimmerman RL, Crystal RG. Role of connective tissue proteases in the pathogenesis of chronic inflammatory lung disease. Environ Health Perspect 55:297–306, 1984.

Galant SP, Rucker RW, Groncy CE, Wells ID, Novey SH. Incidence of serum antibodies to several Aspergillus species and to Candida albicans in cystic fibrosis. Am Rev Respir Dis 114:325–331, 1976.

Gammon RB, Bridges TA, al-Nezir H, Alexander CB, Kennedy JI. Bronchiolitis obliterans organizing pneumonia associated with systemic lupus erythematosus. Chest 102:1171–1174, 1992.

Gan KH, Veeze HJ, van den Ouweland AM, Halley DJ, Scheffer H, van der Hout A, Overbeek SE, de Jongste JC, Bakker W, Heijerman HG. A cystic fibrosis mutation associated with mild lung disease. N Engl J Med 333:95–99, 1995.

Garrick RE, Neilson EG. Anti–basement membrane disease with special reference to Goodpasture's syndrome. In Daniele RP, ed. Immunology and immunologic diseases of the lung. Boston, Mass., Blackwell Scientific Publications, 1988, pp 429–450.

Gaskin K, Gurwitz D, Durie P, Corey M, Levinson H, Forstner G. Improved respiratory prognosis in patients with cystic fibrosis with normal fat malabsorption. J Pediatr 100:857–862, 1982.

Gaynor JW, Bridges ND, Clark BJ, Spray TL. Update on lung transplantation in children. Curr Opin Pediatr 10:256–261, 1998.

Geller DE, Kaplowitz H, Light MJ, Colin AA. Allergic bronchopulmonary aspergillosis in cystic fibrosis: reported prevalence, regional distribution, and patient characteristics. Scientific Advisory Group, Investigators, and Coordinators of the Epidemiologic Study of Cystic Fibrosis. Chest 116:639–646, 1999.

Gephardt GN, Ahmad M, Tubbs RR. Pulmonary vasculitis (Wegener's granulomatosis). Immunohistochemical study of T and B cell markers. Am J Med 74:700–704, 1983.

Ghosal S, Taylor CJ, Colledge WH, Ratcliff R, Evans MJ. Sodium channel blockers and uridine triphosphate: effects on nasal potential difference in cystic fibrosis mice. Eur Respir J 15:146–150, 2000.

Ghose T, Landrigan P, Killeen R, Dill J. Immunopathological studies in patients with farmer's lung. Clin Allergy 4:119–129, 1974.

Gibbons A, Allan JD, Holzel A, McFarlane H. Cell-mediated immunity in patients with cystic fibrosis. Br Med J 1:120–122, 1976.

Girault D, Haloun A, Viard L, Bellon G, Gottrand F, Guillemain R, Lenoir G, Ladurie FL, Plouvier E, Storni V, et al. Sandimmun neoral improves the bioavailability of cyclosporin A and decreases inter-individual variations in patients affected with cystic fibrosis. Transplant Proc 27:2488–2490, 1995.

Goldmann DA, Klinger JD. Pseudomonas cepacia: biology, mechanisms of virulence, epidemiology. J Pediatr 108:806–812, 1986.

Goldstein W, Döring G. Lysosomal enzymes from polymorphonuclear leukocytes and proteinase inhibitors in patients with cystic fibrosis. Am Rev Respir Dis 134:49–56, 1986.

Gonzalez-Crussi F, Hull MT, Grosfeld JL. Idiopathic pulmonary hemosiderosis: evidence of capillary basement membrane abnormality. Am Rev Respir Dis 114:689–698, 1976.

Gonzalez EB, Swedo JL, Rajaraman S, Daniels JC, Grant JA. Ultrastructural and immunohistochemical evidence for release of eosinophilic granules in vivo: cytotoxic potential in chronic eosinophilic pneumonia. J Allergy Clin Immunol 79:755–762, 1986.

Gosset P, Perez T, Lassalle P, Duquesnoy B, Farre JM, Tonnel AB, Capron A. Increased TNF-alpha secretion by alveolar macrophages from patients with rheumatoid arthritis. Am Rev Respir Dis 143:593–597, 1991.

Govan JR. Infection control in cystic fibrosis: methicillin-resistant Staphylococcus aureus, Pseudomonas aeruginosa and the Burkholderia cepacia complex. J R Soc Med 93 (Suppl 38):40–45, 2000.

Graft DF, Mischler E, Farrell PM, Busse WW. Granulocyte chemiluminescence in adolescent patients with cystic fibrosis. Am Rev Respir Dis 125:540–543, 1982.

Grammer LC, Roberts M, Lerner C, Patterson R. Clinical and serologic follow-up of four children and five adults with bird-fancier's lung. J Allergy Clin Immunol 85:655–660, 1990.

Granstrom M, Ericsson A, Strandvik B, Wretlind B, Pavlovskis OR, Berka R, Vasil ML. Relation between antibody response to *Pseudomonas aeruginosa* exoproteins and colonization/infection in patients with cystic fibrosis. Acta Paediatr Scand 73:772–777, 1984.

Grantham JG, Meadows JA III, Gleich GJ. Chronic eosinophilic pneumonia. Evidence for eosinophil degranulation and release of major basic protein. Am J Med 80:89–94, 1986.

Grech V, Vella C, Lenicker H. Pigeon breeder's lung in childhood: varied clinical picture at presentation. Pediatr Pulmonol 30:145-148, 2000.

Greenberger PA. Allergic bronchopulmonary aspergillosis. J Allergy Clin Immunol 74:645–653, 1984.

Greenberger PA, Patterson R. Allergic bronchopulmonary aspergillosis. Model of bronchopulmonary disease with defined serologic, radiologic, pathologic and clinical findings from asthma to fatal destructive lung disease. Chest 91:165S–171S, 1987.

Greenberger PA. Immunologic aspects of lung diseases and cystic fibrosis. JAMA 278:1924–1930, 1997.

Greenberger PA. Allergic bronchopulmonary aspergillosis, allergic fungal sinusitis, and hypersensitivity pneumonitis. Clin Allergy Immunol 16:449–468, 2002.

Gregg RG, Wilfond BS, Farrell PM, Laxova A, Hassemer D, Mischler EH. Application of DNA analysis in a population-screening program for neonatal diagnosis of cystic fibrosis (CF): comparison of screening protocols. Am J Hum Genet 52:616–626, 1993.

Gregory RJ, Rich DP, Cheng SH, Souza DW, Paul S, Manavalan P, Anderson MP, Welsh MJ, Smith AE. Maturation and function of cystic fibrosis transmembrane conductance regulator variants bearing mutations in putative nucleotide-binding domains 1 and 2. Mol Cell Biol 11:3886–3893, 1991.

Griesenbach U, Alton EW. Recent progress in gene therapy for cystic fibrosis. Curr Opin Mol Ther 3:385–389, 2001.

Gross M, Esterly JR, Earle RH. Pulmonary alterations in systemic lupus erythematosus. Am Rev Respir Dis 105:572–577, 1972.

Gudmundsson G, Hunninghake GW. Interferon-gamma is necessary for the expression of hypersensitivity pneumonitis. J Clin Invest 99:2386–2390, 1997.

Gugler E, Pallavicini JC, Swedlow H, Zipkin I, Agnese PA. Immunological studies of submaxillary saliva from patients with cystic fibrosis and from normal children. J Pediatr 73:548–559, 1968.

Guillevin L, Cohen P, Gayraud M, Lhote F, Jarrousse B, Casassus P. Churg-Strauss syndrome. Clinical study and long-term follow-up of 96 patients. Medicine (Baltimore) 78:26–37, 1999.

Gunwar S, Bejarano PA, Kalluri R, Langeveld JP, Wisdom BJ Jr, Noelken ME, Hudson BG. Alveolar basement membrane: molecular properties of the noncollagenous domain (hexamer) of collagen IV and its reactivity with Goodpasture autoantibodies. Am J Respir Cell Mol Biol 5:107–112, 1991.

Guzman J, Wang YM, Kalaycioglu O, Schoenfeld B, Hamm H, Bartsch W, Costabel U. Increased surfactant protein A content in human alveolar macrophages in hypersensitivity pneumonitis. Acta Cytol 36:668–673, 1992.

Hamilos DL, Christensen J. Treatment of Churg-Strauss syndrome with high-dose intravenous immunoglobulin. J Allergy Clin Immunol 88:823–824, 1991.

Hamman L, Rich AR. Acute diffuse interstitial fibrosis of the lungs. Bull Johns Hopkins Hosp 74:117–212, 1944.

Hammond KB, Abman SH, Sokol RJ, Accurso FJ. Efficacy of statewide neonatal screening for cystic fibrosis by assay of trypsinogen concentrations. N Engl J Med 325:769–774, 1991.

Hammond KB, Turcios NL, Gibson LE. Clinical evaluation of the macroduct sweat collection system and conductivity analyzer in the diagnosis of cystic fibrosis. J Pediatr 124:255–260, 1994.

Hamvas A, Nogee LM, Mallory GB Jr, Spray TL, Huddleston CB, August A, Dehner LP, deMello DE, Moxley M, Nelson R, Cole FS, Colten HR. Lung transplantation for treatment of infants with surfactant protein B deficiency. J Pediatr 130:231–239, 1997.

Hansen LP, Jacobsen J, Skytte H. Wegener's granulomatosis in a child. Eur J Respir Dis 64:620–624, 1983.

Hansen PJ, Penny R. Pigeon-breeder's disease: study of the cell-mediated immune response to pigeon antigens by the lymphocyte culture technique. Int Arch Allergy Appl Immunol 47:498–507, 1974.

Hart RJ, Patterson R, Sommers H. Hyperimmunoglobulinemia E in a child with allergic bronchopulmonary aspergillosis and bronchiectasis. J Pediatr 89:38–41, 1976.

Harwood JS, Gould FK, McMaster A, Hamilton JR, Corris PA, Hasan A, Gennery AR, Dark JH. Significance of Epstein-Barr virus status and post-transplant lymphoproliferative disease in pediatric thoracic transplantation. Pediatr Transplant 3:100–103, 1999.

Haslam PL, Turton CW, Lukoszek A, Salsbury AJ, Dewar A, Collins JV, Turner-Warwick M. Bronchoalveolar lavage fluid cell counts in cryptogenic fibrosing alveolitis and their relation to therapy. Thorax 35:328–339, 1980.

Hartling SG, Garne S, Binder C, Heilmann C, Petersen W, Petersen KE, Koch C. Proinsulin, insulin, and C-peptide in cystic fibrosis after an oral glucose tolerance test. Diabetes Res 7:165–169, 1988.

Hauger SB. Guidelines for the care of children and adolescents with HIV infection. Approach to the pediatric patient with HIV infection and pulmonary symptoms. J Pediatr 119:S25–S33, 1991.

Heiner DC, Sears JW, Kniker WT. Multiple precipitins to cow's milk in chronic respiratory disease. A syndrome including poor growth, gastrointestinal symptoms, evidence of allergy, iron deficiency anemia, and pulmonary hemosiderosis. Am J Dis Child 103:634–654, 1962.

Henry M, Bennett DM, Kiely J, Kelleher N, Bredin CP. Fungal atopy in adult cystic fibrosis. Respir Med 94:1092–1096, 2000.

Heritier F, Madden B, Hodson ME, Yacoub M. Lung allograft transplantation: indications, preoperative assessment and postoperative management. Eur Respir J 5:1262–1278, 1992.

Hewitt CJ, Hull D, Keeling JW. Fibrosing alveolitis in infancy and childhood. Arch Dis Child 52:22–37, 1977.

Higenbottam T, Stewart S, Penketh A, Wallwork J. Transbronchial lung biopsy for the diagnosis of rejection in heart-lung transplant patients. Transplantation 46:532–539, 1988.

Hill HR, Warwick WJ, Dettloff J, Quie PG. Neutrophil granulocyte function in patients with pulmonary infection. J Pediatr 84:55–58, 1974.

Hodson ME. Immunological abnormalities in cystic fibrosis: chicken or egg? Thorax 35:801–806, 1980.

Hodson ME. Aerosolized dornase alfa (rhDNase) for therapy of cystic fibrosis. Am J Respir Crit Care Med 151:S70–S74, 1995.

Hodson ME, Turner-Warwick M. Autoantibodies in patients with chronic bronchitis. Br J Dis Chest 70:83–88, 1976.

Hodson ME, Turner-Warwick M. Autoantibodies in cystic fibrosis. Clin Allergy 11:565–570, 1981.

Høiby N, Hertz JB. Precipitating antibodies against *Escherichia coli*, *Bacteroides fragilis* ss. *thetaiotaomicron* and *Pseudomonas aeruginosa* in serum from normal persons and cystic fibrosis patients, determined by means of crossed immunoelectrophoresis. Acta Paediatr Scand 68:495–500, 1979.

Høiby N, Hertz JB. Quantitative studies on immunologically specific and non-specific absorption of *Pseudomonas aeruginosa* antibodies in serum from cystic fibrosis patients. Acta Pathol Microbiol Scand [C] 89:185–192, 1981.

Høiby N, Mathiesen L. *Pseudomonas aeruginosa* infection in cystic fibrosis. Distribution of B and T lymphocytes in relation to the humoral immune response. Acta Pathol Microbiol Scand [B] Microbiol Immunol 82:559–566, 1974.

Høiby N, Olling S. *Pseudomonas aeruginosa* infection in cystic fibrosis. Acta Pathol Microbiol Scand 85:107–114, 1977.

Høiby N, Wiik A. Antibacterial precipitins and autoantibodies in serum of patients with cystic fibrosis. Scand J Respir Dis 56:38–46, 1975.

Holland EJ, Loren AB, Scott PJ, Niwa Y, Yokoyama M. Demonstration of neutrophil dysfunction in the serum of patients with cystic fibrosis. J Clin Lab Immunol 6:137–139, 1981.

Hollsing AE, Granstrom M, Vasil ML, Wretlind B, Strandvik B. Prospective study of serum antibodies to Pseudomonas aeruginosa exoproteins in cystic fibrosis. J Clin Microbiol 25:1868–1874, 1987.

Holzer FJ, Olinsky A, Phelan PD. Variability of airways hyper-reactivity and allergy in cystic fibrosis. Arch Dis Child 56:455–459, 1981.

Holzhauer RJ, Van Ess JD, Schwartz RH. Third component of complement in cystic fibrosis. Am J Hum Genet 28:602–606, 1976.

Hostetler JS, Denning DW, Stevens DA. US experience with itraconazole in *Aspergillus*, *Cryptococcus* and *Histoplasma* infections in the immunocompromised host. Chemotherapy 38(Suppl 1):S12–S22, 1992.

Howatt WF, Heidelberger KP, LeGlovan DP, Schnitzer B. Desquamative interstitial pneumonia. Case report of an infant unresponsive to treatment. Am J Dis Child 126:346–348, 1973.

Howe HS, Boey ML, Fong KY, Feng PH. Pulmonary hemorrhage, pulmonary infarction, and the lupus anticoagulant. Ann Rheum Dis 47:869–872, 1988.

Huddleston CB, Mendeloff EN. Lung transplantation in infants. Semin Thorac Cardiovasc Surg Pediatr Card Surg Annu 4:115–122, 2001.

Hunder GG, McDuffie FC, Hepper NG. Pleural fluid complement in systemic lupus erythematosus and rheumatoid arthritis. Ann Intern Med 76:357–363, 1972.

Hunninghake GW, Fauci AS. Pulmonary involvement in the collagen-vascular diseases. Am Rev Respir Dis 119:471–503, 1979.

Hunninghake GW, Gadek JE, Kawanami O, Ferrans VJ, Crystal RG. Inflammatory and immune processes in the human lung in health and disease: evaluation by bronchoalveolar lavage. Am J Pathol 97:149–206, 1979.

Hunninghake GW, Kawanami O, Ferrans VJ, Young RC, Roberts WC, Crystal RG. Characterization of the inflammatory and immune effector cells in the lung parenchyma of patients with interstitial lung disease. Am Rev Respir Dis 123:407–412, 1981.

Hunninghake GW, Moseley PL. Immunological abnormalities of chronic non-infectious pulmonary diseases. In Bienenstock J, ed. Immunology of the lung and upper respiratory tract. New York, McGraw-Hill, 1984, pp 345–364.

Hutter JA, Scott J, Wreghitt T, Higenbottam T, Wallwork J. The importance of cytomegalovirus in heart-lung transplant recipients. Chest 95:627–631, 1989.

Hyatt RW, Adelstein ER, Halazun JF, Lukens JN. Ultrastructure of the lung in idiopathic pulmonary hemosiderosis. Am J Med 52:822–829, 1972.

Imbeau SA, Cohen M, Reed CE. Allergic bronchopulmonary aspergillosis in infants. Am J Dis Child 131:1127–1130, 1977.

Inoue T, Kanayama Y, Ohe A, Kato N, Horiguchi T, Ishii M, Shiota K. Immunopathologic studies of pneumonitis in systemic lupus erythematosus. Ann Intern Med 91:30–34, 1979.

Inselman LS. Pulmonary disorders in pediatric acquired immunodeficiency syndrome. In Chernick V, Kendig EL, eds. Disorders of the respiratory tract in children, 5th ed. Philadelphia, W. B. Saunders, 1990, pp 991–1003.

Irwin RS, Cottrell TS, Hsu KC, Griswold WR, Thomas MH 3rd. Idiopathic pulmonary hemosiderosis: an electron microscopic and immunofluorescent study. Chest 65:41–45, 1974.

Isles A, Maclusky I, Corey M, Gold R, Prober C, Fleming P, Levison H. *Pseudomonas cepacia* infection in cystic fibrosis: an emerging problem. J Pediatr 104:206–210, 1984.

Jaffe A, Bush A. Cystic fibrosis: review of the decade. Monaldi Arch Chest Dis 56:240–247, 2001.

Jagger KS, Robinson DL, Frantz MN, Warren RL. Detection by enzyme-linked immunosorbent assays of antibody specific for *Pseudomonas* proteinases and exotoxin A in sera from cystic fibrosis patients. J Clin Microbiol 17:55–59, 1982.

Jansen HM, Schutte AJ, van der Giessen M, The TH. Immunoglobulin classes in local immune complexes recovered by bronchoalveolar lavage in collagen vascular diseases. Lung 162:287–296, 1984.

Jederlinic PJ, Sicilian L, Gaensler EA. Chronic eosinophilic pneumonia. A report of 19 cases and a review of the literature. Medicine (Baltimore) 67:154–162, 1988.

Johansen HK, Nir M, Høiby N, Koch C, Schwartz M. Severity of cystic fibrosis in patients homozygous and heterozygous for delta F508 mutation. Lancet 337:631–634, 1991.

Johkoh T, Müller NL, Akira M, Ichikado K, Suga M, Ando M, Yoshinaga T, Kiyama T, Mihara N, Honda O, Tomiyama N, Nakamura H. Eosinophilic lung diseases: diagnostic accuracy of thin-section CT in 111 patients. Radiology 216:773–780, 2000.

Jones MM, Seilheimer DK, Pollack MS, Curry M, Crane MM, Rossen RD. Relationship of hypergammaglobulinemia, circulating immune complexes, and histocompatibility antigen profiles in patients with cystic fibrosis. Am Rev Respir Dis 140:1636–1639, 1989.

Joshi VV, Oleske JM. Pulmonary lesions in children with the acquired immunodeficiency syndrome: a reappraisal based on data in additional cases and follow-up study of previously reported cases. Hum Pathol 17:641–642, 1986.

Kathuria S, Cheifec G. Fatal pulmonary Henoch-Schönlein syndrome. Chest 82:654–656, 1982.

Kaltreider HB. Normal immune responses. In Crystal RG, West JB, et al., eds. The Lung: Scientific Foundations. New York, Raven Press, 1991, pp 499–510.

Katz BZ, Berkman AB, Shapiro ED. Serologic evidence of active Epstein-Barr virus infection in Epstein-Barr virus–associated lymphoproliferative disorders of children with acquired immunodeficiency syndrome. J Pediatr 120:228–232, 1992.

Katz RM, Kniker WT. Infantile hypersensitivity pneumonitis as a reaction to organic antigens. N Engl J Med 288:233–237, 1973.

Kauffman HF, Beaumont F, de Monchy JG, Sluiter HJ, de Vries K. Immunologic studies in bronchoalveolar fluid in a patient with allergic bronchopulmonary aspergillosis. J Allergy Clin Immunol 74:835–840, 1984.

Kawai T, Fujiwara T, Aoyama Y, Aizawa Y, Yamada Y. Diffuse interstitial fibrosing pneumonitis and adenovirus infection. Chest 69:692–694, 1976.

Kearns GL. Hepatic drug metabolism in cystic fibrosis: recent develoments and future directions. Ann Pharmacother 27:74–79, 1993.

Kemp T, Schram-Doumont A, van Geffel R, Kram R, Szpirer C. Alteration of the N-formyl-methionyl-leucyl-phenylalanine–induced response in cystic fibrosis neutrophils. Pediatr Res 20:520–526, 1986.

Kerem E, Corey M, Kerem BS, Rommens J, Markiewicz D, Levison H, Tsui LC, Durie P. The relation between genotype and phenotype in cystic fibrosis—analysis of the most common mutation (?F508). N Engl J Med 323:1517–1522, 1990a.

Kerem E, Bentur L, England S, Reisman J, O'Brodovich H, Bryan AC, Levison H. Sequential pulmonary function measurements during treatment of infantile chronic interstitial pneumonitis. J Pediatr 116:61–67, 1990b.

Khan TZ, Wagener JS, Bost T, Martinez J, Accurso FJ, Riches DW. Early pulmonary inflammation in infants with cystic fibrosis. Am J Respir Crit Care Med 151:1075–1082, 1995.

Kiefer TA, Kesarwala HH, Greenberger PA, Sweeney JR Jr, Fischer TJ. Allergic bronchopulmonary aspergillosis in a young child: diagnostic confirmation by serum IgE and IgG indices. Ann Allergy 56:233–236, 1986.

King KK, Kornreich HK, Bernstein BH, Singsen BH, Hanson V. The clinical spectrum of systemic lupus erythematosus in childhood. Arthritis Rheum 20:287–294, 1977.

Kiper N, Göçmen A, Özçelik U, Dilber E, Anadol D. Long-term clinical course of patients with idiopathic pulmonary hemosiderosis (1979-1994): prolonged survival with low-dose corticosteroid therapy. Pediatr Pulmonol 27:180–184, 1999.

Kitson C, Alton E. Gene therapy for cystic fibrosis. Expert Opin Investig Drugs 9:1523–1535, 2000.

Kjellman B, Elinder G, Garwicz S, Svan H. Idiopathic pulmonary haemosiderosis in Swedish children. Acta Paediatr Scand 73:584–588, 1984.

Knowles MR, Olivier K, Noone P, Boucher RC. Pharmacologic modulation of salt and water in the airway epithelium in cystic fibrosis. Am J Respir Crit Care Med 151:S65–S69, 1995.

Kobayashi I, Ono S, Kawamura N, Okano M, Miyazawa K, Shibuya H, Kobayashi K. KL-6 is a potential marker for interstitial lung disease associated with juvenile dermatomyositis. J Pediatr 138:274–276, 2001.

Koch C, Høiby N. Pathogenesis of cystic fibrosis. Lancet 341:1065–1069, 1993.

Koch C, Høiby N. Diagnosis and treatment of cystic fibrosis. Respiration 67:239–247, 2000.

Koh DM, Hansell DM. Computed tomography of diffuse interstitial lung disease in children. Clin Radiol 55:659–667, 2000.

Konstan MW, Stern RC, Doershuk CF. Efficacy of the Flutter device for airway mucus clearance in patients with cystic fibrosis. J Pediatr 124:689–693, 1994.

Konstan MW, Byard PJ, Hoppel CL, Davis PB. Effect of high-dose ibuprofen in patients with cystic fibrosis. N Engl J Med 332:848–854, 1995.

Kornstein MJ, Pietra GG, Hoxie JA, Conley ME. The pathology and treatment of interstitial pneumonitis in two infants with AIDS. Am Rev Respir Dis 133:1196–1198, 1986.

Krause DS, Theise ND, Collector MI, Henegariu O, Hwang S, Gardner R, Neutzel S, Sharkis SJ. Multi-organ, multi-lineage engraftment by a single bone marrow–derived stem cell. Cell 105:369–377, 2001.

Kronborg G, Hansen MB, Svenson M, Fomsgaard A, Høiby N, Bendtzen K. Cytokines in sputum and serum from patients with cystic fibrosis and chronic Pseudomonas aeruginosa infection as markers of destructive inflammation in the lungs. Pediatr Pulmonol 15:292–297, 1993.

Kuhn C, McDonald JA. The roles of the myofibroblast in idiopathic pulmonary fibrosis. Ultrastructural and immunohistochemical features of sites of active extracellular matrix synthesis. Am J Pathol 138:1257–1265, 1991.

Kuzela L, Vavrecka A, Prikazska M, Drugda B, Hronec J, Senkova A, Drugdova M, Oltman M, Novotna T, Brezina M, Kratky A, Kristufek P. Pulmonary complications in patients with inflammatory bowel disease. Hepatogastroenterology 46:1714–1719, 1999.

Landau LI, Phelan PD. The variable effect of a bronchodilating agent on pulmonary function in cystic fibrosis. J Pediatr 82:863–868, 1973.

Landman S, Burgener F. Pulmonary manifestations in Wegener's granulomatosis. AJR Am J Roentgenol Radium Ther Nucl Med 122:750–757, 1974.

Languepin J, Scheinmann P, Mahut B, Le Bourgeois M, Jaubert F, Brunelle F, Sidi D, de Blic J. Bronchial casts in children with cardiopathies: the role of pulmonary lymphatic abnormalities. Pediatr Pulmonol 28:329–336, 1999.

Larsen GL. Host defense systems of the lung. In Taussig LM, Landau LI, eds. Pediatric respiratory medicine. St. Louis, Mosby, 1999, pp 57–75.

Larson JE, Cohen JC. Cystic fibrosis revisited. Mol Genet Metab 71:470–477, 2000.

Latgé JP. Aspergillus fumigatus and aspergillosis. Clin Microbiol Rev 12:310–350, 1999.

Lau CL, Palmer SM, Posther KE, Howell DN, Reinsmoen NL, Massey HT, Tapson VF, Jaggers JJ, D'Amico TA, Davis RD Jr. Influence of panel-reactive antibodies on posttransplant outcomes in lung transplant recipients. Ann Thorac Surg 69:1520–1524, 2000.

Leahy F, Pasterkamp H, Tal A. Desquamative interstitial pneumonia responsive to chloroquine. Clin Pediatr (Phila) 24:230–232, 1985.

Leatherman JW. Diffuse alveolar hemorrhage in immune and idiopathic disorders. In Lynch JP, DeRemee RA, eds. Immunologically mediated pulmonary diseases. Philadelphia, J. B. Lippincott, 1991, pp 473–498.

Leatherman JW, Davies SF, Hoidal JR. Alveolar hemorrhage syndromes: diffuse microvascular lung hemorrhage in immune and idiopathic disorders. Medicine (Baltimore) 63:343–361, 1984a.

Leatherman JW, Michael AF, Schwartz BA, Hoidal JR. Lung T cells in hypersensitivity pneumonitis. Ann Intern Med 100:390–392, 1984b.

Lebecque P, Leal T, Godding V. [Cystic fibrosis and normal sweat chloride values: a case-report]. Rev Mal Respir 18:443–445, 2001.

Le Clainche L, Le Bourgeois M, Fauroux B, Forenza N, Dommergues JP, Desbois JC, Bellon G, Derelle J, Dutau G, Marguet C, Pin I, Tillie-Leblond I, Scheinmann P, De Blic J. Long-term outcome of idiopathic pulmonary hemosiderosis in children. Medicine (Baltimore) 79:318–326, 2000.

Leitch AG. Pulmonary eosinophilia. Basic Respir Dis 7:1–6, 1979.

Lewis EJ, Schur PH, Busch GJ, Galvanek E, Merrill JP. Immunopathologic features of a patient with glomerulonephritis and pulmonary hemorrhage. Am J Med 54:507–513, 1973.

Lieberman J. Carboxypeptidase B–like activity and C3 in cystic fibrosis. Am Rev Respir Dis 111:100–102, 1975.

Liebow AA, Carrington CB. The eosinophilic pneumonias. Medicine (Baltimore) 48:251–285, 1969.

Liebow AA, Steer A, Billingsley JG. Desquamative interstitial pneumonia. Am J Med 39:396–404, 1965.

Longbottom JL. Allergic bronchopulmonary aspergillosis: reactivity of IgE and IgG antibodies with antigenic components of Aspergillus fumigatus (IgE/IgG antigen complexes). J Allergy Clin Immunol 72:668–675, 1983.

Lopez M, Salvaggio JE. Eosinophilic pneumonias. In Lynch JP, DeRemee RA, eds. Immunologically mediated pulmonary diseases. Philadelphia, J. B. Lippincott, 1991, pp 413–431.

Loughlin GM, Cota KA, Taussig LM. The relationship between flow transients and bronchial lability in cystic fibrosis. Chest 79:206–210, 1981.

Loughlin GM, Taussig LM, Murphy SA, Strunk RC, Kohnen PW. Immune-complex–mediated glomerulonephritis and pulmonary hemorrhage simulating Goodpasture syndrome. J Pediatr 93:181–184, 1978.

Louthrenoo W, Norasetthada A., Khunamornpong S, Sreshthaputra A, Sukitawut W. Childhood Churg-Strauss syndrome. J Rheumatol 26:1387–1393, 1999.

Lyrene RK, Polhill RB Jr, Guthrie LA, Tiller RE. Alternative complement pathway activity in cystic fibrosis. J Pediatr 91:681–682, 1977.

MacFarlane JR, Holman CW. Chylothorax. Am Rev Respir Dis 105:287–291, 1972.

MacFarlane JD, Franken CK, van Leeuwen AW. Progressive cavitating pulmonary changes in rheumatoid arthritis: a case report. Ann Rheum Dis 43:98–101, 1984.

MacLusky I, Levison H. Cystic fibrosis. In Chernick V, Kendig EL, eds. Disorders of the respiratory tract in children. Philadelphia, W. B. Saunders, 1990, pp 692–730.

MacLusky I, Levison H, Gold R, McLaughlin FJ. Inhaled antibiotics in cystic fibrosis: is there a therapeutic effect? J Pediatr 108:861–865, 1986.

Mahadeva R, Webb K, Westerbeek RC, Carroll NR, Dodd ME, Bilton D, Lomas DA. Clinical outcome in relation to care in centres specialising in cystic fibrosis: cross sectional study. BMJ 316:1771–1775, 1998.

Maksymowych W, Russell AS. Antimalarials in rheumatology: efficacy and safety. Semin Arthritis Rheum 16:206–221, 1987.

Mall M, Bleich M, Kuehr J, Brandis M, Greger R, Kunzelmann K. CFTR-mediated inhibition of epithelial Na$^+$ conductance in human colon is defective in cystic fibrosis. Am J Physiol 277:G709–G716, 1999.

Mansfield SG, Kole J, Puttaraju M, Yang CC, Garcia-Blanco MA, Cohn JA, Mitchell LG. Repair of CFTR mRNA by spliceosome-mediated RNA trans-splicing. Gene Ther 7:1885–1895, 2000.

Manthei U, Taussig LM, Beckerman RC, Strunk RC. Circulating immune complexes in cystic fibrosis. Am Rev Respir Dis 126:253–257, 1982.

Marchand E, Reynaud-Gaubert M, Lauque D, Durieu J, Tonnel AB, Cordier JF. Idiopathic chronic eosinophilic pneumonia. A clinical and follow-up study of 62 cases. The Groupe d'Etudes et de Recherche sur les Maladies "Orphelines" Pulmonaires (GERM"O"P). Medicine (Baltimore) 77:299–312, 1998.

Mares DC, Mathur PN. Medical thoracoscopic talc pleurodesis for chylothorax due to lymphoma: a case series. Chest 114:731–735, 1998.

Martinez-Tello FJ, Braun DG, Blanc WA. Immunoglobulin production in bronchial mucosa and bronchial lymph nodes, particularly in cystic fibrosis of the pancreas. J Immunol 101:989–1003, 1968.

Mastella G, Rainisio M, Harms HK, Hodson ME, Koch C, Navarro J, Standvik B, McKenzie SG. Allergic bronchopulmonary aspergillosis in cystic fibrosis. A European epidemiological study. Epidemiologic Registry of Cystic Fibrosis. Eur Respir J 16:464–471, 2000.

Matthay RA, Schwarz MI, Petty TL, Stanford RE, Gupta RC, Sahn SA, Steigerwald JC. Pulmonary manifestations of systemic lupus erythematosus: review of twelve cases of acute lupus pneumonitis. Medicine (Baltimore) 54:397–409, 1975.

Matthews WJ Jr, Williams M, Oliphint B, Geha R, Colten HR. Hypogammaglobulinemia in patients with cystic fibrosis. N Engl J Med 302:245–249, 1980.

Maurer JR. Outcome issues in cystic fibrosis lung transplant recipients. Pediatr Pulmonol S9:199–200, 1993.

Mazer BD, Eigen H, Gelfand EW, Brugman SM. Remission of interstitial lung disease following therapy of associated ulcerative colitis. Pediatr Pulmonol 15:55–59, 1993.

McCarthy DS, Pepys J. Allergic bronchopulmonary aspergillosis. Clinical immunology. 1. Clinical features. Clin Allergy 1:261–286, 1971a.

McCarthy DS, Pepys J. Allergic broncho-pulmonary aspergillosis. Clinical immunology. 2. Skin, nasal and bronchial tests. Clin Allergy 1:415–432, 1971b.

McCarthy DS, Pepys J. Cryptogenic pulmonary eosinophilias. Clin Allergy 3:339–351, 1973.

McCombs RP. Diseases due to immunologic reactions in the lungs (first of two parts). N Engl J Med 286:1186–1194, 1972.

McElvaney NG, Nakamura H, Birrer P, Hébert CA, Wong WL, Alphonso M, Baker JB, Catalano MA, Crystal RG. Modulation of airway inflammation in cystic fibrosis. In vivo suppression of interleukin-8 levels on the respiratory epithelial surface by aerosolization of recombinant secretory leukoprotease inhibitor. J Clin Invest 90:1296–1301, 1992.

McFarlane H, Holzel A, Brenchley P, Allan JD, Wallwork JC, Singer BE, Worsley B. Immune complexes in cystic fibrosis. Br Med J 1:423–428, 1975.

McIntosh I, Cutting GR. Cystic fibrosis transmembrane conductance regulator and the etiology and pathogenesis of cystic fibrosis. FASEB J 6:2775–2782, 1992.

McMahon CJ, Nihill MR, Reber A. The bronchial cast syndrome after the fontan procedure: further evidence of its etiology. Cardiol Young 11:345–351, 2001.

Midulla F, Strappini P, Sandstrom T, Bjermer L, Falasca C, Capocaccia P, Catania S, Soldi E, Pia Villa M, Ronchetti R. Cellular and noncellular components of bronchoalveolar lavage fluid in HIV-1-infected children with radiological evidence of interstitial lung damage. Pediatr Pulmonol 31:205–213, 2001.

Miller RW, Salcedo JR, Fink RJ, Murphy TM, Magilavy DB. Pulmonary hemorrhage in pediatric patients with systemic lupus erythematosus. J Pediatr 108:576–579, 1986.

Mislick KA, Baldeschwieler JD. Evidence for the role of proteoglycans in cation-mediated gene transfer. Proc Natl Acad Sci U S A 93:12349–12354, 1996.

Miyajima M, Suga M, Nakagawa K, Ito K, Ando M. Effects of erythromycin on experimental extrinsic allergic alveolitis. Clin Exp Allergy 29:253–261, 1999.

Moore VL, Fink JN, Barboriak JJ, Ruff LL, Schlueter DP. Immunologic events in pigeon breeders' disease. J Allergy Clin Immunol 53:319–328, 1974.

Morgan JE, Barkman HW, Waring NP. Idiopathic pulmonary fibrosis. Semin Respir Med 5:255–262, 1984.

Morsy MA, Caskey CT. Expanded-capacity adenoviral vectors—the helper-dependent vectors. Mol Med Today 5:18–24, 1999.

Moss RB, Bocian RC, Hsu YP, Wei T, Yssel H. Reduced interleukin-10 production by cystic fibrosis (CF) T cell clones. Am J Resp Crit Care Med 151:A248, 1995.

Moss RB, Hsu YP. Isolation and characterization of circulating immune complexes in cystic fibrosis. Clin Exp Immunol 47:301–308, 1982.

Moss RB, Hsu YP, Lewiston NJ. ^{125}I-Clq-binding and specific antibodies as indicators of pulmonary disease activity in cystic fibrosis. J Pediatr 99:215–222, 1981.

Moss RB, Hsu YP, Sullivan MM, Lewiston NJ. Altered antibody isotype in cystic fibrosis: possible role in opsonic deficiency. Pediatr Res 20:453–459, 1986.

Moss RB, Lewiston NJ. Immune complexes and humoral response to Pseudomonas aeruginosa in cystic fibrosis. Am Rev Respir Dis 121:23–29, 1980.

Moss RB, Lewiston NJ. Immunopathology of cystic fibrosis. In Shapira E, Wilson BG, eds. Immunological aspects of cystic fibrosis. Boca Raton, Fla., CRC Press, 1984, pp 5–27.

Mukhopadhyay S, Singh M, Cater JI, Ogston S, Franklin M, Olver RE. Nebulised antipseudomonal antibiotic therapy in cystic fibrosis: a meta-analysis of benefits and risks. Thorax 51:364–368, 1996.

Müller NL, Ostrow DN. High-resolution computed tomography of chronic interstitial lung disease. Clin Chest Med 12:97–114, 1991.

Murray JF, Mills J. Pulmonary infectious complications of human immunodeficiency virus infection. Part II. Am Rev Respir Dis 141:1582–1598, 1990.

Musk AW, Zilko PJ, Manners P, Kay PH, Kamboh MI. Genetic studies in familial fibrosing alveolitis. Possible linkage with immunoglobulin allotypes (Gm). Chest 89:206–210, 1986.

Nadorra RL, Landing BH. Pulmonary lesions in childhood onset systemic lupus erythematosus: analysis of 26 cases, and summary of literature. Pediatr Pathol 7:1–18, 1987.

Naegel GP, Young KR Jr, Reynolds HY. Receptors for human IgG subclasses on human alveolar macrophages. Am Rev Respir Dis 129:413–418, 1984.

Nair LG, Kurtz CP. Lymphangiomatosis presenting with bronchial cast formation. Thorax 51:765–766, 1996.

Neeld DA, Goodman LR, Gurney JW, Greenberger PA, Fink JN. Computerized tomography in the evaluation of allergic bronchopulmonary aspergillosis. Am Rev Respir Dis 142:1200–1205, 1990.

Nelson LA, Callerame ML, Schwartz RH. Aspergillosis and atopy in cystic fibrosis. Am Rev Respir Dis 120:863–873, 1979.

Nepomuceno IB, Esrig S, Moss RB. Allergic bronchopulmonary aspergillosis in cystic fibrosis: role of atopy and response to itraconazole. Chest 115:364–370, 1999.

Neva FA, Ottesen EA. Tropical (filarial) eosinophilia. N Engl J Med 298:1129–1131, 1978.

Newhouse M, Sanchis J, Bienenstock J. Lung defense mechanisms (second of two parts). N Engl J Med 295:1045–1052, 1976.

Nogee LM, Dunbar AE III, Wert SE, Askin F, Hamvas A, Whitsett JA. A mutation in the surfactant protein C gene associated with familial interstitial lung disease. N Engl J Med 344:573–579, 2001.

Noyes BE, Kurland G, Orenstein DM, Fricker FJ, Armitage JM. Experience with pediatric lung transplantation. J Pediatr 124:261–268, 1994.

O'Brodovich HM, Moser MM, Lu L. Familial lymphoid interstitial pneumonia: a long-term follow-up. Pediatrics 65:523–528, 1980.

O'Connell EJ, Dower JC, Burke EC, Brown AL Jr, McCaughey WT. Pulmonary hemorrhage–glomerulonephritis syndrome; relationship to Goodpasture's syndrome with report of a case in 9-year-old girl. Am J Dis Child 108:302–308, 1964.

Oldham SA, Castillo M, Jacobson FL, Mones JM, Saldana MJ. HIV-associated lymphocytic interstitial pneumonia: radiologic manifestations and pathologic correlation. Radiology 170:83–87, 1989.

Olson J, Colby TV, Elliott CG. Hamman-Rich syndrome revisited. Mayo Clin Proc 65:1538–1548, 1990.

Olson JC, Kelly KJ, Pan CG, Wortmann DW. Pulmonary disease with hemorrhage in Henoch-Schönlein purpura. Pediatrics 89:1177–1181, 1992.

O'Shea PA, Yardley JH. The Hamman-Rich syndrome in infancy: report of a case with virus-like particles by electron microscopy. Johns Hopkins Med J 126:320–336, 1970.

Ostrow D, Cherniack RM. Resistance to airflow in patients with diffuse interstitial lung disease. Am Rev Respir Dis 108:205–210, 1973.

Ottesen EA. Eosinophilia and the lung. In Kirkpatrick CH, Reynolds HY, eds. Immunologic and infectious reactions in the lung. New York, Marcel Dekker, 1976, pp 289–332.

Pai VB, Nahata MC. Efficacy and safety of aerosolized tobramycin in cystic fibrosis. Pediatr Pulmonol 32:314–327, 2001.

Pamukcu A, Bush A, Buchdahl R. Effects of Pseudomonas aeruginosa colonization on lung function and anthropometric variables in children with cystic fibrosis. Pediatr Pulmonol 19:10–15, 1995.

Park S, Nyhan WL. Fatal pulmonary involvement in dermatomyositis. Am J Dis Child 129:723–726, 1975.

Patchefsky AS, Israel HL, Hoch WS, Gordon G. Desquamative interstitial pneumonia: relationship to interstitial fibrosis. Thorax 28:680–693, 1973.

Pathial K, Saff R, Murali P, Splaingard M, Biller J, McCarthy K, Fink J, Greenberger P, Kurup V. Immune responses to *Pseudomonas aeruginosa* in cystic fibrosis. J Allergy Clin Immunol 89:167, 1992.

Patterson R, Roberts M. IgE and IgG antibodies against *Aspergillus fumigatus* in sera of patients with bronchopulmonary allergic aspergillosis. Int Arch Allergy Appl Immunol 46:150–160, 1974.

Patterson R, Schatz M, Fink JN, DeSwarte RS, Roberts M, Cugell D. Pigeon breeder's disease. I. Serum immunoglobulin concentrations; IgG, IgM, IgA and IgE antibodies against pigeon serum. Am J Med 60:144–151, 1976.

Pauwels R, Stevens EM, van der Straeten M. IgE antibodies in bronchopulmonary aspergillosis. Ann Allergy 37:195–200, 1976.

Pennington JE. *Aspergillus* lung disease. Med Clin North Am 64:475–490, 1980.

Pennington JE. Opportunistic fungal pneumonias: *Aspergillus, Mucor, Candida, Torulopsis.* In Pennington JE, ed. Respiratory infections: diagnosis and Management, 2nd ed. New York, Raven Press, 1988, pp 443–456.

Pennington JE, Reynolds HY, Wood RE, Robinson RA, Levine AS. Use of a *Pseudomonas aeruginosa* vaccine in patients with acute leukemia and cystic fibrosis. Am J Med 58:629–636, 1975.

Pepys J. Immunopathology of allergic lung disease. Clin Allergy 3:1–22, 1973.

Pepys J, Simon G. Asthma, pulmonary eosinophilia, and allergic alveolitis. Med Clin North Am 57:573–591, 1973.

Permin H, Skov PS, Norn S, Høiby N, Schiotz PO. Platelet 3H–serotonin releasing immune complexes induced by *Pseudomonas aeruginosa* in cystic fibrosis. Allergy 37:93–100, 1982.

Pervez NK, Kleinerman J, Kattan M, Freed JA, Harris MB, Rosen MJ, Schwartz IS. Pseudomembranous necrotizing bronchial aspergillosis. A variant of invasive aspergillosis in a patient with hemophilia and acquired immune deficiency syndrome. Am Rev Respir Dis 131:961–963, 1985.

Peters SG, McDougall JC, Douglas WW, Coles DT, DeRemee RA. Colchicine in the treatment of pulmonary fibrosis. Chest 103:101–104, 1993.

Phillips BM, David TJ. Pathogenesis and management of arthropathy in cystic fibrosis. J R Soc Med 79:44–50, 1986.

Piedra P, Ogra PL. Immunologic aspects of surface infections in the lung. J Pediatr 108:817–823, 1986.

Pier GB, Grout M, Zaidi TS, Goldberg JB. How mutant CFTR may contribute to *Pseudomonas aeruginosa* infection in cystic fibrosis. Am J Respir Crit Care Med 154:S175–S182, 1996.

Pitcher-Wilmott RW, Levinsky RJ, Matthew DJ. Circulating soluble immune complexes containing *Pseudomonas* antigens in cystic fibrosis. Arch Dis Child 57:577–581, 1982.

Pitt J. Lymphocytic interstitial pneumonia. Pediatr Clin North Am 38:89–95, 1991.

Polley MJ, Bearn AG. Cystic fibrosis: current concepts. J Med Genet 11:249–252, 1974.

Poskitt TR. Immunologic and electron microscopic studies in Goodpasture's syndrome. Am J Med 49:250–257, 1970.

Postma GN, Keyser JS. Management of persistent chylothorax. Ololaryngol Head Neck Surg 116:268–270, 1997.

Prakash UB. Pulmonary manifestations in mixed connective tissue disease. Semin Respir Med 9:318–324, 1988.

Purtilo DT, Brem J, Ceccaci L, Fitzpatrick AJ. A family study of pigeon breeder's disease. J Pediatr 86:569–571, 1975.

Quie PG. Lung defense against infection. J Pediatr 108:813–816, 1986.

Rachelefsky GS, Osher A, Dooley RE, Ank B, Stiehm ER. Coexistent respiratory allergy and cystic fibrosis. Am J Dis Child 128:355–359, 1974.

Ramsey BW, Boat TF. Outcome measures for clinical trials in cystic fibrosis. Summary of a Cystic Fibrosis Foundation consensus conference. J Pediatr 124:177–192, 1994.

Ramsey BW. Management of pulmonary disease in patients with cystic fibrosis. N Engl J Med 335:179–188, 1996.

Ramsey BW, Pepe MS, Quan JM, Otto KL, Montgomery AB, Williams-Warren J, Vasiljev-K M, Borowitz D, Bowman CM, Marshall BC, Marshall S, Smith AL. Intermittent administration of inhaled tobramycin in patients with cystic fibrosis. Cystic Fibrosis Inhaled Tobramycin Study Group. N Engl J Med 340:23–30, 1999.

Rao M, Steiner P, Rose JS, Kassner EG, Kottmeier P, Steiner M. Chronic eosinophilic pneumonia in a one-year-old child. Chest 68:118–120, 1975.

Redding GJ, Fan LL. Idiopathic pulmonary fibrosis and lymphocytic interstitial pneumonia. In Taussig LM, Landau LI, eds. Pediatric respiratory medicine. St. Louis, Mosby, 1999, pp 794–804.

Reed CE, Barbee RA. Pigeon-breeder's lung: a newly observed interstitial pulmonary disease. JAMA 193:261–265, 1965.

Reeder WH, Goodrich BE. Pulmonary infiltration with eosinophilia. Ann Intern Med 36:1217–1240, 1952.

Rees AJ. Pulmonary injury caused by anti–basement membrane antibodies. Semin Respir Med 5:264–272, 1984.

Regan MJ, Hellmann DB, Stone JH. Treatment of Wegener's granulomatosis. Rheum Dis Clin North Am 27:863–886, 2001.

Regelmann WE, Skubitz KM, Herron JM. Increased monocyte oxidase activity in cystic fibrosis heterozygotes and homozygotes. Am J Respir Cell Mol Biol 5:27–33, 1991.

Renzi GD, Lopez-Majano V. Early diagnosis of interstitial fibrosis. Respiration 33:294–302, 1976.

Repetto G, Lisboa C, Emparanza E, Ferretti R, Neira M, Etchart M, Meneghello J. Idiopathic pulmonary hemosiderosis. Clinical, radiological, and respiratory function studies. Pediatrics 40:24–32, 1967.

Reynolds HY. Idiopathic interstitial pulmonary fibrosis. Contribution of bronchoalveolar lavage analysis. Chest 89(3 Suppl):139S–144S, 1986.

Reynolds HY, Atkinson JP, Newball HH, Frank MM. Receptors for immunoglobulin and complement on human alveolar macrophages. J Immunol 114:1813–1819, 1975.

Ricketti AJ, Greenberger PA, Pruzansky JJ, Patterson R. Hyperreactivity of mediator-releasing cells from patients with allergic bronchopulmonary aspergillosis as evidenced by basophil histamine release. J Allergy Clin Immunol 72:386–392, 1983.

Ricketti AJ, Greenberger PA, Patterson R. Serum IgE as an important aid in management of allergic bronchopulmonary aspergillosis. J Allergy Clin Immunol 74:68–71, 1984.

Riordan JR, Rommens JM, Kerem B, Alon N, Rozmahel R, Grzelczak Z, Zielenski J, Lok S, Plavsic N, Chou JL, et al. Identification of the cystic fibrosis gene: cloning and characterization of complementary DNA. Science 245:1066–1073, 1989.

Roberts SR Jr. Immunology and the lung: an overview. Semin Roentgenol 10:7–19, 1975.

Robinson C, Callow M, Stevenson S, Robinson BW, Lake RA. Private specificities can dominate the humoral response to self-antigens in patients with cryptogenic fibrosing alveolitis. Respir Res 2:119–124, 2001.

Rodgers HC, Knox AJ. Pharmacological treatment of the biochemical defect in cystic fibrosis airways. Eur Respir J 17:1314–1321, 2001.

Rogers MF, Thomas PA, Starcher ET, Noa MC, Bush TJ, Jaffe HW. Acquired immunodeficiency syndrome in children: report of the Centers for Disease Control national surveillance, 1982 to 1985. Pediatrics 79:1008–1014, 1987.

Rogers RM, Christiansen JR, Coalson JJ, Patterson CD. Eosinophilic pneumonia. Chest 68:665–671, 1975.

Rommens JM, Iannuzzi MC, Kerem B, Drumm ML, Melmer G, Dean M, Rozmahel R, Cole JL, Kennedy D, Hidaka N, Zsiga M, Buchwald M, Riordan JR, Tsui LC, Collins FS. Identification of the cystic fibrosis gene: chromosome walking and jumping. Science 245:1059–1065, 1989.

Rosenow EC III. The spectrum of drug-induced pulmonary disease. Ann Intern Med 77:977–991, 1972.

Rosenow EC III. Drug-induced hypersensitivity disease of the lung. In Kirkpatrick CH, Reynolds HY, eds. Immunologic and infectious reactions in the lung. New York, Marcel Dekker, 1976, pp 261–287.

Rosenow EC III, O'Connell EJ, Harrison EG Jr. Desquamative interstitial pneumonia in children. Am J Dis Child 120:344–348, 1970.

Rosenstein BJ, Eigen H. Risks of alternate-day prednisone in patients with cystic fibrosis. Pediatrics 87:245–246, 1991.

Rosenstein BJ, Eigen H, Schidlow DV. Alternate-day prednisone in patients with cystic fibrosis. Pediatr Res 33:385A, 1993.

Rosenstein BJ. Cystic fibrosis: other clinical manifestations. In Taussig LM, Landau LI, eds. Pediatric respiratory medicine. St. Louis, Mosby, 1999, pp 1033–1064.

Rottem M, Fauci AS, Hallahan CW, Kerr GS, Lebovics R, Leavitt RY, Hoffman GS. Wegener granulomatosis in children and adolescents: clinical presentation and outcome. J Pediatr 122:26–31, 1993.

Rubio TT, Miles MV, Lettieri JT, Kuhn RJ, Echols RM, Church DA. Pharmacokinetic disposition of sequential intravenous/oral ciprofloxacin in pediatric cystic fibrosis patients with acute pulmonary exacerbation. Pediatr Infect Dis J 16:112–117, 1997.

Rudd RM, Haslam PL, Turner-Warwick M. Cryptogenic fibrosing alveolitis. Relationships of pulmonary physiology and bronchoalveolar lavage to response to treatment and prognosis. Am Rev Respir Dis 124:1–8, 1981.

Rule AH, Lawrence D, Hager HJ, Hyslop N Jr, Schwachman H. IgA: presence in meconium obtained from patients with cystic fibrosis. Pediatrics 48:601–604, 1971.

Saeed MM, Woo MS, MacLaughlin EF, Margetis MF, Keens TG. Prognosis in pediatric idiopathic pulmonary hemosiderosis. Chest 116:721–725, 1999.

Salvaggio JE, deShazo RD. Pathogenesis of hypersensitivity pneumonitis. Chest 89(3 Suppl):190S–193S, 1986.

Sanders A, Crystal RG. Consequences to the lung of specific deficiencies in host defense. In Barnes PJ, Crystal RG, Weibel ER, West JB, eds. The lung: scientific foundations. 2nd ed. Philadelphia, Lippincott-Raven, 1997, pp 2367–2379.

Sanders DY, Huntley CC, Sharp GC. Mixed connective tissue disease in a child. J Pediatr 83:642–645, 1973.

Scadding JG. The bronchi in allergic aspergillosis. Scand J Resp Dis 48:372–377, 1967.

Schatz M, Wasserman S, Patterson R. Eosinophils and immunologic lung disease. Med Clin North Am 65:1055–1071, 1981.

Schatz M, Wasserman S, Patterson R. The eosinophil and the lung. Arch Intern Med 142:1515–1519, 1982.

Schiedner G, Morral N, Parks RJ, Wu Y, Koopmans SC, Langston C, Graham FL, Beaudet AL, Kochanek S. Genomic DNA transfer with a high-capacity adenovirus vector results in improved *in vivo* gene expression and decreased toxicity. Nat Genet 18:180–183, 1998.

Schiller NL, Millard RL. *Pseudomonas*-infected cystic fibrosis patient sputum inhibits the bactericidal activity of normal human serum. Pediatr Res 17:747–752, 1983.

Schiotz PO. Local humoral immunity and immune reactions in the lungs of patients with cystic fibrosis. Acta Pathol Microbiol Scand Suppl 276:1–25, 1981.

Schiotz PO, Clemmensen I, Høiby N. Immunoglobulins and albumin in sputum from patients with cystic fibrosis. A study of protein stability and presence of proteases. Acta Pathol Microbiol Scand [C] 88:275–280, 1980.

Schiotz PO, Egeskjold EM, Høiby N, Permin H. Autoantibodies in serum and sputum from patients with cystic fibrosis. Acta Pathol Microbiol Scand [C] 87:319–324, 1979a.

Schiotz PO, Høiby N. Precipitating antibodies against *Pseudomonas aeruginosa* in sputum from patients with cystic fibrosis: specificities and titres determined by means of crossed immunoelectrophoresis with intermediate gel. Acta Pathol Microbiol Scand 83:469–475, 1975.

Schiotz PO, Høiby N. Precipitating antibodies against *Haemophilus influenzae* and *Staphylococcus aureus* in sputum and serum from patients with cystic fibrosis. Acta Pathol Microbiol Scand [B] 87:345–351, 1979.

Schiotz PO, Høiby N, Juhl F, Permin H, Nielsen H, Svehag SE. Immune complexes in cystic fibrosis. Acta Pathol Microbiol Scand [C] 85:57–64, 1977.

Schiotz PO, Høiby N, Permin H, Wiik A. IgA and IgG antibodies against surface antigens of Pseudomonas aeruginosa in sputum and serum from patients with cystic fibrosis. Acta Pathol Microbiol Scand [C] 87:229–233, 1979b.

Schiotz PO, Nielsen H, Høiby N, Glikmann G, Svehag SE. Immune complexes in the sputum of patients with cystic fibrosis suffering from chronic *Pseudomonas aeruginosa* lung infection. Acta Pathol Microbiol Scand [C] 86:37–40, 1978.

Schiotz PO, Sorensen H, Høiby M. Activated complement in the sputum from patients with cystic fibrosis. Acta Pathol Microbiol Scand [C] 87:1–5, 1979c.

Schlueter DP. Response of the lung to inhaled antigens. Am J Med 57:476–492, 1974.

Schneider RM, Nevius DB, Brown HZ. Desquamative interstitial pneumonia in a four-year-old child. N Engl J Med 277:1056–1058, 1967.

Schofield NC, Davies IR, Cameron IR, Green M. Small airways in fibrosing alveolitis. Am Rev Respir Dis 113:729–735, 1976.

Schuyler M, Salvaggio JE. Hypersensitivity pneumonitis. Semin Respir Med 5:246–254, 1984.

Schuyler MR, Thigpen TP, Salvaggio JE. Local pulmonary immunity in pigeon breeder's disease. A case study. Ann Intern Med 88:355–358, 1978.

Schwartz RH. Serum immunoglobulin levels in cystic fibrosis. Am J Dis Child 111:408–411, 1966.

Schwartz RH, Johnstone DE, Holsclaw DS, Dooley RR. Serum precipitins to *Aspergillus fumigatus* in cystic fibrosis. Am J Dis Child 120:432–433, 1970.

Sedivá A, Lischke R, Simonek J, Tkaczyk J, Vavrova V, Bartosova J, Pohunek P, Bartunkova J, Pafko P. Lung transplantation for cystic fibrosis: immune system and autoimmunity. Med Sci Monit 7:1219–1223, 2001.

Seear M, Hui H, Magee F, Bohn D, Cutz E. Bronchial casts in children: a proposed classification based on nine cases and a review of the literature. Am J Respir Crit Care Med 155:364–370, 1997.

Seear M. Acellular bronchial casts in children after cardiac surgery. Crit Care Med 29:465–466, 2001.

Sekhon HS, Larson JE. In utero gene transfer into the pulmonary epithelium. Nat Med 1:1201–1203, 1995.

Seely JM, Jones LT, Wallace C, Sherry D, Effmann EL. Systemic sclerosis: using high-resolution CT to detect lung disease in children. AJR Am J Roentgenol 170:691–697, 1998.

Semenzato G. Immunology of interstitial lung diseases: cellular events taking place in the lung of sarcoidosis, hypersensitivity pneumonitis and HIV infection. Eur Respir J 4:94–102, 1991.

Serlin SP, Rimsza ME, Gay JH. Rheumatic pneumonia. The need for a new approach. Pediatrics 56:1075–1078, 1975.

Shah A, Pant CS, Bhagat R, Panchal N. CT in childhood allergic bronchopulmonary aspergillosis. Pediatr Radiol 22:227–228, 1992.

Shannon DC, Andrews JL, Recavarren S, Kazemi H. Pigeon breeder's lung disease and interstitial pulmonary fibrosis. Am J Dis Child 117:504–510, 1969.

Shapiro GG, Bamman J, Kanarek P, Bierman CW. The paradoxical effect of adrenergic and methylxanthine drugs in cystic fibrosis. Pediatrics 58:740–743, 1976.

Sharer N, Schwarz M, Malone G, Howarth A, Painter J, Super M, Braganza J. Mutations of the cystic fibrosis gene in patients with chronic pancreatitis. N Engl J Med 339:645–652, 1998.

Sharland M, Gibb DM, Holland F. Respiratory morbidity from lymphocytic interstitial pneumonitis (LIP) in vertically acquired HIV infection. Arch Dis Child 76:334–336, 1997.

Sheikh S, Madiraju K, Steiner P, Rao M. Bronchiectasis in pediatric AIDS. Chest 112:1202–1207, 1997.

Shen J, Brackett R, Fischer T, Holder A, Kellogg F, Michael JG. Specific *Pseudomonas* immunoglobulin E antibodies in sera of patients with cystic fibrosis. Infect Immun 32:967–968, 1981.

Shryock TR, Molle JS, Klinger JD, Thomassen MJ. Association with phagocytic inhibition of anti–*Pseudomonas aeruginosa* immunoglobulin G antibody subclass levels in serum from patients with cystic fibrosis. J Clin Microbiol 23:513–516, 1986.

Sieber OF, Wilska ML, Riggin R. Elevated nitroblue tetrazolium dye reduction test response in acute viral respiratory disease. Pediatrics 58:122–124, 1976.

Silver RM, Miller KS. Lung involvement in systemic sclerosis. Rheum Dis Clin North Am 16:199–216, 1990.

Silverman M, Hobbs FD, Gordon IR, Carswell F. Cystic fibrosis, atopy, and airways lability. Arch Dis Child 53:873–877, 1978.

Simon HU, Plötz SG, Dummer R, Blaser K. Abnormal clones of T cells producing interleukin-5 in idiopathic eosinophilia. N Engl J Med 341:1112–1120, 1999.

Singsen BH, Bernstein BH, Kornreich HK, King KK, Hanson V, Tan EM. Mixed connective tissue disease in childhood. A clinical and serologic survey. J Pediatr 90:893–900, 1977.

Singsen BH, Tedford JC, Platzker AC, Hanson V. Spontaneous pneumothorax: a complication of juvenile dermatomyositis. J Pediatr 92:771–774, 1978.

Singsen BH, Swanson VL, Bernstein BH, Heuser ET, Hanson V, Landing BH. A histologic evaluation of mixed connective tissue disease in childhood. Am J Med 68:710–717, 1980.

Singsen BH, Platzker AC. Pulmonary involvement in the rheumatologic disorders of childhood. In Chernick V, Kendig EL, eds. Disorders of the respiratory tract in children. Philadelphia, W. B. Saunders, 1990, pp 1071–1102.

Skov M, Poulsen LK, Koch C. Increased antigen-specific Th-2 response in allergic bronchopulmonary aspergillosis (ABPA) in patients with cystic fibrosis. Pediatr Pulmonol 27:74–79, 1999a.

Skov M, Pressler T, Jensen HE, Høiby N, Koch C. Specific IgG subclass antibody pattern to Aspergillus fumigatus in patients with cystic fibrosis with allergic bronchopulmonary aspergillosis (ABPA). Thorax 54:44–50, 1999b.

Skov M, Koch C, Reimert CM, Poulsen LK. Diagnosis of allergic bronchopulmonary aspergillosis (ABPA) in cystic fibrosis. Allergy 55:50–58, 2000.

Slavin RG, Laird TS, Cherry JD. Allergic bronchopulmonary aspergillosis in a child. J Pediatr 76:416–421, 1970.

Slavin RG, Bedrossian CW, Hutcheson PS, Pittman S, Salinas-Madrigal L, Tsai CC, Gleich GJ. A pathologic study of allergic bronchopulmonary aspergillosis. J Allergy Clin Immunol 81:718–725, 1988.

Smith A. Pathogenesis of bacterial bronchitis in cystic fibrosis. Pediatr Infect Dis J 16:91–96, 1997.

Smith AL. Antibiotic therapy in cystic fibrosis: evaluation of clinical trials. J Pediatr 108:866–870, 1986.

Smith GJ. The histopathology of pulmonary reactions to drugs. Clin Chest Med 11:95–117, 1990.

Smith JJ, Travis SM, Greenberg EP, Welsh MJ. Cystic fibrosis airway epithelia fail to kill bacteria because of abnormal airway surface fluid. Cell 85:229–236, 1996.

Smith MJ, Morris L, Stead RJ, Hodson ME, Batten JC. Lymphocyte subpopulations and function in cystic fibrosis. Eur J Respir Dis 70:300–308, 1987.

Soergel KH, Sommers SC. Idiopathic pulmonary hemosiderosis and related syndromes. Am J Med 32:499–511, 1962.

Sorensen RU, Stern RC, Polmar SH. Cellular immunity to bacteria: impairment of in vitro lymphocyte responses to Pseudomonas aeruginosa in cystic fibrosis patients. Infect Immun 18:735–740, 1977.

Sorensen RU, Stern RC, Polmar SH. Lymphocyte responsiveness to Pseudomonas aeruginosa in cystic fibrosis: relationship to status of pulmonary disease in sibling pairs. J Pediatr 93:201–205, 1978.

Sorensen RU, Stern RC, Chase P, Polmar SH. Defective cellular immunity to gram-negative bacteria in cystic fibrosis patients. Infect Immun 23:398–402, 1979.

Sorensen RU, Chase PA, Stern RC, Polmar SH. Influence of cystic fibrosis plasma on lymphocyte responses to Pseudomonas aeruginosa in vitro. Pediatr Res 15:14–18, 1981a.

Sorensen RU, Stern RC, Chase PA, Polmar SH. Changes in lymphocyte reactivity to Pseudomonas aeruginosa in hospitalized patients with cystic fibrosis. Am Rev Respir Dis 123:37–41, 1981b.

Sorensen RU, Ruuskanen O, Miller K, Stern RC. B-lymphocyte function in cystic fibrosis. Eur J Respir Dis 64:524–533, 1983.

Sorensen RU, Waller RL, Klinger JD. Cystic fibrosis. Infection and immunity to Pseudomonas. Clin Rev Allergy 9:47–74, 1991.

Sostman HD, Matthay RA, Putman CE. Cytotoxic drug-induced lung disease. Am J Med 62:608–615, 1977.

South MA, Warwick WJ, Wolheim FA, Good RA. The IgA system. 3. IgA levels in the serum and saliva of pediatric patients—evidence for a local immunological system. J Pediatr 71:645–653, 1967.

Specks U, Wheatley CL, McDonald TJ, Rohrbach MS, DeRemee RA. Anticytoplasmic autoantibodies in the diagnosis and follow-up of Wegener's granulomatosis. Mayo Clin Proc 64:28–36, 1989.

Speert DP, Lawton D, Mutharia LM. Antibody to Pseudomonas aeruginosa mucoid exopolysaccharide and to sodium alginate in cystic fibrosis serum. Pediatr Res 18:431–433, 1984.

Spence JE, Buffone GJ, Rosenbloom CL, Fernbach SD, Curry MR, Carpenter RJ, Ledbetter DH, O'Brien WE, Beaudet AL. Prenatal diagnosis of cystic fibrosis using linked DNA markers and microvillar intestinal enzyme analysis. Hum Genet 76:5–10, 1987.

Spino M. Pharmacokinetics of drugs in cystic fibrosis. Clin Rev Allergy 9:169–210, 1991.

Springer C, Maayan C, Katzir Z, Ariel I, Godfrey S. Chloroquine treatment in desquamative interstitial pneumonia. Arch Dis Child 62:76–77, 1987.

Staats BA, Ellefson RD, Budahn LL, Dines DE, Prakash UB, Offord K. The lipoprotein profile of chylous and nonchylous pleural effusions. Mayo Clin Proc 55:700–704, 1980.

Stafford HA, Polmar SH, Boat TF. Immunologic studies in cow's milk–induced pulmonary hemosiderosis. Pediatr Res 11:898–903, 1977.

Stein AA, Manlapas FC, Soike KF, Patterson PR. Specific isoantibodies in cystic fibrosis. A study of serum and bronchial mucus. J Pediatr 65:495–500, 1964.

Steinkamp G, von der Hardt H. Improvement of nutritional status and lung function after long-term nocturnal gastrostomy feedings in cystic fibrosis. J Pediatr 124:244–249, 1994.

Stevens WM, Burdon JG, Clemens LE, Webb J. The 'shrinking lungs syndrome'—an infrequently recognised feature of systemic lupus erythematosus. Aust N Z J Med 20:67–70 1990.

Stiehm ER, Reed CE, Tooley WH. Pigeon breeder's lung in children. Pediatrics 39:904–915, 1967.

Stillwell PC, Norris DG, O'Connell EJ, Rosenow EC III, Weiland LH, Harrison EG Jr. Desquamative interstitial pneumonitis in children. Chest 77:165–171, 1980.

Storey DG, Ujack EE, Rabin HR. Population transcript accumulation of Pseudomonas aeruginosa exotoxin A and elastase in sputa from patients with cystic fibrosis. Infect Immun 60:4687–4694, 1992.

Strauss RG. Complement in cystic fibrosis. Helv Paediatr Acta 34:429–435, 1979.

Strong TV, Smit LS, Turpin SV, Cole JL, Hon CT, Markiewicz D, Petty TL, Craig MW, Rosenow EC 3rd, Tsui LC, et al. Cystic fibrosis gene mutation in two sisters with mild disease and normal sweat electrolyte levels. N Engl J Med 325:1630–1634, 1991.

Strunk RC, Sieber OF, Taussig LM, Gall EP. Serum complement depression during viral lower respiratory tract illness in cystic fibrosis. Arch Dis Child 52:687–690, 1977.

Stuart BO. Deposition and clearance of inhaled particles. Environ Health Perspect 55:369–390, 1984.

Stubblefield C, Murray RL. Making the transition: pediatric lung transplantation. J Pediatr Health Care 14:280–287, 2000.

Sturgill BC, Westervelt FB. Immunofluorescence studies in a case of Goodpasture's syndrome. JAMA 194:914–916, 1965.

Sullivan JF, Dolan TF Jr, Meyers A, Treat K. Use of nitroblue tetrazolium dye test. An aid in managing patients with cystic fibrosis. Am J Dis Child 125:702–704, 1973.

Suszycki LH. Psychological aspects of heart transplantation. Social Work 33:205–209, 1988.

Sweet SC, Spray TL, Huddleston CB, Mendeloff E, Canter CE, Balzer DT, Bridges ND, Cohen AH, Mallory GB Jr. Pediatric lung transplantation at St. Louis Children's Hospital, 1990-1995. Am J Respir Crit Care Med 155:1027–1035, 1997.

Taccetti G, Procopio E, Marianelli L, Campana S; Italian Group for Cystic Fibrosis Microbiology. Allergic bronchopulmonary aspergillosis in Italian cystic fibrosis patients: prevalence and percentage of positive tests in the employed diagnositic criteria. Eur J Epidemiol 16:837–842, 2000.

Tacier–Eugster H, Wuthrich B, Meyer H. Atopic allergy, serum IgE and RAST specific IgE antibodies in patients with cystic fibrosis. Helv Paediatr Acta 35:31–37, 1980.

Talamo RC, Schwartz RH. Immunologic and allergic manifestations. In Taussig LM, ed. Cystic fibrosis. New York, Thieme-Stratton, 1984, pp 175–194.

Tan KK, Trull AK, Hue KL, Best NG, Wallwork J, Higenbottam TW. Pharmacokinetics of cyclosporine in heart and lung transplant candidates and recipients with cystic fibrosis and Eisenmenger's syndrome. Clin Pharmacol Ther 53:544–554, 1993.

Taussig LM. Cystic fibrosis: an overview. In Taussig LM, ed. Cystic fibrosis. New York, Thieme-Stratton, 1984, pp 1–9.

Thomassen MJ, Boxerbaum B, Demko CA, Kuchenbrod PJ, Dearborn DG, Wood RE. Inhibitory effect of cystic fibrosis serum on *Pseudomonas* phagocytosis by rabbit and human alveolar macrophages. Pediatr Res 13:1085–1088, 1979.

Thomassen MJ, Demko CA, Wood RE, Tandler B, Dearborn DG, Boxerbaum B, Kuchenbrod PJ. Ultrastructure and function of alveolar macrophages from cystic fibrosis patients. Pediatr Res 14:715–721, 1980.

Thomassen MJ, Demko CA, Klinger JD, Stern RC. *Pseudomonas cepacia* colonization among patients with cystic fibrosis. A new opportunist. Am Rev Respir Dis 131:791–796, 1985.

Tizzano EF, Buchwald M. Cystic fibrosis: beyond the gene to therapy. J Pediatr 120:337–349, 1992.

Tobin MJ, Maguire O, Reen D, Tempany E, Fitzgerald MX. Atopy and bronchial reactivity in older patients with cystic fibrosis. Thorax 35:807–813, 1980.

Tomashefski JF Jr, Abramowsky CR, Chung-Park M, Wisniewska J, Bruce MC. Immunofluorescence studies of lung tissue in cystic fibrosis. Pediatr Pathol 12:313–324, 1992.

Torres MJ, Girón MD, Corzo JL, Rodriguez F, Moreno F, Perez E, Blanca M, Martinez-Valverde A. Release of inflammatory mediators after cow's milk intake in a newborn with idiopathic pulmonary hemosiderosis. J Allergy Clin Immunol 98:1120–1123, 1996.

Trezise AE, Buchwald M. In vivo cell-specific expression of the cystic fibrosis transmembrane conductance regulator. Nature 353:434–437, 1991.

Tsui LC. The cystic fibrosis transmembrane conductance regulator gene. Am J Respir Crit Care Med 151(3 Pt 2):S47–S53, 1995.

Turner KJ, O'Mahoney J, Wetherall JD. Hypersensitivity studies in asthmatic patients with broncho-pulmonary aspergillosis. Clin Allergy 2:361–372, 1972.

Turner-Warwick M. Philip Ellman lecture. Immunological aspects of systemic diseases of the lungs. Proc R Soc Med 67:541–547, 1974.

Turner-Warwick M. The lung in systemic diseases. In Bienenstock J, ed. Immunology of the lung and upper respiratory tract. New York, McGraw-Hill, 1984, pp 386–396.

Turner-Warwick ME, Haslam PL. Clinical applications of bronchoalveolar lavage: an interim view. Br J Dis Chest 80:105–121, 1986.

Tutor JD, Eid NS. Treatment of idiopathic pulmonary hemosiderosis with inhaled flunisolide. South Med J 88:984–986, 1995.

Ulibarri JI, Sanz Y, Fuentes C, Mancha A, Aramendia M, Sanchez S. Reduction of lymphorrhagia from ruptured thoracic duct by somatostatin (letter). Lancet 336:258, 1990.

Uziel Y, Hen B, Cordoba M, Wolach B. Lymphocytic interstitial pneumonitis preceding polyarticular juvenile rheumatoid arthritis. Clin Exp Rheumatol 16:617–619, 1998.

Valassi-Adam H, Rouska A, Karpouzas J, Matsaniotis N. Raised IgA in idiopathic pulmonary haemosiderosis. Arch Dis Child 50:320–322, 1975.

Valentine VG, Raffin TA. The management of chylothorax. Chest 102:586–591, 1992.

van den Berg JW, Hepkema BG, Geertsma A, Koeter GH, Postma DS, de Boer WJ, Lems SP, van der Bij W. Long-term outcome of lung transplantation is predicted by number of HLA-DR mismatches. Transplantation 71:368–373, 2001.

van der Ent CK, Walenkamp MJ, Donckerwolcke RA, van der Laag J, van Diemen-Steenvoorde R. Pulmonary hemosiderosis and immune complex glomerulonephritis. Clin Nephrol 43:339–341, 1995.

van Straaten HL, Gerards LJ, Krediet TG. Chylothorax in the neonatal period. Eur J Pediatr 152:2–5, 1993.

Van Wye JE, Collins MS, Baylor M, Pennington JE, Hsu Y, Sampanvejsopa V, Moss RB. *Pseudomonas* hyperimmune globulin passive immunotherapy for pulmonary exacerbations in cystic fibrosis. Pediatr Pulmonol 9:7–18, 1990.

Vats KR, Vats A, Kim Y, Dassenko D, Sinaiko AR. Henoch-Schönlein purpura and pulmonary hemorrhage: a report and literature review. Pediatr Nephrol 13:530–534, 1999.

Vlahakis NE, Aksamit TR. Diagnosis and treatment of allergic bronchopulmonary aspergillosis. Mayo Clin Proc 76:930–938, 2001.

Wagener JS, Taussig LM, DeBenedetti C, Lemen RJ, Loughlin GM. Pulmonary function in juvenile rheumatoid arthritis. J Pediatr 99:108–110, 1981.

Wagener JS. Collagen vascular disease. In Taussig LM, Landau LI, eds. Pediatric respiratory medicine. St. Louis, Mosby, 1999, pp 818–829.

Waller RL, Brattin WJ, Dearborn DG. Cytosolic free calcium concentration and intracellular calcium distribution in lymphocytes from cystic fibrosis patients. Life Sci 35:775–781, 1984.

Wallwork JC, Brenchley P, McCarthy J, Allan JD, Moss D, Ward AM, Holzel A, Williams RF, McFarlane H. Some aspects of immunity in patients with cystic fibrosis. Clin Exp Immunol 18:303–320, 1974.

Wallwork JC, McFarlane H. The SIgA system and hypersensitivity in patients with cystic fibrosis. Clin Allergy 6:349–358, 1976.

Walravens PA, Chase HP. The prognosis of childhood systemic lupus erythematosus. Am J Dis Child 130:929–933, 1976.

Wang JL, Patterson R, Mintzer R, Roberts M, Rosenberg M. Allergic bronchopulmonary aspergillosis in pediatric practice. J Pediatr 94:376–381, 1979a.

Wang JL, Patterson R, Roberts M, Ghory AC. The management of allergic bronchopulmonary aspergillosis. Am Rev Respir Dis 120:87–92, 1979b.

Warner JO, Taylor BW, Norman AP, Soothill JF. Association of cystic fibrosis with allergy. Arch Dis Child 51:507–511, 1976.

Warner JO. Lung transplantation. In Taussig LM, Landau LI, eds. Pediatric respiratory medicine. St. Louis, Mosby, 1999, pp 358–363.

Warren CP, Tai E, Batten JC, Hutchcroft BJ, Pepys J. Cystic fibrosis—immunological reactions to *A. fumigatus* and common allergens. Clin Allergy 5:1–12, 1975.

Warren RW. Rheumatologic aspects of pediatric cystic fibrosis patients treated with flouroquinolones. Pediatr Infect Dis J 16:118–122, 1997.

Warwick WJ, Hansen LG. The long-term effect of high-frequency chest compression therapy on pulmonary complications of cystic fibrosis. Pediatr Pulmonol 11:265–271, 1991.

Waters KA, Bale P, Isaacs D, Mellis C. Successful chloroquine therapy in a child with lymphoid interstitial pneumonitis. J Pediatr 119:989–991, 1991.

Watters LC. Genetic aspects of idiopathic pulmonary fibrosis and hypersensitivity pneumonitis. Semin Respir Med 7:317–325, 1986.

Weese WC, Levine BW, Kazemi H. Interstitial lung disease resistant to corticosteroid therapy. Report of three cases treated with azathioprine and cyclophosphamide. Chest 67:57–60, 1975.

Wei L, Vankeerberghen A, Cuppens H, Eggermont J, Cassiman JJ, Droogmans G, Nilius B. Interaction between calcium-activated chloride channels and the cystic fibrosis transmembrane conductance regulator. Pflugers Arch 438:635–641, 1999.

Weller PF. Eosinophilia. J Allergy Clin Immunol 73:1–14, 1984.

Wenzel FJ, Emanuel DA, Gray RL. Immunofluorescent studies in patients with farmer's lung. J Allergy Clin Immunol 48:224–229, 1971.

Wetherill SF, Davies AL, Mayock RL. Chyloptysis. Am J Med 88:437–438, 1990.

Whaley K. Biosynthesis of complement components and the regulatory proteins of the alternative complement pathway by human peripheral blood monocytes. J Exp Med 151:501–516, 1980.

Wheeler WB, Williams M, Matthews WJ Jr, Colten HR. Progression of cystic fibrosis lung disease as a function of serum immunoglobulin G levels: a 5-year longitudinal study. J Pediatr 104:695–699, 1984.

Whitehead B, Scott JP, Helms P, Malone M, Macrae D, Higenbottam TW, Smyth RL, Wallwork J, Elliott M, de Leval M. Technique and use of transbronchial biopsy in children and adolescents. Pediatr Pulmonol 12:240–246, 1992.

Wiedemann HP, Matthay RA. Pulmonary manifestations of the collagen vascular diseases. Clin Chest Med 10:677–722, 1989.

Wiener-Kronish JP, Solinger AM, Warnock ML, Churg A, Ordonez N, Golden JA. Severe pulmonary involvement in mixed connective tissue disease. Am Rev Respir Dis 124:499–503, 1981.

Wiggins J, Sheffield E, Jeffery PK. Bronchial casts associated with lymphatic and pulmonary lymphoid abnormalities. Thorax 44:226–227, 1989.

Wild LG, Lopez M. Hypersensitivity pneumonitis: a comprehensive review. J Investig Allergol Clin Immunol 11:3–15, 2001.

Wilfond BS, Taussig LM. Cystic fibrosis: general overview. In Taussig M, Landau LI, eds. Pediatric respiratory medicine. St. Louis, Mosby, 1999, pp 982–990.

Willoughby WF, Willoughby JB. Immunologic mechanisms of parenchymal lung injury. Environ Health Perspect 55:239–257, 1984.

Wilmott RW. The relationship between atopy and cystic fibrosis. In Moss RB, ed. Clinical reviews in allergy. Vol. 9. *Cystic fibrosis.* Clifton, NJ, Humana Press, 1991, pp 29–46.

Wilmott RW, Amin RS, Colin AA, DeVault A, Dozor AJ, Eigen H, Johnson C, Lester LA, McCoy K, McKean LP, Moss R, Nash ML, Jue CP, Regelmann W, Stokes DC, Fuchs HJ. Aerosolized recombinant human DNase in hospitalized cystic fibrosis patients with acute pulmonary exacerbations. Am J Respir Crit Care Med 153:1914–1917, 1996.

Winnie GB, Cowan RG, Wade NA. Intravenous immune globulin treatment of pulmonary exacerbations in cystic fibrosis. J Pediatr 114:309–314, 1989.

Wisser W, Wekerle T, Zlabinger G, Senbaclavaci O, Zuckermann A, Klepetko W, Wolner E. Influence of human leukocyte antigen matching on long-term outcome after lung transplantation. J Heart Lung Transplant 15:1209–1216, 1996.

Wolfe CA, Hunninghake GW. Vasculitides of the polyarteritis nodosa group. In Lynch JP, DeRemee RA, eds. Immunologically mediated pulmonary diseases. Philadelphia, J. B. Lippincott, 1991, pp 234–249.

Wood RE, Pennington JE, Reynolds HY. Intranasal administration of a *Pseudomonas* lipopolysaccharide vaccine in cystic fibrosis patients. Pediatr Infect Dis 2:367–369, 1983.

Wulffraat NM, de Graeff-Meeder ER, Rijkers GT, van der Laag H, Kuis W. Prevalence of circulating immune complexes in patients with cystic fibrosis and arthritis. J Pediatr 125:374–378, 1994.

Wynants H, Van Gompel A, Morales I, Vervoort T, Ponomarenko N, Surmont I, Bourgeois P, Van den Enden E, Van Marck E, Van den Ende J. The hypereosinophilic syndrome after residence in a tropical country: report of 4 cases. Acta Clin Belg 55:334–340, 2000.

Yamasaki H, Ando M, Brazer W, Center DM, Cruikshank WW. Polarized type 1 cytokine profile in bronchoalveolar lavage T cells of patients with hypersensitivity pneumonitis. J Immunol 163:3516–3523, 1999.

Yankaskas JR, Mallory GB Jr. Lung transplantation in cystic fibrosis: consensus conference statement. Chest 113:217–226, 1998.

Yoshimura K, Nakamura H, Trapnell BC, Dalemans W, Pavirani A, Lecocq JP, Crystal RG. The cystic fibrosis gene has a "housekeeping"-type promoter and is expressed at low levels in cells of epithelial origin. J Biol Chem 266:9140–9144, 1991.

Zabner J, Seiler M, Walters R, Kotin RM, Fulgeras W, Davidson BL, Chiorini JA. Adeno-associated virus type 5 (AAV5) but not AAV2 binds to the apical surfaces of airway epithelia and facilitates gene transfer. J Virol 74:3852–3858, 2000.

Zach MS, Oberwaldner B, Forche G, Polgar G. Bronchodilators increase airway instability in cystic fibrosis. Am Rev Respir Dis 131:537–543, 1985.

Zambie MF, Gupta S, Lemen RJ, Hilman B, Waring WW, Sly RM. Relationship between response to exercise and allergy in patients with cystic fibrosis. Ann Allergy 42:290–294, 1979.

Zapletal A, Houstek J, Samanek M, Copova M, Paul T. Lung function in children and adolescents with idiopathic interstitial pulmonary fibrosis. Pediatr Pulmonol 1:154–166, 1985.

Zeitlin PL. Future pharmacological treatment of cystic fibrosis. Respiration 67:351–357, 2000.

Zielenski J, Tsui LC. Cystic fibrosis: genotype and phenotypic variations. Annu Rev Genet 29:777–807, 1995.

Zimmerman BL, Haller JO, Price AP, Thelmo WL, Fikrig S. Children with AIDS—is pathologic diagnosis possible based on chest radiographs? Pediatr Radiol 17:303–307, 1987.

C H A P T E R

34 Gastroenterologic and Liver Disorders

Gary J. Russell, Athos Bousvaros, and W. Allan Walker

In the past several years, immunology has expanded from the study of lymphocyte biology as a distinct component of host defense to a multidisciplinary field recognizing the complex integration of the immune system with the body as a whole. The importance of the immune system in maintaining the boundary between self and the environment is readily apparent at mucosal epithelial surfaces. A disruption of this balance between antigen exclusion or immune response to antigen uptake may lead to gastrointestinal or even systemic disease.

This chapter first briefly discusses the physiology and development of the mucosal immune system, with emphasis on macromolecular transport, immunoglobulin A (IgA) synthesis, and the role of nutrition in immunity. (For a more detailed review of mucosal immunity, see Chapter 9.) The second part of this chapter reviews gastrointestinal diseases in which immunologic factors play a significant etiologic role (Fig. 34-1).

IMMUNOPHYSIOLOGY OF THE MUCOSAL IMMUNE SYSTEM

Structure of Gut-Associated Lymphoid Tissue

The intestine is challenged with antigenic proteins every day in the form of foods and orally ingested viruses and bacteria. Despite this, clinically significant intestinal inflammation rarely occurs. The intestinal mucosal immune system is able to mount an *immune response* to potentially harmful pathogens and also induce mucosal and systemic *tolerance* to normal bacterial flora and food antigens. The gut epithelium and mucosal lymphoid cells constitute a first line of defense against infection and penetration of potentially harmful macromolecules into the systemic circulation (Sanderson and Walker, 1993).

The population of lymphoid and other immune cells in the intestine is frequently termed *gut-associated lymphoid tissue* (GALT); increasingly, the term *mucosa-associated lymphoid tissue* (MALT) is used to emphasize the interplay between lymphocytes of the gut and other mucosal sites (including respiratory, urinary, and reproductive epithelia) (Kraehenbuhl and Neutra, 1992).

The gut immune system can be arbitrarily divided into two portions (Fig. 34-2). The *organized mucosa-associated lymphoid tissue* (O-MALT, also called the

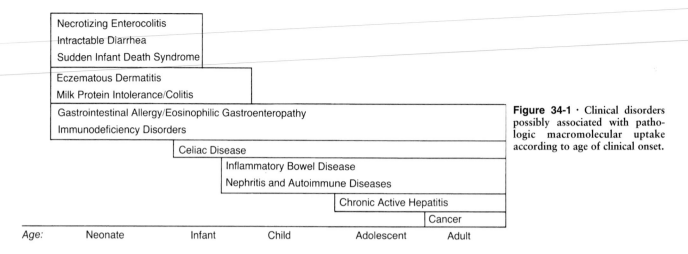

Necrotizing Enterocolitis				
Intractable Diarrhea				
Sudden Infant Death Syndrome				
Eczematous Dermatitis				
Milk Protein Intolerance/Colitis				
Gastrointestinal Allergy/Eosinophilic Gastroenteropathy				
Immunodeficiency Disorders				
	Celiac Disease			
		Inflammatory Bowel Disease		
		Nephritis and Autoimmune Diseases		
			Chronic Active Hepatitis	
				Cancer

Age: Neonate   Infant   Child   Adolescent   Adult

Figure 34-1 · Clinical disorders possibly associated with pathologic macromolecular uptake according to age of clinical onset.

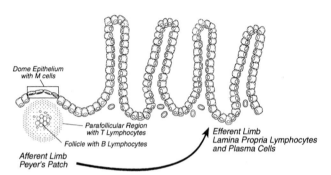

Figure 34-2 · **Components of intestinal host defense.** The afferent limb of the mucosal immune system *(left side of figure)* samples antigen through modified epithelial cells (M cells). Antigen-presenting cells, "naïve" T cells, and B cells within the Peyer's patch sample are activated by antigens taken up by the M cell. In contrast, the efferent limb of the mucosal immune system located in the intestinal lamina propria consists of differentiated "memory" T cells and plasma cells. (From Bousvaros A, Walker WA. Intestinal host defense. In Kirsner J, ed. Inflammatory Bowel Disease, ed 4. Baltimore, Williams & Wilkins, 1995, pp 140–161.)

afferent limb of the mucosal immune system) consists of the dome (follicle-associated) epithelium, Peyer's patches, and mesenteric lymph nodes. Solitary lymphoid aggregates may be seen in the duodenum and jejunum in the human, but Peyer's patches (large groups of lymphoid nodules) are seen almost exclusively in the ileum. Peyer's patches are normally from 0.6 to 3 mm in diameter and are scattered throughout the intestinal lamina propria.

The dome epithelium overlying the Peyer's patches is characterized by a paucity of goblet cells, less intestinal mucin, and the presence of modified epithelial cells *(microfold or M cells)* that are specialized for antigen uptake (Pabst, 1987). These cells are derived from crypt epithelial cells, and their differentiation appears to be directed by factors secreted by lymphocytes in the Peyer's patches (Kerneis et al., 1997).

The putative purpose of the dome epithelium is to provide a portal of entry for antigens to be sampled by antigen-presenting cells (APCs) in the O-MALT, ultimately resulting in activation of B and T cells in the lymphoid follicles and conversion of naïve lymphocytes into memory and effector cells (Kraehenbuhl and Neutra, 1992; Pabst, 1987; Waksman and Ozer, 1976). Regulatory "switch" T cells in the O-MALT may promote B-cell synthesis of immunoglobulin (Kawanishi et al., 1983; Strober and Harriman, 1991).

The *diffuse mucosa-associated lymphoid tissue* (D-MALT, also called the *efferent limb* of the mucosal immune system) consists of lymphocytes widely distributed throughout the intestinal lamina propria and other mucosal sites (see Fig. 34-2). Components of the D-MALT include plasma cells; helper, suppressor, and cytotoxic T cells; and intestinal intraepithelial lymphocytes (IELs). The predominant lymphoid cell type within the lamina propria is IgA-producing plasma cells. The proportion of T cells that are CD4+ in the lamina propria is 60%, compared with 40% CD8+, which is similar to that found in the peripheral circulation; however, the lamina propria CD4+ cells are predominantly CD4+CD45ROhi+ or CD4+Leu-8−, which indicates previous activation, and functionally provide help for immunoglobulin synthesis by B cells (Kanof et al., 1988b; Morimoto et al., 1985).

Other immune cells in the lamina propria, including eosinophils, macrophages, and neutrophils, are not traditionally included in the cells constituting the D-MALT but are important as effectors and regulators of the mucosal inflammatory response.

Components of Intestinal Host Defense

There is now abundant evidence that antigenic macromolecules penetrate the intestinal surface in quantities of immunologic significance (Walker and Isselbacher, 1974; Weiner, 1988). This section focuses on mechanisms by which such antigens and pathogens are degraded, processed, inactivated, and eliminated from the gut before they enter the systemic circulation. Because immunoglobulin A is the principal mucosal antibody (with more than 3 g/day secreted by the human adult intestine), its function is discussed in detail. In addition, because the human responds to most ingested antigens with systemic tolerance, mechanisms of oral tolerance are discussed. Currently recognized components of intestinal host defense are summarized in Figure 34-1 and Table 34-1.

Nonimmunologic Defenses

Nonimmunologic defenses prevent antigen penetration into the systemic circulation by either enzymatic degradation of proteins, intestinal transport out of the lumen, or physical blockage of antigen (see Chapter 10). *Gastric acid* results in a stomach pH cytotoxic to many bacteria and facilitates digestion of proteins by pepsin. Individuals with decreased gastric acid (as a result of medical or surgical reduction of gastric acid output) are more susceptible to gut colonization by pathogenic bacteria (Garvey et al., 1989; Sarker and Gyr, 1992). *Pancreatic secretions,* including proteases, amylase, lipase, and bicarbonate, break down macromolecules and may also have antimicrobial properties (Mett et al., 1984; Saffran et al., 1979). *Intestinal peristalsis* (particularly the spontaneous peristalsis termed the *migrating motor complex*) is important in transporting bacteria out of the bowel, and bacterial overgrowth is common in patients with aperistaltic intestinal "blind loops" or bowel obstruction (Kirsch, 1990; Sarker and Gyr, 1992). The *normal bacterial flora* prevents gut colonization by pathogenic bacteria (e.g., *Clostridium difficile*) and fungi (e.g., *Candida*) through two mechanisms: consumption of intraluminal nutrients and production of volatile fatty acids that inhibit growth of pathogenic bacteria (Hentges, 1986; Tazume et al., 1993).

Physical blockage of antigen passage into the body is prevented by the intestinal mucin layer and the epithelial cell surface barrier. *Intestinal mucins* are highly glycosylated molecules of high molecular weight and consist of a core protein (apomucin) joined to oligosaccharides (including fucose, *N*-acetylglucosamine, and *N*-acetylgalactosamine). Cloning of apomucin genes demonstrates homology between bronchial and intestinal mucins, emphasizing again the presence of a common mucosal immune system (Jany et al., 1991; Kim et al., 1991). Intestinal mucin protects the intestine by multiple mechanisms. First, mucin forms a viscoelastic layer over the intestinal epithelium, serving as a physical barrier to proteins and pathogens. Second, glycoproteins on the mucous coat may preferentially bind pathogenic bacteria, thus competitively inhibiting binding of such bacteria to epithelial cells. Last, mucin may increase antibody concentration over the epithelial cell layer by acting as a matrix to which secretory immunoglobulins can bind, enhancing their effectiveness by preventing rapid loss by normal peristalsis (Snyder and Walker, 1987).

The *intestinal epithelial barrier* is composed principally of five types of cells: enterocytes, goblet cells, IELs, Paneth cells, and neuroendocrine cells (Fig. 34-3) (Pabst, 1987). The enterocytes, joined together by a network of tight junctions, limit antigen passage across the intestine but under certain conditions may take up proteins and present antigenic peptides to T lymphocytes (Bland and Kambarage, 1991). Studies of animals also suggest that during intestinal inflammation, enterocytes can produce cytokines that modulate mucosal immune function (Radema et al., 1991).

Other components of the epithelial cell barrier are also important in preventing infection: goblet cells secrete mucins, and Paneth cells, usually located in the base of crypts to protect intestinal epithelial stem cells, secrete the antimicrobial proteins cryptdins and lysozyme (Selsted et al., 1992). IELs are predominantly CD8[+] cells whose function remains largely unknown but contain cytotoxic granules and under specific conditions have been shown to be cytotoxic to virally infected epithelial cells or suppress immune responses in vitro (Cerf-Bensussan and Guy-Grand, 1991; Ebert, 1990; Hoang et al., 1991; Russell et al., 1993; Sachdev et al., 1993).

TABLE 34-1 · FACTORS PREVENTING ANTIGEN TRANSPORT FROM THE GUT

Nonimmunologic Factors	
Luminal	**Mucosal**
Gastric acid secretion	Intestinal mucin
Intestinal proteolysis	Epithelial cell maturity
Bile acids	
Early enteral nutrition	
Intestinal flora	
Intestinal motility	

Immunologic Factors		
Mucosal	**Passive Defense**	**Hepatic**
Secretory IgA	Transplacental IgG	Reticuloendothelial cells
Other immunoglobulins (IgG, IgM, and IgE)	Breast milk factors (immune/hormonal)	Immune-complex (IgA) clearance
Cell-mediated immunity		Immune modulation

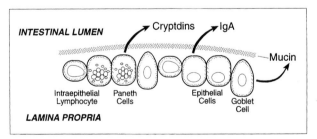

Figure 34-3 · **The gut epithelium in intestinal host defense.** A physical barrier is formed by the enterocytes and their tight junctions that prevents antigen passage into the systemic circulation. In addition, products secreted by the cells of the gut epithelium (including secretory immunoglobulin A transported by the enterocyte, cryptdins synthesized by the Paneth cell, and mucin synthesized by the goblet cell) can prevent invasion by antigens or microbes. (From Bousvaros A, Walker WA. Intestinal host defense. In Kirsner J, ed. Inflammatory Bowel Disease, ed 4. Baltimore, Williams & Wilkins, 1995, pp 140–161.)

Macromolecular Transport Mechanisms

Four mechanisms have been proposed to account for macromolecular transport across the intact epithelial cell barrier (Table 34-2) (Gonnella and Walker, 1987; Sanderson and Walker, 1993; Weiner, 1988). The uptake of macromolecules and microorganisms through the intestinal epithelial barrier primarily occurs through active vesicular transport.

RECEPTOR-MEDIATED ENDOCYTOSIS

Receptor-mediated endocytosis refers to the process initiated by the interaction between an intraluminal macromolecule (ligand) and a specific receptor to which it binds on the enterocyte plasma membrane (Fig. 34-4*A*). The binding stimulates the clustering of additional receptors in a clathrin-coated pit area of the cell, with invagination and internalization of the coated pit, forming a vesicle. Depending on intracellular trafficking, the vesicle and its contents may be either expelled intact from the basolateral membrane of the enterocyte or intracellularly degraded by a lysosome (Walker and Isselbacher, 1974). Intraluminal bacterial pathogens also invade the intestinal barrier by means of receptors present on enterocytes. Recent evidence indicates that *Listeria monocytogenes* express a surface protein, internalin, that recognizes E-cadherin on the basolateral surface of enterocytes to mediate internalization into human epithelial cells (Lecuit et al., 2001).

Receptor-mediated endocytosis is particularly important in the developing animal for uptake of growth factors and antibodies from breast milk. Suckling rodents absorb immunoglobulin G (IgG) in maternal breast milk through Fc receptors located on enterocytes (Rodewald, 1970); a similar receptor has been isolated from fetal human intestine but similar function remains to be demonstrated (Israel et al., 1993). Nerve growth factor and epidermal growth factor (EGF) can also cross the developing epithelium, and specific receptors for EGF have been identified on enterocytes (Sanderson and Walker, 1993; Siminoski et al., 1986; Thompson, 1988). Therefore intestinal uptake of trophic factors and antibodies by the suckling rodent and possibly the human infant may promote intestinal growth and differentiation.

NONSELECTIVE ENDOCYTOSIS

In a second mechanism of macromolecular transport, extracellular macromolecules are nonselectively trapped and internalized through invaginations of noncoated regions of cells (Fig. 34-4*B*). Such a mechanism has been postulated for preferential uptake of macromole-

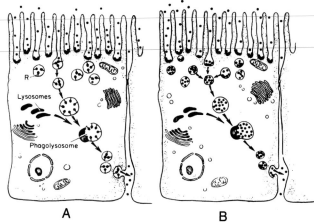

A   B

Figure 34-4 · Mechanisms of macromolecular absorption in the neonatal mammalian intestine. *A*, Selective transport of antigens occurs in the small intestine of the newborn via a specific receptor site (R) present on the microvillus membrane. Antigens thus transported may be protected from intracellular lysosomal digestion because of attachment to the receptor site and would thus be transported in increased quantities out of the cell. *B*, A nonselective uptake and transport of other macromolecules occurs throughout the small intestine of most neonatal animals. Immature intestinal absorptive cells engulf large quantities of macromolecules. After intracellular digestion in phagolysosomes, very small quantities are deposited in the intercellular space. (From Walker WA, Isselbacher KJ. Uptake and transport of macromolecules by the intestine: possible role in clinical disorders. Gastroenterology 67:531–550, 1974.)

cules by microfold cells (M cells). These cells preferentially take up proteins, viruses, and bacteria in the dome epithelium above Peyer's patches (Table 34-3); many pathogens preferentially adhere to M cells through specific receptors for pathogens on the apical surface of M cells (Neutra et al., 1996; Wolf and Bye, 1984). An interaction between a lectin or other adhesion molecule on the surface of the M cell and a corresponding ligand on the viral or bacterial surface may in fact account for this "nonselective endocytosis" (Amerongen et al., 1992). In addition, intraluminal secretory IgA seems to

TABLE 34-3 · MICROORGANISMS AND NONLIVING PARTICLES ADHERENT TO M-CELL APICAL MEMBRANES

Bacteria	Protozoa
Vibrio cholerae	*Cryptosporidium*
Salmonella typhi	
Yersinia enterocolitica	
BCG	Nonliving particles
Campylobacter jejuni	Carbon particles
Shigella flexneri	Latex beads
RDEC-1 strain of *Escherichia coli*	Copolymer microspheres
Viruses	Hydroxyapatite
Reovirus	
Poliovirus	
HIV-1	

BCG = bacille Calmette-Guérin; HIV-1 = human immunodeficiency virus type 1.
From Amerongen MH, Weltzin RW, Mack JA, Winner LS, Michetti P, Apte FM, Kraehenbuhl JP, Neutra MR. M cell–mediated antigen transport and monoclonal IgA antibodies for mucosal immune protection. Ann NY Acad Sci 664:18–26, 1992.

TABLE 34-2 · MACROMOLECULAR TRANSPORT MECHANISMS

1. Receptor-mediated endocytosis
2. Nonselective endocytosis
3. Direct penetration of cell membrane
4. Passage across tight junctions

preferentially adhere to M cells, even though M cells lack Fc receptors (Neutra et al., 1999; Weltzin et al., 1989).

DIRECT PENETRATION

A third means of entry is direct penetration through the epithelial cell membrane. This mechanism may be important for certain bacterial and plant toxins, but its physiologic significance is poorly understood (Goldstein et al., 1979).

PASSAGE ACROSS TIGHT JUNCTIONS (PARACELLULAR PATHWAY)

In the healthy human, only low-molecular-weight molecules can pass across the tight junction between enterocytes. However, passage of larger macromolecules across the gut has been observed in those with intestinal inflammation (including patients with celiac disease, inflammatory bowel disease (IBD), and infectious enteritis), suggesting that inflammation may "loosen" the tight junctions (Hollander, 1992; Turck et al., 1987). Investigators have proposed that relatives of patients with IBD may be predisposed to the development of intestinal inflammation because they have increased intestinal permeability to antigens via the paracellular pathway (May et al., 1993).

Antigen Processing and Immunoglobulin Synthesis

Antigens that have penetrated the intestinal epithelium may provoke an immune response (usually characterized by secretory IgA production) or a state of systemic unresponsiveness (tolerance) to antigen. For an antibody response to antigen to occur, naïve B cells within the Peyer's patch must differentiate, proliferate, and migrate into the lamina propria, where they become immunoglobulin-producing plasma cells (Fig. 34-5). Signals promoting B-cell activation and differentiation include antigen binding to surface immunoglobulins on the B-cell membrane and soluble cytokines (particularly interleukin [IL]-4 and IL-5) secreted by helper T cells (Fig. 34-6) (Abbas, 1988).

Helper (CD4) T cells do not recognize antigen directly but do recognize peptide fragments on the surface of APCs. CD4 cells recognize antigenic peptide in association with major histocompatibility complex (MHC) class II molecules via the T-cell receptor (see Fig. 34-6) (Grey et al., 1989). Macrophages, dendritic cells, and B cells all express surface MHC class II molecules and represent the "professional" APCs within the Peyer's patch. Enterocytes may also express MHC class II molecules on their cell surface when induced, particularly during intestinal inflammation, and can present antigen to T lymphocytes in vitro. Some investigators propose that this pathway of antigen presentation is important in the pathogenesis of mucosal inflammation, but its true significance has not been clarified (Bland and Kambarage, 1991).

The principal immunoglobulin produced by the mucosal immune system is secretory IgA; the plasma

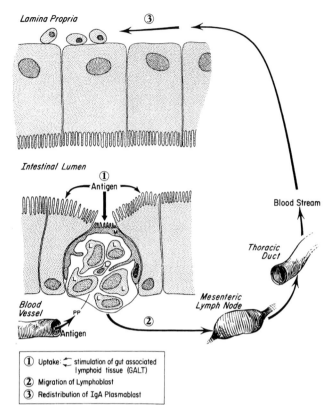

Figure 34-5 · Schematic representation of antigen response of lymphoid tissue located in gut-associated lymphoid tissue (GALT) and of homing of stimulated lymphoid cells to intestinal mucosa. *1*, Antigen is taken up by M cells and, to a lesser degree, by intestinal epithelial cells. This leads to stimulation of cells within the lymphoepithelial complex and within diffuse lymphoid tissue. *2*, After antigen stimulation, cells migrate to mesenteric lymph nodes, where they are "processed" and become lymphoblasts. These lymphoblasts migrate through thoracic duct to systemic circulation, where they "mature." *3*, Lymphocytes then "home" to diffuse lymphoid tissue of the gut, lung, breast, and female reproductive tract. (From Walker WA, Isselbacher KJ. Intestinal antibodies. N Engl J Med 297:767–773, 1977.)

cell ratio of IgA-, IgM-, and IgG-producing cells is 20:3:1, almost the reverse of that in the systemic immune system (Brandtzaeg and Baklien, 1977) (see Chapter 9). B cells stimulated in the Peyer's patches undergo isotype switching to IgA, resulting in the preponderance of mucosal IgA-producing plasma cells. The factors controlling isotype switching probably include cell–cell contact (particularly between CD40 on the B-cell surface and gp39, the CD40 ligand on the T-cell surface), antigenic stimulation itself, and secretion of regulatory "switch factor cytokines" (Fuleihan et al., 1993; Strober and Harriman, 1991).

Mucosally secreted IgA differs from systemic IgA in several aspects. First, whereas systemic IgA is almost exclusively monomeric IgA of the IgA1 subtype, secretory IgA is a dimer (Conley and Delacroix, 1987). Second, secretory IgA (SIgA) is synthesized from both IgA1 and IgA2; the IgA2 present in sIgA may be more resistant to degradation by bacterial proteases (Meyer et al., 1987). The IgA dimer is synthesized within the plasma cell by coupling the constant regions of two IgA molecules to a linking peptide termed J chain. The J

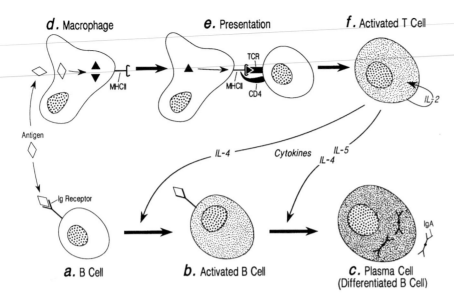

Figure 34-6 · Antigen processing in Peyer's patch. Antigen may bind directly to immunoglobulin on the surface of the B cell or may be endocytosed by an antigen-presenting cell (e.g., a macrophage) and presented to a helper T cell. The antigen presented to the macrophage is located within a cleft in the MHC class II molecule of the macrophage and is bound by the T-cell receptor of the CD4 T cell. The helper T cell then secretes cytokines that promote B-cell differentiation. (From Bousvaros A, Walker WA. Basic gastrointestinal immunity. In Bouchier IA, et al., eds. Gastroenterology: Clinical Science and Practice, ed 2. Philadelphia, WB Saunders, 1993, pp 577–582.)

chain–IgA dimer is secreted by lamina propria plasma cells and binds to the polymeric immunoglobulin receptor (also called *secretory component*, or SC) on the basolateral surface of the enterocyte. The IgA dimer–J chain–SC complex is internalized by the enterocyte and secreted into the intestinal lumen (Ahnen et al., 1985). The cytokines IL-4 and interferon-γ regulate SC expression by the enterocyte and hence may regulate luminal IgA secretion (Philips et al., 1990). Studies of animal models have shown that antigen-specific secretory IgA has potent antimicrobial activity against enteric bacteria and viruses, including *Vibrio cholerae, Salmonella typhimurium,* reovirus, and retroviruses (Kraehenbuhl and Neutra, 1992).

In addition to producing SIgA in the same region as the initial antigenic challenge (i.e., the gut), antigen-stimulated B lymphocytes travel through the mesenteric lymph nodes, thoracic duct, and systemic circulation to other mucosal sites (including bronchi, salivary glands, uterus, biliary tree, and mammary gland), as well as returning to the gut (see Fig. 34-5) (Husband and Gowans, 1977). These migratory B cells may therefore serve to transfer immunologic memory from one mucosal site to another, and antigen-specific IgA produced by these B cells can be complexed to secretory component at other epithelial sites and transported into other secretions.

Kleinman and Walker (1979) postulated an *entero-mammary immune system* in which B cells form IgA to pathogens in the mother's gut and migrate to the mammary gland, where antigen-specific IgA is secreted in breast milk and transferred to the infant (Fig. 34-7).

The Liver: A Second Line of Defense

If an antigen penetrates the gut epithelium and enters the portal circulation, it must pass through the hepatic sinusoids before entering the systemic circulation. The liver Kupffer cells, members of the tissue macrophage family, can phagocytose bacteria, antigens, immune complexes, and tumor cells that have bypassed the intestinal host defenses and entered the portal circulation. Although Kupffer cells do not usually possess specific receptors for bacterial glycoproteins, Kupffer cells can bind fibronectin, the C3b component of complement, and the Fc components of IgG and IgA. These molecules in turn can opsonize bacteria (including Enterobacteriaceae and Streptococci) or bind to food antigens in the intestinal lumen, mucosa, or portal circulation. Therefore antigen–antibody complexes and opsonin-coated bacteria generated in the intestine may be bound through specific Kupffer cell receptors and digested by Kupffer cell lysosomes (Toth and Thomas, 1992). Rodent bile contains high concentrations of sIgA, but biliary IgA is of little functional importance in the human (Kleinman, 1987).

Oral Tolerance

Whereas orally ingested food antigens can generate a mucosal immune response (e.g., SIgA production), a more common systemic response to oral antigen is one of immunologic hyporesponsiveness, or tolerance (see Chapter 8). Oral tolerance is a state of immunologic hyporesponsiveness to a fed antigen to which previous immunologic exposure has occurred. An animal exposed to a tolerance-inducing antigen (tolerogen) will not respond to a more immunogenic form of the antigen given systemically.

The induction of tolerance and the mechanism by which it occurs depends on several factors, including the dose and route of administration of specific antigens (reviewed by Spiekermann and Walker, 2001). Clonal deletion of T lymphocytes may occur centrally during thymic maturation, or antigen-specific deletions of T cells can occur peripherally, usually in response to high-

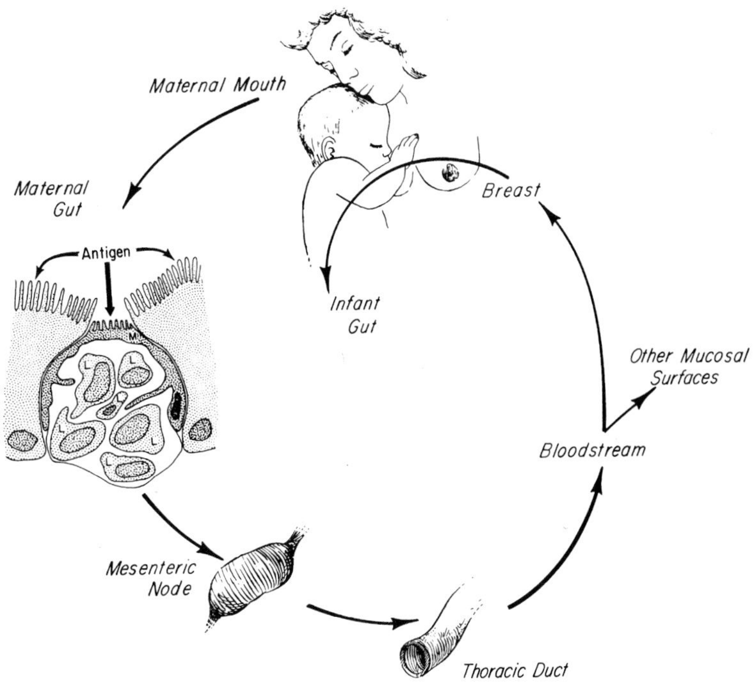

Figure 34-7 · Dietary antigen entering the maternal gut reaches lymphoid follicles through specialized transport cells (M cells). This antigen commits the lymphoblasts to production of specific IgAs, and these then migrate via the mesenteric nodes and thoracic duct into the systemic circulation. During the periods of proper hormonal stimulation, such cells populate the breast and secrete secretory immunoglobulin A (SIgA), which then is ingested by and functions in the infant. T cells, B cells, and macrophages are also extruded into the breast milk and are immunologically active. (From Kleinman RE, Walker WA. The enteromammary immune system: an important new concept in breast milk host defense. Dig Dis Sci 24:876–882, 1979.)

dose antigen, and is mediated by apoptosis mainly through Fas-ligand pathways. High-dose antigen administration may also lead to clonal anergy, in which T cells are unable to secrete IL-2 or proliferate when re-exposed to antigen. This occurs when the T-cell receptor engages the antigen–MHC complex in the absence of a second, or co-stimulatory signal (e.g., B7-CD28 interaction). The T-cell hyporesponsiveness may be overcome by the exogenous administration of IL-2. Clonal anergy usually occurs in helper T cells but may also occur in B cells. The end result is an absence of immunoglobulin-producing cells directed against that specific antigen (Melamed and Friedman, 1993; Mowat, 1987b).

Probably the most important mechanism of oral tolerance is active suppression mediated through suppressive cytokines, especially transforming growth factor-β (TGF-β), secreted mainly by CD4+ cells. Active suppression is favored by the administration of low-dose antigen. Because the immune response is suppressed via secreted cytokines, the suppressive effect may be antigen nonspecific and affect cells within the microenvironment; it has thus been termed *bystander suppression*. The generation of suppressor T cells mediating oral tolerance can be abrogated by the administration of immunosuppressive agents such as cyclophosphamide (Hoyne et al., 1993).

Studies of oral tolerance are largely confined to animal models, but the induction of systemic tolerance by oral feeding of antigen offers promise in the therapy of human autoimmune disease. In mice, orally administered ovalbumin can generate tolerance to intravenous ovalbumin given as early as 1 hour after the oral immunization; this tolerance is in part dependent on the MHC haplotype of the mouse and can be transferred

among syngeneic mice by injecting serum from the orally immunized mouse into an unimmunized mouse (Mowat et al., 1987).

A hypothesis based on these data is that intestinal antigen-processing cells (e.g., macrophages) modify an immunogenic protein (e.g., ovalbumin) into a "tolerogenic" protein that preferentially activates T-suppressor cells in the systemic immune system (Peng et al., 1990). Work by Weiner's group suggests that orally fed myelin basic protein can prevent the development of experimental allergic encephalomyelitis in rats and that tolerance is mediated through the production of immunosuppressive cytokines, including TGF-β (Khoury et al., 1992). After encouraging results of a pilot study of patients with multiple sclerosis, a phase III clinical trial showed no difference in the number of relapses between patients given placebo or myelin (Weiner et al., 1999). Treatments using oral tolerance may therefore be of future therapeutic benefit in human diseases such as multiple sclerosis, rheumatoid arthritis, uveitis, and insulin-dependent diabetes mellitus; clinical trials are currently in progress.

Nutrition and Immunity

Enteral nutrition is important in the development of the neonatal mucosal immune system and is essential in the maintenance of systemic and mucosal immunity in adults. Malnourished children and adults have impaired cell-mediated immunity and increased susceptibility to infections (Keusch, 1986; Wan et al., 1989; see Chapter 23). Properties of enteral nutrition that influence immunity are summarized in Table 34-4. These include stimulation of the mucosal immune system through antigen, provision of trophic factors important in mucosal

TABLE 34-4 · NUTRITIONAL FACTORS INFLUENCING IMMUNITY

1. Protein antigenic stimulation of mucosal B cells
2. Trophic factors
   Nucleotides
   Glutamine
   Epidermal growth factor
   Nerve growth factor
3. Passive immunity from breast milk
   Lactoferrin
   Lysozyme
   Secretory immunoglobulins (principally secretory
     immunoglobulin A)
   Lipases
   Glycoproteins
   Leukocytes
4. Micronutrients
   Zinc
   Copper
   Iron
   Selenium
   Vitamins

From Sanderson IR, Walker WA. Nutrition and immunity. Curr Opin Gastroenterol 7:463–470, 1991; and Slade HB, Schwartz SA. Mucosal immunity: the immunology of breast milk. J Allergy Clin Immunol 80:346–356, 1987.

integrity, transfer of passive immunity through breast milk, and provision of micronutrients important in lymphocyte function (Ferguson, 1994; Sanderson and Walker, 1991).

In rodents and humans, feeding may stimulate the maturation of the sIgA system. Although T and B lymphocytes are present in the human fetal intestinal mucosa as early as 16 to 18 weeks' gestation, the intestinal mucosa of the term neonate contains no IgA-producing plasma cells before 10 days of age (Perkkio and Savilahti, 1980). Both cow's milk protein and protein hydrolysate feeding stimulate IgA plasma cell growth in neonatal mice, but the intact protein stimulates plasma cell development to a greater extent (Sagie et al., 1974). Knox (1986) noted that 2-week-old human infants given enteral feedings had IgA and IgM plasma cells in the intestinal lamina propria, whereas infants not yet fed had a paucity of these cells. Thus dietary antigenic stimulation may be important in promoting mucosal immune maturation.

Trophic factors present in breast milk include epidermal growth factor and nerve growth factor; as stated previously, the neonatal rodent intestine contains specific receptors to transport these substances to the systemic circulation. Other critical trophic substances include dietary nucleotides and the amino acid glutamine (Grimble, 1994). Nunez and colleagues (1990) demonstrated the partial efficacy of nucleotides in promoting epithelial repair in the damaged gut of rodents. Glutamine and nucleotides given to animals receiving total parenteral nutrition increase intestinal villous height, although they do not decrease gut permeability to bacteria (Deitch, 1994; Ogoshi et al., 1985).

Breast milk contains nutrients, growth factors, proteins with antimicrobial properties (including lactoferrin and lysozyme), immunoglobulins (predominantly IgA in the human and IgG in the rodent), and intact leukocytes (including neutrophils, macrophages, and lymphocytes) (Slade and Schwartz, 1987; see Chapter 9). Trophic factors present in breast milk stimulate the maturation of intestinal epithelial function (Heird and Hansen, 1977; Widdowson et al., 1976) and may decrease intestinal permeability to macromolecules (Weaver et al., 1987).

Studies of women immunized with poliovirus support the hypothesis of an enteromammary immune system by demonstrating that virus-specific IgA can be transferred into breast milk (Svennerholm et al., 1981). Prentice and co-workers (1989) measured fecal IgA and lactoferrin in breastfed and bottle-fed Gambian children and found 10-fold higher levels in the stools of breastfed children; they estimated that one third of ingested immunoglobulin escapes digestion. Therefore ingested IgA from breast milk potentially confers intraluminal antimicrobial activity to the entire small bowel and colon.

Specific micronutrients present in enteral nutrition may also promote mucosal immunity. Various studies suggest beneficial effects on immune function from the addition of vitamin A, vitamin E, copper, selenium, iron, and zinc to the diet (Meydani, 1990; Sanderson and Walker, 1991). Infants with primary acrodermatitis enteropathica (AE), an autosomal recessive defect in intestinal zinc absorption, have an increased susceptibility to infection that is correctable with zinc supplementation.

Summary

The control of macromolecular uptake depends on a number of factors within the gut lumen, the mucosal surface, and the intestinal lamina propria. The neonate's intestine may allow increased macromolecular uptake because of decreased gastric acid production, pancreatic function, or epithelial barrier integrity. Nutrition, particularly with mammalian breast milk, confers both antigenic stimulation of the intestine and passive immunity. Immunologic tolerance is essential in the prevention of systemic or mucosal immune responses to dietary antigens, but the cellular and molecular mechanisms resulting in tolerance are just beginning to be unraveled. Disturbances in the permeability of the immature, malnourished, or damaged gut may cause intestinal or systemic disease states as described in the following sections.

ALLERGIC AND INFLAMMATORY CONDITIONS OF THE BOWEL

Necrotizing Enterocolitis

Necrotizing enterocolitis (NEC) is an acute fulminating disease of neonates associated with focal or diffuse ulceration of the distal small intestine and colon, often leading to bowel necrosis or perforation (Santulli et al., 1975). The most common acquired gastrointestinal emergency in the newborn, NEC appears to be a common pathologic response of the immature intestine to many injurious factors. It is primarily a disease of premature infants, occurring in approximately 10% of neonates weighing less than 1500 g. However, 5% to 10% of cases occur in term infants or infants who have not been fed (MacKendrick and Caplan, 1993).

Pathogenesis

The pathophysiology of NEC remains a mystery. Other than their prematurity, no specific risk factors have been identified in infants with low birth weight. A number of factors (including hypoxia/ischemia, hyperosmolar feedings, and intraluminal bacteria) may damage the comparatively immature intestinal barrier, particularly of the premature infant. These multiple insults result in epithelial disruption and permeability to potentially pathogenic bacteria, resulting in a vicious circle leading to gut necrosis (Fig. 34-8).

Prematurity and enteral feedings are the two risk factors most strongly associated with NEC; delay of enteral feedings in the premature infant may delay the onset of NEC, but it will also delay the time of presentation of the disease. Prenatal maternal cocaine use has been identified as a risk factor in term infants, which suggests that the vasoconstrictive properties of cocaine predispose the infant to bowel ischemia (Downing et al., 1991).

Studies of fetal gut blood flow and intestinal maturation in animals provide useful insights into the pathogenesis and potential prevention of NEC. To determine whether episodic mesenteric ischemia of the developing neonatal intestine makes the bowel more permeable to potentially toxic macromolecules, Crissinger and Granger (1989) studied the effects of ischemia and reperfusion of the bowel in developing piglets. Piglets 1 to 30 days of age had similar gut permeability to chromium-51-labeled edetic acid (EDTA) (a small molecule) after their bowels had been subjected to 1 hour of iatrogenic ischemia. However, feeding of cow's milk–based formula to piglets whose intestines were subjected to ischemia and reperfusion for 1 hour caused significantly greater injury in 1-day-old animals than in older animals. These investigators later demonstrated that the lipid fraction of enteral feed in 1-day-old piglets was responsible for the increased permeability of intestinal mucosa after ischemia and reperfusion (Crissinger and Tso, 1992). Thus ischemia combined with feeding potentiates intestinal damage by macromolecules in infant pigs, and triglycerides may potentiate the ischemic damage to the neonatal gut.

Microbial agents are responsible for some of the intestinal damage in NEC. Epidemics of the disease are often reported, although there is no seasonal predilection. The intestinal pneumatosis of NEC is probably due to bacterial fermentation of carbohydrates. Bacterial or viral agents may be isolated from blood or stool of affected infants (Kliegman et al., 1993). Agents commonly reported or isolated from stool or blood include *Klebsiella, Escherichia coli,* rotavirus, *Staphylococcus epidermidis,* and *Clostridium* species (Kliegman and Fanaroff, 1984; Palmer et al., 1989). However, in most cases, no specific infectious pathogen is isolated. Furthermore, it is not clear whether the isolated organisms are the primary cause of bowel damage (perhaps through endotoxin production) or whether they are secondary invaders of a damaged gut.

The role of immature host defenses in the pathogenesis of NEC requires further study. Several pathogens or toxins require contact with a receptor on the mucosal surface to cause damage; for example, rotavirus may bind to intestinal mucins, and cholera toxin binds

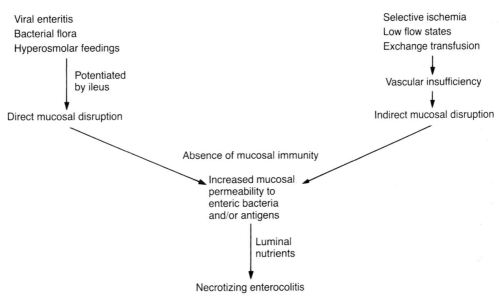

Figure 34-8· **Proposed pathway for the interaction of multiple factors predisposing to the development of necrotizing enterocolitis.** (From Lake AM, Walker WA. Neonatal necrotizing enterocolitis: a disease of altered host defense. Clin Gastroenterol 6:463, 1977.)

to a GM_1 ganglioside on the enterocyte membrane. Diminished degradation or neutralization of these proteins may result in increased binding and intestinal inflammation (Chu and Walker, 1993; Kliegman et al., 1993). The human premature infant has less gastric acid output, less pancreatic enzyme activity, a more permeable gut, and less SIgA than the older infant. Such factors may predispose the neonatal gut to colonization and systemic invasion by viruses or bacteria, with resultant inflammation and sepsis.

Pretreatment of rodent fetuses with either thyroxine or corticosteroids promotes maturation of the gut epithelium, decreases gut permeability, and lessens the occurrence of NEC (Israel et al., 1987, 1990; Pang et al., 1985). Therapeutic attempts to speed gut maturation or to supply exogenous antibody to infants with NEC have met with some success (see later discussion), suggesting that the barrier function of the gut can be augmented pharmacologically.

Inflammatory cytokines may mediate intestinal mucosal damage in NEC. Hsueh and co-workers (1986, 1987) demonstrated that intravenous administration of platelet-activating factor (PAF) in a rat model may cause pathologic changes similar to those seen in NEC. The intestinal damage caused by endotoxin may be blocked by PAF antagonists (Hsueh et al., 1986, 1987). In addition, humans with the disease have significantly higher serum levels of PAF and tumor necrosis factor-α (TNF-α) (Kliegman et al., 1993). Although other cytokines are likely to be important in the pathogenesis of NEC, the role of PAF and TNF-α in promoting the disease warrants further investigation.

In summary, although the exact pathogenesis of NEC is unknown, a combination of bowel immaturity, mesenteric vascular insufficiency, microbial colonization, and early feeding contribute to its development.

Clinical Manifestations

Signs and symptoms of NEC are summarized in Table 34-5. The infant with a mild case has mild abdominal distention, vomiting, or hematochezia; the sick infant with NEC has signs consistent with an acute abdomen, bowel perforation, or sepsis. The clinical staging system of Bell and co-workers (1978), which is still widely used today, utilizes a combination of intestinal and systemic signs plus plain abdominal radiography to grade severity. NEC must be suspected whenever a premature infant exhibits signs of feeding intolerance, regurgitation, apnea, irritability, temperature instability, or hematochezia.

Diagnosis

The diagnosis is then confirmed by a combination of laboratory and radiographic features. A low hematocrit level, elevated white blood cell count, low platelet count, or elevated prothrombin or partial thromboplastin time may be present. The abdominal radiograph may demonstrate pneumatosis intestinalis, gas in the portal venous system, or frank pneumoperitoneum (Fig. 34-9). The pathologic correlate of these radiographic findings is bowel ischemia with intraluminal gas production by microbes or bowel necrosis with perforation. NEC typically involves the distal ileum and ascending colon, although the entire bowel may be involved (Caplan and MacKendrick, 1993; Kliegman, 1993).

Treatment

The primary treatment for NEC is medical and nutritional support; surgical resection of the bowel is

TABLE 34-5 · SIGNS AND SYMPTOMS OF NECROTIZING ENTEROCOLITIS

Mild to Moderate	Severe
Abdominal distention	Peritonitis
Elevated pregavage residuals	Ileus
Vomiting	Acidosis and hyperkalemia
Occult blood in stool	Hematochezia
Temperature instability	Neutropenia and
Coagulopathy	thrombocytopenia
Apnea/bradycardia	Portal venous gas
Abdominal tenderness	Pneumoperitoneum
Dilated bowel on radiography	
Pneumatosis intestinalis	

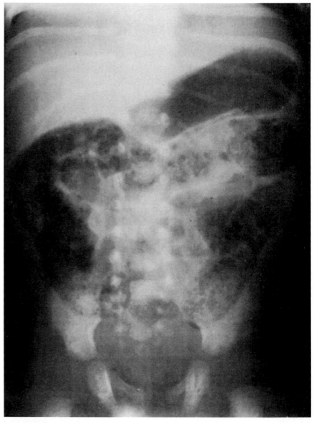

Figure 34-9 · Anteroposterior view of the abdomen of a neonate with abdominal distention and vomiting. The radiograph demonstrates areas of intraluminal air (pneumatosis intestinalis), which confirms necrotizing enterocolitis. (Courtesy of C. C. Roy, M.D., Montreal, Canada.)

reserved for critically ill infants (Table 34-6). Bowel rest up to 3 weeks is recommended for infants with radiographically demonstrated NEC and generally necessitates central venous hyperalimentation. Intravenous antibiotics do not cure the bowel disease but may prevent or treat bacteremia and sepsis. Loss of fluid into the bowel may cause oliguria, hyponatremia, and hypoalbuminemia, and bowel necrosis may cause acidosis and hyperkalemia. To correct these complications, intravenous fluids, albumin, blood, and clotting factors may be required. Infants with clinical or radiographic evidence suggestive of necrotic bowel require laparotomy and bowel resection (Kliegman, 1993).

Prevention

Despite these therapeutic measures, NEC is associated with high morbidity and mortality. Thus efforts to prevent NEC by augmenting intestinal host defenses have been undertaken. Eibl and colleagues (1988) gave premature infants (between 800 and 2000 g) either infant formula alone or formula plus 600 mg of an oral human IgG–IgA preparation. Six cases of NEC occurred in the 91 control infants during refeeding; no cases occurred in the infants receiving oral immunoglobulin. Serum immunoglobulin levels did not differ significantly between the groups, suggesting that the effect of the oral preparation was intraluminal. A similar study showed that oral monomeric IgG can decrease the incidence of the disease in premature infants (Rubaltelli et al., 1991). Enterally administered immunoglobulin could potentially prevent NEC by binding to antigens or microbes intraluminally; such an effect may not occur with donor breast milk because pasteurization may denature antibody.

Another approach to prevention is to accelerate maturation of the infant mucosal barrier by prenatal or postnatal administration of exogenous hormones. Israel and co-workers (1987, 1990) have demonstrated that when either thyroxine or cortisone is injected into pregnant rats, the offspring are less susceptible to ischemic bowel injury and have structurally more mature intestinal mucosal barriers. Oral corticosteroids fed to newborn rats may have a similar effect (Teichberg et al., 1992). A randomized trial of cortisone administration versus placebo administration to 466 premature infants showed that the premature infants receiving cortisone either prenatally or postnatally were less likely to develop NEC (Halac et al., 1990).

Food Allergy

Food allergy is an adverse reaction to a food caused by an immunologic reaction to some component of the food (see Chapter 31). Improved diagnostic techniques enable the clinician to distinguish between true food allergy and reaction to food additives, food intolerance, or an erroneous history. The double-blind, placebo-controlled food challenge is now the gold standard by which the sensitivity and specificity of other diagnostic tests (including skin prick or radioallergosorbent testing) can be measured.

Pathophysiology

At least two types of food allergy are recognized. The first, immediate hypersensitivity, is characterized by clinical symptoms of asthma, urticaria, or anaphylaxis. This is a Gell and Coombs type I hypersensitivity reaction mediated by IgE released when mast cells are degranulated. Although the exact mediators causing food anaphylaxis are unknown, Sampson and co-workers (1989) have identified a histamine-releasing factor that interacts with IgE on the mast cell surface to cause degranulation and release of histamine and prostaglandins.

A second type of food allergy is suggestive of a delayed-type hypersensitivity reaction (Gell and Coombs type IV), inasmuch as children develop symptoms 12 to 72 hours after ingesting the offending food. The symptoms differ from those in type I reactions and include vomiting, colitis, abdominal pain, and atopic dermatitis. This form of food allergy may involve antigen presentation to helper T lymphocytes in the intestinal mucosa, with failure of normal immunoregulatory mechanisms to produce systemic tolerance.

Van Sickle and co-workers (1985) demonstrated increased proliferation in response to milk and soy proteins by peripheral blood T lymphocytes from infants with allergic colitis compared with control infants, suggesting in vivo sensitization to these antigens. In other studies, Kondo and colleagues (1993) and Agata and associates (1992) found that lymphocytes of children with atopic dermatitis and egg hypersensitivity cultured with ovalbumin or egg antigens released interferon-γ and IL-2 in culture supernatants. Thus atopic patients have lymphocytes primed to respond to certain food antigens.

Impaired barrier function of the gut may predispose to food hypersensitivity. Children are at highest risk for developing food allergies in the first year of life, when the mucosal barrier may be more permeable to food

<hr>

TABLE 34-6 · MANAGEMENT OF NECROTIZING ENTEROCOLITIS

Supportive Measures
Nothing by mouth
Parenteral nutrition
Antibiotics
Ventilatory support
Bicarbonate
Fresh frozen plasma
Surgery (if necessary)

Preventive Measures
Oral immunoglobulins A and G
Prenatal/postnatal corticosteroids
Thyroxine (in animal models)
Platelet activating factor antagonist (in animal models)

<hr>

Data from Caplan MS, MacKendrick WM. Necrotizing enterocolitis: a review of pathogenetic mechanisms and implications for prevention. Pediatr Pathol 13:357–369, 1993; Kliegman RM. Neonatal necrotizing enterocolitis. In Wyllie R. Hyams JS, eds. Gastrointestinal Disease: Pathophysiology, Diagnosis, Management. Philadelphia, WB Saunders, 1993, pp 788–798.

antigens. Delaying introduction of highly allergenic and prolonged breastfeeding may reduce the incidence of food allergy in children with a strong family history of atopy. Viral or bacterial infections may damage gut epithelium and increase intestinal macromolecular absorption and can result in postinfectious allergic enteropathy to cow's milk or soy proteins (Harrison et al., 1976; Schrieber and Walker, 1988).

Clinical Manifestations

The incidence of true food allergy in the pediatric population has been estimated to be 2% to 4%. In contrast, histories of childhood "allergies" are reported by the parents of as many as 28% of children. For this reason, the American Academy of Allergy and Immunology and the National Institutes of Health suggest the following nomenclature (Sampson, 1994). *Adverse food reaction* includes any untoward event that follows ingestion of a food and includes *food intolerance* and *food allergy*. Food intolerance can include food poisoning (secondary to bacterial toxins), pharmacologic effects (e.g., reflux or dysrhythmias secondary to caffeine), enzymatic deficiencies (including galactosemia or hypolactasia), or unknown reactions. Food allergies, in contrast, are thought to be true systemic or mucosal immune responses to ingested food antigens and include type I or type IV hypersensitivity reactions. Foods best known to cause these reactions include milk, soy, peanut, egg, and fish (Sampson, 1994). Celiac disease (gluten-sensitive enteropathy) may also be a type IV hypersensitivity reaction (to wheat proteins); it is considered in a separate section.

Clinical manifestations of food hypersensitivity (Table 34-7) include cutaneous (eczema, urticaria), respiratory (rhinitis, asthma), and gastrointestinal reactions (allergic colitis, vomiting, and possibly abdominal pain). Hill and co-workers (1986) have identified three types of milk hypersensitivity: patients in group 1 develop cutaneous reactions within 45 minutes of challenge, those in group 2 develop gastrointestinal symptoms between 45 minutes and 20 hours after challenge, and those in group 3 develop both gastrointestinal and respiratory symptoms more than 24 hours after challenge. This chapter focuses on gastrointestinal manifestations of food allergy; food allergy is also discussed in Chapter 31.

MILK- AND SOY-SENSITIVE ENTEROPATHY

Up to 50% of children with milk allergy develop gastrointestinal symptoms, particularly vomiting or diarrhea. Two common subtypes of this enteropathy,

TABLE 34-7 · CLINICAL MANIFESTATIONS OF FOOD ALLERGY

Asthma	Rhinorrhea
Vomiting	Conjunctivitis
Diarrhea/malabsorption	Urticaria/angioedema
Lactose intolerance	Atopic dermatitis
Abdominal pain	Colic/irritability
Infant colic (questionable)	Migraine headaches
Hematochezia/allergic colitis	Laryngeal edema/anaphylaxis

allergic colitis and postinfectious protein intolerance, are described in the following. Some infants with milk or soy intolerance develop a severe enteropathy in the neonatal period that can be confused with that of infants having either NEC or pyloric stenosis (Schwarzenberg and Whitington, 1983; Snyder et al., 1987). Barium radiography may demonstrate antral narrowing or mucosal thickening of the duodenum and jejunum, and biopsy of an affected area shows a small-bowel eosinophilic infiltrate (Fig. 34-10).

Other infants present in the first months of life with vomiting or chronic diarrhea but without other atopic features; in these patients, celiac disease, giardiasis, cystic fibrosis, or other malabsorptive disorders must be excluded. Biopsies of small intestine in this group may demonstrate partial villous atrophy in a focal or patchy distribution, with or without an eosinophilic infiltrate. In more severe cases, a flat intestinal mucosa resembling that in celiac disease can be seen (Stern, 1991). Similar lesions have been identified with hypersensitivity to soy protein; indeed, 10% to 30% of infants with milk hypersensitivity also react to soy (Ament and Rubin, 1972; Halpin et al., 1977).

ALLERGIC PROCTOCOLITIS OF INFANCY

Infants younger than 1 year of age may present with bloody diarrhea as the only manifestation of protein allergy. This condition occurs most commonly in infants fed cow's milk formula, although colitis can also occur in infants fed soy formula or breast milk (Perisic et al.,

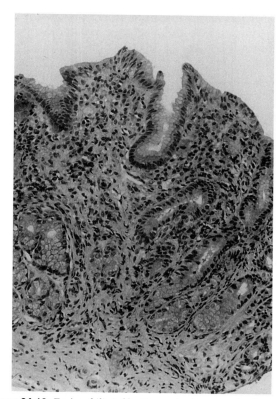

Figure 34-10 · Eosinophilic infiltrate seen in the stomach of a 1-year-old with eosinophilic gastroenteritis. (Courtesy of Dr. Asma Nusrat, Department of Pathology, Children's Hospital, Boston.)

1988; Powell, 1978). Allergic colitis occurs frequently in infants younger than 3 months of age; presentation before 3 days or after 6 months of age is unusual. The patient is typically a term infant who appears healthy, is afebrile, and appears normal on physical examination; there is often a family history of allergy.

The condition must be differentiated from more serious causes of rectal bleeding in the infant, including NEC, infectious colitis, and Hirschsprung's enterocolitis. Flexible sigmoidoscopy with a mucosal biopsy in the symptomatic infant can establish the diagnosis. Endoscopy identifies an erythematous and friable mucosa, and histologic examination of the affected tissue demonstrates a mucosal eosinophilic infiltrate (more than six eosinophils per high-power field) (Odze et al., 1993; Winter et al., 1990). Despite the mucosal eosinophilic infiltrate, eosinophils and neutrophils are rarely seen in the stool.

The infant typically responds promptly to feeding with a casein hydrolysate formula; breastfed infants may respond to a maternal diet in which milk products are strictly avoided (Lake et al., 1982). Often mothers of breastfed infants also have their diets restricted of soy protein, eggs, peanuts and fish.

POSTINFECTIOUS COW'S MILK PROTEIN AND SOY PROTEIN INTOLERANCE

After a viral or bacterial enteric illness, an infant or toddler is at increased risk of developing an enteropathy because of immune hypersensitivity to proteins in milk or soy. In 1976, Harrison and co-workers described 25 children with chronic protracted diarrhea after acute gastroenteritis; all but four were younger than 1 year of age. Small-bowel biopsy demonstrated partial villous atrophy and an inflammatory cell infiltrate. Lactose intolerance was also present but resolved promptly after the illness. These patients improved when fed a protein hydrolysate but redeveloped diarrhea, colitis, urticaria, or wheezing when rechallenged with cow's milk formula (Harrison et al., 1976). Similar illness may occur in infants fed soy formula after enteritis (Iyngkaran et al., 1988).

Excess antigen absorption of ovalbumin has been observed in infants with acute gastroenteritis; Walker-Smith (1986) hypothesized that excess antigen overwhelms the tolerance mechanisms of the gut, leading to systemic and mucosal sensitization and food-sensitive enteropathy. This phenomenon may be less common than previously believed. Hager and colleagues (1987) found enteropathy in only 2 of 24 children younger than 3 months of age who were fed cow's milk formula after a viral infection.

EOSINOPHILIC GASTROENTEROPATHY

Eosinophilic gastroenteropathy is characterized by an eosinophilic infiltrate in one or more parts of the gut, most commonly the gastric antrum, duodenum, or small bowel.

Three forms have been described: *mucosal or submucosal involvement* is characterized by abdominal pain, diarrhea, and protein-losing enteropathy; *muscular involvement* is characterized by bowel thickening or obstruction; and *serosal involvement* is characterized by hypoalbuminemia and abdominal ascitic fluid containing eosinophils.

Clinical features overlap those of milk-sensitive enteropathy, and the two are often confused. Katz and co-workers (1984) have suggested the following characteristics for differentiating between the two entities. Patients with eosinophilic gastroenteropathy are usually older, with a mean age of 4 years. Furthermore, they often have signs of systemic allergy, including rhinitis or urticaria, but a history of food-specific allergy is rarely present. Peripheral blood eosinophilia is seen in 20% to 70% of cases. These patients rarely respond to an elimination diet but respond well to oral corticosteroids, which can then be gradually tapered over time. Case reports suggest that oral disodium cromoglycate may be used to treat this condition (DiGioacchino et al., 1990).

Eosinophilic Esophagitis

Eosinophilic esophagitis is a descriptive histologic diagnosis that may result from mucosal injury as a result of gastric acid reflux or represent an allergic response.

The symptoms of allergic esophagitis and gastroesophageal reflux (GER) can include vomiting, dysphagia, and heartburn. Potential distinguishing features that suggest an allergic etiology of the esophagitis include a history of food allergy associated with asthma or chronic respiratory disease and a family history of atopy (Orenstein et al., 2000; Walsh et al., 1999). Furthermore, there is an incomplete response to therapy for GER and a normal pH probe study indicating the absence of significant gastroesophageal reflux. There may be histologic distinctions as well, including a large number of squamous mucosal eosinophils, preferential localization of eosinophils in the superficial epithelium, and eosinophilic aggregates (which may suggest an allergic esophagitis [Walsh et al., 1999]). The eosinophilic infiltrate of the esophagus is likely mediated by the chemoattractants eotaxin and IL-5 (Furuta, 1998; Furuta and Sherman, 2000).

Because an allergic cause has been suspected, therapeutic responses have been reported with use of elemental diets, systemic corticosteroids, and aerosolized topical steroids (Faubion Jr et al., 1998; Kelly et al., 1995; Liacouras et al., 1998). Recently, aeroallergens have been shown to be an etiology of eosinophilic esophagitis in a murine animal model (Mishra et al., 2001). A respiratory allergen challenge led to epithelial hyperplasia and esophageal eosinophilia, but there was no response to oral allergen challenge and eosinophilic accumulation was ablated in the absence of IL-5 and attenuated without eotaxin (Mishra et al., 2001). It is clear that the presence of eosinophils in the esophageal mucosa is not always the result of GER, and alternative therapies must be considered.

Diagnosis

A combination of history, physical examination, response to elimination diet, and laboratory tests is required to diagnose and treat food allergy. In some cases in which the symptoms are highly suggestive of allergy and the offending agent is easily identified (e.g., in an infant receiving cow's milk formula who has allergic colitis), an empirical dietary elimination or formula change is reasonable. In most cases, however, the diagnosis is not simple and the precipitating agent not obvious. Many diagnostic tests are available to identify the causative food antigens (Table 34-8) (Burks and Sampson, 1992; Van Arsdel and Larson, 1989). Goldman's regimen of eliminating a food and rechallenging with the same food three times is rarely used today because of its difficulty and the risk of exposing an atopic child repeatedly to the same antigen (Goldman et al., 1963).

Skin prick tests and radioallergosorbent testing (RAST) are commonly used in the outpatient setting. Skin tests have an excellent negative predictive value for IgE-mediated food hypersensitivity; that is, if the skin test result is negative, it is highly unlikely (>95%) that the subject will react to that food antigen (Bock et al., 1978; Burks and Sampson, 1992; Sampson and Albergo, 1984). However, positive prick test results correlate poorly with the presence of clinical food allergy. RAST may be performed by nonallergists in the outpatient setting; however, they are somewhat less sensitive and specific than skin tests (Ortolani et al., 1989; Sampson and Albergo, 1984; Wraith et al., 1979). In a study of children with soy hypersensitivity, RAST had a sensitivity of 69%, a specificity of 77%, and a positive predictive value (i.e., likelihood that the patient was truly allergic to soy if the RAST was positive) of only 6% (Giampietro et al., 1992).

Double-blind, placebo-controlled food challenges in the hospital or office are the most definitive and safest way to evaluate patients with food hypersensitivity and to control for confounding factors (e.g., idiopathic urticaria, reactions to food additives, psychogenic influences). In patients with a history of anaphylaxis, personnel trained in resuscitation and use of emergency drugs (including epinephrine and diphenhydramine) must be present. The challenge involves giving increasing amounts of encapsulated lyophilized food protein or placebo in doses ranging from 125 mg to 10 g (Burks and Sampson, 1992). Reactions should be observed by an objective third person unaware of whether the patient receives placebo or antigen. Although the challenges are used primarily in tertiary care centers, protocols for double-blind food challenges in the hospital or office setting are available (Bock et al., 1988; Metcalfe and Sampson, 1990).

. . . .
TABLE 34-8 · DIAGNOSTIC TESTS FOR FOOD ALLERGY

Complete blood count (for peripheral eosinophilia)
Skin testing
Radioallergosorbent (RAST) testing
D-Xylose absorption
Immunoglobulin levels (including immunoglobulin E)
Antigliadin/antiendomysial antibodies (for celiac disease)
Repeated food challenge (Goldman criteria)
Double-blind, placebo-controlled food challenge
Intestinal/colonic biopsy

Treatment

When food allergy is diagnosed, the cornerstone of therapy is the elimination of the offending food. The elimination diet must be strict and often requires the supervision of a registered dietitian, because the offending foods may be present in fillers or additives in processed foods (Leihnas et al., 1987). Most patients have reactions caused by only one or two offending foods, the most common being milk, soy, egg, peanuts, wheat, or fish. However, severe reactions to a great many foods, including rice, are reported (Borchers et al., 1993). Because a milk-allergic infant or child may also react to soy protein, we generally recommend casein hydrolysate formulas for infants with cow's milk intolerance. Mothers who are breastfeeding their infants are encouraged to continue breastfeeding if they restrict their own diet of cow's milk and soy protein, eggs, peanuts, and fish.

For older infants and children, we do not recommend an empirical elimination diet because of the adverse effects on the child's nutrition and growth. Instead, elimination diets should be based on the results of food challenges. Children receiving special diets may require nutritional assessment followed by calcium or vitamin supplementation.

Prevention

Early avoidance of allergenic foods may help prevent the subsequent development of atopic disease in infants at high risk. Zeiger and co-workers (1989) randomly assigned infants of atopic parents to either a regular diet or a restricted diet. The restricted diet consisted of avoidance of maternal ingestion of cow's milk, soy, and peanuts during the third trimester of pregnancy and during lactation and avoidance of infant ingestion of cow's milk, soy, citrus, wheat, peanuts, corn, egg, and fish for the first year of life. The prevalence of atopic disease was 27% in the control group and 16% in the food-restricted group. A similar study was conducted by Sigurs and co-workers (1992), who found a decrease in the percentage of patients with atopic dermatitis but not other disorders. Thus avoidance of antigenic foods in the first year of life may prevent the subsequent development of food allergies.

Prognosis

Most children outgrow their food allergies (except for nut allergies). In our experience, less than 10% of infants with allergic colitis develop adverse reactions when challenged with cow's milk protein at 1 year of age. Infants who have had evidence of an IgE-mediated type I hypersensitivity reaction are at risk for an anaphylactic response to the milk challenge. We thus recommend that for those infants, a challenge be performed under close observation in a physician's office or procedure unit. Bishop and colleagues (1990) reported a long-term study of 100 children with atopic illness (urticaria, eczema, bronchitis, and diarrhea) associated with cow's milk allergy. Of the children, 72% still reacted to milk at 2 years of age, but only 22% of the children reacted to milk at age 6 (Bishop et al., 1990). Thus it may take several years to achieve clinical tolerance. By contrast, children with peanut allergies persist with skin test reactivity and clinical allergy into adolescence (Bock and Atkins, 1989).

Gastroesophageal Reflux

The reflux of small amounts of gastric contents into the lower esophagus is a normal occurrence, particularly after meals. GER is characterized by an increased number or duration of these episodes, the presence of symptoms, and possibly complications.

Clinical Manifestations

Effortless regurgitation is the usual manifestation in infants, whereas older children typically complain of retrosternal burning, epigastric discomfort, and heartburn. In a few patients, symptoms are severe enough to impair weight gain and lead to failure to thrive. In a subset of these infants, peptic esophagitis develops, resulting in hematemesis or occult blood loss and iron deficiency anemia. Esophageal strictures may eventually develop if the child remains untreated.

Less common presentations include recurrent aspiration pneumonia, chronic cough, wheezing (often nocturnal), and asthma (Malroot et al., 1987). Apneic spells in the newborn and sudden infant death syndrome have been ascribed to GER. Pseudoneurologic symptoms, including abnormal posturing (Sandifer's syndrome) and rumination, are rare presentations (Boyle, 1989; Bray et al., 1977). Pathologic reflux is common in children with neurologic disabilities as well as in those with congenital malformations of the esophagus.

Diagnosis

The clinician is confronted with a large number of infants who spit up but are otherwise well. Infants who have normal growth and who do not present with any complications of reflux (i.e., poor weight gain, occult gastrointestinal bleeding, immunodeficiency, anemia, repeated lower respiratory infections, chronic cough, or wheezing) do not require investigation. In addition to infants with these complications, infants with significant neurologic disorders or esophageal anomalies (tracheoesophageal fistula) or those symptomatic beyond 2 years of age require evaluation.

Extended monitoring of the pH of the distal esophagus remains the gold standard in the diagnosis of pathologic reflux. The healthy infant has a higher percentage of acid reflux into the esophagus than the adult; thus caution must be exercised when interpreting pediatric pH studies as being normal or abnormal (Vandenplas et al., 1991). The upper gastrointestinal barium radiographic study is used to rule out anatomic abnormalities (e.g., hiatus hernia, pyloric stenosis, malrotation) or gastric outlet obstruction, but it is a poor test for GER.

Scintigraphic scanning after the patient ingests tracer-labeled milk is a noninvasive technique involving little radiation. It is more sensitive than radiology in the detection of reflux, but its main utility is in the detection of delayed gastric emptying. Esophageal manometry is useful for demonstrating abnormalities of motility or swallowing. GER is associated with transient lower esophageal sphincter relaxation but does not correlate well with basal lower esophageal sphincter pressure (Kawahara, et al., 1997).

Endoscopy and mucosal biopsy demonstrate complications of reflux (esophagitis, strictures, metaplasia, or Barrett's esophagus) and rule out other causes of vomiting (peptic ulcer disease, *Helicobacter pylori* infection, or eosinophilic gastroenteritis). The esophageal histologic findings in a patient with reflux esophagitis include lengthening of the esophageal papillae, hyperplasia of the basal epithelial cell layer, and intraepithelial eosinophils (Vandenplas, 1994). Kelly and co-workers (1995) have proposed that isolated intraepithelial eosinophilia may be caused by food allergy as well as reflux; therefore, as discussed earlier, eosinophilic esophagitis that does not respond to treatment for GER may in fact be related to an ingested or inhaled allergen.

Treatment

Medical management of patients with GER commences initially by recommending that the parents thicken the formula by adding cereal directly to the bottle and offer smaller and more frequent feedings. Positioning of the child (prone, head tilted up) after feedings and during sleep may also be beneficial (Orenstein et al., 1983).

Pharmacotherapy is reserved for either older children or infants with complicated reflux (i.e., children with weight loss, esophagitis, reactive airway disease, apnea, or aspiration). Therapy for GER involves treatment with a prokinetic agent, an antacid, or both. Prokinetic agents currently available include bethanechol and metoclopramide (Reynolds and Putnam, 1992). Antacid therapies include coating agents (e.g., Mylanta), histamine H_2 receptor antagonists (cimetidine, ranitidine, famotidine, and nizatidine), and proton-pump antagonists (esomeprazole, lansoprazole, omeprazole, pantoprazole, and rabeprazole).

Surgery (fundoplication) is reserved for those with severe complications refractory to medical treatment and controls reflux in approximately 90% of patients. Fundoplication has unwanted effects (including delayed gastric emptying or dumping syndrome) in 15% to 20% of patients, so it should be performed only in cases of life-threatening reflux or medical treatment failures (Fung et al., 1990).

Gluten-Sensitive Enteropathy (Celiac Sprue, Celiac Disease)

Gluten-sensitive enteropathy (GSE) is a nonallergic abnormal immunologic response to the ethanol-soluble prolamins of gluten, gliadin, and proline-rich proteins found in wheat, rye, barley, and possibly oats and is characterized clinically by malabsorption and histologically by small-intestinal villous atrophy. A gluten-free diet results in normalization of small-bowel histology and clinical improvement, and rechallenge with gluten causes recurrence of the histologic abnormalities and clinical symptoms.

The relationship of gluten ingestion to celiac disease was astutely deduced in the early 1950s by Willem-Karel Dicke, a Dutch pediatrician, who observed that GSE diminished during the bread shortage of World War II (Dicke et al., 1953; van Berge-Henegouwen and Mulder, 1993). Diagnosis and follow-up of patients with GSE have changed dramatically since the 1970s with the widespread use of noninvasive serologic testing with antigliadin, antireticulin, and antiendomysial and tissue transglutaminase antibodies.

Pathogenesis

The mucosal injury in GSE involves the interaction of genetic and environmental factors (Schuppan, 2000; Trier, 1991). Although genetic factors are probably predominant, ingestion of the gluten proteins is essential for the disease to occur. The toxicity of oat prolamins (avenins) to induce GSE is currently debated. The mechanism by which gluten induces mucosal injury—whether through immunogenicity or in conjunction with direct toxicity of the peptides to the mucosa—is unknown. Both humoral and cell-mediated immune responses are implicated by the induction of autoantibodies and antigen-specific T-cell activation, with an associated alteration in the expression of cytokines in the mucosa dominated by interferon-γ (Nilsen et al., 1998).

There is a 10% incidence of GSE in first-degree relatives of patients with GSE, a 30% concordance in human leukocyte antigen (HLA)-identical siblings, and a 70% concordance among identical twins (Marsh, 1992; Mearin and Pena, 1987; Mylotte et al., 1974). Early epidemiologic studies suggested an association of GSE with the class I MHC antigen HLA-B8 (Auricchio et al., 1988; Falchuk et al., 1972). Subsequently, much stronger associations with certain MHC class II molecules have been observed. More than 90% of GSE patients either have HLA-DR3 or are heterozygous for HLA-DR5/DR7 (Alper et al., 1987; DeMarchi et al., 1979; Ek et al., 1978; Sollid and Thorsby, 1993). The strongest HLA association with GSE is the expression of HLA-DQ2 (HLA-DQα1*0501, HLA-DQβ1*0201) heterodimer in which the two chains are encoded in *cis* (same chromosome) or in *trans* (different chromosome); thus, through linkage, HLA-DQ may associated with HLA-DR5/DR7 or HLA-DR3 (Sollid and Thorsby, 1993).

Gliadin-specific T cells that are restricted by HLA-DQ2 and HLA-DQ8(DQα1*0301, DQβ1*0302) have been identified in the mucosa of patients with GSE (Lundin et al., 1993). Analysis of the motifs of the peptide binding sites of DQ2 and DQ8 suggest a preference for negatively charged residues in the peptide, which may explain the low-affinity binding of gliadin peptides.

Tissue transglutaminase (tTG) is a secreted extracellular enzyme that catalyzes the crosslinking of proteins and has an affinity for gliadin, specifically a "33-mer" gliadin peptide (Shan et al., 2002). Tissue transglutaminase has also been identified as the primary autoantigen for endomysial antibodies in GSE (Dieterich et al., 1997).

tTG deamination of gliadin can result in the conversion of glutamine to glutamate, leading to a large number of negatively charged residues in the peptide. Recent evidence indicates that tTG treatment of gliadin peptides known to be recognized by T-cell clones enhances the reactivity of gliadin-specific, DQ2-and DQ8-restricted T cells (Van de Wal et al., 1998).

Mass spectrometric analysis of peptide has shown that tTG deamination of glutamine residues is selective. Furthermore, several gluten-specific, DQ2-restricted T-cell lines were shown to recognize only two immunodominant peptides that overlap by a seven-residue fragment containing a glutamine that tTG converts to glutamate for T-cell reactivity to occur (Arentz-Hansen et al., 2000). These findings suggest that tTG deamidation of gliadin in the intestinal mucosa could provide a mechanism by which gliadin peptides can bind with high avidity to DQ2 or DQ8 molecules for antigen presentation to T cells in susceptible individuals.

Considering that concordance for GSE is not 100% in HLA-identical siblings and twins, environmental factors must also play a role in its activation (Kagnoff, 1992). Because GSE can present at any time between early infancy and old age, it has been postulated that other antigens may trigger gluten sensitivity in genetically predisposed individuals.

Kagnoff and colleagues (1984) discovered a 12–amino acid sequence homology between A-gliadin and the E1b protein of human adenovirus type 12. These investigators subsequently showed that 16 of 18 patients with celiac disease, compared with 6 of 35 control subjects, had been exposed to this virus (Kagnoff et al., 1987). However, another group has not confirmed this association (Howdle et al., 1989). Although the model of molecular immune mimicry provides an intriguing possibility to explain the variable clinical manifestations of GSE, at this time there is still no compelling evidence for the involvement of viral or nondietary environmental factors in the pathogenesis of GSE.

Another reason only 1% of HLA-DQ carriers develop GSE and that the concordance rate for HLA matched siblings is much lower than that for monozygotic twins may be that there are non–HLA-linked susceptibility genes. However, except for the HLA region of chromosome 6, linkage analysis of different populations has led to contradictory results without identifying relevant loci.

Humoral and cellular immunologic abnormalities are present in the intestinal mucosa of patients with GSE. Increased lamina propria plasma cells and increased mucosal IgA and IgM production are observed. The IgA antibody secreted in GSE is primarily dimeric, whereas monomeric IgA is produced in IBD (Baklien et al., 1977; Colombel et al., 1990). Serum antibodies to gliadin peptides (antigliadin IgG and IgA) and antiendomysial antibodies (IgA) for which tTG is the primary antigen are present in patients with GSE (Ferreira et al., 1992; Levenson et al., 1985). It is unknown whether these antibodies play a pathogenic role in GSE (i.e., through antibody-mediated cellular cytotoxicity) or are simply epiphenomena. They are useful in the diagnosis and monitoring of GSE (see later discussion).

IELs are in close proximity to gut epithelial cells and may be involved in epithelial damage in patients with GSE. The presence of the cytotoxic protein nucleolysin TIA-1 has been demonstrated within the IELs of patients with active GSE; therefore IELs possess cytotoxic molecules that could potentially damage enterocytes (Russell et al., 1993). Spencer and colleagues (1991) have demonstrated that patients with GSE have an increased percentage (up to 30%) of CD3$^+$CD4$^-$CD8$^-$ IELs expressing the γ/δ-T-cell receptor. However, the increase in γ/δ-IEL cells is not specific for GSE, because it is also found in other enteropathies (Halstensen et al., 1989, 1990; Spencer et al., 1989, 1991). Most IELs of patients with GSE bear α/β-T-cell receptors, and these decrease significantly in response to a gluten-free diet, whereas the γ/δ-TCR cells remain stable (Kutlu et al., 1993). Thus both α/β-and γ/δ-IELs are present in the mucosa in GSE, but whether either phenotype mediates intestinal damage is unknown.

In summary, GSE occurs when there is an altered mucosal immune response in genetically susceptible individuals. Whether GSE is caused only by an immunologic response to gluten or in conjunction with direct toxicity of the gluten peptides is unknown.

Clinical Manifestations

The prevalence of celiac disease ranges from 1 in 300 in western Ireland to 1 in 10,000 in other regions. The disease is common in northern Europe and rare in China, Japan, and Africa (Trier, 1991). Variations in prevalence among different geographic regions may relate to the genetic susceptibility of some populations or to a missed or delayed diagnosis as a result of a lack of recognition of the clinical spectrum of the disease.

A more recent study indicates an estimated biopsy-proved prevalence of GSE in Finnish schoolchildren is 1:99 (Maki et al., 2003). A multicenter study in the United States found an overall prevalence of 1:133 in not-at-risk groups recruited from blood donors, schoolchildren, and patients seen in outpatient clinics; however, the diagnosis of GSE was not confirmed by a mucosal biopsy in all patients (Fasano et al., 2003).

Several diseases are associated with GSE, including diabetes mellitus, Down syndrome, and atopic dermatitis (Auricchio et al., 1988; Murphy and Walker, 1991). Selective IgA deficiency is a common association, occurring in 1 of 200 patients with GSE, compared with 1 in 700 in the general population (Cunningham-Rundles, 1988) (see Chapter 14). A study of 75 selective IgA–deficient children found an incidence of GSE near 10% (Savilahti and Pelkonen, 1979).

Patients with GSE may also develop other immunologic disorders, including arthritis, chronic hepatitis, thyroiditis, aphthous ulcers, and pulmonary hemosiderosis (Auricchio et al., 1988). Dermatitis herpetiformis, an immunologically mediated papulovesicular skin disease, is strongly associated with gluten sensitivity, and remission occurs when patients are given a gluten-free diet (Gawkrodger et al., 1988; Reunala et al., 1977). This condition is rare in children (see Chapter 32).

Clinical features of celiac disease are given in Table 34-9. The classical presentation is that of an infant younger than 2 years of age with diarrhea, weight loss, and weakness. However, for the past two decades, this classical presentation has become quite unusual as the age at the time of presentation increases and the symptoms become much milder, such as indigestion for adults or recurrent abdominal pain in children (Maki and Collin, 1997; Maki et al., 1988).

Small children may also present with refusal to feed, constipation, irritability, lethargy, and iron deficiency anemia. Older children may present with short stature, pubertal delay, malaise, or crampy abdominal pain. In adults, amenorrhea, folate deficiency, and peripheral neuropathy have been described. It is now common for the initial symptoms to be nongastrointestinal in nature.

Diagnosis

The diagnosis of celiac disease necessitates a small-bowel biopsy and demonstration of villous atrophy, increased IELs, epithelial destruction, increased crypt mitotic activity, and infiltration of the lamina propria by plasma cells and lymphocytes (Fig. 34-11). The biopsy may be performed either endoscopically or by use of a swallowed small-bowel biopsy capsule passed into the jejunum. Results of endoscopic biopsies of the duodenum correlate well with jejunal histology. Endoscopy can also visualize the gross morphology of the duodenal folds, which may be flattened or scalloped in patients with active GSE.

DIFFERENTIAL DIAGNOSIS

The histologic appearance is not specific to GSE and can be seen in other diseases, such as milk and soy protein intolerance, malnutrition, immunodeficiency, giardiasis, and viral infections. For this reason, before 1990,

TABLE 34-9 · CLINICAL FEATURES OF CELIAC DISEASE

Primary Features	Associated Disorders
Diarrhea	Arthritis
Growth failure	Hepatitis
Anorexia	Pulmonary hemosiderosis
Irritability/lethargy	Diabetes mellitus
Abdominal pain	Thyroid function abnormalities
Constipation	Down syndrome
Pubertal delay	Iritis
Weight loss	Dermatitis herpetiformis
Abdominal distention	Selective IgA deficiency
Buttock wasting	Sarcoidosis
Digital clubbing	IgA nephropathy
Pallor	
Edema	

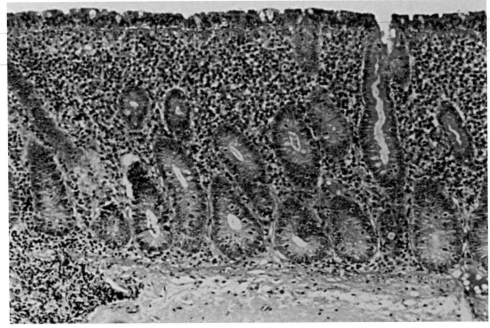

Figure 34-11 · Low-power photomicrograph of a small-bowel biopsy specimen in a patient with celiac disease. Complete villous atrophy, increased mitotic activity in the crypts, and increased cellularity in the lamina propria are seen.

the European Society of Pediatric Gastroenterology and Nutrition (ESPGN) recommended that three small-bowel biopsies be performed to establish the diagnosis: one biopsy at initial presentation, a second after 6 months of a gluten-free diet, and a third after gluten rechallenge (to show that the gluten was truly the offending agent and to exclude transient gluten intolerance) (Walker-Smith et al., 1990). The cost and invasiveness of these repeated procedures led to the widespread use of empirical wheat-free diets. Until recently, noninvasive tests for diagnosis of GSE (Table 34-10) assessed only intestinal mucosal function and lacked sensitivity and specificity for detecting celiac disease.

ANTIGLIADIN, ANTIENDOMYSIAL, AND TISSUE TRANSGLUTAMINASE ANTIBODIES

Assays for serum antigliadin (IgG and IgA enzyme-linked immunosorbent assay [ELISA]) and antiendomysial (immunofluorescence) antibodies have greatly facilitated the diagnosis of GSE. In a study of 340 children with untreated celiac disease, Burgin-Wolff and colleagues (1991) found that the combination of antigliadin IgG and IgA antibodies and antiendomysial IgA antibodies detected GSE in 338 of 340 (99.4%) children with the disease. Therefore, if assays for all three antibodies were negative, GSE was essentially excluded. In this study, the antiendomysial antibody was the most specific, with only 2 false-positive results out of 211; in contrast, the IgG antigliadin antibody had a very high (35%) false-positive rate. A smaller study found the sensitivity and specificity of the antiendomysial antibody alone approached 100% (Ferreira et al., 1992). Although the sensitivity and specificity of the

antiendomysial antibody is very high, it is an IgA antibody and may be negative in those with selective IgA deficiency, which is more common with GSE.

Because tTG is the major antigen recognized by antiendomysial antibodies, ELISA assays to measure tTG antibodies are now available and appear to have a good correlation with the antiendomysial assays; however, they should not be considered equivalent.

We routinely screen all patients suspected of having GSE with antigliadin and antiendomysial or tTG antibodies and perform biopsies for all patients with positive antiendomysial or tTG antibodies. If a patient has a

TABLE 34-10 · DIAGNOSTIC TESTS IN CELIAC DISEASE

Test	Common Finding
Blood count	Microcytic anemia
Blood chemistries	Hypoalbuminemia
	Hypocalcemia
D-Xylose	Poor absorption (1-hour level < 20 mg/dl)
Lactose breath hydrogen test	Lactose intolerance
Fecal fat	Fat malabsorption
Upper gastrointestinal series with small-bowel follow through	Loss of small-bowel pattern Flocculation of barium Bowel dilatation
Antigliadin, antirecticulin, antiendomysial* and anti-tTG antibodies	Elevated titers
Small-bowel biopsy	Villous atrophy

*Most specific antibody for celiac disease.
tTG = tissue transglutaminase.

positive antigliadin IgG and negative antigliadin IgA and antiendomysial IgA antibody, we review the clinical data to determine whether biopsy is warranted. Because selective IgA–deficient patients may not have positive IgA antiendomysial antibodies even if they have celiac disease, quantitative IgA levels are a useful adjunct in the evaluation of the patient in whom GSE is suspected.

Current serologic tests are inadequate to make the diagnosis of GSE alone, and the diagnosis involves lifelong dietary restriction; thus an initial biopsy for every patient with suspected celiac disease remains standard. Antibody titers usually decrease upon institution of a gluten-free diet and increase with gluten rechallenge and may be used to follow disease activity (Burgin-Wolff et al., 1991).

For this reason, the ESPGN has amended its prior recommendation, stating that three biopsies are no longer necessary in every case of GSE (Walker-Smith et al., 1990). Only two criteria were required, which were the presence of clear histologic features of GSE on the first mucosal biopsy and that there was a clear clinical remission on a gluten-free diet.

The need for a second biopsy may be considered when (1) the initial biopsy was done on a child younger than 2 years old; (2) the diagnosis is in doubt, such as with an absent or inadequate initial biopsy; or (3) the patient is noncompliant with the gluten-free diet and there is doubt about the diagnosis and the wish to discontinue all dietary restrictions.

Treatment

Therapy for GSE involves the institution of a strict gluten-free diet and the correction of any nutritional deficiencies caused by malabsorption. Even small amounts of dietary gluten (such as in processed foods) can result in villous inflammation and damage. Consultation with a dietitian and referral to a celiac support group are recommended. Most patients demonstrate some catch-up growth within a year after diagnosis and treatment, although their ultimate height may be less than that of siblings. If symptoms persist or growth remains poor, the patient's dietary compliance should be evaluated, antibody tests or biopsy repeated, and other causes of malabsorption sought.

Adults with celiac disease have a higher incidence of intestinal T-cell lymphoma than the general population (Logan et al., 1989; Nielsen et al., 1985). A gluten-free diet may decrease the risk of this malignancy by minimizing intestinal inflammation, but this has not been proved.

Inflammatory Bowel Disease

IBDs are characterized by persistent chronic intestinal inflammation without an identifiable infectious or dietary cause. In the United States, *IBD* refers to ulcerative colitis (UC) and Crohn's disease (CD). We also discuss Behçet's disease, malakoplakia, and intractable ulcerating enterocolitis of infancy, because these illnesses may have a similar pathophysiology and are often confused clinically with UC and CD. In the United States, 500,000 to 1 million patients are afflicted with either UC or CD. Chapter 35 discusses the rheumatic aspects of these disorders.

Etiology and Pathophysiology

Many factors have been linked with IBD (Table 34-11), but no cause of the disease has been found. Heredity plays a strong role; a patient with UC or CD has a 10% chance of having a first-degree relative with IBD, and concordance among monozygotic twins is approximately 65% for CD and 20% for UC (Yang et al., 1992).

No strong HLA association has been identified in either CD or UC, but some weak associations have been identified. Specifically, whites with UC have an increased prevalence of HLA-B27, HLA-BW35, and HLA-DR2, and whites with CD have an increased incidence of HLA-B2 and HLA-B44 (Schreiber et al., 1992).

Of note, patients with certain genetic syndromes, including Turner's syndrome and Hermansky-Pudlak syndrome, appear to be at increased risk for IBD (Mendeloff and Calkins, 1988). Several patients with both glycogen storage disease type Ib and IBD have also been described (see later discussion).

Numerous organisms, including normal bacterial flora, *E. coli*, atypical mycobacteria, *C. difficile*, and measles virus, have been proposed as causes of IBD. However, no single infectious agent has withstood the test of time as the etiologic agent. The same is true for ingested agents; milk and other foods have been proposed as potential proinflammatory antigens, but little evidence linking dietary substances to exacerbation of IBD exists (Glassman et al., 1990). However, some patients with CD may undergo remission when given an elemental diet, suggesting that elimination of food antigens diminishes intestinal inflammation in CD (Kleinman et al., 1989; Logan et al., 1981; Seidman et al., 1987).

Mucosal immunity may be altered in IBD. Schreiber and co-workers (1992) have proposed that the mucosal immune system in patients with UC and CD is in a heightened state of activation. These and other investigators postulate that enhanced intestinal permeability or antigen presentation by intestinal epithelial cells leads to macrophage activation and IL-1 secretion within mucosal lymphoid aggregates. This in turn results in helper T-lymphocyte secretion of IL-2, IL-4,

TABLE 34-11 · ASSOCIATIONS WITH AND RISK FACTORS FOR INFLAMMATORY BOWEL DISEASE

Genetic	Infections
Jewish ancestry	Atypical mycobacteria
Family history	Enteric bacterial flora
Turner's syndrome	Measles virus
Hermansky-Pudlak syndrome	*Clostridium difficile*
Exogenous Intake	**Immune**
Milk consumption	Altered intestinal permeability
Sugar consumption	Associated autoimmune
Smoking	disorders (e.g., sclerosing
Oral contraceptive pill	cholangitis)

and IL-5; B-cell activation; immunoglobulin production; and recruitment of effector cells (including eosinophils, mast cells, and neutrophils). The inflammatory response results in intestinal epithelial damage, enhanced antigen absorption, and perpetuation of the inflammatory cascade (Fig. 34-12) (Schreiber et al., 1992).

Much evidence supports abnormal immune activation in IBD. First, immunosuppressive agents, including corticosteroids, 6-mercaptopurine, and cyclosporine, are effective therapeutic agents in CD and UC. Second, both diseases are associated with other immune disorders, including peripheral arthritis, chronic active hepatitis, uveitis, and primary sclerosing cholangitis (PSC).

Hollander and colleagues (1986) have demonstrated that some healthy relatives of patients with IBD have increased permeability to macromolecular markers such as lactulose or polyethylene glycol; this may predispose them to IBD. Indeed, some patients with IBD in remission have increased permeability to lactulose, and this may be predictive of disease relapse (Wyatt et al., 1993).

Others have demonstrated that epithelial cells express MHC class II molecules and present antigen in vitro to T lymphocytes; such antigen-presenting activity may be augmented in patients with UC and CD (Bland and Warren, 1986; Mayer and Eisenhardt, 1990; Mayer et al., 1991). Therefore evidence exists for abnormal gut permeability and increased antigen presentation in IBD.

There is other evidence of immune activation in the intestinal mucosa of patients with IBD. Immunohistochemical and flow cytometric studies show increased numbers of activated T cells expressing IL-2 receptors (CD25) in the bowel wall of patients with CD and increased numbers of activated macrophages in the

intestinal mucosa of patients with UC (Choy et al., 1990). Proinflammatory cytokines, including IL-1, IL-2, interferon-γ, IL-6, and IL-8, are elevated in the intestine of patients with IBD (Fais et al., 1991; Mahida et al., 1989; Stevens et al., 1992). IL-8 in particular may be a potent chemotactic factor resulting in neutrophil recruitment. The mucosal plasma cells of patients with IBD have increased local production of IgG and IgA1 (Kett and Brandtzaeg, 1987; Kett et al., 1987). Last, messenger ribonucleic acid (mRNA) for granzyme B, a molecular mediator of damage by cytotoxic T cells, is increased in the mucosa of patients with UC (Stevens et al., 1994). These findings suggest that abnormalities of immune regulation are essential steps in the development of the inflammatory state in CD and UC.

To investigate which cytokine abnormalities cause colitis, researchers have developed several transgenic animals that contract colitis. Sadlack and colleagues (1993) have developed an IL-2–deficient mouse that develops colitis at week 10 of life and whose mucosa contains activated T cells. Similarly, colitis develops in transgenic mice lacking the α/β-T-cell receptor (Mombaerts et al., 1993). An IL-10–deficient mouse develops both colitis and small-bowel lesions (Kuhn et al., 1993).

Last, Hammer and colleagues (1990) have reported a transgenic rat containing multiple copies of the HLA-B27 gene; these rats develop colitis in conjunction with a systemic autoimmune erosive arthropathy. These studies suggest that colitis may be an end result of multiple immune system aberrations rather than a single specific abnormality (Strober and Ehrhardt, 1993).

Circulating autoantibodies to gut epithelium have been implicated in the pathogenesis of IBD. Anticolon

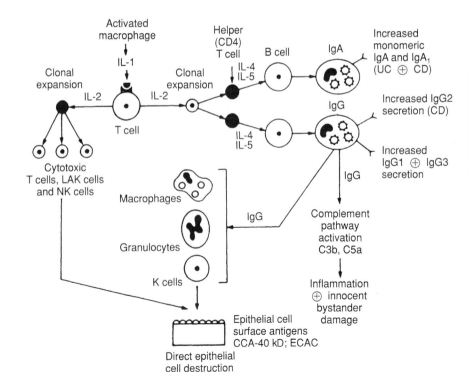

Figure 34-12 · Inflammatory cascade postulated in inflammatory bowel disease. The activated T cell secretes cytokines, causing expansion of T-cell populations (e.g., interleukin [IL]-2) and expansion of B-cell populations (e.g., IL-4, IL-5). Cytokines produced by activated T cells can also stimulate cytotoxic T cells, natural killer (NK) cells, and lymphokine-activated killer (LAK) cells, which can damage gut epithelium. The stimulated B cells mature into plasma cells, produce antibodies, and activate complement, which may further recruit other inflammatory cells (neutrophils, mast cells). Alterations of immunoglobulin A (IgA) and immunoglobulin G (IgG) subclass antibodies may be seen in inflammatory bowel disease. (From Baldassano RN, MacDermott RP. Immunologic aspects of inflammatory bowel disease. Semin Pediatr Gastroenterol Nutr 1:5, 1990.)

antibodies are present in the serum of patients with the disease; however, they are nonspecific and are present in those with other inflammatory colitides (Shorter et al., 1972; Thayer et al., 1969). Das and co-workers (1993) have identified a serum antibody directed against tropomyosin that may be specific for ulcerative colitis.

Serum antineutrophil cytoplasmic antibodies (ANCA) are also found in 60% to 80% of patients with UC; unlike the cytoplasmic ANCA of Wegener's granulomatosis, ANCA of UC are perinuclear (p-ANCA) (Duerr et al., 1991) (see Chapters 33, 35 and 38). Proujansky and colleagues (1993) have shown that, at least in pediatric IBD, serum ANCA are also present in 20% of patients with CD and so do not reliably differentiate between UC and CD.

In summary, host defense abnormalities, including increased gut permeability, increased antigen presentation by enterocytes, T-lymphocyte activation, and alterations in immunoglobulin synthesis, are present in both CD and UC. The genetic factors predisposing to the antigens initiating the intestinal inflammation are largely undefined.

Clinical Manifestations

Despite some similarities, UC and CD must be considered separate entities. CD may involve any part of the gastrointestinal tract from mouth to anus, whereas UC is limited to the large bowel and rectum. Inflammation in CD is transmural and characterized by granulomas, whereas the inflammation in UC is limited to the mucosa and submucosa (Kelts and Grand, 1980). Clinical and pathologic differences between CD and UC are summarized in Table 34-12.

Diagnosis

The diagnosis of CD or UC is established in five separate steps:

1. Clinical suspicion of IBD must be based on identification of suggestive clinical features, particularly growth failure, anemia, abdominal pain, diarrhea, or arthritis.

2. Other infectious (usually bacterial or parasitic) or immune (Behçet's disease, malakoplakia, or chronic granulomatous disease) causes of intestinal inflammation that can mimic the inflammation in UC or CD must be excluded.

3. The disease should be classified as either CD or UC on the basis of laboratory, radiographic, and endoscopic studies; in approximately 10% of cases, this is not possible, and the disease is termed *indeterminate colitis*.

4. The location of the disease should be pinpointed. For UC, this means identifying the segments of the large bowel that are involved; for CD, it requires localizing disease to the mouth, esophagus, stomach, small bowel, colon, or anus.

5. Extraintestinal disease should be sought, including peripheral arthritis (present in 10% to 15% of patients with IBD), liver disease (including chronic active hepatitis and sclerosing cholangitis), eye disease (including episcleritis and uveitis), and skin disease (including pyoderma gangrenosum and erythema nodosum).

A clinical and laboratory evaluation for the patient with suspected UC or CD is given in Table 34-13.

Ulcerative Colitis

Among patients younger than 20 years of age with UC, 50% are older than age 16 and less than 1% are younger than age 5. The most common presentation is a subacute illness with diarrhea, rectal bleeding, weakness, anemia, weight loss, and fever. Stool frequency ranges from 2 to 10 bowel movements per day. A minority of patients present with more severe symptoms, including severe abdominal pain, bloody and mucus-filled diarrhea, tenesmus, leukocytosis, hypoalbuminemia, and bowel wall thickening seen on abdominal radiographs; these symptoms must be differentiated from those of acute infectious colitides such as shigellosis or *Campylobacter* diarrhea (Werlin and Grand, 1977).

Extraintestinal manifestations may also be observed at the time of presentation (Table 34-14). Two forms of

TABLE 34-12 · CLINICAL CHARACTERISTICS OF INFLAMMATORY BOWEL DISEASE

Characteristic	Ulcerative Colitis	Crohn's Disease
Symptoms		
Rectal bleeding	Common	Less frequent
Diarrhea	Often severe	Moderate to absent
Pain	Infrequent	Common
Anorexia	Mild	Often severe
Weight loss	Variable	Common
Extraintestinal symptoms	Not infrequent	Not infrequent
Distribution of the lesions	Colon only; continuous	Throughout the gastrointestinal tract, segmental
Pathologic changes	Mucosal only	Transmural
Clinical Course		
Remissions	Relatively common	Difficult to define
Relapse rate after surgery	None following protocolectomy	70%
Cancer risk	20% per decade of disease after the first decade	20% greater than the population at large

TABLE 34-13 · EVALUATION OF THE PATIENT WITH SUSPECTED INFLAMMATORY BOWEL DISEASE

1. Weight, height, anthropometrics, and bone age
2. Tanner staging
3. Clinical evidence of
   Clubbing
   Iritis
   Mouth ulcers
   Arthritis
   Back pain/sacroiliitis
   Abdominal mass
   Perianal disease—hemorrhoids, fissures, fistulas
4. Laboratory studies
   Stool guaiac (occult blood)
   Complete blood count with differential, reticulocyte count
   Sedimentation rate
   Albumin, total protein
   Transaminases, alkaline phosphatase, bilirubin
   Gamma-glutamyl transpeptidase
   Serum iron, total iron-binding capacity
   Antigliadin, antiendomysial, anti-tTG antibodies (to exclude celiac
      disease)
5. Purified protein derivative, *Candida* skin tests
6. Stool cultures
   Bacteria (including *Escherichia coli* O 157:H7 and *Clostridium difficile*)
   Ova and parasites
   Radiography
   Upper gastrointestinal series (with small-bowel followthrough and antegrade cologram)
   Barium enema (may be useful if colonoscopy unavailable)
7. Flexible sigmoidoscopy or colonoscopy/ileoscopy

tTG = tissue transglutaminase.

TABLE 34-14 · PRESENTING FEATURES OF CROHN'S DISEASE AND ULCERATIVE COLITIS IN CHILDHOOD

Intestinal	Extraintestinal
Crohn's Disease	
Growth failure	Arthritis/arthralgia
Weight loss	Erythema nodosum
Diarrhea	Fever
Abdominal pain	Anorexia
Abdominal mass	Oral ulcers
Rectal bleeding	Anemia
Perianal fissures/fistulas	Pubertal delay
	Clubbing
	Liver disease
	Renal stones (oxalate)
	Uveitis/episcleritis
Ulcerative Colitis	
Diarrhea	Anemia
Rectal bleeding	Fever
Abdominal pain	Arthralgias/arthritis
Cramring/tenesmus	Spondyloarthropathy
Fulminant colitis	Erythema nodosum
Growth failure	Pyoderma gangrenosum
	Liver disease
	Uveitis/episcleritis

arthritis are associated with ulcerative colitis (see Chapter 35). Peripheral arthritis involving the knees, ankles, elbows, and wrists occurs in 10% to 20% of patients, and arthritis tends to wax and wane with disease activity. In contrast, an axial arthritis resembling ankylosing spondylitis occurs in 5% to 10% of patients with UC, progresses despite disease activity, and is associated with HLA-B27 (Gravallese and Kantrowitz, 1988).

Primary sclerosing cholangitis, a progressive inflammation and fibrosis of the bile ducts, occurs in 1% to 2% of patients and may progress to cirrhosis and ultimately require liver transplantation; unfortunately, colectomy does not prevent disease progression (Schrumpf et al., 1988). Erythema nodosum is the most common dermatosis associated with UC and CD in children. Pyoderma gangrenosum is seen rarely in pediatric UC, although it is not uncommon in adults with long-standing UC.

DIAGNOSIS

After infectious agents have been excluded (see Table 34-13), flexible sigmoidoscopy or colonoscopy with biopsy is the most useful diagnostic procedure to establish the diagnosis of UC. Visual inspection of the colon reveals diffuse erythema, mucosal friability with bleeding, loss of the vascular pattern, purulent exudate, and small superficial ulcerations. In contrast to findings in CD, there is continuous involvement of the colon, without skip areas. One of three patterns of disease localization is usually seen: proctitis limited to the rec-

tosigmoid, left-sided colitis from the rectum to the splenic flexure, or pancolitis involving the entire colon. On microscopic examination, a mucosal infiltrate of polymorphonuclear leukocytes with epithelial cell destruction and crypt abscesses is seen; granulomas are absent (Fig. 34-13). Signs of chronic colitis, including mucin depletion and branching of colonic crypts, help differentiate UC from an acute enteritis (Kelts and Grand, 1980; Michener and Wyllie, 1990).

TREATMENT

Therapy for UC is primarily medical and directed at rapidly controlling acute attacks and subsequently maintaining remission. Available therapies are summarized in Table 34-15. Remission is achieved with a potent immunosuppressive agent such as prednisone and maintained with a 5-aminosalicylate derivative (e.g., sulfasalazine or olsalazine sodium [Dipentum]) (Michener and Wyllie, 1990). Corticosteroids must be given cautiously to children and adolescents because of their adverse effects on growth and bone development. Nutritional support may help sustain a patient during an acute flare but will not bring about disease remission. Cyclosporine has been used for patients with severe colitis in an attempt to postpone colectomy (Bousvaros et al., 2000; Ramakrishna et al., 1996; Treem et al., 1991). Oral tacrolimus has been used with favorable results in inducing remissions in steroid-refractory colitis, but it is less effective in maintenance of remissions (Bousvaros et al., 2000).

Surgery is performed in patients who do not respond to or have adverse effects with medical therapy or those who develop colonic epithelial dysplasia and thus are at risk for cancer. Colectomy is curative for patients with UC and may be preferable to protracted medical therapy with corticosteroids or other immunosuppressives.

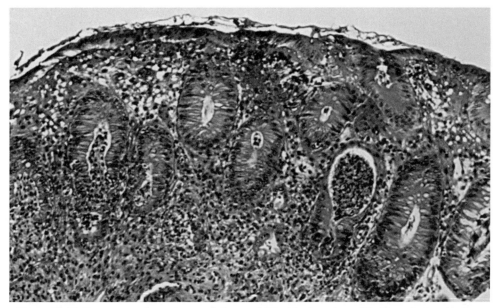

Figure 34-13 · Low-power photomicrograph from a child with ulcerative colitis. The colonic epithelium overlying the crypts is partially denuded, with evidence of mucus depletion in the goblet cells. Several crypt abscesses are present with associated necrosis. The lamina propria shows a dense infiltrate of neutrophils, lymphocytes, and plasma cells.

Crohn's Disease

In contrast to patients with UC, those with CD are more likely to present with protean or subtle symptoms, including growth failure, abdominal pain, anemia, or fever of unknown origin. The prominence of growth failure as a presenting feature of CD cannot be overemphasized. Studies suggest that 50% or more of the patients have short stature and growth retardation (Kirschner et al., 1978). Kanof and colleagues (1988a) retrospectively reviewed growth curves of pediatric patients with CD; one third had an appreciable falloff in height velocity 1 to 2 years before the onset of any gastrointestinal symptoms. The cause of growth failure is unknown, but it is probably decreased caloric intake,

although increased caloric requirements and intestinal malabsorption may be contributing causes. Lenaerts and co-workers (1989) found that one third of pediatric patients with CD had inflammation of the esophagus, stomach, or duodenum; thus upper gastrointestinal tract inflammation may result in the anorexia of CD.

Other atypical presentations of CD include isolated perianal disease, with recurrent skin tags and fistulas in the absence of any bowel disease. Biopsy of a perianal skin tag demonstrates a granuloma in up to 30% of cases. In addition, isolated orofacial granulomatosis may be associated with CD in the absence of any bowel involvement. Buccal swelling, mouth ulcers, cheilitis, and cervical adenopathy may be present and mistaken for symptoms of Melkersson-Rosenthal syndrome or hereditary angioedema (Williams et al., 1991). Granulomatous inflammation of the penis occasionally occurs (Ninan et al., 1992). Extraintestinal manifestations, including arthritis and dermatoses, may also occur; PSC is seen less frequently in CD than in UC.

DIAGNOSIS

The diagnosis is more difficult to establish in CD than in UC. All patients with suspected CD should have an upper gastrointestinal radiographic series with small-bowel followthrough to identify small-bowel nodularity, strictures, or ulceration. In addition, colonoscopy is recommended to look for focal colitis. Finally, consideration must be given to upper endoscopy or directed biopsy of oral or perianal lesions suspected to be lesions of CD. On occasion, the disease presents with acute right lower quadrant pain indistinguishable from that of appendicitis, and the diagnosis is made based on laparotomy; creeping mesenteric fat, adherent intestinal

- -
TABLE 34-15 · THERAPIES FOR CROHN'S DISEASE AND ULCERATIVE COLITIS

1. Corticosteroids
   Prednisone
   Topical steroid enemas
2. 5-Aminosalicylate derivatives
   Sulfasalazine
   Mesalamine
   Olsalazine
   5-Aminosalicylate enemas
3. Antibiotics
   Metronidazole
   Ciprofloxacin
4. Immunosuppressives
   6-Mercaptopurine
   Azathioprine
   Cyclosporine
5. Enteral nutrition
6. Surgery

serosa, and thickened ileum are observed during surgery.

Histologically, CD can be distinguished from UC by the presence of transmural inflammation with fissuring and by the presence of granulomas (Fig. 34-14). Granulomas are present in 50% of surgical resections and 25% of endoscopic biopsy specimens (Jackson and Grand, 1990).

TREATMENT

As with UC, therapy for CD is directed at controlling flares of disease activity. No medication has any proven efficacy in maintaining remission in CD (see Table 34-15). Prednisone has been used for the treatment of acute flares, but many patients are resistant to prednisone or have relapses when therapy is stopped. Accordingly, other immunosuppressive drugs have been used (Ruderman, 1990). In a randomized placebo-controlled crossover study, Present and colleagues (1980) demonstrated that 6-mercaptopurine induced remission and facilitated tapering of corticosteroid use in 70% of patients with active CD. In a similar study, Brynskov and co-workers (1989) used cyclosporine to treat steroid-refractory patients and found a 60% response rate. Oral tacrolimus has also been used with some success (Bousvaros et al., 2000). Cyclosporine works rapidly, with an onset of action within 1 month of initiation of therapy, compared with 3 months for 6-mercaptopurine. Although published experience with immunosuppressives in pediatric CD is limited, the results to date suggest an efficacy similar to that of adult studies (Bousvaros et al., 2000; Markowitz et al., 1990; Ramakrishna et al., 1996; Verhave et al., 1990).

Enteral nutrition is also important in the treatment of patients with CD, improving growth and promoting disease remission. In the recent past, parenteral nutrition was used to improve nutrition before surgery. It is now recognized that enteral nutrition with liquid formulas is equally efficacious for this purpose. Several studies have demonstrated the efficacy of an elemental diet delivered continuously by nasogastric tube to accelerate weight gain and growth velocity (Aiges et al., 1989; Belli et al., 1988; Greenberg et al., 1988; Kleinman et al., 1989). Elemental diets may also bring about disease remission and have been suggested as primary therapy for patients with disease flares (Morin et al., 1982; O'Morain et al., 1984; Sanderson et al., 1987). However, relapses occur quickly when the elemental diet is discontinued. In addition, the unpalatability of the elemental diet and the difficulty of nasogastric tube feeding of children have limited its widespread use. Patients with CD may also develop specific micronutrient deficiencies, including folate, zinc, and vitamin B_{12} deficiencies; therefore blood levels of these nutrients should be monitored (Michener and Wyllie, 1990).

Sulfasalazine and other 5-aminosalicylate (5-ASA) derivatives are commonly used for the treatment in Crohn's colitis. Newer enteric-coated salicylate preparations such as mesalamine (Pentasa) are designed for release into the small bowel, but their efficacy in small-bowel CD has not been established. Antibiotics have also been used. Metronidazole is a useful drug for mild Crohn's ileitis and is the drug of choice for perianal CD. However, its utility is limited because peripheral neuropathy may occur with long-term use (Peppercorn, 1990). Other antibiotics, including ampicillin, tetracycline, and ciprofloxacin, are reported to be efficacious but have not been subjected to controlled studies.

Surgery in CD, unlike in UC, is not curative and is accompanied by a high rate of clinical relapse (50% within 5 years). Surgery is therefore a treatment of last resort, reserved for complications such as stricture, fistula, abdominal abscess, or fulminant colitis. The length of small bowel resected should be as small as possible to minimize the risk of short-bowel syndrome. Data suggest that if surgery is well timed in prepubertal growth-

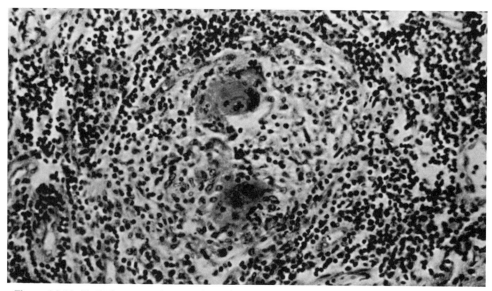

Figure 34-14 · Typical noncaseating granuloma found in Crohn's disease. Note the nodular shape of the lesion made up of epithelioid cells surrounding multinucleated giant cells.

Intestinal Lymphangiectasia

Intestinal lymphangiectasia refers to a primary or secondary impairment of lymphatic drainage variably associated with fat malabsorption and loss of serum proteins and lymphocytes (see Chapter 25). Primary intestinal lymphangiectasia results from lymphatic dysplasia and may occur as an isolated phenomenon or in association with thoracic lymphatic malformations (chylous ascites) or peripheral lymphedema (lymphedema praecox, Milroy's disease) (Hilliard et al., 1990).

In contrast, secondary intestinal lymphangiectasia results from obstruction of lymph flow from the lymphatics and into the heart and may be caused by intestinal inflammatory disorders, increased right-sided heart pressure (e.g., after a Fontan operation for congenital heart disease), obstruction of mesenteric lymphatic outflow (e.g., by intermittent bowel volvulus), or obstruction of the thoracic duct (e.g., by an intrathoracic tumor).

Pathogenesis

The resultant lymphatic obstruction leads to loss of serum proteins and lymphocytes from the bowel, villous blunting (Fig. 34-15), fat and fat-soluble vitamin malabsorption, hypoalbuminemia, hypocalcemia, abdominal pain, and growth failure (Fonkalsrud, 1977; Vardy

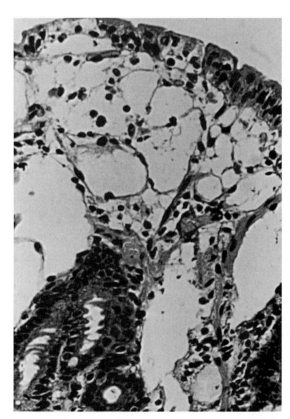

Figure 34-15 · Peroral small-intestinal biopsy specimen from a 2½-year-old patient with intestinal lymphangiectasia, manifested by chronic diarrhea, failure to thrive, hypoproteinemia, and lymphedema of one extremity. Villous architecture is distorted; distended lymphatic channels appear to be bursting through the epithelial cells.

et al., 1975). Immunologic abnormalities are present in severe cases of intestinal lymphangiectasia and are due to the loss of immunoglobulins and lymphocytes into the bowel. Although antibody synthesis remains normal, antibody titers are low because of increased losses (Strober et al., 1967). Defects in cell-mediated immunity include lymphopenia, decreased T-cell numbers, impaired in vitro responses to mitogens and specific antigens, cutaneous anergy, and diminished skin graft rejection (Weiden et al., 1972). Yamamoto and co-workers (1989) identified a patient in whom the peripheral blood was depleted of CD4 T cells, although normal numbers B cells were present; they postulated that this patient may have had a selective impairment of T-cell help.

Clinical Manifestations

The clinical severity of intestinal lymphangiectasia ranges from mild edema with hypoalbuminemia to severe malabsorption requiring parenteral nutrition. In severe cases, growth failure, steatorrhea, chylous ascites, and pleural or pericardial effusions develop. Less common intestinal complications include gastrointestinal bleeding and intestinal ileus (Lenzhofer et al., 1993; Perisic and Kokai, 1991). Despite lymphopenia and hypogammaglobulinemia, severe infections in these patients are rare. However, in one of our patients bacterial sepsis and peritonitis developed, and in another patient fatal fulminant sepsis developed.

Diagnosis

Laboratory studies show hypocalcemia, hypogammaglobulinemia, lymphopenia, and increased 72-hour fecal fat excretion. Radiographic contrast studies show thickened intestinal folds consistent with malabsorption in 50% of the patients. A fecal α_1-antitrypsin level is used to confirm the diagnosis of protein-losing enteropathy (Gleason, 1993). Small-bowel biopsy demonstrates dilated lacteals and distortion of the villous architecture (see Fig. 34-15); several biopsy specimens should be analyzed because of the patchy nature of the lesion.

Treatment

Treatment includes restricting dietary fat, monitoring and correcting deficiencies of fat-soluble vitamins, providing nutritional support, and managing peripheral edema. For infants, Portagen is the formula of choice because it contains no long-chain fat. However, a small amount of long-chain fat should be given enterally (as safflower oil or Lipomul) to prevent essential fatty acid deficiency (Holt, 1964). For older children, a fat-free diet with added medium-chain triglycerides reduces intestinal protein loss, edema, and ascites and corrects albumin and calcium deficiencies (Vardy et al., 1975). In patients with secondary lymphangiectasia, treatment of the underlying cause may reverse the intestinal abnormalities. Some patients with lymphangiectasia after a Fontan operation have improved with corticosteroid therapy (Rothman and Snyder, 1991). Patients with recurrent infections and hypogammaglobulinemia may benefit from intravenous immunoglobulin (IVIG) therapy; however, the half-life of IVIG in these patients is shortened because of intestinal loss.

Acrodermatitis Enteropathica

AE is an autosomal recessive disorder of zinc absorption, manifested in infancy by severe dermatitis, alopecia, diarrhea, and zinc deficiency (Van Wouwe, 1989; see Chapter 23). In addition to the congenital form, the term AE may be applied to secondary zinc deficiency states with similar clinical manifestations. Zinc deficiency in acrodermatitis was first described by Barnes and Moynahan in 1973. Others soon confirmed this observation and described a rapid therapeutic response to oral zinc (Michaelson, 1974; Moynahan, 1974; Nelder and Hambidge, 1975; Thyresson, 1974).

Pathogenesis

Patients with congenital AE have a negative zinc balance and reduced quantities of zinc in the small intestinal mucosa. Although the inherited molecular defect in acrodermatitis is unknown, patients have diminished zinc absorption with a normal diet. Zinc absorption improves when the intraluminal zinc concentration is increased by dietary supplementation.

Acquired zinc deficiency can result from inadequate intake, defective absorption, or excessive loss. Conditions associated with zinc deficiency include CD, intractable diarrhea of infancy, long-term parenteral nutrition with inadequate zinc, high-output ileostomy, celiac disease, and cystic fibrosis (Silverman and Roy, 1983). Infants with inborn errors of metabolism maintained with a nonanimal milk formula or other special formulas may become zinc deficient.

Zinc deficiency has profound effects on the immune system. In murine models, dietary zinc restriction causes thymic atrophy and depresses humoral responses through loss of helper T-cell function. Patients with AE demonstrate increased susceptibility to infection because of depressed humoral and cellular immunity (Good et al., 1979). Findings of autopsies in children demonstrate decreased lymphoid tissue (including Peyer's patches) and thymic abnormalities (Julius et al., 1973; Rodin and Goldman, 1969).

Golden and colleagues (1977, 1978) have shown that the T-cell immunodeficiency of protein-calorie malnutrition (PCM) is associated with zinc deficiency. One patient with acrodermatitis presented with selective IgG deficiency that resolved with zinc supplementation (Wilson et al., 1982). Zinc treatment for PCM enhances delayed cutaneous hypersensitivity and reverses thymic atrophy. However, the sera of patients with acrodermatitis may also contain autoantibodies (including antinuclear antibodies and rheumatoid factor), and these persist despite zinc supplementation (Anttila et al., 1986).

Clinical Manifestations

AE presents in infancy, usually between 4 and 10 weeks of age. The onset is delayed in breastfed infants but occurs several weeks after weaning. Principal findings include intensive acral and orofacial eczematous vesiculopustular dermatitis, progressive alopecia, and diarrhea. Stomatitis, glossitis, photophobia, corneal opacities, blepharitis, conjunctivitis, angular cheilitis with drooling, hoarseness, paronychia, nail dystrophy, and irritability may also occur. Secondary infection often complicates the illness. Secondary zinc deficiency resulting from chronic diarrhea may also cause immune abnormalities; in one case, there was a return of cell-mediated immunity after correction of the zinc deficiency (Oleske et al., 1979).

Diagnosis

The diagnosis of AE is based on the clinical features and the presence of abnormally low plasma levels of zinc (<50 µg/dl). Care must be taken to avoid contamination of the specimen, which can lead to falsely elevated zinc levels (Garretts and Molokhia, 1977). All tubing and glassware should be acid-washed and ordinary rubber stoppers avoided, because commercially available tubes and stoppers (e.g., Vacutainers) contain zinc. Zinc levels in hair are not reliable because they depend on normal growth; in acrodermatitis, hair growth is slow and hair zinc levels may be only slightly depressed. Urinary zinc levels are also abnormally low and return to normal within 2 to 3 weeks after therapy (Nelder and Hambidge, 1975). They correlate well with plasma levels and can be used to monitor therapy. Serum levels are falsely decreased in the presence of hypoalbuminemia. Serum alkaline phosphatase, a zinc-dependent enzyme, is abnormally low in patients with untreated acrodermatitis and returns to normal with zinc therapy.

Treatment

Oral zinc therapy results in both clinical remission and normalization of immune function (Weston et al., 1977). The daily dose of zinc sulfide recommended is 30 to 45 mg (Lungarotti et al., 1976; Silverman and Roy, 1983). No side effects of therapy have been reported.

Prognosis

Oral zinc supplementation must be continued indefinitely in the inborn disorder. Skin improvement begins within several days, with complete healing in weeks. Diarrhea resolves rapidly (1 week), and hair growth recommences within 2 to 3 weeks (Nelder et al., 1978). The prognosis is favorable with therapy, whereas if the patient remains untreated, malnutrition and death may occur, usually by 3 years of age.

Selective IgA Deficiency

Selective IgA deficiency is the most common primary immunodeficiency, with a prevalence as high as 1 in 500 humans (see Chapter 14). The most common gastrointestinal infection associated with IgA deficiency is giardiasis, which may lead to partial villous atrophy and secondary malabsorption (Cunningham-Rundles, 1988; Morgan and Levinsky, 1988; Zinneman and Kaplan, 1972) (Table 34-20). Diagnosis of giardiasis may be difficult; even three stool examinations may miss up to 10% of cases. An ELISA test for *Giardia* antigen that has become available may increase the sensitivity of detection to 98% (Addiss et al., 1991). For the patient in whom giardiasis is suspected but not found, a string test (sampling duodenal fluid by oral ingestion of a string-coated capsule, followed by withdrawal of the string), endoscopy for duodenal aspirate, or an empirical trial of antibiotic therapy should be considered.

Metronidazole, tinidazole, furazolidone, and quinacrine are effective antibiotics for giardiasis, with cure rates in nonimmunocompromised hosts of 60% to 95% (Shepherd and Boreham, 1989). Patients with IgA deficiency often have recurrences, necessitating repeated treatment or treatment of family members and pets. Bacterial overgrowth has also been reported in association with selective IgA deficiency (Pignata et al., 1990).

Patients with selective IgA deficiency have a 10-fold relative risk of developing celiac disease; conversely, 1 in 200 patients with celiac disease has selective IgA deficiency (Collin et al., 1992; Cunningham-Rundles, 1988). Because the antiendomysial antibody used in the diagnosis of celiac disease is an IgA molecule, this test may miss the diagnosis in patients with selective IgA deficiency and celiac disease; in contrast, the IgG class antireticulin antibodies are positive in 94% of patients (Collin et al., 1992). It is unknown whether the increased incidence of celiac disease in patients with selective IgA deficiency represents genetic linkage of two diseases or whether the defect in IgA secretion predisposes to celiac disease. Rarely, idiopathic villous atrophy without celiac disease is seen in patients with selective IgA deficiency.

Food and systemic allergy may also be present in patients with selective IgA deficiency (Ammann and Hong, 1971). Patients have high titers of serum antibodies to milk, as well as increased circulating immune complexes after milk ingestion (Buckley and Dees, 1969; Cunningham-Rundles et al., 1978). However, there is no correlation between these abnormalities and clinical allergy (Cunningham-Rundles, 1988). Lymphoid nodular hyperplasia and sarcoidosis have also been associated with IgA deficiency (Disdier et al., 1991). Finally, there is an increased risk for the development of certain cancers, particularly lymphoma and gastric adenocarcinoma (Cunningham-Rundles et al., 1980).

X-Linked Agammaglobulinemia

X-linked agammaglobulinemia presents with recurrent infections in male infants after 9 months of age as a result of failure of synthesis of all classes of immunoglobulins (see Chapter 13). In a review of 96 patients, Lederman and Winkelstein (1985) found otitis media, sinusitis, pneumonitis, infectious diarrheas, meningitis, and oligoarticular arthritis to be common complications. Furthermore, 10% of patients developed chronic diarrhea, with rotavirus, *Giardia lamblia, Salmonella,* and enteropathogenic *E. coli* the identified pathogens. Other causes of chronic enteritis in patients with X-linked agammaglobulinemia include bacterial overgrowth, *Campylobacter, Cryptosporidium,* coxsackievirus, and poliovirus (Arbo and Santos, 1987; Lederman and Winkelstein, 1985).

An association with sclerosing cholangitis and sprue-like illness has also been noted, but it is unclear whether autoimmune disease is actually increased in these patients (Sisto et al., 1987; Stiehm et al., 1986). In older patients, amyloidosis, atrophic gastritis, pernicious anemia, and gastric adenocarcinomas are seen (Lavilla et al., 1993; Meysman et al., 1993).

Transient Hypogammaglobulinemia of Infancy

Transient hypogammaglobulinemia of infancy is prolonged and exaggerated symptomatic physiologic hypogammaglobulinemia (see Chapters 13 and 22) affecting children between 1 and 3 years of age. This disorder is characterized by low levels of serum IgG or IgG subclasses; IgA or IgM levels may also be decreased. McGeady (1987) has postulated that some of these children develop persistent hypogammaglobulinemia or selective IgA deficiency.

Perlmutter and colleagues (1985) reported 55 patients with transient hypogammaglobulinemia and diarrhea; lactose intolerance, *G. lamblia* infestation, and *C. difficile* infection were frequently identified. Recurrent *C. difficile* infection is particularly difficult to manage in these children and causes either pseudomembranous enterocolitis or chronic diarrhea with failure to thrive (Sutphen et al., 1983). In a survey of 43 infants

---

TABLE 34-20 · GASTROINTESTINAL MANIFESTATIONS OF IMMUNOGLOBULIN A DEFICIENCY

1. None (majority of patients)
2. *Giardia lamblia* infestation (often recurrent)
3. Nodular lymphoid hyperplasia
4. Nonspecific enteropathy ± bacterial overgrowth ± disaccharidase deficiency
5. Increased incidence of circulating antibodies to food antigens
6. Gluten-sensitive enteropathy
7. Pernicious anemia/atrophic gastritis/increased risk of gastric cancer
8. Idiopathic inflammatory bowel disease (Crohn's disease, ulcerative colitis)

and children with *C. difficile* infection, 35% had hypogammaglobulinemia (Gryboski et al., 1991). Patients with hypogammaglobulinemia may lack the ability to make antibodies to *C. difficile* toxin A, the putative mediator of the enteropathy in *C. difficile* colitis (Leung et al., 1991; Triadafilopoulos et al., 1987).

Of patients with transient hypogammaglobulinemia, 50% have histologic small-bowel enteritis, ranging from mild inflammation to complete villous atrophy. Antibiotic therapy or a lactose-free diet benefits those with identifiable microbial pathogens or lactose intolerance. For patients with *C. difficile* infection, vancomycin or metronidazole is used. Recurrence of *C. difficile* infection occurs in 20% to 30% of patients and can be treated with a prolonged, tapering course of vancomycin (Peterson and Gerding, 1990). In addition, IVIG may help prevent recurrences in the immunodeficient patient (Leung et al., 1991). Otherwise, chronic diarrhea may persist for 18 months, and other therapies are rarely necessary (Perlmutter et al., 1985). Some patients have recurrent systemic infections and may benefit from regular IVIG infusions (Benderly et al., 1986; Kosnik et al., 1986).

Common Variable Immunodeficiency

Common variable immunodeficiency (CVID) has an onset in late childhood or adulthood and is characterized by low levels of IgG and the other immunoglobulin classes (see Chapter 13). Recurrent otitis media, bronchitis, pneumonia, and sinusitis are the most common presenting features, but gastrointestinal disease occurs in up to 70% of patients and accounts for much morbidity (Table 34-21) (Hausser et al., 1983). The enteropathy can be either infectious or autoimmune (Sperber and Mayer, 1988).

Giardia is the most common gastrointestinal infectious agent, but *Salmonella, Campylobacter, Cryptosporidium,* or rotavirus may also be implicated (Sperber and Mayer, 1988; Webster, 1980). Nodular lymphoid hyperplasia, defined as multiple discrete lymphoid aggregates in the stomach and small bowel, is detected radiographically or endoscopically in up to 20% of patients and may predispose to either malabsorption or gastrointestinal bleeding (Bastlein et al., 1988; Bennett et al., 1987). Massive nodular lymphoid hyperplasia may develop and be difficult to distinguish from lymphoma. Sander and co-workers (1992), using techniques of in situ hybridization for Epstein-Barr virus and immunohistochemical staining for clonality, concluded that most lymphoid lesions in patients with CVID were benign and not associated with Epstein-Barr virus infection. However, 2 of their 17 patients developed malignant lymphoma. One patient with nodular lymphoid hyperplasia had a clonal B-cell population, but after 4 years of observation, lymphoma has not developed, suggesting that clonality does not necessarily result in malignancy (Laszewski et al., 1990).

An association between CVID and celiac disease exists, but the risk is less than that for patients with selective IgA deficiency (Webster et al., 1981). Idiopathic sprue with subtotal villous atrophy is also reported in patients with no infections and is generally unresponsive to a gluten-free diet (Catassi et al., 1988; Conley et al., 1986). This *hypogammaglobulinemic sprue* is characterized by decreased brush border enzyme activity and lactose intolerance (Dawson et al., 1986).

A granulomatous enteropathy with granulomas scattered throughout the intestine has been reported in adults with CVID (Mike et al., 1991). Patients have a high incidence of gastritis and pernicious anemia–like syndrome, without antibodies to intrinsic factor, gastric parietal cells, or thyroglobulin (Twomey et al., 1970). Other gastrointestinal abnormalities include bacterial overgrowth, aphthous stomatitis, cholelithiasis, malakoplakia, and IBD (Sperber and Mayer, 1988). Severe malabsorption associated with enteropathy in patients with CVID may result in hyperoxaluria, vitamin B_{12} deficiency, and caloric deprivation and may require parenteral nutrition (Bennett et al., 1987).

Hyper-IgM Type 1 Syndrome

Immunodeficiency with hyper-IgM type 1 (HIGM1) is characterized by high serum IgM levels, low IgG and IgA levels, recurrent infections, intermittent leukopenia, lymphoid hyperplasia, and autoimmune disorders (see Chapter 13). Patients with HIGM1 have recurrent oral ulcers and gingivitis (particularly when they are leukopenic) and less commonly have chronic diarrhea and lymphoid nodular hyperplasia. The lymphoid nodular hyperplasia may be massive enough to cause a functional colon obstruction and require steroid therapy. Esophageal histoplasmosis and small-bowel cryptosporidiosis have also been reported (Stiehm et al., 1986; Tu et al., 1991).

Severe Combined Immunodeficiency

Patients with all types of severe combined immunodeficiency (SCID) have profound antibody and T-cell immune defects and present in the first months of life with chronic diarrhea, failure to thrive, and persistent viral or fungal infections (see Chapter 15, 16, and 41). Gastrointestinal illness occurs in 90% of these patients, and intractable diarrhea and oral thrush are common presenting features. Organisms commonly associated

---

TABLE 34-21 · GASTROINTESTINAL MANIFESTATION OF COMMON VARIABLE IMMUNODEFICIENCY

1. Infectious diarrhea (*Giardia*, bacterial, viral)
2. Bacterial overgrowth syndrome
3. Pernicious anemia/atrophic gastritis/gastric carcinoma
4. Nodular lymphoid hyperplasia
5. Gluten-sensitive enteropathy
6. Nonspecific enteropathy/colitis

with illness include rotavirus, *Candida*, cytomegalovirus, and *E. coli*. Chronic viral infection is the most common cause of enteritis (Stephan et al., 1992). Jarvis and co-workers (1983) isolated viral pathogens from the stool in 9 of 12 patients with SCID and chronic diarrhea; the viruses identified included rotavirus, picornavirus, adenovirus type 5, and coxsackievirus A. The viral enteritis was partially or directly responsible for death in 80% of cases. Other, less common causes of enteropathy noted include *Salmonella, Shigella,* and *Cryptosporidium* infections. Although candidiasis rarely involves the intestine, candidal esophagitis should be suspected in infants with SCID who have decreased oral intake (Arbo and Santos, 1987; Stiehm et al., 1986).

In some patients with SCID, enteropathy or colitis occurs in the absence of identifiable infection. Some investigators have postulated that this is an immune-mediated enteritis (S. Strobel, personal communication); however, antienterocyte antibodies or antinuclear cytoplasmic antibodies have not been described in patients with SCID. Gilger and colleagues (1992) used immunostaining to look for extraintestinal rotavirus infection in infants with SCID. Rotaviral particles were found in the kidney and liver of four patients, leading the investigators to postulate that rotavirus may also cause systemic illness.

Bare Lymphocyte Syndrome (MHC Class II Defect)

Another cause of profound cellular immunodeficiency phenotypically similar to SCID is the bare lymphocyte syndrome, the absence of MHC class II molecules on the surface of immune cells (see Chapter 15). In a review of 30 patients with the syndrome (Klein et al., 1993; Touraine et al., 1992), almost all had some form of gastrointestinal illness. Gastrointestinal candidiasis was present in 25 patients, and giardiasis, cryptosporidiosis, and other bacterial enteritides were present. In addition, a high incidence of hepatobiliary abnormalities was noted. Ten patients had evidence of biliary tract disease, including sclerosing cholangitis in four patients (associated with biliary cryptosporidiosis in three of the four). Bacterial cholangitis involving *Pseudomonas, Enterococcus,* and *Streptococcus* was also seen.

Combined Immunodeficiency with Predominant T-Cell Defect

Commonly referred to as *Nezelof syndrome* or *cellular immunodeficiency with immunoglobulins,* combined immunodeficiency with predominant T-cell defect is characterized by absent T-cell function and a variable B-cell defect with some serum immunoglobulin production (Nezelof, 1968) (see Chapter 15). Some of these patients present in late infancy and childhood; others present in early infancy. The literature has limited information regarding their gastrointestinal complications. One older child with a mild variant of Nezelof syn-

drome presented with recurrent chest infections and chronic malabsorption; a mucosal biopsy demonstrated villous atrophy and a mucosal plasma cell infiltrate (Novis et al., 1985).

Chronic Mucocutaneous Candidiasis

Chronic mucocutaneous candidiasis (CMC) is characterized by a diminished T-cell response to candidal antigens and severe local candidiasis. Infants may present with persistent thrush or candidal dermatitis, failure to thrive, and dystrophic nails (see Chapter 17). The principal gastrointestinal complication is candidal esophagitis, which may result in food refusal (Kirkpatrick, 1989). In a series of 43 patients, chronic active hepatitis and giardiasis developed in 5% of the patients (Herrod, 1990). A polyglandular endocrinopathy syndrome characterized by hypoparathyroidism, hypothyroidism, adrenal insufficiency, and pernicious anemia develops in up to 70% of older children. Malabsorption associated with pancreatic insufficiency contributes to the poor weight gain in 10% of patients and requires pancreatic enzyme supplementation (Herrod, 1990).

Chronic Granulomatous Disease

Chronic granulomatous disease (CGD) is caused by an inability of the patient's phagocytes to generate superoxide, leading to infections with catalase-positive organisms, including *Staphylococcus aureus, Serratia, Aspergillus,* and *Nocardia* (Lehrer et al., 1988) (see Chapter 20). The clinical syndrome includes recurrent infections, multifocal abscesses affecting the skin and liver, lymphadenopathy, hepatosplenomegaly, chronic lung disease, and diarrhea.

Small-bowel involvement with inflammatory cells may mimic that in CD, with diarrhea, protein-losing enteropathy, pancolitis, small-bowel obstruction, and fistulizing disease. Multifocal abscesses, giant cells, and noncaseating granulomatous colitis are present on endoscopic biopsy specimens of patients who have colonic inflammation (Isaacs et al., 1985; Werlin et al., 1982). The presence of lipid-containing histiocytes in the mucosa and submucosa of colon biopsy specimens suggests CGD rather than CD (Lindahl et al., 1984; Werlin et al., 1982).

The colitis of patients with CGD may respond to therapy with sulfasalazine or interferon-γ, but surgical resection may be necessary for intractable colitis or acute obstruction (Ezekowitz et al., 1991). High dosages of steroids have also been used to treat patients with intestinal or urinary tract obstruction (Chin et al., 1987).

Leukocyte Adhesion Defect Type 1

Patients with leukocyte adhesion defect type I (LADI) have impaired phagocytic function related to deficiencies of adhesion molecules (CD18/Mac-1) necessary for cell migration and interactions (see Chapters 5 and 20). Necrotic infections of the skin (including pyoderma gangrenosum) and mucous membranes, otitis media, and episodes of microbial sepsis are the principal features (Anderson and Springer, 1987; Voss and Rhodes, 1992). Gastrointestinal complications include intraoral infections and periodontitis, candidal esophagitis, gastritis, appendicitis, NEC, and perirectal abscess (Anderson and Springer, 1987; Roberts and Atkinson, 1990; Todd and Freyer, 1988). Fatal NEC developed in one child at 18 months of age (Hawkins et al., 1992). Therapy includes antibiotic therapy for infections and bone marrow transplantation in severe cases.

Glycogen Storage Disease Type 1b

Patients who have glycogen storage disease (GSD) type 1b present with severe hypoglycemia, failure to thrive, and hepatomegaly (see Chapters 20 and 24). In contrast to those with von Gierke's disease (GSD type 1a), these patients have severe neutropenia and phagocytic dysfunction (Gitzelmann and Bosshard, 1993). GSD type 1a is characterized biochemically by absence of glucose-6-phosphatase activity, and GSD type 1b is characterized by absence of the hepatic glucose-6-phosphate transport protein (Nordlie et al., 1993).

The primary intestinal complication of patients with GSD type 1b is an idiopathic colitis clinically indistinguishable from that in CD (Couper et al., 1991; Roe et al., 1986). The intestinal manifestations develop in late childhood or adolescence and include oral ulceration, perianal infections, anemia, and transmural colonic inflammation with stricturing. This colitis, as well as that in CGD and congenital neutropenia, has led Couper and colleagues (1991) to speculate that neutrophil deficiency or dysfunction predisposes to granulomatous colitis.

Indeed, Roe and co-workers (1992) used granulocyte-macrophage colony-stimulating factor (GM-CSF) in the treatment of two patients with GSD type 1b and noted increased neutrophil counts, decreased sedimentation rates, and decreased bowel inflammation, which suggests that raising the neutrophil count may have a beneficial effect on the bowel lesion.

IMMUNE DISORDERS OF THE LIVER AND BILE DUCTS

Hepatic inflammation arises as an immune response against infectious agents (e.g., in viral hepatitis) or against self-antigens (e.g., in autoimmune chronic active hepatitis). A discussion of viral or other infectious hepatitides can be found elsewhere (Alter and Sampliner, 1989; Balistreri, 1988; Hoofnagle, 1990; Koff, 1993; Krugman, 1992). A partial list of diseases causing chronic hepatitis is given in Table 34-22. We focus on two immune-mediated disorders seen in pediatric patients: autoimmune chronic active hepatitis and primary sclerosing cholangitis (PSC).

TABLE 34-22 · CAUSES OF CHRONIC ACTIVE HEPATITIS

Autoimmune
Type I and type II

Virus-Associated
Hepatitis B
Hepatitis C
Delta hepatitis
Human immunodeficiency virus

Metabolic
Wilson's disease
α_1-Antitrypsin deficiency
Hemochromatosis

Primary Hepatobiliary Disorders
Primary biliary cirrhosis
Sclerosing cholangitis

Drug-Related
Alcoholic liver disease
Alpha-methyldopa
Isoniazid
Phenothiazines
Oxyphenacetin
Nitrofurantoin
Halothane
Sulfonamides
Propylthiouracil

Miscellaneous
Nonalcoholic steatohepatitis

Chronic Active Hepatitis

Chronic active hepatitis (CAH) is a progressive, destructive inflammatory disease characterized by portal tract infiltration with mononuclear cells and destruction of the limiting plate of hepatocytes surrounding the portal tract. In advanced cases, strands of fibrous tissue connecting portal triads (bridging fibrosis), ultimately progressing to macronodular or micronodular cirrhosis, are present (Fig. 34-16). CAH may occur as a result of viral infection, toxin or drug exposure, metabolic disease, or autoimmune hepatitis (see Table 34-22). Autoimmune CAH is characterized by an extensive periportal hepatic infiltrate, the presence of antibodies against different hepatocyte antigens, association with certain HLA antigens, autoimmune diseases, and a good response to immunosuppressive therapy.

Classification

Autoimmune CAH has now been classified into two major types based on clinical features and the types of antibody present (Table 34-23). Type I autoimmune CAH (formerly designated *classical CAH* or *lupoid CAH*) occurs predominantly in young women (often in the second or third decade of life) and is characterized by hypergammaglobulinemia and by antibodies to the cytoskeletal protein F-actin (i.e., anti–smooth muscle antibodies).

In contrast, type II autoimmune CAH occurs predominantly in young children and adolescents. It is characterized by the presence of antibodies to the corticosteroid responsive but in which antibodies to liver antigens are not present (Czaja et al., 1993a).

Pathogenesis

Like other autoimmune disorders, autoimmune CAH tends to occur in genetically susceptible individuals with an aberrant response to target tissue (in this case, the hepatocytes and biliary epithelium). A genetic predisposition to autoimmune CAH can be identified in one third of European and American patients; type I autoimmune CAH has been associated with two HLA types: HLA-A1/B8/DR3 and HLA-DR4 (Czaja et al., 1993b; Donaldson et al., 1991). Autoimmune CAH associated with HLA-DR4 tends to occur in older patients and is more responsive to corticosteroid therapy, but it is unclear whether there is a better long-term prognosis. Japanese patients with autoimmune CAH are more likely to have the HLA-DR4 allele (Maddrey, 1993; Seki et al., 1990).

Many believe that hepatitis C is an important trigger for type II autoimmune CAH. Lenzi and co-workers (1990, 1991) found that 88% of patients with autoimmune CAH type II (with positive anti–LKM-1 antibody) had evidence of prior hepatitis C infection.

Manns (1991) demonstrated a 50% incidence of hepatitis C infection in type II autoimmune CAH, compared with a 0% incidence in type I autoimmune CAH. However, Vergani and Mieli-Vergani (1993) found no association with hepatitis C infection in British patients with autoimmune CAH, leading them to speculate that there is geographic and genetic heterogeneity in autoimmune CAH.

There is even less information on what agents trigger inflammation in type I autoimmune CAH. Vento and co-workers (1991) prospectively monitored 58 healthy relatives of 13 patients with autoimmune CAH type I. Two of the 58 subjects who contracted mild hepatitis A developed type I autoimmune CAH within 5 months of infection. Therefore hepatitis A may be a risk factor for type I autoimmune CAH in genetically predisposed individuals (Vento et al., 1991).

Several authors have postulated that antibodies to actin, cytochromes, and other liver components are important in the immune-mediated liver damage, either

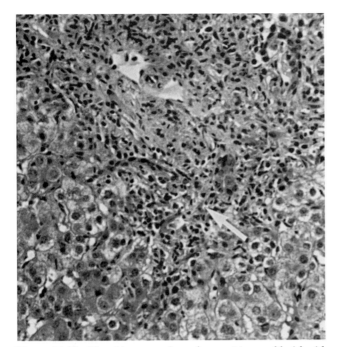

Figure 34-16 · Liver biopsy specimen from a 14-year-old girl with chronic active hepatitis unassociated with hepatitis B. The portal tract area is enlarged and demonstrates fibrosis *(upper center)*. Infiltration of the portal tract by lymphocytes and plasma cells extends beyond the limiting plate, causing piecemeal necrosis *(arrow)*. Hepatocytes surrounding the portal zone demonstrate moderate swelling. (×250.) (Courtesy of P. Brochu, M.D., Montreal, Canada.)

cytochrome P450 component IID6 (anti–liver-kidney microsomal antibodies, anti–LKM-1) (Boyer and Reuben, 1993; Johnson et al., 1991). Both disorders are associated with other autoimmune illness (including thyroiditis, diabetes, and vitiligo), and both respond to immunosuppressive therapy. However, initial reports suggest that type II autoimmune CAH may have a worse prognosis, with 80% progression to cirrhosis after 3 years (Homberg et al., 1987).

Because antibodies to several different liver antigens have been discovered, it is likely that other variants of autoimmune CAH exist (see later discussion). In addition, a form of CAH has been described that is histologically similar to autoimmune CAH and is

TABLE 34-23 · ANTIBODIES PRESENT IN AUTOIMMUNE CHRONIC ACTIVE HEPATITIS (CAH)

Antibody	Antigen	Disease	Comments
Anti–smooth muscle	P-Actin	CAH type I	Also seen in primary biliary cirrhosis
Anti–liver-kidney microsome 1 (anti–LKM-1)	Cytochrome P_{450} IID6	CAH type II	Predominantly in European children, possible association with hepatitis C
Anti–LKM-2	Cytochrome P_{450}-8	Ticrynafen-induced hepatitis	
Anti–LKM-3	Unknown	Delta virus hepatitis (hepatitis D)	
Antinuclear antibodies (ANA)	Nuclear histones	CAH type I	Nonspecific finding
Anti–soluble liver antigen (anti-SLA)	Hepatocyte cytoplasmic protein	CAH type I Other CAH	Seen in CAH I, may also define a third type of CAH

Data from Maddrey WC. How many types of autoimmune hepatitis are there? Gastroenterology 105:1571–1575, 1993; and Johnson PJ, McFarlane IG, Eddleston AL. The natural course and heterogeneity of chronic active hepatitis. Semin Liver Dis 11:187–196, 1991.

directly or through antibody-dependent cytotoxicity (MacFarlane, 1991; Manns, 1991). The nature and significance of the T-cell infiltrate in autoimmune CAH have not yet been determined. Schlaak and colleagues (1993) isolated and cloned the T cells from liver tissues of patients with autoimmune CAH and found the predominant clones isolated to be IL-4–producing CD4 T cells. In contrast, Li and co-workers (1991), analyzing hepatic T cells from liver tissue in a variety of liver diseases, found the proportion of CD8 cells to be increased in autoimmune CAH compared with viral hepatitis.

Clinical Manifestations

Both type I and type II autoimmune CAH are associated with a pronounced female (ranging from 4:1 to 10:1) predominance. Presenting symptoms include fatigue, weakness, jaundice, pruritus, abdominal pain or hepatic tenderness, amenorrhea, arthritis, or rash (Czaja, 1991). Type II autoimmune CAH tends to occur in younger children, whereas type I autoimmune CAH occurs in adolescents and adults; however, there is extensive overlap in the ages of presentation.

Both disorders are associated with other autoimmune disorders, including thyroiditis, diabetes, immune thrombocytopenia purpura, rheumatoid arthritis, IBDs, and hemolytic anemia. Associated autoimmune disease is probably more common in type II autoimmune CAH, occurring in up to 35% of these patients (Homberg et al., 1987).

On physical examination, jaundice, hepatosplenomegaly, acne, palmar erythema, and spider angiomas may be seen; patients with more advanced cases may have ascites or encephalopathy. The serum bilirubin level is usually elevated. Transaminase activities are often 10-fold above normal and commonly exceed 1000 IU/L; alanine aminotransferase activity is usually higher than aspartate aminotransferase activity. In contrast to enzyme levels in PSC, the alkaline phosphatase activity is less elevated than the transaminase activities (Fitzgerald, 1982). Hypergammaglobulinemia is usually pronounced, and in type I autoimmune CAH, the serum IgG level may exceed 4000 mg/dl (Odievre et al., 1983).

Diagnosis

Diagnosis is made by excluding other causes of chronic hepatitis, particularly viral and metabolic liver disease (including Wilson's disease); by determining the presence of specific autoantibodies; by demonstrating a pattern consistent with autoimmune CAH by liver biopsy; and by finding a good response to immunosuppressive therapy. Serologic testing for hepatitis A, B, and C; cytomegalovirus; and Epstein-Barr virus should be done for all patients. To exclude Wilson's disease, ophthalmologic examination for Kayser-Fleischer rings and tests for serum ceruloplasmin and 24-hour urinary copper should be performed, taking into account the fact that copper excretion may be increased in some forms

of chronic liver disease. Deficiency of α_1-antitrypsin should be excluded by obtaining a serum α_1-antitrypsin level and protease inhibitor phenotype. Antinuclear antibody, anti–smooth muscle antibody, and anti–liver-kidney microsomal antibody testing should be performed; the presence of antimitochondrial antibodies may suggest primary biliary cirrhosis. Finally, a liver biopsy should be obtained before starting therapy; this demonstrates a periportal infiltrate of lymphocytes and plasma cells, necrosis of hepatocytes, and in advanced disease, fibrosis or cirrhosis.

Treatment

As soon as the diagnosis is established, therapy should be instituted to slow progression of liver disease. Traditionally, hepatitis must be present for longer than 6 months to be termed *chronic* hepatitis. However, if the clinical picture, serologic testing, and biopsy findings are consistent with autoimmune CAH, it is unwise to delay therapy. Patients receive corticosteroids alone or corticosteroids plus azathioprine (Arasu et al., 1979; Czaja, 1991; Maggiore et al., 1984). A clinical and biochemical response usually occurs within a month, with resolution of fatigue and jaundice, falling transaminase levels, declining levels of IgG, and declining autoimmune antibody levels. Relapse may occur in up to 85% of pediatric patients when steroids are tapered (Maggiore et al., 1984). In adults, a randomized trial showed that azathioprine alone was efficacious in preventing relapse after steroids were tapered (Stellon et al., 1988).

Prognosis

Despite the good initial response to therapy, the long-term prognosis for patients with both type I and type II autoimmune CAH remains guarded. In one series of patients with type I autoimmune CAH, 30% of the patients had cirrhosis upon initial presentation and the 5-year mortality was 13% despite therapy (Keating et al., 1987). Of patients with type II autoimmune CAH, 80% developed cirrhosis within 3 years and mortality was 20% (Homberg et al., 1987). Liver transplantation is of value for patients with autoimmune CAH with advanced liver disease, and recurrence in the transplanted liver is rare.

Primary Sclerosing Cholangitis

PSC is an idiopathic inflammatory disease of the extrahepatic and intrahepatic bile ducts that ultimately results in biliary scarring and stricturing, cholestasis, and hepatic cirrhosis. PSC must be differentiated from chronic cholangitis associated with infectious agents (e.g., cytomegalovirus or *Cryptosporidium*), particularly in patients with HIV infection. Although the pathogenesis of PSC is poorly understood, the association of PSC with IBD and immunodeficiency syndromes in pediatrics suggests an immunologic cause.

Pathophysiology

Suggested causes of PSC include low-grade biliary bacterial infection, abnormal bile acid metabolism, accumulation of a toxin (e.g., copper), viral infection, or ischemia. Another hypothesis suggests that immune-mediated damage to the bile duct occurs in patients with a genetic predisposition. The latter hypothesis is the most likely because toxic, bacterial, or viral causes of biliary injury have largely been excluded (Lindor et al., 1990). The occurrence of PSC in multiple family members suggests a genetic predisposition (Jorge et al., 1987; Quigley et al., 1983). In patients with UC who have the HLA-B8 and HLA-DR3 (DRB1*0301) phenotype, the risk for development of PSC is increased 10-fold (Shepherd et al., 1983). PSC is also associated with HLA-DRW52a (DRB3*0101) and HLA-DR2 (Eddleston and Williams, 1978; Prochazka et al., 1990).

Several humoral and cellular immune abnormalities have been discovered in patients with PSC (Table 34-24). Because most patients with PSC have an associated disease (e.g., UC or histiocytosis), it is difficult to determine whether the reported abnormalities are associated with PSC or with the underlying disease (Chapman, 1991). The best-characterized serum abnormality in patients with PSC is the presence of p-ANCA. About 75% to 90% of patients with PSC have p-ANCA in their serum (Duerr et al., 1991; Mulder et al., 1993; Seibold et al., 1992). This finding is not specific to PSC, because ANCA can also be seen in those with UC or autoimmune CAH (Mulder et al., 1993). The percentage of those expressing ANCA decreases to 40% in patients with PSC without IBD (Seibold et al., 1992).

The liver of patients with PSC demonstrates enhanced expression of MHC class II antigens on biliary tract epithelium, suggesting exchanged antigen presentation or interferon-γ production (Chapman et al., 1988).

Increased numbers of CD8 cells are present in the hepatic and portal infiltrate of patients with PSC (Senaldi et al., 1992); if these cells are cytotoxic T cells, they could cause the observed damage to the biliary tract epithelium.

Clinical Manifestations

PSC can occur at any age; one pediatric series at a large tertiary referral center included 56 cases in 29 years (Debray et al., 1994). Patients may be completely asymptomatic, and the disease may be suspected only because of biochemical abnormalities in high-risk patients (Porayko et al., 1990). Alternatively, patients may present with intermittent jaundice, right upper quadrant abdominal pain, fever, fatigue, weight loss, xanthomas, or ascites. Certain disorders place the pediatric patient at high risk for PSC (Table 34-25). The principal risk factor for the older adolescent is IBD; 1% to 2% of patients with UC develop PSC, and 50% of adults with PSC have IBD. Other associated conditions include histiocytosis X, immunodeficiencies (both cellular and humoral), sickle cell anemia, and psoriasis (Debray et al., 1994; Mowat, 1987a; Sisto et al., 1987).

Diagnosis

Laboratory tests for patients with PSC suggest chronic cholestasis and hepatitis; classically, elevations of alkaline phosphatase and gamma-glutamyl transpeptidase exceed elevations of transaminases. Other signs of cholestasis, including a prolonged prothrombin time, may be seen. Anti–smooth muscle antibodies and antimitochondrial antibodies may be present in a few

TABLE 34-24 · ABNORMALITIES IN PRIMARY SCLEROSING CHOLANGITIS

Abnormality	References
Peripheral Blood	
Perinuclear antineutrophil cytoplasmic antibodies (p-ANCA)	Seibold et al., 1992 Mulder et al., 1993 Duerr et al., 1991
Hypergammaglobulinemia	Chapman et al., 1980 Mowat, 1987a
Antinuclear antibodies	Zauli et al., 1987
Immune complexes	Bodenheimer et al., 1983
Decreased suppressor/cytotoxic (CD8+) cells	Lindor et al., 1987a Snook et al., 1989
Enhanced T-lymphocyte autoreactivity	Lindor et al., 1987b
Tissue	
Increased biliary HLA-DR expression	Chapman et al., 1988 Broome et al., 1990
Inappropriate biliary expression of blood group antigens A and B	Bloom et al., 1993
Increased T lymphocytes	Whiteside et al., 1985
Increased suppressor/cytotoxic (CD8+)	Senaldi et al., 1992
Increased macrophages	

HLA = human leukocyte antigen.

TABLE 34-25 · DISEASES ASSOCIATED WITH PRIMARY SCLEROSING CHOLANGITIS IN CHILDREN AND ADULTS

Inflammatory bowel disease
Histiocytosis X
Cystic fibrosis
Autoimmune, hemolytic anemia
Sickle cell disease
Lupus erythematosus
Vasculitis
Thyroiditis
Celiac disease
Bronchiectasis
Psoriasis
Pancreatitis
Rheumatoid arthritis
Reticular cell sarcoma
Immunodeficiency
    X-linked agammaglobulinemia
    Hyper–immunoglobulin M immunodeficiency
    Pure cellular immunodeficiency
    Combined humoral and cellular immunodeficiency

Data from Sisto A, Feldman P, Garel L, Seidman E, Brochu P, Morin C, Weber AM, Roy CC. Primary scerosing cholangitis in children: study of five cases and review of the literature. Pediatrics 80:918–923, 1987; Debray D, Pariente D, Urvoas E, Hadchouel M, Bernard O. Sclerosing cholangitis in children. J Pediatr 124:49–56, 1994; and Wiesner RH. Primary sclerosing cholangitis. In Schiff L, Schiff ER, eds. Diseases of the Liver, ed 7. Philadelphia, JB Lippincott, 1993, pp 411–426.

patients but occur in low titers (Wiesner and LaRusso, 1980). Liver biopsy may demonstrate periportal inflammation, cholangitis, CAH, or periductular fibrosis; in advanced cases, "onion skin" fibrosis and cirrhosis are seen. The most definitive way of establishing a diagnosis of PSC is by using endoscopic retrograde cholangiopancreatography, which demonstrates segmental stricturing and dilation of the intrahepatic and extrahepatic bile ducts (Wiesner et al., 1985, 1993).

Treatment

When the diagnosis of PSC is established, therapy is directed primarily at symptomatic relief and monitoring for progression to cirrhosis or cholangiocarcinoma. No treatment has been shown to stop the inexorable progression of the biliary inflammation. Ursodeoxycholic acid promotes bile flow, improves the biochemical parameters of cholestasis, and improves clinical symptoms of jaundice and pruritus in patients with PSC (Chazouilleres et al., 1990). An open-label trial of methotrexate in patients with PSC suggested some efficacy, but a randomized trial did not confirm the initial result (Knox and Kaplan, 1994).

In patients with isolated strictures of the bile duct and obstruction, endoscopic stenting of the bile duct or balloon dilation of the stricture may provide long-term symptomatic relief (Martin et al., 1990). Colectomy in patients with UC does not prevent progression of the biliary disease, arguing against a role for colonic bacterial translocation in the pathogenesis of PSC (Cangemi et al., 1989).

The treatment of choice for advanced cases of PSC with cirrhosis and liver failure is liver transplantation, and the 3- and 5-year survival of patients with PSC who undergo liver transplantation is greater than 85% (Goss et al., 1997; McEntee et al., 1991; Narumi et al., 1995; Rand and Whitington, 1992; see Chapter 43). The development of nonanastomotic biliary strictures may indicate recurrence of PSC after transplantation and may occur in 20% of patients; however, it does not have as aggressive disease progression (Angulo and Lindor, 1999; Goss et al., 1997; Graziadei et al., 1999).

Patients with PSC have a 10% to 15% lifetime risk of developing cholangiocarcinoma (De Groen, et al., 1999; Kornfeld et al., 1997) (an incidence of 1.5 percent per year, Berquist et al., 2002) and when detected, precludes liver transplantation.

R E F E R E N C E S

Abbas AK. A reassessment of the mechanisms of T cell-dependent B cell activation. Immunol Today 9:89–94, 1988.

Adachi A, Koenig S, Gendelmann HE, Daugherty D, Gatton-Celii S, Fauci AS, Martin MA. Productive, persistent infection of colorectal cell lines with human immunodeficiency virus. J Virol 61:201–213, 1987.

Addiss DG, Mathews HM, Stewart JM, Wahlquist SP, Williams RM, Finton RJ, Spencer HC, Juranek DD. Evaluation of a commercially available ELISA for *Giardia lamblia* antigen in stool. J Clin Microbiol 29:1137–1142, 1991.

Agata H, Kondo N Fukutomi O, Shinoda S, Orii T. Interleukin-2 production of lymphocytes in food sensitive atopic dermatitis. Arch Dis Child 67:280–284, 1992.

Ahnen DJ, Brown WR, Kloppel TM. Secretory component: the polymeric immunoglobulin receptor. Gastroenterology 89:667–682, 1985.

Aiges H, Markowitz J, Rosa J, Daum F. Home nocturnal supplemental nasogastric tube feedings in growth-retarded adolescents with Crohn's disease. Gastroenterology 97:905–910, 1989.

Alper CA, Fleishnick E, Awdeh Z, Katz AJ, Yunis EJ. Extended major histocompatibility complex haplotypes in patients with gluten-sensitive enteropathy. J Clin Invest 79:251–256, 1987.

Alter MJ, Sampliner RE. Hepatitis C: and miles to go before we sleep. N Engl J Med 321:1538–1540, 1989.

Ament ME, Rubin CE. Soy protein-another cause of the flat intestinal lesion. Gastroenterology 62:227–234, 1972.

Amerongen HM, Weltzin R, Farnet CM, Michetti P, Haseltine WA, Neutra MR. Transepithelial transport of HIV-1 by intestinal M cells. J AIDS 4:760–765, 1991.

Amerongen MH, Weltzin RW, Mack JA, Winner LS, Michetti P, Apter FM, Kraehenbuhl JP, Neutra MR. M cell–mediated antigen transport and monoclonal IgA antibodies for mucosal immune protection. Ann NY Acad Sci 664:18–26, 1992.

Ammann AJ, Hong R. Selective IgA deficiency: presentation of 30 cases and a review of the literature. Medicine (Balt) 50:223–236, 1971.

Anderson DC, Springer TA. Leukocyte-adhesion deficiency: an inherited defect in the Mac-1, LFA-1, and p150,95 glycoproteins. Annu Rev Med 38:175–194, 1987.

Angulo P, Lindor KD. Primary sclerosing cholangitis. 30:323–332, 1999.

Anttila PH, von Willebrand E, Simell O. Abnormal immune responses during hypozincemia in acrodermatitis enteropathica. Acta Paediatr Scand 75:988–992, 1986.

Arasu TS, Wyllie R, Hatch TF, Fitzgerald JF. Management of chronic aggressive hepatitis in children and adolescents. J Pediatr 95:514–522, 1979.

Arentz-Hansen H, Korner R, Molberg O, Quarsten H, Vader W, Kooy YMC, Lundin KEA, Koning F, Roepstorff P, Sollid LM, McAdam SN. The intestinal T cell response to α-gliadin in adult celiac disease is focused on a single deaminated glutamine targeted by tissue transglutaminase. J Exp Med 191:603–612, 2000.

Arbo A, Santos JI. Diarrheal diseases in the immunocompromised host. Pediatr Infect Dis 6:894–906, 1987.

Auricchio S, Greco L, Troncone R. Gluten-sensitive enteropathy in childhood. Pediatr Clin North Am 35:157–187, 1988.

Baklien K, Brandtzaeg P, Fausa O. Immunoglobulins in jejunal mucosa and serum from patients with adult coeliac disease. Scand J Gastroenterol 12:149–159, 1977.

Balistreri WF. Viral hepatitis. Pediatr Clin North Am 35:375–407, 1988.

Barnes PM, Moynahan EJ. Zinc deficiency in acrodermatitis enteropathica: multiple dietary intolerance treated with synthetic diet. Proc R Soc Med 66:325–333, 1973.

Bastlein C, Burlefinger R, Holzberg E, Voeth C, Garbrecht M, Ottenjann R. Common variable immunodeficiency syndrome and nodular lymphoid hyperplasia in the small intestine. Endoscopy 20:272–275, 1988.

Bell MJ, Ternberg JL, Feigin RD, Keating JP, Marshall R, Barton L, Brotherton T. Neonatal necrotizing enterocolitis: therapeutic decisions based on clinical staging. Ann Surg 187:1–7, 1978.

Belli DC, Seidman E, Bouthillier L, Weber AM, Roy CC, Pletincx M, Beaulieu M, Morin CL. Chronic intermittent elemental diet improves growth failure in children with Crohn's disease. Gastroenterology 94:603–610, 1988.

Benderly A, Pollack S, Etzioni A. Transient hypogammaglobulinemia of infancy with severe bacterial infections and persistent IgA deficiency. Isr J Med Sci 22:393–396, 1986.

Benhamou Y, Caumes E, Gerosa Y, Cadranel JF, Dohin E, Katlama C, Amouyal P, Canard JM, Azar N, Hoang C, Le Charpentier Y, Gentilini M, Opolon P, Valla D. AIDS related cholangiopathy: critical analysis of a prospective series of 26 patients. Dig Dis Sci 38:1113–1118, 1993.

Bennett WG, Watson RA, Heard JK, Vesely DL. Home hyperalimentation for common variable hypogammaglobulinemia with malabsorption secondary to intestinal nodular lymphoid hyperplasia. Am J Gastroenterol 82:1091–1095, 1987.

Bergquist A, Ekborn A, Olsson R, Kornfeldt D, Lööf L, Danielsson Å, Hultcrantz R, Lindgrn S, Prytz H, Sandberg-Gertzén H, Almer S, Granath F, Broomé U. Hepatic extrahepatic malignancies in primary sclerosing cholangitis. J Hepatology 36:321–327, 2002.

Biggar WD, Crawford L, Cardella C, Bear RA, Gladman D, Reynolds WJ. Malakoplakia and immunosuppressive therapy. Reversal of clinical and leukocyte abnormalities after withdrawal of prednisone and azathioprine. Am J Pathol 119:5–11, 1985.

Bishop JM, Hill DJ, Hosking CS. Natural history of cow milk allergy: clinical outcome. J Pediatr 116:862–867, 1990.

Bland PW, Kambarage DM. Antigen handling by the epithelium and lamina propria macrophages. Gastroenterol Clin North Am 20:577–596, 1991.

Bland PW, Warren LG. Antigen presentation by epithelial cells of the rat small intestine. II. Selective induction of suppressor T cells. Immunology 58:9–14, 1986.

Bloom S, Heryet A, Fleming K, Chapman RW. Inappropriate expression of blood group antigens on biliary and colonic epithelia in primary sclerosing cholangitis. Gut 34:977–983, 1993.

Bock SA, Atkins FM. The natural history of peanut allergy. J Allergy Clin Immunol 83:900–904, 1989.

Bock SA, Buckley J, Holst A, May CD. Proper use of skin tests with food extracts in diagnosis of food hypersensitivity. Clin Allergy 8:559–564, 1978.

Bock SA, Sampson HA, Atkins FM, Zeiger RS, Lehrer S, Sachs M, Bush RK, Metcalfe DD. Double-blind placebo controlled food challenges as an office procedure: a manual. J Allergy Clin Immunol 82:986–997, 1988.

Bodenheimer HC, La Russo NF, Thayer WP Jr, Charland C, Staples PJ, Ludwig J. Elevated circulating immune complexes in primary sclerosing cholangitis. Hepatology 3:150–154, 1983.

Borchers SD, Friedman RA, McClung HJ. Rice-induced anaphylactoid reaction. J Pediatr Gastroenterol Nutr 15:321–24, 1993.

Boyer JL, Reuben A. Chronic hepatitis. In Schiff L, Schiff ER, eds. Diseases of the Liver. Philadelphia, JB Lippincott, 1993, pp 612–619.

Bousvaros a, Kirschner BS, Werlin SL, Parker-Hartigan L, Daum F, Freeman KB, Balint JP, Day AS, Griffiths AM, Zurakowski D, Ferry GD, Leichtner AM. Oral tacrolimus treatment of severe colitis in children. J Pediatr 137:794–799, 2000.

Boyle JT. Gastroesophageal reflux in the pediatric patient. Gastroenterol Clin North Am 18:315–337, 1989.

Brandtzaeg P, Baklien K. Intestinal secretion of IgA and IgM: a hypothetical model. Ciba Found Symp 46:77–113, 1977.

Bray PF, Herbert JJ, Johnson DG. Childhood gastroesophageal reflux: neurologic and psychiatric symptoms mimicked. JAMA 237:1342–1345, 1977.

Broome U, Galamann H, Hulterantz R, Forsum U. Distribution of HLA-DR, HLA-DP, HLA-DQ antigens in liver tissue from patients with primary sclerosing cholangitis. Scand J Gastroenterol 25:54–58, 1990.

Brynskov J, Freund L, Rasmussen SN, Lauritsen K, Schaffalitsky de Muckadell O, Williams N, MacDonald A, Taunton R, Molina F, Campanini MC, Bianchi P, Ranzi T, Quarto di Palo F, Malchow-Moller A, Thomsen O, Tage-Jensen U, Binder V, Riis P. A placebo-controlled, double-blind, randomized trial of cyclosporine therapy in active chronic Crohn's disease. N Engl J Med 321:845–850, 1989.

Buckley RH, Dees SC. The correlation of milk precipitins with IgA deficiency. N Engl J Med 281:465–469, 1969.

Burgin-Wolff A, Gaze H, Hadziselimovic F, Huber H, Lentze MJ, Nussle D, Raymond-Berthet C. Antigliadin and antiendomysium antibody determination for coeliac disease. Arch Dis Child 66:941–947, 1991.

Burks AW, Sampson HA. Diagnostic approach to the patient with suspected food allergies. J Pediatr 121:S64–S71, 1992.

Cangemi JR, Wiesner RH, Beaver SJ, Ludwig J, MacCarty RL, Dozois RR, Zinsmeister AR, LaRusso NF. Effect of proctocolectomy for chronic ulcerative colitis on the natural history of primary sclerosing cholangitis. Gastroenterology 96:790–794, 1989.

Caplan MS, MacKendrick WM. Necrotizing enterocolitis: a review of pathogenetic mechanisms and implications for prevention. Pediatr Pathol 13:357–369, 1993.

Cappell MS. Hepatobiliary manifestations of the acquired immune deficiency syndrome. Am J Gastroenterol 86:1–15, 1991.

Catassi C, Mirakian R, Natalini G, Sbarbati A, Cinti S, Coppa GV, Giorgi PL. Unresponsive enteropathy associated with circulating enterocyte antibodies in a boy with common variable hypogammaglobulinemia and type 1 diabetes. J Pediatr Gastroenterol Nutr 7:608–613, 1988.

Cello JP, Grendell JH, Basuk P, Simon D, Weiss L, Wittner M, Rood RP, Wilcox CM, Forsmark CE, Read AE, Satow JA, Weikel CS, Beaumont C. Effect of octreotide on refractory AIDS-associated diarrhea. A prospective, multicenter clinical trial. Ann Intern Med 115:705–710, 1991.

Cerf-Bensussan N, Guy-Grand D. Intestinal intraepithelial lymphocytes. Gastroenterol Clin North Am 20:549–576, 1991.

Chajek T. HLA-B51 may serve as an immunogenetic marker for a subgroup of patients with Behçet's syndrome. Am J Med 83:666–672, 1987.

Chapman RW. Role of immune factors in the pathogenesis of primary sclerosing cholangitis. Semin Liver Dis 11:1–4, 1991.

Chapman RW, Marborgh BA, Rhodes JM, Summerfield JA, Dick R, Scheuer PJ, Sherlock S. Primary sclerosing cholangitis—a review of its clinical features, cholangiography, and hepatic histology. Gut 21:870–877, 1980.

Chapman RW, Kelly P, Heryet A, Jewell DP, Fleming KA. Expression of HLA-DR antigens on bile duct epithelium in primary sclerosing cholangitis. Gut 29:422–427, 1988.

Chazouilleres O, Poupon R, Capron JP, Metman EH, Dhumeauz D, Amouretti M, Couzigou P, Labayle D, Trinchet JC. Ursodeoxycholic acid for primary sclerosing cholangitis. J Hepatol 11:120–123, 1990.

Chin TW, Stiehm ER, Falloon J, Gallin JI. Corticosteroids in treatment of obstructive lesions of chronic granulomatous disease. J Pediatr 111:349–352, 1987.

Choy MY, Walker-Smith JA, Williams CB, Macdonald TT. Differential expression of CD25 (interleukin-2 receptor) on lamina propria T cells and macrophages in the intestinal lesions in Crohn's disease and ulcerative colitis. Gut 31:1365–1390, 1990.

Chu SW, Walker, WA. Bacterial toxin interaction with the developing intestine. Gastroenterology 104:916–925, 1993.

Colletti RB, Guillot AP, Rosen S, Bhan AK, Hobson D, Collins AB, Russell GJ, Winter HS. Autoimmune enteropathy and nephropathy with circulating antiepithelial cell antibodies. J Pediatr 118:858–864, 1991.

Collin P, Maki M, Keyrilainen O, Hallstrom O, Reunala T, Pasternack A. Selective IgA deficiency and celiac disease. Scand J Gastroenterol 27:367–371, 1992.

Colombel JF, Mascart-Lemone F, Nemeth J, Vaerman JP, Dive C, Rambaud JC. Jejunal immunoglobulin and antigliadin antibody secretion in active celiac disease. Gut 31:1345–1349, 1990.

Conley ME, Delacroix DL. Intravascular and mucosal immunoglobulin A: two separate systems of immune defense? Ann Intern Med 106:892–899, 1987.

Conley ME, Park CL, Douglas SD. Childhood common variable immunodeficiency with autoimmune disease. J Pediatr 108:915–922, 1986.

Couper R, Kapelushnik J, Griffiths AM. Neutrophil dysfunction in glycogen storage disease Ib: association with Crohn's like colitis. Gastroenterology 100:549–554, 1991.

Crissinger KD, Granger DN. Mucosal injury induced by ischemia and reperfusion in the piglet intestine: influences of age and feeding. Gastroenterology 97:920–926, 1989.

Crissinger KD, Tso P. The role of lipids in ischemia/reperfusion-induced changes in mucosal permeability in developing piglets. Gastroenterology 102:1693–1699, 1992.

Cunningham-Rundles C. Selective IgA deficiency and the gastrointestinal tract. Immunol Allergy Clin North Am 8:435–449, 1988.

Cunningham-Rundles C, Brandeis WE, Good RA, Day NK. Milk precipitins, circulating immune complexes and IgA deficiency. Proc Natl Acad Sci USA 75:3386–3389, 1978.

Cunningham-Rundles C, Pudifin DJ, Armstrong D, Good RA. Selective IgA deficiency and neoplasia. Vox Sang 38:61–67, 1980.

Czaja AJ. Diagnosis, prognosis and treatment of classical autoimmune chronic active hepatitis. In Krawitt EL, Wiesner RH, eds. Autoimmune Liver Diseases. New York, Raven Press, 1991, pp 143–166.

Czaja AJ, Carpenter HA, Santrach PJ, Moore B, Homburger HA. The nature and prognosis of severe cryptogenic chronic active hepatitis. Gastroenterology 104:1755–1761, 1993a.

Czaja AJ, Carpenter HA, Santrach PJ, Moore SB. Significance of HLA DR4 in type I autoimmune hepatitis. Gastroenterology 105:1502–1507, 1993b.

Das KM, Dasgupta A, Mandal A, Geng X. Autoimmunity to cytoskeletal protein tropomyosin. A clue to the pathogenetic mechanism for ulcerative colitis. J Immunol 150:2487–2493, 1993.

Davies G, Evans CM, Shand WA, Walker-Smith JA. Surgery for Crohn's disease in childhood: influence of site of disease and operative procedure on outcome. Br J Surg 77:891–894, 1990.

Dawson J, Bryant MG, Bloom SR, Peters TJ. Jejunal mucosal enzyme activities, regulatory peptides, and organelle pathology of the enteropathy of common variable immunodeficiency. Gut 27:273–277, 1986.

Debray D, Pariente D, Urvoas E, Hadchouel M, Bernard O. Sclerosing cholangitis in children. J Pediatr 124:49–56, 1994.

De Groen PC, Gores GJ, LaRusso NF, Gunderson LL, Nagorney DM. Biliary tract cancers. 341:1368–1378, 1999.

Deitch EA. Bacterial translocation: the influence of dietary variables. Gut 35(Suppl.):S23–S27, 1994.

DeMarchi M, Borelli I, Olivetti E, Richiardi P, Wright P, Ansaldi N, Barbera C, Santini B. Two HLA-D and DR alleles are associated with celiac disease. Tissue Antigens 14:309–316, 1979.

Dicke WK, Weijers HA, van de Kamer JH. Coeliac disease. II. The presence in wheat of a factor having a deleterious effect in cases of coeliac disease. Acta Paediatr Scand 42:34–42, 1953.

Dieterich W, Ehnis T, Bauer M, Donner P, Volta U, Riecken EO, Schuppan D. Identification of tissue transglutaminase as the autoantigen of celiac disease. Nat Med 3:797–801, 1997.

DiGioacchino M, Pizzicannella G, Fini N, Falusca F, Antinucci R, Masci S, Mezzetti A, Marzio L, Cuccurullo F. Sodium cromoglycate in the treatment of eosinophilic gastroenteritis. Allergy 45:161–166, 1990.

Disdier P, Harle JR, Monges D, Chrestian MA, Horschowski N, Weiller PJ. Duodenal sarcoidosis with selective IgA deficiency and lymphoid nodular hyperplasia. Gastroenterol Clin Biol 15:849–851, 1991.

Donaldson PT, Doherty DG, Hayllar KM, McFarlane IG, Johnson PJ, Williams R. Susceptibility to autoimmune chronic active hepatitis: human leukocyte antigens DR4 and A1-B8-DR3 are independent risk factors. Hepatology 13:701–706, 1991.

Downing GJ, Horner SR, Kilbride HW. Characteristics of perinatal cocaine-exposed infants with necrotizing enterocolitis. Am J Dis Child 145:26–27, 1991.

Duerr RH, Targan SR, Landers CJ, La Russo NF, Lindsay KL, Wiesner RH, Shanahan F. Neutrophil cytoplasmic antibodies: a link between primary sclerosing cholangitis and ulcerative colitis. Gastroenterology 100:1385–1391, 1991.

Ebert EC. Intra-epithelial lymphocytes: interferon-gamma production and suppressor/cytotoxic activities. Clin Exp Immunol 82:81–85, 1990.

Eddleston AL, Williams R. HLA and liver disease. Br Med Bull 34:295–300, 1978.

Eibl MM, Wolf HM, Furnkranz H, Rosenkranz A. Prevention of necrotizing enterocolitis in low birth weight infants by IgG-IgA feeding. N Engl J Med 319:1–7, 1988.

Ek J, Albrechtsen D, Solheim BG, Thorsby E. Strong association between the HLA-Dw3–related B cell alloantigen-DRw3 and celiac disease. Scand J Gastroenterol 13:229–233, 1978.

Ellis D, Fisher SE, Smith WI, Jaffe R. Familial occurrence of renal and intestinal disease associated with tissue autoantibodies. Am J Dis Child 136:323–326, 1982.

el-Mouzan MI, Satti MB, al Quorain AA, el-Ageb A. Colonic malacoplakia-occurrence in a family. Report of cases. Dis Colon Rectum 31:390–393, 1988.

Ezekowitz RAB and the International Chronic Granulomatous Disease Cooperative Study Group. A controlled trial of interferon gamma to prevent infection in chronic granulomatous disease. N Engl J Med 324:509–516, 1991.

Fais S, Capobianchi MR, Pallone F, DiMarco P, Boirivant M, Oianzani F, Torsoli A. Spontaneous release of interferon gamma by intestinal lamina propria lymphocytes in Crohn's disease. Kinetics of in vitro response to interferon gamma inducers. Gut 32:403–407, 1991.

Falchuk ZM, Rogentine GN, Strober W. Predominance of histocompatibility antigen HLA-B8 in patients with gluten-sensitive enteropathy. J Clin Invest 51:1602–1605, 1972.

Fasano A, Berti I, Gerarduzzi T, Not T, Colletti RB, Drago S, Elitsur Y, Green PHR, Guandalini S, Hill ID, Pietzak M, Ventura A, Thorpe M, Kryszak D, Fornaroli F, Wasserman SS, Murray JA, Horvath K. Prevalence of celiac disease in at-risk and not-at-risk groups in the United States. A large multicenter study. Arch Intern Med 163:286–292, 2003.

Faubion WA Jr, Perrault J, Burgart LJ, Zein NN, Clawson M, Freese DK. Treatment of eosinophilic esophagitis with inhaled corticosteroids. J Pediatr Gastroenterol Nutr 27:90–93, 1998.

Ferguson A. Immunological functions of the gut in relation to nutritional state and mode of delivery of nutrients. Gut 35(Suppl.):S10–S12, 1994.

Ferreira M, Lloyd Davies S, Butler M, Scott D, Clark M, Kumar P. Endomysial antibody: is it the best screening test for coeliac disease? Gut 33:1633–1637, 1992.

Fitzgerald JF. Chronic hepatitis. Semin Liver Dis 2:282–290, 1982.

Fonkalsrud EW. A syndrome of congenital lymphedema of the upper extremity and associated systemic lymphatic malformations. Surg Gynecol Obstet 145:228–234, 1977.

Fox CH, Kotler D, Tierney A, Wilson CS, Fauci AS. Detection of HIV-1 RNA in the lamina propria of patients with AIDS and gastrointestinal disease. J Infect Dis 159:467–471, 1989.

Fuleihan R, Ramesh N, Loh R, Jahara H, Rosen RS, Chatila T, Fu SM, Stamenkovic I, Geha RS. Defective expression of the CD40 ligand in X chromosome–linked immunoglobulin deficiency with normal or elevated IgM. Proc Natl Acad Sci USA 90:2170–2173, 1993.

Fung KP, Seagram G, Pasieka J, Trevenen C, Machida H, Scott B. Investigation and outcome of 121 infants and children requiring Nissen fundoplication for the management of gastroesophageal reflux. Clin Invest Med 13:237–246, 1990.

Furuta GT. Eosinophils in the esophagus: acid is not the only cause. J Pediatr Gastroenterol Nutr 26:468–471, 1998.

Furuta GT and Sherman P. Eotaxin and eosinophilic homing to the gut. J Pediatr Gastroenterol Nutr 30:229, 2000.

Garretts M, Molokhia M. Acrodermatitis enteropathica without hypozincemia. J Pediatr 91:492–494, 1977.

Garvey BM, McCambley JA, Tuxen DV. Effect of gastric alkalinization on bacterial colonization in critically ill patients. Crit Care Med 17:211–216, 1989.

Gawkrodger DJ, Ferguson A, Barnetson R. Nutritional status in patients with dermatitis herpetiformis. Am J Clin Nutr 48:355–360, 1988.

Giampietro PG, Ragno V, Daniele S, Cantani A, Ferrara M, Businco L. Soy hypersensitivity in children with food allergy. Ann Allergy 69:143–146, 1992.

Gilger MA, Matson DO, Conner ME, Rosenblatt HM, Finegold MJ, Estes MK. Extraintestinal rotavirus infections in children with immunodeficiency. J Pediatr 120:912–917, 1992.

Gitzelmann R, Bosshard NU. Defective neutrophil and monocyte functions in glycogen storage disease type Ib: a literature review. Eur J Pediatr 152(Suppl. 1):S33–S38, 1993.

Glassman MS, Newman LJ, Berezin S, Gryboski JD. Cow's milk protein sensitivity during infancy in patients with inflammatory bowel disease. Am J Gastroenterol 85:838–840, 1990.

Gleason WA. Protein-losing enteropathy. In Hyams JS, Wyllie R, eds. Pediatric Gastrointestinal Disease. Philadelphia, WB Saunders, 1993, pp 536–543.

Golden MH, Jackson AA, Golden BE. Effect of zinc on the thymus of recently malnourished children. Lancet 2:1057–1059, 1977.

Golden MH, Harland PS, Golden BE, Jackson AA. Zinc and immunocompetence in protein-energy malnutrition. Lancet 1:1226–1227, 1978.

Goldman AS, Anderson DW, Sellers WA, Sapperstein S, Kniker WT, Halpern SR. Milk allergy I. Oral challenge with milk and isolated proteins in allergic children. Pediatrics 32:425–443, 1963.

Goldstein JL, Anderson RGW, Brown MS. Coated pits, coated vesicles and receptor-mediated endocytosis. Nature 279:679–685, 1979.

Gonnella PA, Walker WA. Macromolecular absorption in the gastrointestinal tract. Adv Drug Delivery Rev 1:235–248, 1987.

Good RA, Fernandes G, West A. Nutrition, immunity and cancer: a review. Part I: Influence of protein or protein caloric malnutrition and zinc deficiency on immunity. Clin Bull 9:3–12, 1979.

Goss JA, Shackelton CR, Farmer DG, Arnaout WS, Seu P, Markowitz JS, Martin P, Stribling RJ, Goldstein LI, Busuttil RW. Orthotopic liver transplantation for primary sclerosing cholangitits. A 12-year single center experience. Ann Surg 225:472–483, 1997.

Gravallese EM, Kantrowitz FG. Arthritic manifestations of inflammatory bowel disease. Am J Gastroenterol 83:703–709, 1988.

Graziadei IW, Weisner RH, Batts KP, Marotta PJ, LaRusso NF, Porayko MK, Hay JE, Gores GJ, Charlton MR, Ludwig J, Poterucha JJ, Steers JL, Krom RAF. Recurrence of primary sclerosing cholangitis following liver transplantation. Hepatology 29:1050–1056, 1999.

Greenberg GR, Fleming CR, Jeejeebhoy KN, Rosenberg IH, Sales D. Controlled trial of bowel rest and nutritional support in the management of Crohn's disease. Gut 29:1309–1315, 1988.

Grey HM, Sette A, Buus S. How T cells see antigen. Sci Am 261:56–64, 1989.

Grimble GK. Dietary nucleotides and gut mucosal defense. Gut 35(Suppl.):S46–S51, 1994.

Grohmann GS, Glass RI, Pereira HG, Monroe SS, Hightower AW, Weber R, Bryan RT. Enteric viruses and diarrhea in HIV-infected patients. N Engl J Med 329:14–20, 1993.

Gryboski JD, Pellerano R, Young N, Edberg S. Positive role of Clostridium difficile infection in diarrhea in infants and children. Am J Gastroenterol 86:685–689, 1991.

Hager C, Faber J, Kaczuni A, Goldstein R, Levy E, Freier S. Prevalence of postenteritis cow's milk protein intolerance. Isr J Med Sci 23:1128–1131, 1987.

Halac E, Halac J, Begue E, Casanas JM, Indiverdi DR, Petit JF, Figueroa MJ, Olmas JM, Rodriguez LA, Obregon RJ, Martinez NV, Grinblat DA, Vilarrodena HO. Prenatal and postnatal corticosteroid therapy to prevent necrotizing enterocolitis: a controlled trial. J Pediatr 117:132–138, 1990.

Halpin TC, Byrne WJ, Ament ME. Colitis, persistent diarrhea, and soy protein intolerance. J Pediatr 91:404–407, 1977.

Halstensen TS, Scott H, Brandtzaeg P. Intraepithelial T cells of the TCR gamma/delta CD8 negative and V*1/J*1 phenotypes are increased in celiac disease. Scand J Immunol 30:665–672, 1989.

Halstensen TS, Scott H, Brandtzaeg P. Human CD8+ intraepithelial T lymphocytes are mainly CD45A-RB+ and show increased co-expression of CD45RO in celiac disease. Eur J Immunol 20:1825–1830, 1990.

Hammer RE, Maika SD, Richardson JA, Tang JP, Taurog JD. Spontaneous inflammatory disease in transgenic rats expressing HLA-B27 and human $2m: an animal model of HLA-B27 associated human disorders. Cell 63:1099–1112, 1990.

Harfi HA, Akhtar M, Subayti YA, Ali MA, Ferentzi C, Larkworthy W. Gastrointestinal malakoplakia in children. Clin Pediatr (Phila) 24:423–428, 1985.

Harrison M, Kilby A, Walker-Smith J, France N, Wood CB. Cow's milk protein intolerance: a possible association with gastroenteritis, lactose intolerance, and IgA deficiency. BMJ 1:1501–1508, 1976.

Hausser C, Virelizier JL, Buriot D, Griscelli C. Common variable hypogammaglobulinemia in children. Am J Dis Child 137:833–837, 1983.

Hawkins HK, Heffelfinger SC, Anderson DC. Leukocyte adhesion deficiency: clinical and postmortem observations. Pediatr Pathol 12:119–130, 1992.

Heird WC, Hansen IH. Effect of colostrum on growth of intestinal mucosa. Pediatr Res 11:406A, 1977.

Heise C, Dandekar S, Kumar P, Duplantier R, Donovan RM, Halsted CH. Human immunodeficiency virus infection of enterocytes and mononuclear cells in human jejunal mucosa. Gastroenterology 100:1521–1527, 1991.

Hentges DJ. The protective function of the indigenous intestinal flora. Pediatr Infect Dis 5:S17–S20, 1986.

Herrod HG. Chronic mucocutaneous candidiasis in childhood and complications of non-Candida infection. J Pediatr 116:377–382, 1990.

Hill DJ, Firer MA, Shelton MJ, Hosking CS. Manifestations of milk allergy in infancy: clinical and immunologic findings. J Pediatr 109:270–276, 1986.

Hill SM, Milla PJ, Bottazzo GF, Mirakian R. Autoimmune enteropathy and colitis: is there a generalised autoimmune gut disorder? Gut 32:36–42, 1991.

Hilliard RI, McKendry JB, Phillips MJ. Congenital abnormalities of the lymphatic system: a new clinical classification. Pediatrics 86:988–994, 1990.

Hoang P, Dalton HR, Jewell DP. Human colonic intraepithelial lymphocytes are suppressor cells. Clin Exp Immunol 85:498–503, 1991.

Hollander D, Vadheim CM, Brettholz E, Petersen GM, Delahunty T, Rotter JI. Increased intestinal permeability in patients with Crohn's disease and their relatives: a possible etiologic factor. Ann Intern Med 105:883–885, 1986.

Hollander D. The intestinal permeability barrier. Scand J Gastroenterol 27:721–726, 1992.

Holt PR. Dietary treatment of protein loss in intestinal lymphangiectasia. Pediatrics 34:629–635, 1964.

Homberg JC, Abauf N, Bernard O, Islam S, Alvarez F, Khalil S, Poupon R, Darnis F, Levy VG, Grippon P, Opolon P, Bernuau J, Benhamou JP, Alagille D. Chronic active hepatitis associated with anti liver/kidney microsomal antibody type I: a second type of autoimmune hepatitis. Hepatology 7:1333–1339, 1987.

Hoofnagle JH. Chronic hepatitis B. N Engl J Med 323:337–339, 1990.

Howdle PD, Blair Zajdel ME, Smart CJ, Tresdosiewicz LK, Blair GE, Losowsky MS. Lack of serological response to an E1b protein of adenovirus type 12 in celiac disease. Scand J Gastroenterol 24:282–286, 1989.

Hoyne GF, Callow MG, Kuhlman J, Thomas WR. T-cell lymphokine response to orally administered proteins during priming and unresponsiveness. Immunology 78:534–540, 1993.

Hsueh W, Gonzalez-Crussi F, Arroyave JL, Anderson RC, Lee ML, Houlihan WJ. Platelet activating factor induced ischemic bowel necrosis: the effect of PAF antagonists. Eur J Pharmacol 123:79–83, 1986.

Hsueh W, Gonzalez-Crussi F, Hsueh W. Platelet activating factor is an endogenous mediator for bowel necrosis in endotoxemia. FASEB J 1:403–405, 1987.

Husband AJ, Gowans JL. The origin and antigen-dependent distribution of IgA containing cells in the intestine. J Exp Med 148:1146–1160, 1977.

International Study Group for BehHet's Disease. Criteria for diagnosis of Behçet's disease. Lancet 335:1078–1080, 1990.

Isaacs D, Wright VM, Shaw DG, Raafat F, Walker-Smith JA. Chronic granulomatous disease mimicking Crohn's disease. J Pediatr Gastroenterol Nutr 4:498–501, 1985.

Israel EJ, Pang KY, Harmatz PA, Walker WA. Structural and functional maturation of gut mucosal barrier with thyroxine. Am J Physiol 252:G762–G767, 1987.

Israel EJ, Schiffrin E, Carter E, Freiberg E, Walker WA. Prevention of necrotizing enterocolitis in the rat with prenatal cortisone. Gastroenterology 99:1333–1338, 1990.

Israel EJ, Simister N, Freiberg E, Caplan A, Walker WA. Immunoglobulin G binding sites on the human fetal intestine: a possible mechanism for the passive transfer of immunity from mother to infant. Immunology 79:77–81, 1993.

Italian Multicenter Study. Epidemiology and clinical features of pediatric HIV infection: results from an Italian multicenter study on 544 children. Lancet 2:1046–1048, 1988.

Iyngkaran N, Yadav M, Looi L, Boey C, Kam KL, Balabaaskaran S, Puthucheary S. Effect of soy protein on the small bowel mucosa of young infants recovering from acute gastroenteritis. J Pediatr Gastroenterol Nutr 7:68–79, 1988.

Jackson WD, Grand RJ. Crohn's disease. In Walker WA, Durie PR, Walker-Smith JA, Hamilton JR, Watkins JB, eds. Pediatric Gastrointestinal Disease. Philadelphia, BC Decker, 1990, pp 592–608.

Jany BH, Gallup MW, Yan PS, Gum JR, Kim YS, Basbaum CB. Human bronchus and intestine express the same mucin gene. J Clin Invest 87:77–82, 1991.

Jarvis WR, Middleton PJ, Gelfand EW. Significance of viral infections in severe combined immunodeficiency disease. Pediatr Infect Dis 2:187–192, 1983.

Johnson PJ, McFarlane IG, Eddleston AL. The natural course and heterogeneity of chronic active hepatitis. Semin Liver Dis 11:187–196, 1991.

Jorge AD, Esley C, Ahumada J. Family incidence of primary sclerosing cholangitis associated with immunologic diseases. Endoscopy 19:114–117, 1987.

Julius R, Schulkind M, Sprinkle T, Rennert O. Acrodermatitis enteropathica with immune deficiency. J Pediatr 83:1007–1011, 1973.

Kagnoff MF. Celiac disease. A gastrointestinal disease with environmental, genetic, and immunologic components. Gastroenterol Clin North Am 21:405–425, 1992.

Kagnoff MF, Austin RK, Hubert JJ, Bernardin JE, Kusarda DD. Possible role for a human adenovirus in the pathogenesis of celiac disease. J Exp Med 160:1544–1547, 1984.

Kagnoff MF, Paterson YJ, Kumar PJ, Kusarda DD, Carbone FR, Unsworth DJ, Austin RK. Evidence for the role of a human intestinal adenovirus in the pathogenesis of celiac disease. Gut 28:995–1001, 1987.

Kanof M, Lake A, Bayless T. Decreased height velocity in children and adolescents before the diagnosis of Crohn's disease. Gastroenterology 95:1523–1527, 1988a.

Kanof ME, Strober W, Fiocchi C, Zeitz M, James SP. CD4 positive Leu-8 negative helper-inducer T cells predominate in the human intestinal lamina propria. J Immunol 141:3029–3036, 1988b.

Katz AJ, Twarog FJ, Zieger RS, Falchuk ZM. Milk-sensitive and eosinophilic gastroenteropathy: similar clinical features with contrasting mechanisms and clinical course. J Allergy Clin Immunol 74:72–78, 1984.

Kawahara H, Dent J, Davidson G. Mechanisms responsible for gastroesohpageal reflux in children. Gastroenterology 113:399–408, 1997.

Kawanishi H, Saltzman L, Strober W. Mechanisms regulating IgA class-specific immunoglobulin production in gut-associated lymphoid tissues. I. T cells derived from Peyer's patches that switch sIgM B cells to sIgA B cells in vitro. J Exp Med 157:433–450, 1983.

Keating JJ, O'Brien CJ, Stellon AJ, Portmann BC, Johnson RD, Johnson PJ, Williams R. Influence of aetiology, clinical, and histological features on survival in chronic active hepatitis: an analysis of 204 patients. Q J Med 62:59–66, 1987.

Kelly KJ, Lazenby AJ, Rowe PC, Yardley JH, Perman AA, Sampson HA. Eosinophilic esophagitis attributed to gastroesophageal reflux: improvement with an amino acid-based formula. Gastroenterology 109:1503–1512, 1995.

Kelts DG, Grand RJ. Inflammatory bowel disease in children and adolescents. Curr Prob Pediatr 10:5–40, 1980.

Kerneis S, Bogdanova A, Kraehenbuhl J-P, Pringault E. Conversion of Peyer's patch lymphocytes of human enterocytes into M cells that transport bacteria. Science 277:949–952, 1997.

Kett K, Brandtzaeg P. Local IgA subclass alterations in ulcerative colitis and Crohn's disease of the colon. Gut 28:1013–1021, 1987.

Kett K, Rognum TO, Brandtzaeg P. Mucosal subclass distribution of immunoglobulin G-producing cells is different in ulcerative colitis and Crohn's disease of the colon. Gastroenterology 93:919–924, 1987.

Keusch GT. Nutrition and infection. Annu Rev Nutr 6:131–154, 1986.

Khoury SJ, Hancock WW, Weiner HL. Oral tolerance to myelin basic protein and natural recovery from experimental autoimmune encephalomyelitis are associated with downregulation of inflammatory cytokines and differential upregulation of transforming growth factor-beta, interleukin-4, and prostaglandin E expression in the brain. J Exp Med 176:1355–1364, 1992.

Kim YS, Gum JR, Byrd JC, Toribara NW. The structure of human intestinal apomucins. Am Rev Respir Dis 144:S10–S14, 1991.

Kirkpatrick CH. Chronic mucocutaneous candidiasis. Eur J Clin Microbiol Infect Dis 8:448–456, 1989.

Kirsch M. Bacterial overgrowth. Am J Gastroenterol 85:231–237, 1990.

Kirschner BS, Voinchet O, Rosenberg IH. Growth retardation in inflammatory bowel disease. Gastroenterology 75:504–511, 1978.

Klein C, Lisowska-Grospierre L, LeDiest F, Fischer A, Griscelli C. Major histocompatibility class II deficiency: clinical manifestations, immunologic features and outcome. J Pediatr 123:921–928, 1993.

Kleinman RE. The liver and intestinal immunoglobulin A: up from the "minors"? Gastroenterology 93:650–651, 1987.

Kleinman RE, Walker WA. The enteromammary immune system: an important new concept in breast milk host defense. Dig Dis Sci 24:876–882, 1979.

Kleinman RE, Balisteri WF, Heyman MB, Kirschner BS, Lake AL, Motil KJ, Seidman E, Udall JN. Nutritional support for pediatric patients with inflammatory bowel disease. J Pediatr Gastroenterol Nutr 8:8–12, 1989.

Kliegman RM. Neonatal necrotizing enterocolitis. In Wyllie R, Hyams JS, eds. Pediatric Gastrointestinal Disease: Pathophysiology, Diagnosis, Management. Philadelphia, WB Saunders, 1993, pp 788–798.

Kliegman RM, Fanaroff AA. Necrotizing enterocolitis. N Engl J Med 310:1093–1103, 1984.

Kliegman RM, Walker WA, Yolken RH. Necrotizing enterocolitis: research agenda for a disease of unknown etiology and pathogenesis. Pediatr Res 34:701–708, 1993.

Knox WF. Restricted feeding and human intestinal plasma cell development. Arch Dis Child 61:744–749, 1986.

Knox TA, Kaplan MM. A double-blind controlled trial of oral pulse methotrexate therapy in the treatment of primary sclerosing cholangitis. Gastroenterology 106:494–499, 1994.

Koff RS. Viral hepatitis. In Schiff L, Shiff ER, eds. Diseases of the Liver, 7th ed. Philadelphia, JB Lippincott, 1993, pp 492–577.

Kondo N, Fukitomi O, Agata H, Motoyoshi F, Shinoda S, Kobayashi Y, Kuwabara N, Kameyama T, Orii T. The role of T lymphocytes in patients with food sensitive atopic dermatitis. J Allergy Clin Immunol 91:658–668, 1993.

Kornfeld D, Ekbom A, Ihre T. Survival and risk of cholangiocarcinoma in patients with primary sclerosing cholangitis: a population-based study. Scand J Gastroenterol 32:1042–1045, 1997.

Kosnik EF, Johnson JP, Rennels MB, Caniano DA. Streptococcal sepsis presenting as acute abdomen in a child with transient hypogammaglobulinemia of infancy. J Pediatr Surg 21:975–976, 1986.

Kotler DP, Scholes JV, Tierney AR. Intestinal plasma cell alterations in acquired immunodeficiency syndrome. Dig Dis Sci 32:129–138, 1987.

Kraehenbuhl JP, Neutra MR. Molecular and cellular basis of immune protection of mucosal surfaces. Physiol Rev 72:853–879, 1992.

Krugman S. Viral hepatitis: A, B, C, D, E infection. Pediatr Rev 13:203–212, 1992.

Kuhn R, Lohler J, Rennick D, Rajewsky K, Muller W. Interleukin-10 deficient mice develop chronic enterocolitis. Cell 75:263–274, 1993.

Kutlu T, Brousse N, Rambaud C, LeDiest F, Schmitz J, Cerf-Bensussan N. Numbers of T cell receptor alpha/beta but not of TCR gamma/delta intraepithelial lymphocytes correlate with the grade of villous atrophy on a long term gluten free diet. Gut 34:208–214, 1993.

Lake AM, Whittington PF, Hamilton SR. Dietary proteinBinduced colitis in breast-fed infants. J Pediatr 101:906–910, 1982.

Lake-Bakaar G, Quadros E, Beidas S, Elsakr M, Tom W, Wilson DE, Dinscoy HP, Cohen P, Straus EW. Gastric secretory failure in patients with the acquired immunodeficiency syndrome. Ann Intern Med 109:502–504, 1988.

Laszewski MJ, Kemp JD, Goeken JA, Mitros FA, Platz CE, Dick FR. Clonal immunoglobulin gene rearrangement in nodular lymphoid hyperplasia of the gastrointestinal tract associated with common variable immunodeficiency. Am J Clin Pathol 94:338–343, 1990.

Lavilla P, Gil A, Rodriguez MC, Dupla ML, Pintado V, Fontan G. X-linked agammaglobulinemia and gastric adenocarcinoma. Cancer 72:1528–1531, 1993.

Lecuit M, Vandormael-Pournin S, Lefort J, Huerre M, Gounon P, Dupuy C, Babinet C, Cossart P. A transgenic model for Listeriosis: role of internalin in crossing the intestinal barrier. Science 292:1722–1725, 2001.

Lederman HM, Winkelstein JA. X-linked agammaglobulinemia: an analysis of 96 patients. Medicine (Balt) 64:145–156, 1985.

Lee RG. The colitis of Behçet's syndrome. Am J Surg Pathol 10:888–893, 1986.

Lehrer RI, Ganz T, Selsted ME, Babior BM, Curnutte JT. Neutrophils and host defense. Ann Intern Med 109:127–142, 1988.

Leihnas JL, McCaskill C, Sampson HA. Food allergy challenges: guidelines and implications. J Am Diet Assoc 87:604–608, 1987.

Lenaerts C, Roy CC, Vaillancourt M, Weber AM, Morin CL, Seidman E. High incidence of upper gastrointestinal tract involvement in children with Crohn disease. Pediatrics 83:777–781, 1989.

Lenzhofer R, Lindner M, Moser A, Berger J, Schuschnigg C, Thurner J. Acute jejunal ileus in intestinal lymphangiectasia. Clin Invest 71:568–571, 1993.

Lenzi M, Ballardini G, Fusconi M, Cassani F, Selleri L, Volat U, Zauli D, Bianchi FB. Type 2 autoimmune hepatitis and hepatitis C virus infection. Lancet 335:258–259, 1990.

Lenzi M, Johnson PJ, McFarlane IG, Ballardini G, Smith HM, McFarlane BM, Bridger C, Vergani D, Bianchi FB, Williams R. Antibodies to hepatitis C virus in autoimmune liver disease: evidence for geographical heterogeneity. Lancet 338:277–280, 1991.

Leung DY, Kelly CP, Boguniewicz M, Pothoulakis C, LaMont JT, Flores A. Treatment with intravenously administered gamma globulin of chronic relapsing colitis induced by Clostridium difficile toxin. J Pediatr 118:633–637, 1991.

Levenson SD, Austin RK, Dietler MD, Kasarda DD, Kagnoff MF. Specificity of antigliadin antibody in celiac disease. Gastroenterology 89:1–5, 1985.

Li XM, Jeffers LJ, Reddy KR, de Medina M, Silva M, Villanueve S, Klimas NG, Esquenazi V, Schiff ER. Immunophenotyping of lymphocytes in liver tissue of patients with chronic liver diseases by flow cytometry. Hepatology 14:121–127, 1991.

Liacouras CA, Wenner WJ, Brown K, Ruchelli E. Primary eosinophilic esophagitis in children: successful treament with oral corticosteroids. J Pediatr Gastroenterol Nutr 26:380–385, 1998.

Lindahl JA, Williams FH, Newman SL. Small bowel obstruction in chronic granulomatous disease. J Pediatr Gastroenterol Nutr 3:637–640, 1984.

Lindor KD, Wiesner RH, Katzman JA, LaRusso NF, Beaver SJ. Lymphocyte subsets in primary sclerosing cholangitis. Dig Dis Sci 32:720–725, 1987a.

Lindor KD, Wiesner RH, LaRusso NF, Homburger HA. Enhanced autoreactivity of T lymphocytes in primary sclerosing cholangitis. Hepatology 7:884–888, 1987b.

Lindor KD, Wiesner RH, MacCarty RL, Ludwig J, La Russo NF. Advances in primary sclerosing cholangitis. Am J Med 89:73–80, 1990.

Logan RF, Gillon J, Ferrington C, Ferguson A. Reduction of gastrointestinal protein loss by elemental diet in the small bowel. Gut 22:383–387, 1981.

Logan RF, Rifkind EA, Turner ID, Ferguson A. Mortality in celiac disease. Gastroenterology 97:265–271, 1989.

Lundin KEA, Scott H, Hansen T, Paulsen G, Halstensen TS, Fausa O, Thorsby E, Sollid LM. Gliadin-specific, HLA-DQ(α1*0501,β0201) restricted T cells isolated from the small intestinal mucosa of celiac disease patients. J Exp Med 178:187–196, 1993.

Lungarotti MS, Ruffini S, Calbo A, Mariotti G, Ghebreggzabher M, Monaldi B. Treatment of acrodermatitis enteropathica with zinc sulfate. Helv Paediatr Acta 31:117–121, 1976.

MacFarlane IG. Autoimmunity and hepatotropic viruses. Semin Liver Dis 11:223–233, 1991.

MacKendrick W, Caplan M. Necrotizing enterocolitis. Pediatr Clin North Am 40:1047–1059, 1993.

Maddrey WC. How many types of autoimmune hepatitis are there? Gastroenterology 105:1571–1575, 1993.

Maggiore G, Bernard O, Hadchouel M, Hadchouel P, Odievre M, Alagile D. Treatment of autoimmune chronic active hepatitis in childhood. J Pediatr 104:839–844, 1984.

Mahida YR, Wu K, Jewell DP. Enhanced production of interleukin-1 beta by mononuclear cell isolated from mucosa with active ulcerative colitis of Crohn's disease. Gut 30:835–838, 1989.

Maki M, Collin P. Celiac disease. Lancet 349:1755–1759, 1997.

Maki M, Kallonen K, Lahdeaho ML, Visakorpi JK. Changing pattern of childhood coeliac disease in Finland. Acta Paediatr Scand 77:408–412, 1988.

Maki M, Mustalahti K, Kokkonen J, Kulmala P, Haapalahti M, Karttunen T, Ilonen J, Laurila K, Dahlborn I, Hansson T, Hopfl P, Knip M. Prevalence of celiac disease among children in Finland. N Engl J Med 348:2517–2524, 2003.

Malroot A, Vandenplas Y, Verlinden M, Piepsz A, Dab I. Gastroesophageal reflux and unexplained chronic respiratory disease in children. Pediatr Pulmonol 3:208–213, 1987.

Manns MP. Cytoplasmic autoantigens in autoimmune hepatitis: molecular analysis and clinical relevance. Semin Liver Dis 11:205–214, 1991.

Markowitz J, Rosa J, Grancher K, Aiges H, Daum F. Long-term 6-mercaptopurine (6-MP) in adolescents with Crohn's disease. Am J Gastroenterol 94:1347–1351, 1990.

Marsh MN. Gluten, major histocompatibility complex, and the small intestine. Gastroenterology 102:330–354, 1992.

Martin FM, Rossi RL, Nugent FW, Scholz FJ, Jenkins RL, Lewis WD, Gagner M, Foley E, Braasch JW. Surgical aspects of sclerosing cholangitis: results in 178 patients. Ann Surg 212:551–556, 1990.

Martini A, Scotta MS, Notarangelo LD, Maggiore G, Guarnaccia S, DeGiacomo C. Membranous glomerulopathy and chronic small-intestinal enteropathy associated with autoantibodies directed against renal tubular basement membrane and the cytoplasm of intestinal epithelial cells. Acta Paediatr Scand 72:931–934, 1983.

May GR, Sutherland LR, Mengs JB. Is small intestinal permeability really increased in relatives of patients with Crohn's disease? Gastroenterology 104:1627–1632, 1993.

Mayer L, Eisenhardt D. Lack of induction of suppressor T cells by intestinal epithelial cells from patients with inflammatory bowel disease. J Clin Invest 86:1255–1260, 1990.

Mayer L, Eisenhardt D, Salomon P, Bauer W, Plous R, Piccinini L. Expression of class II molecules on intestinal epithelial cells in humans. Differences between normal and inflammatory bowel disease. Gastroenterology 100:3–12, 1991.

McClure J. Malakoplakia of the gastrointestinal tract. Postgrad Med J 57:95–103, 1981.

McEntee G, Wiesner RH, Rosen C, Cooper J, Wahlstorm HE. A comparative study of patients undergoing liver transplantation for primary sclerosing cholangitis and primary biliary cirrhosis. Transplant Proc 23:1563–1564, 1991.

McGeady SJ. Transient hypogammaglobulinemia of infancy: need to reconsider name and definition. J Pediatr 110:47–50, 1987.

McLain BI, Davidson PM, Stokes KB, Beasley SW. Growth after gut resection for Crohn's disease. Arch Dis Child 65:760–762, 1990.

Mearin ML, Pena AS. Clinical indications of HLA typing and measurement of antigliadin antibodies in coeliac disease. Neth J Med 31:279–285, 1987.

Melamed D, Friedman A. Direct evidence for anergy in T lymphocytes tolerized by oral administration of ovalbumin. Eur J Immunol 23:935–942, 1993.

Mendeloff AI, Calkins BM. The epidemiology of idiopathic inflammatory bowel disease. In Kirsner J, Shorter RG, eds. Inflammatory Bowel Disease, ed 3. Philadelphia, Lea & Febiger, 1988, pp 3–34.

Metcalfe DD, Sampson HA. Workshop on experimental methodology for clinical studies of adverse reactions to foods and food additives. J Clin Immunol 86:421–442, 1990.

Mett H, Gyr K, Zak O, Vosbeck K. Duodenopancreatic secretions enhance bactericidal activity of antimicrobial drugs. Antimicrob Agents Chemother 26:35–38, 1984.

Meydani SN. Dietary modulation of cytokine production and biologic functions. Nutr Rev 10:361–369, 1990.

Meyer T, Halter R, Pohlner J. Mechanism of extracellular secretion of an IgA protease by gram-negative host cells. Adv Exp Med Biol 216B:1271–1281, 1987.

Meysman M, Debeuckelaer S, Reynaert H, Schoors DF, Dehou MF, Van Camp B. Systemic amyloidosis-induced diarrhea in sex-linked agammaglobulinemia. Am J Gastroenterol 88:1275–1277, 1993.

Michaelson G. Zinc deficiency in acrodermatitis enteropathica. Acta Derm Venereol (Stockh) 54:377–381, 1974.

Michener WM, Wyllie R. Management of children and adolescents with inflammatory bowel disease. Med Clin North Am 74:103–117, 1990.

Mike N, Hansel TT, Newman J, Asquith P. Granulomatous enteropathy in common variable immunodeficiency: a cause of chronic diarrhea. Postgrad Med J 67:446–449, 1991.

Miller TL, Orav EJ, Martin SR, Cooper ER, McIntosh K, Winter HS. Malnutrition and carbohydrate malabsorption in children with vertically transmitted human immunodeficiency virus infection. Gastroenterology 100:1296–1302, 1991.

Miller TL, Winter HS, Luginbuhl LM, Orav EJ, McIntosh K. Pancreatitis in pediatric human immunodeficiency virus infection. J Pediatr 120:223–227, 1992.

Miller TL, Evans SJ, Orav J, Morris V, McIntosh K, Winter HS. Growth and body composition in children infected with the human immunodeficiency virus-1. Am J Clin Nutr 57:588–592, 1993.

Mirakian R, Richardson A, Milla PJ, Walker-Smith JA, Unsworth J, Savage MO, Bottazzo GF. Protracted diarrhea of infancy: evidence in support of an autoimmune variant. BMJ 293:1132–1136, 1986.

Mishra A, Hogan SP, Brandt EB, Rothenberg ME. An etiological role for aeroallergens and eosinophils in experimental esophagitis. J Clin Invest 107:83–90, 2001.

Mombaerts P, Mizoguchi E, Grusby MJ, Glimcher LH, Bhan AH, Tonegawa S. Spontaneous development of inflammatory bowel disease in T cell receptor mutant mice. Cell 75:275–282, 1993.

Moran CA, West B, Schwartz IS. Malacoplakia of the colon in association with colonic adenocarcinoma. Am J Gastroenterol 84:1580–1582, 1989.

Morgan G, Levinsky RJ. Clinical significance of IgA deficiency. Arch Dis Child 63:579–581, 1988.

Morimoto C, Letvin NL, Distaso JA, Aldrich WR, Schlossman S. The isolation and characterization of the human suppressor-inducer T cell subset. J Immunol 134:1508–1515, 1985.

Morin CL, Roulet M, Roy CC, Weber A, LaPointe N. Continuous elemental enteral alimentation in the treatment of children and adolescents with Crohn's disease. J Parenteral Enteral Nutr 6:194–199, 1982.

Mowat AP. Primary sclerosing cholangitis in childhood. Gastroenterology 92:1226–1235, 1987a.

Mowat AM. The regulation of immune responses to dietary protein antigens. Immunol Today 8:93–98, 1987b.

Mowat AM, Lamont AG, Bruce MG. A genetically determined lack of oral tolerance to ovalbumin is due to the failure of the immune system to respond to intestinally derived tolerogen. Eur J Immunol 17:1673–1676, 1987.

Moynahan EJ. Acrodermatitis enteropathica: a lethal inherited human zinc deficiency disorder. Lancet 2:399–400, 1974.

Mulder AH, Horst G, Haagsma EB, Limburg PC, Kleibeuker JH, Kallenberg CG. Prevalence and characterization of neutrophil cytoplasmic antibodies in autoimmune liver disease. Hepatology 17:411–417, 1993.

Murphy MS, Walker WA. Celiac disease. Pediatr Rev 12:325–330, 1991.

Mylotte M, Egan-Mitchell B, Fottrell PF, McNicholl B, McCarthy CF. Family studies in celiac disease. J Med 43:359–369, 1974.

Narumi S, Roberts JP, Emond JC, Lake J, Ascher NL. Liver transplantation for sclerosing cholangitis. Hepatology 22:451–457, 1995.

Nelder KH, Hambidge KM. Zinc therapy in acrodermatitis enteropathica. N Engl J Med 292:879–882, 1975.

Nelder KH, Hambidge KM, Walravens BA. Acrodermatitis enteropathica. Int J Dermatol 17:380–387, 1978.

Neutra MR, Pringault E, Kraehenbuhl J-P. Antigen sampling across epithelial barriers and induction of mucosal immune responses. Annu Rev Immunol 14:275–300, 1996.

Neutra MR, Mantis NJ, Frey A, Giannasca PJ. The composition and function of M cell apical membranes: implications for microbial pathogenesis. Semin Immunol 11:171–181, 1999.

Nezelof C. Thymic dysplasia with normal immunoglobulins and immunologic deficiency: pure alymphocytosis. Birth Defects 4:104–112, 1968.

Nielsen OH, Jacobsen O, Pedersen ER Rasmussen SN, Petri M, Lauland S, Jarnum S. Non-tropical sprue: malignant diseases and mortality rate. Scand J Gastroenterol 20:13–18, 1985.

Nilsen EM, Jahnsen FL, Lundin KEA, Johansen F-E, Fausa O, Sollid LM, Jahnsen J, Scott H, Brandtzaeg P. Gluten induces an intestinal cytokine response strongly dominated by interferon gamma in patients with celiac disease. Gastroenterology 115:551–563, 1998.

Ninan T, Aggatt PJ, Smith F, Youngson G, Miller ID. Atypical genital involvement in a child with Crohn's disease. J Pediatr Gastroenterol Nutr 15:330–333, 1992.

Ninkovic M. Behçet's syndrome. In Bouchier IA, Allan RN, Hodgson HJ, Keightey MR, eds. Gastroenterology—Clinical Science and Practice. London, WB Saunders, 1993, pp 1247–1254.

Nordlie RC, Sukalskie KA, Johnson WT. Human microsomal glucose-6-phosphatase system. Eur J Pediatr 152(Suppl.):S2–S6, 1993.

Novis BH, Gilinsky NH, Wright JP, Price S, Marks IN. Plasma cell infiltration of the small intestine, recurrent pulmonary infections, and cellular immunodeficiency (Nezelof's syndrome). Am J Gastroenterol 80:891–895, 1985.

Nunez MC, Ayudarte MV, Morales D, Suarez MD, Gil A. Effect of dietary nucleotides on intestinal repair in rats with experimental chronic diarrhea. J Parenteral Enteral Nutr 14:598–604, 1990.

Odievre M, Maggiore G, Homberg JC, Saadoun F, Courouce AM, Yvart J, Hadchouel M, Alagille D. Seroimmunologic classification of chronic hepatitis in 57 children. Hepatology 3:407–409, 1983.

O'Duffy JD, Goldstein NP. Neurological involvement in seven patients with Behçet's disease. Am J Med 61:170–178, 1976.

Odze RD, Bines J, Leichtner AM, Goldman H, Antonioli DA. Allergic proctocolitis in infants: a prospective clinicopathologic biopsy study. Hum Pathol 24:668–674, 1993.

Ogoshi S, Iwasa M, Tamiya T. Effect of nucleotide and nucleoside mixture on rats given total parenteral nutrition after 70% hepatectomy. J Parenteral Enteral Nutr 9:339–342, 1985.

Oleske JM, Westphal ML, Shore S, Gorden D, Bogden JD, Nahmias A. Zinc therapy of depressed cellular immunity in acrodermatitis enteropathica. Its correction. Am J Dis Child 133:915–918, 1979.

O'Morain C, Segal AW, Levi AJ. Elemental diet as primary treatment of acute Crohn's disease: a controlled trial. BMJ 288:1859–1862, 1984.

Orenstein SR, Whittington PF, Orenstein DF. The infant seat as treatment for gastroesophageal reflux. N Engl J Med 309:760–763, 1983.

Orenstein SR, Shalaby TM, Di Lorenzo C, Putnam PE, Sigurdsson L, Kocoshis SA. The spectrum of pediatric eosinophilic esophagitis beyond infancy: a clinical series of 30 children. Am J Gastroenterol 95:1422–1430, 2000.

Ortolani C, Ispano M, Pastorello EA, Ansaloni R, Magri GC. Comparison of results of skin prick tests and RAST in 100 patients with oral allergy syndrome. J Allergy Clin Immunol 83:683–690, 1989.

Pabst R. The anatomic basis for the immune function of the gut. Anat Embryol 176:135–144, 1987.

Palmer SR, Biffin A, Gamsu HR. Outcome of necrotizing enterocolitis. Arch Dis Child 64:388–394, 1989.

Pang KY, Newman AP, Udall JN, Walker WA. Development of gastrointestinal mucosal barrier. VII. In vitro maturation of microvillus surface by cortisone. Am J Physiol 249:G85–G91, 1985.

Patterson BK, Ehrenpreis ED, Yokoo H. Focal enterocyte vacuolization. A new microscopic finding in the acquired immune deficiency syndrome. Am J Clin Pathol 99:24–27, 1993.

Peng HJ, Turner MW, Strobel S. The generation of a tolerogen after the ingestion of ovalbumin. Clin Exp Immunol 81:510–515, 1990.

Peppercorn MA. Advances in drug therapy for inflammatory bowel disease. Ann Intern Med 112:50–60, 1990.

Perisic VN, Kokai G. Bleeding from duodenal lymphangiectasia. Arch Dis Child 66:153–154, 1991.

Perisic VN, Filipovic D, Kokai G. Allergic colitis with rectal bleeding in an exclusively breast-fed neonate. Acta Paediatr Scand 77:163–164, 1988.

Perkkio M, Savilahti E. Time of appearance of immunoglobulin containing cells in the mucosa of the neonatal intestine. Pediatr Res 14:953–955, 1980.

Perlmutter DH, Leichtner AM, Goldmen H, Winter HS. Chronic diarrhea associated with hypogammaglobulinemia and enteropathy in infants and children. Dig Dis Sci 30:1149–1155, 1985.

Peterson LR, Gerding DN. Antimicrobial agents in C. difficile associated intestinal diseases. In Rambaud JC, Ducluzeau R, eds. Clostridium difficile-Associated Intestinal Diseases. New York, Springer-Verlag, 1990, pp 115–127.

Philips JO, Everson MP, Moldoveanu Z, Lue C, Mestecky J. Synergistic effect of IL-4 and IFN-gamma on the expression of polymeric Ig receptor (secretory component) and IgA binding by human epithelial cells. J Immunol 145:1740–1744, 1990.

Pignata C, Budillon G, Monaco G, Nani E, Cuomo R, Parrilli G, Ciccimara F. Jejunal bacterial overgrowth and intestinal permeability in children with immunodeficiency syndromes. Gut 31:879–882, 1990.

Plettenberg A, Stoehr A, Stellbrink HJ, Albrecht H, Meigel W. A preparation from bovine colostrum in the treatment of HIV positive patients with chronic diarrhea. Clin Invest 71:42–45, 1993.

Pol S, Romana CA, Richard S, Amouyal P, Desportes-Livage D, Carnot F, Pays JF, Berthelot P. Microsporidia infection in patients with the human immunodeficiency virus and unexplained cholangitis. N Engl J Med 328:95–99, 1993.

Porayko MK, Wiesner RH, La Russo NF, Ludwig J, MacCarty RL, Steiner BL, Twomey CK, Zinsmeister AR. Patients with asymptomatic primary sclerosing cholangitis frequently have progressive disease. Gastroenterology 98:1594–1602, 1990.

Powell GK. Milk and soy induced enterocolitis of infancy. Clinical features and standardization of challenge. J Pediatr 93:553–560, 1978.

Prentice A, MacCarthy A, Stirling DM, Vasquez-Velasquez L, Ceesay SM. Breast milk IgA and lactoferrin survival in the gastrointestinal tract: a study in rural Gambian children. Acta Paediatr Scand 78:505–512, 1989.

Present DH, Korelitz BI, Wisch N, Glass JL, Sachar DB, Pasternack BS. Treatment of Crohn's disease with 6-mercaptopurine. N Engl J Med 302:981–987, 1980.

Prochazka EJ, Terasaki PI, Park MS, Goldstein LI, Busutil RW. Association of primary sclerosing cholangitis with HLA-DRW 52a. N Engl J Med 322:1842–1844, 1990.

Proujansky R, Fawcett P, Gibney KM, Treem WR, Hyams JS. Examination of anti-neutrophil cytoplasmic antibodies in childhood inflammatory bowel disease. J Pediatr Gastroenterol Nutr 17:193–197, 1993.

Quigley EMM, La Russo NF, Ludwig J, MacSween RNM, Birnie GG, Watkinson G. Familial occurrence of primary sclerosing cholangitis and ulcerative colitis. Gastroenterology 85:1160–1165, 1983.

Radema SA, Vandeventer SJ, Cerami A. Interleukin-1 beta is expressed predominantly by enterocytes in experimental colitis. Gastroenterology 100:1180–1186, 1991.

Ramakrishna J, Langhans N, Calenda K, Grand RJ, Verhave M. Combined use of cyclosporine and azathioprine or 6-mercaptopurine in pediatric inflammatory bowel disease. J Pediatr Gastroenterol Nutr 22:296–302, 1996.

Rand EB, Whitington PF. Successful orthotopic liver transplantation in two patients with liver failure due to sclerosing cholangitis with Langerhans cell histiocytosis. J Pediatr Gastroenterol Nutr 15:202–207, 1992.

Raz I, Okon E, Chajek-Shaul T. Pulmonary manifestations in BehHet's syndrome. Chest 95:585–589, 1989.

Reddy KR, Jeffers LJ. Acquired immunodeficiency syndrome and the liver. In Schiff L, Schiff ER, eds. Diseases of the Liver, ed 7. Philadelphia, JB Lippincott, 1993, pp 1362–1372.

Reunala T, Blomquist K, Tarpila S, Halme H, Kangas K. Gluten-free diet in dermatitis herpetiformis. Clinical response of skin lesions in 81 patients. Br J Dermatol 97:473–480, 1977.

Reynolds J, Putnam P. Prokinetic agents. Gastroenterol Clin North Am 21:567–596, 1992.

Roberts MW, Atkinson JC. Oral manifestations associated with leukocyte adhesion deficiency: a five year case study. Pediatr Dent 12:107–111, 1990.

Rodewald R. Selective antibody transport in the proximal small intestine of the neonatal rat. J Cell Biol 45:635–640, 1970.

Rodin AE, Goldman AS. Autopsy findings in acrodermatitis enteropathica. Am J Clin Pathol 51:315–320, 1969.

Roe TF, Thomas DW, Gilsanz V, Isaacs H, Atkinson JB. Inflammatory bowel disease in glycogen storage disease type Ib. J Pediatr 109:55–59, 1986.

Roe TF, Coates TD, Thomas DW, Miller JH, Gilsanz V. Brief report: treatment of chronic inflammatory bowel disease in glycogen storage disease type Ib with colony-stimulating factors. N Engl J Med 326:1666–1669, 1992.

Rothman A, Snyder J. Protein-losing enteropathy following the Fontan operation: resolution following prednisone therapy. Am Heart J 121:618–619, 1991.

Rubaltelli FF, Benini F, Sala M. Prevention of necrotizing enterocolitis in neonates at risk by oral administration of monomeric IgG. Dev Pharmacol Ther 17:138–146, 1991.

Ruderman WB. Newer pharmacologic agents for the therapy of inflammatory bowel disease. Med Clin North Am 74:133–153, 1990.

Russell, GJ, Nagler-Anderson C, Anderson C, Anderson P, Bhan AK. Cytotoxic potential of intraepithelial lymphocytes. Presence of TIA-1, the cytolytic granule-associated protein, in human intraepithelial lymphocytes in normal and diseased intestine. Am J Pathol 143:350–354, 1993.

Sachdev GK, Dalton HR, Hoang P, DiPaolo MC, Crotty B, Jewell DP. Human colonic intraepithelial lymphocytes suppress in vitro immunoglobulin synthesis by autologous peripheral blood lymphocytes and lamina propria lymphocytes. Gut 34:257–263, 1993.

Sadlack B, Merz H, Schorle H, Schimpl A, Feller AC, Horak I. Ulcerative colitis like disease in mice with a disrupted interleukin-2 gene. Cell 75:253–261, 1993.

Saffran M, Franco-Saenz R, Kong A, Papahadjopoulos D, Szoka F. A model for the study of oral administration of peptide hormones. Can J Biochem 577:548–553, 1979.

Sagie E, Tarabulus J, Maier DM, Freier S. Diet and development of intestinal IgA in the mouse. Isr J Med Sci 10:532–534, 1974.

Sampson HA. Food allergy. In Shils ME, Olson JA, Shike M, eds. Modern Nutrition in Health and Disease. Baltimore, Lea & Febiger, 1994, pp 1391–1398.

Sampson HA, Albergo R. Comparison of results of skin tests, RAST, and double-blind placebo controlled food challenges in children with atopic dermatitis. J Allergy Clin Immunol 74:26–33, 1984.

Sampson HA, Broadbent KR, Bernhisel-Broadbent J. Spontaneous release of histamine from basophils and histamine-releasing factor from patients with atopic dermatitis and food hypersensitivity. N Engl J Med 321:228–232, 1989.

Sander CA, Medeiros LJ, Weiss LM, Yano T, Sneller MC, Jaffe ES. Lymphoproliferative lesions in patients with common variable immunodeficiency syndrome. Am J Surg Pathol 16:1170–1182, 1992.

Sanderson IR, Walker WA. Nutrition and immunity. Curr Opin Gastroenterol 7:463–470, 1991.

Sanderson IR, Walker WA. Uptake and transport of macromolecules by the intestine: possible role in clinical disorders. Gastroenterology 104:622–639, 1993.

Sanderson IR, Boulton P, Menzies I, Walker-Smith JA. Improvement of abnormal lactulose/rhamnose permeability in active Crohn's disease of the small bowel by an elemental diet. Gut 28:1073–1076, 1987.

Sanderson IR, Phillips AD, Spencer J, Walker-Smith JA. Response of autoimmune enteropathy to cyclosporin therapy. Gut 32:1421–1425, 1991a.

Sanderson IR, Risdon RA, Walker-Smith JA. Intractable ulcerating enterocolitis of infancy. Arch Dis Child 66:295–299, 1991b.

Santer R, Lebenthal E. Secretory diarrhea in infancy and childhood. In Lebenthal E, Duffy M, eds. Textbook of Secretory Diarrhea. New York, Raven Press, 1990, pp 337–353.

Santulli TV, Schullinger JN, Heird WC. Acute necrotizing enterocolitis in infancy: a review of 64 cases. Pediatrics 55:376–387, 1975.

Sarker SA, Gyr K. Non-immunological defense mechanisms of the gut. Gut 33:987–993, 1992.

Satti MB, Abu-Melha A. Colonic malakoplakia and abdominal tuberculosis in a child. Dis Colon Rectum 28:353–357, 1985.

Savilahti E, Pelkonen P. Clinical findings and intestinal immunoglobulins in children with partial IgA deficiency. Acta Paediatr Scand 68:513–519, 1979.

Schlaak JF, Lohr H, Gallati H, Meyer zum Buschenfelde KH, Fleischer B. Analysis of the in vitro cytokine production by liver-infiltrating T cells of patients with autoimmune hepatitis. Clin Exp Immunol 94:168–173, 1993.

Schrieber RA, Walker WA. The gastrointestinal barrier: antigen uptake and perinatal immunity. Ann Allergy 61:3–12, 1988.

Schreiber S, Raedler A, Stenson WE, MacDermott RP. The role of the mucosal immune system in inflammatory bowel disease. Gastroenterol Clin North Am 21:451–502, 1992.

Schrumpf E, Fausa O, Elgjo K, Kolmannskog F. Hepatobiliary complications of inflammatory bowel disease. Semin Liver Dis 8:201–209, 1988.

Schuppan D. Current concepts of celiac disease pathogenesis. Gastroenterology 119:234–242, 2000.

Schwarzenberg SJ, Whitington PF. Colonic stricture complicating formula protein intolerance enterocolitis. J Pediatr Gastroenterol Nutr 2:190–192, 1983.

Seibold F, Weber P, Klein R, Berg PA, Wiedmann KH. Clinical significance of antibodies against neutrophils in patients with inflammatory bowel disease and primary sclerosing cholangitis. Gut 33:657–662, 1992.

Seidman EG, Roy CC, Weber AM, Morin CL. Nutritional therapy of Crohn's disease in childhood. Dig Dis Sci 32(Suppl.):82S–88S, 1987.

Seki T, Kiyosawa K, Inoko H, Ota M. Association of autoimmune hepatitis with HLA-Bw54 and DR4 in Japanese patients. Hepatology 12:1300–1304, 1990.

Selsted ME, Miller SI, Henschen AH, Ouellette AJ. Enteric defensins: antibiotic peptide components of intestinal host defense. J Cell Biol 118:929–936, 1992.

Senaldi G, Portman B, Mowat AP, Mieli-Vergani G, Vergani D. Immunohistochemical features of the portal tract mononuclear cell infiltrate in chronic aggressive hepatitis. Arch Dis Child 67:1447–1453, 1992.

Shan L, Molberg O, Parro I, Hausch F, Filiz F, Gray GM, Sollid, LM, Khosla C. Structural basis for gluten intolerance in celiac sprue. Science 297:2275–2278, 2002.

Shepherd HA, Selby WS, Chapman RW, Nolan D, Barbatis C, McGee JO, Jewell DP. Ulcerative colitis and persistent liver dysfunction. Q J Med 52:503–513, 1983.

Shepherd RW, Boreham PFL. Recent advances in the diagnosis and management of giardiasis. Scand J Gastroenterol [Suppl] 169:60–64, 1989.

Shorter RG, Huizenga KA, Spencer RJ. A working hypothesis for the etiology and pathogenesis of inflammatory bowel disease. Am J Dig Dis 17:1024–1032, 1972.

Sigurs N, Hattevig G, Kjellman B. Maternal avoidance of eggs, cow's milk, and fish during lactation: effect on allergic manifestations, skin-prick tests, and specific IgE antibodies in children at age four years. Pediatrics 89:735–739, 1992.

Silverman A, Roy CC. Pediatric Clinical Gastroenterology, ed 3. St. Louis, Mosby, 1983, pp 226-228.

Siminoski K, Gonella P, Bernankke J, Owen L, Neutra M, Murphy R. Uptake and transepithelial transport of nerve growth factor in suckling rat ileum. J Cell Biol 103:1979–1990, 1986.

Sisto A, Feldman P, Garel L, Seidman E, Brochu P, Morin C, Weber AM, Roy CC. Primary sclerosing cholangitis in children: study of five cases and review of the literature. Pediatrics 80:918–923, 1987.

Slade HB, Schwartz SA. Mucosal immunity: the immunology of breast milk. J Allergy Clin Immunol 80:346–356, 1987.

Smith PD, Mai UE. Immunopathophysiology of gastrointestinal disease in HIV infection. Gastroenterol Clin North Am 21:331–345, 1992.

Smith PD, Lane HC, Gill VJ, Manischewitz JF, Quinnan GV, Fauci AS, Masur H. Intestinal infections in patients with the acquired immunodeficiency syndrome: etiology and response to therapy. Ann Intern Med 108:328–333, 1988.

Snook JA, Chapman RW, Sachdev GK, Heryet A, Kelly PM, Fleming KA, Jewell DP. Peripheral blood and portal tract lymphocyte populations in primary sclerosing cholangitis. J Hepatol 9:36–41, 1989.

Snyder JD, Walker WA. Structure and function of intestinal mucin: developmental aspects. Int Arch Allergy Appl Immunol 82:351–356, 1987.

Snyder JD, Rosenblum N, Wershil B, Goldman H, Winter HS. Pyloric stenosis and eosinophilic gastroenteritis in infants. J Pediatr Gastroenterol Nutr 6:543–547, 1987.

Sollid LM, Thorsby E. HLA susceptibility genes in celiac disease: genetic mapping and role in pathogenesis. Gastroenterology 105:910–922, 1993.

Spencer J, Isaacson PG, Diss TC, McDonald TT. Expression of disulfide linked and non disulfide linked forms of the T cell receptor heterodimer gamma/delta in human intraepithelial lymphocytes. Eur J Immunol 19:1335–1338, 1989.

Spencer J, Isaacson PG, McDonald TT, Thomas AJ, Walker SJ. Gamma/delta T cells and the diagnosis of celiac disease. Clin Exper Immunol 85:109–113, 1991.

Sperber KE, Mayer L. Gastrointestinal manifestations of common variable immunodeficiency. Immunol Allergy Clin North Am 8:423–434, 1988.

Spiekermann GM, Walker WA. Oral tolerance and its role in clinical disease. J Pediatr Gastroenterol Nutr 32:237–255, 2001.

Stellon AJ, Keating JJ, Johnson PJ, McFarlane IG, Williams R. Maintenance of remission in autoimmune chronic active hepatitis with azathioprine after corticosteroid withdrawal. Hepatology 8:781–784, 1988.

Stephan JL, Vlekova V, Lediest F, Blanche S, Donadieu J, Saint-Basile G, Durandy A, Griscelli C, Fischer A. Severe combined immunodeficiency: a single-center study of clinical presentation and outcome in 117 patients. J Pediatr 123:564–572, 1992.

Stern M. Gastrointestinal allergy. In Walker WA, Durie PR, Hamilton JR, Walker-Smith JA, Watkins JB, eds. Pediatric Gastrointestinal Disease. Philadelphia, BC Decker, 1991, pp 557–573.

Stevens AC, Walz G, Singaram C, Lipman ML, Zanker B, Muggia A, Antonioli D, Peppercorn MA, Strom TB. Tumor necrosis factor alpha, interleukin-1 beta, and interleukin-6 expression in inflammatory bowel disease. Dig Dis Sci 37:818–826, 1992.

Stevens AC, Lipman M, Spivak J, Peppercorn MA, Strom TB. Heightened perforin and granzyme B but not interleukin 2 mRNA transcripts in active ulcerative colitis colonic specimens. Gastroenterology 106:A778, 1994.

Stiehm ER, Chin TW, Haas A, Peerless AG. Infectious complications of the primary immunodeficiencies. Clin Immunol Immunopathol 40:69–86, 1986.

Strober W, Ehrhardt RO. Chronic intestinal inflammation: an unexpected outcome in cytokine or T cell receptor mutant mice. Cell 75:203–205, 1993.

Strober W, Harriman GR. The regulation of IgA B-cell differentiation. Gastroenterol Clin North Am 20:473–494, 1991.

Strober W, Wochner RD, Carbone PP, Waldmann TA. Intestinal lymphangiectasia: a protein losing enteropathy with hypogammaglobulinemia and impaired homograft rejection. J Clin Invest 46:1643–1656, 1967.

Sutphen JL, Grand RJ, Flores A, Chang TW, Bartlett JG. Chronic diarrhea associated with Clostridium difficile in children. Am J Dis Child 137:275–278, 1983.

Svennerholm AM, Hanson LA, Holmgren J, Jalil F, Lindblad BS, Khan SR, Nilsson A, Svennerholm B. Antibody responses to live and killed poliovirus vaccines in the milk of Swedish women. J Infect Dis 143:707–711, 1981.

Tazume S, Ozawa A, Yamamoto T, Takahashi Y, Takeshi K, Saidi SM, Ichoroh CG, Waiyaki PG. Ecological study on the intestinal bacterial flora of patients with diarrhea. Clin Infect Dis 16:S77–S82, 1993.

Teichberg S, Isolauri E, Wapnir RA, Moyse J, Lifshitz F. Development of the neonatal rat small intestinal barrier to nonspecific macromolecular absorption. II. Role of dietary corticosterone. Pediatr Res 32:50–57, 1992.

Thayer WR Jr, Brown M, Sangree MH, Katz J, Hersh T. *Escherichia coli* O:14 and and colon hemagglutinating antibodies in inflammatory bowel disease. Gastroenterology 57:311–318, 1969.

Thompson JF. Specific receptors for epidermal growth factor in rat intestinal microvillus membranes. Am J Physiol 254:G429–G435, 1988.

Thyresson N. Acrodermatitis enteropathica. Acta Derm Venereol (Stockh) 54:383–386, 1974.

Todd RF, Freyer DR. The CD11/CD18 leukocyte glycoprotein deficiency. Hematol Oncol Clin North Am 2:13–31, 1988.

Toth CA, Thomas P. Liver endocytosis and Kupffer cells. Hepatology 16:255-266, 1992.

Touraine JL, Marseglia GL, Betuel H, Souillet G, Gebuhrer L. The bare lymphocyte syndrome. Bone Marrow Transplant 9(Suppl. 1):54–56, 1992.

Treem WR, Davis PM, Hyams JS. Cyclosporine treatment of severe ulcerative colitis in children. J Pediatr 119:994–997, 1991.

Triadafilopoulos G, Pothoulakis C, O'Brien MJ, LaMont JT. Differential effects of *Clostridium difficile* toxins A and B on rabbit ileum. Gastroenterology 93:273–279, 1987.

Trier JS. Celiac sprue. N Engl J Med 325:1709–1719, 1991.

Tu RK, Peters ME, Gourley GR, Hong R. Esophageal histoplasmosis in a child with immunodeficiency with hyper-IgM. AJR Am J Roentgenol 157:381–382, 1991.

Turck D, Ythier H, Maquet E, Deveaux M, Marchandise X, Farriaux JP, Fontaine G. Intestinal permeability to [15Cr]EDTA in children with Crohn's disease and celiac disease. J Pediatr Gastroenterol Nutr 6:535–537, 1987.

Twomey JJ, Jordan PH, Laughter AH, Meuwissen HJ, Good RA. The gastric disorder of immunodeficient patients. Ann Intern Med 72:499–504, 1970.

Ullrich R, Zeitz M, Heise W, L'age M, Hoffken G, Riecken EO. Small intestinal structure and function in patients affected with human immunodeficiency virus. Ann Intern Med 111:15–21, 1989.

Ullrich R, Zeitz M, Heise W, L'age M, Ziegler K, Bergs C, Riecken EO. Mucosal atrophy is associated with loss of activated T cells in the duodenal mucosa of human immunodeficiency virus infected patients. Digestion 46(Suppl. 2):302–307, 1990.

Unsworth DJ, Hutchins P, Mitchell J, Phillips A, Hindocha P, Holborow J, Walker-Smith JA. Flat small intestinal mucosa and autoimmune antibodies against gut epithelium. J Pediatr Gastroenterol Nutr 1:503–513, 1982.

Van Arsdel PP, Larson EB. Diagnostic tests for patients with suspected allergic disease. Ann Intern Med 110:304–312, 1989.

van Berge-Henegouwen GP, Mulder CJ. Pioneer in the gluten free diet: Willem-Karel Dicke 1905–1962. Gut 34:1473–1475, 1993.

Vandenplas Y. Reflux esophagitis in infants and children: a report from the working group on gastro-oesophageal reflux disease of the European Society of Paediatric Gastroenterology and Nutrition. J Pediatr Gastroenterol Nutr 18:413–422, 1994.

Vandenplas Y, Goyvaerts H, Helven R, Sacre L. Gastroesophageal reflux, as measured by 24-hour pH monitoring, in 509 healthy infants screened for risk of sudden infant death syndrome. Pediatrics 88:834–840, 1991.

Van de Wal Y, Kooy Y, van Veelen P, Pena S, Mearin L, Papadopoulos G, Koning F. Selective deamination by tissue transglutaminase strongly enhances gliadin-specific T cell reactivity. J Immunol 161:1585–1588, 1998.

Van Sickle GJ, Powell GK, McDonald PJ, Goldblum RM. Milk and soy protein–induced enterocolitis: evidence for lymphocyte sensitization to specific food proteins. Gastroenterology 88:1915–1921, 1985.

Van Wouwe JP. Clinical and laboratory diagnosis of acrodermatitis enteropathica. Eur J Pediatr 149:2–8, 1989.

Vardy PA, Lebenthal E, Shwachman H. Intestinal lymphangiectasia: a reappraisal. Pediatrics 55:842-851, 1975.

Vento S, Garofano T, DePerri G, Dolci L, Concia E, Bassetti D. Identification of hepatitis A virus as a trigger for autoimmune chronic hepatitis type I in susceptible individuals. Lancet 337:1183–1187, 1991.

Vergani D, Mieli-Vergani G. Type II autoimmune hepatitis: what is the role of the hepatitis C virus? Gastroenterology 104:1870–1873, 1993.

Verhave M, Winter HS, Grand RJ. Azathioprine in the treatment of children with inflammatory bowel disease. J Pediatr 117:809–814, 1990.

Voss LM, Rhodes KH. Leukocyte adhesion deficiency presenting with recurrent otitis media and persistent leukocytosis. Clin Pediatr 31:442–445, 1992.

Waksman BH, Ozer H. Specialized amplification elements in the immune system. The role of nodular lymphoid organs in the mucous membranes. Prog Allergy 21:1–18, 1976.

Walker WA, Isselbacher KJ. Uptake and transport of macromolecules by the intestine: possible role in clinical disorders. Gastroenterology 67:531–550, 1974.

Walker-Smith JA. Food sensitive enteropathies. Clin Gastroenterol 15:55–69, 1986.

Walker-Smith JA, Guandalini S, Schmitz J, Shmerling D, Visakorpl JK. Revised criteria for the diagnosis of celiac disease. Arch Dis Child 65:909–911, 1990.

Walsh SV, Antonioli DA, Goldman H, Fox V, Bousvaros A, Leichtner AM, Furuta GT. Allergic esophagitis in children: a clinicopathological entity. Am J Surg Pathol 23:390–396, 1999.

Wan JM, Haw MP, Blackburn GL. Nutrition, immune function, and inflammation—an overview. Proc Nutr Soc 48:315–335, 1989.

Weaver LT, Laker MF, Nelson R, Lucas A. Milk feeding and changes in intestinal permeability and morphology in the newborn. J Pediatr Gastroenterol Nutr 6:351–358, 1987.

Webster ADB. Giardiasis and immunodeficiency diseases. Trans R Soc Trop Med Hyg 74:440–443, 1980.

Webster AD, Slavin G, Shiner M, Platts-Mills TA, Asherson GL. Celiac disease with severe hypogammaglobulinemia. Gut 22:153–157, 1981.

Weiden PL, Blaese RM, Strober W, Block JB, Waldmann TA. Impaired lymphocyte transformation in intestinal lymphangiectasia: evidence for at least two functionally distinct populations in man. J Clin Invest 51:1319–1325, 1972.

Weiner HL. Intestinal transport of macromolecules in food. Food Chem Toxicol 26:867–880, 1988.

Weiner HL. Oral tolerance with copolymer 1 for the treatment of multiple sclerosis. Proc Natl Acad Sci USA 96:3333–3335, 1999.

Weltzin RA, Lucia Jandris P, Michetti P, Fields BN, Kraehenbuhl JP, Neutra MR. Binding and transepithelial transport of immunoglobulins by intestinal M cells. J Cell Biol 108:1673–1685, 1989.

Werlin SL, Grand RJ. Severe colitis in children and adolescents: diagnosis, course, and treatment. Gastroenterology 73:828–832, 1977.

Werlin SL, Chusid MJ, Caya J, Oechler HW. Colitis in Chronic granulomatous disease. Gastroenterology 82:328–331, 1982.

Weston WL, Huff JC, Humbert JR, Hambidge KM, Neldner KH, Walravens PA. Zinc correction of defective chemotaxis in acrodermatitis enteropathica. Arch Dermatol 113:422–425, 1977.

Whiteside TL, Lasky S, Si L, VanThiel DH. Immunohistologic analysis of mononuclear cells in liver tissues and blood of patients with primary sclerosing cholangitis. Hepatology 5:468–474, 1985.

Widdowson EM, Colombo VE, Artavans CA. Changes in the organs of pigs in response to feeding for the first 24 hours after birth. II. The digestive tract. Biol Neonate 28:272–281, 1976.

Wiesner RH. Primary sclerosing cholangitis. In Schiff L, Schiff ER, eds. Diseases of the Liver, ed 7. Philadelphia, JB Lippincott, 1993, pp 411–426.

Wiesner RH, LaRusso NF. Clinicopathologic features of the syndrome of primary sclerosing cholangitis. Gastroenterology 79:200–206, 1980.

Wiesner RH, Ludwig J, LaRusso NF, MacCarty RL. Diagnosis and treatment of primary sclerosing cholangitis. Semin Liver Dis 5:241–253, 1985.

Williams AJ, Wray D, Ferguson A. The clinical entity of orofacial Crohn's disease. Q J Med 79:451–458, 1991.

Wilson MC, Fischer TJ, Riordan MM. Isolated IgG hypogammaglobulinemia in acrodermatitis enteropathica: correction with zinc therapy. Ann Allergy 48:288–291, 1982.

Winter HS, Miller TL. Gastrointestinal and nutritional problems in pediatric HIV disease. In Pizzo PA, Wilfert CM, eds. Pediatric AIDS, ed 2. Baltimore, Williams & Wilkins, 1994, pp 513–533.

Winter HS, Antonioli DA, Fukagawa N, Marcial M, Goldman H. Allergy-related proctocolitis in infants: diagnostic usefulness of rectal biopsy. Mod Pathol 3:5–10, 1990.

Wolf JL, Bye WA. The membranous (M) cell and the mucosal immune system. Annu Rev Med 35:95–112, 1984.

Wraith DG, Merret J, Roth A, Yman L, Merrett TG. Recognition of food allergic patients and their allergens by RAST technique and clinical investigation. Clin Allergy 9:25–36, 1979.

Wyatt J, Vogelsang H, Hubl W, Waldjoer T, Lochs H. Intestinal permeability and the prediction of relapse in Crohn's disease. Lancet 341:1437–1439, 1993.

Yamamoto I, Tsutsui T, Mayumi M, Kasakura S. Immunodeficiency associated with selective loss of helper/inducer T cells and hypogammaglobulinemia in a child with intestinal lymphangiectasia. Clin Exp Immunol 75:196–200, 1989.

Yang H, Shohat T, Rotter JI. The genetics of inflammatory bowel disease. In MacDermott R, Stenson W, eds. Inflammatory Bowel Disease. New York, Elsevier, 1992, pp 17–53.

Zauli D, Schrumpf E, Crespi C, Cussani F, Fausa O, Aadland E. An autoantibody profile in primary sclerosing cholangitis. J Hepatol 5:14–17, 1987.

Zeiger RS, Heller S, Mellon MH, Forsythe AB, O'Connor RD, Hamburger RN, Schatz M. Effect of combined maternal and infant food allergen avoidance on development of atopy in early infancy: a randomized study. J Allergy Clin Immunol 84:72–89, 1989.

Zinneman HH, Kaplan AP. The association of giardiasis with reduced secretory immunoglobulin A. Am J Dig Dis 17:793–797, 1972.

C H A P T E R

35

Rheumatic Disorders

Laurie O. Beitz, Laurie C. Miller, and Jane G. Schaller

GENERAL CONSIDERATIONS

The rheumatic diseases can be broadly characterized as inflammatory disorders of connective tissues throughout the body, especially of the musculoskeletal, vascular, and dermal systems. The cause and pathogenesis of most of these illnesses are poorly understood, and the diagnosis of rheumatic illnesses continues to depend on distinctive clinical characteristics in the face of supportive, nonspecific laboratory findings (Table 35-1). Treatment is generally guided by laboratory findings and clinical judgment and aimed at blunting the inflammatory response.

In the past decade, advances in molecular biology, recombinant DNA technology, and sequencing of the human genome have allowed identification of specific proteins involved in the inflammatory response common to so many rheumatic illnesses and have thus given clinicians the ability to treat rheumatic disease more specifically. In the future, use of DNA microarray technology may allow clinicians to predict disease flares and adjust therapy more quickly to limit unwanted side effects of sometimes-toxic drugs. As advances in the basic sciences continue, predicting or preventing disease in susceptible individuals may be possible.

TABLE 35-1 · RHEUMATIC DISORDERS OF CHILDHOOD

Juvenile rheumatoid arthritis
Juvenile spondyloarthropathy syndromes
  Ankylosing spondylitis
  Seronegative enthesopathy
  Arthritis with inflammatory bowel disease
  Reactive arthritis
  Psoriatic arthritis
  Reiter's disease
  Rheumatic fever
Lupus erythematosus and related disorders
  Systemic lupus erythematosus
  Neonatal lupus syndrome
  Mixed connective tissue disease
  Primary antiphospholipid syndrome
Sjögren's syndrome
Dermatomyositis
Vasculitis
  Henoch-Schönlein purpura
  Kawasaki disease
  Takayasu's arteritis
  Wegener's granulomatosis
  Behçet syndrome
Scleroderma
Eosinophilic fasciitis
Pain amplification syndromes

This chapter begins with a discussion of autoimmunity as it applies to the pathogenesis of rheumatic illnesses and is followed by laboratory tests commonly used in rheumatic diseases. Specific rheumatic disease processes are then discussed, and the chapter ends with rheumatic manifestations of infectious illnesses, immune deficiencies, and common pain syndromes.

PATHOGENESIS

All rheumatic illnesses have in common an inflammatory response. During the acute phase of inflammation, increased vascular permeability occurs, followed by phagocyte infiltration, with subsequent recruitment of monocytes/macrophages. These infiltrating cells secrete a variety of acute-phase proteins and cytokines, resulting in systemic responses such as fever. If, however, the acute phase of inflammation is not resolved, chronic inflammation ensues. It is this chronic inflammation that is characteristic of many rheumatic diseases, but how and why the inflammatory response goes unchecked are for the large part unknown.

Many of the rheumatic illnesses are characterized by findings of humoral autoimmunity (autoantibodies) and cellular autoimmunity (cells reactive to body constituents), and these observations have led to speculation that the rheumatic illnesses are caused by autoimmunity. Although this hypothesis has not been well established, much attention has been focused on the contributions of autoimmunity to the pathogenesis of rheumatic illnesses. The following discussion concentrates on mechanisms by which infectious agents, host genetic makeup, and faulty host immune responses may contribute to the development of autoimmunity and to rheumatic disease.

Infections and Autoimmunity

Rheumatic disease often seems to follow infectious illnesses, and multiple theories exist to explain how an infectious agent may elicit an abnormal host immune response resulting in chronic disease, and specifically in autoimmunity.

One hypothesis is that inflammation in general following viral infection can lead to increased expression of co-stimulatory molecules on antigen-presenting cells. This in turn may signal self-reactive lymphocyte clones to expand, resulting in autoimmune disease (von Herrath et al., 1998).

Another hypothesis maintains that molecular cross-reactivity may occur, wherein a microbial antigen appears similar to a human antigen resulting in cross-reactivity and the inability of the host immune system to discriminate foreign from self. Strong evidence suggests that this molecular mimicry contributes to the pathogenesis of chronic Lyme arthritis (Gross et al., 1998), chronic rheumatic heart disease, reactive arthritides after gastrointestinal or genitourinary infections, and HLA-B27–associated arthritides (Albani, 1994).

A third hypothesis provides that infectious illnesses may lead to tissue injury resulting in exposure of normally hidden host antigen. Lymphocytes reactive to a hidden epitope or neoantigen have not been deleted and are activated to expand; consequently autoimmunity ensues. This process occurs in a mouse model of autoimmune myocarditis (Blay et al., 1989). One or more of these processes may be applicable to human rheumatic disease.

Lymphocyte Dysregulation

Dysregulation of B lymphocytes, T lymphocytes, or both may result in autoimmunity. Each individual has immunoglobulin and T-cell receptor genes that encode for reactivity to self. During development, these B and T cells are deleted (programmed cell death or apoptosis) or become anergic (no longer reactive to specific antigen), and the host immune system becomes tolerant to self. This immunologic tolerance occurs both centrally (B cells in the bone marrow and T cells in the thymus) and peripherally (primarily in the lymph nodes and spleen). If self-reactive B or T lymphocytes escape this self-tolerance, autoimmunity may ensue (see Chapter 8).

Many mechanisms contribute to immune tolerance (Fearon and Carroll, 2000; Nemazee, 2000; Shevach, 2000), one of which is deletion of autoreactive B and T lymphocytes through induction of apoptosis. Defects in this process cause systemic autoimmune disease in mice (lpr/lpr and gld/gld mice) that resembles human systemic lupus erythematosus (SLE). These mice exhibit similar autoantibody production and immune complex–mediated organ destruction (nephritis) as do humans with SLE. The lpr/lpr mouse has a defect in the Fas protein, which is a cell surface receptor instrumental in inducing cell death. The gld/gld mouse has a defect in the protein ligand for this receptor, FasL. Both of these defects result in the inability to delete self-reactive T lymphocytes and self-reactive B lymphocytes in the periphery (Takahashi et al., 1994; Watanabe-Fakunaga et al., 1992).

Although the protein defects present in these animals are helpful to the overall understanding of contributing factors to autoimmune disease in general, they fail to explain the cause of human SLE in most patients; some individuals with FAS deficiency, Canale Smith syndrome, do develop SLE (Drappa et al., 1996; Vaishnaw et al., 1999). This is but one mechanism by which lymphocyte-mediated tolerance may be broken, and readers interested in a thorough discussion of lymphocyte-mediated autoimmunity are referred to the cited reviews (Buhl et al., 2000; Freitas and Rocha, 2000; Krammer, 2000; Nemazee, 2000; Shevach, 2000).

Genetic Influences and the Major Histocompatibility Complex

Although the rheumatic diseases do not show Mendelian patterns of inheritance, rheumatic disease in general seems to cluster in families, and identical twins are much more likely to be concordant for autoimmune disease than are dizygotic twins (Ginn et al., 1998; Shamim and Miller, 2000). Although numerous gene loci have been implicated in a variety of rheumatic illnesses (e.g., complement components C2 and C4 in SLE), by far the most important susceptibility genes thus far described are those of the major histocompatibility complex (MHC).

The following discussion addresses the structure and function of the MHC, the general MHC/rheumatic disease susceptibilities, and how genes in the MHC may contribute to the pathophysiology of rheumatic illnesses. More specific MHC/rheumatic disease susceptibilities are discussed in particular disease sections.

MHC Structure and Function

The MHC is made up of class I, class II, and class III molecules and is located on the short arm of chromosome 6. Proteins of the MHC were first recognized as a result of graft rejection, thereby affording them their name (histocompatibility). The genes of the MHC class I and II loci encode the human leukocyte antigens (HLAs) that are necessary for the presentation of foreign peptides to their antigen-specific T lymphocytes. This recognition results in antigen-specific T-cell activation and clearance of cells and organisms bearing the foreign peptides.

Class I MHC molecules are composed of an α chain that binds and presents cytosolic protein antigen and a noncovalently interacting β chain (β2-microglobulin) that functions to stabilize the α chain/peptide complex. The α chains are encoded by multiallelic HLA-A, HLA-B, and HLA-C genes, whereas the nonpolymorphic β chain is encoded by a gene outside the MHC. MHC class I molecules are recognized by $CD8^+$ T cells, predominantly cytotoxic T lymphocytes (CTLs), that and help rid the hosts of intracellular microbes.

MHC class II molecules, termed *HLA-DR, HLA-DQ,* and *HLA-DP,* are composed of two noncovalently interacting highly polymorphic chains, α and β. The peptide-binding domain is formed by extracellular portions of both the α and β chains. Bound peptide (usually from extracellular proteins endocytosed and processed) is presented to $CD4^+$ helper T cells. These helper T cells are then activated for both humoral and cellular immune responses.

MHC and Disease Susceptibility

Certain MHC molecules are found in higher frequencies in individuals diagnosed with particular rheumatic illnesses. The most striking example of an HLA association with rheumatic disease is for the HLA-B27 antigen and ankylosing spondylitis (AS). Among individuals with AS, 90% have the HLA-B27 antigen, and the relative risk of developing AS in an individual positive for B27 is 90 to 100 times greater than that for an individual without this antigen. This striking association, however, is not noted in most other rheumatic illnesses. For example, the relative risk of developing a certain sub-type of juvenile rheumatoid arthritis (JRA) (pauciarticular JRA) if one is DR8 antigen positive is only five times that of those individuals who do not express the DR8 antigen. This means that if the overall risk of developing pauciarticular JRA in a particular population is 1 in 20,000, the child who is DR8 antigen positive now has a risk of 1 in 4000 of developing disease.

Although having a particular MHC background may predispose patients to a particular rheumatic disease, for most illnesses it is a poor predictor of which individual with a particular genotype will actually develop the disease. Relative risks of developing other rheumatic illnesses are listed in Table 35-2 (Cassidy and Petty, 1995; Nepom and Nepom, 1998).

Why are particular HLA antigens associated with rheumatic disease? Several possibilities exist. First, the protein itself may be involved in the disease process, as demonstrated in a rat model of AS. In this model, the human HLA-B27 molecule is expressed in rats, and the rats develop ankylosis of the spine mimicking the human disease (Hammer et al., 1990). Because the only human molecule expressed is the B27 antigen, this points to HLA-B27 as the causative agent of the disease. However, this association has not been shown for other rheumatic diseases in which the HLA associations are much weaker.

For other rheumatic diseases, although the HLA antigen may in some as yet undefined way contribute to the disease process, it is also possible that other genes in the vicinity of the studied gene are causative. This would be a consequence of so-called linkage disequilibrium, wherein one gene is inherited with another at an increased frequency. This may be true in the case of SLE, wherein the C4A allele is inherited with increased frequency with the DR3 haplotype. It may be that the presence of the C4A allele is actually associated with the increase in disease frequency seen in DR3-expressing individuals (Fielder et al., 1983; Howard et al., 1986).

Finally, HLA antigens may be associated with particular rheumatic illnesses as a consequence of similarities between self MHC antigens and antigens from infec-tious agents. The antigen similarities may result in a host autoimmune response after a particular infectious illness. Although many mechanisms are possible, their importance in individual rheumatic illnesses has not been determined.

In summary, although HLA typing may be helpful in trying to identify the potential contributing factors in the pathogenesis of a particular rheumatic disease, HLA typing is not helpful from a clinical or diagnostic stand-point (other than HLA-B27). Although an individual with a particular HLA antigen may be at increased risk of developing disease, most individuals with that HLA type will not develop disease. Furthermore, many individuals with a particular rheumatic illness will not have the most common disease-associated HLA allele(s). Therefore HLA genotyping for most patients with rheumatic illnesses is not indicated from a clinical standpoint.

LABORATORY STUDIES

Many laboratory tests performed in the diagnosis and follow-up of patients with rheumatic conditions are nonspecific and are manifestations of the acute-phase response. Others are found more specifically in particular diseases and are helpful in substantiating suspected rheumatologic disease. The following is a discussion of the most commonly used laboratory tests and how they apply to the classification and treatment of pediatric rheumatic illnesses.

Inflammation and the Acute-Phase Response

Inflammation localized to a particular organ system, or several organ systems or sites, is accompanied by sys-temic changes that have been referred to as the *acute-phase response*. The acute-phase response accompanies both acute and chronic inflammatory conditions, including infection, trauma, tissue hypoperfusion, can-cer, and immune-mediated disease. Because rheumatic diseases are manifested by acute and chronic inflamma-tion, clinical and laboratory changes accompanying the acute-phase response are commonly seen.

Acute-phase proteins are those whose concentrations increase or decrease during the acute-phase response (Table 35-3). These proteins are induced by the action of cytokines, the most important of which are inter-leukin (IL)-1β, IL-6, IL-8, tumor necrosis factor-α (TNF-α), interferon-γ, and transforming growth factor-β (TGF-β) (Gabay and Kushner, 1999). Clinically, the acute-phase response is manifest by constitutional symp-toms such as fever, anorexia, somnolence, and fatigue.

Laboratory findings accompanying the acute-phase response include hematologic abnormalities such as anemia, leukocytosis, and thrombocytosis and decreases in serum iron and zinc concentrations. The most com-mon tests to follow the acute-phase response are the ery-throcyte sedimentation rate (ESR) and the C-reactive protein (CRP).

. . . .

TABLE 35-2 · HLA AND RELATIVE RISK OF RHEUMATIC ILLNESSES

Disease	Antigen	RR
Ankylosing spondylitis	HLA-B27	90–100
Juvenile rheumatoid arthritis		
Systemic onset	HLA-DR4	3
	HLA-DR5	5
	HLA-DR8	4
Polyarticular (RF–)	HLA-DR8	6
Pauciarticular	HLA-DR5	4.5
	HLA-DR8	5
	HLA-DP2.1	4
Juvenile dermatomyositis	HLA-DR3	3
Systemic lupus erythematosus	HLA-DR2	3

RF = rheumatoid factor; RR = relative risk.

TABLE 35-3 · ACUTE-PHASE PROTEIN ALTERATIONS DURING THE ACUTE-PHASE RESPONSE

Increase in the Acute-Phase Response
Complement components (C3, C4, C9, C1 inhibitor, mannose-
  binding lectin)
Fibrinogen
Immune globulins
Ceruloplasmin
Haptoglobin
C-reactive protein
Serum amyloid A
Ferritin

Decrease in the Acute-Phase Response
Albumin
Insulin-like growth factor-1
Thyroxine-binding globulin
Transferrin

Erythrocyte Sedimentation Rate and C-Reactive Protein

ESR and CRP are nonspecific indicators of ongoing inflammation. Many patients with active inflammation, either systemic or localized, exhibit elevated ESR or CRP; however, this is not universally the case. Although ESR and CRP determinations are often helpful in following the effects of treatment, they cannot be used as a sole indicator of disease activity. As the patient's condition improves, the ESR tends to normalize slowly, whereas CRP concentrations change more rapidly (Gabay and Kushner, 1999).

ESR

The ESR is primarily dependent on the concentration of plasma fibrinogen, although other serum proteins may also influence the ESR. Elevations in fibrinogen nonspecifically accompany inflammatory states, thus increasing the ESR. The ESR has advantages over other indictors of inflammation in that it is simple, well tested, inexpensive, and widely available. However, the ESR tends to remain elevated as inflammation resolves, therefore lagging behind the activity of disease.

The ESR is often elevated in anemia; with the use of certain drugs (including heparin and some oral contraceptives); in pregnancy; and in patients with increased quantities of immunoglobulins, such as in multiple myeloma and Waldenström's macroglobulinemia and after intravenous immunoglobulin (IVIG) treatment (Bain, 1983; Burton, 1967; Kauffman et al., 1980; Ozanne et al., 1983; Penchas et al., 1978).

In contrast, the ESR is decreased in patients with polycythemia, sickle cell disease, and other condi-

tions with abnormal red blood cell morphology and in some patients with congestive heart failure and hemodynamic compromise (Haber et al., 1991; Reinhart, 1989). Sex, age, race, and obesity may also affect the ESR (Dalhoj and Wiggers, 1990; Gillum, 1993; Haber et al., 1991).

C-Reactive Protein

CRP is a 27-kD polypeptide that was first identified as a precipitin from the sera of patients with pneumococcal pneumonia, rheumatic fever, and streptococcal infections (Pincus, 1998). Concentrations can increase up to 500-fold in active inflammatory disease and can normalize more quickly than the ESR with a decrease in the inflammatory state. Therefore CRP is more useful in following inflammatory activity than is the ESR, but because of complex methods of detection (immunodiffusion, radioimmunoassay [RIA], and nephelometry), CRP results are not as quickly available. Interestingly, however, CRPs are often normal in active SLE, increasing only with infectious illnesses in these patients (Pereira Da Silva et al., 1980).

Rheumatoid Factors

Classically, rheumatoid factors (RFs) are IgM autoantibodies directed toward the constant region (Fc) of IgG (Milgrom, 1988; Moore and Dorner, 1993; Williams, 1992). RFs were first discovered fortuitously in the sera of adults with classic rheumatoid arthritis (RA) in the 1930s and have now been identified in patients with several other diseases, including tuberculosis, syphilis, hepatitis B, hepatitis C, leukemia, lymphoma, multiple gastrointestinal malignancies, Sjögren's syndrome, SLE, and sarcoid (and in a subset of the healthy population). RF assays are primarily used in the classification of adult RA and to characterize one type of polyarticular JRA. Most children with JRA do not have classic IgM serum RFs, but many may have hidden RFs of poorly defined significance (Moore et al., 1974, 1978).

Several methods exist for the detection of RFs, but the latex agglutination assay is the most common. In this assay, IgG exposing the Fc portion of the molecule is fixed to latex particles, patient sera is added, and if RFs are present, visible agglutination ensues (Fig. 35-1). Dilution of the patient's sera is performed to determine the quantity of reactive antibody present. Recently, enzyme-linked immunosorbent assay (ELISA) methods have been developed to improve the sensitivity of testing, because RFs of the IgG and IgA subclasses agglutinate poorly.

Why RFs occur in RA is speculative. Several hypotheses exist, including the following: (1) RF-producing

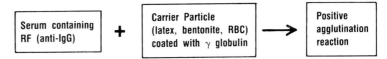

Figure 35-1· Agglutination test to demonstrate anti–gamma globulin antibodies (rheumatoid factors).

B cells may elicit "help" from T cells as a result of binding and processing immune complexes (Carson et al., 1991; Coulie and Van Snick, 1985; Roosnek and Lanzavecchia, 1991; Tighe et al., 1993); (2) RFs may develop as a consequence of cross-reactivity with a foreign infectious antigen; or (3) RFs may develop through anti-idiotypic mimicry of other Fc-binding proteins (such as *Staphylococcus aureus* protein A) (Oppliger et al., 1987; Williams, 1988). Although none have been proven for the human disease, new developments in x-ray crystallography may help sort out the likely culprit(s) (Corper et al., 1997).

The role of classical RFs in disease causation is debatable, but their presence may help characterize the patient's disease state and activity. As RFs form immune complexes with IgG, they may mediate tissue destruction by activating complement and by binding Fcγ receptors on macrophages, resulting in cytokine release. Patients with high RF positivity are more likely to have associated vasculitis (Jodo et al., 1995), and fluctuations in an individual's RF levels correlate with articular disease (Listing et al., 2000; Mottonen et al., 1998; Westedt et al., 1985). Immune complexes containing RFs can be found in diseased synovial tissues and blood vessels from patients with active diseases (Cooke et al., 1975; Johnson and Faulk, 1976; Mannik and Nardella, 1985). Finally, classical RF-negative children with hidden RFs may have more joint inflammation (Moore et al., 1978).

Lupus Erythematosus Cell

The lupus erythematosus (LE) cell was described in the early 1940s by Hargraves, who noted the presence of characteristic inclusion-containing cells in the bone marrow of several patients with SLE (Hargraves, 1969; Hargraves et al., 1948). These cells have also been identified in other body fluids (peritoneal, pericardial, and pleural) of patients with active SLE.

Soon after Hargraves' description of the LE cell, a factor was found to be present in the sera of these SLE patients that induced LE cell formation (Haserick et al., 1950). This factor was determined to be immunoglobulin that reacted with isolated cell nuclei, leading to phagocytosis. The LE factor is now known to be an antinuclear antibody (ANA). Although still available in some laboratories, the LE cell test has for the most part been replaced by more specific tests for ANAs.

Antinuclear Antibodies

The ANAs are antibodies that react with various constituents of cell nuclei. The antigenic targets of ANAs include deoxyribonucleic acid (DNA), histones, non–histone-associated nuclear proteins (RNP, Sm, Ro, La), nuclear enzymes (topoisomerase I and others), and proteins associated with nucleoli and centromeres (Beck, 1969; Friou, 1967; Kunkel and Tan, 1964; Nakamura and Tan, 1978; Notman et al., 1975; Seligmann et al., 1965; Sharp et al., 1976; Tan, 1982; Tan et al., 1982b).

There has been intense research both to determine the specific molecular components of the antigenic targets of ANAs and to determine the characteristics of ANAs (Nakamura and Tan, 1992; Tan, 1989). Despite much new information, the stimuli for production of these autoantibodies and the understanding of their pathogenic role remain an enigma. ANAs of all three major immunoglobulin classes (IgG, IgA, and IgM) have been identified. An individual serum usually contains ANAs reactive with more than one nuclear antigen, resulting from antibody cross-reactivity or the presence of several different ANAs in the same individual.

Laboratory Detection

ANAs are detected with immunofluorescent staining techniques that use a stable source of cell nuclei. Hep2 cells (a human laryngeal carcinoma cell line) are most commonly used today. The technique of detecting ANAs is outlined in Figure 35-2. Fixed cells (nuclear substrate) on a slide are overlaid with the test serum; ANAs in the serum adhere to the cell nuclei. The preparation is washed and layered with a fluorescent-labeled antibody to human immunoglobulin (most commercially available kits use secondary fluorescent antibodies to IgG), which binds to adherent ANAs. Positive preparations appear as fluorescent stained nuclei. Serum containing ANA is generally titered, and the result is reported as the highest dilution at which a positive staining is still detected. The ANA titer in patients with rheumatic disease generally does not correlate well with clinical findings, however, and is usually not helpful in following the course of disease.

Other methods for detecting specific types of ANAs are available. ELISA methods are becoming the most commonly used means of testing for specific autoantibodies (Maddison et al., 1985; Saitta and Keene, 1992). In addition, methods such as counterimmunoelectrophoresis, precipitation in agar gel (Ouchterlony), and passive hemagglutination are sometimes used.

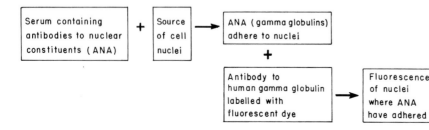

Figure 35-2 · Immunofluorescent method for detection of antinuclear antibodies.

ANA Patterns and Specificities

A variety of patterns of ANA staining are described, including peripheral, homogeneous, speckled, centromere, and nucleolar. The pattern of staining may indicate the type of ANA present and may correlate with a particular disease. A peripheral or homogeneous pattern may be indicative of anti-DNA or histone antibodies, and speckled patterns correlate with anti-Smith (Sm) or RNP specificities (Friou, 1967; Sharp et al., 1976). Nucleolar and centromere staining are often associated with scleroderma (Fritzler et al., 1980; Livingston et al., 1987; Powell et al., 1984).

Determination of the antigen specificities of a patient's ANA may be helpful in the diagnosis of autoimmune diseases. Molecular techniques are used to delineate the specificities of autoantibody reactivity with nuclear antigens. Table 35-4 lists clinically important autoantibody reactivities and their recognized disease associations. Many of the antigen targets of rheumatic autoantibodies are molecules with critical cellular functions. It is unknown whether these molecules are the eliciting immunogens for autoantibody formation or whether these autoantibodies are directly pathogenic based on interaction with these intranuclear antigens (Tan, 1989).

Other important ANA specificities include antibodies reactive with RNA-binding proteins, called Ro/SS-A, La/SS-B, Sm (Smith), and ribonuclear protein (RNP) (see Table 35-4). The Sm and RNP antigens are subcellular particles made up of small nuclear RNA complexed with a set of nuclear nonhistone proteins. These protein and RNA particles have been extensively studied, and their structures have been elucidated through genetic cloning (Craft, 1992; Lerner and Steitz, 1979). Antibodies to Sm are strongly associated with SLE. RNP antibodies were once thought to be diagnostic of mixed connective tissue disease (MCTD) but are also found in SLE and overlap syndromes (Borg et al., 1990; Farber and Bole, 1976; Munieus and Schur, 1983; Sharp et al., 1972; Winn et al., 1979). Titers of these autoantibodies may fluctuate during the course of disease and are rarely useful in the prediction of disease activity.

Ro/SS-A and La/SS-B antibodies are commonly seen in SLE, but the Ro/SS-A antigen was first described in the sera of patients with Sjögren's syndrome (Ben-Chetrit, 1993). The Ro/SS-A autoantigen consists of a 52-kD protein and a 60-kD protein complexed with one of four small RNAs (Harley et al., 1992; Pourmand et al., 1998). The La/SS-B antigen reactivity is with a 50-kD protein that also associates with RNA (St. Clair, 1992). Individuals who have anti-La/SS-B antibodies commonly have anti-Ro/SS-A antibodies, and Ro/SS-A and La/SS-B have been shown to co-localize in the nucleus (Scofield et al., 1999). Both anti-Ro/SS-A and anti-La/SS-B are found in some individuals with SLE, Sjögren's syndrome, subacute cutaneous lupus erythematosus (SCLE), and C2 complement deficiency. These antibodies are strongly associated with the neonatal lupus syndrome (NLS).

Clinical Significance

The detection of ANAs as an isolated laboratory finding is neither diagnostic nor specific for any one disease. ANAs can be detected in 2% to 9% of healthy children (Allen et al., 1991; Kasapcopur et al., 1999; Martini et al., 1989). Cabral and colleagues (1992) found no progression to autoimmune disease among a group of healthy children with positive ANA tests who were carefully followed over an average of 5 years. These data suggest that a child with a positive ANA but no other autoantibodies or clinical findings suggestive of rheumatic illness has little likelihood of developing a rheumatic disease. ANAs are also found in higher frequency among first- or second-degree relatives of patients with rheumatic disease (Miles and Isenberg, 1993).

ANAs are not diagnostic of the presence of a rheumatic disease but do provide valuable information. ANAs are detected in virtually all patients with SLE; the use of human cells for substrate has almost eliminated the occurrence of ANA-negative SLE. ANAs are also routinely found in about 25% of patients with dermatomyositis and in 50% of patients with scleroderma.

ANAs are often found in children with JRA; indeed 50% of young children with pauciarticular-onset disease have detectable ANA, often in low titer (Dracou

---

TABLE 35-4 · AUTOANTIBODY SPECIFICITIES AND DISEASE ASSOCIATIONS

Autoantibody	Disease Association	Specificity
DNA	SLE	dsDNA
RNP	SLE, MCTD	Ribosomal nucleoproteins (70, 30, 22 kD) complexed with U1 snRNA
Sm	SLE	Nucleoproteins (9, 11, 13, 16, 28, 29 kD) complexed with U1, U2, U4-6 snRNAs
Histone	SLE, drug-induced SLE, JRA	H1, H2A, B, H3, H4
Ro (SSA)	SLE, Sjögren's syndrome, neonatal SLE	52- or 60-kD protein complexed with RNA particles
La (SSB)	SLE, Sjögren's syndrome, neonatal SLE	48-kD protein complexed with RNA polymerase proteins
Nucleolar	Scleroderma	RNA Pol 1, fibrillarin
Centromere	Scleroderma, CREST	Centromere proteins (17, 80, 140 kD)
SCL-70	Scleroderma	DNA topoisomerase 1
Jo1	Polymyositis	Histidyl tRNA synthetase
PM-Scl	Overlap polymyositis/scleroderma	Complex of 11 polypeptides

CREST = calcinosis, Raynaud's phenomenon, esophageal motility disorders, sclerodactyly, and telangiectasia; dsDNA = double-stranded DNA; JRA = juvenile rheumatoid arthritis; MCTD = mixed connective tissue disease; SLE = systemic lupus erythematosus; Sn RNA = small nuclear RNA; tRNA = transfer RNA.

et al., 1998; Egeskjold et al., 1982; Garcia-De LaTorre and Miranda-Mendez, 1982; Glass et al., 1980). In these children, the ANA is highly associated with an increased risk for chronic iridocyclitis (Dracou et al., 1998; Glass et al., 1980; Schaller et al., 1974). ANAs are also detected in children with polyarticular-onset JRA.

ANAs are found in a variety of other medical conditions. Patients with bacterial, viral, fungal, or parasitic infections may have a positive ANA that persists for a short time after recovery, and patients taking certain medications may be ANA positive during their therapy. ANAs may also be detected in patients with chronic active (lupoid) hepatitis and malignancies (Doniach et al., 1966; Gurian et al., 1985; Zuber, 1992). Thus the significance of a positive ANA is influenced by the patient's clinical problem.

Anti-DNA Antibodies

Autoantibodies reactive with DNA are detected most often in patients with SLE. Several tests are available. The Farr radioimmunoassay detects anti-DNA antibodies using ammonium sulfate precipitation with radiolabeled DNA. Because it is a fluid-phase assay, it detects high avidity anti-DNA antibodies. The often-used ELISA technique is more sensitive than the Farr assay because it detects lower avidity antibodies and because the reactivity takes place on a solid support (Tipping et al., 1991). The Crithidia assay uses the protozoan *Crithidia luciliae* as a source of double-stranded DNA to detect antibodies by indirect immunofluorescence, similar to that used for the ANA assay (Chubick et al., 1978; Crowe and Kushner, 1977). The Crithidia immunofluorescence assay (IFA) lacks the sensitivity of ELISA but is more specific for DNA.

Clinical Significance

Anti-DNA antibodies are relatively specific for SLE but occur in only about 60% of SLE patients (Schur and Sandson, 1968; Tan et al., 1966; Weinstein et al., 1983). Titers of anti-DNA antibody often correlate with disease activity and can be used to indicate response to therapy or impending disease flare (Rothfield and Stollar, 1967; Ward et al., 1989). Immune complexes containing anti-DNA are found in the glomeruli of patients with nephritis glomerulonephritis, implying a pathologic role.

Antihistone Antibodies

Autoantibodies directed against histones are found in patients with several rheumatic conditions, most commonly SLE and drug-induced SLE. Histones are nuclear proteins that function to form DNA into chromatin structures. There are five types of histones separated into two groups: (1) the core particle histones H2A, H2B, H3, and H4 and (2) H1 and variants. In the nucle-

osome, DNA winds in two superhelical turns around two molecules each of H2A, H2B, H3, and H4; H1 is found associated with the nucleosome in proximity to DNA entering and exiting the nucleosome (Fritzler, 1993; Monestier et al., 1990). Antihistone antibodies are most commonly assayed with ELISA, RIA, or Western blotting using purified histones or chromatin components as antigens. The presence of antihistone antibodies correlates with an ANA with a homogenous or diffuse pattern of immunofluorescence with the hep-2 substrate.

Clinical Significance

Antihistone antibodies are commonly found in drug-induced (especially procainamide, hydralazine, and minocycline) lupus-like illnesses and in SLE (Akin et al., 1998; Ladd et al., 1962; Reinhardt and Waldron, 1954; Shackman et al., 1954). Interestingly, the antibody reactivity to particular histone protein varies from one drug to another and from that found in SLE. In SLE, reactivity is most often observed to H1 and H2B (Gioud et al., 1982; Hardin and Thomas, 1983). There is poor correlation of clinical symptoms or course with the presence of antihistone antibodies. Finally, antihistone antibodies are found in patients with RA, JRA (see later discussion), and primary biliary cirrhosis.

Antineutrophil Cytoplasmic Antibodies

Autoantibodies reactive with neutrophil granules were first described by van der Woude and colleagues in 1985. These antineutrophil cytoplasmic antibodies (ANCAs) were first found in the sera of patients with Wegener's granulomatosis. Since then, there has been intense investigation into the antigenic specificity and clinical applicability of these autoantibodies.

ANCA assays are performed by indirect immunofluorescence using human neutrophils as the substrate and often confirmed with ELISA assays. Two patterns of staining are seen, indicating reactivity with different antigens and correlating with different disease states. The autoantigens to which ANCAs are directed are enzymes in the primary and lysosomal granules of neutrophils; c-ANCAs are directed against proteinase 3, a serine protease, and p-ANCAs are primarily reactive with myeloperoxidase but also react with elastase and lactoferrin (Bini et al., 1992; Falk and Jennette, 1988; Goldschmeding et al., 1990).

Cytoplasmic ANCAs (c-ANCAs) have a diffuse granular reactivity and correlate well with ELISA positivity for proteinase 3, whereas perinuclear ANCAs (p-ANCAs) have staining around the nucleus and are often found nonspecifically in patients with positive ANAs and correlate much less well with ELISA positivity for myeloperoxidase (Merkel et al., 1997). Other recently described proteins with ANCA reactivity include cathepsin G, bacterial/permeability increasing protein (BPI), and azurocidin (Zhao and Lockwood, 1996; Zhao et al., 1995). ELISAs specific for these autoantigens are now performed in some laboratories.

Clinical Significance

The presence of a c-ANCA strongly suggests Wegener's granulomatosis and can be found in 50% to 96% of these patients (Bleil et al., 1991; Nolle et al., 1989). Fluctuations in titers may be useful in following disease activity or predicting flares of disease in patients with Wegener's granulomatosis (Egner and Chapel, 1990; Halma et al., 1990; Tervaert et al., 1990b). Also, c-ANCA can be detected in patients with microscopic polyangiitis and has rarely been reported in Kawasaki disease (KD) (Falk and Jennette, 1988; Harrison et al., 1989; Savage et al., 1989; Tervaert et al., 1991).

The p-ANCAs are less specific than c-ANCAs. Perinuclear ANCA is found in patients with microscopic polyangiitis, necrotizing crescentic glomerulonephritis, and granulomatous vasculitic disorders such as Churg-Strauss syndrome (Halma et al., 1990; Tervaert et al., 1990a). p-ANCA has also been reported in patients with ulcerative colitis, primary sclerosing cholangitis, and autoimmune hepatitis (Hardarson et al., 1993). The IgA isotype of p-ANCA has been reported in patients with Henoch-Schönlein nephropathy (van den Wall Bake, 1989). Both p-ANCA and c-ANCA have been recognized in patients with human immunodeficiency virus (HIV) infection (Klaasen et al., 1992).

Antibodies to Hematopoietic Cell Surface Proteins

Hematopoietic cells such as red cells, platelets, and lymphocytes may be targets for autoantibodies in patients with rheumatic diseases, most commonly in SLE (Karpatkin et al., 1972; Rustagi et al., 1985; Winfield et al., 1992). Red cell antibodies can be detected with the direct antiglobulin test (Coombs' test) (Mongan et al., 1967). However, there are patients with SLE and autoimmune hemolytic anemia who have negative direct Coombs' test results. This circumstance is thought to be a consequence of either low-affinity red cell antibody or red cell antibody of an IgA isotype (Biagi et al., 1999; Kondo et al., 1998; Meyer et al., 1999).

An indirect Coombs' test detects free anti–red cell antibody in the serum. These autoantibodies, when directed against the patient's own red blood cells, result in autoimmune hemolytic anemia, but in such circumstances both the direct and indirect Coombs' test results are positive. A positive direct Coombs' test result is often present in the absence of hemolytic anemia.

Autoantibodies reactive with leukocytes and platelets are also found in patients with SLE.

Antiphospholipid Antibodies

Antiphospholipid antibodies (APLAs) are autoantibodies directed against negatively charged phospholipids alone or in association with other proteins such as B2 glycoprotein-1 (Subang et al., 2000). APLAs include both the lupus anticoagulant and anticardiolipin antibodies, with the former designated by functional assays and the latter by ELISA. APLAs may be found in patients with SLE or unassociated with other disease in the primary antiphospholipid antibody (APLA) syndrome. These antibodies are associated with arterial and venous thrombosis, thrombocytopenia, and recurrent pregnancy loss.

Antiphospholipid antibodies are generally assayed by using a combination of functional coagulation assays or by using the antibodies themselves. Functional tests (measures of lupus anticoagulant activity) include the partial thromboplastin time (PTT), kaolin clotting time, and dilute Russell viper venom time. The lupus anticoagulants function by interfering with one or more of these in vitro phospholipid-dependent tests (coagulation tests that are phospholipid independent, such as the prothrombin time in which commercial reagents contain an excess of phospholipid, are not affected by lupus anticoagulant activity) (Bevers et al., 1991; Grosset and Rodgers, 1999). Several are usually done in combination.

If the PTT is prolonged, a mix of patient plasma and control plasma is done to ensure that a factor deficiency is not present, and then a source of phospholipid is added to overwhelm the antibody, resulting in return of the coagulation times to normal or near normal. This confirms in vitro anticoagulant activity. Next, antibodies to phospholipids or associated proteins are assayed with ELISA. ELISA tests for APLAs are generally directed toward cardiolipin and include antibodies of the IgG, IgM, or IgA isotypes. Another ELISA test assays antibodies reactive to B2 glycoprotein-1 (Alarcon-Segovia and Cabral, 2000). Finally, false-positive syphilis reagin test results are found in patients with antiphospholipid antibodies.

If the APLA syndrome is suspected, both functional coagulation assays (lupus anticoagulant) and ELISA assays should be performed, because APLAs are quite heterogenous and patients may have a an abnormal coagulation time and nondetectable anticardiolipin antibodies or vice versa.

APLAs are present in patients with autoimmune disease and in patients with infections (syphilis, HIV, and others) or malignancy (Kalunian et al., 1988; Love and Santoro, 1990; Sammaritano et al., 1990; Taillan et al., 1989; Vaarala et al., 1986). APLAs are found in 30% to 40% of patients with SLE and when present, especially a high-titer IgG, may indicate an increased risk of thrombosis, thrombocytopenia, hemolytic anemia, stroke, chorea, transverse myelitis, and cardiac valvular disease (Alarcon-Segovia et al., 1989; Asherson and Hughes, 1988; Asherson et al., 1989; Cronin et al., 1988; Ford et al., 1988; Harris et al., 1985; Lavalle et al., 1990).

Immune Complexes

Circulating complexes of antigen and antibody are present in many rheumatic diseases, notably SLE and some forms of vasculitis. Although they participate in disease pathogenesis through tissue deposition and activation of complement, immune complex assays are generally not useful in diagnosis or in following the course of disease.

Various laboratory assays are available for detection of immune complexes; results can be difficult to interpret because of poor standardization and interlaboratory variability. Methods include the following: (1) complement fixation tests, which measure the ability of a serum to consume a standard amount of complement in the presence of aggregates of antigen and antibody; (2) binding of the immune complexes to purified C1q; and (3) the sensitive Raji cell assay in which immune complexes bind to this lymphoblastoid cell that has a high concentration of complement receptors.

Immunoglobulins

Elevated levels of immunoglobulins are often found in the rheumatic diseases in childhood. Patients with SLE often have marked elevations of one or more immunoglobulin classes. Increased levels of immunoglobulins may also occur in JRA, scleroderma, dermatomyositis, and vasculitis and indicate a generalized inflammatory state, without specific diagnostic value. IgE levels may be elevated in vasculitis, particularly in Kawasaki disease (Miyata et al., 1984). Syndromes of depressed or absent antibody production may be associated with rheumatic illnesses as well (see section on immunodeficiencies).

Complement

The complement system is composed of numerous plasma proteins, which act in a network to perform critical biologic functions, including protection from infection by foreign organisms, opsonization of foreign antigens, and clearance of cell debris resulting from cell injury and lysis (Frank, 1992; Nusinow et al., 1985; Schur and Austen, 1972). The complement system can be activated by one of three pathways: the classical pathway, the alternative pathway, and the mannose-binding protein pathway. A complete discussion of the complement system can be found in Chapter 7.

Measurements of complement activity and complement components provide diagnostic information and indicate disease activity in several rheumatic diseases, notably SLE. In diseases characterized by immune complex formation, depression of serum complement indicates active disease. This is particularly true in SLE, serum sickness, poststreptococcal glomerulonephritis, and cryoglobulinemia. Some rheumatic diseases associated with nephritis, including Henoch-Schönlein purpura (HSP), polyarteritis, and Wegener's granulomatosis, are not associated with depression of serum complement; therefore determination of serum complement can have diagnostic utility.

Measurement of the total serum hemolytic complement (CH_{50}) is the most useful laboratory test because it reflects the functional integrity of the entire complement cascade. This test measures the ability of a test serum to hemolyze sensitized (antibody-coated) red blood cells. Measurement of individual complement components, such as C3 and C4, can also be determined by immunodiffusion.

One potential difficulty in the interpretation of complement component levels is that they are increased as acute-phase reactants in the presence of active inflammation. Therefore the actual level may be normal, even with active complement consumption (Frank, 1992; Oppermann et al., 1992). In these situations, assessment of complement breakdown products, such as C3d, may be a more accurate measure of complement activation (Buyon et al., 1992; Rother et al., 1993).

JUVENILE RHEUMATOID ARTHRITIS

JRA, as it is known in North America, is also known as *juvenile idiopathic arthritis, Still's disease, juvenile chronic polyarthritis,* and *juvenile arthritis* in other countries. JRA is a disease characterized by chronic arthritis in children. The arthritis results from inflammation of synovium, the lining tissue of the joints (Fig. 35-3).

The synovitis of JRA is characteristically chronic, lasting weeks, months, or even years. If chronic synovitis persists long enough, damage to articular cartilage and subchondral bone may result, causing permanent joint damage. Damage to joint surfaces and to ligaments and tendons surrounding joints may lead to permanent deformities, such as subluxation, fusion, or joint destruction. Deformities may also result from shortening of muscles and other tissues around arthritic joints (contractures), even in the absence of significant damage to the joints themselves.

Fortunately, many children with chronic arthritis escape without permanent joint damage or deformity, and their disease should not be confused with the classical seropositive RA of adults.

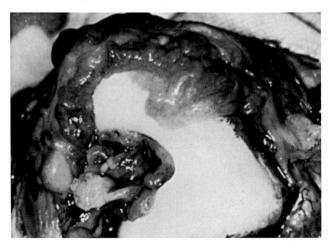

Figure 35-3 · Rheumatoid synovitis, visible in a knee joint undergoing surgery. The synovium is greatly hypertrophied, with formation of grape-like projections (villi) and early extensions over the surface of the articular cartilage (pannus formation).

Historical Aspects

The occurrence of chronic arthritis in children was first described in the English language by the English pediatrician George Frederick Still in 1897. He focused attention on the fact that some children with arthritis have manifestations affecting body systems other than the joints. He was the first to advance the idea that arthritis in children was a different disease than RA in adults. Since Still's first description, many series of children with chronic arthritis have been reported, adding to the clinical spectrum of JRA.

Classification

On careful analysis of large series of children with JRA, several fairly distinct clinical subgroups of disease have emerged, with characteristics generally apparent within 6 months of disease onset (Table 35-5). The criteria proposed by the American College of Rheumatology (ACR) are the most commonly used classification criteria in North America. These classification criteria are used in the discussions that follow. However, because of the nonuniformity of taxonomy internationally, another group of criteria exists.

The International League of Associations for Rheumatology (ILAR) classification criteria were formulated so that international treatment and outcomes studies of children with idiopathic arthritides could be developed. They proposed that the term *juvenile idiopathic arthritis* (JIA) be used for children affected with inflammatory joint disease, and these criteria for classification of arthritic disease in children differ from those of the ACR (Fink, 1995; Petty and Southwood, 1998;

Petty et al., 1998). However, in North America, clinicians have been slow to adopt these criteria.

By the ACR criteria, at least five subgroups of arthritis are easily identified: systemic-onset disease, polyarticular seronegative disease, polyarticular seropositive disease (classical RF negative or positive), pauciarticular disease associated with chronic iridocyclitis (type I), and pauciarticular disease associated with sacroiliitis (type II) (Schaller, 1977d, 1980).

The seropositive polyarticular type of disease is identical to typical adult-onset RA. Seronegative polyarthritis and pauciarticular arthritis associated with sacroiliitis are also recognized in adults. Systemic-onset JRA is rare in adults, however, and pauciarticular disease type I has not been described in adults. It is likely that JRA may be more than one disease, but it is possible that patients with the same basic disease may show several clinical patterns. At any rate, recognition of JRA subgroups is useful in the diagnosis and care of affected children.

Epidemiology

Chronic childhood arthritis rarely occurs in the first year of life but may begin at any time thereafter up to adulthood. There are age differences in onset among the different subgroups: seropositive polyarthritis and pauciarticular disease type II are associated with an older age at onset, seronegative polyarthritis and systemic-onset diseases may begin at any time during childhood (often in young children), and pauciarticular disease type I generally begins before the age of 6 years. Sex ratios also vary among subgroups; there is a strong female preponderance in seronegative polyarthritis,

TABLE 35-5 · SUBGROUPS OF JUVENILE RHEUMATOID ARTHRITIS (JRA)

Subgroup	Percent of JRA Patients	Ratio Girls/Boys	Age at Onset	Joints Affected	Laboratory Tests	Extra-articular Manifestations	Prognosis
Systemic onset	20%	8/10	Any age	Many joints, large and small	ANA negative RF negative	High fever, rash, organomegaly, polyserositis, leukocytosis	25% severe arthritis
Rheumatoid factor negative polyarticular	25%–30%	8/1	Any age	Many joints, large and small	ANA 25% RF negative	Low-grade fever, mild anemia, malaise	10%–15% severe arthritis
Rheumatoid factor positive polyarticular	10%	6/1	Late childhood	Many joints, large and small	ANA 75% RF 100%	Low-grade fever, anemia, malaise; rheumatoid nodules	>50% severe arthritis
Pauciarticular with chronic iridocyclitis (type I)	35%–40%	7/1	Early childhood	Few large joints (hips and sacroiliac joints spared)	ANA 50% RF negative	Few constitutional complaints; chronic iridocyclitis in 50%	Severe arthritis rare; 10%–20% ocular damage from iridocyclitis
Pauciarticular with sacroilitis (type II)	15%–20%	1/10	Late childhood	Few large joints (hip and sacroiliac involvement common)	ANA negative RF negative HLA-B27 75%	Few constitutional complaints; acute iridocyclitis in 5%–10% during childhood	Some will have spondylo-arthropathies as adults

ANA = antinuclear antibody; HLA-B27 = human leukocyte antigen-B27; RF = rheumatoid factor.

seropositive polyarthritis, and pauciarticular disease type I. There is a male preponderance in pauciarticular disease type II. Systemic-onset JRA affects girls and boys equally. These factors are summarized in Table 35-5.

The exact incidence of JRA in the United States is unknown, but it is not rare. It has been estimated that 5% of all chronic inflammatory arthritis begins in children younger than 16 years and that there are about 250,000 affected children in the United States (Gare and Fasth, 1992; Gewanter et al., 1983; Oen and Cheang, 1996; Towner et al., 1983).

Pathogenesis

The cause of JRA is unknown. The histopathology of affected tissues, notably synovial tissues, shows chronic inflammation, with lymphocytes and plasma cells as the chief inflammatory cells. No histologic differences have been reported among synovial tissues from the various JRA subgroups or adult disease (Wynne-Roberts et al., 1978). Affected synovial tissues, studied chiefly in adult RA, may contain organized lymphoid follicles and germinal centers, and plasma cells may be shown by fluorescent antibody or elution techniques to be producing immunoglobulins, including RFs.

There are emerging data to suggest a role for genetic susceptibility factors and immune reactivity in the pathogenesis of JRA. Children with JRA often have a variety of autoantibodies in their serum, although their role in disease onset and pathogenesis is unknown.

Many investigators have searched for specific infectious triggers for JRA. Several viral and bacterial infections are known to be associated with episodes of transient arthritis (Chantler et al., 1985). For example, parvovirus B19, the causative agent of childhood Fifth disease, is associated with transient arthritis similar to JRA (Nocton, 1993). Antibody titers to rubella virus have been found in the sera of children with JRA (Linnemann et al., 1975), and rubella virus has been cultured from their synovial fluid.

Reactive arthritis has a clear association with infectious triggers such as *Chlamydia*, *Yersinia*, *Salmonella*, *Shigella*, and *Campylobacter*. Reactivity of blood and synovial fluid T cells to these bacterial pathogens occur in children with reactive arthritis and in some children with pauciarticular type II JRA (Sieper et al., 1992). These data suggest that exposure to common infectious agents may, in susceptible hosts, result in a chronic arthritis.

Immunogenetics

As increased knowledge has become available concerning the contribution of MHC loci in immune reactivity, interest has focused on whether specific HLA types predispose to autoimmune diseases, including JRA. Reports of JRA occurring in monozygotic twins and siblings (Baum and Fink, 1968; Kapusta et al., 1969; Prahalad et al., 2000) suggest that genetic factors play a

role in susceptibility to JRA. Furthermore, Davies and co-workers (2001) have identified 13 children with a 22q11 deletion (DiGeorge locus) with polyarticular arthritis.

Most studies of HLA associations in JRA have focused on children with the pauciarticular subtype, the most common form of JRA. There is an increase in HLA-A2, HLA-DR11, HLA-DR8, HLA-DR5, and HLA-DPw2 in these patients (Dracou et al., 1998; Glass and Litvin, 1980; Malagon et al., 1992; Nepom and Glass, 1992; Prahalad et al., 2000; Schaller and Hansen, 1982b; Stastny et al., 1992). Correlations of HLA subtype and clinical course of disease to date have been weak and unrevealing.

There is less information concerning HLA associations with other subtypes of JRA. HLA-DR4 occurs more often in children with seropositive polyarticular disease (Nepom et al., 1982), and children with systemic JRA have an increased incidence of HLA-DR4, HLA-DR5, HLA-DR8, and HLA-DPB1. Polyarticular JRA has been associated with HLA-DR4 and DR8 (Barron et al., 1992b; Bedford et al., 1992; Paul et al., 1995).

Systemic-Onset Juvenile Rheumatoid Arthritis

About 20% of JRA children have disease characterized at the onset by prominent extra-articular (systemic) manifestations and arthritis. These include high intermittent fever, rash, hepatosplenomegaly, lymphadenopathy, pericarditis, pleuritis, abdominal pain, leukocytosis, anemia, thrombocytosis, and occasional disseminated intravascular coagulopathy.

Fever is a prominent characteristic, with one or two daily high elevations (39°C to 41.5°C) and subsequent rapid return to normal or subnormal levels (Fig. 35-4). Febrile patients may appear very ill, only to improve dramatically as the fever subsides.

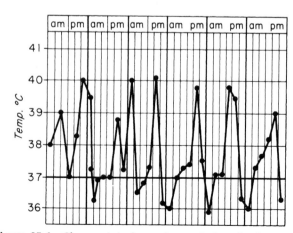

Figure 35-4 · Characteristic fever of systemic juvenile rheumatoid arthritis. High temperature elevations, occurring once or twice daily, are followed by a rapid return to normal or subnormal levels. (From Schaller JG, Beckwith B, Wedgwood RJ. Hepatic involvement in juvenile rheumatoid arthritis. J Pediatr 77:203–210, 1970.)

The rash (Fig. 35-5) characteristic of systemic JRA may be more prominent at times of high fever. Individual lesions are small, evanescent, pale red macules, often with central clearing; they may appear on any part of the body, including the palms and soles. Lesions are occasionally pruritic and often occur in areas of skin trauma, such as scratch marks (Köbner's phenomena or isomorphic response). The rash is more prominent with fever or external application of heat; it generally appears in the evening when the fever is at its maximum and usually disappears by morning (Isdale and Bywaters, 1956; Schaller and Wedgwood, 1970).

Pleuritis and pericarditis are generally mild and often asymptomatic, although some patients may complain of chest pain (Bernstein et al., 1974; Leitman and Bywaters, 1963; Wagener et al., 1981). Occasionally, patients may present with large pericardial effusions leading to cardiac decompensation requiring decompression. Patients with significant effusions may refuse to lie flat and often appear anxious.

Lymphadenopathy and hepatosplenomegaly may be marked, simulating malignancy. There may be mild alternations in liver function tests, which may be associated with active systemic disease; chronic liver disease does not occur (Schaller et al., 1970). When abnormal

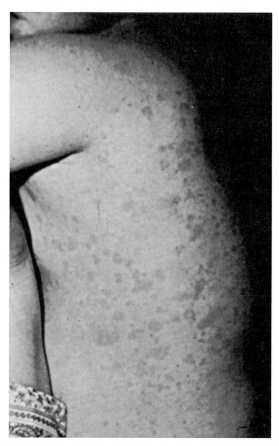

Figure 35-5·Characteristic rash of juvenile rheumatoid arthritis. This rash is also characterized by evanescence and recurrence.

liver function tests are found, the hepatotoxicity of drug therapy resulting from nonsteroidal anti-inflammatory drugs (NSAIDs) or methotrexate must be differentiated from the potentially fatal macrophage activation syndrome (MAS) with fever, elevation of alanine transaminase (ALT) and aspartate transaminase (AST), hypofibrinogenemia, and depression of blood counts (Hadchouel et al., 1985; Prieur and Stephan, 1994). It is rarely seen in patients with active systemic disease.

In the past, some children receiving high-dose salicylates during the systemic phase of the illness developed hepatotoxicity, with dramatic elevation of liver enzymes, hepatic tenderness, and abnormal coagulation profiles (Koff, 1977). This syndrome of disseminated intravascular coagulation has been described in children with systemic JRA and is a potentially fatal complication if not treated promptly with corticosteroids. This syndrome has been reported in a few cases in association with intramuscular gold treatment in children with active systemic disease (Barash et al., 1991; Jacobs et al., 1984; Scott et al., 1985; Silverman et al., 1983).

Severe abdominal pain may occur at times with active systemic JRA, possibly because of mesenteric adenopathy or peritonitis. Peripheral leukocyte counts may be greatly elevated, sometimes exceeding 50,000/mm^3. Severe anemia generally responds to corticosteroid therapy and ultimately to control of the underlying disease. A contributory role of iron deficiency may be present, and in rare cases, severe anemia may be associated with MAS. Therapy for MAS may require immunosuppression (such as with cyclosporine) in addition to corticosteroids and rarely transfusion (Mouy et al., 1996).

Central nervous system (CNS) disease with seizures, behavioral disturbances, and abnormal electroencephalograms have been described (Jan et al., 1972), but whether such events are part of the disease is uncertain.

Growth retardation may accompany long-standing active disease (Bernstein et al., 1977), which may result from the catabolic effects of inflammation, depressed insulin-like growth factor-1 (IGF-1), poor nutritional intake, and prolonged corticosteroid use in children with unremitting disease (Chikanza, 1999).

Joint manifestations at the onset of systemic JRA may include overt arthritis or only myalgia and arthralgia. Children are irritable, seem to hurt all over, and refuse to stand or move about. Joint pain is prominent when the fever is high and may improve when the fever recedes. Systemic manifestations may be so overwhelming that joint problems are initially overlooked. Within a few weeks of onset, however, it usually becomes apparent that the patient has arthritis. Occasionally, overt arthritis does not begin for weeks, months, or even years after systemic manifestations. Multiple joints are generally affected in a polyarticular pattern; a few patients have only a few joints involved.

Systemic manifestations, particularly fever, usually remit after a period of weeks or months. In some patients arthritis becomes chronic, even after systemic manifestations disappear. Systemic manifestations may recur at unpredictable intervals but rarely after late adolescence. Systemic disease is rarely fatal. The major morbidity of systemic-onset JRA lies in the degree and severity of arthritis. Arthritis may involve multiple joints in systemic-onset disease, and 25% of these patients eventually develop progressive arthritis with associated disability.

Polyarticular Juvenile Rheumatoid Arthritis

Seronegative Polyarticular Juvenile Rheumatoid Arthritis

Approximately 20% to 30% of children with JRA have arthritis involving multiple joints within a few months of onset, without prominent systemic manifestations and with negative tests for RFs. Any joint may be affected, except perhaps the lumbothoracic spine. Arthritis may begin in either large joints (knees, ankles, wrists, and elbows) or small joints of the hands (Fig. 35-6) and feet. The cervical spine, temporomandibular joints, and hips are sometimes affected. Joint involvement is usually symmetric. Affected joints are swollen, warm, and tender and have decreased motion or pain on motion. Joint effusions and synovitis are often present. Stiffness of joints after inactivity, particularly in the morning, is characteristic (gelation).

Although extra-articular manifestations are not as dramatic as in systemic-onset JRA, many patients with seronegative polyarthritis have malaise, a low-grade fever, anorexia, growth retardation, irritability, and mild anemia during periods of active disease.

Prognosis is related to the severity and duration of arthritis and the degree of permanent joint damage. Periods of active arthritis may last for months or years and may recur long after seemingly complete remission

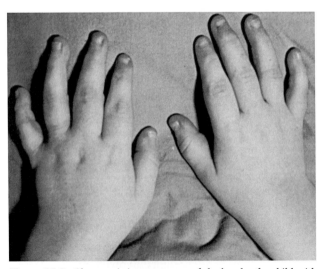

Figure 35-6 · Characteristic appearance of the hands of a child with polyarticular rheumatoid arthritis. The proximal interphalangeal joints are swollen ("spindling"), as are the metacarpophalangeal and wrist joints.

(Jeremy et al., 1968). Most children eventually enter remission or have relatively mild chronic disease and do not develop permanent joint damage or serious disability. A few have severe progressive disease, with joint destruction and permanent disability. Severe hip disease may require joint replacement. Micrognathia with dental deformities and facial asymmetry may result from temporomandibular arthritis in early childhood.

Seropositive Polyarticular Juvenile Rheumatoid Arthritis

About 5% to 10% of children with JRA have polyarticular arthritis associated with positive tests for IgM RFs (seropositivity) based on standard agglutination techniques (Schaller, 1980; Schaller and Hansen, 1982a). RFs are present at disease onset and often remain in high titers. In most seropositive patients, the onset of disease is after 8 years of age. The pattern of joint involvement is similar to that of seronegative polyarthritis and is identical to that in adult-onset RA. The course of arthritis is severe and progressive, with at least 50% of patients (Williams and Ansell, 1985) having poor response to NSAIDs alone. Although long-term studies are not available, the use of biologic agents has seemingly improved the long-term prognosis.

Seropositive patients often have subcutaneous rheumatoid nodules similar to those observed in adults, and a few develop rheumatoid vasculitis. These patients may carry the same HLA type found in adults with RA, HLA-DR4 (Barron et al., 1992b; Nepom et al., 1982). Sjögren's and Felty syndromes have also been described in patients of this subgroup. Patients may have low-grade fever, malaise, weight loss, or growth retardation.

Pauciarticular (Oligoarticular) Juvenile Rheumatoid Arthritis

Approximately 50% of children with JRA have arthritis limited to one or only a few joints during the first 6 months and often during the entire course of their disease. Arthritis generally affects large joints and is spotty rather than symmetric in distribution. It is difficult to define this disease solely by numbers of joints affected; official numbers that are accepted are usually either four or five total joints. This type of disease is referred to as *pauciarticular* (few joint) *arthritis* (Bywaters and Ansell, 1965; Cassidy et al., 1967; Schaller and Hansen, 1982b; Schaller et al., 1974). The clinical appearance of affected joints is similar to that of polyarticular disease, as is the synovial histology. At least two subgroups exist within pauciarticular disease (Schaller and Wedgwood, 1976).

Pauciarticular Arthritis Type I

Dr. Green, an orthopedist at Boston Children's Hospital, was the first to describe pauciarticular type I disease. This subgroup predominantly affects young girls and accounts for about 40% of all JRA cases. Involvement of large joints, particularly the knees, ankles, and elbows, predominates. Small joints of the hands are spared or affected only in a spotty fashion; hip involvement is unusual, and sacroiliitis does not occur. The arthritis may be of long duration but is generally mild. About 80% or more of patients remain with only pauciarticular joint involvement, and prognosis for joint function is good. The remaining develop polyarthritis over the years (pauciarticular to polyarticular course) and may incur joint destruction.

Local bony overgrowth around affected joints may cause growth disturbances, such as inequality of leg lengths; these generally correct with growth, although a lift to the contralateral shoe may be temporarily required to permit normal function. Disabling flexion contractures can occur around affected joints, particularly the knee and elbow, if proper attention is not given to physical therapy.

The main complication in these patients is chronic iridocyclitis (Merriam et al., 1983; Schaller, 1977c; Smiley et al., 1957). Iridocyclitis occurs occasionally in patients with systemic-onset disease or seropositive polyarthritis. Iridocyclitis usually begins insidiously and can be detected early only by using slitlamp examination. One or both eyes may be affected. Unless ocular inflammation is promptly controlled, anterior chamber scarring, secondary glaucoma, cataract formation, and band keratopathy may ensue, with severe or total loss of vision. Reasons for the association of iridocyclitis with pauciarticular arthritis remain unknown, but those who possess the HLA class II gene DRB1* 1104 are at particular risk (Melina-Aldana et al., 1992). Other extra-articular manifestations are uncommon in these patients, although malaise, anorexia, low-grade fever, elevations in ESRs, and mild anemia may occur during periods of active disease.

The outcome for most children with pauciarticular JRA is excellent, but a small percentage of these children progress to a polyarticular course that may be associated with disability and severe disease. It is suggested that up to 10% to 15% of children with pauciarticular JRA eventually develop polyarticular disease (Peterson et al., 1996). There are currently no clinical or genetic parameters to distinguish the children who will progress to a more severe course of disease (Hertzberger-ten Cate et al., 1992).

Pauciarticular Arthritis Type II

Pauciarticular disease type II affects children, usually boys, who tend to be older than 8 years at onset; about 15% of all JRA patients fall into this subgroup. Differentiation of children with this form of JRA and spondyloarthropathy is confusing, because there is considerable overlap between the two groups (Burgos-Vargas, 1993).

In pauciarticular type II disease, large joints, particularly the hips, knees, and ankles, are predominantly affected; metatarsal joints are sometimes involved, and occasional spotty involvement of the upper extremities may occur as well. Hip girdle symptoms are common;

indeed, patients may be rendered nonambulatory by severe hip pain and stiffness. Some patients have radiographic sacroiliitis at the time of onset; this increases with the duration of disease. Sacroiliitis may be silent, may be unassociated with clinical symptoms, or may manifest by hip girdle pain or sacroiliac tenderness.

Enthesopathy (inflammation at the site of tendon insertions into bones) is common and may differentiate these patients from those with other forms of JRA (Jacobs et al., 1982; Rosenberg and Petty, 1982). (See also seronegative enthesopathy and arthropathy syndrome [SEA] under seronegative spondyloarthropathy syndromes.)

The course of pauciarticular disease type II is variable, and the ultimate outcome is not yet defined. Peripheral arthritis may wax and wane over years or remain chronic with little joint destruction. With time, some of these patients develop one of the spondyloarthropathies, such as AS, the spondylitis of inflammatory bowel disease, psoriatic arthritis, or Reiter's disease (Ansell and Wood, 1976; Burgos-Vargas, 1993; Lindsley and Schaller, 1974; Schaller, 1977a; Singsen et al., 1977b). There is often a positive family history of spondyloarthropathy.

Some patients have acute self-limited attacks of iridocyclitis that are rarely associated with permanent ocular damage (Kanski, 1977; Schaller, 1977c; Schaller et al., 1974, 1977). Other extra-articular complaints are not usual, unless features of the spondyloarthropathies appear, such as Reiter's disease or inflammatory bowel disease.

Diagnosis and Laboratory Findings

Diagnosis of JRA rests solely on clinical recognition of the disease (Brewer et al., 1977; Cassidy et al., 1986). The clinician must exclude other disorders associated with arthritis and joint pain, including septic arthritis, osteomyelitis, Lyme arthritis, other rheumatic diseases, inflammatory bowel disease, malignancies, congenital defects of the musculoskeletal system, and numerous noninflammatory conditions of bones and joints (e.g., avascular necrosis of bone, discitis, slipped capital femoral epiphysis, and pain amplification syndromes). Other than radiographic changes of joint destruction occurring late in severe disease, no diagnostic laboratory tests are available; however, laboratory studies are useful in the exclusion of other diseases.

Rheumatoid Factors

RFs are demonstrable in a most adults with RA by standard agglutination techniques, but they are found in JRA patients much less often (Cassidy and Valkenberg, 1967; Hanson et al., 1969; Jeremy et al., 1968; Laaksonen, 1966; Schaller, 1980; Schaller and Hansen, 1982b). RF positivity occurs almost exclusively in children who are older than 8 years at disease onset and who have a form of JRA similar to adult-onset RA. Patients who are seronegative at disease onset do not become seropositive as they get older, even though active disease continues. The presence of RFs detectable by standard agglutination tests correlates with severe joint disease in most patients and with the presence of rheumatoid nodules in both children and adults and with rheumatoid vasculitis in adults (Nepom et al., 1982; Schaller, 1977d, 1977f; Schaller and Hansen, 1982b).

The reasons for negative tests for RFs in most cases of childhood-onset arthritis are unknown. RFs are not seen in systemic JRA or either of the pauciarticular subgroups. Some investigators have reported the presence of "hidden rheumatoid factors" in children with JRA who are seronegative in usual agglutination testing (Moore et al., 1980, 1988). The role of these serum factors is unknown.

Antinuclear Antibodies

ANAs are demonstrable in 20% to 30% of both adults and children with RA (Lawrence et al., 1993; Leak, 1988; Rosenberg, 1988; Schaller et al., 1974). The incidence of ANAs varies among JRA subgroups, but positive tests are found in 25% of children with seronegative polyarthritis, in 50% or more of children with pauciarticular disease type I, and in 75% of patients with seropositive polyarthritis (Schaller, 1977d, 1977f; Schaller and Hansen, 1982b). ANAs are rarely, if ever, found in systemic JRA or pauciarticular disease type II. In general, antibody profiles do not correlate with disease subtype (Szer et al., 1991b).

ANAs occur more often in girls, especially in those with early childhood onset of disease; this is consistent with the subgroup distribution. There is no apparent correlation with severity or duration of disease. ANAs in children with the pauciarticular subtype of JRA, however, are associated with the development of chronic iridocyclitis (Egeskjold et al., 1982; Schaller et al., 1974). Positive tests for ANAs are thus useful in identifying patients who are at risk for this complication. A high prevalence of reactivity against histones among children with JRA, especially those with iridocyclitis, has been described (Leak and Woo, 1991; Monestier et al., 1990; Ostenson, 1989).

Joint Fluid Analysis

Joint fluid analysis is not diagnostic of JRA, but its examination is crucial to exclude septic arthritis (or crystal-induced arthritides such as gout, although rare in children). In JRA, joint fluid is characteristically somewhat turbid and yellow-green in color and contains an increased number of white cells, predominantly polymorphonuclear leukocytes (5000 to 80,000/mm^3 or greater). Synovial histology is not specific but resembles that of other rheumatic diseases; a synovial biopsy is sometimes helpful in excluding chronic septic arthritis, tuberculous arthritis, or rare conditions such as sarcoidosis or synovial tumors.

Acute-Phase Reactants

Acute-phase reactants, such as the ESR and CRP, are increased in many children with active JRA. The ESR is often normal in children with pauciarticular JRA. Tests of acute-phase reactants are not diagnostic and have only limited value in monitoring the course of disease. Mild anemia is common in children with active disease (Koerper et al., 1978); occasionally, children with severe systemic disease may have severe anemia (Schaller, 1977d, 1977f; Schaller and Hansen, 1982b). The nature of the anemia is poorly understood; hypoproliferation of red blood cells, iron deficiency, gastrointestinal blood loss related to medications, and perhaps increased red cell destruction may all play a role. Reports of success in using recombinant erythropoietin in treating the severe anemia of systemic JRA initially looked promising (Fantini et al., 1992), but more recent studies indicate that JRA patients with anemia have normal erythropoietin production but insufficiency of available iron stores for erythrocyte production (Cazzola et al., 1996).

Radiography and Imaging

Radiographs and other imaging techniques may provide useful information in documenting the extent of joint damage in the individual patient. Radiographs taken within the first year or so of disease show only soft tissue swelling, periarticular osteoporosis, and sometimes juxta-articular periostitis; those taken later in severe disease may show evidence of articular damage, including loss of cartilage space and erosions into subchondral bone. With severe joint destruction, deformities and fusion of adjacent bones may occur. Such radiographic changes are characteristic of seropositive RA, particularly in the hands and wrists (Fig. 35-7) (Williams and Ansell, 1985). Chest radiographs may show mild pleuritis and enlargement of the cardiac shadow consistent with pericarditis in children with systemic-onset JRA.

Other imaging techniques such as skeletal scintigraphy (bone scan), ultrasonography, and magnetic resonance imaging (MRI) can also aid in the diagnosis of joint disease in children (Poznanski, 1992). Bone scans are helpful in distinguishing infections of bones or joints and in detecting a malignant process with multiple lesions. Ultrasonography is becoming more and more useful in the diagnosis of arthritic conditions. Ultrasonography is a sensitive way to detect small joint effusions and synovial thickening (especially of hidden joints such as the hip) and is used increasingly as better transducers become available and radiologists become more familiar with the technique (Fig. 35-8) (Szer et al., 1992). MRI is expensive and requires sedation of small children. However, it is a sensitive technique for detecting cartilage loss or bony erosions that are too small to be seen easily in regular radiographs (Poznanski et al., 1988), and synovitis can be detected after intravenous injection of gadolinium (Herve-Somma et al., 1992).

Treatment

Therapy must be designed with the realization that the prognosis for most children with JRA is hopeful,

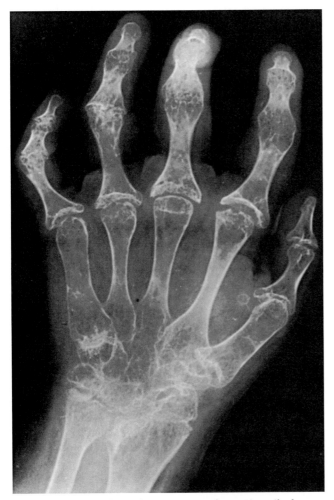

Figure 35-7· Late radiographic appearance of severe juvenile rheumatoid arthritis. There is widespread destruction apparent in the wrist and finger joints, with loss of joint space (articular cartilage), numerous erosions into subchondral bone, and actual fusion of some adjacent bones. Such a radiograph is diagnostic of rheumatoid arthritis, but these changes appear only late in the course of juvenile rheumatoid arthritis. Fortunately, many children with rheumatoid arthritis never incur joint damage severe enough to be visible radiographically.

although for any given patient the outcome and duration of disease are uncertain. With adequate care during periods of active disease, at least 75% of JRA children avoid significant disability. The physician must avoid harmful drugs, as far as possible, and use a good measure of optimism and reassurance to help children and families cope with this sometimes discouraging, but by no means hopeless, disease. Because the cause and pathogenesis of chronic arthritis are poorly understood, therapy is symptomatic, not curative (Schaller, 1993). For those who are severely affected with unremitting symptoms and progressive joint disease and destruction, new biologic agents may be employed. Ancillary measures, such as physical and occupational therapy, are essential. Care must be taken to avoid psychogenic invalidism and to allow normal growth and development.

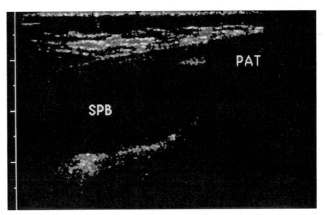

Figure 35-8· Ultrasound of active knee inflammation showing effusion in the suprapatellar bursa (SPB) and synovial overgrowth.

Nonsteroidal Anti-inflammatory Drugs

There are currently a proliferation of NSAIDs used in adults with arthritis, and new agents that preferentially block the production of the inflammatory prostaglandins (COX-2 inhibitors) may afford some gastrointestinal protection for patients requiring chronic NSAID use (Silverstein et al., 2000). However, only aspirin, naproxen, tolmetin, and ibuprofen (and indomethacin after 12 years of age) are currently labeled for use in children in the United States.

Although none of the NSAIDs have been clearly shown to be more effective than salicylates, they may provide the benefit of more convenient dosing schedules. Indomethacin and some of the other nonsteroidal agents are considered useful in the therapy of AS and may be helpful in the treatment of pauciarticular disease type II and the other spondyloarthropathies. Indomethacin is also helpful in the treatment of serositis in children with systemic-onset disease.

Hepatotoxicity may occur with NSAIDs and with salicylates, and liver function tests should be monitored regularly (usually 1 month after initiation and every 6 months thereafter). Salicylates and other nonsteroidal agents are known to cause gastrointestinal side effects in adults, such as gastritis, microscopic blood loss, or frank ulcers. Histamine type 2 receptor blockers, sucralfate, prostaglandin analogs, and proton pump inhibitors may be helpful in this situation. Children also develop gastrointestinal side effects (Mulberg et al., 1993), and complaints of stomach upset or unexplained anemia should prompt evaluation.

Sulfasalazine

Encouraging results in using sulfasalazine in adults with RA and spondyloarthropathies led to trials of this medication in children with JRA. Sulfasalazine is a combination of 5-aminosalicylic acid and sulfapyridine; the salicylate portion is not absorbed in the intestine. Although no placebo-controlled trials have been done, sulfasalazine was effective in open studies in a significant number of children, particularly those with pauciarticular type II disease or spondyloarthropathy (Imundo and Jacobs, 1996; Joos et al., 1991).

The usual maintenance dosage is 50 mg/kg/day, with a maximum daily dose of 2 g. Laboratory monitoring should include a complete blood count (CBC) with platelet count, urinalysis, and liver function tests. Toxicity may include mild gastrointestinal intolerance, leukopenia, or rash, and this medication should not be prescribed to children with glucose-6-phosphate dehydrogenase (G6PD) deficiency. Severe reactions have been reported, particularly in children with systemic-onset disease (Hertzberger-ten Cate and Cats, 1991; Senturk et al., 1997).

Antimalarials (Hydroxychloroquine)

Antimalarials may be useful in some rheumatoid patients but must be given with extreme care to children because of possible irreversible retinal toxicity; antimalarials are also poisons, with no antidote in overdosage. The most frequently reported side effect is corneal deposition of the drug; macular degeneration from retinal deposition is the most severe sequela. Regular monitoring of visual fields and color vision is required. This medication should not be prescribed in children with G6PD deficiency. The usual dosage of hydroxychloroquine (Plaquenil) is 5 to 7 mg/kg/day. Discontinuation of the drug may reverse corneal deposition, but macular degeneration is not reversible and may progress despite drug withdrawal (Aylward, 1993; Mazzuca et al., 1994).

Penicillamine

Penicillamine, another disease-modifying agent used in the treatment of adults with RA, has been studied in children and is thought to have some efficacy in a few patients (Manners and Ansell, 1986). Follow-up studies, however, failed to show efficacy of treatment, and penicillamine in JRA therapy is now only of historical interest (Brewer et al., 1986; van Kerckhove et al., 1988).

Gold

Injections of gold salts were used for patients whose arthritis did not respond to NSAIDs with some effectiveness. However, since the introduction of methotrexate, gold is now rarely used. Gold therapy is reasonably safe if given under careful supervision, but a CBC, platelet count, and urinalysis must be done before each gold injection, as well as a physical examination for evidence of skin or mucosal lesions. Oral gold is not efficacious in childhood arthritis (Giannini et al., 1990).

Methotrexate

In children whose arthritis is refractory to adequate NSAID therapy, methotrexate is the usual therapeutic choice. Methotrexate, given at average dosages of 10 to 15 mg/m^2 once weekly orally (or subcutaneously), is efficacious in many children with persistent disease activity and/or erosive changes (Giannini et al., 1992; Rose, 1990a; Wallace and Sherry, 1992).

The side effects of methotrexate are generally mild and include gastrointestinal upset, oral ulcers, and bone marrow suppression (Cassidy, 1998a; Giannini and Cassidy, 1993). These side effects can be minimized by giving folic acid supplementation or by giving the methotrexate by injection. Elevations of serum transaminases are not uncommon, but severe permanent liver damage has rarely been reported in children, although cases of cirrhosis have been seen in adults (Keim, 1990). With careful laboratory and clinical monitoring, most children tolerate methotrexate well. Severe pulmonary toxicity with fibrosis is an additional rare complication. Pulmonary or liver toxicities have been reported only rarely in children taking methotrexate followed for as long as 5 years (Hashkes et al., 1999; Zisman et al., 2001).

Some investigators advocate higher dosages of methotrexate in children who have an inadequate clinical response to standard dosages (Wallace and Sherry, 1992; Woo et al., 2000).

Cyclosporine

Children with severe polyarticular or systemic-onset disease who do not respond to NSAIDs and methotrexate alone may respond to the addition of cyclosporine at dosages of up to 6 mg/kg/day (Ansell, 1993; Pistoia et al., 1993). Hypertension and renal toxicity are potential complications of therapy, and all children receiving cyclosporine must be monitored carefully (Reiff et al., 1997). Cyclosporine may also be useful treatment in children with chronic iridocyclitis unresponsive to topical steroid and oral methotrexate therapy (Kilmartin et al., 1998).

Mycophenolate Mofetil

Children with severe arthritis or uveitis who do not respond to more conventional therapies may respond to mycophenolate mofetil. No published trials in children have addressed its efficacy in JRA (Gallagher and Bernstein, 1999; Lepore and Kiren, 2000).

Cyclophosphamide

Although studies in adult RA have shown the effectiveness of drugs such as cyclophosphamide, the use in children with JRA remains experimental and is rarely warranted except in extreme and uncontrollable systemic-onset disease (Wallace and Sherry, 1997).

Corticosteroids

Corticosteroids can be dramatic in relieving symptoms and suppressing signs of arthritis, but their long-term use causes significant toxicity (Schaller, 1977g). Corticosteroids do not cure RA; joint destruction may proceed, even during administration. Once started, these drugs may be difficult to discontinue because of severe recurrences of symptoms. Because JRA is usually chronic, corticosteroids may be needed for years and the side effects may be severe. Corticosteroids used alone should be avoided unless all other measures have failed. They are sometimes indicated for severe systemic disease or iridocyclitis. The lowest possible dosages sufficient to relieve symptoms should be used, and long-term use should be avoided. The use of low-dose alternate-day dosing regimens or intermittent intravenous pulse treatments may be effective in treatment and may prevent some of the major side effects.

Various preparations of corticosteroids are also used for intra-articular injection, and for persistent arthritis in the child with pauciarticular disease, they are the treatment of choice. Direct injection of the joint with corticosteroid avoids the systemic toxicity of these agents, and depending on the preparation, relief from a single injection may last as long as 1 year. Triamcinolone hexacetonide (Aristospan) is the preferred agent.

Biologics

Advances in molecular biology and recombinant protein technology have led to the development of new biologic agents for the treatment of inflammatory disease, including JRA. In 1999, the U.S. Food and Drug Administration (FDA) approved the use of etanercept (Enbrel) in children with JRA. Etanercept is a TNF-α receptor-Fc fusion protein that binds to TNF-α, thereby blocking its action; TNF-α is a key cytokine that mediates inflammatory joint disease (Lovell et al., 2000). The usual dosage in children is 0.4 mg/kg twice weekly or 0.8 mg/kg weekly given subcutaneously.

Initial studies in adults have shown fewer erosions and better early outcomes than seen with previous therapies (Bathon et al., 2000). Early toxicity profiles are promising, but there have been several reports of demyelinating disease occurring after initiation of etanercept therapy. Children with frequent or chronic infectious illnesses should not be given this therapy. The long-term risks of immunodeficiency or malignancy in children are unknown (Lovell et al., 2000).

Several other anti–TNF-α agents (infliximab, adalimamab) have also been approved for use in adults. Additionally, an IL-1 receptor antagonist (anakinra) has been developed for use in adults with rheumatoid arthritis. Trials of other biologic agents are currently underway in adults with RA.

Thalidomide

Thalidomide, a biologic response modifier, has been used with success in two children with recalcitrant systemic JRA refractory to conventional drugs, including etanercept (Lehman et al., 2002).

Physical Therapy

Physical therapy is important in preserving range of motion, muscle strength, and endurance. All children with JRA should be started early on a regular program of exercises designed to retain normal joint function, muscle strength, and endurance (Emery and Bowyer,

1991; Klepper, 1999; Rhodes, 1991). Simple measures such as hot baths in the morning may be helpful in relieving joint stiffness. Exercises and judicious splinting may prevent future and correct existing deformities.

Surgery

Orthopedic surgical procedures are occasionally needed. Early prophylactic removal of inflamed synovium (synovectomy) by arthroscopy is of only limited usefulness in children (Granberry, 1977a), although occasional patients treated by an experienced team of surgeons, rheumatologists, and therapists may benefit (Bjornland and Larheim, 1995; Hafner and Pieper, 1995; Pahle, 1996).

Total replacement of damaged joints, particularly hips and knees and more recently elbows, offers hope of rehabilitation for children with severe joint destruction and disability, but only after they have achieved full growth (Boublik et al., 1993; Connor and Morrey, 1998; Lyback et al., 2000; Makai and Vojtek, 1994; Ruddlesdin et al., 1986; Scott; 1990; Singsen et al., 1978).

Soft tissue releases may be useful in alleviating joint contractures unresponsive to physical therapy (Granberry, 1977b; Moreno Alvarez et al., 1992; Rydholm et al., 1986; Witt and McCullough, 1994).

Treatment of Iridocyclitis

Therapy of iridocyclitis should be managed in conjunction with an ophthalmologist. Early recognition of this complication is crucial; for this reason, children with JRA, particularly those with pauciarticular JRA type I, should have quarterly slitlamp examinations (Table 35-6). Topical corticosteroids may be adequate to control ocular inflammation. If not, systemic or locally injected corticosteroids may be tried. Methotrexate may also be beneficial, as may be etanercept (Reiff et al., 2001).

Treatment of Amyloidosis

Chlorambucil has been advocated in the therapy of amyloidosis, a potentially fatal complication that affects as many as 6% of JRA patients in Europe and other parts of the world (David et al., 1993; Schnitzer and Ansell, 1977; Smith et al., 1968). It is rare in the United States.

Autologous Stem Cell Transplantation

Several children with severe, unremitting systemic-onset JRA have undergone autologous stem cell transplants. Although not as risky as allogenic bone marrow transplant, the potential for serious infection still exists. Data as to long-term cure and benefits are not yet available (Tyndall, 1997).

Complications and Prognosis

The morbidity of JRA is determined by the joint damage and the accompanying disability that occurs, as well as visual loss from iridocyclitis. Prognosis varies from subgroup to subgroup. Between 80% and 90% of children with seronegative polyarthritis do well without serious disability in adulthood, although their disease may be active for many years. More than 50% of children with seropositive polyarthritis have persistent destructive arthritis with joint disability.

The acute manifestations of systemic JRA are in themselves rarely a cause of significant long-term morbidity, but 25% of children with systemic JRA develop severe seronegative arthritis with long-term joint disability.

Patients with pauciarticular disease type I have a generally good outlook for joint function, although 20% ultimately develop multiple joint involvement that may be severe. Approximately 30% of children develop chronic iridocyclitis, but with early detection and appropriate therapy, loss of vision is uncommon.

The ultimate prognosis in pauciarticular disease type II is uncertain; a significant number probably have chronic spondyloarthropathy in childhood, although the spondyloarthropathies are usually not associated with severe loss of function.

Overall, a significant number of children with JRA enter remission without significant residual disability. In any given patient, however, the disease is unpredictable, and recurrences may occasionally occur in adulthood after years of remission. Two other causes of long-term morbidity in JRA are iatrogenic damage from drugs, notably corticosteroids, and the psychologic and social disability resulting from chronic disease.

SERONEGATIVE SPONDYLOARTHROPATHIES

Ankylosing Spondylitis

AS is the prototypic spondyloarthropathy. This seronegative inflammatory arthritis primarily involves the axial skeleton and most commonly affects young adult or middle-aged men; however, the onset of AS may occur, usually insidiously, in childhood (Jacobs, 1963b; Ladd et al., 1971; Schaller et al., 1969). In addition to the forme fruste of AS, there are a number of related arthritis syndromes, generally grouped under the heading of *spondyloarthropathies*. These syndromes occur in older children, usually in boys, and are associated with the genetic marker HLA-B27.

In juvenile ankylosing spondylitis (JAS), chronic arthritis of the peripheral joints and axial skeleton occurs, often accompanied by enthesitis. Large joints and joints of the feet are commonly affected, usually in an asymmetric pattern and often with an indolent or transient and recurrent course. Inflammation of the sacroiliac joints must occur by definition, but this finding may be delayed for years, making the early diagnosis difficult. Patients with JAS and AS are generally seronegative for RFs.

Historical and Epidemiologic Aspects

JAS was described in the early 1900s, but diagnostic criteria were not established until 1973 (Moll and Wright, 1973). AS differs from RA in several important aspects, including the classic sacroiliac and lumbosacral involvement, male predominance, familial nature, and lack of RFs. Estimates of the incidence of AS in the adult population range from 1% to 6.7% of the white population (Khan, 1992), and a recent Finish study estimated the incidence of juvenile onset disease at 0.1 in 100,000 children in their population (Gomez et al., 1997). Therefore JAS is considerably less common than JRA.

JAS belongs to a group of related disorders that share genetic features and often occur together in families; these include AS, Reiter's syndrome (RS), inflammatory bowel disease, reactive arthritis, psoriatic arthritis, and the SEA syndrome. All are related by the frequent finding of HLA-B27 in affected individuals (Brewerton et al., 1973a, 1973b, 1974; Morris et al., 1974a, 1974b; Schlosstein et al., 1973). Pauciarticular type II JRA is also logically grouped together with these disorders.

HLA-B27 is found in 90% to 94% of patients with JAS, as compared with 6% to 8% of the general white population (Khan and van der Linden, 1990). Despite this marked HLA association, the relationship of HLA-B27 to disease pathogenesis remains unknown. Infectious agents are suspected as key environmental factors in the development of AS, because AS is related to reactive arthritis and RS in which infections are known triggers (Keat, 1982, 1983). Rats transgenic for human HLA-B27, which are susceptible to spontaneous spondylitis, do not develop AS when maintained in a germ-free environment (Taurog et al., 1994).

Some studies have identified molecular mimicry between HLA-B27 and bacterial agents implicated in spondyloarthropathies (e.g., *Klebsiella* and *Shigella*) (Schwimmbeck et al., 1987), but this has not been proved in either human disease or animal models. Recent attention has been focused on the possibility that the HLA-B27 molecule can misfold, leading to abnormal endoplasmic reticulum processing of the molecule and subsequent susceptibility to disease (Colbert, 2000; Mear et al., 1999).

TABLE 35-6 · RECOMMENDED FREQUENCY OF OPHTHALMOLOGIC EXAMINATIONS FOR CHILDREN WITH JUVENILE RHEUMATOID ARTHRITIS

Risk	Type	Antinuclear Antibody	Age at Onset (yr)	Duration of Disease (yr)
High	Pauci/poly	+	≤7	≤4
Medium	Pauci/poly	+	≤7	>4
	Pauci/poly	−	Any	≤4
	Pauci/poly	+	>7	>4
Low	Systemic	−	Any	Any
	Pauci/poly	+ or −	≤7	>7
	Pauci/poly	+ or −	>7	>4

High-risk groups need ophthalmologic examination every 3 to 4 months, medium risk every 6 months, and low risk yearly.
Pauci = pauciarticular; poly = polyarticular.
From AAP. American Academy of Pediatrics Section on Rheumatology and Section on Ophthalmology. Guidelines for ophthalmologic examinations in children with juvenile rheumatoid arthritis. Pediatrics 92:295–296, 1993.

Clinical Manifestations

Initial joint symptoms in JAS include recurring episodes of pain in the lower back, buttocks, groin, or heels. These early symptoms may be overlooked or misdiagnosed for a long period until more specific symptoms develop. Peripheral joint complaints may be prominent at the onset of disease, making JAS initially indistinguishable from JRA (Garcia-Morteo et al., 1983; Ginsburg and Cohen, 1983; Marks et al., 1982; Schaller, 1977a).

The constellation of clinical clues of male gender, older age of onset, and family history of related disorders should suggest the diagnosis of JAS. Pain and stiffness in the hips is common and often a major source of disability. Axial arthritis involving the sacroiliac joints and lumbar spine develops gradually in children and is not apparent at disease onset. There may be loss of the normal lumbar lordosis, with flattening of the lumbosacral spine and limited forward flexion of the lower spine. Decreased chest expansion related to involvement of the costovertebral joints may be found in early JAS (Schaller et al., 1969). However, recognizing this at onset may be difficult as single measurements are often unhelpful because of individual variation (Burgos-Vargas et al., 1993).

Episodic attacks of acute iritis occur in 5% to 10% of children with JAS (Gargia-Morteo et al., 1983; Marks et al., 1982). Aortitis has been reported in adult patients with long-standing AS; however, aortic valve insufficiency and aortic root dilation have also occasionally been reported in JAS (Bulkley and Roberts, 1973; Gore et al., 1981; Kean et al., 1980; Kim et al., 1997b).

Laboratory and Radiographic Findings

There are no specific laboratory findings in JAS except for its strong association with HLA-B27 with disease. During active disease, mild anemia and an increased ESR may be present. Neither RF nor ANAs are associated with JAS.

Radiologic findings are necessary for the definitive diagnosis of JAS, but these may not be evident for the first several years of disease. Radiographic changes of the sacroiliac joints include sclerosis, erosions of the joint margins, and widening of the joint space; these may progress to narrowing and ankylosis. Computed tomography (CT), MRI scanning, and skeletal scintigraphy are more sensitive than plain radiographs in detecting early disease (Ahlstrom et al., 1990; Bulkley and Roberts, 1973; Gore et al., 1981; Kean et al., 1980; Kim et al., 1997b; Kozin et al., 1981; Russel et al., 1977). Late radiographic changes of the spine include syndesmophyte formation, apophyseal joint fusions, and calcification, with eventual development of "bamboo" spine.

Therapy and Prognosis

The treatment of JAS is similar to that of JRA, with the use of NSAIDs to alleviate pain and stiffness and physical therapy to maintain good posture, muscle strength, and joint function. Some patients with JAS respond particularly well to indomethacin. Sulfasalazine may be useful, although there are no controlled studies of its efficacy (Huang and Chen, 1998). Patients with severe articular disease may require methotrexate or other immunosuppressive agents. Corticosteroids are rarely warranted or effective in JAS.

JAS can enter permanent remission at any stage. Progressive loss of vertebral mobility occurs in some patients, but prognosis for overall function is good if good posture can be maintained. Although the peripheral arthritis of JAS is often benign, some patients develop severe hip disease, with reports of up to 15% of patients requiring total hip replacement (Calin et al., 1988).

Seronegative Enthesopathy and Arthropathy (SEA Syndrome)

Before discussion of the other spondyloarthropathy syndromes in childhood, the syndrome of seronegative enthesopathy and arthropathy (SEA) deserves mention. Although lacking full diagnostic criteria for JAS, there exists a subgroup of children with no serum RF or ANA (seronegative) and with enthesitis (usually of a heel or knee) and lower extremity arthralgia or arthritis. These patients are usually male and commonly HLA-B27 positive. Many of these children go on to develop JAS or another of the spondyloarthropathies. In some, disease remits (Jacobs et al., 1982).

Reiter's Syndrome

RS is defined by the classic triad of arthritis, urethritis, and ocular inflammation. Other common findings include gastroenteritis, mucocutaneous lesions (oral or genital ulcers), and skin rashes (keratoderma blennorrhagicum). The designation "partial Reiter's syndrome" has been proposed for patients who do not fulfill the entire triad but are thought to belong in this disease category (Wilkens et al., 1982). Although RS generally occurs in young men, it has also been described in young women (Kanakoudi-Tsakalidou et al., 1998; Keat, 1983; Leirisalo et al., 1982; Lockie and Hunder, 1971; Rosenberg and Petty, 1979; Singsen et al., 1977b).

Pathogenesis

The cause of RS is unknown, but much evidence suggests that it is postinfectious, or reactive, in nature. In many cases, there is a temporal relationship between the development of RS and enteric infection with *Shigella flexneri, Yersinia enterocolitica, Salmonella enteritidis, Chlamydia trachomatis,* and *Salmonella typhimurium* (Davies et al., 1969; Keat, 1983; Russell, 1977; Smith, 1989). RS also occurs in patients with HIV or acquired immunodeficiency syndrome (AIDS) (Cuellar and Espinoza, 2000; de Mello e Silva and Boulos, 1998).

Clinical Manifestations

The arthritis of RS predominantly affects large joints, particularly of the lower extremities. Sacroiliac joint involvement may occur, with subsequent progression to spondylitis similar to that of classic AS (Oates and Young, 1959; Russell et al., 1977). Prominent systemic complaints of fever, malaise, and weight loss can be present with disease flares. Dysuria is a common complaint suggestive of urethritis, and bilateral acute conjunctivitis is present in two thirds of children at onset (Rosenberg and Petty, 1979). Rarely, aortic insufficiency similar to that of AS has been reported in childhood-onset RS (Hubscher and Susini, 1984).

Treatment

NSAIDs are used for control of pain and stiffness. Local steroid injections are helpful in the treatment of arthritis and enthesitis. If treatment failure occurs with the previously mentioned agents, sulfasalazine may be a useful adjunctive therapy.

Arthritis of Inflammatory Bowel Disease

Arthritis and arthralgia are among the most frequent extra-intestinal complications of inflammatory bowel disease and may be the presenting complaints in some patients (Schaller et al., 1974) (see Chapter 34). Two distinct forms of arthritis are described: peripheral arthritis, often pauciarticular in distribution, and chronic spondylitis, resembling AS. Only the spondylitis of inflammatory bowel disease is associated with HLA-B27 (Brewerton et al., 1974; Morris et al., 1974a).

Occult inflammatory bowel disease should be suspected as an underlying cause of arthritis in children with seronegative arthritis, unexplained anemia, gastrointestinal symptoms, erythema nodosum, growth failure or weight loss, or mucosal ulcerations. The peripheral arthritis of inflammatory bowel disease responds to controlling bowel inflammation, whereas the spondylitis may be progressive.

NSAIDs are the treatment of choice, at times supplemented with sulfasalazine and glucocorticoids, depending on the severity of the arthritis and bowel disease. Infliximab is of proven efficacy in the treatment of inflammatory bowel disease and its associated arthritis (Braun et al., 2001).

Psoriatic Arthritis

A small percentage of children with psoriasis have an associated arthritis, but this is less common than adult psoriatic arthropathy. Arthritis is often mentioned in the context of psoriatic spondyloarthropathy (see Chapter 32) (Lambert et al., 1976; Shore and Ansell, 1982). Two forms of psoriatic arthritis have been described: a peripheral form, either pauciarticular or polyarticular, and a spondylitic form, similar to AS. As with inflammatory bowel disease, the spondylitic form may be associated with HLA-B27, whereas peripheral arthritis in children has been associated with HLA-A2, HLA-B17, and HLA-Cw*0602 (Espinoza et al., 1990; Gladman et al., 1999; Hamilton et al., 1990; Suarez-Almazor and Russell, 1990).

Cutaneous psoriasis may precede arthritis, or there may be a long interval between the onset of arthritis and skin disease (Scarpa et al., 1984). One important clinical finding characteristic of patients with psoriatic arthritis is dactylitis of a single digit, either a finger or toe, caused by inflammation and swelling of the tendon sheath. This is referred to as a "sausage digit" and may help differentiate psoriatic arthritis from JRA. Nail pitting or onycholysis in psoriasis may also be helpful clinical clues.

Treatment includes NSAIDs and in more severe cases glucocorticoids and methotrexate (Kumar et al., 1994). Preliminary evidence suggests that etanercept will be a useful agent for both persistent arthritis and skin disease (Braun et al., 2001; Ogilvie et al., 2001; Yazici et al., 2002).

LUPUS ERYTHEMATOSUS AND RELATED DISORDERS

LE is the prototype of human autoimmune disease. *SLE* refers to LE that can involve multiple organ systems, whereas *discoid lupus erythematosus* (DLE) refers to localized skin disease. SLE has a widely variable presentation, course, and outcome; it may be mild or severe and potentially fatal. The hallmark of SLE is the production of autoantibodies reactive with multiple body tissue constituents, often resulting in end-organ damage. In the past, most children with SLE died of their disease, whereas with modern treatment and disease recognition the prognosis is now good for most patients. Several variants of lupus exist and these are discussed too.

Systemic Lupus Erythematosus

Historical Aspects

The name *lupus*, which derives from the Latin term for wolf, refers to the cutaneous lesions of LE, which can ulcerate and thus resemble the bite of an animal. The skin lesions of LE were recognized as early as the 13th century (Virchow, 1865). In the late 1890s, Sir William Osler recognized that lupus had systemic and cutaneous manifestations. The description of the LE cell by Hargraves and colleagues in 1948 led to the discovery of the prominent role of autoantibodies in patients with SLE.

Epidemiology

The prevalence of SLE is not precisely known; in the United States, it is somewhere between 15 and 50 cases per 100,000 persons. The estimated annual incidence of

SLE in childhood is 0.6 per 100,000 (Denardo et al., 1994; Siegel and Lee, 1973); thus SLE is a relatively uncommon disease. Approximately 20% of SLE cases begin in childhood, with the majority presenting at age 8 or older. SLE rarely is seen in children younger than age 5 (Emery, 1986; Fish et al., 1977; Lehman et al., 1989).

There is a striking female preponderance in SLE; in adults, there are approximately eight women affected to one man. In prepubertal children, the ratio is three girls to one boy affected (Emery, 1986; Kaslow and Masi, 1978; Koster-King et al., 1977; Masi and Kaslow, 1978; Meislin and Rothfield, 1968). These statistics suggest that sex hormones play a role in the susceptibility and development of SLE. Further evidence to support this hypothesis is increased prevalence of Klinefelter's syndrome (XXY) in males with SLE (Stern et al., 1977; Wenkert et al., 1991). In murine SLE, female mice develop earlier and more severe disease. Androgen treatment of female mice ameliorates the onset of nephritis, whereas orchiectomized male mice have earlier, more severe disease (Roubinian et al., 1983).

Racial differences in the distribution of SLE are seen, with a higher incidence among African-American, Hispanic, Native American, and Asian populations (Denardo et al., 1994; Kaslow and Masi, 1978; Koster-King et al., 1977). The reasons for these patterns are unknown.

Genetic influences clearly contribute to susceptibility to SLE. Monozygotic twins have a concordance rate of 25% to 60%, but in dizygotic twins the concordance rate is only 5% (Block et al., 1975, 1976; Brunner et al., 1971; Grennan et al., 1997; Lieberman et al., 1968). There is an increased frequency of SLE among first-and second-degree relatives of SLE patients, with rates of 17% to 27% reported for patients with childhood-onset disease. In addition, positive ANA tests are found in 20% to 30% of unaffected first-degree relatives of lupus patients, compared with less than 5% of controls (Miles and Isenberg, 1993).

Immunogenetics

Histocompatibility antigen associations in SLE have been described (Lindqvist and Alarcon-Riquelme, 1999). Overall, HLA-DR2 and HLA-DR3 are most common, with HLA-DR2 being more prevalent among patients with early-onset SLE (Schur, 1995; Schur et al., 1982; Stastny, 1978). Thus far, there is little evidence to suggest any strong association of HLA haplotypes and specific clinical manifestations of SLE (Hochberg et al., 1985). There is an association noted between certain HLA haplotypes and autoantibody production. The presence of anti-Ro and anti-La antibodies has been associated with HLA-B8/DR3 and HLA-DQw2 and with the co-occurrence of HLA-DR2 and HLA-DR3 (Bell and Maddison, 1980). Other associations include anti–ds-DNA with HLA-DR2 and anti-RNP with HLA-DR4 and HLA-DQw8 (Smolen et al., 1987). Complement loci have also been associated with SLE.

C4A (HLA-C4A*Q0) null alleles are associated with increased risk of SLE (Hong et al., 1994; Ulgaiti and Abraham, 1996), and at least half of individuals with homozygous deficiencies of the early complement components C1q, C4 and C2 have SLE (Schur, 1986; Walport, 1995).

Finally, polymorphisms in Fcγ receptor II and Fcγ receptor III genes have been associated with SLE in particular populations (Hatta et al., 1999; Jiang et al., 2000; Manger et al., 1998; Michel et al., 2000; Oh et al., 1999; Smyth et al., 1997; Tan, 2000; Vyse and Kotzin, 1998; Yap et al., 1999).

Pathogenesis

Although the cause of SLE remains unknown, much is known of its pathogenesis and immune abnormalities. Genetically inherited susceptibility factors contribute to the development of SLE. Hormonal, environmental, or other factors may also trigger or mediate disease, but their relative importance in promoting disease is undefined. A leading hypothesis is that disease-inciting triggers occurring in genetically susceptible individuals incite the production of autoantibodies and autoreactive lymphocytes and the formation of immune complexes that deposit in organs, activate complement, and cause tissue damage.

ROLE OF ABNORMAL B AND T CELLS

Numerous immunologic abnormalities have been described in murine and human SLE. A central feature of SLE is the loss of tolerance to self-antigens, and both B and T cells may play a critical role in initiating and perpetuating escape from tolerance. SLE B cells of patients are hyperactive, spontaneously secreting large amounts of polyclonal immunoglobulin (Blaese et al., 1980; Grondal et al., 2000). Their B cells produce antibodies reactive against self-antigens. These B-cell clones, which are normally deleted, proliferate, undergo somatic mutation, and produce pathogenic autoantibodies (Blaese et al., 1980; Rahman and Isenberg, 1994).

The T-cell system in SLE patients allows the development of autoantibody-producing B cells, although the specific details are not understood. Both abnormal helper and cytotoxic T lymphocytes have been described, as have increased numbers of circulating double-negative T cells (CD4⁻/CD8⁻) (Shivakumar et al., 1989; Zhang et al., 2000).

AUTOANTIBODY FORMATION IN SLE

A key feature of SLE is the production of pathogenic autoantibodies. Whether these antibodies arise nonspecifically as a result of polyclonal activation or are a clonally specific product of selected antigens is unknown (Schwartz and Stollar, 1985). The relationship between lupus autoantibodies and normal protective antibodies has been studied (Shoenfeld et al., 1983). It is known that lupus autoantibodies derive from the same antibody genes used in normal antibody responses. For example, the genes that encode anti-DNA antibodies in autoimmune mice are also present in normal mice (Naparstek et al., 1986). That lupus autoantibodies can arise from somatic mutation of genes used to encode normal antibodies has led to the suggestion that autoantigens are the immune stimuli for the pathogenesis of SLE (Davidson et al., 1987; Shibata et al., 1992).

ROLE OF IMMUNE COMPLEXES

Much of the tissue damage in SLE results from the formation of immune complexes. These complexes are able to bind complement and deposit in tissues such as the renal glomeruli, causing tissue damage (Davis et al., 1978; Koffler et al., 1967; Kohler and Bensel, 1969; Schur and Sandson, 1968). Normally, circulating immune complexes are rapidly cleared by complement receptors on erythrocytes and by fixation to Fc gamma receptors on other cells (Davies et al., 1990). Patients with active SLE have low numbers of CR1 receptors, saturation of available Fc receptors and impaired phagocytic clearance of immune complexes (Kimberly et al., 1983; Walport and Lachmann, 1988; Wilson and Fearon, 1984). Decreased in vitro monocyte Fc gamma receptor numbers is correlated with decreased in vivo macrophage function and increased disease activity (Seres et al., 1998).

These immune complex fixation and clearance abnormalities favor the persistence of free immune complexes and subsequent tissue deposition, although immune complexes can also be formed in situ in patients with SLE (Madaio et al., 1987). The important role of immune complexes and complement in perpetuating the tissue damage in SLE is supported by their presence in affected tissues such as glomeruli and skin (Davis et al., 1978; Koffler et al., 1967, 1969).

The direct role of autoantibodies in pathogenic immune complexes is supported by the elution of anti-DNA antibodies from kidney tissue of patients with active SLE nephritis (Kalunian et al., 1989; Madaio et al., 1987; Winfield et al., 1977) and by the ability to block immune complex deposition and inflammation in the murine kidney with a peptide that binds to immunoglobulins and interfere with Fc gamma receptor recognition (Marino et al., 2000).

Although immune complex levels are often elevated in patients with active SLE, there is no correlation between disease activity and levels of immune complexes.

Clinical Manifestations

LE in childhood is usually systemic, involving multiple organ systems. SLE in children is usually more acute and of greater severity than in adults. Children often present with the sudden appearance of multisystem disease; however, some children may have the insidious onset of vague symptoms before the diagnosis becomes apparent (Cassidy et al., 1977b; Cook et al., 1960; Emery, 1986; Glidden et al., 1983; Gribetz and Henley, 1959; Hagge et al., 1967; Jacobs, 1963a; Lehman et al., 1989; Nepom and Schaller, 1984; Norris et al., 1977; Platt et al., 1982; Wallace et al., 1978; Walravens and Chase, 1976; Zetterstrom and Berglund, 1956). Common

constitutional features include malaise, weight loss, fever, rash, arthritis, and arthralgia.

Cutaneous manifestations usually occur at some time during the course of disease (see Chapter 32). The characteristic facial "butterfly" rash of SLE occurs on the cheeks and over the bridge of the nose, usually sparing the nasolabial folds (Fig. 35-9). The malar rash often has a thickened or scaly quality, and may be photosensitive. Similar macular lesions may involve the extremities and trunk. Distinct purplish erythematous macules may be seen on the palms, soles, or distal digits and are secondary to small vessel vasculitis or thrombosis; infarction of tissue can occur. Raynaud's phenomenon is present in many patients and may precede other symptoms. Erythematous or ulcerative lesions often occur on the oral and nasal mucous membranes. Alopecia, either patchy or generalized, may occur during active disease. Other skin lesions include erythema nodosum, purpura, and erythema multiforme.

Musculoskeletal complaints are common, and arthralgia or arthritis may be the presenting complaints. Severe arthritis may mimic JRA, although the joint involvement is typically nondeforming and rarely erosive. Myositis, with muscle weakness, pain, and elevated muscle enzyme levels occurs in some patients.

Polyserositis (pleuritis, pericarditis, or peritonitis) is common and can be the sole presenting symptom of SLE in children. Cardiac manifestations of SLE include myocarditis, pericarditis, verrucous nonbacterial

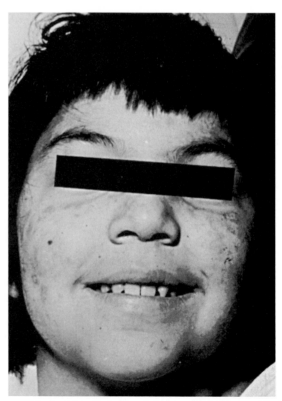

Figure 35-9·Facial rash of systemic lupus erythematosus with characteristic butterfly distribution. This patient also had generalized alopecia and brittle, fragmented hair, which is apparent in the frontal area ("fractured forelocks").

endocarditis (Libman-Sacks endocarditis), and less commonly, myocardial infarction related to coronary artery vasculitis. Cardiac valvular abnormalities and dysfunction occur in active SLE and are best identified with echocardiography (Cervera et al., 1992; Crozier et al., 1990; Galve et al., 1988; Tucker et al., 1992). The increased risk of early atherosclerotic heart disease among some young patients with SLE is likely related to coronary vasculitis, effects of antiphospholipid antibodies, and abnormal lipid profiles resulting from steroid therapy (Homcy et al., 1982; Hosenpud et al., 1983; Urowitz et al., 2000).

Pulmonary manifestations of SLE range from gradual interstitial disease, pneumonitis and pulmonary infiltrates, to pulmonary hemorrhage, a severe complication with high mortality (Delgado et al., 1990; Miller et al., 1986). Renal involvement occurs frequently in children with SLE and represents one of the most serious disease manifestations (Koster-King et al., 1977; Wallace et al., 1979). Signs of renal involvement include abnormal urine sediment with proteinuria, hematuria or cellular casts, hypertension, nephrotic syndrome, or renal insufficiency. Hypertension may be an ominous sign in SLE patients and is often associated with a poor prognosis.

Histopathology of the kidney in more than 50% of cases discloses diffuse proliferative glomerulonephritis, a severe lesion with high potential for progression to renal failure. Progression from mild focal lesions to more severe lesions has been documented in some patients (Garin et al., 1976; Lee et al., 1984; Pollak et al., 1964; Tejani et al., 1983; Woolf et al., 1979). Lupus nephritis is discussed extensively in Chapter 38.

Involvement of the nervous system in SLE is common. Children with SLE may have CNS manifestations at onset (Yancey et al., 1981). Seizures are classic CNS manifestations and are one of the diagnostic criteria (Silber et al., 1984). Intracerebral hemorrhage, thrombosis (especially in association with nephrotic syndrome or antiphospholipid antibodies), and coma may also occur. Peripheral neuritis, cranial nerve abnormalities, and chorea may be seen but are less common (West, 1996). Transverse myelitis, a rare complication of SLE, is associated with the presence of antiphospholipid antibodies in many patients (Provenzale and Bouldin, 1992). Ocular findings may consist of cytoid bodies (resembling cotton wool exudates) secondary to retinal abnormalities, uveitis, or episcleritis.

Hepatosplenomegaly and generalized lymphadenopathy are common. An acute abdominal crisis, caused by vasculitis of the bowel, can occur and have significant morbidity.

Hematologic abnormalities are common and include the anemia of chronic illness, autoimmune hemolytic anemia, leukopenia, lymphopenia, and thrombocytopenia (Budman and Steinberg, 1977). Autoantibodies to red cells, platelets, and lymphocytes may be present. Patients with antiphospholipid antibodies or a lupus anticoagulant often have a prolonged PTT or false-positive Venereal Disease Reference Laboratories (VDRL) test. Clinical manifestations associated with antiphos-

pholipid antibodies include recurrent venous or arterial thrombosis, thrombocytopenia, recurrent spontaneous abortions, transient ischemic attacks, stroke, myocardial ischemia or infarction, and cardiac valvulitis.

Isolated DLE is a chronic skin disease characterized by scarring plaques on the hands and upper body. Isolated discoid lupus rarely affects children and is usually not accompanied by progression to the systemic form of lupus (George and Tunnessen, 1993; Winkelmann, 1968). There is also an increased frequency of discoid lupus in mothers of boys with the X-linked form of chronic granulomatous disease (CGD) (Schaller, 1972) (see Chapter 20).

Diagnosis and Laboratory Findings

The diagnosis of SLE relies primarily on clinical findings of multisystem disease, with confirmation by laboratory and serologic studies. The diagnosis of SLE can be made with 96% sensitivity and specificity when the diagnostic criteria developed by Tan and colleagues (with revisions in 1997) are fulfilled (Table 35-7) (Hochberg et al., 1985; Tan et al., 1982a).

SEROLOGIC STUDIES

Serologic findings provide helpful clues in suggesting and confirming the diagnosis of SLE. The ANA test is the single most useful test for SLE, because it is almost always positive in the presence of active disease. It must be emphasized, however, that ANAs are not specific for SLE. ANA-negative SLE has been described, although its frequency has diminished with the use of the sensitive Hep-2 substrate for ANA testing (Ferreiro et al., 1984; Fessel, 1978). Some ANA-negative patients may have circulating anticytoplasmic antibodies (Provost et al., 1977) or SSA/Ro antibodies (Blomberg et al., 2000).

The presence of antibodies to native DNA is a fairly specific laboratory finding for SLE, because these autoantibodies are rarely seen in other conditions. Not all patients with SLE have detectable anti-DNA antibodies, however, so the lack of these antibodies does not exclude the diagnosis of SLE. In patients with detectable anti-DNA titers, the serum level generally fluctuates with disease activity and provides a clinical marker for treatment response or impending disease flare (Emlen et al., 1986; Pincus et al., 1969, 1971; Schur and Sandson, 1968; Ward et al., 1989). Other serologic abnormalities in SLE include hypergammaglobulinemia, positive RF tests, positive Coombs' test, false-positive serologic test for syphilis, and circulating anticoagulants (antiphospholipid antibodies) (Schur and Sandson, 1968). Organ-specific autoantibodies such as antithyroid antibodies may also be detected.

Serum complement levels are low in patients with active immune complex disease. Measurement of serum complement is useful to follow the course of disease, because levels return to normal as disease activity abates (Appel et al., 1978; Laitman et al., 1989). In patients with SLE whose complement levels remain depressed despite other evidence of improving disease, evaluation

TABLE 35-7 · 1997 REVISED CRITERIA FOR THE CLASSIFICATION OF SYSTEMIC LUPUS ERYTHEMATOSUS (SLE)*

1. Malar rash
2. Discoid lupus rash
3. Photosensitivity
4. Oral or nasal mucocutaneous ulcerations
5. Nonerosive arthritis
6. Nephritis
    Proteinuria >0.5 g/day
    Cellular casts
7. Central nervous system manifestations
    Psychosis
    Seizures
8. Serositis
    Pleuritis or pericarditis
9. Hematologic manifestations
    Coombs'-positive hemolytic anemia
        or
    Lymphopenia <1500 cells/mm^3 or leukopenia
        <4000 cells/mm^3
        or
    Thrombocytopenia
10. Positive antinuclear antibody
11. Positive autoantibodies
    Antibodies to double-stranded DNA or Sm
        or
    Biologic false-positive test for syphilis
        or
    Positive antiphospholipid antibodies

*The presence of 4 of these 11 criteria confers 96% sensitivity and 96% specificity for the diagnosis of SLE.

for a complement deficiency state should be considered (see Chapter 21).

RENAL PATHOLOGY

The histologic classification of renal lesions in patients with SLE can aid in the diagnosis, prognosis, and evaluation of treatment protocols (see Chapter 38). Several different histologic patterns of renal pathology are seen, including mesangial immune deposits with or without proliferation, focal or diffuse proliferative nephritis, or membranous lesions (Baldwin et al., 1970, 1977; Ginzler et al., 1974; Koffler et al., 1967; Lowenstein et al., 1970; Southwest Pediatric Nephrology Group, 1986).

Mesangial or focal proliferative lesions represent milder forms of lupus nephritis, with potential for good response to treatment and outcome. Mild lesions can progress to a more severe form, however, with correspondingly poor outcome.

The diffuse proliferative lesion of lupus nephritis may be associated with severe clinical manifestations, such as hypertension, abnormal urinary sediment, and renal insufficiency (Baldwin et al., 1977; Ginzler et al., 1974).

Membranous lupus nephritis is often characterized by persistent nephrotic syndrome, with risk of subsequent renal failure and catastrophic thrombosis.

The histologic characterization alone may be insufficient to predict response to therapy and outcome (Fries et al., 1978). The degree of chronic changes present in the renal biopsy, as assessed by a chronicity index, is useful to predict potential response to immunosuppressive therapy (Carette et al., 1983) and eventual renal outcome.

OTHER LABORATORY FINDINGS

Acute-phase reactants are present during periods of active disease, although this is not universal. The ESR may be elevated, but this is not generally helpful in following disease activity. Liver function tests are often mildly abnormal during active disease. Patients with SLE appear to be especially sensitive to hepatotoxicity of salicylates; thus transaminase levels must be carefully monitored (Seaman and Ishak, 1974). Myositis may be present, with elevations in serum muscle enzyme levels.

Assessment of organ systems for damage often aids in determining the degree of active disease and guiding therapy. Pulmonary function tests, electrocardiograms, and echocardiography may reveal subtle tissue damage before clinical symptoms (Tucker et al., 1992). Diagnosis of CNS SLE is difficult, because abnormalities of cerebrospinal fluid (CSF), electroencephalograms, CT, or MRI may not correlate well with clinical signs and symptoms (Kelly and Denburg, 1987; Sibitt et al., 1989; West, 1996).

Treatment

Therapy in SLE is initially aimed at reducing inflammation and dampening the immune response. The extent of systemic involvement determines the treatment required in the individual patient, as does the immunologic activity as reflected in serum complement and anti-DNA antibodies. In patients with renal disease, a renal biopsy may be helpful to indicate the severity and activity of disease.

For individuals with mild SLE without nephritis and with normal levels of serum complement, symptomatic therapy with NSAIDs, antimalarials, or possibly low-dose corticosteroids may be sufficient. Careful follow-up, including evaluation of organ status, is crucial to detect early disease flares. For individuals with more severe disease with evidence of organ system damage and low levels of serum complement, aggressive therapy is warranted.

High-dose corticosteroids provide the first line of treatment in patients with active SLE. It is critical to control active disease as quickly and completely as possible to prevent tissue damage. The most useful indication of adequate control of disease is normalization of serum complement levels and decrease of DNA antibodies (Laitman et al., 1989; Schur and Sandson, 1968; Urman and Rothchild, 1977). Whenever possible, once the immunologic activity of the disease is controlled, alternate-day steroid therapy should be attempted to minimize growth retardation and cushingoid features.

Immunosuppressive drugs such as cyclophosphamide, azathioprine, and methotrexate play an important role in the treatment of SLE. These drugs are helpful in controlling active disease in patients with incomplete response to steroids (Carneiro and Sato, 1999); in patients who present with fulminant disease; and in patients with unacceptable side effects of long-term, high-dose steroid treatment.

Of these, cyclophosphamide is most commonly used, especially in severe renal and CNS disease and widespread vasculitis. Long-term outcome in patients with SLE nephritis is improved by intravenous pulse cyclophosphamide treatment in addition to steroids as compared with steroid treatment alone (Austin et al., 1986; Bansal and Beto, 1997; Boumpas et al., 1992; Decker et al., 1975; Lehman et al., 1989). The potential complications and side effects of these medications, however, including severe disseminated infection, possible increased risk of malignancy, and damage to reproductive potential, make careful consideration essential before initiating therapy.

Despite early aggressive treatment, a small subset of individuals have persistent disease marked by organ destruction. For these patients, trials of B-cell depletion with rituximab, autologous bone marrow transplantation or bone marrow ablation induced with cyclophosphamide have been undertaken. Long-term follow-up of these patients helps determine whether long-term remission or disease cure is possible (Balow et al., 2000; Fouillard et al., 1999; Leandro et al., 2002; Traynor and Burt, 1999).

Complications and Prognosis

The prognosis of SLE is related to the extent and severity of systemic involvement in each individual patient. SLE is a potentially fatal disease; however, some patients have relatively mild systemic involvement, which is compatible with long-term, morbidity-free survival. Some patients have prolonged remissions of their disease.

Causes of mortality in SLE have changed with the advent of aggressive treatment for renal disease; fewer patients are developing renal failure, but mortality from fulminant disease, pulmonary hemorrhage, myocardial infarction, and infection still occurs. Infection in particular is emerging as the major cause of morbidity and mortality in patients with SLE as more aggressive immunosuppressive protocols are used in treatment (Lacks and White, 1990). Early atherosclerotic heart disease is emerging as a potential cause of morbidity and mortality among young patients surviving SLE (Homcy et al., 1982; Hosenpud et al., 1983; Zonana-Nachach et al., 2000).

Nonetheless, the prognosis for patients with SLE has greatly improved with 5-year survival in most centers exceeding 90%. Early aggressive therapy and meticulous follow-up are responsible for their improved outlook.

Neonatal Lupus Syndrome

NLS occurs in infants born to mothers with antibodies to Ro(SSA) and/or La(SSB) (see Chapter 32). If these mothers have a rheumatic illness, they more commonly have Sjögren's syndrome than SLE (Schaller, 1977e). A significant portion of mothers have no known rheumatic disease. During gestation, the Ro and La autoantibodies are passed via the placenta to the infants, resulting in transient clinical manifestations of rash and cytopenias and permanent complete congenital heart block. NLS is an important example of organ injury mediated by lupus associated antibodies (Buyon et al., 1998; Reed et al., 1983; Weston et al., 1982).

Pathogenesis and Risk Factors

The clinical manifestations of NLS result from the passage of high titers of anti-Ro and anti-La antibodies from the mother into the developing fetus, with resultant inflammation of tissues such as the heart and skin (Buyon and Winchester, 1990; Harley et al., 1985; Lee and Weston, 1984; Litsey et al., 1985; Reed et al., 1983; Scott et al., 1983; Silverman et al., 1991). The Ro and La antigens are present in high quantities in fetal heart tissue and skin and explain the predilection of involvement of these organs in NLS (Horsfall et al., 1991).

Some, but not all, mothers of infants with NLS have SLE, but a large percentage have no known rheumatic illness (Schaller et al., 1979). Careful questioning of these mothers often reveals rheumatic symptoms, and some of these "well" mothers will develop SLE or Sjögren's syndrome (McCue et al., 1977). Furthermore, not all infants of women with anti-Ro and anti-La are affected with NLS; in fact, most offspring of these women are unaffected. A 1988 study by Lockshin and colleagues (1988) showed that only 10% of infants born to a group of women with SLE and anti-Ro/La antibodies developed NLS and none had heart block. Although there is an increased risk of a second affected infant, the magnitude of this risk is not precisely known.

There have been dizygotic twins of mothers with anti-Ro or anti-La antibodies who were discordant for NLS (Watson et al., 1994). Although anti-Ro and anti-La are the most commonly identified antibodies associated with NLS, several cases associated with anti-RNP (ribonucleoprotein) and anti-Smith antibodies have been reported (Horng et al., 1992; Provost et al., 1987).

The specificities of the autoantibodies involved in NLS have been explored. Antibodies to the Ro antigen are of two types; one to a 52-kD polypeptide and the second to a 60-kD polypeptide. The La antibody is directed to a 48-kD polypeptide. There is a strong association of maternal anti–48-kD La antibody with the development of NLS. The combination of anti–52-kD Ro and anti–48-kD La antibody is strongly associated with the risk of having an affected infant (Buyon et al., 1989; Vianna et al., 1998). Therefore maternal antibody profiles may permit identification of high-risk pregnancies in utero.

Genetic factors of both mothers and infants have been investigated in hopes of defining additional risk factors in the development of NLS. The haplotype of HLA-B8, HLA-DR3, HLA-DQw2, HLA-DRw52 was present in 75% of a group of 20 mothers of infants with NLS in North America (Alexander et al., 1989). In a Japanese cohort, HLA-B*1501 (B62) and Cw*0303 (Cw9) were increased in mothers of children with NLS

(Miyagawa et al., 1997). HLA-DR3 in particular is strongly associated with NLS in mothers with anti-Ro or anti-La antibodies. No infant haplotype was identified that predisposes to NLS.

Clinical Manifestations

The clinical features of neonatal lupus are variable, but most infants have only mild skin findings. In general, infants have either skin or cardiac manifestations; it is rare to find both in the same infant. The skin rash (erythema annulare) is an annular, scaly, erythematous eruption that develops in patches on the face, scalp, extremities, or trunk. The rash is often photosensitive and is similar to lesions of subacute cutaneous lupus (Epstein and Litt, 1961; McCusition and Schoch, 1954; Tseng and Buyon, 1997). The lesions nearly always resolve by 6 to 8 months, coincident with decreasing titers of maternal IgG.

Transient cytopenias can also occur in NLS, with thrombocytopenia most frequently reported. Mild hemolytic anemia and leukopenia can be seen (Seip, 1960; Watson et al., 1988). Less frequently, hepatic abnormalities, hepatosplenomegaly, or severe cytopenias have been reported (Bremers et al., 1979; Draznin et al., 1979; Laxer et al., 1990; Weston et al., 1982).

The most significant manifestation of NLS is complete congenital heart block, because this is a permanent sequela. NLS accounts for most cases of congenital heart block; even when the mother does not have a diagnosed rheumatic condition, she usually has serum anti-Ro or anti-La antibodies. Most infants with congenital heart block require a pacemaker. Overall mortality is as high as 15% to 20% (Buyon et al., 1998; McCue et al., 1977, 1987). Lesser degrees of heart block have been seen in neonatal lupus, with occasional progression (Geggel et al., 1988). Endomyocardial fibroelastosis, myocarditis, or cardiomyopathy has also been reported in neonatal lupus (Hogg, 1957; Hull et al., 1966; Moak et al., 2001).

Prognosis and Treatment

The skin lesions of NLS require no specific treatment; they resolve spontaneously as the maternal autoantibodies disappear from the infant's circulation. No treatment reverses the congenital heart block. Infants with NLS who are seriously ill with evidence of myocardial dysfunction should be considered for aggressive immunosuppressive therapy (Rider et al., 1993; Silverman, 1993). There is controversy over whether identifying infants at risk for NLS in utero and offering aggressive corticosteroid treatment of their mothers (to decrease maternal antibody titers and treat fetal cardiac inflammation) improves neonatal outcome (Buyon et al., 1987; Carreira et al., 1993; Saleeb et al., 1999; Shinohara et al., 1999).

Although most infants with NLS recover without sequelae, a few infants develop SLE later in childhood or early adulthood (Fox et al., 1979; Jackson and Gulliver, 1979; Lanham et al., 1983).

Mixed Connective Tissue Disease

MCTD is an overlap syndrome closely related to SLE. It was first described in 1972 in patients with clinical features of a number of rheumatic conditions who had high titers of antibodies to extractable nuclear antigens, particularly nuclear RNP (Sharp et al., 1972). The variability of clinical manifestations and lack of specificity of anti-RNP antibodies for MCTD have led to difficulties in identifying MCTD as a truly distinct disorder. There remains significant controversy about whether MCTD is a distinctive entity (Black and Isenberg, 1992).

Clinical Manifestations

Clinical features of MCTD combine those of SLE, dermatomyositis, scleroderma, and chronic arthritis (Hoffman and Greidinger, 2000; Oetgen et al., 1981; Sanders et al., 1973; Singsen et al., 1977a). Presentation may mimic any of these disorders; the presence of a high-titer, speckled-pattern ANA and a negative anti-DNA should suggest investigation for the presence of anti-RNP antibodies and further study for clinical features of MCTD (Hoffman et al., 1993).

Polyarthritis may be mild or severe; some patients may develop erosive disease (Catoggio et al., 1983; Halla and Hardin, 1978). Raynaud's phenomenon may be the early presenting feature of MCTD, and scleroderma-like changes of the skin, especially involving distal extremities, can be seen. Some patients have a classic dermatomyositis rash and myositis. Esophageal dysmotility is common and often asymptomatic. Mild pulmonary abnormalities are often present, but severe pulmonary hypertension has also been reported (Derderian et al., 1985; Hoffman and Greidinger, 2000; Prakash et al., 1985; Rosenberg et al., 1979).

Other clinical features include rashes suggestive of SLE, overt vasculitis, fever, lymphadenopathy, organomegaly, thrombocytopenia, and serositis. Early studies suggested that renal disease was less frequent in this group of patients, but this has not proved true on longer follow-up of adult patients (Nimelstein et al., 1980; Singsen et al., 1977a).

Treatment and Prognosis

The treatment of MCTD is similar to that of SLE. Patients with mild disease manifestations may require only NSAIDs, antimalarials, and physical therapy. Patients with severe progressive arthritis can be treated as for JRA with methotrexate, although no formal therapeutic trials have been done. For more severe systemic involvement, corticosteroids or cytotoxic agents may be required. Autologous bone marrow transplant was unsuccessful in one case (Myllykangas-Luosujarvi et al., 2000).

The prognosis of MCTD is variable. Some investigators have reported generally good outcomes (Burdt et al., 1999), but others have reported that many patients evolve over time to a course more consistent with either SLE, scleroderma, or RA and that the mortality is considerably higher than previously thought (Black and Isenberg, 1992; Nimelstein et al., 1980). Since there is potential for long-term morbidity, close follow-up and treatment is warranted.

Primary Antiphospholipid Antibody Syndrome

Patients with the primary (no associated connective tissue disease) APLA syndrome have one or several of the major clinical manifestations of recurrent arterial, venous, or small vessel thrombosis or pregnancy complications (fetal loss, premature births) in association with persistently positive tests for lupus anticoagulant or medium- to high-titer anticardiolipin antibodies (Tanne et al., 2002; Wilson et al., 1999). In children, girls are more commonly affected than boys, and venous thrombosis is more common than arterial (Ravelli et al., 1990).

Children with APLA syndrome may present with unexplained cerebral vascular accidents, myocardial infarction, cardiac valvular disease, or the Budd-Chiari syndrome (Bernstein et al., 1984; Fields et al., 1990; Ravelli et al., 1990; Saca et al., 1994; Sletnes et al., 1992). Rare cases of isolated deep vein thrombosis in children have also been described (Ravelli et al., 1990). In adults, thrombosis tends to recur and is prevented with long-term anticoagulation (most commonly warfarin) (Rosove and Brewer, 1992; Wilson et al., 1999). However, because the recurrence rate for thrombosis in children with APLA syndrome has not been established, the need for long-term anticoagulation is not known.

In considering treatment options in children, one must weigh the possibility of thrombotic recurrences in normotensive nonsmoking children with the possibility of hemorrhagic complications of anticoagulation therapy in children active in sports and play.

SJÖGREN'S SYNDROME

Sjögren's syndrome is a condition affecting multiple exocrine glands, most notably the parotid and lacrimal glands. It may occur as an isolated primary condition or as a secondary manifestation of another illness such as RA or lupus (Anaya et al., 1995; Tomiita et al., 1997). Criteria in adults (San Diego criteria for Sjögren's syndrome [Fox and Saito, 1994]) for definitive diagnosis require signs and symptoms of eye and mouth dryness (SICCA symptoms) (keratoconjunctivitis/xerostomia), autoimmunity (positivity for RF, ANA or anti-SS-A [Ro] or anti-SS-B [La] antibodies), and a characteristic minor salivary gland biopsy showing lymphocytic infiltration. However, these diagnostic criteria are less useful in children because symptoms of dry eyes and mouth are uncommon (Bartunkova et al., 1999) and children present more commonly with parotitis (Bartunkova et al., 1999; Drosos et al., 1997).

RF, ANA, anti-SS-A, and anti-SS-B positivity are common in children, and young women of childbearing age should be counseled as to the potential risk of fetal heart block resulting from placental passage of Ro and La antibodies. Hypergammaglobulinemia is also commonly present (Anaya et al., 1995; Tomiita et al., 1997). Fatigue, arthralgia/arthritis (nonerosive), vasculitis, myalgia/myositis, and Raynaud's phenomena may accompany the glandular features of Sjögren's syndrome.

Treatment depends on the clinical findings. Decreased lacrimal gland secretion is treated with artificial lubricants, and decreased salivary flow is treated with sugar-free lozenges or gum. Fatigue and arthralgia can often be managed with NSAIDs or hydroxychloroquine. Corticosteroids and other agents such as cyclophosphamide are at times required for more fulminant disease with vasculitis or myositis (Chu et al., 1998; Golan et al., 1997; Sato et al., 1993; Yamanishi et al., 1994; Zandbelt et al., 2001).

DERMATOMYOSITIS

Dermatomyositis is a rheumatic disorder characterized by inflammation of striated muscle and specific skin lesions, with occlusive small vessel vasculitis as the characteristic pathologic finding (Ansell, 1984; Banker and Victor, 1966; Bohan and Peter, 1975; Hanson and Kornreich, 1967; Pachman, 1995a; Schaller, 1971; Sullivan et al., 1972, 1977; Wallace et al., 1985). In polymyositis, which is extremely rare in children, cutaneous lesions are lacking.

Pathogenesis

The cause of dermatomyositis is unknown. Humoral and cellular abnormalities have been described and include cytotoxicity of patient lymphocytes and serum to muscle tissue in vitro; excess proliferative responses of peripheral blood mononuclear cells to muscle cells or antigens; and abnormal deposition of complement components, immunoglobulin, and activated leukocytes in muscle tissue (Dawkins and Mastaglia, 1973; Johnson et al., 1972; Kalovidouris et al., 1989; Kissel et al., 1986; Whitaker and Engel, 1972). Increased percentages of CD19+ B cells correlate with increased disease activity in patients with dermatomyositis (Eisenstein et al., 1997).

Various infectious agents, including coxsackievirus, echovirus, picornavirus, retroviruses, and toxoplasmosis, have been proposed, but not proved, to have a role in the pathogenesis of dermatomyositis (Leff et al., 1992; Rosenberg et al., 1989). An increased incidence of HLA-DR3, HLA-B8, HLA-DRB1, and HLA-DQA1 has been found, most strikingly among white patients (Friedman et al., 1983; Malleson, 1990; Pachman et al., 1985; Plamondon et al., 1999; Reed et al., 1991). In one study, children with dermatomyositis were found to have an increased incidence of C4 null genes (Moulds et al., 1990).

Some adult patients with dermatomyositis have associated malignancy, usually carcinomas; the muscle disease may remit with treatment of the tumor (Richardson and Callen, 1989; Sigurgeirisson et al., 1992). This curious relation has not been noted with childhood dermatomyositis.

Clinical Manifestations

The myositis characteristically involves the proximal limb and trunk muscles. Although the disease occasionally presents acutely, more typically weakness develops over weeks to months, and the first symptoms may be decreased endurance or fatigue. Myositis classically involves proximal muscle groups, including the neck, abdominal muscle, shoulder, and hip girdles, more than distal muscles. Involvement of palatal or respiratory muscles may occur as well, with the onset of dysphonia or, less commonly, difficulty swallowing or handling oral secretions. Myalgias, arthralgias, and arthritis may also be present.

The characteristic cutaneous lesions include a violaceous erythema (heliotrope) hue of the upper eyelids and extensor surfaces of the joints, especially the small joints of the hands (Gottron's sign). Dilated periungual capillary loops can readily be seen and may be an accurate indicator of active disease (Nussbaum et al., 1983; Silver and Maricq, 1989). Facial and truncal rashes may also be present.

Vasculitis of the gastrointestinal tract may result in abdominal pain or bleeding, and perforation can occur at any level. Calcinosis of subcutaneous tissue, fascia, and muscle occurs in 20% to 30% of patients and may occur with inadequate early treatment of disease (Bowyer et al., 1983). Other systemic complications of dermatomyositis are exceedingly rare. Cardiac dysrhythmias, pericarditis, tamponade, and myocarditis have been reported. Pronounced weakness may cause restrictive pulmonary disease; interstitial lung disease or pulmonary hemorrhage is uncommon in children. A few children have developed an acquired lipodystrophy associated with insulin resistance and other endocrine abnormalities late in the course of severe disease (Huemer et al., 2001).

Diagnosis

The criteria for the diagnosis of dermatomyositis include the presence of symmetric proximal muscle weakness, characteristic rash, elevated muscle enzyme levels (aldolase, creatine phosphokinase, ALT, AST, and lactate dehydrogenase), myopathic findings on electromyogram, and typical muscle biopsy histology. Serum von Willebrand factor may be increased (Bloom et al., 1995). MRI may also be helpful in assessing extent of disease and localizing areas of inflammation for biopsy (Fig. 35-10) (Bartlett et al., 1999; Rider and Miller, 2000). In patients without typical rash, electromyography (EMG) and biopsy are necessary to exclude other forms of myopathy.

Muscle biopsies show fiber necrosis, variation in fiber size, endothelial swelling, and occlusive vasculitis; perivascular inflammatory infiltrates are minimal as compared with findings in polymyositis. Vasculitis may also be seen in other involved tissues (Crowe et al., 1982). The ESR is often normal. ANAs are sometimes found (Friedman et al., 1983; Mellins et al., 1982; Pachman and Cooke, 1980; Pachman et al., 1985).

In adults with myositis, antibodies to several aminoacyl transfer RNA synthetases have identified patients with an increased risk for interstitial pneumonitis (Dalakas, 1991; Dalakas and Plotz, 1989). These include antibodies to Jo-1 (anti-histidyl tRNA synthetase), PL-7 (anti-threonyl tRNA synthetase), PL-12 (anti-alanyl tRNA synthetase), and anti-isoleucyl and anti-glycyl tRNA synthetases. Autoantibodies to signal recognition peptide are found in adults with polymyositis, as are antibodies to the Pm-Scl antigen (involved in ribosomal RNA processing) and the Mi-2 antigen (part of nucleosome remodeling complex sometimes seen in childhood dermatomyositis) (Targoff, 2000; Targoff et al., 1990).

Analysis of adults with inflammatory myositis has shown that determination of autoantibody reactivity correlated well with specific clinical manifestations and response to therapy (Love et al., 1991; Targoff, 2000). About 10% of children with dermatomyositis test positive for one of these myositis-specific antibodies, most commonly Mi-2 but not the tRNA synthetases as found in 20% to 30% of adults with myositis (Pachman, 1995a, 1995b).

Treatment

Dermatomyositis and polymyositis generally respond well to therapy with corticosteroids and have a good prognosis if treated early and vigorously (Ansell, 1984,

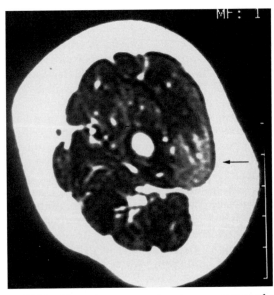

Figure 35-10 · Magnetic resonance imaging appearance of active myositis. Arrow indicates high-intensity signal on T2-weighted images indicative of inflammation.

1992; Hanson and Kornreich, 1967; Mastaglia et al., 1993; Schaller, 1971; Sullivan et al., 1972, 1977). High dosages of oral or intravenous steroids are the usual first choice for treatment (Al-Mayouf et al., 2000).

Additional therapy is necessary for some patients, including those with severe-onset disease (extreme muscle weakness, severe systemic involvement, vasculitis), those with a relapsing course, or those with chronic persistent disease (Malleson, 1990). Adjunctive therapy may also provide significant steroid-sparing effect. Methotrexate is most commonly used, but azathioprine, hydroxychloroquine, and cyclosporine have all been reported to have beneficial effects (Al-Mayouf et al., 2000; Ansell, 1992; Fischer et al., 1979; Heckmatt et al., 1989; Jacobs, 1977; Lueck et al., 1991; Miller et al., 1992b; Olson and Lindsley, 1989; Wallace et al., 1985).

Other treatments, including high-dose IVIG, first reported in adults (Dalakas et al., 1993), have been tried in children with recalcitrant disease, with some promising results (Al-Mayouf et al., 2000; Barron et al., 1992a; Cherin et al., 1991). The mechanism of action of IVIG may be the prevention of deposition of activated complement components in the capillaries of the muscle tissue (Basta and Dalakas, 1994).

A controlled trial of leukapheresis and plasma exchange in 39 adult patients with dermatomyositis or polymyositis found no difference between these treatments and sham pheresis (Miller et al., 1992a).

Physical therapy is an important component of treatment for children with dermatomyositis to maintain range of motion and eventually to improve endurance and muscle strength.

SCLERODERMA

Scleroderma, a disease characterized by hardening of the skin and subcutaneous tissues, occurs in localized forms (morphea, linear scleroderma) and a generalized cutaneous and systemic form (progressive systemic sclerosis [PSS]) (Ansell et al., 1976; Cassidy et al., 1977a; Kornreich et al., 1977; Winkelman et al., 1971).

Clinical Manifestations

The appearance and the histology of cutaneous lesions are similar in the localized and generalized forms. The affected skin becomes shiny, indurated, and eventually bound down to underlying structures; patchy hyperpigmentation or vitiligo may be present. The localized cutaneous forms (morphea, linear scleroderma, and coup de sabre) rarely progress to generalized disease; the relationship between localized cutaneous scleroderma and PSS is not defined.

Systemic manifestations of PSS include involvement of the esophagus, bowel, lung, kidney, and heart (Suarez-Almazor et al., 1985). Raynaud's phenomenon is nearly always present and may precede typical skin changes by months or even years. Capillaroscopy of nail beds has revealed varying patterns of nail fold capillary changes; an active pattern characterized by destruction and loss of capillaries seems to be associated with a rapidly progressive form of the disease as opposed to enlargement and/or telangiectasias, which may herald a milder disease course (Chen et al., 1984; Spencer-Green et al., 1983).

Diagnosis is made on clinical grounds with the aid of laboratory techniques seeking specific organ involvement, such as pulmonary function tests, echocardiography, and esophageal motility studies (Follansbee et al., 1984; Peters-Golden et al., 1984).

Pathogenesis

The pathogenesis of scleroderma is not understood, but a number of immunologic, vascular, and connective tissue abnormalities have been described. Many patients with scleroderma produce antibodies rather specific for these disorders. Anti–topoisomerase I (Scl-70) antibodies are seen in patients with systemic sclerosis.

Patients with a more limited form of scleroderma with subcutaneous calcinosis, Raynaud's phenomenon, esophageal dysmotility, sclerodactyly, and telangiectasias (CREST) Syndrome often have anticentromere antibodies.

Studies of MHC association in scleroderma have shown an increase in HLA-DR1, HLA-DR3, HLA-DR5, HLA-DQA1-0501, and C4 null alleles in particular disease subsets, although results differ among ethnic groups and different countries (Black, 1993; Briggs et al., 1993; Lambert et al., 2000). Finally, women with scleroderma show increased frequency of microchimerism compared with healthy controls (Nelson et al., 1998).

Abnormalities of the microvasculature may play a role in disease pathogenesis. Raynaud's phenomenon, a hyperreactive vascular state, often occurs long before obvious clinical signs of scleroderma, which suggests that vascular changes may take place early in the disease. There is histologic evidence of endothelial cell necrosis early in scleroderma, with arterial intimal proliferation and inflammatory perivascular infiltration (Fleischmajer and Perlish, 1980). Changes in the heterogeneity of type IV collagen occur in the vascular basement membrane; activated complement complexes and complement receptor C5a are noted in the microvasculature from skin biopsies in affected patients (Hoyland et al., 1993; Sprott et al., 2000).

The classic pathologic finding in scleroderma is the increase in normal extracellular matrix and fibrosis. In scleroderma, certain types of collagen are overproduced and the genetic message for these collagen molecules has been shown to be increased. A dinucleotide repeat-haplotype of the COL1A2 type 1 collagen gene in its homozygous form in association with the finding of a positive ANA has been associated with increased frequency of disease (Hata et al., 2000). Cytokines may play a role in abnormal regulation of fibroblasts in scleroderma, but no direct evidence to support this is available (Alecu et al., 1998; Black, 1993).

Several clinical conditions resembling scleroderma have been described. A scleroderma-like state occurs in some patients after bone marrow transplantation (van Vloten et al., 1977), often related to chronic graft-versus-host disease (Jaffe and Claman, 1983). Likewise, symptoms and signs suggestive of scleroderma have been described as part of the Spanish toxic oil syndrome (Kilbourne et al., 1983). There are reports of women with silicone breast implants developing scleroderma (Spiera and Kerr, 1993; Varga et al., 1989); however, a meta-analysis of clinical studies does not support silicone as a causative agent (Janowsky et al., 2000).

Treatment

In contrast to the other rheumatic diseases, scleroderma responds poorly, if at all, to even vigorous therapy with potent anti-inflammatory drugs, such as corticosteroids. Many drugs have been used without success. Drugs such as penicillamine, which result in an increase of soluble collagen components, have been tried, but the results have not been dramatic. Some suggest, however, that treatment with prolonged penicillamine over long periods of time results in improved survival and slows pulmonary involvement (Jimenez and Sigal, 1991). Therapy with chlorambucil has also been proposed, but its efficacy is uncertain (Furst et al., 1989).

Voluntary control of digital temperatures using biofeedback has proved helpful in controlling Raynaud's phenomenon. Nifedipine and other calcium channel blockers are sometimes of value, with action on the vascular abnormalities. Initial trials of calcitonin in localized and diffuse skin disease seemed promising but have since been less so (Hulshof et al., 2000). The efficacy of agents such as recombinant oral bovine type 1 collagen, epoprostenol, and interferons alpha and gamma are under investigation (Black et al., 1999; Grassegger et al., 1998; Hunzelmann et al., 1997; Klings and Farber, 2000; McKown et al., 2000; Vlachoyiannopoulos et al., 1996).

Small studies of methotrexate treatment in systemic sclerosis, localized scleroderma, and widespread morphea are promising (van den Hoogen, 1996; Seyger et al., 1998; Uziel et al., 2000). Both busanten (an endothelin receptor antagonist) and cyclophosphaside have been used with some success in scleroderma associated with lung disease.

With improved knowledge of scleroderma pathogenesis, there is hope for improved therapy.

Prognosis

The prognosis of scleroderma is uncertain. The cutaneous forms are often self-limited but may cause extensive crippling. PSS is inexorably severe but may sometimes develop slowly enough so that the prognosis is not entirely gloomy.

EOSINOPHILIC FASCIITIS

Eosinophilic fasciitis, a rare entity, is characterized by inflammation of the fascia with an eosinophilic infiltrate (Bennett et al., 1977; Grisanti et al., 1989; Michet et al., 1981; Shulman et al., 1979).

Clinical Manifestations

Eosinophilic fasciitis resembles scleroderma in both its diffuse and localized forms, but unlike those disorders, the onset is acute, with widespread inflammation and sclerosis of the deep fascia and without associated Raynaud's phenomenon (Rodnan et al., 1975). Eosinophilic fasciitis can present with hand contractures in childhood (Farrington et al., 1993). Affected fascial tissues are infiltrated with plasma cells, lymphocytes, and often eosinophils. Because fascia is affected and overlying skin is spared, there is often superficial puckering of the skin, with hardening and tenderness of the underlying tissues. The face is characteristically spared; tissues of the limbs and sometimes the trunk are predominantly affected. Visceral involvement is uncommon, but symmetric polyarthritis has been described (Rosenthal and Benson, 1980).

In a number of patients, fasciitis has occurred after vigorous physical activity, suggesting that it may be an aberrant response to the overuse of muscles (Guseva et al., 1986). It has been described after allogeneic bone marrow transplantation (Markusse et al., 1990) in an HLA-identical sibling pair (Thomson et al., 1989) and in association with a T-cell lymphoma (Kim et al., 2000; Masouka et al., 1998).

Diagnosis and Laboratory Findings

No diagnostic laboratory tests are available. ANAs and RFs are generally not present; however, immunoglobulin levels are usually elevated. The clinical picture is reasonably distinctive, although there may be confusion with scleroderma or dermatomyositis. Eosinophilic fasciitis must be differentiated from the eosinophilia-myalgia syndrome related to L-tryptophan ingestion (Silver et al., 1990). Diagnosis rests on demonstration of histologic fasciitis by appropriate deep biopsies. Eosinophilia may be present in either tissue sections or peripheral blood. MRI may be helpful diagnostically and in guiding biopsies (De Clerk et al., 1989).

Treatment and Prognosis

Most patients respond well to corticosteroids. Children with more extensive disease and a younger age of onset appear to have increased risk of development of residual cutaneous fibrosis resembling localized scleroderma (Farrington et al., 1993). Progressive flexion contractures (especially of the small joints of the hands), localized morphea, or carpal tunnel syndrome may occur.

Penicillamine, cimetidine, colchicine, cyclosporine, methotrexate, and chloroquine have been used as therapeutic agents with variable results. Physical and occupational therapy are important to maintain strength, range of motion, and flexibility.

In some patients, prognosis is excellent, with nearly complete resolution over a period of 2 to 5 years (Rodnan et al., 1975). In others, however, systemic involvement similar to that of scleroderma occurs. In a few patients, serious associated disease, such as aplastic anemia or thrombocytopenic purpura, has been described (Kim et al., 1997a; Shulman et al., 1979).

VASCULITIC SYNDROMES

The vasculitides are inflammatory disorders of blood vessels. Inflammation may involve any size vessel and may result in sufficient impairment in blood flow of affected vessels to cause end-organ damage. The exact mechanisms involved in vessel wall inflammation are not fully understood for each specific disease state, but the vasculitides in general are thought to occur by one of several mechanisms, including inflammation secondary to immune complex deposition in the vessel wall, by direct inflammation of a vessel wall itself, and possibly as a direct result of vessel infection. Vasculitis may be isolated or systemic, depending on the disease, and may be acute or chronic.

The two most common vasculitides of childhood are HSP and KD. Less common are polyarteritis nodosa (PAN), Wegener's granulomatosis, Behçet's syndrome, and their variants. Takayasu's arteritis is rarely seen in the pediatric age group. HSP is predominantly a small vessel disease, KD and Wegener's granulomatosis are small to medium vessel diseases, PAN may involve any size vessel except for the aorta, and Takayasu's arteritis affects the aorta and its main branches.

Henoch-Schönlein Purpura

HSP (also known as *anaphylactoid purpura*) is a relatively common form of vasculitis of childhood characterized by purpuric rash, gastrointestinal findings, and renal disease (Allen et al., 1960; Ayoub and Hoyer, 1970; Bywaters et al., 1957; Emery et al., 1977; Vernier et al., 1961) (see Chapters 32, 34, and 38).

Pathogenesis

The cause of HSP is unknown, although numerous antecedent events have been invoked as "triggers," including bacterial or viral infections, drugs, food allergies, vaccination, and malignancy (Maggiore et al., 1984).

Infections have commonly been associated with HSP, and preceding streptococcal infection had been demonstrated in multiple studies, suggesting this as a trigger for some patients with HSP. Later, follow-up studies have found no difference in incidence of streptococcal

disease from that of a control group of healthy children (Al-Sheyyab, et al., 1999; Ayoub and Hoyer, 1970; Bywaters et al., 1957; Sticca et al., 1999). More recently, *Haemophilus parainfluenzae* has been implicated in disease pathogenesis, because IgA immune deposits in the kidneys of 30% of patients were reactive to *H. parainfluenzae* antibodies (Ogura et al., 2000).

Abnormalities in the humoral immune response have also been shown to play a part in HSP pathogenesis based on a number of findings. From 30% to 50% of HSP patients have elevated IgA serum levels (Trygstad and Stiehm, 1971), and increased numbers of IgA-bearing lymphocytes and IgA-containing immune complexes or cryoglobulins are found in the circulation during active disease (Hall et al., 1980; Kauffman et al., 1980; Kuno-Sakai et al., 1979; Saulsbury, 1992). T lymphocytes from HSP patients secrete increased amounts of TGF-β compared with controls (Hall et al., 1980; Kauffman et al., 1980; Kuno-Sakai et al., 1979; Saulsbury, 1992), and B lymphocytes spontaneously synthesize excessive amounts of IgA (Beale et al., 1982).

IgA immune deposits are found in the renal mesangium, skin, and intestinal capillaries (Andre et al., 1980; Conley et al., 1980). How and why abnormal IgA synthesis occurs is unknown, but IgA deposits in patients with HSP are abnormally galactosylated. This may affect normal clearance of IgA immune complexes, resulting in their deposition and triggering a complement-mediated inflammatory response (Ogura et al., 2000).

Finally, increased levels of inflammatory lipid mediators of the cyclo-oxygenase pathway have been found in patients with HSP and may be involved in the pathogenesis of vascular inflammation seen in this disease (Buyan et al., 1994, 1998).

Clinical Manifestations

The clinical picture of HSP is distinctive. A rash of erythematous macules, which may progress to purpura, is invariably present, most commonly over the extensor surfaces of the legs and buttocks but sometimes involving the arms, face, and trunk as well (Fig. 35-11). The rash may initially appear urticarial and may be accompanied by localized edema of the dorsum of the hands, the feet, face, scalp and scrotum. Joint symptoms (arthralgia or arthritis) precede other signs of HSP in 25% of patients. Large joints, especially knees, ankles, wrists, and elbows, are preferentially involved; periarticular swelling and limited joint motion are characteristic findings. The arthritis always resolves completely.

Colicky abdominal pain, often with melena, is the most common gastrointestinal symptom and may precede the rash. In patients who have undergone surgery, purpuric lesions of the small bowel serosa and segmental edema of the bowel walls are found (Martinez-Frontanilla et al., 1984). Generally, the gastrointestinal manifestations of HSP resolve spontaneously; however, intussusception, bowel infarction, and other intestinal complications have been reported.

Renal involvement in HSP ranges from microscopic or gross hematuria to glomerulonephritis, with or

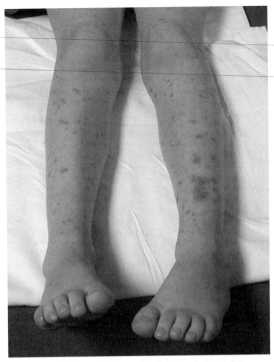

Figure 35-11 · Characteristic rash of Henoch-Schönlein vasculitis. Small erythematous macules, purpuric spots, and petechiae are distributed over the lower extremities. In contrast to the evanescent rash of juvenile rheumatoid arthritis, skin lesions in Henoch-Schönlein vasculitis resolve over a period of days to weeks.

without concomitant nephrotic syndrome. The incidence of renal disease is not known, but significant nephritis is rare and affects children with increasing age and with a history of streptococcal infection. Various series have reported 10% to 90% of patients with HSP have renal manifestations. When renal disease occurs, it generally does so in the first few months of the illness, but later onset after repeated episodes of purpura has been described. Rapidly progressive glomerulonephritis with renal insufficiency can occur (Ansell, 1970; Austin and Balow, 1983; Counahan et al., 1977; Hurley and Drummond, 1972; Kauffman et al., 1980; Levy et al., 1976; Urizar et al., 1968; Vernier et al., 1961) but fortunately is not frequent.

Although the rash, arthritis, and gastrointestinal symptoms may recur episodically, especially in the first month of the disease, renal manifestations may persist for months to years, even in patients who eventually recover completely. Pulmonary, cardiac, and CNS involvement also have rarely been reported in HSP.

Diagnosis and Laboratory Findings

The diagnosis of HSP is clinical and cannot be made in the absence of the characteristic rash. By definition, the purpura is not associated with thrombocytopenia; instead, thrombocytosis is more often observed. Leukocytosis and an elevated ESR are usually seen. Although not usually measured clinically, activation of the alternative complement pathway is reflected in decreased circulating levels of properdin, properdin

convertase, and Factor B (Garcoa-Fuentes et al., 1978). Measurements of CH_{50}, C3, and C4 are normal, but C3d may be increased (Davin et al., 1985). ANAs are not present, but p-ANCA may be found (Zhao et al., 1995).

Treatment and Prognosis

The treatment of HSP is symptomatic. The disease usually resolves in days to weeks. Occasionally, a short course of corticosteroids may be warranted for significant gastrointestinal involvement. Some centers advocate the use of corticosteroids, sometimes supplemented by cytotoxic drugs or plasmapheresis (Faedda et al., 1996; Hattori et al., 1999; Haycock, 1988) to treat rapidly progressive, proliferative, or crescentic glomerulonephritis when there is evidence of renal decompensation (Michael et al., 1967). No controlled studies have been reported, and the number of patients who have received these treatments is small.

The prognosis for patients with HSP is excellent with full recovery without residua occurring in most patients. Many children have recurrences of HSP, with a waxing and waning course over 6 months. The eventual outcome is related to the degree of renal involvement, but even children with severe renal involvement may have complete recovery.

Kawasaki Disease

Kawasaki disease (KD) (formerly called *mucocutaneous lymph node syndrome*) is an acute systemic inflammatory disease affecting infants and young children, first described by Kawasaki in Japan in 1967 (Kawasaki, 1967; Kawasaki et al., 1974). Incidence of KD is estimated at 120 to 150 cases per 100,000 children younger than 5 years, making KD one of the most common vasculitic diseases of childhood (Bell et al., 1983; Burns et al., 2000; Dean et al., 1982; Meade and Brandt, 1982; Melish et al., 1976; Rowley et al., 1988b).

Epidemiology

KD is an illness of young children, with most patients younger than 5 years. The disease is uncommon in teenagers and rare in adulthood. There is a slight male preponderance, with a boy-to-girl ratio of 1.5:1 (Rowley et al., 1988b). KD does not appear to be spread through contact, because it is rare to have multiple cases in a family or school class.

The epidemiologic characteristics of KD are suggestive of an infectious cause, because there are epidemics in different geographic areas and cases are most frequent in the late winter and spring months (Dean et al., 1982; Meade and Brandt, 1982; Rowley et al., 1988a).

Etiology

There is continued speculation about the cause of KD, but infectious triggers are thought to be important because disease comes in epidemic waves and is seen with increased incidence in siblings. Several investigators have suggested that bacterial toxins acting as "superantigens" may be responsible for the selective T-cell subset expansions seen in patients with KD. Both *S. aureus* and *Streptococcus pyogenes* toxins have been implicated (Abe et al., 1993; Yoshioka et al., 1999); in one study, a specific *S. aureus* superantigen-producing strain was been cultured from most children with KD (Leung et al., 1993). However, this has not been confirmed.

Finally, numerous other immunoregulatory abnormalities have been described in the acute stage of KD, including activation of T cells, B cells, monocytes, and macrophages, along with increased production of cytokines and cytokine receptors (interferon-γ, IL-1, TNF-α, IL-6, and IL-2R) (Furukawa et al., 1992; Leung, 1990; Leung et al., 1982; Ono et al., 1985; Terai et al., 1987).

Clinical Manifestations

KD is characterized by prolonged high fever, nonpurulent conjunctivitis, stomatitis, swelling and erythema of hands and feet with subsequent desquamation of the skin (particularly of the distal phalanges, beginning 2 to 3 weeks after onset of the disease), nonsuppurative lymphadenopathy, and polymorphous exanthems. The cardiovascular system is prominently involved in many patients with KD (see later discussion). Other clinical features include arthralgia or arthritis, sterile pyuria, aseptic meningitis, mild hepatitis, hydrops of the gallbladder, and diarrhea.

No specific diagnostic test exists for KD, and diagnosis rests on the fulfillment of criteria developed by the American Heart Association in 1990 as listed in Table 35-8. Fever and at least four of these five features should be present to establish the diagnosis of KD with certainty; however, patients with documented coronary artery disease and fewer than four clinical features are considered to have atypical disease.

Increasingly, cases of atypical KD are being reported, in which patients do not fulfill diagnostic criteria (Levy and Koren, 1990). Most atypical patients are younger than 1 year. Children with a prolonged unexplained febrile illness, particularly with features of desquamating rash, mucosal changes, and thrombocytosis should be investigated for KD with an echocardiogram, in order not to miss an unusual presentation.

TABLE 35-8 · CRITERIA FOR THE DIAGNOSIS OF KAWASAKI DISEASE

Fever for 5 days or more, plus four of the following five:
1. Changes of the peripheral extremities—erythema of the palms and soles, diffuse edema of the hands and feet, subsequent desquamation of the fingertips
2. Polymorphous exanthem
3. Bilateral nonpurulent conjunctival congestion
4. Changes of the lips and oral mucosa—red, dry, cracked lips, strawberry tongue, injection of the oral and pharyngeal mucosa
5. Acute, nonpurulent cervical lymphadenopathy >1.5 cm in size

The clinical criteria for diagnosis of KD are sufficiently nonspecific to possibly include children with other illnesses. Clinicians should take care to exclude infectious diseases, such as measles, streptococcal disease, viral infections, and toxic shock syndrome (Burns et al., 1991).

Cardiovascular manifestations of KD are the most serious, because it is recognized that without treatment up to 2% of children die from the complications of coronary vasculitis such as coronary artery thrombosis and/or myocardial infarction. Coronary aneurysms develop in up to 20% of untreated children with KD (Kato et al., 1979; Koren et al., 1985; Munro-Faure, 1959; Rose, 1990b) and are best diagnosed with echocardiography (Yoshikawa et al., 1979). The size of aneurysms is a helpful prognostic factor; patients who develop giant aneurysms (>8 mm) are at the highest risk for myocardial infarction secondary to thrombosis or stenosis of healing vessels (Nakano et al., 1986; Yoshikawa et al., 1979).

Other cardiovascular manifestations seen less commonly in the acute stage of KD include myocarditis, pericarditis, valvulitis, and dysrhythmias (Dean et al., 1982; Gidding et al., 1986; Imakita et al., 1984; Nakano et al., 1985; van Lier et al., 2000). Even less often, vasculitis and aneurysms affect other medium-sized arteries throughout the body, such as brachial, hepatic, or iliac arteries (Fukushige et al., 1980).

The natural history of coronary artery aneurysms in KD is eventual regression, with 50% resolved by 1 year after onset of disease, as detected on echocardiogram (Akagi et al., 1992; Dean et al., 1982; Takahashi et al., 1987). However, residual abnormalities may remain in these vessels and predispose to future complications (Iemura et al., 2000). Pathologic findings of coronary vessels of children who recovered from KD and died of unrelated causes support these concerns (Fijiwara et al., 1988; Naoe et al., 1987). The coronary arteries of some children with KD and resolved aneurysms have poor vasodilatory responses to infusion of isosorbide dinitrate, suggesting residual dysfunction (Anderson et al., 1985; Iemura et al., 2000; Sugimura et al., 1992).

Increasing numbers of early anginal symptoms, ischemic disease, and sudden death are being reported among patients who have had KD in childhood (Gersony, 1992; Ishiwata et al., 1990; Kohr, 1986; Suzuki et al., 1990; van Lier et al., 2000). Long-term follow-up is necessary to determine the risk of early atherosclerotic heart disease in children with KD (Fulton and Newburger, 2000).

Laboratory Findings

There are no diagnostic laboratory tests for KD. The ESR is elevated, and leukocytosis and anemia are common. Tests for ANA and RFs are negative, but circulating immune complexes have been detected in some patients (Rowley et al., 1988b). Elevated levels of IgE have been reported (Kasakawa and Heiner, 1976). Dramatic elevation of the platelet count is the most helpful laboratory clue, generally occurring in the second week of illness and reaching levels as high as 1 to 2 million/mm^3.

Treatment

The treatment of KD is aimed at preventing or decreasing inflammation of coronary vessels and preventing thrombosis in inflamed vessels. Initially, high-dose salicylate treatment was the only available therapy, used to control fever and to prevent thrombosis (Koren et al., 1985), but salicylate therapy did not prevent the development of coronary aneurysms.

High-dose IVIG has been shown to decrease the incidence of coronary vessel aneurysms, first by Furusho and colleagues in Japan in 1984 and confirmed by the U.S. Multicenter Kawasaki Syndrome studies (Newburger et al., 1991). Treatment with IVIG resulted in rapid clinical improvement and in a decrease in the prevalence of aneurysms and development of giant aneurysms (Chung, 1989; Kato et al., 1979; Rowley et al., 1988a). Further studies have shown that a single infusion of 2 g/kg of IVIG and administration of aspirin (80 to 100 mg/kg/day for 14 days, then 3 to 5 mg/kg/day) is as effective as multiple-day IVIG infusions (Barron et al., 1990; Engle et al., 1989; Newburger et al., 1991). Early use of IVIG (within the first 5 days of illness) is associated with faster recovery and fewer aneurysms (Tse et al., 2002). Partial responding patients may require a second dose of IVIG (Sundel et al., 1993).

Finally, in IVIG-resistant patients, high-dose corticosteroid therapy may be useful (Onouchi and Kawasaki, 1999; Wright et al., 1996). Patients with large aneurysms may benefit from the concomitant use of abciximab, a monoclonal antibody to platelet glycoprotein IIb/IIIa (Williams et al., 2002).

The mechanism of action of IVIG in KD is unknown, with hypotheses including Fc receptor blockade, toxin neutralization, direct inflammatory response blockade, anti-idiotypic effects, or provision of specific antibodies against some as yet unknown pathogen or their superantigens (see Chapter 4).

Polyarteritis Nodosa

Polyarteritis nodosa (PAN) is a diffuse vasculitis that may involve a combination of small, medium, and large arteries; adjacent veins may be involved. PAN is rare in childhood. Antecedent infections may trigger the disease; PAN has been reported to occur in association with hepatitis B and streptococcal infections (Blau et al., 1977; Fink, 1978; Gocke et al., 1970; Jennette et al., 1994; Watts et al., 2000). In some cases, hepatitis B antigen–containing immune complexes are found deposited in affected blood vessels (Gocke et al., 1970). However, most cases of PAN are of unknown cause.

Clinically, multiple organ systems are involved, with skin rash and renal involvement (often manifesting as hypertension) most common. Gastrointestinal involvement may progress to visceral infarction. Neurologic involvement is typically mononeuritis multiplex, although CNS involvement can occur. Skin involvement includes purpura, nodulosis, and livedo reticularis. Vasculitis affecting the testes, epididymis, bladder, or ovaries may occur.

Diagnosis of PAN requires angiography to demonstrate the characteristic aneurysmal dilation of blood vessels or biopsies of affected tissues revealing vasculitis. The prognosis of PAN is much worse than HSP. PAN should be treated with corticosteroids and supplemented as necessary by appropriate cytotoxic therapy.

Takayasu's Arteritis

Takayasu's arteritis, the so-called *pulseless disease* (Shimizu and Sano, 1951), is a chronic inflammatory disorder affecting the aorta and its major branches. It is a rare disorder affecting predominantly women in the second and third decades of life. The incidence in North America has been estimated at fewer than 5 cases/million/year (Hall et al., 1985a). Histologic findings implicate cell-mediated cytotoxicity in the pathogenesis of the disease, because natural killer cells and activated T cells have been found in aortic tissues from patients with active disease (Seko et al., 1994).

Clinically, the disease may present with a variety of complaints. Constitutional symptoms include fever, fatigue, weight loss, myalgia, and arthralgia. Later phases of disease, occlusive symptoms such as visual disturbances, dizziness, syncope, and claudication may be prominent. Hypertension from renal artery stenosis may occur and can result in congestive heart failure.

Physical findings include reduced pulses, especially of the upper extremities, and bruits over affected vessels. For this reason, one should auscultate the carotid, subclavian, and large abdominal vessels because these are the most commonly affected vessels.

Laboratory findings may include a modest leukocytosis and an elevated ESR. However, some patients may have no abnormal findings. Arteriography of the aorta and its branches is helpful in making a diagnosis.

Initial therapy is high-dose corticosteroids, with methotrexate and cyclophosphamide used for persistent or unresponsive disease (Hoffman et al., 1994; Shelhamer et al., 1985). Prognosis is generally good, but the disease course is variable, ranging from spontaneous remission to persistent disease.

Wegener's Granulomatosis

Wegener's granulomatosis is a necrotizing vasculitis associated with granulomas involving the upper and lower respiratory tracts and kidneys (Fauci et al., 1983; Hall et al., 1985b; Orlowski et al., 1978). A possible genetic predisposition has been reported with an increased incidence of HLA-B8, HLA-DR2, HLA-DR9, and HLA-B55 (Elkon et al., 1983; Katz et al., 1979; Nakamaru et al., 1996).

In addition to constitutional symptoms, patients may have sinusitis, serous otitis media, and rhinitis. A saddle-nose deformity may develop. Necrotizing glomeru-lonephritis and pulmonary infiltrates (often asymptomatic) are characteristic. Pulmonary hemorrhage purpura, episcleritis, and neurologic and cardiac involvement may also occur. Laboratory tests for c-ANCAs (Tervaert et al., 1991; van der Wonde et al., 1985) may aid in the diagnosis (Falk and Jennette, 1988).

In the past, Wegener's granulomatosis was nearly always fatal, but early prompt detection and treatment with cyclophosphamide may reverse the disorder (Falk et al., 2000; Fauci et al., 1983; Moorthy et al., 1977; Novack and Pearson, 1971). Limited disease may respond to methotrexate (Lebovics et al., 1992). Rituximab has been successfully used to treat patients with severe, unresponsive disease (Specks et al., 2001).

Behçet's Syndrome

Behçet's syndrome is a vasculitis of both arteries and veins of varying sizes. Patients have recurrent oral aphthous ulcers, with two or more of the following diagnostic clinical features: (1) skin lesions (erythema nodosum, pseudofolliculitis/papulopustular lesions or acneiform nodules), (2) eye disease (anterior or posterior uveitis, cells in the vitreous, or retinal vasculitis), (3) positive pathergy test (erythematous papule (>2 mm) forming at the puncture site when a 20/22-gauge needle is penetrated to a depth of 5 mm (O'Duffy et al., 1998), or (4) recurrent genital ulcerations (ISG, 1990).

Behçet disease is very rare in childhood and is found in highest prevalence in Turkey, Iran, and Japan, where HLA-B5 is commonly associated with the disease (Choukri et al., 2001; Jaber et al., 2001; Kerra et al., 1999; Takano, 1976; Yazici et al., 1977). Other associated findings in Behçet's include arthritis, gastrointestinal inflammation (inflammatory lesions commonly of the terminal ileum and cecum), and CNS involvement, which may be either primarily parenchymal or secondary to major vascular involvement.

Laboratory abnormalities include elevations of ESR and CRP and leukocytosis; RF and ANAs are not common. The aggressiveness of treatment depends on the degree of organ involvement, but generally glucocorticoids, colchicine, or chlorambucil are used to treat most patients. Interferon-α2A, thalidomide, and methotrexate have also been used (Hamuryudan et al., 1998; Hirohata et al., 1998; O'Duffy et al., 1998; Suda, 1999). The disease in general has a relapsing course, with major morbidity attributable to CNS and ocular involvement. Renal amyloidosis may also occur.

SYSTEMIC INFLAMMATORY DISORDERS

Sarcoidosis

Sarcoidosis is a rare systemic granulomatous disorder that may involve multiple organ systems, including the lung, bone, joints, muscle, and blood vessels. The disease is thought to be mediated primarily by CD4[+] T cells, with subsequent recruitment of mononuclear cells (Agostini et al., 2000), which then accumulate in affected tissues and organize into noncaseating granulomas (see Chapter 26 and 33).

Laboratory findings may include increased acute-phase reactants, elevation of angiotensin converting enzyme, and hypercalcemia. ANAs and RFs are generally absent. Frequent clinical characteristics in children include follicular skin rash, uveitis, arthritis, and fever (Hafner and Vogel, 1993). Diagnosis is aided by the finding of noncaseating granulomas on tissue biopsy.

Corticosteroids are the mainstay of treatment, but a variety of immunomodulatory drugs have been used in refractory childhood and adult cases (Shetty and Gedalia, 1998; Vourlekis et al., 2000).

Chronic Recurrent Multifocal Osteomyelitis

Chronic recurrent multifocal osteomyelitis is a noninfectious inflammatory disorder affecting predominantly the metaphyses of bone, although epiphyseal and diaphyseal involvement have been described (Cuende et al., 1995; Schenk et al., 1998). The syndrome was first described in 1972 by Giedion and has since been described in association with inflammatory bowel disease, seronegative spondyloarthropathy, psoriasis, and as part of the synovitis, acne, pustulosis, hyperostosis, and osteitis (SAPHO) syndrome (Bazrafshan and Zanjani, 2000; Beretta-Piccoli et al., 2000; Bergdahl et al., 1979; Bousvaros et al., 1999; Hayem et al., 1999; Kahn, 1993; Omidi and Siegfried, 1998). In a retrospective review of 260 pediatric patients, the average age of onset was 10 years, and females were affected more commonly than males (Beretta-Piccoli et al., 2000).

Clinical Manifestations

Children often complain of pain, tenderness, and swelling at sites of involved bone. Low-grade fever and fatigue may be present, and associated IBD should be suspected in those with significant weight loss or gastrointestinal complaints. Synovitis and various skin abnormalities may be found in those with associated SAPHO syndrome.

Diagnosis and Laboratory Findings

Radiographically, multiple recurrent bone lesions resembling osteomyelitis without an identifiable infectious cause are found. Bone scan is often a helpful adjunct to conventional radiographs in identifying non-symptomatic lesions (Mandell et al., 1998). The ESR and CRP are often elevated, and a mild leukocytosis may be apparent. Biopsy is helpful in differentiating the bone lesions of CRMO from infectious or malignant causes.

Treatment and Prognosis

Most lesions of CRMO heal without specific therapy and result in no long-term morbidity. However, in patients with significant associated pain or frequent recurrence, NSAIDs, glucocorticoids, and a variety of immunomodulating agents have been used with varying success (Andersson, 1995; Girschick et al., 1998; Ishikawa-Nakayama et al., 2000; Nurre et al., 1999).

Chronic Infantile Neurologic Cutaneous and Articular Disease

Chronic infantile neurological cutaneous and articular disease (CINCA), also known as *neonatal onset multisystem inflammatory disease* (NOMID), is a multisystem inflammatory disorder manifested by arthritis and arthropathy, persistent rash, CNS involvement, fever, lymphadenopathy, and splenomegaly. Fewer than 100 cases have been reported in the literature. The pathophysiologic basis of the disease is unknown in half of the cases, and is a result of mutations in the CIAS1 gene in the remaining cases (Aksentijevich et al., 2002).

Clinical Manifestations

Rash is commonly present at birth and usually noted before 6 months of age. The rash may be urticarial, maculopapular, or fixed and tender (erythema nodosum-like) and may persist or recur (Horoupian et al., 1990; Huttenlocher et al., 1995; Lampert, 1986).

Soft tissue swelling and synovitis of multiple joints, including small joints of the hands and feet, knees, elbows, wrists, and ankles, occurs (Hassink and Goldsmith, 1983; Horoupian et al., 1990; Huttenlocher et al., 1995; Lampert, 1986; Yarom et al., 1985), and joint contractures are common. Synovial biopsies have shown both active synovitis and lack thereof (Hassink and Goldsmith, 1983; Yarom et al., 1985); arthrocentesis in some cases shows inflammatory fluid (Hassink and Goldsmith, 1983).

CNS involvement may include sterile meningitis and leptomeningitis, papillitis, seizure disorders, developmental delay, hypotonia, persistently open fontanelle, hydrocephalus, and deafness (Horoupian et al., 1990; Lampert, 1986; Lampert et al., 1975; Yarom et al., 1985).

Fever occurs in most patients, as does lymphadenopathy, splenomegaly, and poor growth.

Diagnosis and Laboratory Findings

Sequencing of the CIAS1 gene may aid in the diagnosis. As in many inflammatory disorders, leucocytosis, anemia, thrombocytosis, hypergammaglobulinemia, and elevation in CRP or ESR are common. The CSF often shows increased protein and neutrophilic pleocytosis. The ANA and RF tests are generally negative.

Treatment and Prognosis

Treatment with NSAIDs has proved inadequate. Gold has been tried without beneficial effects. Steroids at dosages up to 2 mg/kg/day and D-penicillamine at 10 mg/kg/day have in some cases resulted in improvement of symptoms (Hassink and Goldsmith, 1983; Miura et al., 1997; Yarom et al., 1985). Clinical trials using interleukin-1 receptor antagonists are currently underway, and initial results look promising.

Prognosis is variable, but most children are developmentally delayed and growth retarded. Most patients expire before the third decade of life.

PERIODIC FEVER SYNDROMES

Although the genes mutated in several periodic fever syndromes are known, the mechanisms by which the abnormal proteins, or lack of proteins, lead to particular clinical syndromes are not known. Chapter 36 discusses these disorders in detail.

Familial Mediterranean Fever

Familial Mediterranean fever (FMF) is a multisystem, autosomal recessive inherited inflammatory disease characterized by episodes of fever, serositis (especially peritoneal with associated abdominal pain), and arthritis. It occurs predominantly in individuals of Eastern Mediterranean descent. The gene, *MEFV,* has recently been identified and encodes a novel protein whose function has not been well characterized (Balow et al., 1997; FMF, 1997). Long-term prognosis depends on the development of amyloidosis, and daily oral colchicine has been shown to prevent episodes of fever and serositis and to retard the development of amyloidosis (Dinarello et al., 1974; Goldfinger, 1972; Goldstein and Schwabe, 1974; Zemer et al., 1974, 1986). This and other periodic fever syndromes are also discussed in Chapter 36.

Hibernian Fever (TRAPS)

Initially described in a large Irish-Scottish pedigree (McDermott et al., 1999; Mulley et al., 1998), Hibernian fever, an autosomal dominant syndrome, is manifest by longer episodes of fever than FMF and by conjunctivitis, periorbital edema, myalgia, scrotal pain, and inguinal hernias (Centola et al., 1998). Previously known as familial Hibernian fever, this syndrome is now known to result from mutations in the tumor necrosis factor receptor 1 gene. Corticosteroid treatment has proven beneficial, but colchicine has not (Centola et al., 1998). Enbrel has been shown to be a useful steroid-sparing agent in some patients (Drewe et al., 2003).

Hyper-IgD Syndrome

Hyper-IgD syndrome is an autosomally recessive syndrome of recurrent fever, arthralgia, skin rash, headache, abdominal pain, and diarrhea (Wauters et al., 2000). IgD levels are elevated between or during attacks. Febrile episodes tend to be of longer duration than in FMF (3 to 7 days), and amyloidosis does not occur. Patients have mutations in the gene encoding mevalonate kinase. How these mutations result in these clinical manifestations is not understood.

INFECTIOUS ARTHRITIS

Infections of the joint space by bacteria, spirochetes, viruses, fungi, and parasites may all result from hematogenous spread of an organism to the joint or may occur secondary to direct inoculation. Viral arthritides are most commonly transient and nondestructive, whereas those mediated by bacteria, spirochetes, and fungi can result in significant morbidity.

Bacterial Arthritis

Before the widespread use of the *Haemophilus influenzae* vaccine, *H. influenzae* was a common cause of bacterial septic arthritis. The most common etiologic agent today is *S. aureus* followed by group A *Streptococcus* and *Enterobacter* species. Clinically, bacterial septic arthritis is accompanied by systemic illness, including fever and malaise, and the most commonly affected joints are ankles, elbows, hips, and knees. Joints are "hot" and quite tender to palpation and motion. Of note, osteomyelitis often accompanies septic arthritis, and more than one joint can become involved because of hematogenous spread of the infecting organism.

Laboratory abnormalities include elevated synovial fluid white blood cells (WBCs) (commonly more than $100,000/mm^3$) with a predominance of polymorphonuclears (PMNs); culture of joint fluid reveals the offending organism in more than 50% of cases. Culture of other body fluids (especially blood) sometimes reveals the infectious organism when synovial fluid does not.

Treatment is intravenous antibiotics directed toward the offending organism. If infection is highly suspected, and all cultures are negative, coverage must include all likely organisms in a given age group.

Viral Arthritis

Viral arthritis may result from direct infection of synovial tissues, or may be reactive to illness elsewhere. The pathogenesis for most of the viral arthritides are not known. The most common organisms associated with viral arthritis are: parvovirus B19, hepatitis B and C, varicella, rubella, and HIV.

Approximately half of older individuals infected with parvovirus B19 have associated joint symptoms, although the proportion in children is not known. The illness may be reactive, but viral DNA has been found in the synovium of patients with arthritis. All joints can be involved in an oligoarticular or polyarticular course. Symptoms usually resolve within a few weeks, although a small subset go on to have chronic arthritis (Miller, 1998; Scroggie et al., 2000).

The prodromal phase of hepatitis B infection is often characterized by arthralgias of small joints, but frank arthritis of large joint can occur. While viral proteins have been isolated from the joint space, circulating immune complexes are thought to play an important role in the pathogenesis of the joint disease. Symptoms usually resolve by the time clinical hepatitis is recognized (Schnitzer and Penmetcha, 1996). Hepatitis C–associated arthritis is rare but has been associated with small and large joint disease.

Varicella-associated arthritis may occur within a week before the appearance of rash and commonly affects the knee. Virus has been isolated from synovial fluid (Stebbings et al., 1998).

Rubella-associated arthritis most commonly develops in adults and usually affects small joints. Postvaccination arthritis may also occur (Cooper et al., 1969; Farquhar and Corretjer, 1969; Gold, 1969; Lerman et al., 1971; Ogra and Herd, 1971; Speier, 1970). Interestingly, rubella has been isolated from synovial fluid of patients diagnosed with JRA (Chantler et al., 1985).

Finally, about 11% of HIV-infected patients develop arthritis at some time. It may be acute or subacute affecting larger joints of the lower extremities or may be associated with dactylitis and enthesopathy (Reveille, 2000).

In general, treatment is supportive with NSAIDs for pain and discomfort because joint destruction is uncommon. Rarely, perhaps in immunologically susceptible individuals, chronic arthritis ensues (Miller, 1998).

Lyme Disease

Lyme disease is a tickborne illness with multisystem manifestations, including arthritis, caused by a spirochete. There are three different species of *Borrelia* that occur in Europe; only one, *Borrelia burgdorferi*, has been identified in the United States (Baranton et al., 1992). Lyme arthritis was first recognized and described in 1977 in the United States (Steere et al., 1977). Because epidemiologic surveillance of Lyme disease in the United States was initiated by the Centers for Disease Control and Prevention in 1982, increasing numbers of cases have been recognized, and the spirochete has spread geographically. In the United States, Lyme disease is most frequent in coastal New England extending to Virginia and in the northern Midwest.

Clinical Manifestations

Lyme disease occurs in stages, generally described as early localized disease (stage 1), early disseminated disease (stage 2), and late persistent disease (stage 3). Many individuals have only early localized disease, which is either treated successfully or resolves spontaneously. Some patients become symptomatic only in stage 2 or 3, presenting with arthritis, heart block, or neurologic complaints (Cooper and Schoen, 1992; Steere, 1989).

After inoculation through the tick bite, *Borrelia* spreads through the skin to result in the classic skin lesion of Lyme disease, *erythema migrans*. Erythema migrans lesions often begin as a small, red papule and enlarge in a ring-like pattern, with central clearing and an erythematous margin. The lesions can occur anywhere on the body, and multiple lesions are often present (Asbrink, 1991). The skin lesions are often accompanied by mild, flu-like symptoms of fatigue, fever, arthralgia, or headache. Even in untreated patients, the skin lesions resolve over 3 to 4 weeks spontaneously (Steere, 1989; Steere et al., 1983).

Within days to weeks of the early phase of disease, the spirochete spreads hematogenously and results in clinical manifestations involving the heart, nervous system, or musculoskeletal system. Neurologic manifestations occur in 20% of patients, with the most common findings of aseptic meningitis or Bell's palsy. Less often, peripheral neuritis may occur (Finkel and Halpern, 1991; Halpern et al., 1991).

Cardiac manifestations of atrioventricular block, or rarely myocarditis or pericarditis, occur in approximately 10% of patients (Steere et al., 1980). The atrioventricular block resolves with antibiotic treatment of Lyme disease, and therefore patients generally do not require the placement of permanent pacemakers.

Musculoskeletal complaints are common, developing in 60% of patients. An average of 6 months after the onset of the illness, brief recurrent attacks of asymmetric oligoarthritis develop (Eichenfield et al., 1986; Steere et al., 1979). This presentation can mimic that of JRA; therefore Lyme arthritis must be considered in all children with new-onset arthritis.

If untreated, late persistent disease manifests months to years after the onset of disease. Although uncommon, some patients with Lyme disease go on to develop subtle late neurologic findings of encephalomyelitis, polyneuritis, and neurocognitive abnormalities such as memory impairment, behavioral abnormalities, and headache (Bloom et al., 1998; Logigian et al., 1990).

European investigators have described patients with late Lyme disease who present with progressive encephalomyelitis, including paraparesis, ataxia, cognitive and memory impairment, and dementia (Krupp et al., 1991). The demonstration of specific intrathecal production of anti-*Borrelia* antibody or polymerase chain reaction (PCR) identification of *Borrelia* DNA are useful in establishing CNS Lyme disease.

Most patients with Lyme arthritis have complete resolution of their joint disease. However, in some patients, the arthritis may persist for years. Persistent joint disease that responds poorly to antibiotic treatment and becomes erosive (Steere et al., 1987; Szer et al., 1991a) is probably no longer infectious, because patients with this type of joint disease no longer have identifiable *B. burgdorferi* DNA in their synovial fluid (Nocton et al.,

1994). The development of chronic Lyme arthritis in this population is associated with an increased frequency of HLA-DR4 and HLA-DR2, the same genetic haplotypes associated with classic RA (Steere et al., 1979, 1990).

Diagnosis

The diagnosis of Lyme disease rests on serologic determination, because the routine culturing of *Borrelia* is difficult and impractical. Initial serodiagnosis is generally performed using ELISA-based antibody systems; however, there is wide variance of reliability and little standardization among kits and laboratories performing these assays. Therefore Western blot antibody testing is often done for confirmation (Rose et al., 1991; Zoller et al., 1991). IgM and IgG Borrelia titers can help distinguish early active disease from late or previous illness.

Antibodies to *Borrelia* are not detectable during the first several weeks of infection. In addition, early treatment of either tick bites or erythema migrans may abrogate the antibody response, resulting in negative results later in disease. Within 2 to 4 weeks of erythema migrans lesions, IgM anti-*Borrelia* antibodies develop, peak within 6 to 8 weeks, and decline by 4 to 6 months. IgG antibodies develop later, 6 to 8 weeks after onset of illness, and peak within 4 to 6 months. IgG antibodies remain strongly elevated in patients with late persistent disease (Rahn and Malawista, 1991; Sigal, 1992; Steere, 1989).

Treatment

The early manifestations of Lyme disease can be effectively treated in most cases with oral antibiotics (Salazar et al., 1993). Oral doxycycline or amoxicillin is recommended for adults and amoxicillin or erythromycin for children, for a course of 10 to 30 days. CNS disease, cardiac manifestations, or persistent arthritis may require a course of intravenous antibiotics for resolution. Complete resolution of signs and symptoms may not occur for several weeks after a course of therapy, so one should not conclude that the treatment has failed if the individual still has persistent symptoms immediately after treatment.

RHEUMATIC FEVER

Acute rheumatic fever is a poststreptococcal immunologic disease characterized by nonsuppurative inflammation of various tissues, most characteristically the heart (DiSciascio and Taranta, 1980; Feinstein and Spagnuolo, 1962; Kaplan, 1978; Markowitz, 1977; Markowitz and Gordis, 1972; Special Writing Group of the Committee on Rheumatic Fever, 1992).

Historical Aspects

Rheumatic fever was recognized by the ancient Greeks, and its occurrence after pharyngitis was first noted in the 1800s. The relationship of rheumatic fever to strep-

Cellular Deficiencies

A number of patients with Wiskott-Aldrich syndrome develop chronic arthritis and vasculitis (Akman et al., 1998; Preston and Buchanan, 1989). Two patients with Nezelof's syndrome and arthritis have been described (Akman et al., 1998; Schaller et al., 1966) (see Chapter 15). Davies and colleagues (2001) have identified chronic arthritis in 13 patients with a 22q11 deletion (DiGeorge locus); 4 also had IgA deficiency.

PAIN AMPLIFICATION SYNDROMES

Pain in childhood for which no obvious organic pathology is recognized can generally be divided into three major categories: growing pains, reflex sympathetic dystrophy (RSD), and fibromyalgia (diffuse idiopathic pain syndrome of childhood). Hypermobility can also result in nonrheumatic pain.

Growing Pains

Clinical Manifestations

Growing pains generally affect boys and girls equally from the age of 3 to 12. Children commonly complain of aching or cramping pain in the thighs, calves, and shins either late in the evening or upon being awakened during the night but not on waking in the morning. Pain usually lasts for short periods and is relieved by analgesics or massage. Growing pains are never accompanied by limp but may occur after vigorous activity.

Diagnosis and Laboratory Findings

Diagnosis is based on exclusion. The physical examination is completely normal during and between events, and activity should be in no way limited. Results of radiographs and laboratory examinations (including ESR) are all normal.

Treatment and Prognosis

The treatment should be aimed at assuring families that no pathology associated with growing pains has been identified in the long term, despite the fact that the cause of the pain is poorly understood. Analgesics and massage are generally adequate to control symptoms, but if painful episodes occur several nights weekly, premedication before bedtime may avoid nighttime awakening.

Benign Hypermobility Syndrome

Clinical Manifestations

Benign hypermobility is a term coined by Kirk and colleagues (1967) that is used to describe children with musculoskeletal pain associated with generalized joint hypermobility in which no genetic-associated connective tissue abnormalities can be identified. Children older than age 10 are most commonly affected, and girls are affected more commonly than boys. Joints presenting the most frequent complaints are knees, hands, and fingers (Biro et al., 1983). Family history of hypermobility is common (Biro et al., 1983; Jessee et al., 1980).

Diagnosis and Laboratory Findings

Criteria proposed by Carter (1964) and modified by Beighton and colleagues (1973) are often used to establish the diagnosis. Individuals are said to be hypermobile if three of the following five can be performed: (1) passive apposition of the thumb to the flexor surface of the forearm, (2) extension of the wrists and metacarpal phalangeal joints such that the fingers are parallel to the forearm, (3) hyperextension of the elbows (>10 degrees), (4) hyperextension of the knees (>10 degrees), and (5) flexion of the back such that palms can be placed flat on the floor. ANAs and RFs are generally negative, and ESRs are not elevated.

Treatment and Prognosis

Treatment consists of rest, reassurance, physical therapy to strengthen periarticular structures, and NSAIDs as needed for joint discomfort. Ligamentous injuries tend to occur more often in hypermobile individuals, but long-term sequelae in children are generally absent.

Reflex Sympathetic Dystrophy

Children with RSD, also known as *causalgia* or *regional pain syndrome,* complain of constant and increasing pain usually affecting a distal extremity, which far outweighs objective parameters. The usual age of onset is late childhood to adolescence, and females are affected much more commonly than males. Affected children are often high achievers, and psychologic testing of affected individuals and their family members has revealed an abnormal degree of enmeshment (Sherry and Weisman, 1988).

Clinical Manifestations

Clinically, a child complains of pain in the affected body part. Secondary to the pain, the child gets into a vicious cycle of disuse, resulting in abnormal autonomic control in the distribution of the affected area. The limb becomes cool, mottled, and swollen in appearance, and hyperesthesia occurs resulting in further disuse and increasing symptoms. The affected limb is often discolored, and the child may hold the affected limb in a bizarre posture. Passive or active motion is extremely painful.

Diagnosis and Laboratory Findings

Diagnosis is based on a compatible history and physical findings. Localized pain must be present for greater than 1 week in the absence of physical findings to explain the degree of symptoms, and soft tissue swelling, tenderness, and skin color and temperature changes are present. Radiologic abnormalities include increased or decreased uptake on bone scan (Laxer et al., 1985), and eventual osteopenia from disuse. Other laboratory tests are normal (CBC, ESR, other inflammatory indicators).

Treatment and Prognosis

Treatment includes establishing a dialog with the family and an explanation of the cause of the physical findings. Pain control and intense physical therapy must be initiated immediately. Psychologic intervention with counseling for the child and family are often helpful. Prognosis is generally good, but recurrences are common, especially when secondary gain is an issue.

Diffuse Idiopathic Pain Syndrome (Fibromyalgia)

Diffuse idiopathic pain syndrome of childhood (fibromyalgia) is a syndrome of diffuse musculoskeletal pain in the absence of systemic or mechanical disease. Much controversy surrounds the existence of this syndrome as a distinct clinical entity, because the pathophysiologic basis of the disease is not known. Abnormalities in restorative sleep and autonomic nervous function have been described in adults (Bou-Holaigah et al., 1997; Tayag-Kier et al., 2000) and may ultimately be important in understanding the pathogenesis of the disease. As diagnosis is dependent on fairly subjective interpretation of pain at so-called tender points, and because symptoms are often associated with findings of anxiety and depression, practitioners often face difficulties in the diagnosis and management of this syndrome.

Although first recognized in adults, juvenile fibromyalgia has become increasingly recognized over the past half decade in the pediatric population. The juvenile prevalence varies from 1.2% to more than 6% depending on population studied (Buskila, 2000; Clark et al., 1998), with a mean age of onset of symptoms at 13 years of age (Clark et al., 1998). Girls far outnumber boys, and a history of adult family members with fibromyalgia is common (Buskila, 2000).

Clinical Manifestations

Widespread persistent ill-defined musculoskeletal pain for at least 3 months is the hallmark of this syndrome. Patients often complain of constant fatigue and inability to perform normal daily activities. Sleep disturbances are common with difficulty falling asleep, frequent nighttime wakening, fewer hours of total sleep time, and feeling poorly rejuvenated in the morning (nonrestorative sleep) (Tayag-Kier et al., 2000). Patients also commonly complain of headache, stiffness, subjective joint swelling, and dizziness (Gedalia et al., 2000) and often have associated anxiety and/or depression.

TABLE 35-11 · TENDER POINTS (PAIN ON DIGITAL PALPATION) IN FIBROMYALGIA

1. Occiput: at suboccipital muscle insertion
2. Low cervical: anterior aspects of the intertransverse spaces at C5–C7
3. Trapezius: at the midpoint of the upper border
4. Second rib: at the second costochondral junctions
5. Supraspinatus: at origins, above the scapular spine near the medial border
6. Lateral epicondyle: 2 cm distal to the epicondyles
7. Gluteal: in upper outer quadrants of buttocks in anterior fold of muscle
8. Greater trochanter: posterior to the trochanteric prominence
9. Knee: at the medial fat pad proximal to the joint line

Diagnosis and Laboratory Findings

Diagnosis is presently based on the adult classification criteria (reliability in children has not been specifically studied), with at least 3 months of diffuse pain, and 11 of 18 tender points noted on examination (Table 35-11) (Goldenberg, 1998). ESR is in the normal range, and in one U.S. pediatric study, low-titer positive ANAs were common (25%) (Tayag-Kier et al., 2000). Radiologic evaluation, if done to exclude bone or joint pathology, is invariably normal.

Treatment and Prognosis

The treatment of patients with fibromyalgia is difficult, because the patient and family are often unwilling to accept the diagnosis and seek further consultation and diagnostic intervention. Once the diagnosis has been accepted, a combination of psychotherapy with behavioral and educational intervention (Nicassio et al., 1997; Turk et al., 1998) and physical therapy with aerobic and water therapy is often helpful (Gedalia et al., 2000; Mannerkorpi et al., 2000; Ramsay et al., 2000; Rossy et al., 1999). Pharmacologic therapy with low-dose antidepressants (especially tricyclics) before bed often helps with sleep and pain intensity (Arnold et al., 2000; Cassidy et al., 1998b; Fishbain, 2000; Hannonen et al., 1998; O'Malley et al., 2000). Prognosis for children is better than for adults, and greater than half of juvenile patients improve in the long term (Gedalia et al., 2000).

R E F E R E N C E S

AAP. American Academy of Pediatrics Section on Rheumatology and Section on Ophthalmology. Guidelines for ophthalmologic examinations in children with juvenile rheumatoid arthritis. Pediatrics 92:295–296, 1993.

Abe J, Kotzin BL, Meissner C, Melish ME, Takahashi M, Fulton D, Romagne F, Malissen B, Leung DY. Characterization of T cell repertoire changes in acute Kawasaki disease. J Exp Med 177:791–796, 1993.

Agnello V, DeBracco M, Kunkel H. Hereditary C2 deficiency with some manifestations of systemic lupus erythematosus. J Immunol 108:837–840, 1972.

Agostini C, Adami F, Semenzato G. New pathogenetic insights into the sarcoid granuloma. Curr Opin Rheumatol 12:71–76, 2000.

Ahlstrom H, Feltelius N, Nyman R, Hallgren R. Magnetic resonance imaging of sacroiliac joint inflammation. Arthritis Rheum 33:1763–1769, 1990.

Akagi T, Rose V, Benson LN, Newman A, Freedom RM. Outcome of coronary artery aneurysms after Kawasaki disease. J Pediatr 121:689–694, 1992.

Akin E, Miller LC, Tucker LB. Minocycline-induced lupus in adolescents. Pediatrics 101:926–928, 1988.

Akman IO, Ostrov BE, Neudorf S. Autoimmune manifestations of the Wiskott-Aldrich syndrome. Semin Arthritis Rheum 27:218–225, 1998.

Aksentijevich I, Nowak M, Mallah M, Chae JJ, Watford WT, Hofmann SR, Stein L, Russo R, Goldsmith D, Dent P, Rosenberg HF, Austin F, Remmers EF, Balow JE Jr, Rosenzweig S, Komarow H, Shoham NG, Wood G, Jones J, Mangra N, Carrero H, Adams BS, Moore TL, Schikler K, Hoffman H, Lovell DJ, Lipnick R, Barron K, O'Shea JJ, Kastner DL, Goldbach-Mansky R. De novo CIAS1 mutations, cytokine activation, and evidence for genetic heterogeneity in patients with neonatal-onset multisystem inflammatory disease (NOMID): a new member of the expanding family of pyrin-associated autoinflammatory diseases. Arthritis Rheum 46:3340–3348, 2002.

Al-Mayouf S, Al-Mazyed A, Bahabri S. Efficacy of early treatment of severe juvenile dermatomyositis with intravenous methylprednisolone and methotrexate. Clin Rheumatol 19:138–141, 2000.

Al-Sheyyab M, Batieha A, el-Shanti H, Daoud A. Henoch-Schönlein purpura and streptococcal infection: a prospective case-control study. Ann Trop Paediatr 19:253–255, 1999.

Alarcon-Riquelme ME, Alarcon-Segovia D, Loredo-Abdala A, Alcocer-Varela J. T lymphocyte subsets, suppressor and contrasuppressor cell functions, and production of interleukin-2 in the peripheral blood of rheumatic fever patients and their apparently healthy siblings. Clin Immunol Immunopathol 55:120–128, 1990.

Alarcon-Segovia D, Cabral AR. The anti-phospholipid antibody syndrome: clinical and serological aspects. Baillières Best Pract Res Clin Rheumatol 14:139–150, 2000.

Alarcon-Segovia D, Deleze M, Oria C, Sanchez-Guerrero J, Gomez-Pacheco L, Cabiedes J, Fernandez L, Ponce de Leon S. Antiphospholipid antibodies and the antiphospholipid syndrome in systemic lupus erythematosus. Medicine 68:353–365, 1989.

Albani S. Infection and molecular mimicry in autoimmune diseases of childhood. Clin Exp Rheumatol 12:S35–S41, 1994.

Alecu M, Geleriu L, Coman G, Galatescu L. The interleukin-1, interleukin-2, interleukin-6 and tumour necrosis factor alpha serological levels in localised and systemic sclerosis. Rom J Intern Med 36:251–259, 1998.

Alexander EL, McNichall J, Watson RM, Bias W, Reichlin M, Provost TT. The immunogenetic relationship between anti-Ro(SSA)/La(SSB) antibody positive Sjögren's/lupus erythematosus overlap syndrome and the neonatal lupus syndrome. J Invest Dermatol 93:751–756, 1989.

Allen DM, Diamond LK, Howell DA. Anaphylactoid purpura in children (Schönlein-Henoch syndrome). Am J Dis Child 99:833–854, 1960.

Allen RC, Dewez P, Stuart L, Gatenby PA, Sturgess A. Antinuclear antibodies using HEP-2 cells in normal children and in children with common infections. J Paediatr Child Health 27:39–42, 1991.

Alsaeid K, Majeed HA. Acute rheumatic fever: diagnosis and treatment. Pediatr Ann 27:295–300, 1998.

Ammann A, Hong R. Selective IgA deficiency: presentation of thirty cases and review of the literature. Medicine 50:223–236, 1971.

Anaya JM, Ogawa N, Talal N. Sjögren's syndrome in childhood. J Rheumatol 22:1152–1158, 1995.

Anderson TM, Meyer RA, Kaplan S. Long-term echocardiographic evaluation of cardiac size and function in patients with Kawasaki disease. Am Heart J 110:107–115, 1985.

Andersson R. Effective treatment with interferon-alpha in chronic recurrent multifocal osteomyelitis. J Interferon Cytokine Res 15:837–838, 1995.

Andre C, Berthoux FC, Andre F. Prevalence of IgA2 deposits in IgA nephropathies. N Engl J Med 303:1343–1346, 1980.

Annegers JF, Pillman NL, Weidman WH, Kurland LT. Rheumatic fever in Rochester, Minnesota, 1935–1978. Mayo Clin Proc 57:753–757, 1982.

Ansell BM. Henoch-Schönlein purpura with particular reference to the prognosis of the renal lesion. Br J Dermatol 82:211–215, 1970.

Ansell BM. Management of polymyositis and dermatomyositis. Clin Rheum Dis 10:205–213, 1984.

Ansell BM. Juvenile dermatomyositis. J Rheumatol 19(Suppl 33):60–62, 1992.

Ansell BM. Cyclosporin A in paediatric rheumatology. Clin Exp Rheumatol 11:113–115, 1993.

Ansell BM, Nasseh GA, Bywaters EGL. Scleroderma in childhood. Ann Rheum Dis 35:189–197, 1976.

Ansell BM, Wood PH. Prognosis in juvenile chronic polyarthritis. Clin Rheum Dis 2:397–412, 1976.

Appel AE, Sablay LB, Golden RA, Bartland P, Grayzel AI, Bank N. The effect of normalization of serum complement and anti-DNA antibody on the course of lupus nephritis. Am J Med 64:274–283, 1978.

Arnold LM, Keck PE Jr, Welge JA. Antidepressant treatment of fibromyalgia. A meta-analysis and review. Psychosomatics 41:104–113, 2000.

Asbrink E. Cutaneous manifestations of Lyme borreliosis. Scand J Infect Dis 77(Suppl):44–50, 1991.

Asherson RA, Hughes GRV. Antiphospholipid antibodies and chorea. J Rheumatol 15:377–379, 1988.

Asherson RA, Khamashta MA, Ordi-Ros J, Derksen RHWM, Machin SJ, Path FRC, Barquinero J, Outt HH, Harris EN, Vilardell-Torres M, Hughes GRV. The "primary" antiphospholipid syndrome: major clinical and serological features. Medicine 68:366–374, 1989.

Austin HA, Balow JE. Henoch-Schönlein nephritis: prognosis features and the challenge of therapy. Am J Kidney Dis 2:512–520, 1983.

Austin HA, Klippel JH, Balow JE, LeRiche NG, Steinberg AD, Plotz PH, Decker JL. Therapy of lupus nephritis. Controlled trial of prednisone and cytotoxic drugs. N Engl J Med 314:614–619, 1986.

Aylward JM. Hydroxychloroquine and chloroquine: assessing the risk of retinal toxicity. J Am Optom Assoc 64:787–797, 1993.

Ayoub EM, Barrett DJ, Maclaren NK, Krischer JP. Association of class II human histocompatibility leukocyte antigens with rheumatic fever. J Clin Invest 77:2019–2026, 1986.

Ayoub EM, Hoyer J. Anaphylactoid purpura: streptococcal antibody titers and beta$_{ic}$ globulin levels. J Pediatr 75:193–201, 1970.

Bain BJ. Some influences on the ESR and the fibrinogen level in healthy subjects. Clin Lab Haematol 5:45–54, 1983.

Baldwin DS, Gluck MC, Lowenstein J, Gallo GR. Lupus nephritis. Clinical course as related to morphologic forms and their transitions. Am J Med 62:12–30, 1977.

Baldwin DS, Lowenstein J, Rothfield NF, Gallo G, McCluskey RT. The clinical course of the proliferative and membranous forms of lupus nephritis. Ann Intern Med 73:929–942, 1970.

Balow JE, Boumpas DT, Austin HA, 3rd. New prospects for treatment of lupus nephritis. Semin Nephrol 20:32–39, 2000.

Balow JE Jr, Shelton DA, Orsborn A, Mangelsdorf M, Aksentijevich I, Blake T, Sood R, Gardner D, Liu R, Pras E, Levy EN, Centola M, Deng Z, Zaks N, Wood G, Chen X, Richards N, Shohat M, Livneh A, Pras M, Doggett NA, Collins FS, Liu PP, Rotter JI, Kastner DL. A high-resolution genetic map of the familial Mediterranean fever candidate region allows identification of haplotype-sharing among ethnic groups. Genomics 44:280–291, 1997.

Banker BQ, Victor M. Dermatomyositis (systemic angiopathy) of childhood. Medicine 45:261–289, 1966.

Bansal VK, Beto JA. Treatment of lupus nephritis: a meta-analysis of clinical trials. Am J Kidney Dis 29:193–199, 1997.

Baranton G, Postic D, Saint Girons I, Boerlin P, Piffaretti JC, Assous M, Grimont PAD. Delineation of Borrelia burgdorferi sensu stricto, Borrelia garinii sp. nov., and group VS461 associated with Lyme borreliosis. Int J Syst Bacteriol 42:378–383, 1992.

Barash J, Cooper M, Tauber Z. Hepatic, cutaneous and hematologic manifestations in juvenile chronic arthritis. Clin Exp Rheumatol 9:541–543, 1991.

Bardelas J, Winkelstein J, Seto D, Tsai T, Rogol A. Fatal ECHO 24 infection in a patient with hypogammaglobulinemia: relationship to dermatomyositis-like syndrome. J Pediatr 90:396–399, 1977.

Barkley D, Hohermuth H, Howard A, Webster D, Ansell B. IgA deficiency in juvenile chronic polyarthritis. J Rheumatol 6:219–224, 1979.

Barnett E, Winkelstein A, Weinberger H. Agammaglobulinemia with polyarthritis and subcutaneous nodules. Am J Med 48:40–47, 1970.

Barron KS, Murphy DJ, Silverman ED. Treatment of Kawasaki syndrome: a comparison of two dosage regimens of intravenously administered immune globulin. J Pediatr 117:638–644, 1990.

Barron KS, Sher MR, Silverman ED. Intravenous immunoglobulin therapy: magic or black magic. J Rheumatol 19(Suppl 33):94–97, 1992.

Barron KS, Silverman ED, Gonzales JC, Owerbach D, Reveille JD. DNA analysis of HLA-DR, DQ, and DP alleles in children with polyarticular juvenile rheumatoid arthritis. J Rheumatol 19:1611–1616, 1992.

Bartlett ML, Ginn L, Beitz L, Villalba ML, Plotz P, Bacharach SL. Quantitative assessment of myositis in thigh muscles using magnetic resonance imaging. Magn Reson Imaging 17:183–191, 1999.

Bartunkova J, Sediva A, Vencovsky J, Tesar V. Primary Sjögren's syndrome in children and adolescents: proposal for diagnostic criteria. Clin Exp Rheumatol 17:381–386, 1999.

Basta M, Dalakas MC. High-dose intravenous immunoglobulin exerts its beneficial effect in patients with dermatomyositis by blocking endomysial deposition of activated complement fragments. J Clin Invest 94:1729–1735, 1994.

Bathon JM, Martin RW, Fleischmann RM, Tesser JR, Schiff MH, Keystone EC, Genovese MC, Wasko MC, Moreland LW, Weaver AL, Markenson J, Finck BK. A comparison of etanercept and methotrexate in patients with early rheumatoid arthritis. N Engl J Med 343:1586–1593, 2000.

Baum J, Fink C. Juvenile rheumatoid arthritis in monozygotic twins: a case report and review of the literature. Arthritis Rheum 11:33–36, 1968.

Bazrafshan A, Zanjani KS. Chronic recurrent multifocal osteomyelitis associated with ulcerative colitis: a case report. J Pediatr Surg 35:1520–1522, 2000.

Beale MG, Nash GS, Bertorich MJ. Similar disturbances in B cell activity and regulatory T-cell function in Henoch-Schönlein purpura and systemic lupus erythematosus. J Immunol 128:486–491, 1982.

Beck JS. Antinuclear antibodies: methods of detection and significance. Mayo Clin Proc 44:600–619, 1969.

Bedford PA, Ansell BM, Hall PJ, Woo P. Increased frequency of DR4 in systemic onset juvenile rheumatoid arthritis. Clin Exp Rheum 10:189–193, 1992.

Beighton P, Solomon L, Soskolne CL. Articular mobility in an African population. Ann Rheum Dis 32:413–418, 1973.

Bell DA, Maddison PJ. Serologic subsets in systemic lupus erythematosus: the examination of autoantibodies in relationship to clinical features of disease and HLA antigens. Arthritis Rheum 23:1268–1273, 1980.

Bell DM, Morens DM, Holman RC, Hurwitz ES, Hunter MK. Kawasaki syndrome in the United States. Am J Dis Child 137:211–214, 1983.

Ben-Chetrit E. The molecular basis of the SSA/Ro antigens and the clinical significance of their autoantibodies. Br J Rheumatol 32:396–402, 1993.

Bennett RM, Herron A, Keogh L. Eosinophilic fasciitis. Ann Rheum Dis 36:354–357, 1977.

Beretta-Piccoli BC, Sauvain MJ, Gal I, Schibler A, Saurenmann T, Kressebuch H, Bianchetti MG. Synovitis, acne, pustulosis, hyperostosis, osteitis (SAPHO) syndrome in childhood: a report of ten cases and review of the literature. Eur J Pediatr 159:594–601, 2000.

Bergdahl K, Bjorksten B, Gustavson KH, Liden S, Probst F. Pustulosis palmoplantaris and its relation to chronic recurrent multifocal osteomyelitis. Dermatologica 159:37–45, 1979.

Berkel AI, Birben E, Oner C, Oner R, Loos M, Petry F. Molecular, genetic and epidemiologic studies on selective complete C1q deficiency in Turkey. Immunobiology 201:347–355, 2000.

Bernstein B, Takahashi M, Hanson V. Cardiac involvement in juvenile rheumatoid arthritis. J Pediatr 85:313–317, 1974.

Bernstein BH, Stobie D, Singsen BH, Koster-King K, Kornreich HK, Hanson V. Growth retardation in juvenile rheumatoid arthritis (JRA). Arthritis Rheum 20:212–216, 1977.

Bernstein ML, Salusinsky-Sternbach M, Bellefleur M, Esseltine DW. Thrombotic and hemorrhagic complications in children with the lupus anticoagulant. Am J Dis Child 138:1132–1135, 1984.

Berrios X, del Campo E, Guzman B, Bisno AL. Discontinuing rheumatic fever prophylaxis in selected adolescents and young adults. Ann Intern Med 118:401–406, 1993.

Berrios X, Quesney F, Morales A, Blazquez J, Bisno AL. Are all recurrences of "pure" Sydenham chorea true recurrences of acute rheumatic fever? J Pediatr 107:867–872, 1985.

Bevers EM, Galli M, Barbui T, Comfurius P, Zwaal RF. Lupus anticoagulant IgG's (LA) are not directed to phospholipids only, but to a complex of lipid-bound human prothrombin. Thromb Haemost 66:629–632, 1991.

Biagi E, Assali G, Rossi F, Jankovic M, Nicolini B, Balduzzi A. A persistent severe autoimmune hemolytic anemia despite apparent direct antiglobulin test negativization. Haematologica 84:1043–1045, 1999.

Bini P, Gabay JE, Melchior M, Zhou JL, Elkon KB. Antineutrophil cytoplasmic autoantibodies in Wegener's granulomatosis recognize conformational epitope(s) on proteinase 3. J Immunol 149:1409–1415, 1992.

Biro F, Gewanter HL, Baum J. The hypermobility syndrome. Pediatrics 72:701–706, 1983.

Bissenden JG. Transatlantic warning bells sound on rheumatic fever. Brit Med J 296:13, 1988.

Bjornland T, Larheim TA. Synovectomy and diskectomy of the temporomandibular joint in patients with chronic arthritic disease compared with diskectomies in patients with internal derangement. A 3-year follow-up study. Eur J Oral Sci 103:2–7, 1995.

Black C, Isenberg DA. Mixed connective tissue disease—goodbye to all that. Br J Rheumatol 31:695–700, 1992.

Black CM. The aetiopathogenesis of systemic sclerosis. J Intern Med 234:3–8, 1993.

Black CM, Silman AJ, Herrick AI, Denton CP, Wilson H, Newman J, Pompon L, Shi-Wen X. Interferon-alpha does not improve outcome at one year in patients with diffuse cutaneous scleroderma: results of a randomized, double-blind, placebo-controlled trial. Arthritis Rheum 42:299–305, 1999.

Blaese RM, Grayson J, Steinberg AD. Elevated immunoglobulin secreting cells in the blood of patients with active systemic lupus erythematosus: correlation of laboratory and clinical assessment of disease activity. Am J Med 69:345–350, 1980.

Bland EF. Rheumatic fever: the way it was. Circulation 76:1190–1195, 1987.

Blau EB, Morris RF, Yunis EJ. Polyarteritis nodosa in older children. Pediatrics 60:227–234, 1977.

Blay R, Simpson K, Leslie K, Huber S. Coxsackievirus-induced disease. CD4+ cells initiate both myocarditis and pancreatitis in DBA/2 mice. Am J Pathol 135:899–907, 1989.

Bleil L, Manger B, Winkler T, Herrman M, Burmester G, Krapf F, Kalden J. The role of antineutrophil cytoplasm antibodies, anticardiolipin antibodies, von Willebrand factor antigen, and fibronectin for the diagnosis of systemic vasculitis. J Rheumatol 18:1199–1206, 1991.

Block SR, Lockshin MD, Winfield JB, Weksler ME, Imamura M, Winchester RJ, Mellors RC, Christian CL. Immunologic observations on 9 sets of twins either concordant or discordant for SLE. Arthritis Rheum 19:545–554, 1976.

Block SR, Winfield JB, Lockshin MD, D'Angelo WA, Christian CL. Studies of twins with systemic lupus erythematosus. A review of the literature and presentation of 12 additional sets. Am J Med 59:533–552, 1975.

Blomberg S, Ronnblom L, Wallgren AC, Nilsson B, Karlsson-Parra A. Anti-SSA/Ro antibody determination by enzyme-linked immunosorbent assay as a supplement to standard immunofluorescence in antinuclear antibody screening. Scand J Immunol 51:612–617, 2000.

Bloom B, Wyckoff P, Meissner H, Steere A. Neurocognitive abnormalities in children after classic manifestations of Lyme disease. Pediatr Infect Dis J 17:189–196, 1998.

Bloom BJ, Tucker LB, Miller LC, Schaller JG. von Willebrand factor in juvenile dermatomyositis. J Rheumatol 22:320–325, 1995.

Bogner U, Badenhoop K, Peters H, Schmieg D, Mayr W, Usadel K, Schleusener H. HLA-DR/DQ gene variation in nongoitrous autoimmune thyroiditis at the serological and molecular level. Autoimmunity 14:155–158, 1992.

Bohan A, Peter JB. Polymyositis and dermatomyositis. N Engl J Med 292:344–347, 1975.

Bont L, Brus F, Dijkman-Neerincx RH, Jansen TL, Meyer JW, Janssen M. The clinical spectrum of post-streptococcal syndromes with arthritis in children. Clin Exp Rheumatol 16:750–752, 1998.

Borg E, Groen H, Horst G, Limburg P, Wouda A, Kallenberg C. Clinical associations of antiribonucleoprotein antibodies in patients with systemic lupus erythematosus. Semin Arthritis Rheum 20:163–173, 1990.

Botto M. C1q knock-out mice for the study of complement deficiency in autoimmune disease. Exp Clin Immunogenet 15:231–234, 1998.

Botto M, Dell'Agnola C, Bygrave AE, Thompson EM, Cook HT, Petry F, Loos M, Pandolfi PP, Walport MJ. Homozygous C1q deficiency causes glomerulonephritis associated with multiple apoptotic bodies. Nat Genet 19:56–59, 1998.

Bou-Holaigah I, Calkins H, Flynn JA, Tunin C, Chang HC, Kan JS, Rowe PC. Provocation of hypotension and pain during upright tilt table testing in adults with fibromyalgia. Clin Exp Rheumatol 15:239–246, 1997.

Boublik M, Tsahakis PJ, Scott RD. Cementless total knee arthroplasty in juvenile onset rheumatoid arthritis. J Clin Orthop Rel Res 286:88–93, 1993.

Boumpas DT, Austin HA, 3rd, Vaughn EM, Klippel JH, Steinberg AD, Yarboro CH, Balow JE. Controlled trial of pulse methylprednisolone versus two regimens of pulse cyclophosphamide in severe lupus nephritis. Lancet 340:741–745, 1992.

Bousvaros A, Marcon M, Treem W, Waters P, Issenman R, Couper R, Burnell R, Rosenberg A, Rabinovich E, Kirschner BS. Chronic recurrent multifocal osteomyelitis associated with chronic inflammatory bowel disease in children. Dig Dis Sci 44:2500–2507, 1999.

Bowyer SL, Blane CE, Sullivan DB, Cassidy JT. Childhood dermatomyositis: factors predicting functional outcome and development of dystrophic calcification. J Pediatr 103:882–888, 1983.

Braun J, de Keyser F, Brandt J, Mielants H, Sieper J, Veys E. New treatment options in spondyloarthropathies: increasing evidence for significant efficacy of anti-tumor necrosis factor therapy. Curr Opin Rheumatol 13:245–249, 2001.

Bremers HH, Golitz LE, Weston WL, Hays WG. Neonatal lupus erythematosus. Cutis 24:287–290, 1979.

Brewer EJ, Bass J, Baum J, Cassidy JT, Fink C, Jacobs J, Hanson V, Levinson JE, Schaller J, Stillman JS. Current proposed revision of juvenile rheumatoid arthritis criteria. Arthritis Rheum 20(Suppl):195–199, 1977.

Brewer EJ, Giannini EH, Kuzmina N, and Alekseev L. Penicillamine and hydroxychloroquine in the treatment of severe juvenile rheumatoid arthritis. N Engl J Med 314:1270–1276, 1986.

Brewerton D, Hart F, Nicholls A, Caffrey M, James D, Sturrock R. Ankylosing spondylitis and HLA-B27. Lancet 1:904–907, 1973a.

Brewerton D, Nicholls A, Oates J, Caffrey M, Walters D, James D. Reiter's disease and HLA-B27. Lancet 2:996–998, 1973b.

Brewerton DA, Nicholls A, Caffrey M, Walters D, James DC. HLA-B27 and arthropathies associated with ulcerative colitis and psoriasis. Lancet 1:956–958, 1974.

Briggs D, Stephens C, Vaughan R, Welsh K, Black C. A molecular and serologic analysis of the major histocompatibility complex and complement component C4 in systemic sclerosis. Arthritis Rheum 36:943–954, 1993.

Bronze MS, Beachey EH, Dale JB. Protective and heart-cross reactive epitopes located within the NH2 terminus of type 19 streptococcal M protein. J Exp Med 167:1849–1859, 1988.

Brunner CM, Horwitz DA, Davis JS. Identical twins discordant for SLE: an experiment in nature. Arthritis Rheum 14:373, 1971.

Budman DR, and Steinberg AD. Hematologic aspects of systemic lupus erythematosus. Ann Intern Med 86:220–229, 1977.

Buhl AM, Nemazee D, Cambier JC, Rickert R, Hertz M. B-cell antigen receptor competence regulates B-lymphocyte selection and survival. Immunol Rev 176:141–153, 2000.

Bulkley BH, Roberts WC. Ankylosing spondylitis and aortic regurgitation. Circulation 48:1014–1027, 1973.

Burdt MA, Hoffman RW, Deutscher SL, Wang GS, Johnson JC, Sharp GC. Long-term outcome in mixed connective tissue disease: longitudinal clinical and serologic findings. Arthritis Rheum 42:899–909, 1999.

Burgos-Vargas R. Spondyloarthropathies and psoriatic arthritis in children. Curr Opin Rheumatol 5:634–643, 1993.

Burgos-Vargas R, Castelazo-Duarte G, Orozco JA, Garduno-Espinosa J, Clark P, Sanabria L. Chest expansion in healthy adolescents and patients with the seronegative enthesopathy and arthropathy syndrome or juvenile ankylosing spondylitis. J Rheumatol 20:1957–1960, 1993.

Burns J, Kushner H, Bastian J, Shike H, Shimizu C, Matsubara T, Turner C. Kawasaki disease: a brief history. Pediatrics 106:E27, 2000.

Burns JC, Mason WH, Glode MP, Shulman ST, Melish ME, Meissner C, Bastian J, Beiser AS, Myerson HM, Newburger JW. Clinical and epidemiologic characteristics of patients referred for evaluation of possible Kawasaki's disease. J Pediatr 118:680–686, 1991.

Burton JL. Effect of oral contraceptives on erythrocyte sedimentation rate in healthy young women. Brit Med J 559:214–215, 1967.

Buskila D. Fibromyalgia, chronic fatigue syndrome, and myofascial pain syndrome. Curr Opin Rheumatol 12:113–123, 2000.

Buyan N, Erbas D, Akkok N, Oz E, Biberoglu G, Hasanoglu E. Role of free oxygen radicals and prostanoids in the pathogenesis of Henoch-Schönlein purpura. Prostaglandins Leukot Essent Fatty Acids 59:181–184, 1998.

Buyan N, Hasanoglu E, Oguz A, Ercan S. The role of plasma arachidonic acid metabolites in the pathogenesis and the prognosis of Henoch-Schönlein purpura. Prostaglandins Leukot Essent Fatty Acids 50:353–356, 1994.

Buyon JP, Ben-Chetrit E, Karp S, Roubey RAS, Pompeo L, Reeves WH, Tan EM, Winchester R. Acquired congenital heart block: pattern of maternal antibody response to biochemically defined antigens of the SSA/Ro-SSB/La system in neonatal lupus. J Clin Invest 84:627–634, 1989.

Buyon JP, Hiebert R, Copel J, Craft J, Friedman D, Katholi M, Lee LA, Provost TT, Reichlin M, Rider L, Rupel A, Saleeb S, Weston WL, Skovron ML. Autoimmune-associated congenital heart block: demographics, mortality, morbidity and recurrence rates obtained from a national neonatal lupus registry. J Am Coll Cardiol 31:1658–1666, 1998.

Buyon JP, Swersky SH, Fox HE, Bierman FZ, Winchester RJ. Intrauterine therapy for presumptive fetal myocarditis with acquired heart block due to systemic lupus erythematosus. Arthritis Rheum 30:44–49, 1987.

Buyon J, Tamerius J, Belmont H, Abramson S. Assessment of disease activity and impending flare in patients with systemic lupus erythematosus. Comparison of the use of complement split products and conventional measurements of complement. Arthritis Rheum 35:1028–1037, 1992.

Buyon JP, Winchester R. Congenital complete heart block. Arthritis Rheum 33:609–614, 1990.

Bywaters EGL, Ansell BM. Monarticular arthritis in children. Ann Rheum Dis 24:116–122, 1965.

Bywaters EGL, Glynn LE, Zeldis A. Subcutaneous nodules of Still's disease. Ann Rheum Dis 17:278–285, 1958.

Bywaters EGL, Isdale I, Kempton JJ. Schönlein-Henoch purpura evidence for a group A B hemolytic streptococcal etiology. Q J Med 26:161–175, 1957.

Cabral D, Petty R, Fung M, and Malleson P. Persistent antinuclear antibodies in children without identifiable inflammatory rheumatic or autoimmune disease. Pediatrics 89:441–444, 1992.

Calin A, Elswood J, Rigg S, Skevington SM. Ankylosing spondylitis–an analytical review of 1500 patients: the changing pattern of disease. J Rheumatol 15:1234–1238, 1988.

Carette S, Klippel JH, Decker JL, Austin HA, Plotz PH, Steinberg AD, Balow JE. Controlled studies of oral immunosuppressive drugs in lupus nephritis. A long-term follow-up. Ann Intern Med 99:1–8, 1983.

Carneiro JR, Sato EI. Double blind, randomized, placebo controlled clinical trial of methotrexate in systemic lupus erythematosus. J Rheumatol 26:1275–1279, 1999.

Carreira PE, Gutierrez-Larraya F, Gomez-Reino JJ. Successful intrauterine therapy with dexamethasone for fetal myocarditis and heart block in a woman with systemic lupus erythematosus. J Rheumatol 26:1204–1207, 1993.

Carson DA, Chen PP, Kipps TJ. New roles for rheumatoid factor. J Clin Invest 87:379–383, 1991.

Carter CW. Persistent joint laxity and congenital dislocation of the hip. J Bone Joint Surg 46B:40–45, 1964.

Cassidy J, Burt A. Isolated IgA deficiency in juvenile rheumatoid arthritis. Arthritis Rheum 10:272, 1967.

Cassidy J, Burt A, Petty R, Sullivan D. Selective IgA deficiency in connective tissue diseases. N Engl J Med 280:275, 1969.

Cassidy J, Petty R, Sullivan D. Abnormalities in the distribution of serum immunoglobulin concentrations in juvenile rheumatoid arthritis. J Clin Invest 52:1931–1936, 1973.

Cassidy JT. Outcomes research in the therapeutic use of methotrexate in children with chronic peripheral arthritis. J Pediatr 133:179–180, 1998a.

Cassidy JT. Progress in diagnosis and understanding chronic pain syndromes in children and adolescents. Adolesc Med 9:101–114, 1998b.

Cassidy JT, Brody GL, Martel W. Monoarticular juvenile rheumatoid arthritis. J Pediatr 70:867–875, 1967.

Cassidy JT, Levinson JE, Bass JC, Baum J, Brewer EJJ, Fink CW, Hanson V, Jacobs JC, Masi AT, Schaller JG, Fries JF, McShane D, Young E. A study of classification criteria for a diagnosis of juvenile rheumatoid arthritis. Arthritis Rheum 29:274–281, 1986.

Cassidy JT, Petty RE. Textbook of Pediatric Rheumatology. Philadelphia, WB Saunders, 1995.

Cassidy JT, Sullivan DB, Dabich L, Petty RE. Scleroderma in children. Arthritis Rheum 20:351–354, 1977a.

Cassidy JT, Sullivan DB, Petty RE, Ragsdale C. Lupus nephritis and encephalopathy. Prognosis in 58 children. Arthritis Rheum 20:315–322, 1977b.

Cassidy JT, Valkenberg HA. A five-year prospective study of rheumatoid factors tests in juvenile rheumatoid arthritis. Arthritis Rheum 10:83–90, 1967.

Catoggio LJ, Evison G, Harkness JA, Maddison PJ. The arthropathy of systemic sclerosis (scleroderma); comparison with mixed connective tissue disease. Clin Exp Rheumatol 1:101–112, 1983.

Cazzola M, Ponchio L, de Benedetti F, Ravelli A, Rosti V, Beguin Y, Invernizzi R, Barosi G, Martini A. Defective iron supply for erythropoiesis and adequate endogenous erythropoietin production in the anemia associated with systemic-onset juvenile chronic arthritis. Blood 87:4824–4830, 1996.

Centola M, Aksentijevich I, Kastner DL. The hereditary periodic fever syndromes: molecular analysis of a new family of inflammatory diseases. Hum Mol Genet 7:1581–1588, 1998.

Cervera R, Font J, Pare C, Azqueta M, Perez-Villa F, Lopez-Soto A, Ingelmo M. Cardiac disease in systemic lupus erythematosus: prospective study in 70 patients. Ann Rheum Dis 51:156–159, 1992.

Chantler JK, Tingle AJ, Petty RE. Persistent rubella virus infection associated with chronic arthritis in children. N Engl J Med 313:1117–1123, 1985.

Chen ZY, Silver RM, Ainsworth SK, Dobson RL, Rust P, Maricq HR. Association between fluorescent antinuclear antibodies, capillary patterns, and clinical features in scleroderma spectrum disorders. Am J Med 77:812–822, 1984.

Cherin P, Herson S, Wechsler B, Piette J, Bletry O, Coutellier A, Ziza J, Godeau P. Efficacy of intravenous gammaglobulin therapy in chronic refractory polymyositis and dermatomyositis: an open study with 20 adult patients. Am J Med 91:162–168, 1991.

Chikanza IC. Neuroendocrine immune features of pediatric inflammatory rheumatic diseases. Ann NY Acad Sci 876:71–80, 1999.

Chopra P, Narula J, Kumar AS, Sachdeva S, Bhatia ML. Immunohistochemical characterisation of Aschoff nodules and endomyocardial inflammatory infiltrates in left atrial appendages from patients with chronic rheumatic heart disease. Int J Cardiol 20:99–105, 1988.

Choukri F, Chakib A, Himmich H, Hue S, Caillat-Zucman S. HLA-B*51 and B*15 alleles confer predisposition to Behcet's disease in Moroccan patients. Hum Immunol 62:180–185, 2001.

Chu SM, Huang JL, Lin SJ, Hsueh C. Successful treatment of Sjögren's syndrome with cyclophosphamide pulse therapy: report of one case. Zhonghua Min Guo Xiao Er Ke Yi Xue Hui Za Zhi 39:268–270, 1998.

Chubick A, Sontheimer RD, Gilliam JN, Ziff M. An appraisal of tests for native DNA antibodies in connective tissue diseases: clinical usefulness of Crithidia luciliae assay. Ann Intern Med 89:186–192, 1978.

Chung KJ, for the U.S. Multicenter Kawasaki Disease Study. Incidence and prognosis of giant coronary artery aneurysms in Kawasaki disease. Circulation 80:282, 1989.

Clark P, Burgos-Vargas R, Medina-Palma C, Lavielle P, Marina FF. Prevalence of fibromyalgia in children: a clinical study of Mexican children. J Rheumatol 25:2009–2014, 1998.

Colbert RA. HLA-B27 misfolding: a solution to the spondyloarthropathy conundrum? Mol Med Today 6:224–230, 2000.

Colman G, Tanna A, Efstratiou A, Gaworzewska ET. The serotypes of Streptococcus pyogenes present in Britain during 1980-1990 and their association with disease. J Med Microbiol 39:165–178, 1993.

Combined Rheumatic Fever Study Group. A comparison of short-term, intensive prednisone and acetylsalicylic acid therapy in the treatment of acute rheumatic fever. N Engl J Med 272:63–70, 1965.

Congeni B, Rizzo C, Congeni J, Sreenivasan VV. Outbreak of acute rheumatic fever in Northeast Ohio. J Pediatr 111:176–179, 1987.

Conley ME, Cooper MD, Michael AF. Selective deposition of immunoglobulin A, in immunoglobulin A nephropathy, anaphylactoid purpura nephritis, and systemic lupus erythematosus. J Clin Invest 66:1432–1435, 1980.

Connor PM, Morrey BF. Total elbow arthroplasty in patients who have juvenile rheumatoid arthritis. J Bone Joint Surg Am 80:678–688, 1998.

Cook CD, Wedgwood RJ, Craig JM, Hartmann JR, Janeway CA. Systemic lupus erythematosus. Description of 37 cases in children and a discussion of endocrine therapy in 32 of the cases. Pediatrics 26:570–585, 1960.

Cooke TD, Hurd ER, Jasin HE, Bienenstock J, Ziff M. Identification of immunoglobulins and complement in rheumatoid articular collagenous tissues. Arthritis Rheum 18:541–551, 1975.

Cooper JD, Schoen RT. Epidemiology, clinical features, and diagnosis of Lyme disease. Curr Opin Rheumatol 4:520–528, 1992.

Cooper LZ, Ziring PR, Weiss HJ, Matters BA, Krugman S. Transient arthritis after rubella vaccination. Am J Dis Child 118:218–225, 1969.

Corper AL, Sohi MK, Bonagura VR, Steinitz M, Jefferis R, Feinstein A, Beale D, Taussig MJ, Sutton BJ. Structure of human IgM rheumatoid factor Fab bound to its autoantigen IgG Fc reveals a novel topology of antibody-antigen interaction. Nat Struct Biol 4:374–381, 1997.

Coulie PG, Van Snick J. Rheumatoid factor (RF) production during anamnestic immune responses in the mouse. III. Activation of RF precursor cells is induced by their interaction with immune complexes and carrier-specific helper T cells. J Exp Med 161:88–97, 1985.

Counahan R, Winterborn MH, White RHR. Prognosis of Henoch-Schönlein nephritis in children. Brit Med J 6078:11–14, 1977.

Craft J. Antibodies to snRNPs in systemic lupus erythematosus. Rheum Dis Clin North Am 18:311–336, 1992.

Cronin ME, Biswas RM, van der Straeton C. IgG and IgM anticardiolipin antibodies in patients with lupus with anticardiolipin antibody associated clinical syndromes. J Rheumatol 15:795–798, 1988.

Crowe W, Kushner I. An immunofluorescent method using Crithidia lucilliae to detect antibodies to double-stranded DNA. Arthritis Rheum 20:811–814, 1977.

Crowe WE, Bove KE, Levinson JE, Hilton PK. Clinical and pathogenetic implications of histopathology in childhood polydermatomyositis. Arthritis Rheum 25:126–139, 1982.

Crozier IG, Li E, Milne MJ, Nicholls MG. Cardiac involvement in systemic lupus erythematosus detected by echocardiography. Am J Cardiol 65:1145–1148, 1990.

Cuellar ML, Espinoza LR. Rheumatic manifestations of HIV-AIDS. Baillieres Best Pract Res Clin Rheumatol 14:579–593, 2000.

Cuende E, Gutierrez MA, Paniagua G, Feito C, Gonzalez M, Sanchez J. Chronic recurrent multifocal osteomyelitis: report of a case with epiphyseal and metaphyseal involvement. Clin Exp Rheumatol 13:251–253, 1995.

Cunningham MW. Pathogenesis of group A streptococcal infections. Clin Microbiol Rev 13:470–511, 2000.

Cunningham MW, Hall NK, Krisher KK, Spanier AM. A study of anti-group A streptococcal monoclonal antibodies cross-reactive with myosin. J Immunol 136:293–298, 1986.

Cunningham MW, McCormack JM, Talaber LR, Ayoub EM, Muneer RS, Chun LT, Reddy DV. Human monoclonal antibodies reactive with antigens of the group A streptococcus and human heart. J Immunol 141:2760–2066, 1988.

Dajani AS, Bisno AL, Chung KJ, Durack DT, Gerber MA, Kaplan EL, Millard HD, Randolph MF, Shulman ST, Watanakunakorn C. Prevention of rheumatic fever: a statement for health professionals by the Committee on Rheumatic fever, Endocarditis, and Kawasaki disease of the Council on Cardiovascular Disease in the Young, The American Heart Association. Circulation 78:1082–1086, 1988.

Dalakas M, Plotz PH. Current concepts in the idiopathic inflammatory myopathies: polymyositis, dermatomyositis, and related disorders. Ann Intern Med 111:143–157, 1989.

Dalakas M, Illa I, Dambrosia J, Soueidan S, Stein D, Otero C, Dinsmore S, McCrosky S. A controlled trial of high-dose intravenous immune globulin infusions as treatment for dermatomyositis. N Engl J Med 329:1993–2000, 1993.

Dalakas MC. Polymyositis, dermatomyositis, and inclusion-body myositis. N Engl J Med 325:1487–1498, 1991.

Dale JB, Beachey EH. Sequence of myosin-crossreactive epitopes of streptococcal M protein. J Exp Med 164:1785–1790, 1986.

Dalhoj J, Wiggers P. Blood sedimentation rate in healthy persons. Ugeskrift for Laeger 152:456–459, 1990.

David J, Vouyiouka O, Ansell BM, Hall A, Woo P. Amyloidosis in juvenile chronic arthritis: a morbidity and mortality study. Clin Exp Rheumatol 11:85–90, 1993.

Davidson A, Shefner R, Livneh A, Diamond B. The role of somatic mutation of immunoglobulin genes in autoimmunity. Ann Rev Immunol 5:85–108, 1987.

Davies K, Stiehm ER, Woo P, Murray KJ. Juvenile idiopathic polyarticular arthritis and IgA deficiency in the 22q11 deletion syndrome. J Rheumatol 28:2326–2334, 2001.

Davies KA, Hird V, Stewart S, Sivolapenko GB, Jose P, Epenetos AA. A study of in vivo immune complex formation and clearance in man. J Immunol 144:4613–4620, 1990.

Davies NE, Haverty JR, Boatwright M. Reiter's disease associated with shigellosis. Southern Med J 62:1101–1104, 1969.

Davin JC, Vandenbroeck MC, Foidart JB, Mahieu PR. Sequential measurements of the reticulo-endothelial system function in Henoch-Schönlein disease of childhood. Correlations with various immunological parameters. Acta Paediatr Scand 74:201–206, 1985.

Davis JS, Godfrey SM, Winfield JB. Direct evidence for circulating DNA/Anti-DNA complexes in systemic lupus erythematosus. Arthritis Rheum 21:17–22, 1978.

Dawkins RL, Mastaglia FL. Cell-mediated cytotoxicity to muscle in polymyositis. N Engl J Med 288:434–438, 1973.

De Clerck LS, Degryse HR, Wonters E, Van Offel JR, De Schepper AM, Martin JJ, Stevens WJ. Magnetic resonance imaging in the evaluation of patient with eosinophilic fasciitis. J Rheumatol 16:1270–1273, 1989.

De Cunto CL, Giannini EH, Fink CW, Brewer KJ, Person DA. Prognosis of children with poststreptococcal reactive arthritis. Ped Infect Dis J 7:683–686, 1988.

de Mello e Silva AC, Boulos M. Reiter's syndrome and human immunodeficiency virus infection. Rev Hosp Clin Fac Med Sao Paulo 53:202–204, 1998.

Dean AG, Melish ME, Hicks R, Palumbo NE. An epidemic of Kawasaki syndrome in Hawaii. J Pediatr 100:552–557, 1982.

Decker JL, Klippel JH, Plotz PH, Steinberg AD. Cyclophosphamide or azathioprine in lupus glomerulonephritis. A controlled trial: results at 28 months. Ann Intern Med 83:606–615, 1975.

Delgado EA, Malleson PN, Pirie GE, Petty RE. The pulmonary manifestations of childhood onset systemic lupus erythematosus. Semin Arthritis Rheum 19:285–293, 1990.

Denardo BA, Tucker LB, Miller LC, Szer IS, Schaller JG. Demography of a regional pediatric rheumatology patient population. Affiliated Children's Arthritis Centers of New England. J Rheumatol 21:1553–1561, 1994.

Derderian SS, Tellis CJ, Abbrecht PH, Welton RC, Rajagopol HR. Pulmonary involvement in mixed connective disease. Chest 88:45–48, 1985.

Dinarello CA, Wolff SM, Goldfinger SE, Dale DC, Alling DW. Colchicine therapy for familial Mediterranean fever. A double-blind trial. N Engl J Med 291:934–937, 1974.

DiSciascio G, Taranta A. Rheumatic fever in children. Am Heart J 99:635–658, 1980.

Donadi EA, Smith AG, Louzada-Junior P, Voltarelli JC, Nepom GT. HLA class I and class II profiles of patients presenting with Sydenham's chorea. J Neurol 247:122–128, 2000.

Doniach D, Roitt IM, Walker JG, Sherlock S. Tissue antibodies in primary biliary cirrhosis, active chronic (lupoid) hepatitis, cryptogenic cirrhosis and other liver diseases and their clinical implications. Clin Exp Immunol 1:237–262, 1966.

Dracou C, Constantinidou N, Constantopoulos A. Juvenile chronic arthritis profile in Greek children. Acta Paediatr Jpn 40:558–563, 1998.

Drappa J, Vaishnaw AK, Sullivan KE, Chu JL, Elkon KB. Fas gene mutations in the Canale-Smith syndrome, an inherited lymphoproliferative disorder associated with autoimmunity. N Engl J Med 335:1643–1649, 1996.

Draznin TH, Esterly NB, Furey NL, DeBofsky H. Neonatal lupus erythematosus. J Am Acad Dermatol 1:437–442, 1979.

Drewe E, McDermott EM, Powell PT, Isaacs JD, Powell RJ. Prospective study of anti-tumour necrosis factor receptor superfamily 1B fusion protein, and case study of anti-tumour necrosis factor receptor superfamily 1A fusion protein, in tumour necrosis factor receptor associated periodic syndrome (TRAPS): clincal and laboratory findings in a series of seven patients. Rheumatology 42:235–239, 2003.

Drosos AA, Tsiakou EK, Tsifetaki N, Politi EN, Siamopoulou-Mavridou A. Subgroups of primary Sjögren's syndrome. Sjögren's syndrome in male and paediatric Greek patients. Ann Rheum Dis 56:333–335, 1997.

Egeskjold EM, Permin AJH, Hoyeraal HM, Sorenson T. The significance of antinuclear antibodies in juvenile rheumatoid arthritis associated with chronic bilateral iridocyclitis. Acta Paeditr Scand 71:615–620, 1982.

Egner W, Chapel HM. Titration of antibodies against neutrophil cytoplasmic antigens is useful in monitoring disease activity in systemic vasculitides. Clin Exp Immunol 82:244–249, 1990.

Eichenfield AH, Goldsmith DP, Benach JL, Ross AH, Loeb FX, Doughty RA, Athreya BH. Childhood Lyme arthritis: experience in an endemic area. J Pediatr 109:753–758, 1986.

Eisenstein D, O'Gorman M, Pachman L. Correlations between change in disease activity and changes in peripheral blood lymphocyte subsets in patients with juvenile dermatomyositis. J Rheumatol 24:1830–1832, 1997.

El-Demellawy M, El-Ridi R, Guirguis NI, Abdel Alim M, Kotby A, Kotb M. Preferential recognition of human myocardial antigens by T lymphocytes from rheumatic heart disease patients. Infect Immun 65:2197–2205, 1997.

Elkon KB, Sutherland DC, Rees AJ, Hughes GR, Batchelor JR. HLA antigen frequencies in systemic vasculitis: increase in HLA-DR2 in Wegener's granulomatosis. Arthritis Rheum 26:102–105, 1983.

Eltohami EA, Hajar HA, Folger GM Jr. Acute rheumatic fever in an Arabian Gulf country—effect of climate, advantageous socioeconomic conditions, and access to medical care. Angiology 48:481–489, 1997.

Emery H. Clinical aspects of systemic lupus erythematosus in childhood. Pediatr Clin North Am 33:1177–1190, 1986.

Emery H, Larter W, Schaller JG. Henoch-Schönlein vasculitis. Arthritis Rheum 20:385–388, 1977.

Emery HM, Bowyer SL. Physical modalities of therapy in pediatric rheumatic diseases. Rheum Dis Clin of North Am 17:1001–1014, 1991.

Emlen W, Pisetsky DS, Taylor RP. Antibodies to DNA. A perspective. J Pediatr 78:981–984, 1986.

Engle MA, Fatica NS, Bussel JB. Clinical trial of single-dose intravenous gamma globulin in acute Kawasaki disease. Am J Dis Child 143:1300–1304, 1989.

Epstein HC, Litt JZ. Discoid lupus erythematosus in a newborn infant. N Engl J Med 265:1106–1107, 1961.

Espinoza LR, Vasey FB, Oh JH, Wilkinson R, Osterland CK. Association between HLA-BW38 and peripheral psoriatic arthritis. Arthritis Rheum 21:72–75, 1990.

Faedda R, Pirisi M, Satta A, Bosinu L, Bartoli E. Regression of Henoch-Schönlein disease with intensive immunosuppressive treatment. Clin Pharmacol Ther 60:576–581, 1996.

Falk RJ, Jennette JC. Anti-neutrophil cytoplasmic autoantibodies with specificity for myeloperoxidase in patients with systemic vasculitis and idiopathic necrotizing and crescentic glomerulonephritis. N Engl J Med 318:1651–1657, 1988.

Falk RJ, Nachman PH, Hogan SL, Jennette JC. ANCA glomerulonephritis and vasculitis: a Chapel Hill perspective. Semin Nephrol 20:233–243, 2000.

Fantini F, Gattinara M, Gerloni V, Bergoni P, Cirla E. Severe anemia associated with active systemic onset juvenile rheumatoid arthritis successfully treated with recombinant human erythropoietin: a pilot study. Arthritis Rheum 35:724–726, 1992.

Farber SJ, Bole GG. Antibodies to components of extractable nuclear antigen. Clinical characteristics of patients. Arch Intern Med 136:425–431, 1976.

Farquhar JD, Corretjer JE. Clinical experience with Cendehill rubella vaccine in mature women. Am J Dis Child 118:266–268, 1969.

Farrington ML, Haas JE, Nazar-Stewart V, Mellins ED. Eosinophilic fasciitis in children frequently progresses to scleroderma-like cutaneous fibrosis. J Rheumatol 20:128–132, 1993.

Fauci AS, Hayes BF, Katz P, Wolff SM. Wegener's granulomatosis: prospective clinical and therapeutic experience with 85 patients for 21 years. Ann Intern Med 98:76–85, 1983.

Fearon DT, Carroll MC. Regulation of B lymphocyte responses to foreign and self-antigens by the CD19/CD21 complex. Ann Rev Immunol 18:393–422, 2000.

Feinstein AR, Spagnuolo M. The clinical patterns of acute rheumatic fever: a reappraisal. Medicine 41:279–305, 1962.

Feinstein AR, Wood HF, Spagnuolo M, Taranta A, Jonas S, Kleinberg E, Tursky E. Rheumatic fever in children and adolescents. VII. Cardiac changes and sequelae. Ann Intern Med 60(Suppl 5):87–123, 1964.

Ferreiro JE, Reiter WM, Saldana MJ. Systemic lupus erythematosus presenting as a chronic serositis with no demonstrable antinuclear antibodies. Am J Med 76:1100–1105, 1984.

Fessel WJ. ANA-negative systemic lupus erythematosus. Am J Med 64:80–86, 1978.

Fielder AH, Walport MJ, Batchelor JR, Rynes RI, Black CM, Dodi IA, Hughes GR. Family study of the major histocompatibility complex in patients with systemic lupus erythematosus: importance of null alleles of C4A and C4B in determining disease susceptibility. BMJ (Clin Res Ed) 286:425–428, 1983.

Fields RA, Sibbitt WL, Toubbeh H, Bankhurst AD. Neuropsychiatric lupus erythematosus, cerebral infarctions, and anticardiolipin antibodies. Ann Rheum Dis 49:114–117, 1990.

Fijiwara T, Fujiwara H, Nakano H. Pathological features of coronary arteries in children with Kawasaki disease in which coronary arterial aneurysm was absent at autopsy. Circulation 78:345–350, 1988.

Fink CW. Polyarteritis and streptococcal infection. Pediatrics 61:675, 1978.

Fink CW. Proposal for the development of classification criteria for idiopathic arthritides of childhood. J Rheumatol 22:1566–1569, 1995.

Finkel M, Halpern J. Nervous system Lyme borreliosis. Arch Neurol 49:102–107, 1991.

Fischer TJ, Rachelefsky GS, Klein RB, Paulus HE, Stiehm ER. Childhood dermatomyositis and polymyositis: treatment with methotrexate and prednisone. Am J Dis Child 133:386–389, 1979.

Fish AJ, Blau EB, Westberg NG, Burke BA, Vernier RL, Michael AF. Systemic lupus erythematosus within the first two decades of life. Am J Med 62:99–117, 1977.

Fishbain D. Evidence-based data on pain relief with antidepressants. Ann Med 32:305–316, 2000.

Fleischmajer R, Perlish JS. Capillary alterations in scleroderma. J Am Acad Dermatol 2:161–170, 1980.

FMF. A candidate gene for familial Mediterranean fever. The French FMF Consortium. Nat Genet 17:25–31, 1997.

Follansbee WP, Curtiss EI, Medsger TA, Steen VD, Uretsky BF, Owens GR, Rodnan GP. Physiologic abnormalities of cardiac function in progressive systemic sclerosis with diffuse scleroderma. N Engl J Med 310:142–148, 1984.

Ford PM, Ford SE, Lillicrap DP. Association of lupus anticoagulant and severe valvular heart disease in systemic lupus erythematosus. J Rheumatol 15:597–600, 1988.

Fouillard L, Gorin NC, Laporte JP, Leon A, Brantus JF, Miossec P. Control of severe systemic lupus erythematosus after high-dose immunosuppressive therapy and transplantation of CD34+ purified autologous stem cells from peripheral blood. Lupus 8:320–323, 1999.

Fox RI, Saito I. Criteria for diagnosis of Sjögren's syndrome. Rheum Dis Clin North Am 20:391–407, 1994.

Fox RJJ, McCuiston CH, Schoch EPJ. Systemic lupus erythematosus association with previous neonatal lupus erythematosus. Arch Dermatol 115:340, 1979.

Frank M. Detection of complement in relation to disease. J Allergy Clin Immunol 89:641–648, 1992.

Freitas AA, Rocha B. Population biology of lymphocytes: the flight for survival. Annu Rev Immunol 18:83–111, 2000.

Friedman JM, Pachman LM, Maryjowski ML, Radvany RM, Crowe WE, Hanson V, Levinson JE, Spencer CH. Immunogenetic studies of juvenile dermatomyositis: HLA-DR antigen frequencies. Arthritis Rheum 26:214–216, 1983.

Friend P, Repine J, Kim Y, Clawson C, Michael A. Deficiency of the second component of complement (C2) with chronic vasculitis. Ann Intern Med 82:813–816, 1975.

Fries JF, Porta J, Liang HM. Marginal benefit of renal biopsy in systemic lupus erythematosus. Arch Intern Med 138:1386–1389, 1978.

Friou GJ. Antinuclear antibodies: diagnostic significance and methods. Arthritis Rheum 10:151–159, 1967.

Fritzler MJ. Histone antibodies. In Wallace DJ, Hahn BH, eds. Dubois' lupus erythematosus. Philadelphia, Lea and Febiger, 1993, pp 202–215.

Fritzler MJ, Kinsella TD, Garbutt E. The CREST syndrome: a distinct serologic entity with anticentromere antibodies. Am J Med 69:520–526, 1980.

Fukushige J, Nihill MR, McNamara DG. Spectrum of cardiovascular lesions in mucocutaneous lymph node syndrome: analysis of eight cases. Am J Cardiol 45:98–107, 1980.

Fulton DR, Newburger JW. Long-term cardiac sequelae of Kawasaki disease. Curr Rheumatol Rep 2:324–329, 2000.

Furst DE, Clements PJ, Hillis S, Lachenbruch PA, Miller BL, Sterz MG, Paulus HE. Immunosuppression with chlorambucil, versus placebo, for scleroderma. Results of a three-year, parallel, randomized, double-blind study. Arthritis Rheum 32:584–593, 1989.

Furukawa S, Matsubara T, Yabuta K. Mononuclear cell subsets and coronary artery lesions in Kawasaki disease. Arch Dis Child 67:706–708, 1992.

Furusho K, Kamiya T, Nakano H, Kiyosawa N, et al. High-dose intravenous gammaglobulin for Kawasaki disease. Lancet 2:1055–1058, 1984.

Gabay C, Kushner I. Acute-phase proteins and other systemic responses to inflammation. N Engl J Med 340:448–454, 1999.

Gallagher KT, Bernstein B. Juvenile rheumatoid arthritis. Curr Opin Rheumatol 11:372–376, 1999.

Galve E, Candell-Riera J, Pigrau C, Permanyer-Miralda G, Garcia-Del-Castillo H, Soler-Solerl J. Prevalence, morphologic types, and evolution of cardiac valvular disease in systemic lupus erythematosus. N Engl J Med 319:817–823, 1988.

Galvin JE, Hemric ME, Ward K, Cunningham MW. Cytotoxic mAb from rheumatic carditis recognizes heart valves and laminin. J Clin Invest 106:217–224, 2000.

Garcia-De LaTorre I, Miranda-Mendez L. Studies of antinuclear antibodies in juvenile rheumatoid arthritis. J Rheumatol 9:603–606, 1982.

Garcia-Fuentes M, Martin A, Chantler C. Serum complement components in Henoch-Schönlein purpura. Arch Dis Child 53:417–419, 1978.

Garcia-Morteo O, Maldonado-Coco JA, Suarez-Almazor ME. Ankylosing spondylitis of juvenile onset: comparison with adult onset disease. Scand J Rheumatol 12:246–248, 1983.

Gare BA, Fasth A. Epidemiology of juvenile chronic arthritis in Southwestern Sweden: a 5-year prospective population study. Pediatrics 90:950–958, 1992.

Garin EH, Donnelly WH, Fennell RS, Richard GA. Nephritis in systemic lupus erythematosus in children. J Pediatr 89:366–371, 1976.

Gedalia A, Garcia CO, Molina JF, Bradford NJ, Espinoza LR. Fibromyalgia syndrome: experience in a pediatric rheumatology clinic. Clin Exp Rheumatol 18:415–419, 2000.

Geggel RL, Tucker L, Szer I. Postnatal progression from second- to third-degree heart block in neonatal lupus syndrome. J Pediatr 113:1049–1052, 1988.

Gelfand E, Clarkson J, Minta J. Selective deficiency of the second component of complement in a patient with anaphylactoid purpura. Clin Immunol Immunopathol 4:269–276, 1975.

George PM, Tunnessen WWJ. Childhood discoid lupus erythematosus. Arch Dermatol 129:613–617, 1993.

Gersony WM. Long-term issues in Kawasaki disease. J Pediatr 121:731–733, 1992.

Gewanter HL, Roghmann KJ, Baum J. The prevalence of juvenile arthritis. Arthritis Rheum 26:599–603, 1983.

Gewurz A, Lint T, Roberts J, Zeitz H, Gewurz H. Homozygous C2 deficiency with fulminant lupus erythematosus. Arthritis Rheum 21:28–36, 1978.

Giannini EH, Brewer EJ, Kuzmina N. Auranofin in the treatment of juvenile rheumatoid arthritis. Results of the USA-USSR double-blind, placebo-controlled trial. Arthritis Rheum 33:466–476, 1990.

Giannini EH, Brewer EJ, Kuzmina N, Shaikov A, Maximov A, Vorontsov I, Fink CW, Newman AJ, Cassidy JT, Zemel LS. Methotrexate in resistant juvenile rheumatoid arthritis. Results of the USA-USSR double-blind, placebo-controlled trial. N Engl J Med 326:1043–1049, 1992.

Giannini EH, Cassidy JT. Methotrexate in juvenile rheumatoid arthritis. Do the benefits outweigh the risks? Drug Safety 9:325–339, 1993.

Gidding SS, Shulman ST, Ilbawi M, Crussi F, Duffy CF. Mucocutaneous lymph node syndrome (Kawasaki disease): delayed aortic and mitral insufficiency secondary to active valvulitis. J Am Coll Cardiol 7:894–897, 1986.

Giedion A, Holthusen W, Masel LF, Vischer D. Subacute and chronic "symmetrical" osteomyelitis. Ann Radiol (Paris) 15:329–342, 1972.

Gillum RF. A racial difference in erythrocyte sedimentation. J Natl Med Ass 85:47–50, 1993.

Ginn LR, Lin JP, Plotz PH, Bale SJ, Wilder RL, Mbauya A, Miller FW. Familial autoimmunity in pedigrees of idiopathic inflammatory myopathy patients suggests common genetic risk factors for many autoimmune diseases. Arthritis Rheum 41:400–405, 1998.

Ginsburg WW, Cohen MD. Peripheral arthritis in ankylosing spondylitis. A review of 209 patients followed up for more than 20 years. Mayo Clin Proc 58:593–596, 1983.

Ginzler EM, Nicastri AD, Chen CK, Friedman EA, Diamond HS, Kaplant D. Progression of mesangial and focal to diffuse lupus nephritis. Ann Intern Med 291:693–696, 1974.

Gioud M, Kaci MA, Monier JC. Histone antibodies in systemic lupus erythematosus. Arthritis Rheum 25:407–413, 1982.

Girschick HJ, Krauspe R, Tschammler A, Huppertz HI. Chronic recurrent osteomyelitis with clavicular involvement in children: diagnostic value of different imaging techniques and therapy with non-steroidal anti-inflammatory drugs. Eur J Pediatr 157:28–33, 1998.

Gladman DD, Cheung C, Ng CM, Wade JA. HLA-C locus alleles in patients with psoriatic arthritis (PsA). Hum Immunol 60:259–261, 1999.

Glass D, Litvin D. Heterogeneity of HLA associations in systemic onset juvenile rheumatoid arthritis. Arthritis Rheum 23:796–799, 1980.

Glass D, Litvin D, Wallace K, Chylack L, Garovoy M, Carpenter CB, Schur PH. Early onset pauciarticular juvenile rheumatoid arthritis associated with human leukocyte antigen DRw5, iritis, and antinuclear antibodies. J Clin Invest 66:426–429, 1980.

Glass D, Raum D, Gibson D, Stillman JS, Schur PH. Inherited deficiency of the second component of complement. J Clin Invest 58:853–861, 1976.

Glidden RS, Mantzouranis EC, Borel Y. Systemic lupus erythematosus in childhood: clinical manifestations and improved survival in fifty-five patients. Clin Immunol Immunopathol 29:196–210, 1983.

Gocke DJ, Hsu K, Morgan C, Bombardiere S, Lockshin M, Christian CL. Association between polyarteritis and Australia antigen. Lancet 2:1149–1153, 1970.

Golan TD, Keren D, Elias N, Naschitz JE, Toubi E, Misselevich I, Yeshurun D. Severe reversible cardiomyopathy associated with systemic vasculitis in primary Sjögren's syndrome. Lupus 6:505–508, 1997.

Gold JA. Arthritis after rubella vaccination of women. N Engl J Med 281:109, 1969.

Goldenberg D. In Klippel J a DD, ed. Rheumatology. London, Mosby, 1998, pp 4.15.1–4.15.4.

Goldfinger SE. Colchicine for familial Mediterranean fever. N Engl J Med 287:1302, 1972.

Goldschmeding R, Tervaert JW, Gans RO, Dolman KM, van den Ende ME, Kuizinga MC, Kallenberg CG, von dem Borne AE. Different immunological specificities and disease associations of c-ANCA and p-ANCA. Neth J Med 36: 114–116, 1990.

Goldstein I, Rebeyotte P, Parlebas J, Halpern B. Isolation from heart valves of glycopeptides which share immunological properties with streptococcus haemolyticus group A polysaccharides. Nature (London) 219:866–868, 1968.

Goldstein RC, Schwabe AD. Prophylactic colchicine therapy in familial Mediterranean fever. A controlled, double-blind study. Ann Intern Med 81:792–794, 1974.

Gomez KS, Raza K, Jones SD, Kennedy LG, Calin A. Juvenile onset ankylosing spondylitis—more girls than we thought? J Rheumatol 24:735–737, 1997.

Gore JE, Vizcarrondo FE, Rieffel CN. Juvenile ankylosing spondylitis and aortic regurgitation: a case presentation. Pediatrics 68:423–426, 1981.

Granberry G. Soft tissue release in children with juvenile rheumatoid arthritis. Arthritis Rheum 20:565–566, 1977b.

Granberry W. Synovectomy in juvenile rheumatoid arthritis. Arthritis Rheum 20:561–564, 1977a.

Grassegger A, Schuler G, Hessenberger G, Walder-Hantich B, Jabkowski J, MacHeiner W, Salmhofer W, Zahel B, Pinter G, Herold M, Klein G, Fritsch PO. Interferon-gamma in the treatment of systemic sclerosis: a randomized controlled multicentre trial. Br J Dermatol 139:639–648, 1998.

Gray ED, Wannamaker LW, Ayoub EM, El Kholy A, Abdin ZH. Cellular immune responses to extracellular streptococcal products in rheumatic heart disease. J Clin Invest 68:665–671, 1981.

Grayzel AI, Marcus R, Stern R, Winchester RJ. Chronic polyarthritis associated with hypogammaglobulinemia. Arthritis Rheum 20:887–894, 1977.

Grennan DM, Parfitt A, Manolios N, Huang Q, Hyland V, Dunckley H, Doran T, Gatenby P, Badcock C. Family and twin studies in systemic lupus erythematosus. Dis Markers 13:93–98, 1997.

Gribetz D, Henley WL. Systemic lupus erythematosus in childhood. J Mount Sinai Hosp NY 26:289–306, 1959.

Griffiths SP, Gersony WM. Acute rheumatic fever in New York City (1969 to 1988): a comparative study of two decades. J Pediatr 116:882–887, 1990.

Grisanti MW, Moore TL, Osborn TG, Haber PL. Eosinophilic fasciitis in children. Semin Arthritis Rheum 19:151–157, 1989.

Grondal G, Gunnarsson I, Ronnelid J, Rogberg S, Klareskog L, Lundberg I. Cytokine production, serum levels and disease activity in systemic lupus erythematosus. Clin Exp Rheumatol 18:565–570, 2000.

Gross DM, Forsthuber T, Tary-Lehmann M, Etling C, Ito K, Nagy ZA, Field JA, Steere AC, Huber BT. Identification of LFA-1 as a candidate autoantigen in treatment-resistant Lyme arthritis. Science 281:703–706, 1998.

Grosset ABM, Rodgers GM. Acquired coagulation disorders. In Lee GR, ed. Wintrobe's clinical hematology, ed 10. Baltimore, Williams & Wilkins, 1999, pp 1733–1780.

Gu J, Yu B, Zhou J. HLA-DQA1 genes involved in genetic susceptibility to rheumatic fever and rheumatic heart disease in southern Hans. Chung Hua Nei Ko Tsa Chih 36:308–311, 1997.

Gulizia JM, Cunningham MW, McManus BM. Immunoreactivity of anti-streptococcal monoclonal antibodies to human heart valves. Am J Pathol 138:285–301, 1991.

Gurian LE, Rogoff TM, Ware AJ, Jordan RE, Combes B, Gilliam JN. The immunologic diagnosis of chronic active "autoimmune" hepatitis: distinction from systemic lupus erythematosus. Hepatology 5:397–402, 1985.

Guseva NG, Abdykhalykova ZD, Bel'skaia OB, Ivanova MM. Clinical aspects and diagnosis of diffuse eosinophilic fasciitis. Ter Arkh 58:131–135, 1986.

Haber HL, Leavy JA, Kessler PD, Kukin ML, Gottlieb SS, Packer M. The erythrocyte sedimentation rate in congestive heart failure. N Engl J Med 324:353–358, 1991.

Habib GS, Saliba WR, Mader R. Rheumatic fever in the Nazareth area during the last decade. Isr Med Assoc J 2:433–437, 2000.

Hadchouel M, Prieur AM, Griscelli C. Acute hemorrhagic, hepatic, and neurologic manifestations in juvenile rheumatoid arthritis: possible relationship to drugs or infection. J Pediatr 106:561–566, 1985.

Hafez M, Abdalla A, El-Shennawy F, Al-Tonbary Y, Sheaishaa A, El-Moris Z, Tawfik SH, Settien A, El-Khair M. Immunogenetic study of the response to streptococcal carbohydrate antigen of the cell wall in rheumatic fever. Ann Rheum Dis 49:708–714, 1990.

Hafez M, El-Battoty MF, Hawas S, Al-Tonbary Y, Sheishaa A, El-Sallab SH, El-Morsi Z, El-Ziny M, Hawas SE. Evidence of inherited susceptibility of increased streptococcal adherence to pharyngeal cells of children with rheumatic fever. Br J Rheumatol 28:304–309, 1989.

Hafner R, Pieper M. Arthroscopic synovectomy of the knee joint in chronic juvenile arthritis. Z Rheumatol 54:165–170, 1995.

Hafner R, Vogel P. Sarcoidosis of early onset. A challenge for the pediatric rheumatologist. Clin Exp Rheumatol 11:685–691, 1993.

Hagge WW, Burke EC, Stickler GB. Treatment of systemic lupus erythematosus complicated by nephritis in children. Pediatrics 40:822–827, 1967.

Haidan A, Talay SR, Rohde M, Sriprakash KS, Currie BJ, Chhatwal GS. Pharyngeal carriage of group C and group G streptococci and acute rheumatic fever in an Aboriginal population. Lancet 356:1167–1169, 2000.

Hall RP, Lawley TJ, Heck JA. IgA-containing circulating immune complexes in dermatitis herpetiformis, Henoch-Schönlein purpura, systemic lupus erythematosus, and other diseases. Clin Exp Immunol 40:431–437, 1980.

Hall S, Barr W, Lie JT, Stanson AW, Kazmier FJ, Hunder GG. Takayasu arteritis. A study of 32 North American patients. Medicine 64:89–99, 1985a.

Hall SL, Miller LC, Duggan E, Mauer SM, Beatty EC, Hellerstein S. Wegener's granulomatosis in pediatric patients. J Pediatr 106:739–744, 1985b.

Halla JF, Hardin JG. Clinical features of the arthritis of mixed connective tissue disease. Arthritis Rheum 21:497–503, 1978.

Halma C, Daha M, Schrama E, Hermans J, van Es LA. Value of anti-neutrophil cytoplasmic autoantibodies and other laboratory parameters in follow-up of vasculitis. Scand J Rheumatol 19:392–397, 1990.

Halpern J, Volkman D, Wu P. Central nervous system abnormalities in Lyme neuroborreliosis. Neurology 41:1571–1582, 1991.

Hamilton ML, Gladman DD, Shore A, Laxer RM, Silverman ED. Juvenile psoriatic arthritis and HLA antigens. Ann Rheum Dis 49:694–697, 1990.

Hammer R, Maika S, Richardson J, Tang J, Taurog J. Spontaneous inflammatory disease in transgenic rats expressing HLA-B27 and human beta 2m: an animal model of HLA-B27 associated with human disorders. Cell 63:1099–1112, 1990.

Hamuryudan V, Mat C, Saip S, Ozyazgan Y, Siva A, Yurdakul S, Zwingenberger K, Yazici H. Thalidomide in the treatment of the mucocutaneous lesions of the Behcet syndrome. A randomized, double-blind, placebo-controlled trial. Ann Intern Med 128:443–450, 1998.

Hannonen P, Malminiemi K, Yli-Kerttula U, Isomeri R, Roponen P. A randomized, double-blind, placebo-controlled study of moclobemide and amitriptyline in the treatment of fibromyalgia in females without psychiatric disorder. Br J Rheumatol 37:1279–1286, 1998.

Hanson V, Drexler E, Kornreich H. The relationship of rheumatoid factor to age of onset in juvenile rheumatoid arthritis. Arthritis Rheum 12:82–86, 1969.

Hanson V, Kornreich H. Systemic rheumatic disorders ("collagen disease") in childhood. Bull Rheum Dis 17:435–446, 1967.

Hardarson S, LaBrecque DR, Mitros FA, Neil GA, Goeken JA. Antineutrophil cytoplasmic antibody in inflammatory bowel and hepatobiliary diseases. Clin Microbiol Immunol 99:277–281, 1993.

Hardin JA, Thomas JO. Antibodies to histones in systemic lupus erythematosus: Localization of prominent autoantigens on histones H1 and H2B. Proc Natl Acad Sci USA 80:7410–7414, 1983.

Harel L, Zecharia A, Straussberg R, Volovitz B, Amir J. Successful treatment of rheumatic chorea with carbamazepine. Pediatr Neurol 23:147–151, 2000.

Hargraves MM. Discovery of the LE cell and its morphology. Mayo Clin Proc 44:579–599, 1969.

Hargraves MM, Richmond H, Morton R. Presentation of two bone marrow elements, the "tart" cell and the "LE" cell. Mayo Clin Proc 23:25–28, 1948.

Harley JB, Kaine JL, Fox OF, Reichlin M, Gruber B. Ro(SS-A) antibody and antigen in a patient with congenital complete heart block. Arthritis Rheum 28:1321–1325, 1985.

Harley JB, Scofield RH, Reichlin M. Anti-Ro in Sjögren's syndrome and systemic lupus erythematosus. Rheum Dis Clin North Am 18:337–358, 1992.

Harris EN, Asherson RA, Gharavi AE. Thrombocytopenia in SLE and related autoimmune disorders: association with anticardiolipin antibody. Br J Haematol 59:227–230, 1985.

Harrison DJ, Simpson R, Kharbanda R, Abernethy VE, Nimmo G. Antibodies to neutrophil cytoplasmic antigens in Wegener's granulomatosis and other conditions. Thorax 44:373–377, 1989.

Haserick JR, Lewis LA, Bortz DW. Blood factor in acute disseminated lupus erythematosus; determination of gamma globulin as specific plasma fraction. Am J Med Sci 219:660–663, 1950.

Hashkes PJ, Balistreri WF, Bove KE, Ballard ET, Passo MH. The relationship of hepatotoxic risk factors and liver histology in methotrexate therapy for juvenile rheumatoid arthritis. J Pediatr 134:47–52, 1999.

Hassink SG, Goldsmith DP. Neonatal onset multisystem inflammatory disease. Arthritis Rheum 26:668–673, 1983.

Hata R, Akai J, Kimura A, Ishikawa O, Kuwana M, Shinkai H. Association of functional microsatellites in the human type I collagen alpha2 chain (COL1A2) gene with systemic sclerosis. Biochem Biophys Res Commun 272:36–40, 2000.

Hatta Y, Tsuchiya N, Ohashi J, Matsushita M, Fujiwara K, Hagiwara K, Juji T, Tokunaga K. Association of Fc gamma receptor IIIB, but not of Fc gamma receptor IIA and IIIA polymorphisms with systemic lupus erythematosus in Japanese. Genes Immun 1:53–60, 1999.

Hattori M, Ito K, Konomoto T, Kawaguchi H, Yoshioka T, Khono M. Plasmapheresis as the sole therapy for rapidly progressive Henoch-Schönlein purpura nephritis in children. Am J Kidney Dis 33:427–433, 1999.

Haycock GB. The treatment of glomerulonephritis in children. Pediatr Nephrol 2:247–255, 1988.

Hayem G, Bouchaud-Chabot A, Benali K, Roux S, Palazzo E, Silbermann-Hoffman O, Kahn MF, Meyer O. SAPHO syndrome: a long-term follow-up study of 120 cases. Semin Arthritis Rheum 29:159–171, 1999.

Heckmatt J, Saunders C, Peters AM, Rose M, Hasson N, Thompson N, Cambridge G, Hyde SA, Dubowitz V. Cyclosporin in juvenile dermatomyositis. Lancet 8646:1063–1066, 1989.

Herold BC, Shulman ST. Poststreptococcal arthritis. Pediatr Infect Dis J 7:681–682, 1988.

Hertzberger-ten Cate R, Cats A. Toxicity of sulfasalazine in systemic juvenile chronic arthritis. Clin Exp Rheumatol 9:85–88, 1991.

Hertzberger-ten Cate R, Dervlugt BCMD, Van Suijlekomsmit LWA, Cats A. Disease patterns in early onset pauciarticular juvenile chronic arthritis. Eur J Pediatr 151:339–341, 1992.

Herve-Somma C, Touzet P, Lallemand D, Prieur AM. Gd-DOTA enhanced MR imaging in juvenile chronic arthritis (JCA) before and after intraarticular therapy (abstr). J Rheumatol 19:A66, 1992.

Hess EV, Fink CS, Taranta A, Ziff M. Heart muscle antibodies in rheumatic fever and other diseases. J Clin Invest 43:886–893, 1964.

Hicks RM. Rheumatic fever in Hawaii. Arthritis Rheum 20:375–376, 1977.

Hirohata S, Suda H, Hashimoto T. Low-dose weekly methotrexate for progressive neuropsychiatric manifestations in Behcet's disease. J Neurol Sci 159:181–185, 1998.

Hochberg MC, Boyd RE, Ahearn JM, Arnett FC, Bias WB, Provost TT, Stevens MD. Systemic lupus erythematosus: a review of clinic-laboratory features and immunogenetic markers in 150 patients with emphasis on demographic subsets. Medicine 64:285–295, 1985.

Hoffman GS, Leavitt RY, Kerr GS, Rottem M, Sneller MC, Fauci AS. Treatment of glucocorticoid-resistant or relapsing Takayasu arteritis with methotrexate. Arthritis Rheum 37:578–582, 1994.

Hoffman RW, Greidinger EL. Mixed connective tissue disease. Curr Opin Rheumatol 12:386–390, 2000.

Hoffman RW, Cassidy JT, Takeda Y, Smith-Jones EI, Wang GS, Sharp GC. U1-70-kd autoantibody-positive mixed connective tissue disease in children. Arthritis Rheum 36:1599–1602, 1993.

Hogg GR. Congenital acute lupus erythematosus associated with subendocardial fibroelastosis. Am J Clin Pathol 28:648–654, 1957.

Homcy CJ, Liberthson RR, Fallon JT, Gross S, Miller LM. Ischemic heart disease in systemic lupus erythematosus in the young patient: report of 6 cases. Am J Cardiol 49:478–484, 1982.

Hong GH, Kim HY, Takeuchi F, Nakano K, Yamada H, Matsuta K, Han H, Tokunaga K, Ito K, Park KS. Association of complement C4 and HLA-DR alleles with systemic lupus erythematosus in Koreans. J Rheumatol 21:442–447, 1994.

Horng YC, Chou YH, Tsou Yau KI. Neonatal lupus erythematosus with negative anti-Ro and anti-La antibodies: report of one case. Zhonghua Min Guo Xiao Er Ke Yi Xue Hui Za Zhi 33:372–375, 1992.

Horoupian DS, Rapin I, Titelbaum J, Peison B. Infantile inflammatory multisystem disease: clinicopathological findings and review of the literature. Clin Neuropathol 9:170–176, 1990.

Horsfall AC, Venables PJW, Taylor PV, Maini RN. Ro and La antigens and maternal anti-La idiotype on the surface of myocardial fibers in congenital heart block. J Autoimmun 4:165–176, 1991.

Hosenpud JD, Montanaro A, Hart MV, Haines JE, Specht HD, Bennett RM, Kloster FE. Myocardial perfusion abnormalities in asymptomatic patients with systemic lupus erythematosus. Am J Med 77:286–292, 1983.

Hosier DM, Craenen JM, Teske DW, Wheller JJ. Resurgence of acute rheumatic fever. Am J Dis Child 141:730–733, 1987.

Howard PF, Hochberg MC, Bias WB, Arnett FC Jr, McLean RH. Relationship between C4 null genes, HLA-D region antigens, and genetic susceptibility to systemic lupus erythematosus in Caucasian and black Americans. Am J Med 81:187–193, 1986.

Hoyland JA, Newson L, Jayson MI, Freemont AJ. The vascular basement membrane in systemic sclerosis skin: heterogeneity of type IV collagen. Br J Dermatol 129:384–388, 1993.

Huang JL, Chen LC. Sulphasalazine in the treatment of children with chronic arthritis. Clin Rheumatol 17:359–363, 1998.

Hubscher O, Susini JG. Aortic insufficiency in Reiter's syndrome of juvenile onset. J Rheumatol 11:94–95, 1984.

Huemer C, Kitson H, Malleson PN, Sanderson S, Huemer M, Cabral DA, Chanoine JP, Petty RE. Lipodystrophy in patients with juvenile dermatomyositis—evaluation of clinical and metabolic abnormalities. J Rheumatol 28:610–615, 2001.

Hull D, Binns BOA, Joyce D. Congenital heart block and widespread fibrosis due to maternal lupus erythematosus. Arch Dis Child 41:688–690, 1966.

Hulshof MM, Bavinck JN, Bergman W, Masclee AA, Heickendorff L, Breedveld FC, Dijkmans BA. Double-blind, placebo-controlled study of oral calcitriol for the treatment of localized and systemic scleroderma. J Am Acad Dermatol 43:1017–1023, 2000.

Huntley CC, Thorpe DP, Lyerly AD, Kelsey WM. Rheumatoid arthritis with IgA deficiency. Am J Dis Child 113:411–418, 1967.

Hunzelmann N, Anders S, Fierlbeck G, Hein R, Herrmann K, Albrecht M, Bell S, Thur J, Muche R, Adelmann-Grill B, Wehner-Caroli J, Gaus W, Krieg T. Systemic scleroderma. Multicenter trial of 1 year of treatment with recombinant interferon gamma. Arch Dermatol 133:609–613, 1997.

Hurley RM, Drummond KN. Anaphylactoid purpura nephritis: clinicopathological correlations. J Pediatrics 81:904–911, 1972.

Husby G, van de Rijn I, Zabriskie JB, Abdin ZH, Williams RCJ. Antibodies reacting with cytoplasm of subthalamic and caudate nuclei neurons in chorea and acute rheumatic fever. J Exp Med 144:1094–1110, 1976.

Huttenlocher A, Frieden IJ, Emery H. Neonatal onset multisystem inflammatory disease. J Rheumatol 22:1171–1173, 1995.

Iemura M, Ishii M, Sugimura T, Akagi T, Kato H. Long term consequences of regressed coronary aneurysms after Kawasaki disease: vascular wall morphology and function. Heart 83:307–311, 2000.

Imakita M, Sasaki Y, Misugi K, Miyazawa Y, Hyodo Y. Kawasaki disease complicated with mitral insufficiency. Autopsy findings with special reference to valvular lesion. Acta Pathol Jpn 34:605–616, 1984.

Imundo LF, Jacobs JC. Sulfasalazine therapy for juvenile rheumatoid arthritis. J Rheumatol 23:360–366, 1996.

Isdale IC, Bywaters EGL. The rash of rheumatic arthritis and Still's disease. Q J Med 1956:377–387, 1956.

ISG. Criteria for diagnosis of Behcet's disease. International Study Group for Behcet's Disease. Lancet 335:1078–1080, 1990.

Ishikawa-Nakayama K, Sugiyama E, Sawazaki S, Taki H, Kobayashi M, Koizumi F, Furuta I. Chronic recurrent multifocal osteomyelitis showing marked improvement with corticosteroid treatment. J Rheumatol 27:1318–1319, 2000.

Ishiwata S, Nishiyama S, Nakanishi S, Seki A, Watanabe Y, Konishi T, Fuse K. Coronary artery disease and internal mammary artery aneurysms in a young woman: possible sequelae of Kawasaki disease. Am Heart J 120:213–217, 1990.

Jaber L, Weinberger A, Klein T, Yaniv I, Mukamel M. Close association of HLA-B52 and HLA-B44 antigens in Israeli Arab adolescents with recurrent aphthous stomatitis. Arch Otolaryngol Head Neck Surg 127:184–187, 2001.

Jackson R, Gulliver M. Neonatal lupus erythematosus progressing into systemic lupus erythematosus. Br J Dermatol 101:81–83, 1979.

Jacobs J, Berdon W, Johnston A. HLA-B27-associated spondyloarthritis and enthesopathy in childhood: clinical, pathologic, and radiographic observations in 58 patients. J Pediatr 100:521–528, 1982.

Jacobs JC. Systemic lupus erythematosus in childhood. Report of 35 cases with discussion of seven apparently induced by anticonvulsant medication and of prognosis and treatment. Pediatrics 32:257–264, 1963a.

Jacobs JC. Treatment of dermatomyositis. Arthritis Rheum 20:338–341, 1977.

Jacobs JC, Goetzl EJ. "Streaking leukocyte factor," arthritis, and pyoderma gangrenosum. Pediatrics 56:570–578, 1975.

Jacobs JC, Gorin LJ, Hanissian AS, Simon JL, Smithwick EM, Sullivan D. Consumption coagulopathy after gold therapy for juvenile rheumatoid arthritis (Letter). J Pediatr 105:674–675, 1984.

Jacobs P. Ankylosing spondylitis in children and adolescents. Arch Dis Child 38:492–499, 1963b.

Jaffe BD, Claman HN. Chronic graft-versus-host disease (GVHD) as a model for scleroderma. Cell Immunol 77:1–12, 1983.

Jan JE, Hill RH, Low MD. Cerebral complications in juvenile rheumatoid arthritis. Can Med Assoc J 107:623–625, 1972.

Janeway CA, Gitlin D, Craig M, Grice DS. Collagen disease in patients with congenital agammaglobulinemia. Trans Assoc Am Physicians 69:93–97, 1956.

Jankowski J, Crombie I, Jankowski R. Behcet's syndrome in Scotland. Postgrad Med J 68:566–570, 1992.

Janowsky EC, Kupper LL, Hulka BS. Meta-analyses of the relation between silicone breast implants and the risk of connective-tissue diseases. N Engl J Med 342:781–790, 2000.

Jasin HE. Absence of the eighth component of complement (C8) and SLE-like disease. Arthritis Rheum 19:803–804, 1976.

Jennette J, Falk R, Andrassy K, Bacon P, Churg J, Gross W, Hagen E, GS H, Hunder G, Kallenberg CEA. Nomenclature of systemic vasculitides. Proposal of an international consensus conference. Arthritis Rheum 37:187–192, 1994.

Jeremy R, Schaller J, Arkless R, Wedgwood RJ, Healey LA. Juvenile rheumatoid arthritis persisting into adulthood. Am J Med 45:419–434, 1968.

Jessee EF, Owen DS Jr, Sagar KB. The benign hypermobile joint syndrome. Arthritis Rheum 23:1053–1056, 1980.

Jiang Y, Hirose S, Abe M, Sanokawa-Akakura R, Ohtsuji M, Mi X, Li N, Xiu Y, Zhang D, Shirai J, Hamano Y, Fujii H, Shirai T. Polymorphisms in IgG Fc receptor IIB regulatory regions associated with autoimmune susceptibility. Immunogenetics 51:429–435, 2000.

Jimenez SA, Sigal SH. A 15-year prospective study of treatment of rapidly progressive systemic sclerosis with D-penicillamine. J Rheumatol 18:1496–1503, 1991.

Jodo S, Atsumi T, Takeda T, Ogura N, Amasaki Y, Ichikawa K, Tsutsumi A, Mukai M, Onishi K, Fujisaku A, et al. The association of the disease activity of rheumatoid factor positive vasculitis and the level of rheumatoid factor. Nihon Rinsho Meneki Gakkai Kaishi 18:272–281, 1995.

Johnson PM, Faulk WP. Rheumatoid factor: its nature, specificity, and production of rheumatoid arthritis. Clin Immunol Immunopathol 6:414–430, 1976.

Johnson RL, Fink CW, Ziff M. Lymphotoxin formation by lymphocytes and muscle in polymyositis. J Clin Invest 51:2435–2449, 1972.

Joos R, Veys EM, Mielants H, van Werveke S, Goemaere S. Sulfasalazine treatment in juvenile chronic arthritis: An open study. J Rheumatol 18:880–884, 1991.

Kahn MF. Psoriatic arthritis and synovitis, acne, pustulosis, hyperostosis, and osteitis syndrome. Curr Opin Rheumatol 5:428–435, 1993.

Kalovidouris AE, Pourmand R, Passo MH, Plotkin Z. Proliferative response of peripheral blood mononuclear cells to autologous and allogeneic muscle in patients with polymyositis/dermatomyositis. Arthritis Rheum 32:446–453, 1989.

Kalunian KC, Panosian-Sahakian N, Ebling FM, Cohen AH, Louie JS, Kaine J, Hahn BH. Idiotypic characteristics of immunoglobulins associated with human systemic lupus erythematosus. Studies of antibodies deposited in glomeruli of humans. Arthritis Rheum 32:513–522, 1989.

Kalunian KC, Peter JB, Middlekauf HR. Clinical significance of a single test for anticardiolipin antibodies. Am J Med 85:602–608, 1988.

Kanakoudi-Tsakalidou F, Pardalos G, Pratsidou-Gertsi P, Kansouzidou-Kanakoudi A, Tsangaropoulou-Stinga H. Persistent or severe course of reactive arthritis following Salmonella enteritidis infection. A prospective study of 9 cases. Scand J Rheumatol 27:431–434, 1998.

Kanski JJ. Anterior uveitis in juvenile rheumatoid arthritis. Arch Ophthalmol 95:1794–1797, 1977.

Kaplan E, Johnson DR, Cleary PP. Group A streptococcal serotypes isolated from patients and sibling contacts during the resurgence of rheumatic fever in the United States in the mid-1980s. J Infect Dis 159:101–103, 1989.

Kaplan EL. Acute rheumatic fever. Ped Clin North Am 25:817–829, 1978.

Kaplan MH. Immunologic relation of streptococcal and tissue antigens. I. Properties of an antigen in certain strains of group A streptococci exhibiting an immunologic cross-reaction with human tissue. J Immunol 90:595–606, 1963.

Kaplan MH, Meyeserian M, Kushner I. Immunologic studies of heart tissue. IV. Serologic reactions with human heart tissue as revealed by immunofluorescent methods. J Exp Med 113:17–36, 1961.

Kapusta MA, Metrakos JD, Pinsky L. Juvenile rheumatoid arthritis in a mother and her identical twin sons. Arthritis Rheum 12:411–413, 1969.

Karpatkin S, Strick N, Karpatkin M. Cumulative experience in the detection of antiplatelet antibody in 234 patients with idiopathic thrombocytopenic purpura, systemic lupus erythematosus and other clinical disorders. Am J Med 52:776–785, 1972.

Kasakawa S, Heiner DC. Elevated levels of immunoglobulin E in the acute febrile mucocutaneous lymph node syndrome. Pediatr Res 10:108–111, 1976.

Kasapcopur O, Ozbakir F, Arisoy N, Ingol H, Yazici H, Ozdogan H. Frequency of antinuclear antibodies and rheumatoid factor in healthy Turkish children. Turk J Pediatr 41:67–71, 1999.

Kaslow RA, Masi AT. Age, sex and race effects on mortality from systemic lupus erythematosus in the United States. Arthritis Rheum 21:473–479, 1978.

Kato H, Koike S, Yokoyama T. Kawasaki disease: effect of treatment on coronary artery involvement. Pediatrics 63:175–179, 1979.

Katz P, Alling DW, Haynes BF, Fauci AS. Association of Wegener's granulomatosis with HLA-B8. Clin Immunol Immunopathol 14:268–270, 1979.

Kauffman RH, Herrmann WA, Meyer CJ. Circulating IgA-immune complexes in Henoch-Schönlein purpura. Am J Med 69:859–866, 1980.

Kavey RW, Kaplan EL. Resurgence of acute rheumatic fever. Pediatrics 84:585–586, 1989.

Kawasaki T. Acute febrile mucocutaneous syndrome with lymphoid involvement with specific desquamation of the fingers and toes. Arerugi 16:178–222, 1967.

Kawasaki T, Kosaki F, Okawa S, Shigematsu I, Yanagawa H. A new infantile acute febrile mucocutaneous lymph node syndrome (MLNS) prevailing in Japan. Pediatrics 54:271–276, 1974.

Kean WF, Anastassiades TP, Ford PM. Aortic incompetence in HLA-B27-positive juvenile arthritis. Ann Rheum Dis 39:294–295, 1980.

Keat A. HLA-linked disease susceptibility and reactive arthritis. J Infect Dis 5:227–239, 1982.

Keat A. Reiter's syndrome and reactive arthritis in perspective. N Engl J Med 309:1606–1615, 1983.

Keim D, Ragsdale C., Heidelberger K., Sullivan D. Hepatic fibrosis with the use of methotrexate for juvenile rheumatoid arthritis. J Rheumatol 17:846–848, 1990.

Kelly MC, Denburg JA. Cerebrospinal fluid immunoglobulins and neuronal antibodies in neuropsychiatric systemic lupus erythematosus and related conditions. J Rheumatol 14:740–744, 1987.

Kera J, Mizuki N, Ota M, Katsuyama Y, Pivetti-Pezzi P, Ohno S, Inoko H. Significant associations of HLA-B*5101 and B*5108, and lack of association of class II alleles with Behcet's disease in Italian patients. Tissue Antigens 54:565–571, 1999.

Khan MA. An overview of clinical spectrum and heterogeneity of spondyloarthropathies. Rheum Dis Clin North Am 18:1–10, 1992.

Khan MA, van der Linden SM. Ankylosing spondylitis and other spondyloarthropathies. Rheum Dis Clin North Am 16:551–579, 1990.

Khanna AK, Buskirk DR, Williams RCJ, Gibofsky A, Crow MK, Menon A, Fotina M, Reid HM, Poon-King T, Rubinstein P, Zabriskie JB. Presence of a non-HLA B cell antigen in rheumatic fever patients and their families as defined by a monoclonal antibody. J Clin Invest 83:1710–1716, 1989.

Kilbourne EM, Rigau-Perez JG, Heath CWJ, Heath CW Jr, Zack MM, Falk H, Martin-Marcos M, de Carlos A. Clinical epidemiology of toxic-oil syndrome: manifestations of a new illness. N Engl J Med 309:1408–1414, 1983.

Kilmartin D, Forrester J, Dick A. Cyclosporin A therapy in refractory non-infectious childhood uveitis. Br J Ophthalmol 82:737–7742, 1998.

Kim H, Kim MO, Ahn MJ, Lee YY, Jung TJ, Choi IY, Kim IS, Park CK. Eosinophilic fasciitis preceding relapse of peripheral T-cell lymphoma. J Korean Med Sci 15:346–350, 2000.

Kim SW, Rice L, Champlin R, Udden MM. Aplastic anemia in eosinophilic fasciitis: responses to immunosuppression and marrow transplantation. Haematologia (Budapest) 28:131–137, 1997a.

Kim TH, Jung SS, Sohn SJ, Park MH, Kim SY. Aneurysmal dilatation of ascending aorta and aortic insufficiency in juvenile spondyloarthropathy. Scand J Rheumatol 26:218–221, 1997b.

Kimberly RP, Parris TM, Inman RD, McDougal JS. Dynamics of mononuclear phagocyte system Fc receptor function in systemic lupus erythematosus. Relation to disease activity and circulating immune complexes. Clin Exp Immunol 51:261–268, 1983.

Kirk JA, Ansell BM, Bywaters EG. The hypermobility syndrome. Musculoskeletal complaints associated with generalized joint hypermobility. Ann Rheum Dis 26:419–425, 1967.

Kissel JT, Mendell JR, Ramohan KW. Microvascular deposition of complement membrane attack complex in dermatomyositis. N Engl J Med 314:329–334, 1986.

Klaasen RJ, Goldschmeding R, Dolman KM, Vlekke AB, Weigel HM, Eeftinck Schattenkerk JK, Mulder JW, Westedt ML, von dem Borne AE. Anti-neutrophil cytoplasmic autoantibodies in patients with symptomatic HIV infection. Clin Exp Immunol 87:24–30, 1992.

Klepper SE. Effects of an eight-week physical conditioning program on disease signs and symptoms in children with chronic arthritis. Arthritis Care Res 12:52–60, 1999.

Klings ES, Farber HW. IV epoprostenol for systemic sclerosis. Chest 118:881–882, 2000.

Kocak G, Imamoglu A, Tutar HE, Atalay S, Turkay S. Poststreptococcal reactive arthritis: clinical course and outcome in 15 patients. Turk J Pediatr 42:101–104, 2000.

Koerper MA, Stempel DA, Dallman PR. Anemia in patients with juvenile rheumatoid arthritis. J Pediatr 92:930–933, 1978.

Koff RS. Case records of the Massachusetts General Hospital. N Engl J Med 296:1337–1346, 1977.

Koffler D, Agnello V, Carr RI, Kunkel HG. Variable patterns of immunoglobulin and complement deposition in the kidneys of patients with systemic lupus erythematosus. Am J Path 56:305–316, 1969.

Koffler D, Schur PH, Kunkel HG. Immunological studies concerning the nephritis of systemic lupus erythematosus. J Exp Med 126:607–623, 1967.

Kohler PF, Bensel R. Serial complement component alterations in acute glomerulonephritis and systemic lupus erythematosus. Clin Exp Immun 4:191–202, 1969.

Kohr RM. Progressive asymptomatic coronary artery disease as a fatal sequela of Kawasaki disease. J Pediatric 108:256–259, 1986.

Kolble K, Reid KB. Genetic deficiencies of the complement system and association with disease—early components. Int Rev Immunol 10:17–36, 1993.

Komine M, Matsuyama T, Nojima Y, Minoda S, Furue M, Tsuchida T, Sakai S, Ishibashi Y. Systemic lupus erythematosus with hereditary deficiency of the fourth component of complement. Int J Dermatol 31:653–656, 1992.

Kondo H, Kajii E, Oyamada T, Kasahara Y. Direct antiglobulin test negative autoimmune hemolytic anemia associated with autoimmune hepatitis. Int J Hematol 68:439–443, 1998.

Koren G, Rose V, Lavi S. Probable efficacy of high-dose salicylates in reducing coronary involvement in Kawasaki disease. JAMA 254:767–769, 1985.

Kornreich HK, King KK, Bernstein BH, Singsen BH, Hanson V. Scleroderma in childhood. Arthritis Rheum 20:343–350, 1977.

Koster-King K, Kornreich HK, Bernstein BH, Singsen BH, Hanson V. The clinical spectrum of systemic lupus erythematosus in childhood. Arthritis Rheum 20:287–294, 1977.

Kozin F, Carrera GF, Ryan LM, Foley D, Lawson TL. Computed tomography in the diagnosis of sacroiliitis. Arthritis Rheum 24:1479–1485, 1981.

Krammer PH. CD95's deadly mission in the immune system. Nature 407:789–795, 2000.

Krupp L, Masur D, Schwartz J, Coyle P, Langenbach L, Fernquist S, Jandorf L, Halperin J. Cognitive functioning in late Lyme borreliosis. Arch Neurol 48:1125–1129, 1991.

Kumar B, Dhar S, Handa S, Kaur I. Methotrexate in childhood psoriasis. Pediatr Dermatol 11:271–273, 1994.

Kunkel HG, and Tan EM. Autoantibodies and disease. Adv Immunol 4:351–395, 1964.

Kuno-Sakai H, Sakai H, Nomoto Y. Increase of IgA-bearing peripheral blood lymphocytes in children with Henoch-Schönlein purpura. Pediatrics 64:918–922, 1979.

Laaksonen A. A prognostic study of juvenile rheumatoid arthritis. Acta Paediatr Scand 166(Suppl):1–16, 1966.

Lacks S, White P. Morbidity associated with childhood systemic lupus erythematosus. J Rheumatol 17:941–945, 1990.

Ladd JR, Cassidy JT, Martel W. Juvenile ankylosing spondylitis. Arthritis Rheum 14:579–590, 1971.

Laitman RS, Glicklich D, Sablay LB, Grayzel AI, Bartland P, and Bank N. Effect of long-term normalization of serum complement levels on the course of lupus nephritis. Am J Med 87:132–138, 1989.

Lambert JR, Ansell BM, Stephenson E, Wright V. Psoriatic arthritis in childhood. Clin Rheum Dis 2:339–352, 1976.

Lambert NC, Distler O, Muller-Ladner U, Tylee TS, Furst DE, Nelson JL. HLA-DQA1*0501 is associated with diffuse systemic sclerosis in Caucasian men. Arthritis Rheum 43:2005–2010, 2000.

Lampert F. Infantile multisystem inflammatory disease: another case of a new syndrome. Eur J Pediatr 144:593–596, 1986.

Lampert F, Belohradsky BH, Forster C, Eife R, Kollmann D, Stochdorph O, Gokel JM, Meister P, Lampert PW. Letter: Infantile chronic relapsing inflammation of the brain, skin, and joints. Lancet 1:1250–1251, 1975.

Lanham JG, Walport MJ, Hughes GRV. Congenital heart block and familial connective tissue disease. J Rheumatol 10:823–825, 1983.

Lavalle C, Pizzaro S, Drenkard C. A manifestation of systemic lupus erythematosus strongly associated with antiphospholipid antibodies. J Rheumatol 17:34–37, 1990.

Lawrence JM, Moore TL, Osborn TG, Nesher G, Madson KL, Kinsella MB. Autoantibody studies in juvenile rheumatoid arthritis. Semin Arthritis Rheum 22:265–274, 1993.

Laxer RM, Allen RC, Malleson PN, Morrison RT, Petty RE. Technetium 99m-methylene diphosphonate bone scans in children with reflex neurovascular dystrophy. J Pediatr 106:437–440, 1985.

Laxer RM, Roberts EA, Gross KR, Britton JR, Cutz E, Dimmick J, Petty RE, Silverman ED. Liver disease and neonatal lupus eyrthematosus. J Pediatr 116:238–242, 1990.

Leak A. Autoantibody profile in juvenile chronic arthritis. Ann Rheum Dis 47:178–182, 1988.

Leak AM and Woo P. Juvenile chronic arthritis, chronic iridocyclitis, and reactivity to histones. Ann Rheum Dis 50:653–657, 1991.

Leandro MJ, Edwards JC, Cambridge G, Ehrenstein MR, Isenberg DA. An open study of B lymphocyte depletion in systemic lupus erythematosus. Arthritis Rheum 46: 2673–2677, 2003.

Lebovics RS, Hoffman GS, Leavitt RY, Kerr GS, Travis WD, Kammerer W, Hallahan C, Rottem M, Fauci AS. The management of subglottic stenosis in patients with Wegener's granulomatosis. Laryngoscope 102:1341–1345, 1992.

Leddy JP, Griggs RC, Klemperer MR, Frank MM. Hereditary complement (C2) deficiency with dermatomyositis. Am J Med 58:83–91, 1975.

Lee HS, Mujais SK, Kasinath BS, Spargo BH, Katz AI. Course of renal pathology in patients with systemic lupus erythematosus. Am J Med 77:612–620, 1984.

Lee LA, Weston WL. New findings in neonatal lupus syndrome. Am J Dis Child 138:233–236, 1984.

Leff RL, Love LA, Miller FW, Greenberg SJ, Klein EA, Dalakas MC, Plotz PH. Viruses in idiopathic inflammatory myopathies: absence of candidate viral genomes in muscle. Lancet 339:1192–1195, 1992.

Lehman TJA, McCurdy DK, Bernstein BH, King KK, Hanson V. Systemic lupus erythematosus in the first decade of life. Pediatrics 83:235–239, 1989.

Lehman, TJA, Striegel KH, Onel KB Thalidomide therapy for recalcitrant systemic onset juvenile rheumatoid arthritis. J Pediatr 140:125–127, 2002.

Lei B, Mackie S, Lukomski S, Musser JM. Identification and immunogenicity of group A streptococcus culture supernatant proteins. Infect Immun 68:6807–6818, 2000.

Leirisalo M, Skylv G, Kousa M, Voipio-Pulkki LM, Suoranta H, Nissila M, Hvidman L, Nielsen ED, Svejaard A, Tilikainen A, Laitinen O. Follow-up study on patients with Reiter's disease and reactive arthritis with special reference to HLA-B27. Arthritis Rheum 25:249–259, 1982.

Leitman PS, Bywaters EGL. Pericarditis in juvenile rheumatoid arthritis. Pediatrics 32:855–860, 1963.

Leandro MJ, Edwards JC, Cambridge G, Ehrenstein MR, Isenberg DA. An open study of B lymphocyte depletion in systemic lupus erythematosus. Arthritis Rheum 46:2673–2677, 2002.

Lepore L, Kiren V. Autologous bone marrow transplantation versus alternative drugs in pediatric rheumatic diseases. Haematologica 85:89–92, 2000.

Lerman SJ, Nankervis GA, Heggie AD, Gold E. Immunologic response, virus excretion, and joint reactions with rubella vaccine. A study of adolescent girls and young women given live attenuated virus vaccine (HPV-77:DE-5). Ann Intern Med 74:67–73, 1971.

Lerner MR, Steitz JA. Antibodies to small nuclear RNAs complexed with proteins are produced by patients with systemic lupus erythematosus. Proc Natl Acad Sci USA 76:5495–5499, 1979.

Leung DY. Immunologic aspects of Kawasaki syndrome. J Rheumatol 17(Suppl 24):15–18, 1990.

Leung DY, Siegel RL, Grady S, Krensky A, Meade R, Reinherz EL, Geha RS. Immunoregulatory abnormalities in mucocutaneous lymph node syndrome. Clin Immunol Immunopathol 23:100–112, 1982.

Leung DYM, Meissner HC, Fulton DR, Murray DL, Kotzin BL, Schlievert PM. Toxic shock syndrome toxin-secreting Staphylococcus aureus in Kawasaki syndrome. Lancet 342:1385–1388, 1993.

Levy M, Koren G. Atypical Kawasaki's disease: analysis of clinical presentation and diagnostic clues. Pediatr Infect Dis J 9:122–126, 1990.

Levy M, Broyer M, Arsan A. Anaphylactoid purpura nephritis in childhood: natural history and immunopathology. Adv Nephrol 6:183–228, 1976.

Liberman L, Hordof AJ, Alfayyadh M, Salafia CM, Pass RH. Torsade de pointes in a child with acute rheumatic fever. J Pediatr 138:280–282, 2001.

Lieberman E, Heuser E, Hanson V, Kornreich H, Donnell GN, Landing BH. Identical three-year old twins with disseminated lupus erythematosus: one with nephrosis and one with nephritis. Arthritis Rheum 11:22–32, 1968.

Lindqvist AK, Alarcon-Riquelme ME. The genetics of systemic lupus erythematosus. Scand J Immunol 50:562–571, 1999.

Lindsley C, Schaller J. Arthritis associated with inflammatory bowel disease in children. J Pediatr 84:16–20, 1974.

Linnemann CCJ, Levinson JE, Buncher CR, Schiff GM. Rubella antibody levels in juvenile rheumatoid arthritis. Ann Rheum Dis 34:354–358, 1975.

Listing J, Rau R, Muller B, Alten R, Gromnica-Ihle E, Hagemann D, Zink A. HLA-DRB1 genes, rheumatoid factor, and elevated C-reactive protein: independent risk factors of radiographic progression in early rheumatoid arthritis. Berlin Collaborating Rheumatological Study Group. J Rheumatol 27:2100–2109, 2000.

Litsey SE, Noonan JA, O'Connor WN, Cottrill CM, Mitchell B. Maternal connective tissue disease and congenital heart block. Demonstration of immunoglobulin in cardiac tissue. N Engl J Med 312:98–100, 1985.

Livingston JZ, Scott TE, Wigley FM. Systemic sclerosis (scleroderma): clinical, genetic, and serologic subsets. J Rheumatol 14:512, 1987.

Lockie GN, Hunder GG. Reiter's syndrome in children: a case report and review. Arthritis Rheum 14:767–772, 1971.

Lockshin MD, Bonfa E, Elkon K, Druzin ML. Neonatal lupus risk to newborns of mothers with systemic lupus erythematosus. Arthritis Rheum 31:697–701, 1988.

Logigian EL, Kaplan RF, Steere AC. Chronic neurologic manifestations of Lyme disease. N Engl J Med 323:1438–1444, 1990.

Love L, Leff R, Targoff I, Dalakas M, Plotz P, Miller F. A new approach to the classification of idiopathic inflammatory myopathy: myositis-specific autoantibodies define useful homogenous patient groups. Medicine 70:360–374, 1991.

Love PE, Santoro SA. Antiphospholipid antibodies: anticardiolipin and the lupus anticoagulant in systemic lupus erythematosus (SLE) and in non-SLE disorders. Ann Intern Med 112:682–698, 1990.

Lovell DJ, Giannini EH, Reiff A, Cawkwell GD, Silverman ED, Nocton JJ, Stein LD, Gedalia A, Ilowite NT, Wallace CA, Whitmore J, Finck BK. Etanercept in children with polyarticular juvenile rheumatoid arthritis. Pediatric Rheumatology Collaborative Study Group. N Engl J Med 342:763–769, 2000.

Lowenstein J, Rothfield NF, Gallo C, McCluskey RT. The clinical course of proliferative and membranous forms of lupus nephritis. Ann Intern Med 73:929–942, 1970.

Lue HC, Wu MH, Wang JK, Wu FF, Wu YN. Long-term outcome of patients with rheumatic fever receiving benzathine penicillin G prophylaxis every three weeks versus every four weeks. J Pediatr 125:812–816, 1994.

Lueck CJ, Trend P, Swash M. Cyclosporin in the management of polymyositis and dermatomyositis. J Neurol 54:1007–1008, 1991.

Lyback CO, Belt EA, Hamalainen MM, Kauppi MJ, Savolainen HA, Lehto MU. Survivorship of AGC knee replacement in juvenile chronic arthritis: 13-year follow-up of 77 knees. J Arthroplasty 15:166–170, 2000.

Madaio MP, Carlson J, Cataldo J, Ucci A, Migliorini P, Pankewycs O. Murine monoclonal anti-DNA antibodies bind directly to glomerular antigens and form immune deposits. J Immunol 138:2883–2893, 1987.

Maddison PJ, Skinner RP, Vlachoyiannopoulos P. Antibodies to nRNP, Sm, Ro(SSA) and La(SSB) detected by ELISA: their specificity and inter-relations in connective tissue disease sera. Clin Exp Immunol 62:337–345, 1985.

Maggiore G, Martin A, Crifeo S. Hepatitis B virus infection and Schönlein-Henoch purpura. Am J Dis Child 138:681–682, 1984.

Majeed HA, Khuffash FA, Bhatnagar S, Farwana S, Yusuf AR, Yousof AM. Acute rheumatic polyarthritis. Am J Dis Child 144:831–833, 1990.

Makai F, Vojtek R. Implantation of 110 total hip joint endoprosthesis using the Zweymuller method. Acta Chir Orthop Traumatol Cech 61:20–24, 1994.

Malagon C, Vankerckhove C, Giannini EH, Taylor J, Lovell DJ, Levinson JE, Passo MH, Ginsberg J, Burke MJ, Glass DN. The iridocyclitis of early onset pauciarticular juvenile rheumatoid arthritis: outcome in immunogenetically characterized patients. J Rheumatol 19:160–163, 1992.

Malleson PN. Controversies in juvenile dermatomyositis. J Rheumatol 17(Suppl 22):1–6, 1990.

Mandell GA, Contreras SJ, Conard K, Harcke HT, Maas KW. Bone scintigraphy in the detection of chronic recurrent multifocal osteomyelitis. J Nucl Med 39:1778–1783, 1998.

Manger K, Repp R, Spriewald BM, Rascu A, Geiger A, Wassmuth R, Westerdaal NA, Wentz B, Manger B, Kalden JR, van de Winkel JG. Fcgamma receptor IIa polymorphism in Caucasian patients with systemic lupus erythematosus: association with clinical symptoms. Arthritis Rheum 41:1181–1189, 1998.

Manjula BN, Trus BL, Fischetti VA. Presence of two distinct regions in the coiled-coil structure of the streptococcal Pep M5 protein: relationship to mammalian coiled-coil proteins and implications to its biological properties. Proc Natl Acad Sci USA 82:1064–1068, 1985.

Mannerkorpi K, Nyberg B, Ahlmen M, Ekdahl C. Pool exercise combined with an education program for patients with fibromyalgia syndrome. A prospective, randomized study. J Rheumatol 27:2473–2481, 2000.

Manners JP, Ansell BM. Slow acting antirheumatic drug use in systemic onset juvenile chronic arthritis. Pediatrics 77:99–103, 1986.

Mannik M, Nardella FA. IgG rheumatoid factors and self-association of these antibodies. Clin Rheum Dis 11:551–572, 1985.

Marcon MJ, Hribar MM, Hosier DM, Powell DA, Brady MT, Hamoudi AC, Kaplan EL. Occurrence of mucoid M-18 streptococcus pyogenes in a central Ohio pediatric population. J Clin Microbiol 26:1539–1542, 1988.

Marino M, Ruvo M, De Falco S, Fassina G. Prevention of systemic lupus erythematosus in MRL/lpr mice by administration of an immunoglobulin-binding peptide. Nat Biotechnol 18:735–739, 2000.

Markowitz M. The changing picture of rheumatic fever. Arthritis Rheum 20:369–374, 1977.

Markowitz M. The decline of rheumatic fever: role of medical intervention. J Pediatr 106:545–550, 1985.

Markowitz M, Gordis L. Rheumatic fever. Philadelphia, WB Saunders, 1972.

Marks SH, Barnett M, Calin A. A case-control study of juvenile and adult onset ankylosing spondylitis. J Rheumatol 9:739–741, 1982.

Markusse HM, Dijkmans BA, Fibbe W. Eosinophilic fasciitis after allogeneic bone marrow transplantation. J Rheumatol 17:692–694, 1990.

Martinez-Frontanilla LA, Haase GM, Ernster JA. Surgical complications in Henoch-Schönlein purpura. J Ped Surg 19:434–436, 1984.

Martini A, Lorini R, Zanaboni D, Ravelli A, Burgio R. Frequency of autoantibodies in normal children. Am J Dis Child 143:493–496, 1989.

Masi AT, Kaslow RA. Sex effects in systemic lupus erythematosus. Arthritis Rheum 21:480–484, 1978.

Massell BF, Chute CG, Walker AM, Kurland GS. Penicillin and the marked decrease in morbidity and mortality from rheumatic fever in the United States. N Engl J Med 318:280–286, 1988.

Massell BF, Fyler DC, Roy SB. The clinical picture of rheumatic fever. Diagnosis, immediate prognosis course and therapeutic implications. Am J Cardiol 1:436–449, 1958.

Mastaglia FL, Laing BA, Zilko P. Treatment of inflammatory myopathies. Baillieres Clin Neurol 2:717–740, 1993.

Masuoka H, Kikuchi K, Takahashi S, Kakinuma T, Hayashi N, Furue M. Eosinophilic fasciitis associated with low-grade T-cell lymphoma. Br J Dermatol 139:928–930, 1998.

Mazzuca SA, Yung R, Brandt KD, Yee RD, Katz BP. Current practices for monitoring ocular toxicity related to hydroxychloroquine (Plaquenil) therapy. J Rheumatol 21:59–63, 1994.

McCue CM, Mantakas ME, Tingelstad JB, Ruddy S. Congenital heart block in newborns of mothers with connective tissue disease. Circulation 56:82–90, 1977.

McCuistion CH, Schoch EP. Possible discoid lupus erythematosus in newborn infant. Report of a case with subsequent development of acute sytemic lupus erythematosus in mother. Arch Dermatol 70:782–785, 1954.

McCune AB, Weston WI, Lee LA. Maternal and fetal outcome in neonatal lupus erythematosus. Ann Intern Med 106:518–523, 1987.

McDermott MF, Aksentijevich I, Galon J, McDermott EM, Ogunkolade BW, Centola M, Mansfield E, Gadina M, Karenko L, Pettersson T, McCarthy J, Frucht DM, Aringer M, Torosyan Y, Teppo AM, Wilson M, Karaarslan HM, Wan Y, Todd I, Wood G, Schlimgen R, Kumarajeewa TR, Cooper SM, Vella JP, Kastner DL. Germline mutations in the extracellular domains of the 55 kDa TNF receptor, TNFR1, define a family of dominantly inherited autoinflammatory syndromes. Cell 97:133–144, 1999.

McKown KM, Carbone LD, Bustillo J, Seyer JM, Kang AH, Postlethwaite AE. Induction of immune tolerance to human type I collagen in patients with systemic sclerosis by oral administration of bovine type I collagen. Arthritis Rheum 43:1054–1061, 2000.

McLaren MJ, Hawkins DM, Koornhof HJ, Bloom KR, Bramwell-Jones DM, Cohen E, Gale GE, Kannrek K, Lachman AS, Lakier JB, Pocock WA, Barlow JB. Epidemiology of rheumatic heart disease in black school children of Soweto, Johannesburg. Brit Med J 5981:474–478, 1975.

McLaughlin JF, Schaller J, Wedgwood RJ. Arthritis and immunodeficiency. J Pediatr 81:801–803, 1972.

Meade RH, Brandt L. Manifestations of Kawasaki disease in New England outbreak of 1980. J Pediatr 100:558–562, 1982.

Mear JP, Schreiber KL, Munz C, Zhu X, Stevanovic S, Rammensee HG, Rowland-Jones SL, Colbert RA. Misfolding of HLA-B27 as a result of its B pocket suggests a novel mechanism for its role in

susceptibility to spondyloarthropathies. J Immunol 163:6665–6670, 1999.

Mease P, Ochs H, Wedgwood R. Successful treatment of echovirus meningoencephalitis and myositis-fasciitis with intravenous immune globulin therapy in a patient with X-linked agammaglobulinemia. N Engl J Med 304:1278–1281, 1981.

Meislin AG, Rothfield N. Systemic lupus erythematosus in childhood. Pediatrics 42:37–49, 1968.

Melina-Aldana H, Giannini EH, Taylor J, Lovell DJ, Levinson JE, Passo MH, Ginsberg J, Burke MJ, Glass DN. Human leukocyte antigen-DRB1*1104 in the chronic iridocyclitis of pauciarticular juvenile rheumatoid arthritis. J Pediatr 121:56–60, 1992.

Melish ME, Hicks RM, Larson EJ. Mucocutaneous lymph node syndrome in the United States. Am J Dis Child 130:599–607, 1976.

Mellins E, Malleson P, Schaller JG, Hansen J. Childhood dermatomyositis: immunogenetic and family studies. VIII Pan-American Congress of Rheumatology. Arthritis Rheum 25:S151, 1982.

Merino Munoz R, Viota Losada F, Sancho Madrid B, Castro Gussoni C, Garcia-Consuegra Molina J. Rheumatic fever and post-streptococcal arthritis. Clinical review. An Esp Pediatr 35:239–242, 1991.

Merkel PA, Polisson RP, Chang Y, Skates SJ, Niles JL. Prevalence of antineutrophil cytoplasmic antibodies in a large inception cohort of patients with connective tissue disease. Ann Intern Med 126:866–873, 1997.

Merriam JC, Chylack LT, Albert DM. Early-onset pauciarticular juvenile rheumatoid arthritis: a histopathologic study. Arch Ophthalmol 101:1085–1092, 1983.

Meyer F, Garin L, Smati C, Gaspard M, Giannoli C, Rigal D. Application of the gel test using and anti-IgA antiglobulin for the immunologic diagnosis of autoimmune hemolytic anemia with a negative direct Coomb's test. Transfus Clin Biol 6:221–226, 1999.

Michael AF, Vernier RL, Drummond KN, Levitt JI, Herdman RC, Fish AJ, Good RA. Immunosuppressive therapy of chronic renal disease. N Engl J Med 276:817–828, 1967.

Michel M, Piette J, Roullet E, Duron F, Frances C, Nahum L, Pelletier N, Crassard I, Nunez S, Michel C, Bach J, Tournier-Lasserve E. The R131 low-affinity allele of the Fc gamma RIIA receptor is associated with systemic lupus erythematosus but not with other autoimmune diseases in French Caucasians. Am J Med 108:580–583, 2000.

Michet CJJ, Doyle JA, Ginsburg WW. Eosinophilic fasciitis. Mayo Clin Proc 56:27–34, 1981.

Miles S, Isenberg DA. A review of serological abnormalities in relatives of SLE patients. Lupus 2:145–150, 1993.

Milgrom F. Development of rheumatoid factor research through 50 years. Scand J Rheumatol Suppl 75:2–12, 1988.

Miller FW, Leitman SF, Cronin ME, Hicks JE, Leff RL, Wesley R, Fraser DD, Dalakas M, Plotz PH. Controlled trial of plasma exchange and leukapheresis in polymyositis and dermatomyositis. N Engl J Med 326:1380–1384, 1992a.

Miller LC. Infectious causes of arthritis in adolescents. Adolesc Med 9:115–126, 1998.

Miller LC, Gray ED, Regelmann WE. Cytokines and immunoglobulin in rheumatic heart disease: production by blood and tonsillar mononuclear cells. J Rheumatol 16:1436–1442, 1989.

Miller LC, Sisson BA, Tucker LB, DeNardo BA, Schaller JG. Methotrexate treatment of recalcitrant childhood dermatomyositis. Arthritis Rheum 35:1143–1149, 1992b.

Miller RW, Salcedo JR, Fink RJ, Murphy TM, Magilavy DB. Pulmonary hemorrhage in pediatric patients with systemic lupus erythematosus. J Pediatr 108:576–579, 1986.

Miura M, Okabe T, Tsubata S, Takizawa N, Sawaguchi T. Chronic infantile neurological cutaneous articular syndrome in a patient from Japan. Eur J Pediatr 156:624–626, 1997.

Miyagawa S, Fukumoto T, Hashimoto K, Yoshioka A, Shirai T, Shinohara K, Kidoguchi KI, Fujita T. Neonatal lupus erythematosus: haplotypic analysis of HLA class II alleles in child/mother pairs. Arthritis Rheum 40:982–983, 1997.

Miyata K, Kawakami K, Onimaru T, Baba Y, Ono S, Hokonohara M, Yoshinaga M, Terawaki T. Circulating immune complexes and granulocytes chemotaxis in Kawasaki disease. Jpn Circ J 48:1350–1353, 1984.

Moak JP, Barron KS, Hougen TJ, Wiles HB, Balaji S, Sreeram N, Cohen MH, Nordenberg A, Van Hare GF, Friedman RA, Perez M, Cecchin F, Schneider DS, Nehgme RA, Buyon JP. Congenital heart block: development of late-onset cardiomyopathy, a previously underappreciated sequela. J Am Coll Cardiol 37:238–242, 2001.

Moll JMH, Wright V. New York clinical criteria for ankylosing spondylitis. Ann Rheum Dis 32:354–363, 1973.

Moncada B, Day NK, Good RA, Windhorst DB. Lupus-erythematosus-like syndrome with a familiar defect of complement. N Engl J Med 286:689–693, 1972.

Monestier M, Losman JA, Fasy TM, Debbas ME, Massa M, Albani S, Bohn L, Martini A. Antihistone antibodies in antinuclear antibody-positive juvenile arthritis. Arthritis Rheum 33:1836–1841, 1990.

Mongan ES, Leddy JP, Atwater EC, Barnett EV. Direct antiglobulin (Coombs') reactions in patients with connective tissue diseases. Arthritis Rheum 10:502–508, 1967.

Moore T, Dorner RW, Zuckner J. Hidden rheumatoid factor in seronegative juvenile rheumatoid arthritis. Ann Rheum Dis 33:255–257, 1974.

Moore TL, Dorner RW. Rheumatoid factors. Clin Biochem 26:75–84, 1993.

Moore TL, Dorner RW, Osborn TG, Zuckner J. Hidden 19S IgM rheumatoid factors. Semin Arthritis Rheum 18:72–75, 1988.

Moore TL, Dorner RW, Weiss TD. Hidden 19S IgM rheumatoid factor in juvenile rheumatoid arthritis. J Rheumatol 9:599–602, 1980.

Moore TL, Zuckner J, Baldassare AR, Weiss TD, Dorner RW. Complement-fixing hidden rheumatoid factor in juvenile rheumatoid arthritis. Arthritis Rheum 21:935–941, 1978.

Moorthy AV, Chesney RW, Segar WE, Groshong T. Wegener granulomatosis in childhood: prolonged survival following cytotoxic therapy. J Pediatr 91:616–618, 1977.

Moreno Alvarez MJ, Espada G, Maldonado-Cocco JA, Gagliardi SA. Longterm followup of hip and knee soft tissue release in juvenile chronic arthritis. J Rheumatol 19:1608–1610, 1992.

Morris R, Metzger A, Bluestone R, Terasaki P. HL-AW27–a clue to the diagnosis and pathogenesis of Reiter's syndrome. N Engl J Med 290:554–556, 1974a.

Morris RI, Metzger AL, Bluestone R, Terasaki PI. HL-A-W27– a useful discriminator in the arthropathies of inflammatory bowel disease. N Engl J Med 290:1117–1119, 1974b.

Mottonen T, Paimela L, Leirisalo-Repo M, Kautiainen H, Ilonen J, Hannonen P. Only high disease activity and positive rheumatoid factor indicate poor prognosis in patients with early rheumatoid arthritis treated with "sawtooth" strategy. Ann Rheum Dis 57:533–539, 1998.

Moulds JM, Rolih C, Goldstein R, Whittington KF, Warner NB, Targoff IN, Reichlin M, Arnett FC. C4 null genes in American whites and blacks with myositis. J Rheumatol 17:331–334, 1990.

Mouy R, Stephan JL, Pillet P, Haddad E, Hubert P, Prieur AM. Efficacy of cyclosporine A in the treatment of macrophage activation syndrome in juvenile arthritis: report of five cases. J Pediatr 129:750–754, 1996.

Mulberg AE, Linz C, Bern E, Tucker LB, Verhave M, Grand RJ. Identification of nonsteroidal antiinflammatory drug-induced gastroduodenal injury in children with juvenile rheumatoid arthritis. J Pediatr 122:647–649, 1993.

Mulley J, Saar K, Hewitt G, Ruschendorf F, Phillips H, Colley A, Sillence D, Reis A, Wilson M. Gene localization for an autosomal dominant familial periodic fever to 12p13. Am J Hum Genet 62:884–889, 1998.

Munieus EF, Schur PH. Antibodies to Sm and RNP: prognosticators of disease involvement. Arthritis Rheum 26:848–853, 1983.

Munro-Faure H. Necrotizing arteries of the coronary vessels in infancy. Pediatrics 23:914–926, 1959.

Murphy TK, Goodman WK, Ayoub EM, Voeller KK. On defining Sydenham's chorea: where do we draw the line? Biol Psychiatry 47:851–857, 2000.

Myllykangas-Luosujarvi R, Jantunen E, Kaipiainen-Seppanen O, Mahlamaki E, Nousiainen T. Autologous peripheral blood stem cell transplantation in a patient with severe mixed connective tissue disease. Scand J Rheumatol 29:326–327, 2000.

Nakamaru Y, Maguchi S, Takizawa M, Fukuda S, Inuyama Y. The association between human leukocyte antigens (HLA) and cytoplasmic-antineutrophil cytoplasmic antibody (cANCA)-positive Wegener's granulomatosis in a Japanese population. Rhinology 34:163–165, 1996.

Nakamura RM, Tan EM. Recent progress in the study of autoantibodies to nuclear antigens. Hum Pathol 9:85–91, 1978.

Nakamura RM, Tan EM. Update on autoantibodies to intracellular antigens in systemic rheumatic diseases. Clin Lab Med 12:1–23, 1992.

Nakano H, Nojima K, Saito A, Ueda K. High incidence of aortic regurgitation following Kawasaki disease. J Pediatr 107:59–63, 1985.

Nakano H, Saito A, Ueda K, Nojima K. Clinical characteristics of myocardial infarction following Kawasaki disease: report of 11 cases. J Pediatr 108:198–203, 1986.

Naoe S, Takahashi K, Masuda H, Tanaka N. Coronary findings post Kawasaki disease in children who died of other causes. In Shulman S, ed. Kawasaki Disease. New York, Alan R. Liss, 1987, pp 341–346.

Naparstek K, Andre-Schwartz J, Manser T, Wysocki L, Breitman L, Stollar BD, Schwartz RS. A single VH germline gene segment of normal A/J mice encodes autoantibodies characteristic of sytemic lupus erythematosus. J Exp Med 164:614–626, 1986.

Nelson JL, Furst DE, Maloney S, Gooley T, Evans PC, Smith A, Bean MA, Ober C, Bianchi DW. Microchimerism and HLA-compatible relationships of pregnancy in scleroderma. Lancet 351:559–562, 1998.

Nemazee D. Receptor selection in B and T lymphocytes. Annu Rev Immunol 18:19–51, 2000.

Nepom BS, Glass D. Juvenile rheumatoid arthritis and HLA-Report of the Park City III Workshop. J Rheumatol 19:70–74, 1992.

Nepom BS, Schaller JG. Childhood systemic lupus erythematosus. In Cohen A, ed. Progress in clinical rheumatology, I. New York, Grune and Stratton, 1984, pp 33–69.

Nepom BS, Nepom GT, Michelson E, Schaller JG, Antonelli P, Hansen JA. Specific HLA-Dr4 associated histocompatibility molecules characterize patients with juvenile rheumatoid arthritis. J Clin Invest 74:287–291, 1982.

Nepom GT, Nepom B. Genetics of the major histocompatibility complex in rheumatoid arthritis. In Klippel JH, Dieppe PA, eds. Rheumatology. London, Mosby, 1998, pp 5.7.1–5.7.12.

Newburger J, Takahashi M, Beiser A, Burns J, Bastian J, Chung K, Colan S, et al. A single intravenous infusion of gamma globulin as compared with four infusions in the treatment of acute Kawasaki's syndrome. N Engl J Med 324:1633–1639, 1991.

Nicassio PM, Radojevic V, Weisman MH, Schuman C, Kim J, Schoenfeld-Smith K, Krall T. A comparison of behavioral and educational interventions for fibromyalgia. J Rheumatol 24:2000–2007, 1997.

Nimelstein SH, Brody S, McShane D, Holman HR. Mixed connective tissue disease: a subsequent evaluation of the original 25 patients. Medicine 59:239–248, 1980.

Nocton JJ, Dressler F, Rutledge BJ, Rys PN, Persing DH, Steere AC. Detection of Borrelia burgdorferi DNA by polymerase chain reaction in synovial fluid from patients with Lyme arthritis. N Engl J Med 330:229–234, 1994.

Nocton JJ, Miller LC, Tucker LB, Schaller JG. Human parvovirus B19-associated arthritis in children. J Pediatr 122:186–190, 1993.

Nolle B, Specks U, Ludemann J, Rohrbach MS, DeRemee RA, Gross WL. Anticytoplasmic autoantibodies; their immunodiagnostic value in Wegener's granulomatosis. Ann Intern Med 111:28–40, 1989.

Norris DG, Colon AR, Stickler GB. Systemic lupus erythematosus in children. Clin Pediatr 16:774–778, 1977.

Notman DD, Kurata N, Tan EM. Profiles of antinuclear antibodies in systemic rheumatic disease. Ann Intern Med 83:464–469, 1975.

Novack SN, Pearson CM. Cyclophosphamide therapy in Wegener's granulomatosis. N Engl J Med 284:938–942, 1971.

Nurre LD, Rabalais GP, Callen JP. Neutrophilic dermatosis-associated sterile chronic multifocal osteomyelitis in pediatric patients: case report and review. Pediatr Dermatol 16:214–216, 1999.

Nusinow SR, Zuraw BL, Curd JG. The hereditary and acquired deficiencies of complement. Med Clin North Am 69:487–504, 1985.

Nussbaum AI, Silver RM, Maricq HR. Serial changes in nailfold capillary morphology in childhood dermatomyositis. Arthritis Rheum 26:1169–1172, 1983.

O'Duffy JD, Calamia K, Cohen S, Goronzy JJ, Herman D, Jorizzo J, Weyand C, Matteson E. Interferon-alpha treatment of Behcet's disease. J Rheumatol 25:1938–1944, 1998.

O'Malley PG, Balden E, Tomkins G, Santoro J, Kroenke K, Jackson JL. Treatment of fibromyalgia with antidepressants A meta-analysis. J Gen Intern Med 15:659–666, 2000.

Oates JK, Young AC. Sacro-ilitis in Reiter's disease. Brit Med J 1:1013–1015, 1959.

Oen KG, Cheang M. Epidemiology of chronic arthritis in childhood. Semin Arthritis Rheum 26:575–591, 1996.

Oetgen WJ, Boice JA, Lawless OJ. Mixed connective tissue disease in children and adolescents. Pediatrics 67:333–337, 1981.

Ogilvie AL, Antoni C, Dechant C, Manger B, Kalden JR, Schuler G, Luftl M. Treatment of psoriatic arthritis with antitumour necrosis factor-alpha antibody clears skin lesions of psoriasis resistant to treatment with methotrexate. Br J Dermatol 144:587–589, 2001.

Ogra PL, Herd JK. Arthritis associated with induced rubella infection. J Immunol 107:810–813, 1971.

Ogura Y, Suzuki S, Shirakawa T, Masuda M, Nakamura H, Iijima K, Yoshikawa N. Haemophilus parainfluenzae antigen and antibody in children with IgA nephropathy and Henoch-Schönlein nephritis. Am J Kidney Dis 36:47–52, 2000.

Oh M, Petri MA, Kim NA, Sullivan KE. Frequency of the Fc gamma RIIIA-158F allele in African American patients with systemic lupus erythematosus. J Rheumatol 26:1486–1489, 1999.

Olivier C. Rheumatic fever—is it still a problem? J Antimicrob Chemother 45:13–21, 2000.

Olson NY, Lindsley CB. Adjunctive use of hydroxychloroquine in childhood dermatomyositis. J Rheumatol 16:1545–1547, 1989.

Omidi CJ, Siegfried EC. Chronic recurrent multifocal osteomyelitis preceding pyoderma gangrenosum and occult ulcerative colitis in a pediatric patient. Pediatr Dermatol 15:435–438, 1998.

Ono S, Onimaru T, Kawakami K, Hokonohara M, Miyata K. Impaired granulocyte chemotaxis and increased circulatory immune complexes in Kawasaki disease. J Pediatr 106:567–570, 1985.

Onouchi Z, Kawasaki T. Overview of pharmacological treatment of Kawasaki disease. Drugs 58:813–822, 1999.

Oppermann M, Hopken U, Gotze O. Assessment of complement activation in vivo. Immunopharmacol 24:119–134, 1992.

Oppliger IR, Nardella FA, Stone GC, Mannik M. Human rheumatoid factors bear the internal image of the Fc binding region of staphylococcal protein A. J Exp Med 166:702–710, 1987.

Orlowski JP, Clough JD, Dymet PG. Wegener's granulomatosis in the pediatric age group. Pediatrics 61:83–90, 1978.

Ostenson M, Fredriksen K, Kass E, Rekvig O. Identification of antihistone antibodies in subsets of juvenile chronic arthritis. Ann Rheum Dis 48:114–117, 1989.

Osterland CK, Espinoza L, Parker LP, Schur PH. Inherited C2 deficiency and systemic lupus erythematosus: studies on a family. Ann Intern Med 822:323–328, 1975.

Ozanne P, Linderkamp O, Miller FC, Meiselman HJ. Erythrocyte aggregation during normal pregnancy. Am J Obstet Gynecol 147:576–583, 1983.

Ozen S, Besbas N, Saatci U, Bakkaloglu A. Diagnostic criteria for polyarteritis nodosa in childhood. J Pediatr 120:206–209, 1992.

Pachman L. Juvenile dermatomyositis. Pathophysiology and disease expression. Pediatr Clin North Am 42:1071–98, 1995a.

Pachman L. An update on juvenile dermatomyositis. Curr Opin Rheumatol 7:437–441, 1995b.

Pachman LM, Cooke N. Juvenile dermatomyositis: a clinical and immunologic study. J Pediatr 96:226–234, 1980.

Pachman LM, Friedman JM, Maryjowski-Sweeney ML, Jonnason O, Radvany RM, Sharp GC, Cobb MA, Battles ND, Crowe WE, Fink CW, Hanson V, Levinson J, Spencer C, Sullivan D. Immunogenetic studies of juvenile dermatomyositis. III. Study of

antibody to organ-specific and nuclear antigens. Arthritis Rheum 28:151–157, 1985.

Pahle JA. Orthopaedic management of juvenile chronic arthritis (JCA). Z Rheumatol 55:376–387, 1996.

Panush RS, Bianco NE, Schur PH. Serum and synovial fluid IgG, IgA and IgM antigammaglobulins in rheumatoid arthritis. Arthritis Rheum 14:737–747, 1971.

Paul C, Yao Z, Nevinny-Stickel C, Keller E, Schoenwald U, Truckenbrodt H, Hoza J, Suschke HJ, Albert ED. Immunogenetics of juvenile chronic arthritis. I. HLA interaction between A2, DR5/8-DR/DQ, and DPB1*0201 is a general feature of all subsets of early onset pauciarticular juvenile chronic arthritis II. DPB1 polymorphism plays a role in systemic juvenile chronic arthritis. Tissue Antigens 45:280–283, 1995.

Penchas S, Stern Z, Bar-Or D. Heparin and the ESR. Arch Intern Med 138:1864–1865, 1978.

Pereira Da Silva JA, Elkon KB, Hughes GR, Dyck RF, Pepys MB. C-reactive protein levels in systemic lupus erythematosus: a classification criterion? Arthritis Rheum 23:770–771, 1980.

Peters-Golden M, Wise RA, Hochberg MC, Stevens MB, Wigley FM. Carbon monoxide diffusing capacity as predictor of outcome in systemic sclerosis. Am J Med 77:1027–1034, 1984.

Peterson LS, Mason T, Nelson AM, O'Fallon WM, Gabriel SE. Juvenile rheumatoid arthritis in Rochester, Minnesota 1960–1993. Is the epidemiology changing? Arthritis Rheum 39:1385–1390, 1996.

Petty RE, Cassidy JT, Tubergen DG. Association of arthritis with hypogammaglobulinemia. Arthritis Rheum 20:441–443, 1977.

Petty RE, Southwood TR. Classification of childhood arthritis: divide and conquer. J Rheumatol 25:1869–1870, 1998.

Petty RE, Southwood TR, Baum J, Bhettay E, Glass DN, Manners P, Maldonado-Cocco J, Suarez-Almazor M, Orozco-Alcala J, Prieur AM. Revision of the proposed classification criteria for juvenile idiopathic arthritis: Durban, 1997. J Rheumatol 25:1991–1994, 1998.

Pincus T. Laboratory tests in rheumatic disorders. In Klippel JH, Dieppe PA, eds. Rheumatology. London, Mosby, 1998, 2.10.3–2.10.4[AU9].

Pincus T, Hughes GRV, Pincus D, Tina LU, Bellanti JA. Antibodies to DNA in childhood systemic lupus erythematosus. J Pediatr 78:981–984, 1971.

Pincus T, Schur PH, Rose JA, Decker JL, Talal N. Measurement of serum DNA binding activity in systemic lupus erythematosus. N Engl J Med 281:701–705, 1969.

Pistoia V, Buoncompagni A, Scribanis R, Fasce L, Alpigiani G, Cordone G, Ferrarini M, Barrone C, Cottafava F. Cyclosporin A in the treatment of juvenile chronic arthritis and childhood polymyositis-dermatomyositis. Results of a preliminary study [see comments]. Clin Exp Rheumatol 11:203–208, 1993.

Plamondon S, Dent PB, Reed AM. Familial dermatomyositis. J Rheumatol 26:2691–2692, 1999.

Platt JL, Burke BA, Fish AJ, Kim Y, Michael AF. Systemic lupus erythematosus in the first two decades of life. Am J Kidney Dis 2(Suppl 1):212–222, 1982.

Pollak VE, Pirani CL, Schwartz FD. The natural history of the renal manifestations of systemic lupus erythematosus. J Lab Clin Med 63:537–550, 1964.

Pourmand N, Blange I, Ringertz N, Pettersson I. Intracellular localisation of the Ro 52kD auto-antigen in HeLa cells visualised with green fluorescent protein chimeras. Autoimmunity 28:225–233, 1998.

Powell FC, Winkelmann RK, Venencie-LeMarchand F, Spurbeck JL, Schroeter AL. The anticentromere antibody: disease specificity and clinical significance. Mayo Clin Proc 59:700–706, 1984.

Poznanski AK. Radiologic approaches to pediatric joint disease. J Rheumatol 19:78–93, 1992.

Poznanski AK, Glass RBJ, Feinstein KA, Pachman LM, Fisher MR, Hayford JR. Magnetic resonance imaging in juvenile rheumatoid arthritis. Int Pediatr 3:304–311, 1988.

Prahalad S, Ryan MH, Shear ES, Thompson SD, Giannini EH, Glass DN. Juvenile rheumatoid arthritis: linkage to HLA demonstrated by allele sharing in affected sibpairs. Arthritis Rheum 43:2335–2338, 2000.

Prakash UBS, Luthra HS, Divertie MB. Intrathoracic manifestations in mixed connective tissue disease. Mayo Clin Proc 60:813–821, 1985.

Preston SJ, Buchanan WW. Rheumatic manifestations of immune deficiency. Clin Exp Rheumatol 7:547–555, 1989.

Prieur AM, Stephan JL. Macrophage activation syndrome in rheumatic diseases in children. Rev Rheum Ed Fr 61:447–451, 1994.

Provenzale J, Bouldin TW. Lupus-related myelopathy: report of three cases and review of the literature. J Neurol Neurosurg Psychiatry 55:830–835, 1992.

Provost TT, Ahmed AR, Maddison PJ, Reichlin M. Antibodies to cytoplasmic antigens in lupus erythematosus. Serologic marker for systemic disease. Arthritis Rheum 20:1457–1463, 1977.

Provost TT, Watson R, Gammon WR, Radowsky M, Harley JB, Reichlin M. The neonatal lupus syndrome associated with U1RNP (nRNP) antibodies. N Engl J Med 315:1135–1139, 1987.

Quinn RW. Comprehensive review of morbidity and mortality trends for rheumatic fever, streptococcal disease, and scarlet fever: the decline of rheumatic fever. Rev Infect Dis 11:928–953, 1989.

Rahman MA, Isenberg DA. Autoantibodies in systemic lupus erythematosus. Curr Opin Rheumatol 6:468–473, 1994.

Rahn DW, Malawista SE. Lyme disease: recommendations for diagnosis and treatment. Ann Intern Med 114:472–481, 1991.

Rajapakse C, Al Balla S, Al-Dallan A, Kamal H. Streptococcal antibody cross-reactivity with HLA-DR4+ B-lymphocytes. Basis of the DR4 associated genetic predisposition to rheumatic fever and rheumatic heart disease? Br J Rheumatol 29:468–470, 1990.

Rammelkamp CH, Wannamaker LW, Kenny FW. The epidemiology and prevention of rheumatic fever. Bull NY Acad Med 28:321–334, 1952.

Ramsay C, Moreland J, Ho M, Joyce S, Walker S, Pullar T. An observer-blinded comparison of supervised and unsupervised aerobic exercise regimens in fibromyalgia. Rheumatology (Oxford) 39:501–505, 2000.

Ravelli A, Caporali R, Bianchi E, Violi S, Solmi M, Montecucco C, Martini A. Anticardiolipin syndrome in childhood: a report of two cases. Clin Exp Rheum 8:95–98, 1990.

Reed AM, Pachman L, Ober C. Molecular genetic studies of major histocompatibility complex genes in children with juvenile dermatomyositis: increased risk associated with HLA-DQA1 *0501. Hum Immunol 32:235–240, 1991.

Reed BR, Lee LA, Harmon C, Wolfe R, Wiggins J, Peebles C, Weston WL. Autoantibodies to SS-A/Ro in infants with congenital heart block. J Pediatr 103:889–891, 1983.

Regelmann WE, Gray ED, Wanamaker LW, Lebien TW, Mansour M, El Kholy A, Abdin Z. Lymphocyte subpopulations. J Rheumatol 14:23–27, 1987.

Reiff A, Rawlings D, Shaham B, Franke E, Richardson L, Szer I, Bernstein B. Preliminary evidence for cyclosporin A as an alternative in the treatment of recalcitrant juvenile rheumatoid arthritis and juvenile dermatomyositis. J Rheumatol 24:2436–2442, 1997.

Reiff A, Takei S, Sadeghi S, Stout A, Shaham B, Bernstein B, Gallagher K, Stout T. Etanercept therapy in children with treatment-resistant uveitis. Arthritis Rheum 44:1411–1415, 2001.

Reinhardt DJ, Waldron JM. Lupus erythematosus-like syndrome complicating hydralazine (apresoline) therapy. J Am Med Assoc 155:1491–1492, 1954.

Reinhart W. Red blood aggregation and sedimentation: the role of the cell shape. Br J Haematol 73:551–556, 1989.

Reveille JD. The changing spectrum of rheumatic disease in human immunodeficiency virus infection. Semin Arthritis Rheum 30:147–166, 2000.

Rhodes V. Physical therapy management of patients with juvenile rheumatoid arthritis. Phys Ther 71:910–919, 1991.

Rich SS, Gray ED, Talbot R, Martin D, Cairns L, Zabriskie JB, Braun D, Regelmann WE. Cell surface markers and cellular immune response associated with rheumatic heart disease: complex segregation analysis. Genet Epidemiol 5:463–470, 1988.

Richardson JB, Callen JP. Dermatomyositis and malignancy. Med Clin North Am 73:1211–1220, 1989.

Rider L, Miller F. Idiopathic inflammatory muscle disease: clinical aspects. Baillieres Best Pract Res Clin Rheumatol 14:37–54, 2000.

Rider LG, Buyon JP, Rutledge J, Sherry DD. Treatment of neonatal lupus: case report and review of the literature. J Rheumatol 20:1208–1211, 1993.

Rodnan GP, DiBartolomeo AG, Medsger TA. Eosinophilic fasciitis. Report of 7 cases of a newly recognized scleroderma-like syndrome. Arthritis Rheum 18:422–423, 1975.

Roosnek E, Lanzavecchia A. Efficient and selective presentation of antigen-antibody complexes by rheumatoid factor B cells. J Exp Med 173:487–489, 1991.

Rose CD, Fawcett PT, Singsen BH, Dubbs SB, Doughty RA. Use of Western blot and enzyme-linked immunosorbent assays to assist in the diagnosis of Lyme disease. Pediatrics 88:465–470, 1991.

Rose CD, Singsen BH, Eichenfield AH, Goldsmith DP, Athreya BH. Safety and efficacy of methotrexate therapy for juvenile rheumatoid arthritis. J Pediatr 117:653–659, 1990a.

Rose V. Kawasaki syndrome–cardiovascular manifestations. J Rheumatol 17(Suppl 24):11–14, 1990b.

Rosenberg AM. The clinical associations of antinuclear antibodies in juvenile rheumatoid arthritis. Clin Immunol Immunopathol 49:19–27, 1988.

Rosenberg AM, Petty RE. Reiter's disease in children. Am J Dis Child 133:394–398, 1979.

Rosenberg AM, Petty RE. A syndrome of seronegative enthesopathy and arthropathy in children. Arthritis Rheum 25:1041–1047, 1982.

Rosenberg AM, Petty RE, Cumming GR, Koehler BE. Pulmonary hypertension in a child with MCTD. J Rheumatol 6:700–704, 1979.

Rosenberg NL, Rotbart HA, Abzug MJ, Ringel SP, Levin MJ. Evidence for a novel picornavirus in human dermatomyositis. Ann Neurol 26:204–209, 1989.

Rosenfeld SI, Kelly ME, Leddy JP. Hereditary deficiency of the fifth component of complement in man. J Clin Invest 57:1626–1634, 1976.

Rosenthal J, Benson MD. Diffuse fasciitis and eosinophilia with symmetric polyarthritis. Ann Intern Med 92:507–509, 1980.

Rosove MH, Brewer PM. Antiphospholipid thrombosis: clinical course after the first thrombotic event in 70 patients. Ann Intern Med 117:303–308, 1992.

Rossy LA, Buckelew SP, Dorr N, Hagglund KJ, Thayer JF, McIntosh MJ, Hewett JE, Johnson JC. A meta-analysis of fibromyalgia treatment interventions. Ann Behav Med 21:180–191, 1999.

Rother E, Lang B, Coldeway R, Hartung K, Peter HH. Complement split product C3d as an indicator of disease activity in systemic lupus erythematosus. Clin Rheumatol 12:31–35, 1993.

Rothfield NF, Stollar BD. The relation of immunoglobulin class, pattern of anti-nuclear antibody, and complement-fixing antibodies to DNA in sera from patients with systemic lupus erythematosus. J Clin Invest 46:1785–1794, 1967.

Roubinian JR, Talal N, Greenspan JR, Siiteri PK. Effect of castration and sex hormone treatment on survival, anti-nucleic acid antibodies and glomerulonephritis in NZB/NZW F1 mice. J Exp Med 147:1568–1583, 1983.

Rowley AH, Duffy CE, Shulman ST. Prevention of giant coronary artery aneurysms in Kawasaki disease by intravenous gammaglobulin therapy. J Pediatr 113:290–294, 1988a.

Rowley AH, Gonzalez-Crussi F, Shulman ST. Kawasaki syndrome. Rev Infect Dis 10:1–15, 1988b.

Ruddlesdin C, Ansell BM, Arden GP, Swann M. Total hip replacement in children with juvenile chronic arthritis. J Bone Joint Surg 68B:218–222, 1986.

Russell AS. Reiter's syndrome in children following infection with Yersinia enterocolitica and Shigella. Arthritis Rheum 20:471, 1977.

Russell AS, Davis P, Percy JS, Lentle B. The sacroilitis of acute Reiter's syndrome. J Rheumatol 4:293–296, 1977.

Rustagi A, Currie M, Logue G. Complement-activating antineutrophil antibody in systemic lupus erythematosus. Am J Med 78:971–977, 1985.

Ruvalcaba RH, Thuline HC. IgA absence associated with short arm deletion of chromosome No. 18. J Pediatr 74:964–965, 1969.

Rydholm U, Brattstrom H, Lidgren L. Soft tissue release for knee flexion contracture in juvenile chronic arthritis. J Pediatr Orthop 6:448–451, 1986.

Saca LF, Szer IS, Henar E, Nanjundiah P, Haddad ZH, Quismorio FP Jr. Budd-Chiari syndrome associated with antiphospholipid antibodies in a child: report of a case and review of the literature. J Rheumatol 21:545–548, 1994.

Saitta MR, Keene JD. Molecular biology of nuclear autoantigens. Rheum Dis Clin North Am 18:283–310, 1992.

Salazar JC, Gerber MA, Goff CW. Long-term outcome of Lyme disease in children given early treatment. J Pediatr 122:591–593, 1993.

Saleeb S, Copel J, Friedman D, Buyon JP. Comparison of treatment with fluorinated glucocorticoids to the natural history of autoantibody-associated congenital heart block: retrospective review of the research registry for neonatal lupus. Arthritis Rheum 42:2335–2345, 1999.

Sammaritano LR, Gharavi AE, Lockshin MD. Antiphospholipid antibody syndrome: immunologic and clinical aspects. Semin Arthritis Rheum 20:81–96, 1990.

Sanders DY, Huntley CC, Sharp GC. Mixed connective tissue disease in a child. J Pediatr 83:642–645, 1973.

Sanyal SK, Berry AM, Duggal S, Hooja V, Ghosh S. Sequelae of the initial attack of acute rheumatic fever in children from north India. A prospective 5-year follow-up study. Circulation 65:375–379, 1982.

Sargent SJ, Beachey EH, Corbett CE, Dale JB. Sequence of protective epitopes of streptococcal M proteins shared with cardiac sarcolemmal membranes. J Immunol 139:1285–1290, 1987.

Sato M, Takeda A, Honzu H, Saku N, Minato N, Kano S. Adult Still's disease with Sjögren's syndrome successfully treated with intravenous pulse methylprednisolone and oral cyclophosphamide. Intern Med 32:730–732, 1993.

Saulsbury FT. Heavy and light chain composition of serum IgA and IgA rheumatoid factor in Henoch-Schönlein purpura. Arthritis Rheum 35:1377–1380, 1992.

Savage COS, Tizard J, Lockwood JD, Dillon MJ. Antineutrophil cytoplasm antibodies in Kawasaki disease. Arch Dis Child 64:360–363, 1989.

Scarpa R, Oriente P, Pucino A, Torella M, Vigone L, Riccio A, Biondi-Oriente C. Psoriatic arthritis in psoriatic patients. Br J Rheumatol 23:246–250, 1984.

Schaller J, Davis SD, Ching YC, Lagunoff D, Williams CP, Wedgwood RJ. Hypergammaglobulinaemia, antibody deficiency, autoimmune haemolytic anaemia, and nephritis in an infant with a familial lymphopenic immune defect. Lancet 2:825–829, 1966.

Schaller JG. Dermatomyositis. J Pediatr 83:699–702, 1971.

Schaller JG. Illness resembling lupus erythematosus in mothers of boys with chronic granulomatous disease. Ann Intern Med 76:747–750, 1972.

Schaller JG. Ankylosing spondylitis of childhood onset. Arthritis Rheum 20:398–401, 1977a.

Schaller JG. Arthritis and immunodeficiency. Arthritis Rheum 20:443–445, 1977b.

Schaller JG. Iridocyclitis. Arthritis Rheum 20:227–228, 1977c.

Schaller JG. Juvenile rheumatoid arthritis: series I. Arthritis Rheum 20:165–170, 1977d.

Schaller, JG. Lupus phenomena in the newborn. Arthritis Rheum 20:312–314, 1977e.

Schaller JG. The diversity of JRA: a 1976 look at the subgroups of chronic childhood arthritis. Arthritis Rheum 20(Suppl):S52–S61, 1977f.

Schaller JG. Corticosteroids in juvenile rheumatoid arthritis. Arthritis Rheum 20:537–543, 1977g.

Schaller JG. Juvenile rheumatoid arthritis. Pediatr Rev 2:163–174, 1980.

Schaller JG. Therapy for childhood rheumatic diseases. Have we been doing enough? Arthritis Rheum 36:65–70, 1993.

Schaller JG, Beckwith B, Wedgwood RJ. Hepatic involvement in juvenile rheumatoid arthritis. J Pediatr 77:203–210, 1970.

Schaller JG, Bitnum S, Wedgwood RJ. Ankylosing spondylitis with childhood onset. J Pediatr 74:505–515, 1969a.

Schaller JG, Gilliland GC, Ochs HD, Leddy JP, Agodoa LCY, Rosenfeld SI. Severe systemic lupus erythematosus with nephritis in a boy with deficiency of the fourth component of complement. Arthritis Rheum 20:1519–1525, 1977.

Schaller JG, Hansen J. Rheumatoid factor-positive juvenile rheumatoid arthritis: the childhood equivalent of classic adult rheumatoid arthritis. Arthritis Rheum 25:S18, 1982a.

Schaller JG, Hansen J. Early childhood pauciarticular juvenile rheumatoid arthritis: clinical and immunogenetic studies. Arthritis Rheum 25:S63, 1982b.

Schaller JG, Johnson GD, Holborow EJ, Ansell BM, Smiley WK. The association of antinuclear antibodies with the chronic iridocyclitis of juvenile arthritis (Still's disease). Arthritis Rheum 17:409–416, 1974.

Schaller JG, Wallace C, Stamm S, Morgan BC, Patterson M. The occurrence of congenital heart block in infants of mothers with clinical or serological evidence of rheumatic disease. Arthritis Rheum 22:656, 1979.

Schaller JG, Wedgwood RJ. Pruritus associated with the rash of juvenile rheumatoid arthritis. Pediatrics 45:296–298, 1970.

Schaller J, Wedgwood R. Pauciarticular childhood arthritis: identification of two distinct subgroups. Arthritis Rheum 19:820–821, 1976.

Schenk JP, Limberg B, Grauer A, Kauffmann G. Chronic recurrent multifocal osteomyelitis (CRMO). Diaphyseal attack with progressive hyperostosis. Rofo Fortschr Geb Rontgenstr Neuen Bildgeb Verfahr 168:624–627, 1998.

Schlosstein L, Terasaki P, Bluestone R, Pearson C. High association of an HL-A antigen, B27, with ankylosing spondylitis. N Engl J Med 288:704–706, 1973.

Schnitzer TJ, Ansell BM. Amyloidosis in juvenile chronic polyarthritis. Arthritis Rheum 20:245–252, 1977.

Schnitzer TJ, Penmetcha M. Viral arthritis. Curr Opin Rheumatol 8:341–345, 1996.

Schur PH. Inherited complement component abnormalities. Ann Rev Med 37:333–346, 1986.

Schur PH. Genetics of systemic lupus erythematosus. Lupus 4:425–437, 1995.

Schur PH, Austen KF. Complement in the rheumatic diseases. Bull Rheum Dis 22:666–673, 1972.

Schur PH, Meyer I, Garovoy M, Carpenter CB. Associations between systemic lupus erythematosus and the MHC: clinical and immunological considerations. Clin Immunol Immunopathol 24:263–275, 1982.

Schur PH, Sandson J. Immunologic factors and clinical activity in systemic lupus erythematosus. N Engl J Med 278:533–538, 1968.

Schwartz RS, Stollar BD. Origins of anti-DNA antibodies. J Clin Invest 75:321–327, 1985.

Schwimmbeck PL, Yu DT, Oldstone MB. Autoantibodies to HLA B27 in the sera of HLA B27 patients with ankylosing spondylitis and Reiter's syndrome. Molecular mimicry with *Klebsiella pneumoniae* as potential mechanism of autoimmune disease. J Exp Med 166:173–181, 1987.

Scofield RH, Kurien BT, Zhang F, Mehta P, Kaufman K, Gross T, Bachmann M, Gordon T, Harley JB. Protein-protein interaction of the Ro-ribonucleoprotein particle using multiple antigenic peptides. Mol Immunol 36:1093–1106, 1999.

Scott J, Gerber P, Maryjowski MC, Pachman L. Evidence for intravascular coagulation in systemic onset but not polyarticular juvenile rheumatoid arthritis. Arthritis Rheum 28:256–261, 1985.

Scott JS, Maddison PJ, Taylor PV, Esscher E, Scott O, Skinner RP. Connective-tissue disease, antibodies to ribonucleoprotein, and congenital heart block. N Engl J Med 309:209–212, 1983.

Scott RD. Total hip and knee arthroplasty in juvenile rheumatoid arthritis. J Clin Orthop Rel Res 259:83–91, 1990.

Scroggie DA, Carpenter MT, Cooper RI, Higgs JB. Parvovirus arthropathy outbreak in southwestern United States. J Rheumatol 27:2444–2448, 2000.

Seaman WE, Ishak AD. Aspirin-induced hepatotoxicity in patients with systemic lupus erythematosus. Ann Intern Med 80:1–8, 1974.

Segurado OG, Arnaiz-Villena AA, Iglesias-Casarrubios P, Martinez-Laso J, Vicario JL, Fontan G, Lopez-Trascasa M. Combined total deficiency of C7 and C4B with systemic lupus erythematosus (SLE). Clin Exp Immunol 87:410–414, 1992.

Seip M. SLE in pregnancy with haemolytic anemia, leucopenia and thrombocytopenia in the mother and her newborn infant. Arch Dis Child 35:364–366, 1960.

Seko Y, Minota S, Kawasaki A, Shinkai Y, Maeda K, Yagita H, Okumura K, Sato O, Takagi A, Tada Y, et al. Perforin-secreting killer cell infiltration and expression of a 65-kD heat-shock protein in aortic tissue of patients with Takayasu's arteritis. J Clin Invest 93:750–758, 1994.

Seligmann M, Cannat A, Hamard M. Studies on antinuclear antibodies. Ann NY Acad Sci 124:816–832, 1965.

Senturk T, Aydintug AO, Duzgun N, Tokgoz G. Seizures and hepatotoxicity following sulphasalazine administration. Rheumatol Int 17:75–77, 1997.

Seres T, Csipo I, Kiss E, Szegedi G, Kavai M. Correlation of Fc gamma receptor expression of monocytes with clearance function by macrophages in systemic lupus erythematosus. Scand J Immunol 48:307–311, 1998.

Seyger MM, van den Hoogen FH, de Boo T, de Jong EM. Low-dose methotrexate in the treatment of widespread morphea. J Am Acad Dermatol 39:220–225, 1998.

Shackman NH, Swiller AI, Morrison M. Syndrome simulating acute disseminated lupus erythematosus: appearance after hydralazine (apresoline) therapy. J Am Med Assoc 155:1492–1494, 1954.

Shamim EA, Miller FW. Familial autoimmunity and the idiopathic inflammatory myopathies. Curr Rheumatol Rep 2:201–211, 2000.

Sharp GC, Irvin WS, May CM, Holman HR, Mcduffie FC, Hess EV, Schmid FR. Association of antibodies to ribonucleoprotein and Sm antigens with mixed connective tissue disease, systemic lupus erythematosus and other rheumatic diseases. N Engl J Med 295:1149–1154, 1976.

Sharp GC, Irvin WS, Tan EM, Gould RG, Holman HR. Mixed connective tissue disease: an apparently distinct rheumatic disease syndrome associated with a specific antibody to an extractable nuclear antigen (ENA). Am J Med 52:148–159, 1972.

Shelhamer JH, Volkman DJ, Parrillo JE, Lawley TJ, Johnston MR, Fauci AS. Takayasu's arteritis and its therapy. Ann Intern Med 103:121–126, 1985.

Sherry DD, Weisman R. Psychologic aspects of childhood reflex neurovascular dystrophy. Pediatrics 81:572–578, 1988.

Shetty AK, Gedalia A. Sarcoidosis: a pediatric perspective. Clin Pediatr (Phila) 37:707–717, 1998.

Shevach EM. Regulatory T cells in autoimmunity. Ann Rev Immunol 18:423–449, 2000.

Shibata S, Sasaki T, Hatakeyama A, Munakata Y, Hirabayashi Y, Yoshinaga K. Clonal frequency analysis of B cells producing pathogenic anti-DNA antibody-associated idiotypes in systemic lupus erythematosus. Clin Immunol Immunopathol 63:252–258, 1992.

Shimizu K, Sano K. Pulseless disease. J Neuropathol Clin Neurol 1:37–47, 1951.

Shinohara K, Miyagawa S, Fujita T, Aono T, Kidoguchi K. Neonatal lupus erythematosus: results of maternal corticosteroid therapy. Obstet Gynecol 93:952–957, 1999.

Shivakumar S, Tsokos GC, Datta SK. T cell receptor alpha/beta expressing double negative (CD4−/CD8−) and CD4+ T helper cells in human augment the production of pathogenic anti-DNA autoantibodies associated with lupus nephritis. J Immunol 143:103–112, 1989.

Shoenfeld Y, Rauch J, Masicotte I, Datta SK, Andre-Schwartz J, Stollar BD, Schwartz RS. Polyspecificity of monoclonal lupus autoantibodies produced by human-human hybridomas. N Engl J Med 303:414–420, 1983.

Shore A, Ansell BM. Juvenile psoriatic arthritis—an analysis of 60 cases. J Pediatr 100:529–535, 1982.

Shulman LE, Hoffman R, Dainiak N. Antibody-mediated aplastic anemia and thrombocytopenic purpura in diffuse eosinophilic fasciitis. Arthritis Rheum 22:659–661, 1979.

Sibbitt WLJ, Sibbitt RR, Griffey RH, Eckel C, Bankhurst AD. Magnetic resonance and computed tomographic imaging in the evolution of acute neuropsychiatric disease in systemic lupus erythematosus. Ann Rheum Dis 48:1014–1022, 1989.

Siegel M, Lee SL. The epidemiology of SLE. Semin Arthritis Rheum 3:1–54, 1973.

Sieper J, Braun J, Doring E, Wu P, Heesemann J, Trehame J, Kingsley G. Aetiological role of bacteria associated with reactive arthritis in pauciarticular juvenile chronic arthritis. Ann Rheum Dis 51:1208–1214, 1992.

Sigal LH. Current recommendations for the treatment of Lyme disease. Drugs 43:683–699, 1992.

Sigurgeirsson B, Lindelof B, Edhag O, Allander E. Risk of cancer in patients with dermatomyositis or polymyositis. N Engl J Med 326:363–367, 1992.

Silber TJ, Chatoor I, White PH. Psychiatric manifestations of systemic lupus erythematosus in children and adolescents. Clin Pediatr 23:331–335, 1984.

Silver RM, Heyes MP, Maize JC, Quearry B, Vionnet-Fuasset M, Sternberg EM. Scleroderma, fasciitis, and eosinophilia associated with the ingestion of tryptophan. N Engl J Med 322:869–873, 1990.

Silver RM, Maricq HR. Childhood dermatomyositis: serial microvascular studies. Pediatrics 83:278–283, 1989.

Silverman E, Mamula M, Hardin JA, Laxer R. Importance of the immune response to the Ro/La particle in the development of congenital heart block and neonatal lupus erythematosus. J Rheumatol 18:120–124, 1991.

Silverman ED. Congenital heart block and neonatal lupus erythematosus: prevention is the goal. J Rheumatol 20:1101–1104, 1993.

Silverman ED, Miller JJ, Bernstein B, Shafai T. Consumption coagulopathy associated with systemic juvenile rheumatoid arthritis. J Pediatr 103:872–876, 1983.

Silverstein FE, Faich G, Goldstein JL, Simon LS, Pincus T, Whelton A, Makuch R, Eisen G, Agrawal NM, Stenson WF, Burr AM, Zhao WW, Kent JD, Lefkowith JB, Verburg KM, Geis GS. Gastrointestinal toxicity with celecoxib vs nonsteroidal anti-inflammatory drugs for osteoarthritis and rheumatoid arthritis: the CLASS study: a randomized controlled trial. Celecoxib Long-term Arthritis Safety Study. JAMA 284:1247–1255, 2000.

Singsen BH, Bernstein BH, Kornreich HK, King KK, Hansen V. Mixed connective tissue disease in childhood. A clinical and serologic survey. J Pediatr 90:893–900, 1977a.

Singsen BH, Bernstein BH, Koster-King KG, Glovsky MM, Hansen V. Reiter's syndrome in childhood. Arthritis Rheum 20(Suppl):402–407, 1977b.

Singsen BH, Isaacson AS, Bernstein BH, Patzakis MJ, Kornreich HK, King KK, Hansen V. Total hip replacement in children with arthritis. Arthritis Rheum 21:401–406, 1978.

Sletnes KE, Smith P, Abdelnoor M, Arnesen H, Wisloff F. Antiphospholipid antibodies after myocardial infarction and their relation to mortality, reinfarction, and non-haemorrhagic stroke. Lancet 339:451–453, 1992.

Smiley WK, May E, Bywaters EGL. Ocular presentations of Still's disease and their treatment. Ann Rheum Dis 16:371–382, 1957.

Smith ME, Ansell BM, Bywaters EGL. Mortality and prognosis related to the amyloidosis of Still's disease. Ann Rheum Dis 27:137–145, 1968.

Smith RJ. Evidence of Chlamydia trachomata and Ureaplasma urealyticum in a patient with Reiter's disease. J Adolesc Health Care 10:155–159, 1989.

Smolen JS, Klippel JH, Penner E, Reichlin M, Steinberg AD, Chused TM, Scherak O, Graninger W, Hartter E, Zielinski CC, et al. HLA-DR antigens in systemic lupus erythematosus: association with specificity of autoantibody responses to nuclear antigens. Ann Rheum Dis 46:457–462, 1987.

Smyth LJ, Snowden N, Carthy D, Papasteriades C, Hajeer A, Ollier WE. Fc gamma RIIa polymorphism in systemic lupus erythematosus. Ann Rheum Dis 56:744–746, 1997.

Special Writing Group of the Committee on Rheumatic Fever E, and Kawasaki Disease of the Council on Cardiovascular Disease in the Young of the American Heart Association. Guidelines for the diagnosis of rheumatic fever. JAMA 268:2069–2073, 1992.

Speier JE. Complications of rubella vaccination. JAMA 213:2272, 1970.

Specks U, Fervenza FC, McDonald TJ, Hogan MC. Response of Wegener's granulomatosis to anti-CD20 chimeric monoclonal antibody therapy. Arthritis Rheum 44:2836–2840, 2001.

Spencer-Green G, Schlesinger M, Bove KE, Levinson JE, Schaller JG, Hanson V, Crowe WE. Nailfold capillary abnormalities in childhood rheumatic diseases. J Pediatr 102:341–346, 1983.

Spiera H, Kerr LD. Scleroderma following silicone implantation: a cumulative experience of 11 cases. J Rheumatol 20:958–961, 1993.

Sprott H, Muller-Ladner U, Distler O, Gay RE, Barnum SR, Landthaler M, Scholmerich J, Lang B, Gay S. Detection of activated complement complex C5b-9 and complement receptor C5a in skin biopsies of patients with systemic sclerosis (scleroderma). J Rheumatol 27:402–404, 2000.

St. Clair EW. Anti-La antibodies. Rheum Dis Clin North Am 18:359–376, 1992.

Stastny P. HLA-D and Ia antigens in rheumatoid arthritis and systemic lupus erythematosus. Arthritis Rheum 21:5139–5143, 1978.

Stastny P, Fernandez-Vina M, Cerna M, Havelka S, Ivaskova E, Vavrincova P. Sequences of HLA alleles associated with arthritis in adults and children. J Rheumatol 37(Suppl):5–8, 1992.

Stebbings S, Highton J, Croxson MC, Powell K, McKay J, Rietveld J. Chickenpox monoarthritis: demonstration of varicella-zoster virus in joint fluid by polymerase chain reaction. Br J Rheumatol 37:311–313, 1998.

Steere A, Brinckerhoff C, Miller D, Drinker H, Harris E, Malawista S. Association of chronic Lyme arthritis with HLA-DR4 and HLA-DR2 alleles. N Engl J Med 323:219–223, 1990.

Steere A, Malawista S, Snydman D, Shope R, Andiman W, Ross M, Steele F. Lyme arthritis: an epidemic of oligoarticular arthritis in children and adults in three Connecticut communities. Arthritis Rheum 20:7–17, 1977.

Steere A, Schoen R, Taylor E. The clinical evolution of Lyme arthritis. Ann Intern Med 107:725–731, 1987.

Steere AC. Lyme disease. N Engl J Med 321:586–596, 1989.

Steere AC, Bartenhagen NH, Craft JE, Hutchinson GJ, Newman JH, Rahn DW, Sigal LH, Spieler PN, Stenn KS, Malawista SE. The early clinical manifestations of Lyme disease. Ann Intern Med 99:76–82, 1983.

Steere AC, Batsford WP, Weinberg M, Alexander J, Berger HJ, Wolfson S, Malawista SE. Lyme carditis: cardiac abnormalities of Lyme disease. Ann Intern Med 93(Part 1):8–16, 1980.

Steere AC, Gibofsky A, Patarroyo ME, Winchester RJ, Hardin JA, Malawista SE. Chronic Lyme arthritis. Ann Intern Med 90:896–901, 1979.

Stern R, Fishman J, Brusman H, Kunkel HG. Systemic lupus erythematosus associated with Klinefelter's syndrome. Arthritis Rheum 20:18–22, 1977.

Sticca M, Barca S, Spallino L, Livio L, Longhi R. Schönlein-Henoch syndrome: clinical-epidemiological analysis of 98 cases. Pediatr Med Chir 21:9–12, 1999.

Stollerman GH. Global changes in group A streptococcal diseases and strategies for their prevention. Chicago, Yearbook Medical Publishers, 1982.

Stone NM, Williams A, Wilkinson JD, Bird G. Systemic lupus erythematosus with C1q deficiency. Br J Dermatol 142:521–524, 2000.

Suarez-Almazor ME, Cataggio LJ, Maldonado-Cocco JA, R. C, Garcia-Morteo O. Juvenile progressive systemic sclerosis: clinical and serologic findings. Arthritis Rheum 28:699–702, 1985.

Suarez-Almazor ME, Russell AS. Sacroiliitis in psoriasis: relationship to peripheral arthritis and HLA-B27. J Rheumatol 17:804–808, 1990.

Subang R, Levine JS, Janoff AS, Davidson SM, Taraschi TF, Koike T, Minchey SR, Whiteside M, Tannenbaum M, Rauch J. Phospholipid-bound beta 2-glycoprotein I induces the production of anti-phospholipid antibodies. J Autoimmun 15:21–32, 2000.

Suda H. Low-dose weekly methotrexate therapy for progressive neuro-Behcet's disease. Nihon Rinsho Meneki Gakkai Kaishi 22:13–22, 1999.

Sugimura T, Kato H, Inoue O, Takagi J, Fukuda T, Sato N. Vasodilatory response of the coronary arteries after Kawasaki disease: evaluation by intracoronary injection of isosorbide dinitrate. J Pediatr 121:684–688, 1992.

Sullivan DB, Cassidy JT, Petty RE. Dermatomyositis in the pediatric patient. Arthritis Rheum 20:327–331, 1977.

Sullivan DB, Cassidy JT, Petty RE, Burt MT. Prognosis in childhood dermatomyositis. J Pediatr 80:555–563, 1972.

Sundel RP, Burns JC, Baker A, Beiser AS, Newburger JW. Gamma globulin re-treatment in Kawasaki disease. J Pediatr 123:657–659, 1993.

Suzuki A, Kamiya T, Ono Y, Okuno M, Yagihara T. Aorto-coronary bypass surgery for coronary arterial lesions resulting from Kawasaki disease. J Pediatr 116:567–573, 1990.

Szer IS, Taylor E, Steere AC. The long-term course of Lyme arthritis in children. N Engl J Med 325:159–163, 1991a.

Szer IS, Klein-Gitelman M, DeNardo BA, McCauley R. Ultrasonography in the study of prevalence and clinical evolution of popliteal cysts in children with knee effusions. J Rheumatol 19:458–462, 1992.

Szer W, Sierakowska H, Szer IS. Antinuclear antibody profile in juvenile rheumatoid arthritis. J Rheumatol 18:401–408, 1991b.

Taillan B, Roul C, Fuzibet JG. Circulating anticoagulant in patients seropositive for human immunodeficiency virus. Am J Med 87:238, 1989.

Takahashi T, Tanaka M, Brannan CI, Jenkins NA, Copeland NG, Suda T, Nagata S. Generalized lymphoproliferative disease in mice, caused by a point mutation in the Fas ligand. Cell 76:969–976, 1994.

Takahashi M, Mason W, Lewis A. Regression of coronary aneurysms in patients with Kawasaki syndrome. Circulation 75:387–394, 1987.

Takano M. Observations on the course of Behcet's disease—clinical picture and course (author's transl). Nippon Hifuka Gakkai Zasshi 86:309–321, 1976.

Takigawa M, Kanoh T, Imamura S, and Takahashi C. IgA deficiency and systemic lupus erythematosus. Arch Dermatol 112:845–849, 1976.

Tan EM. Autoantibodies to nuclear antigens (ANA), their immunobiology and medicine. Adv Immunol 33:167–240, 1982.

Tan EM. Interactions between autoimmunity and molecular and cell biology. J Clin Invest 84:1–6, 1989.

Tan EM, Cohen AJ, Fries JF. The 1982 revised criteria for the classification of systemic lupus erythematosus. Arthritis Rheum 25:1271–1277, 1982a.

Tan EM, Fritzler MJ, McDougal JS, McDuffie FC, Nakamura RM, Reichlin M, Reimer CB, Sharp GC, Schur PH, Wilson MR, Winchester RJ. Reference sera for antinuclear antibodies. I. Antibodies to native DNA, Sm nuclear RNP, and SS-B/La. Arthritis Rheum 25:1003–1005, 1982b.

Tan EM, Schur PH, Carr RI, Kunkel HG. Deoxyribonucleic acid (DNA) and antibodies to DNA in the serum of patients with systemic lupus erythematosus. J Clin Invest 45:1732–1740, 1966.

Tan SY. Fc gammaRIIa polymorphism in systemic lupus erythematosus. Kidney Blood Press Res 23:138–142, 2000.

Tanne D, D'Olhaberriague L, Trivedi AM, Salowich-Palm L, Schultz LR, Levine SR. Anticardiolipin antibodies and mortality in patients with ischemic stroke: a prospective follow-up study. Neuroepidemiology 21:93–99, 2002.

Taranta A. Relation of isolated recurrences of Sydenham's chorea to preceding streptococcal infections. N Engl J Med 260:1204–1210, 1959.

Targoff IN. Update on myositis-specific and myositis-associated autoantibodies. Curr Opin Rheumatol 12:475–481, 2000.

Targoff IN, Johnson AE, Miller FW. Antibody to signal recognition particle in polymyositis. Arthritis Rheum 33:1361–1370, 1990.

Taurog J, Richardson J, Croft J, Simmons W, Zhou M, Fernandez-Sueiro J, Balish E, Hammer R. The germfree state prevents development of gut and joint inflammatory disease in HLA-B27 transgenic rats. J Exp Med 180:22359–2364, 1994.

Tayag-Kier CE, Keenan GF, Scalzi LV, Schultz B, Elliott J, Zhao RH, Arens R. Sleep and periodic limb movement in sleep in juvenile fibromyalgia. Pediatrics 106:e70, 2000.

Tejani A, Nicastri AD, Chen CK, Fikrig S, and Gurumurthy K. Lupus nephritis in black and Hispanic children. Am J Dis Child 137:481–483, 1983.

Terai M, Kohno Y, Niwa K, Toba T, Sakurai N, Nakajima H. Imbalance among T-cell subsets in patients with coronary arterial aneurysms in Kawasaki disease. Am J Cardiol 60:555–559, 1987.

Tervaert JW, Huitema MG, Hene RJ, Sluiter WJ, The TH, van der Hem GK, Kallenberg CG. Prevention of relapses in Wegener's granulomatosis by treatment based on antineutrophil cytoplasmic antibody titre. Lancet 336:709–711, 1990a.

Tervaert JW, Goldschmeding R, Elema JD, Limburg PC, van der Giessen M, Huitema MG, Koolen MI, Hene RJ, The TH, van der Hem GK, et al. Association of autoantibodies to myeloperoxidase with different forms of vasculitis. Arthritis Rheum 33:1264–1272, 1990b.

Tervaert JW, Limburg PC, Elema JD, Huitema MG, Horst G, The TH, Kallenberg CG. Detection of autoantibodies against myeloid lysosomal enzymes: a useful adjunct to classification of patients with biopsy-proven necrotizing arteritis. Am J Med 91:59–66, 1991.

Thatai D, Turi ZG. Current guidelines for the treatment of patients with rheumatic fever. Drugs 57:545–555, 1999.

Thomson GT, MacDougall B, Watson PH, Chalmers IM. Eosinophilic fasciitis in a pair of sibling. Arthritis Rheum 32:96–99, 1989.

Tighe H, Chen PP, Tucker R, Kipps TJ, Roudier J, Jirik FR, Carson DA. Function of B cells expressing a human immunoglobulin M rheumatoid factor autoantibody in transgenic mice. J Exp Med 177:109–118, 1993.

Tipping PG, Buchanan RC, Riglar AG, Dimech WJ, Littlejohn GO, Holdsworth SR. Measurement of anti-DNA antibodies by ELISA: a comparative study with Crithidia and a Farr assay. Pathology 23:21–24, 1991.

Tomiita M, Saito K, Kohno Y, Shimojo N, Fujikawa S, Niimi H. The clinical features of Sjögren's syndrome in Japanese children. Acta Paediatr Jpn 39:268–272, 1997.

Tontsch D, Pankuweit S, Maisch B. Autoantibodies in the sera of patients with rheumatic heart disease: characterization of myocardial antigens by two-dimensional immunoblotting and N-terminal sequence analysis. Clin Exp Immunol 121:270–274, 2000.

Towner SR, Michet CJ, O'Fallon WM, Nelson AM. The epidemiology of juvenile arthritis in Rochester, Minnesota 1960–79. Arthritis Rheum 26:1208–1213, 1983.

Traynor A, Burt RK. Haematopoietic stem cell transplantation for active systemic lupus erythematosus. Rheumatology (Oxford) 38:767–772, 1999.

Trygstad CW, Stiehm ER. Elevated serum IgA globulin in anaphylactoid purpura. Pediatrics 47:1023–1028, 1971.

Tse SM, Silverman ED, McCrindle BW, Yeung RS. Early treatment with intravenous immunoglobulin in patients with Kawasaki disease. J Pediatr 10:450–455, 2002.

Tseng CE, Buyon JP. Neonatal lupus syndromes. Rheum Dis Clin North Am 23:31–54, 1997.

Tucker LB, Miller LC, Marx G, Dorkin HL, Schaller JG. Cardiopulmonary followup during the course of childhood systemic lupus erythematosus (SLE). Arthritis Rheum 35(Suppl 9):Abstract D81, 1992.

Turk DC, Okifuji A, Sinclair JD, Starz TW. Differential responses by psychosocial subgroups of fibromyalgia syndrome patients to an interdisciplinary treatment. Arthritis Care Res 11:397–404, 1998.

Tyndall A. Hematopoietic stem cell transplantation in rheumatic diseases other than systemic sclerosis and systemic lupus erythematosus. J Rheumatol 48(Suppl):94–97, 1997.

Ulgiati D, Abraham LJ. Comparative analysis of the disease-associated complement C4 gene from the HLA-A1, B8, DR3 haplotype. Exp Clin Immunogenet 13:43–54, 1996.

Urizar RE, Michael AF, Sisson S. Anaphylactoid purpura. II. Immunofluorescent and electron microscopic studies of the glomerular lesions. Lab Invest 19:437–450, 1968.

Urman JD, Rothchild NF. Corticosteroid treatment in systemic lupus erythematosus. Survival studies. JAMA 238:2272–2276, 1977.

Urowitz M, Gladman D, Bruce I. Atherosclerosis and systemic lupus erythematosus. Curr Rheumatol Rep 2:19–23, 2000.

Uziel Y, Feldman BM, Krafchik BR, Yeung RS, Laxer RM. Methotrexate and corticosteroid therapy for pediatric localized scleroderma. J Pediatr 136:91–95, 2000.

Vaarala O, Palusuo T, Kleemola M. Anticardiolipin response in acute infections. Clin Immunol Immunopathol 41:8–15, 1986.

Vaishnaw AK, Toubi E, Ohsako S, Drappa J, Buys S, Estrada J, Sitarz A, Zemel L, Chu JL, Elkon KB. The spectrum of apoptotic defects and clinical manifestations, including systemic lupus erythematosus, in humans with CD95 (Fas/APO-1) mutations. Arthritis Rheum 42:1833–1842, 1999.

Vaisman S, Guasch J, Vignau A, Correa E, Schuster A, Mortimer EA Jr, Rammelkamp CH Jr. Failure of penicillin to alter acute rheumatic valvulitis. JAMA 194:1284–1286, 1965.

van den Hoogen FH, Boerbooms AM, Swaak AJ, Rasker JJ, van Lier HJ, van de Putte LB. Comparison of methotrexate with placebo in the treatment of systemic sclerosis: a 24 week randomized double-blind trial, followed by a 24 week observational trial. Br J Rheumatol 35:364–372, 1996.

van den Wall Bake AWL. IgA class anti-neutrophil cytoplasmic antibodies (IgA-ANCA) in primary IgA nephropathy. Acta Pathol Microbiol Immunol Scand 97(Suppl 6):25–26, 1989.

van der Woude FJ, Rasmussen N, Lobatto S. Autoantibodies against neutrophils and monocytes: tool for diagnosis and marker of disease activity in Wegener's granulomatosis. Lancet 325:425–429, 1985.

van Kerckhove C, Giannini EH, Lovell DJ. Temporal patterns of response to D-penicillamine, hydroxychloroquine, and placebo in juvenile rheumatoid arthritis patients. Arthritis Rheum 31:1252–1258, 1988.

van Lier D, Jorens PG, Cools F, Bossaert LL, Vrints CJ. Successful recovery after ventricular fibrillation in a patient with Kawasaki disease. Resuscitation 44:215–218, 2000.

van Vloten WA, Scheffer E, Dooren LJ. Localized scleroderma-like lesions after bone marrow transplantation in man. A chronic graft-vs-host reaction. Br J Derm 96:337–341, 1977.

Varga J, Schumacher HR, Jimenez SA. Systemic sclerosis after augmentation mammoplasty with silicone implants. Ann Intern Med 111:377–383, 1989.

Veasy LG, Weidmeier SE, Orsmond GS, Ruttenberg HD, Boucek MM, Roth SJ, Tait VF, Thompson JA, Daly JA, Kaplan EL, Hill HR. Resurgence of acute rheumatic fever in the intermountain area of the United States. N Engl J Med 316:421–427, 1987.

Vernier RL, Worthen HG, Peterson RD, Colle E, Good RA. Anaphylactoid purpura; pathology of the skin and kidney and frequency of streptococcal infection. Pediatrics 27:181–193, 1961.

Viana VS, Garcia S, Nascimento JH, Elkon KB, Brot N, Campos de Carvalho AC, Bonfa E. Induction of in vitro heart block is not restricted to affinity purified anti-52 kDa Ro/SSA antibody from mothers of children with neonatal lupus. Lupus 7:141–147, 1998.

Virchow R. Historical note on lupus. Arch Pathol Anat 32:139–143, 1865.

Visentainer JE, Pereira FC, Dalalio MM, Tsuneto LT, Donadio PR, Moliterno RA. Association of HLA-DR7 with rheumatic fever in the Brazilian population. J Rheumatol 27:1518–1520, 2000.

Vlachoyiannopoulos PG, Tsifetaki N, Dimitriou I, Galaris D, Papiris SA, Moutsopoulos HM. Safety and efficacy of recombinant gamma interferon in the treatment of systemic sclerosis. Ann Rheum Dis 55:761–768, 1996.

von Herrath MG, Holz A, Homann D, Oldstone MB. Role of viruses in type I diabetes. Semin Immunol 10:87–100, 1998.

Vourlekis JS, Sawyer RT, Newman LS. Sarcoidosis: developments in etiology, immunology, and therapeutics. Adv Intern Med 45:209–257, 2000.

Vyse TJ, Kotzin BL. Genetic susceptibility to systemic lupus erythematosus. Annu Rev Immunol 16:261–292, 1998.

Wagener JS, Taussig LM, DeBenedetti C. Pulmonary function in juvenile rheumatoid arthritis. J Pediatr 99:108–110, 1981.

Wallace C, Schaller JG, Emery H, Wedgwood R. Prospective study of childhood systemic lupus erythematosus (SLE). Arthritis Rheum 21:599–600, 1978.

Wallace C, Striker G, Schaller JG, Wedgwood RJ, Emery HM. Renal histology and subsequent course in childhood systemic lupus erythematosus (SLE). Arthritis Rheum 22:669, 1979.

Wallace CA, Sherry DD. Preliminary report of higher dose methotrexate treatment in juvenile rheumatoid arthritis. J Rheumatol 19:1604–1607, 1992.

Wallace CA, Sherry DD. Trial of intravenous pulse cyclophosphamide and methylprednisolone in the treatment of severe systemic-onset juvenile rheumatoid arthritis. Arthritis Rheum 40:1852–1855, 1997.

Wallace DJ, Metzger AL, White K. Combination immunosuppressive treatment of steroid resistant dermatomyositis/polymyositis. Arthritis Rheum 28:590–592, 1985.

Wallace MR, Garst PD, Papadimos TJ, Oldfield ECd. The return of acute rheumatic fever in young adults. JAMA 262:2557–2561, 1989.

Walport MJ. Complement deficiency in SLE (abstract). Lupus 4:8, 1995.

Walport MJ, Lachmann PJ. Erythrocyte complement receptor type 1, immune complexes, and the rheumatic diseases. Arthritis Rheum 31:153–158, 1988.

Walravens PA, Chase HP. The prognosis of childhood systemic lupus erythematosus. Am J Dis Child 130:929–933, 1976.

Wannamaker LW. The chain that links the heart to the throat. Circulation 48:9–18, 1973.

Wannamaker LW, Rammelkamp CH, Deny FW, Brink WR, Houser HB, Hahn EO, and Dingle JH. Prophylaxis of acute rheumatic fever by treatment of the preceding streptococcal infection with various amounts of depot penicillin. Am J Med 10:673–695, 1951.

Ward MM, Pisetsky DS, Christenson VD. Antidouble stranded DNA antibody assays in systemic lupus erythematosus: correlations of longitudinal antibody measurements. J Rheumatol 16:609–613, 1989.

Watanabe-Fukunaga R, Brannan CI, Copeland NG, Jenkins NA, Nagata S. Lymphoproliferation disorder in mice explained by defects in Fas antigen that mediates apoptosis. Nature 356:314–317, 1992.

Watson R, Kang JE, Kudak M, Kickler T, Provost TT. Thrombocytopenia in the neonatal lupus syndrome. Arch Dermatol 124:560–563, 1988.

Watson RM, Scheel JN, Petri M, Kan JS, Provost TT, Ratrie H 3rd, Callan NA. Neonatal lupus erythematosus. Report of serological and immunogenetic studies in twins discordant for congenital heart block. Br J Dermatol 130:342–348, 1994.

Watts R, Lane S, Bentham G, Scott D. Epidemiology of systemic vasculitis: a ten-year study in the United Kingdom. Arthritis Rheum 43:414–419, 2000.

Wauters IM, Linskens RK, Stehouwer CD. Periodic fever due to hyper-IgD syndrome. Ned Tijdschr Geneeskd 144:809–811, 2000.

Weinstein A, Bordwell B, Stone B, Tibbetts C, Rothfield NF. Antibodies to native DNA and serum complement (C3) levels. Application to diagnosis and classification of systemic lupus erythematosus. Am J Med 74:206–216, 1983.

Wenkert D, Miller LC, Tucker LB, Szer IS, Schaller JG. Chromosomal abnormalities in boys with systemic lupus erythematosus. Arthritis Rheum 34:169A, 1991.

West SG. Lupus and the central nervous system. Curr Opin Rheumatol 8:408–414, 1996.

Westedt ML, Herbrink P, Molenaar JL, de Vries E, Verlaan P, Stijnen T, Cats A, Lindeman J. Rheumatoid factors in rheumatoid arthritis and vasculitis. Rheumatol Int 5:209–214, 1985.

Weston WL, Harmon C, Peebles C, Manchester D, Franco HL, Huff JC, Norris DA. A serological marker for neonatal lupus erythematosus. Br J Dermatol 107:377–382, 1982.

Whitaker JN, Engel WK. Vascular deposits of immunoglobulins and complement in idiopathic inflammatory myopathy. N Engl J Med 286:333–338, 1972.

WHO SG. Rheumatic fever and rheumatic heart disease. Report of a WHO Study Group. World Health Organ Tech Rep Ser 764:1–58, 1988.

Wilkens RF, Arnett FC, Bitter T. Reiter's syndrome: evaluation of preliminary criteria for definite disease. Bull Rheum 32:31–34, 1982.

Williams RA, Ansell BM. Radiological findings in seropositive juvenile chronic arthritis (juvenile rheumatoid arthritis) with particular reference to progression. Ann Rheum Dis 44:685–693, 1985.

Williams RC Jr. Molecular mimicry and rheumatic fever. Clin Rheum Dis 11:573–590, 1985.

Williams RC Jr. Hypothesis: rheumatoid factors are antiidiotypes related to bacterial or viral Fc receptors. Arthritis Rheum 31:1204–1207, 1988.

Williams RCJ. Rheumatoid factors: historical perspective, origins and possible role in disease. J Rheumol 19(Suppl 32):42–45, 1992.

Williams RV, Wilke VM, Tani LY, Minich LL. Does Abciximab enhance regression of coronary aneurysms resulting from Kawasaki disease? Pediatrics 109:E4, 2002.

Wilson JG, Fearon DT. Altered expression of complement receptors as a pathogenic factor in systemic lupus erythematosus. Arthritis Rheum 27:1321–1328, 1984.

Wilson WA, Gharavi AE, Koike T, Lockshin MD, Branch DW, Piette JC, Brey R, Derksen R, Harris EN, Hughes GR, Triplett DA, Khamashta MA. International consensus statement on preliminary classification criteria for definite antiphospholipid syndrome: report of an international workshop. Arthritis Rheum 42:1309–1311, 1999.

Winfield JB, Faiferman I, Koffler D. Avidity of anti-DNA antibodies in serum and IgG glomerular eluates from patients with systemic lupus erythematosus. Association of high avidity anti native DNA antibody with glomerulonephritis. J Clin Invest 59:90–96, 1977.

Winfield JB, Mimura T, Fernsten PD. Antilymphocyte autoantibodies. In Wallace DJ, Hahn BH, eds. Dubois' Lupus Erythematosus. Philadelphia, Lea & Febiger, 1992, pp 254–259.

Winkelmann RK. Chronic discoid lupus erythematosus in children. JAMA 205:675–678, 1968.

Winkelman RK, Kierland RR, Perry HO, Muller SA, Sams WM. Symposium on scleroderma. Mayo Clin Proc 46:77–134, 1971.

Winn DM, Wolfe JF, Lindberg DA, Fristoe EA, Kingsland L, Sharp GC. Identification of a clinical subset of systemic lupus erythematosus by antibodies to Sm antigen. Arthritis Rheum 22:1334–1337, 1979.

Witt JD, McCullough CJ. Anterior soft-tissue release of the hip in juvenile chronic arthritis. J Bone Joint Surg Br 76:267–270, 1994.

Woo P, Southwood TR, Prieur AM, Dore CJ, Grainger J, David J, Ryder C, Hasson N, Hall A, Lemelle I. Randomized, placebo-controlled, crossover trial of low-dose oral methotrexate in children with extended oligoarticular or systemic arthritis. Arthritis Rheum 43:1849–1857, 2000.

Wood HW, Feinstein AR, Taranta A, Epstein JA, Simpson R. Comparative effectiveness of 3 prophylaxis regimens in preventing streptococcal infections and rheumatic recurrences. Ann Intern Med 60(Suppl 5):31–46, 1964.

Woolf A, Croker B, Osofsky SG, Kredich DW. Nephritis in children and young adults with systemic lupus erythematosus and normal urinary sediment. Pediatrics 64:678–685, 1979.

Wright DA, Newburger JW, Baker A, Sundel RP. Treatment of immune globulin-resistant Kawasaki disease with pulsed doses of corticosteroids. J Pediatr 128:146–149, 1996.

Wurzner R, Orran A, Lalchmann PJ. Inherited deficiencies of the terminal components of human complement. Immunodefic Rev 3:123–147, 1992.

Wynne-Roberts CR, Anderson CH, Turano AM, Baron M. Light and electron-microscopic findings in juvenile rheumatoid arthritis synovium: comparison with normal juvenile synovium. Semin Arthritis Rheum 7:287–302, 1978.

Yamanishi Y, Taooka Y, Mukuzono H, Aoi K, Ishibe Y, Yamana S. Cyclophosphamide-responsive subclinical Sjögren's syndrome in a patient with initial peripheral and central nervous system involvement. Ryumachi 34:633–638, 1994.

Yancey CL, Doughty RA, Athreya BH. Central nervous system involvement in childhood systemic lupus erythematosus. Arthritis Rheum 24:1389–1395, 1981.

Yap SN, Phipps ME, Manivasagar M, Tan SY, Bosco JJ. Human Fc gamma receptor IIA (FcgammaRIIA) genotyping and association with systemic lupus erythematosus (SLE) in Chinese and Malays in Malaysia. Lupus 8:305–310, 1999.

Yarom A, Rennebohm RM, Levinson JE. Infantile multisystem inflammatory disease: a specific syndrome? J Pediatr 106:390–396, 1985.

Yazici H, Akokan G, Yalcin B, Muftuoglu A. The high prevalence of HLA-B5 in Behcet's disease. Clin Exp Immunol 30:259–261, 1977.

Yazici Y, Erkan D, Lockshin MD. Etanercept in the treatment of severe, resistant psoriatic arthritis: continued efficacy and changing patterns of use after two years. Clin Exp Rheumatol 20:115, 2002.

Yoshikawa J, Yanagihara K, Owaki T, Kato H, Takagi Y, Okumachi F, Fukaya T, Tomita Y, Baba K. Cross-sectional echocardiographic diagnosis of coronary artery aneurysms in patients with the mucocutaneous lymph node syndrome. Circulation 59:133–139, 1979.

Yoshioka T, Matsutani T, Iwagami S, Toyosaki-Maeda T, Yutsudo T, Tsuruta Y, Suzuki H, Uemura S, Takeuchi T, Koike M, Suzuki R. Polyclonal expansion of TCRBV2-and TCRBV6-bearing T cells in patients with Kawasaki disease. Immunology 96:465–472, 1999.

Zabriskie JB, Hsu KC, Seegal BC. Heart-reactive antibody associated with rheumatic fever: characterization and diagnostic significance. Clin Exp Immunol 7:147–159, 1970.

Zandbelt MM, van den Hoogen FH, de Wilde PC, van den Berg PJ, Schneider HG, van de Putte LB. Reversibility of histological and immunohistological abnormalities in sublabial salivary gland biopsy specimens following treatment with corticosteroids in Sjögren's syndrome. Ann Rheum Dis 60:511–513, 2001.

Zemer D, Pras M, Sohar E, Modan M, Cabili S, Gafni J. Colchicine in the prevention and treatment of the amyloidosis of familial Mediterranean fever. N Engl J Med 314:1001–1005, 1986.

Zemer D, Revach M, Pras M, Modan B, Schor S, Sohar E, Gafni J. A controlled trial of colchicine in preventing attacks of familial Mediterranean fever. N Engl J Med 291:932–934, 1974.

Zetterstrom R, Berglund G. Systemic lupus erythematosus in childhood. A clinical study. Acta Pediatr 45:189–204, 1956.

Zhang Y, Yasuda T, Wang CR, Yoshimoto T, Nagase H, Takamoto M, Tsubura A, Kimura M, Matsuzawa A. A pivotal role of cell-bound but not soluble CD4 molecules in full development of lupus-like manifestations in MRL-Faslprcg/Faslprcg mice. Clin Exp Immunol 122:124–132, 2000.

Zhao M, Short A, Lockwood C. Antineutrophil cytoplasm autoantibodies and vasculitis. Curr Opin Hematol 2:96–102, 1995.

Zhao MH, Lockwood CM. Azurocidin is a novel antigen for anti-neutrophil cytoplasmic autoantibodies (ANCA) in systemic vasculitis. Clin Exp Immunol 103:397–402, 1996.

Zisman DA, McCune WJ, Tino G, Lynch JP III. Drug-induced pneumonitis: the role of methotrexate. Sarcoidosis Vasc Diffuse Lung Dis 18:243–252, 2001.

Zoller L, Burkard S, Schafer H. Validity of Western immunoblot band patterns in the serodiagnosis of Lyme borreliosis. J Clin Microbiol 29:174–182, 1991.

Zonana-Nacach A, Barr SG, Magder LS, Petri M. Damage in systemic lupus erythematosus and its association with corticosteroids. Arthritis Rheum 43:1801–1808, 2000.

Zuber M. Positive antinuclear antibodies in malignancies. Ann Rheum Dis 51:573–574, 1992.

Periodic Fever Syndromes

Kathryn M. Edwards and Alexander R. Lawton

INTRODUCTION

Periodic fever syndromes "hold a special fascination, not only because of their episodic nature, but because they may provide a window for understanding the regulation of inflammation in a much broader spectrum of clinical settings" (Centola et al., 1998). During the past decade, the genes responsible for two previously reported periodic fever syndromes have been identified, two new periodic syndromes have been defined and the contributing genes characterized, and a new relatively common nonhereditary periodic fever syndrome of childhood has been described. A recent review is also available (Drenth and Van der Meer, 2001). In this chapter, we review these advances.

Historical Aspects

As early as the 17th century, syndromes occurring at specific intervals for many years in otherwise healthy individuals were reported (Reimann, 1951; Reimann and McCloskey, 1974). In the 18th century, a series of articles described regularly recurrent symptoms of arthritis and angioedema. In the 1940s, Hobart Reimann and his colleagues characterized various forms of recurrent disease. By 1948, he proposed using the term *periodic* to indicate episodes recurring at regular intervals. He described a number of patients with periodic fever beginning in infancy, persisting for years to decades, having cycles of fixed duration, and following a benign course (Reimann, 1948).

In 1962, Reimann collected case reports on 52 patients with periodic episodes of fever. Many of these patients had fever recurring in 21- to 28-day intervals with malaise, arthritis, or rash. Several complained of sore throat and cervical lymphadenopathy. Most patients were noted to have leukocytosis, but several also had neutropenia and were later diagnosed with cyclic neutropenia. Reimann suggested that periodic fever was a separate diagnostic entity, unique among other periodic disorders. He stated, "when better known diseases are excluded, recognition of periodic fever obviates continued unnecessary diagnostic effort and expense. The cause is unknown and the treatment ineffective" (Reimann and McCloskey, 1974).

Approach to the Patient

The initial challenge to the clinician evaluating a patient with the complaint of periodic fever is to document the presence of fever and to determine that the fever is indeed periodic. Many children referred for evaluation have inadequately documented fever, multiple self-limited infections, or no fever at the time of referral. Sometimes caretakers have misinterpreted normal temperature fluctuations as fever (Malatack and Long, 1997).

Because body temperature must be evaluated using norms for age and sex, it is often helpful to have the maturational changes in temperature available for reference (Fig. 36-1; Bayley and Stoltz, 1937). For example, during the first 3 years of life, the normal rectal temperature is significantly higher than 98.6°F. For boys at 18 months of age, the mean rectal temperature is 99.9°F, with a standard deviation of 0.68°F; thus a rectal temperature of 101.0°F is less than 2 standard deviations above the mean.

Often, periodic fever in childhood is due to multiple self-limited infections that by chance have occurred with regularity. The onset of repeated episodes of fever may coincide with new infectious exposures in day care

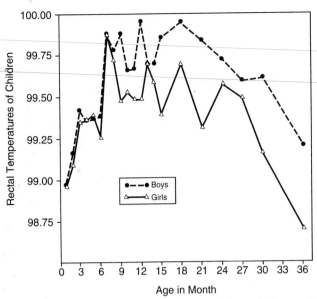

Figure 36-1 · Normal mean rectal temperature is shown for boys and girls through 36 months of age. (Data from Bayley N, Stolz HR. Maturational changes in rectal temperature of 61 infants from 1 to 36 months. Child Dev 8:195–206, 1937.)

or school or may be seen after moving to a new geographic location. The specifics of duration, associated symptoms and signs, and the disparate nature of the illnesses usually indicate that febrile episodes have multiple origins and do not fit into a periodic fever syndrome (Malatack and Long, 1997). A persistent hidden infection is unlikely when periods of fever are separated by days of normal temperature. When a pattern of periodic fever is confirmed, it requires careful assessment. The first question to ask is whether the periodic fever syndrome falls into a hereditary pattern or not. The hereditary patterns are discussed first.

Types of Periodic Fever Syndromes

Hereditary Periodic Fever Syndromes

The hereditary periodic fever syndromes are a group of Mendelian disorders characterized by self-limited episodes of fever accompanied by inflammation of the serosal and synovial membranes without apparent infectious cause (reviewed by Drenth and Van der Meer, 2001). They have been increasingly appreciated during the past few years because of refinements in laboratory and imaging methods used to exclude microbial causes of fever.

Two of the disorders, familial Mediterranean fever (FMF) and hyperimmunoglobulin D with periodic fever syndrome (HIDS), are inherited as autosomal recessive traits. Dominantly inherited hereditary periodic fever syndromes have also been reported in several extended families from different continents and termed familial Hibernian fever and familial periodic fever. These two disorders have recently been shown to have a common

gene defect and the acronym *TRAPS* (TNF receptor 1–associated periodic syndromes) has been proposed to replace the two earlier names.

Another dominantly inherited syndrome is cyclic neutropenia, recently renamed *autosomal dominant cyclic hematopoiesis* and attributed to mutation of the neutrophil elastase gene.

Nonhereditary Periodic Fever Syndrome

The acronym *PFAPA* (periodic fever, aphthous stomatitis, pharyngitis, and cervical adenitis) was coined to describe a fairly common and distinctive childhood syndrome that mimics the symptoms and periodicity of cyclic neutropenia without the hematopoietic fluctuation (Marshall, 1987, Marshall et al., 1989). In contrast to the hereditary syndromes, PFAPA is benign and self-limited and has no apparent genetic linkage (Long, 1999; Padeh et al., 1999; Thomas et al., 1999).

RECESSIVE FORMS OF HEREDITARY PERIODIC FEVER

Familial Mediterranean Fever

FMF is characterized by lifelong recurrence of severe attacks of painful serositis and fever of 38°F or higher. The attacks usually begin in childhood, occur at irregular intervals, and are brief (usually lasting between 12 to 72 hours). Peritonitis is the most common serosal inflammation (95%), followed by arthritis (75%) and unilateral pleuritis (40%). The acute nondeforming arthritis typically involves a single ankle, knee, or hip joint. Uncommon manifestations include an urticarial rash over a painful joint and painful swelling of the scrotum. Lymphadenopathy is not a feature of FMF attacks. Blood leukocytes and acute phase reactants, including fibrinogen, sedimentation rate, C-reactive protein (CRP), and serum amyloid protein, are elevated during attacks (Sohar et al., 1967).

History

The first report of this disease, titled "Benign Paroxysmal Peritonitis" (Siegal, 1945), described five men with recurrent attacks of peritonitis beginning early in life. Episodes were usually accompanied by high fever and sometimes with pleuritic chest pain. One of the five had independent attacks of fever and knee or ankle arthritis lasting 2 to 3 days. All the patients were white, but their ethnic origins were not noted and the hereditary nature of the entity was not appreciated. In 1948, Hobart Reimann included similar patients with "periodic fever and periodic abdominalgia" in his classic description of periodic diseases (Reimann, 1948).

FMF was described in detail and given its current name by Sohar and colleagues in Israel (1967). These investigators determined that the disease was inherited in an autosomal recessive fashion and that it was relatively common in Sephardic Jews (originating from

Mediterranean countries of Africa and southern Europe) but rare in Ashkenazi Jews (coming from eastern Europe). They also noted that amyloidosis was responsible for early death from renal failure in many patients. The name FMF emphasizes the inherited nature of the disease and its high prevalence in Jews, Arabs, and other peoples originating in the Mediterranean basin, but at the cost of disregarding the most characteristic clinical feature, recurrent acute peritonitis.

Because of the resemblance of FMF arthritis to gout, colchicine was introduced as a treatment for FMF as early as 1950. The drug was not effective for acute episodes, but daily prophylactic administration of colchicine was later found to prevent attacks (Goldfinger, 1972) and to avoid the fatal complications of amyloidosis (Zemer et al., 1986).

Clinical Features

The manifestations of FMF in children have been recently reviewed (Ozen, 1999). Severe abdominal pain with peritoneal signs, fever, and prostration occur in 95% of children during an attack. Approximately half of the attacks are associated with arthritis or arthralgia; monoarthritis of the hip, knee, or ankle is most common. Leukocytosis and elevation of acute-phase reactants, including CRP and serum amyloid A (SAA), accompany attacks and usually remit between them.

Livneh and co-workers (1997) have proposed a very detailed set of criteria for diagnosis of FMF. Typical attacks are recurrent (three or more) febrile episodes that last 12 to 72 hours with at least one of the following major criteria: generalized peritonitis; unilateral pleuritis or pericarditis; monoarthritis of hip, knee, or ankle; or temperature greater than 38°C. Incomplete attacks differ in duration, magnitude of fever, and location of serositis.

Minor supporting criteria for diagnosis include exertional leg pain and favorable response to colchicine in this complex diagnostic algorithm. The criteria show a high sensitivity and specificity in ethnic populations in which FMF is common but have not been validated in more diverse populations.

Genetics

The genetic basis of FMF, determined by two positional cloning consortia in 1997, is mutations of a gene designated *MEFV* (for Mediterranean fever) at chromosome 16p13.3 (French FMF Consortium, 1997; International FMF Consortium, 1997). The gene encodes a 3.7-kb transcript expressed predominantly in granulocytes that codes for a protein named pyrin or marenostrin. This protein is a member of the Ro-Ret family of transcription factors, is expressed in the cytoplasm of myeloid cells, and is probably translocated to the nucleus (Centola et al., 1998, 2000; Tidow et al., 2000). The precise anti-inflammatory pathway that the protein triggers has not yet been identified.

At least 14 different mutations of the *MEFV* gene have been described. Investigators at the National Institutes of Health identified eight mutations in a series of 100 patients with FMF, with the most common being V726A, E148Q, and M694V (Centola et al., 1998). In ethnic populations with a high frequency of FMF, about 85% of patients are homozygous or doubly heterozygous for pairs of four common mutations (M694V, M680I, V726A, and M694I), making genetic diagnosis relatively easy (Brik et al., 1999). This is not true in the United States, where it has been estimated that about 40% of carrier chromosomes may have unidentified mutations (Centola et al., 1998). In these cases, the diagnosis is made on clinical grounds.

Treatment

Colchicine at dosages of 1 to 2 mg/day prevents or lessens the frequency and ameliorates attacks of FMF. More important, this treatment prevents renal failure and early death from amyloidosis (Ozen, 1999; Zemer et al., 1986, 1991). Most instances of recurrent attacks or development of amyloidosis are due to poor compliance with colchicine prophylaxis. Adverse reactions to colchicine are uncommon. Treatment begun during childhood does not impair growth, development, or fertility (Zemer et al., 1991). Colchicine is not effective once an attack has begun; indomethacin is considered the most useful anti-inflammatory drug during the acute attack.

The mechanism of action of colchicine in FMF remains to be elucidated, but its efficacy is considered an important diagnostic clue (Livneh et al., 1997; Ozen, 1999). Zemer and colleagues (1991) stated that diagnosis of FMF during childhood is lifesaving because colchicine is such an effective treatment.

Hyperimmunoglobulin D Syndrome and Mevalonic Aciduria

The hyperimmunoglobulin D syndrome (HIDS) and mevalonic aciduria both are disorders associated with mutations of the gene for mevalonate kinase (MVK). Clinically they have distinct features, probably representing different MVK mutations.

Hyperimmunoglobulin D Syndrome

Six patients with a periodic fever syndrome associated with striking increases in the serum concentration of polyclonal immunoglobulin D (IgD) were reported by Van der Meer and others in 1984. By 1996, an international registry had identified a total of 74 patients with a syndrome called HIDS. Most of the patients are Dutch and nearly all are European.

CLINICAL FEATURES

Drench and co-workers reviewed the clinical and laboratory features of 50 HIDS patients in 1994. The median age at onset was 0.5 years. Typical attacks lasted 3 to 7 days and occurred at irregular intervals of 4 to 8 weeks. There was a wide variation in both the frequency and duration of attacks. Computer analysis indicated possible periodicity in only one patient. The severity of attacks diminished as patients aged.

Typical attacks began abruptly with rigors and high fever. Many patients had prodromal symptoms of irritability, malaise, headache, myalgia, vertigo, nasal congestion, and sore throat. Abdominal pain, diarrhea, vomiting, and arthralgias occurred in 70% to 80% of attacks. A number of patients also had exploratory laparotomy secondary to acute abdominal pain. At surgery, mesenteric adenitis and adhesions were often found. Nearly all patients had generalized lymphadenopathy and half had splenomegaly. Macular or maculopapular rash occurred in 80%, and large joint arthritis was seen in nearly 70%. The arthritis was often symmetric and resolved between attacks. No destructive changes occurred, even after repeated episodes.

LABORATORY FEATURES

Laboratory findings include leukocytosis and elevated acute phase reactants, which generally became normal between attacks. IgD concentrations were as high as 5300 IU/ml (758 mg/dl).* Drenth and colleagues (1994) proposed that an IgD concentration of more than 100 IU/ml (e.g., >14 mg/dl) was a requirement for diagnosis. IgA concentrations were increased in 80% and IgG increased in 40% of patients. However, not all patients with the syndrome have high levels of IgD (Drenth and van der Meer, 2001).

GENETICS

Recently, a genome-wide search to map the HIDS gene was undertaken. Two independent groups using different strategies mapped this autosomal recessive genetic disease to chromosome 12q24 and identified the gene for mevalonate kinase (MVK) as the likely candidate (Drenth et al., 1999; Houten et al., 1999). At least eight different mutations or deletions causing partial deficiency of MVK have been described.

Mevalonic Aciduria

Mevalonic aciduria is a rare autosomal recessive disease first described by Hoffman and colleagues in 1986. This organic aciduria is caused by complete absence of functional MVK. This enzyme follows 3-hydroxy-3-methylglutaryl CoA reductase in the biosynthetic pathway of cholesterol and nonsterol isoprenes.

CLINICAL FEATURES

The clinical manifestations of mevalonic aciduria are dysmorphic features, cataracts, progressive psychomotor retardation, lymphadenopathy, hepatosplenomegaly, anemia, and chronic diarrhea. The most severely affected are profoundly retarded and die during infancy. Other patients have moderate mental retardation, cerebellar ataxia, hypotonia, and myopathy. All patients have recurrent crises with fever, vomiting, and diarrhea lasting 4 to 5 days and occurring once or twice a month.

Arthralgia, subcutaneous edema, and maculopapular rash commonly accompany these crises. No metabolic changes have been identified during crises, but the sedimentation rate rapidly increases.

TREATMENT

Crises respond to treatment with corticosteroids. Treatment of a patient with lovastatin lowered the concentration of serum mevalonic acid but also precipitated a febrile episode with profound myopathy (Hoffman et al., 1993).

Summary

In summary, HIDS and mevalonic aciduria represent a spectrum of syndromes caused by partial or complete deficiency of MVK, respectively. The metabolic derangement responsible for the recurrent attacks of fever, abdominal pain, arthritis, and rash in these related diseases has yet to be identified.

DOMINANT FORMS OF PERIODIC FEVER

Familial Hibernian Fever

In 1982, Williamson and colleagues described an Irish family in which 16 members had recurrent attacks of fever, localized myalgia, and painful erythematous rash. They distinguished this illness from other periodic fever syndromes on the basis of its autosomal dominant inheritance pattern and named it familial Hibernian fever (FHF). McDermott and associates (1997) subsequently published a more detailed study of the clinical manifestations in members of the same family.

Clinical Features

Symptoms commonly began during childhood but sometimes not until midlife. Attacks were heterogeneous within individuals and among members of the same immediate family. The most characteristic feature, in addition to fever, was the development of painful erythema and muscle stiffness in an extremity that tended to migrate distally with time. Other common symptoms were abdominal and chest pain, oligoarthralgia, conjunctivitis with or without periorbital edema, painful testicular swelling, and lymphadenopathy. Inguinal hernias occurred in 8 of 10 affected male family members as compared with 1 of 21 unaffected males. Attacks were extremely variable in duration (1 day to several months); a 2- to 3-week course was typical. Frequency of attacks was also variable. Stress, either physical or emotional, seemed to trigger attacks.

Treatment

Attacks of FHF responded promptly to corticosteroid treatment but not consistently to other anti-inflammatory or immunosuppressive drugs. The disease appeared to

---

*1 IU IgD = 1.4 μg; 1 mg IgD = 720 IU.

be benign in most patients. However, secondary amyloidosis occurred in one patient (McDermott et al., 1997).

Familial Periodic Fever

In 1998, Mulley and co-workers reported an autosomal dominant syndrome similar to FHF in an Australian family of Scottish descent and called it familial periodic fever (FPF). Genome-wide searches were begun in the United Kingdom and Australia to map the genes responsible for FHF and FPF. Both groups mapped the responsible gene to chromosome 12p13. Members of the two large FHF and FPF families and members of five smaller families of differing ethnic backgrounds all have mutations in the same gene that codes for the tumor necrosis factor receptor 1 (McDermott et al., 1999).

Tumor Necrosis Factor Receptor 1–Associated Periodic Syndrome (TRAPS)

The name *TRAPS* has been suggested for this dominantly inherited periodic fever syndrome as a replacement for the historical names of FHF and FPF.

Patients with TRAPS have reduced concentrations of soluble p55 TNFR1 between attacks with levels approximating normal resting values during attacks. Monocytes and neutrophils of patients with the mutation C52F have increased membrane concentrations of TNFR1 and normal levels of TNFR2. The defective receptor is able to bind tumor necrosis factor (TNF) with normal affinity. When phagocytes are stimulated with phorbol myristate acetate, there is reduced clearance of the receptor, suggesting that the mutation interferes with shedding of the TNFR1 receptor and prolongs proinflammatory signaling.

McDermott and co-workers (1999) suggested that TRAPS should be designated as an "autoinflammatory" rather than an autoimmune disease.

Cyclic Hematopoiesis

Cyclic hematopoiesis, formerly called cyclic neutropenia, is a rare disorder in which neutrophils disappear from the peripheral blood at intervals of 20 to 22 days. A parallel cycling of platelet numbers and reciprocal fluctuations of both circulating monocytes and reticulocytes is also described. About one third of cases are familial, with an autosomal dominant pattern of inheritance (Palmer et al., 1996; Wright et al., 1981).

History

Leale (1910) described the first case in an infant with recurrent episodes of furunculosis and occasional oral ulcers. Neutropenia was noted, but the periodicity was not. The same patient was followed at Johns Hopkins for more than 10 years and reported by Rutledge and colleagues in 1930. The patient had episodes of malaise, fever, aphthous stomatitis, pharyngitis, and cervical adenitis at intervals of 3 weeks, temporally correlated with disappearance of granulocytes from his peripheral blood. He was well between episodes except for chronic gingivitis. He was able to predict the time of an attack "almost to the day."

Reimann and DeBeradinis (1949) reviewed 15 cases from the literature and added one, establishing cyclic neutropenia as an entity in the collection of periodic diseases. Dale and colleagues have studied this disease for more than a quarter century and have recently determined the responsible gene defect (Dale and Hammond, 1988; Horwitz et al., 1999; Palmer et al., 1996; Wright et al., 1981).

Clinical Features

Clinical manifestations of cyclic hematopoiesis usually begin in childhood, 32% before age 1 year and another 27% by age 5 years (Wright et al., 1981). Recurrent episodes of malaise, fever, aphthous stomatitis, and cervical adenopathy were the characteristic features for each of the eight patients studied at the National Institutes of Health (NIH) and 94% of patients reported in the literature (Wright et al., 1981). Typical attacks begin with a 1- to 3-day prodrome of malaise, during which time the neutrophil count falls. This is followed by development of aphthous ulcerations of buccal mucosa, lips, tongue, and pharynx with tender cervical adenopathy, beginning at the nadir of the neutrophil count and lasting 1 to 3 days. Fever occurs at this time but is often mild and may be absent.

The healing phase, also lasting 1 to 3 days, coincides with a rise of the neutrophil count. In the NIH series, symptoms lasted an average of 5.5 days, with a range of 4 to 8 days (Wright et al., 1981). Children were usually not severely ill and were often thought to have viral syndromes until the agranulocytosis was discovered.

Although serious infections may occur, cyclic hematopoiesis is generally a benign disease, compatible with a long and productive life. Of 18 patients reviewed by Dale and Hammond (1988), 7 had never had a severe infection. Nine patients had common infections such as cellulitis, appendicitis, sinusitis, or pneumonia; one had peritonitis, and one had fatal necrotizing enterocolitis. These authors emphasized that antibiotic treatment was not indicated for typical episodes. The most important infectious risk was bowel perforation, perhaps related to mucosal ulceration permitting bacterial invasion.

Genetics

Autosomal dominant cyclic hematopoiesis is caused by mutations of *Ela2* (19p13.3), the gene encoding neutrophil elastase (Horwitz et al., 1999). Neutrophil elastase is a 25-kD protein synthesized during differentiation of promyelocytes and promonocytes and stored in cytoplasmic granules. It is an important enzyme in tissue destruction mediated by myeloid cells. Homozygous *Ela2*-knockout mice have impaired intracellular killing of bacteria by neutrophils but no abnormality of myeloid cell development or numbers. Heterozygous *Ela2*-mice are normal (Belaaouaj et al., 1998). Thus the pathogenesis of the cycling of hematopoietic cells remains a mystery.

Treatment

Neutropenia may be modified by treatment with granulocyte colony-stimulating factor (G-CSF) or granulocyte-macrophage colony-stimulating factor (GM-CSF). The former has the more powerful effect but exaggerates cycling; the latter raises neutrophil counts modestly while suppressing cycling (Wright et al., 1994). Whether such treatment is needed for a particular patient is a matter of clinical judgment.

PERIODIC FEVER WITH APHTHOUS STOMATITIS, PHARYNGITIS, AND ADENITIS (PFAPA SYNDROME)

History

In 1987, we described a chronic syndrome in 12 children characterized by periodic episodes of high fever lasting for 3 to 6 days and recurring every 3 to 8 weeks, accompanied by aphthous stomatitis, pharyngitis, and cervical adenitis (Marshall et al., 1987). No familial pattern of involvement was identified in these patients. In 1989, the acronym *PFAPA* was coined to describe the entity (Marshall et al., 1989). Additional reports of similar patients appeared from other centers (Abramson et al., 1989; Feder, 1992; Feder et al., 1989; Rubin and Kamani, 1987). Two simultaneously published reports describe larger numbers of PFAPA patients and provide long-term follow-up (Padeh et al., 1999; Thomas et al., 1999).

Clinical Features

Israeli investigators (Padeh et al., 1999) reported 28 patients, 20 of whom were male, with the PFAPA syndrome. In their series the episodes of fever began at 4.2 ± 2.7 years and occurred at mean intervals of 5.1 ± 1.3 weeks. Fever, malaise, tonsillitis with negative throat cultures, and cervical adenopathy were reported in all 28 patients. Aphthous stomatitis occurred in 19, headache in 5, abdominal pain in 5, and arthralgia in 3. Mild hepatosplenomegaly was observed in six patients. Serum IgD was elevated more than 100 U/ml in 12 of 18 patients tested (140.2 ± 62.4 IU/ml). Mild leukocytosis, elevation of the sedimentation rate, and increased serum fibrinogen concentration were found during attacks.

Affected children grew normally, had no associated disease, and had no long-term sequelae. PFAPA was not associated with a particular ethnic group. Attacks resolved spontaneously in 4.3 ± 1.7 days. Attacks could be aborted with a single dose of prednisone (2 mg/kg) at the beginning of the attack in all 15 patients in whom

the medication was tried. In nine patients the syndrome had resolved after a mean duration of 8 ± 2.5 years. In three other patients, tonsillectomy was temporally associated with resolution of the symptoms.

We described the presentation of 94 children with PFAPA and provided long-term follow-up on 83 (Thomas et al., 1999). The sex distribution in our series was 52 males and 42 females. Patients resided in 22 different states in the United States and 3 foreign countries (Sweden, Italy, and Saudi Arabia). Most children were white, with a diverse representation of ethnic backgrounds, including German, English, Irish, Italian, French, Jewish, and American Indian. Two children were black, one was Hispanic, and one was Middle-Eastern. No consistent complications of pregnancy or delivery were reported, and no trends in parental occupations were apparent.

Similar to the report of Padeh and colleagues (1999), our patients' attacks began at a mean of 2.8 years of age, lasted a mean of 4.8 days, and recurred at a mean of 28.2 days (Table 36-1). During episodes, temperatures ranged from 38.9°C to 41.1°C. Additional symptoms are reported in Table 36-2. No patient had documented recurrent pyogenic infections or was given the diagnosis of arthritis, pleuritis, myositis, or menin-

TABLE 36-1 · CHARACTERISTICS OF FEBRILE EPISODES IN CHILDREN WITH PFAPA SYNDROME

Characteristic	Mean (95% Confidence Internal)
Onset of syndrome in years	2.8 (2.4–5.5)
Duration of episodes in days	4.8 (4.5–5.1)
Maximum temperature in degrees centigrade	40.5 (40.4–40.6)
Days temperature > 38.3°C	3.8 (3.5–4.1)
Frequency of episodes per year	11.5 (10.5–12.5)
Symptom-free intervals in days	28.2 (26.0–30.4)

PFAPA = periodic fever, aphthous stomatitis, pharyngitis, and adenitis.
Data from Thomas KT, Feder HM, Lawton AR, Edwards KM. Periodic fever syndrome in children. J Pediatr 135:15–21, 1999.

TABLE 36-2 · SYMPTOMS REPORTED BY PARENTS OF CHILDREN WITH PFAPA SYNDROME

Symptom	Percentage of Children with Symptom
Aphthous stomatitis	67
Pharyngitis	65
Cervical adenopathy	77
Chills	80
Cough	20
Coryza	18
Headache	65
Abdominal pain	46
Nausea	52
Diarrhea	30
Rash	15

PFAPA = periodic fever, aphthous stomatitis, pharyngitis, and adenitis.
Data from Thomas KT, Feder HM, Lawton AR, Edwards KM. Periodic fever syndrome in children. J Pediatr 135:15–21, 1999.

gitis. Many parents commented that these children had fewer common infections than their unaffected siblings.

Telephone follow-up was accomplished in 83 of the 94 patients. The duration of follow-up ranged from 1 month to 9.4 years, with a mean of 3.3 years. The mean age at follow-up was 8.9 years. All children were healthy and exceeded the 5th percentile for height and weight. None had siblings with periodic fever. Five parents stated that they had periodic fevers as young children, but their medical records were not available for review. Of the 83 children, 34 had not had a febrile episode for 1 year or more.

The mean duration of periodic fevers before resolution of symptoms in these patients was 4.5 years. Episodes occurred less frequently before resolution but were otherwise typical. Of the 83 patients, 49 continued to have febrile episodes. In this group the frequency of attacks was bimodal. Thirty-eight children had typical episodes at intervals of 26.4 days, and eleven had had only two to three attacks in the most recent year. The latter children had been having attacks for a mean of 6.8 years. We concluded that this syndrome ends with a decreasing frequency of typical attacks.

Laboratory Features

Laboratory studies were unrevealing. Leukocytosis with a mean leukocyte count of 13,000 (62% polymorphonuclear leukocytes) and an elevated sedimentation rate (mean 41 mm/hr) were noted during the episodes. Immunologic and serologic studies were uniformly nondiagnostic although serum IgD was elevated (more than 100 U/ml) in two thirds of the Isreali series (Padeh et al., 1999). However, IgD levels were normal in 15 of our patients.

Distribution of T lymphocytes was normal in the 12 patients studied. IgD levels were normal in all 15 patients in which they were measured. Imaging studies were all negative.

None of the 10 children from Israel in whom the *MEFV* genetic testing was done were homozygotes or compound heterozygotes for the common mutations; six were found to be heterozygous. The authors speculate that this reflects frequency of *MEFV* mutations in the population studied (Padeh et al., 1999).

Treatment

A number of therapies have been tried. Acetaminophen temporarily reduced fever in 6% and ibuprofen in 33% of our patients. Most patients had received multiple courses of various antibiotics with little therapeutic benefit. A few children have been treated with aspirin, acyclovir, and colchicine, again with no therapeutic benefit.

Most of the patients given corticosteroids had a dramatic resolution of fever and other symptoms, usually within a few hours. Padeh and associates (1999) suggested that a prompt response to a single dose of 2 mg/kg of prednisone is a useful diagnostic test for PFAPA. Brief corticosteroid treatments did not prevent subsequent episodes of fever, but patients continued to respond to steroids during subsequent cycles. Some families reported that the cycles of fever became more closely spaced after steroid therapy, and a few stopped the treatments for this reason.

Symptomatic treatment with short courses of steroids is well tolerated and effective in relieving the distressing symptoms of PFAPA attacks. We recommend a dose of 1 mg/kg prednisone or prednisolone at the beginning of an attack, the same dose on the next morning, and one half of that dose on days 3 and 4. Doses on days 3 and 4 may be omitted in some patients, as determined by trial during subsequent episodes.

Two additional therapies were reported to be beneficial. Cimetidine was associated with resolution of the episodes in 8 of 28 who tried this therapy. Tonsillectomy was associated with total resolution of the symptoms in 7 of 11 subjects, whereas adenoidectomy had no apparent benefit (Thomas et al., 1999).

In summary, PFAPA is not an uncommon cause of periodic fever in children. In some children the syndrome resolves with time, in others the symptoms become more widely spaced, and in others symptoms persist. Long-term sequelae have not been seen. The cause is unknown. Whether the syndrome will be eventually explained on the basis of immune dysregulation or infection or will be attributed to genetic mutations as seen with the hereditary periodic fever syndromes remains to be determined.

REFERENCES

Abramson JS, Givner LB, Thompson JN. Possible role of tonsillectomy and adenoidectomy in children with recurrent fever and tonsillopharyngitis. Pediatrics 8:119–120, 1989.

Bayley N, Stolz HR. Maturational changes in rectal temperature of 61 infants from 1 to 36 months. Child Dev 8:195–206, 1937.

Belaaouaj A, McCarthy R, Baumann M, Gao Z, Ley TJ, Abraham SN, Shapiro SD. Mice lacking neutrophil elastase reveal impaired host defense against gram negative bacterial sepsis. Nat Med 4:615–618, 1998.

Brik R, Shinawi M, Kepten I, Berant M, Gershoni-Baruch R. Familial Mediterranean fever: clinical and genetic characterization in a mixed pediatric population of Jewish and Arab patients. Pediatrics 103:e70, 1999.

Centola M, Aksentijevich I, Kastner DL. The hereditary periodic fever syndromes: molecular analysis of a new family of inflammatory diseases. Hum Mol Genet 7:1581–1588, 1998.

Centola M, Wood G, Frucht DM, Galon J, Aringer M, Farrell C, Kingma DW, Horwitz ME, Mansfield E, Holland SM, O'Shea JJ, Rosenberg HF, Malech HL, Kastner DL. The gene for familial Mediterranean fever, MEFV, is expressed in early leukocyte development and is regulated in response to inflammatory mediators. Blood 15:3223–3231, 2000.

Dale DC, Hammond WPT. Cyclic neutropenia: a clinical review. Blood Rev 2:178–185, 1988.

Drenth JPH, Cuisset L, Grateau G, Vasseur C, van de Velde-Visser SD, de Jong JG, Beckmann JS, van der Meer JW, Delpech M. Mutations in the gene encoding mevalonate kinase cause hyper-IgD and periodic fever syndrome. Nat Genet 22:178–181, 1999.

Drenth J, Hoagsma C, Van der Meer J. Hyperimmunoglobulin D and periodic fever syndrome: the clinical spectrum in a series of 50 patients. Medicine 73:133–44, 1994.

Drenth JPH, van der Meer JWM. Hereditary periodic fever. N Engl J Med 345:1748–1757, 2001.

Feder HM Jr. Cimetidine treatment for periodic fever associated with aphthous stomatitis, pharyngitis, and cervical adenitis. Pediatr Infect Dis J 11:318–321, 1992.

Feder HM, Bialecki CA. Periodic fever associated with aphthous stomatitis, pharyngitis, and cervical adenitis. Pediatr Infect Dis J 8:186–187, 1989.

French FMF Consortium. A candidate gene for familial Mediterranean fever. Nat Genet 17:25–31, 1997.

Goldfinger SE. Colchicine for familial Mediterranean fever. N Engl J Med 287:1302, 1972.

Hoffmann GF, Charpentier C, Mayatepek E, Mancini J, Leichsenring M, Gibson KM, Divry P, Hrebicek M, Lehnert W, Sartor K, et al. Clinical and biochemical phenotype in 11 patients with mevalonic aciduria. Pediatrics 91:915–921, 1993.

Hoffmann GF, Gibson KM, Brandt IK, Bader PI, Wappner RS, Sweetman L. Mevalonic aciduria—an inborn error of cholesterol and nonsterol isoprene biosynthesis. New Engl J Med 314:1610–1614, 1986.

Horwitz M, Benson KF, Person RE, Aprikyan AG, Dale DC. Mutations in the ELA2, encoding neutrophil elastase, define a 21-day biological clock in cyclic haematopoiesis. Nat Genet 23:433–436, 1999.

Houten SM, Kuis W, Duran M, de Koning TJ, van Royen-Kerkhof A, Romeijn GJ, Frenkel J, Dorland L, de Barse MM, Huijbers WA, Rijkers GT, Waterham HR, Wanders RJ, Poll-The BT. Mutations in MVK, encoding mevalonate kinase, cause hyperimmunoglobulinemia D and periodic fever syndrome. Nat Genet 22:175–177, 1999.

International FMF Consortium. Ancient missense mutations in a new member of the RoRet gene family are likely to cause familial Mediterranean fever. Cell 90:797–807, 1997.

Leale M. Recurrent furunculosis in an infant showing an unusual blood picture. JAMA 54:1845–1855, 1910.

Livneh A, Langevitz P, Zemer D, Zaks N, Kees S, Lidar T, Migdal A, Padeh S, Pras M. Criteria for the diagnosis of familial Mediterranean fever. Arthritis Rheum 40:1879–1885, 1997.

Long SS. Syndrome of periodic fever, aphthous stomatitis, pharyngitis, and adenitis. J Pediatr 135:1–4, 1999.

Malatack JJ, Long SS. Fever of unknown origin. In Long SS, Pickering LK, Prober CG, eds. Pediatric Infectious Diseases. Churchill Livingston: New York, 1997, pp 125–133.

Marshall GS, Edwards JM, Butler J, Lawton AR. Syndrome of periodic fever, pharyngitis and aphthous stomatitis. J Pediatr 110:43–46, 1987.

Marshall GS, Edwards KM. PFAPA syndrome. Ped Infect Dis J 8:658–659, 1989.

McDermott MF, Aksentijevich I, Galon J, McDermott EM, Ogunkolade BW, Centola M, Mansfield E, Gadina M, Karenko L, Pettersson T, McCarthy J, Frucht DM, Aringer M, Torosyan Y, Teppo AM, Wilson M, Karaarslan HM, Wan Y, Todd I, Wood G, Schlimgen R, Kumarajeewa TR, Cooper SM, Vella JP, Kastner DL. Germline mutations in the extracellular domains of the 55 kDa TNF Receptor, TNFR1, define a family of dominantly Inherited autoinflammatory syndromes. Cell 97:133–144, 1999.

McDermott MF, McDermott EM, Quane KA, Jones LC, Ogunkolade BW, Curtis D, Waldron-Lynch F, Phelan M, Hitman GA, Molloy MG, Powell RJ. Exclusion of the familial Mediterranean fever locus as a susceptibility region for autosomal dominant familial Hibernian fever. J Med Genet 35:432–434, 1998.

McDermott EM, Smillie DM, Powell RJ. Clinical spectrum of familial Hibernian fever: a 14-year follow-up study of the index case and extended family. Mayo Clin Proc 72:806–817, 1997.

Mulley J, Saar K, Hewitt G, Ruschendorf F, Phillips H, Colley A, Sillence D, Reis A, Wilson M. Gene localization for an autosomal dominant familial periodic fever to 12p13. Am J Hum Genet 62:884–889, 1998.

Ozen S. New interest in an old disease: familial Mediterranean fever. Clin Exp Rheumatol 17:745–749, 1999.

Padeh S, Brezniak N, Zemer D, Pras E, Livneh A, Langevitz P, Migdal A, Pras M, Passwell JH. Periodic fever, aphthous stomatitis, pharyngitis, and adenopathy syndrome: clinical characteristics and outcome. J Pediatr 135:98–101, 1999.

Palmer SE, Stephens K, Dale DC. Genetics, phenotype, and natural history of autosomal dominant cyclic hematopoiesis. Am J Med Genet 66:413–422, 1996.

Reimann HA. Periodic disease: a probable syndrome including periodic fever, benign paroxysmal peritonitis, cyclic neutropenia and intermittent arthralgia. JAMA 136:239–244, 1948.

Reimann HA. Periodic disease. Medicine 30:219–245, 1951.

Reinmann HA. Periodic fever, an entity. A collection of 52 cases. Am J Med Sci 243:162–174, 1962.

Reimann HA, deBerardinis CT. Periodic (cyclic) neutropenia, an entity. Blood 4:1109, 1949.

Reimann HA, McCloskey RV. Periodic fever: diagnostic and therapeutic problems. JAMA 228:1662–1664, 1974.

Rubin LG, Kamani N. Syndrome of periodic fever and pharyngitis. J Pediatr 110:307, 1987.

Rutledge BH, Hansen-Pruss OC, Thayer WS. Recurrent agranulocytosis. Bull Johns Hopkins Hosp 46:369–89, 1930.

Siegal S. Benign paroxysmal peritonitis. Ann Intern Med 23:1–21, 1945.

Sohar E, Gafnl J, Pras M, Heller M. Familial Mediterranean fever: a survey of 470 cases and review of the literature. Am J Med 43:227–253, 1967.

Thomas KT, Feder HM, Lawton AR, Edwards KM. Periodic fever syndrome in children. J Pediatr 135:15–21, 1999.

Tidow N, Chen X, Muller C, Kawano S, Gombart AF, Fischel-Ghodsian N, Koeffler HP. Hematopoietic-specific expression of MEFV, the gene mutated in familial Mediterranean fever, and subcellular localization of its corresponding protein, pyrin. Blood 95:1451–1455, 2000.

van der Meer, Vossen JM, Radi J, van Nieuwkoop JA, Meyer CJ, Lobatto S, van Furth R. Hyperimmunoglobulin D and periodic fever: a new syndrome. Lancet 1:1087–1090, 1984.

Williamson LM, Hull D, Mehta R, Reeves WG, Robinson BH, Toghill PJ. Familial Hibernian fever. Q J Med 204:469, 1982.

Wright DG, Dale DC, Fauci AS, Wolff SM. Human cyclic neutropenia: clinical review and long-term follow-up of patients. Medicine 60:1–13, 1981.

Wright DG, Kenney RF, Oette DH, LaRussa VF, Boxer LA, Malech HL. Contrasting effects of recombinant human granulocyte-macrophage colony stimulating factor (CSF) and granulocyte CSF treatment on the cycling of blood elements in childhood-onset cyclic neutropenia. Blood 84:1257–1267, 1994.

Zemer D, Livneh A, Danyon A, Pras M, Sohar E. Long-term colchicine treatment in children with familial Mediterranean fever. Arthritis Rheum 34:973–977, 1991.

Zemer D, Pras M, Sohar E, Modan M, Cabili S, Gafni J. Colchicine in the prevention and treatment of the amyloidosis of familial Mediterranean fever. N Engl J Med 314:1001–1005, 1986.

CHAPTER

37 Autoimmune Endocrinopathies

William E. Winter and Maria Rita Signorino

AUTOIMMUNITY: AN OVERVIEW

Immune recognition of self-antigens normally results in immunologic tolerance, the process that prevents autoimmunity in health (Delves and Roitt, 2000a, 2000b). Physiologic immune recognition is part of the normal immune response, and pathologic immune recognition with failure of tolerance leads to autoimmunity (Table 37-1) (Theofilopoulos and Dixon, 1982).

Tolerance is primarily a function of T cells and their T-cell receptors (Nossal, 1989). Tolerance in humans is established before birth. In certain animals such as mice, tolerance is not established at birth and can be induced by antigen administration to neonatal mice. The mechanisms of T-cell tolerance include thymic clonal deletion (central T-cell tolerance) and peripheral clonal anergy (peripheral T-cell tolerance).

During T-cell development in the thymus, class I major histocompatibility complex (MHC) and class II MHC self-antigen presentation by thymic nurse epithelial cells to the T-cell receptors of CD4+CD8+ thymocytes induces apoptosis in those developing thymocytes that strongly bind such self-peptides. Apoptosis of such potentially autoreactive cells produces clonal deletion. However, not all self-antigens are expressed in the thymus. Because autoreactive T cells to self-antigens can leave the thymus, extrathymic pathways controlling autoimmunity have evolved (Ramsdell and Fowlkes, 1990). Clonal anergy (Blackman et al., 1990; Kappler et al., 1989; Markmann et al., 1988) occurs in the periphery when autoreactive T cells encounter self-antigens but do not receive all of the normal excitatory signals needed to proliferate and differentiate.

Peripheral anergy results when antigens (e.g., self-peptides) are presented without the proper costimulatory cell surface signals. Specifically, naïve T cells, whose T-cell receptors perceive MHC-presented peptide without concurrent costimulatory signaling through the T-cell surface molecule CD28, are induced to become anergic. In a state of *anergy*, the T cell is not dead; however, the T cell is unresponsive to stimulation even when subsequently restimulated with peptide and B7 from the antigen-presenting cell. B7 is the molecule on antigen-presenting cells that binds to CD28 on T cells that normally provides the second signal. Two varieties of B7 exist: B7.1 (CD80) and B7.2 (CD86). Clear functional differences between B7.1 and B7.2 have not been described at present.

B-cell tolerance can also be considered as occurring in a central compartment and in a peripheral compartment. During B-cell development in the bone marrow (the central compartment), naïve immature B cells that express IgM—but not IgD—on contact with antigen will be tolerized. IgM and IgD are B-cell receptor surface antibodies. The contact event is the actual interaction of the B-cell receptor surface antibody with an epitope of the antigen. If the antigen has many repeating epitopes, the tolerization signal will be sufficiently strong to induce apoptosis in the IgM+IgD− naïve immature B cell. However, if there is a weaker tolerizing signal (e.g., the antigen has few epitopes recognized by the B cell), the IgM+IgD− naïve immature B cell will survive in a nonresponsive state of anergy.

B-cell tolerance to antigen stimulation in the peripheral compartment results from a lack of T-cell help. Whereas antigens with many repeating epitopes can crosslink sur-

TABLE 37-1 CLASSIFICATION OF IMMUNE SELF-RECOGNITION

Physiologic

Class I MHC antigen-directed: CD8 T killer cell: target cell interaction (e.g., lysis of viral-infected cells or aberrant tumor cells)

Class II MHC antigen-directed: Macrophage: CD4 T-cell interaction (e.g., antigen presentation)

Adhesion (addressin) molecules

Pathologic

Autoimmune reactions (autoantibodies, self-reactive cell-mediated immunity)

Autoimmune disease (clinically evident disruption of organ or tissue function and/or structure)

MHC = major histocompatibility complex.

face antibody to elicit an IgM response, T-cell help is required for antigen-stimulated B cells to class switch and undergo affinity maturation. T-cell help occurs via CD40–CD40 ligand interactions and T-cell cytokine elaboration (e.g., IL-4, IL-5) and cytokine contact with B-cell cell surface cytokine receptors. Although IgM might be produced in response to T-independent antigens without T-cell help, T-cell help is required for the development of high-affinity IgG, IgA, or IgE antibody.

Autoimmunity can theoretically develop when tolerance to a self-antigen has not been established or when tolerance to self has been lost or bypassed (Bellgrau and Eisenbarth, 1999; Theofilopoulos, 1995a). Many of these errors may be genetically programmed (Theofilopoulos, 1995b). Failure to acquire tolerance may be due to the following:

1. Failure of clonal deletion of autoreactive cells (failure of central T-cell tolerance)
2. Failure of clonal anergy (failure of peripheral T-cell tolerance)
3. Release of a sequestered antigen to which tolerance has not been developed
4. Alteration of a self-antigen, such that it becomes recognized as nonself
5. Molecular mimicry between an environmental antigen and a self-antigen
6. Aberrant class II MHC expression
7. Superantigen stimulation of otherwise anergic autoreactive clones
8. Polyclonal B-cell stimulation

Failure of peripheral tolerance is a likely explanation for the autoimmune disorders discussed in this chapter that may result from molecular mimicry between an environmental antigen and a self-antigen (Albert and Inman, 1999). In molecular mimicry, damage to the host occurs during the immune response to a microbial invader because the self-antigen is unintentionally targeted. Theoretically, if the self-antigen is in very low concentration and is not expressed in the thymus, the self-antigen may not induce tolerance; however, its low concentration does not induce an immunologic response. In the absence of the environmental cross-reactive epitope, the low-concentration self-antigen is essentially invisible to the immune system. However, when the immunogenic environmental mimic enters the body and stimulates an immune response, the self-antigen is now targeted.

Kaufman and co-workers (1992) have described primary sequence homology between portions of glutamic acid decarboxylase (GAD) (an autoantigen in insulin-dependent diabetes) and the P_2-C protein expressed by coxsackievirus. Likewise, homology between a retroviral protein p73 found in nonobese diabetic mouse islets and insulin has been demonstrated. Rheumatic fever resulting from group A β-hemolytic streptococcal pharyngitis is an excellent example of molecular mimicry leading to an immunologic disease (in this case, to the heart, joints, and basal ganglia). Environmental and genetic factors

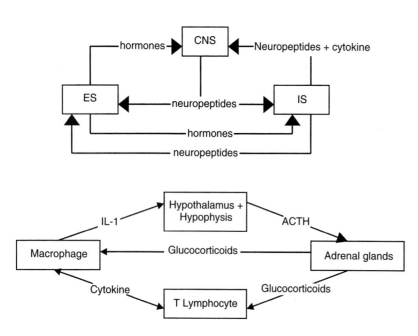

Figure 37-1 · *Top:* The central nervous system (CNS), endocrine system (ES), and immune system (IS) interact through neuropeptides and hormones in maintaining immune homeostasis. *Bottom:* Mechanistically, glucocorticoids produced by the adrenal gland influence T-lymphocyte and macrophage function. Cytokine messages are regularly exchanged between macrophages and T lymphocytes and cytokines such as interleukin-1 (IL-1) secreted by macrophages modify the CNS production of adrenocorticotropic hormone (ACTH).

influence the development of autoimmune disorders, as seen in studies of identical twins. Environmental factors can be intrinsic (e.g., sex hormones and age) or extrinsic (e.g., viral or bacterial infections).

The immune system, the central nervous system (CNS), and the endocrine system are homeostatic systems that collaborate to elicit a balanced immune response by means of messengers such as neuropeptides, hormones, and cytokines (Fig. 37-1). Environmental and genetic factors may interfere with a regulatory circuit, leading to an unbalanced immune response. An example of that interference is the occurrence of macrophage activation syndrome in Epstein-Barr virus infection (Guillaud et al., 1993), in lupus (Javier et al., 1993), and in systemic juvenile rheumatoid arthritis (Imagawa et al., 1997; Mouy et al., 1996; Ravelli et al., 1996). Autoimmune damage to self may trigger a variety of effector pathways (Table 37-2).

Findings that support the hypothesis that a particular disease has an autoimmune cause include the following:

1. Evidence of antiself humoral (e.g., autoantibodies) or cell-mediated autoimmune responses (e.g., lymphocyte proliferation in response to exposure to self-antigens or lymphocytic infiltration of the host target)
2. Ability to transfer disease with either serum or lymphocytes (e.g., usually done in experimental animal models of disease or human disease observed in neonates from transplacentally passed maternal autoantibodies)
3. The ability to prevent, ameliorate, or cure disease with immune intervention therapy (e.g., the use of prednisone in severe cases of systemic lupus erythematosus)
4. Disease recurrence when target tissue, organ, or cells are transplanted into an individual affected by the disease (e.g., recurrence of insulin dependence in a patient with long-standing type 1 diabetes who became initially insulin independent after pancreatic transplantation)

Common findings that provide supportive evidence of an autoimmune cause for a disease include the following:

1. Disease associations with particular human leukocyte antigen (HLA) alleles (e.g., the association of HLA-B27 with ankylosing spondylitis or HLA-DR2 with multiple sclerosis)

2. Disease associations with other autoimmune diseases (e.g., co-existence of autoimmune thyroid disease [AITD] and gastric parietal cell autoimmunity)
3. Increased disease frequency in females (e.g., rheumatoid arthritis and systemic lupus erythematosus)
4. Increased disease frequency in middle age (immunosenescence theory)
5. Associated immune aberrations, such as abnormalities of T-cell subsets, increased levels of activated T cells, hypergammaglobulinemia, or IgA deficiency

The following text covers endocrinopathies resulting from suspected autoimmune processes arranged by the organ affected (Table 37-3). An approach to the patient with autoimmune disorders is discussed in the last section of this chapter.

AUTOIMMUNE DISORDERS OF GLUCOSE METABOLISM INCLUDING THE β CELL, INSULIN, AND THE INSULIN RECEPTOR

Autoimmune abnormalities that perturb glucose metabolism include (1) autoimmune destruction of the β cells causing type 1 diabetes, (2) autoimmune hypoglycemia resulting from spontaneous insulin autoantibodies (IAAs), (3) autoimmunity to the insulin receptor producing the type B acanthosis nigricans-insulin resistance syndrome, and (4) hypoglycemia secondary to insulinomimetic insulin receptor autoantibodies.

Whereas serum autoantibodies to the cytoplasm of α cells and delta cells have been reported in humans (Bottazzo and Lendrum, 1976), neither of these autoimmune conditions produce disease (Del Prete et al., 1978; Winter et al., 1984). Therefore these latter two conditions are not reviewed further. Nonpathologic autoantibodies to circulating glucagon have been described. These autoantibodies may be associated with the use of tolbutamide or methimazole (Baba et al., 1976; Sanke et al., 1983). Likewise, although there was evidence from the 1980s suggesting that a class of autoantibodies directed against β cells may stimulate insulin release (Wilkin et al., 1988), confirmatory studies are lacking and therefore autoimmune stimulation of the β cell

---

TABLE 37-2 · EFFECTOR MECHANISMS IN AUTOIMMUNE DISEASE

Autoantibodies
Complement fixing—cell lysis
Antibody-dependent—cell cytotoxicity
Immune complexes—local and systemic inflammation
Target cell receptor disruption (e.g., myasthenia gravis) or stimulation (e.g., Graves' disease)

Cell-Mediated Autoimmunity
CD8+ T killer cells (cytotoxic T lymphocyte [CTLs]) cell lysis
Macrophage-induced cytokine-mediated cell lysis

TABLE 37-3 · AUTOIMMUNE ENDOCRINOPATHIES

Pancreas
1. Autoimmune diabetes mellitus
2. α-Cell autoimmunity
3. Autoimmune hypoglycemia
4. Type B acanthosis nigricans-insulin resistance syndrome
5. Insulinomimetic insulin receptor autoantibodies
6. Autoimmune β-cell stimulation producing hyperinsulinism

Thyroid
1. Hashimoto's thyroiditis, goitrous and atrophic
2. Graves' disease
3. Thyroid hormone autoantibodies

Adrenal and gonad (Addison's disease and autoimmune hypogonadism)

Anterior pituitary and hypothalamus

leading to hyperinsulinism and hypoglycemia are not addressed further.

Type 1 Diabetes Mellitus

As adopted from the 1997 American Diabetes Association (ADA) guidelines on the diagnosis and classification of diabetes (American Diabetes Association, 2001), type 1 diabetes results from primary β-cell failure producing insulinopenic diabetes. If a specific nonautoimmune cause can be identified (e.g., a genetic, viral, or drug etiology for insulinopenic diabetes), the diabetes is not classified as type 1 diabetes but as *other specific type of diabetes*. When islet autoimmunity is identified before, at the onset of, or after the onset of insulinopenic diabetes, the diabetes can be classified as type 1a or autoimmune type 1 diabetes (Atkinson and Maclaren, 1990; Marx, 1984).

In this chapter, *islet autoimmunity* is used as a generic term indicating that either islet autoantibodies or islet reactive lymphocytes have been detected. *Islet autoantibodies* is also a generic term to include autoantibodies that react either to all cells of the islet or those that react only with the β cells. At present, the only β-cell–specific islet autoantibodies are insulin autoantibodies (IAAs) that bind to circulating insulin. To be exact, in vivo IAAs do not bind to a cell because they bind to an extracellular β-cell product.

In addition to IAA, the most useful islet autoantibodies are those directed against islet cell cytoplasmic autoantigens, glutamic acid decarboxylase (GAD), and an insulinoma-associated protein tyrosine phosphatase (IA-2). In the absence of serologic or cellular immune evidence of islet autoimmunity or a recognized cause of insulinopenic diabetes that falls into the category of other specific types of diabetes, idiopathic insulinopenic type 1 diabetes is classified as type 1b diabetes. There is controversy whether type 1b diabetes is really a separate entity from autoimmune diabetes.

In cases of autoimmune destruction of the pancreatic β cells, the α cells that secrete glucagon, the delta cells that secrete somatostatin, and the pancreatic polypeptide-secreting cells of the islet are undamaged in this highly selective process of β-cell targeting. Severe insulinopenia and secondary hyperglucagonemia produce hyperglycemia and unrestrained fat breakdown, leading to ketosis (Sperling, 1979). When the blood glucose level exceeds the renal threshold, glycosuria occurs, producing polyuria and resultant polydipsia. Marked catabolism leads to weight loss and inanition. Untreated, type 1 diabetes produces ketoacidosis accompanied by declining mentation or frank coma and eventual circulatory failure culminating in death. About 75% of cases of type 1 diabetes present before age 18.

Latent Autoimmune Diabetes of Adulthood

Although type 1 diabetes most commonly presents in the first two decades of life, it can develop at any age. Indeed, cases of *latent autoimmune diabetes of adulthood* are being recognized with increased frequency. Latent autoimmune diabetes of adulthood is the clinical syndrome describing individuals who are initially diagnosed with non–insulin-dependent diabetes yet display islet autoantibody markers and eventually progress to insulin dependence.

In contrast to type 1 diabetes, type 2 diabetes as defined by the 1997 ADA guidelines is a disease of insulin resistance coupled with an inadequate insulin response. Therefore both the β cell and the target tissues display defects. By definition, type 2 diabetes is not caused by autoimmune mechanisms. Insulin levels in type 2 diabetes are not uncommonly above normal; however, despite the hyperinsulinism, if insulin secretion cannot compensate for insulin resistance, decreased insulin action results. Hyperglycemia then ensues as a consequence of decreased insulin action. With persistent hyperglycemia, diabetes is diagnosed.

Type 2 diabetes is predominantly a disease of individuals older than age 40, although increasing numbers of obese children and adolescents are affected with type 2 diabetes (Glaser, 1997; Glaser and Jones, 1996; Jones, 1998). Of all adult type 2 diabetic subjects, 80% or more are obese. Minorities, including Native Americans, African Americans, and Hispanic Americans, are affected more often than whites.

Although the term *latent autoimmune diabetes of adulthood* was born in the 1990s, the recognition that non–insulin-dependent diabetes can be caused by autoimmune β-cell destruction goes back to the late 1970s (Irvine et al., 1977). Latent autoimmune diabetes of adulthood results from slowly progressive autoimmune β-cell destruction (Carlsson et al., 2000). Of patients initially presenting with the phenotype of non–insulin-dependent diabetes, 4% to 17% have serologic evidence of islet autoimmunity in the form of islet cell cytoplasmic autoantibodies (ICAs) (Di Mario et al., 1983; Irvine et al., 1977; Niskanen et al., 1991) or islet cell surface autoantibodies (ICSAs) (Ohgawara and Hirata, 1984).

In the 1990s, when the term *latent autoimmune diabetes of adulthood* was developed, autoantibodies to GAD were noted as a key feature of latent autoimmune diabetes of adulthood (Pietropaolo et al., 2000; Seissler et al., 1998; Tuomi et al., 1993). Although ICA tends to diminish in frequency after the diagnosis of autoimmune diabetes, autoantibodies to GAD (GADAs) are more persistent.

In latent autoimmune diabetes of adulthood, higher ICA titers predict later insulin dependence and a more severe degree of insulinopenia (Betterle et al., 1982; Gray et al., 1980). Autoimmune diabetes masquerading as clinical non–insulin-dependent diabetes is probably as common as classic acute-onset type 1 diabetes. If the frequency of classic acute-onset type 1 diabetes is 1 in 500 and the United States population is 275,000,000, then 550,000 Americans are affected with type 1 diabetes. If non–insulin-dependent diabetes conservatively affects 2% of the general population (5.5 million patients) and 10% of these non–insulin-dependent diabetic patients have β-cell autoimmunity and latent autoimmune diabetes of adulthood, there are 550,000 non–insulin-dependent diabetic patients with latent autoimmune diabetes of adulthood, a figure equal to that for classic type 1 diabetes (Winter et al., 1993).

Type 1 diabetes is usually distinguished from type 2 diabetes on both clinical and immunologic grounds (Table 37-4) (Skyler and Cahill, 1981). In type 1 diabetes, most patients at clinical onset have ICA (70% to 80% ICA-positive) (Neufeld et al., 1980b) and/or GADA (70% to 80% GADA-positive) or autoantibodies to an islet protein tyrosine phosphatase (PTP) (IA-2 autoantibodies [IA-2A] to be discussed later by Rabin et al., 1994). Lesser numbers of new-onset patients (~40%) have IAAs (Atkinson et al., 1986).

Type 1 diabetes is significantly associated with various HLA-DR alleles such as DR3 and DR4 (Cudworth and Wolf, 1982) and various HLA-DQB1 alleles (e.g., DQB1 *0201, DQB1 *0302) and HLA-DQA1 alleles (e.g., DQA1*0501, or DQA1*0301). Type 2 diabetes does not display associations with HLA alleles.

Type 2 Diabetes in Youth and Atypical Diabetes Mellitus of African Americans

Although most cases of acute-onset insulin requiring diabetes are caused by type 1 diabetes, some cases of acute onset diabetes are not caused by autoimmunity. Recognized in the mid-1990s, type 2 diabetes in adolescents can present with diabetic ketoacidosis (Umpierrez et al., 1995). These individuals with youth-onset type 2 are predominantly massively obese, are from Hispanic or African American minority groups, and generally have strong family histories of type 2 diabetes (Pinhas-Hamiel et al., 1996). Other African-American children with acute-onset insulin requiring diabetes have been described with atypical diabetes mellitus (ADM) of African Americans (Winter, 1991; Winter et al., 1987).

ADM is an acute-onset form of childhood diabetes that shifts from an insulin-dependent phenotype at presentation to a non–insulin-dependent phenotype over the first few months to years after diagnosis. In at least three fourths of cases, there is an autosomal dominant family history of similarly affected first-degree relatives. β-Cell function is deficient classifying ADM as a subtype of *maturity-onset diabetes of youth* (MODY) (Winter et al., 1999) that falls into the 1997 ADA classification category of other specific types of diabetes, subtype: genetic defects of the β-cell. In contrast to ADM, white MODY subjects are non–insulin dependent and most closely resemble clinical type 2 diabetes.

Nonatypical MODY can result from one of five molecular diseases involving mutations in hepatocyte nuclear factor-4α (MODY1), glucokinase (MODY2), hepatocyte nuclear factor-1α (MODY3), insulin-promoter factor-1 (IPF1), or hepatocyte nuclear factor 1β (MODY5) (Winter et al., 1999). MODY and ADM subjects lack islet autoantibodies and lack perturbed distributions of HLA alleles. Whereas only 5% of whites with type 1 diabetes lack the high-risk HLA DR3 and DR4 alleles, about 30% of African Americans with youth-onset diabetes lack both DR3 and DR4 (Maclaren et al., 1982; Winter et al., 1987).

ADM subjects differ in several respects from white MODY patients. ADM patients present with severe symptoms, often including ketosis, which requires early insulin therapy that would otherwise be consistent with the diagnosis of type 1 diabetes. White subjects with MODY are usually diagnosed only by oral glucose tolerance testing and do not display ketosis or require insulin treatment (Tattersall, 1974).

Historical Aspects

Insulitis is the histologic appearance of the islets near the time of diagnosis of type 1 diabetes in which the islets are infiltrated with mononuclear cells. These cells are predominantly CD4 and CD8 T cells and macrophages. The classical insulitis lesions observed in the pancreata of newly diagnosed patients with type 1 diabetes were observed as early as 1910 (Cecil, 1910) and were specifically described in 1940 by Von Meyenburg and later confirmed by Gepts (1965). Insulitis was not found in long-standing type 1 diabetes (Gepts and Lecompte, 1981). Disturbed frequencies of HLA alleles were initially observed by Singal and Blajchmann (1973) and were confirmed and expanded by Nerup and associates (1974) and Cudworth and Woodrow (1976).

Bottazzo and associates (1974) described ICAs in patients with autoimmune polyglandular syndromes (APSs), and Lendrum and colleagues (1975) later reported that ICAs were common in patients with type 1 diabetes near the time of diagnosis. Maclaren and Huang (1975) described ICSAs in type 1 diabetic patients. In 1980, these latter investigators reported the presence of anti-insulinoma autoreactive lymphocytes in type 1 diabetic subjects (Maclaren and Huang, 1980). This is some of the earliest evidence that type 1 diabetes results from a cell-mediated attack on the islet β cells.

By the early 1980s, initial studies of immunosuppressive therapy in new-onset type 1 diabetes were reported.

TABLE 37-3 · CLINICAL AND IMMUNOLOGIC COMPARISON OF TYPE 1 AND TYPE 2 DIABETES

	Type 1 Diabetes	Type 2 Diabetes
Clinical		
Age of onset	<18 years old (in 75%)	>40 years
Insulin requiring	+	−
Associated with obesity	−	+
Ketotic	+	−
Family history	+/−	++
Immunologic		
Islet autoantibodies	80%–95% (at diagnosis)	Absent by definition
Association with HLA alleles		
DR3 and DR4	+	−
DQB1*0201,DQB1*0302	+	−

HLA = human leukocyte antigen.

In the mid-1980s through late 1990s, great advances were made in the identification of the autoantigens of type 1 diabetes and studies of the genetics of type 1 diabetes.

Pathogenesis

Almost all cases of type 1 diabetes result from autoimmune destruction of the pancreatic β cells (Atkinson and Maclaren, 1990, 1994; Bottazzo et al., 1984a; Nerup et al., 1983; Winter et al., 1991a) (Fig. 37-2). Cases of nonautoimmune diabetes previously ascribed under the insulin-dependent rubric have been reclassified as other specific types of diabetes. For example, insulinopenic diabetes from toxin ingestion (e.g., the rodenticide Vacor) is classified as *other specific types of diabetes: drug- or chemical-induced diabetes,* severe chronic pancreatitis is classified as *other specific types of diabetes: diseases of the exocrine pancreas,* and viral infection of the β cells is classified as *other specific types of diabetes: infections* (Forrest et al., 1971; Yoon et al., 1979).

There is a significant environmental component in the pathogenesis of type 1 diabetes because identical twin studies show a concordance rate of only one third to one half. A rising incidence of type 1 diabetes has been recognized in several countries (Diabetes Epidemiology Research International Group, 1990; Karvonen et al., 2000; Rewers et al., 1987), which suggests some role for diet or novel infectious agents as initiators or induc-

ers of β-cell autoimmunity. Potential toxins include alloxan, streptozotocin, Vacor (Karam et al., 1980; Kenney et al., 1981; Pont et al., 1979), pentamidine (Hauser et al., 1991), and smoked or cured mutton.

Exposure to cow's milk and bovine serum albumin has been implicated as a potentiator of type 1 diabetes (Karjalainen et al., 1992); however, there is no consensus of opinion on this matter. There are conflicting data whether breastfeeding is protective against type 1 diabetes (Bognetti et al., 1992; Fort et al., 1986; Kyvik et al., 1992; Mayer et al., 1988; Metcalfe and Baum, 1992; Virtanen et al., 1991). Nevertheless, at present, there is no compelling reason to eliminate cow's milk from children's diets (Couper et al., 1999; Maclaren and Atkinson, 1992).

The environmental factors that trigger type 1 diabetes have yet to be identified, but a prior inductive event by an enteroviral infection may be involved (Atkinson and Maclaren, 1994). Although a controversial issue in the lay press, there is no evidence that immunizations predispose to type 1 diabetes (Graves et al., 1999; Hummel et al., 2000).

There is abundant evidence for autoimmunity as the etiologic agent in type 1 diabetes. Humoral and cell-mediated autoimmunity against the islets of Langerhans have been recognized for more than two decades. Insulitis, the pathognomonic inflammatory cell infiltrate observed in type 1 diabetes, has been known for more than 90 years.

ISLET CELL CYTOPLASMIC AUTOANTIBODIES

Islet cell cytoplasmic autoantibodies (ICAs) are detected by indirect immunofluorescence on unfixed sections of human blood group O pancreata. These autoantibodies react with the cytoplasm of islet cells but not their nuclei. Sera from ICA-positive individuals bind to all cells of the islet despite the fact that islet necrosis is limited to β cells. Therefore ICAs are islet specific but not β-cell specific. ICA may represent an epiphenomenon of immune system sensitization after release of sequestered antigens when β cells are damaged by the pathogenic cell-mediated anti–β-cell response that actually causes type 1 diabetes.

ICAs have been reported to react with a sialoglyco-conjugate target antigen (Nayak et al., 1985), as well as with GAD and the islet PTP IA-2 autoantigen. The GAD and IA-2 reactivity of ICAs were described by preabsorbing sera with GAD and IA-2 and then detecting a subsequent diminution or absence of fluorescence produced by the patient's serum. ICAs are polyclonal IgG autoantibodies (Schatz et al., 1988). Quantitation and reproducibility of ICA assays have been assisted by ICA workshops (Gleichmann and Bottazzo, 1987). ICAs are now standardized into Juvenile Diabetes Foundation (JDF) units.

ICAs have been found in 70% to 80% of newly diagnosed white patients with type 1 diabetes (Lendrum et al., 1976; Neufeld et al., 1980b). ICAs are present at diagnosis in only 40% of African Americans with youth-onset diabetes. This suggests that factors other than autoimmunity (e.g., ADM) cause many of the cases

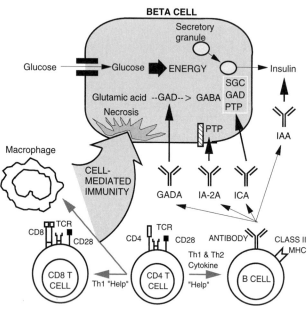

Figure 37-2· Autoimmune reactions in type 1 diabetes. Cell-mediated autoimmunity provided by CD8 T cells and macrophages that are activated by CD4 T helper cells is responsible for β-cell necrosis. B cells in type 1 diabetes produce a variety of nonpathogenic marker autoantibodies directed against the β cell and its products including islet cell cytoplasmic autoantibodies (ICA), insulin autoantibodies (IAA), glutamic acid decarboxylase autoantibodies (GADA), and insulinoma-associated-2 autoantibody (IA-2A). GABA = gamma-aminobutyric acid; PTP = protein tyrosine phosphatase; SGA = sialoglycoconjugate.

of youth-onset diabetes in African Americans (Neufeld et al., 1980a; Winter et al., 1987).

ICAs in nondiabetic individuals predict an increased risk for type 1 diabetes, which is discussed further in the section on natural history (Irvine et al., 1976; Wolf et al., 1981). Following diagnosis, the frequency of ICAs falls; after 5 years, less than 25% of patients remain ICA positive and after 10 years less than 5% remain ICA positive.

Surface antibodies to islet cells (ICSAs) were first identified using a human insulinoma line as a target (Maclaren and Huang, 1980). ICSAs can be demonstrated by indirect immunofluorescence (Lernmark et al., 1978) or by ^{51}Cr release (Eisenbarth et al., 1981) from labeled islets. Most investigators used rat insulinoma cells as targets for ICSAs because of the unavailability of human islet cell lines. ICSAs are carried in the gamma globulin serum fraction; they suppress glucose-stimulated insulin release from isolated murine islets, probably by killing islet cells (Sai et al., 1981), and from intact murine pancreata after perfusion with ICSA-positive sera (Svenningsen et al., 1983). ICSAs can initiate antibody-dependent cellular cytotoxity (Maruyama et al., 1984), and they preferentially bind to β cells rather than to other pancreatic islet cell types (Van Der Winkel et al., 1982). ICSAs are too difficult to measure routinely and thus are not useful for type 1 diabetes risk assessment.

INSULIN AUTOANTIBODIES

Presently, insulin remains the only β-cell product, and thus potential autoantigen, that is absolutely specific to the β cell. In 1983, Palmer and colleagues (1983a, 1983b) demonstrated that insulin was an autoantigen in diabetes. These researchers were able to show that, before exposure to any exogenous insulin, serum from subjects with new-onset type 1 diabetes contained autoantibodies that may immunoprecipitate radioactively labeled insulin. Because such radiobinding immunoprecipitation assays do not distinguish insulin antibodies that occur after insulin administration from spontaneously occurring insulin autoantibodies (IAA), IAA detection should be carried out before therapeutic insulin administration or only after a few days of initiating insulin administration. Although autoreactivity to a circulating protein may appear to be rare among autoimmune diseases, this phenomenon is actually quite common. For example, autoantibodies to thyroid hormone have been reported in AITD.

IAAs are best detected by immunoprecipitation. Modern IAA assays use mono-iodinated A-14 insulin (e.g., ^{125}I is attached to residue 14 of the insulin A chain). Because IAA can be in very low concentration, many laboratories that measure IAA incubate patients' sera with the mono-iodinated A-14 insulin for periods of up to 1 week before the addition of polyethylene glycol to immunoprecipitate the antigen–antibody complexes. Enzyme-linked immunosorbent assays (ELISAs) to measure IAA are strongly discouraged. Many studies have shown that IAAs detected by ELISA do not correlate with an increased risk of developing type 1 diabetes in nondiabetic individuals (Greenbaum et al., 1992; Levy-

Marchal et al., 1991). New "microvolume" IAA assays were introduced in the late 1990s (Naserke et al., 1998).

Before insulin therapy, IAA can be found in subjects with type 1 diabetes (Palmer et al., 1983a; Wilkin et al., 1985). Atkinson and colleagues (1986) found that about 40% of newly diagnosed patients have IAAs. IAAs are much more common in children than in adults before the diagnosis of type 1 diabetes. By themselves, IAAs are minimally predictive of type 1 diabetes because the frequency of IAAs in the population is higher than that of ICAs (Yassin et al., 1991). However, IAAs in conjunction with ICAs greatly improve the predictive value of ICAs for type 1 diabetes (Atkinson et al., 1986). IAAs are more specific than proinsulin autoantibodies for prediction of type 1 diabetes (Williams et al., 1999). IAAs are found in other autoimmune endocrine disorders such as AITD. Cellular reactivity to the insulin β chain has been described (Schloot et al., 1998).

GLUTAMIC ACID DECARBOXYLASE AUTOANTIBODIES

Sera from BioBreeding (BB) rats, nonobese diabetic (NOD) mice, and type 1 diabetic humans can immunoprecipitate unique β-cell proteins (Baekkeskov et al., 1982, 1984; Lernmark and Baekkeskov, 1981) of 64 kD. These 64-kD autoantibodies are at least as common as ICAs at disease onset and are highly predictive of type 1 diabetes (Atkinson et al., 1990). In 1990, Baekkeskov and colleagues identified that the 64-kD autoantigen was the enzyme GAD.

Enzymes that serve as autoantigens in autoimmune disorders are very common (Riley, 1995; Song and Maclaren, 1996); for example, (1) leukocyte myeloperoxidase is an autoantigen in systemic vasculitis, (2) the muscle acetylcholine receptor is an autoantigen in myasthenia gravis, (3) the neuronal presynaptic voltage-gated calcium channel is an autoantigen in Eaton-Lambert syndrome, and (4) elastinolase is an autoantigen in Wegener's granulomatosis.

GAD is found in abundance in several areas of the CNS and catalyzes the conversion of glutamic acid to gamma-aminobutyric acid (GABA), an inhibitory neurotransmitter. In lesser concentrations GAD is found in testes, ovary, adrenal, pituitary, thyroid, islets, and kidney. GAD enzymatic activity is a result of separate GAD enzymes: GAD_{65} (65 kD) and GAD_{67} (67 kD) that are coded by genes on two separate chromosomes. The GAD_{65} gene is located on chromosome 2q31, whereas the GAD_{67} gene is located on chromosome 10p11.2-p12. GAD_{65} and GAD_{67} display 70% amino acid homology. Autoantibodies to both GAD_{65} and GAD_{67} have been detected; however, autoantibodies to GAD_{65} are more common that autoantibodies to GAD_{67}, and thus most GADA assays use GAD_{65} as the target autoantigen (Luhder et al., 1994).

The GAD epitopes recognized by sera from subjects with type 1 diabetes appear to be conformational determinants because such diabetic sera do not recognize linear GAD peptides or denatured GAD. On the other hand, sera from patients with the stiff-man syndrome display high GADA titers and can react with denatured

GAD as observed in Western blots. Stiff-man (or stiff-person) syndrome is a rare neurologic disorder characterized by stiffness. GADAs in humans are only recognized through some form of immunoprecipitation assay. If a radioactive tag is placed on GAD such as ^{125}I by iodination or GAD is synthesized in vitro using a reticulocyte system in the presence of ^{35}S-methionine, the immunoprecipitation assay is termed a radiobinding assay (RBA). The RBAs for GADA are the most popular assays at present.

Cellular reactivity to GAD has been demonstrated by Atkinson and others (1992). Harrison and co-workers (1993) suggested that humoral and cellular reactivity to GAD are inversely related to the risk for type 1 diabetes. This latter issue is controversial.

INSULINOMA ASSOCIATED-2 AUTOANTIBODIES

During the 1980s and 1990s, researchers sought to discover novel autoantibodies by testing sera from type 1 diabetic patients for reactivity to antigens expressed from insulinoma mRNA libraries (Lan et al., 1996). Autoantibodies in type 1 diabetes sera were found to be directed against a protein expressed from an insulinoma mRNA library that they termed insulinoma associated-2 autoantibodies (IA-2A) (Rabin et al., 1994). Analysis of the target autoantigen revealed that IA-2 was a member of the protein tyrosine phosphatase (PTP) family. The PTP family of proteins includes the CD45 as cytoplasmic signal-transducing enzymes. The full-length IA-2 clone encodes a 979-amino acid 106-kD islet-cell autoantigen. By Northern blot analysis, IA-2 is identified in brain, pituitary, adrenal, pancreas, and certain brain tumor cell lines. A smaller portion of the full length mRNA produces an IA-2 protein fragment termed ICA512. Immunoassays for detection of IA-2 have used either the full-size protein (IA-2) or the smaller ICA512 fragment. The gene for IA-2 maps to chromosome 2q35-q36.19. Immunoprecipitation of radiolabeled IA-2 (e.g., a radiobinding assay) is the predominant methodology used to detect IA-2A. Another name for IA-2 is phogrin.

In addition to the IA-2 islet autoantigen, another PTP termed IA-2β also serves as an islet autoantigen. IA-2β is detected using RBA methodologies (Lu et al., 1996). So far no clear advantage has been seen in measuring IA-2β autoantibodies (IA-2βA) over IA-2A.

OTHER AUTOIMMUNE HUMORAL ABNORMALITIES

In addition to the islet cell sialoglycoconjugate, GAD, IA-2, and IA-2β, several other autoantigens have been detected in type 1 diabetes (Table 37-5). Some of these

TABLE 37-5 · AUTOIMMUNITY IN TYPE 1 DIABETES

	Preferred Method of Detection
Humoral Autoimmunity to Islet Cells	
Islet cell cytoplasmic autoantibodies (ICAs)	IFA
GAD autoantibodies (GADAs)	RBA
IA-2 autoantibodies (IA-2As)	RBA
GLUT2 autoantibodies blocking β-cell glucose uptake	Bioassay
52 kD RIN (Rat insulinoma) autoantibodies (anti-rubella virus-related protein)	WB (Karounos et al., 1990)
38-kD autoantibodies	WB (Pak et al., 1990)
Glima 38 autoantibodies	RBA (Aanstoot et al., 1996; Roll et al., 2000)
ICA69 autoantibodies*	WB (Pietropaolo et al., 1993)
Islet-specific monosialoganglioside GM2-1	IDIP (Dionisi et al., 1997)
Humoral Autoimmunity to β-Cell Products	
Insulin autoantibodies (IAAs)	RBA
Proinsulin autoantibodies	RBA
Carboxypeptidase H autoantibodies	WB (Castano et al., 1991)
Humoral Autoimmunity to the Insulin Receptor	
Insulin receptor autoantibodies	RRCA
Nonislet Humoral Autoimmunity	
51-kD aromatic-L-amino-acid decarboxylase AutoAb (1)	(Rorsman et al., 1995)
Chymotrypsinogen-related 30-kD pancreatic AutoAb	WB (Kim et al., 1993)
DNA topoisomerase II autoantibodies	WB (Chang et al., 1996)
Heat shock protein (HSP) autoantibodies*	WB (Atkinson et al., 1991)
SOX-13 autoimmunity	WB (Kasimiotis et al., 2000)
Cellular Autoimmunity	
Cellular autoreactivity to GAD$_{65}$	LPA
Cellular autoreactivity to 38-kD autoantigen (anti-insulin secretory granule protein)	LPA (Roep et al., 1990, 1991)
Cellular autoreactivity to transcription factor jun-B	LPA (Honeyman et al., 1993)
Cellular autoreactivity to imogen-38	LPA (Arden et al., 1996)
Cellular autoreactivity to hsp60	LPA (Abulafia-Lapid et al., 1999)
Cellular autoreactivity to β-lactoglobulin	LPA (Vaarala et al., 1996)

*Controversial.
IDIP = indirect immunoperoxidase technique; IFA = indirect immunofluorescent assay; LPA = lymphocyte proliferation assay (lymphocytes plus antigen; measure ^{3}H-thymidine incorporation or IL-2 release); RBA = radiobinding assay; RRCA = radioreceptor competition assay; WB = Western blot assay; (1) = detected by screening of cDNA expression library with diabetic sera.

autoantigens are islet specific, whereas other autoantigens are not islet specific. Other humoral immune abnormalities include the presence of immune complexes (Virella et al., 1981), antinuclear antibodies, lymphocytotoxic antibodies (Serjeantson et al., 1981), and insulin receptor autoantibodies (Maron et al., 1983).

SPECIFIC T-CELL ABNORMALITIES

Evidence for cell-mediated autoimmunity in type 1 diabetes includes the ability of type 1 diabetes lymphocytes to kill cultured human insulinoma cells in vitro (Maclaren and Huang, 1980). Likewise, in a rat insulinoma system, type 1 diabetes lymphocytes suppress insulin secretion (Boitard et al., 1997). Type 1 diabetes lymphocytes produce macrophage inhibition factor when exposed to islet antigens. Several studies suggest a functional deficiency in regulatory T cells (Lederman et al., 1981; Topliss et al., 1983). In vitro islet cell destruction mediated by immune cells may correlate with clinical disease activity (Charles et al., 1983). Lymphocytes from type 1 diabetic subjects also attach to β cells in vitro (Lang et al., 1987).

Insulitis, a mononuclear cell (lymphocyte and macrophage) infiltrate of the pancreatic islets, is found in at least 60% of patients with type 1 diabetes who come to autopsy within 6 months of diagnosis (Gepts and Lecompte, 1981). Some investigators report insulitis frequencies of 78% to 88% (Foulis and Stewart, 1984; Foulis et al., 1986). Using histochemical staining, as many as 90% of the pancreatic β cells have been destroyed by the time of diagnosis.

In a classic study from Bottazzo and colleagues (1985), a pancreas from a patient newly diagnosed with type 1 diabetes was examined with the use of monoclonal antibody probes. The infiltrating lymphocytes were activated T lymphocytes expressing DR antigen. The T lymphocytes were predominantly of the CD8[+] phenotype, suggesting cell-mediated cytotoxicity as the cause of the β-cell destruction. It is unknown how long insulitis persists after the clinical diagnosis of type 1 diabetes. Hanafusa and co-workers (1983) did not find insulitis in seven type 1 diabetic patients undergoing pancreatic biopsy 2 to 4 months after the onset of type 1 diabetes.

NONSPECIFIC T-CELL ABNORMALITIES

Many other types of cellular immune abnormalities have been described in type 1 diabetes. Type 1 diabetes lymphocytes produce subnormal levels of interleukin (IL)-2 (Rodman, 1984; Zier et al., 1984). In comparison with controls, mitogen-stimulated lymphocytes from subjects with type 1 diabetes provide subnormal cytokine help to B cells (Schatz et al., 1991). Faustman and colleagues (1991) have suggested that class I MHC expression is deficient in type 1 diabetic humans and nonobese diabetic mice.

Before and at the time of diagnosis of type 1 diabetes, peripheral blood activated T cells can be identified (Alviggi et al., 1984; Jackson et al., 1982, 1984) using anti–class II MHC monoclonal and Tac monoclonal antibodies (MAb) (Hayward and Herberger, 1984). The Tac MAb recognizes IL-2 receptors present on activated T cells. Many groups have described abnormalities in the CD4:CD8 ratio (Faustman et al., 1989; Galluzzo et al., 1984; Hitchcock et al., 1986; Horita et al., 1982; Ilonen et al., 1984; Pozzilli et al., 1983). Elevated numbers of natural killer (NK) cells may be present at the time of diagnosis (Pozzilli et al., 1979). The significance and reproducibility of these findings is not established. Litherland and colleagues (1999) have described variations in antigen-presenting cell function in type 1 diabetes and prostaglandin synthase-2 expression.

Bottazzo and co-workers (1983) proposed that endocrine cells that aberrantly express class II MHC molecules foster immunologic suicide by autopresentation of cytoplasmic self-antigens (Londei et al., 1984). However, it is unlikely that aberrant class II MHC expression actually causes autoimmunity. It is more likely that class II MHC expression by non–antigen-presenting cells represents a regulatory action to downregulate an immune response. It is clear that when naïve T cells encounter peptides without the necessary co-stimulatory action of B7, T-cell anergy results. Furthermore, class II MHC molecules present peptides from extracellular antigens and not cytoplasmic antigens. Class II MHC expression does occur on thyroid follicular cells in cases of Hashimoto's thyroiditis and biliary tract epithelial cells in autoimmune biliary cirrhosis.

Other Autoimmune Diseases Associated with Type 1 Diabetes

Type 1 diabetes is associated with other autoimmune endocrine and nonendocrine diseases (Neufeld et al., 1980b). This provides additional evidence that type 1 diabetes is an autoimmune disease. Thyroid microsomal autoantibodies (TMAs) indicative of Hashimoto's thyroiditis are found in 20% to 25% of female patients with type 1 diabetes (Riley et al., 1981). About 10% of male subjects with type 1 diabetes are TMA positive. Approximately 50% of TMA-positive type 1 diabetic subjects go on to have clinical thyroid disease (20% Graves' disease; 80% hypothyroidism).

About 10% of type 1 diabetic patients also have gastric parietal cell autoantibodies (PCAs). These autoantibodies serve as markers for chronic lymphocytic gastritis that can lead to parietal cell destruction with consequent achlorhydria and intrinsic factor deficiency. Subsequently achlorhydria can cause iron malabsorption and iron deficiency anemia (Riley et al., 1982). Prolonged intrinsic factor deficiency leads to vitamin B_{12} deficiency and pernicious anemia in mid to later life (Toh et al., 1997). Thyroid microsomal antibodies (TMAs) and parietal cell autoantibodies occur together in about 5% of type 1 diabetic patients.

Autoimmune Addison's disease occurs in 1 of 300 patients with type 1 diabetes, often in association with thyroid and gastric autoimmunity. Another autoimmune disease occurring in type 1 diabetics is celiac disease.

Genetic Susceptibility to Type 1 Diabetes

Type 1 diabetes is not inherited as a mendelian trait. Furthermore, no single gene allele or molecular mutation is universally detected in patients with type 1 diabetes that is routinely absent in controls. It is suggested that genetic susceptibility to environmental triggers of β-cell autoimmunity is an essential mechanism whereby genes influence the development of type 1 diabetes. As well, polymorphisms in immune system genes (e.g., possibly CLTA-4) and β-cell genes (e.g., insulin) also appear to provide proclivity to type 1 diabetes.

Type 1 diabetes is a polygenic disorder that is believed to be triggered by an environmental insult or insults (Winter et al., 1991b, 1993). More than a dozen genetic loci have been associated with type 1 diabetes (Table 37-6). The combination of polygenicity and suspected environmental influences imply that type 1 diabetes is multifactorial in cause. Earlier-onset type 1 diabetes likely occurs in individuals with a greater genetic load for type 1 diabetes, whereas type 1 diabetes occurs in older individuals with a lesser degree of genetic load for type 1 diabetes after (theoretically) suffering more intense, more frequent, and/or more varied environmental insults. During the pathogenesis of type 1 diabetes, genes and environment interact at several stages in the process, not solely at the time of initiation of β-cell autoimmunity.

Whereas most cases of type 1 diabetes occur sporadically (e.g., the absence of a family history of a similarly affected first-degree relative), 15% of individuals with type 1 diabetes do have a positive family history for type 1 diabetes. First-degree relatives of type 1 diabetic subjects have a 1 in 20 chance of developing type 1 diabetes (5%). An identical twin of an individual affected with type 1 diabetes has a 30% to 50% risk of developing type 1 diabetes. If islet autoimmunity is sought in twins discordant for type 1 diabetes, the nondiabetic twin will frequently display islet autoantibodies. Children of fathers with type 1 diabetes are at higher risk for type 1 diabetes than children of mothers with type 1 diabetes (e.g., 7% vs. 2% risk of type 1 diabetes).

INSULIN-DEPENDENT DIABETES MELLITUS SUSCEPTIBILITY LOCUS 1 (IDDM1)

The first genetic type 1 diabetes susceptibility locus was the HLA complex located on the short arm of chromosome 6. The human MHC contains three classes of genes. Class I MHC molecules include HLA-A, HLA-B, and HLA-C and present cytoplasmic peptides to CD8 T cells. The heterodimer class II MHC molecules include the α and β chains of HLA-DP, HLA-DQ, and HLA-DR that present extracellular and intravesicular peptides to CD4 T cells. Class III MHC molecules have a variety of functions involving the complement system (e.g., C4 and C2), enzymes (e.g., 21-hydroxylase), cytokines (e.g., tumor necrosis factor), and cytoplasmic antigen processing (e.g., large molecular weight proteasome subunits).

The HLA complex is termed *IDDM1* because it is the first susceptibility locus identified for insulin-dependent diabetes. Furthermore, the HLA complex provides the strongest genetic influence for the development of type 1 diabetes. It is estimated that 40% to 50% of genetic susceptibility is supplied by the HLA complex.

HLA molecules may affect genetic susceptibility through several mechanisms (Bottazzo et al., 1984b; Nepom et al., 1998). First, HLA molecules present antigen-derived peptide fragments to T-cell receptors. Specific HLA alleles might be more adept at presenting autoantigens than other alleles and thus elicit a stronger autoimmune response. Alternatively, if self-antigens are presented less efficiently in the thymus, autoimmunity might be more likely. Second, self-antigens, such as the HLA molecules, shape the T-cell receptor repertoire in the thymus as antiself T-cell receptors are eliminated during T-cell ontogeny. Third, other genes in linkage disequilibrium with the HLA alleles may be the real susceptibility genes.

Initial studies indicated that specific HLA-B alleles (e.g., HLA-B8) were associated with type 1 diabetes. With the advent of class II MHC microcytotoxicity typing, HLA-DR alleles were shown to be genetically important. HLA-DR3, HLA-DR4, and to a lesser extent, DR1 are susceptibility alleles for type 1 diabetes. The approximate absolute risks of developing type 1 diabetes is as follows:

General population: 1 in 500
HLA-DR3 positive: 1 in 400
HLA-DR4 positive: 1 in 400
HLA-DR3/4 positive: 1 in 40

Just as some loci provide a proclivity to type 1 diabetes, other alleles are protective of type 1 diabetes. HLA-DR2 and to a lesser extent HLA-DR5 are greatly reduced in type 1 diabetes populations. The specific protective DR2 allele is DRB1*15 (Maclaren et al., 1988). DR7 may also be a risk allele in African Americans. DR9 in the Japanese population replaces DR3 as a risk allele (Kida et al., 1989). Individuals that lack both HLA-DR3 and HLA-DR4 are at reduced risk

TABLE 37-6 · TYPE 1 DIABETES SUSCEPTIBILITY LOCI*

Loci	Location	Gene	Status
IDDM1	**6p21**	**HLA-DR and DQ**	**Confirmed**
IDDM2	**11p15**	**Insulin**	**Confirmed**
IDDM3	15q26	Unknown	Unconfirmed
IDDM4	**11q13**	**Unknown**	**Confirmed**
IDDM5	**6q25**	**Unknown**	**Confirmed**
IDDM6	18q	Unknown	Unconfirmed
IDDM7	2q33	Unknown	Unconfirmed
IDDM8	**6q2**	**Unknown**	**Confirmed**
IDDM9	3q	Unknown	Unconfirmed
IDDM10	10p13-q11	Unknown	Unconfirmed
IDDM11	14q24-q31	Unknown	Unconfirmed
IDDM12	**2q33**	**CTLA-4**	**Confirmed**
IDDM13	2q33	Unknown	Unconfirmed
IDDM15	6q21	Unknown	Unconfirmed

*Confirmed loci are in **bold**.

for type 1 diabetes (1 in 5000). Because HLA-DR α chains are nonpolymorphic, all of the DR susceptibility is provided by the β chains.

More than 95% of white patients with type 1 diabetes express HLA-DR3 or HLA-DR4, in contrast to about 50% of a control population (Cudworth and Wolf, 1982). Nearly 40% of type 1 diabetic patients are HLA-DR3/DR4 heterozygotes. Most of the remainder are HLA-DR3/DRX (25%; X can be any DR allele except DR3 or DR4) or DR4/DRX (30%) positive. Only 3% of the control population are heterozygous for DR3/DR4. Whereas only about 5% of whites with type 1 diabetes lack both HLA-DR3 and HLA-DR4, 30% of young African Americans with acute-onset diabetes lack both of these high-risk alleles for type 1 diabetes (Winter et al., 1987).

In the 1980s, association studies were extended to analyses of the HLA-DQ loci (She, 1996). HLA-DQ α and β chains were both shown to modify susceptibility to type 1 diabetes (Horn et al., 1988; Michelsen and Lernmark, 1987). HLA-DQB1*0302 and HLA-DQB1*0201 were shown to be very important susceptibility alleles. There is tight linkage between DR and DQ alleles: DR4 and DQB1*0302 and DR3 and DQB1*0201 are usually located on the same chromosome. Concerning protective HLA-DQB1 alleles, HLA-DQB1*0602 is distinctly rare in subjects with type 1 diabetes. HLA-DR2 and HLA-DQB1*0602 are linked. Although type 1 diabetes is not a mendelian disease, protective alleles are functionally dominant over susceptibility alleles (Nepom, 1990).

HLA-DQB1 alleles that are risk alleles for type 1 diabetes lack aspartic acid at amino acid 57 in the expressed DQβ chain (Baisch et al., 1990; Morel et al., 1988; Todd et al., 1987). Specific DQα sequences also affect immunodiabetogenesis (Deschamps et al., 1990; Fletcher et al., 1988). Susceptibility DQα chains such as DQA1*0301 and DQA1*0501 display arginine at residue 52. It is postulated that these polymorphisms among susceptibility and resistance alleles influence autoantigen peptide binding or molecular stability (Ettinger et al., 2000; Owerbach et al., 1988).

Family history and HLA can strongly interact. Children who are HLA-identical to their type 1 diabetes sibling will have a 1 in 7 risk of developing type 1 diabetes. This is a 2.9-fold increased risk for type 1 diabetes over the general type 1 diabetes risk in first-degree relatives of about 5% (1 in 20). If a child is HLA-identical to their affected sibling and they share HLA-DR3 and DR4, the risk for type 1 diabetes rises to about 1 in 4. This 25% risk for type 1 diabetes is very similar to the risk of developing type 1 diabetes if one has an affected identical twin (1 in 3 to 1 in 2). This further emphasizes the important role that HLA plays in genetic susceptibility to type 1 diabetes.

Parentage affects susceptibility to type 1 diabetes (Vadheim et al., 1986; Warram et al., 1984). Fathers preferentially pass on HLA-DR4–bearing haplotypes to their offspring, helping to account for the excess risk of type 1 diabetes in the offspring of fathers with type 1 diabetes. Both mothers and fathers with type 1 diabetes preferentially pass on HLA-DR3–bearing haplotypes.

INSULIN-DEPENDENT DIABETES MELLITUS SUSCEPTIBILITY LOCUS 2 (IDDM2)

IDDM2 is the insulin gene located on chromosome 11 (Bain et al., 1992; Bell et al., 1984; Julier et al., 1991). Specifically, the 5' hypervariable region (HVR) influences immunodiabetogenesis. Approximately 500 base pairs upstream of the transcription start site, the HVR consists of variable numbers of 14 to 15 base-pair tandem repeats. HVRs in the population have been classified according to the number of repeats into three classes. The class 1 family has on average 570 base pairs, class 2 has about 1320 base pairs, and class 3 averages 2470 base pairs. In population studies, class 1 alleles occur more commonly in both type 1 and type 2 diabetic subjects than controls.

Recent data suggest that class 1 alleles may be expressed to a lesser degree than the other alleles in the thymus. Therefore if thymic expression is necessary to permit thymic clonal deletion, decreased thymic expression of the insulin gene may lead to thymic evolution of T-cell clones that are reactive to insulin. Again, it is worth noting that insulin is the only β-cell–specific autoantigen identified to date. IDDM1 and IDDM2 interact in providing type 1 diabetes susceptibility (She et al., 1994).

OTHER TYPE 1 DIABETES SUSCEPTIBILITY LOCI

All other loci so far linked to type 1 diabetes have been detected via sib-pair analysis by determining whether siblings affected with the same disorder share specific parental alleles more commonly than one would predict at random. Assuming that both parents are heterozygous and themselves do not share any alleles at a single locus, for a single locus random chance suggests that 25% of their offspring will be identical, 50% will share one allele, and 25% of offspring will share no alleles. When there is significant deviation from the expected, linkage can be established identifying the locus under study as a disease susceptibility locus. Sib-pair analysis does not require that the mode of inheritance of a disorder be specified. The disorder may be mendelian or nonmendelian or dominant or recessive or polygenic in cause. Studying large numbers of affected sib pairs is a powerful tool to study polygenic disorders like type 1 diabetes.

Of the remaining loci (e.g., IDDM3, IDDM4) (Davies et al., 1994), the certainty of linkage of the locus to type 1 diabetes can be expressed as confirmed or unconfirmed. Repeatability of the linkage studies in more than one independent population and strong statistical linkage are necessary to confirm the locus linkage (She and Marron, 1998).

In addition to IDDM1 and IDDM2, there are four other confirmed loci detected via sib-pair analysis: IDDM4, IDDM5, IDDM8, and IDDM12. IDDM4 is located on chromosome 11q13, IDDM5 on chromosome 6q25, and IDDM8 on chromosome 6q2 (Davies et al., 1994; Luo et al., 1996). No candidate genes in these three regions have been identified so far. *IDDM12* on chromosome 2q33 appears to map close to the cytotoxic T-lymphocyte-associated serine esterase-4 gene *(CTLA-4),* but no sequence polymorphisms of CLTA-4 have been identified despite rigorous study (Marron et al., 2000). *CLTA-4* is an excellent candidate gene for autoimmune diseases because *CTLA-4* expression occurs on activated T cells and interaction of *CTLA-4* with B7 from an antigen-presenting cell leads to T-cell downregulation or deactivation. Therefore theoretically, failure to normally downregulate T cells may foster autoimmunity.

Natural History

Type 1 diabetes resembles other autoimmune endocrinopathies in that β-cell destruction proceeds over a period of months to years before clinical presentation (Fig. 37-3) (Gorsuch et al., 1981). As markers of the autoimmune process, ICA, IAA, GADA, and IA-2A are frequently present at diagnosis and can appear months to years before diagnosis (Riley et al., 1984, 1990).

In nondiabetic individuals, the presence of islet autoantibodies predicts an increased risk for the development of type 1 diabetes. An abnormal intravenous glucose tolerance test coupled with the presence of ICA can increase the predictability of developing type 1 diabetes. If low plasma insulin levels are present at times 1 minute plus 3 minutes following the intravenous injection of glucose (e.g., the intravenous glucose tolerance test [IVGTT]) coupled with a positive ICA test, such individuals have a 5-year risk for developing type 1 diabetes of 50% to 60%. It is likely that the 10-year risk for developing type 1 diabetes approaches 100%. Furthermore, the more types of islet autoantibodies that an individual expresses, the higher the risk for the development of type 1 diabetes. A higher titer of ICAs predicts type 1 diabetes better than low-titer ICAs

(Bruining et al., 1984; Riley et al., 1980a). High titers of ICAs are able to fix complement (Bottazzo et al., 1980a), although autoantibodies are not believed to be pathogenic because type 1 diabetes results from cell-mediated β-cell destruction. The predictive value of islet autoantibodies for type 1 diabetes is greater in children than in adults.

THE PREDIABETIC STATE

The prediabetic period can be divided into four stages (Fig. 37-4):

Stage 1. Genetic susceptibility: before there is evidence of islet autoimmunity or metabolic β-cell dysfunction, there is asymptomatic genetic susceptibility (Gutierrez-Lopez et al., 1992; Heimberg et al., 1992).

Stage 2. Following a presumed environmental insult that functions as a trigger for an anti-islet autoimmune response, immune abnormalities (ICA, IAA, GADA, or IA-2A) that indicate islet autoimmunity are now detectable. At this stage, there are still no metabolic perturbations. Islet autoantibodies can be detected very early in life (Ziegler et al., 1999).

Stage 3. β-Cell destruction becomes evident with abnormally low first-phase insulin responses to intravenous glucose (Srikanta et al., 1983a, 1983b, 1983c). In the IVGTT, β-cell function is assessed by measuring the insulin concentrations at 1 and 3 minutes (the first-phase insulin release) following an intravenous glucose injection. In ICA-positive individuals who later display clinical type 1 diabetes, first-phase insulin responses decline at a rate of 20 to 40 mcU/ml per year (Srikanta et al., 1984a, 1984b). Insulin response to intravenous glucagon, arginine, and tolbutamide may be preserved despite deficient insulin secretion to intra-

VARIABLE COURSE OF ISLET AUTOIMMUNITY MARKED BY ISLET AUTOANTIBODIES

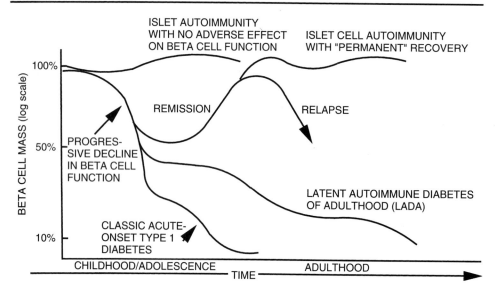

Figure 37-3 · Natural history of β-cell autoimmunity. Some individuals who express islet autoantibodies display no loss of β-cell mass *(top left).* More commonly though, individuals with islet autoantibodies exhibit a progressive decline in β-cell function. Many such individuals will progress to acute-onset type 1 diabetes that presents in childhood or adolescence. Some individuals will enter a remission phase with improved β-cell function, whereas others will slowly progress to type 1 diabetes in adulthood (LADA). Permanent remission, relapse, or progression to type 1 diabetes after an initial remission are possible clinical courses.

PROGRESSIVE NATURAL HISTORY OF PREDIABETES AND TYPE I DIABETES

Figure 37-4 · Prediabetes can be divided into four stages: (1) genetic susceptibility, (2) appearance of islet autoimmunity (islet cell cytoplasmic autoantibodies [ICA], insulin autoantibodies [IAA], glutamic acid decarboxylase autoantibodies [GADA], and insulinoma-associated-2 autoantibody [IA-2A]), (3) abnormal intravenous glucose tolerance test (IVGTT) with low first-phase insulin response, and (4) abnormal oral glucose tolerance test (OGTT). In the natural history of type 1 diabetes, the final stage (stage 5) is the appearance of frank clinical diabetes with symptoms and fasting hyperglycemia.

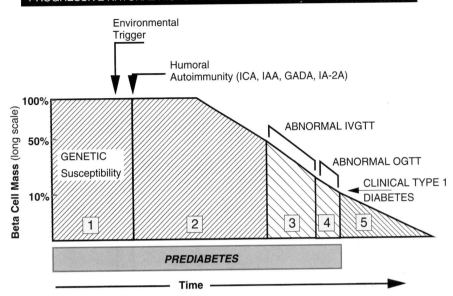

venous glucose (Ganda et al., 1984b). At this stage the patient is clinically asymptomatic.

Stage 4. As a mononuclear cellular islet infiltrate progresses (insulitis), more extensive β-cell destruction occurs. Insulin reserve becomes deficient and oral glucose tolerance deteriorates. Whereas fasting plasma glucose may not be clearly elevated, plasma glucose levels are elevated 2 hours following oral glucose challenge. Once the oral glucose tolerance test is abnormal, the clinical findings of diabetes (polyuria, polydipsia, and weight loss) generally appear within 1 to 2 years.

When prediabetes progresses to clinical type 1 diabetes with typical polyuria, polydipsia, and possible weight loss, the penultimate stage of islet autoimmunity is reached. Diabetes is diagnosed when a plasma or serum glucose measurement indicates hyperglycemia on two different days. However, if ketoacidosis is evident at initial presentation, ketoacidosis by itself is sufficient to warrant the diagnosis of diabetes. *Hyperglycemia* is defined in three possible ways: (1) the fasting plasma glucose is 126 mg/dl or greater; (2) the 2-hour glucose value during an oral glucose tolerance test is 200 mg/dl or greater; and (3) in the presence of symptoms of diabetes, the random plasma glucose is 200 mg/dl or greater.

Patients are said to have been prediabetic only retrospectively when type 1 diabetes develops in people whose ICAs, IAAs, GADAs, or IA-2As are identified before diagnosis. Individuals with humoral islet autoimmunity who do not have diabetes may or may not be prediabetic, because not all autoantibody-positive subjects develop type 1 diabetes. When low titers of ICA are present (e.g., 5 to 10 JDF units), the autoantibodies may disappear spontaneously or may persist at low titers for years or decades without progression to type 1 diabetes, particularly in adults. ICAs do not participate

in β-cell damage; however, they serve as useful markers of β-cell damage. Most researchers use 10 JDF units as the lowest ICA value that is considered to be positive.

Although islet autoantibodies may disappear with time, the body's ability to respond to islet cell antigens can be retained for at least 20 years after diagnosis. This is illustrated in the studies of Sutherland and coworkers (1984a, 1984b) in pancreatic transplantation between sets of identical twins discordant for type 1 diabetes. Immediately after transplantation, all recipient twins showed amelioration of their diabetes with a decline of glucose levels to the normal, nondiabetic range. However, 6 to 8 weeks after transplantation in twins who were not immunosuppressed, insulitis occurred and the recipient twin became frankly diabetic and required insulin treatment. In one of the recipient twins, ICA appeared following the pancreas transplant. This indicates that humoral and cell-mediated autoimmunity was reactivated following re-exposure to the islet cell antigens of the transplanted pancreas. When the recipient twin was immunosuppressed, there was no recurrence of insulitis or diabetes.

Diagnosis

The presence of insulin-dependent, ketosis-prone diabetes in association with ICA, IAA (before insulin treatment), GADA, or IA-2A and type 1 diabetes-associated HLA alleles (e.g., HLA-DR3, HLA-DR4, HLA-DQB1*0201, or HLA-DQB1*0302) is virtually diagnostic of autoimmune type 1 (1a) diabetes. Most clinicians diagnose type 1 diabetes on the basis of its more severe hyperglycemia, ketosis, rapidity of onset, and youth-onset; in contrast, type 2 diabetes is diagnosed when hyperglycemia is less severe, ketosis is generally absent, the onset of the disease is subtle, and affected individuals are usually obese and older than age 40.

Additional supportive evidence for an autoimmune pathogenesis in type 1 diabetes includes:

1. Associated autoantibodies (thyroid microsomal, thyroperoxidase or thyroglobulin, gastric parietal cell, and/or adrenocortical autoantibodies)
2. HLA haplotype sharing with an affected sibling
3. A positive family history of type 1 diabetes in a first-degree relative

As noted previously, when a sibling shares two parental haplotypes with a type-1-diabetes affected sibling, their risk for type diabetes is approximately 1 in 7. If the child shares DR3/4 haplotypes with their affected sibling, the absolute risk for type 1 diabetes rises to 1 in 4. In the absence of serologic evidence of islet autoimmunity (e.g., ICA or IAA), HLA typing by itself has limited use in predicting type 1 diabetes in the general population. However, several research programs are underway that use filter paper polymerase chain reaction (PCR) molecular screening for HLA-DQB1*0201 and HLA-DQB1*0302 as a method to identify individuals who should then undergo further islet autoantibody testing.

Treatment

Since Banting and Best discovered insulin in 1922, the treatment for type 1 diabetes has been subcutaneously injected insulin. Oral hypoglycemic agents have no role in the treatment of type 1 diabetes.

Novel therapies include the following:

1. New approaches to insulin delivery (i.e., insulin pumps, intraportal insulin delivery, closed-loop insulin infusion with glucose sensors, intranasal insulin, inhaled insulin)
2. New insulin analogies (e.g., short-acting lyspro insulin; long-acting glargine [GlyA21,ArgB31,ArgB32] insulin); NN 304, a 14-carbon aliphatic fatty acid acylated insulin analogue]
3. Addition of noninsulin β-cell products to the therapeutic regiment (e.g., amylin; glucagon-like peptide-1 [GLP-1])
4. Immunomodulation (induction of immunologic tolerance) or immunosuppression in pre–type 1 diabetes or in new-onset type 1 diabetes
5. Segmental or whole pancreatic transplantation (Sutherland et al., 1984c)
6. Isolated islet transplantation (Shapiro et al., 2000)
7. Islet stem cell transplantation technologies (Ramiya et al., 2000)
8. Molecular engineering of insulin-responsive non-β cells to create "neo-" β cells

In general, immunosuppression at onset of type 1 diabetes has produced only short-term remission from the requirement to take exogenous insulin in about 50% of patients treated either with cyclosporine (Assan et al., 1985; Bougneres et al., 1980; Stiller et al., 1984) or azathioprine plus glucocorticoids (Harrison et al., 1985; Silverstein et al., 1988). However, these remissions were not permanent and once immunosuppression was discontinued, diabetes recurred. Furthermore, long-term immunosuppression has its own complications that may be similar to or worse than diabetes. Such complications include cyclosporine-induced renal failure (Myers et al., 1984), increased susceptibility to infection, and an increased risk for a lymphoproliferative disorder.

Recognizing that more than 90% to 95% of the β-cell mass has already been destroyed at the time of diagnosis of type 1 diabetes, researchers have turned their attention to the prevention of type 1 diabetes. Susceptibility to type 1 diabetes can be recognized by the detection of the various islet autoantibodies (e.g., identification of pre–type 1 diabetes). As individuals express a greater variety and/or higher concentration of islet autoantibodies, the risk for type 1 diabetes rises. If there is evidence of β-cell dysfunction (e.g., low first-phase insulin response to the injection of intravenous glucose) combined with the presence of ICA, the 5-year risk for developing type 1 diabetes exceeds 50% and likely approaches 100% over 10 years of follow-up in children.

Once pre–type 1 diabetes is diagnosed, researchers have sought methods to interfere with the autoimmune process. Several prevention trials are now underway that attempt to (1) target environmental triggers (e.g., cow's milk avoidance in the Cow's Milk Avoidance Trial), (2) seek to strengthen the β cell against oxidative attack (e.g., nicotinamide in the European Nicotinamide Diabetes Intervention Trial) (Manna et al., 1992), and (3) induce immunologic tolerance and/or rest the β cell (e.g., subcutaneous or oral insulin administration in pre–type 1 diabetes in the Diabetes Prevention Trial-1 [DPT-1] 1993 [Rabinovitch et al., 1998] and intranasal insulin in the Finnish Diabetes Prediction and Prevention Trial [DIPP trial]) (Fuchtenbusch et al., 1998).

There is no clear evidence that cow's milk is a major environmental trigger. Several papers have disputed the claim that nicotinamide is of any benefit in preventing or treating type 1 diabetes (Herskowitz et al., 1989; Vidal et al., 2000).

The results of the subcutaneous-insulin arm of DPT-1, released in the summer of 2001, showed that parenteral insulin was ineffective in preventing type 1 diabetes. Orally administered insulin begun at disease onset is ineffective in changing the disease course over the first 12 months after diagnosis (Pozzilli et al., 2000).

Success in other studies may permit the routine treatment of pre–type 1 diabetic individuals to delay or prevent type 1 diabetes (Pozilli, 1998). Intervention trials must be considered experimental (Rosenbloom et al., 2000). Trials in new-onset type 1 diabetic subjects should not be entirely abandoned. Short-term and relatively nontoxic interventions (e.g., humanized anti–T-cell monoclonal antibodies) should be attempted in such patients. If successful, these interventions may then be studied in the prediabetic subjects.

Prognosis

Before the 1990s, traditional insulin replacement therapy did not prevent significant vascular complications from developing in most patients with type 1 diabetes after 15 to 20 years (Rosenbloom, 1983). Diabetic microvascular disease is a leading cause of blindness and kidney failure. Macrovascular disease results in accelerated atherosclerosis and early myocardial infarction, stroke, and peripheral vascular disease. The Diabetes Control and Complications Trial (DCCT) (1993) demonstrated that good metabolic control lowers the risk for developing microvascular complications by 50% to 60%.

Since then, there has been an emphasis on the need to normalize blood glucose in these patients. With excellent metabolic control, and avoidance of hypertension and hyperlipidemia, the long-term complications can be delayed or eliminated. Because complications do not occur in the absence of overt type 1 diabetes, there is a continued need for prevention or cure.

Autoimmune Hypoglycemia

To a large extent, steroid and thyroid hormones are present in the circulation bound to carrier proteins. In contrast, most protein hormones exist unbound in the circulation except for insulin-like growth factors (somatomedins) and growth hormone. Insulin antibodies develop in diabetic patients treated with exogenous insulin, especially in those without HLA-DR3 alleles. This occurs regardless of the species source of insulin administered—porcine, bovine, or human. These antibodies do not substantially complicate the clinical course of the diabetic patient.

Spontaneously occurring IAAs arising in individuals not exposed to exogenous insulin can occasionally result in spontaneous hypoglycemia or glucose intolerance (Virally et al., 1999). This is termed the *autoimmune hypoglycemia syndrome* or the *insulin autoimmune syndrome* (Uchigata and Hirata, 1999). Autoimmune hypoglycemia is a clinical syndrome of hyperinsulinism in the absence of an insulinoma that is associated with IAAs. Pediatric cases have been reported (Meschi et al., 1992).

Historical Aspects

In 1972, studies from Japan reported IAAs in individuals with hypoglycemia who had not previously been treated with exogenous insulin (Takayama-Hasumi et al., 1990). Autoimmune hypoglycemia has been reported outside of Japan only rarely (Burch et al., 1992; Meschi et al., 1992; Schlemper et al., 1996).

Pathogenesis

A presumed defect in immune surveillance results in the spontaneous production of autoantibodies that bind to circulating insulin and act as carrier proteins for insulin (Goldman et al., 1979). A marked elevation in the total immunoreactive insulin level occurs (Dozio et al., 1998). The large reservoir of circulating autoantibody-bound insulin can spontaneously release insulin, leading to acute elevations in free insulin levels inappropriate for metabolic needs. This can cause hypoglycemia even after feeding. These IAAs can also bind secreted insulin and decrease free insulin in the circulation, thus producing glucose intolerance. Spontaneous IAAs are polyclonal antibodies (Dozio et al., 1991) directed against human insulin and not porcine or bovine insulins.

Other autoimmune diseases (e.g., Graves' disease) may develop in affected patients. Drugs may also elicit insulin autoantibodies, specifically methimazole (Chen et al., 1990; Hirata, 1983) and other drugs containing sulfhydryl groups. A recent study recorded a decrease in IAAs despite continuation of methimazole in a subject with autoimmune hypoglycemia and Graves' disease (Okabe et al., 1999). Japanese investigators have suggested that up to 15% of their patients with spontaneous hypoglycemia have autoimmune hypoglycemia (Takayama and Hirata, 1983; Takayama-Hasumi et al., 1990). The syndrome is associated with HLA-DR4 (Uchigata et al., 1992), especially with the DRB1*0406 subtype that is strongly protective against type 1 diabetes. Although IAAs may also occur in subjects before they exhibit clinical type 1 diabetes, there appears to be no relationship between the two diseases.

Diagnosis and Treatment

Autoimmune hypoglycemia is diagnosed by the findings of hypoglycemia, hyperinsulinism, and insulin antibodies in the absence of prior insulin therapy. Insulinoma should be excluded. Because autoimmune hypoglycemia is antibody-mediated, immunosuppressive therapy may be of benefit, although it has not yet been attempted. Present treatment consists of frequent high-carbohydrate meals and avoidance of fasting.

Acanthosis Nigricans with Insulin Resistance (Type B)

Acanthosis nigricans is a skin condition in which waxy raised pigmented plaques occur, especially about the neck and upper trunk. Insulin resistance in association with acanthosis nigricans has been reported in three forms. One form (type B) is an autoimmune disorder (Flier et al., 1979). In type A disease, there is a primary decrease in insulin receptor number. Most patients with type A insulin resistance are female and display the clinical findings of polycystic ovary disease (i.e., hirsutism and amenorrhea) and accelerated growth. Type C disease is not immunologically mediated, and insulin binding to its receptor is normal, suggesting a nonimmunologic postreceptor defect.

Acanthosis nigricans with insulin resistance (type B) results from spontaneous autoantibodies directed against the insulin receptor that interfere with insulin action (Fig. 37-5) (Kahn et al., 1976). Type B patients may have other findings that suggest abnormal immunoregulation (i.e., antinuclear antibodies, anti-DNA antibodies, periodic hypocomplementemia, hypergammaglobulinemia, and leukopenia). Several patients with type B disease have had ataxia-telangiectasia, systemic lupus erythematosus, scleroderma, or Sjögren's syndrome (Bloise et al., 1989).

CLINICAL CONSEQUENCES OF INSULIN RECEPTOR AUTOANTIBODIES

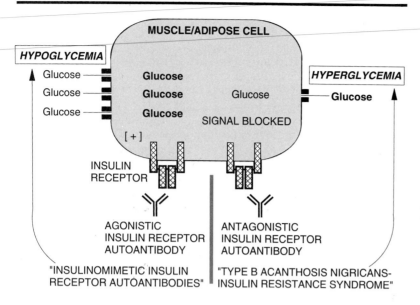

Figure 37-5· Clinical consequences of insulin receptor autoantibodies. Agonistic insulin receptor autoantibodies with insulinomimetic action stimulate muscle and adipose cells to increase glucose removal from the circulation producing hypoglycemia. Not pictured is the effect of agonistic insulin receptor autoantibodies on the liver that would lead to decreased hepatic glucose output similar to the natural action of insulin on the liver. Antagonistic insulin receptor autoantibodies block insulin action leading to decreased glucose clearance by the muscle and adipose cells producing hyperglycemia and the type B acanthosis nigricans-insulin resistance syndrome.

Pathogenesis

The peripheral blood monocytes of type B patients display decreased affinity of insulin for its receptor, whereas insulin receptor number is normal (Flier et al., 1979). In type B disease, the receptor appears to be blocked by the antagonistic autoantibody but not destroyed by the autoantibody, as is the case in myasthenia gravis. In myasthenia gravis, motor end-plate autoantibodies lead to increased receptor turnover, with a net loss in numbers of motor end-plate acetylcholine receptors.

If normal monocytes are incubated with type B sera, insulin binding is blocked, confirming the presence of insulin receptor autoantibodies. Insulin receptor autoantibodies from different individuals may react with different antigenic determinants. In vitro, insulin receptor autoantibody binding may transiently mimic the action of insulin; with chronic exposure, however, the insulin receptor autoantibody antagonizes the metabolic effects of insulin. De Pirro and colleagues (1984) have reported several different insulin receptor autoantibodies in the same patient.

Acanthosis nigricans appears to result from hyperinsulinism, which is a consequence of antagonistic insulin receptor antibodies. Acanthosis nigricans is common in insulin-resistant type 2 diabetic subjects who also display hyperinsulinism. Vitiligo also affects some type B patients. An autoimmune cause for some cases of vitiligo has been well described (Rocha et al., 2000).

Clinical Course

Insulin receptor autoantibodies that block insulin action lead to glucose intolerance and hyperglycemia. Exogenous insulin, in doses exceeding 20,000 units per day, may be ineffective in controlling hyperglycemia. Ketosis is unusual. Insulin resistance produces endogenous hyperinsulinism with insulin levels up to 40,000 IU/ml or higher. Patients may experience symptoms suggestive of hypoglycemia early in the clinical course consistent with the acute in vitro insulinomimetic properties of these antibodies. Because insulin resistance may resolve spontaneously, reports of amelioration of insulin resistance with immunosuppressive therapy are difficult to interpret (Duncan et al., 1983). Upregulation of insulin receptor number may occur as a compensatory phenomenon.

Diagnosis

Patients with insulin-resistant diabetes, immune abnormalities, and acanthosis nigricans must be suspected of having type B disease. Insulin receptor autoantibodies can be identified with radioreceptor binding studies. Other findings may include hypergammaglobulinemia, elevated erythrocyte sedimentation rate, hypocomplementemia, and ANA and anti-DNA antibodies. IAAs are generally not found; if they are present, their titers are usually low.

Treatment and Prognosis

Phenomenal doses of exogenous insulin may be required to control hyperglycemia. Duncan and co-workers (1983) successfully used prednisone in treating a teenaged male with type B disease with severe insulin resistance. Patients with type B insulin resistance have the same potential for long-term complications as patients with type 1 or type 2 diabetes. Further studies concerning the value of immunosuppressive therapy are indicated.

Insulinomimetic Insulin Receptor Autoantibodies

Early in their clinical course, patients with acanthosis nigricans-insulin resistance type B may have symptoms of hypoglycemia (see Fig. 37-5). In 1982, Taylor and associates reported a 60-year-old black woman with spontaneous hypoglycemia resulting from insulinomimetic insulin receptor autoantibodies. Based on these findings, insulin receptor autoantibodies must be considered as a possible cause of hypoglycemia particularly in individuals with autoimmune disease, low insulin levels, and hypoglycemia. Insulinomimetic insulin receptor autoantibodies have been described in a child (Elias et al., 1987) and in adults with lupus erythematosus (Moller et al., 1988; Varga et al., 1990) and Hodgkin's disease (Braund et al., 1987).

AUTOIMMUNE THYROID DISEASE

Autoimmune thyroid disease (AITD) results in a wide clinical spectrum of illness spanning chronic lymphocytic thyroiditis (Dayan et al., 1991) to Graves' disease (Weetman, 2000) (Fig. 37-6). Chronic lymphocytic thyroiditis can be further subdivided into Hashimoto's thyroiditis and atrophic thyroiditis. In Hashimoto's thyroiditis, thyroid follicular cells are destroyed by autoimmune mechanisms. In atrophic thyroiditis, antagonistic thyroid-stimulating hormone (TSH) receptor autoantibodies are at least twice as common as present in Hashimoto's thyroiditis, and these autoantibodies may be responsible for thyroid gland atrophy in atrophic thyroiditis (Akamizu et al., 2000). Hashimoto's thyroiditis is much more common than atrophic thyroiditis. In Graves' disease, thyroid-stimulating immunoglobulins (TSIs) bind to and stimulate the TSH receptor (e.g., agonistic TSH receptor autoantibodies) to release thyroid hormone and produce clinical hyperthyroidism. AITD is common in both children and adults and may even develop before birth (Foley et al., 1994). Autoantibodies to circulating thyroid hormone are also often present in AITD.

Chronic Lymphocytic (Hashimoto's) Thyroiditis

In the broadest sense, a subject with thyroid autoantibodies in the absence of hyperthyroidism can be considered to have chronic lymphocytic thyroiditis, because biopsy studies show a strong correlation between thyroid autoantibodies and histologic chronic lymphocytic thyroiditis. Most cases of chronic lymphocytic thyroiditis are expressed as Hashimoto's thyroiditis with goiter; progressive impairment of thyroid functions may occur, culminating in hypothyroidism. Transient hyperthyroidism can be seen in chronic lymphocytic thyroiditis as a result of thyroid follicular cell destruction with release of thyroid hormone. However, most individuals with chronic lymphocytic thyroiditis are initially euthyroid, but up to 50% will develop hypothyroidism with increasing age and continued thyroid follicular cell destruction (Tunbridge et al., 1981). Chronic lymphocytic thyroiditis is differentiated from colloid goiter by the presence of lymphoid aggregates on biopsy and by the presence of thyroid autoantibodies.

As noted earlier, two forms of chronic lymphocytic thyroiditis are recognized: *goitrous* and *atrophic*. When TSH receptor autoantibodies block TSH binding

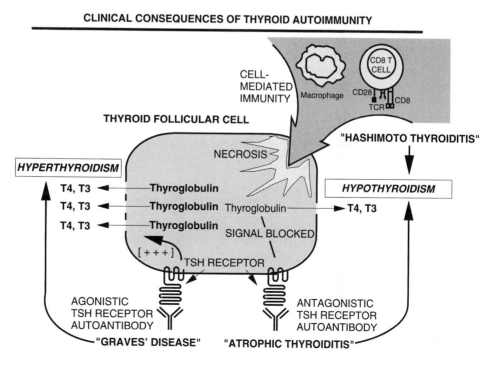

CLINICAL CONSEQUENCES OF THYROID AUTOIMMUNITY

Figure 37-6 · Clinical consequences of thyroid autoimmunity. In Hashimoto's thyroiditis, a cell-mediated autoimmune attack on the thyroid follicular cells by macrophages and CD8 T cells produces necrosis and eventual hypothyroidism (*upper right*). Antagonistic thyroid-stimulating hormone (TSH) receptor autoantibodies block the action of TSH on the thyroid follicular cells producing thyroid gland atrophy and hypothyroidism (atrophic thyroiditis) (*lower right*). In Graves' disease, agonistic TSH receptors stimulate excessive thyroid hormone secretion producing hyperthyroidism (lower left of figure). T_3 = triiodothyronine; T_4 = thyroxine; TCR = T-cell receptor; TSH = thyroid-stimulating hormone.

without stimulating the thyroid, the gland atrophies and produces the same potential for hypothyroidism as seen in goitrous chronic lymphocytic thyroiditis (Hashimoto's thyroiditis) (Okamura et al., 1990). A goiter develops in goitrous Hashimoto's thyroiditis because of lymphocytic infiltration and follicular cell hyperplasia. The latter may be due to growth-promoting thyroid autoantibodies and to pituitary TSH stimulation in the face of diminished glandular function.

Chronic lymphocytic thyroiditis is associated with other autoimmune diseases, including type 1 diabetes, atrophic gastritis/pernicious anemia (Irvine, 1975), vitiligo, and adrenalitis/Addison's disease (Riley et al., 1981). Thyroid autoimmunity, if present, is usually coincident with the onset of type 1 diabetes (Riley et al., 1983). As discussed elsewhere in this chapter, chronic lymphocytic thyroiditis is a component of the APS-2.

Historical Aspects

Hashimoto (1912) identified four elderly patients with lymphocytic thyroiditis in 1901. In 1956, Roitt and associates found high titers of serum TGAs in patients with Hashimoto's thyroiditis. In that same year, Adams and Purves (1956) described a substance in the sera of patients with Graves' disease that was later termed *long-acting thyroid stimulator* (LATS). LATS was the first thyroid-stimulating autoantibody identified.

Pathogenesis

An autoimmune cause for chronic lymphocytic thyroiditis (Strakosch et al., 1982) is suggested by (1) lymphocytic infiltration of the thyroid gland; (2) autoantibodies to the thyroid follicular cells; (3) disordered cell-mediated immunity directed against the thyroid; (4) associated autoantibodies to pancreatic islets, gastric parietal cells, and adrenal gland; and (5) particular HLA associations (Weetman et al., 1990).

Infiltrating lymphocytes are found throughout the thyroid gland in the interfollicular spaces (Hahn et al., 1965). At times, lymphocyte follicles may be formed. Pujol-Borrell and co-workers (1983) reported that lectins can induce HLA-DR expression on thyroid follicular cells, raising the possibility of self-autoantigen presentation by these thyroid cells in affected patients. Thyrocytes express MHC class II antigens in AITDs (Hanafusa et al., 1983).

THYROID AUTOANTIBODIES

Autoantibodies to thyroglobulin (TGAs), follicular cell microsomes (TMAs), and thyroid colloidal antigen have been described (Doniach, 1975). TMAs are cytoplasmic reactive autoantibodies that identify thyroperoxidase (TPO) (Vakeva et al., 1992). TPO catalyzes the conversion of inorganic iodide (I^-) to organic iodine (I^o) that is then covalently bound to the phenolic tyrosine rings of thyroglobulin. TPO is clustered near the apical pole of the thyrocyte (Pinchera et al., 1987).

TGA and TMA can be detected by a variety of methods, including indirect immunofluorescence, hemagglu-

tination, radioimmunoassay, complement fixation, and ELISA techniques. Vakeva and co-workers (1992) have stressed the need to improve TPO autoantibody assays because of frequent false-negative and false-positive results.

The TMA autoantibody reacts with TPO in its native conformation (Berthold et al., 1993). Surface autoantibodies to follicular cells have been observed using suspensions of follicular cells as targets. Antibody-dependent cell-mediated cytotoxicity to these cells has been demonstrated in chronic lymphocytic thyroiditis, but not Graves' disease (Bogner et al., 1984).

It was initially believed that TGA developed because thyroglobulin was released into the circulation following thyroid follicular cell damage, thus exposing the immune system to a previously sequestered antigen. However, sensitive radioimmunoassays have shown that thyroglobulin is present in normal sera, and thus thyroglobulin is not a sequestered antigen. More than 95% of patients with histologic chronic lymphocytic thyroiditis have TMA and/or TGA/TPO autoantibodies, making them excellent markers for chronic lymphocytic thyroiditis (Doniach, 1975). TMA and TPO antibodies are more common at the time of diagnosis, whereas TGAs usually appear later in the disease.

In at least 20% of cases of atrophic chronic lymphocytic thyroiditis, autoantibodies are found that block thyroid cell receptor binding by TSH. Such autoantibodies can cross the placenta and result in congenital hypothyroidism (Iseki et al., 1983; Matsuura et al., 1980; Van Der Gaag et al., 1985a). However, the maternal thyroid autoantibodies (e.g., TMA and TGA) are not increased in frequency in cases of congenital hypothyroidism (Dussault et al., 1980). Transient congenital hypothyroidism may be due to transplacental TSH receptor autoantibodies (Francis and Riley, 1987).

With the use of an assay measuring stimulation of thyroid cell growth in vitro, thyroid growth-promoting antibodies (TGPAs) have been recognized (Valente et al., 1983; Van Der Gaag et al., 1985b). TGPA are sometimes present in both Graves' disease and chronic lymphocytic thyroiditis. These antibodies stimulate tritiated thymidine uptake, a measure of cellular proliferation, without increasing cyclic adenosine monophosphate (cAMP) generation, a measure of TSH-like stimulation. The TSIs stimulate cAMP production and thyroid hormone production and release.

The thyroid Na^+/I^- symporter and megalin (GP330) are two new autoantigens that have been recognized in AITD. Symporters are transporters that move one ion out of a cell in exchange for a second ion moved into the cell. The Na^+/I^- symporter is not believed to be a major thyroid autoantigen because symporter autoantibodies are recognized in only 20% of Graves' disease subjects and 10% of Hashimoto's thyroiditis subjects (Seissler et al., 2000). Megalin, a polyspecific receptor protein, is a multiligand receptor. Antibodies to megalin were found in 50% of subjects with autoimmune thyroiditis and 10% of Graves' disease subjects (Marino et al., 1999).

In the 1980s, researchers believed that the formation of thyroid autoantibodies resulted from deficient T-lymphocyte suppressor numbers and function (Okita et al., 1981a, 1981b). Current theory holds that autoreactive B-cell clones arise frequently but are usually held in check by a lack of T helper cells.

CELLULAR AUTOIMMUNITY

In both Graves' disease and chronic lymphocytic thyroiditis, local infiltrating lymphocytes may be the major source of thyroid autoantibodies (Canonica et al., 1983). Variable numbers of intrathyroidal T and B lymphocytes are seen in both Hashimoto's thyroiditis and Graves' disease (Utiger, 1991). Cell lines derived from autoimmune–thyroid disease thyroid glands display a predominance of CD4+ T cells (Massart et al., 1999) and Th1-like cytokine patterns (Abbas et al., 1996; Drugarin et al., 2000). This suggests that thyroid gland destruction results from a Th1-cell–mediated autoimmune process. In contrast, Graves' disease may result from a predominant Th2 disease with anti-TSH receptor autoantibody production.

Several studies have shown decreased numbers of circulating (Iwatani et al., 1983; Sridama et al., 1982) and intrathyroidal CD8+ or CD4+ CD45RA+ cells (Jansson et al., 1983b; Kawakami et al., 1991). However, Canonica and co-workers (1981) found no T-subset abnormalities. Paschke and associates (1991) recorded increased numbers of intraepithelial CD45RO+ (memory) T lymphocytes and immunoglobulin-producing lymphocytes.

Various cytokines (e.g., IL-1, tumor necrosis factor [TNF], and interferon-gamma [IFN-γ]) can suppress thyroid cell function in vitro (Paolieri et al., 1999; Rasmussen, 2000). In vitro IL-1β stimulates Fas expression on thyroid follicular cells (Giordano et al., 1997). In vivo, apoptosis has been recognized in Hashimoto's thyroiditis glands (Hammond et al., 1997).

HLA Associations and Inheritance of Chronic Lymphocytic Thyroiditis

Although the HLA associations are not as impressive as those in type 1 diabetes, goitrous chronic lymphocytic thyroiditis (Hashimoto's thyroiditis) is associated with an increased frequency of HLA-DR4 (Doniach et al., 1979), and atrophic chronic lymphocytic thyroiditis is associated with HLA-DRB3 (Farid et al., 1981; Weissel et al., 1980). Some studies have implicated HLA-DR5 as a risk allele for chronic lymphocytic thyroiditis instead of HLA-DR4. The HLA-DR3 association with atrophic chronic lymphocytic thyroiditis is of interest because Graves' disease is strongly associated with this HLA allele. This suggests that HLA-DR3 is associated with TSH receptor autoantibody formation that can either stimulate or block the TSH receptor.

Despite the described HLA associations, in multigenerational families with AITD, apparent autosomal dominant inheritance does not cosegregate with HLA haplotype (Gorsuch et al., 1980; Phillips et al., 1990; Roman et al., 1992). HLA type may influence the clinical expression of autosomal dominant thyroid autoimmunity (Wick, 1987) to develop Hashimoto's thyroiditis or Graves' disease when HLA-DR3 is present. DQ alleles may also influence susceptibility to thyroid autoimmunity (Badenhoop et al., 1990).

The pathogenesis of chronic lymphocytic thyroiditis is affected by genetics. Concordance for autoimmune hypothyroidism in female Danish twin pairs was 55% in monozygotic twins versus 0% in dizygotic twins (Brix et al., 2000). Thyroid autoantibody positivity concordance was 80% in monozygotic twins versus 40% in dizygotic twins. Association studies strongly suggest that the CTLA-4 gene located on chromosome 2q33, or genes closely linked to CTLA-4, affect the appearance of Hashimoto's thyroiditis and Graves' disease (Barbesino et al., 2000). The CTLA-4 was previously discussed with reference to T-cell downregulation.

Kotsa and associates (1997) have reported that CTLA-4 allele 106 was increased in autoimmune hypothyroidism. Donner and co-workers (1997a) showed that the alanine CTLA-4 leader sequence polymorphism (threonine/alanine) at amino acid 17 was more common in Hashimoto's thyroiditis (22%) than in controls (15%). Furthermore, a position 318 cytosine/thymine CTLA-4 promoter variant associated with both Graves' disease and Hashimoto's thyroiditis was linked to an exon 1 polymorphism (Braun et al., 1998). Nevertheless, by itself Hashimoto's thyroiditis was not associated with the promoter polymorphism. However, Heward and associates (1999) did not detect a genetic association of the 318 polymorphism with either Graves' disease or autoimmune hypothyroidism.

First reported in 1999, a chromosome 13 locus termed Hashimoto thyroiditis locus-1 (HT-1) was identified in linkage studies (Tomer et al., 1999). This locus was linked to Hashimoto's thyroiditis but not to Graves' disease. In a subset of families, a locus on chromosome 12 was linked to Hashimoto's thyroiditis. One locus on chromosome 6 (AITD locus-1 [AITD-1]) was linked to both Hashimoto's thyroiditis and Graves' disease. This locus was close to, but distinct from, the HLA complex. The Graves' disease-1 locus (GD-1) on chromosome 14 is not linked to Hashimoto's thyroiditis (see following discussion) (Tomer et al., 1998a), nor is the TSH receptor gene associated with either Hashimoto's thyroiditis of Graves' disease (Sunthornthepvarakul et al., 1999).

In summary, AITD including chronic lymphocytic thyroiditis or Graves' disease appears to be inherited as a dominant trait. HLA-DR4 and/or HLA-DR5 are associated with an increased risk for chronic lymphocytic thyroiditis. Loci on chromosomes 2 (CTLA-4) and 13 (HD-1) also influence the development of chronic lymphocytic thyroiditis. Non-MHC regions on chromosome 6 (AITD-1) and chromosome 12 require additional study.

Combined Thyroid and Gastric (Thyrogastric) Autoimmunities

Because of the frequent association of chronic lymphocytic thyroiditis with gastric parietal cell autoimmunity, the term thyrogastric autoimmunity has been coined. The hypothesis is that a single gene outside the HLA complex predisposes to both autoimmune disorders. The expression of this gene is gender-influenced because more women manifest chronic lymphocytic thyroiditis, Graves' disease, and thyroid or gastric autoantibodies. The frequency of TMA and TPO autoantibodies and gastric parietal cell autoantibodies steadily increases with advancing age (Maclaren and Riley, 1985; Mariotti et al., 1992). If the thyrogastric autoimmunity gene frequencies equal the associated autoantibody frequencies fully expressed in the elderly, it may approach 30% of the population.

Because of the frequency of thyrogastric autoantibodies at the time of type 1 diabetes diagnosis, we hypothesize that type 1 diabetic subjects are prematurely expressing their genetic predisposition to thyrogastric autoimmunity. The corollary suggests that thyroid and gastric autoimmunities predispose to type 1 diabetes.

Clinical Manifestations

The most common presenting complaint in AITD is goiter (Reiter et al., 1981). Patients may have difficulty swallowing or a sense of fullness in the neck. Neck pain is more characteristic of acute (bacterial) or subacute (viral) thyroiditis. With extensive destruction of the thyroid follicular cells, a fall in thyroid hormone production elicits the secretion of TSH from the pituitary. This trophic stimulation may further increase the size of the gland. Follicular cell destruction may transiently release excessive amounts of thyroid hormone, producing a temporary hyperthyroidism. Dubbed *Hashitoxicosis* (or *Toximoto* disease), this state is differentiated from Graves' disease by its transient nature and by its relatively low radioactive iodine uptake. Typically, the thyroid scan reveals patchy uptake of iodide in chronic lymphocytic thyroiditis. In chronic lymphocytic thyroiditis, the gland has a pebbly feel, as opposed to the boggy gland of Graves' disease.

With continued destruction of thyroid follicular cells, thyroid hormone production may become deficient despite marked elevations in TSH. Clinical hypothyroidism then develops, often insidiously. Patients with hypothyroidism may manifest brittle hair; dry skin; a puffy, dull appearance; a hoarse voice; bradycardia; constipation; intolerance to cold; and sluggish reflexes. In children, cessation or slowing of growth may be the only manifestation of hypothyroidism.

In some patients, Hashimoto's thyroiditis results only in goiter; in others, it may progress to hypothyroidism. The clinical course may be punctuated by remissions and exacerbations. Permanent remission with disappearance of the goiter is occasionally seen. In adults with chronic lymphocytic thyroiditis, hypothyroidism develops in about 5% per year (Tunbridge et al., 1981).

Postpartum autoimmune thyroiditis affects 5% of all women and 10% of women with type 1 diabetes (Roti and Emerson, 1992; Smallridge, 1996; Stagnaro-Green et al., 2000; Weetman, 1994). There is a highly variable course postpartum that can include hypothyroidism; hyperthyroidism; or sequentially any combination of hypothyroidism, hyperthyroidism, and euthyroidism.

Neonatal thyroid function is unaffected by TMA, TPO, autoantibodies, or TGA that cross the placenta (Dussault et al., 1980). However, TSH receptor autoantibodies that cross the placenta can induce transient neonatal hypothyroidism (Brown et al., 1996; Connors et al., 1986; Francis and Riley, 1987; Iseki et al., 1983).

Diagnosis

Hashimoto's thyroiditis is diagnosed by the presence of goiter and TMAs, TPO autoantibodies, and/or TGAs (Doniach et al., 1979). Occasional patients without these autoantibodies may have autoantibodies to the colloid antigen CA-2 or PCAs. Although their measurement is not widely available, thyroid growth-promoting autoantibodies are supportive of the diagnosis of chronic lymphocytic thyroiditis. Because the treatment for hypothyroidism is simple and straightforward (thyroxine), a thyroid biopsy is rarely indicated. Goiter in Hashimoto's thyroiditis may gradually resolve after thyroid hormone replacement.

Treatment

For goiter unaccompanied by TSH elevation, no therapy is required. However, thyroxine may be administered in an attempt to reduce the size of the goiter. Once the TSH becomes elevated, with or without clinical hypothyroidism, thyroid hormone replacement is indicated (thyroxine, 100 µg/m^2/day). Because of the high efficacy and safety of thyroid hormone therapy, immunomodulatory therapy is not indicated.

Prognosis

For appropriately treated patients, the prognosis for chronic lymphocytic thyroiditis is excellent. However, sometimes the goiter in Hashimoto's thyroiditis may be recalcitrant to hormonal replacement. In adults, untreated hypothyroidism can progress to myxedema with cardiac decompensation and/or coma. In children, the most serious consequence of hypothyroidism is growth retardation. This is in contrast to untreated congenital hypothyroidism in which the most serious consequence is mental retardation. An increased risk of thyroid lymphoma in chronic lymphocytic thyroiditis has been suggested; however, the overall frequency of cancer in patients with chronic lymphocytic thyroiditis is not increased (Holm et al., 1985).

Graves' Disease

Hyperthyroidism is the clinical state resulting from inappropriate and excessive release of thyroid hormone. Graves' disease is present when hyperthyroidism results from stimulatory autoantibodies produced against the TSH receptor (Orgiazzi, 2000; Weetman, 2000). Thyroid autoimmunity (TMA, TPO autoantibodies, and/or TGA), TSIs, and lymphocyte infiltration of the thyroid are the hallmarks of Graves' disease (McKenzie et al., 1975). Exophthalmos and/or proptosis of the eyes is highly associated with Graves' disease but may occur without thyroid enlargement or disease. The third characteristic of Graves' disease, in addition to hyperthyroidism and exophthalmos, is the nonpitting edema of myxedema.

Pathogenesis

An autoimmune cause for Graves' disease is firmly based. Most patients with Graves' disease have thyroid autoantibodies, including TSIs (e.g., LATS), TMAs, TPO autoantibodies, and/or TGAs. Biopsy specimens reveal lymphocytic infiltration of the gland along with diffuse follicular cell hyperplasia and colloid absorption. Aberrant expression of HLA-DR antigens on the surface of the follicular cells in Graves' disease has been described (Hanafusa et al., 1983). However, such ectopic HLA expression is not pathogenic but probably a consequence of local inflammation.

Genetic susceptibility influences the development of Graves' disease. An apparent dominant inheritance of AITD is evident in many families. The AITD can be expressed in terms of chronic lymphocytic thyroiditis or Graves' disease in the same family. The association of HLA-DR3 and Graves' disease is well known. Approximately two of every three patients with Graves' disease carry this HLA-DR allele. Graves' disease is associated with DQA1*0501 in the HLA-DQ region (Yanagawa et al., 1993). In African Americans, the HLA-DRB3*020/DQA1*0501 haplotype has also been associated with Graves' disease (Chen et al., 2000).

Similar to Hashimoto's thyroiditis and type 1 diabetes, CTLA-4 polymorphisms on chromosome 2q33 have been shown to influence the development of Graves' disease (Yanagawa et al., 1995). The 3' untranslated region 106 base-pair allele of the CTLA-4 gene (AT)n microsatellite polymorphism gave a relative risk for Graves' disease of 2.82. As well, the CTLA-4 exon 1, 49 A/G polymorphism (interchanging alanine for threonine) was associated with Graves' disease (Donner et al., 1997b; Heward et al., 1999). Researchers have estimated that 50% of inherited susceptibility to Graves' disease is provided by the CTLA-4 and MHC regions (Vaidya et al., 1999).

Subsequently, a variety of loci have been associated with Graves' disease:

· Graves' disease locus-1 (GD-1) on chromosome 14q31 (Tomer et al., 1997, 1998a)
· GD-2 on chromosome 20q11.2 (Pearce et al., 1999; Tomer et al., 1998b)
· GD-3 on the X chromosome (Tomer et al., 1999)
· IL-4 promoter on chromosome 5q31.1 (Hunt et al., 2000)
· TAP1 and TAP2 on chromosome 6 (Rau et al., 1997)
· IFN-γ on chromosome 12q (Siegmund et al., 1998)
· Vitamin D receptor on chromosome 12q12-q14 (Ban et al., 2000)
· An unnamed Graves' disease susceptibility locus on chromosome 18q21 (Vaidya et al., 2000a)

In summary, whereas the CTLA-4 loci and MHC appear to have the greatest influence on the development of Graves' disease, other loci on multiple chromosomes may also be involved (Gough, 2000).

AUTOANTIBODIES

In most patients with Graves' disease, TSIs can be detected (Orgiazzi, 2000). Several assays have been used. The first were in vivo bioassays that detected the long-acting thyroid stimulator (LATS) TSI, using guinea pigs and mice (Kendall-Taylor, 1975; McKenzie, 1968). The animals were nutritionally iodine depleted, then given thyroid hormone to suppress TSH followed by radioactive iodine, which is taken up by the thyroid gland. Sera from Graves' patients injected into these animals caused the release of increased amounts of ^{131}I from the thyroid. However, the peak response was 10 to 12 hours after injection, significantly delayed from the peak response at 3 hours produced by TSH injection. This delay accounts for the term LATS. This phenomenon was described before LATS's recognition as an autoantibody.

An in vitro variant of this assay measures radioactive iodine release from thyroid slices (Ekins and Ellis, 1975). Cyclic AMP response to TSIs has also been measured in human thyroid cell monolayers (Rapoport et al., 1982). Using cultured human thyroid cells, Rapoport and co-workers (1984) reported a 93% frequency of TSIs in patients with Graves' disease. The failure to find TSIs in all Graves' patients might be the result of bioassay insensitivity (Davies et al., 1983) or the presence of specific human TSIs. Human-specific autoantibodies were initially termed LATS protector, an IgG that blocks LATS neutralization by human thyroid protein (Adams and Kennedy, 1971). TSH receptor autoantibodies can react to different epitopes on the TSH receptor (Dayan et al., 1991; Shishiba et al., 1982); however, most are directed to the extracellular domains of the TSH receptor.

In other assays, radioreceptor techniques are used to measure TSH binding inhibition by sera from Graves' patients (TSH binding inhibitory immunoglobulins [TBII]; Brown et al., 1986). Other assays for TSIs measure colloid droplet formation in follicular cells, glucose oxidation, incorporation of ^{32}P into phospholipids, cAMP accumulation, and adenyl cyclase activity. The lymphocytes infiltrating the thyroid gland may be the chief source of TSIs (Kendall-Taylor et al., 1984).

Carbamizole, a drug that blocks thyroid hormone biosynthesis, may also inhibit thyroid autoantibody production by a suppressive effect on thyroid lymphocytes (McGregor et al., 1980a). However, Jansson and associates (1983a) found intrathyroidal concentrations of methimazole, the breakdown product of carbamizole, to be less immunosuppressive than previously reported (Weiss and Davies, 1981).

CELLULAR AUTOIMMUNITY

Cell-mediated autoimmunity in Graves' disease is suggested by elevated levels of lymphocyte migration inhibition factor (Okita et al., 1981c; Topliss et al., 1983).

Abnormal T-cell numbers or functions have been suggested involving H_2 histamine receptor bearing (Okita et al., 1981a) and/or IgG-Fc receptor bearing T lymphocytes (Mori et al., 1982). Graves' disease appears to result from a CD4 Th2 response against the TSH receptor (Itoh et al., 2000).

Other immune abnormalities in Graves' disease include decreased T-cell numbers with supposed suppressor functions (Okita et al., 1981b; Sridama et al., 1982) and DR-positive T cells (Jackson et al., 1984). However, the cause-and-effect relationship of immune abnormalities to hyperthyroidism has not been firmly established (Grubeck-Loebenstein et al., 1985).

Graves' disease is often associated with other autoimmune diseases, particularly chronic lymphocytic (atrophic) gastritis and type 1 diabetes. Interestingly, in patients with Graves' and type 1 diabetes, the hyperthyroidism often precedes the diabetes (Riley et al., 1981).

Exophthalmos

The relationship of exophthalmos to Graves' disease is controversial (Gorman, 1983; Schifferdecker et al., 1989; Solomon et al., 1977; Weetman, 1991, 1992) but is believed to be immunologically mediated (Bahn, 2000). The two conditions may exist together or independently. The spectrum of such associations is termed thyroid-associated ophthalmopathy (TAO). Some authors suggest that most patients with ophthalmopathy have some form of AITD (Salvi et al., 1990).

Exophthalmos may result from autoimmunity to retrobulbar structures that is independent of Graves' disease. Hyperthyroidism increases sensitivity to endogenous catecholamines. Lid retraction, which can result from the sympathetic effects of hyperthyroidism, should not be confused with exophthalmos resulting from retrobulbar inflammation and lymphocytic infiltration.

An autoimmune cause for the exophthalmos with or without co-existent Graves' disease is postulated (Doniach and Florin-Christensen, 1975). Because the thyroid lymphatic drainage traverses the retro-orbital space, thyroglobulin–antithyroglobulin complexes may be carried to the retro-orbital muscles. Here, they attach to the sarcolemma and, with the participation of complement, induce extraocular muscle damage and inflammation. Thus the retro-orbital extraocular muscles are innocent bystanders to an immune complex disorder generated by the thyroid disease. Sensitized T cells, autoantibody-producing B cells, and other thyroid proteins may also be carried to the retrobulbar space.

Thyroglobulin-containing immune complexes are not the explanation for most cases of exophthalmos (Ohtaki et al., 1981). Indeed, some patients with Graves' disease have no TGAs. Furthermore, exophthalmos is rare in uncomplicated chronic lymphocytic thyroiditis despite a high frequency of TGAs. Autoantibodies to a soluble eye muscle antigen have been detected in up to 75% of patients with Graves' exophthalmos (Kodama et al., 1982). TSH does not interfere with the binding of autoantibodies to the orbital antigens (Waring et al., 1983). The most likely theory of exophthalmos is that retro-orbital tissues express TSH receptors. Next, the TSIs stimulate hyperplasia of the retro-orbital tissues when the TSIs interact with the retro-orbital TSH receptors. Because adipocytes have TSH receptors, TSI stimulation may contribute to exophthalmos by inducing retro-orbital adipose cell hyperplasia.

Other possible causes of exophthalmos include an ophthalmopathic immunoglobulin, as reported by Atkinson and colleagues (1984). Molecular mimicry between thyroid and orbital targets has also been proposed (Wall et al., 1991; Weightman and Kendall-Taylor, 1989). Dobbyns and Wilson (1954) described an exophthalmos-producing substance (EPS) (Der Kinderen, 1967). The sera from Graves' disease patients injected into fish caused exophthalmos. Several other groups confirmed these findings, but the exophthalmos was only transitory and associated with retrobulbar lymph sac distention. EPS is reportedly of pituitary origin.

Multiple autoantigens have been discovered with immunoblotting techniques (e.g., 110 kD, 95 kD, 64 kD, 55 kD, 23 kD) (Bahn et al., 1989; Bernard et al., 1991; Kadlubowski et al., 1987; Kendler et al., 1991). The nature of the orbital antigens continues to be controversial and currently concerns the TSH receptor, a 64-kD autoantigen (Kubota et al., 1998), a 72-kD heat shock protein (Heufelder et al., 1992), and the G2s gene product (Gunji et al., 2000). There is evidence for both CD4 Th1 and CD4 Th2 subset involvement (Aniszewski et al., 2000; Wakelkamp et al., 2000).

The co-existence of Graves' disease and exophthalmos may be much closer than previously recognized. Gamblin and co-workers (1983) sought subclinical ophthalmopathy in Graves' patients and found elevated (>3 mm Hg) intraocular pressure on upward gaze in 76% of their patients. Because only 26% had overt exophthalmos, about 50% had undetected ophthalmopathy. Euthyroid patients with exophthalmos often have thyroid autoantibodies, suggesting a spectrum of co-existent disorders (Ahmann and Burman, 1987). Extreme exophthalmos that threaten vision may be treated with prednisone, orbital irradiation, surgical decompression, and immunomodulatory agents such as nicotinamide (Hiromatsu et al., 1998).

Other Clinical Manifestations

Other than exophthalmos and pretibial myxedema, thyrotoxicosis in Graves' disease does not differ clinically from other forms of hyperthyroidism. Symptoms include fine hair, smooth skin, tachycardia, sweating, diarrhea, weight loss, hyperreflexia, insomnia, and neuropsychologic disorders.

As in Hashimoto's thyroiditis, there may be autosomal dominant inheritance of Graves' disease. Hashimoto's thyroiditis and Graves' disease often co-exist in families, and both are highly associated with gastric parietal cell autoimmunity.

Diagnosis

Graves' disease is diagnosed by the presence of persistent hyperthyroidism with evidence of thyroid autoimmunity. Exophthalmos supports the diagnosis, and a diffusely enlarged thyroid gland is typically found. Because TSIs induce excessive thyroid gland activity, pituitary TSH response to thyrotropin-releasing hormone (TRH) is blunted as a result of negative feedback inhibition. Total and unbound thyroxine (T_4) and triiodothyronine (T_3) are markedly elevated. In cases of iodine deficiency or early Graves' disease, isolated T_3 toxicosis may result with high T_3 but normal T_4 levels (Hollander et al., 1972). Alternatively, if significant nonthyroidal illness co-exists, T_4 may be elevated without elevations of T_3. This may occur because of a relatively deficient T_4 to T_3 conversion, especially in elderly patients. There is a marked predominance of females with Graves' disease; female predominance is usual for most autoimmune disorders except for type 1 diabetes.

The differential diagnosis of hyperthyroidism includes thyrotoxicosis factitia (Mariotti et al., 1982), toxic nodular goiter (Plummer disease), and thyroid neoplasia. Thyrotoxicosis factitia is hyperthyroidism that develops secondary to intended or unintended excess ingestion of exogenous thyroid hormone. Rare cases of TSH-secreting pituitary tumors have been reported (Kourides et al., 1977). In several conditions, high thyroid hormone levels are found in the absence of clinical hyperthyroidism. These disorders fall into two categories: (1) resistance to thyroid hormone (Linde et al., 1982) and (2) elevated levels of circulating thyroid-binding proteins or aberrant carrier proteins. With thyroid hormone resistance, both total and free thyroid hormone levels are elevated, but the patient is clinically euthyroid with normal thyroid-binding globulin (TBG) levels. Defects of the thyroid cell nuclear T_3 receptor explain cases of thyroid hormone resistance.

When there is pituitary thyroid hormone resistance but normal peripheral sensitivity, clinical hyperthyroidism is evident (Novogroder et al., 1977). In such cases it is imperative that a TSH-secreting pituitary adenoma be ruled out with computed tomography (CT) or magnetic resonance imaging (MRI) examination. Total T_4 and T_3 levels can be elevated because of increased thyroid hormone carrier proteins. Here the unbound hormone levels remain normal and the patient is euthyroid. Most commonly, this is the result of a congenital or acquired excess of TBG. TBG elevation can be induced by pregnancy, estrogen administration, and acute liver disease. Congenital TBG excess can be inherited as an autosomal dominant trait.

Rarer syndromes similar to TBG excess include familial dysalbuminemic hyperthyroxinemia (Ruiz et al., 1982) and euthyroid hyperthyroxinemia with abnormal prealbumin (Moses et al., 1982). In these syndromes TBG levels are normal; however, an abnormal albumin or transthyretin (thyroxine-binding prealbumin) carries supranormal amounts of thyroxine, producing an elevation in total T_4 with a normal T_3.

Treatment

Oral antithyroid medications, such as the thioureas propylthiouracil and methimazole, which inhibit thyroid hormone biosynthesis, are used to induce and maintain a clinical remission. Because of their short duration of action (6 to 8 hours), good compliance is crucial. After 1 to 2 years, therapy should be tapered and stopped because 50% of patients with Graves' disease will enter a permanent remission.

Controversy exists as to whether the presence of HLA-DR3 and/or TBII decreases the likelihood of remission (McGregor et al., 1980b). In a prospective study (Allannic et al., 1984), HLA typing did not predict relapse. For those who do experience relapse, radioactive iodine is more efficacious and safer than thyroidectomy (Becker, 1984; Hamburger, 1985). Hypothyroidism is, however, common after radioiodine therapy. In centers skilled in thyroid surgery, thyroidectomy may be preferred.

Exophthalmos may worsen with treatment for hyperthyroidism, especially following ^{131}I ablative therapy. It is unclear whether this is the result of thyroid antigen release or a result of an immunologic alteration with treatment. The treatment of exophthalmos depends on its severity. No treatment is indicated for mild exophthalmos. For advanced or progressing eye disease, oral corticosteroids, orbital irradiation, eye muscle surgery, and orbital decompression are used. Early thyroid hormone replacement following thyroid ablation therapy may minimize the induced exophthalmos.

Prognosis

Untreated, Graves' disease can produce life-threatening, high-output cardiac failure. Similarly, *thyroid storm* can produce heart failure. In addition, hyperthyroidism can produce severe inanition, fatigue, sleeplessness, diarrhea, and personality changes. Appropriately treated, Graves' disease can be controlled or even cured. However, long-term personality changes may persist. Likewise, proptosis may not disappear completely because of fibrosis in the retro-orbital space.

Thyroid Hormone Autoantibodies

Spontaneous anti-T_4 and anti-T_3 autoantibodies can be recognized in Hashimoto's thyroiditis and Graves' disease (Volpe, 1991) but usually have no clinical consequences (Nakamura et al., 1989). Occasionally, such autoantibodies can elevate total thyroid hormone levels without producing clinical disease or can depress free hormone levels, leading to hypothyroidism (Trimarchi et al., 1982). Anti-T_4 autoantibodies may lead to spuriously high unbound T_4 determinations (Fukasawa et al., 1991). Most antithyroid hormone autoantibodies are polyclonal, but oligoclonal and monoclonal autoantibodies have been reported (Moroz et al., 1983). Autoantibodies to bovine TSH (Eto et al., 1984) and human TSH have also been described (Raines et al., 1985).

AUTOIMMUNE DISORDERS OF THE ADRENALS AND GONADS

Because autoimmunity to the adrenal gland and gonads often occurs concomitantly, these autoimmune disorders are discussed together (Muir and Maclaren, 1991).

Addison's Disease

Addison's disease results from the destruction of the adrenal cortex to a degree that clinical problems result from loss of glucocorticoid and mineralocorticoid hormones. Clinical features include weight loss, weakness, fatigue, dehydration, hypoglycemia, and at a late stage, vascular collapse. Although isolated glucocorticoid deficiency can produce hyponatremia, mineralocorticoid deficiency produces hyponatremia and hyperkalemia. A diffuse, muddy hyperpigmentation results from pituitary hypersecretion of adrenocorticotropic hormone (ACTH) and melanocyte-stimulating hormone (MSH), which are stimulatory to melanocytes, in response to cortisol deficiency.

Autoimmune Addison's disease is defined by the absence of known causes of adrenocortical destruction (e.g., tuberculosis, histoplasmosis, hemorrhage, carcinomatosis), the presence of adrenocortical autoantibodies or autoantibodies against steroidogenic enzymes, and lymphocytic infiltration of the adrenal cortices (Betterle et al., 1989; Drexhage, 1999). It is more likely to occur in patients with other autoimmune illnesses (e.g., AITD or type 1 diabetes), especially in those with an HLA phenotype that includes the DR3/DQB1*0201 haplotype.

In other states of adrenocortical insufficiency, such as ACTH deficiency (hypopituitarism), ACTH unresponsiveness, or enzymatic defects of cortisol biosynthesis (congenital adrenal hyperplasia), the term Addison's disease is not applicable because mineralocorticoid secretion is intact. In a study conducted during the 1960s in northeast London, nontuberculous Addison's disease was found at a rate of 27 cases per million (Doniach and Bottazzo, 1981). Second only to iatrogenic adrenocortical suppression from exogenous glucocorticoid administration, autoimmune adrenalitis is the most common cause of Addison's disease.

Premature Gonadal Failure

Autoimmune hypogonadism (gonaditis) is the loss of hormone-producing cells from the ovary or testes. Autoimmune cellular ablation is suggested by loss of follicles from the ovary, lymphocytic infiltrates of either ovary or testis, and the presence of steroidal cell autoantibodies (SCAs) or autoantibodies against steroidogenic enzymes. Affected individuals may have co-existent Addison's disease or other organ-specific autoimmune autoantibodies. Characteristically, acquired hypergonadotropic hypogonadism (with raised plasma follicle-stimulating hormone [FSH] and luteinizing hormone [LH] levels) and infertility result in affected women

(Moncayo and Moncayo, 1992). Male infertility from gonaditis is rare. This may represent the fact that the testes have tremendous spermatogenic capacity, whereas the number of follicles in the ovaries is fixed even before birth.

Gonaditis is usually observed in association with APS-1 but can occur in APS-2 (see later). About 25% of women with autoimmune Addison's disease display amenorrhea and 10% exhibit premature ovarian failure (Gargiulo and Hill, 1999).

Autoimmune Polyglandular Syndromes

In 1981, Neufeld and co-workers proposed that, although many cases of autoimmune Addison's were isolated occurrences, certain cases of Addison's disease presented in association with other immunoendocrinopathies in recognized patterns. The two recurring patterns were termed APS-1 and APS-2 (Table 37-7 and Fig. 37-7).

APS-1 (TYPE 1 APS) AND AUTOIMMUNE POLYENDOCRINOPATHY-CANDIDIASIS-ECTODERMAL DYSTROPHY SYNDROME (APECED)

APS-1 refers to the association of mucocutaneous candidiasis, hypoparathyroidism, and Addison's disease or adrenal autoantibodies (see Chapter 17). Two of three disorders must be present for diagnosis. They usually present in the order stated; if one condition is absent, it only rarely appears at a later date. Another term for APS-1 is APECED (autoimmune polyendocrinopathy-

TABLE 37-7 · AUTOIMMUNE POLYGLANDULAR SYNDROMES

Features	Type 1	Type 2
Early age of onset	+++	+
Onset in midlife	±	+++
Addison's disease	+++	+++
Hypoparathyroidism	+++	−
Chronic mucocutaneous candidiasis	+++	−
Hypogonadism	++	±
Chronic active hepatitis	++	±
Alopecia	++	±
Vitiligo	+	±
Malabsorption syndromes	+	−
Pernicious anemia	++ (juvenile onset)	± (late onset)
Atrophic thyroiditis	−	++
Goitrous thyroiditis	−	+++
Graves' disease	−	+++
Type 1 diabetes	±	+++
Sjögren's syndrome	++	−
Myopathy	+	−
Cholecystokinin deficiency	+	
Immunogenetics	Autosomal recessive (AIRE mutation)	Association of HLA-DR3 and HLA-DR4 with type 1 diabetes

HLA = human leukocyte antigen; − = absent; ± = rarely present; + = occasionally present; ++ = frequently present; +++ = very common or pathognomonic.

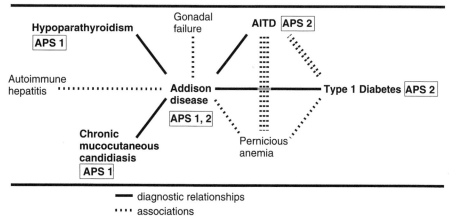

Figure 37-7· Autoimmune polyglandular syndromes (APS): interrelationships. APS-1 consists of two of the three following disorders: Addison's disease (or adrenal autoantibodies), hypoparathyroidism, and chronic mucocutaneous candidiasis. APS-2 consists of Addison's disease (or adrenal autoantibodies) plus autoimmune thyroid disease and/or type 1 diabetes. In addition to these relationships, adrenal autoimmunity is often associated with gonadal failure from autoimmune gonad destruction ("gonaditis"), autoimmune hepatitis, and pernicious anemia. Thyrogastric autoimmunity is a very common association (autoimmune thyroid disease and pernicious anemia), and the strength of this association is indicated by a triple line set. Type 1 diabetes is also strongly associated with thyrogastric autoimmunities (autoimmune thyroid disease and pernicious anemia).

candidiasis-ectodermal dystrophy), emphasizing the multiple autoimmune endocrinopathies associated with ectodermal developmental problems and candidiasis.

APS-1 results from mutations in the autoimmune regulator *(AIRE)* gene (Nagamine et al., 1997) that is believed to encode a transcription factor (Bjorses et al., 1998). When an individual inherits two mutated *AIRE* genes, one from each parent, APS-1 develops, accounting for the autosomal recessive nature of this disorder. As well, males and females are equally commonly affected with APS-1, whereas APS-2 occurs much more commonly in women than in men, similar to most autoimmune diseases. Although an inflammatory parathyroiditis can be observed histologically, there are no reliable indirect immunofluorescent assays for parathyroid autoantibodies. There is a single report of the parathyroid calcium receptor serving as an autoantigen in autoimmune hypoparathyroidism (Li et al., 1996). Cytotoxic parathyroid autoantibodies have been observed (Brandi et al., 1986). In addition, autoantibodies to parathyroid hormone have been described in a variety of clinical circumstances (Cavaco et al., 1999; Juppner et al., 1984).

TYPE 2 APS

APS-2 refers to the association of Addison's disease with Hashimoto's thyroiditis and/or type 1 diabetes (Carpenter et al., 1964). About 50% of patients with Addison's disease have APS-2 (Papadopoulos and Hallengren, 1990). Other autoimmune diseases may occur in association with either APS-1 or APS-2. Cushing syndrome with anti-ACTH receptor autoantibodies has been described (Carstensen et al., 1989; Jones, 1990; Teding van Berkhout et al., 1989; Wilkin, 1990). However, such anti-ACTH receptor autoanti-

bodies are not believed at present to play a pathogenic role in the development of either Addison's disease or Cushing syndrome.

Historical Aspects

In 1849, Thomas Addison, a physician at Guy's Hospital in London, described three patients with severe anemia and loss of the suprarenal capsules. Addison's classic work, published in 1855, reported 11 additional autopsy cases. Four had tuberculosis, four probably had malignancy, and three had unexplained adrenal cortical atrophy. One of the latter three had extensive vitiligo, and perhaps all three had autoimmune disease.

In 1862, Wilks proposed that the suprarenal syndrome that involved vascular collapse should be termed Addison's disease. Nontuberculous Addison's disease was relatively rare. Schmidt (1926) described the concurrence of lymphocytic infiltrates of the thyroid gland and adrenal cortices in autopsies of two patients dying of Addisonian crisis *(Schmidt syndrome)*. In 1928, Brenner identified that Addison's disease results from loss of the adrenal cortex and not the medulla.

Following a report by Beaven and associates (1959), Carpenter and co-workers (1964) described the association between type 1 diabetes and Schmidt syndrome. Doniach and Roitt (1957) provided evidence that these diseases had an autoimmune basis by identifying precipitating autoantibodies to thyroglobulin in patients with Hashimoto's thyroiditis.

Anderson and colleagues (1957) and Blizzard and Kyle (1963) described adrenal autoantibodies in patients with idiopathic Addison's disease. Anderson and others (1968) recognized that some adrenocortical autoantibodies also reacted with steroid hormone-producing gonadal cells, and Irvine and colleagues (1968) reported hypogonadism associated with these antibodies.

Pathogenesis

Early in the course of Addison's disease, *adrenalitis*, a characteristic lymphocytic infiltration of the adrenal cortex, is noted in association with necrosis of adrenocortical cells. As inflammation subsides, fibrosis surrounding regenerating nodules results. Later, complete cortical atrophy with dense fibrosis occurs while the medulla remains relatively intact (Petra and Nerup, 1971). These pathologic changes suggest autoimmune destruction of adrenocortical cells, probably directed against a unique cortical antigen. Also supporting an autoimmune cause is the fact that patients with Addison's disease often have associated disorders such as Hashimoto's thyroiditis. Finally, Addison's disease patients have autoantibodies (Blizzard and Kyle, 1963) and cell-mediated reactions to adrenal tissue. A lymphocytic infiltrate and gonadal autoantibodies are also detected in cases of gonaditis.

ADRENOCORTICAL AUTOANTIBODIES

Adrenal IgG autoantibodies can be detected by indirect immunofluorescence that reacts with a cytoplasmic antigen present in sections of unfixed human adrenal glands (Heinonen and Krohn, 1977). The major adrenocortical autoantigen is 21α-hydroxylase (Peterson et al., 1997). Adrenal cytoplasmic autoantibodies (ACAs) react with all layers of the adrenal cortex but not with the adrenal medulla. These autoantibodies are not pathogenic because they react with a cytoplasmic antigen not present on the surface of adrenal cells. Nonetheless, ACAs are useful markers for the autoimmune process (Leisti et al., 1983). As IgG autoantibodies, they bind complement (Betterle et al., 1983).

The adrenal autoantigens recognized by ACAs have been localized to the microsomes (Bright and Singh, 1990). Detection of adrenal autoantibodies has also been accomplished by a peroxidase-labeled protein A technique (Silva et al., 1998). However, the results of the peroxidase-labeled protein A technique are not fully concordant with those obtained using indirect immunofluorescence.

Autoantibodies to an adrenal cell surface antigen also occur in Addison's disease and were detected in 33 of 38 individuals with adrenocortical cytoplasmic autoantibodies (Khoury et al., 1981). Adrenal cell surface autoantibodies may be pathogenic by complement-dependent lysis or by antibody-dependent cellular cytotoxicity. There is one case of neonatal Addison's disease associated with maternal transplacental adrenocortical autoantibodies (Irvine and Barnes, 1975).

The cytoplasmic adrenocortical autoantigen is organ specific but not species specific. However, human tissue is best for demonstrating ACAs (Elder et al., 1981). The antigen was thought to be a lipoprotein found primarily in adrenocortical cell microsomes (Anderson et al.,

1968). Immunoblotting techniques have demonstrated adrenal autoantigens of 45, 55, and 70 kD (Freeman and Weetman, 1992). Some of these proteins may elicit T-lymphocyte proliferation. The adrenal enzymes 17α-hydroxylase (55 kD) (Krohn et al., 1992) and 21α-hydroxylase (Baumann-Antczak et al., 1992) were shown to be target autoantigens in Addisonian patients with APS-1. Bednarek and colleagues (1992) and Song and associates (1994b) confirmed that 21α-hydroxylase was an autoantigen in Addison's disease. The 21α-hydroxylase autoantibody does not interfere with the enzyme's function in vivo (Boscaro et al., 1996). The side chain cleavage enzyme P450$_{scc}$ (20,22-desmolase) also appears to be an autoantigen in APS-1 but not in isolated Addison's disease (Winqvist et al., 1993).

AUTOANTIBODIES IN ADDISON'S DISEASE

ACAs are rare in the general population (about 0.5%). However, ACAs are common among patients with type 1 diabetes (about 2%) and AITD (about 4%) (Riley et al., 1980b). Because the frequency of autoimmune Addison's disease is estimated at only 1 in 30,000 persons, clinical Addison's disease will not often develop in individuals with the autoantibody. In nontuberculous Addison's disease, adrenal autoantibodies (cytoplasmic type) are present in 38% to 74% of patients (Irvine and Barnes, 1975). The latter figure represents the autoantibody frequency at diagnosis; autoantibodies are less frequent thereafter (Muir and Maclaren, 1991).

Ketchum and associates (1984) found that many asymptomatic patients with ACAs have biochemical evidence for adrenocortical insufficiency. Such patients had elevated basal plasma ACTH levels. Furthermore, their renin levels were elevated when recumbent and when salt intake was unrestricted. An increase in ACTH secretion may temporally compensate for the ongoing autoimmune destruction of adrenocortical cells. Betterle and colleagues (1983) showed that Addison's disease developed in four of nine of their asymptomatic patients with ACA after 1 to 31 months of observation. Clinical disease was more likely to develop in individuals with complement-fixing ACA (Betterle et al., 1983). Scherbaum and co-workers (1982) reported that 10% of women (3 of 30) with ACA and thyroid autoimmunity developed Addison's disease over 3 years of observation. The experience of Riley and associates (1980a) was similar.

Thus, in a certain percentage of patients with ACAs, symptomatic Addison's disease develops each year. With use of a variety of adrenal autoantibody techniques, in up to 50% of asymptomatic autoantibody-positive children, Addison's disease has appeared within 3 years of follow-up (Betterle et al., 1997). Furthermore, 9 of 10 autoantibody-positive children developed Addison's disease over 10 years of follow-up. Furthermore, the single remaining non-Addisonian child did exhibit laboratory evidence of adrenal insufficiency. Higher concentrations of adrenal autoantibodies (both ACA and 21-hydroxylase autoantibodies) predict more severe degrees of adrenocortical impairment and increased risk of progression to Addison's disease (Laureti et al., 1998).

GONADAL AUTOIMMUNE DISORDERS

Steroidal cell autoantibodies (SCAs) closely resemble the ACAs described previously. However, SCAs also react with other steroid hormone-producing cells, including the placental syncytiotrophoblast, the Leydig cells of the testes, the theca interna/granulosa cell layers of the graafian follicles, and the corpora lutea of the ovaries (Jones, 1990; Sotsiou et al., 1980). SCAs are most commonly reported in Addisonian patients with secondary amenorrhea (in up to 60% of patients) (Blizzard et al., 1967; Irvine and Barnes, 1975; Nerup, 1974). Because the steroidal cell antigens are cytoplasmic and not present on the cell membrane, these antibodies are not pathogenic; however, they are markers for an underlying autoimmune process causing gonadal destruction. The target antigens appear to be P450 enzymes involved in sex steroid hormonogenesis. McNatty and colleagues (1975) have described a cytotoxic effect on cultured human granulosa cells by 9 of 23 sera from patients with Addison's disease and ovarian failure.

There is controversy about how commonly SCAs are present in cases of isolated premature ovarian failure. Kirsop and colleagues (1991) found ovary-specific SCAs only rarely in isolated cases of premature ovarian failure, whereas Fenichel and co-workers (1997) identified gonadal autoantibodies in approximately 60% of such cases. In initially asymptomatic patients, ovarian failure is predicted by the finding of SCAs in the patients' sera. In one study, ovarian failure occurred in 100% of SCA-positive women with APS-1 over 12 years of follow-up (Ahonen et al., 1987).

In the absence of associated adrenal autoimmunity, P450$_{scc}$, 17α-hydroxylase, and 21α-hydroxylase autoantibodies are infrequent in subjects with premature gonadal failure (Chen et al., 1996; Reimand et al., 2000). However, 3β-hydroxysteroid dehydrogenase autoantibodies have been detected in at least one study (Arif et al., 1996). Therefore there is controversy as to which steroidogenic enzyme is the major autoantigen in premature gonadal failure. As an aside, circulating autoantibodies to sex steroids have been very rarely reported (Kuwahara et al., 1998).

Cellular Autoimmunity

The early pathologic lesion of Addison's disease is a lymphocytic adrenalitis with inflammation surrounding regenerating nodules. Nerup and colleagues (1969) demonstrated specific antiadrenal cellular hypersensitivity in human Addison's disease using a leukocyte migration inhibition assay. Rabinowe and colleagues (1984) reported activated Ia$^+$ (DR$^+$) T cells in newly diagnosed Addison's disease patients.

In animals, adrenalitis can be induced by immunization with adrenal extracts in Freund's adjuvant. Once induced, adrenalitis can be passively transferred to other animals by immune lymphocytes (Fujii et al., 1992; Levine and Wank, 1968; Witebsky and Milgram, 1962). Despite these clinical and animal observations, proof of a major contribution of T cells in human autoimmune Addison's disease is lacking.

HLA Associations and Genetic Susceptibility

Thompson and colleagues (1975) reported that 70% of patients with Addison's disease were HLA-B8 positive in contrast to 24% of controls. Most patients were also Dw3-positive as determined by mixed leukocyte reaction (MLR) typing.

Maclaren and Riley (1986) found a strong association between Addison's disease and HLA-DR3 and HLA-DR4 antigens reminiscent of the associations seen with type 1 diabetes. However, in patients with Addison's disease and APS-1, the frequencies of HLA-DR antigens were not perturbed. Most of the other patients with isolated Addison's disease or APS-2 had at least one DR3 or DR4 allele. Furthermore, as with type 1 diabetes, a negative association was seen with DR2, DR5, and DR7 alleles. It therefore appears that Addison's disease is HLA associated, except when it is a component of APS-1. Recent studies, however, showed that the HLA-DR4/DQB1*0302 association was entirely a consequence of concurrent pancreatic β-cell autoimmunity (Huang et al., 1996).

Although the HLA-DR3 association with Addison's disease has been recognized for some time, studies in the late 20th century examined *CTLA-4* as a genetic susceptibility locus. In Addison's disease subjects with HLA-DQA1*0501, position 49 A/G site polymorphisms of the *CTLA-4* gene were associated with Addison's disease (Donner et al., 1997a). Concerning the (AT)n microsatellite polymorphism within the *CTLA-4* exon 3, the 106 base-pair allele was more common in English patients with Addison's disease than in controls, but no difference was observed in other ethnic groups (Kemp et al., 1998). A recent study showed that the G allele of the *CTLA-4* A/G polymorphism was associated with isolated Addison's disease and Addison's disease that was part of APS-2 (Vaidya et al., 2000b).

Clinical Manifestations

The clinical picture of Addison's disease is a result of deficiencies in cortisol (the major human glucocorticoid) and aldosterone (the major human mineralocorticoid). Aldosterone deficiency results in urinary sodium loss and potassium retention causing hyponatremia, hyperkalemia, type IV renal tubular acidosis, and fluid depletion. Salt craving may develop, and increased salt intake may keep the patient in electrolyte balance until anorexia or vomiting occurs. Salt depletion leads to hypovolemia, weight loss, hypotension, muscular weakness, fatigue, postural syncope, prerenal azotemia, and as a preterminal event, vascular collapse.

Cortisol deficiency, which may follow aldosterone deficiency, results in adipose wasting, apathy, weakness, deficient energy metabolism with fasting hypoglycemia, ketosis, hypoalaninemia, deficient cortisol response to hypoglycemia, inability to excrete a water load, and impaired response to stress. Gastrointestinal symptoms are common and include anorexia, nausea, vomiting, abdominal pain, and weight loss.

With a lack of negative feedback by cortisol, there is unrestrained secretion of pituitary ACTH and MSH, resulting in the classical muddy hyperpigmentation of the skin and buccal mucosa. Vitiligo is also common and generally believed to have an autoimmune cause (Betterle et al., 1984, 1985). Vitiligo in some patients is associated with autoantibodies to tyrosinase, an enzyme important in melanin formation (Song et al., 1994a).

The evolution of clinical Addison's disease passes through several stages similar to the natural history of type 1 diabetes. These stages include (1) increased renin and normal to low aldosterone, (2) low cortisol response to ACTH infusion, (3) increased basal ACTH concentrations, and eventually, (4) low basal cortisol and aldosterone secretion (Betterle et al., 1988). ACAs and autoantibodies directed against the steroidogenic enzymes precede the first appearance of clinical Addison's disease (Betterle et al., 1989).

Diagnosis

The onset of autoimmune Addison's disease is usually insidious, and the diagnosis may only be made during a crisis situation. In an Addisonian crisis, severe dehydration and vascular collapse develop. The following laboratory values reflect the sodium loss and potassium retention and prerenal azotemia: elevated serum potassium, blood urea nitrogen (BUN), and creatinine; low serum bicarbonate, PCO_2, and pH; normal to low serum sodium; greatly elevated plasma renin and ACTH; hypoglycemia; and inappropriately normal to low plasma cortisol and aldosterone levels. Relative lymphocytosis and modest eosinophilia are also often found.

At an earlier stage, sodium wasting may be reflected by hyperkalemia and mild acidosis and by a subnormal rise of plasma cortisol following ACTH infusion. Persons with adrenocortical autoantibodies without clinical Addison's disease may show elevated basal levels of plasma renin and/or ACTH as the only biochemical evidence of adrenocortical compromise. At diagnosis, adrenocortical autoantibodies are found in about two thirds of patients with idiopathic Addison's disease, and these diminish with time.

The diagnosis of autoimmune hypogonadism is based on the findings of elevated gonadotropin levels (especially FSH) and a characteristic gonadal biopsy or the presence of steroidal cell or steroidogenic enzyme autoantibodies. The gonadal biopsy specimen typically shows lymphocytic infiltration and follicular loss.

Prognosis

The prognosis for well-treated patients is satisfactory. Replacement therapy with 9α-fluorohydrocortisone (0.05 to 0.15 mg/day) and oral hydrocortisone (12 to 15 mg/m²/day in divided doses) is indicated. Extra oral cortisol or parenteral hydrocortisone is given during periods of stress, nausea, and vomiting when the maintenance dose is tripled. In general, the prognosis

depends on the associated disorders. The most significant associated problem in APS-1 is chronic active hepatitis, which often progresses to cirrhosis. Hypocalcemia of concurrent hypoparathyroidism may be masked until initiation of cortisol replacement therapy for Addison's disease. Chronic mucocutaneous candidiasis can lead to cancer of the esophagus. Associated disorders should be sought yearly. For patients with Addison's disease that is not associated with APS-1, thyroid autoantibodies, pancreatic islet autoantibodies, and PCAs should be sought.

AUTOIMMUNE DISORDERS OF THE ANTERIOR PITUITARY AND HYPOTHALAMUS

Anterior Pituitary Autoimmunity

Autoantibodies reacting with the prolactin and/or growth hormone–producing cells of the anterior pituitary have been detected by indirect immunofluorescence in some patients with autoimmune disease (Bottazzo et al., 1975). Such autoantibodies, in concert with reports of lymphocytic hypophysitis (Mayfield et al., 1980), suggest that autoimmunity to certain cells of the anterior pituitary can lead to clinical problems such as mass lesions that may result from lymphocytic infiltration (Supler and Mickle, 1992). Lymphocytic hypophysitis may occur in subjects whose pituitaries were biopsied surgically for evaluation of a pituitary mass lesion (Ruelle et al., 1999). Lymphocytic hypophysitis has been reported in children (Heinze and Bercu, 1997). However, autoimmunity is a rare cause of idiopathic hypopituitarism in children (Maghnie et al., 1995).

Pituitary autoantigens of 40 and 49 kD have been identified via Western blotting, although these proteins were not limited to the pituitary (Crock, 1998). Regarding the 49-kD autoantibody, sera were most commonly positive in subjects with lymphocytic hypophysitis (70%) with lower positive frequencies in individuals with Addison's disease (42%), thyroid autoimmunity (15%), rheumatoid arthritis (13%), and normal subjects (10%). Twenty-eight percent of Swedish patients with hypopituitarism exhibited 49-kD autoantibodies (Stromberg et al., 1998).

Pituitary autoimmunity has also been occasionally implicated in cases of growth hormone deficiency (Bottazzo et al., 1980b) and Sheehan's syndrome (Engelberth et al., 1965). Because some patient's height was increased at diagnosis, Mirakian and co-workers (1982) studied newly diagnosed type 1 diabetic patients for pituitary autoantibodies. More than 15% of such patients tested positive, but no control subject showed positive results. In long-standing type 1 diabetes, only 2% of patients exhibited positive results, suggesting that pituitary autoimmunity may be transient. These findings have yet to be confirmed.

positive type 1 (insulin-dependent) diabetic patients. The Belgian Diabetes Registry. J Clin Endocrinol Metab 84:4062–4067, 1999.

De Pirro R, Roth RA, Rossetti L, Goldfine ID. Characterization of the serum from a patient with insulin resistance and hypoglycemia. Evidence for multiple populations of insulin receptor antibodies with different receptor binding and insulin-mimicking activities. Diabetes 33:301–304, 1984.

Del Prete GF, Tiengo A, Nosadini R, Bottazzo GF, Betterle C, Bersani G. Glucagon secretion in two patients with autoantibodies to glucagon-producing cells. Horm Metab Res 10:260–261, 1978.

Delves PJ, Roitt IM. The immune system. First of two parts. N Engl J Med 343:37–49; 2000a.

Delves PJ, Roitt IM. The immune system. Second of two parts. N Engl J Med 343:108–117, 2000b.

Der Kinderen PJ. EPS, LATS and exophthalmos. In Irvine WJ, ed. Thyrotoxicosis. Baltimore, Williams and Wilkins, 1967, pp 221–234.

Deschamps I, Kahalil I, Lepage V, Gardais E, Hors J. The diagnostic value of DQA-DQB oligonucleotide typing for the prediction of risk of type I diabetes. Diabetes Young 24:14, 1990.

Di Mario U, Irvine WJ, Borsey DQ, Kyner JL, Weston J, Galfo C. Immune abnormalities in diabetic patients not requiring insulin at diagnosis. Diabetologia 25:392–395, 1983.

Diabetes Control and Complications Trial (DCCT) Group. The effect of intensive treatment of diabetes on the development and progression of long-term complications in insulin-dependent diabetes mellitus. The Diabetes Control and Complications Trial Research Group. N Engl J Med 329:977–986, 1993.

Diabetes Epidemiology Research International Group. Secular trends in incidence of childhood IDDM in 10 countries. Diabetes 39:858–864, 1990.

Dionisi S, Dotta F, Diaz-Horta O, Carabba B, Viglietta V, Di Mario U. Target antigens in autoimmune diabetes: pancreatic gangliosides. Ann Ist Super Sanita 33:433–435, 1997.

Dobbyns BM, Wilson LA. An exophthalmos-producing substance in the serum of patients suffering from progressive exophthalmos. J Clin Endocrinol Metab 14:1393–1396, 1954.

Doniach D Humoral and genetic aspects of thyroid autoimmunity. Clin Endocrinol Metab 4:267–285, 1975.

Doniach D, Bottazzo G. Polyendocrine autoimmunity. In Franklin EC, ed. Clinical Immunology Update. New York, Elsevier, 1981, pp 95–102.

Doniach D, Bottazzo GF, Russell RCG. Goitrous autoimmune thyroiditis (Hashimoto's disease). Clin Endocrinol Metab 8:63–80, 1979.

Doniach D, Florin-Christensen A. Autoimmunity in the pathogenesis of endocrine exophthalmos. Med Clin North Am 4:341–350, 1975.

Doniach D, Roitt I. Autoimmunity in Hashimoto's disease and its complications. J Clin Endocrinol Metab 17:1293–1304, 1957.

Donner H, Braun J, Seidl C, Rau H, Finke R, Ventz M, Walfish PG, Usadel KH, Badenhoop K. Codon 17 polymorphism of the cytotoxic T lymphocyte antigen 4 gene in Hashimoto's thyroiditis and Addison's disease. J Clin Endocrinol Metab 82:4130–4132, 1997a.

Donner H, Rau H, Walfish PG, Braun J, Siegmund T, Finke R, Herwig J, Usadel KH, Badenhoop K. CTLA4 alanine-17 confers genetic susceptibility to Graves' disease and to type 1 diabetes mellitus. J Clin Endocrinol Metab 82:143–146, 1997b.

Dozio N, Scavini M, Beretta A, Sarugeri E, Sartori S, Belloni C, Dosio F, Savi A, Fazio F, Sodoyez JC, Pozza G. Imaging of the buffering effect of insulin antibodies in the autoimmune hypoglycemic syndrome. J Clin Endocrinol Metab 83:643–648, 1998.

Dozio N, Sodoyez Goffaux F, Koch M, Ziegler B, Sodoyez JC. Polymorphism of insulin antibodies in six patients with insulin-immune hypoglycaemic syndrome. Clin Exp Immunol 85:282–287, 1991.

Drexhage HA. Autoimmune adrenocortical failure. In Volpe R, ed. Contemporary Endocrinology: Autoimmune Endocrinopathies. Totowa, NJ: Humana Press, 1999, pp 309–336.

Drugarin D, Negru S, Koreck A, Zosin I, Cristea C. The pattern of a T(H)1 cytokine in autoimmune thyroiditis. Immunol Lett 71:73–77, 2000.

Duncan JA, Shah SC, Shulman DI, Siegel RL, Kappy MS, Malone JI. Type b insulin resistance in a 15-year-old white youth. J Pediatr 103:421–424, 1983.

Dussault JH, Letarte J, Guyda H, Laberge C. Lack of influence of thyroid antibodies on thyroid function in the newborn infant and on a mass screening program for congenital hypothyroidism. J Pediatr 96:385–389, 1980.

Eisenbarth GS, Morris MA, Scearance RM. Cytotoxic antibodies to cloned islet cells in serum of patients with diabetes mellitus. J Clin Invest 67:403–408, 1981.

Ekins RP, Ellis SM. The radioimmunoassay of free thyroid hormones in serum. In Robbins J, Braverman LE, eds. Thyroid Research. Amsterdam, Excerpta Medica, 1975, p 597.

Elder M, Maclaren N, Riley W. Gonadal autoantibodies in patients with hypogonadism and/or Addison's disease. J Clin Endocrinol Metab 52:1137–1142, 1981.

Elias D, Cohen IR, Schechter Y, Spirer Z, Golander A. Antibodies to insulin receptor followed by anti-idiotype. Antibodies to insulin in child with hypoglycemia. Diabetes 36:348–354, 1987.

Engelberth O, Jezkova Z, Bleha O, Malek J, Bendl J. Autoantibodies in Scheehan's syndrome. Vnitr Lek 11:737–741, 1965.

Eto S, Fujihira T, Ohnami S, Suzuki H. Autoantibody to bovine TSH in Hashimoto's thyroiditis. Lancet 1:520, 1984.

Ettinger RA, Liu AW, Nepom GT, Kwok WW. Beta 57-Asp plays an essential role in the unique SDS stability of HLA-DQA1*0102/DQB1*0602 alpha beta protein dimer, the class II MHC allele associated with protection from insulin-dependent diabetes mellitus. J Immunol 165:3232–3238, 2000.

Falk RJ, Jennette JC. Anti-neutrophil cytoplasmic autoantibodies with specificity for myeloperoxidase in patients with systemic vasculitis and idiopathic necrotizing and crescentic glomerulonephritis. N Engl J Med 318:1651–1657, 1988.

Farid NR, Sampson L, Moens H, Barnard JM. The association of goitrous autoimmune thyroiditis with HLA-DR5. Tissue Antigens 17:265–268, 1981.

Faustman D, Eisenbarth G, Daley J, Breitmeye J. Abnormal T-lymphocyte subsets in type 1 diabetes. Diabetes 38:1462–1468, 1989.

Faustman D, Li XP, Lin HY, Fu YE, Eisenbarth G, Avruch J, Guo J. Linkage of faulty major histocompatibility complex class I to autoimmune diabetes. Science 254:1756–1761, 1991.

Fenichel P, Sosset C, Barbarino-Monnier P, Gobert B, Hieronimus S, Bene HC, Harter M. Prevalence, specificity and significance of ovarian antibodies during spontaneous premature ovarian failure. Hum Reprod 12:2623–2628, 1997.

Fletcher J, Mijovic C, Odugbesan O, Jenkins D, Bradwell AR, Barnett AH. Trans-racial studies implicate HLA-DQ as a component of genetic susceptibility to type 1 (insulin-dependent) diabetes. Diabetologia 31:864–870, 1988.

Flier JS, Kahn DR, Roth J. Receptors, antireceptor antibodies and mechanisms of insulin resistance. N Engl J Med 330:413–419, 1979.

Foley TP Jr, Abbassi V, Copeland KC, Draznin MB. Brief report: hypothyroidism caused by chronic autoimmune thyroiditis in very young infants. N Engl J Med 330:466–468, 1994.

Forrest JM, Menser MA, Burgess JA. High frequency of diabetes mellitus in young adults with congenital rubella. Lancet 2(7720):332–334, 1971.

Fort P, Lanes R, Dahlem S, Recker B, Weyman Daum M, Pugliese M, Lifshitz F. Breast feeding and insulin-dependent diabetes mellitus in children. J Am Coll Nutr 5:439–441, 1986.

Foulis AK, Liddle CN, Farquharson MA, Richmond JA, Weir RS. The histopathology of the pancreas in Type 1 (insulin-dependent) diabetes mellitus: a 25-year review of deaths in patients under 20 years of age in the United Kingdom. Diabetologia 29:267–274, 1986.

Foulis AK, Stewart JA. The pancreas in recent-onset type 1 (insulin-dependent) diabetes mellitus: Insulin content of islets, insulitis and associated changes in the exocrine acinar tissue. Diabetologia 26:456–461, 1984.

Francis G, Riley W. Congenital familial transient hypothyroidism secondary to transplacental thyrotropin-blocking autoantibodies. Am J Dis Child 141:1081–1083, 1987.

Freeman M, Weetman AP. T and B cell reactivity to adrenal antigens in autoimmune Addison's disease. Clin Exp Immunol 88:275–279, 1992.

Fuchtenbusch M, Rabl W, Grassl B, Bachmann W, Standl E, Ziegler AG. Delay of type I diabetes in high risk, first degree relatives by parenteral antigen administration: the Schwabing Insulin Prophylaxis Pilot Trial. Diabetologia 41:536–541, 1998.

Fujii Y. Kato N, Kito J, Asai J, Yokochi T. Experimental autoimmune adrenalitis: a murine model for Addison's disease. Autoimmunity 12:47–52, 1992.

Fukasawa N, Iitaka M, Hara Y, Yanagisawa M, Hase K, Miura S, Sakatume Y, Ishii J. Studies on thyroid hormone autoantibody (THAA) in 2 cases of Graves' disease with spuriously high free thyroxine values. Nippon Naibunpi Gakkai Zasshi 67:75–83, 1991.

Galluzzo A, Giordino C, Rubino G, Bompiani GD. Immunoregulatory T-lymphocyte subset deficiency in newly diagnosed type-1 (insulin-dependent) diabetes mellitus. Diabetologia 26:426–430, 1984.

Gamblin GT, Harper, DG, Galentine P, Buck DR, Chernow B, Eil C. Prevalence of increased intraocular pressure in Graves' disease-evidence of frequent subclinical ophthalmopathy. N Engl J Med 308:420–424, 1983.

Ganda OP, Srikanta S, Brink SJ, Morris MA, Gleason RE, Soeldner JS, Eisenbarth GS. Differential sensitivity to beta-cell secretagogues in early, type 1 diabetes mellitus. Diabetes 33:516–521, 1984.

Gardner SG, Gale EA, Williams AJ, Gillespie KM, Lawrence KE, Bottazzo GF, Bingley PJ. Progression to diabetes in relatives with islet autoantibodies. Is it inevitable? Diabetes Care 22:2049–2054, 1999.

Gargiulo AR, Hill JA. Autoimmune endocrinopathies in female reproductive dysfunction. In Volpe R, ed. Contemporary Endocrinology: Autoimmune Endocrinopathies. Totowa, NJ, Humana Press, 1999, pp 365–383.

Gepts W. Pathologic anatomy of the pancreas in juvenile diabetes mellitus. Diabetes 14:619–633, 1965.

Gepts W, Lecompte PM. The pancreatic islets in diabetes. Am J Med 70:105–115, 1981.

Giordano C, Stassi G, De Maria R, Todaro M, Richiusa P, Papoff G, Ruberti G, Bagnasco M, Testi R, Galluzzo A. Potential involvement of Fas and its ligand in the pathogenesis of Hashimoto's thyroiditis. Science 275:960–963, 1997.

Glaser NS. Non-insulin-dependent diabetes mellitus in childhood and adolescence. Pediatr Clin North Am 44:307–337, 1997.

Glaser N, Jones KL. Non-insulin-dependent diabetes mellitus in children and adolescents. Adv Pediatr 43:359–396, 1996.

Gleichmann H, Bottazzo GF. Progress toward standardization of cytoplasmic islet cell-antibody assay. Diabetes 36:578–584, 1987.

Goldman J, Baldwin D, Rubenstein AH, Klink DD, Blackard WG, Fisher LK, Roe TF, Schnure JJ. Characterization of circulating insulin and proinsulin-binding antibodies in autoimmune hypoglycemia. J Clin Invest 63:1050–1059, 1979.

Gorman C. Ophthalmopathy of Graves' disease. N Engl J Med 308:453–454, 1983.

Gorsuch AN, Dean BM, Bottazzo GF, Lister J, Cudworth AG. Evidence that type I diabetes and thyrogastric autoimmunity have different genetic determinants. BMJ 280:145–147, 1980.

Gorsuch AN, Spencer KM, Lister J, McNally JM, Dean BM, Bottazzo GF, Cudworth AG. Evidence for a long prediabetic period in type I (insulin-dependent) diabetes mellitus. Lancet 2:1363–1365, 1981.

Gough SC. The genetics of Graves' disease. Endocrinol Metab Clin North Am 29:255–266, 2000.

Graves PM, Barriga KJ, Norris JM, Hoffman MR, Yu L, Eisenbarth GS, Rewers M. Lack of association between early childhood immunizations and beta-cell autoimmunity. Diabetes Care 22:1694–1697, 1999.

Gray RS, Irvine WJ, Cameron EH, Duncan LJ. Glucose and insulin responses to oral glucose in overt non-insulin-dependent diabetics with and without the islet cell antibody. Diabetes 29:312–316, 1980.

Greenbaum CJ, Palmer JP, Kuglin B, Kolb H. Insulin autoantibodies measured by radioimmunoassay methodology are more related to insulin-dependent diabetes mellitus than those measured by

enzyme-linked immunosorbent assay: results of the Fourth International Workshop on the Standardization of Insulin Autoantibody Measurement. J Clin Endocrinol Metab 74:1040–1044, 1992.

Grubeck-Loebenstein B, Derfler K, Kassal H, Knapp W, Krisch K, Liszka K, Smyth PPA, Waldhausl W. Immunological features of nonimmunological hyperthyroidism. J Clin Endocrinol Metab 60:150–155, 1985.

Guillaud R, Schved JF, Gris JC, Chapuis H, Marty-Double C, Astruc J, Lesbros D. Epstein-Barr virus infection and syndrome of inappropriate macrophage activation. Pediatrie 48:459–462, 1993.

Gunji K, De Bellis A, Li AW, Yamada M, Kubota S, Ackrell B, Wengrowicz S, Bellastella A, Bizzarro A, Sinisi A, Wall JR. Cloning and characterization of the novel thyroid and eye muscle shared protein G2s: autoantibodies against G2s are closely associated with ophthalmopathy in patients with Graves' hyperthyroidism. J Clin Endocrinol Metab 85:1641–1647, 2000.

Gutierrez-Lopez MD. Bertera S, Chantres MT, Vavassori C, Dorman JS, Trucco M, Serrano-Rios M. Susceptibility to type 1 (insulin-dependent) diabetes mellitus in Spanish patients correlates quantitatively with expression of HLA-DQ alpha Arg 52 and HLA-DQ beta non-Asp 57 alleles. Diabetologia 35:583–588, 1992.

Hahn HB, Hayles AB, Woolner LB. Lymphocytic thyroiditis in children. J Pediatr 66:73–78, 1965.

Hamburger JI. Management of hyperthyroidism in children and adolescents. J Clin Endocrinol Metab 60:1019–1024, 1985.

Hammond LJ, Lowdell MW, Cerrano PG, Goode AW, Bottazzo GF, Mirakian R. Analysis of apoptosis in relation to tissue destruction associated with Hashimoto's autoimmune thyroiditis. J Pathol 182:138–144, 1997.

Hanafusa T, Pujol-Borrell R, Chiavoto L, Russell RCG, Doniach D, Bottazzo GF. Aberrant expression of HLA DR antigen on thyrocytes in Graves' disease: relevance to autoimmunity. Lancet 2:1111–1115, 1983.

Harrison LC, Colman PG, Dean B, Baxter R, Martin FI. Increase in remission rate in newly diagnosed type I diabetic subjects treated with azathioprine. Diabetes 34:1306–1308, 1985.

Harrison LC, Honyman MC, DeAizpurua HJ, Schmidli RS, Colman PG, Tait BD, Cram DS. Inverse relation between humoral and cellular immunity to glutamic acid decarboxylase in subjects at risk of insulin-dependent diabetes. Lancet 431:1365–1369, 1993.

Hashimoto H. Zur kenntnis der lymphomatosa veranderung der schilddruse (Struma lymphomatosa). Acta Klin Chir 97:219–248, 1912.

Hauser L, Sheehan P, Simpkins H. Pancreatic pathology in pentamidine-induced diabetes in acquired immunodeficiency syndrome patients. Hum Pathol 229:926–929, 1991.

Hayward AR, Herberger M. Culture and phenotype of activated T-cells from patients with type-1 diabetes mellitus. Diabetes 33:319–323, 1984.

Heimberg H, Nagy ZP, Somers G, De-Leeuw I, Schuit FC. Complementation of HLA-DQA and -DQB genes confers susceptibility and protection to insulin-dependent diabetes mellitus. Hum Immunol 33:10–17, 1992.

Heinonen E, Krohn K. Studies on an adrenal antigen common to man and different animals. Med Biol 55:48–53, 1977.

Heinze HJ, Bercu BB. Acquired hypophysitis in adolescence. J Pediatr Endocrinol Metab 10:315–321, 1997.

Herskowitz RD, Jackson RA, Soeldner JS, Eisenbarth GS. Pilot trial to prevent type I diabetes: progression to overt IDDM despite oral nicotinamide. J Autoimmun 2:733–737, 1989.

Heufelder AE, Wenzel BE, Bahn RS. Cell surface localization of a 72 kilodalton heat shock protein in retroocular fibroblasts from patients with Graves' ophthalmopathy. J Clin Endocrinol Metab 74:732–736, 1992.

Heward JM, Allahabadia A, Armitage M, Hattersley A, Dodson PM, Macleod K, Carr-Smith J, Daykin J, Daly A, Sheppard MC, Holder RL, Barnett AH, Franklyn JA, Gough SC. The development of Graves' disease and the CTLA-4 gene on chromosome 2q33. J Clin Endocrinol Metab 84:2398–2401, 1999.

Hirata Y. Methamizole and insulin autoimmune syndrome with hypoglycemia. Lancet 2:1037–1038, 1983.

Hiromatsu Y, Yang D, Miyake I, Koga M, Kameo J, Sato M, Inone Y, Nonaka K. Nicotinamide decreases cytokine-induced activation of orbital fibroblasts from patients with thyroid-associated ophthalmopathy. J Clin Endocrinol Metab 83:121–124, 1998.

Hitchcock CL. Riley WJ, Alamo A, Pyka R, Maclaren NK. Lymphocyte subsets and activation in prediabetes. Diabetes 35:1416–1422, 1986.

Hollander CS, Stevenson C, Mitsuma T, Pineda G, Shenkman L, Silva E. T₃ toxicosis in an iodine-deficient area. Lancet 2:1276–1278, 1972.

Holm L-E, Blomgren H, Lowhagen T. Cancer risks in patients with chronic lymphocytic thyroiditis. N Engl J Med 312:601–604, 1985.

Honeyman MC, Cram DS, Harrison LC: Transcription factor jun-B is target of autoreactive T-cells in IDDM. Diabetes 42:626–630, 1993.

Horita M, Suzuki H, Onodera T, Ginsberg-Fellner F, Fauci AS, Notkins AL. Abnormalities of immunoregulatory T cell subsets in patients with insulin-dependent diabetes mellitus. J Immunol 129:1426–1429, 1982.

Horn GT, Bugawan TL, Long CM, Erlich HA. Allelic sequence variation of the HLA-DQ loci: relationship to serology and insulin-dependent diabetes susceptibility. Proc Natl Acad Sci USA 85:6012–6016, 1988.

Huang W, Connor E, Rosa TD, Muir A, Schatz D, Silverstein J, Crockett S, She JX, Maclaren NK. Although DR3-DQB1*0201 may be associated with multiple component diseases of the autoimmune polyglandular syndromes, the human leukocyte antigen DR4-DQB1*0302 haplotype is implicated only in beta-cell autoimmunity. J Clin Endocrinol Metab 81:2559–63, 1996.

Hummel M, Fuchtenbusch M, Schenker M, Ziegler AG. No major association of breast-feeding, vaccinations, and childhood viral diseases with early islet autoimmunity in the German BABYDIAB Study. Diabetes Care 23:969–974, 2000.

Hunt PJ, Marshall SE, Weetman AP, Bell JI, Wass JA, Welsh KI. Cytokine gene polymorphisms in autoimmune thyroid disease. J Clin Endocrinol Metab 85:1984–1988, 2000.

Ilonen J, Surcel H-M, Mustonen A, Kaar M-L, Akerblom HK. Lymphocyte subpopulations at the onset of type I (insulin-dependent) diabetes. Diabetologia 27:106–108, 1984.

Imagawa T, Katakura S, Mori M, Aihara Y, Mitsuda T, Yokota S. A case of macrophage activation syndrome developed with systemic juvenile rheumatoid arthritis. Ryumachi 37:487–492, 1997.

Irvine W, Chann MMW, Scarth L, Kolb F, Hartog M, Bayliss R, Drury M. Immunologic aspects of premature ovarian failure associated with idiopathic Addison's disease. Lancet 2:883–887, 1968.

Irvine WJ. The association of atrophic gastritis with autoimmune thyroid disease. Clin Endocrinol Metab 4:351–377, 1975.

Irvine WJ, Barnes EW. Addison's disease, ovarian failure and hypoparathyroidism. Clin Endocrinol Metab 4:379–434, 1975.

Irvine WJ, Gray RS, McCallum CJ. Pancreatic islet-cell antibody as a marker for asymptomatic and latent diabetes and prediabetes. Lancet 2:1097–1102, 1976.

Irvine WJ, McCallum CJ, Gray RS, Duncan LJP. Clinical and pathogenic significance of pancreatic islet-cell antibodies in diabetics treated with oral hypoglycemic agents. Lancet 1:1025–1027, 1977.

Iseki M, Shimizu M, Oikawa T, Hojo H, Arikawa K, Ichikawa Y, Momotani N, Ito K. Sequential serum measurements of thyrotropin binding inhibitor immunoglobulin G in transient familial neonatal hypothyroidism. J Clin Endocrinol Metab 57:384–387, 1983.

Itoh M, Uchimura K, Makino M, Kobayashi T, Hayashi R, Nagata M, Kakizawa H, Fujiwara K, Nagasaka A. Production of IL-10 and IL-12 in CD40 and interleukin 4-activated mononuclear cells from patients with Graves' disease. Cytokine 12:688–693, 2000.

Iwatani Y, Amino N, Mori H, Asari S, Izumiguchi Y, Kumahara Y, Miyai K. T lymphocyte subsets in autoimmune thyroid diseases and subacute thyroiditis detected with monoclonal antibodies. J Clin Endocrinol Metab 56:251–4, 1983.

Jackson RA, Haynes BF, Burch WM, Shimizu K, Bowring MA, Eisenbarth GS. Ia+ T cells in new onset Graves' disease. J Clin Endocrinol Metab 59:187–190, 1984.

Jackson RA, Morris MA, Haynes BF, Eisenbarth GS. Increased circulating Ia-antigen bearing T-cells in type I diabetes mellitus. N Engl J Med 306:785–788, 1982.

Jansson R, Dahlberg PA, Johansson H, Lindstrom B. Intrathyroidal concentrations of methimazote in patients with Graves' disease. J Clin Endocrinol Metab 57:129–132, 1983b.

Jansson R, Totterman TH, Sallstrom J, Dahlberg PA. Thyroid-infiltrating T lymphocyte subsets in Hashimoto's thyroiditis. J Clin Endocrinol Metab 56:1164–1168, 1983a.

Javier RM, Sibilia J, Offner C, Albert A, Kuntz JL. Macrophage activation syndrome in lupus Rev Rhum Ed Fr 60:831–835, 1993.

Jones KL. The Cushing syndromes. Pediatr Clin North Am 37:1313–1332, 1990.

Jones KL. Non-insulin dependent diabetes in children and adolescents: the therapeutic challenge. Clint Pediatr Phila 37:103–110, 1998.

Julier C, Hyer RN, Davies J, Merlin F, Soularue P, Briant L, Cathelineau G, Deschamps I, Rotter JI, Froguel P, Boitard C, Bell JI, Lathrop GM. Insulin-IGF2 region on chromosome 11p encodes a gene implicated in HLA-DR4-dependent diabetes susceptibility. Nature 354:155–159, 1991.

Juppner H, Atkinson MJ, Baethke R, Hesch RD. Autoantibodies against parathyroid hormone in a patient with terminal renal insufficiency. Lancet 1:1379–1381, 1984.

Kadlubowski M, Irvine WJ, Rowland AC. Anti-muscle antibodies in Graves' ophthalmopathy. J Clin Lab Immunol 24:105–111, 1987.

Kahn CR, Flier JS, Bar RS, Archer JA, Gorden P, Martin MM, Roth J. The syndromes of insulin resistance and acanthosis nigricans. N Engl J Med 294:739–745, 1976.

Kappler JW, Staerz U, White J, Marrack P. Self-tolerance eliminates T cells specific for Mls-modified products of the major histocompatibility complex. Nature 332:35–45, 1989.

Karam JH, Lewitt PA, Young CW, Nowlain RE, Frankel BJ, Fujiya H, Freedman ZR, Grodsky GM. Insulinopenic diabetes after rodenticide (Vacor) ingestion: a unique model of acquired diabetes in man. Diabetes 29:971–978, 1980.

Karjalainen J, Martin J, Knip M, Ilonen J, Robinson BH, Savilahti E, Akerblom HK, Dosch HM. A bovine albumin peptide as a possible trigger of insulin-dependent diabetes mellitus. N Engl J Med 327:302–307, 1992.

Karlsson FA, Burman P, Loof L, Mardh S. Major parietal cell antigen in autoimmune gastritis with pernicious anemia is the acid-producing H+,K+-adenosine triphosphatase of the stomach. J Clin Invest 81:475–479, 1988.

Karounos DG, Thomas JW. Recognition of common islet antigen by autoantibodies from NOD mice and humans with IDDM. Diabetes 39:1085–1090, 1990.

Karvonen M, Viik-Kajander M, Moltchanova E, Libman I, LaPorte R, Tuomilehto J. Incidence of childhood type 1 diabetes worldwide. Diabetes Mondiale (DiaMond) Project Group. Diabetes Care 23:1516–1526, 2000.

Kasimiotis H, Myers MA, Argentaro A, Mertin S, Fida S, Ferraro T, Olsson J, Rowley MJ, Harley VR. Sex-determining region Y-related protein SOX13 is a diabetes autoantigen expressed in pancreatic islets. Diabetes 49:555–561, 2000.

Kaufman DL, Erlander MG, Clare-Salzler M, Atkinson MA, Maclaren NK, Tobin AJ. Autoimmunity to two forms of glutamate decarboxylase in insulin-dependent diabetes mellitus. J Clin Invest 89:283–292, 1992.

Kawakami A, Eguchi K, Matsunaga M, Tezuka,H, Ueki Y, Shimomura C, Otsubo T, Nakao H, Migita K, Ishikawa N, Itok I, Nagataki S. CD4+CD45RA+ cells (suppressor-inducer T cells) in thyroid tissue from patients with Graves' disease. Acta Endocrinol Copenh 125:687–693, 1991.

Kawasaki E, Eisenbarth GS. High-throughput radioassays for autoantibodies to recombinant autoantigens. Front Biosci 5:E181–E190, 2000.

Kemp EH, Ajjan RA, Husebye ES, Peterson P, Uibo R, Imrie H, Pearce SH, Watson PF, Weetman AP. A cytotoxic T lymphocyte antigen-4 (CTLA-4) gene polymorphism is associated with autoimmune Addison's disease in English patients. Clin Endocrinol (Oxford) 49:609–613, 1998.

Kendall-Taylor P. LATS and human-specific thyroid stimulator; their relation to Graves' disease. Clin Endocrinol Metab 4:319–339, 1975.

Kendall-Taylor P, Knox AJ, Steel NR, Atkinson S. Evidence that thyroid-stimulating antibody is produced in the thyroid gland. Lancet 1:654–656, 1984.

Kendler DL, Rootman J, Huber GK, Davies TF. A 64 kDa membrane antigen is a recurrent epitope for natural autoantibodies in patients with Graves' thyroid and ophthalmic diseases. Clin Endocrinol Oxf 35:539–547, 1991.

Kenney RM, Michaels IA, Flomenbaum NE, Yu GS. Poisoning with N-3-pyridylmethyl-N′-p-nitrophenylurea (Vacor). Immunoperoxidase demonstration of beta-cell destruction. Arch Pathol Lab Med 105:367–370, 1981.

Ketchum CH, Riley WJ, Maclaren NK. Adrenal dysfunction in asymptomatic patients with adrenocortical autoantibodies. J Clin Endocrinol Metab 58:1166–1170, 1984.

Khoury E, Hammond L, Bottazzo G, Doniach D. Surface reactive antibodies to human adrenal cells in Addison's disease. Clin Exp Immunol 45:48–55, 1981.

Kida K, Mimura G, Kobayashi T, Nakamura K, Sonoda S, Inouye H, Tsuji K. Immunogenetic heterogeneity in type I (insulin-dependent) diabetes among Japanese—HLA antigens and organ-specific autoantibodies. Diabetologia 32:34–39, 1989.

Kim YJ, Zhou Z, Hurtado J, Wood DL, Choi AS, Pescovitz MD, Warfel KA, Vandagriff J, Davis JK, Kwon BS. IDDM patients' sera recognize a novel 30-kD pancreatic autoantigen related to chymotrypsinogen. Immunol Invest 22:219–227, 1993.

Kirsop R, Brock CR, Robinson BG, Baber RJ, Wells JV, Saunders DM. Detection of anti-ovarian antibodies by indirect immunofluorescence in patients with premature ovarian failure. Reprod Fertil Dev 3:537–541, 1991.

Kodama K, Sikorska H, Bandy-Dafoe P, Bayly R, Wall JR. Demonstration of a circulating autoantibody against a soluble eye-muscle antigen in Graves' ophthalmopathy. Lancet 2:1353–1356, 1982.

Korponay-Szabo IR, Sulkanen S, Halttunen T, Maurano F, Rossi M, Mazzarella G, Laurila K, Troncone R, Maki M. Tissue transglutaminase is the target in both rodent and primate tissues for celiac disease-specific autoantibodies. J Pediatr Gastroenterol Nutr 31:520–527, 2000.

Kotsa K, Watson PF, Weetman AP. A CTLA-4 gene polymorphism is associated with both Graves disease and autoimmune hypothyroidism. Clin Endocrinol (Oxf) 46:551–554, 1997.

Kourides IA, Ridgeway EC, Weintraub BD, Bigos ST, Gershengorn MC, Maloof F. Thyrotropin-induced hyperthyroidism: use of alpha and beta subunit levels to identify patients with pituitary tumors. J Clin Endocrinol Metab 45:534–543, 1977.

Krohn K, Uibo R, Aavik E. Peterson P, Savilahti K. Identification by molecular cloning of an autoantigen associated with Addison's disease as steroid 17 alpha-hydroxylase. Lancet 339:770–773, 1992.

Kubota S, Gunji K, Ackrell BA, Cochran B, Stolarski C, Wengrowicz S, Kennerdell JS, Hiromatsu Y, Wall J. The 64-kilodalton eye muscle protein is the flavoprotein subunit of mitochondrial succinate dehydrogenase: the corresponding serum antibodies are good markers of an immune-mediated damage to the eye muscle in patients with Graves' hyperthyroidism. J Clin Endocrinol Metab 83:443–437, 1998.

Kuwahara A, Kamada M, Irahara M, Naka O, Yamashita T, Aono T. Autoantibody against testosterone in a woman with hypergonadotropic hypogonadism. J Clin Endocrinol Metab 83:14–16, 1998.

Kyvik KO, Green A, Svendsen A, Mortensen K. Breast feeding and the development of type 1 diabetes mellitus. Diabet Med 9:233–235, 1992.

Lan MS, Wasserfall C, Maclaren NK, Notkins AL. IA-2, a transmembrane protein of the protein tyrosine phosphatase family, is a major autoantigen in insulin-dependent diabetes mellitus. Proc Natl Acad Sci USA 93:636–640, 1996.

Lang F, Maugendr D, Houssaint E, Charbonnel B, Sai P. Cytoadherence of lymphocytes from type I diabetic subjects to insulin-secreting cells, a marker of anti-a-cell cellular immunity. Diabetes 36:1356–1364, 1987.

Laureti S, De Bellis A, Muccitelli VI, Calcinaro F, Bizzarro A, Rossi R, Bellastella A, Santeusanio F, Falorni A. Levels of adrenocortical autoantibodies correlate with the degree of adrenal dysfunction in subjects with preclinical Addison's disease. J Clin Endocrinol Metab 83:3507–3511, 1998.

Lederman MM, Ellner JJ, Rodman HM. Defective suppressor cell generation in juvenile onset diabetes. J Immunol 127:2051–2059, 1981.

Leisti S, Ahonen P, Perheentupa J. The diagnosis and staging of hypercortisolism in progressing autoimmune adrenalitis. Pediatr Res 17:861–867, 1983.

Lendrum R, Walker G, Cudworth AG, Theophanides C, Pyke DA, Bloom A, Gamble DR. Islet-cell antibodies in diabetes mellitus. Lancet 2:1273–1276, 1976.

Lendrum R, Walker G, Gamble DR. Islet-cell antibodies in juvenile diabetes mellitus of recent onset. Lancet 1:880–883, 1975.

Lernmark A, Freedman ZR, Hofmann C, Rubenstein AH, Steiner DF, Jackson RL, Winter RJ, Traisman HS. Islet-cell-surface antibodies in juvenile diabetes mellitus. N Engl J Med 299:375–380, 1978.

Lernmark A, Baekkeskov S. Islet cell antibodies-theoretical and practical implications. Diabetologia 21:431–435, 1981.

Levine S, Wenk E. The production and passive transfer of allergic adrenalitis. Am J Pathol 52:41–44, 1968.

Levy-Marchal C, Bridel MP, Sodoyez-Goffaux F, Koch M, Tichet J, Czernichow P, Sodoyez JC. Superiority of radiobinding assay over ELISA for detection of IAAs in newly diagnosed type I diabetic children. Diabetes Care 14:61–63, 1991.

Li Y, Song YH, Rais N, Connor E, Schatz D, Muir A, Maclaren N. Autoantibodies to the extracellular domain of the calcium sensing receptor in patients with acquired hypoparathyroidism. J Clin Invest 97:910–914, 1996.

Linde R, Alexander N, Island DP, Rabin D. Familial insensitivity of the pituitary and periphery to thyroid hormone: a case report in two generations and a review of the literature. Metabolism 31:510–513, 1982.

Litherland SA, Xie XT, Hutson AD, Wasserfall C, Whittaker DS, She JX, Hofig A, Dennis MA, Fuller K, Cook R, Schatz D, Moldawer LL, Clare-Salzler MJ. Aberrant prostaglandin synthase 2 expression defines an antigen-presenting cell defect for insulin-dependent diabetes mellitus. J Clin Invest 104:515–523, 1999.

Londei M, Lamb JR, Bottazzo GF, Feldman M. Epithelial cells expressing aberrant MHC class II determinants can present antigen to cloned human T cells. Nature 312:639–641, 1984.

Lu J, Li Q, Xie H, Chen ZJ, Borovitskaya AE, Maclaren NK, Notkins AL, Lan MS. Identification of a second transmembrane protein tyrosine phosphatase, IA-2beta, as an autoantigen in insulin-dependent diabetes mellitus: precursor of the 37-kDa tryptic fragment. Proc Natl Acad Sci USA 93:2307–2311, 1996.

Ludemann J, Csernok E, Ulmer M, Lemke H, Utecht B, Rautmann A, Gross WL. Anti-neutrophil cytoplasm antibodies in Wegener's granulomatosis: immunodiagnostic value, monoclonal antibodies and characterization of the target antigen. Neth J Med 36:157–162, 1990b.

Ludemann J, Utecht B, Gross WL. Anti-neutrophil cytoplasm antibodies in Wegener's granulomatosis recognize an elastinolytic enzyme. J Exp Med 171:357–362, 1990a.

Luhder F, Schlosser M, Mauch L, Haubruck H, Rjasanowski I, Michaelis D, Kohnert KD, Ziegler M: Autoantibodies against GAD65 rather than GAD67 precede the onset of type 1 diabetes. Autoimmunity 19:71–80, 1994.

Luo DF, Buzzetti R, Rotter JI, Maclaren NK, Raffel LJ, Nistico L, Giovannini C, Pozzilli P, Thomson G, She JX. Confirmation of three susceptibility genes to insulin-dependent diabetes mellitus: IDDM4, IDDM5 and IDDM8. Hum Mol Genet 5:693–698, 1996.

Maclaren NK, Atkinson MA. Is insulin-dependent diabetes mellitus environmentally induced? N Engl J Med 327:347–349, 1992.

Maclaren NK, Huang S-W. Antibody to cultured human insulinoma cells in insulin-dependent diabetes. Lancet 1:997–999, 1975.

Maclaren NK, Huang S-W. Cell-mediated immunity in insulin dependent diabetes. In Irvine WJ, ed. The Immunology of Diabetes. Edinburgh, Tevoit Scientific Publications, 1980, pp 185–193.

Maclaren N, Lan M, Coutant R, Schatz D, Silverstein J, Muir A, Clare-Salzer M, She JX, Malone J, Crockett S, Schwartz S,

Quattrin T, DeSilva M, Vander Vegt P, Notkins A, Krischer J. Only multiple autoantibodies to islet cells (ICA), insulin, GAD65, IA-2 and IA-2beta predict immune-mediated (Type 1) diabetes in relatives. J Autoimmun 12:279–287, 1999.

Maclaren NK, Riley WJ. Thyroid, gastric, and adrenal autoimmunities associated with insulin-dependent diabetes mellitus. Diabetes Care 8(Suppl 1):34–38, 1985.

Maclaren NK, Riley WJ. Inherited susceptibility to autoimmune Addison's disease is linked to human leukocyte antigens-DR3 and/or DR4. J Clin Endocrinol Metab 62:455–459, 1986.

Maclaren N, Riley W, Rosenbloom A, Elder M, Spillar R, Cuddeback J. The heterogeneity of Black insulin dependent diabetes. Diabetes 31:65A, 1982.

Maclaren N, Riley W, Skordis N, Atkinson M, Spillar R, Silverstein J, Klein R, Vadheim C, Rotter J. Inherited susceptibility to insulin-dependent diabetes is associated with HLA-DR1, while DR5 is protective. Autoimmunity 1:197–205, 1988.

Maghnie M, Cosi G, Genovese E, Manca-Bitti ML, Cohen A, Zecca S, Tinelli C, Gallucci M, Bernasconi S, Boscherini B, Severi F, Arico M. Central diabetes insipidus in children and young adults. N Engl J Med 343:998–1007, 2000.

Maghnie M, Lorini R, Vitali L, Mastricci N, Carra AM, Severi F. Organ-and non-organ-specific auto-antibodies in children with hypopituitarism on growth hormone therapy. Eur J Pediatr 154:450–453, 1995.

Manna R, Migliore A, Martin LS, Ferrara E, Ponte E, Marietti G, Scuderi F, Cristiano G, Ghirlanda G, Gambassi G. Nicotinamide treatment in subjects at high risk of developing IDDM improves insulin secretion. Br J Clin Pract 46:1–9, 1992.

Manns M. Autoantibodies and antigens in liver diseases—updated. J Hepatol 9:272–280, 1989.

Manns MP, Johnson EF. Identification of human cytochrome P450s as autoantigens. Methods Enzymol 206:210–220, 1991.

Marino M, Chiovato L, Friedlander JA, Latrofa F, Pinchera A, McCluskey RT. Serum antibodies against megalin (GP330) in patients with autoimmune thyroiditis. J Clin Endocrinol Metab 84:2468–2474, 1999.

Mariotti S, Martino E, Cupini C, Lasie R, Giani C, Baschieri L, Pinchera A. Low serum thyroglobulin as a clue to the diagnosis of thyrotoxicosis factitia. N Engl J Med 307:410–412, 1982.

Mariotti S, Sansoni P, BarbesinoG, Caturegli P, Monti D, Cossarizza A, Giacomelli T, Passeri G, Fagiolo U, Pinchera A, Franceschi C. Thyroid and other organ-specific autoantibodies in healthy centenarians. Lancet 339:1506–1508, 1992.

Markmann J, Lo D, Naji A, Palmiter RD, Brinster RL, Heber-Katz E. Antigen presenting function of class II MHC expressing pancreatic beta cells. Nature 2:476–479, 1988.

Maron R, Elias D, DeJongh BM, Bruining GF, VanRood JJ, Shechter Y, Cohen IR. Autoantibodies to the insulin receptor in juvenile onset insulin-dependent diabetes. Nature 303:817–818, 1983.

Marron MP, Zeidler A, Raffel LJ, Eckenrode SE, Yang JJ, Hopkins DI, Garchon HJ, Jacob CO, Serrano-Rios M, Martinez Larrad MT, Park Y, Bach JF, Rotter JI, Yang MC, She JX. Genetic and physical mapping of a type 1 diabetes susceptibility gene (IDDM12) to a 100-kb phagemid artificial chromosome clone containing D2S72-CTLA4-D2S105 on chromosome 2q33. Diabetes 49:492–499, 2000.

Maruyama T, Takei I, Matsuba I, Tsuruoka A, Taniyama M, Ikeda Y, Kataoka K, Abe M, Matsuki S. Cell-mediated cytotoxic islet cell surface antibodies to human pancreatic beta cells. Diabetologia 26:30–33, 1884.

Marx JZ. Diabetes—a possible autoimmune disease. Science 225:1381–1383, 1984.

Massart C, Caroff G, Maugendre D, Genetet N, Gibassier J. Peripheral blood and intrathyroidal T cell clones from patients with thyroid autoimmune diseases. Autoimmunity 31:163–174, 1999.

Matsuura N, Yamada Y, Nohara Y, Konishi J, Kasagi K, Endo K, Kojima H, Wataya K. Familial neonatal transient hypothyroidism due to maternal TSH-binding inhibitor immunoglobulins. N Engl J Med 303:738–741, 1980.

Mayer EJ, Hamman RF, Gay EC, Lezotte DC, Savitz DA, Klingensmith GJ. Reduced risk of IDDM among breast-fed children. The Colorado IDDM Registry. Diabetes 37:1625–1632, 1988.

Mayfield RK, Levine, JH, Gordon L, Powers J, Galbraith RM, Rawe SE. Lymphoid adenohypophysitis presenting as a pituitary tumor. Am J Med 69:619–623, 1980.

McGregor AM, Petersen MM, McLachlan SM, Rooke P, Smith BR, Hall R. Carbamizole and the autoimmune response in Graves' disease. N Engl J Med 303:302–307, 1980a.

McGregor AM, Smith BR, Hall R, Petersen MM, Miller M, Dewar PJ. Prediction of relapse in hyperthyroid Graves' disease. Lancet 1:1101–1103, 1980b.

McKenzie JM. Humoral factors in the pathogenesis of Graves' disease. Physiol Rev 48:252–310, 1968.

McKenzie JM, Zakarija M, Bonnyns M. Graves' disease. Med Clin North Am 59:1177–1192, 1975.

McNatty K, Short R, Barnes E, Irvine W. The cytotoxic effect of serum from patients with Addison's disease and autoimmune ovarian failure on human granulosa cells in culture. Clin Exp Immunol 22:378–383, 1975.

Meschi F, Dozio N, Bognetti E, Carra M, Cofano D, Chiumello G. An unusual case of recurrent hypoglycaemia: 10-year follow up of a child with insulin autoimmunity. Eur J Pediatr 151:32–34, 1992.

Metcalfe MA, Baum JD. Family characteristics and insulin dependent diabetes. Arch Dis Child 67:731–736, 1992.

Michelsen B, Lernmark A. Molecular cloning of a polymorphic DNA endonuclease fragment associates insulin-dependent diabetes mellitus with HLA-DQ. J Clin Invest 79:1144–1152, 1987.

Mirakian R, Cudworth AG, Bottazzo GF, Richardson CA, Doniach D. Autoimmunity to anterior pituitary cells and the pathogenesis of insulin-dependent diabetes mellitus. Lancet 1:755–759, 1982.

Moller DE, Ratner RE, Borenstein DG, Taylor SI. Autoantibodies to the insulin receptor as a cause of autoimmune hypoglycemia in systemic lupus erythematosus. Am J Med 84:334–338, 1988.

Moncayo R, Moncayo HE. Autoimmunity and the ovary. Immunol Today 13:255–258, 1992.

Morel PA, Dorman JS. Todd JA, McDevitt HO, Trucco M. Aspartic acid at position 57 of the HLA-DQ_ chain protects against type I diabetes: a family study. Proc Nat Acad Sci USA 85:8111–8115, 1988.

Mori H, Amino N, Iwatani Y, Asari S, Izumiguchi Y, Kumahara Y, Miyai K. Decrease of immunoglobulin G-Fc receptor-bearing T lymphocytes in Graves' disease. J Clin Endocrinol Metab 55:399–402, 1982.

Moroz LA, Meltzer SJ, Bastomsky CH. Thyroid disease with monoclonal (immunoglobulin lambda) antibody to triiodothyronine and thyroxine. J Clin Endocrinol Metab 56:1009–1015, 1983.

Moses AC, Lawlor J, Haddow J, Jackson IMD. Familial euthyroid hyperthyroxinemia resulting from increased thyroxine binding to thyroxine-binding prealbumin. N Engl J Med 306:966–969, 1982.

Mouy R, Stephan JL, Pillet P, Haddad E, Hubert P, Prieur AM. Efficacy of cyclosporine A in the treatment of macrophage activation syndrome in juvenile arthritis: report of five cases. J Pediatr 129:750–754, 1996.

Muir AM, Maclaren NK. Autoimmune diseases of the adrenal glands, parathyroid glands, gonads, and hypothalamic-pituitary axis. Endocrinol Metab Clin North Am 20:619–644, 1991.

Muir A, She JX. Advances in the genetics and immunology of autoimmune polyglandular syndrome II/III and their clinical applications. Ann Med Interne (Paris) 150:301–312, 1999.

Myers BD, Ross J, Newton L, Luetscher J, Perlroth M. Cyclosporin associated chronic nephropathy. N Engl J Med 311:699–705, 1984.

Nagamine K, Peterson P, Scott HS, Kudoh J, Minoshima S, Heino M, Krohn KJ, Lalioti MD, Mullis PE, Antonarakis SE, Kawasaki K, Asakawa S, Ito F, Shimizu N. Positional cloning of the APECED gene. Nat Genet 17:393–398, 1997.

Nakamura S, Sakata S, Komaki T, Kamikubo K, Miura K. Thyroid hormone autoantibodies (THAA) in three sisters: a four-year follow up. J Endocrinol Invest 12:421–427, 1989.

Naserke HE, Dozio N, Ziegler AG, Bonifacio E. Comparison of a novel micro-assay for insulin autoantibodies with the conventional radiobinding assay. Diabetologia 41:681–683, 1998.

Nayak RC, Omar MAK, Rabizadeh A, Srikanta S, Eisenbarth GS. Cytoplasmic islet cell antibodies. Diabetes 34:617–619, 1985.

Nepom G. A unified hypothesis for the complex genetics of HLA associations with IDDM. Diabetes 39:1153–1157, 1990.

Nepom GT, Kwok WW. Molecular basis for HLA-DQ associations with IDDM. Diabetes 47:1177–1184, 1998.

Nerup J. Addison's disease—serological studies. Acta Endocrinol 76:142–160, 1974.

Nerup J, Anderson V, Bendixen G. Antiadrenal cellular hypersensitivity in Addison's disease. Clin Exp Immunol 4:355–358, 1969.

Nerup J, Platz P, Andersen OO. HL-A antigens and diabetes mellitus. Lancet 2:864–866, 1974.

Neufeld M, Maclaren N, Blizzard R. Two types of autoimmune Addison's disease associated with polyglandular syndromes. Medicine 60:355–362, 1981.

Neufeld MR, Maclaren NK, Riley WJ. HLA in American blacks with juvenile diabetes. N Engl J Med 303:111–112, 1980b.

Neufeld M, Maclaren NK, Riley WJ, Lezotte D, McLaughlin JV, Silverstein J, Rosenbloom AL. Islet cell and other organ-specific autoantibodies in U.S. Caucasians and Blacks with insulin-dependent diabetes mellitus. Diabetes 29:589–592, 1980a.

Niskanen L, Karjalaienen J, Sarlund H, Siitonen O, Uusitupa M. Five year follow-up of islet-cell antibodies in type 2 (non-insulin dependent) diabetes mellitus. Diabetologia 34:402–408, 1991.

Nossal GJV. Immunologic tolerance: collaboration between antigen and lymphokines. Science 245:147–153, 1989.

Novogroder M, Utiger R, Boyar R, Levine LS. Juvenile hyperthyroidism with elevated thyrotropin (TSH) and normal 24 hour FSH, LH, GH, and prolactin secretory patterns. J Clin Endocrinol Metab 45:1053–1059, 1977.

Obermayer-Straub P, Manns MP. Autoimmune polyglandular syndromes. Baillieres Clin Gastroenterol 12:293–315, 1998.

Ohgawara H, Hirata Y. Islet cell surface antibodies in diabetes and their possible influence on glucose tolerance. Tohoku J Exp Med 142:211–216, 1984.

Ohtaki S, Endo Y, Horinouchi K, Yoshitake S, Ishikawa E. Circulating thyroglobulin-antithyroglobulin immune complex in thyroid diseases using enzyme-linked immunoassays. J Clin Endocrinol Metab 52:239–246, 1981.

Okabe R, Inaba M, Hosoi M, Ishimura E, Kumeda Y, Nishizawa Y, Morii H. Remission of insulin autoimmune syndrome in a patient with Graves" disease by treatment with methimazole. Intern Med 38:482–485, 1999.

Okamura K, Sato K, Yoshinari M, Ikenoue H, Kuroda T, Nakagawa M, Tsuji H, Washio M, Fujishima M. Recovery of the thyroid function in patients with atrophic hypothyroidism and blocking type TSH binding inhibitor immunoglobulin. Acta Endocrinol Copenh 122:107–114, 1990.

Okita N, How J, Topliss D, Lewis M, Row VV, Volpe R. Suppressor T lymphocyte dysfunction in Graves' disease: role of the H-2 histamine receptor-bearing suppressor T lymphocytes. J Clin Endocrinol Metab 53:1002–1007, 1981a.

Okita N, Row VV, Volpe R. Suppressor T-lymphocyte deficiency in Graves' disease and Hashimoto's thyroiditis. J Clin Endocrinol Metab 52:528–533, 1981b.

Okita N, Topliss D, Lewis M, Row VV, Volpe R. T-lymphocyte sensitization in Graves' and Hashimoto's diseases confirmed by an indirect migration inhibition factor test. J Clin Endocrinol Metab 52:523–527, 1981c.

Orgiazzi J. Anti-TSH receptor antibodies in clinical practice. Endocrinol Metab Clin North Am 29:339–345, 2000.

Owerbach D, Gunn S, Ty G, Wible L, Gabby KH. Oligonucleotide probes for HLA-DQA and DQB genes define susceptibility to type 1 (insulin-dependent) diabetes mellitus. Diabetologia 31:751–757, 1988.

Paja M, Estrada J, Ojeda A, Ramon y Cajal S, Garcia-Uria J, Lucas T. Lymphocytic hypophysitis causing hypopituitarism and diabetes insipidus, and associated with autoimmune thyroiditis, in a non-pregnant woman. Postgrad Med J 70:220–224, 1994.

Pak CY, Cha CY, Rajotte RV, McArthur RG, Yoon JW. Human pancreatic islet cell specific 38 kilodalton autoantigen identified by cytomegalovirus-induced monoclonal islet cell autoantibody. Diabetologia 33:569–572, 1990.

Palmer JP, Asplin CM, Clemons P, Lyen K, Tatpati O, McKnight B, Paquette T. Insulin antibodies in insulin-dependent diabetics before insulin treatment. Science 222:1337–1339, 1983b.

Palmer JP, Asplin CM, Raghu PK, Clemons P, Lyen K, Tatpati O, McKnight B, Paquette T. Anti-insulin antibodies in insulin dependent diabetes before insulin treatment—a new marker for autoimmune B cell damage. Diabetes 32:76A, 1983a.

Paolieri F, Salmaso C, Battifora M, Montagna P, Pesce G, Bagnasco M, Richiusa P, Galluzzo A, Giordano C. Possible pathogenetic relevance of interleukin-1 beta in "destructive" organ-specific autoimmune disease (Hashimoto's thyroiditis). Ann NY Acad Sci 876:221–228, 1999.

Papadopoulos KI, Hallengren B. Polyglandular autoimmune syndrome type II in patients with idiopathic Addison's disease. Acta Endocrinol Copenh 122:472–478, 1990.

Paschke R, Bruckner N, Schmeidl R, Pfiester P, Usadel KH. Predominant intraepithelial localization of primed T cells and immunoglobulin-producing lymphocytes in Graves' disease. Acta Endocrinol Copenh 124:630–636, 1991.

Pearce SH, Vaidya B, Imrie H, Perros P, Kelly WF, Toft AD, McCarthy MI, Young ET, Kendall-Taylor P. Further evidence for a susceptibility locus on chromosome 20q13.11 in families with dominant transmission of Graves' disease. Am J Hum Genet 65:1462–1465, 1999.

Peterson P, Salmi H, Hyoty H, Miettinen A, Reijonen H, Knip M, Akerblom HK, Krohn K. Steroid 21-hydroxylase autoantibodies in insulin-dependent diabetes mellitus. Childhood Diabetes in Finland (DiMe) Study Group. Clin Immunol Immunopathol 82:37–42, 1997.

Petra W, Nerup J. Addison's adrenalitis. Acta Pathol Microbiol Scand 79:381–388, 1971.

Phillips D, McLachlan S, Stephenson A, Roberts D, Moffitt S, McDonald D, Ad'Hiah A, Stratton A, Young E, Clark F, Beever K, Bradbury J, Rees-Smith B. Autosomal dominant transmission of autoantibodies to thyroglobulin and thyroid peroxidase. J Clin Endocrinol Metab 70:742–746, 1990.

Pietropaolo M, Barinas-Mitchell E, Pietropaolo SL, Kuller LH, Trucco M. Evidence of islet cell autoimmunity in elderly patients with type 2 diabetes. Diabetes 49:32–38, 2000.

Pietropaolo M, Castano L, Babu S, Buelow R, Kuo YL, Martin S, Martin A, Powers AC, Prochazka M, Naggert J, Leiter EH, Eisenbath GS. Islet cell autoantigen 69 kD (ICA69). Molecular cloning and characterization of a novel diabetes-associated autoantigen. J Clin Invest 92:359–371, 1993.

Pinchera A, Mariotti S, Chiovato L, Vitti P, Lopez G, Lombardi A, Anelli S, Bechi R, Carayon P. Cellular localization of the microsomal antigen and the thyroid peroxidase antigen. Acta Endocrinol Suppl Copenh 281:57–62, 1987.

Pinhas-Hamiel O, Dolan LM, Daniels SR. Increased incidence of non-insulin dependent diabetes mellitus among adolescents. J Pediatr 128:608–615, 1996.

Pont A, Rubino JM, Bishop D, Peal R. Diabetes mellitus and neuropathy following Vacor ingestion in man. Arch Intern Med 139:185–187, 1979.

Pozzilli P. Prevention of insulin-dependent diabetes mellitus 1998. Diabetes Metab Rev 14:69–84, 1998.

Pozzilli P, Pitocco D, Visalli N, Cavallo MG, Buzzetti R, Crino A, Spera S, Suraci C, Multari G, Cervoni M, Manca Bitti ML, Matteoli MC, Marietti G, Ferrazzoli F, Cassone Faldetta MR, Giordano C, Sbriglia M, Sarugeri E, Ghirlanda G. No effect of oral insulin on residual beta-cell function in recent-onset type I diabetes (the IMDIAB VII). IMDIAB Group. Diabetologia 43:1000–4, 2000.

Pozzilli P, Sensi M, Gorsuch A, Bottazzo GF, Cudworth AG. Evidence of raised K-cell levels in type-1 diabetes. Lancet 2:173–175, 1979.

Pozzilli P, Zuccarini O, Iavicoli M, Andreani D, Sensi M, Spencer KM, Bottazzo GF, Beverly PCL, Kyner JL, Cudworth AG. Monoclonal antibodies defined abnormalities of T-lymphocytes in type 1 (insulin-dependent) diabetes. Diabetes 32:91–94, 1983.

Pujol-Borrell R, Hanafusa T, Chiovata L, Bottazzo GF. Lectin-induced expression of DR antigen on human cultured follicular thyroid cells. Nature 304:71–73, 1983.

Rabin DU, Pleasic SM, Shapiro JA, Yoo-Warren H, Oles J, Hicks JM, Goldstein DE, Rae PM. Islet cell antigen 512 is a diabetes-specific islet autoantigen related to protein tyrosine phosphatases. J Immunol 152:3183–3188, 1994.

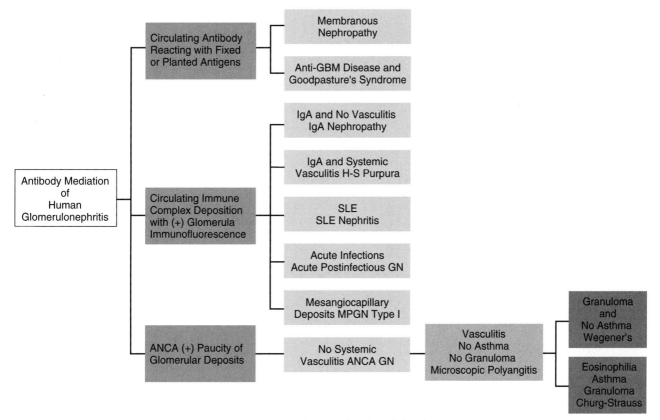

Figure 38-1 · Antibody-mediated renal disorders.

Activated leukocytes are attracted to sites of immune complex deposition and bind to C3 and C4 that are fixed to immune complexes. Also, the membrane attack complex (C5b-9) causes glomerular capillary damage and stimulates granulocytes to produce further inflammatory mediators such as oxidants, proteases, prostaglandins, and cytokines. In anti-GBM nephritis, subendothelial immune complex deposition causes neutrophil exudation. Inflammation can be inhibited by both neutrophil and complement depletion. In contrast, membranous nephritis with subepithelial immune complexes is unaffected by neutrophil depletion, but the inflammatory response is nearly absent in C5-deficient animals (Walport, 1993).

Experimental models of circulating immune complex disease include acute and chronic serum sickness in which rabbits are immunized with bovine serum albumin leading to immune complexes deposition in the subendothelium and mesangium. This mechanism is implicated in the pathogenesis of systemic lupus erythematosus (SLE) nephritis, poststreptococcal glomerulonephritis (PSGN), cryoglobulinemia, and tumor-associated membranous nephropathy (MN). As with deposited antigens, those associated with circulating immune complexes can be endogenous (DNA, immunoglobulins, thyroid antigens, red cell stroma, tumor neoantigens) or exogenous (microbes, soluble foreign serum proteins, chemicals). The antibody-mediated renal disorders are summarized in Figure 38-1.

Cellular Immunity

T-Cell Activation

Integral to activation of the immune system is the interaction of T cells with antigen-presenting cells (APCs), including monocytes, macrophages, dendritic cells, and B cells. T cells recognize, respond to, and remember antigenic challenges in the context of human leukocyte antigen (HLA)-DR (class II) or HLA-A, HLA-B, or HLA-C (class I) antigen presentation. CD4+ T cells interact with HLA-DR, whereas CD8+ T cells interact with HLA-A, HLA-B, and HLA-C. The classic concept of CD4+ T-cell activation involves antigen presentation via HLA-DR molecules on the APC (Fig. 38-2).

Signal 1 follows presentation of antigen through the MHC class II to CD4 cells or MHC class 1 to CD8 cells. Signal 2 is the costimulatory signal given through B7-1/B7-2 to CD28. Signal 3, delivered by cytokines such as interleukin (IL)-2, is given through the tripartite IL-2 receptor on T cells and drives the T cell to divide, resulting in a clonal expansion and differentiation of antigen-reactive cytotoxic lymphocytes.

If signal 1 is delivered alone, anergy (e.g., immune unresponsiveness) and apoptosis are seen. When signals 1 and 2 are given together, an immunizing signal is given to the T cell, resulting in T-cell activation and initiation of cytokine gene transcription and cytokine

T-CELL ACTIVATION BY ANTIGENS

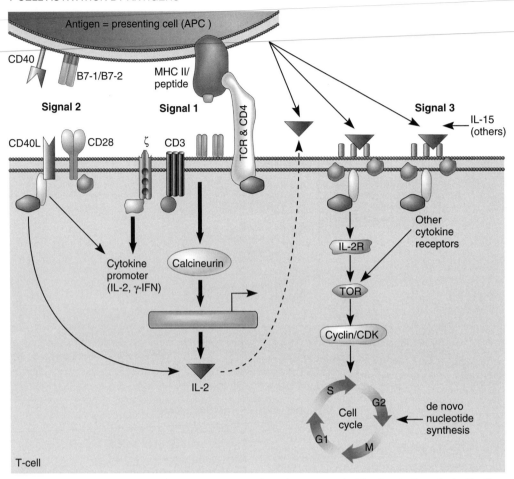

Figure 38-2 · T-cell activation by antigens requires three distinct signals. The first is through the T-cell receptor. Signal 2 provides co-stimulation for signal 1 and initiates IL-2 and other proinflammatory cytokine production. Signal 3 is signaling through the cytokine receptors (i.e., IL-2R), which drive cell proliferation and differentiation.

production. Signal 3 involves the engagement of cytokines with their specific receptors on the T-cell surface, leading to initiation of the cell cycle and cell division. Before division, the T cell must have de novo synthesis of purine and pyrimidine nucleotides. IL-2 is the major cytokine responsible for T-cell differentiation. These events are shown in Figure 38-2.

T-Cell–Mediated Renal Injury

Humoral antibody involvement in renal injury has been suggested both by immunopathologic evidence of antibody and complement deposition in glomeruli and experimental models demonstrating antibody and complement roles in glomerulopathy. Evidence for T-cell–mediated renal injury independent of antibody deposition is provided by nephrotoxic serum nephritis in rats; depletion of CD8+ T cells before administration of serum prevents proteinuria despite an equal amount of antibody in glomeruli of both CD8+ T-cell–depleted rats and controls (Penny et al., 1998). Chickens that undergo neonatal bursectomy that halts B-cell develop-

ment still develop severe proliferative GN following immunization with GBM; T cells accumulate in glomeruli, but anti-GBM antibodies are not present (Cibrik and Sedor, 1998).

The major orchestrator of all immune responses is the CD4+ T cell, and the most promising immunosuppressive strategies disrupt CD4 activation. CD8+ T cells function in a different fashion; they only interact with MHC class I cells presenting foreign antigen and are important in antigen-specific cytotoxic events. In Heymann's nephritis models, CD8+ T-cell–depleted rats did not develop proteinuria despite normal antibody development, nor did they develop T-cell or macrophage infiltrates. Thus CD8+ T cells may be essential to its pathogenesis and a potential target for treatment of idiopathic membranous nephritis.

Interference with T-Cell Activation

Interruption of signal 1 can be accomplished by the immunophilin drugs (cyclosporine A [CSA] and tacrolimus), which interfere with the Ca++/calcineurin pathway of IL-2 gene activation. In addition, monoclonal antibodies to CD3 or CD4 lymphocytes (e.g., OKT3, antithymocyte globulin) and intravenous immunoglobulin (IVIG) treatment can interrupt signal 1 by interfering with the T-cell receptor (TCR) and MHC class II interactions and subsequent signal transduction. Interruption of signal 2 (costimulation of CD28/B7-1, B7-2) without interruption of signal 1 is also an effective way to induce an anergizing signal to the T cell.

Another major costimulatory (signal 2) activity necessary for induction of IL-2 gene activation is the CD40/CD40L interaction; this enhances CD28/B7-1, B7-2 interaction between T cells and the APC. Induction of signal 1 through TCR engagement without signal 2 does not induce an immunizing signal to the T cell; instead it results in anergy and/or clonal deletion of alloreactive T cells. Costimulation (signal 2) is critical for T-cell survival because it induces the expression of anti-apoptotic Bcl-xL gene. CD28 is expressed on 95% of human CD4[+] T cells and 50% of resting CD8[+] T cells. Overexpression is seen with activation.

Another ligand for B7-1/B7-2 is cytotoxic T-cell lymphocyte antigen 4 (CTLA4). This molecule is restricted to activated T cells and serves to downregulate T-cell responses after activation responses have been triggered. CTLA4 knockout mice have a lymphoproliferative phenotype with high levels of autoantibody production and features of autoimmune disease. CD28 knockout mice are deficient in signal 2 and thus exhibit diminished T-cell responses. Experimental autoimmune glomerulonephritis (EAG) in Wister Kyoto rats can be attenuated by CD28/B7 blockade using soluble CTLA4-Ig; this results in decreased autoantibody production, less glomerular cell infiltration, and minimal kidney injury (Reynolds et al., 2000).

Rapamycin, a signal 3 inhibitor, interferes with the initiation of cyclin and cyclin-dependent kinase activation. Further downstream, purine synthesis inhibitors such as mycophenolate mofetil (MMF) act specifically on the lymphocyte-selective enzyme inosine monophosphate dehydrogenase (IMPDH) to inhibit purine synthesis after mitotic signals are sent. There are no data on use of rapamycin in human autoimmune kidney diseases. However, initial animal data have shown paradoxical worsening of experimental immune complex GN (Daniel et al., 2000).

T-helper 1(Th1)/T-helper 2 (Th2) Paradigm in T-Cell Activation

After antigen presentation to T cells, a number of cytokines that regulate subsequent T-cell activation and differentiation are produced. Mosmann and Coffman (1989) demonstrated that cloned CD4[+] T cells from mice and humans can be further divided into two functional subpopulations based on patterns of cytokine secretion.

Th1 cells are defined as those that produce the proinflammatory cytokines IL-2, interferon-γ (IFN-γ), tumor necrosis factor-α (TNF-α), and tumor necrosis factor-β (TNF-β) in response to an antigenic challenge. Th1 cells promote the differentiation of cytotoxic T-cell precursors into fully functional cytotoxic effectors and enhance the production of phlogistic, complement-fixing IgG antibodies (DeKruyff et al., 1989). Th1 cells are important mediators of delayed type hypersensitivity (Cher and Mosmann, 1987). Th1 cells are mediators of effector functions that initiate inflammation and cytodestruction. Th1 cells are important in immune destructive events such as allograft rejection and autoimmune diseases.

In contrast, Th2 cells selectively secrete a distinct pattern of cytokines (IL-4, IL-5, IL-6, and IL-10) in response to antigenic confrontation that direct the synthesis of non-complement-fixing IgG antibodies, IgE, and IgA (Mosmann and Moore, 1991; Mosmann et al., 1990). Th2 cell activation results in little immunogenic inflammation or cytodestructive events.

Both Th1 and Th2 CD4[+] cells are derived from a common precursor, the Th0 cell, and the unique circumstances of the antigenic challenge dictate deviation of the immune response toward a Th1 or Th2 pattern. This deviation is aided by specific cytokines. For example, antigenic encounters that stimulate IL-12 in the APCs (particularly macrophages) result in IFN-γ production by T cells and deviation of the immune response to a Th1 profile, whereas antigenic encounters that induce IL-4/IL-13 deviate the Th0 cells to a Th2 profile. The reciprocal effects that Th1 and Th2 cells can have on each other have also become apparent. In this regard, IFN-γ produced by Th1 cells can inhibit the proliferation of Th2 clones in vitro. Conversely, IL-10 produced by Th2 clones can inhibit the proliferation and secretion of IFN-γ by Th1 clones (Mosmann and Moore, 1991; Scott, 1993).

Holdsworth and co-workers (1999) looked at the Th1-type nephritogenic immune responses as characterized by antigen presentation in the setting of IL-12 expression with IFN-γ and IL-2 production by Th1 cells. The effector responses include T-cell and macrophage accumulation and deposition of Th1 type IgG subclass (IgG1 and IgG3) in glomeruli. Th2 responses include IL-4 and IL-10 production with no T-cell and macrophage responses. Th2-type IgG subclass (IgG4) is deposited in glomeruli.

From these patterns, crescentic and membranoproliferative glomerulonephritis (MPGN) appear to be Th1 directed, with glomerular T cells acting as the predominant initiator of injury. Experimental models of these glomerulonephritides show that administration of Th1 cytokines exacerbates injury, whereas Th2 cytokines attenuate the severity of GN. In contrast, human membranous GN is associated with IgG4 subclass (Th2) deposits with an absence of T cells and macrophages. Administration of Th1 cytokines and inhibition of Th2 cytokines attenuates both immune response and severity of GN. IgA nephropathy and SLE nephritis appear to have both Th1 and Th2 involvement.

The cytokine transforming growth factor-β (TGF-β) may be implicated in the induction of IgA nephropathy. Recent data show that murine B cells deficient in the TGF-β receptor II develop severe IgA deficiency (Cazac and Roes, 2000). Thus overexpression of TGF-β (promoter gene polymorphism), or TGF-β receptor expression on B cells may result in dysregulated IgA production and IgA nephropathy. Crescentic subgroups show evidence of Th1 predominance, whereas membranous lupus nephritis, like idiopathic membranous GN, shows evidence of Th2 predominance. Yap and associates (1999) have shown that IL-13 (Th2) is overexpressed in relapse of minimal change nephropathy of children. IL-13 may increase vascular permeability factor release. Remissions were associated with disappearance of detectable IL-13 levels. In SLE animal models, Th1 immune response appears to induce greater glomerular injury (Holdsworth et al., 1999).

Cytokine-Lymphocyte Interactions in the Treatment of Human Diseases

Robust immune responses are necessary for the maintenance of good health. Undesirable or dysfunctional immune responses can result in diseases such as systemic autoimmunity, allergy, allograft rejection, and nephritogenic immune responses (Strom and Kelley, 1989).

An ideal immunosuppressive agent would selectively block phlogistic cytokine production and deviate T cells to a tolerant or anergic state. T-cell activation involves antigen recognition through the TCR/CD3 complex, and co-stimulatory signals delivered through other receptor and ligand pathways (Harding et al., 1992). This recognition results in the release of proinflammatory cytokines such as IL-2 and IFN-γ. However, TCR recognition of alloantigen alone is not sufficient for robust T-cell activation; T cells must receive one or more costimulatory signals from the APCs to initiate the high level IL-2 production and cell proliferation necessary for T-cell effector functions. Antigen recognition in the absence of costimulation can lead to T-cell anergy or apoptosis (Harding et al., 1992; Tan et al., 1994). A central costimulatory pathway is activated by stimulation of the T cell CD28 receptor by binding to ligands on APCs, notably B7-1/B7-2 and possibly others, resulting in a full immunizing signal to T cells. This leads to increased production and stability of IL-2 transcription and secretion, and cell proliferation.

This pathway, which is CSA resistant, can be specifically and effectively blocked by CTLA4Ig (a soluble recombinant fusion molecule consisting of the extracellular domain of the human T-cell surface receptor CTLA-4 fused to a human IgG chain). CTLA4Ig binds to B7 and other ligands on APCs with high affinity and blocks their interaction with CD28. CTLA4Ig has a 20-fold higher affinity for B7 than does CD28, which allows it to act as a competitive inhibitor of CD28 binding to B7-1/B7-2 with subsequent inhibition of co-activation signals and Th1 cytokine production. Engagement of CTLA4Ig with B7-1 and B7-2 also results in the expression of IL-4 with depressed IL-2 (Th2 >> Th1) (Tan, 1994). This is shown in Figure 38-3.

Although designed for human T cells, CTLA4Ig also binds to murine and rat B7. Thus mixed lymphocyte cultures treated with CTLA4Ig generate reduced levels of IL-2 and decreased proliferation. In vivo, CTLA4Ig blocks T-cell dependent B-cell antibody synthesis and autoimmune GN; it also prevents cardiac allograft rejection in rats and mice (Nishikawa et al., 1994).

Matsumura and co-workers (1995) studied the acute effect of CTLA4Ig on the rejection of rat lung allografts. CTLA4Ig inhibited inflammatory aspects of rat lung acute rejection but did not inhibit cytokine gene activation. Lin and colleagues (1993) showed that a combination of donor spleen cell transfusions and CTLA4Ig resulted in long-term acceptance of cardiac allografts in a mouse model. These animals developed allograft tolerance but retained the ability to reject third-party allografts. Tan (1994) suggested that CTLA4Ig not only results in blocking of the Th1 cytokine profile but deviates the immune response to a Th2 profile. Despite these experimental results, CTLA4Ig has not proved of benefit in human autoimmune disease.

THERAPEUTIC APPLICATION OF CTL4Ig TO AUTOIMMUNITY

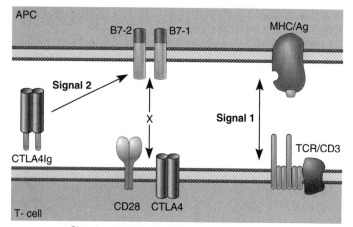

Signal 1 without signal 2 results in:
T-cell anergy Th2 > Th1 apoptosis

Figure 38-3 · CTLA4Ig blocks the co-stimulatory signal provided by CD28-B7-1/B7-2 interactions. This results in incomplete T-cell activation, anergy, and apoptosis.

More promising is the use of anti-CD154 monoclonal antibody, which interferes with the interaction of the co-stimulatory molecules CD40 and CD154. CD154, also known as CD40L or gp39, is found on activated T cells and platelets and is the abnormal molecule in X-linked hyper-IgM syndrome. CD154 binds to CD40 on professional APCs including dendritic cells, B cells, macrophages, and endothelial cells (Bennett et al., 1998; Kirk et al., 1999; Laman et al., 1996; Larsen et al., 1997; Schoenberger et al., 1998). Ligation of CD40 by CD154 (or by anti-CD40 antibodies) results in APC stimulation and secretion of IL-10, TNF-α, and IL-12. Activated endothelial cells are stimulated to secrete chemotactic factors and show increased expression of MHC class II, adhesion molecules, and the costimulatory ligand B7-1 (CD80) and B7-2 (CD86). Thus the CD40–CD154 interaction plays a critical role in T-cell activation.

With bidirectional signaling, APCs are stimulated to become super APCs that stimulate antibody production and enhance cytotoxic CD8+ T-cell development. CD8+ T cells are chemotactically attracted to the sites of immune activation and initiate cytotoxic events that ultimately result in cell death (Fig. 38-4). CD40–CD154 interactions also play a critical role in B cells, activating their class switching from IgM to more phlogistic IgG antibodies. These events are critical for the Th1-directed event of allograft rejection but are also critical for development of T-cell– and B-cell–mediated immune responses of autoimmune diseases.

Blockade of the CD40–CD154 interaction does not substantially interfere with CD4+ T-cell activation but does reduce the number of activated CD8+ cytotoxic T cells and B-cell activation with production of phlogistic antibodies. This may block inflammatory events such as allograft rejection and autoimmune disease (Fig. 38-5).

Kirk and associates (1999) have shown that anti-CD154 monoclonal antibodies prevent acute rejection and result in long-term, rejection-free allograft survival in nonhuman primates. This suggests that costimulatory blockade will result in long-term graft survival in higher animals. Combination therapy with tacrolimus or MMF and steroids actually reduced long-term graft survival. Drugs such as CSA and tacrolimus work by blocking signal 1. Agents that block signal 2 (co-stimulatory blockade) depend on signal 1 without signal 2 to deliver a "death signal" to the T cell, leading to T-cell deletion and a functionally tolerant state. When signal 1 blockers such as tacrolimus are used in combination with anti-CD154, poorer outcomes result because the T-cell death signal is impaired. Thus many current immunosuppressive agents interfere with T-cell activation but do not lead to tolerance. Anti-CD154 is in clinical trials in the United States.

Cytokine/Receptor Gene Polymorphism

Gene Polymorphism

In some genes, nucleic acid sequences are relatively stable, and mutations are uncommon and when they occur, may result in disease. These nonpolymorphic genes are usually present on both somatic chromosomes. By contrast, the sequences of other genes vary considerably among normal individuals. Such genes are polymorphic and each variant is called an *allele*. An individual can have the same allele on both chromosomes of the pair (homozygosity) or two different alleles (heterozygosity). Polymorphism results in structural protein differences, such as variation in eye color (phenotypes).

Polymorphism of the blood group and HLA genes results in multiple allotypes and immune responses after allotransplantation. Variability in promoter and regulatory genes may result in different rates of RNA transcription and protein synthesis, with marked individual variation in protein production. Polymerase chain reaction (PCR) technology has facilitated delineation of

CD40–CD40L: A CRITICAL ROLE FOR STIMULATION OF CD8+ CYTOTOXIC T CELLS AND INDUCTION OF RENAL INJURY

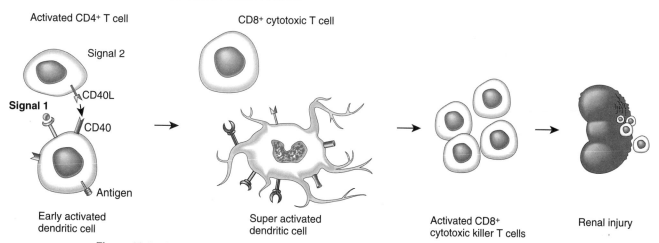

Figure 38-4 · CD154 (CD40L)–CD40 interactions are critical for initiation of allograft rejection and autoimmune disorders.

CD40–CD40L: ANTI-CD40L ANTIBODIES INHIBIT CD8+ T-CELL ACTIVATION AND RENAL INJURY

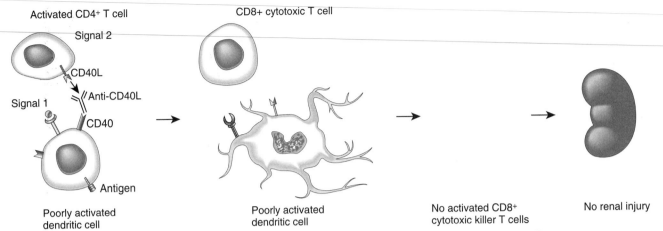

Figure 38-5 · Co-stimulatory blockade with anti-CD154 monoclonal antibody inhibits CD8+ T-cell activation by poorly activating the APCs. This results in poor CD8+ T-cell activation and decreased antibody response. This strategy could offer a focused and less toxic intervention into autoimmune renal diseases.

gene polymorphism phenotypic diversity, for example, the identification of the multiple HLA genotypes and phenotypes now recognized (Grant et al., 1996; Hutchinson, 1999; Jackson et al., 2001; Sankaran et al., 1999; Turner et al., 1997).

Cytokine Gene Polymorphism

Polymorphism in the regulatory regions of specific cytokine genes is associated with decreased or excessive secretion of specific cytokines in response to a particular stimulus (Grant et al., 1996, 1997; Hutchinson, 1999; Reinsomoen, 1999; Sankaran et al., 1999). Cytokine allotypes of TNF-α, IL-10, and TGF-β are associated with acute and chronic graft rejection and autoimmunity.

Tumor Necrosis Factor-α Polymorphisms

TNF-α is a cytokine produced primarily by lipopolysaccharide (LPS)-stimulated macrophages that mediates necrosis of tumors and also has immunoregulatory functions. Bonavida and associates showed that the addition of TNF-α (1 to 10 μg/ml) resulted in a dose-dependent inhibition of pokeweed mitogen (PWM)-induced antibody production by peripheral blood mononuclear cells (PBMCs) (Bonavida, 1991).

Satoh and associates (1989) showed that recombinant TNF-α inhibits the development of autoimmune diabetes mellitus in nonobese diabetic mice (NOD strain) and postulated that their ability to produce TNF-α was correlated with susceptibility to autoimmunity. NOD mice are poor in vitro producers of TNF-α; administration of TNF-α inhibited dysfunctional T-cell activation and prevented development of autoimmunity, possibly by induction of suppressor T cells (Serreze and Leiter, 1988). Others have shown that administration of

TNF-α to NZB × NZW F1 hybrid mice suppressed the progression of murine SLE, again by induction of suppressor cells (Jacob and McDevitt, 1988).

Gross and colleagues (2000) implicated a TNF homolog, zTNF4, in the cause of SLE. This TNF homolog can stimulate human B-cell proliferation, augment IgG production, and enhance B-cell effector functions. They showed that mice transgenic for zTNF4 demonstrate an expansion of splenic B-1a lymphocytes that produce self-reactive IgM antibodies. Glomerular changes that are similar to human SLE develop. Dorner and Putterman (2001) showed that serum zTNF4 levels are elevated in two mouse strains that develop SLE and that the fusion protein TACI-Ig, which binds zTNF4 and inhibits its effects on B cells, suppresses SLE development. Thus interaction of zTNF4 with its receptor TACI on B cells may induce and perpetuate SLE in humans.

TNF-α released at the site of inflammation by macrophages results in endothelial cell activation, upregulation of MHC antigens, increased adhesion molecule expression, vasodilation, and increased vascular permeability, all of which increase the inflammatory response to an allograft by recruiting and activating leukocytes. Plasma levels of TNF-α increase in allograft rejection. Because transcription of TNF-α is also under control of calcineurin and nuclear factor of activated T cells (NF-AT), CSA and tacrolimus can inhibit TNF-α, enhancing their immunosuppressive effects (Reinsomoen, 1999; Sankaran et al., 1999; Turner et al., 1997).

Guanine (G) to adenosine (A) substitution at position 3308 on the TNF-α gene promoter results in alleles TNF1 and TNF2. Expression of the TNF2 allele is associated with a sixfold to sevenfold increase in transcription of TNF-α gene in vitro. Studies in heart, kidney, and lung transplants revealed correlation between high serum TNF-α levels and transplant rejection. One study did not show a direct effect between TNF-α production and rejection episodes; excessive TNF-α production was associated with a higher incidence of steroid-resistant rejection in kidney transplant recipients (Reinsomoen, 1999; Sankaran et al., 1999; Turner et al., 1997). Saito and colleagues (1993) showed that anti–TNF-α antibodies diminish graft rejection in an experimental model of lung transplantation.

Transforming Growth Factor-β Polymorphisms

TGF-β is a cytokine with pleiotropic effects. Receptors for TGF-β are present on most cell types. TGF-β modulates the growth and differentiation of T cells, B cells, natural killer (NK) cells, lymphokine-activated killer (LAK) cells, and monocytes/macrophages (Hooper, 1991; Roberts and Sporn, 1993). TGF-β inhibits T-cell and B-cell activation, and, when antigen is presented in the presence of TGF-β, a Th2 type (tolerogenic) immune response occurs (Matriano et al., 1994). In conjunction with IL-2 and IL-5, TGF-β stimulates IgA production (Lebman et al., 1990). TGF-β1 knockout mice are born without obvious deformities but die at 3 to 4 weeks of age with massive mononuclear infiltration of all organs (Kulkarni and Karlsson, 1993).

The potent immunoregulatory capabilities of TGF-β suggest that it may be useful in regulating dysfunctional immune responses of autoimmune disease. TGF-β may also be of value in the prevention and treatment of acute allograft rejection; rat heart allografts transfected with the human TGF-β gene are not acutely rejected (Qin et al., 1995). These allografts do develop scarring and atypical accelerated chronic rejection. CSA induces TGF-β gene expression while suppressing IL-2 gene expression (Wolf et al., 1995). Tacrolimus (FK-506) is a less potent inducer of TGF-β. TGF-β promotes fibrosis of the kidney and lung in chronic rejection and autoimmune diseases, thus limiting its use in human autoimmunity (Border and Noble, 1995).

The gene encoding TGF-β production is markedly polymorphic, resulting in high and low producer phenotypes (Hutchinson, 1999). In kidney transplant recipients, there was a strong association between high TGF-β production and acute rejection. Many of these individuals also produce high levels of TNF-α. In patients with genotypes associated with increases of both cytokines, the risk of developing two or more acute rejection episodes is increased fourfold ($P < 0.007$) along with resistance to corticosteroids ($P < 0.002$). If the donor is a high TGF-β producer, the steroid-resistant rejection risk was increased even further (Hutchinson, 1999). This may be due to TGF-β–directed induction of CD103 and E-cadherin on cytotoxic T cells and upregulated epithelial cell adhesion molecules, resulting in renal tubular epithelial cell damage and tubulocytolysis (Hadley et al., 1997; Hutchinson, 1999).

Because TGF-β promotes two cardinal features of chronic allograft dysfunction, fibrosis and arteriosclerosis, studies have been done to link the polymorphisms and rate of chronic allograft loss, particularly in lung transplant recipients. Higher levels of TGF-β were associated with lung fibrosis by 6 to 18 months and the high

producer genotype. Patients' deaths were also associated with TGF-β genotypes. The highest TGF-β producers all died within 7 years, whereas 65% of the low producer genotypes still survived at 7 years.

In heart transplant recipients, the presence of a high producer genotype, whether derived from donor or recipient tissues, correlated with the development of transplant coronary artery disease (TCAD). Hutchinson (1999) demonstrated that 90% of patients with the low TGF-β producer genotype were free of TCAD at 7 years, compared with only 39% of the high TGF-β groups. Transplantation from donors that were high TGF-β producers resulted in 40% graft survival at 7 years compared with 75% survival for grafts from donors that were low TGF-β producers.

Interleukin-10 Polymorphisms

IL-10 was originally described as "cytokine synthesis inhibitory factor" because it inhibits the production of Th1 cytokines (Powrie et al., 1993). Human and mouse IL-10 are highly homologous to the Epstein-Barr virus (EBV) gene B-cell replacement factor-1 *(BCRF-1)*, now designated viral-IL-10, or vIL-10 (Hsu et al., 1990). In humans, IL-10 is produced by Th0, Th1, and Th2 CD4+ T cells. IL-10 is also produced by B cells and other cell types.

IL-10 is a pleiotropic cytokine that exerts both immunosuppressive and immunostimulatory effects; its predominant suppressive effect is to inhibit Th1 (IFN-γ and IL-2) cytokine production. In experimental lung transplantation, overexpression of IL-10 occurs in rat strains that develop spontaneous allograft tolerance with suppression of Th1 cytokines. Conversely, in rats that reject allografts, IL-10 expression is reduced (Zuo et al., 1995).

IL-10 downregulates macrophage MHC class II expression, thus limiting their interaction with T cells and NK cells (de Waal Malefyt et al., 1991). IL-10 also inhibits cytokines involved in inflammatory responses including prostaglandin E_2, TNF-α, IL-1, IL-6, and IL-8 (Leeuwenberg et al., 1994; Willems et al., 1994). IL-10 also induces the release of soluble TNF receptors and inhibits the induction of intercellular adhesion molecule (ICAM) and B7 gene expression (Leeuwenberg et al., 1994; Willems et al., 1994). IL-10 induces the expression of IL-1 receptor antagonist (IL-1RA), a potent anti-inflammatory factor. IL-10 also induces the FcRγ I, which enhances antibody-mediated cellular cytotoxicity (ADCC) (de Waal Malefyt et al., 1992).

The potent anti-inflammatory actions of IL-10 may have caused its capture by the EBV to suppress a Th1-mediated inflammation that would jeopardize its survival (Zuo et al., 1995). We have identified vIL-10 expression in fine needle aspiration biopsies (FNAB) of renal allografts from patients with post-transplant EBV-mediated lymphoproliferative disorder (PTLD). After stopping immunosuppressives, vIL-10 expression persists and graft survival is maintained. This overexpression of vIL-10 may suppress Th1 responses to an allograft and to the virus (Nast et al., 1997).

IL-10 induces IgA synthesis in CD40/CD40L-activated B cells (Briere et al., 1994). IL-10 also activates tonsillar and splenic B cells (de Waal Malefyt et al., 1992; Willems et al., 1994). IL-10 knockout mice have normal B-cell and T-cell development and function but develop chronic bowel inflammation resulting from uncontrolled immune reactivity to bowel antigens (Kuhn et al., 1993).

An increased intragraft IL-10 expression is associated with long-term renal graft survival in rodent models. However, high numbers of intragraft IL-10 secreting T cells are present in patients with accelerated vascular rejection resulting from high levels of HLA class II antibodies (Grant et al., 1996; Reinsomoen et al., 1999, Sankaran et al., 1999; Turner et al., 1997).

Three single base substitutions have been described in the IL-10 promoter at positions 1082, 819, and 592. The presence of arginine at position 1082 (IL-10 1*A) is associated with low IL-10 production.

If IL-10 has only inhibitory effects on immune processes involved in rejection, patients with high IL-10 and low TNF-α should have better graft survival. However, Turner and co-workers (1997) found that the IL-10 genotype did not correlate with rejection outcomes, reflecting the diverse roles of IL-10.

Fc Gamma Receptor IIb (FcγRIIb) Polymorphisms

Ravetch and Lanier (2000) found that mice deficient in FcRγIIb (FcγIIb [–/–]) developed a spontaneous autoimmune disease similar to that seen in animals with SLE. They suggest that activation of FcRγIIb (an immunoreceptor tyrosine-based inhibitory motif [ITIM] or inhibitory cell receptor) is responsible for downregulation of undesirable autoimmune responses and that polymorphisms at this locus result in defective FcRγIIB expression.

Nakamura and colleagues (2000) showed that FcRγIIb (–/–) mice developed fulminant anti-GBM disease when immunized with type IV collagen. By contrast, FcRγIIb (+/+) mice develop no immune response to this autoantigen. Pearse and associates (1999) showed that FcRγIIb signaling with co-ligation of the antigen receptor results in B-cell apoptosis. Finally, Samuelsson and co-workers (2001) showed that the immunomodulatory actions of IVIG in a mouse model of autoimmune thrombocytopenia were mediated through activation of FcRγIIb on monocytes and macrophages, suggesting a possible mechanism for the beneficial effects of IVIG in autoimmunity.

NEPHRITIS OF SYSTEMIC LUPUS ERYTHEMATOSUS

SLE is a systemic autoimmune disease with deposition of immune complexes in diverse tissues, including joints, skin, blood vessels, and kidneys (see Chapter 35). In 1902, Sequeira and Balean first described renal involvement in childhood SLE. Currently, one fourth of patients with SLE are children or adolescents and 40% to 80% of them have renal involvement. In lupus nephritis, immune complexes primarily affect glomeruli, but in some patients there is involvement of the interstitium and the vasculature.

The World Health Organization (WHO) classifies renal involvement in SLE into five main morphologic types described on renal biopsy specimens. These include (1) normal glomeruli, (2) mesangial nephropathy, (3) focal proliferative GN, (4) diffuse proliferative glomerulonephritis (DPGN), and (5) membranous nephropathy (MN). Other classifications are the International Study of Kidney Disease in Children (ISKDC) and the Activity/Chronicity Indices. The ISKDC schema includes sclerosing GN and mixed type designations. These newer schemes are useful in choosing optimal treatment.

Clinical Features

Mesangial lupus nephritis, the mildest and perhaps initial form of glomerular injury, may be clinically silent or present with mild hematuria and/or proteinuria. Renal function is usually normal. Focal proliferative nephritis may show nephritic urinary sediment and usually nonnephrotic range proteinuria. Diffuse proliferative nephritis is associated with nephritic and nephrotic syndromes, hypertension, and renal insufficiency, often severe and progressive. MN presents with proteinuria and the overt nephrotic syndrome.

Immunohistology

Immune complexes are deposited in the renal mesangium in all patients with lupus nephritis. The classification of lupus nephritis is based on the degree of immune complex deposition and the cellular infiltrates within the glomerular locations. In mesangial nephritis, IgG, C3, and sometimes C1q are deposited in the mesangium. In other forms of lupus nephritis, IgA, IgG, IgM, and complement components C3 and C1q are deposited. Focal proliferative GN is associated with segmental mesangial proliferation with mesangial deposits, hypercellularity, and segmental capillary necrosis. By definition, less than 50% of glomeruli are involved.

DPGN is characterized by global proliferation and mesangial hypercellularity of greater than 50% of the glomeruli. There is often a monocyte and neutrophil infiltrate. Capillary walls are thickened secondary to large subendothelial deposits termed *wire loop* lesions. Crescent formation is common.

Membranous glomerular nephritis is characterized by uniformly thickened capillary walls with subepithelial and mesangial deposits (Cohen and Nast, 1996).

Pathogenesis

Studies of the pathogenesis of SLE nephritis have used animal models (MRL/1PR mice, NZB × NZW F1 mice) and clinical studies of autoantibodies, cytokines, and HLA types. Some of the autoantibodies of SLE are directed against nucleic acids and proteins of the intracellular transcriptional and translational machinery, but their pathogenic role is unclear. Tsao and co-workers (1990) used the murine lupus model of SLE to examine variable regions of immunoglobulin genes and reported that they are not likely to be responsible for generating pathogenic autoantibodies. It appears that autoantibody production is a regulatory problem.

Suzuki and associates (1990) showed that CD5+ B cells produce anti-DNA antibodies independent of polyclonal activation. Shivakumar and colleagues (1989) identified an unusual population of T cells (TCR α/β cells that are CD4−, CD8−). In patients with SLE, these cells in conjunction with CD4+ T cells induce production of cationic IgG anti-DNA antibodies.

Immune dysregulation in SLE nephritis has been studied by assessing lymphocyte cell surface molecules including the Fas–Fas ligand (FasL) system, which has been implicated in the maintenance of tolerance. Mice with defects in this system develop a lupus-like syndrome. Suzuki and colleagues (1998a) found that 7 of 21 SLE patients had IgG autoantibodies to FasL, suggesting that these autoantibodies interfere with peripheral tolerance by inhibiting FasL-mediated elimination of autoreactive lymphocytes. Nakajima and associates (2000) studied the effect of anti-FasL monoclonal antibody on the development of lupus in NZB/W F1 mice; they found increased IgG1 and IgG2a anti-dsDNA antibody production, but lupus nephritis did not develop.

Other lymphocyte cell surface molecules may be important in the pathogenesis of lupus nephritis, including the CD28 costimulatory molecule and CD40 ligand. Tada and associates (1999) found decreased anti-DNA IgG antibody and IgG rheumatoid factor production in CD28−/− MRL/lymphoproliferative (lpr) mice. Also, there was decreased glomerular deposition of IgG, and GN was significantly retarded. Ma and co-workers (1996) found that CD40L-deficient mice did not develop IgG rheumatoid factor or anti-ds DNA but did have preservation of autoantibody production to ribonucleoproteins, suggesting that different mechanisms may be responsible for the autoantibody production in lpr/lpr mice.

Circulating DNA–anti-DNA complexes and their deposition may play a crucial role in the glomerular injury of SLE nephritis (Fournie, 1998). This is also supported in the MRL mice model of lupus nephritis in which Lake and associates (1988) showed that a monoclonal antibody reactive with single-stranded DNA caused a deterioration in renal function. Fournie and co-workers (1988) also proposed that circulating DNA, possibly in the form of chromatin, is released as a consequence of cytolysis in patients with SLE and that it is immunogenic.

Boes and colleagues (2000) noted that lupus-prone lymphoproliferative (lpr) mice unable to secrete IgM had elevated IgG autoantibodies to dsDNA and histones with increased glomerular immune complex deposition, followed by severe GN and early mortality.

In studying the role of cytokines in SLE, Jacob and McDevitt (1988) found that heritable decrease in the levels of TNF may predispose NZB/NZW F1 mice to develop lupus-like nephritis; replacement with recombinant TNF delayed its development. Similarly, Kontoyiannis and Kollias (2000) noted an emergence of autoreactive lymphocytes in NZB mice who have an engineered heterozygous deficiency of TNF.

Nonimmunologic factors may play a role in SLE pathogenesis. Sex hormones have been implicated in the pathogenesis of murine lupus, and treatment with tamoxifen, an estrogen receptor blocker, resulted in decreased proteinuria and increased survival rate (Wu et al., 2000). Cinotti and Pierucci (1989) suggested that renal impairment in SLE may be mediated by thromboxane A_2 synthesis within the kidney.

Treatment

Most children with nondiffuse proliferative glomerulonephritis (non-DPGN) SLE nephritis respond well to corticosteroid therapy. IV pulse methylprednisolone is used for initial therapy of severe lupus nephritis but is not satisfactory for long-term treatment (Barron et al., 1982). For long-term steroid therapy, alternate-day use is preferable to reduce side effects such as osteoporosis, avascular necrosis of bone, atherosclerosis, and cataracts.

For children with DPGN, IV cyclophosphamide has proved to be effective. Monthly doses of 500 to 1000 mg/m² are recommended. This treatment produces better immunosuppression and less toxicity than does daily oral cyclophosphamide (Austin et al., 1986; McCune et al., 1988). The leukocyte count fall that occurs 10 to 14 days post-treatment should be monitored, and the dose decreased if the white blood cell (WBC) count is less than 2000 cells/mm³ or if the granulocyte count is less than 1000 cells/mm³. Tanganaratchakit and co-workers (1999) gave 31 children with severe proliferative lupus nephritis monthly IV cyclophosphamide for 6 months, followed by repeat infusions every 2 to 3 months for 3 years; they found decreased proteinuria, increased serum albumin, increased creatinine clearance, and increased C3 levels. Cyclophosphamide was given in combination with low-dose oral corticosteroids.

Chan and associates (2000) compared a 12-month course of MMF and steroids with a 6-month course of oral cyclophosphamide and steroids followed by azathioprine (Imuran) and steroids for another 6 months. They found comparable numbers of complete and partial remissions in both groups and less toxicity in the MMF group; however, the relapse rate was slightly higher in the MMF-treated group. Because IV cyclophosphamide (Cytoxan) is superior to oral cyclophosphamide in the treatment of active SLE nephritis, further studies must compare MMF with IV cyclophosphamide.

Others use CSA in SLE nephritis, especially membranous SLE. Favre and colleagues (1989) gave CSA (average of 5 mg/kg/day) in combination with oral steroids to patients with SLE nephritis and found a 90% overall positive response to this regimen, including cessation of proteinuria in those with SLE MN. Tam and associates (2001) also found benefit of CSA in lupus nephritis when used in combination with prednisone and azathioprine. Tacrolimus also has been used in lupus nephritis in NZB × NZWF1 mice, with decreased proteinuria, delayed progression of nephropathy, and prolonged survival (Takabayashi et al., 1989).

IVIG was of benefit in seven patients with membranous and proliferative nephritis (Levy et al., 2000).

Another study showed no significant difference in patients treated with plasmapheresis versus cytotoxic drugs (Derksen et al., 1988), but plasmapheresis was of benefit in a patient with SLE nephritis who developed leukopenia on prednisone and cyclophosphamide (Amato and Salvadori, 1988). Plasmapheresis may be of particular use in patients unable to tolerate cytotoxic drugs and in those who have high circulating immune complex levels or extensive glomerular and interstitial immune complex deposition.

Prognosis

Prognosis in SLE nephritis is dependent on clinical, laboratory, and pathologic features. Persistent proteinuria, hematuria, and decreased renal function suggest a poor prognosis and an indication for further therapy. The renal biopsy classifications of activity and chronicity can also be used to determine prognosis and need for treatment. High-grade proliferation, necrosis, cellular crescents, and extensive immune complex deposition are poor prognostic factors. Low complement and elevated anti-DNA levels are associated with disease flares; persistently abnormal laboratory values are associated with a poor prognosis (Laitman et al., 1989). ESRD occurs in less than 20% of patients. The prognosis is worse in African Americans (Tassiulas et al., 1998).

HENOCH-SCHÖNLEIN PURPURA

Henoch-Schönlein purpura (HSP or anaphylactoid purpura) is a systemic vasculitis of children, characterized by purpuric rash, arthritis, gastrointestinal (GI) hemorrhage, and GN (see Chapters 32, 34, and 35). The peak age is 4 to 5 years, and there is a 2:1 male predominance.

The association of purpura and joint pain was first described by Schönlein in 1837. Henoch in 1899 described skin lesions associated with colicky abdominal pain and GI hemorrhage (Rai et al., 1999). HSP patients have no identifiable autoantibodies but have IgA deposition in the skin and kidneys (Balow, 1998). On renal biopsy, HSP nephritis is indistinguishable from IgA nephropathy, suggesting that the two disorders may be part of a clinicopathologic spectrum, with HSP having extrarenal manifestations not found in IgA nephropathy (see next section).

Clinical Features

The frequency of renal involvement varies depending on the criteria used. Rieu and Noel (1999) reported renal involvement in 33% of HSP children and 63% of HSP adults. Most patients have either no renal involvement or microhematuria and mild proteinuria with normal renal function. The illness may present with macroscopic hematuria followed by microscopic hematuria. Macroscopic hematuria may recur with recurrent purpura or following a URI as in IgA nephropathy patients. Often there is associated proteinuria and sometimes overt nephrotic syndrome. The most severe clinical presentation is a mixed nephritic-nephrotic syndrome with hematuria, renal insufficiency, hypertension, marked proteinuria, and hypoalbuminemia.

Immunohistology

There are two main histologic classifications. The first is based on the degree of mesangial hypercellularity. The second, developed by the ISKDC, relies on the presence of crescents for designating grades of severity (Heaton et al., 1977). Crescents are important prognostic indicators; patients with focal and diffuse proliferation who have greater than 50% crescents on biopsy have worse outcomes (Rai et al., 1999). The diagnostic immunofluorescence (IF) finding is granular mesangial IgA, often accompanied by C3, fibrinogen, light chains, and less frequently IgG and/or IgM (Rieu and Noel, 1999).

Pathogenesis

As with IgA nephropathy, HSP nephritis is characterized by mesangial proliferation and IgA deposition. Miyagawa and co-workers (1989) have described both disorders within the same pedigree. Serum IgA levels may be elevated in both disorders. Similar to IgA nephropathy, the IgA found in mesangial HSP deposits is predominantly IgA1.

Both increased IgA synthesis and decreased clearance may play a role in IgA immune complex deposition. Given the clinical observation of an association between mucosal infection and HSP, a specific antigenic stimuli has been sought, but none have been identified. Lai and colleagues (1987) reported B-cell and T-cell hyperreactivity in vitro to antigenic stimuli from patients with IgA nephropathy and HSP. Other antigens suggested, in addition to microbes, include drugs, malignancies, dietary protein, and extracellular matrix components such as collagen and fibronectin (Rieu and Noel, 1999).

Because the serum IgA1 of IgA nephropathy patients has an altered O-glycosylation, Allen and co-workers (1998) studied HSP patients and found abnormal O-glycosylated IgA1 only in those who had renal involvement. This was not present in other forms of renal disease, supporting a role for abnormal O-glycosylation in both disorders. A defect in β-1,3-galactosyltransferase has been implicated in the hinge region, resulting in a structural change in IgA1 with mesangial deposition and injury (Feehally, 1997).

Treatment

Children with mild proteinuria or microscopic hematuria require no therapy. Although abdominal pain and arthritis respond to corticosteroids, their benefit in HSP renal disease is less clear. It appears that only high doses of corticosteroids are beneficial. In a study of 38 children with severe HSP nephritis, pulse methylprednisolone therapy resulted in less renal disease and decreased chronicity indices on renal biopsy (Niaudet and Habib, 1998).

Bergstein and associates (1998) treated 21 children with severe HSP nephritis with corticosteroids and azathioprine with good results. Foster and co-workers (2000) reported that 20 children (who were given prednisone and azathioprine and studied retrospectively) had no further progression on renal biopsies and improved clinical outcomes.

Rostoker and colleagues (1995b) found a beneficial effect of low-dose IVIG in moderate HSP and IgA nephropathy. Hattori and co-workers (1999) used plasmapheresis in nine children with rapidly progressive HSP nephritis and noted improved renal function with decreased proteinuria in all patients. Three of the nine patients showed rebound proteinuria after completion of the plasmapheresis.

HSP may recur after renal transplantation, resulting in graft loss in 40% of patients. This occurred more frequently with living-donor transplants (Hasegawa et al., 1989). Despite waiting the recommended year from the time of resolution of disease to transplant and despite triple immunosuppressive regimens including CSA, Meulders and associates (1994) found a 30% recurrence rate.

Prognosis

The average duration of HSP is 1 month. Recurrences are common but usually not after 3 months. Urinary abnormalities may persist in some, and a very few may progress to ESRD. Most children with only microscopic hematuria have complete recovery. Patients with heavy proteinuria or nephrotic syndrome have a less favorable outcome.

Histologic patterns that correlate with development of chronic renal failure include a high percentage of crescents, interstitial fibrosis, and extensive mesangial deposits including dense epithelial deposits. Children at highest risk are those with greater than 50% crescents (Rai et al., 1999). Adults are more likely to progress to chronic renal failure than children (Fogazzi et al., 1989).

IgA NEPHROPATHY

IgA nephropathy, first described by Berger and Hinglais in 1968, is an immune complex–mediated GN characterized by deposition of IgA in the glomerular mesangium. IgA nephropathy is the most common form of primary GN in the world, with an increased prevalence in Asia and the Mediterranean region.

IgA deposition is also seen in the nephropathy of Henoch-Schönlein purpura and in other illnesses associated with IgA elevation. IgA nephropathy occurs in all ages but with a peak incidence in the second and third decades. Males are affected two to three times more often than females.

Clinical Features

Children and young adults usually present with microscopic hematuria or "synpharyngitic hematuria," (e.g., macroscopic hematuria concurrent with an upper respiratory tract infection [URI]). After the onset of URI symptoms, the urine becomes red or tea-colored for 1 to 2 days in contrast to the 10- to 14-day period with poststreptococcal nephritis. Overt nephritic syndrome (characterized by hematuria, proteinuria, edema, and hypertension) is rare, as is nephrotic syndrome. The hematuria may last from hours to many days. Although clinical remission occurs in up to one third of patients, complete disappearance of IgA from the glomeruli is rare.

Immunohistology

Immunofluorescent staining of biopsy specimens demonstrates mesangial deposits of IgA often with C3 deposition and sometimes with IgG, IgM, or both. Alternative complement pathway components may also be deposited including properdin, factor H, and the membrane attack complex C5b-9. The presence of minimal or no C1q can be used to differentiate IgA nephropathy from lupus nephritis. Granular deposits of IgA may also be found in capillary walls. Mesangial regions appear widened, with immunoglobulin deposits and increased cellularity. There may be crescents and segmental capsular adhesions or sclerosis with advanced disease associated with heavy proteinuria.

Pathogenesis

The pathogenesis of IgA nephropathy is not known. An association between clinical severity and MHC genes has been made. These include HLA-B35 in France (Berthoux et al., 1988) and HLA-DR4 in Japan (Kashiwabara et al., 1982). In the United States, IgA nephropathy is associated with an increased frequency of the homozygous null C4 phenotypes (Welch et al., 1987). In Europe and the United States, an increase in C3F phenotype was reported (Wyatt et al., 1987). Polymorphism of Ig heavy chain switch region was also reported to be associated with mesangial IgA GN. These findings have not been confirmed. Perhaps these inconsistencies are secondary to ethnic differences, population biases, or disease heterogeneity.

Although a definitive pathogenic antigen in IgA has not been identified, alimentary antigens present in circulating IgA immune complexes are suspect. Viral antigens have also been suspect given the usual temporal association of disease exacerbation and viral infection. Increased titers of herpes simplex virus (HSV), cytomegalovirus (CMV), and EBV have been reported (Nagy et al., 1984). The role of IgA in the pathogenesis of IgA nephropathy has been explored. IgA by itself does not appear to be sufficient to initiate an inflammatory process (Imai et al., 1988). Others have shown that co-deposition of IgG and IgM is necessary for the development of nephritis (Emancipator and Lamm, 1987). Complement activation, predominantly via the alternative pathway, appears to be an important mediator. Cytokines and other inflammatory mediators from infiltrating blood cells and mesangial cells may cause injury with subsequent deposition of extracellular matrix material.

Polymeric IgA1 is the predominant IgA subclass found in the mesangial deposits, and it is more damaging to glomeruli than monomeric IgA1. The IgA deposited may originate from the marrow rather than mucosal sites because IgA production is downregulated in the mucosal lamina propria and upregulated in the marrow. Increased levels of IgA1 are not sufficient to cause IgA nephropathy, because patients with myeloma and human immunodeficiency virus (HIV) infection with high plasma IgA1 levels rarely exhibit glomerular deposits. There is an IgA1 hyperresponsiveness to antigen challenge, and the polymeric IgA1 response may be prolonged as a result of defective isotype switching.

A qualitative abnormality of circulating IgA is probably responsible for its deposition and glomerular injury. There are decreased galactose residues on the O-linked glycans in the hinge region of IgA molecules of patients with IgA nephropathy. This may influence both IgA deposition and subsequent injury by modifying interaction with (1) the antigen binding site (modifying complex formation and affinity); (2) the Fcα receptors on circulating effector cells because the Fc receptor site is located near the hinge region; (3) the Fcα receptors on mesangial cells; (4) the hepatic asialoglycoprotein receptor, a clearance pathway for IgA1; and (5) complement components (Feehally, 1977).

Treatment

In secondary IgA nephropathy, mesangial IgA deposits quickly clear with resolution of the associated medical condition. Primary IgA nephropathy is more difficult to treat. Corticosteroids are of equivocal benefit in both retrospective studies and prospective randomized trials. Pozzi and colleagues (1999) gave patients with moderate proteinuria and normal renal function intravenous (IV) methylprednisolone (three doses of 1 g/day at months 1, 3, and 5) followed by oral prednisone (0.5 mg/kg/day on alternate days for 6 months) and found a better 5-year renal survival in treated patients. Urinary protein excretion decreased rapidly in the steroid group but not in the control group.

Another placebo-controlled, randomized study assessed the effect of fish oil rich in omega 3 fatty acids given for 2 years. Patients with proteinuria of at least 1 g/day who received fish oil had slower decline in creatinine clearance but no attenuation of their proteinuria (Donadio et al., 1994). Administration of IVIG also slowed decline in renal function and decreased proteinuria (Rostoker et al., 1995b). Angiotensin-converting enzyme (ACE) inhibitors also help control blood pressure and protect against sclerosis by decreasing proteinuria and cytokine production.

MMF may be of benefit in the treatment of IgA nephropathy. Ziswiler and associates (1998) showed that MMF decreased mesangial cell proliferation in cell culture and in anti-Thy1.1 nephritic rats. The rats showed decreased extracellular matrix deposition, glomerular hypertrophy, and proteinuria.

Prognosis

IgA nephropathy leads to end-stage renal disease (ESRD) in approximately 33% of patients after 20 years. Another one third of patients have a benign course with microscopic hematuria, a normal serum creatinine, and proteinuria less than 1 g/day. However, patients with a history of macroscopic hematuria, most of whom are younger patients, have a better prognosis. A poor prognosis is associated with hypertension; proteinuria greater than 2 g/24 hours; renal insufficiency at onset; and biopsy findings of sclerosis, interstitial or vascular fibrosis, or extension of IgA deposition to peripheral capillary walls (Bruce, 1998).

IDIOPATHIC MEMBRANOPROLIFERATIVE GLOMERULONEPHRITIS

Membranoproliferative glomerulonephritis (MPGN) is defined microscopically by mesangial proliferation and thickening of the glomerular capillary walls. MPGN occurs as a primary, idiopathic form and as secondary forms associated with other illnesses including viral and bacterial infections, autoimmune diseases, dysproteinemias, chronic liver disease, and thrombotic microangiopathies. MPGN can occur following hepatitis C infection, sometimes associated with cryoglobulinemia. Most cases of MPGN in children are idiopathic, whereas MPGN in adults is usually secondary (D'Agati, 1998).

Idiopathic MPGN is classified morphologically as types I, II, and III. Type I, an immune complex–mediated disease process, has characteristic glomerular lobularity with mesangial proliferation and double contours of the GBM. Type II, also known as dense deposit disease, has a uniformly thickened GBM with electron dense deposits replacing the lamina densa. The GBM may display double contours as well, but they are less well developed (D'Agati, 1998). Type III, often considered a variant of type I or a combination of types I and

II, shows fragmentation of the basement membrane. Some differentiate these into type III and type IV, with type IV being a mixed membranous and proliferative GN.

MPGN usually occurs in older children and adolescents and is uncommon in children younger than age 5. Type I MPGN generally affects a younger population than does type II. Whites are predominantly affected. There are reports of familial clusters. MPGN is more closely associated with activation of the complement system than other forms of renal disease.

Clinical Features

Typically MPGN presents with nephrotic and nephritic features, often both. Two thirds of patients with type I MPGN have the nephrotic syndrome as the dominant feature at clinical presentation (D'Agati, 1998). Other features include asymptomatic hematuria, recurrent episodes of gross hematuria, and subnephrotic range proteinuria. Although MPGN association with systemic disease is less common in children than adults, a search for underlying disease must be undertaken, including tests for antinuclear antibody (ANA), anti-DNA, liver function, cryoglobulins, and hepatitis B and C.

MPGN may present after a respiratory infection, and therefore differentiation from poststreptococcal acute glomerulonephritis (AGN) must be done. Both have hypocomplementemia, but in MPGN it persists beyond 8 weeks, usually with persistent hematuria and proteinuria. C3 is often decreased to a greater extent than is C4 (Varade et al., 1990). Biopsy with IF and electron microscopy is required to confirm the diagnosis and to categorize the type of MPGN, because classification has important prognostic and therapeutic implications.

Immunohistology

Type I MPGN is characterized by a lobular appearance of glomerular tufts with mesangial expansion and hypercellularity. There are double contours of the GBM secondary to peripheral mesangial migration with new subendothelial basement membrane production. Deposits tend to be subendothelial. On IF, C3 is present in the peripheral capillary wall and mesangium. C1q is often present, and sometimes IgG, IgM, and light chains can be seen (Cohen and Nast, 1996).

Type II MPGN is characterized by thickened capillary walls with double contours less prominent than in type I. Deposits are usually intramembranous but may be subepithelial or less commonly in the mesangial and subendothelial areas. On IF, strong staining for C3 of the GBM is seen with segmental thickening of the GBM. Segmental mesangial C3 is also found. IgM and light chains occasionally are noted; C1q is usually absent (Cohen and Nast, 1996).

Type III has features of both types I and II with strong staining for C3. Cohen and Nast (1996) described type III lesions with features of type I with additional subepithelial deposits and basement membrane projections similar to membranous GN.

Pathogenesis

Type I MPGN is associated with circulating immune complexes in greater than 50% of patients; by contrast to type II, no circulating immune complexes are identified and the glomerular deposits consist of only C3, without immunoglobulins (D'Agati, 1998). Type II may be a systemic illness not confined to the kidney because Brach's membrane of the retina has similar deposits (Duvall-Young et al., 1989).

Hypocomplementemia is a hallmark of all types of MPGN; however, type I is generally associated with classic pathway activation and type II with alternative pathway activation (see Chapter 21). In type I, deposited immune complexes activate the classic pathway with subsequent decrease of serum C3 and C4 levels. The patients may have antibodies to C1q that may directly activate the classic pathway.

Tanuma and co-workers (1989) first described the *C4 nephritic factor* (C4NeF), an autoantibody to C4 convertase that stabilizes the enzyme leading to persistent activation of the classic complement pathway in some patients with type I MPGN. Ohi and Yasugi (1994) studied 100 patients with hypocomplementemic MPGN and found that 10 had both *the C3 nephritic factor* (C3NeF) (an autoantibody to the classic pathway enzyme C3 convertase) and C4NeF. These patients were found to have an increased incidence of nephrotic syndrome and a poorer prognosis than patients who were positive to either C3NeF or C4NeF but not to both.

Type II MPGN is associated with activation of the alternative complement pathway with decreased C3 and normal C4 levels. Type II MPGN is also associated with both factor H deficiency and presence of C3NeF. Factor H is essential for inactivating the alternative pathway C3 convertase, C3bBb, which is continuously being formed in vivo. Without factor H, there is increased convertase activity and continued complement activation with resultant hypocomplementemia. Factor H deficiency has also been associated with idiopathic hemolytic uremic syndrome. Irregular expression of factor H by endothelial cells may lead to alternative pathway complement activation and endothelial cell injury (Ault, 2000).

C3NeF stabilizes C3 convertase, so its presence has consequences similar to factor H deficiency. A second form of C3NeF has been described, an IgG that binds to factor H and prevents its inhibitory activity (Williams, 1997).

MPGN type II is often associated with partial lipodystrophy (PLD), characterized by loss of adipose tissue from the face, arms, and upper trunk (Levy et al., 1998). Adipocytes themselves produce complement and can be lysed in vitro by exposure to C3NeF, suggesting a mechanism for PLD and perhaps a mechanism for glomerular damage (Williams, 1997).

Type III MPGN is associated with variable activation of the classic and alternative complement pathways and low levels of terminal complement components. Nephritic factor of the terminal pathway (NFt) is associated with type III MPGN, whereas nephritic factor of the amplification loop (NFa) is associated with type II MPGN (West and McAdams, 1998). The relationship between deposition of terminal complement pathway components in type III MPGN and renal injury remains to be clarified.

Treatment

The usual treatment for idiopathic MPGN is steroids and antiplatelet drugs. For children, alternate-day oral steroids are associated with a 10-year renal survival of 82% (McEnery, 1990). Relapses occurred after discontinuation of glucocorticoids, emphasizing the need for careful monitoring after steroid taper. A prospective, randomized, double-blind, placebo-controlled trial of alternate day prednisone (40 mg/m^2 for 5 years) in children with MPGN and heavy proteinuria identified no significant difference between treatment and control groups at 130 months. However, patients in subcategories types I and III MPGN were shown to have better outcomes than the untreated controls (Tarshish et al., 1992). The value of corticosteroids in adults with primary MPGN is less clear.

Antiplatelet drugs have been used frequently in adults with MPGN. Donadio and associates (1994) reported slower deterioration of glomerular filtration rate (GFR) in patients treated with aspirin and dipyridamole. Zauner and colleagues (1994) reported decreased proteinuria but no change in renal function with these drugs. Alkylating agents such as cyclophosphamide, usually given in combination with steroids, are not more beneficial than steroids alone (Faedda et al., 1994). Erbay and co-workers (1988) reported a modest decrease in proteinuria with the use of CSA and low-dose prednisone.

Prognosis

In type I MPGN, the 10-year renal survival is reported to be 62% to 64% (Cameron et al., 1983; Schmitt et al., 1990). Habib and colleagues (1973b) had previously reported a less favorable outcome for children with type II MPGN, possibly because of an increased number of patients with crescents in their series. More recently, Schwertz and co-workers (1996) reported 10-year renal survival rates for types I, II, and III as 64%, 47%, and 83%, respectively, and the median time to ESRD was 15 years.

Overall, children have a more gradual decline in renal function than do adults, but, after 10 years, their renal survival rates are similar (Cameron et al., 1983). D'Amico (1992) suggested that increased and persistent proteinuria are poor prognostic indicators. Cameron and associates (1983) also reported that the 10-year renal survival rate decreased from 85% to 40% in patients with marked proteinuria. Impaired renal function at presentation is a bad prognostic feature (Valles-Prats et al., 1985), as is hypertension (D'Amico, 1992). Morphologic features associated with a poor outcome include superimposed crescents and/or chronic tubulointerstitial lesions (D'Amico, 1992).

ANTI–GLOMERULAR BASEMENT MEMBRANE NEPHRITIS (GOODPASTURE'S SYNDROME)

Anti-GBM can occur as a renal-limited disease; when combined with pulmonary hemorrhage, it is termed Goodpasture's disease. However, most patients with concurrent pulmonary hemorrhage and GN do not have anti-GBM diseases. Savage and associates (1986) reported two patterns of anti-GBM antibody-mediated disease in the United Kingdom. Young men presented with both pulmonary and renal involvement, whereas women in their 60s presented with nephritis alone. A few cases have been reported in older children. Whites are preferentially affected.

Anti-GBM can occur as recurrent and de novo disease following renal allografts. De novo disease can occur in grafts of Alport's patients; these patients lack the Goodpasture's antigen, a peptide on the $\alpha3$ chain of type IV collagen, predisposing them to an immune response to the newly presented antigen within the allograft.

Clinical Features

Most patients present with rapidly progressive GN, with hematuria, proteinuria, and renal failure over weeks to months. In 75% of patients, hemoptysis may be the presenting symptom (Cohen and Nast, 1996). These patients have an antibody to the alveolar capillary basement membrane. Circulating anti-GBM antibodies are present, and disease activity can be monitored by following the level of this antibody.

Immunohistology

On light microscopy, crescents are present in some or all glomeruli. There are breaks in the basement membrane of Bowman's capsule with cells and fibrin in the surrounding interstitium. The interstitium is usually edematous with a mononuclear cell infiltrate. IF shows linear staining of IgG of the GBM, often accompanied by C3 in a linear, interrupted linear, or globular pattern. Linear IgG staining of the tubular basement membrane is present in 67% of patients (Cohen and Nast, 1996).

Pathogenesis

Antibodies to an epitope on the $\alpha3$ chain of type IV collagen is implicated in the pathogenesis of anti-GBM nephritis. Ryan and co-workers (1998) demonstrated that the amino terminal portion is critical for antibody recognition. Park and colleagues (1998) demonstrated the importance of Fc receptors in the inflammatory cascade; mice deficient in the FcRγ chain survived after administration of anti-GBM antibodies, whereas wild-type mice died with severe GN. Suzuki and associates (1998b) found less renal injury in Fc gamma (−/−) mice but also identified an FcR independent pathway leading to renal injury. This was not attenuated by eliminating complement but may be completely abolished using an angiotensin II type I receptor antagonist. This FcR independent pathway was associated with monocyte/ macrophage accumulation and mesangial expansion.

Hisada and associates (1999) further evaluated the role of angiotensin II in the pathogenesis of anti-GBM nephropathy by comparing angiotensin type Ia receptor (AT1a) deficient mice with wild-type mice challenged with anti-GBM antibody. AT1a-deficient mice had decreased proteinuria and less tissue damage.

Huang and colleagues (1997) studied T cells in glomerular injury of anti-GBM nephritis. CD4+ and CD8+ T-cell inhibition prevented macrophage influx and proteinuria, suggesting that macrophages mediate T-cell renal injury. Similarly, CD28-B7 blockade by CTLA-4-Ig modified autoantibody production, glomerular infiltration, and renal injury in experimental autoimmune glomerulonephritis of rats (Reynolds et al., 2000).

Treatment

Treatment of anti-GBM nephritis consists of removing circulating antibody with plasma exchange and immunosuppression, most commonly corticosteroids and cyclophosphamide in combination with plasma exchange. Response to treatment can be determined by following anti-GBM antibody titers. We have successfully used IVIG for treatment of anti-GBM disease in a renal allograft of a patient with Alport's syndrome.

With therapy, circulating anti-GBM antibody is abolished, but linear antibody may remain fixed within the kidney for a year or more. Most patients do not relapse. However, patients that present with initial azotemia, oliguria or anuria, or extensive crescent formation on renal biopsy usually do not recover renal function (Savage, 1998).

VASCULITIS

Vasculitis encompasses a spectrum of conditions characterized by inflammation of blood vessel walls, associated with rapid progression to renal failure (see Chapter 35). Kidney involvement is usually a necrotizing crescentic GN but also can occur as a result of immune complex syndromes (e.g., HSP and SLE) as noted in Table 38-1. Direct antibody injury to specific antigens of the glomerulus can also elicit a vasculitic response. Anti-GBM disease is the best example of this group,

TABLE 38-1 · IMMUNOLOGIC CAUSES FOR VASCULITIS

Immune complex mediated
  Henoch-Schönlein purpura (systemic IgA-mediated vasculitis)
  Cryoglobulinemic vasculitis
  Systemic lupus erythematosus vasculitis
  Rheumatoid vasculitis
  Polyarteritis nodosa
  Infection-related vasculitis
    Viral (hepatitis C, hepatitis B, parvovirus B19)
    Bacterial (streptococcal)
Antibody-mediated injury
  Goodpasture's syndrome (anti–glomerular basement membrane antibodies)
  Kawasaki disease (antiendothelial cell antibodies)
  Acute vascular rejection of allografts (anti-endothelial cell antibodies)
Antineutrophil cytoplasmic autoantibody-associated/mediated
  Wegener's granulomatosis
  Microsopic polyangiitis
  Churg-Strauss syndrome
T-cell mediated
  Allograft cellular vascular rejection
  Giant-cell (temporal) arteritis
  Takayasu's arteritis

although anti-endothelial cell antibodies have been described in Kawasaki disease (Meroni et al., 1997).

The vasculitic syndromes with renal involvement that occur in childhood include Wegener's granulomatosis, microscopic polyarteritis nodosa, and idiopathic crescentic GN. Classification of these vasculitides is confusing, because there is considerable overlap in symptoms and pathologic findings. However, the identification of ANCAs offers a new understanding of these syndromes. Cell-mediated vasculitis is rare in children, although pediatric Takayasu's arteritis is not uncommon.

Wegener's Granulomatosis and Churg-Strauss Syndrome

The small vessel vasculitides of childhood often have multiorgan involvement, particularly of the kidney, skin, and GI tract. Other manifestations include mononeuritis multiplex of peripheral nerves, necrotizing sinusitis, respiratory tract vasculitis from mucosal angiitis, and pulmonary hemorrhage from necrotizing alveolar capillaritis. These are often referred to as *renal-dermal* or *renal-dermal-sinus* syndromes depending on their clinical manifestations. These features are common to Wegener's granulomatosis and Churg-Strauss syndrome, but in Wegener's granulomatosis there are usually distinctive necrotizing granulomatous lesions of the respiratory tract and orbit.

GN, ranging from minimal renal dysfunction to rapidly progressive irreversible renal failure, is reported in 61% of cases of Wegener's granulomatosis in childhood, although only a minority (9%) have renal involvement at presentation (Rottem et al., 1993). The typical renal histopathology is a pauci-immune necrotizing crescentic GN, often associated with granuloma formation. Patients with Churg-Strauss syndrome usually have asthma and eosinophilia. They may also exhibit clusters of eosinophilic-rich inflammation in the gut and lung.

Microscopic Polyarteritis Nodosa

Microscopic polyarteritis nodosa is a necrotizing vasculitis of small and medium-sized arteries. It occasionally occurs in children but usually affects middle-aged adults. Ozen and associates (1992) reviewed 31 cases of children with polyarteritis nodosa whose major involvement included the kidney and musculoskeletal system and minor involvement included the skin, GI tract, peripheral and central nervous systems, and cardiac and pulmonary systems. Constitutional symptoms, elevation of acute phase reactants, and presence of hepatitis B surface antigen (HBsAg) occurred in some patients.

Renal involvement occurs in 65% of patients and includes proteinuria, hematuria and proteinuria, nephrotic syndrome with hematuria, and rapidly progressive GN. The pathologic findings are similar to those of Wegener's granulomatosis (i.e., a pauci-immune necrotizing crescentic GN).

Idiopathic Crescentic Glomerulonephritis

Idiopathic crescentic GN is a vasculitis of small- to medium-sized vessels that is confined to the kidney and results in a clinical syndrome of rapidly progressive GN in the absence of systemic signs and symptoms. As in Wegener's granulomatosis and microscopic polyarteritis nodosa, renal histopathology reveals a pauci-immune GN.

Pathogenesis

Vasculitis occurs when there is activation of inflammatory mediator within the vessel wall. The initiating events are multiple and usually unknown for most forms of vasculitis (see Table 38-1). An immune response to foreign antigens, such as hepatitis C, hepatitis B, or other infectious agents, in the form of immune complexes or autoantigens is suspected but rarely proved to be the cause in vasculitic disorders.

Pauci-immune vasculitis includes systemic vasculitides that often involve the kidney and have no immune complex or antibody deposits. This group includes microscopic polyangiitis (microscopic polyarteritis), Wegener's granulomatosis, and Churg-Strauss syndrome. All have ANCAs, which activate leukocytes and cause vascular injury.

Although each of these vasculitic syndromes are distinct, the recent description of ANCAs as a serologic marker of vasculitis suggests that they represent a pathologic continuum. ANCAs are autoantibodies directed toward cytoplasmic components of neutrophil primary granules and monocyte lysosomes (Jennette and Falk, 1990). Among patients with pauci-immune crescentic GN, 80% have positive tests for ANCAs; 70% have systemic involvement (i.e., Wegener's granulomatosis or microscopic polyarteritis nodosa), and 30% have idiopathic crescentic GN (Jennette and Falk, 1990).

Two distinct classes of ANCAs are defined by their indirect IF staining patterns. On alcohol-fixed neutrophils, p-ANCAs show perinuclear (p) staining, whereas c-ANCAs demonstrate cytoplasmic (c) staining. Most p-ANCAs are specific for myeloperoxidase, and most c-ANCAs are specific for proteinase-3 (Jennette and Falk, 1990). The pattern of ANCA staining correlates with the distribution of vascular injury.

Among patients with idiopathic crescentic GN without systemic involvement, 83% had p-ANCAs and 17% had c-ANCAs. Among patients with Wegener's granulomatosis with crescentic GN and lung and sinus disease, 90% have c-ANCAs. Both p-ANCAs and c-ANCAs are present in nearly equal frequency in patients with non-Wegener's systemic vasculitis (i.e., microscopic polyarteritis nodosa) (Jennette et al., 1989; Jennette and Falk, 1990).

ANCAs not only are serologic markers for vasculitis but also are implicated in their pathogenesis. Falk and associates (1990) proposed that ANCAs recognize cytoplasmic antigens present on the neutrophil cell surface in response to cytokine-mediated priming. The resulting respiratory burst releases reactive oxygen species and lytic cellular enzymes that damage the vascular endothelial cell. ANCAs damage human endothelial cells in vitro after priming with cytokines and endotoxin (Ewert et al., 1992).

In ANCA-positive GN, the most frequent renal histopathology is a pauci-immune necrotizing crescentic GN, identical to that present in Wegener's granulomatosis, polyarteritis nodosa, and idiopathic crescentic GN. Immunofluorescent and electron microscopic studies show no deposition of immunoproteins. Periglomerular granulomatous response and necrotizing arteritis are present in some renal biopsy specimens.

Treatment

The optimal therapy for these vasculitic syndromes and ANCA-positive pauci-immune necrotizing crescentic GN has not been defined. Cyclophosphamide used with corticosteroids induces remission in Wegener's granulomatosis (Hoffman et al., 1992), systemic necrotizing vasculitis (Fauci et al., 1979), and idiopathic crescentic GN (Kunis et al., 1992). IV pulse methylprednisolone is superior to oral corticosteroids (Bolton and Sturgill, 1989). Oral and IV cyclophosphamide when used with steroids are equally efficacious (Falk et al., 1990). Most treatment regimens include corticosteroids, either oral or IV, and a cytotoxic agent, usually cyclophosphamide. These regimens result in a 70% rate for 2-year patient and renal survival even among patients with systemic involvement (Jennette and Falk, 1990).

Other treatments have included IVIG and plasma-pheresis. IVIG has induced remission in patients resistant to standard therapy (Jayne and Lockwood, 1991; Jayne et al., 1993; Tuso et al., 1992). Plasmapheresis is of little benefit when added to conventional immunosuppressant therapy (Gaskin and Pasey, 2001).

Renal transplantation has been successful in patients with ANCA-associated pauci-immune crescentic necrotizing GN (Montalbert et al., 1980; Morin et al., 1993). However, recurrence of the original disease in the allograft may occur (Jacquot et al., 1990; Oberhuber et al., 1988).

ACUTE POSTSTREPTOCOCCAL GLOMERULONEPHRITIS

AGN is an acute glomerular inflammation that is a delayed sequelae of infection, usually streptococcal. It is characterized by proliferation and inflammation secondary to immune complex deposition within the glomerular capillary walls and the mesangium. It occurs subsequent to infection with certain nephritogenic strains of group A β-hemolytic streptococci or rarely other infections.

These antigens may either bind directly to glomerular sites forming in situ immune complexes or become trapped in the glomeruli as part of circulating immune complexes. Both mechanisms initiate glomerular inflammation, complement activation, and polymorphonuclear leukocyte accumulation. Immunochemical analysis of immune complexes from affected glomeruli has demonstrated bacterial antigens.

Patients with AGN most often have had evidence of a recent infection of the pharynx or skin with group A β-hemolytic streptococci. However, other bacterial, viral, and parasitic agents have been implicated in AGN pathogenesis (Table 38-2). In developed countries, a decline in PSGN and an increase in other infection-related glomerulonephritides, particularly in alcoholics and IV drug abusers, has been observed (Montseny et al., 1995).

PSGN is the most common form of AGN in children. PSGN follows either pharyngeal or skin infection with group A β-hemolytic streptococci. Streptococcal pharyngitis is more common in winter and early spring, whereas impetigo is more common in summer. Only certain serologic types of streptococci known as nephritogenic strains are associated with PSGN. These include protein M types 1, 3, 4, 6, 12, 25, and 49 causing pharyngeal infections and types 2, 49, 55, 57, and 60 causing skin infections. Serotypes 12 (throat) and 49 (skin) are the most common strains causing PSGN (Dodge et al., 1972).

The risk of PSGN following infection with a nephritogenic strain is dependent on environmental, host, and genetic factors. The risk is 10% to 15% during epidemics (Rodriguez-Iturbe, 1984). Subclinical episodes occur more frequently than overt clinical disease. Asymptomatic contacts of PSGN patients may have abnormal urinary findings, most commonly hematuria.

TABLE 38-2 · INFECTIOUS AGENTS ASSOCIATED WITH IMMUNE COMPLEX GLOMERULONEPHRITIS

Bacterial	Parasitic
Group A β-hemolytic streptococci	*Plasmodium malariae*
Staphylococcus aureus	*Toxoplasma*
Staphylococcus epidermidis	*Filaria*
Gram-negative bacilli	*Schistosomia*
Streptococcus pneumoniae	*Trichinella*
Treponema pallidum	*Trypanosome*
Salmonella typhi	**Rickettsial**
Meningococci	Scrub typhus
Leptospirosis	**Fungal**
Viral	*Coccidioides immitis*
Hepatitis B and C	
Cytomegalovirus	
Enteroviruses	
Measles	
Parvovirus	
Oncornavirus	
Mumps virus	
Rubella	
Varicella	

From Moudgil A, Bagga A, Fredrich R, Jordan SC. Post-streptococcal and other infection-related glomerulonephritides. In Greenberg A, Cheung A, Coffman T, Falk R, Jennette J, eds. Primer on Kidney Diseases. San Diego, Academic Press, 1998, pp 193–200.

Pathogenesis

PSGN is mediated by immune complex injury, but the precise identification of the antigens within the nephritogenic immune complexes has not been defined. In the murine model, deposition of streptokinase in the glomeruli is correlated with the development and severity of the nephritis (Nordstrand et al., 1998). Soluble immune complexes may mediate this injury, because PSGN resembles experimental serum-sickness nephritis in rabbits, which is mediated by immune complexes. In experimental serum sickness, a latent period between antigen administration and the appearance of nephritis is similar to the period between the streptococcal infection and the onset of PSGN. Furthermore, the histology of the GBM deposits is similar in both conditions (Fish et al., 1966).

Soluble immune complexes are sometimes present in the serum of patients with PSGN (Tung et al., 1978; Verroust et al., 1979). Streptococcal antigens have occasionally been isolated from the immune complexes deposited in the glomeruli (Seligson et al., 1985) but not always at the site of IgG and C3 deposition (Lange et al., 1983). This may be due to possible denaturation of glomerular antigen or antigen saturation with specific antibody, thus blocking its recognition by antibody probes. Endostreptosin has been identified in the mesangium but not in the humps characteristic of the disease (Lange et al., 1983).

In situ immune complex formation may explain immune glomerular injury in PSGN. Cationic streptococcal antigens fixed to the glomerular capillary wall bind circulating antibody to form immune complexes (Couser and Salant, 1980; Vogt, 1984). These immune complexes initiate complement, kinin, and coagulation activation and release of polymorphonuclear chemotactic factors leading to acute glomerular injury. The erythrogenic toxin type B are responsible for leukocyte infiltration in the rat kidney; human antibodies to erythrogenic toxin B and its precursor are sometimes found in patients with AGN (Romero et al., 1999).

Other factors suspected of a pathogenic role include cellular immunity to GBM antigens (Fillit and Zabriskie, 1984), altered T-cell function (Williams et al., 1981), glomerular localization of T-helper and T-suppressor lymphocytes (Nolasco et al., 1987), and altered C3 synthesis and catabolism (Endre et al., 1984). When type 12 (throat) or type 49 (skin) β-hemolytic streptococcal antigens are administered to experimental animals, no consistent glomerular injury results (Wannamaker and Yasmineh, 1967).

Clinical Features

PSGN is primarily a disease of children between 5 and 15 years of age, occurring more often in males. The onset is abrupt and is preceded by streptococcal pharyngitis or pyoderma by 1 to 4 weeks. Hematuria and edema are the most common clinical features. Coke-colored or reddish brown urine is present in 70%. Microscopic hematuria occurs in all patients. The edema is usually periorbital and worse in the mornings. Weight gain may occur without evidence of edema. The edema is due to excessive fluid accumulation secondary to a reduced GFR, sodium and water retention, and proteinuria. Most patients have a variable degree of oliguria. Anuria is infrequent and if persistent suggests rapidly progressive GN.

Hypertension is usually mild to moderate and is secondary to sodium and water retention. The hypertension may be severe enough to cause encephalopathy, with headache, visual disturbances, coma, or convulsions. Neurologic manifestations may occur, even in the absence of severe hypertension. Circulatory failure with fluid retention may result in dyspnea, orthopnea, cough, cardiomegaly, gallop rhythm, pleural effusions, and pulmonary edema. Pallor is secondary to dilutional anemia and edema. Systemic symptoms such as mild fever, nausea, vomiting, and abdominal pain may be present. Subclinical cases may be discovered by urinalysis of close contacts of overt cases.

Laboratory Diagnosis

Diagnosis of PSGN is based on evidence for previous streptococcal infection, abnormal urinary findings, and very low serum complement levels. Renal biopsy is rarely indicated. Microscope analysis of the urine shows dysmorphic red blood cells, tubular epithelial cells, and granular casts. Mild to moderate proteinuria is usually seen, but nephrotic range proteinuria may also occur. Blood urea nitrogen and serum creatinine levels are usually normal but may occasionally be elevated. Serum albumin levels are usually mildly reduced. A normocytic normochromic anemia is secondary to fluid overload. Shortened erythrocyte survival may occur because of rapid elimination of red cells coated with immune complexes. Thrombocytopenia is rarely reported. Fibrinogen, factor VIII, and plasmin are elevated acutely and correlate with disease activity.

Evidence for Streptococcal Infection

Despite the latent period, throat or skin cultures may show group A streptococci. Family contacts may have positive cultures even in the absence of nephritis. Antibodies against extracellular products of streptococci are indirect evidence of recent infection and include antistreptolysin O (ASO), antistreptokinase, antihyaluronidase (AH), antideoxyribonuclease B (anti-DNAase B), and antinicotyladenine dinucleotidase (anti-NADase). The ASO titer begins to rise 10 to 14 days after streptococcal pharyngitis, peaks at 3 to 4 weeks, and decreases thereafter. Early antibiotic treatment can blunt this rise in titer. The magnitude of the antibody titer has no relationship to the development or severity of nephritis. In streptococcal skin infections, binding of streptolysin to skin lipids may blunt its antibody response, resulting in a low ASO titer. Anti-NADase B and AH occur in 90% of patients with streptococcal skin infections (Dillon and Reeves, 1974).

Abnormalities of Serum Complement

Low hemolytic complement activity (CH_{50}) and C3 levels are seen in 90% to 100% of patients. Decreased C3 levels may be present in contacts despite absence of urinary abnormalities. The early complement components (C1q, C2, C4) may be mildly reduced at the onset of disease. Serum properdin and C5 levels are decreased in 60% of patients, suggesting alternate complement pathway activation. Activation of C3 nephritic factor may be detected initially but is undetectable after C3 levels become normal.

There is no correlation between the depression of serum C3 level and severity of nephritis, and C3 levels return to normal within 6 to 8 weeks in more than 90% of patients. Persistently low C3 levels suggest underlying MPGN, lupus nephritis, and GN associated with endocarditis or occult visceral abscess (Fischel, 1952; Spitzer et al., 1969).

Other Immunologic Abnormalities

Circulating cryoglobulins and immune complexes are found in most patients in the first weeks of the illness. High-molecular-weight fibrinogen complexes are present in severe cases. Circulating antibodies to basement membrane constituents (type IV collagen and laminin) may also be found.

Pathology

Renal biopsy is rarely indicated in PSGN but should be considered in patients with an atypical presentation such as prolonged oliguria, anuria, severe proteinuria, and marked azotemia and in those lacking serologic evidence of preceding streptococcal infection. Biopsy should be undertaken in patients with significant hypertension, persistent gross hematuria after 2 to 3 weeks, persistent proteinuria after 6 months, and persistently low C3 levels. Biopsy is done to assess prognosis or to detect the presence of other underlying glomerular diseases.

The renal histology may show enlarged glomeruli with lobular accentuation of the tufts (Fig. 38-6). There is a diffuse endocapillary and mesangial cell proliferation and infiltration by polymorphonuclear leukocytes, monocytes, and eosinophils within the capillary lumina and mesangium. Epithelial cells are uncommon in the proliferative process, and crescent formation is limited to patients with severe disease. The presence of crescents in 50% or more glomeruli suggests a guarded prognosis.

On electron microscopy, the presence of discrete, electron dense, dome-shaped subepithelial deposits are characteristic (Fig. 38-7). These are present early in the course and decrease after 4 to 6 weeks. Incomplete clinical resolution may occur when they are present in large numbers and in contiguous areas. Mesangial deposits may persist for prolonged periods. Children with the severest symptoms have classic nodular immunoprotein deposits, and those with milder forms of the disease have only focal, interrupted, linear deposition of C3 along the GBM and within the mesangium (Fisher and Reidbord, 1971). Immunofluorescent staining shows deposition of IgG and C3 in a granular pattern along the GBM and in the mesangium.

Prevention and Treatment

No streptococcal vaccine is available. A course of antibiotics should be given to eradicate streptococcus, even without evidence of streptococcal infection. Eradication of the organism in the population is not feasible. Early antimicrobial therapy of patients and family members may prevent the spread of streptococcal infections and may attenuate the severity of PSGN. Widespread use of antimicrobials and better hygiene has markedly reduced the incidence of PSGN in developed countries.

Treatment of acute PSGN is symptomatic. Fluid and sodium restriction, loop diuretics, and antihypertensive therapy may be needed in the acute phase. Restriction of protein may be necessary in the presence of marked azotemia. Hyperkalemia may be treated with ion exchange resins. Occasionally, dialysis is necessary.

Because immunity to streptococcal M protein is type specific and long lasting and nephritogenic serotypes are limited in number, recurrent episodes of PSGN are rare (Roy et al., 1969), and long-term antibiotic prophylaxis is not indicated.

Prognosis

The acute episode of PSGN is usually self-limited; most patients undergo diuresis within 7 to 10 days of the onset of the illness. Hypertension and azotemia subside within 1 to 2 weeks. Serum C3 levels return to normal within 6 to 8 weeks. Hematuria and proteinuria disappear by 6 months in more than 90% of children. Microscopic hematuria may persist for 1 to 2 years. In adults, proteinuria may persist for more than 1 year and occasionally up to 2 years or longer.

In most patients without pre-existing renal disease, heavy proteinuria, or extensive crescentic glomerular lesions, the prognosis is excellent. However, in children with disease severe enough to necessitate hospitalization, the outcome is less favorable. Severe chronic GN

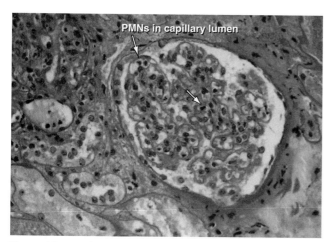

Figure 38-6 · Light microscopy of acute poststreptococcal glomerulonephritis shows a hyper cellular glomerulus with polymorphonuclear leukocytes (PMNs) within the capillary lumen (*arrows*). The adjacent glomerulus, shown in part, has increased endocapillary proliferation, resulting in narrowing of the lumen (H&E stain). (Courtesy Dr. A.H. Cohen.)

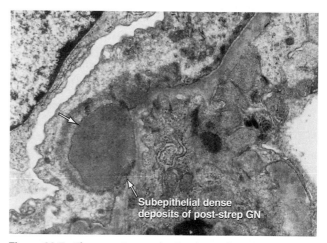

Figure 38-7 · Electron micrograph of a glomerular capillary from a patient with acute poststreptococcal glomerulonephritis shows a large dome-shaped subepithelial electron-dense deposit (*arrows*). (Courtesy Dr. A.H. Cohen.)

does not usually evolve from mild or unrecognized PSGN.

The prognosis in adults is less favorable, and some progress to end-stage renal failure (Vogl et al., 1986). As noted, recurrences are uncommon.

GLOMERULONEPHRITIS ASSOCIATED WITH OTHER INFECTIONS

Glomerulonephritis with Sepsis, Bacterial Endocarditis, and Visceral Abscesses

Glomerulonephritis (GN) may occur following infections other than group A β-hemolytic streptococci (see Table 38-2). Such infectious organisms include *Staphylococcus aureus* and *Staphylococcus epidermidis;* less commonly they include *Streptococcus pneumoniae,* group D streptococci, meningococci, gonococci, and gram-negative rods. These illnesses are increasing, particularly in immunocompromised adults, alcoholics, IV drug abusers, and the elderly (Montseny et al., 1995).

GN may develop following bacterial endocarditis and visceral abscesses. The renal disease in these patients is indistinguishable from PSGN, although the onset may be insidious and the course protracted. The GN is of varying severity, and the biopsy may show focal or diffuse endocapillary proliferation with or without crescents. The total complement and C3 levels are usually decreased. Cryoglobulins and circulating immune complexes are frequently detected.

These patients must be distinguished from PSGN because appropriate antibiotics will lead to resolution of symptoms. Valve replacement surgery may be indicated in patients with bacterial endocarditis. Delay in treatment may lead to incomplete recovery, chronic renal failure, and death.

Shunt Nephritis

GN associated with infected shunts for hydrocephalus, vascular bypass, or venous access is termed shunt nephritis. *S. epidermidis* is the most common organism cultured from the blood or the shunt. Other organisms include *S. aureus* and gram-negative bacteria.

Clinical features are usually indolent and include fever, arthralgia, lethargy, weight loss, pallor, purpuric rash, lymphadenopathy, and hepatosplenomegaly. Patients may have microscopic hematuria, proteinuria, and impaired renal function. Gross hematuria, hypertension, and nephrotic syndrome are uncommon. Serum complement levels are usually low. Factor B and properdin are occasionally decreased, indicating predominant activation of the classic complement pathway. Rheumatoid factor, circulating immune complexes, and cryoglobulins are frequently present.

Renal histology usually shows MPGN or less commonly focal proliferative GN. Renal biopsy is not usu-

ally indicated. Most patients recover with removal of shunts and antibiotic therapy, but some have residual disease.

Glomerulonephritis with Syphilis

Renal involvement may occur in congenital and acquired syphilis, usually presenting with nephrotic syndrome or less commonly with acute nephritis. Other manifestations of congenital syphilis such as hepatosplenomegaly, skin rash, and mucosal involvement are usually present. Complement levels of C1q, C4, C3, and C5 are decreased and return to normal following antibiotic treatment. Complement levels are usually normal in acquired syphilis. MN or diffuse proliferative GN may be present on renal biopsy. Renal disease is probably secondary to an immunologic reaction to treponemal antigens. Antibiotic treatment of both congenital and acquired syphilis usually results in rapid improvement of the renal disease (Hruby et al., 1992).

Glomerulonephritis with Other Bacterial Infections

GN secondary to typhoid fever, brucellosis, and leptospirosis has been described. The nephritis is usually mild, often with minimal hematuria and proteinuria. The absence of bacteriologic and serologic evidence for prior streptococcal illness and the temporal association with these infections should suggest a diagnosis of nonstreptococcal infectious GN.

Glomerulonephritis with Viral Infections

Viral infections are also associated with GN, glomerulosclerosis, and tubulointerstitial lesions. Viruses implicated include hepatitis B, hepatitis C, HIV, parvovirus B19, hantavirus, CMV, and EBV. The association with some is established; in others it is newly recognized. Some patients have concomitant features of systemic infections, whereas in others renal involvement may precede other clinical features or be the sole presenting feature. Diagnosis uses serologic, virologic, or histopathologic analysis by PCR or in situ hybridization.

Ronco and colleagues (1982) suggested several pathogenic mechanisms. First, immune complexes containing either viral antigens or autoantigens rendered immunogenic by the virus may be deposited in the kidney, leading to an inflammatory response. Second, viral antigens may bind to the glomerular structures, resulting in a host antibody or T-cell response to viral antigens or to virus-altered glomerular structures. Finally, viruses may be cytopathic to the glomerular cells or activate cytokines and/or adhesion molecules.

Hantavirus infection, originally described in Korea, is known to cause hemorrhagic fever with renal involvement. A few cases have been described in the United States and other developed countries (Peters et al.,

1999). Hantavirus primarily causes tubulointerstitial nephritis and acute renal failure (ARF). Glomerular mesangial changes may be seen on renal biopsy in some patients.

GN with nephrotic syndrome has been associated with CMV and EBV infection, sometimes following kidney transplantation (Blowey, 1996; Laine et al., 1993). Mesangial lesions and diffuse mesangial sclerosis are found on renal histology.

With new sensitive diagnostic tools such as PCR and in situ hybridization and in situ PCR, other infectious agents will probably be identified.

Glomerulonephritis Associated with Hepatitis B and C

Renal involvement with hepatitis B infection usually results in MN; in addition, MPGN, mesangial proliferative GN, and renal vasculitis have been described. The patients usually present with nephrotic syndrome or less often with AGN. Renal disease may be the sole clinical feature without biochemical features of liver disease. These patients have circulating HBsAg and often circulating hepatitis B e antigen (HBeAg). Serum C3 and C4 levels are usually decreased, and cryoglobulins and circulating immune complexes are often present. Hepatitis B virus (HBV) particles may be seen by electron microscopy in the glomerular capillary wall. HBV DNA has also been detected in the glomerular and tubular epithelial cells (Lai et al., 1996). Patients presenting with the nephrotic syndrome may progress to ESRD. Prognosis is somewhat better in children (Lai et al., 1991; Lin, 1991).

Hepatitis C virus is also associated with GN similar to that with hepatitis B (Gumber and Chopra, 1995). However, hepatitis C is predominantly associated with proliferative GN, whereas hepatitis B is predominantly associated with MN. Figure 38-8 shows

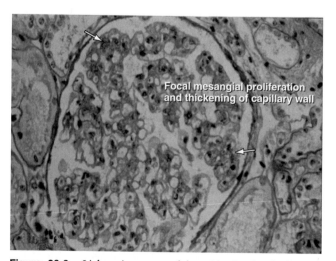

light microscopy of hepatitis C–related GN, illustrating mesangial proliferation and thickening of the GBM in some capillary loops. Clinical findings include systemic features of vasculitis, arthralgias, purpura, hematuria, proteinuria, nephrotic syndrome, and renal insufficiency. Low C3 and circulating cryoglobulins may be present. Hepatitis C virus has been detected in renal biopsies of hepatitis C–associated GN (Rodriguez-Inigo et al., 2000).

Immunosuppressive therapy is contraindicated for hepatitis B– or hepatitis C–associated GN, because it impairs the host's ability to clear the infection and may stimulate viral replication. Some patients, particularly those with hepatitis B–associated GN, may go into spontaneous remission. Antiviral therapy with IFN-α may be useful in clearing viremia and reversing glomerular lesions (Conjeevaram et al., 1995). A combination IFN-α and ribavirin in hepatitis C may reverse the renal lesion (Jefferson and Johnson, 2000).

Human Immunodeficiency Virus–Associated Nephropathy

Renal lesions associated with HIV infection include immune complex–mediated GN, collapsing glomerulopathy (CG), focal segmental glomerulosclerosis (FSGS), and acute renal failure (ARF). Immune complex–mediated GNs, including IgA nephropathy, are observed predominantly in whites, whereas CG and FSGS are more common in blacks (Carbone et al., 1989). Mesangial proliferative GN and immune complex–mediated GN are commonly observed in HIV-infected children, although some develop FSGS and CG (Ray et al., 1998). Others develop MPGN secondary to concomitant hepatitis C. Renal failure generally results from acute tubular injury secondary to drugs, sepsis, and hypotension (Rao and Friedman, 1995). CG and tubular dilation observed in HIV infection is sometimes termed *HIV-associated nephropathy* (HIVAN) (see Chapter 29).

The incidence of HIVAN in autopsy and biopsy varies with geographic location and ethnicity (Carbone et al., 1989). There is no relationship between HIVAN and patient age, duration of HIV infection, or opportunistic infections. About 90% of patients with HIVAN are black, 70% male, and 50% IV drug abusers. Patients with HIVAN have severe nephrotic syndrome and rapidly progress to ESRD. Hypertension is unusual.

Histologic features of HIVAN include a collapsing form of FSGS characterized by focal or complete occlusion of glomerular capillary tufts with hypertrophy and hyperplasia of the overlying visceral epithelial cells. The latter cells may display enlarged vesicular nuclei, mitotic figures, and protein resorption droplets. The severe tubulointerstitial disease is out of proportion to the glomerulosclerosis.

Electron microscopy shows wrinkling of GBM, visceral cell hypertrophy with foot process fusion, and tubuloreticular structures. Proposed mechanisms of

Figure 38-8 · Light microscopy of hepatitis C–related glomerulonephritis showing focal mesangial proliferation *(arrows)* and thickening of the capillary wall (PAS stain). (Courtesy of Dr. A.H. Cohen.)

HIVAN include direct injury to renal epithelial cells by cytopathic effects of viral infection, indirect injury to the kidney by renal uptake of circulating virus, and indirect injury from lymphocytes or monocytes infiltrating the kidney. HIV is present in renal epithelial cells, shown by in situ hybridization and PCR (Bruggeman et al., 2000).

Treatment with antiretrovirals is essential. ACE inhibitors early in the course may be beneficial. Immunosuppressives such as corticosteroids and CSA should be avoided.

Glomerulonephritis Associated with Parvovirus B19

Parvovirus B19 may cause GN in patients with sickle cell disease (SCD) or thrombotic microangiopathy in renal transplant recipients (Murer et al., 2000; Wierenga et al., 1995). Patients with SCD develop proteinuria, nephritic syndrome, and hematuria approximately 1 to 2 weeks after the onset of aplastic crisis. Most progress to chronic renal failure. Focal proliferative GN and FSGS are present in renal biopsies (Wierenga et al., 1995). Parvovirus has also been associated with idiopathic CG and FSGS (Moudgil, 2001; Tanawattanacharoen et al., 2000).

Parvovirus DNA was identified in the blood and renal biopsies of patients with idiopathic CG by PCR. Moudgil and colleagues (2001) found that parvovirus hybridization was localized to the parietal and visceral epithelial and tubular epithelial cells (Fig. 38-9). Direct infection of the renal epithelial cells may be pathogenic and is associated with long-standing viremia in some patients. African Americans seem particularly susceptible.

Specific antiviral therapy is unavailable. However, IVIG may help clear the virus (Mougdil et al., 1997).

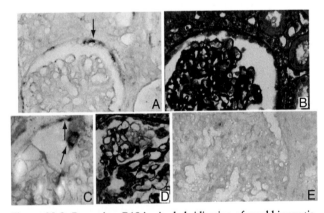

Figure 38-9· **Parvovirus B19 in situ hybridization of renal biopsy tissue from a patient with collapsing glomerulopathy and PV-B19 PCR positivity.** *A,* PV-B19 DNA positivity (parietal epithelial cells) *(arrow).* *C,* Enlarged glomerular epithelial cell *(arrow)* overlying a collapsed segment and adjacent parietal epithelium *(arrowhead),* both infected with PV-B19. *B* and *D,* Compare with periodic acid methenamine silver–stained sections. *E,* Negative controls. (From Moudgil A, Nast CC, Bagga A, Wei L, Nurmamet A, Cohen AH, Jordan SC. Association of parvovirus B-19 infection with idiopathic collapsing glomerulopathy. Kidney Int 59:2126–2133, 2001.)

IDIOPATHIC GLOMERULAR MEMBRANOUS NEPHROPATHY

Membranous nephropathy (MN) is the term used to distinguish thickened GBMs on light microscopy from the normal GBM in most patients with the nephrotic syndrome. Later, with the use of silver stain, the characteristic pattern of projections of the capillary wall, or spikes, was described.

MN is the most common cause of nephrotic syndrome in adults, whereas in children with nephrotic syndrome minimal change disease (see later discussion) is much more common. In the ISKDC, idiopathic membranous GN was found in only 1% of children with nephrotic syndrome (Barnett, 1976). MN can occur at any age. Habib and associates (1973a) reported two cases at 8 and 10 months of age. Adults usually develop idiopathic MN, whereas MN in childhood is usually secondary to systemic illness, notably hepatitis B and SLE.

Clinical Features

The Southwest Pediatric Nephrology study group reported that 45 of 54 MN patients, ranging in age from 6 to 15 years, presented with nephrotic syndrome. Eight presented with asymptomatic proteinuria, and 30 of 54 had microscopic hematuria (Group, 1986). Macroscopic hematuria and isolated microscopic hematuria are rare presentations, and hypertension at onset is uncommon. Renal function is usually normal initially. Serum complement levels are normal in most patients (Trainin et al., 1976).

Immunohistology

Under light microscopy, cellularity is normal, without mesangial cell proliferation, inflammatory cell infiltration, or increase of mesangial matrix. Crescents are only present in rapidly progressive GN. The key finding is a thickened GBM with spikes on silver staining or a vacuolated appearance on tangentially cut sections.

IF reveals a granular capillary wall staining for IgG, C3, and Ig light chains. Mesangial IgG or C1q staining is absent; if present, SLE should be suspected.

Pathogenesis

Initially, MN was thought to be due to the irregular deposition of circulating immune complexes in the GBM. However, the absence of circulating immune complexes and experimental observations suggested that the subepithelial immune deposits form in situ. Heymann nephritis is the characteristic animal model of human MN. The *Heymann nephritis antigen complex*

(HNAC) consists of two glycoproteins, megalin (gp330) and receptor-associated protein. The HNAC is expressed on the surface of glomerular epithelial cells where it is bound by antibody, crosslinked, shed, and then bound to GBM. The human equivalent of this epithelial glycoprotein complex has not been identified.

MN is characterized by glomerular deposits of IgG4 immune complexes, suggesting a Th2-derived defect. Wakui and associates (1999) found high levels of anti-α-enolase in patients with both primary and secondary MN. Because α-enolase antibodies have been reported in Th1-driven autoimmune disorders, MN patients may also have Th1-driven immunopathology.

Terminal complement components may play a major role in the glomerular dysfunction of MN. Proteinuria occurs when the membrane attack complex (C5b-9) is directed at glomerular epithelial cells, producing oxidants, proteases, and TGF-β. Depletion of C6 prevents the development of proteinuria in experimental MN in rats (Baker et al., 1989).

Whereas idiopathic MN may result from in situ immune complex formation, secondary MN results from the deposition of circulating immune complexes containing nonglomerular antigens such as microbial or tumor neoantigens. Lee and Koh (1989) found HBsAg in the immune complexes of MN associated with hepatitis B. Beauvais and co-workers (1989) reported a 7-year-old girl with MN and a benign ovarian tumor who had prompt resolution of the nephrotic syndrome following resection of the tumor.

Treatment

Children with asymptomatic proteinuria may not require treatment because they usually go into spontaneous remission. However, use of ACE inhibitors may decrease the proteinuria and help preserve renal function. Various small trials have demonstrated an approximately 50% reduction in proteinuria in patients treated with ACE inhibitors (Adler and Nast, 1998).

Treatment of children with more significant renal impairment is controversial. The Collaborative Study Group reported less deterioration of renal function in patients treated with 8 weeks of alternate-day prednisone. By contrast, Cattran and colleagues (1989) used alternate-day steroids for 6 months and found no benefit. Ponticelli and co-workers (1997) used IV methylprednisolone for 3 days followed by oral prednisone for 27 days alternating every other month with daily chlorambucil for a total of 6 months. Out of 32 patients, they reported complete remission in 12 and partial remission in 11 with good renal function after 5 years.

CSA has been used in steroid-resistant MN with reduction of proteinuria and remission of nephrotic syndrome. Rostoker and colleagues (1995a) obtained complete remission in 4 of 15 patients and reduction to non-nephrotic range proteinuria in another 7. Relapse occurred in three who were taken off the drug.

Other immunosuppressive drugs used in idiopathic MN include MMF and tacrolimus. Miller and co-workers (2000) used MMF in 16 nephrotic patients with pri-

mary MN; 15 were steroid resistant, 6 had failed cytotoxic agents, and 5 failed CSA. Patients were treated for a mean of 8 months. Overall, 8 patients had a significant decrease in proteinuria and serum cholesterol levels. Kobayashi and colleagues (1998) used tacrolimus on experimental MN in rats with significant reduction of proteinuria.

Nangaku and associates (1996) used IVIG in the Heymann nephritis model of MN and found a 52% reduction in proteinuria. However, subepithelial immune complex deposition and complement levels were not altered. Subsequent in vitro data showed that IgG resulted in reduced C5b-9-induced glomerular epithelial cell lysis, suggesting that IVIG modulates complement-mediated glomerular injury.

Berg and colleagues (1999) found that ACTH improved the serum lipoprotein profiles and glomerular function in MN patients. Treatment of idiopathic MN may retard progression of the disease in some, but who will benefit and the optimal treatment are not established.

Prognosis

Untreated idiopathic MN has a variable outcome. Those presenting with nephrotic syndrome and a normal GFR have a 30% chance of spontaneous complete remission. A spontaneous partial remission with stable GFR occurs in 25%, and persistent nephrotic syndrome with stable or slow loss of GFR occurs in 20% to 25%. The remaining 20% to 25% of MN patients progress to ESRD over a 20- to 30-year period (Adler and Nast, 1998).

Children have better prognoses than do adults. Habib and associates (1973a) reported a 10-year renal survival rate of 90% in 50 pediatric patients, most of whom were treated with cytotoxic drugs and/or prednisone. Other good prognostic factors include female gender; non-nephrotic range proteinuria; absence of focal sclerosis and tubulointerstitial changes; a low ultrastructural stage of the glomerular lesion; and HLA-DR2 rather than DR3, DR5, or B37 (Ponticelli et al., 1989).

MINIMAL CHANGE NEPHROPATHY (NEPHROSIS)

Minimal change nephropathy, or minimal change disease (MCD), is a clinicopathologic syndrome usually associated with the nephrotic syndrome of childhood. The nephrotic syndrome is characterized by marked proteinuria, hypoalbuminemia, edema, and hypercholesterolemia. Although numerous causes for the nephrotic syndrome have been described, all have increased permeability of the glomerular capillary to protein.

Idiopathic MCD of childhood (formerly termed *nephrosis*) is likely an immunologic disease mediated by circulating factor(s) that increase GBM permeability. Other causes of MCD include nonsteroidal anti-inflammatory agents, antibiotic sensitivity, toxins such as mercury and lead, allergic reactions to bee stings, infections such as EBV and HIV, immunizations, and tumors such as Hodgkin's and non-Hodgkin's lymphoma.

Many factors can injure the capillary basement membrane and lead to proteinuria. These include leukocyte lysosomal proteinases, circulating monocytes, chemical mediators, and complement-induced membrane injury. Yap and associates (1999) showed that patients with MCD in relapse had increased blood levels of IL-13. Because IL-13 is elevated in Hodgkin's lymphomas and other lymphomas, it may play a pivotal role in the pathogenesis of MCD.

Diagnosis

MCD is the most common cause of nephrotic syndrome in childhood. It is also termed lipoid or idiopathic nephrosis or nil or minimal lesion nephrotic syndrome. MCD has an abrupt onset and is usually not associated with hypertension or hematuria. If the GFR is depressed, MCD is almost always associated with a low plasma volume and decreased renal perfusion. Urinalysis reveals proteinuria with the absence of formed elements. Serum complement levels are normal, and autoimmune antibodies are also normal. Renal biopsy is usually not indicated in small children because their response to steroids confirms the diagnosis.

Pathogenesis

The cause of MCD is unknown. Light microscopy of biopsy specimens reveals normal or minimally abnormal foot processes and foot process fusion alone; by electron microscopy, no deposition of immune complexes, immunoglobulin, or complement is identified (Siegal et al., 1975). Very low levels of serum immunoglobulins are present, and antibody responses are sometimes decreased, sometimes resulting in a clinically significant immune deficiency with increased susceptibility to bacterial infections (see Chapter 25).

Immunologic abnormalities are not a proven cause of the increased glomerular capillary permeability, but abnormal T-cell function, possibly secondary to elevated lipid levels, has been associated with the nephrotic syndrome. Cytokine abnormalities may also contribute to the development of MCD.

The suggestion that aberrant immune processes are related to the occurrence of MCD is based on its association with certain infections such as HIV and malaria; its remission during measles infection; its association with Hodgkin's disease (with IL-13 over expression), thymoma, bone marrow transplantation, and IFN therapy; and its responsiveness to immunosuppressive medications. The use of immunostimulants such as levamisole may sustain steroid-induced remission. Relapses may be precipitated by viral infections or other immune disorders such as asthma or allergies (Th2 stimuli).

Treatment

The therapy for MCD is corticosteroids, and this is generally highly effective (>95%) in most patients. The good response to corticosteroids is considered diagnostic of MCD. Children usually respond to treatment within 2 weeks, with massive diuresis, weight loss, and disappearance of proteinuria. Other biochemical abnormalities correct with resolution of the nephrotic syndrome.

Patients who respond to steroids with complete remission within 8 to 12 weeks and who have infrequent or no relapses are defined as *steroid sensitive.* Those who have frequent relapses when steroids are tapered are termed *steroid dependent,* and those who fail to respond to steroids at all are termed *steroid resistant.* Steroid-dependent patients often stabilize with reduced or no need for steroids after a 3-month course of cyclophosphamide or chlorambucil. Most steroid-resistant patients do not respond to short courses of cytotoxic drugs but may respond to long-term daily CSA therapy. Bagga and colleagues (1996) found that steroid dependency may be significantly reduced with a 3-month course of MMF.

FOCAL SEGMENTAL GLOMERULOSCLEROSIS

Focal segmental glomerulosclerosis (FSGS) is a clinical and pathologic entity that may occur as a primary or secondary disease. Primary FSGS may initially be confused with MCD, but steroid resistance and progression to ESRD differentiate the two.

Two primary forms of FSGS include IgM nephropathy and collapsing FSGS. Secondary FSGS may occur in nonimmunologic disorders, including unilateral renal agenesis, renal ablation, morbid obesity, reflux nephropathy, cyanotic heart disease, or postnephrectomy. In these secondary cases, hyperfiltration injury may occur with resultant loss of functioning nephrons. Secondary FSGS may also occur in heroin addicts and in patients with HIV infection.

Pathogenesis

The cause of primary FSGS is not known. In addition, the multiple pathologic features of FSGS range from classic focal sclerotic glomeruli surrounded by normal glomeruli to glomerular tip lesions characterized by swelling, vacuolization, and proliferation of epithelial cells progressing to sclerosis and hyalinosis in segments of the glomeruli adjacent to the origin of the proximal tubule.

Another variant of FSGS is associated with focal or global glomerular capillary collapse and sclerosis with visceral epithelial cell swelling. This was first described in HIV-infected patients and was deemed HIV nephropathy. Collapsing FSGS is a malignant form of glomerulosclerosis seen frequently in African-American patients with a rapidly progressing course leading to ESRD.

Not all patients with collapsing FSGS are HIV positive. Moudgil and colleagues (2001) reported that 80% of idiopathic FSGS patients have parvovirus B19 of parietal, visceral, and tubular epithelial cells by in situ hybridization techniques. Thus this virus should be considered in the diagnostic workup of idiopathic FSGS patients.

Dantal and associates (1994) showed that a 50-kD protein was present in the serum of FSGS patients, which was absorbable on protein A but was not an immunoglobulin. Its presence predicted the rapid development of nephrotic syndrome after transplantation. This suggests that FSGS may be caused by a circulating protein that persists even after kidney failure. This factor induces nephrotic syndrome in an allograft that will, if left untreated, progress to ESRD. This factor should be theoretically eliminated by plasma exchange or protein A column absorption, but to date, such therapies have been variably effective.

As previously described, patients with hyperfiltration injury, hyperlipidemia, obesity, or chronic hypoxia may develop FSGS. Thus FSGS is the end result of several distinct pathologic entities with different clinical courses. It is critical to define the cause of FSGS so as to avoid the use of steroids and cytotoxic drugs in patients with nonimmunologic causes.

Diagnosis

The diagnosis of FSGS requires a renal biopsy because there are no distinctive laboratory markers. Complement levels and tests for autoantibodies and other immunologic markers are usually normal. The biopsy reveals classic FSGS or one of the previously described variants. Diagnostic clues to secondary forms of FSGS may include extensive tubulointerstitial nephritis in heroin nephrotoxicity and collapsing FSGS in HIV and parvovirus B19 nephritis. Immunostains for these viruses can confirm the diagnosis. In patients with remnant kidneys and hyperfiltration-induced injury, there is usually less effacement of the GBMs.

Treatment and Prognosis

Most untreated FSGS patients, if left untreated, will progress to ESRD with spontaneous remission uncommon. Patients with collapsing FSGS have more rapid decline in renal function, with progression to ESRD within 1 to 3 years.

Because of the multiple causes for FSGS, therapy is not standardized. Studies before 1985 indicated that only 10% to 30% of FSGS patients responded to steroids or cytotoxic drugs. Thus most nephrologists chose not to treat such patients. Recent trials have indicated that long-term treatment with prednisone and cytotoxic drugs results in a 25% to 60% remission rate. Ponticelli and colleagues (1993) showed that CSA can result in greater than 70% remission rates in both pediatric and adult FSGS patients. However, some patients experience CSA-related nephrotoxicity. Aggressive initial therapy

may not be warranted in mild proteinuria. Treatment with ACE inhibitors alone may decrease proteinuria and minimize sclerosis and reduce the risk of ESRD.

Treatment of secondary FSGS should be aimed at the primary cause. Patients with heroin nephropathy or obesity-related FSGS may experience remissions with cessation of heroin use and weight loss, respectively. Parvovirus-associated FSGS may respond well to IVIG therapy.

REFERENCES

Adler S, Nast C. Membranous nephropathy. In Greenberg A, Cheung A, Coffman T, Falk R, Jennette J, eds. Primer on Kidney Diseases. San Diego, Academic Press, 1998, pp 164–170.

Allen AC, Willis FR, Beattie TJ, Feehally J. Abnormal IgA glycosylation in Henoch-Schönlein purpura restricted to patients with clinical nephritis. Nephrol Dial Transplant 13:930–934, 1998.

Amato M, Salvadori M. Can plasmapheresis improve lupus nephritis without its immunological markers? Nephron 48:252–253, 1988.

Ault BH. Factor H and the pathogenesis of renal diseases. Pediatr Nephrol 14:1045–1053, 2000.

Austin HA, Klippel JH, Balow JE, le Riche NG, Steinberg AD, Plotz PH, Decker JL. Therapy of lupus nephritis. Controlled trial of prednisone and cytotoxic drugs. N Engl J Med 314:614–619, 1986.

Bagga A, Vasudev AS, Moudgil A, Srivastava RN. Peripheral blood lymphocyte subsets in idiopathic nephrotic syndrome of childhood. Indian J Med Res 104:292–295, 1996.

Baker PJ, Ochi RF, Schulze M, Johnson RJ, Campbell C, Couser WG. Depletion of C6 prevents development of proteinuria in experimental membranous nephropathy in rats. Am J Pathol 135:185–194, 1989.

Balow JE. Renal manifestations of systemic lupus erythematosus and other rheumatic disorders. In Greenberg A, Cheung A, Coffman T, Falk R, Jennette J, eds. Primer on Kidney Diseases. San Diego, Academic Press, 1998, pp 208–211.

Barnett H. The natural and treatment history of glomerular disease in children—what can we learn from cooperative studies? In Proceedings of the VIth Congress of the ISN 1976, pp 470–485.

Barron KS, Person DA, Brewer EJ Jr, Beale MG, Robson AM. Pulse methylprednisolone therapy in diffuse proliferative lupus nephritis. J Pediatr 101:137–141, 1982.

Beauvais P, Vuadour G, Boccon Gibod L, Levy M. Membranous nephropathy associated with ovarian tumour in a young girl: recovery after removal. Eur J Pediatr 148:624–625, 1989.

Bennett SR, Carbone FR, Karamalis F, Flavell RA, Miller JF, Heath WR. Help for cytotoxic-T-cell responses is mediated by CD40 signalling. Nature 393:478–480, 1998.

Berg AL, Nilsson-Ehle P, Arnadottir M. Beneficial effects of ACTH on the serum lipoprotein profile and glomerular function in patients with membranous nephropathy. Kidney Int 56:1534–1543, 1999.

Berger J, Hinglais N. Intercapillary deposits of IgA-IgG. J Urol Nephrol 74:694–695, 1968.

Bergstein J, Leiser J, Andreoli SP. Response of crescentic Henoch-Schönlein purpura nephritis to corticosteroid and azathioprine therapy. Clin Nephrol 49:9–14, 1998.

Berthoux FC, Alamartine E, Pommier G, Lepetit JC. HLA and IgA nephritis revisited 10 years later: HLA-B35 antigen as a prognostic factor. N Engl J Med 319:1609–1610, 1988.

Blowey DL. Nephrotic syndrome associated with an Epstein-Barr virus infection. Pediatr Nephrol 10:507–508, 1996.

Boes MT, Schmidt T, Linkeman K, Beaudette BC, Marshak-Rothstein A, Chen J. Accelerated development of IgG autoantibodies and autoimmune disease in the absence of secreted IgM. Proc Natl Acad Sci USA 97:1184–1189, 2000.

Bolton WK, Sturgill BC. Methylprednisolone therapy for acute crescentic rapidly progressive glomerulonephritis. Am J Nephrol 9:368–375, 1989.

Bonavida B. Immunomodulatory effect of tumor necrosis factor. Biotherapy 3:127–133, 1991.

Border WA, Noble NA. Targeting TGF-beta for treatment of disease [letter; comment]. Nat Med 1:1000–1001, 1995.

Briere F, Bridon JM, Chevet D, Souillet G, Bienvenu F, Guret C, Martinez-Valdez H, Banchereau J. Interleukin 10 induces B lymphocytes from IgA-deficient patients to secrete IgA. J Clin Invest 94:97–104, 1994.

Bruce J. IgA nephropathy. In Greenberg A, Cheung A, Coffman T, Falk R Jennette J, eds. Primer on Kidney Diseases. San Diego, Academic Press, 1998, pp 170–175.

Bruggeman LA, Ross MD, Tanji N, Cara A, Dikman S, Gordon RE, Burns GC, D'Agati VD, Winston JA, Klotman ME, Klotman PE. Renal epithelium is a previously unrecognized site of HIV-1 infection. J Am Soc Nephrol 11:2079–87, 2000.

Cameron JS, Turner DR, Heaton J, Williams DG, Ogg CS, Chantler C, Haycock GB, Hicks J. Idiopathic mesangiocapillary glomerulonephritis. Comparison of types I and II in children and adults and long-term prognosis. Am J Med 74:175–192, 1983.

Carbone LV, D'Agati VD, Cheng JT, Appel GB. Course and prognosis of human immunodeficiency virus-associated nephropathy. Am J Med 87:389–395, 1989.

Cattran DC, Delmore T, Roscoe J, Cole E, Cardella C, Charron R, Ritchied S. A randomized controlled trial of prednisone in patients with idiopathic membranous nephropathy. N Engl J Med 320:210–215, 1989.

Cazac BB, Roes J. TGF-beta receptor controls B cell responsiveness and induction of IgA in vivo. Immunity 13:443–451, 2000.

Chan TM, Li FK, Tang CS, Wong RW, Fang GX, Ji YL, Lau CS, Wong AK, Tong MK, Chan KW, Lai KN. Efficacy of mycophenolate mofetil in patients with diffuse proliferative lupus nephritis. Hong Kong-Guangzhou Nephrology Study Group. N Engl J Med 343:1156–1162, 2000.

Chen S, Bacon KB, Li L, Garcia GE, Xia Y, Lo D, Thompson DA, Sinai MA, Yamamoto T, Harrison JK, Feng L. In vivo inhibition of CC and CX3C chemokine-induced leukocyte infiltration and attenuation of glomerulonephritis in Wistar-Kyoto (WKY) rats by vMIP-II. J Exp Med 188:193–198, 1998.

Cher DJ, Mosmann TR. Two types of murine helper T cell clone. II. Delayed-type hypersensitivity is mediated by TH1 clones. J Immunol 138:3688–3694, 1987.

Cibrik D, Sedor J. Immunopathogenesis of renal disease. In Greenberg A, Cheung A, Coffman T, Falk R, Jennette J, eds. Primer on Kidney Diseases. San Diego, Academic Press, 1998, pp 141–149.

Cinotti GA, Pierucci A. Renal effects of nonsteroidal anti-inflammatory drugs and thromboxane receptor antagonists in chronic glomerular disease. Am J Nephrol 9:47–50, 1989.

Cohen A, Nast C. Renal pathology. In Anderson WAD, ed. Anderson's Pathology. St. Louis, Mosby, 1996, pp 2073–2131.

Conjeevaram HS, Hoofnagle JH, Austin HA, Park Y, Fried MW, Di Bisceglie AM. Long-term outcome of hepatitis B virus-related glomerulonephritis after therapy with interferon alfa. Gastroenterology 109:540–546, 1995.

Couser WG, Salant DJ. In situ immune complex formation and glomerular injury. Kidney Int 17:1–13, 1980.

D'Agati V. Membranoproliferative glomerulonephritis. In Greenberg A, Cheung A, Coffman T, Falk R, Jennette J, eds. Primer on Kidney Diseases. San Diego, Academic Press, 1998, pp 153–160.

D'Amico G. Influence of clinical and histological features on actuarial renal survival in adult patients with idiopathic IgA nephropathy, membranous nephropathy, and membranoproliferative glomerulonephritis: survey of the recent literature. Am J Kidney Dis 20:315–323, 1992.

Daniel CR, Ziswiler R, Frey B, Pfister M, Marti HP. Proinflammatory effects in experimental mesangial glomerulonephritis of the agent SDZ RAD, a rapamycin derivative. Exp Nephrol 8:52–62, 2000.

Dantal J, Bigot E, Bogers W, Testa A, Kriaa F, Jacques Y, Hurault de Ligny B, Niaudet P, Charpentier B, Soulillou JP. Effect of plasma protein adsorption on protein excretion in kidney-transplant recipients with recurrent nephrotic syndrome. N Engl J Med 330:7–14, 1994.

DeKruyff RH, Ju ST, Hunt AJ, Mosmann TR, Umetsu DT. Induction of antigen-specific antibody responses in primed and unprimed B cells. Functional heterogeneity among Th1 and Th2 T cell clones. J Immunol 142:2575–582, 1989.

Derksen RH, Hene RJ, Kallenberg CG, Valentijn RM, Kater L. Prospective multicentre trial on the short-term effects of plasma exchange versus cytotoxic drugs in steroid-resistant lupus nephritis. Neth J Med 33:168–177, 1988.

de Waal Malefyt RJ, Haanen J, Spits H, Roncarolo MG, te Velde A, Figdor C, Johnson K, Kastelein R, Yssel H, de Vries JE. Interleukin 10 (IL-10) and viral IL-10 strongly reduce antigen-specific human T cell proliferation by diminishing the antigen-presenting capacity of monocytes via downregulation of class II major histocompatibility complex expression. J Exp Med 174:915–924, 1991.

Dillon HC Jr, Reeves MS, Streptococcal immune responses in nephritis after skin infections. Am J Med 56:333–346, 1974.

Dodge WF, Spargo BH, Travis LB, Srivastava RN, Carvajal HF, DeBeukelaer MM, Longley MP, Menchaca JA. Poststreptococcal glomerulonephritis. A prospective study in children. N Engl J Med 286:273–278, 1972.

Donadio JV Jr, Bergstralh EJ, Offord KP, Spencer DC, Holley KE. A controlled trial of fish oil in IgA nephropathy. Mayo Nephrology Collaborative Group. N Engl J Med 331:1194–1199, 1994.

Dorner T, Putterman C. B Cells, BAFF/zTNF4, TACI, and systemic lupus erythematosus. Arthritis Res 3:197–199, 2001.

Duvall-Young J, MacDonald MK, McKechnie NM. Fundus changes in (type II) mesangiocapillary glomerulonephritis simulating drusen: a histopathological report. Br J Ophthalmol 73:297–302, 1989.

Emancipator SN, Lamm ME. The role of IgG, IgM, and C3 in experimental murine IgA nephropathy. Semin Nephrol 7:286–288, 1987.

Endre ZH, Pussel BA, Charlesworth JA, Coovadia HM, Seedat YK. C3 metabolism in acute glomerulonephritis: implications for sites of complement activation. Kidney Int 25:937–941, 1984.

Erbay B, Karatan O, Duman N, Ertug AE. The effect of cyclosporine in idiopathic nephrotic syndrome resistant to immunosuppressive therapy. Transplant Proc 20:289–292, 1988.

Ewert BH, Jenette JC, Falk RJ. Anti-myeloperoxidase antibodies stimulate neutrophils to damage human endothelial cells. Kidney Int 41:375–383, 1992.

Faedda R, Satta A, Tanda F, Pirisi M, Bartoli E. Immunosuppressive treatment of membranoproliferative glomerulonephritis. Nephron 67:59–65, 1994.

Falk RJ, Terrell RS, Charles LA, Jennette JC. Anti-neutrophil cytoplasmic autoantibodies induce neutrophils to degranulate and produce oxygen radicals in vitro. Proc Natl Acad Sci USA 87:4115–4119, 1990.

Fauci AS, Katz P, Haynes BF, Wolff SM. Cyclophosphamide therapy of severe systemic necrotizing vasculitis. N Engl J Med 301:235–238, 1979.

Favre H, Mieschler PA, Huang YP, Chatelanat F, Mihatsch MJ. Cyclosporin in the treatment of lupus nephritis. Am J Nephrol 9:57–60, 1989.

Feehally J. IgA nephropathy—a disorder of IgA production? Q J Med 90:387–390, 1997.

Fillit HM, Zabriskie JB. New concepts of glomerular injury. Lab Invest 51:117–120, 1984.

Fischel E. Serum complement in acute glomerulonephritis and other renal diseases. Am J Med 12:190–196, 1952.

Fish AJ, Michael AF, Vernier RL, Good, RA. Acute serum sickness nephritis in the rabbit. An immune deposit disease. Am J Path 49:997–1022, 1966.

Fisher ER, Reidbord H. Relationship of antibody localization to lesions in nephrotoxic serum nephritis. Nephron 8:566–74, 1971.

Fogazzi GB, Pasquali S, Moriggi M, Casanova S, Damilano I, Mihatsch MJ, Zuchelloi P, Ponticelli C. Long-term outcome of Schönlein-Henoch nephritis in the adult. Clin Nephrol 31:60–66, 1989.

Foster BJ, Bernard C, Drummond KN, Sharma AK. Effective therapy for severe Henoch-Schönlein purpura nephritis with prednisone and azathioprine: a clinical and histopathologic study. J Pediatr 136:370–375, 2000.

Fournie GJ. Circulating DNA and lupus nephritis. Kidney Int 33:487–497, 1988.

Gaskin G, Pusey CD. Plasmapheresis in antineutrophil cytoplasmic antibody-associated systemic vasculitis. Ther Apher 5:176–181, 2001.

Grant SC, Lsamb WR, Brooks NH, Brenchley PE, Hutchinson IV. Serum cytokines in human heart transplant recipients. Is there a relationship to rejection? Transplantation 62:480–491, 1996.

Gross JA, Johnston J, Mudri S, Enselman R, Dillon SR, Madden K, Xu W, Parrish-Novak J, Foster D, Lofton-day C, Moore M, Littau A, Grossman A, Haugen H, Foley K, Blumberg H, Harrison K, Kindsvogel W, Clegg CH. TACI and BCMA are receptors for a TNF homologue implicated in B-cell autoimmune disease. Nature 404:995–999, 2000.

Group SPNS. Comparison of idiopathic and systemic lupus erythematosus associated membranous glomerulonephritis in children. Am J Kidney Dis 7:115–124, 1986.

Gumber SC, Chopra S. Hepatitis C: a multifaceted disease. Review of extrahepatic manifestations. Ann Intern Med 123:615–620, 1995.

Habib R, Kleinknecht C, Gubler MC. Extramembranous glomerulonephritis in children: report of 50 cases. J Pediatr 82:754–766, 1973a.

Habib RC, Kleinknecht C, Gubler MC, Levy M. Idiopathic membranoproliferative glomerulonephritis in children. Report of 105 cases. Clin Nephrol 1:194–214, 1973b.

Hadley GA, Bartlett ST, Via CS, Rostapshova EA, Moainie S. The epithelial cell-specific integrin, CD103 (alpha E integrin), defines a novel subset of alloreactive CD8+ CTL. J Immunol 159:3748–3756, 1997.

Harding FA, McArthur JC, Gross JA, Raulet DH, Allison JP. CD28-mediated signalling co-stimulates murine T cells and prevents induction of anergy T-cell clones. Nature 356:607–609, 1992.

Hasegawa A, Kawamura T, Ito H, Hasegawa O, Ogawa O, Honda M, Ohara T, Hajikano H. Fate of renal grafts with recurrent Henoch-Schönlein purpura nephritis in children. Transplant Proc 21:2130–2133, 1989.

Hattori M, Ito K, Konomoto T, Kawaguchi H, Yoshioka T, Khono M. Plasmapheresis as the sole therapy for rapidly progressive Henoch-Schönlein purpura nephritis in children. Am J Kidney Dis 33:427–433, 1999.

Heaton JM, Turnet DR, Cameron JS. Localization of glomerular "deposits" in Henoch–Schönlein nephritis. Histopathology 1:93–104, 1977.

Hisada Y, Sugaya T, Yamanouchi M, Uchida H, Fujimura H, Sakurai H, Fukamizu A, Murakami K. Angiotensin II plays a pathogenic role in immune-mediated renal injury in mice. J Clin Invest 103:627–635, 1999.

Hoffman GS, Kerr GS, Leavitt RY, Hallahan CW, Lebovicw RS, Travis WD, Rottem M, Fauci AS. Wegener granulomatosis: an analysis of 158 patients. Ann Intern Med 116:488–498, 1992.

Holdsworth SR, Kitching AR, Tipping PG. Th1 and Th2 T helper cell subsets affect patterns of injury and outcomes in glomerulonephritis. Kidney Int 55:1198–1216, 1999.

Hooper WC. The role of transforming growth factor-beta in hematopoiesis. A review. Leuk Res 15:179–184, 1991.

Hruby Z, Kuzniar J, Rabczynski J, Bogucki J, Steciwko A, Weyde W. The variety of clinical and histopathologic presentations of glomerulonephritis associated with latent syphilis. Int Urol Nephrol 24:541–547, 1992.

Hsu DH, de Waal Malefyt R, Fiorentino DF, Dang MN, Vieira P, de Vries J, Spits H, Mosmann TR, Moore KW. Expression of interleukin-10 activity by Epstein-Barr virus protein BCRF1. Science 250:830–832, 1990.

Huang XR, Tipping PG, Apostolopoulos J, Oettinger C, D'Souza M, Milton G, Holdsworth IV. Mechanisms of T cell-induced glomerular injury in anti-glomerular basement membrane (GBM) glomerulonephritis in rats. Clin Exp Immunol 109:134–142, 1997.

Hutchinson IV. The role of transforming growth factor-beta in transplant rejection. Transplant Proc 31:9S–13S, 1999.

Imai H, Chen A, Wyatt RJ, Rifai A. Lack of complement activation by human IgA immune complexes. Clin Exp Immunol 73:479–483, 1988.

Jackson A, Palmer S, Davis RD, Pappendick A, Pearson E, Savik K, Ormaza S, Hertz M, Dacey M, Miller L, Reinsmoen NL. Cytokine genotypes in kidney, heart, and lung recipients: consequences for acute and chronic rejection. Transplant Proc 33:489–490, 2001.

Jacob CO, McDevitt HO. Tumour necrosis factor-alpha in murine autoimmune 'lupus' nephritis. Nature 331:356–358, 1988.

Jacquot C, Thoua Y, Dupont E, Vereerstraeten P. Recidive de granulomatose de Wegener sur une greffe de rein de cadavre. Nephrologie 11:97–103, 1990.

Jayne DR, Esnault VL, Lockwood CM. ANCA anti-idiotype antibodies and the treatment of systemic vasculitis with intravenous immunoglobulin. J Autoimmun 6:207–219, 1993.

Jayne DR, Lockwood CM. High-dose pooled immunoglobulin in the therapy of systemic vasculitis. Trans Am Assoc Physicians 104:304–312, 1991.

Jefferson JA, Johnson RJ. Treatment of hepatitis C–associated glomerular disease. Semin Nephrol 20:286–292, 2000.

Jennette JC, Falk RJ. Antineutrophil cytoplasmic autoantibodies and associated diseases: a review. Am J Kidney Dis 15:517–529, 1990.

Jennette JC, Wilkman AS, Falk RJ. Anti-neutrophil cytoplasmic autoantibody-associated glomerulonephritis and vasculitis. Am J Pathol 135:921–930, 1989.

Kashiwabara H, Shishido H, Tomura S, Tuchida H, Miyajima T. Strong association between IgA nephropathy and HLA-DR4 antigen. Kidney Int 22:377–382, 1982.

Kirk AD, Burkly LC, Batty DS, Baumgartner RE, Bering JD, Buchanan K, Fechner JH Jr, Germond RL, Kampen RL, Patterson NB, Swanson SJ, Tadaki DK, TenHoor CN, White L, Knechtle SJ, Harlan DM. Treatment with humanized monoclonal antibody against CD154 prevents acute renal allograft rejection in nonhuman primates. Nat Med 5:686–693, 1999.

Kobayashi M, Muro K, Yoh K, Kondoh M, Iwabuchi S, Hirayama K, Ishizu T, Kikuchi S, Yamaguchi N, Koyama A. Effects of FK506 on experimental membranous glomerulonephritis induced by cationized bovine serum albumin in rats. Nephrol Dial Transplant 13:2501–2508, 1998.

Kontoyiannis D, Kollias G. Accelerated autoimmunity and lupus nephritis in NZB mice with an engineered heterozygous deficiency in tumor necrosis factor. Eur J Immunol 30:2038–2047, 2000.

Kuhn R, Lohler J, Rennick D, Rajewsky K, Muller W. Interleukin-10-deficient mice develop chronic enterocolitis. Cell 75:263–274, 1993.

Kulkarni AB, Karlsson S. Transforming growth factor-beta 1 knockout mice. A mutation in one cytokine gene causes a dramatic inflammatory disease. Am J Pathol 143:3–9, 1993.

Kunis CL, Kiss B, Williams G, D'Agati V, Appel GB. Intravenous "pulse" cyclophosphamide therapy of crescentic glomerulonephritis. Clin Nephrol 37:1–7, 1992.

Lai KN, Ho RT, Tam JS, Lai FM. Detection of hepatitis B virus DNA and RNA in kidneys of HBV related glomerulonephritis. Kidney Int 50:1965–1977, 1996.

Lai KN, Lai FM, Chui SH, Chan YM, Tsao GS, Leung KN, Lam C. Studies of lymphocyte subpopulations and immunoglobulin production in IgA nephropathy. Clin Nephrol 28:281–287, 1987.

Lai KN, Li PK, Lui SF, Au TC, Tam JS, Tong KL, Lai FM. Membranous nephropathy related to hepatitis B virus in adults. N Engl J Med 324:1457–1463, 1991.

Laine J, Jalanko H, Holthofer H, Krogerus L, Rapola J, von Willebrand D, Lautenschlager I, Salmela K, Holmberg C. Post-transplantation nephrosis in congenital nephrotic syndrome of the Finnish type. Kidney Int 44:867–874, 1993.

Laitman RS, Glicklich D, Sablay LB, Grayzel AI, Barland P, Bank N. Effect of long-term normalization of serum complement levels on the course of lupus nephritis. Am J Med 87:132–138, 1989.

Lake RA, Staines NA. A monoclonal DNA-binding autoantibody causes a deterioration in renal function in MRL mice with lupus disease. Clin Exp Immunol 73:103–110, 1988.

Laman JD, Claassen E, Noelle RJ. Functions of CD40 and its ligand, gp39 (CD40L). Crit Rev Immunol 16:59–108, 1996.

Lange KG, Seligson G, Cronin W. Evidence for the in situ origin of poststreptococcal glomerulonephritis: glomerular localization of endostreptosin and the clinical significance of the subsequent antibody response. Clin Nephrol 19:3–10, 1983.

Larsen CP, Pearson TC. The CD40 pathway in allograft rejection, acceptance, and tolerance. Curr Opin Immunol 9:641–647, 1997.

Lebman DA, Lee FD, Coffman RL. Mechanism for transforming growth factor beta and IL-2 enhancement of IgA expression in lipopolysaccharide-stimulated B cell cultures. J Immunol 144:952–959, 1990.

Lee HS, Koh HI. Hepatitis B e antigen-associated membranous nephropathy. Nephron 52:356–359, 1989.

Leeuwenberg JF, Jeunhomme TM, Buurman WA. Slow release of soluble TNF receptors by monocytes in vitro. J Immunol 152:4036–4043, 1994.

Levy Y, George J, Yona E, Shoenfeld Y. Partial lipodystrophy, mesangiocapillary glomerulonephritis, and complement dysregulation. An autoimmune phenomenon. Immunol Res 18:55–60,1998.

Levy Y, Sherer Y, Geroge J, Rovensky J, Lukac J, Rauova L, Poprac P, Langevitz P, Fabbrissi F, Shoenfeld Y. Intravenous immuneglobulin treatment of lupus nephritis. Semin Arthritis Rheum 5:321–327, 2000.

Lin CY. Clinical features and natural course of HBV-related glomerulopathy in children. Kidney Int 35:S46–53, 1991.

Lin H, Bolling SF, Linsley PS, Wei RQ, Gordon D, Thompson CB, Turka LA. Long-term acceptance of major histocompatibility complex mismatched cardiac allografts induced by CTLA4Ig plus donor-specific transfusion. J Exp Med 178:1801–1806, 1993.

Ma J, Xu J, Madaio MP, Peng Q, Zhang J, Grewal IS, Flavell RA, Craft J. Autoimmune lpr/lpr mice deficient in CD40 ligand: spontaneous Ig class switching with dichotomy of autoantibody responses. J Immunol 157:417–426, 1996.

Matriano JA, Socarras S, Streilein JW. Cellular mechanisms that maintain neonatally-induced tolerance of class II alloantigens. Evidence that factor-mediated suppression silences cytotoxic T cell activity. J Immunol 153:1505–1514, 1994.

Matsumura Y, Zuo XJ, Prehn J, Linsley PS, Marchevsky A, Kass RM, Matlof JM, Jordan SC. Soluble CTLA4Ig modifies parameters of acute inflammation in rat lung allograft rejection without altering lymphocytic infiltration or transcription of key cytokines. Transplantation 59:551–558, 1995.

McCune WJ, Golbus J, Zeldes W, Bohlke P, Dunne R, Fox DA. Clinical and immunologic effects of monthly administration of intravenous cyclophosphamide in severe systemic lupus erythematosus. N Engl J Med 318:1423–1431, 1988.

McEnery PT. Membranoproliferative glomerulonephritis: the Cincinnati experience–cumulative renal survival from 1957 to 1989. J Pediatr 116:S109–14, 1990.

Meroni PL, Del Papa N, Raschi E, Panzeri P, Borghi MO. Is there any pathogenic role for the anti-endothelial cell antibodies (AECA) in autoimmune vasculitis? J Biol Regul Homeost Agents 11:127–132, 1997.

Meulders Q, Pirson Y, Cosyns JP, Squifflet JP, van Ypersele de Strihou C. Course of Henoch-Schönlein nephritis after renal transplantation. Report on ten patients and review of the literature. Transplantation 58:1179–1186, 1994.

Miller G, Zimmerman R III, Radhakrishnan J, Appel G. Use of mycophenolate mofetil in resistant membranous nephropathy. Am J Kidney Dis 36:250–256, 2000.

Miyagawa S, Dohi K, Hanatani M, Yamanaka F, Okuchi T, Sakamoto K, Ishikawa H. Anaphylactoid purpura and familial IgA nephropathy. Am J Med 86:340–342, 1989.

Montalbert C, Carvallo A, Broumand B, Noble D, Anstine LA, Currier CB Jr. Successful renal transplantation in polyarteritis nodosa. Clin Nephrol 14:206–209, 1980.

Montseny JJ, Meyrier A, Kleinknecht D, Callard P. The current spectrum of infectious glomerulonephritis. Experience with 76 patients and review of the literature. Medicine 74:63–73, 1995.

Morin MP, Thervet D, Legendre C, Pge B, Kreis H, Noel LH. Successful kidney transplantation in a patient with microscopic polyarteritis and positive ANCA. Nephrol Dial Transplant 8:287–288, 1993.

Mosmann TR, Coffman RL. TH1 and TH2 cells: different patterns of lymphokine secretion lead to different functional properties. Annu Rev Immunol 7:145–173, 1989.

Mosmann TR, Moore KW. The role of IL-10 in crossregulation of TH1 and TH2 responses. Immunol Today 12:A49–53, 1991.

Mosmann TR, Schumacher JH, Fiorentino DF, Leverah J, Moore KW, Bond MW. Isolation of monoclonal antibodies specific for IL-4, IL-5, IL-6, and a new Th2-specific cytokine (IL-10), cytokine synthesis inhibitory factor, by using a solid phase radioimmunosorbent assay. J Immunol 145:2938–2945, 1990.

Moudgil A, Bagga A, Fredrich R, Jordan SC. Post-streptococcal and other infection-related glomerulonephritides. In Greenberg A, Cheung A, Coffman T, Falk R, Jennette J, eds. Primer on Kidney Diseases. San Diego, Academic Press, 1998, pp 193–200.

Moudgil A, Nast CC, Bagga A, Wei L, Nurmamet A, Cohen AH, Jordan SC. Association of parvovirus B-19 infection with idiopathic collapsing glomerulopathy. Kidney Int 59:2126–2133, 2001.

Moudgil A, Shidban H, Nast CC, Bagga A, Aswad S, Graham SL, Mendez R, Jordan SC. Parvovirus B19 infection-related complications in renal transplant recipients: treatment with intravenous immunoglobulin. Transplantation 64:1847–1850, 1997.

Murer L, Zachello G, Bianchi D, Dall'Amico R, Montini G, Andreeta B, Perini M, Dossi EC, Zanon G, Zacchello F. Thrombotic microangiopathy associated with parvovirus B 19 infection after renal transplantation. J Am Soc Nephrol 11:1132–1137, 2000.

Nagy J, Uj M, Szucs G, Trinn C, Burger T. Herpes virus antigens and antibodies in kidney biopsies and sera of IgA glomerulonephritic patients. Clin Nephrol 21:259–262, 1984.

Nakajima A, Hirai H, Kayagaki N, Yoshino S, Hirose S, Yagita H, Okumura K. Treatment of lupus in NZB/W F1 mice with monoclonal antibody against Fas ligand. J Autoimmun 14:151–157, 2000.

Nakamura A, Yuasa T, Ujike A, Ono M, Nukiwa T, Ravetch JV, Takai T. Fcgamma receptor IIB-deficient mice develop Goodpasture's syndrome upon immunization with type IV collagen: a novel murine model for autoimmune glomerular basement membrane disease. J Exp Med 191:899–906, 2000.

Nangaku M, Pippin J, Richardson CA, Schulze M, Young BA, Alpers CE, Gordon KL, Johnson RJ, Couser WG. Beneficial effects of systemic immunoglobulin in experimental membranous nephropathy. Kidney Int 50:2054–2062, 1996.

Nast CC, Moudgil A, Zuo XJ, Toyoda M, Jordan SC. Long-term allograft acceptance in a patient with posttransplant lymphoproliferative disorder: correlation with intragraft viral interleukin-10. Transplantation 64:1578–1582, 1997.

Niaudet P, Habib R. Methylprednisolone pulse therapy in the treatment of severe forms of Schönlein-Henoch purpura nephritis. Pediatr Nephrol 12:238–243, 1998.

Nishikawa K, Linsley PS, Collins AB, Stamenkovic I, McCluskey RT, Andres G. Effect of CTLA-4 chimeric protein on rat autoimmune anti-glomerular basement membrane glomerulonephritis. Eur J Immunol 24:1249–1254, 1994.

Nolasco FE, Cameron JS, Hartley B, Coelho A, Hildreth G, Reuben R. Intraglomerular T cells and monocytes in nephritis: study with monoclonal antibodies. Kidney Int 31:1160–1166, 1987.

Nordstrand A, Norgren M, Ferretti JJ, Holm SE. Streptokinase as a mediator of acute post-streptococcal glomerulonephritis in an experimental mouse model. Infect Immun 66:315–321, 1998.

Oberhuber G, Prior C, Bosmuller C, Dietze O, Margreiter R. Early recurrence of Wegener's granulomatosis in a kidney allograft under cyclosporine treatment. Transplant Int 1:49–50, 1988.

Ohi H, Yasugi T. Occurrence of C3 nephritic factor and C4 nephritic factor in membranoproliferative glomerulonephritis (MPGN). Clin Exp Immunol 95:316–321, 1994.

Ozen S, Besbas N, Asstci U, Bakkaloglu A. Diagnostic criteria for polyarteritis nodosa in childhood. J Pediatr 120:206–209, 1992.

Park SY, Ueda S, Ohno H, Hamano Y, Tanaka M, Shiratori T, Yamazaki T, Arase H, Arase N, Karasawa A, Sato S, Ledermann B, Kondo Y, Okumura K, Ra C, Saito T. Resistance of Fc receptor-deficient mice to fatal glomerulonephritis. J Clin Invest 102:1229–1238, 1998.

Pearse RN, Kawabe T, Bolland S, Guinamard R, Kurosaki T, Ravetch JV. SHIP recruitment attenuates Fc gamma RIIB-induced B cell apoptosis. Immunity 10:753–760, 1999.

Penny MJ, Boyd RA, Hall BM. Permanent CD8(+) T cell depletion prevents proteinuria in active Heymann nephritis. J Exp Med 188:1775–1784, 1998.

Peters CJ, Simpson GL, Levy H. Spectrum of hantavirus infection: hemorrhagic fever with renal syndrome and hantavirus pulmonary syndrome. Annu Rev Med 50:531–545, 1999.

Ponticelli C, Passerini P. Membranous nephropathy. In Ponticelli C, Glossock RJ, eds. Treatment of Primary Glomerulonephritis. Oxford Medical Publications, Oxford UK, 1997, pp 46–185.

Ponticelli C, Rizzoni G, Edefonti A, Altieri P, Rivolta E, Rinaldi S, Ghio L, Lusvarghi E, Gusmano R, Locatelli F, et al. A randomized trial of cyclosporine in steroid-resistant idiopathic nephrotic syndrome. Kidney Int 43:1377–1384, 1993.

Ponticelli C, Zuchelli P, Passerini P, Cagnoli L, Cesana B, Pozzi C, Pasquali S, Imbasciati E, Grassi C, Redaelli B, et al. A randomized trial of methylprednisolone and chlorambucil in idiopathic membranous nephropathy. N Engl J Med 320:8–13, 1989.

Powrie F, Menon S, Coffman RL. Interleukin-4 and interleukin-10 synergize to inhibit cell-mediated immunity in vivo. Eur J Immunol 23:3043–3049, 1993.

Pozzi C, Bolasco PG, Fogazzi GB, Andrulli S, Altieri P, Ponticelli C, Locatelli F. Corticosteroids in IgA nephropathy: a randomised controlled trial. Lancet 353:883–887, 1999.

Qin L, Chavin KD, Ding Y Favaro JP, Woodard JE, Lin J, Tahara H, Robbins P, Shaked A, Ho DY, et al. Multiple vectors effectively achieve gene transfer in a murine cardiac transplantation model. Immunosuppression with TGF-beta 1 or vIL-10. Transplantation 59:809–816, 1995.

Rai A, Nast C, Adler S. Henoch-Schönlein purpura nephritis. J Am Soc Nephrol 10:2637–2644, 1999.

Rao TK, Riedman EA. Outcome of severe acute renal failure in patients with acquired immunodeficiency syndrome. Am J Kidney Dis 25:390–398, 1995.

Ravetch JV, Lanier LL. Immune inhibitory receptors. Science 290:84–89, 2000.

Ray PE, Rakusan T, Loechelt BJ, Selby DM, Liu XH, Chandra RS. Human immunodeficiency virus(HIV)-associated nephropathy in children from the Washington, D.C. area: 12 years' experience. Semin Nephrol 18:396–405, 1998.

Reynolds J, Tam FW, Chandraker A, Smith J, Karkar AM, Cross J, Peach R, Sayegh MH, Pusey CD. CD28-B7 blockade prevents the development of experimental autoimmune glomerulonephritis. J Clin Invest 105:643–651, 2000.

Rieu P, Noel LH. Henoch-Schönlein nephritis in children and adults. Morphological features and clinicopathological correlations. Ann Med Intrene 150:151–159, 1999.

Roberts AB, Sporn MB. Physiological actions and clinical applications of transforming growth factor-beta (TGF-beta). Growth Factors 8:1–9, 1993.

Rodriguez-Inigo E, Casqueiro M, Bartolome J, Barat A, Caramelo C, Ortiz A, Albalate M, Oliva H, Manzano ML, Carreno V. Hepatitis C virus RNA in kidney biopsies from infected patients with renal diseases. J Viral Hepat 7:23–29, 2000.

Rodriguez-Iturbe B. Epidemic poststreptococcal glomerulonephritis. Kidney Int 25:129–136, 1984.

Romero M, Mosquera J, Novo E, Fernandez L, Parra G. Erythrogenic toxin type B and its precursor isolated from nephritogenic streptococci induce leukocyte infiltration in normal rat kidneys. Nephrol Dial Transplant 14:1867–1874, 1999.

Ronco P, Verroust P, Morel-Maroger L. Viruses and glomerulonephritis. Nephron 31:97–102, 1982.

Rostoker G, Belghiti D, Ben Maadi A, Remy P, Lang P, Weil B, Lagrue G. Long-term cyclosporin A therapy for severe idiopathic membranous nephropathy. Nephron 63:335–341, 1995a.

Rostoker G, Desveaux-Belghiti D, Pilatte Y, Petit-Phar M, Philippon C, Deforges L, Terzidis H, Intrator L, Andre C, Adnot S. Immunomodulation with low-dose immunoglobulins for moderate IgA nephropathy and Henoch-Schönlein purpura. Preliminary results of a prospective uncontrolled trial. Nephron 69:327–334, 1995b.

Rottem M, Fauci AS, Hallahan CW, Kerr GS, Lebovics R, Leavitt RY, Hoffman GS. Wegener granulomatosis in children and

adolescents: clinical presentation and outcome. J Pediatr 122:26–31, 1993.

Roy S III, Wall HP, Etteldorf JN. Second attacks of acute glomerulonephritis. J Pediatr 75:758–767, 1969.

Rutgers A, Meyers KE, Canziani G, Kalluri R, Lin J, Madaio MP. High affinity of anti-GBM antibodies from Goodpasture and transplanted Alport patients to alpha3(IV)NC1 collagen. Kidney Int 58:115–122, 2000.

Ryan JJ, Mason PJ, Pusey CD, Turner N. Recombinant alpha-chains of type IV collagen demonstrate that the amino terminal of the Goodpasture autoantigen is crucial for antibody recognition. Clin Exp Immunol 113:17–27, 1998.

Saito R, Prehn J, Zuo XJ, Marchevsky A, Castracane J, Waters P, Matloff J, Jordan SC. The participation of tumor necrosis factor in the pathogenesis of lung allograft rejection in the rat. Transplantation 55:967–972, 1993.

Samuelsson A, Towers TL, Ravetch JV. Anti-inflammatory activity of IVIG mediated through the inhibitory Fc receptor. Science 291:484–486, 2001.

Sankaran D, Asderakis A, Ashraf S, Roberts IS, Short CD, Dyer PA, Sinnott PJ, Hutchinson IV. Cytokine gene polymorphisms predict acute graft rejection following renal transplantation. Kidney Int 56:281–288, 1999.

Satoh J, Seino H, Abo T, Tanaka S, Shintani S, Ohta S, Tamura K, Sawai T, Nobunaga T, Oteki T, et al. Recombinant human tumor necrosis factor alpha suppresses autoimmune diabetes in nonobese diabetic mice. J Clin Invest 84:1345–1348, 1989.

Savage CO. Goodpasture's syndrome and antiglomerular membrane disease. In Greenberg A, Cheung A, Coffman T, Falk R, Jennette J, eds. Primer on Kidney Diseases. San Diego, Academic Press, 1998, pp 175–179.

Savage CO, Pusey CD, Bowman C, Rees AJ, Lockwood CM. Antiglomerular basement membrane antibody mediated disease in the British Isles 1980-4. Br Med J Clin Res Ed 292:301–304, 1986.

Schmitt H, Bohle A, Reinke T, Meyer-Eichberger D, Vogl W. Long-term prognosis of membranoproliferative glomerulonephritis type I. Significance of clinical and morphological parameters: an investigation of 220 cases. Nephron 55:242–250, 1990.

Schoenberger SP, Toes RE, van der Voost EI, Offringa R, Melief CJ. T-cell help for cytotoxic T lymphocytes is mediated by CD40-CD40L interactions. Nature 393:480–483, 1998.

Schwertz R, de Jong R, Gretz N, Kirschfink M, Anders D, Scharer K. Outcome of idiopathic membranoproliferative glomerulonephritis in children. Acta Paediatr 85:308–312, 1996.

Scott P. IL-12: initiation cytokine for cell-mediated immunity. Science 260:496–497, 1993.

Seligson G, Lange K, Majeed HA, Deol H, Cronin W, Bovie R. Significance of endostreptosin antibody titers in poststreptococcal glomerulonephritis. Clin Nephrol 24:69–75, 1985.

Serreze DV, Leiter EH. Defective activation of T suppressor cell function in nonobese diabetic mice. Potential relation to cytokine deficiencies. J Immunol 140:3801–3807, 1988.

Shivakumar S, Tsokos GC, Datta SK. T cell receptor alpha/beta expressing double-negative (CD4-/CD8-) and CD4+ T helper cells in humans augment the production of pathogenic anti-DNA autoantibodies associated with lupus nephritis. J Immunol 143:103–112, 1989.

Siegel NJ, Gur A, Krassner LS, Kashgarian M. Minimal-lesion nephrotic syndrome with early resistance to steroid therapy. J Pediatr 87:377–380, 1975.

Spitzer RE, Vallota EH, Forristal J, Sudora E, Stitzel A, Davis NC, West CD. Serum C'3 lytic system in patients with glomerulonephritis. Science 164:436–437, 1969.

Strom TB, Kelley VE. Toward more selective therapies to block undesired immune responses. Kidney Int 35:1026–1033, 1989.

Suzuki N, Ichino M, Mihara S, Kaneko S, Sakane T. Inhibition of Fas/Fas ligand-mediated apoptotic cell death of lymphocytes in vitro by circulating anti-Fas ligand autoantibodies in patients with systemic lupus erythematosus. Arthritis Rheum 41:344–353, 1998a.

Suzuki N, Sakane T, Engleman EG. Anti-DNA antibody production by CD5+ and CD5- B cells of patients with systemic lupus erythematosus. J Clin Invest 85:238–247, 1990.

Suzuki Y, Shirato I, Okumura K, Ravetch JV, Takai T, Tomino Y, Ra C. Distinct contribution of Fc receptors and angiotensin II–dependent pathways in anti-GBM glomerulonephritis. Kidney Int 54:1166–1174, 1998b.

Tada Y, Nagasawa K, Ho A, Morito F, Koarada S, Ushiyama O, Suzuki N, Ohta A, Mak TW. Role of the costimulatory molecule CD28 in the development of lupus in MRL/lpr mice. J Immunol 163:3153–3159, 1999.

Takabayashi K, Koike T, Kurasawa K, Matsumura R, Sato T, Tomioka H, Ito I, Yoshiki T, Yoshida S. Effect of FK-506, a novel immunosuppressive drug on murine systemic lupus erythematosus. Clin Immunol Immunopathol 51:110–117, 1989.

Tam LS, Li EK, Szeto CC, Wong SM, Leung CB, Lai FM, Wong KC, Lui SF. Treatment of membranous lupus nephritis with prednisone, azathioprine and cyclosporin A. Lupus 10:827–829, 2001.

Tan EM. Autoimmunity and apoptosis. J Exp Med 179:1083–1086, 1994.

Tanawattanacharoen S, Falk RJ, Jennette JC, Kopp JB. Parvovirus B19 DNA in kidney tissue of patients with focal segmental glomerulosclerosis. Am J Kidney Dis 35:1166–1174, 2000.

Tanganaratchkit K, Tapaneya-Olarn C, Tapanaya-Olarn W. The efficacy of intravenous pulse cyclophosphamide in the treatment of severe lupus nephritis in children. J Med Assoc Thai 82S:104–140, 1999.

Tanuma Y, Ohi H, Watanabe S, Seki M, Hatano M. C3 nephritic factor and C4 nephritic factor in the serum of two patients with hypocomplementaemic membranoproliferative glomerulonephritis. Clin Exp Immunol 76:82–85, 1989.

Tarshish P, Bernstein J, Tobin JN, Edelmann CM Jr. Treatment of mesangiocapillary glomerulonephritis with alternate-day prednisone–a report of the International Study of Kidney Disease in Children. Pediatr Nephrol 6:123–130, 1992.

Tassiulas IO, Aksentijevich I, Salmon JE, Kim Y, Yaboro CH, Vaughan EM, Davis JC, Scott DL, Austin HA, Klippel JH, Balow JE, Gourley MF, Boumpas DT. Angiotensin I converting enzyme gene polymorphisms in systemic lupus erythematosus: decreased prevalence of DD genotype in African American patients. Clin Nephrol 50:8–13, 1998.

Trainin EB, Boichis H, Spitzer A, Greifer I. Idiopathic membranous nephropathy. Clinical course in children. N Y State J Med 76:357–360, 1976.

Tsao BP, Ebling FM, Roman C, Panosian-Sahakian N, Calame K, Hahn BH. Structural characteristics of the variable regions of immunoglobulin genes encoding a pathogenic autoantibody in murine lupus. Journal of Clinical Investigation 85:530–540, 1990.

Tung KS, Woodroffe AJ, Ahlin TD, Williams RC Jr, Wilson CB. Application of the solid phase C1q and Raji cell radioimmune assays for the detection of circulating immune complexes in glomerulonephritis. J ClinInvest 62:61–72, 1978.

Turner D, Grant SC, Yonan N, Sheldon S, Dyer PA, Sinnott PJ, Hutchinson IV. Cytokine gene polymorphism and heart transplant rejection. Transplantation 64:776–779, 1997.

Tuso P, Moudgil A, Hay J, Goodman D, Kamil E, Koyyana R, Jordan SC. Treatment of antineutrophil cytoplasmic autoantibody-positive systemic vasculitis and glomerulonephritis with pooled intravenous gammaglobulin. Am J Kidney Dis 20:504–508, 1992.

Valles-Prats M, Tovar Mendez JL, Vila Presas J. Glomerulonephritis mesangiocapillary idiopatica. Estudio de 72 cases. Nephrologia 5:17–23, 1987.

Varade WS, Forristal J, West CD. Patterns of complement activation in idiopathic membranoproliferative glomerulonephritis, types I, II, and III. Am J Kidney Dis 16:196–206, 1990.

Verroust P, Ben-Maiz H, Morel-Maroger L, Mahfoud A, Geniteau M, Benayed H, Richet G. A clinical and immunopathological study of 304 cases of glomerulonephritis in Tunisia. Eur J Clin Invest 9:75–79, 1979.

Vogl W, Renke M, Mayer, Eichberger D, Schmit H, Bohle A. Long-term prognosis for endocapillary glomerulonephritis of poststreptococcal type in children and adults. Nephron 44:58–65, 1986.

Vogt A. New aspects of the pathogenesis of immune complex glomerulonephritis: formation of subepithelial deposits. Clin Nephrol 21:15–20, 1984.

Wakui H, Imai H, Komatsuda A, Miura AB. Circulating antibodies against alpha-enolase in patients with primary membranous nephropathy (MN). Clin Exp Immunol 118:445–450, 1999.

Walport M. Complement. In Roitt I, ed. Immunology. London, Mosby, 1993, pp 12.1–12.7.

Wannamaker LW, Yasmineh W. Streptococcal nucleases. I. Further studies on the A,B, and C enzymes. J Exp Med 126:475–496, 1967.

Welch TR, Berry A, Beischel LS. C4 isotype deficiency in IgA nephropathy. Pediatr Nephrol 1:136–139, 1987.

West CD, McAdams AJ. Membranoproliferative glomerulonephritis type III: association of glomerular deposits with circulating nephritic factor-stabilized convertase. Am J Kidney Dis 32:56–63, 1998.

Wierenga KJ, Pattison JR, Brink N, Griffiths M, Miller M, Shah DJ, Williams W, Serjeant BE, Serjeant GR. Glomerulonephritis after human parvovirus infection in homozygous sickle-cell disease. Lancet 346:475–476, 1995.

Willems F, Marchant A, Delville JP, Gerard C, Delvaux A, Velu T, de Boer M, Goldman M. Interleukin-10 inhibits B7 and intercellular adhesion molecule-1 expression on human monocytes. Eur J Immunol 24:1007–1009, 1994.

Williams DG. C3 nephritic factor and mesangiocapillary glomerulonephritis. Pediatr Nephrol 11:96–98, 1997.

Williams RC Jr, Van de Rijn I, Reid H, Poon-King T, Zabriskie JB. Lymphocyte cell subpopulations during acute post-streptococcal glomerulonephritis: cell surface antigens and binding of streptococcal membrane antigens and C-reactive protein. Clin Exp Immunol 46:397–405, 1981.

Wolf G, Thaiss F, Stahl RA. Cyclosporine stimulates expression of transforming growth factor-beta in renal cells. Possible mechanism of cyclosporines antiproliferative effects. Transplantation 60:237–241, 1995.

Wu WM, Lin BF, Su YC, Suen JL, Chiang BL. Tamoxifen decreases renal inflammation and alleviates disease severity in autoimmune NZB/W F1 mice. Scand J Immunol 52:393–400, 2000.

Wyatt RJ, Julian BA, Waldo FB, McLean RH. Complement phenotypes (C3 and C4) in IgA nephropathy. Adv Exp Med Biol 216B:1569–1575, 1987.

Yap HK, Cheung W, Murugasu B, Sim SK, Seah CC, Jordan SC. Th1 and Th2 cytokine mRNA profiles in childhood nephrotic syndrome: evidence for increased IL-13 mRNA expression in relapse. J Am Soc Nephrol 10:529–537, 1999.

Zauner I, Bohler J, Braun N, Grupp C, Heering P, Schollmeyer P. Effect of aspirin and dipyridamole on proteinuria in idiopathic membranoproliferative glomerulonephritis: a multicentre prospective clinical trial. Collaborative Glomerulonephritis Therapy Study Group (CGTS). Nephrol Dial Transplant 9:619–622, 1994.

Ziswiler R, Steinmann-Niggli K, Kappeler A, Daniel C, Marti HP. Mycophenolic acid: a new approach to the therapy of experimental mesangial proliferative glomerulonephritis. J Am Soc Nephrol 9:2055–2066, 1998.

Zuo XJ, Matsumara Y, Prehn J, Saito R, Marchevsky A, Matloff J, Jordan SC. Cytokine gene expression in rejecting and tolerant rat lung allograft models: analysis by RT-PCR. Transpl Immunol 3:151–161, 1995.

CHAPTER 39

Immune-Mediated Hematologic and Oncologic Disorders

Diane J. Nugent and Thomas J. Kunicki

INTRODUCTION

Immunodeficiency, whether congenital or acquired, results in a loss of critical pathways required to maintain a distinction between self and the environment. In attempting to respond to external organisms, patients with immunodeficiencies may trigger a cellular or humoral response that allows the production of self-reactive cells or antibody, normally suppressed in the healthy individual. Many tissues may be targets of these misdirected autoimmune responses, but hematologic and vascular disorders are particularly common.

The inability to downregulate an immune response may also result in sustained polyclonal expansion of cells that should normally undergo apoptosis if not directed against a pathogen. This persistent cellular proliferation increases the likelihood that malignant clones will emerge, especially in the lymphoid compartment. In profound immunodeficiency, individuals are so susceptible to infection that they rarely survive to develop cancer, but in those with less severe conditions associated with a longer life span, there is a high rate of malignancy.

1253

The hematologic and oncologic disorders of immune dysregulation, whether congenital or acquired, may manifest as chronic cytopenias, bone marrow failure, bleeding, or malignancy. When evaluating children with these syndromes, it is critical to incorporate laboratory studies to rule out underlying immunodeficiency. Therapy for autoimmune or malignant disorders in these patients may differ, particularly in the degree of immune suppression and intensity of radiotherapy. This chapter focuses on the common hematologic syndromes and malignancies associated with immunodeficiency or autoimmune disease.

IMMUNE-MEDIATED CYTOPENIAS

Thrombocytopenia, anemia, and neutropenia usually present as isolated immune-mediated cytopenias or in combination, as seen in *Evans's syndrome,* an autoimmune disorder associated with multiple antibodies directed against circulating blood cells. Human immunodeficiency virus (HIV) or Epstein-Barr virus (EBV) infections may also result in autoantibodies directed against platelets, erythrocytes, and less frequently, granulocytes. Clinical features such as adenopathy, fever, splenomegaly, recurrent infection, or failure to thrive usually distinguish a viral process from primary autoimmune disease (Louache and Vainchenker, 1994; Steeper et al., 1989).

Neonatal immune cytopenias may also be secondary to passive antibodies from the mother directed against alloantigens or polymorphic determinants on membrane proteins present in the newborn but not in the mother. Most women produce these antibodies during pregnancy or after exposure to blood products.

IMMUNE THROMBOCYTOPENIC PURPURA

Pathogenesis

Platelets play a central role in the maintenance of normal hemostasis and vascular repair. A decrease in platelet number (e.g., thrombocytopenia) can result in bruising, petechiae, or life-threatening bleeding. Immune-mediated thrombocytopenic purpura (ITP) is perhaps the most common autoimmune disease affecting both adults and children. Patients with ITP develop antibodies that bind to platelet membrane antigens and mediate the rapid destruction of antibody-coated cells in the reticuloendothelial system, particularly in the spleen and liver.

Sensing a decrease in circulating thrombocytes, the bone marrow responds with increased platelet production. The megakaryocytes increase in both number and ploidy to compensate for a shortened platelet life span. The triad of thrombocytopenia, increased platelet production, and decreased platelet survival defines the clinical syndrome of ITP.

Recognition that ITP is an antibody-mediated disease came when Harrington and co-workers (1953)

observed that pregnant women with thrombocytopenia sometimes gave birth to infants with profound—but transient—thrombocytopenia. They postulated that the same plasma factor causing the maternal thrombocytopenia crossed the placenta and resulted in thrombocytopenia in the fetus and, consequently, in the newborn.

To prove that this factor was present in the plasma of thrombocytopenic patients, Harrington infused himself with plasma from a patient with ITP. The results of this infamous experiment left no room for doubt (Altman, 1987): Harrington became acutely thrombocytopenic, with bleeding and a brief seizure, necessitating hospitalization until his platelet count recovered.

Subsequent studies on other volunteers demonstrated that the antiplatelet activity was present in the γ-globulin fraction of ITP plasma (Harrington et al., 1951). Others confirmed that IgG antiplatelet autoantibodies were responsible for the thrombocytopenia in ITP (Shulman et al., 1965).

ITP may occur alone or in association with other conditions such as systemic lupus erythematosus (SLE) or pregnancy. The presentation and prognosis of ITP vary with age, sex, and familial predisposition to autoimmune disease. Even in uncomplicated ITP, there is considerable variation in presentation and prognosis.

Platelet Antibodies in ITP

The presence of platelet-associated immunoglobulin or circulating antiplatelet antibodies has been used to confirm the diagnosis. The sensitivity of the initial assays to assess platelet-bound IgG, IgM, and complement was significantly limited by the fact that the target tissue (i.e., the platelets) was markedly decreased. Moreover, platelets carry an internal pool of IgG in their alpha granules as the result of uptake by the megakaryocyte during platelet production (George et al., 1985, Handagama et al., 1987). In both immune and nonimmune platelet-destruction syndromes, platelet activation triggers the release of alpha granules, increasing the amount of platelet-associated immunoglobulin nonspecifically.

Thus an increase in platelet-associated IgG supports the diagnosis of ITP but may not exclude low-grade platelet consumption from such disorders as hemolytic uremic syndrome, vascular abnormalities (e.g., arterial-venous shunts or hemangiomas), or massive tissue damage as seen with burns or head trauma.

Indirect binding assays to quantitate the amount and type of antibody bound to the platelet or circulating in the plasma have been developed. The relative frequency of Ig isotype and IgG subclass autoantibodies mirrors that found in other autoimmune diseases. The IgG1 and IgG3 subclass antibodies dominate in 60% of patients with ITP, whereas IgG2 and IgG4 are present in 13% and 9% of sera from patients with ITP, respectively (Tijhuis et al., 1991; Winiarski, 1989).

IgM antiplatelet antibodies can also mediate platelet destruction, particularly when they fix complement (Cines et al., 1985; Kayser et al., 1981, Pawha et al.,

1983). The true incidence of IgM antiplatelet autoantibodies is not known because they are rarely studied in sera samples from patients with ITP. One third of children have only IgM antiplatelet antibodies and 20% to 30% have both IgG and IgM. In adults, the frequency of IgM antiplatelet antibodies is 10% or less, which may reflect the relative predominance of chronic ITP in adults.

Platelet-associated complement (C3) is found in approximately 30% to 40% of patients with chronic ITP (Cines and Schreiber, 1979; Hauch and Rosse, 1977).

Platelet Antibodies in Other Disorders

Platelet autoantibodies are often present in collagen-vascular diseases, including SLE, thyroiditis, anticardiolipin syndrome, and primary biliary cirrhosis. Why are platelet antigens such a common target for autoreactive antibodies? Researchers are beginning to examine the role of the platelet itself in triggering such antibodies. The activated platelet shares many of the co-stimulatory receptors present on lymphocytes (e.g., CD40L and CD80) and monocytes (e.g., CD14) (Semple et al., 1996). In an activated state, the platelet itself might substitute for the accessory cells that usually trigger autoantibody production, temporarily bypassing the tightly regulated T- and B-cell idiotypic network.

Semple and colleagues (1996) found that a significant number of children with acute (80%), chronic (71%), or chronic-complex (55%) ITP had platelets that expressed HLA-DR, in contrast to platelets from healthy control subjects and patients with nonimmune thrombocytopenia. Platelets normally express only class I molecules, but in patients with ITP, HLA-DR was variably co-expressed on distinct smaller and larger platelets, along with CD41, CD45, CD14, CD80, and/or glycophorin molecules. Semple and co-workers hypothesized that persistent HLA-DR expression on these young platelets may play a role in the triggering or perpetuation of ITP itself.

The production of autoantibodies is driven and controlled by cellular and soluble regulatory mechanisms. Many investigators have sought evidence of defects of T cells or a predominance of T-helper 1 (Th1) or T-helper 2 (Th2) subsets and their associated cytokines in ITP, but no clear T-cell pattern has been identified. This may reflect the heterogeneous nature of ITP because T-cell dysregulation varies according to age, gender, underlying environmental or viral triggers, and presence or absence of immunodeficiency.

T-Cell Abnormalities

Given the importance of the T-cell receptor (TCR) in other autoimmune diseases, initial studies focused on characterization of γ/δ-TCR use in ITP (Ware and Howard, 1993, 1994). Elevated numbers of γ/δ-TCR–positive T lymphocytes were observed in several patients with acute or chronic ITP. In patients with the highest numbers, the expanded cell population exclusively expressed the surface Vδ2/Vγ9 heterodimer.

Analysis of the nucleotide sequences used by these γ/δ-TCR T cells demonstrated a diverse set of VDJC gene rearrangements, suggesting a superantigen response. The isolation of eight T-cell clones disclosed in vitro proliferation against allogeneic platelets, elevated numbers of Vβ8+ T cells, and IL-2 secretion following platelet stimulation, providing further evidence for T-cell reactivity (Ware and Howard, 1993).

These results provided the first evidence that patients with ITP have platelet-reactive T lymphocytes identifiable at the clonal level, supporting the hypothesis that autoreactive peripheral T lymphocytes may mediate or participate in its pathogenesis.

Kuwana and colleagues (1998) examined in vitro peripheral blood mononuclear cell responses to platelet membrane glycoproteins in 21 patients with chronic ITP or SLE, with or without thrombocytopenia, and in 10 healthy donors. None of the T cells from these subjects responded to the protein complex in its native state, but T cells did respond to reduced or tryptic peptides of the platelet integrin, $\alpha_{IIb}\beta_3$ occurred in nearly all subjects, including those who were healthy. Similar T-cell proliferation in healthy individuals in response to $\alpha_{IIb}\beta_3$ had been described by Filion and co-workers (1996), in 25 healthy people. This implies that autoreactive T cells directed against membrane antigens present on platelets have not been eliminated by intrathymic deletion but are present in a suppressed state in healthy individuals.

In patients with ITP, the T-cell response is class II HLA–restricted; moreover, the responding T cells have a CD4+ phenotype and their lymphoproliferative responses were greater than controls, suggesting in vivo T-cell activation (Filion et al., 1966). None of the peripheral blood mononuclear cells from healthy donors developed a significant titer of IgG anti-$\alpha_{IIb}\beta_3$ antibody, but all exhibited lymphoproliferation to trypsin-digested $\alpha_{IIb}\beta_3$ membrane antigen. Filion and colleagues therefore concluded that CD4+ HLA-DR–restricted T cells to $\alpha_{IIb}\beta_3$ are involved in the production of antiplatelet autoantibody and are implicated in the pathogenesis of chronic ITP.

Cytokines

Cytokines have been measured in ITP to assess the role of Th subsets in the autoimmune process. Most of such studies draw conclusions based on a single cytokine profile that may fluctuate considerably during the course of the illness. In addition, the presence of soluble receptors may cloud the results if they are not assessed at the same time that the cytokines are measured. To distinguish a normal from a pathologic immune response, multiple samples of cytokines and their inhibitors must be obtained over time. The following reports have used multiple samples from patients with chronic or acute ITP and from healthy controls.

Children with ITP have a Th1 type of cytokine response, with very low IL-4 and IL-6 and elevated levels of IL-2, interferon gamma (IFN-γ, and tumor necrosis factor β (TNF-β (Andersson, 1998; Garcia-Suarez et al., 1995). Patients with chronic ITP, patients with malignancy-associated ITP, and patients with autoimmune lymphoproliferative syndrome who have defects in the Fas apoptosis pathway (see Chapter 19) have elevated levels of IL-6, IL-10, IL-11, and IL-13 (Andersson, 1998; Crossley et al., 1996; Dianzani et al., 1997; Erduran et al., 1998; Lazarus et al., 1998). Successful therapy may be associated with changes in the cytokine profile.

Such cytokine profiles have been measured after treatment with intravenous immunoglobulin (IVIG) or anti-D immunoglobulin (Zimmerman et al., 1998). Zimmerman and co-workers (1998) found that children with ITP treated with IVIG and dexamethasone had abnormal T-lymphocyte subsets and depressed in vitro T-lymphocyte proliferation. By contrast, anti-D immunoglobulin treatment did not affect T-cell function, including T-cell subsets; the TCR Vβ repertoire; lymphoproliferative responses to mitogens, antigens, or IL-2; pokeweed mitogen-stimulated IgG synthesis; or T-lymphocyte cytokine mRNA levels.

Bussel and co-workers (1999) compared the changes in IL-6, IL-10, MCP-1, and TNF-α levels after treatment with IVIG and anti-D immunoglobulin in adults with thrombocytopenia. There was an increase in three of four cytokines 2 hours after the administration of anti-D immunoglobulin. MCP-1 increased the most. Following IVIG administration, there was a significant increase in IL-10 levels 4 hours afterwards, but not 2 hours afterwards, and MCP-1 levels increased at 24 hours. No changes were seen in IL-6 or TNF-α. They hypothesized that the early increase in these macrophage-synthesized cytokines after anti-D immunoglobulin was attributable to the interaction of antibody-coated red blood cells (RBCs) with macrophages. The differences between IVIG and anti-D immunoglobulin were presumably attributable to anti-D immunoglobulin creating a very large immune complex with hundreds of antibodies on each RBC.

Humanized monoclonal antibodies to CD40L, CD20, or other accessory molecules have been used to inhibit pathologic autoantibody production (Bussell et al., 2002; George et al., 1999; Stasi et al., 2002). The results of studies of these agents in adults with refractory ITP appear promising.

Clinical Features

Thrombocytopenia lasting less than 6 months is termed *acute ITP*; that lasting longer than 6 months, *chronic ITP*. Children are more likely to develop acute ITP, and in 60% to 75% of these patients, the disorder resolves within 2 to 4 months of diagnosis, regardless of therapy (Lusher et al., 1984; Walker and Walker, 1984). The peak age for acute ITP is 2 to 5 years of age, the time when children experience the greatest frequency of viral infections and when the most common form of childhood leukemia, acute lymphocytic leukemia (ALL), occurs.

Acute ITP of childhood occurs with equal frequency in boys and girls, is seasonal in nature, and often follows a recent infectious exposure or immunization, suggesting a role for viral or bacterial antigens in triggering antiplatelet autoantibody formation (Lusher and Iyer, 1977). There is no familial predisposition in acute childhood ITP.

Chronic ITP is more common in adults (75% to 85% of adult cases) and occurs more frequently in women (3:1 female-to-male ratio), similar to other autoimmune diseases. Chronic ITP is not seasonal and is often associated with nonplatelet autoantibodies (e.g., antinuclear antibodies, anti-DNA, or anticytoskeletal proteins). Furthermore, chronic ITP is more likely to occur in families with an increased incidence of other autoimmune diseases (Lippman et al., 1982; Panzer et al., 1990).

The latter pattern suggests underlying immune dysregulation and, in some cases, a familial predisposition toward autoimmune disease. Unlike the situation in patients with SLE or diabetes mellitus (Steinberg et al., 1991), there is no association with HLA class I or class II HLA-DR, HLA-DP, or HLA-DQ antigens (Gratama et al., 1984; Mayr et al., 1981; Mueller-Eckhardt et al., 1989).

Children with chronic ITP mirror the adult phenotype in that females predominate, and there are no seasonal fluctuations in the onset of disease. In the early stages of chronic ITP, the bone marrow is normal, without the expected expansion of platelet precursors. As the marrow responds to persistent thrombocytopenia, the megakaryocytes increase in number, particularly the early, less-mature cells (ploidy < 4N) that are very large (ploidy > 16N). This pattern is more likely to be seen after 4 weeks of thrombocytopenia and may be present in both immune and nonimmune platelet destruction syndromes. Interestingly, in approximately 15% of adult patients with chronic ITP, the increased number of megakaryocytes may not correlate with increased platelet production (Ballem et al., 1987).

The results of platelet survival studies suggest that antibody binding to platelet antigens on the megakaryocyte may interfere with platelet demargination, or "pinching off" from the megakaryocyte membrane. In ITP, the myeloid and erythroid precursors are normal—both in number and in appearance.

Children younger than 4 years of age with acute ITP often have an increased number of immature lymphocytes in the bone marrow. These cells, which may account for 20% to 30% of nucleated bone marrow cells, express early B-cell markers such as CD10 (CALLA) and CD19 (early B-cell antigen), as is also seen in childhood lymphocytic leukemia (Cornelius et al., 1991). Eosinophilia may also occur in childhood ITP, but its presence has no value in predicting the severity or chronicity of the illness (Lusher and Iyer, 1977; McClure et al., 1975).

Treatment

After the studies by Harrington and colleagues had established the immune nature of ITP, steroids were used to suppress autoantibody production and decrease splenic platelet destruction.

During the 1960s and 1970s, the widespread use of aspirin as an antipyretic resulted in severe platelet dysfunction in ITP, with marked purpura and petechiae despite only moderate thrombocytopenia. Because of mucosal bleeding and a concern for intracranial hemorrhage, many patients were treated with steroids when the platelet count reached 50,000 to 70,000/mm³. Once aspirin was discontinued in general pediatric practice, the occurrence of petechiae, bruising, and intracranial hemorrhage decreased significantly, except in patients with profound thrombocytopenia (<20,000/mm³).

In established ITP with high platelet turnover, the risk of spontaneous intracranial hemorrhage is very low (0.2%). Hence, many physicians chose to observe patients with platelet counts of greater than 20,000/mm³ and institute treatment only when mucosal bleeding is present or when there is significant risk of hemorrhage. Many physicians, to exclude leukemia from the differential diagnosis, performed a bone marrow aspirate before prescribing steroids.

The excellent response of ITP to high-dose IVIG and the demonstration of anti-idiotypic antibodies in these preparations (Berchtold et al., 1989; Imbach et al., 1981) led to its widespread use. IVIG induces a rise in platelet count in most patients regardless of age or etiology of the autoantibody.

Although Fc receptor (FcγRIII) blockade is the chief mechanism for the benefit of IVIG infusions, other mechanisms may also be operative. The response to IVIG in disorders such as Guillain-Barré syndrome or Kawasaki disease suggests alternative mechanisms (see Chapter 4).

Samuellson and colleagues demonstrated that activation of the FcγRIIB molecule is a potent inhibitor of antibody-dependent cell-mediated cytotoxicity in vivo, modulating the activation of FcγRIII on effector cells (Clynes et al., 1999, 2000). Samuellson and co-workers (2001) proved that the administration of clinically protective doses of IVIG prevented platelet consumption triggered by a pathogenic autoantibody. The inhibitory Fc receptor, FcγRIIB, was required for protection, because its disruption by genetic deletion or monoclonal antibody blockade reversed the therapeutic effect of IVIG. IVIG effectiveness was associated with the induction of FcγRIIB on splenic macrophages.

Other agents used to treat ITP, such as anti-D immunoglobulin or rituximab (anti-CD20, an early B-cell antigen), bind to these Fc receptors. The response to these agents depends on the degree of FcγRIII blockade or the upregulation of the FcγRIIB (inhibitory) molecule. Anti-D immunoglobulin decreases antibody-mediated platelet clearance by directly blocking FcγIII receptors, with little effect on inhibitory FcγRII (Bussel, 2000, 2002).

Several authors have shown that polymorphisms found in the FcγIII, FcγRII, and various cytokines may influence the response to therapy (Foster et al., 2001; Fujimoto et al., 2001; Williams et al., 1998). These observations may explain the striking variation in therapeutic effect of each regimen and help to guide the development of agents that modulate Fcγ receptors and cytokines.

Quartier and colleagues (2001) proposed that IVIG and monoclonal antibodies such as anti-CD20 (rituximab) and anti-CD40L exert negative feedback on autoreactive B and T lymphocytes. These treatments may alter T-cell subsets and cytokine production (Tsubakio et al., 1983). Cytokines and their modulating elements are present in IVIG and may influence the course of inflammation and immune dysregulation (Marsh et al., 1998; Sherer et al., 2001).

Immune Deficiency and Immune Thrombocytopenic Purpura

Patients with antibody immunodeficiencies are at particular risk for the development of autoimmunity. Reports of immune-mediated destruction of platelets or RBCs in IgA deficiency date to the 1970s (Ammann and Hong, 1970; Good and Rodey, 1970). Children with IgG subclass deficiencies may also develop autoimmune cytopenias, especially ITP. These immune-mediated cytopenias also occur in common variable immunodeficiency (CVID), DiGeorge syndrome, autoimmune lymphoproliferative syndrome, pregnancy, and infections with HIV or EBV.

Prognosis

In children with acute ITP the prognosis is excellent, with resolution in approximately 85% of patients after 6 months, regardless of the treatment regimen. In the adolescent or adult, there is a greater likelihood that the ITP will become chronic, be associated with other autoimmune disorders, and require aggressive medical therapy or splenectomy. Severe chronic ITP in children and adults has significant morbidity, necessitating costly therapy and time lost from school or work.

AUTOIMMUNE HEMOLYTIC ANEMIA

Pathogenesis

The hallmark of autoimmune hemolytic anemia (AHA) is intravascular or extravascular destruction of antibody-coated RBCs. Intravascular RBC destruction occurs when there is binding of complement components, IgM antibodies, and certain IgG subclass antibody subclasses. Alternatively, *warm* IgG antibodies, which optimally bind at 37° C, mediate extravascular RBC destruction in the spleen. Nearly 70% of all patients with AHA have a warm antibody phenotype.

Typically, IgG-coated erythrocytes attach to macrophages in the spleen, binding to their Fcγ receptors for IgG and C3d. The macrophages then begin clearing the IgG-coated RBCs and, in some cases, pinching off the attached portions of the membrane, creating microspherocytes. If the number of IgG-RBC complexes is large, RBC sequestration and macrophage binding may also occur in the liver, resulting in hepatosplenomegaly. Depending on the duration of hemolysis, the bone marrow responds with increased output of reticulocytes or even nucleated erythrocyte precursors to maintain oxygen-carrying capacity.

Coombs' Tests

In 1945, Coombs and colleagues developed a method to identify free (unbound) anti-erythrocyte antibody in the serum and antibody-coated erythrocytes in the circulation. They developed a high-titered rabbit antihuman immunoglobulin (called *Coombs' reagent*) that could detect antibody-coated RBCs. This reagent binds to the Fc portion of immunoglobulin attached to the RBC membrane, creating bridges between sensitized RBCs and resulting in agglutination. This is the *direct Coombs' test,* or the direct antiglobulin test. The agglutination is graded on a scale of 0 to 4 and roughly correlates with the amount of antibody on the RBC surface.

The *indirect Coombs' test* identifies unbound RBC antibodies in the patient's serum. In this test, the patient's serum is incubated at room temperature and at 37° C with a mixture of type O RBCs containing all Rh and minor blood group antigens. The cells are washed to remove free immunoglobulin, and then the Coombs' reagent is added. Agglutination indicates the presence of anti-erythrocyte antibodies in the patient's serum. The direct and indirect Coombs' tests cannot distinguish between autoantibodies and alloantibodies.

Coombs' tests are used extensively in blood banking to screen donor units for the presence of antibodies (indirect Coombs' test) and to cross-match blood (direct Coombs' test). The indirect Coombs' test is also used to identify maternal Rh antibodies that can cause hemolytic disease of the newborn (HDN).

Coombs' tests are also used to distinguish autoimmune RBC destruction in AHA from hemolysis caused by intrinsic erythrocyte defects.

Classification

Primary or idiopathic AHA occurs spontaneously without other disease or preceding viral infection. Primary AHA is less common than ITP, affecting 1 to 2 individuals per 100,000. It may occur at any age, from infants and toddlers to the elderly. AHA is further classified on the basis of its thermal-binding characteristics, isotype, and antigen specificity of its erythrocyte autoantibody. Knowing these characteristics is critical in determining therapy and prognosis for individual patients.

Erythrocyte Autoantibodies

Thermal-Binding Characteristics

WARM ANTIBODIES

Warm-reactive antibodies optimally bind to RBCs at 37° C; they may also fix complement, depending on the subclass of the IgG antibody. IgG1 alone or in combination with other subtypes makes up 90% of the warm-reactive autoantibodies (Engelfriet et al., 1992; Ishizaka et al., 1967). Warm-reactive antibodies make up 70% of primary AHA but are also found in secondary AHA associated with autoimmune disease, lymphoproliferative syndromes, or various drugs.

COLD ANTIBODIES AND PAROXYSMAL COLD HEMOGLOBINURIA

Cold-reactive antibodies are biphasic IgG antibodies that optimally bind to RBCs at 4° C. They are present in paroxysmal cold hemoglobinuria (PCH) and are also known as *Donath-Landsteiner autoantibodies.* They may be missed in the standard Coombs' tests run at higher temperatures. They are biphasic antibodies that bind to red cells in the cold and then at higher temperatures bind complement, resulting in hemolysis at 37° C.

PCH should be considered whenever the patient has documented hemoglobinuria and has only C3 on the RBC surface. In this setting, the laboratory should be alerted to run an additional assay in which the serum is incubated with RBCs in a melted ice-water bath and then warmed to 37° C. This will result in hemolysis if a cold autoantibody is present (Petz and Garrity, 1980).

In PCH the IgG antibody binds to the RBCs in the colder body regions such as the digits or limbs. Hemolysis occurs when these antibody-coated cells pass into warm regions of the body where complement binding and lysis can occur. PCH is most commonly seen following viral infection or in association with tertiary syphilis. The initial description of this process by Donath and Landsteiner in 1904 was the first report of an autoimmune disease.

Cold agglutinin hemolytic disease is mediated by complement-binding IgM autoantibodies (Bell et al., 1973; Engelfriet et al., 1992). Cold agglutinin AHA may occur as a primary disorder, but it is more commonly associated with lymphoproliferative or infectious diseases.

Antigen Specificities

The erythrocyte antigens at which the antibodies are directed vary greatly in each form of AHA. As erythrocytes age in the circulation, the cell membrane expresses senescent antigens that trigger their clearance by the reticuloendothelial system. Externalized phosphatidylserine on senescent erythrocytes triggers the macrophage to phagocyticize these cells, similar to the removal of other aging or activated circulating cells. As the concentration of oxidized phospholipids on the cell surface reaches a

infusion is inversely proportional to the recipient's isoagglutinin titer (Aster, 1965; Brand et al., 1986; Carr et al., 1990). The otherwise normal survival of platelets that escape initial clearance is best explained by variation in the number of A, B, and H antigens per platelet, unlike the more homogeneous distribution of HLA (Dunstan and Simpson, 1985; Skogen et al., 1988).

Human Platelet Antigens

The increasing number of serologically defined alloantigens of platelets has necessitated the development of a new nomenclature in which each is designated as a human platelet antigen (HPA) (von dem Borne et al., 1980), as shown in Table 39-1. Many of the polymorphisms on a single glycoprotein are linked, and they are best categorized as a limited number of allelic variants (Newman and Valentin, 1995; Newman et al., 1998). By convention, an HPA has been assigned to each alloantigen system in which the serologic difference between alleles has been identified. Of the 10 HPA systems defined to date, 6 are expressed by the integrin-β_3 subunit (HPA-1, HPA-4, HPA-6, HPA-7, HPA-8, and HPA-10w), 2 are localized on the integrin-α_{IIb} subunit (HPA-3 and HPA-9), 1 is found on the integrin-α_2 subunit (HPA-5), and 1 is expressed by the glycoprotein Ibα (HPA-2).

A Leu$_{33}$/Pro$_{33}$ dimorphism of integrin-β_3 defines the HPA-1 alloantigen system. Anti–HPA-1a antibodies clearly have an impact on the function of this receptor. They inhibit clot retraction and platelet aggregation, presumably because they can block the binding of fibrinogen (Furihata et al., 1987; van Leeuwen et al.,

1984). Ryu and colleagues (1990) reported dose-dependent stimulation rather than inhibition of fibrinogen binding induced by anti–HPA-1a. A similar effect has been attributed to other platelet inhibitors, RGD peptides (which interfere with integrin-ligand binding), and certain snake venoms (Du et al., 1991).

Another diallelic human alloantigen system known as *HPA-4a/b* is found on β_3 and is associated with an Arg$_{185}$/Gln$_{185}$ polymorphism (Furihata et al., 1987; Wang, 1992). Given the proximity of the HPA-4a/b polymorphism to the RGD binding domain (residues 109-171) of β_3, it is not surprising that anti–HPA-4a antibodies completely inhibit the aggregation of HPA-4a homozygous platelets (Furihata et al., 1987).

Other cells expressing β_3 as the β subunit of the vitronectin receptor include endothelial cells, fibroblasts, and smooth muscle cells. With β_3, they also express the HPA-1 and HPA-4 epitopes (Giltay et al., 1988, 1989; Kawai et al., 1987; Newman et al., 1986). This may contribute to the heterogeneity of the clinical symptoms in alloimmune-mediated thrombocytopenia.

The sensitization to platelet-specific alloantigens results in two distinct syndromes: neonatal alloimmune thrombocytopenia (NATP) and posttransfusion purpura (PTP).

Neonatal Alloimmune Thrombocytopenia

Maternal sensitization to paternal alloantigens on fetal platelets is the cause of neonatal NATP (Table 39-2). In North America, the alloantigen system most often involved in NATP is HPA-1.

TABLE 39-1 · GENE FREQUENCIES OF THE MAJOR HPA ALLELES

Platelet GP	Alleles	Gene Frequency	HPA Determinants
Integrin-α_2 subunit	Allele 1, Glu$_{505}$	0.39	5a
	Allele 2, Glu$_{505}$	0.53	5a
	Allele 3, Lys$_{505}$	0.076	5b
GP Ib α	Thr$_{145}$-D (short) isoform	0.11 (0.296)	2a
	Thr$_{145}$-C isoform	0.82 (0.539)	2a
	Met$_{145}$-C isoform	<0.01 (<0.01)	2b
	Met$_{145}$-B isoform	0.07 (0.01)	2b
	Met$_{145}$-A (long) isoform	<0.01 (0.155)	2b
GP Ib β	Gly$_{15}$	0.99	Iy^b
	Glu$_{15}$	<0.01	Iy^a
Integrin-α_{IIb} subunit	Val$_{837}$, Ile$_{843}$	0.61	3a, 9a
	Val$_{837}$, Ser$_{843}$	0.36	3b, 9a
	Met$_{837}$, Ser$_{843}$	0.03	3b, 9b
Integrin-β_3 subunit	Leu$_{33}$, Leu$_{40}$, Arg$_{62}$, Arg$_{143}$, Pro$_{407}$, Arg$_{489}$, Arg$_{636}$	0.85	**1a**, 10a, 4a, 7a, 6a, 8a
	Pro$_{33}$, Leu$_{40}$, Arg$_{62}$, Arg$_{143}$, Pro$_{407}$, Arg$_{489}$, Arg$_{636}$	0.15	**1b**, 10a, 4a, 7a, 6a, 8a
	Pro$_{33}$, **Arg$_{40}$**, Arg$_{62}$, Arg$_{143}$, Pro$_{407}$, Arg$_{489}$, Arg$_{636}$	0.005	**1b**, 10a, 4a, 7a, 6a, 8a
	Leu$_{33}$, Leu$_{40}$, **Gln$_{62}$**, Arg$_{143}$, Pro$_{407}$, Arg$_{489}$, Arg$_{636}$	<0.001	1a, **10b**, 4a, 7a, 6a, 8a
	Leu$_{33}$, Leu$_{40}$, Arg$_{62}$, **Gln$_{143}$**, Pro$_{407}$, Arg$_{489}$, Arg$_{636}$	<0.01	1a, 10a, **4b**, 7a, 6a, 8a
	Leu$_{33}$, Leu$_{40}$, Arg$_{62}$, Arg$_{143}$, **Ala$_{407}$**, Arg$_{489}$, Arg$_{636}$	<0.001	1a, 10a, 4a, **7b**, 6a, 8a
	Leu$_{33}$, Leu$_{40}$, Arg$_{62}$, Arg$_{143}$, Pro$_{407}$, **Gln$_{489}$**, Arg$_{636}$	<0.001	1a, 10a, 4a, 7a, **6b**, 8a
	Leu$_{33}$, Leu$_{40}$, Arg$_{62}$, Arg$_{143}$, Pro$_{407}$, Arg$_{489}$, **Cys$_{636}$**	<0.001	1a, 10a, 4a, 7a, 6a, **8b**

Alleles 1, 2, and 3 of integrin-α_2 are defined by several linked dimorphisms that are silent.
Gene frequencies are for Caucasian populations or Japanese populations (in parentheses).
GP = glycoprotein; HPA = human platelet antigen.
Adapted from Newman PJ, Derbes RS, Aster RH. The human platelet alloantigens, P1A1 and P1A2, are associated with a leucine33/proline33 amino acid polymorphism in membrane glycoprotein IIIa, and are distinguishable by DNA typing. J Clin Invest 83:1778–1781, 1989.

TABLE 39-2 · CHARACTERISTICS OF TWO TYPES OF ALLOIMMUNE THROMBOCYTOPENIAS

Neonatal Alloimmune Thrombocytopenic Purpura	Posttransfusion Thrombocytopenic Purpura
Incidence: 1 per 3000; 1 per 2200 births in one prospective study.	Nearly all patients are females previously sensitized by pregnancy or transfusion (<5% were males).
Maternal antibodies produced against paternal antigens on fetal platelets.	Thrombocytopenia usually occurs 1 week after transfusion.
Pathogenesis similar to that of erythroblastosis fetalis, except that 50% of cases occur during first pregnancy.	Homozygous HPA-1b individuals account for a majority (>60%) of cases.
Most frequently implicated antigens are HPA-1a and HPA-5b (United States/Europe).	
When associated with antibody HPA-1a, there is a high-risk association with HLA-DRB3*0101 or HLA-DQB1*02.	High-risk association with HLA-DRB3*0101 or HLA-DQB1*02.
When associated with antibody HPA-6b, there is an increased association with HLA-DRB1*1501, HLA-DQA1*0102, or HLA-DQB1*0602.	Enigmatically, the recipient's antigen-negative platelets are destroyed by autoantibody.

HLA = human leukocyte antigen.

An immune response to HPA-1a is HLA restricted (Reznikoff-Etievant et al., 1981; Valentin et al., 1990). Individuals who are homozygous for Pro_{33} (homozygous HPA-1b) and who develop an antibody to the predominant HPA-1a antigen are almost exclusively HLA-DRB3*0101 (Valentin et al., 1990) or HLA-DQB1*02 (L'Abbé et al., 1992; Maslanka et al., 1996). When the patient is HLA-DRB3*0101, the relative risk is 141, equivalent to that of the HLA-B27–positive individual's relative risk for ankylosing spondylitis (Maslanka et al., 1996).

T cells are the likely candidates for providing HLA-restriction to HPA-1a; furthermore, Maslanka and co-workers (1996) revealed that, in one case of NATP, T cells that share CDR3 motifs could be stimulated by peptides that contain the same Leu_{33} polymorphism recognized by anti–HPA-1a alloantibodies. For another less-frequent antigen, HPA-6b, there appears to be an association between susceptibility and the major histocompatibility complex genes HLA-DRB1*1501, HLA-DQA1*0102, and HLA-DQB1*0602 (Westman et al., 1997).

In a large series of NATP patients, 78% of serologically confirmed cases were associated with anti–HPA-1a and 19% associated with anti–HPA-5b (Mueller-Eckhardt et al., 1989). Other specificities account for less than 5% of cases. NATP has been reported in association with other alloantigens such as HPA-3a, HPA-3b, HPA-1b, or HPA-2b, but this is much less frequent

(Grenet et al., 1965; McGrath et al., 1989; Mueller-Eckhardt et al., 1989; von dem Borne, 1980). Differences in allelic gene frequencies in different racial or ethnic populations influence the frequency of responsiveness to a particular alloantigen.

Table 39-3 summarizes some of the known variations in allelic gene frequencies of different world populations. Thus in the Japanese population, anti–HPA-1a has never been shown to be involved in NATP, but antibodies specific for HPA-4b play a dominant clinical role (Shibata et al., 1986). This is probably because the gene frequency for the HPA-1b allele among the Japanese (0.02) is so much lower than that found in Western populations (0.15). Conversely, the gene frequency of the HPA-4b allele in Japan (0.0083) is higher than that observed in Western populations (<0.001).

Posttransfusion Purpura

PTP can result within 7 to 10 days after an immunogenic blood or platelet transfusion (see Table 39-2). It usually affects previously nontransfused, multiparous women. As with NATP, there is an increased risk of developing PTP among HLA-DR3–positive individuals, and HPA-1a is the target antigen commonly implicated in Western populations (Mueller-Eckhardt et al., 1989; Reznikoff-Etievant et al., 1981).

TABLE 39-3 · GENE FREQUENCIES OF THE MAJOR HPA ALLELES IN VARIOUS WORLD POPULATIONS

HPA	Western	Japan	American Indian	Black	Korea	African American	Finland	Thailand
1a	0.85	0.998	>0.993	0.885	0.995	—	0.86	>0.998
1b	0.15	0.002	<0.007	0.115	0.005	—	0.14	<0.002
2a	0.93	—	0.058	0.852	—	0.82	0.91	0.917
2b	0.07	—	0.042	0.148	—	0.18	0.09	0.083
3a	0.61	—	—	—	—	—	0.59	0.37
3b	0.39	—	—	—	—	—	0.41	0.63
4a	>0.99	0.989	—	—	—	—	—	0.991
4b	<0.01	0.011	—	—	—	—	—	0.009
5a	0.89	—	—	—	—	0.79	0.95	0.973
5b	0.11	—	—	—	—	0.21	0.05	0.027

HPA = human platelet antigen.

Even though antigen-negative, the recipient's platelets in PTP are also cleared from the circulation very rapidly. The exact mechanisms of autoantibody production following exposure to HPA-1a-positive platelets are unknown, but a number of theories exist. First, it has been proposed that during the initial phase of PTP, the patient develops antibodies that recognize framework determinants (i.e., conserved protein structures surrounding the specific polymorphic sites). These antibodies would then react with the framework epitopes of the glycoprotein, including those expressed on the recipient's platelets.

In a second hypothesis, the recipient's antibodies form immune complexes with soluble antigens from the donor platelet that interact with recipient platelets by means of a Fc receptor–dependent mechanism.

Third, soluble antigen from the transfused platelets may be adsorbed on recipient platelets, rendering them positive for the alloantigen. This is a passively acquired form of autoimmunity. Platelet membrane microparticles are known to be a constituent of fresh-frozen plasma and platelet concentrates and seem to be generated in particularly high levels during platelet activation (George et al., 1986). Thus the $\alpha_{IIb}\beta_3$ antigen complex within the microparticles may be adsorbed on recipient platelets.

Isoantibodies Against Platelet Membrane Glycoproteins (GPs)

Sensitization against antigens that are not polymorphic and are universally distributed among all healthy individuals can occur in unique situations, leading to the production of platelet isoantibodies. Isoimmunization occurs when individuals with an inherited deficiency of a membrane glycoprotein, for example, are exposed to multiple platelet transfusions because of their bleeding diathesis. Patients with Glanzmann's thrombasthenia (GT) or Bernard-Soulier syndrome (BSS) fall into this category because the patients either lack the integrin $\alpha_{IIb}\beta_3$ (GT) or glycoprotein Ib-IX-V complex (BSS).

Another example occurs when individuals genetically deficient in glycoproteins (GPIV), for which there is no obvious pathology, are exposed to GPIV through transfusion or pregnancy. Isoantibodies do not distinguish among any of the allelic forms of the glycoprotein in question (e.g., HPA-3 or HPA-1 alloantigens on $\alpha_{IIb}\beta_3$) but react with platelets from any healthy person. Because the patient does not express the platelet glycoprotein that carries the epitope in question, these antibodies do not bind to their own platelets.

HEMOLYTIC DISEASE OF THE NEWBORN (HDN)

Pathogenesis

In hemolytic disease of the newborn, as in NATP, maternal antibody specific for a fetal RBC antigen (not shared by the mother) is passively transferred across the placenta and results in hemolysis. The titer and affinity of the alloantibody may increase with each subsequent pregnancy, resulting in fetal hydrops and even intrauterine death.

HDN was recognized and described at length by French midwives in the early 1600s, but Diamond and colleagues first made the link between hydrops fetalis, neonatal jaundice, and profound anemia and circulating erythroblasts in 1932. In 1939, Levine and Stetson reported that HDN was associated with anti-Rh antibodies in multiparous women who were Rh-negative.

Although there are many antigens on the RBC surface, the proteins in the Rh complex cCdDeE are the most immunogenic, particularly the D antigen (blood groups dD or DD), classically known as the *Rh antigen*. The incidence of HDN varies among different populations based on the frequency of Rh-negative (dd) individuals. The Basque population has a 30% to 35% incidence of Rh negativity, whereas Native Americans have only 1% to 2% incidence of Rh negativity.

Not all Rh-negative women become sensitized during pregnancy with an Rh-positive fetus. As is the case with NATP, other factors such as the comploptype, HLA, and major blood group antigens play a role in sensitization. For example, about 16% of Rh-negative women with ABO-compatible pregnancies develop anti-D immunoglobulin antibodies. In contrast, only 1% to 2% of Rh-negative women become sensitized with an ABO-incompatible pregnancy (e.g., the mother has type O blood, and the fetus has group A or B blood). Presumably, the lower rate is due to rapid hemolysis of fetal cells by maternal anti-A or anti-B isohemagglutinins as they enter the maternal circulation. This observation led to the development of anti-Rh immunoglobulin, which is administered to Rh-negative women during pregnancy and after delivery to eliminate circulating Rh+ fetal cells before sensitization can occur.

When an Rh-negative mother becomes sensitized by exposure to Rh-positive blood, the most common mechanism is fetal-maternal hemorrhage. The greater the hemorrhage, the more likely the sensitization. With subsequent pregnancies, less blood is required to boost the Rh antibody titer. Periodic administration of anti-Rh immunoglobulin during pregnancy is usually adequate to eliminate cells that leak into the maternal circulation from fetal hemorrhage or breaks in the placental barrier.

Another cause of Rh sensitization is exposure to an Rh-positive blood through a transfusion. This is uncommon with current blood-banking practice, but emergency transfusion or exposure to RBCs in platelet concentrates not matched for Rh may sensitize certain individuals.

Finally, the *grandmother theory* proposes that an Rh-negative fetus or newborn is exposed to Rh-positive cells from the mother and becomes sensitized in the perinatal period. Therefore in HDN secondary to Rh antibodies, the fetus's grandmother may have been the original source of RBCs immunizing the Rh-negative mother.

Fetal erythrocyte destruction by maternal antibody is presumed to be secondary to macrophage destruction of antibody-coated cells. To compensate for the severe anemia, extramedullary erythropoiesis ensues in the kidneys, spleen, adrenal glands, and placenta. Erythroblastosis results in the compression and destruction of liver cells, with decreased synthesis of hepatic proteins such as albumin and clotting proteins. The fetus becomes progressively hydropic and may succumb in utero.

With aggressive anti-D immune globulin treatment during and after pregnancy, the frequency of anti-Rh alloantibodies causing HDN is decreasing. Other minor group antigens such as Rh antigens other than D (c, C, e, and E), Kell, Kp, Fy, or S are emerging as causes of HDN. Rh sensitization is still a problem in women not given anti-D immunoglobulin prophylaxis following delivery, miscarriage, or abortion (Lee, 1999; Mollison et al., 1987).

Clinical Features

The delivery of a hydropic infant with anemia, jaundice, and hepatosplenomegaly should prompt an immediate evaluation of maternal blood for anti-RBC alloantibodies (e.g., a positive indirect Coombs' test). Because of profound hypoalbuminemia, massive hepatosplenomegaly, and edema, these infants may require intubation and infusions of blood, albumin, and fresh-frozen plasma to compensate for hepatic dysfunction. The infant's direct Coombs' test is positive for IgG on the erythrocytes. The indirect Coombs' test result is also positive due to passive transfer of maternal anti-RBC antibodies. Although the newborn at delivery may not be severely jaundiced because of maternal clearance of fetal bilirubin, the indirect bilirubin rises rapidly after delivery.

Prenatal blood typing and indirect Coombs' testing are used to identify those expectant mothers who are Rh negative and who have RBC alloantibodies. Amniocentesis is used to monitor the fetus, and ultrasound is used during pregnancy to determine the presence of hydrops. Identification of an infant at risk allows the obstetrician to institute prenatal transfusions and optimize conditions at delivery. Infants of Rh-sensitized mothers are critically ill and may require intensive support for weeks.

Infants of mothers sensitized to other Rh antigens (c, C, e, or E) or the minor group antigens may also be severely anemic and hyperbilirubinemic but are less likely to require intubation. Hydrops fetalis may occasionally be due to sensitization to minor group antigens, usually in multiparous women with anti-c or anti-e alloantibodies.

Once the antibody specificity is known, an exchange transfusion with nonreactive erythrocytes will decrease hemolysis and lower the indirect hyperbilirubin level. If no compatible unit can be identified, washed maternal RBCs can be used. Washing is necessary to remove additional maternal antibody. All blood products should be irradiated to prevent graft-versus-host disease (GVHD).

Treatment

Optimal management of anti-D immunoglobulin (Rh)–mediated erythroblastosis fetalis includes the prevention of sensitization with anti-D immunoglobulin in Rh-negative women carrying Rh-positive infants. Such women should be given anti-D immunoglobulin early in pregnancy and again immediately following delivery because its expanded use has reduced the risk of HDN to less than 1%.

Sensitized women may be candidates for measures to reduce maternal antibody levels. Prenatal plasma exchange will lower the antibody acutely, but it is impractical throughout pregnancy. Maternal IVIG infusions given every 2 weeks, at 1 g/kg dose may be of benefit (Porter et al., 1997; Spong et al., 2001; Voto et al., 1997).

In severe cases, intrauterine transfusions of Rh-negative, irradiated, leukocyte-depleted RBCs will decrease the hemolysis and the erythroblastosis. As the pregnancy progresses, intrauterine transfusions become more risky, so steroids are used to accelerate fetal lung maturation and early induction of labor is undertaken to minimize hydrops.

Once the infant is delivered, measures to minimize hemolysis and prevent hyperbilirubinemia can prevent toxic levels of indirect bilirubin that result in kernicterus with brain damage, deafness, and blindness. Kernicterus is seen with an indirect bilirubin level of greater than 30 mg/dl in a term infant, but it may occur at lower levels if the infant is hypoalbuminemic, acidotic, anemic, or hydropic.

In the delivery room, antigen-negative, washed, and irradiated RBCs can be administered through an umbilical vessel. When stable, an exchange transfusion should be performed to remove antigen-positive erythrocytes and decrease the bilirubin, usually by about 75% of baseline levels.

Infants with HDN who are transfused at birth have a low reticulocyte count for the first 6 to 8 weeks because the high oxygen-carrying capacity of the transfused adult RBCs decreases the stimulus for RBC production. Furthermore, residual Rh antibody may interfere with the infant's RBC production by destroying early RBC precursors and reticulocytes. Thus, these infants may need 1 to 2 additional transfusions before the antibody titer decreases to a level that does not cause hemolysis of newly formed RBCs. Erythropoietin has also been used in infants whose parents object, for religious reasons, to the use of blood products.

Prognosis

Infants with advanced erythroblastosis and hydrops that survive have a protracted stay in the newborn intensive care unit. Prolonged intubation, the use of central catheters, and hyperalimentation place them at high risk for sepsis, thrombosis, and chronic lung disease.

ACQUIRED HEMOPHILIA AND THROMBOPHILIA

Pathogenesis

Patients with immune disorders or malignancy are at increased risk of developing antibodies against clotting proteins. This may result in a bleeding syndrome with autoantibodies to factors VIII, IX, or X. Paradoxically, autoantibodies to phospholipid moieties, such as the lupus anticoagulant and anticardiolipin antibodies, may result in thrombosis caused by the activation of the clotting cascade, increased platelet adhesion, or direct endothelial damage with subsequent clot formation (Harris et al., 2002). These syndromes are rare; in the absence of cancer, pregnancy, or autoimmunity, they are most commonly seen following infections or antibiotic use (Boggio and Green, 2001; Matsumoto et al., 2001). The origin of the autoantibodies is unclear, but it mirrors those antibodies described for ITP and AHA inasmuch as they show significant homology to natural antibodies present in the fetus.

Clinical Features

Patients may present with significant bleeding in joints, muscles, or, most seriously, in the central nervous system (CNS) and gastrointestinal tract. The prothrombin time and partial thromboplastin time are prolonged. The diagnosis of an acquired inhibitor or antibody to a clotting factor is made by mixing the patient's plasma with normal plasma at a 1:1 ratio. With a true factor deficiency, normal plasma will correct the clotting time, but if an inhibitor or autoantibody is present, the partial thromboplastin time (PTT) will not be corrected because the inhibitor or autoantibody will also inhibit that factor in the normal plasma. Further studies to define which factor is targeted should be performed, but treatment can be instituted while awaiting this result.

Spontaneous thrombosis or deep vein thrombosis most often occurs in the legs or at a site of recent trauma. The most serious location is the arterial or venous system of the cerebral nervous system, in which the patient has stroke-like symptoms (e.g., headache, focal weakness, slurred speech, or even seizures or coma). In this setting an immediate magnetic resonance angiography study should be undertaken.

Laboratory studies should include complete blood count to test for occult lymphoid malignancy, a congenital thrombophilia panel to rule out inherited risk factors for thrombosis, and a collagen-vascular disease panel, including lupus anticoagulant and anticardiolipin antibodies.

These tests will dictate the type of treatment used, but often the complete results are not immediately available. Standard anticoagulation can be instituted once the results of the magnetic resonance angiography (MRA) exclude hemorrhage and confirm the presence of thrombosis.

Treatment

The initial goal in the bleeding patient is to affect hemostasis and institute immunosuppressive treatment. A low titer of inhibitor can be neutralized with high doses of recombinant-factor VIII or cryoprecipitate. When this cannot be achieved, related agents that differ immunologically, such as porcine factor VIII, may be given with the hope that the autoantibody is not cross-reactive. Finally, bypassing agents such as activated plasma concentrates or recombinant factor VIIa may also be used. These agents, though costly, are used to control bleeding until immune suppression or plasmapheresis reduces the inhibitor titer and factor replacement can be accomplished.

Plasmapheresis can be used to remove an inhibitor in patients with life-threatening hemorrhage, although pheresis catheter placement has some risk of bleeding. Immune suppression is initiated with cyclophosphamide at moderate to high dosages, but special attention should be paid to the risk of hemorrhagic cystitis. The use of mesna is recommended to prevent this complication. In addition, prednisone at a dosage of 2 mg/kg/day is recommended to initiate and maintain remission for several months.

The initial treatment of thrombosis in patients with lupus inhibitors or anticardiolipin antibodies is directed toward removing the clot with fibrinolytic agents and preventing new clot formation with anticoagulants. If the thrombus is in a life-threatening location such as the lung, tissue plasminogen activator may be used to lyse the clot. Certain clots may require a localized infusion of tissue plasminogen activator, followed by anticoagulation with low–molecular weight heparin. Low–molecular-weight heparin is a good choice because the subcutaneous injections ensure complete absorption and a stable blood level—unlike intravenous heparin infusions, which are frequently interrupted, or the administration of Coumadin, which is not suitable for a patient unable to take oral medications.

Plasmapheresis is usually not necessary in this setting, but immune suppression with corticosteroids is usually started immediately. This is a particularly effective treatment for patients with a lupus anticoagulant or antiphospholipid antibody syndrome. In the patient with thrombosis who has had a stroke and who has anticardiolipin antibodies, with or without vasculitis, daily low-dose aspirin (e.g., 75 mg) may improve long-term survival and decrease the recurrence of CNS thrombosis.

An inherited predisposition to thrombosis is present in patients with factor V Leiden, the prothrombin mutation 20201, or with elevated homocysteine levels. These inherited disorders, when present in a patient with an acquired thrombotic autoantibody, may result in recurrent, severe thrombosis and long-term disability and necessitate lifelong anticoagulation. Other family members should also be tested for the presence of these autosomal dominant clotting disorders.

Prognosis

In the absence of an underlying malignancy or immune disorder, the prognosis for acquired hemophilia is good, with long-term resolution of the antibody in more than 90% of children and 70% of adults. Acquired thrombophilia may persist for a long period, and the sequelae of a stroke or postphlebitic syndrome may result in lifelong disabilities.

AUTOIMMUNE APLASTIC ANEMIA

Pathogenesis

Unlike antibody-mediated destruction of circulating blood cells, which was described in the preceding sections, acquired aplastic anemia appears to be caused by cytotoxic T-cell attack, with the production of Th1 cytokines, not unlike other lymphocyte-mediated organ-specific autoimmune diseases such as diabetes, ulcerative colitis, or multiple sclerosis. The target antigens or triggering events are unknown, but aplastic anemia has been described following viral infections such as hepatitis or in association with other autoimmune diseases—most notably, SLE.

Circulating hematopoietic growth factors and stromal cell function in aplastic anemia are normal, suggesting that early progenitor stem cells are the probable target. Indeed, circulating CD34 stem cells are absent or profoundly decreased in those with aplastic anemia (Marsh, 2000; Young et al., 2000).

In 1970, Mathé and colleagues noted that aplastic anemia improved during conditioning with antithymocyte globulin (ATG). This and other immunosuppressive regimens that target the T lymphocyte have been successful alone or in conjunction with stem cell transplantation (Tsai and Freytes, 1997).

In 1990, Anderson and Weinstein reported the clinical features of transfusion-associated GVHD. In this setting, transfused T lymphocytes attack the recipient's bone marrow and other organs typically affected by GVHD. In transfusion-related GVHD, the bone marrow is recognized as foreign by the infused donor lymphocytes (along with the skin, gut, and liver), in contrast with GVHD following bone marrow transplant (BMT) where the reconstituted bone marrow cells attack the skin, gut, and liver. This model also supports the role of cytotoxic T cells in autoimmune aplastic anemia (Young and Maciejewski, 1997).

A Th1 response was inferred when elevated levels of IFN-γ, IL-2, and TNF were produced in vitro from T cells isolated from the aplastic bone marrow (Sloand et al., 1998; Young and Maciejewski, 1997). These cells suppress hematopoietic colony formation in co-culture with bone marrow cells from healthy individuals. Aplastic anemia induced by alloreactive T cells in animal models may be prevented by pretreatment with a monoclonal antibody to IFN-γ (Sloand et al., 1998). Although not a perfect model for autoimmune aplastic anemia, it shows that modified T-cell responses can affect hematopoietic function.

Verma and colleagues (2002) demonstrated that pharmacologic inhibition of the protein kinase p38 reverses the suppressive effects of IFN-γ and TNF-α on normal human erythroid and myeloid progenitors. They also showed that inhibition of the p38/MAPK-2 signaling cascade strongly enhances hematopoietic progenitor colony formation in cultures of aplastic anemic bone marrow. This suggests that p38/MAPK-2 plays a critical role in the pathogenesis of aplastic anemia, and that selective pharmacologic inhibitors of this kinase may provide an innovative therapeutic approach for aplastic anemia and other cytokine-mediated bone marrow failure syndromes.

Clinical Features

Patients may not be aware of their illness because the anemia occurs slowly, allowing for adaptation to the anemia. Early signs of neutropenia include low-grade fever, mouth sores, and unexplained weight loss. Bruising and petechiae may not occur until the platelet count has fallen to levels less than 20,000/mm³. The progressive anemia may lead to syncope, headaches, or extreme fatigue. When symptoms become apparent, the hemoglobin is usually less than 7.0 g/dl, the absolute neutrophil count is less than 1000/mm³, and the platelets are less than 50,000/mm³.

Immediate admission for a bone marrow biopsy with cytogenetic study of the marrow and peripheral blood is indicated. A bone marrow aspirate is not of value in assessing cellularity of the bone marrow; thus a bone marrow core or biopsy is recommended. Biopsies are also required to rule out myelodysplastic changes, fibrosis, or malignancy.

The incidence of aplastic anemia is low in Europe (~2 cases/million). In developing countries, the incidence is much higher, approaching that of myeloid leukemias in the West (Issaragrisil et al., 1999; Yang and Zhang, 1991). Although a toxic exposure must be suspected, the majority of these cases appear to be idiopathic or triggered by infectious agents, particularly hepatitis in China and Thailand. Hepatitis-associated aplastic anemia may require a different and more conservative approach because of the risks of veno-occlusive disease (VOD) and liver failure associated with the conditioning regimens.

The evaluation excludes paroxysmal nocturnal hemoglobinuria (PNH), which can appear as aplastic anemia (Charles et al., 1996). PNH results from acquired mutations in the phosphatidyl-inositol glycan complementation group A (PIG-A) gene, resulting in hemolysis and an acquired marrow failure syndrome. Diagnostic assays for PNH include hemolytic screens (e.g., Ham's test and complement fixation studies), flow cytometry to measure the expression of CD59 on RBCs, and direct molecular sequencing or probes.

Other studies should include cytogenetics for premalignant disease, such as monosomy 7 or monosomy 5q– DNA breakage studies should be performed on peripheral blood to rule out Fanconi's anemia, particularly if siblings are being considered as bone marrow donors (see Chapter 18).

Autoimmune disease must also be considered because the aplastic anemia of lupus can be treated with immune suppression or steroids alone. These patients are at high risk for renal and pulmonary complications when subjected to transplantation conditioning regimens (Ikehara, 2001; Young and Maciejewski, 1997).

Treatment

In patients with overall marrow cellularity of less than 20% and trilineage failure, one must chose between aggressive immunosuppression alone and immunosuppression with allogeneic BMT. If a full-match sibling is available and there are no major infectious risks such as hepatitis or cytomegalovirus, most centers use conventional bone marrow transplant with ATG, cyclophosphamide, and busulfan, with an overall success rate of 70% to 80%. There is a high rate of GVHD in all patients with aplastic anemia who have transplants, but improved GVHD therapy with cyclosporine, mycophenolate, and tacrolimus has greatly reduced the associated morbidity.

If there is no HLA-identical sibling, immunosuppression with high-dose methylprednisolone, ATG, cyclosporine, and G-CSF is associated with a 60% to 70% success rate. Another less widely used regimen is high-dose cyclophosphamide alone. There is a 30% to 50% incidence of recurrence when immune suppression is used alone, but the patients often respond to retreatment.

These patients lack neutrophils to fight bacterial infections, but lymphocyte and monocyte function is normal or increased in aplastic anemia, unlike patients with malignancies. Immune suppression increases the risk of severe fungal infections (e.g., *Nocardia*, *Aspergillus*, or *Mucor* infections).

When toxicity or treatment failure occurs with immunosuppressive treatment, stem cell transplant from an unrelated matched donor or from a cord blood bank is performed. The risk of graft failure and GVHD should be weighed against the risk of complications such as sepsis or intracranial hemorrhage. Schleuning and colleagues (2000) have recently reviewed novel approaches to transplantation in patients with aplastic anemia, autoimmune disease, or malignancy that may improve their survival.

Patients with elevated liver enzyme levels are at higher risk for complications of transplantation, and thus a conservative approach is indicated. If transplantation is initiated when the liver enzymes are elevated, its success rate is reduced from 80% to 60%–70%. Hematopoietic growth factors are used during the first months following transplantation.

Methylprednisolone and ATG are used only in the first week of therapy, but cyclosporine is recommended for at least 6 months. Bone marrow biopsy should be performed before discontinuing the cyclosporine to confirm the presence of normal cellularity and rule out unrecognized malignancy, PNH, or refractory pure RBC anemia.

Prognosis

Left untreated, 90% of patients with aplastic anemia die within 12 months of presentation, usually from infection or hemorrhage. Significant morbidity related to fully matched allogeneic transplantation may be as high as 30% to 40%, but long-term resolution of the aplastic anemia is close to 80%. Immunosuppression regimens may be effective initially but require repeat courses and carry the risk of serious infection. Unrelated BMT or cord blood transplantation has a high risk of sepsis and GVHD and thus is used only in refractory cases.

PERNICIOUS ANEMIA

Definition

Pernicious anemia (PA) is a megaloblastic anemia caused by a deficiency of vitamin B_{12} resulting from diminished or absent gastric secretion of intrinsic factor (IF). PA is rare in childhood and is most often associated with an underlying immunodeficiency. The presence of parietal cell antibodies, the high incidence of PA in thyroid disease (in which autoimmune phenomena are common), and the lymphocytic infiltration of the stomach wall of patients with PA also suggest the importance of immune factors. PA with gastric achlorhydria has been described in children.

A group of young children with megaloblastic anemia and normal acid secretion has also been identified. In these cases, there is a congenital absence of IF, and both parietal cell and IF antibodies are lacking as a result of an autosomal recessive disorder. They have juvenile PA, differentiated from adult PA, which is characterized by achlorhydria and the presence of parietal cell and IF antibodies. Some children may have the adult type.

In a third form of PA, termed *Imerslund syndrome*, IF is present but the vitamin B_{12}–IF complex is not absorbed from the intestinal lumen (Imerslund and Bjornstad, 1963).

Pathogenesis

IF is a glycoprotein secreted by the parietal cells of the gastric mucosa that binds to the vitamin B_{12} found in most foods of animal origin; it is released during peptic digestion. This complex is intracellularly absorbed within the microvilli and reaches the bloodstream.

Antibodies to parietal cells and IF are detected in the serum and gastric juice of most patients with adult PA. Although parietal cell antibodies are present in approximately 80% of patients, they are nonspecific and are also detected in many healthy subjects. These IgG antibodies are directed against a lipoprotein antigen located on the microvilli of parietal cell secretory canaliculi. Their relationship to gastric inflammation and the development of PA is unclear.

Both IF and parietal cell antibodies can be demonstrated using gastric biopsies (Baur et al., 1968). Gastric IF antibodies are of two types—blocking and binding antibodies, both of which are IgG antibodies. Blocking antibodies combine with IF at or near the vitamin B_{12}–binding site and inhibit the formation of the vitamin B_{12}–IF complex. These antibodies are present in about 60% of patients with PA. Binding antibodies combine with IF at a location remote from the vitamin

B_{12}–binding site and occur in approximately 30% of patients with PA.

Juvenile Pernicious Anemia

Children with juvenile PA have a congenital IF deficiency. This is an autosomal recessive disorder; the heterozygotes manifest no clinical or laboratory abnormalities. In these patients, gastric acid and pepsin secretion is normal. They have no evidence of gastritis, and they lack antiparietal cell or anti-IF antibodies (McIntyre et al., 1965; Miller et al., 1966). Because this disorder shares none of the pathogenetic features of adult PA, it must be considered a separate disorder. These children may develop mild gastritis and reduced gastric acid production if they are not given parenteral maintenance injections of vitamin B_{12} (Lillibridge et al., 1967).

Adult-Type Pernicious Anemia

As a result of the loss of IF-secreting cells from atrophic gastric mucosa, adult-type PA is rare in children. Those factors that lead to gastric atrophy are not known; however, a genetic predisposition is suggested by a higher incidence of PA in the relatives of affected individuals than in the general population. Relatives have an increased incidence of achlorhydria, chronic gastritis, and vitamin B_{12} malabsorption, manifested by a decreased uptake of oral radioactive vitamin B_{12} (Callender and Denborough, 1957).

Adult PA may be due to a genetically determined defect in immunologic tolerance to antigens of the stomach. As a result, committed immunocytes may destroy the gastric mucosa by cell-mediated or antibody-mediated reactions, thus abolishing the parietal cells that synthesize IF. These immune reactions may be initiated spontaneously or as a result of injury to gastric cells by a subclinical infection that renders them antigeneic.

It is of note that PA occurs more frequently in patients with CVID (Conley, 1986). Rheumatoid arthritis and other autoimmune diseases occur frequently in PA (Good et al., 1957). PA often occurs in familial juvenile polyendocrinopathy (see Chapter 37). These children have a genetically determined susceptibility to develop organ-specific autoantibodies; however, many lack parietal cell antibodies, even in the presence of IF antibodies.

Clinical and Laboratory Features

The clinical and laboratory findings in juvenile PA secondary to congenital IF deficiency have been reviewed by Chanarin (1969). Megaloblastic anemia typically occurs between four and 28 months of age; nonetheless, there was one case in a 13-year-old (Lampkin and Schubert, 1968). After a healthy infancy, nonspecific symptoms of pallor, weakness, anorexia, and failure to thrive may develop. Stomatitis develops, and the tongue becomes depapillated. Splenomegaly may also develop. Ataxia, defective speech, loss of vibratory sense, brisk knee jerks, and extensor plantar reflexes may then occur.

The stomach is histologically normal; acid and pepsin secretion is normal (Lillibridge et al., 1967). IF is low to absent, and antibodies to parietal cells and IF are absent. Vitamin B_{12} absorption is impaired and is corrected by the oral administration of IF. Serum vitamin B_{12} levels are markedly reduced.

In children, acquired or adult-type PA usually occurs in late childhood or adolescence. There is usually achlorhydria, absence of IF, and histologic evidence of atrophic gastritis. Antibodies to parietal cells and IF are present. These children should be investigated for the possibility of a coexistent disorder such as familial juvenile polyendocrinopathy (see Chapter 37) or immunodeficiencies such as CVID (see Chapter 13) or mucocutaneous candidiasis (see Chapter 17).

In any child with vitamin B_{12}–responsive megaloblastic anemia, the possibility of generalized intestinal malabsorption (celiac disease), chronic ileal disease (Crohn's disease), congenital or acquired strictures, stagnant loop syndrome, distal ileal resection, or fistulous bypass should be considered. Congenital malabsorption of vitamin B_{12} (Imerslund and Bjornstad, 1963) and transcobalamin II deficiency (Hakami et al., 1971) are rare disorders that must be excluded.

Treatment

Once the diagnosis of PA has been established, parenteral vitamin B_{12} injections are given. Initial doses range from 30 to 1000 μg daily for 7 days. Thereafter, monthly injections of 50 to 1000 μg of B_{12} are continued indefinitely to maintain hematologic and neurologic remission.

IMMUNODEFICIENCY AND MALIGNANCY

Pathogenesis

With successful antibiotic use and immunotherapy, increasing numbers of immunodeficient patients survive beyond the first and second decades of life. Many of these patients then face an increased risk of lymphoproliferative disorders and cancer. The cause of this predisposition is varied and highly dependent on the type of immune deficiency (Gatti and Good, 1971; World Health Organization Scientific Group, 1995).

Cancer, the unregulated proliferation of abnormal cells, may occur as a result of undifferentiated residual embryonic tissue; ineffective DNA repair resulting in the loss of regulatory elements; or malignant conversion of a normal lymphoid response to chronic inflammation or infection. Eventually, these aberrant cells invade healthy tissue or metastasize to vital organs through the blood or lymphatics. By definition, all cancers proliferate and destroy normal organ architecture, but the biology and aggressiveness of each tumor vary greatly depending on its biologic and cytogenetic abnormalities.

The immune system plays a critical role in the recognition and destruction of malignant cells that express novel antigens, oncogene products, or metabolites. Successful elimination of these cells requires an intact immune surveillance system, including identification of the malignant cell; amplification of tumor-specific effector cells; and production of antibodies, cytokines, and chemokines to synergize the destruction of the cancer. Excessive generation of aberrant cells caused by DNA repair defects or disproportionate lymphoproliferation coupled with immunodeficiency may result in the increased incidence of cancer if the primary disease is not corrected with transplantation. Even children successfully treated with BMT may develop malignancy if the underlying defect affects all tissue, as seen in DNA repair disorders.

The most common and pervasive malignancies in immunodeficiencies are lymphoproliferative disorders. Because of polyclonal activation associated with recurrent infections, chromosomal translocations or other cytogenetic abnormalities occur, resulting in clonal evolution from benign hyperplasia into lymphoma or leukemia. Unlike lymphomas in previously well individuals, these same lymphomas in patients with primary immunodeficiency may occur in extranodal sites such as the stomach, small intestine, lung, or CNS (Mentzer et al., 1987).

Immunodeficiency Cancer Registry

A comprehensive database of patients with primary immunodeficiency and malignancy, termed the *Immunodeficiency Cancer Registry*, is maintained by the National Cancer Institute and the National Institute of Allergy and Infectious Diseases. The lymphoproliferative disorders and other tumors most commonly associated with primary immunodeficiencies are summarized in Table 39-4 (Elenitoba-Johnson and Jaffee, 1997; Filipovich et al., 1994; McClain, 1997). Several of these illnesses are associated with increased incidence of malignancy, but the nature and presentation of the tumor or lymphoma vary among syndromes, reflecting the interaction of the cytogenetic abnormalities with each target tissue.

The data in Table 39-4 reflect information collected over a 20-year period starting in 1973. Deficiency of the γc chain of the IL-2 receptor and RAG-1 and RAG-2 recombinase deficiencies are examples of recently delineated molecular mutations that result in severe combined immunodeficiency (see Chapter 15). The occurrence of malignancy and lymphoproliferative disease in these newly described syndromes may further define basic mechanisms leading to cancer in all patients.

Ataxia-telangiectasia

Ataxia-telangiectasia (AT) is an uncommon autosomal recessive genetic disorder characterized by cerebellar ataxia, oculocutaneous telangiectasia, progressive immunodeficiency, and a predisposition to lymphoid malignancy (see Chapter 18).

AT is associated with cytogenetic abnormalities in the ATM gene on chromosome 11 (Gatti et al., 1988, 1991). The mutations occur throughout the coding region of the gene. ATM functions in double-stranded break repair, as occurs in VDJ recombination (Concannon and Gatti, 1997). The ATM gene product is a protein critical for the detection of DNA damage and the control of cell cycle progression.

This gene is homologous with other checkpoint genes, such as phosphatidyl-inositol-3′ kinase activity, and is induced to phosphorylate the tumor suppressor p53 in response to DNA strand–breaking agents (Banin et al., 1998; Savitsky et al., 1995; Shiloh and Rotman, 1996). In its absence, cells cannot arrest mitosis to repair chromosome damage and cannot prevent the spontaneous demise of cells with significant DNA damage (Meyn, 1995).

It is not surprising that defects in this gene result in a high incidence of translocations and inversions. Those involving chromosomes 7 and 14 result primarily in cytogenetic mutations in the TCR and immunoglobulin gene loci and are found in as many as 10% of their circulating T lymphocytes (Savitsky et al., 1995a, 1995b; Taylor et al., 1996). There is a marked disparity in the number of lymphocytes that actually carry a productive rearrangement of their TCR chain or the immunoglobulin molecule, resulting in varying degrees of immunodeficiency in individual patients.

Healthy individuals may have abnormalities associated with gene rearrangements during lymphogenesis, which is, by nature, error-prone, resulting in nonrandom translocations in 1 in every 250 to 500 T cells, as compared with 1 in 10 among T cells exhibiting AT. However, other translocations in patients with AT occur among chromosomes 2p12, 22q11, and 8q24 (c-myc) and may play a role in the high rate of lymphoma. The involvement of c-myc in the translocation and the association of joining signals at the breakpoints suggest that common mechanisms of translocation and oncogene deregulation are involved in B- and T-cell malignancies in AT (Finger et al., 1986).

Because these genetic abnormalities are identical to those in immunocompetent patients with lymphoma, the AT mutations may accelerate or amplify a common mechanism of gene rearrangements during lymphogenesis (Filipovich et al., 1994; Elenitoba-Johnson and Jaffe, 1997).

Large-scale studies have found a 10% to 40% rate of malignancy in AT patients. Greater than 50% of the tumors are lymphomas or leukemia, which is a 70- to 250-fold higher risk for these tumors (Morrell et al., 1986). T-cell tumors are approximately four to five times as common as B-cell tumors. Young adults have a high incidence of T-cell prolymphocytic leukemia with

TABLE 39-4 · MALIGNANCIES ASSOCIATED WITH PRIMARY IMMUNODEFICIENCY DISORDERS

Immunodeficiency	Malignancy (% type)	Characteristics
Ataxia-telangiectasia (30% of reported tumors)	Lymphocytic leukemias (21%)	Myeloid leukemias rare
	T- and B-cell lymphoma (46%)	T-cell tumors 4 times more common than B-cell tumors
	Carcinoma (9%)	Gastric adenocarcinoma; all patients with absent IgA
	Hodgkin's disease (11%)	Primarily lymphocyte-depleted
	Other (13%)	Astrocytomas and medulloblastoma
Common variable immunodeficiency (24% of reported tumors)	Leukemia (7%)	Lymphoid
	Lymphoma (46%)	Multifocal and extranodal; only 25% are EBV positive
	Hodgkin's disease (7%)	May be extralymphatic
	Carcinoma (17%)	Gastric adenocarcinomas
	Other (23%)	Sarcoid-like granulomas
Wiskott-Aldrich syndrome (16% of reported tumors)	Leukemia (9%)	T- and B-cell lymphocytic leukemia
	Lymphoma (76%)	Multifocal and extranodal; 23% CNS
	Hodgkin's disease (4%)	Aggressive; large cell immunoblastic
	Carcinoma (0%)	Nodular sclerosis and lymphocyte-depleted subtypes
	Other (11%)	Kaposi's sarcoma
Severe combined immunodeficiency (8% of reported tumors)	Leukemia (12%)	Lymphoid
	Lymphoma (74%)	Extranodal and 48% multifocal
	Hodgkin's disease (10%)	Poor prognosis
	Carcinoma (2 %)	
	Other (2%)	
IgA deficiency (8% of reported tumors)	Leukemia (0%)	Primarily brain/CNS
	Lymphoma (16%)	Gastric carcinoma with *Helicobacter pylori* infections; carcinomas of thyroid, cervix, and gallbladder; and fibrosarcoma
	Hodgkin's disease (8%)	
	Carcinoma (21%)	
	Other (55%)	
Hypogammaglobulinemia (5% of reported tumors)	Leukemia (33%)	Lymphoid
	Lymphoma (33%)	Multifocal and extranodal, *not* CNS
	Hodgkin's disease (14%)	Poor prognosis
	Carcinoma (14%)	Gastric
	Other (6%)	
Hyper-IgM syndrome (3% of reported tumors)	Leukemia (0%)	Lymph node, CNS, and GI tumors
	Lymphoma (56%)	Poor prognosis is most prevalent; of mixed cellularity
	Hodgkin's disease (25%)	Primary small cell undifferentiated carcinoma of the colon and hepatocellular carcinoma
	Carcinoma (0%)	
	Other (19%)	
Other immunodeficiencies (XLP, hyper-IgE, Bloom and Nijmegen breakage syndromes)	Leukemia (16%)	Lymphoid or myeloid (Hyper-IgE)
	Lymphoma (48%)	Multifocal and extranodal
	Hodgkin's disease (4%)	Mantle cell lymphoma is associated with hyper-IgE syndrome
	Carcinoma (4%)	Nodular sclerosis
	Other (28%)	Gastric, skin, and genitourinary (6% of reported tumors)
All immunodeficiency categories combined (100% of reported tumors)	Leukemia (13%)	B- and T-cell lymphoid leukemias 8% CNS, 9% GI tract, 10% lymph node, and 21% multifocal
	Lymphoma (50%)	Poor prognosis
	Hodgkin's disease (9%)	Mainly gastric adenocarcinoma
	Carcinoma (9%)	Brain tumors and granulomas; sarcoid
	Other tumors (19%)	

CNS = central nervous system; EBV = Epstein-Barr virus; GI = gastrointestinal; XLP = X-linked proliferative syndrome.
Modified from Elenitoba-Johnson KS, Jaffe ES. Lymphoproliferative disorders associated with congenital immunodeficiencies. Semin Diagn Pathol 14:35–47, 1997; Filipovich AH, Mathur A, Kamat D, Kersey JH, Shapiro RS. Lymphoproliferative disorders and other tumors complicating immunodeficiencies. Immunodeficiency 5:91–112, 1994; and McClain KL. Immunodeficiency states and related malignancies. In Walterhouse DO, Cohn SL, eds. Diagnostic and therapeutic advances in pediatric oncology. Boston, Kluwar Academic Publishers, 1997, pp 39–61.

a poor prognosis (Elenitoba-Johnson and Jaffe, 1997; Filipovich et al., 1994). Murine models of AT, with targeted disruption of the ATM gene, result in thymic lymphomas in all affected mice (Barlow et al., 1996; Elson et al., 1996; Xu et al., 1996).

Hodgkin's disease constitutes 10% of the tumors in AT and is generally associated with a lymphocyte-depleted subtype. The median age at diagnosis is 10 years, and there is a 3:2 male predominance. Perhaps due to the histopathologic subtype or ineffective therapy,

the prognosis is poor compared to children who have Hodgkin's disease but a healthy immune system and normal DNA repair.

Although less common, aggressive malignant tumors of B-cell origin are also present in AT and include non-Hodgkin's lymphomas such as Burkitt's lymphoma, diffuse large-cell lymphoma, and immunoblastic B-cell lymphomas. Patients with AT who have these tumors are more likely to have extranodal and multifocal involvement, including CNS or abdominal primary tumors. Unlike the lymphomas in other primary immunodeficiencies, the lymphomas in patients with AT are not always associated with EBV and resemble those in healthy individuals (Elenitoba-Johnson and Jaffe, 1997).

AT patients—many of whom have an IgA deficiency—have an increased incidence of gastric carcinoma, as do patients with selective IgA deficiency but without AT (Bachmeyer et al., 2000; Silvestris et al., 1996). Recurrent gastrointestinal infections with *Giardia lamblia* or *Helicobacter pylori* and coexistent autoimmune diseases may occur in 20% of patients with IgA deficiency and may account for their increased incidence of this adenocarcinoma. Constant antigenic stimulus and inflammation in the gastrointestinal tract may result in the emergence of a malignant clone.

Of interest, patients with AT who have normal levels of IgA have no predisposition to gastric carcinoma (Bachmeyer et al., 2000; Filipovich et al., 1980; Silvestris et al., 1996).

Other solid tumors, including medulloblastomas and gliomas, occur with increased frequency in AT but not at the frequency of lymphoproliferative disorders or gastric carcinoma (Gatti and Good, 1971; Loeb et al., 2000).

Nijmegen Breakage Syndrome

The clinical, immunologic, and chromosomal findings from 42 patients in the Nijmegen breakage syndrome (NBS) registry were recently reviewed (van der Burgt et al., 1996) (see Chapter 18). Although the immunodeficiency and DNA damage resemble those present in AT, the clinical findings are distinct. NBS is a separate entity with its defective gene, *NBS-1,* located on chromosome 8q21.

The gene product nibrin is a novel protein that is a member of the hMre11/hRad50 protein complex and is involved in DNA double-strand break repair (Varon et al., 2001). None of the patients with NBS had signs of cerebellar ataxia, apraxic eye movements, or other neurologic abnormalities, except for twin girls who had clinical symptoms of both NBS and AT (Curry et al., 1989; International Nijmegen Breakage Syndrome Study Group, 2000). Complementation studies assigned these cases to NBS complementation group V1.

Recent observations confirmed a link between NBS and AT based on laboratory observations that the phosphorylation of *NBS-1,* induced by ionizing radiation, requires catalytically active ATM (Zhao et al., 2000). Complexes containing ATM and *NBS*-1 exist in vivo in both untreated cells and cells treated with ionizing radiation. In addition, two residues of *NBS-1* have been identified—Ser 278 and Ser 343—that are phosphorylated in vitro by ATM and whose modification in vivo is essential for the cellular response to DNA damage. Abnormalities activated by DNA damage contribute to oncogenic chromosomal rearrangements that underlie lymphoid malignancies in which there is an absence of normal cell cycle checkpoints.

With increased cell turnover, there is an increased risk of cancer, especially lymphoid malignancies bearing oncogenic immunoglobulin and TCR locus translocations. The frequency of immunodeficiency and malignancy and the percentage of chromosome rearrangements are higher in NBS than in AT. Clinically unaffected relatives of patients with NBS also have an increased risk of cancer (Seemanova, 1990). Twelve of forty-two NBS patients (25% of registry patients) from 1 to 22 years of age had developed lymphoma as of 1996. In addition, one patient each developed a glioma at the age of 12 years, a medulloblastoma at 15 years, and a rhabdomyosarcoma at 4 years of age. In another study, 40% of the patients, primarily of eastern European ancestry, developed cancer before the age of 21 years (International Nijmegen Breakage Syndrome Study Group, 2000).

Investigators have analyzed all 16 exons for mutations of the *NBS-1* gene in 47 children with first relapse of acute lymphocytic leukemia (ALL) (Stumm et al., 2001; Varon et al., 2001). In 7 of 47 children (15%), 4 novel amino acid substitutions were identified. The germline origin of the mutation was confirmed in 3 patients, whereas a somatic mutation was present in the remaining cases. No additional mutations were found on the second allele in any of the 7 patients, suggesting that NBS does not act like a typical tumor suppressor gene. The observed *NBS-1* gene mutations in ALL patients suggest its involvement in the pathogenesis of the disease. In a contrasting study, investigators used a different technique to look for deletions of the *NBS-1* gene in B-cell lymphomas (Stumm et al., 2001). The malignancy was typical of NBS, but no mutations were found, suggesting a different pathophysiology for ALL versus lymphoma in this syndrome.

Other DNA Repair Disorders

An ever-growing number of syndromes are now being reported with immune deficiencies, DNA repair defects, and lymphoproliferative malignancies and cancer (Moses, 2001; van Brabant et al., 2000).

Bloom syndrome (associated with deficient cellular DNA ligase) is characterized by congenital telangiectasia, photosensitivity, growth retardation, immune deficiency, increased susceptibility to infection, and predominantly internal—rather than cutaneous—malignancy (see Chapter 18). The risk of neoplasia, especially leukemia, is greatly increased. Sister-chromatid exchanges occur at an increased frequency and may be detected spontaneously.

The product of the *BLM* gene is a DNA helicase of the RecQ subfamily is critical for maintaining genomic stability. Helicases promote unwinding of double-stranded DNA, and the RecQ subfamily is implicated in DNA repair. Most mutations bring about premature truncation of the protein (Ellis and German, 1996; Kondo et al., 1992).

All children with cancer who have dysmorphic features, neurologic disorders, growth retardation, or a history of immunodeficiency should be studied for DNA repair defects because siblings and parents may have an increased risk of malignancy and thus monitored for this possibility.

Chemotherapy in DNA Repair Disorders

Chemotherapy for patients with DNA repair defects presents a challenge to the oncologist who wishes to treat maximally while minimizing side effects. Radiation and alkylating agents have not been used because of increased risk of toxicity, resulting in poor or partial response to treatment. Recent studies suggest that rather than excluding such therapy altogether, chemotherapy at lower doses may be accomplished (Loeb et al., 2000; Sandoval and Swift, 1998).

In treating nine children with chromosomal breakage syndromes and non-Hodgkin's lymphoma as part of clinical trials in Germany, Seidermann and co-workers (2000) found that alkylating agents and epipodophyllotoxins carried an unacceptable toxicity, but other agents could be used safely with dose adjustments.

Wiskott-Aldrich Syndrome

Wiskott-Aldrich syndrome (WAS) is an X-linked recessive disorder characterized by thrombocytopenia, immunodeficiency, and eczema resulting from mutations of the X-chromosome gene WASP (Wiskott-Aldrich syndrome protein) encoding the WAS protein (Aldrich et al., 1954; Derry et al., 1994; Ochs, 1998; Wiskott, 1936) (see Chapter 17). WAS platelets are small, with a mean platelet volume of less than 7 μm and a "dustlike" appearance on Wright's stain. Circulating lymphocytes also have defective architecture, most likely caused by an abnormality of cell-surface sialoglycoprotein, CD43, which may have a role in T-cell activation and antigen processing (Mentzer et al., 1987; Parkman et al., 1981).

The WAS gene and its protein product, WASP, a 53-kD intracellular hematopoietic cell protein, were described by Derry and colleagues in 1994. Subsequent biochemical studies characterized WASP as a multidomain molecule that helps regulate the actin cytoskeleton (Zhu et al., 1997).

WAS is heterogeneous in severity and course. Shcherbina and co-workers (2001) suggested that the degree of immunodeficiency and the risk of B-cell lymphoma may be related to the presence or absence of WASP and RNA in the lymphocyte subsets. Patients with severe WAS had no measurable WASP in platelets or peripheral mononuclear cells, whereas patients with a moderate WAS phenotype have discordant WASP expression, with T cells expressing WASP and RNA and B cells lacking WASP. The discordant group develops B-cell lymphoma, suggesting that WASP's absence on B cells accelerates lymphoid malignancy.

Baba and colleagues (1999) showed that WASP is both physically associated with Bruton's tyrosine kinase

and can serve as a substrate for it. WASP was transiently tyrosine-phosphorylated after B-cell receptor ligation, suggesting that WASP is located downstream of cytoplasmic tyrosine kinases. This step in B-cell differentiation is one of the many possible roles of WASP, but it suggests a mechanism for the increased rate of lymphoma. Thus testing of WASP expression in lymphocytes is recommended in addition to mutation analysis.

Early BMT to treat WAS reduces the risk of developing malignancy. When the pretransplant conditioning was not fully myeloablative, a chimeric state may develop, with persistent expression of WASP in the patients' own cells and continued predisposition to B-cell malignancy. Long-term survival following non-Hodgkin's lymphoma in children with WAS and the improved survival in children with B-cell acute lymphocytic leukemia (B-ALL) and stage IV B-cell non-Hodgkin's lymphoma (B-NHL) suggest that these cancers should be treated aggressively (Gilson and Taylor, 1999). As with other immunodeficiencies, special attention should be paid to the toxicities of chemotherapy and the increased risk of infection in these patients.

BMT should be considered for patients not transplanted previously, because it may cure WAS and optimize the high-dose chemotherapy.

Common Variable Immunodeficiency

Common variable immunodeficiency (CVID) is an acquired, usually nonfamilial, syndrome characterized by hypogammaglobulinemia, recurrent bacterial infections, and increased occurrence of both autoimmune disease and malignancy (Rosen, 1995) (see Chapter 13). Kinlen and co-workers (1985) reported that patients with hypogammaglobulinemia had a 23-fold increased risk for malignant lymphoma and a 50-fold increased risk for gastric cancer, with the latter especially common in patients with IgA deficiency. Cunningham-Rundles and colleagues (1987) reported a 100-fold increased risk for lymphoma in patients with CVID followed up to 13 years.

These findings are confirmed in the registries for immune deficiency and reports from the 1990s (Filipovich et al., 1994, 1996a, 1996b), in which the rate of lymphoma increased as patients aged. Most patients have non-Hodgkin's lymphomas, but Hodgkin's disease and T-cell lymphoma do occur as well (Durham et al., 1987; Gottesman et al., 1999; Sander et al., 1992). Although not extensively studied, CVID cells may have increased in vitro radiosensitivity, as seen in AT and NBS (Palanduz et al., 1998).

CVID is a heterogeneous illness for which both familial and sporadic patterns of inheritance have been reported. It is variable in severity and onset, suggesting a defect in B-cell regulation rather than an intrinsic B-cell–specific mutation. In contrasting the rate of malignancy in CVID versus that in Bruton's X-linked agammaglobulinemia, it is important to recognize that the Bruton's tyrosine kinase defect of X-linked agammaglobulinemia results in the failure of B-cell precursors to differentiate and proliferate, but T-cell function remains normal (Zenone, 1997).

Some patients with CVID have normal B-cell proliferation but dysregulated immunoglobulin production, whereas others have abnormal T-cell function and cytokine synthesis (Farrant et al., 1994; Kondratenko et al., 1997; Levy et al., 1998; Nonoyama et al., 1994; Webster, 2001). Their B-cell–containing tissue can become hyperplastic as CD19-positive cells may still have the ability to respond to antigen, but they lack the downregulation provided by immunoglobulin feedback.

Given the high rate of malignancy, the mutation(s) responsible for CVID would be helpful in elucidating this link. No animal models or consistent genetic defects have been identified. Abnormalities in T-cell surveillance, cytokine levels, and sensitivity to ionizing radiation may predispose patients to lymphoreticular malignancies following antigen exposure or infection with pathogenic viruses such as EBV. Most patients with CVID have reduced numbers of CD4 cells count and a normal number of CD8 cells (Farrant et al., 1994). In some patients, there is defective TCR signaling and failure of lymphocyte activation following antigen stimulation (Kondratenko et al., 1997; Nordoy et al., 1998). The B cells of some patients with CVID can produce all immunoglobulin isotypes in vitro when stimulated with *Staphylococcus aureus*, Cowan strain in the presence of anti-CD40 antibodies and IL-10 (Nonoyama et al., 1994).

The heterogeneity of CVID precludes a clear link between T- or B-lymphocyte dysfunction and malignancy. However, the persistence of B cells in hyperplastic lymphoid tissue in the absence of T-cell or immunoglobulin downregulation may permit the expansion of malignant lymphoid clones. Gastric carcinoma may result from chronic gastric stimulation, atrophic gastritis, or *H. pylori* colonization.

X-Linked Lymphoproliferative Syndrome

The incidence of X-linked lymphoproliferative syndrome (XLP) is approximately 1 to 3 per million boys. XLP results from a mutation or deletion of the *XLP* (*SAP/SH2D1A*) gene that encodes the T-cell–specific protein SLAM-associated protein (SAP; a protein associated with the signaling lymphocyte activation molecule [SLAM]), a natural inhibitor of SH2 domain–dependent interactions with members of the signaling lymphocyte activation molecule family (Morra et al., 2001; Sayos et al., 1998) (see Chapter 17). This protein is critically important in T-cell signaling because its absence results in the inability to control EBV-induced B-cell proliferation (Coffey et al., 1998).

Although clinically well prior to EBV infection, up to 60% to 75% of XLP patients succumb to fulminant EBV. The immune systems of surviving patients appear to have suffered irreversible damage associated with T- and B-cell defects (Grierson and Purtilo, 1987; Sullivan et al., 1988; Tosato et al., 1995). Although XLP patients have normal numbers of T lymphocytes,

CD8 cells predominate, with a reversal of the CD4/CD8 ratio and, in 30% of the patients, abnormal natural killer cell function. In addition, antibody to EBV-associated nuclear antigen is absent and antibody to capsid antigen decreased.

Between 20% and 35% of survivors develop extranodal non-Hodgkin's B-cell lymphomas with a predilection for the ileocecal region (Thomas et al., 1991). If a diagnosis of XLP can be identified prior to EBV infection, stem cell transplant should be performed (Filipovich et al., 1986, 1994). Seemayer (1995) suggested that BMT after EBV may be successful by using optimal supportive therapy. Treatment with immune modifiers such as acyclovir, IFNs, and IVIG are ineffective in treating the EBV infection (Grierson and Purtilo, 1987; Turner et al., 1992).

DiGeorge Syndrome

As discussed in Chapter 17, DiGeorge syndrome and the related velocardiofacial syndromes are associated with variable degrees of T-cell deficiency, which often improves during the first decade of life. Not typically associated with malignancy, these syndromes may have an increased incidence of B-cell non-Hodgkin's lymphoma with EBV expression (Ramos et al., 1999; Sato et al., 1999). In addition, myeloid leukemia has been reported in twins with a translocation of the mixed lineage leukemia (MLL) promoter region in the genomic region of the 22q11 deletion present in these syndromes (Megonigal et al., 1998).

Summary

The incidence of malignancy in primary immunodeficiency may be further refined as other gene mutations are delineated. Recognition and study of the immune disorders associated with high rates of lymphoid malignancy may provide invaluable insight into their clonal expansion and why they are unable to contain and destroy early cancer cells.

R E F E R E N C E S

Altman LK. Who goes first? The story of self-experimentation in medicine. New York, Random House, 1987, pp 273–283.

Aldrich RA, Steinberg AG, Campbell DC. Pedigree demonstrating a sex-linked recessive condition characterized by draining ears, eczematoid dermatitis, and bloody diarrhea. Pediatrics 13:133–139, 1954.

Ammann AJ, Hong R. Selective IgA deficiency and autoimmunity. Clin Exp Immunol 7:833–838, 1970.

Anderson KC, Weinstein HJ. Transfusion-associated graft-versus-host disease. N Engl J Med 323:315–321, 1990.

Andersson J. Cytokines in idiopathic thrombocytopenic purpura (ITP). Acta Paediatr Suppl 424:61–64, 1998.

Aster RH. Effect of anticoagulant and ABO incompatibility on recovery of transfused human platelets. Blood 26:732–743, 1965.

Baba Y, Nonoyama S, Matsushita M, Yamadori T, Hashimoto S, Imai K, Arai S, Kunikata T, Kurimoto M, Kurosaki T, Ochs HD, Yata J, Kishimoto T, Tsukada S. Involvement of Wiskott-Aldrich syndrome protein in B-cell cytoplasmic tyrosine kinase pathway. Blood 93:2003–2012, 1999.

Bachmeyer C, Monge M, Cazier A, Le Deist F, de Saint Basile G, Durandy A, Fischer A, Mougeot-Martin M. Gastric adenocarcinoma in a patient with X-linked agammaglobulinaemia. Eur J Gastroenterol Hepatol 12:1033–1035, 2000.

Ballem PJ, Segal GM, Stratton JR, Gernsheimer T, Adamson JW, Slichter SJ. Mechanisms of thrombocytopenia in chronic autoimmune thrombocytopenic purpura. Evidence of both impaired platelet production and increased platelet clearance. J Clin Invest 80:33–40, 1987.

Banin S, Moyal L, Shieh S, Taya Y, Anderson CW, Chessa L, Smorodinsky NI, Prives C, Reiss Y, Shiloh Y, Ziv Y. Enhanced phosphorylation of p53 by ATM in response to DNA damage. Science 281:1674–1679, 1998.

Baur S, Fisher JM, Strickland RG, Taylor KB. Autoantibody-containing cells in the gastric mucosa in pernicious anaemia. Lancet 2:887–894, 1968.

Barlow C, Hirotsune S, Paylor RL, Liyanage M, Eckhaus M, Collins F, Shiloh Y, Crawley JN, Ried T, Tagle D, Wynshaw-Boris A. ATM-deficient mice: a paradigm of ataxia telangiectasia. Cell 86:159–171, 1996.

Bell CA, Zwicker H, Sacks HJ. Autoimmune hemolytic anemia: routine serologic evaluation in a general hospital population. Am J Clin Pathol 60:903–911, 1973.

Berchtold P, Dale GL, Tani P, McMillan R. Inhibition of autoantibody binding to platelet glycoprotein IIb/IIIa by anti-idiotypic antibodies in intravenous gammaglobulin. Blood 74:2414–2417, 1989.

Brand A, Sintnicolaas K, Claas FH. Eernisse JG. ABH antibodies causing platelet transfusion refractoriness. Transfusion 26:463–466, 1986.

Boggio LN, Green D. Acquired hemophilia. Rev Clin Exp Hematol 5:389–404, 2001.

Bussel J, Heddle N, Richards C, Woloski M. MCP-1, IL-10, IL-6 and TNFα levels in patients with ITP before and after IV anti-D and IVIG treatments. Blood 94:15a, 1999.

Bussel JB. Fc receptor blockade and immune thrombocytopenic purpura. Semin Hematol 37:261–266, 2000.

Bussel JB. Novel approaches to refractory immune thrombocytopenic purpura. Blood Rev 16:31–36, 2002.

Bux J, Mueller-Eckhardt C. Autoimmune neutropenia. Semin Hematol 29:45–53, 1992.

Bux J, Kober B, Kiefel V, Mueller-Eckhardt C. Analysis of granulocyte-reactive antibodies using an immunoassay based upon monoclonal-antibody-specific immobilization of granulocyte antigens. Transfus Med 3:157–162, 1993.

Bux J, Behrens G, Jaeger G, Welte K. Diagnosis and clinical course of autoimmune neutropenia in infancy: analysis of 240 cases. Blood 91:181–186, 1998.

Bux J, Hofmann C, Welte K. Serum G-CSF levels are not increased in patients with antibody-induced neutropenia unless they are suffering from infectious diseases. Br J Haematol 105:616–617, 1999.

Callender ST, Denborough MA. A family study of pernicious anemia. Br J Haematol 3:88–106, 1957.

Carapella de Luca E, Casadei AM, di Piero G, Midulla M. Bisdomini C, Purpura M. Auto-immune haemolytic anaemia in childhood: follow-up in 29 cases. Vox Sang 36:13–20, 1979.

Carr R, Hutton JL, Jenkins JA, Lucas GF, Amphlett NW. Transfusion of ABO-mismatched platelets leads to early platelet refractoriness. Br J Haematol 75:408–413, 1990.

Cartron J, Fior R, Boue F, Tertian G, Gane P, Cartron JP. Non Hodgkin's lymphoma presenting as neutropenia related to an IgM monoclonal anti-i antibody. Hematol Cell Ther 38:225–230, 1996.

Chanarin I. The megaloblastic anemias. Oxford, England, Blackwell Scientific Publications, 1969.

Charles RJ, Sabo KM, Kidd PG, Abkowitz JL. The pathophysiology of pure red cell aplasia: implications for therapy. Blood 87:4831–4838, 1996.

Cines DB, Wilson SB, Tomaski A, Schreiber AD. Platelet antibodies of the IgM class in immune thrombocytopenic purpura. J Clin Invest 75:1183–1190, 1985.

Cines DB, Schreiber AD. Immune thrombocytopenia. Use of a Coombs antiglobulin test to detect IgG and C3 on platelets. N Engl J Med 300:106–111, 1979.

Clynes R, Maizes JS, Guinamard R, Ono M, Takai T, Ravetch JV. Modulation of immune complex-induced inflammation in vivo by the coordinate expression of activation and inhibitory Fc receptors. J Exp Med 189:179–185, 1999.

Clynes RA, Towers TL, Presta LG, Ravetch JV. Inhibitory Fc receptors modulate in vivo cytotoxicity against tumor targets. Nat Med 6:443–446, 2000.

Coffey AJ, Brooksbank RA, Brandau O, Oohashi T, Howell GR, Bye JM, Cahn AP, Durham J, Heath P, Wray P, Pavitt R, Wilkinson J, Leversha M, Huckle E, Shaw-Smith CJ, Dunham A, Rhodes S, Schuster V, Porta G, Yin L, Serafini P, Sylla B, Zollo M, Franco B, Bentley DR, et al. Host response to EBV infection in X-linked lymphoproliferative disease results from mutations in an SH2-domain encoding gene. Nat Genet 20:129–135, 1998.

Concannon P, Gatti RA. Diversity of ATM gene mutations detected in patients with ataxia-telangiectasia. Hum Mutat 10:100–107, 1997.

Conley ME, Park CL, Douglas SD. Childhood common variable immunodeficiency with autoimmune disease. J Pediatr 108:915–922, 1986.

Coombs RR, Mourant AE, Race RR. A new test for the detection of weak and incomplete Rh agglutinins. Br J Exp Pathol 26:255–268, 1945.

Cornelius AS, Campbell D, Schwartz E, Poncz M. Elevated common acute lymphoblastic leukemia antigen expression in pediatric immune thrombocytopenic purpura. Am J Pediatr Hematol Oncol 13:57–61, 1991.

Costea N, Yakulis VJ, Heller P. Inhibition of cold agglutinins (anti-I) by M. pneumoniae antigens. Proc Soc Exp Biol Med 139:476–479, 1972.

Crossley AR, Dickinson AM, Proctor SJ, Calvert JE. Effects of interferon-alpha therapy on immune parameters in immune thrombocytopenic purpura. Autoimmunity 24:81–100, 1996.

Cunningham-Rundles C, Siegal FP, Cunningham-Rundles S, Lieberman P. Incidence of cancer in 98 patients with common varied immunodeficiency. J Clin Immunol 7:294–299, 1987.

Curry CJ, O'Lague P, Tsai J, Hutchinson HT, Jaspers NG, Wara D, Gatti RA, Hutchinson HT. AT Fresno: a phenotype linking ataxia-telangiectasia with the Nijmegen breakage syndrome. Am J Hum Genet 45:270–275, 1989.

Davies KA, Walport MJ. Processing and clearance of immune complexes by complement and the role of complement in immune complex diseases. In Volanakis JE, Frank MM, eds. The human complement system in health and disease. New York, Marcel Dekker, 1998, p 423.

Deas JE, Janney FA, Lee LT, Howe C. Immune electron microscopy of cross-reactions between Mycoplasma pneumoniae and human erythrocytes. Infect Immun 24:211–217, 1979.

De Angelis V, Biasinutto C, Pradella P, Errante D. Mixed-type auto-immune haemolytic anaemia in a patient with HIV infection. Vox Sang 68:191–194, 1995.

Derry JM, Ochs HD, Francke U. Isolation of a novel gene mutated in Wiskott-Aldrich syndrome. Cell 78:635–644, 1994.

deShazo RH. Immune complex disease. In Goldman A, ed. Cecil textbook of medicine. 21st ed. New York, W. B. Saunders, 2000, pp 1429–1433.

Diamond LK, Blackfan KD, Baty JM. Erythroblastosis fetalis and its association with universal edema of the fetus, icterus gravis neonatorum and anemia of the newborn. J Pediatr 1:269, 1932.

Dianzani U, Bragardo M, DiFranco D, Alliaudi C, Scagni P, Buonfiglio D, Redonglia V, Bonissoni S, Correra A, Dianzani I, Ramenghi U. Deficiency of the Fas apoptosis pathway without Fas gene mutations in pediatric patients with autoimmunity/lymphoproliferation. Blood 89:2871–2879, 1997.

Donath J, Landsteiner K. Über paroxysmale Hämoglobinurie. Munch Med Wochenschr 51:1590–1596, 1904.

Donham JA, Denning V. Cold agglutinin syndrome: nursing management. Heart Lung 14:59–67, 1985.

Du XP, Plow EF, Frelinger AL III, O'Toole TE, Loftus JC, Ginsberg MH. Ligands "activate" integrin alpha IIb β 3 (platelet GPIIb-IIIa). Cell 65:409–416, 1991.

Dunstan RA, Simpson MB. Heterogeneous distribution of antigens on human platelets demonstrated by fluorescence flow cytometry. Br J Haematol 61:603–609, 1985.

Durham JC, Stephens DS, Rimland D, Nassar VH, Spira TJ. Common variable hypogammaglobulinemia complicated by an unusual T-suppressor/cytotoxic cell lymphoma. Cancer 59:271–276, 1987.

Duguesnoy RJ, Anderson AJ, Tomasulo PA, Aster RH. ABO compatibility and platelet transfusions of alloimmunized thrombocytopenic patients. Blood 54:595–599, 1979.

Elder ME. T-cell immunodeficiencies. Pediatr Clin North Am 47:1253–1274, 2000.Elenitoba-Johnson KS, Jaffe ES. Lymphoproliferative disorders associated with congenital immunodeficiencies. Semin Diagn Pathol 14:35–47, 1997.

Ellis NA, German J. Molecular genetics of Bloom's syndrome. Hum Mol Genet 5:1457–1463, 1996.

Elson A, Wang Y, Daugherty CJ, Morton CC, Zhou F, Campos-Torres J, Leder P. Pleiotropic defects in ataxia-telangiectasia protein-deficient mice. Proc Natl Acad Sci USA 93:13084–13089, 1996.

Engelfriet CP, Overbeeke MA, von dem Borne AE. Autoimmune hemolytic anemia. Semin Hematol 29:3–12, 1992.Erduran E, Aslan Y, Aliyazicioglu Y, Mocan H, Gedik Y. Plasma soluble interleukin-2 receptor levels in patients with idiopathic thrombocytopenic purpura. Am J Hematol 57:119–123, 1998.

Evans RS, Takahashi K. Primary thrombocytopenic purpura and acquired hemolytic anemia. Evidence for a common etiology. Arch Intern Med 87:48–54, 1951.

Farrant J, Spickett G, Matamoros N, Copas D, Hernandez M, North M, Chapel H, Webster AD. Study of B and T cell phenotypes in blood of patients with common variable immunodeficiency (CVID). Immunodeficiency 5:159–169, 1994.

Filion MC, Proulx C, Bradley AJ, Devine DV, Sékaly RP, Décary F, Chartrand P. Presence in peripheral blood of healthy individuals of autoreactive T cells to a membrane antigen present on bone marrow–derived cells. Blood 88:2144–2150, 1996.

Filipovich AH, Blazar BR, Ramsay NK, Kersey JH, Zelkowitz L, Harada S, Purtilo DT. Allogeneic bone marrow transplantation for X-linked lymphoproliferative syndrome. Transplantation 42:222–224, 1986.

Filipovich AH, Spector BD, Kersey J. Immunodeficiency in humans as a risk factor in the development of malignancy. Prev Med 9:252–259, 1980.

Filipovich AH, Mathur A, Kamat D, Kersey JH, Shapiro RS. Lymphoproliferative disorders and other tumors complicating immunodeficiencies. Immunodeficiency 5:91–112, 1994.

Filipovich A, Jyonouchi H, Bechtel M, et al. Immune mediated hematologic and oncologic disorders, including Epstein-Barr virus infection. In Stiehm ER, ed. 4th ed. Philadelphia, W. B. Saunders, 1996, pp 855–888.

Filipovich A, Mertens A, Ramsay NK, et al. Lymphoproliferative disorders associated with primary immunodeficiencies. In McGrath I, ed. Non-Hodgkin's lymphoma. 2nd ed. London, England, Edward Arnold, 1996, pp 459–482.

Finger LR, Harvey RC, Moore RC, Showe LC, Croce CM. A common mechanism of chromosomal translocation in T- and B-cell neoplasia. Science 234:982–985, 1986.

Foster CB, Zhu S, Erichsen HC, Lehrnbecher T, Hart ES, Choi E, Stein S, Smith MW, Steinberg SM, Imbach P, Kuhne T, Chanock SJ; The Early Chronic ITP Study Group. Polymorphisms in inflammatory cytokines and Fcγ receptors in childhood chronic immune thrombocytopenic purpura: a pilot study. Br J Haematol 113:596–599, 2001.

Frank MM, Miletic VD, Jiang H. Immunoglobulin in the control of complement action. Immunol Res 22:137–146, 2000.

Fujimoto TT, Inoue M, Shimomura T, Fujimura K. Involvement of Fc gamma receptor polymorphism in the therapeutic response of idiopathic thrombocytopenic purpura. Br J Haematol 115:125–130, 2001.

Furihata K, Nugent DJ, Bissonette A, Aster RH, Kunicki TJ. On the association of the platelet-specific alloantigen, Penᵃ, with glycoprotein IIIa. Evidence for heterogeneity of glycoprotein IIIa. J Clin Invest 80:1624–1630, 1987.

Garcia-Suarez J, Prieto A, Reyes E, Manzano L, Arribalzaga K, Alvarez-Mon M. Abnormal γIFN and αTNF secretion in purified

CD2⁺ cells from autoimmune thrombocytopenic purpura (ATP) patients: their implication in the clinical course of the disease. Am J Hematol 49:271–276, 1995.

Gatti RA, Good RA. Occurrence of malignancy in immuno-deficiency diseases. A literature review. Cancer 28:89–98, 1971.

Gatti RA, Boder E, Vinters HV, Sparkes RS, Norman A, Lange K. Ataxia-telangiectasia: an interdisciplinary approach to pathogenesis. Medicine (Baltimore) 70:99–117, 1991.

Gatti RA, Berkel I, Boder E, Braedt G, Charmley P, Concannon P, Ersoy F, Foroud T, Jaspers NG, Lange K, Lathrop GM, Leppert M, Nakamura Y, O'Connell P, Paterson M, Salser W, Sanal, O, Silver J, Sparkes RS, Susi E, Weeks DE, Wei S, White R, Yoder F. Localization of an ataxia-telangiectasia gene to chromosome 11q22-23. Nature 336:577–580, 1988.

Geissler RG, Kobberling J. Cold agglutinin disease. Klin Wochenschr 66:277–283, 1988.

George JN, Saucerman S, Bainton DF. Immunoglobulin G is a platelet alpha granule–secreted protein. J Clin Invest 76:2020–2025, 1985.

George JN, Pickett EB, Heinz R. Platelet membrane microparticles in blood bank fresh frozen plasma and cryoprecipitate. Blood 68:307–309, 1986.

George J, Raskob G, Bussel J, Cobos E, Green D, Tongol J, Rutherford C, Wasser J, Croft H, Rhinehart S, Oates B, Scaramucci J, Nadeau J. Safety and effect on platelet count of repeated doses of monoclonal antibody to CD40 ligand in patients with chronic ITP. Blood 94:19a, 1999.

Gilson D, Taylor RE. Long-term survival following non-Hodgkin's lymphoma arising in Wiskott-Aldrich syndrome. Clin Oncol (R Coll Radiol) 11:283–285, 1999.

Giltay JC, Leeksma OC, von dem Borne AE, van Mourik JA. Alloantigenic composition of the endothelial vitronectin receptor. Blood 72:230–233, 1988.

Giltay JC, Brinkman HJ, von dem Borne AE. van Mourik JA. Expression of the alloantigen Zwᵃ (or P1ᴬ¹) on human vascular smooth muscle cells and foreskin fibroblasts: a study on normal individuals and a patient with Glanzmann's thrombasthenia. Blood 74:965–970, 1989.

Good RA, Rodey GE. IgA deficiency, antigenic barriers, and autoimmunity. Cell Immunol 1:147–149, 1970.

Good RA, Rotstein J, Mazzitello WF. The simultaneous occurrence of rheumatoid arthritis and agammaglobulinemia. J Lab Clin Med 49:343–357, 1957.

Gottesman SR, Haas D, Ladanyi M, Amorosi EL. Peripheral T cell lymphoma in a patient with common variable immunodeficiency disease: case report and literature review. Leuk Lymphoma 32:589–595, 1999.

Gratama JW, D'Amaro J, de Koning J, den Ottolander GJ. The HLA-system in immune thrombocytopenic purpura: its relation to the outcome of therapy. Br J Haematol 56:287–293, 1984.

Grenet P, Dausset J, Dugas M, Petit D, Badoual J, Tangun Y. Purpura thrombopenique neonatal avec isoimmunisation foeto-maternelle anti-Koᵃ. Arch Fr Pediatr 22:1165–1174, 1965.

Grierson H, Purtilo DT. Epstein-Barr virus infections in males with the X-linked lymphoproliferative syndrome. Ann Intern Med 106:538–545, 1987.

Hakami N, Neiman PE, Canellos GP, Lazerson J. Neonatal megaloblastic anemia due to inherited transcobalamin II deficiency in two siblings. N Engl J Med 285:1163–1170, 1971.

Handagama PJ, George JN, Shuman MA, McEver RP, Bainton DF. Incorporation of a circulating protein into megakaryocyte and platelet granules. Proc Natl Acad Sci USA 84:861–865, 1987.

Harrington WJ, Minnich V, Hollingsworth JW, Moore CV. Demonstration of a thrombocytopenic factor in the blood of patients with thrombocytopenic purpura. J Lab Clin Med 38:1–10, 1951.

Harrington WJ, Sprague CC, Minnich V, Carl MS, Moore CV, Aulvin RC, Dubach R. Immunologic mechanisms in neonatal and thrombocytopenic purpura. Ann Intern Med 38:433–469, 1953.

Harris EN, Peirangeli SS, Gharavi AE. Antiphospholipid syndrome: diagnosis, pathogenesis, and management. J Med Assoc Ga 91:31–34, 2002.

Hauch TW, Rosse WF. Platelet-bound complement (C3) in immune thrombocytopenia. Blood 50:1129–1136, 1977.

Hausler M, Schaade L, Hutschenreuter G, Hannig U, Kusenbach G. Severe cytomegalovirus-triggered autoimmune hemolytic anemia complicating vertically acquired HIV infection. Eur J Clin Microbiol Infect Dis 19:57–60, 2000.

Heegaard NH. Immunochemical characterization of interactions between circulating autologous immunoglobulin G and normal human erythrocyte membrane proteins. Biochim Biophys Acta 1023:239–246, 1990.

Hornig R, Lutz HU. Band 3 protein clustering on human erythrocytes promotes binding of naturally occurring anti-band 3 and anti-spectrin antibodies. Exp Gerontol 35:1025–1044, 2000.

Ikehara S. Treatment of autoimmune diseases by hematopoietic stem cell transplantation. Exp Hematol 29:661–669, 2001.

Imerslund O, Bjornstad P. Familial vitamin B_{12} malabsorption. Acta Haematol 30:1–7, 1963.

Imbach P, Barandun S, d'Apuzzo V, Baumgartner C, Hirt A, Morell A, Rossi E, Schoni M, Vest M, Wagner HP. High-dose intravenous gammaglobulin for idiopathic thrombocytopenic purpura in childhood. Lancet 1:1228–1231, 1981.

International Nijmegen Breakage Syndrome Study Group, The. Nijmegen breakage syndrome. Arch Dis Child 82:400–406, 2000.

Ishizaka T, Ishizaka K, Salmon S, Fudenberg H. Biologic activities of aggregated γ-globulin. 8. Aggregated immunoglobulins of different classes. J Immunol 99:82–91, 1967.

Issaragrisil S, Leaverton PE, Chansung K, Thamprasit T, Porapakham Y, Vannasaeng S, Piankijagum A, Kaufman DW, Anderson TE, Shapiro S, Young NS. Regional patterns in the incidence of aplastic anaemia in Thailand. The Aplastic Anemia Study Group. Am J Hematol 61:164–168, 1999.

Jefferies LC, Carchidi CM, Silberstein LE. Naturally occurring anti-i/I cold agglutinins may be encoded by different VH3 genes as well as the VH4.21 gene segment. J Clin Invest 92:2821–2833, 1993.

Kawai Y, Montgomery RR, Furihata K, Kunicki TJ. Expression of platelet alloantigens on human endothelial cells and HEL cells. Thromb Haemost 58:4, 1987 (abstract).

Kay MM. Generation of senescent cell antigen on old cells initiates IgG binding to a neoantigen. Cell Mol Biol (Noisy-le-grand) 39:131–153, 1993.

Kayser W, Mueller-Eckhardt C, Budde U, Schmidt RE. Complement-fixing platelet autoantibodies in autoimmune thrombocytopenia. Am J Hematol 11:213–219, 1981.

Karpatkin S, Nardi M. Autoimmune anti–HIV-1gp120 antibody with antiidiotype-like activity in sera and immune complexes of HIV-1–related immunologic thrombocytopenia. J Clin Invest 89:356–364, 1992.

Kiefer CR, Snyder LM. Oxidation and erythrocyte senescence. Curr Opin Hematol 7:113–116, 2000.

Kinlen LJ, Webster AD, Bird AG, Haile R, Peto J, Soothill JF, Thompson RA. Prospective study of cancer in patients with hypogammaglobulinaemia. Lancet 1:263–266, 1985.

Kondo N, Motoyoshi F, Mori S, Kuwabara N, Orii T, German J. Long-term study of the immunodeficiency of Bloom's syndrome. Acta Paediatr 81:86–90, 1992.

Kondratenko I, Amlot P, Webster AD, Farrant J. Lack of specific antibody response in common variable immunodeficiency (CVID) associated with failure in production of antigen-specific memory T cells. Clin Exp Immunol 108:9–13, 1997.

König AL, Schabel A, Sugg U, Brand U, Roelcke D. Autoimmune hemolytic anemia caused by IgG lambda-monotypic cold agglutinins of anti-Pr specificity after rubella infection. Transfusion 41:488–492, 2001.

Kuwana M, Kaburaki J, Ikeda Y. Autoreactive T cells to platelet GPIIb-IIIa in immune thrombocytopenic purpura. Role in production of anti-platelet autoantibody. J Clin Invest 102:1393–1402, 1998.

L'Abbé D, Tremblay L, Filion M, Busque L, Goldman M, Décary F, Chartrand P. Alloimmunization to platelet antigen HPA-1a (PI[A1]) is strongly associated with both HLA-DRB3*0101 and HLA-DQB1*0201. Hum Immunol 34:107–114, 1992.

Lach-Trifilieff E, Marfurt J, Schwarz S, Sadallah S, Schifferli JA. Complement receptor 1 (CD35) on human reticulocytes: normal expression in systemic lupus erythematosus and HIV-infected patients. J Immunol 162:7549–7554, 1999.

Lalezari P, Khorshidi M, Petrosova M. Autoimmune neutropenia of infancy. J Pediatr 109:764–769, 1986.

Lampkin BC, Schubert WK. Pernicious anemia in the second decade of life. J Pediatr 72:387–390, 1968.Lazarus AH, Joy T, Crow AR. Analysis of transmembrane signaling and T cell defects associated with idiopathic thrombocytopenic purpura (ITP). Acta Paediatr Suppl 424:21–25, 1998.

Leddy JP, Falany JL, Kissel GE, Passador ST, Rosenfeld SI. Erythrocyte membrane proteins reactive with human (warm-reacting) anti-red cell autoantibodies. J Clin Invest 91:1672–1680, 1993.

Levine P, Stetson RE. An unusual case of intra-group agglutination. JAMA 113:126, 1939.

Levy Y, Gupta N, Le Deist F, Garcia C, Fischer A, Weill JC, Reynaud CA. Defect in IgV gene somatic hypermutation in common variable immuno-deficiency syndrome. Proc Natl Acad Sci USA 95:13135–13140, 1998.

Lillibridge CB, Brandborg LL, Rubin CE. Childhood pernicious anemia. Gastrointestinal secretory, histological, and electron microscopic aspects. Gastroenterology 52:792–809, 1967.

Lippman SM, Arnett FC, Conley CL, Ness PM, Meyers DA, Bias WB. Genetic factors predisposing to autoimmune diseases. Autoimmune hemolytic anemia, chronic thrombocytopenic purpura, and systemic lupus erythematosus. Am J Med 73:827–840, 1982.

Loeb DM, Lederman HM, Winkelstein JA. Lymphoid malignancy as a presenting sign of ataxia-telangiectasia. J Pediatr Hematol Oncol 22:464–467, 2000.

Louache F, Vainchenker W. Thrombocytopenia in HIV infection. Curr Opin Hematol 1:369–372, 1994.

Lusher JM, Iyer R. Idiopathic thrombocytopenic purpura in children. Semin Thromb Hemost 3:175–199, 1977.

Lusher JM, Emami A, Ravindranath V, Warrier AI. Idiopathic thrombocytopenic purpura in children. The case for management without corticosteroids. Am J Pediatr Hematol Oncol 6:149–157, 1984.

Marsh CB, Lowe MP, Rovin BH, Parker JM, Liao Z, Knoell DL, Wewers MD. Lymphocytes produce IL-1beta in response to Fc gamma receptor cross-linking: effects on parenchymal cell IL-8 release. J Immunol 160:3942–3948, 1998.

Marsh JC. Hematopoietic growth factors in the pathogenesis and for the treatment of aplastic anemia. Semin Hematol 37:81–90, 2000.

Maslanka K, Yassai M, Gorski J. Molecular identification of T cells that respond in a primary bulk culture to a peptide derived from a platelet glycoprotein implicated in neonatal alloimmune thrombocytopenia. J Clin Invest 98:1802–1808, 1996.

Matsumoto T, Shima M, Fukuda K, Nogami K, Giddings JC, Murakami T, Tanaka I, Yoshioka A. Immunological characterization of factor VIII autoantibodies in patients with acquired hemophilia A in the presence or absence of underlying disease. Thromb Res 104:381–388, 2001.

Mathé G, Amiel JL, Schwarzenberg L, Choay J, Trolard P, Schneider M, Hayat M, Schlumberger JR, Jasmin C. Bone marrow graft in man after conditioning by antilymphocytic serum. Br Med J 2:131–136, 1970.

Mayr WR, Mueller-Eckhardt G, Kruger M, Mueller-Eckhardt C, Lechner K, Niessner H. HLA-DR in chronic idiopathic thrombocytopenic purpura (ITP). Tissue Antigens 18:56–57, 1981.

McClain KL. Immunodeficiency states and related malignancies. In Walterhouse DO, Cohn SL, eds. Diagnostic and therapeutic advances in pediatric oncology. Boston, Kluwar Academic Publishers, 1997, pp 39–61.

McClure PD. Idiopathic thrombocytopenic purpura in children: diagnosis and management. Pediatrics 55:68–74, 1975.

McGrath K, Minchinton R, Cunningham I, Ayberk H. Platelet anti-Bak[b] antibody associated with neonatal alloimmune thrombocytopenia. Vox Sang 57:182–184, 1989.

McIntyre OR, Sullivan LW, Jeffries GH, Silver RH. Pernicious anemia in childhood. N Engl J Med 272:981–986, 1965.

Megonigal MD, Rappaport EF, Jones DH, Williams TM, Lovett BD, Kelly KM, Lerou PH, Moulton T, Budarf ML, Felix CA. t(11;22)(q23;q11.2) In acute myeloid leukemia of infant twins fuses MLL with hCDCrel, a cell division cycle gene in the genomic region of deletion in DiGeorge and velocardiofacial syndromes. Proc Natl Acad Sci USA 95:6413–6418, 1998.

Mentzer SJ, Remold-O'Donnell E, Crimmins MA, Bierer BE, Rosen FS, Burakoff SJ. Sialophorin, a surface sialoglycoprotein defective in the Wiskott-Aldrich syndrome, is involved in human T lymphocyte proliferation. J Exp Med 165:1383–1392, 1987.

Meyn MS. Ataxia-telangiectasia and cellular responses to DNA damage. Cancer Res 55:5991–6001, 1995.

Mickelson EM, Masewicz SA, Nepom GT, Martin PJ, Hansen JA, Alloreactive T-cell clones identify multiple HLA-DQw3 variants. Hum Immunol 30:32–40, 1991.

Miller DR, Bloom GE, Streiff RR, LoBuglio AF, Diamond LK. Juvenile "congenital" pernicious anemia. Clinical and immunologic studies. N Engl J Med 275:978–983, 1966.

Mittal KK. Human histocompatibility antigens. J Sci Indust Res 38:37–43, 1979.

Mollison PL, Engelfriet CP, Contreras M. Hemolytic disease of the newborn. In Mollison PL, ed. Blood transfusion in clinical medicine. 8th ed. Oxford, Blackwell Scientific, 1987, pp 639–640.

Monroe JG, Silberstein LE. HIV-mediated B-lymphocyte activation and lymphomagenesis. J Clin Immunol 15:61–68, 1995.

Morra M, Howie D, Grande MS, Sayos J, Wang N, Wu C, Engel P, Terhorst C. X-linked lymphoproliferative disease: a progressive immunodeficiency. Annu Rev Immunol 19:657–682, 2001.

Morrell D, Cromartie E, Swift M. Mortality and cancer incidence in 263 patients with ataxia-telangiectasia. J Natl Cancer Inst 77:89–92, 1986.

Moses RE. DNA damage processing defects and disease. Annu Rev Genomics Hum Genet 2:41–68, 2001.

Mueller-Eckhardt C, Kiefel V, Grubert A, Kroll H, Weisheit M, Schmidt S, Mueller-Eckhardt G, Santoso S. 348 cases of suspected neonatal alloimmune thrombocytopenia. Lancet 1:363–366, 1989.

Nasu K. Mycoplasma infection and hemolytic anemia. Nippon Rinsho 9:2545–2549, 1996.

Newman PJ, Derbes RS, Aster RH. The human platelet alloantigens, P1A1 and P1A2, are associated with a leucine33/proline33 amino acid polymorphism in membrane glycoprotein IIIa, and are distinguishable by DNA typing. J Clin Invest 83:1778–1781, 1989.

Newman PJ, Kawai Y, Montgomery RR. Kunicki TJ. Synthesis by cultured human umbilical vein endothelial cells of two proteins structurally and immunologically related to platelet membrane glycoproteins IIb and IIIa. J Cell Biol 103:81–86, 1986.

Newman PJ, Valentin N. Human platelet alloantigens: recent findings. New perspectives. Thromb Haemost 74:234–239, 1995.

Nonoyama S, Farrington M, Ishida H, Howard M, Ochs HD. Activated B cells from patients with common variable immunodeficiency proliferate and synthesize immunoglobulin. J Clin Invest 92:1282–1287, 1993.

Nordoy I, Muller F, Aukrust P, Froland SS. Adhesion molecules in common variable immunodeficiency (CVID)—a decrease in L-selectin–positive T lymphocytes. Clin Exp Immunol 114:258–263, 1998.

Ochs HD. The Wiskott-Aldrich syndrome. Springer Semin Immunopathol 19:435–458, 1998.

Ogasawara K, Ueki J, Takenaka M, Furihata K. Study on the expression of ABH antigens on platelets. Blood 82:993–999, 1993.

Palanduz S, Palanduz A, Yalcin I, Somer A, Ones U, Ustek D, Ozturk S, Salman N, Guler N, Bilge H. In vitro chromosomal radiosensitivity in common variable immune deficiency. Clin Immunol Immunopathol 86:180–182, 1998.

Panzer S, Penner E, Graninger W, Schulz E, Smolen JS. Antinuclear antibodies in patients with chronic idiopathic autoimmune thrombocytopenia followed 2-30 years. Am J Hematol 32:100–103, 1989.

Parkman R, Kenney DM, Remold-O'Donnell E, Perrine S, Rosen FS. Surface protein abnormalities in lymphocytes and platelets from patients with Wiskott-Aldrich syndrome. Lancet 2:1387–1389, 1981.

Pawha J, Giuliani D, Morse BS. Platelet-associated IgM levels in thrombocytopenia. Vox Sang 45:97–103, 1983.

Petz LD, Garratty G. Mechanisms of immune hemolysis. In Acquired immune hemolytic anemias. New York, Churchill Livingstone, 1980, pp 121–142.

Petz LD. Treatment of autoimmune hemolytic anemias. Curr Opin Hematol 8:411–416, 2001.

Porter TF, Silver RM, Jackson GM, Branch DW, Scott JR. Intravenous immune globulin in the management of severe Rh D hemolytic disease. Obstet Gynecol Surv 52:193–197, 1997.

Przybylski GK, Goldman J, Ng VL, McGrath MS, Herndier BG, Schenkein DP, Monroe JG, Silberstein LE. Evidence for early B-cell activation preceding the development of Epstein-Barr virus-negative acquired immunodeficiency syndrome-related lymphoma. Blood 88:4620–4629, 1996.

Quartier P, Brethon B, Philippet P, Landman-Parker J, Le Deist F, Fischer A. Treatment of childhood autoimmune haemolytic anaemia with rituximab. Lancet 358:1511–1513, 2001.

Ramos JT, Lopez-Laso E, Ruiz-Contreras J, Giancaspro E, Madero S. B cell non-Hodgkin's lymphoma in a girl with the DiGeorge anomaly. Arch Dis Child 81:444–445, 1999.

Reznikoff-Etievant MF, Dangu C, Lobet R. HLA-B8 antigens and anti-P1A1 allo-immunization. Tissue Antigens 18:66–68, 1981.

Rhoades CJ, Williams MA, Kelsey SM, Newland AC. Monocyte-macrophage system as targets for immunomodulation by intravenous immunoglobulin. Blood Rev 14:14–30, 2000.

Rosen FS, Cooper MD, Wedgwood RJ. The primary immunodeficiencies. N Engl J Med 333:431–440, 1995.

Ryu T, Davis JM, Schwartz KA. Dose-dependent platelet stimulation and inhibition induced by anti-P1A1 IgG. J Lab Clin Med 116:91–99, 1990.

Samuelsson A, Towers TL, Ravetch JV. Anti-inflammatory activity of IVIG mediated through the inhibitory Fc receptor. Science 291:484–486, 2001.

Sander CA, Medeiros LJ, Weiss LM, Yano T, Sneller MC, Jaffe ES. Lymphoproliferative lesions in patients with common variable immunodeficiency syndrome. Am J Surg Pathol 16:1170–1182, 1992.

Sandoval C, Swift M. Treatment of lymphoid malignancies in patients with ataxia-telangiectasia. Med Pediatr Oncol 31:491–497, 1998.

Savitsky K, Bar-Shira A, Gilad S, Rotman G, Ziv Y, Vanagaite L, Tagle DA, Smith S, Uziel T, Sfez S, et al. A single ataxia telangiectasia gene with a product similar to PI-3 kinase. Science 268:1749–1753, 1995a.

Savitsky K, Sfez S, Tagle DA, Ziv Y, Sartiel A, Collins FS, Shiloh Y, Rotman G. The complete sequence of the coding region of the ATM gene reveals similarity to cell cycle regulators in different species. Hum Mole Genet 4:2025–2028, 1995b.

Sato T, Tatsuzawa O, Koike Y, Wada Y, Nagata M, Kobayashi S, Ishizawa A, Miyauchi J, Shimizu K. B-cell lymphoma associated with DiGeorge syndrome. Eur J Pediatr 158:609–617, 1999.

Sayos J, Wu C, Morra M, Wang N, Zhang X, Allen D, van Schaik S, Notarangelo L, Geha R, Roncarolo MG, Oettgen H, De Vries JE, Aversa G, Terhorst C. The X-linked lymphoproliferative-disease gene product SAP regulates signals induced through the co-receptor SLAM. Nature 395:462–469, 1998.

Schleuning M. Adoptive allogeneic immunotherapy—history and future perspectives. Transfus Sci 23:133–150, 2000.

Seemanova E. An increased risk for malignant neoplasms in heterozygotes for a syndrome of microcephaly, normal intelligence, growth retardation, remarkable facies, immunodeficiency and chromosomal instability. Mutat Res 238:321–331, 1990.

Seemayer TA. X-linked lymphoproliferative disease: twenty-five years after the discovery. Pediatr Res 38:471–478, 1995.

Seidemann K, Henze G, Beck JD, Sauerbrey A, Kuhl J, Mann G, Reiter A. Non-Hodgkin's lymphoma in pediatric patients with chromosomal breakage syndromes (AT and NBS): experience from the BFM trials. Ann Oncol 11:141–145, 2000.

Semple JW, Milev Y, Cosgrave D, Mody M, Hornstein A, Blanchette V, Freedman J. Differences in serum cytokine levels in acute and chronic autoimmune thrombocytopenic purpura: relationship to platelet phenotype and antiplatelet T-cell reactivity. Blood 87:4245–4254, 1996.

Shcherbina A, Miki H, Kenney DM, Rosen FS, Takenawa T, Remold-O'Donnell E. WASP and N-WASP in human platelets differ in sensitivity to protease calpain. Blood 98:2988–2991, 2001.

Sherer Y, Wu R, Krause I, Gorstein A, Levy Y, Peter JB, Shoenfeld Y. Cytokine levels in various intravenous immunoglobulin (IVIg) preparations. Hum Antibodies 10:51–53, 2001.

Shibata Y, Matsuda I, Miyaji T, Ichikawa Y. Yuk^a, a new platelet antigen involved in two cases of neonatal alloimmune thrombocytopenia. Vox Sang 50:177–180, 1986.

Shiloh Y, Rotman G. Ataxia-telangiectasia and the ATM gene: linking neurodegeneration, immunodeficiency, and cancer to cell cycle checkpoints. J Clin Immunol 16:254–260, 1996.

Shulman NR, Marder VJ, Weinrach RS. Similarities between known antiplatelet antibodies and the factor responsible for thrombocytopenia in idiopathic purpura. Ann NY Acad Sci 124:499–542, 1965.

Silberstein LE, Jefferies LC, Goldman J, Friedman D, Moore JS, Nowell PC, Roelcke D, Pruzanski W, Roudier J, Silverman GJ. Variable region gene analysis of pathologic human autoantibodies to the related i and I red blood cell antigens. Blood 78:2372–2386, 1991.

Silberstein LE. Natural and pathologic human autoimmune responses to carbohydrate antigens on red blood cells. Springer Semin Immunopathol 15:139–153, 1993.

Silvestris N, Silvestris F, Russo S, Dammacco F. Common variable immunodeficiency. Recenti Prog Med 87:616–622, 1996.

Skogen B, Rossebo Hansen B, Husebekk A. Havnes T, Hannestad K. Minimal expression of blood group A antigen on thrombocytes from A2 individuals. Transfusion 28:456–459, 1988.

Sloand E, Kim S, Maciejewski JP, Chaudhuri A, Kirby M, Young NS. Presence of intracellular interferon-gamma (IFN-gamma) in circulating lymphocytes and response to immunosuppressive therapy in patients with aplastic anemia. Blood 10 (Suppl 1):158a, 1998.

Spong CY, Porter AE, Queenan JT. Management of isoimmunization in the presence of multiple maternal antibodies. Am J Obstet Gyn 185:276–285, 2001.

Stasi R, Stipa E, Forte V, Meo P, Amadori S. Variable patterns of response to rituximab treatment in adults with chronic idiopathic thrombocytopenic purpura. Blood 99:3872–3873, 2002.

Steeper TA, Horwitz CA, Moore SB, Henle W, Henle G, Ellis R, Flynn PJ. Severe thrombocytopenia in Epstein-Barr virus–induced mononucleosis. West J Med 150:170–173, 1989.

Steinberg AD, Gourley MF, Klinman DM, Tsokos GC, Scott DE, Krieg AM. Systemic lupus erythematosus. Ann Intern Med 115:548–559, 1991.

Stumm M, Neubauer S, Keindorff S, Wegner RD, Wieacker P, Sauer R. High frequency of spontaneous translocations revealed by FISH in cells from patients with the cancer-prone syndromes ataxia telangiectasia and Nijmegen breakage syndrome. Cytogenet Cell Genet 92:186–191, 2001.

Taylor AM, Metcalfe JA, Thick J, Mak YF. Leukemia and lymphoma in ataxia telangiectasia. Blood 87:423–438, 1996.

Thierfelder VS, Pfisterer H. Immunologische aspekte der thrombozyten-transfusion. Blut 18:97–108, 1968.

Thomas JA, Allday MJ, Crawford DH. Epstein-Barr virus–associated lymphoproliferative disorders in immunocompromised individuals. V. The X-linked lymphoproliferative syndrome. Adv Cancer Res 57:337–343, 1991.

Tijhuis GJ, Klaassen RJ, Modderman PW, Ouwehand WH, von dem Borne AE. Quantification of platelet-bound immunoglobulins of different class and subclass using radiolabeled monoclonal antibodies: assay conditions and clinical application. Br J Haematol 77:93–101, 1991.

Tosato G, Taga K, Angiolillo AL, Sgadari C. Epstein-Barr virus as an agent of haematological disease. Ballieres Clin Haematol 8:165–199, 1995.

Tsai TW, Freytes CO. Allogeneic bone marrow transplantation for leukemias and aplastic anemia. Adv Int Med 42:423–451, 1997.

Tsubakio T, Kurata Y, Katagini S, Kanakuna Y, Tamaki T, Kuyama J, Kanayama Y, Yonezawa T, Tarni S. Alteration of T cell subsets and immunoglobulin synthesis in vitro during high-dose gammaglobulin therapy in patients with idiopathic thrombocytopenic purpura. Clin Exp Immunol 53:697–702, 1983.

Tsuchiya Y, Sugai H. The effect of *Mycoplasma pneumoniae* infection on human erythrocytes: changes in osmotic fragility, lipid composition, sialic acid content, Ca^{2+}-ATPase activities, and ATP concentration. Biochem Med 28:256–265, 1982.

Turner AM, Berdoukas VA, Tobias VH, Ziegler JB, Toogood IR, Mulley JC, Skare J, Purtilo DT. Report on the X-linked lymphoproliferative disease in an Australian family. J Paediatr Child Health 28:184–189, 1992.

Uher F, Puskas E, Cervenak J. Beneficial effect of a human monoclonal IgM cryoglobulin on the autoimmune disease of New Zealand black mice. Cell Immunol 206:136–141, 2000.

Valentin N, Vergracht A, Bignon JD, Cheneau ML, Blanchard D, Kaplan C, Reznikoff-Etievant MF, Muller JY. HLA-DRw52a is involved in alloimmunization against PL-A1 antigen. Hum Immunol 27:73–79, 1990.

van Brabant AJ, Stan R, Ellis NA. DNA helicases, genomic instability, and human genetic disease. Annu Rev Genomics Hum Genet 1:409–459, 2000.

van der Burgt I, Chrzanowska KH, Smeets D, Weemaes C. Nijmegen breakage syndrome. J Med Genet 33:153–156, 1996.

van Leeuwen E, Leeksma O, van Mourik J, Engelfriet C. von dem Borne A. Effect of the binding of antiZw^a antibodies on platelet function. Vox Sang 47:280–289, 1984.

Varon R, Reis A, Henze G, von Einsiedel HG, Sperling K, Seeger K. Mutations in the Nijmegen Breakage Syndrome gene (NBS1) in childhood acute lymphoblastic leukemia (ALL). Cancer Res 61:3570–3572, 2001.

Verma A, Deb DK, Sassano A, Kambhampati S, Wickrema A, Uddin S, Mohindru M, Van Besien K, Platanias LC. Cutting edge: activation of the p38 mitogen-activated protein kinase signaling pathway mediates cytokine-induced hemopoietic suppression in aplastic anemia. J Immunol 168:5984–5988, 2002.

von dem Borne AE, von Riesz E, Verheugt F, ten Cate JW, Koppe JG, Engelfriet C, Nijenhuis LE. Bak^a, a new platelet-specific antigen involved in neonatal allo-immune thrombocytopenia. Vox Sang 39:113–120, 1980.

Voto LS, Mathet ER, Zapaterio JL, Orti J, Lede RL, Margulies M. High-dose gammaglobulin (IVIG) followed by intrauterine transfusions (IUTs): a new alternative for the treatment of severe fetal hemolytic disease. J Perinat Med 25:85–88 1997.

Walker RW, Walker W. Idiopathic thrombocytopenic purpura, initial illness and long term follow up. Arch Dis Child 59:316–324, 1984.

Wang R, Furihata K, McFarland JG, Friedman K, Aster RH, Newman PJ. An amino acid polymorphism within the RGD binding domain of platelet membrane glycoprotein IIIa is responsible for the formation of the Pen^a/Pen^b alloantigen system. J Clin Invest 90:2038–2043, 1992.

Ware RE, Howard TA. Phenotypic and clonal analysis of T lymphocytes in childhood immune thrombocytopenic purpura. Blood 82:2137–2142, 1993.

Ware RE, Howard TA. Elevated numbers of gamma-delta (gamma delta+) T lymphocytes in children with immune thrombocytopenic purpura. J Clin Immunol 14:237–247, 1994.

Webster ADB. Common variable immunodeficiency. Immunol Allergy Clin North Am 21:1–22, 2001.

Westman P, Hashemi-Tavoularis S, Blanchette V, Kekomaki S, Laes M, Porcelijn L, Kekomaki R. Maternal DRB1*1501, DQA1*0102,DQB1*0602 haplotype in fetomaternal alloimmunization against human platelet alloantigen HPA-6b (GPIIIa-Gln489). Tissue Antigens 50:113–118, 1997.

Williams Y, Lynch S, McCann S, Smith O, Feighery C, Whelan A. Correlation of platelet Fc gammaRIIA polymorphism in refractory idiopathic (immune) thrombocytopenic purpura. Br J Haematol 101:779–782, 1998.

Winiarski J. IgG and IgM antibodies to platelet membrane glycoprotein antigens in acute childhood idiopathic thrombocytopenic purpura. Br J Haematol 73:88–92, 1989.

Wiskott A. Familiärer, angeborener morbus Werlhofii. Monatschrift Kinderheil 68:212–227, 1936.

WHO Scientific Group. Primary immunodeficiency diseases. Clin Exp Immunol Suppl 1:1–24, 1995.

Xu Y, Ashley T, Brainerd EE, Bronson RT, Meyn MS, Baltimore D. Targeted disruption of ATM leads to growth retardation, chromosomal fragmentation during meiosis, immune defects, and thymic lymphoma. Genes Dev 10:2411–2422, 1996.

Yang C, Zhang X. Incidence survey of aplastic anemia in China. Chin Med Sci J 6:203–207, 1991.

Yayoshi M, Araake M, Hayatsu E, Kawakubo Y, Yoshioka M. Characterization and pathogenicity of hemolysis mutants of *Mycoplasma pneumoniae*. Microbiol Immunol 28:303–310, 1984.

Young NS, Abkowitz JL, Luzzatto L. New insights into the pathophysiology of acquired cytopenias. Hematology (Am Soc Hematol Educ Program) 18–38, 2000.

Young NS, Maciejewski J. The pathophysiology of acquired aplastic anemia. N Engl J Med 336:1365–1372, 1997.

Zenone T, Souillet G. Cancer and primary humoral immunodeficiency Bull Cancer 84:813–821, 1997.

Zhao S, Weng YC, Yuan SS, Lin YT, Hsu HC, Lin SC, Gerbino E, Song MH, Zdzienicka MZ, Gatti RA, Shay JW, Ziv Y, Shiloh Y, Lee EY. Functional link between ataxia-telangiectasia and Nijmegen breakage syndrome gene products. Nature 405:473–477, 2000.

Zhu Q, Watanabe C, Liu T, Hollenbaugh D, Blaese RM, Kanner SB, Aruffo A, Ochs HD. Wiskott-Aldrich syndrome/X-linked thrombocytopenia: WASP gene mutations, protein expression, and phenotype. Blood 90:2680–2689, 1997.

Zimmerman SA, Malinoski FJ, Ware RE. Immunologic effects of anti-D (WinRho-SD) in children with immune thrombocytopenic purpura. Am J Hematol 57:131–138, 1998.

Zuelzer WW, Mastrangelo R, Stulberg CS, Poulik MD, Page RH, Thompson RI. Autoimmune hemolytic anemia. Natural history and viral-immunologic interactions in childhood. Am J Med 49:80–88, 1970.

Zupanska B, Lawkowicz W, Gorska B. Autoimmune hemolytic anemia in children. Br J Haematol 34:511–518, 1976.

CHAPTER

40

Immunologic Disorders of the Nervous System

Kenneth J. Mack and John O. Fleming

The immune system plays an etiologic role in several pediatric neurologic diseases. Despite some overlap it is clinically useful to classify these diseases with respect to the level of the nervous system that they affect (Table 40-1).

INFLAMMATORY MYOPATHIES (DERMATOMYOSITIS AND POLYMYOSITIS)

Historical Aspects

The idiopathic inflammatory myopathies (IMs) of childhood are characterized by chronic skeletal muscle inflammation, resulting in muscle damage and weakness. In 1863, Wagner first described polymyositis (PM). In 1875, Potain described the first case of childhood dermatomyositis (DM). Both disorders are associated with weakness, but the inflammatory changes of PM are limited to muscle, whereas DM involves other tissues, including the skin, heart, lungs, and throat. However, PM is not DM without the rash. DM is the most common IM of childhood, occurring in 1.9 per 1 million children younger than 16 years of age (Symmons et al., 1995). Acute myositis can also occur in childhood and may be associated with a variety of infections, including influenza.

Pathogenesis

The pathogenesis of IMs is unknown, but it is thought that they may result when toxins, medications, or viruses trigger an autoimmune response. The nature of the immune response and the particular targets attacked produce distinctive patterns of immunopathosis and associated clinical findings (see Table 40-1).

DM is the result of small-vessel angiopathy mediated by humoral immunity. Inflammatory elements including CD4$^+$ T cells, B cells, and complement components are restricted to the perivascular region, with little or no lymphocytic invasion within the muscle fascicles themselves. Muscle fiber necrosis occurs at the margins of fascicles, in proximity to the perivascular exudate. The microvasculature is a primary target of an autoimmune response. The myofibrillar injury occurs secondary to small-vessel thrombosis. Similar changes may occur in small nerves, skin, connective tissues, the gastrointestinal tract, and lungs (Dalakas, 1991; Emslie-Smith and Engel, 1990; Engel et al., 1994c; Silver and Mericq, 1989).

Myositis-specific autoantibodies are detectable in 25% to 40% of adults and 11% of children with DM. Antibodies include anti-aminoacyl-tRNA synthetase autoantibodies, anti–signal recognition particle autoantibody, anti–Mi-2 autoantibody, and anti–U5-RNP autoantibody. These specific autoantibodies have some predictive value in the clinical course and prognosis of DM (Rider and Miller, 1997).

By contrast, PM is largely mediated by cellular autoimmunity directed against muscle fibers (Dalakas, 1991; Engel et al., 1994c). Inflammation and necrosis are not limited to the perivascular region as in PM but involve direct invasion of muscle fascicles by inflammatory cells, particularly CD8$^+$ T lymphocytes and macrophages. Predisposition to cytotoxic T-cell attack may be the result of abnormally high expression of class I major histocompatibility antigens in muscle. In fact, T cells derived from muscle biopsy specimens of patients with PM exhibit strong cytotoxic responses to autologous myotubules in vitro (Hohlfield and Engel, 1991).

TABLE 40-1 · NEUROIMMUNOLOGIC DISORDERS

Conditions Primarily Affecting the Peripheral Nervous System	Conditions Primarily Affecting the Central Nervous System
Muscle	**White Matter**
Inflammatory myopathies	Acute disseminated encephalomyelitis
Polymyositis	Optic neuritis
Dermatomyositis	Acute transverse myelitis
Inclusion body myositis	Devic's syndrome
Neuromuscular Junction	Multiple sclerosis
Myasthenia gravis	Acute cerebellar ataxia
Lambert-Eaton myasthenic syndrome	Opsoclonus-myoclonus-ataxia
	Ataxia-telangiectasia
Peripheral Nerve	**Gray Matter**
Guillain-Barré syndrome	Sydenham's chorea
Chronic inflammatory demyelinating polyradiculoneuropathy	Thrombotic thrombocytopenic purpura/hemolytic-uremic syndrome
Bell's palsy	Rasmussen's encephalitis
Other immune-mediated peripheral neuropathies	Paraneoplastic syndromes

The syndromes of myositis associated with known environmental agents are usually not considered to be part of the IMs, but they may occur as a clinically indistinguishable syndrome. In children, common triggers of myositis include infectious agents (influenza, coxsackievirus, human T-lymphotropic virus 1 [HTLV-1], Group A *Streptococcus, Borrelia*), pharmaceuticals, vaccines, growth hormone, and graft-versus-host disease (Rider and Miller, 1997; Rider et al., 1995).

Clinical Features

IMs are characterized by acquired muscular weakness, usually subacute in onset, with variable accompanying features that clinically differentiate the subtypes.

Dermatomyositis

Dermatomyositis (DM) can occur at any age, but most cases occur in children 3 to 10 years of age (this disorder is also covered in Chapter 35). The onset of weakness is usually insidious and often associated with prominent muscle aching, stiffness, and systemic features such as malaise or fever. The discomfort and irritability are usually prominent enough to justify the aphorism that in children, misery plus weakness equals DM. Weakness is usually proximal and greater in the legs than the arms, but younger children may have generalized weakness. Muscles may be tender and slightly indurated, and contractures are often present early (Hanissian et al., 1983). The ocular and facial muscles are rarely affected.

The skin manifestations of DM are variable. The classical skin manifestations include a purplish discoloration of the eyelids (heliotrope rash), often associated with scaling and periorbital edema. The classic heliotrope rash may require weeks to months to develop. A similar rash with even more prominent scaling may occur over pressure areas such as the knees, elbows, and malleoli of the ankles, and characteristic papular scaling may involve the dorsal surfaces of the fingers over the interphalangeal joints (Gottron's papules). Other dermatologic findings are the presence of a subtle reticular, sun-sensitive rash on the face, neck, and anterior chest (*V* sign); on the shoulders and upper back (shawl sign); and on the extensor surfaces of the arms, occasionally punctuated by fine telangiectasia, atrophy, and dyspigmentation (poikiloderma) (Amato and Barohn, 1997; Callen, 2000).

The esophagus is involved in 20% of patients with DM, which typically results in dysphagia and delayed gastric emptying. Occasionally, the myocardium may be involved, resulting in arrhythmias, pericarditis, myocarditis, and congestive heart failure. Pulmonary interstitial fibrosis may develop in 10% of patients. Subcutaneous calcification occurs in half of children with DM. Malignant disease is more typically associated with adult-onset cases rather than childhood cases. Abdominal pain, arthralgias, fever, hoarseness, and melena also occur (Amato and Barohn, 1997; Callen, 2000; Pachman et al., 1998).

Polymyositis

Patients with childhood PM exhibit similar clinical features, particularly with respect to the insidious onset (over weeks to months) of proximal weakness and muscle tenderness. Malaise and mild fever are variable. Distal and facial weakness may also be seen but are not as prominent as proximal weakness. The reflexes are preserved. Systemic complaints may be minimal, but dysphagia occurs in one third of patients. Cardiac involvement, polyarthritis, and interstitial lung disease are also seen. Slowly evolving PM can readily be mistaken for limb-girdle muscular dystrophy. Periods of spontaneous arrest and remission are observed (Amato and Barohn, 1997; Mastaglia and Ojeda, 1985a, 1985b).

Associated Disorders

In addition to DM and PM, other myositis syndromes are recognized (Table 40-2). *Overlap myositis* occurs when criteria are met for both myositis and other connective tissue diseases. For instance, DM has been asso-

TABLE 40-2 · FEATURES OF INFLAMMATORY MYOPATHIES

Entity	Clinical
Dermatomyositis (DM)	Most common inflammatory myopathy. Involves muscular and systemic findings.
Polymyositis	Myositis without typical rash of DM. Different mechanism than DM, however.
Overlap myositis	Criteria are met for both myositis and another connective tissue disease, such as scleroderma or lupus.
Orbital myositis	Involves periorbital muscles and presents with limitation of gaze, periorbital pain, proptosis.
Cancer-associated myositis	Typically seen within 2 years of cancer diagnosis. Responds to steroids.
Focal or nodular myositis	Focal pain or swelling, or both.
Proliferative myositis	Presents as painless mass in a muscle. Treated by surgical excision.
Inclusion body myositis	Slowly progressive, characteristic biopsy findings, responds poorly to treatment.
Dermatomyositis sine myositis	Cutaneous manifestations of DM without obvious myositis. Myositis may occur up to 4 years after onset of skin findings.
Eosinophilic myositis	Eosinophilic infiltrates on biopsy.
Granulomatous myositis	Granulomas prominent in biopsy specimen. May be associated with sarcoid myositis.
Congenital/infantile myositis	Generalized areflexia, weakness, and hypotonia. The clinical appearance is that of severe congenital myopathy or spinal muscular atrophy; muscle biopsy is essential to diagnose this treatable disorder.
Acute myositis of childhood	Typically, calf pain after viral prodrome. Elevated creatine phosphokinase. Natural history is rapid recovery.

Adapted from Rider and Miller (1997).

ciated with scleroderma and mixed connective tissue disease (Mastaglia and Ojeda, 1985a, 1985b; Tymms and Webb, 1985). PM is frequently associated with autoimmune diseases such as systemic lupus erythematosus (SLE), rheumatoid arthritis, and Sjögren's syndrome (Mimori, 1987; Tymms and Webb, 1985). Up to 6% of children with myositis may fall into this category.

Patients with *ocular myositis* can have limitations of gaze and periorbital pain. *Cancer-associated myositis* can occur with leukemia, lymphoma, and other malignancies. The onset is often within 2 years of the cancer diagnosis and is steroid-responsive. *Focal or nodular myositis* occurs as focal pain and swelling. *Proliferative myositis* manifests as a painless mass, typically on the extremities. Childhood lesions are well demarcated, and treatment is by surgical excision. *Inclusion body myositis* only rarely occurs in childhood and is manifested by indolent proximal weakness and rimmed vacuoles on a trichrome muscle biopsy specimen (Lotz et al., 1989).

DM sine myositis has the cutaneous manifestations of DM without muscle involvement. However, in DM, myositis may occur up to 4 years after skin involvement. *Eosinophilic myositis* is associated with prominent eosinophilia on the muscle biopsy specimen and the peripheral smear. *Granulomatous myositis* may be associated with sarcoidosis or may be idiopathic in nature.

Congenital/infantile myositis is a striking disorder of infants who have generalized areflexia, weakness, and hypotonia, often so marked as to require resuscitation and ventilatory support. The clinical appearance is that of severe congenital myopathy or spinal muscular atrophy; muscle biopsy is essential to diagnose this treatable disorder (Roddy et al., 1986; Shevell et al., 1990; Thompson, 1982). *Benign acute childhood myositis* may also occur in association with a viral infection and typically involves the calves; recovery occurs within a week (Mackay et al., 1999)

Adults with DM have an increased risk of neoplasm (i.e., tumors occur in 15%; Callen 1988; Dalakas, 1991; Engel et al., 1994c; Richardson and Callen, 1989), but no such association has yet been documented for children. Childhood DM is occasionally associated with X-linked agammaglobulinemia (see Chapter 13).

Diagnosis

The differential diagnoses of inflammatory myopathies include inherited and metabolic diseases of muscle, disorders of the neuromuscular junction, diseases of the motor neurons or peripheral nerves, and weakness associated with endocrinopathies. Genetic disorders of muscle, including muscular dystrophies and myopathies, are rarely associated with fever and muscle pain and may exhibit relentless progression as compared with the fluctuating course frequently observed in inflammatory myopathies. As noted, limb-girdle muscular dystrophy is particularly difficult to distinguish from both PM and inclusion body myositis when the toxic symptoms are minimal. Congenital myositis must be distinguished from spinal muscular atrophy and congenital myopathies.

Disorders of the neuromuscular junction, such as myasthenia gravis (MG), are marked by fatigable weakness and prominent involvement of the ocular and facial muscles. Lower motor neuron diseases are distinguished by the absence or reduction of deep tendon reflexes; upper motor neuron diseases, by long-tract signs; and peripheral neuropathy, by sensory changes. Endocrinopathies, such as thyrotoxicosis, usually cause widespread systemic disturbances, in addition to weakness. *Toxoplasma gondii* infestation may occasionally produce a condition resembling DM or PM (Topi et al., 1979). Viral myositis, especially that caused by influenza or coxsackievirus B, may closely resemble DM.

A diagnosis of IM is established after consideration of the clinical features, muscle enzyme determinations, electrodiagnostic test results, and muscle biopsy specimens (Dalakas, 1991). For DM, the diagnostic features include (1) proximal symmetric weakness, (2) typical rash, (3) increased creatine kinase (CK; i.e., 5 to 50 times normal), (4) typical electromyographic findings, and (5) typical results from biopsy. A diagnosis is established when four or more of these features are present.

CK is released from injured muscle cells, but the CK elevation corresponds only roughly with the clinical course. Thus because CK elevation occurs in 90% of patients, this is a sensitive and reliable screen for muscle injury. CK elevation corresponds only roughly with the clinical course and thus is nonspecific.

The electromyogram usually depicts typical myopathic features, including insertional activity; fibrillation; and positive waves at rest with limited-duration, low-amplitude polyphasic potentials during voluntary contraction. However, the electromyogram may also be normal/nondiagnostic in 20% of patients.

Muscle biopsy should be undertaken in all patients in whom there is a suspicion of IM, and an analysis of the biopsy specimen will usually permit a definitive diagnosis in 80% of patients. Rarely, the results of the biopsy may fail to show cellular infiltrates in active IM; in this case, a biopsy performed at another site should be considered (Pachman et al., 1998).

Treatment

Prednisone is the mainstay of treatment for DM and is used in other IMs. This treatment has reduced DM mortality from 30% to less than 5%. Moreover, early prednisone therapy reduces contracture formation and calcinosis. Most authorities advocate the use of high-dose prednisone each morning, with dosages ranging from 1 to 2.5 mg/kg/day. After approximately 6 weeks, the dose is slowly tapered, with the clinical response dictating the dose reduction. Therapy must be continued for long periods, usually for 1 or more years. Response is best judged in terms of a combination of muscle strength and CK levels (Amato and Barohn, 1997; Huber et al., 2000; Kokontis and Gutmann, 2000; Rider and Miller, 1997).

Prednisone may paradoxically increase weakness as a result of *steroid myopathy* (Dalakas, 1991). In some patients, it may be difficult to distinguish between increased disease activity and prednisone toxicity; in this case, the pattern of response to past treatment should be carefully reviewed. On occasion, the dose of prednisone must be raised or lowered arbitrarily; in such circumstances, the response over several weeks will usually dictate the correct therapeutic course to follow.

The response of PM to prednisone is less clear, and remissions may occur even without therapy. Congenital/infantile myositis is clearly steroid-responsive, but prednisone should be tapered aggressively to prevent side effects such as infection.

Physical therapy is an important part of the first-line management of myositis. Physical therapy helps to restore muscle strength and endurance and to prevent the development of contractures (Rider and Miller, 1997).

Up to 20% of children with DM do not improve significantly while taking prednisone. Immunosuppressive agents should be considered for these children and for patients who have poorly responsive PM, who have inclusion body myositis, or who experience unacceptable prednisone toxicity (Engel et al., 1994c). Methotrexate is effective in 75% of resistant DM or PM cases (Hanissian et al., 1983; Miller et al., 1983). Treatment should be started immediately in very ill patients, since many weeks may elapse before improvement is seen. Azathioprine may also be effective. Pulse methylprednisolone and cyclosporine have also been advocated (Kokontis and Gutmann, 2000; Laxer et al., 1987). Unfortunately, many studies are retrospective studies of a small number of patients, so information is needed on what is the optimal second-line approach in DM.

A small, controlled double-blind study has shown that high-dose intravenous immunoglobulin (IVIG) is a safe and effective treatment for DM, and open trials have suggested that IVIG treatment may be effective in PM as well (Dalakas et al., 1993; Sansome and Dubowitz, 1995). Recent studies have suggested a daily dose of 400 mg/kg per day for 5 days, followed by monthly 3-day courses for 3 to 6 months (Kokontis and Gutmann, 2000).

Prognosis

IMs are serious conditions for which aggressive treatment is warranted. Most patients with DM and PM improve with prednisone therapy, but many require long-term treatment. Patients with pulmonary involvement or extensive gastrointestinal ulceration have particularly poor prognoses (Callen, 2000). In one multicenter retrospective study, 37% of patients had a monocyclic course, but most (63%) had a chronic, continuous (or polycyclic) course. Of the patients followed up for at least 3 years, 40% still had rash, 23% reported continued weakness, and 35% continued to take medications (Huber et al., 2000). Recent work with myositis-specific autoantibodies may improve the ability to prognosticate (Rider and Miller, 1997).

MYASTHENIA GRAVIS

Myasthenia gravis (MG) is a disorder characterized by weakness associated with fatigue of the voluntary muscles (i.e., worsening weakness with repetitive activity) and by the striking tendency to recover motor power after rest or the administration of anticholinesterase medications. These symptoms typically result from an autoimmune response in which antibodies are produced against nicotinic *a*cetyl*ch*oline *r*eceptors (AChRs) in skeletal muscle.

Several major types of MG may be distinguished (Table 40-3). Engel (1992, 1994a) and Drachman (1994) have provided comprehensive reviews.

Historical Aspects

In 1672, Sir Thomas Willis first described "asthenia of voluntary muscle" with recovery on resting. Jolly (1895) named the syndrome *myasthenia gravis pseudoparalytica*. In 1901, Laquer and Diegert described tumors of the thymus in patients with MG, yet a possible link between this immunologically central organ and the pathogenesis of MG was not considered until relatively recently. Simpson (1960) suggested an autoimmune pathogenesis on the basis of a clinical and pathologic study of 440 patients who had MG. Nastuk and coworkers (1960) described the fluctuation of serum complement with exacerbations and remissions of MG, which suggested an antigen-antibody interaction.

Strauss and colleagues (1960) used immunofluorescent and complement-fixation techniques to show that the γ-globulin from patients with MG binds to muscle. Fambrough and colleagues (1973) first demonstrated a

TABLE 40-3 · CLASSIFICATION OF MYASTHENIA GRAVIS (MG)

Type	Onset	Etiology
Neonatal	Birth	Adoptive transfer of anti-AChR antibodies from mother; MG is transient.
Congenital*	Birth	Genetic defects in neuromuscular junction; weakness is usually permanent; and anti-AChR antibodies are absent.
Juvenile	Early childhood or puberty	Autoimmune; anti-AChR antibodies are pathogenic.
Adult	After puberty	Autoimmune; anti-AChR antibodies are pathogenic.

*Congenital myasthenic syndromes have traditionally been classified as variants of MG, but these syndromes have a genetic, rather than immune, pathogenesis (Engel, 1992). For this reason, congenital myasthenic syndromes should be distinguished from MG nosologically, even though the clinical distinction may be difficult to make. Most genetic myasthenic syndromes are apparent at birth, but some patients may have an onset in childhood or adult life.
AchR = acetylcholine receptor; MG = myasthenia gravis.

decrease in AChRs in MG. These seminal findings have influenced much of MG research in subsequent decades.

Coincident with the understanding of the pathophysiology, treatments have changed. Acetylcholinesterase inhibitors were used in the 1950s, prednisone and thymectomy in the 1970s, and plasma exchange and IVIG in the 1980s (Kissel and Franklin, 2000)

Pathogenesis

Acetylcholine Receptor

Normal voluntary motor activity depends on the release of acetylcholine (ACh) by presynaptic nerve terminals at the neuromuscular junction. These terminals abut nicotinic receptors for AChRs, which are grouped on postsynaptic folds on the muscle surface. When sufficient ACh is bound to the AChR, intracellular events leading to muscle contraction occur. Normally, this reaction is rapidly terminated by extracellular acetylcholinesterase, which degrades residual synaptic ACh. This action clears the neuromuscular junction, which again becomes receptive to new signals and the effective modulation of motor activity.

The AChR itself consists of an aggregate of five types of polypeptide subunits. Each AChR contains two α-subunits, one β-subunit, one δ-subunit, and one γ-or ε-subunit (Drachman, 1994). The α-subunits contain the sites that actually bind molecules of ACh; these sites are the antigenic targets most frequently recognized by anti-AChR antibodies. Ultrastructural studies have shown that each AChR has a central pit, probably the channel through which cations flow after ACh-mediated activation.

The basic defect in all forms of MG (except congenital MG or the familial myasthenic syndromes; see later discussion) is a reduction in number of the postsynaptic receptors of the neuromuscular junction (Engel, 1992), the result of the action of autoantibodies.

Anti-AChR Antibodies

The central role of antibodies to AChR has been shown in clinical studies of patients with MG and in experimental models of animals with MG. Antibody to AChR can be detected in approximately 84% of patients with MG (Engel, 1992). Ig from patients with MG causes weakness and AChR depletion on passive transfer to mice (Engel, 1992). Moreover, the adoptive transfer of peripheral blood lymphocytes from patients with MG (even from patients who are seronegative for anti-AChR antibodies) induces MG and anti-AChR antibodies in recipient immunodeficient mice (Martino et al., 1993). Taken together, this evidence indicates that the autoimmune effector mechanisms in MG are primarily humoral.

Despite these observations, the relationship between clinical MG and anti-AChR antibodies is not simple. As noted, approximately 16% of patients with clear-cut MG are seronegative when tested with commercially available assays. In certain subsets of patients who have MG, such as those with exclusively ocular manifestations, the pro-

portion of patients who are seronegative may be as high as 50%. In addition, among different patients, anti-AChR titers correlate poorly with clinical severity.

Nonetheless, in an individual patient, a substantial reduction in antibody titer over time usually is associated with clinical improvement (Engel, 1992). These discrepancies may reflect technical factors in the assay for anti-AChR antibody, the effects of anti-AChR antibodies of different fine specificities, the sequestration of antibody at the neuromuscular junction, or the existence of different subtypes of MG, including some in which the disorder is either not autoimmune or in which antibody is directed against antigenic determinants other than the AChRs.

Anti-AChR antibodies may exert their effect in MG by at least three mechanisms (Drachman, 1994; Engel, 1992). First, binding of the antibody to AChR may directly affect its function as a mediator between nerve impulse and muscle contraction; second, antibody cross-linking of AChR may increase receptor degradation and depletion; third, the antibody-AChR interaction may bind complement, with subsequent damage to the AChR-containing postsynaptic membrane folds.

The central role of anti-AChR antibodies in MG is generally accepted, but the putative factors that may initiate or trigger MG, such as viral infections and thymic myoid cells, are poorly understood. Molecular mimicry between the AChR and microbial (especially viral) antigenic determinants may exist and could trigger an autoimmune reaction (Carrieri et al., 1999; Drachman, 1994); however, surgically removed thymus glands with MG have no evidence of viral infection (Aoki et al., 1985). The proximity of thymic myoid cells to thymic centers for T lymphocyte production may result in sensitization to muscle cell antigens, as noted earlier.

A third consideration is based on the observation that low levels of anti-AChR antibodies and AChR-specific T-helper cells can be detected in apparently healthy individuals (Melms et al., 1993). These findings prompted the suggestion that a "few cells secreting antibodies at subpathologic levels could be a normal occurrence and that activation and expansion of these clones may be involved in initiation of the MG disease process" (Mittag et al., 1984). MG developing after bone marrow transplantation may be a result of such clonal expansion of normal cells under unusual circumstances (Smith et al., 1983).

The Thymus and Cell-Mediated Immunity

Humoral immunity clearly predominates as the autoimmune effector mechanism in MG, but a significant role for cell-mediated immunity and the thymus, particularly during the inductive phase of the illness, has been proposed (Drachman, 1994; Wekerle, 1993). Thus lymphocytes are common in MG muscle biopsy specimens, and the thymus is histologically abnormal in 70% to 90% of patients with MG (Castleman, 1966). Because myoid, or musclelike, cells are present in the thymus, the presence of these AChR-bearing cells and lymphocytes in the thymus during the maturation of the immune system may initiate autoimmunity in MG.

In view of the production of anti-AChR antibodies in MG, one might expect thymic cells to have an excess of T-helper cells. Evidence of this has been sought but has only inconsistently been found (Seybold and Lindstrom, 1982). The favorable clinical response to thymectomy supports the role of the thymus in MG pathogenesis (Gronseth and Barohn, 2000).

Genetic and Disease Associations

MG has a modest association with HLA antigens B8 and DRw3 and a strong—but unconfirmed—association with DQw2 (Drachman, 1994). Family studies have revealed a prevalence of MG in the relatives of as much as 2% of patients with congenital and juvenile MG, prompting the observation that those "who are most genetically prone to develop myasthenia do so early in life" (Bundey et al., 1972).

Adult patients with MG have an increased incidence of thyroid disease, rheumatoid arthritis, SLE, and pernicious anemia, all autoimmune disorders. Monozygotic and dizygotic twins have concordance rates of approximately 40% and 0%, respectively. These observations suggest that both genetic and environmental factors are involved in the development of MG.

Clinical Features

The hallmark of MG is excessive fatigability. Variable weakness manifests differently in each subtype of MG (see Table 40-3).

Neonatal Myasthenia Gravis

In *neonatal MG*, weakness develops transiently in 10% to 25% of children born to mothers who are myasthenic as a result of the passive transfer of maternal antibodies to the fetal circulation (Barlow, 1981; Fenichel, 1978; Morel et al., 1988). The factors that make one fetus more vulnerable than another are unknown. Thus the chances of delivering an affected child may vary from pregnancy to pregnancy for any given mother. Therefore every newborn of a woman with MG should be considered at risk and observed meticulously.

Neonatal MG most frequently develops the day after birth, but it may occur as late as 1 week of age. The signs of neonatal MG include weak sucking, crying, and swallowing; facial diplegia; respiratory difficulty; extremity weakness; hypotonia; and depressed reflexes. Unlike the manifestations in adults, ptosis and ophthalmoplegia are rare in neonatal MG. Neonatal MG may also occur in mothers with latent or undiagnosed MG.

Congenital Myasthenia Gravis

Several different *congenital* myasthenic syndromes resembling neonatal MG that do not appear to share the immune mechanisms have been discovered (i.e., AChR antibodies are not found, and infants are not responsive to immunotherapy). Thus other forms of myasthenia may occur in the neonatal period that are hereditary rather than autoimmune.

Several features help to distinguish congenital myasthenic syndromes from neonatal MG, including the following: (1) a nonmyasthenic mother, (2) the lack of antibodies to AchR, (3) a relatively benign course involving mostly the ocular muscles, and (4) a high incidence of affected family members (Engel, 1992, 1994b; Fenichel, 1978). Drawing this distinction is important because the treatment of the 2 conditions differs.

Juvenile Myasthenia Gravis

Juvenile MG is so similar to adult MG in its manifestations that most authorities consider the conditions to be one disease with different ages of onset (Lisak and Barchi, 1982).

Diagnosis

The diagnosis of MG is usually apparent from the clinical features of weakness and fatigability, especially when symptoms are maximal at the end of the day or after exercise. Confirmation of the diagnosis should be sought by assessing serum anti-AChR antibodies and neuromuscular function, the latter by the edrophonium chloride (Tensilon) test and repetitive nerve stimulation (the Jolly test) (Engel, 1992; Linton and Philcox, 1990). The Tensilon test may be negative in some cases of MG, especially in the ocular form. Anti-AChR antibodies are demonstrable in most patients with MG, but seronegative patients do respond to immunotherapy. An ice test can also be used, in which ice is applied to a ptotic eye for 2 minutes. Two or more millimeters of improvement is considered a positive result, with 80% of patients with MG having this response (Golnik et al., 1999).

Electromyographic testing with repetitive stimulation at low frequencies (2-3 Hz) should be performed and is one of the most reliable ways to diagnose MG. This should also be done at high frequency (20 Hz) if some other neuromuscular blockade syndrome (e.g., botulism) is suspected. A decremental response (>20% amplitude reduction of the muscle-evoked potential) is observed at either frequency in MG. This can be seen even in children whose clinical manifestations of MG are confined to the extraocular muscles, especially if the extensor digitorum brevis muscles are studied. Resolution of the abnormality with edrophonium administration is diagnostic. In obscure cases, single-fiber electromyography, in vitro microelectrode studies of neuromuscular transmission, and immunocytochemical analyses may be necessary (Engel, 1992).

A search for the presence of thymoma in juvenile and adult MG should be undertaken through the use of chest radiographs and computed tomography or magnetic resonance imaging (MRI) of the superior mediastinum (Linton and Philcox, 1990).

The differential diagnoses of MG include all conditions causing acute or subacute weakness (see Guillain-

Barré syndrome [GBS] later in this chapter). The important diseases to exclude are neurasthenia, botulism, brainstem lesions, acquired myopathies, and *Lambert-Eaton myasthenic syndrome* (LEMS; detailed later in this chapter).

The lack of objective clinical and laboratory findings, in addition to the presence of variable, "give-way" weakness at the bedside, usually indicate neurasthenia. Botulism typically has an abrupt onset, accompanying gastrointestinal symptoms, and prominent visual findings, including abnormal or absent pupillary responses to light. Brainstem lesions usually produce widespread lower cranial nerve dysfunction associated with definite signs of central nervous system (CNS) involvement, such as involvement of long–motor and sensory tracts. Thyroiditis or hyperthyroidism may mimic or co-exist with MG; recognition of these is important because thyroid abnormalities may exacerbate MG (Drachman, 1994).

Exogenous substances may produce illnesses resembling MG, such as a prolonged myasthenic state that may occur after neuromuscular blockade (Benzing et al., 1990). Other exogenous substances to consider include arthropod, snake, and insect venoms; trimethadione and phenytoin; aminoglycosides and polymyxins; magnesium; and quinine and carnitine (Bazzato et al., 1981; Masters et al., 1977; Swift, 1981; Wittbrodt, 1997).

Treatment

Treatment depends on the type and severity of MG (Engel, 1992, 1994a; Lindstrom et al., 1988; Linton and Philcox, 1990; Lisak and Barchi, 1982; Shah and Lisak, 1993). Neonatal MG is treated with supportive care and anticholinesterase drugs; neostigmine, 0.05 mg intramuscularly before feedings, is often sufficient. Because neonatal MG is transient and disappears when the passively transferred maternal anti-AChR antibodies are metabolized, the amount of medication should be gradually diminished to prevent cholinergic overdose. Exchange transfusions may be useful in severe cases (Pasternak et al., 1981).

Juvenile and adult forms of MG are the result of ongoing humoral immunopathogenesis. Current treatments have had limited study in controlled clinical trials (Engel, 1992). There are, however, several accepted approaches.

Anticholinesterase Drugs

First, many mild cases and patients with exclusively ocular manifestations will respond adequately to anticholinesterase agents such as neostigmine or pyridostigmine. This treatment increases the half-life of ACh within the synaptic cleft, thereby increasing the likelihood of binding to the sparse postsynaptic receptors. Common side effects include nausea, vomiting, intestinal cramping, bradycardia, and diaphoresis. Long-term anticholinesterase therapy carries the theoretical risk of additional injury to the motor end plate (Hudson et al., 1978).

Thymectomy

If an adequate trial of anticholinesterase treatment is not effective (an adequate trial may require up to a year), thymectomy should be considered in most adults, many children, and a few elderly patients (the latter reservation is because of increased complications and limited benefit). Early thymectomy apparently has no adverse effects on the maturation of the immune system (Seybold et al., 1971) and results in clinical remission in as much as two thirds of children with MG (Aicardi, 1992). Some clinicians believe that thymectomy should be put off until after puberty if possible (Drachman, 1994). A recent evidence-based review by the American Academy of Neurology concluded that in nonthymomatous autoimmune MG, thymectomy is recommended as an option to increase the probability of remission or improvement (Gronseth and Barohn, 2000).

Immunosuppressives and IVIG

Other therapies include plasmapheresis, alternate-day corticosteroids, IVIG, and immunosuppressives (e.g., azathioprine, cyclosporine) (Ciafaloni et al., 2000; Drachman, 1994; Palace et al., 1998). IVIG, in particular, shows promise because of its ease, safety, and efficacy (Drachman, 1994; Selcen et al., 2000), and the response rate is similar—but slower—to that of plasma exchange (Howard, 1998). Azathioprine as adjunctive therapy to alternate-day prednisolone is associated with fewer treatment failures, longer remissions, and fewer side effects than prednisolone alone (Palace et al., 1998). Cyclosporine has a high rate of clinical improvement, but with the side effects of elevated serum creatinine (28%) and malignancy (11%) (Ciafaloni et al., 2000).

Cholinergic Crisis

Patients with MG may experience a sudden, severe worsening with respiratory and bulbar compromise, called *crisis*. Crisis may be caused by excessive *(cholinergic crisis)* or insufficient *(myasthenic crisis)* anticholinesterase medication, the initiation of corticosteroid therapy, physical or emotional stress, concurrent infection, or the administration of drugs such as aminoglycosides, quinidine, procainamide, phenytoin, chlorpromazine, D-penicillamine, neuromuscular blocking agents, and others (Wittbrodt, 1997). Because deterioration may rapidly develop into a life-threatening state, patients with significant worsening, particularly of bulbar or respiratory function, are at risk of crisis and should immediately be admitted to an intensive care unit.

The edrophonium test was formerly used to distinguish crisis caused by undermedication from that resulting from overmedication, yet all authorities currently recommend admitting the patient to an intensive care unit, stopping anticholinesterase treatment for 48 to 72 hours, providing respiratory support if needed, and searching for a reversible precipitant of the crisis. After stabilization, treatment may include reinstitution of anticholinesterase medication, plasmapheresis, IVIG, and corticosteroids (Fink, 1993; Lisak and Barchi, 1982).

In children with MG who respond poorly to immunotherapy, have a family history of neuromuscular disorder, lack antibodies to AChR, or have a dysmorphic appearance, a congenital myasthenic syndrome should be considered. Congenital myasthenic conditions may be caused by diverse defects in the neuromuscular apparatus (Engel, 1992). Furthermore, the response to therapy varies widely in these patients, and in some instances, conventional treatment may result in clinical worsening. When a congenital myasthenic syndrome is suspected, referral to a specialized center is advisable.

Prognosis

Jolly (1895) introduced the term *gravis* to emphasize the poor outlook in untreated MG. With modern therapy, the prognosis is relatively good, but mortality rates still range from 3% to 30%. In contrast, 30% of children experience spontaneous remission, particularly those with MG confined to the extraocular muscles (Aicardi, 1992; Engel, 1994a; Evoli et al., 1998). With the use of thymectomy and immunosuppression, remission is seen in 60% of juvenile patients (Lindner et al., 1997).

LAMBERT-EATON MYASTHENIC SYNDROME

Lambert-Eaton myasthenic syndrome (LEMS) is usually associated with a malignancy, often small-cell carcinoma of the lung (Engel, 1994b; O'Neill et al., 1988). LEMS usually occurs in adults; however, two apparently similar, but rare, illnesses have been described in children: (1) a congenital myasthenic syndrome (Bady et al., 1987) and (2) a juvenile form with features of limb-girdle distributed myopathy and LEMS (Husain et al., 1989). Neither has been associated with malignancy.

Unlike those with MG, patients with LEMS usually do not have prominent ocular symptoms and they often develop increased strength with repetitive effort (Eaton and Lambert, 1957). Electrophysiologic studies reveal incremental evoked muscle responses at high rates of repetitive stimulation (>50 Hz) in contrast to the decremental responses characteristic of MG.

LEMS in adults is associated with antibodies directed against P/Q-type voltage–gated calcium channels and synaptotagmin on the presynaptic nerve terminals of the neuromuscular junctions (Lang et al., 1993; Takemori et al., 2000; Wray and Porter, 1993).

The treatment of LEMS has been reviewed by Posner (1991) and Engel (1992, 1994b). In general, antitumor therapy and alternate-day prednisone are recommended for neoplastic LEMS, and azathioprine and alternate-day prednisone are recommended for non-neoplastic LEMS. Plasmapheresis may also be of benefit. Treatment with 3,4-diaminopyridine may also lead to increased release of ACh and symptomatic improvement (Newsom-Davis, 2001).

GUILLAIN-BARRÉ SYNDROME

Historical Aspects

Guillain-Barré syndrome (GBS) is characterized by progressive motor weakness and areflexia. Sensory, autonomic, and brainstem findings also occur. Landry first described this syndrome in 1859; it was described later by French army neurologists Guillain, Barré, and Strohl in 1916. Their observation that this weakness occurred with "albuminocytologic dissociation" (i.e., an elevated cerebrospinal fluid [CSF] protein with a normal CSF cell count) allowed this entity to be distinguished from polio and other neuropathies (see the review by Ropper and Kehne, 1985)

Pathogenesis

GBS is believed to be an autoimmune-mediated process. Several infections—Epstein-Barr virus, cytomegalovirus (CMV), mycoplasma, and *Campylobacter*—and immunizations have been known to precede the illness (Stratton et al., 1994). GBS is generally thought of as a demyelinating process; however, more recently, an axonal form of GBS has been described after a diarrhea illness secondary to *Campylobacter* infection (Griffin et al., 1995). Occasionally, surgery is noted to be a precipitating factor. To date, treatment has been primarily aimed at immunomodulation, with either IVIG or plasmapheresis being the most effective forms of therapy.

In the demyelinating form of GBS, demyelination and mononuclear infiltration are seen. Lymphocytes and macrophages surround endoneural vessels and cause an adjacent demyelination. These lesions can be discrete and are scattered through the peripheral nervous system, but there may be a predilection for inflammation of the nerve roots (Ropper, 1992). The conduction block and demyelination of the motor nerves result in the progressive weakness present in this syndrome. Similarly, the involvement of the sensory nerves leads to pain and paresthesias.

Many authors believe that the mechanism of disease involves an abnormal T-cell response, precipitated by an infection (Ropper and Kehne, 1985). A variety of specific antigens may be involved in this response, including myelin P2 and GM1 ganglioside, P2, GM1, and GQ1 gangliosides (Rostami, 1993).

Recently, epidemics of GBS were noted to occur annually in the rural north of China, particularly during the summer months. This has been associated with *Campylobacter jejuni* infection; many of these patients have antiglycolipid antibodies (Griffin et al., 1995; Ho et al., 1995). In this axonal form of GBS, biopsy specimens reveal Wallerian-like degeneration of fibers in the ventral and dorsal nerve roots, with only minimal demyelination or lymphocytic infiltration (Griffin et al., 1996). These axonal lesions affect both sensory and motor fibers. This form of GBS has been associated with *Campylobacter* infection, but it appears to be a rare complication of such infection (McCarthy et al., 1999).

Clinical Features

Patients with GBS have weakness and unsteadiness (ataxia). The weakness typically starts in the lower extremities and ascends into the upper extremities. This progression may extend from hours to days to weeks. Pain and dysesthesias are also noted, particularly in children. Pain may be the initial manifestation in almost half of children (Bradshaw and Jones, 1992; Delanoe et al., 1998). Often these symptoms will follow an illness or an immunization given within 2 to 4 weeks of symptom onset.

During the physical examination, an ascending motor weakness with areflexia is noted. This tends to be symmetric and usually begins in the legs. Occasionally, autonomic instability (26%), ataxia (23%), and cranial nerve findings (35%-50%) are seen. The latter findings are probably seen more frequently in children than in adults with this syndrome (Bradshaw and Jones, 1992; Delanoe et al., 1998).

The autonomic neuropathy involves both the sympathetic and parasympathetic systems. Manifestations can include orthostatic hypotension, pupillary dysfunction, sweating abnormalities, and sinus tachycardia (England, 1990).

Miller-Fisher syndrome is a variant also seen in children and manifested as ophthalmoplegia, ataxia, and areflexia with relatively little weakness. This syndrome has been associated with antibodies to ganglioside GQ1b (Marks et al., 1977; Ropper, 1992).

Diagnosis

Laboratory evaluation reveals an elevated CSF protein level without pleocytosis, but it may not be seen in the first 48 hours of symptoms. After several days, abnormalities in conduction velocities, F waves, and compound motor action potential can be seen in electrophysiologic studies. Lumbosacral MRI may demonstrate enhancement of the nerve roots.

The differential diagnoses of GBS in childhood include other disorders of progressive, symmetric weakness. Botulism should be a consideration, particularly in infants. In botulism there is also involvement of the extraocular muscles and constipation. In addition, when ophthalmoplegia is present, MG is a consideration. Nerve conduction velocity and electromyographic findings can help one distinguish among these conditions. Conditions similar to GBS can occur in certain infections such as Lyme disease and human immunodeficiency virus. In these latter cases, the lumbar puncture will typically reveal CSF pleocytosis.

Patients with myelopathies can sometimes have progressive weakness, and the physical examination (or spinal MRI) should help differentiate a spinal cord syndrome from a diffuse neuropathy. Other acute neuropathies from lead, heavy metals, or vincristine also cause a predominantly motor neuropathy. Tick bites can also cause ascending paralysis; children should be searched for ticks if they have these symptoms. Often there is dramatic improvement after tick removal. Finally, a patient with organophosphate poisoning may have the signs and symptoms of GBS.

Treatment

IVIG is often used to treat GBS. IVIG seems most helpful in reducing the severity of the disease and the duration of symptoms. The long-term outcome, however, may not be affected. Several regimens have been used. One regimen includes daily IVIG for 5 days at a dosage of 0.4 gm/kg/day, which results in a clinical improvement in a mean of 2 to 3 days after the start of therapy (Abd-Allah et al., 1997). Others advocate the use of 2 gm/kg of IVIG given as a single dose (Zafeiriou et al., 1997).

Plasmapheresis is also an option. Studies in children making use of both historical and case controls indicate that plasmapheresis may decrease the severity and shorten the duration of GBS (Epstein and Sladky, 1990; French Cooperative Group, 1997; Lamont et al., 1991). The results of plasmapheresis and IVIG seem similar, with possibly fewer side effects seen with IVIG (Bril et al., 1996; Van der Meche and Schmitz, 1992).

Steroids have been used to treat GBS, yet current data suggest there is no benefit with the use of these agents (Hughes and van der Meche, 2000).

Vital signs and respiratory capacity should be monitored. When vital capacity falls below 15 ml/kg of body weight, arterial Po_2 falls below 70 mm/Hg, or there is significant fatigue, then intubation and mechanical ventilation may be necessary (Ropper and Kehne, 1985). Orthostatic hypotension and urinary retention may also occur during the acute phase of the illness. Attention should also be paid to possible decubitus ulcers and contractures in severely ill patients or in those who have a prolonged course. Long-term physical therapy may be beneficial to patients during the recovery phase of the illness.

Prognosis

Most children with GBS fully recover. The recovery period is longer than the onset period, often requiring weeks to months, with a median recovery time of 7 months (Bradshaw and Jones, 1992). In another series, the median time from the onset of symptoms to the first recovery was 17 days; to walk unaided, 37 days; and to be symptom free, 66 days (Korinthenberg and Monting, 1996). Adults with the axonal form of GBS have a poorer prognosis, with a median time to walking with assistance of approximately 32 days (Ho et al., 1997).

The most serious complication occurs with weakness of the breathing muscles. Many seriously affected individuals—up to 16% in one series (Korinthenberg and Monting, 1996)—will need respiratory support. During the progression of the disease, attention should be paid to the child's respiratory status, and measurements of vital capacity, for example, can provide objective data.

Recurrences in children are uncommon. Some children may have a chronic progressive course, whereas others may have recurrences or relapses. At a long-term follow-up examination, 93% were free of symptoms and the remainder were able to walk unaided (Korinthenberg and Monting, 1996).

CHRONIC INFLAMMATORY DEMYELINATING POLYRADICULONEUROPATHY

Children with chronic inflammatory demyelinating polyradiculoneuropathy (CIDP) experience a subacute onset of symmetrical weakness that progresses over at least 2 months. CIDP exhibits a close clinical, immunologic, and pathologic resemblance to GBS. Unlike GBS, CIDP usually has an indolent onset and a progressive or relapsing course. GBS typically is associated with spontaneous recovery and a lack of responsiveness to corticosteroids; almost paradoxically, CIDP is responsive to corticosteroids but has a relatively poorer long-term prognosis (Connolly, 2001; Dyck et al., 1993; Parry, 1993).

Historical Aspects

In 1958, Austin defined the picture of acquired recurrent polyneuropathy and demonstrated its susceptibility to glucocorticoid treatment. Dyck and colleagues (1968) reported the frequent occurrence of elevated CSF protein levels in chronic relapsing neuropathy, and Borit and Altrocchi (1971) documented the presence of lymphocytic infiltrates in roots and peripheral nerves.

The term *chronic inflammatory polyradiculoneuropathy* was used first by Dyck and colleagues (1975) to characterize 53 patients with relapsing, slow monophasic, relapsing-progressive, or steadily progressive forms of acquired nonfamilial neuropathy. In 1984, Dyck and Arnason acknowledged the demyelinating nature of this disorder by proposing the current definition for CIDP (see also the review by Maimone, 2001).

Pathogenesis

The pathologic features of CIDP include mononuclear infiltration of the peripheral nerves, segmental demyelination, and onion-bulb formation. The pathology of CIDP resembles that of GBS or acute IDP in segmental demyelination but differs in the amount of remyelinative onion-bulb formation surrounding axons and in the relative paucity of inflammatory cells, consistent with the chronicity of the process (Barohn et al., 1989; Dyck et al., 1993; Prineas and McLeod, 1976).

Ganglioside, sulfatide, acidic glycolipids, proliferating nonmyelinating Schwann cells, and β-tubulin autoantibodies have been found in adults with CIDP (Connolly, 2001). Fifty percent of patients with GBS and 35% of patients with CIDP have autoantibodies to peripheral myelin protein 22 (Gabriel et al., 2000). Nevertheless, the exact mechanism of CIDP demyelinization is not known (Lisak and Brown, 1987; Rostami, 1993).

As many as 20% to 30% of patients with CIDP studied with MRI and electroencephalography, in terms of evoked responses, exhibit CNS involvement (Ohtake et al., 1990), but pathologic confirmation is lacking. Occasionally, patients have features of CIDP and multiple sclerosis (MS) (Dyck et al., 1993; Thomas and Walker, 1987).

Other rare, chronic immune-mediated polyneuropathies of childhood (Linington and Brostoff, 1993) include neuropathies associated with neoplasms, lymphoma, leukemia, and polycythemia vera (McLeod, 1993a, 1993b); monoclonal gammopathies (Kyle and Dyck, 1993); systemic vasculitides (Chalk et al., 1993); and idiopathic inflammatory conditions (Smith et al., 1993). In some of these disorders, autoantibodies can be identified in the serum or CSF or by immunohistochemical study of peripheral nerve biopsy specimens.

Clinical Features

CIDP is characterized by symmetrical proximal and distal weakness and sensory loss; however, other variants do exist (Saperstein et al., 2000). The two mandatory clinical research criteria for CIDP include progressive or relapsing motor and sensory dysfunction of more than one limb and hyporeflexia or areflexia that usually involves all four limbs (AAN Taskforce, 1991). The onset of symptoms may begin as early as infancy; the symptoms include gait difficulties, fatigue, dysesthesia, and sensory loss.

Diagnosis

During the symptomatic phase of CIDP, the CSF is acellular with an elevated protein level often exceeding 100 mg/dl (Dalakas and Engel, 1981). Motor nerve conduction velocities are slow, and sensory potentials typically are absent (Barohn et al., 1989; Dyck et al., 1975).

The differential diagnoses include (1) hereditary sensory-motor neuropathies, (2) toxic neuropathies, (3) monoradicular or polyradicular gammopathies, and (4) polyneuropathy associated with systemic autoimmune or inflammatory conditions. The electrophysiologic findings of conduction block, temporal dispersion, and focal slowing distinguish CIDP from most heritable neuropathies (Uncini et al., 1991); in difficult cases, it may be necessary to establish the correct diagnosis by performing a nerve biopsy.

Treatment

Corticosteroid therapy for CIDP is of benefit to both children and adults (Uncini et al., 1991). Prednisone at dosages of 1.5 to 2.0 mg/kg/day is a typical initial therapy. Prednisone is tapered to alternate-day therapy over several weeks and then tapered off over several additional weeks. Almost all children respond to steroids, but some may relapse during the taper, necessitating retreatment and slower tapering. Functional recovery is expected in 50% to 80% of patients (Dyck et al., 1993).

The adverse effects of chronic steroid administration have prompted the use of plasmapheresis and IVIG as alternatives. Beydoun and associates (1990) report that plasmapheresis for children with CIDP is safe and effective. Controlled trials have shown the benefit of IVIG use in patients with CIDP (Mendell et al., 2001; Van Doorn et al., 1990). Case reports have described the benefits of azathioprine, cyclophosphamide, and cyclosporine; these drugs are reserved for refractory cases (Parry, 1993). Some authors advocate IVIG or plasmapheresis as initial therapy (Connolly, 2001; Dyck et al., 1993).

Prognosis

Two common clinical courses are described in children. One is a monophasic course in which progression to maximal weakness occurs within a 3-month period. This group responds well to steroids and has a good prognosis. In the other group, the disease presents more gradually and has a relapsing-remitting course and therefore a poorer prognosis (Connolly, 2001; Nevo et al., 1996; Ryan et al., 2000).

BELL'S PALSY

Historical Aspects

Acute idiopathic dysfunction of the facial nerve (usually postinfectious), is called Bell's palsy (BP) after Sir Charles Bell, who first described the condition in 1821. Facial nerve abnormalities include (1) decreased facial motor movement (e.g., facial expression, lid closure), (2) denervation of the tensor tympani (resulting in inability to dampen the eardrum to loud noises), (3) decreased taste sensation of the anterior two thirds of the tongue, and (4) abnormal lacrimal and salivary function.

Pathogenesis

The acute pathologic course of BP is inflammatory, with nerve swelling and compression. Histologic studies of the facial nerve during the acute stage of BP have revealed signs of edema, perivascular, perineurial, lymphocytic, and macrophage infiltration of the nerve, and axonal changes (Liston and Kleid, 1989).

Various reports have noted an association between acute facial palsy and several viruses, including herpes simplex virus 1, varicella-zoster virus, human herpesvirus 6, human herpesvirus 7, CMV, Epstein-Barr virus, coxsackie, influenza, polio, and mumps (Bauer and Coker, 1996; Pitkaranta et al., 2000). Varicella-zoster virus and herpes simplex virus are considered to be the major causes of BP (Furuta et al., 2000). Herpes simplex virus 1 DNA can be detected in 77% of patients with BP (Murakami et al., 1996). In patients without HSV, 29% had detectable varicella-zoster virus reactivation (Furuta et al., 2000).

Clinical Features

As with GBS and acute disseminated encephalomyelitis (detailed later in this chapter), BP often follows an upper respiratory illness (60%). Most cases are unilateral, but asymmetric bilateral BP is occasionally encountered. Facial weakness is often heralded by ear pain (50%). The majority of patients (90%) have a decreased ipsilateral stapes reflex; approximately 25% have impaired taste perception; and 10% have a loss or significant decrease of ipsilateral tearing or submandibular salivary flow (Adour et al., 1978).

The clinical features of BP include impairment of voluntary movement of facial and platysmal muscles, and on attempting to close the eye, the eyeball is diverted upward and outward (called *Bell's phenomenon*). With a lesion proximal to the geniculate ganglion, there may be decreased tearing in the affected eye. When the chorda tympani is affected, there may be a decrease in salivation and taste in the anterior two thirds of the tongue (Russel, 2001).

The peripheral white blood cell count and sedimentation rate are normal, but CSF pleocytosis and the elevation of CSF protein and IgG may be present; these findings are consistent with transient inflammation and blood-brain barrier disturbance. Lyme titers should also be obtained in at-risk individuals.

Late complications of BP usually do not occur until 3 to 4 months after the onset of the facial paralysis. The most common late complication is contracture, which is commonly accompanied by synkinesis (Adour et al., 1978). Ptosis of the eyebrow may require surgical correction if severe. The last late complication to develop is gustatory (or crocodile) tearing, in which there is aberrant regeneration of secretory fibers to the lacrimal glands, resulting in tearing of the eyes during eating. Gustatory tearing usually does not occur until 4 months after the onset of BP.

Treatment and Prognosis

Symptomatic therapy with artificial tears and eye patches should be used for incomplete eye closure. Attention should be paid to the possibility of an ophthalmic herpes infection. The American Academy of Neurology has recently reviewed the use of steroids, acyclovir, and facial nerve decompression for BP. They concluded that steroids are probably effective and acyclovir (combined with prednisone) may be effective in improving facial functional outcomes (Grogan and Gronseth, 2001).

Full recovery occurs in approximately 80% to 90% of patients, but 10% may have a recurrence. Recovery usually occurs 4 to 6 months after the onset of symptoms (May and Klein, 1991).

ACUTE DISSEMINATED ENCEPHALOMYELITIS

Historical Aspects

Illnesses resembling *acute disseminated encephalomyelitis* (ADEM) were first recognized in the 19th century by Osler and others, who were struck by the circumstance of an occasional child who developed severe, acute, multifocal encephalitis that was followed by a remarkable recovery. Many cases occurred during the influenza epidemic after World War I. The characteristic pathologic features in these patients were also seen in children after common exanthems or vaccinations (Greenfield, 1930).

Pathogenesis

The prominent pathologic features of ADEM are perivenular inflammatory infiltration and periaxial demyelination—that is, the destruction of myelin with relative preservation of nerve fiber axons (Allen and Kirk, 1992). These findings resemble those for multiple sclerosis (MS) and distinguish it from viral encephalitis. Several pathologic stages are recognized, including (1) venular hyperemia; (2) perivascular and subendothelial inflammatory cell infiltration and edema; (3) vascular necrosis; (4) demyelination with or without hemorrhage; and (5) astrocytic response with remyelination and gliosis.

The initial infiltrate consists of polymorphonuclear leukocytes, but over time, lymphocytes predominate. As demyelination occurs, microglial cells become admixed with lymphocytes, as do phagocytes containing lipid byproducts of myelin degradation. Meningeal inflammation may also be found. Brain involvement is symmetric. Reactive changes in the spleen have also been demonstrated (Turnbull and McIntosh, 1926). In severe cases, there are disseminated hemorrhages, a syndrome called *acute hemorrhagic encephalopathy*.

The possibility that a CNS viral infection causes ADEM is suggested by its occurrence after viral infection and by the induction of experimental encephalomyelitis by viruses. Before widespread immunization, measles was the most common prodromal illness; ADEM occurred in 1 of 800 cases of measles. ADEM can also occur after herpes simplex encephalitis (Koenig et al., 1979), and many other DNA and RNA viruses have also been associated with ADEM.

The occurrence of ADEM after the administration of vaccine, including rabies, pertussis, measles, tetanus, and influenza vaccines; spirochetal illnesses (e.g., Lyme disease); and noninvasive bacteria (e.g., *Bordetella pertussis*) suggests that ADEM is not associated with productive infection (Fenichel, 1982). More likely, these exposures mimic critical CNS antigens and induce immune injury. Similar immune injury and demyelination occur during subacute and chronic CNS infections caused by herpes simplex virus (Sarchielli et al., 1993); HTLV-1 (tropical spastic paraparesis) (Tachi et al., 1992); and human immunodeficiency virus (acquired immunodeficiency virus) (Rhodes, 1993).

Vascular changes may precede an inflammatory perivenular exudate and demyelination, mimicking the vasculitis of serum sickness and immune complex disease. Injury to capillary vascular endothelial cells at the capillary level may result in impairment of the blood-brain barrier. A role for adhesion molecules in the vascular phase of ADEM has been proposed. They may attract inflammatory cells and may have either positive or negative consequences depending on whether the cells clear infection or aggravate inflammatory demyelination (Simmons and Cattle, 1992). Enhanced expression of adhesion molecules occurs during experimental relapsing autoimmune encephalomyelitis (Cannella et al., 1990).

Circulating immune complexes are present in some children with ADEM, resulting in immune complex injury to some organs, with myalgia, rash, and proteinuria (Stricker et al., 1992).

The pathologic changes in ADEM resemble those of experimental allergic encephalomyelitis (EAE) (Rivers et al., 1933). In this model, CNS demyelination is induced by repeated inoculation with "encephalitogenic" antigens (e.g., whole spinal cord homogenate, myelin basic protein, or proteolipid protein) into a susceptible animal. The resulting illness, EAE, shares many pathologic features with human demyelinating diseases, including ADEM and MS (Waksman and Adams, 1955).

Wekerle and coworkers (1994) believe the major lessons gained from the study of EAE are that the CNS is not a privileged or isolated immunologic site; that activated T cells penetrate the blood-brain barrier; and that autoaggressive, anti-CNS T cells exist. However, the triggers that activate autoaggressive T cells during naturally occurring demyelination in animals and humans have not been identified. There is growing evidence that autoaggressive T cells may have restricted T-cell receptor gene usage and epitope specificity. Finally, Wekerle and coworkers (1994) pointed out that EAE can be initiated by injections of several different CNS antigens, not only of myelin basic protein.

Clinical Features

ADEM usually occurs 2 to 20 days after a febrile illness (Miller et al., 1957; Scott, 1967). ADEM is more common in winter, when childhood respiratory and gastrointestinal viral illnesses are prevalent. ADEM typically begins in children recovering from a viral illness who abruptly develop irritability and lethargy. Most children have fever during the viral prodrome; at the onset of ADEM itself, fever is variable. Approximately 15% of affected children have no prodrome. In a few children, there may be a prolonged fever of unknown origin. Diffuse neurologic signs develop rapidly, along with mental status changes and long-tract signs. Seizures occur in 25%. All portions of the CNS may be involved, but the optic nerves and spinal cord are most commonly affected (Patel and Friedman, 1997; Rust, 2000).

Diagnosis

The evaluation of children with ADEM is initially aimed at excluding other causes of diffuse CNS dysfunction such as intoxication, infection (e.g., encephalitis, parasitic conditions), and systemic vasculitis. Before MRI, the diagnostic test of choice, was developed, encephalitis was difficult to distinguish from ADEM. On T2-weighted MRI of patients with ADEM, there are multiple areas of increased signal intensity, characteristically at the gray-white junction. When these signs are present, the differential diagnosis is narrowed to ADEM, MS, or SLE (Kesselring et al., 1990; Valk and van der Knapp, 1989). The clinical course and ancillary tests can usually distinguish these conditions.

Other laboratory tests of value include the electroencephalogram (EEG) and CSF analysis. The EEG usually depicts slowing while the patient is awake; the absence of slowing suggests an ultimate diagnosis of MS. The CSF in ADEM is suggestive of an inflammatory reaction, with elevated IgG, oligoclonal bands, and moderate lymphocytosis (Valk and van der Knapp, 1989).

Treatment

Large controlled trials have not been performed, but most clinicians favor corticosteroids for the treatment of ADEM. A clinical response may occur within hours of the initiation of therapy, particularly when high-doseage (i.e., 15-20 mg/kg/day) IV methylprednisolone is used. Relapse may occur when steroids are tapered; some relapsing children respond well to a slower taper, but a few may require prolonged steroid therapy (i.e., over months or years) (Apak et al., 1999; Rust, 2000).

In patients resistant to high-dose corticosteroids, the use of plasmapheresis, IVIG, or cyclosporine may be used (Pradhan et al., 1999; Stricker et al., 1995).

Prognosis

The outlook for complete recovery is excellent. Some older series report a 10% mortality rate, but only 2% of patients in more recent series have died from ADEM-related complications (Rust, 2000). Recovery is unre-

lated to the severity of the initial signs, and complete recovery may even occur in patients who are blind, comatose, and quadriparetic at the nadir of ADEM. Prognosis is poorest in children under 2 years of age, many of whom have persistent motor and mental defects. These patients may display generalized abnormalities on MR images and are sometimes labeled as having acute toxic encephalopathy. For older children, fixed deficits are uncommon.

After 10 years, approximately 25% of patients with ADEM develop MS. Patients with ADEM are more likely to develop MS if they are (1) afebrile, (2) have no mental status change, (3) have no prodromal viral illness or immunization, (4) have no generalized slowing on encephalograms, and (5) have abnormal CSF (Rust, 2000).

OPTIC NEURITIS

Clinical Features

Childhood optic neuritis (ON) may be an isolated finding or may be associated with other inflammatory and demyelinative illnesses. The clinical and laboratory findings from some children with ADEM and a few children with GBS are consistent with those of ON; also, ON commonly is the presenting symptom of MS. In addition, ON may be associated with transverse myelitis, a combination called *Devic's syndrome (DS)*. The frequency and age at diagnosis of patients with isolated ON (rare in the first years of life, more common in patients 6-14 years old) are similar to those of patients with ADEM. In approximately 70% of children, visual loss occurs days to weeks after a viral illness (especially measles, mumps, and varicella) or immunization (Morales et al., 2000; Purvin et al., 1988; Riikonen, 1989).

Diagnosis

The diagnosis of ON is made on the basis of acute, unilateral diminution in visual acuity not attributed to nutritional deficiency, ischemia, vasculitis, compressive lesions, or genetic causes (e.g., Leber's hereditary optic atrophy). ON can usually be diagnosed when characteristic clinical findings are present, so an extensive evaluation is rarely indicated (Beck et al., 1992). When a progressive course, associated neurologic signs, or other orbital findings suggest optic nerve compression, MRI should be performed.

Treatment and Prognosis

The treatment of ON is controversial. The standard of care in North America is IV methylprednisone (Kaufman et al., 2000). This will hasten visual recovery, but it may not affect its ultimate course.

ON may recur, and some children with ON will develop MS. The precise likelihood of MS developing in infants and children with ON is not known but is lower than in adolescents or adults with ON. The risk for MS is higher in unilateral ON and is rare in bilateral ON (Parkin et al., 1984). In one series, 50% of children with ON with poor or incomplete visual recovery were ultimately diagnosed as having MS (Good et al., 1992). Other studies have revealed a 0% to 60% risk of MS after childhood ON in patients followed up for 8 to 18 years (Kriss et al., 1988; Morales et al., 2000; Parkin et al., 1984; Riikonen et al., 1988).

Pediatric ON is usually associated with visual recovery, but a significant number (22%) may remain visually impaired (Brady et al., 1999). When ON is associated with ADEM or GBS, visual recovery is likely and the neurologic prognosis is dependent on the underlying syndrome. Normal MRI results and a history of preceding infection within 2 weeks of symptom onset are associated with a better outcome. Younger patients are more likely to have bilateral disease and a better visual prognosis (Brady et al., 1999; Lucchinetti et al., 1997).

ACUTE TRANSVERSE MYELITIS

Clinical Features

Acute transverse myelitis (ATM) is a disorder manifesting as CNS dysfunction at a discrete level of the spinal cord. It manifests as paraplegia with or without sensory symptoms and bladder dysfunction. The onset of symptoms occurs over hours to a week (Knebusch et al., 1998). ATM often occurs days to weeks after an infection, as a complication of vaccination, or as a manifestation of Lyme disease (Byrne and Waxman, 1990; Rousseau et al., 1986; Tyler et al., 1986). ATM may occur as an isolated finding or in association with features suggestive of GBS, ADEM, or MS. The pathologic features of ATM consist of perivenular inflammatory changes with demyelination similar to that of ADEM; in severe cases, spinal cord necrosis may occur (Aicardi, 1992).

Diagnosis

A diagnosis of ATM is made through the exclusion of tumor, compressive injury, vascular malformation, hemorrhage, stroke, infection, and radiation injury. MRI with gadolinium enhancement is indicated for imaging the spinal cord. With contrast enhancement, neuroimaging may show changes at the appropriate spinal level and cord swelling (Miller et al., 1987). MRI may disclose clinically silent lesions; the significance of these findings in children is uncertain, and their presence does not necessarily necessitate a diagnosis of MS. In some cases, myelography may be useful.

Lyme disease, syphilis, parasitic infection (cysticercosis), herpes simplex, varicella, and acquired immunodeficiency virus must be considered; serologic studies and CSF sampling are helpful. CSF pleocytosis is present in 25%, and increased CSF protein is present in 50% of

patients (Aicardi, 1992). Tropical spastic paraparesis, a progressive myelopathy caused by HTLV-1 infection, occurs in children and may produce MRI changes indistinguishable from those of ATM, but HTLV-1 lesions often are disseminated throughout the cord (Link et al., 1989; Newton et al., 1987); also, the clinical course of HTLV-1 myelopathy is slower than that of ATM.

Treatment and Prognosis

No therapy, including corticosteroids, has proved efficacious in the treatment of ATM. Nonetheless, in severe cases, IV corticosteroids are often used, sometimes with a dramatic response. Otherwise, management is supportive.

Some degree of recovery occurs in 80% to 90% of children, but this may require weeks to months. Approximately 50% of children with ATM have an excellent recovery; however, 10% to 20% develop cord necrosis and remain severely paralyzed (Berman et al., 1981; Ropper and Poskanzer, 1978). The most important prognostic factor is acuteness of onset; recovery is poor with a hyperacute onset. Ultimately, a diagnosis of MS is made in approximately 10% of adults who experience ATM; the occurrence of MS after isolated childhood ATM is exceptional (Aicardi, 1992).

DEVIC'S SYNDROME

The combination of ON and ATM, first described by Devic in 1894, is called *neuromyelitis optica*, or *Devic's syndrome (DS)*. The signs of ON and ATM may develop simultaneously or in rapid succession, often after a viral illness or immunization. ON is often bilateral, and funduscopic changes of papillitis are frequently present. The clinical features are otherwise similar to the conditions in isolation. The clinical syndrome is distinct, and the differential diagnoses include only other inflammatory CNS demyelinating disorders (e.g., ADEM and MS) (Haslam, 1987). Features that help distinguish DS from typical MS include more than 50 cells/ml in the CSF, a normal initial brain MRI, and lesions extending over 3 or more vertebral segments on spinal cord MRI (Wingerchuk et al., 1999).

As in ON and ATM, corticosteroid therapy is often used, particularly when optic nerve or spinal cord swelling is marked and when the cervical cord dysfunction is severe or when respiratory symptoms occur. The prognosis may be more guarded for each component of DS than for ON and ATM occurring in isolation (Whitham and Brey, 1985).

MULTIPLE SCLEROSIS

Multiple sclerosis (MS), also known as *disseminated sclerosis* or *sclérose en plaques*, is the principal immune-mediated demyelinating disease of humans (Matthews, 1991). Primarily a disorder of young adults, MS has been pathologically verified in infancy (Hanefeld et al., 1993; Shaw and Alvord, 1987). In childhood, however, MS is less common than ADEM. MS and ADEM may be difficult to distinguish, particularly at the onset of symptoms.

Historical Aspects

The pathologic lesions of MS were reported by Cruveilhier and Carswell in the early 19th century. In 1849, Frerichs first made a clinical diagnosis of MS. Charcot (1868) distilled these observations into a coherent and recognizable clinical entity. A detailed account of the history of MS is available (Murray, 2000).

Pathogenesis

MS primarily affects young adults (Sadovnick and Ebers, 1993). The peak age of onset is 25 to 30 years. In one study, only 125 of 4632 patients (3%) had an onset before age 16 years; the mean age of onset in these patients was 13 years, and only eight had signs or symptoms before age 11 (Duquette et al., 1987). The female-to-male ratio is 2:1, and whites are at greater risk than blacks.

The risk of MS is related to the latitude in which individuals spend their childhood; that is, the risk increases in proportion to the distance from the Equator.

A viral pathogenesis of MS is suggested by several lines of evidence (Johnson, 1994). First, the results of epidemiologic tests suggest exposure to an environmental agent that parallels the prevalence of common viral infections. Second, the CSF Ig from patients with MS may have antibodies to several viruses, notably measles virus; also, viruses have occasionally been isolated from MS tissue. Third, certain animal viruses, such as visna, Theiler's, and canine distemper viruses, cause similar demyelinating diseases (Dal Canto, 1990).

Several MS clusters and epidemics provide support for an infectious pathogenesis and genetic susceptibility (Sadovnick and Ebers, 1993). The introduction of MS to the Faroe Islands during World War II suggests that an infectious agent was introduced to a genetically susceptible population. Some infections, such as human herpesvirus 6, have been associated with both ADEM and MS (Campadelli-Fiume et al., 1999). Chlamydia is present in a high percentage of patients with MS, as well as in patients with other neurologic disorders (Gieffers et al., 2001).

Racial variation in MS susceptibility also suggests that there is a genetic aspect to MS. There is also a small, but definite, increase in MS risk among close relatives of index patients. In approximately 10% to 15% of patients with MS, another family member also has MS. Overall, the risk of MS in relatives of an index patient is approximately 0.5% for offspring, 0.6% for parents, 1.2% for siblings, 2% to 4% for dizygotic twins, and 25% to 27% for monozygotic twins (Ebers, 1994a; Mumford et al., 1994).

These studies indicate the importance of genetics in MS susceptibility; however, because concordance in monozygotic twins is considerably less than 100%, environmental factors remain important. Phillips (1993), using a mathematical model, concluded that genetic susceptibility is attributable to 10 to 15 interacting genes.

Pathology

The characteristic MS pathologic lesions are small areas of perivenular demyelination and large plaques of confluent demyelination with relative axon sparing (Allen, 1991; Allen and Kirk, 1992; Prineas, 1990; Raine, 1994). The perivenular demyelination resembles that present in ADEM. The demyelination coalesces to form the typical macroscopic MS plaques. These well-demarcated plaques may be located in any area of the CNS but have a predilection for white matter in the periventricular zones, centrum semiovale, optic nerves, and spinal cord. Axonal damage and lesion heterogeneity can also be present.

Microscopically, these acute plaques have intense cellular infiltrates with lymphocytes, plasma cells, reactive astrocytes, microglia, and macrophages present. Older plaques appear quiescent, with severe loss of myelin and myelin-producing oligodendroglial cells. Established plaques are sclerotic, with reactive astrocytosis. Plaques of varying activity occur in every case. Remyelination occurs, but these areas are particularly susceptible to recurrent demyelination. Electron microscopy depicts demyelination at the margins of active MS plaques; destruction and engulfment of the myelin sheaths occurs outward to inward.

Clinical Features

Children and adolescents with MS have a variety of symptoms and signs and may have a relapsing-remitting or a primary progressive course. In the more common relapsing-remitting group, symptoms appear over several days, may last for weeks, and then gradually resolve. In the primary-progressive course, symptoms constantly progress over years (Pinhas-Hamiel et al., 1998; Simone et al., 2000).

Initially, MS is difficult to distinguish from ADEM. Ultimately, approximately 25% of children with ADEM develop MS (Rust, 2000). The most common initial manifestation of MS is a sensory disturbance (26%). Other features include ON (17%), other visual disturbances (e.g., diplopia or blurred vision; 17%), pure motor disturbance (11%), abnormal gait (8%), cerebellar ataxia or combined sensorimotor disturbances (5%), myelitis (3%), vestibular abnormalities (2%), and sphincter disturbances (1%) (Duquette et al., 1987; Ghezzi et al., 1997; Ruggieri et al., 1999).

In a comparison of children with ADEM with those with MS, patients with ADEM were more likely to have a predemyelinating infectious disease, polysymptomatic presentation, pyramidal signs, encephalopathy, and bilateral ON. Seizures occurred only in the ADEM group, and unilateral ON occurred only in the studied MS group (Dale et al., 2000)

Diagnosis

The main diagnostic criteria of MS consist of two or more flares and clinical evidence of two or more neurologic lesions (McDonald et al., 2001). The diagnosis requires temporal and spatial dissemination of lesions, exclusion of other illness, and a clinical course typical of MS (i.e., relapsing-remitting, primary progressive, secondary progressive, or progressive-relapsing). Laboratory tests, such as brain imaging and CSF analysis, assist in ascertaining a diagnosis.

Rudick and colleagues (1986) studied patients misdiagnosed with MS and suggested some findings that cast doubt on an MS diagnosis: (1) absence of eye findings (optic nerve or oculomotor), (2) absence of clinical remissions, (3) localized disease, (4) absence of sensory or bladder abnormalities, and (5) absence of CSF abnormalities.

The differential diagnoses of MS include focal conditions, multifocal diseases, and systemic degenerative diseases. Focal conditions to be excluded are tumors of the optic nerve, hypothalamus, or sella turcica; Arnold-Chiari malformation, brainstem glioma; spinal cord tumors; vascular malformations; syrinx; and arachnoiditis. Multifocal diseases to be excluded are SLE, sarcoidosis, Behçet's syndrome, Lyme disease, moyamoya disease, granulomatous angiitis, and central-type neurofibromatosis. Degenerative diseases to be excluded are metabolic ataxias, spinocerebellar degeneration, late-onset leukodystrophies, mitochondrial cytopathies, and beriberi. Vitamin B_{12} deficiency, an important condition to exclude in adult MS, is rare in children.

Ancillary evaluations for MS entail (1) neuroimaging, particularly MRI, (2) CSF testing, and (3) evoked-potential studies. In children with MS, the lymphocyte count of the CSF is usually 50 to 100 cells/mm³, higher than that present in adults (Hanefeld et al., 1993; Rust et al., 1988; Whitaker et al., 1990). CSF myelin basic protein levels are elevated in 70% to 90% of acute MS exacerbations, but this is a nonspecific abnormality (Cohen et al., 1980). CSF Ig abnormalities (i.e., with respect to the IgG index, IgG synthetic rate, light-chain levels, and oligoclonal bands) are present in 85% to 90% of children with clinically definite MS (Boutin et al., 1988; Hanefeld et al., 1993) and in 25% to 30% of patients with possible or suspected MS (Francis et al., 1991).

Treatment

In the United States, there are four Food and Drug Administration–approved drugs for the treatment of MS. These include two forms of recombinant human interferon (interferon β-1a, Avonex; interferon β-1b [Betaseron]), a synthetic co-polymer (glatiramer acetate, Copaxone), and a chemotherapeutic agent (mitoxantrone, Novantrone).

The mechanisms of benefit of type 1 interferons in MS are unknown, but they may be related to the production of cytokines, which down-regulate inflammatory responses, inhibit cellular traffic across the blood-brain barrier, direct actions on glial cells, or inhibit viruses residing in the CNS. Interferon β-1a has been shown to have a positive effect on the time of the first neurologic event to the time of conversion to clinically definite MS. It may also decrease disease progression in patients with relapsing-remitting MS (Comi et al., 2001; PRISMS Study Group, 2001).

Glatiramer acetate is a co-polymer of four amino acids, combined approximately in proportion to the number of these constituents in the encephalogenic determinants of myelin basic protein. Glatiramer may function as a decoy molecule for antigen-presenting cells or may decrease the activity of myelin-specific T cells. Use of this agent reduces the relapse rate and plaque burden observed on MR images (Johnson et al., 2000).

Supportive measures include antispasticity medications, urologic management, control of pain, and psychological support (Matthews, 1991). In severe cases in which rapid deterioration is occurring, the use of cyclophosphamide, cyclosporine, methotrexate, azathioprine, and IVIG may be helpful, but benefit is uncertain (Ebers, 1994b).

Prognosis

An early age of onset of MS has not been associated with worse disease (Liguori et al., 2000). The "5-year rule" (Kurtzke et al., 1985) states that the degree of disability after 5 years correlates well with the degree of disability at 10 and 15 years. Because most pediatric patients have few fixed defects after 5 years, the prognosis is relatively good. In patients with T2-weighted lesions on head MRI at their initial presentations, the presence of new T2 lesions at a follow-up examination altered the risk of MS within 1 year (55% vs. 5%; Brex et al., 2001)

ACUTE CEREBELLAR ATAXIA

Clinical Features

Batten first described acute cerebellar ataxia (ACA) in 1907. ACA is most often recognized as a sudden disturbance of gait and balance. Gait ataxia of gait is the most prominent sign of ACA, but appendicular ataxia and nystagmus also occur. The ataxia appears anywhere from immediately after the illness to 6 weeks after the illness.

ACA usually develops days to weeks after a viral illness, particularly chickenpox. In the largest series (Connolly et al., 1994), 26% of patients had chickenpox, 3% had Epstein-Barr virus infection, 49% had other viral illnesses, 19% had no prodrome, and 3% developed ACA after immunizations. Other preceding infections include measles, mumps, herpes simplex virus, coxsackievirus, echovirus, poliovirus, *Mycoplasma pneumoniae*, and *Legionella pneumophila* (Aicardi, 1992; Kuban et al., 1983).

ACA usually occurs in children between 2 and 5 years of age and is rare in adolescents and adults. Epstein-Barr virus infection and immunizations are the most common causes in these older patients (Connolly et al., 1994). Some ataxia is seen in all children who have ACA, and 20% to 50% of patients are unable to walk. Finger dysmetria is seen in two thirds of these children but is strikingly mild compared with the gait ataxia (Connolly et al., 1994). Nystagmus was present in less than 20% of the patients studied by Connolly (1994), whereas 45% of the patients studied by Weiss and Carter (1959) had nystagmus. Transient behavioral alterations and school difficulties are seen in at least one third of children with ACA.

Laboratory studies reveal mild CSF pleocytosis. Neuroimaging studies typically yield normal results, but, occasionally, abnormal signals can be seen in the cerebellum.

Given the variety of antecedents, it is likely that a common immunoinflammatory process mediates ACA. In this respect, a recent report has identified antineuronal antibodies in ACA after Epstein-Barr virus infection (Ito et al., 1994). CSF pleocytosis occurs in 25% to 50% of children, almost always with a lymphocytic predominance (Connolly et al., 1994; Weiss and Carter, 1959). The CSF IgG index is elevated in 50% of these children, and oligoclonal bands are present in 10% to 17%.

Treatment and Prognosis

Ninety percent of children will completely recover from the ataxia, typically within the first few months after the onset of the disease. However, supportive therapy is needed. One fifth of children experience transient behavioral or intellectual problems (see the extensive review by Connolly et al., 1994). In rare patients without complete recovery, atrophy of the cerebellar hemispheres or other conditions such as cerebellar tumor, opsoclonus-myoclonus ataxia (OMA), or intoxication should be expected.

OPSOCLONUS-MYOCLONUS ATAXIA

Historical Aspects

Opsoclonus-myoclonus (OMA) is a rare syndrome that has generated great interest because of its association with neuroblastoma. It consists of opsoclonus (or "dancing eyes"), myoclonus, and ataxia and occurs in infants, with sudden onset. It appears in the literature with the names *myoclonic encephalopathy of infancy, Kinsbourne syndrome, infantile polymyoclonia,* and "dancing eyes" syndrome. The initial report of six patients (Kinsbourne, 1962) has been supplemented by more than 100 additional case reports (Lott and Kinsbourne, 1986), some with long-term follow-up.

Pathogenesis

The syndrome may be idiopathic, viral, or neuroblastoma-related. Idiopathic OMA and neuroblastoma-related OMA may be distinct entities or may represent immunologic reactions of varying effectiveness against neuroblastoma formation. In the published literature, the incidence of neuroblastoma associated with OMA is approximately 50%; however, because of a selection bias in favor of reporting cases associated with neuroblastoma, the true incidence of associated neuroblastoma is probably much lower (Lott and Kinsbourne, 1986).

Patients with OMA generate an immune response against a variety of brain antigens (Connolly et al., 1997; Pranzatelli, 1992). It is probable that neuroblastoma (or viral antigens) and the cerebellum are joint targets of an immunologic attack. Some adults with paraneoplastic OMA develop antibodies to the RNA-binding protein *Nova-1* (Jensen et al., 2000). To date, this antibody has not been found in the childhood version of OMA. Other as-yet-unidentified antibrain antibodies can be seen in childhood cases of OMA (Antunes et al., 2000). In one large series, most patients with childhood OMA that was associated with neuroblastoma exhibited diffuse and extensive lymphocytic infiltration with lymphoid follicles in their primary tumors, supporting an immune-mediated mechanism for this syndrome (Cooper et al., 2001).

Clinical Features

Onset usually occurs between the ages of 6 and 18 months but can occur up to 36 months of age. The onset of myoclonus is acute, often occurring after a nonspecific respiratory or gastrointestinal illness, and reaches maximal intensity in 2 to 7 days. The myoclonic movements are intense and brief with continual shock-like muscular contractions, irregularly timed and of variable amplitude. They are widely distributed across muscle groups, asymmetric, increased by startle, present at rest, and abolished only by deep sleep. Rarely, choreoathetosis may also be seen.

Abnormal eye movements (opsoclonus) temporally unrelated to the myoclonus consist of rapid (up to 8 displacements or rotations/second), irregular, conjugate ocular movements, mainly horizontal, but also vertical and diagonal. The eye movements are exacerbated by the same stimuli as the myoclonus, and some authors consider opsoclonus to be the ocular equivalent of myoclonus.

Patients may also experience cognitive and mood changes that persist past the myoclonic stage of illness.

Diagnosis

The diagnosis is a clinical one. Myoclonus should be distinguished from infantile spasms and myoclonic epilepsy. Opsoclonus should be distinguished from nystagmus or the rotatory eye movements of *Pelizaeus-Merzbacher* disease. The differential diagnoses of opsoclonus include posterior fossa tumor, ACA, encephalitis, and spasmus nutans.

When OMA is associated with a neuroblastoma, neurologic symptoms may occur months before a tumor if found. Fifty percent of reported tumors are localized to the thorax. Imaging studies of the chest have the highest diagnostic yield, followed by abdominal studies. Urinary catecholamines are rarely diagnostic. Electroencephalograms are normal. Anti-Hu antibodies were seen in 10 of 64 patients with neuroblastoma but were not specific for the development of OMA (Antunes et al., 2000).

Treatment

Success of treatment ranges from complete recovery in 3 months to persistence over several years, with the latter course more frequently noted. Incomplete recovery may be followed by relapse related to an infection or the discontinuation of effective therapy. Most patients exhibit a remarkable response to adrenocorticotropic hormone (ACTH) or corticosteroid therapy, but it is not clear which treatment is more beneficial. Usually 20 to 40 U/day of ACTH or 5 to 20 mg of prednisolone are needed for therapeutic benefit, with the dose titrated downward to a level below which symptoms appear.

Prognosis

Approximately half of patients are left with sequelae such as mental retardation, dysarthria, learning disabilities, or attention-deficit/hyperactivity disorder. Patients with neuroblastoma have slightly less-serious sequelae. Neuroblastoma associated with myoclonic encephalopathy has a more favorable prognosis than neuroblastoma without the neurologic syndrome (Altman and Baehner, 1976).

ATAXIA-TELANGIECTASIA

Historical Aspects

Ataxia-telangiectasia (AT) is an autosomal-recessive immunodeficiency associated with prominent neurologic features, including cerebellar ataxia, choreoathetosis, and dystonia. It is also discussed in Chapters 18, 24, and 39. In 1926, Syllaba and Henner first described the association of ocular and cutaneous telangiectasias with chorea. In 1941, Madame Louis-Bar reported an association between progressive cerebellar ataxia and bilateral oculocutaneous telangiectasia. Boder and Sedgwick introduced the term *ataxia-telangiectasia* in 1958. These authors recognized the familial nature of AT and proposed an autosomal-recessive mode of inheritance.

Pathogenesis

The gene responsible for AT has been cloned (see Chapter 18). The gene, called *AT mutated*, is a kinase that may be involved in cell-cycle control, DNA repair, and the prevention of programmed cell death (Savitsky et al., 1995). In vitro, the cells derived from patients with AT have defective DNA repair capability when exposed to irradiation. Heterozygotes for the AT gene (present in approximately 1% of the general population) may be at increased risk for cancer, particularly female breast cancer (Janin et al., 1999).

The cerebellar and extrapyramidal systems of the brain are the most severely affected. Macroscopically, the cerebellum is usually grossly atrophic (Gatti et al., 1991), most prominently throughout the vermis. Microscopically, atrophy affects all layers of the cerebellar cortex. Other pathologic changes include cortical atrophy, diffuse gliosis, and degeneration of anterior horn cells (de Leon et al., 1976). The neuronal degeneration may be a result of both accumulated DNA damage and defects in neurogenesis (McKinnon, 2001).

Clinical Features

AT is a multisystem disease affecting both the nervous system and the immune system. Soon after beginning to walk, children can develop progressive ataxia and choreoathetotic movements of their extremities. There is typically a loss of deep-tendon reflexes, dysarthria, and oculomotor apraxia. The children often require constant use of a wheelchair during their second decade of life.

In addition to their neurologic symptoms, the children have prominent telangiectasias, most prominently seen in the bulbar conjunctiva or on the skin. The child with AT may have frequent sinus and pulmonary infections. Sera have decreased IgA and IgE levels and elevated α-fetoprotein levels. In addition, impaired T-cell function and atrophy of the thymus gland are seen.

Care should be taken to minimize x-rays in these patients, because their cells are hypersensitive to ionizing radiation. Neuroimaging reveals atrophy of the cerebellar hemispheres and vermis, but white matter abnormalities mimicking leukodystrophy or primary demyelinating disease have been described (Ciemins and Horwitz, 2000).

These patients have a nearly 100-fold increased risk for malignancy and should be carefully monitored for their presence (see Chapter 39). Heterozygotes for the AT gene have nearly a sevenfold risk of increased malignancies (Swift et al., 1987).

Diagnosis

A diagnosis is made primarily on the basis of the history and the physical examination. Other than their neurologic symptoms, these children will also have prominent telangiectasias that can be most easily seen in the conjunctiva and skin. α-Fetoprotein levels are highly elevated, but difficult to interpret, in patients younger than age 2 years. The diagnosis is often difficult to make before the age of 5 years, and many children will experience symptoms for several years before a definitive diagnosis is made (Cabana et al., 1998).

Treatment and Prognosis

The treatment is supportive. Infections can be treated with antibiotics and IVIG. Care should be taken to avoid radiography, because their cells are hypersensitive to ionizing radiation. As noted the patients should be carefully monitored for malignancies. Live-virus vaccines should not be used (Pohl et al., 1992). Genetic counseling should be provided for the families of patients with this autosomal recessive disorder.

Prognosis is poor, with relentless progression. Children lose the ability to walk independently in their second decade of life. Death may occur in adolescence or early adulthood because of malignancy or pulmonary infection.

SYDENHAM'S CHOREA

Historical Aspects

Sydenham's chorea (SC; St. Vitus' dance) was first described by Sydenham in 1684 (Swann, 1753). A century later, it was recognized as the major neurologic manifestation of rheumatic fever. St. Vitus was originally designated the protector of the faithful from the dancing manias of the Middle Ages. St. Vitus later lost his protector status when his name became synonymous with the chorea of acute rheumatic disease.

Pathogenesis

Rheumatic fever, an inflammatory disease that affects the heart, joints, CNS, and subcutaneous tissue, typically follows group A β-hemolytic streptococcal (GABHS) pharyngitis (see Chapter 35).

SC presumably results from an immune response to streptococcal antigens. Serum Igs from patients with SC bind to caudate and subthalamus brain tissue in direct proportion to the clinical severity of the chorea (Bronze and Dale, 1993; Husby et al., 1976; Swedo, 1994). Antineuronal antibodies may be associated with other childhood movement disorders, such as Tourette's syndrome and motor or vocal tics (Kiessling et al., 1993).

Limited autopsy studies have disclosed mild neuronal injury and perivascular inflammatory infiltrates. The pathologic course of SC involves the caudate and subthalamic nuclei, cerebral cortex, trigeminal nerve, geniculate ganglion, and medullary hypoglossal nucleus. With neurologic symptoms there is arteritis of small meningeal and cortical vessels, embolism, and, rarely, meningoencephalitis with perivascular and diffuse round cell infiltration of the gray and white matter.

Clinical Features

The onset of SC is usually subtle, beginning with clumsiness, restlessness, fidgeting, and fatigue. The chorea is characterized by quick, uncoordinated motions (often occurring unilaterally), whereas the athetosis is writhing in nature. Speech is dysarthric. Emotional lability may be prominent. Psychological manifestations include emotional lability, nightmares, poor attention span, and obsessive-compulsive symptoms (Swedo, 1994).

Onset occurs between 5 and 15 years of age, and the sex ratio is approximately 50:50 until puberty, when females become affected twice as often as males. There may be a positive family history for rheumatic fever. The chorea can lag behind the etiologic streptococcal infection by 1 to 6 months, so antistreptococcal titers may be negative (Ayoub and Wannamaker, 1966). A physical examination discloses hypotonia and spooning of the hands.

The clinical course worsens for several weeks and then gradually improves over several months. The symptoms are often short lived, but can be quite debilitating. Relentless deterioration should suggest an alternative diagnosis (e.g., SLE, Wilson's disease, and Tourette's syndrome). Commonly prescribed drugs—such as phenytoin, female sex hormones (or pregnancy) and thyroid hormones (which sensitize postsynaptic striatal dopamine receptors), decongestants (sympathomimetic or anticholinergic), and d-amphetamine—may induce chorea at low doses in patients with a history of SC.

Diagnosis

A diagnosis is made on the basis of the acute onset of symptoms (chorea) with a history of a recent streptococcal infection. Antistreptolysin O (ASO) titers may be elevated but are not specific to SC. Recently, MRI studies have shown an increase in T2 signal intensity in the basal ganglia after symptoms appear (Kienzle et al., 1991). These signal abnormalities occur contralateral to the affected extremities in children with hemichorea and gradually resolve after the movements cease. The mechanism for the increased signal may be either a breakdown of the blood-brain barrier (as in an arteritis) or, alternatively, an area of local inflammation.

Treatment and Prognosis

Treatment for SC has included bed rest, diazepam, haloperidol, carbamazepine, valproate, baclofen, and steroids, but their efficacy has not been well established.

Many of these medications may be more useful in attenuating the chorea; they are less successful in dealing with the psychological symptoms.

Because of the high incidence of associated rheumatic heart disease, penicillin or other antibiotic prophylaxis is indicated until at least adulthood and during childbearing years.

The natural history of SC is that one quarter to one third of patients who have chorea but no other signs of rheumatic fever will eventually develop rheumatic heart disease. If other manifestations of rheumatic fever occur at any time, the risk of heart disease is greatly increased (Aron et al., 1965). The course of the disease is *subacute*. Often, chorea and associated findings disappear by 1 month and invariably are gone by 2 years after onset. Approximately 20% of patients develop a second episode of chorea, usually within 2 years of the first attack (Nausieda et al., 1983).

Uncomplicated SC is usually a benign, self-limited disorder of the CNS, but minimal neurologic sequelae may remain. Mild motor abnormalities, such as choreiform movements, hypotonia, intention tremor, and impaired fine and gross motor abilities, have been found 20 years after the initial episode (Bird et al., 1976; Nausieda et al., 1983). Psychiatric symptoms are more frequent in patients evaluated two or three decades after the onset of SC (Freeman et al., 1965).

PEDIATRIC AUTOIMMUNE NEUROPSYCHIATRIC DISORDER

Pathogenesis

As early as 1929, it was noted that some children with obsessive-compulsive disorder (OCD) or tics, or both, had symptom exacerbations triggered by GABHS infection or other infections (Garvey et al., 1999; Singer, 1999). A proposed mechanism is that the GABHS infection triggers antibodies that cross-react with the basal ganglia of genetically susceptible hosts, leading to OCD or tics, or both (Garvey et al., 1998).

The proposed relationship between *pediatric autoimmune neuropsychiatric disorders associated with Streptococcus* (PANDAS) and GABHS is controversial. In one prospective study, OCD symptoms were seen in 16% of rheumatic fever patients with chorea, but in no patients without chorea (Asbahr et al., 1998). B-lymphocyte antigen D8/17 is expressed in nearly all patients with rheumatic fever. In PANDAS, 85% of the children also express this marker, as compared with 17% of healthy children (Murphy et al., 1997; Swedo et al., 1997). This latter association suggests a similar predisposition to poststreptococcal autoimmunity.

Singer and colleagues (1998) have reported antineuronal antibodies from patients with Tourette's syndrome to human putamen. These antigens were 83 kd, 67 kd, and 60 kd and are present in the synaptosomal fraction. The identities of the specific antigens are still unknown.

Clinical Features

In PANDAS the symptom onset is triggered by GABHS infection or pharyngitis. In addition to tics and OCD, many of the patients described in the literature have emotional lability, separation anxiety, nighttime fears and bedtime rituals, cognitive deficits, oppositional behaviors, and motoric hyperactivity (Swedo et al., 1998). Abrupt tic onset or an exacerbation of tics associated with a streptococcal infection (11%) or any infection (18%) is not uncommon in patients with tic disorders (Singer et al., 2000).

Treatment

One controlled study of penicillin prophylaxis reported that it failed to prevent either the exacerbation of symptoms or the frequency of infections (Garvey et al., 1999). An open-label trial of plasma exchange also failed to show benefit in a group of five patients with OCD without streptococcal exacerbations (Nicolson et al., 2000).

In contrast, either plasma exchange or IVIG benefits the symptoms of patients with severe infection-triggered exacerbations of OCD or tic disorders (Perlmutter et al., 1999). Because these studies have limited controls and draw from highly select populations, many authors suggest that treatment be given to patients only as part of controlled double-blind protocols (Singer, 1999).

THROMBOTIC THROMBOCYTOPENIC PURPURA/HEMOLYTIC-UREMIC SYNDROME

Historical Aspects and Pathogenesis

Thrombotic thrombocytopenic purpura (TTP) was first described by Moschcowitz in 1925 and is characterized by fever, hemolytic anemia, renal failure, and neurologic dysfunction. The pathologic features consist of thrombotic microangiopathy characterized by microvascular lesions with platelet aggregation. TTP/hemolytic-uremic syndrome (HUS) may occur spontaneously or may be secondary to inflammatory diseases (e.g., rheumatoid arthritis, polyarteritis nodosa, SLE, Sjögren's syndrome), lymphoma, endocarditis, and drugs and poisons (sulfa, iodine, contraceptives) (Remuzzi and Bertani, 1988).

Clinical Features

In children, TTP/HUS is often preceded by an infection, usually with diarrhea. The most common associated pathogens are *Escherichia coli* O157:H7 as well as *Shigella, Salmonella, Yersinia*, and *Campylobacter* (Shapiro, 2001).

Symptoms of TTP/HUS develop over 7 to 10 days. Purpura is one of the initial findings in more than 90%

of patients; fever is usually present early. Hemorrhages (retinal, choroidal, nasal, gingival, gastrointestinal, and genitourinary), pallor, abdominal pain, arthralgia, and pancreatitis may develop. Neurologic findings include fatigue, confusion, headache, and visual and language dysfunction. Because TTP/HUS primarily affects the microvasculature, major strokelike events are uncommon.

Laboratory findings include microangiopathic hemolytic anemia, thrombocytopenia, proteinuria, and microscopic hematuria. Pathologic findings include capillary and arteriolar thrombi.

Diagnosis

Diagnosis requires the presence of at least two major criteria (e.g., thrombocytopenia, microangiopathic anemia, and neurologic dysfunction) and two minor criteria (e.g., fever, renal dysfunction, and circulating thrombi) (Ridolfi and Bell, 1981). HUS may have these same findings and seems to be a continuum with TTP.

Treatment and Prognosis

Plasmapheresis is the standard of care. Other treatment modalities include the infusion of fresh-frozen plasma, antiplatelet therapy, corticosteroids, and splenectomy (Symonette and Garner, 2001). The prognosis for patients with TTP/HUS is guarded. A successful outcome is associated with early diagnosis and prompt treatment (Scully, 1994).

Survival has increased from 5% to 80% during the past few decades with the use of plasma infusion and plasma exchange (Symonette and Garner, 2001).

RASMUSSEN'S ENCEPHALITIS

Historical Aspects and Pathogenesis

Rasmussen's encephalitis (RE) is a rare progressive gray matter disease of children (Rasmussen et al., 1958; Vining et al., 1993) that manifests in the first decade of life and is characterized by intractable focal epilepsy (epilepsia partialis continua), progressive hemiparesis, cerebral atrophy, and dementia.

This pathology often consists of microglial nodules with perivascular cuffs of small lymphocytes and monocytes (Hart et al., 1998). Numerous viruses have been implicated in its pathogenesis, including CMV, herpes simplex, Epstein-Barr virus, and Russian spring-summer tick-borne encephalitis.

Of particular note, Rogers and associates (1994) attempted to raise antibodies to recombinant glutamate receptors (GluR) in rabbits and observed that some rabbits developed anorexia and seizures. Pathologic findings in the rabbits resembled those of RE in humans. Subsequent studies showed that only rabbits immunized with one of the five GluR subtypes (GluR3) were affected. These investigators then found anti-GluR3 antibodies in two of four patients with RE. Plasma exchange performed in one child with RE resulted in a decrease in GluR3 antibody titer, decreased seizure frequency, and improved neurologic function.

Antibodies to another synaptic protein, *munc-18*, have also been found in a patient with RE (Yang et al., 2000). Some patients with RE are found to have a second underlying pathosis such as tumor or tuberous sclerosis, in addition to the characteristic inflammatory changes (Hart et al., 1998).

Clinical Features

This syndrome typically affects children between 1 and 16 years of age. Often there is a viral prodrome before the start of the seizures. The seizures are progressive, often focal, and can eventually turn into epilepsia partialis continua. Progressive intellectual impairment and hemiparesis develop with time (Andermann and Hart, 2001; Topcu et al., 1999).

Diagnosis

A diagnosis is made on the basis of a history of progressive medically intractable focal seizures and progressive hemiparesis. Cortical and caudate atrophy is seen on MR images but may lag behind the clinical progression. The results of CSF studies can be abnormal, with mild pleocytosis and an increase in protein. Positive CSF viral study results for herpes or CMV are occasionally seen. Testing for anti-GluR3 antibodies has limited sensitivity, because not all patients with RE will have detectable antibodies to GluR3.

Treatment and Prognosis

Conventional therapy consists of anticonvulsant medication and resection of the involved tissue (Vining et al., 1993). The best outcomes occur with hemispherectomy of the affected side. Antiviral, IVIG, or corticosteroid therapies may be helpful (Hart et al., 1994; Leach et al., 1999); however, many patients have only temporary improvement. Left untreated, many cases eventually burn themselves out, but the patient is left with significant neurologic impairment (Andermann and Hart, 2001).

R E F E R E N C E S

AAN Taskforce. Research criteria for diagnosis of chronic inflammatory demyelinating polyneuropathy (CIDP). Report from an Ad Hoc Subcommittee of the American Academy of Neurology AIDS Task Force. Neurology 41:617–618, 1991.

Abd-Allah SA, Jansen PW, Ashwal S, Perkin RM. Intravenous immunoglobulin as therapy for pediatric Guillain-Barré syndrome. J Child Neurol 12:376–380, 1997.

Adour KK, Byl FM, Hilsinger RL Jr, Kahn ZM, Sheldon MI. The true nature of Bell's palsy: analysis of 1000 consecutive patients. Laryngoscope 88:787–801, 1978.

Aicardi J. Diseases of the Nervous System in Childhood. London, Mac Keith Press, 1992.

Allen IV. Pathology of multiple sclerosis. In Matthews WB, ed. McAlpine's multiple sclerosis, 2nd ed. Oxford, Churchill Livingstone, 1991, pp 341–378.

Allen IV, Kirk J. Demyelinating diseases. In Adams JH, Duchen LW, eds. Greenfield's neuropathology. New York, Oxford University Press, 1992, pp 447–620.

Altman AJ, Baehner RL. Favorable prognosis for survival in children with coincident opso-myoclonus and neuroblastoma. Cancer 37:846–852, 1976.

Amato AA, Barohn RJ. Idiopathic inflammatory myopathies. Neurol Clin 15:615–648, 1997.

Andermann F, Hart Y. Rasmussen syndrome. In Gilamn, S, ed. Medlink neurology. San Diego, Medlink Corporation. Available at www.medlink.com. 2001.

Antunes NL, Khakoo Y, Matthay KK, Seeger RC, Stram DO, Gerstner E, Abrey LE, Dalmau J. Antineuronal antibodies in patients with neuroblastoma and paraneoplastic opsoclonus-myoclonus. J Pediatr Hematol Oncol 22:315–320, 2000.

Aoki T, Drachman DB, Asher DM, Gibbs CJ Jr, Bahmanyar S, Wolinsky JS. Attempts to implicate viruses in myasthenia gravis. Neurology 35:185–192, 1985.

Apak RA, Kose G, Anlar B, Turanli G, Topaloglu H, Ozdirim E. Acute disseminated encephalomyelitis in childhood: a report of 10 cases. J Child Neurol 14:198–201, 1999.

Aron AM, Freeman JM, Carter S. The natural history of Sydenham's chorea. Am J Med 38:83–95, 1965.

Asbahr FR, Negrao AB, Gentil V, Zanetta DM, da Paz JA, Marques-Dias MJ, Kiss MH. Obsessive-compulsive and related symptoms in children and adolescents with rheumatic fever with and without chorea: a prospective 6-month study. Am J Psychiatry 155:1122–1124, 1998.

Austin JH. Recurrent polyneuropathies and their corticosteroids treatment; with five-year observations of a placebo-controlled case treated with corticotrophin, cortisone, and prednisone. Brian 81:157–192, 1958.

Ayoub EM, Wannamaker LW. Streptococcal antibody titers in Sydenham's chorea. Pediatrics 38:946–56, 1966.

Bady B, Chauplannaz G, Carrier H. Congenital Lambert-Eaton myasthenic syndrome. J Neurol Neurosurg Psychiatry 50:476–478, 1987.

Barlow CF. Neonatal myasthenia gravis. Am J Dis Child 135:209, 1981.

Barohn RJ, Kissel JT, Warmolts JR, Mendell JR. Chronic inflammatory demyelinating polyradiculoneuropathy. Clinical characteristics, course, and recommendations for diagnostic criteria. Arch Neurol 46:878–884, 1989.

Batten FE. A case of acute ataxia. Trans Clin Soc London 40:276–277, 1907.

Bauer CA, Coker NJ. Update on facial nerve disorders. Otolaryngol Clin North Am 29:445–454, 1996.

Bazzato G, Coli U, Landini S, Mezzina C, Ciman M. Myasthenia-like syndrome after D,L—but not L—carnitine. Lancet 1:1209, 1981.

Beck RW, Cleary PA, Anderson MM Jr, Keltner JL, Shults WT, Kaufman DI, Buckley EG, Corbett JJ, Kuppersmith MJ, Miller NR, Savino PJ, Guy JA, Trobe JD, McCrary JA, Smith CH, Chrousos GA, Thompson S, Katz BJ, Brodsky MC, Goodwin JA, Atwell CW. A randomized, controlled trial of corticosteroids in the treatment of acute optic neuritis. The Optic Neuritis Study Group. N Engl J Med 326:581–588, 1992.

Benzing G 3rd, Iannaccone ST, Bove KE, Keebler PJ, Shockley LL. Prolonged myasthenic syndrome after one week of muscle relaxants. Pediatr Neurol 6:190–196, 1990.

Berman M, Feldman S, Alter M, Zilber N, Kahana E. Acute transverse myelitis: incidence and etiologic considerations. Neurology 31:966–971, 1981.

Beydoun SR, Engel WK, Karofsky P, Swartz MU. Long-term plasmapheresis therapy is effective and safe in children with chronic relapsing dysimmune polyneuropathy. Rev Neurol (Paris) 146:123–127, 1990.

Bird MT, Palkes H, Prensky AL. A follow-up study of Sydenham's chorea. Neurology 26:601–606, 1976.

Boder E, Sedgwick RP. Ataxia-telangiectasia: a familial syndrome of progressive cerebellar ataxia, oculocutaneous telangiectasia and frequent pulmonary infection. Pediatrics 21:526–554, 1958.

Borit A, Altrocchi PH. Recurrent polyneuropathy and neurolymphomatosis. Arch Neurol 24:40–49, 1971.

Boutin B, Esquivel E, Mayer M, Chaumet S, Ponsot G, Arthuis M. Multiple sclerosis in children: report of clinical and paraclinical features of 19 cases. Neuropediatrics 19:118–123, 1988.

Bradshaw DY, Jones HR Jr. Guillain-Barré syndrome in children: clinical course, electrodiagnosis and prognosis. Muscle Nerve 15:500–506, 1992.

Brady KM, Brar AS, Lee AG, Coats DK, Paysse EA, Steinkuller PG. Optic neuritis in children: clinical features and visual outcome. J AAPOS 3:98–103, 1999.

Brex PA, Miszkiel KA, O'Riordan JI, Plant GT, Moseley IF, Thompson AJ, Miller DH. Assessing the risk of early multiple sclerosis in patients with clinically isolated syndromes: the role of follow up MRI. J Neurol Neurosurg Psychiatry 70:390–393, 2001.

Bril V, Ilse WK, Pearce R, Dhanani A, Sutton D, Kong K. Pilot trial of immunoglobulin versus plasma exchange in patients with Guillain-Barré syndrome. Neurology 46:100–103, 1996.

Bronze MS, Dale JB. Epitopes of streptococcal M proteins that evoke antibodies that cross-react with human brain. J Immunol 151:2820–828, 1993.

Bundey S, Doniach D, Soothill JF. Immunological studies in patients with juvenile-onset myasthenia gravis and in their relatives. Clin Exp Immunol 11:321–332, 1972.

Byrne TN, Waxman SG. Spinal cord compression: diagnosis and principles of management. Philadelphia, F. A. Davis, 1990, pp 229–231.

Cabana MD, Crawford, TO, Winkelstein JA, Christensen JA, Lederman HM. Consequences of the delayed diagnosis of ataxia-telangiectasia. Pediatrics 102:98–100, 1998.

Callen JP. Malignancy in polymyositis/dermatomyositis. Clin Dermatol 6:55–63, 1988.

Callen JP. Dermatomyositis. Lancet 355:53–57, 2000.

Campadelli-Fiume G, Mirandola P, Menotti L. Human herpesvirus 6: An emerging pathogen. Emerg Infect Dis 5:353–366, 1999.

Cannella B, Cross AH, Raine CS. Upregulation and coexpression of adhesion molecules correlate with relapsing autoimmune demyelination in the central nervous system. J Exp Med 172:1521–1524, 1990.

Carrieri PB, Marano E, Perretti A, Caruso G. The thymus and myasthenia gravis: immunological and neurophysiological aspects. Ann Med 31 Suppl 2:52–56, 1999.

Castleman B. The pathology of the thymus gland in myasthenia gravis. Ann NY Acad Sci 135:496–505, 1966.

Chalk CH, Dyck PJ, Conn DL. Vasculitic neuropathy. In Dyck PJ, ed. Peripheral neuropathy. 3rd ed. Philadelphia, Saunders, 1993, pp 1424–1435.

Charcot JM. Histologie de la sclrose en plaques. Gaz Hop (Paris) 41:554–566, 1868.

Ciafaloni E, Nikhar NK, Massey JM, Sanders DB. Retrospective analysis of the use of cyclosporine in myasthenia gravis. Neurology 55:448–450, 2000.

Ciemins JJ, Horowitz AL. Abnormal white matter signal in ataxia telangiectasia. AJNR Am J Neuroradiol 21:1483–485, 2000.

Cohen SR, Brooks BR, Herndon RM, McKhann GM. A diagnostic index of active demyelination: myelin basic protein in cerebrospinal fluid. Ann Neurol 8:25–31, 1980.

Comi G, Filippi M, Barkhof F, Durelli L, Edan G, Fernandez O, Hartung H, Seeldrayers P, Sorensen PS, Rovaris M, Martinelli V, Hommes OR, Early Treatment of Multiple Sclerosis Study Goup. Effect of early interferon treatment on conversion to definite multiple sclerosis: a randomised study. Lancet 357:1576–1582, 2001.

Connolly AM, Dodson WE, Prensky AL, Rust RS. Course and outcome of acute cerebellar ataxia. Ann Neurol 35:673–679, 1994.

Connolly AM, Pestronk A, Mehta S, Pranzatelli MR 3rd, Noetzel MJ. Serum autoantibodies in childhood opsoclonus-myoclonus syndrome: an analysis of antigenic targets in neural tissues. J Pediatr 130:878–884, 1997.

Connolly AM. Chronic inflammatory demyelinating polyneuropathy in childhood. Pediatr Neurol 24:177–182, 2001.

Cooper R, Khakoo Y, Matthay KK, Lukens JN, Seeger RC, Stram DO, Gerbing RB, Nakagawa A, Shimada H. Opsoclonus-myoclonus-ataxia syndrome in neuroblastoma: histopathologic features—a report from the Children's Cancer Group. Med Pediatr Oncol 36:623–629, 2001.

Dalakas MC, Engel WK. Chronic relapsing (dysimmune) polyneuropathy: pathogenesis and treatment. Ann Neurol 9 Suppl:134–145, 1981.

Dalakas MC. Polymyositis, dermatomyositis and inclusion-body myositis. N Engl J Med 325:1487–1498, 1991.

Dalakas MC, Illa I, Dambrosia JM, Soueidan SA, Stein DP, Otero C, Dinsmore ST, McCrosky S. A controlled trial of high-dose intravenous immune globulin infusions as treatment for dermatomyositis. N Engl J Med 329:1993–2000, 1993.

Dal Canto MC. Experimental models of virus-induced demyelination. In Cook SD, ed. Handbook of multiple sclerosis. New York, M. Dekker, 1990, pp 63–100.

Delanoe C, Sebire G, Landrieu P, Huault G, Metral S. Acute inflammatory demyelinating polyradiculopathy in children: clinical and electrodiagnostic studies. Ann Neurol 44:350–356, 1998.

Dale RC, de Sousa C, Chong WK, Cox TC, Harding B, Neville BG. Acute disseminated encephalomyelitis, multiphasic disseminated encephalomyelitis and multiple sclerosis in children. Brain 123:2407–422, 2000.

De Leon GA, Grover WD, Huff DS. Neuropathologic changes in ataxia-telangiectasia. Neurology 26:947–951, 1976.

Devic ME. Myelite subaigu complique de nevrite optique. Bull Medical (Paris) 8:1033, 1894.

Drachman DB. Myasthenia gravis. N Engl J Med 330:1797–1810, 1994.

Duquette P, Murray TJ, Pleines J, Ebers GC, Sadovnik D, Weldon P, Warren S, Paty DW, Upton A, Hader W, Nelson R, Auty A, Neufeld B, Meltzer C. Multiple sclerosis in childhood: clinical profile in 125 patients. J Pediatr 111:359–363, 1987.

Dyck PJ, Gutrecht JA, Bastron JA, Karnes WE, Dale AJ. Histologic and teased-fiber measurements of sural nerve in disorders of lower motor and primary sensory neurons. Mayo Clin Proc 43:81–123, 1968.

Dyck PJ, Lais AC, Ohta M, Bastron JA, Okazaki H, Groover RV. Chronic inflammatory polyradiculoneuropathy. Mayo Clin Proc 50:621–637, 1975.

Dyck PJ, Arnason BG. Chronic inflammatory demyelinating polyradiculoneuropathy. In: Dyck PJ, ed. Peripheral neuropathy. 2nd ed. Philadelphia. W.B. Saunders, 1984, pp 2101–2114.

Dyck PJ, Prineas J, Pollard J. Chronic inflammatory demyelinating polyradiculoneuropathy. In Dyck PJ, ed. Peripheral neuropathy, 3rd ed. Philadelphia. Saunders, 1993, pp 1498–1517.

Eaton LM, Lambert EH. Electromyography and electrical stimulation of nerves in diseases of the motor unit: observations on a myasthenic syndrome associated with malignant tumors. JAMA 163:1117–1124, 1957.

Ebers GC. Genetics and multiple sclerosis: an overview. Ann Neurol 36 Suppl:S12–S14, 1994.

Ebers GC. Treatment of multiple sclerosis. Lancet 343:275–279, 1994.

Emslie-Smith AM, Engel AG. Microvascular changes in early and advanced dermatomyositis: a quantitative study. Ann Neurol 27:343–356, 1990.

Engel AG. Myasthenia gravis and syndromes. In Rowland LP, DiMauro S, eds. Handbook of clinical neurology. New York, Elsevier, 1992, pp 391–455.

Engel AG. Acquired autoimmune myasthenia gravis. In Engel AG, Franzini-Armstrong C, eds. Myology. New York, McGraw-Hill, 1994a, pp 1769–1797.

Engel AG. Myasthenic syndromes. In Engel AG, Franzini-Armstrong C, eds. Myology. New York, McGraw-Hill, 1994b, pp 1798–1835.

Engel AG, Hohlfield R, Banker BQ. Inflammatory myopathies. In Engel AG, Franzini-Armstrong C, eds. Myology. New York, McGraw-Hill, 1994c, pp 1335–1383, 1994c.

England JD. Guillain-Barré syndrome. Annu Rev Med 41:1–6, 1990.

Epstein MA, Sladky JT. The role of plasmapheresis in childhood Guillain-Barré syndrome. Ann Neurol 28:65–69, 1990.

Evoli A, Batocchi AP, Bartoccioni E, Lino MM, Minisci C, Tonali P. Juvenile myasthenia gravis with prepubertal onset. Neuromuscul Disord 8:561–567, 1998.

Fambrough DM, Drachman DB, Satyamurti S. Neuromuscular junction in myasthenia gravis: decreased acetylcholine receptors. Science 182:293–295. 1973.

Fenichel GM. Clinical syndromes of myasthenia in infancy and childhood. Arch Neurol 35:97–103, 1978.

Fenichel GM. Neurological complications of immunization. Ann Neurol 12:119–128, 1982.

Fink ME. Treatment of the critically ill patient with myasthenia gravis. In Ropper AH. Neurological and Neurosurgical Intensive Care. New York, Raven Press, pp. 351–62, 1993.

Francis GS, Antel JP, Duquette P. Inflammatory demyelinating diseases of the central nervous system. In Bradley WG, Daroff RB, Fenichel GM, Marsden DC, eds. Neurology in clinical practice. Boston, Butterworth-Heinemann, 1991, pp. 1133–1166.

Freeman JM, Aron AM, Collard JE, MacKay MC. The emotional correlates of Sydenham's chorea. Pediatrics 35:42–48, 1965.

French Cooperative group on Plasma Exchange in Guillain-Barré Syndrome. Appropriate number of plasma exchanges in Guillain-Barré syndrome. Ann Neurol 41:298–306, 1997.

Furuta Y, Ohtani F, Mesuda Y, Fukuda S, Inuyama Y. Early diagnosis of zoster sine herpete and antiviral therapy for the treatment of facial palsy. Neurology 55:708–710, 2000.

Gabriel CM, Gregson NA, Hughes RA. Anti-PMP22 antibodies in patients with inflammatory neuropathy. J Neuroimmunol 104:139–146, 2000.

Garvey MA, Giedd J, Swedo SE. PANDAS: the search for environmental triggers of pediatric neuropsychiatric disorders. Lessons from rheumatic fever. J Child Neurol 13:413–423, 1998.

Garvey MA, Perlmutter SJ, Allen AJ, Hamburger S, Lougee L, Leonard HL, Witowski ME, Dubbert B, Swedo SE. A pilot study of penicillin prophylaxis for neuropsychiatric exacerbations triggered by streptococcal infections. Biol Psychiatry 45:1564–1571, 1999.

Gatti RA, Boder E, Vinters HV, Sparkes RS, Norman A, Lange K. Ataxia-telangiectasia: an interdisciplinary approach to pathogenesis. Medicine (Baltimore) 70:99–117, 1991.

Ghezzi A, Deplano V, Faroni J, Grasso MG, Liguori M, Marrosu G, Pozzilli C, Simone IL, Zaffaroni M. Multiple sclerosis in childhood: clinical features of 149 cases. Mult Scler 3:43–46, 1997.

Gieffers J, Pohl D, Treib J, Dittmann R, Stephan C, Klotz K, Hanefeld F, Solbach W, Haass A, Maass M. Presence of Chlamydia pneumoniae DNA in the cerebral spinal fluid is a common phenomenon in a variety of neurological diseases and not restricted to multiple sclerosis. Ann Neurol 49:585–589, 2001

Golnik KC, Pena R, Lee AG, Eggenberger ER. An ice test for the diagnosis of myasthenia gravis. Ophthalmology 106:1282–1286, 1999.

Good WV, Muci-Mendoza R, Berg BO, Frederick DR, Hoyt CS. Optic neuritis in children with poor recovery of vision. Aust N Z J Ophthalmol 20:319–323, 1992.

Greenfield JG. Acute disseminated encephalomyelitis and sequel to influenza. J Pathol Bacteriol 33:453–462, 1930.

Griffin JW, Li CY, Ho TW, Xue P, Macko C, Gao CY, Yang C, Tian M, Mishu B, Cornblath DR. Guillain-Barré syndrome in northern China. The spectrum of neuropathological changes in clinically defined cases. Brain 118:577–595, 1995.

Griffin JW, Li CY, Ho TW, Tian M, Gao CY, Xue P, Mishu B, Cornblath DR, Macko C, McKhann GM, Asbury AK. Pathology of the motor-sensory axonal Guillain-Barré syndrome. Ann Neurol 39:17–28, 1996.

Grogan PM, Gronseth GS. Practice parameter: Steroids, acyclovir, and surgery for Bell's palsy (an evidence-based review): report of the Quality Standards Subcommittee of the American Academy of Neurology. Neurology 56:830–836, 2001.

Gronseth GS, Barohn RJ. Practice parameter: thymectomy for autoimmune myasthenia gravis (an evidence-based review): report of the Quality Standards Subcommittee of the American Academy of Neurology. Neurology 55:7–15, 2000.

Guillain G, Barré JA, Strohl A. Sur un syndrome de radiculonévrite avec hyperalbuminose du liquide cephalo-rachidien sans reaction cellulaire: Remarques sur les caractères cliniques et graphiques des réflexes tendineux. Bull Soc Med Hop (Paris) 40:1462–1470, 1916.

Hanefeld FA, Christen HJ, Kruse B, Bauer HJ. Childhood and juvenile multiple sclerosis. In Bauer HJ, Hanefeld FA, eds. Multiple sclerosis: its impact from childhood to old age. Philadelphia, W. B. Saunders, 1993, pp 14–52.

Hanissian AS, Masi AT, Pitner SE, Cape CC, Medsger TA Jr. Polymyositis and dermatomyositis in children: an epidemiologic and clinical comparative analysis. J Rheumatol 9:390–394, 1982.

Hart YM, Cortez M, Andermann F, Hwang P, Fish DR, Dulac O, Silver K, Fejerman N, Cross H, Sherwin A, Caraballo R. Medical treatment of Rasmussen's syndrome (chronic encephalitis and epilepsy): effect of high-dose steroids or immunoglobulins in 19 patients. Neurology 44:1030–1036, 1994.

Hart YM, Andermann F, Robitaille Y, Laxer KD, Rasmussen T, Davis R. Double pathology in Rasmussen's syndrome: a window on the etiology? Neurology 50:731–735, 1998.

Haslam RHA. Multiple sclerosis: experience at the Hospital for Sick Children. Int Pediatr 2:163–167, 1987.

Ho TW, Mishu B, Li CY, Gao CY, Cornblath DR, Griffin JW, Asbury AK, Blaser MJ, McKhann GM. Guillain-Barré syndrome in northern China. Relationship to Campylobacter jejuni infection and anti-glycolipid antibodies. Brain 118:597–605, 1995.

Ho TW, Li CY, Cornblath DR, Asbury AK, Griffin JW, McKhann GM. Patterns of recovery in the Guillain-Barré syndromes. Neurology 48:695–700, 1997.

Hohlfeld R, Engel AG. Coculture with autologous myotubes of cytotoxic T cells isolated from muscle in inflammatory myopathies. Ann Neurol 29:498–507, 1991.

Howard JF Jr. Intravenous immunoglobulin for the treatment of acquired myasthenia gravis. Neurology 51:S30–S36, 1998.

Huber AM, Lang B, LeBlanc CM, Birdi N, Bolaria RK, Malleson P, MacNeil I, Momy JA, Avery G, Feldman BM. Medium- and long-term functional outcomes in a multicenter cohort of children with juvenile dermatomyositis. Arthritis Rheum 43:541–549, 2000.

Hudson CS, Rash JE, Tiedt TN, Albuquerque EX. Neostigmine-induced alterations at the mammalian neuromuscular junction. II. Ultrastructure. J Pharmacol Exp Ther 205:340–356, 1978.

Hughes RA, van der Meche FG. Corticosteroids for treating Guillain-Barré syndrome. Cochrane Database Syst Rev 2:CD001446, 2000.

Husby G, van der Rijn I, Zabriskie JB, Abdin ZH, Williams RC Jr. Antibodies reacting with cytoplasm of subthalamic and caudate nuclei neurons in chorea and acute rheumatic fever. J Exp Med 144:1094–1110, 1976.

Husain F, Ryan NJ, Hogan GR. Concurrence of limb-girdle muscular dystrophy and myasthenia gravis. Arch Neurol 46:101–102, 1989.

Ito H, Sayama S, Irie S, Kanazawa N, Saito T, Kowa H, Haga S, Ikeda K. Antineuronal antibodies in acute cerebellar ataxia following Epstein-Barr virus infection. Neurology 44:1506–1507, 1994.

Janin N, Andrieu N, Ossian K, Lauge A, Croquette MF, Griscelli C, Debre M, Bressac-de-Paillerets B, Aurias A, Stoppa-Lyonnet D. Breast cancer risk in ataxia telangiectasia (AT) heterozygotes: haplotype study in French AT families. Br J Cancer 80:1042–1045, 1999.

Jensen KB, Dredge BK, Stefani G, Zhong R, Buckanovich RJ, Okano HJ, Yang YY, Darnell RB. Nova-1 regulates neuron-specific alternative splicing and is essential for neuronal viability. Neuron 25:359–371, 2000.

Johnson RT. The virology of demyelinating diseases. Ann Neurol 36:S54–60, 1994.

Johnson KP, Brooks BR, Ford CC, Goodman A, Guarnaccia J, Lisak RP, Myers LW, Panitch HS, Pruitt A, Rose JW, Kachuck N, Wolinsky JS. Sustained clinical benefits of glatiramer acetate in relapsing multiple sclerosis patients observed for 6 years. Copolymer 1 Multiple Sclerosis Study Group. Mult Scler 6:255–266, 2000.

Jolly F. Ober myasthenia gravis pseudoparalytica. Berl Klin Wochenschr 32:1–7, 1895.

Kaufman DI, Trobe JD, Eggenberger DO, Whitaker JN. Practice parameter: The role of corticosteroids in the management of acute monosymptomatic optic neuritis. Neurology 54:2039–44, 2000.

Kesselring J, Miller DH, Robb SA, Kendall BE, Moseley IF, Kingsley D, du Boulay EP, McDonald WI. Acute disseminated encephalomyelitis. MRI findings and the distinction from multiple sclerosis. Brain 113:291–302, 1990.

Kienzle GD, Breger RK, Chun RW, Zupanc ML, Sackett JF. Sydenham chorea: MR manifestations in two cases. AJNR Am J Neuroradiol 12:73–76, 1991.

Kiessling LS, Marcotte AC, Culpepper L. Antineuronal antibodies in movement disorders. Pediatrics 92:39–43, 1993.

Kissel JT, Franklin GM. Treatment of myasthenia gravis: A call to arms. Neurology 55:3–4, 2000.

Knebusch M, Strassburg HM, Reiners K. Acute transverse myelitis in childhood: nine cases and review of the literature. Dev Med Child Neurol 40:631–639, 1998.

Koenig H, Rabinowitz SG, Day E, Miller V. Post-infectious encephalomyelitis after successful treatment of herpes simplex encephalitis with adenine arabinoside: ultrastructural observations. N Engl J Med 300:1089–1093, 1979.

Kokontis L, Gutmann L. Current treatment of neuromuscular disease. Arch Neurol 57:939–943, 2000.

Korinthenberg R, Monting JS. Natural history and treatment effects in Guillain-Barré syndrome: a multicentre study. Arch Dis Child 74:281–287, 1996.

Kriss A, Francis DA, Cuendet F, Halliday AM, Taylor DS, Wilson J, Keast-Butler J, Batchelor JR, McDonald WI. Recovery after optic neuritis in childhood. J Neurol Neurosurg Psychiatry 51:1253–1258, 1988.

Kuban KC, Ephros MA, Freeman RL, Laffell LB, Bresnan MJ. Syndrome of opsoclonus-myoclonus caused by Coxsackie B3 infection. Ann Neurol 13:69-71, 1983.

Kurtzke JF. Epidemiology of multiple sclerosis. In Vinken PJ, Bruyn GW, Klawans HL, eds. Handbook of clinical neurology, Vol. 47. New York, Elsevier Science Publishers, 1985, pp 259–287.

Kyle RA, Dyck PJ. Neuropathy associated with the monoclonal gammopathies. In Dyck PJ, ed. Peripheral neuropathy, 3rd ed. Philadelphia, W. B. Saunders, 1993, pp 1275–1287.

Lamont PJ, Johnston HM, Berdoukas VA. Plasmapheresis in children with Guillain-Barré syndrome. Neurology 41:1928–1931, 1991.

Landry O. Note sur la paralysic ascendante aigue. Gaz Hebd Med Chir 6:472–474, 1859.

Lang B, Johnston I, Leys K, Elrington G, Marqueze B, Leveque C, Martin-Moutot N, Seagar M, Hoshino T, Takahashi M, Sugimori M, Cherksey BD, Llinas R, Newson-Davis J. Antibody specificities in Lambert-Eaton myasthenic syndrome. Ann NY Acad Sci 681:382–393, 1993.

Laxer RM, Stein LD, Petty RE. Intravenous pulse methylprednisolone treatment of juvenile dermatomyositis. Arthritis Rheum 30:328–334, 1987.

Leach JP, Chadwick DW, Miles JB, Hart IK. Improvement in adult-onset Rasmussen's encephalitis with long-term immunomodulatory therapy. Neurology 10:738–742, 1999.

Liguori M, Marrosu MG, Pugliatti M, Giuliani F, DeRoberts F, Cocco E, Zimatore GB, Livrea P, Trojano M. Age at onset in multiple sclerosis. Neurol Sci 21:S825–S829, 2000.

Lindner A, Schalke B, Toyka KV. Outcome in juvenile-onset myasthenia gravis: a retrospective study with long-term follow-up of 79 patients. J Neurol 244:515–520, 1997.

Lindstrom J, Shelton D, Fujii Y. Myasthenia gravis. Adv Immunol 42:233–284, 1988.

Linington C, Brostoff SW. Peripheral nerve antigens. In Dyck PJ, ed. Peripheral neuropathy, 3rd ed. Philadelphia, W. B. Saunders, 1993, pp 404–417.

Link H, Cruz M, Gessain A, Gout O, De The G, Kam-Hansen S. Chronic progressive myelopathy associated with HTLV-I: oligoclonal IgG and anti-HTLV-I IgG antibodies in cerebrospinal fluid and serum. Neurology 39:1566–1572, 1989.

Linton DM, Philcox D. Myasthenia gravis. Dis Mon 36:593–637, 1990.

Lisak RP, Barchi RL, eds. Myasthenia gravis. Philadelphia, W. B. Saunders, 1982.

Lisak RP, Brown MJ. Acquired demyelinating polyneuropathies. Semin Neurol 7:40–48, 1987.

Liston SL, Kleid MS. Histopathology of Bell's palsy. Laryngoscope 99:23–26, 1989.

Lott I, Kinsbourne M. Myoclonic encephalopathy of infants. Adv Neurol 43:127–136, 1986.

Lotz BP, Engel AG, Nishisno H, Stevens JC, Litchy WJ. Inclusion body myositis. Observations in 40 patients. Brain 112:727–42, 1989.

Lucchinetti CF, Kiers L, O'Duffy A, Gomez MR, Cross S, Leavitt JA, O'Brien P, Rodriguez M. Risk factors for developing multiple sclerosis after childhood optic neuritis. Neurology 49:1413–1418, 1997.

Mackay MT, Kornberg AJ, Shield LK, Dennett X. Benign acute childhood myositis: laboratory and clinical features. Neurology 53:2127–2131. 1999.

Maimone D. Chronic inflammatory demyelinating polyneuropathy. In: Gilman S, editor. MedLink Neurology. San Diego, MedLink Corporation. Available at www.medlink.com. Accessed August 18, 2003.

Marks HG, Augustyn P, Allen RJ. Fisher's syndrome in children. Pediatrics 60:726–729, 1977.

Martino G, Grimaldi LM, Wollmann RL, Bongioanni P, Quintans J, Arnason BG. The hu-SCID myasthenic mouse. A new tool for the investigation of seronegative myasthenia gravis. Ann NY Acad Sci 681:303–305, 1993.

Mastaglia FL, Ojeda VJ. Inflammatory myopathies: Part 1. Ann Neurol 17:215–227, 1985a.

Mastaglia FL, Ojeda VJ. Inflammatory myopathies: Part 2. Ann Neurol 17:317–323, 1985b.

Masters CL, Dawkins RL, Zilko PJ, Simpson JA, Leedman RJ. Penicillamine-associated myasthenia gravis, antiacetylcholine receptor and antistriational antibodies. Am J Med 63:689–694, 1977.

Matthews WB, ed. McAlpine's multiple sclerosis, 2nd ed. Edinburgh, Churchill Livingstone, 1991.

May M, Klein SR. Differential diagnosis of facial nerve palsy. Otolaryngol Clin North Am 24:613–645, 1991.

McCarthy N, Andersson Y, Jormanainen V, Gustavsson O, Giesecke J. The risk of Guillain-Barré syndrome following infection with Campylobacter jejuni. Epidemiol Infect 122:15–17, 1999.

McDonald WI, Compston A, Edan G, Goodkin D, Hartung HP, Lublin FD, McFarland HF, Paty DW, Polman CH, Reingold SC, Sandberg-Wollheim M, Sibley W, Thompson A, van den Noort S, Weinshenker BY, Wolinsky JS. Recommended diagnostic criteria for multiple sclerosis: guidelines from the International Panel on the diagnosis of multiple sclerosis. Ann Neurol 50:121–127, 2001.

McKinnon PJ. Ataxia telangiectasia: new neurons and ATM. Trends Mol Med 7:233–234, 2001.

McLeod JG. Paraneoplastic neuropathies. In Dyck PJ, ed. Peripheral neuropathy, 3rd ed. Philadelphia, W. B. Saunders, 1993a, pp 1583–1590.

McLeod JG. Peripheral neuropathy associated with lymphomas, leukemias, and polycythemia vera. In Dyck PJ, ed. Peripheral neuropathy. Philadelphia, W. B. Saunders, 1993b, pp 1591–1598.

Melms A, Malcherek G, Schoepfer R, Sommer N, Kalbacher H, Lindstrom J. Acetylcholine receptor-specific T cells are present in the normal immune repertoire. A study with recombinant polypeptides of the human acetylocholine receptor alpha-subunit. Ann NY Acad Sci 681:310–312, 1993.

Mendell JR, Barohn RJ, Freimer ML, Kissel JT, King W, Nagaraja HN, Rice R, Campbell WW, Donofrio PD, Jackson CE, Lewis RA, Shy M, Simpson DM, Parry GJ, Rivner MH, Thornton CA, Bromberg MB, Tandan R, Harati Y, Giuliani MJ; Working Group on Peripheral Neuropathy. Randomized controlled trial of IVIG in untreated chronic inflammatory demyelinating polyradiculoneuropathy. Neurology 56:445–449, 2001.

Miller DH, McDonald WI, Blomhardt LD, du Boulay GH, Halliday AM, Johnson G, Kendall BE, Kingsley DP, MacManus DG, Moseley IF, Rudge P, Sandercock PA. Magnetic resonance imaging in isolated noncompressive spinal cord syndromes. Ann Neurol 22:714–723, 1987.

Miller G, Heckmatt JZ, Dubowitz V. Drug treatment of juvenile dermatomyositis. Arch Dis Child 58:445–450, 1983.

Miller HG, Stanton JB, Gibbons JL. Acute disseminated encephalomyelitis and related syndromes. Br Med J 1:668–671, 1957.

Mimori T. Scleroderma-polymyositis overlap syndrome. Clinical and serologic aspects. Int J Dermatol 26:419–425, 1987.

Mittag TW, Xu X, Moshoyiannis H, Kornfeld P, Genkins G. Analysis of false negative results in the immunoassay for anti-acetylcholine receptor antibodies in myasthenia gravis. Clin Immunol Immunopathol 31:191–201, 1984.

Morales DS, Siatkowski RM, Howard CW, Warman R. Optic neuritis in children. J Pediatr Ophthalmol Strabismus 37:254–259, 2000.

Morel E, Eymard B, Vernet-der Garabedian B, Pannier C, Dulac O, Bach JF. Neonatal myasthenia gravis: a new clinical and immunologic appraisal on 30 cases. Neurology 38:138–142, 1988.

Moschcowitz E. An acute febrile pleiochromic anemia with hyaline thrombosis of the terminal arterioles and capillaries. Arch Intern Med 36:89–95, 1925.

Mumford CJ, Wood NW, Kellar-Wood H, Thorpe JW, Miller DH, Compston DA. The British Isles survey of multiple sclerosis in twins. Neurology 44:11–15, 1994.

Murakami S, Mizobuchi M, Nakashiro Y, Doi T, Hato N, Yanagihara N. Bell palsy and herpes simplex virus: identification of viral DNA in endoneurial fluid and muscle. Ann Intern Med 124:27–30, 1996.

Murphy TK, Goodman WK, Fudge MW, Williams RC, Ayoub EM, Dalal M, Lewis MH, Zabriskie JB. B lymphocyte antigen D8/17: a peripheral marker for childhood-onset obsessive-compulsive disorder and Tourette's syndrome? Am J Psychiatry 154:402–407, 1997.

Murray JT. The history of multiple sclerosis. In: Burks JS, Johnson KP, eds. Multiple sclerosis: diagnosis, medical management and rehabilitation. New York, Demos, 2000, pp 1–32, 2000.

Nastuk WL, Plescia OJ, Osserman KE. Changes in serum complement activity in patients with myasthenia gravis. Proc Soc Exp Biol Med 105:177–184, 1960.

Nausieda PA, Bieliauskas LA, Bacon LD, Hagerty M, Koller WC, Glantz RN. Chronic dopaminergic sensitivity after Sydenham's chorea. Neurology 33:750–754, 1983.

Nevo Y, Pestronk A, Kornberg AJ, Connolly AM, Iqbal I, Shield LK. Childhood chronic inflammatory demyelinating neuropathies: clinical course and long-term follow-up. Neurology 47:98–102, 1996.

Newsom-Davis J. Lambert-Eaton myasthenic syndrome. Curr Treat Options Neurol 3:127–131, 2001.

Newton M, Cruickshank K, Miller D, Dalgleish A, Rudge P, Clayden S, Moseley I. Antibody to human T-lymphotropic virus type 1 in West-Indian-born UK residents with spastic paraparesis. Lancet 1:415–416, 1987.

Nicolson R, Swedo SE, Lenane M, Bedwell J, Wudarsky M, Gochman P, Hamburger SD, Rapoport JL. An open trial of plasma exchange in childhood-onset obsessive-compulsive disorder without poststreptococcal exacerbations. J Am Acad Child Adolesc Psychiatry 39:1313–1315, 2000.

Ohtake T, Komori T, Hirose K, Tanabe H. CNS involvement in Japanese patients with chronic inflammatory demyelinating polyradiculoneuropathy. Acta Neurol Scand 81:108–112, 1990.

O'Neill JH, Murray NM, Newsom-Davis J. The Lambert-Eaton myasthenic syndrome. A review of 50 cases. Brain 111:577–596, 1988.

Pachman LM, Hayford JR, Chung A, Daugherty CA, Pallansch MA, Fink CW, Gewanter HL, Jerath R, Lang BA, Sinacore J, Szer IS, Dyer AR, Hochberg MC. Juvenile dermatomyositis at diagnosis: clinical characteristics of 79 children. J Rheumatol 25:1198–1204, 1998.

Palace J, Newsom-Davis J, Lecky B. A randomized double-blind trial of prednisolone alone or with azathioprine in myasthenia gravis. Myasthenia Gravis Study Group. Neurology 50:1778–1783, 1998.

Parkin PJ, Hierons R, McDonald WI. Bilateral optic neuritis. A long-term follow-up. Brain 107:951–964, 1984.

Parry GJ. Guillain-Barré syndrome. New York, Thieme Verlag, 1993.

Pasternak JF, Hageman J, Adams MA, Philip AG, Gardner TH. Exchange transfusion in neonatal myasthenia. J Pediatr 99:644–646, 1981.

Patel SP, Friedman RS. Neuropsychiatric features of acute disseminated encephalomyelitis: a review. J Neuropsychiatry Clin Neurosci 9:534–540, 1997.

Perlmutter SJ, Leitman SF, Garvey MA, Hamburger S, Feldman E, Leonard HL, Swedo SE. Therapeutic plasma exchange and intravenous immunoglobulin for obsessive-compulsive disorder and tic disorders in childhood. Lancet 354:1153–1158, 1999.

Phillips JT. Genetic susceptibility models in multiple sclerosis. In Rosenberg RN, ed. The molecular and genetic basis of neurological disease. Boston, Butterworth-Heinemann, 1993, pp 41–46.

Pinhas-Hamiel O, Barak Y, Siev-Ner I, Achiron A. Juvenile multiple sclerosis: clinical features and prognostic characteristics. J Pediatr 132:735–737, 1998.

Pitkaranta A, Piiparinen H, Mannonen L, Vesaluoma M, Vaheri A. Detection of human herpesvirus 6 and varicella-zoster virus in tear fluid of patients with Bell's palsy by PCR. J Clin Microbiol 38:2753–2755, 2000.

Pohl KR, Farley JD, Jan JE, Junker AK. Ataxia-telangiectasia in a child with vaccine-associated paralytic poliomyelitis. J Pediatr 121:405–407, 1992.

Posner JB. Paraneoplastic syndromes. Neurol Clin 9:919–936, 1991.

Potain CE. Morve chronique de forme anormale. Bull Soc Hop Paris 12:314, 1875.

Pradhan S, Gupta RP, Shashank S, Pandey N. Intravenous immunoglobulin therapy in acute disseminated encephalomyelitis. J Neurol Sci 165:56–61, 1999.

Pranzatelli MR. The neurobiology of the opsoclonus-myoclonus syndrome. Clin Neuropharmacol 15:186–228, 1992.

Prineas JW, McLeod JG. Chronic relapsing polyneuritis. J Neurol Sci 27:427–458, 1976.

Prineas JW. Pathology of multiple sclerosis. In Cook SD, ed. Handbook of multiple sclerosis. New York, M. Dekker, 1990, pp 187–218.

PRISMS Study Group and the University of British Columbia MS/MRI Analysis Group. PRISMS-4: Long-term efficacy of interferon-beta-1a in relapsing MS. Neurology 56:1628–1636, 2001.

Purvin V, Hrisomalos N, Dunn D. Varicella optic neuritis. Neurology 38:501–503, 1988.

Raine CS. The Dale E. McFarlin Memorial Lecture: the immunology of the multiple sclerosis lesion. Ann Neurol 36:S61–S72, 1994.

Rasmussen T, Olszewski J, Lloyd-Smith D. Focal seizures due to chronic localized encephalitis. Neurology 8:435–445, 1958.

Remuzzi G, Bertani T. Thrombotic thrombocytopenic purpura, hemolytic uremic syndrome, and acute cortical necrosis. In Schrier RW, Gottschalk CW, eds. Diseases of the kidney, 4th ed. Boston, Little, Brown, 1988, pp 2301–2348.

Rhodes RH. Histopathologic features in the central nervous system of 400 acquired immunodeficiency syndrome cases: implications of rates of occurrence. Hum Pathol 24:1189–1198, 1993.

Richardson JB, Callen JP. Dermatomyositis and malignancy. Med Clin North Am 73:2111–120, 1989.

Rider LG, Okada S, Sherry DD, et al. Epidemiologic features and environmental exposures associated with illness onset in juvenile idiopathic inflammatory myopathy. Arthritis Rheum 38 (suppl):362, 1995.

Rider LG, Miller FW. Classification and treatment of the juvenile idiopathic inflammatory myopathies. Rheum Dis Clin North Am 23:619–655, 1997.

Ridolfi RL, Bell WR. Thrombotic thrombocytopenic purpura. Report of 25 cases and review of the literature. Medicine (Baltimore) 60:413–428, 1981.

Riikonen R, Donner M, Erkkila H. Optic neuritis in children and its relationship to multiple sclerosis: a clinical study of 21 children. Dev Med Child Neurol 30:349–359, 1988.

Riikonen R. The role of infection and vaccination in the genesis of optic neuritis and multiple sclerosis in children. Acta Neurol Scand 80:425–431, 1989.

Rivers TM, Sprunt DH, Berry G. Observations on attempts to produce disseminated encephalomyelitis in monkeys. J Exp Med 58:39–53, 1933.

Roddy SM, Ashwal S, Peckham N. Infantile myositis: a case diagnosis in neonatal period. Pediatr Neurol 2:241–244, 1986.

Rogers SW, Andrews PI, Gahring LC, Whisenand T, Cauley K, Crain B, Hughes TE, Heinemann SF, McNamara JO. Antibodies to glutamate receptor GluR3 in Rasmussen's encephalitis. Science 265:648–651, 1994.

Ropper AH, Poskanzer DC. The prognosis of acute and subacute transverse myelopathy based on early signs and symptoms. Ann Neurol 4:51–59, 1978.

Ropper AH, Kehne SM. Guillain-Barré syndrome: management of respiratory failure. Neurology 35:1662–1665, 1985.

Rostami AM. Pathogenesis of immune-mediated neuropathies. Pediatr Res 33:S90–S94, 1993.

Rousseau JJ, Lust C, Zangerle PF, Bigaignon G. Acute transverse myelitis as presenting neurological feature of Lyme disease. Lancet 2:1222–1223, 1986.

Rudick RA, Schiffer RB, Schwetz KM. Multiple sclerosis. The problem of incorrect diagnosis. Arch Neurol 43:578–583, 1986.

Ruggieri M, Polizzi A, Pavone L, Grimaldi LM. Multiple sclerosis in children under 6 years of age. Neurology 53:478–484, 1999.

Russel JW. Bell's Palsy. In Gilman S, editor. MedLink Neurology. San Diego: MedLink Corporation. Available at www.medlink.com. Accessed August 18, 2003.

Rust RS Jr, Dodson WE, Trotter JL. Cerebrospinal fluid IgG in childhood: the establishment of reference values. Ann Neurol 23:406–410, 1988.

Rust RS. Multiple sclerosis, acute disseminated encephalomyelitis, and related conditions. Semin Pediatr Neurol 7:66–90, 2000.

Ryan MM, Grattan-Smith PJ, Procopis PG, Morgan G, Ouvrier RA. Childhood chronic inflammatory demyelinating polyneuropathy: clinical course and long-term outcome. Neuromuscul Disord 10:398–406, 2000.

Sadovnick AD, Ebers GC. Epidemiology of multiple sclerosis: a critical review. Can J Neurol Sci 20:17–29, 1993.

Sansome A, Dubowitz V. Intravenous immunoglobulin in juvenile dermatomyositis—four year review of nine cases. Arch Dis Child 72:25–28, 1995.

Saperstein DS, Katz JS, Amato AA, Barohn RJ. Clinical spectrum of chronic acquired demyelinating polyneuropathies. Muscle Nerve 24:311–324, 2000.

Sarchielli P, Trequattrini A, Usai F, Murasecco D, Gallai V. Role of viruses in the etiopathogenesis of multiple sclerosis. Acta Neurol (Napoli) 15:363–381, 1993.

Savitsky K, Sfez S, Tagle DA, Ziv Y, Satiel A, Collins Fs Shiloh Y, Rotman G. The complete sequence of the coding region of the ATM gene reveals similarity to cell cycle regulators in different species. Hum Mol Genet 4:2025–2032, 1995.

Scott TF. Postinfectious and vaccinal encephalitis. Med Clin North Am 51:701–717, 1967.

Scully RE. Case records of the Massachusetts General Hospital. Case 33C1994. N Engl J Med 331:661–667, 1994.

Selcen D, Dabrowski ER, Michon AM, Nigro MA. High-dose intravenous immunoglobulin therapy in juvenile myasthenia gravis. Pediatr Neurol 22:40–43, 2000.

Seybold ME, Howard FM Jr, Duane DD, Payne WS, Harrison EG Jr. Thymectomy in juvenile myasthenia gravis. Arch Neurol 25:385–392, 1971.

Seybold ME, Lindstrom JM. Immunopathology of acetylcholine receptors in myasthenia gravis. Springer Semin Immunopathol 5:389–412, 1982.

Shah A, Lisak RP. Immunopharmacologic therapy in myasthenia gravis. Clin Neuropharmacol 16:97–103, 1993.

Shapiro W. Hemolytic-uremic syndrome. eMedicine Journal 2(6), 2001.

Shaw CM, Alvord EC Jr. Multiple sclerosis beginning in infancy. J Child Neurol 2:252–256, 1987.

Shevell M, Rosenblatt B, Silver K. Carpenter S, Karpati G. Congenital inflammatory myopathy. Neurology 40:1111–1114, 1990.

Silver RM, Maricq HR. Childhood dermatomyositis: serial microvascular studies. Pediatrics 83:278–283, 1989.

Simmons RD, Cattle BA. Sialyl ligands facilitate lymphocyte accumulation during inflammation of the central nervous system. J Neuroimmunol 41:123–130, 1992.

Simone IL, Carrara D, Tortorella C, Ceccarelli A, Livrea P. Early onset multiple sclerosis. Neurol Sci 21:S861–S863, 2000.

Simpson JA. Myasthenia gravis: a new hypothesis. Scott Med J 5:419–436, 1960.

Singer HS, Giuliano JD, Hansen BH, Hallett JJ, Laurino JP, Benson M, Kiessling LS. Antibodies against human putamen in children with Tourette syndrome. Neurology 50:1618–1624, 1998.

Singer HS. PANDAS and immunomodulatory therapy. Lancet 354:1157–1158, 1999.

Singer HS, Giuliano JD, Zimmerman AM, Walkup JT. Infection: a stimulus for tic disorders. Pediatr Neurol 22:380–383, 2000.

Smith CI, Aarli JA, Biberfeld P, Bolme P, Christensson B, Gahrton G, Hammarstrom L, Lefvert AK, Lonnqvist B, Matell G, Pirskanen R, Ringden OI, Svanborg E. Myasthenia gravis after bone-marrow transplantation. Evidence for a donor origin. N Engl J Med 309:1565–1568, 1983.

Smith BE, Windebank AJ, Dyck PJ. Nonmalignant inflammatory sensory polyganglionopathy. In Dyck PJ, ed. Peripheral neuropathy, 3rd ed. Philadelphia, WB Saunders, 1993, pp 1525–1531.

Stratton KR, Howe CJ, Johnston RB Jr. Adverse events associated with childhood vaccines other than pertussis and rubella. Summary of a report from the Institute of Medicine. JAMA 271:1602–1605, 1994.

Strauss AJ, Seegal BC, Hsu KC, Burkholder PM, Nastuk WL, Osserman KE. Immunofluorescence demonstration of a muscle-binding complement-fixing serum globulin fraction in myasthenia gravis. Proc Soc Exp Biol Med 105:184–191, 1960.

Stricker RB, Miller RG, Kiprov DD. Role of plasmapheresis in acute disseminated (postinfectious) encephalomyelitis. J Clin Apheresis 7:173–179, 1992.

Swann J. The entire works of Dr. Thomas Sydenham. London, E. Cave, 1753.

Swedo SE. Sydenham's chorea. A model for childhood autoimmune neuropsychiatric disorders. JAMA 272:1788–1791, 1994.

Swedo SE, Leonard HL, Mittleman BB, Allen AJ, Rapoport JL, Dow SP, Kanter ME, Chapman F, Zabriskie J. Identification of children with pediatric autoimmune neuropsychiatric disorders associated with streptococcal infections by a marker associated with rheumatic fever. Am J Psychiatry 154:110–112, 1997.

Swedo SE, Leonard HL, Garvey M, Mittleman B, Allen AJ, Perlmutter S, Lougee L, Dow S, Zamkoff J, Dubbert BK. Pediatric autoimmune neuropsychiatric disorders associated with streptococcal infections: clinical description of the first 50 cases. Am J Psychiatry 155:264–271, 1998.

Swift TR. Disorders of neuromuscular transmission other than myasthenia gravis. Muscle Nerve 4:334–353, 1981.

Symmons DP, Sills JA, Davis SM. The incidence of juvenile dermatomyositis: results from a nation-wide study. Br J Rheumatol 34:732–736, 1995.

Symonette D, Garner LM. Thrombocytopenic purpura. eMedicine Journal 2(5), 2001.

Tachi N, Watanabe T, Wakai S, Sato T, Chiba S. Acute disseminated encephalomyelitis following HTLV-I associated myelopathy. J Neurol Sci 110:234–235, 1992.

Takamori M, Komai K, Iwasa K. Antibodies to calcium channel and synaptotagmin in Lambert-Eaton myasthenic syndrome. Am J Med Sci 319:204–208, 2000.

Thomas PK, Walker RW, Rudge P, Morgan-Hughes JA, King RH, Jacobs JM, Mills KR, Ormerod IE, Murray NM, McDonald WI. Chronic demyelinating peripheral neuropathy associated with multifocal central nervous system demyelination. Brain 110:53–76, 1987.

Thompson CE. Infantile myositis. Dev Med Child Neurol 24:307–313, 1982.

Topi GC, D'Alessandro L, Catricala C, Zardi O. Dermatomyositis-like syndrome due to *Toxoplasma*. Br J Dermatol 101:589–591, 1979.

Topcu M, Turanli G, Aynaci FM, Yalnizoglu D, Saatci I, Yigit A, Genc D, Soylemezoglu F, Bertan V, Akalin N. Rasmussen encephalitis in childhood. Childs Nerv Syst 15:395–402, 1999.

Turnbull HM, McIntosh J. Encephalomyelitis following vaccination. Br J Exp Pathol 7:181–222, 1926.

Tyler KL, Gross RA, Cascino GD. Unusual viral causes of transverse myelitis: hepatitis A virus and cytomegalovirus. Neurology 36:855–858, 1986.

Tymms KE, Webb J. Dermatopolymyositis and other connective tissue diseases: a review of 105 cases. J Rheumatol 12:1140–1148, 1985.

Uncini A, Parano E, Lange DJ, De Vivo DC, Lovelace RE. Chronic inflammatory demyelinationg polyneuropathy in childhood: clinical and electrophysiological features. Childs Nerv Sys 7:191–196, 1991.

Valk J, van der Knapp MS. Magnetic resonance of myelin, myelination, and myelin disorders. Berlin, Springer-Verlag, 1989, pp 206–214.

Van der Meche FG, Schmitz PI. A randomized trial comparing intravenous immune globulin and plasma exchange in Guillain-Barré syndrome. Dutch Guillain-Barré Study Group. N Engl J Med. 326:1123–1129, 1992.

Van Doorn PA, Rossi F, Brand A, van Lint M, Vermeulen M, Kazatchkine MD. On the mechanism of high-dose intravenous immunoglobulin treatment of patients with chronic inflammatory demyelinating polyneuropathy. J Neuroimmunol 29:57–64, 1990.

Vining EP, Freeman JM, Brandt J, Carson BS, Uematsu S. Progressive unilateral encephalopathy of childhood (Rasmussen's syndrome): a reappraisal. Epilepsia 34:639–650, 1993.

Wagner E. Fall einer seltnen Muskelkrankheit. Arch Heilk 4:282–283, 1863.

Waksman BH, Adams RD. Allergic neuritis: an experimental disease of rabbits induced by the injection of peripheral nervous tissue and adjuvants. J Exp Med 102:213–235, 1955.

Weiss S, Carter S. Course and prognosis of acute cerebellar ataxia in childhood. Neurology 9:711–712, 1959.

Wekerle H. The thymus in myasthenia gravis. Ann NY Acad Sci 681:47–55, 1993.

Wekerle H, Kojima K, Lannes-Vieira J, Lassmann H, Linington C. Animal models. Ann Neurol 36:S47–S53, 1994.

Whitaker JN, Benveniste EN, Zhou S. Cerebrospinal fluid. In Cook SD, ed. Handbook of multiple sclerosis. New York, Marcel Dekker, 1990, pp 251–270.

Whitham RH, Brey RL. Neuromyelitis optica: two new cases and review of the literature. J Clin Neuroophthalmol 5:263–269, 1985.

Willis T. De anima brutorum. Oxford, England: Theatro Sheldoniano, 404–406, 1672.

Wingerchuk DM, Hogancamp WF, O'Brien PC, Weinshenker BG. The clinical course of neuromyelitis optica (Devic's syndrome). Neurology 53:1107–1114, 1999.

Wittbrodt ET. Drugs and myasthenia gravis. An update. Arch Intern Med 157:399–408, 1997.

Wray D, Porter V. Calcium channel types at the neuromuscular junction. Ann NY Acad Sci 681:356–367, 1993.

Yang R, Puranam RS, Butler LS, Qian WH, He XP, Moyer MB, Blackburn K, Andrews PI, McNamara JO. Autoimmunity to munc-18 in Rasmussen's encephalitis. Neuron 28:375–383, 2000.

Zafeiriou DI, Kontopoulos EE, Katzos GS, Gombakis NP, Kanakoudi FG. Single dose immunoglobulin therapy for childhood Guillain-Barré syndrome. Brain Dev 19:323–325, 1997.

CHAPTER

41 Infection in the Compromised Host

James D. Cherry and Jaime G. Deville

PREVENTION OF INFECTION IN THE COMPROMISED CHILD

Certain inherited and acquired disorders are frequently associated with infections by organisms that produce no significant disease in most healthy individuals. The infections in compromised hosts are caused by organisms indigenous to the host or commonly found in the environment and are frequently referred to as *opportunistic infections* (Bode et al., 1974; Feigin and Shearer, 1975a, 1975b; Hart et al., 1969; Hewitt and Sanford, 1974; Klainer and Beisel, 1969; Patrick et al., 1998; Young et al., 1974). The clinical evaluation and treatment of immunologically compromised children with possible opportunistic infection are now frequent occurrences.

It is important to emphasize that the relationship among the host and the exogenous and endogenous microbial surroundings is a dynamic one. Specific microbial virulence can be expressed only in comparative terms because of daily variations in the total spectrum and concentration of microorganisms to which the host is exposed and the changes in host defense mechanisms.

Pathogenicity, which is the capacity of a microorganism to cause disease, is not an absolute term. Frequently, highly "pathogenic" microorganisms do not cause disease in exposed "susceptible" individuals, and, on other occasions, "nonpathogens" cause disease in "normal, healthy" persons. In addition to the risks of opportunistic infection, the compromised child is susceptible to all microorganisms to which healthy children are susceptible, and the illnesses in the compromised children are frequently more severe and protracted.

Infections in compromised children have always occurred, but their relative importance has increased steadily over the last 45 years. The major change over time has been in the specific microorganisms causing fatalities and the fact that in the past, compromised children frequently died as the result of their first systemic infections. Today, compromised children have a history of survival from repeated serious infections.

A major problem of the present era is the large number of infections in the compromised host that are hospital acquired. These nosocomial infections tend to be more difficult to manage because they are caused by microorganisms from the hospital environment that frequently are resistant to conventional antimicrobial therapy (Edmond et al., 1999; Eickhoff, 1972, 1975; Hewitt and Sanford, 1974; Huskins and Goldmann, 1998; Moore, 1974; Neu, 1984; Sattler et al., 2000; Turnidge and Bell, 2000; Wagenlehner and Naber, 2000; Westwood et al., 1974).

INFECTION IN CHILDREN COMPROMISED BY ANATOMIC DEFECTS

Opportunistic infections frequently are associated with the following anatomic defects: (1) dermal sinus tracts defects, (2) congenital and acquired cardiac defects, (3) urinary tract abnormalities, and (4) cleft palate. The microorganisms responsible for infections in children with anatomic defects and an approach to treatment and prevention are presented in Table 41-1.

Dermal Abnormalities of the Craniospinal Axis

Congenital dermal abnormalities of the craniospinal axis are more common than generally appreciated (Givner and Kaplan, 1993; Powell et al., 1975). Approximately 1% of children have midline defects; fortunately, only a small fraction of these defects communicate with the central nervous system (CNS) and become infected. Powell and colleagues (1975) reviewed the literature and found reports detailing 110 infections of the dermal sinuses. The most common infectious agents were those of a healthy bowel or

---

TABLE 41-1 · INFECTION IN THE HOST COMPROMISED BY ANATOMIC DEFECTS

Predisposing Causes	Opportunistic Organisms Isolated Most Frequently	Approach to Treatment of Infections	Prevention of Infections
Dermal abnormalities of the craniospinal axis	*Corynebacterium* sp., *Proteus* sp., *Escherichia coli*, *Staphylococcus epidermidis*, *Staphylococcus aureus*, diphtheroids, *Pseudomonas aeruginosa*, *Alcaligenes faecalis*, *Bacteroides* sp., *Haemophilus aphrophilus*, and *Streptococcus* sp.	1. Gram stain smear and culture of lesion drainage and cerebrospinal fluid 2. Incision and drainage if abscess present 3. Before identification of an organism, immediate therapy with systemic antibiotics (choice made on basis of results of Gram stain); if etiologic agent in doubt, antibiotic therapy should include coverage for *S. aureus*, *S. epidermidis*, *Corynebacterium* sp., and *Enterobacteriaceae* 4. Repair of defect	1. Careful evaluation of all skin defects 2. Surgical repair of all defects that might communicate with the central nervous system
Cardiac defects	*Streptococcus viridans* group, *Streptococcus pneumoniae*, other streptococci, enterococci, *S. aureus*, *S. epidermidis*, *Neisseria* sp., many gram-negative bacilli, *Candida sp.*, *Aspergillus* sp., *H. aphrophilus*, *Corynebacterium* sp., *Burkholderia cepacia*, *Aerococcus viridans*, and *Aspergillus fumigatus*	1. Multiple blood specimens for culture before therapy 2. Penicillin therapy for susceptible (MIC ≤ 0.2 μg/ml penicillin G) *Streptococcus* viridans group; ampicillin or vancomycin and an aminoglycoside for enterococci and resistant viridans group streptococcus; penicillinase-resistant penicillin or vancomycin for *Staphylococcus* sp.	1. Prophylactic administration of recommended antibiotics during dental and other procedures resulting in extensive bacteremia*
Obstructive lesions of the urinary tract	*E. coli* and other gram-negative bacilli; enterococci and *S. epidermidis*	1. Smear and quantitative culture of urine 2. Urologic evaluation and corrective surgery 3. Antibiotic therapy on the basis of the results of culture	1. Corrective surgery 2. Prophylactic antibiotics
Cleft palate	*E. coli* and other gram-negative bacilli; *H. influenzae*, *Streptococcus* sp., and *S. aureus*	1. Culture of ear drainage 2. Antibiotic therapy based on culture data 3. Tympanostomy tube insertion	1. Tympanostomy tube insertion 2. Prophylactic antibiotics 3. Surgical repair of cleft palate

*Data from Dajani AS, Bisno AL, Chung KJ, Durack DT, Freed M, Gerber MA, Karchmer AW, Millard HD, Rahimtoola S, Shulman ST, Watanakunakorn C, Taubert KA. Prevention of bacterial endocarditis. Recommendations by the American Heart Association. JAMA 264:2919–2922, 1990.
MIC = minimum inhibitory concentration.

skin flora (see Table 41-1). Some infections were nosocomial.

Because the morbidity and mortality from dermal sinus tract infections are great, prevention by surgical correction is indicated whenever defects are noted. An approach to therapy is listed in Table 41-1.

Cardiac Defects

Children with congenital and acquired heart disease may develop acute or subacute bacterial endocarditis. The most common etiologic agents include viridans group streptococci, *Streptococcus pneumoniae*, other non–β-hemolytic streptococci, enterococci, *Staphylococcus aureus*, and *Staphylococcus epidermidis* (Bhat et al., 1996; Brook, 1999; Caldwell et al., 1971; Elward et al., 1990; Johnson and Rhodes, 1982; Kramer et al., 1983; Martin et al., 1997; Mendelsohn and Hutchins, 1979; Noel et al., 1988; Saiman et al., 1993; Stanton et al., 1984; Starke, 1998; Van Hare et al., 1984).

Subacute bacterial endocarditis in children with congenital cardiac defects has also been reported in association with other opportunistic organisms, including *Haemophilus aphrophilus* (Johnson and Rhodes, 1982); *Neisseria* sp. (Brodie et al., 1971; Scott, 1971); diphtheroids (Merzbach et al., 1965; Van Hare et al., 1984); *Moraxella* (Christensen and Emmanouilides, 1967); *Enterobacter* sp. (Caldwell et al., 1971; Stanton et al., 1984); *Pseudomonas* sp. (Johnson and Rhodes, 1982; Kramer et al., 1983); *Escherichia coli* (Johnson and Rhodes, 1982); *Klebsiella pneumoniae* (Stanton et al., 1984); *Candida sp.* (Mendelsohn and Hutchins, 1979; Saiman et al., 1993); *Serratia* sp. (Stanton et al., 1984); *Haemophilus* sp. (Blair and Weiner, 1979; Stanton et al., 1984); Kingella kingae (Odum et al., 1984); β-hemolytic streptococci groups B, C, and G (Goldberg et al., 1985; Saiman et al., 1993); *Aspergillus* sp. (Barst et al., 1981; Saiman et al., 1993); *Actinobacillus actinomycetemcomitans* (Van Hare et al., 1984); and *Acinetobacter* calcoaceticus (Malik, 1995).

In addition to microbial infections within the heart, infants with congenital heart disease have an increased risk of severe illness when infected with respiratory syncytial virus (Hall, 1998; MacDonald et al., 1982). An approach to prevention and treatment is presented in Table 41-1.

Urinary Tract Abnormalities

Obstructive lesions of the urinary tract increase the risk of infection significantly. In addition to the usual gram-negative enteric microorganisms that cause urinary tract infections in children without demonstrable structural malformations, organisms of low virulence, such as *S. epidermidis,* are noted in infections in children with obstructive defects (Deinard and Libit, 1972).

Cleft Palate

Otitis media is an almost-universal complication of cleft palate (Paradise, 1976; Paradise and Bluestone, 1974; Paradise et al., 1969; Sancho Martin et al., 1997). The increased susceptibility in children with cleft palate is thought to be attributable to anatomical factors, such as a craniofacial skeleton deviation, and a functional impairment of the opening mechanisms of the eustachian tube (Kemaloglu et al., 1999). There has been little microbiologic study of otitis media in children with cleft palates. Because otitis media occurs in early infancy in these children, *E. coli* and other gram-negative bacilli are frequent pathogens as well as *Haemophilus influenzae*, *S. pneumoniae*, and *S. aureus*.

INFECTION IN CHILDREN COMPROMISED BY CHANGES IN OR PROCEDURES THAT BYPASS THE SKIN OR MUCOUS MEMBRANE BARRIERS

The skin and mucous membranes represent important barriers to infection. The intact skin generally resists infection by organisms that may contaminate it, and few microorganisms are able to penetrate it (Aly et al., 1972, 1975; Burtenshaw, 1948; Cooperstock, 1992). Situations in which the skin or mucous membrane barriers to infection have been compromised and thereby predispose the host to opportunistic infection are presented in Table 41-2.

Catheters

Intravascular Catheters

In the present era, the care of the majority of hospitalized children involves the use of one or more intravascular catheters, and these catheters are the most common cause of nosocomial bacteremias (Maki and Band, 1981). Catheter types include peripheral intravenous (IV) catheters, short-term arterial and central venous lines, long-term cuffed silicone central lines such as Broviac and Hickman catheters, and implanted venous access systems.

Opportunistic infections occur with all intravascular access lines (Adams et al., 1980; Band and Maki, 1979, 1980; Begala et al., 1982; Buxton et al., 1979; Daghistani et al., 1996; Dawson et al., 1991; Decker and Edwards, 1988; Flynn et al., 1987a, 1988; Freeman et al., 1990; Furfaro et al., 1991; Gorelick et al., 1991; Ingram et al., 1991; Jarvis, 1987; Jarvis et al., 1983; Moyer et al., 1983; Palmer, 1984; Press et al., 1984; Rhame et al., 1979; Richet et al., 1990; Riikonen et al., 1993; Rupar et al., 1990; Severien and Nelson, 1991; Shinozaki et al., 1983; Tomford et al., 1984; Wang et al., 1984; Wurzel et al., 1988).

In simple (noncuffed) catheters, infections are classified as exit-site infections (local infection at the point

TABLE 41-2 · INFECTION IN THE CHILD COMPROMISED BY PROCEDURES THAT BYPASS THE SKIN OR MUCOUS MEMBRANE BARRIERS

Predisposing Causes	Opportunistic Organisms Isolated Most Frequently	Approach to Treatment of Infections	Prevention of Infections
Intravenous catheters	*Staphylococcus epidermidis, Staphylococcus aureus, Enterococcus* sp., *Streptococcus* sp., *Bacteroides* sp., *Escherichia coli, Acinetobacter* sp., *Pseudomonas* sp., *Citrobacter* sp., *Klebsiella* sp., *Enterobacter* sp., *Bacillus* sp., *Serratia* sp., *Cryptococcus* sp., *Candida* sp., *Malassezia furfur, Corynebacterium* sp., and *Mycobacterium* sp.	1. Removal of catheter, if possible, especially with persistently positive blood culture or clinical signs suggesting persistent infection 2. Aspiration of blood through the line and peripheral blood culture 3. Culture of tip of removed catheter 4. Culture of infusing solution 5. Culture of skin at site of insertion 6. If patient is febrile, start therapy with a penicillinase-resistant penicillin or vancomycin and an aminoglycoside; consider addition of a third-generation cephalosporin 7. Examination of catheter tip for a thrombus by ultrasonography 8. If thrombus is present, prolonged antimicrobial therapy will be necessary; line will need to be removed frequently 9. Tunnel infections may need surgical excision and prolonged antimicrobial therapy	1. When possible, use of scalp vein needles rather than plastic catheters 2. Frequent change of intravenous site and administration set 3. Use of surgical preparation before placing catheter 4. Fewer infections occur with subcutaneous ports than with external catheters 5. Intravenous antibiotic prophylaxis preoperatively 6. Adequate staff training in the care of indwelling catheters 7. Line preferably placed in the upper body
Urinary catheters	Gram-negative enteric bacilli, *Pseudomonas* sp., *Serratia* sp., *Acinetobacter* sp., *S. epidermidis, Candida* sp., *Alcaligenes* sp., *Enterococcus* sp., and *Proteus mirabilis*	1. Gram-stain smear, culture of urine, and culture of blood 2. Removal of catheter, if possible 3. If patient is febrile, immediate therapy with systemic antibiotics (choice made on basis of Gram stain). Frequently, therapy includes an aminoglycoside 4. Treat *Proteus* sp., even if patient is symptom-free, to prevent calculi 5. If removal of catheter is not possible, local therapy with either continuous antibiotic or acetic acid bladder irrigation	1. Careful attention to sterile technique during catheter insertion 2. Use of a closed drainage system or continuous bladder irrigation with acetic acid or antibiotic solution
Inhalation therapy equipment	*S. aureus, Streptococcus pneumoniae*, other streptococci, *Haemophilus influenzae, Pseudomonas* sp., *Serratia* sp., *Klebsiella pneumoniae, Acinetobacter* sp., *Flavobacterium* sp., *Alcaligenes* sp., and other gram-negative bacilli	1. Culture from patient's respiratory tract 2. Initial therapy usually includes an aminoglycoside and a third-generation cephalosporin	1. Use of a specific regimen for cleaning inhalation therapy equipment and maintaining airway catheters 2. Infection control protocols to monitor associated infections

where the catheter exits the skin), septic infections, or combination infections. Cuffed catheters also are associated with exit-site and septic infections; in addition, they also may have tunnel infections (infections of the subcutaneous tract that extends proximally from the skin exit site to the point at which the catheter enters the vein) (Decker and Edwards, 1988).

Bacteremia or fungemia with organisms commonly found on the skin has been reported in 0.4% to 5% of patients with simple IV catheters (Harbin and Schaffner, 1973; Maki et al., 1973a). The rate of septicemia associated with prolonged IV catheterization for providing total nutrition parenterally has been even higher (Begala et al., 1982; Daghistani et al., 1996; Decker and Edwards, 1988; Goldman and Maki, 1973; Press et al., 1984; Riikonen et al., 1993; Wurzel et al.,

1988). *S. epidermidis, S. aureus, Streptococcus* group D and *Streptococcus viridans* group, *Bacillus* sp., *Pseudomonas* sp., *Bacteroides* sp., *Serratia, Citrobacter, Enterobacter* sp., *Acinetobacter* sp., and other organisms have been recovered from patients receiving total parenteral alimentation (Boeckman and Krill, 1970; Curry and Quie, 1971; Decker and Edwards, 1988; Dillon et al., 1973; Dudrick et al., 1968; Groff, 1969; Rodrigues et al., 1971; Saleh and Schorin, 1987). Tissue invasion by fungi has been documented; *Candida albicans* and *Torulopsis glabrata* appear to be the principal offenders (Freeman and Litton, 1974). Broviac catheter–related outbreaks of sepsis caused by *Malassezia furfur* in infants receiving IV fat emulsions have been described (Azimi et al., 1988; Powell et al., 1984).

Bacteremia related to IV therapy may occur even if local signs of inflammation are absent. Frequently, however, signs of inflammation, thrombosis, or purulent material are present at the site of catheterization. When positive cultures or clinical signs suggest infection resulting from IV therapy with short-term catheters (noncuffed), the therapy should be discontinued immediately. Therapy may be re-established at another site, if necessary. After the removal of a contaminated IV catheter, bacteremia or fungal septicemia may resolve spontaneously without specific antimicrobial therapy. When positive cultures or clinical signs suggest persistent infection, appropriate antimicrobial drugs should be administered.

Central venous lines with Broviac and Hickman catheters are usually left in place for considerable periods of time. Infection rates in different studies have varied from 0.47 to 7.59 per 1000 catheter-use days (Begala et al., 1982; Decker and Edwards, 1988; Press et al., 1984; Wurzel et al., 1988). Reported rates of bacteremia in neonates with central venous catheters have been as high as 42% (Maas et al., 1998).

Press and associates (1984) have shown that exit-site infections in patients with Hickman catheters usually can be cured with antibiotics alone without removal of the catheter. They also noted that tunnel infections usually necessitate catheter removal. They suggest that exit-site and tunnel infections be treated with antibiotics. Removal of the catheter should be considered if clinical improvement (i.e., no persistence of fever, bacteremia, and local inflammation) has not occurred after 48 hours of treatment.

Our experience with patients receiving total parenteral nutrition who are immunocompetent but have bacteremia is that they frequently can be cured with appropriate antimicrobial treatment without removal of the line. However, some tunnel infections may require surgical excision and prolonged antimicrobial therapy (Ward et al., 1999).

Routine replacement of all apparatus used for IV administration every 72 hours can decrease significantly the hazard of extrinsic contamination (Maki et al., 1987; Snydman et al., 1987). All bottles containing fluids for IV administration should be inspected immediately before use for cracks and turbidity. When peripheral IV administration is required, a small needle rather than a plastic catheter should be used; the use of needles has been associated with a lower incidence of septicemia and phlebitis than has the use of catheters (Crossley and Matsen, 1972; Peter et al., 1972).

Topical antibiotic preparations applied repeatedly to the site of catheter insertion have been widely used to prevent infections. Some studies have suggested benefit from this procedure, yet there is the added risk of infection with more-resistant bacterial strains (Maki et al., 1973a). In a multicenter, randomized trial (Garland et al., 2001), a chlorhexidine-impregnated dressing was applied or a povidone-iodine skin scrub was administered to the central venous catheter site in patients admitted to neonatal intensive care units. Catheter-tip colonization rates were slightly lower in the chlorhexidine group

(15% vs. 24%). However, contact dermatitis requiring discontinuation of the chlorhexidine-impregnated dressings developed in 15% of neonates with a birth weight below 1000 g, and the rates of catheter-related bloodstream infection and of bloodstream infection without source were similar in both groups.

Guidelines for the prevention of infections of arterial lines have been described in detail by Mermel and Maki (1989) and Shinozaki and associates (1983). Recommendations for the prevention of nosocomial intravascular device–related infections have been issued by the Centers for Disease Control and Prevention (Pearson, 1996).

IV catheter–associated sepsis may be caused by the infusion of contaminated IV fluids. Infection related to contaminated IV fluids has been caused by *Enterobacter cloacae, Enterobacter agglomerans, Pseudomonas* sp., *Citrobacter freundii, Klebsiella* sp., *Serratia* sp., and yeasts (Jarvis et al., 1983; Maki et al., 1973a, 1976). Nosocomial infection outbreaks with *E. agglomerans* and *E. cloacae* have been related to fluid contamination during the manufacturing process.

Urinary Catheters

The use of indwelling urinary catheters is a common cause of opportunistic infection, and these infections may lead to bacteremia and septicemia (Kunin and McCormack, 1966; Lohr et al., 1989; Meanes, 1991; Stamm, 1975; Wagenlehner and Naber, 2000; Wong and Hooton, 1981). Many infections are asymptomatic (Tambyah and Maki, 2000a). There is poor correlation between pyuria and catheter-associated urinary tract infection (Tambyah and Maki, 2000b). In addition to common gram-negative enteric bacteria, many highly resistant organisms such as *Pseudomonas* sp., *Acinetobacter, Achromobacter, Candida,* and *Serratia* have been incriminated frequently (Ederer and Matsen, 1972; Maki et al., 1973b; Schonebeck, 1972). Some approaches to the prevention and treatment of catheter-associated urinary tract infections are presented in Table 41-2.

Inhalation Therapy

Nosocomial pneumonias are common in immunocompromised patients, and the most common associated factor is mechanical ventilation. The incidence, risk factors, and etiologic agents of these pneumonias have been well studied in adults, but few recent studies have been conducted in pediatric intensive care units (Barzilay et al., 1988; George, 1993; Kollef, 1993; Leu et al., 1989; Nielsen et al., 1992; Rello et al., 1991). Fayon and colleagues (1997) presented data on 960 consecutive children admitted to a pediatric intensive care unit who required intubation and mechanical ventilation. They excluded patients with pre-existing respiratory infections. Seventeen instances of bacterial tracheitis (1.8%) and 12 instances (1.3%) of bacterial pneumonia occurred. *S. aureus* and enteric gram-negative bacilli were the most common pathogens. One death was attributed to bacterial pneumonia. Tullu and associates (2000) found endotracheal tube colonization in 70 of 88 (80%) intubated patients and a nosocomial pneumonia rate of 7.96 cases per 100 intubation days.

The etiologic diagnosis of pulmonary infections in patients receiving ventilation is difficult because of contamination by oropharyngeal flora. In a study in baboons, Johanson and colleagues (1988) found that tracheal aspirates revealed 78% of the organisms found in lung tissue, but false-positive cultures occurred frequently. *S. aureus*, *S. pneumoniae*, other streptococci, *H. influenzae*, *Pseudomonas aeruginosa*, *Serratia marcescens*, *Acinetobacter* sp., *Flavobacterium* sp., *Achromobacter* sp., *K. pneumoniae*, and other gram-negative bacilli have been the most commonly implicated organisms (Edmondson et al., 1966; Mertz et al., 1967; Nielsen et al., 1992; Pierce et al., 1970; Reinhardt et al., 1980; Rello et al., 1991; Sanders et al., 1970).

In the past, contaminated reservoir nebulizers were a problem, but with present-day cleaning and maintenance programs, this source of infection is uncommon. However, when an outbreak occurs in an intensive care unit, specimens for culture should be obtained from the equipment (e.g., reservoirs) and the techniques of respiratory therapists and others caring for airway catheters should be reviewed. Specific regimens for the cleaning and maintenance of inhalation therapy equipment (particularly nebulizers and tubing) should be adopted and continuously used.

Surgery

Opportunistic infections are common in patients who have undergone a surgical procedure (Belio-Blasco et al., 2000; Centers for Disease Control and Prevention [CDC], 1981; Cruse, 1981; Cruse and Foord, 1980; Davis et al., 1984; Horan et al., 1993; Keita-Perse et al., 1998; Olson and O'Conner-Allen, 1989; Riley, 1969; Sleigh and Peutherer, 1988). The patient undergoing surgery is compromised primarily because of the disruption of the skin and mucous membrane protective barriers, but other aspects of therapy, such as the use of IV and urinary catheters and inhalation therapy devices, also contribute to the overall infection risk. A discussion of infection in patients who have undergone surgery is presented in Chapter 30.

General Surgery

Wound infection is the most common opportunistic problem in patients who have undergone surgery. The incidence of wound infection varies greatly among different centers and in the type of surgery performed. In "clean" surgical cases, the incidence of wound infection can be expected to be between 2% and 5%. In a prospective study of 849 patients, Davis and colleagues (1984) reported a "clean" surgical wound infection rate of 3.1%. Davenport and Doig (1993) reported an infection rate of 20.7% in contaminated wounds and 11.1% in "clean" wounds, in 1433 surgical incisions in 1094

neonates. Length of incision, duration of procedure, and intraoperative contamination were associated with a higher incidence of wound infection. There was no association between gestational age and incidence of infection. Staphylococci were the most frequently isolated organisms in all categories. The most common etiologic agents and an approach to prevention are presented in Table 41-3.

When a postoperative fever develops in a child, infection by opportunistic microorganisms must be considered. Appropriate cultures and serologic tests are mandatory to establish an etiologic diagnosis. The many types and varied nature of the opportunistic organisms that produce disease postoperatively prevent the suggestion of a single specific antibiotic regimen as appropriate for all patients.

Cerebrospinal Fluid Shunts

Odio and associates (1984) reviewed the records of 516 cerebrospinal fluid (CSF) shunt procedures performed in 297 patients from 1975 through 1981. There were three ventriculoatrial (VA) and 513 ventriculoperitoneal (VP) shunt procedures. Fifty-nine shunt infections (11%) occurred in 50 (17%) of the children. Staphylococci accounted for 75% of the infections, with *S. epidermidis* being more common than *S. aureus*. There were 11 (19%) infections with gram-negative bacilli, and two or more pathogens were isolated in 15% of the infections. In a more recent study involving 273 VP and 75 VA shunts in children, the infection rate was 8% (Kontny et al., 1993). The rate of infection was 13.6% for operations lasting more than 90 minutes and 5.2% for those under 30 minutes.

In a report of 299 children with CSF shunt insertions and revisions, Kulkarni and colleagues (2001) noted that 31 patients (10.4%) developed shunt infections. The presence of a postoperative CSF leak and a gestational age of less than 40 weeks at the time of surgery were both associated with an increased risk of shunt infection.

Most shunt infections are caused by microorganisms considered to be normal flora of the skin. The recovery of such organisms from the CSF, the shunt, or the blood of patients with shunts should be regarded as presumptive evidence of infection. There has been a recent rise in fungal shunt infections (Montero et al., 2000; Nguyen and Yu, 1995). Chiou and colleagues (1994) reported that 8 of 48 (17%) shunt infections seen in children were attributable to fungal pathogens. Interestingly, all fungal infections occurred in premature infants. Hypocomplementemic glomerulonephritis is a well-recognized complication of shunt infection (Black et al., 1965; McKenzie and Hayden, 1974; Stickler et al., 1968). Most commonly, *S. epidermidis* has been implicated as the organism associated with this syndrome.

Fever is an almost universal manifestation of shunt infection. Erythema of the skin overlying the tubing used for diversion of the CSF is virtually diagnostic of infection. Children with infection of VA shunts generally have bacteremia, whereas patients with infection of

VP shunts rarely have positive blood cultures and may have negative CSF cultures. Thus when fever is observed in a child with a VA shunt, multiple blood cultures should be obtained, because generally they will permit an etiologic diagnosis. Direct aspiration of the shunt reservoir or valve is a helpful procedure for establishing the diagnosis of an infection of the shunt in patients who are not receiving antibiotics.

Patients with infected shunts should be treated with antibiotics directed specifically toward the offending organisms. Before the isolation and identification of the etiologic agent, treatment should include coverage for *Staphylococcus* sp., diphtheroids, and *Bacillus* sp. (Nydahl and Hall, 1965; Odio et al., 1984; Schoenbaum et al., 1975; Shurtleff et al., 1974; Walters et al., 1984; Yogev, 1985).

Because most strains of *S. epidermidis* are resistant to methicillin, an initial treatment regimen of vancomycin and an aminoglycoside is suggested. It is occasionally possible to successfully treat shunt infections with antibiotics alone, but it is usually safer and necessary to remove the infected shunt (Odio et al., 1984; Walters et al., 1984; Yogev, 1985).

The temporal association of surgery with infection of VA and VP shunts with *S. epidermidis* and *S. aureus* (Odio et al., 1984; Schoenbaum et al., 1975) suggests that the administration of antistaphylococcal antibiotics prophylactically in the perioperative period may be warranted.

In one uncontrolled study of 80 adult patients, shunt infection was reduced from 19% to 3% when a regimen of parenteral methicillin, followed by oral dicloxacillin, was used (Salmon, 1972). Odio and associates (1984) noted infections in 38% of 89 procedures in which prophylaxis was not used but in only 6% of 427 procedures when prophylaxis was performed. Schoenbaum and colleagues (1975) and Yogev (1985) also noted lower infection rates when prophylactic antistaphylococcal antibiotics were administered.

In contrast, others (Naito et al., 1973; Tsingoglou and Forrest, 1971) have not noted benefits when prophylactic antibiotics were used. Langley and associates (1993) performed a meta-analysis on the efficacy of antimicrobial prophylaxis, and they concluded that perioperative use of antimicrobial agents significantly reduces the risk of infection.

Cardiac Surgery

Cardiac surgery has been associated with a significant risk of postoperative infection resulting from opportunistic microorganisms. *S. aureus* and *S. epidermidis*, *Salmonella*, *Serratia*, diphtheroids, *Acinetobacter lwoffi*, *Enterobacter* sp., *Pseudomonas* sp., *C. albicans*, and *Aspergillus* are the opportunists that have been implicated most frequently (Bernhard, 1975; Boyce et al., 1990; Brandt and Swahn, 1960; Fisher et al., 1981; Flynn et al., 1987b; Griffin et al., 1973; Kammer and Utz, 1974; Koiwai and Nahas, 1956; Pike et al., 1951; Shafer and Hall, 1970; Watanakunakorn et al., 1968; Wilhelmi et al., 1987; Wilson et al., 1975).

Delayed sternal closure is a frequent method used by surgeons to prevent postoperative cardiac and respiratory compromise. Tabbutt and colleagues (1997) reviewed 178 pediatric patients between 1992 and 1995 who underwent median sternotomy and were left with open sternums postoperatively. They found seven cases of mediastinitis (3.9%) and clinical evidence of surgical site infections in 12 patients (6.7%). More recently, Mehta and colleagues (2000) reviewed 202 median sternotomies performed between 1996 and 1998. They found 10 patients with sternal wound infections (5%); six of the infections were considered superficial, and four infections were deep-seated. *S. aureus* was isolated from the wounds of six patients; other organisms encountered were *P. aeruginosa* and *H. influenzae* non–type B. An approach to the prevention and treatment of infections in patients undergoing cardiac surgery is presented in Table 41-3.

Burns

Thermal injury is, unfortunately, commonplace and is associated with significant morbidity and mortality in children (see Chapter 30). Opportunistic infection accounts for approximately half of all burn-associated fatalities (Feller and Crane, 1970; MacMillan, 1980). A burn destroys the normal skin barrier to infection, allowing normal skin bacteria and environmental contaminants a portal of entry (Pruitt et al., 1984). In addition, abnormalities in neutrophil function in patients with burns have been noted (Alexander et al., 1971). The killing of *Staphylococcus* and *Pseudomonas* organisms by neutrophils was less efficient than was the killing of *Serratia* and streptococci. Alexander (1971a) also noted a circadian periodicity of neutrophil function; that is, the time of day at which activity was minimal could be associated with an increased risk of sepsis in the burned patient.

In addition to neutrophil dysfunction, burn injury may be associated with abnormal vascular responses, diminished uptake of particles by the reticuloendothelial system, abnormal responses to antigens, and delayed rejection of homografts (Alexander, 1971a; Pruitt et al., 1984) (see Chapter 29).

Before the antibiotic era, infections with *Streptococcus pyogenes* were of most importance in patients with burns (Alexander, 1971b). Associated with the frequent use of penicillin therapy in patients with burns, streptococcal complications were controlled, but penicillin-resistant strains of *S. aureus* became a problem.

After the introduction and widespread use of penicillinase-resistant penicillins and cephalosporins, staphylococcal infections decreased in prominence in patients with burns and gram-negative organisms became the predominant pathogens. Septicemia with *P. aeruginosa* was frequent. Since the early 1980s, however, methicillin-resistant strains of staphylococci have developed, and because of this, sepsis caused by staphylococcal infection is again a major problem.

Rodgers and colleagues (2000) reported a prospective study of 70 pediatric patients hospitalized for burns.

TABLE 41-3 · INFECTION IN THE CHILD COMPROMISED BY SURGICAL PROCEDURES

Type of Surgery	Opportunistic Organisms Isolated Most Frequently	Approach to Treatment of Infections	Prevention of Infections
General surgery	*Staphylococcus aureus, Staphylococcus epidermidis, Streptococcus* sp., *Escherichia coli, Clostridia* sp., *Klebsiella pneumoniae, Enterobacter* sp., *Pseudomonas* sp., *Proteus* sp., other gram-negative bacilli, *Bacteroides* sp., and other anaerobes, *Candida* sp., and other fungi; Pasteurella multocida, *Bacillus subtilis, Alcaligenes faecalis*, and *Aeromonas hydrophila*	1. Gram stain smear; culture from wound and blood specimens for culture 2. Withhold antibiotic therapy until specimens for culture obtained	1. Discourage use of prophylactic antibiotics unless they have been demonstrated to be useful in controlled trials for particular surgical condition 2. Discourage unnecessary use of urinary and intravenous catheters and respirators 3. Careful attention to aseptic techniques 4. Routine hospital surveillance of surgical infections
CSF shunts	*S. epidermidis, S. aureus, Bacillus* sp., diphtheroids, and gram-negative enteric bacilli	1. Gram stain smear and cultures of CSF, blood, and shunt 2. In patients with a ventriculoatrial shunt, obtain multiple blood specimens for culture 3. Immediate therapy with vancomycin and an aminoglycoside; possible change of antibiotic therapy after culture results 4. Direct aspiration of shunt reservoir or valve 5. Removal of infected shunt	1. Prophylactic administration of a penicillinase-resistant penicillin or cefazolin during the perioperative period
Burns	*Streptococcus* sp., *Staphylococcus* sp., *Pseudomonas* sp., *Serratia* sp., *A. hydrophila, Klebsiella* sp., *Flavobacterium* sp., *Enterobacter* sp., *Escherichia coli, Proteus* sp., *Providencia* sp., *Enterococcus* sp., *Candida* sp., *Mucor* sp., *Aspergillus* sp., *Geotrichum, Helminthosporium, Alternaria, Fusarium, Cryptococcus*, herpes simplex virus, and varicella-zoster virus	1. Burn wound biopsy specimen and blood specimens for culture 2. If patient febrile or toxic, immediate therapy with a penicillinase-resistant penicillin or vancomycin and an aminoglycoside 3. Use of IVIG in selected patients 4. Early wound closure	1. Low-dose prophylaxis with penicillin 2. Careful cleaning of the burned skin and meticulous protective care 3. Anticipatory treatment for invading and translocating organisms
Cardiac surgery	*S. aureus, S. epidermidis,* diphtheroids, *Acinetobacter* sp., *Serratia* sp., *Pseudomonas* sp., *Candida* sp., *Aspergillus* sp., *Salmonella* sp., and *Enterobacteriaceae*	1. Multiple blood specimens for culture before therapy	1. Prophylactic administration of a penicillinase-resistant penicillin or cefazolin during the perioperative period 2. Prophylaxis is started immediately before the operative procedure, repeated during prolonged procedures, and continued for no more than 24 hours postoperatively to minimize occurrence of microbial resistance

CSF = cerebrospinal fluid; IVIG = intravenous immunoglobulin.

Nineteen patients (27%) had 39 infectious complications; of these, one third were catheter-related septicemia, one third involved the burn wound (six episodes of burn sepsis, five of graft loss, and two of cellulitis), and the remaining third involved other sites (six episodes of pneumonia; three of urinary tract infection; two of bacteremia; and one each of endocarditis, otitis media, myocardial abscess, and toxin-mediated syndrome). The most common pathogen was *S. aureus* (46%), followed by coagulase-negative staphylococci (10%), *P. aeruginosa* (10%), *Enterococcus* sp. (10%), and *E. coli* (7%). The main risk factors for infections were the depth and extent of the injury and the mechanism of burn (i.e., flame or inhalation).

Septicemia in children with burns also has been related to *S. epidermidis, Serratia* sp., *Aeromonas hydrophila, Klebsiella* sp., *Enterobacter* sp., *Flavobacterium* sp., *Pseudomonas* sp., *E. coli, Proteus* sp., *Providencia* sp., *Candida* sp., *Mucor, Aspergillus* sp., *Geotrichum, Helminthosporium, Alternaria, Fusarium*, and *Cryptococcus* (Abramovsky et al., 1974; Alexander and Meakins, 1972; Benjamin et al., 1970; Foley, 1969; MacMillan, 1980; Peterson and Baker, 1959; Phillips et al., 1974; Pruitt et al., 1984; Rabin et al., 1961;

Sheridan et al., 1993; Spebar and Lindberg, 1979; Tredget et al., 1992). Viral invasion of the burned area also may occur; children with burns are particularly susceptible to herpes simplex infection (Sheridan et al., 2000). In addition, Linnemann and MacMillan (1981) noted that 22% of pediatric burn patients had serologic evidence of cytomegalovirus infections. Bale and colleagues (1990) reported that 52% of cytomegalovirus-seropositive burn patients had a fourfold or greater rise in cytomegalovirus antibody titers during their hospitalization and that 19% of cytomegalovirus-seronegative patients seroconverted. Airway injury associated with smoke inhalation may lead to invasive pulmonary disease and bacteremia (Dietrich et al., 1990).

An approach to the treatment and prevention of opportunistic infections in children with burns is presented in Table 41-3 (Alexander, 1971b; MacMillan, 1980; Pruitt et al., 1984; Shuck, 1972).

INFECTION IN CHILDREN COMPROMISED BY INHERITED DISORDERS OF IMMUNITY

Disorders of Polymorphonuclear Leukocyte Function or Number

The development of the polymorphonuclear phagocytic system is presented in Chapter 5, and the pathophysiology and clinical aspects of these disorders are presented in Chapter 20.

Chronic Granulomatous Disease of Children

The clinical manifestations of chronic granulomatous disease (CGD) include marked lymphadenopathy, pneumonitis, suppuration of nodes, hepatomegaly, dermatitis, splenomegaly, liver and perianal abscesses, diarrhea, genitourinary granulomata, and osteomyelitis, particularly of the small bones of the hands and feet (Johnston and Baehner, 1971; Mills and Quie, 1980; Quie and Hetherington, 1984; Tauber et al., 1983).

This condition is caused by an inherited disorder of phagocyte function caused by mutations in genes encoding for proteins that constitute the major component of the phagocyte-NADPH-oxidase system (Curnutte, 1993a). The phagocytes from these patients are unable to generate superoxide anions and other microbicidal oxygen metabolites, resulting in severely impaired intracellular killing of catalase-positive microorganisms (see Chapter 20).

Bacteria such as S. pneumoniae and S. pyogenes do not cause unusual difficulty in patients with CGD because they generate hydrogen peroxide but not catalase. In contrast, catalase-positive organisms such as S. aureus and gram-negative enteric bacteria are troublesome. S. aureus has been frequently isolated from patients with this disease.

Systemic abscesses and other infections with organisms of low virulence such as Enterobacter sp., E. coli,

S. epidermidis, Serratia sp., Pseudomonas sp., Proteus sp., Salmonella sp., Candida sp., and Aspergillus sp. are common (Johnston and Baehner, 1971; Lazarus and Neu, 1975). Infections with Torulopsis sp., Hansenula polymorpha, Pneumocystis jiroveci (carinii), Streptococcus intermedius, Nocardia sp., Actinomyces israelii, Alcaligenes faecalis, Chromobacterium sp., Acinetobacter sp., and Mycobacterium fortuitum have also been reported (Chusid et al., 1975; Gallin et al., 1983; Johnston and Baehner, 1971; Lazarus and Neu, 1975; McGinnis et al., 1980; Mills and Quie, 1980; Quie and Hetherington, 1984; Tauber et al., 1983; Walzer et al., 1973). Disseminated infection with bacillus Calmette-Guérin (BCG) has been noted in three immunized children with CGD (Esterly et al., 1971; Verronen, 1974).

In recent years, Aspergillus sp. has emerged as a predominant pathogen in patients with CGD. It accounts for approximately 20% of major infections in patients with CGD and is associated with 50% of deaths (Mouy et al., 1989).

A registry of patients with CGD was established in the United States by Winkelstein and colleagues (2000). Of 386 patients, 259 have the X-linked form, 81 have one of several autosomal recessive forms, and in 368 patients the inheritance mode is unknown. The authors estimated that the incidence of CGD is between 1/200,000 and 1/250,000 live births. The most prevalent infections are pneumonia (79%), suppurative adenitis (53%), subcutaneous abscess (42%), liver abscess (27%), osteomyelitis (25%), and sepsis (18%).

Aspergillus sp. is the most common cause of pneumonia, and S. aureus is the predominant pathogen isolated in suppurative adenitis, subcutaneous abscesses, and liver abscesses. Serratia is the most common pathogen isolated in patients with osteomyelitis, and Salmonella is the most common cause of sepsis. Since the registry was established in 1993, the most common causes of death have been pneumonia or sepsis resulting from Aspergillus sp. (23 patients) or Burkholderia cepacia (12 patients). Fifteen percent of patients had gastric outlet obstruction, and 10% had urinary tract obstruction.

Patients with the X-linked form have a worse prognosis than patients with autosomal recessive forms; 21.2% of registry patients with the X-linked form, compared with 8.6% of those with the autosomal recessive forms, died. Patients with the X-linked form were also diagnosed earlier (3.0 vs. 7.8 years) and had a significantly higher prevalence of sepsis (21% vs. 10%), perirectal abscesses (17% vs. 7%), suppurative adenitis (59% vs. 32%), gastric outlet obstruction (19% vs. 5%), and urinary tract obstruction (11% vs. 3%) than did patients with autosomal recessive forms.

The treatment of infection in patients with CGD must be dictated by the organisms producing the infections and their sensitivity patterns. In patients with suspected sepsis, treatment parenterally with a semisynthetic penicillinase-resistant penicillin and with an aminoglycoside antibiotic such as gentamicin is recommended until the results of cultures are available. Drainage of abscesses is imperative. Aspergillus infections should be treated vigorously with amphotericin B or itraconazole. Antibiotic therapy must be continued for extended periods of time as dictated by the course of infection. Rifampin may be particularly effective in some patients because it may exert a bactericidal effect intracellularly (Ezer and Soothill, 1974; Jacobs and Wilson, 1983). Isoniazid, fosfomycin, clindamycin, trimethoprim-sulfamethoxazole, and chloramphenicol also readily cross cellular membranes and inhibit intracellular bacteria, so they also could be useful when infecting organisms are sensitive (Gmunder and Seger, 1981; Hoger et al., 1985; Jacobs and Wilson, 1983; Quie, 1973).

In this regard, Thompson and Soothill (1970) noted clinical improvement in two children with CGD who were treated with isoniazid and para-aminosalicylic acid, despite the fact that neither was affected by known mycobacterial agents.

Granulocyte infusions have been suggested as an adjunct to therapy in life-threatening infections (Gallin et al., 1983; Raubitschek et al., 1973; Tauber et al., 1983). Corticosteroids in conjunction with antimicrobial therapy have been used to reduce obstruction caused by inflammation in three patients with CGD (Chin et al., 1987; Quie and Belani, 1987).

Attempts at prevention of infection in children with CGD have been disappointing. Live bacterial vaccines such as BCG should be avoided. Twenty-five years ago, continuous antibiotic therapy prophylactically was advocated (Ammann and Wara, 1975; Johnston et al., 1975; Phillapart et al., 1972). In nine patients with CGD, nafcillin therapy appeared to reduce the number of infectious episodes (Phillapart et al., 1972).

Lazarus and Neu (1975) pointed out that the majority of fatalities in children with CGD were attributable to gram-negative bacilli, a finding in contrast to those of Phillapart and colleagues. Furthermore, Lazarus and Neu suggested that some of these deaths may have been caused by changes in the flora of children treated prophylactically with penicillinase-resistant penicillins.

In another study reported in 1975, the number of infectious episodes and the severity of bacterial infections were reduced in four of five children with CGD who were placed on long-term sulfisoxazole treatment (Johnston et al., 1975). The decrease in the number of infections was out of proportion to the demonstrable direct antibacterial effect of the drug. There was a modest enhancement of the bactericidal activity of leukocytes in all five patients in the presence of sulfisoxazole, but studies of phagocytosis-associated oxidative metabolism in patients' cells have not revealed a metabolic basis for improved killing. Two children with CGD who were followed up by one of us also appeared to benefit from continuous sulfisoxazole prophylactic administration.

There have been several reports of prophylactic success with trimethoprim-sulfamethoxazole (Frayha and Biggar, 1983; Gallin et al., 1983; Kobayashi et al., 1978; Margolis et al., 1990; Mendelsohn and Berant, 1982; Tauber et al., 1983). In contrast, no benefit from either clofazimine or co-trimoxazole treatment was noted in one child with CGD (McCrae and Raeburn, 1972).

Anderson (1981) noted that the administration of oral ascorbate in three children resulted in slight increases in neutrophil hexose monophosphate shunt staphylocidal activity and a reduction in the occurrence of obvious infections. Foroozanfar and associates (1983) treated three patients with ascorbate for 8 months and were unable to document any improvement in the intracellular killing of microorganisms, which is in contrast to Anderson's findings.

The most common agent used today for chemoprophylaxis is trimethoprim-sulfamethoxazole. It has broad activity against pathogens encountered in CGD, is lipophilic and therefore concentrates inside cells, does not affect anaerobic bowel flora, and thus is well tolerated (Seger et al., 1981).

Itraconazole has been a major advance in the treatment of *Aspergillus* infections in CGD (Neijens et al., 1989) and perhaps is also useful as a prophylactic agent (Mouy et al., 1994).

Relatively recently, in vitro and in vivo studies have shown that interferon-γ can partially correct the metabolic defect in the phagocytes of patients with CGD (Curnutte, 1993b; Mühlebach et al., 1992; Sechler et al., 1988). In a controlled trial involving 128 patients with CGD, it was found that interferon-γ therapy was effective in reducing the frequency of serious infections (International Chronic Granulomatous Disease Cooperative Study Group, 1991). Patients were treated with interferon-γ (50 μg/m^2 of body surface area) three times a week.

Bone marrow transplantation has been successfully undertaken in several patients (see Chapter 43). In one patient, improvement persisted for 3 years (Gallin et al., 1983; Tauber et al., 1983). Another patient had stable neutrophil engraftment for 7 years after bone marrow transplantation (Leung et al., 1999). An 8-year-old with invasive aspergillosis unresponsive to amphotericin B and interferon-γ treatment underwent bone marrow transplantation, in addition to the administration of granulocyte colony-stimulating factor. The clinical and biologic signs of infection started to improve 7 days after transplantation. Two years after transplantation, the patient was well, with full immune reconstitution and no sign of *Aspergillus* infection (Ozsahin et al., 1998). However, morbidity, mortality, and graft failure rates remain high in patients with CGD, except in those with an HLA antigen–identical sibling donor (Leung et al., 1999).

Hyperimmunoglobulin E (Job's) Syndrome

Hyperimmunoglobulin E recurrent-infection syndrome (hyper-IgE, or Job's syndrome) was first described in fair, redhaired girls who developed repeated episodes of "cold" staphylococcal abscesses of the skin, subcutaneous tissue, or lymph nodes (Davis et al., 1966; Donabedian and Gallin, 1983; Quie and Hetherington, 1984) (see Chapter 17). It has been described in both sexes and often has an autosomal dominant mode of inheritance.

Infections are also caused by *C. albicans, H. influenzae, S. pyogenes,* gram-negative pathogens, and other fungi (Shyur and Hill, 1991). Skin infections are frequent and first occur in infancy. They include furunculosis, cold abscesses, and cellulitis. Pulmonary infections are frequent and severe, again most commonly because of *S. aureus.* Oral moniliasis, chronic nail infections, deep-seated *Candida* infections, and *Aspergillus* and *Cryptococcus* infections have been reported (Erlewyn-Lajeunnesse, 2000; Stone and Wheeler, 1990; van der Meer et al., 1998).

Peripheral stem cell transplantation was performed in a 46-year-old man who had a history of hyper-IgE syndrome and had developed a B-cell lymphoma. After engraftment, the symptoms of hyper-IgE syndrome disappeared. Unfortunately, the patient later died of interstitial pneumonia (Nester et al., 1998).

When patients known to have Job's syndrome are infected, appropriate cultures should be obtained and initial treatment with a semisynthetic penicillinase-resistant penicillin should ensue. Continuous antibiotic therapy prophylactically with a penicillinase-resistant penicillin is a worthwhile approach in the severely affected child. Hattori and colleagues (1993) reported on a 13-year-old boy who had marked clinical improvement with trimethoprim-sulfamethoxazole therapy; associated with this clinical improvement was an improvement in neutrophil function and a decrease in serum IgE concentration.

Glucose-6-Phosphate Dehydrogenase Deficiency

The leukocytes of patients with glucose-6-phosphate dehydrogenase deficiency are unable to kill *S. aureus, E. coli,* or *Serratia* normally (Cooper et al., 1972) (see Chapter 20). Acute anemia has been reported during infections with hepatitis A, cytomegalovirus, Epstein-Barr virus, and parvovirus B19 (Garcia et al., 1987; Nibu et al., 1989; Rosenbloom et al., 1988; Siddiqui and Khan, 1998). The treatment and prevention of clinical infections should be similar to those used in CGD.

Chédiak-Higashi Syndrome

Chédiak-Higashi, an inherited autosomal recessive disorder, is associated with recurrent pyogenic infection. Patients with this syndrome have infections similar to those in CGD *(S. aureus, Serratia);* in addition, they experience recurrent infections with catalase-negative organisms (Ammann and Wara, 1975). Infection with Epstein-Barr virus has resulted in lymphoproliferative disease caused by chronic active infection (Kinugawa, 1990; Merino et al., 1986).

Treatment must be based on the recovery of the etiologic agents and the determination of their sensitivity patterns. In the septic child, initial therapy with a penicillinase-resistant penicillin and an aminoglycoside antibiotic such as gentamicin is recommended. The use of low-dose penicillin or trimethoprim-sulfamethoxazole prophylaxis should be considered in patients with recurrent infections with sensitive organisms. Affected children may also benefit from pneumococcal vaccine. Bone marrow transplantation may be lifesaving (Patrick and Slobod, 1998).

Neutropenia

Congenital neutropenia may occur as an isolated deficit, with aplastic anemia, or in some patients with agammaglobulinemia or other immunodeficiency diseases (Baehner, 1972; Feigin and Shearer, 1975a, 1975b; Kauder and Mauer, 1966) (see Chapters 20 and 39). Neutropenia associated with pancreatic insufficiency and malabsorption also is a well-defined clinical syndrome (Shmerling et al., 1969). Cyclic neutropenia is another syndrome in which circulating white blood cells are depressed at intervals of approximately 3 weeks, and this is associated with aphthous stomatitis and fever (Wright et al., 1981; see Chapter 36). Almost all reported fatal infections in patients with cyclic neutropenia have been caused by *Clostridium* sp. (Bar-Joseph et al., 1997).

Acquired neutropenias are a more common clinical problem than is congenital disease. They most frequently are associated with drug administration. Acquired neutropenia also may be associated with overwhelming infection, collagen disease, allergic disorders, neoplasms, myelophthisic disorders, hypersplenism, and radiation. Viral infections with parvovirus B19, Epstein-Barr virus, cytomegalovirus, and human immunodeficiency virus 1 (HIV-1) have been associated with neutropenia (Gautier et al., 1997; Hermans et al., 1999; Herrod et al., 1985; Ivarsson and Ljung, 1988; Kuritzkes, 2000).

McClain and colleagues (1993) found evidence of parvovirus B19 infection in 15 of 19 children with neutropenia of more than 3 months' duration. Nine of the children had antineutrophil antibodies, suggesting that infection with parvovirus B19 may trigger immune-mediated chronic neutropenia in children.

In all neutropenic syndromes except cyclic neutropenia, severe pyogenic infections are the rule. Infection with common pathogens is the usual occurrence, but sepsis caused by opportunistic organisms such as *Acinetobacter* sp., *Serratia* sp., *Pseudomonas* sp., *S. epidermidis,* and fungi is also frequent.

Atraumatic *Clostridium septicum* infection is a rare cause of sepsis in children, but it has a very high mortality rate. All reported pediatric cases have occurred in patients with neutropenia. Approximately 30% of described cases have occurred in children with cyclic neutropenia, and the remainder have been associated with chemotherapy (Bar-Joseph et al., 1997).

Prevention of infections in the patient with neutropenia is a formidable challenge. As in Chédiak-Higashi syndrome, prophylaxis with low-dose penicillin or trimethoprim-sulfamethoxazole may be useful in children with congenital neutropenia who have recurrent infections with sensitive organisms.

The treatment of infections in children with neutropenia is dependent on data derived from cultures taken before therapy. In treating infections with

Pseudomonas sp. and other gram-negative bacilli, it is important to use two synergistic antimicrobial agents, including a β-lactam and an aminoglycoside. The clinical manifestations of infections in patients with neutropenia are different from those in patients without neutropenia. Sickles and colleagues (1975) noted that exudation, fluctuation, ulceration or fissure, local heat, swelling, and regional adenopathy were less commonly found in patients with malignancies who were profoundly granulocytopenic than in similar patients without granulocytopenia. Only erythema and local pain or tenderness were common findings in both patients with and without granulocytopenia. The response to therapy in children with neutropenia generally is slower than that in healthy children.

Treatment with a single bactericidal broad-spectrum agent (monotherapy) has been advocated as initial empiric therapy for febrile episodes in neutropenic cancer patients. Ceftazidime has been the agent most commonly used (Morgan et al., 1983). Recent data suggest that cefepime has equivalent efficacy and may also reduce the subsequent need for more-extensive antimicrobial treatment (Kebudi et al., 2001; Mustafa et al., 2001). For a selected low-risk subpopulation, outpatient management with either IV ceftriaxone or ceftazidime or oral ciprofloxacin has been suggested (Mullen et al., 1999; Petrilli et al., 2000)

Patients with either congenital or acquired neutropenia may respond to granulocyte-macrophage colony-stimulating factors or granulocyte colony-stimulating factors (Dale, 1994, Dale et al., 1995; Welte et al., 1990). Patients have been treated with granulocyte colony-stimulating factors for more than 3 years without adverse effects.

Splenic Deficiency

The pathophysiology of splenic deficiency is discussed in Chapters 5 and 30. The major cause of splenic deficiency is surgical removal, but congenital asplenia and splenosis also occur (Pedersen, 1983). In patients with splenic deficiency disorders, there is an increased susceptibility to overwhelming infection with *S. pneumoniae*, *Neisseria meningitidis*, and *H. influenzae*. Rarely, other streptococci, *Staphylococcus* sp., *E. coli*, *Klebsiella*, *Salmonella*, and *P. aeruginosa* cause septicemia (Chilcote et al., 1976; Walker, 1976).

In endemic areas, persons with splenic deficiency are also at increased risk of severe and often-fatal infections with *Plasmodium* and *Babesia* spp. protozoan diseases (Editorial, 1976; Katz, 1982). Hatcher and associates (2001) recently noted that 12 of 34 patients with babesiosis had undergone splenectomies. This confirms an earlier observation by Rosner and colleagues (1984), who observed that one third of all reported cases of babesiosis occurred in individuals who had undergone splenectomy. It should be noted that in areas in which malaria is endemic, infection with *Babesia* spp. is often not recognized because its clinical presentation closely resembles that of malaria.

Standard therapy for babesiosis is a combination of clindamycin and quinine taken for 7 to 10 days (Krause, 1998). In a recent study, Krause and colleagues (2000) found that atovaquone and azithromycin had an efficacy similar to that of clindamycin and quinine. They suggested that the atovaquone-azithromycin combination was a useful alternative because it caused fewer adverse reactions than clindamycin and quinine. The prevention of Babesia infections is extremely important in patients with asplenia. Areas in which ticks, deer, and mice thrive—especially tall grass and brush—should be avoided. Protective clothing and the use of tick repellents are recommended for people who have contact with the foliage endemic to their areas. A search of the body for ticks should be carried out after exposure, and ticks should be removed as soon as possible.

The pneumococcus is the major risk in children with asplenia. The experience to date suggests that, although splenectomy increases the risk of infection in all persons, susceptibility is in large part influenced by the underlying disease state for which splenectomy was performed. Until recently, the pneumococcus has been highly susceptible to penicillin and therefore penicillin prophylaxis has been recommended. Most authorities agree that asplenic children with malignancies, thalassemia, histiocytosis, and other debilitating diseases should be placed on prophylactic penicillin. In children in whom splenectomy was performed because of trauma, there is less agreement with regard to prophylaxis.

We recommend that children under the age of 3 years undergo prophylaxis; in older children, the parents should be offered an option. If prophylaxis is undertaken, it must be emphasized to the parents that haphazard compliance is probably worse than no antibiotic administration.

If a continuous prophylactic regimen is not instituted, the parents should have a supply of amoxicillin/clavulanate potassium (Augmentin) readily available. At the first sign of respiratory illness, the patient's physician should be contacted and Augmentin therapy (40 mg/kg/day, based on the amoxicillin component in divided doses every 8 hours) immediately instituted. It should be emphasized that all febrile illnesses must be considered potentially serious and immediate medical attention sought.

For prophylaxis, oral penicillin G two times a day should be used. Children under 5 years of age should receive 200,000 U/dose; for those older than 5 years of age, 400,000 U/dose. Alternatively, oral penicillin V can be used (125 mg twice daily for children younger than 5 years of age and 250 mg twice daily for older children).

In recent years, there has been a worldwide increase in pneumococci that are resistant to penicillin (Friedland et al., 1993; Jacobs, 1992; Klugman et al., 1990; Rauch et al., 1990; Tan et al., 1993). The majority of so-called resistant strains are intermediately resistant (i.e., with minimum inhibitory concentrations of 0.1 to 1 μg/ml), but some are highly resistant (>1 μg/ml); some of these latter strains are also resistant to third-generation cephalosporins. Whether this resistance will make present penicillin prophylaxis ineffective is not known at this time. In the past, when sepsis was a possibility, immediate therapy with a third-generation cephalosporin was recommended. At present, because of the possibility of highly resistant organisms, we recommend the use of IV vancomycin (40 mg/kg/day every 6 hours), in addition to third-generation cephalosporin (cefotaxime 200 mg/kg/day every 6 hours).

Infants with asplenia should receive their scheduled immunizations, including *H. influenzae* type B and pneumococcal conjugate vaccines (American Academy of Pediatrics, 2000f). Older children should receive polyvalent pneumococcal polysaccharide vaccine and quadrivalent meningococcal polysaccharide vaccine.

Sickle Cell Disease and Other Hemoglobinopathies

An increased incidence of pneumonia, osteomyelitis, meningitis, and genitourinary infections caused by *S. pneumoniae*, *H. influenzae*, *Salmonella* sp., *Edwardsiella tarda*, and *Mycoplasma* sp. has been described in children with hemoglobinopathies (Barrett-Connor, 1971; Rubin et al., 1968; Sachs et al., 1974; Shulman et al., 1972; Wong et al., 1992). Aspects of pathophysiology are discussed in Chapter 24.

All children at appropriate ages should be given pneumococcal, meningococcal, and *H. influenzae* type B vaccines. There are data that support the use of pneumococcal conjugate vaccine at 2, 4, 6, and 12 to 15 months of age, followed by 23-valent pneumococcal polysaccharide vaccine at 24 months of age (O'Brien et al., 2000). The treatment of bacterial infections in children with sickle cell disease requires an aggressive approach. Before therapy, cultures of blood, stool, throat, and bone and joint lesions, if present, should be obtained. In the toxic child, initial therapy with cefotaxime and vancomycin is indicated. In the older child with pneumonia, therapy with erythromycin or tetracycline for M. *pneumoniae* should also be started.

B-Cell Immunodeficiencies

The prototype B-cell deficit is X-linked agammaglobulinemia (Bruton, 1952); this and other B-cell immunodeficiencies are discussed in Chapter 13. Opportunistic infections occur because the lack of secretory antibody allows infection of mucosal surfaces, and this infection can spread systemically because of the absence of serum cytotoxic or neutralizing antibody or an antibody that participates in antibody-dependent cellular cytotoxicity (Stiehm et al., 1986). The lack of antibody-antigen interaction may lead to impaired complement activation, decreased chemotaxis, and a deficiency of opsonization and phagocytosis of microorganisms.

The following clinical illness categories are manifestations of B-cell immunodeficiencies: recurrent pneumonia and otitis media, pharyngitis-tonsillitis, sinusitis, bronchiectasis, conjunctivitis, rhinitis, meningitis, septicemia, persistent infectious diarrhea and viral encephalitis, viral hepatitis, cholangitis, paralytic poliomyelitis, *Mycoplasma* arthritis, and chronic cystitis and urethritis (Hausser et al., 1983; Stiehm et al., 1986).

Before the advent of Ig replacement therapy, patients with X-linked agammaglobulinemia had early onset, recurrent severe infections caused by encapsulated bacteria such as *S. pneumoniae*, *S. aureus*, *H. influenzae*, *N. meningitidis*, and *P. aeruginosa* (Gitlin et al., 1959; Hermaszewski and Webster, 1993; Ochs and Smith, 1996). Severe, recurrent, or chronic infections more recently have been noted with other bacteria, viruses, protozoa, and *Mycoplasma* spp. (Erlendsson et al., 1985; Ponka et al., 1983; Saulsbury et al., 1980; Sloper et al., 1982; Stiehm et al., 1986; Wilfert et al., 1977).

In Table 41-4, a list of opportunistic infectious agents in B-cell deficiency states is presented. Particularly troublesome have been enteroviral syndromes such as chronic encephalitis, dermatomyositis, and vaccine-induced paralytic poliomyelitis. In a recent study of 31 hospitalized boys with X-linked agammaglobulinemia, it was found that approximately half had bacterial pneumonias (Quartier et al., 1999). Other bacterial infections observed in this study were sepsis, meningitis, arthritis, osteomyelitis, and cellulitis; aseptic arthritis was the most common nonbacterial infection. In Table 41-4, a general approach to the treatment and prevention of infections in B-cell immunodeficiencies is presented.

The availability of IVIG has had a major impact on the treatment and prevention of infections in children with B-cell deficiencies (Liese et al., 1992; Yap, 1993). The routine prophylactic use of IVIG has decreased the incidence of acute bacterial infections from 0.40 per patient year to 0.06 per patient year (Quartier et al., 1999).

T-Cell Immunodeficiencies

There are many T-cell immunodeficiencies; these are described in Chapters 15 through 18; HIV-1 infection is discussed in Chapter 29. The prototype T-cell deficiency is thymic aplasia (DiGeorge syndrome), in which there is failure of development of the third and fourth pharyngeal pouches (DiGeorge, 1968); patients with this syndrome may have a marked T-cell defect, but their Ig levels are usually not depressed. In contrast, children with severe combined immunodeficiency syndrome have marked defects of both the B-cell and T-cell systems (Buckley, 1983; Rosen et al., 1984).

Severe infections in children with T-cell immunodeficiencies can be generated by organisms that cause common illnesses in healthy children. In addition, children with T-cell defects may contract severe disease from opportunistic infections with organisms that rarely cause disease in healthy hosts. Infectious agents that frequently cause disease in children with T-cell immunodeficiencies are presented in Table 41-4.

There are several unique infections in T-cell deficiency states (Hughes, 1993; Stiehm et al., 1986). Chronic diarrhea is caused by *Cryptosporidium* sp., *Giardia*

TABLE 41-4 · INFECTION IN THE HOST COMPROMISED BY B- AND T-CELL IMMUNODEFICIENCY SYNDROMES

Immunodeficiency Syndrome	Opportunistic Organisms Isolated Most Frequently	Approach to Treatment of Infections	Prevention of Infections
B-cell immunodeficiences	Encapsulated bacteria (*Streptococcus pneumoniae, Staphylococcus aureus, Haemophilus influenzae,* and *Neisseria meningitidis*), *Pseudomonas aeruginosa, Campylobacter* sp., enteroviruses, rotaviruses, *Giardia lamblia, Cryptosporidium* sp., *Pneumocystis jiroveci (carinii), Ureaplasma urealyticum,* and *Mycoplasma pneumoniae*	1. IVIG 200–800 mg/kg 2. Vigorous attempt to obtain specimens for culture before antimicrobial therapy 3. Incision and drainage if abscess present 4. Antibiotic selection on the basis of sensitivity data	1. Maintenance IVIG for patients with quantitative and qualitative defects in IgG metabolism (200–800 mg/kg q3–5wk) 2. In chronic recurrent respiratory disease, vigorous attention to postural drainage 3; in selected cases (recurrent or chronic pulmonary or middle ear), prophylactic administration of ampicillin, penicillin, or trimethoprim-sulfamethoxazole
T-cell immunodeficiencies	Encapsulated bacteria (*S. pneumoniae, H. influenzae, S. aureus*), facultative intracellular bacteria (*Mycobacterium tuberculosis,* other *Mycobacterium* sp., and *Listeria monocytogenes*); *Escherichia coli; Pseudomonas aeruginosa; Enterobacter* sp.; *Klebsiella* sp.; *Serratia marcescens; Salmonella* sp.; *Nocardia* sp.; viruses (cytomegalovirus, herpes simplex virus, varicella-zoster virus, Epstein-Barr virus, rotaviruses, adenoviruses, enteroviruses, respiratory syncytial virus, measles virus, vaccinia virus, and parainfluenzae viruses); protozoa (*Toxoplasma gondii* and *Cryptosporidium* sp.); and fungi (*Candida* sp., *Cryptococcus neoformans, Histoplasma capsulatum,* and *Pneumocystis jiroveci [carinii]*)	1. Vigorous attempt to obtain specimens for culture before antimicrobial therapy 2. Incision and drainage if abscess present 3. Antibiotic selection on the basis of sensitivity data 4. Early antiviral treatment for herpes simplex, cytomegalovirus, and varicella-zoster viral infections 5. Topical and nonadsorbable antimicrobial agents frequently are useful	1. Prophylactic administration of trimethoprim-sulfamethoxazole for prevention of *P. carinii* pneumonia 2. Oral nonadsorbable antimicrobial agents to lower concentration of gut flora 3. No live virus vaccines or bacillus Calmette-Guérin vaccine 4. Careful tuberculosis screening

IVIG = intravenous immunoglobulin.

lamblia, and rotaviruses, and chronic pulmonary infection is caused by respiratory syncytial virus, parainfluenza viruses, cytomegalovirus, and adenoviruses. Persistent *C. albicans* infections involving the mucous membranes, scalp, skin, and nails occur in chronic mucocutaneous candidiasis.

Males with X-linked lymphoproliferative syndrome have a specific immune defect to Epstein-Barr virus (see Chapter 17). When a person is infected with this virus, a severe or fatal infection occurs because of a killer cell response directed against both infected and uninfected cells (Sullivan et al., 1983). Recently, it has been proposed that 2B4 surface molecules that have reverted inhibitory action are responsible for the inability of natural killer cells to kill Epstein-Barr virus–infected cells (Parolini et al., 2000). Cord blood stem cell transplantation has been successfully undertaken to reconstitute the immune system in two brothers with X-linked lymphoproliferative syndrome before they were exposed to Epstein-Barr virus (Ziegner et al., 2001).

Children with cartilage-hair hypoplasia, a rare autosomal recessive disorder with short-limbed dwarfism, are particularly susceptible to severe varicella-zoster and vaccinia infections (Hong et al., 1972) (see Chapter 17). In a report of 108 patients with cartilage-hair hypoplasia,

it was noted that 56% had been unusually susceptible to infections and 5.5% had died of primary infectious complications (Makitie and Kaitila, 1993). In children with combined immunodeficiency, death has followed immunization with live viral vaccines or with BCG (Hitzig et al., 1968; Rosen and Janeway, 1964).

An approach to treatment and prevention of infections in patients with T-cell immunodeficiencies is presented in Table 41-4.

Selective IgA Deficiency

Selective IgA deficiency (see Chapter 14) occurs in approximately one in 700 persons. Many afflicted persons are healthy; others have recurrent respiratory or gastrointestinal infection, or both (Burgio et al., 1980; Shyur and Hill, 1991). A 20-year follow-up study of 159 blood donors with primary selective IgA deficiency who were initially healthy revealed that those who had severe deficiency (IgA < 5 mg/dl) had a higher incidence of pneumonia and other respiratory infections than those with values that were above 80 mg/dl (Koskinen, 1996). Infections in children with selective IgA deficiency should be treated vigorously with specific antimicrobial agents indicated by appropriate cultures. Immune serum globulin treatment is contraindicated in selective IgA deficiency because the product contains insufficient amounts of IgA for adequate replacement but sufficient amounts to sensitize the patient so that anti-IgA antibodies develop.

Complement Immunodeficiencies

Complement immunodeficiencies are described in detail in Chapter 21. The complement deficiencies C2, C3, C5, C6, C7, and C8 have been associated with disseminated and recurrent infections with encapsulated and other bacterial organisms (Goldstein and Marder, 1983; Hyatt et al., 1981; McBride et al., 1991; Shyur and Hill, 1991; Stiehm et al., 1986). Specific organisms include S. pneumoniae, S. pyogenes, H. influenzae, N. meningitidis, Neisseria gonorrhoeae, S. aureus, Salmonella typhi, E. coli, other gram-negative enteric bacteria, Proteus sp., Pseudomonas sp., and Klebsiella sp. Illnesses have included septicemia, meningitis, pneumonia, sinusitis, endocarditis, and arthritis.

Patients with known infection-associated complement defects should be treated vigorously and for an extended duration with an appropriate antibiotic such as cefotaxime at the onset of febrile illnesses. Appropriate cultures before therapy will dictate further therapy. In life-threatening instances, the administration of complement-containing plasma may be beneficial. Children of appropriate age will benefit from pneumococcal, H. influenzae type B, and meningococcal vaccines.

Cystic Fibrosis

Children with cystic fibrosis experience premature death owing to pulmonary insufficiency, which results from chronic pulmonary infection (see Chapter 33). In these children, infections caused by S. aureus, P. aeruginosa, coliform bacteria, and Haemophilus sp. are common. The management of infection in children with cystic fibrosis is a major and continuous challenge. The early acquisition of P. aeruginosa infection is associated with increased morbidity and mortality (Nixon et al., 2001); the acquisition of mucoid strains is particularly associated with a worse outcome (Parad et al., 1999).

Recently, other bacterial species have been recognized in association with a poor outcome in patients with cystic fibrosis. The most prominent of these are Burkholderia cepacia and Stenotrophomonas maltophilia (LiPuma, 2000). In the antibiotic era, the longevity of children with cystic fibrosis has increased substantially. However, the exact role of antibiotics in this increased survival period is not clear. Several different methods of antibiotic administration are used at different cystic fibrosis centers, and there are few differences in outcome among these centers. At some centers, continuous prophylaxis with oral or aerosolized antibiotics is used. At other centers, antibiotics are used only at times of exacerbation of pulmonary symptoms.

There is little evidence to support the concept that continuous aerosolized and oral antibiotic prophylaxis diminishes the presence of pulmonary infection more than could be achieved by meticulous attention to pulmonary toilet without continuous antibiotic administration. Continuous administration of antibiotics (orally or by the aerosol route) may predispose the patient to colonization and infection with saprophytic strains of bacteria, which are resistant to multiple antibiotics.

The issue of antimicrobial resistance is even more important today because patients with cystic fibrosis live longer, and therefore more antimicrobial courses are given. Methicillin-resistant S. aureus is increasingly found in patients with cystic fibrosis (Miall et al., 2001). Ramsey and colleagues (1999) reported the results of two multicenter, placebo-controlled trials of inhaled tobramycin given intermittently in 4-week cycles. There was a moderate improvement in forced expiratory volume in the treatment group. However, patients were followed for only 24 weeks, so the long-term benefits, if any, remain unknown. In addition, there was an increase in the proportion of strains of Pseudomonas resistant to tobramycin observed during the study period.

We believe it is best to use antibiotics in children with cystic fibrosis at times when respiratory-related changes (e.g., fever, increased sputum, and increased breathing difficulty) occur. Therapy should be guided by sputum cultures, but in many instances of minor respiratory worsening, patients often will improve somewhat while taking antibiotics that would not be expected to be effective on the basis of sensitivity data. Oral cephalosporins, penicillinase-resistant penicillins, sulfonamides, ampicillin, and quinolones all enjoy frequent use. In children with greater clinical deterioration, parenteral antibiotics are indicated. If culture reveals a predominant growth of coagulase-positive staphylococci, a penicillin such as oxacillin is indicated. In the usual situation in which P. aeruginosa is the major organism in the sputum, therapy should include an aminoglycoside antibiotic to which the pathogen is sensitive. At the present time, gentamicin with ceftazidime or piperacillin is a satisfactory regimen. Sensitivity testing always should be performed so that when resistance to gentamicin is noted, another aminoglycoside (e.g., tobramycin or amikacin) can be used.

Diabetes Mellitus

Children and adults with diabetes mellitus have a decreased resistance to bacterial and fungal infections (see Chapter 25). Pyelonephritis and perinephric abscesses caused by S. aureus and S. epidermidis, E. coli, and Proteus have been reported frequently (McCabe, 1972; Vejlsgaard, 1973). The increased incidence of bacteremia and pyelonephritis in patients with diabetes may be attributable, in part, to a greater frequency of hospitalization and catheterization.

Infection by Mucor, C. glabrata, and Candida sp. has been noted with greater frequency in children with diabetes mellitus than in the healthy host. It is of interest that *Mucor* (Baker and Severance, 1948; Marks et al., 1970; Martin et al., 1954) was not reported in the United States until 1943, shortly after the introduction of antibiotic therapy, but diabetes mellitus and other diseases associated with an increased risk of *Mucor* infection have been present for centuries (Gregory et al., 1943). This suggests that the increased frequency of fungal disease is related to the repeated use of antibiotics. The management of infection in children with diabetes depends on careful attention to even trivial infections. Cultures should be done and appropriate antibiotic therapy instituted.

INFECTION IN CHILDREN COMPROMISED BY ACQUIRED DISORDERS OF IMMUNITY

Malignancy

In children with cancer, infection is a major problem and also may be a terminal event (Brown, 1984; Chanock and Pizzo, 1997; Friedman et al., 1984; Hughes et al., 1984; Jackson et al., 1982; Katz and Mustafa, 1993; Koll and Brown, 1993; Kosmidis, 1980; Lewis et al., 1985; Miser and Miser, 1980; Nachman and Honig, 1980; Pizzo et al., 1991a, 1991b; Saarinen, 1984; Siegel et al., 1980; Steele, 1985; Wong and Ogra, 1983; see also Chapter 26).

In general, children with solid tumors have less frequent, less severe infections than do children with lymphoproliferative diseases (Hughes et al., 1974; Levine et al., 1974; Nachman and Honig, 1980). Hughes and colleagues (1974), in a study of 482 children with malignancies, noted that infection was most common in children with leukemia and least common in those with Wilms' tumor. Disseminated infections were more likely in lymphoproliferative diseases, whereas localized infections were more frequent with solid tumors. In an analysis of fever and neutropenia in children with neoplastic disease, Nachman and Honig (1980) noted an infection rate of 36.7% in children with leukemia, whereas the rate was only 15% in children with solid tumors. Septicemia occurred in 58.3% of the children with leukemia and in 35.7% of those children with solid tumors. In contrast, 42.8% of infections in children with solid tumors were pulmonary, whereas lung infections accounted for only 25% of the infections in children with leukemia.

However, in a recent prospective study, Auletta and colleagues (1999) reported similar infection rates in patients with solid tumors and leukemia (0.66 and 0.68 per 100 patient days, respectively).

Therapeutic maneuvers that are associated with a minimal risk of infection in the healthy host become significant hazards to children with cancer. IV fluids, scalp vein needles, indwelling IV and urinary catheters, transfusions, and the use of respirators all have been associated with opportunistic infection in children with cancer. Bronchial or urinary tract obstruction by tumor growth also may predispose them to infection.

Chemotherapy may be complicated by gangrenous stomatitis and necrotizing enteropathy, which may be associated with septicemia due to gram-negative or anaerobic organisms. Rectal fissures and perirectal abscesses may serve as sources of infection in children with cancer, and fatal infections have developed in patients with Hodgkin's disease after splenectomy performed for staging of the disease.

The single most important factor that predisposes patients with cancer to infection is granulocytopenia (Auletta et al., 1999; Bodey et al., 1966; Hughes, 1971; Katz and Mustafa, 1993; Rolston, 1999; Viscoli et al., 1999). In an extensive study, Bodey (1984) noted that the incidence of infectious episodes in persons with leukemia increased with decreasing blood granulocyte levels.

An absolute neutrophil count of 500 cells/mm^3 is a critical value. Below this value, the risk of infection is high. In addition, the duration of granulocytopenia is directly related to the risk of developing infection. Bodey and associates (1966) demonstrated that the risk and severity of infection is highest in patients with profound (<100 cells/mm^3) and prolonged (lasting more than 14 days) neutropenia.

Granulocytopenia in patients with cancer may be related to their primary disease or may be the result of the therapy provided. In some cases, neutrophil function may be impaired in children with leukemia both in relapse and in remission, even though the number of circulating leukocytes is normal (Skeel et al., 1971; Strauss et al., 1970). Decreased chemotaxis and digestive capacity of neutrophils have been reported in patients with Hodgkin's disease and myelocytic leukemia (Holland et al., 1971; Rosner et al., 1970).

Lymphopenia or a deficiency in T-lymphocyte function, or both, may contribute to the development of viral or fungal disease in patients with cancer (Bodey et al., 1966; Levy and Kaplan, 1974). Patients with lymphoma are particularly susceptible to infection produced by facultative intracellular organisms, and in these individuals, macrophage function may be altered (Sinkovics and Smith, 1970).

No reduction in the concentration of serum Igs or complement components has been noted in most patients with leukemia or lymphoma, other than that induced by chemotherapy (Gooch and Fernbach, 1971; Ragab et al., 1970). The levels of specific antibodies, however, may be decreased. In children with acute leukemia who were receiving combination chemotherapy, heat-stable opsonins specific for *P. aeruginosa* fell precipitously, whereas those specific for *S. epidermidis* remained unchanged (Wollman et al., 1975).

Because of the extensive immunologic defects in children with malignancies, the spectrum of agents associated with opportunistic infections is great and involves both aerobic and anaerobic gram-positive and gram-negative bacteria, fungi, viruses, and protozoa. The incidence of infections caused by specific microbial agents varies among geographic areas and hospital centers and during different time periods in the same location.

A listing of the more usual causative agents in serious infections, in addition to an approach to infection prevention and treatment, is presented in Table 41-5. In an analysis of fatal infections in children with leukemia, Hughes (1971) noted that gram-negative bacillary organisms were the etiologic agents in more than half of the study group. *P. aeruginosa* was the most common etiologic agent noted. Surprisingly, one fifth of the infections were attributable to *C. albicans* and only 17 of the 199 infections were attributable to *S. aureus*. There were 11 terminal viral infections, and eight fatalities were caused by protozoa.

TABLE 41-5 · INFECTION IN THE HOST COMPROMISED BY MALIGNANCY, IMMUNOSUPPRESSION, OR TRANSPLANTATION

Category	Opportunistic Organisms Isolated Most Frequently	Approach to Treatment of Infections	Prevention of Infections
Malignancy	Bacteria—*Pseudomonas aeruginosa* and other sp., *Escherichia coli*, *Enterobacter* sp., *Klebsiella* sp., *Acinetobacter* sp., *Proteus* sp., *Serratia* sp., other gram-negative bacilli, *Bacteroides* sp. and other anaerobes, *Staphylococcus aureus*, *Staphylococcus epidermidis*, *Streptococcus* sp., enterococci, diphtheroids, *Listeria* sp., *Haemophilus influenzae*, *Salmonella* sp., and *Mycobacterium tuberculosis* and other *Mycobacterium* sp. Fungi—*Candida albicans* and other *Candida* sp., *Aspergillus* sp., *Cryptococcus neoformans*, *Histoplasma capsulatum*, *Fusarium* sp., *Pneumocystis jiroveci (carinii)*, *Trichosporon beigelii*, *Curvularia* sp., and *Mucor* sp. Viruses—Varicella-zoster virus, cytomegalovirus, herpes simplex, hepatitis B and C, Epstein-Barr, adenoviruses, measles, and papovavirus Parasites—*Toxoplasma gondii*, *Cryptosporidium* sp., and *Strongyloides stercoralis*	1. Obtain appropriate Gram stain smears and specimens for culture (blood, urine, CSF, intravenous sites, and wounds), even of minor lesions, before the onset of therapy 2. When possible, choose antibiotic combinations for specific etiologic agents (use bactericidal rather than bacteriostatic antibiotics) 3. With the occurrence of fever (three oral temperature readings of 38°C in a 24-hour period or a single temperature of ≥38.5°C), initiate empiric antimicrobial therapy; several regimens have been successful; a cost-effective approach is monotherapy with ceftazidime 4. Once therapy has been begun, allow ample time for effect; therapy should rarely last fewer than 7 days; in patients with neutropenia, continue therapy until the absolute neutrophil count is >500 cells/mm³ 5. Institute empiric therapy with antifungal agents in patients who are neutropenic with fever that is unresponsive to antibiotics	1. Prophylactic administration of trimethoprim-sulfamethoxazole to prevent *Pneumocystis carinii* pneumonia 2. Avoidance of unnecessary hospitalization 3. Avoidance of antibiotics and catheters unless specifically indicated 4. Routine surveillance culture specimens (throat, stool, and axilla) at regular intervals may be useful 5. Use of VZIG, IG, or IVIG (measles), in addition to HBIG, if exposed 6. Use of pneumococcal, *H. influenzae* type B, and influenza vaccines 7. Use of acyclovir (250 mg/M² q8h) in herpes simplex B–seropositive patients during intensive therapy for acute leukemia 8. Administration of varicella vaccine in children with acute lymphocytic leukemia in remission who have not had varicella
Immunosuppression	Same as Malignancy above	Same as Malignancy above	1. Avoidance of unnecessary hospitalization 2. Avoidance of antibiotics and catheters unless specifically indicated 3. Use of VZIG, IG, or IVIG (measles), in addition to HBIG, if exposed
Transplantation	Same as Malignancy above, plus: Bacteria—*Listeria monocytogenes* Viruses—Parainfluenzae, respiratory syncytial, and parvovirus B19 Fungi—*Coccidioides immitis* and *Blastomyces dermatitidis*	Same as Malignancy above, plus: Use of ganciclovir preemptive/early therapy for cytomegalovirus infections	Same as Malignancy above, plus: 1. Reduction of total bowel flora of microorganisms with nonadsorbable antibiotics 2. Removal of dietary items that may contain significant microbial contamination 3. When blood products are necessary, use (if possible) cytomegalovirus-seronegative products in patients who are cytomegalovirus-seronegative 4. Consideration of prophylactic ganciclovir in cytomegalovirus-seropositive transplant recipients or when the donor was seropositive and the recipient was seronegative

CSF = cerebrospinal fluid; HBIG = hepatitis B immune globulin; IG = human immune serum globulin; IV = intravenous; IVIG = human intravenous immune serum globulin; VZIG = varicella-zoster immune globulin.

In contrast with the findings of Hughes (1971), Saarinen (1984) surveyed infections in 100 children with acute lymphoblastic leukemia in Helsinki, Finland, and noted a total absence of disseminated candidiasis, a relative infrequency of gram-negative septicemia and a predominance of septicemias caused by gram-positive organisms. In 165 septic episodes in pediatric patients with leukemia and lymphoma at Memorial Sloan-Kettering Cancer Center, the most common etiologic agents were the following: *S. viridans*, 16.3%; *E. coli*, 15.2%; *Serratia* sp., 12.1%; *S. epidermidis*, 11.5%; *P. aeruginosa*, 9.1%; fungi, 7.3%; *Klebsiella* sp., 5.5%; and *S. aureus*, 4.9% (Brown, 1984).

Recently, Viscoli and colleagues (1999) presented prospective data from 18 centers, encompassing 191 bloodstream infections in children with malignancies; two thirds of all episodes occurred in neutropenic children. Forty-five percent of infections were caused by gram-positive pathogens, 41% by gram-negative bacteria, 9% by fungi, and 5% were polymicrobial infections. The main risk factor was the presence of an indwelling catheter. Mortality was higher in patients with neutropenia than in patients without neutropenia (15% vs. 4%) and in recipients of bone marrow transplant (21%); in children with acute leukemia (11%) or solid tumors (6%), mortality was also lower than in those with neutropenia. Patients with fungal infections had a higher mortality (22%) than patients with gram-positive (11%) or gram-negative bacteremias (6%).

Recent changes in the patterns of infections in patients with malignancies are (1) an increase in infections caused by gram-positive cocci (coagulase-negative staphylococci, *Streptococcus* sp., and *Enterococcus* sp.), (2) a decrease in infections caused by *E. coli* and an increase in infections by other *Enterobacteriaceae* (e.g., *Klebsiella* sp., *Enterobacter* sp., and *Serratia* sp.) and non–*Enterobacteriaceae*-fermentatitive and nonfermentative bacilli, and (3) the emergence of multiple-resistant infectious organisms (Koll and Brown, 1993).

In leukemia, the cause of fever and presumed infection is associated with the stage of disease (Kosmidis et al., 1980). At the time of diagnosis of leukemia, the cause of fever is found in only approximately one third of patients. Of the infections documented, approximately one third are bacterial and two thirds are viral. During induction therapy, fever is usually caused by bacterial infection. During remission, most fevers are attributable to viral infections; during relapse, febrile episodes are most commonly caused by viruses, bacteria, and fungi. Documented bacterial and fungal septic episodes virtually always are associated with severe neutropenia. Pneumonia caused by *P. jiroveci (carinii)* usually does not occur early in the course of childhood malignant disease but is noted during remission and relapse (Siegel et al., 1980).

Immunosuppression

Immunosuppressive therapy is used in a large number of human diseases, such as rheumatoid arthritis and other connective tissue diseases, inflammatory bowel disease, chronic active hepatitis, several hematologic diseases, nephrotic syndrome and nephritis, many allergic conditions, and a large number of other poorly understood illnesses (Skinner and Schwartz, 1972). Immunosuppressive therapy is also used in organ transplantation, and drugs that cause immunosuppression are an integral part of cancer chemotherapy. Opportunistic infection in malignancies has been presented earlier in this chapter, and infection problems related to organ transplantation are covered in a subsequent section of this chapter.

Infections are responsible for significant morbidity and mortality in children undergoing immunosuppressive therapy (see Chapter 27). The incidence of infections and their etiology and severity are dependent on both the basic underlying disease process and the immunosuppressive agents used.

Experimental evidence suggests that predisposition to infection in patients who have been immunosuppressed with steroids is a reflection of a multifaceted derangement of the normal mechanisms of host resistance. This may include depression of leukocyte chemotaxis and local inflammatory responses, interference with the acquisition or expression of cell-mediated functions, impairment of phagocytosis and killing of bacteria, and depression of interferon synthesis (Claman, 1972; Dale and Petersdorf, 1973; Didonato et al., 1996; Ward, 1966; Zurier and Weissman, 1973).

Nitrogen mustard, cyclophosphamide, busulfan, and chlorambucil (biologic alkylating agents); cytosine arabinoside, 5-fluorouracil, azathioprine, 6-mercaptopurine, and 6-thioguanine (antimetabolites); methotrexate (a folic acid antagonist); and cyclosporine all interfere with the replication of cells. These drugs may suppress primary and secondary antibody responses and delayed hypersensitivity in some individuals (Schwartz, 1965; Steinberg et al., 1972; see also Chapter 27).

It is clear that immunosuppressive therapy increases the general risk of opportunistic infection, but it is difficult to quantitate this risk and to separate it from the risk associated with the disease for which immunosuppression was undertaken. For example, a short course of corticosteroid therapy in asthma is of little increased risk to the patient. In contrast, the risk is considerably greater in the child receiving long-term therapy for an illness such as systemic lupus erythematosus.

The spectrum of possible opportunistic infection associated with immunosuppression includes all the microorganisms listed in Table 41-5. The possibilities in any specific patient depend on his or her endogenous and exogenous surroundings at the time of suppressive therapy. The nonhospitalized child is particularly at extra risk to common viral and bacterial contagious diseases and to factors associated with the home environment (e.g., bacteria and viruses from household pets, fungi in the soil). In contrast, the frequently hospitalized child has a much greater risk of systemic infection with nosocomial, highly resistant bacteria.

It should be remembered that all live viral vaccines generally are contraindicated in immunosuppressed children. An approach to the prevention and treatment of infections is presented in Table 41-5.

Transplantation

Organ and tissue transplantation in children is presented in detail in Chapter 43. Opportunistic infections are common in recipients of transplant and are a threat both to the patient's life and the survival of the transplanted tissue. Immunosuppressive therapy is an integral part of the process of transplantation; predictably, infections after transplantation are similar to those associated with immunosuppression. In addition, the transplantation process per se and the rejection process predispose the host to infection, particularly with viruses. Infection risks and the microorganisms involved are also related to the organ or tissue being transplanted (renal, liver, heart, or bone marrow).

A general listing of the causes of infection and an approach to prevention and treatment are presented in Table 41-5.

Kidney Transplantation

Renal transplantation in children is presently very successful, with 1-, 2-, and 5-year graft survival rates of 91%, 87%, and 77%, respectively, for living-related kidney transplants and 81%, 75%, and 61%, respectively, for cadaveric kidney transplants (Benfeld et al., 1999). However, infections are common and are a major cause of morbidity and mortality (Brayman et al., 1992; Harmon, 1991; Najarian et al., 1986; Potter et al., 1986; Smith and McDonald, 2000).

Early infections after transplantation are most often bacterial and involve the urinary tract, the graft and wound site, vascular catheters, and the lungs (Deen and Blumberg, 1993; So and Simmons, 1992). Urinary tract infections are most common and are attributable to *E. coli* and other gram-negative bacilli, enterococci, and coagulase-negative staphylococci.

Late-onset infections involve a multitude of opportunistic agents. Predisposing factors include immunosuppression, graft rejection, and antibiotics. The etiologic agents of most importance are cytomegalovirus, Epstein-Barr virus, herpes simplex virus, varicella virus, *Candida* sp., *Aspergillus* sp., *Mycobacterium* sp., *Toxoplasma gondii*, and *P. jiroveci (carinii)*. Deaths are often attributable to polymicrobial infections involving cytomegalovirus and bacterial, fungal, or parasitic agents.

Cytomegalovirus is the most common viral opportunistic infection in the recipient of a transplant (Kanj et al., 1996). Cytomegalovirus infection can be a primary infection when a seronegative recipient receives a kidney from a seropositive donor or it can be reinfection in seropositive recipients. Several approaches have been used to prevent cytomegalovirus infections. These include IVIG, cytomegalovirus Ig, high-dose oral acyclovir, and ganciclovir (Conti et al., 1993; Pakkala et al., 1992; Prokurat et al., 1993; Snydman, 1993; So and Simmons, 1992; Turgeon et al., 1998; Werner et al., 1993), in addition to the use of seronegative blood products. The use of antiviral prophylaxis with ganciclovir has been beneficial, but the best way to use this drug remains a matter of controversy.

The two most common approaches are universal prophylaxis and pre-emptive therapy. Universal prophylaxis involves the prolonged use of ganciclovir in all recipients of transplants, regardless of the risk of cytomegalovirus disease. Pre-emptive, or early, therapy uses ganciclovir in recipients of transplants when early replication of cytomegalovirus is detected, in an attempt to stop the progression of asymptomatic infection into cytomegalovirus disease. The relative advantages and limitations of both methods remain controversial matters (Singh et al., 2000).

The main unresolved issues related to pre-emptive therapy are its efficacy, the optimal surveillance strategies, the reliability of the diagnostic tools, the cost of prophylaxis, the potential for emergence of resistant viral strains, the impact on indirect sequelae, and the epidemiology of cytomegalovirus disease. Neither universal prophylaxis nor pre-emptive therapy appears to be ideal. The lack of carefully planned studies in the target population remains a major problem.

Liver Transplantation

Today, liver transplantation offers hope to children with acute fulminant hepatic failure and end-stage chronic liver disease (Kuhls and Leach, 1992; Yamanaka et al., 2000). Of children receiving transplants, 70% to 90% survive for 1 year and long-term survivals are common. However, serious infections after transplantation occur in 40% to 70% of pediatric patients and infection is the leading cause of death (Andrews et al., 1987; Hiatt et al., 1987; Vacanti et al., 1987; Yamanaka et al., 2000; Zitelli et al., 1987).

Children with liver transplants have similar risks of infection as other recipients of solid-organ transplants. In addition, they have an added risk from the gastrointestinal flora, which is in direct contact with the biliary drainage system, and the frequent occurrence of postoperative biliary stasis or vascular insufficiency, or both, resulting in ischemia in a segment of the liver.

Common locations of infection in children with liver transplants are the wound, the central venous catheter, the liver, the extrahepatic intra-abdominal region, the urinary tract, and the lung. The major causes of liver and extrahepatic intra-abdominal infections are bacteria and include gram-negative enteric bacilli, *P. aeruginosa*, streptococci, enterococci, and enteric anaerobes. Anaerobes are the most prevalent organisms in the flora of the large bowel, but they are a relatively infrequent cause of post-transplantation infection. Infections caused by *Candida* sp. also are common. Cytomegalovirus and adenoviruses also may cause hepatitis.

Infections related to immunosuppression are similar to those in other recipients of transplants and include viruses (e.g., cytomegalovirus, varicella-zoster, Epstein-Barr, herpes simplex, adenoviruses, parvovirus B19, respiratory viruses, hepatitis viruses, human herpesvirus 6), protozoa (*T. gondii* and *Cryptosporidium parvum*), and endogenous fungi and bacteria (*Histoplasma capsulatum*, *P. jiroveci (carinii)*, *Mycobacterium tuberculosis*, and other *Mycobacterium* sp.) (Kuhls and Leach, 1992;

Lautenschlager et al., 2000; Nour et al., 1993; Younes et al., 2000). Cytomegalovirus infection was discussed in the kidney transplantation section of this chapter.

The rate of infections after liver transplantation can be reduced by using perioperative antibiotics intravenously, nonabsorbable antibiotics orally, seronegative blood products, and perhaps high-dose acyclovir (Bailey et al., 1993; Mollison et al., 1993; Saliba et al., 1993; Singh et al., 2000; Smith et al., 1993; Turgeon et al., 1998).

Heart Transplantation

Compared with renal, liver, and bone marrow transplantation, the experience in children with heart transplantation is relatively limited (Fricker et al., 1987; Gajarski et al., 1998; Green et al., 1989; Kaplan, 1992; Schowengerdt et al., 1997). Children with heart transplants have similar risks of infections resulting from immunosuppression as do recipients of liver transplants.

The most important early postoperative infections are similar to those that are associated with other major thoracic surgeries, including pneumonia, mediastinitis, lung abscess, and wound infections. Common causative organisms include *Pseudomonas* sp. and other gram-negative bacilli, *Staphylococcus* sp., streptococci, and other organisms of the upper respiratory tract flora.

Respiratory viruses (respiratory syncytial virus, influenza viruses, and adenoviruses) are also an important cause of morbidity and mortality during the early postoperative period. Late infections in patients with heart transplants are similar to those that occur in recipients of liver transplants. The approach to cytomegalovirus infection in those with heart transplants is similar to that discussed previously in the kidney transplantation section of this chapter.

Bone Marrow Transplantation

Infection and graft-versus-host disease and the interaction between these two factors are the major sources of morbidity and mortality in recipients of bone marrow transplants (Hiemenz and Greene, 1993; Sable and Donowitz, 1994; Walter and Bowden, 1995; Wasserman et al., 1988; Winston et al., 1979; Zaia, 1992). The major difference between bone marrow transplantation and solid organ transplantation is the occurrence of neutropenia in all recipients of bone marrow transplants.

There is an extensive literature related to the prevention and treatment of infections in bone marrow transplantation; however, there are few studies that deal exclusively with children. This is an important omission because, in general, children tolerate many antimicrobial agents, such as aminoglycosides and amphotericin B, better than do adults and also accept certain unpleasant regimens, such as the oral use of nonabsorbable antibiotics, with better compliance.

The infection risks in bone marrow transplantation can be separated into four time periods:

1. Pretransplantation
2. Pre-engraftment
3. Early postengraftment
4. Late postengraftment

The occurrence of infection during the pretransplantation period depends on the underlying condition and its stage of treatment. Neutropenia is the main defect. The most common infections are bacteremias and septicemias caused by aerobic gram-negative bacilli and local infections (skin, soft tissue, intraoral, and urinary), which result from cutaneous local flora.

The pre-engraftment period begins with the onset of neutropenia, lasts 4 to 6 weeks, and is always associated with mucositis. Bacterial infections predominate during this period. In the past, the most common systemic infections were caused by gram-negative bacilli, either from the patient's enteric flora or from the hospital environment. Infection with these organisms is still common, but in recent years, there has been an increase in aerobic gram-positive coccal infections attributable to *S. aureus*, *S. epidermidis*, streptococci, and enterococci. Opportunistic fungal infections also occur, with those attributable to *Candida* sp. being most common. Severe hemorrhagic mucositis caused by the reactivation of latent herpes simplex virus is also common.

The early postengraftment period, which lasts for approximately 1 to 3 months after transplantation, is indicated by absolute neutrophil count values increasing to higher than 500 cells/mm³. With the recovery from neutropenia, the risk of gram-negative and gram-positive bacterial sepsis is reduced. During this period, there is severe combined immunodeficiency; this problem may be complicated by graft-versus-host disease and its treatment. A major problem in this period is the reactivation of latent cytomegalovirus or primary infection in a previously cytomegalovirus-seronegative patient. The manifestations of cytomegalovirus infection include asymptomatic virus shedding, fever, hepatitis, leukopenia, thrombocytopenia, gastrointestinal disease, and pneumonia.

Other infectious risks during this period are attributable to adenoviruses, Epstein-Barr virus, influenza viruses, human herpesvirus 6, parvovirus B19, parainfluenza viruses, respiratory syncytial virus, JC virus, BK virus, *Candida sp.*, *Aspergillus* sp., and other environment fungi, *P. jiroveci (carinii)*, and *T. gondii*.

The late post-engraftment period is complicated by chronic graft-versus-host disease and its treatment. A major problem in this period is the reactivation of latent varicella-zoster virus and frequent dissemination of the disease. The approach to cytomegalovirus infection in bone marrow transplantation is similar to that discussed in the kidney transplantation section earlier in this chapter. Another risk factor that must be considered during this period is infection caused by encapsulated organisms such as *S. pneumoniae, H. influenzae,* and *N. meningitidis.*

The approach to prevention and treatment of infections in recipients of bone marrow transplants is outlined in Table 41-5. Hemorrhagic mucositis can be prevented by the prophylactic use of acyclovir, and *P. carinii* pneumonia can be prevented by the prophylactic use of trimethoprim-sulfamethoxazole. The use of clotrimazole troches or nystatin has reduced the frequency and severity of oropharyngeal candidiasis, and the use of oral nonabsorbable antimicrobials has reduced the occurrence of sepsis attributable to gram-negative bacilli.

The empiric treatment of febrile episodes with broad-spectrum antibiotics and of persistent fevers with amphotericin B has decreased the rates of morbidity and mortality during the period of neutropenia.

Acquired Immunodeficiency Syndrome

By definition, acquired immunodeficiency syndrome (AIDS) occurs when an HIV-infected person has an opportunistic infection or evidence of severe immunosuppression (Table 41-6) (CDC, 1987, 1992, 1994). In Chapter 29, the historical, epidemiologic, and immunologic aspects of HIV infections in children are presented. In this chapter, specific infections and their diagnosis and treatment in HIV-infected children are discussed.

Patients with AIDS have a broad-based immunodeficiency that involves the following cells: T cells, macrophages, monocytes, B cells, and natural killer cells (Flynn and Shenep, 1992; Hanson and Shearer, 1998). Combined effects include depletion of CD4 lymphocytes, diminished or absence of delayed-type hypersensitivity, decreased production of interleukin-2 and interferon-γ, depletion of T cells, impaired chemotaxis and phagocytosis, decreased specific antibody response to specific antigen challenge, hypergammaglobulinemia, and impaired cytotoxicity.

The classification system for HIV infection in children younger than 13 years of age is presented in Table 41-6. The clinical categories for children with HIV infection are presented in Table 41-7, and conditions included in the 1993 AIDS surveillance case definition for adolescents and adults are presented in Table 41-8.

Today almost all new HIV infections in young children in industrialized countries are a result of the antenatal or peripartum transmission of the virus from an infected mother. However, transmission through breast-feeding continues to occur in many areas of the world.

Clinical manifestations of illness in children infected with HIV can be due to the primary HIV infection, the exaggerated and persistent effects of a congenital infection (e.g., cytomegalovirus, *T. gondii*), the exaggerated and often persistent effects of a regular human pathogen (e.g., respiratory syncytial virus), exaggerated anatomically localized infections (e.g., otitis media), and true opportunistic infections with organisms that do not cause disease in healthy hosts (Barnett et al., 1992; Chandwani et al., 1990; Falloon et al., 1989; Flynn and Shenep, 1992; Frenkel et al., 1990; Hanson, 1993; Hanson and Shearer, 1998; Hoyt et al., 1992; Krasinski et al., 1988; Leggiadro et al., 1991; Leibowitz et al., 1990, 1991, 1993; Lewis et al., 1992; Mitchell et al., 1990; Oleske et al., 1983; Principi et al., 1991; Rubinstein, 1983; Rutstein et al., 1993; Scott, 1991; Scott et al., 1984; Shannon and Ammann, 1985; Vandersteenhoven et al., 1992; Vernon et al., 1988).

Eighty percent of untreated HIV-infected newborns have clinical manifestations of disease during the first 24 months of life (Scott, 1991). Initial manifestations may be nonspecific and include hepatomegaly or splenomegaly, or both; generalized lymphadenopathy; failure to thrive; and developmental delay.

Recurrent bacterial infections with common pediatric pathogens (*H. influenzae* type B, *S. pneumoniae*,

TABLE 41-6 · CLINICAL AND IMMUNOLOGIC CLASSIFICATION OF PEDIATRIC HIV INFECTION IN CHILDREN YOUNGER THAN 13 YEARS OF AGE*

	Clinical Classifications[†]				Immunologic Categories					
					Age-Specific CD4+ T-Lymphocyte Count and Percentage of Total Lymphocytes[‡]					
					<12 mo		1–5 yr		6–12 yr	
Immunologic Definitions	N	A	B[§]	C[§]	mm³	%	mm³	%	mm³	%
1: No evidence of suppression	N1	A1	B1	C1	≥1500	≥25	≥1000	≥25	≥500	≥25
2: Evidence of suppression	N2	A2	B2	C2	750–1499	15–24	500–999	15–24	200–499	15–24
3: Severe suppression	N3	A3	B3	C3	<750	<15	<500	<15	<200	<15

*Modified from Centers for Disease Control and Prevention. 1994 revised classification system for human immunodeficiency virus infection in children less than 13 years of age: official authorized addenda: human immunodeficiency virus infection codes and official guidelines for coding and reporting ICD-9-CM. MMWR 43(RR-12):1–19, 1994.
[†]Children whose HIV infection status is not confirmed are classified by using this grid with a letter E (for perinatally exposed) placed before the appropriate classification code (e.g., EN2)."
[‡]To convert values in microliters to Système International units (×109/L), multiply by 0.001.
[§]Lymphoid interstitial pneumonitis in category B or category C is reportable to state and local health departments as acquired immunodeficiency syndrome (see Table 41-7 for further definition of clinical categories).
A = mild signs and symptoms; B = moderate signs and symptoms; C = severe signs and symptoms; HIV = human immunodeficiency virus; N = no signs or symptoms.
Modified from American Academy of Pediatrics. Human immunodeficiency virus infection. In Pickering L, ed. 2000 Red Book: Report of the Committee on Infectious Diseases, 25th ed. Elk Grove Village, IL, American Academy of Pediatrics, 2000, Table 3.25, p 327.

TABLE 41-7 · CLINICAL CATEGORIES FOR CHILDREN YOUNGER THAN 13 YEARS OF AGE WITH HIV INFECTION

Category N: Not Symptomatic
Children who have no signs or symptoms considered to be the result of HIV infection or have only one of the conditions listed in Category A

Category A: Mildly Symptomatic
Children with two or more of the conditions listed but none of the conditions listed in Categories B and C
· Lymphadenopathy (>0.5 cm at more than two sites; bilateral at one site)
· Hepatomegaly
· Splenomegaly
· Dermatitis
· Parotitis
· Recurrent or persistent upper respiratory tract infection, sinusitis, or otitis media

Category B: Moderately Symptomatic
Children who have symptomatic conditions other than those listed for Category A or C that are attributed to HIV infection
· Anemia (hemoglobin, <8 g/dl [<80 g/L]), neutropenia (white blood cell count, <1000/μl [<1.0 × 109/L]), or thrombocytopenia (platelet count, <100 × 103/μl [<100 × 109/L]), or all, persisting for >30 days
· Bacterial meningitis, pneumonia, or sepsis (single episode)
· Candidiasis or oropharyngeal (thrush), persisting (>2 mo) in children older than 6 mo of age
· Cardiomyopathy
· Cytomegalovirus infection, with onset before 1 mo of age
· Diarrhea, recurrent or chronic
· Hepatitis
· HSV stomatitis, recurrent (more than two episodes within 1 year)
· HSV bronchitis, pneumonitis, or esophagitis with onset before 1 mo of age
· Herpes zoster (shingles) involving at least two distinct episodes or more than one dermatome
· Leiomyosarcoma
· Lymphoid interstitial pneumonia or pulmonary lymphoid hyperplasia complex
· Nephropathy
· Nocardiosis
· Persistent fever (lasting >1 mo)
· Toxoplasmosis, onset before 1 mo of age
· Varicella, disseminated (complicated chickenpox)

Category C: Severely Symptomatic
· Serious bacterial infections, multiple or recurrent (i.e., any combination of at least two culture-confirmed infections within a 2-yr period), of the following types: septicemia, pneumonia, meningitis, bone or joint infection, or abscess of an internal organ or body cavity (excluding otitis media, superficial skin or mucosal abscesses, and indwelling catheter-related infections)
· Candidiasis, esophageal or pulmonary (i.e., involving the bronchi, trachea, or lungs)
· Coccidioidomycosis, disseminated (at site other than or in addition to lungs or cervical or hilar lymph nodes)
· Cryptococcosis, extrapulmonary
· Cryptosporidiosis or isosporiasis with diarrhea persisting >1 mo
· Cytomegalovirus disease with onset of symptoms after 1 mo of age (at a site other than liver, spleen, or lymph nodes)
· Encephalopathy (at least one of the following progressive findings present for at least 2 mo in the absence of a concurrent illness other than HIV infection that could explain the findings):
  (1) Failure to attain or loss of developmental milestones or loss of intellectual ability, verified by standard developmental scale or neuropsychological tests
  (2) Impaired brain growth or acquired microcephaly demonstrated by head circumference measurements or brain atrophy demonstrated by computed tomography or magnetic resonance imaging (serial imaging required for children younger than 2 yr of age)
  (3) Acquired symmetric motor deficit manifested by two or more of the following: paresis, pathologic reflexes, ataxia, or gait disturbance
· HSV infection causing a mucocutaneous ulcer that persists for longer than 1 mo or bronchitis, pneumonitis, or esophagitis for any duration affecting a child older than 1 mo of age
· Histoplasmosis, disseminated (at a site other than or in addition to lungs or cervical or hilar lymph nodes)
· Kaposi's sarcoma
· Lymphoma, primary, in brain
· Lymphoma, small, noncleaved cell (Burkitt's), or immunoblastic, or large-cell lymphoma of B-cell or unknown immunologic phenotype
· *Mycobacterium tuberculosis*, disseminated or extrapulmonary
· *Mycobacterium*, other species or unidentified species, disseminated (at a site other than or in addition to lungs, skin, or cervical or hilar lymph nodes)
· *Pneumocystis jiroveci (carinii)* pneumonia
· Progressive multifocal leukoencephalopathy
· *Salmonella* (nontyphoid) septicemia, recurrent
· Toxoplasmosis of the brain with onset after 1 mo of age
· Wasting syndrome in the absence of a concurrent illness other than HIV infection that could explain the following findings:
  (1) Persistent weight loss >10% of baseline
  (2) Downward crossing of at least two of the following percentile lines on the weight-for-age chart (e.g., 95th, 75th, 50th, 25th, 5th) in a child 1 yr of age or older
  (3) <5th percentile on weight-for-height chart on two consecutive measurements, ≥30 days apart PLUS
    (a) Chronic diarrhea (i.e., at least two loose stools per day for >30 days)
    (b) Documented fever (for >30 days, intermittent or constant)

Modified from Centers for Disease Control and Prevention. 1994 revised classification system for human immunodeficiency virus infection in children less than 13 years of age: Official authorized addenda: Human immunodeficiency virus infection codes and official guidelines for coding and reporting ICD-9-CM. MMWR 43(RR-12):1–19, 1994.
HIV = human immunodeficiency virus; HSV = herpes simplex virus.

TABLE 41-8 · CONDITIONS INCLUDED IN THE 1993 AIDS SURVEILLANCE CASE DEFINITION

Candidiasis of bronchi, trachea, or lungs
Candidiasis, esophageal
Cervical cancer, invasive*
Coccidioidomycosis, disseminated or extrapulmonary
Cryptococcosis, extrapulmonary
Cryptosporidiosis, chronic intestinal (>1 mo duration)
Cytomegalovirus disease (other than liver, spleen, or nodes)
Cytomegalovirus retinitis (with loss of vision)
Encephalopathy, HIV-related
Herpes simplex: chronic ulcer(s) (>1 mo duration) or bronchitis, pneumonitis, or esophagitis
Histoplasmosis, disseminated or extrapulmonary
Isosporiasis, chronic intestinal (>1 mo duration)
Kaposi's sarcoma
Lymphoma, Burkitt's (or equivalent term)
Lymphoma, immunoblastic (or equivalent term)
Lymphoma, primary, of brain
Mycobacterium avium complex or *Mycobacterium kansasii,* disseminated or extrapulmonary
Mycobacterium tuberculosis, any site (pulmonary* or extrapulmonary)
Mycobacterium, other species or unidentified species, disseminated or extrapulmonary
Pneumocystis jiroveci (carinii) pneumonia
Pneumonia, recurrent*
Progressive multifocal leukoencephalopathy
Salmonella septicemia, recurrent
Toxoplasmosis of brain
Wasting syndrome caused by HIV

*Added in the 1993 expansion of the AIDS surveillance case definition.
AIDS = acquired immunodeficiency syndrome; HIV = human immunodeficiency virus.
From Centers for Disease Control and Prevention. 1993 revised classification system for HIV infection and expanded surveillance case definition for AIDS among adolescents and adults. MMWR 41(RR-17):15, 1992.

S. aureus, and *Salmonella* sp.) are common. Septicemia is most common; other illnesses include pneumonia, meningitis, urinary tract infection, osteomyelitis, septic arthritis, and deep-seated abscesses. Also common are otitis media, sinusitis, and skin infections that do not respond as well to conventional antimicrobial therapy as do similar infections in children without HIV infections.

Case reports of new opportunistic infections and unusual clinical manifestations of known pathogens are being reported every day (Di John et al., 1990; Friedland et al., 1992; Glaser et al., 1994; Gradon et al., 1992; Hughes and Parham, 1991; Kline and Dunkle, 1988; Lacroix et al., 1988; Markowitz et al., 1988; Silliman et al., 1993; Wong and Ross, 1988). For example, fatal cases of both measles pneumonia and varicella encephalitis without rash have been reported (Markowitz et al., 1988; Silliman et al., 1993).

Farm animals and pets may be a source of unusual infections in patients with AIDS (Glaser et al., 1994). Of particular risk is bacillary angiomatosis caused by *Bartonella henselae* and *Bartonella quintana,* which can be acquired from cats, and cutaneous granulomas caused by *Mycobacterium marinum,* which can be acquired from fish tanks.

Other illnesses in patients with AIDS may include toxic shock syndrome, supraglottitis, very late onset group B streptococcal infection, severe molluscum contagiosum,

disseminated Acanthamoeba infection, and septicemia caused by *Moraxella catarrhalis* (Di John et al., 1990; Friedland et al., 1992; Hughes and Parham, 1991; Kline and Dunkle, 1988; Lacroix et al., 1988; Wong and Ross, 1988). Gradon and associates (1992) presented a review of unusual opportunistic pathogens in patients with AIDS by anatomic location of the infections.

Prevention of Infection

The approach to the prevention and treatment of infections in HIV-infected children is continually changing (the therapy of the primary HIV infection is presented in Chapter 29, and a summary of available antiretroviral agents is presented in Table 41-9). Children with HIV infections should receive all regularly scheduled immunizations, except that inactivated polio vaccine rather than oral polio vaccine should be given (American Academy of Pediatrics, 2000a). In addition, family members who are to be immunized should also receive inactivated polio vaccine rather than oral polio vaccine. Children with HIV infections should also receive a yearly influenza immunization. Recently, the use of varicella vaccine has been suggested in HIV-infected children in CDC class NI and AI (see Table 41-6) who have mild or no symptoms (American Academy of Pediatrics, 2000a, 2000e).

Because inadequate immune responses after measles immunization in HIV-infected children are common, children exposed to measles should be given human immune globulin prophylaxis (0.5 ml/kg; maximum, 15 ml/kg) unless they are routinely receiving IVIG and have received a dose within 3 weeks of exposure. If HIV-infected children experience an injury with a wound classified as tetanus-prone, they should receive tetanus immune globulin (human), regardless of their vaccination status.

P. jiroveci (carinii) pneumonia is the most important HIV-associated opportunistic infection in children. Infection with this agent is often fatal, and the median survival time after successful treatment of a first episode is less than 4 months in infants and children. Therefore prophylaxis is a high priority (CDC, 1995). Because *P. jiroveci (carinii)* pneumonia occurs early in life and because HIV infection is often difficult to diagnose during early infancy, prophylaxis must be initiated in the first few months of life and often before HIV infection has been definitively diagnosed. Recommendations for the initiation of *P. jiroveci (carinii)* pneumonia prophylaxis are presented in Table 41-10. Drug regimens for prophylaxis are presented in Table 41-11. The mainstay of prophylaxis is trimethoprim-sulfamethoxazole, but aerosolized pentamidine in older children and dapsone, atovaquone, and IV pentamidine are also effective (Abrams, 2000; Carr et al., 1993; Hand et al., 1994; Kletzel et al., 1991; Orcutt et al., 1992; Stavola and Noel, 1993).

IVIG Prophylaxis

Because children with AIDS have defective humoral and cellular immunities, IVIG has been used prophy-

TABLE 41-9 · ANTIRETROVIRAL AGENTS*

Class	Agent	Dosage	Side Effects
Nucleoside reverse transcriptase inhibitors			Lactic acidosis/severe hepatomegaly with steatosis, including fatal cases, have been reported with the use of these agents alone or in combination with other antiretrovirals. A majority of cases have been in women. Obesity and prolonged nucleoside exposure may be risk factors.
	Abacavir	16 mg/kg/day q12h PO	*Most frequent:* Nausea, vomiting, headache, fever, rash, anorexia, and fatigue. Approximately 5% of adults and children receiving abacavir develop a potentially fatal hypersensitivity reaction. Symptoms include fever, fatigue, malaise, nausea, vomiting, diarrhea, and abdominal pain. Physical findings include lymphadenopathy, ulceration of mucous membranes, and maculopapular or urticarial skin rash. The hypersensitivity reaction can occur without a rash. Laboratory abnormalities include elevated liver function test results, elevated creatine kinase, elevated creatinine, and lymphopenia. This reaction generally occurs in the first 6 weeks of therapy. In patients suspected of having a hypersensitivity reaction, abacavir should be discontinued and not restarted, because hypotension and death have occurred at rechallenge. *Uncommon:* Diarrhea, pancreatitis, increased liver enzymes, elevated blood glucose, elevated triglycerides, and lactic acidosis.
	Didanosine	240 mg/m^2/day q12h PO	*Most frequent:* Diarrhea, abdominal pain, nausea, and vomiting. *Unusual (more severe):* Peripheral neuropathy (dose-related), electrolyte abnormalities, and hyperuricemia. *Uncommon:* Pancreatitis (dose-related, less common in children than adults), increased liver enzymes, and retinal depigmentation.
	Lamivudine	8 mg/kg/day q12h PO	*Most frequent:* Headache, fatigue, nausea, diarrhea, skin rash, and abdominal pain. *Unusual (more severe):* Pancreatitis (primarily seen in children with advanced HIV infection receiving multiple other medications), peripheral neuropathy, decreased neutrophil count, and increased liver enzymes.
	Stavudine	2 mg/kg/day q12h PO	*Most frequent:* Headache, gastrointestinal disturbances, and skin rashes. *Uncommon (more severe):* Peripheral neuropathy and pancreatitis. *Other:* Increased liver enzymes.
	Tenofovir (nucleotide analogue)	300 mg q24h PO (for adolescents; pediatric dose not adequately established)	*Most frequent:* Nausea, diarrhea, asthenia, headache, vomiting, flatulence, abdominal pain, and anorexia. Bone abnormalities (e.g., reduced bone density) and renal toxicity have been observed in animal studies.
	Zalcitabine	0.03 mg/kg/day q8h PO	*Most frequent:* Headache, gastrointestinal disturbances, and malaise. *Unusual (more severe):* Peripheral neuropathy, pancreatitis, hepatic toxicity, oral ulcers, esophageal ulcers, hematologic toxicity, and skin rashes.
	Zidovudine	480 mg/m^2/day q12h PO	*Most frequent:* Hematologic toxicity, including granulocytopenia and anemia, and headache. *Unusual:* Myopathy, myositis, and liver toxicity.
Non-nucleoside reverse transcriptase inhibitors	Delavirdine	400 mg q8h PO (for adolescents; pediatric dose not adequately established)	*Most frequent:* Headache, fatigue, gastrointestinal complaints, and rash (may be severe).
	Efavirenz	600 mg q24h PO (for adolescents; pediatric dose not adequately established)	*Most frequent:* Skin rash; central nervous system (e.g., somnolence, insomnia, abnormal dreams, confusion, abnormal thinking, impaired concentration, amnesia, agitation, depersonalization, hallucinations, euphoria), symptoms primarily reported in adults; increased aminotransferase levels, teratogenic in primates (use in pregnancy should be avoided, and women of childbearing potential should undergo pregnancy testing before initiating therapy).
	Nevirapine	120 mg/m^2/day q24h PO over first 14 days, then 240–400 mg/m^2/day q12h PO	*Most frequent:* Skin rash (some severe and life-threatening, including Stevens-Johnson syndrome), sedative effect, headache, diarrhea, and nausea. *Unusual:* Elevated liver enzymes and, rarely, hepatitis.
Protease inhibitors	Amprenavir	45 mg/kg/day q12h PO	*Most frequent:* Vomiting, nausea, diarrhea, perioral paresthesias, and rash. *Unusual (more severe):* Life-threatening rash, including Stevens-Johnson syndrome in 1% of patients. *Rare:* Increased cholesterol levels, new-onset diabetes mellitus, hyperglycemia, exacerbation of pre-existing diabetes mellitus, hemolytic anemia, and spontaneous bleeding in persons with hemophilia.

Continued

TABLE 41-9 · ANTIRETROVIRAL AGENTS*—cont'd

Class	Agent	Dosage	Side Effects
	Indinavir	1500 mg/m²/day q8h PO (under study)	*Most frequent:* Nausea, abdominal pain, headache, metallic taste, dizziness, and asymptomatic hyperbilirubinemia (10%). *Unusual (more severe):* Nephrolithiasis (4%) and exacerbation of chronic liver disease. *Rare:* Spontaneous bleeding episodes in persons with hemophilia; hyperglycemia; ketoacidosis; diabetes; and hemolytic anemia.
	Lopinavir-ritonavir	600/150 mg/m²/day q12h PO	*Most frequent:* Nausea, vomiting, diarrhea, headache, abdominal pain, rash, and asthenia. *Less common:* Body pain, imsomnia. *Rare:* Spontaneous bleeding episodes in those with hemophilia; pancreatitis; increased levels of triglycerides and cholesterol, hyperglycemia; ketoacidosis; diabetes; and hepatitis.
	Nelfinavir	110 mg/kg/day q12h PO	*Most frequent:* Diarrhea. *Less common:* Asthenia, abdominal pain, rash, and exacerbation of chronic liver disease. *Rare:* Spontaneous bleeding episodes in those with hemophilia; hyperglycemia; ketoacidosis; and diabetes.
	Ritonavir	800 mg/m²/day q12h PO, beginning at 500 mg/m²/day q12h PO and increasing stepwise over 5 days	*Most frequent:* Nausea, vomiting, diarrhea, headache, abdominal pain, and anorexia. *Less common:* Circumoral paresthesias and increase in liver enzymes. *Rare:* Spontaneous bleeding episodes in persons with hemophilia; pancreatitis; increased levels of triglycerides and cholesterol; hyperglycemia; ketoacidosis; diabetes; and hepatitis.
	Saquinavir	1200 mg q8h PO (soft-gel capsules, adolescents)	*Most frequent:* Diarrhea, abdominal discomfort, headache, nausea, paresthesias, and skin rash. *Less common:* Exacerbation of chronic liver disease. *Rare:* Spontaneous bleeding episodes in those with hemophilia; hyperglycemia; ketoacidosis; and diabetes.

*Consult drug product information sheets (package inserts) and other sources for more complete administration and drug interaction data.
HIV = human immunodeficiency virus.
Adapted in part from: Guidelines for the Use of Antiretroviral Agents in Pediatric HIV Infection, HIV/AIDS Treatment Information Service (ATIS), January 7, 2000.

TABLE 41-10 · RECOMMENDATIONS FOR PCP PROPHYLAXIS AND CD4⁺ MONITORING FOR HIV-B–EXPOSED INFANTS AND HIV-INFECTED CHILDREN BY AGE AND HIV INFECTION STATUS

Age	HIV Infection Status	PCP Prophylaxis	CD4⁺ Monitoring
Birth to 4–6 wk	HIV-exposed	No prophylaxis	1 mo
4–6 wk to 4 mo	HIV-exposed	Prophylaxis	3 mo
4–12 mo	HIV-infected or indeterminate	Prophylaxis	6, 9, and 12 mo
4–12 mo	HIV infection reasonably excluded	No prophylaxis	None
1–5 yr	HIV-infected	Prophylaxis if: CD4⁺ count is <500 cells/mm³ or CD4⁺ percentage is <15%‡	Every 3–4 mo*
6–12 yr	HIV-infected	Prophylaxis if: CD4⁺ count is <200 cells/mm³ or CD4⁺ percentage is <15%‡	Every 3–4 mo*

*More frequent monitoring (i.e., monthly) is recommended for children whose CD4⁺ counts or percentages are approaching the threshold at which prophylaxis is recommended.
†Children 1–2 years of age who were receiving PCP and had a CD4⁺ count of <750 cells/mm³ or a percentage of <15% at <12 mo of age should continue prophylaxis.
‡Prophylaxis should be considered on a case-by-case basis for children who might otherwise be at risk for PCP, such as children with rapidly declining CD4⁺ counts or percentages or children with category C conditions (see Chapter 18 and Table 18-3). Children who have had PCP should receive lifelong PCP prophylaxis.
HIV = human immunodeficiency virus; PCP = *Pneumocystis jiroveci (carinii)* pneumonia.
Adapted from Centers for Disease Control and Prevention. Revised guidelines for prophylaxis against *Pneumocystis jiroveci (carinii)* pneumonia for children. MMWR 44(RR-4):1–11, 1995.

TABLE 41-11 · MEDICATIONS FOR PROPHYLAXIS AGAINST PCP IN HIV-INFECTED CHILDREN

Medication	Dosing Schedule	Adverse Events
TMP-SMX	150 mg TMP/M^2/day bid PO on 3 consecutive days; 150 mg TMP/M^2/day bid PO on consecutive days; 150 mg TMP/M^2/day bid PO daily; or 150 mg TMP/M^2/day bid PO on 3 alternating days	Rash, Stevens-Johnson syndrome, neutropenia, thrombocytopenia, aplastic and megaloblastic anemia, renal impairment, and abnormal liver function test results
Dapsone	2 mg/kg PO daily (maximum, 100 mg)	Rash, pruritus, methemoglobinemia, and hemolytic anemia; screen for glucose-6-phosphate dehydrogenase deficiency
Inhaled pentamidine	300 mg pentamidine isethionate inhaler every 28 days (children >5 yr of age)	Cough, bronchospasm, increased risk of extrapulmonary PCP
IV pentamidine	4 mg/kg IV q2–4wk	Hypoglycemia, hyperglycemia, hypotension, hypocalcemia, rash, nephrotoxicity, pancreatitis, and cardiac arrhythmia
Atovaquone	30 mg/kg PO daily (maximum, 1500 mg); not yet approved for children	Rash, gastrointestinal intolerance, and diarrhea

HIV = human immunodeficiency virus; PCP = *Pneumocystis jiroveci (carinii)* pneumonia; TMP-SMX = trimethoprim-sulfamethoxazole.
From Abrams EJ. Opportunistic infections and other clinical manifestations of HIV disease in children. Pediatr Clin North Am 47:79–108, 2000.

lactically and is recommended by the Working Group on Antiretroviral Therapy: National Pediatric HIV Resource Center (1993). IVIG is recommended for children with hypogammaglobulinemia (IgG < 250 mg/ml) and recurrent serious bacterial infections and for children who cannot form antibodies to common antigens such as measles. The IVIG dosage is 400 mg/kg every 4 weeks (American Academy of Pediatrics, 2000a).

Other Prophylactic Measures

Prophylaxis or maintenance therapy should also be used in the following instances (CDC, 1993b):

1. For household or day care contact with active tuberculosis, treat with isoniazid for 9 to 12 months (if there is a known exposure to a drug-resistant strain, a multidrug regimen is necessary).
2. Varicella-zoster immune globulin should be administered to those exposed to varicella-zoster or herpes-zoster.
3. Those treated for cytomegalovirus infection should undergo a maintenance regimen with ganciclovir or foscarnet.
4. Patients treated for cryptococcal meningitis should undergo maintenance therapy with oral fluconazole.
5. Patients with persistent or recurrent mucocutaneous candidiasis should undergo maintenance therapy with topical clotrimazole; if this measure fails, use ketoconazole or fluconazole.
6. Patients treated for ocular or CNS toxoplasmosis should undergo maintenance therapy with daily pyrimethamine-sulfadiazine and folinic acid.
7. Patients with frequently recurring severe herpes simplex infections should be given oral acyclovir daily.
8. Children treated for disseminated *Mycobacterium avium* complex infections should remain on lifelong prophylaxis with azithromycin or clarithromycin and rifabutin.

Malnutrition

Children with chronic severe malnutrition are immunologically compromised and frequently experience opportunistic infections (see Chapter 23). In children with protein-calorie malnutrition, the following immunologic defects have been noted: decreased concentrations of C1q, C1s, C3, C5, C6, C8, C9, and C3 proactivator; depression in T-cell function; defective intracellular bacterial killing by leukocytes; and significant reductions in the migration of polymorphonuclear leukocytes to the sites of inflammation (Chandra, 1972; Ferguson et al., 1974; Freyre et al., 1973; Geefhuysen et al., 1971; Neumann, 1981; Neumann et al., 1975; Sellmeyer et al., 1972; Seth and Chandra, 1972; Smythe et al., 1971; Yoshida et al., 1967).

These deficits, acting alone or in concert, undoubtedly predispose these children to infection with opportunistic microorganisms. In addition, infections with normal pathogens can frequently be expected to be more severe than in the immunologically competent host.

Serum Ig deficiencies have not been found consistently, but deficits in specific antibody responses despite normal or elevated total serum Igs have been observed (Cannon, 1945; Work et al., 1973). A transient deficiency of nasal secretory IgA has been reported in malnourished children in Thailand (Sirisinha et al., 1975). Cellular immunity, serum complement activity, and polymorphonuclear leukocyte function return to normal with nutritional restoration.

Children with protein-calorie malnutrition are particularly susceptible to severe and progressive measles virus infection and disseminated herpes simplex virus infection. Severe and protracted bacterial urinary tract, pulmonary, and gastrointestinal infections are common, as are chronic diarrheas caused by parasites. Particularly troublesome are infections with gram-negative enteric bacilli and *M. tuberculosis* infections

(Becker et al., 1963; Faber, 1938; James, 1972; Morley, 1969; Phillips and Wharton, 1968).

Nephrotic Syndrome

Before the use of antibiotics and corticosteroids, primary or spontaneous peritonitis caused by *S. pneumoniae*, group A streptococci, staphylococci, and *H. influenzae* type B was a relatively common and often-fatal complication of nephrotic syndrome (see Chapter 25). Primary peritonitis is often the clinical presentation that leads to the diagnosis of nephrotic syndrome (Chuang et al., 1999; Markenson et al., 1999). Peritonitis caused by these microorganisms still occurs in the antibiotic and corticosteroid era, yet systemic infection attributable to gram-negative bacilli has been observed with increasing frequency (Wilfert and Katz, 1968).

Patients with nephrotic syndrome have been found to have cellular and humoral immune defects and decreased bacterial killing by neutrophils (Yetgin et al., 1980). Infants with nephrotic syndrome should receive their pneumococcal conjugate vaccine series, and older children should receive pneumococcal polysaccharide vaccine (Fikrig et al., 1978).

Uremia

Renal failure is associated with an increased risk of infection with opportunistic organisms (Haag-Weber and Hörl, 1993; Welt et al., 1970). Common offending microorganisms include *Enterobacter*, *Staphylococcus*, *Serratia*, *Bacteroides*, *Candida*, *Mucor*, herpesviruses, and *Pneumocystis*.

Reasons for the increased propensity for infection have been sought (see Chapter 25). Lymphopenia has been observed frequently; a depressed and delayed response to tuberculin, coccidioidin, histoplasmin, *Candida*, trichophytin, and mumps, in addition to impaired allograft rejection have also been reported in patients who were uremic (Dammin et al., 1957; Kirkpatrick et al., 1964; Lang et al., 1966; Riis and Stougaard, 1959). The inability of lymphocytes to proliferate in response to antigens has been well documented and has been related in part to a plasma factor in patients with uremia (Elves et al., 1966; Ming et al., 1968; Silk, 1967). The increased risk of infection with saprophytic fungi, herpesviruses, and *Pneumocystis* in patients with uremia may be related to the depression of T-cell function.

Ig concentrations generally have been normal. Polymorphonuclear leukocyte production is apparently normal, but a defect in the early phase of the acute inflammatory response has been suggested (Haag-Weber and Hörl, 1993; Wilson et al., 1965).

Exudative Enteropathy

When an excessive loss of protein occurs in the gastrointestinal tract, a significant reduction in albumin and γ-globulin, particularly IgG, may be noted (see Chapters 4, 25, and 34). Disorders in which exudative enteropathy has been noted include acute gastrointestinal infection, Menetrier's disease (protein loss with giant hypertrophy of the gastric mucosa), gluten-induced enteropathy, intestinal lymphangiectasia, kwashiorkor, Hirschsprung's disease, gastrointestinal neoplasms, allergic gastroenteritis, regional enteritis, ulcerative colitis, jejunal malformations, gastrocolic fistula, angioneurotic edema, postgastrectomy syndrome, congestive heart failure, constrictive pericarditis, and aminopterin administration (Feigin and Shearer, 1975a, 1975b; Waldmann, 1966; Waldmann and Schwab, 1965). Infection related specifically to the IgG deficiency is rare.

In patients with intestinal lymphangiectasia, however, hypogammaglobulinemia may be accompanied by lymphopenia and skin anergy; furthermore, impaired homograft rejection has been documented in these individuals (Strober et al., 1967; Weiden et al., 1972). The increased susceptibility of some of these children to infection is related to the loss of Igs and lymphocytes, with disruption of the normal circulation of small lymphocytes from the blood into lymphoid tissues and back to the blood (Gatti et al., 1970). Persistent giardiasis in children with this disease has resolved, with improvement in the clinical and immunologic status of the patient (Feigin and Shearer, 1975a, 1975b).

Inflammatory Bowel Disease

Granulomatous colitis and ulcerative colitis (see Chapter 34) per se do not appear to predispose the host to opportunistic infection. When those disorders are treated with corticosteroids, however, opportunistic infection with bacteria, viruses, fungi, and parasites may occur. Infection is usually systemic, but *Candida* endophthalmitis (localized infection) has been noted in a child who was receiving corticosteroids for ulcerative colitis (Haning et al., 1973).

Inflammatory Disease of Connective Tissue

Abnormalities in Igs and antibodies that react with body tissue constituents or with other Igs (e.g., rheumatoid factors) have been noted in patients with collagen diseases (see Chapter 35). When opportunistic infections with *Candida*, *Aspergillus*, *Mucor*, and *Pneumocystis* occur in patients with connective tissue disorders, they are most likely related to the administration of corticosteroids and other immunosuppressive agents (Klainer and Beisel, 1969). Infection with *Pseudomonas*, *Listeria*, *Staphylococcus*, *Serratia*, diphtheroids, *Nocardia*, *Candida*, *Aspergillus*, *Cryptococcus*, *Mucor*, cytomegalovirus, varicella-zoster virus, and *Pneumocystis* may be seen in patients with significant involvement of the reticuloendothelial system (Feigin and Shearer, 1975a, 1975b).

INFECTION IN THE NEWBORN

From an immunologic point of view, all newborns (full-term and premature) can be considered to be compromised (see Chapter 22). Most neonatal infections are opportunistic in that the principal offending microorganisms are those that are readily cultured from the exogenous and endogenous environments of healthy individuals. Specific immunodeficiencies of newborns are presented in Chapters 13 and 22.

The greatest infection risk for the newborn is the surrounding environment, and an important defect that the infant at birth has is the total lack of microbial flora. Natural antibiosis and competitive inhibition among organisms are important host defense mechanisms that are not available to the newborn. The events leading to the acquisition of a flora are critical in the determination of which infants will become infected. In general, the infant who receives a balanced dose of organisms from the mother runs a lower risk of infection than the infant heavily colonized with a single organism from the environment.

In recent years, IVIG has been used in several controlled and uncontrolled studies to treat and prevent infections in low-birth-weight infants (Baker et al., 1992; Hill, 1993; Kinney et al., 1991; Magny et al., 1991; National Institutes of Health Consensus Conference, 1990; Weisman et al., 1992). These studies were reviewed at a National Institutes of Health Consensus Conference in 1989 and more recently by Hill (1993). Of six prophylaxis studies, two disclosed marginal benefit; four of five treatment studies revealed benefit. One treatment study in animals indicated that the IVIG impaired the antibacterial activity of antibiotics in animals infected with group B streptococci (Kim, 1989).

A meta-analysis of prospective and retrospective, small and large trials (Jenson and Pollock, 1998) revealed a marginal, but significant, benefit of prophylactic IVIG administered shortly after birth in preventing early onset sepsis in premature low-birth-weight newborns. The expense of this agent for the extensive premature newborn population, given its minimal benefit, does not appear justified.

Similarly, the data regarding therapy are such that it should not be used routinely but perhaps should be reserved for specific individual patients.

GENERAL APPROACH TO TREATMENT OF INFECTION IN THE COMPROMISED HOST

The general principles of diagnosis and treatment of opportunistic infections are the same as those applied when infections are caused by organisms normally considered to be pathogenic. The possibility of opportunistic infections can be anticipated in association with certain clinical situations, and the physician can frequently predict the types of organisms that may be responsible for specific infections that are suspected or observed. The physician must alert the laboratory to the possibility of opportunistic infection, and, in turn, the microbiologist must not regard the isolation of a normally saprophytic microorganism as a contaminant, particularly if it is recovered repeatedly from specimens obtained from the same patient.

It is important to emphasize that the relationship between a microorganism and the host is a dynamic one. Virulence can be expressed only in comparative terms because of daily variations in the mechanisms of host defense and the microorganisms to which the host is exposed. Any microorganism can produce disease in an appropriate host.

Opportunistic microorganisms do not produce disease in a haphazard manner. Thus diagnosis and treatment need not be initiated haphazardly. For example, in the compromised host with an indwelling venous catheter, periodic blood specimens should be obtained for culture and the site of insertion of the catheter should be examined carefully. The tip of the catheter should be cultured routinely on removal. Similarly, cultures of sputum or tracheal aspirates should be obtained repeatedly in children who have a tracheostomy and who are undergoing inhalation therapy. In this manner, the physician can detect sequential changes in the microbial flora of the patient. Cultures of this type assume special importance in children who are immunosuppressed, because, in these individuals, the usual clinical signs of infection may be absent.

Once appropriate cultures and the results of serologic tests designed to establish an etiologic diagnosis have been obtained from the immunologically compromised child, therapy should be initiated immediately in most instances. Before the identification of a specific infectious agent, initial treatment must be guided by the underlying disease process with which the patient is afflicted and the types of organisms that most commonly are responsible for infection in these individuals (see Tables 41-1 through 41-5, 41-7, and 41-8). When a specific organism is recovered and specific sensitivities are obtained, therapy may be changed accordingly.

Approach to Diagnosis

Serious infections in compromised children usually have only a limited number of clinical manifestations (e.g., fever, respiratory distress, abdominal distress, neurologic complaints, skin and soft tissue lesions, and bone or joint complaints) and sites of infection (e.g., causing septicemia, pneumonia, peritonitis or abdominal abscess, meningitis or brain abscess, skin cellulitis and ulcers, soft tissue abscess, arthritis, and osteomyelitis). However, each clinical category of infection can be attributable to a multitude of different microorganisms, including common bacteria, mycobacteria, fungi, parasites, and viruses. In the preceding sections and the tables of this chapter, the various microorganisms most frequently associated with opportunistic infections in children with specific immunologic defects are presented.

Septicemia

Fever is a frequent occurrence in hospitalized children with severe combined immunodeficiencies, malignancies, and immunosuppression; in most instances, this fever is attributable to septicemia. The approach to diagnosis should be easy, but all too frequently, undue delay occurs because of failure to collect appropriate cultures. Multiple blood cultures should be obtained.

In addition to blood cultures, cultures from all other possible sites of infection should be obtained. Cutdown sites, IV catheters, tracheal aspirates, and the urine should be cultured.

Pneumonia

Pneumonia is the second most common problem in compromised patients, and all too frequently, antibiotics are prescribed before appropriate cultures are obtained. Because many children with pneumonia caused by opportunistic microorganisms also have septicemia, multiple blood cultures should be obtained. In addition, tracheal aspirates or sputum smears and cultures should be obtained. In virtually all instances in which pleural fluid is visible by means of radiography, thoracentesis should be performed. In many instances in which only "pleural thickening" is observed, thoracentesis reveals 1 or 2 ml of diagnostically useful fluid.

In many instances, more invasive diagnostic study is indicated (Commers et al., 1984; Dichter et al., 1993; Johanson et al., 1988; Prober et al., 1984). The nature of subsequent studies depends on the skill of the physician's consulting services. Diagnostic bronchoscopy with bronchoalveolar lavage or direct lung tap frequently is rewarding. Open lung biopsy is often necessary.

Other Infections

Arthritis, osteomyelitis, cellulitis, and abscess areas should be needled for culture before therapy. Frequently, these culture attempts are facilitated by having a small amount of saline in the syringe. If the tap is dry, the saline can be pushed into and withdrawn from the site of suspected infection. Cerebrospinal fluid should be obtained for culture whenever there is the slightest suspicion of CNS infection.

Handling of Cultures

Positive cultures are the hallmark of therapeutic success. Frequently, extensive and invasive surgical procedures are performed for diagnosis and the specimens are then handled improperly. All cultures obtained from deep sites should be inoculated into aerobic and anaerobic bacterial media and into fungal and mycobacterial media. Multiple smears should be made and treated with the Gram, methenamine silver, hematoxylin-eosin, Ziehl-Neelsen, or other appropriate tissue stains. For specimens obtained from the lung and urine, cerebrospinal fluid, and, frequently, blood, viral cultures and direct antigen tests (i.e., polymerase chain reaction and hybridization assays) also are indicated.

Approach to Therapy

Empiric Treatment for the Neutropenic Febrile Cancer or Bone Marrow Transplant Patient

After the initial collection of appropriate cultures, all neutropenic cancer and bone marrow transplant patients with fever of unknown origin should be started immediately on empiric antimicrobial therapy (Bodey, 1984; Chastagner et al., 2000; Cherry, 1983; Fanci et al., 2000; Frazier et al., 1984; Katz and Mustafa, 1993; Pizzo, 1993; Pizzo et al., 1991a; Sable and Donowitz, 1994; Winston et al., 1984; Zaia, 1992). Empiric therapy must consist of broad-spectrum agents because the variation of types of organisms and their susceptibility patterns are legion (see Table 41-5). There are many possible empiric antimicrobial regimens.

In the past, we suggested the use of an aminoglycoside (amikacin, gentamicin, netilmicin, or tobramycin) in combination with either an anti-*Pseudomonas* penicillin (azlocillin, carbenicillin, ticarcillin, mezlocillin, or piperacillin) or a third-generation cephalosporin and a penicillinase-resistant penicillin (nafcillin or oxacillin). More recent experience indicates that empiric therapy can be simplified and made less costly by the use of ceftazidime monotherapy (Pizzo, 1993; Pizzo et al., 1991a).

After the results of cultures and sensitivity tests are obtained, the antimicrobial regimen can be altered. Combination treatment (an anti-*Pseudomonas* penicillin and an aminoglycoside) should be used for gram-negative bacillary infections. For infections with gram-positive cocci, a narrow-spectrum penicillin, penicillinase-resistant penicillin (depending on sensitivity of the organism), or vancomycin is adequate for the treatment of the infection. However, it has been noted on occasion that in immunocompromised patients treated initially with single narrow-spectrum drugs, secondary gram-negative bacterial infections develop. Because of this problem, it may be important to administer an aminoglycoside and ceftazidime along with the specific treatment for the gram-positive organism.

When cultures do not reveal a bacterial etiology for the fever and a patient remains febrile while undergoing ceftazidime monotherapy, further empiric treatment must be considered. After additional cultures, we would suggest adding an aminoglycoside, and perhaps vancomycin, to the regimen. With continued fever, empiric antifungal treatment must be considered. We would suggest the routine empiric administration of amphotericin B if fever has persisted for more than 7 days; amphotericin B should be added to the regimen at an earlier time if the patient's clinical condition is deteriorating.

The duration of antimicrobial treatment in the neutropenic cancer or bone marrow transplantation patient is not well established. If the child remains neutropenic, therapy should be continued for at least 7 days after the temperature has returned to normal. However, because relapse or re-infection is common, it is frequently recommended that once treatment is started, it be continued until the child is no longer neutropenic (i.e., absolute granulocyte count $\geq$ 500 cells/mm^3) (Pizzo et al., 1984).

In recent years, there has been a search for alternative less costly approaches for treatment of infections in the low-risk neutropenic patients. Bash and colleagues (1994) reported successful early discharge of hospitalized patients with localized infections, before recovery of neutrophil counts above 500 cells/mm^3. The criteria for low-risk classification used in this study were absence of fever, negative cultures, control of local infection, evidence indicating bone marrow recovery, and good clinical appearance.

Shenep and colleagues (2001) compared oral cefixime with continuous IV vancomycin, ticarcillin, and tobramycin in 200 episodes of fever and neutropenia that occurred in 156 children, once these patients had negative cultures after 48 hours of initial therapy. Failure to respond to therapy was defined by documented or suspected bacterial infection, recurrent fever, or discontinuation of assigned therapy for any reason before neutropenia resolved. The rates of treatment failure were similar in both groups (28% vs. 27%).

Aquino and associates (2000) successfully used oral ciprofloxacin in febrile neutropenic children who were considered low-risk. These low-risk children were older than 12 months, had neutrophil counts of more than 100 cells/mm^3, had their malignancy in remission, were not ill-appearing, and had reliable parents.

Bacterial Infections

Selected antimicrobial agents useful for the treatment of severe bacterial infections in children who are compromised immunologically are presented in Table 41-12. Both the dosage and usual susceptible organisms are listed. Frequently, in seriously ill children, antibiotic

TABLE 41-12 · SELECTED AGENTS USEFUL IN TREATING SEVERE BACTERIAL INFECTIONS IN IMMUNOLOGICALLY COMPROMISED CHILDREN*

Agent	Dosage	Usual Susceptible Organisms	Comments
Amikacin	15–40 mg/kg/day (420–1100 mg/M^2/day) q8h IM or intravenously (30-min infusion)	*Enterobacter* sp., *Escherichia coli, Klebsiella pneumoniae, Proteus* sp., *Providencia* sp., *Serratia* sp., *Acinetobacter* sp., *Pseudomonas* sp., nontuberculous mycobacteria	Measurement of blood levels 1 hr and 8 hr (peak and trough) after administration frequently necessary to ensure adequate concentration without toxicity
Ampicillin	100–300 mg/kg/day (2.8–8.4 g/M^2/day) q4h IM or intravenously (5-min infusion)	Enterococci, streptococci, *Listeria monocytogenes, E. coli, Proteus mirabilis, Salmonella* sp., *Shigella* sp., *Haemophilus influenzae*	When administered in conjunction with an aminoglycoside, synergism frequently occurs
Ampicillin-sulbactam	As per ampicillin	Organisms susceptible to ampicillin plus β-lactamase–producing (but not methicillin-resistant) *Staphylococcus aureus, H. influenzae, Moraxella catarrhalis, Neisseria gonorrhoeae, E. coli, Proteus* sp., and some anaerobes, including *Bacteroides fragilis*	Most useful as monotherapy of potential polymicrobial infections such as intra-abdominal, gynecologic, or soft tissue infections Drug of choice for IV therapy of infected human or animal bites
Azithromycin	10 mg/kg/day (280 mg/M^2/day) (day 1) intravenously or PO; 5 mg/kg/day (140 mg/M^2/day) on subsequent days	Legionella sp., Chlamydia trachomatis, *S. aureus* (methicillin-sensitive), *Streptococcus* sp., *Enterococcus* sp., *N. gonorrhoeae*, anaerobic cocci, *Campylobacter jejuni, H. influenzae, Bacteroides* sp., *Mycobacterium leprae, Mycobacterium kansasii, Mycobacterium avium/intracellulare, Corynebacterium* sp., *L. monocytogenes, Clostridium perfringens, Peptococcus, Peptostreptococcus, Bordetella pertussis, M. catarrhalis, Pasteurella multocida*	
Aztreonam	90–120 mg/kg/day (2.6–3.4 g/M^2/day) q6–8h IM or intravenously	Most aerobic gram-negative bacteria; virtually devoid of activity against aerobic gram-positive and anaerobic organisms	Useful when gram-negative aerobic bacteria are resistant to cephalosporins, penicillins, and aminoglycosides; superinfection with gram-positive organisms is a problem
Cefazolin	25–50 mg/kg/day (0.7–1.4 g/M^2/day) q6h IM or intravenously (5-min infusion)	*S. aureus, Staphylococcus epidermidis*, group A β-hemolytic streptococci, *Streptococcus pneumoniae*	When administered in conjunction with an aminoglycoside, synergism frequently occurs

Continued

TABLE 41-12 · SELECTED AGENTS USEFUL IN TREATING SEVERE BACTERIAL INFECTIONS IN IMMUNOLOGICALLY COMPROMISED CHILDREN*—cont'd

Agent	Dosage	Usual Susceptible Organisms	Comments
Cefotaxime	100–200 mg/kg/day (2.8–5.6 g/M²/day) q6–8h intravenously (10- to 20-min infusion)	Most gram-positive and gram-negative aerobes except *L. monocytogenes* and enterococci	
Ceftriaxone	50–100 mg/kg/day (1.4–2.8 g/M²/day) q12h intravenously (10- to 20-min infusion)	Similar to cefotaxime	
Cefuroxime	100–200 mg/kg/day q6–8h intravenously (10- to 20-min (2.8–6.7 g/M²/day) infusion)	Most gram-positive cocci (except enterococci), *H. influenzae, Neisseria meningitidis*	
Chloramphenicol	50–100 mg/kg/day (1.4–2.8 g/M²/day) q6h PO or IV (30-min infusion)	*Salmonella* sp., *Shigella* sp., *H. influenzae,* anaerobes, gram-negative bacilli	
Ciprofloxacin	20–30 mg/kg/day (560–840 mg/M²/day) q12h IV or PO	*Enterococcus faecalis, Staphylococcus* sp., *Citrobacter* sp., *Enterobacter cloacae, E. coli, H. influenzae, Haemophilus parainfluenzae, Klebsiella pneumoniae, Morganella morganii, Proteus* sp., *Providencia* sp., *P. aeruginosa, Serratia marcescens*	Not approved for patients <18 yr of age; causes arthropathy in juvenile animals
Clarithromycin	15 mg/kg/day (420 mg/M²/day) q12h PO; 10–30 mg/kg/day (280–840 mg/M²/day) q12h PO for *M. avium–intracellulare*	*Legionella* sp., *C. trachomatis, S. aureus* (methicillin-sensitive), *Streptococcus* sp., *Enterococcus* sp., *N. gonorrhoeae,* anaerobic cocci, *C. jejuni, H. influenzae, Bacteroides* sp., *Mycobacterium leprae, M. kansasii, M. avium* Bintracellulare, *Corynebacterium* sp., *L. monocytogenes, C. perfringens, Peptococcus, Peptostreptococcus, B. pertussis, M. catarrhalis, P. multocida*	
Clindamycin	10–40 mg/kg/day (280–1120 mg/M²/day) q6h IM or IV (30-min infusion)	Anaerobes	
Dalfopristin-quinupristin	15–22.5 mg/kg/day (420–630 mg/M²/day) q8–12h IV	*Enterococcus faecium*	Not approved for patients <16 yr of age
Erythromycin	30–50 mg/kg/day (840–1400 mg/M²/day) q6h PO or IV (1-hr infusion)	*Mycoplasma pneumoniae, Chlamydia* sp., *Legionella* sp., *S. aureus, Streptococcus* sp., *B. pertussis*	
Ethambutol	25 mg/kg/day (700 mg/M²/day) for 2 mo, then 15 mg/kg/day (420 mg/M²/day) PO	*Mycobacterium tuberculosis,* atypical mycobacteria	Used in conjunction with isoniazid, rifampin, and pyrazinamide
Gentamicin	5–7.5 mg/kg/day (140–210 mg/M²/day) q8h IM or IV (30-min infusion)	*Enterobacter* sp., *E. coli, K. pneumoniae, Proteus* sp., *Providencia* sp., *P. aeruginosa, Citrobacter* sp., *Serratia* sp.	Blood levels 1 hr and 8 hr (peak and trough) after administration frequently necessary to ensure adequate concentration without toxicity
Imipenem-cilastatin	40–60 mg/kg/day (1.1–1.7 g/M²/day)	Active against most gram-positive cocci and gram-negative bacilli	Not approved for children; useful for organisms resistant to cephalosporins, penicillins, and aminoglycosides; usually used in conjunction with an aminoglycoside; has propensity to induce seizures
Isoniazid	10–20 mg/kg/day (280–560 mg/M²/day) (maximum, 500 mg/day) PO or IM	*M. tuberculosis,* atypical mycobacteria	Used in conjunction with ethambutol, streptomycin, rifampin, and pyrazinamide
Kanamycin	15–20 mg/kg/day (420–560 mg/M²/day) q8h IM or intravenously (30-min infusion)	*Enterobacter* sp., *E. coli, K. pneumoniae, Proteus* sp., *Providencia* sp., *Serratia* sp., *Acinetobacter* sp.	

TABLE 41-12 · SELECTED AGENTS USEFUL IN TREATING SEVERE BACTERIAL INFECTIONS IN IMMUNOLOGICALLY COMPROMISED CHILDREN*—cont'd

Agent	Dosage	Usual Susceptible Organisms	Comments
Linezolid	0–11 yr: 30 mg/kg/day (840 mg/M^2/day) q8h PO or IV ≥12 yr: 600 mg q12h PO or IV	Broad gram-positive spectrum; *S. aureus* including methicillin-resistant strains, *S. epidermidis*, *Streptococcus* sp. including penicillin- and cephalosporin-resistant pneumococcal strains, enterococci including penicillin- and vancomycin-resistant strains, also *Corynebacterium* spp., *Bacillus* spp., *L. monocytogenes*, *M. catarrhalis*, *Chlamydia pneumoniae*, and mycobacteria	
Meropenem	60–120 mg/kg/day (1.7–3.4 g/M^2/day) q8h IV	Similar to imipenem-cilastatin	Safety and efficacy are established in children >3 mo old
Metronidazole	15–50 mg/kg/day (420–1400 mg/M^2/day) q6h intravenously or PO	Most anaerobes	
Mezlocillin	300 mg/kg/day (8.4 g/M^2/day) q4–6h IV (10- to 20-min infusion)	Many *Bacteroides* species and other anaerobes; with gentamicin, amikacin, or tobramycin for *Pseudomonas aeruginosa* and other gram-negative bacilli	Should always be used with an aminoglycoside antibiotic
Nafcillin	100–200 mg/kg/day (2.8–5.6 g/M^2/day) q4–6h IM or IV (5-min infusion)	*S. aureus*	
Norfloxacin	400 mg q12h PO	Similar to ciprofloxacin	Not approved for patients <21 yr of age; causes arthropathy in juvenile animals
Ofloxacin	400–800 mg/day q12h PO	*C. trachomatis*; otherwise, similar to ciprofloxacin	Not approved for children; causes arthropathy and osteochrondrosis of juvenile animals
Oxacillin	100–200 mg/kg/day (2.8–5.6 g/M^2/day) q4–6h IM or intravenously (5-min infusion)	*S. aureus*	
Penicillin	50,000–300,000 U/kg/day (1.4–8.4 million U/M^2/day) q4h IM or IV (5-min infusion)	*Streptococcus* sp., *Neisseria* sp., *Clostridium* sp., *P. multocida*, oropharyngeal anaerobes, *Streptococcus moniliformis*	
Piperacillin	200–300 mg/kg/day (5.6–8.4 g/M^2/day) q4h IM or IV (30-min infusion)	Many *Bacteroides* species and other anaerobes; with gentamicin, amikacin, or tobramycin for *P. aeruginosa* and other gram-negative bacilli	Should always be used in combination with aminoglycoside
Piperacillin-tazobactam	As per piperacillin	Extends the spectrum of piperacillin to include β-lactamase–producing strains of methicillin-susceptible *S. aureus* and many members of *Enterobacteriaceae*	
Pyrazinamide	20–30 mg/kg/day (560–840 mg/M^2/day) or 20 mg/kg (560 mg/M^2) twice weekly PO	*M. tuberculosis*, atypical mycobacteria	Use in mycobacteria infections with resistant organisms in conjunction with other agents
Rifampin	10–20 mg/kg/day (280–560 mg/M^2/day) (maximum 600 mg/day) PO	*M. tuberculosis*, atypical mycobacteria	For tuberculosis, use in conjunction with isoniazid, pyrazinamide, streptomycin, and ethambutol
Streptomycin	15–30 mg/kg/day (420–840 mg/M^2/day) IM	*M. tuberculosis*, atypical mycobacteria	Used in three- or four-drug therapy with isoniazid, rifampin, pyrazinamide, and ethambutol; has synergistic role in therapy of bacterial endocarditis
Tetracycline	20–40 mg/kg/day (560–1120 mg/M^2/day) q6h PO or IV (2-hr infusion)	*M. pneumoniae*, *Chlamydia* sp.	

Continued

TABLE 41-12 · SELECTED AGENTS USEFUL IN TREATING SEVERE BACTERIAL INFECTIONS IN IMMUNOLOGICALLY COMPROMISED CHILDREN*—cont'd

Agent	Dosage	Usual Susceptible Organisms	Comments
Ticarcillin	200–300 mg/kg/day (5.6–8.4 g/M²/day) q4–6h IV (10- to 20-min infusion)	Many *Bacteroides* species and other anaerobes; with gentamicin, amikacin, or tobramycin for *Pseudomonas aeruginosa* and other gram-negative bacilli	Should always be used with an aminoglycoside antibiotic
Ticarcillin-potassium clavulanate	As per ticarcillin	Extends the spectrum of ticarcillin to include β-lactamase–producing strains of methicillin-susceptible *S. aureus*, *H. influenzae*, *E. coli*, *K. pneumoniae*, and *B. fragilis*	
Tobramycin	3–5 mg/kg/day (84–140 mg/M²/day) q8h IM or IV (30-min infusion)	*Enterobacter* sp., *E. coli*, *K. pneumoniae*, *Proteus* sp., *Providencia* sp., *Serratia* sp., *Acinetobacter* sp., *Pseudomonas* sp., *Citrobacter* sp.	Blood levels 1 hr and 8 hr (peak and trough) after administration frequently necessary to ensure adequate concentration without toxicity
Trimethoprim-sulfamethoxazole	Trimethoprim 10–20 mg/kg/day (280–560 mg/M²/day) Sulfamethoxazole 50–100 mg/kg/day (1.4–2.8 g/M²/day) q12h PO or IV	*Providencia* sp., *Salmonella* sp., *Serratia* sp., *Shigella* sp., *E. coli*, *Klebsiella* sp., *Enterobacter* sp., *Morganella morganii*, *Proteus* sp., *H. influenzae*, *Shigella flexneri*, *Shigella sonnei*	Useful when organisms resistant to aminoglycosides
Trisulfapyrimidines	120 mg/kg/day (3.4 g/M²/day) q6h PO for 4 wk	*Nocardia*	
Vancomycin	40–60 mg/kg/day (1200–1800 mg/M²/day) q6h IV (30-min infusion)	*S. aureus*, *S. epidermidis*, *Streptococcus* sp., enterococci, *Clostridium difficile*	For treatment of an enterococcal infection, used with an aminoglycoside antibiotic; for *C. difficile* enteritis, administered 50 mg/kg/day PO

*Consult drug product information sheets (package inserts) and other sources for more complete administration and toxicity data. Some doses and administration suggestions in this table may be different from those recommended by the manufacturer.
Data from Nelson JD. Pocketbook of pediatric antimicrobial therapy, 14th ed. Baltimore, Williams & Wilkins, 2000; and Feigin RD, Cherry JD. Textbook of pediatric infectious diseases, 4th ed. Philadelphia, WB Saunders, 1998.

therapy must be started before culture results are available. Because gram-negative bacillary infections are most common in compromised children, and because many such infections are hospital-acquired, the likelihood of resistance to many drugs is great. Thus initial therapy should provide broad bactericidal coverage (as aforementioned).

In Table 41-12, antimicrobial dosage is listed by square meter as well as by kilogram. This is of little importance with penicillins and cephalosporins but can be very important with aminoglycoside antibiotics. Children who are underweight for their age tend to have relatively greater blood volumes and extracellular fluid spaces than their weights would indicate. Therefore dosages calculated by kilogram nearly always will be too low. Underdosage is a common occurrence with aminoglycoside therapy in children with cystic fibrosis. In addition, because the gap between effective therapeutic and toxic levels of aminoglycoside antibiotics is small, it is imperative to determine peak and trough blood levels when these drugs are administered. The specific in vitro sensitivity of the infectious agent for which treatment is provided also must be determined.

Pseudomonas infections should always be treated with both an aminoglycoside and an anti-*Pseudomonas* penicillin or ceftazidime because significant synergism has been described. Anti-*Pseudomonas* penicillins should not be used as single drugs in the treatment of *Pseudomonas* infections because therapeutic results have been disappointing and resistance rapidly develops. Trimethoprim-sulfamethoxazole on occasion can be life-saving in illnesses that are caused by multiresistant gram-negative bacillary infections.

When anaerobic infections are suspected, chloramphenicol, clindamycin, or metronidazole should be added to the therapeutic regimen.

Vancomycin is a useful drug that should be administered to patients with multiresistant staphylococcal, enterococcal, and streptococcal infections and in serious streptococcal and staphylococcal infections in allergic individuals. Agents such as dalfopristin-quinupristin and linezolid are alternatives in vancomycin-resistant strains, and when vancomycin is not tolerated. *M. pneumoniae* infections are frequently of greater severity in compromised patients and should be treated vigorously with erythromycin, clarithromycin, or azithromycin.

Tuberculosis in compromised patients frequently is far advanced before it is recognized by the physician. In addition, the emergence of tuberculosis caused by drug-resistant *M. tuberculosis* is a major problem (CDC, 1993a). At present, a four-drug regimen with isoniazid, rifampin, pyrazinamide, and streptomycin or ethambutol is recommended for initial empiric treatment. A total of 1 year of therapy is the minimum recommended in such situations.

Viral Infections

Viral infections are responsible for considerable morbidity and mortality in compromised children. Specific antiviral therapy is still at a rudimentary stage of development in contrast to antibacterial therapy, but there is much that can be offered to the patient. Useful therapeutic agents are listed in Table 41-13. Topical ophthalmic preparations of acyclovir, idoxuridine, trifluridine, and vidarabine have all been shown to be effective in treating acute keratoconjunctivitis and recurrent epithelial keratitis caused by herpes simplex virus. No topical antiviral agent is presently useful for treating recurrent skin herpes simplex viral infections.

The use of amantadine or rimantadine in early influenza A infection would appear to be supported by adequate scientific data, and in the clinical situation in which influenza A infection is suspected, this therapy is recommended. The newer neuraminidase inhibitors, such as zanamivir and oseltamivir are active against both influenza A and B and have been approved for use in children.

Routine immunization with inactivated influenza vaccine is recommended in most immunocompromised children.

TABLE 41-13 · SELECTED AGENTS USEFUL IN TREATING VIRAL INFECTIONS, EXCEPT HIV, IN IMMUNOLOGICALLY COMPROMISED CHILDREN*

Type	Agent	Dosage and Method of Administration	Susceptible Viruses	Comments
Topical	Acyclovir	Eye: 5% ointment q3–4h	Herpes simplex, varicella-zoster	
	Idoxuridine	Eye: 0.1% solution q1h; 0.5% ointment, q4h	Herpes simplex	
	Trifluridine	Eye: 1% solution q2h (maximum, 9 drops/eye/24 hr)	Herpes simplex	
	Vidarabine	Eye: 3% ointment, 1/2," 5 times/day	Herpes simplex, varicella-zoster	
Systemic	Acyclovir	15–45 mg/kg/day (420–1350 mg/M²/day) q8h IV (1-hr infusion)	Herpes simplex and varicella-zoster	
	Amantadine	1–9 yr: 4.4–8.8 mg/kg/day (125–250 mg/M²/day) q12h PO (maximum, 150 mg/day) 9–12 yr: 100 mg PO q12h	Influenza A	
	Cidofovir	Induction: 5 mg/kg IV once with hydration/ probenecid Maintenance: 3 mg/kg/wk IV with hydration/ probenecid	Cytomegalovirus retinitis	
	Famciclovir	750–2250 mg/kg/day q8–12h PO	Herpes simplex	
	Foscarnet	180 mg/kg/day (5 g/M²/day) IV q8h for 14–21 days, then 60–120 mg/kg/day (1.7–2.4 g/M²/day) q24h for maintenance	Cytomegalovirus	
	Ganciclovir	10 mg/kg/day (300 mg/M²/day) IV q12h for 14–21 days 5 mg/kg/day (150 mg/M²/day) IV q24h for long-term suppression 10 mg/kg/day (300 mg/M²/day) IV q12h for 1 wk, then 5 mg/kg/day (150 mg/M²/day) IV q24h for prophylaxis	Cytomegalovirus	
	Oseltamivir	<15 kg: 30 mg PO q12h 15–23 kg: 45 mg PO q12h 23–40 kg: 60 mg PO q12h >40 kg: 75 mg PO q12h	Influenza A and B	
	Ribavirin	Administered by aerosol generator (6 g in 300 ml of sterile water) 12–18 hours' exposure/day	Respiratory syncytial virus	In vitro studies have shown efficacy against influenza, parainfluenza, and measles virus; clinical studies of this agent for treatment of influenza and parainfluenza virus are in progress
	Rimantidine	5 mg/kg/day (150 mg/M²/day) q12h Maximum dose: <10 yr, 150 mg/day; ≥10 yr, 200 mg/day	Influenza A	Approved for prophylactic use
	Valacyclovir	500–1000 mg PO q12h	Herpes simplex	Approved for adolescents
	Vidarabine	15–30 mg/kg/day (420–840 mg/M²/day; 12-hr infusion) for 10–14 days	Herpes simplex, varicella-zoster	
	Zanamivir	10 mg inhaled q12h	Influenza A and B	Approved for ages ≥12 yr

*Consult drug product information sheets (package inserts) and other sources for more complete administration and toxicity data. Some doses and administration suggestions in this table may be different from those recommended by the manufacturer.
HIV = human immunodeficiency virus.
Data from Nelson JD. Pocketbook of pediatric antimicrobial therapy, 14th ed. Baltimore, Williams & Wilkins, 2000; Feigin RD, Cherry JD. Textbook of pediatric infectious diseases, 4th ed., Philadelphia, WB Saunders, 1998; and American Academy of Pediatrics. Antiviral drugs. In Pickering L, ed. 2000 Red Book: Report of the Committee on Infectious Diseases, 24th ed. Elk Grove Village, IL, American Academy of Pediatrics, 2000, pp 675–657.

Ribavirin, administered through an aerosol generator, appears to be therapeutically effective in respiratory syncytial and influenza viral infections in immunocompetent children and adults. Gelfand and colleagues (1983) and McIntosh and associates (1984) reported encouraging results in three children with severe combined immunodeficiency syndromes infected with respiratory syncytial virus or parainfluenza virus type 3.

Mucocutaneous herpes simplex viral infections are common in immunocompromised children; they are frequently severe and chronic, being the cause of significant morbidity (Bryson, 1984; Wong and Hirsch, 1984). These infections can be treated successfully with acyclovir. Similarly, both exogenous (varicella) or endogenous (zoster or disseminated zoster) infections with varicella-zoster virus can be treated effectively with acyclovir. Cytomegalovirus infections should be treated with ganciclovir. In addition to treatment, recurrences of illness caused by herpes simplex virus can be prevented by the prophylactic use of acyclovir. Maintenance therapy with ganciclovir is used to prevent recurrence of the clinical manifestations of cytomegalovirus infection in severely immunosuppressed patients.

Fungal Infections

Fungal infections are a major cause of death in compromised children. In many instances, vigorous antibiotic therapy has been carried out, but extensive fungal infection is found at autopsy. In particular, *Candida* overgrowth is common in compromised patients receiving antibiotic therapy. This overgrowth should be treated vigorously with topical agents because it is quite probable that dissemination can be reduced. Useful antifungal agents are listed in Table 41-14.

TABLE 41-14 · SELECTED AGENTS USEFUL IN TREATING FUNGAL INFECTIONS IN IMMUNOLOGICALLY COMPROMISED CHILDREN*

Type	Agent	Dosage and Method of Administration	Susceptible Fungi	Comments
Topical	Nystatin	Cream, ointment, powder, oral suspension, and oral tablets; vaginal tablets, 100,000 to 1 million U/day qid	*Candida* sp.	
	Clotrimazole	1% ointment or solution bid to qid	*Candida* sp., dermatophytes	
	Ketoconazole	2% cream bid to qid	*Candida* sp., dermatophytes	
Systemic	Amphotericin B deoxycholate	0.8–1.5 mg/kg/day (22–42 mg/M²/day) qd or qod IV (3- to 4-hr infusion)	*Aspergillus* sp., *Blastomyces, Candida* sp., *Coccidioides immitis, Cryptococcus neoformans, Histoplasma capsulatum, Mucor, Paracoccidioidomycosis, Phaeohyphomycosis, Zygomycosis*	In children, an initial dose of 0.25 mg/kg is usually well tolerated, increasing by 0.25 mg/kg daily until 1.0 mg/kg is reached; in severely ill patients, the first 4 doses can be given 6 hr apart, then adjusted to qd or qod
	Amphotericin B lipid complex	5 mg/kg/day IV (2-hr infusion)	Same as Amphotericin B deoxycholate	
	Amphotericin B cholesteryl sulfate	3–6 mg/kg/day IV (infused at 1 mg/kg/hr)	Same as Amphotericin B deoxycholate	
	Liposomal amphotericin B (AmBisome)	5 mg/kg/day (1- to 2-hr infusion) (AmBisome)	Same as Amphotericin B deoxycholate	
	Caspofungin acetate	70 mg/day IV (day 1), 50 mg/day subsequent days	Invasive aspergillosis	Not adequately studied in patients <18 yr
	Fluconazole	6–12 mg/kg/day (168–336 mg/M²/day) IV or PO	Mucosal candidiasis, cryptococcal meningitis, *Candida* urinary tract infection	
	Flucytosine	50–150 mg/kg/day (1.4–4.2 g/M²/day) q6h PO	*Candida* sp., *Cryptococcus neoformans*	Used in conjunction with amphotericin B
	Itraconazole	200 mg PO once or twice daily for adults; dose for children not established	*Aspergillus* sp., *Blastomyces dermatitidis, C. immitis, Cryptococcus neoformans*	
	Ketoconazole	3.3–6.6 mg/kg/day (100–200 mg/M²/day) qd PO	*B. dermatitidis, Candida* sp., *C. immitis, H. capsulatum, Paracoccidioides brasiliensis, C. neoformans, Pseudallescheria boydii*	Drug of choice for chronic mucocutaneous candidiasis
	Miconazole	20–40 mg/kg/day (600–1200 mg/M²/day) IV q8h (30- to 60-min infusion)	*Candida* sp.	

*Consult drug product information sheets (package inserts) and other sources for more complete administration and toxicity data.
Data from Nelson JD. Pocketbook of pediatric antimicrobial therapy, 14th ed., Baltimore, Williams & Wilkins, 2000; Feigin RD, Cherry JD. Textbook of pediatric infectious diseases, 4th ed., Philadelphia, WB Saunders, 1998; and American Academy of Pediatrics. Antifungal drugs for systemic fungal infections. In Pickering L, ed. 2000 Red Book: Report of the Committee on Infectious Diseases, 24th ed. Elk Grove Village, IL, American Academy of Pediatrics, 2000, pp 668–672.

For systemic fungal disease, the most effective agent is amphotericin B. This is a drug with considerable toxicity, but with judicious use, it can be highly effective. In children, in whom renal functional abnormalities are usually less of a problem, dosage can frequently be pushed higher and treatment continued longer than in adult patients. When amphotericin B is used, it is important to determine blood concentrations of amphotericin B and the sensitivity of the fungus. These tests are not performed in many hospital laboratories, but they are available in reference laboratories. After institution of therapy with amphotericin B, it should be continued for at least 3 weeks and usually for at least 6 weeks.

Flucytosine is also a potent antifungal agent. However, in our experience, it has proved disappointing when used as the single therapeutic agent, because resistance rapidly ensues (Rinaldi, 1998). In therapy for *Candida* infections, we frequently use both amphotericin B and flucytosine together.

Fluconazole, itraconazole, and ketoconazole are three antifungal agents that, when used on the basis of sensitivity studies, can frequently be used in place of amphotericin B. In particular, itraconazole has been used successfully in invasive *Aspergillus* sp. infections and fluconazole in disseminated *Coccidioides immitis* infections. Fluconazole is also effective in cryptococcal meningitis.

Lipid-complexed formulations of amphotericin B licensed in the United States include colloidal dispersion (Amphotec), lipid complex (Abelcet), and liposomal (AmBisome). All are significantly less nephrotoxic than amphotericin B. They require higher doses to achieve similar efficacy in laboratory animals. Acute infusion-related reactions occur with all three formulations but are generally less frequent and severe with Abelcet and AmBisome than with amphotericin B deoxycholate. They appear to be equivalent to amphotericin B deoxycholate in terms of efficacy (Blau and Fauser, 2000; Wingard et al., 2000), but further randomized trials are needed.

The use of these agents should be restricted to patients who have poor baseline renal function or those patients who experienced either unacceptable nephrotoxicity or intractable infusion-related reactions. Another barrier has been the high cost of these preparations, which has ranged between thirtyfold and sixtyfold higher than amphotericin B deoxycholate.

Parasitic Infections

The major parasitic infections causing opportunistic infection in immunologically compromised children are caused by *P. jiroveci* (*carinii*: now classified as a fungi), *T. gondii,* and *Cryptosporidium* sp. Occasionally, *Entamoeba histolytica, Isospora belli, Cyclospora cayetanensis,* and *Giardia* are also problems. Selected agents useful in treating parasitic infections in immunologically compromised children are presented in Table 41-15.

PREVENTION OF INFECTION IN THE COMPROMISED CHILD

Prevention of infection in the compromised child varies with the nature and degree of the individual defect (see Tables 41-1 through 41-5). For example, children with splenic deficiency syndromes need only to be vaccinated against encapsulated organisms and to undergo specific antibiotic prophylaxis against selected bacteria, and patients with simple Ig deficiency need only replacement therapy. However, prevention of infection in the more severely compromised child (e.g., the immunosuppressed, a transplant recipient, or a child with combined immunodeficiency) requires considerable organization and expense. Frequently, ill-advised preventive measures can lead to greater opportunistic infection rather than protection.

Baseline Studies

In newly acquired immunologic defects and hereditary defects, it is important to determine the past microorganism experience of the patient, in addition to that of close family contacts. A generous amount of serum should be obtained for routine serologic baseline value determinations at the time, and the majority of the specimen should be saved for future comparative study. The following baseline antibody studies should be performed: Toxoplasma, cytomegalovirus, herpes simplex, varicella-zoster virus, and measles. A tuberculin and *Candida* skin test should be performed, and tuberculin testing of family members also should be carried out frequently.

Surveillance Cultures

When patients with severe immunodeficiencies with neutropenia are seen initially, baseline cultures of throat and stool should be obtained to determine the levels of bacterial and fungal flora. The throat and urine specimens should be cultured for viruses in patients with B-cell and those with T-cell immunodeficiencies.

Stool examination for ova and parasites also is indicated. In severely compromised children, routine culture monitoring should frequently be continued, because changes in flora can be used to predict forthcoming disease.

Immunization

After historic and serologic data are obtained, many active and passive immunologic procedures can be useful (see Chapter 42). Inactivated polio and influenza vaccines should be administered to all patients. Passive immunization with varicella-zoster immune globulin or other γ-globulins should be used after known exposures. Tetanus and diphtheria immunizations should be kept up to date.

TABLE 41-15 · AGENTS USEFUL IN TREATING SELECTED PARASITIC INFECTIONS IN IMMUNOLOGICALLY COMPROMISED CHILDREN*

Parasitic Agent	Therapy of Choice and Dose	Comments
Babesia sp.	Clindamycin 20 mg/kg/day q6h PO or IV and quinine 25 mg/kg/day q6–8h PO for 7–10 days	
Entamoeba histolytica (severe infection)	Metronidazole 35–50 mg/kg/day (1000–1400 mg/M²/day) q8h PO for 10 day or Dehydroemetine 1.0–1.5 mg/kg/day (29–41 mg/M²/day) (maximum, 90 mg) q12h IM for 5 days or Either drug followed by Iodoquinol 40 mg/kg/day (1.1 g/M²/day) q8h PO for 20 day or If hepatic abscess: Chloroquine phosphate 10 mg base/kg (maximum, 300 mg base) (290 mg/M²/day) q24h PO for 2–3 wk	Dehydroemetine available from Centers for Disease Control and Prevention
Giardia lamblia	Quinacrine HCl 6 mg/kg/day (170 mg/M²/day) q8h PO (maximum, 300 mg/day) for 7 days	Alternative therapies: metronidazole and furazolidine
Isospora belli	TMP-SMX 10 mg TMP and 50 mg SMX/kg/day (280 mg TMP and 1400 mg SMX/M²/day) q6h PO for 10 days, then 5 mg TMP and 25 mg SMX/kg/day q12h PO for 3 wk	
Malaria	Chloroquine-sensitive parasites: Chloroquine phosphate or sulfate 25 mg/kg of base (500 mg of phosphate provides approximately 300 mg of chloroquine base) given in 4 doses over 3 days Chloroquine-resistant parasites: Quinine sulfate 25 mg/kg/day (up to 650 mg) q8h PO for 7–10 days, mefloquine 15 mg/kg (up to 1250 mg) as a single dose, and halofantrine 8 mg/kg q6h for 3 doses, repeated 7 days later for nonimmune patients, and Fansidar (25 mg of pyrimethamine and 500 mg of sulfadoxine) as a single dose (two to three tablets for children 15 years and older, two tablets for children 9–14 years of age, one tablet for children 4–8 yr of age, ½ tablet for children 1–3 yr of age, and ¼ tablet for infants)	
Pneumocystis jiroveci (carinii)	See Table 40-10	
Strongyloides stercoralis	Thiabendazole 50 mg/kg/day (1400 mg/M²/day) q12h PO, maximum dose 3000 mg/day for 2 days (5 days or longer for disseminated disease)	Clarithromycin proved effective in adults
Toxoplasma gondii	Pyrimethamine 2 mg/kg/day (60 mg/M²/day) q12h PO for 3 days, then 1 mg/kg/day (maximum 25 mg/day) × 4 wk plus Sulfadiazine 100–200 mg/kg/day (2.8–5.4 g/M²/day) q6h PO × 4 wk	
Cryptosporidium sp.	Spiramycin 100 mg/kg/day (2400 mg/M²/day) q6h PO	Spiramycin is an investigational drug, and no data related to children are available; octreotide may control diarrhea; paromomycin and azithromycin also possibly effective

*Consult drug product information sheets (package inserts) and other sources for more complete administration and toxicity data.
Data from Nelson JD. Pocketbook of pediatric antimicrobial therapy, 14th ed. Baltimore, Williams & Wilkins, 2000; Feigin RD, Cherry JD. Textbook of pediatric infectious diseases, 4th ed. Philadelphia, WB Saunders, 1998; and American Academy of Pediatrics. Drugs for parasitic infections. In Pickering L, ed. 2000 Red Book: Report of the Committee on Infectious Diseases, 24th ed. Elk Grove Village, IL, American Academy of Pediatrics, 2000, pp 693–725.

General Care of Severely Compromised Patients

Patients with immunologic defects should not have undue exposure when being treated at home. Patients should be discouraged from having contact with pets and should avoid crowds and other situations that may involve heavy exposure to potentially infectious microorganisms. In the hospital, protective care should be practiced. Some protective care practices place considerable restrictions on the patient, visitors, and the medical staff. Poorly carried out protective care procedures are frequently worse than no protective care procedures at all.

In general, immunocompromised children should be cared for with infection precautions that are not different from routine good patient-care techniques (Garner and Simmons, 1983). For these children, routine techniques must be emphasized and enforced. All personnel and others having contact with the child must wash their hands before, during, and after patient care. Immunocompromised children should be separated from patients who are infected or who have conditions that result in infection transmission. Private rooms should be used whenever possible.

The hallmark of good protective care is handwashing. Unfortunately, in many elaborate settings, this is overlooked or is performed improperly. There are two types of handwashing. The first is the surgical scrub; the second is a quick wash designed only to remove surface bacteria likely to have been picked up from recent contact. Except when certain procedures (e.g., catheter insertion) are to be carried out, the single quick wash is all that should be done (Sprunt et al., 1973; Steere and Mallison, 1975). This is particularly important for persons spending a considerable amount of time with the child in protective care. If their hands contain normal flora, they are less likely to become heavily colonized with more resistant gram-negative bacillary organisms from the hospital environment.

Frequently used, masks offer little in the way of protective care. The mask that remains on for a prolonged period of time concentrates organisms, so that if it is touched (e.g., rubbing the nose), it creates a greater hazard than no mask at all.

Because opportunistic infections with hospital organisms are the major problem in the severely compromised individual, protective practices should be directed against these agents. Hospital equipment involved in multiple patient use must be carefully monitored. This equipment includes respirators, ophthalmoscopes, pumps, stands, thermometers, and so on. Other environmental sources of gram-negative organisms, including flower vases, improperly maintained soap dispensers, water-surrounded bar soap, and raw fruits and vegetables, should be monitored carefully.

Second only to handwashing in the success of protective care is the exclusion of personnel and visitors who are disseminators of microorganisms. All persons with respiratory illnesses or cutaneous lesions of any sort should not be allowed in the room of an immunocompromised patient.

Prophylactic Antimicrobial Agents

There is considerable controversy related to the role of prophylactic antimicrobial agents in the prevention of opportunistic infections, but it is clear that, in some instances, they have a place. In patients with urinary catheters, serious systemic infections can be prevented by using a continuous bladder rinse with either a neomycin-polymyxin or a 0.25% acetic acid solution.

Silver and sulfa compounds can be useful locally in reducing systemic infections in burn patients. Nonabsorbable antibiotics can be used to reduce the total number of organisms in the gastrointestinal tract; this would appear to be useful in patients undergoing transplantation.

The systemic use of antibiotics can be expected to be successful prophylactically when a particular drug is used to prevent infections with one or two specific organisms. Penicillin administration can be used to prevent pneumococcal infections in individuals with asplenia and streptococcal infection at the time of dental surgery in persons with cardiac defects. Prevention of staphylococcal infection of prostheses (heart valves, CNS shunts) with oxacillin or nafcillin administration may be possible. Prophylactic administration of trimethoprim-sulfamethoxazole is useful for the prevention of Pneumocystis infections in children undergoing immunosuppressive therapy.

The administration of acyclovir orally to adults with leukemia and after bone marrow transplantation has been successful in preventing troublesome cutaneous herpes simplex virus lesions (Anderson et al., 1984; Wade et al., 1984).

As discussed earlier, recipients of transplants are routinely given prophylaxis or early/pre-emptive therapy against cytomegalovirus. The use of polymerase chain reaction–based techniques has allowed for early detection in many patients (Meuleman et al., 2000, Singh et al., 2000).

Prophylactic IVIG

IVIG is highly effective in patients with agammaglobulinemia. Recent studies indicate its usefulness in selected children with HIV infections (see Chapter 29).

REFERENCES

Abramowsky CR, Quinn D, Bradford WD, Conant NF. Systemic infection by *Fusarium* in a burned child. The emergence of a saprophytic strain. J Pediatr 84:561–564, 1974.

Abrams EJ. Opportunistic infections and other clinical manifestations of HIV disease in children. Pediatr Clin North Am 47:79–108, 2000.

Adams JM, Speer ME, Rudolph AJ. Bacterial colonization of radial artery catheters. Pediatrics 65:94–97, 1980.

Alexander JW. Immunological considerations in burn injury and the role of vaccination. In Stone HH, Polk HC, eds. Contemporary burn management. Boston, Little, Brown & Co, 1971a, pp 265–280.

Alexander JW. Control of infection following burn injury. Arch Surg 103:435–441, 1971b.

Alexander JW, Dionigi R, Meakins JL. Periodic variation in the antibacterial function of human neutrophils and its relationship to sepsis. Ann Surg 173:206–213, 1971.

Alexander JW, Meakins JL. A physiological basis for the development of opportunistic infections in man. Ann Surg 176:273–287, 1972.

Aly R, Maibach HI, Shinefield HR, Strauss WG. Survival of pathogenic microorganisms on human skin. J Invest Dermatol 58:205–210, 1972.

Aly R, Maibach HI, Rahman R, Shinefield HR, Mandel AD. Correlation of human in vivo and in vitro cutaneous antimicrobial factors. J Infect Dis 131:579–583, 1975.

Academy of Pediatrics. Human Immunodeficiency Virus Infection. In Pickering LK, ed. 2000 Red Book: Report of the Committee on Infectious Diseases, 25th ed. Elk Grove Village, IL, American Academy of Pediatrics, 2000a, pp 325–350.

American Academy of Pediatrics. Antiviral drugs. In Pickering LK, ed. 2000 Red Book: Report of the Committee on Infectious Diseases, 25th ed. Elk Grove Village, IL, American Academy of Pediatrics, 2000b, pp 675–677.

American Academy of Pediatrics. Drugs of choice for invasive and other serious fungal infections. In Pickering LK, ed. 2000 Red Book: Report of the Committee on Infectious Diseases, 25th ed. Elk Grove Village, IL, American Academy of Pediatrics, 2000c, pp 670–672.

American Academy of Pediatrics. Drugs for parasitic infections. In Pickering LK, ed. 2000 Red Book: Report of the Committee on Infectious Diseases, 25th ed. Elk Grove Village, IL, American Academy of Pediatrics, 2000d, pp 694–725.

American Academy of Pediatrics. Committee on Infectious Diseases. Varicella vaccine update. Pediatrics 105:136–141, 2000e.

American Academy of Pediatrics. Committee on Infectious Diseases. Policy Statement: recommendations for the prevention of pneumococcal infections, including the use of pneumococcal conjugate vaccine (Prevnar), pneumococcal polysaccharide vaccine and antibiotic prophylaxis. Pediatrics 106:362–366, 2000f.

Ammann AJ, Wara DW. Evaluation of infants and children with recurrent infection. Curr Prob Pediatr 5:34–37, 1975.

Anderson H, Scarffe JH, Sutton RN, Hickmott E, Brigden D, Burke C. Oral acyclovir prophylaxis against herpes simplex virus in non-Hodgkin lymphoma and acute lymphoblastic leukaemia patients receiving remission induction chemotherapy. A randomised double blind, placebo controlled trial. Br J Cancer 50:45–49, 1984.

Anderson R. Assessment of oral ascorbate in three children with chronic granulomatous disease and defective neutrophil motility over a 2-year period. Clin Exp Immunol 43:180–188, 1981.

Andrews W, Fyock B, Gray S, Coln D, Hendrickse W, Siegel J, Belknap B, Hogge A, Benser M, Kennard B, Stewart S, Albertson N. Pediatric liver transplantation: the Dallas experience. Transplant Proc 19:3267–3276, 1987.

Aquino VM, Herrera L, Sandler ES, Buchanan GR. Feasibility of oral ciprofloxacin for the outpatient management of febrile neutropenia in selected children with cancer. Cancer 88:1710–1714, 2000.

Auletta JJ, O'Riordan MA, Nieder ML. Infections in children with cancer: a continued need for the comprehensive physical examination. J Pediatr Hematol Oncol 21:501–508, 1999.

Azimi PH, Levernier K, Lefrak LM, Petru AM, Barrett T, Schenck H, Sandhu AS, Duritz G, Valesco M. Malassezia furfur: a cause of occlusion of percutaneous central venous catheters in infants in the intensive care nursery. Pediatr Infect Dis J 7:100–103, 1988.

Baehner RL. Disorders of leukocytes leading to recurrent infection. Pediatr Clin North Am 19:935–956, 1972.

Bailey TC, Ettinger NA, Storch GA, Trulock EP, Hanto DW, Dunagan WC, Jendrisak MD, McCullough CS, Kenzora JL, Powderly WG. Failure of high-dose oral acyclovir with or without immune globulin to prevent primary cytomegalovirus disease in recipients of solid organ transplants. Am J Med 95:273–278, 1993.

Baker CJ, Melish ME, Hall RT, Casto DT, Vasan U, Givner LB. Intravenous immune globulin for the prevention of nosocomial infection in low-birth-weight neonates. The Multicenter Group for the Study of Immune Globulin in Neonates. N Engl J Med 327:213–219, 1992.

Baker RD, Severance AO. Mucormycosis with report of acute mycotic pneumonia (abstract). Am J Pathol 24:716–717, 1948.

Bale JF Jr, Kealey GP, Massanari RM, Strauss RG. The epidemiology of cytomegalovirus infection among patients with burns. Infect Control Hosp Epidemiol 11:17–22, 1990.

Band JD, Maki DG. Infections caused by arterial catheters used for hemodynamic monitoring. Am J Med 67:735–741, 1979.

Band JD, Maki DG. Steel needles used for intravenous therapy. Morbidity in patients with hematologic malignancy. Arch Intern Med 140:31–34, 1980.

Bar-Joseph G, Halberthal M, Sweed Y, Bialik V, Shoshani O, Etzioni A. Clostridium septicum infection in children with cyclic neutropenia. J Pediatr 131:317–319, 1997.

Barnett ED, Klein JO, Pelton SI, Luginbuhl LM. Otitis media in children born to human immunodeficiency virus–infected mothers. Pediatr Infect Dis J 11:360–364, 1992.

Barrett-Connor E. Bacterial infection and sickle cell anemia. An analysis of 250 infections in 166 patients and a review of the literature. Medicine (Baltimore) 50:97–112, 1971.

Barst RJ, Prince AS, Neu HC. Aspergillus endocarditis in children: case report and review of the literature. Pediatrics 68:738, 1981.

Barzilay Z, Mandel M, Keren G, Davidson S. Nosocomial bacterial pneumonia in ventilated children: clinical significance of culture-positive peripheral bronchial aspirates. J Pediatr 112:421–424, 1988.

Bash RO, Katz JA, Cash JV, Buchanan GR. Safety and cost effectiveness of early hospital discharge of lower risk children with cancer admitted for fever and neutropenia. Cancer 74:189–196, 1994.

Becker W, Naude DT, Kipps A, McKensie D. Virus studies in disseminated herpes simplex infections associated with malnutrition in children. S Afr Med J 37:74–76, 1963.

Begala JE, Maher K, Cherry JD. Risk of infection associated with the use of Broviac and Hickman catheters. Am J Infect Control 10:17–23, 1982.

Belio-Blasco C, Torres-Fernandez-Gil MA, Echevarria-Echarri JL, Gomez-Lopez LI. Evaluation of two retrospective active surveillance methods for the detection of nosocomial infection in surgical patients. Infect Control Hosp Epidemiol 21:24–27, 2000.

Benfield MR, McDonald R, Sullivan EK, Stablein DM, Tejani A. The 1997 annual renal transplantation in children report of the North American Pediatric Renal Transplant Cooperative Study (NAPRTCS). Pediatr Transplant 3:152–167, 1999.

Benjamin RP, Callaway L, Conant NF. Facial granuloma associated with Fusarium infection. Arch Dermatol 101:598–600, 1970.

Bernhard VM. Management of infected vascular prostheses. Surg Clin North Am 55:1411–1417, 1975.

Bhat AW, Jalal S, John V, Chat AM. Infective endocarditis in infants and children. Indian J Pediatr 63:204–209, 1996.

Black JA, Challacombe DN, Ockenden BG. Nephrotic syndrome associated with bacteraemia after shunt operations for hydrocephalus. Lancet 2:921–924, 1965.

Blair DC, Weiner LB. Prosthetic valve endocarditis due to Haemophilus parainfluenzae biotype II. Am J Dis Child 133:617–618, 1979.

Blau IW, Fauser AA. Review of comparative studies between conventional and liposomal amphotericin B (Ambisome) in neutropenic patients with fever of unknown origin and patients with systemic mycosis. Mycoses 43:325–332, 2000.

Bode FR, Pare JA, Fraser RG. Pulmonary diseases in the compromised host. A review of clinical and roentgenographic manifestations in patients with impaired host defense mechanisms. Medicine (Baltimore) 53:255–293, 1974.

Bodey GP. Antibiotics in patients with neutropenia. Arch Intern Med 144:1845–1851, 1984.

Bodey GP, Buckley M, Sathe YS, Freireich EJ. Quantitative relationships between circulating leukocytes and infection in patients with acute leukemia. Ann Intern Med 64:328–340, 1966.

Boeckman CR, Krill CE Jr. Bacterial and fungal infections complicating parenteral alimentation in infants and children. J Pediatr Surg 5:117–126, 1970.

Boyce JM, Potter-Bynoe G, Opal SM, Dziobek L, Medeiros AA. A common-source outbreak of Staphylococcus epidermidis infections among patients undergoing cardiac surgery. J Infect Dis 161:493–499, 1990.

Brandt L, Swahn G. Subacute bacterial endocarditis due to coagulase negative Staphylococcus albus. Acta Med Scand 166:125–132, 1960.

Brayman KL, Stephanian E, Matas AJ, Schmidt W, Payne WD, Sutherland DE, Gores PF, Najarian JS, Dunn DL. Analysis of infectious complications occurring after solid-organ transplantation. Arch Surg 127:38–48, 1992.

Brodie E, Adler JL, Daly AK. Bacterial endocarditis due to an unusual species of encapsulated Neisseria. Neisseria mucosa endocarditis. Am J Dis Child 122:433–437, 1971.

Brook MM. Pediatric bacterial endocarditis. Treatment and prophylaxis. Pediatr Clin North Am 46:275–287, 1999.

Brown AE. Neutropenia, fever, and infection. Am J Med 76:421–428, 1984.

Bruton OC. Agammaglobulinemia. Pediatrics 9:722–727, 1952.

Bryson YJ. The use of acyclovir in children. Pediatr Infect Dis 3:345–348, 1984.

Buckley RH. Immunodeficiency. J Allergy Clin Immunol 72:627–641, 1983.

Burgio GR, Duse M, Monafo V, Ascione A, Nespoli L. Selective IgA deficiency: clinical and immunological evaluation of 50 pediatric patients. Eur J Pediatr 133:101–106, 1980.

Burtenshaw JML. The autogenous disinfection of the skin. Dermatology 158–185, 1948.

Buxton AE, Highsmith AK, Garner JS, West CM, Stamm WE, Dixon RE, McGowan JE Jr. Contamination of intravenous infusion fluid: effects of changing administration sets. Ann Intern Med 90:764–768, 1979.

Caldwell RL, Hurwitz RA, Girod DA. Subacute bacterial endocarditis in children. Current status. Am J Dis Child 122:312–315, 1971.

Cannon PR. The relationship of protein metabolism to antibody production and resistance to infection. Adv Protein Chem 135–154, 1945.

Carr A, Penny R, Cooper DA. Efficacy and safety of rechallenge with low-dose trimethoprim-sulphamethoxazole in previously hypersensitive HIV-infected patients. AIDS 7:65–71, 1993.

Centers for Disease Control and Prevention. National nosocomial infections study report: annual summary, 1978, issued March 1981.

Centers for Disease Control and Prevention. Classification system for human immunodeficiency virus (HIV) infection in children under 13 years of age. MMWR Morb Mortal Wkly Rep 36:225–230, 235–236, 1987.

Centers for Disease Control and Prevention. 1993 revised classification system for HIV infection and expanded surveillance case definition for AIDS among adolescents and adults. MMWR Recomm Rep 41:1–19, 1992.

Centers for Disease Control and Prevention. Initial therapy for tuberculosis in the era of multidrug resistance. Recommendations of the Advisory Council for the Elimination of Tuberculosis. MMWR Recomm Rep 42:1–8, 1993a.

Centers for Disease Control and Prevention. Recommendations on prophylaxis and therapy for disseminated Mycobacterium avium complex for adults and adolescents infected with human immunodeficiency virus. U.S. Public Health Service Task Force on Prophylaxis and Therapy for Mycobacterium avium Complex. MMWR Recomm Rep 42:14–20, 1993b.

Centers for Disease Control and Prevention. 1994 revised classification system for human immunodeficiency virus infection in children less than 13 years of age. MMWR 43 (RR-12):1–19, 1994.

Centers for Disease Control and Prevention. 1995 revised guidelines for prophylaxis against Pneumocystis carinii pneumonia for children infected with or perinatally exposed to human immunodeficiency virus. National Pediatric and Family HIV Resource Center and National Center for Infectious Diseases, Centers for Disease Control and Prevention. MMWR Recomm Rep 44(RR-4):1–11, 1995.

Chandra RK. Immunocompetence in undernutrition. J Pediatr 81:1194–1200, 1972.

Chandwani S, Borkowsky W, Krasinski K, Lawrence R, Welliver R. Respiratory syncytial virus infection in human immunodeficiency virus–infected children. J Pediatr 117:251–254, 1990.

Chanock SJ, Pizzo PA. Infectious complications of patients undergoing therapy for acute leukemia: current status and future prospects. Semin Oncol 24:132–140, 1997.

Chastagner P, Plouvier E, Eyer D, Plesiat P, Lozniewski A, Sommelet D. Efficacy of cefepime and amikacin in the empiric treatment of febrile neutropenic children with cancer. Med Pediatr Oncol 34:306–308, 2000.

Cherry JD. Selection of antimicrobial agents for initial treatment of suspected septicemia in infants and children. Rev Infect Dis 5:S32–S39, 1983.

Chilcote RR, Baehner RL, Hammond D. Septicemia and meningitis in children splenectomized for Hodgkin's disease. N Engl J Med 295:798–800, 1976.

Chin TW, Stiehm ER, Falloon J, Gallin JI. Corticosteroids in treatment of obstructive lesions of chronic granulomatous disease. J Pediatr 111:349–352, 1987.

Chiou CC, Wong TT, Lin HH, Hwang B, Tang RB, Wu KG, Lee BH. Fungal infection of ventriculoperitoneal shunts in children. Clin Infect Dis 19:1049–1053, 1994.

Christensen CE, Emmanouilides GC. Bacterial endocarditis due to "Moraxella new species I". N Engl J Med 277:803–804, 1967.

Chuang TF, Kao SC, Tsai CJ, Lee CC, Chen KS. Spontaneous bacterial peritonitis as the presenting feature in an adult with nephrotic syndrome. Nephrol Dial Transplant 14:181–182, 1999.

Chusid MJ, Parrillo JE, Fauci AS. Chronic granulomatous disease. Diagnosis in a 27-year-old man with Mycobacterium fortuitum. JAMA 233:129–156, 1975.

Claman HN. Corticosteroids and lymphoid cells. N Engl J Med 287:388–397, 1972.

Commers JR, Robichaud KJ, Pizzo PA. New pulmonary infiltrates in granulocytopenic cancer patients being treated with antibiotics. Pediatr Infect Dis 3:423–428, 1984.

Conti DJ, Freed BM, Lempert N. Prophylactic immunoglobulin therapy improves the outcome of renal transplantation in recipients at risk for primary cytomegalovirus disease. Transplant Proc 25:1421–1422, 1993.

Cooper MR, DeChatelet LR, McCall CE, LaVia MF, Spurr CL, Baehner RL. Complete deficiency of leukocyte glucose-6-phosphate dehydrogenase with defective bactericidal activity. J Clin Invest 51:769–778, 1972.

Cooperstock MS. Indigenous flora in host economy and pathogenesis. In Feigin RD, Cherry JD, eds. Textbook of pediatric infectious diseases, 3rd ed. Philadelphia, W. B. Saunders, 1992, pp 91–119.

Crossley K, Matsen JM. The scalp-vein needle. A prospective study of complications. JAMA 220:985–987, 1972.

Cruse P. Wound infection surveillance. Rev Infect Dis 3:734–737, 1981.

Cruse PJ, Foord R. The epidemiology of wound infection. A 10-year prospective study of 62,939 wounds. Surg Clin North Am 60:27–40, 1980.

Curnutte JT. Chronic granulomatous disease: the solving of a clinical riddle at the molecular level. Clin Immunol Immunopathol 67:S2–S15, 1993a.

Curnutte JT. Conventional versus interferon-gamma therapy in chronic granulomatous disease. J Infect Dis 167:S8–S12, 1993b.

Curry CR, Quie PG. Fungal septicemia in patients receiving parenteral hyperalimentation. N Engl J Med 285:1221–1225, 1971.

Daghistani D, Horn M, Rodriguez Z, Schoenike S, Toledano S. Prevention of indwelling central venous catheter sepsis. Med Pediatr Oncol 26:40–58, 1996.

Dajani AS, Bisno AL, Chung KJ, Durack DT, Freed M, Gerber MA, Karchmer AW, Millard HD, Rahimtoola S, Shulman ST, Watanakunakorn C, Taubert KA. Prevention of bacterial endocarditis. Recommendations by the American Heart Association. JAMA 264:2919–2922, 1990.

Dale DC. Potential role of colony-stimulating factors in the prevention and treatment of infectious diseases. Clin Infect Dis 18:S180–S188, 1994.

Dale DC, Liles WC, Summer WR, Nelson S. Review: granulocyte colony-stimulating factor—role and relationships in infectious diseases. J Infect Dis 172:1061–1075, 1995.

Dale DC, Petersdorf RG. Corticosteroids and infectious diseases. Med Clin North Am 57:1277–1287, 1973.

Dammin GJ, Cough NP, Murray JE. Prolonged survival of skin homografts in uremic patients. Ann NY Acad Sci 64:967–976, 1957.

Davenport M, Doig CM. Wound infection in pediatric surgery: a study in 1,094 neonates. J Pediatr Surg 28:26–30, 1993.

Davis SD, Schaller J, Wedgwood RJ. Job's Syndrome. Recurrent, "cold," staphylococcal abscesses. Lancet 1:1013–1015, 1966.

Davis SD, Sobocinski K, Hoffmann RG, Mohr B, Nelson DB. Postoperative wound infections in a children's hospital. Pediatr Infect Dis 3:114–116, 1984.

Dawson S, Pai M, Smith S, Rothney M, Ahmed K, Barr R. Right atrial catheters in children with cancer: a decade of experience in the use of tunnelled, exteriorized devices at a single institution. Am J Pediatr Hematol Oncol 13:126–129, 1991.

Decker MD, Edwards KM. Central venous catheter infections. Pediatr Clin North Am 35:579–612, 1988.

Deen JL, Blumberg DA. Infectious disease considerations in pediatric organ transplantation. Semin Pediatr Surg 2:218–234, 1993.

Deinard AS, Libit SA. Coagulase-negative Staphylococcus bacteriuria in a child. Pediatrics 49:300–302, 1972.

Didonato JA, Saatcioglu F, Karin M. Molecular mechanisms of immunosuppression and anti-inflammatory activities by glucocorticoids. Am J Respir Crit Care Med 154:S11–S15, 1996.

Dichter JR, Levine SJ, Shelhamer JH. Approach to the immunocompromised host with pulmonary symptoms. Hematol Oncol Clin North Am 7:887–912, 1993.

Dietrich MC, Gerding RL, Kumar ML. Branhamella catarrhalis pneumonia with bacteremia in a pediatric patient with smoke inhalation. J Burn Care Rehabil 11:71–73, 1990.

DiGeorge AM. Congenital absence of the thymus and its immunologic consequences: concurrence with congenital hypoparathyroidism. In Bergsma D, Good RA, eds. Immunologic deficiency diseases in man. New York, The National Foundation-March of Dimes, 1968, pp 116–123.

Di John D, Krasinski K, Lawrence R, Borkowsky W, Johnson JP, Schieken LS, Rennels MB. Very late onset of group B streptococcal disease in infants infected with the human immunodeficiency virus. Pediatr Infect Dis J 9:925–928, 1990.

Dillon JD Jr, Schaffner W, Van Way CW 3rd, Meng HC. Septicemia and total parenteral nutrition. Distinguishing catheter-related from other septic episodes. JAMA 223:1341–1344, 1973.

Donabedian H, Gallin JI. The hyperimmunoglobulin E? recurrent-infection (Job's) syndrome. A review of the NIH experience and the literature. Medicine (Baltimore) 62:195–208, 1983.

Dudrick SJ, Wilmore DW, Vars HM, Rhoads JE. Long-term total parenteral nutrition with growth, development, and positive nitrogen balance. Surgery 64:134–142, 1968.

Ederer GM, Matsen JM. Colonization and infection with Pseudomonas cepacia. J Infect Dis 125:613–618, 1972.

Editorial: Infective hazards of splenectomy. Lancet 1:116–178, 1976.

Edmond MB, Wallace SE, McClish DK, Pfaller MA, Jones RN, Wenzel RP. Nosocomial bloodstream infections in United States hospitals: a three-year analysis. Clin Infect Dis 29:239–244, 1999.

Edmondson EB, Reinarz JA, Pierce AK, Sanford JP. Nebulization equipment. A potential source of infection in gram-negative pneumonias. Am J Dis Child 111:357–360, 1966.

Eickhoff TC. Hospital infections. Disease of the Month. Chicago, Year Book Medical Publishers, 1972.

Eickhoff TC. Nosocomial infections. Am J Epidemiol 101:93–97, 1975.

Elves MW, Israels MC, Collinge M. An assessment of the mixed leukocyte reaction in renal failure. Lancet 1:682–685, 1966.

Elward K, Hruby N, Christy C. Pneumococcal endocarditis in infants and children: report of a case and review of the literature. Pediatr Infect Dis J 9:652–657, 1990.

Erlendsson K, Swartz T, Dwyer JM. Successful reversal of echovirus encephalitis in X-linked hypogammaglobulinemia by intraventricular administration of immunoglobulin. N Engl J Med 312:351–353, 1985.

Erlewyn-Lajeunesse MD. Hyperimmunoglobulin-E syndrome with recurrent infection: a review of current opinion and treatment. Pediatr Allergy Immunol 11:133–141, 2000.

Esterly JR, Sturner WQ, Esterly NB, Windhorst DB. Disseminated BCG in twin boys with presumed chronic granulomatous disease of childhood. Pediatrics 48:141–144, 1971.

Ezer G, Soothill JF. Intracellular bactericidal effects of rifampicin in both normal and chronic granulomatous disease polymorphs. Arch Dis Child 49:463–466, 1974.

Faber K. Tuberculosis and nutrition. Acta Tuberc Scand 12:287–335, 1938.

Falloon J, Eddy J, Wiener L, Pizzo PA. Human immunodeficiency virus infection in children. J Pediatr 114:1–30, 1989.

Fanci R, Paci C, Martinez RL, Fabbri A, Pecile P, Leoni F, Longo G. Management of fever in neutropenic patients with acute leukemia: current role of ceftazidime plus amikacin as empiric therapy. J Chemother 12:232–239, 2000.

Fayon MJ, Tucci M, Lacroix J, Farrell CA, Gauthier M, Lafleur L, Nadeau D. Nosocomial pneumonia and tracheitis in a pediatric intensive care unit: a prospective study. Am J Respir Crit Care Med 155:162–169, 1997.

Feigin RD, Shearer WT. Opportunistic infection in children I. In the compromised host. J Pediatr 87:507–514, 1975a.

Feigin RD, Shearer WT. Opportunistic infection in children. II. In the compromised host. J Pediatr 87:677–694, 1975b.

Feller I, Crane KH. National Burn Information Exchange. Surg Clin North Am 50:1425–1436, 1970.

Ferguson AC, Lawlor GJ, Neumann CG, Oh W, Stiehm ER. Decreased rosette-forming lymphocytes in malnutrition and intrauterine growth retardation. J Pediatr 85:717–723, 1974.

Fikrig SM, Schiffman G, Phillipp JC, Moel DI. Antibody response to capsular polysaccharide vaccine of Streptococcus pneumoniae in patients with nephrotic syndrome. J Infect Dis 137:818–821, 1978.

Fisher MC, Long SS, Roberts EM, Dunn JM, Balsara RK. Pseudomonas maltophilia bacteremia in children undergoing open heart surgery. JAMA 246:1571–1574, 1981.

Flynn DM, Weinstein RA, Nathan C, Gaston MA, Kabins SA. Patients' endogenous flora as the source of "nosocomial" Enterobacter in cardiac surgery. J Infect Dis 156:363–368, 1987a.

Flynn PM, Shenep JL, Stokes DC, Barrett FF. In situ management of confirmed central venous catheterrelated bacteremia. Pediatr Infect Dis J 6:729–734, 1987b.

Flynn PM, Van Hooser B, Gigliotti F. Atypical mycobacterial infections of Hickman catheter exit sites. Pediatr Infect Dis J 7:510–513, 1988.

Flynn PM, Shenep JL. Acquired immunodeficiency syndrome. In Patrick CC, ed. Infections in immunocompromised infants and children. New York, Churchill Livingstone, 1992, pp 161–177.

Foley FD. The burn autopsy. Fatal complications of burns. Am J Clin Pathol 52:11–13, 1969.

Foroozanfar N, Lucas CF, Joss DV, Hugh-Jones K, Hobbs JR. Ascorbate (1 g/day) does not help the phagocytic killing defect of X-linked chronic granulomatous disease. Clin Exp Immunol 51:99–102, 1983.

Frayha HH, Biggar WD. Chronic granulomatous disease of childhood: a changing pattern? J Clin Immunol 3:287–291, 1983.

Frazier JP, Kramer WG, Pickering LK, Culbert S, Brandt K, Frankel LS. Antimicrobial therapy of febrile children with malignancies and possible sepsis. Pediatr Infect Dis 3:40–45, 1984.

Freeman JB, Litton AA. Preponderance of gram-positive infections during parenteral alimentation. Surg Gynecol Obstet 139:905–908, 1974.

Freeman J, Goldmann DA, Smith NE, Sidebottom DG, Epstein MF, Platt R. Association of intravenous lipid emulsion and coagulase-negative staphylococcal bacteremia in neonatal intensive care units. N Engl J Med 323:301–308, 1990.

Frenkel LD, Gaur S, Tsolia M, Scudder R, Howell R, Kesarwala H. Cytomegalovirus infection in children with AIDS. Rev Infect Dis 12:S820–S826, 1990.

Freyre EA, Chabes A, Poemape O, Chabes A. Abnormal Rebuck skin window response in kwashiorkor. J Pediatr 82:523–526, 1973.

Fricker FJ, Griffith BP, Hardesty RL, Trento A, Gold LM, Schmeltz K, Beerman LB, Fischer DR, Mathews RA, Neches WH, Park SC, Zuberbuhler JR, Lenox CC, Bahnson HT. Experience with heart transplantation in children. Pediatrics 79:138–146, 1987.

Friedland LR, Raphael SA, Deutsch ES, Johal J, Martyn LJ, Visvesvara GS, Lischner HW. Disseminated Acanthamoeba infection in a child with symptomatic human immunodeficiency virus infection. Pediatr Infect Dis J 11:404–407, 1992.

Friedland IR, Shelton S, Paris M, Rinderknecht S, Ehrett S, Krisher K, McCracken GH Jr. Dilemmas in diagnosis and management of cephalosporin-resistant Streptococcus pneumoniae meningitis. Pediatr Infect Dis J 12:196–200, 1993.

Friedman LE, Brown AE, Miller DR, Armstrong D. Staphylococcus epidermidis septicemia in children with leukemia and lymphoma. Am J Dis Child 138:715–719, 1984.

Furfaro S, Gauthier M, Lacroix J, Nadeau D, Lafleur L, Mathews S. Arterial catheter–related infections in children. A 1-year cohort analysis. Am J Dis Child 145:1037–1043, 1991.

Gajarski RJ, Smith EO, Denfield SW, Rosenblatt HM, Kearney D, Frazier OH, Radovancevic B, Price JK, Kertesz NJ, Towbin JA. Long-term results of triple-drug-based immunosuppression in nonneonatal pediatric heart transplant recipients. Transplantation 65:1470–1476, 1998.

Gallin JI, Buescher ES, Seligmann BE, Nath J, Gaither T, Katz P. NIH conference. Recent advances in chronic granulomatous disease. Ann Intern Med 99:657–674, 1983.

Garcia S, Linares M, Colomina P, Miguel A, Miguel A. Cytomegalovirus infection and aplastic crisis in glucose-6-phosphate dehydrogenase deficiency. Lancet 2:10–15, 1987.

Garland JS, Alex CP, Mueller CD, Otten D, Shivpuri C, Harris MC, Naples M, Pellegrini J, Buck RK, McAuliffe TL, Goldmann DA, Maki DG. A randomized trial comparing povidone-iodine to a chlorhexidine gluconate-impregnated dressing for prevention of central venous catheter infections in neonates. Pediatrics 107:1431–1436, 2001.

Garner JS, Simmons BP. Guideline for isolation precautions in hospitals. Infect Control 4:245–325, 1983.

Gatti RA, Stutman O, Good RA. The lymphoid system. Annu Rev Physiol 32:529–546, 1970.

Gautier E, Bourhis JH, Bayle C, Cartron J, Pico JL, Tchernia G. Parvovirus B19 associated neutropenia. Treatment with Rh G-CSF. Hematol Cell Ther 39:85–87, 1997.

Geefhuysen J, Rosen EU, Katz J, Ipp T, Metz J. Impaired cellular immunity in kwashiorkor with improvement after therapy. Br Med J 4:527–529, 1971.

Gelfand EW, McCurdy D, Rao CP, Middleton PJ. Ribavirin treatment of viral pneumonitis in severe combined immunodeficiency disease. Lancet 2:732–733, 1983.

George DL. Epidemiology of nosocomial ventilator–associated pneumonia. Infect Control Hosp Epidemiol 14:163–169, 1993.

Gitlin D, Janeway CA, Apt L, Craig JM. Agammaglobulinemia. In Lawrence HS, ed. Cellular and humoral aspects of the hypersensitive states; a symposium held at the New York Academy of Medicine. New York, P.B. Hoeber Medical Division, Harper & Row, 1959, pp 375–441.

Givner LB, Kaplan SL. Meningitis due to *Staphylococcus aureus* in children. Clin Infect Dis 16:766–771, 1993.

Glaser CA, Angulo FJ, Rooney JA. Animal-associated opportunistic infections among persons infected with the human immunodeficiency virus. Clin Infect Dis 18:142–144, 1994.

Gmunder FK, Seger RA. Chronic granulomatous disease: mode of action of sulfamethoxazole/trimethoprim. Pediatr Res 15:1533–1537, 1981.

Goldberg P, Shulman ST, Yogev R. Group C streptococcal endocarditis. Pediatrics 75:114–116, 1985.

Goldmann DA, Maki DG. Infection control in total parenteral nutrition. JAMA 223:1360–1364, 1973.

Goldstein IM, Marder SR. Infections and hypocomplementemia. Annu Rev Med 34:47–53, 1983.

Gooch WM 3rd, Fernbach DJ. Immunoglobulins during the course of acute leukemia in children. Effects of various clinical factors. Cancer 28:984–989, 1971.

Gorelick MH, Owen WC, Seibel NL, Reaman GH. Lack of association between neutropenia and the incidence of bacteremia associated with indwelling central venous catheters in febrile pediatric cancer patients. Pediatr Infect Dis J 10:506–510, 1991.

Gradon JD, Timpone JG, Schnittman SM. Emergence of unusual opportunistic pathogens in AIDS: a review. Clin Infect Dis 15:134–157, 1992.

Green M, Wald ER, Fricker FJ, Griffith BP, Trento A. Infections in pediatric orthotopic heart transplant recipients. Pediatr Infect Dis J 8:87–93, 1989.

Gregory JE, Golden A, Haymaker W. *Mucor*mycosis of the central nervous system: a report of 3 cases. Bull Johns Hopkins Hosp 73:405–419, 1943.

Griffin JR, Pettit TH, Fishman LS, Foos RY. Blood-borne *Candida* endophthalmitis. A clinical and pathologic study of 21 cases. Arch Ophthalmol 89:450–456, 1973.

Groff DB. Complication of intravenous hyperalimentation in newborns and infants. J Pediatr Surg 4:460–464, 1969.

Haag-Weber M, Hörl WH. Uremia and infection: mechanisms of impaired cellular host defense. Nephron 63:125–131, 1993.

Hall CB. Respiratory syncytial virus. In Feigin RD, Cherry JD, eds. Textbook of pediatric infectious diseases, 4th ed. Philadelphia, W. B. Saunders, 1998, pp 2041–2054.

Hand IL, Wiznia AA, Porricolo M, Lambert G, Caspe WB. Aerosolized pentamidine for prophylaxis of *Pneumocystis carinii* pneumonia in infants with human immunodeficiency virus infection. Pediatr Infect Dis J 13:100–104, 1994.

Haning HA, Johnston R, Touloukian R, Margolis CZ. Successfully treated *Candida* endophthalmitis in a child. Pediatrics 51:1027–1031, 1973.

Hanson IC, Shearer WT. AIDS and other acquired immunodeficiency diseases. In Feigin RD, Cherry JD, eds. Textbook of pediatric infectious diseases, 4th ed. Philadelphia, W. B. Saunders, 1998, pp 954–979.

Hanson IC. Respiratory infections in HIV-infected children. Immunol Allergy Clin North Am 13:205–217, 1993.

Harbin RL, Schaffner W. Septicemia associated with scalp-vein needles. South Med J 66:638–640, 1973.

Harmon WE. Opportunistic infections in children following renal transplantation. Pediatr Nephrol 5:118–225, 1991.

Hart PD, Russell E Jr, Remington JS. The compromised host and infection: II. Deep fungal infection. J Infect Dis 120:169–191, 1969.

Hatcher JC, Greenberg PD, Antique J, Jimenez-Lucho VE. Severe babesiosis in Long Island: review of 34 cases and their complications. Clin Infect Dis 32:1117–1125, 2001.

Hattori K, Hasui M, Masuda K, Masuda M, Ogino H, Kobayashi Y. Successful trimethoprim-sulfamethoxazole therapy in a patient with hyperimmunoglobulin E syndrome. Acta Paediatr 82:324–326, 1993.

Hausser C, Virelizier JL, Buriot D, Griscelli C. Common variable hypogammaglobulinemia in children. Clinical and immunologic observations in 30 patients. Am J Dis Child 137:833–837, 1983.

Hermans P, Sommereijns B, Van Cutsem N, Clumeck N. Neutropenia in patients with HIV infection: a case control study in a cohort of 1403 patients between 1982 and 1993. J Hematother Stem Cell Res 8:S23–S32, 1999.

Hermaszewski RA, Webster AD. Primary hypogammaglobulinaemia: a survey of clinical manifestations and complications. Q J Med 86:31–42, 1993.

Herrod HG, Wang WC, Sullivan JL. Chronic T-cell lymphocytosis with neutropenia. Its association with Epstein-Barr virus infection. Am J Dis Child 139:405–407, 1985.

Hewitt WL, Sanford JP. Workshop on hospital-associated infections. J Infect Dis 130:680–686, 1974.

Hiatt JR, Ament ME, Berquist WJ, Brems JF, Brill JE, Colonna JO 2nd, el Khoury G, Quinones WJ, Ramming KP, Vargas JH, Busuttil RW. Pediatric liver transplantation at UCLA. Transplant Proc 19:3282–3288, 1987.

Hiemenz JW, Greene JN. Special considerations for the patient undergoing allogeneic or autologous bone marrow transplantation. Hematol Oncol Clin North Am 7:961–1002, 1993.

Hill HR. Intravenous immunoglobulin use in the neonate: role in prophylaxis and therapy of infection. Pediatr Infect Dis J 12:549–559, 1993.

Hitzig WH, Barandun S, Cottier H. Die schweizerische form der agammaglobulinamie. Ergeb Inn Med Kinderheilkd 27:79–154, 1968.

Hoger PH, Seger RA, Schaad UB, Hitzig WH. Chronic granulomatous disease: uptake and intracellular activity of fosfomycin in granulocytes. Pediatr Res 19:38–44, 1985.

Holland JF, Senn H, Banerjee T. Quantitative studies of localized leukocyte mobilization in acute leukemia. Blood 37:499–511, 1971.

Hong R, Ammann AJ, Huang S, Levy RL, Davenport G, Bach ML, Bach FH, Bortin MM, Kay HEM. Cartilage-hair hypoplasia: effect of thymus transplants. Clin Immunol Immunopathol 1:15–26, 1972.

Horan TC, Culver DH, Gaynes RP, Jarvis WR, Edwards JR, Reid CR. Nosocomial infections in surgical patients in the United States, January 1986 June 1992. National Nosocomial Infectious Surveillance (NNIS) System. Infect Control Hosp Epidemiol 14:73–80, 1993.

Hoyt L, Oleske J, Holland B, Connor E. Nontuberculous mycobacteria in children with acquired immunodeficiency syndrome. Pediatr Infect Dis J 11:354–360, 1992.

Hughes WT. Fatal infections in childhood leukemia. Am J Dis Child 122:283–287, 1971.

Hughes WT, Feldman S, Cox F. Infectious diseases in children with cancer. Pediatr Clin North Am 21:583–615, 1974.

Hughes WT. Hematogenous histoplasmosis in the immunocompromised child. J Pediatr 105:569–575, 1984.

Hughes WT, Parham DM. Molluscum contagiosum in children with cancer or acquired immunodeficiency syndrome. Pediatr Infect Dis J 10:15–26, 1991.

Hughes WT. Prevention of infections in patients with T cell defects. Clin Infect Dis 17:S368–S371, 1993.

Huskins WC, Goldmann DA. Prevention and control of nosocomial infections in hospitalized children. In Feigin RD, Cherry JD, eds.

Textbook of pediatric infectious diseases, 4th ed. Philadelphia, W. B. Saunders, 1998, pp 2585–2602.

Hyatt AC, Altenburger KM, Johnston RB Jr, Winkelstein JA. Increased susceptibility to severe pyogenic infections in patients with an inherited deficiency of the second component of complement. J Pediatr 98:417–419, 1981.

Ingram J, Weitzman S, Greenberg M, Parkin P, Filler R. Complications of indwelling venous access lines in the pediatric hematology patient: a prospective comparison of external venous catheters and subcutaneous ports. Am J Pediatr Hematol Oncol 13:130–136, 1991.

International Chronic Granulomatous Disease Cooperative Study Group, The. A controlled trial of interferon gamma to prevent infection in chronic granulomatous disease. N Engl J Med 324:509–516, 1991.

Ivarsson SA, Ljung R. Neutropenia and congenital cytomegalovirus infection. Pediatr Infect Dis J 7:436–437, 1988.

Jackson ME, Wong KY, Lampkin B. Pseudomonas aeruginosa septicemia in childhood cancer patients. Pediatr Infect Dis 1:239–241, 1982.

Jacobs MR. Treatment and diagnosis of infections caused by drug-resistant Streptococcus pneumoniae. Clin Infect Dis 15:119–127, 1992.

Jacobs RF, Wilson CB. Activity of antibiotics in chronic granulomatous disease leukocytes. Pediatr Res 17:916–919, 1983.

James JW. Longitudinal study of the morbidity of diarrheal and respiratory infections in malnourished children. Am J Clin Nutr 25:690–694, 1972.

Jarvis WR. Epidemiology of nosocomial infections in pediatric patients. Pediatr Infect Dis J 6:344–351, 1987.

Jarvis WR, Highsmith AK, Allen JR, Haley RW. Polymicrobial bacteremia associated with lipid emulsion in a neonatal intensive care unit. Pediatr Infect Dis 2:20–38, 1983.

Jenson HB, Pollock BH. The role of intravenous immunoglobulin for the prevention and treatment of neonatal sepsis. Semin Perinatol 22:50–63, 1998.

Johanson WG Jr, Seidenfeld JJ, Gomez P, De Los Santos R, Coalson JJ. Bacteriologic diagnosis of nosocomial pneumonia following prolonged mechanical ventilation. Am Rev Respir Dis 137:259–264, 1988.

Johnson CM, Rhodes KH. Pediatric endocarditis. Mayo Clin Proc 57:86–94, 1982.

Johnston RB Jr, Baehner RL. Chronic granulomatous disease: correlation between pathogenesis and clinical findings. Pediatrics 48:730–739, 1971.

Johnston RB Jr, Wilfert CM, Buckley RH, Webb LS, DcChatelet LR, McCall CE. Enhanced bactericidal activity of phagocytes from patients with chronic granulomatous disease in the presence of sulphisoxazole. Lancet 1:824–827, 1975.

Kammer RB, Utz JP. Aspergillus species endocarditis. The new face of a not so rare disease. Am J Med 56:506–521, 1974.

Kanj SS, Sharara AI, Clavien PA, Hamilton JD. Cytomegalovirus infection following liver transplantation: review of the literature. Clin Infect Dis 22:537–549, 1996.

Kaplan SL. Heart transplants: infections in immunocompromised infants and children. In Patrick CC, ed. Infections in immunocompromised infants and children. New York, Churchill Livingstone, 1992, pp 251–260.

Katz JA, Mustafa MM. Management of fever in granulocytopenic children with cancer. Pediatr Infect Dis J 12:330–337, 1993.

Katz M. Babesiosis. Pediatr Infect Dis 1:219–220, 1982.

Kauder E, Mauer AM. Neutropenias of childhood. J Pediatr 69:147–157, 1966.

Kebudi R, Gorgun O, Ayan I, Gurler N, Akici F, Toreci K. Randomized comparison of cefepime versus ceftazidime monotherapy for fever and neutropenia in children with solid tumors. Med Pediatr Oncol 36:434–441, 2001.

Kemaloglu YK, Kobayashi T, Nakajima T. Analysis of the craniofacial skeleton in cleft children with otitis media with effusion. Int J Pediatr Otorhinolaryngol 47:57–69, 1999.

Keita-Perse O, Edwards JR, Culver DH, Gaynes RP. Comparing nosocomial infection rates among surgical intensive-care units: the importance of separating cardiothoracic and general surgery

intensive-care units. Infect Control Hosp Epidemiol 19:260–261, 1998.

Kim KS. High-dose intravenous immune globulin impairs antibacterial activity of antibiotics. J Allergy Clin Immunol 84:579–588, 1989.

Kinney J, Mundorf L, Gleason C, Lee C, Townsend T, Thibault R, Nussbaum A, Abby H, Yolken R. Efficacy and pharmacokinetics of intravenous immune globulin administration to high-risk neonates. Am J Dis Child 145:123–138, 1991.

Kinugawa N. Epstein-Barr virus infection in Chediak-Higashi syndrome mimicking acute lymphocytic leukemia. Am J Pediatr Hematol Oncol 12:182–186, 1990.

Kirkpatrick CH, Wilson WEC, Talmadge DW. Immunologic studies in human organ transplantation. I. Observation and characterization of suppressed cutaneous reactivity in uremia. J Exp Med 119:727–742, 1964.

Klainer AS, Beisel WR. Opportunistic infection: a review. Am J Med Sci 258:431–456, 1969.

Kletzel M, Beck S, Elser J, Shock N, Burks W. Trimethoprim-sulfamethoxazole oral desensitization in hemophiliacs infected with human immunodeficiency virus with a history of hypersensitivity reactions. Am J Dis Child 145:142–189, 1991.

Kline MW, Dunkle LM. Toxic shock syndrome and the acquired immunodeficiency syndrome. Pediatr Infect Dis J 7:736–738, 1988.

Klugman KP. Pneumococcal resistance to antibiotics. Clin Microbiol Rev 3:171–196, 1990.

Kobayashi Y, Amano D, Ueda K, Kagosaki Y, Usui T. Treatment of seven cases of chronic granulomatous disease with sulfamethoxazole-trimethoprim (SMX-TMP). Eur J Pediatr 127:247–254, 1978.

Koiwai EK, Nahas HC. Subacute bacterial endocarditis following cardiac surgery. AMA Arch Surg 73:272–278, 1956.

Koll BS, Brown AE. Changing patterns of infections in the immunocompromised patient with cancer. Hematol Oncol Clin North Am 7:753–769, 1993.

Kollef MH. Ventilator-associated pneumonia. A multivariate analysis. JAMA 270:1965–1970, 1993.

Kontny U, Hofling B, Gutjahr P, Voth D, Schwarz M, Schmitt HJ. CSF shunt infections in children. Infection 21:89–92, 1993.

Koskinen S. Long-term follow-up of health in blood donors with primary selective IgA deficiency. J Clin Immunol 16:165–170, 1996.

Kosmidis HV, Lusher JM, Shope TC, Ravindranath Y, Dajani AS. Infections in leukemic children: a prospective analysis. J Pediatr 96:814–819, 1980.

Kramer HH, Bourgeois M, Liersch R, Kuhn H, Nessler L, Meyer H, Sievers G. Current clinical aspects of bacterial endocarditis in infancy, childhood, and adolescence. Eur J Pediatr 140:253–259, 1983.

Krasinski K, Borkowsky W, Bonk S, Lawrence R, Chandwani S. Bacterial infections in human immunodeficiency virus infected children. Pediatr Infect Dis J 7:323–328, 1988.

Krause PJ. Babesiosis. In Feigin RD, Cherry JD, eds. Textbook of pediatric infectious diseases, 4th ed. Philadelphia, W. B. Saunders, 1998, pp 2432–2437.

Krause PJ, Lepore T, Sikand VK, Gadbaw J Jr, Burke G, Telford SR 3rd, Brassard P, Pearl D, Azlanzadeh J, Christianson D, McGrath D, Spielman A. Atovaquone and azithromycin for the treatment of babesiosis. N Engl J Med 343:1454–1458, 2000.

Kuhls TL, Leach CT. Infections in pediatric liver transplant recipients. In Patrick CC, ed. Infections in immunocompromised infants and children. New York, Churchill Livingstone, 1992, pp 231–250.

Kulkarni AV, Drake JM, Lamberti-Pasculli M. Cerebrospinal fluid shunt infection: a prospective study of risk factors. J Neurosurg 94:195–201, 2001.

Kunin CM. Detection, Prevention and Management of Urinary Tract Infections; A Manual for the Physician, Nurse, and Allied Health Worker. Philadelphia, Lea & Febiger, 1972.

Kunin CM, McCormack RC. Prevention of catheter-induced urinary-tract infections by sterile closed drainage. N Engl J Med 274:1155–1161, 1966.

Kuritzkes DR. Neutropenia, neutrophil dysfunction, and bacterial infection in patients with human immunodeficiency virus disease: the role of granulocyte colony-stimulating factor. Clin Infect Dis 30:256–260, 2000.

Lacroix J, Gauthier M, Lapointe N, Ahronheim G, Arcand P, Girouard G. *Pseudomonas aeruginosa* supraglottitis in a six-month-old child with severe combined immunodeficiency syndrome. Pediatr Infect Dis J 7:739–741, 1988.

Lang PA, Ritzmann SE, Merian FL, Lawrence MC, Levin WC, Gregory R. Cellular evolution in induced inflammation in uremic patients. Tex Rep Biol Med 24:107–111, 1966.

Langley JM, LeBlanc JC, Drake J, Milner R. Efficacy of antimicrobial prophylaxis in placement of cerebrospinal fluid shunts: meta-analysis. Clin Infect Dis 7:98–103, 1993.

Lautenschlager I, Linnavuori K, Hockerstedt K. Human herpesvirus-6 antigenemia after liver transplantation. Transplantation 69:2561–2566, 2000.

Lazarus GM, Neu HC. Agents responsible for infection in chronic granulomatous disease in childhood. J Pediatr 86:415–417, 1975.

Leggiadro RJ, Kline MW, Hughes WT. Extrapulmonary cryptococcosis in children with acquired immunodeficiency syndrome. Pediatr Infect Dis J 10:658–662, 1991.

Leibovitz E, Cooper D, Giurgiutiu D, Coman G, Straus I, Orlow SJ, Lawrence R. Varicella-zoster virus infection in Romanian children infected with the human immunodeficiency virus. Pediatrics 92:838–842, 1993.

Leibovitz E, Rigaud M, Chandwani S, Kaul A, Greco MA, Pollack H, Lawrence R, Di John D, Hanna B, Krasinski K, Borkowsky W. Disseminated fungal infections in children infected with human immunodeficiency virus. Pediatr Infect Dis J 10:888–894, 1991.

Leibovitz E, Rigaud M, Pollack H, Lawrence R, Chandwani S, Krasinski K, Borkowsky W. *Pneumocystis carinii* pneumonia in infants infected with the human immunodeficiency virus with more than 450 CD4 T lymphocytes per cubic millimeter. N Engl J Med 323:531–533, 1990.

Leu H-S, Kaiser DL, Mori M, Woolson RF, Wenzel RP. Hospital-acquired pneumonia. Attributable mortality and morbidity. Am J Epidemiol 129:1258–1267, 1989.

Leung T, Chik K, Li C, Shing M, Yuen P. Bone marrow transplantation for chronic granulomatous disease: long-term follow-up and review of literature. Bone Marrow Transplant 24:567–570, 1999.

Levine AS, Schimpff SC, Graw RG Jr, Young RC. Hematologic malignancies and other marrow failure states: progress in the management of complicating infections. Semin Hematol 11:141–202, 1974.

Levy R, Kaplan HS. Impaired lymphocyte function in untreated Hodgkin's disease. N Engl J Med 290:181–186, 1974.

Lewis IJ, Hart CA, Baxby D. Diarrhoea due to Cryptosporidium in acute lymphoblastic leukemia. Arch Dis Child 60:60–62, 1985.

Lewis LL, Butler KM, Husson RN, Mueller BU, Fowler CL, Steinberg SM, Pizzo PA. Defining the population of human immunodeficiency virus infected children at risk for *Mycobacterium avium intracellulare* infection. J Pediatr 121:677–683, 1992.

Liese JG, Wintergerst U, Tympner KD, Belohradsky BH. High-vs low-dose immunoglobulin therapy in the long-term treatment of X-linked agammaglobulinemia. Am J Dis Child 146:33–59, 1992.

Linnemann CC Jr, MacMillan BG. Viral infections in pediatric burn patients. Am J Dis Child 135:750–753, 1981.

LiPuma JJ. Expanding microbiology of pulmonary infection in cystic fibrosis. Pediatr Infect Dis J 19:473–474, 2000.

Lohr JA, Donowitz LG, Sadler JE 3rd. Hospital-acquired urinary tract infection. Pediatrics 83:193–199, 1989.

Maas A, Flament P, Pardou A, Deplano A, Dramaix M, Struelens MJ. Central venous catheter-related bacteraemia in critically ill neonates: risk factors and impact of a prevention programme. J Hosp Infect 40:211–224, 1998.

MacDonald NE, Hall CB, Suffin SC, Alexson C, Harris PJ, Manning JA. Respiratory syncytial viral infection in infants with congenital heart disease. N Engl J Med 307:397–400, 1982.

MacMillan BG. Infections following burn injury. Surg Clin North Am 60:185–196, 1980.

Magny JF, Bremard-Oury C, Brault D, Menguy C, Voyer M, Landais P, Dehan M, Gabilan JC. Intravenous immunoglobulin therapy for prevention of infection in high-risk premature infants: report of a multicenter, double-blind study. Pediatrics 88:437–443, 1991.

Maki DG, Goldman DA, Rhame FS. Infection control in intravenous therapy. Ann Intern Med 79:867–887, 1973a.

Maki DG, Hennekens CG, Phillips CW, Shaw WV, Bennett JV. Nosocomial urinary tract infection with *Serratia marcescens*: an epidemiologic study. J Infect Dis 128:579–587, 1973b.

Maki DG, Rhame FS, Mackel DC, Bennett JV. Nationwide epidemic of septicemia caused by contaminated intravenous products. I. Epidemiologic and clinical features. Am J Med 60:471–485, 1976.

Maki DG, Band JD. A comparative study of polyantibiotic and iodophor ointments in prevention of vascular catheterrelated infection. Am J Med 70:739–744, 1981.

Maki DG, Botticelli JT, LeRoy ML, Thielke TS. Prospective study of replacing administration sets for intravenous therapy at 48-vs 72-hour intervals. 72 hours is safe and cost-effective. JAMA 258:1777–1781, 1987.

Malik AS. *Acinetobacter* endocarditis in children: a case report and review of the literature. Infection. 23:306–309, 1995.

Makitie O, Kaitila I. Cartilage-hair hypoplasia—clinical manifestations in 108 Finnish patients. Eur J Pediatr 152:211–217, 1993.

Margolis DM, Melnick DA, Alling DW, Gallin JI. Trimethoprim-sulfamethoxazole prophylaxis in the management of chronic granulomatous disease. J Infect Dis 162:723–726, 1990.

Markenson DS, Levine D, Schacht R. Primary peritonitis as a presenting feature of nephrotic syndrome: a case report and review of the literature. Pediatr Emerg Care 15:407–409, 1999.

Markowitz LE, Chandler FW, Roldan EO, Saldana MJ, Roach KC, Hutchins SS, Preblud SR, Mitchell CD, Scott GB. Fatal measles pneumonia without rash in a child with AIDS. J Infect Dis 158:480–483, 1988.

Marks MI, Langston C, Eickhoff TC. *Torulopsis glabrata*—an opportunistic pathogen in man. N Engl J Med 283:1131–1135, 1970.

Martin FP, Lukeman JM, Ranson RF, Geppert LJ. Mucormycosis of central nervous system associated with thrombosis of the internal carotid artery. J Pediatr 44:437–516, 1954.

Martin JM, Neches WH, Wald ER. Infective endocarditis: 35 years of experience at a children's hospital. Clin Infect Dis 24:669–675, 1997.

McBride SJ, McCluskey DR, Jackson PT. Selective C7 complement deficiency causing recurrent meningococcal infection. J Infect 22:273–276, 1991.

McCabe WR: Pyelonephritis. In Hoeprich PD, ed. Infectious diseases: a guide to the understanding and management of infectious processes. Hagerstown, MD, Medical Dept., Harper & Row, 1972, pp 507–521.

McClain K, Estrov Z, Chen H, Mahoney DH Jr. Chronic neutropenia of childhood: frequent association with parvovirus infection and correlations with bone marrow culture studies. Br J Haematol 85:57–62, 1993.

McCrae WM, Raeburn JA. Chronic granulomatosus disease: an attempt to stimulate phagocytic activity. Lancet 1:1370–1371, 1972.

McGinnis MR, Walker DH, Folds JD. *Hansenula polymorpha* infection in a child with chronic granulomatous disease. Arch Pathol Lab Med 104:290–292, 1980.

McIntosh K, Kurachek SC, Cairns LM, Burns JC, Goodspeed B. Treatment of respiratory viral infection in an immunodeficient infant with ribavirin aerosol. Am J Dis Child 138:305–308, 1984.

McKenzie SA, Hayden K. Two cases of "shunt nephritis." Pediatrics 54:806–808, 1974.

Meares EM Jr. Current patterns in nosocomial urinary tract infections. Urology 37:91–92, 1991.

Mehta PA, Cunningham CK, Colella CB, Alferis G, Weiner LB. Risk factors for sternal wound and other infections in pediatric cardiac surgery patients. Pediatr Infect Dis J 19:1000–1004, 2000.

Mendelsohn G, Hutchins GM. Infective endocarditis during the first decade of life. An autopsy review of 33 cases. Am J Dis Child 133:619–622, 1979.

Mendelsohn HB, Berant M. Chronic granulomatous disease: a new clinical variant. Acta Paediatr Scand 71:869–872, 1982.

Merino F, Henle W, Ramirez-Duque P. Chronic active Epstein-Barr virus infection in patients with Chediak-Higashi syndrome. J Clin Immunol 6:299–305, 1986.

Mermel LA, Maki DG. Epidemic bloodstream infections from hemodynamic pressure monitoring: signs of the times. Infect Control Hosp Epidemiol 10:47–53, 1989.

Mertz JJ, Scharer L, McClement JH. A hospital outbreak of Klebsiella pneumonia from inhalation therapy with contaminated aerosol solutions. Am Rev Respir Dis 95:454–460, 1967.

Merzbach D, Freundlich E, Metzker A, Falk W. Bacterial endocarditis due to Corynebacterium. J Pediatr 67:792–796, 1965.

Meuleman N, Debruyne JM, Jacquy C, Bron D. Incidence of CMV infection and CMV disease in allogeneic transplanted patients; From no prophylaxis to preemptive treatment. Exp Hematol 28:1501, 2000.

Miall LS, McGinley NT, Brownlee KG, Conway SP. Methicillin-resistant Staphylococcus aureus (MRSA) infection in cystic fibrosis. Arch Dis Child 84:160–162, 2001.

Mills EL, Quie PG. Congenital disorders of the functions of polymorphonuclear neutrophils. Rev Infect Dis 2:505–517, 1980.

Ming PL, Ming SC, Dammin GJ. Effect of uremia and azathioprine on lymphocyte response to phytohemagglutinin. Pediatr Proc 27:432, 1968.

Miser JS, Miser AW. Staphylococcus aureus sepsis in childhood malignancy. Am J Dis Child 134:831–833, 1980.

Mitchell CD, Erlich SS, Mastrucci MT, Hutto SC, Parks WP, Scott GB. Congenital toxoplasmosis occurring in infants perinatally infected with human immunodeficiency virus 1. Pediatr Infect Dis J 9:512–518, 1990.

Mollison LC, Richards MJ, Johnson PD, Hayes K, Munckhof WJ, Jones R, Dabkowski PD, Angus PW. High-dose oral acyclovir reduces the incidence of cytomegalovirus infection in liver transplant recipients. J Infect Dis 168:721–724, 1993.

Montero A, Romero J, Vargas JA, Regueiro CA, Sanchez-Aloz G, De Prados F, De la Torre A, Aragon G. Candida infection of cerebrospinal fluid shunt devices: report of two cases and review of the literature. Acta Neurochir (Wien) 142:67–74, 2000.

Moore WL Jr. Nosocomial infections: an overview. Am J Hosp Pharm 31:832–838, 1974.

Morgan G, Duerden BI, Lilleyman JS. Ceftazidime as a single agent in the management of children with fever and neutropenia. J Antimicrob Chemother 12 Suppl A:347–351, 1983.

Morley D. Severe measles in the tropics. I. Br Med J 1:297–300, 1969.

Moyer MA, Edwards LD, Farley L. Comparative culture methods on 101 intravenous catheters. Routine, semiquantitative, and blood cultures. Arch Intern Med 143:66–69, 1983.

Mouy R, Fischer A, Vilmer E, Seger R, Griscelli C. Incidence, severity, and prevention of infections in chronic granulomatous disease. J Pediatr 114:555–560, 1989.

Mouy R, Veber F, Blanche S, Donadieu J, Brauner R, Levron JC, Griscelli C, Fischer A. Long-term itraconazole prophylaxis against Aspergillus infections in thirty-two patients with chronic granulomatous disease. J Pediatr 125:998–1003, 1994.

Mühlebach TJ, Gabay J, Nathan CF, Erny C, Dopfer G, Schroten H, Wahn V, Seger RA. Treatment of patients with chronic granulomatous disease with recombinant human interferon-gamma does not improve neutrophil oxidative metabolism, cytochrome b558 content or levels of four anti-microbial proteins. Clin Exp Immunol 88:203–206, 1992.

Mullen CA, Petropoulos D, Roberts WM, Rytting M, Zipf T, Chan KW, Culbert SJ, Danielson M, Jeha SS, Kuttesch JF, Rolston KV. Outpatient treatment of fever and neutropenia for low risk pediatric cancer patients. Cancer 86:126–134, 1999.

Mustafa MM, Carlson L, Tkaczewski I, McCracken GH Jr, Buchanan GR. Comparative study of cefepime versus ceftazidime in the empiric treatment of pediatric cancer patients with fever and neutropenia. Pediatr Infect Dis J 20:362–369, 2001.

Nachman JB, Honig GR. Fever and neutropenia in children with neoplastic disease: an analysis of 158 episodes. Cancer 45:407–412, 1980.

Naito H, Toya S, Schizawa H, Iizaka Y, Tsukumo D. High incidence of acute postoperative meningitis and septicemia in patients undergoing craniotomy with ventriculoatrial shunt. Surg Gynecol Obstet 137:810–812, 1973.

Najarian JS, So SK, Simmons RL, Fryd DS, Nevins TE, Ascher NL, Sutherland DE, Payne WD, Chavers BM, Mauer SM. The outcome of 304 primary renal transplants in children (1968-1985). Ann Surg 204:246–258, 1986.

Neijens HJ, Frenkel J, de Muinck Keizer-Schrama SM, Dzoljic-Danilovic G, Meradji M, van Dongen JJ. Invasive Aspergillus infection in chronic granulomatous disease: treatment with itraconazole. J Pediatr 115:1016–1019, 1989.

Nester TA, Wagnon AH, Reilly WF, Spitzer G, Kjeldsberg CR, Hill HR. Effects of allogeneic peripheral stem cell transplantation in a patient with job syndrome of hyperimmunoglobulinemia E and recurrent infections. Am J Med 105:16–24, 1998.

Neu HD. Unusual nosocomial infections. Dis Mon 30:16–18, 1984.

Neumann CG. Malnutrition and infection. In Powanda MC, Canonico PG, eds. Infection, the physiologic and metabolic responses of the host. Amsterdam, Elsevier/North-Holland Biomedical Press, 1981, pp 320–357.

Neumann CG, Lawlor GJ Jr, Stiehm ER, Swenseid ME, Newton C, Herbert J, Ammann AJ, Jacob M. Immunologic responses in malnourished children. Am J Clin Nutr 28:89–104, 1975.

Nguyen MH, Yu VL. Meningitis caused by Candida species: an emerging problem in neurosurgical patients. Clin Infect Dis 21:323–327, 1995.

Nibu K, Matsumoto I, Yanai F, Nunoue T. Aplastic crisis due to human parvovirus B19 infection in glucose-6-phosphate dehydrogenase deficiency. Nippon Ketsueki Gakkai Zasshi 52:1117–1121, 1989.

Nielsen SL, Roder B, Magnussen P, Engquist A, Frimodt-Moller N. Nosocomial pneumonia in an intensive care unit in a Danish university hospital: incidence, mortality and etiology. Scand J Infect Dis 24:65–70, 1992.

NIH consensus conference. Intravenous immunoglobulin. Prevention and treatment of disease. JAMA 264:3189–3193, 1990.

Nixon GM, Armstrong DS, Carzino R, Carlin JB, Olinsky A, Robertson CF, Grimwood K. Clinical outcome after early Pseudomonas aeruginosa infection in cystic fibrosis. J Pediatr 138:699–704, 2001.

Noel GJ, O'Loughlin JE, Edelson PJ. Neonatal Staphylococcus epidermidis right-sided endocarditis: description of five catheterized infants. Pediatrics 82:234–239, 1988.

Nour B, Green M, Michaels M, Reyes J, Tzakis A, Gartner JC, McLoughlin L, Starzl TE. Parvovirus B19 infection in pediatric transplant patients. Transplantation 56:835–838, 1993.

Nydahl BC, Hall WH. The treatment of staphylococcal infection with nafcillin with a discussion of staphylococcal nephritis. Ann Intern Med 63:27–43, 1965.

O'Brien KL, Swift AJ, Winkelstein JA, Santosham M, Stover B, Luddy R, Gootenberg JE, Nold JT, Eskenazi A, Snader SJ, Lederman HM. Safety and immunogenicity of heptavalent pneumococcal vaccine conjugated to CRM(197) among infants with sickle cell disease. Pediatrics 106:965–972, 2000.

Ochs HD, Smith CI. X-linked agammaglobulinemia. A clinical and molecular analysis. Medicine (Baltimore) 75:287–299, 1996.

Odio C, McCracken GH Jr, Nelson JD. CSF shunt infections in pediatrics. A seven-year experience. Am J Dis Child 138:110–138, 1984.

Odum L, Jensen KT, Slotsbjerg TD. Endocarditis due to Kingella kingae. Eur J Clin Microbiol 3:263–266, 1984.

Oleske J, Minnefor A, Cooper R Jr, Thomas K, dela Cruz A, Ahdieh H, Guerrero I, Joshi VV, Desposito F. Immune deficiency syndrome in children. JAMA 249:234–259, 1983.

Olson MM, Allen MO. Nosocomial abscess. Results of an eight-year prospective study of 32,284 operations. Arch Surg 124:356–361, 1989.

Orcutt TA, Godwin CR, Pizzo PA, Ognibene FP. Aerosolized pentamidine: a well-tolerated mode of prophylaxis against Pneumocystis carinii pneumonia in older children with human immunodeficiency virus infection. Pediatr Infect Dis J 11:290–294, 1992.

Ozsahin H, von Planta M, Muller I, Steinert HC, Nadal D, Lauener R, Tuchschmid P, Willi UV, Ozsahin M, Crompton NE, Seger RA. Successful treatment of invasive aspergillosis in chronic granulomatous disease by bone marrow transplantation, granulocyte colony-stimulating factor-mobilized granulocytes, and liposomal amphotericin-B. Blood 92:2719–2724, 1998.

Pakkala S, Salmela K, Lautenschlager I, Ahonen J, Hayry P. Anti-CMV hyperimmune globulin prophylaxis does not prevent CMV disease in CMV-negative renal transplant patients. Transplant Proc 24:283–284, 1992.

Palmer DL. Microbiology of pneumonia in the patient at risk. Am J Med 76:53–60, 1984.

Parad RB, Gerard CJ, Zurakowski D, Nichols DP, Pier GB. Pulmonary outcome in cystic fibrosis is influenced primarily by mucoid *Pseudomonas aeruginosa* infection and immune status and only modestly by genotype. Infect Immun 67:4744–4750, 1999.

Paradise JL, Bluestone CD, Felder H. The universality of otitis media in 50 infants with cleft palate. Pediatrics 44:35–42, 1969.

Paradise JL, Bluestone CD. Early treatment of the universal otitis media in infants with cleft palate. Pediatrics 53:48–54, 1974.

Paradise JL. Management of middle ear effusions in infants with cleft palate. Ann Otol Rhinol Laryngol 85:28–58, 1976.

Parolini S, Bottino C, Falco M, Augugliaro R, Giliani S, Franceschini R, Ochs HD, Wolf H, Bonnefoy JY, Biassoni R, Moretta L, Notarangelo LD, Moretta A. X-linked lymphoproliferative disease. 2B4 molecules displaying inhibitory rather than activating function are responsible for the inability of natural killer cells to kill Epstein-Barr virus-infected cells. J Exp Med 192:337–346, 2000.

Patrick CC, Slobod KS. Opportunistic infections in the compromised host. In Feigin RD, Cherry JD, eds. Textbook of pediatric infectious diseases, 4th ed. Philadelphia, WB Saunders, 1998, pp 980–994.

Pearson ML. Guideline for prevention of intravascular device-related infections. Part I. Intravascular device-related infections: an overview. The Hospital Infection Control Practices Advisory Committee. Am J Infect Control 24:262–277, 1996.

Pedersen FK. Postsplenectomy infections in Danish children splenectomized 1969-1978. Acta Paediatr Scand 72:589–595, 1983.

Peter G, Lloyd-Still JD, Lovejoy FH Jr. Local infection and bacteremia from scalp vein needles and polyethylene catheters in children. J Pediatr 80:78–83, 1972.

Peterson JE, Baker TJ. An isolate of *Fusarium roseum* from human burns. Mycologia 51:453–456, 1959.

Petrilli AS, Dantas LS, Campos MC, Tanaka C, Ginani VC, Seber A. Oral ciprofloxacin vs. intravenous ceftriaxone administered in an outpatient setting for fever and neutropenia in low-risk pediatric oncology patients: randomized prospective trial. Med Pediatr Oncol 34:87–91, 2000.

Philapart AI, Colodny AH, Baehner RL. Continuous antibiotic therapy in chronic granulomatous disease: preliminary communication. Pediatrics 50:923–925, 1972.

Phillips I, Wharton B. Acute bacterial infections in kwashiorkor and marasmus. Br Med J 1:407–409, 1968.

Phillips JA, Bernhardt HE, Rosenthal SG. *Aeromonas hydrophila* infections. Pediatrics 53:110–112, 1974.

Pierce AK, Sanford JP, Thomas GD, Leonard JS. Long-term evaluation of decontamination of inhalation-therapy equipment and the occurrence of necrotizing pneumonia. N Engl J Med 282:528–531, 1970.

Pike RM, Schulze ML, McCullough M. Isolation of *Mima polymorpha* from a patient with subacute bacterial endocarditis. Am J Clin Pathol 21:1094–1096, 1951.

Pizzo PA. Management of fever in patients with cancer and treatment-induced neutropenia. N Engl J Med 328:1323–1332, 1993.

Pizzo PA, Commers J, Cotton D, Gress J, Hathorn J, Hiemenz J, Longo D, Marshall D, Robichaud KJ. Approaching the controversies in antibacterial management of cancer patients. Am J Med 76:436–449, 1984.

Pizzo PA, Rubin M, Freifeld A, Walsh TJ. The child with cancer and infection. I. Empiric therapy for fever and neutropenia, and preventive strategies. J Pediatr 119:679–694, 1991a.

Pizzo PA, Rubin M, Freifeld A, Walsh TJ. The child with cancer and infection. II. Nonbacterial infections. J Pediatr 119:845–857, 1991b.

Ponka A, Tilvis R, Kosunen TU. Prolonged campylobacter gastroenteritis in a patient with hypogammaglobulinaemia. Acta Med Scand 213:159–160, 1983.

Potter D, Feduska N, Melzer J, Garovoy M, Hopper S, Duca R, Salvatierra O Jr. Twenty years of renal transplantation in children. Pediatrics 77:465–470, 1986.

Powell DA, Aungst J, Snedden S, Hansen N, Brady M. Broviac catheterrelated *Malassezia furfur* sepsis in five infants receiving intravenous fat emulsions. J Pediatr 105:987–990, 1984.

Powell KR, Cherry JD, Hougen TJ, Blinderman EE, Dunn MC. A prospective search for congenital dermal abnormalities of the craniospinal axis. J Pediatr 87:744–750, 1975.

Press OW, Ramsey PG, Larson EB, Fefer A, Hickman RO. Hickman catheter infections in patients with malignancies. Medicine (Baltimore) 63:189–200, 1984.

Principi N, Marchisio P, Tornaghi R, Onorato J, Massironi E, Picco P. Acute otitis media in human immunodeficiency virus–infected children. Pediatrics 88:566–571, 1991.

Prober CG, Whyte H, Smith CR. Open lung biopsy in immunocompromised children with pulmonary infiltrates. Am J Dis Child 138:60–63, 1984.

Prokurat S, Drabik E, Grenda R, Vogt E. Ganciclovir in cytomegalovirus prophylaxis in high-risk pediatric renal transplant recipients. Transplant Proc 25:2577, 1993.

Pruitt BA Jr, McManus AT. Opportunistic infections in severely burned patients. Am J Med 76:146–154, 1984.

Quartier P, Debre M, De Blic J, de Sauverzac R, Sayegh N, Jabado N, Haddad E, Blanche S, Casanova JL, Smith CI, Le Deist F, de Saint Basile G, Fischer A. Early and prolonged intravenous immunoglobulin replacement therapy in childhood agammaglobulinemia: a retrospective survey of 31 patients. J Pediatr 134:589–596, 1999.

Quie PG. Infections due to neutrophil malfunction. Medicine (Baltimore) 52:411–417, 1973.

Quie PG, Hetherington SV. Patients with disorders of phagocytic cell function. Pediatr Infect Dis 3:272–380, 1984.

Quie PG, Belani KK. Corticosteroids for chronic granulomatous disease. J Pediatr 111:393–394, 1987.

Rabin ER, Lundberg GD, Mitchell ET. Mucormycosis in severely burned patients: report of two cases with extensive destruction of the face and nasal cavity. N Engl J Med 264:1286–1289, 1961.

Ragab AH, Lindqvist KJ, Vietti TJ, Choi SC, Osterland CK. Immunoglobulin pattern in childhood leukemia. Cancer 26:890–894, 1970.

Ramsey BW, Pepe MS, Quan JM, Otto KL, Montgomery AB, Williams-Warren J, Vasiljev-K M, Borowitz D, Bowman CM, Marshall BC, Marshall S, Smith AL. Intermittent administration of inhaled tobramycin in patients with cystic fibrosis. Cystic Fibrosis Inhaled Tobramycin Study Group. N Engl J Med 340:23–30, 1999.

Raubitschek AA, Levin AS, Stites DP, Shaw EB, Fudenberg HH. Normal granulocyte infusion therapy for aspergillosis in chronic granulomatous disease. Pediatrics 51:230–233, 1973.

Rauch AM, O'Ryan M, Van R, Pickering LK. Invasive disease due to multiply resistant *Streptococcus pneumoniae* in a Houston, Tex, day-care center. Am J Dis Child 144:923–927, 1990.

Reinhardt DJ, Kennedy C, Malecka-Griggs B. Selective nonroutine microbial surveillance of in-use hospital nebulizers by aerosol entrapment and direct sampling analyses of solutions in reservoirs. J Clin Microbiol 12:199–204, 1980.

Rello J, Quintana E, Ausina V, Castella J, Luquin M, Net A, Prats G. Incidence, etiology, and outcome of nosocomial pneumonia in mechanically ventilated patients. Chest 100:439–444, 1991.

Rhame FS, Maki DG, Bennett JV. Intravenous cannula–associated infections. In Bennett JV, Brachman PS, eds. Hospital infections. Boston, Little, Brown & Co., 1979, pp 433–442.

Richet H, Hubert B, Nitemberg G, Andremont A, Buu-Hoi A, Ourbak P, Galicier C, Veron M, Boisivon A, Bouvier AM, Ricome JC, Wolff MA, Pean Y, Berardi-Grassias L, Bourdain JL, Hautefort B, Laaban JP, Tillant D. Prospective multicenter study of vascular-catheter–related complications and risk factors for positive central-catheter cultures in intensive care unit patients. J Clin Microbiol 28:2520–2525, 1990.

Riikonen P, Saarinen UM, Lahteenoja K-M, Jalanko H. Management of indwelling central venous catheters in pediatric cancer patients with fever and neutropenia. Scand J Infect Dis 25:357–364, 1993.

Riis P, Stougaard J. The peripheral blood leukocytes in chronic renal insufficiency. Dan Med Bull 6:85–90, 1959.

Riley HD Jr. Hospital-associated infections. Pediatr Clin North Am 16:701–734, 1969.

Rinaldi M. Antifungal agents. In Feigin RD, Cherry JD, eds. Textbook of pediatric infectious diseases, 4th ed. Philadelphia, W. B. Saunders, 1998, pp 2697–2706.

Rodgers GL, Mortensen J, Fisher MC, Lo A, Cresswell A, Long SS. Predictors of infectious complications after burn injuries in children. Pediatr Infect Dis J 19:990–995, 2000.

Rodrigues RJ, Shinya H, Wolff WI, Puttlitz D. *Torulopsis glabrata* fungemia during prolonged intravenous alimentation therapy. N Engl J Med 284:540–541, 1971.

Rolston KV. New trends in patient management: risk-based therapy for febrile patients with neutropenia. Clin Infect Dis 29:515–521, 1999.

Rosen FS, Janeway CA. Dangers of vaccination in lymphopenic infants. Pediatrics 33:310–311, 1964.

Rosen FS, Cooper MD, Wedgwood RJ. The primary immunodeficiencies. N Engl J Med 311:235–242, 300–310, 1984.

Rosenbloom BE, Weingarten S, Rosenfelt FP, Weinstein IM. Severe hemolytic anemia due to glucose-6-phosphate dehydrogenase deficiency and Epstein-Barr virus infection. Mt Sinai J Med 55:404–405, 1988.

Rosner F, Valmont I, Kozinn PJ, Caroline L. Leukocyte function in patients with leukemia. Cancer 25:835–842, 1970.

Rosner F, Zarrabi MH, Benach JL, Habicht GS. Babesiosis in splenectomized adults. Review of 22 reported cases. Am J Med 76:696–701, 1984.

Rubin HM, Eardley W, Nichols BL. *Shigella sonnei* osteomyelitis and sickle-cell anemia. Am J Dis Child 116:83–87, 1968.

Rubinstein A. Acquired immunodeficiency syndrome in infants. Am J Dis Child 137:825–827, 1983.

Rupar DG, Herzog KD, Fisher MC, Long SS. Prolonged bacteremia with catheter-related central venous thrombosis. Am J Dis Child 144:879–882, 1990.

Rutstein RM, Cobb P, McGowan KL, Pinto-Martin J, Starr SE. *Mycobacterium aviumintracellulare* complex infection in HIV-infected children. AIDS 7:507–512, 1993.

Saarinen UM. Severe infections in childhood leukemia. A follow-up study of 100 consecutive ALL patients. Acta Paediatr Scand 73:515–522, 1984.

Sable CA, Donowitz GR. Infections in bone marrow transplant recipients. Clin Infect Dis 18:273–284, 1994.

Sachs JM, Pacin M, Counts GW. Sickle hemoglobinopathy and *Edwardsiella tarda* meningitis. Am J Dis Child 128:387–388, 1974.

Saiman L, Prince A, Gersony WM. Pediatric infective endocarditis in the modern era. J Pediatr 122:847–853, 1993.

Saleh RA, Schorin MA. *Bacillus* sp. sepsis associated with Hickman catheters in patients with neoplastic disease. Pediatr Infect Dis J 6:851–856, 1987.

Saliba F, Eyraud D, Samuel D, David MF, Arulnaden JL, Dussaix E, Mathieu D, Bismuth H. Randomized controlled trial of acyclovir for the prevention of cytomegalovirus infection and disease in liver transplant recipients. Transplant Proc 25:1444–1445, 1993.

Salmon JH. Adult hydrocephalus. Evaluation of shunt therapy in 80 patients. J Neurosurg 37:423–428, 1972.

Sancho Martin I, Villafruela Sanz MA, Alvarez Vicent JJ. Incidence and treatment of otitis with effusion in patients with cleft palate. Acta Otorrinolaringol Esp 48:441–445, 1997.

Sanders CV Jr, Luby JP, Johanson WG Jr, Barnett JA, Sanford JP. *Serratia marcescens* infection from inhalation therapy medications: nosocomial outbreak. Ann Intern Med 73:15–21, 1970.

Sattler CA, Mason EO Jr, Kaplan SL. Nonrespiratory *Stenotrophomonas maltophilia* infection at a children's hospital. Clin Infect Dis 31:1321–1330, 2000.

Saulsbury FT, Winkelstein JA, Yolken RH. Chronic rotavirus infection in immunodeficiency. J Pediatr 97:61–65, 1980.

Schoenbaum SC, Gardner P, Shillito J. Infections of cerebrospinal fluid shunts: epidemiology, clinical manifestations, and therapy. J Infect Dis 131:543–552, 1975.

Schonebeck J. Asymptomatic candiduria. Prognosis, complications and some other clinical considerations. Scand J Urol Nephrol 6:136–146, 1972.

Schowengerdt KO, Naftel DC, Seib PM, Pearce FB, Addonizio LJ, Kirklin JK, Morrow WR. Infection after pediatric heart transplantation: results of a multiinstitutional study. The Pediatric Heart Transplant Study Group. J Heart Lung Transplant 16:1207–1216, 1997.

Schwartz RS. Immunosuppressive drugs. Prog Allergy 9:246–303, 1965.

Scott GB. HIV infection in children: clinical features and management. J Acquir Immune Defic Syndr 4:109–115, 1991.

Scott GB, Buck BE, Leterman JG, Bloom FL, Parks WP. Acquired immunodeficiency syndrome in infants. N Engl J Med 310:76–81, 1984.

Scott RM. Bacterial endocarditis due to *Neisseria flava*. J Pediatr 78:673–675, 1971.

Sechler JMG, Malech HL, White CJ, Gallin JI. Recombinant human interferon-gamma reconstitutes defective phagocyte function in patients with chronic granulomatous disease of childhood. Proc Natl Acad Sci USA 85:4874–4878, 1988.

Seger RA, Baumgartner S, Tiefenauer LX, Gmunder FK. Chronic granulomatous disease: effect of sulfamethoxazole/trimethoprim on neutrophil microbicidal function. Helv Paediatr Acta 36:579–588, 1981.

Sellmeyer E, Bhettay E, Truswell AS, Meyers OL, Hansen JD. Lymphocyte transformation in malnourished children. Arch Dis Child 47:429–435, 1972.

Seth V, Chandra RK. Opsonic activity, phagocytosis, and bactericidal capacity of polymorphs in undernutrition. Arch Dis Child 47:282–284, 1972.

Severien C, Nelson JD. Frequency of infections associated with implanted systems vs cuffed, tunneled Silastic venous catheters in patients with acute leukemia. Am J Dis Child 145:1433–1438, 1991.

Shafer RB, Hall WH. Bacterial endocarditis following open heart surgery. Am J Cardiol 25:602–607, 1970.

Shannon KM, Ammann AJ. Acquired immune deficiency syndrome in childhood. J Pediatr 106:332–342, 1985.

Shenep JL, Flynn PM, Baker DK, Hetherington SV, Hudson MM, Hughes WT, Patrick CC, Roberson PK, Sandlund JT, Santana VM, Sixbey JW, Slobod KS. Oral cefixime is similar to continued intravenous antibiotics in the empirical treatment of febrile neutropenic children with cancer. Clin Infect Dis 32:36–43, 2001.

Sheridan RL, Ryan CM, Pasternack MS, Weber JM, Tompkins RG. Flavobacterial sepsis in massively burned pediatric patients. Clin Infect Dis 17:185–187, 1993.

Sheridan RL, Schulz JT, Weber JM, Ryan CM, Pasternack MS, Tompkins RG. Cutaneous herpetic infections complicating burns. Burns 26:621–624, 2000.

Shinozaki T, Deane RS, Mazuzan JE, Hamel AJ, Hazelton D. Bacterial contamination of arterial lines. A prospective study. JAMA 249:223–225, 1983.

Shmerling DH, Prader A, Hitzig WH, Giedion A, Hadorn B, Kuhni M. The syndrome of exocrine pancreatic insufficiency, neutropenia, metaphyseal dysostosis and dwarfism. Helv Paediatr Acta 24:547–575, 1969.

Shuck JM. Infection control in burns?? Topical and systemic. Surg Clin North Am 52:1425–1438, 1972.

Shulman ST, Bartlett J, Clyde WA Jr, Ayoub EM. The unusual severity of mycoplasmal pneumonia in children with sickle-cell disease. N Engl J Med 287:164–167, 1972.

Shurtleff DB, Foltz EL, Weeks RD, Loeser J. Therapy of *Staphylococcus epidermidis*: infections associated with cerebrospinal fluid shunts. Pediatrics 53:55–62, 1974.

Shyur SD, Hill HR. Immunodeficiency in the 1990s. Pediatr Infect Dis J 10:595–611, 1991.

Sickles EA, Greene WH, Wiernik PH. Clinical presentation of infection in granulocytopenic patients. Arch Intern Med 135:715–719, 1975.

Siddiqui T, Khan AH. Hepatitis A and cytomegalovirus infection precipitating acute hemolysis in glucose-6-phosphate dehydrogenase deficiency. Mil Med 163:434–435, 1998.

Siegel SE, Nesbit ME, Baehner R, Sather H, Hammond GD. Pneumonia during therapy for childhood acute lymphoblastic leukemia. Am J Dis Child 134:28–34, 1980.

Silk MR. The effect of uremic plasma on lymphocyte transformation. Invest Urol 5:195–199, 1967.

Silliman CC, Tedder D, Ogle JW, Simon J, Kleinschmidt-DeMasters BK, Manco-Johnson M, Levin MJ. Unsuspected varicella zoster virus encephalitis in a child with acquired immunodeficiency syndrome. J Pediatr 123:418–422, 1993.

Singh N, Paterson DL, Gayowski T, Wagener MM, Marino IR. Cytomegalovirus antigenemia directed pre-emptive prophylaxis with oral versus I.V. ganciclovir for the prevention of cytomegalovirus disease in liver transplant recipients: a randomized, controlled trial. Transplantation 70:717–722, 2000.

Sinkovics JG, Smith JP. Septicemia with *Bacteroides* in patients with malignant disease. Cancer 25:663–671, 1970.

Sirisinha S, Suskind R, Edelman R, Asvapaka C, Olson RE. Secretory and serum IgA in children with protein-calorie malnutrition. Pediatrics 55:166–170, 1975.

Skeel RT, Yankee RA, Henderson ES. Hexose monophosphate shunt activity of circulating phagocytes in acute lymphocytic leukemia. J Lab Clin Med 77:975–984, 1971.

Skinner MD, Schwartz RS. Immunosuppressive therapy. N Engl J Med 287:221–227, 281–286, 1972.

Sleigh JD, Peutherer JF. Changing patterns of bacterial and viral infections in surgery. Br Med Bull 44:403–422, 1988.

Sloper KS, Dourmashkin RR, Bird RB, Slavin G, Webster AD. Chronic malabsorption due to cryptosporidiosis in a child with immunoglobulin deficiency. Gut 23:80–82, 1982.

Smith JM, McDonald RA. Progress in renal transplantation for children. Adv Ren Replace Ther 7:158–171, 2000.

Smith SD, Jackson RJ, Hannakan CJ, Wadowsky RM, Tzakis AG, Rowe MI. Selective decontamination in pediatric liver transplants. A randomized prospective study. Transplantation 55:1306–1309, 1993.

Smythe PM, Brereton-Stiles GG, Grace HJ, Mafoyane A, Schonland M, Coovadia HM, Loening WE, Parent MA, Vos GH. Thymolymphatic deficiency and depression of cell-mediated immunity in protein-calorie malnutrition. Lancet 2:939–943, 1971.

Snydman DR. Review of the efficacy of cytomegalovirus immune globulin in the prophylaxis of CMV disease in renal transplant recipients. Transplant Proc 25:25–26, 1993.

Snydman DR, Donnelly-Reidy M, Perry LK, Martin WJ. Intravenous tubing containing burettes can be safely changed at 72-hour intervals. Infect Control 8:113–116, 1987.

So SKS, Simmons RL. Infections following kidney transplantation in children. In Patrick CC, ed. Infections in immunocompromised infants and children. New York, Churchill Livingstone, 1992, pp 215–230.

Spebar MJ, Lindberg RB. Fungal infection of the burn wound. Am J Surg 138:879–882, 1979.

Sprunt K, Redman W, Leidy G. Antibacterial effectiveness of routine hand washing. Pediatrics 52:264–271, 1973.

Stamm WE. Guidelines for prevention of catheter-associated urinary tract infections. Ann Intern Med 82:386–390, 1975.

Stanton BF, Baltimore RS, Clemens JD. Changing spectrum of infective endocarditis in children. Analysis of 26 cases, 1970-1979. Am J Dis Child 138:720–725, 1984.

Starke JR. Infective endocarditis. In Feigin RD, Cherry JD, eds. Textbook of pediatric infectious diseases, 4th ed. Philadelphia, W. B. Saunders, 1998, pp 315–338.

Stavola JJ, Noel GJ. Efficacy and safety of dapsone prophylaxis against *Pneumocystis carinii* pneumonia in human immunodeficiency virus–infected children. Pediatr Infect Dis J 12:644–647, 1993.

Steele RW. Infection in the immunocompromised host. Pediatr Infect Dis 4:309–314, 1985.

Steere AC, Mallison GF. Handwashing practices for the prevention of nosocomial infections. Ann Intern Med 83:683–690, 1975.

Steinberg AD, Plotz PH, Wolff SM, Wong VG, Agus SG, Decker JL. Cytotoxic drugs in treatment of nonmalignant diseases. Ann Intern Med 76:619–642, 1972.

Stickler GB, Shin MH, Burke EC, Holley KE, Miller RH, Segar WE. Diffuse glomerulonephritis associated with infected ventriculoatrial shunt. N Engl J Med 279:1077–1082, 1968.

Stiehm ER, Chin TW, Haas A, Peerless AG. Infectious complications of the primary immunodeficiencies. Clin Immunol Immunopathol 40:69–86, 1986.

Stone BD, Wheeler JG. Disseminated cryptococcal infection in a patient with hyperimmunoglobulinemia E syndrome. J Pediatr 117:92–95, 1990.

Strauss RR, Paul BB, Jacobs AA, Simmons C, Sbarra AJ. The metabolic and phagocytic activities of leukocytes from children with acute leukemia. Cancer Res 30:80–88, 1970.

Strober W, Wochner RD, Carbone PP, Waldmann TA. Intestinal lymphangiectasia: a protein-losing enteropathy with hypogammaglobulinemia, lymphocytopenia and impaired homograft rejection. J Clin Invest 46:1643–1656, 1967.

Tabbutt S, Duncan BW, McLaughlin D, Wessel DL, Jonas RA, Laussen PC. Delayed sternal closure after cardiac operations in a pediatric population. J Thorac Cardiovasc Surg 113:886–893, 1997.

Tambyah PA, Maki DG. The relationship between pyuria and infection in patients with indwelling urinary catheters: a prospective study of 761 patients. Arch Intern Med 160:673–677, 2000a.

Tambyah PA, Maki DG. Catheter-associated urinary tract infection is rarely symptomatic: a prospective study of 1,497 catheterized patients. Arch Intern Med 160:678–682, 2000b.

Tan TQ, Mason EO Jr, Kaplan SL. Penicillin-resistant systemic pneumococcal infections in children: a retrospective case-control study. Pediatrics 92:761–767, 1993.

Tauber AI, Borregaard N, Simons E, Wright J. Chronic granulomatous disease: a syndrome of phagocyte oxidase deficiencies. Medicine (Baltimore) 62:286–309, 1983.

Thompson EN, Soothill JF. Chronic granulomatous disease: quantitative clincopathological relationships. Arch Dis Child 45:24–32, 1970.

Tomford JW, Hershey CO, McLaren CE, Porter DK, Cohen DI. Intravenous therapy team and peripheral venous catheter–associated complications. A prospective controlled study. Arch Intern Med 144:1191–1194, 1984.

Tredget EE, Shankowsky HA, Joffe AM, Inkson TI, Volpel K, Paranchych W, Kibsey PC, Alton JD, Burke JF. Epidemiology of infections with *Pseudomonas aeruginosa* in burn patients: the role of hydrotherapy. Clin Infect Dis 15:941–949, 1992.

Tsingoglou S, Forrest DM. A technique for the insertion of Holter ventriculoatrial shunt for infantile hydrocephalus. Br J Surg 58:367–372, 1971.

Tullu MS, Deshmukh CT, Baveja SM. Bacterial nosocomial pneumonia in Paediatric Intensive Care Unit. J Postgrad Med 46:18–22, 2000.

Turgeon N, Fishman JA, Basgoz N, Tolkoff-Rubin NE, Doran M, Cosimi AB, Rubin RH. Effect of oral acyclovir or ganciclovir therapy after preemptive intravenous ganciclovir therapy to prevent cytomegalovirus disease in cytomegalovirus seropositive renal and liver transplant recipients receiving antilymphocyte antibody therapy. Transplantation 66:1780–1786, 1998.

Turnidge JD, Bell JM. Methicillin-resistant *Staphylococcus aureus* evolution in Australia over 35 years. Microb Drug Resist 6:223–229, 2000.

Vacanti JP, Lillehei CW, Jenkins RL, Donahoe PK, Cosimi AB, Kleinman R, Grand RJ, Cho SI. Liver transplantation in children: the Boston Center experience in the first 30 months. Transplant Proc 19:3261–3266, 1987.

van der Meer JW, Bont L, Verhage J. *Aspergillus* infection in patients with hyperimmunoglobulin E syndrome. Clin Infect Dis 27:13–37, 1998.

Vandersteenhoven JJ, Dbaibo G, Boyko OB, Hulette CM, Anthony DC, Kenny JF, Wilfert CM. Progressive multifocal leukoencephalopathy in pediatric acquired immunodeficiency syndrome. Pediatr Infect Dis J 11:232–237, 1992.

Van Hare GF, Ben-Shachar G, Liebman J, Boxerbaum B, Riemenschneider TA. Infective endocarditis in infants and children during the past 10 years: a decade of change. Am Heart J 107:1235–1240, 1984.

Vejlsgaard R. Studies on urinary tract infections in diabetics. 3. Significant bacteriuria in pregnant diabetics and in matched controls. Acta Med Scand 193:337–341, 1973.

Vernon DD, Holzman BH, Lewis P, Scott GB, Birriel JA, Scott MB. Respiratory failure in children with acquired immunodeficiency syndrome and acquired immunodeficiency syndromerelated complex. Pediatrics 82:223–228, 1988.

Verronen P. Case report. Presumed disseminated BCG in a boy with chronic granulomatous disease of childhood. Acta Paediatr Scand 63:627–630, 1974.

Viscoli C, Castagnola E, Giacchino M, Cesaro S, Properzi E, Tucci F, Mura RM, Alvisi P, Zanazzo G, Surico G, Bonetti F, De Sio L, Izzi G, Di Cataldo A, Ziino O, Massolo F, Nardi M, Santoro N, Binda S. Bloodstream infections in children with cancer: a multicentre surveillance study of the Italian Association of Paediatric Haematology and Oncology. Supportive Therapy Group-Infectious Diseases Section. Eur J Cancer 35:770–774, 1999.

Wade JC, Newton B, Flournoy N, Meyers JD. Oral acyclovir for prevention of herpes simplex virus reactivation after marrow transplantation. Ann Intern Med 100:823–828, 1984.

Wagenlehner FM, Naber KG. Hospital-acquired urinary tract infections. J Hosp Infect 46:171–181, 2000.

Waldmann TA. Protein-losing enteropathy. Gastroenterology 50:422–443, 1966.

Waldmann TA, Schwab PJ. IgG (7S gamma globulin) metabolism in hypogammaglobulinemia: studies in patients with defective gamma globulin synthesis, gastrointestinal protein loss, or both. J Clin Invest 44:1523–1533, 1965.

Walker W. Splenectomy in childhood: a review in England and Wales, 1960–4. Br J Surg 63:36–43, 1976.

Walter EA, Bowden RA. Infection in the bone marrow transplant recipient. Infect Dis Clin North Am 9:823–847, 1995.

Walters BC, Hoffman HJ, Hendrick EB, Humphreys RP. Cerebrospinal fluid shunt infection. Influences on initial management and subsequent outcome. J Neurosurg 60:1014–1021, 1984.

Walzer PD, Schultz MG, Western KA, Robbins JB. *Pneumocystis carinii* pneumonia and primary immune deficiency diseases of infancy and childhood. J Pediatr 82:416–422, 1973.

Wang EE, Prober CG, Ford-Jones L, Gold R. The management of central intravenous catheter infections. Pediatr Infect Dis 3:110–113, 1984.

Ward MS, Lam KV, Cannell PK, Herrmann RP. Mycobacterial central venous catheter tunnel infection: a difficult problem. Bone Marrow Transplant 24:325–329, 1999.

Ward PA. The chemosuppression of chemotaxis. J Exp Med 124:209–226, 1966.

Wasserman R, August CS, Plotkin SA. Viral infections in pediatric bone marrow transplant patients. Pediatr Infect Dis J 7:109–115, 1988.

Watanakunakorn C, Carleton J, Goldberg LM, Hamburger M. *Candida* endocarditis surrounding a Starr-Edwards prosthetic valve. Recovery of *Candida* in hypertonic medium during treatment. Arch Intern Med 121:243–245, 1968.

Weiden PL, Blaese RM, Strober W, Block JB, Waldmann TA. Impaired lymphocyte transformation in intestinal lymphangiectasia: evidence for at least two functionally distinct lymphocyte populations in man. J Clin Invest 51:1319–1325, 1972.

Weisman LE, Stoll BJ, Kueser TJ, Rubio TT, Frank CG, Heiman HS, Subramanian KN, Hankins CT, Anthony BF, Cruess DF, Hemming VG, Fischer GW. Intravenous immune globulin therapy for early-onset sepsis in premature neonates. J Pediatr 121:434–443, 1992.

Welt LG, Black HR, Krueger KK. Symposium on uremic toxins. Arch Intern Med 126:773–780, 1970.

Welte K, Zeidler C, Reiter A, Muller W, Odenwald E, Souza L, Riehm H. Differential effects of granulocyte-macrophage colony-stimulating factor and granulocyte colony-stimulating factor in children with severe congenital neutropenia. Blood 75:1056–1063, 1990.

Werner BG, Snydman DR, Freeman R, Rohrer R, Tilney NL, Kirkman RL. Cytomegalovirus immune globulin for the prevention of primary CMV disease in renal transplant patients:

analysis of usage under treatment IND status. The Treatment IND Study Group. Transplant Proc 25:1441–1443, 1993.

Westwood JC, Legace S, Mitchell MA. Hospital-acquired infection: present and future impact and need for positive action. Can Med Assoc J 110:769–774, 1974.

Wilfert CM, Katz SL. Etiology of bacterial sepsis in nephrotic children, 1963–1967. Pediatrics 42:840–843, 1968.

Wilfert CM, Buckley RH, Mohanakumar T, Griffith JF, Katz SL, Whisnant JK, Eggleston PA, Moore M, Treadwell E, Oxman MN, Rosen FS. Persistent and fatal central-nervous-system ECHOvirus infections in patients with agammaglobulinemia. N Engl J Med 296:1485–1489, 1977.

Wilhelmi I, Bernaldo de Quiros JC, Romero-Vivas J, Duarte J, Rojo E, Bouza E. Epidemic outbreak of *Serratia marcescens* infection in a cardiac surgery unit. J Clin Microbiol 25:1298–1300, 1987.

Wilson WEC, Kirkpatrick CH, Talmage DW. Suppression of immunologic-responsiveness in uremia. Ann Intern Med 62:1–14, 1965.

Wilson WR, Jaumin PM, Danielson GK, Giuliani ER, Washington JA II, Geraci JE. Prosthetic valve endocarditis. Ann Intern Med 82:751–756, 1975.

Wingard JR, White MH, Anaissie E, Raffalli J, Goodman J, Arrieta A. A randomized, double-blind comparative trial evaluating the safety of liposomal amphotericin B versus amphotericin B lipid complex in the empirical treatment of febrile neutropenia. L Amph/ABLC Collaborative Study Group. Clin Infect Dis 31:1155–1163, 2000.

Winkelstein JA, Marino MC, Johnston RB Jr, Boyle J, Curnutte J, Gallin JI, Malech HL, Holland SM, Ochs H, Quie P, Buckley RH, Foster CB, Chanock SJ, Dickler H. Chronic granulomatous disease. Report on a national registry of 368 patients. Medicine (Baltimore) 79:155–169, 2000.

Winston DJ, Gale RP, Meyer DV, Young LS. Infectious complications of human bone marrow transplantation. Medicine (Baltimore) 58:1–31, 1979.

Winston DJ, Ho WG, Champlin RE, Gale RP. Infectious complications of bone marrow transplantation. Exp Hematol 12:205–215, 1984.

Wollman MR, Young LS, Armstrong D, Haghbin M. Anti-*Pseudomonas* heat-stable opsonins in acute lymphoblastic leukemia of childhood. J Pediatr 86:376–381, 1975.

Wong DT, Ogra PL. Viral infections in immunocompromised patients. Med Clin North Am 67:1075–1092, 1983.

Wong ES, Hooton TM. Guideline for prevention of catheter-associated urinary tract infections. In Guidelines for the Prevention and Control of Nosocomial Infections. U.S. Department of Health and Human Services, Centers for Disease Control and Prevention, 1981, pp 1–5.

Wong KK, Hirsch MS. Herpes virus infections in patients with neoplastic disease. Diagnosis and therapy. Am J Med 76:464–478, 1984.

Wong VK, Ross LA. *Branhamella catarrhalis* septicemia in an infant with AIDS. Scand J Infect Dis 20:559–560, 1988.

Wong WY, Overturf GD, Powars DR. Infection caused by *Streptococcus pneumoniae* in children with sickle cell disease: epidemiology, immunologic mechanisms, prophylaxis, and vaccination. Clin Infect Dis 14:1124–1136, 1992.

Work TH, Ifekwunigwe A, Jelliffe DB, Jelliffe P, Neumann CG. Tropical problems in nutrition. Ann Intern Med 79:701–711, 1973.

Wright DG, Dale DC, Fauci AS, Wolff SM. Human cyclic neutropenia: clinical review and long-term follow-up of patients. Medicine (Baltimore) 60:1–13, 1981.

Wurzel CL, Halom K, Feldman JG, Rubin LG. Infection rates of Broviac-Hickman catheters and implantable venous devices. Am J Dis Child 142:536–540, 1988.

Yamanaka J, Lynch SV, Ong TH, Fawcett J, Robinson HE, Beale K, Balderson GA, Strong RW. Surgical complications and long-term outcome in pediatric liver transplantation. Hepatogastroenterology 47:1371–1374, 2000.

Yap PL. Prevention of infection in patients with B-cell defects: focus on intravenous immunoglobulin. Clin Infect Dis 17:S372–S375, 1993.

Yetgin S, Gur A, Saatci U. Non-specific immunity in nephrotic syndrome. Acta Paediatr Scand 69:21–24, 1980.

Yogev R. Cerebrospinal fluid shunt infections: a personal view. Pediatr Infect Dis 4:113–118, 1985.

Yoshida T, Metcoff J, Frenk S, De la Pena C. Intermediary metabolites and adenine nucleotides in leukocytes of children with protein-calorie malnutrition. Nature 214:525–526, 1967.

Younes BS, McDiarmid SV, Martin MG, Vargas JH, Goss JA, Busuttil RW, Ament ME. The effect of immunosuppression on posttransplant lymphoproliferative disease in pediatric liver transplant patients. Transplantation 70:94–99, 2000.

Young RC, Bennett JE, Geelhoed GW, Levine AS. Fungemia with compromised host resistance: a study of 70 cases. Ann Intern Med 80:606–612, 1974.

Zaia JA. Infections associated with bone marrow transplantation. In Patrick CC, ed. Infections in immunocompromised infants and children. New York, Churchill Livingstone, 1992, pp 261–276.

Ziegner UH, Ochs HD, Schanen C, Feig SA, Seyama K, Futatani T, Gross T, Wakim M, Roberts RL, Rawlings DJ, Dovat S, Fraser JK, Stiehm ER. Unrelated umbilical cord stem cell transplantation for X-linked immunodeficiencies. J Pediatr 138:570–573, 2001.

Zitelli GJ, Gartner JC, Malatack JJ, Urbach AH, Miller JW, Williams L, Kirdpatrick B, Breinig MK, Ho M. Pediatric liver transplantation: patient evaluation and selection, infectious complications, and life-style after transplantation. Transplant Proc 19:3309–3316, 1987.

Zurier RB, Weissman G. Anti-immunologic and anti-inflammatory effects of steroid therapy. Med Clin North Am 57:1295–1307, 1973.

CHAPTER

Active and Passive Immunization in the Prevention of Infectious Diseases

Heidi Schwarzwald and Mark W. Kline

Prevention of disease through immunization predates knowledge of infection or immunology by many centuries. Inoculation of smallpox material intranasally in an effort to prevent smallpox was first noted in 590 BC in the Sung Dynasty (Dixon, 1962). From such empiric beginnings are derived current immunization practices, built on a long history of painstaking observation, intuition, and scientific experiment. This chapter summarizes present practices, underlying theories, and future directions of immunization.

Current immunization practice is based on immunologic aspects of the host response, the state of microbiologic technology, the restraints of practicality and economics, and ethical and medicolegal considerations. Immunizations can change the world. The elimination of smallpox is the most recent chapter of a 2500-year history of vaccination, which has included all of the aforementioned factors (Fenner, 1982).

Immunization played a vital part in the dramatic decrease in deaths from infectious diseases among American children who were observed during the 20th century. At the beginning of the century, leading causes of child mortality included diphtheria, measles, pneumonia and influenza, and pertussis. Between 1980 and 1998, the percentage of child deaths attributable to infectious diseases declined from more than 60% to just 2% (Guyer et al., 2000). Immunization programs in the United States have been highly successful for two reasons: (1) the nationwide Childhood Immunization Initiative, begun in 1977, effectively mobilized the public and private sectors, and (2) subsequent state laws required routine immunizations for admission to school (Centers for Disease Control and Prevention [CDC], 1982b). All states and the District of Columbia now have such laws, and more than 95% of children entering school have routinely received the recommended immunizations. Unfortunately, immunization levels among preschool-aged children are considerably lower (CDC, 1992). The recent resurgence of measles in the United States is attributable largely to failure to vaccinate children at the recommended age of 12 to 15 months (National Vaccine Advisory Committee, 1991).

The decrease in the natural occurrence of vaccine-preventable diseases has increased the visibility of the rare adverse reactions to vaccination. For the benefit of society, state laws require childhood immunization. Those who suffer serious sequelae from immunization may seek compensation through a judicial system that does not allow optimal recourse for the injured or for the private manufacturers and suppliers of immunizing agents. The result has been ever-increasing costs of vaccination and a reluctance on the part of manufacturers to continue producing vaccines.

A National Childhood Vaccine Injury Compensation Act was passed by the United States Congress in 1986. It sought to improve record keeping about vaccine administration and complications, to provide parents or guardians with standardized statements on the benefits and risks of vaccines, and to establish a federal Vaccine Injury Compensation Program (Peter, 1992). An additional goal was to stabilize vaccine supply and cost (Smith, 1988). Since the act was passed, the number of vaccine injury cases in the civil courts has declined and vaccine prices have stabilized.

Other standard pediatric immunization practices have recently been summarized (American Academy of Pediatrics, 2003; CDC, 2000a).

ACTIVE IMMUNIZATION

Exposure to an infectious agent initiates a variety of cellular and molecular responses. Collectively, these responses are termed the *active immune response,* which is usually characterized by (1) specificity, (2) variety, (3) a molecular sequence, and (4) memory. In some cases, such as the mechanisms of pertussis immunity, these elements are not well understood. In other cases, such as the immunoglobulin G (IgG) toxin-neutralizing antibody response in tetanus, the mechanism has been well characterized.

The specificity of an active immune response is related to unique antigenic structures of the infectious agent or one of its chemical products. After immunization, a variety of antibodies are synthesized and directed against a limited number of antigens present on the immunizing substance. On exposure to an antigen, B lymphocytes multiply and produce immunoglobulin molecules, which can react with the antigen or a portion of the antigen; this is the *primary response.* T lymphocytes are also stimulated and influence the capacity of B

lymphocytes to respond to the antigen. These cells do not elaborate antibody but do contain an antigen recognition mechanism. Sensitized T cells are capable of effective immunologic action directly by means of the cell-mediated immune response. They may also influence other cells (macrophages or granulocytes) and release lymphokines, such as interleukin-2 and interferon. The role of the cell-mediated immune response to some immunizing agents has been increasingly recognized.

After initial antigen challenge, both B and T cells are capable of memory, as manifested by the continued presence of active immunity beyond the original exposure and the development of a secondary (anamnestic) response. The latter is characterized by rapid response to re-exposure of greater magnitude than that observed in the primary response, often to a lesser quantity of antigen.

To be useful, a vaccine must stimulate B cells, T cells, or both to a degree sufficient to produce effective resistance against a virulent agent. Attenuated measles virus fulfills this criterion and offers protection against natural measles. By contrast, the parainfluenza virus vaccines fail to evoke active immunity despite demonstration of some immunologic responses (Fulginiti et al., 1969).

In addition, memory T and B cells must be stimulated to ensure long-lasting, even lifelong, immunity. Lifelong immunity can occur after certain immunizations, such as with attenuated measles virus vaccine, whereas other immunizations, such as pertussis, have relatively short-lived immunity, probably as a result of inadequate memory stimulation. Thus the goal in most immunizations is to mimic natural immunity by evoking an active immune response similar to that following natural infection.

PASSIVE IMMUNIZATION

Passive immunity is achieved by antibody administration. Passive immunity occurs in infancy by transplacental transfer of maternal IgG antibody, which affords temporary protection against some infectious diseases. Once the maternal IgG disappears, the infant is susceptible unless he or she has already developed active immunity.

Medical practice has long sought to mimic this model of passive immunity. Initially, animal antisera were raised against specific infectious agents and infused into susceptible individuals on exposure to the infectious agent or after disease was established. Only limited success was achieved with this method, especially if done late in incubation or after the appearance of the disease. A further limitation was the hypersensitivity to animal antigens evoked in many humans.

Human Gamma Globulin

During World War II, human immune serum globulin (ISG) from pooled adult plasma became available and was used in the prevention of poliomyelitis, measles, and hepatitis. Later, gamma globulin derived from plasma lots selected for their high titer of a specific antibody or from subjects deliberately immunized or convalescing from disease was prepared. These special ISGs are useful in the prevention of tetanus, hepatitis B, varicella-zoster virus infection (chickenpox), and several other disorders.

Human gamma globulin preparations intended for intramuscular administration (ISG, IG) are concentrated solutions of electrophoretically similar globulins, usually prepared by cold alcohol fractionation (Cohn method). They contain high concentrations of IgG molecules with minimal amounts of IgA and IgM. A spectrum of antibodies generally is represented based on the immunologic experience of the adults from whom the pool of plasma was obtained. These preparations contain aggregates of IgG that can cause anaphylactoid reactions if given intravenously.

A number of intravenous immunoglobulin (IVIG) products are licensed for use in the United States. Three general strategies—enzymatic degradation, chemical modification, and physical purification—have been used to eliminate aggregated IgG from these preparations. Each IVIG lot is derived from thousands of adult donors. In addition, special hyperimmune IVIGs are available or are in development, most notably for immunocompromised patients at risk for cytomegalovirus, varicella-zoster, respiratory syncytial virus, or *Pseudomonas* infection.

Whenever gamma globulin is administered simultaneously with an immunizing antigen, active immunity may be suppressed. The specific antibody in the gamma globulin combines with the antigen to reduce the net amount of antigen given. In addition, central inhibition of antibody synthesis by the passive antibody may occur, necessitating additional doses of antigen.

Animal Sera

Another way to transfer passive immunity is by administering sera prepared from animal sources, usually horses. These preparations differ not only in their antibody content but also in their specific antigenic composition.

The chief disadvantage of antiserum is the risk of serum reactions, both immediate and delayed. This possibility must be considered each time horse serum is used. Appropriate medications to treat anaphylactic shock, including epinephrine drawn up in a syringe for instant administration, should be readily available. The possibility of serum sickness that may develop later should also be kept in mind.

Before animal serum is administered, the following steps are completed (Table 42-1):

1. A careful history of previous use of horse serum products and of subsequent reactions is sought.
2. A history of other allergies or allergic symptoms from contact with horses or horse dander is sought. Although this history is rarely elicited, it can serve as a warning to proceed with extreme caution.
3. Skin or conjunctival tests are performed.

TABLE 42-1 · STEPS NECESSARY BEFORE HORSE SERUM ADMINISTRATION

History—Specific Inquiries
1. Allergy in general
2. Receipt of horse serum in past
3. Allergic reaction to horse serum or to other horse antigen (e.g., dander)

Skin Tests*
1. Scratch test first; intradermal test if scratch test is negative
2. Administer
   a. 0.1 ml of 1:100 saline dilution of serum to be used; reduce dose to 0.05 ml of 1:1000 in allergic individuals
   b. Appearance of wheal in 10 to 30 minutes indicates hypersensitivity

Procedure
1. History and skin tests negative
   a. Give appropriate intramuscular dose *or*
   b. Give 0.5 ml serum intravenously in 10 ml saline; with no reaction in 30 minutes, give remainder of dose as 1:20 dilution
2. History or skin test positive
   a. Give 1.0 ml of 1:10 dilution subcutaneously; with no reaction proceed as in 3a
3. History and skin test positive:[†]
   a. Use only if imperative
   b. Give 0.05 ml of 1:20 dilution subcutaneously
   c. With no reaction, increase dose every 15 minutes as follows:
      (1) 0.1 ml of 1:10 dilution
      (2) 0.3 ml of 1:10 dilution
      (3) 0.1 ml of undiluted
      (4) 0.2 ml of undiluted
      (5) 0.5 ml of undiluted
      (6) Remainder of dose

*Conjunctival tests are unreliable because of irritant effect.
[†]If a positive reaction occurs at any stage, reduce dose by half.
ID = intradermal; IM = intramuscular; SC = subcutaneous.
Adapted from American Academy of Pediatrics. Report of Committee on Infectious Diseases. The Red Book. Evanston, IL, American Academy of Pediatrics, 2000.

Because a severe reaction occasionally ensues from the testing procedure, one should be prepared to intervene. Most experts believe that conjunctival testing cannot be used because the irritant effect of the material placed in the conjunctival sac often produces a false-positive reaction. For this reason, skin tests using 0.1 ml of a 1:100 saline dilution of the serum injected intradermally are preferred. In allergic individuals, the dose is reduced to 0.05 ml of a 1:1000 dilution. The appearance of a wheal in 10 to 30 minutes indicates hypersensitivity.

If there is no history of allergy and no reaction to the serum, the appropriate intramuscular dose of the horse serum can be given. For intravenous administration, 0.5 ml of serum in 10 ml of fluid is given initially; if no reaction occurs within 30 minutes, the remainder of the dose is given in a 1:20 dilution. If the patient has a history of allergy or a positive reaction to the skin test but the use of serum is imperative, desensitization must be accomplished. Initially, 0.05 ml of a 1:20 dilution is given subcutaneously. If there is no reaction, the dose is increased every 15 minutes as follows: 0.1 ml of a 1:10 dilution, 0.3 ml of a 1:10 dilution, 0.1 ml undiluted, 0.2 ml undiluted, 0.5 ml undiluted; finally, the remainder of the dose is administered. If an adverse reaction develops at any step, the dose should be reduced by one half. If this fails to stop reactivity, the preparation cannot be used.

VACCINE DEVELOPMENT AND USE

The Ideal Vaccine

The ideal immunizing agent has the following characteristics:

1. The antigen is pure and defined.
2. The specific response protects the individual against the disease.
3. The antigen is given in a simple, painless, one-step procedure.
4. The protection afforded is lifelong without the need for boosters.
5. There are no adverse immediate or long-range side effects.
6. The vaccine is acceptable to recipients and parents or guardians.
7. The vaccine is inexpensive.

The degree to which a vaccine fulfills these characteristics is the major issue confronting the practitioner in selection or use of a vaccine. As increasing numbers of vaccines, antisera, and gamma globulin preparations become available, the physician must assess the value of each preparation before using it for the individual patient.

The product brochure carries a complete description of the product and its use. The recommendations of the Committee on Infectious Diseases of the American Academy of Pediatrics (The Red Book) and the Advisory Committee on Immunization Practices of the CDC (Morbidity and Mortality Weekly Report) should be consulted. Whenever a new vaccine is introduced, these sources offer an authoritative description of the product, the positive and negative attributes, and recommendations for its use in children and in adults.

Vaccine Composition

There is no typical vaccine, but the following categories of components are listed:

1. *The principal antigen:* This may be whole bacteria, bacterial products (e.g., toxins, hemolysins), whole viruses, or substructures of viruses.
2. *Host-derived antigens:* These are proteins or other constituents of host tissue that are carried along with or intimately associated with viral particles.
3. *Altered antigens:* These are denatured proteins and other substances that result from the viral infection of the cells on which the virus is grown.
4. *Preservatives and stabilizers:* These are chemical compounds added to prevent bacterial growth or to stabilize the antigen (e.g., thimerosal [Merthiolate], glycerin).
5. *Antibiotics:* Trace amounts may be present in viral vaccines from the media used in their growth. The

same vaccine from different manufacturers may contain different antibiotics.
6. *Menstruum:* The fluid phase of the vaccine suspension or solution may consist of saline or a complex tissue culture medium.
7. *Unwanted or unknown constituents:* Despite elaborate precautions in preparing vaccines, viruses or other unwanted antigens may be present.
8. *Adjuvant:* This is a substance, such as alum, aluminum phosphate, or aluminum hydroxide, that enhances the antigenicity of the principal antigen. Adjuvants often retain the antigen at the depot site and release it slowly.

This list points out the complexities of some vaccines and the difficulty in attributing an unusual reaction to a specific component.

Specific Antigens

Antigens vary in their ability to stimulate the desired immunologic response. For a given antigen, the response is variable, with some individuals responding poorly and a few not at all. Some children who receive a vaccine under optimal circumstances simply do not respond and contract the disease on exposure. This failing should not condemn the vaccine for other children, because it can protect most.

In general, adjuvant (depot type) vaccines are preferred over fluid vaccines because they provide more prolonged immunity, greater antigenic stimulation, and fewer systemic effects. For example, diphtheria with tetanus and pertussis (DTP) vaccine stimulates prolonged antitoxin production against diphtheria and tetanus and enhances the antibody response to pertussis, particularly in early infancy (Kendrick, 1943). Fluid or aqueous preparations may achieve earlier immunity and are less likely to produce local reactions at the injection site but generally offer no clinically significant advantages.

A great deal of research is currently looking at developing vaccine antigens based on incorporating into the host DNA encoding the desired antigen. In animal models, this approach has provoked both humoral and cell-mediated responses. It is hoped that this approach will allow the development of safe vaccination (e.g., tuberculosis, HIV).

Dose of Vaccine

Most vaccine schedules are determined by trial and error until an appropriate dose is selected. What is sought is a dose large enough to produce the desired immune response in most or all recipients yet small enough to be harmless, economical, and easy to administer. Although it is tempting to reduce the usual dose for reasons of economy, convenience, or comfort, this practice may result in inadequate immunization. Increasing the dose may be accompanied by toxic effects or unwanted complications.

Route of Immunization

The route of vaccine administration is a critical determinant of both effectiveness and safety and may determine the type and duration of immunologic response. For example, an intramuscular injection of inactivated poliomyelitis virus vaccine induces serum antibody production and systemic immunity. However, it fails to evoke local antibody in the form of secretory IgA and thus does not prevent subsequent gastrointestinal infection.

Live, attenuated oral polio vaccine induces both local gastrointestinal and systemic antibody production; therefore immunization by the oral route may be preferred. Oral or intramuscular administration of a vaccine meant to be given subcutaneously may result in ineffective immunization. Occasionally, the side effects of a subcutaneous vaccine may be diminished by intracutaneous inoculation, but this should be done only if the efficacy of this route has been established. In general, strict adherence to the recommended dose and route is advisable.

Timing of Immunization

In a disease prevalent in infants (e.g., pertussis), immunization must be undertaken early enough to be effective and preventive yet late enough that an adequate immune response occurs. Thus epidemiologic factors of the disease help determine the timing of vaccine administration.

Some circumstances warrant administration of vaccine coincident with or shortly after exposure. Rabies immunization at the time of a bite is the prime example, but live measles virus (LMV) vaccination in a just-exposed susceptible person also can be done (Fulginiti, 1964). The incubation period of rabies is long (weeks to months), providing ample time to actively immunize an exposed individual. The incubation period of natural measles is about 11 days, and that of the attenuated virus infection is 7 days (Katz et al., 1960), so the vaccine must be given within a few days of exposure.

With some vaccines, booster doses are required if long-term immunity is to be maintained. The precise timing of these additional doses is determined by both theory and experience. Some vaccines require multiple, frequent doses over the life span of an individual (e.g., cholera). Others can be given infrequently at long intervals (e.g., yellow fever). In general, inactivated vaccines require repetitive administration, whereas live vaccines do not. In general, intervals between multiple doses of an antigen (e.g., oral polio vaccine [OPV]) that are longer than those recommended do not lead to a reduction in overall immunity achieved at the completion of the immunization series. Usually, it is not necessary to restart an interrupted series or to add doses in addition to those recommended. In contrast, the provision of multiple vaccine doses of an antigen at less than the recommended interval may lessen the immune response; doses given at less than the recommended interval

should not be counted as part of the primary series. Accurate record keeping on the part of physicians is imperative, and an up-to-date immunization record should be kept by parents (American Academy of Pediatrics, 2003).

Combination of Antigens

Vaccines are often combined to facilitate immunization. Early studies suggested the following:

1. There were limits to the responsiveness of an individual to multiple antigens.
2. Specific vaccine combinations, particularly viral vaccines, were mutually inhibitory, thus diminishing their efficacy.
3. Additive adverse effects were likely to occur.

However, experience with certain vaccine combinations has failed to substantiate these theoretical risks. Thus DTP and oral poliovirus vaccines, a combination of six antigens, are given together with no decrease in immune response or increase in adverse consequences. Measles, mumps, and rubella virus vaccines can be administered together, without adverse consequences or diminished effect. It is essential that only proven combinations be used; there is no guarantee of efficacy or safety if the physician mixes in a single syringe other combinations from components designed for individual use.

Rapid sequential administration of certain vaccines has the potential for viral interference. For example, live measles vaccine given 1 week before smallpox vaccine inhibited the latter to some extent (Merigan et al., 1965). Thus care must be taken to observe acceptable intervals between vaccines. For viral vaccines, interferon stimulation and subsequent viral inhibition is a potential problem. In general, 4 weeks or more should separate administrations of live virus vaccine.

Safety of Vaccines

Most available vaccines are generally safe and effective. Undesirable side effects can be anticipated in a small number of patients with any of the available vaccines; a small but definite risk is associated with the administration of every immunizing agent. The benefits to the child as well as to society and the risks of vaccine administration should be explained to parents, patients, or both before vaccine administration, and informed consent should be obtained.

The risk of adverse reactions associated with vaccine administration always must be compared with the risk of natural acquisition of the disease and its complications. For example, primary immunization with OPV in individuals older than age 18 is associated with a definite risk of vaccine-associated poliomyelitis. Because this risk may be greater than the risk of naturally acquiring the disease, such immunization is not recommended routinely. Similarly, because pertussis acquired by individuals older than 6 years of age carries with it a relatively small risk of morbid complications, immunization is not recommended for older children and adults.

To improve overall knowledge about adverse reactions, all temporally associated events severe enough to require the patient to seek medical attention should be evaluated and reported in detail to local and state health officials, as well as the vaccine manufacturer. Often, cause-and-effect relationships are impossible to establish when untoward events occur after immunization.

Scientific trials designed to document the incidence and nature of adverse reactions to already available or newly introduced vaccines are of critical importance to ensure a scientific rationale for vaccine use recommendations and to ensure optimal public and professional vaccine acceptance.

Vaccine Administration

Injectable vaccines should be administered at a body site relatively free from risk of nerve or vascular injury. The best sites for intramuscular or subcutaneous injections are the anterolateral thigh (in infants) and the deltoid area of the upper arm (in older children and adults). Intragluteal injections carry the risk of damage to the sciatic nerve.

Vaccines containing adjuvants must be injected deep into a large muscle mass; subcutaneous or intracutaneous injection or leakage should be avoided because of the risk of local irritation, inflammation, and necrosis. Vaccines requiring intramuscular injection include DTP, DT (diphtheria and tetanus, pediatric), Td (diphtheria and tetanus, adult), hepatitis B, and rabies (human diploid cell). Immunoglobulin preparations also require intramuscular injection.

Contraindications for Vaccines

Contraindications to live virus vaccine administration include conditions associated with high risk for replication of viruses. Immunodeficient patients are at risk, especially those with profound B- or T-cell defects. Both congenital and acquired immunodeficiencies (e.g., acquired immunodeficiency syndrome [AIDS], lymphomas, immunosuppressive therapy) are associated with such risks.

Severe reactions, such as extreme somnolence, seizures, or high fever, may represent a contraindication to subsequent immunization with the same antigen. Because scientific data do not support their safety or efficacy, fractional doses of the immunizing agent that elicited the reaction are not recommended to complete an immunization schedule. Minor illness is not an indication for deferral of childhood immunizations, regardless of the degree of accompanying fever (American Academy of Pediatrics, 2003).

Allergic diseases may pose special problems in immunization. Certain vaccine antigens produced in biologic systems containing allergenic substances (e.g., antigens derived from embryonated chick eggs) may cause hypersensitivity reactions, including anaphylaxis, when the final vaccine dose contains a substantial amount of the allergen (e.g., yellow fever vaccine) (CDC, 1983c). Influenza vaccine antigens, although prepared from viruses grown in embryonated eggs, are highly purified during preparation and only rarely have been associated with hypersensitivity reactions. Similarly, hypersensitivity reactions to measles vaccine rarely have been reported in persons with anaphylactic hypersensitivity to eggs. A history of ability to eat eggs without anaphylaxis excludes most individuals at risk for hypersensitivity reactions to measles, mumps, or influenza vaccines.

Some vaccines contain preservatives or trace amounts of antibiotics (e.g., neomycin) to which individuals may be hypersensitive. Patients with known anaphylactic hypersensitivity to preservatives or antibiotics indicated in the package inserts should not receive these vaccines.

Because of theoretical risks to the developing fetus, live viral vaccines are usually not recommended for pregnant women or those likely to become pregnant within 3 months after receiving the immunizing agent. With respect to some of these vaccines (e.g., rubella, measles, and mumps), pregnancy is an absolute contraindication. Other agents, such as yellow fever and oral polio vaccines, can be given safely to pregnant women who are at substantial risk of exposure to natural infection. When vaccine must be given during pregnancy, a reasonable precaution is to wait until the second or third trimester to minimize concerns about teratogenicity (CDC, 1983c). Further specific information about immunization of pregnant women is provided with each immunizing agent discussed in this chapter.

RECOMMENDATIONS FOR VACCINES IN COMMON USE

Diphtheria Immunization

Rationale for Active Immunization

Historically, diphtheria has always represented a potentially serious pediatric disease. In the prevaccine era, 5% to 10% of reported respiratory cases were fatal, and the highest case-fatality ratios were in very young and elderly patients. The introduction of diphtheria toxoid more than half a century ago has led to a dramatic reduction in the incidence of diphtheria in the United States. More recently, no more than five cases have been reported annually (Vitek and Wenger, 1999).

However, diphtheria may continue to represent a potentially significant public health issue because (1) serologic surveys in the United States suggest that many adults are not currently immunized adequately (Crossley et al., 1979) and (2) adequate immunization does not completely eliminate the potential for transmission of *Corynebacterium diphtheriae* (Miller et al., 1972). Moreover, epidemic diphtheria continues to occur in various other parts of the world, including the newly independent states of the former Soviet Union.

Diphtheria is caused by infection with *C. diphtheriae*. Multiplication of the organism is less important than the local elaboration and systemic distribution of a powerful exotoxin. Toxin production is associated with strains of the organism infected with a specific bacteriophage.

Immunity to diphtheria depends on the presence of adequate levels of circulating antitoxin. Neutralization of diphtheria toxin prevents the severe manifestations of disease and helps reduce infection. Because the toxin plays a major role in permitting the bacterium to establish itself in the host, neutralization by antitoxin reduces infectious risk and also prevents the severe manifestations of disease. Immunization stimulates the formation of circulating antitoxin and sensitizes the immune system so that additional antitoxin can be synthesized rapidly.

Immunizing Antigen

The immunizing antigen is a toxoid prepared by chemical alteration of toxin to remove its toxicity but maintain antigenicity. Diphtheria toxoid is available at two levels of potency, regular (D) and adult (d) and in combination with tetanus (T) as DT (diphtheria and tetanus, pediatric) or Td (diphtheria and tetanus, adult), and with tetanus and acellular pertussis (DTaP). Primary immunization of children younger than 7 years is accomplished with preparations containing 7 to 25 Lf units of toxoid, the regular toxoid dose (DT or DTaP).

Because this antigen concentration is too toxic for older children and adults, a preparation containing no more than 2 Lf of toxoid is given (Td) after age 6. These antigens are absorbed to an alum-type adjuvant to provide maximal stimulation. A fluid toxoid is also available but rarely indicated or used. Toxoid should be given deep into a large muscle mass (CDC, 1981).

Immunity

Immunization of children with diphtheria toxoid does not provide 100% protection but instead brings about a 5-fold to 10-fold reduction in incidence of subsequent disease. Furthermore, few severe (or fatal) cases of diphtheria occur among fully immunized individuals.

Immunity is correlated with the presence of circulating antitoxin, which can be precisely measured only in specialized laboratories but is not practical for routine testing. In past years, the Schick test has been used to estimate the amount of circulating antitoxin. Diphtheria toxin (0.1 ml) and a toxoid control are injected intradermally at different sites. A positive test, consisting of erythema and more than 10-mm induration at the site of toxin injection in 48 to 96 hours and little or no reaction at the control site, indicates susceptibility to diphtheria. A hypersensitivity reaction, indicated by equivalent reactions to toxoid and control, is occasionally noted.

Diphtheria immunity is of longer duration than previously thought. Booster doses used to be recommended every 4 to 6 years; it is now believed that 10-year intervals are adequate.

Vaccine Use

The CDC (2000a) and American Academy of Pediatrics (2000) have made the following recommendations for use of DTP.

PRIMARY IMMUNIZATION IN INFANCY

Three 0.5-ml doses of DTaP are given intramuscularly at 2-month intervals, beginning as early as 2 months of age. Additional DTaP doses are given at the age of 15 to 18 months and 4 to 6 years (Table 42-2).

PRIMARY IMMUNIZATION AFTER 6 YEARS OF AGE

Primary immunization is accomplished with two 0.5-ml doses of tetanus toxoid combined with the lower adult dose of diphtheria toxoid (Td) given at least 4 weeks apart and followed by a booster 1 year later.

RECALL IMMUNIZATION

Tetanus toxoid should be given with diphtheria toxoid as Td every 10 years. If a dose is given sooner as part of wound management (Td is preferred over tetanus toxoid alone), the next booster is not needed for 10 years thereafter.

LAPSED IMMUNIZATION

If doses are missed in the primary series, regardless of the interval, additional doses are given until a primary series of doses is completed. Interruption of the

TABLE 42-2 · IMMUNIZATION SCHEDULE SUGGESTED FOR HEALTHY INFANTS AND CHILDREN*

Age	Immunization
At birth	HBV
1–2 mo	HBV
2 mo	DTaP, HbCV, IPV, PCV
4 mo	DTaP, HbCV, IPV, PCV
6 mo	DTaP, HbCV[†], PCV
6–18 mo	HBV, IPV
12–15 mo	MMR, HbCV[†], VVV, PCV
15–18 mo	DTaP or DTP
4–6 yr	DTaP or DTP, IPV
11–12 yr	MMR[‡]
14–16 yr	Td

*See text for more detail.
[†]The first two vaccine doses are given at 2 and 4 months of age. If either HbOC or PRP-T is used, a third dose is given at age 6 months. A booster vaccination is given at 12 to 15 months of age.
[‡]The second dose of MMR can be given at school entry rather than at age 11 to 12 years.
DTaP = diphtheria, tetanus, and acellular pertussis; DTaP = diphtheria, tetanus, and acellular pertussis; HbCV = *H. influenzae* type b conjugate vaccine; HBV = hepatitis B vaccine; MMR = measles, mumps, and rubella vaccine; IPV = inactivated polio vaccine; PCV = pneumococcal conjugate vaccine; Td = diphtheria and tetanus vaccine for adults; VVV = varicella virus vaccine.
Adapted from American Academy of Pediatrics. In 2003 Red Book: Report of the Committee on Infectious Diseases, 26th ed. Elk Grove Village, IL, American Academy of Pediatrics, 1994.

recommended schedule or delay in administering subsequent doses during primary immunization does not reduce ultimate immunity; there is no need to restart a series regardless of the time elapsed between doses.

SPECIAL CIRCUMSTANCES

Household contacts of patients with suspected respiratory diphtheria should receive an injection of a diphtheria toxoid–containing preparation appropriate for age and should be evaluated closely. Those who have previously received at least three doses of diphtheria toxoid, including at least one dose during the previous 5 years, need not be vaccinated.

In addition, asymptomatic unimmunized or inadequately immunized household contacts should receive prompt chemoprophylaxis with either an intramuscular injection of benzathine penicillin (600,000 units for children younger than 6 years old and 1.2 million units for those 6 years or older) or a 7-day course of erythromycin. Primary immunization should be completed in all persons who have received fewer than the recommended number of vaccine doses. For patients convalescing from diphtheria infection, complete active immunization should be performed because infection does not necessarily confer immunity. The only specific contraindication to diphtheria toxoid administration is a history of neurologic or severe hypersensitivity reaction following a previous dose. Vaccination should be deferred during acute illness with high-grade fever.

The use of equine diphtheria antitoxin in unimmunized diphtheria contacts generally is not recommended because of the potential for immediate hypersensitivity reactions. However, for treatment of infected individuals (except those with cutaneous diphtheria), administration of antitoxin should be considered (American Academy of Pediatrics, 2003). The dose of antitoxin is empiric and should be administered as soon as diphtheria is diagnosed, even before positive cultures are obtained. Suggested doses are as follows:

· Pharyngeal or laryngeal diphtheria (<48 hours)—20,000 to 40,000 units
· Nasopharyngeal—40,000 to 60,000 units
· Extensive disease present for more than 72 hours—80,000 to 120,000 units
· Brawny neck edema—80,000 to 120,000 units

These doses are empiric and may be modified depending on the site and size of the membrane, the severity of symptoms, and the duration of illness. Cervical adenitis often reflects toxin absorption; soft and diffuse adenopathy indicates moderate to severe toxicity.

Before antitoxin is administered, sensitivity tests must be done. A 1:10 dilution of antitoxin in the eye or a 1:100 dilution in the skin is used. Desensitization is accomplished as previously described. Antimicrobial therapy must not be substituted for antitoxin; instead, the antitoxin and antibiotics should be used together.

Tetanus Immunization

Rationale for Active Immunization

Tetanus is caused by the neurotoxicity of a potent exotoxin elaborated by *Clostridium tetani*, a ubiquitous organism found throughout nature and particularly in animal excreta. *C. tetani* remains in the spore form until entry into a wound. The spores germinate if an anaerobic environment is established. Common circumstances that lead to tetanus infection include the following:

· Contamination of the umbilicus of the neonate, especially in areas of the world where poultices of animal dung are applied to the stump
· Wounds that result in pockets of anaerobiosis (the wound may be trivial or obvious)
· Insect bites
· Contaminated surgical wounds, particularly those exposed to gastrointestinal contents

Routine immunization of civilian populations in the United States with tetanus toxoid has resulted in a dramatic decrease in the incidence of tetanus. Of further importance has been the near-elimination of neonatal tetanus in the United States, although it continues to represent a significant cause of morbidity and mortality in many parts of the world. Most tetanus cases in the United States now occur in individuals older than age 50, and in virtually all cases, the disease has been reported only in unimmunized or inadequately immunized individuals (CDC, 1981). Because it provides long-lasting protection and is relatively safe in human populations, tetanus toxoid has proved to be a nearly ideal immunizing agent.

Immunization is aimed at stimulating the development of antitoxin similar to that in diphtheria immunization. Tetanus is also prevented by prompt and appropriate treatment of injuries and wounds, rather than relying on immunization. Immunization against tetanus provides personal protection but does not provide community protection.

Immunizing Antigen

Tetanospasmin, the toxin of *C. tetani*, is modified by chemical treatment to provide a stable nontoxic agent for immunization. A potent antigen with minimal toxicity, tetanus toxoid is used alone or in combination with diphtheria (DT, Td) and pertussis vaccine (DTaP). It is one of the most effective vaccine antigens, and a complete primary series provides long-lasting immunity.

Because toxoid evokes a potent antibody response, too-frequent immunizations can result in severe local necrotic Arthus reactions. The high levels of serum antibody result in antigen–antibody complexes at the injection site, with resultant inflammation and vasculitis.

Immunity

The presence of antitoxin appears to be the sole factor in protection from the disease. As little as 0.01 IU/ml of antitoxin is protective (Goldsmith et al., 1962). Primary immunization is so effective that values above this protective level have been observed as long as 35 years after primary immunization (Peebles et al., 1969). Furthermore, a booster dose results in a brisk anamnestic response. Although it may not always be necessary, 10-year boosters are recommended to maintain protective levels of antitoxin.

Vaccine Use

The CDC (2000a) and American Academy of Pediatrics (2000) have made the following recommendations for tetanus toxoid.

PRIMARY IMMUNIZATION IN INFANCY

Three doses of tetanus toxoid, usually as DTaP, are administered intramuscularly at 2-month intervals, beginning as early as 2 months of age. Booster doses are given at 15 to 18 months and 4 to 6 years of age (see Table 42-2).

PRIMARY IMMUNIZATION AT 7 YEARS OF AGE OR OLDER

Two doses of either tetanus toxoid alone (0.5 ml) or as Td are administered 2 months apart. A booster dose is given 6 months to 1 year later.

LAPSED IMMUNIZATION

If doses are missed, the next dose in the series is administered regardless of interval. It is not necessary to begin the series anew.

RECALL IMMUNIZATION

Tetanus toxoid (Td) should be given every 10 years to maintain immunity. Usually, a booster dose is given when the child enters school and every 10 years thereafter. If a dose is administered sooner as part of wound management, the next routine booster is not needed until 10 years later. In the United States, when the risk of neonatal tetanus is significant, antenatal immunization is recommended for previously unimmunized pregnant women using two properly spaced doses of Td. Booster injections of Td may be used in previously immunized pregnant women. In other regions of the world, adsorbed preparations containing higher concentrations of tetanus toxoid may be available for use in the antenatal immunization of previously unimmunized mothers (CDC, 1981, 1985; Chen et al., 1983).

IMMUNIZATION ASSOCIATED WITH WOUND MANAGEMENT OR TETANUS INFECTION

Active immunization may not be necessary as part of wound management for trauma or injury (Table 42-3). Adequate primary immunization provides sufficient protective titers of antitoxin for at least 10 years and ensures prompt, anamnestic responses to booster injections for several years longer (Peebles et al., 1969). The prolonged immunity afforded, in addition to the known increased incidence of hypersensitivity reactions

TABLE 42-3 · RECOMMENDED USE OF TETANUS TOXOID AND TETANUS IMMUNE GLOBULIN IN WOUND MANAGEMENT

History of Tetanus Immunization (Doses)	Clean, Minor Wounds		Tetanus-Prone* Wounds	
	Td[†]	TIG[‡]	Td	TIG
Uncertain, less than three	Yes[§]	No	Yes[¶]	Yes
Three or more	No[§]	No	No[¶]	No

*Tetanus-prone generally refers to wounds that yield anaerobic conditions or are incurred under conditions in which exposure to tetanus species is probable (puncture wound, severe necrotizing soft tissue wound, or wound contaminated with animal excreta).
[†]Tetanus and diphtheria toxoids (DT recommended for children younger than 7 years).
[‡]Human tetanus immunoglobulin (250 to 500 units intramuscularly).
[§]Unless more than 10 years since the last dose.
[¶]Unless more than 5 years since the last dose.
Td = diphtheria and tetanus vaccine for adults; TIG = tetanus immune globulin vaccine.
Modified from American Academy of Pediatrics. 2003 Red Book: Report of the Committee on Infectious Diseases, 26th ed. Elk Grove Village, IL, American Academy of Pediatrics, 2003.

associated with frequent booster injections, supports a conservative approach to the use of tetanus toxoid in wound management. Specific recommendations depend on the individual's immunization status, the nature of the wound, and the duration of time before evaluation and treatment of the injury. In individuals who are immunized adequately, it is not necessary to provide tetanus toxoid more than every 5 years.

Tetanus immunoglobulin (TIG) is indicated only for individuals who have received fewer than two previous doses of tetanus toxoid or those in whom a tetanus-prone wound has been unattended for more than 24 hours. Generally, DT (Td in patients 7 years of age and older) is recommended for wound prophylaxis instead of tetanus toxoid alone to ensure additional immunity to diphtheria (American Academy of Pediatrics, 2000). Subsequent to prophylaxis, primary immunization should be completed in those incompletely immunized.

The exact dose of TIG for therapeutic use is unknown. At least 140 U/kg given intramuscularly is recommended, with larger doses used in more severe cases. Patients convalescing from tetanus infection should receive active immunization because infection often does not confer immunity (CDC, 1981).

Adverse Effects of Immunization

Tetanus toxoid is an extremely safe biological and is rarely associated with local or systemic reactions. A local Arthus reaction may occur if too many doses are given (Edsall et al., 1967). A history of neurologic or severe hypersensitivity reactions to tetanus toxoid–containing preparations contraindicates subsequent tetanus toxoid use; skin testing may be helpful in the rare patient demonstrating a severe allergic reaction (Jacobs et al., 1982).

Pertussis Immunization

Rationale for Active Immunization

Pertussis (whooping cough) continues to account for significant morbidity and mortality among pediatric patients worldwide, including in the United States. Serious complications (e.g., seizures, encephalopathy, and not uncommonly, death) still occur, especially in children younger than 1 year. Thus primary prevention programs in the United States emphasize early active immunization of all infants.

Since the introduction of pertussis vaccine in the United States in the 1940s, a dramatic decline in the incidence of clinical pertussis has been documented. Whereas more than 265,000 pertussis cases, including 7518 deaths, were reported in the United States in 1934, only 103 pertussis deaths were reported during the 1990s (Vitek et al., 2003).

Recent epidemiologic studies have clearly demonstrated the protective efficacy of pertussis vaccine in the United States. In one study (Broome and Fraser, 1981), attack rates among household contacts younger than 10 years of age declined from 67% for unvaccinated individuals to 4% for those who had received three or more vaccinations (calculated vaccine efficacy of 94% for children younger than 5 years of age).

Because children in the United States do not receive three doses of vaccine until 6 months of age under the current vaccination schedule, not all cases of pertussis are preventable. However, the morbidity of clinical disease among incompletely immunized infants and children is related inversely to the number of vaccine doses they have received (CDC, 1982e). Furthermore, the risk of infection in infants younger than 6 months old may be reduced indirectly by achieving high levels of immunity in household contacts.

Concerns about pertussis vaccine toxicity and controversies about the relative risks and benefits of routine immunization have diminished vaccine acceptance rates in other countries. For example, in the United Kingdom, accounts of neurologic sequelae associated with vaccine use accounted for a drop in vaccine acceptance rates from 77% in 1974 to 30% in 1978. Not unexpectedly, an outbreak of 102,500 cases of pertussis with 36 fatalities occurred in that country during 1977 to 1979 (Miller et al., 1982). Vaccine acceptance in Japan dropped from 77% in 1974 to 13% in 1976 after two fatalities were associated with vaccine use. Only 393 pertussis cases and no deaths had been reported in that country in 1974, but 13,000 cases and 41 deaths were reported in 1979 (Kanai, 1980).

Such experience clearly indicates that although immunization with the whole-cell pertussis vaccine is associated with a measurable risk (Cody et al., 1981), this risk is far outweighed by the benefit of disease prevention (Hinman and Koplan, 1984). An acellular vaccine developed in Japan appears to have equal efficacy but fewer side effects compared with conventional whole-cell vaccines (Sato et al., 1984).

Immunizing Antigen

The pertussis vaccine in use for many years consisted of killed whole *Bordetella pertussis* and fragments of organisms. The precise antigen responsible for protection is unknown. New pertussis vaccines, composed of purified components of *B. pertussis* rather than whole-cell vaccines prepared from inactivated organisms, have been licensed for use in the United States (Peter, 1992). These new vaccines are termed *acellular* pertussis vaccines (aP).

Potency of pertussis vaccine is a critical issue. The standard test is a mouse-protective model developed in the 1940s that correlates well with human protection. Vaccines used in England and elsewhere before 1968 were of low potency as measured by this procedure (Stewart, 1977). The poor results of immunization in England that led to the suggestion that pertussis vaccine be abandoned were probably a result of ineffective vaccine. Potent vaccine, as judged by mouse-protective units, is capable of providing active immunity and 85% to 90% protection when 12 protective units are administered in three equal doses given at 4- to 8-week intervals (Broome and Fraser, 1981).

Acellular pertussis vaccines can be administered alone or in combination with diphtheria and tetanus toxoid (DTaP). Acellular pertussis vaccines contain one or more immunogens derived from *B. pertussis* organisms, including pertussis toxoid, filamentous hemagglutinin, fimbrial proteins, and pertactin. As of 2003, five acellular pertussis vaccines have been licensed in the United States and four have been licensed for use in infants and children in the standard vaccine schedule.

Immunity

Although several antigens have been isolated from *Bordetella pertussis,* and several antibodies occur after immunization, the precise mechanism of immunity is unknown. Almost total protection has been associated with high antibody titers (>1:320) in humans and monkeys (Sako, 1947). However, some protection (approximately 60%) occurs at serum antibody levels below this and may even occur in the absence of antibody. Thus a role for cell-mediated immunity may exist.

Solid immunity usually follows natural disease, although second cases of proven disease have occurred. Protection after receiving the vaccine is relatively short-lived, so adults likely to be at risk (e.g., health personnel) need booster doses of vaccine to maintain immunity.

Complicating the assessment of vaccine efficacy is the occurrence of pertussis caused by agents other than *B. pertussis* (Lewis et al., 1973). Parapertussis may account for up to 2% of cases attributed to pertussis. There is no cross-immunity between these organisms. Adenoviruses and other viral agents may also cause pertussis-like syndromes. Thus evaluation of the efficacy of pertussis vaccine necessitates precise laboratory diagnosis.

Vaccine Use

The American Academy of Pediatrics (2000) and the CDC (2000a) have made the following recommendations for pertussis vaccination.

PRIMARY IMMUNIZATION IN INFANCY

Pertussis vaccine is usually combined with diphtheria and tetanus toxoids as DTaP. Each dose of DTaP contains 4 units of pertussis vaccine. Three doses of DTaP (a total of 12 units) are given intramuscularly at 2-month intervals, beginning at 2 months of age; a booster is given at 15 to 18 months of age (see Table 42-2). Routine recall booster doses are suggested when the child enters school. For the fourth and fifth doses, a tetra-immune combination of DTaP and *Haemophilus influenzae* b (Hib) may be used if desired.

PRIMARY IMMUNIZATION AFTER 6 YEARS OF AGE

A somewhat similar schedule of primary immunization can be used for children not immunized in early infancy and those younger than 7 years. Because of the risks of pertussis immunization and the overall decreased morbidity from pertussis in older individuals, pertussis vaccine is generally recommended only for children younger than 7 years. The adult diphtheria and tetanus toxoids (Td) preparation may be used for older patients.

SPECIAL CIRCUMSTANCES

In areas of high endemicity or during epidemics, immunization can begin earlier; the vaccine (DTaP or pertussis, adsorbed) is begun at 4 to 6 weeks of age, and three doses are given 1 month apart. Rarely, in severe epidemics affecting very young infants, pertussis immunization can be initiated in the first few days or weeks of life.

During pertussis outbreaks, certain exposed individuals require special consideration. Close contacts who are younger than 7 years (e.g., siblings, classmates) and who were previously immunized but have not received a pertussis immunization within the last 6 months should be reimmunized. In this setting, chemoprophylaxis with oral erythromycin also can be considered, especially in children younger than 1 year of age and in unimmunized patients.

Although pertussis vaccine is not recommended routinely for persons older than 7 years, a booster dose (0.25 ml of pertussis vaccine, adsorbed) can be given to older patients with chronic pulmonary disease who are exposed to pertussis or to health care personnel exposed during outbreaks. Prophylactic chemotherapy can also be considered in such persons. Chemotherapy of the index case may decrease the period of infectivity, but it will not alleviate the clinical course. Individuals who recover from bacteriologically confirmed pertussis require no further pertussis immunization (American Academy of Pediatrics, 2000).

After intimate exposure to pertussis or during epidemics, children younger than 7 years should receive a 0.5-ml dose. Older patients should receive a half-dose (0.25 ml) of either DTaP or pertussis adsorbed vaccine.

Adverse Effects of Immunization

Both local and systemic adverse effects may occur after the administration of preparations containing pertussis vaccine. Reported reactions after the use of DTaP or DT cannot be related certainly to the pertussis component. However, given that the incidence of adverse reactions after administration of pediatric diphtheria and tetanus toxoids is markedly less, most serious adverse reactions to DTP are more likely to be from the pertussis vaccine than from the toxoid components (Cody et al., 1981).

Local reactions to DTP, including erythema, swelling, and pain, are seen in about two thirds of recipients and occur more commonly with repeated immunization. These adverse effects are significantly less frequent with DTaP.

Occasionally, a sterile abscess may develop at the injection site. Systemic reactions, such as slight to moderate fever, can occur in DTaP recipients. Systemic reactions can be accompanied by mild lethargy, irritability, or vomiting. Such symptoms usually appear within hours and last 1 to 2 days after immunization (American Academy of Pediatrics, 2000).

More serious but very rare systemic reactions include persistent crying, pronounced fever ($\geq 40.5°C$), seizures, and collapse or shocklike states during which the infant is pale, hypotonic, and unresponsive. Such symptoms characteristically occur within hours after vaccination and last several minutes to hours. Affected infants generally recover completely. The rates of all these uncommon, but potentially serious, adverse events appear to be significantly less following DTaP than after DTP.

The significance of vaccine reactions in terms of permanent neurologic sequelae is not well defined. The National Childhood Encephalopathy Study performed in the United Kingdom estimated that the risk of an acute neurologic disorder occurring in a previously healthy child within 7 days of DTP immunization was 1 per 110,000 doses administered, with sequelae persisting at least 1 year in 1 per 310,000 doses administered (Miller et al., 1981).

Precise estimates of the risk of serious reactions to pertussis vaccine are difficult to determine because the incidence of temporally related reactions is so low that it is difficult to differentiate them from the background incidence of similar syndromes seen in unvaccinated children. Adsorbed vaccines are associated with fewer reactions than those without adjuvant, and reaction rates vary among preparations from different manufacturers of pertussis vaccine. DTaP is associated with lower rates of local reactions, fever, and common systemic reactions than is DTP.

Precautions and Contraindications

Most reactions following DTP or DT administration do not represent contraindications to further pertussis vaccination. When reactions that do not contraindicate further pertussis immunization occur, some health care providers divide the remaining inoculations into multiple small doses. No definitive clinical or serologic studies to evaluate the efficacy of such schedules or the effects on the subsequent frequency and severity of adverse reactions have been performed. Thus the use of fractional doses cannot be recommended at this time (Barkin et al., 1984). Physicians should encourage parents to report adverse reactions temporally related to vaccine administration.

Each of the following reactions to pertussis vaccine represents an absolute contraindication to subsequent pertussis immunization:

· An immediate anaphylactic reaction
· Encephalopathy within 7 days

Should the following adverse events occur with acellular pertussis vaccination, subsequent vaccination should be considered carefully. These events were once considered absolute contraindications, but because they have not been proved to cause permanent sequelae, they are now considered precautions (American Academy of Pediatrics, 2000):

· Fever 40.5°C or greater within 48 hours
· Persistent screaming or crying for 3 hours or more or an unusual, high-pitched cry
· Collapse or shocklike state
· Convulsions with or without fever occurring within 72 hours after immunization

Children younger than 7 years in whom further pertussis vaccine is contraindicated may complete the necessary immunization schedule with the DT preparation (American Academy of Pediatrics, 2000).

Seizures following pertussis immunization occur more commonly in those with a history of a previous seizure disorder, but they appear to be similar to febrile seizures and are associated with a benign outcome (Cody et al., 1981; Hirtz et al., 1983). Pertussis immunization should be deferred in patients with a seizure disorder until it can be determined that there is no evidence of evolving neurologic disease. Patients with stable neurologic disorders, including well-controlled seizures, may receive pertussis vaccine. Furthermore, a family history of seizures or other neurologic disease is not a contraindication to pertussis immunization.

Poliomyelitis Immunization

Rationale for Immunization

The efficacy of primary prevention through active immunization is perhaps most convincingly demonstrated by the near-extinction of poliomyelitis in the United States since the introduction of polio vaccines. In contrast to the prevaccine era, when more than 18,000 cases of paralytic disease occurred in the United States each year, the last case of poliomyelitis attributable to indigenously acquired, wild-type poliovirus occurred in 1979. Only a single case of imported wild-type poliomyelitis has been observed (in 1993). Since 1979, all other cases of paralytic poliomyelitis (approximately eight per year) have been vaccine associated (American Academy of Pediatrics, 2000).

Active immunity can be achieved with either inactivated or attenuated poliovirus vaccines. For maximal effectiveness, polio immunization must involve a large segment of the population, which reduces the spread of wild poliovirus in the community and provides protection to unimmunized individuals. This so-called herd immunity may be more theoretical than practical because unimmunized individuals remain susceptible and wild poliovirus may not be totally eliminated.

The relative safety and efficacy of the inactivated versus the live, attenuated poliovirus vaccine is a topic of controversy among scientists, laypeople, and politicians (Nightingale, 1977). Proponents of using inactivated polio vaccine (IPV) have suggested that IPV, which does not cause vaccine-associated disease, should replace OPV as the vaccine of choice in the United States (Salk, 1980b). Before the introduction of OPV from 1961 to 1963, IPV, which had been available since 1955, had reduced the incidence of paralytic polio by more than 90% (Salk, 1980a). Furthermore, other countries, such as Sweden (Bottiger, 1984), Finland (Lapinieimu, 1984), and the Netherlands (Bijkerk, 1984), achieved eradication of indigenous polio with the use of IPV exclusively.

The American Academy of Pediatrics (2000) now recommends an all IPV vaccine schedule for routine immunization of infants and children in the United States.

OPV should be used only in the following circumstances in the United States unless otherwise contraindicated:

· Mass vaccination campaigns to control outbreaks of paralytic poliomyelitis
· Unimmunized children who will be traveling to areas where poliomyelitis is endemic and who do not have enough time to receive at least two IPV vaccines (i.e., 4 weeks before travel)
· Children whose parents do not accept the current vaccine schedule, but OPV is only recommended for the third or fourth dose or both

OPV remains the vaccine of choice for global eradication, in part because its ability to induce local (mucosal) immunity and its ability to contribute to herd immunity by secondarily immunizing some contacts.

Immunizing Antigens

INACTIVATED POLIOVIRUS VACCINES

A polyvalent vaccine containing formalin-inactivated poliovirus types 1, 2, and 3 grown in monkey kidney tissue culture was introduced into the United States in 1955 (Salk and Salk, 1977). This conventional IPV was widely used until the OPV became available during the period from 1961 to 1964. A method of producing a more potent IPV with greater antigenic content was developed in 1978 and led to the newly licensed IPV, which is produced in human diploid cells (Bernier, 1986; Von Seefried et al., 1984). This enhanced-potency IPV, which is manufactured and distributed by Connaught Laboratories Ltd., is currently recommended when IPV immunization is indicated (CDC, 1987). Stringent manufacturing and testing precautions have made it highly unlikely that the infamous "Cutter incident," in which recipients developed poliomyelitis because of a failure to inactivate live poliovirus in certain batches, can recur.

ATTENUATED ORAL POLIOVIRUS VACCINE

Trivalent OPV (TOPV) is a mixture of polioviruses types 1, 2, and 3, grown either in monkey kidney tissue culture or human-fetal-diploid tissue culture (CDC, 1982g; Sabin, 1984). Usually, the dose of type 2 poliovirus is reduced to equalize the antigenicity with types 1 and 3. Monovalent OPV containing a single poliovirus type is usually reserved for epidemics and is stockpiled for this purpose.

Immunity

There are two phases of poliovirus immunity: a mucosal phase and a systemic phase (Nathanson and Bodian, 1962; Ogra et al., 1968). Secretory immunoglobulin A (SIgA) poliovirus antibody, the chief component of topical mucosal immunity in the pharynx and possibly in the intestinal mucosa, neutralizes poliovirus and either prevents or limits infection. Serum antibody also provides protection, and titers are correlated with immunity to systemic disease.

Systemic immunity follows both IPV and OPV immunization and natural disease, and local immunity occurs after OPV immunization. Thus wild poliovirus may replicate asymptomatically in the gastrointestinal tract of IPV recipients despite the presence of serum antibody.

Poliovirus immunity is type specific and, following natural disease, is lifelong. OPV is also associated with prolonged immunity and perhaps is lifelong. IPV results in seroconversion in 99% to 100% of recipients after three doses. Like OPV, immunity is prolonged and perhaps lifelong (American Academy of Pediatrics, 2000).

Vaccine Use

For primary immunization of infants with IPV, doses of vaccine are recommended at 2 and 4 months of age, with a third dose at 6 to 18 months of age (American Academy of Pediatrics, 2003; CDC, 1999a). An additional dose is recommended before the child enters school (i.e., at 4 to 6 years of age). If the third dose is given after the child is 4 years old, a fourth dose is not necessary (see Table 42-2).

In cases in which the time interval between the doses of the primary series has been longer than recommended, no additional doses are required and primary immunization may be resumed after any time lapse. Children and adolescents who were not immunized in infancy should receive an initial dose of IPV, followed by another dose 1 month later and a third dose before entering school.

In the United States, routine immunization of adults 18 years of age or older is not necessary because most adults are immune and little or no transmission of wild poliovirus occurs. Persons traveling to countries where poliomyelitis may be epidemic or endemic and health care workers in close contact with patients who may excrete poliovirus should be vaccinated. In these instances, a single booster dose of IPV may be given to those who previously have completed a primary series. Incompletely immunized adults should complete the primary series IPV. Three 0.5-ml subcutaneous doses of enhanced-potency IPV are recommended. The first two doses are given at intervals of 1 to 2 months, followed by a third dose 6 to 12 months after the second dose.

Precautions and Contraindications

TOPV use is contraindicated in individuals with altered immune states, including those with suspected or proven primary immunodeficiency (both humoral and cellular immunodeficiency disease), human immunodeficiency virus (HIV) infection, or malignancy or those receiving immunosuppressive therapy (corticosteroids, cytotoxic agents, or radiation therapy). Enhanced-potency IPV should be given if immunization is necessary. TOPV should not be given to household contacts of immunodeficient patients. Administration of TOPV to even healthy hospitalized children is not advisable because of the inherent risks to immunocompromised patients in that setting. TOPV and IPV administration during pregnancy should be avoided. If immediate protection against poliomyelitis is needed, IPV is recommended. Because conventional and enhanced-potency IPV contains streptomycin and neomycin, neither preparation should be administered to individuals demonstrating anaphylactic hypersensitivity to these antibiotics (American Academy of Pediatrics, 2000).

Measles (Rubeola) Immunization

Rationale for Active Immunization

Measles virus produces a severe systemic infection involving multiple organs that lasts for 7 days or more. Complications are common; 5% to 15% develop bacterial infections and 1 in 1000 patients develops encephalitis (Kempe and Fulginiti, 1964). In developing countries, morbidity and mortality from measles remain high. Worldwide, approximately 1 million children die each year as a result of measles. The highest occurrence and death rates affect children younger than 1 year.

The licensure and distribution of killed (1963), live (Edmonston B) (1963), and further attenuated measles vaccines (1965) has had a staggering impact on the prevalence of measles and its associated morbidity and mortality in the United States. The U.S. Department of Health, Education and Welfare (now Health and Human Services; HHS) predicted the elimination of indigenous measles in the United States by October 1, 1982 (CDC, 1978b). Although this goal was not realized, the incidence of measles in the United States was reduced by 99.7% from the prevaccine era in which some 500,000 cases were reported each year (CDC, 1984d; Hinman et al., 1983).

A major factor for the successful measles immunization effort in the United States was new state legislation to enforce immunization requirements for school entrance. By the 1982–1983 school year, 97% of children entering school had documented measles immunity. Most of the 1163 measles cases recognized in 1983 occurred in a limited number of outbreaks, largely among susceptible preschool or college-aged individuals who were not affected directly by existing state laws (CDC, 1984d). From 1983 to 1991, a steady increase in the incidence of measles in the United States was observed, primarily due to low vaccination rates among preschool children in urban areas (American Academy of Pediatrics, 2003). Since 1992, the incidence of measles has decreased secondary to increased efforts to vaccinate preschoolers.

Immunizing Antigens

KILLED MEASLES VIRUS VACCINE

Although no longer available in the United States, killed measles virus (KMV) vaccine has been administered to more than 600,000 children, and its adverse effects are still being observed. KMV vaccine was prepared by inactivating live virus grown in tissue culture and adding adjuvant (Fulginiti et al., 1963). The usual series consisted of two or three doses of KMV vaccine followed by boosters of KMV or a dose of LMV vaccine.

KMV vaccine produced only short-lived antibody production (Fulginiti et al., 1963). After 6 months, KMV recipients exposed to attenuated measles vaccine developed local reactions (heat, induration, pain, and rash at the inoculation site) or systemic reactions (fever, regional adenopathy, headache, and malaise) (Fulginiti et al., 1968). Exposure to wild virus resulted in bizarre atypical eruptions (peripheral accentuation and onset of the rash, vesicles, petechiae, and purpura), severe systemic manifestations (fever, headache, and lethargy), and organ involvement (pneumonia, serositis, pleuritis, peritonitis, and central nervous system symptoms) (Fulginiti et al., 1967; Rauh and Schmidt, 1965). Extremely high antibody titers were also noted. This *atypical measles syndrome* can occur up to 17 years or more after administration of KMV vaccine.

LIVE MEASLES VIRUS VACCINE

Two types of LMV vaccine have been developed. The original LMV vaccine was developed by Enders and colleagues (1960) from the Edmonston strain of measles virus isolated by Enders. An attenuated Edmonston B virus, obtained after many passages in chick embryo tissue culture, produced mild symptoms and reliable immunity. However, the 15% incidence of rash and 80% incidence of fever were judged too severe. Thus injection of human measles immunoglobulin (MIG) at a different site was given to reduce the incidence of rash and fever without significantly reducing immunogenicity.

Schwarz (1964) developed a second attenuated virus through further passages in chick embryo tissue culture. This *further attenuated measles virus* (FAMV) produces fewer febrile and exanthematous reactions, but antibody levels are lower and decrease more rapidly than with the Edmonston B vaccine. Despite these lower antibody responses, the vaccine appears to be equally protective against measles. FAMV vaccine does not require the simultaneous administration of MIG.

Although millions of children received these vaccines, the vaccine available today in the United States is the Moraten strain developed by Merck, Sharp and Dohme (Hilleman et al., 1968a). It resembles the Schwarz strain and is considered an FAMV.

LMV vaccine is supplied in lyophilized form for reconstitution just before immunization. The manufacturer's directions should be followed explicitly in its storage, reconstitution, and administration. The virus is fragile and can be inactivated if any of these steps are omitted or changed. Heating the vaccine, adding improper diluent, using glass syringes, and mixing with immunoglobulin all may inactivate the virus and result in vaccine failure. Before reconstitution, LMV vaccine must be stored between 2°C and 8°C or colder and protected from light, which inactivates the virus. LMV vaccine is most often used in combination with mumps and rubella vaccines.

Immunity

Recovery from measles is independent of antibody formation, inasmuch as agammaglobulinemic patients with intact cell-mediated immunity usually have a normal course of measles (Good et al., 1962). However, immunity to measles on subsequent exposure is well correlated with the presence of antibody. Other factors, notably cell-mediated immunity, may be important, but antibody alone seems sufficient because passive administration of antibody can prevent measles in a susceptible patient. Thus antibody acts to prevent infection while cell-mediated immunity acts to resolve the infection.

Immunity following natural measles is lifelong, as evidenced by measles in isolated communities in which individuals have been exposed at intervals as long as 65 years apart (Christensen et al., 1953). Immunity after LMV immunization is probably equivalent to that resulting from natural disease. Although vaccine-induced antibody titers are lower than those following natural disease, persistence of protective titers at least 16 years after vaccine administration has been demonstrated (Krugman, 1983). Furthermore, more than 20 years have elapsed since FAMV has been in use, and immunity and protection have been sustained during this period.

When measles occurs in vaccine recipients, one of the following factors is usually the cause:

· *Administration of LMV vaccine before 15 months of age:* LMV vaccine was originally recommended for infants 12 months of age and younger; it is now known that LMV vaccine may be ineffective because of persistent maternal antibody, even though it is undetected in the infant's serum. If LMV is given with immunoglobulin or before 1 year of age, the likelihood of vaccine failure is increased. As many as 35% of infants given LMV vaccine at 9 months of age may not be immunized. The data are conflicting regarding the efficacy of immunization at 12 months of age. Some studies show failure rates of 15% to 22% at 12 months of age, and others show a failure rate as low as 3% to 5% (Krugman, 1977; Wilkins and Wehrle, 1978; Yeager et al., 1977).

· *Use of impotent vaccine:* Several factors, as previously mentioned, may result in LMV vaccine inactivation before administration.
· *The natural failure rate:* LMV vaccine does not immunize all recipients; 3% to 5% may not develop antibody despite potent vaccine and optimal technique.
· *True vaccine failure:* Studies by Cherry and colleagues (1972, 1973) suggest that true vaccine failures occur; that is, vaccine-induced immunity wanes with time. This seems to be rare and accounts for only occasional failure.

Vaccine Use

For primary immunization, a single dose of FAMV (Moraten or Attenuvax) is given subcutaneously at 12 to 15 months of age or older (see Table 42-2). A second vaccine dose is recommended either at the time of school entry or at entry to junior high school or middle school (i.e., at 11 or 12 years of age) (American Academy of Pediatrics, 2003; CDC, 1989). FAMV vaccine can be given most conveniently by a measles, mumps, and rubella (MMR) combination vaccine, although monovalent and measles and rubella (MR) preparations are also available. The antibody responses to MMR vaccine may be inhibited for up to several months after administration of immunoglobulin (Siber et al., 1993).

Adults born before 1957 can be considered immune. Those who have not had clinical measles documented by a physician or who have not had IMV should receive a single dose of FAMV vaccine. Any child immunized before 12 months of age, at a time when persistence of maternal antibody may have interfered with successful immunization, should be reimmunized with FAMV vaccine. During outbreaks, when the likelihood of exposure is high, infants as young as 6 months of age should be immunized. These children then should be revaccinated at 15 months and 11 or 12 years of age. Wilkins and Wehrle (1978) noted, however, that patients initially vaccinated before 1 year of age may respond poorly to subsequent revaccination.

Individuals previously immunized with KMV vaccine or those who received a vaccine of unknown type before 1968 should be reimmunized with FAMV vaccine, even if a dose of LMV was given within 3 months after a killed or unknown vaccine type. These children may experience untoward reactions to LMV vaccine and are susceptible to atypical measles on exposure to wild virus. Thus discussion with parents and consent for further measles vaccination should be obtained. These chil-

dren should then be given a single cutaneous dose of FAMV. In 10% to 50% of children, local heat, induration, and tenderness occur. In 3% to 10% of children, systemic symptoms of fever, malaise, and regional adenopathy occur (Fulginiti et al., 1969). No evidence of an enhanced risk of vaccine-associated reactions exists for those receiving LMV vaccine after previous LMV immunization or natural measles infection (CDC, 1982c).

If an unimmunized child is exposed to measles, prompt LMV administration may prevent measles. This protection occurs because LMV has a shorter incubation period than natural measles (7 as opposed to 11 days). LMV given within 72 hours of exposure can provide protection. If exposure does not result in infection, immunization protects against future infection.

Human immune serum globulin (ISG), which can prevent or modify disease if given within 6 days of exposure, is indicated for susceptible household contacts younger than 1 year of age who are at highest risk for complications. Then, FAMV vaccine should be given at least 3 months later, when passive measles antibody titers have waned and the child is at least 15 months old. HISG can be given to exposed immunocompromised hosts (CDC, 1982c).

Children who received their original LMV vaccination before 12 months of age should be given a second dose of LMV after 15 months of age because protection from the first dose is uncertain. Considerable confusion exists about the necessity for reimmunizing children who previously received their LMV vaccine at 12 months of age. Because the data are conflicting and the risk appears small, routine reimmunization is not recommended. If risk for natural disease is high, reimmunization may be warranted.

In measles epidemics or endemic areas of the world, newborn infants are at high risk. Under these circumstances, infants should be given LMV vaccine as early as 6 months of age. Some of these infants are not successfully immunized because of the immunosuppressive effect of transplacental antibody, so they should be reimmunized at or after 15 months of age. For individuals who cannot be given LMV vaccine because of an underlying disease, a preventive dose of HISG can be given when necessary.

Precautions and Contraindications

Certain precautions must be observed with LMV vaccine. Because disseminated disease and death can result from LMV given to patients with depressed cellular immunity, live, attenuated measles vaccine should not be administered to individuals with suspected or proven primary immunodeficiency disease or to those who have disorders or who are taking therapeutic regimens associated with secondary immunodeficiency states, with the exception of HIV infection (or AIDS). Severe and even fatal measles has occurred among HIV-infected children.

Therefore measles immunization is recommended at the usual ages for individuals with asymptomatic HIV infection and for those with symptomatic infection who are not severely immunocompromised (American Academy of Pediatrics, 1999). Severely immunocompromised HIV-infected infants, children, and adults should not receive measles-containing vaccine because vaccine-related pneumonitis has been reported under these circumstances.

The LMV used for immunization is not communicable. Therefore contacts of immunocompromised patients should be vaccinated to prevent the spread of natural measles to such patients. Although no direct evidence demonstrates that LMV vaccine is harmful to the pregnant female or her fetus, it should not be administered to pregnant women because of the theoretical risk of fetal infection associated with a live virus vaccine.

Because measles vaccination may diminish cutaneous manifestations of cell-mediated immunity temporarily, a tuberculin test performed several days to 6 weeks after immunization may yield a false-negative result. Although natural measles infection may exacerbate tuberculosis, no evidence exists that measles vaccination is associated with such an effect. Thus tuberculin skin testing is not a prerequisite for LMV immunization because the risk of natural measles far outweighs the theoretical hazard of exacerbating undiagnosed tuberculosis (CDC, 1982c).

Acute illness with high-grade fever justifies postponement of LMV administration, but commonly observed minor respiratory illness associated with low-grade fever does not preclude immunization. LMV immunization also should be postponed for 3 months in persons who have received whole blood, plasma, or ISG, because these products may contain sufficient measles antibody to neutralize the vaccine virus.

Measles vaccine contains chick embryo tissue culture protein. Children with egg allergies are at low risk for anaphylactic reaction to measles-containing vaccines. However, in a study of 54 egg-allergic patients, none had an immediate or delayed adverse reaction to MMR (James et al., 1995). Because measles vaccine preparations contain neomycin, patients with a history of anaphylactic reaction to neomycin should not receive measles vaccine.

Passive Immunization

Human immune serum globulin (ISG) contains a variable amount of measles antibody. MIG contained 4000 measles virus–neutralizing units per milliliter, but it is no longer available.

ISG can be used to prevent or modify measles in exposed, susceptible individuals. Regardless of vaccination status, symptomatic HIV-infected persons who are exposed to measles also should receive ISG prophylaxis. Prevention with a dose of 0.25 ml/kg or 0.5 ml/kg (immunocompromised hosts; maximum dose of 15 ml) is recommended, followed by LMV immunization (if not already done) in 5 or 6 months.

ISG is given intramuscularly deep in a large muscle mass; no more than 5 ml is given at one site (American Academy of Pediatrics, 2000).

Rubella (German Measles) Immunization

Rationale for Active Immunization

Largely as a consequence of a major epidemic in the United States in 1964 (>20,000 cases of congenital rubella), active immunization programs with attenuated rubella vaccines were initiated in 1969 in hopes of preventing an epidemic expected in the early 1970s. A decision at the time to immunize all children 1 to 12 years old represented an attempt to reduce the reservoir and transmission of wild rubella virus and, secondarily, to diminish the risk of rubella in susceptible pregnant women. Subsequently, high rates of infantile immunization with rubella vaccine (as a component of MMR) have resulted in a marked decrease in the incidence of rubella and congenital rubella in the United States (American Academy of Pediatrics, 2003). Nevertheless, outbreaks of rubella still occur occasionally, predominately among unimmunized young adults (Danovaro-Holliday et al., 2000).

Immunizing Antigens

Live, attenuated rubella vaccines licensed for use in the United States in 1969 included HPV-77:DE-5, grown in duck embryo tissue culture; HPV-77:DK-12, grown in dog kidney tissue culture (neither was available after 1979); and Cendehill, grown primarily in rabbit kidney cells and not available after 1976. RA 27/3 (rubella abortus, 27th specimen, third extract) prepared in human diploid tissue culture is the only vaccine now available in the United States. This live, attenuated vaccine induces higher antibody titers that more closely parallel the immune response following natural infection than previous vaccines (Lerman et al., 1981; Orenstein et al., 1984). Monovalent and combination preparations—including MR, rubella and mumps, and MMR vaccines—are available. The MMR combination vaccine is used for routine infant immunization programs. Rubella vaccine must be kept at 2°C to 8°C or colder during storage and should be protected from light to avoid virus inactivation. Once reconstituted, it should be used within 8 hours.

Immunity

At least 95% of susceptible vaccinees 12 months of age or older develop antibody titers that are protective, although not as high as those resulting from natural infection. The exact duration of protection is uncertain, but antibody levels have waned only slightly after 10 years in the initial group of children receiving the RA 27/3 vaccine (Herrman et al., 1982). Lifelong protection against clinical reinfection, subclinical viremia, or both probably results from a single dose of vaccine early in childhood. Therefore routine rubella reimmunization is not recommended.

In some cases, vaccinees exposed to natural rubella develop a rise of antibody titer unassociated with clinical symptoms. This reinfection (with a fourfold or greater rise of rubella hemagglutination-inhibition [HAI] antibody titer) is associated only rarely with viremia. Significant pharyngeal shedding also is observed infrequently. Similarly, reinfection can be observed in individuals with previous natural rubella. Cell-mediated immunity is probably responsible for recovery from and immunity to rubella; this is emphasized by the fact that infection has occurred in individuals with circulating antibody.

Infants with congenital rubella may have persistent viremia despite high levels of transplacentally acquired serum antibodies. Persistent rubella infection may result from direct viral infection of lymphocytes, rendering them unresponsive to rubella antibody. When lymphocyte infection ends, cell-mediated immunity is restored and the virus is eradicated.

The fetus initially offers no defense to the virus, but with persistence of the virus, specific IgM antibody develops. Thus the neonate with congenital rubella has both virus and antibody present. A syndrome analogous to subacute sclerosing panencephalitis has been observed following congenital rubella (Townsend et al., 1975). This suggests that rubella virus becomes latent in brain cells, despite a persistent and brisk antibody response.

Vaccine Use

For primary immunization, any child from 12 months old to prepuberty is a candidate for rubella immunization. The American Academy of Pediatrics (2000) recommends immunization at 12 to 15 months of age along with measles vaccination (see Table 42-2). In conjunction with the recently recommended two-dose measles immunization schedule, two doses of rubella vaccine are now recommended (American Academy of Pediatrics, 2003). There is a need to identify unimmunized children on entry into school and at intervals thereafter. All states have adopted mandatory rubella immunization as part of their health code.

Concerns about potential transmission of disease from immunized children to susceptible contacts (including pregnant women) have not been supported by studies of susceptible household contacts. Therefore susceptible children whose household contacts are pregnant can be vaccinated (CDC, 1984i).

Rubella vaccine is given as a single subcutaneous injection of the antigen (0.5-ml dose given subcutaneously) or as part of a combined vaccine (such as MMR).

Rubella vaccine also should be administered to adolescent and adult women of childbearing age who have not been previously immunized. Premarital screening, routine gynecologic examinations, and the immediate postpartum period are excellent settings for immunization. Rubella vaccine should not be given 2 weeks before to 3 months after administration of HISG. If it is given after the administration of anti-Rho (D) immunoglobulin or blood products, seroconversion should be documented 6 to 8 weeks after vaccination. When practical, potential vaccinees can be screened for susceptibility. However, vaccination of women of childbearing age is justifiable and may be preferable without prior serologic testing in women not known to be pregnant. There is no increased risk of complications in individuals who are vaccinated but already immune.

Women of childbearing age should be vaccinated only when they deny being pregnant and after they are counseled not to become pregnant for 3 months after vaccination. The theoretical risks to the fetus should be explained to them (discussed later).

Students or employees of childbearing age in educational or training institutions, such as colleges and military installations, should be considered for immunization on the basis of prior documented vaccination or serologic testing. Individuals working in hospitals or other health care facilities or in any setting where women of childbearing age congregate should be immunized to avoid transmission to susceptible women. Men need not receive routine serologic screening before immunization.

During rubella outbreaks, all susceptible individuals should be vaccinated promptly, except those for whom live viral vaccine is contraindicated. Although immunization after exposure probably does not prevent illness, it is not harmful and, if natural infection does not occur, vaccination ensures future immunity. International travelers should have documented rubella immunity.

Adverse Effects of Vaccine

Rubella vaccines generally are well tolerated. Rash, fever, or lymphadenopathy may occur in susceptible children. Arthralgia and arthritis occur in 0.5% of all children immunized (American Academy of Pediatrics, 2003). The arthritis can occur several weeks after immunization, so its association with the vaccine is often overlooked. Because symptoms resemble rheumatoid arthritis or other related disorders, costly diagnostic evaluations often are undertaken. Arthralgia and arthritis are more common in older girls and women; 10% to 30% of these recipients experience these complications.

Unusual pain syndromes rarely occur in recipients of rubella vaccine. Nonlocalized pain about the joints of the upper and lower extremities is believed to be caused by neuropathy induced by the vaccine. Two forms have been described: one involves the arms, with severe recurrent pain, usually at night, and the other involves the legs, with pain relieved by crouching (catcher's crouch syndrome). The time of onset is variable but can be as late as 70 days after vaccination. Episodes recur at varying intervals; one patient in Arizona had recurrent symptoms in the lower extremities for almost 2 years.

In a report of 214 susceptible women who inadvertently received a live, attenuated rubella vaccine within 3 months before or after conception and carried their pregnancy to term, none of their infants had defects compatible with congenital rubella syndrome, although a small number showed serologic evidence of intrauterine infection (CDC, 1984j). Because rubella virus has been isolated from the products of conception of women vaccinated during pregnancy, continued caution with respect to vaccination during pregnancy is advised.

However, based on the available evidence, the CDC (1984i) suggests that inadvertent rubella vaccination during pregnancy does not ordinarily represent a reason to consider interruption of pregnancy.

Precautions and Contraindications

Specific contraindications of live rubella vaccine administration include the following:

· Pregnancy
· Immunodeficiency states (malignancy, primary immunodeficiency disease, immunosuppressive or corticosteroid therapy, and radiation therapy)
· Severe febrile illness
· Known history of anaphylactic reaction to neomycin, a component of the vaccine

Mumps Immunization

Rationale for Active Immunization

Mumps is a viral disease of glandular tissue mostly affecting preteenagers. It usually is mild but can be severe, and complications occur often enough to warrant immunization. Mumps is a risk for postpubertal boys, because 20% develop orchitis, a painful, incapacitating disease, although sterility is extremely rare (Candel, 1951).

Mumps is a leading cause of clinical meningoencephalitis and, in even greater numbers, a cause of subclinical meningoencephalitis (Wilfert, 1969). Mumps has also been suspected as a cause of juvenile diabetes mellitus based on its predilection for infecting the pancreas and the concordance between waves of mumps infection followed by juvenile diabetes mellitus 2 to 4 years later (Sultz et al., 1975).

Originally, there was some reluctance to recommend routine mumps vaccination for all infants; authorities preferred instead to restrict its use to prepubertal boys and susceptible men. Since 1967, these restraints have been modified, accounting for a marked reduction in epidemic parotitis. In most states, immunity to mumps is required for school entry; states without this requirement have a twofold higher incidence of reported mumps than those that have this legislation.

Immunizing Antigen

A mumps virus isolated from Dr. Maurice Hilleman's daughter, Jeryl Lynn (hence the term *Jeryl Lynn strain*), was attenuated by passage in chick embryo tissue culture (Hilleman et al., 1968b) and used for the vaccine. After testing in 6000 children, it was licensed in 1967.

It produces no significant symptoms, and more than 96% of recipients develop antibody titers (lower than that following natural infection), which persist for more than 15 years (CDC, 1982d, 1983a, 1984e). Reported clinical vaccine efficacies have ranged from 75% to 90% (CDC, 1982d, 1983a, 1984e). A lack of immunity after mumps immunization can be caused by improp-

erly stored vaccine. Before reconstitution, mumps vaccine must be stored at 2°C to 8°C or colder and protected from light. After reconstitution, the vaccine should be used within 8 hours or discarded.

Immunity

Mumps is one of the few viruses for which cell-mediated immunity can be evaluated, because mumps virus antigen injected intradermally provokes a delayed hypersensitivity response. Although the exact role of cell-mediated immunity is unknown, there is evidence that it plays a role in the disease as well as in recovery. Immunity is associated with the presence of serum antibody that occurs following natural disease or vaccination. Two or more episodes of mumps are best explained by other viral agents that produce parotitis.

Vaccine Use

For primary immunization in infants, mumps virus vaccine is routinely included in pediatric immunization schedules (American Academy of Pediatrics, 2003; CDC, 2000a). A single dose of mumps vaccine, either alone or as MMR, is injected subcutaneously at 12 to 15 months of age. A second dose of MMR is now recommended at 4 or 5 years of age (American Academy of Pediatrics, 2000).

Mumps virus vaccine can be administered to boys and men. A history of mumps can be misleading, because other viruses can produce parotitis. Furthermore, failure to recall mumps is no guarantee that one has not been infected; in fact, 30% of childhood mumps cases are asymptomatic.

Susceptible individuals exposed to mumps, particularly adolescent boys or men, can be immunized with mumps vaccine, but there is no guarantee that mumps will be averted. However, if mumps does not occur, the individual is protected against subsequent exposures.

Precautions and Contraindications

The use of mumps vaccine is associated with few side effects. The frequency of reported central nervous system dysfunction after vaccination may be even lower than the observed background rate in the unimmunized. Anyone with a history of anaphylactic reaction to egg ingestion should be vaccinated only with extreme caution. Individuals with histories of nonanaphylactic reactions to egg ingestion or allergies to chicken or feathers are not at increased risk of vaccine-associated reactions. A person with a history of anaphylactic reaction to neomycin, which is present in the vaccine, should not be vaccinated. However, those with cutaneous hypersensitivity (contact dermatitis) to neomycin may be vaccinated.

Because of the theoretical risk of fetal damage, mumps vaccine should not be administered to pregnant women. Lymphoreticular or other generalized malignancy and primary or secondary immunodeficiency states represent other specific contraindications for this live viral vaccine. Because infection after vaccination is noncommunicable, mumps vaccine may be given to susceptible close contacts of immunosuppressed patients to help reduce the likelihood of exposure to natural measles. Mumps vaccination generally should be avoided in patients with acute illness and high-grade fever. In addition, it should not be given until 3 months after the administration of ISG because passively acquired antibody may interfere with the active immune response.

Haemophilus influenzae Type B Immunization

Rationale for Active Immunization

In the pre-vaccine era, Hib was the leading cause of bacterial meningitis in the United States, accounting for half of all cases. More than 90% of meningitis cases from Hib occurred in children younger than 5 years (11,000 cases annually). Among these cases, 80% occurred in children younger than 2 years, and most of these were in children younger than 18 months old. The peak attack rate occurs in children 6 to 8 months old. Hib meningitis is fatal in 3% to 10% of cases, and neurologic sequelae occur in 20% to 35% of survivors. Hib also was the primary cause of epiglottitis and a common cause of sepsis, pneumonia, septic arthritis, and cellulitis in children, accounting for about 7300 cases of nonmeningeal invasive disease annually (Cochi et al., 1985).

The advent of immunization against Hib, first with the purified capsular polysaccharide vaccine and subsequently with various conjugate vaccines, has markedly changed the epidemiology of invasive Hib disease over the past 15 years.

Immunizing Antigens

HAEMOPHILUS TYPE B POLYSACCHARIDE VACCINE

The first Hib vaccine, licensed for use in the United States in April 1985, contained the purified Hib capsular polysaccharide polyribosyl-ribitol phosphate (PRP) (b-CAPSE I vaccine, Praxis Biologics). Development of this vaccine was based on observations that serum antibodies directed against PRP provide protection against Hib disease. Whereas the protective level of Hib capsular antibody in the unimmunized may be greater than 0.15 µg/ml, data suggest that a serum level of at least 1.0 µg/ml 3 weeks after immunization correlates with subsequent protection (Kaythy et al., 1983).

As with other polysaccharide vaccines, immunogenicity of the Hib vaccine in children is age dependent. Vaccine responsiveness increases markedly at about 16 to 20 months of age. Protective antibody levels are observed after vaccination in 45% of children 12 to 17 months old, 75% of vaccinees 18 to 23 months old, and 90% of those 24 to 35 months old. Furthermore, the duration of protective antibody levels is related to the age of vaccinees. In persons vaccinated before 18 months of age, serum antibody levels are less than protective within 6 months. Protective antibody levels remain for at least 1½ but not 3½ years after immunization in those 18 to 35 months of age, whereas protective levels remain at least 3½ years in those vaccinated at 3 to 5 years of age (Kaythy et al., 1984).

The clinical efficacy of the first-generation Hib PRP vaccine was prospectively evaluated in Finland in a double-blind study (Peltola et al., 1977a) on children 3 to 71 months of age. In this study, approximately 50,000 children received an Hib vaccine similar to that later licensed in the United States and 50,000 received group A meningococcal vaccine. Protection was correlated with the production of an anticapsular antibody concentration that exceeded 1.0 µg/ml in serum obtained 3 weeks after immunization.

In children immunized at 18 to 71 months of age, the protective efficacy was 90%; among those immunized at 18 to 23 months of age, the small number of cases in the vaccine and the control group precluded a definitive conclusion. In 8453 children immunized at 2 years of age (24 to 35 months), the efficacy was 80% (Daum and Granoff, 1985). No efficacy was observed in children 3 to 17 months.

These data led the Committee on Infectious Diseases to recommend immunization with PRP for all children at 24 months of age. The results of postmarketing case-control studies after licensure in 1985 indicated that PRP is effective, although its efficacy in 2-year-old American children may be lower than that found in Finland. Lack of efficacy was reported in Minnesota (Osterholm et al., 1987), and several investigators have suggested that an excess of infections occurred during the week after immunization with PRP (Black et al., 1987; CDC, 1988).

HAEMOPHILUS TYPE B CONJUGATE VACCINE (DIPHTHERIA TOXOID CONJUGATE)

With the ultimate goal of providing an effective vaccine for infants and younger children, Schneerson and co-workers (1980) covalently linked the capsular polysaccharide of H. influenzae to a protein carrier. Several manufacturers have prepared conjugate vaccines suitable for use in children. The first of these, the diphtheria toxoid conjugate vaccine (PRP-D), is approved for use in children 12 months of age or older. The immunogenicity of PRP-D is significantly greater than that observed with PRP in children 18 months of age or older (Berkowitz et al., 1987; CDC, 1982e, 1988; Pincus et al., 1982).

During 1990, the U.S. Food and Drug Administration (FDA) approved two Hib conjugate vaccines for use in infants 2 months of age and older. The carrier protein for one (HbOC) is a nontoxic mutant diphtheria toxin, whereas the carrier for the other vaccine (PRP-OMP) consists of an outer membrane protein complex of Neisseria meningitidis. Approval was based in part on a review of two large studies in the United States that demonstrated the protective efficacy of these vaccines (Black et al., 1991; Santosham et al., 1991). In one of these studies, more than 20,000 infants were given

HbOC vaccine at 2, 4, and 6 months of age. Three cases of invasive Hib disease occurred among infants who had received only one dose of vaccine; invasive disease was not reported in any infant who had received at least two doses.

Another Hib conjugate vaccine, which uses tetanus toxoid as the carrier protein (PRP-T), has been approved for use in infants as young as 2 months of age. In addition, the oligosaccharide conjugate vaccine (HbOC) has been combined with DTaP for ease of administration to young infants.

Vaccine Use

The routine schedule for Hib immunization during infancy is shown in Table 42-2. The same conjugate vaccine should be used for all doses administered to infants younger than 12 months of age. Only HbOC, PRP-OMP, or PRP-T should be given to children younger than age 12 months. The first two vaccine doses are given at 2 and 4 months of age. If either HbOC or PRP-T is used, a third dose is given at age 6 months. A booster vaccination is given at 12 to 15 months of age.

Unimmunized children between the ages of 15 and 60 months should receive one dose of any licensed conjugate vaccine. Immunization against Hib generally is not indicated in children older than age 5; however, a single dose of any licensed conjugate vaccine is recommended for children older than age 5 who have chronic illnesses associated with an increased risk of Hib disease. Unimmunized children younger than 24 months of age who experience invasive Hib disease should be immunized beginning 1 to 2 months after recovery from the acute illness. Children who have such disease at 24 months of age or older generally do not require immunization because of natural disease-induced immunity.

All of the conjugate vaccines appear to be safe and well tolerated. No increased incidence of invasive Hib disease in the weeks after immunization has been reported.

Pneumococcal Immunization

Rationale for Active Immunization

Pneumococcal infections are common and account for considerable morbidity in healthy children. Although there are 83 pneumococcal serotypes, only a few account for more than 80% of pneumococcal infections, which include otitis media, pneumonia, bacteremia, and meningitis. The highest rates of invasive pneumococcal disease occur among children younger than 2 years. Furthermore, penicillin resistance, including strains resistant to multiple antibiotics, has been described.

These events give emphasis to an immunologic approach for the control of pneumococcal infections. Some children are particularly susceptible to severe or even fatal pneumococcal infection, including those with functional or anatomic asplenia (e.g., congenital absence, surgical removal, or sickle cell anemia with autosplenectomy), nephrotic syndrome, or congenital or acquired immunodeficiencies (American Academy of Pediatrics, 2000).

Until recently, pneumococcal vaccination was available only as a 23-valent polysaccharide vaccine (PPV23) and was recommended only for high-risk individuals older than age 2 years. In 2000, a seven-valent pneumococcal polysaccharide conjugate vaccine (PCV7) became available, and it is recommended for all infants and children aged 2 to 24 months.

Immunizing Agents

A polyvalent pneumococcal vaccine containing a purified polysaccharide antigen derived from the capsules of 14 of the 83 individual strains of pneumococci was licensed for use in the United States in 1977. In 1983, it was replaced by a 23-valent vaccine, each dose of which contains 25 µg of each polysaccharide antigen (as compared with its predecessor, which contained a 50 µg dose of each antigen). This new vaccine confers protective levels of antibodies to a larger number of serotypes while providing less total polysaccharide and, possibly, fewer irritants and pyrogens (Robbins et al., 1983). The 23 serotypes contained in the vaccine are responsible for more than 88% of cases of pneumococcal bacteremia in the United States.

In February 2000, a seven-valent pneumococcal conjugate vaccine (PCV7) that includes seven purified capsular polysaccharides of *S. pneumoniae,* each coupled with a nontoxic variant of diphtheria toxin, CRM 197, became available. The conjugation of polysaccharides to proteins alters the nature of the immune system's response (i.e., from T-lymphocyte independent to T-lymphocyte dependent). Hence, infants and children younger than 2 years of age exhibit a substantial primary humoral response to PCV7, as opposed to the ineffective response seen in this age group to PPV23. The serotypes contained in the PCV7 are the seven most common serotypes isolated from the blood or cerebrospinal fluid of children younger than 6 years (CDC, 2000b).

Immunity

Polysaccharide-protein conjugate vaccine induces type-specific antibodies that bind to polysaccharide on the surface of bacteria and enhance opsonization and phagocytosis. After three doses of PCV7, 92% to 100% (varied by serotype) of children had 0.15 µg/ml or more of type-specific antibody (CDC, 2000b). Although the level of antibody activity that correlates with protection against pneumococcal disease is unknown, the presence of type-specific antibody to capsular polysaccharide is associated with protection among adults. Whether vaccination confers lifelong immunity remains to be determined.

Clinical trials in healthy adults in South Africa (Austrian et al., 1976; Smit et al., 1977) and in New Guinea (Riley et al., 1977) have demonstrated the

23-valent vaccine's high efficacy (serologic response and prevention of disease secondary to vaccine serotypes). Although the duration of protection afforded by the vaccine is unknown, persistence of antibodies has been demonstrated 5 years after immunization.

Vaccine Use

All children younger than 23 months of age should be vaccinated with PCV7. Newborns should begin the primary vaccine series at age 2 months, with two subsequent doses at 2-month intervals. A fourth dose should be given at 12 to 15 months of age. Infants between the ages of 6 and 12 months who are receiving the primary series of PCV7 require only three doses of the vaccine. Two doses should be administered 2 months apart, followed by a dose at age 12 to 15 months. Children 12 to 24 months of age require two doses two months apart. Children 24 to 59 months with the following conditions should receive PCV7 and PPV23 (although not simultaneously):

· Sickle cell disease or other sickle cell hemoglobinopathies; congenital or acquired asplenia, or splenic dysfunction
· Infection with HIV
· Other immunocompromising conditions (e.g., leukemias, congenital immunodeficiencies, nephrotic syndrome)
· Chronic illness (e.g., cyanotic congenital heart disease, chronic pulmonary disease, diabetes mellitus)

In addition, PPV23 should be given to children with cerebrospinal fluid leaks. PCV7 should also be considered for children aged 24 to 59 months of Alaskan Native, American Indian, or African-American descents, as well as those who attend group day-care centers. For healthy children aged 24 to 59 months, one dose of PCV7 is adequate. For those with "high-risk" conditions (just listed), two doses 2 months apart are recommended.

Previous vaccination with PCV7 is not a contraindication to vaccination with PPV23. However, PCV7 and PPV23 should not be administered at the same time. Immunization should be separated by 2 months. A single 0.5-ml dose given subcutaneously or intramuscularly of PPV23 is recommended for high-risk patients older than 24 months of age. Vaccine should be administered at least 2 weeks before elective splenectomy and as long as possible before planned immunosuppressive therapy. Vaccine is also recommended for adults who are at increased risk of pneumococcal disease and its complications, including those with chronic cardiopulmonary, hepatic, or renal disease, as well as healthy individuals 65 years and older.

Revaccination with PPV23 should be considered after 3 to 5 years for children younger than age 10 years (at revaccination), children at risk for severe pneumococcal infection (e.g., patients with asplenia), and patients who have rapid disappearance of antipneumococcal antibody after vaccination (e.g., patients with sickle cell anemia, nephrotic syndrome, or renal failure, and transplant recipients). Revaccination also should be considered for older children and adults at high risk for pneumococcal infections who were vaccinated previously at age 6 or younger (American Academy of Pediatrics, 2003).

Adverse Effects of Active Immunization

The most common adverse effects associated with PCV7 included erythema at the injection site, mild to moderate fever, fussiness, drowsiness, or decreased appetite. Adverse reactions associated with initial vaccination with PPV23 include the following:

· Erythema and pain at the injection site in half of the recipients
· Fever, myalgia, and severe local reactions in less than 1% of recipients
· Severe systemic reactions in approximately 5 per 1 million doses administered

Hepatitis B Immunization

Rationale for Active Immunization

Hepatitis B is reported in about 16,000 persons annually in the United States (CDC, 1994). About 1% of reported cases are associated with fulminant disease and death. Approximately 1 million people in the United States are chronic carriers of hepatitis B, and many will ultimately develop cirrhosis or hepatic carcinoma.

Children become infected with hepatitis B in a variety of ways. The risk of perinatal hepatitis B infection among infants born to mothers with hepatitis B ranges from 10% to 85%, depending on maternal factors. Infants with perinatal hepatitis B infection have a 90% risk of chronic infection, and up to 25% die of chronic liver disease.

Because selective screening of pregnant women fails to identify a high percentage of those infected with hepatitis B, universal screening of all pregnant women for hepatitis B is recommended (CDC, 1991). The continuing occurrence of hepatitis B infections despite the availability of an effective vaccine since 1982 has led to a recommendation for universal childhood immunization against hepatitis B (American Academy of Pediatrics, 1992; CDC, 1991).

Immunizing Antigen

The first licensed hepatitis B vaccine was a suspension of inactivated and purified plasma–derived hepatitis B surface antigen. It is no longer produced in the United States, and its use is limited to hemodialysis patients, immunocompromised hosts, and persons with known allergy to yeast. The plasma-derived vaccine is immunogenic, effective, and safe.

The available recombinant hepatitis B vaccines are produced using hepatitis B surface antigen synthesized by *Saccharomyces cerevisiae* (baker's yeast), into which a plasmid containing the hepatitis B surface antigen gene has been inserted. The purified product is obtained by lysis of the yeast and chemical and physical separation.

Hepatitis B vaccines contain 10 to 40 μg of hepatitis B surface antigen protein per milliliter after adsorption to aluminum hydroxide (0.5 mg/ml). Because of increasing concern regarding mercury exposure in children, thimerosal (a mercury-based compound) is no longer used in any of the pediatric hepatitis B vaccines licensed in the United States (CDC, 2000c). The yeast protein content is 5% or less of the final product.

A three-dose schedule of recombinant hepatitis B vaccine produces adequate antibody responses in 90% to 95% of healthy recipients. Field trials of the vaccines licensed in the United States have shown 80% to 95% protective efficacy. The most common side effect is soreness at the injection site; hypersensitivity to yeast or thimerosal has been reported.

Vaccine Use

Primary immunization against hepatitis B should be administered using a three-dose schedule beginning in early infancy (American Academy of Pediatrics, 2003; CDC, 2000a). The first vaccine dose can be administered at birth before hospital discharge; subsequent doses are administered at 1 to 2 and 6 to 18 months of age. Alternatively, the three vaccine doses can be administered at 1 to 2, 4, and 6 to 18 months of age. Because hepatitis B vaccine can be administered simultaneously with other vaccines, the latter schedule has the advantage of minimizing the required number of health care visits.

In addition to its routine use during infancy, hepatitis B immunization is recommended for all adolescents who have not been immunized. Hepatitis B vaccine is also indicated in certain other groups at high risk for hepatitis B infection:

1. Adolescents who have multiple sex partners or who are injecting drugs and those who reside in communities where such activity is prevalent
2. Persons with occupational risk for infection (health care or public safety workers)
3. Clients and staff of institutions for the developmentally disabled
4. Hemodialysis patients
5. Recipients of certain blood products (e.g., clotting factor concentrates)
6. Household contacts and sex partners of chronic hepatitis B carriers
7. Adoptees from countries where hepatitis B infection is endemic
8. International travelers
9. Users of injection drugs
10. Sexually active homosexual and bisexual men
11. Sexually active heterosexual men and women
12. Inmates of long-term correctional facilities

A three-dose vaccine schedule similar to that used during infancy is recommended.

The doses of recombinant hepatitis B vaccines used in children and adults vary by patient age and the vaccine preparation used; package inserts should be consulted.

The immunogenicity and efficacy of hepatitis B vaccines in hemodialysis patients are lower than those seen in healthy individuals; thus larger doses of the standard recombinant or plasma-derived vaccines should be used. A more concentrated formulation of recombinant vaccine (Recombivax HB) is also available for use in dialysis patients. Vaccine is administered intramuscularly. In older children and adults, the deltoid area of the upper arm is the recommended site for vaccination because of reduced immunogenicity when vaccine is administered in the buttocks. The anterolateral thigh is preferred for infants.

The schedules outlined previously are appropriate only for hepatitis B pre-exposure prophylaxis. Postexposure prophylaxis entails administration not only of hepatitis B vaccine but also of hepatitis B immunoglobulin (HBIG).

In the case of infants born to mothers with hepatitis B infection, HBIG (0.5 ml intramuscularly) should be administered as soon as possible after birth (preferably within 12 hours). In addition to HBIG, hepatitis B vaccination should be initiated within 7 days (preferably within 12 hours) of birth. The first dose of hepatitis B vaccine can be given simultaneously with HBIG, provided it is given with a separate syringe and at a different body site.

Influenza Immunization

Influenza outbreaks occur each year in the United States, and the potential for epidemic (pandemic) spread of this disease in susceptible human populations is well recognized. Periodic minor antigenic shifts of influenza A or B virus account for most influenzal disease yearly; these outbreaks generally are limited in magnitude, although the extent of morbidity and mortality remains unacceptably high. Major antigenic changes of influenza A virus, as occurred in 1957 and 1958 (Asian strain) and again in 1968 and 1969 (Hong Kong variant), account for pandemic spread of disease associated with greater overall morbidity and mortality in highly susceptible populations.

With respect to most prevailing influenza A and B viruses in civilian populations, primary prevention with available vaccines has been directed only at individuals and patient groups at high risk as a result of underlying systemic disease. Prophylaxis may be achieved in the most cost-effective manner by vaccinating individuals in whom there is a higher than average potential for infection and in whom infection can have severe consequences (CDC, 1993a; Glezen, 1980; Glezen et al., 1983; Paisley et al., 1978). Difficulties in identifying new antigenic variants (multiple minor variants may be prevalent simultaneously) and the subsequent preparation, testing, and provision of new vaccines have precluded routine mass immunization for most influenza strains.

Before 2003, only inactivated vaccines were licensed for prevention of influenza. Since their introduction more than 40 years ago, refinements in their production have largely eliminated the toxic manifestations commonly observed after vaccination in the past. After receiving the vaccine by parenteral administration, nearly all young adults develop hemagglutination-inhibition antibody titers that are likely to be protective. If provided under optimal conditions (i.e., at an appropriate time and against the prevailing influenzal strain), these vaccines can reduce the incidence of disease by 75% to 80% (Glezen, 1980).

Unfortunately, protection afforded by inactivated vaccine is transient; yearly injections are necessary even when no significant antigenic changes of a prevailing influenzal strain have occurred. As a result of rapid and repeated changes in policy, health care personnel should refer to current statements by the CDC published periodically in *Morbidity and Mortality Weekly Report*.

Intranasal vaccination with a live, attenuated, cold-adapted recombinant influenza virus vaccine (FluMist) was licensed in the United States in 2003 for low-risk subjects aged 5 to 50. Its acceptance by the public was disappointing. This vaccine is well tolerated and protects healthy adults and children against influenza.

Recent studies report that a combination of intranasal and intramuscular vaccination may improve immune responses against influenza (Keitel et al., 2001).

Vaccine Use

Available inactivated vaccines include whole, intact virus particles and split-product preparations derived by disrupting whole virus with organic solvents. In newer preparations, immunogenicity and reactogenicity of split and whole virus vaccines have been shown to be similar in adults, but field studies of the efficacy of split-product vaccines in children are lacking. Because protective influenza vaccines must contain strains antigenically similar to those strains expected to be prevalent during a given respiratory season, the formulation of vaccines is changed periodically. Recommended formulations generally include multivalent products containing recent antigenic variants of influenza A and influenza B strains.

Influenza vaccine is recommended for patients 6 months of age or older who are at high risk for disease, for their medical care personnel, and for anyone who wishes to decrease the risk of illness from influenza. Annual vaccination against influenza is recommended for individuals at high risk of lower respiratory tract complications or death following influenza infection.

These high-risk groups have been further classified on the basis of priority into defined target groups for which vaccination is most necessary and include the following:

1. Persons 65 years or older
2. Residents of nursing homes and other long-term care facilities
3. Adults and children with chronic disorders of the pulmonary or cardiovascular systems, including children with asthma
4. Adults and children who have required regular medical follow-up or hospitalization during the preceding year because of chronic metabolic disease, renal dysfunction, hematoglobinopathies, or immunosuppression
5. Children and teenagers who are receiving long-term aspirin therapy and therefore may be at risk for Reye syndrome

Medical personnel can transmit influenza infections to their high-risk patients while they are themselves incubating an infection, undergoing subclinical infection, or working despite the existence of symptoms (Glezen, 1980). The potential for introducing influenza to high-risk groups with compromised cardiopulmonary or immune systems or to infants in neonatal intensive care units should be reduced by vaccination programs targeted at medical personnel. Annual influenza vaccination of physicians, nurses, and other personnel who have extensive contact with high-risk patient groups is recommended.

Persons who provide essential community services (e.g., fire and police department personnel, health care workers), although not at increased risk of serious influenzal disease, may be offered vaccine to minimize disruption of services during outbreaks. Furthermore, any person wishing to reduce the risk of acquiring influenza infections should be vaccinated.

Current influenza vaccines generally are well tolerated; less than one third of vaccines have been reported to develop local redness or induration for 1 to 2 days at the injection site. Systemic reactions, including fever, chills, headache, and malaise, although uncommon, most often affect children who have had no previous exposure to the influenza virus antigens contained in the vaccine.

These reactions, attributable to influenza antigens, generally begin 6 to 12 hours after vaccination and persist for only 1 to 2 days. As a result of its diminished potential for causing febrile reactions, only split (subviron) vaccine is recommended for use in children younger than 13 years.

However, a single dose of split-product vaccine may be significantly less immunogenic than a single dose of whole virus preparation. Therefore the administration of two doses of the available split-product vaccine separated by at least 4 weeks is recommended for children who have not received vaccines previously (American Academy of Pediatrics, 2003). Variable immunogenicity of influenza vaccine has been reported among immunocompromised individuals, including those with malignancy; successful immunologic responses in these populations are most likely to occur when these individuals have been immunized with antigenically similar influenzal strains (Gross et al., 1978; Lange et al., 1979).

The recommended dose of split-product influenza vaccine is 0.25 ml for patients 6 to 35 months of age and 0.5 ml for older patients. Whole virus vaccine preparations should be administered as a 0.5-ml dose. The vaccines should be administered into the deltoid muscle when possible. Infants and young children can be vaccinated in the anterolateral thigh muscle.

Chemoprophylaxis or chemotherapy also should be considered, but it should not replace active immunization against influenza. Both amantadine and rimantadine are approved for prophylaxis of influenza A virus infections in children and adults. Rimantadine is as effective as amantadine and has fewer side effects (e.g., agitation, insomnia, seizures). Neither are effective against influenza B. Two other antivirals, both neuramidase inhibitors, can also be used during the first 2 days of infection. These are zanamivir inhaled powder (approved for children > 6 years) and oral oseltamivir (for children > 1 year).

Antiviral therapy should be considered for use during influenza A outbreaks in the following situations (CDC, 1993a).

- When the vaccine may be relatively ineffective or unavailable
- As an adjunct to late immunization of high-risk individuals until the immune response to the vaccine has developed (a period of 6 weeks for primary immunization of young children [two doses of vaccine, 4 weeks apart] and 2 weeks for booster immunization)
- To supplement protection afforded by vaccination of high-risk patients in whom a poor immunologic response may be expected
- To protect those few high-risk individuals for whom influenza vaccine is contraindicated because of anaphylactic hypersensitivity or a previous severe reaction to influenza vaccine
- To protect high-risk patients in the hospital from developing nosocomial influenza A infection
- As chemoprophylaxis of medical personnel who have extensive contact with high-risk patients but have not been vaccinated

Amantadine or rimantadine also should be considered for therapeutic use in high-risk patients (regardless of vaccine status) who develop an illness compatible with influenza during a period of influenza A activity in the community. In such patients, the drug should be given within 24 to 48 hours after the onset of illness and continued for 48 hours after the resolution of symptoms. Amantadine should be used with caution in patients with impaired renal function or active seizure disorders. Use of amantadine or rimantadine in infants younger than 1 year of age has not been evaluated adequately.

Precautions and Contraindications

Because influenza vaccine is prepared in embryonated chick eggs, persons with known anaphylactic hypersensitivity to egg protein should not be vaccinated. Even though current influenza vaccines contain only a small quantity of egg protein, severe hypersensitivity reactions occur rarely and probably are attributable to sensitivity to residual egg protein (CDC, 1993a). Despite concerns about a theoretical risk of vaccine-associated Guillain-Barré syndrome, there is essentially no risk of developing the syndrome after vaccination.

Hepatitis A Immunization

Rationale for Active Immunization

Hepatitis A is the most prevalent form of infectious hepatitis in the United States. In 2001, 10,600 cases of hepatitis A were reported to the CDC; the death rate from fulminant hepatitis A was estimated to be about 0.7%. The cost associated with hepatitis A infection is about $200 million annually.

Hepatitis A infection is acquired via fecal–oral transmission. Poor sanitation, contamination of drinking water, and improper sewage disposal contribute to spread of the virus. As a consequence, the incidence and age at acquisition of hepatitis A vary greatly in different geographic locales. In the developing world, acquisition of hepatitis A in childhood is the rule, whereas only about 40% of U.S. residents are infected with the virus by age 20 years (CDC, 1994). About one in five reported cases in the United States occurs in children younger than 10 years. Because asymptomatic disease is common in children, case report data undoubtedly underestimate the true prevalence of infection in the pediatric age group.

Children often are implicated in transmission of hepatitis A to older siblings and adults. Icterus is observed in 70% to 80% of young adults with hepatitis A infection. In contrast, 10% or fewer of children younger than 5 years become icteric.

Immunizing Antigen

Hepatitis A vaccine is prepared by propagation of human-derived virus strain HM175 in human diploid cells, followed by purification and inactivation with formalin. Each 1-ml adult dose of vaccine contains not less than 1440 ELISA units (EL.U.) of viral antigen, adsorbed on aluminum hydroxide. Each 0.5-ml pediatric dose of vaccine contains not less than 360 EL.U. of viral antigen, also adsorbed on aluminum hydroxide. The vaccine contains 2-phenoxyethanol as a preservative.

Two inactivated hepatitis A vaccines, including the currently licensed product, have been demonstrated to be highly efficacious in placebo-controlled trials in children older than age 2 (Innis et al., 1994; Werzberger et al., 1992). The vaccines are usually associated with only mild local reactions; systemic reactions are very rare. Vaccination appears to be protective for at least 3 years, and extrapolation models suggest protection for a minimum of 10 years (Berger and Just, 1992; CDC, 1994).

Vaccine Use

Hepatitis A vaccine is administered intramuscularly. The deltoid region of the upper arm is the preferred site of injection; gluteal injection may result in a suboptimal antibody response. Primary vaccination of adults consists of a single adult vaccine dose (1440 EL.U.). Primary vaccination of children aged 2 to 18 years consists of a single pediatric vaccine dose (360 EL.U.).

A booster dose, given 6 to 12 months after the initiation of primary vaccination, is recommended for both adults and children to ensure high anti–hepatitis A antibody titers.

Immunocompromised individuals may not develop adequate antibody titers in response to routine vaccination. Such individuals may require additional vaccine doses.

Hepatitis A immunization is indicated for adults and children at least 2 years of age who desire protection against hepatitis A. Individuals who are at high risk for hepatitis A and therefore might be particularly good candidates for vaccination include the following:

1. Travelers to areas endemic for hepatitis A
2. Military personnel, hospital personnel, and food handlers
3. Individuals residing in areas of high endemicity
4. Certain ethnic and geographic populations that experience cyclic hepatitis A epidemics, including Native Americans and Alaskan natives
5. Other high-risk individuals, including homosexual males, users of illicit injectable drugs, and residents of a community experiencing a hepatitis A outbreak
6. Individuals exposed to hepatitis A (ISG should be given concomitantly)
7. Individuals with chronic liver disease

Varicella Virus Immunization

Rationale for Active Immunization

About 3.9 million cases of varicella (chickenpox) occur annually in the United States (American Academy of Pediatrics, 1995). Varicella typically occurs in children younger than 10 years, but 5% to 10% of adults are susceptible.

Most cases of varicella in otherwise healthy children are self-limited and free of complications. Possible complications include bacterial superinfection, Reye syndrome, pneumonitis, and encephalitis. The CDC receives reports of about 90 fatal cases of varicella annually in the United States, mostly in otherwise healthy children.

Severe varicella infections are observed with increased frequency in certain groups of individuals, including adults as well as children immunocompromised by cancer chemotherapy, corticosteroid therapy, or congenital or acquired immunodeficiency states. A congenital varicella syndrome occurs in about 2% of infants born to mothers who have varicella in the first or second trimester of pregnancy.

The economic costs associated with varicella are substantial. In a study published in 1985, it was estimated that the annual health care costs for varicella were $399 million (Preblud et al., 1985). A cost-benefit analysis published in 1994 concluded that routine varicella vaccination at 1 year of age could result in savings of $384 million annually in the United States (Lieu et al., 1994).

Immunizing Antigen

The vaccine is a cell-free, live, attenuated preparation of the Oka strain of varicella-zoster virus. The virus was obtained initially from a child with natural varicella and was propagated sequentially in human embryonic lung cell cultures, embryonic guinea pig cell cultures, and human diploid cell cultures. Each 0.5-ml vaccine dose contains a minimum of 1350 plaque-forming units of varicella-zoster virus.

Varicella vaccine is supplied as a lyophilized product containing sucrose, phosphate, glutamate, and processed gelatin as stabilizers as well as trace amounts of neomycin. It must be stored frozen at a temperature of 15°C (+5°F) or colder. The storage life is up to 18 months. To ensure viral potency, vaccine must be administered within 30 minutes of reconstitution.

The vaccine is efficacious in adults and children 1 year of age or older. All studies demonstrate high rates of protection against severe disease (>95% protection after household exposure) (American Academy of Pediatrics, 1995). Vaccinees, as compared with unvaccinated children, experience much milder cases of varicella, with fewer skin lesions, reduced fever, and more rapid recovery. During 8 years of study, the annual rate of varicella among vaccinees has averaged from less than 1% to 3% after exposure to wild virus, compared with an annual rate of 7% to 8% in unvaccinated children (Asano et al., 1985; Watson et al., 1993). Waning immunity has not been demonstrated.

Adverse events occur uncommonly after varicella immunization and consist predominantly of mild maculopapular or varicelliform rash (<10% of vaccine recipients) and mild local reactions at the injection site (about 20% of children and 25% to 35% of adolescents and adults). Zoster occurs with lower frequency after immunization than after natural disease and reported cases have been mild. Transmission of vaccine strain varicella-zoster virus by vaccinees is a theoretical possibility. Clinical cases of varicella from contact with healthy vaccinees have not been reported. Spread of vaccine virus by vaccinees with leukemia and vaccine-associated rash has been reported; contact cases had subclinical or mild illness (Tsolia et al., 1990).

Vaccine Use

Varicella vaccine is now recommended for all children at 12 months of age (American Academy of Pediatrics, 2000). Varicella vaccine is administered subcutaneously. The outer aspect of the upper arm (deltoid) is the preferred site of injection. Primary immunization of children 12 months to 12 years consists of a single 0.5-ml vaccine dose. Individuals 13 years or older should receive two 0.5-ml vaccine doses separated by at least 4 to 8 weeks.

Varicella vaccine may be given simultaneously with MMR vaccine, but separate syringes and injection sites should be used. If not done simultaneously, administration of varicella vaccine and MMR should be separated by an interval of at least 1 month. There is no evidence to suggest that varicella vaccine and any other routine vaccines interact in any way that would adversely affect immune responses to vaccination.

Varicella vaccination is contraindicated in the following individuals (American Academy of Pediatrics, 1995):

1. Immunocompromised children, including those with congenital immunodeficiency, blood dyscrasias, leukemia, lymphoma, HIV infection, and malignancy for which they are receiving immunosuppressive therapy. Exceptions include children with acute lymphocytic leukemia in remission for at least 1 year and a lymphocyte count greater than 700/µl as well as asymptomatic HIV-infected children with CD4 lymphocyte cell percentages greater than 25. Children with acute lymphocytic leukemia (ALL) can obtain vaccine through a research protocol, and children infected with HIV should receive two doses of the vaccine 1 month apart.
2. Individuals who have been receiving high-dose systemic corticosteroids for more than 1 month.
3. Pregnant women.
4. Individuals with a history of anaphylactoid reactions to neomycin.

The American Academy of Pediatrics recommends administration of varicella vaccine to susceptible children within 72 hours and possibly up to 120 hours after varicella exposure. This may prevent or significantly modify disease, unless the child was exposed at the same time as the index case. There is no evidence to suggest that administration of the varicella vaccine during the prodromal stage of illness increases the risk for vaccine-associated adverse events or increases the severity of natural disease (American Academy of Pediatrics, 2003).

The vaccine should not be administered within 5 months of receipt of IVIG or other blood products. Because of the theoretical risk of vaccine-associated Reye syndrome, the manufacturer recommends avoidance of salicylates for 6 weeks after immunization.

VACCINES INFREQUENTLY INDICATED FOR SELECTED INDIVIDUALS

Anthrax Vaccine

Anthrax is of public health importance only to select, high-risk, occupationally related segments of the U.S. population. The vaccine is currently recommended for individuals whose work involves production quantities or concentrations of *B. anthracis* cultures or those engaged in activities with a high potential for aerosol production. Vaccination is no longer recommended routinely for veterinarians or persons working with imported animal products (CDC, 2000e).

Of primary importance in the prevention of this disease is a continued awareness of the potential for transmission of anthrax to those at risk and surveillance of anthrax disease among animal populations.

Frequent cleaning of working facilities, decontamination of potentially contaminated raw materials, and optimal personal hygiene are other effective preventive measures.

Anthrax vaccine is available from the Michigan Department of Public Health, Lansing, or through the CDC (1984a). It consists of an aluminum hydroxide–adsorbed concentrate of protective antigen prepared from a nonencapsulated strain of *B. anthracis* (Puziss and Wright, 1963). Field trials using similar vaccines in human populations have demonstrated their effectiveness (92%), with minimal local reactions (Brachman et al., 1962). Anthrax vaccine should be considered for individuals with high-risk occupations. A basic series consists of six 0.5-ml injections given subcutaneously, the first three at 2-week intervals and the next three at 6-month intervals. When continued occupation-associated exposure is anticipated, booster injections (0.5 ml) are recommended yearly (CDC, 1984a).

BCG Vaccine

Tuberculosis remains a serious public health problem in the United States. Nevertheless, the overall prevalence of tuberculosis is not sufficient to justify routine primary prevention through active immunization programs. Efforts to recognize and control tuberculosis in the United States are directed primarily at the early identification and treatment of active cases, followed by surveillance of closely related individuals and the institution of appropriate preventive measures for those at high risk.

In only selected instances, the risk of exposure to recognized cases is significant enough to consider primary immunization with bacille Calmette-Guérin (BCG) vaccine. Of importance to the pediatrician is the risk to infants born to tuberculous mothers or to those living in a household with an identified tuberculous individual (Avery and Wotsdorf, 1968).

BCG is a live, attenuated strain derived from *Mycobacterium bovis*. All available BCG vaccines are derived from the original strain but vary in their immunogenic and reactogenic properties. Efficacy trials before 1955 of previously available liquid BCG vaccines demonstrated variable efficacy from 0% to 80% (Clemens et al., 1983; Luelmo, 1982), but freeze-dried preparations available in the United States represent further attenuated strains; their efficacy has not been demonstrated in controlled clinical trials.

BCG preparations have been associated with localized reactions (ulceration, lymphadenitis, or both in 1% to 10%) and osteomyelitis (1 per 1 million vaccinees and possibly higher in newborns). Fatal or disseminated BCG infection (1 to 10 per 10 million vaccinees) occurs almost exclusively in immunocompromised children (CDC, 1979).

BCG administration represents only an ancillary measure in the public health armamentarium designed to identify, treat, and prevent tuberculosis in the United

States. Individuals with negative tuberculin skin tests who have had or are likely to have repeated exposure to untreated or ineffectively treated, sputum-positive pulmonary tuberculosis are candidates for BCG. Immunization should be considered for those at risk in well-defined communities or groups in which high infectivity rates have been demonstrated and in which therapeutic or preventive measures are difficult to implement (e.g., medically indigent or migrant populations). Some health care workers may be at increased risk of repeated exposure, especially those working in settings where the prevalence of tuberculosis is relatively high (CDC, 1979; Thompson et al., 1979).

Vaccination with BCG should be considered only for uninfected children who are at unavoidable risk for continued exposure to tuberculosis and for whom other prevention strategies are not feasible. Recommended vaccine recipients include infants and children who have negative tuberculin skin tests, who live in households with repeated or persistent exposure to infectious cases of tuberculosis, and who live in groups with a rate of new tuberculous infections exceeding 1% per year if other control strategies have failed (American Academy of Pediatrics, 2000).

BCG should be given only to individuals who have a negative skin test to 5 tuberculin units (TU) of tuberculin purified protein derivative (PPD). Preparations available in the United States can be administered either percutaneously or intradermally.

Recommended dosages are 0.05 ml for infants younger than 1 month of age and 0.1 ml for older infants, children, and adolescents. Recipients of BCG should have follow-up tuberculin skin tests 2 to 3 months later to establish that tuberculin sensitivity has been acquired; failure to react dictates the need for another BCG injection. In general, the tuberculin reaction to BCG vaccine measures 7 to 15 mm of induration and diminishes gradually over 5 years.

BCG should not be administered to individuals with primary or secondary immunodeficiency states, including chronic granulomatous disease. Leukemia, lymphoma, or other generalized malignancies; HIV infection; immunosuppressive therapy (cytotoxic agents, corticosteroids, or irradiation); disseminated skin infections; and burns all constitute specific contraindications to BCG administration. Although no harmful effects of BCG have been documented in the fetus, it is reasonable to avoid vaccination during pregnancy unless an immediate excessive risk of exposure is unavoidable.

Subsequent to immunization with BCG, it may be difficult to distinguish between a tuberculin reaction representing acquired tuberculous suprainfection and persisting postvaccination sensitivity. Because the degree and duration of protection against tuberculous disease afforded by BCG is uncertain, a positive tuberculin reaction must always be suspected to be disease related, especially if a recent exposure to active tuberculosis is identified (American Academy of Pediatrics, 2003; CDC, 1979; Fox and Lepow, 1983).

Cholera Vaccine

Cholera vaccines are of limited value. Only rare cases of cholera have been recognized in the United States in the past decade, although it remains a significant public health concern in African and Asian countries. Even in these countries, however, the risk to American travelers is low, and persons following tourist itineraries who use standard accommodations are at virtually no risk. A traveler's best protection against contracting cholera is to avoid food and water that may be contaminated. Cholera vaccination is indicated only for travelers to countries that require evidence of cholera vaccination for entry, although the World Health Organization no longer recommends cholera vaccination for any travelers.

The available vaccines are phenol-inactivated suspensions of several strains of Vibrio cholerae. In field trials conducted in cholera-endemic regions, these vaccines have been shown to be only about 50% effective in reducing the incidence of clinical illness for 3 to 6 months after vaccination (CDC, 1978a, 1984b, 1984c).

Travelers to countries that have entry requirements should obtain a validated international certificate of vaccination documenting receipt of vaccine 6 days to 6 months before entry. Most city, county, and state health departments can validate certificates. Only a single dose is needed to satisfy international health regulations for most countries.

A full primary series, recommended only for special high-risk groups working and living in endemic areas, includes two subcutaneous or intramuscular doses administered 1 week to 1 month or more apart. The dose depends on the patient's age (6 months to 4 years, 0.2 ml; 5 to 10 years, 0.3 ml; older than 10 years, 0.5 ml). The vaccine also can be administered intradermally (0.2 ml) to individuals 5 years or older. These doses are appropriate for all primary and booster immunizations. Booster doses are recommended at 6 months after primary immunization and at 6-month intervals thereafter when necessary. Vaccine is not recommended for infants younger than 6 months.

Cholera and yellow fever vaccinations should be separated by at least 3 weeks. If time constraints preclude this, they can be given simultaneously (CDC, 1978a, 1984b; Felsenfeld et al., 1973).

Side effects of cholera vaccine include fever; malaise; headache; and tenderness, erythema, and induration at the injection site for 1 or 2 days. Serious reactions after cholera vaccine are rare but contraindicate revaccination.

Meningococcal Vaccine

Significant morbidity and mortality secondary to Neisseria meningitidis (purulent meningitis or septicemia) occur disproportionately in children; those younger than 5 years account for half of all cases (CDC, 1993b), with the peak age of incidence and mortality occurring during the first year of life. Serogroups B and C account for about 90% of the cases (CDC, 1993b). In children younger than 5 years, serogroup B can account for more than 70% of meningococcal disease (Band et al., 1983).

Routine immunization of civilians against meningococcal disease is not recommended for several reasons:

1. The overall risk of acquiring meningococcal disease in civilian populations is low.
2. No vaccine is currently available for serogroup B.
3. The current vaccines may be of little benefit in those at highest risk (infants).

Routine vaccination is recommended only for those who may be at high risk for meningococcal disease because of an underlying abnormality, such as deficiency of the terminal components of serum complement (Ellison et al., 1983) or anatomic or functional asplenia (CDC, 2000d) (see Chapters 21, 24, and 30). Immunization of college students also is recommended. In addition, immunization may be beneficial for travels to countries known to have hyperendemic or epidemic meningococcal disease caused by a vaccine-preventable serogroup (A, C, Y, and W-135).

However, preventive measures must be considered for selected contacts of identified meningococcal cases. Significant secondary attack rates occur in susceptible household contacts (3 per 1000); during epidemic conditions, household secondary attack rates can reach 10% (Meningococcal Disease Surveillance Group, 1976; Munford et al., 1974). Other selected groups, including contacts of cases in day-care centers (Jacobson et al., 1977) or schools (Feigin et al., 1982) and hospital personnel who have intimate contact with patients before antimicrobials are administered, also may be at high risk (American Academy of Pediatrics, 2000).

Active immunization should be considered to control epidemic outbreaks of meningococcal disease. Although chemoprophylaxis is the primary means of limiting the spread of sporadic disease, active immunization of close contacts also can be considered in such cases, especially when additional cases are likely to occur during an extended period (American Academy of Pediatrics, 2003). About half of secondary household cases occur 5 days or more after the primary case (Greenwood et al., 1978), thereby allowing time for benefit from vaccination. Furthermore, unless chemoprophylaxis completely eliminates the transmission of N. meningitidis within an "epidemiologic unit" (clearly, often not possible), additional secondary cases among susceptible individuals will occur if active immunization is not provided.

Immunizing Antigens

Four preparations derived from the capsular polysaccharides of N. meningitidis are licensed for use in the United States: group A, group C, bivalent A/C, and quadrivalent A/C/Y/W-135. The meningococcal vaccines consist of 50 µg of each respective capsular polysaccharide and induce group-specific antibody or

antibodies within 1 week after parenteral administration; the duration of protection is unknown. Occasional untoward reactions have been reported and consist primarily of localized erythema and tenderness (American Academy of Pediatrics, 2003; Hankins et al., 1982).

Serogroup A vaccine has been shown under epidemic conditions to be effective in infants and children 3 months to 5 years old in Finland and has also been shown to be highly effective and safe in Egyptian school children 6 to 15 years old (Wahdan et al., 1973).

Serogroup C vaccine, used during a Brazilian epidemic, was protective in children 24 to 35 months old but not in those younger than 24 months (Taunay et al., 1974). These observations are in agreement with other investigations that have demonstrated a strong age-dependent association with serum antibody response (Gold et al., 1979; Kaythy et al., 1980; Wilkins and Wehrle, 1979).

The capsular polysaccharides of serogroups Y and W135 are safe and immunogenic in children older than 2 years, although clinical efficacy has not been demonstrated for these antigens. Controlled trials using meningococcal vaccines in household or day-care contacts of sporadic cases have not been performed, so their ultimate protective value in this setting is unknown.

Recently, studies have examined candidate meningococcal vaccines that use the same protein conjugate approach used with success for prevention of Hib and pneumococcal disease. These studies suggest that conjugate meningococcal vaccines may be useful in the immunization of even very young infants.

Vaccine Use

The quadrivalent meningococcal vaccine should be administered subcutaneously in a single 0.5-ml dose. Routine immunization is not recommended for civilian populations because of insufficient evidence of its value when the overall risk of infections is low. Routine immunization using the quadrivalent vaccine is recommended only for certain high-risk groups, including those with deficiencies of the terminal components of serum complement and those with anatomic or functional asplenia (CDC, 2000d).

When an outbreak of meningococcal disease occurs, the etiologic serogroup should be determined, and if represented in the vaccine, the population at risk should be immunized. Definition of the presence and scope of epidemics when they occur should be carried out in conjunction with local health authorities or officials at the CDC before extensive vaccination. When sporadic cases of meningococcal disease are identified, vaccination in addition to chemoprophylaxis should be considered for household or day-care contacts, especially when cases occur over an extended period.

Vaccination of individuals before travel to countries where epidemic meningococcal disease is present also should be considered. The quadrivalent vaccine is given to all United States military recruits. Although the meningococcal polysaccharide vaccines may be safe to give pregnant women, they should not be administered because of theoretical considerations unless there is a substantial risk of disease. Children first immunized before age 4 should be considered for revaccination after they are 2 or 3 years old if they remain at high risk. The necessity of revaccinating older patients currently is not known.

Plague Vaccine

Plague is an enzootic infection of many wild rodent species in several parts of southwestern United States. Its occurrence in U.S. human populations is of increasing public health importance; more cases (40) were reported in 1983 than in any previous year since 1920 (CDC, 1984g). The control of epizootic plague and control measures directed against the vector (Oriental rat flea, *Xenopsylla cheopsis*) represent the most important prevention program against human plague, but active immunization is of additional protective value in select high-risk persons.

A formaldehyde-inactivated *Yersinia pestis* vaccine is licensed for use in the United States (CDC, 1982f). Adequate serologic responses have been demonstrated in 83%, 90%, and 90% of adult volunteers after one, two, and three doses (1 ml each) of vaccine, respectively (Bartelloni et al., 1973). Immunization is associated with a reduced incidence and severity of clinical plague following exposure. Vaccine administration is recommended for the following groups:

· Laboratory and field personnel working with *Y. pestis* organisms resistant to antimicrobial agents
· Persons engaged in aerosol experiments with *Y. pestis*
· Persons engaged in field operations in areas where plague is enzootic and where prevention of exposure is not possible (e.g., disaster areas)

Plague vaccination should also be considered for the following groups (CDC, 1982f, 1984f):

· Laboratory personnel regularly working with *Y. pestis* or plague-infected rodents
· Persons whose vocations bring them into regular contact with wild rodents or rabbits in areas with enzootic plague
· Persons traveling to plague endemic areas, especially if travel is not limited to urban areas

Primary immunization consists of three intramuscular doses of vaccine for both adults and children. Generally, a second dose is given 4 weeks after the initial dose, and the third dose is given 4 to 12 weeks after the second dose. If an accelerated schedule is required, three doses can be administered at least 1 week apart. Three booster doses should be given at approximately 6-month intervals under circumstances of continuing plague exposure. Subsequently, booster doses at 1- to 2-year intervals should provide good protection under most circumstances.

Persons exposed to patients with known plague pneumonia or to *Y. pestis* aerosol in the laboratory should be given a 7- to 10-day course of antimicrobial therapy (tetracycline, chloramphenicol, or streptomycin) regardless of their previous immunization history.

Primary immunization may result in mild systemic symptoms, such as general malaise, headache, fever, and mild lymphadenopathy, or local erythema and induration at the injection site in approximately 10% of recipients, especially with repeated injections. Sterile abscesses or hypersensitivity reactions (urticaria or reactive airway symptoms) have been reported rarely. Severe local or systemic reactions to plague vaccine contraindicate revaccination.

Plague vaccine should not be administered to individuals with a known hypersensitivity to any of the vaccine constituents, such as beef protein, soy, casein, or phenol. Because safety of plague vaccine administered during pregnancy has not been established, it should not be used unless there is substantial risk of infection (CDC, 1982f).

Rabies Vaccine

Although human rabies occurs rarely in the United States, some 25,000 individuals each year require prophylaxis after known or potential exposure to rabies. Carnivorous wild animals (skunks, foxes, coyotes, raccoons, and bats) account for about 85% of proven cases of animal rabies in the United States; the prevalence of rabies among these animal populations has increased in recent years. Domestic animals (dogs and cats) represent only a small proportion of proven rabid animals, but they account for most postexposure courses of rabies prophylaxis given annually (Helmick, 1983). Rodents (squirrels, hamsters, gerbils, rats, and mice) and lagomorphs (rabbits and hares) are rarely infected and have not been associated with rabies in the United States (Mann, 1983).

Only 36 cases of human rabies were reported in the United States from 1980 to 1997 (American Academy of Pediatrics, 2000). This exceedingly low incidence attests to the efficacy of postexposure prophylaxis using the recommended vaccine and immunoglobulin preparations. In fact, rabies has not been reported in any patient who has received currently recommended postexposure prophylaxis.

Although rabies is associated with an almost universally fatal outcome, the need for prophylaxis should be evaluated carefully, because available prophylactic methods are rarely complicated by severe adverse reactions. However, the longer treatment is postponed, the less likely it is to be effective.

Human Diploid Cell Vaccines

The human diploid cell vaccines (HDCVs) was licensed for use in the United States in 1980. HDCV is supplied as 1.0-ml single-dose vials of lyophilized vaccine with accompanying diluent. It is administered intramuscularly, generally in the deltoid area. These preparations represent a significant advantage over previous vaccines (inactivated duck embryo and nervous tissue–derived vaccines no longer available in the United States) with respect to immunogenicity, reaction rates, and convenience. Essentially all recipients develop protective antibody titers that persist for at least 2 years.

Local reactions (pain, erythema, or swelling) occur in 25% of recipients, and mild systemic reactions (nausea, abdominal pain, headache, or myalgia) have been noted in about 20%. Systemic and occasionally severe allergic reactions have been reported to occur at a rate of 1 per 1000 HDCV doses administered to more than 400,000 individuals (CDC, 1984k). Transient neuroparalytic reactions have been observed even less commonly, at 1 per 170,000 vaccinees worldwide.

Two other human rabies vaccines, rabies vaccine absorbed (RVA) and purified chick embryo cell (PCEC) vaccine, also are approved for use in the United States.

Rabies Immunoglobulin and Antiserum

Antirabies human immune serum globulin (RIG) concentrated by cold ethanol fractionation from plasma of hyperimmunized human donors is available from Cutter Laboratories (Hyperrab) and Merieux Institute (Imogam). The content of rabies-neutralizing antibody is standardized to contain 150 IU/ml. It is supplied in 2-ml (300 IU) and 10-ml (1500 IU) vials for pediatric and adult use, respectively. Antirabies serum (ARS), available from Selavo, is a concentrated serum obtained from hyperimmunized horses. Neutralizing antibody content is standardized to contain 1000 IU per vial.

RIG is well tolerated in most recipients, although local pain and low-grade fever may result. Anaphylaxis, angioneurotic edema, or other systemic reactions have not been reported. However, ARS produces serum sickness in approximately 40% of adult recipients, and in a small number of children, anaphylactic reactions occur. Therefore, although RIG and ARS are both effective, RIG is the product of choice and is recommended unless unavailable. When ARS must be used, the patient must be tested for sensitivity to equine serum (Hattwick et al., 1974) (see Chapter 4).

Vaccine and Rabies Immunoglobulin Use

POSTEXPOSURE PROPHYLAXIS

Recommendations for the management of individuals following possible exposure to rabies include meticulous attention to flushing and cleaning of the wound with soap and water and active immunization and passive immunoglobulin administration. The need for preventive measures must be individualized. This decision depends on circumstances precipitating the exposure; the species, clinical state, and availability of the animal inflicting the wound; and the local prevalence of rabies in animal populations. Bites or nonbite exposures (scratches, abrasions, open wounds, or mucous membranes contaminated with saliva) must be considered significant.

A combination of active and passive immunization almost always is indicated for the treatment of bites and nonbite exposures inflicted by rabid animals, as well as by those suspected of being rabid (American Academy of Pediatrics, 2000; CDC 1999b) (Table 42-4). When possible, the brains of wild animals (skunks, foxes, coyotes, raccoons, and bats) or symptomatic dogs or cats implicated in an exposure should be examined for evidence of rabies at the CDC.

Active and passive immunization always should be initiated promptly, and vaccine administration should be discontinued only if laboratory results are negative. Individuals exposed to healthy dogs or cats that are available for observation do not require immediate prophylactic treatment. Implicated healthy domestic dogs or cats should be quarantined and observed by a veterinarian for at least 10 days; if suggestive symptoms develop, the exposed individuals should begin postexposure prophylaxis promptly, and the brain of the animal should be examined. An unknown (escaped) animal must be regarded as rabid (see Table 42-4).

TABLE 42-4 · RABIES POSTEXPOSURE PROPHYLAXIS GUIDE

Animal Type	Evaluation and Disposition of Animal	Postexposure Prophylaxis Recommendations
Dogs and cats	Healthy and available for 10 days of observation	Do not begin prophylaxis unless animal develops symptoms of rabies[*]
	Rabid or suspected rabid[†]	Immediate vaccination and RIG
	Unknown (escaped)	Consult public health officials for advice
Skunks, raccoons, bats, foxes, and most other carnivores; woodchucks	Regarded as rabid unless geographic area is known to be free of rabies or until animal proven negative by laboratory tests[†]	Immediate vaccination and RIG
Livestock, ferrets, rodents, and lagomorphs (rabbits and hares)	Consider individually	Consult public health officials; bites of squirrels, hamsters, guinea pigs, gerbils, chipmunks, rats, mice, other rodents, rabbits, and hares almost never require antirabies treatment

[*]During the 10-day holding period, treatment with RIG and vaccine should be initiated at the first sign of rabies in the biting dog or cat. The symptomatic animal should be killed immediately.
[†]The animal should be killed and tested as soon as possible. Holding for observation is not recommended. Vaccination is discontinued if immunofluorescent test of the animal is negative.
RIG = human rabies immune globulin vaccine.
Adapted from American Academy of Pediatrics. In 2003 Red Book: Report of the Committee on Infectious Diseases, 26th ed. Elk Grove Village, IL, American Academy of Pediatrics, 2003.

Vaccine must be provided as early as possible but should be used regardless of the time interval after exposure. After initial vaccine administration, four additional 1.0-ml intramuscular doses are given at 3, 7, 14, and 28 days. An immunization series should be initiated and completed with one vaccine product (HDCV, RVA, or PCEC). Routine serologic testing is not indicated after postexposure prophylaxis and is reserved only for those whose immune response may be impaired by primary disease or by immunosuppressive therapy. Pregnancy is not a contraindication to rabies prophylaxis.

RIG is administered only once, at the beginning of antirabies prophylaxis, to provide immediate passive protection until adequate antibody titers are achieved from active HDCV immunization. If not administered initially together with the vaccine, RIG can be given up to 8 days afterward; it is not indicated after that, because antibody responses to the vaccine have likely occurred. The recommended dose of RIG is 20 IU/kg. About half the dose of RIG should be infiltrated into the area surrounding the wound and the remainder administered intramuscularly.

PRE-EXPOSURE PROPHYLAXIS

Active immunization for pre-exposure prophylaxis in high-risk groups (veterinarians, animal handlers, selected laboratory workers, persons visiting countries where rabies is endemic, and persons whose pursuits may involve frequent contact with rabid animals) should be considered.

For this purpose, an initial 1.0-ml intramuscular injection of HDCV is given followed by a second dose 7 days later and a third injection 3 weeks after the second. Under conditions of continued exposure, booster doses should be given or serologic testing performed as recommended (CDC, 1984h). Pre-exposure prophylaxis also can be given using the Merieux Institute HDCV preparation packaged for intradermal use; a series of 0.1-ml doses is administered in the lateral aspect of the upper arm, following a schedule similar to that recommended for intramuscular administration (CDC, 1983b).

Routine postvaccination serology after pre-exposure prophylaxis is necessary only for those suspected of being immunosuppressed. In individuals who have received adequate pre-exposure prophylaxis, postexposure prophylaxis consists of two 1.0-ml intramuscular doses of HDCV; the first dose is administered at the time of the exposure and a second dose 3 days later. RIG is not required under these circumstances.

Typhoid Vaccine

The overall prevalence of typhoid fever is significantly lower in the United States than in highly endemic countries, but the potential for importation from Central and South America is well recognized. Most of the 350 to 600 cases reported annually in the United States since 1963 have been acquired during foreign travel (CDC, 1982a; Taylor et al., 1983). The gradual elimination of typhoid fever in the United States during the past half-century reflects improved public health measures, including optimal sanitation methods and identification and reporting of affected individuals. Active immunization with typhoid vaccine represents only an ancillary preventive public health measure to be used in selected settings to prevent transmission from known infected individuals.

Immunizing Antigens

Two typhoid vaccines are available in the United States for civilian use. The older of the two is a heat-phenol–inactivated preparation for parenteral administration. A live, attenuated vaccine prepared from the Ty21a strain of *Salmonella typhi* recently has become available. This vaccine can be administered orally. Unfortunately, data concerning its efficacy and safety for children younger than 6 years are limited, and it is not yet recommended for use in this age group.

In field trials, the parenteral vaccine and the Ty21a vaccine have had similar efficacy. Unfortunately, protection depends somewhat on the challenge inoculum. Demonstrated protection to small inocula of *S. typhi* can be overcome with a high-inoculum challenge.

Vaccine Use

Specific indications for typhoid vaccination in the United States include household or other intimate exposure to a known typhoid carrier and foreign travel to areas where typhoid fever is endemic.

Yellow Fever Vaccine

Because yellow fever does not occur in the United States, prevention is considered only for purposes of international travel. As is true for other arboviral diseases, urban disease can be prevented best by suppressing or eradicating mosquito vectors. Another effective preventive measure is to immunize persons living in or traveling to areas where yellow fever is endemic (CDC, 1984l).

Immunizing Antigen

The yellow fever vaccine (YFV) licensed in the United States is a live, attenuated preparation derived from the 17D viral strain prepared in chick embryos (CDC, 1984l). In contrast to the previously used Dakar strain preparation, the 17D strain has been associated only rarely with significant neurologic complications (two cases of encephalitis following administration of 34 million doses of vaccine). Mild side effects, including low-grade fever, headache, and myalgia, have been observed in 2% to 5% of recipients. Immediate hypersensitivity reactions, including rash, urticaria, and reactive airway symptoms, are extremely uncommon (<1 per 1 million doses) and occur primarily in individuals with histories of egg allergy (CDC, 1984l).

Immunity after vaccination with the 17D strain virus has been demonstrated to persist for more than 10 years (Rosenzweig et al., 1963; Wisseman and Sweet, 1962).

Vaccine Use

YFV is recommended for individuals older than 9 months who are traveling to or reside in areas of yellow fever endemicity (parts of Africa and South America). Vaccination for international travel is required by local health regulations in individual countries. To obtain an international certificate of vaccination, a YFV approved by the World Health Organization and administered at a designated YFV center is required. Such centers in the United States can be located by contacting state and local health departments.

Primary immunization consists of a single, subcutaneous injection of 0.5 ml reconstituted, freeze-dried vaccine for both adults and children. Revaccination is required no more frequently than every 10 years. In preparation for imminent travel, other live virus vaccines can be given at a different site simultaneously with YFV; if not given on the same day, the administration of multiple live virus vaccines should be separated by at least 4 weeks.

Cholera vaccine and YFV administration should be separated by at least 3 weeks; if time constraints preclude this, they can be given simultaneously (Felsenfeld et al., 1973).

A prospective study of individuals given YFV and commercially available immunoglobulin indicated no attenuation of the immune response to YFV compared with controls (CDC, 1984l).

Precautions and Contraindications

Although no adverse effects of YFV on the developing fetus have been demonstrated, vaccine administration to pregnant women should be avoided. Pregnant women and infants younger than 9 months should be considered for vaccination only when travel to high-risk areas is required and high-level protection against mosquito exposure is not feasible. As is true of other live viral vaccines, YFV should not be administered to patients with altered immune states as a result of underlying disease or immunosuppressive therapy.

Documented hypersensitivity to eggs is a contraindication to vaccination. However, experience in the armed forces suggests that allergy sufficiently severe to preclude vaccination is uncommon and occurs only in those individuals who are unable to eat eggs. If international quarantine regulations represent the only reason to immunize a patient known to be hypersensitive to eggs, attempts should be made to obtain a waiver. If immunization of an individual with a questionable history of egg hypersensitivity is considered essential because of a high-risk of exposure, an intradermal skin test may be given as directed in the YFV package insert (CDC, 1984l).

INVESTIGATIONAL ACTIVE IMMUNIZING AGENTS

Human Immunodeficiency Virus Vaccines

Several candidate HIV vaccines are undergoing clinical trials. A vaccine to HIV has proved incredibly challenging. Subtype diversity and the complex interaction of the virus with the immune system have hampered early attempts at vaccine development. In addition, there is a shortage of good animal models for study. Most of these vaccines are genetically engineered products based on the HIV envelope proteins gp120 and gp160. Several groups have also used newer DNA technology to boost the potency of vaccines. HIV vaccine development has focused not only on prevention of infection but also on slowing of immune attrition in individuals already infected with the virus (see Chapter 29).

More than 70 different vaccines are currently in phase I trials. Phase II/III vaccine studies are currently being planned in sub-Saharan Africa. Several have already commenced in the United Kingdom and Kenya, using healthy volunteers.

Cytomegalovirus Vaccine

About 1% of newborns in the United States are infected congenitally with cytomegalovirus (CMV), and 10% to 20% of these manifest significant neurologic defects. Certain allograft recipients are also at high risk for severe CMV disease; at least 90% of renal transplant patients excrete CMV postoperatively. The development of CMV vaccines has been targeted at diminishing morbidity associated with CMV disease in these and other high-risk patient groups.

Live, attenuated vaccines, passaged in human tissue culture, have been developed and tested in Britain (AD 169 strain) (Stern, 1984) and the United States (Towne strain) (Plotkin et al., 1984). Following subcutaneous administration to healthy volunteers, both humoral and cell-mediated immune responses are observed. However, the duration of the immune response or protection afforded is unknown.

Controlled trials have demonstrated that the use of CMV vaccine in seronegative renal transplant candidates may not diminish the rate of CMV infection after transplantation but may decrease the severity of acquired CMV disease. Viremia or shedding of vaccine-type CMV has not been demonstrated after immunization, and adverse reactions to the vaccine are limited to minor local reactions.

Before CMV vaccine can be used on a large scale, studies are required to evaluate if vaccine-induced antibody in pregnant women reduces the risk of disease in offspring. Furthermore, the protective efficacy of the vaccines against multiple strains of CMV and the possible risks of latent infection or oncogenesis associated with vaccination need to be defined.

Rotavirus Vaccine

Rotavirus is one of the most common causes of severe diarrhea in children worldwide. In developing countries, it can be a major cause of diarrhea and death. In August 1998, a rhesus rotavirus tetravalent vaccine was approved for use in children by the U.S. Food and Drug Administration. This vaccine was administered orally. However, subsequently the vaccine was voluntarily withdrawn from the market because the vaccine was found to be associated with an increase risk of intussusception.

Group B Streptococcal Vaccine

Group B *Streptococcus* (GBS) is the leading cause of neonatal sepsis and meningitis. Morbidity and mortality rates remain high despite the use of antimicrobials and intensive supportive care. Serotype III is responsible for about two thirds of all GBS infections in infants. Although less information is available about other serotypes, high titers of transplacental antibody to type III GBS capsular polysaccharide prevents the development of disease in exposed neonates.

Because high levels of maternal type-specific anti-GBS antibody should protect full-term newborns, immunization of pregnant women with purified type-specific vaccine has been considered as an approach to control of GBS infections. In general, the immunogenicity of purified GBS capsular polysaccharide has been disappointing, with response rates of 40% to 80% in nonimmune adults (Baker and Kasper, 1985). However, one study (Baker et al., 1988) reported that type III vaccine was tolerated well by pregnant women and that opsonically active antibody could be demonstrated in their infants.

Tularemia Vaccine

Human tularemia occurs primarily in the south central United States, where the disease is enzootic in both domestic and wild animals. Prevention of human disease depends on the prevention of transmission either (1) directly from infected animals (rabbits, squirrels, skunks, muskrats, woodchucks, coyotes, and others) or animal products or (2) indirectly from infected vector insects (e.g., ticks or deer flies). Active immunization rarely is indicated except in high-risk settings, such as persons engaged in laboratory work involving *Francisella tularensis* (American Academy of Pediatrics, 2000).

A live, attenuated tularemia vaccine for intradermal use is available in the United States as an investigational product from the CDC. In laboratory workers, vaccine administration has reduced the incidence of typhoidal tularemia and the severity of ulceroglandular disease (Burke, 1977), but its efficacy in the prevention of naturally occurring disease is unknown.

PASSIVE IMMUNIZATION AGENTS

Varicella-Zoster Immunoglobulin

Early studies demonstrated the efficacy of zoster immunoglobulin (ZIG), prepared from patients convalescing from herpes zoster, in preventing chickenpox among exposed, susceptible, healthy or high-risk children when administered within 72 hours after exposure. The scarcity of plasma from patients convalescing from zoster used to prepare ZIG resulted in a limited supply of this material. Thus techniques were developed to prepare a globulin of similar potency from plasma of normal donors with high varicella-zoster antibody. This varicella-zoster immunoglobulin (VZIG) is available in ample supply in the United States.

Since VZIG became available for use in 1978, both serologic and clinical evaluations have demonstrated that the product is equivalent to ZIG in preventing or modifying clinical disease in susceptible immunocompromised patients exposed to varicella. VZIG (human) is a sterile, 10% to 18% solution of the globulin fraction of human plasma (primarily IgG) in 0.3 molar glycine stabilizer and 1:10,000 thimerosal preservative. It is prepared by Cohn ethanol precipitation. This product is available through regional distribution centers in conjunction with the American Red Cross and from hospital pharmacies.

VZIG Use

The appropriateness of VZIG administration after a known or suspected exposure to varicella depends on the susceptibility of the exposed individual, whether the exposure is likely to result in infection, and whether the exposed individual is at high risk for complications of varicella.

Both normal and immunocompromised adults and children who have had clinical varicella based on a carefully obtained history can be considered immune. Bone marrow transplant recipients, however, represent an exception to this rule. Because subclinical primary infections rarely occur (estimated to be <5% of infections among normal children), children younger than 15 years without histories of clinical varicella should be considered susceptible unless serologic studies demonstrate adequate immunity. Most healthy adults with negative or unknown histories of clinical varicella are probably immune, based on very low attack rates of varicella in adult populations after household or hospital exposure.

Multiple serologic techniques have been developed to determine susceptibility to varicella. The complement-fixing test is the most commonly available serologic assay, but its overall usefulness is limited by its lack of sensitivity and specificity, as well as the fact that about two thirds of patients lack detectible complement-fixing antibody to varicella within a year after clinical infection. Other more sensitive assays—including fluorescent antibody membrane antigen (FAMA), immune adherence hemagglutination assay (IAHA), enzyme-linked immunosorbent assay (ELISA), and neutralization anti-

TABLE 42-5 · RECOMMENDATIONS FOR USE OF VARICELLA-ZOSTER IMMUNE GLOBULIN (VZIG)

Exposure Criteria*
1. One of the following types of exposure to persons with chickenpox or zoster:
   a. Continuous household contact
   b. Playmate contact (generally >1 hour of play indoors)
   c. Hospital contact (in same two- to four-bed room or adjacent beds in a large ward or prolonged face-to-face contact with an infectious staff member or patient)

and

2. Time elapsed after exposure is such that VZIG can be administered within 96 hours but preferably sooner

Candidates for VZIG†
1. Susceptible to varicella-zoster (see text)
2. Significant exposure, as listed above
3. Age <15 years; administration to immunocompromised adolescents and adults and to other older patients on an individual basis (see text)
4. One of the following underlying illnesses or conditions:
   a. Leukemia or lymphoma
   b. Congenital or acquired immunodeficiency, including the acquired immunodeficiency syndrome
   c. Immunosuppressive treatment
   d. Newborn of mother who had onset of chickenpox within 5 days before delivery or 48 hours after delivery
   e. Premature infant (≥28 weeks' gestation) whose mother has no history of chickenpox
   f. Premature infants (<28 weeks' gestation or ≤1000 g) regardless of maternal history

*Patients must meet both criteria.
†Patients must meet both exposure criteria above.
Adapted from Centers for Disease Control and Prevention. MMWR 33(7):84–100, 1984; and American Academy of Pediatrics. In 2003 Red Book: Report of the Committee on Infectious Diseases, 26th ed. Elk Grove Village, IL, American Academy of Pediatrics, 2003

body assay—are not generally available and have not been fully evaluated, especially in immunocompromised populations. Furthermore, even sensitive antibody assays may not be useful in assessing the likelihood that neonates and young infants exposed to varicella will develop clinical disease.

Exposure criteria for which VZIG is indicated among susceptible individuals at risk for severe varicella infection include one of the following types of exposure to persons with chickenpox or zoster:

· Continuous household contact
· Playmate contact (generally >1 hour of play indoors)
· Hospital contact (in same two- to four-bed room or adjacent beds in a large ward or prolonged face-to-face contact with an infectious staff member or patient)
· Newborn contact (newborn of mother who had onset of chickenpox ≤5 days before delivery or within 48 hours after delivery)

Each of these criteria is contingent on the possibility that VZIG can be administered within 96 hours (preferably sooner) after the earliest known exposure.

Specific recommendations for use of VZIG among persons meeting appropriate exposure criteria are outlined in Table 42-5. In general, patients receiving

monthly doses of IVIG should be protected and do not require VZIG. However, VZIG should be considered if exposure occurs more than 3 weeks after the most recent dose of immunoglobulin or if the patient has advanced HIV disease with a markedly depressed CD4+ lymphocyte count.

VZIG in Infants and Children

IMMUNOCOMPROMISED CHILDREN

Passive immunization of susceptible immunocompromised children following significant exposure to chickenpox or zoster represents the most important use of VZIG. This includes children with primary immunodeficiency disorders or neoplastic diseases and children whose treatment is considered immunosuppressive.

NEWBORNS OF MOTHERS WITH VARICELLA

VZIG is indicated for newborns of mothers who develop chickenpox within 5 days before or 48 hours after delivery. Infants of mothers who develop clinical varicella more than 5 days before delivery are thought to be protected from varicella complications by transplacentally acquired maternal antibody. No evidence exists to suggest that infants born to mothers who develop varicella more than 48 hours after delivery are at increased risk for serious complications.

POSTNATAL EXPOSURE OF NEWBORN INFANTS

Premature infants exposed to varicella postnatally should be evaluated on an individual basis. Because the risk of complications from postnatally acquired varicella in the premature infant is unknown, it is reasonable to administer VZIG to exposed premature infants whose mothers have negative or uncertain histories of varicella exposure; these infants should be considered at risk as long as they are hospitalized. All exposed infants less than 28 weeks' gestation or with a birth weight of 1000 g or less should receive VZIG regardless of maternal history because of the uncertainty of acquiring transplacental maternal antibody. Full-term infants who develop varicella after postnatal exposure are not known to be at increased risk for complications of chickenpox as compared with older children, so VZIG is not recommended for full-term infants regardless of the mother's immune status.

VZIG in Adults

IMMUNOCOMPROMISED ADULTS

Complications of varicella in immunocompromised adults are substantially greater than in normal individuals. Most (85% to 95%) immunocompromised adults with negative or unknown histories of previous varicella are immune. Nonetheless, adults who are believed to be susceptible and who have had significant exposures should receive VZIG.

HEALTHY ADULTS

Varicella can be severe in healthy adults. Epidemiologic and clinical studies indicate that healthy adults who develop varicella have a 9- to 25-fold greater risk of complications, including death, than do healthy children. Most adults with negative or uncertain histories of varicella are immune, so a decision to administer VZIG to an adult must be individualized. If sensitive laboratory screening tests for varicella are available, they might be used to determine susceptibility if time permits.

PREGNANT WOMEN

Some investigators have recommended VZIG administration for pregnant women with negative or uncertain histories of varicella who were exposed significantly in the first or second trimester to try to prevent congenital varicella syndrome or in the third trimester to prevent neonatal varicella. However, no evidence exists that administering VZIG to a susceptible pregnant woman prevents viremia, fetal infection, or congenital varicella syndrome. Thus the primary (perhaps only) indication for VZIG in pregnant women is to prevent varicella complications in a susceptible adult rather than to prevent intrauterine infection.

VZIG in Hospital Settings

Health care personnel with negative or uncertain histories of chickenpox should be evaluated in a manner similar to that for other adults. If possible, sensitive laboratory tests for determining susceptibility can be used to assess candidacy for VZIG and to determine possible work restrictions that may be necessary during the incubation period, especially when large numbers of individuals have been exposed.

Ideally, all health care personnel caring for patients with varicella or zoster should be immune. Other control measures to prevent or control nosocomial varicella outbreaks include (1) strict isolation precautions, (2) isolation of exposed patients, and (3) early discharge, when possible.

Potentially susceptible hospital personnel with significant exposure should not have direct patient contact from approximately the 10th through the 21st day after exposure, the period during which chickenpox may occur. These control measures should apply regardless of whether potentially susceptible exposed personnel or patients receive VZIG.

Data on clinical attack rates and incubation periods of varicella following VZIG administration in this setting are lacking. However, studies of immunocompromised children with negative histories of varicella treated with VZIG who have had intense exposures, such as in a household setting, demonstrate that about one third to one half develop clinical varicella and might be infectious. Furthermore, VZIG may prolong the average incubation period in immunocompromised patients from 14 to 18 days, but the vast number of cases occur within 28 days of exposure in immunocompromised, VZIG-treated patients. Thus personnel who receive VZIG should probably not work in patient areas for 10 to 28 days after exposure if no illness occurs, and patients who receive VZIG should be isolated during this interval if early discharge is not possible.

VZIG Administration

VZIG is of maximum benefit when administered as soon as possible after a presumed exposure but may be effective when given as late as 96 hours after exposure. No evidence exists documenting the usefulness or efficacy of VZIG in treating clinical varicella or zoster or in preventing disseminated zoster. The duration of protection afforded by VZIG administration is uncertain, but based on the known half-life of immunoglobulin (approximately 3 weeks), high-risk patients who are reexposed more than 3 weeks after a previous dose of VZIG should receive another full dose.

VZIG is supplied in vials containing 125 units per vial (1.25 ml). The generally recommended dose is 125 units per 10 kg (22 lb) of body weight up to a maximum of 625 units (five vials). However, the minimum dose recommended is 125 units, and fractional doses are not advised. Some investigators recommend exceeding a total dose of 625 units in some immunocompromised adults. VZIG should be administered intramuscularly, as directed. It should never be administered intravenously.

Adverse reactions to VZIG administration are rare; local discomfort, pain, redness, or swelling occurs at the injection site in about 1% of recipients. Less frequent systemic reactions, such as gastrointestinal symptoms, malaise, headaches, rash, or respiratory symptoms, occur in approximately 0.2% of recipients. Severe reactions, such as angioneurotic edema and anaphylactic shock, have been reported rarely (<0.1%). When VZIG is indicated for patients with severe thrombocytopenia or any other coagulation disorder that would generally contraindicate intramuscular injections, the expected benefits should outweigh the risks.

Human Immune Serum Globulin

There are only a few well-accepted indications for ISG (e.g., immunodeficiency, hepatitis A prophylaxis, and measles prophylaxis). In most situations for which its use is considered, either ISG or IVIG can be used. However, ISG has advantages in terms of cost and ease of administration (see Chapter 4).

Hepatitis A Virus Prophylaxis

The value of ISG in the prevention or attenuation of hepatitis A virus (HAV) infection is well established (Krugman and Ward, 1961–1962). Individuals exposed to HAV are afforded protection against symptomatic disease by the prompt administration of ISG by the intramuscular route. It is recommended for all household contacts as soon as possible after exposure. The use of ISG more than 2 weeks after exposure or after the onset of illness is not recommended. Serologic testing is not generally indicated because it may delay the administration of ISG.

ISG is also recommended for contacts of HAV cases occurring in day-care centers. If a case is identified in a child, a staff member, or the household of two or more families of attendees, ISG 0.02 ml/kg should be given to all children and staff. In custodial institutions, such as those for the mentally challenged, HAV infection is highly transmissible; when outbreaks occur, residents and staff having close personal contact with identified patients should receive 0.02 ml/kg of ISG (American Academy of Pediatrics, 2003).

Exposures to HAV in classrooms or other places in schools generally do not represent significant risk for infection. ISG is not generally indicated, except in the unusual instance of a school-centered epidemic, for which ISG is recommended for close contacts of identified patients. Similarly, routine administration of ISG to hospital personnel caring for patients with HAV is not indicated. Rather, emphasis should be placed on handwashing and proper isolation procedures in the management of patients.

In most cases, the source of food- or water-borne HAV epidemics is usually recognized too late for ISG to be effective. However, if administered within 2 weeks after ingestion of identified HAV-contaminated water or food, it may be effective.

ISG is generally not indicated in newborn infants whose mothers had HAV during pregnancy, unless the mother is jaundiced and otherwise actively symptomatic at the time of delivery. Although administration of 0.02 ml/kg ISG is recommended in this setting, adequate documentation of its value is lacking.

In most cases, tourist travel does not require the prophylactic administration of ISG. However, individuals traveling to underdeveloped areas, such as tropical rural villages, should receive 0.02 ml/kg ISG if they anticipate staying less than 3 months. Those who require long-term protection should receive 0.06 ml/kg ISG and should receive additional booster doses every 4 to 5 months or receive the hepatitis A vaccine. ISG can be given with hepatitis A vaccine if the traveler will be exposed before the 1 month needed to ensure immunity from the vaccine (American Academy of Pediatrics, 2003).

Measles Prophylaxis

Human ISG has been shown to prevent or modify clinical measles in susceptible individuals when given within 6 days of exposure. The recommended dose of ISG is 0.25 ml/kg (or a maximum dose of 15 ml). It may be especially indicated for susceptible household contacts of measles patients, particularly contacts younger than 1 year, for whom the risk of complications is highest. Live measles vaccine should then be given about 3 months later, when measles antibody titers have diminished, if the child is then at least 15 months old.

Immunocompromised children should receive 0.5 ml/kg ISG after measles exposure (or a maximum dose of 15 ml). Although ISG usually prevents measles in susceptible healthy children following exposure, it may not be effective in certain children with acute leukemia or other conditions associated with altered immunity. A child regularly receiving intramuscular or intravenous ISG preparations for the treatment of antibody immunodeficiency need not receive additional prophylaxis if exposed to measles.

Other Considerations Regarding Human Immune Serum Globulin

Human ISG is sometimes used in circumstances in which only questionable or no proof of efficacy exists. For example, massive doses of ISG have been used in an attempt to prevent rubella in recently exposed pregnant women. However, there is little evidence that even 20 to 40 ml of ISG offers any protection. Similarly, there is no evidence for efficacy of ISG in the management or treatment of asthma or severe allergic diathesis, burn patients, or most acute infections, including severe, even life-threatening bacterial or viral diseases. Of particular importance is the lack of efficacy of ISG in the management of undifferentiated recurrent upper respiratory tract infections.

Adverse reactions to ISG are largely limited to the discomfort or pain experienced on administration. Severe systemic reactions are uncommon, but anaphylaxis and collapse have been reported. A higher risk of systemic reactions is associated with inadvertent intravenous administration, so ISG should always be given intramuscularly in a large muscle mass and not by any other route. Mild systemic symptoms (e.g., fever, chills, sweating) are sometimes observed in individuals receiving repeated doses.

Because ISG preparations contain trace amounts of IgA, persons who are selectively IgA deficient may develop IgA antibodies and have systemic symptoms (e.g., chills, fever, shocklike symptoms) in response to subsequent doses of ISG, plasma, or whole blood transfusions (American Academy of Pediatrics, 2003).

Special Human Immune Serum Globulins

Special human immune serum globulin preparations differ from ISG only with respect to the selection of donors. Individuals known to have high titers of a specific desired antibody are selected for preparation of these products as compared with random selections of adults for ISG. Available special ISGs include (1) hepatitis B immunoglobulin (see hepatitis B vaccine), (2) RIG (see rabies vaccine), (3) TIG (see tetanus vaccine), (4) VZIG, (5) cytomegalovirus IVIG, and (6) Rh immunoglobulin (Rho-Gam), and respiratory synctial virus IVIG (RSV-IGIV [Respigam]; see Chapter 4).

Respiratory Syncytial Virus Prophylaxis

Two products are currently available to prevent respiratory syncytial virus (RSV) infection: respiratory syncytial virus immunoglobulin intravenous (RSV-IGIV) and palivizumab, a humanized mouse monoclonal antibody that is given intramuscularly. Both have been approved for prevention of RSV in certain high-risk infants and children. RSV-IGIV is given once per month just before and monthly during RSV season at a dose of 15 ml/kg. Palivizumab (Sgnagis) is given monthly during the RSV season at a dose of 15 mg/kg intramuscularly.

Palivizumab is often preferred because of its ease of administration, safety, and efficacy. RSV prophylaxis is recommended for infants and children younger than 24 months with chronic lung disease requiring treatment (including bronchopulmonary dysplasia) and infants born prematurely. The duration of therapy will be determined by gestational age, with those born earlier requiring longer therapy.

Although not studied in randomized controlled studies, in immunocompromised patients receiving standard IVIG monthly, physicians may consider substituting RSV-IGIV during RSV season. RSV-IVIG is contraindicated in children with cyanotic congenital heart disease. Studies are ongoing evaluating palivizumab in this population.

Palivizumab does not interfere with the response to vaccines. However, infants and children receiving RSV-IGIV should delay vaccination with varicella vaccine and MMR vaccine for 9 months following the final dose of RSV-IGIV.

Intravenous Immunoglobulin

A complete discussion of the use of IVIG in immunodeficiency and autoimmune and inflammatory diseases is given in Chapters 4 and 12.

R E F E R E N C E S

American Academy of Pediatrics. Universal hepatitis B immunization. Pediatrics 89:795–800, 1992.

American Academy of Pediatrics. Recommendations for the use of live attenuated varicella vaccine. Pediatrics 95:791–796, 1995.

American Academy of Pediatrics, Committee on Infectious Diseases and Committee on Pediatric AIDS. Measles immunization in HIV-infected children. Pediatrics 103:1057–1060, 1999.

American Academy of Pediatrics. In Pickering LK, ed. Red Book: 2003 Report on the Committee on Infectious Disease, 26th ed. EIK Grove Village, IL, American Academy of Pediatrics, 2003.

Asano Y, Nagai T, Miyata T. Long-term protective immunity of recipients of the Oka strain of live varicella vaccine. Pediatrics 75:667–671, 1985.

Austrian R, Douglas RM, Schiffman G, Coetzee AM, Koornhof HJ, Hayden-Smith S, Reid RDW. Prevention of pneumococcal pneumonia by vaccination. Trans Assoc Am Phys 89:184–192, 1976.

Avery ME, Wofsdorf J. Diagnosis and treatment: approaches to newborn infants of tuberculous mothers. Pediatrics 42:519–522, 1968.

Baker CJ, Kasper DL. Group B streptococcal vaccines. Rev Infect Dis 7:458–467, 1985.

Baker CJ, Rench MA, Edwards MS, Carpenter RJ, Hays BM, Kasper DL. Immunization of pregnant women with a polysaccharide vaccine of group B streptococcus. N Engl J Med 319:1180–1185, 1988.

Band JD, Chamberland ME, Platt T, Weaver RE, Thornsberry C, Fraser DW. Trends in meningococcal disease in the United States, 1975–1980. J Infect Dis 148:754–758, 1983.

Barkin RM, Samuelson JS, Gotlin LP. DTP reactions and serologic response with a reduced dose schedule. J Pediatr 105:189–194, 1984.

Bartelloni PJ, Marshall JD Jr, Cavanaugh DC. Clinical and serological responses to plague vaccine U.S.P. Milit Med 138:720–722, 1973.

Berger R, Just M. Vaccination against hepatitis A: control 3 years after the first vaccination. Vaccine 10:295, 1992.

Berkowitz CD, Ward JI, Meier K, Hendley JC, Brunnell PA, Barkin RA, Zahradnik J, Samuelson J, Gorden L. Safety and immunogenicity of Haemophilus influenzae type b polysaccharide and polysaccharide diphtheria toxoid conjugate vaccines in children 15–24 months. J Pediatr 110:509–514, 1987.

Bernier FH. Improved inactivated poliovirus vaccine: an update. Pediatr Infect Dis 5:289–292, 1986.

Bijkerk H. Surveillance and control of poliomyelitis in the Netherlands. Rev Infect Dis 6(Suppl.):S451–S456, 1984.

Black SB, Shinefield HR. Northern California Permanente Medical Care Program, Departments of Pediatrics Vaccine Study Group. b-Capsia I. Haemophilus influenzae, type b, capsular polysaccharide vaccine safety. Pediatrics 79:321–325, 1987.

Black SB, Shinefield HR, Fireman B, Hiatt R, Polen M, Vittinghoff E. Efficacy in infancy of oligosaccharide conjugate Haemophilus influenzae type b (HbOC) vaccine in a United States population of 61,080 children. Pediatr Infect Dis J 10:97–104, 1991.

Bottiger M. Long-term immunity following vaccination with killed poliovirus vaccine in Sweden, a country with no circulating poliovirus. Rev Infect Dis 6(Suppl.):S548–S551, 1984.

Brachman PS, Gold H, Plotkin SA, Fekety FR, Werrin M, Ingraham NR. Field evaluation of a human anthrax vaccine. Am J Public Health 52:632–645, 1962.

Broome CV, Fraser DW. Pertussis in the United States, 1979: a look at vaccine efficacy. J Infect Dis 144:187–190, 1981.

Burke DS. Immunization against tularemia: analysis of the effectiveness of live Francisella tularensis vaccine in prevention of laboratory-acquired tularemia. J Infect Dis 135:55–60, 1977.

Candel S. Epididymitis in mumps, including orchitis: further clinical studies and comments. Ann Intern Med 34:20–24, 1951.

Centers for Disease Control and Prevention. Cholera vaccine. MMWR 27(20):173–174, 1978a.

Centers for Disease Control and Prevention. Goal to eliminate measles from the United States. MMWR 27(41):391, 1978b.

Centers for Disease Control and Prevention. BCG vaccines. MMWR 28(21):241–244, 1979.

Centers for Disease Control and Prevention. Diphtheria, tetanus and pertussis: guidelines for vaccine prophylaxis and other preventive measures. MMWR 30(32):392–407, 1981.

Centers for Disease Control and Prevention. Annual summary. MMWR 31(54):142–144, 1982a.

Centers for Disease Control and Prevention. Childhood immunization initiative, United States—5-year follow-up. MMWR 31(17):231–232, 1982b.

Centers for Disease Control and Prevention. Measles prevention. MMWR 31(17):217–231, 1982c.

Centers for Disease Control and Prevention. Mumps vaccine. MMWR 31(46):617–625, 1982d.

Centers for Disease Control and Prevention. Pertussis surveillance. MMWR 31(25):333–336, 1982e.

Centers for Disease Control and Prevention. Plague vaccine. MMWR 31(22):301–304, 1982f.

Centers for Disease Control and Prevention. Poliomyelitis prevention. MMWR 31(3):22–34, 1982g.

Centers for Disease Control and Prevention. Efficacy of mumps vaccine—Ohio. MMWR 32(30):391–398, 1983a.

Centers for Disease Control and Prevention. Field evaluations of pre-exposure use of human diploid cell rabies vaccine. MMWR 32(46):601–603, 1983b.

Centers for Disease Control and Prevention. General recommendations on immunization. MMWR 32(1):1–17, 1983c.

Centers for Disease Control and Prevention. Anthrax and anthrax vaccine—adult immunization. MMWR 33(1S):33S–34S, 1984a.

Centers for Disease Control and Prevention. Practices Advisory Board—adult immunization. MMWR 33(1S):28S–29S, 1984b.

Centers for Disease Control and Prevention. Cholera—healthy information for international travel 1984. MMWR 33:70–71, 1984c.

Centers for Disease Control and Prevention. Measles—United States, 1983. MMWR 33(8):105–108, 1984d.

Centers for Disease Control and Prevention. Mumps outbreak—New Jersey. MMWR 33(29):421–430, 1984e.

Centers for Disease Control and Prevention. Plague—adult immunization. MMWR 33(1S):29S–30S, 1984f.

Centers for Disease Control and Prevention. Plague in the United States, 1983. MMWR 33(1S):15S–21S, 1984g.

Centers for Disease Control and Prevention. Rabies prevention—United States, 1984. MMWR 33(28):393–408, 1984h.

Centers for Disease Control and Prevention. Rubella prevention. MMWR 33(22):301–318, 1984i.

Centers for Disease Control and Prevention. Rubella vaccination during pregnancy—United States, 1971–1983. MMWR 33(26):365–373, 1984j.

Centers for Disease Control and Prevention. Systemic allergic reactions following immunization with human diploid cell rabies vaccine. MMWR 33(14):185–187, 1984k.

Centers for Disease Control and Prevention. Yellow fever vaccine. MMWR 32(52):679–688, 1984l.

Centers for Disease Control and Prevention. Diphtheria, tetanus, and pertussis: guidelines for vaccine prophylaxis and other preventive measures. MMWR 34(27):405–426, 1985.

Centers for Disease Control and Prevention. Poliomyelitis prevention: enhanced-potency inactivated poliomyelitis vaccine. MMWR 36(22):139–140, 1987.

Centers for Disease Control and Prevention. Update prevention of *Haemophilus influenzae* type b disease. MMWR 37(2):13–16, 1988.

Centers for Disease Control and Prevention. Measles prevention: recommendations of the Immunization Practices Advisory Committee (ACIP). MMWR 38(S-9):1–18, 1989.

Centers for Disease Control and Prevention. Hepatitis B virus: a comprehensive strategy for eliminating transmission in the United States through universal childhood vaccination. MMWR 40 (RR-13):1–25, 1991.

Centers for Disease Control and Prevention. Retrospective assessment of vaccination coverage among school-aged children—selected U.S. cities, 1991. MMWR 41:103–107, 1992.

Centers for Disease Control and Prevention. Prevention and control of influenza. Part I. Vaccines. MMWR 42(RR-6):1–14, 1993a.

Centers for Disease Control and Prevention. Laboratory-based surveillance for meningococcal disease in selected areas—United States, 1989–1991. MMWR 42(SS-2):21–30, 1993b.

Centers for Disease Control and Prevention. Hepatitis surveillance report no. 55. Atlanta, Centers for Disease Control and Prevention, 1994.

Centers for Disease Control and Prevention. Recommendations of the Advisory Committee on Immunization Practices: revised recommendations for routine poliomyelitis vaccination. MMWR 48(27): 590, 1999a.

Centers for Disease Control and Prevention. Human rabies prevention—United States, 1999. Recommendations of the Advisory Committee on Immunization Practices. MMWR 8(48): 1-21, 1999b.

Centers for Disease Control and Prevention. Recommended childhood immunization schedule—United States, 2000. MMWR 49(2): 35-38, 2000a.

Centers for Disease Control and Prevention. Preventing pneumococcal disease among infants and young children. MMWR 49(RR-9), 2000b.

Centers for Disease Control and Prevention. Notice to readers: update: expanded availability of thimerosal preservative-free hepatitis B vaccine MMWR 49(28);642-651, 2000c.

Centers for Disease Control and Prevention. Prevention and control of meningococcal disease. Recommendations of the Advisory Committee on Immunization Practices (ACIP). MMWR 49(7): 1-10, 2000d.

Chen ST, Edsall G, Peel MM, Sinnathvray TA. Timing of antenatal tetanus immunization for effective protection of the neonate. Bull WHO 61:159–165, 1983.

Cherry JD, Feigin RD, Lobes LA, Hinthorn DR, Shackelford PG, Shirley RH, Lins RD, Choi CS. Urban measles in the vaccine era: a clinical epidemiologic and serologic study. J Pediatr 81:217–230, 1972.

Cherry JD, Feigin RD, Shackelford PG, Hinthorn DR, Schmidt RR. A clinical and serologic study of 103 children with measles vaccine failure. J Pediatr 82:802–808, 1973.

Christensen PE, Schmidt H, Bang HO, et al. An epidemic of measles in Southern Greenland in 1951. Acta Med Scand 144:430–450, 1953.

Clemens JD, Chuong JJH, Feinstein AR. The BCG controversy: a methodological and statistical reappraisal. JAMA 249:2362–2369, 1983.

Cochi SL, Broome CV, Hightower AW. Immunization of U.S. children with *Haemophilus influenzae* type B polysaccharide vaccine: a cost-effectiveness model of strategy assessment. JAMA 253:521–529, 1985.

Cody CL, Baraff LJ, Cherry JD, March SM, Manclark CR. Nature and rates of adverse reactions associated with DTP and DT immunizations in infants and children. Pediatrics 68:650–660, 1981.

Crossley K, Irvine P, Warren JB, Lee BK, Mead K. Tetanus and diphtheria immunity in urban Minnesota adults. JAMA 242:2298–2300, 1979.

Danovaro-Holliday MC, LeBaron CW, Allensworth C, Raymond R, Borden TG, Murray AB, Icenogle JP, Reef SE. A large rubella outbreak with spread from the workplace to the community. JAMA 284:2733–2739, 2000.

Daum RS, Granoff DM. A vaccine against *Haemophilus influenzae* type b. Pediatr Infect Dis 4:355–357, 1985.

Dixon CW. Smallpox. London, JA Churchill, 1962.

Edsall G, Elliott MW, Peebles TC, Levine L, Eldred MC. Excessive use of tetanus toxoid boosters. JAMA 202:17019, 1967.

Ellison RT III, Kohler PF, Curd JG, Judson FN, Keller LB. Prevalence of congenital or acquired complement deficiency in patients with sporadic meningococcal disease. N Engl J Med 308:913–916, 1983.

Enders JF, Katz SL, Milovanovic MW, Holloway A. Studies on an attenuated measles virus vaccine. I. Development and preparation of the vaccine. N Engl J Med 263:153–159, 1960.

Feigin RD, Baker CJ, Herwaldt LA, Lampe RM, Mason EO, Whitney SE. Epidemic meningococcal disease in an elementary school classroom. N Engl J Med 307:1255–1257, 1982.

Felsenfeld O, Wolf RH, Gyr K, Grant LS, Dutta NK, Zarifi AZ, Zafari Y. Simultaneous vaccination against cholera and yellow fever. Lancet 1:457–458, 1973.

Fenner F. Global eradication of smallpox. Rev Infect Dis 4:916–922, 1982.

Fox AS, Lepow ML: Tuberculin skin testing in Vietnamese refugees with a history of BCG vaccination. Am J Dis Child 137:1093–1094, 1983.

Fulginiti VA. Simultaneous measles exposure and immunization. Arch Ges Virusforsch 16:300–304, 1964.

Fulginiti VA, Arthur JH, Pearlman DS. Altered reactivity to measles virus: local reactions following attenuated measles virus immunization in children who previously received a combination of inactivated and attenuated vaccines. Am J Dis Child 115:671–675, 1968.

Fulginiti VA, Arthur JH, Pearlman S, Kempe CH. Altered reactivity to measles virus: skin test reactivity and antibody response to measles virus antigens in recipients of killed measles virus vaccine. J Pediatr 75:609–616, 1969.

Fulginiti VA, Eller JJ, Downie AW. Altered reactivity to measles virus: atypical measles in children previously immunized with inactivated measles virus vaccines. JAMA 202:1075–1078, 1967.

Fulginiti VA, Leland OS, Kempe CH. Evaluation of measles immunization methods. Am J Dis Child 105:509, 1963.

Glezen WP. Consideration of the risk of influenza in children and indications for prophylaxis. Rev Infect Dis 2:408–420, 1980.

Glezen WP, Frank AL, Taber LH, Tristan MP, Vallbona C, Paredes A, Allison JE. Influenza in childhood. Pediatr Res 17:1029–1032, 1983.

Gold R, Lepow ML, Goldschneider I, Draper TF, Gotschlich EC. Kinetics in antibody production of group A and group C meningococcal polysaccharide vaccines and administered during the first six years of life: prospects for routine immunization of infants and children. J Infect Dis 140:690–697, 1979.

Goldsmith S, Rosenberg E, Pollaczek EH. A study of the antibody response to a dose of tetanus toxoid. N Engl J Med 267:485–487, 1962.

Good RA, Kelly WD, Rotstein J, Varco RL. Immunologic deficiency diseases. Progr Allergy 6:187–319, 1962.

Greenwood BM, Hassan-King M, Whittle HC. Prevention of secondary cases of meningococcal disease in household contacts by vaccination. Br Med J 1:1317–1319, 1978.

Grenier B, Hamza B, Biron G, Xueref C, Viarme F, Roumiantzeff M.

Gross PA, Lee H, Wolff JA, Hall CB, Minnefore AB, Lazicki ME. Influenza immunization in immunosuppressed children. J Pediatr 92:30–35, 1978.

Guyer B, Freedman MA, Strobino DM, Sondik EJ. Annual summary of vital statistics: trends in the health of Americans during the 20th century. Pediatrics 106:1307–1317, 2000.

Hankins WA, Gwaltney JM Jr, Hendley JO, Farquhar JD, Samuelson JS. Clinical and serological evaluation of a meningococcal polysaccharide vaccine: groups A, C, Y and W 135(41306). Proc Soc Exp Biol Med 169:54–57, 1982.

Hattwick MAW, Rubin RH, Music S, Sikes RK, Smith JS, Gregg MB. Postexposure rabies prophylaxis with human rabies immune globulin. JAMA 227:407–410, 1974.

Helmick CG. The epidemiology of human rabies postexposure prophylaxis, 1980–1981. JAMA 250:1990–1996, 1983.

Herrman KL, Halstead SB, Wiebenga NH. Rubella antibody persistence after immunization. JAMA 247:193–196, 1982.

Hilleman M, Buynak EB, Weibel RE. Development and evaluation of the Moraten measles virus vaccine. JAMA 206:487–491, 1968a.

Hilleman MR, Buynak EB, Weibel RE, Stokes J Jr. Live, attenuated mumps-virus vaccine. N Engl J Med 278:227–232, 1968.

Hinman AR, Orenstein WA, Bloch AB, Bart KJ, Eddins, DL, Amler RW, Kirby CD. Impact of measles in the United States. Rev Infect Dis 5:439–444, 1983.

Hinman AR, Koplan JP. Pertussis and pertussis vaccine. Reanalysis of benefits, risks, and costs. JAMA 251:3109–3113, 1984.

Hirtz DG, Nelson KB, Ellenberg JH. Seizures following childhood immunizations. J Pediatr 102:14–18, 1983.

Innis BL, Snitbhan R, Kunasol P. Protection against hepatitis A by inactivated vaccine. JAMA 271:1328–1334, 1994.

Jacobs RL, Lowe RS, Lanier BQ. Adverse reactions to tetanus toxoid. JAMA 247:40–42, 1982.

Jacobson JA, Filice GA, Holloway JT. Meningococcal disease in day-care centers. Pediatrics 59:299–300, 1977.

James JM, Burks AW, Roberson PK, Sampson HA. N Engl J Med 332:1262–1266, 1995.

Kanai K: Japan's experience in pertussis epidemiology and vaccination in the past thirty years. Jpn J Med Sci Biol 33:107–143, 1980.

Katz SL, Enders JF, Holloway A. Studies on attenuated measles virus vaccine. VIII. General summary and results of vaccination. N Engl J Med 263:180, 1960.

Kaythy H, Karanko V, Peltola H. Serum antibodies after vaccination with Haemophilus influenzae type b capsular polysaccharide and responses to reimmunization: no evidence of immunologic tolerance or memory. Pediatrics 74:857–865, 1984.

Kaythy H, Karanko V, Peltola H, Sarno S, Makela PH. Serum antibodies to capsular polysaccharide vaccine in group A Neisseria meningitidis followed for three years in infants and children. J Infect Dis 142:861–868, 1980.

Kaythy H, Peltola H, Karanko V. The protective level of serum antibodies to the capsular polysaccharide of Haemophilus influenzae type b. J Infect Dis 147:1100, 1983.

Kempe CH, Fulginiti VA. The pathogenesis of measles virus infection. Arch Ges Viruforsch 16:103–128, 1964.

Kendrick P. A field study of alum-precipitated combined pertussis vaccine and diphtheria toxoid for active immunization. Am J Hyg 38:193–202, 1943.

Keitel, WA, Thomas RC, Nino, D, Huggins, LL, Six, HR, Quarles, JM, Couch, RB. Immunization against influenza: comparison of various topical and parenteral regimens containing inactivated and/or live attenuated vaccines in health adults. J Infect Dis 183:329–332, 2001.

Krugman S. Present status of measles and rubella immunization in the United States: a medical progress report. J Pediatr 90:1–5, 1977.

Krugman S. Further-attenuated measles vaccine: characteristics and use. Rev Infect Dis 5:477–481, 1983.

Krugman S, Ward R. Infectious hepatitis: current status of prevention with gamma globulin. Yale J Biol Med 34:329–333, 1961–1962.

Lange B, Shapiro SA, Waldman MTG, Proctor E, Arbeter A. Antibody responses to influenza immunization of children with acute lymphoblastic leukemia. J Infect Dis 140:402–406, 1979.

Lapinleimu K. Elimination of poliomyelitis in Finland. Rev Infect Dis 6(Suppl.):S457–S460, 1984.

Lerman SJ, Bollinger M, Brunken JM. Clinical and serologic evaluation of measles, mumps, and rubella (HPV-77: DE-5 and RA 27/3) virus vaccines, singly and in combination. Pediatrics 68:18–22, 1981.

Lewis FA, Gust ID, Bennett MM. On the etiology of whooping cough. J Hyg 71:139, 1973.

Lieu T, Cochi SL, Black SB. Cost-effectiveness of a routine varicella vaccination program for U.S. children. JAMA 271:375–381, 1994.

Luelmo F. BCG vaccination. Am Rev Resp Dis 125(Suppl.):70–73, 1982.

Mann JM. Systematic decision-making in rabies prophylaxis. Pediatr Infect Dis 2:162–167, 1983.

Meningococcal Disease Surveillance Group. Meningococcal disease: secondary attack rate and chemoprophylaxis in the United States, 1974. JAMA 235:261–265, 1976.

Merigan TC, Petralli JK, Wilbur J. Circulating human interferon induced by measles vaccination and its in vitro antiviral efficacy (abstract). Clin Res 13:197, 1965.

Miller DL, Alderslade R, Ross EM. Whooping cough and whooping cough vaccine: the risks and benefits debate. Epidemiol Rev 41:1–24, 1982.

Miller DL, Ross EM, Alderslade R, Bellman MH, Rawson NSB. Pertussis immunization and serious acute neurological illness in children. Br Med J 282:1595–1599, 1981.

Miller LW, Older JJ, Drake J, Zimmerman S. Diphtheria immunization: effect upon carriers and the control of outbreaks. Am J Dis Child 123:197–199, 1972.

Munford RS, Taunay A deE, de Morais JS, Fraser DW, Feldman RA. Spread of meningococcal infection within households. Lancet 1:1275–1278, 1974.

Nathanson N, Bodian D. Experimental poliomyelitis following intramuscular virus infection. III. The effect of passive antibody on paralysis and viremia. Bull Johns Hopkins Hosp 111:198–220, 1962.

National Vaccine Advisory Committee. The measles epidemic: the problems, barriers, and recommendations. JAMA 266:1547–1552, 1991.

Nightingale E. Recommendations for a national policy on poliomyelitis vaccination. N Engl J Med 297:249–253, 1977.

Ogra PL, Karzon DT, Righthand F. Immunoglobulin response in serum and secretions after immunization with live and inactivated polio vaccine and natural infection. N Engl J Med 279:893–900, 1968.

Orenstein WA, Bart KJ, Hinman HR, et al. The opportunity and obligation to eliminate rubella from the United States. JAMA 251:1988–1994, 1984.

Osterholm MT, Rambeck JH, White KE. Lack of protective efficacy and increased risk of disease within 7 days after vaccination associated with Haemophilus influenzae type b (Hib) polysaccharide (PS) vaccine use in Minnesota (abstract). Abstracts of the 27th ICAAC, New York, 1987.

Paisley JW, Bruhn FW, Lauer BA, McIntosh K. Type A2 influenza viral infections in children. Am J Dis Child 132:34–36, 1978.

Peebles TC, Levine L, Eldred MC, Edsall G. Tetanus-toxoid emergency boosters: a reappraisal. N Engl J Med 280:575–581, 1969.

Peltola H, Kaythy H, Sivonen A, Makela PH. Haemophilus influenzae type b capsular polysaccharide vaccine in children: A double-blind field study of 100,000 vaccines 3 months to 5 years of age in Finland. Pediatrics 60:730–737, 1977a.

Peter G. Childhood immunizations. N Engl J Med 327:1794–1800, 1992.

Pincus DJ, Morrison D, Andrews C, Lawrence E, Sell SH, Wright PF. Age-related response to two Haemophilus influenzae type b vaccines. J Pediatr 100:197–201, 1982.

Plotkin SA, Smiley ML, Friedman HM, Starr SE, Fleischer GR, Wlodaver G, Dafoe DC, Friedman AD, Grossman RA, Bahker CF. Prevention of cytomegalovirus disease by Towne strain live attenuated vaccine. In Plotkin SA, Michelson S, Pagano JS, Rapp F, eds. CMV: Pathogenesis and Prevention of Human Infection. New York, Alan R. Liss, 1984, pp 271–284.

Preblud SR, Orenstein WA, Koplan JP, Bart KJ, Hinman AR. A benefit-cost analysis of a childhood vaccination program. Postgrad Med J 61:17–22, 1985.

Puziss M, Wright GG. Studies on immunity in anthrax. X. Gel-Absorbed protective antigen for immunization of man. J Bacteriol 85:230–236, 1963.

Rauh LW, Schmidt R. Measles immunization with killed virus vaccine. Am J Dis Child 109:232–234, 1965.

Riley ID, Tarr PI, Andrews M, Pfeiffer M, Howard R, Challands P, Jennison G, Douglas RM. Immunization with a polyvalent pneumococcal vaccine: reduction of adult respiratory mortality in a New Guinea highlands community. Lancet 1:1338–1341, 1977.

Robbins JB, Austrian R, Lee C-J, Rastogi SC, Schiffman G, Henrichsen J, Makela PH, Broome CV, Facklam RR, Tiesjema RH, Parke JC Jr. Consideration for formulating the second-generation pneumococcal capsular polysaccharide vaccine with emphasis on the cross-reactive types within groups. J Infect Dis 148:1136–1159, 1983.

Rosenzweig EC, Babione RW, Wisseman CL Jr. Immunological studies with group B arthropod-borne viruses. IV. Persistence of yellow fever antibodies following vaccination with 17D strain yellow fever vaccine. Am J Trop Med Hyg 12:230–235, 1963.

Sabin AB. Strategies for elimination of poliomyelitis in different parts of the world with use of oral poliovirus vaccine. Rev Infect Dis 6(Suppl.):S391–S396, 1984.

Sako W. Studies on pertussis immunization. J Pediatr 30:29–40, 1947.

Salk D. Eradication of poliomyelitis in the United States. II. Experience with killed poliovirus vaccine. Rev Infect 2:243–257, 1980a.

Salk D. Eradication of poliomyelitis in the United States. III. Polio vaccines—practical considerations. Rev Infect Dis 2:258–273, 1980b.

Salk J, Salk D. Control of influenza and poliomyelitis with inactivated vaccines. Science 195:834–847, 1977.

Santosham M, Wolff M, Reid R, Hohenboken M, Bateman M, Goepp J, Cortese M, Sack D, Hill J, Newcomer W, Capriotti L, Smith J, Owen M, Gahagan S, Hu D, Kling R, Lukacs L, Ellis RW, Vella PP, Calandra G, Matthews H, Ahonkhai V. The efficacy in Navaho infants of a conjugate vaccine consisting of Haemophilus influenzae type b polysaccharide and Neisseria meningitidis outer-membrane protein complex. N Engl J Med 324:1767–1772, 1991.

Sato Y, Kimura M, Fukumi H. Development of a pertussis component vaccine in Japan. Lancet 1:122–126, 1984.

Schneerson R, Barrera O, Sutton A, Robbins JB. Preparation, characterization and immunogenicity of Haemophilus influenzae type b polysaccharide protein conjugates. J Exp Med 152:361–376, 1980.

Schwarz AJ. Immunization against measles: development and evaluation of a highly attenuated live measles vaccine. Ann Pediatr (Stockh) 202:241–252, 1964.

Siber GR, Werner BG, Halsey NA, Reid R, Almeido-Hill J, Garrett SC, Thompson C, Santosham M. Interference of immune globulin with measles and rubella immunization. J Pediatr 122:204–211, 1993.

Smit P, Oberholzer D, Hayden-Smith S, Koornhof HJ, Hilleman MR. Protective efficacy of pneumococcal polysaccharide vaccines. JAMA 238:2613–2616, 1977.

Smith MH. National Childhood Vaccine Injury Compensation Act. Pediatrics 82:264–269, 1988.

Stern H. Live cytomegalovirus vaccination of healthy volunteers: Eight-year follow-up studies. In Plotkin SA, Michelson S, Pagano JS, Rapp F, eds. CMV: Pathogenesis and Prevention of Human Infections. New York, Alan R Liss, 1984, pp 263–269.

Stewart GT. Vaccination against whooping cough: efficacy versus risks. Lancet 1:234–239, 1977.

Sultz HA, Hart BA, Zielezny M. Is mumps virus an etiologic factor in juvenile diabetes mellitus? J Pediatr 86:654–656, 1975.

Taunay A deE, Galvao PA, de Morais JS, Gotschlich EC, Feldman RA. Disease prevention by meningococcal serogroup C polysaccharide vaccine in preschool children: results after eleven months in São Paulo, Brazil. Pediatr Res 8:429, 1974.

Taylor DN, Pollard RA, Blake PA. Typhoid in the United States and the risk to the international traveler. J Infect Dis 148:599–602, 1983.

Thompson NJ, Glassroth JL, Snider DE Jr, Farer LS. The booster phenomenon in serial tuberculin testing. Am Rev Respir Dis 119:587–597, 1979.

Townsend JT, Baringer JR, Wolinsky JS. Progressive rubella panencephalitis: late onset after congenital rubella. N Engl J Med 292:990–993, 1975.

Tsolia M, Gershon A, Steinberg S, Gelb L. Live attenuated varicella vaccine: evidence that the virus is attenuated and the importance of skin lesions in transmission of varicella-zoster virus. J Pediatr 116:184–189, 1990.

Vitek C, Wenger J. Diphtheria. Bull WHO 76: 129–130, 1998.

Vitek CR, Pascual FB, Baughman AL, Murphy TV. Increase in deaths from pertussis among young infants in the United States in the 1990s. Pediatr Infect Dis J 22:628–634, 2003.

von Seefried A, Chun JH, Grant JA, Letvenuk L, Pearson EW. Inactivated poliovirus vaccine and test development at Connaught Laboratories Ltd. Rev Infect Dis 6(Suppl. 2):S345–S349, 1984.

Wahdan MH, Rizk F, El-Akkad AM, El Ghoroury AA, Hablas R, Girgis NI, Amer A, Boctar W, Sippel JE, Gotschlich EC, Triav R, Sanborn WR, Cvjetanovic B. A controlled field trial of a serogroup A meningococcal polysaccharide vaccine. Bull WHO 48:667–673, 1973.

Watson BM, Piercy SA, Plotkin SA, Starr SE. Modified chickenpox in children immunized with the Oka/Merck varicella vaccine. Pediatrics 91:17–22, 1993.

Werzberger A, Mensch B, Kuter B. A controlled trial of a formalin-inactivated hepatitis A vaccine in healthy children. N Engl J Med 327:453–457, 1992.

Wilkins J, Wehrle PF. Additional evidence against measles vaccine administration to infants less than 12 months of age: altered immune response following active/passive immunization. J Pediatr 94:865–869, 1979.

Wilkins J, Wehrle PFA. Evidence for reinstatement of infants 12–14 months of age into routine measles immunization programs. Am J Dis Child 132:164–166, 1978.

Wisseman CL Jr, Sweet BH. Immunological studies with group B arthropod-borne viruses. III. Response of human subjects to revaccination with 17D strain yellow fever vaccine. Am J Trop Med Hyg 11:570–575, 1962.

Yeager AS, Davis JH, Ross LA. Measles immunization: successes and failures. JAMA 237:347–351, 1977.

CHAPTER

43

Transplantation

Rebecca H. Buckley

HISTORICAL ASPECTS

Although replacement of injured or diseased parts of the body with those of others has been an aspiration of many from ancient times, this feat was accomplished only within the past 50 years. This achievement followed recognition of the immunologic nature of graft rejection, first demonstrated by the skin grafting experiments of Medawar (1944). He showed that the first skin graft from an unrelated donor was rejected more rapidly and that autologous grafts were never rejected. Medawar (1946) later demonstrated that injections of leukocytes sensitized the recipient to subsequent skin grafts from the leukocyte donor and inferred from this that leukocytes carried transplantation antigens.

Prior to 1955, only isolated reports of attempted (largely unsuccessful) organ transplants had appeared in the scientific literature. Since then, the explosive growth of transplantation is attested by the fact that by 2001, 535,075 kidney transplants had been reported from 588 transplant centers worldwide, along with 117,984 stem

1400

cell transplants from 249 centers, 61,195 heart transplants from 236 centers, 100,179 liver transplants from 235 centers, 17,002 pancreas or pancreas–kidney transplants from 163 centers, 297 intestinal transplants from 10 centers, and 16,432 lung or heart–lung transplants from 120 centers, for a total of 848,164 transplants in the last half century (Cecka and Terasaki, 2002).

Organ and tissue transplantations have the greatest potential application to pediatrics, because fatal or debilitating disease of single organs is more common in young patients. In addition to the proven usefulness of renal transplantation for renal failure; bone marrow transplantation for immunodeficiency, aplastic anemia, leukemia, and inborn errors of metabolism; liver transplantation for biliary atresia; and skin transplantation for burns, other organs, and tissues have also proved successful in children, including transplantation of the lungs and the heart, the parathyroids, and the pancreas.

Since the last edition of this book, another major therapeutic advance occurred in that reinfusions of autologous marrow cells transfected with normal genes corrected both X-linked and adenosine deaminase (ADA)-deficient severe combined immunodeficiency (SCID) (Aiuti et al., 2002; Hacein-Bey-Abina et al., 2002). However, serious adverse events in two such patients have halted further such attempts at therapy.

Despite progress in the technical aspects of organ transplantation and in the development of immunosuppressive agents capable of preventing early organ graft rejection, the histocompatibility barrier still limits the long-term survival rate of solid organ graft recipients and is of major importance in all aspects of bone marrow transplantation. However, an insufficient number of donor organs is the larger problem for solid organ transplantation.

This chapter presents current knowledge of the major transplantation antigens, cells, antibodies, and types of reactions responsible for graft rejection; the methods available for identifying such antigens and for matching donor and recipient; the means by which the immune response can be manipulated to control graft rejection; and the clinical experience with various organ and tissue grafting in pediatrics.

HISTOCOMPATIBILITY ANTIGENS AND DONOR–RECIPIENT PAIRING

The Major Histocompatibility Complex

Transplantation or histocompatibility antigens are those antigens present on tissue cells that are capable of inducing an immune response in a genetically dissimilar (allogeneic) recipient, resulting in their rejection. Much of the information on histocompatibility antigens came initially from studies in inbred strains of mice, in which at least 30 independently segregating genetic loci encoding for such antigens were identified (Klein, 1975). Their gene products are called *alloantigens,* because they occur as genetically dissimilar forms within the species. Early on, it was noted that although genetic disparity between donor and recipient mice for any of these loci led to eventual graft rejection, differences in the H-2 genetic complex resulted in the most rapid and vigorous rejection. Thus the H-2 complex was identified as the major histocompatibility complex (MHC) of mice; loci coding for antigens evoking weaker responses were termed *minor* loci.

In every mammalian species that has been studied subsequently, a single genetic complex has been found to encode histocompatibility antigens with rejection-inducing potency similar to those of H-2. Examples of MHCs in other species include the B complex in chickens, the AgB complex in rats, the DLA complex in dogs, the SLA locus in swine, the RhL-A complex in monkeys, and the H-1 complex in rabbits. Each MHC is genetically complex because it includes many different loci, each encoding separate cell surface proteins, and because these loci demonstrate extreme polymorphism.

The Human Major Histocompatibility Complex: HLA

Recognition of the genetic region encoding the human major histocompatibility complex in 1967 (Bach and Amos, 1967) was the result of a 15-year effort by many investigators throughout the world and was a major breakthrough for clinical organ and tissue transplantation. Similarities between histocompatibility antigens of animals and humans began to be appreciated when Amos (1953) identified transplantation antigens on mouse leukocytes by leukoagglutination and Dausset (1954) found that 90% of 60 multitransfused humans had leukocyte agglutinins in their sera. Dausset then correctly deduced that leukocyte alloantigens present in transfused blood were frequently responsible for alloimmunization against human histocompatibility antigens.

A far more common cause of such alloimmunization was appreciated in 1958, however, when Payne and Rolfs (1958) and van Rood and co-workers (1958) independently demonstrated alloantibodies to human leukocyte antigens (HLAs) in sera from multiparous women. It was later recognized that such antibodies are also found in the sera of recipients of tissue or organ grafts.

In 1968, Amos and Bach presented convincing evidence for the existence of a single chromosomal region controlling the inheritance of the major human histocompatibility antigens; they showed that compatibility by leukocyte typing correlated with compatibility in mixed leukocyte culture (MLC) in pairs of siblings from seven large families.

The World Health Organization (WHO) Nomenclature Committee in 1968 proposed that the leukocyte antigens controlled by the closely linked genes of the human MHC be designated by the letters *HLA.* This committee has convened every 2 to 3 years since. At each meeting, new genes, alleles, and antigens were identified. Thus a very large number of genes have been found within the HLA region over the past 36 years, and enormous strides have been made in understanding the serology, biochemistry, and biologic functions of their gene products (Bodmer et al., 1999; Klein and Sato, 2000a, 2000b; Schreuder et al., 2001).

Nomenclature, Location, and Structure

The multiple genetic loci of the human MHC reside on the short arm of chromosome 6 (Fig. 43-1). The HLA complex contains in excess of 200 genes, more than 40 of which encode leucocyte antigens (Forbes and Trowsdale, 1999; Klein and Sato, 2000a). They and their cell surface and soluble protein products are divided into three classes (I, II, and III) on the basis of their tissue distribution, structure, and function (Bodmer et al., 1999; Klein and Sato, 2000a, 2000b). Class I and II genes encode for HLA cell surface antigens, which are codominantly expressed, and class III for several components of the complement system; all share important roles in immune function.

CLASS I MHC ANTIGENS

Class I MHC antigens are present on all nucleated cells and are each composed of a 45-kD α heavy chain encoded by genes of the HLA-A, HLA-B, or HLA-C loci on chromosome 6 and associated noncovalently with a 12-kD protein, β$_2$-microglobulin (β$_2$m) encoded by a gene on chromosome 15 (Klein and Sato, 2000a). The α chains are composed of approximately 340 amino acid residues that form three extracellular domains, a transmembrane part, and an intracytoplasmic tail (Fig. 43-2). The β chain (β$_2$m) is nonpolymorphic and consists entirely of a single extracellular domain of 100 amino acids.

The alloantigenic activity of class I antigens is determined exclusively by hypervariable regions of the N-terminal domains of the 45-kD α heavy chain (Klein and Sato, 2000a). These proteins, similar to products of the K and D loci in the mouse, are now recognized as the principal targets for CD8+ cytotoxic T cells (Klein and Sato, 2000a).

CLASS II MHC ANTIGENS

By contrast, MHC class II antigens have a more limited tissue distribution and are expressed only on B lymphocytes, monocyte–macrophages, Langerhans cells, dendritic cells, endothelium, activated T lymphocytes, and epithelial cells (Klein and Sato, 2000b). Each is a heterodimer composed of noncovalently associated α and β chains of approximately 230 amino acids encoded by

genes of the HLA-D region. The α chains have a molecular mass between 29 and 34 kD; the β chains, between 25 and 28 kD. Both chains form two extracellular domains, a transmembrane part, and an intracytoplasmic tail (see Fig. 43-2). Class II MHC molecules present antigenic peptides to CD4+ T-helper lymphocytes.

The genetic organization of the HLA loci is depicted schematically in Figure 43-1. In addition to the well-known HLA class I A, B, and C genes shown, there are seven more class I genes—HLA-E, HLA-F, HLA-G, HLA-H, HLA-J, HLA-K, and HLA-L—and five class II "families" of genes—referred to as HLA-DM, HLA-DO, HLA-DP, HLA-DQ, and HLA-DR (Table 43-1) (Bodmer et al., 1999; Klein and Sato, 2000b; Schreuder et al., 2001). Each of the latter families includes at least one α gene and one or more β genes. Thus, because genes of two separate MHC loci encode the α and β chains of each family's heterodimer, one cannot refer simply to "the" DR, DQ, or DP genes, for example, but must also specify the α or β chain gene. Only the DP and DQ α chains are polymorphic; the DR α chain shows no variation. One nonpolymorphic α gene and nine β genes have been identified in the DR family.

In most DR haplotypes (see following discussion), the product of the α gene associates on the cell surface with the product of the DRβ1 gene to form the DR αβ1 heterodimer. The DRβ1 genes are highly polymorphic; there are 271 alleles encoding for variations on the classic DR antigens (Bodmer et al., 1999; Schreuder et al., 2001). The DRβ3 allele encodes additional "supertypic" DR molecules, variations on DR52, and the DRβ4 allele for variations on DR53. DR52 occurs with DR3, DR5, DR6, and DR8 and DR53 with DR4, DR7, and DR9. DRβ 2 and DR 6-9 genes are not expressed and are referred to as *pseudogenes* (see Table 43-1) (Klein and Sato, 2000b).

The DQ gene family contains two α chain genes, of which one is very polymorphic, and three β chain genes, one of which encodes the presently recognized DQ antigens. DQ antigens are referred to as being *supertypic* to DR antigens. This means that whenever a particular DQ specificity is present, any one of several DR specificities may be present. For example, all Caucasians who are DR1, DR2, or DRw6 positive are also DQ1 positive. It is generally considered that DQ is the homolog of murine I-A and DR the homolog of murine I-E.

The DP family has two α and two β genes; only one of each has an expressed gene product. Finally, there are other genes within the HLA region, including DOB,

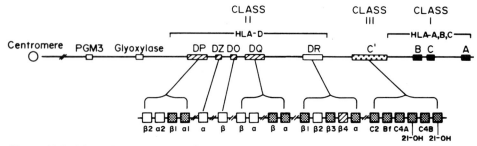

Figure 43-1 · Schematic representation of the human leukocyte antigen (HLA) region on the short arm of chromosome 6. Open squares in the HLA-D region represent genes that may not be expressed.

not possible to detect all parental HLA antigens by serotyping. Nonetheless, observations on the intrafamilial reaction patterns usually permit genotyping even when all antigens are not identified.

Molecular Typing

SEQUENCE-SPECIFIC OLIGONUCLEOTIDE GENOTYPING

Sequence-specific oligonucleotide (SSO) genotyping permits far more precise and detailed HLA typing than can be achieved with serologic or lymphocyte functional typing methods. It is carried out on polymerase chain reaction (PCR)-amplified DNA by oligonucleotide hybridization. A number of variations on this technique have been developed, but a particularly useful semiautomated method was developed by Cros and colleagues (1992). This consists of PCR amplification of DNA from lysed cells, followed by sequence-specific oligonucleotide probe (SSOP) typing using microtiter plates or paper strips, followed by automatic colorimetric reading. The entire typing assay can be completed in less than 4 hours and has been validated on more than 1000 haplotypes in prospective DR typing of patients and their potential donors (Cros et al., 1992). It is simple enough for routine laboratory use.

SEQUENCE-SPECIFIC PRIMER TYPING

Molecular typing can also be performed with PCR amplification of purified DNA, using sequence-specific primers (SSP) for each HLA gene being tested and gel analysis. A version of this is termed Reference Strand Mediated Conformation Analysis (RSCA), which differs in that HLA type is assigned on the basis of accurate measurement of conformation-dependent DNA mobility in polyacrylamide gel electrophoresis (PAGE) (Arguello and Madrigal, 1999).

UNIVERSAL HETERODUPLEX GENERATOR CROSS-MATCHING

Another DNA-based matching technique is that of universal heteroduplex generator (UHG) cross-matching (Clay et al., 1994). UHG is a rapid and simple method of screening prospective bone marrow donors for HLA-DPβ1 compatibility with the recipient. The method relies on the visual comparison of PCR heteroduplex banding patterns on nondenaturing polyacrylamide minigels. It determines whether pairs or groups of samples are HLA-DPβ1 matched or mismatched, but it does not permit direct assignment of HLA-DPβ1 alleles. In a comparative study with SSO typing, 52 of 56 (93%) pairs showed concordant findings in UHG cross-matching (Clay et al., 1994).

Lymphocyte-Defined Antigen Typing

Lymphocyte-defined HLA class II antigens are detected through their stimulatory capacity in the mixed leukocyte reaction (MLR). This test is performed by mixing blood leukocytes from donor and recipient in tissue culture for 5 to 6 days and noting, through ^{3}H-thymidine incorporation, the amount of DNA synthesis; the latter indicates the degree of reactivity of the two cell populations against alloantigens of each other (Bach and Hirschhorn, 1964; Bain et al., 1964).

In actual practice, the bidirectional response in an MLR is usually prevented so that the reactivity of each cell population can be measured separately. This is accomplished by pretreating one population of cells with either x-irradiation or mitomycin C to arrest DNA synthesis and cell division, the so-called one-way MLR (Amos and Bach, 1968). The treated cells are still alive, with HLA class II membrane antigens intact, and hence are able to stimulate the untreated lymphoid cell population. The responding cell population is composed entirely of T lymphocytes, whereas the stimulating cells consist of B lymphocytes and monocytes, both of which bear HLA class II antigens.

The one-way MLR is used in intrafamilial typing to confirm that siblings who appear HLA-identical based on serotyping are also identical for T-lymphocyte–defined antigens. Although the precision of molecular typing in matching within families usually obviates the need for direct MLR testing, MLR testing can detect other class II antigen differences when unrelated donors are matched only for A, B, and DR antigens (Mickelson et al., 1994).

Cross-Matching

Serologic cross-matching is a form of matching the donor and recipient and is of particular importance to the success of primarily vascularized grafts, such as kidney and heart. Serum from the prospective recipient is tested against cells from the potential donor for the presence of antibodies to red blood cell and/or HLA antigens. The two-stage microlymphocytotoxicity test is usually used to detect the latter.

In most transplant centers, patients awaiting kidney or heart transplants are screened monthly for serum anti-HLA antibodies to a reference cell panel. This cross-match should also be performed near the time of the actual transplant, because these antibodies can form within a short period, particularly if the recipient is receiving blood transfusions. Conversely, the reactivity of sera from such patients can diminish despite their once having had a high titer (Sanfilippo et al., 1984).

The presence of such antibodies correlates with hyperacute renal graft rejection (Kissmeyer-Nielsen et al., 1966). For this reason, a positive serologic cross-match has been considered an absolute contraindication to renal transplantation. However, not all lymphotoxic antibodies in patients with positive cross-matches are directed against class I HLA antigens. Some appear to have specificities for only class II antigens on B lymphocytes, and a number of renal allografts have been successfully carried out in their presence (Carpenter and Morris, 1978).

Reed and co-workers (1987) demonstrated that the presence of anti-anti-HLA (i.e., anti-idiotypic) antibodies (shown by blocking of lymphocytotoxic activity of anti-donor HLA antibody) correlated well with graft acceptance, whereas the presence of anti-anti-anti-HLA antibodies that potentiated the cytotoxic activity of anti-donor HLA antibodies correlated with graft rejection.

Value of HLA Typing in Clinical Organ Transplantation

Most of the information concerning the usefulness of HLA typing in clinical transplantation has come from renal, bone marrow, and corneal transplantation. Although typing for intrafamilial transplants of all types is of great value, the usefulness of HLA typing in cadaveric kidney grafting has been a point of much controversy since cyclosporine became available (Kahan, 1999). Although short-term survival rates did not appear to be that different for closely or poorly matched cadaveric kidneys, the degree of HLA matching correlates with long-term survival. Renal grafts from HLA-identical sibling donors have a 10-year survival rate of about 74%; those from "6 antigen"–matched cadavers, 57% (65% if identical by DNA typing); those from family members sharing one haplotype, 54%; and those from HLA-mismatched cadaveric donors, 40% (Cecka, 2002).

Data from the London Transplant Group indicate that matching for B locus antigens is more important than matching for A locus antigens (Festenstein et al., 1986). The advantage of matching for HLA-B and HLA-DR in cadaveric renal transplantation was also supported in a worldwide survey by Opelz (1987) and in a similar analysis by the Eurotransplant group (van Rood, 1987). HLA matching is particularly important in patients who have become presensitized to MHC antigens before renal transplantation or in patients undergoing a second transplant, because 45% of patients with early rejection of primary grafts become sensitized to HLA antigens and reject most subsequent transplants (Barber et al., 1985; Perdue, 1985).

In regard to corneal grafts, HLA matching usually does not influence the rate of rejection; the exception is high-risk patients who have severely vascularized corneas or who have had two or more previous grafts (Sanfilippo et al., 1986).

Prior to 1980, strict HLA matching was crucial for successful bone marrow transplantation, because both graft rejection and lethal graft-versus-host (GVH) reactions are common complications. Until 1980, usually only HLA-identical siblings could be bone marrow donors; rarely, other relatives (e.g., parents, cousins) were found to be identical for class II HLA antigens when there had been consanguineous marriages (Mickelson et al., 1976). Fortunately, the development of techniques to rigorously deplete post-thymic T cells from donor marrow has permitted numerous successful half-matched marrow transplants with no or minimal GVH disease over the past two decades (Buckley et al., 1999; Myers et al., 2002).

HLA and the Immune Response

Class I and II chains of HLA molecules are structurally closely related to each other and to many other recognition structures of the immune system (Parham, 1999). The domains closest to the cell membrane ($I\alpha_3$, β_2m, $II\alpha_2$, and $II\beta_2$) show strong sequence homologies (see Fig. 43-2). They also have sequences similar to those found in immunoglobulin heavy and light chains, in the α, β, and γ chains of the T-cell receptor, and in CD3, CD4, and CD8 T-cell surface antigens. Because of their shared sequence homologies, these molecules have been designated as members of the *immunoglobulin gene superfamily* (Fig. 43-4) (Klein and Sato, 2000a; Parham, 1999). These closely related molecules may have evolved from a common ancestral gene.

Evidence that products of MHC genes are involved in immune responsiveness was first presented in 1969 by McDevitt and Chinitz; they described linkage of so-called MHC immune response (Ir) genes in mice to defects in responsiveness to certain antigens. MHC gene products are involved in most, if not all, responses to T-dependent antigens. Soluble antigens must first be

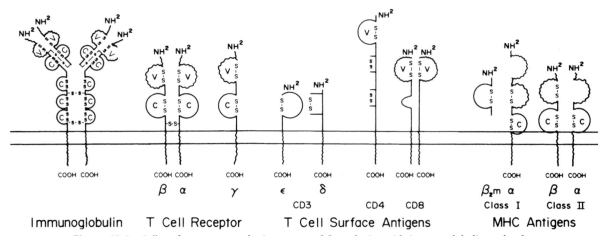

Figure 43-4 · Cell surface receptors sharing structural homologies with immunoglobulin molecules. Other candidates include intracellular adhesion molecules (ICAMs), such as I-CAM and N-CAM.

processed and degraded by antigen-presenting cells (APCs; macrophages, dendritic cells, or B cells) and a resulting peptide presented in the groove of an HLA class II antigen to a T lymphocyte capable of recognizing that peptide before a proliferative response is elicited (Klein and Sato, 2000a). Thus the HLA molecule serves as a crucial component of recognition units responsible for immune cell interaction and T-lymphocyte activation.

Although self-HLA molecules do not normally stimulate a response by autologous T cells, when a foreign antigenic peptide is associated with self class I or II antigens on target cells or APCs, an autologous T-cell receptor capable of recognizing that peptide in the context of self-MHC interacts with the APC and a signal is sent to the nucleus of that T cell to become activated (Fig. 42-5). Foreign antigens on the cell surface with autologous class I molecules are recognized by CD8+ cytotoxic T cells; antigens associated with class II molecules are recognized by CD4+ helper/inducer T cells (Klein and Sato, 2000a).

Thus these self-HLA antigens serve as both restricting and regulating molecules, because the T cells do not recognize soluble foreign antigens on cells that do not bear self-HLA antigens, and the HLA antigen class with which the foreign antigen is associated determines which type of T-cell function is activated. By contrast, foreign HLA antigens alone appear to be sufficient to activate receptors on CD4+ T cells to cause them to proliferate and on CD8+ T cells to make them become cytolytic for cells bearing those foreign antigens (Krensky, 1985).

Further restrictions imposed by the MHC are conferred on pre-T cells while they are differentiating in the thymus (Klein and Sato, 2000a). Studies using irradiated parental or F_1 hybrid mice reconstituted with bone marrow cells from the F_1 hybrid indicate that MHC antigens of the recipient (those on recipient epithelial and dendritic cells within the thymus) influence the differentiating T cells to have restricted cytotoxic T-cell activity against virus-infected tissues (Zinkernagel et al., 1978).

Indeed, the genetic environment in which T cells develop is crucial. Haploidentical stem cells that enter the thymus of a human recipient with SCID develop into thymocytes that are positively selected by HLA antigens on thymic epithelial cells and on resident dendritic cells so that they learn to recognize foreign antigens in the context of HLA antigens present on recipient antigen-presenting cells; those not selected die by apoptosis (Roberts et al., 1989). The positively selected cells are then negatively selected by the infant's self-peptides in the clefts of the HLA antigens so that cells with the potential to react against the recipient are deleted (Schiff and Buckley, 1987).

HLA and Disease Associations

Since the relationships between H-2 phenotypes and the susceptibility of mice to virus-induced tumors were established (Lilly et al., 1964), there has been considerable interest in the association of HLA phenotypes and disease susceptibility in humans. These associations may provide information relevant to the pathogenesis, diagnosis, and genetics of the disease.

Since 1967, a large number of diverse diseases have been found to be associated with increased or decreased frequencies of various HLA antigens (Table 43-4) (Klein and Sato, 2000b). These include autoimmune diseases (Flavell and Hafler, 1999), infectious diseases (Hill, 1998), primary immunodeficiencies (Volanakis et al., 1992; Vorechovsky et al., 1999), and various forms of malignancy, all of which are considered immunologic diseases. However, associations have also been reported between HLA antigens and conditions such as narcolepsy and hemochromatosis, which have no immunologic basis.

Narcolepsy

Narcolepsy results from a mutation in the gene encoding the hypocretin type 2 receptor *(HCRTR2)* (Chemelli et al., 1999; Lin et al., 1999). This prevents normal binding of hypocretins (or orexins—neuropeptides from the lateral hypothalamus) to the receptor. The *HCRTR2* gene is located on chromosome 6 near DQB1*0602 and DQA1*0102 alleles. Because this was a recent mutation, the mutated gene has not become separated from these DQ alleles by crossing over, accounting for the very high association of narcolepsy with these two alleles (Klein and Sato, 2000b).

Hemochromatosis

Hemochromatosis is caused by mutations in an MHC class I α chain gene whose product has lost its ability to bind antigenic peptides and has acquired a new function—an ability to form complexes with the transferrin receptor. However, even though this α chain gene product has a nonimmune function, it still must associate with β_2m to perform that function. The mutation in the α chain gene, *HFE*, destroys its protein's ability to associate with β_2m, which prevents transport of the α chain–transferrin receptor complex to the cell surface (Feder et al., 1996). Thus patients with this mutation do

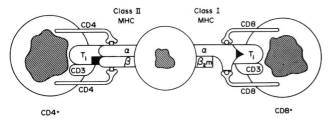

Figure 43-5 · Schematic of cell–cell interactions involving the T-cell receptor (TI), HLA class I and II molecules, and T-cell surface antigens CD4 and CD8.

TABLE 43-4 · MOST COMMON HUMAN LEUKOCYTE ANTIGEN (HLA) AND DISEASE ASSOCIATIONS

Disease	Associated HLA Molecule*	Relative Risk[†]
Ankylosing spondylitis	B27	87.4
Reactive arthropathy, Reiter's syndrome	B27	37
Acute anterior uveitis	B27	>20
Rheumatoid arthritis	DR4	4.2
Behçet's syndrome	B51	3.8
Systemic lupus erythematosus	DR3	5.8
Insulin-dependent diabetes mellitus	DR3	3.3
	DQB1*0201	2.4
	DR4	6.4
	DQB1*0302	9.5
	DR2	0.19
	DRB*1501[‡]	
	DRB*0101[‡]	
	DQ8	14
	DQB1*0602	0.15
Addison's disease	DR3	6.3
Graves' disease	DR3	3.7
Hashimoto's disease	DR11	3.2
Postpartum thyroiditis	DR4	5.3
Celiac disease	DR3	10.8
	DQ2	>250
	DQB1*0201[‡]	
	DQA1*0501[‡]	
	DR7,11	6.0–10.0
	DR7, DQB1*0201[‡]	
	DR11, DQA1*0501[‡]	
Dermatitis herpetiformis	DR3	15.9
Sicca syndrome	DR3	9.7
Myasthenia gravis	DR3	2.5
	B8	3.4
Idiopathic membranous glomerulonephritis	DR3	12.0
Goodpasture's syndrome	DR2	15.9
Multiple sclerosis	DR2	4.1
	DRB1*1501[‡]	
	DRB5*1101[‡]	
	DQB1*0602[‡]	
Pemphigus vulgaris (among Ashkenazi Jews)	DR4	14.4
Narcolepsy	DQ6	>38
Psoriasis vulgaris	Cw6	13.3
Birdshot retinochoroidopathy	A29	109

*Symbols with asterisks indicate alleles, and symbols without asterisks indicate serologically defined antigens. For each disease, the marker or markers with the strongest associations are given. In many cases in which it is difficult to decide whether HLA-DR or HLA-DQ markers are responsible for the association, both markers are given.

[†]The relative risk indicates the frequency of a disease in persons with the HLA marker as compared with persons without the marker. A positive association (i.e., when the HLA marker is more frequent in persons with the disease than in those without it) is indicated by a relative risk of more than one, a negative association by a relative risk of less than 1.0, and no association by a relative risk of 1.0.

[‡]The risk has not been assessed separately for this allele.

Modified from *Klein J, Sato A. The HLA system. Second of two parts. N Engl J Med 343:782–786. 2000.*

not have this complex on the surfaces of their duodenal crypt cells and absorb two to three times more iron from food than do people without that mutation. The mutation in *HFE* is in linkage disequilibrium with the HLA-A*03 allele, with which hereditary hemochromatosis was originally found to be associated.

Malaria

An example of an infectious disease in which protection from severe complications is associated with particular HLA antigens is malaria. Disease severity was found to be associated with a lower than normal frequency of the HLA-B*53 allele (Hill, 1999). Evidence has been obtained that HLA-B*53 molecules bind peptides processed from the malaria circumsporozoite protein and present them to CD8+ T cells, whose progeny attack the liver-stage parasites, thus reducing disease severity (Hill, 1999). Persons possessing the class II HLA-DRB1*13302/DQB1*0501 haplotype also appear less likely to develop severe anemia in malaria (Klein and Sato, 2000b).

Hepatitis B

A significant excess of HLA-DR7 and a significant deficiency of HLA-DR2 have been found in patients with chronic persistent hepatitis B virus infection (Almarri and Batchelor, 1994). In addition, the allele DRβ1*1302 was associated with protection against persistent hepatitis B virus infection among both children and adults in Gambia (Thursz et al., 1995).

Autoimmune Diseases

Multiple studies have shown that persons who have certain HLA alleles have a higher risk of specific autoimmune diseases than persons who lack these alleles (Flavell and Hafler, 1999; Thorsby, 1997; Tiwari and Terasaki, 1985). Although the HLA and autoimmune disease associations reported are all statistically significant and some are particularly striking, the magnitudes of the risk vary greatly (Klein and Sato, 2000b; Thorsby, 1997).

An example of this is the association of HLA-DR4 with rheumatoid arthritis (Nepom et al., 1987). Although this association has been reported in numerous studies and multiple ethnic groups, one fourth to one third of individuals affected with rheumatoid arthritis do not have the HLA-DR4 antigen and, among those who do, there is evidence for an effect of specific combinations of other MHC alleles with DR4 (Nepom et al., 1987).

Reasons for the lack of complete correlation include the possibility that the MHC genes are not themselves responsible for the disease susceptibility but are closely linked to the as-yet unidentified disease-causing genes, as illustrated by the narcolepsy gene mutation noted previously (Chemelli et al., 1999). Furthermore, the disease may also be affected by genes outside the MHC and by environmental factors. Another likely possibility is that the disease under question, although phenotypically homogeneous, may be genetically heterogeneous.

Ankylosing Spondylitis

Of all the associations between autoimmune diseases and HLA alleles, the strongest is that between HLA-B27 and ankylosing spondylitis (see Table 43-4) (Feltkamp et al., 1996). Of Caucasians with the latter disease, 90% carry the HLA-B27 allele, whereas the frequency in the general Caucasian population is around 9%. Lopez and associates (1993) reported finding two CTL T-cell clones with the same T-cell receptor that had cross-reactivity between HLA-B27 and HLA-DR2 as a result of a shared structural motif between HLA-B27 and the DR2 β5*0101 chain. The authors postulated that HLA-B27 spondyloarthropathies may be the product of an autoimmune T-cell response against a tissue-specific peptide specifically presented by HLA-B27 in joint tissues. In other studies, rats made transgenic for two human genes, *HLA-B27* and *β2M*, spontaneously developed inflammatory disease that resembled human spondyloarthropathies (Taurog et al., 1993).

Insulin-Dependent Diabetes Mellitus

It has been known for some time that type 1 insulin-dependent diabetes mellitus (IDDM) is closely associated with positivity for HLA-DR3 and/or HLA-DR4 antigens and negativity for HLA-DR2, but this is not absolute (Wolf et al., 1983). These and several other HLA antigens associated with IDDM are listed in Table 43-4 and discussed in Chapter 37.

Convincing evidence for a role for HLA antigens in the pathogenesis of IDDM comes from recent studies of inbred mice whose own class II genes had been replaced by human HLA-DQA1*0301 and HLA-DQB1*0302 genes and whose pancreatic cells had been made to express the human B7 molecule (Wen et al., 2000). Spontaneous diabetes developed in these mice, implicating the HLA-DQ8 molecule, which consists of the α and β polypeptide chains encoded by the HLA-DQA1*0301 and HLA-DQB1*0302 genes, in the pathogenesis of this disease. Further studies of this type should clarify some of the currently weak associations of MHC antigens with other diseases.

GRAFT REJECTION

Mechanisms of Graft Rejection

Role of Lymphatics

Adequate lymphatic drainage of the graft site is necessary for graft sensitization. This was illustrated by the experiment of Barker and Billingham (1967), who raised skin flaps connected by narrow pedicles that contained arteries and veins alone or arteries, veins, and lymphatics. Skin allografts placed on the flaps connected by all three vessels were destroyed in the usual length of time, whereas those placed on flaps without a lymphatic supply persisted as long as the flaps were viable. When another graft from the same donor was placed elsewhere on that host, the graft on the skin flap was promptly rejected, showing that lymphatics are not needed for graft rejection once sensitization occurs.

Although blood vessels transport the effectors of rejection and vascular destruction is a prominent feature of rejection, vascular alterations are not essential for rejection because cytolysis can occur within Millipore chambers containing only immunocytes and target cells.

Events of Rejection

Histologic studies of skin grafts have provided most of the knowledge of the events of graft rejection. Within a few days after a histoincompatible skin graft is made, vascularization of the graft bed occurs and the site appears to be healing. A few days later, however, the grafted tissue appears darker; by the sixth day, there is vascular dilation and tortuosity, with perivascular accumulation of MNCs. These processes continue until thrombosis of the vascular supply occurs, the cellular infiltrate extends throughout the graft, and complete rejection occurs, usually after 10 to 11 days.

The rejection process begins much earlier for a second graft from the same donor. Rejection begins just at the time vascular connections are established and is usually complete in 7 days or less. In an even more rapid form of rejection, the *white graft phenomenon*, vascularization does not occur at all.

Although MNC infiltration is a prominent feature of rejection, the extent of damage does not always correlate with the degree of infiltration; indeed, the more rapid the rejection, the less the infiltrate. Conversely, slowly rejecting grafts may have intense accumulations of MNCs (and even plasma cells) (the *blue graft phenomenon*) (Eichwald et al., 1966). Kidney graft rejection is accomplished by subendothelial depositions on the capillary basement membrane and infiltration of lymphoid cells, plasma cells, and macrophages. The extent of rejection is best correlated with the proportion of nonviable cells in the grafted tissue.

Role of Antibody

Because the cellular infiltrates in most rejected grafts resemble those of delayed hypersensitivity reactions and because graft rejection capability can be passively transferred with lymphoid cells but not with serum antibody even in large doses, investigators formerly believed that graft rejection was mediated solely through the action of the small lymphocyte. The relatively intact capacity of patients with congenital X-linked agammaglobulinemia to reject allografts also attests to the major role of thymus-dependent immunity.

This view was modified when cytotoxic antibodies were found in recipients of allogeneic grafts and when less-than-perfect correlation was found between the MNC infiltration and the degree of rejection. The strongest evidence for a role for antibody in graft rejection is the hyperacute rejection of primarily vascularized organs, such as the kidney and heart. Humoral antibodies can be demonstrated in recipients undergoing these reactions (Kissmeyer-Nielsen et al., 1966).

These antibodies combine with HLA antigens on endothelial cells, with subsequent complement fixation and accumulation of polymorphonuclear cells. Endothelial damage then occurs, probably as a result of enzymes released from polymorphonuclear leukocytes; platelets then accumulate, thrombi develop, and the result is renal cortical necrosis or myocardial infarction.

Cellular Basis of Graft Rejection

Results from both in vitro studies in humans and in vivo investigations in animals of cellular responses to MHC-encoded alloantigens support roles for both CD4[+] T-helper and CD8[+] cytotoxic T lymphocytes, as well as macrophages, in the rejection process (Bach and Sachs, 1987). When different combinations of class I and class II antigen-bearing cells in MLR and cell-mediated lympholysis (CML) experiments were used, it was learned that both helper and cytotoxic lymphocytes collaborate in the generation of cytotoxic responses.

Over the past two decades, considerably more information has accrued about the nature of this collaboration and the rejection response in general (Suthanthiran and Strom, 1994). It is known that allograft rejection results from the coordinated activation of alloreactive T cells and APCs. Although acute rejection is a T-cell–dependent process, the destruction of the allograft results from a broad array of effector mechanisms. Cell–cell interactions and the release by primed T-helper

cells of multiple types of cytokines (interleukin [IL]-2, IL-4, IL-5, IL-7, IL-10, and IL-15; tumor necrosis factor-α [TNF-α]; and interferon-γ [IFN-γ]) recruit not only immunocompetent donor-specific CD4[+] T cells, CD8[+] cytotoxic T cells, and antibody-forming B cells but also nonspecific inflammatory cells, which form the majority of cells infiltrating an allograft (Suthanthiran and Strom, 1994).

The initial event occurs when the recipient's T-cell receptors recognize either the donor's foreign HLA molecules on donor APCs within the graft (direct presentation) or peptides from the donor's released HLA molecules on the recipient's APCs (so-called indirect presentation) (Gould and Auchincloss, 1999).

Signal Transduction

On stimulation with antigens, the T-cell receptor/CD3/CD4 or CD8 complex physically associates with several intracellular protein tyrosine kinases. Tyrosine phosphorylation activates the coenzyme phospholipase Cγ1 to hydrolyze phosphatidylinositol 4,5-biphosphate and the generation of inositol 1,4,5-triphosphate and diacylglycerol. In the presence of intracellular calcium mobilized by inositol triphosphate, diacylglycerol binds to and activates protein kinase C, which promotes the expression of several nuclear regulatory proteins and causes transcriptional activation and expression of genes central to T-cell division (such as the genes encoding IL-2 and its receptor) (Suthanthiran and Strom, 1994).

One of the participants in the signal transduction process is *calcineurin*, a calcium- and calmodulin-dependent serine-threonine phosphatase. Inhibition of calcineurin's phosphatase activity is the mechanism of action of cyclosporine and tacrolimus (FK-506), two potent immunosuppressive agents that have played major roles in the success of allografting over the past two decades (Kahan, 1999).

Co-stimulatory Signals

Stimulation of CD4[+] T cells through their antigen receptor is not sufficient to initiate T-cell activation unless co-stimulation is provided by interaction of other ligand-receptor pairs present on the surfaces of T cells and APCs during their encounter. Some of these interactive pairs include the T-cell surface molecule, CD2, and its ligand, CD58 on APCs; CD11a/CD18:CD54; CD5:CD72; CD40 ligand:CD40; and CD28:CD80 or CD86.

Unless signals are provided through one or more of these receptor-ligand interactions (particularly through CD40L:CD40 and CD28:CD80 or CD86) or by cytokines (e.g., IL-1 and IL-6 from the APC), CD4[+] T-cell anergy or tolerance induction occurs when the T-cell receptor interacts with the APC (Demirci et al., 2002). Thus T-cell accessory proteins and their ligands on APCs are target molecules for antirejection therapy. If co-stimulation does occur, the CD4[+] T cell becomes activated, which leads to stable transcription of genes important in T-cell activation.

Role of CD8 Cells

CD8+ T cells recognize antigenic peptides displayed on MHC class I molecules and represent a major cytotoxic T-effector cell (CTL) population in graft rejection. Donor class I molecules on donor APC in the graft directly activate CTLs. However, CD8 activation also requires a co-stimulatory second signal and an IL-2 signal. It has been shown that activation of CD8+ CTLs is highly dependent on signaling through the common γ chain (γc) of multiple cytokine receptors, whereas this is not true for activation of CD4+ T cells (Demirci et al., 2002). Activated CD8+ T cells proliferate and mature into specific alloreactive clones capable of releasing granzyme (serine esterase), perforin, and toxic cytokines (e.g., TNF-α).

Other Effector Mechanisms

As noted earlier, cyclosporine and tacrolimus interfere significantly with the activation process initiated by interaction of APCs with the T-cell receptor and many of the co-stimulatory molecules. An exception, however, is the CD28:CD80 or CD86 co-stimulatory pathway, which is independent of protein kinase C and calcium but can also lead to stable transcription of the IL-2 gene and other activation genes. That pathway is resistant to inhibition by cyclosporine and tacrolimus. Stimulation of the B cell by antigen occurs through its antigen receptor (i.e., surface immunoglobulin), but co-stimulation is also required for B-cell activation. This co-stimulation can be provided by cytokines released by T cells or through many of the same T-cell protein-ligand pairs important in T-cell–APC co-stimulation, because these ligands are also present on B cells.

Once T-cell activation has occurred, autocrine T-cell proliferation continues as a consequence of the expression of the IL-2 receptor. Interaction of IL-2 with its receptor triggers the activation of protein-tyrosine-kinases and phosphatidylinositol-3-kinase, resulting in translocation into the cytosol of an IL-2 receptor–bound serine-threonine kinase, Raf-1. This in turn leads to the expression of several DNA-binding proteins, such as c-jun, c-fos, and c-myc, and to progression of the cell cycle (Suthanthiran and Strom, 1994). The consequence of all of these events is the development of graft-specific, infiltrating cytotoxic T cells. Cytokines from the T cells also activate macrophages and other inflammatory leukocytes and cause upregulation of HLA molecules on graft cells. The activated T cells also stimulate B cells to produce antigraft antibodies. Ultimately, all of these cellular and humoral factors destroy the graft.

Nonspecific Immunosuppression

Because there is no method to suppress the host's immune response to antigens of the graft while simultaneously maintaining other immune responses, rejection must be prevented by nonspecific immunosuppressive agents. The development of immunosuppressive strategies over the past four decades reflects enormous progress in understanding the cellular and molecular mechanisms that mediate allograft rejection (Hong and Kahan, 2000). The success of transplantation between an unrelated donor and recipient can be attributed to implementation of these strategies.

However, because these agents depress both specific and nonspecific immunity, they render the recipient more susceptible to infection and malignancy. Indeed, infection is the most important cause of transplant recipient mortality. Thus all patients must have their immunosuppressive regimen fine-tuned to prevent rejection while minimizing the risk of infection. Too large a dose and infection supervenes; too small a dose and the graft is rejected.

The immunosuppressive agents used in most centers for nearly two decades were corticosteroids, azathioprine, and cyclosporine. Several new agents have been introduced over the past few years: mycophenolate mofetil, which has a similar but more effective mode of action to that of azathioprine; tacrolimus, which has a mode of action and side effects similar to those of cyclosporine; and sirolimus, which blocks IL-2–induced T-cell cycle progression (Table 43-5; see Chapter 27).

Immunosuppressive agents can be categorized on the basis of whether they (1) interrupt lymphocyte cell division, (2) deplete lymphocytes, (3) interfere with lymphocyte maturational events, (4) interfere with

TABLE 43-5 · NONSPECIFIC IMMUNOSUPPRESSIVE AGENTS

Drug	Mechanism of Action	Outcome	Adverse Effects
Steroids	Binds cytosolic receptors and heat shock proteins	Blocks transcription of cytokine genes, IL-1, IL-2, IL-3, IL-6, TNF-α, and IFN-γ	Hypertension, glucose intolerance, dyslipidemia, osteoporosis
Cyclosporine	Binds cyclophilin, inhibits calcineurin, blocks cytokine production	Inhibits IL-2 production, stimulates TGF-β production	Nephrotoxicity, hypertension, dyslipidemia, glucose intolerance
Tacrolimus	Binds FKBP-12, inhibits calcineurin, blocks cytokine production	Inhibits IL-2 production	Similar to cyclosporine but less hirsutism/gum enlargement, increased incidence of diabetes
Azathioprine	Inhibits purine synthesis	Blocks DNA and RNA synthesis	Marrow suppression
Mycophenolate mofetil	Inhibits inosine monophosphate dehydrogenase	Blocks de novo pathway of purine synthesis (selective for lymphocytes), blocks glycosylation	Diarrhea, leukopenia but less than with azathioprine
Sirolimus	Binds FKBP-12, blocks p70 S6 kinase	Blocks IL-2–induced cell cycle progression	Hyperlipidemia, mild thrombocytopenia

immune cell co-stimulation, (5) modulate ischemia-reperfusion injury, or (6) facilitate induction of tolerance (Hong and Kahan, 2000). They can also be grouped into those used for induction therapy, for prophylaxis against rejection, for reversal of acute rejection episodes, or for maintenance immunosuppression. These agents are also discussed in Chapter 27.

Corticosteroids

On entering the cell, steroids bind to a specific intracellular receptor. The steroid-receptor complex then enters the nucleus, interacting with glucocorticoid reactive elements (GRE) within the DNA sequences of a variety of gene promoters, such as the enhancer regions of IL-1, IL-2, IL-3, IL-6, TNF-α, and IFN-γ, decreasing synthesis of these cytokines (see Table 43-5). Steroids thus dampen APC functions and thereby interfere with allorecognition.

Prednisone is used as part of the induction therapy in most renal transplantations, beginning with a dosage of 2 mg/kg/day; this may be continued indefinitely but at a progressively lower dosage. In children, every effort is made to eventually achieve an alternate-day regimen or discontinue the regimen altogether. Intravenous injection of prednisolone at a high dosage (20 to 30 mg/kg) is particularly valuable in reversing acute organ rejection crises (Bell et al., 1971); the steroid is usually given for three doses on consecutive or alternate days. However, as noted in the following section, a lower dosage is usually used for pediatric patients (Ettenger et al., 1990).

Cytotoxic Agents

The cytoxic agents are a complex and heterogeneous group of chemicals, each having different biochemical effects at various points in the cell cycle (see Table 43-5). Nevertheless, all of these agents affect the structure or properties of DNA. The most common cytotoxic agents follow:

· The purine antagonists, 6-mercaptopurine (6-MP), azathioprine (Imuran), and mycophenolate mofetil (CellCept)
· Methotrexate, a folic acid antagonist
· Cyclophosphamide (Cytoxan), an alkylating agent similar to nitrogen mustard

Purine Antagonists (6-Mercaptopurine, Azathioprine, and Mycophenolate Mofetil)

For two decades, azathioprine was the most widely used immunosuppressive agent in transplantation, although its therapeutic index is no higher than that of 6-MP, from which it differs by an imidazole ring. It damages cells because its metabolites are incorporated into purine nucleotides, which inhibits de novo nucleoside synthesis and thereby blocks proliferation of immunocompetent lymphoid cells. Its major effect is on T cells,

and there is a lesser effect on B cells (Bach and Strom, 1985). Until the availability of cyclosporine, azathioprine was used by almost all renal transplant centers as the principal immunosuppressive agent, usually in combination with prednisone.

More recently, mycophenolate mofetil has essentially replaced azathioprine, because it has a similar but more effective mode of action. It inhibits inosine monophosphate dehydrogenase and thus blocks de novo purine synthesis. The drug is given orally at dosages of 1500 to 3000 mg/day. It has much less marrow toxicity and is non-nephrotoxic; side effects include mild diarrhea and some leukopenia (Hong and Kahan, 2000).

In centers that still use azathioprine, a high dosage (5 mg/kg/day) is used for 2 preoperative and the first 2 postoperative days, tapering to a maintenance dosage of 1.5 mg/kg/day by 1 week. The intravenous dose is half the oral dose. Because bone marrow toxicity is a major side effect of azathioprine administration, hemoglobin levels, white blood cell (WBC) counts, and platelet counts must be followed closely (daily during the first 2 weeks, several times a week for the next 2 to 3 months, and at lesser intervals thereafter). WBC counts of 4000/mm^3 or less are an indication for temporarily withholding the drug. Recovery usually occurs within 2 to 3 days. The drug can also lead to hepatotoxicity, usually manifested by mild to marked jaundice but occasionally manifested only by elevated liver enzymes (Bach and Strom, 1985).

Fludarabine phosphate has recently been used as a component of nonmyeloablative conditioning for bone marrow transplantation (see following discussion) (Gaspar et al., 2002). The active metabolite of this drug inhibits DNA polymerase alpha, ribonucleotide reductase, and DNA primase, thus inhibiting DNA synthesis.

Methotrexate

Because methotrexate (a folic acid antagonist) is excreted by the kidneys, there has been reluctance to use it in kidney transplantation. Methotrexate has been used most successfully in the prevention of graft-versus-host disease (GVHD) in patients with aplastic anemia or leukemia who are undergoing bone marrow transplantation (Thomas et al., 1975).

Cyclophosphamide and Busulfan

Cyclophosphamide, an alkylating agent, is an effective substitute for azathioprine in renal and liver transplantation, offering the advantage of lessened liver toxicity (Bach and Strom, 1985). The dosage is usually half that of azathioprine. The same precautions should be followed with regard to monitoring blood counts because leukopenia is common. Cyclophosphamide at high dosages has been especially useful in conditioning patients for acceptance of bone marrow transplants (Santos, 1974).

Busulfan, another alkylating agent, is commonly used at high dosages together with cyclophosphamide to cause marrow ablation before bone marrow transplantation (Blazar et al., 1985). Because these two agents at high dosages are toxic to the liver, lungs, and other organs and cause infertility, there has been considerable interest in using nonmyeloablative regimens for recipients who already have organ damage, who are older, or who have nonmalignant conditions.

Antilymphocyte and Antithymocyte Globulins (ALG, OKT3, and ATG)

Antibodies from animals immunized with human lymphoid cells are useful agents for induction therapy as well as for reversal of acute rejection episodes (see Table 43-5) (Russell and Cosimi, 1979). They consist of the IgG fraction of sera from horses or rabbits immunized with either lymphoid cells (antilymphocyte globulin, ALG) or thymocytes (antithymocyte globulin, ATG, Thymoglobulin), or murine monoclonal antibodies to T-cell surface antigens (anti-CD3, OKT3) (Cosimi et al., 1981).

Administration of horse, rabbit, or murine antilymphocyte antibodies has been followed by the so-called cytokine storm from the release of intracellular cytokines. OKT3 initially activates T cells, resulting in release of IL-2 and TNF-α. This causes fever, chills, myalgias, and aseptic meningitis. Sensitization to these animal proteins can also result in urticaria, serum sickness, chills, fever, and/or anaphylaxis. These reactions are more common if treatment is interrupted and reinstituted or if continued for long periods.

In general, ALG, ATG, and OKT3 decrease the onset, severity, and number of rejection episodes. Such antibodies are particularly useful in reversing acute graft rejection that occurs in the first 2 weeks. However, antibodies to the foreign epitopes on these molecules eventually develop in the recipient, including anti-idiotypic antibodies, thereby causing their immune elimination and reducing their efficacy as immunosuppressive agents (Hong and Kahan, 2000).

Monoclonal Antibodies to Cytokine Receptors

Prevention of graft rejection has also been approached by inhibiting cytokines from interacting with their receptors. Chimeric or humanized murine anti–IL-2 receptor α chain antibodies have been developed for clinical use (Kahan et al., 1994; Vincenti et al., 1998) (see Table 4-8 and 27-3). The advantage of these monoclonal antibodies to the IL-2 receptor α chain is that such molecules are present only on activated T lymphocytes; therefore the main effect is on T cells, possibly activated by graft antigens. Thus, even if IL-2 is synthesized by these activated T cells, the anti–IL-2 receptor α chain antibodies would interfere with the binding of IL-2 to its receptor, preventing an autocrine response to IL-2 by cells bearing this receptor.

Cyclosporine and Tacrolimus

The main action of cyclosporine and tacrolimus (FK-506) is to prevent the synthesis of IL-2 and other cytokines produced by T cells activated by allografts (see Table 43-5). A fungal metabolite of *Tolyplocadium inflatum*, cyclosporine is a neutral, hydrophobic, cyclical peptide containing 11 amino acids. It was recognized as a potentially valuable immunosuppressive agent in the late 1970s and has been used extensively in human organ transplantation for the past two decades (Kahan, 1989). Because of its extreme hydrophobicity, the drug must be dissolved in oil for administration; however, a reliably absorbed oral form of the drug is available (Kahan et al., 1994). Cyclosporine is noncytotoxic and nonmyelosuppressive.

Cyclosporine's hydrophobicity allows it to readily penetrate cell membranes to gain access to and bind to the cytoplasmic isomerase protein, cyclophilin. The complex then inhibits calcineurin, an intracellular phosphatase critical for the translocation of signals from the T-cell receptor to the nucleus. In this manner, it blocks transcription of the IL-2 gene. Thus its predominant immunosuppressive effect is produced by blocking IL-2 synthesis and IL-2 receptor expression. In addition, cyclosporine also blocks the synthesis of other cytokines and thereby interferes with activated CD4+ T-helper lymphocyte function (Kahan, 1989). As a consequence, T-cell proliferation and differentiation of precursor cytotoxic lymphocytes are blocked.

Tacrolimus (FK-506) is a macrolide compound isolated from the fungus *Streptomyces tsukubaensis* that has potent immunosuppressive properties (Kino et al., 1987). Tacrolimus binds to a cytoplasmic isomerase protein in the same way cyclosporine does, but to a different one—the FK-binding protein (FK-BP-12) (see Table 43-5). The complex formed inhibits calcineurin in the same manner as does the cyclosporine/cyclophilin complex to prevent T-cell receptor signal transduction to the nucleus. Tacrolimus thus inhibits synthesis of IL-2, IL-3, IFN-γ, and other cytokines, just as cyclosporine does. However, it was found to be 100 times more potent than cyclosporine as an immunosuppressive agent (Kinoet al., 1987; The U.S. Multicenter FK-506 Liver Study Group, 1994).

In a study comparing tacrolimus and cyclosporine for liver transplantation, 1-year patient survival rates were similar (88%) and graft survival rates were not significantly different (82% and 79%, respectively) (The U.S. Multicenter FK-506 Liver Study Group, 1994).

Tacrolimus was associated with significantly fewer episodes of acute corticosteroid-resistant or refractory rejection, but there were side effects that necessitated discontinuation of the drug. The most serious side effects were nephrotoxicity and neurotoxicity. More recently, hypertrophic cardiomyopathy has been associated with the use of tacrolimus in pediatric transplant patients; the condition resolved after reducing the dosage, discontinuing the drug, or changing to cyclosporine (Atkison et al., 1995).

Sirolimus

Sirolimus (SRL, rapamycin, Rapamune) has a structure similar to that of tacrolimus, and its activity is dependent on its binding to FK-BP-12. However, the complex formed does not inhibit calcineurin but rather prevents the phosphorylation of p70^{S6} kinase, which blocks signal transduction from many cell surface cytokine receptors, including IL-2R, IL-4R, IL-15R, and IL-10R (see Table 43-5) (Kahan et al., 1991). Both in vitro and in vivo studies have shown a synergistic effect of SRL with cyclosporine, as would be expected because SRL prevents cytokine receptor signaling and cyclosporine inhibits cytokine production (Kahan et al., 1991; Stepkowski and Kahan, 1991).

Combination Therapy

From the preceding discussion, it can be appreciated that no agent is the perfect nonspecific immunosuppressive drug. Antilymphocyte antibodies, nucleoside synthesis inhibitors, steroids, cyclosporine (or tacrolimus), anti-IL-2Rα, and sirolimus all affect allorecognition and antigen-driven T-cell proliferation at different points in the T-cell activation process. Newer agents with similar actions are already under trial.

Thus the combined use of several of these types of agents provides a synergistic rather than a mere additive effect (Hong and Kahan, 2000). As a result, lower dosages of each of the agents can be used, with a resulting reduction in drug toxicity. Although the use of this multipronged strategy will provide more effective immunosuppression and enhance graft survival, it will also increase the risk of opportunistic infections and malignancy.

Specific Immunosuppression

Specific immunosuppression is defined as suppression of the host's (and/or donor's, in the case of bone marrow transplantation) immune response against donor (and/or host in marrow transplantation) alloantigens without suppression of responses to other antigens.

Tolerance

Tolerance (specific immunologic unresponsiveness) is an induced state that occurs as a consequence of specific deletion or suppression of a clone of cells that react with a specific antigen (Dresser and Mitchison, 1968; see Chapter 8). Most attempts to achieve specific immunosuppression have been directed toward manipulation of either graft antigens or the specific antigen receptors on cells capable of mediating rejection. The antigen receptors include both T- and B-cell (e.g., antibody) receptors.

The first example of specific immunosuppression was the "neonatal tolerance" observed by Billingham and colleagues (1953). They injected adult bone marrow cells intravenously into neonatal mice and found that such animals, even as adults, would accept donor-type skin grafts indefinitely. Although this is not feasible in humans, other approaches designed to induce specific immunosuppression show promise.

Modification of the antigenicity of endocrine tissues (thyroid, pancreatic islet cells) by culturing the tissues before transplantation has resulted in indefinite graft survival across the MHC or even across species in experimental animals (Bowen et al., 1980; Lacy et al., 1979; Lafferty et al., 1976; Sollinger et al., 1976). The mechanism of this modification is not completely clear, but it appears to be due to loss of cells rich in class II MHC antigens (dendritic and other APCs). This possibility is supported further by the studies of Faustman and associates (1981), who obtained extended survival of pancreatic islets treated with anti-Ia antibodies. Thus it may be possible to avoid an effective immune response against a tissue if class II antigens are absent.

Other studies in experimental animals have shown that avoidance of class II antigens is sufficient for acceptance of grafts of only certain tissues, namely primarily vascularized organs, such as the kidney (Pescovitz et al., 1984), and not others, namely skin, where class I differences led to rejection (Kortz and Sachs, 1987). The liver appears to be capable of long-term acceptance, even in the face of disparities of antigens of both MHC classes.

Another means of inducing specific immunosuppression in animals is to administer antigen after a nonspecific immunosuppressive agent, such as ALG (Monaco and Wood, 1970) or azathioprine (Tyler et al., 1987). The fact that reduced dosages or, in some cases, actual discontinuation of immunosuppressive agents still allows for successful maintenance of renal or hepatic allografts suggests that some degree of specific tolerance may be induced in human organ transplantation (Starzl and Zinkernagel, 2001).

There has been considerable interest in the possibility of inducing tolerance by using agents designed to interfere with interaction of co-stimulatory molecules while still allowing antigen to be presented to the T-cell receptor by B cells or other APCs. Among the ones that have seemed promising is an IgG conjugate of a CD28 homolog (co-stimulatory T-lymphocyte antigen-4 Ig [CTLA-4Ig] that blocks the interaction of CD28 on T cells with CD80 or CD86 on APCs). This induced tolerance to xenogeneic human pancreas islets in experimental animals.

Even more effective than CTLA-4Ig were anti-CD154 antibodies to prevent the interaction of CD154 with CD40 on B cells. However, because thrombotic events occurred during the clinical trials, the trials were discontinued (Hong and Kahan, 2000).

In human trials using CTLA-4Ig, unfractionated bone marrow from haploidentical donors was co-cultured with irradiated blood cells from the recipients in the presence of CTLA-4Ig for 36 hours before infusion of the marrow cells into the recipients (Guinan et al., 1999). Of 11 evaluable patients, there was acute GVHD confined to the gastrointestinal tract in 3 and there were no deaths from GVHD.

Enhancement

Enhancement is a form of antibody-mediated specific immunosuppression first appreciated when it was noted that administration of an antibody to a tumor prevented its rejection (Kaliss, 1958). In this phenomenon, antiserum to the graft blocks the response of host lymphoid cells to the grafted tissues; in bone marrow transplantation, donor serum blocks the attack of grafted immunocompetent cells against host tissues. This is thought to be the mechanism underlying the beneficial effect of donor-specific blood transfusions used in some centers to improve outcomes in haploidentical renal transplantation (Salvatierra et al., 1987; Tyler et al., 1987).

The mechanism of enhancement is unknown. The antibody may interfere with recognition of antigenic determinants by nonimmune lymphocytes (afferent inhibition), may have a direct effect on the immunocyte (central inhibition), or may mask the antigen (efferent inhibition). The existence of active enhancement tends to preclude afferent inhibition, because both sensitized lymphocytes and blocking factors coexist. Moreover, tolerance following enhancement can be transferred by cells and not serum from enhanced animals (French and Batchelor, 1972). Unfortunately, enhancement has not been successful for prolonging survival of grafts other than kidney or in species other than the rat.

Prior Bone Marrow Transplantation

A final possible means of specifically modifying the host's immune response for organ grafting is that of first performing bone marrow transplantation from the prospective donor to the host. Thus far, this has been done primarily in experimental animals, for obvious reasons (e.g., danger to the host of immunosuppression for marrow acceptance and the risk of a GVH reaction). Nevertheless, if rigorous T-cell depletion of donor marrow is used, a GVH reaction can be prevented, as already demonstrated for animals (Muller-Ruchholtz et al., 1976) and humans (Buckley et al., 1999). Depletion of donor marrow T cells and ablation of host immune cells by conditioning regimens led to incomplete immunoreconstitution because the T cells that arose matured in a thymus that was histoincompatible with donor marrow B cells and APCs (Singer et al., 1981).

This problem has been circumvented experimentally by using total lymphoid irradiation (i.e., the long bones are shielded from irradiation) (Slavin et al., 1978) or by reconstituting total-body irradiated animals with a mixture of T-cell–depleted syngeneic and allogeneic bone marrow cells (Ildstad and Sachs, 1984). Both techniques have led to mixed chimeras. In the latter case, the animals were tolerant to donor grafts, lacked GVHD, and were completely immunologically reconstituted. The first method was not successful in sensitized hosts, but the second method was successful (Sachs, 1987).

Regardless of the mechanism of specific immunosuppression, the development of a predictable means of inducing unresponsiveness only to the foreign histocompatibility antigens of the grafted tissue cells would represent a major breakthrough for the field of organ and tissue transplantation.

Differences in Tissue Acceptability

As already alluded to earlier, certain allogeneic tissues are accepted better than others (Russell and Cosimi, 1979). These differences may be due to the following:

· Variation in the degree of expression of HLA antigens on certain tissues
· The presence of unique or special antigens on certain tissues
· Differences in the resistance to immune attack of various tissues
· Differences in the anatomic site to which the tissue is transplanted

Because lymphocytes are particularly rich in HLA antigens, several approaches have been used to reduce their number in grafted organs or tissues. These include radiation or perfusion of kidneys and culturing of endocrine tissues (e.g., pancreas, thyroid) (Lafferty et al., 1976).

Differentiation antigens or other unique antigens may exist on cells from certain tissues (e.g., liver, lung) that evoke a strong immune reaction; their importance in clinical organ transplantation is not yet known. Certain cells (e.g., chondrocytes) are less susceptible to rejection than others. By contrast, some organs (e.g., the heart) are rejected more readily (Russell and Cosimi, 1979). Finally, the site of grafting is important because allografts survive longer in "privileged" sites, such as the anterior chamber of the eye, the interior of the brain, and probably the interior of the testis. Grafts in these sites may be protected by a diminished blood supply or a lessened traffic of lymphoid cells.

The liver is also considered a "protected" organ to some extent. This has been attributed to the fact that the liver bears "nonprofessional" APCs that cannot deliver critical signals, either because of their failure to produce co-stimulatory cytokines, such as IL-1, IL-6, and IL-12, or because of the absence of CD80/86 or CD40 (Starzl and Zinkernagel, 2001).

PEDIATRIC RENAL TRANSPLANTATION

Overview

At one time, children were considered poor candidates for renal transplantation because of (1) the surgical technical problems of small vessels and donor organ–recipient size disparities and (2) growth impairment, orthopedic complications, and psychosocial problems resulting from the high-dose steroids required to prevent rejection. That kidney transplantation can be carried out successfully in children, however, has been repeatedly established at many centers over the past four decades; survival and graft function have been comparable with those in adults (Benfield et al., 1999; Cecka, 2002; Dall'Amico et al., 2001; Kari et al., 1999; Moudgil and Jordan, 1999; Smith and McDonald, 2000).

At present, there are more than 15,000 functioning renal allografts in children worldwide (Benfield et al., 1999). The increased number of kidney transplants performed in children over the past two decades has paralleled the dramatic increase in renal transplantation in adults worldwide during that period (Cecka, 2002).

Despite spectacular improvement in dialysis techniques and the availability of this form of therapy to very young infants (Nevins and Kjellstrand, 1983), renal transplantation remains the treatment of choice for end-stage renal disease (ESRD) in patients of nearly all ages (Benfield et al., 1999; Cecka, 2002). A successful kidney transplant brings about improvements in overall body function and in the quality of life that cannot be achieved with even the most advanced dialysis techniques.

There is no lack of patients for such transplants. Estimates of new cases of ESRD range from 1.5 to 3 per million people annually. In the United States, between 360 and 720 infants and children are newly diagnosed as having ESRD each year (Ettenger et al., 1990).

Indications

The three main causes of ESRD in infants and children, in descending order of frequency, are glomerulopathies of various types, congenital hypoplasia-dysplasia, and obstructive uropathy (Benfield et al., 1999). In the January 1997 report of the North American Pediatric Renal Transplant Cooperative Study (NAPRTCS), covering the years 1987 to 1996 (Benfield et al., 1999), of the disorders that led to ESRD and transplantation, structural and developmental anomalies of aplasia, dysplasia, and obstructive uropathy accounted for more than 1500 patients.

Focal segmental glomerulosclerosis (FSGS) was the most common cause of renal failure and transplantation among acquired diseases (Benfield et al., 1999). Wilms' tumor is the principal malignancy seen in the pediatric age group, but this indication for transplantation accounts for less than 5% of those performed (Ettenger et al., 1990).

The only patients with ESRD who should be excluded from consideration for kidney transplantation are those with malignancy that cannot be brought under control or those with debilitating irreversible brain injury (Benfield et al., 1999; Humar et al., 2001). Thus neither age nor pre-existing illness, such as diabetes or collagen-vascular disease, is an absolute contraindication to transplantation (Humar et al., 2001).

Donor Selection

Rates of Success

As discussed previously, renal transplant procedures are most successful when related donors are involved. In the January 1997 report of NAPRTCS, data were analyzed on 4898 patients who received 5362 transplants (Benfield et al., 1999). Graft survival was 90% at 1 year and 74% at 6 years for living donor kidneys and was 80% at 1 year and 58% at 6 years for cadaveric donor patients. The most common cause for graft failure was chronic rejection (30%). Many factors have contributed to these improvements, including improved surgical techniques (Adams et al., 2001) and better approaches to prevent graft rejection (Ettenger, 1998; Hong and Kahan, 2000).

For recipients of living donor grafts, relative risk (RR) factors for graft survival were African-American race (RR = 2.1, $P < 0.001$) and greater than five prior transfusions (RR = 1.6, $P < 0.001$). Prophylactic anti–T-cell antibody also reduced the risk of graft failure (RR = 0.76, $P = 0.009$). For recipients of cadaver kidneys, risk factors were recipient age younger than 2 years (RR = 2, $P < 0.001$), donor age younger than 6 years (RR = 1.3, $P = 0.005$), and absence of induction T-cell antibody (RR = 1.31, $P < 0.001$) (Benfield et al., 1999).

Clearly, HLA matching improves the outcome of renal grafts, not only when related donors are available but also when cadaver kidneys are used (Cecka, 2002). Because of the ethical problems surrounding the use of minors as donors, HLA-identical sibling transplant procedures are not performed as often with minor donors as from adult donors. As mentioned, the donor of the organ graft should not possess either A or B blood group antigens if that antigen is absent in the recipient (Breimer et al., 1987). In addition, living donors with hypertension should not be used. Finally, the serologic cross-match between the recipient's current serum and the donor's lymphocytes must be negative to minimize the chance of hyperacute rejection from preformed antileukocyte antibodies (Cicciarelli and Teraski, 1983).

Transplantation in Infants Younger Than Age 1

Prior to 1985, renal transplantation in infants younger than 1 year of age had generally met with dismal success, with only 2 of 13 reported cases surviving with functioning grafts (Ettenger and Fine, 1986). Most of those had received cadaver kidneys, and many were from anencephalic donors. However, an analysis of the experience with 30 renal transplants into infants younger than 1 year at the University of Minnesota between the years of 1984 and 1999 revealed that the outcome was comparable to that in all other age groups (Humar et al., 2001).

Pretransplant Dialysis

The development within the last two decades of improved dialysis techniques has been of major importance to successful renal transplantation in children (Nevins and Kjellstrand, 1983). The objective of dialysis is to correct electrolyte imbalances and reduce the blood urea nitrogen (BUN) to 50 to 70 mg/dl, thus avoiding a marked diuresis in the immediate post-transplantation period. Hemodialysis should be performed 24 to 36 hours before transplantation of a kidney from a related donor. Although this is usually not possible when cadaver donors are used, the technique of continuous ambulatory peritoneal dialysis (CAPD) developed over the past several years has yielded results comparable with those for hemodialysis (Ettenger et al., 1990).

Surgical Procedures

For adults and most children, the renal transplant operation has become standardized (Simmons and Najarian, 1984). The earlier practice of removing the patient's diseased kidneys 2 to 3 weeks before transplantation has not been carried out routinely in recent years, except in patients with hypertension or infection; nephrectomy is now performed at the time of transplantation.

For children who weigh 15 kg or more, an extraperitoneal surgical approach is made. The donor renal vein and artery are anastomosed end-to-end to the recipient's distal inferior vena cava and distal aorta or common iliac artery, respectively. One of the major advances has been in overcoming the technical problems of transplanting adult kidneys into small children (Humar et al., 2001; So et al., 1986).

For infants and children who weigh less than 15 kg, the kidney is transplanted intraperitoneally. Results of kidney transplantation in small children have improved considerably with the consistent use of the aorta and the distal caval vein to perform vascular anastomoses (Adams et al., 2001).

Immunosuppressive Regimens

Until cyclosporine became available in the early 1980s, most centers used a combination of azathioprine (Imuran), at initial dosages of 3 to 5 mg/kg/day and maintenance dosages of 2 to 3 mg/kg/day, and prednisone, at initial dosages of 1 to 3 mg/kg/day (or 70 to 100 mg/M^2/day) and maintenance dosages of 0.2 to 0.3 mg/kg/day, to prevent graft rejection. Beginning in 1983 and 1984, many centers began to use cyclosporine (in lieu of azathioprine) and lower dosages of prednisone for immunosuppression (Ettenger, 1998).

Although cyclosporine showed clear superiority over azathioprine as an initial immunosuppressive agent, its major side effect in children as well as adults has been nephrotoxicity (Ettenger et al., 1990). Neurotoxicity has also occurred (Kahan, 1989). Cyclosporine has been given at varying dosages at different centers but has generally been given intravenously over 2 to 3 hours in doses of 3 to 10 mg/kg during or just after transplantation and of 7.5 to 10 mg/kg on the day after. It was then subsequently administered orally at dosages of 15 to 17.5 mg/kg/day, given as a single dose or in two divided doses for 1 to 2 weeks. It was then gradually tapered to 6 to 12.5 mg/kg/day by 9 weeks, depending on signs of toxicity or rejection and blood levels. Alternately, it was given on the basis of body surface area (500 mg/M^2 daily, reducing by 50 mg/M^2 weekly to 300 mg/M^2). Trough blood levels are monitored with a radioim-

munoassay, and dosages are adjusted to maintain them above 200 ng/ml.

Prednisone is given in a dose of 0.5 mg/kg on the day of transplantation and gradually reduced to 0.1 to 0.2 mg/kg/day by 12 weeks. In some centers, prednisone is discontinued 4 or 5 months after transplantation; in others, a maintenance dose is given on an alternate-day schedule (Benfield et al., 1999; Ettenger et al., 1990).

In the January 1997 report of NAPRTCS, covering the years 1987 to 1996 (Benfield et al., 1999), 89% of patients with a functioning graft continued to receive cyclosporine 5 years after transplantation and 84% of patients continued to receive azathioprine, whereas 26% of patients received alternate-day steroid therapy 4 years after transplantation. Polyclonal T-cell antibody ATG/ALG was used for induction in 37% of the living donor recipients and in 47% of the cadaver donor recipients, and the monoclonal T-cell antibody, OKT3, was used for induction in 12% of the living related donor recipients and in 19% of the cadaveric donor recipients.

As discussed earlier, improved understanding of graft rejection mechanisms and the development of several new agents now permit a multipronged attack on the rejection process. This has resulted in better patient and graft survivals with less toxicity. Thus the combined use of several of these agents provides a synergistic rather than a mere additive effect (Hong and Kahan, 2000). In many centers, the induction agents consist of one of the anti–IL-2Rα chain antibodies, Daclizumab or basiliximab, along with steroids, mycophenolate mofetil (instead of azathioprine), and tacrolimus instead of cyclosporine. Some are combining tacrolimus with steroids and sirolimus (Shapiro et al., 2002).

In the past, acute rejection episodes were treated with intravenous pulses of methylprednisolone as high as 30 mg/kg/day for 3 days (Bell et al., 1971). However, Kauffman and colleagues (1979) found pulses of 3 mg/kg to be equally effective, so most centers now use lower steroid dosages. The major reason is the recognition of the deleterious effects of high cumulative dosages of corticosteroids (Ettenger et al., 1990). Among the most useful agents have been either ALG or ATG for 5 days or OKT3 (2.5 to 10 mg/day for 1 to 14 days). ATG is usually effective only for reversing rejection episodes in low-risk patients (i.e., those with living-related donor kidneys or 6 antigen–matched cadaveric kidneys), but OKT3 may reverse rejection crises in high-risk patients who are resistant to high-dose methylprednisolone and/or ATG (Leone et al., 1987).

Post-transplantation Problems

Rejection

Rejection is the most common problem during the 3 months immediately after transplantation (Ettenger et al., 1990; McEnery et al., 1992). Except for hyperacute rejection, most such episodes can be partially or completely reversed by one of the earlier-mentioned immunosuppressive agents. Rejection episodes are classified as follows (Table 43-6):

TABLE 43-6 · SOLID ORGAN REJECTION PATTERNS, EXAMPLE: RENAL

Type	Time after Transplant	Signs and Symptoms	Rapidity of Onset	Immune Component	Pathology	Treatment (% Success)
Hyperacute	<24 hr	Fever, anuria	Hours	Antibody and complement	PMN deposition and thrombosis	None (0%)
Accelerated	3–5 days	Fever, graft swelling, oliguria, tenderness	1 day	Non–complement-fixing antibody	Vascular disruption, hemorrhage	ALG, ATG, anti-CD3 (60%)
Acute	6–90 days	Oliguria, salt retention, graft swelling, tenderness, sometimes fever	Days to weeks	T cells and antibody	Tubulitis, endovasculitis	Steroids, ALG, ATG, anti-CD3 (60-90%)
Chronic	>60 days	Edema, hypertension, proteinuria, occasional hematuria	Months to years	Antibody	Vascular onion skinning	None (0%)

· *Hyperacute rejection* occurs within the first 48 hours after the anastomosis in recipients with preformed antileukocyte antibodies. It is characterized by fever and anuria. The binding of cytotoxic antibodies to the vascular endothelium activates complement with subsequent aggregation of neutrophils and platelets, resulting in thrombosis. This is an irreversible event, and the only treatment option is immediate transplant removal.

· *Accelerated rejection* occurs on the third to the fifth day after transplantation. It is accompanied by fever, graft swelling, oliguria, and tenderness. It is thought to be mediated by non–complement-fixing antibodies to antigens present in the donor kidney. Histopathologically it is characterized by vascular disruption with hemorrhage. The most effective treatment is antilymphocyte reagents with or without plasmapheresis; these have a success rate of about 60% in reversing this process.

· *Acute rejection,* the most common form, is due to a primary allogeneic response occurring within the first 6 to 90 days after transplantation. It is mediated by both T cells and antibodies that cause "tubulitis" and vasculitis, respectively. High-dose pulse steroids and antilymphocyte reagents are effective in reversing the T-cell response about 80% to 90% of the time, but antilymphocyte antibodies reverse the vasculitis only about 60% of the time.

· *Chronic rejection* occurs when the tenuous graft tolerance is disturbed, 2 months or more after transplantation. It is characterized by marked proteinuria, occasional hematuria, hypertension, and nephrotic syndrome. The primary mediator of this type of rejection is antibody. Histopathologically, there is vascular onion skinning. A kidney biopsy is usually necessary to distinguish rejection from cyclosporine or tacrolimus nephrotoxicity. There is no effective treatment.

Graft loss accounts for most prolonged hospital stays for renal transplant patients (Arbus et al., 1993). Most of these patients receive a second kidney. Subsequent grafts from living donors have an improved survival, but those from cadavers do not (Cecka, 2002; Tejani et al., 1993).

Other problems of the immediate post-transplantation period include acute tubular necrosis (particularly if cadaver kidneys are used and the ischemic time is prolonged), ureteral leaks (Ehrlich, 1984), and recurrence of the hemolytic-uremic syndrome, especially in patients who are treated with cyclosporine (Leithner et al., 1985). Hypertension, if present before transplantation, is eventually ameliorated, although it usually persists for the first 6 months and may persist in a mild form indefinitely.

Primary Disease Recurrence

Recurrence of the primary renal disease in the grafted kidney does occur, but the overall frequency is low (Cameron, 1982; Laine et al., 1993). The diseases most likely to recur fall into three categories:

· Primary glomerulonephritis (particularly focal glomerulosclerosis with the nephrotic syndrome)
· Systemic diseases that involve the kidney (mainly insulin-dependent diabetes mellitus, systemic lupus erythematosus, and Henoch-Schönlein purpura)
· Metabolic diseases (e.g., cystinosis and oxalosis)

Because of the low frequency of recurrence of these primary diseases, none is a contraindication for renal transplantation (Cecka, 2002; McEnery et al., 1992).

Growth Retardation

Growth retardation is a major problem in pediatric renal transplantation (Fine, 1997; Sanchez et al., 1998). Initially, this is a result of the ESRD itself. Despite successful renal transplantation, growth failure is perpetuated by immunosuppressive regimens that use high-dose steroids.

Another contributing factor is the recipient's age. When transplantation is performed shortly before puberty, growth spurts fostered by normally functioning grafts have usually led to epiphyseal closure, so true catch-up growth and normal adult stature rarely occur. The lower-dose and/or alternate-day steroid regimens that have been used more recently have improved growth rates and prevented other unwanted steroid side effects (Turenne et al., 1997). In addition, significant amelioration of this problem is accomplished by early transplantation, particularly during the first year of life (Humar et al., 2001). With combination immunosuppressive regimens using alternate-day steroids or discontinuing steroids a few months post-transplantation, lessened growth failure can be expected without compromised graft survival (Fine, 1997).

Finally, studies have shown a sustained improvement in height and maintenance of bone mass when growth hormone therapy was administered to renal transplant recipients (Sanchez et al., 2002). However, bone formation rates did not increase with growth hormone treatment.

Orthopedic Problems

Orthopedic problems in renal transplantation include slipped femoral epiphyses, spontaneous fractures, and aseptic necrosis, all of which may lead to crippling deformities. Osteoporosis may result in axial compression fractures and osteonecrosis of the lower extremities (Ruderman et al., 1979). The cause of osteoporosis is uncertain but may be related to steroid therapy, antecedent uremia, inactivity, and renal osteodystrophy. Secondary hyperparathyroidism does not usually necessitate parathyroidectomy at the time of transplantation, because it can be managed with a low-calcium, high-phosphate diet and eventually subsides spontaneously.

Psychiatric Problems

Psychiatric problems are common in pediatric renal transplantation, particularly in adolescents, in large part because of their obesity, Cushingoid changes, and loss of physical attractiveness. The latter problems have not been completely obviated by cyclosporine and steroid reduction, because hirsutism and a disproportionate Cushingoid appearance have been observed in patients receiving cyclosporine. Suicide is not uncommon.

Other Problems

Other nonimmunologic causes of death include electrolytic imbalance, infection, pulmonary embolism, cerebral hemorrhage, recurrence of Wilms' tumor, and reticulum cell sarcoma of the brain. However, infection is the most common cause of death, in large part a result of the immunosuppression.

Prognosis

Despite the sequelae of rejection, recurrence of disease, growth retardation, and orthopedic and psychiatric problems, renal transplantation is clearly as successful in children as in adults, and there is strong support for its continued and expanded use in pediatric ESRD (Benfield et al., 1999; Humar et al., 2001).

PEDIATRIC LIVER TRANSPLANTATION

Historical Aspects

Liver transplantation had its inception in 1963, when Starzl and co-workers (1987) replaced the diseased liver of a 3-year-old child who had extrahepatic biliary atre-

sia. Although that patient died, subsequent successes have established liver transplantation as standard therapy for a variety of advanced chronic liver diseases in both children and adults (Jain et al., 2002). At present, at least 235 centers worldwide are performing liver transplants and, by 2001, a total of 100,179 transplants had been performed (Cecka and Terasaki, 2002). Infants and children account for approximately 15% of all recipients (Jain et al., 2002).

High mortality was common before the 1980s because of surgical technical and organ preservation problems, choice of recipients with hopelessly advanced disease, overwhelming infection, and graft rejection. Since 1983, however, 1-year survival rates have increased from 25% to 78%, depending on the age and health of the recipient, the underlying condition, and various clinical considerations. This improvement has resulted not only from better surgical techniques but, most important, from the use of cyclosporine (Starzl et al., 1987).

Indications

Liver transplantation is indicated in the following situations (Mowat, 1987):

· Chronic end-stage liver disease
· Fulminant acute liver failure
· Cancer limited to the liver

The most common causes of chronic end-stage liver disease in children include (1) the biliary atresia syndromes (accounting for nearly 50% of all transplant operations); (2) metabolic diseases (representing roughly 25%), such as α_1-antitrypsin deficiency, Wilson's disease, Crigler-Najjar syndrome, tyrosinemia, glycogen storage disease types I and IV, protoporphyria, sea-blue histiocyte syndrome and others; (3) bile duct hypoplasia; (4) Byler's familial cholestasis; and (5) chronic active hepatitis (Starzl et al., 1987). Infants with newborn liver failure have undergone successful allogeneic liver transplants (Lund et al., 1993).

Fulminant hepatitis and primary hepatic tumors (hepatoblastomas, hepatocellular tumors, and cholangiocarcinomas) are rare indications for liver transplantation in children. Hepatocellular carcinoma is often a result of maternal transmission of hepatitis B; for two such infants, the procedure was successful and there was no tumor recurrence; however, there was a recurrence of hepatitis B infection (Yandza et al., 1993).

The difficult clinical problem is to select patients who are not too ill to survive the procedure but who are sufficiently ill to warrant a high-risk procedure. Practically, patients who meet two of the following four criteria are considered candidates (van Thiel, 1985):

· A total bilirubin of 15 mg/dl or greater
· A prothrombin time greater than the control by 5 seconds and uncorrectable with vitamin K
· A serum albumin level of 2.5 g/dl or lower
· Hepatic encephalopathy that prevents normal function despite optimal medical therapy

Preoperative Evaluation

The potential recipient should be evaluated carefully to make certain that the underlying cause of the liver failure has been diagnosed accurately, to ascertain that hydration is adequate, to assess renal status, to determine whether encephalopathy is present, and to identify any potential source of infection. Angiography, ultrasound, Doppler computed tomography (CT), and magnetic resonance imaging (MRI) can be used to evaluate whether vascular or biliary abnormalities are present.

Of particular importance is the determination of patency of the portal vein. If the portal vein is thrombosed, perfusion of the graft can be accomplished by means of a vascular graft; however, this greatly increases the surgical complexity and failure rate of the transplant procedure.

Donor Operation

Current organ preservation and surgical techniques limit the time possible for donor organ storage to 6 to 12 hours at most, with best results in those held for less than 6 hours (Starzl et al., 1987). Especially in the pediatric age group, good matching of donor and recipient size is mandatory for surgical implantation of the orthotopic (same site) graft. Donor weight limits are usually set at 30% below to 10% above the recipient's weight. This narrow range markedly reduces the number of potential appropriate organ donors for children. Because of these considerations, decisions regarding suitability of the organ are based only on the potential donor's ABO blood type, human immunodeficiency virus (HIV) antibody status, organ size, liver function tests, and stability of the heart-beating cadaver. Usually, neither HLA matching nor serologic cross-matching is considered.

Proper harvest of the donor liver is crucial, because the liver cannot tolerate either warm or cold ischemia as well as a donor kidney can. Multiple organs are usually harvested from a single heart-beating cadaver. The liver is dissected first, followed by the kidneys and the heart. After the initial dissection of all organs, the abdominal viscera are perfused through the aorta with cold intracellular electrolyte (Collins') solution while the heart is perfused to induce cardioplegia. Rapid core cooling of the liver and kidneys is accomplished in this fashion, which practically eliminates any period of warm ischemia. Livers harvested in this manner will function if reimplanted within 8 to 12 hours.

Recipient and Transplant Operations

Removal of the diseased liver is often the most difficult aspect of orthotopic liver transplantation, which in its totality is one of the most technically demanding of all surgical procedures. Because of problems such as portal hypertension, coagulation defects, and metabolic imbalances, the major intraoperative problems are hemodynamic and metabolic, with hyperkalemic cardiac arrest remaining a major risk. During hepatectomy, the entire venous return from the abdominal viscera and from the lower half of the body is clamped off. This technique produces two deleterious effects; it significantly reduces overall cardiac output and produces marked venous hypertension in the splanchnic and renal circulations.

In adults and larger children, this problem is diminished by constructing a veno-venous bypass wherein the blood in the portal vein and inferior vena cava is shunted through a centrifugal pump similar to those used in cardiopulmonary bypass and returned to the superior vena cava via the axillary vein. Although this procedure increases the technical complexity of the operation, it greatly diminishes the fluid accumulation in the splanchnic bed and diminishes the incidence of renal failure postoperatively.

In smaller children with vessels that are too small to cannulate and bypass effectively, reliance is placed on the natural collateral venous circulation. Younger infants naturally tolerate this type of clamping better. Unlike the situation in adults, prior abdominal surgery has little overall impact on the prognosis in pediatric liver transplantation.

Although all of the operative steps, up to actual removal of the liver, can be performed in the recipient while the donor organ is in transit, the recipient's hepatectomy is not done until the donor organ arrives in the operative suite. Suprahepatic vena caval and portal venous donor–recipient anastomoses are performed first to re-establish portal blood flow and end the cold ischemia time. End-to-end hepatic artery and infrahepatic vena caval anastomoses are done next, then end-to-end choledochostomy is performed. Assessment of allograft function begins during the operation with assessment of bile output and correction of coagulation factor deficiencies.

Immunosuppression and Postoperative Care

As with renal transplantation, combined therapy attacking several facets of the potential rejection process is used for liver transplantation. Anti-IL-2Rα antibodies are given intravenously on the day of the transplant, followed by tacrolimus at a dosage of usually 0.05 mg/kg every 12 hours intravenously initially, then orally at 0.12 mg/kg every 12 hours thereafter plus mycophenolate mofetil and steroids tapered slowly over a year.

Major postoperative problems may occur (1) immediately (0 to 24 hours), (2) early (24 to 48 hours), (3) subacutely (2 to 12 days), or (4) later (13 days and beyond) (van Thiel, 1985). Fluid overload is the most common immediate problem, and hepatic arterial or portal vein thrombosis is the major early complication (usually signaling graft failure). Biliary leaks are the next most common early or subacute problem. Infection and renal dysfunction may also occur subacutely. Graft rejection or viral hepatitis is a late complication.

A form of chronic rejection, the *vanishing bile duct syndrome*, has been correlated with a complete mismatch for class I antigens (Donaldson et al., 1987). Patients without serious complications are ordinarily hospitalized for 3 weeks, are then followed closely as outpatients, and can return home by 6 weeks. Most patients have excellent graft function, with serum bilirubin and transaminase values in the normal or moderately elevated range.

Prognosis

As already noted, 1-year survival rates after liver transplantation have improved dramatically since 1983. In general, most programs achieve 75% to 80% 1-year survival rates in children. From March 1981 to April 1998, 808 children received liver transplants at Children's Hospital of Pittsburgh (Jain et al., 2002). All patients were followed until March 2001, with a mean follow-up of 12.2 ± 3.9 years. There were 405 female (50.2%) and 403 male (49.8%) recipients. Mean age at transplant was 5.3 ± 4.9 years (mean 3.3; range 0.04 to 17.95), with 285 children (25.3%) being younger than 2 years of age at transplant. Cyclosporine was used for immunosuppression before November 1989 in 482 children (50.7%), but all 326 subsequent recipients (40.3%) were given tacrolimus.

Overall patient survival at 1, 5, 10, 15, and 20 years was 77.1%, 72.6%, 69.4%, 65.8%, and 64.4%, respectively. There was no difference in survival for male or female patients at any time point. A significant decrease in survival was seen with cyclosporine-based immunosuppression (71.2%, 68.1%, 65.4%, and 61%) versus tacrolimus-based immunosuppression (85.8%, 84.7%, 83.3%, and 82.9%) at 1, 3, 5, and 10 years, respectively ($P = 0.0001$). The mean annual death rate beyond 2 years after transplantation was 0.47%, with the mean annual death rate for patients who received tacrolimus-based immunosuppression being significantly lower than that for those who received cyclosporine-based immunosuppression (0.14% vs. 0.8%; $P = 0.001$).

In the Pittsburgh study, the overall 20-year actuarial survival for pediatric liver transplantation was 64% (Jain et al., 2002). Survival has increased by 20% in the last 12 years with tacrolimus-based immunosuppression. Although this improvement may be the result of several factors, retransplantation as a result of acute or chronic rejection has been completely eliminated in patients treated with tacrolimus.

Acute rejection episodes occur in approximately two thirds of patients in the first 6 months; these usually subside after 3 days of high-dose methylprednisolone (Solu-Medrol), but some patients require OKT3 or ATG therapy for reversal. In the Pittsburgh study, the most common etiologies of graft loss were hepatic artery thrombosis (33.4%), acute or chronic rejection (26.6%), and primary nonfunction (16.7%) (Jain et al., 2002). Of note, retransplantation for graft loss because of acute or chronic rejection occurred only in those patients who received cyclosporine-based immunosuppression at Pittsburgh (Jain et al., 2002).

Causes of death include acute and chronic rejection, infection, vascular surgical complications, liver infarction, and cerebrovascular accidents. Patients with cholestatic chronic liver disease or end-stage liver disease caused by metabolic disorders, such as α_1-antitrypsin deficiency, survive longer than those with fulminant liver failure or postnecrotic cirrhosis (e.g., postneonatal hepatitis, chronic active hepatitis) (Belle et al., 1995).

There is considerable controversy over whether to operate on patients with chronic hepatitis B infections. In a retrospective study of European patients who were hepatitis B surface antigen (HBsAg) positive at the time of transplantation, survival was 75% at 1 year and 63% at 3 years; most patients were given long-term immunoprophylaxis with anti-HBs immune globulin, but the risk of recurrent infection at 3 years was 50% (Samuel et al., 1993).

Patients with malignancy fare least well, with less than a 50% 2-year survival. In one French study, patients who received liver transplants before age 2 had poor growth velocity by the third year after transplantation (Codoner-Franch et al., 1994); however, the authors found that long-term improvement in height usually occurred in most patients when surgery took place after age 2 years, particularly if the patients were kept on an alternate-day steroid regimen.

Chimerism

Chimerism, the presence of genetically different components within an animal or person, is an interesting phenomenon that has been reported after liver transplantation with increasing frequency (Starzl and Zinkernagel, 2001; Starzl et al., 1992a, 1992b, 1994). GVH reactions have long been known to occur in some liver transplant recipients. One such patient was investigated after recovery from GVH-mediated myelosuppression and found to have donor-type stem cells (Collins et al., 1993).

This phenomenon was also extensively investigated by PCR analysis of tissues from two patients with type IV glycogen storage disease and from one with type I Gaucher's disease 26 to 91 months after surgery (Starzl et al., 1994). Donor-type HLA-DR DNA was found in the heart of both patients with glycogen storage disease; in the skin of one; and in the skin, intestine, blood, and bone marrow of the patient with Gaucher's disease. The cardiac deposits of amylopectin in the patients with type IV glycogen storage disease and the lymph node deposits of glucocerebroside in the patient with Gaucher's disease were reportedly dramatically reduced. The authors concluded that systemic microchimerism occurs after allogeneic liver transplantation and that this can ameliorate pancellular enzyme deficiencies.

In addition to stem cells, however, the liver is also a source of many other hematopoietic cell lineages; thus it is not clear that all of the chimeric cells arose from hepatic stem cells. The authors also speculate that the chimerism, which they think may occur almost uniformly in liver transplant recipients, also accounts for tolerance of the recipient to the liver and resultant graft acceptance (Starzl et al., 1992a, 1992b). They point out that a number of liver transplant recipients have discontinued their immunosuppressive drugs altogether without graft rejection (Starzl and Zinkernagel, 2001; Starzl et al., 1992b).

Liver Transplantation from Living-Related Donors

As is the case for all solid organ transplantation, lack of suitable donors is a major problem for liver transplantation. Xenotransplantation is being explored as an alternative, but there have been no successes yet. Since 1988, this problem has been approached at several centers by partial hepatectomies of living-related donors (Yamaoka et al., 1993). In a report from Japan (Yamaoka et al., 1993), 73 living-related transplants had been given to 72 patients, and 59 recipients were alive and well with the original graft and normal liver function at follow-ups 3 to 47 months afterward. The left lateral segment was used in 46 cases, the left lobe in 25 cases, and the right lobe in one case. Donor safety is much greater with use of the left lateral segment; the recipients undergo total hepatectomies.

PEDIATRIC HEART TRANSPLANTATION

The first human heart transplant was performed in December 1967. By 2001, 61,195 heart transplantations had been reported to the International Heart Transplantation Registry (Cecka and Terasaki, 2002). More than 2000 patients have been pediatric recipients (Azeka et al., 2002; Bauer et al., 2001; Dellgren et al., 2001; Laks et al., 2001; Towbin, 2002; Vricella et al., 2002), and most of these operations have been performed since 1983.

Indications

The various forms of cardiomyopathy are the most common pediatric indications for heart transplantation, followed by congenital heart disease. Congenital heart disease includes hypoplastic left-sided heart syndrome and other forms of complex congenital heart defects.

Absolute contraindications include the presence of active uncontrolled infection in the recipient, insulin-dependent diabetes mellitus, active or recent malignancy, gastroduodenal ulcer, a positive serologic HLA cross-match, ABO incompatibility, elevated pulmonary arterial resistance, HIV antibodies, and significant chronic end-organ dysfunction (Ardehali et al., 1994; Breen et al., 1993; Michler et al., 1993). Patients with increased pulmonary vascular resistance are referred for heart–lung transplantation.

As with other forms of organ transplantation, a paucity of available organs is a major limitation, particularly in the pediatric age group. The cardiac allografts are selected by matching ABO blood group and approximate body weight and heart size. However, there have been a few successful ABO mismatched heart transplants in young infants who do not have high titers of isohemagglutinins (West et al., 2001). Contraindications for donation include the presence of severe cardiac disease and unresolved systemic infection. A history of resuscitation or the receipt of inotropic agents is not necessarily an exclusion.

Immunosuppression

Modern immunosuppressive regimens for heart transplantation are similar in many respects to those already described for renal and hepatic grafts. Usually, an anti–IL-2R alpha chain monoclonal antibody is given for induction therapy on the day of the transplant along with high-dose (10 mg/kg) intravenous methylprednisolone. Prednisone is given postoperatively at 3 mg/kg/day and maintained at 0.1 mg/kg/day orally; it is discontinued after the first normal findings from an endomyocardial biopsy. Tacrolimus is then begun as the primary immunosuppressive agent (Armitage et al., 1993). In some centers, mycophenolate mofetil has also been used as part of the combination of immunosuppressive agents. High-dose methylprednisolone, ALS/ATG, or OKT3 monoclonal antibody has been used to treat acute rejection episodes, and methotrexate or total lymphoid irradiation has been used for chronic rejection (Chinnock et al., 1993).

Complications

Post-transplantation complications include (1) hemodynamic problems during the first few days, (2) rejection episodes, and (3) side effects of immunosuppression. Hemodynamic problems are more likely to occur if there is increased pulmonary arterial resistance or if the donor heart is in less than optimal condition.

Rejection episodes can be diagnosed with endomyocardial biopsy (Caves et al., 1973). The frequency of rejection is greatest within the first 6 months after transplantation. Although the frequency of rejection episodes may not be diminished by the newer immunosuppressive agents, their severity has been. The result is that many fewer hearts have been lost to this complication (Armitage et al., 1993).

A retrospective analysis by Opelz and Wujciak (1994) revealed that graft survival in heart transplantation was significantly influenced by the extent of HLA compatibility. In addition, use of a male donor heart into a female recipient has also been associated with a higher incidence of rejection (Kawauchi et al., 1993).

Postoperative pulmonary hypertension can be a major cause of early death after heart transplantation, particularly in older children and especially in those with congenital heart disease who received a graft that had been preserved more than 6 hours (Fukushima et al., 1994).

Because a much lower dosage of steroids is required with tacrolimus immunosuppression, the frequency of infectious complications is lower. This is particularly true because steroids have been discontinued altogether in a number of patients (Armitage et al., 1993; Canter et al., 1994). Nevertheless, bacterial, fungal, and viral infections still occur with significant frequency (Miller et al., 1994).

Viral infections, such as cytomegalovirus (CMV) and hepatitis, represent the major cause of morbidity in pediatric transplant patients and account for 19% of all deaths (Bernstein, 1993; Elkins et al., 1993; Miller et al., 1994). CMV accounts for 25% of serious infections and occurs either as a primary infection or as a reactivation.

Lymphomas have developed in a number of patients receiving cyclosporine and azathioprine plus antilymphocyte antibodies for rejection episodes (Opelz and Henderson, 1993). The tumors have often regressed after a reduction or discontinuation of these immunosuppressive agents.

Prognosis

Since the introduction of cyclosporine 20 years ago, the results of cardiac transplantation have improved greatly. The International Heart Transplantation Registry has shown a 71% 4-year survival rate for patients receiving cyclosporine- or tacrolimus-based, triple-immunosuppression therapy, compared with a 41% survival rate for those given immunosuppression with only azathioprine and prednisone (Kaye, 1993). Survival, however, is influenced by the age of the recipient; patients younger than age 40 have a better survival rate.

Especially impressive have been results of cardiac transplantation procedures performed in newborn infants or in infants in the first year of life (Assaad, 1993; Bailey et al., 1993; Zales and Stapleton, 1993).

The largest experience with infant transplant surgery has been at Loma Linda, California (Assaad, 1993; Bailey et al., 1993), where 140 transplants were performed in 139 infants from 1985 until 1993. These patients ranged in age from 3 hours to 12 months. Overall survival was 83%, with 5-year actuarial survival at 80%; 5-year survival of 60 newborn recipients was 84%.

At the University of Giessen in Germany, 82 heart transplants were performed in 80 infants and children from 1988 to 2001 (Bauer et al., 2001). Diagnoses before transplant were hypoplastic left-sided heart syndrome (n = 43), cardiomyopathy (n = 19), endocardial fibroelastosis (n = 6), and other complex congenital heart diseases (n = 12). Sixty-one patients were younger than 1 year at transplantation. Overall survival rate was 79% at 1 year and 73% at 5 and 10 years. Twenty patients died after transplantation from the following

causes: rejection (eight patients), right ventricular failure (four patients), transplant coronary artery disease (two patients), and other causes (six patients). In the majority of patients, somatic growth was not impaired and renal function was reduced (but stable). Two patients developed post-transplant lymphoproliferative disease, which was treated successfully. Major long-term morbidity was neurologic deficit—severe in three patients and minor in six.

In summary, heart transplantation in infants and children can be performed with good early and late results (Bauer et al., 2001). However, neurologic problems are significant (Fleisher et al., 2002).

HEART–LUNG AND LUNG TRANSPLANTATION

By 2001, combined heart and lung transplants had been performed successfully at 78 institutions in 2722 patients of all ages who had both end-stage heart and lung disease (Cecka and Terasaki, 2002). The indications are congenital heart disease, primary pulmonary hypertension, cystic fibrosis, and other end-stage lung diseases.

Heart–lung transplantation has been used most successfully in the treatment of cystic fibrosis (Vricella et al., 2002) and has become an established form of treatment over the past few years. Sixty-four patients with cystic fibrosis underwent heart–lung transplantation (n = 22, 34.4%) or bilateral lung transplantation (n = 42, 65.6%) at Stanford between 1988 and 2000. The actuarial survival rates at 1, 3, 5, and 10 years were 93.2%, 77.7%, 61.8%, and 48.1%, respectively, with no significant difference between bilateral lung transplantation and heart–lung transplantation.

The major hospital complications were pneumonia (n = 11, 17.2%) and bleeding (n = 8, 12.5%). Freedom from acute lung rejection beyond 1 year was 47.7%. Obliterative bronchiolitis accounted for 8 (50.0%) of 16 late deaths. Patients with immunodeficiency disorders who have end-stage lung disease and cor pulmonale may also be candidates for a transplant.

As of 2001, 13,710 lung transplantations in children and adults were reported to the World Transplant Registry from 120 centers (Cecka and Terasaki, 2002). From 1990 to 2002, 207 isolated lung transplants were performed on 190 children younger than age 18 at St. Louis Children's Hospital, representing the single largest series of lung transplants in children (Huddleston et al., 2002). Of the patients, 32 were younger than 1 year of age, 22 were 1 to 5 years of age, 32 were 5 to 10 years of age, and 121 were 10 to 18 years old.

The groups by major diagnostic category were cystic fibrosis (n = 89), pulmonary vascular disease (n = 44), bronchiolitis obliterans (n = 21), pulmonary alveolar proteinosis (n = 12), pulmonary fibrosis (n = 15), and other (n = 26). The average age at the time of transplant was 9.5 ± 5.9 years (range 36 days to 18 years).

Overall survival was 77% at 1 year, 62% at 3 years, and 55% at 5 years. The most common cause of early deaths was graft failure (13/25, 52%). The most common causes of late death were bronchiolitis obliterans (35/61, 57%), infection (13/61, 21%), and post-transplant malignancies (11/61, 18%). No patient died of acute rejection. In those who survived for more than 3 months (mean follow-up 3.5 years, range 3 months to 11 years), the overall rate of occurrence of bronchiolitis obliterans was 46% (80/175) and the overall incidence of post-transplant malignancies was 14% (24/175). Major risk factors for the development of bronchiolitis obliterans were age older than 3 years, more than two episodes of acute rejection, and organ ischemic time longer than 180 minutes (Huddleston et al., 2002).

Thus lung transplantation in children is a high-risk but viable treatment for end-stage pulmonary parenchymal and vascular disease. The major hurdle to overcome in long-term survival is bronchiolitis obliterans.

Donor organ availability is an even greater problem for heart–lung and lung transplantation than for other organs and tissues, because both heart and lungs must be normal. If the recipient's heart is normal, it can be used as a donor heart for a second patient. There is an extreme scarcity of healthy donor lungs because pulmonary edema, aspiration, and pneumonia commonly occur in brain-dead patients.

As a potential means of providing organs for more patients, some have advocated single-lung transplantation. Single-lung transplantation has been advocated for adult patients with end-stage emphysema or pulmonary fibrosis. A combined liver, heart, and lung transplantation was performed successfully in a patient who had primary biliary cirrhosis and primary pulmonary hypertension (Wallwork et al., 1987). Lung transplantation is also discussed in Chapter 33.

TRANSPLANTATION OF PANCREATIC TISSUE

Indications

Even though endocrine deficiencies can be treated with hormone administration, permanent cure can theoretically be achieved through organ or tissue transplantation. This is particularly attractive in diabetes, because, despite insulin administration, it is a leading cause of uremia and blindness and remains the third leading cause of death in the United States (Tyden et al., 1986).

As with other forms of organ transplantation, the past four decades have witnessed a tremendous increase in transplantation of the pancreas. From 1966 to 2001, 4086 pancreatic transplants and 12,916 combined kidney and pancreas transplants were reported to the World Transplant Directory (Cecka and Terasaki, 2002). In addition, there have been pancreas–liver, pancreas–kidney–liver, and pancreas–heart transplants.

There appears to be a beneficial effect from combining pancreas and kidney transplantation in diabetic patients, because most such recipients have irreversible renal disease. In those dually grafted, cadaver renal graft functional rates at 1 year were comparable to those in diabetic patients who were given only renal grafts. Moreover, the dually transplanted patients were found to have no further deterioration in retinopathy or neuropathy.

The best current immunosuppressive regimens include combinations of tacrolimus, mycophenolate mofetil, and prednisone (Stratta, 1999).

Prognosis

Clearly, the results of pancreatic transplantation have improved with time, with 1-year graft survival rates rising from 42% prior to 1978 to 70% to 80% in 2001 (Sutherland et al., 2001). The improvement is largely due to the introduction of calcineurin inhibitors as well as other newer immunosuppressive agents (Oh et al., 2001; Stratta, 1999). In addition, the major technical problem of what to do with the exocrine ducts has been successfully overcome by anastomosing them to the bladder; the earlier practice of enteric drainage resulted in lower graft survival rates (Sutherland et al., 1994).

TRANSPLANTATION OF PARATHYROID TISSUE

Autotransplantation of parathyroid tissue is useful in the treatment of primary (Ross et al., 1986) and secondary hyperparathyroidism (Saxe, 1984; Sitges-Serra and Caralps-Riera, 1987; Wells et al., 1978). In this procedure, a total parathyroidectomy is performed and the extirpated glands are sliced into small (1×2 mm) pieces and placed in culture medium. Some 20 to 25 such pieces are then implanted into a site on the volar surface of the nondominant forearm. The remaining pieces are frozen for future use (Durando et al., 1993). The incidence of hypoparathyroidism after total parathyroidectomy plus autotransplantation has ranged from 13% to 40%, however, and there have been several cases of late graft failure (Sitges-Serra and Caralps-Riera, 1987).

SKIN TRANSPLANTATION

The principal indication for a skin allograft is a burn affecting more than 80% of the body surface, an invariably fatal injury. In these patients, the burn sites are covered with cultured allogeneic epidermal cells grown from cadaveric skin (Madden et al., 1986) and whatever autologous skin is available. Culturing the epidermal cells eventually results in loss of DR antigen expression (Hefton et al., 1984). Wound healing is significantly hastened for first- and second-degree burns but not for third-degree burns (Madden et al., 1986). It is possible that the allografted cells survive only temporarily and that they are gradually replaced by autologous epidermal cells (Madden et al., 1986).

BONE TRANSPLANTATION

Bone transplantation has been used primarily to replace large segments of the long bones or the pelvis with non-viable allogeneic bone in patients with bone tumors. In several series, success rates as high as 89% have been reported (Czitrom et al., 1986; Friedlander et al., 1983). No immunosuppression or HLA donor typing is used.

BONE MARROW TRANSPLANTATION

Historical Aspects

The observation by Lorenz and co-workers (1952) that lethally irradiated animals could be reconstituted by bone marrow cells stimulated attempts to apply this therapy to patients with bone marrow failure. However, such transplants were initially successful only in identical twins (Pillow et al., 1966); this changed in the late 1960s with the discovery of the human MHC (Amos and Bach, 1968).

Since 1955, more than 118,000 bone marrow transplantations have been performed worldwide at 249 centers in the treatment of more than 50 different fatal diseases (Cecka and Terasaki, 2002). Most of these transplants have been autologous, with 25,000 to 35,000 such transplants performed annually, compared with approximately 15,000 allogeneic transplants done annually. Approximately 30% of the transplants have been performed in children, where they have been more successful than in adults. Over the past decade, granulocyte colony-stimulating factor (G-CSF) mobilized stem cells in peripheral blood have often been used instead of bone marrow cells, particularly for autologous transplants and in older recipients. Another source of stem cells is umbilical cord blood (Barker and Wagner, 2002).

The objective of bone marrow or any other form of *hematopoietic stem cell transplantation* is to replace defective, absent, or malignant cells of the recipient with normal replicating hematopoietic and immunocompetent cells. Normal bone marrow contains self-replicating cells that can give rise to erythrocytes, granulocytes, cells of the monocyte-macrophage lineage, megakaryocytes, and immunocompetent T, B, and NK cells (Brenner et al., 1993; Wu et al., 1967; 1968).

Problems Unique to Bone Marrow Transplantation

Certain unique problems distinguish bone marrow transplantation from grafting of solid organs, such as the kidney, liver, and heart. The first problem is that immunocompetent cells in both the recipient and in the donor marrow or blood have the potential of rejecting each other, resulting in graft rejection on the one hand and GVHD on the other (Martin et al., 1987). The second concern is that successful unfractionated marrow or blood stem cell grafting usually requires strict donor and recipient MHC class II antigen compatibility to minimize such reactions (Martin et al., 1987).

Finally, except for patients with SCID, complete DiGeorge anomaly, or identical twin donors, even HLA-identical recipients have to be pretreated with lethal doses of irradiation or cytotoxic agents and usually myeloablative agents as well to prevent graft rejection (Martin et al., 1987). Immunosuppressive agents commonly used to ensure the acceptance of solid organ grafts have deleterious effects on the very cells one is trying to engraft in patients with genetically determined immunodeficiency. Therefore immunosuppressive and myeloablative agents must be given *before* infusion of the marrow to avoid injury to the donor cells.

Indications

Diseases treated successfully with allogeneic bone marrow transplantation include the following (Good and Verjee, 2001):

- Radiation injury
- Primary immunodeficiencies
- Hematologic abnormalities: hemoglobinopathies, aplastic anemia, multiple myeloma, and leukemia
- Solid tumors, such as neuroblastoma and non-Hodgkin's lymphoma
- A number of inborn errors of metabolism

In addition, autologous marrow transplantation has been used in conjunction with lethal irradiation or chemotherapy in the treatment of patients with some hematologic malignancies (Woods et al., 2001), solid tumors (Montuoro et al., 2000; Nieboer et al., 2001), or breast cancer and is the most common type of bone marrow transplant being performed at present.

The rationale for bone marrow transplantation in leukemia is the hope that the leukemic cells can be reduced or eliminated with irradiation or chemotherapy and that the grafted allogeneic normal cells can then reject any remaining leukemic cells (Weiden et al., 1979). This concept of adoptive immunotherapy for leukemia, although supported by higher recurrence rates in identical twin transplants (Fefer et al., 1977; Gale and Champlin, 1984), is challenged by reports of patients in whom allogeneic engraftment was achieved but who had recurrences of their leukemia and of patients in whom the leukemia recurred in cells of donor type (Thomas, 1987; Thomas et al., 1975). Nevertheless, transplants into leukemic recipients using T-cell–depleted marrow have been associated with a higher degree of leukemia recurrence (Maraninchi et al., 1987).

Prevention of Rejection

Factors influencing the likelihood of engraftment include the following:

- The degree of immunoincompetence of the recipient
- The degree of MHC disparity of donor and recipient

· The degree of presensitization of the recipient to the histocompatibility antigens of the donor
· The number of marrow cells administered
· The pretransplant immunosuppression given to the recipient
· Whether T-cell depletion techniques are used

As already noted, unfractionated bone marrow or peripheral blood transplantation is unique in its requirement for MHC class II antigen compatibility. However, even MHC-compatible donor marrow or blood will be rejected unless the recipient is immunosuppressed or profoundly immunodeficient. Such rejection probably occurs on the basis of non-MHC minor locus (possibly including unique self-peptides) histocompatibility antigen differences. Unfractionated marrow or peripheral blood cells can become engrafted in HLA-disparate recipients if they lack cellular immunity, but fatal GVHD can be anticipated.

Presensitization of dogs to donor antigens by blood transfusion increases the likelihood of rejection of DLA-identical marrow (Martin et al., 1987). Thus prospective marrow recipients should not receive blood transfusions from potential sibling donors or from other family members because these will increase the risk of sensitization to minor locus antigens not controlled by the MHC.

Between 3 and 10.9×10^8/kg of nucleated marrow cells are required to achieve engraftment in aplasia and leukemia (Martin et al., 1987). By contrast, patients with SCID have required far fewer cells; as few as 4×10^6 unfractionated nucleated marrow cells per kilogram recipient body weight have resulted in immunologic reconstitution (O'Reilly et al., 1984). The difference is undoubtedly due to the presence of ample hematopoietic cells other than lymphocytes in the unconditioned SCID recipients, whereas the conditioning regimens in leukemia and aplasia leave the marrow devoid of cellular elements. However, despite receiving much higher numbers of T-cell–depleted marrow cells, some patients with non-SCID T-cell deficiency have not achieved engraftment (Berthet et al., 1994; O'Reilly et al., 1986).

The pretransplant conditioning agents used most widely have been x-irradiation, procarbazine, cyclophosphamide, busulfan, melphalan, fludarabine, and ATG. In nonmalignant conditions, such as aplasia or immunodeficiency, preparation of the recipient need be directed only at immunosuppression and "spacing" (i.e., making room in the marrow for donor cells). Thus total-body irradiation (TBI) required to eradicate malignant cells is not necessary.

Preparation of patients with acute leukemia or other malignancies for marrow transplantation is more complex because 1000 to 1200 rad of TBI is usually used to eradicate the tumor cells (Martin et al., 1987). A combination of 2 to 4 mg/kg of busulfan daily for 4 days, followed by 50 mg/kg cyclophosphamide daily for 2 days, has been commonly used to condition nonmalignant disorders (Blazar et al., 1985). A similar regimen has also been used by Tutschka (1986) for leukemia patients as an alternative to TBI and cyclophosphamide, resulting in considerably less morbidity in the early post-transplant period, no increase in leukemia recurrence, and better survival rates.

Marrow Transplant Procedure

Unfractionated bone marrow transplantation is the simplest of all transplantation procedures, offering little risk to the donor, because it involves removal of a tissue that is readily regenerated. The bone marrow cells are usually obtained by aspiration with a 14- or 16-gauge needle from multiple sites along both iliac crests, over the length of the sternum, or (in children) from the upper one third of the tibia while the donor is under general anesthesia (Martin et al., 1987; Thomas et al., 1975). The aspirate is placed in heparinized tissue culture medium, then passed through metal screens with diminishing apertures to remove bone spicules. Nucleated marrow cells are then enumerated and given intravenously in a manner similar to that of a blood transfusion.

Graft-versus-Host Reactions

GVH reactions are the major barrier to widespread successful application of bone marrow or peripheral blood stem cell transplantation to the treatment of many different diseases (Ferrara and Deeg, 1991; Glucksberg et al., 1974; Martin et al., 1987; O'Reilly, 1987; Parkman, 1991). The principal reason for this is that the recipient with a lethal T-cell defect (or one made equally T-cell–deficient by irradiation or chemotherapy) cannot reject bone marrow, matched or mismatched (Ferrara and Deeg, 1991). By contrast, engrafted genetically different immunocompetent donor T cells recognize foreign HLA antigens on the recipient's cells and respond to them (Ferrara and Deeg, 1991; Glucksberg et al., 1974; Parkman, 1991). In the case of unfractionated marrow or peripheral blood cell transplants from HLA-D–mismatched donors, this reaction of the donor T lymphocytes against the recipient is almost invariably fatal.

GVH reactions are usually mild and self-limited in infants with SCID who are not given pretransplant immunosuppression and who receive unfractionated HLA-identical related marrow (Parkman, 1991). However, in 60% of recipients given pretransplant irradiation or immunosuppressive drugs, GVH reactions are moderate to severe and they are fatal in 15% to 20% despite HLA identity (Glucksberg et al., 1974; Martin et al., 1987). This is likely a result of recognition by donor T cells of recipient minor locus histocompatibility or Y chromosome–associated transplantation antigens, because a significantly higher incidence of GVHD occurs in male aplasia and immunodeficient patients given MHC-matched unfractionated female marrows than in patients receiving MHC- and sex-matched marrows (Bortin and Rimm, 1977; Martin et al., 1987).

The severity of GVH reactions increases with the recipient's age (Parkman, 1991; Storb et al., 1986), the use of HLA-matched unrelated donors, and if a related donor is not HLA-identical, with the degree of genetic disparity unless that donor's marrow is rigorously T-cell–depleted (Buckley et al., 1999).

Clinical Features of GVH Reactions

Acute GVH reactions begin 6 days or more after transplantation (or after transfusion in the case of nonirradiated blood products) (Schroeder, 2002). Such reactions include fever, a morbilliform maculopapular erythematous rash, and severe diarrhea (Glucksberg et al., 1974). The rash becomes progressively confluent and may involve the entire body surface; it is both pruritic and painful and eventually leads to marked exfoliation. Eosinophilia and lymphocytosis develop, followed shortly by hepatosplenomegaly, exfoliative dermatitis, protein-losing enteropathy, bone marrow aplasia, generalized edema, marked susceptibility to infection, and death (Gratama et al., 1987; Parkman, 1991; Skinner et al., 1986).

Skin biopsy specimens reveal basal vacuolar degeneration or necrosis, spongiosis, single-cell dyskeratosis, eosinophilic necrosis of epidermal cells, and a dermal perivascular round cell infiltration (Deeg and Henslee-Downey, 1990; Woodruff et al., 1976). Similar necrotic changes occur in the liver and intestinal tract and eventually in most other tissues.

Grading of Acute GVH Reactions

Grading of the severity of acute GVHD is based on the severity and number of organ systems involved (Glucksberg et al., 1974; Thomas et al., 1975). The four categories generally defined are as follows:

Grade 1: 1+ to 2+ skin rash without gut involvement and with no more than 1+ liver involvement.

Grade 2: 1+ to 3+ skin rash with either 1+ to 2+ gastrointestinal involvement or 1+ to 2+ liver involvement or both.

Grade 3: 2+ to 4+ skin rash with 2+ to 4+ gastrointestinal involvement with or without 2+ to 4+ liver involvement. Decrease in performance status and fever also characterize grades 2 and 3, with increasing severity per stage.

Grade 4: The pattern and severity of GVHD is similar to those in grade 3 with extreme constitutional symptoms.

If the patient does not die and if the acute GVH reaction persists, the reaction is termed *chronic* after 100 days. Chronic GVH disease may evolve from acute GVH reactions or may develop in the absence of or after resolution of acute GVHD. It occurs in approximately 45% to 75% of conditioned patients receiving matched bone marrow transplants (Lee et al., 2002b; Visentainer et al., 2002; Zecca et al., 2002). Skin lesions of chronic GVHD resemble scleroderma, with hyper-keratosis, reticular hyperpigmentation, atrophy with ulceration, and fibrosis and limitation of joint movement. Other manifestations include the sicca syndrome, and/or disordered immunoregulation—as evidenced by autoantibody and immune complex formation and polyclonal and monoclonal hyperimmunoglobulinemia, idiopathic interstitial pneumonitis, and frequent infections. Currently there is no grading of the severity of chronic GVHD, although there are proposals for such grading (Akpek, 2002).

Treatment of GVH Reactions

Many regimens have been used to mitigate GVH reactions in both MHC-incompatible and MHC-compatible bone marrow transplants. In MHC-compatible bone marrow transplants into patients with SCID or complete DiGeorge anomaly, it is not usually necessary to give immunosuppressive agents to prevent or mitigate GVHD, although occasionally steroids are used to treat more severe forms of the condition. However, for unfractionated HLA-identical marrow transplants for patients for whom pretransplant chemotherapy is given to prevent rejection, it is necessary to use prophylaxis against GVHD.

Patients are usually given methotrexate (15 mg/M^2 on the first day after transplantation and 10 mg/M^2 on the third, sixth, and eleventh days and weekly thereafter until day 100) and cyclosporine daily for 6 months (Kumar et al., 2002; Martin et al., 1987; Parkman, 1991; Storb et al., 1986). However, newer immunosuppressive regimens, including the use of mycophenolate mofetil with methotrexate and cyclosporine, are being investigated (Wang et al., 2002).

Once GVHD has become established, it is extremely difficult to treat. Antithymocyte serum, steroids, anti–IL-2R α chain (CD25) antibodies, mycophenolate mofetil, and murine monoclonal antibodies to human T-cell surface antigens have ameliorated some, but the course has been inexorably fatal in others similarly treated (Koc et al., 2002; Martin et al., 1987; Ogawa et al., 2002; Parkman, 1991).

The best approach to GVH reactions is a preventive one. The agents already mentioned have not prevented GVH reactions entirely; moreover, in children with genetically determined severe T-cell deficiency, these agents adversely affect the immune cells one is trying to engraft. By far, the best preventive approach is the removal of all post-thymic T cells from the donor marrow or blood (see later discussion).

Post-transplantation Problems

Multiple problems occur during the post-transplantation period, particularly in chemoablated or irradiated patients. Thus bone marrow or blood stem cell transplantation that requires conditioning with these agents should be carried out only by teams experienced in giving them.

Anemia and Thrombocytopenia

Multiple red blood cell and platelet transfusions are usually necessary for chemoablated or irradiated patients during the 7 to 20 days before engraftment occurs. All transfusions that contain immunocompetent cells should be irradiated with from 1500 to 4000 rad to prevent GVH reactions (Martin et al., 1987), and if the recipient is CMV-seronegative, the transfusion should be from CMV-seronegative donors (Tutschka, 1986). Family members can be used as blood donors during this period; they are preferred because using blood of a relative minimizes the risk of hepatitis and CMV infections. Platelets from an HLA-matched sibling are preferred, inasmuch as they are not as subject to immune elimination as are randomly selected platelets.

Infection

The immunodeficiency (Graze and Gale, 1979; Noel et al., 1978) that occurs in the post-transplantation period for patients who have had conditioning regimens, regardless of whether GVHD is present, is responsible for the high incidence of infections in those patients during the first 100 days after marrow cell infusion (Martin et al., 1987; Skinner et al., 1986). Another contributing factor is the profound granulocytopenia that occurs in conditioned patients for 11 to 18 days after transplantation. Fortunately, the use of recombinant G-CSF has reduced the severity of this problem. The advent of GVHD prolongs the impaired immunity (Graze and Gale, 1979; Noel et al., 1978) and further heightens the susceptibility to infection. Protective isolation is necessary, and most transplant groups use isolation units (Martin et al., 1987). Because such hosts are highly susceptible to opportunistic viral, fungal, and facultative intracellular microorganisms, untreatable infections commonly develop (Skinner et al., 1986).

The most problematic infectious agents include *Candida albicans*, *Aspergillus*, *Pneumocystis carinii*, CMV, herpes simplex, varicella-zoster virus, Epstein-Barr virus (EBV), parainfluenza 3, enteroviruses, and adenoviruses (Skinner et al., 1986). Bacterial infections with high-grade pathogens also occur but, if identified in time, can usually be treated effectively with antibiotics.

Trimethoprim-sulfamethoxazole has vastly reduced the mortality from *P. carinii* pneumonia and is an effective prophylactic agent for this infection. Long-term therapy with ribavirin has provided some amelioration of parainfluenza 3 infections in SCID recipients. Acyclovir is highly effective in treating varicella-zoster and herpes simplex infections and may have some prophylactic effect for EBV infections. Ganciclovir and intravenous immunoglobulin with high titers of anti-CMV antibody (CytoGam) have ameliorated CMV infections.

Nevertheless, little other than the development of normal host T-cell function will abrogate ongoing infections with CMV, EBV, parainfluenza 3 virus, enteroviruses, and adenoviruses (DeVoe et al., 1985).

Infections often lead to death before successful engraftment can occur; this is particularly true if severe GVH reactions occur.

Veno-occlusive Disease

Veno-occlusive disease (VOD) is a major cause of mortality following conditioning regimens that use cytoreductive agents that damage hepatic vascular endothelium (DeLeve et al., 2002; Eltumi et al., 1993). Distinguishing VOD from other causes of liver damage can be difficult after bone marrow transplantation, particularly when thrombocytopenia poses an unacceptable risk for diagnostic percutaneous liver biopsy in the early post-transplant period.

The diagnosis is usually made based on clinical criteria; however, studies suggest that monitoring for plasminogen activator inhibitor-1 (PAI-1) antigen can be used as a diagnostic marker as well as a severity predictor of VOD after allogeneic bone marrow transplantation (Lee et al., 2002a).

Identification of Engraftment

Four types of markers are used to identify donor cells in marrow recipients:

- Chromosomal differences (Korver et al., 1987; Van Den Berg et al., 1994)
- Erythrocyte and leukocyte antigens
- Serum allotypes (Korver et al., 1987)
- DNA sequence polymorphisms (Ginsburg et al., 1985)

If the donor and recipient are of the opposite sex, karyotypic markers or fluorescence in situ hybridization (FISH) can detect donor T cells by 2 weeks after grafting, even earlier in unfractionated marrow transplants. Serum immunoglobulin allotypic markers are useful in documenting chimerism of B cells; however, a far more useful approach is to establish EBV-transformed B-cell lines, which can be used for karyotyping, FISH, or restriction fragment length polymorphism (RFLP) analyses. The advantage of RFLP analyses is that they do not require cell division, so the origin of even nondividing cells, such as monocytes or natural killer (NK) cells, can be determined (Ginsburg et al., 1985).

Time to Immune Reconstitution

The time course of immune reconstitution varies according to the following:

- Whether the donor marrow is depleted of T cells
- Whether immunosuppressive agents are administered after transplantation to prevent GVH reactions
- Whether GVHD develops

Normal T- and B-cell function can be seen by 12 days or earlier after the administration of unfractionated HLA-identical marrow cells or cord blood transplants to infants with SCID (DeVoe et al., 1985; Sindel et al., 1984). On the other hand, T-cell function does not develop until 90 to 120 days after the administration of

T-cell–depleted haploidentical marrow cells, and B-cell function may require 2 or 3 years or longer to develop (Buckley et al., 1986, 1999; Myers et al., 2002).

In matched marrow transplants into patients with leukemia or aplasia or into any patients who require conditioning and GVHD prophylaxis, the period of immunodeficiency can be prolonged well beyond 100 days (Graze and Gale, 1979; Noel et al., 1978). NK-cell function appears earlier than T-cell function, at around 4 to 8 weeks (Rooney et al., 1986). When T cells do appear, they may present with normal subset populations (Buckley et al., 1986, 1999) or with a profound CD4 deficiency and CD8 predominance if GVHD is present (Janossy et al., 1986).

Early development of antibody production has been achieved by immunizing the donor of unfractionated HLA-identical bone marrow or blood transplants and the recipient with an antigen or vaccine shortly before chemoablated transplants; the antibody is produced by adoptively transferred donor B cells (Lum et al., 1988).

HLA-Identical Bone Marrow Transplantation for Severe T-Cell Immunodeficiency

The only adequate therapy for most patients with severe forms of cellular immunodeficiency is immunologic reconstitution by transplantation of immunocompetent tissue. Although fetal liver and thymus appeared ideal for this because they have very low GVH potential (Uphoff, 1958) and are rich in precursors of immune cells, their success in conferring immune function on such patients was, at best, only 10% to 15% (Buckley et al., 1976; O'Reilly, 1987). Moreover, the immune function that developed was incomplete and unsustained.

Shortly after the discovery of HLA in 1967 (Bach and Amos, 1967), immune function was conferred in two patients with invariably fatal genetically determined immunodeficiency diseases by transplanting into them HLA-identical allogeneic bone marrow cells (Bach et al., 1968; Gatti et al., 1968). One patient had SCID (Gatti et al., 1968), and the other had Wiskott-Aldrich syndrome (Bach et al., 1968).

The correction of those two very different defects, as well as the subsequent correction of many other types of primary immunodeficiency by bone marrow transplantation, has taught us that the defects in most such conditions are intrinsic to cells of one or more hematopoietic lineages. Thus bone marrow or peripheral blood stem cells have been and remain the tissues of choice for immunoreconstitution (Buckley and Fischer, 1999).

Until 1980, only HLA-identical unfractionated bone marrow could be used for this purpose because of the lethal GVHD that ensued if mismatched donors were used (Bortin and Rimm, 1977). In most cases, both T- and B-cell immunity have been reconstituted by such fully matched transplants, with evidence of function detected very soon after unfractionated bone marrow transplantation (DeVoe et al., 1985; Good, 1987; O'Reilly et al., 1984; Sindel et al., 1984).

Analysis of the genetic origins of the immune cells in the engrafted patients has revealed that although the T cells are all of donor origin, the B cells in approximately half are those of the recipient (Buckley et al., 1999; Myers et al., 2002; O'Reilly et al., 1984). Initially, it was considered that bone marrow was effective in conferring immunity in patients with SCID because it provided normal stem cells, but it is apparent from the later experience with T-cell–depleted marrow (Buckley et al., 1986, 1999; Myers et al., 2002) that the early restoration of immune function in unfractionated HLA-identical marrow transplants is by adoptive transfer of mature T and B cells in the donor marrow (DeVoe et al., 1985; Sindel et al., 1984).

As noted previously, however, unfractionated bone marrow transplantation has not been possible for more than 85% of the immunodeficient patients who could have benefited, because they had no HLA-identical donors (Buckley et al., 1999; Myers et al., 2002). As a consequence, most such patients died (Bortin and Rimm, 1977).

HLA-Haploidentical Bone Marrow Transplantation for Severe T-Cell Deficiency

Historical Aspects

Because of the infrequent availability of HLA-matched sibling donors for patients with lethal T-cell defects, many approaches were tried to avoid lethal GVHD when mismatched donors were used. From 1968 to 1980, all of these methods were unsuccessful except for fetal tissue transplants, which gave only marginal and unsustained immunologic improvement (Bortin and Rimm, 1977). However, the fact that totally HLA-disparate fetal liver cells could correct the immune defect in a few such patients without causing GVH reactions gave hope that HLA-disparate marrow stem cells could do the same if all donor post-thymic T cells could be removed.

Early success in T-cell depletion was achieved in experimental animals by treating donor marrow or spleen cells with anti–T-cell antisera or agglutinating the unwanted cells with plant lectins (Muller-Ruchholtz et al., 1976; Reisner et al., 1978). The remaining immature marrow or splenic non-T cells restored lymphohematopoietic function to lethally irradiated MHC-disparate recipients without lethal GVH reactions.

Methods of T-Cell Depletion

SOYBEAN LECTIN AND SHEEP ERYTHROCYTE AGGLUTINATION

Following these leads, methods were developed to deplete post-thymic T cells from human marrow. The most widely used and successful method for accomplishing this involves agglutination of most mature marrow cells with soybean lectin and subsequent removal of T cells from the unagglutinated marrow by sheep erythrocyte rosetting and density-gradient centrifugation

(Reisner et al., 1983; Schiff et al., 1987). Patients treated with haploidentical (i.e., half-matched) parental stem cells prepared by this method have had minimal or no GVH reactions (Buckley et al., 1986, 1999; Fischer et al., 1986a; Myers et al., 2002; O'Reilly et al., 1986).

MONOCLONAL ANTIBODY AND COMPLEMENT LYSIS

A second method of depleting post-thymic T cells from donor marrow or peripheral blood involves incubating the donated cells with monoclonal antibodies to human T cells plus a source of complement (Filipovich et al., 1984; Reinherz et al., 1982; Waldmann et al., 1984). Antibodies used for this purpose have included T12, Leu 1, CT-2, and CamPATH-1. T-cell depletion may not be as effective with this approach, possibly because of modulation of T-cell antigens from the surface of the T cells without destroying them. As a consequence, somewhat more frequent and severe GVHD has been observed.

SHEEP ERYTHROCYTE AGGLUTINATION

A final approach has been to use sheep erythrocyte rosette depletion alone to remove T cells from haploidentical donor marrow (Fischer et al., 1986a, 1986b). Because different centers have used different numbers of rosette depletions and different methods of modifying the sheep red blood cells (i.e., no modification, neuraminidase, or aminoethylisothiuroniun treatment), it has been difficult to evaluate whether this approach is as effective as the others in removing post-thymic T cells. In one center, only a single rosetting step is done, with the intent of leaving a few post-thymic T cells (Fischer et al., 1986a). GVH reactions are then modulated by giving the recipient cyclosporine continuously for various time periods after the transplantation.

Time Course and Nature of Engraftment

The time to development of immune function following haploidentical stem cell grafts is quite different from that after unfractionated HLA-identical marrow. Lymphocytes with mature T-cell phenotypes and functions fail to rise significantly until 3 to 4 months after transplantation; normal T-cell function is reached between 4 and 7 months (Buckley et al., 1986, 1999; Myers et al., 2002). B-cell function develops much more slowly, averaging 2 to 2.5 years for normalization in some; many do not develop B-cell function altogether, despite normal T-cell function (Buckley et al., 1986, 1999; Myers et al., 2002). Genetic analyses of the lymphocytes from such chimeric patients have revealed all T cells to be genetically donor, whereas the B cells and APCs almost always remain those of the recipient (Buckley et al., 1986, 1999; Myers et al., 2002).

These observations indicate that the thymic microenvironment of most infants with SCID is capable of differentiating half-matched normal stem cells to mature and functioning T lymphocytes that can cooperate effectively with host B cells for antibody production (Buckley et al., 1999; Myers et al., 2002; Patel et al.,

2000). Thus the genetic defect in most does not involve the thymus (Fig. 43-6).

Studies of these chimeric children reveal that the genetically donor cells that matured from stem cells to functioning mature T cells in the patient are tolerant of host class I and II HLA antigens and become autoreactive against the original donor's MNCs (Schiff and Buckley, 1987). In addition, my associates and I (Roberts et al., 1989) have found that some cloned tetanus toxoid-specific T cells from these chimeras prefer host APCs (i.e., they are "educated" to recognize host as self), as has been noted in murine models (Singer et al., 1981). The finding that functioning B cells are those of the host indicates that the genetic defect does not affect the B cells in some of these patients (Buckley et al., 1986, 1999; Myers et al., 2002).

Bone Marrow Transplantation in Immunodeficiency Diseases

Although precise figures are not available, more than 1200 patients worldwide with different forms of genetically determined immunodeficiency have been given bone marrow transplants over the past four decades in attempts to correct their underlying immune defects. From 1968 to 1977, only 14 (or 29%) of 48 infants with SCID were long-term survivors of successful HLA class II compatible bone marrow transplants (Bortin and Rimm, 1977). Possibly because of earlier diagnosis before untreatable opportunistic infections develop, the results have improved considerably over the last two decades (Antonine et al., 2003; Buckley et al., 1999; Haddad et al., 1998; Myers et al., 2002).

In a worldwide survey I conducted from 1994 to 1997, with subsequent additions of published cases from the literature, I found that 239 of 302 (79%) of patients with primary immunodeficiency transplanted with HLA-identical marrow over a period of 29 years were surviving. This is similar to the survival rate in European transplant centers for 1968 to 1999 (Antoine et al., 2003).

Severe Combined Immunodeficiency

Bone marrow transplantation has been more widely applied and more successful in infants with SCID than in any other primary immunodeficiency (see Chapter 15). Because SCID infants lack T cells, there is no need to give pretransplant chemotherapy. In the same survey and literature review, only 126 SCIDs were reported as having received HLA-identical marrow, and 106 (84%) were surviving. By contrast, 477 SCID infants had received haploidentical marrow, and 301 (63%) survived worldwide; however, the haploidentical transplants were not depleted of T cells until after 1980.

Nevertheless, this is a major accomplishment, because SCID is 100% fatal without marrow transplantation or, in the case of ADA-deficient SCID, enzyme-replacement therapy. The latter is helpful for only a small percentage of SCID patients, because ADA-deficiency accounts for only approximately 15%

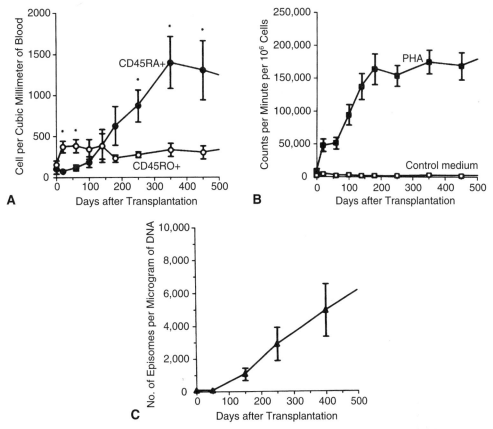

Figure 43-6 · Memory (CD45RO⁺) versus naïve (CD45RA⁺) T cells (panel A), T-cell proliferation in response to phytohemagglutinin (panel B), and T-cell receptor excision circles (TRECs) (panel C) after bone marrow transplantation with T-cell–depleted HLA-identical (7) or haploidentical (71) related bone marrow stem cells into infants with SCID without pretransplant chemoablation or post-transplant GVHD prophylaxis. The findings indicate that thymic processing is crucial for the development of new T cells from normal allogeneic stem cells in these SCID infants. (From Patel DD, Gooding ME, Parrott RE, Curtis KM, Haynes BF, Buckley RH. Thymic function after hematopoietic stem cell transplantation for the treatment of severe combined immunodeficiency. N Engl J Med 342:1325–1332, 2000, with permission.)

of SCID cases (Buckley et al., 1997, 1999; Stephan et al., 1993).

Only 17 SCID patients were reported to have received matched unrelated donor (MUD) transplants, and 12 (71%) were surviving. Six SCID patients were reported as having received related or unrelated cord blood transplants, and five were surviving.

A longitudinal study of 193 European SCID patients who had received haploidentical T-cell–depleted bone marrow transplants (a majority of whom had received pretransplant chemotherapy) revealed that only 92 (48%) were long-term survivors (Haddad et al., 1998). These results are similar to those from another center that routinely uses pretransplant chemotherapy, where only 46% were surviving (Smogorzewska et al., 2000). Thus survival rates are superior in centers that do not use pretransplant chemotherapy.

A retrospective analysis by the European Group for Bone Marrow Transplantation and the European Society for Immunodeficiency of the influence of the SCID phenotype on the outcome of haploidentical marrow transplants found the disease-free survival to be significantly better for patients with B⁺ SCID (60%) than

for those with B⁻ SCID (35%) (P = 0.002) (Bertrand et al., 1999). However, in the United States, 12 of 16 (75%) infants with the B⁻ Athabascan form of SCID due to Artemis deficiency were reported as surviving following bone marrow transplantation (O'Marcaigh et al., 2001) (see Chapter 15).

Over the past two decades, my associates and I have transplanted 134 infants with SCID, and 103 of these (77%) are currently surviving from 1 month to 21.8 years after transplantation. With the exception of three infants who also received cord blood transplants, no pretransplant conditioning was given. HLA-identical donors were available for only 15 patients; all of the 15 survive today with functioning grafts. Half-matched related donor stem cells prepared by the soy lectin, SRBC rosetting T-cell depletion technique were used in 119 SCID patients, and 88 (74%) of these patients survive today. Survival rates were similar whether the patients were ADA normal (77%) or ADA deficient (75%), and there was no significant difference in disease-free survival for B⁺ versus B⁻ SCID. More important, our studies have shown that such transplants can provide normal numbers of T cells and normalize T-cell function in all known molecular types of SCID (Buckley, 2000, 2001, 2002) (Fig. 43-7).

Despite the fact that all SCID infants have vestigial thymi, we have recently demonstrated that the T cells that emerge after transplantation in these chimeras are thymically derived (Myers et al., 2002; Patel et al., 2000). They are CD45RA⁺ and contain extra chromosomal DNA circles formed during intrathymic T-cell development (T-cell receptor excision circles [TRECs]) (see Fig. 43-6). Before transplantation, neither the few host T cells that are present nor any transplacentally transferred maternal T cells contain TRECs, and they are CD45RO⁺. However, after transplantation, both CD45RA⁺ and TREC-containing T cells gradually emerge, coinciding with the development of T-cell function.

Most impressive is the fact that 36 of 37 (97%) infants in whom we have performed transplantation during the first 3.5 months of life currently survive (Fig. 43-8) (Buckley, 2001; Buckley et al., 1999). Thus there appears to be no advantage in performing such transplants in utero (Flake et al., 1996; Wengler et al., 1996) as opposed to performing them soon after birth (Myers et al., 2002). In utero transplants also carry the risks associated with injecting the fetus and the inability to detect GVHD during gestation.

Wiskott-Aldrich Syndrome

The second largest group of immunodeficiency patients who have received bone marrow transplants since 1968 are those with the Wiskott-Aldrich syndrome (Brochstein et al., 1991; Filipovich et al., 2001; Lenarsky et al., 1993; Miano et al., 1998; Ozsahin et al., 1996; Parkman et al., 1978; Rumelhart et al., 1990) (see Chapter 17). In a recent report from the International Bone Marrow Transplant Registry, 170 patients with Wiskott-Aldrich syndrome had been transplanted, and the 5-year probability of survival (95% confidence interval) for all subjects was 70% (63% to 77%) (Filipovich et al., 2001). Probabilities differed by donor type: 87% (74% to 93%) with HLA-identical sibling donors, 52% (37% to 65%) with other related donors, and 71% (58% to 80%) with MUDs (*P* = 0.0006). Boys who had received a MUD transplant before age 5 had survival rates similar to those in boys who received HLA-identical sibling transplants.

The fact that all such patients require myeloablation and cytoreduction to prevent graft rejection, that they have been multiply transfused with allogeneic platelets before transplantation resulting in resistance to engraftment, that many have developed chronic herpesvirus infections before transplantation, and that they are prone to develop malignancy are all likely contributing factors to their failure to survive the 3 to 4 months required for stem cells to mature to functioning T cells from a T-cell–depleted marrow graft. Many of the deaths were from EBV-associated B-lymphocyte lymphoproliferative disorders (Fischer et al., 1994).

Combined Immunodeficiency

Patients with combined immunodeficiencies (CIDs) characterized by less severe T-cell defects than in SCID constitute the third largest group of patients who have received bone marrow transplants since 1968 (Berthet et al., 1994). Some of these are termed *T-cell deficiency* or *Nezelof syndrome* (see Chapter 15). Of 65 patients, 33 (51%) so treated were reported as surviving. HLA-identical marrow transplants were clearly more successful (13 of 17 [76%]) than T-cell–depleted haploidentical (15 of 38 [39%]) (Lanfranchi et al., 2000) or MUD adult marrow (0 of 2) transplants, but 5 of 7 recipients of cord blood transplants were surviving (Knutsen and Wall, 1999).

Omenn Syndrome

Forty-five patients with Omenn syndrome were reported in the literature (Fischer et al., 1994; Gomez et al., 1995; Lanfranchi et al., 2000; Loechelt et al., 1995) (see Chapter 15) or to me as having received marrow transplants since 1968, and 23 (51%) were alive at the

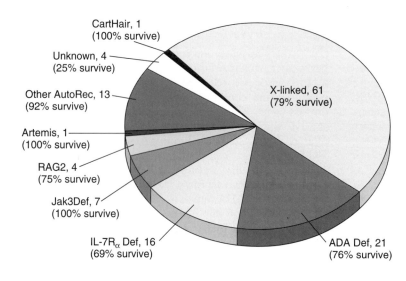

Figure 43-7 · Survival rates for bone marrow transplants given to 128 infants with different types of SCID showing that bone marrow transplantation is effective for all known genetic types.

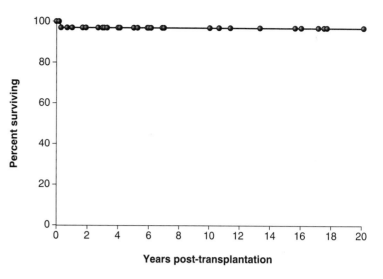

Figure 43-8 · Kaplan-Meier survival curve for 37 consecutive infants with SCID at my institution who received bone marrow transplants from HLA-identical (*n* = 5) or haploidentical (*n* = 32) donors before they were 3.5 months old without pretransplantation chemoablation or post-transplantation GVHD prophylaxis. Thirty-five (97%) infants survived for 1 month to 21.5 years after transplantation. The one death occurred from a cytomegalovirus infection.

time. As with the other non-SCID defects, however, the greatest success was with HLA-identical sibling transplants, 9 of 12 (75%) of whom were surviving, whereas only 11 of 27 (41%) haploidentical marrow and 3 of 6 (50%) MUD marrow recipients were alive.

Leukocyte Adhesion Deficiency Type 1

Of 33 patients with leukocyte adhesion deficiency type 1 (LAD1), 25 (76%) were alive after bone marrow transplantation at the time of the survey and review (Fischer et al., 1994; Lanfranchi et al., 2000; LeDeist et al., 1989; Thomas et al., 1995b). All types of marrow transplantation were successful in this condition: 6 of 8 (75%) HLA-identical sibling transplants, 15 of 21 (71%) T-cell–depleted haploidentical marrow transplants, 2 of 2 (100%) MUD adult marrow transplants, and 2 of 3 (67%) cord blood transplants.

MHC Antigen Deficiency Syndromes

Of 26 patients with bare lymphocyte syndrome, 14 (54%) were reported as being alive after having received marrow transplants (Canioni et al., 1997; Fischer et al., 1994; Klein et al., 1995). These included 4 of 9 (44%) who received HLA-identical sibling marrow, but only 7 of 20 (35%) who received T-cell–depleted haploidentical marrow, 2 of 2 (100%) who received MUD marrow, and 1 of 1 (100%) who received a related cord blood transplant (Bonduel et al., 1999; Canioni et al., 1997; Casper et al., 1990a; Fischer et al., 1994).

Chediak-Higashi Syndrome

Of 23 patients with Chediak-Higashi syndrome who received bone marrow transplants, 18 (78%) were reported to be alive (Fischer et al., 1986a, 1994; Haddad et al., 1995; Liang et al., 2000). These included 10 of 12 (83%) who received HLA-identical sibling marrow, 1 of 5 (20%) who received haploidentical marrow, and 6 of 6 (100%) who received MUD marrow.

Chronic Granulomatous Disease

Of 29 patients with chronic granulomatous disease (CGD) who had received bone marrow transplants, 21 (72%) were reported as surviving, and a majority of these were chimeric (Hobbs et al., 1992; Leung et al., 1999; Nagler et al., 1999; Ozsahin et al., 1998; Rappeport et al., 1982). The overall survival figures include 19 of 26 (72%) HLA-identical sibling marrow recipients and 3 of 4 (75%) MUD marrow recipients (Hobbs et al., 1992; Seger and Ezekowitz, 1994; Watanabe et al., 2001).

Some success has been reported in treating patients with CGD with the "minitransplant" approach using HLA-identical sibling donors and non-myeloablative conditioning (Horwitz et al., 2001; Nagler et al., 1999). Seger and associates (2002) have summarized the European experience using myeloablative conditioning. In 27 cases (including 25 children) survival occurred in 23 of 27, and 22 were cured of their disease.

DiGeorge Syndrome

Eleven patients with the complete DiGeorge syndrome were reported to me as undergoing marrow transplantation, while four more underwent fetal thymus or cultured mature thymic tissue transplantation. The only survivors were two of the three who received unfractionated HLA-identical sibling marrow (Goldsobel et al., 1987), and two of two who were recipients of explants of cultured thymic epithelium. Goldsobel and associates in 1987 identified from the literature 26 more as having undergone fetal thymus or cultured thymic epithelial transplantation, and at the time of their review, only 8 were alive and well.

Bensoussan and associates (2002) report memory T-cell reconstitution in a 4-year-old boy with complete DGS using peripheral blood mononuclear cells from an HLA-identical sister using no preconditioning and GVH prophylaxis. More recently Markert and associates (1999, 2003) have used cultured allogeneic postnatal cultured thymus tissue transplants in 12 infants with complete DiGeorge syndrome. Seven have survived, six have developed antigen-specific T-cell proliferative responses, and three have intact B-cell function.

Other Primary Immunodeficiencies

Other disorders treated successfully with bone marrow transplantation include the following: X-linked hyper-IgM (13 of 21 surviving) (Duplantier et al., 2001; Fasth, 1993; Khawaja et al., 2001; Scholl et al., 1998; Thomas et al., 1995a; Ziegner et al., 2001), reticular dysgenesis (12 of 21 surviving) (Bertrand et al., 2002; De Santes et al., 1996; Knutsen and Wall, 1999), purine nucleoside phosphorylase (PNP) deficiency (3 of 8 surviving) (Broome et al., 1996; Carpenter et al., 1996), cartilage hair hypoplasia (4 of 7 surviving), X-linked lymphoproliferative syndrome (6 of 9 surviving) (Gross et al., 1996; Pracher et al., 1994; Williams et al., 1993; Ziegner et al., 2001), pigmentary dilution (Griscelli's) syndrome (3 of 7 surviving) (Schneider et al., 1990), IL-2 deficiency (2 of 2 surviving) (Berthet et al., 1994), common variable immunodeficiency (CVID) (0 of 4 surviving); chronic mucocutaneous candidiasis (0 of 1 surviving); ataxia-telangiectasia (0 of 4 surviving), and Fas (CD95) deficiency (1 of 1 surviving) (Benkerrou et al., 1997).

My associates and I have also performed transplantations in 51 patients with non-SCID immunodeficiency, with the following survival rates: 11 of 26 (42%) with CID, 5 of 7 (71%) with LAD, 2 of 2 (100%) with Chediak-Higashi syndrome, 2 of 2 (100%) with CGD, 1 of 1 (100%) with ZAP-70 deficiency, 4 of 7 (57%) with Omenn syndrome, 2 of 3 (67%) with PNP deficiency, 1 of 2 (50%) with Wiskott-Aldrich syndrome, 1 of 1 (100%) with X-linked hyper-IgM, and 1 each with Griscelli's syndrome and IFN-γR2 deficiency, neither of whom survived.

Bone Marrow Transplantation in Malignancy

The success of marrow transplantation in curing malignancy depends on a number of factors, the most important of which include the type of malignant disease, the stage of that disease, and the age of the recipient (Thomas, 1987). Although autologous and syngeneic (identical twin) marrow have been used successfully in the treatment of various forms of solid organ malignancy, by far, the greatest experience and success in the treatment of leukemia has been with allogeneic bone marrow (Martin et al., 1987; O'Reilly, 1987; Rowlings et al., 1993; Thomas, 1987).

In contrast to the success noted previously with T-cell–depleted haploidentical marrow in treating infants with SCID, this approach has been confounded by resistance to engraftment and leukemia recurrence when applied to the treatment of malignancies (Maraninchi et al., 1987). Thus most successful allogeneic bone marrow transplants for malignant diseases have been with unfractionated HLA-identical marrow.

However, because only 25% to 30% of patients have HLA-identical siblings, alternative donor types have been sought (Bleakley et al., 2002; Ohnuma et al., 2002). Surprisingly, unfractionated marrow from family donors who share one genetically identical HLA haplotype but whose other haplotype differs from the patient's other haplotype by only one HLA locus has achieved results similar to those with marrow from HLA-matched sibling donors in the treatment of patients with malignancy (Beatty et al., 1985).

A possible breakthrough was reported in solving the graft failure repeatedly seen with T-cell–depleted haploidentical marrow infusions for leukemia. Aversa and colleagues (1994) from Italy found that by (1) increasing the size of the graft inoculum 7-fold to 10-fold by adding G-CSF–mobilized haploidentical donor peripheral blood stem cells (depleted of T cells by soy lectin/sheep erythrocyte rosetting) to similarly T-cell–depleted donor marrow cells and (2) using a highly immunosuppressive and myeloablative conditioning regimen (single fraction fast total body irradiation, ATG, cyclophosphamide, and thiotepa), they achieved engraftment in 16 of 17 patients with end-stage chemoresistant leukemia. Nine patients died from transplant-related toxicity and two relapsed, but six were alive and event free after a median follow-up of 230 days. Higher probabilities of relapse (60% to 70%) account for lower survival rates for patients with end-stage leukemia (10% to 20%) and advanced Hodgkin's disease or lymphomas (15% to 20%) (Thomas, 1987).

Another approach to using histoincompatible bone marrow for leukemia or lymphoma patients has involved the co-culture of irradiated blood cells from the recipient with haploidentical bone marrow cells in the presence of CTLA-4Ig in vitro to inhibit co-stimulation by CD28 and B7 and to create "anergic" T cells (Guinan et al., 1999). Of 12 patients so treated, 5 were alive and in remission 4.5 to 29 months after transplantation of the "anergic" bone marrow. No deaths occurred from GVHD.

A recent study of long-term survival and late deaths in 6691 patients who had received allogeneic bone marrow transplantation as treatment for acute myelogenous or lymphoblastic leukemia or CML and who were free of their original disease 2 years later revealed that the disease is probably cured at that point (Socie et al., 1999). However, for many years after transplantation, the mortality among these patients was higher than that in a normal population. The best survival rates (50% to 70%) with the lowest probability of relapse (20%) occurred in patients younger than 20 years who had acute nonlymphocytic leukemia (ANL) transplanted in first remission and in patients with CML transplanted in chronic phase (Goldman et al., 1986; Sharathkumar et al., 2002).

Clearly, HLA-identical bone marrow transplantation is the treatment of choice for all of these patients. These statistics were upheld by those from analyses by European Leukemia Cooperative Groups (Zittoun et al., 1995) on transplants in patients with acute myelogenous leukemia and by the International Bone

Marrow Transplant Registry on 16,905 allogeneic marrow transplants for any disease reported over a 20-year period (Rowlings et al., 1993). However, the long-term survival after allogeneic bone marrow transplantation is confounded by problems of chronic GVHD (Socie et al., 1999).

For patients with acute myelogenous leukemia during the first complete remission, the projected rate of disease-free survival at 4 years was 55% for allogeneic transplantation, 48% for autologous transplantation, and 30% for intensive chemotherapy (Mehta et al., 2002; Zittoun et al., 1995). For the autologous transplants (done when there is no HLA-identical donor), autologous remission marrow is purged with 4-hydroperoxycyclophosphamide, cryopreserved, and then reinfused after the patient has been given intensive cytoreductive therapy (Miller et al., 2001).

For patients with CML, the 3-year leukemia-free survival rate was 57% for transplantations done in the first chronic phase, 41% for those in accelerated or second chronic phase, and 18% for those in more advanced disease (Rowlings et al., 1993). Success in this group of patients has continued to improve (Ji et al., 2002; Okamoto et al., 2002; Sharathkumar et al., 2002).

Because approximately 45% of patients with acute lymphoblastic leukemia (ALL) have been cured with combination chemotherapy (Rivera et al., 1993) and the probability of event-free survival has steadily increased with advances in this therapy (to a recent high of 71%), most of these patients do not undergo bone marrow transplantation. However, a number of such patients have received transplants in second remission when they were in good condition and the prognosis was known to be poor with chemotherapy alone (Barrett et al., 1994; Bleakley et al., 2002; Uderzo, 2000; Woolfrey et al., 2002).

In an analysis comparing data in the International Bone Marrow Transplant Registry on such transplants with results of continued chemotherapy in children with ALL treated by the Pediatric Oncology Group, Barrett and colleagues (1994) found that the mean probability of a relapse at 5 years was significantly lower among the transplant recipients than among the chemotherapy recipients (45% vs. 80%). At 5 years, the probability of leukemia-free survival was higher after transplantation than after chemotherapy (40% vs. 17%). These figures have continued to improve (Bleakley et al., 2002; Uderzo, 2000; Woolfrey et al., 2002).

Indications for Autologous Marrow Transplantation

Data from the International Bone Marrow Transplant Registry indicate that the use of autologous bone marrow or (more commonly) mobilized peripheral blood infusions is now more than double that of allogeneic bone marrow transplants (Rowlings et al., 1993). The most common indications for autologous marrow or blood infusions include non-Hodgkin's lymphoma, multiple myeloma, breast cancer, Hodgkin's disease, other cancers, and acute myelogenous leukemia (Ball et al., 2000; Mak et al., 2000; Montuoro et al., 2000).

Bone Marrow Transplantation in Aplastic Anemia

Both identical twin and unfractionated HLA-identical marrow have effected cures of severe marrow aplasia (Casper et al., 1990b; Pillow et al., 1966). The fact that more than 50% of adult patients with this condition improve dramatically after immunosuppressive therapy (ATG/ALG, cyclosporine, and/or androgens) suggests that immunologic mechanisms have an etiologic role in some forms of aplasia. In children, however, most cases appear to be caused by stem cell abnormalities, as evidenced by the fact that HLA-identical bone marrow transplantation is far more successful than immunosuppressive therapy (Bacigalupo et al., 2000; Ballester and Elfenbein, 1994; Casper et al., 1990b).

During the past decade, many transplant centers have reported favorable outcomes of matched marrow transplants in children; long-term disease-free survival increased from 47% in 1978 to 1980 to between 70% and 80% in the more recent larger series (Bacigalupo et al., 2000; Casper et al., 1990b; Horowitz, 2000). Therefore bone marrow transplantation should be considered the treatment of choice for children with severe aplastic anemia (especially those younger than 6 years) if an HLA-identical sibling donor is available.

For patients without an HLA-identical sibling or who are older than 40 years, immunosuppressive therapy is the treatment of choice, because non–HLA-identical grafts have had very poor outcome (Bacigalupo et al., 2000; Casper et al., 1990b; Ellis et al., 2002). However, even if a favorable response occurs after immunosuppressive therapy, the actuarial incidence of relapse is 35% and there is an increased incidence of clonal hematopoietic disorders (Ballester and Elfenbein, 1994; Schrezenmeier et al., 1993).

Multiple transfusions before marrow transplantation should be avoided if marrow transplantation is a possibility, because transfusions can sensitize the recipient. Use of more intense conditioning regimens, including radiation, as well as large numbers of marrow cells ($>4 \times 10^8$ cells/kg) has helped overcome this problem (Casper et al., 1990b; Gaziev et al., 1999).

Bone Marrow Transplantation in Hemoglobinopathies, Osteopetrosis, and Metabolic Storage Diseases

Bone marrow transplantation has been highly effective for the treatment of homozygous β-thalassemia, with survival rates reaching 70% to 80% for marrow transplants from HLA-identical siblings (Boulad et al., 1998; Ghavamzadeh et al., 1998; Lucarelli et al., 2002; Mentzer and Cowan, 2000). Increasing age, the presence of portal fibrosis, and increasing serum ferritin were significantly associated with reduced probability of survival ($P = 0.0047$, $P = 0.016$, and $P = 0.024$, respectively) (Ghavamzadeh et al., 1998).

Recently, good success has been achieved by using MUDs who shared extended haplotypes with the recipients, offering another option when an HLA-identical sibling donor is not available (La Nasa et al., 2002). Likewise, HLA-identical bone marrow transplantation has also been very successful for patients with sickle cell disease; 59 patients are known to have been treated, and 55 were surviving, with 50 of those free of sickle cell disease (Walters et al., 2001).

The European Bone Marrow Transplantation Group reported on 69 patients with autosomal recessive osteopetrosis who were given HLA-identical or haploidentical bone marrow transplants between 1976 and 1994 (Gerritsen et al., 1994). Recipients of genotypically HLA-identical marrow had an actuarial probability for 5-year survival, with osteoclast function, of 79%. Recipients of phenotypically HLA-identical marrow from a related or unrelated donor had an actuarial probability for 5-year survival, with osteoclast function, of 38%, and those who received HLA-haploidentical marrow from a related donor had an actuarial probability for 5-year survival, with osteoclast function, of only 13%.

More recently, however, there has been much greater success with haploidentical transplants performed in patients with this condition (Andolina et al., 2000; Schulz et al., 2002). Success has also been obtained with MUD and cord blood transplants (Eapen et al., 1998; Locatelli et al., 1997).

Other diseases treated successfully with bone marrow transplantation include histiocytosis X (Ringden et al., 1987), paroxysmal nocturnal hemoglobinuria (Antin et al., 1985), Fanconi's anemia, congenital aregenerative anemias, acute myelofibrosis, four types of polysaccharidoses, Gaucher's disease (Chan et al., 1994), metachromatic leukodystrophy, thrombocytopenia-absent radii syndrome (Brochstein et al., 1992), and other mucolipidoses (Krivit and Whitley, 1987; O'Reilly et al., 1984).

Nonmyeloablative Bone Marrow Transplantation

In patients with pre-existing organ damage, significant morbidity and mortality is seen with traditional conditioning regimens that use busulfan and cyclophosphamide or irradiation. Because of this, there has been increasing interest in developing conditioning regimens that are less toxic (Barta et al., 2001; Feinstein et al., 2001; Gaspar et al., 2002; Horwitz et al., 2001; Mielcarek et al., 2002; Nagler et al., 1999; Pulsipher and Woolfrey, 2001; Woolfrey et al., 2001). This has been accomplished with either total-lymphoid irradiation or a combination of nucleoside analogs and antilymphocyte antibody preparations.

Although these regimens are significantly less cytotoxic than high-dose alkylating agents and TBI, they are profoundly immunosuppressive. Opportunistic infections such as the reactivation of CMV remain clinical obstacles when nonmyeloablative stem cell transplants are performed using these agents, especially in elderly and previously immunosuppressed patients. GVHD prophylaxis with cyclosporine and methotrexate, with added mycophenolate mofetil in some cases, has been necessary because GVHD is common after nonmyeloablative transplantation.

Nonmyeloablative bone marrow transplantation has been used successfully for patients with chronic granulomatous disease when HLA-identical sibling donors were available (Horwitz et al., 2001; Nagler et al., 1999). The conditioning regimens used were fludarabine, busulfan, and ATG in 1 case (Nagler et al., 1999) and cyclophosphamide, fludarabine, and ATG in 10 cases (Horwitz et al., 2001); 7 of the 11 were surviving with mixed chimerism and good health.

Gaspar and associates (2002) at Great Ormand Street, United Kingdom, have reported on the outcomes of their treatment of 21 patients with a variety of different immunodeficiencies using four different nonmyeloablative conditioning regimens: (1) fludarabine/melphalan/ATG or Campath 1H ($n = 16$), (2) fludarabine/cyclophosphamide/Campath 1H ($n = 1$), (3) TBI/CyA/MMF ($n = 1$), or (4) fludarabine/melphalan/busulphan/ATG ($n = 3$). In 13 cases matched ($n = 9$) and 1 antigen mismatched ($n = 4$), unrelated donors were used, and in 8 cases transplants from matched siblings ($n = 4$), 1 antigen-mismatched sibling ($n = 1$), matched parent ($n = 1$), and haploidentical parents ($n = 3$) were performed. At a median follow-up of 13 months, 19 of 21 (90%) patients were still alive after transplantation. Despite using T-cell–replete grafts and unrelated donor grafts in the majority of patients, there was no evidence of significant organ disease. Immune reconstitution in terms of $CD3^+$ and $CD4^+$ T-cell recovery and function was reported to be equivalent in comparison with a historical cohort (Gaspar et al., 2002).

Placental Blood Transplantation

Unfractionated cord blood, which is a rich source of stem cells, is an alternative source of hematopoietic stem cells for transplantation (Barker and Wagner, 2002). More than 1500 cord blood transplants have been performed for a variety of malignant and genetic diseases since the first successful transplant in a patient with Fanconi's anemia was reported (Gluckman et al., 1989).

Part of the rationale for using cord blood is that the incidence and severity of GVHD appears to be lower than with unfractionated adult MUD transplants, even when there is only partial matching (Barker and Wagner, 2002). The time to search for an unrelated cord blood donor is also less than that for a MUD adult donor.

Several successes with cord blood transplantation from HLA-identical siblings or MUDs have been reported in patients with genetic and immunodeficiency disorders—including LAD, X-linked lymphoproliferative syndrome (XLP), PNP, CID, Wiskott-Aldrich syndrome, and X-linked hyper-IgM (Ohnuma et al., 2002;

Stary et al., 1996; Vowels et al., 1993; Wagner et al., 1995; Ziegner et al., 2001). However, as compared with MUD adult donors, the graft failure rate is higher with cord blood transplantation. There is also a longer period before neutrophil engraftment and a much longer period of thrombocytopenia (100 days) than after HLA-identical related or MUD unfractionated marrow transplants (Barker et al., 2001).

The problem with both matched unrelated adult bone marrow donors and unrelated cord blood donors is that because humans are an outbred population, the matching can never be perfect. Minor locus histocompatibility antigen differences are also much more likely to be present than in the related setting, resulting in a high probability of GVHD. GVHD prophylaxis is routinely given after transplants from either type of unrelated donor, and this is continued for many months. If a patient with primary immunodeficiency is already infected, these drugs make them even more at risk for demise from these agents.

In addition, most of the current protocols for cord blood transplantation call for pretransplant conditioning regardless of the underlying diagnosis of the patient. The conditioning, together with GVHD prophylaxis, contributes to a long period of impaired immunity after transplantation. For those who survive, however, these conditioning and immunosuppressive agents do not prevent eventual new T-cell development, although GVHD may prevent such development (Weinberg et al., 2001).

REFERENCES

Adams J, Gudemann C, Tonshoff B, Mehls O, Wiesel M. Renal transplantation in small children—a comparison between surgical procedures. Eur Urol 40:552–556, 2001.

Aiuti A, Slavin S, Aker M, Ficara F, Deola S, Mortellaro A, Morecki S, Andolfi G, Tabucchi A, Carlucci F, Marinello E, Cattaneo F, Vai S, Servida P, Miniero R, Roncarolo MG, Bordignon C. Correction of ADA-SCID by stem cell gene therapy combined with nonmyeloablative conditioning. Science 296:2410–2413, 2002.

Akpek G. Clinical grading in chronic graft-versus-host disease: is it time for change? Leuk Lymphoma 43:1211–1220, 2002.

Almarri A, Batchelor JR. HLA and hepatitis B infection. Lancet 344:1194–1195, 1994.

Amos DB. The agglutination of mouse leukocytes by iso-immune sera. Br J Exp Path 34:464–470, 1953.

Amos DB, Bach FH. Phenotypic expressions of the major histocompatibility locus in man (HL-A): leukocyte antigens and mixed leukocyte culture reactivity. J Exp Med 128:623–637, 1968.

Amos DB, Seigler HF, Southworth JG, Ward FE. Skin graft rejection between subjects genotypes for HLA. Transplant Proc 1:342–346, 1969.

Andolina M, Maximova N, Rabusin M, Vujic D, Bunjevacki G, Vidali C, Beorchia A. Haploidentical bone marrow transplantation in leukemia and genetic diseases. Haematologica 85:37–40, 2000.

Antin JH, Ginsburg D, Smith BR, Nathan DG, Orkin SH, Rappeport JM. Bone marrow transplantation for paroxysmal nocturnal hemoglobinuria: eradication of the PNH clone and documentation of complete lymphohematopoietic engraftment. Blood 66:1247–1250, 1985.

Antoine C, Muller S, Cant A, Cavazzana-Calvo M, Veys P, Vossen J, Fasth A, Heilmann C, Wulffraat N, Seger R, Blanche S, Friedrich W, Abinun M, Davies G, Bredius R, Schulz A, Landais P, Fischer A; European Group for Blood and Marrow Transplantation; European Society for Immunodeficiency. Long-term survival and transplantation of haemopoietic stem cells for immunodeficiencies: report of the European experience 1968–1999. Lancet 361:553–560, 2003.

Arbus GS, Sullivan EK, Tejani A. Hospitalization in children during the first year after kidney transplantation. Kidney Int 44:83–86, 1993.

Ardehali A, Laks H, Drinkwater DC, Ziv ET, Sorensen TJ, Hamilton MA, Warner-Stevenson L, Moriguchi JB, Kobashigawa JA. Cardiac transplantation at UCLA. Clinical Transplants 10:119–128, 1994.

Arguello JR, Madrigal JA. HLA typing by Reference Strand Mediated Conformation Analysis (RSCA). Rev Immunogenet 1:209–219, 1999.

Armitage JM, Fricker FJ, del Nido P, Startzl TE, Hardesty RL, Griffith BP. A decade (1982 to 1992) of pediatric cardiac transplantation and the impact of FK 506 immunosuppression. J Thor Cardiovasc Surg 105:464–473, 1993.

Assaad A. Post-transplantation management of the newborn and the immunosuppressive role of prostaglandin E1. J Heart Lung Transplant 12:191–194, 1993.

Atkison P, Joubert G, Barron A, Grant D, Paradis K, Seldman E, Wall W, Rosenberg H, Howard J, Williams S, Stiller C. Hypertrophic cardiomyopathy associated with tacrolimus in paediatric transplant patients. Lancet 345:894–896, 1995.

Aversa F, Tabilio A, Terenzi A, Velardi A, Falzetti F, Giannoni C, Iacucci R, Zei T, Martelli MP, Gambelunghe C, Rossetti M, Caputo P, Latini P, Aristei C, Raymondi C, Reisner Y, Martelli MF. Successful engraftment of T-cell–depleted haploidentical "three-loci" incompatible transplants in leukemia patients by addition of recombinant human granulocyte colony-stimulating factor-mobilized peripheral blood progenitor cells to bone marrow inoculum. Blood 84:3948–3955, 1994.

Azeka E, Marcial MB, Jatene M, Auler JO, Ramires JA. Eight-year experience of pediatric heart transplantation: Clinical outcome using non-invasive methods for the evaluation of acute rejection. Pediatr Transplant 6:208–213, 2002.

Bach FH, Albertini RJ, Joo P, Anderson JL, Bortin MD. Bone marrow transplantation in a patient with the Wiskott-Aldrich syndrome. Lancet 2:1364–1366, 1968.

Bach FH, Amos DB. Hu-1: major histocompatibility locus in man. Science 156:1506–1508, 1967.

Bach FH, Hirschhorn K. Lymphocyte interaction, a potential histocompatibility test in vitro. Science 143:813–814, 1964.

Bach FH, Sachs DH. Transplantation immunology. N Engl J Med 317:489–492, 1987.

Bach JF, Strom TB. The mode of action of immunosuppressive Drugs. New York, Elsevier, 1985.

Bacigalupo A, Oneto R, Bruno B, Socie G, Passweg J, Locasciulli A, van Lint MT, Tichelli A, McCann S, Marsh J, Ljungman P, Hows J, Marin P, Schrezenmeier H. Current results of bone marrow transplantation in patients with acquired severe aplastic anemia. Report of the European Group for Blood and Marrow transplantation. On behalf of the Working Party on Severe Aplastic Anemia of the European Group for Blood and Marrow Transplantation. Acta Haematol 103:19–25, 2000.

Bailey LL, Gundry SR, Razzouk AJ, Wang N, Sciolaro CM, Chiavarelli M. Bless the babies: one hundred fifteen late survivors of heart transplantation during the first year of life. J Thoracic Cardiovas Surg 105:805–815, 1993.

Bain B, Magdalene RV, Lowenstein L. The development of large immature mononuclear cells in mixed leukocyte cultures. Blood 23:108–116, 1964.

Ball ED, Wilson J, Phelps V, Neudorf S. Autologous bone marrow transplantation for acute myeloid leukemia in remission or first relapse using monoclonal antibody-purged marrow: results of phase II studies with long-term follow-up. Bone Marrow Transplant 25:823–829, 2000.

Ballester OF, Elfenbein GJ. A rational appraisal of bone marrow transplantation and immunosuppressive therapy for severe aplastic anemia. Cancer Control 1:208–212, 1994.

Barber WH, Curtis JJ, Whelchel JD, Luck RG, Diethelm AG. Outcome of second kidney allografts following failure of transplants from living-related donors. Transplantation 40:225–228, 1985.

Barker CF, Billingham RE. The role of regional lymphatics in the skin homograft response. Transplantation 5:962–966, 1967.

Barker JN, Davies SM, DeFor T, Ramsay NK, Weisdorf DJ, Wagner JE. Survival after transplantation of unrelated donor umbilical cord blood is comparable to that of human leukocyte antigen-matched unrelated donor bone marrow: results of a matched-pair analysis. Blood 97:2957–2961, 2001.

Barker JN, Wagner JE. Umbilical cord blood transplantation: current state of the art. Curr Opin Oncol 14:160–164, 2002.

Barrett AJ, Horowitz MM, Pollock BH, Zhang M-J, Bortin MM, Buchanan GR, Camitta BM, Ochs J, Graham-Pole J, Rowlings PA, Rimm AA, Klein JP, Shuster JJ, Sobocinski KA, Gale RP. Bone marrow transplants from HLA-identical siblings as compared with chemotherapy for children with acute lymphoblastic leukemia in a second remission. N Engl J Med 331:1253–1258, 1994.

Barta A, Denes R, Masszi T, Remenyi P, Batai A, Torbagyi E, Sipos A, Lengyel L, Jakab K, Gyodi E, Reti M, Foldi J, Paldi-Haris P, Avalos M, Paloczi K, Fekete S, Torok J, Hoffer I, Jakab J, Varadi G, Kelemen E, Petranyi G. Remarkably reduced transplant-related complications by dibromomannitol non-myeloablative conditioning before allogeneic bone marrow transplantation in chronic myeloid leukemia. Acta Haematol 105:64–70, 2001.

Bauer J, Thul J, Kramer U, Hagel KJ, Akinturk H, Valeske K, Schindler E, Bohle RM, Schranz D. Heart transplantation in children and infants: short-term outcome and long-term follow-up. Pediatr Transplant 5:457–462, 2001.

Beatty PG, Clift RA, Mickelson EM, Nisperos B, Flournoy N, Martin PJ, Sanders JE, Stewart P, Buckner CD, Storb R, Thomas ED, Hansen JA. Marrow transplantation from related donors other than HLA-identical siblings. N Engl J Med 313:765–771, 1985.

Bell PRF, Calman KC, Wood RFM, Briggs JC, Paton AM, MacPherson SG. Reversal of acute clinical and experimental organ rejection using large doses of intravenous prednisolone. Lancet 1:876–888, 1971.

Belle SH, Beringer KC, Detre KM. An update on liver transplantation in the United States: Recipient characteristics and outcome. Clin Transpl 19–33.

Benfield MR, McDonald R, Sullivan EK, Stablein DM, Tejani A. The 1997 annual renal transplantation in children report of the North American Pediatric Renal Transplant Cooperative Study (NAPRTCS). Pediatr Transplant 3:152–167, 1999.

Benkerrou M, Le Deist F, De Villartay JP, Caillat-Zucman S, Rieux-Laucat F, Jabado N, Cavazzana-Calvo M, Fischer A. Correction of Fas (CD95) deficiency by haploidentical bone marrow transplantation. Eur J Immunol 27:2043–2047, 1997.

Bensoussan D, Le Deist F, Latger-Cannard v, Gregoire MJ, Avinens O, Feugier P, Bourdon V, Andre-Botte C, Schmitt C, Jonveaux P, Eliaou JF, Stoltz JF, Bordigoni P. T-cell immune constitution after peripheral blood mononuclear cell transplantation in complete DiGeorge syndrome. Br J Haematol 117:899–906, 2002.

Bernstein D. Update on cardiac transplantation in infants and children. Critical Care Med 21:354–355, 1993.

Berthet F, Le Deist F, Duliege AM, Griscelli C, Fischer A. Clinical consequences and treatment of primary immunodeficiency syndromes characterized by functional T and B lymphocyte anomalies (combined immune deficiency). Pediatrics 93:265–270, 1994.

Bertrand Y, Landais P, Friedrich W, Gerritsen B, Morgan G, Fasth A, Cavazzana-Calvo M, Porta F, Cant A, Espanol T, Muller S, Veys P, Vossen J, Haddad E, Fischer A. Influence of severe combined immunodeficiency phenotype on the outcome of HLA non-identical T cell-depleted bone marrow transplantation. J Pediatr 134:740–748, 1999.

Bertrand Y, Muller SM, Casanova JL, Morgan G, Fischer A, Friedrich W. Reticular dysgenesis: HLA non-identical bone marrow transplants in a series of 10 patients. Bone Marrow Transplant 29:759–762, 2002.

Billingham RE, Brent L, Medawar PB. Actively acquired tolerance of foreign cells. Nature 172:603–606, 1953.

Blazar DR, Ramsay NKC, Kersey JH, Krivit W, Arthur DC, Filipovich AH. Pretransplant conditioning with busulfan (Myleran) and cyclophosphamide for non malignant diseases. Assessment of engraftment following histocompatible allogeneic bone marrow transplantation. Transplantation 39:597, 1985.

Bleakley M, Shaw PJ, Nielsen JM. Allogeneic bone marrow transplantation for childhood relapsed acute lymphoblastic leukemia: comparison of outcome in patients with and without a matched family donor. Bone Marrow Transplant 30:1–7, 2002.

Bodmer JG, Marsh SG, Albert ED, Bodmer WF, Bontrop RE, Dupont B, Erlich HA, Hansen JA, Mach B, Mayr WR, Parham P, Petersdorf EW, Sasazuki T, Schreuder GM, Strominger JL, Svejgaard A, Terasaki PI. Nomenclature for factors of the HLA system, 1998. Tissue Antigens 53:407–446, 1999.

Bonduel M, Pozo A, Zelazko M, Raslawski E, Delfino S, Rossi J, Figueroa C, Sackmann MF. Successful related umbilical cord blood transplantation for graft failure following T cell-depleted non-identical bone marrow transplantation in a child with major histocompatibility complex class II deficiency. Bone Marrow Transplant 24:437–440, 1999.

Bortin MM, Rimm AA. Severe combined immunodeficiency disease. Characterization of the disease and results of transplantation. JAMA 238:591–600, 1977.

Boulad F, Giardina P, Gillio A, Kernan N, Small T, Brochstein J, Van Syckle K, George D, Szabolcs P, O'Reilly RJ. Bone marrow transplantation for homozygous beta-thalassemia. The Memorial Sloan-Kettering Cancer Center experience. Ann NY Acad Sci 850:498–502, 1998.

Bowen KM, Andrus L, Lafferty KJ. Successful allotransplantation of mouse pancreatic islets to non-immunosuppressed recipients. Diabetes 29S:98–104, 1980.

Breen TJ, Keck B, Hosenpud JD, White R, Daily OP. Thoracic Organ Transplants in the United States from October 1987 through December 1992: A Report from the UNOS Scientific Registry for Organ Transplants. Clin Transpl 3:37–45, 1993.

Breimer ME, Brynger H, Le Pendu J, Oriol R, Rydberg L, Samuelsson BE, Vinas J. Blood group ABO incompatible kidney transplantation biochemical and immunochemical studies of blood group A glycolipid antigens in human kidney and characterization of the antibody response (antigen specificity and antibody class) in O recipients receiving A2 grafts. Transplant Proc 19:226–230, 1987.

Breimer ME, Brynger H, Rydberg L, Samuelsson BF. Transplantation of blood group A2 kidneys to O recipients. Biochemical and immunological studies of blood group A antigens in human kidneys. Transplant Proc 17:2640–2643, 1985.

Brenner MK, Rill DR, Holladay MS, Heslop HE, Moen RC, Buschle M, Krance RA, Santana VM, Anderson WF, Ihle JN. Gene marking to determine whether autologous marrow infusion restores long-term haemopoiesis in cancer patients. Lancet 342:1134–1137, 1993.

Brochstein J, Gillio AP, Ruggerio M. Marrow transplantation from HLA-identical or haploidentical donors for correction of Wiskott-Aldrich syndrome. J Pediatr 119:907–912, 1991.

Brochstein JA, Shank B, Kernan NA, Terwilliger JW, O'Reilly RJ. Marrow transplantation for thrombocytopenia-absent radii syndrome. J Pediatr 121:587–589, 1992.

Broome CB, Graham ML, Saulsbury FT, Hershfield MS, Buckley RH. Correction of purine nucleoside phosphorylase deficiency by transplantation of allogeneic bone marrow from a sibling. J Pediatr 128:373–376, 1996.

Buckley RH. Primary immunodeficiency diseases due to defects in lymphocytes. N Engl J Med 343:1313–1324, 2000.

Buckley RH. Advances in the understanding and treatment of human severe combined immunodeficiency. Immunol Res 22:237–251, 2001.

Buckley RH. Primary cellular immunodeficiencies. J Allerg Clin Immunol 109:747–757, 2002.

Buckley RH, Fischer A. Bone marrow transplantation for primary immunodeficiency diseases. In Ochs H, Smith E, and Puck J, eds. Primary immunodeficiency diseases: a molecular and genetic approach. New York and Oxford, Oxford University Press, 1999, pp 459–475.

Buckley RH, Schiff RI, Schiff SE, Markert ML, Williams LW, Harville TO, Roberts JL, Puck JM. Human severe combined immunodeficiency (SCID): genetic, phenotypic and functional diversity in 108 infants. J Pediatr 130:378–387, 1997.

Buckley RH, Schiff SE, Sampson HA, Schiff RI, Markert ML, Knutsen AP, Hershfield MS, Huang AT, Mickey GH, Ward FE. Development of immunity in human severe primary T cell deficiency following haploidentical bone marrow stem cell transplantation. J Immunol 136:2398–2407, 1986.

Buckley RH, Schiff SE, Schiff RI, Markert L, Williams LW, Roberts JL, Myers LA, Ward FE. Hematopoietic stem cell transplantation for the treatment of severe combined immunodeficiency. N Engl J Med 340:508–516, 1999.

Buckley RH, Whisnant KJ, Schiff RI, Gilbertsen RB, Huang AT, Platt MS. Correction of severe combined immunodeficiency by fetal liver cells. N Engl J Med 294:1076–1081, 1976.

Cameron JS. Glomerulonephritis in renal transplants. Transplantation 34: 237–245, 1982.

Canioni D, Patey N, Cuenod B, Benkerrou M, Brousse N. Major histocompatibility complex class II deficiency needs an early diagnosis: report of a case. Pediatr Pathol Lab Med 17:645–651, 1997.

Canter CE, Moorhead S, Saffitz JE, Huddleston CB, Spray TL. Steroid withdrawal in the pediatric heart transplant recipient initially treated with triple immunosuppression. J Heart Lung Transplant 13:74–80, 1994.

Carpenter CB, Morris PJ. The detection and measurement of pretransplant sensitization. Transplant Proc 10:509–513, 1978.

Carpenter PA, Ziegler JB, Vowels MR. Late diagnosis and correction of purine nucleoside phosphorylase deficiency with allogeneic bone marrow transplantation. Bone Marrow Transplant 17:121–124, 1996.

Casper JT, Ash RA, Kirchner P, Hunter JB, Havens PL, Chusid MJ. Successful treatment with an unrelated donor bone marrow transplant in an HLA-deficient patient with severe combined immune deficiency ("bare lymphocyte syndrome"). J Pediatr 116:262–265, 1990a.

Casper JT, Truitt RR, Baxter-Lowe LA, Ash RC. Bone marrow transplantation for severe aplastic anemia in children. Am J Ped Hem-Onc 12:434–448, 1990b.

Caves PK, Stinson EB, Billingham ME, Rider AK, Shumway NE. Diagnosis of human cardiac allograft rejection by serial cardiac biopsy. J Thorac Cardiovasc Surg 66:461–466, 1973.

Cecka JM. The UNOS renal transplant registry. Clin Transpl 1–20, 2002.

Cecka JM, Terasaki PI. Clin Transpl 2001, Los Angeles, UCLA Immunogenetics Center, 2002, pp 809–834.

Ceppellini R, Bigliani S, Curtoni ES, Leigheb G. Experimental allotransplantation in man. II. The role of A1, A2 and B antigens. III. Enhancement by circulating antibody. Transplant Proc 1:390–394, 1969.

Chan KW, Wong LTK, Applegarth D, Davidson AGF. Bone marrow transplantation in Gaucher's disease: effect of mixed chimeric state. Bone Marrow Transplant 14:327–330, 1994.

Chemelli RM, Willie JT, Sinton CM, Elmquist JK, Scammell T, Lee C, Richardson JA, Williams SC, Xiong Y, Kisanuki Y, Fitch TE, Nakazato M, Hammer RE, Saper CB, Yanagisawa M. Narcolepsy in orexin knockout mice: molecular genetics of sleep regulation. Cell 98:437–451, 1999.

Chinnock RE, Baum MF, Larsen R, Bailey L. Rejection management and long term surveillance of the pediatric heart transplant recipient: the Loma Linda experience. J Heart Lung Transplant 12:255–264, 1993.

Cicciarelli J, Teraski P. Sensitization patterns in transfused kidney transplant patients and their possible role in kidney graft survival. Transplant Proc 15:1208–1211, 1983.

Clay TM, Culpan D, Howell WM, Sage DA, Bradley BA, Bidwell JL. UHG crossmatching—a comparison with PCR-SSO typing in the selection of HLA-DPB1–compatible bone marrow donors. Transplantation 58:200–207, 1994.

Codoner-Franch P, Bernard O, Alvarez F. Long term follow-up of growth in height after successful liver transplantation. J Pediatr 124:368–373, 1994.

Collins RH, Anastasi J, Terstappen LWM, Nikaein A, Feng J, Fay JW, Klintmalm G, Stone MJ. Brief report: Donor-derived long term multilineage hematopoiesis in a liver transplant recipient. N Engl J Med 328:762–770, 1993.

Cosimi AB, Colvin RB, Burton RC, Rubin RH, Goldstein G, Kung PC, Hansen WP, Delmonico FL, Russell PS. Use of monoclonal antibodies to T-cell subsets for immunologic monitoring and treatment in recipients of renal allografts. N Engl J Med 305:308–314, 1981.

Cros P, Allibert P, Mandrand B, Tiercy J-M, Mach B. Oligonucleotide genotyping of HLA polymorphism on microtitre plates. Lancet 340:870–873, 1992.

Czitrom AA, Langer F, McKee N, Gross AE. Bone and cartilage allotransplantation. A review of 14 years of research and clinical studies. Clin Orthop 208:141–145, 1986.

Dall'Amico R, Ginevri F, Ghio L, Murer L, Perfumo F, Zanon GF, Berardinelli L, Basile G, Edefonti A, Garavaglia R, Damiani B, Valente U, Fontana I, Bertipaglia M, Cardillo M, Scalamogna M, Zacchello G. Successful renal transplantation in children under 6 years of age. Pediatr Nephrol 16:1–7, 2001.

Dausset J. Leuco-agglutinins. IV. Leuco-agglutinins and blood transfusion. Vox Sang 4:190–198, 1954.

Dausset J, Rapaport FT. The role of ABO erythrocyte groups in human histocompatibility reactions. Nature 209:209–211, 1966.

De Santes KB, Lai SS, Cowan MJ. Haploidentical bone marrow transplants for two patients with reticular dysgenesis. Bone Marrow Transplant 17:1171–1173, 1996.

Deeg HJ, Henslee-Downey PJ. Management of acute graft-versus-host disease. Bone Marrow Transplant 6:1–8, 1990.

DeLeve LD, Shulman HM, McDonald GB. Toxic injury to hepatic sinusoids: sinusoidal obstruction syndrome (veno-occlusive disease). Semin Liver Dis 22:27–42, 2002.

Dellgren G, Koirala B, Sakopoulus A, Botta A, Joseph J, Benson L, McCrindle B, Dipchand A, Cardella C, Lee KJ, West L, Poirier N, Van Arsdell GS, Williams WG, Coles JG. Pediatric heart transplantation: improving results in high-risk patients. J Thorac Cardiovasc Surg 121:782–791, 2001.

Demirci G, Gao W, Zheng XX, Malek TR, Strom TB, Li XC. On CD28/CD40 ligand costimulation, common gamma-chain signals, and the alloimmune response. J Immunol 168:4382–4390, 2002.

DeVoe PW, Buckley RH, Shirley LR, Darby CP, Ward FE, Mickey GH, Raab-Traub N, Vandenbark GH. Successful immune reconstitution in severe combined immunodeficiency despite Epstein-Barr virus and cytomegalovirus infections. Clin Immunol Immunopathol 34:48–59, 1985.

Donaldson PT, O'Grady J, Portmann B, Davis H, Alexander GJM, Neuberger J, Thick M, Calne RY, Williams L. Evidence for an immune response to HLA class I antigens in the vanishing bileduct syndrome after liver transplantation. Lancet 1:945–948, 1987.

Dresser DW, Mitchison NA. The mechanism of immunological paralysis. Adv Immunol 8:120–181, 1968.

Duplantier JE, Seyama K, Day NK, Hitchcock R, Nelson RP, Jr., Ochs HD, Haraguchi S, Klemperer MR, Good RA. Immunologic reconstitution following bone marrow transplantation for X-linked hyper IgM syndrome. Clin Immunol 98:313–318, 2001.

Durando R, Palestini N, Mazzucco G. Parathyroid transplantation and cryopreservation techniques. Minerva Chir 48:1307–1311, 1993.

Eapen M, Davies SM, Ramsay NK, Orchard PJ. Hematopoietic stem cell transplantation for infantile osteopetrosis. Bone Marrow Transplant 22:941–946, 1998.

Ehrlich RM. Surgical complications of renal transplantation. Ann Intern Med 100:246–257, 1984.

Eichwald EJ, Wetzel B, Lustgraaf EC. Genetic aspects of second-set skin grafts in mice. Transplant 4:260–273, 1966.

Elkins CC, Frist WH, Dummer JS, Stewart JR, Merrill WH, Carden KA, Bender HW. Cytomegalovirus disease after heart transplantation: Is acyclovir prophylaxis indicated? Ann Thoracic Surg 56:1267–1273, 1993.

Ellis RJ, Kahn Q, Skikne BS, Mayo MS, Allgood JW, Bodensteiner DM, Deauna-Limayo D, Cook JD. A retrospective analysis of long-term survival in severe aplastic anemia patients treated with allogeneic bone marrow transplantation or immunosuppressive therapy with antithymocyte globulin and cyclosporin A at a single institution. Mil Med 167:541–545, 2002.

Eltumi M, Trivedi P, Hobbs JR, Portmann B, Cheeseman P, Downie C, Risteli J, Risteli L, Mowat AP. Monitoring of veno-occlusive disease after bone marrow transplantation by serum aminopropeptide of type III procollagen. Lancet 342:518–521, 1993.

Ettenger RB. New immunosuppressive agents in pediatric renal transplantation. Transplant Proc 30:1956–1958, 1998.

Ettenger RB, Fine RN. Pediatric renal transplantation. In Garovoy MR, Guttmann RD, eds. Renal Transplantation. New York, Churchill Livingstone, 1986, pp 399–435.

Ettenger RB, Rosenthal JT, Marik J. Cadaver renal transplantation in children: results with long-term cyclosporine immunosuppression. Clin Tranplant 4:329–336, 1990.

Fasth A. Bone marrow transplantation for hyper-IgM syndrome. Immunodeficiency 4:323, 1993.

Faustman D, Hauptfeld V, Lacy P, Davie J. Prolongation of murine islet allograft survival by pretreatment of islets with antibody directed to determinants. Proc Natl Acad Sci USA 78:5156–5159, 1981.

Feder JN, Gnirke A, Thomas W, Tsuchihashi Z, Ruddy DA, Basava A, Dormishian F, Domingo R, Jr., Ellis MC, Fullan A, Hinton LM, Jones NL, Kimmel BE, Kronmal GS, Lauer P, Lee VK, Loeb DB, Mapa FA, McClelland E, Meyer NC, Mintier GA, Moeller N, Moore T, Morikang E, Wolff RK. A novel MHC class I-like gene is mutated in patients with hereditary haemochromatosis. Nat Genet 13:399–408, 1996.

Fefer A, Buckner CD, Thomas ED, Cheever MA, Clift RA, Glucksberg H, Neiman PE, Storb R. Cure of hematologic neoplasia with transplantation of marrow from identical twins. N Engl J Med 297:146–148, 1977.

Feinstein L, Sandmaier B, Maloney D, McSweeney PA, Maris M, Flowers C, Radich J, Little MT, Nash RA, Chauncey T, Woolfrey A, Georges G, Kiem HP, Zaucha JM, Blume KG, Shizuru J, Niederwieser D, Storb R. Nonmyeloablative hematopoietic cell transplantation. Replacing high-dose cytotoxic therapy by the graft-versus-tumor effect. Ann NY Acad Sci 938:328–337, 2001.

Feltkamp TE, Khan MA, Lopez de Castro JA. The pathogenetic role of HLA-B27. Immunol Today 17:5–7, 1996.

Ferrara JL, Deeg HJ. Graft-versus-host disease. N Engl J Med 324:667–674, 1991.

Festenstein H, Doyle P, Holmes J. Long-term follow-up in London transplant group recipients of cadaver renal allografts. N Engl J Med 314:7–14, 1986.

Filipovich AH, Stone JV, Tomany SC, Ireland M, Kollman C, Pelz CJ, Casper JT, Cowan MJ, Edwards JR, Fasth A, Gale RP, Junker A, Kamani NR, Loechelt BJ, Pietryga DW, Ringden O, Vowels M, Hegland J, Williams AV, Klein JP, Sobocinski KA, Rowlings PA, Horowitz MM. Impact of donor type on outcome of bone marrow transplantation for Wiskott-Aldrich syndrome: collaborative study of the International Bone Marrow Transplant Registry and the National Marrow Donor Program. Blood 97:1598–1603, 2001.

Filipovich AH, Vallera DA, Youle RJ, Quinones RR, Neville DM Jr, Kersey JH. Ex-vivo treatment of donor bone marrow with anti-T-cell immunotoxins for prevention of graft-versus-host disease. Lancet 1:469–472, 1984.

Fine RN. Growth post renal-transplantation in children: lessons from the North American Pediatric Renal Transplant Cooperative Study (NAPRTCS). Pediatr Transplant 1:85–89, 1997.

Fischer A, Durandy A, De Villartay JP, Vilmer E, Le Deist F, Gerota I, Griscelli C. HLA-haploidentical bone marrow transplantation for severe combined immunodeficiency using E rosette fractionation and cyclosporine. Blood 67:444–449, 1986a.

Fischer A, Griscelli C, Friedrich W, Kubanek B, Levinsky R, Morgan G, Vossen J, Wagemaker G, Landais P. Bone marrow transplantation for immunodeficiencies and osteopetrosis: European survey, 1968–1985. Lancet 2:1080–1084, 1986b.

Fischer A, Landais P, Friedrich W, Gerritsen B, Fasth A, Porta F, Vellodi A, Benkerrou M, Jais JP, Cavazzana-Calvo M, Souillet G, Bordigoni P, Morgan G, Van Dijken P, Vossen J, Locatelli F, di Bartolomeo P. Bone marrow transplantation (BMT) in Europe for primary immunodeficiencies other than severe combined immunodeficiency: a report from the European Group for BMT and the European Group for Immunodeficiency. Blood 83:1149–1154, 1994.

Flake AW, Roncarolo MG, Puck JM, Almeida-Porada G, Evans MI, Johnson MP, Abella EM, Harrison DD, Zanjani ED. Treatment of X-linked severe combined immunodeficiency by in utero transplantation of paternal bone marrow. N Engl J Med 335:1806–1810, 1996.

Flavell RA, Hafler DA. Autoimmunity. Curr Opin Immunol 11:635–707, 1999.

Fleisher BE, Baum D, Brudos G, Burge M, Carson E, Constantinou J, Duckworth J, Gamberg P, Klein P, Luikart H, Miller J, Stach B, Bernstein D. Infant heart transplantation at Stanford: growth and neurodevelopmental outcome. Pediatrics 109:1–7, 2002.

Forbes SA, Trowsdale J. The MHC quarterly report. Immunogenetics 50:152–159, 1999.

French ME, Batchelor JR. Enhancement of renal allografts in rats and man. Transplant Rev 13:115–141, 1972.

Friedlander GE, Mankin HJ, Sell KW. Osteochondral allografts. Biology, banking and clinical applications. Boston, Little, Brown, 1983.

Fukushima N, Gundry SR, Razzouk AJ, Bailey LL. Risk factors for graft failure associated with pulmonary hypertension after pediatric heart transplantation. J Thor Cardiovasc Surg 107:985–989, 1994.

Gale RP, Champlin RE. How does bone marrow transplantation cure leukaemia? Lancet 2:28–30, 1984.

Gaspar HB, Amrolia P, Hassan A, Webb D, Jones A, Sturt N, Vergani G, Pagliuca A, Mufti G, Hadzic N, Davies G, Veys P. Non-myeloablative stem cell transplantation for congenital immunodeficiencies. Recent Results Cancer Res 159:134–142, 2002.

Gatti RA, Meuwissen HJ, Allen HD, Hong R, Good RA. Immunological reconstitution of sex-linked lymphopenic immunological deficiency. Lancet 2:1366–1369, 1968.

Gaziev D, Giardini C, Galimberti M, Lucarelli G, Angelucci E, Polchi P, Baronciani D, Erer B, Sotti G. Bone marrow transplantation for transfused patients with severe aplastic anemia using cyclophosphamide and total lymphoid irradiation as conditioning therapy: long-term follow-up from a single center. Bone Marrow Transplant 24:253–257, 1999.

Gerritsen EJA, Vossen JM, Fasth A, Friedrich W, Morgan G, Padmos A, Vellodi A, Porras O, O'Meara A, Porta F, Bordigoni P, Cant A, Hermans J, Griscelli C, Fischer A. Bone marrow transplantation for autosomal recessive osteopetrosis. J Pediatr 125:896–902, 1994.

Ghavamzadeh A, Nasseri P, Eshraghian MR, Jahani M, Baybordi I, Nateghi J, Khodabandeh A, Sadjadi AR, Mohyeddin M, Khademi Y. Prognostic factors in bone marrow transplantation for beta thalassemia major: experiences from Iran. Bone Marrow Transplant 22:1167–1169, 1998.

Ginsburg D, Antin JH, Smith BR, Orkin SH, Rappeport JM. Origin of cell populations after bone marrow transplantation. Analysis using DNA sequence polymorphisms. J Clin Invest 75:596–603, 1985.

Gluckman E, Broxmeyer HA, Auerbach AD, Friedman HS, Douglas GW, Devergie A, Esperou H, Thierry D, Socie G, Lehn P. Hematopoietic reconstitution in a patient with Fanconi's anemia by means of umbilical-cord blood from an HLA-identical sibling. N Engl J Med 321:1174–1178, 1989.

Glucksberg H, Storb R, Fefer A, Buckner CD, Neiman PE, Clift RA, Lerner KG, Thomas ED. Clinical manifestations of graft-versus-host disease in human recipients of marrow from HLA-matched sibling donors. Transplantation 18:295–304, 1974.

Goldman JM, Apperley JF, Jones L, Marcus R, Goolden AWG, Batchelor R, Hale G, Waldmann H, Reid CD, Hows J, Gordon-Smith E, Catovsky D, Galton DAG. Bone marrow transplantation for patients with chronic myeloid leukemia. N Engl J Med 314:202–207, 1986.

Goldsobel AB, Haas A, Stiehm ER. Bone marrow transplantation in DiGeorge syndrome. J Pediatr 111:40–44, 1987.

Gomez L, Le Deist F, Blanche S, Cavazzana-Calvo M, Griscelli C, Fischer A. Treatment of Omenn syndrome by bone marrow transplantation. J Pediatr 127:76–81, 1995.

Good RA. Bone marrow transplantation symposium: bone marrow transplantation for immunodeficiency diseases. Am J Med Sci 294:68–74, 1987.

Good RA, Verjee T. Historical and current perspectives on bone marrow transplantation for prevention and treatment of immunodeficiencies and autoimmunities. Biol Blood Marrow Transplant 7:123–135, 2001.

Gould DS, Auchincloss H Jr. Direct and indirect recognition: the role of MHC antigens in graft rejection. Immunol Today 20:77–82, 1999.

Graff R, Bailey DW. The non-H2 histocompatibility loci and their antigens. Transplant Rev 15:26–49, 1973.

Gratama JW, Zwaan FE, Stijnen T, Weijers TF, Weiland HT, D'Amaro J, Hekker AC, The TH, de Gast GC, Vossen JM. Herpes-virus immunity and acute graft-versus-host disease. Lancet 1:471–474, 1987.

Graze PR, Gale RP. Chronic graft-versus-host disease: a syndrome of disordered immunity. Am J Med 66:611–620, 1979.

Gross TG, Filipovich AH, Conley ME, Pracher E, Schmiegelow K, Verdirame JD, Vowels M, Williams LL, Seemayer TA. Cure of X-linked lymphoproliferative disease (XLP) with allogeneic hematopoietic stem cell transplantation (HSCT): report from the XLP registry. Bone Marrow Transplant 17:741–744, 1996.

Guinan EC, Boussiotis VA, Neuberg D, Brennan LL, Hirano N, Nadler LM, Gribben JG. Transplantation of anergic histoincompatible bone marrow allografts. N Engl J Med 340:1704–1714, 1999.

Hacein-Bey-Abina S, Le Deist F, Carlier F, Bouneaud C, Hue C, De Villartay JP, Thrasher AJ, Wulffraat N, Sorensen R, Dupuis-Girod S, Fischer A, Davies EG, Kuis W, Leiva L, Cavazzana-Calvo M. Sustained correction of X-linked severe combined immunodeficiency by ex vivo gene therapy. N Engl J Med 346:1185–1193, 2002.

Haddad E, Landais P, Friedrich W, Gerritsen B, Cavazzana-Calvo M, Morgan G, Bertrand Y, Fasth A, Porta F, Cant A, Espanol T, Muller S, Veys P, Vossen J, Fischer A. Long-term immune reconstitution and outcome after HLA-nonidentical T-cell-depleted bone marrow transplantation for severe combined immunodeficiency: a European retrospective study of 116 patients. Blood 91:3646–3653, 1998.

Haddad E, Le Deist F, Blanche S, Benkerrou M, Rohrlich P, Vilmer E, Griscelli C, Fischer A. Treatment of Chediak-Higashi syndrome by allogenic bone marrow transplantation: report of 10 cases. Blood 85:3328–3333, 1995.

Hefton JM, Amberson JB, Biozes DG, Weksler ME. Loss of HLA expression by human epidermal cells after growth in culture. J Invest Derm 83:48–50, 1984.

Hill AV. The immunogenetics of human infectious diseases. Annu Rev Immunol 16:593–617, 1998.

Hill AV. The immunogenetics of resistance to malaria. Proc Assoc Am Physicians 111:272–277, 1999.

Hobbs JR, Monteil M, McCluskey DR, Jurges E, Eltuni M. Chronic granulomatous disease, 100% corrected by displacement bone marrow transplantation from a volunteer unrelated donor. Eur J Pediatr 15:806, 1992.

Hong JC, Kahan BD. Immunosuppressive agents in organ transplantation: past, present, and future. Semin Nephrol 20:108–125, 2000.

Horowitz MM. Current status of allogeneic bone marrow transplantation in acquired aplastic anemia. Semin Hematol 37:30–42, 2000.

Horwitz ME, Barrett AJ, Brown MR, Carter CS, Childs R, Gallin JI, Holland SM, Linton GF, Miller JA, Leitman SF, Read EJ, Malech HL. Treatment of chronic granulomatous disease with nonmyeloablative conditioning and a T-cell-depleted hematopoietic allograft. N Engl J Med 344:881–888, 2001.

Huddleston CB, Bloch JB, Sweet SC, De La MM, Patterson GA, Mendeloff EN. Lung transplantation in children. Ann Surg 236:270–276, 2002.

Humar A, Arrazola L, Mauer M, Matas AJ, Najarian JS. Kidney transplantation in young children: should there be a minimum age? Pediatr Nephrol 16:941–945, 2001.

Ildstad ST, Sachs DH. Reconstitution with syngeneic plus allogeneic or xenogeneic bone marrow leads to specific acceptance of allografts or xenografts. Nature 307:168–170, 1984.

Jain A, Mazariegos G, Kashyap R, Kosmach-Park B, Starzl TE, Fung J, Reyes J. Pediatric liver transplantation. A single center experience spanning 20 years. Transplantation 73:941–947, 2002.

Janossy G, Prentice HG, Grob JP, Ivory K, Tidman N, Grundy J, Favrot M, Brenner MK, Campana D, Blacklock HA, Gilmore MJML, Patterson J, Griffiths PD, Hoffbrand AV. T lymphocyte regeneration after transplantation of T cell depleted allogeneic bone marrow. Clin Exp Immunol 63:577–586, 1986.

Ji SQ, Chen HR, Wang HX, Yan HM, Pan SP, Xun CQ. Comparison of outcome of allogeneic bone marrow transplantation with and without granulocyte colony-stimulating factor (lenograstim) donor-marrow priming in patients with chronic myelogenous leukemia. Biol Blood Marrow Transplant 8:261–267, 2002.

Kahan BD. Cyclosporine. N Engl J Med 321:1725–1738, 1989.

Kahan BD. Cyclosporine: a revolution in transplantation. Transplant Proc 31:14S-15S, 1999.

Kahan BD, Chang JY, Sehgal SN. Preclinical evaluation of a new potent immunosuppressive agent, rapamycin. Transplantation 52:185–191, 1991.

Kahan BD, Dunn J, Fitts C, Van Buren D, Wombolt D, Pollak R, Carson R, Alexander JW, Chang C, Choc M. The Neoral formulation: improved correlation between cyclosporine trough levels and exposure in stable renal transplant recipients. Transplant Proc 26:2940–2943, 1994.

Kaliss N. Immunological enhancement of tumor homografts in mice. A review. Cancer Res 18:992–1003, 1958.

Kari JA, Romagnoli J, Duffy P, Fernando ON, Rees L, Trompeter RS. Renal transplantation in children under 5 years of age. Pediatr Nephrol 13:730–736, 1999.

Kauffman HP, Stormstad AS, Sampson D, Stawicki AT. Randomized steroid therapy of human kidney transplant rejection. Transplant Proc 11:36–38, 1979.

Kawauchi M, Gundry SR, Alonso de Begona J, Fullerton DA, Razzouk AJ, Boucek MM, Nehlsen-Cannarella S, Bailey LL. Male donor into female recipient increases the risk of pediatric heart allograft rejection. Ann Thoracic Surg 55:716–718, 1993.

Kaye MP. Pediatric thoracic transplantation: the world experience. J Heart Lung Transplant 12:344–350, 1993.

Khawaja K, Gennery AR, Flood TJ, Abinun M, Cant AJ. Bone marrow transplantation for CD40 ligand deficiency: a single centre experience. Arch Dis Child 84:508–511, 2001.

Kino T, Hatanaka H, Miyata S. FK-506, a novel immunosuppressant isolated from a Streptomyces II. Immunosuppressive effect of FK-506 in vitro. J Antibiot (Toyko) 40:1256–1265, 1987.

Kissmeyer-Nielsen F, Olsen S, Petersen VP, Fjeldborg O. Hyperacute rejection of kidney allografts associated with pre-existing humoral antibodies against donor cells. Lancet 2:662–665, 1966.

Klein C, Cavazzana-Calvo M, Le Deist F, Jabado N, Benkerrou M, Blanche S, Lisowska-Grospierre B, Griscelli C, Fischer A. Bone marrow transplantation in major histocompatibility complex class II deficiency: a single center study of 19 patients. Blood 85:580–587, 1995.

Klein J. Biology of the mouse histocompatibility complex: principles of immunogenetics applied to a single system. Berlin, Springer, 1975.

Klein J, Sato A. The HLA system. First of two parts. N Engl J Med 343:702–709, 2000a.

Klein J, Sato A. The HLA system. Second of two parts. N Engl J Med 343:782–786, 2000b.

Knutsen AP, Wall DA. Kinetics of T-cell development of umbilical cord blood transplantation in severe T-cell immunodeficiency disorders. J Allergy Clin Immunol 103:823–832, 1999.

Koc S, Leisenring W, Flowers ME, Anasetti C, Deeg HJ, Nash RA, Sanders JE, Witherspoon RP, Storb R, Appelbaum FR, Martin PJ. Therapy for chronic graft-versus-host disease: a randomized trial comparing cyclosporine plus prednisone versus prednisone alone. Blood 100:48–51, 2002.

Kortz EO, Sachs DH. Mechanisms of specific transplantation tolerance induction by vascular allografts across a class I difference in miniature swine. Transplant Proc 19:861–863, 1987.

Korver K, De Lange GG, Langloid van den Bergh R, Schellekens PTA, Van Loghem E, van Leeuwen F, Vossen JM. Lymphoid chimerism after allogeneic bone marrow transplantation. Transplantation 44:643–650, 1987.

Krensky AM. The human cytolytic T lymphocyte response to transplantation antigens. Pediatr Res 19:1231–1234, 1985.

Krivit W, Whitley CB. Bone marrow transplantation for genetic diseases. N Engl J Med 316:1985–1087, 1987.

Kumar S, Wolf RC, Chen MG, Gastineau DA, Gertz MA, Inwards DJ, Lacy MQ, Tefferi A, Litzow MR. Omission of day +11 methotrexate after allogeneic bone marrow transplantation is associated with increased risk of severe acute graft-versus-host disease. Bone Marrow Transplant 30:161–165, 2002.

La Nasa G, Giardini C, Argiolu F, Locatelli F, Arras M, De Stefano P, Ledda A, Pizzati A, Sanna MA, Vacca A, Lucarelli G, Contu L. Unrelated donor bone marrow transplantation for thalassemia: the effect of extended haplotypes. Blood 99:4350–4356, 2002.

Lacy PE, Davie JM, Finke EH. Prolongation of islet allograft survival following in vitro culture (24° C) and a single injection of anti-lymphocyte serum. Science 204:312–313, 1979.

Lafferty KJ, Bootes A, Dart G, Talmage DW. Effect of organ culture on the survival of thyroid allografts in mice. Transplantation 22:138–149, 1976.

Laine J, Jalanko H, Holthofer H, Krogerus L, Rapola J, von Willebrand E, Lautenschlager I, Salmela K, Holmberg C. Post-transplantation nephrosis in congenital nephrotic syndrome of the Finnish type. Kidney Int 44:867–874, 1993.

Laks H, Marelli D, Odim J, Fazio D. Heart transplantation in the young and elderly. Heart Fail Rev 6:221–226, 2001.

Lanfranchi A, Verardi R, Tettoni K, Neva A, Mazzolari E, Pennacchio M, Pasic S, Ugazio AG, Albertini A, Porta F. Haploidentical peripheral blood and marrow stem cell transplantation in nine cases of primary immunodeficiency. Haematologica 85:41–46, 2000.

LeDeist F, Blanche S, Keable H. Successful HLA non-identical bone marrow transplantation in three patients with leukocyte adhesion deficiency. Blood 74:512, 1989.

Lee JH, Lee KH, Lee JH, Kim S, Seol M, Park CJ, Chi HS, Kang W, Kim ST, Kim WK, Lee JS. Plasminogen activator inhibitor-1 is an independent diagnostic marker as well as severity predictor of hepatic veno-occlusive disease after allogeneic bone marrow transplantation in adults conditioned with busulphan and cyclophosphamide. Br J Haematol 118:1087–1094, 2002a.

Lee SJ, Klein JP, Barrett AJ, Ringden O, Antin JH, Cahn JY, Carabasi MH, Gale RP, Giralt S, Hale GA, Ilhan O, McCarthy PL, Socie G, Verdonck LF, Weisdorf DJ, Horowitz MM. Severity of chronic graft-versus-host disease: association with treatment-related mortality and relapse. Blood 100:406–414, 2002b.

Leithner C, Sinzinger H, Pohanka E, Schwarz M, Kretschmer G, Syre G. Occurrence of hemolytic uremic syndrome under cyclosporine treatment: accident or possible side effect mediated by a lack of prostacyclin-stimulating plasma factor. Transplant Proc 15:2787–2789, 1985.

Lenarsky C, Weinberg K, Kohn DB, Parkman R. Unrelated donor bone marrow transplantation for Wiskott-Aldrich syndrome. Bone Marrow Transplant 12:145–147, 1993.

Leone MR, Alexander SR, Barry JM, Henell K, Funnell MB, Goldstein G, Norman DJ. OKT3 monoclonal antibody in pediatric kidney transplant recipients with recurrent and resistant allograft rejection. J Pediatr 111:45–50, 1987.

Leung TF, Chik KW, Li CK, Shing MMK, Yuen PMP. Bone marrow transplantation for chronic granulomatous disease: long-term follow-up and review of the literature. Bone Marrow Transplant 24:567–570, 1999.

Liang JS, Lu MY, Tsai MJ, Lin DT, Lin KH. Bone marrow transplantation from an HLA-matched unrelated donor for treatment of Chediak-Higashi syndrome. J Formos Med Assn 99:499–502, 2000.

Lilly F, Boyse EA, Old LI. Genetic basis of susceptibility to viral leukaemogenesis. Lancet 2:1207–1209, 1964.

Lin L, Faraco J, Li R, Kadotani H, Rogers W, Lin X, Qiu X, de Jong PJ, Nishino S, Mignot E. The sleep disorder canine narcolepsy is caused by a mutation in the hypocretin (orexin) receptor 2 gene. Cell 98:365–376, 1999.

Locatelli F, Beluffi G, Giorgiani G, Maccario R, Fiori P, Pession A, Bonetti F, Comoli P, Calcaterra V, Rondini G, Severi F.

Transplantation of cord blood progenitor cells can promote bone resorption in autosomal recessive osteopetrosis. Bone Marrow Transplant 20:701–705, 1997.

Loechelt BJ, Shapiro RS, Jyonouchi H, Filipovich AH. Mismatched bone marrow transplantation for Omenn syndrome: a variant of severe combined immunodeficiency. Bone Marrow Transplant 16:381–385, 1995.

Lopez D, Barber DF, Villadangos JA, Lopez de Castro JA. Cross-reactive T cell clones from unrelated individuals reveal similarities in peptide presentation between HLA-B27 and HLA-DR2. J Immunol 150:2675–2686, 1993.

Lorenz E, Cogdon C, Uphoff D. Modification of acute radiation injury in mice and guinea pigs by bone marrow injection. Radiology 58:863–877, 1952.

Lucarelli G, Andreani M, Angelucci E. The cure of thalassemia by bone marrow transplantation. Blood Rev 16:81–85, 2002.

Lum LG, Noges JE, Beatty P, Martin PJ, Deeg J, Doney KC, Loughran T, Sullivan KM, Witherspoon RP, Thomas ED, Storb R. Transfer of specific immunity in marrow recipients given HLA-mismatched, T cell-depleted, or HLA-identical marrow grafts. Bone Marrow Transplant 3:399–406, 1988.

Lund DP, Lillehei CW, Kevy S, Perez-Atayde A, Maller E, Treacy S, Vacanti JP. Liver transplantation in newborn liver failure: treaatment for neonatal hemochromatosis. Transplant Proc 25:1068–1971, 1993.

Madden MR, Finkelstein JL, Staiano-Coico L, Goodwin LW, Shires GT, Nolan EE, Hefton JM. Grafting of cultured allogeneic epidermis on second and third degree burn wounds on 16 patients. J Trauma 26:955–962, 1986.

Mak YK, Chan CH, Chu YC, Chen YT, Lau CK, Lau JS. Autologous bone marrow transplantation for patients with acute myeloid leukaemia: prospective follow-up study. Hong Kong Med J 6:37–42, 2000.

Maraninchi D, Blaise D, Rio B, Leblond V, Dreyfus F, Gluckman E, Guyotat D, Pico JL, Michallet M, Ifrah N, Bordigoni A. Impact of T cell depletion on outcome of allogeneic bone marrow transplantation for standard risk leukaemias. Lancet 2:175–178, 1987.

Markert ML, Boeck A, Hale LP, Kloster AL, McLaughlin TM, Batchvarova MN, Douek DC, Koup RA, Kostyu DD, Ward FE, Rice HE, Mahaffey SM, Schiff SE, Buckley RH, Haynes BF. Transplantation of thymus tissue in complete DiGeorge syndrome. N Engl J Med 341:1180–1189, 1999.

Markert ML, Sarzotti M, Ozaki DA, Sempowski GD, Rhein ME, Hale LP, Le Deist F, Alexieff MJ, Li J, Hauser ER, Haynes BF, Rice HE, Skinner MA, Mahaffey SM, Jaggers J, Stein LD, Mill MR. Thymus transplantation in complete DiGeorge syndrome: immunologic and safety evaluations in 12 patients. Blood 102:1121–1130, 2003.

Marsh SG. Nomenclature for factors of the HLA system, update March 2002. Tissue Antigens 59:239–240, 2002.

Martin PJ, Hansen JA, Storb R, Thomas ED. Human marrow transplantation: an immunological perspective. Adv Immunol 40:379–438, 1987.

McDevitt HO, Chinitz A. Genetic control of the antibody response: relationship between immune response and histocompatibility (H-2) type. Science 163:1207–1208, 1969.

McEnery P, Stablein D, Arbus G, Tejani A. Renal transplantation in children. N Engl J Med 326:1727–1732, 1992.

Medawar PB. The behaviour and fate of skin autografts and skin homografts in rabbits. J Anat 78:176–199, 1944.

Medawar PB. Immunity to homologous grafted skin. II. The relationship between antigens of blood and skin. Br J Exp Pathol 27:15–24, 1946.

Mehta J, Powles R, Sirohi B, Treleaven J, Kulkarni S, Saso R, Tait D, Singhal S. Does donor-recipient ABO incompatibility protect against relapse after allogeneic bone marrow transplantation in first remission acute myeloid leukemia? Bone Marrow Transplant 29:853–859, 2002.

Mentzer WC, Cowan MJ. Bone marrow transplantation for beta-thalassemia: the University of California San Francisco experience. J Pediatr Hematol Oncol 22:598–601, 2000.

Miano M, Porta F, Locatelli F, Miniero R, La Nasa G, di Bartolomeo P, Giardini C, Messina C, Balduzzi A, Testi AM,

Garbarino L, Lanino E, Crescenzi F, Zecca M, Dini G. Unrelated donor marrow transplantation for inborn errors. Bone Marrow Transplant 21(Suppl. 2):S37–S41, 1998.

Michler RE, Chen JM, Mancini DM, Reemtsma K, Rose EA. Sixteen years of cardiac transplantation: the Columbia-Presbyterian Medical Center experience 1977 to 1993. Clin Transpl 9:109–118, 1993.

Mickelson EM, Fefer A, Storb R, Thomas ED. Correlation of the relative response index with marrow graft rejection in patients with aplastic anemia. Transplantation 22:294–330, 1976.

Mickelson EM, Guthrie LA, Etzioni R, Anasetti C, Martin PJ, Hansen JA. Role of the mixed lymphocyte culture (MLC) reaction in marrow donor selection: matching for transplants from related haploidentical donors. Tissue Antigens 44:83–92, 1994.

Mielcarek M, Sandmaier BM, Maloney DG, Maris M, McSweeney PA, Woolfrey A, Chauncey T, Feinstein L, Niederwieser D, Blume KG, Forman S, Torok-Storb B, Storb R. Nonmyeloablative hematopoietic cell transplantation: status quo and future perspectives. J Clin Immunol 22:70–74, 2002.

Miller CB, Rowlings PA, Zhang MJ, Jones RJ, Piantadosi S, Keating A, Armitage JO, Calderwood S, Harris RE, Klein JP, Lazarus HM, Linker CA, Sobocinski KA, Weisdorf D, Horowitz MM. The effect of graft purging with 4–hydroperoxycyclophosphamide in autologous bone marrow transplantation for acute myelogenous leukemia. Exp Hem 29:1336–1346, 2001.

Miller LW, Naftel DC, Bourge RC, Kirklin JK, Brozena SC, Jarcho J, Hobbs RE, Mills RM. Infection after heart transplantation: a multiinstitutional study. J Heart Lung Transplant 13:381–393, 1994.

Monaco AP, Wood ML. Studies on heterologous antilymphocyte serum in mice. VII. Optimal cellular antigen for induction of immunologic tolerance with antilymphocyte serum. Transplant Proc 2:489–496, 1970.

Montuoro A, Lalle M, Ingletto D. Autologous bone marrow transplantation as consolidation therapy in newly diagnosed non-Hodgkin's lymphoma: long-term outcome. Int J Oncol 17:771–775, 2000.

Moudgil A, Jordan SC. Renal transplantation in infants and children. Indian J Pediatr 66:263–275, 1999.

Mowat AP. Liver disorders in children: the indications for liver replacement in parenchymal and metabolic diseases. Transplant Proc 19:3236–3241, 1987.

Muller-Ruchholtz W, Wottge HU, Muller-Hermelink HK. Bone marrow transplantation in rats across strong histocompatibility barriers by selective elimination of lymphoid cells in donor marrow. Transplant Proc 8:537–541, 1976.

Myers LA, Patel DD, Puck JM, Buckley RH. Hematopoietic stem cell transplantation for severe combined immunodeficiency in the neonatal period leads to superior thymic output and improved survival. Blood 99:872–878, 2002.

Nagler A, Ackerstein A, Kapelushnik J, Or R, Naparstek E, Slavin S. Donor lymphocyte infusion post-non-myeloablative allogeneic peripheral blood stem cell transplantation for chronic granulomatous disease. Bone Marrow Transplant 24:339–342, 1999.

Nepom GT, Hansen JA, Nepom BS. The molecular basis for HLA class II associations with rheumatoid arthritis. J Clin Immunol 7:1–7, 1987.

Nevins TE, Kjellstrand CM. Hemodialysis for children—a review. Int J Pediatr Nephrol 4:155–169, 1983.

Nieboer P, de Vries EG, Mulder NH, Sleijfer DT, Willemse PH, Hospers GA, Gietema JA, Sluiter WJ, Der Graaf WT. Long-term haematological recovery following high-dose chemotherapy with autologous bone marrow transplantation or peripheral stem cell transplantation in patients with solid tumours. Bone Marrow Transplant 27:959–966, 2001.

Noel DR, Witherspoon RP, Storb R, Atkinson K, Doney K, Mickelson EM, Ochs HD, Warren RP, Weiden PL, Thomas ED. Does graft-versus-host disease influence the tempo of immunologic recovery after allogeneic human marrow transplantation? An observation on 56 long term survivors. Blood 51:1087–1105, 1978.

Ogawa H, Soma T, Hosen N, Tatekawa T, Tsuboi A, Oji Y, Tamaki H, Kawakami M, Ikegame K, Murakami M, Fujioka T, Kim EH, Oka Y, Sugiyama H. Combination of tacrolimus, methotrexate, and methylprednisolone prevents acute but not chronic graft-versus-host disease in unrelated bone marrow transplantation. Transplantation 74:236–243, 2002.

Oh JM, Wiland AM, Klassen DK, Weidle PJ, Bartlett ST. Comparison of azathioprine and mycophenolate mofetil for the prevention of acute rejection in recipients of pancreas transplantation. J Clin Pharmacol 41:861–869, 2001.

Ohnuma K, Isoyama K, Nishihira H. Cord blood transplantation from HLA-mismatched unrelated donors. Leuk Lymphoma 43:1029–1034, 2002.

Okamoto S, Watanabe R, Takahashi S, Mori T, Izeki T, Nagayama H, Ishida A, Takayama N, Yokoyama K, Tojo A, Asano S, Ikeda Y. Long-term follow-up of allogeneic bone marrow transplantation after reduced-intensity conditioning in patients with chronic myelogenous leukemia in the chronic phase. Int J Hematol 75:493–498, 2002.

O'Marcaigh AS, DeSantes K, Hu D, Pabst H, Horn B, Li L, Cowan MJ. Bone marrow transplantation for T-B-severe combined immunodeficiency disease in Athabascan-speaking native Americans. Bone Marrow Transplant 27:703–709, 2001.

Opelz G. HLA matching and transplant survival. Effect of HLA matching in 10,000 cyclosporin-treated cadaver kidney transplants. Transplant Proc 19:92–102, 1987.

Opelz G, Henderson R. Incidence of non-Hodgkin lymphoma in kidney and heart transplant recipients. Lancet 342:1514–1516, 1993.

Opelz G, Wujciak T. The influence of HLA compatibility on graft survival after heart transplantation. N Engl J Med 330:816–819, 1994.

O'Reilly RJ. Current developments in marrow transplantation. Transplant Proc 19:92–102, 1987.

O'Reilly RJ, Brochstein J, Collins N, Keever C, Kapoor N, Kirkpatrick D, Kerman N, Dupont B, Burns J, Reisner Y. Evaluation of HLA-haplotype disparate parental marrow grafts depleted of T lymphocytes by differential agglutination with a soybean lectin and E rosette depletion for the treatment of severe combined immunodeficiency. Vox Sang 51:81–86, 1986.

O'Reilly RJ, Brochstein J, Dinsmore R, Kirkpatrick D. Marrow transplantation for congenital disorders. Semin Hematol 21:188–221, 1984.

Ozsahin H, Le Deist F, Benkerrou M, Cavazzana-Calvo M, Gomez L, Griscelli C, Blanchi S, Fischer A. Bone marrow transplantation in 26 patients with Wiskott-Aldrich syndrome from a single center. J Pediatr 129:238–244, 1996.

Ozsahin H, von Planta M, Muller I, Steinert HC, Nadal D, Lauener R, Tuchschmid P, Willi UV, Ozsahin H, Crompton NE, Seger RA. Successful treatment of invasive aspergillosis in chronic granulomatous disease by bone marrow transplantation, granulocyte colony-stimulating factor-mobilized granulocytes, and liposomal amphotericin-B. Blood 92:2719–2724, 1998.

Parham P. Genomic organization of the MHC: structure, origin and function. Immunol Rev 167:5–379, 1999.

Parkman R. Human graft-versus-host disease. Immunodef Rev 2:253–264, 1991.

Parkman R, Rappeport J, Geha R, Belli J, Cassady R, Levey R, Nathan DG, Rosen FS. Complete correction of the Wiskott-Aldrich syndrome by allogenic bone-marrow transplantation. N Engl J Med 298:921–927, 1978.

Patel DD, Gooding ME, Parrott RE, Curtis KM, Haynes BF, Buckley RH. Thymic function after hematopoietic stem-cell transplantation for the treatment of severe combined immunodeficiency. N Engl J Med 342:1325–1332, 2000.

Payne R, Rolfs MR. Fetomaternal leukocyte incompatibility. J Clin Invest 37:1756–1763, 1958.

Perdue ST. Risk factors for second transplants 1985. In Terasaki PI, ed. Clinical Kidney Transplants. Los Angeles, UCLA Tissue Typing Laboratory, 1985, pp 191–203.

Pescovitz MD, Thistlethwaite JR, Auchincloss H, Ildstad ST, Sharp TG, Terrill R, Sachs DH. Effect of class II antigen matching on renal allograft survival in miniature swine. J Exp Med 160:1495–1508, 1984.

Pillow RP, Epstein RB, Buckner CD, Giblett ER, Thomas ED. Treatment of bone marrow failure by isogeneic marrow infusion. N Engl J Med 275:94–97, 1966.

Pracher E, Panzer-Grumayer ER, Zoubek A, Peters C, Gadner H. Successful bone marrow transplantation in a boy with X-linked lymphoproliferative syndrome and acute severe infectious mononucleosis. Bone Marrow Transplant 13:655–658, 1994.

Pulsipher MA, Woolfrey A. Nonmyeloablative transplantation in children. Current status and future prospects. Hematol Oncol Clin North Am 15:809–834, 2001.

Rappeport JM, Newburger PE, Goldblum RM, Goldman AS, Nathan DG, Parkman R. Allogeneic transplantation for chronic granulomatous disease. J Pediatr 101:952–955, 1982.

Reed E, Hardy M, Benvenisty A, Lattes C, Brensilver J, McCabe R, Reemstma K, King DW, Suciu-Foca N. Effect of antidiotypic antibodies to HLA on graft survival in renal allograft recipients. N Engl J Med 316:1450–1455, 1987.

Reinherz EL, Geha R, Rappeport JM, Wilson M, Penta AC, Hussey RE, Fitzgerald KA, Daley JF, Levine H, Rosen FS, Schlossman SF. Reconstitution after transplantation with T-lymphocyte-depleted HLA haplotype-mismatched bone marrow for severe combined immunodeficiency. Proc Natl Acad Sci USA 79:6047–6051, 1982.

Reisner Y, Itzicovitch L, Meshorer A, Sharon N. Hematopoietic stem cell transplantation using mouse bone marrow and spleen cells fractionated by lectins. Proc Nat Acad Sci USA 75:2933–2936, 1978.

Reisner Y, Kapoor N, Kirkpatrick D, Pollack MS, Cunningham-Rundles S, Dupont B, Hodes MZ, Good RA, O'Reilly RJ. Transplantation for severe combined immunodeficiency with HLA-A, B, D, DR incompatible parental marrow cells fractionated by soybean agglutinin and sheep red blood cells. Blood 61:341–348, 1983.

Ringden O, Ahstrom L, Lonnqvist B, Baryd I, Svedmyr E, Gahrton G. Allogeneic bone marrow transplantation in a patient with chemotherapy-resistant progressive histiocytosis X. N Engl J Med 316:733–735, 1987.

Rivera GK, Pinkel D, Simone JV, Hancock ML, Crist WM. Treatment of acute lymphoblastic leukemia—30 years' experience at St. Jude Children's Research Hospital. N Engl J Med 329:1289–1295, 1993.

Roberts JL, Volkman DJ, Buckley RH. Modified MHC restriction of donor-origin T cells in humans with severe combined immunodeficiency transplanted with haploidentical bone marrow stem cells. J Immunol 143:1575–1579, 1989.

Rooney CM, Wimperis JZ, Brenner MK, Patterson J, Hoffbrand AV, Prentice HG. Natural killer cell activity following T cell depleted allogeneic bone marrow transplantation. Br J Haematol 62:413–420, 1986.

Ross AJ, Cooper A, Attie MF, Bishop HC. Primary hyperparathyroidism in infancy. J Pediatr Surg 21:493–499, 1986.

Rowlings PA, Horowitz MM, Armitage JO, Gale RP, Sobocinski KA, Zhang M-J, Bortin MM. Report from the International Bone Marrow Transplant Registry and the North American Autologous Bone Marrow Transplant Registry. Clin Transpl 101–108, 1993.

Ruderman RJ, Poehling GG, Gray R, Nardone M, Goodman W, Seigler HF. Orthopedic complications of renal transplantation in children. Transplant Proc 11:104–106, 1979.

Rumelhart SL, Trigg ME, Horowitz SD, Hong R. Monoclonal antibody T-cell-depleted HLA-haploidentical bone marrow transplantation for Wiskott-Aldrich syndrome. Blood 75:1031–1035, 1990.

Russell PS, Cosimi AB. Transplantation. N Engl J Med 301:470–479, 1979.

Sachs DH. Specific immunosuppression. Transplant Proc 19:123–127, 1987.

Salvatierra O, Melzer J, Vincenti F, Amend WJC, Tomianovich S, Potter D, Husing R, Garovoy M, Feduska NJ. Donor-specific blood transfusions versus cyclosporine—the DST story. Transplant Proc 19:160–166, 1987.

Samuel D, Muller R, Alexander G, Fassati L, Ducot B, Benhamou J-P, Bismuth H. Liver transplantation in European patients with the hepatitis B surface antigen. N Engl J Med 329:1842–1847, 1993.

Sanchez CP, Kuizon BD, Goodman WG, Gales B, Ettenger RB, Boechat MI, Wang Y, Elashoff R, Salusky IB. Growth hormone and the skeleton in pediatric renal allograft recipients. Pediatr Nephrol 17:322–328, 2002.

Sanchez CP, Salusky IB, Kuizon BD, Ramirez JA, Gales B, Ettenger RB, Goodman WG. Bone disease in children and adolescents undergoing successful renal transplantation. Kidney Int 53:1358–1364, 1998.

Sanfilippo F, MacQueen JM, Vaughn WK, Foulks GN. Reduced graft rejection with good HLA-A and B matching in high risk corneal transplantation. N Engl J Med 315:29–35, 1986.

Sanfilippo F, Vaughn WK, Spees EK, Bollinger RR. Cadaver renal transplantation ignoring peak reactive sera in patients with markedly decreasing pre-transplant sensitization. Transplantation 38:119–124, 1984.

Santos GW. Immunosuppression for clinical marrow transplantation. Semin Hematol 11:341–351, 1974.

Saxe A. Parathyroid transplantation: a review. Surgery 95:507–526, 1984.

Schiff SE, Buckley RH. Modified responses to recipient and donor B cells by genetically donor T cells from human haploidentical bone marrow chimeras. J Immunol 138:2088–2094, 1987.

Schiff SE, Kurtzberg J, Buckley RH. Studies of human bone marrow treated with soybean lectin and sheep erythrocytes: stepwise analysis of cell morphology, phenotype and function. Clin Exp Immunol 68:685–693, 1987.

Schneider LC, Berman RS, Shea CR, Perez-Atayde AR, Weinstein H, Geha RS. Bone marrow transplantation (BMT) for the syndrome of pigmentary dilution and lymphohistiocytosis (Griscelli's syndrome). J Clin Immunol 10:146–153, 1990.

Scholl PR, O'Gorman MR, Pachman LM, Haut P, Kletzel M. Correction of neutropenia and hypogammaglobulinemia in X-linked hyper-IgM syndrome by allogeneic bone marrow transplantation. Bone Marrow Transplant 22:1215–1218, 1998.

Schreuder GM, Hurley CK, Marsh SG, Lau M, Maiers M, Kollman C, Noreen HJ. The HLA Dictionary 2001: a summary of HLA-A, -B, -C, -DRB1/3/4/5 and -DQB1 alleles and their association with serologically defined HLA-A, -B, -C, -DR and -DQ antigens. Eur J Immunogenet 28:565–596, 2001.

Schrezenmeier H, Marin P, Raghavachar A, McCann S, Hows J, Gluckman E, Nissen C, van't Veer-Korthof ET, Hinterberger LW, van Lint MT, Frickhofen N, Bacigalupo A. Relapse of aplastic anaemia after immunosuppressive treatment: a report from the European Bone Marrow Transplantation Group SAA Working Party. Br J Haematol 85:371–377, 1993.

Schroeder ML. Transfusion-associated graft-versus-host disease. Br J Haematol 117:275–287, 2002.

Schulz AS, Classen CF, Mihatsch WA, Sigl-Kraetzig M, Wiesneth M, Debatin KM, Friedrich W, Muller SM. HLA-haploidentical blood progenitor cell transplantation in osteopetrosis. Blood 99:3458–3460, 2002.

Seger RA, Ezekowitz RAB. Treatment of chronic granulomatous disease. Immunodeficiency 5:113–130, 1994.

Seger RA, Gungor T, Belohradsky BH, Blanche S, Bordigoni P, DiBartolomeo P, Flood T, Landais P, Muller S, Ozsahin H, Passwell JH, Porta F, Slavin S, Wulffraat N, Zintl F, Nagler A, Cant A, Fischer A. Treatment of chronic granulomatous disease with myeloblative conditioning and an unmodified hemopoietic allograft: a survey of the European experience, 1985–2000. Blood 100:4344–4350, 2002.

Shapiro R, Scantlebury V, Jordan M, Vivas C, Jain A, Hakala T, McCauley J, Johnston J, Randhawa P, Fedorek S, Gray E, Chesky A, Dvorchik I, Donaldson J, Fung J, Starzl T. A pilot trial of tacrolimus, sirolimus, and steroids in renal transplant recipients. Transplant Proc 34:1651, 2002.

Sharathkumar A, Thornley I, Saunders EF, Calderwood S, Freedman MH, Doyle J. Allogeneic bone marrow transplantation in children with chronic myelogenous leukemia. J Pediatr Hematol Oncol 24:215–219, 2002.

Simmons RL, Najarian JS. Kidney transplantation. Manual of Vascular Access, Organ Donation, and Transplantation. New York, Springer-Verlag, 1984, pp 292–328.

Simpson E, Roopenian D. Minor histocompatibility antigens. Curr Opin Immunol 9:655–661, 1997.

Sindel LJ, Buckley RH, Schiff SE, Ward FE, Mickey GH, Huang AT, Naspitz C, Koren H. Severe combined immunodeficiency with natural killer cell predominance: abrogation of graft-versus-host disease and immunologic reconstitution with HLA-identical bone marrow cells. J Allergy Clin Immunol 73:829–836, 1984.

Singer A, Hathcock KS, Hodes RJ. Self-recognition in allogeneic radiation bone marrow chimeras. A radiation-resistant host element dictates the self specificity and immune response gene phenotype of T helper cells. J Exp Med 153:1286–1301, 1981.

Sitges-Serra A, Caralps-Riera A. Hyperparathyroidism associated with renal disease. Surg Clin North Am 67:359–377, 1987.

Skinner J, Finlay JL, Sondel PM, Trigg ME. Infectious complications in pediatric patients undergoing transplantation with T lymphocyte-depleted bone marrow. Pediatr Infect Dis 5:319–324, 1986.

Slavin S, Reitz B, Bieber CP, Kaplan HS, Strober S. Transplantation tolerance in adult rats using total lymphoid irradiation: permanent survival of skin, heart, and marrow allografts. J Exp Med 147:700–707, 1978.

Smith JM, McDonald RA. Progress in renal transplantation for children. Adv Ren Replace Ther 7:158–171, 2000.

Smogorzewska EM, Brooks J, Annett G, Kapoor N, Crooks GM, Kohn DB, Parkman R, Weinberg KI. T cell depleted haploidentical bone marrow transplantation for the treatment of children with severe combined immunodeficiency. Arch Immunol Ther Exp (Warsz) 48:111–118, 2000.

So SKS, Mauer SM, Nevins TE, Fryd DS, Sutherland DER, Ascher NL, Simmons RL, Najarian JS. Current results in pediatric renal transplantation at the University of Minnesota. Kidney Int 30:25–30, 1986.

Socie G, Stone JV, Wingard JR, Weisdorf D, Henslee-Downey PJ, Bredeson C, Cahn JY, Passweg JR, Rowlings PA, Schouten HC, Kolb HJ, Klein JP. Long-term survival and late deaths after allogeneic bone marrow transplantation. Late Effects Working Committee of the International Bone Marrow Transplant Registry. N Engl J Med 341:14–21, 1999.

Sollinger HW, Burkholder PM, Rasmus WR, Bach FH. Prolonged survival of xenografts after organ culture. Surgery 81:74–79, 1976.

Stary J, Bartunkova J, Kobylka P, Vavra V, Hrusak O, Calda P, Kral V, Svorc K. Successful HLA-identical sibling cord blood transplantation in a 6-year-old boy with leukocyte adhesion deficiency syndrome. Bone Marrow Transplant 18:249–252, 1996.

Starzl TE, Demetris AJ, Murase N, Ildstad S, Ricordi C, Trucco M. Cell migration, chimerism and graft acceptance. Lancet 339:1579–1582, 1992a.

Starzl TE, Demetris AJ, Trucco M, Ramos H, Zeevi A, Rudert WA, Kocova M, Ricordi C, Ildstad S, Murase N. Systemic chimerism in human female recipients of male livers. Lancet 340:876–877, 1992b.

Starzl TE, Demetris AJ, Trucco M, Ricordi C, Ildstad S, Terasaki PI, Murase N, Kendall RS, Kocova J, Rudert WA, Zeevi A, van Thiel D. Chimerism after liver transplantation for type IV glycogen storage disease and type I Gaucher's disease. N Engl J Med 328:745–749, 1994.

Starzl TE, Esquivel C, Gordon R, Todo S. Pediatric liver transplantation. Transplant Proc 19:3230–3235, 1987.

Starzl TE, Zinkernagel RM. Transplantation tolerance from a historical perspective. Nat Rev Immunol 1:233–239, 2001.

Stephan JL, Vlekova V, Le Deist F, Blanche S, Donadieu J, de Saint-Basile G, Durandy A, Griscelli C, Fischer A. Severe combined immunodeficiency: a retrospective single-center study of clinical presentation and outcome in 117 cases. J Pediatr 123:564–572, 1993.

Stepkowski SM, Kahan BD. Rapamycin and cyclosporine synergistically prolong heart and kidney allograft survival. Transplant Proc 23:3262–3264, 1991.

Storb R, Deeg HJ, Whitehead J, Appelbaum F, Beatty P, Bensinger W, Buckner CD, Clift R, Doney K, Farewell V, Hansen J, Hill R, Lum L, Martin P, McGuffin R, Sanders J, Stewart P, Sullivan K, Witherspoon R, Yee G, Thomas ED. Methotrexate and cyclosporine compared with cyclosporine alone for prophylaxis of acute graft versus host disease after marrow transplantation for leukemia. N Engl J Med 314:729–735, 1986.

Stratta RJ. Review of immunosuppressive usage in pancreas transplantation. Clin Transpl 13:1–12, 1999.

Sullivan KA, Amos DB. The HLA system and its detection. In Rose NR, Friedman H, Fahey JL, eds. Manual of Clinical Laboratory Immunology. Washington, DC, American Society for Microbiology, 1986, pp 835–846.

Suthanthiran M, Strom TB. Renal transplantation. N Engl J Med 331:365–394, 1994.

Sutherland DE, Gruessner RW, Gruessner AC. Pancreas transplantation for treatment of diabetes mellitus. World J Surg 25:487–496, 2001.

Sutherland DER, Moudry-Munns K, Gruessner A. Pancreas Transplant Results in United Network for Organ Sharing (UNOS) United States of American (USA) Registry with a Comparison to Non-USA Data in the International Registry. In Terasaki PI, Cecka JM, eds. Clinical Transplants 1993. Los Angeles, UCLA Tissue Typing Laboratory, 1994, pp 47–70.

Taurog JD, Maika SD, Simmons WA, Breban M, Hammer RE. Susceptibility to inflammatory disease in HLA-B27 transgenic rat lines correlates with the level of B27 expression. J Immunol 150:4168–4178, 1993.

Tejani A, Stablein D, Fine R, Alexander S. Maintenance immunosuppression therapy and outcome of renal transplantation in North American children—a report of the North American Pediatric Renal Transplant Cooperative Study. Pediatr Nephrol 7:132–137, 1993.

Terasaki PI, McClelland JD. Microdroplet assay of human serum cytotoxins. Nature 206:998–1000, 1964.

The U.S. Multicenter FK506 Liver Study Group. A comparison of tacrolimus (FK506) and cyclosporine for immunosuppression in liver transplantation. N Engl J Med 331:1110–1115, 1994.

Thomas C, de Saint Basile G, Le Deist F, Theophile D, Benkerrou M, Haddad E, Blanche S, Fischer A. Brief report: correction of X-linked hyper-IgM syndrome by allogeneic bone marrow transplantation. N Engl J Med 333:426–429, 1995a.

Thomas C, LeDeist F, Cavazzana-Calvo M, Benkerrou M, Haddad E, Blanche S, Hartmann W, Friedrich W, Fischer A. Results of allogeneic bone marrow transplantation in patients with leukocyte adhesion deficiency. Blood 86:1629–1635, 1995b.

Thomas ED. Marrow transplantation for malignant disease. Am J Med Sci 294:75–79, 1987.

Thomas ED, Storb R, Clift RA, Fefer A, Johnson L, Neiman PE, Lerner KG, Glucksberg H, Buckner CD. Bone marrow transplantation. N Engl J Med 292:823–843, 1975.

Thorsby E. HLA associated diseases. Hum Immunol 53:1–11, 1997.

Thursz MR, Kwiatkowski D, Allsopp CEM, Greenwood BM, Thomas HC, Hill AVS. Association between an MHC Class II allele and clearance of hepatitis B virus in the Gambia. N Engl J Med 332:1065–1069, 1995.

Tiwari JL, Terasaki PI. HLA and disease associations. New York, Springer-Verlag, 1985.

Towbin JA. Cardiomyopathy and heart transplantation in children. Curr Opin Cardiol 17:274–279, 2002.

Turenne MN, Port FK, Strawderman RL, Ettenger RB, Alexander SR, Lewy JE, Jones CA, Agodoa LY, Held PJ. Growth rates in pediatric dialysis patients and renal transplant recipients. Am J Kidney Dis 30:193–203, 1997.

Tutschka PJ. Diminishing morbidity and mortality of bone marrow transplantation. Vox Sang 51:87–94, 1986.

Tyden G, Lundgren G, Ost L, Kojima Y, Gunnarsson R, Ostman J, Groth CG. Progress in segmental pancreatic transplantation. World J Surg 10:404–409, 1986.

Tyler JD, Anderson CB, Sicard GA. Interleukin 2 response inhibition following donor specific transfusions given with azathioprine. Transplant Proc 19:258–261, 1987.

Uderzo C. Indications and role of allogeneic bone marrow transplantation in childhood very high risk acute lymphoblastic leukemia in first complete remission. Haematologica 85:9–11, 2000.

Uphoff DE. Preclusion of secondary phase of irradiation syndrome by inoculation of fetal hematopoietic tissue following lethal total body X irradiation. J Natl Cancer Inst 20:625–632, 1958.

Van Den Berg H, Vossen JM, van den Bergh RL, Bayer J, van Tol MJD. Detection of Y chromosome by in situ hybridization in combination with membrane antigens by two-color immunofluorescence. Lab Invest 64:623–628, 1994.

van Rood JJ. Prospective HLA typing is helpful in cadaveric renal transplantation. Transplant Proc 19:139–143, 1987.

van Rood JJ, Eernisse JG, van Leewen A. Leukocyte antibodies in sera from pregnant women. Nature 181:1735–1736, 1958.

van Thiel DH. Liver transplantation. Pediatr Ann 14:474–480, 1985.

Vincenti F, Kirkman R, Light S, Bumgardner G, Pescovitz M, Halloran P, Neylan J, Wilkinson A, Ekberg H, Gaston R, Backman L, Burdick J. Interleukin-2–receptor blockade with daclizumab to prevent acute rejection in renal transplantation. Daclizumab Triple Therapy Study Group. N Engl J Med 338:161–165, 1998.

Visentainer JE, Lieber SR, Persoli LB, Souza Lima SC, Vigorito AC, Aranha FJ, Eid KA, Oliveira GB, Miranda EC, de Souza CA. Correlation of mixed lymphocyte culture with chronic graft-versus-host disease following allogeneic stem cell transplantation. Braz J Med Biol Res 35:567–572, 2002.

Volanakis JE, Zhu Z-B, Schaffer FM, Macon KJ, Palermos J, Barger BO, Go R, Campbell RD, Schroeder HW, Cooper MD. Major histocompatibility complex class III genes and susceptibility to immunoglobulin A deficiency and common variable immunodeficiency. J Clin Invest 89:1914–1922, 1992.

Vorechovsky I, Webster AD, Plebani A, Hammarstrom L. Genetic linkage of IgA deficiency to the major histocompatibility complex: evidence for allele segregation distortion, parent-of-origin penetrance differences, and the role of anti-IgA antibodies in disease predisposition. Am J Hum Genet 64:1096–1109, 1999.

Vowels MR, Tang RL, Berdoukas V, Ford D, Thierry D, Purtilo D, Gluckman E. Brief Report: Correction of X-linked lymphoproliferative disease by transplantation of cord blood stem cells. N Engl J Med 329:1623–1625, 1993.

Vricella LA, Karamichalis JM, Ahmad S, Robbins RC, Whyte RI, Reitz BA. Lung and heart-lung transplantation in patients with end-stage cystic fibrosis: the Stanford experience. Ann Thorac Surg 74:13–17, 2002.

Wagner JE, Kernan NA, Steinbuch M, Broxmeyer HE, Gluckman E. Allogeneic sibling umbilical-cord-blood transplantation in children with malignant and non-malignant disease. Lancet 346:214–219, 1995.

Waldmann H, Polliak A, Hale G, Or R, Cividalli G, Weiss L, Weshler Z, Samuel S, Manor D, Brautbar C, Rachmilewitz EA, Slavin S. Elimination of graft-versus-host disease by in vitro depletion of alloreactive lymphocytes with a monoclonal rat anti-human lymphocyte antibody (CAMPATH-1). Lancet 2:483–486, 1984.

Wallwork J, Williams R, Calne RY. Transplantation of liver, heart and lungs for primary biliary cirrhosis and primary pulmonary hypertension. Lancet 2:182–184, 1987.

Walters MC, Patience M, Leisenring W, Rogers ZR, Aquino VM, Buchanan GR, Roberts IA, Yeager AM, Hsu L, Adamkiewicz T, Kurtzberg J, Vichinsky E, Storer B, Storb R, Sullivan KM. Stable mixed hematopoietic chimerism after bone marrow transplantation for sickle cell anemia. Biol Blood Marrow Transplant 7:665–673, 2001.

Wang J, Song X, Zhang W, Tong S, Hou J, Chen L, Lou J, Li H, Ding X, Min B. Combination of mycophenolate mofetil with cyclosporine A and methotrexate for the prophylaxes of acute graft versus host disease in allogeneic peripheral stem cell transplantation. Zhonghua Yi Xue Za Zhi 82:507–510, 2002.

Watanabe C, Yajima S, Taguchi T, Toya K, Fujii Y, Hongo T, Ohzeki T. Successful unrelated bone marrow transplantation for a patient with chronic granulomatous disease and associated resistant pneumonitis and Aspergillus osteomyelitis. Bone Marrow Transplant 28:83–87, 2001.

Weiden PL, Flournoy N, Thomas ED, Prentice R, Fefer A, Buckner CD, Storb R. Antileukemic effect of graft-versus-host disease in human recipients of allogeneic marrow grafts. N Engl J Med 300:1068–1073, 1979.

Weinberg K, Blazar BR, Wagner JE, Agura E, Hill BJ, Smogorzewska M, Koup RA, Betts MR, Collins RH, Douek DC. Factors affecting thymic function after allogeneic hematopoietic stem cell transplantation. Blood 97:1458–1466, 2001.

Wells SA, Stirman JA, Bolman RM, Gunnells JC. Transplantation of the parathyroid glands. Clinical and experimental results. Surg Clin North Am 58:391–402, 1978.

Wen L, Wong FS, Tang J, Chen NY, Altieri M, David C, Flavell R, Sherwin R. In vivo evidence for the contribution of human histocompatibility leukocyte antigen (HLA)-DQ molecules to the development of diabetes. J Exp Med 191:97–104, 2000.

Wengler GS, Lanfranchi A, Frusca T, Verardi R, Neva A, Brugnoni D, Giliani S, Fiorini M, Mella P, Guandalini F, Mazzolari E, Pecorelli S, Notarangelo LD, Porta F, Ugazio AG. In-utero transplantation of parental CD34 haematopoietic progenitor cells in a patient with X-linked severe combined immunodeficiency (SCIDX1). Lancet 348:1484–1487, 1996.

West LJ, Pollock-Barziv SM, Dipchand AI, Lee KJ, Cardella CJ, Benson LN, Rebeyka IM, Coles JG. ABO-incompatible heart transplantation in infants. N Engl J Med 344:793–800, 2001.

Williams LL, Rooney CM, Conley ME, Brenner MK, Krance RA, Heslop HE. Correction of Duncan's syndrome by allogeneic bone marrow transplantation. Lancet 342:587–588, 1993.

Wolf E, Spencer KM, Cudworth AG. The genetic susceptibility to type I (insulin-dependent) diabetes: analysis of the HLA-DR association. Diabetologia 24:224–230, 1983.

Woodruff JM, Hansen JA, Good RA, Santos GW, Slavin RE. The pathology of the graft-versus-host reaction (GVHR) in adults receiving bone marrow transplants. Transplant Proc 8:675–684, 1976.

Woods WG, Neudorf S, Gold S, Sanders J, Buckley JD, Barnard DR, Dusenbery K, DeSwarte J, Arthur DC, Lange BJ, Kobrinsky NL. A comparison of allogeneic bone marrow transplantation, autologous bone marrow transplantation, and aggressive chemotherapy in children with acute myeloid leukemia in remission. Blood 97:56–62, 2001.

Woolfrey A, Pulsipher MA, Storb R. Nonmyeloablative hematopoietic cell transplant for treatment of immune deficiency. Curr Opin Pediatr 13:539–545, 2001.

Woolfrey AE, Anasetti C, Storer B, Doney K, Milner LA, Sievers EL, Carpenter P, Martin P, Petersdorf E, Appelbaum FR, Hansen JA, Sanders JE. Factors associated with outcome after unrelated marrow transplantation for treatment of acute lymphoblastic leukemia in children. Blood 99:2002–2008, 2002.

Wu AM, Till JE, Siminovitch L, McCulloch EA. A cytological study of the capacity for differentiation of normal hemopoietic colony-forming cells. J Cell Physiol 69:177–184, 1967.

Wu AM, Till JE, Siminovitch L, McCulloch EA. Cytological evidence for a relationship between normal hematopoietic colony-forming cells and cells of the lymphoid system. J Exp Med 127:455–464, 1968.

Yamaoka Y, Tanaka K, Ozawa K. Liver transplantation from living-related donors. Clin Transpl 16:179–184, 1993.

Yandza T, Alvarez F, Laurent J, Gauthier F, Dubousset A-M, Valayer J. Pediatric liver transplantation for primary hepatocellular carcinoma associated with hepatitis virus infection. Transplant Int 6:95–98, 1993.

Zales VR, Stapleton PL. Neonatal and infant heart transplantation. Pediatr Clin North Am 40:1023–1046, 1993.

Zecca M, Prete A, Rondelli R, Lanino E, Balduzzi A, Messina C, Fagioli F, Porta F, Favre C, Pession A, Locatelli F. Chronic graft-versus-host disease in children: incidence, risk factors, and impact on outcome. Blood 100:1192–1200, 2002.

Ziegner UH, Ochs HD, Schanen C, Feig SA, Seyama K, Futatani T, Gross T, Wakim M, Roberts RL, Rawlings DJ, Dovat S, Fraser JK, Stiehm ER. Unrelated umbilical cord stem cell transplantation for X-linked immunodeficiencies. J Pediatr 138:570–573, 2001.

Zinkernagel RM, Callahan GN, Klein J, Dennert C. Cytotoxic T cells learn specificity for self H-2 during differentiation in the thymus. Nature 271:251–253, 1978.

Zittoun RA, Maandelli F, Roel-Willemze R, de Witte T, Labar B, Resegotti L, Leoni F, Damasio E, Visani G, Papa G, Caronia F, Hayat M, Stryckmans P, Rotoli B, Leoni P, Peetermans ME, Dardenne M, Vegna ML, Petti MC, Solbu G, Suciu S. Autologous or allogeneic bone marrow transplantation compared with intensive chemotherapy in acute myelogenous leukemia. N Engl J Med 332:217–223, 1995.

TABLE A1-1 · HUMAN LEUKOCYTE DIFFERENTIATION ANTIGENS—cont'd

Monoclonal Antibody Cluster Designation	Leukocyte Distribution	Function of Antigen	Molecular Weight ($\times 10^3$)
CD213a1	—	IL-13R α1	—
CD213a2	—	IL-13R α2	—
CDw217	—	IL-17R	—
CD220	—	Insulin R	—
CD221	—	IGF1 R	—
CD222	Leukocytes	Mannose-6-phosphate/IGF2 R; internalizes extracellular ligands into lysosomes	250
CD223	—	LAG-3	—
CD224	—	γ-Glutamyl transferase	—
CD225	—	Leu13	—
CD226	T, NK, platelets, monocytes; some thymocytes, B	Cell adhesion	65
CD227	Act T, monocytes hematopoietic, some B	Surface mucin glycoprotein protects, modifies cell adhesion; tumor marker in serum	300–700
CD228	—	Melanotransferrin	—
CD229	—	Ly9	—
CD230	—	Prion protein	—
CD231	T-ALL cells	TALLA-1 marker	150
CD232	—	VESPR	—
CD233	—	Band 3	—
CD243	—	Fy-glycoprotein	—
CD235a	—	Glycophorin A	—
CD235b	—	Glycophorin B	—
CD235ab	—	Glycophorin A/B crossreacting	—
CD236	—	Glycophorin C/D	—
CD236R	—	Glycophorin C	—
CD238	—	Kell	—
CD239	—	B-CAM	—
CD240CE	—	Rh30CE	—
CD240D	—	Rh30D	—
CD240DCE	—	Rh30D/CE crossreacting	—
CD241	—	RhAg	—
CD242	—	ICAM-4	—
CD243	Progenitor cells	MDR-1	—
CD244	NK	2BR	—
CD245	T	P220/240	—
CD246	T	Anaplastic lymphoma kinase	—
CD247	T	Zeta chain of TCR	—

Act = activated; ADP = adenosine diphosphate; Ag = antigen; B = B cell; B-CAM = basal cell adhesion molecule; CALLA = common acute lymphoblastic leukemia antigen; CCR = receptor for chemokines with 4-6 cysteines, the N-terminal/2 being adjacent; CEA = carcinoembryonic antigen; CLL = chronic lymphocytic leukemia; CTLA-4 = cytotoxic T lymphocyte-associated antigen 4; CXCR = receptor for chemokines with 4-6 cysteines distinguished by one intervening variable amino acid; DC-LAMP = dendritic cell-specific lysosome-associated, membrane glycoprotein; DC-SIGN = dendritic cell-specific ICAM-3 grabbing nonintegrin; DEC 205 = membrane protein found on dendritic and thymic epithelial cells; EBV = Epstein-Barr virus; endo = endothelium; eosin = eosinophil; EPC-R = endothelial protein C receptor; H-CAM = homing cell adhesion molecule; HEV = high endothelial venules; HIV = human immunodeficiency virus; ICAM = intracellular adhesion molecule; Ig = immunoglobulin adhesion molecule; IGF1-R = insulin-like growth factor 1 receptor; IL = interleukin; KIR = killer cell immunoglobulin-like receptor; LAG3 = lymphocyte activation gene 3; LAMP = lysosome-associated membrane protein; LFA = leukocyte function–associated; LPS = lipopolysaccharide; lymph = lymphocytes; Mφ = macrophage; MAb = monoclonal antibody; Mel-CAM = invasion/metastasis-related melanoma cell adhesion molecule; MDR-1 = multidrug resistance-1 protein; MHC = major histocompatibility complex; N-CAM = neural cell adhesion molecule; NK = natural killer cell; NKG2A = natural killer cell glycoprotein 2A-NK inhibitory receptor; OX-2 = orexin receptor type 2; PDGF = platelet-derived growth factor; PEN5 = sulfated poly-N-lactosamine epitope on NK cells; PMN = polymorphonuclear cells; RHAMM = receptor for hyaluronic acid–mediated motility; SIRPα = signal regulatory phosphatase binding protein α; T = T cell; TACE = TNF-α–converting enzyme; T-ALL = T-cell acute lymphoblastic leukemia; TALLA-1 = T-cell acute lymphoblastic leukemia antigen 1; TAPA = target of antiproliferative antibody; TCR = T-cell receptor; TGF = transforming growth factor; TNF = tumor necrosis factor; V-CAM = vascular cell adhesion molecule; VESPR = viral-encoded Semaphorin receptor; VLA = very late activation.

The values separated by a semicolon represent unreduced versus reduced forms.

R E F E R E N C E S

Barclay AN, Birkeland ML, Brown MH, Beyers AD, Davis SJ, Somoza C, Williams AF. The leucocyte antigen facts book. London, Academic Press, 1993.

PROW, Protein Reviews on the Web. *http://www.ncbi.nlm.nih.gov/prow/* (comprehensive list of CDs, including new ones, from the Seventh Workshop on Human Leucocyte Differentiation Antigens [HLDA], Harrogate, England, June 20-24, 2000).

Zola H, Swart B, Boumsell L, Mason DY. Human leukocyte differentiation antigen nomenclature: update on CD nomenclature. Report of IUIS/WHO subcommittee. J Immunol Methods 275:1–8, 2003.

Principal Human Cytokines and Chemokines

Susan F. Plaeger

TABLE A2-1 · PRINCIPAL HUMAN CYTOKINES AND CHEMOKINES

Cytokine	Immune Cells That Secrete	Immune Target Cells	General Function in Immune System	Association with Pathology/Therapeutic Potential	Comments
IL-1	MO, T, B lymphs, NK, PMN	T, B lymphs, MO, PMN	Major pro-inflammatory cytokine; cell activation and induction of effector function	Increased in chronic inflammation, autoimmune disease, inhibitors, or antagonists used as therapeutics	2 proteins (α, β) with same receptors; IL-1 receptor antagonist competes for binding
IL-2	T, B lymphs	T, B lymphs, NK, MO, PMN	T-cell activation, clonal expansion, induction of apoptosis, development of CTL; activates NK, B, MO, and PMN	Therapeutic use in cancer, immune deficiency, and transplantation; potential vaccine adjuvant to enhance Th1 response	Th1-associated cytokine
IL-3	Activated T cells, mast cells	Hematopoietic stem and progenitor cells, PML, MO, mast cells	Synergizes with IL-5 and GM-CSF for myeloid cell proliferation and differentiation	Therapeutic use in pancytopenia and bone marrow failure	Shared functions and receptor subunit with other hematopoietic cytokines IL-5 and GM-CSF
IL-4	T lymphs	B and T lymphs, NK, MO, progenitor cells, mast cells	B-cell activation, enhances expression of IgG1 and IgE, regulates expression of CD23 on lymphs and MO; drives Th2 response; mast cell growth factor	Therapeutic use in malignancy, therapeutic use of antagonists in asthma and inflammatory and autoimmune disease	Th2-associated cytokine
IL-5	T lymphs	Eosinophils, basophils (B lymphs)	Regulates eosinophil expansion and chemotaxis	Induces eosinophilic airway inflammation; potential therapeutic use of antagonists in asthma	Functional synergy with IL-13
IL-6	T, B lymphs, MO	B, T lymphs, NK, thymocytes	Pro-inflammatory cytokine; broad effects on cell growth, differentiation, and activation	Therapeutic use in multiple myeloma; dysregulation associated with autoimmune disease	Growth factor for certain malignant cells
IL-7	Bone marrow, thymic stroma	B, T lymphs, NK, MO, thymocytes	Early T-cell development; regulator of peripheral T-cell homeostasis and expansion and memory cell survival	Therapeutic use in immune restoration for T-cell depletion (chemotherapy, HIV)	Originally known as lymphopoietin-1
IL-8	T lymphs, MO, PMN	PMN	Induced by proinflammatory cytokines; mediator of acute inflammation, leukocyte activation, chemotaxis, and adhesion	Potential therapeutic use of inhibitors in lung disease and injury	Member of CXC chemokine family; also known as CXCL8
IL-9	T lymphs	T, B lymphs, mast cells, thymocytes	Mast cell growth and differentiation; T-cell cytokine production, B-cell IgE production and eosinophil maturation	Potential therapeutic use of inhibitors in asthma	Synergizes with IL-4, IL-5, and IL-13

Continued

TABLE A2-1 · PRINCIPAL HUMAN CYTOKINES AND CHEMOKINES—cont'd

Cytokine	Immune Cells That Secrete	Immune Target Cells	General Function in Immune System	Association with Pathology/Therapeutic Potential	Comments
IL-10	T lymphs, mast cells	T, B lymphs, MO, thymocytes	Limits inflammatory responses through effects on MO; strongly inhibits IL-12; regulates growth and differentiation of B, T (including Treg), NK, mast cells, and PMN	Potential therapeutic use in infectious disease and autoimmunity; inhibitors have potential for treatment of immunopathology	Several viral homologs
IL-11	Stromal cells	Bone marrow progenitors	Stimulates hematopoiesis, regulates mϕ proliferation and differentiation	Therapeutic use in thrombocytopenia	Shares biologic activities with IL-6
IL-12	B lymphs, MO, PMN	DC, MO, PMN	Drives Th1 development; proinflammatory cytokine; induces production of IFN-γ and other cytokines by NK and T cells; links innate and adaptive immunity	Therapeutic potential in infectious/parasitic diseases and cancer; potential vaccine adjuvant	Synergizes with IL-18 and IL-12 family members = IL-23 and IL-27
IL-13	T lymphs	MO/Mϕ, B cells, DC	B-cell proliferation and class-switching (see IL-4); enhances adhesion molecules and class II MHC expression on MO/Mϕ; activation of eosinophils and mast cells	Therapeutic potential of inhibitors in allergy and asthma, Hodgkin's disease, and other malignancies	Functional synergy with IL-4
IL-14	T cells; malignant B cells	B cells	Induction of B cell proliferation; inhibition of Ig secretion; selective expansion of B cell subpopulations	May play a role in growth of NHL-B	Also known as high-molecular weight B-cell growth factor
IL-15	Mϕ Human stromal cells, MO	T, NK cells T, B lymphs, monocytes, NK cells, endothelial cells, mast cells, granulocytes	T-cell proliferation, and maturation and survival of memory T cells, inhibits T-cell apoptosis; essential for NK-cell development, survival, and function, including induction of IFN-γ production	Increased in HTLV-1–associated diseases; may play a role in inflammatory autoimmune diseases	Synergizes with IL-18 and IL-21 in enhancing IFN-γ gene expression
IL-16	CD4, CD8 T cells	CD4 T cells, MO	Regulates CD4 T-cell recruitment, activation, and the switch from immune to inflammatory phenotype	Increased in asthma and inflammatory autoimmune diseases; inhibits HIV-1 replication	Receptor = CD4
IL-17	CD4 and CD8 T cells (predominantly memory phenotype)	T-cell lines, Mϕ, neutrophils	Pro-inflammatory cytokine; chemoattractant for neutrophils; regulation of hematopoiesis	May promote allograft rejection; cartilage destruction in arthritis	IL-17B and IL-17C related structurally and functionally; homolog encoded by HVS-13
IL-18	Activated Mϕ	T, NK cells	Enhances T- and NK cell maturation, cytokine production, and cytolytic activity; can promote Th1 or Th2 maturation depending on cytokine milieu	Potential as vaccine adjuvant and in tumor immunotherapy; enhances resistance to intracellular pathogens	Synergizes with IL-15 and IL-21 in enhancing IFN-γ gene expression; formerly called IFN-γ–inducing factor
IL-19	Activated MO, B cells	Unknown; works on MO in vitro	Probably participates in the regulation of the inflammatory response; induces apoptosis and growth inhibition	Possible use of IL-19 agonist as anti-inflammatory	IL-10 family, helical structure
IL-20	Keratinocytes	Keratinocytes	Probably modulates inflammatory response in the skin	Potential treatment for psoriasis	IL-10 family; helical structure
IL-21	Activated T cells	B, T, NK cells	Induces IFN-γ production, involved in NK-cell development and differentiation, co-stimulation of B and T cells	Possible use as immunomodulator	Synergizes with IL-15 and IL-18 in enhancing IFN-γ gene expression

TABLE A2-1 · PRINCIPAL HUMAN CYTOKINES AND CHEMOKINES—cont'd

Cytokine	Immune Cells That Secrete	Immune Target Cells	General Function in Immune System	Association with Pathology/Therapeutic Potential	Comments
IL-22	Activated T, NK cells	Hepatocytes	Probable role in regulating inflammatory response; induces expression of genes for acute-phase proteins	None known	IL-10 family, helical structure, formerly IL-TIF
IL-23	Antigen-presenting cells	Memory CD4 T cells	Promotes Th1 function; induces IFN-γ and cell proliferation	Could enhance resistance to intracellular pathogens	Similarities to IL-12 in signal transduction
IL-24	Activated PBMC (Th2 and MO)	Tumor cells	Possible tumor suppressor; induces tumor cell apoptosis and growth inhibition	Potential as anticancer agent	IL-10 family; helical structure, YLDV encodes viral homology; formerly MDA-7
IL-25	CD4 T cells, mast cells	Th2 cells	Stimulates production of IL-4, IL-5, and IL-13; induces Th2 responses	May be related to allergic-type inflammatory responses	Structurally—but not functionally—related to IL-17
IL-26	T cells (over expressed in HVS-transformed T cells)	Unknown	Unknown	Possible role in malignant transformation	Formerly AK155
IL-27	Activated APC	CD4 T cells	May be involved in early Th1 initiation, before IL-12		IL-12 family member
IL-28	Activated PBMC	Virus-infected cell lines	Has antiviral function similar to type I IFNs	Induced by viral infection and poly IC	Has members A and B
IL-29	Activated PBMC	Virus-infected cell lines	Has antiviral function similar to type I interferons	Induced by viral infection and poly IC	None
IFN-α, β	MO/Mφ, B, NK cells	DC, MO, NK	Antiviral effects, regulate innate and adaptive immune responses, upregulate MHC expression	Therapeutic use in MS and other autoimmune diseases, hepatitis C, tumors	Production triggered by Toll-like receptors
IFN-γ	T cells (Th1) NK	T, B lymphs, MO, NK	Cell activation differentiation; up-regulation of MHC; cytolytic potentiator, antibody isotype selection	Therapeutic potential as antiviral (<IFN-α or β), antiprotozal; effective in treatment of certain malignancies, chronic granulomatous disease	Th1-associated cytokine
TNF-α, β	MO, T, NK cells	Leukocytes, vascular endothelium	Major pro-inflammatory cytokine, antitumor effects	Therapeutic use in cancer but associated with severe toxicity; use of inhibitors and antagonists in autoimmune diseases, sepsis, and toxic shock	Production triggered by Toll-like receptors
GM-CSF, G-CSF	MO/Mφ, T cells	MO, PMN	Stimulates myelopoiesis and myeloid cell function; recruits stem cells; pro-inflammatory cytokine	Therapeutic use for neutropenia, mobilization of HSC; potential vaccine adjuvant	
M-CSF	MO/Mφ	MO, mφ	Stimulates MO function	Potential therapeutic use in infectious disease	T cells, PMN
TGF-β	Platelets, MO	T, B lumphs, NK, thermocytes, MO	Suppression of proliferation and inflammation; chemoattractant; suppression of cytotoxic function; downregulation of antibody secretion (IgG, IgM); up-regulation of IgA	Therapeutic potential in wound healing, auto-immune disease, transplant rejection; inhibitors for glomerulonephritis	5 isoforms
CXC (α) chemokines (IL-8, GRO family, SDF-1)	T cells, PMN, eosinophils, mast cells	T cells, PMN	Chemoattraction and/or cell activation	Inhibits entry of X4-type HIV-1	Receptors = CXCR1 through CXCR5

Continued

TABLE A2-1 · PRINCIPAL HUMAN CYTOKINES AND CHEMOKINES—cont'd

Cytokine	Immune Cells That Secrete	Immune Target Cells	General Function in Immune System	Association with Pathology/Therapeutic Potential	Comments
CC (β) chemokines (MIP-1α β; RANTES; MCP 1-3; eotaxin)	T cells, PMNs, eosinophils, mast cells	T cells, NK, dendritic cells, mφ, eosinophils, basophils	Cell adhesion Chemoattraction Cell activation	Inhibits entry of R5-type HIV-1; may mediate allergic and autoimmune diseases	Receptors = CCR1 through CCR9
C chemokine (lympho-tactin) and CX3C chemokine (fractalkine = CXCL1)	T cells, PMNs, eosinophils, mast cells	T cells, NK T cells; MC	Cell adhesion Chemoattraction Cell activation	Lymphotactin may have antitumor and antiviral effects	Receptors = XCR1 and CX3CR1

See footnote to Table A1-1 for abbreviations; MO = monocytes.

REFERENCES

Brombacher F, Kastelein RA, Alber G. Novel IL-12 family members shed light on the orchestration of Th1 responses. Trends Immunol 24:207–212, 2003.

Blumberg H, Conklin D, Xu W, Grossmann A, Brender T, Carollo S, Eagan M, Foster D, Haldeman BA, Hammond A, Haugen H, Jelinek L, Kelly JD, Madden K, Maurer MF, Parrish-Novak J, Prunkard D, Sexson S, Sprecher C, Waggie K, West J, Whitmore TE, Yao L, Kuechle MK, Dale BA, Chandrasekher YA. Interleukin 20: discovery, receptor identification, and role in epidermal function. Cell 104:9–19, 2001.

Cruikshank WW, Kornfeld H, Center DM. Interleukin-16. J. Leukoc Biol 67:757–766, 2000.

Davies DR, Wlodawer A. Cytokines and their receptor complexes. FASEB J 9:50–56, 1995.

Fort MM, Cheung J, Yen D, Li J, Zurawski SM, Lo S, Menon S, Clifford T, Hunte B, Lesley R, Muchamuel T, Hurst SD, Zurawski G, Leach MW, Gorman DM, Rennick DM.. IL-25 induces IL-4, IL-5, and IL-13 and Th2-associated pathologies in vivo. Immunity 15:985–995, 2001.

Foster PS, Martinez-Moczygemba M, Huston DP, Corry DB. Interleukins-4, -5, and -13: emerging therapeutic targets in allergic disease. Pharmacol Ther 94:253–264, 2002.

Gately MK. Interleukin-12: A recently discovered cytokine with potential for enhancing cell-mediated immune responses to tumors. Cancer Invest 11:500–506, 1993.

Giri JG, Ahdieh M, Eisenman J, Shanebeck K, Grabstein K, Kumaki S, Namen A, Park LS, Cosman D, Anderson D. Utilization of the β and γ chains of the IL-2 receptor by the novel cytokine IL-15. EMBO J 13:2822–2830, 1994.

Greaves DR, Schall TJ. Chemokines and myeloid cell recruitment. Microbes Infect 2:331–336, 2000.

Hamilton JA. GM-CSF in inflammation and autoimmunity. Trends Immunol 23:403–408, 2002.

Herbert CA, Baker JB. Interleukin-8: A review. Cancer Invest 11:743–750, 1993.

Holland G, Zlotnik A. Interleukin-10 and cancer. Cancer Invest 11:751–758, 1993

Hunter CA, Reiner SL. Cytokines and T cells in host defense. Curr Opin Immunol 12:413–418, 2000.

Johnson CS. Interleukin-1: Therapeutic potential for solid tumors. Cancer Invest 11:600–608, 1993.

Johnson HM, Bazer FW, Szente BE, Jarpe MA. How interferons fight disease. Sci Am 28:68–75, 1994.

Lankford CS, Frucht DM. A unique role for IL-23 in promoting cellular immunity. J Leukoc Biol 73:49–56, 2003.

Liao YC, Liang WG, Chen FW, Hsu JH, Yang JJ, Chang MS. IL-19 induces production of IL-6 and TNF-α and results in cell apoptosis through TNF-α. J Immunol 169:4288–4297, 2002.

Lindeman A, Mertelsmann R. Interleukin-3: Structure and function. Cancer Invest 1:609–623, 1993.

Lotz M. Interleukin-6. Cancer Invest 1:732–742, 1993.

Mahanty S, Nutman TB. The biology of interleukin-5 and its receptor. Cancer Invest 11:624–634, 1993.

Moore KW, de Waal Malefyt R, Coffman RL, O'Garra A. Interleukin-10 and the interleukin-10 receptor. Annu Rev Immunol 19:683–765, 2001.

Nakanishi K, Yoshimoto T, Tsutsui H, Okamura H. Interleukin-18 regulates both Th1 and Th2 responses. Annu Rev Immunol 19:423–474, 2001.

Neben S, Turner K. The biology of interleukin 11. Stem Cells Dayton 11:156–162, 1993.

Parrish-Novak J, Dillon S, Nelson A, Hammond A, Sprecher C, Gross JA, Johnston J, Madden K, Xu W, West J, Schrader S, Burkhead S, Heipel M, Brandt C, Kuijper JL, Kramer J, Conklin D, Presnell SR, Berry J, Shiota F, Bort S, Hambly K, Mudri S, Clegg C, Moore M, Grant FJ, Lofton-Day C, Gilbert T, Rayond F, Ching A, Yao L, Smith D, Webster P, Whitmore T, Maurer M, Kaushansky K, Holly RD, Foster D. Interleukin 21 and its receptor are involved in NK cell expansion and regulation of lymphocyte function. Nature 408:57–63, 2000.

Renauld JC, Houssiau F, Louahed J, Vink A, Van Snick J, Uyttenhove C. Interleukin-9. Adv Immunol 54:79–97, 1993.

Rubin JT. Interleukin-2: Its biology and clinical application in patients with cancer. Cancer Invest 11:460–469, 1993.

Sheppard P, Kindsvogel W, Xu W, Henderson K, Schlutsmeyer S, Whitmore TE, Kuestner R, Garrigues U, Birks C, Roraback J, Ostrander C, Dong D, Shin J, Presnell S, Fox B, Haldeman B, Cooper E, Taft D, Gilbert T, Grant FJ, Tackett M, Krivan W, McKnight G, Clegg C, Foster D, Klucher KM. IL-28, IL-29 and their class II cytokine receptor IL-28R. Nat Immunol 4:63–68, 2003.

Strengell M, Matikainen S, Siren J, Lehtonen A, Foster D, Julkunen I, Sareneva T. IL-21 in synergy with IL-15 or IL-18 enhances IFN-γ production in human NK and T cells. J Immunol 170:5464–5469, 2003.

Trinchieri G. Interleukin-12 and the regulation of innate resistance and adaptive immunity. Nat Rev Immunol 3:133–146, 2003.

Waldmann T. The contrasting roles of IL-2 and IL-15 in the life and death of lymphocytes : implications for the immunotherapy of rheumatological diseases. Arthritis Res 4 Suppl 3:S161–167, 2002.

Witowski J, Pawlaczyk K, Breborowicz A, Scheuren A, Kuzlan-Pawlaczyk M, Wisniewska J, Polubinska A, Friess H, Gahl GM, Frei U, Jorres A. IL-17 stimulates intraperitoneal neutrophil infiltration through the release of GROα chemokine from mesothelial cells. J Immunol 165:5814–5821, 2000.

Xie MH, Aggarwal S, Ho WH, Foster J, Zhang Z, Stinson J, Wood WI, Goddard AD, Gurney AL. Interleukin (IL)-22, a novel human cytokine that signals through the interferon receptor–related proteins CRF2-4 and IL-22R. J Biol Chem 275:31335–31339, 2000.

Zlotnik A, Morales J, Hedrick JA. Recent advances in chemokines and chemokine receptors. Crit Rev Immunol 19:1–47, 1999.

Index

Page numbers followed by f indicate figures; t, tables.